Oxford Textbook of

Rheumatology

Indexer Newgen Imaging Systems (P) Ltd
Production Manager Kate Martin
Design Manager Andrew Meaden
Typographer Jonathan Coleclough
Publisher Helen Liepman

The Editors and Publishers would like to thank the following companies whose generous support has enabled us to produce the colour illustrations in the book:

Wyeth Pharmaceuticals

Aventis

Schering Plough Ltd

Oxford Textbook of
Rheumatology
Third Edition

Edited by

David A. Isenberg
Centre for Rheumatology/Bloomsbury Rheumatology Unit, Middlesex Hospital, University College London, London, UK

Peter J. Maddison
Department of Rheumatology, Ysbyty Gwynedd, Bangor, UK

Patricia Woo
Centre for Adolescent and Paediatric Rheumatology, The Windeyer Institute of Medical Sciences, University College London, London, UK

David Glass
Division of Rheumatology, Cincinnati Children's Hospital Medical Center, Cincinnati, USA

and

Ferdinand C. Breedveld
Rheumatology, Divisie 2, Medical Faculty, University of Leiden, Leiden, The Netherlands

OXFORD
UNIVERSITY PRESS

OXFORD
UNIVERSITY PRESS

Great Clarendon Street, Oxford OX2 6DP

Oxford University Press is a department of the University of Oxford.
It furthers the University's objective of excellence in research, scholarship, and education by publishing worldwide in

Oxford New York

Auckland Cape Town Dar es Salaam Hong Kong Karachi
Kuala Lumpur Madrid Melbourne Mexico City Nairobi
New Delhi Shangai Taipei Toronto

With offices in
Argentina Austria Brazil Chile Czech Republic France Greece
Guatemala Hungary Italy Japan South Korea Poland Portugal
Singapore Switzerland Thailand Turkey Ukraine Vietnam

Oxford is a registered trade mark of Oxford University Press in the UK and in certain other countries

Published in the United States
by Oxford University Press Inc., New York

First edition published 1993
Second edition published 1998
Third edition published 2004
Reprinted 2005

British Library Cataloguing in Publication Data

Data available

ISBN 0 19 850948 0

10 9 8 7 6 5 4 3 2

Typeset by Newgen Imaging Systems (P) Ltd, Chennai, India
Printed in Italy
on acid-free paper by Lego Print s.r.l.

Summary of contents

Contents

Section 6 The scope of rheumatic disease

Preface to the third edition

The third edition of the *Oxford Textbook of Rheumatology* sets out to capture the excitement evident to most rheumatologists as the 'bench to bedside' concept genuinely delivers new drugs for the treatment of rheumatic diseases. Although we have endeavoured to keep the best ideas and section layout of the first two editions, the pace of change in methods of assessment, our understanding of immunopathology, and imaging have demanded many changes to this edition. Most obviously we now welcome Ferdinand Breedveld as the fifth editor. Ferdinand brings us a wealth of experience as a clinician-scientist who reflects the growing importance of Europe as the source of ideas and clinical trials in rheumatology. As in the second edition, we have had a turnover of some 25 per cent of chapter authors to try and capture the best possible selection of leaders in their field and those who deliver their chapters on time!

This third edition provides a new section on health outcomes in the rheumatic diseases ranging widely from rehabilitation to problems with sexuality and the economics of caring for patients with arthritis. The chapters on vasculitides have been significantly revised and there are new chapters on the problems of adolescence macrophage activation syndrome and management issues in patients with rheumatoid arthritis and systemic lupus erythematosus. Many chapters have sections examining the use of the new biological therapies and we have encouraged more management algorithms.

However, we do not see the need to make this textbook ever larger in size. The availability of the internet to most rheumatologists makes vast reference lists unnecessary. However, we have aimed to provide rather more than a mere shortlist of advised reading. Our authors have been asked to quote key and around 100 useful overview references per chapter.

We believe the *Oxford Textbook of Rheumatology* has an established place in world rheumatology and hope that this third edition will be a welcome and timely addition to the library of those training in rheumatology, established rheumatologists, and scientists interested in the subject.

Finally, we wish to pay tribute to Barbara Ansell who died recently. She truly put paediatric rheumatology on the map and made several contributions to the first and second editions. She influenced our decision to make the difference in rheumatological diseases as they present in different age groups a major feature of this textbook.

The Editors also wish to acknowledge the outstanding contribution of Peter Renton who died, prematurely, during the production of this edition.

London, UK DI
Bangor, UK PM
London, UK PW
Cincinnati, USA DG
Leiden, The Netherlands FB
January 2004

Preface to the second edition

Four years ago, in 1993, the first edition of this textbook was published to considerable acclaim. The many rapid developments in the basic science of rheumatology, imaging of joints, bones, and soft tissues, and exciting advances in treatment for some of the previously most intractable rheumatic diseases, have persuaded us that a second edition is timely and will contain sufficient new material both to stimulate and inform the reader.

The second edition has benefited, we believe, from the rearrangement of some chapters, the expansion of many others which have been brought up to date, and the addition of several completely new chapters. Our contributors have also been asked to provide expanded reference lists to facilitate access to the original sources. This approach ensures freshness of ideas and style, which is complemented by the improved quantity and quality of the colour figures. We also wished to make this a textbook to which rheumatologists could refer as a guide to their management of both the common and more unusual rheumatic conditions. To facilitate this aim, algorithms of optimal treatment are provided in the clinical chapters with additional practical management suggestions, including a section on joint and soft tissue injection.

The textbook has been designed as an attractive and informative manual for rheumatology trainees, full-time clinicians, and academic rheumatologists. We have encouraged our authors to express their opinions freely, to bring areas of dispute into the open, and to present a balanced view overall. As in the first edition, this volume places special emphasis upon the perspective of the age of the patient when dealing with the presentation of various rheumatic conditions, and a number of chapters focus on paediatric rheumatology. Another important emphasis in this edition is on the overlap of rheumatology with other subspecialties. This is provided by a series of chapters co-authored by rheumatologists and colleagues with expertise in a wide range of related conditions.

It has been both a challenge and a pleasure for us to edit the second edition which we hope will build on the clarity and standards of production of the first.

Peter Maddison
David Isenberg
Patricia Woo
David Glass

Preface to the first edition

These are exciting times for the study of rheumatology. Current research, incorporated in this textbook and integral to the editors' enthusiasm for their project, continuously increases our knowledge of the molecular basis of many of the rheumatic diseases. These advances more than justify a new textbook written to complement the successful *Oxford Textbook of Medicine.* As with the other volumes in this series, it is designed to be comprehensive and sufficient for both the trainee and the general physician who require up-to-date information.

The book begins with the variations in presentation of rheumatic symptoms at different ages. There follow chapters dealing with those syndromes, which are not easy to classify and which may be best considered as regional. Although the aetiology of these syndromes is still incomplete they are such a significant part of practice that they demand comprehensive cover. Special emphasis has been placed on back symptomatology both in children and in adults as this problem represents an especially large part of rheumatological practice. Chapters in the third part of Section 1 then discuss rheumatic disease in relation not only to general (internal) medicine but also to other specialties, including psychiatry, anaesthesia, obstetrics, and ophthalmology. The text provides both a comprehensive account of these extensive and pervasive interactions and more focused discussions, either on an area of particular interest to the authors or of special clinical interest; hence the variety of approaches ranges from the general view to the in-depth analysis of a specialist topic.

The next two sections, dealing primarily with basic science, include conceptual advances of relevance to rheumatology and provide an understanding of the rationale for newer therapies being introduced into clinical practice. We have not attempted to replace basic science textbooks; rather we have indicated good reviews on specific topics, concentrating in our volume on how the different areas interact within the context of rheumatic diseases. For example, genetic abnormalities of collagen are described in relation to diseases of cartilage and bone. The joint is treated as a functional unit, and its physiological and biomechanical disturbances are described in the context of a variety of diseases. Parts of the immune system currently thought to be important in the pathogenesis of chronic inflammation are highlighted in some detail. The sections finish with a review of available and innovative ways of controlling inflammation.

Volume 1 concludes with discussion of clinical laboratory practices. Considerable advances have been made in developing laboratory and imaging techniques for clinical assessment. In this section, guidance is given on the selection of appropriate investigations as well as an indication of future developments.

Volume 2 contains the necessary systematic and comprehensive review of the rheumatic diseases. We have tried to encompass rheumatic diseases met throughout the world together with their epidemiological and environmental influences. To this end, authors have been selected who have appropriate clinical experience and established reputations in teaching and research. Colour has been used in this volume to enhance the clinical descriptions while the authors provide a personal as well as an informative approach to management. The final section deals with the important aspects of surgery and rehabilitation. A comprehensive review of surgical techniques has not been attempted. Rather, the major principles have been established to enable appropriate referral as well as the early recognition of complications of surgery.

Throughout the text, considerable emphasis is placed on the age of presentation, thus ensuring that a paediatrician faced with a rheumatological problem is well catered for. Referencing has been selective rather than exhaustive; with the knowledge that computer searches are widely available, we feel that the space may be better used for clinical description.

No project of this magnitude is complete without acknowledgements. We would like to thank the staff of Oxford University Press for their unfailing help. Thanks are also due to our staff, Sheena Stewart, Carolyn Keith Haun, Louise Kittredge, Geraldine Brown, Ann Maitland, and Kate Young for their invaluable assistance in preparing the text.

Peter Maddison
David Isenberg
Patricia Woo
David Glass

Contributors

Sanjiv N. Amin Consultant Rheumatologist, Bombay Hospital and Medical Research Center, Mumbai, India
6.2.7 Mycobacterial diseases

Andrew A. Amis Orthopaedic Biomechanics, Departments of Mechanical Engineering and Musculoskeletal Surgery, Imperial College, London, UK
3.8 Biomechanics of articulations and derangements in disease

Janice R. Anderson Consultant Neuropathologist, Addenbrooke's Hospital, Cambridge, UK
5.7 Histopathology

John Baum Professor Emeritus of Medicine and Paediatrics, Department of Medicine, University of Rochester School of Medicine and Dentistry, New York, USA
2.4 Rheumatic disease and sexuality

Robert M. Bernstein 23 Anson Road, Manchester, UK
6.18.2 Rheumatic complications of drugs and toxins

Johannes W.J. Bijlsma Rheumatologist, Professor and Head of the Department of Rheumatology and Clinical Immunology, University Medical Center Utrecht, Utrecht, The Netherlands
6.13.1 Fibromyalgia and diffuse pain syndromes—adult onset

Allan I. Binder Consultant Rheumatologist, Lister Hospital, East & North Herts NHS Trust, Stevenage, UK
1.3.11 An anaesthetic perspective
6.17.2 Cervical pain syndromes
7.3 Corticosteroid injection therapy

Sarah J. Bingham Academic Unit of Musculoskeletal Disease, Department of Rheumatology, Leeds General Infirmary, Leeds, UK
6.3.3 Rheumatoid arthritis—management

Howard A. Bird Clinical Pharmacology Unit, Chapel Allerton Hospital, Leeds, UK
5.1 Acute phase response
5.2 Biochemistry

Carol M. Black Professor of Rheumatology, Royal Free and University College Medical School, London, UK
6.7 Scleroderma and related disorders in adults and children

David Blake Royal National Hospital for Rheumatic Diseases, Upper Borough Walls, Bath, UK
3.5 The physiology of the joint and its disturbance in inflammation

Emilio Bouza Professor and Chief, Department of Clinical Microbiology and Infectious Diseases, Hospital General Universitario 'Gregorio Marañón', Complutense, University of Madrid, Madrid, Spain
6.2.3 Osteomyelitis and associated conditions

Ferdinand C. Breedveld Head, Department of Rheumatology, Leiden University Medical Center, Leiden, The Netherlands
4.5.3 Immunosuppressive and other drugs—monotherapy versus combination therapy

Barry Bresnihan Consultant Rheumatologist and Professor of Rheumatology, St Vincent's University Hospital, Dublin, Ireland
3.6 Synovial pathology
6.12.6 Sarcoidosis

Petr Broulík Professor of Medicine, 3rd Department of Internal Medicine of First Medical School, Charles University, Prague, Czech Republic
1.3.8 The endocrine system

Kay Brune Friedrich Alexander University, Erlangen–Nurnberg, Erlangen, Germany
4.5.1 Non-steroidal anti-inflammatory drugs—old and new

Anthony M.J. Bull Lecturer, Imperial College, London, UK
3.8 Biomechanics of articulations and derangements in disease

Gerd-Rüdiger Burmester Charité University Hospital, Humboldt University of Berlin, Berlin, Germany
6.2.4 Lyme disease

Carolyn P. Cacho Assistant Professor of Medicine, UHC-MP, Case Western Reserve School of Medicine, Ohio, USA
1.3.13 The kidney

Andrei Calin Consultant Rheumatologist, Royal National Hospital for Rheumatic Diseases, Bath, UK
6.4.3 Ankylosing spondylitis

Evan Calkins 3799 Windover Drive, Hamburg, New York, USA
1.1.4 The geriatric age group

Jeffrey P. Callen Professor of Medicine (Dermatology), Chief, Division of Dermatology, University of Louisville School of Medicine, Louisville, USA
6.12.4 Panniculitis
6.12.5 Neutrophilic dermatoses

Simon Carette Head, Division of Rheumatology, University Health Network (Western Division), University of Toronto, Toronto, Canada
1.2.2.1 The upper limbs in adults

Tim Cawston University of Newcastle, The Medical School, Newcastle-upon-Tyne, UK
6.14 Osteoarthritis

Ann E. Clarke Immunology/Epidemiology, Montreal General Hospital, Montreal, Canada
2.5 The economics of the musculoskeletal diseases

Justin P. Cobb Orthopaedic Department, University College London Hospitals, London, UK
7.1 Surgery in adults

Philip G. Conaghan Senior Lecturer and Honorary Consultant Rheumatologist, University of Leeds, Leeds General Infirmary, Leeds, UK
5.6.1 Imaging in adults

Cyrus Cooper Professor of Rheumatology and Director of Research, University of Southampton School of Medicine, Southampton, UK
6.1.1 Epidemiology and the rheumatic diseases

Marjonne C.W. Creemers Rheumatologist, University Medical Center Nijmegen, Nijmegen, The Netherlands
6.3.2 Rheumatoid arthritis—the clinical picture

B. Dasgupta Department of Rheumatology, Southend General Hospital, Westcliff on Sea, Essex
6.10.6 Polymyalgia rheumatica

Kevin A. Davies Professor of Medicine, Brighton and Sussex Medical School, Brighton, UK
4.1 Cells, cytokines, and other mediators

Yaël A. de Man ErasmusMC, University Medical Centre Rotterdam, Rotterdam, The Netherlands
1.3.1.1 Pregnancy
1.3.1.2 Antirheumatic drugs in pregnancy and lactation

Fabrizio De Benedetti Dirigente Medico, IRCCS Bambino Gesù, Rome, Italy
1.1.7 Growth and skeletal maturation

Christopher P. Denton Senior Lecturer/Consultant Rheumatologist, Royal Free Hospital, London, UK
6.7 Scleroderma and related disorders in adults and children

Stanley C. Deresinski Assistant Chief of Infectious Diseases, Santa Clara Valley Medical Center, California, USA
6.2.10 Fungal arthritis

Michael Doherty Academic Rheumatology, University of Nottingham, City Hospital, Nottingham, UK
6.14 Osteoarthritis

Frances Dormon Consultant, Anaesthetics and Intensive Care, Poole Hospital NHS Trust, Poole, Dorset, UK
1.3.11 An anaesthetic perspective

Erkki Eerola Head of Laboratory, Turku University, Turku, Finland
1.3.6 The gastrointestinal tract

Michael R. Ehrenstein Senior Lecturer, Middlesex Hospital, University College London, London, UK
6.6.1 Systemic lupus erythematosus in adults—clinical features and aetiopathogenesis

M. Shirley Emerson 74 Cavendish Avenue, Cambridge, UK
7.5 Sports injuries

Paul Emery Leeds General Infirmary, Leeds, UK
6.3.3 Rheumatoid arthritis—management

Adel G. Fam Sunnybrook and Women's College, Health Sciences Center, University of Toronto, Toronto, Canada
1.2.2.1 The upper limbs in adults

Bruno Fautrel Assistant Professor, Hôpital Pitié-Salpêtrière, University Paris VI—Pierre et Marie Curie, Paris, France
2.5 The economics of the musculoskeletal diseases

Marc Feldmann Head of Division, Kennedy Institute of Rheumatology Division, Imperial College School of Medicine, Hammersmith, London, UK
6.3.1 Immunopathogenesis of rheumatoid arthritis

Iain T. Ferguson Consultant Neurologist, Department of Neurology, North Bristol NHS Trust, Frenchay Hospital, Bristol, UK
1.3.3 Neurological complications

Daniel Fishman Consultant Physician and Rheumatologist, Luton and Dunstable Hospital NHS Trust, Luton, UK
1.3.7 Liver, spleen, and pancreas

Berit Flatø Senior Consultant, Rikshospitalet University Hospital, Oslo, Norway
1.2.1.2 Spinal problems in children

Øystein Førre Center for Rheumatic Diseases, The National Hospital, Oslo, Norway
1.2.1.2 Spinal problems in children

Andrew O. Frank Arthritis Centre, Northwick Park Hospital, Harrow, UK
1.2.1.1 Spinal problems in adults

Patricia A. Fraser Director, Pediatric Rheumatology, Brigham and Women's Hospital, Boston, USA
6.1.2 Epidemiology of rheumatic diseases in selected non-European populations

İzzet Fresko Associate Professor, Cerrahpasa Medical Faculty, Istanbul, Turkey
6.10.8 Behçet's syndrome

Patrick J. Gallagher University Microbiology and Pathology Department, Southampton General Hospital, Southampton
5.7 Histopathology

Carlos Garcia-Porrua Rheumatology Staff Member, Hospital Xeral-Calde, Lugo, Spain
6.10.7 Other vasculitides including small-vessel vasculitis

J.S. Hill Gaston Professor of Rheumatology, University of Cambridge School of Clinical Medicine, Addenbrooke's Hospital, Cambridge, UK
6.4.5 Reactive arthritis and enteropathic arthropathy

Rinie Geenen Psychologist, Assistant Professor, Utrecht University, Utrecht, The Netherlands
6.13.1 Fibromyalgia and diffuse pain syndromes—adult onset

Allan Gibofsky Professor of Medicine and Public Health, Weill Medical College of Cornell University, Attending Rheumatologist, Hospital for Special Surgery, Adjunct Faculty, The Rockefeller University, New York, USA
6.2.12 Rheumatic fever

Dafna D. Gladman Professor of Medicine, University of Toronto, Senior Scientist, Toronto Western Research Institute, University Health Network, Toronto Western Hospital, Toronto, Ontario, Canada
6.4.4 Psoriatic arthritis

David Glass Professor of Pediatrics, Cincinnati Children's Hospital Medical Center, Ohio, USA
3.1 Genomics and its relevance to rheumatology

Miguel A. Gonzalez-Gay Rheumatology Staff Member, Hospital Xeral-Calde, Lugo, Spain
6.10.7 Other vasculitides including small-vessel vasculitis

Elizabeth M. Graham Consultant Medical Ophthalmologist, St Thomas' Hospital, London, UK
1.3.12 The eye

Ian D. Griffiths Consultant Rheumatologist and Senior Clinical Lecturer, Freeman Hospital, Newcastle-upon-Tyne, UK
1.2.3 Extra-articular features of rheumatic diseases

Alexei Grom Cincinnati Children's Hospital Medical Center, Ohio, USA
6.12.7 Macrophage activation syndrome

Wolfgang L. Gross Professor and Chief, University of Leubeck, Department of Rheumatology, Clinic of Rheumatology bad Bramstedt Lubeck, Germany
6.10.2 Clinical features of primary ANCA-associated vasculitis

Richard Haigh Consultant Rheumatologist, Royal Devon and Exeter Hospital (Wonford), Exeter, UK
2.2 Rehabilitation of adults

Renate Häfner Pediatric Rheumatologist, Rheumaklinik für Kinder und Jugendliche, Garmisch-Partenkirchen, Germany
2.3 Rehabilitation of children

Christine Hall Department of Radiology, Great Ormond St Hospital for Children, London, UK
6.16.4 Diseases of bone and cartilage in children

Frances C. Hall ARC Rheumatology Lecturer, University of Cambridge, School of Clinical Medicine, Addenbrooke's Hospital, Cambridge, UK
4.3 Specific immune responses

Timothy E. Hardingham Professor of Biochemistry, Wellcome Trust Centre for Cell-Matrix Research, University of Manchester, Director, UK Centre for Tissue Engineering, Universities of Manchester and Liverpool Office, School of Biological Sciences, Manchester, UK
3.3 Articular cartilage

Mark Harries Northwick Park and St Marks NHS Trust, Harrow, UK
7.4 Sports medicine

D.O. Haskard Director, The Eric Bywaters Centre, BHF Cardiovascular Medicine Unit, Imperial College London, Hammersmith Hospital, London, UK
4.2 Leucocyte trafficking in inflammation

P.N. Hawkins Professor of Medicine, Royal Free and University College Medical School, London, UK
6.12.1 Amyloidosis

J. Mieke Hazes ErasmusMC, University Medical Centre Rotterdam, Rotterdam, The Netherlands
1.3.1.1 Pregnancy
1.3.1.2 Antirheumatic drugs in pregnancy and lactation

Diane Hebert Director, Renal Transplantation, The Hospital for Sick Children, Ontario, Canada
6.6.3 Paediatric systemic lupus erythematosus

Simon M. Helfgott Assistant Professor of Medicine, Harvard Medical School, Boston, Attending Rheumatologist, Brigham and Women's and Massachusetts General Hospitals, Boston, USA
1.3.14 Psychiatric issues in rheumatology

Burkhard Hinz Friedrich Alexander University, Erlangen–Nurnberg Erlangen, Germany
4.5.1 Non-steroidal anti-inflammatory drugs—old and new

Peter Hollingworth North Bristol NHS Trust, Southmead Hospital, Westbury on Trym, Bristol, UK
1.3.3 Neurological complications

J. Lawrence Houk Professor of Clinical Medicine, University of Cincinnati Center, Cincinnati, USA
5.5 Joint fluid

Pearl Huey Head Biomedical Scientist, Immunology, Ysbyty Gwynned, Bangor, UK
5.4 Serological profile

Graham R.V. Hughes Lupus Research Unit, The Rayne Institute, London, UK
6.6.4 The antiphospholipid antibody syndrome

David A. Isenberg Arthritis Research Campaign Diamond Jubilee Professor of Rheumatology, The Middlesex Hospital, University College London, London, UK
1.3.5 The respiratory system
6.6.1 Systemic lupus erythematosus in adults—clinical features and aetiopathogenesis
6.6.2 SLE—management in adults

Mary Anne Jackson Chief, Section of Pediatric Infectious Diseases, Children's Mercy Hospital, Missouri, USA
6.2.2 Pyogenic arthritis in children

Johannes W.G. Jacobs Rheumatologist, Associate Professor, Department of Rheumatology and Clinical Immunology, University Medical Center Utrecht, Utrecht, The Netherlands
6.13.1 Fibromyalgia and diffuse pain syndromes—adult onset

David Jayne Consultant in Nephrology, Addenbrooke's Hospital, Cambridge, UK
6.10.3 Treatment of primary ANCA-associated vasculitis

Malcolm I.V. Jayson The Gate House, 8 Lancaster Road, Didsbury, Manchester, UK
6.17.1 Intervertebral disc disease and other mechanical disorders of the back

J.R. Jenner Rheumatology Department, Addenbrooke's NHS Trust, Cambridge
7.5 Sports injuries

Adrian Jones Consultant Rheumatologist, Nottingham City Hospital, Nottingham, UK
6.14 Osteoarthritis

David A. Jones Professor of Sport and Exercise Sciences, The University of Birmingham, Birmingham, UK
3.7 Skeletal muscle physiology and damage

Shubhada Kalke Consultant Rheumatologist, Lilavati Hospital, Mumbai, India
6.10.6 Polymyalgia rheumatica

Gary M. Kammer Wake Forest University School of Medicine, Winston-Salem, NC, USA
1.3.13 The kidney

Thomas Kamradt Deutsches Rheumaforschungszentrum, Schumannstrasse 21/22, Berlin, Germany
6.2.4 Lyme disease

Amy H. Kao Rheumatology Research Instructor, University of Pittsburgh School of Medicine, Pittsburgh, PA, USA
1.3.4 The cardiovascular system

Carol A. Kemper Assistant Chief of Infectious Diseases, Santa Clara Valley Medical Center, California, USA, and an Associate Clinical Professor of Medicine, Stanford University, California, USA
6.2.10 Fungal arthritis

Edward C. Keystone Mount Sinai Hospital, Toronto, Canada
4.5.3 Immunosuppressive and other drugs—monotherapy versus combination therapy

Munther A. Khamashta Lupus Research Unit, Rayne Institute, St Thomas Hospital, London, UK
6.6.4 The antiphospholipid antibody syndrome

John R. Kirwan Consultant and Reader in Rheumatology, Bristol Royal Infirmary, Bristol, UK
4.5.2 The place of glucocorticoids in the management of rheumatic disease

Andreas Krause Immanuel Hospital, Berlin, Germany
6.2.4 Lyme disease

Weitse Kuis Professor of Paediatrics, UMC—Wilhelmina Children's Hospital, Utrecht, The Netherlands
6.4.2 Spondyloarthritis in childhood

Pnina Langevitz Clinical Professor of Medicine, Sackler Faculty of Medicine, Tel-Aviv University, Head, Rheumatic Disease Unit, Sheba Medical Center, Tel-Hashomer, Israel
6.12.2 Familial Mediterranean fever

Tal Laor Department of Radiology, Cincinnati Children's Hospital Medical Center, Ohio, USA
5.6.2 Imaging in children

C.B.D. Lavy Associate Professor, University of Malawi College of Medicine, Malawi
7.1 Surgery in adults

Ronald M. Laxer Division of Rheumatology, The Hospital for Sick Children, Toronto, Canada
6.5.2 Systemic-onset juvenile chronic arthritis

Alison M. Leak Queen Elizabeth the Queen Mother Hospital, Margate, UK
1.3.12 The eye

Keng Hong Leong Consultant Rheumatologist, Gleneagles Medical Centre, Singapore
6.12.10 Hyperlipidaemias

Geoffrey O. Littlejohn Associate Professor and Director of Rheumatology, Monash University at Monash Medical Centre, Melbourne, Australia
6.18.1 Complex regional pain syndrome (algodystrophy/reflex sympathetic dystrophy syndrome)

Avi Livneh Associate Professor of Medicine, Sackler Faculty of Medicine, Tel-Aviv University, Head, Medicine, Sheba Medical Center, Tel-Hashomer, Israel
6.12.2 Familial Mediterranean fever

C.R. Lovell Department of Dermatology, Royal United Hospital, Bath, UK
1.3.2 The skin and rheumatic disease

Peter J. Maddison Consultant Rheumatologist and Professor of Joint and Muscle Disorders, School of Sport, Health and Exercise Science, University of Wales, Bangor, Ysbyty Gwynedd, UK
1.3.2 The skin and rheumatic disease
5.4 Serological profile
6.12.9 Multicentric reticulohistiocytosis
6.16.3 Miscellaneous disorders of bone, cartilage, and synovium

Mohamad Maghnie Dirigente Medico, Department of Paediatrics, IRCCS S. Matteo, Pavia, Italy
1.1.7 Growth and skeletal maturation

Sir Ravinder N. Maini Emeritus Professor of Rheumatology, The Kennedy Institute of Rheumatology, Faculty of Medicine, Imperial College of Science, Technology and Medicine, Hammersmith, London, UK
6.3.1 Immunopathogenesis of rheumatoid arthritis

Susan Manzi Associate Professor of Medicine and Epidemiology, University of Pittsburgh School of Medicine and Graduate School of Public Health, Pittsburgh, USA
1.3.4 The cardiovascular system

Paul Mapp Senior Research Fellow, University of Bath, Claverton Down, Bath, UK
3.5 The physiology of the joint and its disturbance in inflammation

Alberto Martini Professor and Head, University of Genova, IRCCS G, Genova, Italy
1.1.7 Growth and skeletal maturation
6.3.4 Polyarticular rheumatoid factor positive (seropositive) juvenile idiopathic arthritis

Michael F. McDermott Reader in Molecular Medicine, Barts and the London, Royal London Hospital, London, UK
6.12.3 Periodic fevers

Janet E. McDonagh ARC Senior Lecturer in Paediatrics and Adolescent Rheumatology, Institute of Child Health, Birmingham Children's Hospital, Birmingham, UK
1.1.3 Adolescence and transition

Neil John McHugh Consultant Rheumatologist, Royal National Hospital for Rheumatic Diseases, Bath, UK
6.11 Overlap syndromes in adults and children
6.12.10 Hyperlipidaemias

Elizabeth D. Mellins Associate Professor of Pediatrics, Stanford University School of Medicine, California, USA
6.5.1 Juvenile idiopathic arthritis

Herman Mielants Professor of Rheumatology, University Hospital, Gent, Belgium
6.4.1 Spondyloarthropathy, undifferentiated spondyloarthritis, and overlap

Marc L. Miller Rheumatology Associates, Portland, USA
6.2.1 Pyogenic arthritis in adults

Timo Möttönen Assistant Professor, Head of Division of Rheumatology, Turku University Central Hospital, Paimio, Finland
1.3.6 The gastrointestinal tract

Haralampos M. Moutsopoulos Professor and Director, Department of Pathophysiology, Athens, Greece
6.9 Sjögren's syndrome

Kathleen Mulligan Research Fellow, Centre for Behavioural and Social Sciences in Medicine, University College London, London, UK
1.1.6 Psychological aspects of rheumatic disease

Patricia Munoz Associated Professor of Medical Microbiology, Infectious Disease Consultant, Hopital General Universitario 'Gregorio Marañón', University of Madrid, Madrid, Spain
6.2.3 Osteomyelitis and associated conditions

Kevin J. Murray Paediatric Rheumatologist, Princess Margaret Hospital for Children, and Senior Lecturer, School of Paediatrics and Child Health, University of Western Australia, Perth, Australia
6.13.3 Pain syndromes—childhood onset

Stanley J. Naides Thomas B Hallowell Professor of Medicine, Professor of Microbiology and Immunology and Pharmacology, Pennsylvania State University, College of Medicine, Milton S. Hershey Medical Center, Pennsylvania, USA
6.2.5 Viral arthritis

Stanton Newman Professor of Health Psychology and Director, Centre for Behavioural and Social Sciences in Medicine, University College London, London, UK
1.1.6 Psychological aspects of rheumatic disease

Claes Nordborg Institute of Laboratory Medicine, Department of Pathology, Sahlgrenska University Hospital, Göteborg, Sweden
6.10.5 Large vessel vasculitis/giant cell arteritis

Elisabeth Nordborg Senior Consultant, Huddinge University Hospital, Stockholm, Sweden
6.10.5 Large vessel vasculitis/giant cell arteritis

Andrew S. O'Connor Instructor in Medicine, Division of Nephrology, Case Western Reserve University School of Medicine, MetroHealth Medical Center, Ohio, USA
1.3.13 The kidney

Seza Ozen Kuleli sok 9/2, Gazi Osman Pasa 06700, Ankara, Turkey
6.10.9 Vasculitis in children

Lauren M. Pachman Professor of Pediatrics, Feinberg School of Medicine, Northwestern University, Interim-Director Disease Pathogenesis Program, CMIER, Chicago, USA
6.8.2 Polymyositis and dermatomyositis in children

Gabriel S. Panayi ARC Professor of Rheumatology, King's College London, Guy's Hospital, London, UK
4.5.4 Future targeted therapies

S.E. Papapoulos Department of Endocrinology and Metabolic Diseases, Leiden University Medical Centre, Leiden, The Netherlands
6.16.2 Paget's disease of bone

Eliseo Pascual Profesor Titular de Reumatología, Hospital General Universitario de Alicante, Alicante, Spain
6.2.8 Brucellar arthritis

Yusuf I. Patel Consultant Physician/Rheumatologist, Hull Royal Infirmary, Kingston-upon-Hull, UK
6.2.9 Parasitic involvement

Reijo Peltonen Turku University Central Hospital, Turku, Finland
1.3.6 The gastrointestinal tract

John R. Penrod Immunology/Epidemiology, Montreal General Hospital, Montreal, Canada
2.5 The economics of the musculoskeletal diseases

Ross E. Petty 1A19 B.C. Children's Hospital, Vancouver, Canada
1.1.2 The child

F. Michael Pope Consultant Dermatologist, West Middlesex University Hospital, Professor of Medical Genetics and Honorary Consultant Clinical Geneticist, Institute of Medical Genetics, University of Wales College of Medicine and University Hospital of Wales, Cardiff, Professor of Connective Tissue Matrix Genetics and Head of Connective Tissue Genetics Group, King's College, London, UK
3.2 Molecular abnormalities of collagen and connective tissue

Mordechai Pras Professor of Medicine, Sackler Faculty of Medicine, Tel-Aviv University Head, Heller Institute of Medical Research, Sheba Medical Center, Tel-Hashomer, Israel
6.12.2 Familial Mediterranean fever

Anne-Marie F. Prieur Specialist of Paediatrics, Hôpital Necker Enfants-Malades, Paris, France
6.5.3 Rheumatoid factor-negative polyarthritis in children ('seronegative polyarthritis')
6.12.8 The chronic, infantile, neurological, cutaneous, and articular syndrome

J.F. Quignodon Paediatric Radiologist, Hôpital des Enfants Malades, Paris, France
5.6.2 Imaging in children

Mark A. Quinn Academic Unit of Musculoskeletal Disease, Department of Rheumatology, Leeds General Infirmary, Leeds, UK
6.3.3 Rheumatoid arthritis—management

Anisur Rahman Senior Lecturer in Rheumatology, University College London, London, UK
6.6.2 SLE—management in adults

Niels Rasmussen Rigshospitalet, Copenhagen, Denmark
6.10.3 Treatment of primary ANCA-associated vasculitis

Angelo Ravelli Dirigente Medico I livello, Pediatria II, IRCCS G. Gaslini, Genova, Italy
1.2.2.3 The arm and leg in children

J.P.D. Reckless Consultant Physician, Diabetes, Endocrinology and Metabolism, Directorate of Medicine, Royal United Hospital, Bath, UK
6.12.10 Hyperlipidaemias

David M. Reid Professor of Rheumatology, University of Aberdeen, Aberdeen, UK
6.16.1 Osteoporosis and osteomalacia

Eva Reinhold-Keller Senior Registrar, University of Lubeck, Lubeck, Germany
6.10.2 Clinical features of primary ANCA-associated vasculitis

Peter Renton* Consultant Radiologist, Institute of Orthopaedics UCL, Royal National Orthopaedic Hospital, London, UK
5.6.1 Imaging in adults

Malcolm P. Rogers Associate Clinical Professor of Psychiatry, Harvard Medical School, Attending Psychiatrist, Brigham and Women's Hospital, Department of Psychiatry, Boston, USA
1.3.14 Psychiatric issues in rheumatology

Ann K. Rosenthal Rheumatology Section /cc-111W, Zablocki VAMC, Milwaukee, USA
6.15 Crystal arthropathies

Joan M. Round Department of Sport & Exercise Sciences, The University of Birmingham, Edgbaston, Birmingham, UK
3.7 Skeletal muscle physiology and damage

Anthony S. Russell Professor of Medicine and Head, University of Alberta, Heritage Medical Research Center, Edmonton, Canada
1.1.1 The adult patient

Christy I. Sandborg Pediatric Immunology, CCSR, Stanford, USA
6.5.1 Juvenile idiopathic arthritis

Vivian E. Saper Clinical Associate Professor, Stanford University School of Medicine, California, USA
6.5.1 Juvenile idiopathic arthritis

Hans-Georg Schaible Institut für Physiologie, Universität Jena, Jena, Germany
3.9 The neurophysiology of pain

Rayfel Schneider Head, Division of Rheumatology, Hospital for Sick Children, Toronto, Canada
6.5.2 Systemic-onset juvenile chronic arthritis

Susan C. Scholes Senior Research Associate, School of Engineering, University of Durham, Durham, UK
3.8 Biomechanics of articulations and derangements in disease

David G.I. Scott Consultant Rheumatologist and Honorary Professor—UEA, Norfolk and Norwich University Hospital, Norwich, UK
6.10.1 Classification and epidemiology of vasculitis
6.10.4 Secondary vasculitis and vasculitis mimics

Geoffrey Scott Consultant Microbiologist, University College London Hospitals, London, UK
5.3 Microbiology and diagnostic serology

G.H. Sebag Chef de Service, Imagerie Pediatrique, Hôpital Robert Debre, Paris, France
5.6.2 Imaging in children

David D. Sherry Professor and Clinical Director, Rheumatology, The Children's Hospital of Philadelphia, Philadelphia, USA
6.5.1 Juvenile idiopathic arthritis

* It is with regret that we must report the death of Peter Renton during the preparation of this Textbook.

Michael Shipley Centre for Rheumatology/Bloomsbury Rheumatology Unit, London, UK
6.13.2 Local pain syndromes—adult onset

David M. Siegel Professor of Paediatrics and Medicine, Chief, Division of Paediatric Rheumatology and Immunology, New York, USA
2.4 Rheumatic disease and sexuality

Earl D. Silverman Division of Rheumatology, The Hospital for Sick Children, Toronto, Canada
6.6.3 Paediatric systemic lupus erythematosus

Robert W. Simms Clinical Director, Rheumatology, Professor of Medicine, Boston University School of Medicine, Massachusetts, USA
1.2.2.2 The lower limbs in adults

Roger Smith Nuffield Orthopaedic Centre NHS Trust, Oxford, UK
3.4 Bone in health and disease

Alexander Kai-Lik So Chef du service de rhumatologie, Médecine physique et réhabilitation, Hôpital Nestlé, Lausanne, Switzerland
1.3.10 Haematology

Roger Sørensen Senior Consultant, Rikshospitalet University Hospital, Oslo, Norway
1.2.1.2 Spinal problems in children

Enrique Roberto Soriano Consultant Rheumatologist, Hospital Italiano de Buenos Aires, Buenos Aires, Argentina
6.11 Overlap syndromes in adults and children

Taunton R. Southwood Professor of Paediatrics, Birmingham Children's Hospital, Birmingham, UK
6.4.2 Spondyloarthritis in childhood

Marianne Spamer Chief Physiotherapist, Rheumaklinik für Kinder und Jugendliche, Garmisch-Partenkirchen, Germany
2.3 Rehabilitation of children

Stephen G. Spiro UCLH NHS Trust, London, UK
1.3.5 The respiratory system

Cliff R. Stevens Senior Lecturer, Department of Medical Sciences, University of Bath, Bath, UK
3.5 The physiology of the joint and its disturbance in inflammation

Thomas Stoll Medical Director, aarReha Schinznach, Specialist Clinic for Rheumatology, Physical Medicine and Rehabilitation and Center for Osteoporosis, Schinznach–Bad, Switzerland
2.1 Outcome assessment in rheumatology

Gerold Stucki Professor of Physical Medicine and Rehabilitation, University Hospital of Munich, Munich, Germany
2.1 Outcome assessment in rheumatology

Malcolm Swann Consultant Orthopaedic Surgeon, Windsor, UK
7.2 Surgery in children

Douglas S. Swanson Assistant Professor of Pediatrics, Children's Mercy Hospital, Missouri, USA
6.2.2 Pyogenic arthritis in children

Deborah P.M. Symmons ARC Epidemiology Unit, University of Manchester, Manchester, UK
1.3.9 Links between malignant disease and musculoskeletal conditions

Paul Peter Tak Division of Clinical Immunology and Rheumatology, Academic Medical Center, University of Amsterdam, Amsterdam, The Netherlands
3.6 Synovial pathology

Ira N. Targoff Professor of Medicine, University of Oklahoma Health Sciences Center, Veterans Affairs Medical Center, and Assistant Member, Oklahoma Medical Research Foundation, Oklahoma, USA
6.8.1 Polymyositis and dermatomyositis in adults

Douglas Thompson Principal Biochemist, The General Infirmary, Leeds, UK
5.1 Acute phase response
5.2 Biochemistry

Susan D. Thompson Research Associate Professor, Cincinnati Children's Hospital Medical Center, University of Cincinnati, Cincinnati, USA
3.1 Genomics and its relevance to rheumatology

Athanasios G. Tzioufas Associate Professor, Department of Pathophysiology, Athens, Greece
6.9 Sjögren's syndrome

Anthony Unsworth Chairman, School of Engineering, Director, Centre for Biomedical Engineering, University of Durham, Durham, UK
3.8 Biomechanics of articulations and derangements in disease

Peter van Riel Professor of Rheumatology, Head of Department of Rheumatology, University Hospital Nijmegen, Njimegen, The Netherlands
1.1.5 Principles of examination

Leo B.A. van de Putte Professor of Medicine and Rheumatology, University Medical Center Nijmegen, Nijmegen, The Netherlands
6.3.2 Rheumatoid arthritis—the clinical picture

Wim B. van den Berg Professor of Experimental Rheumatology, University Medical Center Nijmegen, Nijmegen, The Netherlands
4.4 Animal models of arthritis

Patrick Venables Professor of Viral Immunorheumatology, The Kennedy Institute of Rheumatology Division, Imperial College School of Medicine, London, UK
6.2.6 HIV and other retroviruses

Jiří Vencovský Professor of Medicine, Institute of Rheumatology, Prague, Czech Republic
1.3.8 The endocrine system

Eric Veys Professor and Chief of the Department of Rheumatology, University Hospital, Gent, Belgium
6.4.1 Spondyloarthropathy, undifferentiated spondyloarthritis, and overlap

Russell Viner Consultant in Adolescent Medicine and Endocrinology, UCL Hospitals and Great Ormond Street Hospital, The Middlesex Hospital, London, UK
1.1.3 Adolescence and transition

Stefania Viola Dirigente Medico I Livello, IRCCS G. Gaslini, Genova, Italy
1.2.2.3 The arm and leg in children

Karen Walker-Bone University of Southampton School of Medicine, Southampton, UK
6.1.1 Epidemiology and the rheumatic diseases

Mary Chester M. Wasko Associate Professor of Medicine, University of Pittsburgh School of Medicine, Pittsburgh, USA
1.3.4 The cardiovascular system

Richard A. Watts Consultant Rheumatologist, Ipswich Hospital NHS Trust, Ipswich, UK
6.10.1 Classification and epidemiology of vasculitis
6.10.4 Secondary vasculitis and vasculitis mimics

A.D.B. Webster Consultant Immunologist, Academic Head of Department, University College London (Royal Free Campus), London, UK
6.2.11 Immunodeficiency

Johann Delf Witt Department of Orthopaedics, Middlesex Hospital, London, UK
7.2 Surgery in children

Patricia Woo Professor of Paediatric Rheumatology, Centre for Adolescent and Paediatric Rheumatology, The Windeyer Institute of Medical Sciences, University College London, London, UK
3.1 Genomics and its relevance to rheumatology
4.1 Cells, cytokines, and other mediators
6.16.4 Diseases of bone and cartilage in children

B.P. Wordsworth Seddon Ward, Nuffield Orthopaedic Centre, Headington, Oxford, UK
4.3 Specific immune responses

Hasan Yazici Professor and Chief, Cerrahpasa Medical Faculty, Istanbul, Turkey
6.10.8 Behçet's syndrome

Pierre Youinou Laboratoire d'Immunologie, Centre Hospitalier Regional et Universitaire, France
6.9 Sjögren's syndrome

Adam Young Rheumatology Department, St Albans City Hospital, St Albans, UK
5.8 Electrophysiology

Sebahattin Yurdakul Professor, Cerrahpasa Medical Faculty, Istanbul, Turkey
6.10.8 Behçet's syndrome

John B. Zabriskie Assistant Professor and Head, Laboratory of Clinical Microbiology/Immunology, Rockefeller University, New York, USA
6.2.12 Rheumatic fever

1

Clinical presentation of rheumatic disease

1 Clinical presentation of rheumatic disease

1.1 Clinical presentations in different age groups

1.1.1 The adult patient

Anthony S. Russell

Introduction

In rheumatology, as in other subspecialties, the very core of medical practice is the consultation, during which the physician advises the patient about diagnostic and therapeutic procedures. The physician recognizes that patients may believe they come 'for a blood test', or 'for an X-ray', or 'for treatment'. What the patient has come for, in fact, is advice, which may incorporate some if not all of the patient's expectations. This chapter explores the problems the rheumatologist meets in attempting to fulfil these expectations.

In locomotor disease, it is not uncommon to meet patients who bring what can best be described as a loosely tied bundle of complaints that they wish to transfer to the doctor for instant solution. Trying to help, they may often have diagnostic suggestions, which they believe will ease this task. These suggestions may be of diverse origins and doubtful practicality often compounded by information from the communications media. The physician, a pragmatist by training and experience, should use these suggestions judiciously to direct the patient along the correct diagnostic and therapeutic pathway.

The experienced rheumatologist often makes a diagnostic and therapeutic management plan by an intuitive process in the first moments of meeting the patient. Dissection of this intuitive exercise is difficult. But, nevertheless, central to this process is the differentiation of systemic from local disease and serious from minor illness. Systemic disease is suggested by the patient looking ill, weight loss, dyspnoea, fever, neuropathy, lymphadenopathy, splenomegaly, rash, anaemia, raised erythrocyte sedimentation rate or C-reactive protein, and abnormal urinalysis.

The interview and examination that follow the initial contact serve to confirm or deny the initial impression. Any surprises that may arise have to be integrated by a feedback mechanism into the continuing process of assessment. For example, the discovery of significant weight loss in a patient who sounded as though he had a rotator cuff syndrome will cause reflection and reassessment. Indeed, this is the mechanism by which physicians develop their clinical expertise and continue to learn (Schon 1987). One important purpose of the interview and physical examination, apart from identification of specific problems, is to gain the patient's confidence and thereby encourage compliance with the suggested investigations and treatment. The patient needs to know that the physician is considering all possibilities and is making a thorough assessment, not only of the presenting complaints, but also of the patient's overall physical and mental state. The difference in emphasis of the approach used in children and in elderly people will be discussed in Chapters 1.1.2 and 1.1.4.

Before the history and physical examination

The process of evaluation begins even before the patients begin to give their history. After reading the physician's referral letter and any accompanying documentation, our own initial assessment begins in the waiting room (Table 1).

Many important signs may be noticed when asking for the patient. An accompanying friend or relative may respond, leading a disabled or reluctant patient forward and apparently wishing to take charge of the proceedings. Observation of such interpersonal reactions forms a significant part of the assessment. We also see whether the patient rises from a chair with difficulty, owing to weakness or stiffness, and how he or she walks towards us. Is a walking aid being used? If so, does it seem to be needed? On introduction, with a normal handshake, is there a flinch? Does the gait change in the walk from the waiting to the examining room? What is the patient's general demeanour? Even before the history taking begins, areas of focus will have already been intuitively defined. These will subsequently be organized in a systematic manner.

History

When taking the history, the physician should, in due course, attempt to focus the patient's complaints into a differential diagnostic scheme. It is obviously important to determine where the complaints are situated. Are they localized or generalized, episodic, constant, or progressive? Is there any

Table 1 Pre-consultation intuitive observations

Clinical problem	Possible diagnosis
Painful foot, elderly woman on diuretics	Gout
Young, sexually active; hot swollen joint	Gonococcal arthritis
Headache with diffuse aches and pains in an elderly person	Polymyalgia rheumatica
Antinuclear antibody-positive, but no symptoms	Referring physician's dilemma, not the patient's
On allopurinol with high uric acid but no arthritis	Not gout
Post-pubertal male with low back pain	Ankylosing spondylitis
Woman, 6 weeks post-partum; small joint arthritis	Rubella vaccination; rheumatoid arthritis

Note: Intuitive diagnoses must be constantly subject to reflection and reassessment.

diurnal variation and what, if any, are the aggravating or alleviating factors? In many conditions it is often possible to establish a fairly firm diagnosis from the history alone and, when symptoms are episodic, such a working diagnosis will have to suffice until the patient is seen during a symptomatic period. A 'wait and see' approach is not uncommon in rheumatology but the rationale must be carefully explained to the patient. Thus, the described pattern of joint involvement and characteristic symptoms will often allow the diagnosis of acute gout or palindromic rheumatism to be made with confidence, awaiting objective confirmation during the next episode.

Specific symptoms to be asked for include arthralgias, myalgias, joint swelling, morning stiffness, Raynaud's phenomenon, and skin rashes and paraesthesias.

If there is suspicion of a systemic disease, a full systematic medical inquiry must be embarked upon and any significant symptoms noted. Figure 1 shows what we believe to be the key points in our own intuitive diagnostic process. This becomes modified by the statistics of disease likelihood in our practice. Even if the problem appears to be localized, one must be conscious of the fact that systemic diseases (rheumatic and non-rheumatic) often present with local symptoms, for example, carpal tunnel syndrome in rheumatoid arthritis and hypothyroidism (Table 2).

Pain and stiffness

The majority of adult patients seeking a rheumatological consultation complain of pain and/or stiffness. The pain is usually localized descriptively to their joints, muscles, or bones and the clinician has to determine whether this localization is correct.

It is important to bear in mind that patients are not usually familiar with anatomy and physiology, and that it is often impossible, for example, to elucidate an anatomically correct description of pain and paraesthesias due to compression of the median nerve from a patient with pain in the hand and forearm. Similarly, patients may complain of pain in the hip 'right in the joint' and when asked to indicate the site of the pain, they will point to the greater trochanter or gluteal region, not the groin.

Nevertheless, if a patient presents with a somewhat localized problem (e.g. forearm pain with use), close attention to the anatomical peculiarities of the region and the relevant symptoms and signs will generally provide a clear diagnosis. Localized problems may be multifocal, suggesting a generalized disorder, but a careful examination (e.g. for bursitis and for tendinitis) after the history will help in this distinction. It is important to be wary of the diagnosis of diffuse or even focal osteoarthritis as the cause of symptoms, even when there may be supporting radiographic evidence. Although this condition may be present, it may not be the predominant cause of symptoms (Table 3).

Pain is defined by the patient's subjective description. The clinician's task is to characterize this in terms that are in common medical usage. As indicated, the starting point is to describe localization. The quality, intensity, duration, and type of onset, as well as provoking, aggravating, or alleviating factors must be determined, together with the presence of a diurnal variation. However, such technical terms are usually best avoided with the patient. Important and revealing questions are 'What brings on the pain?', 'What can you do to relieve it?'. Having become familiar with the customary responses to such questions the rheumatologist is more alert to the patient who seems unable or even unwilling to describe the problem clearly. It is often helpful to try and reproduce the symptoms by manipulation or pressure, particularly when the patient appears unable to pinpoint the location without help. Thus, forearm pain on gripping tightly may help

Table 2 Primarily non-rheumatic illnesses presenting in the rheumatology clinic

Symptom/sign	Illness
Weight loss/bone pain	Multiple myeloma
Carpal tunnel syndrome	Acromegaly Hypothyroidism Amyloid
Bone pain	Secondary tumour
Vasculitis (polyarteritis nodosa)	Hepatitis
Stiffness and difficulty in walking	Parkinson's disease
Chronic synovitis with bowel problems	Inflammatory bowel disease
Stiff fingers, shoulder pain	Diabetic cheiroarthropathy

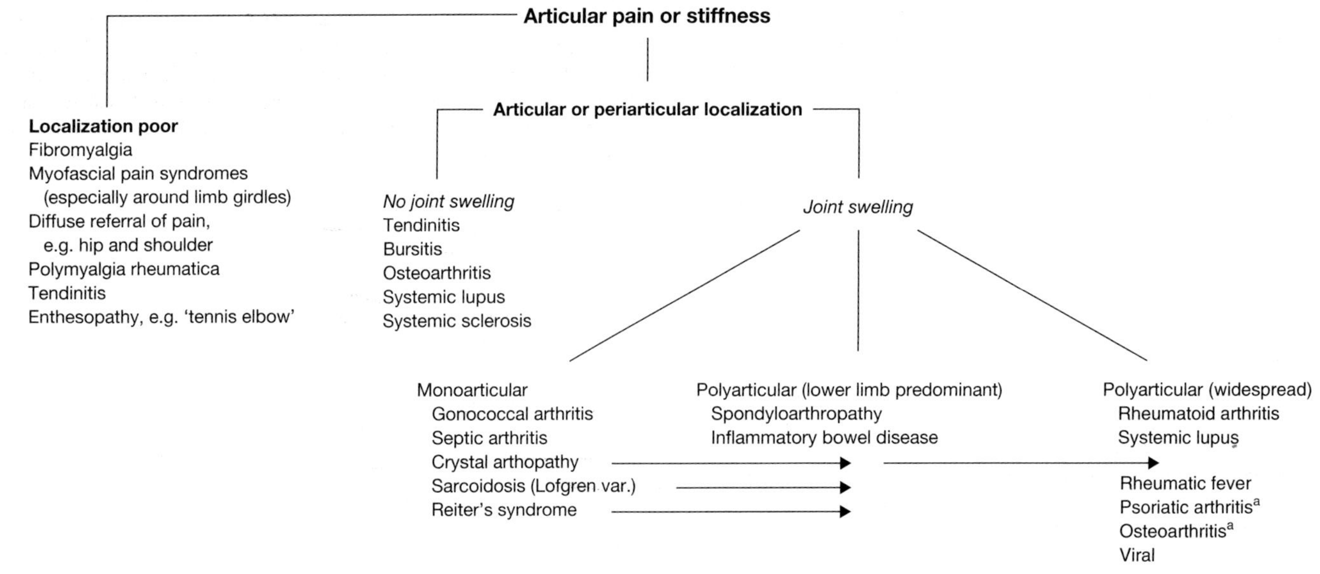

[a] Psoriatic arthropathy and osteoarthritis in an inflammatory phase may have a similar distribution and discrimination may be difficult.

Fig. 1 Aspects of differential diagnosis in rheumatology.

Table 3 Clinical pointers in syndromes where pain is poorly localized

Diagnosis	Clinical pointer
Periarticular shoulder pain	Referred to deltoid insertion
Tennis and golfer's elbow	Diffuse forearm pain on gripping
Carpal tunnel	Nocturnal paraesthesiae, often diffuse
Flexor tenosynovitis	Triggering and/or finger pain on gripping (pulp-pinch sign positive)
de Quervain's tenosynovitis	Positive Finkelstein test
Mechanical back pain	Tenderness over gluteals and sacroiliac ligaments frequent
Spondylitic back pain	Minimal sacroiliac or gluteal tenderness; morning stiffness marked
Trochanteric bursitis	Nocturnal pain when lying on that side; focal, point tenderness
Hip synovitis	Usually groin and outer-thigh pain, occasionally elsewhere
Anserine bursitis	Often nocturnal medial knee pain if knees are touching; localized tenderness

Note: Other, better localized syndromes, e.g. calcaneal bursitis, plantar fasciitis, infrapatellar bursitis should be immediately apparent on examination of the painful area.

distinguish the tender origin of the common extensor in a patient with tennis elbow from a similarly tender trigger point found in fibromyalgia.

While the spread of pain outside the usual limits may reflect intensity, this rarely proves a problem with a superficial pain, which is commonly well localized; thus gout or septic arthritis may be associated with severe pain but the origin is obvious. A glomus tumour of the nail bed may cause considerable proximal radiation of pain but examination should localize the source. To locate the source of pain of deeper or visceral origin may be much more difficult because of the phenomenon of 'referral'. Some patterns of referred pain are precise and well known, for example, shoulder pain from a diaphragmatic lesion or gallbladder; arm and/or neck pain from myocardial ischaemia. Others are more variable. Thus, the presence of sciatica may reflect nerve-root compression from a lumbar disc but much more commonly represents a referred distribution of pain from one or more regions around the lumbar spine. Experiments involving threads left temporarily after surgery around painful sensory structures or involving injection of hypertonic saline into ligaments and facetal joint structures have shown referral of pain from the lumbar spine into gluteal areas, to the posterior thigh, and even down the calf (Kellgren 1977). Involvement of the upper half of the lumbar spine tends to be referred to the anterior thigh. The only way to distinguish clearly true sciatica from such referred pain is on the basis of neurological signs, as associated symptoms (e.g. a cough or sneeze impulse) may be found with either. Sometimes, the pain may be remarkably well localized but again at a point distant from the exciting lesion; thus interscapular pain may be seen with postural/mechanical problems in the cervical spine, and anterior chest pain in relation to inflammation involving the mid-dorsal spine. Sometimes, relatively focal or diffuse tenderness may be associated with such referred pain syndromes. Pain referral may prove confusing to the physician but it is also often difficult to explain to a patient with, for example, pain well localized to the deltoid insertion that it is coming from a pericapsular lesion of the shoulder joint. Equally, deep visceral pain, such as a penetrating duodenal ulcer, may of course be referred to skeletal structures. Because of potentially similar patterns of pain referral a differentiation between skeletal and true visceral pain may have to be made on grounds other than the location of the discomfort.

Quality of pain

Skeletal pain may be caused by a variety of problems ranging from ischaemia, inflammation, and nerve entrapment to central factors that lead to a perception of pain where no evident peripheral causes exist. Quite apart from aggravating or relieving factors, the quality of the pain may provide diagnostic pointers. Thus, a burning pain in the feet, especially at night, may suggest a neuropathy. The pain of rheumatoid arthritis is usually steady and aching, not agonizing, excruciating, or terrifying. Such descriptions in a patient with rheumatoid arthritis would suggest an alternative explanation, for example sepsis, fracture, nerve entrapment, or non-organic causes. Chronic pain syndromes are well recognized but their underlying nature remains controversial. Because of overlapping and insufficient criteria a single individual may be designated by one physician as having a myofascial pain, by another as referred pain with secondary depression, and by a third as a (non-organic, i.e.) central, pain syndrome. The descriptions used by patients with central pain tend to be extreme and we find that to have patients complete instruments such as the McGill pain questionnaire is helpful as a teaching aid in illustrating to students the range of terms used. Some of the terms from that questionnaire, which distinguish between central or non-organic pain include flickering, shooting, lancinating, lacerating, crushing, seating, placing, unbearable, exhausting, terrifying, tearing and peripheral or organic pain syndromes include pounding, jumping, pricking, sharp, pinching, hot, tender, nagging, spreading, annoying, tiring, fearful, and tight. Similar expressions are chosen by patients with fibromyalgia, which is one reason for its earlier name of 'pain magnification syndrome', but also by those with causalgia, reflex sympathetic dystrophy, and occasionally even periarticular shoulder pain. In addition, some individuals or groups of individuals tend to use these extreme terms out of a sense of frustration or anxiety, or because of ethnic convention (Zborowski 1952), and risk being labelled as neurotic because of them, when the presence of organic disease may be missed. The reality of such pain of central origin has often been dramatically demonstrated by the stage hypnotist with a variety of forms of post-hypnotic suggestion. The severe quality of the rare thalamic pain syndrome is also well recognized. It is notable that Mark et al. (1960) observed, with stereotactic thalamic surgery, that in some, pain sensation could be abolished without loss of the unpleasant emotional effect and in others the emotional effect may disappear and yet the pain remain without its unpleasant qualities. Some of our current pharmacotherapeutic approaches reflect these findings. Therapy that is less conventional may have even more dramatic affects. Organic pain—for example, hot metal or hand immersion at 4°C for 45 min—can be blocked both from consciousness and from detection by electroencephalography during some forms of meditation. The block appears to be below the level of the cortex (Davidson and Goleman 1977). While the various central pain syndromes may respond to narcotic analgesics, this is for us an inappropriate approach both because it decreases the production of endorphins and because it is likely to cement the abnormal pain-behaviour patterns. Furthermore, no clearcut improvements in function have been demonstrated as a result of narcotic use. Some of these patients have post-traumatic pain syndromes with associated medicolegal implications. In any event, as a group they form a large proportion of patients in many rheumatological practices. It is clear that we still need better criteria both for diagnosis and classification of pain syndromes, as well as better approaches to treatment.

Stiffness

Stiffness is an important symptom in rheumatological disease. Typically, patients with rheumatoid arthritis complain of peripheral joint stiffness present for more than 30 min after awakening and recurring after periods of immobility. Patients with peripheral joint osteoarthritis may also have morning stiffness. This is usually of shorter duration but may also recur after rest. Peripheral stiffness may reflect non-articular inflammation and can be marked, as in plantar fasciitis, but is unusual with lesions around the shoulder. Stiffness for less than 5 min is generally of minor significance but could represent, for example, flat feet. Mechanical disorders of the lumbar spine may be associated with morning stiffness of short duration (less than 15 min) whereas patients with ankylosing spondylitis may say that their stiffness persists for several hours. Stiffness present for many hours, and even 'all day', in the absence of gross physical findings usually points to a functional condition such as fibromyalgia.

Is there a history of joint swelling or not?

The cardinal observation made by rheumatologists is that of joint swelling but patients can be amazingly unreliable, in being able to describe joint swelling. This is most notorious in fibromyalgia and it is critical to be able to distinguish arthralgias, which may include a variety of lesions of bursas, tendons, and tendon sheaths, from true arthritis (i.e. a swollen joint observed by a physician). It is, therefore, a critical part of the subsequent examination to confirm the presence or absence of joint swelling (see below).

Comment

In addition to focusing on differential diagnosis, the history and presentation of symptoms should give the first indication of how patients should be given advice. Some people will often make light of severe rheumatoid arthritis whereas in another circumstance a patient with fibromyalgia will say that they cannot carry out mundane tasks because of 'knives twisting in the muscles'. The physician's task is to ameliorate disease and to provide advice that will allow both types of patient to carry on with normal lives. The stoical patient may elicit a more sympathetic response from the physician but complaints from a medically trivial condition are no less valid or worthy of attention.

Physical examination

The physician recognizes disease entities from the physical findings in addition to symptoms and needs to integrate these two sets of data. Pain may be localized to joints, the spine, soft tissue, muscle, or bone. If it is localized in joints, can swelling be observed? If so, is the swelling severely inflammatory, moderately inflammatory, or non-inflammatory? This issue of joint swelling and its nature is one of the most critical aspects of the rheumatological examination and is reflected in the importance of teaching proper techniques for the 'wipe' or 'bulge' test in the knee, the proper palpation of the interphalangeal joints, metatarsophalangeal joints, etc. It is perhaps due to inability to assess swelling in the hip joint that the assessment of the range of motion is most important in this joint. The pattern of joint involvement is very important: is it monoarticular, polyarticular, symmetrical, asymmetrical, widespread, or restricted to lower extremities? Is there a surrounding cellulitis? Severe monoarticular arthritis with or without surrounding cellulitis suggests a crystal-induced arthritis, septic arthritis, sometimes Reiter's syndrome, gonococcal arthritis, or the Lofgren variant of sarcoidosis. These conditions may affect more than one joint, in which case the distribution is usually asymmetrical and, in gout, may involve contiguous joints of the same limbs. Widespread inflammatory joint swelling of moderate or severe degree may be seen in rheumatoid arthritis, psoriatic arthritis, polyarticular crystal-deposit disease, systemic lupus erythematosus, and other diffuse diseases of connective tissue; systemic conditions such as Whipple's disease may also present in this fashion. Joint swelling, without much evidence of inflammation, usually indicates osteoarthritis, which may involve distal and proximal finger joints—a classical feature of this predominantly female familial condition. Involvement of the metacarpophalangeal joints, especially if seen with chondrocalcinosis, should suggest the possibility of previously unrecognized haemochromatosis in the family, and premature osteoarthritis in a variety of joints makes one also consider conditions such as alcaptonuria, Wilson's disease, or epiphyseal dysplasias.

During the course of the examination, obvious findings may give substantial clues to the diagnosis. The facial rash of systemic lupus erythematosus, the scaling skin lesions accompanying psoriatic arthritis, and the specific lesion associated with Lyme arthritis are examples that readily come to mind and are discussed further in Chapter 1.3.2.

Tests

Think hard before you order them, inappropriate testing causes more problems than it solves.

Many of the tests that are available (see Section 4) are often abnormal in a range of rheumatic and non-rheumatic diseases and so, for example, the commonly used rheumatoid factor and antinuclear antibody tests are rarely sufficient in themselves to arrive at a precise diagnosis. Clinical experience teaches that the results of laboratory tests must be interpreted with caution and with continual reference to the clinical presentation. This is not because the tests used in the rheumatology subspecialty are less reliable than those of other disciplines but they are less specific and, more importantly, as many of these diseases are uncommon, the history and physical examination remain pre-eminent. Most of us would request a recent full blood picture and urinalysis on every patient, regardless of diagnosis. The erythrocyte sedimentation rate is still used by many despite the recognized pitfalls of false positive and negative results. The CRP is technically easier and may reflect the same issues. It nevertheless remains difficult to support a diagnosis of polymyalgia rheumatica, for example, with a relatively normal sedimentation rate or CRP; on the other hand, it is comfortably reassuring to see a normal result in a patient in whom we have found no evidence of inflammatory disease. Selective lymphopaenia of less than 1000/ml is the poor man's indication of systemic lupus or a recent virus infection. Thrombocytosis is common in active rheumatoid arthritis and the vasculitides.

As with other tests, it is important to know why the test is being ordered and what influence the result will have on diagnosis and management. A test for rheumatoid factor may be ordered in a patient with clinically obvious nodular rheumatoid arthritis not for diagnosis but for better definition of the condition. A serum uric acid level is of no value in the diagnosis of gout; there are simply too many non-gout individuals with raised levels and too many normal levels seen even during the acute attack to make this helpful. It is, nevertheless, an effective way to monitor compliance with hypouricaemic therapy. In a patient with mechanical back symptoms it is clear that a raised uric acid or a positive rheumatoid factor, for example, are not going to influence diagnostic considerations; they should, therefore, not have been ordered.

A consideration of pre- and post-test probabilities is critical. A positive fluorescent antinuclear antibody (FANA) test is about 97 per cent specific and 99 per cent sensitive for systemic lupus erythematosus. These figures sound, and are, excellent but it remains true that as systemic lupus has a prevalence of around 0.1 per cent of the population or even less, there are, in a given population, more normal people positive for antinuclear antibody than there are lupus patients. A 97 per cent specificity is as good as can be achieved and in many laboratories it is very much lower than this, for example, 75 per cent. This variability of the local specificity must be known; nevertheless, despite even a 97 per cent specificity, the majority of individuals with a positive antinuclear antibody in a randomly screened population will not have systemic lupus. On the other hand, if a patient with photosensitivity, leucopaenia, and an abnormal urinary sediment has a positive antinuclear antibody, one can be virtually certain that the diagnosis is systemic lupus. Using Bayes' theorem, it has often been calculated that if the pre-test probability, that is the clinical likelihood, of a given patient having systemic lupus is over 50 per cent, a positive antinuclear antibody will increase this likelihood to near certainty. If one orders the test 'as a screen' in a patient who has no clinical evidence of lupus, for example a tennis elbow, where the pre-test likelihood of lupus is minimal, then a positive test will have no real import on this probability, perhaps increasing it to about 2 per cent, that is still 50 : 1 against the diagnosis of systemic lupus erythematosus. This would surely argue against ever doing the test as a screen. In the management of diffuse disease of connective tissue it is important to establish the broad category of the disease which is being treated but the precise subcategory may be therapeutically unimportant. For example, a serological diagnosis of mixed connective tissue disease (MCTD) should not prevent routine urinalysis and aggressive treatment of any renal or any other end-organ involvement. 'Anti-ENA' antibody tests (antibodies to extractable nuclear antigen) are often performed in patients with a positive FANA. Their role should surely be to help delineate clinical subtypes of disease where this information will be of help, either therapeutically or prognostically.

Sometimes laboratory tests may be helpful in reducing the need for more invasive procedures. Thus, a positive test for antineutrophil cytoplasmic antibodies in a patient with features of Wegener's granulomatosis may make a biopsy unnecessary. Similarly, anti-Jo-1 antibodies in a patient with muscle weakness and elevated enzymes may not only help avoid a biopsy but give potentially important prognostic information.

If a young male complains of nocturnal low back pain with stiffness lasting more than 1 h in the morning with a restricted range of flexion in the lumbar spine, would testing for HLA-B27 be at all helpful? Under normal circumstances it would not. One would check the pelvic radiograph—it would be very uncommon, even in early ankylosing spondylitis, to see normal sacroiliac joints. Although, as routine interpretation is notoriously unreliable it is a good idea to develop the expertise to review these personally. In the late teens and early twenties and, of course, in children, the radiographs can be difficult to interpret and here B27 typing may be helpful. Recent studies suggest T_2-weighted fat suppressed MRI images may also be helpful in delineating sacroiliac inflammation. In a relative of a B27 ankylosing spondylitis proband, a negative B27 test indicates that any back symptoms are very unlikely to be ankylosing spondylitis related, just as a positive test in this context, even with normal radiographs, may suggest a forme fruste of the disease.

Problems of interpretation of the findings also abound in radiography. Mild asymptomatic radiographic changes are frequent, especially in the lumbar spine but also in the knee. It is easy to ascribe symptoms to these changes when examination would reveal an anserine bursitis or a similar localized, readily treatable problem. A more critical problem has arisen because of 'false positive' findings, for example, of disc protrusion, seen with computed tomography and with magnetic resonance imaging of the lumbar spine. Thus, a high proportion of asymptomatic subjects will have one or more abnormalities evident. This means that little reliance can be placed on these findings in symptomatic subjects unless the findings clearly fit with an anatomical lesion predictable with reasonable probability from the clinical examination. These investigations become useful in the management of patients with back pain only if it is important to clearly delineate either the nature of the pathological process or the extent and location of a lesion, for example, prior to a surgical intervention or, more questionably, for medicolegal requirements.

It is tempting for the inexperienced to place more weight on test results than on clinical judgement; all rheumatologists see too many patients with minor problems where a consultation has been stimulated by a positive but inappropriate test. Thus, from a diagnostic perspective, tests are ordered where they can help support or deny the clinical impression. A further indication would be to follow a patient's progress. For example, in the treatment of patients with rheumatoid arthritis progression of erosive changes may, by themselves, influence therapeutic decisions. Bone mineral density measurements may be helpful in the diagnosis of demineralization. They will be indicated primarily when the results will help the patient or physician reach a therapeutic decision. Thus, if the patient is to be started on medication anyway, for example, following a low trauma fracture, there is little or no point in ordering the test.

A management plan and the individual patient

It is clear that any management plan depends on the underlying disease process and the extent of its progression in the individual patient. Other factors are important in involving the management plan which certainly include compliance, geographic issues, age of patient, psychological status, history of other conditions including upper gastrointestinal problems like peptic ulceration. There is now a consensus that the earlier remittive therapy is instituted in rheumatoid arthritis, the more likely it is to be successful. Thus, we would argue that at least all seropositive patients should be started on a remittive agent as soon as the diagnosis is made without a demonstration of the inefficacy of non-steriodal anti-inflammatory drugs alone. Similarly, the longer lupus nephritis has gone untreated, the more refractory it seems to be to treatment, which hastens our decision to add cytotoxic therapy to the management of this condition.

In elderly patients, or those with impaired renal function from other causes, we check the serum creatinine before and either 2 or 7 days after the institution of therapy with non-steroidal anti-inflammatory drugs, depending on the drug half-life. Similarly, in elderly patients or in those who have had significant gastrointestinal haemorrhage or perforation, we would either combine use of such non-steroids with gastric protection or use Cox-2 specific agents. In rheumatoid arthritis, this is a further argument in favour of the early use of remittive agents. In localized but painful conditions such as tendinitis and bursitis, it is more economical for the patient to be treated with local steroid injections where appropriate rather than by oral non-steroidal drugs, although it may be less convenient for the physician. The expected treatment benefits should not be outweighed by difficulties in complying with the suggested therapeutic programme. For example, geographical considerations may be important in the decision whether to use a parenteral or oral remittive agent in rheumatoid arthritis. It is most important that the relative risks and benefits of treatment be most carefully explained to the patient, with supporting written information provided. Except in life-threatening or rapidly crippling conditions it is wise to allow the patient a waiting period for discussion with family members and the referring physician rather than to try to persuade a reluctant patient to accept your suggestions. One phrase we find useful in this circumstance is 'If I or one of my family members had your disease, and another rheumatologist were to suggest this course of treatment, I would have no hesitation in accepting it'.

In any management plan for patients with rheumatological disease, a careful assessment must be made of the relative architectural, mechanical, and inflammatory components. All of these must be seen in the context of the patient's general health. Generally speaking, architectural problems may benefit from surgical solutions and secondary mechanical problems, such as muscle weakness, are susceptible to physical therapy. In rheumatoid arthritis, seriously disabling problems in the feet and ankles can be prevented by the provision of adequate transverse and longitudinal supports for the metatarsal arches, combined with suitable footwear. Surgery does not necessarily pose any increased risk in elderly patients, if risk factors such as electrolyte imbalance, heart failure, or arrhythmia can be corrected or treated. It is most important to determine that surgical correction of the musculoskeletal problem, in, for example, a painful unstable knee, will improve the patient's quality of life. There may be little point in giving a patient a perfectly stable, painless joint if exercise distance cannot be significantly increased due to cardiac, respiratory, or peripheral vascular problems. Under these circumstances it may be more practical simply to provide an external brace. Similarly, age can be an important consideration in any plan for staged orthopaedic surgery accompanied by the necessary long periods of rehabilitation between procedures. Such a treatment plan, which may extend over several months or years, may be entirely sensible for patients in their 40s or 50s whose life expectancy is 20 or 30 years. It is unlikely to improve the overall quality of life for someone of 80 years whose life expectancy is less.

If someone's life expectancy is very short because of, say, terminal malignant disease, we may choose to prescribe steroids for their rheumatoid arthritis, but we have on occasion been surprised at the length of the terminal illness, which has allowed serious steroid complications to arise.

Conclusions

Finally, it should be remembered that the ability to recognize a seriously ill patient before a specific diagnosis is as important for rheumatologists as for all other physicians. While this remains part of the art of medicine, it is also a reason for the triggering of appropriate perceptive questions, even to patients who may at first sight appear to have minor disease.

References

Davidson, R.J. and Goleman, D.J. (1977). The role of attention in meditation and hypnosis: a psychobiologic perspective on transformations of consciousness. *International Journal of Clinical Experimental Hypnosis* **15**, 291–308.

Kellgren, J.H. (1977). The anatomical source of back pain. *Rheumatology and Rehabilitation* **16**, 7–12.

Mark, V.H., Irvin, F.R., and Hackett, T.P. (1960). Clinical aspects of stereotactic thalomotomy in the human. 1. The treatment of chronic severe pain. *Archives of Neurology* **3**, 351–67.

Schon, D.A. *Educating the Reflective Practitioner: Toward a New Design for Teaching and Learning in the Professions.* San Francisco CA: Jossey-Bass, 1987.

Zborowski, M. (1952). Cultural components in responses to pain. *Journal of Social Issues* **8**, 17–30.

1.1.2 The child

Ross E. Petty

Introduction

Rheumatic complaints in childhood are common, but usually short-lived, and most are ultimately inconsequential (Apley 1976). It may be difficult, however, to differentiate definitively such problems from those associated with long-term illness. A full discussion of childhood rheumatic diseases is beyond the scope of this chapter and summaries of many of the important entities are provided in later chapters or other sources (Cassidy and Petty 2001; Petty and Cabral 2002).

Classification and epidemiology

There is a paucity of valid data on the incidence and prevalence of rheumatic disease in childhood, and such data as exist show wide variations. This is due, in part, to difficulties in classifications and their application.

Classifications of childhood arthritis

There are three major sets of criteria for the classification of chronic childhood arthritis: the American College of Rheumatology (ACR) criteria for juvenile rheumatoid arthritis (JRA) (Brewer et al. 1977), the European League Against Rheumatism (EULAR) criteria for juvenile chronic arthritis (JCA) (European League Against Rheumatism 1977); and the International League of Associations for Rheumatology (ILAR) criteria for juvenile idiopathic arthritis (JIA) (Fink 1995; Petty et al. 1998, 2002). They are as follows:

ACR criteria (JRA)	EULAR criteria (JCA)	ILAR criteria (JIA)
Pauciarticular	Pauciarticular	Oligoarthritis Persistent Extended
Polyarticular	Polyarticular RF− Polyarticular RF+	Polyarthritis RF− Polyarthritis RF+
Systemic	Systemic Psoriatic Ankylosing spondylitis	Systemic arthritis Psoriatic arthritis Enthesitis related Undefined arthritis

All are based on the behaviour of the disease at onset (within the first 6 months). They apply to patients with onset of arthritis before the sixteenth birthday, and rely principally on clinical characteristics. To meet ACR and ILAR criteria arthritis must persist for at least 6 weeks; in EULAR criteria, the arthritis must persist for at least 3 months. They include similar groups of patients, but the ILAR criteria are most inclusive and most specific, and include a number of characteristics that may exclude a patient from any specific category (Table 1). The ILAR criteria have been revised twice by an international committee of paediatric rheumatologists in an ongoing process of evidence-based modifications.

Other classifications of importance

The criteria for the seronegative enthesitis and arthritis (SEA) syndrome (Rosenberg and Petty 1982) identify children who, although they do not currently fulfil criteria for the diagnosis of ankylosing spondylitis, are likely to do so in the future (Burgos-Vargas and Clarke 1989; Cabral et al. 1992b). Similarly, criteria for the diagnosis of juvenile psoriatic arthritis (The Vancouver Criteria) (Southwood et al. 1989) facilitate early identification of children with this type of arthritis. These criteria sets have largely been superseded by the ILAR criteria for JIA.

The only other diagnostic criteria that have been developed for the classification or diagnosis of childhood rheumatic diseases are those for acute rheumatic fever (Special Writing Group of the American Heart Association 1992) and those for Kawasaki disease (Sekiguchi et al. 1985). Both of these criteria sets have reasonably high sensitivity, but lower specificity. In addition, the strict application of the Kawasaki criteria could lead to the exclusion of children whose later disease course (i.e. the development of coronary artery aneurysms) indicates that they had Kawasaki disease.

Criteria for the diagnosis or classification of other chronic rheumatic diseases of childhood either do not exist, have been adopted in whole or in part from criteria for the classification of diseases in adults, as for systemic lupus erythematosus (Tan et al. 1982; Hochberg 1997), the vasculitides (Jennette et al. 1994), or dermatomyositis (Bohan and Peter 1975), or have not been widely used in clinical practice. The criteria for dermatomyositis and the vasculitides, in particular, require validation in paediatric patients. A recent report (Moenkemoeller et al. 2001) noted that few paediatric rheumatologists rely on the Bohan and Peter criteria for the diagnosis of juvenile dermatomyositis, but no other criteria have been formally proposed.

Frequencies of childhood rheumatic diseases

It is a common perception that rheumatic diseases are rare in childhood and adolescence. As a result, consideration of such a diagnosis may be inappropriately delayed. In fact, a significant fraction of adults with rheumatic diseases have onset of the disease in childhood, and a number of important conditions occur almost exclusively in the paediatric age range including rheumatic fever, Henoch–Schönlein purpura, and Kawasaki disease. Thus, up to one-fifth of all patients with systemic lupus erythematosus or dermatomyositis/polymyositis have onset of their disease before age 17 years. Onset of disease in childhood occurs in 5–10 per cent of individuals with

Table 1 The ILAR criteria for classification of the juvenile idiopathic arthritides

Category	Definition	Exclusions
Oligoarthritis	Arthritis in less than five joints during the first 6 months of disease Persistent: never more than four joints Extended: More than four joints *after* the first 6 months of disease	1,2,3,4,5
Polyarthritis RF+	Arthritis in five or more joints during the first 6 months of disease, with positive RF tests (×2)	1,2,3,5
Polyarthritis RF−	Arthritis in five or more joints during the first 6 months of disease, with negative RF test	1,2,3,4,5
Systemic arthritis	Arthritis with fever of >2 weeks duration, documented to be quotidian for at least 3 days, and accompanied by one or more of: a. Evanescent, non-fixed rash b. Hepatomegaly or splenomegaly c. Serositis d. Generalized lymphadenopathy	1,2,3,4
Psoriatic arthritis	Arthritis + psoriasis, or Arthritis with one or more of: a. Dactylitis b. Nail pitting or onycholysis c. Psoriasis in a first degree relative	2,3,4,5
Enthesitis-related arthritis	Arthritis and enthesitis, or Arthritis *or* enthesitis with one or more of: a. Sacroiliac joint tenderness and/or inflammatory lumbosacral spinal pain b. HLA B27 positivity c. Acute symptomatic uveitis d. First degree relative with HLA B27 associated disease e. Onset of arthritis in a boy over the age of 8 years	1,4,5
Undefined arthritis	A child with arthritis who meets criteria for more than one category or for no category	

Exclusions
1. Psoriasis in the patient or first degree relative
2. Arthritis in an HLA B27 positive male with onset after 8 years of age
3. Ankylosing spondylitis, enthesitis related arthritis, sacroiliitis with inflammatory bowel disease, Reiter's syndrome, or acute anterior uveitis in a first degree relative
4. Presence of IgM rheumatoid factor on at least two occasions more than 3 months apart
5. The presence of systemic JIA

Source: Adapted from Petty and Southwood (1997, 2002).

one of the more chronic arthropathies such as ankylosing spondylitis and rheumatoid arthritis, whereas gout and scleroderma are almost non-existent in childhood. It is likely that these estimates represent minima because, particularly in diseases such as oligoarticular-onset juvenile chronic arthritis, many children have remission of the disease in childhood. A population-based study by Manners and Diepeveen (1996) suggested that the prevalence of chronic arthritis in 12-year-old Australian school children was actually much higher (400/100 000) than suspected.

Table 2 Relative frequencies of childhood rheumatic diseases: data from National Registries in Europe and North America

Diagnosis	%
JRA[a]	
Systemic	11.2
Polyarticular	23.2
Oligoarticular	44.4
JPsA[b]	5.2
JAS	2.5
Undifferentiated spondyloarthropathy	10.4
Reiter's syndrome	<1
Arthritis with inflammatory bowel	2.1

[a] Includes JRA (ACR criteria) and JCA (EULAR criteria).
[b] Vancouver criteria.
Source: Modified from Cassidy and Petty (2001).
Data derived from Bowyer et al. (1996); Malleson et al. (1996); and Symmons et al. (1996).

Some rheumatic diseases occur almost exclusively in those under 16 years of age. Included in this category are oligoarticular onset juvenile idiopathic arthritis with uveitis, systemic onset juvenile idiopathic arthritis, acute rheumatic fever (at least in North America and Europe), and, among the vasculitides, Henoch–Schönlein purpura and Kawasaki disease. In contrast, certain rheumatic diseases almost never occur in childhood. Included in this group are gout, calcium pyrophosphate deposition disease, polymyalgia rheumatica, and primary osteoarthritis.

The actual frequencies of each of the types of arthritis in a community is difficult to ascertain. A Finnish study (Kunnamo et al. 1986) indicates that acute, presumably post-viral arthritis of the hip or knee accounts for three-quarters of all children with arthritis; chronic childhood arthritis accounts for approximately one-fifth. Children with other rheumatic disease were not included in this study. The overall impression is, however, that the annual incidence of significant joint inflammation or infection involves approximately 1 in 1000 children and that chronic arthritis occurs in 1 in 5000 children per year. Three national registries of childhood rheumatic disease have provided a good estimate of the relative frequencies of a range of childhood rheumatic diseases in the United States (Bowyer et al. 1996), Canada (Malleson et al. 1996), and the United Kingdom (Symmons et al. 1996) (Table 2). Data from registries or large surveys in other parts of the world are not available. There is strong indication, however, that ethnogeographical parameters strongly influence disease subtype incidence. Oligoarticular JIA is, for example, much less common in series of children reported from India, whereas systemic onset disease, in particular, is more common (Chandrasekaran et al. 1996; Seth et al. 1996). Certain of the vasculitides (Kawasaki disease, Takayasu's arteritis) are much more prevalent in Japan than in Europe or North America. Rheumatic fever is by far the most important rheumatic disease in the developing world, but is quite uncommon in North America and Europe. Thus, the spectrum of rheumatic disease in the paediatric population varies considerably depending on the part of the world being studied.

Age at presentation

Many of the rheumatic diseases of childhood have characteristic ages at onset (Fig. 1) and consideration of the age of the child at onset of symptoms can be of value in diagnosis. For this purpose, four age groups can be considered. Rare syndromes that make their appearance in the neonatal period include neonatal lupus, chronic inflammatory neurocutaneous and articular syndrome (CINCA), episodic fever syndromes, and infantile sarcoidosis. In early childhood (1–4 years) oligoarticular JIA, juvenile psoriatic arthritis, Kawasaki disease, and septic arthritis are most frequent. In mid-childhood (7–9 years)

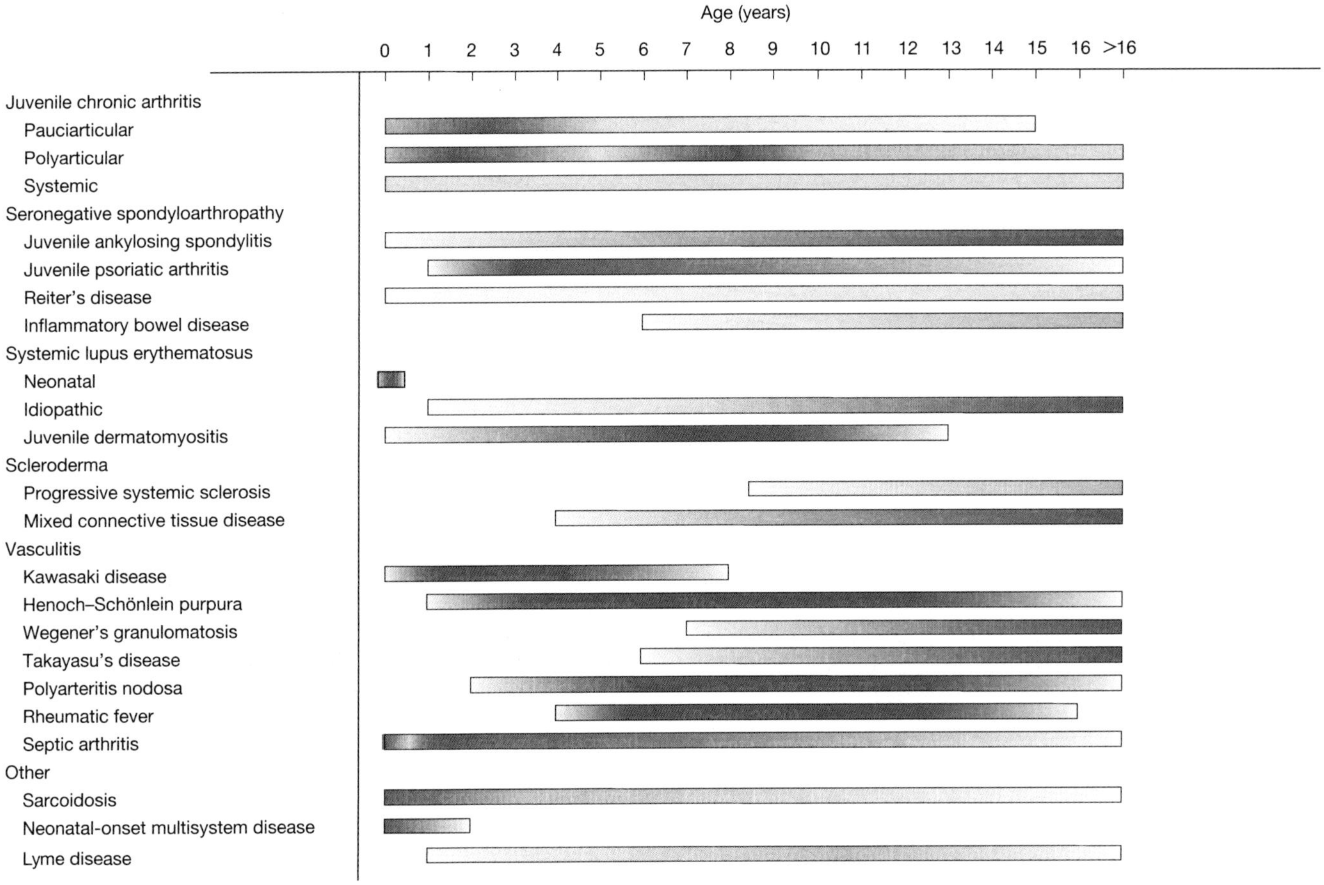

Fig. 1 Characteristic ages of onset of rheumatic diseases of childhood.

polyarticular JIA and ankylosing spondylitis begin to be seen, and juvenile dermatomyositis, Henoch–Schönlein purpura, and polyarteritis nodosa have their peak frequencies. In late childhood and adolescence, enthesitis related arthritis (ankylosing spondylitis) (in boys) and systemic lupus erythematosus (in girls) show a marked increase, and the rare vasculitis syndromes such as Wegener's granulomatosis and Takayasu's arteritis occur.

Influence of gender

Consideration of the sex of the child may help in formulating the differential diagnosis (Fig. 2). The most striking differential sex ratios are in the predominance of juvenile ankylosing spondylitis in boys and of systemic lupus erythematosus in girls. In systemic lupus, the sex ratio is closer to unity in the very young, however (Cassidy et al. 1977).

Growth and development

Important age-related characteristics of the patient affect the physician's approach to rheumatic disease in childhood. Some of the most important are briefly discussed here.

Psychosocial and educational considerations

Chronic illness can have a major impact on the quality of life of the child and family (Quirk and Young 1990). It is often useful for the health care team to meet with the family as a whole to acknowledge this fact and to educate other family members about the health problems faced by the child. An extensive guide for families with children who have arthritis is an important resource (Tucker et al. 1996). The physician must establish a professional relationship not only with the child, but also with the parents. Equally importantly, the physician must recognize the primacy of the patient, even the very young patient, and every reasonable attempt must be made to incorporate the child into the process of obtaining a history and explaining the findings of the physical examination and laboratory investigations. Throughout childhood the roles of child and parent change, and adolescents must be expected to assume increasing responsibility for their health and medical care. The older teenager should be given the opportunity to visit the physician without the parent.

The school is one of the child's most important environments: it is to the child what the workplace is to the adult. Attention to school performance, both academic and social, is critical to the development of a complete picture of the child's health, and in children with functional musculoskeletal pain it is often the key to understanding the cause of the distress. The cooperation of teachers and counsellors in facilitating compliance with medications that are taken during school hours, in modifying physical education programmes, and in ensuring the optimal participation of the child with a rheumatic disease in all classroom activities is a vital component of the child's long-term management.

A comprehensive team approach will help address the broad areas of concern to the older child and adolescent, including self-esteem, sexuality, and educational and vocational goals. The timing of transition from a paediatric to an adult health care setting varies with the patient, physician, and availability of appropriate facilities. In general, children are seen in paediatric clinics until they complete secondary education, enter college or

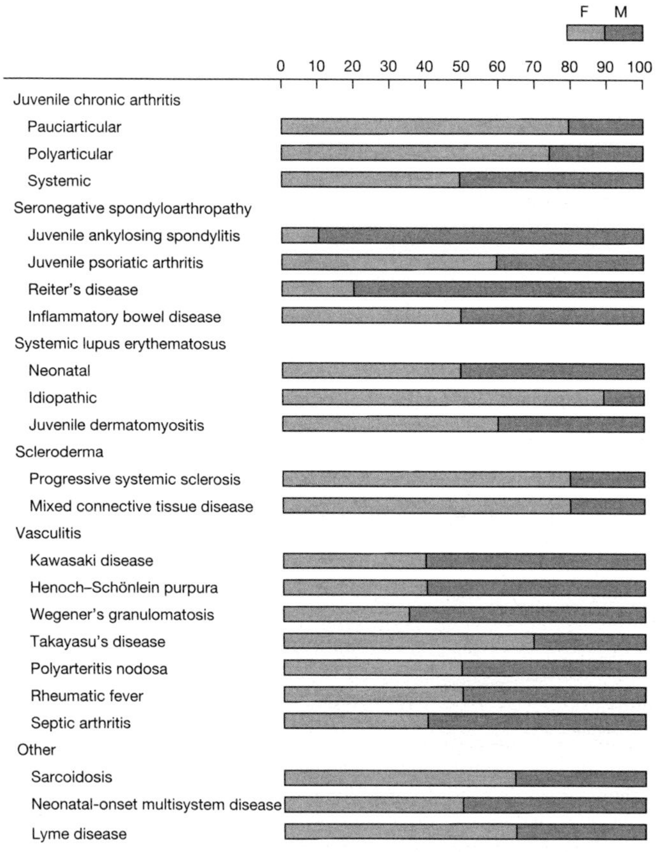

Fig. 2 Differences in frequency of rheumatologic diseases in boys and girls.

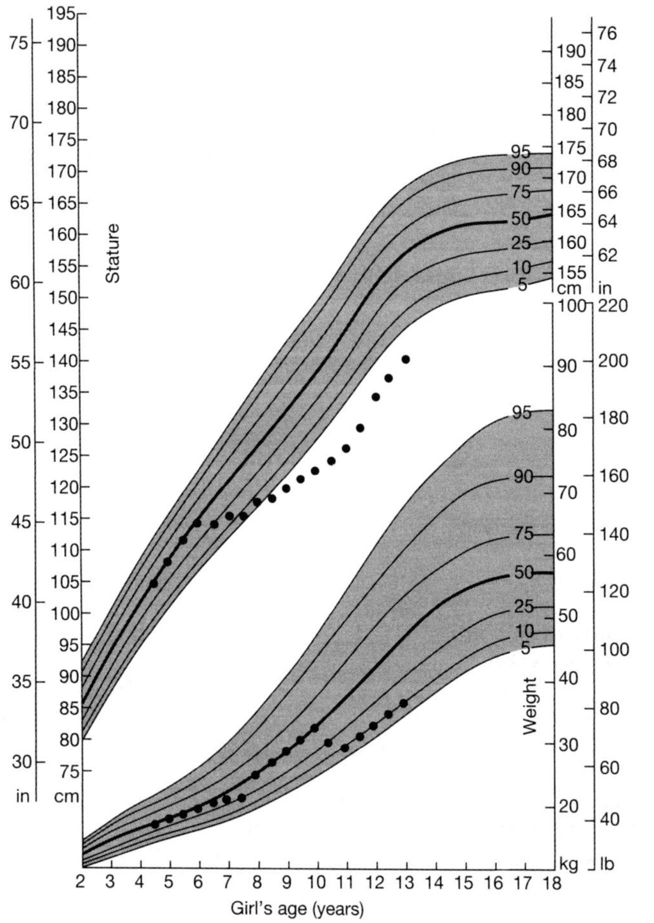

Fig. 3 Growth record of child with polyarticular juvenile idiopathic arthritis of onset age 5.5 years and severe active disease until age 8 years. The disease was controlled with corticosteroids between 8 and 10 years of age. The disease was in remission age 11–13 years during which time corticosteroids were discontinued.

university, or join the workforce. A transition clinic in which the expertise of both paediatric and adult rheumatologists is available is an ideal way to facilitate successful entry into the adult medical care setting. From the psychosocial aspect, a 21-year-old patient with a 15-year history of a chronic disease is very different from a 21-year-old patient in whom a similar disease has just begun. Little is known about the best way to provide care for adults with childhood onset of chronic illnesses. Transition clinics will help provide this much needed information (Foster and Marshall 2000).

Motor development

Recognition of the range of normal motor development in the young child is essential for interpretation of findings on physical examination and functional assessment. There is considerable normal variation in the age at which individual developmental milestones are achieved. The following should be used as guidelines only (Vaughan and Litt 1992):

Age (months)	Milestone achieved by this age
7	Independent sitting
10	Crawling
12	Cruising, walking with one hand held
15	Walking alone, crawling up stairs
18	Running stiffly
24	Running well; walking up and down stairs one step at a time
30	Jumping
36	Walking up stairs alternating feet; rides tricycle
48	Hopping on one foot
60	Skipping

Delay in such achievement may occur in a child with any chronic disease, and may be accentuated in the child with disease affecting the musculoskeletal system, the function of which is the basis for the estimation of developmental stages. Although developmental delay is common in chronically ill children, milestones are eventually achieved.

Physical growth

Chronic inflammatory disease of the musculoskeletal system, and the side-effects of its therapy sometimes have profound effects on physical growth. Careful documentation of height and weight should be made at each encounter and compared to growth curves for healthy children of the same sex and age. In so doing it is important to consider genetic influences and record the parents' height and weight. Sequential measurements ensure not only that the child's height and weight are appropriate for age and sex, but also that the velocity of growth is normal. A growth curve of a child with severe polyarticular JIA is shown in Fig. 3. When the disease was controlled, growth velocity increased and a final height close to the expected value was achieved. This is not always the case, however, and severe stunting may result from disease or from prolonged high dosage of glucocorticoids. Growth failure may be a serious psychologic issue for the adolescent whose peers are growing at a normal rate. Attempts to accelerate growth by giving nutritional supplements or growth hormone have met with limited success, and feasibility and cost often preclude their use (Davies et al. 1994).

Table 3 Normal sexual development (Tanner Stages)

Stage	Pubic hair	Penis	Testes
Boys			
1	None	Preadolescent	Preadolescent
2	Scant, long, straight	Slightly enlarged	Slightly enlarged
3	Dark, starts to curl	Longer	Larger
4	Coarse, curly	Broader, glans enlarges	Larger, scrotum dark
5	Spreads to thighs	Adult	Adult

Stage	Pubic hair	Breasts
Girls		
1	None	Preadolescent
2	Scant, straight, medial margin of labia	Small mound; areolar diameter increased
3	Darker, starts to curl	Breasts and areolae enlarged; no contour separation
4	Coarse, curly	Areola and papilla form secondary mound
5	Spreads to thighs	Nipple projects; areola part of breast contour

Sexual maturation

Sexual maturation may be delayed as a consequence of chronic inflammation, although very rarely, rheumatic disease can be associated with Turner's syndrome (Zulian et al. 1998) or Klinefelter's syndrome (Gilliland and Stashower 2000) in which delayed sexual maturation reflects the effect of the underlying chromosomal abnormalities. The normal development of secondary sexual characteristics is shown in Table 3. In boys, the genitalia may reach Tanner Stage 2 any time after the age of 9 years, but may not do so until ages 14 or 15 years. Complete genital maturity (Tanner 5) may occur before the age of 13, but may not occur until 18 years of age (Marshall and Tanner 1986). Axillary hair develops approximately a year after the appearance of pubic hair and facial hair begins to grow in male a year after the appearance of axillary hair. Menarche occurs at approximately 12.5–13 years of age in North America and Europe, followed after a year or more by development of the breasts and the appearance of pubic and axillary hair (Marshall and Tanner 1986). Delay or irregularity of menstruation is characteristic of adolescent girls who have active inflammatory disease (Fraser et al. 1988).

In addition to indicating the presence of chronic inflammatory disease, delay in sexual maturation is sometimes a source of anxiety for the adolescent. The physician or nurse should raise these issues with adolescent patients if they do not initiate the discussion. The adolescent should understand the reason for delay in sexual development, and be assured that it is almost certain that normal sexual development will eventually occur. Concerns about fertility, and in girls, the ability to deliver a baby, should be recognized and discussed with an obstetrician. Late sequelae of childhood arthritis on sexual and reproductive function have been documented (Ostensen et al. 2000). Questions of inheritance of the rheumatic disease are often raised and require answers as permitted by the limited information available.

Assessment

History and physical examination

The history and physical examination provide most of the diagnostic information in children with rheumatic diseases; the laboratory provides limited help. The history should be obtained from both the care-giver (parent or other adult) and child. Even a young child may be capable of giving a more accurate history of the symptom than the parent. It is, after all, the child, not the *parent* who has the disease.

Rheumatic diseases are systemic disorders and a complete physical examination should be performed, during which the child's comfort, modesty, and dignity must be respected. Appropriate gowns, shorts, and private changing space should be provided, and the child's wish about having the parent present should be honoured. The child's permission to examine him or her should be sought informally. Experienced physicians will identify the 'examinable moment' when the child has gained sufficient confidence in the examiner and acceptance of the environment that useful, trauma-free examination is possible. Reassurance should be given that the examination will not continue if it causes pain and, if possible, examination of the painful areas should be left to the last. In small children, examination may begin by observing the child at play or moving about the room. Examination of the joints may begin with the child in the mother's lap.

Age-related normal variations in physical examination must be taken into account:

Position and range of motion: In full-term newborns, the elbows, knees, and hips do not fully extend. In the young child, and even the adolescent, hyperextension at the knees and elbows is often greater than in the adult. In other ways, however, normal adult range is achieved by approximately 3 or 4 years. Asymmetry of range at any age should be considered to be abnormal.

The appearance of flat feet results from the distribution of fat and limited muscle development in the child up to the age of 5 or 6 years. In the absence of symptoms no investigation or treatment is needed.

Alignment of the legs is a frequent source of parental concern, and age-dependent characteristics should be identified (Salenius and Vankka 1975). From birth until 2 years of age it is normal to have symmetrical genu varus. From 2 to 5 years of age, mild genu valgum may occur. At no time should the degree of valgus or varus exceed 10 degrees, and it should be bilaterally symmetrical.

Muscle strength: Evaluation of muscle strength in the child may be difficult because of age-related differences, and difficulty gaining the child's cooperation in the examination of individual muscle groups, particularly in very young children. Myometry can be used in older children, but repeated evaluation by the same well-trained examiner (usually a physiotherapist), using a standard muscle grading system, is probably the best way of evaluating muscle strength over time.

Ambulation: Cruising (walking while holding on to a hand or to furniture) develops by 12 months of age, and independent walking should occur by 15 months, often earlier. Until the age of 3 years the stance is broad-based in relation to pelvic width, the knee may not be fully extended and the ankle may be plantar flexed at foot-strike (Sutherland et al. 1980). The ability to climb stairs one at a time develops at about 2 years of age; by 3 years of age the child can usually go up and down stairs, alternating feet. Walking on tiptoe is not abnormal for a child who has just begun to walk. This pattern should disappear by the age of 2 years, however. If it persists beyond this age, causes such as spasticity, muscle weakness or tethered cord should be considered.

A limp (asymmetry of gait) may result from structural asymmetry, muscle weakness, or pain. Painful causes of limps include (Hensinger 1986; Petty 1994):

Back	Trauma, spondylolysis or spondylolisthesis
	Inflammation (discitis, spondylitis)
	Infection (osteomyelitis)
	Tumours (osteoid osteoma, malignancy)
Sacroiliac joint	Trauma
	Septic sacroiliitis
	Inflammatory sacroiliitis
Hip	Transient synovitis
	Legg–Perthes' disease
	Slipped capital femoral epiphysis
	Chronic synovitis (JIA)
	Myalgia (dermatomyositis)
	Congenital dysplasia or dislocation
Knee	Hypermobility, patellar dislocation
	Osgood–Schlatter disease

	Inflammatory enthesitis
	Osteochondritis dissecans
	Torn meniscus
	Chronic synovitis (JIA)
Ankle and foot	Hypermobility, trauma, including stress fracture and footwear problems
	Enthesitis
	Chronic synovitis (JIA)

Functional assessment

Age-related functional assessment can be documented with tools specifically developed for this purpose. The juvenile arthritis functional assessment scale (JAFAS) for children older than 7 years (Lovell at al. 1989), can be administered in a few minutes in the outpatient setting, and has been shown to have excellent reliability and validity. The juvenile arthritis functional assessment report (JAFAR) (Howe et al. 1991) provides similar information but is completed by the patient and/or parent. The juvenile arthritis self-report index (JASI) (Wright et al. 1994) focuses on a broad range of physical activities in children with arthritis over the age of 8 years. A number of other functional assessment tools are available and have been recently reviewed (Duffy and Lovell 2001).

Diagnosis of childhood rheumatic diseases

The child with musculoskeletal pain

The very young child may not complain of having pain, but may alter the manner in which he or she uses a limb. The child may refuse to use one arm or leg, or may regress in major motor milestones. For example, a child who is an established walker may, for no apparent reason, stop walking or develop a limp or other alteration of gait. Until fine motor movement of hands has developed, it may be difficult to notice the subtle functional effects of arthritis in the joints of the hands and fingers. Preference for the use of one hand before the age of 2–4 years, when 'handedness' normally develops, suggests the possibility of an abnormality of the underused arm.

Localization of the source of the pain to bone, joint, or soft tissues facilitates appropriate investigations. Young children often localize pain poorly and the physician must carefully identify the area of discomfort by palpation and observation. The child's behaviour is the most important indicator of the presence of absence of pain. The child may not admit to pain but will withdraw the limb or appear anxious when the affected part is examined. Observation of the child's facial expression during examination is very important, as is the parent's interpretation of the child's response. Visual tools to assess pain such as that shown in Fig. 4 may be useful, especially in following change over time (McGrath and Unruh 1987).

The presence of an identifiable time of onset may suggest trauma or infection; chronic arthritis most frequently has an insidious onset, especially in the very young child. Diurnal variation in symptoms is significant, but in the infant or young child this may be difficult to identify, although observant parents will report that the limp or distress is most marked on awakening.

Trauma is seldom the cause of persisting joint pain or swelling in the young child. If the physician considers trauma to be the cause of a child's persisting complaints, non-accidental abuse should be considered.

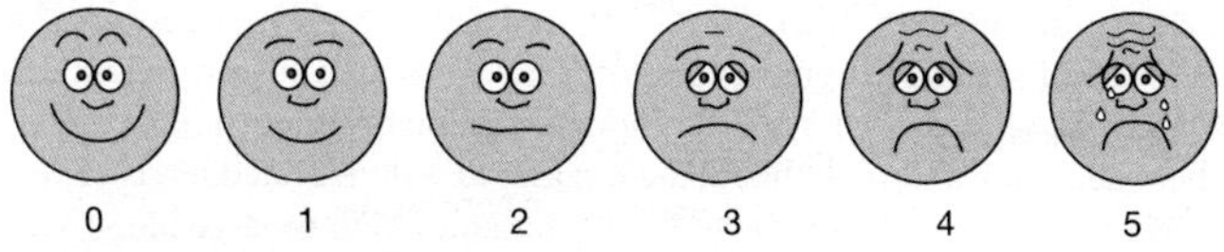

Fig. 4 Pain assessment in children—faces rating scale.

Occasionally children who engage in sports such as gymnastics, or football have activity-related injuries that cause chronic pain, often in the back.

The child with back pain

Back pain is an uncommon complaint, particularly in young children, and should always be thoroughly investigated as the underlying cause may require prompt, specific therapy. Pain may be referred from the back to the thigh, from the sacroiliac joint to the buttocks, or from the hip to the knee. Pain in the absence of tenderness in the painful site suggests that it may be referred from another site. Important causes of back pain in children and adolescents are listed in Table 4.

Pattern of joint involvement

Using knowledge of the relative frequencies of individual rheumatic diseases, the age of the child at the onset of symptoms, and the sex of the child, coupled with the pattern of joint involvement and the character of extra-articular signs and symptoms, it is possible to make some informed guesses about the likely diagnosis of a specific rheumatic disease. Certain patterns of these clinical characteristics are illustrated below.

- Acute onset of large joint monoarthritis in a young girl should be considered to be oligoarticular-onset JIA unless there is evidence of infection.
- At any age and in either sex, a pattern of scattered, asymmetrical large and small joint oligoarthritis or limited polyarthritis suggests the possibility of juvenile psoriatic arthritis.
- Oligoarthritis of large joints of the lower extremity, *especially with enthesitis*, in an older boy suggests a seronegative spondyloarthropathy such as enthesitis-related arthritis.

Table 4 Back pain in children and adolescents

Pain in the back
Acute trauma
  Fracture, dislocation, haematoma
  Spondylolysis, spondylolisthesis
Tumour
  Benign (osteoid osteoma)
  Malignant (reticulum cell sarcoma, metastatic neuroblastoma, leukaemia, lymphoma)
Infection
  Discitis
  Vertebral osteomyelitis
Osteoporosis
Scheuermann's disease (painful adolescent kyphosis)
Fibromyalgia

Pain in the sacroiliac joints
Septic sacroiliitis
Spondyloarthropathy

Pain in the pelvis
Osteomyelitis
Tumour (usually osteogenic sarcoma or Ewing's sarcoma)

Cause	Peak age (year)	Usual site
Relationship to age and site		
Discitis	1–3	L4–5 or L3–4
Osteomyelitis	<12	Any site
Scheuermann's disease	13–17	Lower thoracic or upper lumbar
Osteoid osteoma	10–30	Posterior elements of vertebrae
Spondylolysis	10–20	L5–S1
Metastatic neuroblastoma	<10	Multiple
Inflammatory sacroiliitis	>12	Unilateral or bilateral
Osteogenic sarcoma	10–20	Ilium
Ewing's sarcoma	10–20	Ilium

- The onset of polyarthritis in a teenage girl should suggest the possibility of systemic lupus erythematosus as well as polyarticular JIA.
- Isolated hip joint pains may be caused by toxic synovitis, Legg–Perthes' disease, a slipped capital femoral epiphysis, or less likely, by chronic inflammatory arthritis, probably enthesitis-related arthritis.
- An older child or young adolescent male with low back pain may have enthesitis-related arthritis, but mechanical causes, infection, or malignancy are more likely.

The child with monoarticular arthritis

Among the presentations of arthritis in childhood, monoarticular arthritis is particularly problematic. In a child with acute onset of monoarthritis, the initial differential diagnosis includes infection (septic arthritis and/or osteomyelitis), trauma (accidental or non-accidental), and malignancy (especially leukaemia, neuroblastoma) or, in the older child, osteogenic sarcoma. Chronic monoarthritis may represent oligoarticular JIA, enthesitis-related arthritis, psoriatic arthritis, or possibly tuberculosis. Additionally, a number of rare disorders may mimic chronic monoarticular inflammatory arthritis. These include intra-articular haemangiomas, osteochondritis dissecans (especially at the knee), synovial chondromatosis, lipomatosis arborescens, villonodular synovitis, osteoid osteomas, and discoid meniscus.

Localized growth disturbances are characteristic of the effect of joint inflammation in the child whose epiphyses have not yet fused. In general, the bones adjacent to an inflamed joint grow more rapidly, and in consequence, the affected digit or limb is longer. If this occurs in a single knee, an inequality of leg length results.

The child with muscle weakness

Muscle weakness is common in children with inflammatory musculoskeletal diseases, although its detection and quantitation may be difficult because of age-related developmental differences in normal muscle strength. Observation of the child at play, of the manner in which he or she gets up from sitting and lying position, and of the ability to stand on tiptoes, heels, and squat, and recover from a squat all provide useful clues to the presence of muscle weakness. The child with weakness of trunk muscles, as seen in dermatomyositis, may have to roll over on the side or abdomen in order to assume a sitting position from a supine position. The child with weakness of the hip girdle may be unwilling to squat and unable to stand upright after a squat without exhibiting Gower's sign. Observation of the gait for a wide base or Trendelenburg sign may suggest weakness of the hip girdle muscles. It may be difficult to pick up the young child with weakness of the shoulder girdle because of the instability of the upper trunk. The presence of head lag when lifting the child from the supine to sitting position suggest weakness of the neck flexors. With experience and patience the physician or physiotherapist can demonstrate muscle weakness of a grade of more by formal testing in the child over 3–4 years of age. Prolonged muscle weakness without muscle wasting is unlikely to be the result of organic disease. Assessment of muscle strength should also include a neurological examination. Asymmetric weakness is not likely to result from an inflammatory myositis such as dermatomyositis, or from a primary myopathy. Weakness of one limb or muscle group is most likely to reflect a peripheral neuropathic lesion or inflammation in a major joint such as hip, knee, or ankle. Sacroiliitis or *osteoid osteoma in the femoral neck* can cause severe weakness of the proximal thigh and wasting of muscle. Symmetrical proximal weakness accompanied by muscle tenderness strongly suggests dermatomyositis, and the presence of classical cutaneous changes and elevated muscle enzymes would confirm that diagnosis and differentiate it clinically from primary myopathies.

The child with fever of unknown origin

Elucidation of the cause of *fever* of *unknown origin* may be difficult. The child who has a history of weeks or even months of fever without discernable cause should be evaluated first to exclude the possibility of occult infection or malignancy (especially leukaemia or lymphoma). Complete blood count, bone marrow biopsy, chest radiograph, and abdominal ultrasound are appropriate initial investigations. A technetium bone scan and gallium scan may also be indicated. Bacterial endocarditis should be excluded by blood cultures and echocardiography.

The onset of systemic juvenile idiopathic arthritis may be characterized by fever and rash before the development of joint disease. It is very unusual, however, for arthritis to lag more than a few weeks behind the onset of the systemic features of this disease, and a diagnosis of systemic onset JIA in the absence of arthritis should always be tentative. The presence of pleural or pericardial effusions, splenomegaly, anaemia, leucocytosis, and elevated ESR, together with a quotidian fever and characteristic evanescent macular rash would support the possibility of this diagnosis.

Fever with weight loss, with or without gastrointestinal disturbances, erythema nodosum, arthritis, or arthralgia, suggests the possibility of inflammatory bowel disease. In such instances there may be anaemia, leucocytosis, hypoalbuminaemia, and marked elevation of the ESR. Definitive diagnosis requires biopsy of the colon or small bowel.

Children with vasculitis may have only fever and elevation of indicators of inflammation without objective physical signs. Indirect evidence of vasculitis may be obtained by demonstration of antibody to neutrophil cytoplasmic antigens (ANCA), high levels of von Willebrand factor (Factor VIII-related antigen), abnormalities on Doppler ultrasonography of large arteries, magnetic resonance arteriography, or contrast arteriography. Evidence of coronary arteritis in children with Kawasaki disease is shown by echocardiography. Hypertension or haematuria suggests the presence of renal arterial or glomerular disease. Deficiencies in peripheral pulses suggest the possibility of Takayasu's arteritis. In polyarteritis, the presence of painful subcutaneous nodules, characteristically in the calf or sole of the foot provide the opportunity for definitive excisional biopsy.

Recent advances in molecular biology have made possible the specific identification of some of the rare causes of fever of unknown origin in children (Frenkel and Kuis 2002). Genetic diagnosis of familial Mediterranean fever, hyper IgD syndrome with mevalonate kinase deficiency, and TNF alpha receptor associated period syndrome (TRAPS) is now possible. Disorders such as periodic fever, adenitis, pharyngitis, and aphthous stomatitis (PFAPA) syndrome likely represent several similar disorders, and no genetic mutation has yet been identified (see also Chapter 6.12.3).

Laboratory investigations

Laboratory evaluation of the child with a rheumatic disease serves three functions: to provide or exclude evidence of inflammation, to provide evidence of diagnostic significance, and to exclude non-rheumatic diseases.

In screening for evidence of inflammation, the white blood cell count and differential, haemoglobin, platelet count, and erythrocyte sedimentation rate (ESR) or C-reactive protein usually suffice. A low platelet count in the presence of an elevated ESR should prompt consideration of an underlying malignancy. In acute Kawasaki disease, the platelet count may exceed one million. Decreased serum albumin suggests the possibility of underlying inflammatory bowel disease in a child with arthritis. In a child with a fever of unknown origin and an elevated ESR but no abnormalities on physical examination, inflammatory bowel disease, polyarteritis nodosa or occult malignancy should be considered.

Tests that have diagnostic specificity are few in number. Although antinuclear antibody (ANA) is present in many children with a wide variety of rheumatic disease, it occurs in non-rheumatic disease as well (Cabral et al. 1992a). If clinically indicated, the antigenic specificity of the ANA should be determined. Antibody to double-stranded DNA or the extractable nuclear antigens SS/A (Ro), SS/B (La), and Sm is highly suggestive of a diagnosis of systemic lupus erythematosus. Antibodies to cardiolipin are strongly associated with systemic lupus erythematosus but are found in other rheumatic and non-rheumatic diseases as well. Elevated levels of von Willebrand factor occur in patients with inflammation of large blood vessels. ANCAs are most commonly found in vasculitides such as Wegener's granulomatosis (cANCA) and polyarteritis nodosa (pANCA).

Studies of the sensitivity and specificity of testing for rheumatoid factor in the child have shown unequivocally that it has little value as a diagnostic test (Eichenfield et al. 1986).

Some laboratory investigations are useful in excluding rather than diagnosing disease. Normal white blood cell and platelet counts, ESR, and C-reactive protein make the possibility of a malignant, rheumatic, or infectious disease very unlikely. If abnormal, radiographs are very helpful in delineating disease; when they are normal, however, recent onset pathology cannot be excluded. Technetium bone scans are very useful in this situation, and a normal three phase bone scan virtually excludes bone or joint disease in a child with undiagnosed musculoskeletal pain.

Summary

The child with a rheumatic disease is often a diagnostic and therapeutic challenge. An effective approach to diagnosis requires a careful history, and a physical examination that takes into account normal age-related variations, which may otherwise be misleading. Management requires an understanding that the child is rapidly growing and changing physically, psychologically, and socially. It requires recognition of the child's place as a member of a family and the impact of chronic disease on all family members. Problems related to psychosocial and educational development, challenges in school, and the possibility of limitations on employment necessitate management by a well coordinated team of health professionals. Attention to these features of care are all the more important because, with few exceptions, rheumatic disease of childhood are as yet incurable, although in many instances effective control is possible and the child is able to lead a happy fulfilling childhood and adulthood.

References

Apley, J. (1976). Limb pains with no organic disease. *Clinics in Rheumatic Diseases* **2**, 487–91.

Bohan, A. and Peter, J.B. (1975). Polymyositis and dermatomyositis. *New England Journal of Medicine* **292**, 344–7, 403–7.

Bowyer, S., Roettcher, P., and the members of the Pediatric Rheumatology Database Research Group (1996). Pediatric rheumatology clinic populations in the United States: results of a 3 year survey. *Journal of Rheumatology* **23**, 1968–74.

Brewer, E.J., Bass, J., Baum, J., Cassidy, J.T., Fink, C., Jacobs, H., Hanson, V., Levinson, J.E., Schaller, J., and Stillman, J.S. (1977). Current proposed revision of JRA criteria. *Arthritis and Rheumatism* **20** (Suppl.), 194–9.

Burgos-Vargas, R. and Clarke, P. (1989). Axial involvement in the seronegative enthesopathy and arthropathy syndrome and its progression to ankylosing spondylitis. *Journal of Rheumatology* **16**, 192–7.

Cabral, D.A., Petty, R.E., Fung, M., and Malleson, P.N. (1992a). Persistent antinuclear antibodies in children without identifiable inflammatory, rheumatic or autoimmune disease. *Pediatrics* **89**, 441–4.

Cabral, D.A., Petty, R.E., and Oen, K.G. (1992b). SEA syndrome revisited: a long-term followup of children with a syndrome of seronegative enthesopathy and arthropathy. *Journal of Rheumatology* **19**, 1282–5.

Cassidy, J.T. and Petty, R.E. *Textbook of Pediatric Rheumatology* 4th edn. Philadelphia PA: W.B. Saunders Company, 2001.

Cassidy, J.T., Sullivan, D.B., Ragsdale, C.G., and Petty, R.E. (1977). Lupus nephritis and encephalopathy. Prognosis in 58 children. *Arthritis and Rheumatism* **20** (Suppl.), 315–22.

Chandrasekaran, A.N., Rajendran, C.P., and Madhavan, R. (1996). Juvenile rheumatoid arthritis—Madras experience. *Indian Journal of Pediatrics* **63**, 501–10.

Davies, U.M., Rooney, M., Preece, M.A., Ansell, B.M., and Woo, P. (1994). Treatment of growth retardation in juvenile chronic arthritis with recombinant human growth hormone. *Journal of Rheumatology* **21**, 153–8.

Duffy, C.M. and Lovell, D.J. (2001). Assessment of health status, function and outcome. In *Textbook of Pediatric Rheumatology* 4th edn. (ed. J.T. Cassidy and R.E. Petty), pp. 178–87. Philadelphia PA: W.B. Saunders Company.

Eichenfield, A.H., Athreya, B.H., Doughty, R.A., and Cebul, R.D. (1986). Utility of rheumatoid factor in the diagnosis of juvenile rheumatoid arthritis. *Pediatrics* **78**, 480–4.

European League Against Rheumatism (EULAR) *Bulletin 4. Nomenclature and Classification of Arthritis in Children.* Basel: National Zeitung AG Basel, 1977.

Fink, C.W. (1995). Proposal for the development of classification criteria for idiopathic arthritides of childhood. *Journal of Rheumatology* **22**, 1566–9.

Foster, H. and Marshall, N. (2000). JCA in adult life: a study of long-term outcome in patients with JCA or adult RA. *Clinical Rheumatology* **19**, 326–9.

Fraser, P.A., Hoch, S., Erlandson, D., Partridge, R., and Jackson, J.M. (1988). The timing of menarche in juvenile rheumatoid arthritis. *Journal of Adolescent Health Care* **9**, 483–7.

Frenkel, J. and Kuis, W. (2002). Overt and occult rheumatic diseases: the child with chronic fever. *Best Practice Research in Clinical Rheumatology* **16**, 443–69.

Gilliland, W.R. and Stashower, M.E. (2000). Klinefelter's syndrome and systemic lupus erythematosus. *Clinical and Experimental Rheumatology* **18**, 107–9.

Hensinger, R.N. (1986). Limp. *Pediatric Clinics of North America* **33**, 1355–64.

Hochberg, M.C. (1997). Updating the American College of Rheumatology revised criteria for the classification of systemic lupus erythematosus. *Arthritis and Rheumatism* **40**, 1725.

Howe, S., Levinson, J., Shear, E., Hartner, S., McGirr, G., Schulte, M., and Lovell, D. (1991). Development of a disability measurement tool for juvenile rheumatoid arthritis—the Juvenile Arthritis Functional Assessment Report for children and their parents. *Arthritis and Rheumatism* **34**, 873–80.

Jennette, J.C., Falk, R.J., Andrassy, K., Bacon, P.A., Churg, J., Gross, W.L., Hagan, E.C., Hoffman, G.S., Hunder, G.G., Kallenberg, C.G.M., McClusky, R.T., Sinico, R.A., Rees, A.J., van Es, L.A., Waldherr, R., and Wijk, A. (1994). Nomenclature of systemic vasculitides. Proposal of an international consensus conference. *Arthritis and Rheumatism* **37**, 187–92.

Kunnamo, I., Kallio, P., and Pelkonen, P. (1986). Incidence of arthritis in urban Finnish children. *Arthritis and Rheumatism* **19**, 1232–8.

Lovell, D.J., Howe, S., Sheare, E., Hartner, S., McGirr, G.F., Schulte, M., and Levinson, J. (1989). Development of a disability measurement tool for juvenile rheumatoid arthritis. The juvenile arthritis functional assessment scale. *Arthritis and Rheumatism* **32**, 1390–5.

Malleson, P.N., Fung, M.Y., and Rosenberg, A.M. (1996). The incidence of pediatric rheumatic diseases: results of the Canadian Pediatric Rheumatology Association Disease Registry. *Journal of Rheumatology* **23**, 1981–7.

Manners, P.J. and Diepeveen, D.A. (1996). Prevalence of juvenile chronic arthritis in a population of 12-year-old children in urban Australia. *Pediatrics* **98**, 84–90.

Marshall, B. and Tanner, J.M. (1986). Puberty. In *Human Growth, A Comprehensive Treatise* 2nd edn. (ed. F. Falkner and J.M. Tanner), pp. 171–209. New York: Plenum.

McGrath, P.J. and Unruh, A.M. *Pain in Children and Adolescents.* New York: Elsevier, 1987.

Moenkemoeller, K., Petty, R.E., Malleson, P.N., Cabral, D.A., and Tucker, L.B. (2001). What criteria do pediatric rheumatologists use to make the diagnosis of juvenile dermatomyositis (JD). *Arthritis and Rheumatism* **44** (Suppl.), S293.

Ostensen, M., Almberg, K., and Koksvik, H.S. (2000). Sex, reproduction, and gynaecological disease in young adults with a history of juvenile chronic arthritis. *Journal of Rheumatology* **27**, 1783–7.

Petty, R.E. (2001). Limp. In *Handbook of Pediatric Emergencies* 3rd edn. (ed. G.A. Baldwin), pp. 397–401. Philadelphia PA: Lippincott Williams & Wilkins.

Petty, R.E. and Cabral, D.A. (2002). Baillière's Clinics in Rheumatology. *Pediatric Rheumatology.*

Petty, R.E., Southwood, T.R., Baum, J., Bhettay, E., Glass, D.N., Manners, P., Maldonado-Cocco, J., Suarez-Almazor, M., Orozco-Alcala, J., and Prieur, A.-M. (1998). Revision of the proposed classification criteria for juvenile idiopathic arthritis. Durban, 1997. *Journal of Rheumatology* **25**, 1991–4.

Petty, R.E., Southwood, T.R., Baum, J., Glass, D.N., Manners, P., Maldonado-Cocco, J., Suarez-Almazor, M., Orozco-Alcala, J., Prieur, A.-M., and Woo, P. (2002). Second revision of the ILAR criteria for the classification of juvenile idiopathic arthritis: Edmonton 2001 (in preparation).

Quirk, M.E. and Young, M.H. (1990). The impact of JRA on children, adolescents, and their families. Current research and implications for future studies. *Arthritis Care and Research* **3**, 36–43.

Rosenberg, A.M. and Petty, R.E. (1982). A syndrome of seronegative enthesopathy and arthropathy in children. *Arthritis and Rheumatism* **25**, 1041–7.

Salenius, P. and Vankka, E. (1975). The development of the tibiofemoral angle in children. *Journal of Bone and Joint Surgery* **57A**, 259–61.

Sekiguchi, M., Takao, A., Endo, M., Asai, T., and Kawasaki, T. (1985). On the mucocutaneous lymph node syndrome or Kawasaki disease. In *Progress in Cardiology* Vol. 13 (ed. P.N. Yu and J.F. Goodwin), p. 97. Philadelphia PA: Lea and Febiger.

Seth, V., Kabra, S.K., Semwal, O.P., and Jain, Y. (1996). Clinico-immunological profile in juvenile rheumatoid arthritis—Indian experience. *Indian Journal of Pediatrics* **63**, 293–300.

Southwood, T.R., Petty, R.E., Malleson, P.N., Delgado, E.A., Hunt, D.W., Wood, B., and Schroeder, M.-L. (1989). Psoriatic arthritis in children. *Arthritis and Rheumatism* **32**, 1007–13.

Special Writing Group of the American Heart Association (1992). Guidelines for the diagnosis of rheumatic fever. *Journal of the American Medical Association* **268**, 2069–73.

Sutherland, D.H., Ohlsen, R., Cooper, L., and Woo, S.-L.-Y. (1980). The development of the mature gait. *Journal of Bone and Joint Surgery* **62A**, 336–53.

Symmons, D.P., Jones, M., Osborne, J., Sills, J., Southwood, T.R., and Woo, P. (1996). Pediatric rheumatology in the United Kingdom. Data from the British Pediatric Rheumatology Group National Diagnostic Register. *Journal of Rheumatology* **23**, 1975–80.

Tan, E.M., Cohen, A.S., Fries, J.F., Masi, A.T., McShane, D.J., Rothfield, N.F., Schaller, J.G., Talal, N.B., and Winchester, R.J. (1982). The 1982 revised criteria for the classification of systemic lupus erythematosus. *Arthritis and Rheumatism* **25**, 1271–7.

Tucker, L.B., DeNardo, B.A., Stebulis, J.A., and Schaller, J.G. *Your Child with Arthritis*. Baltimore MD: Johns Hopkins University Press, 1996.

Vaughan, V.C. III and Litt, L.F. (1992). Assessment of growth and development. In *Textbook of Pediatrics* 14th edn. (ed. R.E. Behrman), pp. 32–43. Philadelphia PA: W.B. Saunders Company.

Wright, V.F., Law, M., Crombie, V., Goldsmith, C.H., and Dent, P. (1994). Development of a self-report functional status index for juvenile rheumatoid arthritis. *Journal of Rheumatology* **21**, 536–44.

Zulian, F., Schumacher, H.R., Calore, A., Goldsmith, D.P., and Athreya, B.H. (1998). Juvenile arthritis in Turner's syndrome: a multicenter study. *Clinical and Experimental Rheumatology* **16**, 489–94.

1.1.3 Adolescence and transition

Janet E. McDonagh and Russell Viner

Introduction

Since the second edition of this textbook in which the concept of transition was limited to a few sentences, adolescent rheumatology has gathered momentum and now necessitates a whole chapter! Transition has now become a quality issue in the care of young people with chronic illness (Viner 1999). This chapter will highlight some of these needs and detail some models of care and strategies in their management.

Adolescence, literally the process of becoming an adult, is a difficult period of human development to precisely define chronologically, reflected in the numerous definitions currently prevalent in the literature: World Health Organization: 10–20 years (WHO 1993); Society for Adolescent Medicine: 10–25 years (Society for Adolescent Medicine 1995). The onset of adolescence is easy to define in terms of biology—that is, the onset of puberty. The entry into adulthood is less easy and more often carries a legal non-biological definition in terms of the age of consent which itself can vary from one country to the next. Chronological definitions take little account of the developmental changes at the heart of the concept of adolescence, and the most useful way of thinking about adolescence is as a biopsychosocial development process leading to functionally independent adult life.

Biological development includes sexual maturation and growth. Psychological development is driven by increasing myelination and maturation of the central nervous system, and results in the development of abstract thinking and a more complete personal identity. In contrast to the biological and psychological changes, which are fairly universal, the social changes of adolescence are largely culturally determined. In Western cultures, the social 'tasks' of adolescence are concerned with establishing relationships outside the family, achieving independence from parents, and establishing financial (i.e. vocational) independence. These processes are outlined in Table 1.

In adolescent rheumatology, an awareness of the interdependence of these tasks and processes in addition to a working knowledge of adolescent development and culture are vital for appropriate management of these young people. As young people with a chronic rheumatic illness negotiate the transition from home to independent living, from school to further education and/or job, they also need to negotiate the transition from paediatric to adult health care.

Adolescence and chronic rheumatic illness

Rheumatic disease spectrum during (and beyond) adolescence

Over one-fourth of all juvenile idiopathic arthritis (JIA) subtypes present during adolescence, particularly enthesitis-related JIA and rheumatoid factor positive polyarticular JIA. Some rheumatic diseases typically present during adolescence, for example, idiopathic pain syndromes, systemic lupus erythematosus (SLE), spondylolysis/listhesis, idiopathic Raynaud's.

Childhood-onset rheumatic disease is not confined to the childhood years and does not always 'burn out' with or without adult sequelae. Follow-up studies in JIA report a third of young people continue to have active inflammation into adulthood and 60 per cent have some impairment in activities of daily living (David et al. 1994; Gare and Fasth 1995; Petersen et al. 1997; Ruperto et al. 1997; Oen et al. 2002; Packham and Hall 2002a; Foster et al. 2003). Although reports vary, many point to a less than perfect outcome for young people with JIA. Despite good educational achievement there are reports of higher levels of unemployment in UK JIA populations (Martin and Woo 1997; Packham and Hall 1999, 2002b). Petersen et al. (1997) reported more fatigue, lower health perception, level of exercise, physical functioning in a case control study of young adults with JIA. Wirrel et al. (1995) reported young adults with JIA to have lower perceived social functioning, which was unrelated to the level of disability or disease subtype.

Another shared concern of paediatric and adult rheumatologists is osteoporosis. The greatest increase in bone mineral content during life occurs during the adolescent years—between 11 and 14 years in girls and between 13 and 17 years in boys (Pepmueller et al. 1996)—and ceases in the mid-20s. Young adults who have higher peak bone mass are likely to be at lower risk of developing osteoporosis in later life. It is therefore important for those caring for children and young people, to recognize the important potential window of opportunity for primary preventive strategies earlier in life before peak bone mass is attained. This is particularly important when there is any relative impairment in bone formation such as occurs in JIA (Kotaniemi et al. 1999; Zak et al. 1999; Haugen et al. 2000; Henderson et al. 2000) which will then have an accentuated effect during adolescent years when bone acquisition would normally be at its maximum. Zak et al. (1999) demonstrated that adult patients (male and female) with a history of JIA also have reduced bone mineral density and increased bone turnover compared with healthy controls matched for age, sex, height, and weight.

Low back pain in adolescence has been linked with continuing pain in adulthood. Students who had low back pain at age 14 were more likely to have back pain 25 years later than students who did not have it

Table 1 Biopsychosocial development during adolescence

	Biological	Psychological	Social
Early adolescence	Early puberty *Girls* Breast bud and pubic hair development (Tanner Stage 2) Initiation of growth spurt *Boys* Testicular enlargement, beginning of genital growth (Stage 2)	Thinking remains concrete but with development of early moral concepts Progression of sexual identity development: Development of sexual orientation—possibly by experimentation Possible homosexual peer interest Reassessment and restructuring of body image in face of rapid growth	Realization of differences from parents Beginning of strong peer identification Early exploratory behaviours (smoking, violence)
Mid adolescence	*Girls* Mid to late puberty (Stage 4–5) and completion of growth Menarche (Stage 4 event) Development of female body shape with fat deposition *Boys* Mid puberty (Stages 3 and 4) Spermarche and nocturnal emissions Voice breaking Initiation of growth spurt (Stage 3–4)	Emergence of abstract thinking although ability to imagine future applies to others rather than self (self seen as 'bullet-proof') Growing verbal abilities; adaptation to increasing educational demands Conventional morality (identification of law with morality) Development of fervently held ideology (religious/political)	Establishment of emotional separation from parents Strong peer group identification Increased health risk behaviours (smoking, alcohol, drugs, sexual exploration) Heterosexual peer interests develop Early vocational plans Development of an educational trajectory; early notions of vocational future
Late adolescence	*Boys* Completion of pubertal development (Stage 5) Continued androgenic effects on muscle bulk and body hair	Complex abstract thinking Post-conventional morality (ability to recognize difference between law and morality) Increased impulse control Further completion of personal identity Further development or rejection of ideology and religion—often fervently	Further separation from parents and development of social autonomy Development of intimate relationships—initially within peer group, then separation of couples from peer group Development of vocational capability, potential or real financial independence

(Harreby et al. 1995). Prevention of back pain in youth may potentially contribute to the prevention of back pain in adulthood with all the significant associated morbidity associated with the latter.

Another significant group of patients in adolescent rheumatology are those with chronic idiopathic pain syndromes. Outcome data varies in the literature from favourable (Bushkila et al. 1995; Sherry 2000) to unfavourable (Flato et al. 1997). There is no prospective data of the outcome of this group of patients into adulthood yet. A recent outcome study of another chronic pain syndrome in children, that is, headache reported increased risk of recurring headache in adulthood in addition to other physical (including back pain) and psychiatric symptoms (Fearon and Hotopf 2001). Prospective studies of chronic idiopathic pain syndromes into adulthood are awaited with interest.

Adolescence and chronic illness

Many of the problems in the management of rheumatological conditions in adolescence are not unique but are common to all chronic illness in adolescence. Chronic illness management and adolescent development have reciprocal adverse effects on each other. A chronic condition may retard adolescent development, producing pubertal and growth delay, delayed social independence, poor body and sexual self-image, and educational and vocational failure. On the other hand, the imperatives of adolescent development (the search for identity and independence, immature abstract thinking including poor future thinking, etc.) make chronic illness management problematic through poor adherence to medical regimens and 'risky' health behaviours. Health risk behaviours such as smoking, alcohol, and drug use are as common in adolescents with chronic illness or disability as in the general population. A few studies involving adolescent patients with JIA have reported significant alcohol use (Timko et al. 1992; Nash et al. 1998). However, Timko et al. (1992) also reported that after 1 year of disease, patients were less involved in substance abuse than their healthy siblings (see also Nash et al. 1998; Hargrave et al. 1999). More studies in specific populations of chronic rheumatic illnesses are needed.

One of the most challenging aspects of chronic rheumatic illnesses for both the young person and the rheumatology team is the uncertainty. There are still few, true predictive factors in many of these conditions and although there are the so-called 'disease-modifying drugs', there are few cures. Young people at this time of their lives are searching for a sense of control yet face a life with an apparent uncontrollable, living with chronic illness. They long for independence yet may still be dependent on their family for activities of daily living. Having a chronic illness makes you *more* dependent on your family at a time you should be less dependent.

Adolescents are also searching for their own, individual identity. Increasing importance of their peer group characterizes adolescence. Yet how can young people who have a chronic illness be the same as their healthy peers? Adolescence is also a time of ambivalence and 'changing minds and opinions' with young people longing to express themselves yet not really sure how. This can be difficult in the health care setting with concerned parents and knowledgeable experts demanding 'air time' for their own viewpoints.

Comparison of paediatric, adolescent, and adult rheumatology

Professionals who have worked in paediatric, adolescent, and adult healthcare soon realize the important differences in clinical practice and the different skills required in caring for adolescents and their families, particularly those with chronic illnesses. These differences require focus on spectrum of disease, impact of disease, growth and development, consultation dynamics, communication, decision-making processes, role of parent and/or family, generic health issues, and adherence issues.

Table 2 Useful interview strategies with young people

Give choices 'Do you want to start the therapy this month or next month?' 'Which test will we do first?'
Decriminalize non-adherence 'All young people find it hard to take all their prescribed treatments. How often do you manage to take all your medications?' 'Which pills do you find it easiest or most difficult to take? . . . We'll concentrate on those'
Give time for decision-making 'You don't need to decide which treatment to start today. I will write to you with the list of options, give you time to think about it and I will phone you next week and we can discuss it again'
Open-ended questions: 'What are you most concerned about?'
Posing hypothetical situations—'Some young people with (disease) worry about . . .; do you ever worry about this?'
Problem solving: 'What might you do if your friends are drinking alcohol at a party and you are still taking methotrexate?'
The 'positive sandwich' technique *Positive slice:* Initial praise for adherence with regimen *Negative filling:* Express concern that the young person e.g. may be drinking more alcohol than he/she should on a particular therapy. Give appropriate explanation and rationale for limiting alcohol intake *Positive slice:* Further praise that the young person has been honest
The brief intervention strategy (or the gentle nagging approach!) e.g. if concern regarding smoking habit *Initial visit:* How many are you smoking? Document without further comment *Next visit:* Are you still smoking *n* cigarettes? Document without further comment *Next visit:* Are you still smoking *n* cigarettes? Have you tried cutting down? and so on . . .
Goal setting with them
Drawing up contracts with them
Prioritize therapies
Negotiation: e.g. time-out periods during each week free of home exercise routines, etc.
See young people by themselves 'We routinely see young people by themselves as well as with their parents from 13–14 years up' (These remarks are directed to the young person AND parents!)

Growth and development

In paediatrics, the growth and development of the young person contrasts with the aging and senescence of adult rheumatology. Adolescence is a critical time period in development, which may be disrupted by a chronic illness. The reciprocal influences of a chronic illness are on adolescent development (physical, cognitive, and psychosocial) as mentioned above and need to be addressed by multidisciplinary rheumatology teams. Evidence suggests that both paediatricians and adult physicians are poor at monitoring growth and pubertal development in chronic illness. Continued attention is required to these variables well into the early 20s (Ghosh et al. 1998).

Consultation dynamics

The paternalistic triangular model that characterizes paediatric care with parent, professional, and child evolves during adolescence until the horizontal adult relationship of patient and professional is achieved. Communication and counselling skills are important aspects of training for those working with this age group, and there is evidence from randomized trials that these skills *can* be learned (Sanci et al. 2000).

Table 3 Useful strategies for adolescent rheumatology service development

I. Personnel Continuity of care at consecutive appointments regarding personnel Identify key person Offer professional of preferred gender when feasible Involvement of the whole team, e.g. rheumatology secretaries trained to take messages, etc. from young people Use of peers in disease education programmes Use of role models Preparation for independent visits Advisory panel of young people for service developments, etc.
II. Administrative Notebook for questions to bring to clinic Information sheets specifically written for young people, prepared with their active input Letter to patient reiterating the information exchanged during each clinic visit and suggesting issues that need further discussion/review at the next visit
III. Environmental Dedicated clinic and waiting area Rooms available for young person and parent to be seen independently Careful arrangement of the chairs in the clinic room—ideally have young person sitting in direct eye contact with the health professional and have parent out of direct range

It is important for health professionals in the adult specialties to remember that the impact of rheumatic disease for a young person without memory of a healthy childhood differs significantly from an adult with a healthy childhood and disease onset in middle age. Although family support is important whatever the age of the patient, there are potential negative as well as positive consequences. As self-advocacy is encouraged and evolves in the young person, so the parents must take an increasingly secondary role in consultations and learn to 'let go'. The healthcare setting must remain inclusive yet acknowledge the changing roles of parent and child. This can be very challenging to the health professional!

Communication skills

Acquiring mastery of such consultations requires communication skills and strategies, which may vary depending on the subject matter and circumstance. There are no absolutes but some useful ones are listed here as examples (Table 2).

Once again, a working understanding of adolescent development is important for those professionals dealing with young people. As they mature, young people normally develop from using emotional strategies (such as wishful thinking or resignation) to problem-solving strategies. Chronic illness can interfere with this development or cause the adolescent to regress in this respect. Unpredictable diseases such as JIA or SLE tend to encourage the use of emotion-focused coping strategies. Emotion-based coping strategies are related to self-reports of depression, anxiety, and substance abuse in adolescents whereas with a problem-based approach fewer emotional and behaviour problems are reported (Eiser 1990).

There are also personnel, administrative, and environmental strategies that can be usefully employed in the adolescent healthcare setting (see Table 3).

What young people want

Involvement of young people in developing age- and developmentally appropriate health services is vital and increasingly recognized. Several surveys have highlighted what the young people want from rheumatology services. Young people in the United Kingdom request information about their disease and treatment options; counselling about personal relationships; early career counselling; and information about financial benefits

(Foster 1998). In Canada, they wanted: to be involved in decision-making about their disease; educated about new research developments; and understand medication side effects. In addition, there was interest in learning how to manage pain, tiredness, and disease flares as well as learning more about the disease. Other concerns include their future ability to have children (Lang et al. 1998).

Requests for career counselling are not so very different from the needs of their healthy peers. Job security and future employment are included in the top five concerns of healthy 15–16 year olds in the United Kingdom (Oakley et al. 1995).

Transition—principles

Transition is an important part of quality care that attempts to encompass the needs of young people with chronic illness and/or disability. Transition is most usefully defined, as 'a multi-faceted, active process that attends to the medical, psychosocial and educational/vocational needs of adolescents as they move from child to adult centred care' (Blum et al. 1993). The aims of transition are:

(i) To provide co-ordinated, uninterrupted health care which is age-appropriate, developmentally appropriate, and comprehensive;

(ii) To promote skills in communication, decision-making, assertiveness, and self-care;

(iii) To enhance sense of control and independence in health care.

It is vital to stress that transition is a process *not* an event. Transfer to adult care is an event, which is part of the transition process. Transition must be a planned with preparation starting early. In a US report, the reasons for failure of transition into adult health care system was firstly financial and secondly lack of planning (Blum and Okinow 1993). This has also been highlighted in several UK-based studies of physically disabled young people (Bax et al. 1998; Florentino et al. 1998). The unpredictability of many chronic illnesses can further accentuate the negative effects of deficient transition planning. If transition is 'forced' at a time when the young person is ill prepared, their perceived lack of control and choices is further accentuated. Successful transition becomes less likely.

In keeping with the concept of transition being a process, there is no age cut-off for the end of transition or the event of transfer to adult care. The essence of timing in all aspects of transition is that of flexibility. Timing of events within the transitional process must be individualized for each patient (Table 4). Any plan for transition and transfer should be regularly reviewed particularly in the context of an unpredictable chronic disease. Discussion and preparation for transition needs relative disease remission and transfer should not be implemented during an 'active' phase of their disease.

The concept of transition implies movement from one place to another and successful transition requires active involvement and commitment from both places, that is, paediatric and adult rheumatology teams. Transfer must be synonymous with bridging the gap and not passing the buck (Viner 1999).

Table 4 Timings and key elements within a transitional care programme

Timing of transition and transfer
Chronological age
Maturity
Current medical status
Adherence to therapy
Independence in health care
Preparation
Readiness of the young person
Availability of an appropriate adult rheumatologist
Key elements of a transitional care programme in rheumatology
Transition policy agreed by all members of the multidisciplinary team and target adult rheumatology services
Preparation period for patient and parent
Education programme for patient and parent
Flexible policy on timing of events
Network of relevant local agencies and target adult services
Administrative support
Liaison personnel in paediatric and/or adult teams
Key person identified for each individual patient

Transition models

Various models for transition have been reported (Rettig and Athreya 1991; Chamberlain and Rooney 1996) and are largely dependent on local resources, geographical variables, and the type of health service provision in the particular country. Transition models can be a single step from paediatric to adult or have an intermediary step of either a transition clinic, or a specific adolescent clinic or indeed have two intermediary steps of adolescent clinic to young adult clinic. The latter is particularly pertinent to rheumatology where the average age of an adult rheumatology clinic is often well into middle age! Other variations of transition models include disease specific as opposed to generic adolescent clinics, the latter recognizing that many issues facing adolescents with chronic illness are generic. Transition models may be centred on primary, secondary, or tertiary care. Finally where paediatric and adult specialties exist within the same hospital site, transition models can be single site as compared to the more practically challenging split-site models required by stand-alone paediatric hospitals.

Whatever the model, there are some principles of transition common to all. The key players in the process are first and foremost the young persons themselves. Young people both on an individual level as well as in an advisory and consultative level should participate in the development of adolescent services. Other key players include their family, the primary health care team, the multidisciplinary rheumatology team, the education services, social services, and voluntary organizations.

The key elements of a transitional care programme (Table 4) include a preparation period and education programme for both the young person and their parents. A policy on timing of events during the transitional process is useful in acknowledging the importance of flexibility as highlighted above. Co-ordination of both transition and eventual transfer is integral to the success of the process as is an interested and capable adult service. Establishing a local network of interested and committed professionals is vital for the success of a transitional care programme. Adequate administrative support for transitional care must not be underestimated. This in turn facilitates effective communication between all professionals involved in the transition process, integral to success. Key liaison personnel who can bridge the gap between the paediatric and adult service both for the patient on an individual basis as well as the multidisciplinary teams are very useful particularly in split-site models.

Unfortunately, the evidence base for effective transitional care is limited in rheumatology as is the case in most other specialties! An audit of adolescent rheumatology services in the United Kingdom highlighted the heterogeneity and relative paucity of services for this age group in the United Kingdom (McDonagh et al. 2000). In the only textbook specifically addressing adolescent rheumatology, Rettig and Athreya (1998) detail an example of a transition intervention plan with a transition skills checklist. The same authors have reported improved follow-up when a co-ordinated transitional care programme was implemented (Rettig and Athreya 1991). There is also evidence to support the benefits of co-ordinated transitional care programmes in other chronic illnesses, for example, diabetes (Salmi et al. 1986; Sawyer 1998) and cystic fibrosis (Nasr et al. 1992).

It is unlikely that there is a universal transition prescription for rheumatology patients and each is likely to be an individualized plan, which will vary between patients, diseases, as well as between centres.

Transitional care for parents of young people with chronic rheumatic conditions

One of the basic tenets of a transitional care programme is that it is inclusive of the family, not exclusive. The positive, affirming role of the family must not be forgotten in the attempts to engender increasing adolescent independence. Family connectedness, family role models, family concern for the well-being of the child, and autonomy at home are all factors identified that foster resilience in children and should be encouraged and affirmed (Patterson and Blum 1996), especially during adolescence and transition.

Just as the young person with a chronic rheumatic condition is negotiating the tasks and transitions detailed above, their parent(s) is also having to negotiate the transition of being a parent of a dependent child with a chronic illness to a parent of an independent young adult with a chronic illness—not always easy. In one study, although parents of non-disabled patients with JIA denied any impact of the disease on their child, they still had lower expectations for their education compared to their healthy siblings (McAnarney et al. 1974). Only 17 per cent of parents expected their non-disabled child with JIA to go to university compared to 73 per cent of their healthy siblings (McAnarney et al. 1974). When 100 adolescents with chronic illness and/or physical disabilities were studied, their lack of career maturity and paucity of early work experience related to their parents view that the mean age for first work experience should be 16 years or older (White et al. 1990). This is compared to reports of 50 per cent healthy 13 year olds are involved in work experience outside their home (Phillips and Sandston 1990). Parental expectations for their child with a chronic illness and/or disability are therefore important areas to address during the transition period, as they may be too high or too low. Such issues need sensitivity of approach.

Parents too need a preparation period for transition and transfer. Programmes should facilitate parental understanding of adolescent development and the dynamic role of parents in transition. Parents can be helped to encourage involvement of their son/daughter in decision-making from early age, to ensure attainment of functional living skills and development of autonomy and self-advocacy skills similar to their peers. Some parents find it difficult to trust their son/daughter to tell the health professional everything unless they (the parent) remain in the room to remind them or ask the question for them. It is sometimes helpful to suggest the young person prepares for the hospital visit with their parent the day before and make a list of questions that both the young person and the parent want to ask. The young person can then bring this in with them as an aide memoire. In this way, young people can practice remembering and asking questions without their parents around, thereby gaining confidence and self-advocacy skills. This strategy also allows time for another team member to see the parents independently of their son or daughter as parents too may have questions they would prefer not to ask in front of their child. Concluding the visit with a meeting with the parents as well as the young person is often a good interim measure until all parties are confident that independent visits are inclusive and a positive step forward. As part of this process, parents need to be helped to become more aware of resources available in their local community and encouraged to facilitate career exploration for their young person.

Transitional care issues

So what are the issues in a transitional care programme beyond controlling the disease and pain management, etc?

Disease education

If the young persons have had their disease since early childhood, much of the initial disease education may have been primarily directed to the parents. This may explain in part the significant level of inaccuracies and misunderstandings reported in long-term clinic attendees (Berry et al. 1993). Berry et al. (1993) also reported that adolescents with JIA were still at the concrete operational stage of cognitive development rather than the more adult abstract stage, a factor that must be considered by professionals providing disease education for young people. Requests for disease education also appear in many surveys of adolescent clinics highlighting the need for a continuing education process. Issues irrelevant at the age of 9 may be major concerns by the age of 15 years to a young person with a chronic rheumatic illness.

Generic health education

Generic health issues also need to be borne in mind especially as many adult health-promoting behaviours become established in adolescence, which is therefore an important time for intervention. A useful acronym is listed below.

H Home
E Education, exercise
A Activities
D Drugs and alcohol, diet
S Sexual health

Adolescents with chronic illness report more age-related concerns than their healthy peers: acne, alcohol and drug, periods, headaches, anxiety, contraception, insomnia, worry about height and weight and sexual health (Carroll et al. 1983). It is important therefore for health professionals to ensure they are being addressed by someone, especially as 75 per cent of such patients will have at least two rheumatology visits per year with 61.4 per cent having at least two other health-related visits per year (Timko et al. 1992).

In the area of sexual health, chronically ill adolescents become sexually active at rates comparable to healthy teenagers (Choquet et al. 1997; Packham and Hall 2002c). A trend to increased pelvic inflammatory disease in young female adults with JIA has recently been reported (Ostensen et al. 2000) and should be borne in mind in view of the of the increasing incidence of sexually transmitted infections in teenagers (Coleman and Schofield 2001). It is concerning that in a recent paper it was not felt relevant to counsel males regarding unprotected sexual intercourse (Britto et al. 2000)! Chronic illnesses and/or their therapy may cause delayed puberty and some of the drugs frequently used in these conditions are teratogenic and/or affect fertility. If the patient is pubertal and such drugs, for example, cyclophosphamide are contemplated, storage of sperm or eggs must be considered. Cervical screening is also important in sexually active female patients. Cervical atypia has been reported in SLE patients, the exact nature of the relationship, however, is still unclear (Blumenfeld et al. 1994).

Studies in young adults with JIA have further highlighted sexual health as a potentially neglected area. Increased metorrhagia and surgery for polycystic ovaries in young adults with JIA has been reported (Ostensen et al. 2000). In the latter study, young female adults with JIA had similar attitudes to sexual activity, contraception, wish for children, age at first child, and similar fertility but had increased problems conceiving and increased miscarriage rates (Ostensen et al. 2000).

Although severe non-remitting disease may reduce the wish for children (Ostensen 1991), young people with JIA are also concerned that they may 'pass it on to their children' (Ostensen et al. 2000). Some young adults with JIA report having been advised against conception by their doctors (Ostensen 1991; Petersen et al. 1997; Ostensen et al. 2000).

A lack of a serious relationship with the opposite sex has been reported in significant proportions of selected JIA populations (Ungerer et al. 1988; David et al. 1994; Ostensen et al. 2000). Of some concern are reports that young adult males with JIA have greater difficulty than both healthy males and female patients in establishing relationships with the opposite sex with a trend towards lower sexual activity (Ostensen et al. 2000). This is against a background of increasing public concern of the lack of male role models for today's young men. With this in mind, it may be important to reflect on the impact of an often female predominant paediatric rheumatology multidisciplinary team on the adolescent male patient with JIA.

Substance abuse is another area at risk of neglect in the adolescent rheumatology clinic. Timko et al. (1992) studied substance use in adolescents with JIA and their healthy siblings and reported similar rates at baseline but after 1 year of disease, patients with JIA were less involved. In another study of adolescents with JIA (mean age 13.9 years), Nash et al. (1998) reported 30.7 per cent of patients were drinking alcohol, including 23.5 per cent who were on methotrexate. The average age of initiation of alcohol use in this population was 13.6 years and 37 per cent of alcohol users were also smokers. Interestingly there was no significant difference in alcohol use between methotrexate and non-methotrexate patients! The use of other illicit substances was reported by 13.4 per cent of patients at some time but surprisingly no marijuana use was reported! It is important not to isolate rheumatological problems from generic health issues. Frequent drunkenness, early initiation, and drinking can predict serious alcohol problems in adulthood. Furthermore, teenagers are more likely to have casual sex, are less likely to use a condom when under the influence of alcohol.

Cigarette smoking has both generic and specific importance. For those patients with SLE or on long-term steroid therapy, the risk of premature atheroslerosis must be borne in mind during adolescence with respect to primary preventive measures including smoking, dietary lipids, etc. (Ilowite 2000).

Britto et al. (2000) recently highlighted the nature of some of the barriers to appropriate counselling of sexual activity (and alcohol use—see later) amongst adolescents with JIA. These barriers included availability of time, discomfort of the rheumatologist with the subject area, ambivalence of the rheumatologist to the role, and the perceived lack of applicability (Britto et al. 2000).

Just as parents may be reluctant to address the topic of sexuality with their healthy children, never mind their child with JIA (Zuengler and Neubeck 1983), so are many health professionals who have been involved with a young person with JIA since early childhood. To consider discussing such subjects as sexual activity and alcohol use in the rheumatology clinic needs preparation of both the patient and their family. Such consultations require settings conducive to confidentiality, physician comfort, good interagency relationships (re-counselling), and above all confidence in the young person of the professional. Seeing the young person independently from the parents can be conducive for such conversations and confidences (see below), as does continuity of the same professional over consecutive visits. Sometimes, the offer of such time will not be taken up at the first visit but often at a subsequent visit when the young person feels more confident with the professional. With respect to sexual activity, often the 'open model' approach (i.e. recognition of sexuality but encouragement to postpone until older) is more realistic than the 'closed model' (i.e. abstinence as the only choice). Problem-solving, negotiating, and communication skills are all part of this education process. The role of peer educators is an exciting development in this area. Care must also be taken not to assume heterosexuality in discussions regarding sexual health and homosexuality issues may need to be considered in this age group. Cultural and religious sensitivity in the area of sexual health and alcohol and drug use must be remembered and respected by the multidisciplinary team.

Although younger children may comply with home exercise programmes supervised by their eagle-eyed parents, adolescents often admit to poor adherence to such regimented programmes. Klepper et al. (1992) reported reduced fitness in children with polyarticular JIA compared to controls though lack of fitness was not associated with the activity of the arthritis. In a case–control study of young adults with JIA, in addition to a lower health perception, lower levels of physical functioning and higher levels of fatigue, a lower level of general exercise was observed in the adults with JIA compared to their healthy peers (Petersen et al. 1997). Conversely, greater levels of exercise are associated with well-being and long-term functioning in patients with chronic conditions (Stewart et al. 1994). A further issue is the importance of weight-bearing exercise in many chronic rheumatic conditions like JIA in view of the risk of premature osteoporosis (Kotaniemi et al. 1999). Making a regular exercise programme attractive to young people is therefore a challenge to rheumatology physiotherapists! Normalizing it into a regular visit to the local gym with their peers helps both their physical fitness level as well as their social life!

Self-advocacy issues

Seeing the young person independently from the parent may help provide the privacy for such discussions of generic health concerns such as those detailed above, for example, sexual health, alcohol use, with the assurance of confidentiality. In a study of adolescents in primary care, confidentiality was their major priority when surveyed as to the most important attributes of an adolescent friendly practice (Jacobson and Owen 1993). However, in the studies reported to date, the majority of young people are not seen independently in adolescent rheumatology clinics (Timko et al. 1992; Nash et al. 1998; Britto et al. 2000). This is in contrast to their 'healthy peers'. In primary healthcare, young people in the United Kingdom on average go to the general practitioner or family doctor on their own by age 14–15 years (Jacobson and Owen 1993) and in another study, 50 per cent of 15 year olds (M > F) did so (Balding 1991). Independent visits can be difficult to contemplate for both the young person and their parent(s). Preparation and planning is vital for success, for example, at age 11–12 years the concept is introduced—'in a year or so, you may feel able to come in to see the doctor on your own . . .'. At future visits they can therefore practice taking a lead in the consultation, practice remembering their medication, preparing lists of questions, making their own appointments. By the age of 13–14, both the young persons and their parents will then feel ready to be seen independently for some future consultations.

Independent visits are only part of the process of the young person becoming a good self-advocate. Other aspects include a full understanding of the illness, involvement in decision-making, self-medication, adherence, etc. As mentioned above, the healthcare setting is a safe and often familiar area to practice self-advocacy skills, for example, communication skills, independent living skills, accessing the health service, which are in turn, important for success in independent living and the workplace.

Finally, anyone who cares for adolescents should be aware of legislation concerning this age group in their country. One should always aim for parallel consent, that is, consent from both young person and parent/guardian, even when the young person can consent without parental consent during adolescence. Early involvement in decision-making is important for all young people with a chronic illness and/or disability and simple acknowledgements of this, for example, co-signing consent forms for joint injection procedures, etc. are important messages for both the young persons and their parents.

Vocational issues

Adolescents spend the majority of their waking hours in school and it is therefore important that as well as addressing health needs, transitional care addresses vocational needs. In many countries, early adolescence often includes a transfer to a different school. Secondary level schools are often significantly larger and require multiple changes between classes with more teachers to inform about a chronic illness and/or disability. Academic as well as sport-related demands often increase during this period as well as peer pressure and potential for bullying. Many rheumatic conditions and/or their therapies may contribute to visible manifestations of their illness, for example, growth retardation. A recent study in the United Kingdom suggested that short children are more likely to be bullied than their taller peers and also reported a degree of social isolation—the result or possibly the cause of their victimization (Voss and Mulligan 2000).

Information needs of the teachers need to be addressed particularly those of the head of year and the physical education teacher (Mukherjee et al. 2000). It is important for health professionals to explore with the young person, their family, and their teachers, the impact of a chronic illness and/or disability in specific areas with respect to the school day: education, environmental considerations, medical needs, and activities of daily living. This process should also take place in preparation for the move from secondary to further education and/or employment (Edelman et al. 1998). Discussions with the young person and their family should emphasize strengths rather than limitations and aim for inclusion rather than exclusion. Self-advocacy and involvement in decision-making are as important in the school as in the healthcare setting.

Despite these concerns, educational achievement in JIA is generally good: [secondary (Miller et al. 1982; Petersen et al. 1997); university (Hill et al. 1976; White and Shear 1992)] although there may be higher rates of unemployment (Martin and Woo 1997; Packham and Hall 1999, 2002b). Vocational readiness is an important concept to consider as it addresses both educational achievement as well as prior work experience, psychological aspects like self-esteem, expectations of the young person as well as those of their family, their teachers, and their healthcare team. An important question in the adolescent rheumatology clinic to ask is 'what do you want to be when you leave school and what do you need to do it?' Knowledge of resources as well as societal attitudes towards chronic illness and/or disability are also factors involved in vocational readiness. In a study of 100 adolescent with chronic illness and/or physical disabilities including patients with JIA, the lack of career maturity and work experience of the young person was related to their parents' view that the mean age for first work experience should be greater than 16, the earliest permitted school leaving age in the United Kingdom (White et al. 1990). Of eight adolescent rheumatology clinics in the United Kingdom, only half had access to disability employment officers (McDonagh et al. 2000).

Independence in daily living

The first 'work' experiences of children are often within the context of the family with household chores. Long-term studies have shown that the early incorporation of a child with disabilities into household chores is key for fostering competence and responsibility (Werner and Smith 1992). Patterson and Blum (1996) reported that involvement in household chores was one of several factors associated with resilience in young people with disabilities. One of the questions in the Childhood Health Assessment Questionnaire (CHAQ) (Singh et al. 1994) incorporates this—'Is your child able to do household chores?' Preliminary results from a study at the author's (JMcD) institution of 100 consecutive outpatients attending a UK paediatric rheumatology clinic (mean age 11.5 years, range 7–16) reported 10 patients who answered 'not applicable'. These patients were significantly less disabled than those who acknowledged difficulty with household chores ($p = 0.0002$) and were more likely to be male [odds ratio = 8.89 (95% CI 1.56–50.5)] and have systemic onset JIA [odds ratio = 4.8 (95% CI 1.0–23)]. Lack of involvement in household chores was therefore not explained by age or the presence of more disabling disease. Other influences such as gender and diagnosis appear to be important and need to be borne in mind when addressing this aspect of management of JIA.

Becoming independent in activities of daily living even with the use of aids and/or appliances is important and regular review of such patients by an occupational therapist is important.

Being able to drive a car enhances a young person's independence. Adjustments to the car may be required if there is significant deformity. In the United Kingdom, certain young people in receipt of high-level disability living allowance can learn to drive at age 16, 1 year before their healthy peers.

Adherence issues

The terms adherence and compliance tend to be used interchangeably although the former is now preferred as the term compliance implies paternalism, coercion, and/or acquiescence. Recently compliance has been defined as an active, intentional and responsible process of care in which the individual works to maintain his or her health in close collaboration with healthcare personnel (Kyngas et al. 2000). This highlights that compliance or adherence is more than just a behaviour coinciding with medical advice and that an active commitment to care on the part of the individual is emphasized. Non-adherence (or non-compliance) is often thought as a major defining characteristic of adolescent patients yet 25–95 per cent of adults have been reported to be non-adherent (Stewart and Claff 1972)! There is little good evidence to show that young people are less adherent than adults. Data shows that adherence to medication varies from 55 to 95 per cent in JIA populations and from 46 to 86 per cent for adherence to physiotherapy (Kroll et al. 1999).

In any discussion regarding non-adherence in adolescent rheumatology, it is important to reflect on what young people with chronic rheumatic diseases have to face. They often face long-term therapeutic regimens. In addition the benefit of drug therapy is not immediately apparent. They often have to continue medication even when they feel well. Many drug regimens also required regular monitoring. All of these factors potentially lead to restrictions on leisure time, personal freedom, and peer interactions. Non-adherent behaviour may be the only control mechanism open to the young person and/or be a simple wish to be heard and to take an active role in the decision making.

Doctors assume that poor disease control reflects poor adherence, although there is evidence that this assumption is often false (Du Pasquier-Fediaevsky and Tubiana-Rufi 1999). It is important to acknowledge that adolescents are often differentially adherent to different parts of their regimen, that is, they take some treatments faithfully and refuse to take others at all. Rather than 'non-adherent', young people are often faithfully adherent to a regimen of their own choosing. This is why exploring young people's health goals is central to improving control of chronic conditions.

Addressing non-adherence in the clinic setting should never be about identifying 'poor' adherence. Instead various considerations should be borne in mind in terms of health beliefs, previous experiences (first- or second-hand), disease duration, reality factors in terms of inter-relationships with the rheumatology team members, maturity, etc. (Kroll et al. 1999). Litt and Cuskey (1981) found an earlier age at disease onset and long treatment duration correlated with medication adherence independent of current disease severity. Adolescents with onset before the age of nine displayed significantly more adherence problems than adolescents with later onset (Litt and Cuskey 1981). The role of the family is also important in adherence during adolescence. Degotardi et al. (1996) reported that differences in family coping strategies accounted for variance in treatment adherence among 15 adolescents aged 11–14. One of the common misunderstandings in dealing with non-adherence is that explanation about the rationale of therapy will suffice. Demonstrating how the young person can become an active partner in self-management is imperative and strategies such as contracting, etc. can facilitate this (Table 5). Finally, the quality of the relationship between the health professional and the young person—the therapeutic alliance—is an important, yet often underestimated, determinant of adherence.

Table 5 Handy hints to improve adherence

Decriminalize non-adherence
Explore 'differential' non-adherence—i.e. that adherence may be different for each different medical
Simplify therapy regime
Encourage taking pills in the morning rather than the evening (this actually makes a difference!)
Consider therapy regime in context of lifestyle of patient, e.g. school-day, etc.
Prioritize exercises
Normalize when at all possible e.g. exercise in local gym
Draw up a realistic contract with the young person
Education including rationale of therapy
Involve in decision-making about therapy
Offer choices even if limited

Active participation of young people

One of the tenets of adolescent healthcare is active participation of the young people themselves both in terms of the consultation as well as in the capacity of advisors and educators themselves.

Summer camps offer adolescents with chronic rheumatic diseases an opportunity to be outdoors, participate either as campers or counsellors and improve their self-image. In one study, campers improved during a 7-day camping experience in both self-image and locus of control (Stefl et al. 1996). Repeat campers did even better. In addition to physical and psychosocial benefits, the campers gain independence from parents and can meet new friends that may share their health-related problems. Increasing independence will in turn foster disease-management capabilities (Stefl et al. 1996).

Conventional approaches to promote emotional well-being in young people with chronic illness and/or disability often includes referral to psychology services. Peer support may be another means of promoting well-being for such young people and may represent another critical component of any program designed to promote successful transition of youth with special health needs from adolescents to independence and adulthood. The Chronic Illness Peer Support (ChIPS) program is one such programme, developed in Australia which aims to promote positive adjustment to chronic illness by bringing together young people facing similar circumstances (Olsson et al. 2000).

Peer-led programmes in school sex education have been reported to produce behavioural changes that lead to health benefit (Mellanby et al. 1995). Peer education programmes within the context of adolescent rheumatology may also have similar benefit.

Barriers to transition

Unfortunately, various barriers to transition can be identified.

The young person

The young person may have a long and close relationship with the paediatric team since disease onset which they are reluctant to give up. They may feel safe with the familiar and scared of the unknown—a new hospital, a new team, etc. These young people may also be less mature than their peers, more dependent on their parents and be non-adherent with their therapy. They may still have 'paediatric' medical problems such as pubertal delay and growth retardation, the management of which may be unfamiliar to adult teams.

The family of the young person

Likewise, the family of the young person may have a similarly close relationship with the pediatric team with less confidence in the adult team and may not understand the importance of age-appropriate care for adults. The family may be overprotective of their dependent young person and may resist the attempts of the healthcare team to enhance the self-advocacy of their child if not adequately prepared.

The paediatric rheumatology team

The paediatric team may also not be confident about the adult team's management of conditions that have important differences from their adult counterparts. They too may rather enjoy the comfort of long-term clinic attendees and postpone the transition and transfer process!

The adult rheumatology team

The adult team may indeed have no confidence or training in looking after childhood onset disease. They may assume such diseases are the same as their adult counterparts and forget both the differences in disease manifestations and impact of childhood onset disease. They may also feel that paediatric care is too paternalistic and be reluctant to acknowledge the process of transition.

Many of the barriers detailed above are attitudinal and all those involved in transitional care need to examine their personal or professional strengths, unexplored biases, and ultimate goals prior to active involvement in a transitional care programme. There needs to be an acknowledgment of differences in practice philosophies and style between paediatric and adult teams with the necessary planning, preparation, and coordination. As health professionals, we need to learn how to shift the expert model and become enablers of young people and their families. We need to encourage more horizontal than vertical communication in our clinics from an early age and start to alter our institutions to enable self-advocacy whatever the age of our patients.

The future

Transitional care in rheumatology as in other chronic illness specialties, is an area ripe for further research. What types of transition models are most effective for which conditions and for which patients? Do different models of transitional care produce equivalent medical and psychological outcomes? Which patient characteristics (medical, social, psychological) identify those who need a transitional programme? Do all patients need one? Are different models required for different diseases or are the majority of issues generic to all young people with a chronic disease? What is the relative cost-effectiveness of each model? Perhaps the next edition of this textbook will have some reference to an evidence base for the answers of at least some of these questions.

References

Balding, J. *Young People into the Nineties. Doctor and Dentist. Book 1.* Exeter: Schools Health Education Unit, University of Exeter, 1991.

Bax, M.C., Smyth, D.P., and Thomas, A.P. (1998). Health care of physically handicapped young adults. *British Medical Journal* **296**, 1153–5.

Berry, S.L. et al. (1993). Conceptions of illness by children with juvenile rheumatoid arthritis: a cognitive developmental approach. *Journal of Pediatric Psychology* **18**, 83–97.

Blum, R.W. and Okinow, N.A. *Teenagers at Risk—A National Perspective of State Level Services for Adolescents with Chronic Illnesses or Disabilities.* Minneapolis: National Center for Youth with Disabilities, 1993.

Blum, R.W. et al. (1993). Transition from child-centred to adult health-care systems for adolescents with chronic conditions. A position paper of the Society for Adolescent Medicine. *Journal of Adolescent Health* **14**, 570–6.

Blumenfeld, Z., Lorber, M., Yoffe, N., and Scharf, Y. (1994). Systemic lupus erythematosus: predisposition for uterine cervical dysplasia. *Lupus* **3**, 59–61.

Britto, M.T. et al. (2000). Improving rheumatologists screening for alcohol use and sexual activity. *Archives of Pediatric and Adolescent Medicine* **154**, 478–83.

Bushkila, D., Neumann, L., Hershman, E., Gedalia, A., Press, J., and Sukenik, S. (1995). Fibromyalgia syndrome in children—an outcome study. *Journal of Rheumatology* **22**, 525–8.

Carroll, G., Massarelli, E., Opzoomer, A., Pekeles, G., Pedneault, M., Frappier, J.Y., and Onetto, N. (1983). Adolescents with chronic disease: are they receiving comprehensive health care? *Journal of Adolescent Health Care* **17**, 32–6.

Chamberlain, M.A. and Rooney, C.M. (1996). Young adults with arthritis: meeting their transitional needs. *British Journal of Rheumatology* **35**, 84–90.

Choquet, M., Fediaevsky, L.D.P., and Manfredi, R. (1997). Sexual behaviour among adolescents reporting chronic conditions: a French national survey. *Journal of Adolescent Health* **20**, 62–7.

Coleman, J. and Schofield, J. *Key Data on Adolescence.* Brighton: Trust for the Study of Adolescence, 2001.

David, J., Cooper, C., Hickey, L., Lloyd, J., Dore, C., McCullough, C., and Woo, P. (1994). The functional and psychological outcomes of juvenile chronic arthritis in young adulthood. *British Journal of Rheumatology* **33**, 876–81.

Degotardi, P., Revenson, T.A., and Ilowite, N. (1996). Family coping, adaptation and treatment compliance in juvenile rheumatoid arthritis. *Arthritis and Rheumation* **24** (Suppl. 1), 5.

Du Pasquier-Fediaevsky, L. and Tubiana-Rufi, N. (1999). Discordance between physician and adolescent assessments of adherence to treatment: influence of HbA1c level. The PEDIAB Collaborative Group. *Diabetes Care* **9**, 1445–9.

Edelman, A., Schyler, V., and White, P. *Maximizing Success for Young Adults with Chronic Health-Related Illnesses: Transition Planning for Education After High School.* Washington DC: HEATH Resource Center, American Council on Education, 1998.

Eiser, C. (1990). Psychological effects of chronic disease. *Journal of Child Psychology and Psychiatry* **31**, 85–98.

Fearon, P. and Hotopf, M. (2001). Relation between headache in childhood and physical and psychiatric symptoms in adulthood: national birth cohort study. *British Medical Journal* **322**, 1145–8.

Flato, B., Aasland, A., Vandvik, I.H., and Forre, O. (1997). Outcome and predictive factors in children with chronic idiopathic musculoskeletal pain. *Clinical and Experimental Rheumatology* **15**, 569–7.

Florentino, L., Datta, D., Gentle, S., Hall, D.M.B., Harpin, V., Phillips, D., and Walker, A. (1998). Transtion from school to adult life for physically disabled young people. *Archives of Diseases in Children* **79**, 306–11.

Foster, H.E. *Young Adults with Juvenile Chronic Arthritis: Beyond the Transition.* Park City IV UT: Abstract, 1998.

Foster, H.E., Marshall, N., Myers, A., Dunkley, P., and Griffiths, I.D. (2003). Outcome in adults with juvenile idiopathic arthritis. *Arthritis and Rheumatism* **48**, 767–75.

Gare, B.A. and Fasth, A. (1995). The natural history of juvenile chronic arthritis. A population based cohort study. II. Outcome. *Journal of Rheumatology* **22**, 308–19.

Ghosh, S., Drummond, H., and Ferguson, A. (1998). Neglect of growth and development in the clinical monitoring of children and teenagers with inflammatory bowel disease: review of case records. *British Medical Journal* **317**, 120–1.

Hargrave, D.R., McMaster, C., O'Hare, M.M., and Carson, D.J. (1999). Tobacco smoke exposure in children and adolescents with diabetes mellitus. *Diabetic Medicine* **16**, 31–4.

Harreby, M. et al. (1995). Are radiologic changes in the thoracic and lumbar spine of adolescents risk factors for low back pain in adults? A 25 year prospective cohort study of 640 school children. *Spine* **20**, 2298–302.

Haugen, M. et al. (2000). Young adults with juvenile arthritis in remission attain normal peak bone mass at the lumbar spine and forearm. *Arthritis and Rheumatism* **43**, 1504–10.

Henderson, C.J. et al. (2000). Total-body bone mineral content in non-corticosteroid-treated postpubertal females with juvenile rheumatoid arthritis. *Arthritis and Rheumatism* **43**, 531–40.

Hill, R., Herstein, A., and Walters, K. (1976). Juvenile rheumatoid arthritis: follow-up into adulthood—medical, sexual and social status. *Canadian Medical Association Journal* **114**, 790–6.

Ilowite, N.T. (2000). Premature atherosclerosis in systemic lupus erythematosus. *Journal of Rheumatology* **27** (Suppl. 58), 15–19.

Jacobson, L. and Owen, P. (1993). Study of teenage care in one general practice. *British Journal of General Practitioners* **43**, 349.

Klepper, S., Darbee, J., Effgenr, S.K., and Singsen, B.H. (1992). Physical fitness levels in children with polyarticular juvenile rheumatoid arthritis. *Arthritis Care and Research* **5**, 93–100.

Kotaniemi, A. et al. (1999). Weight-bearing physical activity, calcium intake, systemic glucocorticoids, chronic inflammation and body constitution as determinants of lumbar and femoral bone mineral in juvenile chronic arthritis. *Scandinavian Journal of Rheumatology* **28**, 19–26.

Kroll, T., Barlow, J.H., and Shaw, K. (1999). Treatment adherence in juvenile rheumatoid arthritis—a review. *Scandinavian Journal of Rheumatology* **28**, 10–18.

Kyngas, H.A., Kroll, T., and Duffy, M.E. (2000). Compliance in adolescent with chronic diseases: a review. *Journal of Adolescent Health* **26**, 379–88.

Lang, B., MacNeill, Bruce, B., and Gordon, K. Assessing the needs of adolescents with rheumatic diseases: implications for the development of transition clinics. Park City IV UT: Abstract, 1998.

Litt, I.F. and Cuskey, W.R. (1981). Compliance with salicylate therapy in adolescents with juvenile rheumatoid arthritis. *American Journal of Diseases in Children* **135**, 434–6.

Martin, K. and Woo, P. (1997). Outcome in juvenile chronic arthritis. *Revue de Rhumatica (English edition)* **10**, S242.

McAnarney, E.R., Pless, I.B., Satterwhite, B., and Friedman, S.B. (1974). Psychological problems of children with chronic juvenile arthritis. *Pediatrics* **53**, 523–8.

McDonagh, J.E., Foster, H., Hall, M.A., and Chamberlain, M.A. on behalf of the BPRG (2000). Audit of rheumatology services for adolescents and young adults in the UK. *Rheumatology* **39**, 596–602.

Mellanby, A.R., Phelps, F.A., Crichton, N.J., and Tripp, J.H. (1995). School sex education: an experimental programme with educational and medical benefit. *British Medical Journal* **311**, 414–17.

Miller, J., Spitz, P., Simpson, U., and Williams, G. (1982). The social function of young adults who had arthritis in childhood. *Journal of Paediatrics* **100**, 378–82.

Mukherjee, S., Lightfoot, J., and Sloper, P. *Improving Communication Between Health and Education for Children with Chronic Illness or Physical Disability.* University of York: Social Policy Research Unit, 2000.

Nash, A.A., Britto, M.T., Lovell, D.J., Passo, M.H., and Rosenthal, S.L. (1998). Substance use among adolescents with JRA. *Arthritis Care and Research* **11**, 391–6.

Nasr, S.Z., Campbell, C., and Howatt, W. (1992). Transition program from paediatric to adult care for cystic fibrosis patients. *Journal of Adolescent Health* **13**, 682–5.

Oakley, A., Bendelow, G., Barnes, J., Buchanan, M., and Nasseem Hussain, O.A. (1995). Health and cancer prevention: knowledge and beliefs of children and young people. *British Medical Journal* **310**, 1029–33.

Oen, K., Malleson, P.N., Cabral, D.A., Rosenberg, A.M., Petty, R.E., and Cheang, M. (2002). Disease course and outcome of juvenile rheumatoid arthritis in a multicenter cohort. *Journal of Rheumatology* **29**, 1989–99.

Olsson, C.A., Sawyer, S.M., and Boyce, M. (2000). What are the special needs of chronically ill young people? *Australian Family Physician* **29**, 299–300.

Ostensen, M. (1991). Counselling women with rheumatic disease—how many children are desirable? *Scandinavian Journal of Rheumatology* **20**, 121–6.

Ostensen, M., Almberg, K., and Koksvik, H.S. (2000). Sex, reproduction and gynecological disease in young adults with a history of juvenile chronic arthritis. *Journal of Rheumatology* **27**, 1783–7.

Packham, J.C. and Hall, M.A. (1999). Long-term outcome of juvenile idiopathic arthrits, education and employment status. *Archives of Diseases in Children* **80** (Suppl. 1), P22.

Packham, J.C. and Hall, M.A. (2002a). Long-term follow-up of 246 adults with juvenile idiopathic arthritis: functional outcome. *Rheumatology* **4**, 1428–35.

Packham, J.C. and Hall, M.A. (2002b). Long-term follow-up of 246 adults with juvenile idiopathic arthritis: education and employment. *Rheumatology* **41**, 1436–9.

Packham, J.C. and Hall, M.A. (2002c). Long-term follow-up of 246 adults with juvenile idiopathic arthritis: social function, relationships and sexual activity. *Rheumatology* **41**, 1440–3.

Patterson, J. and Blum, R.J. (1996). Risk and resilience among children and youth with disabilities. *Archives of Pediatric and Adolescence Medicine* **150**, 692–8.

Pepmueller, P., Cassidy, J., Allen, S., and Hillman, L. (1996). Bone mineralisation and bone mineral metabolism in children with juvenile rheumatoid arthritis. *Arthritis and Rheumatism* **39**, 746–57.

Petersen, L.S., Mason, T., Nelson, A.M., Fallon, W., and Gabriel, S.E. (1997). Psychosocial outcomes and health studies in adults who have had juvenile arthritis: a controlled population based study. *Arthritis and Rheumatism* **40**, 2235–40.

Phillips, S. and Sandston, K.L. (1990). Parental attitudes toward work. *Youth and Society* **22**, 160.

Rettig, P. and Athreya, B.H. (1991). Adolescents with chronic disease: transition to adult health care. *Arthritis Care and Research* **4**, 174–80.

Rettig, P. and Athreya, B.H. (1998). Leaving home—preparing the adolescent with arthritis for coping with independence in the adult rheumatology world. In *Adolescent Rheumatology* (ed. D.A. Isenberg and J. Miller), pp. 341–9. London: Martin Dunitz.

Ruperto, N., Levinson, J.E., Ravelli, A., Shear, E.S., Tague, B.L., Murray, K., Martini, A., and Giannini, E.H. (1997). Long-term health outcomes and quality of life in American and Italian inception cohort of patients with juvenile rheumatoid arthritis. I. Outcome status. *Journal of Rheumatology* **24**, 945–51.

Salmi, J., Huuponen, T., Oksa, H., Oksala, H., Koivula, T., and Raita, P. (1986). Metabolic control in adolescent insulin-dependent diabetics referred from pediatric to adult clinic. *Annals of Clinical Research* **4**, 174–80.

Sanci, L.A., Coffey, C.M., Veit, F.C., Carr-Gregg, M., Patton, G.C., Day, N., and Bowes, G. (2000). Evaluation of the effectiveness of an educational intervention for general practitioners in adolescent health care: randomised controlled trial. *British Medical Journal* **320**, 224–30.

Sawyer, S.M. (1998). The process of transition to adult health care services. In *Diabetes and the Adolescent* (ed. G. Werther and J. Court). Melbourne: Blackwell.

Sherry, D.D. (2000). An overview of amplified musculoskeletal pain syndromes. *Journal of Rheumatology* **58**, 44–8.

Singh, G., Athreya, B., Fries, J., Goldsmith, D.P., and Ostrov, B.E. (1994). Measurement of health status in children with juvenile rheumatoid arthritis. *Arthritis and Rheumatism* **37**, 1761–9.

Society for Adolescent Medicine (1995). A position statement of the Society for Adolescent Medicine. *Journal of Adolescent Health* **16**, 413.

Stefl, M.E., Shear, E.S., and Levinson, J.E. (1996). Summer camps for juveniles with rheumatic disease: do they make a difference? *Arthritis Care and Research* **9**, 35–41.

Stewart, A.L., Hays, R.D., Wells, K.B., Rogers, W.H., Spritzer, K.L., and Greenfield, S. (1994). Long-term functioning and well-being outcomes associated with physical activitiy and exercise in patients with chronic conditions in the Medical outcomes study. *Journal of Clinical Epidemiology* **47**, 719–30.

Stewart, R.B. and Claff, L.E. (1972). Review of medication errors and compliance in ambulatory patients. *Clinical Pharmacology and Therapy* **13**, 463–5.

Timko, C., Stovel, K.W., Moos, R.H., and Miller, J.J. (1992). Adaptation to juvenile rheumatic disease: a controlled evaluation of functional disability with a one-year follow-up. *Health Psychology* **11**, 67–76.

Ungerer, J.A., Horgan, B., Chaitow, J., and Campion, G.D. (1988). Psychosocial functioning in children and young adults with juvenile arthritis. *Pediatrics* **81**, 195–202.

Viner, R.M. (1999). Transition from paediatric to adult care. Bridging the gaps or passing the buck? *Archives of Diseases in Children* **81**, 271–5.

Voss, L.D. and Mulligan, J. (2000). Bullying in school: are short pupils at risk? Questionnaire study in a cohort. *British Medical Journal* **320**, 612–13.

Werner, E.E. and Smith, R.S. *Overcoming the Odds: High Risk Children from Birth to Adulthood.* Ithaca NY: Cornell University Press, 1992.

White, P.H. and Shear, E.S. (1992). Transition/job readiness for adolescents with juvenile arthritis and other chronic illnesses. *Journal of Rheumatology* **19**, 23–7.

White, P.H. et al. (1990). Career maturity in adolescents with chronic illness. *Journal of Adolescent Health Care* **11**, 372.

Wirrell, E., Long, B., and Canfield, C. (1995). Social outcome in young adults with juvenile arthritis: implication for the development of transition clinics. *Arthritis and Rheumation* **38**, S184.

World Health Organisation. *The Health of Young People.* Geneva: WHO, 1993.

Zak, M. et al. (1999). Assessment of bone mineral density in adults with a history of juvenile chronic arthritis: a cross sectional long-term follow-up study. *Arthritis and Rheumatism* **42**, 790–8.

Zuengler, K.L. and Neubeck, G. (1983). Sexuality: developing togetherness. In *Stress and the Family* (ed. H. McCubben), pp. 41–3. New York: Bruner/Mazel.

Appendix

Examples of resources on the world-wide web

- Arthritis

  www.arc.org.uk
  —Website of the Arthritis Research Campaign in the UK
  —Leaflet 'Arthritis in teenagers' now online

- Generic health issues

  www.teenagehealthfreak.com—UK based
  www.lifebytes.gov.uk—UK based; for 11–14 year olds
  www.mindbodysoul.gov.uk—UK based; for 14–16 year olds
  www.youthealth.com—For 6–14 year olds

- Career websites for young people with chronic illness and/or disability

  www.cando.lancs.ac.uk—UK based careers advisory network on opportunities for disabled young people
  www.familyfundtrust.org—UK based charity Family Fund Trust website. Choices and challenges for young disabled people after the age of 16
  www.skill.org.uk—UK based National Bureau for Students with Disabilities
  www.connexions.gov.uk—Careers advice and more for young people aged 13–19 years in England and Wales

- Computer access

  www.abilitynet.org.uk—UK based charity with aim to make the benefits of using computers available to disabled children and adults

- Disability websites

  www.drc-gb.org
  —UK Disability Rights Commission
  —Good links

- Transition websites—US based

  http://chs.ky.gov/commissionkids/transition.htm
  http://depts.washington.edu/healthtr/—the adolescent health transition project at the university of Washington
  www.communityinclusion.org/transition/familyguide.html
  www.hctransitions.ichp.edu
  Key recent adolescent health and transition documents
  'Bridging the Gaps. Health Care for Adolescents' (June 2003). Available at www.rcpch.ac.uk/publications/recent_publications/Adol.pdf
  A multimethod review to identify components of practice which may promote continuity in the transition from child to adult care for young people with chronic illness or disability. Forbes A, While A, Ullman R, Lewis S, Mathes L, Griffiths P. London, NCCSDO, 2002. Available in full on www.sdo.lshtm.ac.uk/publications.htm/
  American Academy of Pediatrics et al. (2002). A consensus statement on health care transitions for young adults with special health care needs. Pediatrics 110,1304–6. http://pediatrics.aappublications.org/

1.1.4 The geriatric age group

Evan Calkins

Introduction

Dr T. Franklin Williams (1986) has referred to care of older people as 'the fruition of the clinician'. Challenging, as it does, the physician's understanding of human biology, and people, as we age, geriatric practice calls upon the best that a physician has to offer. This is particularly true as it relates to the musculoskeletal system. Second only to maintenance of cognitive capacity, preservation of physical function, sufficient to enable one to remain independent in the community, is, for most older people, the most prized component of an effective, happy old age. If one couples this with the fact that musculoskeletal diseases are the most frequent cause of the complaints of older people, exceeding, in frequency, diseases of all other organ systems, one gains an appreciation of the importance of rheumatology in caring for older people.

Rheumatologic practice with older patients differs from that with persons at mid-life in many ways, including the physiological, anatomic, and psychological characteristics of the patients, the array of diseases, treatment goals, and the approach to management. This chapter will, first, summarize aspects of the biology of ageing that underlie these differences.

Secondly, we will consider implications of the biology of ageing on rheumatologic practice in a general sense, that is, the 'geriatric perspective'. Thirdly, we will review how the process of ageing influences the diagnosis and management of several conditions frequently seen in a rheumatology/geriatric consulting practice. Space limitations will prevent consideration of specific age-related aspects of other important but less frequent entities.

The biology of ageing

Ageing—a continuum

Ageing is a continuous life-long process. Rapid changes occur during early life and extend through youth and adolescence. Most functions achieve their peak by the time the person reaches his/her mid-20s. From then on, the physiologic capacity of almost all organs, and the organism as a whole, undergoes progressive decline (Sehl and Yates 2001). Although the reasons for this decline are not yet understood fully, they are known to include prolonged exposure to toxins (such as silica and cigarettes), dietary habits, illnesses in youth that predispose to problems in old age (such as rheumatic fever, poliomyelitis, or congenital laxity of connective tissue), lifetime patterns of physical inanition and genetic predisposition. Factors that tend to decrease the slope of decline include education, a lifetime pattern of exercise, a happy marriage, and an optimistic personality with strong coping skills (Vaillant and Mukemal 2001).

Due to wide variations in these and other factors, there is marked variability among individuals as we age. A study of centenarians is showing that there is a small percentage of older people who are able to retain physiologic function into their second century. However, the pattern described above pertains to most older people and has general applicability to medical practice.

The lifetime course of bone density, described in Chapter 3.4 of this book, illustrates how characteristics instilled at conception, and experiences and habits during early and mid-life, have a direct bearing on health in old age. Another illustration of age-related physiologic decline is muscle strength. Most individuals achieve their greatest level of muscle strength in their mid-20s. For the average person, this level remains fairly constant until about age 45, at which time significant declines usually occur (Pendergast et al. 1993). Increases in strength, well above the average, can be achieved by vigorous physical training. However, once the new level of muscle and cardiovascular/pulmonary function has been achieved, declines occur inexorably with time and advancing age. The ability of properly designed resistance exercises to achieve short-term enhancement of strength is retained throughout most and probably all of life. However, even with continued exercises, declines occur with time. Thus, ageing is a lifetime experience. Many of the problems encountered by older people have a direct relationship to lifestyle patterns and events during youth and mid-life.

Loss of reserve capacity: frailty and fragility

For each organ system there is a minimal level of function that is necessary to sustain life. The difference between this functional level and the maximal level that can be achieved by the particular individual, at his or her stage of life, represents the reserve capacity of a given organ system—a capacity not needed in ordinary daily life that can be called upon in response to a sudden stress such as an overwhelming infection or severe injury. Young people, with functional capacity four to ten times that required to sustain life, have extensive physiologic reserves and can usually respond even to major physical stresses. In old age, however, the reserve capacity of a given organ system shrinks markedly.

When, eventually, the functional capacity of a given system falls below the minimal level required for preservation of life, the individual attempts to restore homeostasis by enlisting other organ systems to compensate. For example, in a person with severe pulmonary emphysema, as lung function reaches this critical point, the muscles of respiration respond by hyperventilation; soon they, too, can no longer sustain the respiratory function necessary for survival. The individual then experiences a cascade of organ failure leading to death.

Reflecting, in part, this concept of multiple organ failure, most persons aged 75 years and older suffer from multiple chronic diseases. Gruenberg (1977) has pointed out that medical science has succeeded, at least for the time being, in preventing or treating many of the acute life-threatening illnesses, such as serious infection, but has, as yet, had limited success in preventing or curing many of the chronic diseases such as osteoarthritis or macular degeneration of the eye—diseases that do not kill but linger on to collect, in multiples, as one ages (van den Akker et al. 1998). The presence of multiple diseases in almost all patients, aged 75 years and older, has major implications for diagnosis and treatment of rheumatic and other diseases.

Despite the problems mentioned above, most older people, when questioned, regard themselves to be in good health, and often seem that way to others. Some are able to maintain particularly demanding schedules, such as serving as a conductor of a symphony orchestra. When challenged by significant additional stress, however, they are at risk of 'falling apart', like a piece of porcelain. This characteristic, shared by most older people aged 80 and older, has been termed 'frailty' (Fried et al. 2001). I suggest, however, that the term 'fragility' may be more appropriate.

Implications for rheumatologic practice

Six areas of particular importance will be discussed: (i) fragility and the role of rheumatology, (ii) prevention of acute stresses, (iii) differential diagnosis in the setting of multiple diseases, (iv) use of drugs in older people, and (v) age-related psychological issues.

Can rheumatology play a role in preventing frailty and fragility?

Essential to the ability of older people to withstand the threats of frailty and loss of independence is maintenance of good relatively pain-free function of their joints and muscles. For most people, this involves an ability to walk. Patients who are unable to walk can draw benefits from regular exercise to the upper body through use of dumbbells, for example. This, too, requires good function of hands and shoulders. The role of rheumatology in enabling older people to maintain overall physical capacity is one of the greatest contributions that the field can make to older people. The staff of the Hospital for Special Surgery in New York City have expressed this theme in referring to themselves as 'specialists in mobility'.

There is now good evidence that a sustained level of physical activity among older people yields important benefits in deferring disability, fostering independence, and prolonging life (see Table 1).

While there is abundant evidence concerning the short-term benefits of specific exercise programmes in enhancing functional capacity of older people, documentation that these benefits will result in long-term gains will require additional study. Further information is needed concerning the specific exercises that are most effective for individual groups of patients; issues of motivation and organization need to be addressed, and controlled outcome studies are required. Based on our present knowledge, the US Department of Health and Human Services (1996) recommends that 'every adult should accumulate 30 minutes or more of moderate-intense physical activity on most if not all days of the week'. The big question remains: how to motivate people to do it?

Role of rheumatology in prevention of acute stresses

A second way in which rheumatologists can contribute to longer, more effective life of older people is by helping them to avoid some of the major 'setbacks', which challenge an older person's diminishing functional reserve.

Table 1 Examples of evidence concerning benefits of maintenance of physical function in old age

Objective measurements of mobility predict: Ability to carry out instrumental activities of daily living Extent of reliance on the health care system (Judge et al. 1996) Likelihood of admission to a nursing home (Guralnik et al. 1994) Duration of life (Guralnik et al. 1994; Soderlin et al. 1998)
Loss of capacity in four out of six instrumental activities of daily living, together with cognitive loss at advancing age, are the most important predictors of an adverse outcome following hospital admission, including longer hospital stay and increased chance of in-hospital mortality (Sager et al. 1996; Soderlin et al. 1998)
Increased levels of physical activity decrease the risk of heart attack in college alumni (Paffenberger et al. 1978)
Well-designed resistance exercises can produce improved muscle strength even in frail nursing home residents (Fisher et al. 1991), and improvements in physical function, joint mobility, and decreased pain and disability in patients with osteoarthritis (Ettinger et al. 1997) and rheumatoid arthritis (van den Endy et al. 2000)
Walking more than 2 miles per day reduces mortality rate (Hakim et al. 1998)

Osteoporotic fractures provide a good example. Nearly one out of two women will have an osteoporotic fracture at some point during their life. This is true for 13 per cent of men. The risk of death from the fracture per se is small—for a 50-year-old woman in good general health and fitness it is only 5 per cent during the first year after fracture. The risks escalate markedly in persons of advancing age, especially individuals with numerous comorbidities, decreased cognitive capacity, and decreased prefracture level of physical function (National Osteoporosis Foundation 1998). Thus, the average risk of dying during the first year after fracture, for a woman aged 50 or higher, is 24 per cent following a fracture of hip or femur, only one-third if the patients regain their pre-fracture level of function. Data suggest that intensive programmes of physical therapy would improve the chance of regaining independent physical function and also survival. Death rates are higher for men than for women. For women the risk of death from an osteoporotic fracture exceeds the risk of death from carcinoma of the breast (Cummings et al. 1989).

Despite recent increases in knowledge concerning osteoporosis, the majority of patients with this condition are not aware that they have the disease and are not receiving treatment. Patients with arthritis are at a greater risk for osteoporosis than the population as a whole, not only because of their relative immobility, but also because a number of the drugs utilized, especially corticosteroids and immunosuppressive drugs, contribute to bone loss. Rheumatologists have a special obligation and opportunity to see that guidelines for osteoporosis diagnosis and management are carried out, especially for patients receiving corticosteroid therapy (Saag et al. 1998). Regular swimming is good for joint flexibility but does not have the benefit on bone density that is achieved by walking.

A second condition leading to serious fractures and consequent stress in older people is that of falls. On the average, 30 per cent of people aged 65 and older fall each year, some falling many times. In older people, approximately 12 per cent of falls result in serious soft tissue injury or fracture (King and Tinetti 1995). The frequency of falls and the likelihood of serious injury increase substantially in persons 75 years of age and older.

While most cases of frequent falls are due to multifactorial issues, two or three specific problems often predominate. Examples include a foot drop or weakness of quadriceps muscles or hip flexors, neurological changes interfering with balance, consumption of drugs that decrease response time, hazards in the home, failing eyesight, painful, awkwardly functioning joints, and generalized weakness. Rheumatologists are in an excellent position to conduct comprehensive falls assessments on individual patients, to highlight the major underlying causes, and to recommend therapy. Even in instances in which it is not possible to achieve specific functional improvement, so long as the older person has reasonable cognitive function, with minimental status of 20 or higher (Folstein et al. 1975), a detailed explanation of the reasons for the falls, and suggestions concerning potential compensatory actions are frequently followed by a significant decrease in the number of falls.

Multiple disease

The fact that older patients suffer from multiple diseases presents one of the most unique and also challenging aspects of rheumatologic practice in older people (van den Akker et al. 1998). The symptoms of rheumatic disease are, themselves, relatively non-specific. In the young person, with recent onset of musculoskeletal complaints, the product of these symptoms usually permits the physician to identify, as the cause, a single rheumatologic or non-rheumatologic entity. In old people, many diseases, not formally regarded as rheumatic in nature, will express themselves, at least in part, by musculoskeletal manifestations mimicking those seen in specific rheumatologic diseases. An example is polyarthritis, often resembling rheumatoid arthritis, occurring in association with or secondary to carcinomatosis, Hodgkin's disease, and various forms of lymphoma, sarcoidosis, or tuberculosis. Another example is myopathy, resembling polymyositis, due to cholesterol-lowering drugs (Pierce et al. 1990). Indeed, many older people have multiple rheumatologic or musculoskeletal diseases (polymyalgia rheumatica or fibromyalgia in a patient with clinical and radiologic evidence of cervical spondylosis will serve as an example). The physician should not be led to erroneous conclusions by focusing on the stigmata (whether physical, radiologic, or laboratory) of a given 'obvious' disease, while missing the subtle clues to the presence of a separate disorder that may be the cause of his or her current symptoms.

Multiple drugs

With the multiple medications many older people consume, in response to their multiplicity of diseases and complaints, including the increasing consumption of herbal medications (often concealed from the physician), the issue of multiple drugs emerges as a major problem in the treatment of older people. There are a number of characteristics of older people that make it difficult to predict with certainty a person's response to a given agent. For example, many, probably most older people, despite normal values for blood urea nitrogen and serum creatinine, will have a significant reduction in renal function as assessed by creatinine clearance, and a corresponding decrease in the clearance of many drugs. Similarly, many older people will exhibit altered capacity for catabolism of drugs in their liver, sometimes due to the toxic effect of medication. Many agents commonly used in rheumatologic practice, such as methotrexate, NSAIDs, allopurinol, probenecid, and hydroxychloroquine, have the capacity to cause liver damage. Other agents, including some of the above, have the capacity for causing renal damage as well. It is important to order routine liver and kidney profiles at intervals of 3–6 months in all patients receiving treatment with drugs that have the capacity for yielding either liver or kidney damage and even small changes must be taken seriously.

For these and other reasons, most older people exhibit significant alterations in pharmacokinetics (absorption, distribution, protein-binding, catabolism, and excretion) and pharmacodynamics (end organ responsiveness) as compared with younger individuals (Hanlon et al. 2001). In addition, the multiplicity of drugs taken by many patients increases the likelihood of drug interaction. Therefore, the response of an older person to a given drug is far less predictable than is true with younger individuals and the potential for upsetting the delicate balance that I have termed 'fragility' is very great.

Some of the approaches that have proved helpful in decreasing the risk of adverse drug effects in older people are:

- Obtain list of all current medications, including over the counter preparations, and document any adverse reaction that may have occurred.
- Limit number of drugs. Use non-pharmacologic treatment when appropriate.

- Identify mode of excretion, detoxification, and drug interactions of all drugs you use.
- Reduce dosage for older patients. Start treatment with even lower dosage. Instruct patients about possible side-effects.
- Obtain appropriate pre-treatment laboratory data to assess risk of therapy and provide baseline for identification of possible future toxicity.
- Define specific goals for each drug used. Discontinue drug if goal not achieved.
- If toxic effects ensue to drug A, it is better to shift to another agent (B), than to add a drug to offset the toxic effects of drug A.

Although these recommendations relate to all medications, they are especially relevant to the wide range of agents used in rheumatologic practice.

Psychosocial factors

The most common and, probably, most devastating loss for older people, often but not always associated with advanced age, is that of cognitive capacity. The extent of this loss is not readily apparent. Older patients are very good at concealing it. Physicians seldom include objective assessment of cognitive capacity as part of their physical examination and frequently overlook losses that have a significant effect on the person's ability to comply with medication regimens and rehabilitation guidelines. Assessments of cognitive capacity can easily be performed through a series of simple questions requiring not more than 10 min (Folstein et al. 1975). In addition to Alzheimer's disease and multi-infarct dementia, there are a number of other causes of cognitive failure in older people, some of which are reversible, at least on a short-term basis. These include depression, delirium (often secondary to infection or inappropriate medication), hyperthyroidism or myxoedema, hypercalcaemia, and vitamin B12 deficiency. Depression has been shown to be present in approximately 20 per cent of patients in an ambulatory care practice, including those with rheumatic diseases, and is often accompanied by changes in cognition. Good objective means for identification of depression in a clinic population have been designed (Yesavage et al. 1983; Mulrow et al. 1995), and should be more widely used. Chronic anxiety and panic attacks, frequently experienced by older patients, are readily amenable to appropriate therapy.

Older patients also experience serious social losses. These include loss of a job, decreased income, death of friends, possible death of a spouse, children moving away, and possible relocation from the house one has occupied for 40–50 years. Despite these losses, essentially all older patients adhere, fiercely, to two goals: ability to live independently in the community and retention of a measure of control. They are aided by two assets, experience and social skills, that they have acquired since childhood. It is fascinating to see how different people use these two resources to fend off or compensate for the often staggering social and physical losses, sometimes maintaining their proud independence into their early 90s. Others, endowed with a less flexible, resourceful, and determined psychological makeup, crumple at an earlier age in the face of far less formidable losses and obstacles. The way a patient responds to the challenge of musculoskeletal disease has a great deal to do with the outcome. Therefore, attention to the psychological and social aspects of a given patient emerge as major considerations in a rheumatologic practice with older people.

Application of general principles to specific diseases

Rheumatoid arthritis

Rheumatoid arthritis (RA) is a fairly frequent entity in the older population. Focusing on a population of patients aged 65–79, Engel et al. (1966) determined that the frequency of 'definite rheumatoid arthritis' [by the criteria of Ropes et al. (1958)] was 49/1000 women and 18/1000 men. In a total population, the frequency was 16/1000 women and 7/1000 men.

In the patient aged 65 and older, RA brings to the primary care physician and consulting rheumatologist one of two divergent clinical presentations and therapeutic challenges. One is the patient with long-standing RA who has grown old with his or her disease. The second is the patient with new onset polyarthritis, presenting features consistent with or suggestive of RA. The relative frequency of these two presentations in clinical practice depends on whether the physician is working at a major medical centre or in a community site. With the development and increased utilization of new disease modifying and immuno-regulatory agents, new approaches to reconstructive surgery, and improved physician and patient education, the number and severity of patients in the former category will almost surely decrease. However, many patients with disease onset 10–30 years ago still present themselves to the rheumatologist in the advanced stages of the disease. The concepts of management of a patient who has grown old with his or her disease are outlined in Table 2.

Most points in Table 2, while important, are self-evident and will not be discussed further. Among comorbid diseases, two that have a major impact on the symptoms of RA are hyper- and hypothyroidism. The presence of either of these diseases in patients with RA may mimic or accentuate the symptoms of active disease. Hyperthyroidism will lead to or accentuate weight loss, fatigue, and other constitutional symptoms; hypothyroidism also contributes to fatigue, and to a particular pattern of stiffness that needs to be differentiated from the stiffness of RA or Parkinson's disease. Because these conditions are easily overlooked, a TSH and T4 should always be included in the standard battery of tests undertaken in patients with new onset RA or recently exacerbated disease.

Another entity to which the physician must be on guard is that of atlanto-axial instability or subluxation, a not in-frequent concomitant of RA in older patients. This condition brings serious risk of disastrous and sometimes fatal damage to the spinal cord, especially during manipulation of the head in the course of trachial intubation in preparation for anaesthesia (Stevens et al. 1971; Mikulowski et al. 1975). In patients with destructive forms of RA, it is important to obtain appropriate neck X-rays to assess the risk of this condition and, if present, either to alert the anaesthesiologist to the risk, or arrange neck surgery before other procedures are undertaken.

Restorative surgery

Consistent with the goal of enhanced mobility, surgical replacement of knees, hips, shoulders, and elbows, and reconstruction of hands and wrists has become a major component of care for older people with advanced RA.

Table 2 Management of the older patient with long-standing RA

Assess the functional status, including joint damage, systemic organ function, and nutritional status; search for comorbid disease
Assess the degree of activity of the rheumatoid process
Identify the nature and cause of new symptoms. Are they due to RA or a comorbid condition
Assess psychological status with special reference to depression and dementia
Analyse the pattern of social support and available funding
Assess the home environment (accessibility, functionality, and safety)
Planning: together with the patient, and, with the patient's consent, family, define both short-term and long-term treatment goals
Treat comorbid disease
Treat active RA, if still present, using drugs sparingly and appropriately; avoid drug interaction
Design rehabilitative programme, including exercises and orthopedic aspects
Be alert to possible setbacks such as atlanto-occipital subluxation
Communicate with patient, family, and other care providers; patient education

The outcomes of these procedures vary markedly among individual patients; those with a positive attitude and determination to optimize their physical mobility usually do well. The referring physician should be aware, however, of the very considerable stress imposed by both knee and hip replacements. As an example, a 76-year-old man entered the surgical amphitheater with a haemoglobin level of 16 g per cent. Two hours later, following insertion of bilateral knee replacements and two transfusions, his haemoglobin level had fallen to 8. Fortunately, he did not sustain a cardiovascular or cerebral vascular event, and achieved an excellent outcome.

New onset RA in older people

Although the frequency of new onset acute arthritis increases as people age, reaching a peak in patients in their early 70s (Gabriel et al. 1999), the frequency of the diseases that often masquerade as RA escalates even more rapidly. Thus, the differential diagnosis of older patients with new onset polyarthritis often becomes very difficult (see Table 3).

It is not surprising, therefore, that the published reports of new onset RA in the older population (typically defined as persons age 60 and older), have yielded conflicting results. Some reports conclude that patients with 'elderly onset RA' have a more benign prognosis than younger patients, and may even represent a different subset of the disease (Deal et al. 1985). Others conclude that older-onset patients have a more destructive form of the disease. After a meta-analysis of the literature, Kavanaugh (1997) concluded that the differences are explainable on the basis of increased comorbidity and frailty among the older population.

Earlier, the accepted approach to treatment of RA involved gradual escalation in power and potential toxicity of medications—the 'pyramid approach'. This, together with all elements of the conservative regimen and use of the less toxic disease modifying agents, such as hydroxychloraquine, provided abundant opportunity to consider, further, the diagnosis of the individual patient before the time when one needed to make a decision concerning use of the major disease-remitting agents. More recently, with clearer emphasis on the value of instituting powerful disease modifying agents at the onset of illness (van de Putte and Weinblatt 1995), this 'consideration period' becomes markedly compressed, and difficulties in diagnosis in older patients, early in their disease, lead to more serious problems in designing treatment.

Two factors that play a major role in determining the future outlook of a patient and guide the decision-making process are the presence or absence of rheumatoid factor and the age of the patient. In a fascinating duo of articles, Van Schaardenberg et al. (1993a) focused attention first on patients with new onset RA aged 60 years and older. Patients were considered seropositive if they had latex fixation titres 1 : 160 or greater (before 1984) or 12.5 i.u. or greater from 1984 onwards. During a follow-up period averaging 5.6 years, seropositive patients in the 60+ age group exhibited a much more adverse course than those with seronegative disease, with far higher frequency of major (sometimes fatal) gastrointestinal complications, greater comorbidity, and a five-fold increase in mortality. Glennas et al. (2000) studied patients with average age of 72 with new onset polyarthritis and also found that those with seropositive disease had a much more severe course than seronegative patients, with a 12-fold increase in 5-year mortality rate.

In contrast, when Van Shaardenburg et al. (1993b) addressed a population of patients with RA with either new-onset or established disease who had survived to age 85 and older, the rheumatoid factor no longer held adverse connotations. The prevalence of rheumatoid factor in the patients with RA (27 per cent) was no greater than that in the general population of similar age, and was not associated with more severe disease. It seems likely that the divergent views of authors describing 'new onset RA in the older age group', relate in part to three factors: (i) uncertainty in diagnostic criteria, (ii) failure to differentiate clearly those with seropositive and seronegative disease, and (iii) failure to differentiate patients in the various age brackets referred to by the term 'older'.

The data summarized above, together with undocumented clinical experience, suggest that the management of new onset RA in older people should be tailored to a number of factors including the patient's age, status regarding rheumatoid factor, physical functional capacity, comorbidity, and psychosocial factors. The approach followed in our clinic will serve as an example. The workup starts with a detailed history, complete physical examination, and appropriate laboratory tests:

- Obtain always or almost always
  - Complete blood cell count and differential
  - Erythrocyte sedimentation rate and/or C-reactive protein
  - Biochemical screen, including renal and liver function and serum calcium
  - Serum uric acid
  - Urinalysis
  - Radiographs of hands and other involved joints
- Obtain if appropriate
  - ANA screen. If elevated, follow up with ANA titre, anti-dsDNA, and other antinuclear and anticytoplasmic antibodies and complement levels as appropriate
  - Rheumatoid factor, chest radiograph
  - T4, thyroid stimulating hormone
  - Synovial fluid examination for culture, crystals and cell count
  - Serum creatine kinase, aldolase, and lipase
  - Antibodies to Borrelia burgdorferi (ELISA or Western blot)
  - Stool leucocyte count, haemoccult examinations
  - Other diagnostic studies: Schirmer's test, serum protein electrophoresis and immunofixation, electromyography, bone scan, MRI, CT scan, dual energy X-ray absorptiometry, biopsy of skin, muscle, kidney, lacrimal gland, etc.

For older patients in the age group 60–70 who experience new onset polyarthritis having the characteristics of RA, especially those with seropositive disease, the treatment is similar to that currently employed for younger persons with new onset disease, that is, initial treatment with NSAIDs (watching carefully for evidence of GI toxicity), a well-designed programme of rest, exercise, and supportive care, progressing rapidly to an appropriate DMARD, hydroxychloroquine or sulfasalazine or, for those with more active disease, methotrexate. Recently, combinations of two or three agents have proved effective.

Introduction of the immunomodulatory agents, especially the TNF inhibitors etanercept and infliximab, has provided an important new dimension of therapy for patients with severe active RA, ulcerative colitis, and the spondyloarthropathies. Unfortunately, the effectiveness and safety of these agents in patients aged 70 and older, as compared with other forms of therapy, has not yet, to our knowledge, been documented by controlled studies. The agents are, however, already receiving extensive use, with good

Table 3 Reasons why differential diagnosis of new onset polyarthritis in patients aged 65+ is frequently difficult

Increased age-related frequency of other diseases that may masquerade as RA [inflammatory osteoarthritis, polymyalgia rheumatica, fibromyalgia, gout, RS_3PE syndrome (McCarty et al. 1985), and polyarthritis associated with malignancy]
Lack of assistance from ARA and ACR criteria for classification of RA (Ropes et al. 1958; Arnett et al. 1988). These were designed to assist in outcome studies, and not specifically as diagnostic aids. Few patients aged 75+ were included in the population on which they were derived. The time required for the full criteria to be achieved is inconsistent with the need for prompt diagnosis in clinical practice
Many patients initially classified as having RA, even in 'definite' RA by Ropes Criteria (1958), prove, in time, to have other less threatening causes for their polyarthritis (Lawrence and Bennett 1960; Eidler and Hulsemann 1989)
Many people, aged 60+, without any evidence of a rheumatic disease, exhibit levels in erythrocyte sedimentation rate and rheumatoid factor that would be regarded as abnormal in a younger population (Wernick 1989)

to excellent clinical responses in many patients, including those in the 60–70 age group. Because of the inconvenience of biweekly subcutaneous injections, infliximab is frequently the agent of choice. However, the need to lie still, in a reclining position, for $2\frac{1}{2}$–3 h while receiving the infliximab infusions is proving difficult for many older patients.

These optimistic reports, moreover, are tempered by the serious threat of infection due to reduction in the patient's immune competence. Although the frequency of intercurrent acute illnesses does not appear to be increased following use of these drugs, deaths due to overwhelming infection are being reported. An even more serious complication is wide dissemination of latent tuberculosis and chronic fungal infection. A recent warning issued by Centocor, Inc., distributors of infliximab in the United States, recommends that 'all patients being considered for treatment with this agent should receive a tuberculin skin test and, if positive, initiation of therapy should be deferred pending appropriate anti-tuberculosis therapy'. The warning also states: 'Special attention to the balance between the benefits and risks of therapy should be provided for patients with comorbid chronic illnesses, such as diabetes mellitus, and also for patients who have resided in regions where histoplasmosis is endemic'. In view of the marked increase in frequency of concomitant chronic diseases in older patients, and the patient's age-related decrease in immune competence, use of these agents should be undertaken with great care. Further objective study of the risk–benefit ratio is needed.

For all older patients, sudden disruption of their pattern of life creates hazards of depression and 'failure to thrive'. Therefore, if a good clinical response cannot be achieved easily and rapidly (within a few weeks), by one of the above approaches, institution of small doses of corticosteroids should be considered seriously.

Approach to the very old and frail

For people aged 75, 80, and older with new onset arthritis, especially those with multiple comorbid diseases and significant physical or cognitive incapacity, the goal of returning the patient to his or her previous level of functional capacity in the shortest possible period of time becomes especially important. In our view, in many, possibly most patients in this group, prednisone should be introduced at the outset, in doses of 4–6 mg/day. NSAIDs will, in most cases, be less effective, and the toxicity in the patients of this age group, especially those with seropositive disease, is significant. Appropriate disease modifying agents are introduced gradually and, if appropriate, sequentially. However, the chief goal is to re-establish physical function and a 'normal' pattern of life. The issue of possible long-term sequellae of the rheumatoid process is far less important at this age. Although the adverse prognosis described by Van Schaardenburg et al. (1993a,b) and Glennas et al. (2000) in seropositive patients in the young-old group appears no longer to be operative by age 85, it is not clear at what age the presence of rheumatoid factors becomes less relevant, nor the reasons why.

Polymyalgia rheumatica

Polymyalgia rheumatica (PMR) is common among the older population, with an annual incidence in persons aged 50 and older of 54.8/100 000 (Salvarani et al. 1995a; Salvarani et al. 1995b). Occurring in a ratio of women to men of 1.3, its frequency in patients in this age group (7/1000), approximates that of RA. The prevalence escalates logarithmically with age from 20/100 000 at age 50–54 years to 320/100 000 at age 60–64, 1180/100 000 at age 70–74, and 2580/100 000 at age 80–84 (Salvarani et al. 1995a,b; Lawrence et al. 1998).

The onset of PMR may be gradual or acute, often occurring following a viral or viral-like illness. The chief manifestations are aching and severe morning stiffness of the neck, upper back, shoulders or proximal regions of the arms, and/or pelvic girdle or proximal regions of the thighs, accompanied by severe fatigue and, at times, low-grade fever. The stiffness occurs predominantly in the morning, lasting 30 min or more, but is frequently present throughout the day and night. Because of pain on movement, the patient experiences what she or he interprets as weakness. Objective testing of the affected areas usually discloses marked tenderness but only moderate weakness. Because of the stiffness and pain on motion, the patient may not be able to lift a coffee cup to his or her lips or manipulate a steering wheel. At night, the patient may find it impossible to roll over in bed without a push from his or her bed partner.

MRI and ultrasonography have shown that the major cause of the pain and stiffness is inflammation of subacromial, subdeltoid, and other bursae, often with accumulation of fluid (Pavlica et al. 2000). Inflammation of extensor tendon sheaths of the hand and arm may also be present, causing severe tenderness. Importantly, and in sharp distinction from RA, the fingers themselves are not involved. This produces a clinical picture similar to and possibly identical with RS_3PE syndrome (remitting seronegative symmetrical synovitis with pitting oedema) (McCarty et al. 1985). This syndrome, occurring primarily in men, may also be seen independently or in association with ankylosing spondylitis, sarcoidosis, and haematologic malignancies. The HLA-B27 antigen is often present.

The most consistent laboratory abnormality in PMR is an elevated erythrocyte sedimentation rate (ESR). In one series (Kyle et al. 1989) the value ranged between 32 and 138 mm in 1 h, with a mean of 70.21 mm in 1 h (Westergren). These values are not significantly different from those encountered in giant cell arteritis. In a percentage of cases, estimated between 7 and 22 per cent (Ellis and Ralston 1983), however, the ESR is normal or falls below 30 mm in 1 h.

The response of patients with PMR to moderate doses of prednisone (10–15 mg/day) is dramatic and provides an important additional clue to diagnosis. One strategy that has proved useful involves careful observation of a patient's response following administration of 15 mg of prednisone a day for 3 days. Patients with PMR usually exhibit marked decrease of symptoms on the day following the initiation of corticosteroid. Patients with rheumatoid arthritis will also improve, but the improvement is rarely evident before the third day.

Continuing therapy is best provided by prednisone, initially in a dosage between 7 and 12 mg/day. The dose should be tapered, very gradually, using the ESR and/or C reactive protein and the clinical symptoms as a guide. While it is usually possible to discontinue the medication within $1\frac{1}{2}$ years of onset, there are some patients in whom continued therapy, in a dose of 5 or 6 mg/day, is required to maintain the patient in an asymptomatic state. Initial treatment with higher doses of prednisone does not decrease the overall duration of treatment required. Physicians caring for patients with PMR must always be on the alert for the possible development of giant cell (temporal) arteritis.

Temporal arteritis

Temporal arteritis (TA), also referred to as giant cell arteritis (GCA), cranial arteritis, and granulomatous arteritis, is by no means infrequent among older people. In the study in Olmsted County, its annual incidence rate was 17.8 cases/100 000, with a prevalence rate of active or remittant cases of 2/1000 (Salvarani et al. 1995b). This is approximately one-fifth the estimated prevalence rate for RA in the same county (Gabriel et al. 1999).

In the office practice of rheumatology, temporal arteritis is one of the few entities, if not the only one, that requires rapid and decisive action based almost entirely on clinical judgement, resembling, in this regard, the decisional priorities of the surgeon. The consequences of a clinical decision that the patient either has or is at high risk for having temporal arteritis are significant, involving a surgical referral for a temporal artery biopsy and, in all probability, initiation of prednisone in doses of 60–80 mg/day. For older people, the prospect of any biopsy is a threatening one, bringing with it an association with malignancy. For any older person to be placed on prednisone in this dose carries inherent risks, including GI bleeding, hypertension, glucose intolerance, and psychological side-effects. Except for people with specific contraindications, prednisone therapy in this dose should always be accompanied by cimetadine or a similar agent to reduce gastric acidity, and the patient should be alerted to watch for appearance of black stools. For prevention of loss of bone matrix, the patient should also be placed on an antiresorptive medication, ideally a bisphosphonate, and calcium and vitamin D. These additional medications bring their own share of potential complications, especially in patients who may already be receiving a number of other drugs for comorbid disease. Therefore, a decision that the patient has or is at risk for having temporal arteritis leads to significant consequences for the immediate management of the patient. This, of course, has to be balanced against the significant risk of blindness or other vascular complications if the temporal arteritis goes untreated. The key, therefore, lies in making the correct diagnosis on clinical grounds.

Although the precise nature of the association between PMR and temporal arteritis is not understood, there is a significant relationship. Between 10 and 18 per cent of patients with PMR also exhibit CGA (Salvarani et al. 1995a,b); 41 per cent of patients with CGA exhibit clinical manifestations of PMR (Salvarani and Hunder 1999).

Thus, in all patients with PMR one must be on the constant look out for clues to the presence of temporal arteritis. Guidelines for the classification of temporal arteritis have been developed (Hunder et al. 1990). Unfortunately, as with other classification guidelines, the application of these to clinical practice is far from perfect. While many patients with temporal arteritis exhibit clinical manifestations consistent with PMR, this is not always the case. Twenty-four per cent of the patients described by Salvarani and Hunder (1999) exhibited arthritis of the knee, wrist, and ankle and also metacarpopharyngeal joints and proximal interphalangeal joints, quite distinct from that seen in polymyalgia rheumatica. Six met the ACR criteria for classification of RA (Arnett et al. 1988). Other patients have no arthritis at all.

Faced with this dilemma, it is our practice to maintain a high level of suspicion in patients with major or minor musculoskeletal symptoms resembling PMR or rheumatoid-like arthritis whose erythrocyte sedimentation rate and/or C-reactive protein concentration is at a level clearly out of proportion to the extent of musculoskeletal inflammation. Because of the association of giant cell arteritis with elevated platelet counts (Lincoff et al. 2000), we follow this value also. We watch carefully for symptoms or signs relevant to the temporal artery, such as tenderness, headache, or alterations in vision, especially generalized dimness or 'zigzag lines'. If any of these occur, the patient is started immediately on high doses of prednisone and arrangements are made for a confirmatory temporal artery biopsy. It should be noted, however, that values for ESR reaching as high as 120 mm in 1 h occur in other entities as well, including multiple myeloma and enteropathic spondyloarthropathy.

Fibromyalgia

Fibromyalgia is a poorly understood condition that affects people of all ages, with a seven-fold predominance in women. In a community-based population, Wolfe et al. (1995) found a total prevalence of 34/1000 in women, and 5/1000 in men (approximately equal to that of 'definite' RA), with an approximately seven-fold increase in prevalence from ages 18–29 to 70–79, and a slight decrease in those 80 and older. Because the condition is often triggered by a severe auto accident or other major trauma, the patients may be given a diagnosis of 'post-traumatic syndrome'.

Fibromyalgia is typically slow in onset, occurring, gradually, over the course of weeks, rather than hours, as in the case of gout, or days as in the case of PMR. In addition to pain involving, at times, any or all regions of the body, the majority of patients also experience morning stiffness, difficulty both in falling asleep and in remaining in sleep throughout the night, and extreme fatigue. Most patients with the disease are significantly depressed. The weakness is profound, resembling what one sees in chronic fatigue syndrome, with which fibromyalgia is closely associated. Although not mentioned widely in the literature, many patients with fibromyalgia will admit to fainting spells if asked specifically. Significant postural hypotension is frequently seen. Many patients also exhibit symptoms of irritable bowel syndrome.

On physical examination, the most characteristic clinical feature is the presence of 'tender points' (Wolfe et al. 1995). These are sharply localized areas of tenderness which may occur at any area of the body, most often the upper back, shoulders, arms adjacent to the elbows, and legs adjacent to the knees. The localized nature of the tenderness is important. A typical 'tender point' is so sharply localized that, if one moves one's finger a $\frac{1}{2}$ in. in any direction, the tenderness is no longer perceived.

Our understanding of the pathogenesis and treatment of fibromyalgia is still in the process of evolution. Treatment, at present, involves four components: drugs, physical modalities, psychological therapy and 'alternative medicine'. The approach to pharmacotherapy, which has achieved greatest use, especially in young people and those of mid-life, is a combination of amitriptyline and cyclobenzaprine. Amitriptyline is prescribed in doses from 10 to 25 mg at bed time, increasing, gradually, to 75 mg/day (25 mg in the a.m. and 50 mg at supper or bedtime). Later, cyclobenzaprine is added, in a starting dose of 10 mg, increasing, gradually, to 20–30 mg/day if tolerated. Because of risk of adverse effects of amitriptyline in older people, especially falls, the drug should be used with caution in patients in this age group. NSAIDs are relatively ineffective. Traditional physical therapy often makes the condition worse, at least at the onset. Many patients, however, describe benefits from gentle stretching exercises.

Psychological therapy, focusing on patient education and coping skills training, is gaining increasing attention. Several small-scale studies, both controlled and sequential, have documented the effectiveness of this approach in patients with fibromyalgia (Sandstrom and Keefe 1998) and also with irritable bowel syndrome, a closely related entity.

Frustrated by lack of knowledge and, often, interest on their condition by most physicians, many fibromyalgia patients rely, extensively, on non-traditional therapy, chiefly chiropractic, herbs, relaxation techniques, and massage. Information for patients on this approach is readily available on the Internet and in several books on the topic. An estimated 30 per cent of individuals, aged 65 and older, utilize alternative medicine. The majority do not report this use to their physicians. While few of these methodologies have been subjected to controlled study, reports from individual patients describe benefits from several of them, especially massage therapy and muscle relaxation techniques.

Whatever treatment is employed, an essential ingredient of success is determination by the patient to get better (i.e. clear establishment of a patient-based 'locus of control'), especially if accompanied by genuine interest and encouragement by the physician.

Gout

The frequency of gout in older patients approximates that of RA (7.2/1000 in men; 4.8/1000 in women) (Lawrence et al. 1998). Gout in older people is substantially different from that in younger persons. Attacks may occur in a wide range of joints, including knees, wrists, ankles, shoulders, and small joints of the hand, resembling RA. Frequently, several joints are involved at the same time. Although the involvement is typically asymmetrical, that is not always the case. Gout frequently occurs simultaneously with other musculoskeletal disorders.

Careful history will often reveal that the patient experiences an aura or premonition that an acute attack is about to occur, hours or even a day or two before it actually ensues. Key features in the diagnosis include the remarkable speed with which the attack, once underway, moves on to its maximal intensity (usually within 6–8 h) and the striking degree of tenderness of the involved joint. Unfortunately, in recent years, at least in the United States, uric acid determinations are no longer included as part of the panel of tests routinely obtained under the heading 'Comprehensive Metabolic Labs'. Therefore, uric acid determinations should be requested, specifically, in all patients with new onset arthritis. However, patients with acute gouty arthritis may, at one time or another, have serum urate values within the normal range. Full confirmation of the diagnosis can only be obtained by demonstration of uric acid crystals in the synovial fluid or a gouty tophus.

The treatment of gout in older people is similar to that in younger persons. Determination of the precise dose of colchicine that will be effective in prevention of acute attacks requires a careful process of titration. The goal is to identify a good dose just short of that which will induce diarrhoea or soft stool. It may range between one tablet (0.6 mg) every other day or every third day, to one tablet one day and two the next, or even two tablets a day. If the titration is carefully done, colchicine, maintained on a long-term basis, will prevent gout in over 90 per cent of patients.

The treatment of acute gouty arthritis in older patients is best accomplished either by a short course of a non-steroidal drug, such as rofecoxib, naproxen, or indomethacin, or by prednisone 20 mg initially, with reductions over the course of a week. The use of large doses of colchicine to *treat* acute gout is no longer appropriate, especially in older patients, because of the serious side-effects to the large doses required.

Initiation of allopurinol therapy should only be undertaken after one has demonstrated a programme of colchicine dosage that will effectively inhibit acute attacks. The reason is that there is a tendency, early in the course of allopurinol therapy, for an increase in the frequency of acute gouty attacks and one needs to be well equipped to prevent these before starting new medication. Allopurinol is a potentially toxic drug and should be prescribed with care (Smith et al. 2000). As a consultant rheumatologist, one may be referred a patient from a primary care physician who is utilizing the appropriate agents in a good or excellent way, yet the patient still manifests severe articular complaints. In this case, it is important that one look, carefully, for other causes for these symptoms.

Osteoarthritis

Although early evidence of osteoarthritis occurs in many young people in their early 20s, the frequency of the condition escalates markedly in advancing years. In a population-based cohort of patients, age 70 years, Bergstrom (1986a,b) found osteoarthritis of the knee to be present, on clinical grounds, in 12 per cent of the sample (19 per cent of the men and 16 per cent of the women). Radiographic changes consistent with this diagnosis were present in 26 per cent of men and 15 per cent of women (20 per cent of the total population). By age 79, however, the frequency of clinically evident osteoarthritis in the survivors had decreased from 12 to 6 per cent. Frequency of radiographic changes consistent with this diagnosis had decreased from 20 to 13 per cent. Since it seems highly unlikely that the radiologic changes are reversible, this suggests that osteoarthritis may be associated with a decreased life span. In view of the threat of osteoarthritis on a person's physical function and the benefits of exercise on overall health, this conclusion is not totally illogical. A recent study has added support to this hypothesis (Cerhan et al. 1995).

The concepts of comprehensive care, described earlier in this chapter for RA (Table 2), including psychosocial factors, the issue of multiple disease and guidelines for safe use of drugs, are as appropriate in patients with osteoarthritis as in those with RA or other chronic forms of arthritis. Evidence of the benefits of well defined exercises, both an aerobic and aerobic, is increasingly solid (Ettinger et al. 1997). Although many physicians are reluctant to accept it, the use of continuous low-dose narcotic therapy is currently being explored (Roth et al. 2000). Other modalities include diet therapy, topical agents, acupuncture, transcutaneous nerve stimulation, pulsed electro-magnetic fields, heat and cold, non-traditional medication, and nutritional supplements such as glucosamine/chondroitin sulfate (Felson et al. 2000; Gloth 2001). Clinical experience is showing what appear to be important benefits of the latter agent in some patients (and also animals). However, there are, as yet few objective studies of the indications for or effectiveness of any of these modalities. A great deal of additional work needs to be done.

Dermatomyositis–polymyositis

These conditions, occurring in young as well as old, are much less frequent than those that have been given greatest attention in this chapter. However, they occupy an important place in geriatric rheumatology for three reasons. First, the conditions need to be considered in the differential diagnosis of other more frequent entities characterized by diffuse pain, stiffness, and a sense of weakness, such as PMR. Second, the occurrence of the conditions, especially in older people, is associated with a markedly increased risk of malignant disease—a 6.2-fold increased risk in patients with polymyositis, 2.6-fold in those with dermatomyositis, and 2.4-fold for inclusion body myositis (Buchbinder et al. 2001). All patients diagnosed with these diseases, especially older patients, should be reviewed, carefully, for the presence of malignant disease. Third, with the increased use of cholesterol-lowering agents, there is a significant incidence of toxic myositis and, at times, rhabdomyolysis, resembling that seen in dermatomyositis (Pierce et al. 1996). The condition may follow use of most or all of the statin drugs. It has been described in 30 per cent of patients taking lovastatin in combination with immunosuppressive drugs, 5 per cent of those taking lovastatin and gemfibrozil and many patients taking a statin drug alone. The condition is associated with a marked increase in creatinine phosphokinase resembling that seen in polymyositis–dermatomyositis (with a mean increase of 10-fold, occasionally reaching 100-fold).

Summary

Important points to remember—special characteristics of older patients

Most older people function reasonably well and independently in community settings, usually belittling and concealing their functional limitations. Nevertheless, most of them suffer from and have learned to adapt to, multiple chronic illnesses. Whether due to these illnesses or to the process of ageing, most older persons have little remaining functional reserve. A seemingly minor event, such as a fall or mild infection, may lead to a crescendo of organ failure and death.

Despite this generalization, and their rather similar appearance, older people differ from one another in specific functional capacity, as well as experience and personality, to a greater extent than younger persons.

Most older people value preservation of function and independence over duration of life. Because of the threat to functional independence implicit with many musculoskeletal disorders, treatment modalities to enhance function, even at some risk, should not be overlooked.

Preventive care, at all levels, and a balanced consideration of psychosocial and medical issues emerge as the keys to successful care of older people.

Use of drugs, especially multiple drugs, in older patients is a double-edged sword, and a frequent cause of avoidable decline.

In view of the escalating incidence of malignant disease in patients of advanced years, and their protean manifestations, the physician should be alert to the possible presence of these disorders, especially in the patients experiencing new onset of musculoskeletal symptoms. Complete physical exam, including breast, lymph nodes, abdomen, and rectal exam and appropriate laboratory investigation should be part of every work up for an older patient with new onset rheumatic disease.

References

Arnett, F. et al. (1988). The American Rheumatism Association 1987 revised criteria for the classification of rheumatoid arthritis. *Arthritis and Rheumatism* **31**, 315–24.

Bergstrom, G. et al. (1986a). Prevalence of rheumatoid arthritis, osteoarthritis, chondrocalcinosis and gouty arthritis at age 79. *Journal of Rheumatology* **13**, 527–34.

Bergstrom, G. et al. (1986b). Joint disorders and ages 70, 75 and 79 years—a cross sectional comparison. *British Journal of Rheumatology* **25**, 333–41.

Buchbinder, R., Forbes, A., Hale, S., Dennett, Y., and Giles, G. (2001). Incidence of malignant disease in biopsy-proven inflammatory myopathy. *Annals of Internal Medicine* **134**, 1087–95.

Cerhan, J.R., Wallace, R.B., El-Khoury, G.Y., Moore, T.E., and Long, C.R. (1995). Decreased survival with increased prevalence of full-body radiologically defined osteoarthritis in women. *American Journal of Epidemiology* **141**, 225–34.

Cummings, S.R., Black, D.M., and Rubin, S.M. (1989). Life time risks of hip, Colles', or vertebral fracture and coronary heart disease among white postmenopausal women. *Archives of Internal Medicine* **149**, 2445–8.

Deal, C.L. et al. (1985). The clinical features of elderly-onset rheumatoid arthritis. A comparison with younger-onset disease of similar duration. *Arthritis and Rheumatism* **28**, 987–94.

Eidler, H. and Hulsemenn, J.L. (1989). Benign polyarthritis and undifferentiated arthritis. An epidemiologic tera incognita. *Scandinavian Journal of Rheumatology* **S79**, 13–20.

Ellis, M.E. and Ralston, S. (1983). The ESR in the diagnosis and management of polymyalgia rheumatica/giant cell arteritis syndrome. *Annals of the Rheumatic Diseases* **43**, 163–70.

Engel, A., Roberts, J., and Burtch, T.A. (1966). Rheumatoid arthritis in adults: United States 1960–1962. *Vital and Health Statistics, Series 1: Programs and Collection Procedures* **11** (17), 1–43.

Ettinger, W.H. et al. (1997). A randomized trial comparing aerobic exercise and resistance exercise with a health education program in older adults with knee osteoarthritis. *Journal of the American Medical Association* **277**, 25–31.

Felson, D.T. et al. (2000): Osteoarthritis: new insights. Part 2: Treatment approaches. *Annals of Internal Medicine* **133**, 726–37.

Fisher, N.M., Pendergast, D.R., and Calkins, E. (1991). Muscle rehabilitation in impaired nursing home resident. *Archives of Physical Medicine and Rehabilitation* **72**, 118–25.

Fried, L.P. et al. (2001). Frailty in older adults: evidence for a phenotype. *Journal of Gerontology Medical Sciences* **56a**, m146–56.

Gabriel, S.E., Crowson, C.S. and O'Fallon, W.M. (1999). The epidemiology of rheumatoid arthritis in Rochester, Minnesota, 1955–1985. *Arthritis and Rheumatism* **42**, 415–20.

Glennas, A., Kvien, T.K., Andrup, O., Karstensen, B., and Munthe, E. (2000). Recent onset arthritis in the elderly: a 5 year longitudinal observational study. *Journal of Rheumatology* **27**, 101–8.

Gloth, F.M. (2001). Pain management in older adults: prevention and treatment. *Journal of the American Geriatrics Society* **49**, 188–99.

Gruenberg, E.M. (1977). The failure of success. *Milbank Memorial Fund Quarterly—Health and Society* **55**, 3–24.

Guralnik, J.M. et al. (1994). A short physical performance battery assessing lower extremity function: association with self-reported disability and prediction of mortality and nursing home admission. *Journal of Gerontology* **49**, m85–94.

Hakim, A.A. et al. (1998). Effects of walking on mortality among nonsmoking retired men. *New England Journal of Medicine* **338**, 94–9.

Hanlon, J.T., Schmader, K.E., Ruby, C.M., and Weinberger, M. (2001). Suboptinal prescribing in older inpatients and outpatients. *Journal of the American Geriatrics Society* **49**, 200–9.

Hunder, G.G. et al. (1990). The American College of Rheumatology 1990 criteria for the classification of giant cell arteritis. *Arthritis and Rheumatism* **33**, 122–8.

Judge, J.O., Schechtman, K., and Cress, E. (1996). The relationship between physical performance measures and independence in instrumental activities of daily living. The FICSIT Group. Frailty and injury: cooperative studies of intervention trials. *Journal of the American Geriatrics Society* **44**, 1332–41.

Kavanaugh, A.F. (1997). Rheumatoid arthritis in the elderly: is it a different disease? *American Journal of Medicine* **103** (6A), 40S–8S.

King, M.B. and Tinetti, M.E. (1995). Falls in community-dwelling older persons. *Journal of the American Geriatrics Society* **43**, 1146–54.

Kyle, V., Cawston, T.E., and Hazleman, B. (1989). ESR and C-reactive protein in the assessment of polylmyalgia rheumatica-giant cell arteritis on presentation and during follow-up. *Annals of Rheumatic Diseases* **48**, 667–71.

Lawrence, J.S. and Bennett, P.H. (1960). Benign polyarthritis. *Annals of the Rheumatic Diseases* **19**, 20–30.

Lawrence, R.C. et al. (1998). Estimates of the prevalence of arthritis and selected musculoskeletal disorders in the United States. *Arthritis and Rheumatism* **41**, 778–99.

Lincoff, N.S., Erlich, P.D., and Brass, L.S. (2000). Thrombocytosis in temporal arteritis. Rising platelet counts: a red flag for giant cell arteritis. *Journal of Neuro-Ophthalmology* **20**, 67–72.

McCarty, D.J. et al. (1985). Remitting sero-negative symmetrical synovitis with pitting edema. RS_3PE syndrome. *Journal of the American Medical Association* **254**, 2763–7.

Mikulowski, P., Wollheim, F.A., Rotmil, P., and Olsen, J. (1975). Sudden death in rheumatoid arthritis with atlanto-axial dislocation. *Acta Medica Scandinavica* **198**, 445–51.

Mulrow, C.D., Williams, J.W., Gerety, M.B., Ramirez, G., Monteil, O.M., and Kerber, C. (1995). Case-finding instruments for depression in primary care settings. *Annals of Internal Medicine* **122**, 913–21.

National Osteoporosis Foundation (1998). Ostoporosis: review of evidence for prevention, diagnosis, and treatment and cost-effective analysis; status report. *Osteoporosis International* (Suppl. 4), S1–2.

Paffenberger, R.S., Jr., Wing, A.L., and Hyde, R.T. (1978). Physical activity as an index of heart attack risk in college alumni. *American Journal of Epidemiology* **108**, 161–75.

Pavlica, P. et al. (2000). Magnetic resonance imaging in the diagnosis of PMR. *Clinical and Experimental Rheumatology* **18** (Suppl. 29), S38–9.

Pendergast, D.R., Fisher, N.M., and Calkins, E. (1993). Cardiovascular, neuromuscular and metabolic alterations with age leading to frailty. *Journal of Gerontology* **48**, 61–7.

Pierce, R., Wysowski, D.L., and Gross, T.P. (1990). Myopathy and rhabdomyolysis associated with lovastatin-gemfibrozil combination therapy. *Journal of the American Medical Association* **264**, 71–5.

van den Akker, M., Buntinx, F., Metsemakers, J.F., Roos, S., and Knottnerus, J.A. (1998). Multimorbidity in general practice: prevalence, incidence, and determinants of co-occurring chronic and recurrent diseases. *Journal of Clinical Epidemiology* **51** (5), 367–75.

van de Putte, L.B.A. and Weinblatt, M.E. (1995). Radical interventions in early rheumatoid arthritis. The case for enteric-coated sulphasalizine, methotrexate and combined regimines. A workshop held in Camagli, Italy, September, 1994. *British Journal of Rheumatology* **34** (Suppl. 2) (entire volume).

Ropes, M.W., Bennett, G.A., Cobb, S., Jacox, R., and Jessar, R. (1958). 1958 Revision of diagnostic criteria for rheumatoid arthritis. *Bulletin on the Rheumatic Diseases* **9**, 175–6.

Roth, S.H. et al. (2000). Around-the-clock, controlled-release oxycodone therapy for osteoarthritis-related pain: placebo-controlled trial and long-term evaluation. *Archives of Internal Medicine* **160**, 853–60.

Saag, K.G. et al. (1998). Alendronate for the prevention and treatment of glucocorticoid-induced osteoporosis. *New England Journal of Medicine* **339**, 292–9.

Sager, A., Rudberg, M.A., Jalaluddin, M., Frank, T., Inouye, S.K., Landefeld, C.S., Siepens, H., and Winograd, C.H. (1996). Hospital admission risk profile (HARP): identifying older patients at risk for functional decline following acute medical illness and hospitalization. *Journal of the American Geriatrics Society* **44**, 251–7.

Salvarani, C. and Hunder, G.G. (1999). Musculoskeletal manifestations in a population-based cohert of patients with giant cell arteritis. *Arthritis and Rheumatism* **42**, 1259–66.

Salvarani, C., Gabriel, S.E., O'Fallon, W.M., and Hunder, G.G. (1995a). Epidemiology of polymyalgia rheumatica in Olmsted County, Minnesota, 1970–1991. *Arthritis and Rheumatism* **38**, 369–73.

Salvarani, C., Gabriel, S.E., O'Fallon, W.M., and Hunder, G.G. (1995b). The incidence of giant cell arteritis in Olmsted County: apparent fluctuations in a cyclic pattern. *Annals of Internal Medicine* **123**, 192–4.

Sandstrom, M.J. and Keefe, F.J. (1998). Self-management of fibromyalgia: the role of formal coping skills training and physical exercise training program. *Arthritis Care Research* **11**, 432–47.

Sehl, M. and Yates, F. (2001). Kinetics of human aging. I. Rates of decline between ages 30 and 70 years in healthy people. *Journal of Gerontology—Biological Sciences* **56A**, B198–208.

Smith, P., Karlson, N., and Nair, B.R. (2000): Quality use of allopurinol in the elderly. *Journal of Quality in Clinical Practice* **20** (1), 42–3.

Soderlin, M.K., Nieminen, P., and Hakala, M. (1998). The functional status predicts mortality in a community based rheumatoid arthritis population. *Journal of Rheumatology* **25**, 1895–909.

Stevens, J.C., Cartilage, N.E.F., Saunders, M., Applebee, A., Hall, M., and Shaw, D.A. (1971). Atlanto axial subluxation and cervical myelopathy in rheumatoid arthritis. *Quarterly Journal of Medicine* **40**, 391–408.

US Department of Health and Human Services. *Physical Activity and Health: A Report of the Surgeon General.* Atlanta GA: US Department of Health and

Human Services, Center for Disease Control and Prevention. National Center for Chronic Disease Prevention and Health Promotion, 1996.

Vaillant, G.E. and Mukemal, K. (2001). Successful aging. *American Journal of Psychiatry* **158**, 839–40.

Van den Endy, C.H. et al. (2000). Effective intensive exercise on patients with active rheumatoid arthritis: a randomized clinical trial. *Annals of the Rheumatic Diseases* **59**, 615–21.

Van Schaardenburg, D., Hazes, J.M., de Boer, A., Zwinderman, A.H., Meijers, K.A., and Breedveld, F.C. (1993a). Outcome of rheumatoid arthritis in relation to age and rheumatoid factor at diagnosis. *Journal of Rheumatology* **20**, 45–52.

Van Schaardenburg, D., Lagaay, A.M., Breedveld, F.C., Hijmans, W., and Vandenbroucke, J.P. (1993b). Rheumatoid arthritis in a population of persons aged 85 years and over. *British Journal of Rheumatology* **32**, 104–9.

Wernick, R. (1989). Avoiding laboratory tests' misinterpretation in geriatric rheumatology. *Geriatrics* **44**, 61–80.

Williams, T.F. (1986). Geriatrics: the fruition of the clinician reconsidered. *The Gerontologist* **26**, 345–9.

Wolfe F. et al. (1990). The American College of Rheumatology, 1990 Criteria for the classification of fibromyalgia: report of the multicenter criteria committee. *Arthritis and Rheumatism* **33**, 160–72.

Wolfe, F., Ross, K., Anderson, J., Russell, I.J., and Hebert, L. (1995). The prevalence and characteristics of fibromyalgia in the general population. *Arthritis and Rheumatism* **38**, 19–28.

Yesavage, J.A. et al. (1983). Development and validation of a geriatric depression screening scale—a preliminary report. *Journal of Psychiatric Research* **17**, 37–49.

1.1.5 Principles of examination

Peter van Riel

General principles

The examination of the musculoskeletal system can be considered under two headings: (i) the systematic screening of virtually all the accessible joints of the body to identify abnormalities and establish their distribution; (ii) the more detailed analysis of an abnormal joint or group of joints with specific attention for signs of inflammation, deformities, and loss of function. The screening is intended to be brief but comprehensive and efficient. It can be accomplished in a few minutes and should be part of the routine examination taught to all medical students.

The patient is best examined lying comfortably on a couch or bed for most of the examination, but sitting up for the shoulders and neck, and standing for the final stages of examining the feet and the movements of the back. Walking should be observed, either at the start in the outpatient clinic or at the end of the examination if the patient is already undressed and in bed. In a very young child, much of the examination can be carried out while he or she sits on the parent's lap.

The examination starts most logically with the hands, the calling cards of many of the rheumatic diseases, then moves up the arms to the joints of the shoulder girdle and the jaw, down the spine from the neck to the coccyx and on to the legs, finishing with the toes.

The same basic pattern governs the examination of the most of the joints: inspection, palpation, and establishing the range of movement. This pattern is altered for some parts, for example, the back, in the interests of efficiency.

It is important to realize that sometimes pain in a certain joint is being caused by a process outside the musculoskeletal system. For instance, a patient with a malignant tumour in the lung can have complains of severe pain in the shoulder. This is also called 'referred pain', in this case no abnormalities will be found by examining the painful joint.

Inspection (Table 1)

Where a joint is paired, both should be exposed to allow comparison of the two sides. Redness overlying a joint is an important indicator of acute inflammation, as in gout or septic arthritis. Any skin rash, subcutaneous nodules, cysts, scars, or evidence of local infection are noted. Muscle wasting is often associated with joint disease, but may be masked by joint swelling. Swelling or deformity should be sought. Discrepancies in limb or digit length may indicate growth problems secondary to inflammation, as in juvenile chronic arthritis.

Palpation (Table 2)

Temperature change is assessed relative to the same joint on the other side, or to surrounding normal skin. The back of the hand is rapidly moved between the areas to be compared. Errors may occur if one side has been kept warmer by a bandage, glove, or splint.

Tenderness is elicited with firm pressure along the joint margins, and over tendons and ligaments. This should be carried out with the examiner's eyes on those of the patient, rather than on the joint, so as to pick up the first signs of discomfort.

Swelling noted on inspection is palpated, to answer the question: 'Is this swelling bone, soft tissue, or fluid?' Bony swelling is especially a feature of osteoarthritis. Other causes are new bone formation with psoriatic arthritis, Charcot's joints, and callus formation after a fracture. Soft tissue swelling about a joint is most often synovial. The consistency of synovial swelling is more doughy than bouncy, like foam rubber. Where synovial fluid and synovial swelling coexist, the fluid can be pushed away or aspirated, allowing the synovium to be palpated. Fluid is recognizable for its incompressibility. Palpating a lax effusion is easy, because the fluid can be pushed from one part of the joint to another (fluctuation). A tense effusion can be recognized by its 'bouncy' quality, like a firm rubber ball.

Joint noises are frequently better felt than heard. Loud cracks and snaps, particularly on pulling the fingers or rotating the ankles, may be quite normal. Pulling the fingers creates a vacuum and the popping sound represents the sudden development of a gas cavity in the joint fluid. The snap on rotating an ankle is related to the slipping of one tendon over another. Similar, harmless snapping and crunching noises occur when the head is extended and rotated from side to side, or the shoulders are braced back and rotated.

Velvet crepitations are too soft to be audible, but may be felt. They occur when the joint contains small particles of proteinaceous material, most typically in rheumatoid arthritis. Crepitus in the joint of a patient with osteoarthritis feels like a dull, coarse crunching, and is caused by irregularities in the cartilage.

Table 1 Inspection of joints

Colour
Skin or other local changes
Muscle wasting
Swelling
Deformity

Table 2 Palpation of joints

Temperature
Tenderness
Swelling Bone Soft tissue Fluid
Crepitus

Eburnation crepitus is both heard and felt, occurring when the cartilage has been destroyed and the two bony surfaces are in contact. The name means 'turning to ivory' and the sound is thought to be similar to that of ivory grinding on ivory. Most often it emanates from the hip or the knee, and then care is needed to work out which is the affected joint as the vibrations are well transmitted up or down the femur. To demonstrate eburnation crepitus, the examiner lays a hand on the joint and asks the patient to move it. Passive movement may fail to elicit the sign because the joint surfaces are not so closely opposed when the muscles are relaxed.

Range of movement

The patient is usually first asked to move the joint actively. If a full range of active movement can be carried out without discomfort, there is rarely any need to proceed to passive movement. If the patient is unable to carry out the full range of active movement, then the passive movements will be most informative. In general, where active and passive restriction are the same, limitation of movement will reflect one of the following: inflammation of a joint; contracture of the tendons or ligaments surrounding the joint; destruction of bone or cartilage in the joint. Restriction of active but not passive movement indicates rupture or inflammation of a tendon, muscle weakness, or failure of the nerve supply to the muscle.

The 'normal' range of movement must be interpreted with caution. There is much variation in joint mobility with age and race, and from individual to individual. The figures commonly given are those considered to be at the lower end of the usual range. An excessive range of movement in otherwise normal joints is referred to as the hypermobility syndrome. An excessive range in diseased joints reflects damage to the articular surfaces or the capsule and ligaments, leading to instability.

The systematic survey

The whole patient (Table 3)

Rheumatic diseases are often multisystem in their effects, and many systemic diseases will present with rheumatic complaints. The discussion of the examination of the other systems in the body is outside the scope of this chapter, but it should be remembered that the examination of the musculoskeletal system is only one aspect of the careful and comprehensive history-taking and general physical examination that makes up the assessment of the patient with rheumatic symptoms.

Posture and gait

It is instructive to observe how the patient gets off a chair and starts moving after a period of inactivity. Gelling, or stiffness after inactivity, is a common feature of many arthritic conditions. Posture may give a clue to disorders of the back, and gait to problems in the lower limbs. Watching the patient undress is a valuable opportunity for observing whether there are difficulties. In a paediatric setting, quiet observation of the child at play can be extremely valuable in discovering whether a limb is being protected.

Table 3 Observing the whole patient

Dress: unkempt or neat
Shoes: high fashion or slippers
Getting out of chair: use of arms, help
Walking aids: stick, frame
First steps: gelling phenomenon
Gait: antalgic, waddling
Posture: erect, kyphotic, hangdog
Undressing: trouble with buttons, jacket

The hands

Screening

Inspect the hands, back and front. Palpate each of the finger joints in turn, one hand at a time, moving from the distal row proximally, including the thumbs, checking for tenderness or swelling. Ask the patient to make the hands into fists and straighten them out again. Offer the patient two fingers to grip each side and assess grip strength.

Inspection (Table 4)

Nails

The nails may show the pitting or lifting from the nail bed (onycholysis) typical of psoriasis, nail-fold infarcts typical of vasculitis, or the shaggy cuticles and periungual erythema of dermatomyositis. Dilated capillary loops in the nail fold can be seen with the naked eye, though more easily with a magnifying glass, and tend to accompany certain rheumatic diseases, for example systemic sclerosis and dermatomyositis.

Skin

A rash on the backs of the hands may be due to psoriasis or to dermatomyositis, best distinguished from each other by the distribution. Dermatomyositis tends to affect the extensor surfaces of the joints in a neat and symmetrical fashion while psoriasis is more likely to be distributed at random across the hand. Palmar erythema is common in patients with connective tissue diseases, and is frequently different in nature from the palmar erythema of pregnancy or liver disease, looking more mottled and indeed more like palmar livedo reticularis than erythema. This appearance seems to be associated with systemic vasculitis.

Muscle wasting

This is common whenever joints are inflamed, but attention should be paid to any significant patterns of muscle wasting, such as the wasting of the thenar eminence in carpal tunnel syndrome, which spares only the adductor pollicis, visible as a band parallel to the wrist. Wasting of

Table 4 Inspecting the hands

Nails Pitting Onycholysis Splinter haemorrhages Shaggy cuticles Nailfold infarcts Periungual erythema Dilated capillary loops
Skin Rash of psoriasis, dermatomyositis Vitiligo Purpura Raynaud's colour changes Infarcts Tophi Calcinosis Waxy thickening Nodules Palmer erythema
Muscles Wasting
Tendons Swelling of sheath Rupture Displacement
Joints Swelling Deformity

opponens pollicis commonly accompanies osteoarthritis of the first carpometacarpal joint.

Tendon involvement

Tenosynovitis of the flexor tendons may be seen as a fullness in the palm. It may be differentiated from Dupuytren's contracture by the absence of skin tethering over the surface, and the presence of crepitus on flexing the fingers. To detect crepitus of the flexor tendon, the examiner places the index and middle fingers over the course of the tendon, with the thumb on the back of the hand exerting firm pressure. The patient is then asked to make a fist, and crepitus or nodularity may be felt as the tendon moves within its sheath. The procedure is repeated for each of the flexor tendons in turn.

Trigger finger occurs when the finger locks in flexion, but can be passively (albeit painfully) straightened. This is caused by a nodule on the tendon passing through a stricture in the tendon sheath. The weaker extensor muscles are unable to pull the nodule back through the same obstruction. The nodule is usually to be found in the palm just proximal to the metacarpal head, but will only be detected during active movement of the affected digit. Tendon involvement may also be recognized in the fingers by pinching the thickened soft tissues at the palmar surface of the base of each finger.

Swelling

The hands may look generally puffy with no localization of this over joints. This is especially common in mixed connective tissue disease or early systemic sclerosis, where the hands may resemble a bunch of sausages, and also occurs with systemic lupus erythematosus, dermatomyositis, polymyalgia rheumatica, reflex sympathetic dystrophy, and with early rheumatoid arthritis.

Where only one or two fingers have a diffuse, cylindrical swelling, not centred on a joint, we speak of a 'sausage' digit. These may represent swelling of the flexor tendon, as in the seronegative spondyloarthropathies (particularly in psoriatic arthritis), diffuse soft tissue inflammation as in gout, or infection as in leprosy or tuberculosis.

Synovial swelling in the proximal interphalangeal joints is sometimes called spindling because of the fusiform appearance. Osteoarthritis causes a swelling of these joints that is bony and irregular, occasionally with effusions.

Distribution

The distribution of joint swelling gives an immediate clue to the diagnosis. Swelling predominantly of the terminal (distal) interphalangeal joints indicates osteoarthritis, psoriatic arthritis, or occasionally gout. Osteoarthritis also predominantly affects the first carpometacarpal joint, an articulation spared by most other arthropathies. The joint looks to be squared, because of osteophyte formation, wasting of the surrounding muscles, and adduction of the thumb. Rheumatoid arthritis has a predilection for the second and third metacarpophalangeal joints, as well as the proximal interphalangeal joints.

Deformities

Note deformities such as swan neck, boutonnière, ulnar drift, and Z thumbs. Palmar subluxation of the metacarpophalangeal joints is often mistaken for synovial swelling, but the exposed metacarpal heads are rounded and bony on palpation. Palmar subluxation is easily confirmed by running a finger along the back of the patient's hand and fingers to assess whether the phalanges are on the same plane as the metacarpals. Wherever deformities are found, assess whether they are reversible, either actively or passively.

Range of movement

The patient should be able to make a fist, burying the fingertips in the palm, a movement that requires 90° of flexion in each of the three phalangeal joints. Hypermobility is indicated by more than 90° extension in the metacarpophalangeal joints and ability to approximate thumb to forearm, passively.

The wrist

Screening

Inspect both wrists, front and back, and palpate the joint line for tenderness or swelling. Ask the patient to press both palms together and bring the elbows out at right angles in the 'prayer position'. Then reverse the position with the backs of the hands together to demonstrate palmar flexion (Figs 1 and 2). If the hands, wrists, or elbows are deformed, this test cannot be carried out. In this case, assess the range of active and passive movement at each wrist in turn.

Swelling

In rheumatoid arthritis, exuberant soft tissue swelling may be seen, originating either from the wrist joint itself or from the synovial tendon sheaths, and spreading both sides of the extensor pollucis retinaculum. An undulating swelling of the ulnar border of the wrist is a particular feature of rheumatoid arthritis. The undulations are the result of synovial swelling pushing its way through the fibres of the extensor retinaculum. This appearance is associated with an increased risk of rupture of the fourth and fifth extensor digitis tendons. Synovial proliferation is less often visible on the palmar aspect of the joint, although sometimes a visible fullness extends under the flexor retinaculum and into the palm.

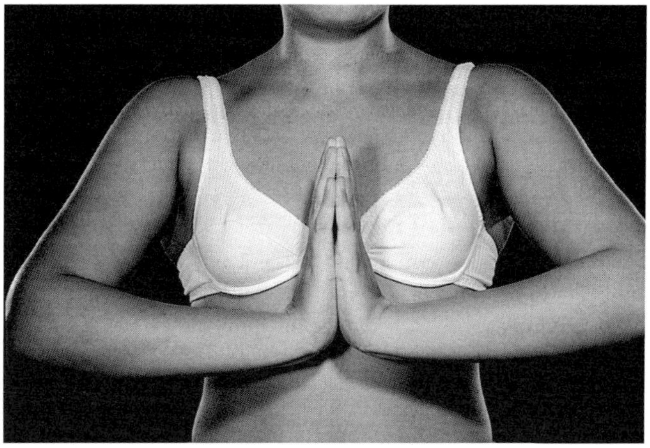

Fig. 1 The 'prayer position', demonstrating wrist dorsiflexion. (Photography in this and other figures in this chapter by courtesy of Eric Leung, The Photography and Illustration Centre, University College London.)

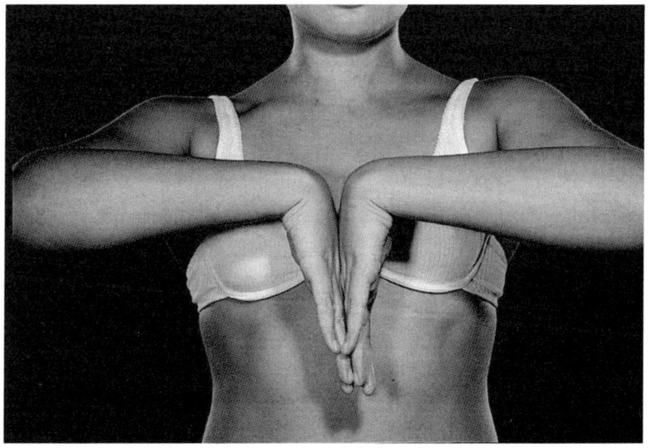

Fig. 2 The reversed 'prayer position', demonstrating wrist palmar flexion.

Swelling of the wrist joint is associated with compression of the median nerve in the carpal tunnel. Particular attention should be paid to looking for evidence of this complication.

Inflammation of the abductor pollicis longus tendon at the wrist (de Quervain's tenosynovitis) is best diagnosed by inspecting the wrists from the radial side, with the palms together and any watches or bracelets removed. Unilateral swelling may then easily be seen, extending from the first carpometacarpal joint proximally. The diagnosis can be confirmed using Finkelstein's test. In this the patient is asked to bring the thumb across the palm and clasp the fingers around it. The examiner holds the clenched fist and tweaks it sharply in an ulnar direction, putting a sudden but not excessive pull on the inflamed tendon. This elicits a sharp pain, and should be done with care, watching the patient's face for signs of discomfort.

Quervain's tenosynovitis can occur as a result of repetitive strain injuries (RSI). RSI is a group of disorders often affecting the tendons, muscles, and joints of the upper limbs that develop as a result of repetitive movements, awkward postures, and force (Table 5).

Deformity

Deformity of the wrist joint usually takes the form radiair deviation (with ulnair deviation of the fingers in the MCP joints) and palmar subluxation, owing to the stronger pull of the flexor than the extensor muscles of the forearm. Prominence of the lower end of the ulna is also common, because synovial proliferation at the inferior radioulnar joint weakens the ligaments and allows the bone to ride up in a deformity that may be either fixed or mobile. When the bone is mobile it is often painful, giving rise to the 'piano-key' sign, whereby pressure on the bone leads to the production of an audible protest from the patient.

Range of movement

The 'prayer position' normally allows 90° of passive palmar and dorsiflexion. The active range is 20° less in each direction.

The elbow

Screening

Ask the patient to fold the arms across the chest. Compare the elbow joints in this position. Inspect the extensor surface of each. Ask the patient to extend and flex the elbows, then with the elbows flexed and held against the sides, to show in turn the palms and the backs of the hands.

Inspection

Inspecting the elbows is a fruitful source of clues to the diagnosis in many rheumatic diseases. Rheumatoid nodules, gouty tophi, tendon xanthomata, olecranon bursitis, and the rash of psoriasis or of dermatomyositis may all be detected by a glance at the extensor surface of the elbow, just distal to the olecranon. The joints are most easily compared with the elbows flexed and the arms folded.

Table 5 Repetitive strain injuries

Hand and wrist
De Quervain's tenosynovitis
Trigger finger
Elbow
Epicondylitis lateralis
Epicondylitis medialis
Shoulder and neck
Trapezius myalgie
Rotator cuff tendinitis
Cervical syndrome

Palpation

Palpation for synovial proliferation or joint effusion is best done in the groove between the lateral epicondyle and the olecranon process. The radioulnar joints are frequently involved in rheumatoid arthritis, leading to loss of pronation and supination. The examiner places one thumb on the radial head and the other on the inferior radioulnar joint at the wrist, then passively pronates and supinates the patient's forearm, feeling for crepitus in one or both joints.

Tenderness of the lateral or medial epicondyles and the muscles inserting into them is found in 'tennis' or 'golfer's elbow', respectively. To confirm, the patient is asked to clench the fist and to extend or flex the wrist against resistance. These manoeuvres should cause pain at the affected muscle insertion.

Range of movement

Flexion is usually limited by the interposition of soft tissues, and should be about 150°. Extension beyond −10° implies hypermobility. Pronation and supination take place at the superior and inferior radioulnar joints and must be done with the elbows flexed to exclude movement at the shoulder joint. The hands can normally be fully supinated and pronated.

The shoulder girdle

The three shoulder-girdle joints are best considered together, as all three work together in movements of the shoulder, and pain from all three is felt around the shoulder and upper arm. Acromioclavicular pain is usually felt at the tip of the shoulder. Pain in the glenohumeral joints is most often felt over the deltoid muscle and midhumerus. The manubriosternal joint is often swollen and sometimes painful in rheumatoid arthritis and in seronegative spondyloarthritis.

Screening

Inspect the shoulder girdles both from the front and the back. Palpate the sternoclavicular and acromioclavicular joints for tenderness or swelling, then the glenohumeral joints starting from the anterior joint line, across the subacromial bursa, and on to the posterior joint line. Ask the patient to raise the arms sideways above the head, clasp the hands behind the neck with elbows well back, then clasp them behind the back as far up as possible (Figs 3 and 4).

A common source of error lies in what seems to be the attraction of symmetry. The patient with one stiff shoulder will often respond to a request to raise both arms by lifting both to the limit of the range of the abnormal shoulder, thereby giving the impression that both are stiff. It is worth encouraging the patient to make sure that the maximum range of each joint is being demonstrated.

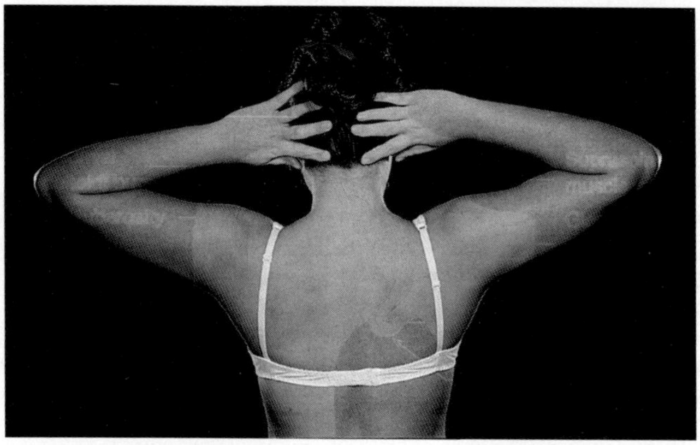

Fig. 3 Clasping the hands behind the neck to demonstrate external rotation.

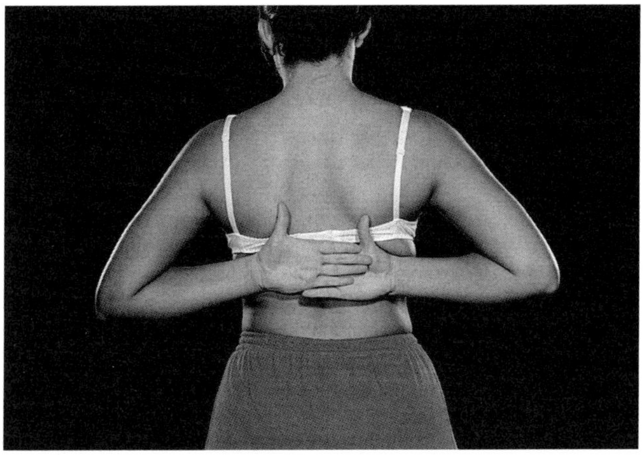

Fig. 4 Raising the hands as high as possible behind the back. The opposite scapula can usually just be reached.

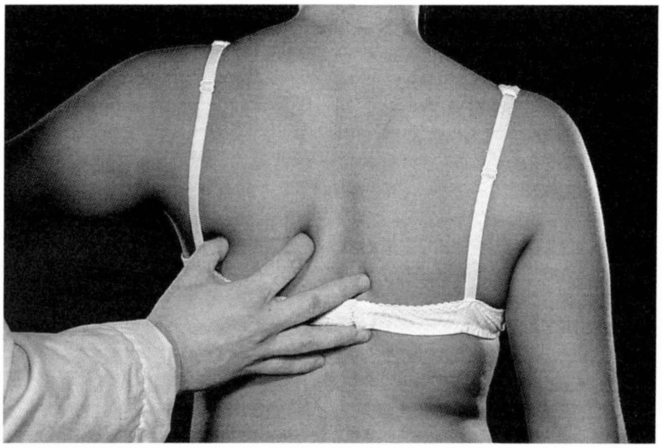

Fig. 5 Fixing the inferior angle of the scapula, while passively abducting the arm, to demonstrate true glenohumeral movement.

The sternoclavicular joint

The sternoclavicular joint is often neglected, despite the fact that it is frequently affected in a variety of arthropathies, including polymyalgia rheumatica, rheumatoid arthritis, the seronegative spondyloarthropathies, and septic arthritis. Pain is rarely localized to the joint, even when there is obvious swelling and redness, but is referred to the upper arm. Palpation should include the inner end of the clavicle and the articular surface of the manubrium, directly below it. Pain can best be elicited by asking the patient to brace the shoulders forward and back, or to shrug the shoulders up and down, movements which do not involve the glenohumeral joint. If these movements are painful but external rotation of the shoulder is not, there is strong evidence of sternoclavicular disease.

The acromioclavicular joint

The acromioclavicular joint is near the surface and can easily be seen and palpated if swollen. Passive adduction of the arm across the chest will often cause pain if the joint is inflamed. There may be a painful arc on abduction above 90°.

The shoulder (glenohumeral) joint

Inspection

Wasting of muscles should be noted both from the front and the back.

Swelling of the shoulder joint is not always obvious. A shoulder effusion in a patient with rheumatoid arthritis may give that shoulder a more normal-looking contour. Rupture of the shoulder capsule may lead to fluid tracking down to the upper arm.

A dislocated shoulder may appear square and dropped, while in rheumatoid arthritis the shoulders appear both square (due to muscle wasting) and raised, owing to upward subluxation of the humeral heads as a result of dysfunction of the rotator cuff and muscle contracture.

Palpation

A shoulder effusion is best felt by placing the thumb in front and the fingers behind the joint and fluctuating the fluid back and forth across the shoulder. Tenderness may be elicited over the whole line of the joint in capsulitis or inflammatory arthritis, or may be localized where there is an isolated lesion of the tendon. Inflammation of the long head of biceps gives tenderness in the bicipital groove anteriorly, while supraspinatus tendinitis causes tenderness in the subacromial bursa.

Rupture of the long head of biceps is best appreciated by asking the patient to contract the muscle against resistance. The affected muscle will form a ball (the 'Popeye sign').

Movements of the shoulder girdle

Although individual arcs of movement may be attributed to each of the three joints of the shoulder girdle, in practice they work smoothly together when the arm is raised. The sternoclavicular joint is the single point of bony connection between the arm and the trunk, and allows considerable movement of the clavicle, which in turn acts as a strut to add freedom of movement to the arm. The acromioclavicular joint has less movement, but allows for rotation of the scapula on the thorax.

Pure glenohumeral movement can be isolated from movement of the scapula across the thorax by fixing the inferior angle of the scapula with one hand and passively abducting the arm with the other (Fig. 5). Normally, the scapula starts to move at 30° of abduction, but if it is fixed at least 90° of glenohumeral movement is possible. Passive external rotation is another reliable measure of pure glenohumeral movement. Restriction of this movement is a first sign of inflammation of the glenohumeral joint. The last few degrees of abduction may be lost in patients with a painful neck lesion.

Passive movements should always be checked if the active range is incomplete. Loss of active and passive range in equal measure suggests intracapsular disease such as arthritis or adhesive capsulitis ('frozen shoulder'). Loss of active more than passive movement, accompanied by pain, suggests a lesion of tendon or rotator cuff. Limitation or weakness of active movement with a full and pain-free passive range suggests muscular or neurological disease.

The painful arc

During abduction of the arm, pain may be experienced in an arc, above or below which movement is pain free. The most common cause is supraspinatus tendinitis. In this condition pain occurs somewhere in the arc from 60 to 100° as the greater tuberosity impinges on the acromion, pinching the supraspinatus tendon. The pain may be severe enough to prevent abduction. The patient is often able to elevate the arm fully by forward flexion, but if asked to take it down sideways, will complain of pain as the upper limit of the painful arc is reached. A painful arc above 90° occurs in acromioclavicular disease.

Resisted movements

Specific tendon lesions can be identified by using resisted movements to elicit pain. Pain on resisted abduction suggests a supraspinatus lesion. Pain on resisted external rotation suggests an infraspinatus lesion. Pain on resisted internal rotation suggests a subscapularis lesion (Fig. 6).

Range of movement

Movement at the shoulder comprises forward flexion to 180°, abduction to 180°, extension to 45°, and rotation to 70° internally and externally.

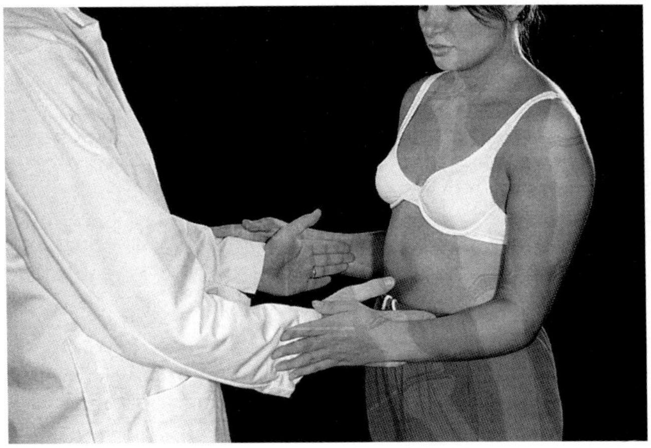

Fig. 6 Testing resisted internal rotation of the shoulder.

Movement at the sternoclavicular joint includes protraction and retraction of the clavicle in an arc of 60°, and elevation of the clavicle to 60°.

The temporomandibular joint

Screening

Palpate the joints for tenderness or swelling and ask the patient to open the mouth wide.

These joints are most frequently involved in rheumatoid arthritis but other inflammatory arthropathies may also affect them. The complaint is of pain on chewing or yawning and sometimes of pain in the ear. The joints rarely look abnormal, but there is local tenderness and pain on opening the jaws. Normally, it is possible for the fully open jaws to accommodate the middle three digits of the patient's hand, held vertically between the teeth. Restricted mouth opening from disease of the temporomandibular joints, may be differentiated from that caused by scleroderma by inspecting the lips, which will be drawn tight in scleroderma.

Micrognathia occurs as a result of temporomandibular joint inflammation in childhood, as in juvenile chronic arthritis (juvenile rheumatoid arthritis). Premature closure of the epiphysis leads to failure of normal development of the mandible.

The cervical spine

Screening

Inspect posture: palpate the spinous processes for tenderness and alteration of the normal curve; ask the patient to flex, extend, rotate, and laterally flex the neck to left and right. It is important to remember that the detailed examination of the neck should not be considered complete until a neurological assessment has also been made.

Inspection

Neck posture may indicate underlying disease. A poking chin with dorsal kyphosis often accompanies cervical spondylosis. Acute torticollis can be recognized as the patient enters the room, one sternocleidomastoid muscle in spasm and the head tilted to the side and slightly rotated. The patient with rheumatoid arthritis will often have lost neck height and there may be a lateral asymmetry if there has been softening and erosion of bone.

Palpation

Palpation of the neck should include the occipital ridge, the spinous processes, and the paravertebral muscles overlying the facet joints. The occipital ridge is frequently tender in cervical spondylosis, especially over the greater occipital nerve. The spinous processes normally form a lordotic arc, with C2 and C7 being prominent at either end of the curve. Loss of lordosis or even a reversed curve can be appreciated by palpation. Palpation of the paravertebral muscles may reveal spasm in any case of neck pain, but especially after a whiplash injury or in cases of headache and neck pain related to stress. Through the paravertebral muscles, the facet joints can be felt, and tenderness or swelling elicited. Each pair of facet joints should be palpated in turn.

Range of movement

The patient should be able to touch the chin to the chest, tip the head back until the forehead and nose are parallel to the ceiling, and rotate in each direction to 70°. Lateral flexion is normally 45° each side, and this movement is lost early in ankylosing spondylitis. Passive neck movements are not a part of the routine examination, as neck instability is a feature of the rheumatic diseases.

Lhermitte's sign is more correctly a symptom. The patient complains of paraesthesia down the body on flexing the neck. It is sometimes present in cases of compression of the cervical cord, especially in rheumatoid arthritis. The examiner should not attempt to elicit this sign by forcible neck flexion.

The thoracic spine

Screening

Inspect the thoracic spine for swellings or deformities; palpate the spinous processes in turn; assess chest expansion. It is important to remember that the detailed examination of the thoracic spine should not be considered complete until a neurological assessment, including all four limbs, has also been made.

Inspection

This will reveal postural abnormality such as kyphosis or scoliosis. Destruction or collapse of vertebrae may lead to a sharply angled kyphosis, or angular gibbus, most often seen in tuberculosis. Kyphosis in adolescents suggests Scheuermann's disease. Scoliosis may be developmental, in which case there is usually some rotation of the ribs, which can be exaggerated by asking the patient to bend forward so that the rotation is more easily appreciated. Scoliosis resulting from muscle spasm becomes less obvious on forward flexion.

Palpation

The spinous processes and paravertebral muscles are next palpated, especially for tenderness. Recent collapse of a vertebra, malignant deposits, or vertebral osteomyelitis all produce local or 'point' tenderness. If direct pressure over the spinous process is insufficient to elicit this, it is worth trying percussion, laying two fingers over each process in turn and striking these with the fist, gently at first, then more firmly if no discomfort is elicited. Tenderness of the upper thoracic vertebrae and the paravertebral muscles is a common feature of thoracic spondylosis.

Range of movement

Rotation is best assessed with the patient seated to fix the pelvis and is usually 45°. Flexion is most easily measured with a tape measure. Distraction on flexion between marks made at C7 and T12 is normally at least 2.5 cm. Costovertebral movement is measured by chest expansion at the level of the nipples, usually more than 7 cm.

The lumbar spine

Screening

Inspect the standing patient from behind; palpate for tenderness or muscle spasm; ask them to touch the toes, lean back, and bend from side to side. With four fingers along the lumbar spine, assess whether movement is taking place at the lumbar spine rather than the hips. It is important to remember that the detailed examination of the lumbar spine should not be considered complete until a neurological assessment of the lower limbs has been made. This may conveniently be done as an intrinsic part of the examination of the back, which takes place in three positions as indicated in Table 6 and below.

Table 6 Examination of the lumbar spine

The patient standing
1. Inspect
—Posture
—Deformity
2. Palpate
—Muscle spasm
3. Move
—Flexion
—Extension
—Lateral flexion
—Rotation
4. Walk
—Heels
—Tiptoes
The patient lying face up
1. Straight-leg raise
2. Reflexes
—Knee jerks
—Ankle jerks
—Plantars
3. Power
—Toe flexion, extension
—Foot inversion, eversion
—Ankle flexion, extension
—Knee flexion, extension
—Hip flexion, extension
4. Sensation
—Dermatomes L1–S1
The patient lying face down
1. Palpation
—Spinous processes
—Paravertebral muscles
—Sacroiliac joints
—Coccyx
2. Femoral stretch test
3. Sensation
—Dermatomes S2–S5
4. Buttock tone (+rectal examination)

Examination

The patient standing

The examiner inspects the back for abnormality of posture or deformity, such as scoliosis or kyphosis, then palpates the paravertebral muscles for evidence of spasm. Palpation for tenderness is best left until the patient is lying down.

The patient is then asked to carry out the movements outlined in Table 6. Forward flexion and extension are relatively more restricted in the patient with a mechanical back pain, while lateral flexion is the first to be lost in ankylosing spondylitis. Schober's test is a useful method of measuring lumbar flexion, especially in ankylosing spondylitis. Using a tape measure, the examiner makes two marks, one 5 cm below the level of the sacroiliac dimples and one 10 cm above. The patient bends forward and the examiner measures the distance between the marks. Distraction of at least 5 cm is normal.

Asking the patient to take a few steps on the heels and toes is a crude but useful test of power in the legs and feet, and at the same time the buttocks can be inspected for any evidence of a Trendelenburg sign (dipping down of the pelvis when the ipsilateral foot is raised from the ground) suggesting muscle weakness.

The patient lying face up

Straight-leg raise (Lasègue's sign) The patient lies supine while the examiner grasps one of the ankles and raises it from the couch, keeping the knee straight with a hand on the knee, and watching the patient's face for any sign of discomfort (Fig. 7). Normally 80–90° can be attained without discomfort, depending on the tightness of the hamstrings. Irritation of the dural sleeve of any of the nerve roots contributing to the sciatic nerve will result in pain when the sciatic nerve is put on the stretch, and a much reduced straight-leg raise on the affected side. The usual cause of this is a prolapsed lumbar disc protruding posterolaterally. Bilateral reduction in straight-leg raising implies a central disc prolapse. To distinguish between sciatic irritation and hip disease, the leg is raised with the knee flexed. This will now be painless in sciatic irritation, but just as uncomfortable in hip disease.

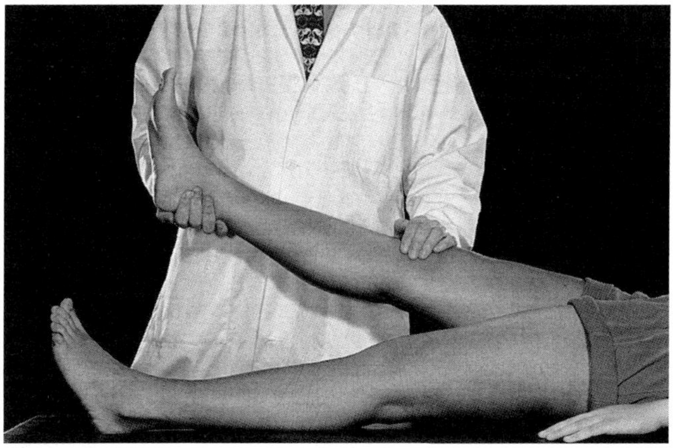

Fig. 7 The straight leg raise.

The sciatic stretch test may be useful in distinguishing sciatic irritation from tight hamstrings if the straight-leg raise is reduced. Once the limit of straight-leg raising is established, the leg is lowered a fraction until the pain is relieved. Now the examiner dorsiflexes the foot. If the pain was due to sciatic irritation, it returns.

After the straight-leg raise, the examiner tests the knee, ankle, and plantar reflexes. Testing power in each of the major muscle groups of the legs, especially the hip muscles, may cause difficulties if the patient is in pain. It may be necessary to reassess the patient after adequate control of the pain. Sensation to light touch and pinprick is next elicited, following a dermatomal pattern over the anterior aspects of both legs and the soles of the feet.

The patient lying face down

It is important to have the couch flat, with pillows removed to avoid painful hyperextension. A pillow under the patient's abdomen will usually increase comfort and render the examination easier. The examiner palpates each spinous process in turn, gently at first, then increasing the pressure by using one hand laid on the other. Then the examiner palpates for tenderness in the paravertebral muscles, the posterior iliac crests, and over the sacrum and coccyx. Coccygeal tenderness may also be felt by a rectal examination. Point tenderness is a feature of local infection or malignancy. More diffuse tenderness is common in patients with mechanical back pain.

The femoral stretch test is the parallel of the straight leg-raising test, putting the femoral nerve roots on the stretch. The examiner takes the prone patient's ankle in one hand, flexing the knee to 90°, and raising the bent leg to extend the hip (Fig. 8). Pain during this manoeuvre may indicate a lesion of a high lumbar disc or hip disease.

Loss of sensation around the saddle area is an important clue to the presence of cauda equina lesions and should always be tested for. Buttock tone is assessed by asking the patient to pinch the cheeks of the buttocks together as hard as possible, and palpating the two sides. A rectal examination is helpful where there is any hint of a lesion of the cauda equina, to assess sphincter tone and sensation, in addition to its importance as part of the general assessment of the patient.

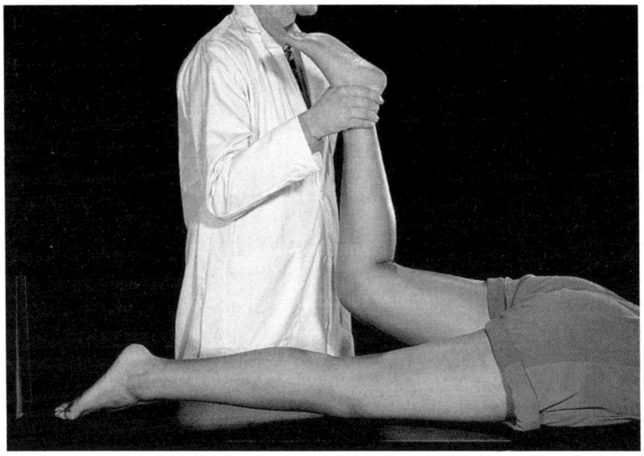

Fig. 8 The femoral stretch test.

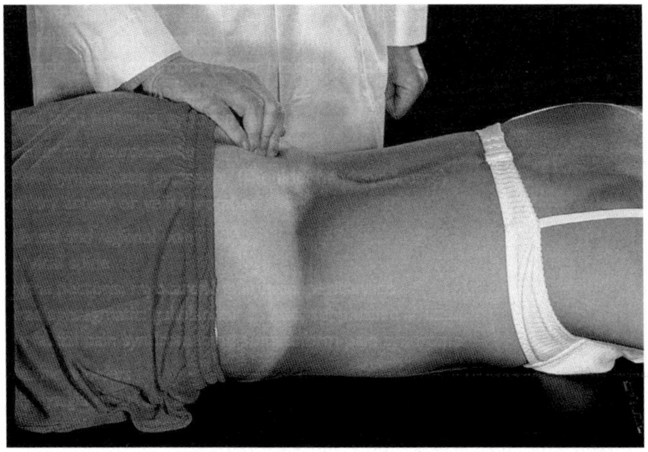

Fig. 9 Palpating over the sacroiliac joint.

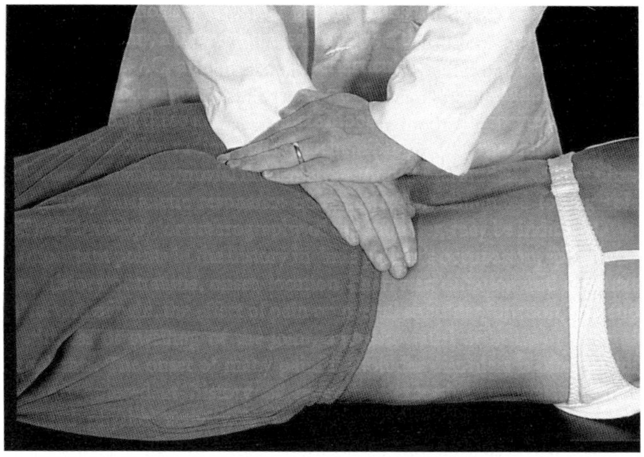

Fig. 10 Stressing the sacroiliac joints from the back.

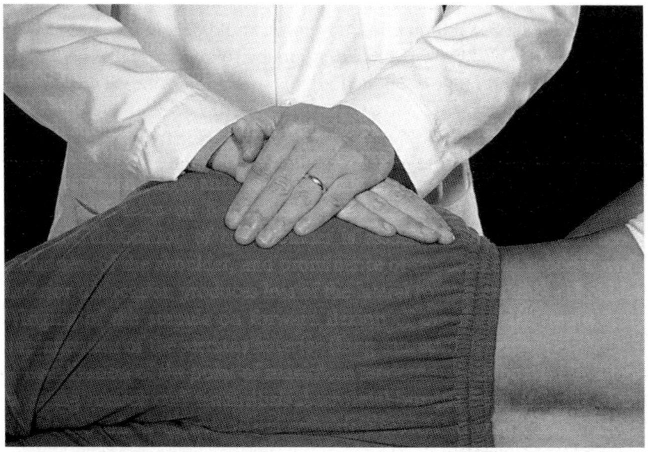

Fig. 11 Stressing the sacroiliac joints from the side.

The sacroiliac joints

Screening

Inspect and palpate the joints from behind (Fig. 9), and stress them by pressure on the sacrum; roll the patient on one side and press again over the uppermost iliac crest.

Inspection and palpation

Inspecting the joints from behind may reveal evidence of swelling or deformity, especially in tuberculous infection. Palpation is best done with the four fingers of the hand along the length of the joint. Nodules of tender fibrofatty tissue often overlie the joints, and are of no significance except that they are often found in patients with chronic back pain. Bony fusion of the joints in ankylosing spondylitis obliterates the joint line. The synovial portion of the joint lies too deep to be felt under normal circumstances.

Range of movement

Moving the sacroiliac joints is not easy, as there is only a small amount of rotational glide, but they may be stressed by a variety of manoeuvres. The simplest method is to press firmly on the sacrum while the patient lies on the front, then on the pelvic brim as he or she lies on the back and on the side (Figs 10 and 11). If the sacroiliac joints are inflamed, these manoeuvres may elicit pain. Instability of the sacroiliac joints, especially post-partum, may cause pain, which is aggravated when the patient is asked to stand on one leg. Sometimes the excessive movement can be appreciated by placing one finger on each side of the joint as the patient makes the manoeuvre.

The hip

Screening

Inspect leg length and position. Grasp the leg at knee and ankle, with the knee flexed; now flex the hip as far as it will go. Return the hip to 90° of flexion and test internal and external rotation using the foot as a pointer and the knee as a pivot (Fig. 12). Straighten the leg, grasp the opposite iliac crest, and test abduction and adduction with the pelvis thus fixed (Fig. 13).

Inspection

The gait is particularly important in the assessment of the lower limb joints. The patient with a fixed flexion deformity of the hips throws the spine into an exaggerated lordosis to compensate. The patient with weak hip muscles walks with a waddle, and the one with a painful hip walks in such a way as to spend the least time possible on the painful leg, leaning to the opposite side, often with a walking-stick. This is called the antalgic gait.

Inspection of the hips should always include comparison of leg lengths and attention to the position of the leg. The leg that is short and externally rotated suggests a fractured neck of femur, or a legacy of juvenile chronic arthritis. Failure to observe the back of the hips may mean that the evidence of previous surgery is missed.

Palpation

Palpation of the hip is difficult because the joint is so deep, although occasionally an effusion can be detected by fluctuation just beneath the inguinal ligament. A psoas abscess may cause a very painful, stiff hip with spasm that cannot be overcome without anaesthesia. The psoas abscess will eventually point as a mass below the inguinal ligament. The greater trochanteric bursa lies over the greater trochanter and if it is inflamed, tenderness can easily be elicited with the patient lying on the unaffected side.

Range of movement

Flexion, 110°; extension, −30°; abduction, 50°; adduction, 30°; internal and external rotation, each 45°.

A fixed flexion deformity can be demonstrated with Thomas' test. The patient lies supine and one knee and hip are flexed until any lumbar lordosis has been obliterated. Flexion of the other hip during this manoeuvre indicates a fixed flexion deformity of that hip.

A catch for the inexperienced is the patient with a painful knee that is held in flexion. Attempts to straighten the knee in the bed are unsuccessful because of pain, and yet no other abnormality is seen in the knee. This patient probably has disease of the hip, with a fixed flexion deformity and pain referred to the knee. If the examiner were to straighten the knee while maintaining a flexed hip, a full range of movement would be found in most cases.

Rotation may also be tested in extension, by rolling the leg. Where both hips have a limited range of abduction, it is useful to record the maximum distance between the two medial malleoli. Extension of the hip is best measured with the patient lying on the side or prone.

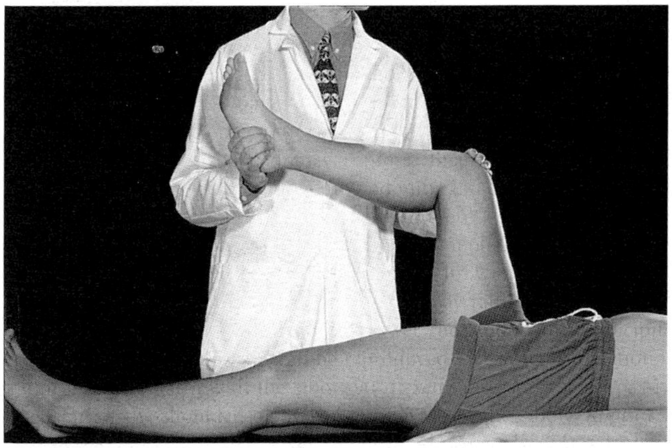

Fig. 12 Testing hip rotation using the foot as a pointer.

The knee

Screening

Inspect for swelling, abnormal alignment, or quadriceps wasting. Palpate for tenderness, effusion, popliteal cyst. Flex and extend. Test ligament stability.

Inspection

Knee swellings can be recognized by fullness of the suprapatellar pouch and obliteration of the hollows either side of the patella. Quadriceps wasting may be masked by swelling of the knee and measurement of quadriceps bulk should be made above the upper limit of the suprapatellar bursa. Deformities may be varus or valgus, forward or backward slip.

Palpation

Tenderness of the medial collateral ligaments occurs early in osteoarthritis, followed by the development of a tender bony ridge as osteophytes develop.

A knee effusion can be demonstrated in one of three ways, depending on the quantity of fluid present, as follows.

(i) A small effusion can be milked from one side of the patella to the other in the 'bulge sign'. Any fluid in the medial side of the joint is swept firmly upward and laterally into the suprapatellar pouch. Then the back of the hand presses firmly and sharply on the lateral side of the joint. When a small effusion is present, a bulge will appear on the medial side of the joint as the fluid returns.

(ii) A moderate effusion is best detected by eliciting the 'patellar tap' (Fig. 14). One hand is placed on the suprapatellar pouch, the finger, and thumb exerting side-to-side pressure, squeezing any fluid in the pouch to the retropatellar space. The patella is then sharply depressed with the fingers of the other hand, so that it floats through the fluid to strike the lower end of the femur. This sharp tap will not be felt if the undersurface of the patella is covered with synovial pannus, which acts as a blanket to muffle the impact. A tap may be felt in the absence of fluid if intra-articular fat is squeezed behind the patella.

(iii) A large, tense effusion can be confirmed by fluctuation across the joint, from one side of the patella to the other.

A cyst of the calf or popliteal fossa is often easier to feel than see, and has the consistency of a firm rubber ball.

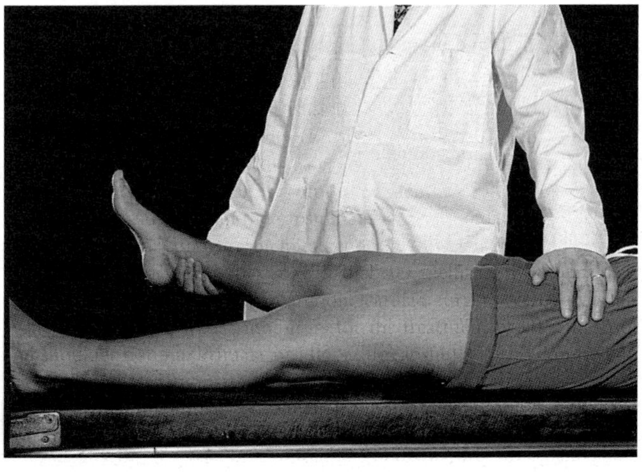

Fig. 13 Abducting the hip, with the pelvis fixed.

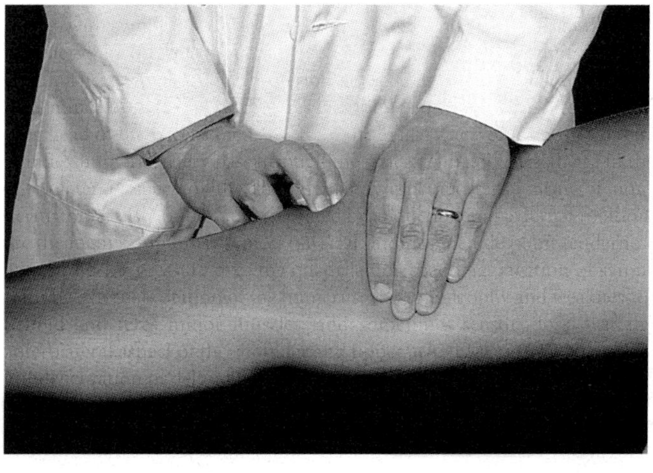

Fig. 14 Eliciting a patellar tap.

The patellar compression test

The patient lies supine with the quadriceps relaxed. The examiner presses the patella firmly distally between finger and thumb. The patient is then asked to push the knee hard into the bed. If this causes pain or crepitus it suggests retropatellar disease, such as chondromalacia patellae in the young or osteoarthritis in the elderly.

Testing stability

To test the cruciate ligaments the examiner grasps the leg just below the knee, with both hands, and exerts pressure first anteriorly, then posteriorly (flexion?). To test the medial and lateral collaterals the examiner raises the patient's leg, supported with the fingers of one hand under the knee, holding it slightly flexed, and the other under the ankle (Fig. 15). Then pressure is exerted with the heel of each hand, producing a stress across the knee joint, centred on the ligament to be tested.

McMurray's sign

This is a test for cartilage tears. The patient lies supine and the examiner grasps the knee in one hand and the ankle in the other. The examiner then flexes the knee fully, internally rotates the lower leg as far as it will go, and slowly straightens the knee. Then the test is repeated with external rotation. If the hand over the knee detects a clunk on straightening, accompanied by wincing or other expression of pain from the patient, the test is positive.

Range of movement

Extension, 0°; flexion, 135°. Hyperextension can be tested by holding the knee firmly on the bed and lifting the ankle. Extension beyond −10° is abnormal.

The ankle joint

Screening

Inspect for swelling or deformity. Palpate the anterior joint line for tenderness, swelling. Assess dorsiflexion and plantar flexion.

Swelling can be detected anteriorly, between the malleoli, where it has the appearance and feeling of a 'spare tyre', quite unlike the diffuse swelling of ankle oedema. Swelling behind the lateral malleolus suggests peroneal tendinitis. Synovitis of the extensor tendons results in swelling both above and below the extensor retinaculum.

Range of movement

Dorsiflexion, −20°; plantar flexion, 70°.

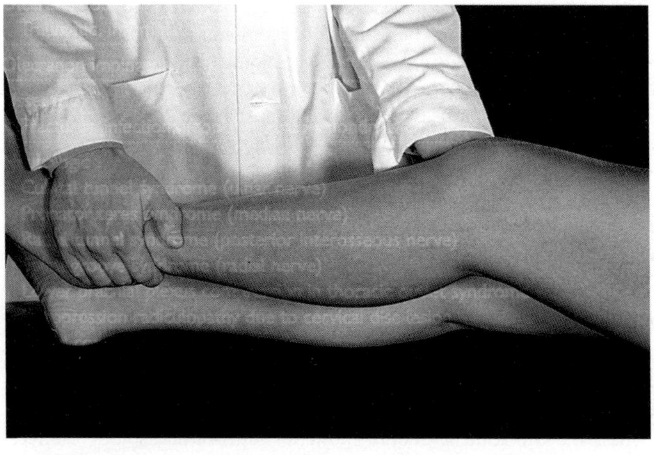

Fig. 15 Testing for lateral collateral ligament stability at the knee.

The subtalar (talocalcaneal) joint

Screening

Inspect for varus or valgus deformity of the hindfoot. Grasp the heel and assess inversion and eversion (Fig. 16).

Swelling is seen below the malleoli. This joint is prone to symptomless involvement, especially in rheumatoid arthritis and juvenile chronic arthritis. Tali pes valgus deformity usually results, and is best appreciated from behind, with the patient standing.

Range of movement

Inversion, 25°; eversion, 15°.

The heel and foot

Screening

Inspect both the dorsal and plantar aspects of the foot, and the back of the heel. Palpate the Achilles tendon insertion, the plantar fascia insertion (Fig. 17), and the metatarsophalangeal joints. Apply torsion to the midfoot to test movement in the midtarsal joints.

Painful feet may be caused by vascular or neurological lesions. The peripheral pulses and sensation should always be assessed, and search made for ulcers, sinuses, or skin infarcts. Occasionally a prolapsed lumbar disc will present with foot pain without back pain or sciatica.

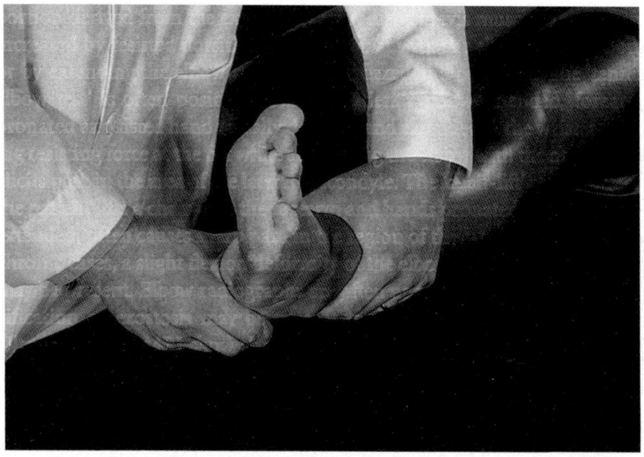

Fig. 16 Testing subtalar movement.

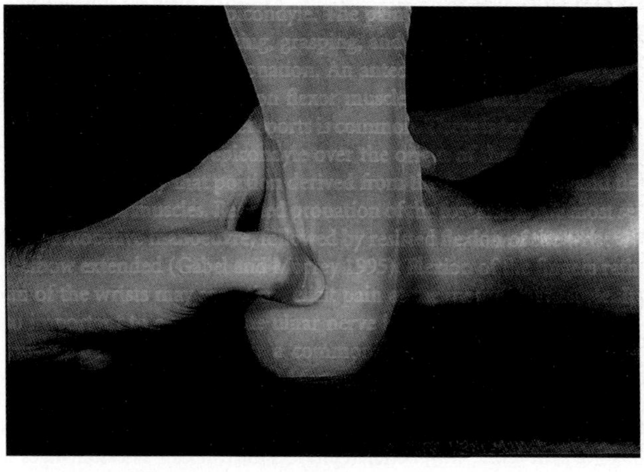

Fig. 17 Eliciting tenderness over the plantar fascia insertion.

The Achilles tendon

This is inspected from behind, either with the patient standing or lying prone. Thickening, tenderness, and rupture can be detected. With rupture, the patient may have difficulty in standing on tiptoe at first, though fibrosis later occurs, rendering the movement possible. The Achilles tendon is a common site for traumatic bursas related to pressure from shoes, rheumatoid nodules, gouty tophi, and tendon xanthomata.

Heel

Heel pain is commonly due to plantar fasciitis. The heel can be inspected from below with the patient lying down. It is unusual to see swelling or discoloration, though the affected side often feels firmer. Tenderness is elicited by pressure directly crianal from the centre of the heel and by pressure from side to side at the level of the anterior margin of the calcaneum.

Midfoot

The naviculocuneiform joint is subject to osteoarthritis and is often found to show bony enlargement.

The sole

Callosities under the metatarsal heads develop when the metatarsophalangeal joints are subluxated. The rash of psoriasis or keratoderma blennorrhagica may be detected on the soles. Perforating foot ulcers may be a sign of systemic disease.

The arches

Flattening of the transverse or longitudinal arches is best seen with the patient standing. Pes cavus should also be assessed while standing.

The toes

Inspect the toes for deformities such as hallux valgus, clawing, overlapping toes, undersized toes. In rheumatoid arthritis, fibular drift of the toes is common. Clawed toes press on the uppers of shoes and callosities form over the proximal interphalangeal joints. 'Sausage toes' suggest Reiter's disease, gout, or psoriatic arthropathy. A bursa between the joints will spread the toes. Diffuse swelling over the metatarsophalangeal joints may be easier to feel than see; tenderness may be elicited by palpating each joint individually. Beware of squeezing the forefoot, as this can cause severe pain if the joints are inflamed.

Standardized quantification

Rheumatologists are more and more aware that standardized instruments are useful and even required for the evaluation of disease progress and treatment efficacy in rheumatic patients. Measures that are reproducible, valid, and sensitive to relevant changes are recommended for clinical trials, but also increasingly in daily clinical practice.

Several devices have been developed and validated to quantify for instance range of motion, muscle strength, and skin elasticity. Furthermore, indices are developed that combine clinical assessments into a single outcome measure.

Below we shall discuss some frequently used/widely known devices, tests and indices in rheumatology.

Devices and tests

Skin

Skin elasticity can be assessed with a cutometer SEM 474 or 575. This cutometer exerts a controlled vacuum force on a skin area using a 2 or 8 mm probe. In systemic scleroderma it showed good correlation with the subjective skin score, with better reproducibility. It can assess changes in skin extensibility over time, and may be useful in monitoring the disease and its treatment.

In scleroderma skin thickness can be measured using several tests: the maximal oral opening, and the distance between third finger and the distal palmar crease in full flexion respectively extension (flexion/extension index).

For the assessment of skin temperature several devices have been developed. Infrared thermography is the most frequently reported, especially for the evaluation of Raynaud's phenomenon (primary, or secondary due to systemic sclerosis). Other rheumatic aspects that can be evaluated with thermography are (large) changes in the degree of joint synovitis in rheumatoid arthritis. This latter evaluation is rarely used because the additional value to clinical examination is relatively small, and a temperature-controlled room is required.

Muscles

Muscle strength—both isometric and isokinetic—can be assessed using dynamometers produced by several manufacturers. Rheumatoid arthritis patients show decreased muscle strength compared to healthy controls. For patient or trial evaluation no standards for muscle strength assessments are recommended. The reliability and validity of the different dynamometers are still to be determined. Grip strength is the most frequently assessed aspect, although the type of instrument used is not standardized. A special sphygmomanometer with its own manometer is most convenient, though a small cuff attached to a standard mercury manometer is also satisfactory. The cuff is inflated to 30 mmHg and the patient squeezes it with one hand. The maximum reading achieved in three attempts is recorded.

Muscle tenderness can be measured, for example, in fibromyalgia, using a dolorimeter (or palpometer). The dolorimeter (Fisher or Chatillon) consists of a flat circular rubber probe of varying diameters, attached to a spring loaded gauge. The probe is placed on a skin area, and the minimum pressure is recorded that provokes tenderness. However, the validity of the dolorimeter compared to a manual tender point examination is disputed.

Joints

Joint tenderness is usually ascertained by manual pressure on the joint margins, or by passive movement for less palpable joints. These methods show large interobserver variation because the pressure is not standardized. A more reproducible device for the assessment of tenderness might be a dolorimeter, as is used to record muscle tenderness. The validity and feasibility of this instrument for the quantification of joint tenderness needs still further confirmation.

Nowadays, joint swelling can be ascertained with several imaging techniques, such as ultrasonography and MRI, although these methods are not feasible and too costly for daily clinical practice. Swelling of superficial joints is mostly assessed by manual palpation. The Ring Size is a useful objective device for recording changes in proximal interphalangeal joint swelling. The smallest size that will slip easily over the joint is recorded.

Range of motion: for accurate measurement of angles of movement or degrees of deformity a goniometer is necessary. It is useful to have a long-limbed one for large joints and a smaller one for joints of hands and feet. The limbs of the goniometer should be lined up along the long axis of the joint, the hinge on the joint line, and the maximum angles of flexion and extension recorded. The position of the joint in the extended anatomical position is taken as zero, and further extension is recorded as a minus value. A spirit-level inclinometer is also available for measuring angles of spinal movement.

For the spinal and chest mobility several tests are described that are frequently used in ankylosing spondylitis:

- Occiput-wall-distance, measured in centimetre with the patient standing as erect as possible with heels and back against the wall.
- Chest expansion, assessed as the difference in centimetre between the circumference of the chest at nipple line on full inspiration and full expiration.
- Schober 10 cm test (measured in centimetre), with the patient erect, mark the skin at the level of the posterior superior iliac spines (dimples of venus) and another 10 cm above in the midline. Ask the patient to bend maximally forward without bending the knees.

- Fingertip-to-floor-distance, recorded as the distance in centimetre between the third finger and the floor with the patient bending forward maximally, without flexing the knees.
- Lumbar lateral flexion, measured as a percentage of the body height.

Indices

Below we report some examples of indices frequently used to quantify musculoskeletal pathology in rheumatic diseases.

Skin

Skin score

In patients with systemic sclerosis the severity of skin thickness is determined by physical examination of several specified sites. Each site is graded on a three- or four-point scale, and to obtain a total skin score all scores are summed.

Tendons

The enthesis index (in ankylosing spondylitis) combines the degree of tenderness (0, 1, 2, 3) on pressure on several enthesis sites. It ranges from 0 to 90. It can discriminate between patients with high and low disease activity, and has moderate/good reproducibility.

Muscles

The muscle strength index is the mean score of standardized isometric extension and flexion strength of the knee and elbow joints. The index is reliable and correlates with self-reported functional disability and radiological damage in rheumatoid arthritis.

The tender point score is an index of 18 selected points which are frequently tender on pressure in patients with fibromyalgia. The score is moderately reliable as diagnostic criterion, and is moderately responsive to perceived symptomatic change.

Joints

Joint counts

Several joint counts have been developed, counting a varying number of joints that are tender and/or swollen. Examples frequently used in rheumatoid arthritis are the 28-joint count for pain and for swelling, the 68-joint count for pain, and the 66-joint count for swelling. The Ritchie articular index is a method of recording activity in rheumatoid arthritis by means of grading the tenderness to firm pressure or pain on movement in 53 joints, divided over 26 units, with a score ranging from 0 to 78. The articular index developed by Thompson and Kirwan comprises 38 joints, scored for the presence of tenderness and swelling, and weighted for surface area. In a comparative study it was concluded that no joint count was superior, and therefore the most simple method, the ungraded 28 joint count recommended.

The Root joint index is a summation of pain severity in shoulders and hips by palpation and/or passive movement, used in ankylosing spondylitis.

Further reading

Arnold, M.H., Preston, S.J., Beller, E.M., and Buchanan, W.W. (1989). Infra-red surface thermography. Evaluation of a new radiometry instrument for measuring skin temperature over joints. *Clinical Rheumatology* **8**, 225–30.

Atkins, C.J., Zielinski, A., Klinkhoff, A.V., Chalmers, A., Wade, J., Williams, D., Schulzer, M., and Della-Cioppa, G. (1992). An electronic method for measuring joint tenderness in rheumatoid arthritis. *Arthritis and Rheumatism* **35**, 407–10.

Bland, J.H. *Rheumatism of the Cervical Spine.* London: W.B. Saunders, 1987.

Cott, A., Parkinson, W., Bell, M.J., Adachi, J., Bedard, M., Cividino, A., and Bensen, W. (1992). Interrater reliability of the tender point criterion for fibromyalgia. *Journal of Rheumatology* **19**, 1955–9.

Cyriax, J. *Textbook of Orthopaedic Medicine Diagnosis of Soft Tissue Lesions* Vol. 1. London: Baillière Tindall, 1982.

Creemers, M.C., van't Hof, M.A., Franssen, M.J., van de Putte, L.B., Gribnau, F.W., and van Riel, P.L. (1996). Disease activity in ankylosing spondylitis: selection of a core set of variables and a first set in the development of a disease activity score. *British Journal of Rheumatology* **35** (9), 867–73.

Dieppe, P.A., Bacon, P.A., Bamji, A.N., and Weist, J., ed. (1986). The clinical evaluation of the rheumatic diseases. In *Slide Atlas of Rheumatology*, pp. 1.2–1.16. London: Gower Medical Publishing.

Dunkl, P.R., Taylor, A.G., McConnell, G.G., Alfano, A.P., and Conaway, M.R. (2000). Responsiveness of fibromyalgia clinical trial outcome measures. *Journal of Rheumatology* **27**, 2683–91.

Edgar, M.A. and Park, W.M. (1974). Induced pain patterns on passive straight-leg-raising in lower lumbar disc protrusion. *Journal of Bone and Joint Surgery* **56B**, 658.

Enomoto, D.N., Mekkes, J.R., Bossuyt, P.M., Hoekzema, R., and Bos, J.D. (1996). Quantification of cutaneous sclerosis with a skin elasticity meter in patients with generalized scleroderma. *Journal of the American Academy of Dermatology* **35**, 381–7.

Finkelstein, H. (1930). Stenosing tenovaginitis at the radial styloid process. *Journal of Bone and Joint Surgery* **12**, 509.

Grieve, G. (1971). The hip. *Physiotherapy* **57**, 212.

Khostanteen, I., Tunks, E.R., Goldsmith, C.H., and Ennis, J. (2000). Fibromyalgia: can one distinguish it from simulation? An observer-blind controlled study. *Journal of Rheumatology* **27**, 2671–6.

Klenerman, L. (1991). Examination of the foot. In *The Foot and its Disorders* 2nd edn. (ed. L. Klenerman), pp. 27–31. Oxford, England: Blackwell Scientific Publications.

Larson, R.L. and Grana, W.A., ed. *The Knee: Form, Function, Pathology and Treament.* Philadelphia PA: W.B. Saunders, 1993.

MacDonald, A.G., Land, D.V., and Sturrock, R.D. (1994). Microwave thermography as a noninvasive assessment of disease activity in inflammatory arthritis. *Clinical Rheumatology* **13**, 589–92.

Magee, D.J. *Orthopedic Physical Assessment.* Philadelphia PA: W.B. Saunders, 1987.

Moll, J. and Wright, V. (1987). Measurement of spinal movements. In *The Lumbar Spine and Back Pain* 3rd edn. (ed. M.I.V. Jayson), pp. 215–34. Edinburgh: Churchill Livingstone.

Nikkels-Tassoudji, N., Henry, F., Pierard-Franchimont, C., and Pierard, G.E. (1996). Computerized evaluation of skin stiffening in scleroderma. *European Journal of Clinical Investigation* **26**, 457–60.

Prevoo, M.L., van Riel, P.L., van't Hof, M.A., van Rijswijk, M.H., van Leeuwen, M.A., Kuper, H.H., and van de Putte, L.B. (1993). Validity and reliability of joint indices. A longitudinal study in patients with recent onset rheumatoid arthritis. *British Journal of Rheumatology* **32** (7), 589–94.

Riel van, P.L.C.M., Gestel van, A.M., and Scott, D.L. (2000). EULAR handbook of clinical assessments in rheumatoid arthritis. *Van Zuiden Communications bv Alphen aan den Rijn*, ISBN 90-75141-90-4.

Ritchie, D.M. et al. (1968). Clinical studies with an articular index for the assessment of joint tenderness in patients with RA. *Quarterly Journal of Medicine* **37**, 393–406.

Rudge, S.R., Swannell, A.J., Rose, D.H., and Todd, J.H. (1982). The clinical assessment of sacro-iliac joint involvement in ankylosing spondylitis. *Rheumatology Rehabilitation* **51**, 15.

Schumacher, R.H. and Gall, E.P. *Rheumatoid Arthritis: An Illustrated Guide to Pathology, Diagnosis and Management.* Philadelphia PA: J.B. Lippincott, 1998.

Stickland, A. (1984). Examination of the knee joint. *Physiotherapy* **70**, 144.

Stucki, G., Schonbachler, J., Bruhlmann, P., Mariacher, S., Stoll, T., and Michel, B.A. (1994). Does a muscle strength index provide complementary information to traditional disease activity variables in patients with rheumatoid arthritis? *Journal of Rheumatology* **21**, 2200–5.

Thompson, P.W., Silman, A.J., Kirwan, J.R., and Currey, H.L.F. (1987). Articular indices of joint inflammation in rheumatoid arthritis. *Arthritis and Rheumatism* **30**, 618–23.

Wolfe, F. (1997). The relation between tender points and fibromyalgia symptom variables: evidence that fibromyalgia is not a discrete disorder in the clinic. *Annals of the Rheumatic Diseases* **56**, 268–71.

Yocum, L.A. (1983). Assessing the shoulder: history, physical examination, differential diagnosis, and special tests used. *Clinical Sports Medicine* **2**, 281.

1.1.6 Psychological aspects of rheumatic disease

Stanton Newman and Kathleen Mulligan

Introduction

Treatment for most rheumatic conditions tends to revolve around attempting to manage and control the symptoms, and reduce the disabling consequences of the illness. The main thrust of treatment has been pharmacological or surgical (e.g. joint replacement), but also includes a range of non-medical interventions such as physiotherapy, pain control, weight-loss regimens, and self-management courses.

The shift from cure to management in rheumatological conditions mirrors the general shift in industrial societies from acute care to the management and treatment of chronic illness. This has been accompanied by an increasing focus on the psychological and social aspects surrounding chronic illnesses. Most chronic rheumatological conditions require major psychological adaptation as individuals face a lifetime of painful and increasingly disabling illness without prospect of a cure. They have to take regular medication and face the possibility of major surgery some time in their lives. Not only do individuals have to come to terms with the symptoms and treatment; but have to adapt to altered life plans, reduced employment prospects, and uncertainty about the future course of the disease and its impact on their lives.

Impact of rheumatological disorders on the individual

Introduction

Terminology continues to cast a cloud over the understanding of this domain of research. Various different and often overlapping terms are commonly used to refer to the more general consequences of rheumatological diseases on the individual. These terms include health status, functional status, impairment, disability, handicap, quality of life, and activities of daily living. The term quality of life has been used to accommodate all of these dimensions but has also on occasions been used to refer to a more limited domain such as mood state and psychiatric disturbance. In this chapter, 'quality of life' will be used to refer to composite measures of functional ability, mood and psychiatric state, and lifestyle. In studies where composite measures of the quality of life have been used, significant associations have been found with levels of disability (see, e.g., Bendtsen and Hornquist 1993).

The majority of studies of chronic disease in general and rheumatological disorders in particular have, however, tended to examine specific aspects of quality of life: physical function, symptoms, social and psychological well being (Fitzpatrick et al. 1992a). The focus on different areas of functioning enables the specific impact of the illness on different areas of life to be examined. The divisions of quality of life into symptoms, physical functioning, social functioning, and psychological well being will be used in this chapter, although it must be recognized that this does impose arbitrary boundaries in relation to the realities of chronic illness for the individual (Newman et al. 1996).

Symptoms

Pain

Pain is customarily ranked as the most important symptom for adults with rheumatoid arthritis (Gibson and Clark 1985) and concerns about being free of pain are patients' primary concerns (Deyo 1988). Pain reports have been found to differ between sexes, with women reporting more pain than men, and those with rheumatoid arthritis (RA) reporting higher levels of pain than those with osteoarthritis (OA) (Affleck et al. 1999). The extent of pain is related to general measures of physical disability. Using the functional classes (Steinbrocker et al. 1949), Parker et al. (1988a) found that patients classified as functional class III ('functional capacity quite limited') reported more pain and that a greater area of their body was painful, in contrast to those from classes I and II. Clinical measures of disease activity or damage have, in general, not been found to predict the extent of pain reported by individuals with RA. In the study by Parker et al. (1988a), clinical variables such as erythrocyte sedimentation rate, Ritchie articular index, grip strength, walking speed, and morning stiffness were only able to account for 3 per cent of the variance in pain scores. In contrast, sociodemographic factors such as age and income were reasonable predictors of pain. In OA, Creamer et al. (1999) found that pain was not predicted by radiographic severity as measured by Kellgren and Lawrence grade but pain severity was related to osteophyte score in patients with OA of the knee. They also found a relationship between pain severity and years of formal education and helplessness as well as body mass index (BMI). Other studies, discussed further below, emphasize the importance of psychological variables such as 'self-efficacy' (Buescher et al. 1991) and coping (Newman et al. 1990) as mediators of reports of the extent of pain.

Melzack (1975) reported that patients with arthritis used words like aching, exhausting, and rhythmic to describe the quality of their pain and more than one-third mentioned gnawing, annoying, and constant. Other research has suggested that patients use terms such as throbbing and burning, but do not use terms such as scalding, drilling, or cutting (Wagstaff et al. 1985). Pain quality, however, appears to be dependent on activity, with pain at rest described as 'throbbing' or 'aching', and pain on movement described as 'shooting' and 'spreading' (Papageorgiou and Badley 1989).

Stiffness

In contrast to pain, stiffness has been subjected to less research and its qualities less understood. For example, it is unclear whether it can be clearly distinguished from pain by individuals with rheumatological conditions. In one study the term stiffness was described as limitations in movement (Rhind et al. 1980) and in another, individuals with RA referred to stiffness as resistance to movement and limited range of movement (Helliwell 1995).

Because of its temporal nature, individuals who are able to adjust their timetable to accommodate early-morning stiffness may be more able to deal with the problems of stiffness in arthritis. The ability to be flexible in work has been shown to be important and for many who have early-morning stiffness rescheduling their day is one way of dealing with this aspect of stiffness.

Fatigue

Fatigue is a primary symptom of rheumatoid arthritis and in some studies was found to be the most severe symptom (Fitzpatrick et al. 1992b). It tends to fluctuate with the characteristics of the disease as well as increase in times of emotional distress (Tack 1990). Wolfe et al. (1996) found that clinically important levels of fatigue were present in more than 41 per cent of patients with RA or OA and 76 per cent of those with fibromyalgia. Fatigue is also a major symptom of systemic lupus erythematosus and in some studies was the most problematical aspect of the illness (Shortall et al. 1995).

In both RA and systemic lupus erythematosus, fatigue is associated with sleep difficulties, and with mood problems, in particular depression (Basia 1995; McKinley et al. 1995; Shortall et al. 1995). In RA, fatigue has also been associated with functional disability, and pain as well as with a lower haematocrit (Basia 1995). Determining the causal direction of these influences is difficult, but McKinley et al. (1995) suggest that the experience of fatigue in systemic lupus erythematosus is best understood by the impact of the disease mediated through sleep and emotional difficulties.

Physical functioning

Prevalence of disability

Population surveys of disability arising from musculoskeletal disorders estimate 5–8 per cent of individuals experience substantial disability

(Badley 1992), with arthritis identified as the most common cause of disability (Martin et al. 1988). Most surveys show an age-related increase in disability (e.g. Badley and Tennant 1993).

In population studies that have specifically examined rheumatic conditions, differences in the numbers and level of disability in different types of rheumatic disease have been found. Badley and Tennant (1993) found that OA and back disorders were the most common cause of disablement in rheumatic disease, but those with RA had the highest level of disability.

Reporting disability

Many techniques for assessing disability rely on self-reports of individual capability and these may be coloured by an individual's psychological state. For example, individuals who are depressed may underestimate their abilities. Studies have shown that self-reports of functional performance are related to other factors such as mental health and also health perceptions (Spiegel et al. 1988). Self-perceptions of health appear in turn to be related to demographic factors such as education as well as physical activity and depression (Guccione et al. 1995).

Among young children who have juvenile RA a problem exists as to whether their information correlates with that obtained from a parent. Doherty et al. (1993), using a formal questionnaire (the Child Health Assessment Questionnaire), found a relatively good concordance between assessments of their disability and pain made by young individuals with RA and those made by their parents.

Predicting disability

Determining what factors are associated with disability in rheumatic diseases may guide clinicians to potential areas of intervention. There are significant differences in the health status of individuals with rheumatological illnesses despite appearing similar on clinical criteria. This has led to the view that one needs to incorporate both biological and psychosocial factors when looking at predictors of disability. Studies that have used both clinical and psychosocial variables have been able to achieve much greater levels of prediction of health status than those using disease measures alone. One study (Lorish et al. 1991) examined and followed 155 patients with RA and examined the association of clinical and psychosocial factors with physical disability. Cross-sectional step-wise regression analysis showed that the two sets of variables combined accounted for 54 per cent of the variance at baseline and 35 per cent at 12-month follow-up. The psychological measure of helplessness in this study added significantly to the ability to predict disability independent of disease severity. The importance of mood was demonstrated in another study where depressed RA patients were found to be more impaired in their daily functioning than non-depressed patients (Katz and Yelin 1993).

Leigh and Fries (1992) made an 8-year follow-up study and Eberhardt and Fex (1995) a 5-year follow-up study on individuals with early RA. Both these studies found the level of disability at outset of the study was the most important predictor of future disability, as had been reported previously (Wolfe and Cathey 1991). Women were found to be more disabled than men (see also Thompson and Pegley 1991) although what factors are included in the assessment of disability appears to influence the likelihood of finding sex differences in disability. While studies have demonstrated a gender difference on the Health Assessment Questionnaire, the Groningen Activity Restriction Scale appears to show smaller sex differences (Doeglas et al. 1995a).

Other sociodemographic factors are important predictors of disability. Leigh and Fries (1992) found that older patients and those who were single at the time of the first assessment showed increasing disability over time. Evers et al. (1998) reported that a smaller social network at baseline was related to a decrease in mobility at 1-year follow-up. These findings emphasize the role and importance of social support as buffers against disability in rheumatic disease.

Level of pain, global health status, and number of working hours assessed at the outset were also predictive of disability 8 years later (Leigh and Fries 1992). The investigators offer two explanations to account for this last finding. First, and most obvious, is that individuals with lower levels of disability would be more likely to be in work. The second explanation is more psychological and interprets the increase in disability through the effects of unemployment on self-esteem and depression and the health-protective effects of employment. Further longitudinal study is required to see which of these explanations is the more accurate.

Higher levels of education have also been found to be associated with lower levels of disability (Pincus and Callahan 1985; Eberhardt and Fex 1995). One interpretation of this finding is that higher levels of education are associated with more 'white collar' work and higher incomes, and as a result, better work and social conditions. Education may therefore be a marker of the importance of social factors on the course of disability in RA.

Social functioning

Employment and work

Rheumatoid arthritis has a dramatic impact on employment, with in one study over half of individuals with RA who worked before the onset of the disease stopping work within 10 years of diagnosis (Yelin et al. 1980). In another study (Barrett et al. 2000), 39 per cent had work disability after 10 years. Work performance and occupational status are affected by rheumatoid arthritis even soon after it has been diagnosed. Doeglas et al. (1995b) found that 90 per cent of a group who had been diagnosed 2 years previously, had either given up work or had made changes in their work because of their RA. In ankylosing spondylitis (AS) rates of employment were found to be 15.4 per cent lower for men and 5.2 per cent lower for women than the general population (Boonen et al. 2001). Ward and Kuzis (2001) found 13.2 per cent of individuals with AS to develop permanent work disability.

The effects of arthritis on employment have a considerable impact on income. In one study in the United States, men with RA had 48 per cent and women 27 per cent of the income of those without the disease (Mitchell et al. 1988). A prospective 18 year study found that over the course of their RA, family income of the work disabled reduced by 35 per cent (Wolfe and Hawley 1998). The absence of paid employment for individuals with RA appears to have an independent effect on symptoms and mood. Fifield et al. (1991) assessed 723 RA patients and found that those without paid employment reported higher levels of pain and depression, even when confounding factors such as disease severity were controlled.

The nature of work appears to be an important predictor of the likelihood of retaining employment. Those in professional or managerial occupations are more likely to stay in employment after the onset of RA (Callahan et al. 1992). This is reflected in the finding that the social characteristics of work, in particular being able to control the pace of work and being self-employed, had greater explanatory power than the four best medical variables in predicting continuing work (Yelin et al. 1980). Doeglas et al. (1995b) found an association between educational level and remaining in employment despite RA. They attribute this to the nature of work performed by the more highly educated. In their study 32 per cent on the non-manual workers and 80 per cent of the manual workers with RA had left their jobs. Ward and Kuzis (2001) also found that significant risk factors for permanent work disability among men with AS were older age of disease onset, lower education level, and having had more physically demanding jobs. Lower levels of education, higher disease activity at diagnosis and higher physical job demands were also among significant predictors of early work disability in people with systemic lupus erythematosus (Partridge et al. 1997).

The problem of employment for individuals who have juvenile RA revolves around making the transition between the relatively sheltered world of education to the world of work. Programmes have been devised to assist this transition. One report of a programme indicates a high level of training and education as well as high levels of employment for individuals with juvenile RA (White and Shear 1992). In the sample of 242, the majority of whom had juvenile RA, 27 per cent had completed 4 years of college education, which was well above that achieved by the general population

(9 per cent), and only 6 per cent were unemployed. In contrast, Peterson et al. (1997) reported significantly lower levels of employment in adults who had had juvenile RA than in age and sex matched controls.

It is not only in paid employment that work disability is found. In a study by Reisine et al. (1987) many women with RA reported limitations in cleaning the house (73 per cent), in laundry work (65 per cent), and shopping (61 per cent). More importantly, RA appeared to affect the ability to perform the nurturing roles such as giving attention and support to other household members and maintaining family ties with others outside the household such as relatives and friends. Allaire et al. (1991) found that women with mild RA spent as much time on household work as a control group, but accomplished less in that time. Women with more severe RA did less housework and spent less time on housework than those in the mild and non-RA groups, but this reduction was compensated for by their families, who spent on average 7 hours more time per week on household chores.

Family relationships

Rheumatoid arthritis

Studies on the frequency of divorce in arthritis are inconclusive (Anderson et al. 1985; Fitzpatrick 1993). Early studies suggested an increased frequency of divorce in RA but later studies have tended to find similar rates of divorce to those of the general population (Hull 1988; Hawley et al. 1991).

It is clear, however, that difficulties in relationships do arise when one partner has arthritis. In some cases these appear to come out of a decreased interest in sexual relations (Reisine et al. 1987). Other issues that appear to create some difficulties in relationships include problems of dependency, shared problems of isolation, and reduced income (Locker 1983; Williams 1987). Specific symptoms such as pain may lead to increased levels of irritability and bad temper which may have an impact on the relationships. There is, however, little apparent loss of the quality of close relationships when assessed from the perspective of the person with RA. Fitzpatrick et al. (1988) found little or no difference in how individuals with RA rate the quality of their close relationship. They also found no reduction in the quality of the relationship in those who had more severe disease.

Social relationships

Social relationships appear to be more at risk than close relationships in arthritis. Individuals with RA reduce their social contacts with others (Deyo et al. 1982). Over time, as disability increases, individuals with arthritis have fewer opportunities for contact with friends and acquaintances and also derive less satisfaction with these relationships (Fitzpatrick et al. 1988). With progression and reduced mobility, social contacts become even more difficult and social withdrawal may arise in some individuals. The social withdrawal may not, however, simply be attributable to increasing disability. Some individuals may withdraw socially in order to avoid the stigma and embarrassment associated with RA (Williams and Wood 1988; Locker 1989).

Psychological well-being

The bulk of research has assessed depression and depressed mood and relatively little attention has been directed to other areas of mood such as anxiety and positive mood.

Prevalence of depression

The reported prevalence of clinical depression in RA ranges between 8 and 22 per cent in different studies (Creed 1990). While this is higher than in the general population, similar rates have been found in other chronic illnesses (Frank et al. 1988; Murphy et al. 1988; DeVellis 1993). Thus, the increased levels of depression that occur in RA appear to reflect the general effects of a chronic illness.

Hawley and Wolfe (1993) compared the incidence of depression and depressed mood in individuals with a variety of rheumatic conditions. They found no evidence to support the notion that patients with RA, in comparison to individuals with other rheumatological conditions, have a particular propensity to develop depression. Rates of depression were, however, higher in fibromyalgia (Hawley and Wolfe 1993). Wolfe and Skevington (2000) reported no difference in levels of depression between RA and OA. Aasland et al. (1997), in a 9-year follow-up of 52 people with juvenile chronic arthritis, found that none met the DSMIII-R criteria for depressive disorder.

Factors associated with depression and low mood

A number of studies have attempted to identify the factors that lead to depression in rheumatic disease. While a simple interpretation might be that those with more severe disease are more likely to be depressed or have low mood, no direct relation between markers of the severity of arthritis and clinical depression or depressed mood has been found (McFarlane and Brooks 1988; Newman et al. 1989; Creed 1990; Blalock and DeVellis 1992). The most important predictor of depression and depressed mood in adults with RA and in juvenile arthritis appears to be disability (Newman et al. 1989; David et al. 1994). The research therefore suggests that two of the consequences of arthritis, depression and disability, are associated with each other but that neither is linked with clinical markers of the severity or activity of the disease. These associations serve to emphasize that how individuals respond to and experience their arthritis may be very different from what would be expected from clinical measures of the disease. It is also interesting that psychological status among patients with rheumatic disease remains fairly stable over time in spite of worsening disease severity (Wolfe 1999).

In studies of individuals with arthritis, pain is commonly associated with depression and/or distress (e.g. Hawley and Wolfe 1988; Smedstad et al. 1995, 1997). It is commonly thought that the direction of this association is of pain causing the mental distress, although it could well be the opposite, that individuals who are distressed report higher levels of pain. Smedstad et al. (1997) attempted to develop a causal model of the temporal relationship between pain, disability, and distress but did not obtain consistent results.

The impact of RA and its symptoms is mediated through a number of psychological and social factors. Notable amongst these are coping responses and social supports, which are discussed below, but other important factors include social isolation and economic resources (Newman et al. 1989).

An important consideration is how low mood or depression may affect other aspects of the quality of life. Depressed mood is generally associated with dramatically reduced perceptions of quality of life (Sensky and Catalan 1992) and individuals with high levels of depression may restrict their social activities and become isolated. High levels of depression may also affect the individual's perceptions of their functioning and thus their self-reports of their functional status may be worse (Spiegel et al. 1988; Brooks et al. 1990; Guccione et al. 1995). These interactions between mood and other measures underlie the importance of studies that are conducted longitudinally and can examine causal direction between variables.

Impact of psychological variables on health status and well-being

A simple model of arthritic disease and its consequences would suggest a linear relation leading from disease to disablement and psychological well-being. The research findings suggest that this simple model is untenable and that the consequences of arthritis are dependent upon how individuals interpret their illness, how others respond to their needs, and aspects of their environment. A number of psychological concepts have been used in attempting to account for the mediation between disease and its consequences, and it is to these that we now turn.

Coping

The term coping refers to what individuals attempt to do to limit the impact of a stress such as arthritis (see Newman and Revenson 1993). This work may be divided into studies that have examined coping with arthritis in general and those that have focused on coping with specific symptoms, such as pain.

Many studies have used variants of the Ways of Coping Scale (Folkman and Lazarus 1980; Folkman and Lazarus 1988) to assess coping with RA in general. The questionnaire has eight sub-scales divided between two broad classifications of coping: problem-focused coping (e.g. 'Come up with a couple of solutions to the problem') and emotion-focused coping (e.g. 'I am changing or growing as a person in a good way'). A number of studies have used this questionnaire and found that patients with RA who use the coping strategy of cognitive restructuring ('attempts to seek new meaning in their situation') had better psychological well-being (Felton et al. 1984; Parker et al. 1988b; Manne and Zautra 1989). Those who used the coping strategy of wishful thinking (e.g. 'Wish that the situation would go away or somehow be over with') tended to have worse psychological well-being (Felton et al. 1984; Parker et al. 1988b; Manne and Zautra 1989; Long and Sangster 1993). Using a questionnaire designed specifically to assess coping with RA, Newman et al. (1990) used a cluster analysis to divide patients into distinct groups according to how they attempted to cope with their disease. The groups defined in this way did not differ on clinical measures of disease. One group, which tended to be the most open and active in the manner in which they attempted to deal with the stresses of arthritis, had significantly lower scores on measures of pain, stiffness, and disability, and better psychological well-being. The findings suggest that how individuals attempt to deal with their arthritis, in terms of actions and thoughts, has an impact on psychological well-being, symptom reporting, and disability.

Some studies have examined the ways in which individuals with arthritis cope with pain. One important coping strategy is the perception of control over pain, which leads to higher levels of psychological well being and lower levels of disability (Beckham et al. 1991). Keefe et al. (1989) found that high scores on the 'catastrophising scale' of the Coping Strategies Questionnaire were associated with poorer outcomes on measures of disability and psychological well-being 6 months later. In a study by Evers et al. (1998), a deterioration in functional status after 1 year could be predicted by the passive pain coping strategies of resting and worrying. Longitudinal research with the Vanderbilt Pain Management Inventory has demonstrated that active coping strategies lead to more favourable outcomes and passive strategies unfavourable outcomes; passive coping during periods of high pain may be particularly detrimental to psychological well-being (Brown and Nicassio 1987; Brown et al. 1989). When Covic et al. (2000) used this measure, they found that passive coping mediated between disability and pain and between disability and depression.

Taken together, these studies confirm that the psychological responses to arthritis and its symptoms are important determinants of health status. Both the disease and the psychological processes of trying to deal with arthritis are not static. This implies an approach to understanding the consequences of arthritis which accepts that both the disease and coping with the disease change over time. The research also opens up the possibility that psychological interventions to alter coping behaviour may be able to reduce the impact of arthritis.

Social comparison

Individuals' attempts to cope with the stresses of their arthritis take place in a social context. Part of the processes associated with coping involves making comparisons with others in order to provide a reference point to evaluate one's relative position. Social comparison constitutes a part of the coping mechanism used by some individuals. It is particularly important when the means to change the situation are not available (Wills 1987). In the context of arthritis, individuals frequently compare themselves with others who have arthritis. Research on the social comparison process suggests that individuals with RA do predominantly tend to make comparisons with those in a worse state and that this type of comparison is associated with better psychological well being (Affleck et al. 1988; DeVellis et al. 1990).

Social support

The process of dealing with the stresses caused by arthritis frequently involves others as potential providers of both practical help and emotional support. The term 'social support' refers to the process by which interpersonal relationships promote well being and protect people from a decline in health. In healthy individuals, social support reduces morbidity and mortality (Berkman 1985), particularly at times when they are facing stressful life circumstances (Cohen 1988), and improves mental health (Kessler and McLeod 1985).

Eliciting social support is one coping strategy that many individuals use. This is dependent upon having people in the environment from whom support may be elicited. These include family, friends, health care professionals, and patients' groups. These individuals and groups may provide emotional support by offering a receptive ear when individuals are upset as well as practical support such as assistance and advice about how to deal with a problem.

A large number of studies show the importance of social support. At the simplest level, married people with RA show slower progression in their disability than those without partners (Ward and Leigh 1993). Other studies have shown that individuals with RA who have more social contacts have lower levels of depression (Newman et al. 1990). Most studies of social support, however, suggest that the number of individuals with whom one has contact is less important than the belief that one has adequate support available. These studies have demonstrated that those individuals with RA who perceive greater social support exhibit greater self-esteem (Fitzpatrick et al. 1988) and life satisfaction (Smith et al. 1991), are better adjusted (Affleck et al. 1988), show less depression (Fitzpatrick et al. 1991; Doeglas et al. 1994), and cope better with their arthritis (Manne and Zautra 1990). The important role of the individuals' judgement of their social support parallels findings in both epidemiological studies and studies in other illnesses.

It is important to recognize that the provision of support implies shared understandings of need, what is required, when it is required, and an ability to negotiate the provision of support at a time when the provider is ready to offer it (Newman et al. 1996). This process takes place within a reciprocal relationship in which the individual with RA is also a support provider. Given these factors it is not surprising that some social support may have negative effects (Revenson et al. 1991). Although in some cases the negative effects may be intended. The relation between negative social support and coping efficacy was well demonstrated in a study by Manne and Zautra (1989), who found a direct relation between spouses' critical comments and wives' coping and adaptation to their RA. Patients with critical spouses tended to engage in more wishful thinking, which led to poorer psychological outcomes. The authors argue that spouses' criticism 'may encourage ineffective and even harmful coping strategies'. Patients who perceived their spouses as supportive engaged more in cognitive restructuring and information seeking, strategies that proved to be more adaptive in dealing with the stresses of arthritis. Kraaimaat et al. (1995) report similar findings but found that spousal criticism led to anxiety in men and both anxiety and depression in women.

Some researchers have looked at the impact of different types of social support and found that not all elements of support lead to improved health status or psychological well-being in individuals with arthritis. Taal et al. (1993) found that while emotional support was not positively related to health status, practical support was and Doeglas et al. (1994) found that receiving greater amounts of emotional support had a negative effect on some aspects of psychological well-being. These findings suggest that to understand fully the impact of social support in arthritis further research needs to examine the nature of the support provided, who provides it, and when it is provided.

Control, self-efficacy, and perceived competence

Individuals hold beliefs about their health and what they are able to do about the course of their arthritis. The role of these more general beliefs are considered next.

Beliefs about whether and who may influence the course of health and illness in the future have been widely studied. This concept, known as health locus of control, has three dimensions. The internal health locus of control (IHLC) is the belief that the individual has an influence over future health and illness; the chance health locus of control (CHLC) is the belief that fate and chance will determine future health and illness, and 'powerful other' health locus of control (POHLC) is the belief that others such as healthcare professionals will wield an important influence on future health and illness (Wallston et al. 1978). This concept usefully identifies that individuals with arthritis who join self-help groups have higher IHLC scores (Volle et al. 1990).

Early cross-sectional research suggested that high IHLC beliefs had positive effects on psychological well-being in RA and OA (Wallston 1993). Later studies have shown the issue about control to be more complex. A study that distinguished between control over treatment and control over symptoms found that personal control over treatment was associated with higher psychological well-being while perceptions of greater control over symptoms by healthcare providers were associated with lower psychological well being (Affleck et al. 1987). A later study by the same group (Tennen et al. 1992) showed that patients who believed they had control over their pain (IHLC) at the beginning of an intensive daily study reported less pain. More interestingly, it appeared that when individuals believed they could control their pain but were thwarted by higher levels of pain than expected, they become distressed. These studies clearly demonstrate that perceptions of personal control over arthritis do not necessarily lead to improved outcomes.

Perceived competence and self-efficacy are terms used to describe individuals' beliefs that they have the skills to be able to deal effectively with issues in the environment. It has been argued that these beliefs act as a mediator between measures of disease and adaptation. One study (Smith et al. 1991) found that, levels of competence acted as a mediator between levels of disease, perceptions of control and social support on the one hand, and life satisfaction and depression on the other. Patients with higher self-efficacy have been found to display fewer pain behaviours (Buescher et al. 1991) have less depression (Lorig et al. 1989a) and disability (Shoor and Holman 1984). Brekke et al. (2001), in a study of 815 RA patients, found a significant correlation between baseline self-efficacy score and favourable changes in health status over 2 years. Self-efficacy has also been found to predict outcome of self-management interventions (Buckelow et al. 1996; Rhee et al. 2000).

Intervention studies

Studies have demonstrated how psychological factors mediate between the disease on the one hand and outcomes on the other. These investigations have led to the development of intervention studies, which attempt to modify individuals' understanding, beliefs, coping styles, and social supports in order to influence psychological well-being and health status. The use of psychosocial interventions in arthritis has seen considerable development over the last 20 years. Historically, RA was the main target of interventions but they are now more widely available for other rheumatic diseases. In many of these interventions, participants receive not only disease information but are also taught a range of skills to help enhance their ability to manage their disease. Several different approaches have been used and the interventions vary in a number of ways.

Information about arthritis is a small but significant component that appears integral to most intervention studies. Reviews of the effects of information have found increases in knowledge among the participants (Lorig et al. 1987) but there is little evidence to support the view that the provision of general information alone has any impact on behaviour or results in any benefits to individuals with arthritis (DeVellis and Blalock 1993).

Most psychosocial interventions for rheumatic disease use a number of different components. Which components are included partly reflects the theoretical framework being used. Interventions that are based on social learning theory aim to enhance patients' self-efficacy (confidence) to manage their disease. Others have attempted to influence how individuals think about their symptoms and disability and use a cognitive–behavioural framework. Some aim to improve patients' ability to enrol social support. The interventions may include training in cognitive pain management, joint protection, exercise, communication skills, and problem-solving, amongst others. Unfortunately, published reports give only scant descriptions of intervention content so it is frequently not possible to identify their detail. In order to advance our understanding of the impact of interventions it is necessary for detailed descriptions of the content and manner of delivery of interventions to be documented and made available.

Whilst most interventions are delivered by health professionals in either an individual or group format and usually take place in a hospital setting, others have been delivered by telephone or using a self-instruction manual or computer program. The most well known amongst psychosocial interventions in arthritis is the Arthritis Self-Management Programme (ASMP). This programme differs from many others in that it is community based and delivered by trained lay leaders who themselves have arthritis (Lorig 1995). Most other interventions have been designed for a single rheumatic disease but ASMP groups can include people with different types of arthritis. More recently the programme has broadened yet further to include people with a variety of different chronic conditions (Lorig et al. 1999b).

Psychosocial intervention studies typically measure several potential outcome variables. Early studies often measured knowledge, but while knowledge is necessary, it would appear to be insufficient to change behaviour. Although many studies have measured depression, most participants do not score highly on measures of depression on entry into the study creating the problem of floor effects. The most important outcomes for individuals with arthritis are pain and disability. These are appropriate outcomes for psychosocial interventions as they have been shown to be influenced by psychological factors.

Participants in psychosocial interventions do not undergo a drug wash-out period before commencing the study, therefore any effect found is in addition to that already being achieved by medication. A number of reviews have reported the beneficial effects of these types of interventions on pain, disability, and depression (Lorig et al. 1987; Mullen et al. 1987; Hirano et al. 1994; Hawley 1995; Taal et al. 1997). An advantage of psychosocial interventions is that they do not have harmful side effects but overall, their beneficial impact tends to be fairly modest. It remains necessary to establish the most effective elements of these interventions and to systematically evaluate their benefits across a wider range of patients and outcomes.

It is unlikely that a single type of intervention will show benefits for all patients on all outcomes. Clear differences have been demonstrated on different outcomes; Keefe et al. (1996), in a spouse-assisted coping skills training programme for OA knee, found improvement in pain but not physical disability. Conversely, Taal et al. (1993), in a 5-week programme for people with RA, found improvement in disability but not pain. These examples highlight that it is important to consider what aspects of different interventions appear to be most beneficial for different outcomes. Given that the interventions typically combine several different components it would require a systematic series of studies to compare different permutations of these components to tackle this question.

The ASMP requires special mention as it is the most widely used psychosocial intervention and has been the subject of several studies. Several evaluations of the ASMP have used single groups assessed prior to and following the intervention. Where randomized controlled trials (RCT) have been performed with the ASMP the results are mixed. Lorig et al. (1986) found changes in exercise and relaxation behaviour but no effect on pain, disability or number of physician visits. A larger trial with over 800 participants (Lorig et al. 1989b) found improvements in knowledge, pain, and behaviours after 4 months but no impact on disability or depression. A Spanish variant of the ASMP found improvements in pain, self-efficacy and motion exercise after 4 months but no effects on aerobic exercise, general health status, depression, or drug and health care utilization (Lorig et al. 1999a). This variant of the ASMP did find an improvement in disability and it may be that inclusion of exercise practice in class, which is not usually part of the ASMP, had a beneficial effect. An RCT in the United Kingdom (Barlow et al. 2000) found improvement in self-efficacy, cognitive symptom management, dietary habit, communication with physician, fatigue, anxiety, depression, and positive mood but did not show an impact on negative affect, pain, disability, or GP visits.

The question of whether a single intervention can be used with all types of rheumatic disease or whether different interventions work better in some than others, needs to be addressed. Most interventions are used for a single condition and are not tested with other forms of rheumatic disease. In general, the interventions in OA seem to have better outcomes than those in RA but it is not clear if this is because they use different components or if OA is more amenable to change. A further complication is that the OA studies tend to be larger and therefore less likely to be under-powered. The ASMP uses mixed groups and in the most recent RCT (Barlow et al. 2000), there was little difference in outcome between OA and RA.

Conclusion

Research on the psychological factors associated with arthritis has shown that attempts to predict disability and psychological well being in individuals with arthritis need to incorporate how individuals perceive their arthritis, how they try to deal with the stresses it creates, as well as factors in their social environments. This area of research and its resulting interventions are likely to lead to important findings in the future but a clear focus on the contents of the interventions, the group to which they are applied as well as the methodology of studies, will be required for a greater understanding of psychosocial interventions in musculoskeletal conditions.

References

Aasland, A., Flato, B., and Vandvik, I.H. (1997). Psychosocial outcome in juvenile chronic arthritis: a nine-year follow-up. *Clinical and Experimental Rheumatology* **15**, 561–8.

Affleck, G., Tennen, H., Pfeiffer, C., and Fifield, J. (1987). Appraisals of control and predictability in adapting to a chronic disease. *Journal of Personality and Social Psychology* **53**, 273–9.

Affleck, G., Pfeiffer, C., Tennen, H., and Fifield, J. (1988). Social support and psychosocial adjustment to rheumatoid arthritis. *Arthritis Care and Research* **1**, 71–7.

Affleck, G. et al. (1999). Everyday life with osteoarthritis or rheumatoid arthritis: independent effects of disease and gender on daily pain, mood, and coping. *Pain* **83**, 601–9.

Allaire, S.H., Meenan, R.F., and Anderson, J.F. (1991). The impact of rheumatoid arthritis on the household work performance of women. *Arthritis and Rheumatism* **34**, 669–78.

Anderson, K., Bradley, L., Young, L., McDaniel, L., and Wise, C. (1985). Rheumatoid arthritis: review of psychological factors related to etiology, effects and treatment. *Psychological Bulletin* **98**, 358–7.

Badley, E. (1992). The impact of musculoskeletal disorders on the Canadian population. *Journal of Rheumatology* **19**, 337–40.

Badley, E.M. and Tennant, A. (1993). Impact of disablement due to rheumatic disorders in a British population: estimates of severity and prevalence from the Calderdale Rheumatic Disablement Survey. *Annals of the Rheumatic Diseases* **52**, 6–13.

Barlow, J.H., Turner, A.P., and Wright, C.C. (2000). A randomised controlled study of the Arthritis Self-Management Programme in the UK. *Health Education Research* **15** (6), 665–80.

Barrett, E.M., Scott, D.G., Wiles, N.J., and Symmons, D.P. (2000). The impact of rheumatoid arthritis on employment status in the early years of the disease: a UK community-based study. *Rheumatology* **39**, 1403–9.

Basia, L. (1995). Comparison of self reported fatigue in rheumatoid arthritis and controls. *Journal of Rheumatology* **22**, 639–43.

Beckham, J.C. et al. (1991). Pain coping strategies in rheumatoid arthritis. *Behaviour Therapy* **22**, 113–24.

Bendtsen, P. and Hornquist, J.O. (1993). Severity of rheumatoid arthritis, function and quality of life: subgroup comparisons. *Clinical and Experimental Rheumatology* **11**, 495–502.

Berkman, L.F. (1985). The relationship of social networks and social support to morbidity and mortality. In *Social Support and Health* (ed. S. Cohen and S.L. Syme), pp. 243–62. New York: Academic Press.

Blalock, S.J. and DeVellis, R.F. (1992). Rheumatoid arthritis and depression: an overview. *Bulletin of the Rheumatic Diseases* **41**, 6–8.

Boonen, A. et al. (2001). Employment, work disability, and work days lost in patients with ankylosing spondylitis: a cross sectional study of Dutch patients. *Annals of the Rheumatic Diseases* **60**, 353–8.

Brekke, M., Hjortdahl, P., and Kvien, T.K. (2001). Self-efficacy and health status in rheumatoid arthritis: a two-year longitudinal observational study. *Rheumatology* **40**, 387–92.

Brooks, B., Jordan, J., Divinew, G., Smith, K., and Neelon, F. (1990). The impact of psychologic factors on measurement of functional status. *Medical Care* **28**, 793–804.

Brown, G.K. and Nicassio, P.M. (1987). Development of a questionnaire for the assessment of active and passive coping strategies in chronic pain patients. *Pain* **31**, 53–63.

Brown, G.K. et al. (1989). Pain coping strategies and depression in rheumatoid arthritis. *Journal of Consultative Clinical Psychology* **57**, 652–7.

Buckelew, S.P. et al. (1996). Self-efficacy predicting outcome among fibromyalgia subjects. *Arthritis Care and Research* **9**, 97–104.

Buescher, K.L. et al. (1991). Relationship of self efficacy to pain behaviour. *Journal of Rheumatology* **18**, 968–72.

Callahan, L., Bloch, D., and Pincus, T. (1992). Identification of work disability in rheumatoid arthritis. *Journal of Clinical Epidemiology* **45**, 127–38.

Cohen, S. (1988). Psychosocial models of the role of social support in the etiology of physical disease. *Health Psychology* **7**, 269–97.

Covic, T., Adamson, B., and Hough, M. (2000). The impact of passive coping on rheumatoid arthritis pain. *Rheumatology* **39**, 1027–30.

Creamer, P., Lethbridge-Cejku, M., and Hochberg, M.C. (1999). Determinants of pain severity in knee osteoarthritis: effect of demographic and psychosocial variables using 3 pain measures. *Journal of Rheumatology* **26** (8), 1785–92.

Creed, F. (1990). Psychological disorders in rheumatoid arthritis: a growing consensus. *Annals of the Rheumatic Diseases* **49**, 808–12.

David, J. et al. (1994). The functional and psychological outcomes of juvenile chronic arthritis in young adulthood. *British Journal of Rheumatology* **33**, 876–81.

DeVellis, B.M. (1993). Depression in rheumatological diseases. In *Psychological Aspects of Rheumatic Disease; Ballière's Clinical Rheumatology* Vol. 7, Part 2 (ed. S. Newman and M. Shipley), pp. 241–58. London: Baillière Tindall.

DeVellis, R. and Blalock, S. (1993). Psychological and educational interventions to reduce arthritis disability. In *Psychological Aspects of Rheumatic Disease; Ballière's Clinical Rheumatology* Vol. 7, Part 2 (ed. S. Newman and M. Shipley), pp. 397–416. London: Baillière Tindall.

DeVellis, R., Holt, K., and Renner, B. (1990). The relationship of social comparison to rheumatoid arthritis symptoms and affect. *Basic and Applied Social Psychology* **11**, 1–18.

Deyo, R.A. (1988). Measuring the quality of life of patients with rheumatoid arthritis. In *Quality of Life: Assessment and Application* (ed. S.R. Walker and R.M. Rosser), p. 205. Lancaster: MTP.

Deyo, R.A., Inui, T., Leininger, J., and Overman, S. (1982). Physical and psychosocial function in rheumatoid arthritis. *Archives of Internal Medicine* **142**, 879–82.

Doeglas, D. et al. (1994). Social support, social disability and psychological well being in rheumatoid arthritis. *Arthritis Care and Research* **7**, 10–15.

Doeglas, D. et al. (1995a). The assessment of functional status in rheumatoid arthritis: a cross cultural, longitudinal comparison of the Health Assessment Questionnaire and the Groningen Activity Restriction Scale. *Journal of Rheumatology* **22**, 1834–43.

Doeglas, D. et al. (1995b). Work disability in early rheumatoid arthritis. *Annals of the Rheumatic Diseases* **54**, 455–60.

Doherty, E., Yanni, G., Conroy, R.M., and Bresnihan, B. (1993). A comparison of child and parent ratings of disability and pain in juvenile chronic arthritis. *Journal of Rheumatology* **20**, 1563–6.

Eberhardt, K. and Fex, E. (1995). Functional impairment and disability in early rheumatoid arthritis—development over 5 years. *Journal of Rheumatology* **22**, 1037–42.

Evers, A.W.M., Kraaimaat, F.W., Geenan, R., and Bijlsma, J.W.J. (1998). Psychosocial predictors of functional change in recently diagnosed rheumatoid arthritis patients. *Behaviour Research and Therapy* **36**, 179–83.

Felton, B. et al. (1984). Stress and coping in the explanation of psychological adjustment among chronically ill adults. *Social Science and Medicine* **18**, 889–98.

Fifield, J., Reisine, S.T., and Grady, K. (1991). Work disability and the experience of pain and depression in rheumatoid arthritis. *Social Science and Medicine* **33**, 579–85.

Fitzpatrick, R. (1993). The measurement of health status and quality of life in rheumatoid arthritis. In *Psychological Aspects of Rheumatic Disease; Ballière's Clinical Rheumatology* Vol. 7, Part 2 (ed. S. Newman and M. Shipley), pp. 297–317. London: Baillière Tindall.

Fitzpatrick, R., Newman, S., Lamb, R., and Shipley, M. (1988). Social relationships and psychological well-being in rheumatoid arthritis. *Social Science and Medicine* **27**, 399–403.

Fitzpatrick, R., Newman, S., Archer, R., and Shipley, M. (1991). Social support, disability and depression: a longitudinal study of RA. *Social Science and Medicine* **33**, 605–11.

Fitzpatrick, R., Fletcher, A., Gore, S., Jones, D., Spieglehalter, D., and Cox, D. (1992a). Quality of life measures in health care. I: Applications and issues in assessment. *British Medical Journal* **305**, 1074–7.

Fitzpatrick, R., Ziebland, S., Jenkinson, C., and Mowat, A. (1992b). A generic health status instrument in the assessment of rheumatoid arthritis. *British Journal of Rheumatology* **31**, 87–90.

Folkman, S. and Lazarus, R. (1980). An analysis of coping in a middle-aged community sample. *Journal of Health and Social Behaviour* **21**, 219–39.

Folkman, S. and Lazarus, R.S. *Manual for the Ways of Coping Questionnaire.* Palo Alto CA: Consulting Psychologists Press, 1988.

Frank, R. et al. (1988). Depression in rheumatoid arthritis. *Journal of Rheumatology* **15**, 920–5.

Gibson, T. and Clark, B. (1985). Use of simple analgesics in rheumatoid arthritis. *Annals of the Rheumatic Diseases* **44**, 27–9.

Guccione, A. et al. (1995). The correlates of health perceptions in rheumatoid arthritis. *Journal of Rheumatology* **22**, 432–9.

Hawley, D.J. (1995). Psycho-educational interventions in the treatment of arthritis. *Baillière's Clinical Rheumatology* **9**, 803–23.

Hawley, D.J. and Wolfe, F. (1988). Anxiety and depression in patients with rheumatoid arthritis. *Journal of Rheumatology* **15**, 932–41.

Hawley, D.J. and Wolfe, F. (1993). Depression is not more common in rheumatoid arthritis: a 10-year longitudinal study of 6153 patients with rheumatic disease. *Journal of Rheumatology* **20**, 2025–31.

Hawley, D.J. et al. (1991). Marital status in rheumatoid arthritis and other rheumatic disorders: a study of 7293 patients. *Journal of Rheumatology* **18**, 654–60.

Helliwell, P.S. (1995). The semiology of arthritis: discriminating between patients on the basis of their symptons. *Annals of the Rheumatic Diseases* **54**, 924–6.

Hirano, P.C., Laurent, D.D., and Lorig, K. (1994). Arthritis patient education studies, 1987–1991: a review of the literature. *Patient Education and Counseling* **24**, 9–54.

Hull, R.G. (1988). Outcome in juvenile arthritis. *British Journal of Rheumatology* **27**, 66–71.

Katz, P. and Yelin, E. (1993). Prevalence and correlates of depressive symptoms among persons with rheumatoid arthritis. *Journal of Rheumatology* **20**, 790–6.

Keefe, F.J. et al. (1989). Coping with rheumatoid arthritis pain: catastrophising as a maladaptive strategy. *Pain* **37**, 51–6.

Keefe, F.J., Caldwell, D.S., Baucom, D., Salley, A., Robinson, E., Timmons, K., Beaupre, P., Weisberg, J., and Helms, M. (1996). Spouse-assisted coping skills training in the management of osteoarthritic knee pain. *Arthritis Care and Research* **9**, 279–91.

Kessler, R.C. and McLeod, J.D. (1985). Social support and mental health in community samples. In *Social Support and Health* (ed. S. Cohen and S.L. Syme), pp. 219–40. New York: Academic Press.

Kraaimaat, F. et al. (1995). Association of social support and the spouse's reaction with psychological distress in male and female patients with rheumatoid arthritis. *Journal of Rheumatology* **22**, 644–8.

Leigh, P.J. and Fries, J.F. (1992). Predictors of disability in a longitudinal sample of patients with rheumatoid arthritis. *Annals of the Rheumatic Diseases* **51**, 581–7.

Locker, D. *Disability and Disadvantage: The Consequences of Chronic Illness.* London: Tavistock, 1983.

Locker, D. (1989). Coping with disability and handicap. In *Disablement in the Community* (ed. D. Patrick and H. Peach), pp. 176–96. Oxford: Oxford University Press.

Long, B.C. and Sangster, J.L. (1993). Dispositional optimism/pessimism and coping strategies: predictors of psychosocial adjustment of rheumatoid and osteoarthritis patients. *Journal of Applied Social Psychology* **23**, 1069–91.

Lorig, K. *Arthritis Self-Help Course. Leader's Manual and Reference Materials.* Atlanta GA: Arthritis Foundation, 1995.

Lorig, K., Feigenbaum, P., Regan, C., Ung, E., Chastain, R.L., and Holman, H.R. (1986). A comparison of lay-taught and professional-taught arthritis self-management courses. *Journal of Rheumatology* **13**, 763–7.

Lorig, K., Konkol, L., and Gonzolez, V. (1987). Arthritis patient education: a review of the literature. *Patient Education and Counselling* **10**, 207–52.

Lorig, K., Chastain, R.L., Ung, E., Shoor, S., and Holman, H.R. (1989a). Development and evaluation of a scale to measure perceived self-efficacy in people with arthritis. *Arthritis and Rheumatism* **32**, 37–44.

Lorig, K., Seleznick, M., Lubeck, D., Ung., Chastain, R.L., and Holman, H.R. (1989b). The beneficial outcomes of the Arthritis Self-Management Course are not adequately explained by behavior change. *Arthritis and Rheumatism* **32**, 91–5.

Lorig, K., Gonzalez, V.M., and Ritter, P. (1999a). Community-based Spanish language arthritis education program. A randomized trial. *Medical Care* **9**, 957–63.

Lorig, K. et al. (1999b). Evidence suggesting that a chronic disease self-management program can improve health status while reducing hospitalization. *Medical Care* **37**, 5–14.

Lorish, C.D., Abraham, N., and Austin, J.E.A. (1991). Disease and psychosocial factors related to physical functioning in rheumatoid arthritis. *Journal of Rheumatology* **18**, 1150–7.

McFarlane, A.C. and Brooks, P. (1988). An analysis of the relationship between psychological morbidity and disease activity in rheumatoid arthritis. *Journal of Rheumatology* **15**, 926–31.

McKinley, P., Ouellette, S.C., and Winkel, G. (1995). The contributions of disease activity, sleep patterns, and depression to fatigue in systemic lupus erythematosus. *Arthritis and Rheumatism* **38**, 826–34.

Manne, S. and Zautra, A. (1989). Spouse criticism and support: their association with coping and psychological adjustment among women with rheumatoid arthritis. *Journal of Personal and Social Psychology* **56**, 608–17.

Manne, S. and Zautra, A. (1990). Couples coping with chronic illness: women with rheumatoid arthritis and their healthy husbands. *Journal of Behavioural Medicine* **13**, 327–43.

Martin, J., Meltzer, H., and Elliott, D. *The Prevalence of Disability Among Adults.* London: HMSO, 1988.

Melzack, R. (1975). The McGill Pain Questionnaire—major properties and scoring methods. *Pain* **1**, 277–99.

Mitchell, J., Burkhauser, R., and Pincus, T. (1988). The importance of age, education and comorbidity in the substantial earnings losses of individuals with symmetric polyarthritis. *Arthritis and Rheumatism* **31**, 348–57.

Mullen, P.D., Laville, E.A., Biddle, A.K., and Lorig, K. (1987). Efficacy of psychoeducational interventions on pain, depression, and disability in people with arthritis: a meta-analysis. *Journal of Rheumatology* **14** (Suppl. 15), 33–9.

Murphy, S. et al. (1988). Psychiatric disorder and illness behaviour in rheumatoid arthritis. *British Journal of Rheumatology* **27**, 357–63.

Newman, S. and Revenson, T.A. (1993). Coping with rheumatoid arthritis. In *Psychological Aspects of Rheumatic Disease (Vol. 7) (Issue 2) Baillière's Clinical Rheumatology* (ed. S. Newman and M. Shipley), pp. 259–80. London: Baillière Tindall.

Newman, S.P., Fitzpatrick, R., Lamb, R., and Shipley, M. (1989). The origins of depressed mood in rheumatoid arthritis. *Journal of Rheumatology* **16**, 740–4.

Newman, S. et al. (1990). Patterns of coping in rheumatoid arthritis. *Psychology and Health* **4**, 187–200.

Newman, S., Fitzpatrick, R., Revenson, T.A., Skevington, S., and Williams, G. *Understanding Rheumatoid Arthritis.* London: Routledge, 1996.

Papageorgiou, A.C. and Badley, E.M. (1989). The quality of pain in arthritis: the words patients use to describe overall pain and pain in individual joints at rest and on movement. *Journal of Rheumatology* **16**, 106.

Parker, J. et al. (1988a). Pain in rheumatoid arthritis: relationship to demographic medical and psychological factors. *Journal of Rheumatology* **15**, 433.

Parker, J. et al. (1988b). Coping strategies in rheumatoid arthritis. *Journal of Rheumatology* **15**, 1376–83.

Partridge, A.J. et al. (1997). Risk factors for early work disability in systemic lupus erythematosus: results from a multicenter study. *Arthritis and Rheumatism* **40**, 2199–206.

Peterson, L.S., Mason, T., Nelson, A.M., O'Fallon, W.M., and Gabriel, S.E. (1997). Psychosocial outcomes and health status of adults who have had juvenile rheumatoid arthritis. *Arthritis and Rheumatism* **40**, 2235–40.

Pincus, T. and Callahan, L.F.C. (1985). Formal education as a marker for increased mortality and morbidity in rheumatoid arthritis. *Journal of Chronic Diseases* **38**, 973–84.

Reisine, S., Goodenow, C., and Grady, K. (1987). The impact of rheumatoid arthritis on the homemaker. *Social Science and Medicine* **25**, 89–96.

Revenson, T.A., Schiaffino, K.M., Majerovitz, S.D., and Gibofsky, A. (1991). Social support as a double-edged sword: the relation of positive and problematic support to depression among rheumatoid arthritis patients. *Social Science and Medicine* **33**, 801–13.

Rhee, S.H. et al. (2000). Stress management in rheumatoid arthritis: what is the underlying mechanism? *Arthritis Care and Research* **13**, 435–42.

Rhind, V.M., Bird, H.A., and Wright, V. (1980). Comparison of clinical assessments of disease activity in rheumatoid arthritis. *Annals of the Rheumatic Diseases* **39**, 135–7.

Sensky, T. and Catalan, J. (1992). Asking patients about their treatment. *British Medical Journal* **305**, 1109–10.

Shoor, S.M. and Holman, H.R. (1984). Development of an instrument to explore psychological mediators of outcome in chronic arthritis. *Transactions of the Association of American Physicians* **97**, 325–31.

Shortall, E., Isenberg, D., and Newman, S.P. (1995). Factors associated with mood and mood disorders in SLE. *Lupus* **4**, 272–9.

Smedstad, L. et al. (1995). The relationship between pain and sociodemographic variables, anxiety, and depressive symptoms in rheumatoid arthritis. *Journal of Rheumatology* **22**, 514–20.

Smedstad, L.M., Vaglum, P., Moum, T., and Kvien, T.K. (1997). The relationship between psychological distress and traditional clinical variables: a 2 year prospective study of 216 patients with early rheumatoid arthritis. *British Journal of Rheumatology* **36**, 1304–11.

Smith, C.A., Dobbins, C.J., and Wallston, K.A. (1991). The mediational role of perceived competence in psychological adjustment to rheumatoid arthritis. *Journal of Applied Social Psychology* **21**, 1218–47.

Spiegel, J. et al. (1988). What are we measuring? An examination of self-reported functional status measures. *Arthritis and Rheumatism* **31**, 721–8.

Steinbrocker, O., Traeger, C., and Battman, R. (1949). Therapeutic criteria in rheumatoid arthritis. *Journal of the American Medical Association* **140**, 659–62.

Taal, E. et al.(1993). Health status, adherence with health recommendations, self-efficacy and social support in patients with rheumatoid arthritis. Special issue: psychosocial aspects of rheumatic diseases. *Patient Education and Counseling* **20**, 63–76.

Taal, E., Riemsma, R.P., Brus, H.L.M., Seydel, E.R., Rasker, J.J., and Wiegman, O. (1993). Group education for patients with rheumatoid arthritis. *Patient Education and Counseling* **20**, 177–87.

Taal, E., Rasker, J.J., and Wiegman, O. (1997). Group education for rheumatoid arthritis patients. *Seminars in Arthritis and Rheumatism* **26**, 805–16.

Tack, B. (1990). Fatigue in rheumatoid arthritis. *Arthritis Care and Research* **3**, 65–70.

Tennen, H. et al. (1992). Perceiving control, construing benefits, and daily processes in rheumatoid arthritis. *Canadian Journal of the Behavioral Sciences* **24**, 186–203.

Thompson, P.W. and Pegley, F.S. (1991). A comparison of disability measured by the Stanford Health Assessment Questionnaire disability scales (HAQ) in male and female rheumatoid outpatients. *British Journal of Rheumatology* **30**, 298–300.

Volle, B., Wiedenbusch, S., and Lohaus, A. (1990). Psychological correlates of self help group membership in patients with rheumatic diseases. *Psychotherapie, Psychosomatik Medizinische Psychologie* **40**, 230–7.

Wagstaff, S., Smith, O.V, and Wood, P.H.N. (1985). Verbal pain descriptors used by patients with arthritis. *Annals of the Rheumatic Diseases* **44**, 262–5.

Wallston, K. (1993). Psychological control and its impact in the management of rheumatological disorders. In *Psychological Aspects of Rheumatic Disease; Baillière's Clinical Rheumatology* Vol. 7, Part 2 (ed. S. Newman and M. Shipley), pp. 281–95. London: Baillière Tindall.

Wallston, K.A., Wallston, B., and DeVellis, R.F. (1978). Development of the multidimensional health locus of control scale (MHLC). *Health Education Monographs* **6**, 160–70.

Ward, M. and Leigh, P. (1993). Marital status and the progression of functional disability in patients with rheumatoid arthritis. *Arthritis and Rheumatism* **36**, 581–92.

Ward, M.M. and Kuzis, S. (2001). Risk factors for work disability in patients with ankylosing spondylitis. *Journal of Rheumatology* **28**, 315–21.

White, P. and Shear, E.S. (1992). Transition/job readiness for adolescents with juvenile arthritis and other chronic illness. *Journal of Rheumatology* **19**, 23–7.

Williams, G.H. (1987). Disablement and the social context of daily activity. *International Disability Studies* **9**, 97–102.

Williams, G.H. and Wood, P.H.N. (1988). Coming to terms with chronic illness: the negotiation of autonomy in rheumatoid arthritis. *International Disability Studies* **10**, 128–32.

Wills, T.A. (1987). Downward comparison as a coping mechanism. In *Coping with Negative Life Events* (ed. C.R. Snyder and C.E. Ford), pp. 243–68. New York: Plenum.

Wolfe, F. (1999). Psychological distress and rheumatic disease. *Scandanavian Journal of Rheumatology* **28**, 131–6.

Wolfe, F. and Cathey, M. (1991). The assessment and prediction of functional disability in rheumatoid arthritis. *Journal of Rheumatology* **18**, 1298–306.

Wolfe, F. and Hawley, D.J. (1998). The longterm outcomes of rheumatoid arthritis: work disability: a prospective 18 year study of 823 patients. *Journal of Rheumatology* **25**, 2108–17.

Wolfe, F. and Skevington, S.M. (2000). Measuring the epidemiology of distress: the rheumatology distress index. *Journal of Rheumatology* **27**, 2000–9.

Wolfe, F., Hawley, D.J., and Wilson, K. (1996). The prevalence and meaning of fatigue in rheumatic disease. *Journal of Rheumatology* **23**, 1407–17.

Yelin, E. et al. (1980). Work disability in rheumatoid arthritis: effects of disease, social and work factors. *Annals of Internal Medicine* **93**, 551–6.

1.1.7 Growth and skeletal maturation

Fabrizio De Benedetti, Mohamad Maghnie, and Alberto Martini

Normal growth

Normal growth is a complex process that involves a number of interacting forces, including genetic mechanisms, tissue-specific factors, hormone regulators, nutrition, psycho-social and economic influences.

Despite the fact that the growth process is multifactorial, children normally grow in a remarkably predictable manner. Deviation from a normal pattern of growth represents a primary and important manifestation of a wide variety of disease processes involving both endocrine and non-endocrine organs. The accurate assessment of growth is therefore of cardinal importance in the care of children.

Growth stages

Growth occurs at different rates during intrauterine life, infancy, childhood, and adolescence prior to its cessation with the attainment of adult stature, sexual maturation, and reproductive function. During the embryonic period the foetus grows primarily by a cellular multiplication showing an extraordinary and spectacular linear growth rates (MacGillivray 1995; Reiter and Rosenfeld 1998). The size of full-term newborn is influenced by the size of the mother, the uterine size, the placenta organ, and gender. Any disturbance of early placental growth due to embryologic abnormalities, infections, or vascular insults may cause permanent growth retardation. The linear growth and weight gain continue at a remarkable rate during the first year of life with a deceleration and stabilization by the age of 2 years at a rate which is characteristic of the childhood years. Adolescence is the last period of major growth being the time of onset of puberty highly variable in healthy children, reflecting the concept of a 'tempo of growth' or rate of maturation, as emphasized by Tanner (1990).

Testicular enlargement is followed by the onset of penis growth while pubic hair appears at approximately 12.5–13 years; the first signs of axillary and facial hair occur between 14.5 and 15 years. The first ejaculation of seminal fluid and nocturnal emissions occur at approximately 14 years of age. Adult height in males is usually attained by age 18, growth cessation occurs first in the hands and feet, followed by the legs, trunk, and shoulder girdle (Reiter and Rosenfeld 1998). About two-thirds of girls start to develop breasts at the average of 11 years before pubic hair growth commences, but the remainder show pubic hair growth first or at the same time. Pubic hair development is more rapid, averaging 2.5 years to reach the adult form. Development of the mature breast takes an average of 4 years. Menarche most commonly occurs in Tanner Stage 4, but in one-fourth of girls occurs in Stage 3 (Tanner 1990). The age of peak height velocity is relatively earlier in the course of puberty in girls and nearly always precedes the menarche, but by a rather variable interval which averages about a year.

Measurement of growth

Length and height

Assessment of growth requires accurate and reproducible determinations of height. Supine length is routinely measured in children less than 2 years of age and standing height is assessed in older children. The inaccuracies in measuring length in infants are often obscured by the rapid skeletal growth during this period. For measurement of supine length, it is best to use a firm box with an inflexible board against which the head lies, with a movable footboard on which the feet are placed perpendicular to the plane of the supine length of the infant. Optimally, the legs should be fully extended, and the head should be positioned in the 'Frankfort plane', with the line connecting the outer canthus of the eyes and the external auditory meatus perpendicular to the long axis of the trunk (Buckler 1997).

In children able to stand independently, the Harpenden stadiometer is the best readily available instrument. It has a rigid horizontal wooden headboard which moves up and down a rigid backboard on miniature rollers and has a display counter from which the observer can read the height directly. However, if alternative equipment must be used, a rigid horizontal wooden headboard must be incorporated. The traditional measuring device of a flexible arm mounted to a weight balance is notoriously unreliable and does not provide accurate serial measurements. The technique for measuring height is also of critical importance. The subject's shoes and socks must be removed, not only because they will affect the height of the subject but also they may conceal slight raising of the heels. The child should be fully erect, with the head in the 'Frankfort plane'; the back of the head, thoracic spine, buttocks, and heels should touch the vertical axis of the stadiometer, and the heels should be together. While the subject is in this position, he is instructed to take a deep breath and stand tall while keeping his heels flat on the ground. Height determinations should be performed by a trained individual, ideally at the same time of day and by the same one to eliminate interobserver variability, because standing height may undergo diurnal variation as much as 20 mm (Strickland and Shearin 1972). Lengths and height should be measured in triplicate with a variation of less than 3 mm; the mean height is recorded. Height velocity at a minimum interval of 6 months is advisable for meaningful computation. Data gathered over 12 months is preferable so that seasonal variation of growth rate is included.

Sitting height

The most accurate means of measuring sitting height is by using the Harpenden sitting height table. This equipment is usually considered too expensive and a cheaper alternative is an anthropometer (Harpenden). Sitting height is an appropriate alternative in the subjects with muscle weakness, hip, and/or knee contracture or disproportionate growth (spine deformity, vertebral collapses, etc.). To obtain the actual sitting height, the height of the sitting platform is subtracted from the total height of the subject sitting upon it. Published standards exist for the body proportion measurements, which must be evaluated to the patient's age (Tanner 1990).

Growth charts

Evaluation of a child's height must be performed in the context of normal standards. The growth assessment in a clinical setting is most commonly related to the Tanner–Whitehouse standards for British children or to the standards for American children. Most American paediatric endocrine clinics continue to use the cross-sectional data provided by the National Center for Health statistics (Reiter and Rosenfeld 1998). These data are useful in computing standard deviation (SD) scores, which are more helpful. A height SD score for age is calculated as follows: SD scores equal height minus mean height for normal children at this age and sex divided by the SD of height for normal children at this age and sex. The reference curves for stature, length and weight most widely used in the United Kingdom were based on data published in 1966 (Tanner 1990). New charts have recently been published based on data acquired since 1980 by Freeman et al. (1995). They have the additional advantage of being more nationally representative as the measurements were derived from seven UK sources on white children; unfortunately these new charts are based exclusively on cross-sectional data, which do not demonstrate the growth pattern typical of the individual at the time of rapidly changing growth rate in puberty. A number of European countries also have their own national standards.

Skinfold measurements

Skinfold callipers are used for these measurements which show the thickness of subcutaneous tissue and reflect primarily fat. The Holtain and Harpenden varieties apply a constant pressure of 10 g/mm^2 over a measuring range of 0–48 mm and the measurements can be estimated to 0.1 mm. The most commonly measured sites are the triceps and subscapular which probably reflect best the body fat component as a whole. The triceps skinfold is measured at a marked midpoint in the mid-posterior line of the left upper arm between the acromion and the olecranon processes with the arm extended and hanging loosely at the side. The subscapular measurement is estimated, taking a vertical skinfold, directly below the angle of the left scapula. This technique is not easy mastered and is subject to error even with very skilled operators.

Accuracy with experienced observers is of the order of ± 5 per cent but readings vary considerably with different observers. Serial observations should preferably be undertaken by the same person. Percentile charts for boys and girls for triceps and subscapular skinfolds have been already reported (Buckler 1997).

Body mass index

This index, which derived by dividing the weight in kilograms by the square of the height in metres, is a reasonable index of the degree of fatness of an adult individual. Although extremes of high or low body mass index (BMI) are likely to be indicative of excessive obesity or leanness in children, lesser deviations do not necessarily have this implication and interpretation of the values must be cautious. BMI in the growing child must be evaluated on the basis of centile charts, and British charts have been recently published (Cole et al. 1995). A number of European countries have their own national standards. These BMI charts are based on cross-sectional data and, as with height, the normal child's values will not adhere to a centile through puberty.

Pubertal development

Assessment of pubertal development has been made systematic by Tanner (1990) in such a thorough and practical fashion that it has become the standard for assessment worldwide (Tables 1 and 2). Assessment of the stage of pubertal development is enormously important, not only for the recognition of large changes in the size and functional structure of the reproductive organs themselves, but also the major changes in hormonal and growth potential associated with the various pubertal stages. The interpretation of pubertal staging is somewhat subjective and imprecise, and reports from different centres show considerable variations. There is great variation not only in the ages at which stages of puberty take place, but also in their duration and in the order in which they occur.

The first signs of puberty in females are the appearance of breast buds and the beginning of growth spurt at the average of 11 years of age followed by the pubic hair at 11.5 years, menarche at 12.5 years, and axillary hair at 12.5–13 years. This latter almost invariably occurs after the attainment of peak growth velocity observed at 12 years. Slower rates of linear growth continue after menarche until age 16–17 years, when epiphyseal fusion occurs. Unlike females, the sequence of physiologic events and their relation to the hormonal changes are different in males who begin their growth spurt approximately 1 year after the first signs of testicular enlargement and achieve greater peak at age 14. In the average male, testicular size increases at age 12 years and represents, together with axillary sweat and body odour, the first signs of adolescence.

This can be quantitatively assessed by comparison with a Prader orchidometer (Zachmann et al. 1974), either visually or by palpation. The information required is merely whether the testis has grown to a larger than pre-pubertal size (1–4 ml) and a testis volume over 4 ml is the first indication that puberty has started.

Table 1 Stages of puberty in females as described by Tanner

Tanner stage	Pubic hair	Breast development
1	No pubic hair	Pre-adolescent
2	Sparse growth of slightly pigmented downy hair chiefly along the labia	Breast bud stage. Elevation of the breast and papilla as a small mound. Enlargement of the areola diameter
3	Hair darker, coarser, and more curled, spreading sparsely over the junction of the pubes	Further enlargement and elevation of the breast and areola, with no separation of their contours
4	Hair adult type, but covering a considerably smaller area than adult. No spread to the medial surface of the thighs	Projection of the areola and papilla above the level of the breast
5	Adult feminine triangle and spread to the medial surface of the thighs	Mature stage, projection of the papilla alone due to recession of the areola

Table 2 Stages of puberty in males as described by Tanner

Tanner stage	Pubic hair	Genital development stage
1	No pubic hair	The testes, scrotum, and penis are about the same size and proportions as in early childhood
2	Sparse growth of slightly pigmented downy hair chiefly at the base of the penis	Enlargement of the scrotum and testes. The skin of the scrotum reddens and changes in texture. Little or no enlargement of the penis
3	Hair darker, coarser, and more curled, spreading sparsely over the junction of the pubes	Lengthening of the penis. Further growth of the testes and scrotum
4	Hair adult type, but covering a considerably smaller area than adult. No spread to the medial surface of the thighs	Increase in breadth of the penis and development of the glans. The testes and scrotum are larger; the scrotum darkens
5	Adult distribution, spread to the medial surface of the thighs	Adult size

Skeletal maturation/height prediction/target height

The skeletal maturation (bone age) can be assessed by evaluation of the size, shape, and the ossification centres in the epiphyses. To minimize X-ray exposure, the left hand is the most commonly used for radiographic study. The carpal, metacarpal, and phalangeal epiphyses are compared with the published standards of Greulich and Pyle (1959) obtained on healthy children at different ages. It is not clear what factors determine this normal maturational pattern, but genes and hormones are involved. In children with mineralization problems, skeletal dysplasia, chronic articular inflammation, cautious interpretation of bone age is advisable.

Prediction of estimated adult height based on bone age and height can be made from the Bayley and Pinneau predictive tables (Bayley and Pinneau 1952). Height prediction cannot be made accurately in children with pathologic growth, or chronic inflammation or treated with corticosteroids.

Since genetic factors are important determinants of growth and height potential, it is useful to assess a patient's stature relative to that of siblings and parents by the midparental height (Tanner 1990). The child's predicted adult height may be related to a 'parental target height' namely the mean parental height with the addition or substraction of 6.5 cm for boys and girls, respectively. The 2 SD range for this calculated parental target height is about $\pm$10 cm.

Hormonal control of growth processes

In infancy, growth is primarily dependent on nutrition, whereas during childhood growth hormone (GH) is the major determinant of growth. Sex hormones and GH control the adolescent growth spurt. Normal thyroid function is essential to each of these stages of growth. Insulin and glucocorticoids influence carbohydrate, fat, and protein metabolism; provide sources of energy needed for growth; and exert a permissive influence on the anabolic actions of GH.

The GH secretion is regulated primarily by two hypothalamic hormones; somatostatin (SRIH) which inhibits, and growth hormone releasing hormone (GHRH) which stimulates GH secretion. Release of the hypothalamic hormones is in turn regulated by biogenic amines derived from neurosecretory neurons in the central nervous system. The pulsatile pattern characteristic of GH secretion largely reflects the combination of a rise in GHRH and a decline in SRIH. The synthesis and secretion of GH are also regulated by the insulin-like growth factor (IGF) peptides.

Under physiologic conditions, the pituitary gland secretes approximately eight discrete peaks of GH every day. In children and young adults, approximately 50–75 per cent of the daily production of GH occurs during the early night-time hours that follow the onset of deep sleep. Approximately 50 per cent of GH in circulation is bound to a high-affinity GH binding protein (GHBP) which is identical to the extracellular domain of the GH receptor. Most of the remaining GH in circulation is free.

Growth hormone actions

The physiological actions of GH are pleiotropic and involve multiple organs and physiological systems. GH exerts many metabolic effects that persist throughout life. GH is essentially an anabolic hormone, inducing positive nitrogen balance and protein synthesis in muscle. Because GH enhances amino acid uptake into skeletal muscle, it has been suggested that this tissue is the primary target of the physiological effects of GH; it remains controversial whether the effects of GH on nitrogen balance are direct or mediated by IGF-I. Systemic administration of GH stimulates longitudinal bone growth and skeletal muscle growth, whereas treatment with IGF-I increases the size of lymphoid tissues (spleen and thymus) and kidney. GH has a more robust effect than IGF-I on longitudinal bone growth in animals, and the effects of these factors may be additive (Le Roith et al. 2001).

GH has a lipolytic action on fat and muscle, whereby circulating FFA and glycerol levels rise after acute administration of GH. This effect is apparently mediated by the inhibition of lipoprotein lipase, an enzyme involved in lipid accumulation in adipocytes, and represents a major effect of GH on metabolic intermediates (Ottosson et al. 1991). GH administration also causes mild reductions in low-density lipoprotein cholesterol levels and small elevations in high-density lipoprotein cholesterol.

Evidence for synthesis of GH in a number of extrapituitary sites, including the lateral hypothalamus, lymphocytes, thymocytes, neutrophils, the placenta, and both normal and neoplastic tissue has been reported. These findings suggest that GH may have local paracrine/autocrine effects that might be distinct from, or in addition to, its classic effects that are known to be mediated by circulating IGF-I (Le Roith et al. 2001).

The IGF system

According to the somatomedin hypothesis, the anabolic actions of GH are mediated through the IGF peptides (Daughaday and Rotwein 1989). IGF-I is a member of the IGF family of growth factors and related molecules. The IGF family comprises ligands (IGF-I, IGF-II, and insulin), six well characterized binding proteins (IGFBP-1 through -6), and cell surface receptors that mediate the actions of the ligands (IGF-I receptor, insulin receptor, and the IGF-II mannose-6-phosphate receptor).

IGF-I plays an important role in both embryonic and post-natal growth. Mice carrying null mutations in the IGF-I gene are born small and grow very poorly post-natally. Since GH and GH receptor gene-deleted mice have relatively normal birth weights, this strongly supports a GH-independent effect of IGF-I in embryonic growth. Moreover, plasma IGF-I levels in humans correlate with body size. Infusions of rhIGF-I also enhance body weight and size in a number of models, further suggesting a role for circulating IGF-I in growth (Le Roith et al. 2001).

Naturally occurring mutations in the IGF system have proved to be extremely rare. A single patient with both intrauterine and post-natal growth retardation has been found with a deletion of the IGF-I gene (Woods et al. 1996). Since the low levels of circulating IGF-I are associated with high GH levels, this strongly supports the somatomedin hypothesis. Recent experiments using transgenic and gene-deletion technologies have attempted to answer many of the questions about the role of circulating IGF-I. In the liver-specific IGF-I gene-deleted mouse model, post-natal growth and development are normal despite the marked reduction in circulating IGF-I and IGF-binding protein levels (Le Roith et al. 2001). In plasma, the majority of the IGFs exist as 150 kDa complex composed of the IGF molecule, IGF binding protein 3, and the acid labile subunit. The inactivation of both liver IGF-I and the acid labile sub-unit genes cause a marked reduction in serum IGF-I and post-natal growth retardation demonstrating that plasma IGF-I is needed for normal growth (Yakar et al. 2001).

Thyroid hormone and gonadal steroids

Thyroid hormone by itself does not fulfil the criteria needed to classify it as true growth-promoting hormone because it is unable to stimulate cellular multiplication directly if growth hormone is absent. Nevertheless, the importance of these hormones has been demonstrated in studies which showed that maximal GH stimulation of tissues requires the presence of thyroxine. Thus, normal thyroid function is a fundamental requirement for a normal growth process.

The growth spurt of puberty is dependent mainly on gonadal steroids and GH; adrenal steroids are probably not essential. Studies indicate that males experience rapid growth during puberty because of androgen-mediated enhancement of GH secretion; this in turn stimulates increased production of IGF-I and accounts for the elevated levels observed in adolescence (Parker et al. 1984). Oestrogens have less growth-promoting capacity than androgens, yet are capable of accelerating the pace of osseous maturation.

Growth abnormalities in juvenile idiopathic arthritis

Growth abnormalities occur frequently in childhood rheumatic diseases. They may be secondary to the inflammatory process as well as to the treatment with glucocorticoids. While in patients with diseases such as juvenile dermatomyositis or systemic lupus erythematosus treatment with glucocorticoids are usually the main factor responsible for growth retardation, the abnormalities of growth in patients with juvenile idiopathic arthritis (JIA), and in particular with the systemic onset form, may be secondary to both mechanisms.

Growth disturbances are frequent complications of JIA and have been noted in many early studies. A 'general arrest of somatic growth' has been reported in the original description of the disease by G.F. Still in 1897, and later was re-emphasized by a study by Kuhns and Swaim, who described three types of growth disorders in JIA: generalized retardation of body growth, persistence of infantile proportions and asymmetry of growth (Kuhns and Swaim 1932).

Local disturbance in growth

Local disturbance of growth occurs at sites of inflammation resulting in either overgrowth or undergrowth of the juxta-articular bone. Overgrowth is due to accelerated development of ossification centres, possibly related to inflammation-induced increased vascularization and growth factor release. Undergrowth is secondary to growth centre damage or premature fusion of epiphyseal plates. Anomalies in growth and morphogenesis of skeletal segments are a peculiar aspect of childhood chronic arthritis and result not only from inflammation of joints and periarticular tissues but also from anomalous traction, on growing structures, secondary to muscular spasm and periarticular fibrosis. They are worse in children with early onset of arthritis and active disease.

Overgrowth is particularly common in the lower limbs, and less frequent in the wrists. Asymmetric knee involvement often results in lengthening of the affected leg with leg-length inequality (Fig. 1). Proper recognition and treatment of this discrepancy is important because, if left untreated, it can result in compensatory, functional scoliosis of the spine. Enlargement and squaring of the epiphyses is common at carpal and tarsal level.

Undergrowth may involve several sites. When extremities are involved, it may be symmetric resulting in small hands or feet, or it may be isolated with selective brachydactyly. Arthritis of the wrist may cause growth failure of the ulnar head with shortened ulna and ulnar deviation of the carpus. Unilateral involvement of the temporomandibular joint may result in mandibular asymmetry, and bilateral involvement may cause marked micrognatia (Fig. 2). Similarly, involvement of the cervical spine, which is frequent in patients with JIA, may cause undergrowth of the vertebral bodies resulting ultimately in a short neck. A characteristic developmental anomaly of the hip is often observed in children with early onset of arthritis. It includes enlargement and flattening of the femoral head, incompletely covered by an underdeveloped acetabulum, and a short, squat, valgus, and anteverted femoral neck.

Generalized disturbance in growth

Decrease in linear growth occurs during periods of active disease, particularly in severe systemic JIA. Treatment with glucocorticoids, at high doses

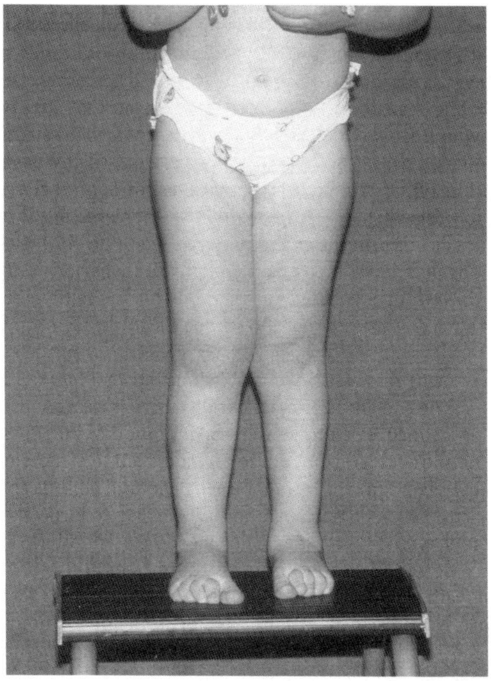

Fig. 1 Leg-length inequality due to persistent arthritis of the right knee with subsequent overgrowth of the right leg.

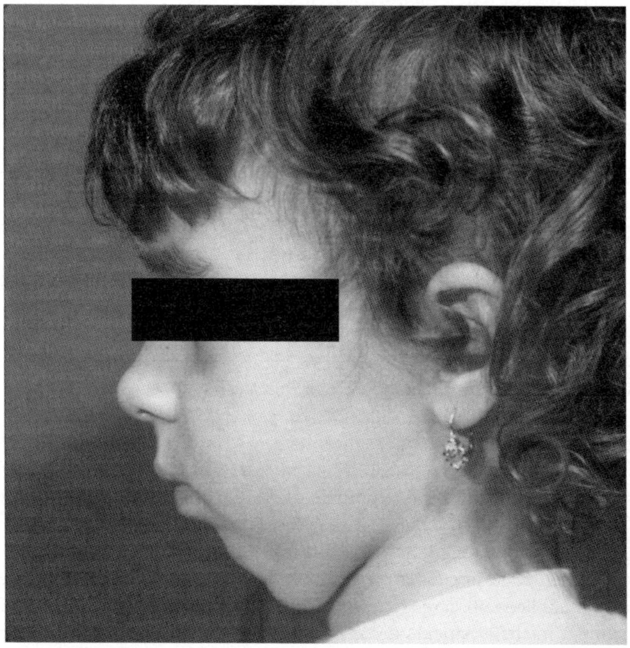

Fig. 2 Arthritis of both temporomandibular joints resulting in micrognatia and retrognatia with an anterior open underbite.

and for prolonged periods of time, also results in growth impairment. Although catch-up growth may occur during remission, children that have undergone prolonged arrest or retardation of growth rarely return to their previous growth percentile; therefore growth retardation may be a permanent sequela in children with very active disease.

In 1956, Ansell and Bywaters found that in patients with JIA decreased linear growth was associated with long duration of active disease even in patients not receiving glucocorticoids (Ansell and Bywaters 1956). Treatment with glucocorticoids worsened this problem. These findings were confirmed by Laaksonen (1966). The frequency and severity of growth retardation is variable in different series. A follow-up evaluation of JIA patients at 5–7.5 years showed that approximately 30 per cent of them were below the third percentile (Bernstein et al. 1977). The growth defect appears to be particularly frequent in patients with systemic or severe polyarticular JIA, while it is significantly less common in oligoarticular JIA (Bacon and White 1987). In a study on adults who had been affected with JIA, short stature (less than fifth percentile) was observed in 50 per cent of patients with systemic JIA and in 16 per cent of those with polyarticular JIA (Lovell and White 1991). Similarly, Bernstein et al. (1977) found the highest degree of growth failure in systemic JIA.

Growth hormone and IGF studies in JIA

Studies of growth hormone secretion in patients with JIA generally report normal GH secretion (Sturge et al. 1970; Butenandt et al. 1974; Allen et al. 1991; Touati et al. 1998; Al-Mutair et al. 2000). Study of 24-h GH secretion in children with JIA and severe growth retardation revealed normal pulsatile patterns of GH secretion, and the mean and median levels were comparable to that of healthy children with short stature (Davies et al. 1994).

Levels of IGF-I JIA are reduced or normal (Bennett et al. 1988; Allen et al. 1991; Davies et al. 1994). In a study of 15 systemic JIA patients and 79 normal children, the serum IGF-I level was lower than the mean normal values for age, irrespective of steroid therapy (Bennett et al. 1988). Furthermore, IGF-I showed a significant negative correlation with erythrocyte sedimentation rate as a measure of disease activity but no correlation with growth rate. In contrast, in the study by Aitman et al. (1989) of 32 children with JIA with growth ranging from normal to severe retardation, serum IGF levels showed significant correlation with height and to lesser extent with height velocity. Like IGF-I, reduced IGFBP-3 levels have been reported in children with juvenile chronic arthritis (Davies et al. 1997; Touati et al. 1998).

Inflammatory cytokines and growth

Several observations suggest that a factor produced during inflammation is responsible for the growth defect, and for the abnormalities in the IGF-I system. In addition to the previously mentioned association of growth retardation with long lasting active disease, Ansell and Bywaters (1956) found that many of the younger children showed normal or even accelerated growth during remission and that they could even reach normal height if premature epiphyseal fusion had not occurred. Bernstein et al. (1977) compared the growth rate in patients with systemic JIA and in patients with systemic lupus erythematosus treated with equivalent dose of glucocorticoids and found that the former had significantly more growth impairment. More recently patients with JIA treated with recombinant growth hormone the growth velocity during treatment was satisfactory in under 50 per cent of the patients and was inversely correlated with C-reactive protein concentrations (Davies et al. 1994). The direct link between chronic inflammation and stunted growth has been demonstrated by the observation that transgenic mice who overexpress the proinflammatory cytokine IL-6 show a marked decrease in growth rate leading to a 30–50 per cent reduction in the adult size (De Benedetti et al. 1997). Increased levels of IL-6 are found in patients with JIA. Prominent production of IL-6 is a characteristic feature of systemic JIA, the JIA onset form in which growth retardation is by far more frequent, and appears to explain several, if not all, the clinical and laboratory manifestation of the disease (De Benedetti and Martini 1998).

The effect of IL-6, as well as of other proinflammatory cytokines (see below), on somatic growth may be mediated through effects on the GH/IGF-I axis. Indeed, IL-6 transgenic mice with a growth defect have abnormalities of the IGF-I system similar to those present in patients with systemic JIA (Table 3) (De Benedetti et al. 1997, 2001). This supports a relationship between abnormalities of the IGF-I system and increased IL-6 production. An inverse correlation of IL-6 levels with IGF-I and IGFBP-3 levels has been found in patients with systemic JIA (De Benedetti et al. 1997, 2001).

Table 3 The GH/IGF-I system in the IL-6 transgenic mice with growth defect and in children with systemic juvenile idiopathic arthritis (s-JIA), Crohn's disease (Crohn's), cystic fibrosis (CF), and with AIDS. *In vivo* effects of the inflammatory cytokines interleukin-6 (IL-6), interleukin-1 (IL-1), and tumour necrosis factor (TNF) on the GH/IGF-I system in experimental animals

	IL-6 transgenic mice	s-JIA	Crohn's	CF	AIDS	IL-6	IL-1	TNF
GH levels	Normal	Normal	Normal	Normal	Normal/low	Normal	Unknown	Normal
IGF-I levels	Decreased	Decreased	Decreased	Decreased	Decreased	Decreased	Decreased	Decreased
ALS levels	Normal	Normal	Decreased	Decreased	Decreased	Normal	Decreased	Unknown
IGFBP-3 levels	Decreased	Decreased	Normal	Unknown	Unknown	Decreased	Normal	Normal
IGFBP-3 proteolysis	Increased	Increased	Increased	Unknown	Increased	Increased	Normal	Normal

Experiments in the IL-6 transgenic mice have shown that the decrease in IGF-I levels is not due to decreased liver IGF-I production, but rather to shortened half-life. This is secondary to impaired formation of the heterotrimeric complex comprising IGF-I, IGFBP-3, and the acid labile subunit (ALS), which constitutes a long-lasting reservoir of circulating IGF-I. Impaired formation of the complex is due to the reduction in intact active IGFBP-3. The reduction in IGFBP-3 appears to be secondary to proteolytic degradation by a metalloproteinase directly induced by IL-6 (De Benedetti et al. 2001).

Overproduction of IL-6 may represent a generalized mechanism by which chronic inflammation affects growth. Indeed, in addition to JIA, stunted growth is a complication of other chronic inflammatory diseases or of diseases characterized by severe recurrent infections, such as Crohn's disease, cystic fibrosis, chronic granulomatous disease, and AIDS. In these conditions, growth impairment was found to be associated with the inflammatory activity of the disease or with the severity and frequency of infections. Increased IL-6 production has been demonstrated in AIDS and in Crohn's disease, and evaluation of the GH/IGF-I axis has shown abnormalities similar to those found in systemic JIA and in the IL-6 transgenic mice (Beattie et al. 1998; Bannerjee et al. 2000; De Martino et al. 2000) (Table 3).

Incidentally, in addition to IL-6, IL-1 and tumour necrosis factor (TNF) affect the GH/IGF-I axis as well. However, the abnormalities of the GH/IGF-I axis induced by IL-1 or TNF are different from those induced by IL-6 (De Benedetti et al. 1997, 2001) (Table 3) and moreover there does not exist, to the best of our knowledge, an animal model that, in the same way as for IL-6, can prove a link between stunted growth and a chronic overproduction of IL-1 and/or TNF-α.

Besides their effects on growth through endocrine mechanisms via the GH/IGF-I axis the inflammatory response may also affect the processes of bone formation at the cartilage plate. The formation of bone in cartilage plates is a process involving continuous apposition of bone tissue by osteoblasts and its continuous remodelling by osteoclasts. Factors influencing this equilibrium may affect bone growth. The inflammatory cytokines IL-6, IL-1, and TNF have been shown to induce osteoclast differentiation and activation. Although their role in osteoporosis has been demonstrated both *in vitro* and *in vivo* (Manolagas and Jilka 1995), their effects on bone growth via osteoclast activation and differentiation has yet to be clearly proven. The recent identification of new molecules involved in osteoclast activation and differentiation may also provide the basis for an additional mechanism through which a chronic proinflammatory immune response may affect growth (Suda et al. 2001). Osteoblasts have been shown to express RANKL [receptor activator of nuclear factor (NF)-kappaB ligand], a member of the TNF family, as a membrane bound factor in response to several osteotropic factors. RANKL interacts with RANK [receptor activator of nuclear factor (NF)-kappaB], a TNF receptor family member, expressed by osteoclast precursors and this interaction causes osteoclast differentiation and activation. This interaction is regulated by osteoclastogenesis inhibitory factor (OCIF, also called OPG) which acts as a secreted decoy receptor for RANKL. Recent data suggest that inflammatory cytokines affects the expression of RANK, RANKL, and OPG. Moreover activated T lymphocytes have been shown to express RANKL, and may directly interfere with the cross-talks between osteoblasts and osteoclasts, therefore affecting bone formation (Takayanagi et al. 2000).

Glucocorticoids and growth

Glucocorticoid therapy is an essential treatment modality in various chronic inflammatory and immune-mediated diseases in childhood. Long-term, high-dose glucocorticoid medication in children leads inevitably to growth failure and protein catabolism. Children treated with hydrocortisone for adrenal disorders have growth decline within 3 months when given doses only two or three times greater than the physiologic production rate for cortisol. At prednisone doses more than 0.35 mg/kg day, the growth velocity did not increase during rhGH therapy (Rivkees et al. 1994).

Recent evidence indicates that these effects are partially mediated by alterations at the level of growth hormone secretion, growth receptor expression and the IGF system. The growth-depressing effects of glucocorticoids are certainly multifactorial and involve suppression of pituitary GH release, by stimulating release of somatostatin from the hypothalamus; down-regulation of hepatic GH receptors; inhibition of IGF bioactivity, by the induction of IGF inhibitors; a complex alteration of the IGFBP serum profile; and a direct suppressive effect on tissue matrix production.

GH secretion

Short-term incubation of human pituitary cells with glucocorticoids *in vitro* inhibits the GH release stimulated by GH-releasing hormone (Ceda et al. 1987). Glucocorticoids have also been found to have a dual effect on stimulated GH secretion *in vivo*. Acute administration of glucocorticoids has a permissive effect on GH secretion and it has been used as an alternative test for the diagnosis of GH deficiency. In contrast, chronic administration of glucocorticoids leads to a suppression of the pituitary response to most pharmacological and physiological stimulants but not to the arginine-induced GH secretion in humans (Gacs et al. 1973; Miell et al. 1988).

GH receptor

Experimental evidence has shown that long-term exposure to pharmacological doses of glucocorticoids suppresses hepatic GH receptor (GHR) expression. Treatment of uraemic rats and controls with methylprednisolone reduces the levels of circulating GH-binding protein (GHBP) derived from the extracellular domain of the GHR by proteolytic cleavage (Tönshoff et al. 1994).

In patients receiving glucocorticoids after renal transplantation, a significant reduction in circulating GHBP levels compared with age-matched controls has been observed (Tönshoff and Mehls 1994). Subcutaneous GH treatment in these patients did not increase the reduced plasma levels of GHBP suggesting that long-term exposure to glucocorticoids reduces the tissue sensitivity to GH by downregulation of the receptor. Recently it has been demonstrated that dexamethasone regulates GHR expression at several levels. Post-transcriptionally, dexamethasone favours GHR pre-mRNA splicing to truncated GHR mRNA. The latter isoform represents the inactive receptor which lacks the intracellular signalling domain (Vottero et al. 2000).

IGF system

The levels of IGF-I in the serum of children with Cushing's syndrome were reported to be similar to those of age-matched controls, although the growth rate of these patients averaged only 1.4 cm/year (Gourmelen et al. 1982).

Similarly, circulating immunoreactive IGF-I levels in children with renal transplants who are treated with glucocorticoids are within the normal range (Tönshoff et al. 1993). These results indicate that hypercortisolism growth failure cannot simply be attributed to IGF deficiency. Under experimental conditions, 6 days of dexamethasone treatment in rats with an intact pituitary did not change serum IGF-I concentrations, but significantly reduced hepatic and tibial IGF-I mRNA levels (Luo and Murphy 1989). Furthermore, in hypophysectomized rats, pre-treatment with a single dose of dexamethasone reduced GH induction of IGF-I mRNA expression, which is not reflected by changes in serum IGF-I levels (Luo and Murphy 1989).

Although glucocorticoids do not consistently reduce circulating immunoreactive IGF-I levels under clinical conditions, they inhibit serum IGF bioactivity possibly by the induction of IGF inhibitors. The latter, with a molecular weight of 12–20 kDa, differ from IGFBPs in several ways, but have not been fully characterized; they could potentially alter the distribution between the 'free' and 'bound' forms of IGF (Chen et al. 2001).

GH treatment in JIA

There are several studies where growth hormone treatment was used in different treatment regimens in children with JIA and stunted growth (Ward et al. 1966; Sturge et al. 1970; Butenandt et al. 1974; Allen et al. 1991; Svantesson 1991; Davies et al. 1994, 1997; Touati et al. 1998; Al-Mutair et al. 2000). GH treatment was first advocated even before the era of recombinant GH by Ward et al. (1966). An increase of growth velocity was reported in most cases with a great variability between patients. Davies et al. showed significant linear growth of 3–5 cm during 1 year's treatment with GH. GH hormone treatment withdrawal was followed by a return of growth velocity to pre-treatment values (Touati et al. 1998), while sustained growth was reported after 2 years of treatment in a small series of patients (Al-Mutair et al. 2000).

GH treatment seems to be effective in counteracting the harmful effects of glucocorticoid treatment on growth and metabolism in children with JIA without side-effects at the doses used. Several questions, however, are still to be answered including the timing of GH treatment, the dosage, the duration, the long-term safety, and what are the benefits for adult height.

References

Aitman, T.J. et al. (1989). Serum IGF-I levels and growth failure in juvenile chronic arthritis. *Clinical and Experimental Rheumatology* **7**, 557–61.

Allen, R.C. et al. (1991). Insulin-like growth factor and growth hormone secretion in juvenile chronic arthritis. *Annals of the Rheumatic Diseases* **50**, 602–6.

Al-Mutair, A. et al. (2000). Efficacy of recombinant human growth hormone in children with juvenile rheumatoid arthritis and growth failure. *Journal of Pediatric Endocrinology and Metabolism* **13**, 899–905.

Ansell, B.M. and Bywaters, E.G.L. (1956). Growth in Still's disease. *Annals of the Rheumatic Diseases* **15**, 295–319.

Bacon, M.C. and White, P. (1987). A new approach to the assessment of growth in JRA. *Arthritis and Rheumatism* **30**, S132.

Bannerjee, K. et al. (2000). Relationship of changes in IGF-I, IGFBP-3, ALS and leptin to inflammatory and nutritional markers during enteral feeding in children with Crohn's disease. Program of the 39th Annual Meeting of the European Society for Paediatric Endocrinology (ESPE), Brussels, p. 63 (abstract), 2000.

Bayley, N. and Pinneau, S. (1952). Tables for predicting adult height from skeletal age. *Journal of Pediatrics* **40**, 423–41.

Beattie, R.M. et al. (1998). Responsiveness of IGF-I and IGFBP-3 to therapeutic intervention in children and adolescents with Crohn's disease. *Clinical Endocrinology Oxford* **49**, 483–9.

Bennet, A.E. et al. (1988). Insulin-like growth factors I and II in children with systemic onset juvenile arthritis. *Journal of Rheumatology* **15**, 655–8.

Bernstein, B.H. et al. (1977). Growth retardation in juvenile rheumatoid arthritis (JRA). *Arthritis and Rheumatism* **20**, 212–16.

Buckler, J.M.H. *A Reference Manual of Growth and Development* 2nd edn. UK: Blackwell Science Ltd, 1997.

Butenandt, O. et al. (1974). Growth hormone studies in patients with rheumatoid arthritis with or without glucocorticoid therapy. *European Journal of Pediatrics* **118**, 53–62.

Ceda, G.P. et al. (1987). Glucocorticoid modulation of growth hormone secretion *in vitro*. Evidence for a biphasic effect on GH-releasing hormone mediated release. *Acta Endocrinologica* **104**, 465–9.

Chen, C. et al. (2001). Discovery of a series of nonpeptide small molecules that inhibit the binding of insulin-like growth factor (IGF) to IGF-binding proteins. *Journal of Medical Chemistry* **44**, 4001–10.

Cole, T.J. et al. (1995). Body mass index reference curves for the UK, 1990. *Archives of Disease in Childhood* **73**, 25–9.

Daughaday, W.H. and Rotwein, P. (1989). Insulin-like growth factors I and II. Peptide, messenger ribonucleic acid and gene structures, serum and tissue concentrations. *Endocrine Review* **10**, 68–91.

Davies, U.M. et al. (1994). Treatment of growth retardation in juvenile chronic arthritis with recombinant growth hormone. *Journal of Rheumatology* **21**, 153–8.

Davies, U.M. et al. (1997). Juvenile rheumatoid arthritis: effects of desease activity and recombinant human growth hormone on insulin-like growth factor 1, insulin-like growth factor binding proteins 1 and 3, and osteocalcin. *Arthritis and Rheumatism* **40**, 332–40.

De Benedetti, F. and Martini, A. (1998). Is systemic juvenile rheumatoid arthritis an interleukin-6 mediated disease? *Journal of Rheumatology* **25**, 203–7.

De Benedetti, F. et al. (1997). IL-6 causes growth impairment in transgenic mice through a decrease in insulin-like growth factor-I: a model for stunted growth in children with chronic inflammation. *Journal of Clinical Investigation* **99**, 643–50.

De Benedetti, F. et al. (2001). Effect of interleukin-6 on IGFBP-3. A study in interleukin-6 transgenic mice and in patients with systemic juvenile idiopathic arthritis. *Endocrinology* **142**, 4818–26.

De Martino, M. et al. (2000). Interleukin-6 release by cultured peripheral blood mononuclear cells inversely correlates with height velocity, bone age, insulin-like growth factor-I, and insulin-like growth factor binding protein-3 serum levels in children with perinatal HIV-1 infection. *Clinical Immunology* **94**, 212–18.

Freeman, J.V. et al. (1995). Cross-sectional stature and weight reference curves for the UK, 1990. *Archives of Disease in Childhood* **73**, 17–24.

Gacs, G. et al. (1973). Growth hormone secretion in children during corticosteroid treatment. Responses to arginine. *Hormone and Metabolic Research* **5**, 106–8.

Gourmelen, M. et al. (1982). Serum somatomedin/insulin-like growth factor (IGF) and IGF carrier levels in patients with Cushing's syndrome or receiving glucocorticoid therapy. *Journal of Clinical Endocrinology and Metabolism* **54**, 885–92.

Greulich, W.W. and Pyle, S.E. *Radiographic Atlas of Skeletal Development of the Hand and Wrist* 2nd edn. Standford CA: Stanford University Press, 1959.

Kuhns, J.G. and Swaim, L.T. (1932). Disturbances in growth in chronic arthritis in children. *American Journal of Diseases of Children* **43**, 1180–3.

Laaksonen, A.L. (1966). A prognostic study of juvenile rheumatoid arthritis. Analysis of 544 cases. *Acta Pediatrica Scandinavica* (Suppl.), 1–163.

Le Roith, D. et al. (2001). The somatomedin hypothesis: 2001. *Endocrine Review* **22**, 53–74.

Lovell, D.J. and White, P.H. (1990). Growth and nutrition in juvenile rheumatoid arthritis. In *Pediatric Rheumatology Update* (ed. P. Woo, B.M. Ansell, and P.H. White), pp. 47–57. New York: Oxford University Press.

Luo, J. and Murphy, L.J. (1989). Dexamethasone inhibits growth hormone induction of insulin-like factor-I (IGF-I), messenger ribonucleic acid (mRNA) in hypophysectomized rats and reduces IGF-I mRNA abundance in the intact rat. *Endocrinology* **125**, 165–71.

MacGillivray, M.H. (1995). Disorders of growth and development. In *Endocrinology and Metabolism* (ed. P. Felig, J.D. Baxter, and L.A. Frohman), pp. 1619–73. New York: McGraw-Hill.

Manolagas, S.C. and Jilka, R.L. (1995). Bone marrow, cytokine and bone remodelling. Emerging insights into the pathophysiology of osteoporosis. *New England Journal of Medicine* **332**, 305–11.

Miell, J.P. et al. (1988). Effects of dexametasone on GHRH, arginine and dopaminergic stimulated GH secretion and total plasma IGF-I concentration in normal male volunteers. *Journal of Clinical Endocrinology and Metabolism* **72**, 675–81.

Ottosson, M. et al. (1991). Growth hormone inhibits lipoprotein lipase activity in human adipose tissue. *Journal of Clinical Endocrinology and Metabolism* **80**, 936–41.

Parker, M.W. et al. (1984). Effect of testosterone on somatomedin-C concentrations in pre-pubertal boys. *Journal of Clinical Endocrinology and Metabolism* **58**, 87–90.

Reiter, E.O. and Rosenfeld, R.G. (1998). Normal and aberrant growth. In *Williams Textbook of Endocrinology* (ed. J.D. Wilson, D.W. Foster, H.M. Kronenberg, and P.R. Larsen), pp. 1427–507. Philadelphia PA: W.B. Saunders.

Rivkees, S.A. et al. (1994). Prednisone dose limitation of growth hormone treatment of steroid-induced growth failure. *Journal of Pediatrics* **125**, 322–5.

Strickland, A.L. and Shearin, R.N. (1972). Diurnal height variation in children. *Pediatrics* **80**, 1023–7.

Sturge, R.A. et al. (1970). Cortisol and growth hormone secretion in relation to linear growth: patients with Still's disease on different therapeutic regimens. *British Medical Journal* **3**, 547–51.

Suda, T. et al. (2001). The molecular basis of osteoclast differentiation and activation. *Novartis Foundation Symposia* **232**, 235–47.

Svantesson, H. (1991). Treatment of growth failure with human growth hormone in patients with juvenile chronic arthritis. A pilot study. *Clinical Experimental Rheumatology* **9** (Suppl.), 47–50.

Takayanagi, H. et al. (2000). T-cell-mediated regulation of osteoclastogenesis by signalling cross-talk between RANKL and IFN-gamma. *Nature* **408**, 600–5.

Tanner, J.M. *Foetus into Man*. Cambridge MA: Harvard University Press, 1990.

Tönshoff, B. and Mehls, O. (1994). Use of rhGH post transplant in children. In *Pediatric Renal Transplantation* (ed. A.H. Tejani, R.N. Fine), pp. 441–60. New York: Wiley.

Tönshoff, B. et al. (1993). Efficacy and safety of growth hormone treatment in short children with renal allografts: three year experience. *Kidney International* **44**, 199–207.

Tönshoff, B. et al. (1994). Reduced hepatic growth hormone (GH) receptor gene expression and increased plasma Gh binding protein in experimental uremia. *Kidney International* **45**, 1085–92.

Touati, G. et al. (1998). Beneficial effects of one-year growth hormone administration in children with juvenile chronic arthritis on chronic seroid therapy. *Journal of Clinical Endocrinology and Metabolism* **83**, 403–9.

Vottero, A. et al. (2000). Transcriptional and translational regulation of the splicing isoforms of the GH receptor by glucocorticoids. *Hormone Research* **53** (Suppl. 2), 7.

Ward, D.J. et al. (1966). Corticosteroid-induced dwarfism in Still's disease treated with growth hormone: clinical and metabolic effects during hydroxyproline excretion in two cases. *Annals of the Rheumatic Disease* **26**, 416–20.

Woods, K.A. et al. (1996). Intrauterine growth retardation and postnatal growth failure associated with deletion of the insulin-like growth factor I gene. *New England Journal of Medicine* **335**, 1363–7.

Yakar, S. et al. (2001). Inactivation of both liver IGF-I and the acid labile subunit genes cause a marked reduction in serum IGF-I and postnatal growth retardation. The Endocrine Society's 83rd Annual Meeting, Denver, Co (Abstract OR5-5), 2001.

Zachmann, M. et al. (1974). Testicular volume during adolescence. *Helvetica Paediatrica Acta* **29**, 61.

1.2 Common clinical problems

1.2.1 Spinal problems

1.2.1.1 Spinal problems in adults

Andrew O. Frank

Introduction

Definition of low back pain is difficult (Spitzer et al. 1987). In this chapter, the term 'low back pain' applies to pain localized to the lumbar spine or refers into the leg or foot, where other specific causal conditions have been excluded. As pain from non-disc structures, such as facet joints, causes pain that may refer to the distal leg and foot, the term 'leg pain' is used, not sciatica.

Terms used in this chapter, modified from the Quebec Task Force (Spitzer et al. 1987), are defined below:

- Acute pain—pain free at onset, lasting 0–7 days.
- Acute on chronic pain—significant exacerbation of pre-existing pain.
- Subacute pain—7 days to 3 months.
- Chronic pain—over 3 months.
- Chronic pain syndrome—psychological and social consequences of chronic pain.
- Intractable pain—failed conservative treatment for chronic pain.
- Back school—treatment programme emphasising educational management.
- Intensive rehabilitation—multiprofessional combination of skills and therapeutic modalities.
- Lumbar segment—two adjacent vertebrae and their intervening soft tissues (Waddell 1982).

The precise timings suggested in this paper are less important than understanding that underlying spinal (dys)function changes over time. Health workers must adopt strategies that allow for this.

Many patients are out of work, taking medication and making demands on primary and secondary health care and the private sector, including

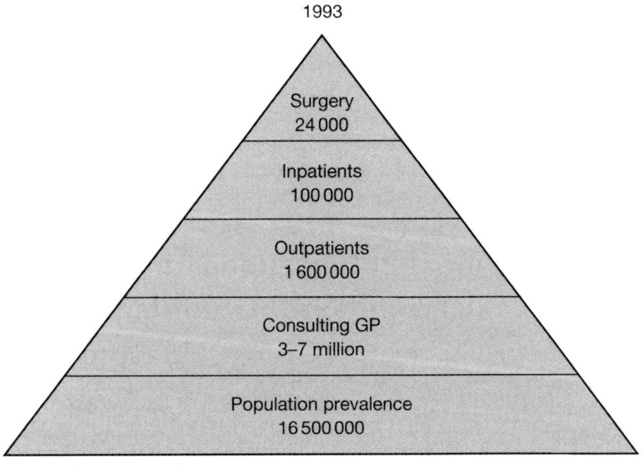

Fig. 1 Estimated annual health care for back pain in 1993. Report from the Clinical Standards Advisory Group Committee 1994 (United Kingdom).

orthodox and heterodox practitioners [Fig. 1; Clinical Standards Advisory Group (CSAG) 1994a].

The estimated losses due to the back pain epidemic are:

- 90 days sickness absence, 1994–1995, 1995–1996, 1997–1998 [British Society of Rehabilitation Medicine (BSRM) 2000];
- £90 090 million lost output, 1997–1998 (Maniadakis and Gray 2000);
- 8.2–12 million GP consultations annually (Maniadakis and Gray 2000; CSAG 1994b);
- 1.7–2.4 million hospital outpatient consultations annually (Maniadakis and Gray 2000; CSAG 1994b);
- 70 000 Hospital inpatient episodes, 1994–1995 (Maniadakis and Gray 2000).

Most clinicians assume a biomechanical basis for spinal pain, although we seldom understand why some patients suffer worse than others. Explanations may be found in factors such as the elasticity of the soft tissue spinal support structures, biochemistry of the disc, and the shape and size of the spinal canal. The dorsal horn of the spinal cord and areas of the brain involved in intractable back pain have been discussed by Jayson (Jayson 1994).

Doctors used to treating better-understood disease processes may have difficulty treating patients with spinal pain. There are few objective physical signs and no laboratory investigations to confirm precise cause and severity. Availability of magnetic resonance imaging (MRI) and computed tomographic (CT) scanning is helping, but does not help patients with minor symptoms. Doctors have had difficulty inspiring confidence in patients, who may seek help from heterodox practitioners. Our inability to help back pain sufferers is reflected in the large number of therapies available (Table 1). Medical training hinders satisfactory approaches by concentrating on the exclusion of pathology. Patients need understanding of their problems, alleviation of their symptoms, and encouragement that activity is therapeutic.

Individuals' attitudes, strengths, and weaknesses reflect their response to pain, reactions of family and colleagues, ability to fight to prevent recurrences, etc. Thus, a positive attitude is required from professional advisors from the initial acute attack onwards. The two important questions in back pain management are, when to take control of the pain from the patient and when and how to return control to them?

Person management is a prerequisite to back pain management and translating rehabilitation philosophy into back pain practice. Most attacks are self-limiting and of short duration, but recur. Recurrent episodes may require additional therapy, organized through hospital. A combination of the measures outlined in Table 1 may be needed, but most episodes are resolved or alleviated within a year. Patients who do badly should be considered as having failed conservative treatment and require different management strategies (see 'intractable back pain'). Management of lumbar disc disease is discussed in Chapter 6.17.1.

Table 1 Therapeutic options

General measures	Strict bed rest	1
	Local spinal support—corset	1–3
	Avoid aggravating factors	1–4
	Adjustment of life style	1–4
	Stop smoking	1–4
Physical measures	Mobilization techniques	1–3
	Exercises	1–4
	Postural training and self-care education	1–4
	Proprioceptive strapping	1–3
	Hydrotherapy	1–4
	Soft tissue techniques—massage	1–3
	Electro-therapy	1–3
	Transcutaneous electrical nerve stimulation (TENS)	3–4
	Acupuncture	1–4
Medication		
Oral	Pure analgesia	1–3
	Non-steroidal anti-inflammatory drugs (NSAIDs)	1–3
	Muscle relaxants	1
	Tricyclic drugs	3–4
Injection	Local or epidural steroid with local anaesthetic	1–3
	Dextrose-glycerine-phenol into soft tissues	3–4
Long-term measures	Cognitive behavioural therapy (CBT)	1–4
Psychological	Development of coping strategies	2–4
	Couple therapy	3–4
	Phobia management	3–4
	Sensory deprivation	3–4
	Self-help group	2–4
	Management of depression	
Psychiatric	Post-traumatic distress	2–4
	General toughening up programme	3–4
Intensive rehabilitation	Work hardening	3–4
	Sports injury approach	3–4
	Spinal education	3–4
	Functional restoration	3–4

Note: 1, acute low back pain; 2, subacute low back pain; 3, chronic low back pain; 4, chronic pain syndrome.
Source: Modified from Frank and Hills (1989).

The spine

The spine is complex, constituting 139 joints, 24 discs, numerous bursae, supporting ligaments, and muscles. The five lumbar vertebrae are linked by intervertebral discs anteriorly, two synovial facet joints posteriorly and supporting structures, including ligaments and muscles. Pain, a subjective symptom, may arise from any of these structures and is the cardinal feature of spinal disorders. The lumbar spine is designed to take the weight of the upper body with less facility for movement, whilst still protecting the spinal cord.

Non-specific low back pain (NSLBP), that is, no specific pathological (as opposed to degenerative) process can be attributed, may occur at any age. Under the age of 25, congenital factors are often involved, such as hypermobility or abnormal boney segments and the size and shape of the spinal canal (Porter et al. 1978). Disc lesions are more likely in early middle life and the aftermath of disc disease may lead to osteoarthrosis of the facet joints. In old age, osteoarthritis may be compounded by osteoporosis, particularly in women. Facetal osteoarthritis rarely precedes disc disease.

The lower cervical and lower lumbar segments take the majority of mechanical stress and lesions at these sites often coexist. The spine must be considered as a whole, so advice given for one area does not aggravate another. This chapter concentrates on pain from the lower spine, as these problems have a greater effect on the economy through sickness absence from work. Difficulties assessing studies on low back pain therapy are reviewed elsewhere (Spitzer et al. 1987). Randomized, controlled trials have shown benefits for patients and particular attention has been paid to reviewing such studies (see 'Cochrane reviews').

Epidemiology

Scale of the problem

Low back pain has enormous economic consequences; costs to the National Health Service (NHS) in 1993 are estimated at £481 million (CSAG 1994a). Indirect costs were estimated to exceed £5 billion for lost work and Social Security benefits alone (Fig. 2).

International comparisons within the Organization for Economic Co-operation and Development (OECD) suggest back pain accounts for 1–2 per cent of gross national product in Europe and the United States,

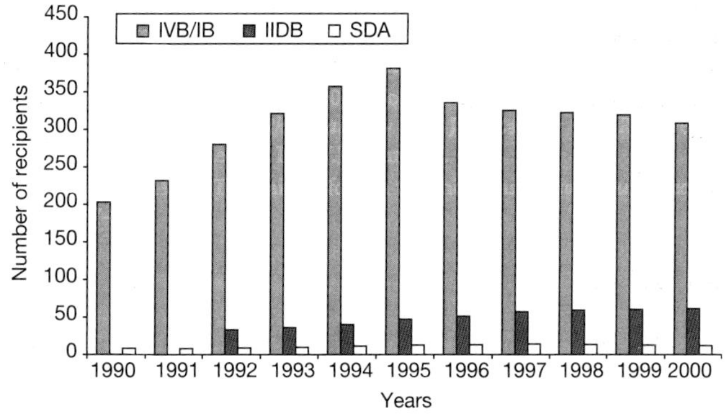

Fig. 2 Number of working age recipients of United Kingdom social security benefits for back incapacities (000s): 1990–2000. Published by kind permission of the Department of Work and Pensions, 2002; IVB/IB, Invalidity benefit/Incapacity benefit; IIDB, Industrial Injuries Disablement Benefit; SDA, Severe Disability Allowance.

with about 10 per cent direct and 90 per cent indirect costs (Norlund and Waddell 2000). Low back pain is one of the commonest causes of absence through illness in western societies and has been reported from many countries with differing cultures; however, disabling back pain is predominantly a feature of western society. The back pain epidemic did not exist in the United Kingdom until legislated social support became available. It is possible that factors relating to urbanization and industrialization are relevant. One hypothesis is that the medical, legal, and insurance environment of developed countries may actually contribute to the problem (back pain) rather than relieve it. This idea may be painful for societies whose laws are based on caring concepts.

In 1993, out of an estimated 2.4 million outpatient referrals, 100 000 people were admitted to hospital for spinal pain in England, Scotland, and Wales, of which about 3 per cent were cervical. Approximately 12 000 operations are performed on lumbar discs annually in the United Kingdom (CSAG 1994a), with less than 2000 fusions. In the United States about 200 000 surgical procedures involving lumbar disc excision are performed each year. Of these, as many as 30 000 are unsuccessful, joining the high-cost, high-demand, and highly emotional subset of the low back disabled. The chances of an individual having back surgery are six times greater in North America than Europe, with documented variations in disc excision rates across the United States of nearly twofold.

Low back pain is a relatively small cause of permanent severe disability; nonetheless, consequences for employment and health care are enormous. Back pain is one of the commonest causes of inability to work through illness in the United Kingdom, with a total work incapacity estimated at 90 million days in Britain annually between 1994 and 1998 (BSRM 2000). These calculations ignore the effects on individuals, their families and of litigation.

Prevalence

In the United Kingdom, the point prevalence of back pain is 14 per cent, period prevalence is 39 per cent in 1 month, 40 per cent in 1 year, and lifetime prevalence is 58 per cent (CSAG 1994a; Boucher 1999). This is lower than in many high-income countries, but also lower than some populations in Indonesia and Nigeria.

In the United States, cumulative lifetime prevalence of episodes lasting two or more weeks is approximately 14 per cent, with a point prevalence of 7 per cent at any moment in time. Of those reporting an episode of 2 weeks or more, one-third had pain lasting less than 1 month, one-third had pain lasting 1–5 months, and one-third had pain lasting 6 months or more.

The cumulative lifetime prevalence was greatest in the white population, varied by region in the United States and with the degree of education (greater prevalence with less education). The greatest prevalence is between the ages of 45 and 64. Onset of NSLBP is uncommon after the mid-50s. Mechanical back pain in children and adolescents is common, but rarely severe, and usually solved by life style advice.

Sex

There may be differences of spinal structure in males and females. Back pain is equally prevalent in both sexes, although the clinical course is different. More men require surgery, possibly because disc disease is more prevalent in men, whilst more women attend pain clinics. Males are more likely to suffer back pain bringing them to the health care system for help, but females are more likely to have pain that lingers into chronicity (Fordyce et al. 1986). It is unclear whether these differences are physically, psychologically, or socially based. In men, the only proven socio-economic link with back pain is manual labour. Women with no formal educational qualifications, or who live in households in the lowest-income category, are more likely to have back pain.

Nearly half of all pregnant women suffer back, or posterior pelvic, pain during pregnancy, often losing time from work. Pregnancy contributes to low back pain, with abortions and live births being associated. Hormonal changes are important, as they influence development of osteoporosis. One-third of British women aged 16–34 thought their back pain started during pregnancy or childbirth. There is no evidence that epidural analgesia leads to post-puerperal back pain.

Occupation

The relationship between low back pain and occupation has been recognized since 1705. Jobs requiring physically heavy work, static work postures, frequent bending and twisting, repetitive heavy lifting, forceful movements, repetitive work, and vibrations predispose to low back pain (Vingard and Nachemson 2000). Psychological factors are implicated, such as monotony and dissatisfaction at work (Vingard and Nachemson 2000). Those who 'hardly ever' enjoy their job are 2.5 times more likely to report back injury than those who 'almost always' enjoy their job (Bigos et al. 1991). Nurses are at high risk of back injury, the most at risk are aides and auxiliaries, doing the most physical work and least for registered nurses. Nursing auxiliaries have a greater incidence of back pain than construction workers, garbage collectors, and truck drivers (Kaplan and Deyo 1987).

Risk of recurrent attacks and returning to work

Five per cent of back pain sufferers aged 16–64 took time off work during the previous month because of back pain (Boucher 1999). Factors influencing a return to work are sex, duration of sick leave, reported need for analgesics, pain in the dorsal and cervical regions of the spine (in addition to lumbar pain), negative attitudes to their own capabilities, and after-work fatigue. Residual pain in the leg and positive clinical signs on returning to work, longer sickness absence, and two or more previous attacks are also associated with recurrences. The recurrence rate of occupational back pain may rise to 33 per cent at 3 years. Men have a higher chance of recurrence, drivers the highest recurrence rate, and nurses the highest average number of recurrences. Falls are associated with longer periods of absence from the current attack and higher rates of recurrence.

Caldwell and Glanville followed 373 patients under the age of 40 presenting to General Practitioners (GPs) or hospital consultants in 1963 (Caldwell and Glanville 1980):

- 11 per cent had single attacks, most lasting less than 2 weeks;
- 33 per cent had no time off work due to back pain;
- 3.3 per cent of men gave up work or took early retirement;
- 21 per cent changed job;
- 10 per cent took a reduction in working hours;
- 19 per cent of men and 10 per cent of women had loss of income or potential income.

In Sweden, Bergquist-Ullman showed that, in a population of workers at the Volvo plant (Bergquist-Ullman 1972):

- 35 per cent had pain for less than 1 month;
- 87 per cent had pain for less than 3 months;
- 4 per cent had pain at 1 year;
- 60 per cent had recurrences during the first year.

A history of low back pain, requiring time off work, remains the most useful predictor of future episodes.

Other social factors

Back pain sufferers are commonly from social and economic situations that are below average. A greater proportion suffer from drug and alcohol abuse. Divorces and family problems are more frequent and educational level is often lower (Croft and Rigby 1994). It is difficult to assess whether factors are primary or secondary and the relationship with smoking and occupation is unclear.

Risk factors

Smoking is a weak risk factor for back pain, relating to prolapsed lumbar intervertebral disc, the first attack, and the severity of low back pain. A dose–effect relationship exists between severity of back pain, number of cigarettes smoked, and duration of smoking. Explanations include, impaired blood supply to the involved spinal segment, carbon monoxidaemia, coughing and ergonomic factors related to smoking, attitude, lifestyle, and behaviour patterns.

Vibrations around 5 Hz are the most troublesome, explaining back pain in those spending prolonged periods driving. A mismatch between physical stress and strength predisposes to back problems. People under the age of 60 admitted to hospital for a traffic accident or fall have a 7 per cent chance of developing low back pain. Links between injury and subsequent symptoms are often not obvious to the patient.

Health associations

Previous hospital admissions or operations are frequent in those with a first episode of low back pain. Cardiovascular and gastrointestinal symptoms are more common in those with narrow spinal canals. Those with wider canals had more post-school qualifications. The association between a smaller canal and impairment of health may result from an adverse environment that affects growing systems early in life (Porter and Oakshot 1994). The associations with smoking (see above) may be linked with atherosclerosis of the abdominal aorta. Kauppila et al. (1994) examined 86 males at autopsy, comparing the radiological evidence of disc degeneration with atherosclerosis of the abdominal aorta. They postulated that stenosis of the ostia of the segmental arteries may play a part in lumbar disc degeneration.

The nature of back pain

Examples of causes of low back pain are:

- Mechanical—muscles, ligaments, degenerative joints, discs, nerve compression, root or cauda equina, inflammatory ankylosing spondylitis, or rheumatoid arthritis.
- Infection—bacterial osteomyelitis, tuberculous osteomyelitis, epidural abscess, and brucellosis.
- Neoplasm—multiple myeloma, lymphoma, secondary cancer, and primary cancer (rare).
- Bone disease—osteoporosis, osteomalacia, and Paget's disease.
- Other—gynaecological, neurological, renal, sickle cell disease, and vascular claudication.

Over 90 per cent of low back pain episodes may be considered idiopathic when non-spinal conditions (e.g. arthritis of the hip, proximal myopathy) and spinal pathology have been excluded. The important questions relate to whether pain, which arises from the lumbar segment, does or does not involve the nerve root. Many treatments for low back pain are based on the assumption that it is usually associated with excessive mechanical stress at work or leisure, normal stresses on degenerate discs and facet joints, or poorly resolved acute episode (Frank and Hills 1989).

Doctors and therapists have concentrated on physical measures to alleviate the problem, with attention paid to psychological approaches to management. Whilst this is aimed at those with prolonged and chronic low back pain, Fordyce has used the behavioural approach to back pain management in acute situations (Fordyce et al. 1986). The longer an episode continues, the more important it is to manage individuals and their problems. Most programmes for chronic back pain sufferers and back schools have an emphasis on psychological management.

Few studies have followed patients over many years. In contrast to the pessimistic outcome of Caldwell and Glanville (1980), Wilson and Wilson (1964) studied 117 employees 10 years after an episode of back pain. Fifty-two per cent had no time off work over 10 years (including 50 per cent of the heavy manual workers), although more than 80 per cent of those at greatest risk had recurrences. Only 13 patients were referred to hospital after failed therapy at work and two patients changed job. They conclude patients should be treated optimistically and not given bed rest or referral to hospital, if this could be avoided. Waddell (1987) views the back pain epidemic as being contributed to by doctors prescribing rest and social concepts of disability, contrasting the traditional medical model of illness with a psychosocial model (Plate 1).

It is argued that the reduction of claims for incapacity benefits for back pain (Fig. 2) reflects political decisions concerning eligibility as much as better management of acute NSLBP by health professionals.

The view that most attacks of NSLBP are self-limiting and of short duration has been challenged by Von Korff et al. (1993), who followed patients in primary care for 1 year. Sixty-nine per cent of patients with recent onset pain had had pain in the previous month and 82 per cent of those had pain for more than 6 months.

A positive attitude is essential, minimizing rest and medication (Von Korff et al. 1994). For an individual who has had a major episode of back pain, the risk of a recurrent attack is always present. Advise on the importance of adopting strategies that minimize the risks of such attacks must be given, such advise could include avoiding prolonged leaning forward, long-distance driving, uneven loading of spine, or overstretching. Patients should also be encouraged to use small lumbar supports in seats, frequently change posture, and take regular exercise.

Differential diagnosis

General considerations

A strictly medical approach to back pain management is disadvantageous, concentrating on excluding other diseases presenting as spinal pain and not dedicating time to helping patients understand their problem and how they can best be helped. Whilst the measures outlined in Table 3 help, the patient must grasp control of the situation. Attitudes towards avoiding aggravating factors, exercise, and a positive approach are as important as physical management (Frank and Hills 1989).

It is important to balance identifying treatable organic pathology, avoiding unnecessary and costly investigation. Pattern recognition of common presentations of low back pain helps with this. Common features of NSLBP include:

- central pain, usually over L5;
- leg pain;
- unilateral or bilateral buttock pain;
- episodic or cyclical pain in the middle years of life;
- arises from L3–S1;
- early morning stiffness or pain eases when up and about;
- relationship to posture (sitting or standing still aggrevates and is eased by walking).

NSLBP should be positively diagnosed rather than being diagnosed by exclusion. Leg pain is a common presentation, usually felt within the sciatic distribution on the lateral border of the calf or foot, although this is rarer. There is often a history of pain radiating up to the buttock or back. Sometimes, paraesthesiae gives a clue to the nature of the underlying pain in the presence of atypical leg pain. The three patient groups to consider are those with NSLBP (backache), nerve root compression, and back pain caused by other conditions (CSAG 1994a). More complex algorhithms can be consulted (Waddell 1982; Gavin and Wiesel 1991) and fuller reviews of the differential diagnosis are available (Bogduk 1992).

Thoracic pain is less common than lumbar or cervical pain and requires investigation (CSAG 1994a). In older patients, kyphosis is usually due to degenerative disease of the thoracic spine, but collapse may be due to osteoporosis, or more rarely, myeloma, or secondary malignancy.

Investigations—exclusion of other pathology

Age is important. Before the age of 25, X-rays are necessary to exclude congenital disorders, such as spondylolisthesis (Waddell 1982). Inclusion of the sacroiliac joints helps exclude ankylosing spondylitis. The sudden onset of new, or different, low back pain after the age of 55 warrants investigation. In 900 patients presenting to orthopaedic back clinics, 46 per cent of those over 55 had a definite abnormality, including 11 per cent with malignant disease (Waddell 1982). A series from a rheumatology service found only 8 per cent of patients had a specific pathology with metabolic bone disease predominating (Frank et al. 2000).

Most patients with back pain will not require investigation to exclude pathology. X-rays are helpful for reassurance that serious pathology is not present, explaining mechanical factors to the patient and assisting physiotherapists. Usually blood tests are not helpful, but erythrocyte sedimentation rate is the most helpful screening test (Waddell 1982).

Table 2 Guidelines for radiological investigation

First attack of pain	
Age 25–55	Pain resolving within 3 months—no X-ray needed, static after 6 weeks, consider a long lateral[a]
Age 0–25	Pain resolving within 3 months—no X-ray needed, static after 6 weeks—AP and lateral[a]
Age over 55	Pain resolving within 3 months—no X-ray needed, unresolved after 6 weeks—AP and lateral
Atypical pain	Well localized-CT scan or MRI if available
Atypical pain	Not well localized—bone scan. If positive, CT and/or biopsy under imaging control (or open)
Discogenic disease	Well localized (one or two adjacent levels)[b] Surgery being considered, CT scan or MRI if available[a]
Intractable mechanical low back pain	Stimulation followed by local anaesthetic and/or steroid into one or more facet joints to localize source of pain but may have no therapeutic potential[c]
Second attack of pain	If similar to previous episode—no X-rays needed If different in character or level, as above
Indications for radiology in psycho-social management	Plain films for visual display of structural normality or abnormality when explaining the mechanical nature of back pain CT or MRI to define presence or absence of discogenic disease for prognostic reasons

[a] If sacroiliitis suspected, dedicated views of sacroiliac joints (SIJ), MRI, or CT scan may confirm if SIJ is normal on AP film.

[b] Occasionally radiculography needed preoperatively, particularly if non-invasive investigations have suggested multilevel disease and MRI not available.

[c] Discography seldom used now for such purposes.

Cancer

Those with a history of cancer frequently suffer from mechanical low back pain. As X-rays may not show deposits till late in the disease, a bone scan is often a helpful investigative tool, unless the level of the lesion is clearly established on clinical grounds when CT or MRI scanning is appropriate (Table 2).

Leg pain

Leg pain does not necessarily reflect nerve root pain. It can arise from the facet joint and most structures within a segment. Leg pain caused by root irritation is more clearly defined, sharper, and often has an element of paraesthesiae (Waddell 1982).

Extraspinal causes of pain

Three per cent of apparent back troubles presented at an orthopaedic clinic are due to extraspinal causes, such as retroperitoneal or pelvic pathology, hip disease, peripheral vascular disease, or primary neurological disease (Waddell 1982). Pelvic pathology is not easy to exclude on history as many women notice their pain to be more severe in the last few days of their menstrual cycle, easing off on the first or second day of their period. This is also described in women with neck pain or headaches and is non-specific. Where there is doubt, abdominal and pelvic examinations are required.

Spinal causes

Children and adolescents usually require investigation. Acute pain may be caused by spondylolisthesis, or a developing scoliosis warranting referral to a specialist orthopaedic clinic. Adolescent discitis may cause severe pain and is often only diagnosed retrospectively.

Spondylolisthesis is common and unrelated to low back pain. At the L5/S1 level it is stable and does not require follow-up. At the L4/L5 level, however, instability diagnosed by lateral lumbar spine views in flexion and extension may develop and sometimes requires fusion, particularly if root involvement is present. Spondylolisthesis may cause stenosis at the level of slip.

Lumbar disc disease

The most frequent major pathology seen in back pain clinics. Physicians must ensure they are not missing nerve root compression that would benefit from decompression, when leg pain usually dominates back pain. The presence of symptoms correlating with objective physical signs (loss of sensation, power, and/or reflexes), confirmed by imaging, suggests that surgery should be 95 per cent successful. A central disc prolapse may give bilateral leg pain in the absence of demonstrable signs and with a normal straight leg raise test. Sphincter disturbances may reflect spinal cord compression and often require emergency treatment.

Spinal stenosis

Spinal stenosis is a symptom complex of root pain, sensory, or motor symptoms that start during walking and pass off within 5 min of sitting down or flexing the spine. Symptoms are aggravated by extension (Waddell 1982) and are associated with a congenitally narrow spinal canal. Additional pathology often develops in later life, such as posteriorly protruding discs, osteoarthritis of the facet joints, and hypertrophy of the soft tissues (e.g. ligamentum flavum) to compress the cauda equina. Predominately lateral compression, usually due to bony outgrowths from osteoarthritis of the facet joint, is lateral canal stenosis. There may be narrowing of the exit foramen, compressing the root and resulting, when bilateral, in a trifoliate shape to the canal (Fig. 3).

Infections

Brucellosis appears in those working in abattoirs, or with animals. Back pain is generalized with evidence of systemic disease. Most infections of the

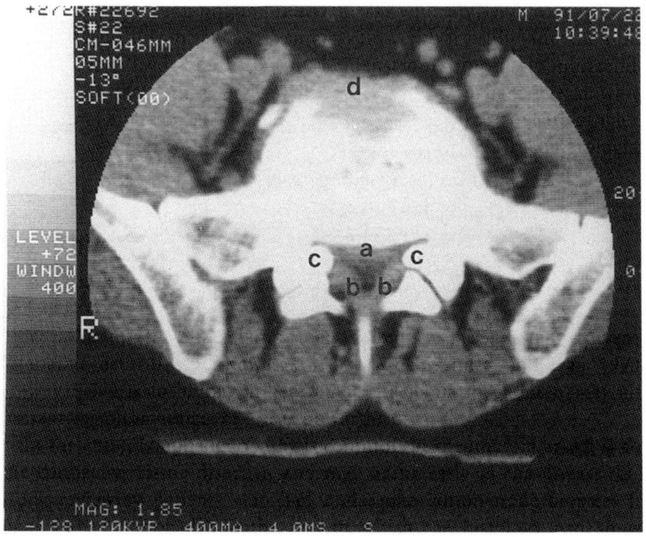

Fig. 3 Spinal stenosis secondary to a combination of a degenerate disc protruding posteriorly and laterally (a) and hypertrophy of the ligamenta flava (b) in an individual with OA of the facet joints intruding into the lateral recesses (c) to produce the symptoms of spinal stenosis. The anterior margin of the disc is degenerate (d).

spine are localized and give rise to constant pain often in an unusual or atypical site.

Tuberculosis affects the lower thoracic or upper lumbar vertebrae and must always be considered for populations at risk for this disease: those who arrived from the Indian subcontinent within the last decade, the frail or elderly, and those who have been immunocompromised, from therapy or other reasons.

This contrasts with degenerative lumbar disease that usually affects the L5/S1, L4/L5 levels, or, less commonly, L3/4. Where suspicion exists, without localizing plain X-ray changes, or clinical level, a bone scan may help, although it is not 100 per cent positive. If a level is suspected, CT or MRI will confirm abnormalities. Biopsy, under radiological guidance, or open, will usually provide microbiological and histological evidence of the causal organism. Confirmation of tuberculosis is not always obtained and a trial of antituberculous chemotherapy is needed.

Tumours

Primary tumours of the spine are rare. Exclusion of benign tumours may require myelography, or MRI. Secondary tumours are due to myeloma, lymphoma, or carcinoma. Features suggestive of malignancy include, absence of typical features, unremitting pain in atypical or multiple sites, pain unrelated to movement or posture, generalized bone pain, systemic or constitutional symptoms, elevated erythrocyte sedimentation rate (ESR), and the patient is over 55 with no previous similar episodes. Routine haematology and biochemistry usually confirm disseminated disease. Radiology will follow the pattern outlined above for infection (Table 2).

Ankylosing spondylitis

A common condition presented in back pain clinics and presents at a younger age than mechanical or degenerative back pain. Stiffness is a cardinal symptom, particularly in the morning, relieved by movement and exercise. Early diagnosis is important as treatment differs from NSLBP and because of family and other associations. Vigorous exercise programme maintains spinal movement, preventing spinal contracture, and may inhibit calcification at the enthesis.

Non-steroidal anti-inflammatory drugs (NSAIDs) get good results, particularly if a long-acting preparation is taken after food last thing at night, inhibiting early morning pain and stiffness. This facilitates early morning exercise programmes. In the early stages, plain X-rays of the spine and sacroiliac joints are normal, and CT or MRI of sacroiliac joints may show early erosive change. Bone scans are less specific. The disease can include localized calcified segments of the spine or neck, although this is rare.

Genetic predisposition to the disease is indicated by the presence of the B 27 genotype. This is not diagnostic, but may be helpful in those patients with a suspicious clinical picture and negative investigations. Its absence does not exclude the diagnosis.

Bone disease

Metabolic diseases of bone are the commonest pathology found in back pain clinics (Frank et al. 2000). Osteoporosis must be considered in women with early menopause, or other risk factors (see Chapter 6.16.1). In older patients, collapse is usually due to osteoporosis, but myeloma and secondary malignancy need exclusion (Table 2). Osteoporosis secondary to steroid use is common, particularly in older women with polymyalgia rheumatica or arteritis.

Osteomalacia is seen in vegetarian immigrants, when women may also spend time indoors. Elevated alkaline phophatase, in the presence of normal liver function tests, confirms diagnosis, but low vitamin D levels with compensatory high parathyroid hormone levels are frequently seen without an elevated alkaline phosphatase.

Paget's disease is destructive when infection and tumour lie within the differential and biopsy is sometimes required. More frequently, it is found on X-ray when its significance is uncertain. Activity may be demonstrated on bone scan and with an elevated alkaline phosphatase. Sickle cell disease must also be considered in populations at risk.

Referred pain to head thorax and abdomen

Presentations of spinal pain include pain in occiput to bifrontal areas (headaches), arms, chest wall (common cause of non-cardiac chest pain), loins (often mistaken for kidney pain), groin, and femoral and sciatic distribution. Facial pain may arise from involvement of the upper cervical segments. Dizziness is frequent and not always be due to vertebro-basilar insufficiency. Pain radiating to the shoulders may contribute to symptom complexes associated with capsulitis or painful arc syndromes, perhaps by involvement of the sympathetic nerves. It is more frequent in those with narrow cervical canal diameters. Similarly, epicondylitis and carpal tunnel syndromes are associated with narrow cervical canal diameters. Pain may refer to the anterior chest wall where it is often superficial, unilateral, and associated with tenderness. This is a common cause of visits to accident and emergency departments through fear of ischaemic heart disease.

Acute abdominal pain, referred from the spine, is a diagnosis of exclusion. A history of pain radiating from or to the spine may be obtained. Sometimes the pain can be reproduced by rotation of the spine, or spinal palpation or mobilization.

Prevention

Primary prevention

Stress management programmes at three high-risk work sites have reduced the number of accidents and related costs. A review of ergonomic changes in the US railroad industry has shown low back injuries are the most common and most costly, in terms of compensation and productivity. Corrective measures resulted in low back injuries and lost work days falling to zero and absenteeism falling from 4 to 1 per cent (BSRM 2000). Ergonomic approaches to minimising back injuries in the Railroad Industry include:

- storing tools and materials off the ground (between knee and shoulder height);
- heavier items stored at knuckle height;

- winches used to lift and handle heaviest equipment;
- worktables, dollies and carts used to carry heavy parts and tools.

Teaching and social support may not be enough to alter behaviour, but in a hospital environment teaching, alongside ward instruction on lifting techniques, may change behaviour of nurses in the short term. Publicity, with positive messages about back pain, improves population and family doctor beliefs and influences medical management, reducing disability and workers compensation costs.

Secondary prevention

This topic is addressed in the sections on 'Back schools' and 'Intensive rehabilitation'. The combination of intensive physical training, behavioural principles, and attention to working environment appears to be effective. Back schools are most effective in the work environment (Weiser and Cedraschi 1992; van Tulder et al. 1999b).

Tertiary prevention

Studies reporting follow-up data of 6 months duration may be considered preventive (Weiser and Cedraschi 1992). At 6 and 12 months, patients given cognitive therapy, relaxation, and cognitive therapy with relaxation, all improved significantly compared to a waiting list control group. Intensive rehabilitation embracing biopsychosocial models appears effective if more than 100 h of treatment are provided (Guzman et al. 2001), although vocational outcomes and cost effectiveness are unproven.

Specially trained physiotherapists reduce the amount of back pain during pregnancy, sick leave during pregnancy, and postpartum back pain. Specially shaped pillows reduce pregnancy back pain.

Acute low back pain

Correct management of acute back pain in primary care is crucial to prevention of long-term pain and disability (CSAG 1994a). Guidelines for the initial management have been issued by many bodies concentrating on the initial triage of patients [Agency for Health Care Policy and Research (AHCPR) 1994; CSAG 1994a; Chartered Society of Physiotherapy 1994; Waddell et al. 1999; Carter and Birrell 2000; Klein et al. 2000]. Guidelines do not have to be adhered to, particularly if they contrast with patient preferences. Advice on history, examination, and key management is given in Table 3.

The provision of literature reinforces advice given, gives specific recommendations on pain management, prevents unnecessary treatment (Roland and Dixon 1989), counters medicalization by challenging conventional beliefs about back pain, reduces harmful beliefs, and reduces disability (Burton et al. 1999).

The longer someone is off work with back pain, the lower their chance of returning to work (CSAG 1994a). In the absence of root signs or other pathology, advise is that:

- backache is rarely due to serious disease, most people have not damaged their spine;
- most patients do not require X-rays and blood tests;
- most severe back pain improves in a few days or weeks;
- milder symptoms may persist after a few months;
- recurrences are common;
- symptoms may persist at one year, but most can continue with normal activities;
- activity is helpful;
- clicks are not harmful;
- severity of pain does not equal severity of cause (serious illness).

Analgesia assists this active policy, as will the reassurance given by the physical assessment performed by the family practitioner. Rest is best in the position of maximum comfort (Frank 2001a).

Table 3 The initial consultation for acute back pain

History	Listen to site and character of the pain
Examination	Ask patient to show you the site of pain (characteristic hand movements are particularly helpful if there are language barriers) Check for obvious spinal deformity, spasm, or gross loss of movement Check straight leg raise, reflexes, and sensation if leg pain symptoms present
Management	Explanation and information, e.g. The Back Book (Roland et al. 1996; Buchbinder et al. 2001) Explore the patient's specific fears, reassure if appropriate (Frank 2001a; Grogan et al. 2000): Serious illness very unlikely X-rays and blood tests unlikely to be needed Severe back pain improves in days-weeks; milder symptoms may persist for a few months Recurrences are common Minimize rest and encourage resumption of normal activity, including work, patient must take *active* part in recovery Advise regular and not 'as needed' analgesia—may enable activities to be maintained Offer early review if the pain is uncontrolled

Note: Ensure the patient feels comfortable with your actions and plans.

Most patients are able to travel to the office or clinic. Those unable to do so will be physically ill, have severe discogenic pain with probable root pain, or major psychological issues. The frail or elderly may warrant a visit at home by the primary care team. Mobility, emotional, environmental, and social factors are all more easily assessed during a home visit leading to better advise on pain management.

Medication

Medication is important as severe pain inhibits activity and a speedy return to work (Table 4). Drugs minimize unnecessary rest to control pain. Trials with the simplest analgesics, usually paracetamol, may be adequate. NSAIDs often help, particularly in obtaining sufficient duration of analgesia for a good sleep. Short courses may be no more risky than prescribing stronger opiate derivatives, although increased vigilance is necessary. Ibuprofen is safer than any other NSAID in terms of its gastro-intestinal toxicity. Ketoprofen does not influence control of hypertension and is well tolerated by an elderly population. Care must be taken with smokers, those with a history of dyspepsia, or elderly people. Inability to control pain at home without using strong opiates is an indication for admission to hospital. Further information is available in standard reviews/texts (AHCPR 1994; Cherkin et al. 1998; Frank 2001a).

Drugs

Ensuring compliance and getting people back to work cannot be done if they are in severe pain. It is important to assess when, how much, and for how long medication should be prescribed to obtain the best balance of benefit versus risk. The big risk is people taking unnecessary rest to control pain that could be helped by analgesics, enhancing ability to regain normal activity patterns quickly. NSAIDs are often the only non-opiate derivatives available giving analgesia that lasts through the night.

Antidyspeptic medication

Many suffer side-effects from the gastro-intestinal tract when taking NSAIDs. Whilst omitting drugs giving side-effects is best policy, sometimes this is not in the patient's best interest. In these situations, men or older

Table 4 Oral medication used in back pain

Standard analgesics	Paracetamol, dextropropoxyphene, codeine, and dihydrocodeine or in compound preparation formulation (paracetamol and dextropropoxyphene), (paracetamol and codeine), (paracetamol and dihydrocodeine); long-acting compound preparations, e.g. ibuprofen or dihydrocodeine and codeine
Non-steroidal anti-inflammatory drugs (NSAIDs)	
Mostly cyclo-oxygenase 1 (COX-1) inhibition	Proprionic acid derivatives, e.g. ibuprofen, naproxen Others, e.g. soluble aspirin, diclofenac nabumetone, etodolac, meloxicam
Some COX-2 inhibition	Celecoxib, nimesulide, rofecoxib
COX-2 inhibitors	
Strong analgesics	
Moderately potent	Meptazinol, nefopam, pentazocine
Potent	buprenorphine, tramadol
Very potent	Diamorphine or morphine (not appropriate for use in primary care)
Other	Muscle relaxants or mild tranquilizers, e.g. diazepam for 5–7 days (acute back pain only) Tricyclic antidepressant compounds, e.g. amitriptyline, dothiepin, lofepramine (chronic pain only)

women may be helped by taking misoprostol separately, or combined with NSAIDs. 'Pro-preparations' may have fewer side-effects, or side-effects may be minimized by prescribing acid suppression tablets. Where gastric pathology has been confirmed, for example, erosions, proton pump inhibitors are the best option. If duodenal pathology is present, H2 receptor antagonists may be preferred.

If preparations containing paracetamol are insufficient, NSAIDs may be augmented by powerful analgesia, for example, nefopam, meptazinol, or tramadol. Many require only mild analgesics (e.g. compound paracetamol preparations). Antiemetics are helpful in those inclined to vomit after medication, as vomiting inhibits healing and aggravates pain. Opiates should rarely be prescribed in the home for acute or chronic back pain. Failure to control pain with these measures requires admission to hospital.

Anti-spasm medications may be used in the first few days together with NSAIDs (Cherkin et al. 1998). Benzodiazepine drugs may be of value for a maximum of 1 week for those having difficulty resting. They may facilitate a good night's sleep, essential for coping with subsequent pain. Those with a history of mood disorders, insomnia, or dependency are treated more safely with a tricyclic compound with sedative properties, for example, amitriptyline.

Injections

Most interest has been in the effect of local injections of lignocaine and/or corticosteroid around the area of maximal tenderness, the disc or facet joint. There is no evidence that they offer benefit (Nelemans et al. 1999), but injections have been effective combined with manipulation. Injections by the epidural route are discussed in the section on 'Intractable pain'.

Bed rest

In the absence of nerve root irritation minimal rest is encouraged (Allen et al. 1999), usually in the position of maximum comfort. Flexing hips and knees tilts the pelvis, flattening the lordos with reduction of pain intensity (Fig. 4). Supporting the hip and knee of the affected leg with cushions or pillows, or sleeping in a chair may be appropriate for femoral root irritation, although sitting often aggravates acute pain.

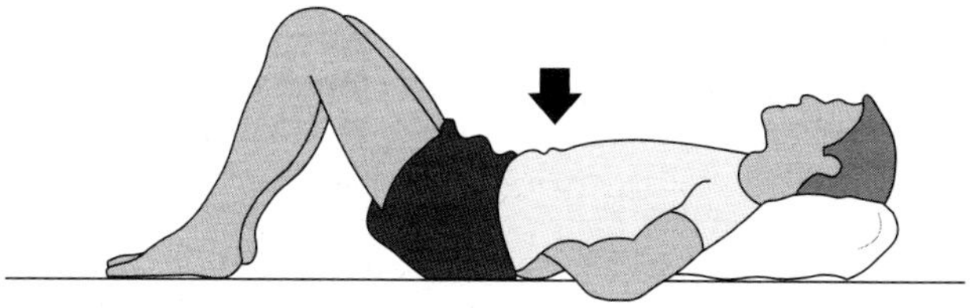

Fig. 4 Flattening of the lumbar lordos is often helpful in easing pain following an acute attack. Some exercises encourage adoption of this position (reproduced by kind permission of the Northwick Park Hospital Department of Physiotherapy).

For those with very severe attacks of pain, or the elderly, attention must be paid to good-quality rest and adequate support during mobilization. Mattress should not sag, height of bed should be appropriate, and walking sticks or elbow crutches should help take stress off the spine.

Mobilization after bed rest

A corset may facilitate initial mobilization. Social services or rehabilitation staff may provide blocks to raise chair or bed, or appropriate chair and toilet raise to facilitate mobility at home. Prolonged bed rest is particularly inadvisable for the very old; joints stiffen up and osteoporosis is encouraged. For this group of back sufferers, domiciliary physiotherapy greatly improves confidence and self-image. A commode by the bed is essential to prevent long walks to the toilet. Stairs may become a major barrier to health if the toilet is upstairs. The elderly often have coincidental urinary problems related to diuretics. Stairs cause strain to the spine and legs, reduced by banisters, having a bed downstairs, using of a commode, etc. (Frank and Hills 1989; Turner-Stokes and Frank 1992).

When improving, physiotherapy is usually helpful, except when symptoms are exacerbated due to sitting whilst travelling to hospital. If there is involvement of an L5 or S1 root, domiciliary therapy may still be advised.

Physical management

Considerable evidence supports the role of physical therapy in acute and subacute back pain (Frank and De Souza 2001). Increased compliance, with better results from physiotherapy, can be obtained by simultaneous use of complementary literature and a planned review of patients after treatment. There is no role for exercise, other than continuing normal activities, in acute back pain (Maher et al. 1999; van Tulder et al. 2000a).

Chiropractic, osteopathic manipulation, manipulation by physical therapists, psychological management with more supervision and planned withdrawal of treatment (behavioural group), McKenzie techniques of passive extension and postural correction, graded activity programmes with behavioural therapy, and behavioural support in a sports injury approach (Mitchell and Carmen 1994) can reduce pain, disability, compensation and disability award costs, and even work absence. Corsets should be reserved for those with failed manual therapy (Frank and Hills 1989).

Reviews of manipulative treatment show manipulation may speed recovery of acute backache (Frank 1993b; Shekelle 1994), although there is no universal agreement in view of the poor quality of some of the studies (Assendelft and Lankhorst 1998). A novel approach by Fordyce (1986) compared traditional and behavioural methods of treating acute back pain of 10 days duration or less. At 9–12 months, those given more supervision and planned withdrawal of treatment (behavioural group) were less sick and claimed less impairment than the group able to control their own schedules of medication, activity, exercise, and follow up (traditional group). This shows the benefit of taking control of acute back pain from the patient and giving it to the therapist.

As cervical symptoms often co-exist with low back symptoms, advice about physical and ergonomic measures must be appropriate for all parts of the spine. Lying prone may help some people with low back pain, but aggravate neck problems.

The elderly

The deleterious effect of musculoskeletal disorders in elderly people is well known. A recent review of patients referred to my back clinic revealed 15 per cent were over the age of 65. Some had major degenerative problems (spinal stenosis and root compression). Many had additional medical problems that complicated their management, for example, cardiac and gastrointestinal diseases, peripheral arthritis, and cervical degenerative problems (Frank et al. 2000). The differential diagnosis can be difficult in old age when acute pain may be due to osteoporotic collapse, aggravations of disc, or facetal degenerative disease.

If rest is required, attention must be paid to resting posture. Usually avoiding sitting, taking pressure off protruding bony points, and adequate support must be given during mobilization. Sitting is preferable if the femoral roots are involved. Advice is given by the domiciliary physiotherapy service, social services, or the hospital occupational therapy service and can include:

- the matress should not sag, nor be too hard;
- appropriate height of bed for transfers;
- domiciliary physiotherapy;
- blocks to raise chairs or bed;
- toilet height for transfers;
- teaching self-care;
- the need for a bedside commode;
- banisters;
- helping hands.

For older people with acute or chronic back pain, a visit to the home by a physician or member of the primary care or community team is an ideal method of teaching self-care. Self-care is not successfully learnt away from home. A simple check is needed to ensure tasks can be performed without placing unnecessary stress on the spine. This encourages a speedier resolution of pain and minimizes the risk of recurrence if the advice is understood and maintained by the patient and their partner, friend, or care assistant.

Chronic low back pain

Exercises

Exercise regimes aim to increase range of movement, strengthen muscles, stretch tightened structures, and help the patient to toughen up physically and mentally. Exercise helps with subacute and chronic pain and the prevention of NSLBP (Maher et al. 1999; van Tulder et al. 2000b). Exercises, combined with behavioural methods, are more effective than exercises alone, both are more effective than inaction (Turner et al. 1990). Behavioural principles also reduce sickness behaviour and get people back to work quicker (Lindstrom et al. 1992). Aerobic exercise is increasingly recommended and has been shown to augment the benefits of an English back school (Frost et al. 1995). There is a suggestion that specific muscle strengthening or aerobic fitness training may improve job satisfaction amongst nurses, as well as decreasing the duration of back pain.

Intensive outpatient physical retraining consisting of pain relief, mobilization, increasing movement, muscle strengthening, and work conditioning reduces sickness absence. The increased costs to health care were more than offset by savings in 'wages loss cost' (Mitchell and Carmen 1994). This is seen as an essential part of intensive rehabilitation (Fig. 5).

Manual therapy and manipulation

Manual therapy, including manipulation, is effective in reducing pain of longer duration (Blomberg et al. 1992; Koes et al. 1992; Shekelle 1994; Meade et al. 1995). Meade et al. showed this technique was most beneficial for chronic or severe pain (Meade et al. 1995). These studies are open to many interpretations, but lead this author to conclude these forms of

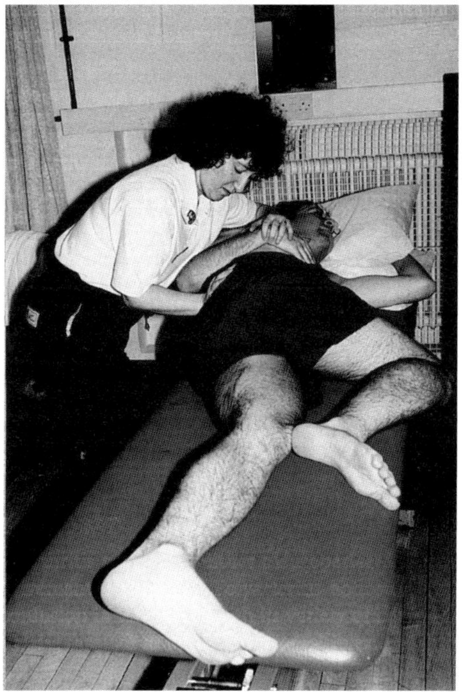

Fig. 5 Mobilization or manipulation of the lumbar spine is helpful in reducing morbidity and duration of symptoms in acute and chronic, but not intractable, low back pain (reproduced by kind permission of the Northwick Park Hospital Department of Physiotherapy).

therapy are effective. The beneficial effects on the economy of 'a few days' reduction of sickness absence by more effective means of treatment are potentially enormous.

Other physical treatments

Posture training supports may be more appropriate than ordinary corsets to help those with a kyphosis and may be useful adjuncts to physical management. Traction is rarely useful and bed rest in traction is not recommended (CSAG 1994a).

Heterodox management

Use of complementary and alternative medicines is increasing and they are more likely to be used by the more highly educated (Palinkas et al. 2000). Some forms have a fair evidence base, for example, chiropractic (Meade et al. 1995; Assendelft and Lankhorst 1998). Others (e.g. acupuncture) remain to be proved helpful (van Tulder et al. 1999a). Whilst there are risks attached to acupuncture, these are rare in the hands of medical practitioners. The public should be safeguarded against unproven and potentially harmful techniques. Doctors should not recommend heterodox treatment unless the practitioner is a member of a recognized professional association. Patients like massage, but its effects are seldom sustained and it cannot be recommended.

Medication

Although the risk of serious side-effects with NSAIDs is probably less than 2 per cent, attempts to wean patients off them are worthwhile, giving patients the opportunity to have 5–10 day courses of these drugs to relieve acute pain.

Long-term analgesia may encourage sedation or effect the gastrointestinal tract and many patients discontinue their use. Having a bottle of tablets at hand that are known to be effective is prudent. The knowledge that they are available helps counter fear of aggravation from activity and may inhibit the risks of depression (Frank and Hills 1989).

A major advance in managing chronic pain is the use of tricyclic antidepressant compounds (TCA), particularly in neuropathic pain (McQuay and Moore 1997; Sindrup and Jensen 1999). The mode of action is unclear, although increasing the serotonergic uptake in the central nervous system has been suggested. Evidence supporting TCA use for those without nerve involvement in the absence of depression is small. The sedative side-effects can be useful in those with disturbed sleep and may facilitate relaxation. Appropriate warnings about sedation, a dry mouth, and interference with driving must be given. Patients need reassurance that TCAs are neither addictive nor being prescribed for psychiatric purposes. Gradual withdrawal is recommended.

Intractable low back pain

Some patients have persistant disabling pain despite the above measures. Having excluded spinal and non-spinal pathology and direct nerve root involvement, patients should be considered as having failed conservative treatment. The term intractable low back pain is used to differentiate failed conservative management from chronic pain, which may never have been treated before, or chronic pain syndrome when changes in behaviour are apparent (Frank 1993b). Up to 10 per cent may have major underlying medical problems (Wiesel et al. 1988; Frank et al. 2000).

It must be determined whether physical or psychological factors dominate, usually both are present (Frank and Hills 1989). They are described separately for clarity, but both aspects must be managed, as in most back schools and rehabilitation programmes.

Physical management

Clues that physical aspects are important lie in the pattern of pain. When episodic or related to movement or posture, physical issues probably dominate. Often faulty posture causes abnormal stress on normal tissue, or recurrent stress on degenerate structures within the lumbar segment. Management consists of education into relevant mechanical and ergonomic factors. Physical issues can include:

- repetative lifting or bending;
- inappropriate bed or mattress;
- sleeping in an inappropriate position;
- sitting for long perionds, especially driving;
- stopping exercise regime or medication when improved;
- generally unfit.

Sleep patterns are important, after checking that bedding and mattress are satisfactory (Frank and Hills 1989), it must be established whether sleep loss is due to insomnia (e.g. thinking about social problems), pain, depression, and post-traumatic distress.

Physical measures

Transcutaneous electrical nerve stimulation (TENS) is widely used to try to control pain where conservative measures were unsuccessful and surgery not contemplated. If successful, TENS is continued at home with patients having their own machine. Pain clinics and some physiotherapy departments now frequently offer acupuncture. Currently, it is not possible to predict who will do well with TENS or acupuncture, and evidence of efficacy is lacking in spite of considerable research (van Tulder et al. 1999a; Milne et al. 2001).

Medication

There is little evidence that local injections are of benefit (Nelemans et al. 2001). Sclerosants may be helpful if combined with manipulation (Ongley et al. 1987). Opiates, steroids, and local anaesthetics have all been administered epidurally. The use of morphine for the treatment of post-operative pain is unhelpful and hazardous. Epidural steroids help to reduce post-operative pain following laminectomy and sometimes with root compression. The use of epidural local anaesthetic has been reviewed with and without steroids and evidence of efficacy remains unconvincing (Rozenberg et al. 1999; Nelemans et al. 2001).

Psychological and social management

Some patients present with pain that is continuous and does not alter over the 24-h period often claim to have suffered non-stop pain for many years (Frank et al. 2000). Many are suffering from pain or illness behaviour syndrome (Waddell 1987) or learned helplessness. Examination reveals signs not compatible with the disability described and pattern of pain may be non-anatomical. Examination is often accompanied by over-reaction, exaggerated gestures of pain, distraction, pain on simulated rotation, regional weakness, or sensory and superficial and non-anatomical tenderness (Main and Waddell 1998).

Constant, 24-h pain suggests depression. If pain disturbs sleep, a long-acting NSAID or codeine preparation may be helpful. Asking 'what do you think about when you lie awake?' may give clues about social factors influencing the causes or consequences of the pain (Fig. 6). Other important variables including irritability and somatization are also important.

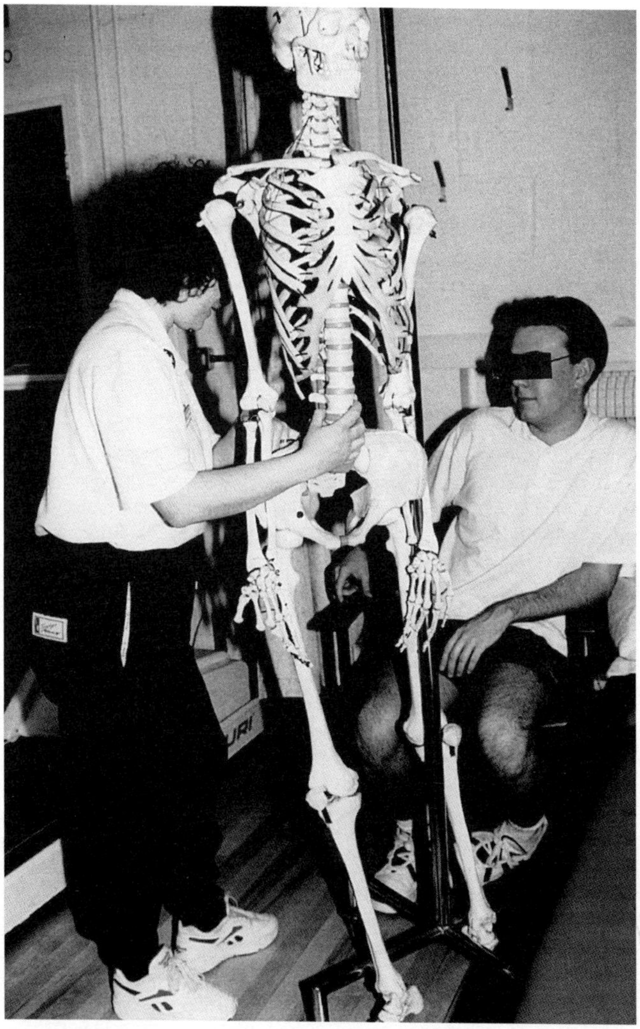

Fig. 6 Patient education has been shown to reduce back pain (reproduced by kind permission of the Northwick Park Hospital Department of Physiotherapy).

Patients may admit to problems consequent to loss of earnings, changing marital or sexual relations. Not all patients can continue a normal sexual relationship when in severe pain, but many can be helped by the intelligent use of positioning (Frank 2001a). Often unrealistic fears exist (Grogan et al. 2000). The effect on the partner cannot be over-stressed, particularly if over-protection or excessive sympathy has encouraged adoption of a sick patient role. Other strains may be placed on marital and family relationships (Frank and Hills 1989). Where the marital relationship has been difficult prior to the onset of back pain, the pain may be the final blow to the marriage. A list of possible psychological barriers is given in Table 5.

Trauma and litigation

Autopsies after road traffic accidents have shown haemorrhage into the outer annulus of the disc, haemarthroses, and capsular or synovial tears to the facet joints, in addition to traumatic herniation of the disc, explaining much previously unexplained pain. The psychological consequences of road traffic accidents have been largely ignored in the past. Mayou et al. (1993) have shown that mood disturbances, severe horrific intrusive memories of the accident, and travel anxiety persist 1 year on. In a small series of patients involved in litigation, irritability, tearfulness, sleep disturbance, and travel anxiety occurred in over half of the sample (Frank 1993a).

Trauma remains a complicating issue when distress is commonly seen and symptoms fail to resolve. The reasons are unclear and do not always revolve around litigation, although they can do. Negative attitudes may play a part, such as bitterness and an inability to understand 'why me?'. Depression may go undetected and phobias may develop.

Factors hampering resolution of disability when litigation is involved include the need to persuade doctors that their injuries are serious, compensation vindicates patients who blame third parties, fears that a return to work would compromise their safety, use of disability to avoid difficult situations, and financial anxieties (Teasell and White 1994).

There is abundant evidence that settlement of litigation does not relieve symptoms (Anonymous 1989), but the uncertainty surrounding litigation is unhelpful. Once medical reports have been obtained, patients can be assured that the basis for a settlement is likely and they must now concentrate on positive matters.

Table 5 Psychological barriers to successful outcome

Fear
Medication
Drug dependency
Side-effects
Effectiveness will mask pain/creating further damage
Physical activity
Will increase pain particularly during recovery
Cause, e.g. cancer, multiple sclerosis
Consequences
Loss of job (status and poverty)
Disability (e.g. in a wheelchair)
Clicks in the back—frightened of damage to spine
Effects on the family (particularly partner)
Potential to develop learned helplessness or pain behaviour
Psychiatric considerations
Depression
Phobic disorders
Substance abuse, e.g. alcohol
Post-traumatic psychological distress
Previous psychiatric history
Other
Job dissatisfaction
Litigation/compensation; assessment of intractable pain/pain behaviour; pain management
Surgery

Rehabilitation

Hypnosis, relaxation, and sensory deprivation may have small adjunctive roles as part of rehabilitation or pain management. Other psychological factors are listed in Table 5. Many are amenable to psychological or psychiatric intervention. Often back pain sufferers and their families can learn to cope with life again through literature, group work, or specialist counselling.

Psychologists have an important role helping patients cope with pain. Groups help in boosting confidence through sharing experiences and realizing they are not alone in their suffering. Cognitive behavioural therapy (CBT) is the cornerstone of psychological pain management. CBT analyses thoughts negatively influencing behaviour and addresses dysfunction caused by false beliefs (van Tulder et al. 2000c).

Psychologists also advise rehabilitation teams on behavioural approaches to management combining physical and behavioural approaches (Fordyce et al. 1986; Turner et al. 1990; Lindstrom et al. 1992; Klaber Moffett et al. 1999). Incorporation of behavioural therapy into early physical management offers hope of reducing morbidity of pain behaviour. Pre-existing psychopathology is frequent in those requiring intensive rehabilitation and does not hamper treatment if taken into account. The results of physically demanding programmes vary between individuals with different psychological profiles (Harkapaa et al. 1991; Talo et al. 1992).

Back schools

A back school is any programme with an educational content, varying from one-session outpatient programmes to inpatient programmes (Harkapaa et al. 1990). Back schools, with or without concurrent therapy, have been shown to decrease back pain and disability. Those in occupational settings are effective, but cost-effectiveness is unknown (van Tulder et al. 1999b). The best-rated study is discussed below (Harkapaa et al. 1990). Results are short term and success at changing human behaviour long term (over a year) continues to escape us. Non-compliance and relapse remain major problems.

Intensive rehabilitation

For a failure of conservative or surgical management, rehabilitation programmes often involve multiprofessional input covering physical, psychosocial, educational, and vocational components. Intensive rehabilitation includes the long term measures in Table 1, these factors should be part of any back pain programme. Programmes should embrace concepts of sports injury approach (Mitchell and Carmen 1994), functional restoration (Schonstein et al. 2000), and work hardening (Schonstein et al. 2000), as well as intensive rehabilitation (Harkapaa et al. 1990).

There is evidence that inpatient rehabilitation is superior to outpatient rehabilitation at reducing pain and disability whilst enhancing compliance. Intensive rehabilitation is one of the few indications for admitting patients to hospital. Evidence suggests that intensive, multiprofessional programmes encouraging individuals to ignore pain, toughen up and taking away control of pain before giving control back are cost effective. Long-term benefits have been demonstrated in terms of reduced sickness absence (Bendix et al. 1998).

Education and self-care

The first presentation of back pain is an opportunity to illustrate to patient and family common precipitating factors for back pain episodes (e.g. a trivial bending episode, possibly related to twisting). A demonstration of correct lifting techniques is important. Whilst squatting is usually recommended (to avoid bending the trunk with straight legs), this is awkward and inappropriate for older people. Approaching the floor from the kneeling position can overcome this and some (if not using helping hands) may find using their arms to assist rising helpful. The combination of arthritis of the large joints of the legs and back pain is particularly disabling. Helping hands help avoid bending (Fig. 7).

Use of educational booklets, such as The Back Book, have decreased fear avoidance scores and reduced back disability (Burton et al. 1999). Other booklets have reduced reconsultations with back pain, referrals to hospital consultants, referrals for physiotherapy, admissions to hospital and laminectomies (Roland and Dixon 1989).

In acute stages, patients often prefer professionals to take responsibility for their back care, which is therapeutic (Fordyce et al. 1986). This responsibility has to be transferred back if pain becomes chronic and intractable. Ultimately the individual is responsible for keeping physically fit, maintaining their exercise programme, and remaining relaxed to avoid physically and ergonomically stressing the spine.

Living with low back pain

It is common for patients to have persistent low back pain, in spite of many forms of therapy. Some patients conclude that they can live with their pain. Others can be helped to that conclusion, particularly if they are convinced they have received good treatment, their specific fears have been addressed, and disease has been excluded.

(a) (b)

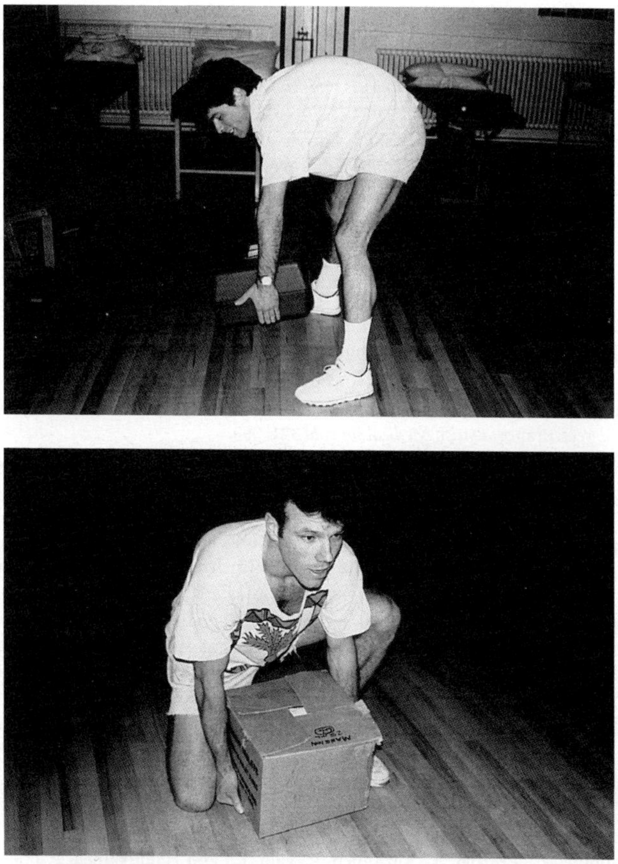

Fig. 7 (a) Incorrect lifting technique: the lumbar lordosis is lost with maximal stress being placed on the spine; (b) correct lifting technique: use of the kneeling position minimizes strain on the back and is more stable than lifting from squatting or bending; painful knees from osteoarthritis or other causes prevent this and increase patient's disability (reproduced by kind permission of the Northwick Park Hospital Department of Physiotherapy).

Mechanical stress on the spine can be minimized by simple advice. Incorporation of such advice into everyday life can remove triggering factors perpetuating the current episode or precipitating a recurrence. Details of bedding, mattresses, chairs, and cars have been outlined elsewhere (Frank and Hills 1989). The importance of avoiding prolonged sitting must be stressed. Avoiding rushing about, relaxing, and planning activities reduces the risk of doing everyday tasks in a harmful way.

The development of coping strategies is important. Those with pain resulting from trauma (particularly at work) may benefit from professional psychological advice. Some individuals find sharing experiences with fellow sufferers, in a counsellor run group setting, helpful. Others may join branches of voluntary bodies (e.g. Backcare). The National Ankylosing Spondylitis Society has developed groups that have a very physically orientated approach to their group meetings. Many appreciate further information about their condition provided by booklets from charities (e.g. The Arthritis Research Campaign).

Return to work

Vocational rehabilitation

A minority of low back pain patients may be off sick for prolonged periods and have difficulty returning to work. Problems arise from the fear that work will aggravate pain or cause it to recur, prolonged adoption of the patient role, discouraging a positive approach to work, and loss of self-discipline leading to poor time-keeping, lack of stamina, and strength due to prolonged inactivity (BSRM 2000).

Such people can be helped by intensive rehabilitation with a behavioural approach. Table 6 gives a list of ways that employers and health professionals can help with vocational rehabilitation. Returning to work may require working with pain, developing physical stamina, and addressing

Table 6 Helping back pain sufferers back to work (BSRM 2000)

Employer's role	Take an interest in the patient—contact them When they are off sick—offer support Offer assistance of the Occupational Health Service if available Offer ergonomic advice at the work site Ensure the line manager or supervisor understands the situation (British Society of Rehabilitation Medicine 2000) Allow a phased return to work Facilitate travel at non-peak times Minimize stress Accept that the patient may need less demanding work short term both physically and emotionally
Health professionals	Advise partner on Encouraging a return to activities Specifying any risk factors Discourage excessive protection Discuss the 'side-effects' of being 'off sick' Encourage a positive view of work Liaise with employers Encourage the patient to accept that returning to work is unlikely to aggravate the cause of the pain Offer analgesia to facilitate getting fitter and to lessen pain at work Consider a surgical corset or a weight-lifters belt if physically demanding work Offer support for after return to work to ensure work patterns safely re-established if no occupational health service

fear. Sessions of therapy should be increased to mimic a full day at work, reassuring both patient and staff that a return to work is viable. Ideally, such programmes should include CBT to develop coping strategies. When a rehabilitation programme clarifies that individuals are unable to return to work, referral to the Government Employment Agency or vocational councillor is essential. In the United Kingdom, the Disability Employment Adviser can discuss alternative work with employer's, which should be within the patient's capabilities.

It is critical to avoid the principle of 'health getting it right before employment agencies can intervene' (BSRM 2000). Restoration of confidence and alleviation of the fear of returning to work is achieved by a programme of planned withdrawal of support, preferably linked to a phased return to work planned between therapist and employer. This can occur whilst off sick as part of rehabilitation. The cost-effectiveness of such approaches has been poorly evaluated, but non-surgical treatment of chronic pain returns patients to work. Increased rates of return to work are due to treatment and the benefits of treatment not being temporary (Cutler et al. 1994).

The important principle is to enable those with pain to keep working, even if with reduced duties, to prevent sickness absence and reduce the likelihood of needing long-term state benefits.

References

Agency for Health Care Policy and Research, Bigos, S., Bowyer, O., Breen, G., Brown, K., Deyo, R., and Haldeman, S.E., ed. *Acute Low Back Problems in Adults. Clinical Practice Guideline Number 14: Acute Low Back Problems in Adults: Assessment and Treatment. Quick Reference Guide for Clinicians Number 14: Understanding Low Back Problems. Patient Guide.* AHCPR/PUB-95-0642, pp.1–200. Atlanta GA: Agency for Toxic Substances and Disease Registry, 1994.

Allen, C., Glasziou, P., and Del Mar, C. (1999). Bed rest: a potentially harmful treatment needing more careful evaluation. *Lancet* **354**, 1229–33.

Assendelft, W. and Lankhorst, G. (1998). Effectiveness of manipulative therapy in low back pain: systematic literature reviews and guidelines are inconclusive. *Nederlands Tijdschrift voor Geneeskunde* **142**, 684–7.

Bendix, A., Bendix, T., Haestrup, C., and Busch, E. (1998). A prospective randomised 5 year follow-up study of functional restoration in chronic low back pain patients. *European Spine Journal* **7**, 111–19.

Bergquist-Ullman, M. (1972). Acute low back pain in industry. A controlled prospective study with special reference to therapy and confounding factors. *Acta Orthopaedica Scandinavica* **170**, 1–117.

Bigos, S., Battie, M., Spengler, D., Fisher, L., Fordyce, W., Hansson, T., Nachemson, A., and Wortley, M. (1991). A prospective study of work perceptions and psychosocial factors affecting the report of back injury. *Spine* **16**, 1–6.

Blomberg, S., Svardsudd, K., and Mildenberger, F. (1992). A controlled, multicentre trial of manual therapy in low back pain: initial status, sick leave and pain score during follow-up. *Scandinavian Journal of Primary Health Care* **10**, 170–8.

Bogduk, N. (1992). The sources of low back pain. In *The Lumbar Spine and Back Pain* 4th edn. (ed. M. Jayson), pp. 61–88. Edinburgh: Churchill Livingstone.

Boucher, A. The prevalence of back pain in Great Britain. http://www.doh.gov.uk/public/backpain.htm. London: Department of Health, 1999.

British Society of Rehabilitation Medicine. *Vocational Rehabilitation: The Way Forward.* London: British Society of Rehabilitaton Medicine, 2000.

Buchbinder, R., Jolley, D., and Wyatt, M. (2001). Population based intervention to change back pain beliefs and disability: three part evaluation. *British Medical Journal* **322**, 1516–20.

Burton, A., Waddell, G., Tillotson, K., and Summerton, N. (1999). Information and advice to patients with back pain can have a positive effect: a randomized controlled trial of a novel educational booklet in primary care. *Spine* **24**, 2484–91.

Caldwell, J. and Glanville, H. The industrial and social implications of low back pain 1963–1980. *Report to the European Coal and Steel Community, Luxemberg and the DHSS, London,* 7245.50.8.004, pp. 1–61. Southampton: University of Southampton, 1980.

Carter, J. and Birrell, L. *Occupational Health Guidelines for the Management of Low Back Pain at Work: Evidence Review and Recommendations.* London: Faculty of Occupational Medicine, 2000.

Chartered Society of Physiotherapy. *Guide to the Management of Low Back Pain for General Practitioners.* London: Chartered Society of Physiotherapy, 1994.

Cherkin, D., Wheeler, K., Barlow, W., and Deyo, R. (1998). Medication use for low back pain in primary care. *Spine* **23**, 607–14.

Clinical Standards Advisory Group—Chairman Prof. M. Rosen. *Back Pain,* pp. 1–89. London: HMSO, 1994a.

Clinical Standards Advisory Group. *Epidemiology Review: the Epidemiology and Cost of Low Back Pain,* pp. 1–72. London: HMSO, 1994b.

Croft, P. and Rigby, A. (1994). Socioeconomic influences on back problems in the community in Britain. *Journal of Epidemiology and Community Health* **48**, 166–70.

Cutler, R., Fishbain, D., Rosomoff, H., Abdel-Moty, E., Khalil, T., and Rosomoff, R. (1994). Does nonsurgical pain center treatment of chronic pain return patients to work? A review and meta-analysis of the literature. *Spine* **19**, 643–52.

Anonymous (1989). Risk factors for back trouble (Editorial). *Lancet* **1**, 1305–6.

Fordyce, W., Brockway, J., Bergman, J., and Spengler, D. (1986). Acute back pain: a control-group comparison of behavioural vs traditional management methods. *Journal of Behavioural Medicine* **9**, 127–40.

Frank, A. (1993a). Psychiatric consequences of road traffic accidents—often disabling and unrecognised (letter). *British Medical Journal* **307**, 1283.

Frank, A. (1993b). Low back pain—regular review. *British Medical Journal* **306**, 901–9.

Frank, A., De Souza, L., McAuley, J., Sharma, V., and Main, C. (2000). A cross-sectional survey of the clinical and psychological features of low back pain and consequent work handicap: use of the Quebec Task Force Classification. *International Journal of Clinical Practice* **54**, 639–44.

Frank, A. *Low Back Pain: Diagnosis and Management.* London: Current Medical Literature, 2001a.

Frank, A. and De Souza, L. (2001). Conservative management of low back pain. *International Journal of Clinical Practice* **55**, 21–31.

Frank, A. and Hills, J. (1989). Spinal pain. In *Disabling Diseases. Physical, Environmental and Psychosocial Management* (ed. A. Frank and G. Maguire), pp. 41–78. Oxford: Heinemann Medical Books.

Frost, H., Klaber Moffett, J., Moser, J., and Fairbank, J. (1995). Evaluation of a fitness programme for patients with chronic low back pain. A randomised controlled trial. *British Medical Journal* **310**, 151–4.

Gavin, M. and Wiesel, S. (1991). Low back pain. *Current Opinion in Rheumatology* **3**, 65–70.

Grogan, E., Frank, A., and Keat, A. (2000). Patients in rheumatology clinics need reassurance. *British Medical Journal* **321**, 300.

Guzman, J., Esmail, R., Karjalainen, K., Malmivaara, A., Irvin, E., and Bombardier, C. (2001). Multidisciplinary rehabilitation for chronic low back pain: systematic review. *British Medical Journal* **322**, 1511–16.

Harkapaa, K., Mellin, G., Jarvikoski, A., and Hurri, H. (1990). A controlled study on the outcome of inpatient and outpatient treatment of low back pain. *Scandinavian Journal of Rehabilitation Medicine* **22**, 181–8.

Harkapaa, K., Jarvikoski, A., Mellin, G., Hurri, H., and Luoma, J. (1991). Health locus of control beliefs and psychological distress as predictors for treatment outcome in low back pain patients: results of a 3 month follow-up of a controlled intervention study. *Pain* **46**, 35–41.

Jayson, M. (1994). Mechanisms underlying chronic back pain. Studies are looking at the brain and spinal cord. *British Medical Journal* **309**, 681–2.

Kaplan, R. and Deyo, R. (1987). Back pain in hospital workers. In *SPINE: State of the Art reviews: Occupational Back Pain* (ed. R. Deyo), pp. 61–73. Philadelphia PA: Hanley and Belsus.

Kauppila, L., Penttila, A., Karhunen, P., Lalu, K., and Hannikainen, P. (1994). Lumbar disc degeneration and atherosclerosis of the abdominal aorta. *Spine* **19**, 923–9.

Klaber Moffett, J., Torgerson, D., Bell-Syer, S., Jackson, D., Llewlyn-Phillips, H., Farrin, A., and Barber, J. (1999). Randomised controlled trial of exercise for low back pain: clinical outcomes, costs, and preferences. *British Medical Journal* **319**, 279–83.

Klein, B., Radecki, R., Foris, M., Feil, E., and Hickey, M. (2000). Bridging the gap between science and practice in managing low back pain: a comprehensive spine care system in a health maintenance organisation setting. *Spine* **25**, 738–40.

Koes, B., Bouter, L., van Mameren, H., Essers, A., Verstegen, G., Hofhuizen, D., Houben, J., and Knipschild, P. (1992). Randomised clinical trial of manipulative therapy and physiotherapy for persistent back and neck complaints: results of one year follow-up. *British Medical Journal* **304**, 601–5.

Lindstrom, I., Ohlund, C., Eek, C., Wallin, L., Peterson, L., and Nachemson, A. (1992). Mobility, strength, and fitness after a graded activity program for patients with subacute low back pain. A randomised prospective clinical study with a behavioural therapy approach. *Spine* **17**, 641–9.

Maher, C., Lattimer, J., and Refshaute, K. (1999). Prescription of activity for low back pain: what works? *The Australian Journal of Physiotherpy* **45**, 121–32.

Main, C. and Waddell, G. (1998). Spine update: behavioural responses to examination: a reappraisal of the interpretation of 'non-organic signs'. *Spine* **23**, 2367–71.

Maniadakis, N. and Gray, A. (2000). The economic burden of back pain in the United Kingdom. *Pain* **84**, 95–103.

Mayou, R., Bryant, B., and Duthie, R. (1993). Psychiatric consequences of road traffic accidents. *British Medical Journal* **307**, 647–51.

McQuay, H. and Moore, R. (1997). Antidepressants and chronic pain: effective analgesia in neuropathic pain and other syndromes. *British Medical Journal* **314**, 763–4.

Meade, T., Dyer, S., Browne, W., and Frank, A. (1995). Randomised comparison of chiropractic and hospital outpatient management of low back pain: results from extended follow up. *British Medical Journal* **311**, 349–51.

Milne, S., Welch V., Brosseau, L., Shea, B., Tugwell, P., and Wells, G. (2001). Transcutaneous elecrtical nerve stimulation (TENS) for chronic low back pain. In *The Cochrane Database of Systematic Reviews* Issue 2, CD003008. Oxford: Update Software.

Mitchell, R. and Carmen, G. (1994). The functional restoration approach to the treatment of chronic pain in patients with soft tissue and back injuries. *Spine* **19**, 633–42.

Nelemans, P., de Bie, R.A., de Vet, H.C., and Strumans, F. (1999). Injection therapy for subacute and chronic benign low back pain. In *The Cochrane Database of Systematic Reviews* Issue 2, CD001824. Oxford: Update Software.

Nelemans, P., deBie, R., deVet, H., and Strumans, F. (2001). Injection therapy for subacute and chronic benign low back pain (Cochrane Review). *Spine* **26**, 501–15.

Norlund, A. and Waddell, G. (2000). Cost of back pain in some OECD countries. In *Neck and Back Pain: the Scientific Evidence of Causes, Diagnosis and Treatment* (ed. A. Nachemson and E. Jonsson), pp. 421–5. Philadelphia PA: Lippincott, Williams & Wilkins.

Ongley, M., Klein, R., Dorman, T., EEk, B., and Hubert, L. (1987). A new approach to the treatment of chronic low back pain. *Lancet* 143–6.

Palinkas, L., Kabongo, M., and Surf Net Study Group (2000). The use of complementary and alternative medicine by primary care patients. *The Journal of Family Practice* **49**, 1121–30.

Porter, R., Hibbert, C., and Wicks, M. (1978). The spinal canal in symptomatic disc lesions. *The Journal of Bone and Joint Surgery* **60-B**, 485–7.

Porter, R. and Oakshot, G. (1994). Spinal stenosis and health status. *Spine* **19**, 901–3.

Roland, M., Waddell, G., Klaber Moffett, J., Burton, A., Main, C., and Cantrell, T. *The Back Book.* Norwich: The Stationary Office, 1996.

Roland, M. and Dixon, M. (1989). Randomized controlled trial of an educational booklet for patients presenting with back pain in general practice. *The Journal of The Royal College of General Practitioners* **39**, 244–6.

Rozenberg, S., Dubourg, G., Khalifa, P., Paolozzi, L., Maheu, E., and Ravaud, P. (1999). Efficacy of epidural steroids in low back pain and sciatica. A critical appraisal by a French Task Force of randomized trials. Critical Analysis Group of the French Society of Rheumatology *Revue de Rhumatisme (English Edition)* **66**, 79–85.

Schonstein, E., Kenny, D., Keating, J., and Koes, B. *Work Conditioning, Work Hardening and Functional Restoration for Workers with Back and Neck Pain (Cochrane Protocol).* Oxford: Update Software, 2000.

Shekelle, P. (1994). Spine update—spinal manipulation. *Spine* **19**, 858–61.

Sindrup, S. and Jensen, T. (1999). Efficacy of pharmacological treatments of neuropathic pain: an update and effect related to mechanism of drug action. *Pain* **83**, 389–400.

Spitzer, W., LeBlanc, F., and Dupuis, M. (1987). Scientific approach to the assessment and management of activity-related spinal disorders. A monograph for clinicians. Report of the Quebec Task Force on spinal disorders. *Spine* **12** (Suppl. 17), S1–59.

Talo, S., Rytokoski, U., and Puukka, P. (1992). Patient classification, a key to evaluate pain treatment: a psychological study in chronic low back pain patients. *Spine* **17**, 998–1011.

Teasell, R. and White, K. (1994). Clinical approaches to low back pain. Part 2: Management, sequelae, and disability and compensation. *Canadian Family Physician* **40**, 490–5.

Turner, J., Clancy, S., McQuade, K., and Cardenas, D. (1990). Effectiveness of behavioural therapy for chronic low back pain: a component analysis. *Journal of Consulting and Clinical Psychology* **58**, 573–9.

Turner-Stokes, L. and Frank, A. (1992). Urinary incontinence among patients with arthritis. *Journal of the Royal Society of Medicine* **85**, 389–93.

van Tulder, M., Cherkin, D., Berman, D., Lao, L., and Koes, B. (1999a). Acupuncture for low back pain. In *Cochrain Database of Systematic Reviews* Issue 2, CD001351. Oxford: Update Software.

van Tulder, M., Esmail, R., Bombardier, C., and Koes, B. (1999b). Back schools for non-specific low back pain. In *Cochrane Database of Systematic Reviews* Issue 2, CD000261. Oxford: Update Software.

van Tulder, M., Malmivaara, A., Esmail, R., and Koes, B. (2000a). Exercise therapy for low back pain: a systematic review within the framework of the Cochrane Collaboration Back Review Group. *Spine* **25**, 2784–96.

van Tulder, M., Malmivaara, A., Esmail, R., and Koes, B. (2000b) Exercise therapy for low back pain. In *Cochrane Database of Systematic Reviews* Issue 2, CD000335. Oxford: Update Software.

van Tulder, M., Ostelo, R., Vlaeyen, J., Linton, S., Morley, S., and Assendelft, W. (2000c). Behavioral treatment for chronic low back pain: a systematic review within the framework of the Cochrane Back Review Group. *Spine* **26**, 270–81.

Vingard, E. and Nachemson, A. (2000). Work-related influences on neck and low back pain. In *Neck and Back Pain: The Scientific Evidence of Causes, Diagnosis and Treatment* (ed. A. Nachemson and E. Jonsson), pp. 97–126. Philadelphia PA: Lippincott, Williams & Wilkins.

Von Korff, M., Deyo, R., Cherkin, D., and Barlow, W. (1993). Back pain in primary care. Outcomes at one year. *Spine* **18**, 855–62.

Von Korff, M., Barlow, W., Cherkin, D., and Deyo, R. (1994). Effects of practice style in managing back pain. *Annals of Internal Medicine* **121**, 187–95.

Waddell, G. (1982). An approach to backache. *British Journal of Hospital Medicine* **28**, 187 (See also pp. 190–1, 193–4).

Waddell, G. (1987). A new clinical model for the treatment of low back pain. 1987 Volvo award in clinical sciences. *Spine* **12**, 632–44.

Waddell, G., McIntosh, A., Hutchinson, A., Feder, G., and Lewis, M. *Low Back Pain Evidence Review* pp. 1–34. London: Royal College of General Practitioners, 1999.

Weiser, S. and Cedraschi, C. (1992). Psychosocial issues in the prevention of chronic low back pain—a literature review. *Clinical Rheumatology* **6**, 657–84.

Wiesel, S., Feffer, H., and Borenstein, D. (1988). Evaluation and outcome of low back pain of unknown etiology. *Spine* **13**, 679–80.

Wilson, R. and Wilson, S. (1964). A ten year follow-up of cases of low back pain. *The Practitioner* **192**, 657–60.

1.2.1.2 Spinal problems in children

Berit Flatø, Roger Sørensen, and Øystein Førre

Introduction

Children with spinal problems present with deformity, back pain, limping, systemic features, neurological disturbances, or a combination of these factors.

Deformity

Scoliosis or kyphosis is frequently asymptomatic and may be detected by a teacher, physician, physiotherapist, or relative.

Back pain

The number of children with back pain seen in hospitals is low, and in orthopaedic or paediatric rheumatology practices it accounts for 2–3 per cent of admissions (Turner et al. 1989; Malleson et al. 1996). On the other hand, back pain is found in 20–30 per cent of the children and adolescents in the general population (Fairbank et al. 1984; Balague et al. 1988; Salminen et al. 1992a; Burton et al. 1996; Taimela et al. 1997; Gunzburg et al. 1999; Troussier et al. 1999). Spinal symptoms are rarely seen in children under the age of 10 years, but approximately 30 per cent of the adolescents have experienced low back pain (Balague et al. 1988; Taimela et al. 1997).

While back pain is frequently mechanical or idiopathic in adult patients, children, and particularly preadolescents, admitted for back pain, often have an underlying organic condition. A specific cause has been found in 52–85 per cent of children admitted to the orthopaedic clinic (Turner et al. 1989; Richards et al. 1999). On the other hand, Feldman et al. (1995) identified a pathological condition in only 22 per cent of 226 schoolchildren using single photon emission computed tomography (SPECT). Differences in the definition of back pain, the selection of patients and the age at onset influence the number of times a detectable underlying pathological process is found. Deformity (Table 1) and back pain (Table 2) in children have multiple causes, including congenital disorders, trauma, inflammatory rheumatic diseases, infections, neoplasms, and non-specific factors.

History

A detailed history should be obtained with emphasis on possible pathological processes (Table 3). The age of the child may help in differentiating between disorders. In general, young children are more likely to have an underlying infection or tumour than adolescents, who tend to have less severe disorders, such as spondylolysis or Scheuermann kyphosis. There is often a history of trauma in children with musculoskeletal symptoms. However, this may reflect the frequency of trauma in the paediatric population in general rather than the frequency of trauma as a cause of back pain.

Questions about the onset, duration, frequency, and intensity of the pain are important. Mild pain associated with physical activities that has been present for a short time may represent muscle strain or overuse. Pain that persists for weeks or months following active athletic training may represent an underlying spondylosis or spondylolisthesis. The presence of constant, progressive pain, particularly if present at night and unrelieved by rest or mobilization suggests a tumour or infection. Morning stiffness and

Table 1 Major causes of spinal deformity in children

Structural scoliosis
Idiopathic
Neuromuscular
Congenital
Infection
Related to spondylolysis
Tumours
Non-structural
Postural
Limb length discrepancy
Nerve root irritation
Kyphosis
Postural
Scheuermann disease
Congenital

Table 2 Causes of back pain in children

Developmental
Painful scoliosis
Spondylolysis and spondylolisthesis
Scheuermann disease
Infection
Discitis
Vertebral osteomyelitis
Spinal epidural abscess
Inflammation
Juvenile arthritis
Osteoporosis
Mechanical
Herniated disk
Muscle strain
Fractures
Neoplasms
Benign (osteoid osteomas, osteoblastoma, aneurysmal bone cyst)
Malignant (leukaemia, lymphoma, sacroma)
Visceral
Pyelonephritis, appendicitis, retroperitoneal abscess

Table 3 Approach to the child's spinal pain or deformity

History
Onset, duration, frequency, intensity, location, and radiation of discomfort
Constitutional symptoms
Morning stiffness
Trauma
Continence of bladder and bowel
Family history of related symptoms
Examination
General screening
Posture
Anterior and lateral flexion
Joint examination
Neurological examination
Laboratory evaluation
Complete blood count
C-reactive protein or erythrocyte sedimentation rate (HLA-B27, antinuclear antibody, rheumatoid factor)
Imaging
Plain radiographs, anterioposterior, lateral (and oblique) view
Technetium bone scans
Single photon emission computed tomography
CT or MRI

improvement on mobilization suggests an inflammatory rheumatic disease. Inflammatory processes are usually relieved by non-steroidal anti-inflammatory drugs (NSAIDs), but aspirin and NSAIDs also relieve the pain associated with tumours like osteoid osteoma. Neurological symptoms, such as radicular pain, paraesthesia, and changes in sphincter control, should be noted, although these symptoms are uncommon in children.

Changes in the general health of the patient, like fever, malaise, lethargy, or weight loss, may indicate a malignant, infectious, or inflammatory aetiology. A limp or refusal to walk may be the first manifestation of a spinal disorder particularly in young children. Abdominal pain may also be the presenting symptom. Furthermore, referred back pain may be a presenting feature of renal disease, gastrointestinal disorders, abdominal processes, pneumonia, or gynaecological disorders in children.

Scoliosis is usually pain-free. The combination of pain and scoliosis indicates an underlying pathology, such as neoplasm, infection, or a prolapsed intervertebral disc.

Physical examination

A general examination, assessments of the spine and peripheral joints and a neurological examination should be performed (Table 3). The spinal examination should include an assessment of posture, alignment, and skin conditions. The spine should be examined from the posterior and lateral viewpoints and leg length discrepancies and pelvic asymmetry should be determined. The forward bending test assesses thoracic and lumbar asymmetry and spinal flexibility. The modified Schober method has been found to be useful in distinguishing between normal and reduced anterior lumbar flexion in children and adolescents (Fig. 1) (Macrae and Wright 1969; Burgos-Vargas et al. 1985). Values of at least 6 cm in boys and 5 cm in girls are considered normal (Burgos-Vargas et al. 1985; Salminen et al. 1992b). The range of lateral movement is another useful measure (Domjan et al. 1990). This is found to be at least 10 per cent of body height in normal young adults (Fig. 2). Spinal stiffness may indicate an inflammatory process, infection, or neoplasms. Palpation may help to localize the lesion to paravertebral musculature or midline spinous processes.

Neurological abnormalities, such as limping, disturbed sensation, muscle weakness, or reflex changes are associated with nerve root compression. Limited strait leg raising indicates compression of the spinal cord or nerve roots. The test is positive when passive supine raising of the straight leg to less than 60° of hip flexion aggravates pain that radiates below the knee. The presence of clonus and an abnormal Babinski reflex may indicate a central abnormality, while asymmetry in abdominal reflexes may be found in patients with spinal cord abnormalities like syringomyelia.

Imaging

Plain radiographs are consistently the most important imaging method and should always be reviewed before requisitioning more advanced methods (Richards et al. 1999). If scoliosis or kyphosis is present, erect radiographs should be taken. Anterior and lateral views of the entire spine are useful for examinating children with low back pain, particularly those under the age of 5 years. Deformities, fractures, pars defects, disc space narrowing, destructive radio-dense or radio-lucent lesions are examples of abnormalities that can be detected. Additional oblique views may provide further information of bone pathology.

If the pain persists and plain radiographs and neurological examinations are normal, a technetium bone scan should be performed. A bone scan is sensitive to reactive processes, such as infections, inflammation, occult fractures, and tumours and is particularly useful in young children who are unable to localize the pain. SPECT may give a more precise localization of a lesion within the spine and is superior to bone scan in detecting spondylolysis (Bodner et al. 1988).

Magnetic resonance imaging (MRI) is the optimal method for assessing spinal cord tumours, discitis, and herniated discs. This examination should be performed prior to bone scan if a neurological abnormality is present. However, care must be taken not to interpret normal MRI scans as

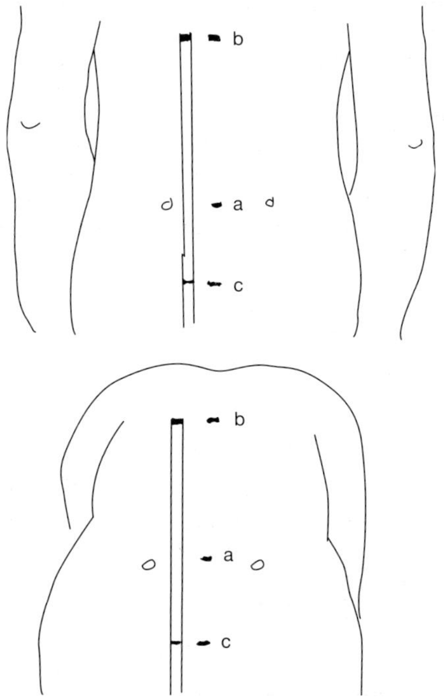

Fig. 1 Measuring anterior spinal flexion. With the child standing upright, marks are made on the skin overlying the lumbosacral junction, a; 10 cm above, b; and 5 cm below this point, c. The child is asked to bend forward as far as possible without bending the knees. The Schober measure is the distance from b to c in the forward bending position minus the distance in the upright position (Macrae and Wright 1969).

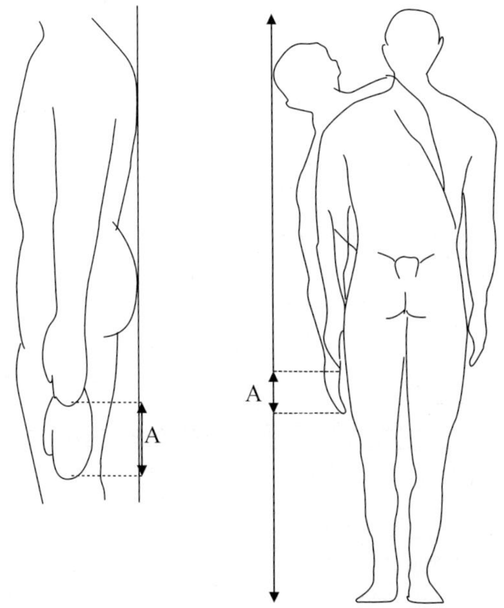

Fig. 2 Measuring spinal lateral flexion. The patient stands against a wall with the arms and fingers stretched. The difference between the mark of the tip of the third finger in the upright and maximal lateral flexion is measured (A). A distance (A) longer than 10% of the body height is considered to be normal (Domjan et al. 1990).

pathological in the developing child (Richards et al. 1999). MRI signals of the discs, end plates, and vertebral bodies in the normal paediatric spine change dramatically with age. Bone tumours and fractures may also be seen on MRI, but computer tomography (CT) remains the best method for determining the extent of osseous abnormalities that are identified on plain radiographs or bone scans (Petrus and Nelson 1998).

Laboratory evaluation

A complete blood count, C-reactive protein (CRP), and an erythrocyte sedimentation rate (ESR) are the most useful screening laboratory tests in children and adolescents with back pain. Otherwise the history and physical examination will dictate the appropriate laboratory tests. If a rheumatological disorder is suspected, testing for HLA-B27, antinuclear antibodies, and rheumatoid factor may be indicated.

Non-specific low back pain

The annual incidence of non-specific low back pain in schoolchildren is 10–22 per cent (Table 4) (Nissinen et al. 1994; Burton et al. 1996; Kujala et al. 1997; Ehrmann-Feldman 1998), and a lifetime prevalence of approximately 30–50 per cent have been found in most studies of schoolchildren (Table 5) (Fairbank et al. 1984; Balague et al. 1988; Turner et al. 1989; Salminen et al. 1992a; Burton et al. 1996; Malleson et al. 1996; Taimela et al. 1997; Gunzburg et al. 1999; Troussier et al. 1999). The prevalence increases with the age of the child, from 6–20 per cent in the 10-year-old schoolchildren to 20–70 per cent in the 15-year-old schoolchildren (Balague et al. 1988; Taimela et al. 1997; Troussier et al. 1999). A very low 1-year prevalence (1 per cent) in 7-year-old children was found in a nation wide cohort-based Finnish study (Taimela et al. 1997).

An increased prevalence among girls has been found in most studies (Balague et al. 1988; Troussier et al. 1999), but some authors report no gender differences (Fairbank et al. 1984; Taimela et al. 1997). Adolescent low back pain has been associated with familial clustering, physical inactivity, sport injuries, decreased trunk muscle strength, and psychosocial factors (Fairbank et al. 1984; Balague et al. 1988; Kujala et al. 1997; Taimela et al. 1997; Troussier et al. 1999).

The clinical significance of non-specific low back pain in schoolchildren is unclear. Most patients have self-limiting symptoms (Taimela et al. 1997). Recurrent or continuous symptoms were found to be present in one-third of the children with low back pain in Finland, increasing with the age of the child (Salminen et al. 1992a,b; Taimela et al. 1997). Children and adolescents with low back pain are rarely admitted to paediatric rheumatology or orthopaedic centres (Turner et al. 1989; Malleson et al. 1996). Compared with schoolchildren without back pain, adolescents with low back pain have been found to have an increased frequency of low back pain, hospital admissions, and decreased work capacity due to low back pain in adulthood (Harreby et al. 1996). In a hospital based study, half of 37 children admitted for chronic non-specific musculoskeletal pain had persistent pain and disability 10 years after the onset of symptoms (Flatø et al. 1997). Thus, even though most schoolchildren with non-specific spinal symptoms have mild, self-limiting pain, there is a subgroup of children with more chronic and severe symptoms persisting into adulthood.

Scoliosis

Scoliosis represents alterations in normal spinal alignment in the anterioposterior plane that always involve a rotational malalignment of the vertebra. This rotational malalignment of the vertebra results in rib rotation when the curve is in the thoracic area. With forward bending, the ribs are rotated posteriorly (hump) on the convexity of the curvature and anteriorly (valley) on the concavity (Fig. 3). The degree of curvature is measured on anterioposterior radiographs from the inferior to the superior end vertebra involved (Fig. 4). The frequency of scoliosis is approximately 3 per cent in schoolchildren. Most scoliotic deformities are idiopathic.

Table 4 The incidence of low back pain in children

Author	Publication year	*n*	Age in years	Country	Source	One year incidence (%)
Nissinen et al.	1994	859	13	Finland	Population	18
Burton et al.	1996	216	12–16	England	Population	12–22
Kujala et al.	1997	98	10–16	Finland	Athletes and non-athletes	11
Ehrmann-Feldman	1998	377	14	Canada	Population	17

Table 5 The prevalence of low back pain in children

Author	Publication year	*n*	Age in years	Country	Source	Prevalence (%)
Turner et al.	1989	61	<15	England	Dep. of orthopedic	2
Malleson et al.	1996	3362	2–18	Canada	Paed. Rheum. Clin.	3
Fairbank et al.	1984	446	13–17	England	Population	26
Balague et al.	1988	1715	7–16	Swiss	Population	33
Salminen et al.	1992	1503	14	Finland	Population	18
Burton et al.	1996	216	11–15	England	Population	12–50
Taimela et al.	1997	1171	7–16	Finland	Population	1–18
Gunzburg et al.	1999	392	9	Belgium	Population	36
Troussier et al.	1999	972	9–17	France	Population	33

(a)

(b)

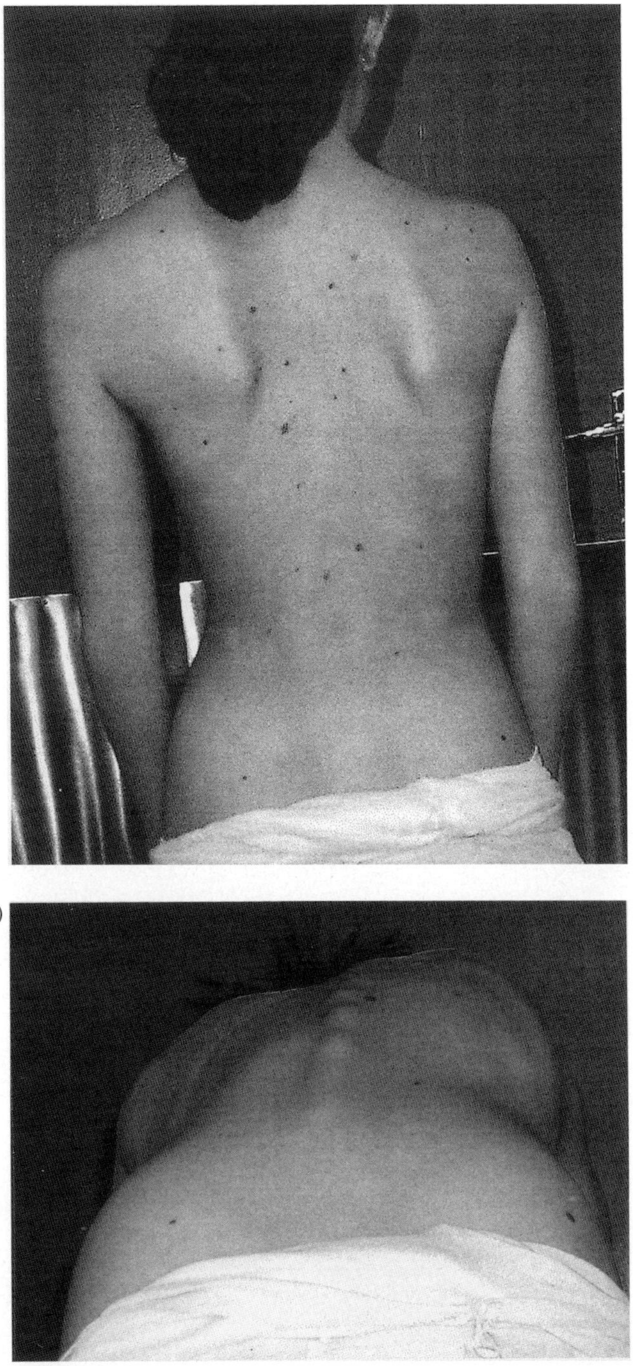

Fig. 3 (a) Idiopathic scoliosis in a 14-year-old girl. (b) With forward bending a hump is seen on the concavity of the curvature.

Idiopathic scoliosis

Approximately 20 per cent of children with scoliosis have other family members with the same condition. However, the exact cause is unknown. The incidence is slightly higher in girls than in boys, and the deformity more often progresses and requires treatment in girls. Scoliosis most frequently occurs in adolescents (adolescent form), but may also present before the age of 3 years (infantile form) or between 4 and 10 years (juvenile form). A thoracic curve that is convex toward the right is the most common pattern.

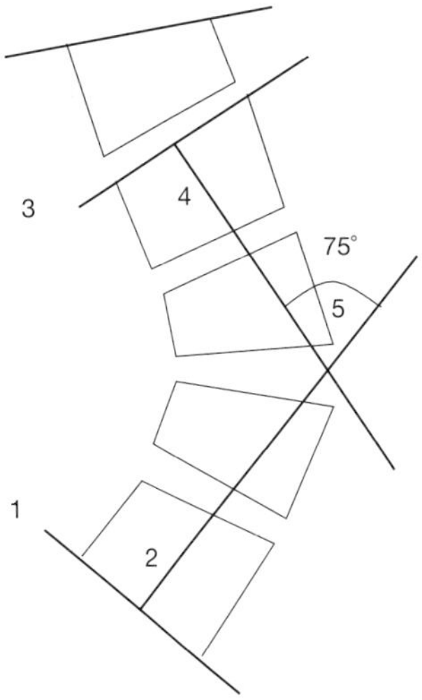

Fig. 4 Measurement of the degree of scoliosis by the Cobb method: 1, the lowest vertebra whose bottom tilts to the concavity of curve; 2, the erect perpendicular to line 1; 3, the highest vertebra whose top tilts to the concavity of curve; 4, the drop perpendicular to line 3; 5, the intersecting angle. Curves less than 20° are considered to be mild, 20–40° are moderate, and above 40° are severe (McCarthy 1994).

The possibility of progression increases with younger age, thoracic left curves and greater curves. Idiopathic scoliosis is usually painless and the presence of back pain and a left thoracic curve is associated with an increased incidence of intraspinal pathology (Table 2). However, in a recent study of 2442 adolescents with scoliosis, some back pain was present in 32 per cent (Ramirez et al. 1997). Only 9 per cent of those with pain had an identifiable underlying condition. The pain was mild, non-specific, intermittent and resolved with rest. When persistent, severe pain is present in combination with scoliosis, the possibility of an associated condition must be thoroughly investigated. These children should be evaluated with MRI.

The treatment of progressive idiopathic scoliosis is bracing or surgery. Other methods are ineffective. The risk of progression depends on several factors like age and the location and magnitude of the curve. Usually curves between 25° and 45° are treated with bracing and those greater than 45° by surgery in skeletally immature patients.

Congenital and neuromuscular scoliosis

Congenital scoliosis depends on a partial or complete failure of formation or segmentation of vertebra. Congenital genitourinary malformations occur in 20 per cent of children with congenital scoliosis, and renal ultrasonography should be performed in all patients. Congenital heart disease may also be associated. Spinal dysraphism occur in approximately 20 per cent of the patients (see 'Spina bifida and spinal dysraphism' below). Congenital scoliosis may occur in association with syndromes such as Klippel-Feil syndrome and myelodysplasia. The risk of progression depends on the growth potential of the malformed vertebra.

Neuromuscular scoliotic deformity is associated with neuromuscular disorders like cerebral palsy, muscular dystrophy, spinal muscular atrophy, and myelodysplasia. Progression is usually continuous once scoliosis begins. The magnitude of the deformity depends on the severity of the condition and how the weakness has progressed.

Radiographs should include anterioposterior and lateral standing and sitting views of the entire spine. MRI is the method of choice in evaluating the possibility of spinal dysraphism. Early diagnosis and prompt treatment of progressive curves are essential because of the risk of rapid progression (McMaster 1994). Orthotic treatment is of limited value and surgical treatment is usually indicated in progressive congenital and neuromuscular scolioses.

Compensatory scoliosis

Leg-length discrepancies result in pelvic obliquity that can appear clinically as scoliosis, but it disappears with forward bending.

Kyphosis

Kyphosis refers to a round-back deformity with increased angulations in the thoracic or thoracolumbal spine in the sagittal plane.

Scheuermann kyphosis

Scheuermann disease is one of the most common causes of spinal deformity and back pain in children and adolescents. The disorder is seen in 3–5 per cent of adolescents in the general population, usually those between 13 and 17 years of age (Lowe 1990). The aetiology is mainly unknown. Histological studies show vertebral end plate and growth cartilage anomalies. Mild or no symptoms are seen in the scolioses located in the high- and mid-thoracic region. Approximately 70 per cent of patients with kyphosis in the low thoracic and lumbar spine have continuous back pain (Murray et al. 1993).

The physical examination demonstrates an increased thoracic kyphosis that cannot be corrected and usually a compensatory lumbar hyperlordosis. The classical radiographic findings include kyphosis exceeding 45° (normal range 20–45°), wedging of at least 5° in three adjacent vertebra, vertebral end plate irregularities, disc space narrowing, and occasionally protrusion of disc material into the vertebral body (Schmorl's nodes). The clinical and functional outcome was benign in a 32-year follow-up of 61 patients with Scheuermann disease (Murray et al. 1993).

Exercises to stretch the hamstrings and lumbodorsal region and to strengthen the abdominal muscles may improve symptoms, but will not correct the kyphosis. Brace treatment may inhibit progression of the curve. Surgical intervention is rarely indicated, but may be considered if there are large or progressive deformities (>70°) or continuous pain, or if the patient is greatly concerned about their appearance.

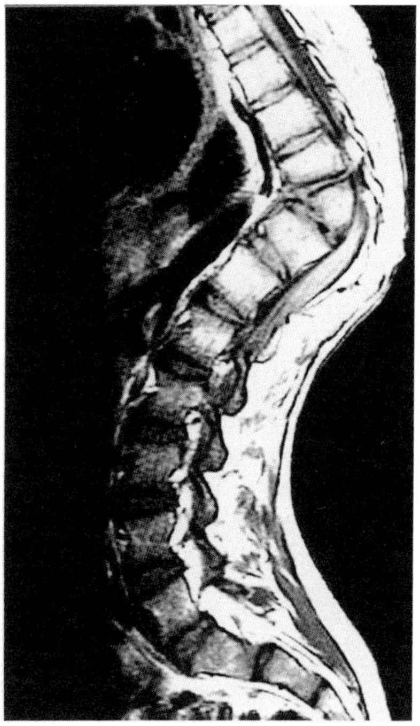

Fig. 5 Lateral magnetic resonance imaging of a 13-year-old boy with congenital kyphosis.

Congenital kyphosis

Congenital kyphosis is due to vertebral malformation (Fig. 5). The more severe deformities are usually recognized at birth and progress rapidly. Other less severe deformities may not appear until years later. Once progression begins, it does not cease until growth ends. A progressive deformity may result in paraplegia. Thus, early diagnosis and admission to specialized care are important. Treatment, when necessary, is operative, because other methods are ineffective.

Postural kyphosis

Postural kyphosis is secondary to bad posture. The diagnosis is based on the adolescent's ability to correct the rounded back voluntarily. No abnormalities are present radiographically.

Spondylolysis and spondylolisthesis

Spondylolysis is a defect in the pars interarticularis of the vertebra. The defect probably represents a stress fracture. Spondylolisthesis refers to a forward slippage away from the next caudal vertebra. Spondlylosis is most common at L5 and spondylolisthesis usually occurs with L5 slipping forward on S1 (Fig. 6).

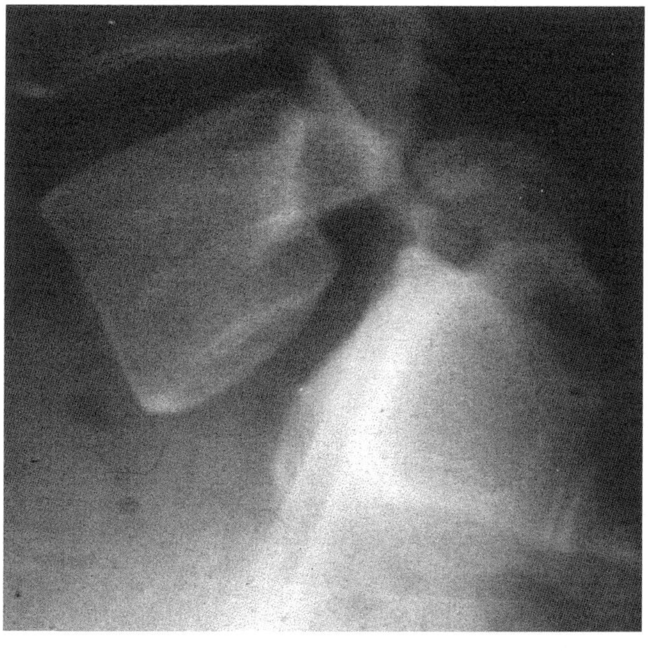

Fig. 6 Spondylolysis and spondylolisthesis (L5–S1) in a 15-year-old girl.

Slippage caused by spondylolysis is the most common form of spondylolisthesis (isthmic spondylolisthesis). Spondylolysis with or without spondylolisthesis has been found to affect 4 per cent of preschool children, increasing to 6 per cent at age 18 (Fredrickson et al. 1984). The proportion of spondylolysis patients who have slippage is not known, but this condition has been reported to develop in up to 74 per cent. Pars defects are half as common in girls as in boys, but spondylolisthesis is four times more common in girls (Lonstein 1999).

The causes of spondylolysis and spondylolisthesis include hereditary factors, congenital predisposition, trauma, posture, growth, and biomechanical factors. Repetitive micro-trauma and hyperextensions are thought to explain the higher incidence among athletes, football players, and weightlifters. The patients frequently present in adolescence with midline low lumbar pain related to activity and relieved by rest.

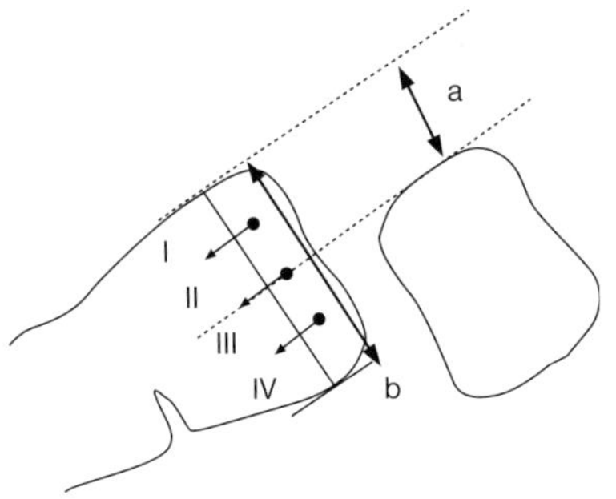

Fig. 7 Spondylolisthesis measured as the percentage slip of L5 on S1 (a/b). The grade of slippage ranges from I (≤25%) to IV (>75%) (McCarthy 1994).

On examination, the pain can be reproduced by hyperextension of the spine. In most cases (90 per cent), the slippage has already occurred at the time of the initial examination. There may be a palpable step between the area of the unaffected lumbar spine and the affected area. Standing anterio-posterior and lateral radiographs are usually diagnostic. Additional oblique views may increase the sensitivity of plain radiographs. CT may be necessary to better define the disorder. MRI may be useful in the early diagnosis of spondylolisthesis and for the evaluation of nerve roots.

A progressing slippage occurs in a low percentage of the cases, most often during the adolescent growth spurt. Repeated radiographs are needed until the end of puberty. If the slippage is more than 25 per cent (grade II or more), a warning not to participate in contact sports or sports with lumbar hyperextension may be considered (Fig. 7). Conservative management with exercises and braces is successful if treatment is started in the early stage. Surgical fusion is indicated for skeletally immature patients if slipping is progressive or greater than 50 per cent (grade III or IV) (Morita et al. 1995).

Spondylolisthesis may also be due to a congenital deficiency (dysplastic spondylolisthesis). This includes a dysplastic, elongated pars interarticularis with facets that subluxate at the L5–S1 level. These patients are more prone to recurrent symptoms and deformity than those with isthmic spondylolisthesis. In addition to these factors, degenerative and traumatic changes may cause spondylolisthesis.

Infectious spondylitis

Infectious spondylitis includes discitis, vertebral osteomyelitis, non-specific spondylitis, and sacroiliac joint infections. Bacteraemia from multiple possible causes (urinary tract infections, otitis, pneumonia, etc.) is thought to initiate the process. The infections may arise in the vertebral end plate and spread to the intervertebral disc space, and can develop into vertebral osteomyelitis (Correa et al. 1993). In contrast to adult patients, discitis predominates and true vertebral osteomyelitis is rare in children because discs are more vascular in childhood. The most common organism is *Staphylococcus aureus* followed by salmonella and streptococcus. *Mycobacterium tuberculosis* may also cause spondylitis. The most common sites of infectious spondylitis is the lumbar spine, but it may also be located in the thoracic, cervical, and lumbosacral areas. There are two peak age periods: one at the age of 6 months to 4 years and another between 10 and 14 years.

Symptoms will depend on the age of the child (Correa et al. 1993). Under the age of 3 years, crawling without any lumbar lordosis, limping or loss of the ability to walk or stand are presenting symptoms. Children aged between 3 and 8 years present with primary abdominal symptoms. Older children may be able to localize the back pain and stand with an abnormal posture. Systemic symptoms with fever are frequently seen.

Physical examination typically reveals a rigid lumbar spine, pain on flexion, tenderness over the area involved, and positive straight leg test. CRP and ESR are significantly elevated in most patients. The white blood cell count may be elevated and blood cultures may be positive.

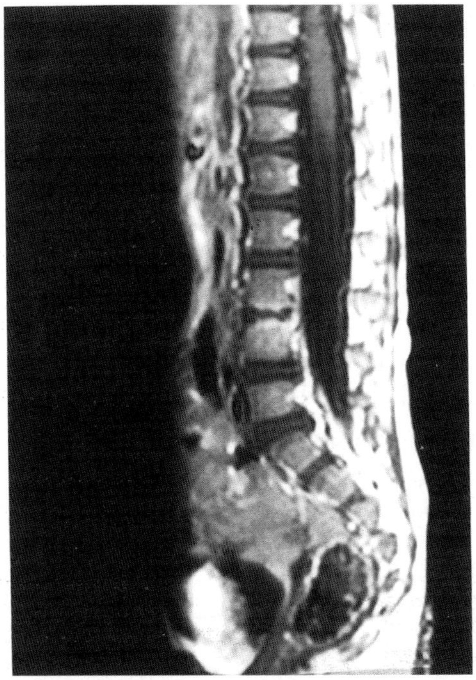

Fig. 8 A 2-year-old girl with discitis and vertebral osteomyelitis at the L2–L3 level. The child presented with a painful back and inability to walk. Magnetic resonance imaging demonstrated narrowing of the disc space and the end plates are irregular. There is oedema of the adjacent part of the vertebral bodies involved.

Plain radiographs are usually normal early on, but disc space narrowing and irregularities in the adjacent vertebra may develop later during the disease course. Bone scan can help to localize the process. MRI gives the best picture of the pathology (Fig. 8). Needle aspiration or biopsy is reserved for children who do not respond to treatment, are systemically ill, or live in environments where tuberculosis or other unusual infections are found (Richards et al. 1999). Symptoms usually resolve rapidly with intravenous antibiotics. These should be continued for 1–2 weeks followed by oral antibiotics for an additional 4 weeks. Bracing may be indicated to avoid the development of kyphosis. Surgery with debridement is rarely necessary.

Herniated disc

Lumbar intervertebral disc herniation, although common in adults, is infrequent in children. The onset of symptoms in childhood or adolescence is reported in 1–4 per cent of patients with disc herniation (Martinez-Lage et al. 1997; Richards et al. 1999). Likewise, between 1 and 3 per cent of children and adolescents with back pain are reported to have herniated nucleus prolepses, mostly after the age of 11 years. However, the diagnosis is difficult to establish in children. In a prospective study utilizing MRI, abnormal spinal findings were found in as many as 42 per cent of 40 adolescents with low back pain (Erkintalo et al. 1995).

The L4–L5 and L5–S1 levels are the most common location of disc herniation. The symptoms may arise from the damaged disc complex, but posterior displacement of these structures into the spinal canal may also cause pain (Mason 1999). Low back pain with sciatica and scoliosis are the most frequent findings. There may be lumbar rigidity and a positive straight leg raising test.

Females predominate in the younger age group while males predominate after the age of 16 years. Adolescents with early disc degenerative changes are at greater risk for suffering from low back pain in adult life than those without disc abnormalities (Salminen et al. 1995).

Plain radiographs are of limited value because disc space narrowing is a rare manifestation in children. MRI is helpful, but care must be taken not to misdiagnose normal changes in the developing spine.

Patients without nerve root impingement should be given non-surgical treatment, including a short period of bed rest, medication (analgesics, muscle relaxants, and/or NSAIDs), and exercises. There are few long-term studies of conservative treatment of disc herniation in children, but approximately 50 per cent of the patients improve without surgical intervention (Martinez-Lage et al. 1997; Richards et al. 1999). The indications for surgical treatment include significant neurological deficits or pain that does not respond to conservative treatment. Surgical treatment is effective in the vast majority of children and adolescents with disc herniation.

Spinal problems in inflammatory rheumatic diseases

Inflammatory synovitis frequently affects the spine in children with juvenile idiopathic arthritis (JIA) (Burgos-Vargas and Vazquez-Mellado 1995; Laiho et al. 2001; Flatø et al. 2002a,b). The axial involvement differs in the subtypes of JIA. The frequency of affection of the sacroiliac joints are increased in enthesitis related and psoriatic arthritis, while the cervical spine is the most frequent site of spine involvement in rheumatoid factor positive and negative polyarthritis, persistent and extended oligoarthritis, and systemic arthritis.

Sacroiliitis as seen in ankylosing spondylitis is characterized by clinical and radiographic signs of arthritis in the sacroiliac joint (Fig. 9). However, peripheral arthritis usually precedes sacroiliitis by several years. Burgos-Vargas and Vazquez-Mellado (1995) found that 15 per cent of 225 Mexican JIA patients developed ankylosing spondylitis during at least 10 years of follow-up. Although rare in the first years of disease, most patients had lumbar pain and stiffness more than 7 years after disease onset. In a recent study of 314 Norwegian JIA patients, the cervical spine was the most frequent site of spine involvement (Table 6) (Flatø et al. 2002a,b). In this study, 6 per cent of the JIA patients had radiographically demonstrated sacroiliitis at follow-up 12–25 years after disease onset. Chronic low back pain and restricted lumbar mobility was common in the patients with, but not those without, sacroiliitis. Alternating buttock pain and night pain were the most characteristic complaints in patients with sacroiliitis.

Radiographic abnormalities of the thoracic and lumbar spine are rarely seen in children with sacroiliitis. The typical finding of 'bamboo spine' and calcification of the spinal ligaments is generally not seen in children. Sacroiliitis is associated with HLA-B27, male gender, late onset of the arthritis, and hip involvement (Burgos-Vargas and Vazquez-Mellado 1995; Flatø et al. 2002a). A higher frequency of sacroiliitis is seen in childhood arthritides related to enthesitis (70–90 per cent), psoriasis (30 per cent), inflammatory bowel disease (30–50 per cent), and Reiter's disease (Burgos-Vargas and Clark 1989; Hamilton et al. 1990; Cabral et al. 1992; Flatø et al. 2002b).

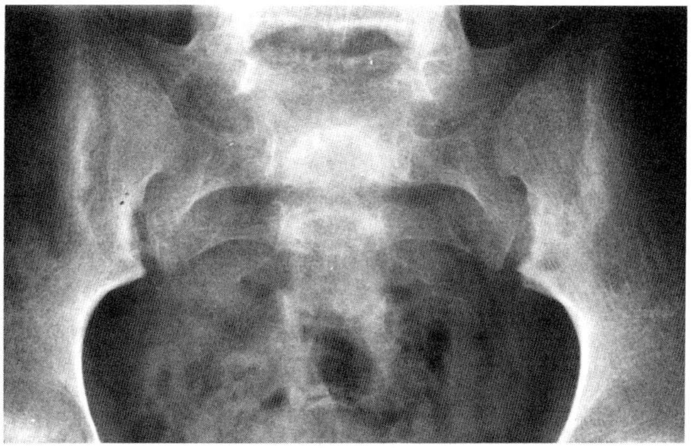

Fig. 9 Bilateral radiographic sacroiliitis in a 13-year-old boy with a 17-month history of peripheral arthritis and low back pain. Note the widening, indistinct lateral margins, and lateral sclerosis of the sacroiliac joints, particularly the lower parts. Radiographs of the same patient 7 months earlier demonstrated normal sacroiliac joints.

Table 6 The frequency of spinal symptoms during 15 years of disease course in patients with juvenile idiopathic arthritis

	% of total no. of JIA pts (*n* = 314)	% of pts with sacroiliitis (*n* = 20)	% of pts without sacroiliitis (*n* = 294)	*P* of pts with versus without sacroiliitis
Cervical pain	32	35	32	NS
Cervical stiffness	37	40	37	NS
Reduced cervical rotation	36	60	38	NS
Stiffness of the lower back	16	55	13	<0.001
Episodic low back pain	32	60	30	0.006
Low back pain not relieved by rest	9	46	6	<0.001
Low back pain relived by mobility	6	30	5	<0.001
Effect of NSAID	8	25	7	0.004
Buttock pain	9	40	7	<0.001
Alternating buttock pain	4	30	2	<0.001
Back pain at night	8	45	6	<0.001
Up at night because of back pain	3	20	2	<0.001
Reduced anterior flexion	32	75	30	<0.001
Reduced lateral spinal flexion	33	70	31	<0.001

Results of a study of a cohort of 314 patients with juvenile idiopathic arthritis followed up 15 years after disease onset (Flatø et al. 2002a,b). NS = not statistically significant; pts = patients.

NSAIDs have a good effect on back pain and stiffness in spondyloarthritis of childhood (see Chapter 6.4.2). Active physical and occupational therapy is important. The goal of the therapy is the maintenance of normal range of motion and strength. The children should be encouraged to participate in sport and other everyday activities as much as they want.

Cervical involvement is common in rheumatoid factor negative and positive polyarthritis, persistent and extended oligoarthritis, and systemic juvenile arthritis, particularly in the polyarticular subtypes. Neck pain and decreased range of movement have been found in 30 per cent of these JIA patients (Flatø et al. 2002b, 2003). Recently, Laiho et al. (2001) found radiographic cervical changes in 86 per cent of 42 children with severe refractory JIA. Young children may not complain of neck pain and yet lose significant range of motion. The spine involvement almost always starts at the C2–C3 level. The inflammation may hamper the growth of the vertebral bodies and intervertebral discs. Radiologically, loss of sharp margins at the articular facets may be seen initially, to be followed later by erosions, joint space narrowing and fusion of vertebrae (Copley and Dormans 1998). The odontoid (dens axis) may be eroded due to synovial hypertrophy. The loss of dens axis as a functional peg, may cause atlantoaxial subluxation (see 'Atlantoaxial instability' below). Cervical involvement is associated with micrognatia.

The treatment of cervical involvement in JIA includes NSAIDs and physical and occupational therapy (see Chapter 6.5.1). JIA patients with neck stiffness or pain should have flexion-extension radiographs taken at intervals to monitor disease progression. Careful planning of any surgical procedure is important. Stiff cervical collars and surgical corrections may be needed (see 'Atlantoaxial instability' below). Special consideration should be given to children with both JIA and Down syndrome, as both conditions may contribute to cervical instability.

Svantesson et al. (1981) examined the spines of 320 juvenile rheumatoid arthritis patients in Sweden and found structural scoliosis in 5 per cent, which is considerably more frequent than in the normal population.

Osteoporosis, vertebral compression fractures, and infections due to persistently active disease and/or treatment occur in JIA (see 'Osteoporosis' below).

The spine is not a primary area of involvement of the disease process in juvenile systemic lupus erythematosus, dermatomyositis, systemic sclerosis, mixed connective tissue disease, or vasculitis syndromes. However, back pain in these patients needs to be evaluated carefully with a view to the possibility of infections, vertebral compression fractures, serositis, haemorrhages, or tumours.

Back pain is present in 20–40 per cent of children with chronic idiopathic musculoskeletal pain (Sherry et al. 1991; Flatø et al. 1997). In these children, any organic causes of the symptoms should be eliminated followed by a comprehensive treatment program including physical and occupational therapy and sometimes psychiatric evaluations.

Atlantoaxial instability

Atlantoaxial or atlantooccipital instability may be due to inflammatory rheumatic diseases, congenital anomalies (aplasia, hypoplasia, Down syndrome, skeletal dysplasia, Klippel-Feil syndrome and inborn errors of metabolism), inflammatory processes of the retro pharyngeal or pharyngeal spaces, or to trauma (Copley and Dormans 1998). The mechanism may be an abnormal dens axis (odontoid process), laxity of the transverse ligament, or fractures. Instability may produce spinal cord compression and neurologic signs, spontaneously or after minor trauma. The symptoms and signs may range from neck pain and limited range of motion to paraesthesia of the upper extremities, distal muscle weakness, sleep apnoea, torticollis, or quadriplegia.

Anterioposterior and lateral radiographs may confirm the diagnosis. Flexion and extension lateral positions are useful to evaluate instability, but the child must be conscious, cooperative, not very young, and have no trauma or neurological deficit. The distance of the posterior margin of the anterior arch of the atlas (C1) to the front of dens axis (C2) (antlantodens interval) is less than 4–5 mm in children and 3 mm in adults (Fig. 10). When the atlantodens interval exceeds 10–12 mm, all ligaments have failed. The distance between the posterior margin of the axis body and the posterior atlas arch (anteroposterior canal diameter) helps to determine the risk of cord compression, which is

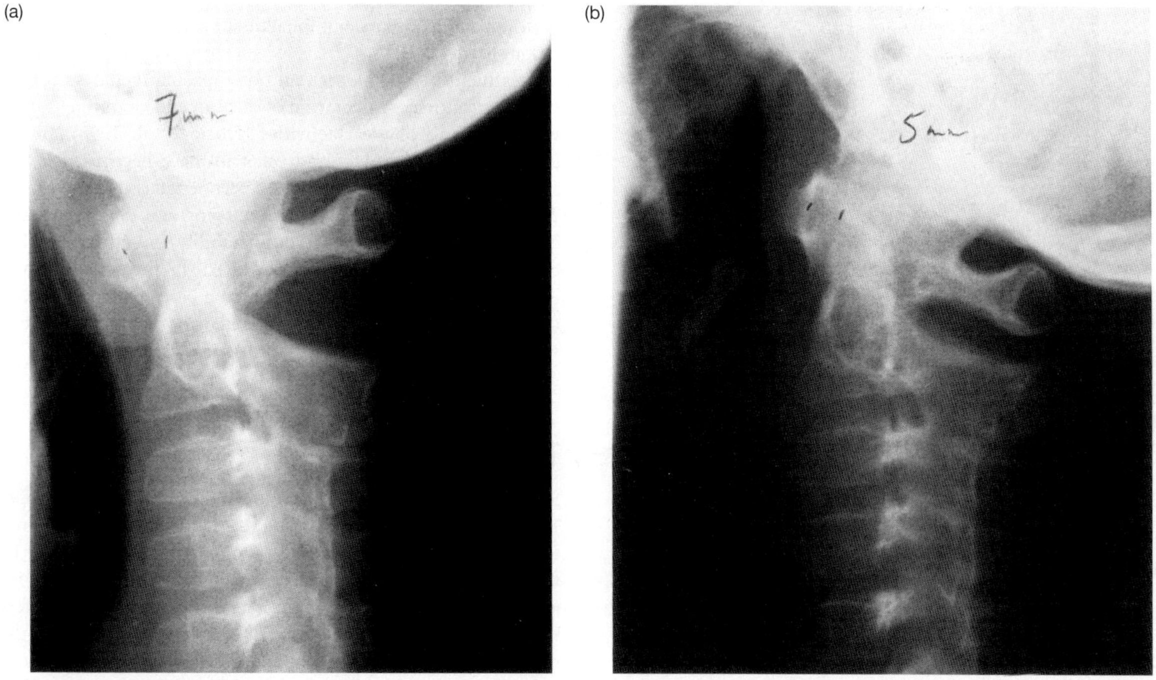

Fig. 10 Anterior atlantoaxial subluxation in a 13-year-old boy with systemic onset juvenile idiopathic arthritis. The atlantodens interval is 7 mm in flexion (a) and 5 mm in extension (b). Note also the bony ankylosis of C2–C6.

usually at a distance of more than 18 mm (Copley and Dormans 1998). Open mouth anterioposterior radiographs may be needed to visualize rotary displacement. CT scans and MRI may delineate bone abnormalities and cord involvement.

Brace reduction and immobilization for approximately 3 months may permit healing. Although rare in children, unstable atlantoaxial or atlantooccipital dislocations may require a posterior fusion of the upper cervical spine.

Juvenile osteoporosis and osteopaenia

Osteoporosis is characterized by loss of bone mass and micro-architectural structure of the skeleton, which leads to bone fragility and risk of fractures (Henderson et al. 2000). The World Health Organization defines osteoporosis as bone mineral density less than 2.5 standard deviations below the mean. Trabecular bone is more affected by osteoporosis than cortical bone. Therefore, the spine, which mainly consists of trabecular bone, is a prime target for disorders causing osteoporosis.

Osteopaenia means low bone mineral content for age, and is defined as bone mineral density between 1 and 2.5 standard deviations below the mean. Bone mass increases throughout childhood, reaching peak levels by late adolescence. Skeletal maturation in children is dependent upon bone formation exceeding resorption, whereas these two fundamental processes are closely balanced in adults. Low peak bone mass in young adults increases the risk of developing osteoporosis later in life (Cassidy 1999).

Bone mass can be reliably assessed by bone densitometry techniques, including single-photon absorptiometry, dual-photon absorptiometry, and quantitative CT. Routine radiographs permit limited assessment of osteoporosis. However, vertebral wedging or collapse may be present (Fig. 11). Involvement of multiple vertebrae in the thoracic and lumbar spine occurs in severe cases.

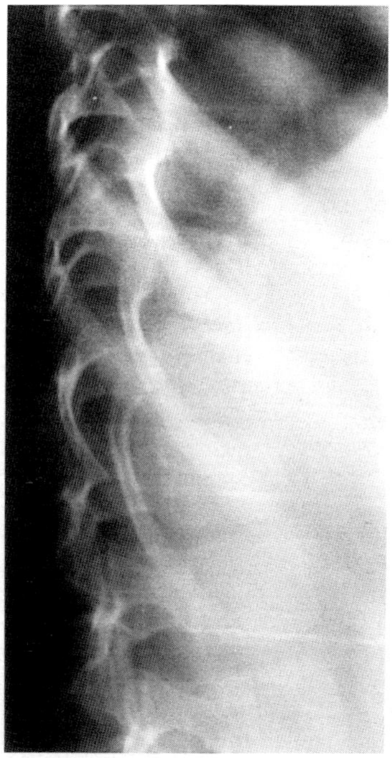

Fig. 11 Osteoporosis in a 5-year-old boy with active systemic juvenile idiopathic arthritis. After 3 months on corticosteroids he developed thoracic back pain. Standing lateral radiographs demonstrate osteoporosis and severe collapse of vertabrae Th6. There are also compression fractures of Th11, Th12, and L1.

Pain in the back and/or lower extremities is a typical symptom. The child may walk with a limp or stiff-legged gait. Kyphosis is also common.

Osteopaenia and osteoporosis in children may be caused by medications. Corticosterioids have been shown to increase the tendency to develop osteoporosis. Decline in bone mass has been correlated with daily steroid dose, duration of treatment, and cumulative dose (Trapani et al. 1998; Haugen et al. 2000). Osteoporosis is also secondary to a range of different conditions. In JIA, approximately 30 per cent of the patients have osteopaenia or osteoporosis (Haugen et al. 2000; Henderson et al. 2000). Young adults with persistent JIA have reduced peak bone mass compared with healthy controls (Haugen et al. 2000). Likewise, young adults with juvenile systemic lupus erythematosus seem to have lower bone mineral density than controls (Trapani et al. 1998). Osteopaenia and osteoporosis in patients with juvenile rheumatic diseases may be a result of poor growth and nutritional status, delayed pubertal development, the disease itself, and the effect of corticoid treatment (Trapani et al. 1998; Haugen et al. 2000; Henderson et al. 2000).

A number of metabolic bone disorders may cause osteoporosis (Docio et al. 1998). Screening tests including serum calcium, phosphate, alkaline phosphatase, parathyroid hormone, calcitonin, 25-hydroxyvitamin D, and 1,25-hydroxyvitamin D, are recommended. Cushing's syndrome, hyperthyreosis diabetes mellitus, and other endocrine disorders are well-known causes of osteoporosis. Osteogenesis imperfecta typically leads to fractures during infancy, blue sclerae, and gracile bones. Other genetic disorders like Down's syndrome and Turner's syndrome are associated with osteopaenia, but these conditions rarely cause osteoporosis during childhood. Amenorrhoea and anorexia nervosa are frequent causes of low bone mineral density in adolescence (Sambrook and Naganathan 1997). Due to the consequences of delayed diagnoses, it is important to exclude leukaemia or lymphoma in a child with generalized osteoporosis (Santangelo and Thomson 1999). Lysinuric protein intolerance, homocystinuria, and hyperimmunoglobulina E syndrome must also be considered.

Juvenile idiopathic osteoporosis is a rare paediatric bone disorder. This primary type of osteoporosis is diagnosed after possible secondary forms have been excluded. The hallmarks of the disorder are generalized osteoporosis that presents during prepuberty and usually remits during puberty. There is usually pain in the back or lower extremities and an increased frequency of fractures that cease after the onset of puberty. Reconstruction of bone apparently occurs, but the ultimate bone density has not been assessed in long-term studies.

Treatment of osteoporosis and osteopaenia includes avoidance of contributing factors, consideration of calcium and vitamin D supplement, and weight-bearing physical activities (Docio et al. 1998). Biphosphonates, palmidronate, calcitonin, and calcitriol have been used in children, but such use must still be regarded as experimental (Marder et al. 1982; Krassas 2000; Shaw et al. 2000). Close monitoring and evaluations are needed in order to establish the long-term tolerability and efficacy of these drugs in children. A lumbosacral corset may be tried if the patient's main complaint is low back pain. If kyphosis is present a brace may minimize progression of the deformity. A total-contact spinal orthosis is contraindicated because of the risk of accentuated osteoporosis and deformity.

Tumours

Spinal tumours are relatively rare in children, accounting for approximately 10 per cent of childhood spinal cord lesions. In 45 children with primary tumours, Beer and Merezes (1997) found that 64 per cent of the tumours were benign and 36 per cent were malignant. Back pain (79 per cent) and neurological deficits (74 per cent) were the most frequent presenting features. Tumour excision was achieved in 80 per cent of the patients, recurrence rate was 13 per cent and mortality 7 per cent. Painful scoliosis, radicular pain, night pain that awakens the child from sleep, effectiveness of NSAIDs or aspirin, and stiffness are classic and common findings in children with spinal neoplasms. Abnormalities on plain radiographs have

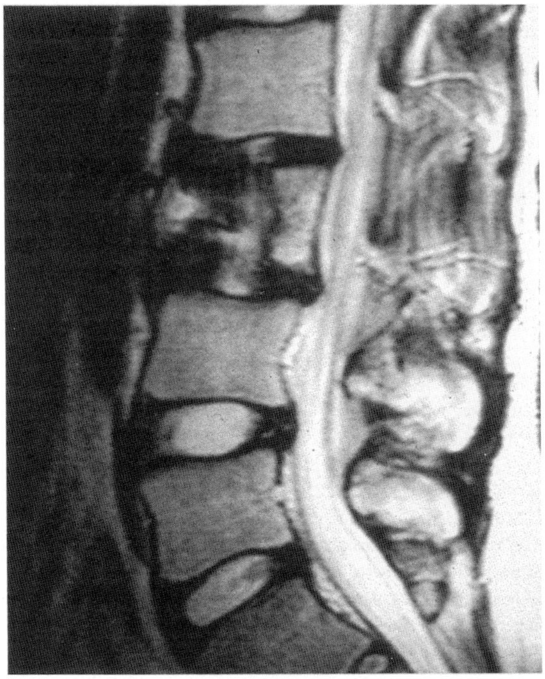

Fig. 12 Magnetic resonance imaging showing Ewing's sarcome at the L3 in a 13-year-old boy.

been found in up to 98 per cent of the cases during the disease course, but the radiographs may be negative at disease onset. Bone scan and MRI are indicated (Fig. 12).

Benign tumours of the spine have a strong predilection for the posterior vertebral elements. The most common benign tumours are osteoid oateoma and osteoblastoma. The histology of these lesions is identical, and they can only be differentiated by the size. Osteoid osteomas are less than 1.5 cm in diameter and osteoblastomas are lager than 1.5 cm. Symptoms usually start after the age of 10 years and the male to female ratio is 2 : 1. In a retrospective study of 44 museums cases and 421 cases from the literature, Saifuddin et al. (1998) found scoliosis in 63 per cent. Tumours were usually located on the concave side of the scoliosis, most frequently at the thoracic and lumbar levels. Surgical excision is the treatment of choice, and complete resection and stabilisation should be the aim.

Other benign tumours include anaurysmal bone cysts and eosinophil granulomas (histocystosis). The onset of symptoms may be triggered by collapse, fracture, or deformity of the vertebra.

Primary malignant tumours in the spine include leukaemia, Ewing's sarcoma, and lymphoma. Metastatic lesions include neuroblastoma, rhabdomyosarcoma, Wimps tumour, retinoblastoma, and teratoblastoma. Intractable back pain, night pain, and constitutional findings should alert the examiner to the possibility of a malignant process.

Trauma

Sport injuries, motor-vehicle accidents, fall from height, and child abuse are common causes of spine injuries in children (McMahon et al. 1997; Copley and Dormans 1998). Such injuries may go unrecognized and only present with a vague history of back pain. The incidence of spinal fractures in childhood is not known, but these fractures are thought to account for 2–3 per cent of all injuries in children (Richards et al. 1999). Twenty per cent of these patients have neurological deficits.

Plain radiographs are the primary method of detection. The injuries most commonly affect the vertebral bodies, with anterior compression and notching near the superior end plates. Narrowing of disc space or a true fracture dislocation may be seen. MRI and CT can provide a more accurate and detailed picture. These changes must be differentiated from normal developmental changes that occur in the growing vertebra.

Spinal cord injury without radiographic evidence of fracture or dislocation is a feature that is unique in children under the age of 10 years. This injury most commonly affects the cervical cord. Plain radiographs are negative, but MRI may be a useful diagnostic tool. Possible mechanisms are traction, contusion, cord rupture, traumatic infarction, blunt abdominal trauma, interference of the vascular supply, and soft tissue enfolding. Upto 70 per cent of the patients have paraplegia (Richards et al. 1999). Slipped vertebral apophysis is another injury that is unique in children.

If spinal injury due to high-energy trauma is suspected, the child should be immobilized. If a stable fracture is present, the treatment is symptomatic, but if the fracture is unstable or the spinal cord compressed, surgical treatment is needed. The use of corticosteroids is believed to improve outcomes in children with spinal cord injuries. Considerable efforts must be made to prevent spinal deformity (Bergstrøm et al. 1999).

Healing of an unstable pelvic fracture in malposition with asymmetry has been shown to have a poor outcome. Spinal cord injuries in young children have been found to cause more severe scoliosis than injuries occurring at an older age (Bergstrøm et al. 1999). A history of childhood abuse seems to be related to poorer socio-economic prognosis compared with other chronic spinal disorder patients (McMahon et al. 1997).

Torticollis

Torticollis means twisted neck. The most common causes are muscular torticollis (due to *in utero* malposition, difficult delivery, or sternocleideomastoid muscle compartment syndrome), rotary fixation (due to injury or upper respiratory tract infection), congenital anomalies, and posterior fossa tumours. The child presents with the ear pulled down towards the clavicle. The range of motion is limited.

A potential underlying disorder must be ruled out. In muscular torticollis, passive stretching will usually be effective in restoring the range of motion in children under the age of 1 year. Surgical management includes releasing all restricting bands involving the sternocleideomastoid muscle and other neck structures.

Spina bifida and spinal dysraphism

Spina bifida (myelomeningocele) is a major birth defect resulting from failure of the neural tube to close in the developing foetus. It is associated with varying degrees of neurological impairment, from complete paralysis to minimal or no motor deficit. Approximately half of the cases are caused by nutritional deficiency (folic acid) (Sarwark 1996). The remaining cases are inherited. Paralytic scoliosis develops in 40–60 per cent of the patients.

Spina bifida occulta is fairly common and is not associated with any symptoms or cord involvement in the majority of patients. This bony anomaly may be associated with neural anomaly causing spinal dysraphism. In spinal dysraphism, clinical signs and symptoms of a tethered cord develop, including leg weakness, deformities like leg length inequality and pes cavus, spasticity, contractures, rapid progression of scoliosis, back pain, and change in urodynamics (Sarwark 1996). It may be associated with cutaneous manifestations such as a hairy patch, dimple, haemangioma, lipoma, or area of atrophic skin. MRI usually shows dural scarring, and neurosurgical treatment is needed.

Conclusion

Back pain is common in schoolchildren, and only infrequently require referral to a paediatric rheumatology or an othopaedic centre. In contrast to back pain in adults, back pain in children and adolescents often indicates serious underlying pathology, particularly when the back pain is associated with deformity or the child is young. A variety of disorders may account for back pain and deformity in children and adolescents. Some of these may result in severe morbidity if they are not properly diagnosed and treated. A careful medical history, complete clinical examination, and appropriate imaging and laboratory studies are essential.

References

Balague, F., Dutoit, G., and Waldburger, M. (1988). Low back pain in schoolchildren. An epidemiological study. *Scandinavian Journal of Rehabilitation Medicine* **20**, 175–9.

Beer, S.J. and Menezes, A.H. (1997). Primary tumors of the spine in children. Natural history, management, and long-term follow-up. *Spine* **22**, 649–58.

Bergstrøm, E.M. et al. (1999). The effect of childhood spinal cord injury on skeletal development: a retrospective study. *Spinal Cord* **37**, 838–46.

Bodner, R.J. et al. (1988). The use of single photon emission computed tomography (SPECT) in the diagnosis of low-back pain in young patients. *Spine* **13**, 1155–60.

Burgos-Vargas, R. and Clark, P. (1989). Axial involvement in the seronegative enthesopathy and arthropathy syndrome and its progression to ankylosing spondylitis. *Journal of Rheumatology* **16**, 192–7.

Burgos-Vargas, R., Lardizabal-Sanabria, J., and Katona, G. (1985). Anterior spinal flexion in healthy Mexican children. *Journal of Rheumatology* **12**, 123–5.

Burgos-Vargas, R. and Vazquez-Mellado, J. (1995). The early clinical recognition of juvenile-onset ankylosing spondylitis and its differentiation from juvenile rheumatoid arthritis. *Arthritis and Rheumatism* **38**, 835–44.

Burton, A.K., Clarce, R.D., McClune, T.D., and Tillotson, K.M. (1996). The natural history of low back pain in adolescents. *Spine* **21**, 2323–8.

Cabral, D.A., Oen, K.G., and Petty, R.E. (1992). SEA syndrome revisited: a longterm followup of children with a syndrome of seronegative enthesopathy and arthropathy. *Journal of Rheumatology* **19**, 1282–5.

Cassidy, J.T. (1999). Osteopenia and osteoporosis in children. *Clinical and Experimental Rheumatology* **17**, 245–50.

Copley, L.A. and Dormans, J.P. (1998). Cervical spine disorders in infants and children. *Journal of the American Academy of Orthopedic Surgeons* **6**, 204–14.

Correa, A.G., Edwards, M.S., and Baker, C.J. (1993). Vertebral osteomyelitis in children. *Paediatric Infectious Disease Journal* **12**, 228–33.

Docio, S. et al. (1998). Seasonal deficiency of vitamin D in children: a potential target for osteoporosis-preventing strategies? *Journal of Bone and Mineral Research* **13**, 544–8.

Domjan, L. et al. (1990). A simple method for measuring lateral flexion of the dorsolumbar spine. *Journal of Rheumatology* **17**, 663–5.

Ehrmann-Feldman, D. *Risk Factors for the Development of Low Back Pain in Adolescents.* Thesis, McGill University, Montreal, 1998.

Erkintalo, M.O. et al. (1995). Development of degenerative changes in the lumbar intervertebral disc: results of a prospective MR imaging study in adolescents with and without low-back pain. *Radiology* **2**, 529–33.

Fairbank, J.C.T. et al. (1984). Influence of anthropometric factors and joint laxity in the incidence of adolescent back pain. *Spine* **9**, 461–4.

Feldman, D.S., Wright, J.G., and Hedden, D.M. (1995). Back pain in children and adolescents. *Orthopedic Transactions* **19**, 350.

Flatø, B. et al. (1997). Outcome and predictive factors in children with chronic idiopathic musculoskeletal pain. *Clinical and Experimental Rheumatology* **15**, 569–77.

Flatø, B. et al. (2002a). Spinal problems in juvenile idiopathic arthritis. *Scandinavian Journal of Rheumatology* **31** (Suppl. 117), 25.

Flatø, B. et al. (2002b). The influence of patient characteristics, disease variables and HLA alleles on the development of radiographic sacroiliitis in juvenile idiopathic arthritis. *Arthritis and Rheumatism* **46**, 986–94.

Flatø, B. et al. (2003). Prognostic factors in juvenile rheumatoid arthritis: a case control study revealing early predictors and outcome after 14.9 years. *Journal of Rheumatology* **30** (2), 386–93.

Fredrickson, B.E. et al. (1984). The natural history of spondylolysis and spondylolisthesis. *Journal of Bone and Joint Surgery—American* **66**, 699–707.

Gunzburg, R. et al. (1999). Low back pain in a population of school children. *European Spine Journal* **8**, 439–43.

Hamilton, M.L., Gladman, D.D., Shore, A., Laxer, R.M., and Silverman, E.D. (1990). Juvenile psoriatic arthritis and HLA antigens. *Annals of the Rheumatic Diseases* **49**, 694–7.

Harreby, M. et al. (1996). Epidemiological aspects and risk factors for low back pain in 38-year-old men and women: a 25-year prospective cohort study of 640 school children. *European Spine Journal* **5**, 312–18.

Haugen, M. et al. (2000). Young adults with juvenile arthritis in remission attain normal peak bone mass at the lumbar spine and forearm. *Arthritis and Rheumatism* **43**, 1504–10.

Henderson, C.J. et al. (2000). Total-body bone mineral content in non-corticosteroid-treated postpubertal females with juvenile rheumatoid arthritis: frequency of osteopenia and contributing factors. *Arthritis and Rheumatism* **43**, 531–40.

Krassas, G.E. (2000). Idiopathic juvenile osteoporosis. *Annals of the New York Academy of Sciences* **90**, 409–12.

Kujala, U.M. et al. (1997). Lumbar mobility and low back pain during adolescence. A longitudinal three-year follow-up study in athletes and controls. *American Journal of Sports Medicine* **25**, 363–8.

Laiho, K., Hannula, S., Savolainen, A., and Kauppi, M. (2001). Cervical spine in patients with juvenile chronic arthritis and amyeloidosis. *Clinical and Experimental Rheumatology* **19**, 345–8.

Lonstein, J.E. (1999). Spondylolisthesis in children. Cause, natural history, and management. *Spine* **24**, 2640–8.

Lowe, T.G. (1990). Scheuermann disease. *Journal of Bone and Joint Surgery—American* **72**, 940–5.

Macrae, I.F. and Wright, V. (1969). Measurement of back movement. *Annals of the Rheumatic Diseases* **28**, 584–9.

Malleson, P.N., Fung, M.Y., and Rosenberg, A.M. (1996). The incidence of childhood rheumatic diseases: results from the Canadian Paediatric Rheumatology Association Disease Registry. *Journal of Rheumatology* **23**, 1981–7.

Marder, H.K. et al. (1982). Calcitriol deficiency in idiopathic juvenile osteoporosis. *American Journal of Diseases of Children* **136**, 914–17.

Martinez-Lage, J.F. et al. (1997). Disc protrusion in the child. Particular features and comparison with neoplasms. *Childs Nervous System* **13**, 201–7.

Mason, D.E. (1999). Back pain in children. *Paediatric Annals* **28**, 727–38.

McCarthy, R.E. (1994). Evaluation of the patient with deformity. In *The Paediatric Spine: Principles and Practice* (ed. S.L. Weinstein), pp. 185–226. New York: Raven Press.

McMahon, M.J. et al. (1997). Early childhood abuse in chronic spinal disorder patients. A major barrier to treatment success. *Spine* **22**, 2408–15.

McMaster, M.J. (1994). Evaluation of the patient with deformity. In *The Paediatric Spine: Principles and Practice* (ed. S.L. Weinstein), pp. 227–44. New York: Raven Press.

Morita, T. et al. (1995). Lumbar spondylolysis in children and adolescents. *Journal of Bone and Joint Surgery—British* **77**, 620–5.

Murray, P.M., Weinstein, S.L., and Spratt, K.F. (1993). The natural history and long-term follow-up of Scheuermann kyphosis. *Journal of Bone and Joint Surgery—American* **75**, 236–48.

Nissinen, M. et al. (1994). Antrophometric measurements and the incidence of low back pain in a cohort of pubertal children. *Spine* **18**, 8–13.

Petrus, L.V. and Nelson, M.D., Jr. (1998). Current role of CT in paediatric neuroimaging. *Neuroimaging Clinics of North America* **8**, 685–93.

Ramirez, N., Johnston, C.E., and Browne, R.H. (1997). The prevalence of back pain in children who have idiopathic scoliosis. *Journal of Bone and Joint Surgery—American* **79**, 364–8.

Richards, B.S., McCarthy, R.E., and Akbarnia, B.A. (1999). Back pain in childhood and adolescence. *Instructional Course Lectures* **48**, 525–42.

Saifuddin, A. et al. (1998). Osteoid osteoma and osteoblastoma of the spine. Factors associated with the presence of scoliosis. *Spine* **23**, 47–53.

Salminen, J.J., Pentti, J., and Terho, P. (1992a). Low back pain and disability in 14-year-old schoolchildren. *Acta Paediatrica* **81**, 1035–9.

Salminen, J.J., Maki, P., Oksanen, A., and Pentti, J. (1992b). Spinal mobility and trunk muscle strength in 15-year-old schoolchildren with and without low-back pain. *Spine* **17**, 405–11.

Salminen, J.J., Erkintalo, M., Laine, M., and Pentti, J. (1995). Low back pain in the young. A prospective three-year follow-up study of subjects with and without low back pain. *Spine* **20**, 2101–7.

Sambrook, P.N. and Naganathan, V. (1997). How do we manage specific types of osteoporosis? *Baillières Clinical Rheumatology* **11**, 597–612.

Santangelo, J.R. and Thomson, J.D. (1999). Childhood leukemia presenting with back pain and vertebral compression fractures. *American Journal of Orthopedics (Chatham, NJ)* **28**, 257–60.

Sarwark, J.F. (1996). Spina bifida. *Paediatric Clinics of North America* **43**, 1151–8.

Shaw, N.J., Boivin, C.M., and Crabtree, N.J. (2000). Intravenous pamidronate in juvenile osteoporosis. *Archives of Disease in Childhood* **83**, 143–5.

Sherry, D.D. et al. (1991). Psychosomatic musculoskeletal pain in childhood: clinical and psychological analyses of 100 children. *Paediatrics* **88**, 1093–9.

Svantesson, H., Marhaug, G., and Haeffner, F. (1981). Scoliosis in children with juvenile rheumatoid arthritis. *Scandinavian Journal of Rheumatology* **10**, 65–8.

Taimela, S., Kujala, U.M., Salminen, J.J., and Viljanen, T. (1997). The prevalence of low back pain among children and adolescents. A nationwide, cohort-based questionnaire survey in Finland. *Spine* **22**, 1132–6.

Trapani, S., Civinini, R., Ermini, M., Paci, E., and Falcini, F. (1998). Osteoporosis in juvenile systemic lupus erythematosus: a longitudinal study on the effect of steroids on bone mineral density. *Rheumatology International* **18**, 45–9.

Troussier, B. et al. (1999). Back pain and spinal alignment abnormalities in schoolchildren. *Revue Du Rhumatisme, English Edition* **66**, 370–80.

Turner, P.G., Green, J.H., and Galasko, C.S.B. (1989). Back pain in childhood. *Spine* **14**, 812–14.

1.2.2 Regional problems

1.2.2.1 The upper limbs in adults

Adel G. Fam and Simon Carette

Applied anatomy

Shoulder

Shoulder movements are a synthesis of motion at four articulations: glenohumeral, acromioclavicular, sternoclavicular, and scapulothoracic (Polley and Hunder 1978; Williams et al. 1989).

The sternoclavicular joint is a simple spheroidal joint between the medial end of the clavicle and the manubrium sternum and first costal cartilage. An intra-articular fibrocartilaginous disc divides the joint into two cavities. The joint capsule is reinforced by the anterior and posterior sternoclavicular ligaments.

The acromioclavicular joint is a spheroidal joint between the lateral end of the clavicle and the acromion. An intra-articular fibrocartilaginous disc divides the joint into two compartments. The joint capsule is strengthened by the superior and inferior acromioclavicular ligaments. The coracoclavicular ligament (conoid and trapezoid parts) extends between the distal clavicle and the coracoid process of the scapula. It stabilizes both the clavicle and scapula, and maintains a close relation between the two bones during shoulder movements, thus limiting scapular rotation around the acromioclavicular joint. A subcutaneous, usually non-communicating bursa may be present over the joint.

Movements at the sternoclavicular and acromioclavicular joints enable slight rotation of the clavicle along its long axis, and allow elevation or depression (as in shoulder shrugging), and flexion or extension (as in forward or backward thrusting) of the shoulder girdle.

The glenohumeral joint is a ball-and-socket articulation between the glenoid fossa of the scapula and the humeral head (Fig. 1). The lax articular capsule, and the small area of contact between the shallow glenoid cavity and the spheroidal humeral head, permit a wide range of movements. The stability of the joint depends upon a number of static and dynamic stabilizers. Static stabilizers include the capsule, glenoid labrum, and ligaments (glenohumeral and coracohumeral). The capsule has two apertures: one for the long head of the biceps tendon and the other for the subscapularis bursa. Dynamic stabilizers play a greater part in the stability of the shoulder, and include two musculotendinous layers: an inner stratum, made of the rotator cuff muscles (supraspinatus, infraspinatus, teres minor, and subscapularis), and the tendon of the long head of the biceps, and an outer stratum made of the deltoid, teres major, pectoralis major, latissimus dorsi, and trapezius muscles.

The muscles of the inner stratum stabilize and retain the humeral head in the glenoid cavity during shoulder movements, while simultaneously providing abduction (through the supraspinatus, which inserts into the superior part of the greater tuberosity), external rotation (through the infraspinatus and teres minor, which insert into the posterior aspect of the greater tuberosity), and internal rotation (through the subscapularis, which inserts into the lesser tuberosity). At the initiation of shoulder abduction, the rotator cuff muscles and the long head of the biceps tendon depress and fix the humeral head against the glenoid cavity to counteract the upward pull of the more powerful deltoid muscle. The mechanism whereby these two groups of muscles combine to produce abduction, the one elevating (deltoid muscle) and the other stabilizing the humeral head (rotator cuff and biceps tendons), is termed 'force-couple'.

The muscles of the outer stratum are the prime movers of the shoulder, although the trapezius acts through movements of the scapula and clavicle. These muscles provide abduction, flexion, extension, adduction and some degree of rotation, and together with the rotator cuff muscles (which provide more rotation of the humeral head) permit a wide range of movement at the shoulder.

The coracoacromial arch (coracoid, coracoacromial ligament, and acromion) acts as a secondary socket for the humeral head under which the rotator cuff tendons and long head of the biceps tendon glide, with the subacromial bursa lying in between. The arch protects the humeral head and the rotator cuff from direct trauma. The subacromial bursa facilitates movements of the greater tuberosity beneath the rigid coracoacromial arch during shoulder abduction, and acts as a cushion minimizing the impingement of the supraspinatus, infraspinatus, teres minor, and long head of the biceps tendons on the undersurface of the acromion during abduction (Fig. 1). The bursa, which extends beneath the deltoid (subdeltoid part), communicates with the cavity of the glenohumeral joint in about one-third of adults. The synovium of the shoulder has two extracapsular outpouchings: the synovial tendon sheath of the long head of the biceps tendon, and the subscapularis bursa lying beneath the subscapularis tendon (Fig. 2).

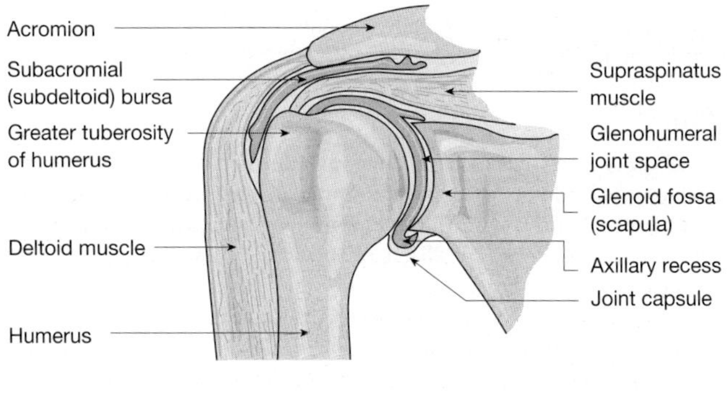

Fig. 1 The shoulder.

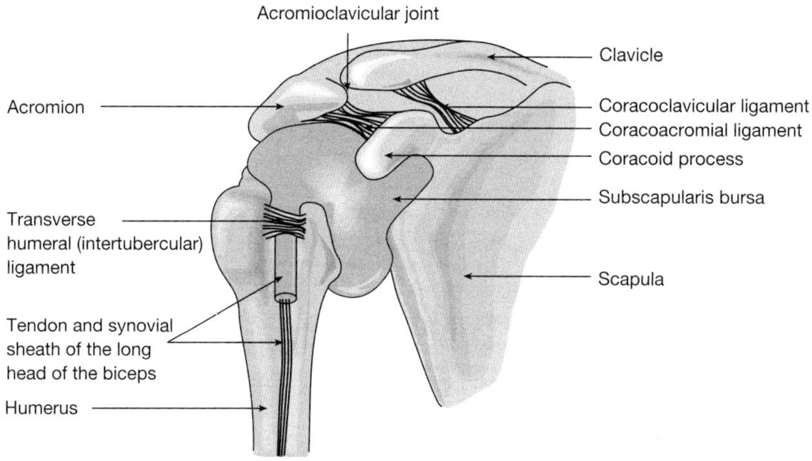

Fig. 2 The shoulder (synovial membrane and its outpouchings).

The subcoracoid bursa lies between the shoulder capsule and coracoid process, but it rarely communicates with the subacromial bursa.

Scapulothoracic articulation

The scapula is connected to the posterior aspect of the chest wall by the axioappendicular muscles. The scapula provides the origin for the rotator cuff muscles and deltoid, and the trapezius inserts into its superior aspect. Scapulothoracic movements, including rotation, elevation, depression, protrusion, retraction, and circumduction, are important for the normal functioning of the shoulder.

Shoulder abduction involves synchronous movements of the glenohumeral, sternoclavicular, and acromioclavicular joints and rotation of the scapula on the chest wall. The initial 30° of abduction, achieved by contraction of the supraspinatus, takes place at the glenohumeral joint with little movement of the scapula. Beyond 30°, an approximate 2 : 1 ratio exists between movements at the glenohumeral joint and the scapula. The combined movement is referred to as the 'scapulohumeral rhythm'. Abduction of the shoulder (normal range, 180°) is associated with external rotation of the humerus. The prime movers are the supraspinatus and deltoid muscles. The flexors of the shoulders (normal range, 180°) are the deltoid and coracobrachialis muscles. The normal range of shoulder adduction across the front of the chest is about 50°. The pectoralis major muscle is the main adductor. The normal range of extension (posterior flexion) is about 50°. The latissimus dorsi, teres major, and deltoid muscles are the principal extensors. With the shoulder abducted to 90° and the elbow flexed at a right angle, the normal range of internal and external rotation is 90° each. The normal range of external rotation with the elbow placed by the side at the waist is about 45°, and internal rotation is to 55° (before its motion is stopped by the body), or to 120° if the patient can reach behind the back to touch the inferior angle of the opposite scapula. The prime movers of internal rotation are subscapularis, and pectoralis major. The infraspinatus and teres minor are the main external rotators.

Elbow

The elbow is a relatively stable hinge joint formed by the humeroulnar (trochleo–ulnar), humeroradial (capitelloradial), and proximal radio–ulnar articulations (Fig. 3), with the trochleo–ulnar being the principal joint (Polley and Hunder 1978; Williams et al. 1989). The stability of the joint depends on its congruity, anterior capsule, and ulnar and radial collateral ligaments. The common flexor tendon (pronator teres, flexor carpi radialis, palmaris longus, flexor carpi ulnaris, and flexor digitorum superficialis) takes origin from the medial epicondyle of the humerus. The common extensor tendon (brachioradialis, extensor carpi radialis longus and brevis, extensor digitorum communis, and anconeus) originates from the lateral epicondyle. The annular ligament is a strong, cup-shaped band that encircles the radial head at the proximal radio–ulnar joint. The paraolecranon grooves are the depressions between the ulnar olecranon process and the medial and lateral epicondyles. The ulnar nerve runs in a groove (cubital tunnel) behind the medial epicondyle.

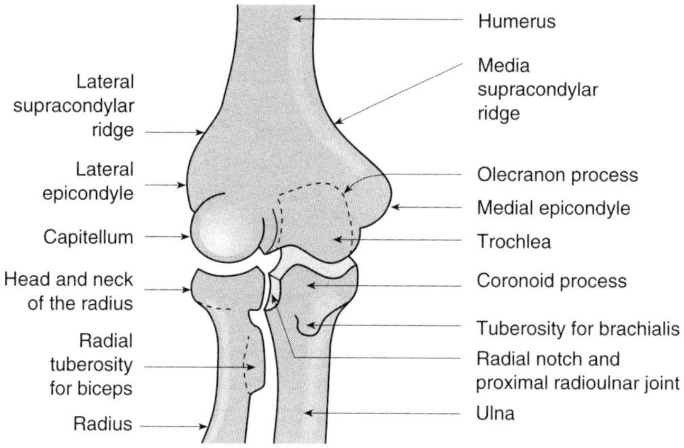

Fig. 3 The elbow.

The trochleo–ulnar, capitelloradial, and proximal radio–ulnar joints share a common synovial cavity. The subcutaneous olecranon bursa overlies the olecranon process but does not communicate with the joint.

The neutral position or position of complete extension of the elbow is designated 0°. Some normal individuals (particularly muscular athletes) lack 5–10° of full extension, while others (particularly women) may demonstrate 5–10° of hyperextension. The normal range of flexion at the cubital (humeroulnar and humeroradial) joint is 150–160°. The brachialis, biceps, and brachioradialis muscles are the main elbow flexors. Extensors of the elbow include the triceps and anconeus muscles.

Due to the oblique shape of the trochlea, extension of the elbow is associated with slight lateral (valgus) angulation of 5–15°. This is known as the 'carrying angle' of the elbow. The normal angle is about 5° in men and 10–15° in women. During flexion of the elbow, the ulna becomes more parallel with the humerus.

Pronation of forearm and hand (palm of the hand turned backward) to 90°, and supination (palm turned forward) to 90° occur at the proximal and distal radio–ulnar joints. During these movements the radial head pivots on

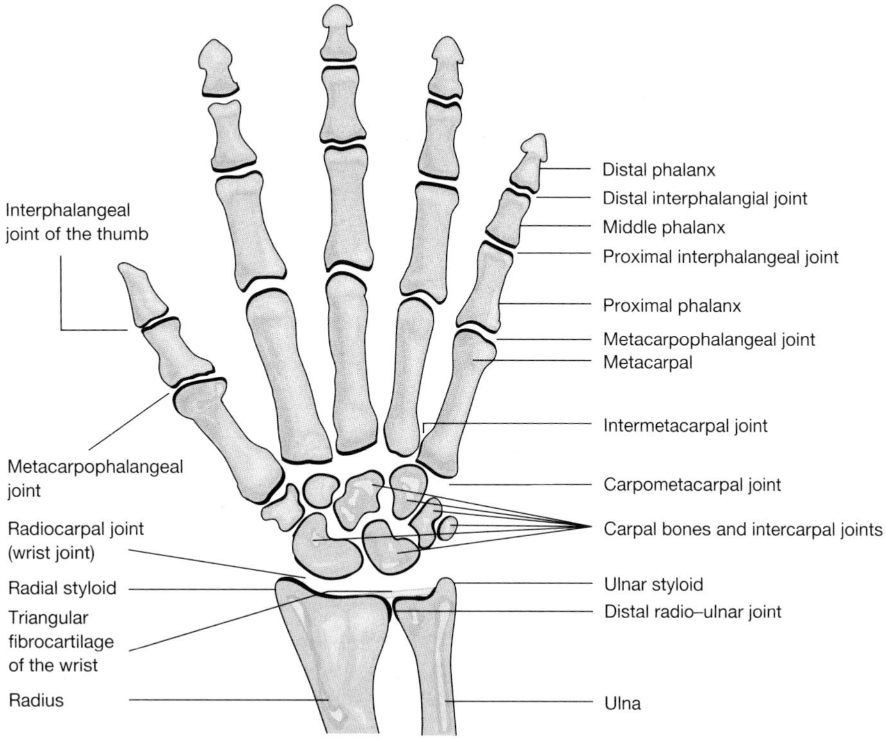

Fig. 4 Bones and joints of the wrist and hand.

the capitellum while the distal radius rotates around the ulna. The biceps and supinator muscles are the primary supinators of the radio–ulnar joints, and the pronator teres and pronator quadratus are the principal pronators.

Wrist (radiocarpal) joint

This is an ellipsoid joint between the distal radius and articular disc proximally and the scaphoid, lunate, and triquetrum distally (Fig. 4) (Polley and Hunder 1978; Williams et al. 1989). The articular capsule is strengthened by the radiocarpal (dorsal and palmar) and collateral (radial and ulnar) ligaments. The articular disc, or triangular fibrocartilage of the wrist, joins the radius to the ulna. Its base is attached to the ulnar border of the distal radius and its apex to the base of the ulnar styloid process. The synovial cavity of the distal radio–ulnar joint is L-shaped and extends distally beneath the triangular fibrocartilage but is usually separated from the radiocarpal joint.

The radiocarpal, intercarpal, midcarpal (located between the proximal and distal rows of the carpal bones), carpometacarpal, and intermetacarpal joints often intercommunicate through a common synovial cavity (Fig. 4).

The carpal bones form a volarly concave arch or carpal tunnel: pisiform and hook of the hamate on the ulnar side, and scaphoid tubercle and crest of the trapezium on the radial side. The four bony prominences are joined by the flexor retinaculum (transverse carpal ligament), which forms the roof of the carpal tunnel. The palmaris longus (absent in 10–15 per cent of the population) partly inserts into the flexor retinaculum and partly fans out into the palm forming the palmar aponeurosis (fascia). The aponeurosis divides distally into four digital slips that attach to the finger flexor tendon sheaths, metacarpophalangeal joint capsules, and proximal phalanges (Polley and Hunder 1978; Williams et al. 1989). Tendons crossing the wrist are enclosed for part of their course in tenosynovial sheaths. The common flexor tendon sheath encloses the long flexor tendons of the fingers (flexor digitorum superficialis and flexor digitorum profundus) and extends from approximately 2.5 cm proximal to the wrist crease to the mid-palm. It runs with the flexor pollicis longus tendon sheath and the median nerve through the carpal tunnel (Fig. 5). The tendon sheath of the little finger is usually continuous with the common flexor sheath. The flexor pollicis longus

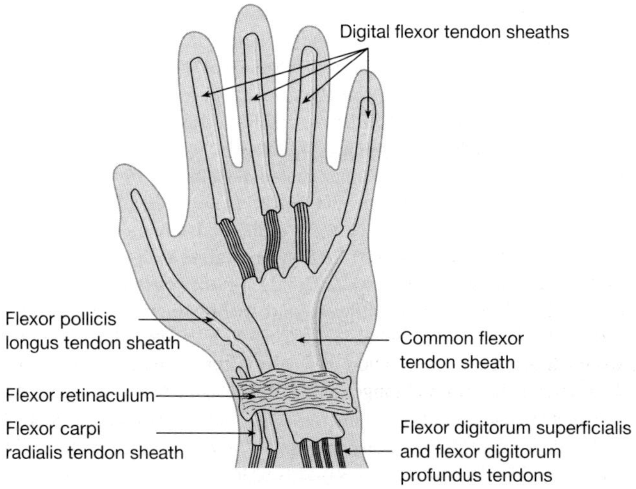

Fig. 5 Flexor tendon sheaths of the wrist and hand.

tendon to the thumb runs through a separate tenosynovial sheath, but may join the common flexor sheath. The flexor carpi radialis is invested in a short tendon sheath as it crosses the volar aspect of the wrist between the split radial attachment of the flexor retinaculum. The flexor retinaculum straps down the flexor tendons as they cross at the wrist. The ulnar nerve, artery, and vein cross over the retinaculum but are sometimes covered by a fibrous band—the superficial part of the transverse carpal ligament—to form the ulnar tunnel or Guyon's canal.

On the dorsum of the wrist, the extensor tendons pass through six tenosynovial, fibro-osseous tunnels beneath the extensor retinaculum (dorsal carpal ligament); abductor pollicis longus and extensor pollicis brevis, usually in a single sheath (first extensor compartment, most radial); extensor carpi radialis longus and brevis; extensor pollicis longus; extensor digitorum communis and extensor indicis proprius; extensor digiti minimi;

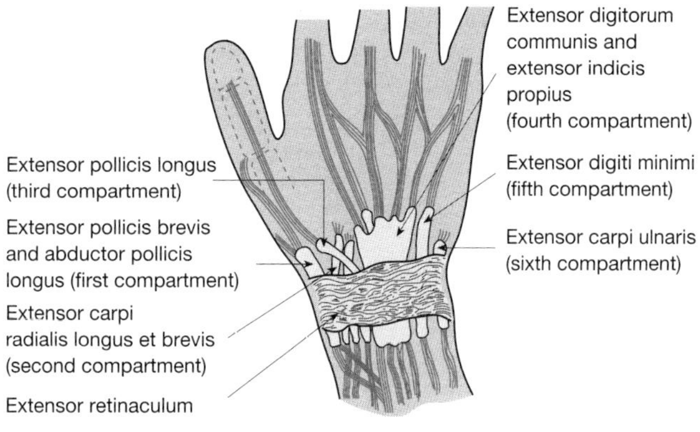

Fig. 6 Extensor tendon sheaths of the wrist.

and extensor carpi ulnaris (sixth extensor compartment, most ulnar) (Fig. 6). Each tenosynovial sheath extends about 2.5 cm proximally and distally from the retinaculum. The extensor retinaculum, by its deep attachments to the distal radius and ulnar, binds down and prevents bowstringing of the extensor tendons as they cross the wrist.

Movements of the wrist include palmar flexion (flexion), dorsiflexion (extension), ulnar deviation, radial deviation, and circumduction. The intercarpal joints contribute to wrist movements, particularly palmar flexion. Prime wrist palmar flexors are flexor carpi radialis, flexor carpi ulnaris, and palmaris longus. The prime dorsiflexors are the extensor carpi radialis longus and brevis, and the extensor carpi ulnaris.

The first carpometacarpal joint is a saddle-shaped, very mobile joint between the trapezium and the base of the first metacarpal. It allows 40–50° of thumb flexion–extension (parallel to the plane of the palm) and 40–70° of adduction–abduction (perpendicular to the plane of the palm). These movements are important in bringing the thumb into opposition with the fingers.

The metacarpophalangeal joints are modified hinge joints that lie about 1 cm distal to the knuckles (metacarpal heads) (Fig. 4). Their capsule is strengthened by the radial and ulnar collateral ligaments on the sides and by the palmar (volar) plate on the volar surface. The collateral ligaments are loose in the neutral position, allowing radial and ulnar deviations, but become tight in the fully flexed position preventing side-to-side motion (referred to as 'sagittal cam effect'). The deep transverse metacarpal ligament joins the volar plates of the second to fifth metacarpophalangeal joints. The metacarpophalangeal joint of the thumb is large and has two sesamoid bones overlying its volar surface.

Where the long extensor tendon of the digit reaches the metacarpal head it is joined by the tendons of the interossei and lumbricales, and it expands over the dorsum of the metacarpophalangeal joint and digit to form the extensor hood or expansion (Fig. 7). The expansion divides over the dorsum of the proximal phalanx into an intermediate slip, which is inserted principally into the base of the middle phalanx, and two collateral slips, which are inserted into the base of the distal phalanx.

The first metacarpophalangeal joint permits 50–70° palmar flexion and 10–30° dorsiflexion. Radial and ulnar deviations are limited to less than 10–20°. The other metacarpophalangeal joints allow 90° palmar flexion, 30° dorsiflexion, and 35° of radial and ulnar movements. The extensor pollicis brevis, extensor indicis proprius, extensor digitorum communis, and extensor digiti minimi dorsiflex the metacarpophalangeal joints. The palmar flexors are the flexor pollicis brevis, lumbricales, interossei, and flexor digiti minimi brevis assisted by the long flexors. Radial and ulnar movements of the second to fifth metacarpophalangeal joints are a function of the intrinsic muscles.

The interphalangeal joints

The proximal and distal interphalangeal joints of the fingers and the interphalangeal joints of the thumbs are hinge joints (Fig. 4). Their capsules are

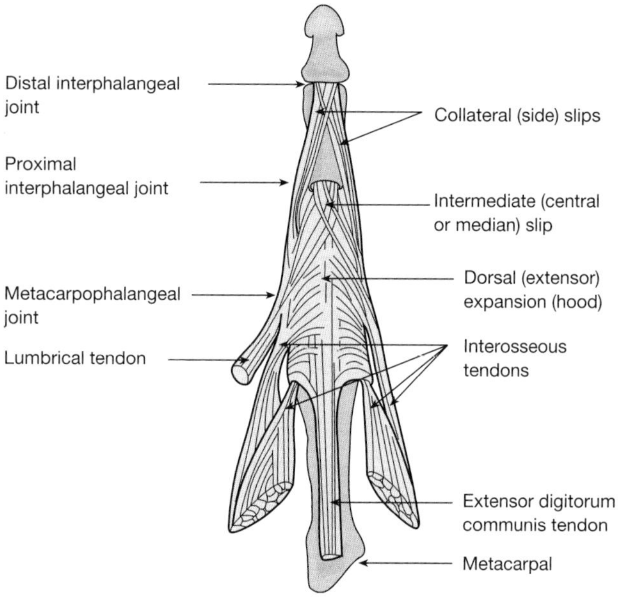

Fig. 7 Extensor expansion of the finger.

strengthened by the collateral ligaments on the sides and by the volar plate on the palmar surface. The volar plates serve to limit hyperextension, particularly at the proximal interphalangeal joints. Unlike the metacarpophalangeal joints, the radial and ulnar collateral ligaments remain taut in all positions, providing side-to-side stability throughout the range of movement.

The flexor tendon sheaths for the fingers enclose the flexor digitorum superficialis and profundus tendons to their insertions on the middle and distal phalanges, respectively. The sheaths extend from just proximal to the metacarpophalangeal joints to the bases of the distal phalanges (Fig. 5). The flexor pollicis longus tendon sheath of the thumb extends proximally to the carpal tunnel. The flexor sheath of the little finger is often continuous with the common flexor tendon sheath of the wrist. Segmental condensations, or annular pulleys, in the digital flexor sheaths prevent bowstringing of the tendons, and are mechanically critical for full digital flexion (Polley and Hunder 1978; Williams et al. 1989)

The proximal interphalangeal joints do not normally hyperextend. They allow 100–120° palmar flexion. The distal interphalangeal joints permit 50–80° palmar flexion and 5–10° dorsiflexion. The interphalangeal joint of the thumb allows 80–90° palmar flexion and 20–35° dorsiflexion. The flexor digitorum superficialis flexes the proximal interphalangeal joints, and the flexor digitorum profundus flexes the distal interphalangeal joints of the fingers. The prime dorsiflexors are the interossei and lumbrical muscles. The flexor pollicis longus flexes the interphalangeal joint of the thumb and the extensor pollicis longus dorsiflexes the joint.

General considerations and differential diagnosis of regional rheumatic pain syndromes of the upper extremities in adults

Differential diagnosis of shoulder pain

Pain in the shoulder region is relatively common, and may reflect a multitude of conditions (Table 1). The pain may have its origin in the glenohumeral (GH), acromioclavicular (AC) or sternoclavicular (SC) joints, or periarticular structures (rotator cuff tendons, bicipital tendon, subacromial bursa, capsule),

Table 1 Classification of shoulder disorders

Intrinsic disorders
Articular
Arthritis of GH or AC joints: traumatic, rheumatoid, psoriatic, enteropathic, spondylitic, osteoarthritic, and crystal-induced
Glenohumeral instability and rotator cuff tear arthropathy
Traumatic lesions of capsule, ligaments, glenoid labrum (Bankart's lesion)
Periarticular
Rotator cuff tendonitis/impingement syndrome
Rotator cuff tears
Bicipital tendonitis/rupture long head of biceps tendon
Subacromial bursitis
Adhesive capsulitis (frozen shoulder)
Osseous
Humeral head osteonecrosis
Skeletal metastases, multiple myeloma, lymphoma
Fractures, infections, hyperparathyroidism, osteolysis of distal clavicle
Extrinsic disorders
Neurologic
Suprascapular neuropathy
Acute brachial plexus neuritis (upper brachial plexus)
Quadrilateral space syndrome (axillary nerve)
Thoracic outlet syndrome (lower brachial plexus)
Compression radiculopathy
Spinal cord tumours, syringomyelia
Vascular and neurovascular
Reflex sympathetic dystrophy (shoulder-hand syndrome)
Axillary artery or vein thrombosis
Referred and regional pain
Cervical spine
Angina pectoris, myocardial infarction, pericarditis
Infradiaphragmatic: gallbladder disease, subphrenic abscess
Myofascial pain syndrome and somatoform pain syndrome
Systemic disorders
Polymyalgia rheumatica
Polymyositis, dermatomyositis
Hypothyroidism
Fibromyalgia

or be referred from the cervical spine (often felt at the supraspinatus region), thoracic outlet, diaphragm (often felt at the tip of the shoulder), brachial plexus, suprascapular nerve, nerve roots, spinal cord, or vascular structures, or be part of a systemic condition. Recent studies have emphasized the significant interobserver disagreement in classifying the most common disorders of the shoulder (Bamji et al. 1996; DeWinter et al. 1999).

Periarticular disorders are by far the most common cause of shoulder pain in adults. A combination of factors, both extrinsic and intrinsic to the rotator cuff have been implicated in the development of tendinopathy (Tytherleigh-Strong et al. 2001) The anatomical configuration of the shoulder joint is such that during abduction, the rotator cuff and long biceps tendon are subjected to impingement between the greater tuberosity of the humerus and the coracoacromial arch. Excessive or repetitive overhead activities can lead to tendinitis and tears of the rotator cuff that compromises its function as a stabilizer and depressor of the humeral head. This results in chronic GH instability, superior migration of the humeral head, due to unopposed upward pull of the deltoid, and further impingement on both the rotator cuff and long biceps tendon. Osteophytes on the inferior surface of the AC joint can also aggravate this impingement. Thus, the spectrum of the chronic impingement syndrome ranges from mild tendonitis of the rotator cuff, with or without inflammation of the adjacent subacromial bursa, to bicipital tendinitis, rotator cuff tears, rupture of the long head of the biceps tendon, and chronic GH instability with secondary osteoarthritis of the GH joint ('rotator cuff tear arthropathy').

Accurate diagnosis of shoulder pain depends upon an understanding of the basic anatomy, a detailed clinical history, a thorough physical examination of the GH, AC, and SC joints, periarticular structures, cervical spine, nerve and blood supplies, and a few carefully selected diagnostic studies. Included among these are: a complete blood count, erythrocyte sedimentation rate, shoulder radiographs, biochemical profile, rheumatoid factor, and when available synovial fluid analysis. Additional studies, such as ultrasonography, magnetic resonance imaging (MRI), computed tomography (CT), arthroscopy, or arthrography of the shoulder, may be indicated.

Important points in the history include patient's occupation, sport activities, history of trauma, onset, location, character, duration and modulating factors of pain, the effect of pain on overall shoulder function, presence of stiffness or swelling of the joint, and associated arthritic or systemic complaints. The onset of many painful shoulder disorders is often insidious. An antecedent history of repetitive, excessive, unaccustomed or overhead physical activity, is particularly useful in diagnosing shoulder tendonitis due to an overuse syndrome. A careful occupational history is important for determining whether the shoulder tendonitis is work-related, either as a cumulative trauma disorder or an acute injury. Abnormal tensile stresses exceeding the elastic limits of tendons can lead to cumulative microfailure of the molecular links between tendon fibrils, a phenomenon referred to as 'fibriller creep'. With aging, tendons become less flexible and less elastic, making them more susceptible to injury and tears. A short-ended musculotendinous unit, from lack of regular stretching exercises, is also more prone to injury.

Both shoulders are examined with the patient either sitting or standing. Effusion of the GH joint due to arthritis, produces a diffuse swelling of the shoulder which bulges anteriorly. Chronic GH subluxation, due to trauma, rotator cuff tears or hemiparesis, produces sagging of the shoulder. Posterior dislocation of the shoulder is associated with loss of anterior roundness of the shoulder, and prominence of the coracoid process, while anterior dislocation produces loss of the lateral roundness of the shoulder. Winging of the scapula on forward flexion of the shoulder results from impingement of the serratus anterior (long thoracic) nerve.

Localization of the point of maximum tenderness is important in differentiating rotator cuff tendinitis/subacromial bursitis from arthritis of the GH or AC joints. *Glenohumeral arthritis* is associated with diffuse tenderness over the joint, global restriction of movements, and sometimes an effusion. Rheumatoid arthritis, spondyloarthropathies, crystal-induced arthritidies, including that due to the deposition of basic calcium crystals (Milwakee shoulder), are the most common causes of inflammatory glenohumeral arthritis. *Rotator cuff tendinitis/subacromial bursitis*, by contrast, is characterized by tenderness localized to the rotator cuff and greater tuberosity, and painful shoulder movements, particularly on active abduction between 60 and 120° (painful arc), rotation, and sometimes when lowering the arm. Night pain on rolling on the affected side, and pain on resisted movement of the affected tendon, are common. The 'supraspinatus or empty can sign' is often positive: pain on resisted elevation of the arm to 90° midway between abduction and forward flexion with the thumb pointing downward in internal rotation. In Neer's 'impingement sign', the examiner's hand forward flexes the patient's arm while the other hand restricts scapular rotation. Shoulder pain in the overhead position near full flexion constitutes a positive test. In 'Hawkins–Kennedy impingement sign', the humerus is both forward flexed to 90° and forcibly internally rotated by the examiner, causing impingement of the greater tuberosity against the anterior acromion with reproduction of the patient's pain.

Calcification of the cuff tendons may be asymptomatic, but can present as an acute condition in the younger patient, or as a chronic calcific tendonitis associated with aching pain and symptoms of impingement. In *acute calcific tendinitis*, the onset is often explosive, with severe pain, exquisite tenderness, muscle spasm, and marked painful restriction of all shoulder movements. An acute *subacromial bursitis* may also be present when calcific material ruptures into the adjacent bursa, causing bursal fluid distension, just anterior and lateral to the acromion when the shoulder is extended. Shoulder radiographs may appear either normal, or show oval or round calcific deposits in the region of the rotator cuff tendons, particularly that of the supraspinatus. These deposits often disappear following resolution of an attack of acute calcific tendonitis/bursitis. In chronic tendonitis, the presence of sclerosis, cystic changes, and osteophytes of the greater tuberosity is suggestive of chronic impingement and insertional damage.

Rotator cuff tears can be partial or complete, acute or chronic. They are further classified as small (<1 cm), medium (1–3 cm), large (3–5 cm), and massive (>5 cm) (Synder 1993). In young adults, acute tears can result from direct trauma, unexpected falls or a sport injury. In older patients, minor less severe trauma, superimposed on an already degenerated cuff tendon from chronic impingement and age-related attritional changes, can lead to partial tears. Clinical features include shoulder pain on abduction, night pain, varying degrees of weakness of abduction and external rotation, local tenderness, and loss of movement. The supraspinatus and other impingement signs are usually positive. In *complete supraspinatus tears*, the 'drop-arm' sign is positive: inability to actively maintain 90° of passive shoulder abduction. *Partial rotator cuff tears* due to chronic impingement, are associated with persistent shoulder pain on abduction and external rotation, night pain, restriction of movements, varying degrees of weakness of abduction and external rotation, and localized wasting of supraspinatus and infraspinatus muscles. Subacromial crepitus and rupture of the long biceps tendon are often present. Radiographic findings include sclerosis and cystic degeneration of the greater tuberosity, superior migration of the humeral head with narrowing of the subacromial space (less than 6 mm indicates a tear), and secondary glenohumeral osteoarthritis. Ultrasonography and magnetic resonance imaging are very helpful in confirming the diagnosis of rotator cuff tear and they have replaced arthrography as the diagnostic modality of choice (Swen et al. 1998). Both have high and equivalent sensitivity and specificity for the detection of full-thickness tears (Swen et al. 1999). Their accuracy is much less for partial-thickness tears.

Bicipital tendonitis is often related to chronic impingement of the bicipital tendon on the acromion (Murthi et al. 2000). The long biceps tendon becomes fibrotic, frayed, and may rupture. Bicipital tendonitis usually occurs in association with rotator cuff tendonitis and glenohumeral instability. Primary, isolated, isolated bicipital tendonitis is rare, and develops as an overuse injury due to repetitive stresses applied to the tendon in certain sports such as weight lifting and ball throwing. The pain is felt over the anterior aspect of the shoulder but may radiate into the biceps muscle. Localized tenderness is present over the tendon in the bicipital groove. Bicipital tendon pain can be reproduced by resisted supination of the pronated forearm with the elbow 90° flexed (Yergason's sign), passive extension of the shoulder, or by resisted flexion of the elbow. *Rupture of the long biceps tendon* typically occurs at the superior edge of the bicipital groove. It produces a characteristic bulbous bunching up of the lateral half of the biceps belly, best seen with resisted elbow flexion and supination ('Popeye sign').

Adhesive capsulitis or frozen shoulder is associated with diffuse pain and tenderness in the deltoid area, night pain, and progressive equal limitation of both active and passive movements with a capsular pattern: external rotation more than; abduction more than; internal rotation (Hulstyn and Weiss 1993; Noel et al. 2000). Disuse atrophy of the deltoid and scapular muscles may be present. Adhesive capsulitis is rare before the age of 40 years, and is bilateral in about 15 per cent of patients. A period of immobility of the shoulder is the most commonly identified predisposing factor. The onset is insidious, and the capsulitis is often secondary to rotator cuff tendonitis, rotator cuff tears, bicipital tendonitis, or glenohumeral arthritis. The condition may also coexist with diabetes mellitus, hypothyroidism, lung carcinoma, myocardial infarction, cardiac surgery, cerebrovascular events, the use of protease inhibitors for the treatment of HIV infection, and shoulder trauma. Primary or idiopathic capsulitis is rare. Limited histological studies demonstrate an initial phase with increased vascularity, sparse chronic inflammatory cellular infiltrate, and fibroblastic proliferation. This is followed by fibrous thickening and contraction of the capsular folds, recesses, and surrounding ligamentous structures. The capsule often adheres to the humeral neck, and the axillary pouch becomes obliterated causing restricted movements (Neviaser 1987). Double-contrast arthrography is diagnostic, showing a marked decrease in the joint volume to under 10 ml (normal values: 20–25 ml), loss of normal axillary recess, and reduced filling of the bicipital tendon sheath. Dynamic sonography, demonstrating limitation of sliding movements of the supraspinatus tendon during abduction of the arm, is a reliable, non-invasive, rapid technique for the diagnosis of this disorder (Ryu et al. 1993). MRI may show postgadolimium enhancement of the joint capsule and synovial membrane (Emig et al. 1995).

Chronic glenohumeral instability and rotator cuff tear arthropathy (rotator cuff-deficient osteoarthritic shoulder) results from chronic impingement with tears of the capsule, rotator cuff, and biceps tendon. It is characterized by abnormal motion of the humeral head relative to the glenoid fossa during active shoulder movements, associated with a long history of progressive pain that is worse at night, and is intensified by GH movements. There is often atrophy of the supraspinatus and infraspinatus muscles, weakness of external rotation and abduction, and limitation of active and passive shoulder movements, especially external rotation and abduction. Patients may also complain of 'the shoulder slipping or going out of joint' during abduction or external rotation. An effusion and crepitus of the GH joint may be present. The 'anterior and posterior drawer's or glide sign' is positive: excessive forward and backward motion of the humeral head and proximal humerus on the glenoid fossa. The 'sulcus sign' may be present: applying distal traction on the upper arm produces a palpable gap between the humeral head and the acromium.

Arthritis of the AC joint produces pain, tenderness, swelling, and sometimes crepitus localized to the joint. In the 'cross-arm AC loading test', shoulder abduction to 90° and then adduction across the chest at shoulder height, reproduces the AC joint pain.

Of the neurologic causes of shoulder pain (Table 1), two conditions merit special comment: acute brachial plexus neuritis and quadrilateral space syndrome. *Acute brachial plexus neuritis (acute brachial plexitis or brachial neuralgic amyotrophy or Parsonage–Turner syndrome)* is an uncommon disorder affecting adults, particularly men (Misomore and Lehman 1996). It is characterized by a rapid onset of severe burning shoulder and upper arm pain, followed in a few days by profound upper arm weakness and atrophy affecting multiple muscles supplied by the upper brachial plexus: supraspinatus, infraspinatus, deltoid, and sometimes biceps. The course of the neuritis is usually one of gradual recovery in 3–4 months. MRI of the shoulder and upper arm may within days, reveal denervation of affected muscles with high signal intensity on T_2-weighted images. Electromyography (EMG), conducted 3–4 weeks after the onset, often shows signs of denervation of muscles supplied by the upper brachial plexus. The multiple nerve involvement distinguishes acute brachial neuritis from *cervical radiculopathy* where the pain, parasthesia, and weakness are usually restricted to a single nerve root.

Quadrilateral space syndrome is a rare condition affecting active young adults, with symptoms caused by compression by fibrous bands of the axillary nerve in the quadrilateral space (Lester et al.1999; Chautems et al. 2000). The space lies inferoposterior to the GH joint, and is bounded by teres minor muscle superiorly, teres major inferiorly, humerus laterally, and long head of the triceps medially. Both the axillary nerve and posterior circumflex humeral artery pass through the space. Pain and parasthesia in the anterolateral aspect of the shoulder and upper posterior arm, of non-dermatomal distribution, excacerbated by abduction and external rotation, are the main symptoms. Typical physical findings include point tenderness with posterior pressure over the quadrilateral space, aggravation of symptoms by external rotation of the humerus, variable atrophy and weakness of deltoid and teres minor muscles, and sometimes sensory loss over the anterolateral aspect of the shoulder and upper arm. EMG is usually normal but denervation of deltoid muscle may be present. MRI of the quadrilateral space often shows no abnormality but may reveal atrophy of deltoid and teres minor. Arteriography, or MRI-angiography may reveal occlusion of the posterior circumflex humeral artery when the arm is abducted and externally rotated. In thoracic outlet syndrome, by contrast, there are symptoms of compression of both the lower brachial plexus and the subclavian artery. The latter can be demonstrated by dynamic arteriography or MRI-angiography. Adson's manoeuvre is often positive: disappearance of ipsilateral radial pulse when patient abducts, extends and externally rotates the shoulder while taking a deep breath and rotating the head maximally towards the side being tested.

Differential diagnosis of elbow pain

Pain in the elbow is a relatively frequent symptom of diverse causes (Table 2). The pain may arise from the elbow or proximal radioulnar joints, periarticular structures (tendons, ligaments, muscle groups or olecranon bursa), or be referred from the cervical spine, nerve roots, brachial plexus, peripheral nerves, shoulder, or wrist. Periarticular disorders are again the most frequent causes of elbow pain (Putnam and Cohen 1999).

Precise diagnosis of elbow pain depends on a complete history, and a thorough examination of the elbow, shoulder, wrist, cervical spine, nerve and vascular supplies (Colman and Strauch 1999). Diagnostic studies, including radiography, ultrasonography, diagnostic joint or bursal needle aspiration, CT, MRI, arthroscopy, EMG, and nerve conduction studies, may be required. Helpful points in the history include onset, exact location, nature, and duration of elbow pain, aggravating and relieving factors, history of antecedent trauma or unaccustomed, repetitive or excessive sport or occupational elbow activities, effects of pain and stiffness on elbow function, and history of elbow swelling and its location. Parasthesias or muscle weakness are clues to a nerve entrapment syndrome or cervical radiculopathy.

The elbow is examined for swelling, tenderness and its location, varus, valgus or flexion deformity, and for fluid distension and tenderness of the olecranon bursa. Arthritis of the elbow and proximal radioulnar joints is associated with joint line tenderness, diffuse swelling with obliteration of the paraolecranon grooves, and restriction of elbow flexion and of radio-ulnar supination and pronation. An elbow effusion produces fluctuant swelling in the lateral and medial paraolecranon grooves. Ulnar and radial ligamentous stabilities are assessed with the patient's elbow flexed 10–20° in order to unlock the olecranon process from its fossa.

Table 2 Classification of elbow disorders

Category	Disorders
Articular	Arthritis of elbow and proximal radioulnar joints: traumatic, rheumatoid, psoriatic, osteoarthritic, gouty, septic
	Traumatic lesions of capsule and ligaments
Periarticular tendinitis	Lateral epicondylitis (tennis elbow)
	Medial epicondylitis (golfer's elbow)
	Bicipital insertional tendinitis
	Triceps tendonitis and dislocating or snapping medial triceps
	Brachialis tendinitis
Olecranon bursitis	Traumatic, inflammatory, septic
Olecranon impingement syndrome	
Osseous	Fractures, infection, neoplasms, osteochondritis dissecans
Neurologic	Cubital tunnel syndrome (ulnar nerve)
	Pronator teres syndrome (median nerve)
	Radial tunnel syndrome (posterior interosseous nerve)
	Spiral groove syndrome (radial nerve)
	Lower brachial plexus compression in thoracic outlet syndrome
	Compression radiculopathy due to cervical disc lesion
	Spinal cord tumours, syringomyelia
Miscellaneous	Reflex sympathetic dystrophy syndrome
	Fibromyalgia
	Somatoform pain syndrome (psychogenic regional pain syndrome)

Lateral epicondylitis (tennis elbow) is one of the most common painful lesions of the upper extremity. It affects 1–3 per cent of the adult population, mostly between 40 and 60 years of age (Gabel 1999). The dominant arm is most frequently involved. Although about 40 per cent of tennis players suffer with lateral epicondylitis, less than 10 per cent of patients in clinical practice acquire the disorder through playing tennis. The exact mechanism of lateral epicondylitis is not entirely clear. It is generally regarded as a cumulative trauma overuse disorder due to repetitive mechanical overloading of the common extensor tendon, particularly of the portion derived from the extensor carpi radialis brevis. Histopathological studies of involved tendons show fibroblastic and vascular hyperplasia (angiofibroblastic degeneration) and disorganized collagen. Acute and chronic inflammatory cells are rarely seen and this is why the term epicondylosis rather than epicondylitis has been recommended by some authors (Kraushaar and Nirschl 1999). In late stages, fibrosis, soft matrix, and osseous calcifications can be seen.

The onset is often insidious, and bilateral involvement is not uncommon. A rapid onset following a direct blow to the lateral epicondyle or a sports-related injury is more frequent in the younger, more active patient. Pain is localized to the lateral epicondyle but may extend both distally and proximally. It is made worse by handshakes, turning doorknobs, carrying a briefcase, lifting or gripping, resulting in restricted hand activities. Localized tenderness is present just distal, medial, and slightly anterior to the lateral epicondyle, over the common extensor tendon particularly that portion derived from the extensor carpi radialis brevis muscle. The pain is increased by resisted dorsiflexion of the wrist with the elbow in extension, or by extending the elbow with the wrist flexed and pronated. The 'tennis elbow test' is often positive: with the patient's elbow extended, forearm pronated and fisted hand radially deviated and extended at the wrist, applying resisting force at the fist while supporting the elbow with the other hand elicits pain in the area of the lateral epicondyle. The 'chair-lift' test, in which the patient lifts a chair with the forearm and hands pronated and the elbow extended, often causes sharp pain in the region of the lateral epicondyle. In chronic cases, a slight flexion deformity of the elbow, and a weak hand grip may be present. Elbow radiographs are often normal, but periarticular calcification or exostosis may be present in those with chronic symptoms. Ultrasound and MRI show abnormalities in most patients, including partial and complete tendon tears, particularly in young athletes with acute onset of symptoms (Warhold et al. 1993; Connell et al. 2001). MRI in patients with chronic symptoms can also demonstrate signs of tendon degeneration (Schenk and Dalinka 1997).

Medial epicondylitis (golfer's elbow) is five to eight times less common than lateral epicondylitis (Gabel and Morrey 1999). It commonly occurs in individuals who overuse their arms, and its pathology is essentially similar to that of tennis elbow. It is characterized by insidious onset of aching pain in the area of the medial epicondyle. The pain may spread down the forearm, and is increased by lifting, grasping, and activities that require rapid wrist flexion and forearm pronation. An antecedent history of cumulative repetitive strain of the common flexor muscles of the forearm in golfing, baseball pitching, and racquet sports is common. There is tenderness at and just distal to the medial epicondyle over the origin of the common flexor tendon, particularly that portion derived from the pronator teres and flexor carpi radialis muscles. Resisted pronation of the forearm is the most sensitive provocative manoeuvre, followed by resisted flexion of the wrist with the elbow extended (Gabel and Morrey 1995). Flexion of the fingers rather than of the wrists may sometime elicit pain at the medial epicondyle. It is also important to examine the ulnar nerve in the cubital tunnel as a concomitant ulnar neuropathy is a common finding associated with a less favourable prognosis (Gabel and Morrey 1995).

Olecranon bursitis, whether traumatic, inflammatory (e.g. rheumatoid arthritis, gouty, psoriatic arthritis), or septic, is associated with local pain, tenderness, and fluid distension of the olecranon bursa (Fam 1992). Movements of the elbow joint are usually unimpaired and painless.

Peribursal cellulitis is characteristic of septic bursitis. Non-septic olecranon bursitis can result from either a discrete injury, for example, an acute blow (traumatic olecranon bursitis), or from repetitive, minor, or occult trauma to the elbow, for example, excessive leaning (idiopathic olecranon bursitis, 'student's elbow', 'dialysis elbow'). Septic olecranon bursitis usually result from the direct introduction of bacteria through a skin abrasion. It typically occurs in otherwise healthy adult men engaged in physical work involving frequent trauma to the elbows (e.g. plumbers, miners, gardeners, construction workers, etc.). *Staphylococcus aureus* is the most common pathogen.

Olecranon impingement syndrome, is a traumatic lesion characterized by aching posterior elbow pain increased by elbow extension. Recurrent 'clicking' or 'locking' with terminal extension of the elbow, crepitus, and a mechanical extension block, are common. Radiographs may show osteophytes of both the olecranon process and fossa.

Tendinitis of the biceps tendon insertion into the radial tuberosity is a less frequent cause of anterior elbow pain. It typically occurs in individuals engaged in repetitive elbow flexion and forearm supination, as in weight lifting, bowling, and gymnastics. It is associated with local tenderness and sometimes swelling of the distal biceps tendon. The pain is increased by resisted flexion and supination of the forearm and by full elbow extension. An elbow flexion deformity may develop in advanced cases.

Triceps tendonitis, is characterized by posterior elbow pain, increased by resisted elbow extension. There is localized tenderness, and sometimes swelling of the triceps tendon near its insertion into the olecranon process. Triceps tendonitis typically affects adult men in the setting of repetitive elbow extension, as in heavy manual work, boxing, or weight lifting.

The cubital tunnel syndrome is due to ulnar nerve entrapment within its groove behind the medial epicondyle. It may result from repetitive trauma, occupational strains, or sport activities such as skiing, throwing, or racquet sports. It is characterized by medial elbow pain, parasthesias along the ulnar aspect of forearm into the ring and little fingers, and sometimes a weak hand grip with fatique and clumsiness. Tenderness is often present over the ulnar nerve, and Tinel's sign is usually positive. Atrophy of the hypothenar muscles with weakness of index pinch may also be present. Electrophysiologic studies are often diagnostic.

The pronator teres syndrome is often a cumulative repetitive strain disorder, due to entrapment of the median nerve as it passes through the humeral and ulnar heads of the pronator teres muscle. Anterior elbow pain, made worse by resisted pronation of the forearm, and distal paresthesias in the distribution of the median nerve, are characteristic symptoms. A positive 'papal sign' may be present: weak palmar flexion of index and middle fingers resulting in finger extension in the resting position. The diagnosis can be confirmed by nerve conduction studies.

The radial tunnel syndrome is due to entrapment of the deep branch of the radial nerve (posterior interosseous nerve), as it passes through the arcade of Frohse, a fibrous arc formed by the proximal margin of the superficial head of the supinator muscle (Rosenbaum 1999). It occurs most often in adults who overuse their arm in vocational or recreational activities. The syndrome is associated with lateral elbow pain that radiates into the dorsal forearm, and is increased by activities involving repetitive supination of forearm and hand. Typical findings include tenderness where the radial nerve crosses the head of the radius, a positive Tinel's sign on tapping the nerve distal and anterior to the lateral epicondyle, and pain on resisted supination of the forearm with the elbow extended and the wrist palmar flexed. A flexion force applied against the middle finger extension distal to the PIP joint may induce pain in the extensor muscles of the proximal forearm. Weakness of the wrists and fingers dorsiflexors may be present.

Differential diagnosis of wrist and hand pain

Painful disorders of the wrist and hand are a relatively common presentation in rheumatologic, orthopaedic, and plastic surgery practices (Table 3). The pain may have its origin in the bones and joints of the wrist and hand, periarticular structures (subcutaneous tissue, palmar fascia, tendon sheaths, ligaments), nerve roots, peripheral nerves, or vascular structures of the hand, or it may be referred from the cervical spine, thoracic outlet, or elbow.

Table 3 Classification of disorders of wrist and hand

Articular
Arthritis of wrist, MCP, PIP, DIP joints: trauma, RA, OA, psoriatic, remitting seronegative symmetric synovitis with pitting edema (RS_3PE)
Joint neoplasms
Periarticular
Subcutaneous: rheumatoid nodules, tophi, glomus tumor of nail bed, hereditary angio-oedema, infections
Palmar fascia: Dupuytren's contracture
Tendon sheath:
Wrist extensor tenosynovitis, including de Quervain's tenosynovitis
Wrist common flexor tenosynovitis
Thumb/finger flexor digital tenosynovitis (trigger thumb/finger)
Pigmented villonodular tenosynovitis (giant cell tumor of tendon sheath)
Acute calcific periarthritis: wrist, MCP, PIP, DIP
Ganglion
Osseous
Fracture, infections, neoplasms, osteonecrosis of lunate (Kienbock's disease), and of scaphoid (Preiser's disease), os centrale carpi, hamato-lunate impingement
Neurologic
Nerve entrapment syndromes:
Median nerve:
Carpal tunnel syndrome (at wrist)
Pronator teres syndrome (at pronator teres)
Anterior interosseous nerve syndrome
Ulnar nerve:
Cubital tunnel syndrome (at elbow)
Guyon's canal syndrome (at wrist)
Radial nerve:
Spiral groove syndrome
Posterior interosseous nerve (radial tunnel syndrome)
Superficial branch of radial nerve (Wartenberg's or bracelet syndrome)
Lower brachial plexus: thoracic outlet syndrome
Cervical nerve roots: herniated cervical disc
Focal hand dystonia
Spinal cord tumours, syringomyelia
Vascular and neurovascular
Vasospastic disorders (Raynaud's), and vasculitis
Reflex sympathetic dystrophy (shoulder-hand syndrome, causalgia)
Referred
Cervical spine disorders
Cardiac: angina pectoris
Elbow disorders

A history of repetitive, excessive, or unaccustomed physical activity, is particularly important in diagnosing wrist, thumb, or finger tenosynovitis due to an overuse syndrome. The wrist and hand are examined for clubbing, subcutaneous nodules, tophi, osteoarthritic Heberden's and Bouchard's nodes, ischemic digital ulcers, pitted scars, nailfold infarcts, sclerodactyly, telangiectasia, periungual erythema, or psoriatic skin/nail lesions.

Wrist (radiocarpal) arthritis produces painful restriction of all movements, and a diffuse swelling with tender synovial thickening, just distal to the radius and ulna. The presence of fluctuance indicates a large effusion: pressure bidigitally with one hand on one side of the joint produces a fluid wave transmitted to the second hand placed on the opposite side of the wrist. *Extensor wrist tenosynovitis*, by contrast, presents as a superficial, linear, tender, dorsal swelling conforming to the affected tendon sheath, and extending beyond the joint margins. When the fingers are actively extended, the distal margin of the swelling moves proximally and folds in, like a sheet being tucked under a mattress (tuck sign). *Common flexor wrist tenosynovitis* presents as a tender swelling on the volar aspect of the wrist and distal forearm, just proximal to the carpal tunnel. A tendon crepitus may be palpable, and movements of the involved tendons are painful.

The wrist is a common site for ganglia. A *ganglion* is a relatively painless, mucin-filled, uni- or multilocular cyst attached to a joint capsule, tendon, or tendon sheath.

Wrist deformities are frequent in rheumatoid and other inflammatory arthritides. These include volar subluxation of the carpus with a visible step at the radiocarpal joint, carpal collapse with loss of carpal height to less than half the length of the third metacarpal, and radial deviation of the carpus from the axis of the wrist and hand. *Chronic synovitis and instability of distal radiocarpal joint* produces dorsal subluxation of the ulnar head with a 'piano-key' movement on downward pressure. Entrapment of the median nerve within the carpal tunnel (*carpal tunnel syndrome*) is characterized by pain, parasthesia, or sensory loss in the median nerve distribution, nocturnal exacerbation of symptoms, and sometimes motor loss and atrophy of the thenar muscles. Percussion of the median nerve at the flexor retinaculum just radial to the palmaris longus tendon at the distal wrist crease (Tinel's sign), produces parasthesias in the median nerve distribution: thumb, index and middle finger and radial half of ring finger. Sustained palmar flexion of the wrist for 30–60 s may induce finger parasthesias (Phalen's wrist flexion sign). If the wrist cannot be flexed because of arthritis, pressure over the median nerve for 30 s often produces the same effect. Median nerve conduction time is usually abnormal.

MCP synovitis produces a diffuse swelling of the joint that may obscure the ulnar valleys between the knuckles. *MCP joint deformities* include ulnar drift, volar subluxation (often visible as a step), and flexion deformities. *Synovitis of the PIP joint* produces a fusiform or spindle-shaped finger. To detect an effusion, compression of the joint using the thumb and forefinger of one hand produces ballooning or a hydraulic lift sensed by the other hand, (balloon sign). Unlike PIP synovitis, *dorsal knuckle pads* produce a non tender thickening of the skin localized to the dorsal surface of the PIP joints. A *finger swan-neck deformity* consists of hyperextension of the PIP joint and palmar flexion of the DIP joint. In *'boutonniere' finger deformity* there is flexion of the PIP joint and hyperextension of the DIP joint. A *Z deformity of the thumb* consists of flexion of the MCP joint and hyperextension of the IP joint. *Telescoped shortening of one or more digits*, produced by osteolysis of the phalanges secondary to psoriatic or rheumatoid arthritis, is often associated with concentric wrinkling of the skin (opera-glass hand).

Flexor tendon entrapment of the digits also known as *trigger or snapping finger (or thumb)* occurs in 2–3 per cent of non-diabetic adults. The pathological lesion is hypertrophy and fibrocartilaginous metaplasia of the ligamentous layer of the tendon sheath at the level of the first annular pulley that overlies the metacarpophalangeal joint, resulting in stenosis of the fibro-osseous canal and mechanical entrapment of the tendon (Moore 2000). A nodular thickening of the tendon often develops at the site of stenosis; this interferes mechanically with the normal gliding of the tendon, resulting in pain over the area of the pulley and 'snapping', 'triggering', or 'catching' of the finger or thumb. Pain over the sheath with resisted flexion, and pain on stretching the tendon passively in extension, are common. Intermittent locking of the digit in flexion may also develop, particularly upon arising in the morning. Examination reveals tenderness over the area of the proximal pulley, linear swelling of the flexor tendon sheath, tendon crepitus, and, often, limitation of digital flexion and extension. A nodular tendon swelling can often be palpated in the palm just proximal to the MCP joint (opposite the proximal annular pulley of the sheath), as it moves during finger or thumb flexion and extension. One digit is often affected, usually the thumb, middle, or ring fingers in that order. Most cases of flexor tendon entrapment are idiopathic although overuse trauma of the hands from repetitive gripping activities, has been implicated in some cases. Patients with diabetes mellitus and rheumatoid arthritis are at increased risk and the condiiton appears to be more common also in patients with carpal tunnel syndrome, Dupuytren's disease, and hypothyroidism.

de Quervain's stenosing tenosynovitis of the common tendon sheath of the abductor pollicis longus (APC) and extensor pollicis brevis (EPB), is characterized by pain over the radial aspect of the wrist, aggravated by thumb movements during pinching, grasping, or lifting (Moore 1997). Despite its name, there is usually no histological evidence of inflammation in either the tendons or their sheath. Instead, the pathology lies in the extensor retinaculum that covers the first compartment of the wrist, which is thickened and causes tendon entrapment (Moore 1997). The concept that de Quervain's tenosynovitis is caused by occupational or avocational repetitive movement of the thumb has recently been challenged (Kay 2000). de Quervain's tenosynovitis has also been associated with rheumatoid arthritis, psoriatic arthritis, direct trauma, pregnancy, and during the post-partum period. The affected tendon sheath is tender and often swollen 1–2 cm proximal to the radial styloid. Finkelstein's test is positive: passive ulnar deviation of the wrist with the fingers flexed over the thumb placed in the palm, stretches the APC and EPB tendons, and reproduces the pain over the radial side. A tendon crepitus is often palpable. de Quervain's tenosynovitis is sometimes confused with the *intersection syndrome:* tenosynovitis of the extensor carpi radialis longus and brevis at their intersection with the tendons of the abductor pollicis longus and flexor pollicis brevis. Unlike de Quervain's tenosynovitis, the intersection syndrome is associated with pain, tenderness, swelling, and sometimes crepitus over the dorsoradial aspect of the distal forearm, about 4 cm proximal to the wrist joint.

Nodular thickening and contracture of the palmar fascia or *Dupuytren's contracture* can lead to disabling flexion deformities of the ring, and less commonly, little, middle; and index fingers (Rayan 1999a, b). In most patients, Dupuytren's contracture affects the ulnar side of both hands. The ring finger is usually affected first, followed by the small finger, then the thumb, middle finger, and the index fingers in decreasing order of frequency. Fibrous nodules, composed of whorls of proliferating fibroblasts and myofibroblasts in the superficial layers of the palmar fascia, are the earliest abnormality. The formation of these nodules result in puckering, dimpling, and tethering of the overlying skin. There is usually little pain initially. However, after a variable period of months or years, the aponeurotic thickening may extend distally to involve the digits. The fingers become fixed at the metacarpophalangeal joints by taut fibrous bands radiating from the plamar fascia (Fig. 8), and the hand cannot be placed flat on a table (positive 'table top' test). Although there is no direct involvement of the joints and tendons, progressive flexion deformity of the fingers can lead to severe functional impairment.

Focal hand dystonia is a repetitive strain injury that may occur in musicians, particularly guitar players. Uncontrollable movements when trying to perform a common target task, is the main symptom. There is uncontrollable contraction of both the extensors and flexors usually of a finger, with loss of the graded fine motor control of the digit. There are no objective findings but the diagnosis can be confirmed by EMG showing co-contractions of the extensors and the flexors, due to loss of reflex inhibition between the agonists and antagonists.

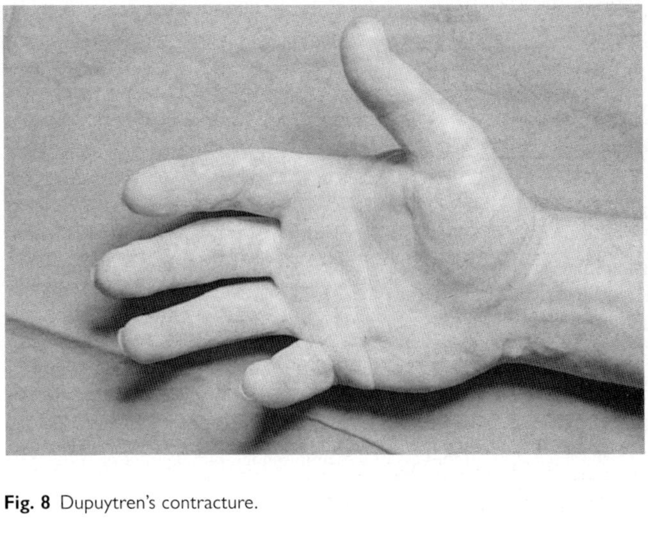

Fig. 8 Dupuytren's contracture.

References

Bamji, A.N., Erhardt, C.C., Prive, C.R., and Williams, P.L. (1996). The painful shoulder: can consultants agree? *British Journal of Rheumatology* **35**, 1172–4.

Chautems, R.C., Glauser, T., Waeber-Fey, M.C., Rostan, O., and Barraud, G.E. (2000). Quadrilateral space syndrome: case report and review of the literature. *Annals of Vascular Surgery* **14**, 673–6.

Colman, W.W. and Strauch, R.J. (1999). Physical examination of the elbow. *Orthopedic Clinics of North America* **30**, 15–20.

Connell, D., Burke, F., Coobes, S., McNealy, S., Freeman, D., Pryde, D., and Hoy, G. (2001). Sonographic examination of lateral epicondylitis. *American Journal of Rheumatology* **176**, 777–82.

DeWinter, A.F., Jans, M.P., Scholten, R.J., Deville, W., van Schaardenburg, D., and Bouter, L.M. (1999). Diagnostic classification of shoulder disorders: interobserver agreement and determinants of disagreement. *Annals of the Rheumatic Diseases* **58**, 272–7.

Emig, E.W., Schweitzer, M.E., Karasick, D., and Lubowitz, J. (1995). Adhesive capsulitis of the shoulder: MR diagnosis. *American Journal of Roentgenology* **164**, 1457–9.

Fam, A.G. (1992). Bursitis and tendinitis: a practical approach to diagnosis. *Geriatrics* **8**, 35–42.

Gabel, G.T. and Morrey, B.F. (1995). Operative treatment of medial epicondylitis. Influence of concomitant ulnar neuropathy at the elbow. *Journal of Bone and Joint Surgery of America* **77**, 1065–9.

Gabel, G.T. (1999). Acute and chronic tendinopathies at the elbow. *Current Opinion in Rheumatology* **11**, 138–43.

Hulstyn, M.J. and Weiss, A.-P.C. (1993). Adhesive capsulitis of the shoulder. *Orthopedic Reviews* **22**, 425–33.

Kay, N.R. (2000). De Quervain's disease. Changing pathology or changing perception? *Journal of Hand Surgery of Britain* **25**, 65–9.

Kraushaar, B.S. and Nirschl, R.P. (1999). Tendinosis of the elbow (tennis elbow). Clinical features and findings of histological, immunohistochemical, and electron microscopic studies. *Journal of Bone and Joint Surgery of America* **81**, 259–78.

Lester, B., Jeong, G.K., Weiland, A.J., and Wickiewicz, T.L. (1999). Quadrilateral space syndrome: diagnosis, pathology, and treatment. *American Journal of Orthopedics* **28**, 718–22.

Misomore, G.W. and Lehman, D.E. (1996) Parsonage–Turner syndrome (acute brachial neuritis). *Journal of Bone and Joint Surgery of America* **78**, 1405–8.

Moore, J.S. (1997). de Quervain's tenosynovitis. Stenosing tenosynovitis of the first dorsal compartment. *Journal of Occupational and Environmental Medicine* **39**, 990–1002.

Moore, J.S. (2000). Flexor tendon entrapment of the digits (trigger finger and trigger thumb). *Journal of Occupational and Environmental Medicine* **42**, 526–45.

Murthi, A.M., Vosburgh, C.L., and Neviaser, T.J. (2000). The incidence of pathologic changes of the long head of the biceps tendon. *Journal of Shoulder and Elbow Surgery* **9**, 382–5.

Neviaser, T.J. (1987) Adhesive capsulitis. *Orthopedic Clinics of North America* **18**, 439–43.

Noel, E., Thomas, T., Schaeverbeke, T., Thomas, P., Bonjean, M., and Revel, M. (2000). Frozen shoulder. *Joint of Bone and Spine* **67**, 393–400.

Polley, H. and Hunder, G. (1978). The shoulder, elbow, wrist, carpal, metacarpophalangeal, proximal and distal interphalangeal joints. In *Rheumatologic Interview and Physical Examination of the Joints* 2nd edn. pp. 55–148. Philadelphia PA: W.B. Saunders.

Putnam, M.D. and Cohen, M. (1999). Painful conditions around the elbow. *Orthopedic Clinics of North America* **30**, 109–18.

Rayan, G.M. (1999a). Palmar fascial complex anatomy and pathology in Dupuytren's disease. *Hand Clinic* **15**, 73–86.

Rayan, G.M. (1999b). Clinical presentation and types of Dupuytren's disease. *Hand Clinic* **15**, 87–96.

Rosenbaum, R. (1999). Disputed radial tunnel syndrome. *Muscle and Nerve* **22**, 960–7.

Ryu, K.N., Lee, S.W., Rhee, Y.G., and Lim, J.H. (1993). Adhesive capsultis of the shoulder joint: usefulness of dynamic sonography. *Journal of Ultrasound Medicine* **12**, 445–9.

Schenk, M. and Dalinka, M.K. (1997). Imaging of the elbow. An update. *Orthopedic Clinics of North America* **28**, 517–35.

Snyder, S.J. (1993). Evaluation and treatment of the rotator cuff. *Orthopedic Clinics of North America* **24**, 173–92.

Swen, W.A., Jacobs, J.W., Neve, W.C., Bal, D., and Bijlsma, J.W. (1998). Is sonography performed by the rheumatologist as useful as arthrography executed by the radiologist for the assessment of full thickness rotator cuff tears? *Journal of Rheumatology* **25**, 1800–6.

Swen, W.A., Jacobs, J.W., Algra, P.R., Manoliu, R.A., Rijkmans, J., Willems, W.J., and Bijlsma, J.W. (1999). Sonography and magnetic resonance imaging equivalent for the assessment of full-thickness rotator cuff tears. *Arthritis and Rheumatism* **42**, 2231–8.

Tytherleigh-Strong, G., Hirahara, A., and Miniaci, A. (2001). Rotator cuff disease. *Current Opinion of Rheumatology* **13**, 135–45.

Warhold, L.G., Osterman, A.L., and Skirven, T. (1993). Lateral epicondylitis: how to treat it and prevent recurrence. *Journal of Musculoskeletal Medicine* **10**, 55–73.

Williams, P.L., Warwick, R., Dyson, M., and Bannister, L.H. (ed.) (1989). Joints of the upper limb. *Gray's Anatomy* 37th edn. pp. 499–516. Edinburgh: Churchill Livingstone.

1.2.2.2 The lower limbs in adults

Robert W. Simms

Applied anatomy

The hip

The hip joint is a diarthrodial ball-and-socket joint comprising the head of the femur and the acetabulum of the pelvis (Fig. 1). The acetabular cavity is a horseshoe shaped cavity made by the ilium, ischium, and pubis to accommodate the head of the femur. Below the centre of the cavity is a fat pad lined with synovium. The glenoid labrum or lip, a circular fibrocatilagenous rim, forms an additional reinforcement to the hip joint. The transverse ligament bridges the lower portion of a gap in the labrum and gives rise to the

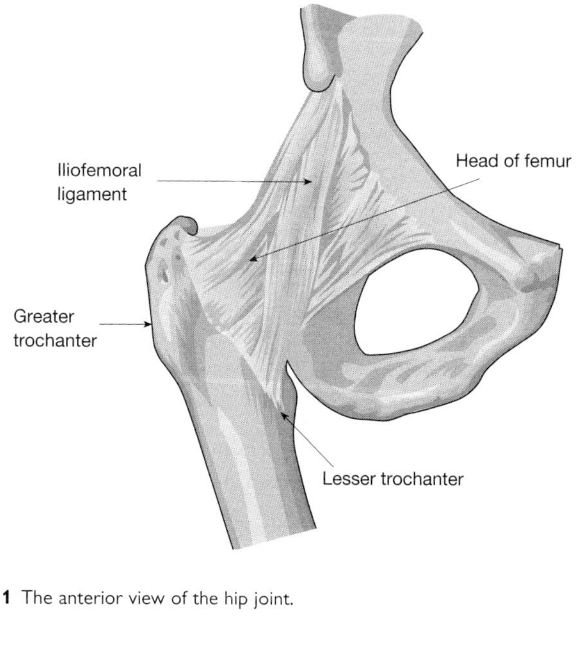

Fig. 1 The anterior view of the hip joint.

ligamentum teres, an intracapsular ligament attached to a small depression in the head of the femur. This supplies it with blood vessels that provide nutrients to a small area of the head of the femur. The head of the femur is lined with hyaline cartilage varying in thickness. It is thickest over the superior and posterior aspects (3 mm) and thinnest at the lateral margins (2–2.5 mm). The capsule of the hip is a dense, fibrous structure, lined by synovial membrane and attached to the acetabulum, labrum, and transverse ligament. The capsule is also reinforced by three ligaments.

A number of bursae have been identified on or about the hip joint (Figs 2 and 3). The most important clinically are the trochanteric bursae, the iliopectineal or iliopsoas bursae, and the ischiogluteal bursae (Larsson and Baum 1986). The trochanteric bursae comprises three bursae, the gluteus maximus is clinically the most important bursa (Fig. 2). The iliopectineal or iliopsoas bursa lies anteriorly between the psoas muscle and the joint capsule. The ischiogluteal bursa lies over the ischeal tuberosity and facilitates gliding of the gluteus maximus.

Hip joint movement is facilitated by several powerful muscle groups. Flexion is accomplished by the iliopsoas, with accessory function of the rectus femoris, pectineus, sartorius, and adductor longus. Extension is accomplished by the gluteus maximus and hamstrings, with accessory function by the ischial head of the adductor magnus. Abduction is accomplished by the gluteus medius, with accessory function by the gluteus minimus. Adduction is accomplished by the adductor magnus, with accessory function by the adductor longus, adductor brevis, pectineus, and gracilis. External rotation is accomplished by the gluteus maximus, quadratus femoris, and piriformis, with accessory function by the sartorius and gracilis. Internal rotation is accomplished by the gluteus minimus, with accessory function by the gluteus maximus, gluteus medius, adductor longus, adductor brevis, adductor magnus, pectineus, iliacus, and psoas. Normal hip range of motion varies with the manner in which it is examined. With the knee in flexion, the hip can be flexed to 120°. With the knee extended, the hip can be flexed to only about 90°, limited by the pull of the hamstrings. Internal rotation is normally 40° with external rotation to 45°. Abduction is normally 45° and adduction 20–30°.

The normal gait cycle involves two phases, the stance phase and the swing phase (Morris et al. 1994) (Fig. 4). The stance phase begins with heal contact. Full weight bearing begins with forefoot contact and ends with heel lift. The stance phase then ends with lift off and starts the swing phase. The swing phase then continues until heel contact and the cycle repeats. Under normal conditions the stance phase comprises approximately 65 per cent of the gait cycle. Hip disorders may cause the patient to walk with a shortened stance phase or with an antalgic gait since he/she will try to minimize the time spent on full weight bearing. Chronic hip disorders frequently produce weakness of the gluteus medius or a Trendelenberg gait. Here, hip abduction is impaired and the pelvis on the opposite side drops during the stance phase. The body leans toward the diseased side when weight bearing is on the diseased hip.

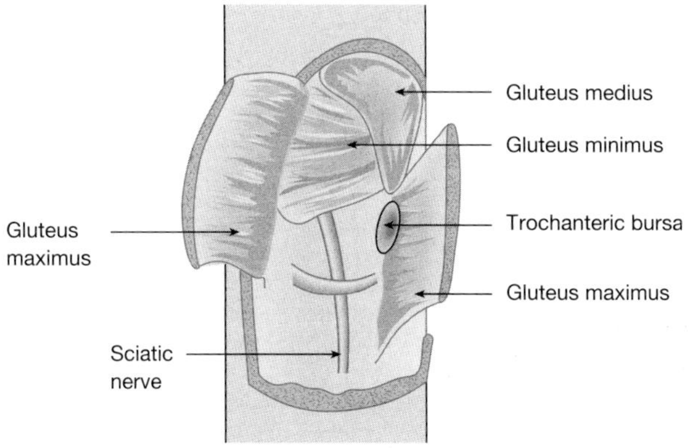

Fig. 2 The posterior view of the hip joint.

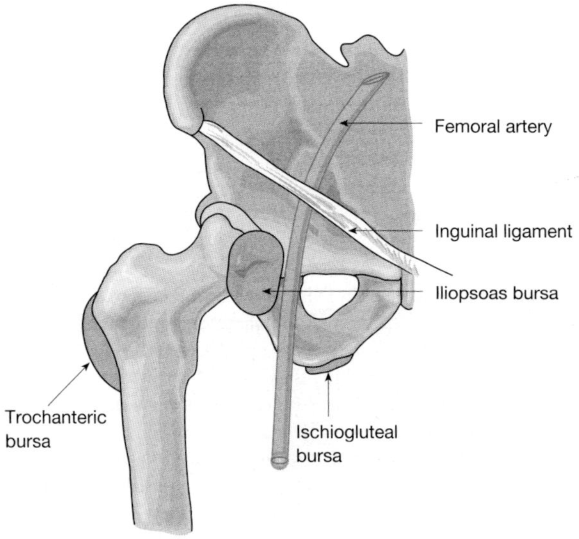

Fig. 3 The bursae of the hip joint.

The knee

The knee is the most complex and largest joint in the human body (Fig. 5). It is a modified hinge joint, capable of flexion, extension, and rotation, with three compartments: the medial, the lateral tibiofemoral, and the patellofemoral. Stability is provided by the cruciate ligaments and menisci and the capsule with its associated capsular ligaments.

The menisci or semilunar cartilages (Fig. 6) are crescent-shaped structures consisting of fibrocartilage, which transmit up to 70 per cent of the force through the tibiotalar joint and also have a lubricating role. They are predominately avascular, although the peripheral 10–30 per cent and the anterior and posterior horns receive blood supply from the geniculate vessels and, therefore, have the capability for repair. The remainder of the menisci receive nutrients passively from the synovial fluid.

The anterior and posterior cruciate ligaments, together with the medial and lateral collateral ligaments, are accessory ligaments of the capsule of the knee. The anterior and posterior cruciate ligaments cross each other within the joint and are formed by twisting rope-like fibres of collagen. The

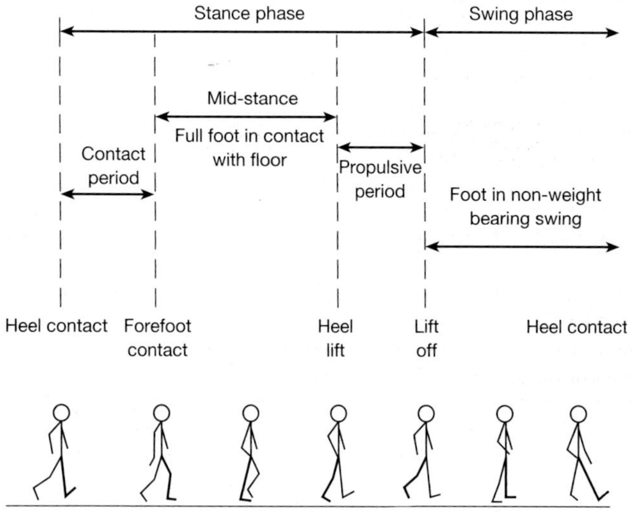

Fig. 4 The gait cycle.

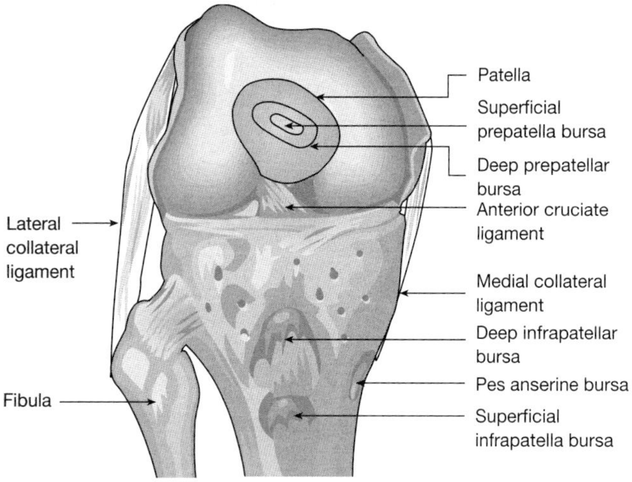

Fig. 5 The anterior view of the knee joint with associated bursae.

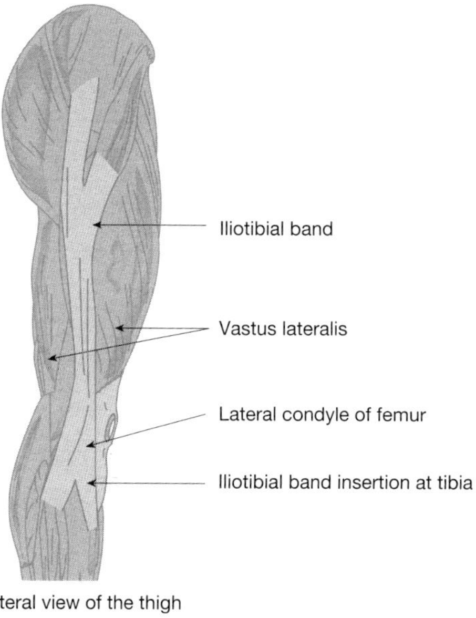

Fig. 7 The iliotibial band.

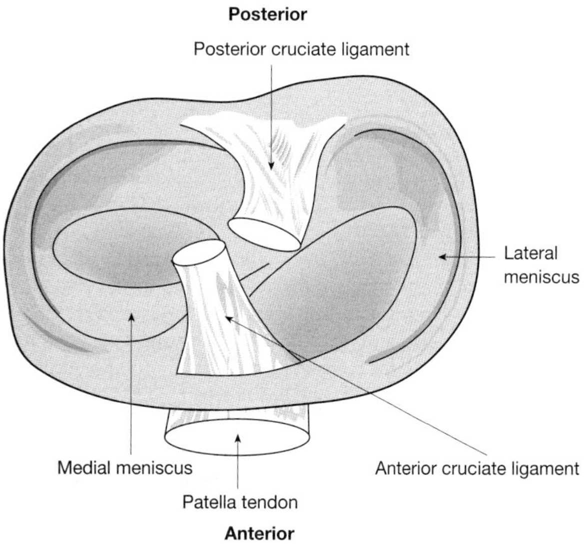

Fig. 6 The meniscii of the knee.

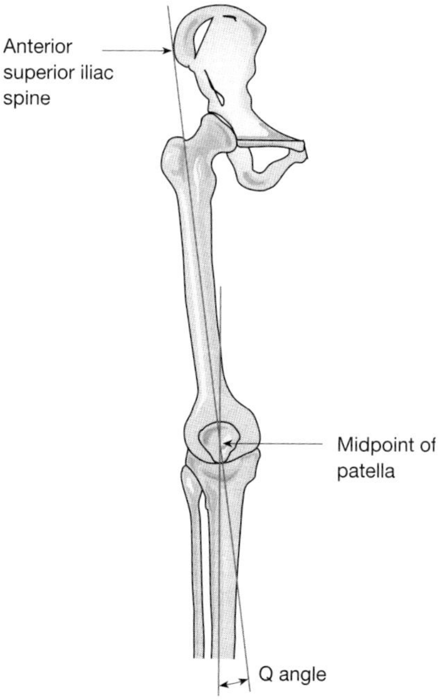

Fig. 8 The patella Q angle.

cruciate ligaments are the principal knee stabilizers in the anteroposterior plane with the anterior cruciate preventing anterior slippage of the femur and the posterior cruciate preventing posterior slippage. The cruciates also provide rotational stability. The collateral ligaments provide medial and lateral stability. The iliotibial band (Fig. 7) is a fascial band connecting the ilium with the lateral tibia and contributes to the lateral stability of the knee.

The patella is the largest sesamoid bone in the human body and its undersurface possesses the thickest articular cartilage. The primary function of the patella is to increase the lever arm of the quadriceps. The stability of the patella is provided statically by the trochlea of the femur and the undersurface of the patella. Dynamic stability is provided predominately by the extensor mechanism. There is considerable variation in the articular anatomy of the patella. The most common shape is a relatively larger lateral facet when compared to the medial facet. The shape of the femoral trochlea also varies considerably from shallow and broad to deeply V shaped. The quadriceps mechanism and its attachment to the knee is complex. Most anterior is the rectus femoris that inserts anteriorly to the patella. Medially the vastus medialis inserts at an angle of 60–70° and provides dynamic medial stability for the patella. This counteracts the lateral dynamic force on the patella from the majority of the quadriceps mechanism, which is a consequence of the normal slight varus angulation of the lower leg in relation to the femur. Patellar tracking is influenced by the direction of pull of the quadriceps and the position of attachment of the patellar tendon into the tibial tubercle (Tria et al. 1992). This relationship is expressed by the patella Q angle (Fig. 8), which is the angle formed by a line between the centre of the patella extending proximally to the anterosuperior iliac spine and extending distally to the centre of the tibal tubercle. The normal Q angle is 10° in men and 15° in women. Femoral neck anteversion and external tibial torsion increases the Q angle, whereas, femoral neck retroversion and internal tibial torsion decreases the Q angle (Tria et al. 1992). An excessive Q angle may predispose to patella subluxation or dislocation, since, as the Q angle increases, the patella tends to track more laterally.

There are a number of bursae surrounding the knee joint. Anteriorly is the subcutaneous, prepatellar bursa, which lies over the lower pole of the patella. Inferiorly are the infrapatellar bursae, the superficial and deep infrapatellar bursae. Medial and inferior to the joint is the pes anserine bursa, which lies between the medial collateral ligament and the insertion of the adductor muscles of the thigh, the sartorius, gracilis, and semitendinosus. Posteriorly is the gastrocnemius–semimembranous bursa, a complex structure comprising three components, a base, the medial extent between the heads of the gastrocnemius and the semimembranous muscle, and a small subfascial extension. In over 50 per cent of individuals over the age of 50 years there is communication between the gastrocnemius–semimembranous bursa and the knee joint (Canoso 1981). When a communication exists, synovial fluid from any aetiology may enter the bursa. If a large volume of synovial fluid expands into the gastrocnemius–semimembranous bursa suddenly it may bulge into the popliteal fossa, or rupture into the calf producing the so-called ruptured Baker's cyst or pseudothrombophlebitis (Rauschning 1980).

The foot and ankle

The foot comprises 26 bones, 38 muscles, and a variable number of sesamoids held together by 125 interconnecting ligaments and must absorb up to six times the body's weight with each step (Fig. 9). The foot is divided into three sections; the forefoot, the midfoot, and the hindfoot. The forefoot consists of the five metatarsals and is separated from the midfoot by the tarsometatarsal joint of Lisfranc. The midfoot contains three cuneiforms, the navicular, and the cuboid and is separated from the hindfoot by the transverse midtarsal joint. The hindfoot consists of the calcaneus and the talus.

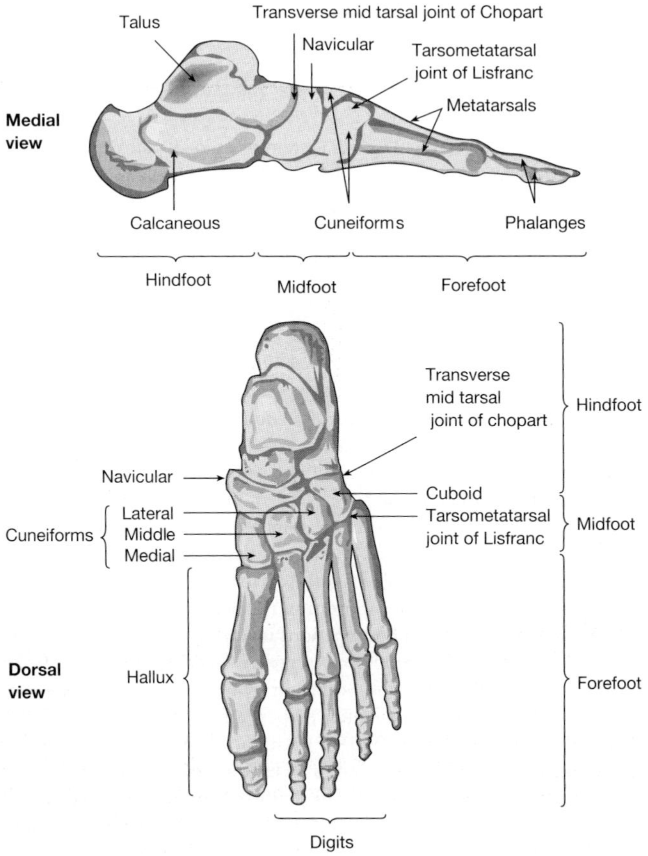

Fig. 9 The bones of the foot.

The ankle joint comprises three articulations, the tibiotalar joint, the subtalar joint, and the talonavicular joint. The tibiotalar joint is the result of the articulation of the dome of the talus, the roof or plafond of the distal tibia, and the distal tibiofibular joint. In addition to the complex set of ligaments, the joint is stabilized medially by the distal tibia, the medial malleolus, and the distal lateral fibula forming the lateral malleolus. Motion at the tibiotalar joint consists of 20° dorsiflexion and 50° plantar flexion.

The subtalar joint is composed of the articulation of the calcaneous and talus, is surrounded by its own distinct capsule, and does not articulate with other joints. Normal range of motion is 5° of inversion and 5° of eversion. The subtalar joint provides inversion and eversion of the heel for walking on uneven terrain. The transverse midtarsal joint of Chopart is composed of the talonavicular joint and the calcaneocuboid joint and permits multiaxial motion, inversion and eversion of the midfoot and forefoot and, to a lesser degree, dorsiflexion and plantar flexion, and abduction and adduction. It is stabilized by the bifurcate ligament. The tarsometatarsal joint of Lisfranc comprises the interconnected second to fifth tarsometatarsal joints. A complex set of ligaments on their dorsal and plantar aspects provide stability.

The metatarsophalangeal joints are analogous to the metacarpophalangeal joints of the hands and are stabilized by the deep transverse metatarsal ligament and the plantar ligaments. The first metatarsophalangeal joint plays a critical role in normal gait. Under most conditions, 65–75° of dorsiflexion of the hallux on the first metatarsal is required for normal gait and for the hallux to function in propulsion (Mahan 1994). Disorders such as hallux valgus and hallux rigidus affect gait adversely by limiting dorsiflexion of the first metatarsophalangeal joint.

The interphalangeal joints of the toes consist of hinge joints, stabilized by collateral ligaments and a plantar capsular ligament with a fibrous plate. The plantar aponeurosis, or plantar fascias, runs from the plantar aspect of the calcaneous to the region of the metatarsal heads. The superficial layer blends with subcutaneous tissue, whereas the deep layer joins the deep transverse metatarsal ligament and the flexor tendons.

Attached to the foot and ankle are the tendons of the extrinsic muscles, which form *four* compartments in the lower leg: the anterior compartment containing the dorsiflexors or extensors of the foot and ankle, the lateral compartment containing the peroneal muscles acting as plantar flexors and abductors, and the superficial and deep posterior compartment containing the plantar flexors. Posterior to the ankle is the Achilles tendon, formed by the conjoined tendons of the gastrocnemius and the soleus muscles, which functions to plantar flex the foot. Medially at the ankle is the tibialis posterior tendon complex passing underneath the flexor retinaculum posterior to the medial malleolus. Between the sheaths of the flexor digitorum longus and the flexor hallucis longus tendons lies the posterior tibial artery and nerve within the tarsal tunnel. Tenosynovitis of either the tibialis posterior, flexor hallucis longus, or flexor digitiorum longus tendons may produce functional compression of the posterior tibial nerve producing tarsal tunnel syndrome (Grumbine et al. 1990). The tibialis posterior is the principal inverter of the foot and maintains the longitudinal arch by its insertion to the navicular and medial and intermediate cuneiforms, and bases of the second, third, and fourth metatarsals (Sarrafian et al. 1983). Laterally at the ankle, passing under the superior and inferior peroneal retinacula, is the common sheath of the peroneus longus and brevis tendons, which are the principal everters and abductors of the foot (Fig. 10). Anteriorly, the extrinsic extensor tendons of the foot pass under the fibrous superior and inferior extensor retinacula.

There are several pertinent bursae of the foot and ankle, the retrocalcaneal bursa (Fig. 11) lies between the calcaneus and the Achilles tendon. This bursa has a synovial lining which abuts the Achilles fat pad. Anteriorly, the bursal wall is composed of fibrocartilage and posteriorly is contiguous with the Achilles tendon (Canoso et al. 1984; Frey et al. 1992). The bursa itself is horseshoe shaped with the average length of the legs measuring 22 mm and the width 4 mm, with the width of the body measuring 8 mm

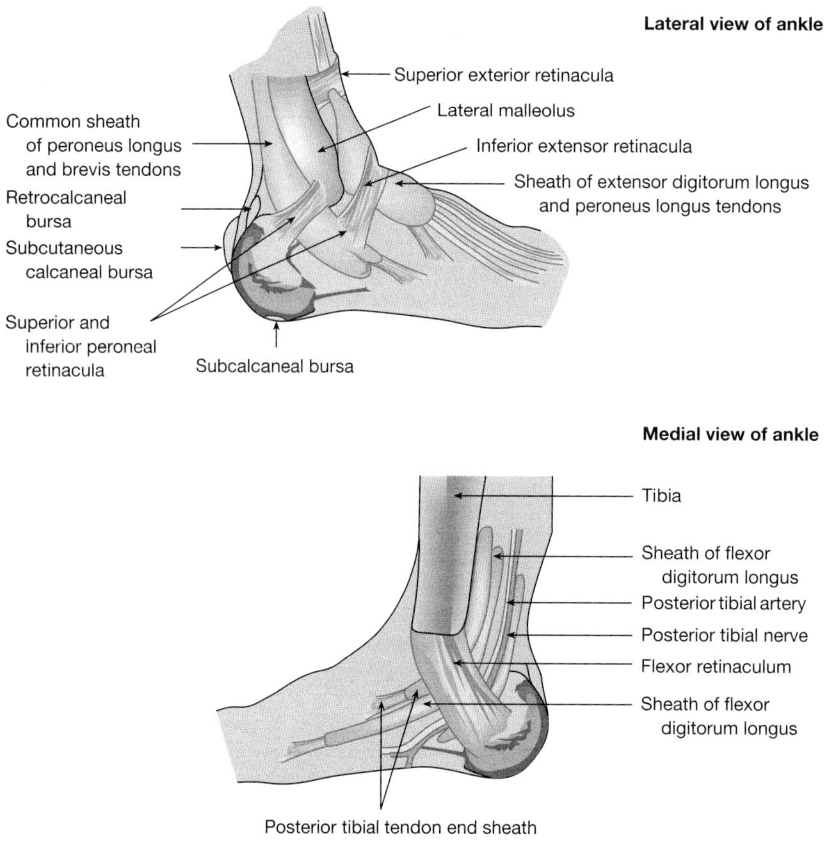

Fig. 10 The ankle: lateral and medial views.

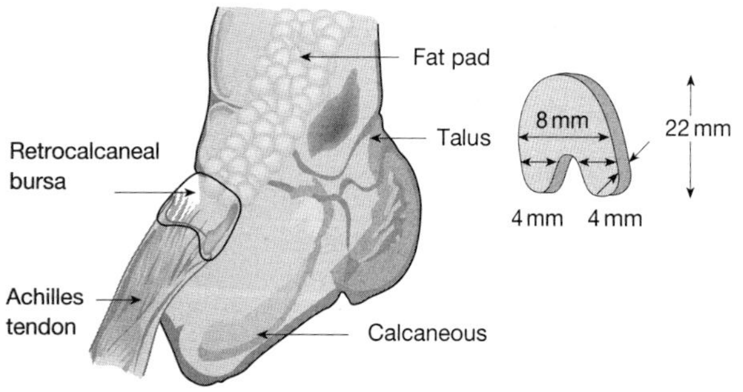

Fig. 11 The retrocalcaneal bursa.

(Frey et al. 1992). Between the skin and the Achilles tendon is the subcutaneous calcaneal bursa. At the plantar aspect of the midcalcaneous is the subcalcaneal bursa.

General approach

Lower extremity regional pain syndromes are common in rheumatology and orthopaedic practices. A detailed survey and examination of soft tissue abnormalities in 123 unselected medical students revealed that approximately 10 per cent had bursitis, tendinitis, or chondromalacia patellae (Raskin and Lawless 1982). Lower extremity regional pain conditions often present a challenge to the clinician because of complexity, frequent confusion with other conditions, and lack of precise diagnostic tests. However, careful history and physical examination combined with knowledge of the relevant anatomy will generally permit identification. Table 1 provides a classification of the regional disorders of the lower extremity based on location.

Many conditions producing lower extremity regional pain are bursal disorders. Bursae are synovial-lined sacs that facilitate tissue gliding. Bursae are generally either divided into deep or subcutaneous. Subcutaneous bursae overlie bony prominences and permit skin movement without undue stretching and tearing and develop after birth (Canoso and Yood 1979; Canoso 1981). Deep bursae are located between divergently pulling tendons, or between tendons and bone and form in early fetal development. Normal bursal fluid has characteristics similar to synovial fluid, a high content of hyaluronic acid, low leucocyte count ($<300/mm^3$) with a predominance of mononuclear cells (Canoso 1981; Canoso et al. 1983). A variety of disorders can affect bursae, including trauma, infection, and systemic or metabolic conditions, such as rheumatoid arthritis or gout. Septic subcutaneous bursitis is particularly important to exclude. Subcutaneous bursae around the knee are the most common sites of infection. Prepatellar bursitis is the second most common form of septic bursitis behind olecranon bursitis, accounting for 27 per cent of 49 cases of septic bursitis in one series (Raddatz et al. 1987). Identifiable risk factors for septic bursitis include skin breakdown, trauma, immunosuppression (diabetes, concurrent immunosuppressive medication), and occupations involving frequent or sustained pressure on bursae, such as roofing or carpentry (Raddatz et al. 1987). By far the most common organism responsible for septic bursitis is *Staphylococcus aureus*, accounting for approximately 80 per cent of cases (Ho et al. 1978; Ho and Ticer 1979; Raddatz et al. 1987). Aspiration of symptomatic subcutaneous bursae is generally required to exclude infection. In the case of the prepatellar bursa, aspiration should be performed on the lateral site of the bursa to prevent a chronic draining sinus that can occur if aspiration is performed over the apex of the bursa. Bursal fluid leucocyte counts that exceed $5000/mm^3$ should be suspected of being septic and empirical antibiotic coverage directed against *S. aureus* should be considered. Optimal treatment

Table 1 Classification of painful lower limb disorders

Articular	Traumatic, inflammatory, degenerative, infectious, and crystalline arthritis
Periarticular	
Hip	Trochanteric bursitis
	Ischiogluteal bursitis
	Iliopsoas bursitis
Knee	Prepatellar bursitis
	Infrapatellar bursitis
	Anserine bursitis
	Gastrocnemius–semimembranous bursitis (Baker's cyst)
	Iliotibial band syndrome
	Pelligrini–Stieda syndrome
	Plica syndrome
	Patellofemoral pain
	Sinding–Larsen–Johansson disease
	Mechanical derangements
Foot	Achilles tendinitis
	Retrocalcaneal bursitis
	Subcalcaneal bursitis
	Plantar fascitis
	Metatarsalgia
Osseous	Avascular necrosis, regional osteoporosis, neoplasm, infection
Neurological	
Nerve entrapment syndromes	
Lateral cutaneous nerve of the thigh	Meralgia paraesthetica
Lumbar nerve roots	Lumbar disc herniation
Posterior tibial nerve	Tarsal tunnel syndrome
Neurovascular	
Compartment syndromes	
Vasculitis	
Reflex sympathetic dystrophy	
Arterial and venous thrombosis	
Referred and miscellaneous pain	
Lumbar spine disorders with lumbar radiculopathy	
Intrapelvic and retroperitoneal disorders	
Femoral hernias	
Abdominal aortic aneurysm	
Fibromyalgia syndrome	

consists of frequent aspiration until no fluid reaccumulates and either oral or intravenous antibiotics (Ho and Su 1981). The length of time required to achieve culture sterility with antibiotic therapy was correlated with the duration of symptoms prior to diagnosis in one series. In patients treated within 2 weeks from the onset of symptoms, culture sterility occurred within 1 week of therapy, while longer duration of symptoms was associated with delayed response (Ho and Su 1981).

Hip pain

Trochanteric bursitis

There are three bursae in the greater trochanteric region of the hip. The largest and most important clinically is the gluteus maximus bursa separating the fibres of the gluteus maximus from the greater trochanter (Larsson and Baum 1986). The other two bursae lie between the greater trochanter and gluteus medius and greater trochanter, respectively. Patients with trochanteric bursitis present with a deep, aching pain over the lateral upper thigh, often intensified by walking, but may be worse at night, especially when the patient is lying on the affected side. The course is variable with an acute phase lasting several days followed by gradual improvement and resolution over a period of days or weeks. In some cases the course may be protracted with symptoms persisting for months. The diagnosis is confirmed with palpation of the posterior aspect of the greater trochanter, causing local tenderness in this area. Resisted abduction of hip on the affected side may also be painful.

The aetiology of trochanteric bursitis is unknown; however, potential risk factors include local trauma, overuse activities, and leg length discrepancies (primarily on the side with the longer leg). These factors are thought to lead to increased tension of the gluteus maximus on the iliotibial band producing bursal inflammation. The differential diagnosis of trochanteric bursitis includes lumbar radiculopathy (particularly the L1 and L2 nerve roots), meralgia paraesthetica (entrapment of the lateral cutaneous nerve of the thigh as it passes under the inguinal ligament), true hip joint disease, and intra-abdominal pathology. These potentially confounding conditions can be excluded by careful history and physical examination.

Trochanteric bursitis is treated by avoiding aggravating activity and local injection of a long-acting corticosteroid. Referral to physical therapy in resistant cases may be helpful, particularly for exercises to stretch the iliotibial band.

Ischiogluteal bursitis

The ischiogluteal bursa lies over the ischeal tuberosity (Fig. 3). In the sitting position, the gluteus maximus slides superiorly exposing the isheal tuberosity to potential friction. Repeated leg flexion and extension in the sitting position or prolonged sitting on hard surfaces may lead to ischiogluteal bursitis, also known as 'weavers bottom'. The ischiogluteal bursa may become infected (Lambie et al. 1989). Diagnosis is by characteristic history and eliciting tenderness on palpation of the ischeal tuberosity with the patient lying supine and with the hip and knee flexed. Treatment consists of using a cushioning 'doughnut' seat and performing trunk and knee-to-chest stretches while lying on the cushion. A local injection of corticosteroid is useful in refractory cases, although care should be taken to avoid the sciatic nerve, lateral to the ischiogluteal bursa.

Iliopsoas bursitis

The iliopsoas bursa (also called the iliopectineal bursa) lies over the anterior surface of the hip joint (Fig. 3). In most cases of reported iliopsoas bursitis, communication between the hip joint and the bursa occurs, either due to pre-existing communication (which occurs in approximately 15–20 per cent of normal cases) and associated excessive synovial fluid accumulation or rupturing of the hip joint capsule (Canoso 1981). The condition is associated with a number of hip disorders including osteoarthritis, rheumatoid arthritis, synovial chrondromatosis, pigmented villonodular synovitis, osteonecrosis, and septic arthritis (Letourneau et al. 1991; Manueddu et al. 1991; Generini et al. 1993; Broadhurst 1995; Flanagan et al. 1995). Patients present with an inguinal mass, often painful and may be associated with secondary femoral vein obstruction or femoral nerve compression (Lavyne et al. 1982; Savarese et al. 1991). Diagnosis is by computer tomography (CT) and treatment of the underlying hip disorder is generally sufficient, although surgical excision is sometimes required.

Knee pain

Knee pain is among the most common articular complaints and non-arthritic conditions are particularly prevalent, in younger patients.

Adolescence (see also Chapter 1.2.2.3)

There are a variety of knee pain syndromes unique to this age group (10–18 years). Osgood–Schlatter disease is one such condition and presents with activity-related pain around the tibial tubercle. This condition is thought to result from submaximal, repetitive tensile stresses acting on the immature junction of the patellar ligament, tibial tubercle, and tibia, causing mild avulsion injury, followed by failed osseous repair with cartilage and bone proliferation (Ogden and Southwick 1976; Kujala et al. 1985). Pain is intermittent and increases with activity, especially kneeling, squatting, or jumping. Athletically active boys were found to have a fivefold risk of Osgood–Schlatter disease compared to inactive controls and an increased Q angle has also been associated with Osgood–Schlatter disease (Kujala et al. 1985). The tibial tubercle is swollen with local tenderness and approximately 50 per cent have a discrete ossicle at the tibial tubercle. Radiographs of the knee exclude tumours and infection. Treatment with ice, anti-inflammatory agents, an appropriately contoured knee pad, and maintainance of hamstring and quadriceps flexibility are usually sufficient to control symptoms that may take up to 12 months to resolve. Progressive or disabling symptoms may require immobilization for 7–10 days.

Sinding–Larsen–Johansson disease is another cause of anterior knee pain similar to Osgood–Schlatter disease, except that tenderness is localized to the inferior pole of the patella, or the junction of the quadriceps tendon and the patella (Medlar and Lyne 1978). This condition is thought to be the result of persistent traction at the cartilagenous junction of the patella and the patella ligament and radiographs may show ossification at this point. The treatment programme outlined for Osgood–Schlatter disease is followed for management of Sinding–Larsen–Johansson disease.

Prepatellar bursitis

Prepatellar bursitis presents as a painful, red, swelling anterior to the kneecap most often seen in people who kneel a lot, for example, roofers, or carpet fitters (Raddatz et al. 1987). Active knee extension is usually quite painful although passive knee flexion is only minimally limited. Infection and gout are excluded by aspirating bursal fluid. Most cases are resolved by resting and avoiding sustained kneeling. Septic bursitis is usually due to *S. aureus* and requires antibiotic therapy as well as repeated drainage if fluid reaccumulates (Ho et al. 1978; Ho and Su 1981; Raddatz et al. 1987; Kerr 1993). Rarely, recurrent episodes of inflammation require surgical excision of the bursa (Kerr 1993).

Infrapatellar bursitis

The deep infrapatellar bursa lies between the upper portion of the tibial tuberosity and patellar ligament and is separated from the knee joint synovium by a fat pad (Fig. 5). The risk factors for the development of infrapatellar bursitis are the same as prepatellar bursitis (Taylor 1989; Meys et al. 1992) and presents in a similar fashion. The location of swelling and tenderness is in the soft tissues on either side of the patellar ligament proximal to its insertion on the tibial tubercle. Inflammation in this bursa is more difficult to detect than in a subcutaneous bursa (Taylor 1989).

Anserine bursitis

The anserine bursa lies under and about the pes anserinus, the insertion of the thigh adductor complex consisting of the sartorius, gracilis, and semitendinosus muscles (Fig. 5) about 5 cm below the medial aspect of the joint space. Anserine bursitis is a term loosely applied to pain and associated local tenderness in this region, although 'medial ligament' syndrome and pes anserinus tendinitis may be impossible to separate. Nocturnal pain, often leading to the use of a pillow between the knees, is characteristic. Fluid distention and palpable masses are rare (Voorneveld et al. 1989; Zeiss et al. 1993). Women seem more likely to develop anserine bursitis, perhaps because of a broader pelvic area and more tensio caused by greater angulation of the adductors at the knee joint (Larsson and Baum 1985). Obesity and osteoarthritis of the knees are predisposing factors (Larsson and Baum 1985). Optimal treatment includes local corticosteroid injections mixed with local anaesthetic.

Gastrocnemius–semimembranous bursitis (Baker's cyst)

Synovitis in the knee can lead to leakage into the popliteal space when a communication exists in the gastrocnemius–semimembranous bursa which occurs in 40 per cent of normal adults and increases in frequency with age (Morris et al. 1994). Symptoms include fullness and tightness in the popliteal space that increases with walking. A Baker's cyst is detected by palpation of fullness in the medial third of the popliteal fossa, although there is wide variation in size, ranging from politeal cysts to large calf cysts (Smith et al. 1988). Baker's cysts become softer with semiflexion and harder with extension of the knee (Foucher's sign) (Wigley 1982). Knee effusions are generally present, although they can be small and often overlooked. Baker's cysts may dissect into the muscles of the calf, simulating thrombophlebitis (Hench et al. 1966). The presence of crescent bruising beneath the medial malleolus, the 'haemorrhagic crescent sign', is felt to be a useful clinical clue to the presence of popliteal cyst rupture or calf haematoma (Kraag et al. 1976). Rupture of a Baker's cyst is confirmed by Doppler ultrasound, excluding thrombophlebitis of the popliteal vein (Fam et al. 1982). Attention must be directed to the soft tissue plains of the calf where dissecting fluid is generally seen. Rupture of a Baker's cyst can cause associated thrombophlebitis or compressive neuropathy due to extensive venous or neural compression (Nakano 1978).

Treatment requires treating the cause of excess or abnormal synovial fluid production. Management includes aspiration of the knee joint with synovial fluid analysis and culture. Direct posterior aspiration should not be performed because of the neurovascular structures. In non-infectious synovitis of the knee, intra-articular instillation of corticosteroid is effective.

Iliotibial band syndrome (Runner's knee)

The iliotibial band is a fascial band connecting the ilium with the lateral tibia (Fig. 7). Repetitive flexion and extension, particularly with high intensity running causes inflammation of the iliotibial band or its associated bursa (Sutker 1981; Martens et al. 1989). Excessive foot pronation, resulting in tightening of the iliotibial band and increased friction across the femoral epicondyle has also been proposed as a cause (Bouche et al. 1994). Examination reveals tenderness localized to the lateral femoral condyle approximately 2 cm above the joint line, pain with weight bearing on the knee flexed 30–40°, and a positive Ober test (the patient lies on his or her side with the lower leg flexed to eliminate lordosis of the lumbar spine, the knee of the upper leg is flexed to 90°, and the thigh is abducted and extended, a positive test occurs when the hip remains abducted when the examiner's supporting hand is removed). Treatment consists of rest, locally applied heat, and orthotics when excessive foot pronation is present. Occasionally, a local injection of corticosteroid into the painful area is required . Partial resection of the iliotibial band over the lateral femoral condyle is reserved for the most resistant cases (Martens et al. 1989).

Pelligrini–Stieda disease

This is a calcification of haematoma at the femoral insertion of the medial collateral ligament following injury, identifible by radiographs. Valgus stress to the knee causes local tenderness and pain. The condition is self-limiting and treatment consists of rest, non-steroidal anti-inflammatory drugs (NSAIDs), and, occasionally, local corticosteroid injection.

Plica syndrome

Synovial plica are folds of the synovium, remnants of the embryonic development of the synovial sac that are found in approximately 50 per cent of cadaveric knees (Galloway and Jokl 1990). Arthroscopy and direct visualization of these structures have implicated synovial plica in previously undiagnosed knee symptoms (Patel 1978). Pathological plica result from two mechanisms:

- direct trauma causing haemorrhage, oedema, and progressive fibrosis;
- overuse, associated with minor irregularities in knee mechanics causing progressive inflammation with recurrent synovitis, oedema, and fibrosis (O'Dwyer and Peace 1988; Tindel and Nisonson 1992).

Patients with symptomatic plica feel snapping or popping in the knee at particular degrees of flexion. Medial plica are most often implicated as a cause of knee symptoms, presumably occurring when the plica rubs across the femoral condyle (Galloway and Jokl 1990). Examination reveals tenderness at the joint line and palpation of the plica, especially with the knee in 20° of flexion. Most patients respond to a combination of quadriceps strengthening and flexibility exercises with anti-inflammatory medication. Surgical resection is sometimes advocated, but is controversial (Tindel and Nisonson 1992).

Internal derangements

Internal derangements refer to disruption of ligaments and menisci function, most often the result of significant, often athletic, trauma. Acute meniscal injury in young adults is usually the result of a twisting force applied to the weight bearing knee resulting in a longitudinal tear, which, if it is large enough, causes the knee to lock (a 'bucket-handle' tear). Degenerative tears are more frequent in older adults and consist of radial tears. Chronic tears of this nature may occur without trauma, but are generally accompanied by the knee locking or giving way. Examination generally reveals pain with forced extension and normal, or mildly reduced, flexion. McMurray's test (flexing and extending the knee while the tibia is internally and then externally rotated with a positive test indicated by pain and an associated click) may be helpful if positive, but is relatively insensitive (Gillies and Seligson 1979; Simonsen et al. 1984). In the United States, magnetic resonance imaging (MRI) is used to diagnose suspected meniscal tears and help plan therapy. Early studies with MRI suggested a relatively high rate of false positive findings. Although improved technology and experience appears to be improving this, there may be substantial variation in accuracy among centres (Reicher et al. 1986; Fischer et al. 1991; Watt 1991). Symptomatic peripheral tears (i.e. the outer one-third) of the meniscus in the young adult are generally repaired. Partial menisectomy is recommended if tears involve the avascular inner two-thirds of the meniscus. Non-operative treatment can be considered for older patients with a degenerative meniscal tear, although arthroscopic resection may be required for persistent symptoms. Total menisectomy is avoided since long-term follow-up studies demonstrate high rates of osteoarthritis following this procedure (Cooper 1995).

Patellofemoral pain syndrome

Chondromalacia patellae has been used synonymously with patellofemoral pain, but this is no longer recommended given the almost universal presence of asymptomatic cartilage changes on the medial facet of the patella and the observation that most individuals with anterior knee symptoms have normal articular surfaces (Griffiths and Pinder 1981; Kelly and Insall 1992; Tria et al. 1992). Chrondromalacia patellae is now used for gross pathological observation made operatively or at autopsy (Tria et al. 1992), while patellofemoral pain should be used to describe ill-defined, anterior knee pain.

Patellofemoral pain syndrome is poorly localized, anterior knee pain, frequently accompanied by the 'grab' sign (patients cover the entire front of the knee with the hand when asked to identify the location of the discomfort). Pain frequently occurs after prolonged sitting with flexed knees, the 'theatre' sign. Physical examination may reveal tenderness of the medial or lateral facets of the patella, pain with compression of the patella on the femoral condyle, or a patellar 'shrug' sign (pain when pressure is applied to the patella while the patient contracts the quadriceps). An abnormally increased Q angle (greater than 15° in males and greater than 20° in females) appears to predispose to patellofemoral pain. Patellofemoral pain syndrome is thought to result from either anatomical abnormalities or repetitive micro-trauma to the patella surface. Standard radiographs are not helpful in the evaluation of anterior knee pain, particulary for patellar tracking, since most tracking abnormalities occur during dynamic use. Non-operative treatment of idiopathic anterior knee pain is successful in 75–90 per cent of patients (Tria et al. 1992). Treatment modalities include avoidance of overuse, exercises, orthoses, and anti-inflammatory medications.

Lower leg pain

Medial tibial stress syndrome or shin splints

The term 'shin splints' has been used to describe a painful distal medial tibial pain condition common to novice runners and other repetitive weight-bearing athletes, such as gymnasts and football players. The condition has been variously attributed to periostitis, or disruption of the tibial attachment of the soleus, or medial tibial stress syndrome (Mubarek et al. 1982; Michael and Holder 1985). 'Shin splints' has been used by some to encompass all types of pain involving the lower leg, and should be avoided as a diagnostic term as stress fractures and compartment syndromes may cause pain in similar locations. Medial tibial stress syndrome pain typically occurs transiently after the inciting athletic activity, but may be constant in severe cases. The condition is precipitated most commonly as the result of training errors, such as rapid increases in volume or intensity of training. Physical examination reveals tenderness along the medial aspect of the distal tibia and in more severe cases may include soft tissue swelling. Plain radiographs are negative or may show mild periosteal reaction along the medial tibia. MRI should be considered in refractory or severe cases to exclude tibial stress fractures or a compartment syndrome. Treatment consists of rest or reduction in training volume. Orthoses are recommended for associated hyperpronation of the forefoot, which may be a contributing factor.

Compartment sydromes of the lower leg

The lower leg is anatomically divided into four compartments: anterior, lateral, superficial, and deep posterior. Small increases in muscle volume may cause increased pressure within the compartment because of the unique bone and fascial boundaries. Acute compartment syndromes of the lower leg result in sudden and generally irreversible increases in compartmental pressure with neural and vascular compromise. More common are chronic compartmental sydromes, which are reversible and seen in weight bearing athletes, such as runners and often results from training errors (Styf et al. 1987; Pedowitz et al. 1990). The symptoms consist of exercise-induced pain in the affected compartment. Physical examination at rest is typically normal, but local tenderness may be present during or immediately after exercise. Radiographs are negative, MRI may show oedema within the affected compartment or muscle. The diagnosis can be confirmed by direct intracompartmental pressure measurement using a specialized needle pressure gauge inserted into the symptomatic compartment. Treatment consists of activity modification or rest and NSAIDs. Rarely, compartmental release is required.

Foot pain

Heel pain

The most common causes of heel pain are Achilles tendinitis, retrocalcaneal bursitis, and plantar fasciitis. Achilles tendinitis is generally caused by repetitive trauma and microscopic tears of the tendon at the calcaneous (Puddu et al. 1976). Achilles tendinitis may be seen in patients with seronegative spondyloarthropathies without a history of overuse. The usual presentation is gradual onset of pain with foot push off. Physical examination reveals tenderness and occasionally thickening of the tendon. Rest, anti-inflammatory medication, heel lift gentle stretching exercises, and local heat application are effective treatment measures. The Achilles tendon is vulnerable to rupture in the elderly.

The retrocalcaneal bursa resides between the Achilles tendon and a fat pad posterior to the talus (Fig. 11). Retrocalcaneal bursitis is associated with posterior heel pain made worse with passive dorsiflexion of the ankle and may be associated with tender swelling on both sides of the tendon insertion (Canoso et al. 1984; Frey et al. 1992). Causes include repetitive trauma due to athletic activity, rheumatoid arthritis, and all the seronegative spondyloarthropathies (Hernandez et al. 1991; Goldenstein-Schainberg et al. 1992). Treatment is the same as for Achilles tendinitis, although cautious use of local corticosteroid injection may be necessary in resistant cases.

Plantar fasciitis is attributed to repetitive microtrauma to the attachment of the plantar fascia at the calcaneous producing periostitis and degenerative changes in the origin of the plantar fascia (Kwong et al. 1988; Karr 1994). Localized pain with weight bearing on the undersurface of the heel is typical with tenderness over the anteromedial portion of the plantar surface of the calcaneous, worsening on passive dorsiflexion of the toes. Radiographs may show a plantar calcaneal spur. Associated conditions include enthesopathy due to any of the seronegative spondyloarthropathies (Gerster 1980). Subcalcaneal or infracalcaneal bursitis is similar to plantar fasciitis, but passive dorsiflexion of toes does not increase symptoms. Treatment consists of a heel pad or cushion, rest, application of local heat, and anti-inflammatory agents. Local injection of corticosteroid at the insertion of the plantar fascia may be useful. The vast majority of patients respond to these conservative measures. Surgical approaches, such as fasciotomy and spur excision, may be required in resistant cases (Karr 1994).

Metatarsalgia

Metatarsalgia is the symptom of pain across the plantar surface of one or more metatarsophalangeal joints and may be due to diverse causes, including muscle imbalance, fat pad atrophy, Morton's neuroma, hallux valgus or rigidus, callosities, flat (pes planus) or cavus foot, arthritis of the metatarsophalangeal joints, intermetatarsophalangeal bursitis, tarsal tunnel syndrome, and arterial insufficiency. Symptomatic treatment for patients with muscle imbalance and fat pad atrophy includes the use of a metatarsal pad and flexion exercises. Arch supports are recommended for patients with flat or pronated feet.

Hallux valgus and rigidus are deformities of the great toe producing pain in the first metatarsophalangeal joint. It is caused by narrow foot wear, high heels, or osteoarthritis of the first metatarsophalangeal joint (Caughlin 1984). Often associated with bursitis over the medial aspect of the metatarsophalangeal joint, altered weight bearing may result in secondary callosities under the second metatarsophalangeal joint and a hammer toe deformity of the second toe (Schoenhaus and Cohen 1992). Treatment consists of the use of accommodating footwear and a bunion pad. Surgical correction may be required for resistant cases or marked deformities.

Hallux rigidus produces progressive pain and loss of motion in the first metatarsophalangeal joint. The causes are multiple and include osteoarthritis of the first metatarsophalangeal and congenital deformities of the hallux (Mahan 1994). Treatment is designed to reduce the need for first metatarsophalangeal dorsiflexion and consists of wide, stiff soled shoes. Surgical procedures such as the bunionectomy, implant arthroplasties, and first metatarsophalangeal fusion are advocated for severe cases (Mahan 1994).

Morton's neuroma is a common cause of foot pain, caused by neurofibroma, or perineural fibrosis of the large superficial branch of the external plantar nerve between the metatarsal heads (Miller 1987). The most common cause is repetitive microtrauma of the common digital nerve. The typical presentation is paraesthesias or dysaesthesias in interdigital web spaces, particularly between the third and fourth interspaces. Pain is increased by weight bearing, or tight-fitting footwear. Examination reveals interspace tenderness with palpation. The diagnosis may be confirmed with an injection of 1 per cent lidocaine into the interspace, relieving symptoms almost immediate. Treatment consists of using low heel and wider width footwear. Local injection of corticosteroids or surgical resection may be required in resistant cases (Miller 1987).

Tarsal tunnel syndrome refers to compression of the posterior tibial nerve (Fig. 10). It has diverse aetiologies, including mechanical factors and synovitis of the ankle (Grabois et al. 1981; Grumbine et al. 1990). Typical presentation is with dysaesthesias involving the plantar aspect of the foot often more prominent at night. Examination reveals a Tinel's sign with percussion of the flexor retinaculum. Reduced vibratory sensation and decreased two-point discrimination may be present on the plantar aspect of the foot and toes. The diagnosis of tarsal tunnel syndrome may be confirmed by nerve conduction studies documenting delay in conduction of the posterior tibial nerve across the ankle (Goodgold et al. 1965). MRI may also be useful in the evaluation of the relevant anatomical structures (Erickson et al. 1990). Treatment consists of local corticosteroid injection, use of NSAIDs, and orthotic devices. Surgical decompression of the posterior tibial nerve is reserved for resistant cases.

References

Bouche, R., Sullivan, K., and Ichikawa, D. (1994). Athletic injuries. In *Disorders of the Lower Extremities. Musculoskeletal* (ed. L. Oloff), pp. 234–59. Philadelphia PA: W.B. Saunders.

Broadhurst, N. (1995). Iliopsoas tendinitis and bursitis. *Australian Family Physician* **24**, 1303.

Canoso, J. (1981). Bursae, tendons, and ligaments. *Clinics in Rheumatic Diseases* **7**, 189–221.

Canoso, J. and Yood, R. (1979). Reaction of superficial bursae in response to specific disease stimuli. *Arthritis and Rheumatism* **22**, 1361–4.

Canoso, J., Stack, M., and Brandt, K. (1983). Hyaluronic acid content of deep and subcutaneous bursae of man. *Annals of the Rheumatic Diseases* **43**, 308–12.

Canoso, J., Wohlgethan, J., Newberg, A., and Goldsmith, M. (1984). Aspiration of the retrocalcaneal bursae. *Annals of the Rheumatic Diseases* **43**, 308–12.

Caughlin, M. (1984). Hallux valgus: causes, evaluation and treatment. *Postgraduate Medicine* **75**, 174–87.

Cooper, C. (1995). Epidemiology of osteoarthritis. In *Rheumatology* (ed. J. Klippel and P. Dieppe), pp. 7:3.1–7:3.4. St. Louis MO: Mosby.

Erickson, S., Quinn, S., and Kneeland, J. (1990). MR imaging of the tarsal tunnel and related spaces: normal and abnormal findings with anatomic correlation. *American Journal of Radiology* **155**, 323–8.

Fam, A., Wilson, S., and Holmberg, S. (1982). Ultrasound evaluation of popliteal cysts in osteoarthritis of the knee. *Journal of Rheumatology* **9**, 428–34.

Fischer, S., Fox, J., Pizzo, W.D., Friedman, M., Snyder, S., and Ferkel, R. (1991). Accuracy of diagnoses from magnetic resonance imaging of the knee. *Journal of Bone and Joint Surgery* **73A**, 1–10.

Flanagan, F.L., Sant, S., Coughlan, R.J., and O'Connell, D. (1995). Symptomatic enlarged iliopsoas bursae in the presence of a normal plain hip radiograph. *British Journal of Rheumatology* **34**, 365–9.

Frey, C., Rosenberg, Z., Shereff, M., and Kim, H. (1992). The retrocalcaneal bursa: anatomy and bursography. *Foot and Ankle* **13**, 203–7.

Galloway, M. and Jokl, P. (1990). Patella plica syndrome. *Annals of Sports Medicine* **5**, 38–41.

Generini, S. and Matucci-Cerinic, M. (1993). Iliopsoas bursitis in rheumatoid arthritis. *Clinical and Experimantal Rheumatology* **11**, 549–51.

Gerster, J. (1980). Plantar fasciitis and Achilles tendinitis among 150 cases of seronegative spondarthritis. *Rheumatology and Rehabilitation* **19**, 218–22.

Gillies, H. and Seligson, D. (1979). Precision in the diagnosis of meniscal lesions: a comparison of clinical evaluation, arthrography and arthroscopy. *Journal of Bone and Joint Surgery* **61A**, 343–6.

Goldenstein-Schainberg, C., Homsi, C., Rodrigues Pereira, R.M., and Cossermelli, W. (1992). Retrocalcaneal bursitis in juvenile chronic arthritis. *Annals of the Rheumatic Diseases* **51**, 1162–3.

Goodgold, J., Kopell, H., and Spielholz, N. (1965). Tarsal tunnel syndrome: objective diagnostic criteria. *New England Journal of Medicine* **273**, 742–5.

Grabois, M., Puentres, J., and Lidsky, M. (1981). Tarsal tunnel syndrome in rheumatoid arthritis. *Archives of Physical and Medical Rehabilitation* **62**, 401–3.

Griffiths, I. and Pinder, I. (1981). Chondromalacia patella: a clinical and arthroscopic study. *Annals of the Rheumatic Diseases* **40**, 617–25.

Grumbine, N., Radovic, P., Parsons, R., and Scheinin, B. (1990). Tarsal tunnel syndrome: comprehensive review of 87 cases. *Journal of the American Podiatry Association* **80**, 457–61.

Hench, P., Reid, R., and Reames, P. (1966). Dissecting popliteal cyst simulating thrombophlebitis. *Annals of Internal Medicine* **64**, 1259–64.

Hernandez, P.A., Hernandez, W.A., and Hernandez, A. (1991). Clinical aspects of bursae and tendon sheaths of the foot. *Journal of the American Podiatry Association* **81**, 366–72.

Ho, G. and Su, E. (1981). Antibiotic therapy of septic bursitis. *Arthritis and Rheumatism* **24**, 905–11.

Ho, G. and Ticer, A. (1979). Comparison of nonseptic and septic bursitis. *Archives of Internal Medicine* **139**, 1269–73.

Ho, G., Tice, A., and Kaplan, S. (1978). Septic bursitis in the prepatellar and olecranon bursae. *Annals of Internal Medicine* **89**, 21–7.

Karr, S. (1994). Subcalcaneal heel pain. *Orthopedic Clinics of North America* **25**, 161–75.

Kelly, M. and Insall, J. (1992). Historical perspectives of chondromalacia patellae. *Orthopedic Clinics of North America* **23**, 517–21.

Kerr, D.R. (1993). Prepatellar and olecranon arthroscopic bursectomy. *Clinical Sports Medicine* **12**, 137–42.

Kraag, G., Thevathasan, E., Gordon, D., and Walker, I. (1976). The hemorrhagic crescent sign of acute synovial rupture. *Annals of Internal Medicine* **85**, 477–8.

Kujala, U., Kvist, M., and Heinonen, O. (1985). Osgood–Schlatter's disease in adolescent atheletes: retrospective study of incidence and duration. *American Journal of Sports Medicine* **13**, 236–41.

Kwong, P., Kay, D., and Voner, R. (1988). Plantar fasciitis: mechanics and pathomechanics of treatment. *Clinical Sports Medicine* **7**, 119–26.

Lambie, P., Kaufman, R., and Beardmore, T. (1989). Septic ischial bursitis in systemic lupus erythematosus presenting as a perirectal mass. *Journal of Rheumatology* **16**, 1497–9.

Larsson, L. and Baum, J. (1985). The syndrome of anserina bursitis: an overlooked diagnosis. *Arthritis and Rheumatism* **28**, 1062–5.

Larsson, L. and Baum J. (1986). The syndromes of bursitis. *Bulletin of Rheumatic Diseases* **36**, 1–8.

Lavyne, M., Voorhies, R., and Coll, R. (1982). Femoral neuropathy caused by an iliopsoas bursal cyst. *Journal of Neurosurgery* **56**, 584–6.

Letourneau, L., Dessureault, M., and Carette, S. (1991). Rheumatoid iliopsoas bursitis presenting as unilateral femoral nerve palsy. *Journal of Rheumatology* **18**, 462–3.

Mahan, K. (1994). Joint preservation techniques in hallux limitus/rigidus repair. In *Musculoskeletal Disorders of the Lower Extremities* (ed. L. Oloff). Philadelphia PA: W.B. Saunders.

Manueddu, C.A., Hoogewoud, H.M., Balague, F., and Waldeburger, M. (1991). Infective iliopsoas bursitis. A case report. *International Orthopaedics* **15**, 135–7.

Martens, M., Librecht, P., and Burssens, A. (1989). Surgical treatment of the iliotibial band friction syndrome. *American Journal of Sports Medicine* **17**, 651–4.

Medlar, R. and Lyne, E. (1978). Sinding-Larsen-Johansson disease. *Journal of Bone and Joint Surgery* **60**, 1113–9.

Meys, E., Michaux, L., Lambert, M., Triki, R., and Nagant de Deuxchaisnes, C. (1992). Septic *Streptococcus milleri* prepatellar bursitis. *Clinical Rheumatology* **11**, 109–11.

Michael R.H. and Holder L.E. (1985). The soleus syndrome, a cause of medial tibial stress (shin splints). *American Journal of Sports Medicine* **13**, 87–94.

Miller, S. (1987). Morton's neuroma: a syndrome. In *Comprehensive Textbook of Foot Surgery* (ed. E. McGlamry), pp. 38–57. Baltimore MD: Williams and Wilkins.

Morris, J., Berenter, R., and Kosai, D. (1994). Biomechanics of musculoskeletal diseases. In *Musculoskeletal Disorders of the Lower Extremities* (ed. L. Oloff), pp. 65–82. Philadelphia PA: W.B. Saunders.

Mubarak, S.J., Gould, R.N., and Lee, Y.R. (1982). The medial tibial sydrome. *American Journal of Sports Medicine* **10**, 201–5.

Nakano, K. K. (1978). Entrapment neuropathy from Baker's cyst. *Journal of the American Medical Association* **239**, 135.

O'Dwyer, K. and Peace, P. (1988). The plica syndrome. *Injury* **19**, 350–61.

Ogden, J. and Southwick, W. (1976). Osgood–Schlatter's disease and tibial tuberosity development. *Clinical Orthopedics* **116**, 180–6.

Patel, D. (1978). Arthroscopy of the plicae: synovia folds and their significance. *American Journal of Sports Medicine* **6**, 217–28.

Pedowitz R.A., Hargens A.R., and Murabek J.J. (1990) Modified criteria for the objective diagnosis of chronic compartment syndrome at the leg. *American Journal of Sports Medicine* **18**, 35–40.

Puddu, G., Ippolito, E., and Postacchini, F. (1976). A classification of Achilles tendon disease. *American Journal of Sports Medicine* **4**, 145–51.

Raddatz, D., Hoffman, G., and Franck, W. (1987). Septic bursitis: presentation, treatment and prognosis. *Journal of Rheumatology* **14**, 1160–3.

Raskin, R. and Lawless, O. (1982). Articular and soft tissue abnormalities in a 'normal' population. *Journal of Rheumatology* **9**, 284–8.

Rauschning, W. (1980). Anatomy and function of the communication between knee joint and popliteal bursae. *Annals of the Rheumatic Diseases* **39**, 354–8.

Reicher, M., Hartzman, S., Duckwiler, G., Bassett, L., Anderson, L., and Gold, R. (1986). Meniscal injuries: detection using MR imaging. *Radiology* **159**, 753–7.

Sarrafian, S. *Anatomy of the Foot and Ankle: Descriptive, Topographic, Functional.* Philadelphia PA: Lipincott, 1983.

Savarese, R.P., Kaplan, S.M., Calligaro, K.D., and DeLaurentis, D.A. (1991). Iliopectineal bursitis: an unusual cause of iliofemoral vein compression. *Journal of Vascular Surgery* **13**, 725–7.

Schoenhaus, H. and Cohen, R. (1992). Etiology of the bunion. *Journal of Foot Surgery* **31**, 25–9.

Simonsen, O., Jensen, J., Mouritsen, P., and Lauritzen, J. (1984). The accuracy of clinical examination of injury of the knee joint. *Injury* **16**, 96–101.

Smith, T., Shawe, D., Crawley, J., and Gumpel, J. (1988). Use of single photon emission computed tomography (SPECT) to study the distribution of Yttrium-90 in patients with Baker's cysts and persisitent synovitis of the knee. *Annals of the Rheumatic Diseases* **47**, 553–8.

Styf, J.A., Surkula, D., and Korner, L.M. (1987). Intramuscular pressure and muscle blood flow during exercise in chronic compartment syndrome. *Journal of Bone and Joint Surgery (British)* **69**, 301–5.

Sutker, A. (1981). Iliotibial band syndrome in distance runners. *Physical Sports Medicine* **9**, 69–73.

Taylor, P. (1989). Inflammation of the deep infrapatellar bursa of the knee. *Arthritis and Rheumatism* **32**, 1312–14.

Tindel, N. and Nisonson, B. (1992). The plica syndrome. *Orthopedic Clinics of North America* **23**, 613–18.

Tria, A., Palumbo, R., and Alicea, J. (1992). Conservative care for patellofemoral pain. *Orthopedic Clinics of North America* **23**, 545–54.

Voorneveld, C., Arenson, A., and Fam, A. (1989). Anserine bursal distention: diagnosis by ultrasonography and computed tomography. *Arthritis and Rheumatism* **32**, 1335–8.

Watt, I. (1991). Magnetic resonance imaging in orthopaedics. *Journal of Bone and Joint Surgery* **73-B**, 539–50.

Wigley, R. (1982). Popliteal cysts: variations on a theme of Baker. *Seminars in Arthritis and Rheumatism* **12**, 1–10.

Zeiss, J., Coombs, R.J., Booth, R.L., Jr, and Saddemi, S.R. (1993). Chronic bursitis presenting as a mass in the pes anserine bursa: MR diagnosis. *Journal of Computer Assisted Tomography* **17**, 137–40.

1.2.2.3 The arm and leg in children

Angelo Ravelli and Stefania Viola

Musculoskeletal problems occur frequently in the paediatric age group, but information on their incidence and prevalence is scarce. Musculoskeletal complaints were the second most common recorded complaint after headache in a questionnaire survey of school-aged children. Paediatric rheumatology registries from four countries on three continents list 14–21 per cent of patients as having musculoskeletal pain or a chronic pain syndrome.

In the evaluation of a child with a musculoskeletal complaint, the examiner must first clarify if the problem is local or part of a systemic process and, if local, whether it involves the periarticular structures (tendons, ligaments, bursas), intra-articular structures, or is due to referred pain from another source.

There are multiple causes of regional musculoskeletal pain, which include both serious conditions, such as infections and malignancy, as well as self-limited problems such as bursitis and tendonitis. Thus, in any one area of the body, the differential diagnosis of a pain syndrome can be extensive.

The age of the child at the time the painful condition started will help focus on the possible causes. Indeed, certain conditions are seen most commonly in particular age groups; for example, hip pain presenting in a 5–10-year-old is likely to be Legg–Calvé–Perthes's disease, whereas similar pain in an adolescent is most likely to be due to a slipped capital femoral epiphysis. A common cause of regional musculoskeletal pain is trauma. Other physical signs of injury such as bruising and swelling often direct the assessment towards a search for a fracture, tendon injury, or tear. Constitutional complaints and signs, such as fever, anorexia, malaise, and weight loss, in association with a regional pain syndrome draw attention towards the possibility of infection, malignancy, or other systemic disease. Recurrent, predictable symptoms following a specific activity suggest local ligamentous or bursal inflammation or internal derangement of the joint, and may be seen more often in active children with hypermobile joints.

Equally important is the intensity, timing, and location of the pain because this information may help define its cause. Severe, constant pain with constitutional symptoms brings infection and malignancy to the top of the differential diagnostic list. Milder pain or no pain associated with upper or lower extremity disease (e.g. limp) is often seen in chronic arthritis due to juvenile arthritis or aseptic necrosis. Morning pain associated with morning stiffness is highly suggestive of a chronic inflammatory condition such as juvenile idiopathic arthritis, whereas pain occurring at night without constitutional symptoms may be due to an osteoid osteoma or growing pains.

As mentioned earlier, the physician should attempt to discern the anatomical location of the pain syndrome. The examiner often needs to know the local anatomy to determine if the painful process is periarticular, intra-articular, or referred from another area. Periarticular pain is often worse at the end of the day and occasionally keeps the child awake at night. Last, but not least, inquiry into family history should be made. Known inherited diseases in families very often give a clue to the child's current, local musculoskeletal problem, such as sickle-cell disease or haemophilia.

An accurate physical examination to localize the problem is a key to finding the cause of the pain. Examine the areas for local tenderness, swelling, range of motion, and muscle size and symmetry. Also look for growth abnormalities that can occur in chronic conditions. On physical examination, periarticular disorders or referred pain syndromes, in contrast to intra-articular disorders, will often result in localized tenderness and the active range of motion of the joint will be less than the passive range of motion.

The arm

The shoulder

Pain is the most frequent symptom of an inflammatory process of the shoulder. Shoulder complaints in children can resemble those seen in adults. For example, subdeltoid bursitis and bicipital tendinitis are also seen in children. Anatomically, the subdeltoid bursa lies next to the supraspinatus tendon making it difficult clinically to separate out which structure is inflamed. Both result in pain in the lateral aspect of the shoulder worsened by raising the child's hand above his or her head or resisting adduction of the shoulder.

Bicipital tendonitis causes pain in the anterior aspect of the shoulder on resisted forward flexion of the shoulder. Pain can also be elicited by having the child supinate the flexed forearm against the examiner's resisting hand. This manoeuvre is called Yergason's sign.

The elbow

In the elbow, children present with particular problems not seen in adults. A common injury in the preschool-aged child is the nursemaid's elbow, or pulled elbow, a result of a strong pull on the forearm or wrist which tears the annular ligament surrounding the radial neck The child presents with a painful flexed and pronated elbow and the radiographic examination is normal.

'Little-league' elbow is most commonly seen in baseball pitchers between 9 and 13 years of age and is most likely due to an overuse syndrome. Pain and swelling may be localized to the medial, lateral, or posterior aspect of the elbow region. The most common site is in the medial epicondyle; fragmentation and/or calcification in the soft tissue is sometimes visible on the plain radiograph. Tennis elbow can also occur in middle to late childhood.

Avascular necrosis can occur in childhood in multiple locations. Panner's disease is an avascular necrosis of the capitellum of the humerus; it occurs most often in middle or late childhood. The child may complain of pain and have swelling around the elbow with slight loss of motion, but the diagnosis is made by the sclerosis and irregularity of the capitellum on radiography. Comparison views of the opposite elbow are helpful in diagnosing mild instances.

Olecranon bursitis is rarer than prepatellar bursitis of the knee because the olecranon bursa develops between the ages of 7 and 10 years and the prepatellar bursa develops at a younger age. Pain and swelling of the olecranon bursa can be secondary to infection or idiopathic inflammation found in students or sports enthusiasts such as gymnasts, weight lifters, or wrestlers.

The wrist and hand

Wrists and hands can be affected by several abnormalities. Some of them can be due to congenital diseases. Madelung deformity is a congenital lesion inherited as an autosomal dominant trait, which is bilateral and more common in females. Clinical manifestations become evident between 8 and 12 years of age with a visible prominence on the dorsal and ulnar side of the wrist. There is limited range of motion, joint instability, and pain. The lesion retards the development of the ulnar and volar aspects of the distal radial physis, with resultant displacement and bowing of the distal radio that becomes shortened. Roentgenograms confirm the diagnosis. Treatment includes relief of pain and poor function with conservative therapy. Surgery is not needed for all patients; when necessary it is delayed until 11–13 years of age.

A condition that may be familial in some cases is Thiemann's disease. It is an osteochondrosis caused by osteonecrosis of the phalangeal epiphyses, possibly secondary to trauma. There is a progressive, painless enlargement during adolescence of the epiphyses of the proximal interphalangeal joints of the hands and the interphalangeal joints of the first toes. Radiologically there is irregularity of the epiphysis of the digits.

Another condition of probably congenital origin is the 'familial hypertrofic synovitis': it is an arthropathy characterized by flexion contractures of the fingers ('trigger fingers'), which appears during the first few months of life, and non inflammatory joint effusions. There is neither pain nor systemic manifestations. Ollier's disease is a multiple enchondromatosis that commonly affects the hands and feet, which at clinical presentation can be mistaken for arthritis.

Pachydermodactily is a rare condition that has been mainly reported in male patients around the age of puberty. It produces diffuse bulbous swelling of the skin around the dorsal aspect and sides of the proximal phalanx and proximal interphalangeal joints of the fingers. It is frequently associated with mechanical trauma of the fingers in subjects who have the habit of rubbing and gripping their fingers unconsciously. Pachydermoperiostosis is characterized by the onset (usually in adolescent boys) of 'spadelike' enlargement of the hands and feet, sometimes accompanied by pain along the distal long bones.

Regional pain disorders of the wrist and hand are often secondary to fractures in childhood. Fractures of the distal forearm are very common in children and fractures of the carpal bones are rare. The most common carpal fracture is a fracture of the navicular and it is seen in adolescents. The trigger thumb seen in children mimics trigger finger in the adult in its presenting signs and symtoms as do de Quervain stenosing tenosynovitis and carpal tunnel syndrome.

Diabetic cheiroarthropathy, though rare in diabetic adults, is commonly seen in adolescents with onset of diabetes in early childhood. The adolescent presents with painless thickening and tightening of the soft tissues around the fingers resulting in progressive stiffness and flexion contractures, first of the distal interphalangeal joints and the proximal interphalangeal joints. Another disorder, reflex sympathetic dystrophy (algodystrophy), can occur in the upper or lower extremity. It is discussed below as it may occur more commonly in the lower extremity in children.

A deforming arthropathy, mainly of the hands, named Jaccoud's arthropathy, has been described in 2–4 per cent of adult patients, and occasionally children, with systemic lupus erythematosus. It is characterized by severe deformities of the hands with multiple subluxations, little or no pain, and usually well-preserved function. Radiographic studies generally do not show evidence of bone or cartilage damage.

Raynaud phenomenon is characterized by the triple-phase sequence of blanching, cyanosis, and erythema, occurring spontaneously or in response to cold or physical or emotional stress. These changes may be restricted to a single digit, may be unilateral or bilateral, and usually spare the thumb. Colour changes may be accompanied by paraesthesias, numbness, or pain (especially during the erythematous phase). Raynaud phenomenon occurs in 90 per cent of children with diffuse cutaneous systemic scleroderma and is often the initial symptom of the disease, preceding other manifestations in some instances by years. At variance, idiopathic Raynaud disease is uncommon in childhood, with the exception of the familial benign variety.

The leg

Generalized leg pains are very frequent in childhood and the most common causes are growing pains, shin splints, and stress fractures. Growing pain occurs in approximately 10–20 per cent of school-aged children and young adolescents. It has an aching or sometimes crampy quality and is usually localized to both lower extremities, most often in the thigh, shin, or calf. The pain is never associated with a limp and often occurs in the evening and can interrupt sleep. The child is completely normal by the morning and all laboratory and radiographic investigations are normal. The term 'growing pains' is a misnomer; the aetiology of this disorder is unknown and it occurs after the time of most rapid growth.

Shin splints result in pain after activity that is relieved by rest. The pain occurs along the medial or lateral tibial shaft and is thought to be due to microtears of muscle, tendons, and ligaments, muscle inflammation, periostitis, and muscle compartment syndromes. A similar pain syndrome is found with stress fractures. These occur anywhere in the weight-bearing skeleton but are most common in the diaphysial region of the tibia. They present with localized pain that worsens with activity. Plain radiographs will often be negative until new bone formation occurs, which may take at least 2 weeks. A technetium bone scan can be positive much earlier and will differentiate this condition from shin splints which should have negative radiographic studies.

Unequal leg length can be an important sign of a regional musculoskeletal disorder. Leg length inequality is defined as greater than 2-cm difference between the length of the legs and can result in a limp, scoliosis, and leg or back pain. The leg length discrepancy can be due to overgrowth early in childhood or early epiphyseal closure in adolescence. Some causes are hemihypertrophy, fractures, infections, tumours, intra-articular abnormalities in the hip, knee, or feet (such as juvenile arthritis or avascular necrosis), and neurological disorders such as poliomyelitis. Accurate measurements of the true or apparent discrepancy in the leg length can be difficult and often the best determination is done by plain radiographs of the pelvis centred at the level of the femoral heads when the child is standing.

Regional pain syndromes are much more common in the lower than in the upper extremities. The most common presentation is that of a limp. Abnormalities in the pelvis or back such as discitis or spinal cord lesions can refer pain to the lower extremities. Similarly, hip inflammation may refer pain to the knee. If, on examining the painful area, no focal abnormalities are found, a referral source for the pain should be suspected.

The hip

Pain from the hip region is usually localized to the anterior groin, around the greater trochanter, and down the anterolateral thigh to the knee. The differential diagnosis of hip pain includes tumours of the pelvis, spine, or proximal femur, infections of the hip joint, discitis, congenital dislocation, Legg–Calvé–Perthes's disease, slipped capital femoral epiphysis, and toxic or transient synovitis of the hip.

The most common disorder causing hip pain in children is transient synovitis of the hip. It is a self limited inflammatory condition that has no known cause and generally has a very good clinical outcome. Transient synovitis of the hip may develop anytime, but the peak age is between 3 and 6 years. At least half of children have or recently have had a form of upper respiratory illness. The most common presentation is unilateral hip pain and the leg is usually held in flexion, with slight abduction and external rotation. Occasionally a fever is present. The complete blood count and sedimentation rate are usually normal, but occasionally the latter can be elevated. Ultrasonography is extremely accurate in detecting intracapsular effusion. The majority of children are better in 2–3 weeks. Oral anti-inflammatory medication in appropriate dosage, may reduce the pain and are recommended; bedrest may be necessary to achieve pain relief. Transient synovitis of the hip is a diagnosis of exclusion and more serious diagnoses, such as aseptic necrosis, Lyme disease, or poststreptococcal arthritis, must be ruled out.

Legg–Calvé–Perthes's disease is an idiopathic avascular necrosis of the femoral head that is seen in children between 5 and 10 years of age. It is about four times more common in boys than in girls and affects both hips in 10–15 per cent of cases. It has been noted that children with the disease have delayed skeletal maturation and reduced height. Children with Perthes' disease present with pain and/or a limp; the pain may be localized to the groin, but frequently the pain may be referred to the thigh or knee. Range of motion testing of the hip in the supine position, especially extreme rotation or abduction, may elicit pain. Radiographs taken shortly after the onset of symptoms are often normal, but later radiographs show a progression through four stages [Fig. 1(a)]: (i) an initial stage, at which there may be a small ossific nucleus, widening of the joint space, irregularity of the physis, and a subchondral radiolucent area; (ii) a fragmentation stage, at which the bony epiphysis begins to fragment and there are patchy areas of increased radiolucency and radiodensity; (iii) a reossification stage, at which normal bone density develop in previously radiolucent areas, and abnormalities of the shape of the femoral head and neck appear; (iv) the healed stage, at which the bone density is normal but the head is left with residual deformities. These changes may take several years to complete. Bone scans and magnetic resonance imaging studies have a greater sensivity for the detection of early disease than do plain radiographs. Treatment aims at improving the range of motion of the affected hips and containing the hip within the acetabulum by either non-operative or operative means.

Slipped capital femoral epiphysis is the gradual or abrupt slippage of the femoral neck anteriorly and superiorly from the femoral head through the growth plate. It affects most commonly overweight boys in early to mid-adolescence. Most cases are unilateral, but up to one-third will be bilateral The most frequent symptoms at presentation are pain and altered gait. The pain occurs either deep in the groin or along the distal medial thigh and knee. The pain is usually present during walking and is accentuated by running and jumping. Physical examination usually demonstrates a loss of internal rotation of the affected hip, diminished flexion, atrophy of the thigh, if symptoms have been long standing, and shortening of the leg. A pathognomonic sign for this condition is seen when flexing of the involved hip will produce a concomitant external rotation of the hip. Slipped capital femoral epiphysis is associated with endocrine disorders. The diagnosis can be missed unless both anteroposterior and lateral radiographic views are taken as a mild slip can be missed on an anteroposterior view [Fig. 1(b)].

Treatment of a slipped capital femoral epiphysis in the early stages is aimed at preventing further slip and correction of the deformity while minimizing the risk of avascular necrosis and condrolysis. If the slip of the femoral head is minimal (<1 cm in the lateral projection) surgical stabilization is the best treatment. It is more difficult to find agreement in the literature as to the best surgical approach if the slip is chronic and greater than 1 cm.

Acute chondrolysis of the hip can occur as idiophatic or secondary to other pathology as Perthes' disease or slipped capital femoral epiphysis. There is hip pain and limitation of movement in association with radiographic evidence of progressive loss of articular cartilagine. Many children have minimal symptoms on long-term follow-up; in those children with persistent symptoms there is progressive loss of joint space and eventual anchilosis. Congenital dislocation and subluxation of the hip are quite common with a prevalence of 1.5 per 1000 live births. Girls are affected eight times more commonly than boys and the dislocation is bilateral in 50 per cent. It is important to make the diagnosis early in the new-born period so as to lessen the long-term sequelae, which often result in a total replacement. Barlow's manoeuvre of flexion, adduction, and axial pressure in a posterior direction can demonstrate dislocation occuring in the hip. Another physical sign which is significant at any age is shortening of the affected femur. This can be detected when both hips are flexed to 90° with the child lying down on his or her back; the knee on the side of the affected hip is lower than its normal counterpart. If children are not diagnosed until a later age, they present with painful weight bearing and limited range of motion in the affected hip. Radiographic studies may be diagnostic and the examiner must rely on the physical examination to make the diagnosis.

As in adults, trochanteric bursitis or inflammation of the fascia lata overlying the greater trochanter occurs in children. The pain is localized over the greater trochanter and is worse with walking or lying on the affected side. The pain can be reproduced if pressure is applied to the lateral aspect of the greater trochanter or the fascia lata is put on stretch.

The knee

Recurrent patellar dislocation is most commonly seen in adolescence to young adulthood. The disorder is thought to result from malalignment and/or instability of the patellofemoral joint. It may be associated with a congenital abnormality of the patella (unifaceted or bibartite patella), of the femoral condyles (shallow intercondylar groove), or of the patellar ligament (lateral attachment). Symptoms include dull or aching knee pain most commonly with activity such as climbing stairs or squatting and, when the symptoms are severe, there may be intermittent giving way or buckling of

(a) (b)

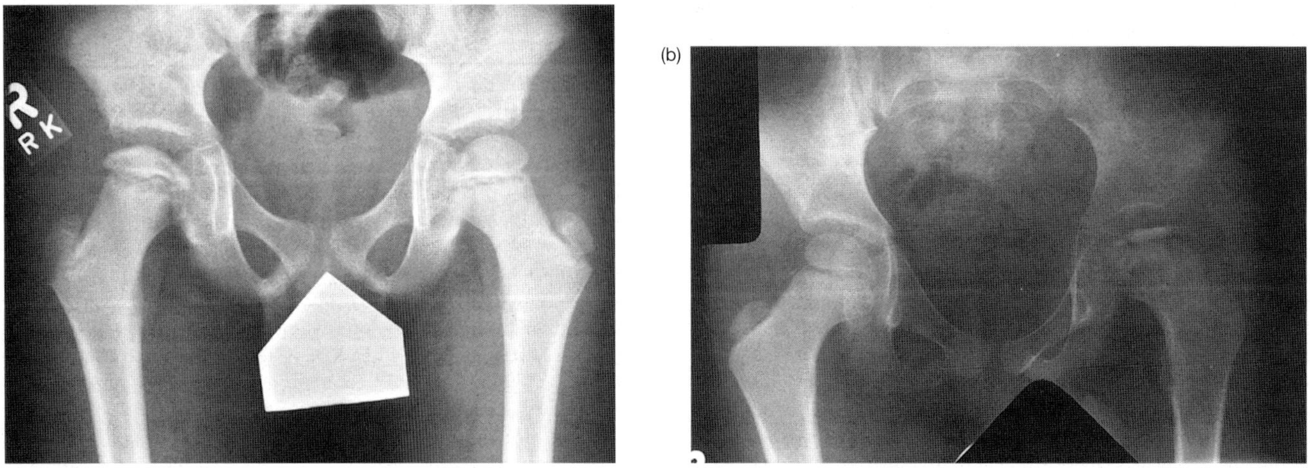

Fig. 1 (a) Legg–Calvé–Perthes's disease—8-year-old child with flattened dense right femoral head characteristic of femoral capital collapse from ischaemic necrosis or Legg–Calvé–Perthes's disease. (b) Slipped capital femoral epiphysis—12-year-old, overweight boy. In the anteroposterior view, note the widening of the growth plate and blurring of the metaphyseal side of the growth plate of the left femoral head.

the knee due to quadriceps weakness. Repeated episodes of dislocation lead to premature degeneration of the articular cartilage of the patellofemoral joint. Locking of the knee is more consistent with an internal derangement or meniscal disorder of the knee. Pain can be precipitated if the patella is compressed or restrained when the quadriceps is contracting. Atrophy of the vastus medialis, patella alta, increased genua valgus, femoral anteversion, and hypermobility are also seen. Laboratory tests are normal. Radiographs are normal unless there is significant malalignment. Arthroscopic examination of the knee reveals fissuring, fibrillation, and fragmentation of the retropatellar anterior cartilage. Mild patellofemoral pain can be improved by a programme of isometric exercises, designed both to stretch the tight iliotibial band and to strengthen the hamstrings and quadriceps muscle. If exercises fail, surgery must be considered.

The mediopatellar plica syndrome causes pain with flexion of the knee. A plica is an abnormal synovial band that originates in the suprapatellar area and extends down to the medial side of the knee. It can become trapped between the tibia and femur resulting in pain, giving way, and locking of the knee. Erosion of the cartilage may eventually occur. The condition is diagnosed by arthroscopy; if necessary, resection can be performed at the same time.

The fat-pad syndrome or Hoffa's disease is characterized by intermittent pain and swelling in the anterior knee joint underneath the patellar tendon. Singling–Larsen–Johanssen disease is an osteochondrosis caused by repeated trauma to the inefrior pole (secondary ossification center) of the patella which occurs in adolescence; it results in pain at the insertion of the patellar tendon where it attaches to the patella and is worsened by activity. Treatment consists of rest or reduction in physical activity that involve the leg. Radiographs show calcification at the insertion of the patellar tendon.

Internal derangement of the knee can be secondary to a meniscal tear, torn cruciate ligament, or loose body within the knee joint. A child with a meniscal tear presents with a significant past history of trauma. No matter what the aetiology, locking, giving way, pain and intermittent swelling are found in association with the presence of foreign bodies within the joint space.

Genu recurvatum may be part of a generalized hypermobility syndrome or may occur as an isolated phenomenon. Symptomatic genu recurvatum occurs most commonly in adolescent girls: symptoms are worse with standing or walking and are relieved by rest.

Genu varum (bowed legs) is normal in children under age 2 years. The most common pathological condition that can cause genu varum is Blount's disease. Blount's disease is a disorder of the posterior or the medial tibial physis and those most commonly affected are black males. Radiographs show diminished height of the medial tibial plateau [Fig. 2(a)].

Osgood–Schlatter disease, osteochondritis of the tibial tubercle, is thought to be an overuse syndrome involving the attachment of the patellar tendon to the tibial tubercle and is often caused by recurrent microtrauma. This condition is seen in preadolescence and adolescence and is more common in males. There is pain and swelling around the tibial tubercle which is worsened by strenuous physical activity. Radiographs may be normal in the early stages but can show slight avulsion or fragmentation of the tubercle or both. Ultrasonography can help in identifying the lesion. This condition is usually mild and often asymptomatic. If the pain is significant or recurrent, restriction of activity or immobilization of the knee may be necessary.

Osteochondritis dissecans is a condition in which there is partial or complete separation of articular cartilage with or without involvement of the subchondral bone. The inner aspect of the distal femoral medial condyle is the most commonly affected area [Fig. 2(b)]; however, osteochondritis dissecans of the dome of the talus, the capitellum, or the patella also occurs commonly. It is characterized by activity-related pain, sometimes with recurrent bland effusion. Magnetic resonance imaging may become the method of choice for staging the lesion. If the articular cartilagine is intact, the treatment consists of restricting activity to the child's tolerance level. Healing can take up to several months. If the fragment is loose, arthroscopy to remove small pieces or surgery to replace significant bony components should be undertaken.

(a)
(b)
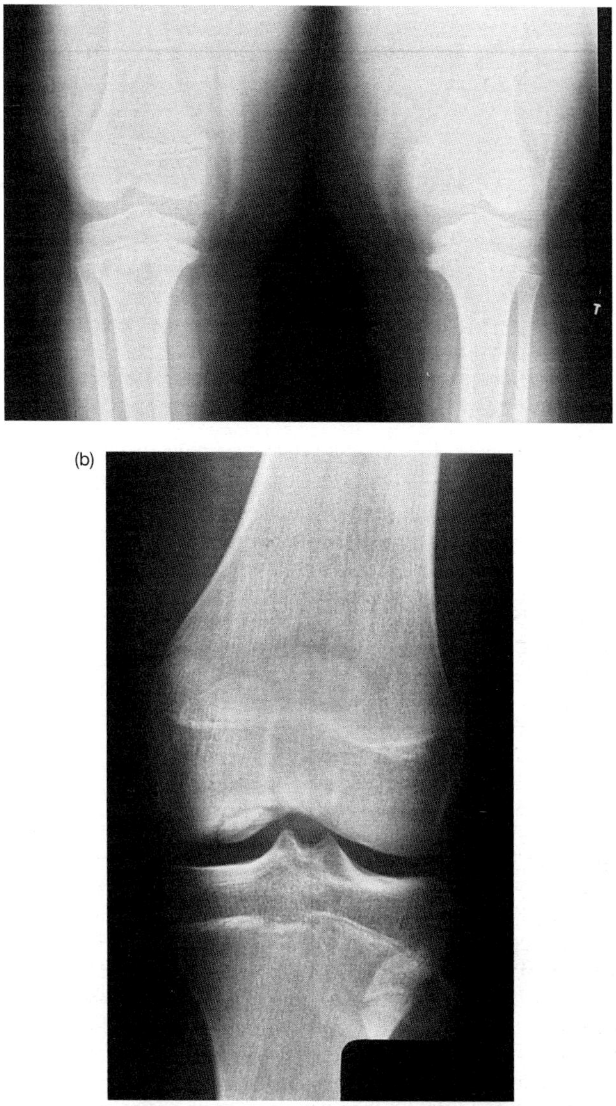

Fig. 2 (a) Blount's disease—4-year-old child with a varus configuration of the right knee. The height of the medial tibial plateau appears to be diminished with sclerosis of the medial tibial metaphysis. (b) Osteochondritis dissecans—12-year-old adolescent with a dense ovoid subchondral body on the medial femoral chondyle next to the interchondylar notch.

Another regional condition is a Baker's or popliteal cyst. This is a cystic mass filled with synovial fluid or gelatinous fluid resembling that in ganglion cysts of the wrist. This cystic mass can arise from the joint itself or from the semimembranosus bursas. A cyst in a child is usually a self-limited condition, resolving spontaneously over several months. In contrast to Baker's cysts seen in adults, Baker's cysts in children are not usually associated with intra-articular pathology, and thus investigation of the knee of an asymptomatic child with a Baker's cyst is often unhelpful. However, in juvenile idiopathic arthritis large synovial cysts may appear in the popliteal space and may dissect into the calf. Ultrasound or magnetic resonance imaging will aid in their correct diagnosis.

There are two benign tumours that must be considered in the differential of regional musculoskeletal pain of the knee; pigmented villonodular synovitis and synovial chrondromatosis. Both occur in teenagers and affect the knee most commonly. Pigmented villonodular synovitis results in a bloody arthrocentesis and has a characteristic histopathology including a cellular infiltrate of the synovium with haemosiderin-laden stromal cells. It is thought that pigmented villonodular synovitis represents a benign tumour of uncertain aetiology. This condition is unusual in chilhood but may appear as a recurrent swelling in the knee or ankle. Treatment of the lesion often requires surgical excision.

Synovial chondromatosis is a condition in which intrasynovial cartilaginous nodules develop and may project into the joint space, resulting in symptoms of pain and locking. Unless the nodules calcify, this diagnosis must be made by arthroscopy.

Prepatellar bursitis is a common problem of the periarticular region of the knee in adults. It can occur in children, but is much less common than in adults. Because of its superficial location, it is often inflamed secondary to a bacterial infection from a nearby cellulitis.

The ankle and foot

Foot pain in young children is rare; it becomes more common as the child grows older. Foot discomfort in children can be divided into the following categories; hypermobile flat feet, trauma, infections, apophysitis, neurological disorders, tumours, and bony abnormalities such as avascular necrosis and tarsal or subtalar coalition.

Flat feet are common in infants and common in children. It can be described as a loss of the longitudinal arch of the weight-bearing foot joint. Pain is unusual and, if it occurs, it is located in the arch, on the medial side of the ankle, or at the insertion of the plantar fascia at the metatarsal heads or calcaneus. If pain is present it is important to distinguish between a flexible planovalgus (flat) foot and a peroneal spastic flat foot. A flexible flat foot is supple with full ankle and subtalar joint motion and the arch is restored when one stands on the toes. In the peroneal spastic flat foot, ankle motion is normal but there is limited inversion and eversion of the foot and/or subtalar joint. Also the arch is not restored when not weight bearing. Peroneal spastic flat foot may be caused by a tarsal coalition or by inflammatory arthritis. Tarsal coalition is the leading cause of peroneal spastic flat foot.

Calcaneonavicular coalition is most common and the next most common is the talocalcaneal coalition which is seen most often between the ages of 12 and 16 years and is best demonstrated by computed tomography scan. Although flat feet do not require treatment, some children present with painful flat feet, although it is less common. Most of these are older, and the examiner should identify the location of the pain. Generally, the pain is either lateral in the area of the subtalar joint and the sinus tarsi or over the heelcord and heelcord insertion. In checking range of motion, if the subtalar joint is stiff one must think of a tarsal coalition. A stiff or painful subtalar joint can also indicate a juvenile idiopathic arthritis. If the pain is posterior a thight heelcord is usually present and can be treated with stretching and anti-inflammatory agents.

Flexible flat foot or hypermobile pes planus is a normal part of the development of the foot. At the age of 1 year when the child starts to walk the midfoot is flat to the floor due to normal ligamentous laxity. The foot usually develops the normal longitudinal arch by 5 years. Children with flexible flat feet due to ligamentous laxity form a good arch when standing on tiptoe. No treatment with corrective shoes is thought necessary for the asymptomatic flat foot. Occasionally, the hypermobile flat foot may result in pain at the medial side of the arch on weight bearing. Mild genovalgus, slight flexion of the knees and hips, as well as lordosis can occur due to this pes planus and result in lower extremity pain. Often mild symptoms can be improved with a moulded insert.

Another cause of painful flat feet is the hypermobile foot with a short Achilles' tendon. The diagnosis is made when dorsiflexion of the ankle with an inverted foot does not reach 90°. Heel-cord stretching exercises are usually helpful. Rarely, an accessory navicular will result in foot pain necessitating its excision. An accessory navicular is found in 50 per cent of all feet; most are asymptomatic.

The most common non-neuromuscular cause of the rigid flat foot in the 8–16-year-old age group is tarsal coalition which occurs when two or more of the tarsal bones are joined, either by a bony bar or a fibrocartilaginous bridge. Clinically the adolescent has a rigid flat foot associated occasionally with peroneal spasm. The coalitions are diagnosed by radiography but special views are often needed to demonstrate the coalition; for example, an oblique view of the hindfoot is necessary to demonstrate a calcaneonavicular bar.

In adolescents a common cause of foot pain is stress fractures of the second and third metatarsal shafts. Like other stress fractures, they may be difficult to see early in the radiographs. They can either be documented by a technetium bone scan or callus formation on a plain radiograph can be awaited. This takes approximately 3 weeks to form.

There are three tendon–bone junctions in the foot that present problems in preadolescents. Calcaneal apophysitis (Sever's disease) occurs in both girls and boys between the ages of 8 and 10 years, usually in those who are just beginning to play competitive sports. The pain localizes to the insertion of the Achilles' tendon where it inserts on to the calcaneus, and adolescents with this condition often have difficulty walking on their heels. Radiographs are normal, often showing a dense fragmented calcaneal apophysis, which is a normal finding at this age. A second condition seen in children aged 10–12 years is swelling and pain at the insertion of the peroneus brevis into the apophysis of the base of the fifth metatarsal. There can be a secondary ossification centre in the apophysis and this can cause pain, particularly if narrow shoes are worn. Finally, an accessory navicular bone can result in foot pain. In 75 per cent of cases an accessory navicular will fuse with the main navicular bone. Pain can occur over the accessory navicular and is usually relieved with rest.

Reflex sympathetic dystrophy can occur in the hand but is much more common in the foot. This condition is often initiated by trauma and presents with a diffusely swollen, painful foot. The pain is worse at night and is not relieved by rest. Often the symptoms appear out of proportion to the physical findings. As the condition progresses, the foot can become hypersensitive and demonstrate vascular changes such as being cool, sweaty, and swollen; finally, muscle wasting and contractures can develop if no treatment with physiotherapy is begun. Radiographs can show osteopenia and diffuse increased uptake is found in a technetium bone scan.

Two painful conditions of the foot are due to avascular necrosis; Kohler's disease and Freiberg's infraction. Kohler's disease is an osteochondrosis of the tarsal navicular bone that occurs in girls and boys between the ages of 4 and 6 years. Pain with exercise slowly develops over the tarsal navicula and radiographs demonstrate a 'pancake' condition of the navicula. Freiberg's infarction is aseptic necrosis of the metatarsal head and most commonly affects the head of the second metatarsal. Very active adolescent girls are most affected and pain is localized to the metatarsal head involved.

There are many tendinous attachments and bursas around the foot and inflammation, such as plantar fasciitis, 'pump bumps' underneath the bursa near the insertion of the Achilles' tendon on the calcaneus, and Achilles' tendonitis due to type IIa or IV hyperproteinaemia, are often seen in many of these structures. Similarly, bunions or hallux valgus are most common in adolescence but occur in all age groups. Many of these conditions are described elsewhere as they are more common in adults.

In adolescents, a common cause of foot pain is stress fractures of the second and third metatarsal shafts. Like other stress fractures they may be difficult to see early in the radiographs. They can either be documented by a technetium bone scan.

Generalized conditions that can present as regional musculoskeletal pain syndromes

There are several systemic conditions that can present to the rheumatologist with regional muscoloskeletal complaints. It is only after a careful, general examination that the systemic condition may be revealed.

One example is hypermobility, which occurs in 12–19.5 per cent of the population. Joint laxity predisposes periarticular structures to injury resulting in musculoskeletal pain around one or several joints. This painful syndrome is more common in girls with a family history of hypermobility. Mild joints effusions may be observed. Reassurance is the initial treatment of hypermobility. Pain due to joint laxity is also a feature of other inherited disorders of joint laxity, such as Marfan's syndrome, Ehlers–Danlos syndrome, and Larsen's syndrome.

Disorders that result in acquired hypomobility result in joint contractures and little signs of inflammation are found. The mucopolysaccharidoses and mucolipidoses can present with limited motion of the fingers and, occasionally, other joints. Fabry's disease requires the attention of a rheumatologist because patients with this disease develop degenerative changes and flexion contractures of the fingers. Severe, burning pain in the fingers and toes occurs in 80 per cent of children or young adults with Fabry's disease. Gaucher's disease also has hip and knee pain as a component of the syndrome.

Stickler's dysplasia is a heterogenous group of disorders with an autosomal dominant pattern of inheritance. Ankle, knee, and wrists become enlarged in childhood and cause intermittent arthralgias. Joint enlargement can be misdiagnosed as juvenile idiopathic arthritis and may be associated with a marfanoid body habitus with congenital hyperextensibility of the joints. The epiphyseal dysplasia syndromes can result in pain around or in a joint and a plain radiograph assists in the diagnosis. Another genetic syndrome that often presents with regional musculoskeletal pain is sickle-cell disease. Synovial, capsular, and tendon infarction can occur in sickle-cell disease resulting in joint pain.

Haemarthrosis is a hallmark of haemophilia. Haemorrhages into the elbows, knees, and ankles cause pain and swelling and limited movement of the joints; this may be induced by minor trauma, but often appear to be spontaneous. Repeated haemorrhages may produce degenerative changes, with osteoporosis, muscle atrophy and, ultimately, a fixed, unusable joint.

Fibromyalgia occurs in the paediatric age group. This condition usually presents as diffuse musculoskeletal aching in a 9–15-year-old complaining of fatigue. There is a preponderance of girls. The diagnosis is one of exclusion and is based on the demonstration of tender points often found in periarticular locations associated with bursas, epicondyles, and insertion of tendons. Occasionally the child complains of pain in only one or two of these periarticular areas and the cause of the regional pain syndrome is revealed only after looking for multiple tender points. Myopathies can also present as leg aching or tenderness and should be considered in the differential diagnosis of regional pain syndromes.

Conditions associated with hyperostosis often result in regional pain syndromes. Primary hypertrophic osteoarthropathy is an autosomal dominant disorder seen in adolescent boys with 'spade-like' enlargement of the hands and feet and pain in the distal long bones. Secondary hypertrophic osteoarthropathy is associated most commonly with malignancy but can occur in pulmonary disease (cystic fibrosis, infections, fibrosis), cardiovascular disease (subacute bacterial endocarditis, cyanotic congenital heart disease), gastrointestinal disease (inflammatory bowel disease, bacterial or parasitic colitis, subphrenic abscess, cirrhosis), and endocrine (thyroid) conditions. Most children present with clubbing of the fingers, periostitis and pain in the long bones, and arthritis of the large joints. Infantile cortical hyperostosis of Caffey's disease is an uncommon disease with hyperostosis in which a child has a symmetrical painful enlargement of the mandible or shoulder girdles or long bones. It is self-limiting and usually occurs before 6 months of age.

Another cause of pain in the lower limbs may be the 'growing pains'. Most growing pains occur in pre-school to school-aged children. The pain is sometimes crampy, often deep in the thigh, shin, or calf or behind the knee. They occur frequently in the evening or at night and often interrupt sleep. The pathophysiology of the pain is unknown; gentle massage with or without analgesics is usually effective.

A syndrome of juvenile-onset diabetes mellitus, short stature and tightening of the skin and soft tissues leading to contractures of the finger joints has been described. Winchester's syndrome, a form of multicentric osteolysis, begins at about 6 weeks of age with restricted joint mobility, swelling and pain of the proximal interphalangeal joints and enlargement of the wrists. Osteoporosis, bone erosion, and atlantoaxial subluxation are characteristic radiographic findings.

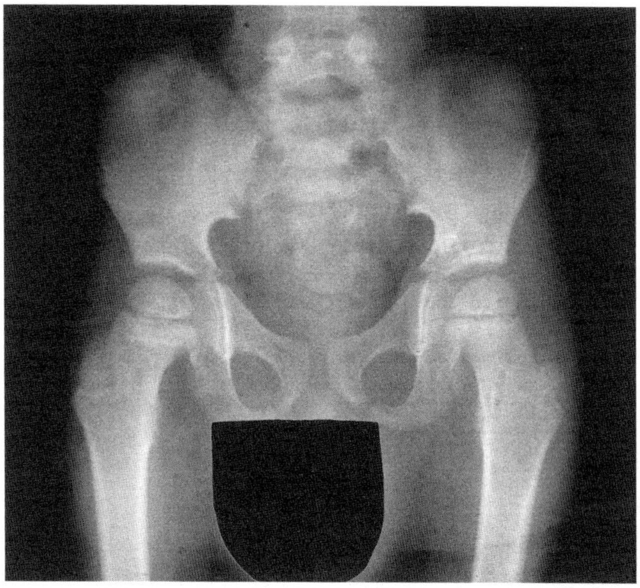

Fig. 3 Multiple osteolytic bone lesions of the pelvis and the femoral heads in a child with chronic recurrent multifocal osteomyelitis.

The idiophatic osteolyses are grouped according to the area affected: phalangeal, carpal-tarsal, or multicentric. Familial acro-osteolysis is inherited as an autosomal trait and becomes apparent at about 3 years of age. The carpus or tarsus alone may be affected, or the bones of the hands, feet, elbows and knees may be involved. The onset can mimic juvenile idiopathic arthritis in that affected areas are swollen and warm. Radiographs show progressive bone lysis and destruction of the involved joints. Spontaneous remissions during the young adult years are characteristic.

Chronic recurrent multifocal osteomyelitis is a rare chronic inflammatory process of bone, characterised by multiple and often symmetrical sites of osseous involvement, periodic exacerbations and remissions and failure to isolate pathogens from the affected areas (Fig. 3). It may lead to episodic bone pain, with each episode varying in duration and location. In children with back pain magnetic resonance imaging may lead to discover unsuspected vertebral lesions. In as many as 20 per cent of patients, bone lesions may be associated with a sterile palmo-plantar pustulosis.

Erythromelalgia is a rare condition which is characterized by burning pain in the hands and feet, relieved by cold. Aspirin can dramatically reduce the pain.

Another rare syndrome that can be mistaken for growing pains is restless legs syndrome. It consists of a feeling of discomfort in and an inability to keep from moving the legs at night after resting or going to bed. Periodic movements of the limbs during sleep are common. They usually last less than a minute and rarely cause the child to awaken.

General bibliography

Craig, L. and Goldberg, M.J. (1993). Foot and leg problems. *Pediatrics in Review* **14**, 395–400.

Hoffinger, S.A. (1996). Evaluation and management of pediatric foot deformities. *Pediatric Clinics of North America* **43**, 1091–111.

Jacobs, J.C., ed. *Pediatric Rheumatology for the Practitioner*. New York: Springer, 1993.

Koop, S. and Quanbeck, D. (1996). Three common causes of childhood hip pain. *Pediatric Clinics of North America* **43**, 1053–66.

Prieur, A.M. (1990). Miscellaneous conditions associated with musculoskeletal complaints in children. *Current Opinion in Rheumatism* **2**, 824–31.

Renshaw, T.S. *Pediatric Orthopedics*. Philadelphia PA: W.B. Saunders, 1986.

Sherry, D.D. and Malleson, P.N. (2001). Nonrheumatic musculoskeletal pain. In *Textbook of Pediatric Rheumatology* (ed. J.T. Cassidy and R.E. Petty), pp. 362–80. Philadelphia PA: W.B. Saunders.

Wilkings, K.E. (1988). The painful foot in the child. *Instruction Course Lectures* **37**, 77–85.

1.2.3 Extra-articular features of rheumatic diseases

Ian D. Griffiths

Introduction

The diagnosis and management of the rheumatic diseases remains a stimulating challenge. Systemic diseases often present under a rheumatological guise and; the subject of this section; rheumatic diseases may present in non-rheumatological fashion. Today, rheumatological diseases rank second as the cause of fever of unknown origin (FUO) in Europe and the United States (Davies and Finch 2001).

Some of the rheumatic disorders, such as the connective tissue diseases are by their nature multisystem and it is not surprising that they may present with organ involvement other than the musculoskeletal system. This chapter does not attempt to catalogue all the extra-articular features encountered in the rheumatic diseases but focus on the problem of underlying rheumatic diseases that may present in a non-rheumatological fashion. In practice this may occur either before the rheumatic features have manifested themselves, when the non-articular features clinically dwarf the rheumatic symptoms, or when the underlying rheumatic disease produces only mild symptoms or subtle joint manifestations.

Arguably, the most critical factor in establishing the diagnosis at presentation is the competence of the attending doctor in obtaining a history and performing an examination that will elicit features of the underlying musculoskeletal disorder (Doherty et al. 1990). Failure to identify a musculoskeletal disorder, or to recognize its relevance in the context of the overall clinical picture, is more than an 'academic' nicety. It was perhaps disappointing to read in a 1997 article on the assessment of a patient with FUO 'The history of joint pains is intriguing but non-specific. If she had had overt arthritis I would be interested in examining her for rheumatic diseases' (Berkwits and Gluckman 1997) and reflects the continuing need to promote routine examination of the musculoskeletal system as the 'fifth system'. Most clinicians have experience of patients who have been invasively (and expensively) investigated for symptoms, signs, or laboratory abnormalities which could have been readily accounted for if the underlying diagnosis had been recognized. More alarming are the patients who have been inappropriately treated because of the failure to recognise an associated rheumatological disorder (e.g. lymph node biopsies that have been misclassified and subsequently treated as lymphoma by the pathologist who was not made aware of the coexisting diagnosis of rheumatoid arthritis).

The development of medical specialization means that undifferentiated diseases or non-specific laboratory abnormalities, such as a raised erthrocyte sedimentation rate (ESR), may be directed to a wide variety of disciplines depending upon the predominant symptoms and local practice. There remains a tendency in standard medical textbooks to underrecognize the frequency with which non-specific systemic features, such as fever or weight loss, may be the presenting feature of a rheumatic disorder.

This chapter considers 'extra-articular' presentation of musculoskeletal disorders under three broad headings: general systemic features, specific systems, and clinical patterns. Often, patients will present with an acute or subacute multisystem illness of which arthritis or arthralgia are a feature.

General systemic features

These are frequently present in inflammatory joint and connective tissue disorders (Table 1). It is often the combination of features that suggests an underlying cause, for example, swinging fever and transient rash in adult onset Still's disease. Similarly, in the non-inflammatory disorders, the coexistence of problems may point towards a diagnosis, for example, lethargy and poor sleep patterns in fibromyalgia. This section considers some of the more common systemic problems.

Table 1 Generalized systemic features which may be the presenting feature of rheumatological disorder

Systemic feature	Rheumatological disorder	Prevalence of systemic features (%)
Weight loss	Rheumatoid arthritis	10
	Polymyalgia rheumatica	50
	Connective tissue disorders	20
	Sjögren's syndrome	10
	Chronic infectious arthritis (e.g. tuberculosis)	50
	Multicentric reticulohistiocytosis	30
	Wegener's granulomatosis	40
Fever (children)	Juvenile idiopathic arthritis (systemic)	90
	Septic arthritis	90
	Chronic infectious arthritis (e.g. tuberculosis)	70
	Rheumatic fever	90
	Kawasaki's disease	90
	Familial Mediterranean fever	90
	Hyper IgD syndrome	90
	TRAPS	90
	Reactive arthritis	30
Fever (adult)	Rheumatoid arthritis	10
	Polymyalgia/temporal arteritis	15
	Adult onset Still's disease	100
	Reactive arthritis	10
	Behçet's	10
	Seronegative spondyloarthritis	5
	Connective tissue diseases	60
	Acute and chronic septic arthritis	80
	Multicentric reticulohistiocytosis	30
	Lyme disease	40
Malaise	Fibromyalgia	80
	Primary Sjögren's syndrome	70
	Polymyalgia/temporal arteritis	60
	Connective tissue disorders	50
	Rheumatoid arthritis	40
Lymphadenopathy	Rheumatoid arthritis	60
	Connective tissue disorders	40
	Juvenile idiopathic arthritis (systemic)	90
	Primary Sjögren's syndrome	40

Fever

Pyrexia is a common feature of many rheumatic disorders that have an inflammatory component (Plate 2 and Fig. 1), including viral arthritis, septic arthritis, crystal induced arthritis, chronic inflammatory joint disease, connective tissue disorders, and vasculitis (Pinals 1994). In most of these cases the associated rheumatic disorder will be apparent; the major exception is septic arthritis in a young child, where the presentation may be as non-specific as the 'irritable, febrile child'.

Fever as an early or presenting feature of a rheumatic disease is more difficult to evaluate. Fever patterns can be considered as:

(i) intermittent, when the temperature is swinging but returns to normal between episodes;

(ii) remittent, when the temperature varies but does not return to normal;

(iii) sustained, when no variation occurs.

If no cause is found for a fever of 38.3°C or above persisting for 3 weeks after 1 week of investigation, it is usually labelled as fever of unknown origin (FUO) (Petersdorf and Beeson 1961). Several reviews of patients presenting with FUO show that rheumatological disorders remain a common underlying cause, accounting for between 8 and 38 per cent of cases, second only to infection (Knockaert et al. 1992). The most frequent rheumatological disorders were temporal arteritis and SLE. A similar pattern emerged when patients with intermittent fever of unknown origin were studied but in that group an underlying disorder was found less frequently (Knockaert et al. 1993).

Intermittent fever

If sepsis has been excluded intermittent fever with temperatures of 39°C or above occurring in the later afternoon to evening and returning to normal by morning, so called quotidian fever, is very suggestive of systemic onset juvenile idiopathic arthritis in the child or adult onset Still's disease. The finding of the typical evanescent macular rash at the height of the fever would further support the diagnosis. The fever may precede the arthritis in both juvenile and adult forms of the disease, sometimes by many months, causing diagnostic problems (Martin et al. 1994). Approximately 10 per cent of fevers of unknown origin in children are eventually found to be associated with juvenile idiopathic arthritis.

In adults, there is often a considerable delay before the diagnosis of adult onset Still's is established (Wouter and Van de Putte 1986; Pouchot et al. 1991). Several reasons exist for this; the patient often presents as a fever of unknown origin to the general medical department, other 'non-articular' features may dominate the clinical picture, for example deranged liver function tests, or pleuropericardial disease. While no diagnostic tests exist, certain laboratory features support the diagnosis, including a marked leucocytosis, very high acute phase reactants, and a marked elevation of the serum ferritin (>1000 μg/l); and the absence of any of these features weighs strongly against the diagnosis of adult onset Still's disease.

The hereditary disorders associated with periodic fever, such as familial Mediterranean fever (FMF), Hibernian fever, and hyper-IgD syndrome, have undergone major advances in the understanding of their pathogenesis since the discovery of the FMF gene in 1997, and subsequently the gene abnormalities associated with hyper-IgD syndrome and Hibernian fever. All the disorders tend to start in childhood and are characterized by episodic fever associated with multiorgan involvement of which serositis, arthritis, and cutaneous involvement are most common feature. Hibernian fever is autosomal dominant and was originally diagnosed in families of Irish/Scottish descent. It is also known as TRAPS (TNF receptor associated periodic syndromes) and gene mutations in the soluble TNFR have been described in a widening range of ethnic groups, including Finnish, French, Australian, North American, and Arab (see later chapters on FMF and periodic fevers).

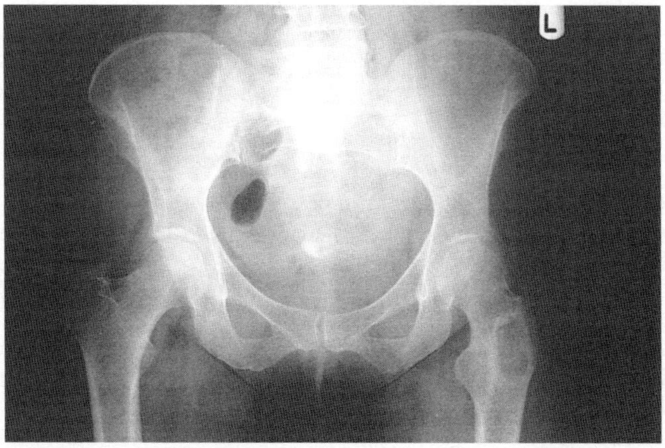

Fig. 1 A 60-year-old woman who presented with left hip pain, weight loss, and low grade pyrexia. Radiographs show erosion in the left greater trochanter and calcified pyometrium. Aspiration and culture of the left greater trochanter bursa revealed *Mycobacterium tuberculosis*.

Continuous or remittent fever

Continuous or remittent fever is an integral feature of some forms of chronic infectious disorders associated with arthritis, for example brucellosis and Lyme disease (O'Connell 1995), and certain forms of vasculitis, for example, Kawasaki's syndrome. The more complex situation arises in the patient with a low grade pyrexia, often with a raised ESR, and in whom infection and neoplasia has been excluded. Rheumatological disorders that can be easily overlooked include Reiter's syndrome, particularly in the younger adult and there is a lack of recognition of the sometimes severe systemic nature of Reiter's syndrome. Moreover, Reiter's syndrome increasingly presents as an 'incomplete' form and the precipitating event may be overlooked, particularly if it was a transient gastrointestinal disturbance. The clinical finding of an enthesitis, sacroiliitis, or asymptomatic oral ulcers would support the diagnosis.

In the middle-aged to elderly population, temporal arteritis, polymyalgia rheumatica, and primary Sjögren's syndrome may present as low grade pyrexia with elevated ESR, with little evidence of the underlying disorder. Specific enquiry about dry eyes and mouth coupled with a simple bedside screening test (e.g. Schirmer's test) may help and the striking diurnal symptoms of polymyalgia may suggest the diagnosis. Elderly onset rheumatoid arthritis may also present as FUO, often associated with other constitutional features such as weight loss and fatigue (Bajocchi et al. 2000). Although this section is not aimed at discussing the differential diagnosis of arthritis plus fever, it should be noted that the country of origin of the person will influence the possible diagnosis—for example, in a community study of children in Turkey, FMF was found to be more prevalent than juvenile idiopathic arthritis (Ozen et al. 1998) and HIV-associated rheumatic diseases usually with lymphadenopathy and weight loss are common in sub-Sharian Africa (Stein and Davis 1996).

Weight loss

Managing musculoskeletal disorders is hampered by the lack of objective, numerical clinical measurements. Weight is a simple measure and weight loss at the onset or during the early stages of several inflammatory joint diseases is not uncommon (Fig. 2).

There is no agreed definition of significant weight loss. Working definitions have included weight loss of 2 kg or more, or a decrease of 10 per cent in body weight. It is rare to have weight loss greater than 10 kg due to arthritis. However, in one series 13 per cent of women with rheumatoid arthritis lost more than 15 per cent of their initial body weight (Munro and Capell 1997). The weight loss tends to plateau after a few months, unlike

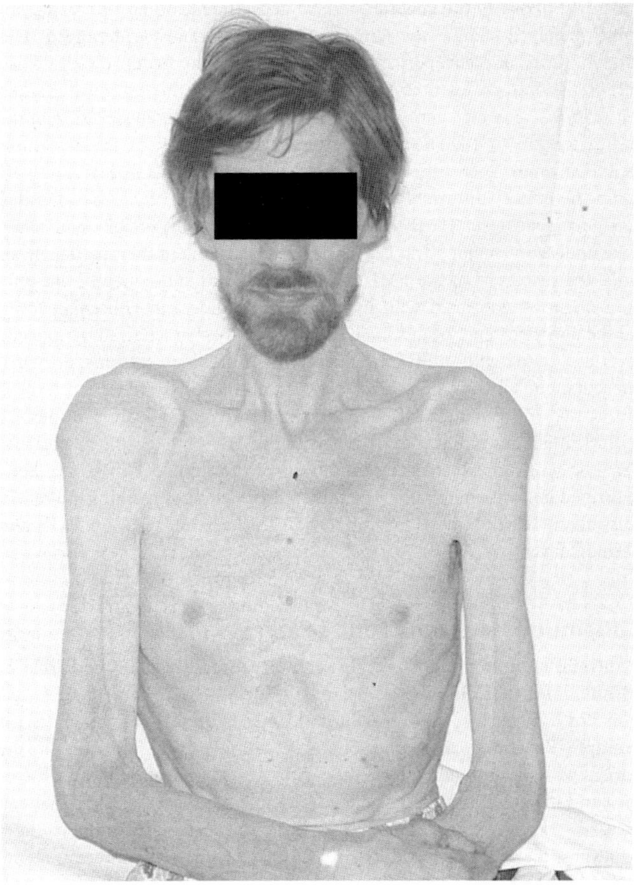

Fig. 2 Profound weight loss in a man with inflammatory polyarthritis, subcutaneous nodules, and low grade persistent pyrexia. The final diagnosis, on histology, was multicentric reticulohistiocytosis.

that associated with malignancy or endocrine disease. Calculation of body mass index [weight (kg)/ height $(m)^2$] offers standardization and in children weight needs to be routinely plotted on growth charts.

In clinical practice, weight loss is most commonly encountered as an early feature of rheumatoid arthritis. It occurs particularly in elderly onset rheumatoid arthritis, being present in 50 per cent of subjects in this age group in one series (Terkeltaub et al. 1983). Often the articular features are mild and atypical. The weight loss is often associated with other systemic features, such as lymphadenopathy and low grade pyrexia (Bajocchi et al. 2000), suggesting a wide range of diagnostic possibilities, particularly lymphoma. There is the suggestion that reduction of lean body mass in rheumatoid arthritis may be related to tumour necrosis factor-α levels (Roubenoff et al. 1992). Munro and Capell (1997) found that 13 per cent of a rheumatoid arthritis population fell into the lowest 5th centile for BMI for the general population. Patients with the greatest weight loss had significantly higher HAQ, ESR, and lower albumin than the other patients.

However, as may be expected, weight loss is not confined to rheumatoid arthritis and can occur in association with any inflammatory joint or connective tissue disorder. It is particularly in the elderly (if associated with rather non-specific symptoms such as in polymyalgia rheumatica, polyarteritis nodosa, or a related inflammatory vasculitis) that the major diagnostic dilemmas emerge, especially in relationship to underlying neoplasms. The evaluation depends upon detailed clinical, radiological, and laboratory assessment, which should include routine urine testing, full blood count, erythrocyte sedimentation rate (or other measure of acute phase response), biochemical profile (including thyroid function and protein electrophoresis), autoantibodies (including antineutrophil cytoplasmic antibodies), and a chest radiograph. Neoplasms which in their turn may mimic musculoskeletal disorders include carcinoma of the bronchus, renal carcinoma, lymphomas, and primary and secondary neoplasms of bone.

Other disorders of the gastrointestinal tract that may present with musculoskeletal features and weight loss include inflammatory bowel disease, Whipple's disease, and adult coeliac disease. A seronegative relapsing oligoarthritis precedes the weight loss and diarrhoea in most cases of Whipple's disease (Puechal 2001). The identification of the organism, *Tropheryma whippellii*, a PCR method for demonstrating bacterial ribosomal RNA at sites of inflammation, a technique of culturing *T. whippellii*, and the development of serological tests for IgG and IgM antibodies to *T. whippellii* all suggest that the clinical spectrum of Whipples disease will be intensively re-evaluated particularly as the serological tests suggest the organism may be ubiquitous (Swartz 2000). It is often the presence of an unusual feature, for example, the failure of an iron deficiency anaemia to respond to oral iron or reticulin or endomysial antibody that suggests adult coeliac disease.

True weight loss in children due to juvenile idiopathic arthritis or related disorders is extremely uncommon, but a downward drift to lower percentile lines on both weight and height growth curves is frequent in active disease. Cabrel and Tucker (1999) reviewed 29 children who were ultimately diagnosed with malignancy but who had been initially referred to rheumatology departments. Common clinical features included weight loss (42 per cent), fever (54 per cent), and fatigue (50 per cent). Features considered atypical for inflammatory arthritis included nocturnal fever in 14 per cent.

Malaise, lethargy, and fatigue

These symptoms give rise to difficulties in medical definition but are frequent clinical complaints. In practice, fatigue is considered to be present and pathological if it causes disability and is unrelieved by rest. While common and well-recognized accompaniments of chronic inflammatory joint and connective tissue disorders, they may be the presenting or sole clinical feature of some disorders that fall within the rheumatological spectrum. Arbitrarily they have been divided on the basis of a normal ESR and raised ESR.

Normal erythrocyte sedimentation rate

Fibromyalgia is probably the most common associated problem. The subject is typically a middle-aged woman with a non-restorative sleep pattern and diffuse pains in a girdle distribution with multiple symmetrical tender points. Clinically, overlap seems to exist with other syndromes, where profound tiredness and lethargy may exist in the absence of clear physical or laboratory abnormalities, in particular the chronic fatigue syndromes (Goldenberg 1993; Straus 1996). Metabolic and endocrine disorders such as periodic hypokalaemic paralysis, Addison's disease, and hypothyroidism need be excluded.

Raised erythrocyte sedimentation rate

Primary Sjögren's syndrome frequently presents under this guise, and lethargy is well recognized as one of the most distressing features (Barendregt et al. 1998). There are no specific features in the history to point to the diagnosis and the patient just complains of intense fatigue. Sleep disturbance may be found but is not as consistent a finding as in fibromyalgia, indeed Sjögren's patients may often sleep for several hours in the afternoon and again through the night. Trigger points are not usually present in Sjögren's syndrome; Giles and Isenberg (2000) finding that only 12 per cent of their primary Sjögren's patients fulfil the criteria for fibromyalgia, otherwise the sex and age distribution is very similar to fibromyalgia. As well as the raised ESR, polyclonal hypergammaglobulinaemia and serological abnormalities such as rheumatoid factor, antinuclear factor, and anti-Ro/La antibodies are often present.

Although less common, profound lethargy with a raised ESR may be the presenting features of bacterial endocarditis, polyarteritis (and the other vasculitides), cryoglobulinaemia, Waldenstrom's macroglobulinaemia, polymyalgia, temporal arteritis and a wide variety of malignancies of which lymphoma, bronchogenic neoplasm, and renal cell carcinoma are probably the most commonly encountered as presenting under a rheumatological guise.

Lymphadenopathy

This alarming finding may occur as a presenting feature in both children and adults.

In children, generalized lymphadenopathy is usual in systemic juvenile idiopathic arthritis and Kawasaki's disease (Bissenden and Hall 1990). However, it has to be remembered that leukaemia in children may also present as polyarthralgia or a true polyarthritis.

In the adult, lymphadenopathy is common in rheumatoid arthritis and the connective tissue disorder, and may occur early in the disease. One study reviewing patients who had undergone lymph node biopsies for unexplained lymphadenopathy and in which the histology had shown reactive hyperplasia, found that one-third of them developed a connective tissue disorder within a year of biopsy (Kelly and Malcolm 1987). A more common clinical problem arises when marked lymphadenopathy develops in a patient with connective tissue disease or rheumatoid arthritis. If, on clinical grounds, it is felt desirable to have a lymph node biopsy to exclude neoplastic disease, then it is important that the histopathologist is informed about the associated connective tissue disorder, as the histological differential diagnosis of marked reactive hyperplasia and giant follicular cell lymphoma may be difficult (Kelly et al. 1987).

Persistent lymphadenopathy above the clavicles usually causes greatest clinical concern. A review of 13 patients with a variety of rheumatological disorders, who had lymph node biopsies of either supraclavicular or cervical lymph nodes because of persisting lymphadenopathy, failed to detect changes other than 'reactive' hyperplasia in any of the biopsies (Kelly et al. 1987). However, lymphadenopathy associated with an atypical seronegative polyarthritis can arise in a wide variety of disorders including angio-immunoblastic lymphadenopathy, lymphoma, sarcoidosis, and Whipple's disease. In these disorders, lymph node biopsy is usually required to establish a diagnosis: in angio-immunoblastic lymphadenopathy, fever and a pleomorphic rash may also occur but the absence of leucocytosis and relentlessly progressive nature of the disease tends to separate it from adult onset Still's disease (Layton et al. 1998).

Specific systems

This section considers some individual systems and their disorders that may be the presenting feature of an underlying rheumatological disorder. It cannot be completely comprehensive as anecdotal reports exist about virtually all known medical disorders being associated with one or other rheumatological condition. It attempts to identify those non-articular 'rheumatological' disorders that are commonly seen either prior to or in a very early stage of the rheumatic disease process (Table 2).

Mucocutaneous systems

Ocular system

The commonest disorder is acute anterior uveitis occurring in association with spondyloarthropathies or reactive arthritis. Other eye problems which should prompt a clinical/serological evaluation for a rheumatological disorder include chronic anterior uveitis (pauciarticular juvenile idiopathic arthritis), uveitis (Behçet's syndrome), episcleritis (relapsing polychondritis), keratoconjunctivitis sicca (primary Sjögren's syndrome), visual loss (temporal arteritis), and cortical blindness (systemic lupus erythematosus), peripheral ulcerative keratitis or 'corneal melt' (rheumatoid arthritis).

Oropharyngeal system

Presenting disorders include xerostomia (primary Sjögren's syndrome), painful oral ulceration (Behçet's syndrome and systemic lupus erythematosus), painless oral ulceration (reactive arthritis), and apparent 'toothache' (temporomandibular joint involvement). Occasionally, apparently unrelated events may suggest a rheumatological disorder (e.g. severe dental caries and primary Sjögren's syndrome, macroglossia and amyloidosis).

Cutaneous system

The vast range of cutaneous features associated with rheumatological disorders is dealt with in Chapter 1.3.2. Table 2 lists some cutaneous disorders that may be the presenting feature of rheumatological disorders. In clinical practice, Raynaud's, psoriasis, various rashes, and vasculitis are the most commonly encountered.

Cardiovascular system

Table 2 lists cardiovascular problems that may be the presenting features. Again, in clinical practice, the most commonly seen are pericarditis (with rheumatoid arthritis, systemic lupus erythematosus, and systemic juvenile idiopathic arthritis) (Kelly et al. 1990), valvular heart disease (with systemic lupus erythematosus and spondyloarthropathies), peripheral ischaemia (with polyarteritis and other forms of medium/large vasculitis) and congenital complete heart block (with maternal, Ro-positive, systemic lupus erythematosus /Sjögren's syndrome) (McCredie et al. 1990). Approximately half the mothers of children born with congenital complete heart block will develop a connective tissue disorder, of which Sjögren's syndrome is the most frequent.

Cardiomyopathies (e.g. with amyloid, polymyositis, and scleroderma) tend to occur late in the natural history of the underlying disease.

Respiratory system

Lung and respiratory tract involvement is common to many rheumatological disorders and breathlessness is a common presenting feature. In clinical practice the most frequently encountered are pleural disease (rheumatoid arthritis and systemic lupus erythematosus), pulmonary fibrosis (rheumatoid arthritis and connective tissue disorders), asthma (Churg–Strauss vasculitis), pulmonary opacities on routine chest radiography (rheumatoid arthritis nodules, Wegener's granulomatosis), bronchial 'irritability' (Sjögren's syndrome), and recurrent thromboembolic disease with antiphospholipid syndrome. Sinus disorders with Wegener's granulomatosis are common.

Gastrointestinal system

Although the associations of rheumatic diseases and gastrointestinal disorders, particularly infectious and chronic inflammatory diseases, is well established, it is more common to see these problems causing diagnostic confusion because of their rheumatological presentation—for example, Crohn's disease, where the gastrointestinal features may be less apparent in the early stages.

Areas of overlap encountered in clinical practice tend to relate to abdominal pain arising from spinal disease, mesenteric vasculitis, polyserositis (e.g. familial Mediterranean fever), or abnormal biochemical tests (particularly liver function tests) detected on 'routine' tests and secondary to an underlying chronic inflammatory rheumatological disease, and apparent bowel disturbance in the irritable bowel/fibromyalgia overlapping group of patients (Wolfe 1989).

Dysphagia in systemic sclerosis is very rarely a presenting complaint.

Urogenital and renal systems

Renal system

Kidney involvement; in the form of microscopic haematuria or proteinura, hypertension or renal failure; is frequently the presenting feature of the

Table 2 Specific system involvement that may be the presenting feature of an underlying rheumatological disorder

System	Involvement	Associated disorder
Ocular		
Blindness/loss of acuity	Cortical involvement	Systemic lupus erythematosus
	Retinal artery thrombosis	Temporal arteritis
	Hyperviscosity syndrome	Primary Sjögren's syndrome
		Secondary Sjögren's syndrome
	Chronic uveitis	Pauciarticular juvenile chronic arthritis
		Behçet's syndrome
Red, painful eye	Acute anterior uveitis	Reiter's syndrome
		Ankylosing spondylitis
		Seronegative spondyloarthritis
		Behçet's syndrome
	Episcleritis	Rheumatoid arthritis
		Relapsing polychondritis
Dry eye	Keratoconjunctivitis	Primary Sjögren's syndrome
		Secondary Sjögren's syndrome
Diplopia		Temporal arteritis
		Systemic lupus erythematosus
		Wegener's granuloma
Changes in sclera pigment	Black	Alkaptonuria (ochronosis)
	Blue	Osteogenesis imperfecta
		Scleromalacia
Proptosis		Wegener's granuloma
Oral		
Painful, oral ulcers		Behçet's syndrome
		Systemic lupus erythematosus
		Stevens–Johnson syndrome
Painless, mucosal erosions		Reiter's syndrome
Dry mouth (xerostomia)		Primary Sjögren's syndrome
		Secondary Sjögren's syndrome
'Toothache'		Temporomandibular joint disease
		Wegener's granulomatosis
Recurrent oral candida		Primary Sjögren's syndrome
Extensive dental caries		Primary Sjögren's syndrome
Limited mouth opening		Systemic sclerosis
		Temporomandibular joint disease
Strawberry tongue		Kawasaki's disease
Cutaneous		
Head and neck	Alopecia	Systemic lupus erythematosus
	Psoriasis	Psoriatic arthritis
	Periorbital rash	Dermatomyositis
	Malar rash	Systemic lupus erythematosus
	Telangiectasia	Systemic sclerosis/CREST syndrome
	Photosensitive	Systemic lupus erythematosus
	Inflammation of pinna	Relapsing polychondritis
	Ear nodules	Tophaceous gout
Hands	Raynaud's	Connective tissue disease
	Nail pitting/onycholysis	Psoriatic arthritis
	Splinter haemorrhages	Rheumatoid arthritis
	Nail-fold infarcts	Connective tissue disorders
	Palmar erythema	Rheumatoid arthritis
	Subcutaneous calcinosis	Systemic sclerosis/CREST syndrome
	Osler's nodes	Connective tissue disorders
	Digit infarction	Polyarteritis
		Systemic sclerosis
	Periungual nodules	Multicentric reticulohistiocytosis
	Knuckle pads	Dupuytren's contracture
	Gottron's sign (collodion)	Dermatomyositis
	Desquamation	Kawasaki's disease
		Reiter's syndrome
Trunk and upper arms	Macular rash	Systemic juvenile chronic arthritis
		Systemic lupus erythematosus
		Rubella arthritis
		Parvovirus arthritis
		Kawasaki's disease
	Papular rash	Behçet's syndrome
	Erythema marginatum	Rheumatic fever
	Subcutaneous nodules	Rheumatoid arthritis
		Rheumatic fever
		Tophaceous gout
		Multicentric reticulohistiocytosis
		Churg–Strauss vasculitis
		Xanthoma (hyperlipidaemic arthritis)
	Vitiligo	Systemic lupus erythematosus
	Increased pigmentation	Haemachromatosis
	Urticaria	Rheumatoid arthritis
		Connective tissue disease
	'Paniculitis' (can occur anywhere)	Eosinophiliic fasciitis
		Systemic lupus erythematosus
		Weber–Christian disease
	Acne fulminans	Pustuloarthritis
Lower limbs and feet	Livedo reticulosis	Connective tissue disease
		Relapsing polychondritis
	Purpura	Henoch–Schönlein disease
		Cryoglobulinaemia
		Primary Sjögren's syndrome
	Erythema nodosum	
	Varicose veins	Hypermobility syndrome (and variants)
	Keratoderma blennorrhagia	Reiter's disease
		Pustula psoriasis
	Infarction	Polyarteritis (and variants)
		Rheumatoid arthritis
	Vasculitic ulcers	Rheumatoid arthritis
		Connective tissue diseases
	Pyoderma gangrenosum (can occur at any site)	Rheumatoid arthritis
		Seronegative spondyloarthritis
Genital	Circinate balanitis	Reiter's syndrome
	Vaginal ulceration	Behçet's syndrome
	Vaginal dryness	Primary Sjögren's syndrome
Gastrointestinal	Dysphagia	Sjögren's syndrome
		Systemic sclerosis/CREST syndrome
	Abdominal pain	Mesenteric vasculitis (polyarteritis nodosa)
		Pancreatitis (systemic lupus erythematosus/ Sjögren's syndrome)
		Referred pain (thoracic spine)
	Bowel disturbance	Crohn's disease (spondyloarthritis)
		Irritable bowel (fibromyalgia)
		Malabsorption (Whipple's disease)
		Diarrhoea (ulcerative colitis; ischaemic colitis; systemic sclerosis)
	Abnormal liver function	Rheumatoid arthritis
		Sjögren's syndrome
		Systemic lupus erythematosus

Table 2 Continued

System	Involvement	Associated disorder
		CREST/primary biliary cirrhosis overlap
		Juvenile chronic polyarthritis
	Splenomegaly	Rheumatoid arthritis
		Systemic juvenile chronic arthritis
Respiratory	Upper airway disease	Rheumatoid arthritis (cricoarytenoid)
		Wegener's granuloma
		Primary Sjögren's syndrome
		Relapsing polychondritis
	Obstructive lung disease	Churg–Strauss vasculitis
	Interstitial lung disease:	
	Pulmonary fibrosis	Rheumatoid arthritis
		Connective tissue disorders
		Sjögren's syndrome
		Sarcoidosis
		Ankylosing spondylitis
	Restrictive defects	Systemic lupus erythematosus (shrinking lung)
		Ankylosing spondylitis
	Pulmonary opacities	Rheumatoid arthritis
		Caplan's syndrome
		Wegener's granuloma
	Pleural disease	Rheumatoid arthritis
		Connective tissue disease (mainly systemic lupus erythematosus)
		Thromboembolic (antiphospholipid syndrome)
		Familial Mediterranean fever
	Pulmonary hypertension	Systemic sclerosis
		Antiphospholipid syndrome
Cardiovascular	Thrombotic and thromboembolic	Antiphospholipid syndrome
		Systemic lupus erythematosus
	Pericardial	Juvenile chronic arthritis
		Rheumatic fever
		Rheumatoid arthritis
		Systemic lupus erythematosus
	Myocarditis	Polymyositis
		Rheumatic fever
		Amyloidosis
		Haemochromatosis
	Endocarditis	Systemic lupus erythematosus
		Rheumatic fever
	Valvular heart disease	Rheumatoid arthritis
		Ankylosing spondylitis
		Rheumatic fever
		Systemic lupus erythematosus
		Antiphospholipid syndrome
		Hypermobility syndrome
	Conduction defects	Maternal systemic lupus erythematosus with anti-Ro antibodies
		Rheumatoid nodules
	Coronary arteritis	Kawasaki's disease
		Polyarteritis nodosa
	'Anterior chest pain'	Seronegative spondyloarthritis
		Reiter's syndrome
		Teitze's syndrome
		Thoracic spine disease

Table 2 Continued

Nephrological/ urogenital		
Renal	Glomerulonephritis	Systemic lupus erythematosus
		Polyarteritis
		Relapsing polychondritis
		Cryoglobulinaemia
		Wegener's granulomatosis
	Interstitial nephritis	Primary Sjögren's syndrome
		Gout
	'Arteritis'	Systemic sclerosis
Collecting system	Renal calculi	Gout/hyperuricaemia
Bladder		Systemic sclerosis
Urethra	Urethritis	Reiter's syndrome
	Genital ulceration	Gonococcal
		Behçet's syndrome
Recurrent spontaneous abortion		Antiphospholipid syndrome
		Systemic lupus erythematosus
Impotence		Systemic sclerosis
		Large-vessel vasculitis
Neurological		Systemic lupus erythematosus
Psychiatric and disorders of cognitive function		
Involuntary movement	Epilepsy	Systemic lupus erythematosus
		Polyarteritis
	Chorea	Systemic lupus erythematosus
		Rheumatic fever
Focal cerebral disorders		Systemic lupus erythematosus
		Polyarteritis
		Behçet's syndrome
		Temporal arteritis
		Hyperviscosity syndromes
Cranial nerve lesions		Systemic lupus erythematosus
		Temporal arteritis
		Sarcoid
		Behçet's syndrome
Paraplegias		Cervical spondylosis
		Intervertebral disc lesions
		Rheumatoid arthritis
		Systemic lupus erythematosus
		Ossification of posterior longitudinal ligament
Neuropathies	Vasculitis	Rheumatoid arthritis
		Polyarteritis nodosa
		Relapsing polychondritis
	Entrapment	Inflammatory polyarthritis
		Diffuse idiopathic skeletal hyperostosis
		Osteoarthritis
	Nerve root	Prolapsed vertebral disc
		Spondylosis
		Cervical rib
Headache		Cervical spondylosis
		Temporal arteritis
		Systemic lupus erythematosus
		Fibromyalgia
		Hyperviscosity
		Behçet's syndrome

CREST, Calcinosis, Raynaud's (o)esophageal dysphagia, sclerodactyly, telangiectasia syndrome.

connective tissue disorders (e.g. systemic lupus erythematosus, polyarteritis). Renal tubular acidosis (detected either clinically as secondary osteomalacia or biochemically) may be a presenting feature of primary Sjögren's syndrome (Maher 1989). Renal calculi may develop prior to clinical gout. Acute hypertensive renal failure can be the presenting feature of systemic sclerosis. Conversely, renal carcinoma may present under a 'rheumatological' guise, often mimicking polymyalgia rheumatica.

Male urogenital tract

Urethritis is the rule with both gonococcal and non-gonococcal sexually acquired arthritis. It may also occur in reactive arthritis secondary to gastrointestinal infections. Balanitis occurs and may reoccur in Reiter's syndrome without fresh exposure to infectious agents (Fisk 1982).

Impotence is a rare presenting feature of large vessel vasculitis (mimicking the Le Riche syndrome) and is not uncommon in systemic sclerosis. Peyronies' disease associates with other disorders of collagen deposition (e.g. Dupuytren's contracture, knuckle pads, and systemic sclerosis).

Female urogenital tract

Probably the most common presenting disorders are dyspareunia (with primary Sjögren's syndrome), recurrent spontaneous abortion (with the antiphospholipid syndrome) (Hughes 1983; Hughes et al. 1989), vaginal ulceration (Behçet's), and vaginal prolapse (hypermobility syndrome and its variants) (Al Rawi and Al Rawi 1982).

Neurological system

Disorders affecting this system are frequently the presenting complaint in rheumatological disease.

The wide diversity of neurological features occurring in systemic lupus erythematosus is well recognized. Entrapment neuropathies, most often carpal tunnel, is a presenting complaint in inflammatory joint disease. Mononeuritis is common in polyarteritis. Headaches are a feature of temporal arteritis and cervical spondylosis. Migraine occurs more commonly in systemic lupus erythematosus and Sjögren's syndrome (Pal et al. 1989). Spastic quadriplegia may be the presenting feature of cervical spondylosis and ossification of the posterior longitudinal ligament, particularly in Japanese subjects.

Clinical patterns

The varied nature of clinical medicine means that every physician will have anecdotes about bizarre presentations of relatively common disorders.

Certain patterns of disease occur sufficiently frequently that the confirmation or exclusion of an underlying 'rheumatological' disorder is essential. The commonest problems encountered in the United Kingdom are described below.

Children

The ill, febrile child with a rash suggests the need to exclude systemic juvenile idiopathic arthritis. Recognition of significant articular pathology is not easy in a small, unhappy, and irritable child.

Young women

Multisystem disease in young women should always raise the possibility of systemic lupus erythematosus. It is in this group that serological tests are most likely to be helpful.

Young men

Reactive arthritis, either sexually or gastrointestinally acquired, frequently causes a systemic illness of greater severity than is usually described by medical textbooks. In an ill, febrile young man with weight loss and a subacute history, a careful search for clues (e.g. mild back pain and stiffness, a single swollen metatarsal phalangeal joint or toe, or tenderness under the calcanum may provide clinical pointers).

Middle-aged women

Three main diagnostic groups may present in a 'non-rheumatological guise'.

Rheumatoid arthritis presents not infrequently in a non-articular fashion. Pulmonary or pleuropericardial involvement tends to be the most frequent manifestation.

Two disorders may present as marked malaise or lethargy associated with other non-specific symptoms. The symptom complex of 'fibromyalgia' is suggested by the finding of multiple tender points and normal screening laboratory investigations. Primary Sjögren's syndrome often also presents in this non-specific fashion. Specific questions about ocular and oral dryness suggest the diagnosis and laboratory investigations (particularly raised ESR, positive antinuclear antibodies and rheumatoid factor, and Ro or La antibodies) are often surprisingly abnormal against a relatively normal physical examination.

Middle-aged men

Rheumatoid arthritis presenting either pleuropericardial disease or pulmonary involvement is common. Polyarteritis nodosum may also cause diagnostic confusion in this group with its variety of clinical features ranging from malaise through to mononeuritis multiplex.

Elderly women

Two disorders commonly cause diagnostic confusion—polymyalgia rheumatica when it presents as a systemic disease with malaise, weight loss, and FUO (Myklebus and Gran 1996).

Secondly, tophaceous gout is increasingly common in the elderly female taking diuretics. The lesions on the distal interphalangeal joints are often diagnosed as Heberden's nodes and ulcerating lesions adjacent to the first metatarsal phalangeal joint attributed to either vascular insufficiency or trophic changes.

Elderly men

Extra-articular presentation of rheumatic disorders is less common in this age group. More commonly one encounters the reverse situation of non-rheumatological disorders (particularly neoplastic) presenting under a rheumatological guise of either joint or bone pain of a paraneoplastic syndrome.

Conclusions

The recognition of an underlying rheumatological diagnosis as the cause of non-articular disease is not merely an academic exercise. To overlook certain diagnoses (e.g. systemic lupus erythematosus or temporal arteritis) may have severe consequences in terms of morbidity and mortality. Furthermore, to pursue increasingly invasive investigations in a patient with fibromyalgia exposes them to all the risks of iatrogenesis.

Ultimately, the establishment of the underlying cause usually depends upon clinical acumen, often helped by maintaining an 'open mind' when diagnostic uncertainty exists, and the passage of time.

References

Al Rawi, Z.S. and Al Rawi, Z.T. (1982). Joint hypermobility in women with genital prolapse. *Lancet* **i**, 1439–41.

Bajocchi, G., La Corte, R., Locapato, A., Govoni, M., and Trotta F. (2000). Elderly onset RA: clinical aspects. *Clinical and Experimental Rheumatology* **18**, 549–50.

Barendregt, P.J. et al. (1998). Fatigue in primary Sjögren's syndrome. *Annals of the Rheumatic Diseases* **57**, 291–5.

Berkwits, M. and Gluckman, S. (1997). Seeking an expert interpretation. *New England Journal of Medicine* **337**, 1682–4.

Bissenden, J.G. and Hall, S. (1990). Kawaski syndrome: lessons for Britain. *British Medical Journal* **300**, 1025–6.

Cabral, D.A. and Tucker, L.B. (1999). Malignancies in children who initially present with rheumatic complaints. *Journal of Paediatrics* **134**, 53–7.

Davies, G.R. and Finch, R.G. (2001). Fever of unknown origin. *Clinical Medicine* **1**, 177–9.

Doherty, M., Abawi, J., and Pattrick, M. (1990). Audit of medical inpatient examination: a cry from the joint. *Journal of the Royal College of Physicians* **24**, 115–8.

Fisk, P. (1982). Reiter's disease. *British Medical Journal* **284**, 3–4.

Giles, I. and Isenberg, D. (2000). Fatigue in primary Sjögren's syndrome: is there a link with the fibromyalgia syndrome? *Annals of the Rheumatic Diseases* **59**, 875–8.

Goldenberg, D.L. (1993). Fibromyalgia, chronic fatigue syndrome and mycofacial pain syndrome. *Current Opinion in Rheumatology* **5**, 199–208.

Hughes, G.R.V. (1983). Thrombosis, abortion, cerebral disease and the lupus anti-coagulant. *British Medical Journal* **287**, 1088–9.

Hughes, G.R.V., Asherson, R.A., and Khamashta, M.A. (1989). Anti-phospholipid syndrome: linking many specialties. *Annals of the Rheumatic Diseases* **48**, 355–6.

Kelly, C.A. and Malcolm, A.J. (1987). The significance of hyperplastic lymphadenopathy. *British Journal of Hospital Medicine* **37**, 159–60.

Kelly, C.A., Malcolm, A., and Griffiths, I.D. (1990). Chronic pericardial disease in patients with rheumatoid arthritis. *Quarterly Journal of Medicine* **277**, 461–70.

Kelly, C.A., Bourke, J.P., Malcolm, A., and Griffiths, I.D. (1987). Lymphadenopathy in rheumatic patients. *Annals of the Rheumatic Diseases* **46**, 224–7.

Knockaert, D.C., Vanneste, L.J., and Bobbaers, H.J. (1993). Recurrent or episodic fever of unknown origin. *Medicine* **72**, 184–96.

Knockaert, D.C., Vanneste, L.J., Vanneste, S.B., and Bobbaers, H.J. (1992). Fever of unknown origin in the 1980s. *Archives of Internal Medicine* **152**, 51–5.

Layton, M.A., Musgrove, C., and Dawes, P.T. (1998) Polyarthritis, rash and lymphadenopathy: case reports of two patients with angioimmunoblastic lymphadenopathy presenting to a rheumatology clinic. *Clinical Rheumatology* **17**, 148–51.

Maher, E.R. (1989). Renal tubular acidosis. *British Journal of Hospital Medicine* **42**, 116–19.

Martin, K., Davies, E.G., and Axford, J.S. (1994). Fever of unknown origin in childhood: difficulties in diagnosis. *Annals of the Rheumatic Diseases* **53**, 429–33.

McCredie, M., Celermajor, J., Sholler, G., Kelly, D., Chivers, T., Wang, Y., and Schrieber, L. (1990). Case control study of C.C.H.B.: association with maternal antibodies to Ro and La. *British Journal of Rheumatology* **29**, 10–14.

Munro, R. and Capell, H. (1997). The prevalence of low body mass in rheumatoid arthritis: association with the acute phase response. *Annals of the Rheumatic Diseases* **56**, 326–9.

Myklebust, G. and Gran, J.T. (1996). A prospective study of 287 patients with polymyalgia rheumatica and temporal arteritis. *British Journal of Rheumatology* **35**, 1161–68.

O'Connell, S. (1995). Lyme disease in the United Kingdom. *British Medical Journal* **310**, 303–8.

Ozen, S., Karaaslan, Y., Ozdemir, O., Saatai, U., Bakkaloglu, A., Koroglu, E., and Tezcan, S. (1998). Prevalence of juvenile chronic arthritis and FMF in Turkey: a field study. *Journal of Rheumatology* **25**, 2445–9.

Pal, B., Gibson, C., Passmore, J., Griffiths, I.D., and Dick, W.C. (1989). A study of headaches and migraine in Sjögren's syndrome and other rheumatic disorders. *Annals of the Rheumatic Diseases* **48**, 312–16.

Petersdorf, R.G. and Beeson, P.B. (1961). Fever of unexplained origin: report on 100 cases. *Medicine* **40**, 1–30.

Pinals, R.S. (1994). Polyarthritis and fever. *New England Journal of Medicine* **330**, 769–74.

Pouchot, J. et al. (1991). Adult Still's disease: manifestations, disease course and outcome in 62 patients. *Medicine* **70**, 118–36.

Puechal, X. (2001). Whipple's disease and arthritis. *Current Opinion in Rheumatology* **13**, 74–9.

Roubenoff, R., Roubenoff, R.A., Ward, L., Hollands, S., and Hellman, D. (1992). Rheumatoid cachexia: depletion of lean body mass in rheumatoid arthritis. Possible association with tumour necrosis factor. *Journal of Rheumatology* **19**, 1505–10.

Stein, C.M. and Davis, P. (1996). Arthritis associated with HIV infection in Zimbabwe. *Journal of Rheumatology* **23**, 506–11.

Straus, S.E. (1996). Chronic fatigue syndrome. *British Medical Journal* **313**, 831–2.

Swartz, M.N. (2000). Whipple's disease—past, present and future. *New England Journal of Medicine* **342**, 648–50.

Terkeltaub, R., Esdaile, J., De'Cary, F., and Tannenbaum, H. (1983). A clinical study of older age rheumatoid arthritis with comparison to a younger onset group. *Journal of Rheumatology* **10**, 418–24.

Wolfe, F. (1989). The fibromyalgia syndrome. *Rheumatic Disease Clinics of North America* **15**, 1–18.

Wouter, J. and Van de Putte, L. (1986). Adult onset Still's disease; clinical and laboratory features, treatment and progress of 45 cases. *Quarterly Journal of Medicine* **61**, 1055–65.

1.3 Views from different perspectives

1.3.1 Pregnancy and lactation

1.3.1.1 Pregnancy

Yaël A. de Man and J. Mieke Hazes

Introduction

Pregnancy has an important impact on many rheumatic diseases. This may be either a dramatic improvement like in rheumatoid arthritis (RA) or a deterioration as in systemic lupus erythematosus (SLE). In addition, the disease may influence the outcome of the pregnancy by causing recurrent spontaneous abortions, still birth, or congenital abnormalities. The changes in the course of rheumatic diseases during pregnancy can be explained by the major changes in the immune system of the mother in order to enable her to maintain the partially non-self foetus. The immunological phenomena that are part of the rheumatic diseases may influence the pregnancy itself and the health of the foetus.

As soon as a patient indicates that she wants to become pregnant, the physician needs to pay extra attention. The medication has to be changed often and the physician should be alert to potential decreased fertility or frequent early miscarriages. Sometimes the gynaecologist has to be consulted at an early stage. Depending on the underlying disease, the frequency of the clinic visits has to be increased to monitor the woman and foetus in close cooperation with a specialized obstetrician. The delivery can cause problems either for the mother or for the child and needs specialist supervision. After delivery, breastfeeding and the risk of a flare in some of the rheumatic diseases require adjustments of the medication. Additional non-medical measures might be needed to lighten the physical task of the mother in caring for her baby. This chapter deals with the influence of pregnancy on the course and outcome of the rheumatic diseases, the effect of the rheumatic diseases on the course and outcome of the pregnancy for mother (obstetric complications), and child, fertility and disease management before, during, and after pregnancy.

Rheumatoid arthritis

Effect of pregnancy on maternal disease

Amelioration of signs and symptoms of RA during pregnancy is a consistent finding throughout the RA literature, starting with the classical observation by Hench (1938). The improvement of RA occurs in about 75 per cent of the patients. In retrospective studies, improvement of the arthritis is reported in 54–83 per cent (Nelson and Ostensen 1997), in prospective studies in 66–86 per cent (Nelson and Ostensen 1997; Barret et al. 1999). The most recent and largest study showed widespread variability of disease response during pregnancy with 16 per cent of the patients experiencing a complete remission (Barret et al. 1999) in contrast to the high remission rate of 53 per cent reported by Nelson and Ostensen (1997). The reported amelioration of RA in pregnancy is probably an underestimation of the favourable effect of pregnancy as patients will diminish or stop their antirheumatic medication during gestation. The improvement of RA starts in the first trimester of the pregnancy to reach its peak in the second and third trimesters.

RA typically deteriorates after delivery starting in the first month post-partum. After 3–4 months post-partum, most women will experience disease recurrence. Upto 90 per cent of the women will get active disease after childbirth, irrespective of whether they had a remission during pregnancy or not (Nelson and Ostensen 1997).

Prediction of the pregnancy effect on RA

The disease response during previous pregnancies is predictive for the disease response in subsequent pregnancies (Nelson and Ostensen 1997; Barret et al. 1999). The post-partum flare—or the absence of a post-partum flare—cannot be predicted. Presence of rheumatoid factor, age, disease duration, functional class, or parity have no influence on the RA response during or after pregnancy.

Pregnancy in relation to onset and outcome of RA

RA onset

Women who never had children have an approximately two-fold risk of developing RA compared to women who have children (Hazes et al. 1990; Spector et al. 1990; Nelson and Ostensen 1997). This conclusion can also be reversed by stating that women who have been pregnant have an approximately two-fold reduced risk of developing RA compared to nulliparous women. Notably, one hardly sees women develop RA during pregnancy, but the onset of RA in the post-partum period is a well-known phenomenon. This has been confirmed in several studies showing a reduced risk of onset during pregnancy, odds ratios between 0.2 and 0.6, and an increased risk of onset in the 3-month post-partum period, odds ratios between 3.4 and 5.6 (Silman et al. 1992; Lansink et al. 1993; Nelson and Ostensen 1997). Breastfeeding, in particular after the first pregnancy, has been implicated as being responsible for the increased risk of RA onset after pregnancy or for the post-partum flare in established RA (Brennan and Silman 1994; Barret et al. 2000). Whether pregnancy really reduces the risk of RA or just delays the onset of symptoms through its ameliorating effect on the disease is still debated, though the latter explanation appears the most acceptable. There are some studies that question a reduced lifetime risk of RA due to pregnancy or breastfeeding (Hernandez-Avila et al. 1990; Brun et al. 1995).

Outcome of RA

Patients often ask whether pregnancy will affect the ultimate outcome of their disease. The amelioration during pregnancy and post-partum flare appear to have no net effect on the prognosis of RA (Nelson and Ostensen 1997). In the only prospective study trying to answer this question, a trend was found to a more favourable outcome in patients who had ever been pregnant compared to women who were never pregnant; this trend was, however, not significant (Drossaers-Bakker et al. 2002).

Table 1 summarizes the clinical observations in relation to RA and pregnancy.

Mechanisms explaining the favourable effect of pregnancy

The possible mechanisms by which pregnancy decreases disease activity in RA have intrigued doctors and scientists for many decades with no conclusive explanation till now. Doctors have tried to copy the favourable effect by treating patients with blood, placental products, or serum from pregnant women without much success. The hormonal, immunological, and biochemical changes during pregnancy have all been considered as possible causes of the pregnancy-induced remission in RA (Nelson and Ostensen 1997; Kanik and Wilder 2000). Increased serum cortisol concentrations did not explain the amelioration of RA probably because the concomitant elevation of steroid binding globulin. The elevated levels of sex hormones also could not satisfactorily explain the pregnancy-induced remission in RA. Treatment with female hormones exerts no or only a modest effect on disease activity in RA (Kanik and Wilder 2000). Many other hormones are increased during pregnancy. The hormonal shifts are associated with shifts in cytokine profiles. Pregnancy is characterized by a decreased production of T-helper1 (Th1) associated cytokines (like IL-1 and interferon-gamma), an increased production of Th2 associated cytokines (like IL-4 and IL-10) and decreased production of proinflammatory cytokines (TNF-alpha, IL-12) (Kanik and Wilder 2000). Since RA is marked by a Th1 cytokine profile, a shift towards a Th2 cytokine profile during pregnancy is an attractive explanation for a pregnancy-induced remission in RA. Exposure of foetal (paternal) non-self HLA antigens to the mother is also implicated in the causation of pregnancy induced amelioration of RA. Disparity of maternal–foetal HLA-DR and particularly HLA-DQ correlated with amelioration of the arthritis during pregnancy (Nelson and Ostensen 1997). These findings fit well with the fact that not all patients will improve

Table 1 Clinical observations in relation to RA and pregnancy

Issues	Clinical observation
During pregnancy	
Disease activity	Amelioration or remission in about 75% (peak third trimester)
Onset RA	A two- to five-fold decreased risk to develop RA during pregnancy in healthy women
Obstetric problems (pre-eclampsia)	None, or probably none
Foetal outcome	No significant differences compared to healthy women and their babies
Delivery	No problems, unless severe hip arthritis
Post-partum	
Disease activity	Flare in 90% of patients within 6 months
Breastfeeding	Breastfeeding may increase the risk to develop (two- to five-fold) or deteriorate RA post-partum
Maternal care	Need for extra assistance for mother and child
Long-term (>10 years)	No adverse effect but also no apparent favourable effect
Fertility	Equal to healthy women
Fecundity	Possibly decreased

during pregnancy and that a favourable response in a previous pregnancy will predict a similar response in a subsequent pregnancy. The studies till now are, however, not conclusive (Van der Horst-Bruinsma et al. 1998; Brennan et al. 2000).

Changes in the levels of α-2 pregnancy-associated protein (PAG) parallel the timing of arthritis amelioration during, and return after, pregnancy and are therefore also indicated as a possible explanation for the pregnancy-induced changes in RA. The studies on this topic are also not conclusive (Nelson and Ostensen 1997). Recently, a correlation was found between the increase during pregnancy and decrease post-partum of glycosylation of IgG and the clinical course of RA in that period (Alavi et al. 2000), though the significance of this finding is still not clear. Table 2 summarizes the possible mechanisms that account for the pregnancy effect on disease activity of RA.

Fertility

Women with RA were found to have smaller family sizes than controls, which could not be attributed to lower fertility (Nelson and Ostensen 1997). Women with RA appear to need a longer time to conceive (lower fecundity). Many possible explanations have been put forward such as ovulatory dysfunction, tubal abnormalities, antibodies to spermatozoa, and hormonal disturbances. Another reason for delayed conception could be a decrease in the frequency of intercourse owing to pain from the arthritis. The physician should be aware of the potential increased time to conception because of pain or low fecundity in order to timely discuss the issue with the woman and, if necessary, refer her to a gynaecologist. Patients often stop or lower their antirheumatic medication the moment they seriously make efforts to get pregnant. When it takes a long time before the woman conceives—or knows she cannot conceive—she is also without adequate antirheumatic medication for an unnecessarily long time, a situation that should be avoided.

Obstetric problems and foetal outcome

Labour and delivery are usually uneventful in women with RA and there is no increased risk of foetal loss, prematurity, or low birth weight. There is one study showing a higher risk for pre-eclampsia among patients with inflammatory arthritis compared to the general population (Skomsvoll et al. 2000). In that study, the case group did not only include RA but also ankylosing spondylitis (AS) and juvenile idiopathic arthritis (JIA), which prohibits specific conclusions for RA. In rare cases, a normal vaginal delivery is not possible because of severe hip arthritis. If a caesarean section under general anaesthesia is required, special precaution has to be taken in case of atlanto-axial subluxation of the spine.

Table 2 Possible mechanisms that account for the pregnancy effect on disease activity of RA

Mechanisms	Account for amelioration of RA
Hormonal	
Cortisol	Probably not; serum levels rise along with steroid binding globulin
Female sex hormones	Explain insufficiently the amelioration of RA and when given as a treatment it has at the most a modest effect on disease activity
Immunological	
Cytokines	
Shift in Th1 (IL1 and INF-γ) and Th2 (IL-4 and IL-10) cytokine profiles	Possible; not yet determined for well defined RA patients
Decreased pro-inflammatory (TNF-α, IL-12)	Possible; not yet determined for well defined RA patients
Maternal–foetal HLA disparity HLA–DR, HLA–DQ	Possible HLA–DQ correlates, but there are conflicting results in literature
Biochemical	
Increased α-2 pregnancy-associated protein (PAG) levels	Possible; changes in PAG parallels the timing of amelioration and deterioration of RA during pregnancy
Increased glycosylation of IgG	Possible; levels change along with the clinical course

Ankylosing spondylitis

Effect of pregnancy on maternal disease

Unlike the pregnancy effects in RA, disease activity in AS does not substantially change during pregnancy. Amelioration of the disease is found in 20–31 per cent, aggravation in 28–33 per cent, and no change in 33–60 per cent. A post-partum aggravation of AS is seen in 45–87 per cent of the women depending on whether women were studied retrospectively or prospectively (Ostensen 1992; Gran and Ostensen 1998; Ostensen and Ostensen 1998). In retrospect, women tend to forget their post-partum deterioration. The differences in the percentages are due to the heterogeneity of the studied populations. In general, spinal disease remains unchanged during pregnancy while peripheral arthritis and uveitis are suppressed during gestation and tend to exacerbate after delivery. The post-partum flare correlates with the disease activity during conception (Ostensen and Ostensen 1998).

Prediction of pregnancy effect on AS

Improvement of AS activity during pregnancy—if any—is predicted by a history of peripheral arthritis. Women carrying a female foetus appear to fare better than women pregnant with a male foetus (Ostensen and Ostensen 1998). This effect may be attributed to hormonal differences in pregnancies of a male or female child. Patients who get pregnant during active disease tend to have active disease in the post-partum period and—in case of spinal disease—will also experience many problems during pregnancy because of unchanged or even aggravated disease activity. Patients with predominantly spinal disease are therefore advised not to get pregnant during a very active period of their disease. Post-partum flares in AS have no relation with breastfeeding or the return of menses after delivery (Ostensen 1992).

Pregnancy in relation to the onset of AS

The onset of AS symptoms typically occurs at the childbearing age. Consequently, the onset of AS around pregnancy would not be rare. Ostensen and Ostensen (1998) found a pregnancy-related onset of AS in 21 per cent of 939 studied patients. For AS not associated with psoriasis or inflammatory bowel disease, the onset of AS seems to be slightly more often in the post-partum period than during pregnancy. This slightly increased onset post-partum can be explained in several ways: (i) high physical demands on the mother in caring for her new-born; (ii) a methodological flaw, comparing the 9 months risk of onset during pregnancy with the 6 months post-partum risk; (iii) a real increased post-partum risk of onset of AS. The risk of pregnancy-related onset of AS—if any—appears to be low.

Fertility

In a large multinational study, women with AS had 2.4 pregnancies per woman, with an average of two children per woman (Ostensen and Ostensen 1998). These figures do not differ from the situation in the general population of those countries, indicating that there is no decreased fertility in AS.

Obstetric problems and foetal outcome

Foetal outcome is not compromised in AS (Gran and Ostensen 1998; Ostensen and Ostensen 1998). Women with AS have no increased risk for foetal loss, prematurity, or low birth weight. Delivery may be a problem in advanced hip disease. This is, however, rarely the case in this age group and a normal vaginal delivery can be expected. Caesarean section was reported more frequently in AS women (28 per cent) than expected from the figures reported for healthy women in North America and Europe (Ostensen and Ostensen 1998). In 58 per cent, AS was mentioned as the reason for the caesarean section. The decision to perform a caesarean section may be influenced by the inclination of the obstetrician to choose primary surgical delivery for women with inflammatory joint disease of the pelvic region and not by actual peri-partum problems.

Juvenile idiopathic arthritis

The onset of JIA is by definition before the childbearing age, so all patients will be confronted with the possible effects of their disease on reproduction and fertility. In a recent study, at least one-third of female JIA patients were advised against having children, in particular by doctors (Ostensen et al. 2000). There are no good reasons for such negative advice, however, since the outcome of pregnancy in JIA is good.

Effect of pregnancy on maternal disease

The effect of pregnancy on disease activity in JIA is very similar to that in RA (Ostensen 1997; Musiej-Nowakowska and Ploski 1999; Ostensen et al. 2000). About 60 per cent of the patients will experience amelioration and 10–20 per cent an aggravation. The favourable effect of pregnancy on disease activity is pre-eminently seen in patients with polyarticular disease, although patients with pauciarticular disease also showed a high remission rate of the disease during pregnancy (Musiej-Nowakowska and Ploski 1999). The remission rate during pregnancy of systemic disease is generally much lower than the remission rate of the other forms of JIA.

Post-partum flares are common, even in women who did not have a change in their disease activity during pregnancy. In about 60 per cent, the disease will flare in the post-partum period, mostly in the first 6 months after delivery. In the study of pauciarticular JIA (Musiej-Nowakowska and Ploski 1999) the post-partum flare seemed to be predicted by active disease before pregnancy and by breastfeeding. The flare related to breastfeeding occurred only when the breastfeeding was stopped. Analogous to RA, the experience of previous pregnancies appears to predict the response of the disease to subsequent pregnancies.

Pregnancy complications and foetal outcome

Pregnancy generally passes without extra problems. Consequences of the JIA influence the mode of delivery; severe hip involvement may prevent normal vaginal delivery. This problem is probably encountered more often in JIA than in RA because of the relative long duration of the disease in JIA. Similarly, patients with JIA may have more problems in caring for their babies than RA patients because of the more extensive joint impairments.

Early case series showed no evidence of adverse foetal outcome in terms of increased abortion rate, still birth, pre-term birth, or intrauterine growth retardation. In a recent controlled study, however, a significantly higher rate of miscarriages was seen in JIA patients than in healthy controls, 20.8 and 9.5 per cent, respectively (Ostensen et al. 2000).

Fertility

Fertility appears to be normal in JIA, but patients report more difficulties in getting pregnant during 1 year of unprotected intercourse than healthy controls (Ostensen et al. 2000). The lower chance to conceive (fecundity) may be due to the higher frequency of gynaecological problems that were also found more often in the JIA patients than in the healthy controls. Ultimately, the number of pregnancies was similar for JIA and healthy controls with an average of 2.3 pregnancy per woman.

Systemic lupus erythematosus

In pregnancies associated with SLE both maternal and foetal problems are common. Maternal disease outcome and maternal obstetric complications will be discussed separately from foetal and neonatal outcome (Table 3).

The maternal perspective

Effect of pregnancy on maternal disease: lupus flare

Despite all the conflicting results in the literature, there is some agreement that the frequency of flares is higher in pregnant than in non-pregnant SLE patients (Khamashta et al. 1997; Petri 1997; Georgiou et al. 2000). Considering the often heterogeneous patient populations studied and the very different ways flares were assessed, the similarity of the results in the different studies support the clinical impression that SLE patients tend to

Table 3 Consequences of pregnancy in SLE

Consequences	Risk factors
Maternal perspective	
Effect of pregnancy on SLE flares	
(a) More than two-fold risk of flares	Active disease before conception
(b) No time preference of flares	
(c) Flares not more severe than outside pregnancy	
Effect of SLE on pregnancy: obstetric complications	
(a) Hypertension	Renal flare, prednisone
Pre-eclampsia	Renal flare, prednisone
(b) Thrombosis	
—deep venous thrombosis	Antiphospholipid syndrome
—stroke	Antiphospholipid syndrome
(c) Diabetes mellitus	Prednisone
Hyperglycaemia	Prednisone
Bladder infections	Medications?
(d) Premature rupture of membranes	Probably multifactorial
More frequent caesarean section	Multifactorial
(e) Rare obstetric complications (uterine rupture, bilateral retinal detachment during labour, severe retinopathy, HELLP)	Renal flare, APLS, and medication
Foetal perspective	
(a) Overall a two-fold risk of foetal loss	
(b) First trimester	
—probable increased frequency of spontaneous abortions	Active disease? APLS?
(c) Second and third trimesters	
—increased frequency of foetal loss	Antiphospholipid syndrome (particularly in LA) Low renal function Low serum C3
(d) Pre-term birth and intrauterine growth retardation	
—24–59% pre-term deliveries	Active disease in general Renal disease and hypertension Prednisone Poor obstetric history (anticoagulant therapy because of antiphospholipid syndrome)
Neonatal outcome	
(a) Neonatal lupus syndrome	
Transient	
—skin rashes	Anti-SSA/Ro and Anti-SSB/La
—cytopaenias	
—hepatosplenomegaly	
—myocarditis/pericarditis	
Permanent	
—complete heart block	Anti-SSA/Ro and Anti-SSB/La

flare during pregnancy. In nearly all studies the frequencies of flares during pregnancy were higher than 57 per cent, with flare rates ranging from 0.06 to 0.136 per patient-month, compared to very consistent flare rates in control groups of 0.039–0.054 per patient-month. The flares during pregnancy are not more severe than outside pregnancy and they mostly affect the skin and the joints (Khamastha et al. 1997; Georgiou et al. 2000), though others found less musculoskeletal flares and more renal and haematologic flares (Petri 1997). One should realize that the frequency, nature, and severity of the flares are not only determined by pregnancy itself but also by the change in medication because of the pregnancy. The disease manifestations, the pregnancy, and the medication together will determine the morbidity of mother and child. Hypertension develops frequently during pregnancy as well as mild oedema and proteinuria and may progress into (pre)eclampsia mimicking a flare of the disease. In general, pregnancy does not lead to worsening of renal function in patients with previous lupus nephritis, but the combination of pre-eclampsia and renal disease may rapidly lead to serious morbidity requiring clear differentiation between a renal flare and (pre)eclampsia and subsequent adequate therapy; high dose immunosuppression or delivery, respectively.

Prediction of lupus flare

A flare can occur at any time during pregnancy or the puerperium. There is no specific post-partum risk of a flare. It is not possible to predict when or if an individual patient will flare and what the nature of the flare will be, though quiescent disease in the year prior to conception seems to be associated with fewer disease flares during pregnancy (Mascola and Repke 1997). Low-dose prednisone (10 mg/day) does not prevent flares occurring. Close monitoring of the patient during the whole pregnancy and the puerperium is necessary, since most patients can or will not plan their pregnancy exclusively after a year without disease activity.

Mechanisms explaining pregnancy flares

During pregnancy, strong hormonal and immunologic changes are required to permit the woman to carry a child that is partly non-self. SLE is strongly associated with female sex hormones since the female to male ratio of SLE is about 10 : 1. In particular, female sex hormones will rise during pregnancy, which in turn stimulate prolactin production. Prolactin is known to be an immunomodulator with multiple effects on the immune system. Prolactin receptors are expressed in a number of cells, including T- and B-lymphocytes, and belong to the family of cytokine receptors. Prolactin levels were found to be associated with SLE activity in some studies, but not in others (Khamastha et al. 1997; Petri 1997).

In contrast with the possibly favourable effect in RA, the shift from Th1 to Th2 cytokines in pregnancy may be deleterious in SLE. The Th2 cytokines are responsible for the humoral immunity and a shift towards a Th2 cytokine profile may therefore worsen an antibody-mediated disease like SLE.

Obstetric complications

Obstetric morbidity is a serious problem in SLE. Obstetric morbidity is higher in lupus patients than in controls. In particular, hypertension, pre-eclampsia, diabetes mellitus, hyperglycaemia, and bladder infections are common with a four- to six-fold increased risk compared to controls (Petri 1997). Corticosteroid therapy strongly contributes to this comorbidity, particularly in patients taking more than 10 mg/day. Lupus patients are more likely to have premature rupture of membranes and they require also more frequently caesarean sections. The rare, but more serious obstetric complications are uterine rupture, bilateral retinal detachment during labour, severe retinopathy, deep venous thrombosis, and stroke (associated with secondary antiphospholipid syndrome, APLS) and the HELLP syndrome (haemolysis, elevated liver enzymes, and low platelets). The APLS-associated complications can occur in patients who are already receiving antithrombotic treatment. Women with APLS and a previous arterial thromboembolism should be discouraged to become pregnant because of the high risk of recurrent thromboembolism, even with anticoagulant treatment (Petri 1997; Welsch and Branch 1997). A substantial proportion of all thrombotic events in women with APLS occurs during pregnancy or in the post-partum period.

Fertility

SLE does not apparently affect fertility, unless patients have been treated previously with cyclophosphamide. Despite the fact that women who have, or later develop, SLE are at greater risk of pregnancy loss, their ultimate family size is comparable to that of healthy controls (Hardy et al. 1999). However, infertility may be a factor in a small group of women with high levels of APL antibodies seeking help for inability to conceive (Meng and Lockshin 1999). Some clinicians recommend that infertile women with APLS should be treated with heparin/aspirin when they are undergoing *in vitro* fertilization. In particular, women with APL antibodies against phosphatidylethanolamine (PE) or phosphatidylserine (PS) appear to have low success rates with *in vitro* fertilization. In these women, treatment with intravenous immunoglobulin might help if heparin/aspirin fails.

The foetal perspective

Foetal loss

There is an increased foetal loss in SLE pregnancies, in particular in the second trimester. Most studies report foetal loss in 20–30 per cent of the SLE pregnancies, which is more than a twofold risk of foetal loss compared to controls (Mascola and Ropke 1997; Petri 1997; Welsch and Branch 1997; Hardy et al. 1999; Georgiou et al. 2000). Secondary APLS is strongly associated with foetal loss in the second trimester, but not with foetal loss in the first trimester. The risk of foetal loss in APLS is strong for the presence of lupus anticoagulant (LA) (odds ratio 27.7), but less strong for anticardiolipin (odds ratio 1.7). Other risk factors for foetal loss are impaired renal function and active disease, for example, measured by low serum C3 (Petri 1997; Georgiou et al. 2000).

Pre-term birth

The rate of pre-term delivery in SLE patients ranges from 24 to 59 per cent. Disease activity, measured with whatever marker for SLE activity, is probably the most important risk factor for pre-term birth (Petri 1997). Renal disease with proteinuria in the nephrotic range and hypertension are particularly important in causing prematurity. High prednisone doses either as a marker of active (renal) disease, or by a direct effect contributes to the prematurity risk. In addition, poor obstetric history also predicts pre-term birth. Prematurity in SLE is often multifactorial and preventive measures should include optimal antihypertensive treatment, treatment of SLE activity and treatment of secondary APLS.

Women with SLE are also at risk for foetal growth impairment and foetal distress caused by placental insufficiency. Placental pathology in SLE patients is characterized by decidual vasculopathy and infarction. The latter feature in particular can be extensive in APLS patients (Meng and Lockshin 1999).

Neonatal outcome

Women with circulating anti-52 kDa SSA/Ro or SSB/La antibodies are at risk of having a child with neonatal lupus syndrome. Transient symptoms of neonatal lupus are rash, cytopenias, hepatosplenomegaly, and myocarditis/pericarditis. A permanent, and potentially lethal, manifestation of neonatal lupus is complete congenital heart block. Mortality in congenital heart block may accumulate to 20 per cent *in utero*. Of the new-born babies with a congenital heart block 64 per cent need a pacemaker (Tseng and Buyon 1997). The risk of having a subsequent child with congenital heart block appears to be between 12 and 16 per cent (Meng and Lockshin 1999). Series of foetal echocardiograms are indicated between weeks 16 and 24 of gestation to follow the foetal cardiac function in women with anti-SSA/Ro, anti-SSB/La antibodies or with a previous child with congenital heart block. Oral dexamethasone and/or plasmapheresis have been used to attenuate or to reverse the serious complication of congenital heart block *in utero* with varying degree of success (Tseng and Buyon 1997; Neiman et al. 2000).

Patient management with SLE pregnancy

Successful pregnancies are now possible in 85 per cent of the women with SLE. This is only made possible through partnership between expert rheumatologists, obstetricians, and neonatologists. SLE still carries a high risk for adverse pregnancy outcome. Counselling and obstetric care ideally begins before conception (Mascola and Repke 1997). Risk factors can be assessed and treatment can be optimized aiming at a quiescent disease at least 6 months before conception. A series of laboratory assessments will provide the baseline measures for further follow up during pregnancy and the potential risk factors for adverse outcome (Table 4). In normal pregnancy the C3 and C4 should rise. Monthly monitoring—if necessary more often—by rheumatologist, obstetrician, and possibly other specialists may pick up important change that have to be acted upon. Particular attention has to be given to disease flare, renal deterioration, hypertension, and adverse foetal development. The medication has to be adapted to the patient's needs depending on disease activity, prior obstetric history, presence of APLS, presence of anti-SSA/Ro or anti-SSB/La antibodies, and the course of the present pregnancy. Management of lupus flares can be problematic because of the limitations on medications that can be used safely during pregnancy. Mild flares can be treated with prednisone, although high doses of prednisone are not favoured because of the increased risk of obstetric problems and pre-term birth. For moderate to major flares intravenous methylprednisolone pulse therapy, 1000 mg/day, for 3 days may be an option combined with azathioprine, which has been used without much problem in lupus flares during pregnancy. Hydroxychloroquine has been shown to control disease activity during pregnancy and can be continued during pregnancy in SLE without harm to the foetus (Mascola and Repke 1997; Petri 1997). Treatment with NSAIDs after the second trimester is not advised because of the potential adverse effect on the foetal renal and cardiac system. The preferred treatment for APLS nowadays is a combination of low-dose aspirin and low-molecular-weight heparin that can be given for the duration of pregnancy (Petri 1997; Welsch and Branch 1997). The use of prednisone to prevent APLS complications is not advocated anymore because of the lack of effect and the risk of prednisone associated obstetric complications such as diabetes mellitus, hypertension, pre-eclampsia, and pre-term delivery (Table 3). Antihypertensive treatment is often necessary in lupus pregnancy but should not be too aggressive because of the differential effect on maternal hypertension and placental blood flow. Antihypertensives that are most commonly used in SLE pregnancies include methyldopa, hydralazine, and—in more severe hypertension—labetolol. Patients who are chronically on thiazide diuretics or nifedipine because of renal disease could potentially remain on these drugs if closely monitored. ACE inhibitors should be stopped because of effects on foetal kidney development (Mascola and Repke 1997).

Prednisone and hydrocortisone are inactivated in the placenta and therefore have little effect on the foetus. Dexamethasone and betamethasone do cross the placenta in an unmetabolized form and are therefore used if the foetus has to be treated, for example, in case of anti-SSA/Ro or anti-SSB/La foetal myocardiopathy.

Approaching delivery, the team has to include a neonatologist. Obstetric management during labour is not dissimilar from normal pregnancy care. Stress dose steroids should be administered to patients who are on prolonged courses of steroids. Any antithrombotic therapy should be stopped if labour is imminent. Because of the high-risk nature of SLE pregnancies, the rate of caesarean sections will be higher than usual. The usual precautions for anaesthesia and surgery should be taken in case of prednisone and/or anticoagulant use. After delivery the newly born baby has to be observed for signs and symptoms of neonatal lupus. There are no objections against breastfeeding, unless certain medications prevent it because of risk for the baby.

Table 4 Baseline laboratory assessments in SLE-pregnancy

Investigations	Parameter
Immunological	ANA titre
	Anti-dsDNA and titre
	Anti-SSA/Ro
	Anti-SSB/La
	Anticardiolipin IgM and IgG
	Lupus anticoagulant (LA)
	Complement levels: C3, C4, and CH50
Haematological and chemical	Haemoglobin
	Haematocrit
	Leucocytes
	Platelets
	Full serum electrolyte panel
	Serum creatinine
	Liver enzymes
	Glucose
Urinalysis	24 h creatinine clearance
	24 h total protein
	Sediment

Scleroderma

Effect of pregnancy on maternal disease

Pregnancy in general does not change the disease status of scleroderma. The few studies that systematically evaluated the disease status during pregnancy reported no change in 72–88 per cent, improvement in 5–14 per cent, and worsening in 7–14 per cent of scleroderma patients (Steen 1997; Sampaio-Barros et al. 2000). Scleroderma symptoms such as oedema, arthralgias, gastrointestinal reflux, and mild shortness of breath are also common in normal pregnancy. Raynaud's phenomenon usually improves, but will come back after delivery. Hypertension, a frequent symptom during pregnancy, should be aggressively treated, since renal crisis is the most serious complication of scleroderma and cause of death in scleroderma pregnancies. The presence of hypertension and proteinuria related to pre-eclampsia could be confused with a renal crisis and it may be difficult to distinguish between the presence of pre-eclampsia or scleroderma renal crisis per se or a renal crisis in scleroderma induced by pregnancy. Recent studies showed far fewer episodes of renal crises than earlier anecdotal case reports (Steen 1997; Sampaio-Barros et al. 2000). Women with symptoms of scleroderma of less than 4 years, those with diffuse cutaneous scleroderma and those who have antitopoisomerase antibodies (anti-Scl70) have a greater risk of aggressive disease than those with longstanding disease with anticentromere antibodies (Steen 1997). Women with early progressive disease are therefore more at risk of renal crisis during pregnancy than women with limited scleroderma or longstanding stable disease. Prednisone therapy is another precipitating factor for renal crisis in scleroderma and should therefore be avoided, particularly during pregnancy. The overall outcome of scleroderma is not influenced by pregnancy; the 10-year cumulative survival for women with and without a pregnancy was similar (Table 5).

Pregnancy in relation to onset of scleroderma

There is no relation between the onset of scleroderma and pregnancy. The disease can develop during as well as outside pregnancy with similar risks. Parity has been implicated in the causation of scleroderma through persistent, HLA similar (but not entirely identical), foetal microchimerism disrupting the maternal immunoregulatory mechanisms (Nelson 2002). Parous women and women who had abortive pregnancy, however, were found to have three-fold decreased risk of scleroderma compared to nulliparous women, which excludes the possibility of pregnancy itself being a risk factor for the development of scleroderma (Pisa et al. 2002).

Fertility

The most recent studies show no evidence of decreased fertility in scleroderma (Steen and Medsger 1999), though older studies suggested that

Table 5 Clinical observations in relation to scleroderma and pregnancy

Issues	Clinical observation
During pregnancy	
Disease activity	No change in 72–88%, 5–14% improvement, 7–14% worsening Only Raynaud's phenomenon usually improves
Onset scleroderma	No relation between the timing of onset and pregnancy Parous women have threefold decreased risk of developing scleroderma
Obstetric problems Measures —Need frequent evaluations of blood pressure, urinalysis and foetal growth by ultrasound —Prednisone is contraindicated	Hypertension: treat aggressively Renal crises: most serious complication that can cause death in scleroderma patients. Must be treated with ACE-inhibitor —Risk factors of renal crisis: early progressive disease (<4 year), diffuse cutaneous scleroderma, presence of antitopoisomerase antibodies (anti-Scl70) and prednisone therapy —Low risk of renal crisis: longstanding disease with anticentromere antibodies Pre-eclampsia; difficult to distinguish from renal crisis in scleroderma induced by pregnancy
Foetal outcome	Slightly increased risk of prematurity and miscarriages in diffuse scleroderma
Delivery	Caution with the use of beta-adrenergic agonists to prevent pre-term labour, because of its potential side-effects of myocardial ischaemia and pulmonary oedema In case of general anaesthesia difficult intubation because of restricted scleroderma mouth Special care needed for surgical repair of caesarean wound and episiotomy
Post-partum	
Disease activity	Raynaud's comes back
Long-term (>10 years)	Overall outcome and 10-year cumulative survival is not influenced by pregnancy
Fertility	No evidence of decreased fertility in scleroderma patients

fertility was decreased (Steen 1997). Patients with systemic sclerosis are more often nulliparous than controls. When nulliparity was adjusted for number of women who never married, women who were sexually active, and women who chose not to have children, the differences from the controls disappeared. Only 2–5 per cent of both the scleroderma and control women who attempted to become pregnant was unsuccessful. All other determinants of fertility were also similar in both groups (Steen and Medsger 1999).

Foetal outcome

Pregnancy outcome in scleroderma is variable but the overall adverse pregnancy outcome rate is increased in most case-control studies (Steen 1997). Scleroderma patients are more likely to have adverse pregnancy outcome after disease onset than before, in particular, prematurity. An increased rate of miscarriages and prematurity is reported especially in patients with longstanding diffuse scleroderma but not in limited scleroderma. Recent studies show, however, more favourable pregnancy outcomes in scleroderma than the older case series (Steen and Medsger 1999). The current consensus is that the overall success of pregnancy in scleroderma is good, and only in the diffuse disease is there a slight increased risk of adverse pregnancy outcome, in particular, prematurity.

Patient management of scleroderma pregnancy

The overall outcome of pregnancy in scleroderma is favourable though, in the individual patient, the risk of maternal harm and foetal prematurity may be substantial. Careful management of the pregnant scleroderma patient is therefore indicated. Patients with early diffuse scleroderma should wait to become pregnant until their disease stabilizes and the risk of renal crisis has decreased. Patients with longstanding diffuse systemic sclerosis and extensive organ involvement have to be assessed regarding the risk of serious health problems during the physical demands of pregnancy. When cardiac, renal, or lung function are greatly impaired the patient should be strongly advised against pregnancy. This decision is based on the abnormalities found and is independent of the fact that scleroderma is the cause of these abnormalities.

Management of the pregnant scleroderma patient includes frequent evaluation of blood pressure, urinalysis, and foetal growth by ultrasound. Prednisone therapy is contraindicated because of the risk of a renal crisis. Patients with diffuse scleroderma are advised to monitor their blood pressure very frequently, if possible several times a week, by home monitoring. Even a slight elevation in blood pressure compared to previous levels should be considered potentially serious and be treated promptly. In case of (suspicion of) a renal crisis the first choice of treatment is an ACE inhibitor; this could make the difference in the life or death of the mother and the foetus. ACE inhibitors have been reported to cause foetal abnormalities, but successful use in pregnancies has been documented. The risk of renal failure and foetal loss may outweigh the risk of the birth defects associated with the use of ACE inhibitors and justify the use of these drugs in pregnancy of a scleroderma patient.

Antacids and antireflux measures can manage common problems such as oesophageal dysmotility. The use of histamine blockers and proton pump blockers has not been reported to cause significant problems in pregnancy.

The risk of pre-term labour, in particular in diffuse scleroderma, is increased. The use of beta-adrenergic agonists to prevent pre-term labour particularly in this patient group should be used with great caution, because of the potential side effects of myocardial ischaemia and pulmonary oedema. Before delivery venous access should be secured because of the potential difficulties finding access in the taut skin. General anaesthesia should be avoided because of the difficulties in intubating a scleroderma patient with a minimal mouth opening and the risk of aspiration. An epidural block can normally be used without problem. If a caesarean section is indicated, the wound normally heals without difficulty if care is taken in the surgical repair. The same applies for an episiotomy incision.

If the baby is born full term, no special care has to be taken.

Dermatomyositis/polymyositis

Pregnancy in dermatomyositis (DM) or polymyositis (PM) is infrequent because of the rarity of the disease and the late age at onset. In over 85 per cent of the patients, the disease starts after childbearing age. The knowledge about pregnancy in DM/PM, is based on some case series and several case reports (Mintz 1989; Harris et al. 1995; Kanoh et al. 1999) and can best be divided into: (i) influence of pregnancy on childhood DM/PM; (ii) influence of pregnancy on adult DM/PM; and (iii) onset of DM/PM related to pregnancy (Table 6).

Maternal disease and pregnancy outcome

All reported cases of childhood DM/PM started their pregnancy in an inactive phase of their disease. Two patients had an abortion (one spontaneously, one induced) and a flare post-abortion. Of the remaining eight patients, only two (25 per cent) flared during pregnancy. Seven out of 10 patients (70 per cent) had full term new-borns. One baby was born prematurely. In adult DM/PM, 88 per cent of the patients remained stable during pregnancy and the corticosteroid dosages were not changed. The pregnancy outcome was worse than in childhood DM/PM with only 50 per cent full-term newborns. Of eight pregnancies two ended with an abortion, one in pre-term birth and one in neonatal death of a pair of twins.

Risk for adverse outcome of pregnancy

It appears that the outcome is best in mothers with inactive disease ($n = 12$), with 72 per cent full term birth, 11 per cent spontaneous abortions and no pre-term birth (when excluding the induced abortion). In active disease ($n = 14$) the outcome is worse with only 47 per cent full-term birth, 33 per cent foetal loss, and 13 per cent premature birth. The babies did not show any sign of an autoimmune disease.

Onset of DM/PM during pregnancy

There are several case reports of DM/PM starting during pregnancy, mostly in the first, sometimes in the second and rarely in the third trimester (Mintz 1989; Harris et al. 1995). The group of patients with onset of DM/PM during pregnancy has the poorest outcome of pregnancy with over 50 per cent foetal death. Conversely, pregnancy appeared to have a negative influence on the disease in the mother, with very active therapy-resistant disease during pregnancy. In some of these cases, patients showed remarkable post-partum remissions.

Table 6 Clinical observations in relation to dermatomyositis/polymyositis and pregnancy

Issues	Clinical observation
Child DM/PM	
Risk of flare during pregnancy	Low
Foetal outcome	Favourable
Adult DM/PM	
Risk of flare during pregnancy	Low
Foetal outcome	Moderate-poor (±50% at term) Risk factor for adverse outcome: active disease at start of pregnancy
Onset of DM/PM during pregnancy	
Risk of uncontrollable disease	High
Foetal outcome	Moderate-poor (±50% adverse outcome) Remarkable post-partum remission reported

Primary Sjögren's syndrome

There are few studies on pregnancy in primary Sjögren's syndrome. Fertility, parity, and sexual activity of patients with primary Sjögren's syndrome do not appear to differ from that of the healthy population. There are, however, some contradictory results on the risk of foetal loss (Skopouli et al. 1994; Julkunen et al. 1995). In some studies the risk of foetal loss is approximately two-fold increased and comparable to that of SLE, while in other studies no such risk is observed. Foetal growth retardation and preterm birth are not problems in primary Sjögren's syndrome. APLS antibodies or antibodies to SSA/Ro or SSB/La appeared to play no major role in the increased risk of foetal loss in Sjögren's patients. There may be the risk of congenital heart block, but only few prospective data are available.

Rare diseases

Adult onset Still's disease

Reviewing the scarce case reports, pregnancy seems to have no effect on adult onset Still's disease, and conversely, adult onset Still's disease has no obvious influence on pregnancy, foetal growth, or infant maturity and health (Le Loët et al. 1993).

Vasculitis syndromes

Polyarteritis nodosa

Polyarteritis nodosa (PAN) developing during pregnancy has an extremely bad prognosis. All seven women diagnosed during gestation or in the immediate post-partum period died within 6 weeks post-partum (Klipple and Riordan 1989; Ramsey-Goldman 1998). This grave prognosis may be explained to a certain extent by difficulties in diagnosing PAN in the setting of pregnancy and by the very active disease during pregnancy. Pregnant women with a known, quiescent PAN have a much better prognosis, with only one in four women experiencing an exacerbation. Perinatal outcome was surprisingly good, with approximately 70 per cent survival of the child.

Wegener's granulomatosis

Upto 26 pregnancies have now been reported in Wegener's granulomatosis (WG) of which 10 occurred during or immediately after pregnancy (Ramsey-Goldman 1998; Auzary et al. 2000). If the disease is inactive prior to pregnancy the chance of disease activation during pregnancy is not particularly high and the foetal outcome is generally favourable. In contrast, obstetric problems, such as pre-eclampsia, prematurity, and foetal deaths occurred when maternal disease was not controlled.

Takayasu arteritis

Pregnancy does not seem to worsen Takayasu arteritis, although symptoms common to both the disease and pregnancy—such as hypertension and abdominal discomfort—have to be correctly interpreted (Sharma et al. 2000). There is an increased risk of foetal loss, intrauterine growth retardation, and pre-term birth. All patients with poor perinatal outcome had abdominal aortic involvement and a significant delay in seeking medical attention.

Behçet's disease

In women with Behçet's disease, convincing reports of both pregnancy-related flares and remissions, mainly of mucocutaneous involvement, are found in the literature. Gestational exacerbations of the more serious manifestations of

Behçet's including major eye problems, vasculitis, and CNS disease are uncommon. Also, foetal development and survival is generally good in Behçet's syndrome (Klipple and Riordan 1989).

The general advice for management of pregnancy in a vasculitis syndrome is that pregnancy should be planned during a remission of the disease. If vasculitis activity reappears, rigorous treatment of the vasculitis is required in order to protect mother and child against serious morbidity and mortality. If necessary, cyclophosphamide pulse therapy in the second and third trimesters should be considered as a therapeutic option, since maximal suppression of the vasculitis activity is the goal.

References

Alavi, A. et al. (2000). Immunoglobulin G glycosylation and clinical outcome in rheumatoid arthritis during pregnancy. *Journal of Rheumatology* **27** (6), 1379–85.

Auzary, C. et al. (2000). Pregnancy in patients with Wegener's granulomatosis: report of five cases in three women. *Annals of the Rheumatic Diseases* **59** (10), 800–4.

Barrett, J.H. et al. (1999). Does rheumatoid arthritis remit during pregnancy and relapse postpartum? Results from a nationwide study in the United Kingdom performed prospectively from late pregnancy. *Arthritis and Rheumatism* **42** (6), 1219–27.

Barrett, J.H. et al. (2000). Breast-feeding and postpartum relapse in women with rheumatoid and inflammatory arthritis. *Arthritis and Rheumatism* **43** (5), 1010–15.

Brennan, P. and Silman, A. (1994). Breast-feeding and the onset of rheumatoid arthritis. *Arthritis and Rheumatism* **37** (6), 808–13.

Brennan, P. et al. (2000). Maternal–fetal HLA incompatibility and the course of inflammatory arthritis during pregnancy. *Journal of Rheumatology* **27** (12), 2843–8.

Brun, J.G. et al. (1995). Breast feeding, other reproductive factors and rheumatoid arthritis. A prospective study. *British Journal of Rheumatology* **34** (6), 542–6.

Drossaers-Bakker, K.W. et al. (2002). Pregnancy and oral contraceptive use do not significantly influence outcome in long term rheumatoid arthritis. *Annals of the Rheumatic Diseases* **61** (5), 405–8.

Georgiou, P.E. et al. (2000). Outcome of lupus pregnancy: a controlled study. *Rheumatology (Oxford)* **39** (9), 1014–19.

Gran, J.T. and Ostensen, M. (1998). Spondyloarthritides in females. *Baillières Clinical Rheumatology* **12** (4), 695–715.

Hardy, C.J. et al. (1999). Pregnancy outcome and family size in systemic lupus erythematosus: a case–control study. *Rheumatology (Oxford)* **38** (6), 559–63.

Harris, A. et al. (1995). Dermatomyositis presenting in pregnancy. *British Journal of Dermatology* **133** (5), 783–5.

Hazes, J.M. et al. (1990). Pregnancy and the risk of developing rheumatoid arthritis. *Arthritis and Rheumatism* **33** (2), 1770–5.

Hench, P.S. (1938). The ameliorating effect of pregnancy on chronic atrophic (infectious rheumatoid) arthritis, fibrositis, and intermittent hydrarthrosis. *Proceedings Staff Meetings Mayo Clinic* **13**, 161–17.

Hernandez Avila, M. et al. (1990). Reproductive factors, smoking, and the risk for rheumatoid arthritis. *Epidemiology* **1** (4), 285–91.

Julkunen, H. et al. (1995). Fetal outcome in women with primary Sjögren's syndrome. A retrospective case–control study. *Clinical and Experimental Rheumatology* **13** (1), 65–71.

Kanik, K.S. and Wilder, R.L. (2000). Hormonal alterations in rheumatoid arthritis, including the effects of pregnancy. *Rheumatic Disease Clinics of North America* **26** (4), 805–23.

Kanoh, H. et al. (1999). A case of dermatomyositis that developed after delivery: the involvement of pregnancy in the induction of dermatomyositis. *British Journal of Dermatology* **141** (5), 897–900.

Khamashta, M.A., Ruiz-Irastorza, G., and Hughes, G.R. (1997). Systemic lupus erythematosus flares during pregnancy. *Rheumatic Disease Clinics of North America* **23** (1), 15–30.

Klipple, G.L. and Riordan, K.K. (1989). Rare inflammatory and hereditary connective tissue diseases. *Rheumatic Disease Clinics of North America* **15** (2), 383–98.

Lansink, M. et al. (1993). The onset of rheumatoid arthritis in relation to pregnancy and childbirth. *Clinical and Experimental Rheumatology* **11** (2), 171–4.

Le Loët, X. et al. (1993). Adult onset Still's disease and pregnancy. *Journal of Rheumatology* **20** (7), 1158–61.

Mascola, M.A. and Repke, J.T. (1997). Obstetric management of the high-risk lupus pregnancy. *Rheumatic Disease Clinics of North America* **23** (1), 119–32.

Meng, C. and Lockshin, M. (1999). Pregnancy in lupus. *Current Opinion in Rheumatology* **11** (5), 348–51.

Mintz, G. (1989). Dermatomyositis. *Rheumatic Disease Clinics of North America* **15** (2), 375–82.

Musiej-Nowakowska, E. and Ploski, R. (1999). Pregnancy and early onset pauciarticular juvenile chronic arthritis. *Annals of the Rheumatic Disease* **58**, 475–80.

Neiman, A.R. et al. (2000). Cutaneous manifestations of neonatal lupus without heart block: characteristics of mothers and children enrolled in a national registry. *Journal of Pediatrics* **137** (5), 674–80.

Nelson, J.L. (2002). Pregnancy and microchimerism in autoimmune disease: protector or insurgent? *Arthritis and Rheumatism* **46** (2), 291–7.

Nelson, J.L. and Ostensen, M. (1997). Pregnancy and rheumatoid arthritis. *Rheumatic Disease Clinics of North America* **23** (1), 195–212.

Ostensen, M. (1992). The effect of pregnancy on ankylosing spondylitis, psoriatic arthritis, and juvenile rheumatoid arthritis. *American Journal of Reproductive Immunology* **28** (3–4), 235–7.

Ostensen, M. (1997). Problems related to pregnancy in patients with juvenile chronic arthritis. *Revue du Rhumatisme (English Edition)* **64** (Suppl. 10), 196S–7S.

Ostensen, M. and Ostensen, H. (1998). Ankylosing spondylitis—the female aspect. *Journal of Rheumatology* **25** (1), 120–4.

Ostensen, M., Almberg, K., and Koksvik, H.S. (2000). Sex, reproduction, and gynecological disease in young adults with a history of juvenile chronic arthritis. *Journal of Rheumatology* **27** (7), 1783–7.

Petri, M. (1997). Hopkins Lupus Pregnancy Center: 1987 to 1996. *Rheumatic Disease Clinics of North America* **23** (1), 1–13.

Pisa, F.E. et al. (2002). Reproductive factors and the risk of scleroderma: an Italian case-control study. *Arthritis and Rheumatism* **46** (2), 451–6.

Ramsey-Goldman, R. (1998). The effect of pregnancy on the vasculitides. *Scandinavican Journal of Rheumatolgy Supplement* **107**, 116–17.

Sampaio-Barros, P.D., Samara, A.M., and Marques Neto, J.F. (2000). Gynaecologic history in systemic sclerosis. *Clinical Rheumatology* **19** (3), 184–7.

Sharma, B.K., Jain, S., and Vasishta, K. (2000). Outcome of pregnancy in Takayasu arteritis. *International Journal of Cardiology* **75** (Suppl. 1), S159–62.

Silman, A., Kay, A., and Brennan, P. (1992). Timing of pregnancy in relation to the onset of rheumatoid arthritis. *Arthritis and Rheumatism* **35** (2), 152–5.

Skomsvoll, J.F. et al. (2000). Pregnancy complications and delivery practice in women with connective tissue disease and inflammatory rheumatic disease in Norway. *Acta Obstetrica et Gynecologica Scandinavica* **79** (6), 490–5.

Skopouli, F.N. et al. (1994). Obstetric and gynaecological profile in patients with primary Sjögren's syndrome. *Annals of the Rheumatic Diseases* **53** (9), 569–73.

Spector, T.D., Roman, E., and Silman, A.J. (1990). The pill, parity, and rheumatoid arthritis. *Arthritis and Rheumatism* **33** (6), 782–9.

Steen, V.D. (1997). Scleroderma and pregnancy. *Rheumatic Disease Clinics of North America* **23** (1), 133–47.

Steen, V.D. and Medsger, T.A., Jr. (1999). Fertility and pregnancy outcome in women with systemic sclerosis. *Arthritis and Rheumatism* **42** (4), 763–8.

Tseng, C.E. and Buyon, J.P. (1997). Neonatal lupus syndromes. *Rheumatic Disease Clinics of North America* **23** (1), 31–54.

Van der Horst-Bruinsma, I.E. et al. (1998). Influence of HLA-class II incompatibility between mother and fetus on the development and course of rheumatoid arthritis of the mother. *Annals of the Rheumatic Diseases* **57** (5), 286–90.

Welsch, S. and Branch, D.W. (1997). Antiphospholipid syndrome in pregnancy. Obstetric concerns and treatment. *Rheumatic Disease Clinics of North America* **23** (1), 71–84.

1.3.1.2 Antirheumatic drugs in pregnancy and lactation

J. Mieke Hazes and Yaël A. de Man

Introduction

The inflammatory rheumatic diseases predominantly affect women, often in the childbearing years. Antirheumatic drugs are necessary to control the disease and many times the medication cannot be stopped in pregnancy because of risk of a disease flare potentially threatening the health of mother and child. Some drugs appear to be safe during pregnancy, though an association between drugs and malformations is hard to totally exclude. It therefore seems prudent to stop all medications during pregnancy if possible. In general, the outcome for mother and child is best if pregnancy occurs in a period of disease remission (Mascola and Repke 1997). Often, pregnancy will or cannot be planned in a period of remission or, conversely, the disease will flare during pregnancy and the doctor will face the question which antirheumatic drugs to use during pregnancy. The most critical phase for the foetal outcome in relation to use of medication is in the first weeks of pregnancy during conception, embryogenesis, and organogenesis. It is important therefore that a pregnancy is carefully planned and the antirheumatic medication is adapted as soon as the patient seriously wishes to conceive.

There are virtually no controlled data on the safety of drug use during pregnancy, since pregnant women are always excluded from randomized controlled trials. Placental transfer has been described for the majority of antirheumatic drugs. The foetal concentrations of drugs can vary considerably compared to the maternal concentrations depending on the type and dosage of the drug, duration of treatment, and timing. Both protein binding and hepatic metabolism in the foetus differ from those in the mother and depend on the stage of development of the foetus. The first trimester and the few weeks before delivery are the most vulnerable periods for the foetus: the former because of the early foetal development and the potential risk of malformations during foetal organogenesis (teratogenesis), the latter because of the risk of functional abnormalities and post-natal problems in the neonate due to exposure to a specific drug.

Knowledge about safety for mother and child during pregnancy comes from observations during long-term clinical experience, case series, and case reports. The last of these tends to overestimate adverse effects of drugs on the foetus due to publication bias. Animal studies may provide some guidance in the usage of drugs during pregnancy though they cannot be easily extrapolated to the human situation. Physicians should be aware of the potential adverse effects of antirheumatic drugs during conception, pregnancy, and lactation, and should carefully weigh the risks and the benefits of these medications for mother and child. Comprehensive management of the patient starting before conception is prerequisite for an optimal outcome. This chapter describes what is known about the effects of antirheumatic drugs on fertility, conception, pregnancy, and lactation for both mother and child. This information is summarized in Tables 1–6. This chapter is based on some excellent reviews (Esplin and Branch 1997; Ramsey-Goldman and Schilling 1997; Ostensen and Ramsey-Goldman 1998; Janssen and Genta 2000; Ostensen 2001) and the information from the Micromedex on drugs during pregnancy and lactation (Micromedex 2002).

General considerations of antirheumatic treatment during pregnancy

Treatment of (rheumatoid) arthritis

The majority of the patients with rheumatoid arthritis (RA) improve during pregnancy and in most cases the antirheumatic treatment can be stopped as soon as the woman becomes pregnant. The same applies for arthritis symptoms in other rheumatic diseases, such as juvenile idiopathic arthritis and peripheral arthritis in spondyloarthropathies (Nelson and Ostensen 1997). Cytotoxic drugs have to be stopped before conception, because of the teratogenic effect on the foetus. This holds for both male and female patients. In case of an arthritis flare during pregnancy, the symptoms can often be safely controlled with intra-articular steroids, non-steroidal anti-inflammatory drugs (NSAIDs) or, if necessary, low dose oral prednisone.

Treatment of systemic lupus erythematosus (SLE) and other systemic diseases during pregnancy

SLE and other systemic rheumatic diseases should be planned when the disease is quiescent. Similar to RA treatment with cytotoxic drugs should be stopped several months before conception because of the teratogenic effect on the foetus. In SLE, there is a possible risk of a flare during pregnancy and

Table 1 Use of NSAIDs and corticosteroids in pregnancy

	Aspirin		Inhibitors		
	High dose	Low dose	Non-selective COX	COX-2 selective	Corticosteroids
Fertility	No effect	May promote embryo implantation	Probably no effect	Unknown	No effect
Teratogenicity	Possibly not	No	Possibly not	Unknown	High dose: possibly risk of oral clefts
Late pregnancy	Contraindicated for bleeding risk and foetal renovascular complications	For complicated SLE and positive effect on hypertension and preeclampsia	Contraindicated	Probably as non-selective COX-inhibitors	Maternal: obstetric complications Child: hypercortisolism
Risk/benefit ratio[a]	Negative	Positive	Neutral–negative (third trimester)	Negative because of unknown data	Neutral–positive depending on disease
FDA category[b]	C–D (third trimeter)	—	B–D (third trimeter)	C	B
Breast-feeding[c]	Unsafe	With caution	Usually compatible	Unknown	Compatible up to dose 20 mg/day

[a] Positive, disease is worse than the drug; neutral, always better to stop the drug if possible; negative, drug is always worse than the disease.

[b] FDA category: A, no foetal risk in controlled studies; B, no risk in animals, no controlled human studies; or abnormalities in animal studies but not in controlled human studies; C, studies show teratogenic or embryocidal effects in animals, but no controlled human studies; or no studies are available in either human or animals; D, positive evidence for foetal abnormalities but potential benefits may outweigh potential risks; X, contra-indicated.

[c] According to the Micromedex (2002) advice.

Table 2 Use of conventional DMARDs in pregnancy

	Hydroxychloroquine	Sulfasalazine	Gold	D-Penicillamine
Fertility	No effect	Females no effect Males reversible infertility	No effect	Unknown
Teratogenicity	Probably not in average dose	No	Probably not (little data)	Definite: physical defects, tissue abnormalities
Late pregnancy	No problems	No problems	Little data	Connective tissue abnormalities (cutis laxa)
Risk/benefit ratio[a]	Positive in SLE	Positive	Neutral	Negative
FDA category[b]	C (in high doses)	B	C	D
Breast-feeding[c]	Use with caution	Use with caution	Use with caution	No reports of use

[a] Positive, disease is worse than the drug; neutral, always better to stop the drug if possible; negative, drug is always worse than the disease.

[b] FDA category: A, no foetal risk in controlled studies; B, no risk in animals, no controlled human studies; or abnormalities in animal studies but not in controlled human studies; C, studies show teratogenic or embryocidal effects in animals, but no controlled human studies; or no studies are available in either human or animals; D, positive evidence for foetal abnormalities but potential benefits may outweigh potential risks; X, contra-indicated.

[c] According to the Micromedex (2002) advice.

Table 3 Use of cytotoxic medications in pregnancy

	MTX	Azathioprine	Cyclophosphamide
Fertility	Female: no effect Male: oligospermia	Possibly no effect	Definite adverse effect Infertility: increased risk with high cumulative doses and age >31 years
Teratogenicity	Definite: ossification and neural tube defects	Possibly not	Definite: facial cleft, limb defects, craniofacial dysmorphism
Late pregnancy	Growth retardation and myelosuppression	Variety of adverse effects; foetal immunosuppression	Myelotoxicity and growth retardation
Risk/benefit ratio[a]	Negative	Neutral–positive depending on disease	Negative in first trimester Neutral–positive in second half of pregnancy depending on disease
FDA category[b]	X (high doses)	D	D
Breast-feeding[c]	Contra-indicated	No data	Contra-indicated

[a] Positive, disease is worse than the drug; neutral, always better to stop the drug if possible; negative, drug is always worse than the disease.

[b] FDA category: A, no foetal risk in controlled studies; B, no risk in animals, no controlled human studies; or abnormalities in animal studies but not in controlled human studies; C, studies show teratogenic or embryocidal effects in animals, but no controlled human studies; or no studies are available in either human or animals; D, positive evidence for foetal abnormalities but potential benefits may outweigh potential risks; X, contra-indicated.

[c] According to the Micromedex (2002) advice.

treatment may be necessary. Both the disease and the treatment may harm mother and child. It can be difficult to interpret whether an adverse outcome of mother or child is due to the disease manifestations or to the drug treatment (see also Chapter 1.3.1.1). A rheumatologist and an obstetrician with expertise in treating these kinds of patient should frequently see every mother with SLE throughout pregnancy (Petri 1997).

Aspirin

Aspirin is the oldest and most commonly used NSAID and is the most often researched NSAID during pregnancy. In high doses it has adverse effects on both mother and child, whereas in low doses it is safe.

Effects on the mother

High doses of aspirin in the third trimester inhibit uterine contractility and prolong labour and gestation. Labour may be complicated by pre- and postpartum haemorrhage. Low-dose aspirin appears to be safe and is even of benefit in patients at risk for pregnancy-induced hypertension and preeclampsia. Low-dose aspirin is prescribed in patients with SLE and antiphospholipid syndrome at risk for recurrent foetal loss.

Effects on the child

There are several conflicting reports on teratogenicity of high doses of aspirin in the first trimester of pregnancy in animals as well in humans (Esplin and Branch 1997; Ostensen 1998; Ostensen and Ramsey-Goldman 1998; Janssen and Genta 2000; Ginsberg et al. 2001; Micromedex 2002). There is no evident teratogenic effect of low dose aspirin. High doses of aspirin in the perinatal period lead to clotting defects in mother and child through irreversible binding to platelet cyclooxygenase enzymes. The mother can experience increased blood loss during delivery. An increased incidence of intra-cerebral haemorrhage in the newborns exposed to aspirin in the last weeks before delivery has been reported (Esplin and Branch 1997; Ostensen 1998; Ostensen and Ramsey-Goldman 1998). This problem has been found in newborns exposed to a total of 325–650 mg/day within 1 week prior to delivery. Nowadays, more than 10 000 pregnancies

Table 4 Use of new antirheumatic drugs in pregnancy

	Cyclosporine	Leflunomide	TNF-blockade
Fertility	No effect	Not known	Not known
Teratogenicity	Probably not	Definite in animals; human not known	Possibly not
Late pregnancy	Growth retardation Prematurity	Not known	Not known
Risk/benefit ratio[a]	Negative–neutral depending on disease	Negative	Possibly neutral–positive
FDA category[b]	C	X	B (etanercept)[c] B (infliximab)
Breast-feeding[d]	Contra-indicated	Contra-indicated	No data

[a] Positive, disease is worse than the drug; neutral, always better to stop the drug if possible; negative; drug is always worse than the disease.

[b] FDA category: A, no foetal risk in controlled studies; B, no risk in animals, no controlled human studies; or abnormalities in animal studies but not in controlled human studies; C, studies show teratogenic or embryocidal effects in animals, but no controlled human studies; or no studies are available in either human or animals; D, positive evidence for foetal abnormalities but potential benefits may outweigh potential risks; X, contra-indicated.

[c] High doses of these drugs have been tested in animals, without leading to teratogenicity, controlled human studies have not been done.

[d] According to the Micromedex (2002) advice.

Table 5 Use of miscellaneous antirheumatic drugs in pregnancy

	Paracetamol	Intravenous immunoglobulins	Colchicine
Fertility	No effect	Probably no effect	Probably no effect
Teratogenicity	No	No effect	Probably not
Late pregnancy	No problems	No problems	No problems
Risk/benefit ratio[a]	Neutral–positive	Neutral–positive depending on disease	Positive depending on disease
FDA category[b]	B	C	C
Breast-feeding[c]	Compatible	Unknown, probably compatible	Compatible

[a] Positive, disease is worse than the drug; neutral, always better to stop the drug if possible; negative, drug is always worse than the disease.

[b] FDA category: A, no foetal risk in controlled studies; B, no risk in animals, no controlled human studies; or abnormalities in animal studies but not in controlled human studies; C, studies show teratogenic or embryocidal effects in animals, but no controlled human studies; or no studies are available in either human or animals; D, positive evidence for foetal abnormalities but potential benefits may outweigh potential risks; X, contra-indicated.

[c] According to the Micromedex (2002) advice.

have been exposed to 60–80 mg/day of aspirin that has been shown to have a positive effect on interleukin-3, a cytokine that affects pregnancy and foetal development. No adverse effect of low-dose aspirin of 80 mg/day or lesser on clotting ability, renal function, or ductus arteriosus in the newborn has been demonstrated. Doses up to 80 mg/day of aspirin can be used safely throughout pregnancy.

Breast-feeding

Aspirin is found in breast milk up to approximately 20 per cent of the amount ingested by the mother. Peak salicylate concentrations in milk occur about 2 h after peak serum levels in the mother. In case of high anti-inflammatory doses of aspirin ingested by the mother the child is potentially at risk of developing salicylate intoxication and bleeding problems during lactation. It is therefore recommended that aspirin can be used during breast-feeding, but with caution and in low doses.

NSAIDs

The most commonly used antirheumatic drugs during pregnancy are NSAIDs. They readily cross the placenta and block prostaglandin synthesis in a variety of foetal tissues. Because of the prostaglandin blocking effect NSAIDs have been used for pregnancy related indications such as premature labour, polyhydramnion, and pregnancy-induced hypertension.

Far less information is available on the relatively new NSAIDs and pregnancy than on aspirin and pregnancy. The risk of NSAIDs during pregnancy is best researched for indomethacin, sulindac, naproxen, ibuprofen, ketoprofen, and diclofenac (Ostensen 1998; Ostensen and Ramsey-Goldman 1998), mostly because of their ability to suppress premature labour. The potential adverse effects of NSAIDs in pregnancy have been described most extensively for indomethacin (Norton 1997), though these adverse effects have also been reported to a certain extent for the other NSAIDs. The potential side effects of NSAIDs in pregnancy are linked to their ability to inhibit prostaglandin synthesis. Dose, duration, and period of gestation are important determinants of the extent of these effects.

Effects on the mother

There is some evidence that women who have problems in conceiving should stop NSAIDs when attempting to become pregnant because of the findings in a variety of animal models indicating that prostaglandin inhibitors block blastocyst implantation (Janssen and Genta 2000). Ingestion of NSAIDs near term will significantly delay and prolong labour. There is a serious risk of increased maternal blood loss at delivery. If NSAIDs are stopped at least 1 month before the expected delivery these problems can be avoided.

Effects on the child

NSAIDs can cross the placenta and have been detected in foetal tissues (Siu et al. 2000). A recent study reported no increased risk for any congenital malformation with NSAID use in early pregnancy. But when controlled for maternal age, parity, and smoking habits, in a small number of women there was an increased risk for cardiac defects and of oral facial clefts (Ericson and Kallen 2001). The general opinion is that NSAIDs can be continued during conception and the first two trimesters of pregnancy when necessary to control maternal disease (Ostensen 1998, 2001; Ostensen and Ramsey-Goldman 1998; Janssen and Genta 2000; Micromedex 2002).

NSAIDs administered in the last trimester of pregnancy can cause premature constriction of the ductus arteriosus, pulmonary hypertension, impaired renal function, a reduction in foetal urine output, and oligohydramnion. These effects are reversible if the NSAID is stopped (Rein et al. 1999). Due to the effect on platelets, NSAIDs administered in the perinatal period can cause intracerebral haemorrhage in the child. Discontinuation of NSAIDs 6–8 weeks before delivery is considered safe. Theoretically the effects of the new COX-2 selective inhibitors on the duration of labour and clotting function should be less compared to that of the non-selective COX inhibitors. The effects on the foetal vasculature and renal function are, however, the same as for the non-selective COX inhibitors and for the benefit of the child discontinuation of any NSAID 6–8 weeks prior to the expected delivery is warranted. Because of the lack of data on these new drugs, the COX-2 selective inhibitors are better avoided in pregnant women altogether.

Breast-feeding

Because breast milk has a pH of 6.9–7.6, weak acids are ionized so drugs such as NSAIDs are not readily distributed into the breast milk. Trace amounts of naproxen, piroxicam, ibuprofen, and diclofenac have been reported in breast milk (Janssen and Genta 2000; Micromedex 2002). NSAID use is considered compatible with breast-feeding, though some NSAIDs (indomethacin, sulindac) circulate enterohepatically and should therefore be avoided. NSAIDs are contraindicated in the jaundiced neonate

Table 6 Summary of recommendations

1. Aspirin

Low dose, ≤ 80 mg/day of aspirin can be used safely throughout pregnancy without evident risk of foetal malformations, clotting problems in either mother or child, or abnormality in foetal renal function or premature closure of the ductus arteriosus. Cautious use of low dose of aspirin during breast-feeding will not adversely affect the child. High, anti-inflammatory doses of aspirin should be avoided during all stages of pregnancy, in particular in the last trimester

2. NSAIDs

NSAIDs can be safely used in the first and second trimester of pregnancy, if necessary to control maternal disease. There is no consistent reported risk of foetal malformation. NSAIDs should be stopped in the last 6–8 weeks of pregnancy because of the prostaglandin inhibiting effects on mother and child potentially leading to a delayed labour, renal, and vascular effects on the child and perinatal bleeding in mother and child. NSAIDs with a short half-life and inactive metabolites, such as ibuprofen, flurbiprofen, and diclofenac may be used more safely, in particular during breast-feeding (Spigset and Hagg 2000). Since only trace amounts of NSAIDs will appear in breast milk, breast-feeding is recommended to be compatible with NSAID use. There is a lack of data on the new COX-2 selective inhibitors in pregnancy and their use in pregnant or lactating women should be avoided

3. Corticosteroids

Low dose of prednisone is considered safe in pregnancy for both mother and child. High doses (1–2 mg/kg/day) should be avoided during the first trimester because of the possible risk of oral cleft in the child. The fluorinated corticosteroids, dexamethasone, and betamethasone, will pass the placenta and are only used to treat the foetus, if necessary. The lowest possible dose of prednisone needed to control the maternal disease should be used to minimize the risk for gestational diabetes and hypertension. Calcium supplementation for prevention of osteopaenia is advisable. Emergency surgery, cesarean section and prolonged labour are indications for 'stress doses' of corticosteroids. Breast-feeding is compatible with prednisone doses up to 20 mg/day, 3–4 h before actual breast-feeding

4. Antimalarials

The favourable effects of hydroxychloroquine in preventing flares in SLE outweigh the potential risk for the unborn child. No adverse effects on the child have been found in the doses of hydroxychloroquine of 200–400 mg/day commonly used to treat the rheumatic diseases. Breast-feeding should be undertaken cautiously because of the long elimination half-life and the risk of accumulation

5. Sulfasalazine

Sulfasalazine can be safely used prior to and during all stages of pregnancy. Males who wish to produce offspring should stop the drug because of its adverse effect on spermatozoa. This effect is reversible after discontinuation of the drug. Breast-feeding is compatible with sulfasalazine treatment though should be advised with caution because of the rare event that the mother is a slow acetylator

6. Gold

Common practice is to continue gold treatment until pregnancy is recognized and then stop the treatment. There seems no risk of foetal malformation, although this is based on very limited information. Gold therapy is compatible with breast-feeding, but it seems most prudent to avoid nursing because of the possible toxic effect on the infant

7. Penicillamine

Penicillamine should be stopped in women who wish to become pregnant because of the serious risk of congenital malformations and the far better alternatives available for the treatment of the rheumatic diseases during pregnancy

8. Methotrexate

Methotrexate is contra-indicated in the treatment of the rheumatic diseases during pregnancy. The rate of abortion and congenital abnormalities is significantly increased particularly with exposure during the first trimester. Strict contraception is needed when a patient is on methotrexate. Fertility appears not to be adversely effected by prior methotrexate use. Women and men who wish to conceive have to stop methotrexate treatment 4–6 months prior to conception. Continuation of folate supplementation is advised to prevent adverse outcome due to folic deficiency. Breast-feeding is contra-indicated because of excretion of methotrexate in breast milk

9. Azathioprine

Women with severe rheumatic diseases that are otherwise hard to control may use azathioprine during pregnancy. No apparent congenital malformations are known with doses of azathioprine up to approximately 2 mg/kg/day. Exposure to azathioprine throughout pregnancy may lead to immunosuppression and low blood cell counts in the neonate. Strict adjustment of the azathioprine dosage to maintain normal maternal blood cell counts may prevent neonatal abnormalities. Breast-feeding is not recommended

10. Cyclophosphamide

Cyclophosphamide treatment leads to infertility in particular after cumulative doses and in patients aged over 30 years. Cryopreservation of semen and oocytes can help to preserve the changes of future offspring. Oral contraception is advised to possibly protect ovarian function during cyclophosphamide treatment. Adequate contraception is anyhow necessary because of the teratogenicity of the drug. Exposure to cyclophosphamide during the first trimester of pregnancy leads to congenital malformation and should be avoided. Treatment with cyclophosphamide during the second half of pregnancy may be considered in case of severe, life threatening disease of the mother. Breast-feeding is contra-indicated

11. Cyclosporine A

Cyclosporine is apparently not associated with congenital malformation, but can cause prematurity and intra-uterine growth retardation. Long-term effect of intrauterine exposure is not known. It is generally advised not to use cyclosporine during pregnancy unless the severity of the maternal disease urges to do so. Breast-feeding should be discouraged in women using cyclosporine

12. Leflunomide

Leflunomide is contra-indicated during pregnancy and safe contraception during its use is warranted. Due to the long half-life and slow elimination time, leflunomide should be washed out in both male and female patients who wish to conceive. The wash-out procedure consists of 8 g of cholestyramine three times daily for 11 days, followed by two separate tests to verify whether the drug has been eliminated. If blood levels remain high the procedure has to be repeated. Without a wash-out the levels of leflunomide may stay too high for pregnancy for up to 2 years. Breast-feeding is considered unsafe

13. Colchicine

Colchicine is considered safe during pregnancy as well as during breast-feeding. Fertility is probably not decreased with the possible exception of males taking colchicine because of Behçet's disease because of their property to displace bilirubin and by that increasing the risk of kernicterus.

Paracetamol (acetaminophen)

Paracetamol is the most widely used analgesic during pregnancy. Therapeutic doses are safely used during pregnancy without apparent adverse affects on mother or child. The drug is distributed in breast milk in amount ranging from approximately 1–2 per cent of the maternal dose (Micromedex 2002). The usage of paracetamol during pregnancy and breast-feeding is considered safe (Spigset and Hagg 2000).

Since paracetamol is only a moderate painkiller without anti-inflammatory properties the drug is for most pregnant women with an active rheumatic disease often not sufficient to treat the maternal disease.

Glucocorticoids

Glucocorticoid therapy is the mainstay treatment for SLE during pregnancy and is also a popular choice in joint diseases when NSAIDs are insufficient to control the arthritis. Many potentially serious adverse effects of high dose corticosteroids in pregnancy have been reported for both mother and child, although one should realize that active SLE per se, for which the corticosteroids are prescribed, may equally well be the culprit of the observed adverse effects (see Chapter 1.3.1.1). The non-fluorinated steroid preparations such as prednisone, prednisolone, and methylprednisolone are the drugs of choice to treat active maternal disease. They are metabolized by placental 11-hydroxygenase, and the foetus is exposed to only 10 per cent of the maternal dose. If the foetus has to be treated, for example, in case of immature lungs or foetal carditis due to anti-SSA/SSB antibodies, fluorinated corticosteroids such as dexamethasone and betamethasone are preferred because they are less well metabolized in the placenta and higher doses are available to the foetus.

Effects on the mother

All the well-known side effects of corticosteroids may be more marked when used during pregnancy. Pregnancy is associated with hypertension, hyperglycaemia, striae, osteopenia, and immunosuppression, the risk of these conditions will be enhanced by corticosteroid use. Premature rupture of the membranes has been observed during steroid use, although the causative role of corticosteroids cannot be separated from the possible role of a flare of the underlying rheumatic disease.

Effects on the child

Exposure to corticosteroids during pregnancy has been studied in various animal species resulting in reports on deleterious effects on the offspring, including cleft palate. In the human series, no evidence was found for congenital abnormalities due to corticosteroid use in pregnancy (Esplin and Branch 1997; Ostensen and Ramsey-Goldman 1998; Janssen and Genta 2000; Ostensen 2001). However, in a meta-analysis of epidemiological studies an increased risk for oral clefts after exposure to corticosteroids during the first trimester was found (Park-Wyllie et al. 2000). There are some case reports on masculinization of female infants, growth restriction, neonatal cataract, and adrenal suppression in children exposed to high doses of corticosteroid before birth (Ostensen 2001).

Breast-feeding

The dose of corticosteroids found in breast milk is negliglible when the mother receives prednisone 20 mg or less. Abstaining from breast-feeding in the 3–4 h after the mother has taken her medication can minimize the dose received by the infant (Micromedex 2002).

Chloroquine and hydroxychloroquine

Most observations of the effects of antimalarials during pregnancy have been made in women taking malaria prophylaxis with chloroquine. Hydroxychloroquine is widely used in the treatment of rheumatic diseases. The use of antimalarials in RA is relatively easy to avoid but it is a mainstay of treatment in many patients with SLE and can help to prevent flares during pregnancy.

Effects on the mother

Knowledge is now accumulating about hydroxychloroquine exposure in pregnant SLE patients (Buchanan et al. 1996; Parke and West 1996; Janssen and Genta 2000; Ostensen 2001). A double blind, placebo-controlled trial of hydroxychloroquine in lupus pregnancy was published recently (Levy et al. 2001). Discontinuation of hydroxychloroquine may precipitate a flare of the SLE with harmful consequences for mother and child. For both it appears to be better to continue the hydroxychloroquine therapy during pregnancy since women on hydroxychloroquine experienced less disease activity and better neonatal outcome than women who stopped hydroxychloroquine (Levy et al. 2001).

Effects on the child

Chloroquine crosses the placenta and accumulates preferentially in melanin-containing structures in the foetal uveal tract and inner ear. In animal models, abnormalities of the foetal eye have been reported as well as in some infants who had been exposed to higher than the daily recommended dose of chloroquine throughout pregnancy (Ostensen and Ramsey-Goldman 1998; Ostensen 2001). No increase in the rate of congenital abnormalities, prematurity, or foetal growth restriction was found in a cohort study of 169 pregnancies of women exposed to chloroquine 300 mg/week for malaria prophylaxis as compared to a four times larger control group.

In the last few years, it has become apparent that hydroxychloroquine used in doses of 200–400 mg/day to prevent SLE flare carries no risk of congenital malformation or adverse neonatal outcome (Buchanan et al. 1996; Parke and West 1996; Klinger et al. 2001; Levy et al. 2001; Motta et al. 2002). Discontinuation of hydroxychloroquine in controlled SLE runs the risk of flares and consequently harms the child. It is therefore advised not to stop hydroxychloroquine during gestation. Moreover, due to the very long elimination time of hydroxychloroquine, the foetus will still be exposed to the drug long after the mother has stopped taking the drug.

Breast-feeding

Low concentrations of hydroxychloroquine are found in breast milk. Although hydroxychloroquine is considered compatible with breast-feeding, the slow elimination rate and the potential accumulation of a toxic amount of hydroxychloroquine in the infant, breast-feeding should be undertaken with caution (Micromedex 2002).

Sulfasalazine

Sulfasalazine is an effective treatment for RA in a daily dose up to 3 g/day. About 30 per cent of the drug is absorbed in the small intestine; the other 70 per cent passes into the colon where it is cleaved into 5-aminosalicylic acid and sulfapyridine. Sulfasalazine and sulfapyridine cross the placenta and foetal blood concentrations will come close to maternal concentrations. The 5-amino salicylic acid has very limited placental transfer. There are data available for the safe use of sulfasalazine in over 2000 pregnancies of women with inflammatory bowel disease (Rains et al. 1995). There is no reason to assume that the safety of sulfasalazine in pregnant women with arthritis would prove to be different from its safety in pregnant women with inflammatory bowel disease.

Effects on the mother

Sulfasalazine does not adversely affect fertility in women and can therefore safely be prescribed in women who wish to become pregnant. If the arthritis is not adequately controlled after conception the drug can be continued during gestation without problems. In contrast to the situation in women, men have decreased fertility with sulfasalazine due to oligospermia, impaired sperm motility, and an increase in abnormal spermatozoa (Rains et al. 1995; Janssen and Genta 2000). The decreased fertility has been shown reversible when treatment with the drug is discontinued.

Effects on the child

The wealth of data regarding pregnancy and sulfasalazine use in inflammatory bowel disease shows no increased rate of congenital malformation, prematurity or low gestational weight (Rains et al. 1995; Ostensen and Ramsey-Goldman 1998; Janssen and Genta 2000). Theoretically, sulfasalazine may increase the risk of kernicterus when used near term because of its bilirubin-displacing ability. Severe neonatal jaundice, however, has never been reported in connection with maternal sulfasalazine use.

Sulfasalazine is thought to have an effect on folate metabolism and may cause folate deficiency. Folate supplementation would seem prudent both prior to and during pregnancy in women taking sulfasalazine (Janssen and Genta 2000; Rains et al. 1995). Nowadays, folate supplementation is recommended for all women considering pregnancy.

Breast-feeding

Sulfasalazine concentrations in breast milk may reach 40–50 per cent of the concentration found in the mother. Sulfasalazine use is considered compatible with breast-feeding. Substantial adverse effects have been published in some infants, probably because of high drug concentrations in the mother due to slow acetylation. It has been advised to use sulfasalazine with caution during breast-feeding (Micromedex 2002).

Gold

Intramuscular gold has been used extensively to treat RA in the past, although the data on its use during pregnancy are very limited (Esplin and Branch 1997; Ostensen and Ramsey-Goldman 1998; Janssen and Genta 2000; Ostensen 2001). Gold is not one of the first choice drugs for RA anymore, but it may still be an alternative drug in the treatment of arthritis of women or men who choose to have offspring.

Effects on the mother

Rheumatologists often advise their patients to continue gold therapy until pregnancy is recognized and then stop the injections. One approach in long-term gold treatment is to give monthly injections on the first day of menses. Gold does not seem to impair fertility in either women or men. Data on gold therapy during pregnancy, albeit scarce, does not reveal adverse effects on the mother. Generally, the drug can be stopped during gestation because of the favourable effect of pregnancy itself on the arthritis.

Effects on the child

The limited data on possible adverse effects of gold treatment on the foetus are conflicting and uncontrolled. Gold compounds cross the placenta and are found in foetal tissues. In over 100 reports on gold therapy during pregnancy, no congenital malformations have been observed (Ostensen 2001). One case of multiple foetal malformations in a mother who received aurothiomalate has been reported, though a causal relationship between the malformations and the drug was disputed. To date, little is known about the effect of oral gold (auranofin) on the human foetus, but no abnormalities occurred in the few pregnancy reported during oral gold treatment.

Breast-feeding

Gold is excreted in human breast milk in significant amounts. There have been reports of skin rash, nephritis, hepatitis, and blood dyscrasias in children of mothers treated with gold injections while nursing their infants (Janssen and Genta 2000; Micromedex 2002). Although gold is usually considered compatible with breast-feeding, caution is recommended because of the long retention of gold in the body and the potential toxic effects in the infant.

Penicillamine

Penicillamine is used in the treatment of RA and scleroderma. Its popularity is, however, waning because of a wider choice of more effective treatments, in particular for RA. The possible risks of this drug during pregnancy definitely outweigh the benefits (Ostensen and Ramsey-Goldman 1998; Janssen and Genta 2000; Ostensen 2001). In contrast, the use of penicillamine in Wilson's disease is crucial for a successful outcome of pregnancy in this disease. Therefore, knowledge about the teratogenicity of penicillamine mainly comes from the experience in the treatment of pregnant women with Wilson's disease.

Effects on the child

In animals as well as in humans a variety of connective tissue abnormalities have been found in the neonates, including cutis laxa, physical defects such as wide nasal bridge, low set ears, flattened face, club feet, inguinal hernia, congenital hip dislocation, and ventricular septal defects have been reported (Micromedex 2002). There are also reports on favourable outcomes of pregnancy after prenatal exposure to penicillamine, which make its use acceptable for women with Wilson's disease. The risks of penicillamine during pregnancy are not acceptable for women with a rheumatic disease, for them the risk/benefit ratio is much too high.

Breast-feeding

There are no reports on breast-feeding and mothers on penicillamine should not nurse their infants (Micromedex 2002).

Methotrexate

Methotrexate (MTX) is the mainstay drug in the treatment of RA and is also frequently used in many other rheumatic diseases. It is the drug of choice in early RA and patients of child-bearing age will often be on MTX treatment (Bresnihan 2001).

The experience with MTX during pregnancy mainly comes from women treated with high dose MTX often in combination with other cytotoxic drugs, and from women who have taken the drug to terminate pregnancy, for example, because of an ectopic pregnancy. Also, some very small series of pregnancies exposed to low-dose MTX have been published (Esplin and Branch 1997; Ostensen and Ramsey-Goldman 1998; Janssen and Genta 2000; Ostensen 2001). An extensive review on the effects of MTX on pregnancy, fertility, and lactation was published in 1999 (Lloyd et al. 1999).

Effects on the mother

MTX does not impair fertility, even in high doses. Oligospermia has been reported, though further studies showed no long-term effects on ovarian or testicular function (Lloyd et al. 1999). The presence of MTX in liver tissue has been reported up to 116 days after MTX exposure. The duration of spermatogenesis is approximately 74 days. Consequently, a period of 6 months off MTX therapy seems safe for men before attempting conception.

MTX is a strong abortifacient and has been used for that purpose. It can be expected that exposure to low dose MTX in early pregnancy will lead to an increased abortion rate. In small series of patients exposed to low dose MTX in the first trimester there was indeed an increase in the abortion rate (Ostensen and Ramsey-Goldman 1998; Lloyd et al. 1999; Janssen and Genta 2000; Ostensen 2001). Because of the embryotoxicity, women of child bearing age on MTX must use adequate contraception. Women who wish to conceive must stop MTX at least 3–4 months prior to conception and folate supplementation is best continued to avoid folic depletion.

Effects on the child

MTX treatment is associated with increased risk of congenital malformation. Women who wish to continue pregnancy when exposed to MTX in the first trimester have a 20–30 per cent chance of an abnormal child (Lloyd et al. 1999). The MTX-induced congenital defects are similar to those produced by aminopterin, another folic antagonist. The defects to be expected with severe folate deficiency include neural tube defects resulting in anencephaly, hydrocephaly, meningomyelocele, and ossification defects resulting in craniofacial and limb defects.

Developmental delay has also been reported (Del Campo et al. 1999). The most vulnerable period for the development of foetal malformations is 6–8 weeks of gestation (Lloyd et al. 1999). Women who wish to continue pregnancy having had exposure during the first trimester of pregnancy should be offered treatment with folinic acid in order to minimize MTX effects on the foetus. MTX exposure in the second and third trimesters of pregnancy is associated with growth retardation and myelosuppression (Del Campo et al. 1999; Lloyd et al. 1999; Janssen and Genta 2000).

Breast-feeding

MTX is excreted in breast milk in low concentrations and may accumulate in neonatal tissues. Breast-feeding is contra-indicated because of potentially severe problems in the neonatal infant (Janssen and Genta 2000; Micromedex 2002).

Azathioprine

Experience of azathioprine exposure during pregnancy is derived mainly from the treatment of transplantation patients complemented by some reports of treatment in SLE and inflammatory bowel disease (Ramsey-Goldman and Schilling 1997; Ostensen and Ramsey-Goldman 1998; Janssen and Genta 2000; Ostensen 2001; Micromedex 2002). Azathioprine crosses the placenta, but the foetal liver lacks the enzyme inosate pyrophophorylase and is therefore unable to convert azathioprine to its active and more toxic metabolite, 6-mercaptopurine. This foetal enzyme deficiency theoretically protects the foetus from any teratogenic effect of azathioprine in early pregnancy.

Effects on the mother

There seems to be no adverse effect on fertility and no increase in the abortion rate in women exposed to azathioprine. This drug is used to preserve allografts or to control systemic autoimmune disease. The choice to continue treatment during pregnancy is dependent on the need to treat maternal disease.

Effects on the child

No predominant or specific pattern of malformation has been identified during 40 years of experience. There are some reports of congenital malformations, but a causal relationship with azathioprine is hard to prove. Women with abnormal babies took significantly higher doses of azathioprine than women with normal babies, suggesting some risk for congenital deformities with increasing doses of azathioprine (Janssen and Genta 2000; Ostensen 2001; Micromedex 2002). Exposure throughout pregnancy has been associated with a variety of adverse effects including thymic atrophy, intra-uterine growth retardation, foetal immunosuppression, foetal pancytopaenia, and chromosomal aberrations. Often, the mother received several drugs and it was not possible to blame either one of the drugs or the underlying disease for the adverse effects on the child. It has been suggested that adjustment of the azathioprine dosage to maintain normal maternal blood cell counts might prevent neonatal cytopenias.

Breast-feeding

Low concentrations of azathioprine have been found in breast milk. Breast-feeding is not recommended because of the potential adverse effects for the child.

Cyclophosphamide

Cyclophosphamide is an alkylating agent only used in rheumatology to treat severe, potentially life threatening disease. The observations of cyclophosphamide exposure during pregnancy are predominantly in women with malignancies (Esplin and Branch 1997; Ramsey-Goldman and Schilling 1997; Ostensen and Ramsey-Goldman 1998; Janssen and Genta 2000; Ostensens 2001; Micromedex 2002).

Effects on the mother

The adverse effect of cyclophosphamide on fertility in both men and women is well recognized. The key risk factors for ovarian failure after cyclophosphamide exposure are age 31 years or more, total doses of more than 10 g and treatment greater than 15 pulse cycles (Esplin and Branch 1997; Janssen and Genta 2000). Men who start cyclophosphamide treatment have the option of cryopreservation of their semen. Cryopreservation of oocytes is much more complicated and often not possible due to the underlying disease. Inhibition of ovulation, for example, by oral contraceptives is believed to protect ovarian follicle viability. Adequate contraception during cyclophosphamide therapy is necessary because of the teratogenic effects of the drug.

Effects on the child

Both in animals and in humans congenital malformations and changes in the foetal genome have been found when exposed to cyclophosphamide in the first trimester of pregnancy, although normal newborns have also been reported. Abnormalities include facial clefts, limb reduction defects, and craniofacial dysmorphisms. Exposure of the foetus to cyclophosphamide in second half of pregnancy may lead to myelotoxicity of the foetus and growth retardation. It is not established whether the latter adverse effect is due to the underlying disease or to the drug. The risk/benefit ratio may permit cyclophosphamide treatment in the second half of pregnancy in case of severe systemic disease of the mother.

Breast-feeding

Cyclophosphamide has been found in substantial amounts in human breast milk. Breast-feeding is therefore unsafe for the newborn child.

Cyclosporine

More than 600 pregnancies exposed to cyclosporine have been reported, mainly in transplant recipients (Olshan et al. 1994; Ostensen and Ramsey-Goldman 1998; Janssen and Genta 2000; Ostensen 2001; Tendron et al. 2002; Micromedex 2002).

Effects on the mother

There is no indication that cyclosporine impairs human fertility. In case of rheumatoid arthritis the drug can be stopped before pregnancy and, if necessary, replaced by an alternative drug more compatible with pregnancy. When the woman is treated because of systemic disease the possible benefits of the treatment have to be weighted against the possible harm the drug can caused during pregnancy. Renal impairment and hypertension are of particular concern during pregnancy.

Effects on the child

Cyclosporine crosses the placenta and foetal levels may reach between 37 and 64 per cent of the maternal plasma levels. It has been shown to have embryotoxic and fetotoxic effects in animals, but only at supra-therapeutic dose levels. In women receiving an average dose of cyclosporine of 5 mg/kg/day during pregnancy no increased rate of congenital malformations was seen. The major problems were prematurity and low birth weight in approximately 50 per cent of the pregnancies. It is difficult to estimate what the independent contribution of cyclosporine treatment to these pregnancy problems is, since concomitant medication or the underlying disease may cause these problems as well. The effects of foetal exposure to cyclosporine in the long term are not known.

Breast-feeding

Cyclosporine is excreted in human breast milk, therefore breast-feeding should be avoided.

Leflunomide

Leflunomide is a new drug amongst the medications to treat arthritis. There are no data published on leflunomide exposure during human pregnancy (Prakash and Jarvis 1999; Janssen and Genta 2000; Ostensen 2001). Animal data indicate that exposure to leflunonide during pregnancy has teratogenic and foetotoxic effects at normal therapeutic levels. The malformations observed include anophthalmia, micro-ophthalmia, and hydrocephalus. In addition, embryolethality and reduced foetal weight were noted in animals. Due to the long half-life and slow elimination time, leflunomide should be washed out in both male and female patients who wish to conceive (Table 6). Distribution of leflunomide into breast milk is unknown.

TNF-α blockade

TNF-α inhibition is becoming increasingly popular in the treatment of various rheumatic diseases, in particular, rheumatoid arthritis. Only a very few reports on human pregnancies exposed to TNF-α inhibitors are known (Janssen and Genta 2000; Ostensen 2001; Micromedex 2002).

Etanercept

Soluble TNF-α receptor crosses the placenta in mice, but does not impair foetal development. Studies in rats and rabbits did not find teratogenicity or fetotoxicity with doses by far exceeding the therapeutic human doses. Because of insufficient data in humans it is advised to abstain from pregnancy while on etanercept treatment. No data are available on breast-feeding, but immunoglobulins are known to be excreted in human milk. Because of the potential for serious adverse effects in nursing infants breast-feeding should be discouraged during etanercept treatment.

Infliximab

In mice, no embryo- or foetotoxicity was noted. Only one case of exposure to infliximab in early pregnancy in a woman with inflammatory bowel disease and an adverse outcome (prematurity and death) was reported (Srinivasan 2001). The patient had active disease at time of conception that also may explain the adverse outcome of the pregnancy. Initial observations in a series of human pregnancies exposed to infliximab in the first trimester did not show an increase in birth defects or adverse pregnancy outcomes (Ostensen 2001). Since the safety of infliximab during pregnancy has not been sufficiently documented, safe contraception is recommended during its use. No data are available on excretion in human milk and breast-feeding is therefore considered unsafe.

Intravenous immunoglobulins

Intravenous immunoglobulins are sometimes used in specific autoimmune conditions such as antiphospholipid syndrome, myositis, and autoimmune thrombocytopenia. Information regarding teratogenicity in animals is limited. In humans, immunoglobulins will cross the placenta after 32 weeks of pregnancy. No harmful effects to the foetus have been reported. Care has to be taken to prevent hepatitis virus transfer through the infusion. If necessary for the treatment of the mother, intravenous immunoglobulins may be administered during pregnancy without apparent adverse effect to the foetus. There seems to be no harm in breast-feeding during intravenous immunoglobulins therapy, because of transfer of protective immunoglobulins to the child.

Colchicine

Colchicine is mainly used for gout, which is very uncommon in women of child-bearing age. It is also used in conditions such as Behçet's disease.

Effects on the mother

In high doses, colchicine arrests mitosis through an inhibitory effect on microtubuli. Theoretically colchicine may induce infertility. In males an increased frequency of oligospermia and azoospermia has been found in patients with Behcet's disease but not in patients with familial Mediterranean fever (FMF) during treatment with colchicine (Ben-Chetrit and Levy 1998). In women the fertility rate appears to remain normal when on colchicine. With colchicine treatment FMF patients seem to have even higher fertility and better pregnancy outcome than without treatment due to a better control of the disease.

Effects on the child

Colchicine has been found to be teratogenic in mice and transplacental passage has been described in humans (Ben-Chetrit and Levy 1998; Ostensen and Ramsey-Goldman 1998; Micromedex 2002). In humans treated with colchicine during pregnancy—mainly because of FMF—no increase in the rate of congenital malformations, miscarriages or stillbirths was seen. A slight increase in trisomy 21 was noted in the FMF patients using colchicine during pregnancy, though this was ascribed to a probably slight increased risk for this abnormality in FMF itself (Ben-Chetrit and Levy 1998).

Breast-feeding

Colchicine is excreted in human milk reaching similar levels to that in the serum of the mother (Ben-Chetrit and Levy 1998; Micromedex 2002). However, the estimated daily amount of colchicine ingested by the nursing infant was at least 10 times less than the therapeutic dose (per kilogram) given to the mother. Breast-feeding is considered safe for the child.

References

Ben-Chetrit, E. and Levy, M. (1998). Colchicine: 1998 update. *Seminars in Arthritis and Rheumatism* **28** (1), 48–59.

Bresnihan, B. (2001). Treating early rheumatoid arthritis in the younger patient. *Journal of Rheumatology* **62** (Suppl.), 4–9.

Buchanan, N.M. et al. (1996). Hydroxychloroquine and lupus pregnancy: review of a series of 36 cases. *Annals of the Rheumatic Diseases* **55** (7), 486–8.

Del Campo, M. et al. (1999). Developmental delay in foetal aminopterin/methotrexate syndrome. *Teratology* **60** (1), 10–12.

Ericson, A. and Kallen, B.A. (2001). Nonsteroidal anti-inflammatory drugs in early pregnancy. *Reproductive Toxicology* **15** (4), 371–5.

Esplin, M.S. and Branch, D.W. (1997). Immunosuppressive drugs and pregnancy. *Obstetric and Gynecological Clinics of North America* **24** (3), 601–16.

Ginsberg, J.S., Greer, I., and Hirsh, J. (2001). Use of antithrombotic agents during pregnancy. *Chest* **119** (Suppl. 1), 122S–131S.

Janssen, N.M. and Genta, M.S. (2000). The effects of immunosuppressive and anti-inflammatory medications on fertility, pregnancy, and lactation. *Archives of Internal Medicine* **160** (5), 610–19.

Klinger, G. et al. (2001). Ocular toxicity and antenatal exposure to chloroquine or hydroxychloroquine for rheumatic diseases. *Lancet* **358** (9284): 813–14.

Levy, R.A. et al. (2001). Hydroxychloroquine (HCQ) in lupus pregnancy: double-blind and placebo-controlled study. *Lupus* **10** (6), 401–4.

Lloyd, M. et al. (1999). The effects of methotrexate on pregnancy, fertility and lactation. *Quarterly Journal of Medicine* **92** (10), 551–63.

Mascola, M.A. and Repke, J.T. (1997). Obstetric management of the high-risk lupus pregnancy. *Rheumatic Disease Clinics of North America* **23** (1), 119–32.

Micromedex (2002) *Micromedex® Healthcare Series* Vol. 112 Colorado: Micromedex, G.V. (edition expires 6/2002).

Motta, M. et al. (2002). Antimalarial agents in pregnancy. *Lancet* **359** (9305), 524–5.

Nelson, J.L. and Ostensen, M. (1997). Pregnancy and rheumatoid arthritis. *Rheumatic Disease Clinics of North America* **23** (1), 195–212.

Norton, M.E. (1997). Teratogen update: fetal effects of indomethacin administration during pregnancy. *Teratology* **56** (4), 282–92.

Olshan, A.F., Mattison, D.R., and Zwanenburg, T.S. (1994). International Commission for Protection Against Environmental Mutagens and Carcinogens. Cyclosporine A: review of genotoxicity and potential for adverse human reproductive and developmental effects. Report of a Working Group on the genotoxicity of cyclosporine A, August 18, 1993. *Mutation Research* **317** (2), 163–73.

Ostensen, M. and Ramsey-Goldman, R. (1998). Treatment of inflammatory rheumatic disorders in pregnancy: what are the safest treatment options? *Drug Safety* **19** (5), 389–410.

Ostensen, M. (1998). Nonsteroidal anti-inflammatory drugs during pregnancy. *Scandinavian Journal of Rheumatology* **107** (Suppl.), 128–32.

Ostensen, M. (2001). Drugs in pregnancy. Rheumatological disorders. *Best Practice Research Clinics in Obstetrics and Gynaecology* **15** (6), 953–69.

Parke, A. and West, B. (1996). Hydroxychloroquine in pregnant patients with systemic lupus erythematosus. *Journal of Rheumatology* **23** (10), 1715–18.

Park-Wyllie, L. et al. (2000). Birth defects after maternal exposure to corticosteroids: prospective cohort study and meta-analysis of epidemiological studies. *Teratology* **62** (6), 385–92.

Petri, M. (1997). Hopkins Lupus Pregnancy Center: 1987 to 1996. *Rheumatic Disease Clinics of North America* **23** (1), 1–13.

Prakash, A. and Jarvis, B. (1999). Leflunomide: a review of its use in active rheumatoid arthritis. *Drugs* **58** (6), 1137–64.

Rains, C.P., Noble, S., and Faulds, D. (1995). Sulfasalazine. A review of its pharmacological properties and therapeutic efficacy in the treatment of rheumatoid arthritis. *Drugs* **50** (1), 137–56.

Ramsey-Goldman, R. and Schilling, E. (1997). Immunosuppressive drug use during pregnancy. *Rheumatic Diseases Clinics of North America* **23** (1), 149–67.

Rein, A.J. et al. (1999). Contraction of the fetal ductus arteriosus induced by diclofenac. Case report. *Fetal Diagnosis and Therapy* **14** (1), 24–5.

Siu, S.S., Yeung, J.H., and Lau, T.K. (2000). A study on placental transfer of diclofenac in first trimester of human pregnancy. *Human Reproduction* **15** (11), 2423–5.

Spigset, O. and Hagg, S. (2000). Analgesics and breast-feeding: safety considerations. *Paediatric Drugs* **2** (3), 223–38.

Srinivasan, R. (2001). Infliximab treatment and pregnancy outcome in active Crohn's disease. *American Journal of Gastroenterology* **96** (7), 2274–5.

Tendron, A., Gouyon, J.B., and Decramer, S. (2002). In utero exposure to immunosuppressive drugs: experimental and clinical studies. *Pediatric Nephrology* **17** (2), 121–30.

1.3.2 The skin and rheumatic disease

C.R. Lovell and Peter J. Maddison

Introduction

Why is it important to examine the skin in a patient with arthritis? The skin is the most accessible organ for clinical examination and investigation. Pattern recognition of skin lesions is valuable in the diagnosis and prognosis of underlying joint disease. Often, the skin bears the brunt of toxicity from antirheumatic drugs.

Joint abnormalities may be mirrored by similar changes in the skin. For example, joint hypermobility and skin hyperextensibility coexist in heritable disorders of connective tissue, such as the Ehlers–Danlos syndrome. Cutaneous erythema and hyperpigmentation may overlie an inflamed joint. Furthermore, many patterns of cutaneous involvement are highly specific to certain arthropathies, such as the characteristic erythematous eruption of erythema marginatum in rheumatic fever (Plate 3), the 'butterfly' facial erythema of acute lupus erythematosus and erythema chronicum migrans following infection with *Borrelia burgdorferi*, which can result in Lyme disease.

The degree and extent of skin lesions can be of prognostic importance, for example the cutaneous vasculitis and nodules in rheumatoid disease.

Finally, several antirheumatic drugs produce highly specific, and potentially serious, cutaneous reactions that require accurate diagnosis and prompt management.

This chapter comprises:

(i) A brief outline of the major descriptive terms used in dermatology and the simple investigations required to make a firm dermatological diagnosis.

(ii) The differential diagnoses of important cutaneous abnormalities.

(iii) Aspects of treatment of the skin in rheumatic disorders.

(iv) Cutaneous side-effects of commonly used antirheumatic drugs.

The approach to the patient with skin lesions

History

A careful history should include the following features:

(i) duration of the eruption;

(ii) duration of individual lesions (e.g. weals in simple urticaria individually last less than 24 h, whereas they persist for two or more days in urticarial vasculitis);

(iii) timing of lesions (e.g. the eruption of Still's disease is typically worse in the early afternoon, and evening);

(iv) seasonal variation of lesions (e.g. 'summer' vasculitis);

(v) the relation of skin lesions to joint disease (e.g. scattered gonococcal pustules occurring with flitting arthritis in the bacteraemic phase);

(vi) whether the skin lesions occur singly or in crops, as in Henoch–Schönlein purpura;

(vii) where the lesions occur;

(viii) do lesions blister or crust? (Remember that many infiltrated or hyperkeratotic lesions may be described as 'blisters' by the patient. True blisters are seen in some drug reactions, notably fixed drug eruption and erythema multiforme. Superficial blisters rupture early, leaving eroded areas, as in penicillamine-induced pemphigus.);

(ix) whether lesions itch;

(x) whether lesions are tender;

(xi) are lesions caused or aggravated by light? (Several drugs cause photosensitivity and cutaneous lupus typically occurs on areas of sun exposure.);

(xii) whether there is cold sensitivity—enquire about features of Raynaud's phenomenon;

(xiii) whether there is orogenital ulceration of recent onset;

(xiv) a careful history of present and recent drug therapy.

Examination

The skin should be examined in a good, preferably natural, light. A torch and pocket magnifying glass are invaluable. Since some skin lesions are transient, repeated examination of the skin may be necessary. A dermatoscope can be helpful to examine the fine details, particularly of pigmented lesions.

Note the distribution and morphology of individual lesions. Knowledge of a few technical terms is essential (Table 1).

The regional distribution of lesions

Scalp

Look for alopecia. Is it diffuse or localized? Is it non-scarring (the scalp itself looks normal) or scarring (Plate 4) (when there are inflammatory changes around hair follicles and evidence of cutaneous atrophy or sclerosis). Look for the well-demarcated areas of scaling typical of psoriasis.

Face

(i) Look for evidence of photosensitivity [which classically spares the 'shaded' areas such as the nasolabial folds, eyelids, chin, and Wilkinson's triangle (behind the ears)].

Table 1 Important descriptive terms in dermatology

Term	Definition	Examples
Macule	A flat, impalpable area of altered skin colour	A *café-au-lait* spot
Papule	A lump smaller than 0.5–1 cm diameter	A viral wart
Nodule	A lump smaller than 0.5–1 cm diameter	An epidermoid ('sebaceous') cyst
Plaque	A slightly raised, circumscribed area, often disc shaped	Plaque psoriasis
Vesicle	A small blister (fluid-filled lesion), less than 0.5 cm diameter	Herpes simplex
Bulla	A blister greater than 0.5 cm diameter	A friction blister
Pustule	An accumulation of pus in the skin	Folliculitis
Erosion	A loss of epidermis that heals without scarring	An abrasion
Ulcer	A defect or loss of dermis and epidermis produced by sloughing of necrotic tissue	Pyoderma gangrenosum
Telangiectasia	Visibly dilated, small vascular lesions that blanch on pressure	'Spider naevi'
Purpura	Extravasation of blood, leaving cutaneous areas of discoloration, which does not blanch on pressure; small lesions are termed petechiae (1–2 mm diameter) Larger areas of extravasation of blood are termed ecchymoses	Traumatic bruising
Erythema	Redness	
Violaceous	Purplish hue	Lichen planus
Weal	A transient are of dermal oedema which produces a white or skin-coloured papule or nodule surrounded by a 'flare' of erythema	Urticaria
Atrophy	Skin thinning with reduction of recognizable structures and perhaps translucency	
Poikiloderma	Atrophy with telangiectasia	Radiotherapy scars, dermatomyositis
Alopecia	Loss of hair. It may be localized (e.g. alopecia areata) or diffuse (e.g. systemic lupus erythematosus or iron deficiency). Scarring alopecia, with destruction of hair follicles, is a feature of discoid lupus affecting the scalp	
Onycholysis	Increased free edge of the nail	Psoriasis, Raynaud's phenomenon

(ii) Is there periorbital oedema or the 'heliotrope' violaceous erythema characteristic of dermatomyositis?

(iii) Examine the nose for infiltration (e.g. lupus pernio in sarcoidosis). Inability to evert the lower eyelid is an early feature of systemic sclerosis.

(iv) Look inside the mouth for ulcers and the lace-like white streaks of oral lichen planus (Plates 5 and 6).

Ears

These are an important site for discoid lupus erythematosus (Plate 7), gouty tophi, and, occasionally, rheumatoid nodules.

Hands and feet

(i) A photosensitive eruption spares the finger webs and palms. The distribution of erythema on the backs of the fingers helps to distinguish systemic lupus erythematosus from dermatomyositis (Plate 8).

(ii) In a patient with Raynaud's phenomenon, evidence of ulceration of fingertips, atrophy of finger pulps, induration, and tethering of skin indicates systemic sclerosis. Later features include telangiectasia and calcinosis.

(iii) Look for palmar erythema, especially seen in rheumatoid disease.

(iv) Examine the soles for keratoderma blennorrhagica or localized pustular psoriasis.

Nails

(i) Look for onycholysis, pitting, salmon patches, and subungual hyperkeratosis (typical of psoriasis) (Plates 9–11).

(ii) Examine the nailfolds for periungual erythema, digital vasculitis, periungual papules (e.g. in multicentric reticulohistiocytosis), and paronychia (Plate 12).

(iii) It is helpful to assess the nailfold capillaries with an ophthalmoscope set at 40 dioptres (∞10), applying a drop of oil to the cuticle. Capillaroscopy (see below under Investigation) is a useful investigation.

(iv) Examine the whole body, including the natal cleft and umbilicus (common sites for psoriasis). Look for penile or vulval ulceration, which, like oral ulceration, may be asymptomatic.

For further reading, see Ashton (1995) and Lovell et al. (1990).

Investigation

Routine histological examination of a formalin-fixed skin biopsy may provide considerable useful information (Harrison 1980). The histological features of many lesions are diagnostic, for example, the palisading granulomas seen in rheumatoid nodules and 'liquefaction degeneration' in cutaneous lupus. Where possible, take an elliptical biopsy across the edge of an early lesion, following skin folds. The biopsy should be at least 10 × 5 mm, unless this is undesirable cosmetically. Include subcutaneous fat in the biopsy. (This is especially important if a panniculitis is suspected, and allows easier closure of the wound.) Use a skin hook or the tip of a needle to lift the end of the biopsy, avoiding forceps trauma. Close the wound with 4/0 or 5/0 silk or prolene. A 5-mm punch biopsy may be adequate for small lesions. Mount the biopsy on filter paper to ensure correct orientation for sectioning. Special stains may be indicated, for example, a mucin stain for dermatomyositis. An elastin stain may show the depletion of normal connective tissue structures in localized scleroderma or systemic sclerosis.

Direct skin immunofluorescence is of particular value in lupus erythematosus and in the investigation of blistering disorders. The lupus band test (granular deposition of immunoglobulins at the dermoepidermal junction) is positive in lesional skin in discoid lupus erythematosus and negative in normal skin. It may be negative in early subacute cutaneous lupus erythematosus. In systemic lupus erythematosus, the lupus band test is positive in clinically non-involved skin in 70 per cent of cases, particularly if the biopsy is taken from a sun-exposed site such as the extensor forearm. A punch biopsy is usually adequate for direct immunofluorescence and should be snap-frozen immediately in liquid nitrogen or despatched to the laboratory in appropriate transport medium.

Several non-invasive techniques can be used to measure tissue perfusion in the skin, including laser-Doppler flowmetry, transcutaneous oxygen-pressure measurement, thermography, and capillary microscopy. Thermography, using an infrared radiometer or liquid crystal contact, is a useful non-invasive technique in the assessment of Raynaud's phenomenon. Digital blood flow can be measured in a resting state or following a mild thermal stress. Thermography can be used to measure the degree of severity of Raynaud's phenomenon and its response to therapy; it may help to distinguish primary Raynaud's phenomenon from that secondary to connective tissue disease (Will et al. 1992).

In connective tissue diseases, local vascular changes can be studied by capillary microscopy of the nailfold. This area is easily accessible for examination and the arrangement of the capillaries in the nailfold allows the visualization of the complete capillary loop. In addition, vascular abnormalities appear earlier in the course of the disease than at other sites of the skin of the finger. The morphology of skin capillaries can be studied directly with an ordinary light microscope. Capillaroscopy has been coupled with a videophotometric system and used with computer software to analyze the number and morphology of capillary loops as well as blood-cell velocity under various physiological conditions including local cold exposure (Fagrell et al. 1988).

Morphological changes in capillaries seen in primary Raynaud's approximate those seen in normal individual but the blood-cell velocity is decreased markedly after exposure to cold (Jacohs et al. 1987). Characteristic structural abnormalities are found to a much greater extent in connective tissue diseases such as systemic sclerosis, overlap syndromes (including 'mixed connective tissue disease'), and dermatomyositis. They include enlargement of capillary loops (a non-specific finding in idiopathic Raynaud's phenomenon) and, particularly in systemic sclerosis, deformed capillary loops, segmental (or rarely diffuse) loss of capillaries, new capillary formation leading to excessive branching (arborization), and haemorrhage into the nailfold. Their presence in patients presenting with Raynaud's has prognostic significance (Houtman et al. 1986).

These changes are dynamic, especially in dermatomyositis. Rapid evolution of structural changes, especially loss of capillaries, is linked with a poor prognosis in systemic sclerosis (Maricq 1988).

Differential diagnosis of common physical signs

Erythema

The red face

Photosensitivity, for example drug-induced subacute and acute cutaneous lupus erythematosus may cause diffuse facial erythema. An important cause of photosensitivity is polymorphic light eruption (Plate 13), which affects 10 per cent of Caucasian females but typically spares the face and hands (Ros and Wennersten 1986).

Papules

Telangiectatic papules are found in rosacea and papular lupus erythematosus. These may need to be distinguished by skin biopsy. Papules occur around the alae nasi and lips in sarcoid (Plate 14), particularly in the Afro-Caribbean patient, and in multicentric reticulohistiocytosis.

'Heliotrope'

Violaceous erythema and oedema affect both eyelids in dermatomyositis. Episodic oedema of eyelids, and swollen tongue and lips are characteristic of angioedema, which may be a presenting feature of systemic lupus erythematosus.

'Slapped cheek' erythema

This is characteristic of erythema infectiosum (due to parvovirus infection) (Anderson et al. 1983).

Strawberry erythema of the tongue and lips

This occurs in streptococcal infections. In Kawasaki disease, erythema can be generalized or localized, typically affecting the hands and feet with subsequent desquamation; red dry fissured lips and a 'strawberry tongue' are characteristic.

Exanthem

(i) Maculopapular eruptions are typical of viral infections. The circumscribed pink macules of rubella tend to start on the face, and later become confluent and spread to the limbs. In erythema infectiosum, the 'slapped cheek' erythema is followed by a reticulate eruption starting on the buttocks and spreading distally.

(ii) The 'raindrop' erythematous lesions of guttate psoriasis occur on the trunk and limbs and may follow a streptococcal sore throat. Scaling may be minimal.

(iii) Widespread erythema may be a feature of a connective tissue disease, particularly dermatomyositis, in which dusky erythema occurs on light exposed areas and extensor surfaces, later developing telangiectasia and atrophy (poikiloderma).

(iv) An evanescent, non-pruritic, pinkish maculopapular eruption occurs on the trunk and limbs in Still's disease. Often it is most marked in the late afternoon, and evening at the height of fever.

(v) In rheumatic fever, annular erythematous lesions enlarge to form large figurate patches within hours.

(vi) Erythema chronicum migrans, the characteristic skin lesion of Lyme disease, is a solitary, annular lesion gradually expanding around the site of a tick bite (Plate 15) (Steere 1989).

(vii) Many drugs cause a generalized maculopapular eruption (see below).

Localized erythema

Periarticular erythema may be seen around inflamed joints in rheumatoid disease and is a feature of gout and septic arthritis. Erythema may occur over early Heberden's nodes.

Erythroderma

Generalized erythema may be a presenting feature of psoriasis, particularly in the elderly male (Plate 16). It may also be caused by drugs.

Scaling skin

Scaling is caused by easily detachable keratin, and is due to disordered regulation of epidermal turnover. Any acute inflammation may cause scaling related to the intensity of inflammation, for example, after gout and drug-induced exanthems. Scaling is characteristic of the different forms of psoriasis and is seen also in lupus erythematosus, particularly discoid forms (Plate 17). In the 'psoriasiform' subset of subacute lupus erythematosus, there is a rim of scale at the periphery of the lesion. A scaling psoriasiform eruption ('mechanics hands') on the palms and fingers is characteristically seen in patients with polymyositis associated with anti-Jo-1 antibodies (Mitra et al. 1994) (Plate 18).

Blisters and pustules

Blisters are a feature of pemphigus and pemphigoid, which may be drug-induced. Bullous lesions occur rarely in morphoea, lichen sclerosus et atrophicus, and lupus erythematosus. Epidermolysis bullosa acquisita, characterized by skin fragility, blisters, and milia, may presage the development of systemic lupus erythematosus (Boh et al. 1990). Similar lesions are seen in porphyria cutanea tarda and 'pseudoporphyrias' associated with non-steroidal anti-inflammatory drugs. Widespread bullae are seen in drug-induced erythema multiforme; typical 'target lesions' are seen, particularly on the hands and feet (Plate 19). Drug-induced toxic epidermal necrolysis is characterized by widespread shedding of skin. Fixed drug eruptions may be bullous; they tend to recur at the same site after repeated exposure to the drug.

Pustules may be localized to the hands and feet, as in Reiter's syndrome. Localized forms of pustular psoriasis can be indistinguishable. Generalized pustulation may be seen in pustular vasculitis, Behçet's syndrome, intestinal bypass syndromes, and gonococcal bacteraemia, where they may be scanty. Severe pustular acne and hidradenitis suppurativa, a chronic pustular eruption of the flexures, may be associated with inflammatory arthritis. SAPHO syndrome encompasses patients with acneiform lesions and palmoplantar pustulosis associated with multifocal aseptic osteomyelitis and synovitis. Early lesions of pyoderma gangrenosum and leucocytoclastic vasculitis may be pustular. Subcorneal pustular dermatosis (Sneddon–Wilkinson disease) has been reported as typical of rheumatoid disease (Butt and Burge 1995). Pustules are seen in Behçet's syndrome and a pustule at the site of venepuncture is a helpful diagnostic sign (pathergy test).

Plaques

Plaques on extensor surfaces and the scalp are characteristic of chronic psoriasis. The infiltrated plaques of sarcoidosis occur typically at the anterior scalp margin. Xanthelasmas are a feature of multicentric reticulohistiocytosis and hyperlipidaemias. Plaques of discoid lupus erythematosus are characterized by hyperkeratosis and scarring with 'tintack' scales. Plum-coloured plaques (Plate 20) occur, especially around the neck and upper trunk, in Sweet's syndrome (acute neutrophilic dermatitis) (van den Driesch 1994). A characteristic neutrophilic eruption is seen in rheumatoid arthritis (Scherbenske et al. 1989). Histologically, it is difficult to distinguish from Sweet's syndrome. Indurated, tender areas are a feature of panniculitis and erythema nodosum. Localized plaques of morphoea are initially typically violaceous and later become ivory-white and sclerotic. Lesions resembling linear scleroderma are seen in melorheostosis (Wagers et al. 1972). Urticarial plaques may be a feature of vasculitis and familial Mediterranean fever.

Connective tissue naevi present in childhood as firm, skin-coloured or yellowish nodules or plaques distributed asymmetrically on the trunk and proximal limbs. In the Buschke–Ollendorf syndrome, they are associated with radiological features of osteopoikilosis (Fig. 1) (Verbov and Graham 1972).

Papules and nodules

Important causes are summarized in Table 2.

Purpura and telangiectasia

Impalpable purpuric lesions may be due to diminished numbers of platelets or their dysfunction, for example idiopathic thrombocytopenic purpura or drug-induced marrow aplasia. Trauma, including battering and sports injuries, causes ecchymoses. The 'talon noir', a black area of subcutaneous haemorrhage, occurs on the heel typically in tennis and squash players and may be misdiagnosed as a malignant melanoma. Similarly, splinter haemorrhages and ecchymoses under nails may be due to trauma. The 'crescent sign' occurs typically over the medial or lateral malleoli after a ruptured Baker's cyst. Purpura and ecchymoses are also a feature of corticosteroid toxicity, Ehlers–Danlos syndrome, and haemophilia. Perifollicular haemorrhages occur in scurvy.

Palpable purpura reflects vasculitis, including drug-induced vasculitis and the hypergammaglobulinaemic purpura associated with Sjögren's syndrome. Remember that a recent bruise can also be palpable and painful! The matt telangiectasia of hereditary haemorrhagic telangiectasia is indistinguishable from those seen in systemic sclerosis. Telangiectasia and atrophy (poikiloderma) are characteristic of dermatomyositis.

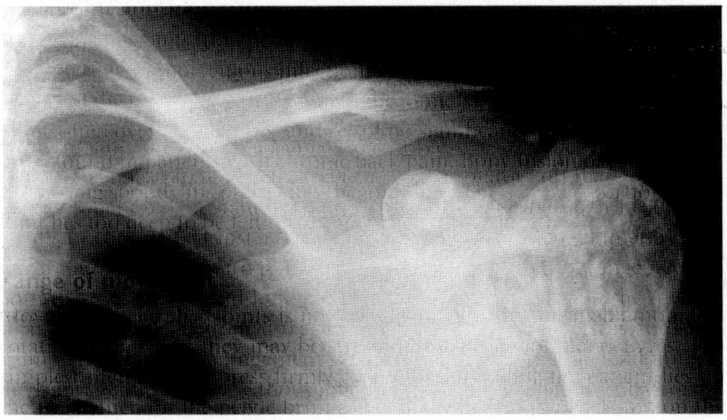

Fig. 1 Osteopoikilosis: note stippling of bone, especially adjacent to joint (photograph by courtesy of Dr G. Evison).

Ulcers

Cutaneous ulceration may have more than one cause in connective tissue diseases. Thus, in rheumatoid arthritis, punched-out ulcers due to vasculitis are common, particularly on the lower limbs. Venous hypertension may play a part in the immobile patient and ulceration may occur over nodules on pressure points. Rheumatoid arthritis is an important cause of pyoderma gangrenosum, which presents as an indurated, expanding, plum-coloured plaque or an acne-like pustule; this ulcerates early and the resulting crater has irregular, 'undermined', thickened, bluish margins. The ulcers may be multiple and heal with considerable scarring. Pyoderma gangrenosum can occur in association with other inflammatory disorders such as Behçet's syndrome.

Neurotropic ulceration occurs rarely in rheumatoid disease, in association with mononeuritis multiplex and severe vasculitis. Foot ulceration may occur with Charcot joints in the patient with syphilis. Similar changes occur in the upper limb in syringomyelia. Cranial arteritis may cause ulceration on the scalp and tongue.

Superficial erosions may be due to pemphigus or more commonly to scratching; in the absence of an obvious dermatosis, pruritus may be due to metabolic causes such as low serum iron or bile-salt retention.

Fingertip ulceration occurs in systemic sclerosis, leaving brownish scars. Severe widespread ulceration may develop rapidly in a child with active dermatomyositis, and reflects the underlying vasculopathy.

Orogenital ulceration

It is important to remember that aphthous ulcers are common in the general population.

In Behçet's syndrome, oral and genital ulcers tend to be more severe and persistent, each lesion often lasting several weeks. They tend to heal with scarring. The ulceration in Reiter's syndrome is typically superficial and painless. Oral lesions of discoid lupus erythematosus occur on the vermilion border and oral mucosa. They are dull red and may have radiating white streaks similar to lichen planus. Oral and palatal ulceration is common in systemic lupus erythematosus and reflects disease activity. Bullous disorders, particularly erythema multiforme, are associated with orogenital involvement. Oral ulceration is common in patients on methotrexate and also occurs following therapy with non-steroidal anti-inflammatory drugs. Gold therapy causes a punctate stomatitis.

Ulceration of part of the tongue may occur in cranial arteritis. A 'geographical' tongue is generally a normal variant, but can occur in psoriasis and Reiter's syndrome.

Pigmentary changes

Relevant causes of hyper- and hypopigmentation are listed in Table 3. Yellow–brown infiltrated lesions include xanthomas and xanthelasmas. Granulomas, such as sarcoid nodules, are dull yellowish on pressure. Rippled yellow streaks occur around the neck and inner arms in pseudoxanthoma elasticum.

Table 2 Papules and nodules

Colour	Diagnosis	Site	Tenderness	Clinical significance
Skin-coloured	Rheumatoid papules and nodules	Extensor surfaces/ pressure points	Sometimes	Seropositive rheumatoid arthritis. May perforate, producing sinuses and fistulae. Similar nodules may occur in systemic lupus erythematosus
	Gouty tophi	Extensor surfaces/ pressure points	No	Elderly patients on diuretics
	Myxoid cyst	Distal phalanges	No	Sporadic, may be multiple. Often associated grooving of the nail
	Giant cell tumour	Phalanges	No	Often multiocular. No significant disease association
	Aponeurotic fibromas	Palmar/plantar fascia	Sometimes in early stages	Associated with Dupuytren syndrome
	Knuckle pads	Extensor surface of digits	Sometimes in early stages	Associated with Dupuytren syndrome
	Prayer nodules	Pressure points	No	Similar lesions are seen on the dorsa of feet in hypermobile young females
	Molluscum fibrosum	Elbows/knees	No	Ehlers–Danlos syndrome
	Epithelioid cell sarcoma	Palm and flexor aspect of finger	Yes	May ulcerate early. Slow-growing. Needs early adequate excision
	Nodular vasculitis	Shins, inner upper arms, overlying arteries	Yes	Polyarteritis nodosa
Erythematous	Urticaria (usually plaques)	Any	Not usually (pruritic)	Evanescent (less than 24 h). Blanch on pressure. Acute attacks may be associated with arthralgia
	Urticarial vasculitis	Any	Yes	Last more than 24 h. Tend to result in painful bruising. Look for underlying connective tissue disease
	Papular lupus erythematosus	Light exposed areas (especially face, neck and upper trunk)	No	May be the only cutaneous manifestation of lupus erythematosus. Difficult to distinguish from rosacea
	Guttate psoriasis	Widespread, especially on trunk	No	May be associated with psoriatic arthritis
Purple/ violaceous	Lichen planus	Any, especially on flexor wrists and lower shins	No. Often pruritic	Idiopathic or drug-induced. Histology characteristic
	Sarcoid	Any, especially truncal. May occur in scars, e.g. venepuncture sites	No	Other features of sarcoidosis, e.g. bone disease, dactylitis
	Erythema nodosum	Limbs	Yes	Associations include sarcoidosis, post-streptococcal infection, inflammatory bowel disease, drugs
	Kaposi sarcoma	Lower limbs	Rarely	Typical of 'benign' form in elderly Jewish individuals
		Generalized		Typically associated with AIDS
	Palpable purpura	Lower limbs	Yes	Underlying small-vessel vasculitis
Yellow/white	Xanthomas	Especially palmoplantar	Sometimes	Associated hyperlipidaemia and synovitis
	Xanthelasma palpebrarum	Facial, especially around eyelids	No	May form plaques. Retinal changes
	Calcification	Extensor surfaces/ pressure points	Sometimes	Dermatomyositis (especially in children)
	Tophi	Extremities, especially over Heberden's nodes	No	Elderly patients on diuretics

Induration or thickening of skin or subcutis

Diffuse cutaneous sclerosis is the hallmark of systemic sclerosis, where it typically affects the extremities and face, spreading proximally. In generalized morphoea, the sclerosis tends to be truncal, with sparing of the areolae; sometimes a typical violaceous margin is seen.

Scleroderma-like changes occur in several metabolic disorders, including phenylketonuria, scurvy, and porphyria cutanea tarda, where cutaneous sclerosis occurs in light-exposed areas. Several industrial chemicals trigger scleroderma-like syndromes.

Solid oedema and sclerosis of the limbs occur in the eosinophilia–myalgia syndrome associated with L-tryptophan ingestion (Connolly et al. 1990). Stiff swollen fingers, resembling acrosclerosis, occur in rheumatoid arthritis and in overlap connective tissue syndromes. Stiff skin and joint contractures occur rarely in diabetes mellitus. Scleroedema of Buschke affects the upper trunk and neck; the skin can be 'wrinkled' over the indurated subcutis. Fibrotic induration of the lower legs occurs in lipodermatosclerosis ('champagne-bottle legs'), associated with chronic venous stasis. Malignant infiltration of the skin, overlying lung or breast carcinoma, causes extensive erythema and induration (carcinoma erysipelatoides). Gross skin thickening, forming deep folds, is associated with thickened digits in pachydermoperiostosis (Fam et al. 1983).

Table 3 Cutaneous hyper- and hypopigmentation

Colour	Causes	Site	Other features
Hyperpigmentation (grey/black)	Postinflammatory hyperpigmentation	Over inflamed joints and diffusely, e.g. systemic sclerosis	
	Ochronosis	Cartilage, especially on nose and ears	Alkaptonuria or drug-induced, e.g. antimalarials
	Fixed drug eruption	Any, especially on head and genitalia	Often asymptomatic. Recurs in the same site on re-exposure to the drug
	Haemochromatosis	Diffuse	Hypertrophic osteoarthropathy due to calcium pyrophosphate deposition
Hypo- or depigmentation (white)	Postinflammatory depigmentation	Various	Frequently seen in resolving psoriasis
	Lichen sclerosus et atrophicus	Genitalia or trunk	May be associated morphoea or organ-specific autoimmune disease
	Degos syndrome (malignant atrophic papulosis)	Anywhere, especially on proximal limbs	Pink or red papules are followed by a 'porcelain'-like scaling lesion and eventually a telangiectatic scar. Rare, but associated with a high mortality, usually due to intestinal crises
	Connective tissue disease, especially dermatomyositis	Scalp and upper back	A characteristic feature in the Afro-Caribbean
	Sarcoid	Anywhere, particularly on neck and trunk	A characteristic feature in the Afro-Caribbean
	Leprosy (tuberculoid)	Any; typically solitary	Anaesthetic, with decreased sweat production and loss of hair within the lesion

Hair abnormalities

Increased hair growth (hypertrichosis) occurs over sites of hyperaemia such as arteriovenous fistulas and chronically inflamed joints. Drugs, such as corticosteroids, penicillamine, and cyclosporin, and metabolic disorders, such as porphyria cutanea tarda, cause hypertrichosis.

Treatment of cutaneous manifestations of rheumatic diseases

The skin has the advantage of being accessible to topical therapy; high concentrations of otherwise toxic agents can be achieved in the epidermis and superficial dermis. Percutaneous absorption of drugs is affected by many factors, including inflammation of the skin and site variation in the density of dermal connective tissue and epidermal thickness. The most important topical agents in this context are corticosteroids, which are available in bewildering variety. They can be classified in four main groups: mild, moderately potent, potent, and very potent (Table 4).

Topical sunscreens are also important, particularly in individuals with connective tissue disease. Several are freely available and a few may be had on prescription. The sun protection factor is the ratio of the dose of a particular wavelength of ultraviolet (UV)B irradiation that causes minimum erythema with sunscreen over that without sunscreen. Most sunscreens protect the skin adequately from short wavelengths of UV (UVC and UVB) but are inadequate against long-wavelength UV (UVA), which contributes to photoageing, and visible light. There is no internationally agreed standard for measuring the degree of protection against UVA or visible light although recent attempts have been made such as a 'star system' and various *in vitro* models (Lim et al. 2001). In recent years, sunscreens are becoming available that contain micromized particles of titanium dioxide or zinc oxide. These preparations block a wider spectrum of light than those that rely on chemical absorption at a specific wavelength. However, individual preference is important; it is essential that the patient is willing to use the preparation regularly.

Table 4 Relative potencies of some commonly used topical corticosteroids

Potency	Pharmacological name	Trade name
Mild	Hydrocortisone 0.1–2.5%	Various
	Fluocinolone acetomide 0.0025%	Synalar 1:10
Moderate	Clobetasone butyrate 0.05%	Eumovate
	Desoxymethasone 0.05%	Stiedex LP
	Flurandrenolone 0.0125%	Haelan
Potent	Betamethasone valerate 0.025%	Betnovate RD
	Betamethasone valerate 0.05%	Betnovate
	Desoxymethasone 0.25%	Stiedex
	Fluocinomide 0.05%	Metosyn
	Hydrocortisone 17-butyrate 0.1%	Locoid
	Mometasone furoate 0.1%	Elocon[a]
	Fluticasone propionate 0.05%	Cutivate[b]
	Betamethasone dipropionate 0.05%	Diprosalic[c]
	Fluclorolone acetomide 0.025%	Topilar
	Beclomethasone dipropionate 0.025%	Propaderm
	Budesonide 0.025%	Preferid
Very potent	Clobetasol propionate 0.05%	Dermovate
	Mometasone furoate 0.1%	Elocon
	Flurandrenolone-impregnated tape	Haelan tape—for hospital use only

[a] Claimed to be once-daily treatment.

[b] Claimed to cause less suppression of hypothalamopituitary–adrenal axis.

[c] Addition of salicylic acid to formulation makes it useful in hyperkeratosic lesions, e.g. verrucous lupus erythematosus.

Note: Combined steroid/antiseptic preparations are available for infected lesions and steroid/tar preparations for use in inflamed or superficial psoriasis.

Systemic agents, such as β-carotene, are somewhat photoprotective.

Cosmetic camouflage is particularly effective for vascular lesions, such as matt telangiectasia in systemic sclerosis.

Treatment of cutaneous ulceration requires careful assessment of the causes and correction of contributory factors such as severe anaemia.

Large, punched-out ulcers reflect necrotizing vasculitis and justify aggressive immunosuppressive therapy. Most vasculitic ulcers are clean and require minimal local interference. Excessive slough can be removed by surgical debridement or the application of a preparation such as Varidase® (streptokinase/streptodornase powder for preparing topical solutions). Clean indolent ulcers should respond to hydrocolloid dressings. Sometimes admission to hospital is necessary, often for long periods. Grafting has been found to be necessary on occasion. There are reports of the beneficial use of methotrexate in intractable rheumatoid ulcers.

Rapidly expanding ulcers with a bluish 'undermined' edge should raise the possibility of pyoderma gangrenosum. This requires specific therapy; usually prednisolone (40–60 mg/day) results in rapid healing. Stubborn lesions may require intralesional triamcinolone. Milder forms of pyoderma gangrenosum sometimes respond to minocycline (100 mg twice daily). Other therapeutic agents include clofazimine, dapsone, cyclosporin, and tacrolimus.

Digital ulceration occurs with Raynaud's phenomenon, particularly in systemic sclerosis. Patients should avoid excessive manicuring of the cuticles. Digital ulcers can be treated with a topical antimicrobial. Hydrocolloids or occlusive dressings can be helpful.

Management of specific disorders

Cutaneous lupus

A moderate to very potent steroid ointment is generally necessary for chronic discoid lesions, even on the face. Stubborn lesions may even require polythene occlusion. For small lesions, flurandrenolone tape can be cut to size. Prolonged use of topical corticosteroids produces telangiectasia and cutaneous atrophy. Rarely, intralesional triamcinolone (10 mg/ml) is necessary, particularly for lesions on the ears and nose. Injections should be directed as superficially as possible, but even so there is still a risk of atrophic scarring. Disfiguring lesions may respond well to excision and grafting or even dermabrasion. CO_2 laser therapy is an alternative destructive technique (Henderson and Odom 1986).

Sunscreens should be used regularly and, in some cases of subacute cutaneous lupus (Plate 21), may be the only therapy required.

In many patients, systemic therapy is necessary. Antimalarials are the drugs of choice, either hydroxychloroquine (400 mg daily) or chloroquine (200 mg daily). Mepacrine may be preferred, although it causes yellow discoloration of the skin and sclerae in therapeutic doses (Plate 22). (This may enhance the photoprotective effect of the drug.) A combination of two antimalarials may have a synergistic effect without necessarily increased toxicity, although this observation has not yet been confirmed in a controlled study. Other drugs used in cutaneous lupus include clofazimine (100 mg daily), dapsone (50–100 mg daily), azathioprine (Askinoff et al. 1988), and oral gold (6 mg daily). Aromatic retinoids such as acetretin (50–75 mg daily) (Ruzicka et al. 1988) decrease hyperkeratosis and can be used together with antimalarials. Increasingly, thalidomide is used in patients with resistant skin disease (Stevens et al. 1997) and may be particularly effective for chilblain lupus or lupus profundus. It is unusual for systemic steroids to be necessary for cutaneous lesions alone.

Dermatomyositis

Cutaneous features of dermatomyositis can occur in the absence of musculoskeletal changes. Extensive skin lesions can be treated with a moderately potent topical steroid. Sunscreens are important. Systemic treatment is usually required. Mild cases respond well to antimalarials but most require corticosteroids, initially in moderately high doses (1 mg/kg body weight) with an immunosuppressive agent, such as methotrexate, as a steroid-sparing agent.

Scleroderma

Localized forms of scleroderma (e.g. morphoea) are often self-limiting, although a topical corticosteroid or occasionally intralesional triamcinolone may help. Extensive lesions may require systemic therapy. There are anecdotal reports of efficacy with penicillamine and sulfasalazine. Methotrexate has been used with encouraging results in children with linear morphoea (*en coup de sabre*). Phototherapy with PUVA and, more recently, UVA1 are reported to be effective in localized and systemic scleroderma (Camacho et al. 2001). Severe hemifacial atrophy and ossifying lesions may respond well to plastic surgical reconstruction, sometimes with tissue expansion (Handfield-Jones et al. 1988).

Treatment of the skin lesions in systemic sclerosis is generally supportive, and includes emollients, and treatment of digital ulcers.

Itch is often a major symptom in patients with systemic sclerosis. Its cause is unclear. Symptomatic treatments include the use of emollients such as aqueous cream or emulsifying ointment, applied directly to the skin or as soap substitutes; these also counteract dryness of the skin. Sedative antihistamines may help, as may topical preparations such as 1–2 per cent menthol in aqueous cream, or even topical corticosteroids.

Digital ulcers may respond to topical nitroglycerine or stable prostaglandins. In severe digital ulceration, or incipient gangrene of a digit, intravenous infusions of vasodilators such as prostaglandin E_1 or prostacyclin may be helpful.

Psoriasis

Superficial lesions (e.g. guttate psoriasis) respond to topical tar preparations, the topical vitamin D analogue, calcipotriol, or dilute corticosteroids. Potent steroids should not be used. Dithranol is used for thicker plaques. Its use should be supervised carefully as it is irritant and stains skin and clothing. Several different concentrations and bases are available. Initially a weak preparation (e.g. 0.1 per cent) can be used as short-contact therapy and washed off after 30–120 min. The strength and duration of therapy can be increased gradually. Dithranol must not be used on the flexures or face. Often admission or day-centre therapy is necessary. Narrow-band ultraviolet B (TL-01) is highly effective in guttate psoriasis and as part of a combined approach in chronic plaque psoriasis.

A minority of patients with extensive or unstable disease (e.g. generalized pustular psoriasis) will require second-line therapy. This includes drugs such as etretinate and acetretin, aromatic retinoids related to vitamin A. They are teratogenic and may cause hypercholesterolaemia and hypertriglyceridaemia. Methotrexate, in low weekly dosage (5–15 mg) is especially useful in erythrodermic or generalized pustular psoriasis, particularly in elderly people. Since the drug appears to be more hepatotoxic in patients with psoriasis than those with rheumatoid disease, most dermatologists would carry out routine liver biopsies in psoriatic patients under 65 years on long-term methotrexate therapy. Hydroxyurea (0.5–1.5 g) is sometimes of value in a proportion of patients; although it may cause short-term marrow toxicity, fatalities are rare (Layton et al. 1989). There are encouraging results from cyclosporin, initially 3–5 mg/kg per day, in patients with severe disease (Ellis et al. 1991), although the long-term renal toxicity of the drug is uncertain. Regular monitoring should include measurement of blood pressure, serum creatinine and measurement of glomerular filtration rate in high risk patients. Patients with localized pustular psoriasis should be encouraged to give up smoking. The imidazole liarozole is useful in patients with resistant palmoplantar pustulosis (Bhushan et al. 2001). Anti-TNF alpha antagonists can induce dramatic remissions in patients with severe psoriasis (Oh et al. 2000).

PUVA (psoralen + UVA) is valuable in recalcitrant psoriasis of hands and feet or in some individuals with widespread disease. It is particularly effective in combination with low-dose retinoids (Saurat et al. 1988). PUVA is potentially carcinogenic to the skin, particularly in patients who have previously received other carcinogens such as methotrexate.

Antimalarials should not be used in psoriatic arthritis, as they may exacerbate cutaneous psoriasis.

Cutaneous side-effects of antirheumatic therapy

Skin lesions are common in patients receiving antirheumatic therapy. They are often non-specific and trivial, although sometimes they may be severe enough to warrant stopping the drug. In the following we list important cutaneous adverse effects of the different forms of antirheumatic therapy (Breathnach and Hintner 1992; Lovell and Maddison 1992).

Non-steroidal anti-inflammatory drugs

(i) Non-specific exanthems/morbilliform eruptions are common.

(ii) Generalized exfoliative dermatitis is rare (has been caused by phenylbutazone, oxyphenbutazone, and indomethacin).

(iii) Photoallergic reactions (e.g. caused by fenbufen, piroxicam).

(iv) Photo-onycholysis, skin fragility in light exposed sites, and features resembling porphyria cutanea tarda appear to be a direct phototoxic effect of drugs. These effects were seen typically with benoxaprofen, but can occur with other non-steroidal anti-inflammatory drugs. Pseudoporphyria typically occurs with naproxen.

(v) Acneiform lesions (e.g. caused by naproxen).

(vi) Stomatitis has been reported with indomethacin.

(vii) Urticaria may be immunologically mediated (e.g. caused by diclofenac, mefanamic acid) or may be a pharmacological effect of the drug (typically aspirin in patients with nasal polyposis).

(viii) Erythema multiforme and toxic epidermal necrolysis (Plate 23) (Korstanje 1995) (e.g. caused by fenbufen, benoxaprofen, piroxicam, sulindac, and especially phenylbutazone, oxyphenbutazone, and diclofenac, where it has been fatal).

(ix) Fixed drug eruptions (Plate 24). One or more well-demarcated erythematous lesions, sometimes with blistering, resolve, leaving persistent, dusky grey-black pigmented areas. The eruption occurs at the same site, with or without further lesions, on re-exposure to the drug. Systemic symptoms are few, if any, and re-exposure to the drug is justifiable if diagnostically necessary. Oxyphenbutazone is a classical cause, although a non-pigmenting fixed drug eruption has been reported due to piroxicam.

(x) Several topically applied non-steroidals (e.g. ketoprofen) cause allergic contact dermatitis and photoallergic contact dermatitis.

(xi) Purpura may be due to thrombocytopaenia (e.g. caused by fenoprofen, phenylbutazone) or allergic vasculitis (e.g. caused by phenylbutazone, naproxen).

Gold

Cutaneous reactions occur at any stage of treatment in 25 per cent more of patients on intramuscular gold salts; they may require cessation of therapy. A high incidence of mucocutaneous side-effects appears to be linked with therapeutic efficacy. Gold-salt dermatitis appears to be related to HLA class I B35 antigen. Oral gold (auranofin) causes similar, although less severe, toxic reactions to intramuscular gold. Important side-effects include the following.

(i) Pruritus.

(ii) Non-specific maculopapular/morbilliform eruptions—these may progress to fatal erythroderma if the drug is continued.

(iii) An eczematous or pityriasis rosea-like eruption. Even in relatively banal eruptions, histology may reveal striking features resembling lichen planus. Typical lichen planus (Plate 25) may develop, with hyperkeratotic changes, especially in the scalp, sometimes causing scarring alopecia.

(iv) Intramuscular gold therapy may reactivate pre-existing nickel sensitivity (e.g. to jewellery).

(v) Punctuate or aphthous stomatitis (common, may be the only adverse effect).

(vi) Purpura due to thrombocytopaenia or (rarely) vasculitis.

(vii) Erythema multiforme and toxic epidermal necrolysis (rare).

(viii) Prolonged gold therapy may cause slate-grey pigmentation (chrysiasis), especially in light-exposed sites.

D-Penicillamine

Many adverse effects from this drug are similar to those seen in gold therapy. An urticarial or morbilliform eruption is common early in therapy, although usually it can be avoided by a 'go low, go slow' dose regimen.

Immunologically mediated skin reactions may mimic inflammatory dermatoses such as lichen planus. The eruptions may persist for several years after the drug is discontinued. Typical cicatricial pemphigoid may occur, with the development of fibrous conjunctival bands (synechiae). Pemphigus foliaceus is the most common pattern induced by penicillamine; it may be mild and the crusted erythematous truncal lesions may mimic eczema (Plate 26). However, direct immunofluorescence of uninvolved skin reveals the characteristic intercellular deposition of IgG. More rarely, the drug may induce pemphigus vulgaris, in which flaccid bullae rupture to form extensive eroded areas of skin. Oral lesions and vulvovaginitis may occur. Penicillamine may precipitate lesions closely resembling morphoea, systemic sclerosis, dermatomyositis, and both discoid and systemic lupus erythematosus. Antibodies to native DNA are found, unlike in other forms of drug-induced lupus. Other inflammatory adverse effects include thrombocytopaenic purpura, stomatitis, glossitis, and alopecia.

Penicillamine has a profound effect on connective tissue proteins: it inhibits collagen synthesis and cleaves newly formed intermolecular cross-links; it also stimulates elastin synthesis. Although effects on connective tissue are generally associated with the high doses used in metabolic disorders such as Wilson's disease, elastosis perforans serpiginosa has been reported in one child receiving penicillamine for rheumatoid arthritis. Typical features include serpiginous and annular crusted plaques on the limbs. Histological changes include transepidermal elimination of elastin. Pseudoxanthoma elasticum-like changes and elastosis may occur in relatively low doses (e.g. 750 mg/day).

Sulfasalazine

Eruptions caused by the sulfapyridine moiety are typical of those induced by sulfonamides in general. They include:

(i) leucocytoclastic vasculitis;

(ii) photosensitivity;

(iii) a pruritic, scaly, maculopapular eruption (common)—desensitization may be possible;

(iv) a lupus-like syndrome;

(v) erythema multiforme/toxic epidermal necrolysis (rare).

Antimalarials

Reactions include:

(i) diffuse grey itchy pigmentation, especially in light-exposed areas;

(ii) blackish pigmentation (especially nose and ears) due to acquired ochronosis—nails may also be affected;

(iii) bright yellow pigmentation (mepacrine);

(iv) bleaching of red or blonde hair;

(v) photosensitivity or exacerbation of porphyria cutanea tarda;

(vi) exacerbation of psoriasis;

(vii) toxic epidermal necrolysis (rare);

(viii) lichenoid eruptions (rare);

(ix) a generalized pustular eruption (hydroxychloroquine).

Corticosteroids

Reactions include:

(i) atrophy, telangiectasia, and easy bruising;

(ii) increased risk of cutaneous sepsis;

(iii) dermal atrophy, causing dimpled scars—this may follow injudicious local infiltration with corticosteroids.

Immunosuppressive drugs

Reactions include:

(i) Opportunistic infections (e.g. multiple warts and molluscum contagiosum lesions) may follow chronic immunosuppressive therapy (e.g. with azathioprine and methotrexate).

(ii) Cytotoxic agents cause alopecia.

(iii) Pigmentation of skin and nails occurs with cyclophosphamide.

(iv) Hypersensitivity reactions to azathioprine may present as an exanthem or generalized urticarial eruption.

(v) Orogenital ulcers occur typically with methotrexate.

Anti-TNF drugs

Anaphylaxis can follow infusion of TNF-alpha antagonists, for example, infliximab. Other adverse effects include flushing, hyperhidrosis, an urticarial eruption and, rarely, a lupus-like syndrome (Shakoor et al. 2002).

Some key points for skin manifestations of rheumatic diseases (Table 5)

Table 5 Important clinical points

1. Examine skin thoroughly, including nailfolds, genitalia, and feet. Examine oral mucosa
2. Stress the importance of photoprotection
3. Do not be afraid to use potent topical corticosteroids in cutaneous lupus—but keep under review
4. Do not overtreat cutaneous lupus with systemic therapy
5. Consider skin biopsy if there is diagnostic difficulty—try to biopsy an early lesion and orientate correctly
6. In any rash that does not fit a precise pattern—consider a drug cause

References

Anderson, M.J. et al. (1983). Human parvovirus, the cause of erythema infectiosum (fifth disease). *Lancet* **ii**, 1378–81.

Ashton, R.E. (1995). Teaching non-dermatologists to examine the skin: a review of the literature and some recommendations. *British Journal of Dermatology* **132**, 221–5.

Askinoff, R., Werth, V.P., and Franks, A.G., Jr. (1988). Resistant discoid erythematosus of palms and soles: successful treatment with azathioprine. *Journal of the American Academy of Dermatology* **19**, 961–5.

Baron, E.D. and Stevens, S.R. (2002). Sunscreens and immune protection. *British Journal of Dermatology* **146**, 933–7.

Boh, E., Roberts, L.J., Lieu, T-S., Gammon, W.R., and Sontheimer, R.D. (1990). Epidermolysis bullosa acquisita preceding the development of systemic lupus erythematosus. *Journal of the American Academy of Dermatology* **22**, 587–93.

Breathnach, S.M. and Hintner, H. *Adverse Drug Reactions and the Skin.* Oxford: Blackwell Scientific, 1992.

Butt, A. and Burze, S.M. (1995). Sneddon–Wilkinson disease in association with rheumatoid arthritis. *British Journal of Dermatology* **132**, 313–15.

Camacho, N.R. et al. (2001) Medium-dose UVA1 phototherapy in localized scleroderma and its effect on CD34-positive dendritic cells. *Journal of the American Academy of Dermatology* **45**, 697–9.

Connolly, S.M. et al. (1990). Scleroderma and L-tryptophan: a possible explanation of the eosinophilia–myalgia syndrome. *Journal of the American Academy of Dermatology* **23**, 451–7.

van den Driesch, P. (1994). Sweet's syndrome (acute febrile neutrophilic dermatosis). *Journal of the American Academy of Dermatology* **31**, 535–56.

Ellis, C.N. et al. (1991). Cyclosporin for plaque-type psoriasis. Results of a multidose, double-blind trial. *New England Journal of Medicine* **324**, 277–84.

Fagrell, B., Eriksson, S.E., Malmstrom, S., and Sjolund, A. (1988). Computerised data analysis of capillary blood cell velocity. *International Journal of Microcirculation Clinical and Experimental* **7**, 276–81.

Fam, A.G., Chin-Sang, H., and Ramsay, C.A. (1983). Pachydermoperiostosis: scintigraphic, thermographic, plethysmographic, and capillaroscopic observations. *Annals of the Rheumatic Diseases* **42**, 98–102.

Handfield-Jones, S.E. et al. (1988). Ossification in linear morphoea with hemifacial atrophy—treatment by surgical excision. *Clinical and Experimental Dermatology* **13**, 385–8.

Harrison, P.V. (1980). A guide to skin biopsies and excisions. *Clinical and Experimental Dermatology* **5**, 235–45.

Henderson, D.L. and Odom, J.C. (1986). Laser treatment of discoid lupus erythematosus. *Lasers in Surgical Medicine* **6**, 12–15.

Houtman, P.M., Kallenberg, C.G.M., Fidler, V., and Wouda, A.A. (1986). Diagnostic significance of nailfold capillary patterns in patients with Raynaud's phenomenon. *Journal of Rheumatology* **13**, 556–63.

Jacohs, M.J.H.M., Breslau, P.J., Slaaf, D.W., Reneman, R.S., and Lemmens, J.A.J. (1987). Nomenclature of Raynaud's phenomenon—a capillary microscopic and hemorheologic study. *Surgery* **101**, 136–45.

Korstanje, M.J. (1995). Drug-induced mouth disorders. *Clinical and Experimental Dermatology* **20**, 10–18.

Layton, A.M. et al. (1989). Hydroxyurea in the management of therapy-resistant psoriasis. *British Journal of Dermatology* **121**, 647–53.

Lebwohl, M. et al. (2003). An international, randomized, double-blind placebo-controlled phase 3 trial of intramuscular alefacept in patients with chronic plague psoriasis. *Archives of Dermatology* **139**, 719–27.

Lim, H.W. et al. (2001). American Academy of Dermatology Consensus Conference on UVA protection of sunscreens: summary and recommendations. *Journal of the American Acadamy of Dermatology* **44**, 505–8.

Lovell, C.R. and Maddison, P.J. (1992). Rheumatoid arthritis and the skin. In *Recent Advances in Dermatology* (ed. R.H. Champion and R.J. Pye), pp. 1–16. London: Churchill Livingstone.

Lovell, C.R., Maddison, P.J., and Campion, G.V. *The Skin in Rheumatic Disease.* London: Chapman and Hall Medical, 1990.

Maricq, M.R. Raynaud's phenomenon and microvascular abnormalities in scleroderma (systemic sclerosis). In *Systemic Sclerosis: Scleroderma* (ed. M.I.V. Jayson and C. M. Black), pp. 151–66. Chichester: Wiley, 1988.

Mitra, D., Lovell, C.L., MacLeod, T.I.F., Tan, R.S.H., and Maddison, P.J. (1994). Clinical and histological features of 'mechanic's hands' in a patient with antibodies to Jo-1—a case report. *Clinical and Experimental Dermatology* **19**, 146–8.

Oh, C.J. et al. (2000). Treatment with anti-tumor necrosis factor alpha (TNF-alpha) monoclonal antibody dramatically decreases the clinical activity of psoriasis lesions. *Journal of the American Academy of Dermatology* **42**, 829–30.

Ros, A. and Wennersten, G. (1986). Current aspects of polymorphous light eruptions in Sweden. *Photodermatology* **3**, 298–302.

Ruzicka, T., Meurer, M., and Bieber, T. (1988). Efficacy of acetretin in the treatment of cutaneous lupus erythematosus. *Archives of Dermatology* **124**, 897–902.

Saurat, J-H. et al. (1988). Randomised double-blind multicentre study comparing acetretin–PUVA, etretinate–PUVA and placebo–PUVA in the treatment of severe psoriasis. *Dermatologica* **177**, 218–24.

Scherbenske, J.M. et al. (1989). Rheumatoid neutrophilic dermatitis. *Archives of Dermatology* **125**, 1105–8.

Shakoor, N., Michalska, M., Harris, J.A., and Block, J.A. (2002). Drug-induced systemic lupus erythematosus associated with etanercept therapy. *Lancet* **359**, 579–80.

Steere, A.C. (1989). Lyme disease. *New England Journal of Medicine* **321**, 586–96.

Stevens, R.J., Andujar, C., Edwards, C.J., Ames, P.R.J., Barwick, A.R., Khamashta, M.A., and Hughes, G.R.V. (1997). Thalidomide in the treatment of the cutaneous manifestations of lupus erythematosus: experience in sixteen consecutive patients. *British Journal of Rheumatology* **36**, 353–59.

Verbov, J. and Graham, R. (1972). Buschke–Ollendorff syndrome: disseminated dermofibrosis with osteopoikilosis. *Clinical and Experimental Dermatology* **11**, 17–26.

Wagers, L.T., Young, A.W., and Ryan, S.F. (1972). Linear melorheostotic scleroderma. *British Journal of Dermatology* **86**, 297–301.

Will, R.K., Ring, E.F.J., Clarke, A.K., and Maddison, P.J. (1992). Infrared thermography: what is its place in rheumatology in the 1990's? *British Journal of Rheumatology* **31**, 337–44.

1.3.3 Neurological complications

Iain T. Ferguson and Peter Hollingworth

Introduction

When acute, as in cervical cord compression, neurological complications are among the few rheumatological emergencies. When they cause a gradual functional decline, they may be misconstrued as deterioration of the arthritis. Either way, the addition of weakness or sensory symptoms to an already painful, stiff limb may result in severe disability. Drugs used in the treatment of rheumatic diseases (Mastaglia 1989) can themselves cause neurological side-effects (Table 1). Coincidental neurological diseases must be considered in the differential diagnosis and some neurological disorders have musculoskeletal manifestations (Table 2) (Figs 1 and 2). Such is the interplay between rheumatological and neurological disorders that the rheumatologist must be alert to the diagnostic pitfalls they present (Table 3).

Accurate assessment of power, tone, reflexes, or the plantar response may be impossible in a limb already weak, stiff, or deformed from arthritis, so recognition of these complications demands a high index of suspicion and help from sophisticated investigations.

The recognition of patterns of symptoms and signs is necessary in forming a diagnosis (Box 1).

Weakness patterns

The distribution of weakness is important. Symmetrical, proximal weakness suggests muscle disease but other causes should be considered (Table 4). Difficulty getting out of a chair, climbing stairs, lifting objects from a high shelf, or brushing hair are common.

In upper motor neurone disease, shoulder abductors and arm extensors are affected more than the flexors, whereas in the legs the flexors are affected more than the extensors. Hyper-reflexia, hypertonia, and an extensor plantar response are usually present.

Myasthenia gravis is characterized by fluctuating weakness with fatiguability. The weakness tends to be proximal and associated with diplopia and dysarthria towards the end of the day. Symptomatic myasthenia responding to intravenous edrophonium can occur in polymyositis, where a reduced number of acetylcholine receptors has been demonstrated. Penicillamine may produce myasthenia responsive to the edrophonium test. Antibodies to acetylcholine receptors are present and recovery usually follows withdrawal of the drug. The Eaton–Lambert syndrome, with painful, proximal muscle weakness, is not associated with antibodies to acetylcholine receptors. Three-quarters of males and 30 per cent of females will have an underlying carcinoma. Electromyography is diagnostic.

Distal weakness usually results from disease of peripheral nerves, either of their roots or a polyneuropathy. Involvement of specific muscle groups may allow precise anatomical localization (Guarantors of Brain 1988). Weakness of one limb is usually neurogenic, except for tendon rupture. The differential diagnosis includes motor neurone disease, neuralgic amyotrophy, and early fascioscapulohumeral dystrophy. Hysterical or non-organic weakness is commonly superimposed on organic disease (Marsden 1986). Features include:

- great display of effort to little effect;
- intermittent or jerky weakness;
- simultaneous contraction of agonist and antagonist muscles;
- failure of stabilizing or synergistic muscles to contract when testing limb power;

Table 1 Neurological side-effects of drugs used for rheumatic disorders

Side-effect	Drugs
Aseptic meningitis	Sulindac, Ibuprofen, Tolmetin } in systemic lupus erythematosus
Benign intracranial hypertension	Steroids, especially on withdrawal in children
Chorea	Cimetidine
Confusion	Chloroquine, indomethacin, and other NSAIDs[a]
Cortical blindness	Salicylates
Delirium	Cimetidine and chloroquine
Depression	Indomethacin and other NSAIDs
Dizziness	Many NSAIDs
Encephalopathy	Methotrexate
Extrapyramidal disorders	Chloroquine
Fits	Allopurinol, chlorambucil, cimetidine, cyclosporin (in renal failure), indomethacin, methotrexate
Guillain–Barré syndrome	Penicillamine
Hallucinations	Cyclosporin methotrexate
Headache	NSAIDs, especially at the start of treatment, notably: indomethacin, ketoprofen, diclofenac, ibuprofen
Muscle cramps	Cimetidine, gold salts, penicillamine
Myasthenia gravis	Penicillamine: chloroquine unmasks myasthenia
Myopathies	Cimetidine, chloroquine (painful), colchicine, steroids (chronic, painless)[b]
Myositis	Penicillamine (painful)
Optic neuropathy	Ibuprofen, indomethacin, penicillamine
Ototoxicity	Chloroquine, indomethacin, naproxen, salicylates
Peripheral neuropathy	
Sensorimotor	Chlorambucil, chloroquine (>0.5 g daily), colchicine, indomethacin, gold salts, penicillamine
Predominantly motor	Cimetidine, dapsone, gold salts, sulindac
Predominantly sensory	Sulindac
Personality change	Steroids
Psychosis	Chloroquine, dextropropoxyphene, indomethacin, steroids
Taste impairment or distortion	Allopurinol, azathioprine, penicillamine, gold salts, salicylates
Tremor	Cimetidine, cyclosporin, indomethacin, steroids

[a] NSAID, non-steroidal anti-inflammatory drug.

[b] Especially fluorinated steroids (triamcinolone, betamethasone, dexamethasone) or prednisolone >40 mg/day: severe wasting, late loss of reflexes, normal muscle enzymes, type IIb fibre atrophy.

Table 2 Neurological disorders presenting with rheumatic symptoms (see also Table 3)

Neurological disorders	Rheumatic symptoms and signs
Parkinson's disease	Painful, stiff shoulder, arm or hand; less frequently lower limb
Multiple sclerosis	Stiff (spastic) legs may be confused with or coincide with cervical spondylitic myelopathy
Spinal cord tumour	Radicular pain with aching, stiff legs; legs feel swollen with dorsal column involvement
Dorsal root entry-zone lesion (e.g. multiple sclerosis, tumour, neurosyphilis)	'Lighting' limb pains
Motor neurone disease	Wasted hand, confused with T1 root lesion from cervical spondylosis
Syringomyelia, tabes dorsalis, primary sensory neuropathy, diabetes	Neuropathic joints; swollen fingers (*main en courgette*) with syringomyelia
Hereditary sensorimotor neuropathy (Charcot–Marie–Tooth)	Pes cavus
Myotonias	Stiff hands, often worse in cold
Myasthenia	Weak, sometimes aching muscles, may be confused with polymyositis

- inconsistencies in performance: for example, the patient may have weak quadriceps when lying on the couch yet be able to walk, squat, or jump normally.

Muscle pain

When at rest, this is rarely from primary muscle disease. Exertion pain is commonly non-organic, once peripheral vascular disease has been excluded. However, McArdle's disease (mild myophosphorylase deficiency) and phosphofructokinase deficiency should be considered if the pain is in the calves, increases with further exertion, and leads to myoglobulinuria. The ischaemic lactate test, electromyography, and muscle biopsy are necessary for diagnosis.

Muscle twitching

Fasciculation is painless, visible, muscle contractions of small groups of muscle fibres, often felt by the patient. It is benign in the absence of weakness or wasting which, if present, suggests anterior horn cell disease or motor neuropathy. Fibrillation is contraction of single fibres seen in the tongue or exposed muscle, and may be recorded by electromyography. Myokymia is a slower or coarse contraction of bands of muscle fibres, most often seen in healthy individuals. Facial myokymia can occur in brain-stem multiple sclerosis and Whipple's disease.

Contractures

These occur in both neurogenic and myopathic muscle disease; Duchenne muscular dystrophy, spinal muscular atrophy, and Friedreich's ataxia are common causes. They may develop rapidly in acute polymyositis.

Reflex patterns

Deep tendon reflexes may be absent at joints stiffened by arthritis. The plantar response may be difficult to assess in hallux valgus or after Keller's operation. Absent ankle jerks after the age of 60 is often normal. Exaggerated reflexes, especially with clonus, point to an upper motor-neurone lesion. Absent or depressed reflexes occur in peripheral neuropathies. A combination of an absent segmental reflex and hyper-reflexia below that level, as in the inverted supinator sign (absent biceps and supinator jerk but present triceps jerk, indicating a C5/6 cord lesion), is of considerable localizing value. In polymyositis, the reflexes may be increased, possibly because of muscle spindle hyperexcitability secondary to inflammation.

Sensory patterns

Sensory loss may be the most important clue to involvement of the nervous system in patients with arthritis. The distribution and type of sensory deficit usually permits anatomical localization (Guarantors of Brain 1988); for example, anaesthesia of the little finger and ulnar half of the ring finger and palm, extending no further than the wrist crease, indicates an ulnar nerve lesion rather than a C8 radiculopathy.

Knowledge of key dermatomes and the area supplied by peripheral nerves is essential. Loss of pain and temperature with sparing of joint position sense points to a cord or brain-stem lesion. Cervical cord compression from atalantoaxial subluxation may be confused with a peripheral neuropathy, as the sensory loss can be in a glove-and-stocking distribution, perhaps from cord ischaemia. As sensory examination is subjective, electrophysiological testing may be the only way to determine the site of nerve damage.

Central nervous system involvement in rheumatic diseases

Fortunately, central nervous system complications are a common manifestation of only the rarer rheumatic diseases. Most are mild and self limiting, but some have devastating consequences. Difficulties abound in understanding these complications as there is a dearth of agreed diagnostic criteria, specific signs, laboratory tests, or imaging techniques. When a patient with a rheumatic disease disorder develops central nervous system disease, one should ask whether it is:

(i) a direct complication and, if so, is it residual or progressive;

(ii) secondary to another complication, such as uraemia, infection, or hypertension;

(iii) a side-effect of therapy, such as steroid psychosis or drug-induced systemic lupus erythematosus;

(iv) non-organic, such as hysteria or depression;

(v) coincidental, such as a cerebral thrombosis from atheroma.

The most common and closely studied central nervous system disorders that present to the rheumatologist occur in systemic lupus erythematosus (Adelman et al. 1986) and the allied lupus-like and antiphospholipid syndrome (Asherson et al. 1989). Details are given in the appropriate chapters but how these concern the neurologist will be considered in depth here.

Neuropsychiatric systemic lupus erythematosus (see Chapter 6.6.1)

The incidence of neuropsychiatric systemic lupus erythematosus may be as high as 50 per cent (Hanly et al. 1992) but the incidence of serious complications, as opposed to minor psychiatric disturbance, is far less. The most common features are depression, fits, and headaches, although virtually every manifestation of central nervous system disease has been described (Singer and Denburg 1990), including subtle cognitive defects in memory, intellect, and learning (Hanly et al. 1994). Most victims are young women. It usually occurs when the systemic lupus erythematosus is active and early in its course, though some patients have had seizures for years before the patient presents with other manifestations.

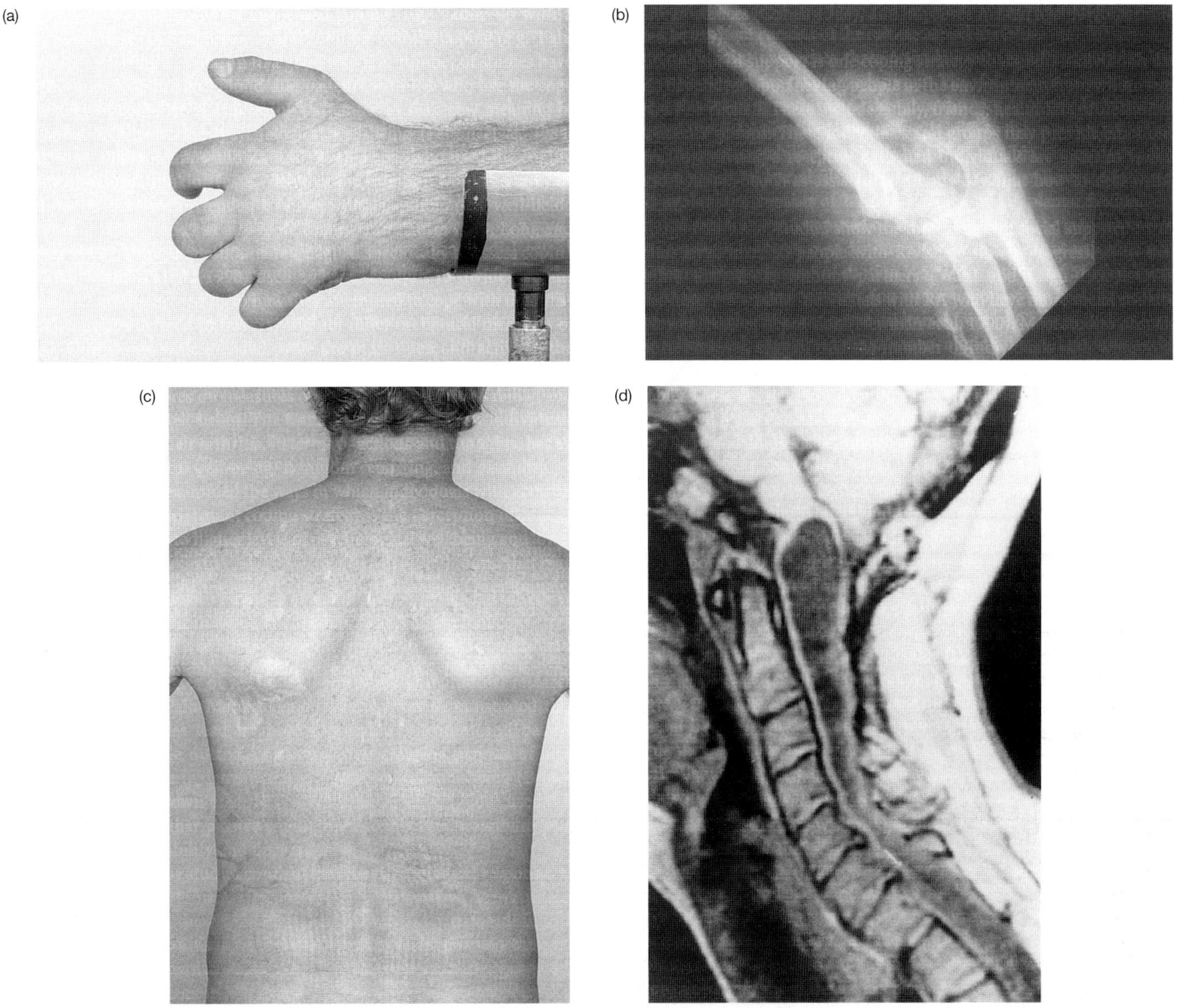

Fig. 1 Syringomyelia.

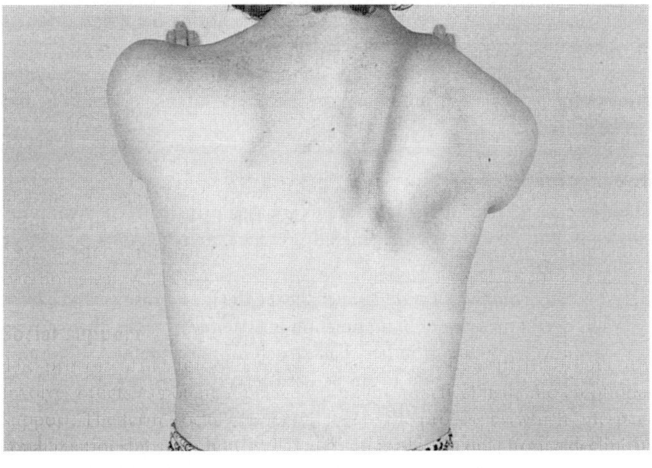

Fig. 2 Neuralgic amyotrophy with winging of the scapula.

Pathogenic factors

(i) Antineuronal antibodies, directed notably against the cytoskeletal neurofilaments, tend to be associated with diffuse neuropsychiatric systemic lupus erythematosus (Robbins et al. 1988).

(ii) IgG anticardiolipin antibodies occur in patients with antiphospholipid syndrome and in 20–50 per cent with systemic lupus erythematosus. By their action on platelet and endothelial cells, they predispose to thrombosis of arteries, veins, and venous sinuses as well as cross-reacting with sphingolipids. They tend to be associated focal lesions in neuropsychiatric lupus (McHugh et al. 1988).

(iii) Vegetations on the aortic and mitral valves of some patients carrying anticardiolipin antibodies might be a source of emboli to the brain, causing transient ischaemic attacks, strokes, or dementia (Asherson and Lubbe 1988).

(iv) Cerebral vasculitis, causing ischaemia, oedema, and infarction is rare.

(v) Antiribosomal P antibodies might be associated with lupus psychosis and severe lupus depression. An initial study (Bonfa et al. 1987) found

Table 3 Some important points to remember

Cerebral
'Transient cerebral ischaemic attacks' may be focal seizures with an underlying structural abnormality
Migraine and other headaches are a common early symptom of systemic lupus erythematosus
Posture deformities are common in Parkinson's disease, e.g. torticollis, scoliosis, hand and foot dystonias
Causes of stroke in young adults
A cause is identified in half. Thrombosis and embolism are implicated in 60% and haemorrhage in the remainder
1. Cardiac: valvular disease, e.g. Libman Sacks endocarditis or atrial myxoma, cardiomyopathy, e.g. AL amyloidosis
2. Haematological (increased clotting tendency): hyperviscosity syndrome, protein C and S deficiencies, thrombotic thrombocytopaenia, antiphospholipid syndrome
3. Arteritis, e.g. polyarteritis nodosa, Wegener's granulomatosis, Takayasu's arteritis
4. Carotid or vertebral artery dissection
5. Venous sinus thrombosis
6. Metabolic and hormonal, e.g. contraceptive pill, pregnancy, diabetes mellitus
7. Infection, e.g. syphilis, mucomycosis
8. Drugs, e.g. amphetamines, heroin, cocaine
Spinal cord
A sensation of walking through quicksand, wet legs, a feeling of being encased in plaster are symptoms often associated with spinal cord disease
Cervical cord compression may produce glove-and-stocking sensory loss, mimicking peripheral neuropathy
Bilateral hand sensory symptoms may be due to cervical cord disease, rather than bilateral mononeuropathies
Syringomyelia may present with Chacot joints and swollen fingers (Fig. 1)
Cauda equina
Pre- and post-exercise examination may be helpful in patients with lumbar canal stenosis. In upper motor neurone disease, signs may also be more apparent after exercise
Peripheral nerve
Sensory 'splitting' of the fourth finger usually indicates median or ulnar mononeuropathy rather than a radiculopathy. Persistent symptoms following carpal tunnel decompression may be due to an incorrect diagnosis or ineffective decompressive procedure. Nerve conduction studies can be helpful
Early decompression of an acute common peroneal nerve entrapment syndrome may be effective
Neuralgic amyotrophy
This may present with shoulder pain (Fig. 2)
Muscle
A false-positive edrophonium test mimicking myasthenia may occur in polymyositis, some motor neuropathies, and motor neurone disease
Too early and rapid reduction in steroids in polymyositis may cause a relapse
Hyperthyroidism may give rise to profound hyper-reflexia, increased muscle tone, and proximal muscle weakness simulating central nervous system disease
Hypothyroidism may cause a raised serum creatinine phosphokinase, mild weakness, and muscle cramps

Box 1 Important points for the rheumatologist to remember

1. Joint damage often prevents a meaningful clinical assessment of neurological symptoms, so special investigations are usually necessary.
2. Beware of attributing deteriorating function to progression of joint disease in rheumatoid arthritis: consider superimposed neurological complications.
3. Be alert to hysteria, mimicking neurological disease, coexisting with rheumatological or organic neurological diseases.
4. The differential diagnosis of cerebral lupus includes complications of lupus uraemia, sepsis and hypertensive encephalopathy, and side-effects of drugs in its treatment.
5. Cervical myelopathy and rheumatoid arthritis is suggested by deteriorating function, 'electric shocks' in the arms; recently worsening of neck pain.
6. Mononeutritis multiplex may progress rapidly and is a rheumatological emergency.
7. Entrapment neuropathies are the commonest neurological complication of rheumatic diseases.

that 90 per cent of those suffering from lupus psychosis carried high levels of these antibodies, and that the levels of these antibodies rose before or during the psychotic episode, suggesting both a diagnostic and predictive value in measuring anti-P antibodies.

However, half of all the lupus patients in this study who carried anti-P antibodies did not suffer from lupus psychosis and subsequent studies have given conflicting results , either confirming or refuting the initial findings or suggesting an association of raised levels of these antibodies with severe lupus depression. Until the position is clarified, single or sequential measurement of anti-P antibodies is felt to be of no value (Teh and Isenberg 1992).

Investigations

The diagnosis of neuropsychiatric lupus is based principally on symptoms and signs, but the most useful, generally available investigations (Schrieber et al. 1988) are listed below.

(i) *Formal neuropsychological testing.* May be the most sensitive and clinically useful measure of brain function in systemic lupus erythematosus; it measures function rather than structural abnormalities, it is non-invasive, objective, and it can be used serially (Ginsburg et al. 1992). Shortened versions of these tests are available (Jacobs et al. 1977).

(ii) *Magnetic resonance imaging.* Three distinct patterns detected by increased intensity of T_2 weighted images are recognized (Molad et al. 1992).

Table 4 Causes of proximal weakness in adults

Inherited
Limb girdle, facioscapulohumeral, scapuloperoneal syndromes
Glycogen and lipid storage disorders
Mitochondrial myopathies
Familial periodic paralysis
Myotonic dystrophies
Metabolic causes
Osteomalacia
Hypo- and hyperkalaemia
Hypomagnesaemia
Endocrine causes
Hyper- and hypothyroidism
Cushing's disease
Hypopituitarism
Acromegaly
Hyper- and hypoparathyroidism
Primary hyperaldosteronism
Lower motor neurone disorders
Guillain–Barré syndrome
Diabetic amyotrophy
Motor neurone disease
Carcinomatous neuromyopathy
Syringomyelia
Cauda equina compression
Other
Polymyositis, dermatomyositis, and overlap syndromes
Myasthenia gravis and Eaton–Lambert syndrome
Inflammatory myopathies: viral, bacterial, sarcoidosis
Drug induced (see Table 1), including alcohol

Note: Upper motor neurone disorders from whatever cause may present with proximal muscle weakness.

(a) Small, multifocal lesions in the white matter, not detected on computed tomography probably represent microinfarcts or demyelination.

(b) Large lesions, also in the white matter and evident on computed tomography, are infarcts.

(c) Large lesions in the grey matter, not evident on computed tomography, are caused by oedema. The lesions may resolve or evolve to infarction (Sibbitt et al. 1989).

Magnetic resonance imaging also detects intracranial catastrophes such as cerebral venous thrombosis, haematoma, abscess, and tumour. Patients with focal neurological findings or seizures are more likely to have abnormalities detected by magnetic resonance imaging than computed tomography, but it cannot diagnose neuropsychiatric lupus in the absence of clinical features.

(iii) *Electroencephalography.* Abnormalities are found in 80 per cent. Focal changes are associated with fits and focal neurological deficits, and diffuse changes with organic brain syndrome. Serial evaluation may monitor disease activity in response to treatment (Ritchlin et al. 1992).

(iv) *Anticardiolipin antibody.* This may be associated with thromboses or emboli that may warrant anticoagulation (Asherson and Lubbe 1988).

(v) *Echocardiography.* Valvular vegetations as a possible source of emboli may be demonstrated if anticardiolipin antibodies are present.

Analysis of cerebrospinal fluid is important to exclude infectious meningitis. In acute, unstable, catastrophic central nervous system disease, computed tomography scanning will identify haemorrhage, large infarction, abscess, or tumour. Blood levels of anti-DNA antibody, complement, and immune complexes do not correlate with neuropsychiatric lupus. Less requently available but useful investigations are positron emission tomography, which detects reduced cerebral metabolism (Stoppe et al. 1990), and single-photon-emission tomography which detects abnormalities of cerebral blood flow (Nossent et al. 1991).

Differential diagnosis

Exclusion of the many complications of systemic lupus erythematosus or its treatment which have central nervous system manifestations is imperative (Futran et al. 1986). These include:

- septicaemia;
- intracranial sepsis;
- accelerated atherosclerosis;
- hypertensive encephalopathy;
- uraemic encephalopathy;
- psychiatric disorders;
- emboli from valvular vegetations;
- drug side-effects especially steroid psychosis;
- multifocal leucoencephalopathy.

Treatment

Most patients have mild, self-limiting disease that does not warrant treatment. Corticosteroids and cytotoxic drugs are often given for serious manifestations but their value is unproved. Patients receiving more than 100 mg/day of prednisolone for more than a month are at greater risk of dying from infection than neuropsychiatric lupus (Sargent et al. 1975). The evolution of irreversible lesions on serial magnetic resonance imaging could be an indicator for starting treatment, which should be early to prevent progression or new lesions developing (Sibbitt et al. 1989).

It is imperative to consider whether other factors are contributing to the clinical picture that would respond to different treatment. These include:

- subdural haematoma;
- persistent intracerebral haemorrhage causing symptoms and signs;
- some patients with chorea from antiphospholipid syndrome have strokes that may be prevented by prophylactic warfarin or aspirin;
- multiple emboli associated with valvular vegetations in antiphospholipid syndrome causing ischaemic attacks or multi-infarct dementia also respond to the above regimen;
- organic depression can respond to antidepressants.

Antiphospholipid syndrome (see Chapter 6.6.4)

Anticardiolipin antibody appears to be responsible for the thrombotic and, possibly, embolic manifestations that occur in systemic lupus erythematosus, lupus-like syndromes, and antiphospholipid syndrome. Most patients have a history of a multiplicity of seemingly unrelated disorders, notably livedo reticularis, hypertension, and a history of deep venous thromboses (Asherson et al. 1989). Antiplatelet drugs or anticoagulation may be indicated. The principal neurological manifestations are:

(i) cerebral thromboses;

(ii) progressive dementia, either in isolation or associated with repeated cerebrovascular accidents resulting from multiple emboli that arise from cardiac vegetations;

(iii) transient ischaemic attacks;

(iv) chorea, sometimes in pregnancy or as a harbinger of a stroke;

(v) global amnesia;

(vi) transverse myelitis (see below).

Other connective tissue diseases

Central nervous system disease occurs in polyarteritis nodosa, Wegener's granulomatosis, mixed connective tissue disease, scleroderma, Sjögren's

Table 5 Other rheumatic diseases with central nervous system manifestations

Behçet's syndrome	Recurrent neurological symptoms, principally brain-stem
Hyperviscosity syndrome	The rheumatological associations are Sjögren's syndrome and rheumatoid arthritis; diverse symptoms occur often with confusion, ataxia, and visual symptoms; retinopathy may be marked with engorged fundal veins
Lyme disease	Early: aseptic meningitis Late: 15% develop a fluctuating meningoencephalitis with cranial nerve lesions
Sarcoidosis	Cranial nerve lesions, aseptic meningitis, fits, hydrocephalus
Takayasu's arteritis	Carotid or vertebrobasilar ischaemia (see below) Retinopathy with arteriovenous anastomoses around the disc
Whipple's disease	Slow progression of apathy, personality change, memory loss, or hypersomnia. Occasionally, cranial nerve lesions, facial myokymia, focal, motor, or sensory signs

syndrome (Hietaharju et al. 1992), and giant cell arteritis, but far less frequently than in systemic lupus erythematosus or antiphospholipid syndrome. Cranial nerve lesions (see below) may predominate. Vasculitis, anticardiolipin antibodies, and overlap with systemic lupus erythematosus are the principal factors (Shannon and Goetz 1989). Other rheumatic disorders may have central nervous system manifestations (Table 5).

Brain-stem syndromes

The brain-stem comprises the mid-brain, pons, and medulla. It conducts the major motor and sensory tracts and gives rise to all the cranial nerves except the olfactory and optic. The vertebrobasilar arteries supply the brain-stem and the cerebellum, as well as the cerebrum via the circle of Willis. The features of brain-stem disease are:

- bilateral motor or sensory long-tract signs;
- crossed (face/limb) motor or sensory signs;
- dissociated pain and temperature loss;
- cerebellar signs;
- stupor or coma;
- dysconjugate eye movements; nystagmus;
- Horner's syndrome;
- unilateral deafness, deafness, or pharyngeal weakness (these cranial nerves are not affected by single hemispheric disease);
- bulbar weakness.

The principal rheumatological associations are:

(i) vertebrobasilar insufficiency;

(ii) inflammatory conditions, notably Behçet's disease and connective tissue diseases;

(iii) platybasia from vertical and atlantoaxial subluxation or Paget's disease.

Vertebrobasilar insufficiency occurs in cervical spondylosis, atlantoaxial subluxation, giant cell arteritis, and Takayasu's arteritis. Its manifestations are myriad but the principal features are diplopia, circumoral numbness, dysarthria, and ataxia. Symptoms are often provoked by moving the head (Brust 1989).

Cranial nerve palsies

These occur in brain-stem disease or as a cranial neuropathy. They may be single or multiple. The notable associations are:

- brainstem disease (see above);
- connective tissue diseases: any nerve may be affected, in any combination, but notably trigeminal neuropathy in scleroderma and mixed connective tissue disease;
- giant cell arteritis: optic; occulomotor;
- Lyme disease: multiple;
- sarcoidosis: facial; optic chiasm;
- Whipple's disease: multiple.

Spinal cord disease

Only cervical myelopathy consequent to rheumatoid arthritis or cervical spondylosis presents to the rheumatologist with any frequency. Other causes usually affect the thoracic or lumbar cord. These include:

- cervical disc prolapse;
- cervical spondylosis;
- Paget's disease;
- rheumatoid arthritis;
- spinal tuberculosis;
- staphylococcal discitis.

Most result from compression of the cord or its blood supply by vertebral structures, so neck or back pain are usually, but not always, found in association with spastic weakness of the limbs and radicular signs at this level.

Magnetic resonance imaging has major advantages over other forms of imaging as it distinguishes the cord from other structures and identifies compression from soft tissues, such as rheumatoid pannus. It can be performed with the neck in flexion, and axial views show irreversible changes such as myelomalacia. Magnetic resonance imaging uses non-ionizing radiation and the contrast medium, gadolinium, is not toxic.

Cervical myelopathy and rheumatoid arthritis

While subluxation of the cervical spine is common in rheumatoid arthritis (25–36 per cent) (Winfield et al. 1981) cervical myelopathy is rare and mostly in those with long-standing, crippling disease. Half will die within 5 years, often from unrelated causes (Nakano 1975). Compression is usually at the craniocervical junction from anterior or vertical atlantoaxial subluxation, and less frequently from subaxial subluxation. Compression may not occur with large displacements when the canal is roomy, or it may be caused by pressure from pannus, evident on magnetic resonance imaging (Komusi et al. 1985), with only small displacements. In half, the myelopathy progresses unless halted by surgery.

Recognition of this potentially fatal complication is often delayed for months, thereby jeopardizing surgical success, as functional decline is usually so insidious it may be dismissed as deterioration of the arthritis.

A high degree of suspicion is necessary and the principal indicators that should alert the rheumatologist are:

(i) recent (less than 18 months) neck pain or occipital neuralgia;

(ii) paraesthesias or numbness in the limbs or trunk, 'electric-shocks' on neck movement such as lifting the head off the pillow or reading;

(iii) the patient's own account of diminished motor ability or documented change since the last examination (Crockard et al. 1985).

Paraesthesias may be in a glove-and-stocking distribution that could be mistaken for a peripheral neuropathy. Patients with spinothalamic involvement often describe sensations of heat or cold. Posterior column symptoms include sensations of the leg being encased in plaster or walking through quicksand. Spastic weakness may affect arms or legs. Compression of vertebral arteries may cause symptoms of vertebrobasilar insufficiency. Sphincter disturbance, usually urinary retention, occasionally occurs. An acute quadriparesis may follow a fall, whiplash injury, or forcible hyperextension during anaesthesia.

Manubriosternal joint subluxation in rheumatoid arthritis is associated with major deformities of the cervical spine, perhaps from the weight of the head causing chronic flexion of the neck (Khong and Rooney 1982).

Recognition of cord compression and assessment of its progression relies heavily on the history: evaluation of motor signs is difficult with destroyed joints and sensory symptoms are often patchy and transient. Demonstration of obscure 'textbook' signs of atlantoaxial instability may entertain, but do not guide management.

Surgical decompression may halt deterioration of the myelopathy and is recommended even in the relatively symptomless patient (Agarwal et al. 1992). Subaxial subluxation may need stabilization at the same time or may develop later (Henderson et al. 1993).

Other causes of atlantoaxial subluxation include Jaccoud's arthropathy complicating systemic lupus erythematosus (Babini et al. 1990), ankylosing spondylitis (Hunter 1989), juvenile chronic arthritis, Down syndrome, Klippel–Feil malformation, multiple epiphyseal dysplasia, and rheumatic fever.

Myelopathy caused by cervical spondylosis

Complaints of difficulty climbing stairs, heaviness, stiffness or dragging of the legs, suggesting spastic weakness, in a patient with neck pain, should alert the rheumatologist to this complication. Other symptoms include paraesthesias, numbness or aching of the legs, or weakness of the arms. Sphincter disturbance is rare. A history of recurrent brachial neuralgia is uncommon in these patients.

Neurological signs are always present; 80 per cent have weakness, either of the arms or a para-, hemi-, or quadriparesis, with hyper-reflexia in most and an extensor plantar response in half. Hand muscles may atrophy and mimic syringomyelia. Fasciculation, attributed to interference with the descending blood supply to the lumbar segment, is sometimes present in the legs and can confuse the diagnosis with amyotrophic lateral sclerosis. The most useful clinical sign is sensory loss in the arms in a dermatomal pattern, but the usual picture is patchy sensory loss in the arms sometimes in a glove distribution, together with a combination of dorsal column and/or spinothalamic tract involvement in the legs, usually without a clear sensory level. Cord damage is chiefly at levels C4–C7 and results from a combination of direct pressure from osteophytes, disc degeneration or ligamentous hypertrophy, trauma during neck movement, and interference with the spinal blood supply. Magnetic resonance imaging and where it is contraindicated computed tomography myelography are the preferred investigations.

Surgical decompression with bone fusion may help to prevent further neurological deterioration. The best results are from patients with a short history treated early. Surgery improves only half (Rowland 1989); untreated most patients are little changed after many years. Alternative or additional disorders may be present (atheroma of the vertebral and carotid arteries, multiple sclerosis, amyotropic lateral sclerosis, neurosyphilis and (rarely) spinal tumours).

Transverse myelitis in systemic lupus erythematosus or antiphospholipid syndrome

The onset of this rare complication is dramatic with paraesthesias, numbness, and weakness ascending over hours to a thoracic level, and always associated with loss of sphincter function. Magnetic resonance imaging can be useful in the diagnosis and monitoring of these patients (Boumpas et al. 1990; Lavalle et al. 1990). Even high-dose prednisolone does not affect the poor prognosis, but improvement has been reported following pulse intravenous methylprednisolone followed by repeated pulses of intravenous cyclophosphamide (Barile and Lavalle 1992).

Cauda equina syndrome

This rare complication of ankylosing spondylitis develops after more than two decades, often when the disease is clinically inactive. Arachnoiditis causes adhesions resulting in an enlargement of the caudal sac and arachnoid cysts causing pressure erosion of the adjacent bone and damage to the cauda equina. The principal presenting features are sensory with paraesthesias, pain or numbness in the perineum, buttocks, or lower limbs. Sometimes there is sphincter disturbance and, later, motor impairment. Computed tomography may be diagnostic. Decompression of the cyst, either at laminectomy or by shunting, has variable success (Tyrrell et al. 1994).

Peripheral nervous system involvement in rheumatic diseases

Radicular pain

The most common causes of radicular pain in rheumatological practice are cervical spondylosis and lumbar disc disease (Bland 1990), which are described in detail elsewhere. However, several points should be stressed.

(i) Arm and leg pains associated with spinal disease are often wrongly attributed to nerve root (radicular) compression. In fact, the pain is commonly referred from muscles, tendons, joint capsules, and ligaments. This pain is perceived away from the site of origin; it radiates widely (from the cervical spine to the hand, arm, chest, and scapula regions; from the lumbar spine to the sacroiliac region, buttocks, and posterior thigh) in a poorly localized, non-dermatomal distribution, more proximally than distal. It is felt as a deep, aching pain and is not associated with neurological signs (Bland 1990).

(ii) Radicular pain is less common. It arises from compression (or ischaemia) of the dorsal roots or their ganglia from osteophytes, disc herniation, oedema, or fibrous tissue. Radicular pain follows a dermatomal pattern, it is perceived as sharp and lancinating, and is usually exacerbated by movement of the spine, coughing, or sneezing. Paraesthesias in a dermatomal distribution are often associated. Signs of nerve root compression or irritation are usually present (Fig. 3). Dermatomal numbness or myotomal weakness may occur.

(iii) Soft tissue rheumatism in the arm (shoulder lesions, epicondylitis, carpal tunnel syndrome, de Quervain's tenosynovitis) are strongly associated with cervical spondylosis, possibly unmasked by radicular compression in the neck.

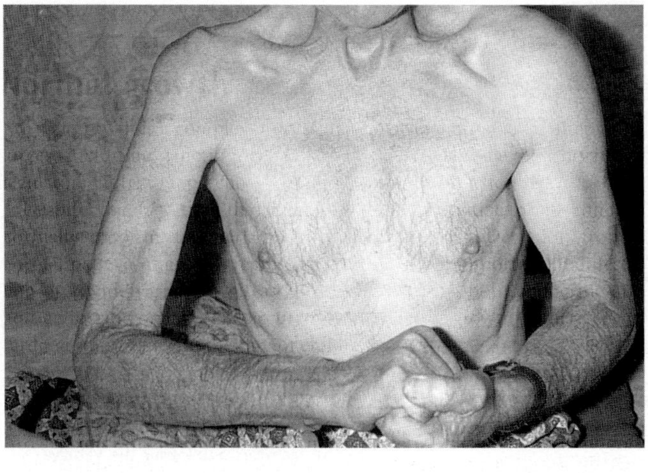

Fig. 3 A right cervical 5th and 6th nerve root lesion with wasted biceps.

(iv) Compression of the lumbar nerve root from disc herniation is too frequently diagnosed. The straight leg raising test is specific, but only under the age of 30, and only for L5/S1 lesions; for higher lesions the femoral stretch test is indicated. The straight leg raising test is deemed positive only when it is restricted to less than 40° by the radicular pain. A crossed, straight leg raising test is even more specific; radicular pain is felt on the affected side when the contralateral leg is lifted. Loss, but not depression, of a reflex is a valuable localizing sign.

(v) Radicular pain may be mistaken as arising from other structures sharing the same dermatomes; for example C5 as shoulder pain, thoracic nerves as angina or pleurisy, L3 as hip pain, L5 as knee or ankle pain.

Peripheral neuropathies

Several kinds of peripheral neuropathy (Asbury and Gilliatt 1984) complicate rheumatic diseases (Table 6) but may be overlooked if the resulting pain or weakness is taken as reflecting joint disease. Neuropathies may also be manifestations of another complication, for example, uraemic neuropathy in systemic lupus erythematosus, a side-effect of therapy such as gold salts, or coincidental such as diabetic or alcoholic neuropathy. Subclinical neuropathy may be unmasked by a second insult, so dual pathology, such as entrapment neuropathy together with polyneuropathy, should be considered. Confirmation is by electrodiagnostic studies. A nerve biopsy occasionally aids diagnosis particularly in localized vasculitis.

Entrapment neuropathies

In patients with joint disease, peripheral nerves may be damaged by pressure from deformed joints or periarticular structures, by callipers, or from the operating table. The onset is usually insidious, with pain, paraesthesias, or weakness. The differential diagnosis includes other causes of regional pain, such as brachial neuralgia, mononeuritis multiplex complicating vasculitis, and reflex sympathetic dystrophy. Confirmation is by electrodiagnosis.

Conservative treatment includes removal of the offending callipers, rest, splints, and steroid injections. Surgical decompression or transposition may be necessary for persistent pain or if motor signs develop.

Table 6 Peripheral neuropathies

Type	Clinical features
Polyneuropathy	Distal sensory and motor impairment; arreflexia
Sensory	Glove-and-stocking distribution of pain, paraesthesia, or numbness; typically starts in the feet and only affects the hands when it has risen to the level of the knees
	The pain is spontaneous or touch-induced; often the threshold to pain or touch is delayed but has an exaggerated response
	Paraesthesias are usually perceived as tingling or as tight bands
	Sensory loss may be all modalities, large fibre only (position and vibration), or small fibre only (pain and temperature)
Motor	Distal weakness, with depressed reflexes, wasting, and occasionally, fasciculation
Mononeuropathy including entrapment neuropathies	Loss of single peripheral nerve function
Mononeuritis multiplex	Involvement of two or more nerves; usually indicative of a systemic disease, notably vasculitis
Autonomic neuropathy	Postural hypotension, impotence, flushing, sweating, loss of sinus arrhythmia, loss of reactive tachycardia following the Valsalva manoeuvre; abnormal gut motility

Only those entrapment neuropathies relevant to the rheumatologist will be considered here.

Median nerve

Pressure on the median nerve in the carpal tunnel causes tingling, pain, or numbness in the radial three and a half digits, sometimes radiating up to, or even above, the elbow. It is commonly present at night, which can be relieved by exercising the hand or hanging it out of bed. Symptoms sometimes persist through the day so the patient cannot manipulate small objects and drops things. Signs may be absent. When present, sensory loss is confined to the median nerve distribution, with blunting of touch and pinprick in the radial three and a half digits. Symptoms may be provoked by Tinel's sign (tapping the nerve at the volar surface of the wrist) or Phalen's sign (sustained flexion at the wrist). Thenar weakness or wasting is a late feature.

Common causes include family history, obesity, fluid retention from pregnancy, arthritis, Colles, or scaphoid fractures. Acromegaly, hypothyroidism, amyloidosis, or chronic haemodialysis are rare. (Gossett et al. 1998).

Anterior interosseous nerve

Pressure at the elbow of this branch of the median nerve results in weakness of the deep flexors of the thumb, index, and middle fingers, with pain in the forearm but without sensory signs. The characteristic sign is loss of normal thumb–index pincer movement.

Ulnar nerve

Pressure behind the medial epicondyle of the elbow produces numbness in the ulnar one and a half digits and the corresponding side of the hand, but not proximal to the wrist, which differentiates it from a C8 radiculopathy. The intrinsic muscles of the hand and the deep flexors of the ring and little fingers may be weak. Occasionally, the ulnar nerve may be trapped in Guyon's canal at the wrist. Motor loss is then confined to the intrinsic muscles of the hand, and sensory loss to the palmar aspect of the ulnar side of the hand. The deep palmar motor branch may become compressed by repetitive trauma for example, using a chisel, and present with wasting of small hand muscles without sensory loss. This can be confused with motor neurone disease.

Posterior interosseous nerve

Entrapment at the elbow of this branch of the radial nerve causes weakness of extension of all fingers and may be mistaken for tendon ruptures. Sensory symptoms are absent.

Thoracic outlet compression syndrome

The lower elements of the brachial plexus, derived from the C8 and T1 roots, are compressed in isolation or together with the brachial artery and vein at the thoracic outlet. Various structures in this region have been implicated—cervical rib, scalenus anterior, pectoralis minor, and a costoclavicular band—each with its own name and operation. In reality, the evidence is usually lacking and the syndrome is far less common than is diagnosed (Bland 1990).

Presentation is often with pain, paraesthesias, and numbness in the ulnar side of the hand and forearm associated with vasomotor changes and wasting of the thenar emminence. The various provocative tests described are now discounted. Confirmation requires arteriography and electrodiagnostic studies.

Sciatic nerve

This may be trapped by the piriformus muscle causing pain in the lateral thigh, foot drop, and an absent ankle jerk. Compression by a Baker's cyst gives only the motor signs.

Lateral cutaneous nerve of thigh

Tight clothes or obesity can compress this nerve as it passes under the inguinal ligament causing pain, paraesthesias, and numbness in the outer side of the thigh (meralgia paraesthetica), which may be mistaken for hip pain, an L3 root lesion, or trochanteric bursitis.

Common peroneal nerve

Where it winds around the head of the fibula, this nerve is vulnerable to pressure from the joint, callipers, or the operating table. Foot drop and weakness of eversion are associated with sensory loss on the dorsum of the foot.

Posterior tibial nerve

Compression occurs in the tarsal tunnel behind the medial malleolus causing pain and tingling in the sole on standing or at night.

Autonomic neuropathy

A mild and possibly clinically irrelevant autonomic neuropathy has been demonstrated in rheumatoid arthritis (Toussirot et al. 1993), systemic lupus erythematosus (Liote and Osterland 1994), CREST syndrome (Hermosillo et al. 1994), and systemic sclerosis (Dessein et al. 1992). Familial amyloid neuropathy is often associated with severe autonomic involvement.

Peripheral neuropathies in particular diseases

Rheumatoid arthritis

Carpal tunnel syndrome may be the presenting feature of rheumatoid arthritis, but other neuropathies usually develop in established disease (Good et al. 1965). Entrapment neuropathies are the most frequent and may be multiple. An indolent pure sensory neuropathy is also common. The mechanism is unknown. The sensory loss in atlantoaxial subluxation may mimic a polyneuropathy in the arms. A rare but serious problem is mononeuritis multiplex, usually where there is also clinical and serological evidence of vasculitis. The nerves of the upper arm and thigh are vulnerable because of their sparse supply of nutrient arteries. The onset is usually sudden, with dermatomal pain and paraesthesias followed within hours by weakness. Additional nerves are involved asymmetrically over days or weeks.

Polyarteritis nodosa

Mononeuritis multiplex (see above) occurs in 50–70 per cent of patients, sometimes as a presenting feature, but typically in the systemically ill patient with multisystem disease (Conn and Dyck 1975). The kidneys are usually involved. Lesions may summate to resemble a polyneuropathy. Occasionally a peripheral sensory neuropathy slowly develops (see Table 6).

Sjögren's syndrome

Mild or subclinical, motor, or sensory neuropathy occurs in one-fifth of patients. Mononeuritis multiplex is rare and usually associated with frank vasculitis; anti-Ro is over represented in this group (Binder et al. 1988).

Scleroderma

A mild sensorineuropathy has been described (Schady et al. 1991). A parasympathetic autonomic neuropathy, evident on cardiovascular tests, is reported to be common and arguably related to the Raynaud's syndrome, oesophageal dysmotility, and bowel disturbance (Hermosillo et al. 1994). Carpal tunnel syndrome is the only other peripheral neuropathy reported with any frequency; fibrosis following surgical decompression may worsen the symptoms. Subacute combined degeneration of the cord is reported in vitamin B_{12} deficiency consequent to sclerodermatous bowel involvement (Lee et al. 1984).

Systemic lupus erythematosus

Mild peripheral neuropathies, mostly sensory, occur particularly during active disease. Mononeuritis multiplex is uncommon.

L-Tryptophan toxicity

Before this drug was withdrawn, several cases were described of a vasculitis associated with eosinophilic myositis and neuropathy.

Other rheumatological disorders

Mixed connective tissue disease, Churg–Strauss syndrome, amyloidosis, sarcoidosis, Wegener's granulomatosis, cryoglobulinaemia, Lyme disease, and giant cell arteritis may all be complicated by peripheral neuropathies.

References

Adelman, D.C., Saltiel, E., and Klinenberg, J.R. (1986). The neuropsychiatric manifestations of systemic lupus: an overview. *Seminars in Arthritis and Rheumatism* **15**, 185–99.

Agarwal, A.K., Peppelman, W.C., Kraus, D.R., Pollock, B.H., Stolzer, B.L., Eisenbeis, C.H., and Donaldson, W.F. (1992). Recurrence of cervical spine instability in rheumatoid arthritis following previous fusion: can disease progress be prevented by early surgery? *Journal of Rheumatology* **19**, 1364–70.

Asbury, A.K. and Gilliatt, R.W. *Peripheral Nerve Disorders: A Practical Approach.* London: Butterworths, 1984.

Asherson, R.A. and Lubbe, W.F. (1988). Cerebral and valve lesions in systemic lupus erythematosus: association with antiphospholipid antibodies (editorial). *Journal of Rheumatology* **15**, 539–43.

Asherson, R.A., Khamashta, M.A., and Ordis-Ros, J. (1989). The 'primary' antiphospholipid syndrome: major clinical and serological features. *Medicine* **68**, 366–77.

Babini, S.M., Maldonado Cocco, J.A., Babini, J.C., de la Sota, M., Arturi, A., and Marcos, J.C. (1990). Atlantoaxial subluxation in systemic lupus erythematosus: further evidence of tendinous alterations. *Journal of Rheumatology* **17**, 173–7.

Barile, L. and Lavalle, C. (1992). Transverse myelitis in systemic lupus erythematosus—the effect of I.V. pulse methylprednisolone and cyclophosphamide. *Journal of Rheumatology* **19**, 370–2.

Binder, A., Snaith, M.C., and Isenberg, D. (1988). Sjögren's syndrome: a study of its neurological complications. *British Journal of Rheumatology* **27**, 275–80.

Bland, J.H. (1990). Cervical and thoracic pain including thoracic outlet syndrome and brachial neuritis. *Current Opinion in Rheumatology* **2**, 242–52.

Bonfa, E., Golombek, S.J., Kaufman, L.D., Skelly, S., Weissbach, H., Brot, N., and Elkon, K.B. (1987). Association between lupus psychosis and anti-ribosomal P protein antibodies. *New England Journal of Medicine* **317**, 265–71.

Boumpas, D.T., Patronas, M.J., Dalakas, M.C., Hakim, C.A., Klippel, J.H., and Balow, J.E. (1990). Acute transverse myelitis in systemic lupus erythematosus: magnetic resonance imaging a review of the literature. *Journal of Rheumatology* **17**, 89–92.

Brust, J.C.M. (1989). Cerebral infarction. In *Merritt's Textbook of Neurology* (ed. L.P. Rowland), pp. 206–14. Philadelphia PA: Lea and Febiger.

Conn, D.C. and Dyck, P.J. (1975). Angiopathic neuropathy in connective tissue diseases. In *Peripheral Neuropathy* (ed. P.J. Dyck, P.K. Thomas, and E.H. Leubert), pp. 1149–65. Philadelphia PA: W.B. Saunders.

Crockard, H.A., Essigman, W.K., Stevens, J.M., Pozo, J.L., Ransford, A.O., and Kendall, B.E. (1985). Surgical treatments of cervical cord compression in rheumatoid arthritis. *Annals of the Rheumatic Diseases* **44**, 809–16.

Dessein, P.H., Joffe, B.I., Metz, R.M., Millar, D.L., Lawson, M., and Stanwix, A.E. (1992). Autonomic dysfunction in systemic sclerosis: sympathetic activity and instability. *American Journal of Medicine* **93**, 143–50.

Futran, J., Shore, A., Murray, B., Urowitz, M.B., and Grossman, H. (1986). Subdural haematoma in systemic lupus erythematosus. Report and review of the literature. *Journal of Rheumatology* **14**, 378–81.

Ginsburg, K.S., Wright, E.A., Larson, M.C., Fossel, A.H., Albert, M., Schur, P.H., and Liang, M.H. (1992). A controlled study of the prevalence of cognitive dysfunction in randomly selected patients with systemic lupus erythematosus. *Arthritis and Rheumatism* **35**, 776–82.

Good, A.F., Christopher, R.P., Koepke, G.H., Bender, L.F., and Tarter, M. (1965). Peripheral neuropathies associated with rheumatoid arthritis: a clinical and electrodiagnostic study of 70 cases in rheumatoid arthritis. *Annals of Internal Medicine* **63**, 87.

Gossett, J.F. and Chance, P.F. (1998). Is there a familial carpal tunnel syndrome? An evaluation and literature review. *Muscle and Nerve* **21**, 1533–6.

Guarantors of Brain. *Aids to the Investigation of Peripheral Nerve Injuries.* London: Baillière Tindall, 1988.

Hanly, J.G., Walsh, N.M.G., and Sangalang, V. (1992). Brain pathology in systemic lupus erythematosus. *Journal of Rheumatology* **19**, 732–41.

Hanly, J.G., Fisk, J.D., Sherwood, G., and Eastwood, B. (1994). Clinical course of cognitive dysfunction in systemic lupus erythematosus. *Journal of Rheumatology* **21**, 1825–31.

Henderson, F.C., Geddes, J.F., and Crockard, H.A. (1993). Neuropathology of the brain stem and spinal cord in end-stage rheumatoid arthritis: implications for treatment. *Annals of the Rheumatic Diseases* **52**, 629–37.

Hermosillo, A.G., Ortiz, R., Dayaque, J., Casanova, J.M., and Martinez-Lavin, M. (1994). Autonomic dysfunction in diffuse scleroderma vs CREST: an assessment of computerised heart rate variabilities. *Journal of Rheumatology* **21**, 1849–54.

Hietaharju, A., Korpela, M., Ilonen, J., and Frey, H. (1992). Nervous system disease, immunological features and HLA phenotype in Sjögren's syndrome. *Annals of the Rheumatic Diseases* **51**, 506–9.

Hunter, T. (1989). The spinal complications of ankylosing spondylitis. *Seminars in Arthritis and Rheumatism* **19**, 172–82.

Jacobs, J.W., Bernard, M.R., Delgado, A., and Strain, J.J. (1977). Screening for organic mental syndrome in the mentally ill. *Annals of Internal Medicine* **86**, 40–6.

Khong, T.K. and Rooney, P.J. (1982). Manubrio-sternal joint subluxation in rheumatoid arthritis. *Journal of Rheumatology* **9**, 712–15.

Komusi, T., Munro, T., and Harth, M. (1985). Radiologic review: the rheumatoid cervical spine. *Seminars in Arthritis and Rheumatism* **14**, 187–95.

Lavalle, C., Pizarro, S., Drenkard, L., Sanchez-Guerrero, J., and Alarcon-Segovia, D. (1990). Transverse myelitis: a manifestation of systemic lupus erythematosus strongly associated with antiphospholipid antibodies. *Journal of Rheumatology* **17**, 34–7.

Lee, P., Bruni, J., and Sukenik, S. (1984). Neurological manifestations of systemic sclerosis (scleroderma). *Journal of Rheumatology* **11**, 480–3.

Liote, F. and Osterland, C.K. (1994). Autonomic neuropathy in systemic lupus erythematosus: Cardiovascular autonomic fuction assessment. *Annals of the Rheumatic Diseases* **53**, 671–4.

McHugh, N.J., Maymo, J., Skinner, R.P., James, I., and Maddison, P.J. (1988). Anticardiolipin antibodies, livedo reticularis and major cerebrovascular and renal disease in systemic lupus erythematosus. *Annals of the Rheumatic Diseases* **47**, 110–15.

Marsden, C.D. (1986). Hysteria—a neurologist's view. *Psychological Medicine* **16**, 277–88.

Mastaglia, F.L. (1989). Iatrogenic (drug-induced) disorders of the nervous system. In *Neurology and General Medicine* (ed. M.J. Aminoff), pp. 505–32. New York: Churchill Livingstone.

Molad, Y., Siddi, Y., Gornish, M., Lerner, M., Pinkhas, J., and Weinberger, A. (1992). Lupus anticoagulant: correlation with magnetic resonance imaging of brain lesions. *Journal of Rheumatology* **19**, 556–61.

Nakano, K.K. (1975). Neurological complications of rheumatoid arthritis. *Orthopaedic Clinics of North America* **6**, 861–81.

Nossent, J.C., Hovestadt, A., Schonfeld, D.H.W., and Swaak, A.J.E. (1991). Single-photon-emission computed tomography of the brain in the evaluation of cerebral lupus. *Arthritis and Rheumatism* **34**, 1397–403.

Ritchlin, C.T., Chabot, R.J., Alper, K., Buyon, J., Belmont, H.M., Roueby, R., and Abramson, S.B. (1992). Quantitative electroencephalograpy. *Arthritis and Rheumatism* **35**, 1330–42.

Robbins, M.L., Kornguth, S.E., Bell, C.L., Kalinke, D.E., England, D., Turski, P., and Graziazo, F.M. (1988). Anti-neurofilament antibody evaluation in neuropsychiatric systemic lupus erythematosus. *Arthritis and Rheumatism* **31**, 623–31.

Rowland, L.P. (1989). Myelopathy caused by cervical spondylosis. In *Merritt's Textbook of Neurology* (ed. L.P. Rowland), pp. 409–11. Philadelphia PA: Lea and Febiger.

Sargent, J.S., Lockshin, M.D., Klempner, M.S., and Lipsky, B.A. (1975). Central nervous system disease in systemic lupus erythematosus. *American Journal of Medicine* **58**, 644–54.

Schady, W., Sheard, A., Hassell, A., Holt, L., Jason, M.I.V., and Klimiuk, P. (1991). Peripheral nerve dysfunction in scleroderma. *Quarterly Journal of Medicine* **80**, 661–75.

Schrieber, L., McCredie, M., Tugwell, P., and Brook, M. (1988). An evaluation of the role of laboratory investigations in establishing a diagnosis of CNS lupus. *British Journal of Rheumatology* **27**, 138–42.

Shannon, K.M. and Goetz, G.G. (1989). Connective tissue diseases and the nervous system. In *Neurology and General Medicine* (ed. M.J. Aminoff), pp. 389–413. New York: Churchill Livingstone.

Sibbitt, W.L., Sibbitt, R.R., Griffey, R.H., Eckel, C., and Bankhurst, A.D. (1989). Magnetic resonance and CT imaging in the evaluation of acute neuropsychiatric disease in systemic lupus erythematosus. *Annals of the Rheumatic Diseases* **48**, 1014–22.

Singer, J. and Denburg, J.A. (1990). Diagnostic criteria for neuropsychiatric systemic lupus erythematosus: the results of a consensus meeting. *Journal of Rheumatology* **17**, 1397–402.

Stoppe, G., Wildhagen, K., Seidel, J.W., Meyer, G.J., Schober, O., Heintz, P., Kunkel, H., Deicher, H., and Hundeshagen, H. (1990). Positron emission tomography in neuropsychiatric lupus erythematosus. *Neurology* **40**, 304–8.

Teh, L.S. and Isenberg, D.A. (1994). Anti ribosomal P protein antibodies in systemic lupus erythematosus. *Arthritis and Rheumatism* **37**, 307–15.

Toussirot, E., Serratrice, G., and Valentin, P. (1993). Autonomic nervous system involvement in rheumatoid arthritis. 50 cases. *Journal of Rheumatology* **20**, 1508–14.

Tyrrell, P.N.M., Davies, A.M., and Evans, N. (1994). Neurological disturbances in ankylosing spondylitis. *Annals of the Rheumatic Diseases* **53**, 714–17.

Winfield, J., Cook, D., Brook, A.S., and Corbett, M. (1981). A progressive study of the radiological changes in the cervical spine in rheumatoid disease. *Annals of the Rheumatic Diseases* **40**, 109–14.

1.3.4 The cardiovascular system

Susan Manzi, Amy H. Kao, and Mary Chester M. Wasko

Cardiovascular manifestations of the rheumatic diseases include pericardial, myocardial, coronary, and valvular diseases as well as conduction system abnormalities. In certain rheumatic conditions, cardiac complications can also involve the aortic root. These manifestations typically result from inflammatory and immunologic damage, and, in some cases, subsequent fibrosis. The prevalence and relative importance of the various cardiovascular complications varies among the rheumatic diseases, as illustrated in Table 1.

Pericardial diseases

The variability in reported prevalence of pericardial disease in rheumatic conditions is partially attributable to the methods used to document it and whether symptomatic or asymptomatic cases are included. Pericarditis with or without effusion is the most recognized cardiovascular manifestation of systemic lupus erythematosus (SLE); the reported prevalence ranges from 12 to 48 per cent (Moder et al. 1999). Clinical (symptomatic) pericarditis is estimated to occur in 25 per cent of SLE patients at some point in their disease course. Asymptomatic pericardial effusions are clearly more common than clinical pericarditis. In a study of 100 unselected patients with SLE, approximately 40 per cent had pericardial effusions detected using echocardiography (Badui et al. 1985). A combined autopsy series revealed pericardial involvement in 62 per cent of patients with SLE (Doherty and Siegel 1985). Cardiac tamponade can be a complication of drug-induced lupus and has been reported as an initial manifestation of SLE in several cases. Pericardial thickening may be seen in nearly 30 per cent of patients with SLE; however, constrictive pericarditis is rare.

Analysis of pericardial fluid in acute lupus pericarditis typically reveals elevated white blood cell count, elevated protein, normal glucose, and low complement levels. Antinuclear antibodies, anti-double-stranded DNA antibodies, and lupus erythematosus cells are sometimes present. However, the presence of antinuclear antibodies in pericardial fluid is not specific for SLE and may be seen in other connective tissue diseases or may arise from

Table 1 Cardiac manifestations of rheumatic diseases

	Pericardial disease	Myocardial disease	Valvular disease	Aortic root disease	Coronary disease	Conduction system disease
Ankylosing spondylitis	+	+	++	++		+
Behçet's disease	+		+	+	+	
Churg–Strauss syndrome		+			+	
Giant cell arteritis		+	+	++	+	
Kawasaki's disease					+++	
Neonatal lupus erythematosus		+				++
Polyarteritis nodosa					+	
Polymyositis/dermatomyositis	+	+				+
Reiter's syndrome			+	+		
Rheumatoid arthritis	+++	+	+	+	++	
Adult Still's disease	++	+				+
Systemic lupus erythematosus	+++	+	++		++	+
Systemic sclerosis	++	++				++
Takayasu's arteritis		+	++	+++	+	+
Wegener's granulomatosis					+	

Note: Plus signs range from +++ (commonly seen) to + (rarely reported) associations with the indicated rheumatic disease.

a neoplastic or paraneoplastic origin. Pericarditis in lupus patients rarely has an infectious aetiology.

Pericarditis is the most common form of cardiac involvement in rheumatoid arthritis (RA) (Corrao et al. 1995). Autopsy studies have detected chronic pericardial disease in up to 50 per cent of patients (Bonfiglio and Atwater 1969). The vast majority of these are not diagnosed before death. Clinical pericarditis has been reported in up to 3 per cent of RA patients, though the true incidence is not known (Gordon et al. 1973). Estimates vary with the prospective versus retrospective nature of study and the methods used to diagnose pericardial disease. In one large retrospective study of 41 patients with clinical rheumatoid pericarditis at a tertiary care center, median RA disease duration was 9 years at time of diagnosis (Hara et al. 1990). A positive rheumatoid factor was noted in seven-eighths of patients, and subcutaneous nodules were seen in about two-thirds of the cohort. Most patients in this series had acute pericarditis. Among the 41 patients, the most common symptoms were dyspnoea/orthopnoea (32), typical pericardial pain (27), and peripheral oedema (19). Examination abnormalities suggestive of pericarditis were found in 34 patients, and echocardiographic findings typical of pericardial inflammation were found in 30. In the eight patients having pericardiocentesis, six had serosanguineous fluid; glucose values were variable. While cardiac compression is seen in less than half of patients with acute pericarditis, it carries a mortality approaching 100 per cent (Hara et al. 1990).

Those with symptomatic rheumatoid pericarditis may present with insidious manifestations of pericardial constriction (McRorie et al. 1997). This has been reported as a complication in 10–24 per cent of patients with a prior history of pericarditis (Hara et al. 1990). Clinically, this condition may mimic congestive heart failure, including the presence of pleural effusions and pulmonary infiltrates. In fact, the diagnosis of constrictive pericarditis may be delayed for months, since many patients will initially respond to medical therapy for biventricular fluid overload.

Rarely, RA patients may develop purulent pericarditis as a complication of infection at a remote site (Martin et al. 1996). This complication has been reported in patients treated with corticosteroids and other immunosuppressive drugs for active joint or extra-articular disease. Typical findings of pyogenic infection, such as fever and leucocytosis, may not be present. For these reasons, diagnostic pericardiocentesis is warranted in the immunocompromised patient with a pericardial effusion. If severe or unrelenting pericardial chest pain is present, or an effusion persists in the setting of immunosuppressive therapy, infectious pericarditis must be ruled out. Pyogenic pericarditis is associated with major morbidity and mortality (Martin et al. 1996).

In systemic sclerosis (SSc), clinically symptomatic pericardial disease (5–16 per cent) is much less common than pericardial involvement at autopsy (33–72 per cent) (Deswal and Follansbee 1996). Clinical manifestations include acute pericarditis, arrhythmias, sudden cardiac death, or chronic pericardial effusions. Large pericardial effusions that can lead to cardiac tamponade are associated with poor outcomes including renal crisis. Patients with other rheumatologic disorders such as polymyositis, mixed connective tissue disease, adult Still's disease (33–37 per cent) (Pouchot et al. 1991), Behçet's disease (Ghate and Jorizzo 1999), and, rarely, ankylosing spondylitis may also present with pericarditis.

Signs and symptoms of acute pericarditis include a characteristic positional precordial or substernal chest pain, fever, tachycardia, and decreased heart sounds. Sometimes a pericardial rub can be heard. Pulsus paradoxus, a drop of systolic blood pressure 10 mmHg or greater during each inspiratory cycle, is a characteristic sign of impending tamponade.

Electrocardiography (EKG) may reveal changes suggestive of pericarditis, such as depression of the PR segment, elevation of the ST segment, inversion of T waves, or atrial arrhythmias (atrial flutter or fibrillation). If the pericardial effusion is large with impending tamponade, electrical alternans, an EKG pattern of alternating increases and decreases in QRS voltage with or without T-wave elevation, can be seen. Frequently, the only detectable clinical findings are enlargement of the cardiac silhouette by chest radiography and pericardial effusion by echocardiography. Echocardiography is the diagnostic test of choice in determining the presence and size of an effusion and the features suggestive of cardiac tamponade, such as collapse of the right ventricle during diastolic filling. A right heart catheterization is sometimes required to confirm tamponade physiology and reveals equalization of pressures. Imaging with computed tomography (CT) or magnetic resonance imaging (MRI) can help distinguish between pericardial fluid and fibrosis.

Non-steroidal anti-inflammatory agents have been beneficial in treating symptomatic cases, but systemic corticosteroid treatment (prednisone, 20–60 mg daily) and other systemic immunosuppression may be needed in refractory or severe cases. Asymptomatic pericardial effusions do not require treatment unless they are associated with tamponade physiology. Rarely, invasive procedures such as pericardiocentesis, or pericardial window are needed. If cardiac catheterization confirms equalization of pressures in all four cardiac chambers during diastole in the absence of a pericardial effusion, pericardial stripping is indicated (McRorie et al. 1997).

Myocardial diseases

Myocardial disease and myocarditis

Congestive heart failure has been reported in approximately 10 per cent of SLE patients (Badui et al. 1985). Whereas some cases are due to myocarditis, many are due to ischaemic heart disease, hypertension, renal failure, valvular disease, or toxicity from medications. There are also case reports of unusual causes of myocardial dysfunction in patients with SLE, such as acute myocarditis with localized left ventricular aneurysm, acute hemorrhagic myocarditis with thrombocytopaenia, and calciphylaxis-induced cardiomyopathy with chronic renal failure and secondary hyperparathyroidism. Subclinical myocarditis is more prevalent than clinically apparent disease. Whereas clinical myocarditis was reported in 14 per cent of a consecutive series of SLE patients, autopsy series suggest a prevalence of 40–50 per cent (Badui et al. 1985; Doherty and Siegel 1985).

Myocardial dysfunction in SLE from any of the aetiologies discussed above can result in a dilated cardiomyopathy characterized by enlargement of all heart chambers. In contrast, hypertrophic cardiomyopathy involving the left ventricle typically develops in SLE patients with long-standing hypertension. More recently, echocardiographic studies in SLE have demonstrated common abnormalities in both systolic and diastolic left ventricular function that can be progressive and often related to hypertension and coronary artery disease (Winslow et al. 1993).

Clinically recognized myocarditis in RA is extremely rare. Autopsy studies have documented nonspecific myocarditis and granulomatous lesions of the myocardium (Ind and Lewis 1984). Conduction system abnormalities attributed to occult myocardial disease are infrequent, but have been described. Variable atrioventricular block and substernal chest pain in a seropositive RA patient without evidence of myocardial ischaemia completely resolved with high-dose steroids; he had nodulosis and a prior gastrocnemius muscle biopsy showing inflammatory infiltrates, but vasculitis was not described (Newman and Cooney Jr. 1980). While congestive heart failure accounts for significant morbidity and mortality in RA, ischaemic cardiomyopathy due to atherosclerotic coronary artery disease and hypertensive cardiomyopathy rather than myocarditis have been implicated as the underlying mechanism of cardiac dysfunction (Mutru 1989; Wallberg-Jonsson 1997).

Myocardial fibrosis is the hallmark of cardiac involvement in SSc (Deswal and Follansbee 1996; Clements 2000). The fibrosis is typically patchy and widely distributed throughout both ventricles. These fibrotic deposits can cause systolic and diastolic dysfunction and can also produce arrhythmias when they involve the cardiac conduction system. Although congestive heart failure may occur in advanced disease, the systolic dysfunction is most often clinically occult. Follansbee et al. (1993) reported that although only 15 per cent of 26 patients had clinical evidence of myocardial dysfunction or abnormal left ventricular ejection fraction at rest, 46 per cent had an abnormal ejection fraction response to exercise. The myocardial fibrosis seen in patients with SSc may result from intermittent ischaemia, either from vasospasm or microvascular disease. Echocardiographic studies in SSc suggest that both right and left ventricular dysfunction is common. Right heart failure is typically due to primary or secondary (pulmonary fibrosis) pulmonary hypertension. Less commonly, cardiomyopathy in SSc may be caused by an inflammatory myocarditis. Myocarditis is more frequent in those patients with SSc who have features of polymyositis and skeletal muscle disease (myositis).

Myocarditis associated with polymyositis and dermatomyositis is seen in up to 3 per cent of patients and may be present in 30 per cent at autopsy (Denbow et al. 1979). Myocardial fibrosis, necrosis, and overt carditis with inflammatory infiltrates can be seen histopathologically (Lie 1995). Myocardial involvement most prominently results in conduction disturbances, but rarely will cause congestive heart failure.

In diseases where aortic root involvement and chronic aortic insufficiency can be seen, such as ankylosing spondylitis, giant cell arteritis, and Takayasu's arteritis, left ventricular hypertrophy and a subsequent dilated cardiomyopathy may develop. Myocarditis is rare in ankylosing spondylitis and has been infrequently reported in adult-onset Still's disease (Pouchot et al. 1991).

Symptoms of myocardial dysfunction include dysponea, tachycardia, arrhythmias, and in some cases congestive heart failure. Although echocardiography can detect abnormalities in cardiac function, it cannot accurately determine the aetiology. There are no typical findings on EKG and cardiac enzymes may be normal in cases of myocarditis. Endomyocardial biopsy remains the technique of choice in diagnosing myocarditis; however, the procedure is invasive and subject to sampling error. Non-specific histologic findings of myocarditis include focal areas of fibrosis and mild perivascular lymphocytic infiltration of the myocardium. There are several promising investigational, non-invasive techniques for diagnosing myocarditis. ^{111}In-antimyosin Fab imaging uses a specific marker for myocellular injury and has potential to be a reasonable screening test in patients with suspected myocardial involvement (Morguet et al. 1995). Focal myocardial enhancement on MRI with T1 spin echo may support a diagnosis of myocarditis (Roditi 2000).

Acute myocarditis is typically treated with systemic corticosteroids. Congestive heart failure from cardiomyopathy is treated similarly to heart failure from all causes with afterload-reducing agents, diuretics, and inotropics as indicated. Other treatable causes of congestive heart failure, such as progressive renal failure and uncontrolled hypertension, should not be overlooked.

Aortic involvement

Ankylosing spondylitis is one of the inflammatory diseases that mainly affects the aortic root. Proximal aortitis can lead to aortic root thickening and dilatation and aortic and mitral regurgitation. Aortitis and aortic valvulitis are thought to be unrelated to clinical features of ankylosing spondylitis except for duration of the disease (Roldan et al. 1998b). Diseases of the aortic wall can also result from the inflammatory process of Takayasu's arteritis, giant cell arteritis, and reactive arthritis, as well as from inherited connective tissue disorders such as Marfan's syndrome, Ehlers–Danlos syndrome, and osteogenesis imperfecta.

A potential life-threatening complication of aortic root disease is aortic dissection. Marfan's syndrome accounts for 3–5 per cent of aortic dissections (Westaby 1995). Eighty to ninety per cent of patients present with severe pain localized to the lumbar region, anterior chest, or abdomen. A total of 15–20 per cent of patients may present with neurologic findings and vascular compromise.

Rheumatoid aortitis is a rare entity. Due to potential confusion between the spondyloarthropathies and classical RA in the older rheumatology literature, early case reports may not represent true aortitis associated with RA. Nevertheless, a 1989 case series of 10 patients with aortitis on autopsy indicates that this complication of RA, although infrequent, does occur (Gravallese et al. 1989). These were noted amongst 188 consecutive RA cases examined at autopsy; 60 cases had histology of the aorta available. No cases were suspected antemortem, though three patients were known to have aortic aneurysms. Nine of the 10 patients had seropositive nodular disease; mean disease duration was 9.6 years. None had evidence of infectious aortitis; vasculitis of the aortic branches was noted in four patients. In three cases, aortitis retrospectively was considered a clinically significant factor in the patients' demise: two with congestive heart failure, one from a ruptured aortic aneurysm. In patients with severe, seropositive disease, this entity may cause haemodynamic compromise and be fatal.

Valvular diseases

Libman–Sacks endocarditis, also known as marantic endocarditis or noninfectious verrucous vegetations, was first described in 1924. More than one-half of SLE patients have abnormal valves, but most are not clinically significant. Clinical examination is not always helpful in detecting abnormal valves since the associated murmur may be soft or inaudible. Echocardiography can usually distinguish Libman–Sacks lesions from infectious endocarditis and rheumatic valvular disease. Libman–Sacks lesions occur most frequently on the mitral valve and affect both surfaces of the leaflets as well as the rings and the commissures. In contrast, infective vegetations are almost always located at the leaflet's line of closure and show vibratory or rotatory motion independent of the leaflet motion. Rheumatic valvular disease has leaflet thickening localized to the leaflet tips and a marked degree of chordal thickening, fusion, tethered motion, and calcification. The prevalence of Libman–Sacks vegetations in SLE ranges from less than 10 per cent by transthoracic echocardiography to 30 per cent by transoesophageal echocardiography (Roldan et al. 1996). A definitive diagnosis can be made only on pathologic examination of the affected valve.

Immunoglobulins have been detected in the lesions of Libman–Sacks vegetations, suggesting that these lesions may result from endocardial damage mediated by immune complexes. These complexes may contribute to the deposition of fibrin-platelet thrombi in layers causing the subsequent scarring and deformity of the valves. It is unclear whether antiphospholipid antibodies play a role in the pathogenesis of Libman–Sacks endocarditis. Approximately 32 per cent of patients with primary antiphospholipid syndrome have Libman–Sacks lesions as detected by echocardiography (Reisner et al. 2000). However, Libman–Sacks endocarditis is also commonly found in SLE patients without anticardiolipin antibodies.

In RA, clinically significant valvular heart disease is uncommon. Patients with seropositive nodular joint disease comprise the majority of those affected. Case reports of aortic insufficiency requiring replacement suggest that granulomatous, nodular type valve involvement accounts for the valve lesions in some but not all patients (Newman and Cooney Jr. 1980).

Most echocardiographic evaluations of patients with RA indicate that, in an unselected cohorts, prevalent valvular heart disease is more common than in controls (Corrao et al. 1995; Wislowska et al. 1998). Mitral valve disease is the most commonly noted valvular abnormality on transthoracic examination, with both mitral insufficiency and mitral valve prolapse being reported. Valvular abnormalities detected by transoesophageal echocardiography are extremely common and occur twice as often as in controls. Guedes et al. (2001) documented mitral regurgitation in 80 per cent of 30 unselected RA patients, compared with only 37 per cent of controls ($p < 0.001$). Aortic insufficiency was noted in 33 per cent of the RA patients, but was no more frequent than in the controls. Valve thickening accounted for the majority of aortic and mitral regurgitation, though round mitral images, presumed to be nodules, could be visualized in two patients. All patients were asymptomatic. One longitudinal study over 4 years demonstrated resolution of mitral valve findings in a subset of patients, though the significance of this is unknown (Nomeir et al. 1979). Efforts to correlate echocardiographic findings with clinical features of RA have shown no consistent correlation with ischaemic heart disease, RA duration, disease severity, seropositivity, or other extra-articular involvement (Nomeir et al. 1979).

In summary, valvular heart disease, particularly mitral insufficiency due to valvular thickening, is more prevalent by echocardiography in RA patients than the general population or comparison groups referred for echocardiography. However, nodular lesions account for a minority of valvular dysfunction, and these lesions are rarely of clinical significance.

Valvular and aortic root disease associated with ankylosing spondylitis includes aortic valvulitis resulting in cusp thickening and retraction, thickening of the aorto-mitral junction (subaortic bump) with mitral regurgitation, proximal aortitis leading to aortic root thickening and dilatation and aortic regurgitation (Roldan 1998a). Aortitis, valvulitis, and regurgitation are generally mild and clinically silent, with prevalence rates less than 10 per cent. Other conditions associated with aortic insufficiency that typically result from aortic root inflammation, dilatation, dissection, or deformity of the leaflets are reactive arthritis, giant cell arteritis, Takayasu's arteritis, Behçet's disease, and other connective tissue diseases such as Marfan's syndrome and Ehlers–Danlos syndrome. Echocardiographic and autopsy studies have suggested minor, if any, increased cardiac valvular involvement in SSc and polymyositis/dermatomyositis.

There is no direct evidence that treatment with corticosteroids or cytotoxic therapy can prevent valvular damage; however, the decline in prevalence of Libman–Sacks lesions at autopsy following the introduction of corticosteroids from approximately 59 to 35 per cent supports a possible indirect beneficial role. The valvular abnormalities seen in rheumatic diseases may predispose to bacterial endocarditis, thus prophylactic antibiotics should be used for dental or surgical procedures with an increased risk of transient bacteraemia.

Coronary artery disease

Clinical manifestations of coronary artery disease in rheumatologic disorders can result from atherosclerosis and thrombosis, arteritis, and/or vasospasm.

Coronary atherosclerotic disease

Cardiovascular disease accounts for considerable morbidity and mortality in patients with SLE and RA. A striking feature of most patients with SLE that experience ischemic heart disease is their young age. Women with SLE aged 35–44 are 50 times more likely to have a myocardial infarction than their non-lupus counterparts, whereas women with SLE aged 45–64 are only two to four times more likely (Manzi et al. 1997). The mean age at the first coronary atherosclerotic disease (CAD) event among SLE patients is 48–49 years. The prevalence of myocardial infarction, angina, and sudden cardiac death ranges from 6 to 10 per cent (Manzi et al. 1997); however, the true prevalence of subclinical CAD in patients with SLE is unknown. Urowitz et al. (1976) first emphasized the importance of CAD as a cause of mortality when they described the bimodal mortality pattern in SLE. Mortality due to CAD accounts for up to 30 per cent of all deaths in patients with SLE (Ward et al. 1995).

Most studies have documented an increased mortality in RA. Lifespan in patients with RA is shortened by 2.5–18 years, with variations in estimates attributed to community-based versus hospital-based studies (Wolfe et al. 1994; Myllykangas-Luosujärvi et al. 1995). Cardiovascular disease accounts for roughly 50 per cent of deaths in patients with RA, with most deaths attributed to myocardial infarction or congestive heart failure (Mutru et al. 1989; Wolfe et al. 1994; Myllykangas-Luosujärvi et al. 1995).

Autopsy studies in SLE have suggested a paucity of overt vasculitis and a high frequency of atherosclerotic coronary disease and small vessel intimal thickening in young patients (Fukumoto et al. 1987). Similarly, coronary artery disease in RA appears to result from accelerated atherosclerosis rather than active arteritis or vasospasm, although information from autopsy specimens is limited. The reason for the escalation of atherosclerosis in SLE and RA is not clear, though it is likely multifactorial (Table 2).

Increases in traditional risk factors such as hypercholesterolemia, hypertension, smoking, diabetes mellitus, and sedentary lifestyle have been recognized as potential contributors to premature coronary disease in SLE and RA. In SLE, renal disease with resulting hypertension also likely plays a role in accelerated atherogenesis. Recent evidence suggests, however, that the increased risk of coronary heart disease in SLE cannot be fully accounted for by traditional risk factors and that the underlying SLE disease and/or its treatment likely play a role (Esdaile et al. 2001).

Inherent abnormalities of lipid metabolism in RA patients may increase susceptibility to atherosclerosis. Serum concentrations of lipoprotein A [Lp(a)], a suspected independent risk factor for atherosclerosis, are elevated in RA patients compared with controls. The S3 Apo(a) phenotype was twice as prevalent in an RA cohort, independent of HLA–DR4 status, and may explain in part the Lp(a) elevations (Asanuma et al. 1999). Other patterns

Table 2 Potential factors contributing to cardiovascular disease in SLE and RA

Traditional cardiovascular risk factors	Disease or treatment related	Immunologic/ inflammatory[a]
Hypertension	Elevated homocysteine	Proinflammatory cytokines[b]
Hyperlipidaemia	Glucocorticoid use	Complement-fixing immune complexes
Diabetes mellitus	Renal disease (SLE)	CD4+ T cells (RA)
Smoking	Seropositive disease (RA)	B cell–T cell interactions (SLE)
Obesity		Antiphospholipid antibodies
Sedentary lifestyle		

[a] The immunologic/inflammatory processes involve endothelial activation and upregulation of adhesion molecules.

[b] Including TNF-α in RA.

Table 3 Cardiovascular disease risk management strategies

Physician awareness
Recognize increased risk
Be suspicious of new onset chest pain
Patient education
Minimize traditional cardiovascular risk factors
Control hypertension
Treat hyperlipidaemia
Maintain normoglycaemia
Encourage smoking cessation
Suggest weight loss programmes for obesity
Initiate appropriate exercise programmes
Address disease-specific potential risk factors
Reduce homocysteine levels (consider folate supplementation)
Minimize glucocorticoid use
Recognize thrombotic potential (antiphospholipid antibodies) and initiate aspirin or anticoagulants
Low threshold for cardiac evaluation

of lipid metabolism that might predispose to atherosclerosis have been noted in RA patients with active synovitis. When compared with healthy controls, they have alterations in lipoprotein lipase mass and activity (Wallberg-Jonsson et al. 1996). Low levels of Apo A1 and HDL-cholesterol, both risk factors for atherosclerosis, have been documented in untreated RA patients with active joint disease (Park et al. 1999). Recent work has supported these findings. In early, untreated RA, both total and HDL-cholesterol are depressed; antirheumatic therapy resulted in an increase in both levels, with the most rapid rise in HDL-cholesterol somewhat paradoxically noted in those patients receiving corticosteroid therapy (Boers et al. 2001). These studies suggest that unfavourable lipid profiles in RA are in part a function of active inflammatory disease, and may be corrected with disease-modifying therapy, including corticosteroids.

Medications used to treat SLE and/or RA may also contribute to accelerated atherosclerosis by increasing the influence of traditional risk factors. Specifically, non-steroidal anti-inflammatory drug (NSAID) therapy may cause chronic increases in blood pressure with cumulative effects over time. Aspirin therapy was first noted to confer possible cardiovascular protection in RA men in the 1970s (Linos et al. 1978). More recent use of traditional NSAIDs with relatively long half-lives, such as naproxen, appears to have provided protection from ischaemic cardiovascular disease via their antiplatelet effects (Watson et al. 2001).

Cholesterol metabolism may be altered unfavourably by chronic use of corticosteroids or favourably by chronic use of antimalarials. Methotrexate use has been associated with increased cardiovascular morbidity and mortality in a Scandinavian cohort of RA patients; the mechanism for such association is not known, but may be due to alterations in homocysteine metabolism (Landewe et al. 2000). Hyperhomocysteinaemia is associated with an increased risk of coronary artery disease, cerebrovascular accidents, and carotid vascular disease (Landewe et al. 2000). Hyperhomocysteinaemia is noted in RA patients treated with methotrexate without concomitant folate supplementation, though no increase in cardiovascular events has yet been recognized in this group (Trujillo-Martin et al. 2000). More recently, however, methotrexate use has been associated with improved cardiovascular mortality in a cohort of patients with RA (Choi et al. 2002). Elevated serum homocysteine levels associated with arterial thrombosis were documented in a population of SLE patients (Petri et al. 1996). The reasons for hyperhomocysteinaemia in SLE are unclear and may be related to diet or treatment.

Other SLE and RA disease-specific factors independent of treatment are also suspected. Atherosclerosis, SLE, and RA are now recognized as systemic chronic inflammatory diseases and share pathogenic mechanisms (Manzi and Wasko 2000). Inflammation at the site of vascular injury is thought to mediate atherogenesis by increasing the permeability, adhesiveness, and prothrombotic properties of the endothelium (Ross 1999).

Factors related to SLE that may contribute to vascular injury include immune complexes, viruses, and toxins such as homocysteine. Deposition of complement-fixing immune complexes on the endothelium triggers upregulation of adhesion molecules such as E-selectin and intercellular and vascular cell adhesion molecules on the endothelial cell surface. In addition, the interaction between CD40 and CD40L involved in autoantibody production in SLE may affect the vascular endothelium triggering an inflammatory response. The importance of immunologic factors in atherogenesis is further supported by studies on antiphospholipid antibodies in SLE, which have been associated with thromboembolic events, stroke, and foetal loss. Evidence indicates that these antibodies may also promote atherosclerosis (Vaarala 2000).

In RA, immunologic components of atherosclerotic plaque and rheumatoid joint disease are strikingly similar, leading to speculation that smouldering or overtly active rheumatoid synovitis may account for accelerated vascular plaque formation and rupture (Pasceri and Yeh 1999; Weyand et al. 2001).

Rheumatic disease patients with ischaemic heart disease have presenting signs and symptoms not unlike those without an underlying autoimmune illness. However, the differential diagnosis of chest pain in SLE and RA is extensive, and other causes are usually entertained initially. These include upper gastrointestinal pathology associated with NSAID use, disease-related costochondral pain or, less commonly, pleuropericarditis, and osteoporotic rib fractures. The prompt diagnosis of ischaemic heart disease in the younger patient requires an astute physician with an awareness of increased risk. Like the standard management of patients with increased risk of CAD, a full cardiac workup is indicated for young patients with unexplained non-pleuritic chest pain, chest pressure, or dyspnoea on exertion. Stress thallium scans, dobutamine echocardiography, and coronary angiography can define the severity of involvement. Physical limitations may require pharmacologic rather than standard exercise stress testing.

Table 3 illustrates the strategies for managing CAD risk. In both SLE and RA, treatment of ischaemic heart disease should be directed at minimizing traditional risk factors for atherosclerosis. These include aggressive blood pressure control, lipid-lowering agents where indicated, and an individualized exercise regimen to increase aerobic fitness, tailored to accommodate physical limitations of the rheumatoid patient. Theoretically beneficial recommendations, as yet not assessed, include the prophylactic benefit of folate supplementation with or without concomitant methotrexate therapy for cardiovascular protection. Daily low-dose aspirin is indicated in any patient with prior cardiovascular event, though the risk of gastrointestinal toxicity is probably increased when administered with daily NSAID therapy. The risks versus benefits of empiric low-dose aspirin in the asymptomatic RA patient on COX-2 inhibitors have not yet been determined.

Measures to minimize glucocorticoid dose may also be beneficial. Newer biological therapies directed at reducing endothelial activation and upregulation of adhesion molecules and other mechanisms specific to the pathogenesis of SLE and RA may provide added reduction in the number of cardiovascular events by more effectively controlling inflammation and reducing corticosteroid requirements.

The growing use of non-invasive vascular imaging in the detection of subclinical CAD may improve our ability to identify patients at high risk for having a clinical event (e.g. myocardial infarction) (Manzi et al. 2000). The current trend in vascular imaging focuses on measuring early structural and functional properties of the vascular system rather than measuring flow-limiting vessel stenosis because current evidence suggests that most myocardial infarctions result from occlusion of a vessel that had previously shown stenosis of less than 50 per cent on angiography or in areas supplied by coronary arteries without critical stenosis (Manzi et al. 2000). A plaque that does not cause significant stenosis may rupture, leading to unstable angina, myocardial infarction, or sudden death. Atherosclerotic plaques that are prone to rupture, dubbed 'vulnerable' plaques, are thought to have characteristic structural, cellular, and molecular features. Thallium scanning and dual-isotope myocardial perfusion imaging, which rely on perfusion abnormalities, may underestimate atherosclerotic disease and risk for future myocardial infarction. In contrast, coronary artery scanning by electron beam CT detects coronary calcification, which is thought to be an accurate marker of the burden of coronary atherosclerosis. B-mode carotid ultrasound, which measures intima media thickness and degree of carotid plaque, is another modality for detecting subclinical cardiovascular disease. B-mode ultrasound and electron beam CT are widely used in epidemiological studies evaluating the prevalence and associated risk factors of subclinical atherosclerosis in population-based samples, and more recently have been applied in lupus populations. Limited evidence suggests that there is a significant amount of coronary calcification detected by electron beam CT in female patients with SLE (Manzi et al. 2000). In contrast to a prevalence of 6–10 per cent for clinical coronary events in patients with SLE, two studies report evidence of subclinical vascular disease detected by B-mode carotid ultrasound in up to 40 per cent of patients (Manzi et al. 1999; Roman et al. 2001).

The prevalence of atherosclerotic coronary artery disease in other rheumatic diseases, including SSc and polymyositis/dermatomyositis, is not increased above expected frequencies.

Coronary arteritis

Coronary arteritis, a pathologic diagnosis in SLE and RA, is distinctly uncommon and an unusual cause for myocardial ischaemia and/or infarction. Patients present with symptoms of obstructive atherosclerotic coronary disease, making premortem diagnosis extremely difficult. Among one series of 47 autopsied patients with RA, coronary vasculitis was not specifically evaluated. However, of the 10 patients with acute myocardial infarction in the month prior to death, atherosclerotic lesions were grossly apparent and considered the cause of coronary occlusion. Histologic examination for evidence of vasculitis was not performed. Although evidence of vasculitis in other organ systems may favour a diagnosis of coronary arteritis in an SLE or RA patient with symptoms of ischaemic heart disease, the absence of this does not preclude the diagnosis. A recent comparison of RA patients with and without rheumatoid vasculitis indicated a slightly increased risk of death in the vasculitis group (adjusted hazard ratio 1.26, 95 per cent CI 0.79–2.01); the only vasculitis-associated death, however, was a myocardial infarction diagnosed at post-mortem examination (Voskuyl et al. 1996). In the RA or SLE patient with new onset angina or congestive heart failure and underlying vasculitis, coronary arteritis should be considered in the differential diagnosis.

Vasculitis affecting the ascending aorta in Takayasu's arteritis can extend into the proximal segment or ostium of the coronary arteries causing proximal stenosis and leading to angina and myocardial infarction (Longo and Remetz 1998). The distal coronary arteries usually do not manifest arteritis. There have also been reports of coronary arteritis in other vasculitides associated with aortitis, including giant cell arteritis and Behçet's disease. Systemic necrotizing vasculitis due to polyarteritis nodosa, Wegener's granulomatosis, or Churg–Strauss syndrome can involve the coronary vessels causing fibrinoid necrosis of arterioles, venules, and capillaries (Frustaci et al. 1998). Clinical manifestations include acute myocardial infarction, angina, and congestive heart failure. Kawasaki disease, an acute vasculitis in children, typically causes coronary artery changes 3–14 days after the onset; coronary aneurysms are the most common and serious complication. About 20–25 per cent of untreated patients with Kawasaki disease develop these coronary artery lesions. Among patients with Kawasaki disease, myocardial infarction occurs in 1.9 per cent of all patients and in 39 per cent of those with persistent aneurysms (Kato et al. 1996).

Coronary arteritis can be detected on coronary angiography, which may reveal aneurysms, a rare finding except in Kawasaki disease, or rapidly progressive stenotic lesions on serial angiograms. The distinction between coronary atherosclerosis and arteritis is important since treatment of arteritis with increased corticosteroid dose can worsen the risk factors in patients with atherosclerotic disease. Anticoagulation or antiplatelet therapy has been used in patients with arteritis to reduce the risk of thrombotic occlusion.

Coronary vasospasm and microvascular disease

Microvascular coronary disease is a recognized entity in SLE (Doherty and Siegel 1985). Histologic changes of the intramural coronary vessels reveal hyalinization and microthrombi. Microvascular disease may result in angina-like chest pain in the setting of insignificant coronary artery disease, and has been implicated as a potential aetiology for lupus cardiomyopathy. Intramural coronary artery disease is considered the most common primary cardiac disease in SSc. Thallium perfusion scans are abnormal in over 70 per cent of patients with SSc. These defects likely reflect microvascular changes since the prevalence of extramural atherosclerotic coronary artery disease in SSc is not increased compared with the general population.

While myocardial Raynaud's phenomenon has been postulated as a contributing factor to cardiac perfusion defects in SSc, the available findings suggest that it is different from peripheral Raynaud's. In SSc patients with myocardial ischaemia, the small arteries of the heart infrequently demonstrate narrowing, which is in contrast to the significant anatomic narrowing of the peripheral arteries (Follansbee et al. 1990). Because Raynaud's phenomenon in SLE and RA patients is usually mild and likely vasospastic rather than vasculopathic in origin, one might suspect that vasospasm of the coronaries has little to no clinical significance. However, systematic investigation has not been pursued.

Conduction abnormalities

Cardiac rhythm and conduction abnormalities can occur in SLE; however, the direct relationship to the underlying disease is unclear. Many times the arrhythmias reflect ischaemic heart disease or cardiomyopathy. More recently, evidence suggests that heart rate variability in SLE may be related to cardiac autonomic dysfunction (Lagana et al. 1996).

Conduction abnormalities in SLE are most commonly recognized as a manifestation of neonatal lupus. Congenital heart block can occur in children born to mothers with anti-SSA antibodies with or without lupus and results from transplacental passage of maternal anti-SSA antibodies (Buyon et al. 1989). Congenital heart block with or without associated myocarditis is diagnosed *in utero*, usually between 22 and 24 weeks gestation or shortly after birth. Approximately 40–70 per cent of babies with heart block will require pacemaker placement. Clinicians should monitor pregnancies at high risk for congenital heart block with close foetal heart rate checks and foetal echocardiography. Dexamethasone therapy may be warranted when intrauterine bradycardia is detected and when signs of heart failure are present. Conduction system abnormalities have been rarely described in patients with RA.

Conduction system disease is common in SSc with a prevalence of electrocardiographic abnormalities in as many as 50 per cent of patients (Deswal and Follansbee 1996). The frequency of arrhythmias increases if 24-h ambulatory monitoring is used. Unlike supraventricular arrhythmias, ventricular ectopy is strongly associated with mortality and sudden death.

Patchy myocardial fibrosis involving the conduction system accounts for a significant percentage of these conduction system abnormalities. Similarly, myocardial fibrosis resulting from myocarditis in patients with polymyositis and dermatomyositis can present as cardiac conduction disturbances, most commonly left anterior hemiblock and right bundle branch block.

The second most common cardiac disease in ankylosing spondylitis, after aortitis and aortic regurgitation, is conduction system disease, caused by subaortic fibrosis extending into the base of the septum resulting in atrioventricular block. Few reported cases of Takayasu's arteritis are associated with complete atrioventricular block from fibrosis of the conduction system. Infiltrative diseases such as sarcoidosis and amyloidosis also induce arrhythmias by involving the myocardium or conduction system. Sudden death due to ventricular arrhythmias or heart block accounted for 30–65 per cent of mortality in an autopsy series of cardiac sarcoidosis (Perry and Vuitch 1995). In general, there are no disease specific treatments for conduction system involvement; patients are treated in the standard fashion with antiarrhythmic drugs and pacemakers as appropriate.

In summary, the prevalence and relative importance of the various cardiovascular complications differ among the numerous rheumatic diseases. However, a common underlying finding is that subclinical cardiac complications are more prevalent than clinically evident disease. Recent evidence indicates that one of the most recognized cardiovascular manifestations resulting in serious morbidity and mortality is coronary artery disease in rheumatic diseases such as SLE and RA. The first step in appropriately managing the patient is awareness of the increased risk. Prompt recognition of ischaemic heart disease can be a clinical challenge in those rheumatic disease patients who are relatively sedentary and who have other common aetiologies for chest pain. With emerging evidence that atherogenesis is an immune and inflammatory process, the rheumatic diseases are becoming models for investigation of the pathogenesis of atherosclerotic cardiovascular disease.

Acknowledgments

This work was supported by the Lupus Foundation of America, Western Pennsylvania Chapter; the Arthritis Foundation, Western PA Chapter; the American Heart Association; NIH-MAC P60-AR-44811; NIH R01 AR46588; NIH K24 AR02213; NIH K23 R47571. Portions of this information concerning cardiovascular complications associated with SLE are found in Kao and Manzi (2002). The authors would like to thank Janice Sabatine, PhD, for editorial assistance.

References

Asanuma, Y. et al. (1999). Serum lipoprotein(a) and apolipoprotein(a) phenotypes in patients with rheumatoid arthritis. *Arthritis and Rheumatism* **42**, 443–7.

Badui, E. et al. (1985). Cardiovascular manifestations in systemic lupus erythematosus. Prospective study of 100 patients. *Angiology* **36**, 431–41.

Boers, M. et al. (2001). Corticosteroids and cholesterol levels in early RA. *Arthritis and Rheumatism* **44** (Suppl. 9), S53 (Abstract 2).

Bonfiglio, T. and Atwater, E.C. (1969). Heart disease in patients with seropositive rheumatoid arthritis; a controlled autopsy study and review. *Archives of Internal Medicine* **124**, 714–19.

Buyon, J.P. et al. (1989). Acquired congenital heart block. Pattern of maternal antibody response to biochemically defined antigens of the SSA/Ro–SSB/La system in neonatal lupus. *Journal of Clinical Investigation* **84**, 627–34.

Choi, H.K. Hernan, M.A., Seeger, J.D., Robins, J.M., and Wolfe, F. (2002). Methotrexate and mortality in patients with rheumatoid arthritis: a propective study. *Lancet* **359**, 1173–7.

Clements, P.J. (2000). Systemic sclerosis (scleroderma) and related disorders: clinical aspects. *Baillières Best Practice and Research in Clinical Rheumatology* **14**, 1–16.

Corrao, S. et al. (1995). Cardiac involvement in rheumatoid arthritis: evidence of silent heart disease. *European Heart Journal* **16**, 253–6.

Denbow, C.E. et al. (1979). Cardiac involvement in polymyositis: a clinicopathologic study of 20 autopsied patients. *Arthritis and Rheumatism* **22**, 1088–92.

Deswal, A. and Follansbee, W.P. (1996). Cardiac involvement in scleroderma. *Rheumatic Diseases Clinics of North America* **22**, 841–60.

Doherty, N.E. and Siegel, R.J. (1985). Cardiovascular manifestations of systemic lupus erythematosus. *American Heart Journal* **110**, 1257–65.

Esdaile, J.M. et al. (2001). Traditional Framingham risk factors fail to fully account for accelerated atherosclerosis in systemic lupus erythematosus. *Arthritis and Rheumatism* **44**, 2331–7.

Follansbee, W.P. et al. (1990). A controlled clinicopathologic study of myocardial fibrosis in systemic sclerosis (scleroderma). *Journal of Rheumatology* **17**, 656–62.

Follansbee, W.P., Zerbe, T.R., and Medsger, T.A., Jr. (1993). Cardiac and skeletal muscle disease in systemic sclerosis (scleroderma): a high risk association. *American Heart Journal* **125**, 194–203.

Frustaci, A. et al. (1998). Necrotizing myocardial vasculitis in Churg–Strauss syndrome: clinicohistologic evaluation of steroids and immunosuppressive therapy. *Chest* **114**, 1484–9.

Fukumoto, S. et al. (1987). Coronary atherosclerosis in patients with systemic lupus erythematosus at autopsy. *Acta Pathologica Japonica* **37**, 1–9.

Ghate, J.V. and Jorizzo, J.L. (1999). Behçet's disease and complex aphthosis. *Journal of the American Academy of Dermatology* **40**, 1–18.

Gordon, D.A., Stein, J.L., and Broder, I. (1973). The extra-articular features of rheumatoid arthritis. A systematic analysis of 127 cases. *American Journal of Medicine* **54**, 445–52.

Gravallese, E.M. et al. (1989). Rheumatoid aortitis: a rarely recognized but clinically significant entity. *Medicine (Baltimore)* **68**, 95–106.

Guedes, C. et al. (2001). Cardiac manifestations of rheumatoid arthritis: a case–control transesophageal echocardiography study in 30 patients. *Arthritis and Rheumatism* **45**, 129–35.

Hara, K.S. et al. (1990). Rheumatoid pericarditis: clinical features and survival. *Medicine (Baltimore)* **69**, 81–91.

Ind, P.W. and Lewis, P. (1984). Systemic hypertension in the rheumatic diseases. In *Butterworths International Medical Reviews. Rheumatology* (ed. B.M. Ansell and P.A. Simkin), pp. 186–212. London: Butterworths.

Kao, A.H. and Manzi, S. (2002). How to manage patients with cardiopulmonary disease? *Baillieres Best Practise and Research in Clinical Rheumatology* **16**, 211–27.

Kato, H. et al. (1996). Long-term consequences of Kawasaki disease. A 10- to 21-year follow-up study of 594 patients. *Circulation* **94**, 1379–85.

Lagana, B. et al. (1996). Heart rate variability and cardiac autonomic function in systemic lupus erythematosus. *Lupus* **5**, 49–55.

Landewe, R.B. et al. (2000). Methotrexate effects in patients with rheumatoid arthritis with cardiovascular comorbidity. *Lancet* **355**, 1616–17.

Lie, J.T. (1995). Cardiac manifestations in polymyositis/dermatomyositis: how to get to heart of the matter. *Journal of Rheumatology* **22**, 809–11.

Linos, A. et al. (1978). Effect of aspirin on prevention of coronary and cerebrovascular disease in patients with rheumatoid arthritis. A long-term follow-up study. *Mayo Clinic Proceedings* **53**, 581–6.

Longo, M.J. and Remetz, M.S. (1998). Cardiovascular manifestations of systemic autoimmune diseases. *Clinics in Chest Medicine* **19**, 793–808, x.

Manzi, S. and Wasko, M.C. (2000). Inflammation-mediated rheumatic diseases and atherosclerosis. *Annals of the Rheumatic Diseases* **59**, 321–5.

Manzi, S. et al. (1997). Age-specific incidence rates of myocardial infarction and angina in women with systemic lupus erythematosus: comparison with the Framingham Study. *American Journal of Epidemiology* **145**, 408–15.

Manzi, S. et al. (1999). Prevalence and risk factors of carotid plaque in women with systemic lupus erythematosus. *Arthritis and Rheumatism* **42**, 51–60.

Manzi, S. et al. (2000). Vascular imaging: changing the face of cardiovascular research. *Lupus* **9**, 176–82.

Martin, J.C., Harvey, J., and Dixey, J. (1996). Chest pain in patients with rheumatoid arthritis. *Annals of the Rheumatic Diseases* **55**, 152–3.

McRorie, E.R. et al. (1997). Rheumatoid constrictive pericarditis. *British Journal of Rheumatology* **36**, 100–3.

Moder, K.G., Miller, T.D., and Tazelaar, H.D. (1999). Cardiac involvement in systemic lupus erythematosus. *Mayo Clinic Proceedings* **74**, 275–84.

Morguet, A.J. et al. (1995). Indium-111-antimyosin Fab imaging to demonstrate myocardial involvement in systemic lupus erythematosus. *Journal of Nuclear Medicine* **36**, 1432–5.

Mutru, O. et al. (1989). Cardiovascular mortality in patients with rheumatoid arthritis. *Cardiology* **76**, 71–7.

Myllykangas-Luosujärvi, R. et al. (1995). Cardiovascular mortality in women with rheumatoid arthritis. *Journal of Rheumatology* **22**, 1065–7.

Newman, J.H. and Cooney, L.M., Jr. (1980). Cardiac abnormalities associated with rheumatoid arthritis: aortic insufficiency requiring valve replacement. *Journal of Rheumatology* **7**, 375–8.

Nomeir, A.M., Turner, R.A., and Watts, L.E. (1979). Cardiac involvement in rheumatoid arthritis. Followup study. *Arthritis and Rheumatism* **22**, 561–4.

Park, Y.B. et al. (1999). Lipid profiles in untreated patients with rheumatoid arthritis. *Journal of Rheumatology* **26**, 1701–4.

Pasceri, V. and Yeh, E.T. (1999). A tale of two diseases. Atherosclerosis and rheumatoid arthritis. *Circulation* **100**, 2124–6.

Perry, A. and Vuitch, F. (1995). Causes of death in patients with sarcoidosis. A morphologic study of 38 autopsies with clinicopathologic correlations. *Archives of Pathology and Laboratory Medicine* **119**, 167–72.

Petri, M. et al. (1996). Plasma homocysteine as a risk factor for atherothrombotic events in systemic lupus erythematosus. *Lancet* **348**, 1120–4.

Pouchot, J. et al. (1991). Adult Still's disease: manifestations, disease course, and outcome in 62 patients. *Medicine (Baltimore)* **70**, 118–36.

Reisner, S.A. et al. (2000). Echocardiography in nonbacterial thrombotic endocarditis: from autopsy to clinical entity. *Journal of the American Society of Echocardiography* **13**, 876–81.

Roditi, G.H., Hartnell, G.G., and Cohen, M.C. (2000). MRI changes in myocarditis—evaluation with spin echo, cine MR angiography and contrast enhanced spin echo imaging. *Clinical Radiology* **55**, 752–8.

Roldan, C.A. (1998a). Valvular disease associated with systemic illness. *Cardiology Clinics* **16**, 531–50.

Roldan, C.A. et al. (1998b). Aortic root disease and valve disease associated with ankylosing spondylitis. *Journal of the American College of Cardiology* **32**, 1397–404.

Roldan, C.A., Shively, B.K., and Crawford, M.H. (1996). An echocardiographic study of valvular heart disease associated with systemic lupus erythematosus. *New England Journal of Medicine* **335**, 1424–30.

Roman, M.J. et al. (2001). Prevalence and relation to risk factors of carotid atherosclerosis and left ventricular hypertrophy in systemic lupus erythematosus and antiphospholipid antibody syndrome. *American Journal of Cardiology* **87**, 663–6, A11.

Ross, R. (1999). Atherosclerosis—an inflammatory disease. *New England Journal of Medicine* **340**, 115–26.

Trujillo-Martin, E. et al. (2000). Plasma homocysteine levels in patients with rheumatoid arthritis treated with methotrexate: effect of folic acid supplementation. *Arthritis and Rheumatism* **43** (Suppl. 9), S342 (Abstract 1651).

Urowitz, M.B. et al. (1976). The bimodal mortality pattern of systemic lupus erythematosus. *American Journal of Medicine* **60**, 221–5.

Vaarala, O. (2000). Autoantibodies to modified LDLs and other phospholipid–protein complexes as markers of cardiovascular diseases. *Journal of Internal Medicine* **247**, 381–4.

Voskuyl, A.E. et al. (1996). The mortality of rheumatoid vasculitis compared with rheumatoid arthritis. *Arthritis and Rheumatism* **39**, 266–71.

Wallberg-Jonsson, S. et al. (1996). Lipoprotein lipase in relation to inflammatory activity in rheumatoid arthritis. *Journal of Internal Medicine* **240**, 373–80.

Wallberg-Jonsson, S., Ohman, M.L., and Dahlqvist, S.R. (1997). Cardiovascular morbidity and mortality in patients with seropositive rheumatoid arthritis in Northern Sweden. *Journal of Rheumatology* **24**, 445–51.

Ward, M.M., Pyun, E., and Studenski, S. (1995). Causes of death in systemic lupus erythematosus. Long-term followup of an inception cohort. *Arthritis and Rheumatism* **38**, 1492–9.

Watson, D.J. et al. (2001). Reduced risk of thromboembolic events with naproxen in rheumatoid arthritis patients in the UK general practice research database. *Arthritis and Rheumatism* **44** (Suppl. 9), S372 (Abstract 1918).

Westaby, S. (1995). Management of aortic dissection. *Current Opinion in Cardiology* **10**, 505–10.

Weyand, C.M. et al. (2001). T-cell immunity in acute coronary syndromes. *Mayo Clinic Proceedings* **76**, 1011–20.

Winslow, T.M. et al. (1993). The left ventricle in systemic lupus erythematosus: initial observations and a five-year follow-up in a university medical center population. *American Heart Journal* **125**, 1117–22.

Wislowska, M., Sypula, S., and Kowalik, I. (1998). Echocardiographic findings, 24-hour electrocardiographic Holter monitoring in patients with rheumatoid arthritis according to Steinbrocker's criteria, functional index, value of Waaler-Rose titre and duration of disease. *Clinical Rheumatology* **17**, 369–77.

Wolfe, F. et al. (1994). The mortality of rheumatoid arthritis. *Arthritis and Rheumatism* **37**, 481–94.

1.3.5 The respiratory system

Stephen G. Spiro and David A. Isenberg

Introduction

The lungs and the chest wall are commonly affected by several of the rheumatological conditions. The involvement may be a direct manifestation of disease or it may be indirect as a result or complication of treatment. This chapter will detail the common symptoms of pulmonary diseases and show how often these are implicated in rheumatological conditions. The role of radiography and physiological tests in the assessment of these conditions will then be described. Finally, there is advice on which investigations should be carried out, together with a discussion on the treatment of pulmonary infections related to rheumatological disorders. A synopsis of how these disorders can affect the different respiratory structures is given in Table 1.

Respiratory symptoms

Cough

Most rheumatological conditions that affect the lungs cause cough (Fig. 1). The airways can be involved in a variety of ways. It was once considered that asthma was more common in patients with rheumatoid arthritis, but there now seems no particular association except that of two relatively common conditions. Chronic bronchitis is likely to occur in patients who smoke.

Asthmatics will complain of waking during the night to cough, usually with a tight or wheezy chest. They will often be worse early in the morning and after exercise, exposure to cold air, pungent smells, and other chemical irritants. The diagnosis is seldom obscure and responds promptly to inhaled β_2-sympathomimetic agonists. In adults, asthma is associated more with cough and mucus (often yellow due to an increase in eosinophils) rather than wheezy breathlessness. The patient with chronic bronchitis will, by definition, have morning cough and sputum for three consecutive months for at least 2 years. He or she will be prone to acute exacerbations with infection, producing larger than usual quantities of yellow or green sputum, and needs antibiotics for control. Gradually deteriorating exercise tolerance will follow, especially if smoking does not cease.

Chronic bronchial sepsis (or bronchiectasis) with persistent cough and the production of more than 30 ml of purulent sputum a day is found in some patients with rheumatoid arthritis. There is an increased incidence of bronchiectasis in these patients and the typical radiographic features are usually confined to just one or two lobes. Occasionally, cough with purulent sputum is an immunological reaction to the underlying condition, usually rheumatoid arthritis, but also occurs with inflammatory bowel disease. In

Table 1 Respiratory associations of the rheumatic disorders

	Airways	Alveolae	Pulmonary vessels	Pleura	Chest wall/muscle
Rheumatoid arthritis	Bronchitis Bronchiectasis Obliterative bronchiolitis	Pneumonia Fibrosing alveolitis Alveolitis Nodules	Hypertension	Pleurisy Effusion Empyema	
Systemic lupus erythematosus		Pneumonia Fibrosing alveolitis Atelectasis	Hypertension	Pleurisy Effusion	Shrinking lungs with high diaphragms
Systemic sclerosis	Bronchiectasis	Fibrosing alveolitis Aspiration pneumonia	Hypertension		'Encased' chest
Sjögren's syndrome	Bronchitis	Fibrosing alveolitis Lymphoma			
Dermatomyositis		Aspiration pneumonia			Myopathy
Polymyocytis		Fibrosing alveolitis			
Ankylosing spondylitis		Upper lobe fibrosis			Costovertebral joint fixation
Behçet's syndrome		Haemorrhage	Aneurysm		
Pulmonary vasculitides		Nodules			
Relapsing polychondritis	Upper airway narrowing				

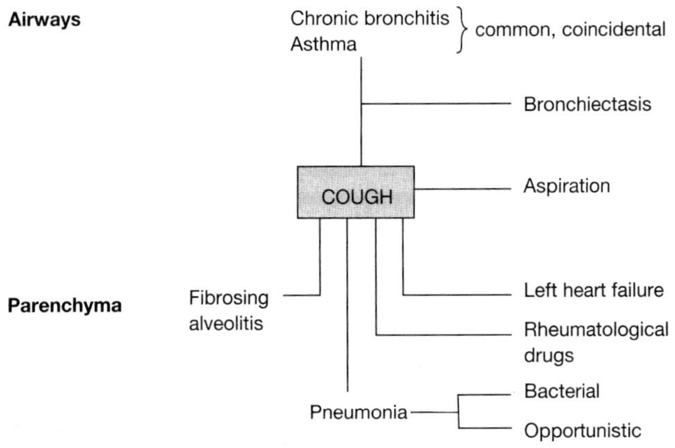

Fig. 1 The causes of cough.

these patients the symptoms respond dramatically to cortico-steroids and not just antibiotics.

The development of parenchymal disease is almost universally associated with a persistent, dry, irritating cough, worse with exercise.

Fibrosing alveolitis occurs in association with several of the rheumatic disorders including rheumatoid arthritis, systemic sclerosis, Sjögren's syndrome, and systemic lupus (Table 1). There are no clinical, physiological, radiological, or histopathological differences between 'lone' cryptogenic fibrosing alveolitis (with or without associated rheumatoid factor) and the alveolitis in patients with rheumatic diseases. The pathogenesis is uncertain—it is possible that the alveolitis develops as a reaction to immune complexes deposited in the pulmonary capillaries. Limitations on exercise imposed by the joint disease may explain why some of these patients present relatively late with their respiratory symptoms, although florid fibrosing alveolitis with positive rheumatoid factor can herald the onset of rheumatoid arthritis and precede the joint manifestations by months or years. Usually, however, it is the patients with more severe rheumatoid arthritis who develop pulmonary fibrosis. In addition to cough, other clinical features include finger clubbing in up to 70 per cent of patients, bilateral inspiratory basal crackles, and, late in the disease, cyanosis.

The physiological and radiological features of fibrosing alveolitis are described below. However, the symptoms of cough together with infiltrates on the chest radiograph may also indicate a drug-induced pneumonitis (e.g. gold, cyclophosphamide, methotrexate), pneumonia (common in patients with chronic diseases, especially if also on corticosteroid or other immunosuppressive therapy), left ventricular failure (more likely on steroids or some non-steroidal anti-inflammatory drugs; and in old age), and opportunistic infections associated with the primary autoimmune rheumatic disorder or the consequence of its therapy.

The treatment of cough can be difficult but is helped greatly if the cause is identified. Asthma responds promptly and well to inhaled steroids with additional β_2-agonists when necessary. Chronic bronchitis improves on stopping smoking, and most exacerbations respond rapidly to conventional oral antibiotics. The treatment of fibrosing alveolitis is unsatisfactory, although initially oral corticosteroids improve the cough, but may be withdrawn if lung function does not improve in order to prevent long-term steroid side-effects. Cough suppressants such as pholcodeine or codeine linctus in sufficiently large doses are a boon at night. In the most refractory cases, nebulized bupivacaine local anaesthetic solution (0.03 per cent) can be helpful for a few hours, but patients risk aspiration and must avoid eating when their larynx is anaesthetized.

Cough, especially in association with purulent secretions and radiographic pulmonary infiltrations, can be caused by aspiration of stomach and oesophageal contents in systemic sclerosis. The high incidence of oesophageal reflux, especially when the patient is supine, can cause major problems with pulmonary infection, particularly by anaerobic organisms.

Breathlessness

Breathlessness is a common feature of most pulmonary conditions and causes associated with connective tissue disorders can be listed (Fig. 2).

Airways

Asthma, chronic bronchitis, and bronchiectasis, if sufficiently severe, will result in breathlessness on exertion and in asthmatics at rest as well.

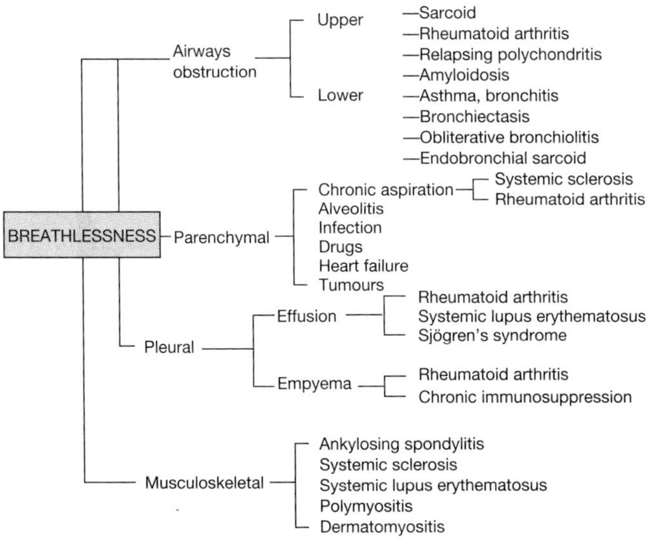

Fig. 2 The causes of breathlessness.

Upper airways obstruction will, because of its dominant effect on airways resistance, readily cause dyspnoea. Collapse of the cartilaginous support of the trachea and main bronchi in relapsing polychondritis can cause great difficulty with both inspiration and expiration and will be associated with loud, harsh wheezing, and dyspnoea. This rare syndrome is often also associated with a deep, bovine cough. Endobronchial sarcoidosis or laryngeal infiltration by sarcoid can result in severe upper airways obstruction and breathlessness, particularly on exertion. Minor degrees of upper airways obstruction have been reported in up to 18 per cent of autopsies in patients with rheumatoid arthritis. Synovitis of the cricoarytenoid joint may cause supraglottic narrowing and also hoarseness and breathlessness.

Obliterative bronchiolitis has been recognized more recently to complicate rheumatoid arthritis. It is rare and can be rapidly fatal, although in most, whilst the condition seems to be of sudden onset and rapidly progressive, it becomes stable leaving the patient to suffer severe exertional dyspnoea with grossly reduced lung function. Pathologically the small airways (less than 3 mm in diameter) are narrowed or obliterated by a chronic inflammatory process with fibrotic scar formation. Wheezing is not a symptom but on examination high-pitched, end-inspiratory, basal squeaks are often readily audible. The condition responds poorly to corticosteroid or other therapy.

Parenchymal disease

These complications include fibrosing alveolitis, pulmonary infections, aspiration, drug-induced pneumonitis, heart failure, and acute manifestations such as acute lupus pneumonia. The history and the radiographic appearances are sometimes helpful but often frustratingly non-specific. The history may be of more importance, for example, drug history, rate of onset of symptoms, and chest pain. Often a diagnosis is made only on lung biopsy (see below).

Sarcoidosis is often associated with widespread pulmonary infiltration, predominantly in the mid and upper zones. However, this is rarely accompanied by physical signs or breathlessness. Late progressive fibrotic changes in sarcoidosis cause shrinkage of the upper lobes with subsequent distortion of the lower lobes, and dyspnoea can develop.

Pleural disease

Pleural effusion

This is the most common respiratory sign in patients with rheumatoid arthritis. It is regarded generally as the only complication of rheumatoid arthritis to be more common in men. It is usually asymptomatic, although there can be pleuritic pain, dyspnoea, and fever. Although the effusions are usually small and unilateral, they can be large and bilateral. Large pleural effusions with dyspnoea are also occasionally seen in systemic lupus, although classically the effusions are small. It is more common in lupus to obtain a history of pleuritic chest pain and breathlessness with no visible effusion. Aspiration of an effusion is required usually to exclude infection or malignancy. The fluid is characteristically clear coloured, an exudate (protein greater than 30 g/l) with, in rheumatoid arthritis, a very low or unrecordable glucose concentration. The concentrations of lactate dehydrogenase and cholesterol are raised. Rheumatoid factor is detected frequently in the fluid. Pleural biopsy is rarely helpful, with non-specific features of chronic inflammation only. If the effusions fail to resolve, or relapse after drainage, oral corticosteroids may be rapidly effective. It is rare to have to resort to surgical pleurectomy.

Empyema

Empyema is relatively common in patients with rheumatoid arthritis. This usually is secondary to long periods of corticosteroid therapy, but is seen less often in other autoimmune rheumatic disorders that are similarly treated. Breathlessness is common, as is a fever with malaise and weight loss. The diagnosis is established on aspiration of turbid fluid containing pus cells. The fluid should be cultured for aerobic and anaerobic organisms as well as tuberculosis. The empyema should be treated intensively, with local drainage as well as systemic antibiotics. Rib resection should be done early to facilitate drainage if intercostal tube drainage is not effective. A decortication may be necessary when the infection has resolved as a thick residual pleural cortex can cause severe restriction of movement of the underlying lung. Ideally, surgical decortication should be done at least 6 weeks after the infection has resolved, thus allowing the underlying lung tissue to heal and making surgery easier and less traumatic.

Chest wall disease

Breathlessness can be caused by the patient's inability to ventilate the lungs adequately. Gross restriction of the chest wall can occur in advanced systemic sclerosis and in ankylosing spondylosis. In the presence of normal lung fields on a chest radiograph, musculoskeletal causes of dyspnoea are often overlooked and psychogenic reasons may have to be considered. However, clinical examination of the patient and appropriate lung function tests should leave the physician in little doubt as to the correct cause.

Weakness of the respiratory muscles is often insidious and difficult to detect unless there is obvious wasting of other muscle groups such as in the upper limb girdle. Again, lung function tests are extremely helpful but the physician should be alert to the possibility of muscle weakness. In systemic lupus, the contractile properties of the diaphragm are sometimes impaired, allowing it to keep its curved shape and resulting in lungs that look small radiographically on full inspiration. In polymyositis and dermatomyositis, the well-recognized proximal myopathy often extends to involve the respiratory muscles.

Rarer causes of dyspnoea

These include pulmonary haemorrhage in Behçet's syndrome, usually due to a leaking aneurysm of a pulmonary artery, or bleeding from a pulmonary infiltration subsequent to the pneumonitis occasionally seen in this condition.

Tumours can develop in some autoimmune rheumatic disorders, particularly rheumatoid arthritis and Sjögren's syndrome, and less frequently dermatomyositis. Lymphoma can develop as a result of long-term immunosuppressive therapy. For a detailed review see Rapti et al. (1998).

Radiological aspects

There is a plethora of pulmonary abnormalities providing a large differential diagnosis for radiographic shadowing in association with connective tissue diseases (Fig. 3). Some of these are detailed next.

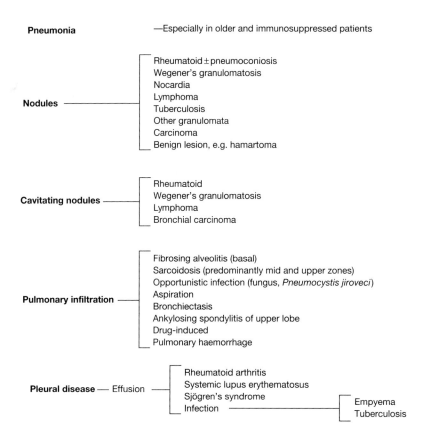

- **Pneumonia** —Especially in older and immunosuppressed patients
- **Nodules**
  - Rheumatoid ± pneumoconiosis
  - Wegener's granulomatosis
  - Nocardia
  - Lymphoma
  - Tuberculosis
  - Other granulomata
  - Carcinoma
  - Benign lesion, e.g. hamartoma
- **Cavitating nodules**
  - Rheumatoid
  - Wegener's granulomatosis
  - Lymphoma
  - Bronchial carcinoma
- **Pulmonary infiltration**
  - Fibrosing alveolitis (basal)
  - Sarcoidosis (predominantly mid and upper zones)
  - Opportunistic infection (fungus, *Pneumocystis jiroveci*)
  - Aspiration
  - Bronchiectasis
  - Ankylosing spondylitis of upper lobe
  - Drug-induced
  - Pulmonary haemorrhage
- **Pleural disease** — Effusion
  - Rheumatoid arthritis
  - Systemic lupus erythematosus
  - Sjögren's syndrome
  - Infection
    - Empyema
    - Tuberculosis

Fig. 3 The radiological abnormalities of rheumatic diseases.

Pulmonary nodules

Although the most common cause of a round lesion on the chest radiograph is a bronchial carcinoma and the next most common a benign lesion such as a hamartoma, there are several rheumatological causes or associations with pulmonary nodules.

In rheumatoid arthritis, nodules histologically identical to subcutaneous necrobiotic nodules can occur. They tend to be peripheral, and can increase in size, remain static, or disappear (Fig. 4). They can also cavitate and they can occasionally cause a pneumothorax. When single, the differential diagnosis will include another benign lesion, a bronchogenic carcinoma, tuberculosis, or another granuloma (Fig. 3). The diagnosis is often elusive, although occasionally fine-needle aspiration of the lesion yields granulation tissue suggestive of a necrobiotic nodule.

Caplan's syndrome occurs when simple coal-workers' pneumoconiosis, or another pneumoconiosis, is complicated by the development of rheumatoid nodules, which are visible on the chest radiograph. These often arise in crops and may sometimes enlarge rapidly.

Nodular shadowing can occur in Wegener's granulomatosis, often as the only abnormality associated with malaise, fever, and a high erythrocyte sedimentation rate. The antineutrophil cytoplasmic antibody test is usually positive. The nodules can enlarge rapidly, become multiple, and cavitate producing relatively large, thin-walled lesions (Fig. 5). Diagnosis by fibreoptic transbronchial lung biopsy is unusual as a moderately large artery is required to provide evidence of vasculitis. Open lung biopsy is usually necessary if tissue for diagnosis is required.

Nocardia, a variety of the Actinomycetaceae, can develop as an opportunistic infection in patients on prolonged immunosuppressive therapy. They form single or multiple nodules, which may cavitate. Usually extrapulmonary lesions soon develop, as, for example, in joints and the subcutaneous tissues.

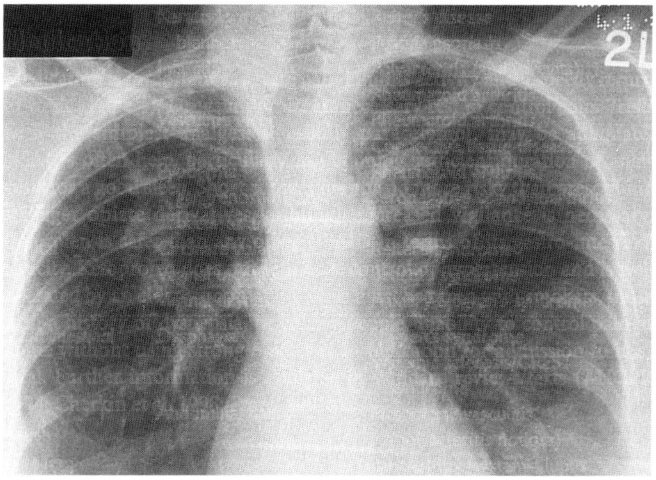

Fig. 4 Necrobiotic nodules with bilateral effusions (the right is subpulmonary) in a case of rheumatoid arthritis.

It is often impossible to distinguish a malignant from a benign nodule. This is particularly the case for pulmonary metastases, which are often spherical with smooth margins. If they are multiple and occur in a range of sizes, then malignant disease is probable.

The classical malignant primary tumour will have an irregular margin with 'sun ray' spicules radiating out into the surrounding parenchyma. The presence of flecks of calcium cannot guarantee benign disease. Computed tomography (CT) often identifies subpleural nodules invisible

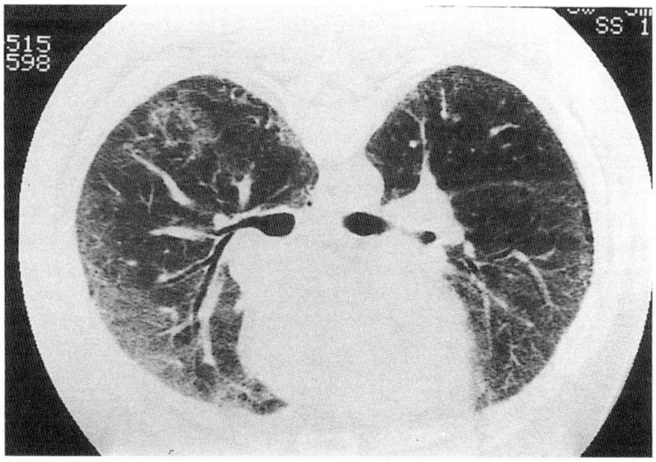

Fig. 5 Prone, high-resolution CT at the level of the carina. Diffuse parenchymal opacification in a subpleural distribution. This pattern is seen during the desquamative phase of fibrosing alveolitis.

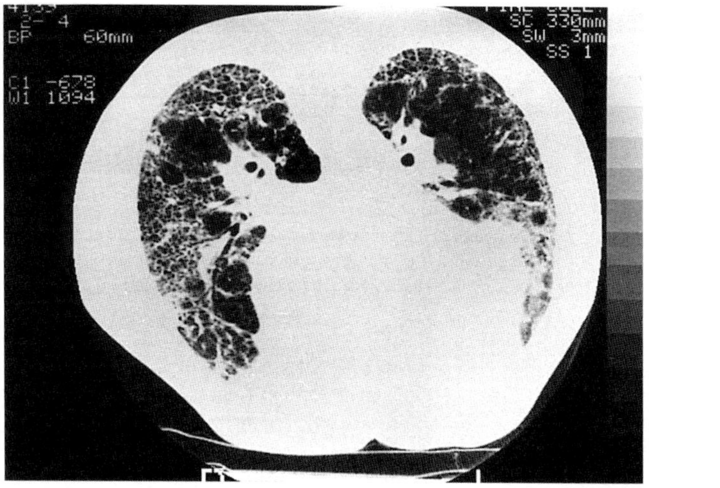

Fig. 6 Prone, high-resolution CT through the lower lobes. There is a reticular pattern in a subpleural distribution representing established fibrosis in a case of systemic sclerosis.

on routine chest radiographs. The likelihood of malignant origin will increase if the nodules are greater than 10 mm in diameter. Most subpleural nodules are granulomata, that is old tuberculosis or sarcoid, and in the United States may often be due to fungal disease such as histoplasmosis or coccidioidomycosis.

Hyperinflated lungs

These occur only in some cases of obliterative bronchiolitis, unless there is emphysema as an independent feature in a patient who also happens to have a connective tissue disorder. The lung fields in obliterative bronchiolitis are clear, with no other specific features. They are, however, often of normal size and appearance.

Small lungs

This appearance occurs in lupus; bilateral diaphragmatic weakness prevents the diaphragms from shortening and 'flattening' on inspiration, and both diaphragms remain elevated and deeply domed. There may be linear atelectatic shadows in the lower lobes, particularly above the diaphragm as a consequence of the basal hypoventilation. There is an apparent mediastinal widening in these patients but only as a consequence of the volume loss and not due to mediastinal disease.

Parenchymal shadowing

Diffuse, predominantly basal, reticulonodular shadowing, possibly with overall reduction in lung volume, is typical of fibrosing alveolitis. This occurs in association with rheumatoid arthritis, systemic lupus, systemic sclerosis, and Sjögren's syndrome. The appearances are non-specific and identical to those cases of lone fibrosing alveolitis. Interstitial lung disease in rheumatoid arthritis correlates with the severity of joint disease, ranging from an incidence of just 1 per cent in mild rheumatoid arthritis to a 30–40 per cent association in patients with severe joint deformity. The interstitial infiltrates are depicted radiographically as small, irregular shadows or opacities, predominantly at the lung bases. These shadows are also termed reticulonodular densities, ground-glass densities, or increased interstitial markings. Eventually, the infiltrates extend to the upper lung fields. They can occasionally respond remarkably well to treatment with corticosteroids. If the interstitial fibrosis progresses, it can develop areas of honeycombing comprising round or polygonal air cysts with well-defined walls and measuring less than 5 mm in diameter. The cysts may eventually become confluent, forming large destructive cavities in the subpleural regions. Rupture can cause pneumothorax.

High-resolution CT scanning provides an 'early warning' means of assessing the lungs. In a study of 17 patients with early scleroderma, it was shown that 15 (88 per cent) had a variety of abnormalities, especially subpleural cysts and honeycombing (Warrick et al. 1991). In contrast, the plain chest radiograph was abnormal in only 10 cases (59 per cent). Similarly changes consistent with rheumatoid-associated lung disease, notably interstitial fibrosis, were detected in patients with rheumatoid arthritis at a time when the chest radiograph was often normal (Fewins et al. 1991). This form of scanning also facilitates the precise distribution of alveolitis and the extent of any lung fibrosis and destruction (Figs 5 and 6).

Other causes of diffuse pulmonary infiltrates include:

(i) Sarcoidosis. The shadowing is usually more nodular and spares the lung bases. It is often associated with bilateral hilar lymphadenopathy, few symptoms, and commonly no decrease in lung size.

(ii) Infection. Opportunistic infection with fungi can also cause diffuse shadowing. However, the lesions are often more nodular and, although usually affecting more than one lobe, are often focal.

(iii) Polyarteritides. In polyarteritis nodosa a peripheral, soft, ill-defined, predominantly apical and/or mid-zone shadowing can develop, usually in association with an elevated peripheral eosinophil count. This 'pulmonary eosinophilia' can also be associated with pleural or pericardial effusions and is very responsive to corticosteroid therapy. It is similar to a hypersensitivity drug reaction within the lung such as occurs with gold salts (Fig. 7).

(iv) Upper lobe fibrosis is seen in ankylosing spondylosis, with contracture of the upper lobes and upward traction of the hilas. Eventually the upper lobes may cavitate. Apical pleural thickening may also develop and be extensive.

(v) Cavitation in the upper lobes, and to a lesser extent the mid-zones, amongst florid scarring is also seen in sarcoidosis. This progressive course of sarcoid usually develops after the bilateral hilar lymphadenopathy has regressed. In both sarcoidosis and ankylosing spondylosis the cavities can become colonized by *Aspergillus* spp. to form mycetomata. These semisolid masses appear to 'sit' in the cavity surrounded by a halo of air, a characteristic appearance. Serum aspergillal precipitins will be strongly positive.

(vi) Focal intrapulmonary shadowing can occur after aspiration of gastric contents. Classically, aspiration happens when the subject is lying prone and the inhaled contents run posteriorly to the posterior segment of

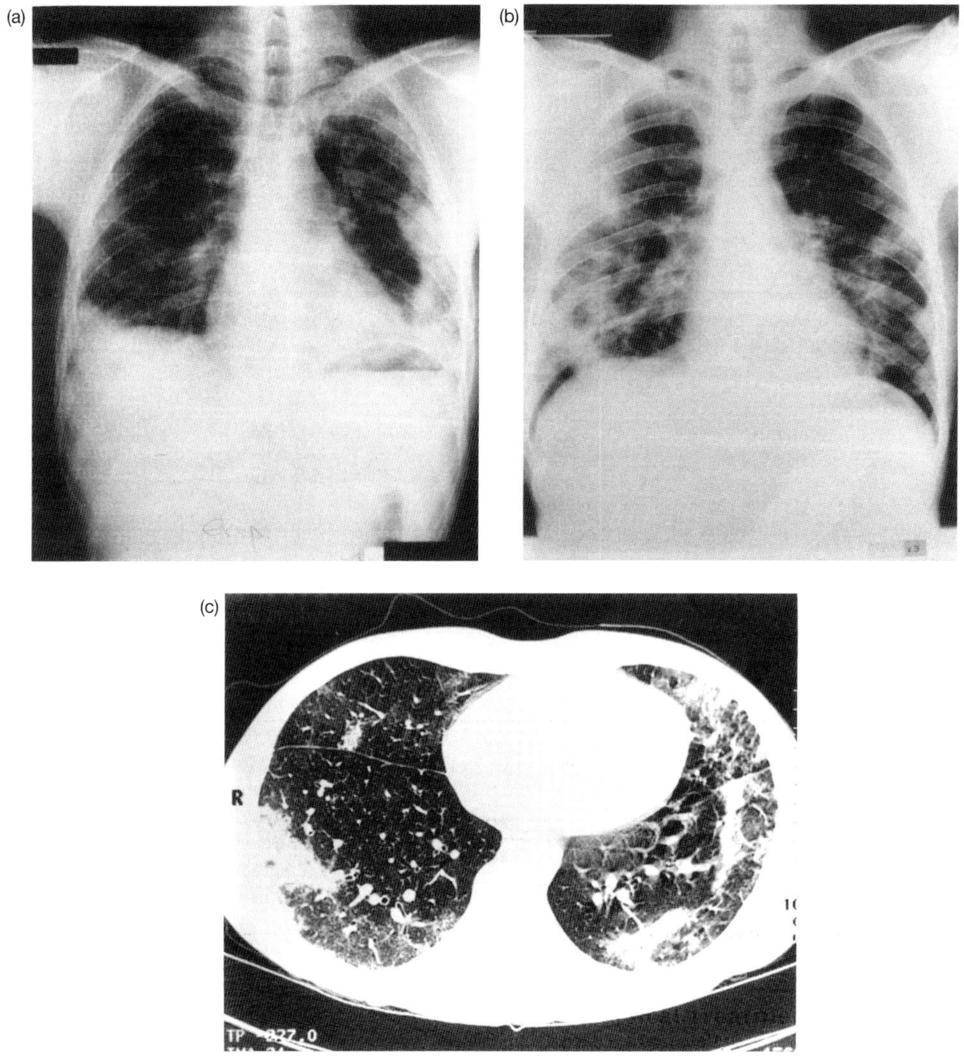

Fig. 7 Bilateral soft ill-defined peripheral shadowing typical of pulmonary eosinophilia. (a) Cleared with 7 days of oral steroids. (b) Recurrence 9 months later. (c) CT showing peripheral distribution of shadowing at both bases.

the upper lobes or apical segment of the lower lobes. Consolidation will be concurrent with the symptoms and signs of infection. Aspiration of anaerobic organisms is frequent and can cause pulmonary cavities. However, there can also be aspiration into basal segments, especially if it is associated with gross dysphagia as in advanced systemic sclerosis.

(vii) Bronchiectasis is recognized by peribronchial thickening causing 'tram-lines' on the chest radiograph due to a widened lumen and the thickened bronchial walls. Cystic changes can also be detected in cases where the damage is extensive. The lesions are patchy but usually confined to the middle and lower lobes.

Rare causes of pulmonary infiltrations will include acute exacerbations of lupus, a lymphoid tumour in, for example, Sjögren's syndrome, and intrapulmonary haemorrhage in a vascular disorder such as polyarteritis, Wegener's granulomatosis, or Behçet's syndrome.

Pleural disease

Pleural thickening is very unusual in autoimmune rheumatic disorders but pleural effusions are moderately common, especially in rheumatoid arthritis. They also occur in lupus and Sjögren's syndrome, and can reach considerable size.

Pulmonary function tests

Pulmonary function tests are not diagnostic but provide invaluable information as to the pattern and extent of an abnormality. They should be carried out early in any patient with pulmonary complications so that a baseline can be established and followed in order to evaluate the response to therapy, or assist in making decisions when to start therapy.

Spirometry

This is a simple test for almost any patient. It requires some co-operation for maximal inspiration and forced expiration until 'empty'.

The forced expiratory manoeuvre measures the forced expired volume in 1 s (FEV_1) and the forced vital capacity (FVC). The FEV_1/FVC ratio, expressed as a percentage, should be greater than 75 per cent, but falls with normal ageing to 65 per cent at 70 years. Figure 8 shows typical obstructive and restrictive patterns of spirometry. The obstructive pattern, with a proportionately greater decrease in FEV_1 than FVC, is found in all types of airflow obstruction. In pulmonary infiltrative conditions with or without fibrosis the FEV_1 is preserved relatively (although reduced) compared to the FVC. This results in an FEV_1/FVC ratio of greater than 80 per cent, but with reduced absolute values, the extent depending on the severity of the lesion.

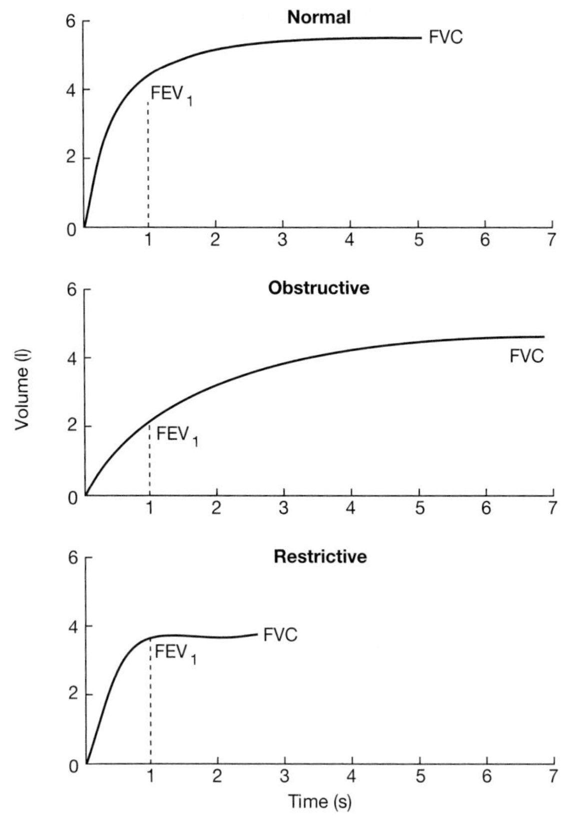

Fig. 8 Normal, obstructive, and restrictive patterns of spirometry.

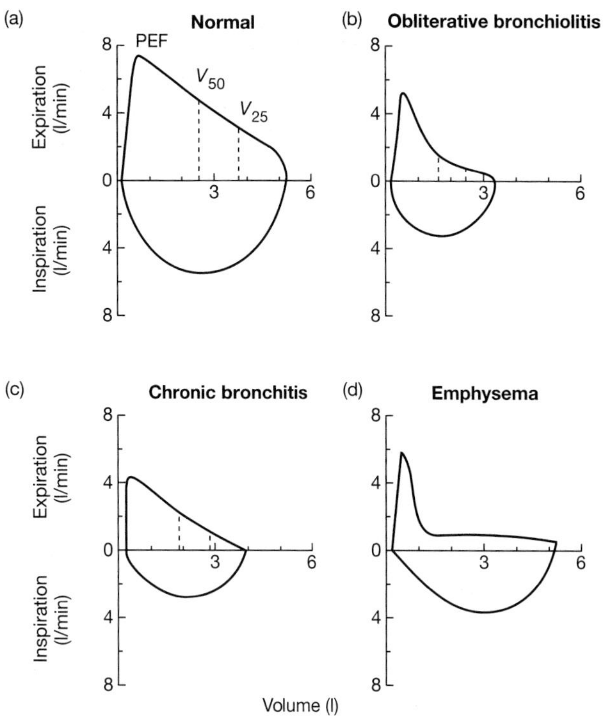

Fig. 9 A normal flow volume curve. During expiration flow reaches an immediate peak (peak expiratory flow) and gradually falls to zero at residual volume. Flow rates at 50 and 25 per cent of the vital capacity are shown. (b) Reduced flows and small vital capacity in obliterative bronchiolitis. (c) 'Volume-dependent' reduction in expiratory flows in chronic bronchitis. (d) 'Pressure-dependent' reduction in expiratory flow in emphysema.

In patients with stiff chest walls or weak muscles, the pattern of spirometry is also restrictive, with reduction in both FEV_1 and FVC. The FEV_1/FVC per cent is not always increased as the elastic recoil pressures within the lung remain normal in contrast to parenchymal diseases.

Peak expiratory flow (PEF)

This is the most commonly tested lung function and yet is not particularly sensitive. The PEF is the instantaneous flow rate during the first 10 msec of expiration after a maximum inspiration. It is a measure of airflow obstruction, dominated by flow from the upper airways. The PEF is of little value in restrictive pulmonary conditions as the airways are normal. However, where upper airways obstruction is suspected the PEF is reduced severely. An indication that there may be obstruction in the trachea, carina, or main bronchi can be deduced if the ratio of FEV_1 (ml) to the PEF (l/min) is greater than 10.

Flow volume curves

The envelope of expiratory flow from total lung capacity (TLC) to residual volume (RV) and then back in again to TLC can be simply captured as flow versus volume (Fig. 9). This provides a sensitive measure of peak flow and expiratory flow. Flows along subsections of the vital capacity—usually at 25 and 50 per cent above the residual volume ($V_{25} : V_{50}$) are measured and compared to age- and sex-matched normal values. These flow rates represent flow in the small airways and are reduced especially when generalized obstruction predominates. In rheumatological medicine a good example is found in obliterative bronchiolitis (Fig. 9) where flow at V_{50} and V_{25} is reduced especially compared to the FEV_1 and PEF when expressed as the percentage predicted. Pressure-dependent collapse (as in emphysema), that is decreased recoil causing collapse of major airways on forced expiration (Fig. 9), is especially prominent in relapsing polychondritis where the trachea collapses during expiration. Flow volume curves give little information in patients with parenchymal disease.

The flow volume loop is also particularly useful for detecting upper airways obstruction. The site of the lesion and whether it is fixed or variable will affect the shape of the flow volume loop.

Total respiratory pressures

Classically patients with weakness of the respiratory muscles will show reduced spirometric and PEF values. However, this is not diagnostic as it fails to differentiate between muscle weakness and reduced lung volumes secondary to parenchymal disease. The strength of the respiratory muscles is best and simply measured by the maximum inspiratory and expiratory mouth pressures.

If pure diaphragmatic weakness or paralysis is suspected, then spirometry done with the patient first lying and then standing can be most useful. A drop in vital capacity by up to 40 per cent can occur when lying flat if the diaphragm is non-functioning. This is due to the abdominal contents moving towards the chest unopposed when the patient lies flat. This is a remarkably reproducible test.

Thoracic lung volumes

Measurement of TLC and RV in patients with restrictive lung disease is very important before treatment and should be closely followed during therapy. Lung volumes can be measured either by the wash-out (or wash-in) method of using an inert gas as by body plethysmography. In restrictive conditions both RV and TLC will be reduced. However, in patients with muscle weakness, RV may be reduced but TLC can be reasonably normal.

Diffusing capacity

The magnitude of carbon monoxide gas transfer (*TL*CO) depends on the volume of the pulmonary capillary bed and the matching between the distribution of ventilation and perfusion within the lungs. The test is done with the subject inspiring a known concentration of carbon monoxide and of an inert gas, helium. As the helium is not absorbed, the change in its concentration in the expired sample will provide a measure of the volume of alveolar gas into which the gas mixture was inspired (alveolar volume, V_A). If the quality of uptake of carbon monoxide per unit of lung is desired, then dividing the *TL*CO by the V_A will provide the carbon monoxide transfer coefficient (*K*CO), a quantitative assessment of the efficacy of uptake by the lung and alveolar capillaries of carbon monoxide per litre of lung volume.

The *TL*CO is reduced when:

(i) The alveolar capillaries are reduced in number, for example, in emphysema, pulmonary fibrosis, pulmonary embolic disease, and pulmonary hypertension.

(ii) There is an increased ventilation/perfusion mismatch as occurs in pneumonia, infection, and infiltrates, and sometimes in pulmonary oedema.

(iii) There is a reduction in haemoglobin content in the blood.

(iv) The patient is a heavy smoker with high levels of carboxyhaemoglobin.

The *TL*CO is increased when:

(i) There is a redistribution of ventilation/perfusion ratios enabling more capillary blood to come into contact with inspired gas as sometimes happens in asthma.

(ii) There is alveolar haemorrhage increasing the amount of haemoglobin available to carbon monoxide in the alveoli.

(iii) Polycythaemia increases the level of available haemoglobin in the capillaries.

Walking tests

Assessment of the functional ability of an individual in a manner that uses a normal, habitual activity is very useful. In patients with joint disease, formal treadmill or cycle ergometric exercise testing is often not possible. However, a walking test may be feasible. The subject is asked to walk up and down a corridor of known length or other suitable enclosed space for 2, 6, or 12 min watched by a technician who measures the distance walked and uses standard terms of encouragement at regular intervals. After a practice walk, a second walk distance is recorded. This is often up to 30 per cent longer than the initial distance walked, as the patient develops confidence in the test and his or her ability. Extra information can be obtained, for example, by attaching a portable pulse oximeter to the finger or ear to measure oxygen saturation during the walk. The test is highly reproducible after the test practice walk.

Differences in pulmonary function in the context of rheumatological diseases are summarized in Fig. 10. As indicated earlier, serial performance of these tests provides a useful way of assessing response to therapy. Thus, Akesson and colleagues demonstrated that cyclophosphamides increased vital capacity and static lung compliance in 18 patients with scleroderma who had lung disease (Akesson et al. 1994).

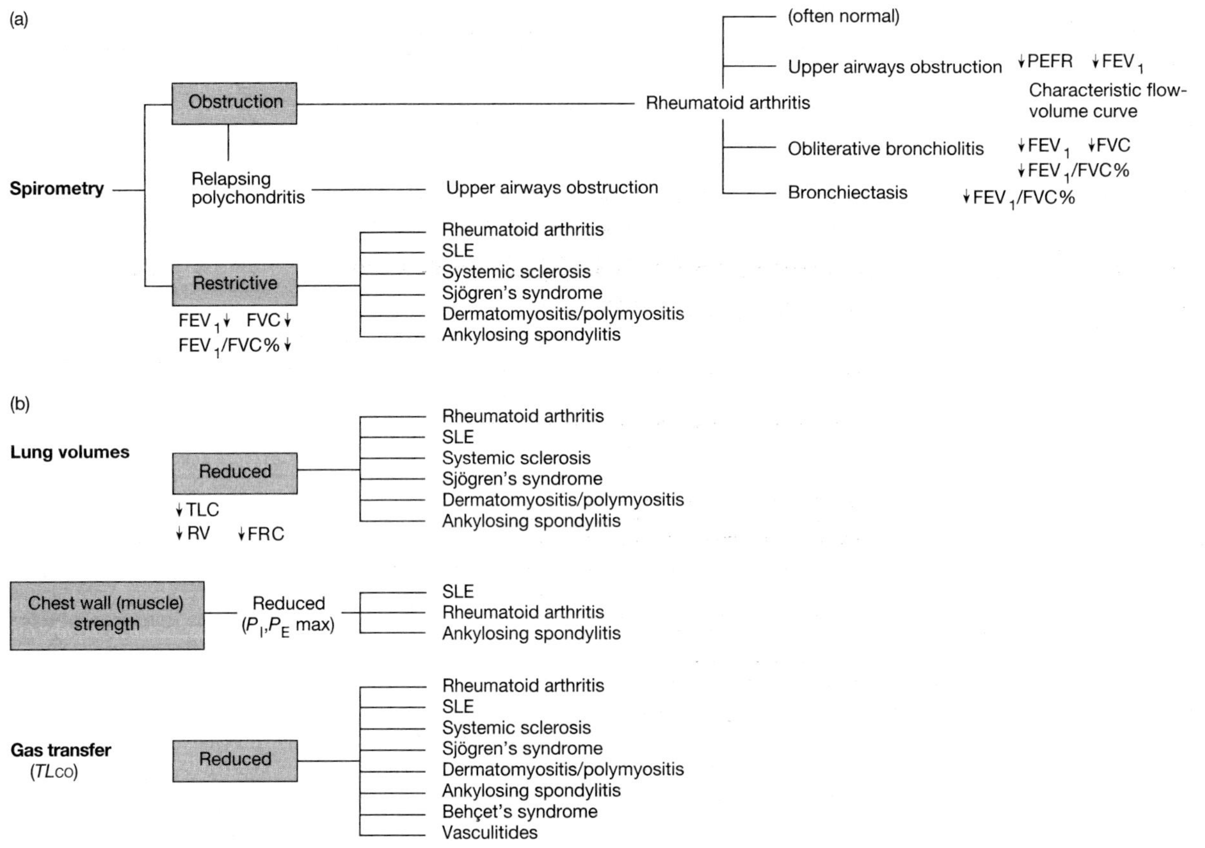

Fig. 10 A summary of pulmonary function in rheumatological diseases. PEFR, peak expiratory flow rate; FEV_1, forced expiratory volume in 1 s; FVC, forced vital capacity; TLC, total lung capacity; RV, residual volume; FRC, functional residual capacity; P_1 max, maximal inspiratory mouth pressure; P_E max, maximal expiratory mouth pressure.

Bronchoscopy, lavage, biopsy, and other diagnostic tests

Lung biopsy

Open lung biopsy remains the best method for providing tissue for histopathological diagnosis of chronic infiltrative lung diseases, and a review of several series gave a diagnosis in 94 per cent of cases (Gaensler and Carrington 1980). However, this procedure is not routinely performed, particularly when the association between the joint disease and the presence of pulmonary infiltration is both typical and as expected. The ultimate answer will be the response to any attempted therapy. A survey in the United Kingdom reviewed the case notes of 200 patients with cryptogenic fibrosing alveolitis, of whom 119 cases had only a clinical diagnosis—based on typical physical signs. Only 15 patients underwent an open lung biopsy, 35 bronchoalveolar lavage, and 66 transbronchial biopsy (Johnson et al. 1993). More recent studies, mainly in patients with cryptogenic fibrosing alveolitis, have again raised doubts as to the value of histological specimens from open lung biopsy providing an accurate guide to prognosis and response to therapy (Nicholson et al. 2000).

If open lung biopsy is done, it is usually through a minithoracotomy and by video-assisted thoracotomy (VATS) and at least two areas of lung are sampled. In general, the right middle lobe and the lingula are avoided as it is claimed by some that fibrosis occurs more readily in these areas. Similarly, there is little value in removing a piece of grossly fibrotic lung as it will be histologically less helpful. A moderately involved and an apparently uninvolved piece of lung should be sampled. In general, open lung biopsy is a safe procedure and has very little deleterious effect on lung function whether carried out by an open or VATS procedure (Daniil et al. 2000). The alternative to open lung biopsy is a transbronchial lung biopsy via the fibreoptic bronchoscope. While this is usually simple, with few complications (e.g. pneumothorax), the biopsies suffer from being very small and probably are not representative of a diffuse, chronic process. Four to six biopsies are recommended, all from one lung to avoid the risk of bilateral pneumothoraces, but from more than one segment whenever possible. Non-specific reactions and non-diagnostic microscopic appearances may be misleading (Wall et al. 1981).

Computed tomography

In patients who present with interstitial infiltration together with an obvious autoimmune rheumatic disease, the need to obtain pulmonary histology is less urgent or potentially helpful. High-resolution CT has been shown to be a good predictor of lung histology in systemic sclerosis, and can discriminate between fibrotic and inflammatory histology (Wells et al. 1992). Furthermore, high resolution CT in patients with systemic sclerosis can identify different patterns of the disease; that is ground-glass pattern, mixed, or predominantly reticular patterns—the latter being the most abnormal. These patterns correlate strongly with lung function, especially gas transfer (TL_{CO}). Responses to therapy were seen most commonly in patients with a ground-glass appearance on high resolution CT, and least in those with a reticular CT appearance (Wells et al. 1993b).

Another potentially useful predictor of prognosis is the rate of clearance of technetium labelled diethylene-triamine-pentacetae (99mTc-DTPA) from the lung. Those patients with interstitial lung disease who had normal clearances had stable disease, whilst those with rapid clearances had deteriorating disease. There was no association between rates of clearance and the likelihood of responding to corticosteroid treatment (Wells et al. 1993a), and this was not influenced by any association of the fibrosing alveolitis with an autoimmune rheumatic disease.

Bronchoalveolar lavage

Lavage allows examination of the cellular and non-cellular elements present on the epithelial surface of the alveolar space. It does not truly sample the lung parenchyma; however, in some studies there has been good correlation between the type and the number of inflammatory cells obtained by lavage and those obtained by diagnostic lung biopsy (Reynolds 1987).

The technique does, however, have serious shortcomings both in its diagnostic value and as a tool for following disease activity. There is no satisfactory consensus on what constitutes a 'routine' analysis of fluid from bronchoalveolar lavage. Total and differential cell counts, frequently with identification of T-lymphocyte subsets by monoclonal antibody techniques, are usually made. Fluid from a non-smoker normally contains 85–90 per cent macrophages, 7–12 per cent lymphocytes, and 0.1 per cent neutrophils (Reynolds 1987). Patients may be classified as having a neutrophil alveolitis or a lymphocyte alveolitis based on an increase in the percentage of neutrophils or lymphocytes. A neutrophil alveolitis is often seen in cryptogenic fibrosing alveolitis, histiocytosis X, and in smokers; a lymphocytic alveolitis is commonly seen in sarcoidosis, hypersensitivity alveolitis, and granulomatous infections. However, there is marked overlap.

The value of bronchoalveolar lavage in the serial follow-up of lesions is not yet established with confidence. However, a study that included a subgroup of patients with rheumatoid arthritis associated with fibrosing alveolitis showed a link between a response to steroids and a decrease in neutrophils in the lavage (Turner-Warwick and Haslam 1987).

In patients suspected of pulmonary infections, especially by opportunistic organisms, bronchoalveolar lavage has a distinct role. On failing to make a diagnosis from sputum, or in the absence of sputum, a lavage via fibreoptic bronchoscopy in patients with pulmonary infiltrates can reveal fungi, *Pneumocystis carinii*, cytomegalovirus, Nocardia, tuberculosis, and other bacteria.

In patients suspected of drug-induced pulmonary shadowing, bronchoalveolar lavage may have a role but often the cell counts are non-specific. Data are too scanty to confirm the use of lavage as a diagnostic tool for drug-induced pathology.

Transbronchial lung biopsy also can provide findings suggestive of drug eruptions—with type I pneumonocyte desquamation and type II cell dysplasia. Hypersensitivity reactions may produce granulomas, interstitial eosinophilic infiltration, or granulation tissue as seen in some drug-induced organizing pneumonias.

Vascular studies

With the identification in the mid-1980s of clinical syndromes associated with the presence of antiphospholipid antibodies, much interest has focused on clotting abnormalities in the lungs of patients with underlying rheumatic disease. The widespread availability of ventilation/perfusion ratio (V/Q) scanning, CT and magnetic resonance imaging scans, and the more specialized pulmonary angiograms and digital subtraction angiography have greatly facilitated the ability to demonstrate the presence of pulmonary emboli and infarction. The association of antiphospholipid antibodies with deep venous thrombosis and thromboembolic pulmonary hypertension seems to be better documented in patients with the primary antiphospholipid antibody syndrome (Asherson et al. 1989) than in patients with systemic lupus erythematosus (Gulko et al. 1993).

Although much less common, pulmonary arterial aneurysms have been demonstrated in approximately 1 per cent of patients with Behçet's syndrome (Hamuryudan et al. 1994). Haemoptysis is the usual presenting symptom and the prognosis is often poor.

Pulmonary infections (Table 2)

The rheumatological conditions have a considerable association with pulmonary infection, probably because they induce host-defence defects within the immune system. In systemic lupus, many aspects of the immune system have been reported to be abnormal. These include the antibacterial activity of the alveolar macrophages, defects in the Fc receptor function of the macrophages, and diminished clearance of immune complexes by macrophages.

Table 2 Pulmonary infections in rheumatology

Bacteria
Gram-negative bacilli
Klebsiella pneumoniae
Escherichia coli
Pseudomonas aeruginosa
Gram-positive bacteria
Streptococcus pneumoniae
Staphylococcus aureus
Haemophilus influenzae
Legionella pneumophilia
Fungi
Aspergillus
fumigatus
flavus
niger
Phycomycetes
Histoplasma capsulatum
Coccidioides immitis
Cryptococcus neoformans
Nocardia asteroides
Tuberculosis
M. tuberculosis
M. kansasii
M. avium-intracellulare
M. xenopii
Pneumocystis jiroveci
Viruses
Cytomegalovirus
Herpes simplex
Herpes varicella-zoster

Defects have also been described in the chemotactic and phagocytic activity of both polymorphonuclear neutrophils and blood monocytes. Lymphopaenia is common, and T-lymphocytes, especially T-suppressors, are decreased.

Patients with rheumatoid arthritis have a predisposition to pleuropulmonary infection. A twofold rise in pneumonia was found when patients with rheumatoid arthritis were compared to those with degenerative joint disease; deaths due to respiratory infection were four times more frequent than expected.

The drugs used to treat rheumatic diseases also adversely affect the host defence system; the complex and many effects of glucocorticoids have been described by Cupps and Fauci (1982). Cyclophosphamide affects virtually all components of the cellular and humoral immune response. The drug acts primarily during the S phase of the cell cycle and so all rapidly dividing cells are involved. B-lymphocyte depletion occurs early and antibody production can also be inhibited. Azathioprine also inhibits both humoral and cell-mediated immunity, and suppresses the numbers of both T- and B-lymphocytes. Methotrexate is a folic acid antagonist that interferes with transport of carbon fragments required for thymidine synthesis; DNA synthesis and cellular proliferation are inhibited.

Specific infections

Bacteria

Gram-negative bacteria (*Klebsiella pneumoniae, Escherichia coli*, and *Pseudomonas aeruginosa*) are frequent causes of pneumonias in patients with autoimmune rheumatic disorders. The high frequency of these infections is probably related to the ease with which Gram-negative bacteria colonize the upper respiratory tract in patients with serious or debilitating conditions.

As far as Gram-positive bacteria are concerned, the incidence of pneumococcal infections in this group of patients is probably no higher than in the general population. *Staphylococcus aureus* is a common cause of death in patients with systemic lupus (Hellman et al. 1987).

Infection with *Legionella* spp. is more frequent than normal in immunocompromised patients and those on immunosuppressive medication; 95 per cent will be caused by *Legionella pneumophilia*, and occasional cases by *L. micdadei*. The radiographic features of Legionella pneumonia will usually be indistinguishable from those of the other bacterial pneumonias. However, confusion, prostration, hyponatraemia, and disturbance of liver function are more common. Standard bacterial cultures will be unhelpful but cultures in specific media may provide a diagnosis within 2–7 days. Indirect immunofluorescence antibody techniques are positive in 70–90 per cent of cases at 10 days.

Fungal infections

Aspergillus

Aspergillus causes two types of infection in patients with autoimmune connective diseases. *Aspergillus* spp. frequently colonize cavities in patients with chronic fibrotic lung disease. In the autoimmune rheumatic diseases, these include sufferers from type III sarcoidosis and, occasionally, patients with upper lobe fibrosis secondary to ankylosing spondylosis. Usually, the mycetoma remains asymptomatic but it can cause large haemoptyses. Should haemoptyses develop, resection will be difficult because of the surrounding fibrosis and scarring, with extensive adhesion to the chest wall, and the probability of poor overall lung function. Embolization of bronchial arteries by selective angiography is the treatment of choice and is successful in approximately half of cases.

Invasive aspergillosis is a much more lethal condition. Patients prone to this complication are those with severe defects in both cellular immunity and granulocyte neutrophil count and function. Other factors include cytotoxic or corticosteroid therapy, recent broad-spectrum antibiotic therapy, and severe neutropaenia. Over 90 per cent of cases occur in association with the treatment of haematological malignancies or with organ transplantation. The most common initial finding is fever, usually with a patchy bronchopneumonia on the chest radiograph. However, the radiograph can also show nodular infiltration, lobar consolidation, cavitating lesions, or a diffuse miliary or interstitial pattern. Progressive parenchymal necrosis due to invasion of blood vessels by the fungus can cause cavitation with rapid colonization by a mycetoma. The propensity to invade vessels predisposes to death from massive haemoptysis.

The diagnosis of invasive aspergillosis is difficult. Bronchoscopy with lavage is seldom helpful but transbronchial biopsy will produce fungal hyphae in 40–70 per cent of cases. The mortality is in excess of 80 per cent, but starting treatment early and restoring the immune function may improve survival. Amphotericin B is the mainstay of therapy and the addition of 5-fluorocytosine is probably helpful. The renal toxicity of amphotericin is a serious potential problem, particularly if there is underlying renal disease. Liposomal amphotericin B with higher local deposition and activity is valuable in patients not tolerant of the conventional drug.

Phycomycetes

These non-septate fungi cause infection much less commonly than aspergillus. They also have a propensity to infect the lung and the central nervous system, and invade the vasculature. The diagnosis is usually by transbronchial lung biopsy. Untreated the mortality rate is nearly 100 per cent. Amphotericin B is the recommended treatment.

Cryptococcus neoformans

This organism usually invades the central nervous system but pulmonary involvement can arise, either in conjunction with infection of the central nervous system or in isolation (Kerkering et al. 1981). In up to a quarter of cases there may be no symptoms, only the incidental findings on a chest radiograph. A nodular lesion (single or multiple) is common but alveolar infiltrates are also often found. Sputum culture is positive in up to one-third of cases of cryptococcal pneumonia. Transbronchial lung biopsy is positive in up to half of cases presenting with infiltration, but nodular lesions usually require open lung biopsy for diagnosis.

(Histoplasmosis and coccidiomycosis also occur in endemic areas but are rare.)

Nocardia asteroides

Nocardiosis can complicate autoimmune rheumatic disease, particularly lupus. Prompt diagnosis is critical as the infection disseminates rapidly to cause death. Early treatment can cure up to 80 per cent of cases. Pulmonary involvement usually predominates, with an abnormal chest radiograph in 70 per cent of cases. Multiple nodular densities with or without cavitation are characteristic. A percutaneous fine-needle aspiration biopsy is diagnostic in up to 80 per cent of cases. Treatment with trimethoprim–sulfamethoxazole is highly effective.

Mycobacterial infections

Both typical and atypical mycobacterial infections occur in patients with autoimmune rheumatic disorders. The clinical features are often nonspecific and pulmonary infiltration common, usually lacking the classical cavitating appearance found in the non-immunosuppressed. A high degree of suspicion is required. Sputum smears are the investigation of choice but, if negative, alveolar lavage can provide a diagnosis in up to 80 per cent of cases (Stover et al. 1984). *Mycobacterium tuberculosis* is sensitive to standard antituberculous therapy—rifampicin, isoniazid, and pyrazinamide—with the prospect of cure in more than 80 per cent. The cure rates for atypical mycobacteria infection are always considerably lower.

Pneumocystis jiroveci

Although the prevalence of *P. jiroveci* pneumonia has increased dramatically in some populations over the last few years, it is still an unusual opportunistic pathogen in patients with autoimmune rheumatic disorders. Nevertheless, one should be aware of the small possibility of it arising and a bronchoalveolar lavage will almost invariably provide a positive diagnosis if the organism is present. Therapy comprises 2 weeks of intravenous trimethoprim, 20 mg/kg per day, with sulfamethoxazole, 100 mg/kg per day, followed by a week of conventional oral trimethoprim and sulfamethoxazole therapy. If trimethoprim and sulfamethoxazole therapy is not possible, then pentamidine isoethionate, 4 mg/kg per day intravenously for 3 weeks, is effective.

Viral infections

Infections with cytomegalovirus, herpes simplex, and herpes varicella zoster are more of a problem in patients with severe and sustained defects in cellular immunity, that is, after organ transplantation, in human immunodeficiency virus-positive patients, and in sufferers from haematological malignancies. Nevertheless, these infections occasionally occur in people with connective tissue disorders, especially if taking immunosuppressive therapy.

Drug-induced pulmonary reactions

The disorders caused by the drugs used in autoimmune rheumatic disorders can be grouped as shown in Table 3. The range of such disorders is clearly wide and they mimic pulmonary reactions to the diseases themselves or other causes of pulmonary damage. There is very little that is helpful in the clinical manifestations, laboratory findings, or radiographic appearances specifically to suggest a drug-induced problem. Several patterns of radiographic abnormality occur, including increased interstitial markings, reticulonodular patterns, and alveolar infiltrates, often bilateral and most common in the lower lung fields.

Pulmonary function tests tend to show a restrictive defect with a reduced *T*Lco unless the drug causes a problem that purely affects the airways. Lung biopsy may demonstrate characteristic changes and exclude infection. Interstitial and alveolar inflammation is characterized by mononuclear cell infiltrates. Epithelial abnormalities include proliferation of both type I and type II pneumonocytes, with some dysplastic changes. In those with an acute hypersensitivity reaction, bronchiolitis, giant cells, granuloma formation, and an eosinophil infiltration may develop.

The precise prevalence of clinical manifestations that complicate drug therapy is not established. However, some associations are particularly well founded. For example, Chakravarty and Webley (1992) reported that

Table 3 Clinical manifestations of drug-induced pulmonary disease

Drug	Common usage	Pneumonitis	Pulmonary complications		Bronchiolitis obliterans	Non-cardiogenic pulmonary oedema	Pulmonary/renal syndrome
			Fibrosis	Bronchospasm			
NSAIDs/salicylates	Virtually any form of arthritis	−	−	+	−	+	−
Sulfasalazine	Rheumatoid arthritis, psoriatic arthritis	+	+	−	+	−	−
Colchicine	Gout	−	−	−	−	+	−
Gold	Rheumatoid arthritis	+	−	−	+	−	−
D-penicillamine	Rheumatoid arthritis	+	−	−	+	−	+
Methotrexate	Rheumatoid arthritis, psoriatic arthritis	+	+	−	−	+	−
Cyclophosphamide	Vasculitis, renal and central nervous system lupus, Wegener's granulomatosis	+	+	−	−	+	−
Chlorambucil	Rheumatoid arthritis, amyloid	+	+	−	−	−	−
Azathioprine	Rheumatoid arthritis, systemic lupus erythematosus	+	+	−	−	−	−

46 per cent of patients treated with gold and 21 per cent treated with D-penicillamine developed a restrictive defect within 2 years of the onset of therapy. The chest radiographs often shows dense reticulonodular infiltrates, often basal, and occasionally with pleural fluid. Other features of gold toxicity may be evident elsewhere. Treatment is a combination of stopping therapy and adding corticosteroids and gives excellent results (Israel-Biet et al. 1991).

Methotrexate may cause pneumonitis. This complication has been estimated to occur in 7 per cent of patients receiving methotrexate for either neoplastic or non-neoplastic disorders (Cooper et al. 1986). In a case–control study, however, no overt risk factors for the development of pneumonitis could be identified (Carroll et al. 1994). Even standard-dose regimens of methotrexate (<20 mg/week) can cause toxicity. Presentation of this complication is non-specific with cough, dyspnoea, and pulmonary crackles. Response is usual if the methotrexate is discontinued and high-dose steroids started. The steroids can be withdrawn once maximal improvement is achieved (Hargreaves et al. 1992; Imokawa et al. 2000).

Care should be taken if patients develop bronchospasm in relation to salicylates or non-steroidal anti-inflammatory drugs. These episodes usually arise early in treatment with these drugs and can even be seen after a single dose. The episodes can rapidly worsen and death may occur if the drug is continued.

Important points to remember

(i) Rheumatoid diseases are associated predominantly with parenchymal infiltration, but airway, pleural, and musculoskeletal involvement are well recognized.

(ii) Breathlessness may be due to upper airways obstruction or weak muscles or an immobile chest wall. A normal chest radiograph does not eliminate a respiratory cause of dyspnoea.

(iii) High-resolution CT provides clinical patterns of distribution of changes due to fibrosing alveolitis. The grading of those changes correlate to histological appearances and prognosis.

(iv) Lung function tests should include measurement of gas transfer, assessment of upper airway function (flow volume curves) and, where indicated, measurement of total respiratory inspiratory and expiratory mouth pressures.

(v) Open lung biopsy rarely provides information that is not intuitive from high-resolution CT and lung function tests. It is more important where a non-associated cause is suspected, for example, infection.

(vi) Drugs used by rheumatologists can cause pulmonary disease.

(vii) Infection is relatively common and a diagnosis should be sought, even if invasive tests are necessary.

References

Akesson, A., Scheja, A., Ludin, A., and Wollheim, F.A. (1994). Improved pulmonary function in systemic sclerosis after treatment with cyclophosphamide. *Arthritis and Rheumatism* **37**, 729–35.

Asherson, R.A. et al. (1989). The 'primary' antiphospholipid syndrome: major clinical and serological features. *Medicine* **68**, 366–74.

Carroll, G.J., Thomas, R., Phatouros, C.C., Atchison, M.H., Leslie, A.L., Cook, N.J., and D'Souza, I. (1994). Incidence, prevalence and possible risk factors for pneumonitis in patients with rheumatoid arthritis receiving methotrexate. *Journal of Rheumatology* **21**, 51–4.

Chakravarty, K. and Webley, M.A. (1992). A longitudinal study of pulmonary function in patients with rheumatoid arthritis treated with gold and D-pencillamine. *British Journal of Rheumatology* **31**, 829–33.

Cooper, J.D., White, D.A., and Matthey, R.A. (1986). Drug-induced pulmonary disease. *American Review of Respiratory Diseases* **133**, 321–40.

Cupps, T.R. and Fauci, A.S. (1982). Corticosteroid-mediated immunoregulation in man. *Immunology Review* **65**, 133–55.

Daniil, Z., Gichrist, F.C., Marciniak, S.J., Pantelidis, P., Goldstraw, P., Pastorino, U., and Du Bois, R.M. (2000). The effect of lung biopsy on lung function in diffuse lung disease. *European Respiratory Journal* **16**, 67–73.

Fewins, H.E., McGowan, I., Whitehouse, G.H., Williams, J., and Mallyar, R. (1991). High definition computed tomography in rheumatoid arthritis associated pulmonary disease. *British Journal of Rheumatology* **30**, 214–16.

Gaensler, E.A. and Carrington, C.B. (1980). Open biopsy for chronic diffuse infiltrative lung disease: clinical, roentgenographic and physiologic correlations in 502 patients. *Annals of Thoracic Surgery* **30**, 411–26.

Gulko, P.S., Reville, J.D., Koopman, W., Burgurd, S.L., Bartolucci, A.A., and Alarcon Segovia, G.S. (1993). Anticardiolipin antibodies in systemic lupus erythematosus: clinical correlates, HLA associations and impact on survival. *Journal of Rheumatology* **20**, 1684–93.

Hamuryudan, V., Yurkakul, S., Moral, F., Numan, F., Tüzün, H., Tüzüner, N., Mat, C., Tüzün, Y., Özyazgan, Y., and Yazici, H. (1994). Pulmonary arterial aneurysms in Behçet's syndrome: a report of 24 cases. *British Journal of Rheumatology* **33**, 48–51.

Hargreaves, M.R., Mowat, A.G., and Benson, M.K. (1992). Acute pneumonitis associated with low dose methotrexate treatment for rheumatoid arthritis: report of five cases and review of published reports. *Thorax* **47**, 628–33.

Hellman, D.B., Petri, M., and Whiting-O'Keefe, Q. (1987). Fatal infections in systemic lupus erythematosus: the role of opportunistic organisms. *Medicine* **66**, 341–8.

Imokawa, S., Colby, T.V., Leslie, K.O., and Helmers, R.A. (2000). Methotrexate pneumonitis: review of the literature and histopathological findings in nine patients. *European Respiratory Journal* **15**, 373–81.

Israel-Biet, D., Labrune, S., and Huchon, G.J. (1991). Drug induced lung disease. 1990 review. *European Respiratory Journal* **4**, 465–78.

Johnson, D.A., Gomm, S.A., Kalra, A., Woodcock, A.A., Evans, C.C., and Hind, C.R.K. (1993). The management of cryptogenic fibrosing alveolitis in three regions in the United Kingdom. *European Respiratory Journal* **6**, 891–3.

Kerkering, T.M., Duma, R.J., and Shadomy, S. (1981). The evolution of pulmonary cryptococcosis. *Annals of Internal Medicine* **94**, 611–16.

Nicholson, A.G., Colby, T.V., Du Bois, R.M., Hansell, D.M., and Wells, A.U. (2000). The prognostic significance of the histological pattern of interstitial pneumonia in patients presenting with the clinical entity of cryptogenic fibrosing alveolitis. *American Journal of Respiratory and Critical Care Medicine* **162**, 2213–17.

Rapti, A., Devi, B.S., Spiro, S.G., and Isenberg, D.A. (1998). The respiratory system in rheumatoid diseases. In *Auto-immune Aspects of Lung Disease* (ed. D.A. Isenberg and S.G. Spiro), pp. 23–52. Basel: Birkhaus.

Reynolds, H.Y. (1987). Bronchoalveolar lavage. *American Review of Respiratory Disease* **135**, 250–63.

Stover, D.E., Zaman, M.B., Hajdu, S.J., Lange, M., Gold, J., and Armstrong, D. (1984). Bronchoalveolar lavage in the diagnosis of diffuse pulmonary infiltrates in the immunosuppressed host. *Annals of Internal Medicine* **101**, 1–7.

Turner-Warwick, M. and Haslam, P. (1987). The value of serial bronchoalveolar lavages in assessing the clinical progress of patients with cryptogenic fibrosing alveolitis. *American Review of Respiratory Diseases* **135**, 26–34.

Wall, C.P., Gaensler, E.A., Carrington, C.B., and Hayes, J.A. (1981). Comparison of transbronchial and open biopsies in chronic infiltrative lung diseases. *American Review of Respiratory Diseases* **123**, 280–5.

Warrick, J.H., Bhalla, M., Schabel, S.I., and Silver, R.M. (1991). High resolution computed tomography in early scleroderma lung disease. *Journal of Rheumatology* **18**, 1520–7.

Wells, A.U., Hansell, D.M., Corrin, B., Harrison, N.K., Goldstraw, P., and Black, C.M. (1992). High resolution computed tomography as a predictor of lung histology in systemic sclerosis. *Thorax* **47**, 738–42.

Wells, A.U., Hansell, D.M., Harrison, N.K., Lawrence, R., Black, C.M., and Dubois, R.M. (1993a). Clearance of inhaled ^{99m}Tc-DTPA predicts the clinical course of fibrosing alveolitis. *European Respiratory Journal* **4**, 797–802.

Wells, A.U., Hansell, D.M., Rubens, M.B., Cullinan, P., Black, C.M., and Dubois, R.M. (1993b). The predictive value of appearance on thin-section computed tomography in fibrosing alveolitis. *American Review of Respiratory Diseases* **148**, 1076–82.

1.3.6 The gastrointestinal tract

Erkki Eerola, Reijo Peltonen, and Timo Möttönen

Introduction

In 1672 Sydenham and in 1743 Ives described arthritis in patients with dysentery. By the end of the nineteenth century arthritis was connected to shigellosis and inflammatory gut diseases. Since then, knowledge about interactions between rheumatic and gastroenterologic disorders has greatly increased. Associations may be aetiologic as in enterogenic reactive arthritides or without a causative link as in many gastrointestinal (GI) and rheumatic diseases with manifestations in both systems. Sometimes, it is even difficult to decide to which category a disease should belong. The cellular and molecular mechanisms of inflammation and tissue damage are basically similar both in chronic inflammatory joint and bowel diseases (Parke 1993). The same drugs can sometimes be used to treat diseases of both systems or gastrointestinal and rheumatic manifestations of the same disease. An important association is also the large number of GI adverse effects of rheumatological medications.

Gastroenterological disorders with rheumatic manifestations

GI diseases with rheumatic associations are listed in Table 1. The closest association is naturally in enteropathic arthropathies, which by definition are associated with GI disorders. In patients with inflammatory bowel disease, the prevalence of arthritic manifestations is reported to be about 20 per cent, peripheral enthesiopathy to occur in 6 per cent and clubbing of fingers in 8–11 per cent. However, the actual prevalence of rheumatic manifestations is probably higher. On the other hand, up to 50–60 per cent of patients with spondyloarthropathy has gut inflammation (Braun and Sieper 1999). In some of the enteropathic arthropathies, rather convincing evidence of aetiologic association does exist. Antigenic material of intestinal microbial origin has been demonstrated in the synovial samples of the patients with reactive arthritis after Yersinia and Salmonella enteric infections (Granfors et al. 1989, 1990). Another aetiologically significant finding is the identification of the causative agent of Whipple's disease (*Tropheryma whippelii*) from the duodenal samples of the patients (Relman et al. 1992). Intestinal bypass surgery is a an example of an operation leading to microbiological changes in the gut and finally to arthritis in a large number of patients. The most definitive the aetiological link is, however, in purulent or viral arthritides, when intestinal pathogens are isolated in affected joints.

Hepatic disorders with rheumatic manifestations include viral hepatitides (A, B, and C), autoimmune hepatitis, some cirrhotic disorders (cryptogenic and primary biliary cirrhoses), and storage diseases (Wilson's disease and haemochromatosis). Recently, hepatitis C virus (HCV) has received most of the attention. There is a strong association between HCV and mixed cryoglobulinaemia. In addition, suggested HCV-related autoimmune rheumatic disorders include sicca syndrome, rheumatoid arthritis (RA), polyarteritis nodosa, poly/dermatomyositis, and fibromyalgia (Ferri and Zignego 2000).

Paraneoplastic rheumatic manifestations may be induced by several malignancies including GI cancers and lymphomas. Autoimmunity is the most common, but not the only possible mechanism involved. Such rheumatic syndromes as asymmetric polyarthritis in the elderly with explosive onset, RA with monoclonal gammopathy, Sjögren's syndrome with monoclonality, hypertrophic osteoarthropathy, dermatomyositis, polymyalgia rheumatica with atypical features, palmar fasciitis and arthritis syndrome, and chronic erythema nodosum are particularly suggestive for occult malignancies (Naschitz 2001). An extensive search for malignancies in rheumatic syndromes is usually considered not cost-effective, but in these syndromes it may be feasible. Rheumatic syndromes may also increase the risk of cancer. Such syndromes include RA, Felty's syndrome, dermatomyositis, temporal arteritis, and systemic sclerosis (Naschitz et al. 1999).

Gastrointestinal manifestations of rheumatic diseases

GI manifestations of rheumatic diseases are listed in Table 2.

Rheumatoid arthritis

The most common GI manifestations in the patients suffering from RA are gastric erosions and ulcerations caused by drug therapy. A common manifestation of the disease itself is oesophageal dysmotility, but it is usually benign and rarely causes serious complications or even dysphagia or heartburn. A potentially serious GI manifestation is rheumatoid vasculitis, which has been estimated to affect 0.1 per cent of patients, but may be considerably more common. With complications such as ischaemic cholecystitis, appendicitis, pancolitis, bowel ulcerations, infarction, perforation, and massive bleeding the mortality is high. Amyloidosis has also been considered a rare complication. Amyloidosis as a cause of death in juvenile RA is reported to have decreased from 42 per cent in the 1970s to 17 per cent in the 1980s (Savolainen and Isomäki 1993). Aggressive treatment with immunosuppressive agents may be the reason for this decline in mortality. Rectal biopsy or subcutaneous fat biopsy gives a 75 per cent diagnostic yield for amyloidoisis, but lip biopsy may be even better.

Scleroderma

GI manifestations are common in scleroderma, occurring in 50–90 per cent of patients. They may precede the skin involvement, but usually, when the GI tract is affected, the disease process is diffuse with multiple levels of involvement. The disease is characterized by mononuclear cell infiltrates, collagen deposition, and small vessel vasculitis in the skin and internal organs (Abu-Shakra et al. 1994). The most common symptoms are heartburn and dysphagia, and the most frequent manifestations of the disease include oesophageal dysmotility and lower oesophageal sphincter laxity. Small bowel involvement occurs in 17–50 per cent of patients. These manifestations often include segmental dilatation, atony, pseudo-obstruction, and bacterial overgrowth of the small bowel (10 per cent). The reported frequency of colonic involvement varies between 10 and 50 per cent; constipation in about 30 per cent and wide mouth diverticula in over 28 per cent. Other colonic complications such as telangiectasis, pseudo-obstruction, and volvulus are rare and each of them occurs in about 1 per cent of patients.

Systemic lupus erythematosus

The most common GI manifestation of systemic lupus erythematosus is abdominal pain. Nausea, anorexia, or vomiting affects over 50 per cent of patients. Diarrhoea may affect 5–25 per cent of patients. In systemic lupus, liver disease is not considered to be one of the most serious problems but it has been reported in 20 per cent and some biochemical evidence of hepatobiliary involvement in over 50 per cent of patients. Ascites occurs in 10 per cent of patients and can be caused by peritoneal or mesenteric vasculitis, pancreatitis, serositis, nephrotic syndrome, or cardiac failure. Vasculitis is one of the most serious GI manifestations of lupus. It affects only 2 per cent of patients, but has a mortality rate of 50 per cent. It may result in colonic perforation, which has been reported to be responsible for about 27 per cent of deaths occurring in patients with lupus.

Sjögren's syndrome

Xerostomia is one of the two major symptoms of Sjögren's syndrome. Dysphagia is reported in two-thirds of the patients. Abnormalities of oesophageal motility are seen in about 36 per cent and oesophageal webs in up to 10 per cent of patients. Impairment of pancreatic exocrine function is common. Sjögren's syndrome is associated with primary biliary cirrhosis.

Table 1 Gastrointestinal disorders with rheumatic manifestations

GI disorder	Rheumatic manifestation	Association
Enteropathic arthropathies		
Enteric infection	Enterogenic reactive arthritis and Reiter's syndrome	Aetiologic. Arthritis in 2% of the patients with enteric infections (20% in HLA-B27-positive). Most common causative agents: *Salmonella, Shigella, Yersinia, Cambylobacter, Clostridium difficile*
Inflammatory bowel disease	Arthritic manifestations: 20%	Same inflammatory mechanisms
Crohn's disease	Peripheral arthritis: 17–20% Ankylosing spondylitis: 6–13% Radiological sacroiliitis: 26%	Histologic evidence of gut inflammation in 50–60% of patients with spondyloarthropathy
Ulcerative colitis	Peripheral arthritis: 17–20% Ankylosing spondylitis: 7% Radiological sacroiliitis: 16%	
Whipple's disease	Migratory polyarthritis: >60% *Tropheryma whippelii*, identified in duodenal tissue of the patients Diarrhoea: >75%	Aetiologic agent, *Tropheryma whippelii*
Intestinal bypass surgery (Ross et al. 1989)	Symmetrical arthralgia or polyarthritis: 6–52%	Intestinal bacterial overgrowth (+ other blind loop syndromes)
Coeliac disease (Collin et al. 1995; Lubrano et al. 1996)	Arthritis: 7–26%, without gluten-free diet up to 50%	Increased intestinal permeability and increased antigen absorption. Gluten-free diet improves arthritis
Infective arthritides		
Enteric bacteria	Septic arthritis, osteomyelitis	Aetiologic. *Salmonella, Pseudomonas*, or other Gram-negative bacilli in 9–17%
Enteric viruses	Arthritis rarely: 0.13%	Enteroviruses (Coxsackie, Echo) isolated in joints
Hepatic disorders		
Hepatitis A	Prodromal arthralgia: 14% Arthritis or vasculitis only rarely	Aetiologic
Hepatitis B	Prodromal arthralgia: 10–25% and arthritis: 10% Polyarteritis nodosa	Aetiologic
Hepatitis C (Buskila 2000)	Mixed cryoglobulinaemia: 10–50% Arthralgia: 10% Arthritis: 4%	Aetiologic
Primary biliary cirrhosis	Polyarthritis: 19% Scleroderma: 18% Secondary Sjögren's syndrome: 50% (Tsianos et al. 1990)	Autoimmune manifestations
Chronic active hepatitis	Polyarthralgia or arthritis: 25–50%	Autoimmune manifestation
Cryptogenic cirrhosis	Arthralgia or arthritis: 3%	
Wilson's disease	Osteoarthritis: 50% of adults Chondrocalcinosis	Copper storage disease
Haemochromatosis	Non-inflammatory chronic polyarthropathy: 50% Chondrocalcinosis	Iron storage disease
Paraneoplastic manifestations		
GI malignancies	GI cancers and lymphomas able to induce various paraneoplastic rheumatic manifestations (Naschitz et al. 1999)	Autoimmune manifestation Metastatic and other mechanisms

Vasculitides

Vasculitis is one of the pathogenetic mechanisms by which rheumatic diseases, such as RA and lupus, cause serious GI manifestations. The frequency of GI manifestations in diseases which in the first place are regarded as vasculitides varies widely. In Behçet's syndrome, vasculitic oral ulcers constitute a major diagnostic criterium. In Wegener's granulomatosis, the occurrence of GI vasculitis is 5 per cent and in some other vasculitic diseases it is even lower. However, GI vasculitis is common in polyarteritis nodosa (80 per cent), Henoch–Schönlein purpura (68 per cent), and Churg–Strauss syndrome (42 per cent) (see Fig. 1).

Gastrointestinal side-effects of rheumatic drug treatment

GI side-effects of rheumatic drug treatment are listed in Table 3.

Non-steroidal anti-inflammatory drugs and coxibs

Non-steroidal anti-inflammatory drugs (NSAIDs) have improved the quality of life for patients with arthritis for over 90 years. They are some of the most commonly used drugs throughout the world, and the annual

Table 2 Gastrointestinal manifestations of rheumatologic diseases

Disease	Abnormality	Manifestation
Rheumatoid arthritis	Temporomandibular arthritis	Impaired mastication
	Oesophageal dysmotility	Dysphagia, reflux
	GI vasculitis (0.1%)	Buccal ulcers, abdominal pain, ulceration, acalculous cholecystitis, bowel infarction, perforation
	Amyloidosis	Pseudo-obstruction, malabsorption, intestinal ulceration and infarction, protein-losing enteropathy, gastric outlet obstruction, hepatic dysfunction
	Portal hypertension (Felty's syndrome)	Splenomegaly, variceal hemorrhage
	Liver involvement (Felty's syndrome)	Enzyme and histological abnormalities (in upto 65% of patients)
	Hepatosplenomegaly	Non-specific hepatosplenomegaly
	Sjögren's (sicca) syndrome	
Scleroderma	Reduced oral aperture	Difficulties to eat
	Oesophageal dysmotility (87%)	Heartburn and dysphagia (79%) (Abu-Shakra et al. 1994), reflux (66%), ulceration, strictures, fistulae, Barrett's metaplasia (38%)
	Delayed gastric emptying (75%)	Gastric retention, worsened reflux
	Intestinal fibrosis and dysmotility (88%)	Malabsorption (5%), constipation (30%), pseudo-obstruction (<1%), intussusception, volvulus (1%), pneumatosis intestinalis
	Pseudo- and wide-mouth diverticulae (28%)	Haemorrhage, stasis, bacterial overgrowth (10%)
	Arteritis (rare)	Intestinal thrombosis, infarction, pancreatic necrosis
	Pancreatitis	Calcific pancreatitis, exocrine pancreatic insufficiency
	Hepatic cirrhosis	Primary biliary cirrhosis
SLE	Oesophageal dysmotility	Dysphagia, reflux
	GI vasculitis (2%)	Buccal ulcers, ileocolitis, gastritis, ulceration, perforation, intussusception, pneumatosis intestinalis, pancreatitis
	Protein-losing enteropathy	Hypoalbuminaemia
	Peritonitis	Ascitis (10%), polyserositis, bacterial superinfection
	Hepatosplenomegaly (30%)	Non-specific hepatosplenomegaly
Polymyositis–dermatomyositis	Skeletal muscle dysfunction	Aspiration, impaired deglutition
	Disordered motility	Dysphagia, pharyngeal atonia, heartburn, delayed gastric emptying, constipation, colonic dilatation, diverticula
	Vasculitis (rare)	Mucosal ulcerations, perforation, pneumatosis intestinalis
Mixed connective tissue disease	Hypomotility	Dysphagia, reflux, stricture, gastric bezoars, pseudo-obstruction
	Vasculitis (rare)	Ulceration, perforation, pancreatitis
Sjögren's syndrome	Dessiccation of membranes	Xerostomia, oral fissures, dysphagia
	Oesophageal webs (10%)	Dysphagia (>60%)
	Gastric atrophy/infiltrates	Gastric masses, dyspepsia, nausea
	Pancreatitis	Pain, exocrine pancreatic insufficiency, hyperamylasemia (25%)
	Hepatic dysfunction	Hepatomegaly (25–28%), elevated enzymes (25%)
	Hepatic cirrhosis	Primary biliary cirrhosis/cryptogenic
	Malabsorption	
Polyarteritis nodosa	Vasculitis (mesenteric vasculitis in 80%)	Buccal ulcers, cholecystitis (17%), bowel infarction, perforation, appendicitis, pancreatitis, strictures, chronic wasting syndrome
Churg–Strauss syndrome	GI vasculitis (42%)	Haemorrhage, ulcerations, infarction, perforation
	Eosinophilic gastritis	Gastric masses
Henoch–Schönlein purpura	GI vasculitis (68%)	Intussusception, ulcers, cholecystitis, haemorrhage, infarction, perforation, appendicitis
Wegener's granulomatosis	GI vasculitis (<5%)	Cholecystitis, appendicitis, ileocolitis, bowel infarction
Cryoglobulinaemia	GI vasculitis (rare)	Infarction, ischaemia
	Splenomegalia: upto 50%	
	Hepatic involvement: 62–88%	
Behçet's syndrome	Mucosal ulcerations (vasculitis)	Buccal ulcers, GI inflammation, intestinal ulcers and haemorrhage, perforation, pyloric stenosis, rectal ulcers
	Amyloidosis	Complications as in rheumatoid arthritis (above)
Reactive arthritis and ankylosing spondylitis	Infective diarrhoea	Usually asymptomatic
	Ileocolonic inflammation	
	Amyloidosis	
Marfan/Ehlers–Danlos syndromes	Defective collagen	Megaesophagus, hypomotility, giant diverticula, malabsorption, megacolon, perforation, arterial rupture
Whipple's disease	Infection due to *Tropheryma whippelii*	Diarrhoea, steatorrhoea (75%), abdominal pain
Kawasaki disease	GI vasculitis	Abdominal pain, intestinal obstruction, non-infective diarrhoea
Giant cell arteritis	GI vasculitis	Intestinal vasculitis/ischaemia

Modified from Ryan and Sleisenger 1993.

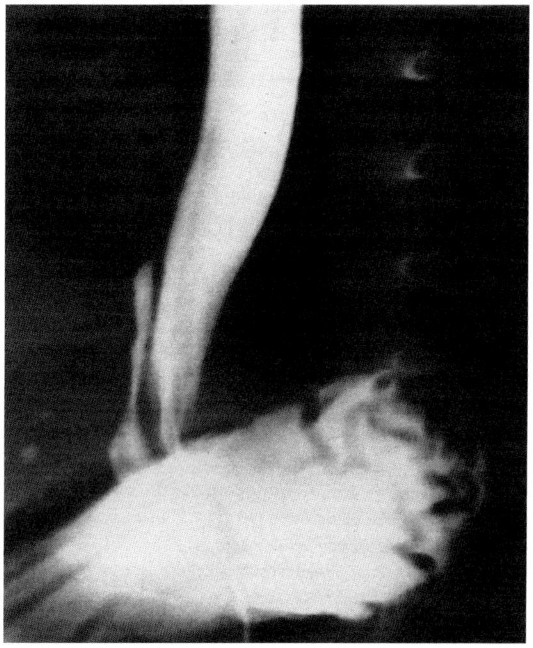

Fig. 1 Perforated lower oesophagus in a patient with dermatomyositis.

increase in prescriptions is about 5 per cent. Unfortunately they also cause a higher number of adverse effects than any other class of drug. NSAIDs are able to induce mucosal damage in every part of the GI tract from oesophagus to rectum, but most of the serious damage occurs in the gastroduodenal region. The mechanisms involved are believed to be direct topical injury and systemic prostaglandin inhibition. It is the prostaglandin inhibition which is also responsible for the anti-inflammatory effect of the drugs and therefore all NSAIDs have the potential to initiate serious GI events. Endoscopic studies have shown that virtually every subject develops gastroduodenal mucosal injury after a single 650–1350 mg dose of acetylsalicylic acid. NSAIDs can cause ultrastructural damage of the gastric epithelium within minutes and gross subepithelial haemorrhages and erosions within hours of ingestion (Plate 27). With long-term treatment 50–75 per cent of patients develop mucosal damage, and 10–37 per cent gastroduodenal ulcers, a value over 5–15-fold greater than would be expected in a healthy population. The risk is directly dose-related. However, only approximately 30–40 per cent of patients receiving long-term treatment with NSAIDs have symptoms of dyspepsia and in as many as 58 per cent of subjects with a life-threatening complication, the complication itself has been the presenting manifestation of NSAID injury without prior dyspepsia as a warning. The annualized incidence rate of symptomatic GI ulcers and ulcer complications in NSAID users ranges from 2 to 4 per cent.

NSAIDs inhibit prostaglandin synthesis by blocking cyclooxygenase (COX) enzymes. At least two different cyclooxygenases exist, COX-1 and COX-2. Tissue expression of the COX-1 isoform is constitutive, suggesting that this enzyme synthesizes prostanoids responsible for physiologic 'housekeeping' functions including GI mucosal protection, while COX-2 seems to be responsible for peripheral inflammatory responses. At therapeutic doses, all currently available NSAIDs inhibit both of the COX isoenzymes. Recently, a new class of COX-2 specific drugs, coxibs (celecoxib and rofecoxib) has been approved for the treatment of osteoarthritis and RA in many countries. According to the recent studies celecoxib and refecoxib, at dosages greater than those indicated clinically, were associated with a lower incidence of symptomatic ulcers and ulcer complications compared with NSAIDs at standard dosages. In addition, in the coxib-treated patients, significantly fewer patients discontinued the treatment as a result of GI symptoms than in the NSAIDs groups (Bombardier et al. 2000; Silverstein et al. 2000).

Table 3 Gastrointestinal side effects of rheumatic drug treatment

Disease	Symptom
NSAIDs	Nausea Oesophagitis Non-ulcer dyspepsia Peptic ulcer Hepatic enzyme abnormalities Ileopathy with malabsorption and protein losing enteropathy Increased intestinal permeability Intestinal ulceration, stricture, obstruction, and perforation
Chloroquines	Anorexia, nausea, vomiting, diarrhoea
Gold	Buccal ulcers (5–20%) Hepatic enzyme abnormalities, cholestatic jaundice, hepatic necrosis Diarrhoea (44%, the most common GI side-effect of gold) Gold enterocolitis (enteritis, diarrhoea, fever, eosinophilia, megacolon)
Sulfasalazine	Nausea, vomiting, dyspepsia, malaise, anorexia, abdominal pain, indigestion (common), diarrhoea Colonic inflammation, mucosal ulceration, bloody diarrhoea (resembling ulcerative colitis) Hepatic enzyme abnormalities, granulomatous hepatitis, severe hepatitis and necrosis Cholestasis Pancreatitis
D-Penicillamine	Dysgeusia (abnormalities of taste) (2–25% in the first 3–6 months), oral ulcers, nausea, anorexia, abdominal pain (8–35%) Diarrhoea (occasionally) Hepatic enzyme abnormalities (>5%), toxic hepatitis, hepatic necrosis, Cholestatic jaundice Acute haemorrhagic colitis (rare)
Methotrexate	Nausea, vomiting, diarrhoea, stomatitis Liver enzyme abnormalities Hepatic fibrosis
Azathioprine	Nausea, vomiting (common), diarrhoea (<1%) Stomatitis Liver enzyme abnormatities
Leflunomide	Vomiting, stomatitis, diarrhoea, weight loss, liver enzyme abnormalities
Cyclosporine	Nausea, vomiting, gum hyperplasia (4–12%), diarrhoea Abnormal liver function
Chlorambusil	Nausea, vomiting Stomatitis
Cyclophosphamide	Nausea, vomiting, diarrhoea Stomatitis Hepatic abnormalities
Corticosteroids	Peptic ulcer with NSAIDs, pancreatitis

Oesophageal injury has been reported rarely and seems to come from direct topical irritation of NSAIDs. Asymptomatic, small intestinal enteropathy is seen in 60–70 per cent of patients with long-term treatment. It is associated with mild blood loss (1–10 ml/day) and increased intestinal permeability. Colonic injury occurs less frequently, but may be serious with perforations and bleeding. NSAIDs have been linked to development of collagenous colitis or colitis resembling inflammatory bowel disease. The drugs are also known to exacerbate pre-existing inflammatory bowel disease. Rectal administration may cause proctitis. Reversible elevations in liver enzymes are seen in about 5 per cent, and monitoring them may be necessary when NSAID therapy is initiated. Serious complications and deaths from hepatic damage are rare. It should be realized that neither subjective symptoms nor endoscopic evidence of injury reliably predict the development of serious complications. In order to decrease the incidence of untoward GI events induced by NSAIDs high-risk patients must be identified. Risk factors for gastroduodenal injury include age over 60 years, chronic use of NSAIDs, history of peptic ulcer, previous NSAID gastroduodenal intolerance, recent upper abdominal pain due to NSAIDs, multiple NSAID use, cardiovascular or other chronic disease in addition to arthritis, and use of multiple concurrent medications especially corticosteroids. If high-risk patients must be treated with NSAIDs, either the lowest possible dose, an alternative non-NSAID analgesic, or coxibes are recommended. If a NSAID is used, a coadministration of misoprostol should be considered. Misoprostol is a synthetic prostaglandin E1 analogue and so far the only prophylactic agent that is unequivocally effective in protecting duodenal mucosa as well as the stomach from NSAID-induced injury. Prophylactic use of high dose H2 blockers and proton pump inhibitors (e.g. omeprazole) seems to offer protection against NSAID-induced ulcers. However, even misoprostol cannot be relied upon to prevent more than 40 per cent of serious upper GI complications, and the drug has not been proven to reduce the number of deaths. The treatment of GI injury includes withholding NSAIDs and administering H2 blockers or proton pump inhibitors (Lichtenstein et al. 1995).

For a long time, it was believed that DMARDs were many times more toxic than NSAIDs. In fact, because of the high frequency of GI problems with NSAIDs, there are no substantial differences in toxicity between the two drug categories and the order in which the drugs are initiated in rheumatic diseases should be carefully considered (Fries et al. 1991).

Disease-modifying antirheumatic drugs

Chloroquines and corticosteroids have a low number of GI side-effects. The main GI problems commonly associated with the use of corticosteroids are peptic ulceration (especially when used with NSAIDs), gastric haemorrhage, intestinal perforation, and pancreatitis. The risk of corticosteroids alone causing peptic ulcers is estimated to be very small or absent and this concern should not inhibit the use of small or moderate doses of steroids, for example, in RA.

GI side-effects of disease modifying antirheumatic drugs (DMARDs) occur most frequently in treatment with oral gold compounds, over 600 events per 1000 patient-years. With intramuscular gold the incidence is only one-tenth of that, but the complications appear to be more serious (Fries et al. 1991). Diarrhoea is the most common GI manifestation of oral gold therapy (44 per cent). It responds well to dosage reduction and often declines even with continued use. Although serious GI complications are rare, gold enterocolitis has been reported. Diarrhoea should therefore never be overlooked during any kind of gold therapy.

Sulfasalazine has a good GI safety profile. Dyspepsia, nausea, abdominal discomfort, and mucosal ulceration are the most common side-effects of the therapy. Hepatic injuries, even massive liver necrosis, have been reported. Pancreatitis, cholestasis, and inflammatory diarrhoea are also rare complications.

Penicillamine is responsible for over 100 GI adverse events per 1000 patient-years. GI pain or diarrhoea occurs in 8–35 per cent of patients. Taste abnormalities are experienced by 2–25 per cent of patients within the first 3–6 months. The symptom is dose related and usually subsides within a few months of treatment.

Methotrexate and azathioprine have been reported to cause over 200 GI adverse effects per 1000 patient-years (Fries et al. 1991). In a long-term study, methotrexate caused nausea and/or GI distress in 65 per cent of patients, mouth ulceration or soreness in 55 per cent, and liver enzyme elevation in up to 88 per cent at some time during the treatment. Serious or potentially serious liver abnormalities have been reported in 12 per cent of patients. Hepatic and GI toxicity has resulted in discontinuation of therapy in 16 per cent of patients treated with methotrexate.

Leflunomide, a novel immunomodulator for the treatment of RA, inhibits de novo pyrimidine synthesis, resulting in an inhibition of actively dividing lymphocytes. GI disturbances, diarrhoea, nausea, mouth ulceration, and weight loss as well as elevated liver enzyme levels (about as frequent as with methotrexate), are associated with the therapy of leflunomide.

Half of patients given cyclophosphamide complain of nausea, vomiting, or diarrhoea, and stomatitis also is common. Liver enzyme abnormalities are often seen. Serious hepatotoxicity, however, is uncommon; a few cases of hepatic necrosis have been reported.

Diet and rheumatic diseases

RA and many other systemic rheumatic diseases remain illnesses of unknown causes for which current therapy is often inadequate. This easily leads patients to seek alternative remedies, prominent among which are dietary manipulations. From the 1980s there has been a renewed scientific interest in the topic. Dietary therapies can be divided into three categories: elimination, supplementation, and oral tolerization. Very often, the diets tried by patients are both supplementary and eliminative at the same time. The main approaches are fasting, vegetarian diet, dietary supplementation with vitamins, oils, trace elements, or various antioxidants, exclusion of specific food substances suspected of causing food allergy, intolerance or of triggering attacks of illness, and a variety of 'fad diets' focusing on special food items such as Brewer's yeast, garlic, ginger, or bromelaine, etc. One investigational diet, elemental diet, has shown to be beneficial in some experiments. In spite of some positive reports, the overall conclusion is that dietary therapy for arthritis should still be considered investigational. Many diets also require careful nutritional supervision to avoid malnutrition (Henderson and Panush 1999).

Supplementation therapy

Supplementation therapy is based on the findings showing low serum levels of certain minerals in RA patients and on the concept that certain oils, vitamins, and minerals have anti-inflammatory effect. Some supplements do have mild anti-inflammatory effect, but none has been shown to exert any disease modifying effect. One diet suitable for those, who cannot or do not want to use NSAIDs, is fish-enriched diet and/or T-3 fatty acid supplementation. It also provides some cardiovascular benefit. Trace elements or antioxidants as supplements to a balanced diet seem unnecessary with a possible exception of vitamin E, which may have some analgesic effect (Mangge et al. 1999).

Elimination therapy

The idea of elimination diet is based mainly on the concept of possible food allergy and exclusion of provocative items from the diet. There is some evidence suggesting that eliminating specific food items may be reasonable in a small subset of patients whose rheumatic disease appears to deteriorate from allergic reactions to such items as milk, eggs, chocolate, wheat, beans, fish, etc. However, the most commonly tried eliminative diet is probably a short period of fasting with or without a prolonged vegetarian diet. In spite of some encouraging results, the clinical effectiveness of this approach remains still to be proven.

Oral tolerization

Tolerization therapy refers to the decreased systemic responsiveness to the antigen following oral exposure to that antigen. Results from studies with collagen type II in preventing autoimmune disorders and modulating ongoing disease justify further efforts to determine efficacy and to identify which patients may have a good response to such therapy (Henderson and Panush 1999).

Intestinal microbiology and rheumatic diseases

The intestinal microbial flora is not essential for life. Animals free from microbes and on adequate nutrition live more than 30 per cent longer than colonized animals. Although the relationship between host and normal flora is truly symbiotic, it is evident that intestinal bacteria may have either beneficial or harmful effects on the host, depending on the bacterial species and available substrates for their metabolism.

The idea that intestinal bacteria might be associated with RA is essentially derived from the association between GI disease and arthritis and from the fact that several intestinal bacteria cause reactive arthritis. Another reason for associating intestinal bacteria and RA is the fact that the genetic component of this disease is unlikely to be greater than 30 per cent, and there are no obvious environmental factors that explain the remaining 70 per cent of cases (Silman 1991). Furthermore, the gut flora can modify induction of arthritis induced experimentally by streptococcal cell wall extracts (van den Broek et al. 1992) and pristane (Thompson and Elson 1993). Also a germfree state prevents the development of arthritis in transgenic rats (Taurog et al. 1994). However, there is no definitive proof of a primary role for the gut in the pathogenesis of RA. If the link is substantiated, the therapeutic implications would be considerable.

The main reasons for the difficulties encountered in studies on the association of RA and the intestinal microbial flora have been the enormous complexity of the latter and the inadequacy of traditional methods to study it (Woese 1987; Relman et al. 1993). Each gram of wet faeces contains 10^{10}–10^{12} bacteria recoverable by traditional bacteriological methods. The estimate of the number of bacterial species in the human intestine is more than 400 detected by culture methods (Moore and Holdeman 1974). Based on the studies which have relied on cloned or amplified 16S rRNA molecules using broad-range oligonucleotides environmental microbiologists postulate that most of the extant microorganisms (more than 80 per cent) remain unidentified, because of the insensitivity of bacterial cultures. The same may apply to the commensal microbial flora endogenous to humans (Relman et al. 1993).

No definite connection between any microbe and RA is ever made. In addition, no finding, direct or indirect, has generally been approved to connect RA to any microbe or any type of infection. The connection between RA and some (intestinal) microbe is based on one of the following findings. Quantitative culture of intestinal bacteria showing increased amount of some species in patients with RA. Presence of higher amounts of antibodies against some microbes in RA patients when compared to controls. Chemical analyses of intestinal content showing differences in some components between RA patients and controls. Demonstrating a connection of some treatment between its clinical outcome and the change of intestinal flora it has caused. Change of diet or fasting has a positive effect in some patients on the clinical picture of RA. In these patients the response can be linked to change in the intestinal flora (Kjeldsen-Kragh et al. 1991; Peltonen et al. 1994, 1997). Of individual bacterial species found in the stool samples *Streptococcus agalactiae, Yersinia enterocolitica, Klebsiella pneumoniae*, and *Clostridium perfringens* have earlier been linked to RA, but no positive proof has been shown. Increased levels of antibodies against *Proteus mirabilis* have been found in RA patients, and the therapeutic effect of vegan diet has been associated with the decrease in the antibody levels (Kjeldsen-Kragh et al. 1993). However, none of these findings have been generally accepted to have a marked role on the aetiology or pathogenesis of RA. One marked reason for this speculative attitude has been the inability to explain the findings and their possible mechanism in the pathogenesis of RA. Recently, however, new data have been obtained by molecular methods. Gas chromatography of bacterial cellular fatty acids, analysed directly from stool samples demonstrates that the intestinal flora is changed in RA (Eerola et al. 1994), the change is mainly in the anaerobic flora, and the beneficial effect of dietary treatment in RA is linked to changes in the intestinal flora (Peltonen et al. 1994, 1997). New studies with fluorescent, species-specific DNA probes have confirmed these findings at the species level. Another approach is based not on specific bacterial species or overall changes in the intestinal microflora but on the translocation of bacterial arthritogenic antigens from the gut.

Non-viable bacterial antigens have been detected in rheumatoid synovial effusions (Bartholomew and Bartholomew 1979). As the translocation of viable bacteria from the gut to extraintestinal sites is not a rare phenomenon, it is quite feasible that debris (including peptidoglycan) from bacteria normally present in the GI tract also traverses the gut–blood barrier and stimulates the immune system. This idea is supported by experimental findings that bacterial cell wall material injected into rats can induce arthritis (Simelyte et al. 2000). The normal intestinal flora harbours a sufficiently diverse population of bacteria to produce the peptidoglycan–polysaccharide polymers capable of inducing arthropathic responses in the host. In a susceptible person, arthritis might result from the accumulation of a certain threshold concentration of these arthropathic polymers in the joint. This accumulation might be accelerated greatly when the intestinal epithelium is damaged (Stimpson et al. 1986). Alterations in the intestinal flora have also been proposed to influence on the permeability of the epithelium and absorbtion of the bacterial peptidoglycan. As in the case of bacterial cell wall material, these peptidoglycan–polysaccharide complexes produced by the human intestinal flora can also induce arthritis when injected subcutaneously into rats (Simelyte et al. 2000).

Conclusions on the aetiological role of the intestinal microbial flora in RA have remained limited over the years. Intestinal absorption of antigens and other noxious substances from intestinal microbes may play an important role in a multifactorial aetiopathogenesis of RA. Since arthropathies could be indirect consequences of change in the resident bacterial population in the gut, the same may be applicable to RA. At present, there is interest on the subject but little firm evidence that intestinal microbes or their products are aetiologically important in RA.

References

Abu-Shakra, M., Guillemin, F., and Lee, P. (1994). GI manifestations of systemic sclerosis. *Seminars in Arthritis and Rheumatism* **24**, 29–39.

Bartholomew, L.E. and Bartholomew, F.N. (1979). Antigenic bacterial polysaccharide in rheumatoid synovial effusions. *Arthritis and Rheumatism* **22**, 969–77.

Bombardier, C. et al. (2000). Comparison of upper GI toxicity of refecoxib and naproxen in patients with rheumatoid arthritis. *New England Journal of Medicine* **343**, 1520–8.

Braun, J. and Sieper, J. (1999). Rheumatologic manifestations of GI disorders. *Current Opinion in Rheumatology* **11**, 68–74.

van den Broek, M.F. et al. (1992). Gut flora induces and maintains resistance against streptococcal cell wall-induced arthritis in F344 rats. *Clinical and Experimental Immunology* **88**, 313–17.

Buskila, D. (2000). Hepatitis C-associated arthritis. *Current Opinion in Rheumatology* **12**, 295–9.

Collin, P. et al. (1994). Coeliac disease—associated disorders and survival. *Gut* **35**, 1215–18.

Eerola, E. et al. (1994). Intestinal flora in early rheumatoid arthritis. *British Journal of Rheumatology* **33**, 1030–8.

Ferri, C. and Zignego, A.L. (2000). Relation between infection and autoimmunity in mixed cryoglobulinemia. *Current Opinion in Rheumatology* **12**, 53–60.

Fries, J.F., Williams, C.A., and Bloch, D.A. (1991). The relative toxicity of nonsteroidal anti-inflammatory drugs. *Arthritis and Rheumatism* **34**, 1353–60.

Granfors, K. et al. (1989). Yersinia antigens in synovial-fluid cells from patients with reactive arthritis. *New England Journal of Medicine* **320**, 216–21.

Granfors, K. et al. (1990). Salmonella lipopolysaccharide in synovial cells from patients with reactive arthritis. *New England Journal of Medicine* **335**, 685–8.

Henderson, C.J. and Panush, R.S. (1999). Diets, dietary supplements, and nutritional therapies in rheumatic diseases. *Rheumatic Disease Clinics of North America* **25**, 937–68.

Kjeldsen-Kragh, J. et al. (1991). Controlled trial of fasting and one-year vegetarian diet in rheumatoid arthritis. *Lancet* **ii**, 899–902.

Kjeldsen-Kragh, J. et al. (1993). Anti-proteus antibody titres in rheumatoid arthritis patients during a controlled clinical trial of fasting and one-year vegetarian diet. *Revista Española de Reumatologia* **20** (Suppl. 1), 471.

Lichtenstein, D.R., Syngal, S., and Wolfe, M.M. (1995). Nonsteroidal anti-inflammatory drugs and the GI tract. *Arthritis and Rheumatism* **38**, 5–18.

Lubrano, E., Ciacci, C., Ames, P.R.J., Mazzacca, G., Oriente, P., and Scarpa, R. (1996). The arthritis of coeliac disease: prevalence and pattern in 200 adult patients. *British Journal of Rheumatology* **35**, 1314–18.

Mangge, H., Hermann, J., and Schauenstein, K. (1999). Diet and rheumatoid arthritis—a review. *Scandinavian Journal of Rheumatology* **28**, 201–9.

Moore, W.E.C. and Holdeman, L.V. (1974). Special problems associated with isolation and identification of intestinal bacteria in fecal flora studies. *American Journal of Clinical Nutrition* **27**, 1450–5.

Naschitz, J.E. (2001). Rheumatic syndromes: clues to occult neoplasia. *Current Opinion in Rheumatology* **13**, 62–6.

Naschitz, J., Rosner, I., Rozenbaum, M., Zuckerman, E., and Yeshurun, D. (1999). Rheumatic syndromes: clues to occult malignancies. *Seminars in Arthritis and Rheumatism* **29**, 43–55.

Parke, A.L. (1993). GI disorders and rheumatic diseases. *Current Opinion in Rheumatology* **5**, 79–84.

Peltonen, R. et al. (1994). Changes of faecal flora in rheumatoid arthritis during fasting and one-year vegetarian diet. *British Journal of Rheumatology* **33**, 638–43.

Peltonen, R. et al. (1977). Faecal microbial flora and disease activity in rheumatoid arthritis during a vegan diet. *British Journal of Rheumatology* **36**, 64–8.

Relman, D. et al. (1992). Identification of the uncultured bacillus of Whipple's disease. *New England Journal of Medicine* **327**, 293–301.

Relman, D.A. (1993). The identification of uncultured pathogens. *Journal of Infectious Diseases* **168**, 1–8.

Ross, C.B., Scott, H.W., and Pincus, T. (1989). Jejunoileal bypass arthritis. *Bailliere's Clinical Rheumatology* **3**, 339–54.

Ryan, J.C. and Sleisenger, M.H. (1993). Effects of systematic and extraintestinal disease on the gut. In *GI Disease* (ed. M.H. Sleisenger and J.S. Fordtran). Philadelphia PA: W.B. Saunders.

Savolainen, H.A. and Isomäki, H.A. (1993). Decrease in the number of deaths from secondary amyloidosis in patients with juvenile rheumatoid arthritis. *Journal of Rheumatology* **20**, 1201–3.

Silman, A.J. (1991). Is rheumatoid arthritis an infectious disease? (Editorial.) *British Medical Journal* **303**, 200–1.

Silverstein, F.E. et al. (2000). GI toxicity with celecoxib versus nonsteroidal anti-inflammatory drugs for osteoarthritis and rheumatoid arthritis. The CLASS study: a randomized controlled trial. *Journal of the American Medical Association* **284**, 1247–55.

Simelyte, E. et al. (2000). Bacterial cell wall-induced arthritis: chemical composition and tissue distribution of four Lactobacillus strains. *Infection and Immunity* **68**, 3535–40.

Stimpson, S.A. et al. (1986). Arthropatic properties of cell wall polymers from normal flora bacteria. *Infectious Immunology* **51**, 240–9.

Taurog, J.D. et al. (1994). The germfree state prevents development of gut and joint inflammatory disease in HLA-B27 transgenic rats. *Journal of Experimental Medicine* **180**, 2359–64.

Thompson, S.T. and Elson, C.J. (1993). Susceptibility to pristane-induced arthritis is altered with changes in bowel flora. *Immunology Letters* **36**, 227–32.

Woese, C.R. (1987). Bacterial evolution. *Microbiological Reviews* **51**, 221–71.

1.3.7 Liver, spleen, and pancreas

Daniel Fishman

The spleen

Functional anatomy

The normal spleen weighs between 100 and 200 g and is not clinically detectable. Its blood supply derives from the distal branches of the splenic artery, a branch of the coeliac artery. The splenic artery also supplies the body and tail of the pancreas and part of the stomach.

Splenic white pulp is composed of a periarteriolar lymphatic sheath, which is subdivided into a T-cell domain (periarteriolar) and B-cell domain (the follicles and perifollicular marginal zone). Surrounding the white pulp is the red pulp, a network of macrophage-laden stromal cords, and vascular sinuses. These function as a filtration system, removing abnormal erythrocytes, granulocytes, and platelets. They are responsible for the cellular destruction in autoimmune cytopaenias, during some immune complex diseases, and in hypersplenism.

The spleen sequesters granulocytes and up to 45 per cent of the total number of circulating platelets. The size of this pool is determined by splenic blood flow and the intrasplenic platelet transit time. Antigen presentation (notably bacterial polysaccharides) occurs within the spleen.

Rheumatoid arthritis

Splenomegaly is a common feature of uncomplicated rheumatoid arthritis (RA). Clinically detectable splenomegaly is present in 5–10 per cent of patients, but it may be detected by radionuclide scanning in up to 58 per cent of patients with active RA. Patients with active RA take longer to clear ^{99}Tc-labelled, heat-damaged autologous erythrocytes than those with inactive disease. This impairment of splenic reticuloendothelial function fluctuates during the course of the disease.

Spontaneous and post-traumatic splenic rupture may occur in seropositive, erosive, nodular RA. Histological examination reveals palisading fibroblasts, lymphocytes, neutrophils, and foamy histiocytes at the site of the rupture.

Felty's syndrome

The association of RA with splenomegaly and neutropaenia occurs in less than 1 per cent of patients, mainly women. It has been reported in children with both seropositive and seronegative arthritis, and in adults may appear prior to the development of arthritis.

Splenomegaly results from an increase in the splenic red pulp, with associated sinus hyperplasia and a prominent macrophage population. The presence of hyaline arteriosclerosis, endothelial hyperplasia, and an increased elastin content in the lamina of the splenic follicular arteries, suggests the presence of portal hypertension. Splenic size does not correlate with the degree of haematological abnormality. Moreover, neutropaenia is not solely the result of increased phagocytosis by splenic macrophages, as splenectomy is beneficial in only a proportion of patients. This may be due to the inadequate clearance of all functional splenic material, such as accessory spleens and remnants from traumatic splenic rupture.

Splenectomy

Recurrent neutropaenic sepsis, intractable leg ulcers, or severe anaemia or haemorrhage requiring transfusions may all respond to splenectomy. Indeed, the inflammatory arthritis itself can remit after splenectomy. An enlarged spleen may even spontaneously return to normal, following which Felty's syndrome can enter remission.

Safer alternatives to surgical splenectomy are splenic artery ligation, splenic irradiation, or partial splenic embolization (Nakamura et al. 1994).

Rheumatoid arthritis and Felty's syndrome, and their respective drug therapies, both confer an increased risk of infection. Splenectomy increases this risk, especially from pneumococci, even when the individual has previously been vaccinated. Rapidly fatal overwhelming post-splenectomy infection may present with non-specific signs, followed rapidly by the development of septicaemic shock and disseminated intravascular coagulation. To prevent this, polyvalent pneumococcal vaccination should be given 1 month before elective surgery, augmented by penicillin V, 250 mg twice daily.

Splenic abscess

Splenic abscesses result from haematogenous spread from other septic foci. The patient typically presents with a pain-free, non-specific febrile illness, in the context of Felty's syndrome or RA. Abdominal CT and isotope scanning may demonstrate wedge shaped splenic infarctions, although an unsuspected abscess can be discovered at splenectomy. Pre- or intraoperative rupture of the splenic abscess usually proves to be fatal.

Asplenia

The appearance of hyposplenism on the blood film of patients with RA is a predictor of asplenia on ultrasound or technetium scanning. These patients require prophylaxis against pneumococcal infection.

Large granular lymphocyte (LGL) syndrome

LGL syndrome is a rare, low-grade malignancy associated with bone marrow infiltration by LGL, neutropaenia, and splenomegaly. The spleen demonstrates a characteristic lymphoid infiltration of the red pulp chords, often with prominent germinal centres. One-third of patients develop RA (pseudo-Felty's syndrome). However, the arthritis in LGL syndrome is rarely severe, erosive, or associated with other extra-articular features. The spleen is the major reservoir of LGL, hence splenectomy is contraindicated as it may exacerbate LGL syndrome.

Sjögren's syndrome

Splenomegaly has been reported in 15.6 per cent of patients with Sjögren's syndrome and RA, compared to 5.6 per cent of patients with rheumatoid arthritis alone, and 3.7 per cent of patients with sicca symptoms alone (Webb et al. 1975). Splenomegaly was more frequent in patients with smooth muscle or mitochondrial antibodies. In primary Sjögren's syndrome the development of splenomegaly correlated with the presence of anti-Ro and anti-La antibodies.

Systemic lupus erythematosus (SLE)

Lupus splenomegaly develops as a result of lymphoid hyperplasia, enlargement of the white pulp lymphoid follicles, and an accumulation of red pulp periarteriolar macrophages and plasma cells. It is frequently associated with hepatomegaly and when developing in the context of a lupus flare it usually resolves with corticosteroid therapy. Occasionally, massive idiopathic splenomegaly develops in a female patient.

The pathognomonic histological feature of splenic involvement in SLE is the onion-skin lesion of periarterial fibrosis, observed in up to 83 per cent of cases at post-mortem. Multiple concentric layers of periarteriolar hyalinized collagen, which may calcify, develop around penicillary or follicular arteries. Other commonly observed features are capsulitis and small infarctions, secondary to thrombosis. They occur in association with a raised titre of anti-cardiolipin antibodies or the lupus anticoagulant. The pain of splenic infarction is usually felt in the left upper quadrant and may refer to the left shoulder tip, mimicking a pulmonary embolus. There may be splenic tenderness and an overlying rub. Complete splenic infarction develops after coeliac artery thrombosis, splenic artery thrombosis (when pancreatic infarction also occurs), or splenic vein thrombosis.

Very rare splenic complications include spontaneous rupture of an apparently normal spleen, and lymphocytoplasmic malignant lymphoma of the spleen, associated with the lupus anticoagulant and anticardiolipin antibodies (Ciaudo et al. 1991).

Splenic function

In mild to moderate lupus, ^{99m}Tc-labelled sulfur colloid uptake correlates directly with serum IgM level, and inversely with anti-DNA antibody titre (Wilson et al. 1989). The serum IgM level therefore represents an indirect measurement of splenic function.

The defective splenic phagocytic function in lupus is potentially the result of saturation of the splenic reticuloendothelial system by immune complexes. Despite an increase in splenic blood flow during active lupus there is a strongly positive correlation between disease activity, immune complex levels, and prolonged clearance of IgG-sensitized, ^{51}Cr-labelled autologous erythrocytes (Hamburger et al. 1982).

Splenic atrophy

Splenic atrophy leads to the features of hyposplenism on the peripheral blood film (Howell–Jolly bodies, Pappenheimer bodies, spherocytes, target cells, and poikilocytes) and functional asplenia (the failure to accumulate ^{99m}Tc-sulfur colloid in the spleen). Splenic atrophy in SLE is detectable in about 4 per cent of patients by screening for hyposplenism. An atrophic spleen is not necessarily nonfunctional, and may still be responsible for clinically significant cytopaenias.

Asplenic or hyposplenic lupus patients are at considerable risk of death from pneumococcal or salmonella septicaemia (Uthman et al. 1996), and they should be vaccinated with polyvalent pneumococcal vaccine. Patients with SLE in general produce a lower titre of antipneumococcal antibodies following vaccination than do normal individuals, so should be considered for revaccination after 6 years.

Splenectomy is of benefit to some patients with autoimmune cytopaenias and antiphospholipid-associated thrombocytopaenia, unresponsive to immunosuppression (Hakim et al. 1998).

Wegener's granulomatosis

Prior to the introduction of effective immunosuppressive therapy, splenic pathology in Wegener's granulomatosis was frequently observed at post-mortem. Splenomegaly with capsular adhesions was common, with the occasional observation of splenic artery or vein thromboses. Splenic necrosis was usually associated with extensive arteritis and disseminated visceral granulomata.

Clinically significant splenic involvement in Wegener's granulomatosis, in the form of spontaneous rupture or massive necrosis, is now rare. Incidental splenic lesions may be detected during ultrasound or CT scans on adjacent areas. Their hypodense nature suggests they are infarctions secondary to active vasculitis, which can resolve with treatment.

Splenic function

Splenomegaly associated with active disease is usually accompanied by impaired clearance of antibody-coated, or heat-damaged, red cells. As in RA and SLE, immune complexes may be responsible for the observed impairment of splenic function. These disappear within a few days of treatment, when splenic function also improves.

Other vasculitides

The main splenic complication of classical polyarteritis nodosa is atraumatic rupture, caused by a leaking splenic artery aneurysm. Acute fibrinoid vasculitis may result in a subcapsular infarction, but splenic abscess formation is very rare. Splenic granulomas and vasculitis occur commonly in Churg–Strauss syndrome.

Juvenile idiopathic arthritis

Splenomegaly is very common in systemic arthritis, affecting 50–75 per cent of children. It is present in 36–75 per cent of cases of adult-onset disease (Laxer and Schneider 1993), where it may be due to massive granulocytic infiltration.

Miscellaneous conditions

Splenomegaly in systemic sclerosis occurs in conjunction with portal hypertension and leucopaenia. Typical 'onion-peeled' splenic arteries are found on histology. Splenomegaly has been reported in eosinophilic fasciitis and rarely in Lyme disease. Amyloidosis, secondary to chronic inflammatory arthritis, frequently affects the spleen. It is a major complication of familial Mediterranean fever, but clinical splenomegaly is a variable feature. AL amyloidosis with infiltrative splenomegaly may require splenectomy for life-threatening splenic haemorrhage. Ultrasonographic splenomegaly occurs in 16 per cent of males with Behçet's disease (especially in childhood-onset disease), where it may be due to amyloidosis, Budd–Chiari syndrome, or splenic vein thrombosis. Gaucher's disease (acid glucosidase deficiency) results in the deposition of glucosyl ceramide in the spleen. The resulting hypersplenism causes haematological abnormalities that are reversible with enzyme replacement therapy. Splenectomy may advance the skeletal damage, so it is only indicated for massive splenomegaly or severe haematological complications.

The pancreas

Primary pancreatic disease

From a rheumatological perspective it is important to note that the pain of pancreatic carcinoma is diffuse, may be posture related, and in one-quarter of patients presents as thoraco-lumbar back pain. It may also present with the pancreatitic arthritis syndrome.

Pancreatitic arthritis syndrome

The syndrome of acute arthritis, painful subcutaneous nodules, and medullary bone necrosis complicates 2–3 per cent of cases of pancreatitis. The typical patient is male, around 50 years old, with a history of alcohol abuse, previous acute or chronic pancreatitis, cholelithiasis, or pancreatic carcinoma (especially acinar cell). It has also been observed with pancreatic calculi, after pancreatic trauma, in ischaemic pancreatitis, and with pancreatic duct arterio-venous fistulae.

Arthritis occurs in two-thirds of those with extra-abdominal manifestations of pancreatitis. It may be a presenting feature in one-fourth to one-third of all cases and has preceded the abdominal symptoms by up to 3 weeks. The pattern of arthritis is highly variable, but typically affects the ankles, knees, elbows, metacarpophalangeal, and foot joints.

The synovial fluid from an affected joint is yellow, turbid, or creamy in appearance (rarely it is clear) with a supernatant of fatty droplets. Microscopy reveals a low white cell count, with abundant droplets of necrotic fat, which may appear as strongly birefringent microspherules ('liquid lipid crystals') with a Maltese cross appearance that may be mistaken for urate crystals.

Arthritis is not a primary inflammatory synovitis, but rather results from the presence of high concentrations of free fatty acids within the joint. These are probably released into the joint following hydrolysis and necrosis of periarticular fat by blood borne pancreatic lipase. This may gain access to adipose tissue through the action of pancreatic proteolytic enzymes, also released into the circulation during acute pancreatitis. Intra-articular complement is reduced, and the intra-articular amylase concentration may be higher than that found in normal serum (Hammond and Tesar 1980).

Metastatic (disseminated) fat necrosis almost invariably accompanies arthritis, resulting in raised, tender erythematous nodules predominantly found on the lower limbs. They resemble nodular panniculitis, but frequently break down and discharge a tenacious, milky white exudate, rich in triglycerides, and heal without scarring. Like arthritis, they are the result of subcutaneous fat hydrolysis. The histological appearances are distinct: there is panniculitis with lobular fat necrosis, which is quite unlike the interlobular fibrous septal necrosis of the panniculitis of erythema nodosum. There are 'ghost cells' with dark, thickened cell walls and no nuclei, a peripheral inflammatory infiltrate and fine basophilic granular material is present in the cytoplasm and around necrotic cells. There may also be secondary haemorrhage and calcification.

The appearance of disseminated fat necrosis may predate the onset of abdominal symptoms by up to 3 weeks. In one series 40 per cent of patients with fat necrosis secondary to pancreatitis, and 80 per cent of those with fat necrosis secondary to pancreatic carcinoma, presented without abdominal symptoms (Hughes et al. 1975).

Other features of pancreatitic arthritis include: mental state changes, eosinophilia (more common where there is an underlying pancreatic carcinoma), polyserositis, and lesions in the metaphysis or diaphysis of long bones. These bone lesions are the result of intramedulary fat necrosis and fat embolism leading to bone infarction. Inflammatory changes in the intramedulary blood vessels, or vascular occlusion from surrounding interosseous oedema, may all lead to further aseptic necrosis (Waterlot et al. 1984). Plain radiographs reveal small lytic lesions in the cortex of long bones or vertebrae after 3–6 weeks. Magnetic resonance imaging of the lesions demonstrates a low signal on T_1 weighted images and a heterogeneous signal on T_2 weighted images, indicative of osteonecrosis, marrow oedema, and overlying soft tissue change [Fig. 1(a) and (b) (Watts et al. 1993)].

Pancreatitic arthritis also occurs in children, when it is almost always post-traumatic. Where no clear history of trauma is apparent non-accidental injury must be considered. It must be differentiated from other conditions such as multicentric osteomyelitis, juvenile idiopathic arthritis (JIA), or hereditary/idiopathic lipodystrophy (a cause of panniculitis, fat atrophy, venous disease, myopathy, and hepatomegaly). As in the adult disease arthritis may develop up to 3 weeks after the initial injury. Radiological evidence of diaphyseal lytic lesions and periosteal new bone formation appears 4–8 weeks later, but changes may be seen earlier on a bone scan. Subcutaneous fat necrosis occurs less frequently than in adults and the overall prognosis is good.

The treatment of pancreatitic arthritis should be aimed at reducing the degree of pancreatic inflammation and thereby the leakage of pancreatic enzymes into the systemic circulation. Aspiration of the affected joint, with corticosteroid injection, is helpful for the arthritis. When severe, disseminated fat necrosis may respond to systemic corticosteroids, although the risk of exacerbating the underlying pancreatitis is unclear.

Rheumatoid arthritis

In uncomplicated RA, asymptomatic hyperamylasaemia occurs in 13 per cent of patients (Tsianos et al. 1984). Similarly asymptomatic exocrine dysfunction has been detected in 35 per cent of patients. Clinically significant pancreatic involvement is rare. Systemic rheumatoid vasculitis involving the visceral circulation may lead to infarction of the pancreas, gallbladder, or intestine. The patient may present with only vague abdominal pain and diarrhoea. Angiography, CT scanning, or a laparotomy, is required to confirm the diagnosis.

Sjögren's syndrome

Impaired pancreatic exocrine function, leading to pancreatic insufficiency, occurs in up to half of all cases of both primary and secondary Sjögren's syndrome. Asymptomatic hyperamylasaemia and an elevated immunoreactive trypsin are frequently found in patients with a disease duration of more than 10 years, especially in those with primary disease (Griffiths and Walker 1983). Although diabetes mellitus is no more common than expected, impaired glucose tolerance is a frequent finding.

A few patients with a combination of Sjögren's syndrome, primary biliary cirrhosis, and pancreatitis have been described. The occasional patient with primary sclerosing cholangitis may display pancreatic dysfunction due to Sjögren's syndrome.

Pancreatic histological changes in Sjögren's syndrome range from relatively minor lymphocytic infiltration with parenchymal atrophy, mild pancreatitis, and fat necrosis, to significant atrophy with necrotizing arteritis. Antibodies to pancreatic duct cells, that cross-react with lachrymal and salivary duct cells, have been demonstrated in 33 per cent of patients with

(a)

(b)

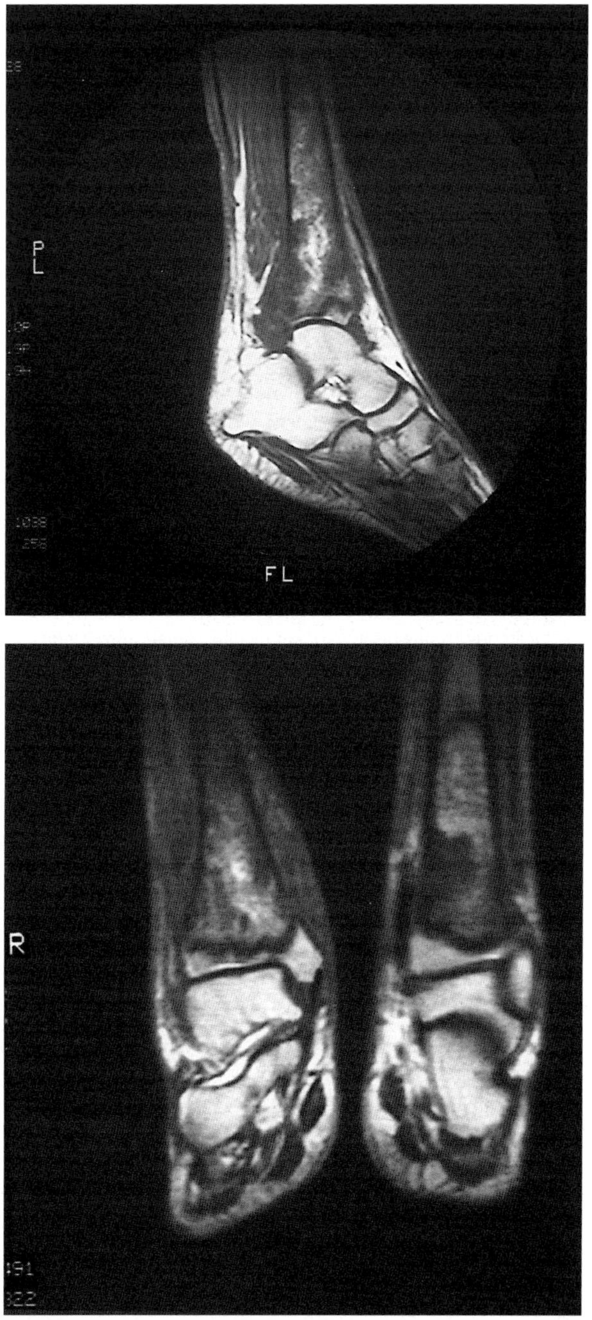

Fig. 1 (a) Sagittal T_1 weighted and (b) coronal proton density MRI of the ankle of a patient with asymptomatic pancreatitis, metastatic fat necrosis, and polyarthritis. Multiple low signal areas within the distal tibia, which expand the posterior cortex, are osteonecrotic lesions. Further abnormal areas, lateral to the tibia, are regions of subcutaneous fat necrosis. [From Watts et al. (1993). Reproduced with kind permission of the author and journal editor.]

Sjögren's syndrome, and 25 per cent of RA patients (Gobelet et al. 1983). These may be responsible for the sub-clinical pancreatic damage, but the degree of pancreatic abnormality is independent of the extent of salivary gland damage.

Systemic lupus erythematosus

Gastrointestinal involvement in lupus develops in 35–40 per cent of patients at some point in their disease. Pancreatic vasculitis, as with vasculitis affecting the other visceral organs, presents with an acute abdomen and is usually seen only in the context of a generalized systemic vasculitis, which frequently proves fatal. Ischaemic damage and necrosis may be widespread, including ulceration of the intestine, gallbladder, and pancreatitis, with fat necrosis and haemorrhage. Even in the absence of clinical pancreatitis, 25 per cent of lupus patients have abnormal pancreatic function tests, and over 30 per cent have hyperamylasaemia. Sub-acute or chronic pancreatitis occurs in 5–10 per cent of patients, but acute pancreatitis is rare.

The two main drugs used in the treatment of SLE, corticosteroids and azathioprine, have both been implicated in the development of pancreatitis. Whilst pancreatitis has been associated with both an increase and a decrease in steroid dose, it is the disease per se that is probably the most important aetiological factor. Elements such as ischaemia due to vasculitis and hypotension have been proposed, as have autoimmune mechanisms involving immune complex deposition and complement activation in pancreatic vessels. There are no significant autoantibody or HLA associations for lupus complicated by pancreatitis.

Systemic sclerosis

There is a generalized reduction in secretions from the stomach, biliary tree, and pancreas in systemic sclerosis, with evidence of asymptomatic pancreatic dysfunction in up to 61 per cent of patients. Clinically significant pancreatic complications are very rare, but fatal pancreatic necrosis due to arteritis can develop. Most reported cases of pancreatitis have occurred in patients with limited cutaneous disease (CREST syndrome).

Dermatomyositis

Pancreatitis is a rare complication of active childhood-onset dermatomyositis, which responds to immunosuppression and general supportive treatment. Childhood pancreatitis may also be due to SLE, Henoch–Schönlein purpura, polyarteritis nodosa, Kawasaki disease, and Crohn's disease. It must be considered in any child with abdominal pain, and as in the adult disease the serum amylase may be normal.

Kawasaki disease

Gastrointestinal involvement in Kawasaki disease occurs in one-third of patients. Liver dysfunction is a more common feature of this disease than pancreatitis, which must be differentiated from Reye's syndrome. Vasculitis of medium-sized pancreatic arteries, and inflammatory changes in medium and large veins, has been found at post-mortem. These changes are analogous to the vasculitis observed in the coronary arteries. Symptomatic pancreatitis only develops rarely, and then it might present before the typical signs of Kawasaki disease appear.

Wegener's granulomatosis

Clinically significant pancreatic involvement in Wegener's granulomatosis is rare, although histological evidence of pancreatic vasculitis was recorded in 9.3 per cent of historical post-mortem cases. This figure has presumably been reduced by the introduction of more effective immunosuppressive therapy.

On occasion Wegener's granulomatosis may mimic pancreatic carcinoma, by presenting with acute pancreatitis due to compression of the pancreatic duct by a mass of inflammatory tissue within the head of the pancreas. It recurs when the primary disease reactivates (Kemp et al. 1990). Parotid gland involvement by Wegener's granulomatosis is associated with pancreatic involvement. Systemic corticosteroids improve Wegener's-associated pancreatitis, which supports a vasculitic aetiology to this complication.

Behçet's disease

The pancreatitis of Behçet's disease results from pancreatic vasculitis, which settles with immunosuppression.

Polyarteritis nodosa

Although two-thirds of patients have mesenteric and renal aneurysms, clinically significant pancreatitis is a rare feature of classical polyarteritis nodosa. Massive haemorrhagic infarction of the pancreas presents as an acute abdomen.

Drugs

Pancreatitis is a recognized side-effect of the use of all of the non-steroidal anti-inflammatory drugs, especially sulindac and phenylbutazone. Several of the disease-modifying antirheumatic drugs also cause pancreatitis. Oral and intramuscular gold both cause a systemic cell mediated hypersensitivity reaction, similar to that seen in the liver. A syndrome of fever, rash, and an elevated IgE may accompany an attack of acute pancreatitis; which usually responds to withdrawal of the drug. Idiosyncratic hypersensitivity to azathioprine may result in pancreatitis, hepatotoxicity, and acute renal failure. Cyclosporin may also induce pancreatitis.

Steroid therapy itself is possibly associated with pancreatitis. The mechanisms are unknown but may include an increased viscosity of pancreatic secretions, hyperlipidaemia, fluid and electrolyte imbalance, hypersensitivity, or intravascular coagulation.

The liver

Clinically significant hepatic involvement in the rheumatic diseases is relatively rare. When detected it is more likely to be due to the effects of anti-rheumatic drugs than due to the disease itself. In addition, primary hepatic diseases, such as primary biliary cirrhosis, chronic active hepatitis, and haemochromatosis, all present with non-specific rheumatic symptoms.

Rheumatoid arthritis

Clinically detectable hepatomegaly is an occasional finding in active RA. However, scintigraphic scanning with technetium^{99m} sulfur colloid reveals hepatomegaly in one-fourth of cases. These patients are more frequently seropositive. Splenomegaly is not necessarily a coincident feature.

Rheumatoid liver

Mild to moderate abnormalities in liver function commonly accompany active RA (rheumatoid liver). Serum gamma glutamyl transferase is elevated in around 50 per cent of patients with active disease, hepatic alkaline phosphatase is elevated in up to 50 per cent and the aminotransferases are elevated in 15 per cent. A liver biopsy is generally unhelpful in this context, as it usually reveals only the features of non-specific, reactive hepatitis, that is, fatty change, Kupffer cell hyperplasia and a mild portal tract mononuclear cell infiltrate. Parenchymal inflammatory cell infiltration is rare, and definable chronic liver disease only occurs in 13 per cent of cases. There is no correlation between any parameter of liver function tests and the observed structural abnormality. However, the changes in liver function reflect the inflammatory component of the disease: the elevation in alkaline phosphatase correlates with disease activity and the abnormalities improve as the disease remits. Patients with polymyalgia rheumatica and seronegative arthritis display similar abnormalities, suggesting that abnormal liver function is a common feature of systemic inflammatory disease.

The elevation in plasma alkaline phosphatase also correlates with the amount of coincident lachrymal and salivary gland dysfunction in patients with sicca features. A cross reactivity between salivary and biliary antigens has been proposed as the mechanism for this correlation.

The historical observation that RA and JIA remit when the patient becomes jaundiced from viral hepatitis remains to be explained. A reduction in hepatic corticosteroid metabolism has been suggested. A safe and effective therapeutic exploitation of this phenomenon has not been forthcoming.

Structural abnormalities

Post-mortem studies of patients with RA dying prior to the widespread use of methotrexate, reveal the prevalence of clinically insignificant mild, diffuse hepatic fibrosis to be 11 per cent. Severe fibrosis is only present in the few cases with pre-morbid alcoholic liver disease or viral hepatitis. During the development of the American College of Rheumatology guidelines for monitoring in methotrexate-treated RA, eight histological studies involving 295 patients were reviewed for the presence of abnormalities in pre-treatment liver biopsies (Kremer et al. 1994). Only one case of cirrhosis (0.3 per cent) and 11 cases of mild fibrosis (4 per cent) were detected.

Other histological abnormalities found in the rheumatoid liver include sinusoidal dilatation, portal tract fibrosis, amyloid deposits, and lipogranulomas containing gold. These residues from intramuscular gold therapy may remain for many years. They appear on CT scanning as areas of high attenuation in the liver parenchyma. Compared to their frequency in other visceral organs, intrahepatic rheumatoid nodules are exceptionally rare.

Intrahepatic haemorrhage is a severe, life-threatening complication of rheumatoid vasculitis, also complicating mild, seronegative disease. It presents with right upper quadrant pain, hepatomegaly, hepatocellular dysfunction, and may progress to hypovolaemic shock and capsular rupture. The bleeding source is a large vessel affected by arteritis: there is transmural fibrinoid necrosis with thrombosis, aneurysmal dilatation, and focal rupture. Intra-arterial corticosteroids or hepatic artery embolization or ligation may control the bleeding.

Nodular regenerative hyperplasia

First described in a patient with Felty's syndrome, this is an uncommon hepatic abnormality, characterized by irregular hepatic nodulosis. It is most frequently found in association with seropositive RA and Felty's syndrome, notably where extra-articular features such as vasculitis are prominent. Patients with Felty's syndrome may also display portal fibrosis, and have varying degrees of liver dysfunction and portal hypertension.

Nodular regenerative hyperplasia has also been reported in SLE, Sjögren's syndrome, primary antiphospholipid syndrome, diffuse and limited cutaneous systemic sclerosis, polyarteritis nodosa, myeloproliferative disorders, neoplasia, endocrine disorders, renal failure, and following prolonged corticosteroid therapy.

The clinical features of nodular regenerative hyperplasia vary from none, to liver failure. However, the liver function tests are often abnormal, usually with an elevation in alkaline phosphatase, but the synthetic function of the liver remains intact. Pancytopaenia may also occur. Half of the patients present with complications of portal hypertension, such as bleeding oesophageal varicies, ascities, or hepatic encephalopathy. The clinical course is usually benign, but varices, hepatic rupture, or hepatic failure can be life-threatening.

The histology of nodular regenerative hyperplasia is distinctive, with obliteration of the small portal veins and atrophy of hepatocytes in some lobules, and regenerative nodule formation in others. Unlike cirrhosis, there are no internodular fibrous septae, the architectural framework of the liver is preserved, and the nodules do not form around central veins. There is little or no inflammatory infiltration. The diffusely distributed nodules expand to compress the surrounding normal liver parenchyma. Within the nodule, the hepatocytes display the regenerative features of double nuclei, prominent nucleoli, and the occasional mitotic feature.

The nodules are about 0.5 cm in diameter. As the width of a core of liver tissue obtained using a standard liver biopsy needle may be less than this, the nodular nature of the tissue obtained may not be recognized. An open wedge biopsy may therefore be required to make the diagnosis accurately.

Nodular regenerative hyperplasia probably develops as a result of liver regeneration following ischaemic injury. There is a significant reduction in the number of small portal veins, small intrahepatic arteries, and bile ducts in liver biopsies of patients with nodular regenerative hyperplasia. The obliteration of the small portal vein in the nodule may be due to arteritis in its neighbouring small artery, with thrombosis and fibrous obliteration causing the loss of the vein and the subsequent development of portal hypertension. In the non-vasculitic conditions associated with nodular regenerative hyperplasia, widespread thrombosis in the intrahepatic portal vein radicals could lead to portal tract ischaemia. This mechanism is supported by the occasional association of nodular regenerative hyperplasia occurring with pulmonary hypertension, caused by recurrent pulmonary emboli or pulmonary vasculitis. In general, the localized loss of small portal veins may cause irregular ischaemic atrophy, with compensating regenerative hyperplasia in areas of intact circulation. Progression of this sequence may lead to the characteristic histological appearance of 'waves of regeneration' within the liver.

Interleukin-6 (IL-6) is required for hepatocyte proliferation and reconstitution of the liver mass after partial hepatectomy. Overexpression of IL-6 and its receptor, IL-6R, in transgenic mice causes hepatocellular hyperplasia in a pattern identical to human nodular regenerative hyperplasia (Maione et al. 1998). High levels of serum IL-6 are found in plasma cell Castleman's syndrome, where nodular regenerative hyperplasia and sinusoidal dilatation are sometimes observed. Removal of the Castleman's tumour, or treatment with anti-IL-6 antibodies relieves the associated cholestasis.

The management of nodular regenerative hyperplasia may include splenectomy, but more frequently a splenorenal or mesocaval shunt is required to alleviate the portal hypertension. Oesophageal varicies are managed by band ligation or sclerotherapy. Patients in liver failure have been successfully transplanted.

Juvenile idiopathic arthritis

Clinically insignificant abnormalities of liver function sometimes occur in the oligo- or polyarticular forms of JIA, but are more frequent in systemic arthritis. A mild to moderate elevation in the serum transaminases frequently accompanies the hepatomegaly that is present in up to 75 per cent of cases, but it is rarely clinically significant. Some patients have elevated liver enzymes without hepatomegaly. Hypoalbuminaemia is another of the common abnormalities observed during active disease, all of which improve during remission.

Liver biopsies from children with massive, painful hepatomegaly reveal periportal infiltration by mononuclear inflammatory cells, mild fatty changes, intrahepatic cholestasis, and Kupffer cell hyperplasia. Fibrotic changes occur after acute hepatitis and sub-massive hepatic necrosis. Very rarely, systemic arthritis is complicated by chronic, mild, persistent or recurrent inflammatory liver disease with focal necrosis. Fatal hepatic failure from acute inflammatory necrosis may occur.

Similar biochemical and histological abnormalities occur in adult-onset Still's disease, the analogous condition starting in adulthood. In this disease, the abnormally elevated levels of alkaline phosphatase and the transaminases also regress with therapy. Serum ferritin is also significantly elevated. This feature can be useful in establishing the diagnosis, as it is often elevated out of proportion to the increase in the rest of the acute phase reactants (Fautrel et al. 2001).

If systemic arthritis is complicated by viral or drug-induced hepatitis, a resolution of the systemic features and arthritis may occur. The erythrocyte sedimentation rate falls as the hepatitis develops and the systemic disease remits. With the resolution of the hepatitis the reverse is observed. Such remissions usually last for 4–8 weeks, but in exceptional cases remission can be for up to 5 years (Kornreich et al. 1971).

The use of methotrexate in the management of JIA is increasing. The dose is based on body surface area, and is proportionally greater than that given to adults with RA. However, abnormalities on liver biopsy appear less commonly than in adults and significant fibrosis is almost non-existent. Obesity and serial enzyme abnormalities correlate with the Roenigk grade (Hashkes et al. 1999), so the recommendations for the monitoring of adults treated with methotrexate are being applied to children.

The drugs particularly implicated as causing acute hepatic dysfunction in systemic arthritis, which may lead to a brief resolution in systemic symptoms, are salicylates, indomethacin, and gold. However, gold therapy is now contra-indicated in systemic arthritis because of the risk of precipitating acute macrophage activation syndrome (haemophagocytic syndrome).

Macrophage activation syndrome

Acute macrophage activation syndrome may be precipitated by the introduction of new drugs, such as gold (especially following the second or third injection), penicillamine and anti-inflammatories, or viral infections, especially infectious mononucleosis. Patients present with a fever, rash, lymphadenopathy, marked hepatosplenomegaly, elevated liver enzymes, and a pancytopaenia. A consumption coagulopathy, with marked hypofibrinogenaemia may develop. The liver biopsy appearance of a proliferation of cytologically benign histiocytes, actively phagocytosing erythrocytes, platelets, or polymorphonuclear leucocytes, is pathognomonic. Successful treatment with ciclosporin underlines the importance of abnormal T-cell function in the pathogenesis of the disease.

Granulomatous diseases

Sarcoidosis in pre-school children presents with rashes, uveitis, or arthritis. The liver and spleen are involved in half of the cases. About 20–30 per cent have hepatomegaly with cholestasis, a raised alkaline phosphatase, and non-caseating granulomas on liver biopsy. Hepatic granulomata also occur in familial granulomatous arthritis (Blau syndrome), an autosommal dominant disease characterized by granulomatous synovitis, a papuloerythematous rash, uveitis, cyst-like synovial lesions, and camptodactyly.

Systemic lupus erythematosus and antiphospholipid syndrome

The frequency with which clinically significant liver disease occurs in SLE is variable. Miller et al. (1984) found only two out of 260 patients to have hepatomegaly or jaundice directly attributable to lupus. However, 20 patients had a disease-related elevation in alkaline phosphates and serum transaminases, up to five times that of normal. Runyon et al. (1980) found that 18 per cent of 238 patients had evidence of liver disease. Of these, 24 per cent were jaundiced and 39 per cent had hepatomegaly. Where available, liver histology revealed a wide range of abnormalities, including cirrhosis, chronic active hepatitis, granulomatous hepatitis, chronic persistent hepatitis, and steatosis. Three patients died from liver failure.

Systemic lupus erythematosus may be associated with primary biliary cirrhosis, and a clear distinction from autoimmune hepatitis, which often displays features of SLE, is frequently difficult. Most authorities believe that autoimmune ('lupoid') hepatitis is a form of chronic active hepatitis, with features of rheumatoid arthritis, Sjögren's syndrome, and Hashimoto's thyroiditis.

Intrahepatic veno-occlusive disease, hepatic infarction, and Budd–Chiari syndrome are all features of the antiphospholipid syndrome. Nodular regenerative hyperplasia can develop in both systemic lupus erythematosus and primary antiphospholipid syndrome associated with intrahepatic thrombosis. Severe lupus vasculitis may result in intrahepatic haematomas following the rupture of a vasculitic vessel.

Systemic sclerosis

A variety of hepatic abnormalities occur in systemic sclerosis: calcification, gall bladder fibrosis, hepatic portal tract fibrosis, lupoid hepatitis, portal cirrhosis, and primary biliary cirrhosis (especially in the limited cutaneous form). Nodular regenerative hyperplasia is rare in diffuse systemic sclerosis, but does occur in the limited cutaneous form, where vasospastic visceral Raynaud's phenomenon has been proposed to be the precipitating ischaemic injury. A single case of eosinophilic fasciitis with focal hepatitis has been reported.

Sjögren's syndrome

Liver abnormalities are commonly observed in Sjögren's syndrome. Up to 20 per cent of patients have hepatomegaly, and elevations in the plasma alkaline phosphatase and gamma glutamyl transpeptidase enzymes occur frequently. Likewise, sicca features are common in patients with autoimmune hepatitis and primary biliary cirrhosis.

Behçet's disease

Behçet's disease is a vasculitis of large and medium sized arteries which has the potential to result in aneurysmal dilatation and rupture of hepatic and renal arteries. The development of nodular regenerative hyperplasia in Behçet's disease is probably related to hepatic ischaemia secondary to vasculitis.

Drugs

Non-steroidal anti-inflammatory drugs

As a class, all the non-steroidal anti-inflammatory drugs are hepatotoxic. Specifically, meloxicam can induce an acute cytolytic hepatitis associated with antinuclear antibodies. Diclofenac can cause a syndrome of thrombocytopaenia, renal insufficiency, and hepatotoxicity, similar to thrombotic thrombocyotpaenic purpura, which responds to steroids.

Methotrexate

Experience gained from its use in the treatment of psoriasis demonstrated that methotrexate could cause significant hepatotoxicity after a cumulative dose of around 1.5 g. Hence, routine liver biopsy was advocated and a histological grading scale was developed (Table 1, Roenigk et al. 1988). However, rheumatological experience is that serious hepatic side effects are quite rare, and routine liver biopsies are now only performed under special circumstances (e.g. persistent elevations in the aminotransferases or a falling serum albumin concentration) (Kremer et al. 1994). However, liver biopsy is an invasive procedure, with a significant morbidity and mortality. It rarely demonstrates significant fibrotic change or cirrhosis, and there is only a slight increase in the incidence of portal tract inflammatory infiltration and fatty change in post-treatment biopsies. Older age and longer disease duration make these changes more likely. Pre-treatment liver biopsies are of no benefit in predicting subsequent fibrosis or cirrhosis.

Co-morbidities such as diabetes mellitus, obesity, Felty's syndrome, congestive cardiac failure, and pulmonary fibrosis increase the incidence of clinically significant liver dysfunction. Abnormalities on liver biopsy, whilst not necessarily clinically significant, are usually predictable by careful monitoring of routine liver function tests. Folic acid supplementation normalizes persistently elevated serum transaminases associated with chronic methotrexate therapy.

Gold

Gold therapy induces mild to moderate abnormalities in liver biopsy samples (Roenigk grade I to IIIB), even though liver function tests usually remain normal. Whilst gold can cause a severe, potentially fatal, hepatonecrosis, a more common side-effect is intrahepatic cholestasis. This develops either very early on in treatment, or after 12 weeks. There is often an accompanying eosinophilia. The ensuing elevation in alkaline phosphatase may continue for some weeks after the other liver enzymes return to normal. Unlike gold-induced thrombocytopaenia and nephrotoxicity, patients with this hepatic toxicity syndrome do not carry the DR3 allele.

Table 1 Grading scheme for histological liver abnormalities, developed originally for psoriasis patients receiving methotrexate (Roenigk et al. 1988)

Grade I	Normal, possibly with mild fatty change, anisonucleosis and mild portal inflammation
Grade II	Grade I with severe, spotty hepatocellular necrosis
Grade IIIA	Mild portal fibrosis, with or without fibrotic septa extending into the lobule
Grade IIIB	Piecemeal necrosis or moderate-to-severe septal fibrosis with portal bridging
Grade IV	Frank cirrhosis

Azathioprine

Azathioprine-induced hepatic veno-occlusive disease usually occurs in the context of renal transplantation or liver disease, but may complicate rheumatoid arthritis. The patient presents with jaundice, hepatomegaly, and ascities. Liver biopsy demonstrates hepatic congestion, non-thrombotic occlusion of centrilobular vessels, periventricular necrosis and fibrosis, and perisinusoidal fibrosis with sinusoidal dilatation. Azathioprine may also induce cholestatic hepatitis, peliosis hepatis, fibrosis, and nodular regenerative hyperplasia.

Miscellaneous

Leflunomide is associated with reversible liver enzyme abnormalities in 63 per cent of patients treated in combination with methotrexate, and severe hepatic toxicity (including grade IV cirrhosis) can develop. However, combining cyclosporin with methotrexate does not appear to cause significant liver enzyme abnormalities, at least in the short term (hepatic damage with cyclosporin alone is rare). Combining hydroxychloroquine with methotrexate may lead to an improvement in the liver function test abnormalities present during monotherapy with the latter drug. Hepatic damage is rarely encountered with the antimalarials. Colchicine is associated with severe hepatitis if used in excessive doses. Hepatitis may also occur as part of the syndrome of severe hypersensitivity reaction to Allopurinol.

D-penicillamine

D-penicillamine can cause liver dysfunction, with an elevation in lactate dehydrogenase, alkaline phosphatase, and aminotransaminases. These changes are reversible on discontinuing the drug. Structural abnormalities, such as mild inflammatory changes or toxic liver necrosis, are rare.

Sulfasalazine

Sulfasalazine commonly produces small, clinically insignificant elevations in the liver transaminases. On occasion, it may induce a hypersensitivity-type reaction, with severe hepatic dysfunction and bone marrow suppression. If withdrawal of the drug and corticosteroid therapy is ineffective, high-dose intravenous immunoglobulin therapy has been reported to be of benefit (Huang et al. 1998).

Infection

'Parasitic rheumatism' is an asymmetrical reactive, seronegative arthritis, which may be unresponsive to conventional therapies (Bocanegra and Vasey 1993). Eradicating the precipitating parasitic infestation, such as intrahepatic hydatid disease (Echinococcosis), relieves the arthritis.

Acute hepatitis B arthritis is a transient, symmetrical, small joint synovitis, occurring in around 25 per cent of patients during the pre-icteric phase of the disease. However, hepatitis B may also induce a chronic polyarthritis mimicking RA, which is unresponsive to therapy (Csepregi et al. 2000). Affected patients may be more at risk of methotrexate-induced liver disease. Hence, in the course of investigating a patient with presumed rheumatoid arthritis, any significant liver function test abnormality should be investigated with hepatitis serology and a liver biopsy. Antiviral therapy alone ameliorates the arthritis.

Hepatic hypertrophic osteoarthropathy

Hepatic hypertrophic osteoarthropathy is characterized by a periosteal reaction affecting the shafts of long bones. Very rarely it is also associated with a very painful arthritis. This commonly affects the knees, where recalcitrant effusions develop, but the elbows, wrists, and ankles are also affected. It frequently presents at the time of acute liver decompensation. Resolution is only achieved after a successful liver transplantation (Pitt et al. 1994).

Polyarteritis nodosa

Both classical and microscopic polyarteritis nodosa commonly affect the hepatic vessels. Hepatomegaly occurs in up to half of the patients, as do abnormalities of the liver function tests. However, liver biopsies usually show only non-specific changes. Potential complications include hepatic artery aneurysms that may rupture and lead to an intrahepatic haematoma or hepatic rupture. Necrotizing arteritis may result in thrombosis and hepatic infarction. Ischaemic cholangitis is usually a post-mortem finding and not clinically significant. Acalculous cholecystitis is rare.

Churg–Strauss syndrome

Unlike the high frequency of splenic involvement in this disease, the liver is almost never affected, except by the very rare association of primary biliary cirrhosis.

Wegener's granulomatosis

At least half of the patients with this disease have hepatomegaly, and three-fourths have an elevated plasma alkaline phosphatase.

Giant cell arteritis/polymyalgia rheumatica

Hepatomegaly is not an uncommon feature of these associated diseases. The plasma alkaline phosphatase may be considerably raised, and granulomas or hepatic arteritis can be observed in liver biopsies.

Dermatomyositis and polymyositis

Hepatic involvement in dermatomyositis usually takes the form of metastases from the tumour responsible for triggering the myositis. However, hepatomegaly and liver function test abnormalities do occur in primary dermatomyositis, and primary biliary cirrhosis occurs in association with polymyositis.

Mixed connective tissue disease

Individual cases of associations with primary biliary cirrhosis and autoimmune hepatitis have occurred.

References

Bocanegra, T.S. and Vasey, F.B. (1993). Musculoskeletal syndromes in parasitic diseases. *Rheumatic Diseases Clinics of North America* **19** (2), 505–13.

Ciaudo, M. et al. (1991). Lupus anticoagulant associated with primary malignant lymphoplasmacytic lymphoma of the spleen: a report of four patients. *American Journal of Hematology* **38**, 271–6.

Csepregi, A. et al. (2000). Chronic seropositive polyarthritis associated with hepatitis B virus-induced chronic liver disease: a sequel of virus persistence. *Arthritis and Rheumatism* **43** (1), 232–3.

Fautrel, B. et al. (2001). Diagnostic value of ferritin and glycosylated ferritin in adult onset Still's disease. *Journal of Rheumatology* **28** (2), 322–9.

Gobelet, C. et al. (1983). A controlled study of the exocrine pancreatic function in Sjögren's syndrome and rheumatoid arthritis. *Clinical Rheumatology* **2** (2), 139–143.

Griffiths, I.D. and Walker, D.J. (1983). The role of the laboratory in rheumatology. Other organs. *Clinics in Rheumatic Diseases* **9** (1), 257–69.

Hakim, A.J., Machin, S.J., and Isenberg, D.A. (1998). Autoimmune thrombocytopaenia in primary antiphospholipid syndrome and systemic lupus erythematosus: the response to splenectomy. *Seminars in Arthritis and Rheumatism* **28**, 20–5.

Hamburger, M.I. et al. (1982). A serial study of splenic reticuloendothelial system Fc receptor functional activity in systemic lupus erythematosus. *Arthritis and Rheumatism* **25**, 48–54.

Hammond, J. and Tesar, J. (1980). Pancreatitis-associated arthritis. Sequential study of synovial fluid abnormalities. *Journal of the American Medical Association* **244** (7), 694–6.

Hashkes, P.J. et al. (1999). The relationship of hepatotoxic risk factors and liver histology in methotrexate therapy for juvenile rheumatoid arthritis. *Journal of Pediatrics* **134** (1), 47–52.

Huang, J.L. et al. (1998). Successfully treated sulphasalazine-induced fulminant hepatic failure, thrombocytopenia and erythroid hypoplasia with intravenous immunoglobulin. *Clinical Rheumatology* **17** (4), 349–52.

Hughes, S.H., Apisarnthanarax, P., and Mullins, F. (1975). Subcutaneous fat necrosis associated with pancreatic disease. *Archives of Dermatology* **111** (4), 506–10.

Kemp, J.A., Arora, S., and Fawaz, K. (1990). Recurrent acute pancreatitis as a manifestation of Wegener's granulomatosis. *Digestive Diseases and Sciences* **35** (7), 912–15.

Kornreich, H., Malouf, N.N., and Hanson, V. (1971). Acute hepatic dysfunction in juvenile rheumatoid arthritis. *Journal of Pediatrics* **79** (1), 27–35.

Kremer, J.M. et al. (1994). Methotrexate for rheumatoid arthritis. Suggested guidelines for monitoring liver toxicity. *Arthritis and Rheumatism* **37** (3), 316–28.

Laxer, R. and Schneider, R. (1993). Systemic-onset juvenile chronic (rheumatoid) arthritis and adult-onset Still's disease. In *Oxford Textbook of Rheumatology* (ed. P. Maddison, D. Isenberg, P. Woo, and D. Glass), pp. 722–33. Oxford: Oxford Medical Publications.

Maione, D. et al. (1998). Coexpression of, IL-6 and soluble, IL-6R causes nodular regenerative hyperplasia and adenomas of the liver. *EMBO Journal* **17** (19), 5588–97.

Miller, M.H. et al. (1984). The liver in systemic lupus erythematosus. *Quarterly Journal of Medicine* **53** (211), 401–9.

Nakamura, H. et al. (1994). Partial splenic embolization for Felty's syndrome: a 10-year followup. *Journal of Rheumatology* **21**, 1964–6.

Pitt, P. et al. (1994). Hepatic hypertrophic osteoarthropathy and liver transplantation. *Annals of the Rheumatic Diseases* **53** (5), 338–40.

Roenigk, H.H., Jr. et al. (1988). Methotrexate guidelines: revised. *Journal of the American Academy of Dermatology* **6** (2), 145–55.

Runyon, B.A., LaBrecque, D.R., and Anuras, S. (1980). The spectrum of liver disease in systemic lupus erythematosus. Report of 33 histologically-proved cases and review of the literature. *American Journal of Medicine* **69** (2), 187–94.

Tsianos, E.B. et al. (1984). Serum isoamylases in patients with autoimmune rheumatic diseases. *Clinical and Experimental Rheumatology* **2** (3), 235–8.

Uthman, I. et al. (1996). Autosplenectomy in systemic lupus erythematosus. *Journal of Rheumatology* **23**, 1806–10.

Waterlot, Y., Peretz, A., and Cauchie, P. (1984). Febrile polyarthritis and cutaneous nodules. An unusual presentation of a pancreatitis. *Clinical Rheumatology* **3** (4), 521–3.

Watts, R.A. et al. (1993). Fat necrosis. An unusual cause of polyarthritis. *Journal of Rheumatology* **20** (8), 1432–5.

Webb, J. et al. (1975). Liver disease in rheumatoid arthritis and Sjögren's syndrome. Prospective study using biochemical and serological markers of hepatic dysfunction. *Annals of the Rheumatic Diseases* **34**, 70–81.

Wilson, W.A. et al. (1989). Scintigraphic quantitation of splenic function in, S.L.E: correlation with IgM levels in serum. *Clinical and Experimental Rheumatology* **7**, 251–5.

Further reading

Fishman, D. and Isenberg, D.A. (1997). Splenic involvement in rheumatic diseases. *Seminars in Arthritis and Rheumatism* **27** (3), 141–5.

Watts, R.A. and Isenberg, D.A. (1989). Pancreatic disease in the autoimmune rheumatic disorders. *Seminars in Arthritis and Rheumatism* **19** (3), 158–65.

Weinblatt, M.E., Tesser, J.R., and Gilliam, J.H. (1982). The liver in rheumatic diseases. *Seminars in Arthritis and Rheumatism* **11** (4), 339–405.

1.3.8 The endocrine system

Jiří Vencovský and Petr Broulík

Endocrine diseases are frequently associated with clinical rheumatic syndromes. These are mediated by altered hormone production that leads to a disturbed behaviour of connective tissue cells and to changes in the synthesis of their products. All musculoskeletal structures, including bone, cartilage, synovium, tendons, ligaments, and muscles, can be involved in processes triggered by the endocrine disorder and its related disturbances of homeostasis (Lioté and Orcel 2000). Some osteoarticular disorders can resolve or largely improve after treatment of the endocrine disease; however, some persistence either due to the irreversible changes or unbalanced disease management may occur.

Thyroid disease

Increased incidence of *thyroiditis* was described in patients with primary Sjögren's syndrome and their family members, in systemic lupus erythematosus, mixed connective tissue disease, and scleroderma. Conversely, patients with autoimmune thyroid disease have high prevalence of subclinical Sjögren's syndrome, which was found in 24 per cent. Women with rheumatoid arthritis have either hypothyroidism or Hashimoto's thyroiditis three times more frequently than non-inflammatory controls. Two studies with disparate results looked at thyroid dysfunction in polymyalgia rheumatica-giant cell arteritis. Clinically significant hypothyroidism is more common in this disease, whereas mild biochemical and antibody abnormalities are not.

Rheumatic manifestations of hypothyroidism and hyperthyroidism are summarized in Table 1.

Hypothyroidism

Hypothyroid arthropathy manifests as swelling, stiffness, and arthralgias, which affect most typically knees, metacarpophalangeal, proximal interphalangeal, and metatarsophalangeal joints. Joint effusions, synovial thickening, and ligamentous laxity can be seen, but joint tenderness and signs of inflammation are usually absent (Bland et al. 1979). Knee synovial effusions can be bilateral with occasional popliteal cysts (Dorwart and Schumacher 1975). Synovial fluid demonstrates large volumes, normal or slightly elevated cell counts, normal mucin clots, normal total protein concentration, increased hyaluronic acid concentration, and markedly increased viscosity. Radiographic findings show joint space narrowing and loose bodies without osteophytes. Bland et al. (1979) found osteoporosis with occasional erosions, rare avascular necrosis, and occasional crumbling and fragmentation. Osteonecrosis of the hip has been described and this, as well as other features of myxedematous arthropathy, was proposed to be associated with hypercholesterolaemia in hypothyroidism. In the original description of hypothyroid arthropathy by Bland et al. (1979), all 11 patients' signs and symptoms resolved after 4–12 months of treatment with thyroid replacement.

Table 1 Rheumatic manifestations of thyroid disease

Hypothyroidism
Hypothyroid arthropathy—swelling, stiffness, knee effusions
Inflammatory arthritis—RA-like, associated with Hashimoto's thyroiditis
Flexor tendon synovitis (hands)
Hyperuricaemia, hypothyroidism frequent in gouty arthritis
Carpal tunnel syndrome
Myopathy—weakness, slowed movement, muscle enlargement, cramps
Chondrocalcinosis? CPPD crystals, without pseudogout attacks
Skeletal abnormalities in children
Hyperthyroidism
Thyroid acropachy—swelling, clubbing, periosteal new formation
Periarthritis of the shoulder
Osteoporosis
Myopathy—proximal weakness, respiratory muscles may be affected

Inflammatory arthritis resembling rheumatoid arthritis may be associated with Hashimoto's disease and hypothyroidism (Leriche and Bell 1984). Seropositive cases represent probable coincidence with rheumatoid arthritis. Seronegative polyarthritis and oligoarthritis patients have milder clinical course, frequent spontaneous remissions, absence of bone erosions, low synovial fluid level of interleukin-1β, and increased frequency of HLA–DR3 (Punzi et al. 1997). This arthritis is probably independent of thyroid dysfunction and shows a clinical pattern similar to the arthritis usually found in connective tissue diseases.

Flexor tendon synovitis of the hands was found in four out of 12 patients with hypothyroidism (Dorwart and Schumacher 1975). The same authors described radiographic findings of *chondrocalcinosis* in seven out of 12 myxedematous patients and presence of CPPD crystals in six out of nine effusions. However, recent case–control studies did not confirm this association. Job-Deslandre et al. (1993) found chondrocalcinosis in 17 out of 100 hypothyroid patients compared with 10 in 100 controls. This difference was not significant. No attacks of pseudogout were observed.

Hyperuricaemia was believed to be associated with hypothyroidism; however, newer studies are conflicting. Conversely, Erickson et al. (1994) found hypothyroidism in 15 per cent of prospectively examined patients with gouty arthritis; rates being 2.5 times greater in women and six times greater in men that found in controls. The prevalence of hypothyroidism in the retrospective group was even higher: 20 per cent overall, 40 per cent in women, and 15 per cent in men. Screening for hypothyroidism in all patients with gouty arthritis should be considered.

Carpal tunnel syndrome was reported in myxedematous patients in approximately 7 per cent of cases. Dorwart and Schumacher (1975) described it in 50 per cent of their patients; however, this study was biased, because eight of 12 patients were examined for rheumatic complaints. Frymoyer and Bland (1973) reviewed 49 patients with carpal tunnel syndrome and found that five had myxoedema. Compression of median nerve by deposits of mucinous material in the tunnel, flexor tendon synovitis, and neuronal metabolic dysfunction, all contribute to the development of the syndrome.

Hypothyroid myopathy is characterized by proximal weakness, fatigue, slowed movement and reflexes, stiffness, myalgia, myoedema, and, less commonly, muscle enlargement (Kocher–Debre–Semelaigne syndrome) and cramps (Hoffman syndrome) (Klein et al. 1981). Muscle stiffness, aching, and slight weakness are present in the majority of hypothyroid patients and occasionally are the only indication of thyroid disease. Serum CK activity is elevated in most hypothyroid patients. Serum myoglobin is elevated in proportion to the severity of hypothyroidism. CK levels correct rapidly with thyroid replacement. Creatine excretion is not usually elevated. The EMG findings are variable. Usually the EMG is normal or low-amplitude polyphasic motor unit potentials are seen. Muscle biopsy findings are often normal, although atrophy, hypertrophy or necrosis of fibres, increased number of nuclei, ring fibres, glycogen accumulation, and increased interstitial connective tissue may be seen. Ultrastructural studies show mitochondrial swelling and inclusions, myofibrillar disorganization, dilation of sarcoplasmic reticulum, and T-tubule proliferation. The differential diagnosis includes polymyalgia rheumatica, fibromyalgia, drug-induced muscular disorder, and polymyositis.

Slipping of femoral capital epiphysis may be found in children with acquired hypothyroidism.

Hyperthyroidism

Thyroid acropachy is a rare condition characterized by painless soft tissue swelling of the hands and feet with clubbing and periosteal new bone formation. Stiffness is common. The classical description of acropachy included exophthalmos and pretibial myxoedema. The diaphyseal bone formation of 'soap bubbly' appearance is best noticed on the radial aspects of second and third metacarpals (Kinsella and Black 1968). Acropachy occurs in patients with treated Graves' disease, sometimes with a long interval between the onsets of the two conditions. Symptoms may diminish over years whether or not thyroid function is corrected.

Periarthritis of the shoulder was reported in 6.7 per cent of patients with Graves' disease, 3.3 per cent with toxic adenomatous goitre, and 1.7 per cent with non-toxic goitre. Symptoms may be related to periarthritic calcifications. The condition may be resistant to treatment, unless euthyroid state is achieved.

Endogenous hyperthyroidism is associated with *low bone mineral density* in most studies (Greenspan and Greenspan 1999). In a prospective epidemiological study of a large cohort of white women older than 65 years of age, a history of hyperthyroidism was associated with a 1.8 relative risk of hip fracture. Osteoporosis related to Graves' disease is reversible and bone mineral density increases significantly after 12 months antithyroid therapy.

The effect of thyroid hormone therapy on bone mineral density in patients who receive thyroxin is still controversial. It seems that replacement therapy, that is, the administration of a dose compensating a deficient secretion and maintaining a normal TSH level, does not have a deleterious effect on bone mass. Patients taking suppressive doses (>1.6 μg/kg) have significantly lower bone mineral density compared with non-users. Estrogens can be considered and were shown to stop loss of bone mineral density in these patients.

Thyrotoxic *myopathy* occurs in approximately 67 per cent of patients (Kaminski and Ruff 1994). Weakness is primarily proximal and is often out of proportion to the amount of muscle wasting. Fatigue and exercise intolerance are common complaints; respiratory insufficiency can occur. Bulbar muscles and oesophagus may be involved. CK and myoglobin are usually normal. Creatine excretion is elevated. EMG shows short and polyphasic motor unit potentials in proximal muscles. Biopsy may show atrophy of both fibre types.

Parathyroid disease

Hyperparathyroidism

Primary hyperparathyroidism is a relatively common endocrine disorder, which in 80 per cent of cases is caused by a single adenoma arising in one of the four parathyroid glands.

It mainly affects middle-aged adults and occurs more frequently in females than in males. Most cases are asymptomatic and usually detected on routine biochemical screening. Classical primary hyperparathyroidism is characterized by frank hypercalcaemia and hypercalciuria, often with phosphate depletion, as well as by clinical features such as urolithiasis, renal injury, and skeletal effects ranging from osteoporosis to osteitis fibrosa. Despite the absence of classical features, even asymptomatic primary hyperparathyroidism is known to affect the skeleton. The classical form of primary hyperparathyroidism is rarely seen. Instead, we typically see a disorder that is asymptomatic in 80 per cent of cases.

The bone disease that occurs as a manifestation of hyperparathyroidism has four main features: subperiosteal resorption of distal phalanges and clavicles, generalized decalcification, bone cysts, and the so-called brown tumours. The bone disease results in many types of deformities—bending of the long bones and deformities of the pelvis. Preferential loss of cortical bone in primary hyperparathyroidism is compatible with the known physiological effects of parathormone.

Patients with hyperparathyroidism often have articular symptoms involving the knees, shoulders, and hands. Rheumatic symptoms develop in approximately half of all patients with primary hyperparathyroidism.

There is a certain relationship between primary hyperparathyroidism and crystal-induced arthropathies. Calcium pyrophosphate deposition disease is a condition in which calcium pyrophosphate dihydrate crystals are deposited in joint articular cartilage, menisci and synovium. The main clinical presentations of calcium pyrophosphate dihydrate crystals are chondrocalcinosis (calcification of cartilage), pseudogout, acute joint inflammation due to crystal induced synovitis, and pyrophosphate arthropathy—degenerative joint disease similar to osteoarthritis.

In patients with hyperparathyroidism, *chondrocalcinosis* is relatively common finding with a reported prevalence of 18–40 per cent (McGill et al. 1984). This disease is often asymptomatic. Higher serum levels of parathyroid hormone and calcium, as well as a larger size of parathyroid gland correlate with the development of chondrocalcinosis. The prevalence of chondrocalcinosis in the hyperparathyroid patients sharply increases with age.

Pseudogout is defined as recurrent acute inflammatory arthritis due to intrasynovial deposition of calcium dihydrate crystals. An attack of pseudogout may offer a clue to the presence of an unsuspected metabolic disease such as primary hyperparathyroidism (Geelhoed and Kelly 1989). Acute arthritis develops rapidly, the joint becoming red, swollen, warm, and painful. The acute attack is usually confined to a single joint. The knee is the joint most often affected, but the disease may occur in the wrist, hand, ankle, and other joints. The post-operative attacks were seen most commonly on or after the second day after parathyroidectomy and were associated with the lowest point in serum calcium levels (Geelhoed and Kelly 1989). The diagnosis is proved by aspiration of joint synovial fluid and identification of calcium pyrophosphate dihydrate crystals. Acute arthritis after parathyroidectomy is most likely pseudogout. An attack of pseudogout may therefore be one of the most common post-operative complications of parathyroid surgery in the elderly.

Some patients with primary hyperparathyroidism have *pyrophosphate arthropathy*, a progressive destructive accelerated form of osteoarthritis. This is a relatively common osteoarthritis-like degenerative joint disease, which affects elderly individuals. Fewer white cells and polymorphs are seen but pyrophosphate crystals are present. Calcium pyrophosphate crystal deposition may also rarely present clinically as other forms of arthritis. These include a severe destructive neuropathic-like arthropathy, pseudorheumatoid polyarticular arthritis, polymyalgia rheumatica-like disease, and destructive changes in the spine. The diagnosis of chronic pyrophosphate arthropathy is established on the basis of the clinical and radiological features as well as examination of synovial fluid. When X-rays display ordinary osteoarthritis, arthrocentesis makes the diagnosis thanks to the identification of calcium pyrophosphate crystals by polarizing microscope. Large joints are usually involved but the disease can impair the spine, small joints, and tendon sheaths or synovial bursae. One can even see articular destruction. Thus, the condition of certain patients may resemble those with rheumatoid arthritis.

Erosive arthropathy of the hands and wrists has been recognized in patients with primary and secondary hyperparathyroidism (Resnick 1974). The erosions are not inflammatory and result from resorption and collapse of subchondral bone, with subsequent changes in the overlying cartilage. Unlike in rheumatoid arthritis, erosions are predominantly on the ulnar aspect of the joints, the joint space is not narrowed significantly, and the proximal interphalangeal joints are affected less often. Intraarticular and periarticular erosions of the head of humerus (*shoulder arthropathy*) were described in six patients who had been on chronic long-term haemodialysis with secondary hyperparathyroidism (Nussbaum and Doppman 1982). A similar arthropathy occurs in patients with primary hyperparathyroidism. No calcium deposits are seen in the shoulder joint and patients are asymptomatic. Joint lesions are postulated to result from a direct effect of parathyroid hormone on collagen, causing ligamentous laxity and joint instability.

The classic *neuromuscular syndrome* of primary hyperparathyroidism with its attendant potential for myopathy has virtually disappeared. A poorly characterized sense of weakness and easy fatigability reported by a substantial number of patients is clearly not related to classical neuromuscular disease. The results suggest that the neurologic component of primary hyperparathyroidism should be included among those features of the disease that have changed along with other aspects of the clinical profile of primary hyperparathyroidism (Silverberg et al. 1999).

An association between primary hyperparathyroidism and gout has been reported. Arthritis clinically indistinguishable from gout and accompanied by high serum uric acid levels has been seen in hyperparathyroidism (Bhalla 1986). In some of these patients, the arthritis become manifested only following parathyroidectomy. The proper diagnosis of gout and pseudogout leads to correct treatment. The two disorders can be easily confused and misdiagnosed in certain situations. Thus, synovial fluid aspiration and microscopic synovial fluid analysis should be done (Beutler and Schumacher 1994). In 14 of the 53 tested patients with primary hyperparathyroidism serum urate was increased above normal limits. Six months after parathyroidectomy serum urate fell significantly. Serum urate levels did not correlate with the severity of skeletal changes expressed by serum B-ALP (activity of osteoblasts) and urinary excretion of hydroxyproline. These results suggest that parathormone does not increase the part of the urate pool coming from the nucleic acids of the increased bone metabolism (Broulik et al. 1987).

Renal osteodystrophy represents a complex disorder of bone metabolism resulting from the many derangements that occur during the course of chronic renal failure. The various types of renal osteodystrophy found in patients with end-stage renal failure are hyperparathyroid bone disease, adynamic bone lesion, osteomalacia, and mixed renal osteodystrophy. Hyperparathyroid bone disease is the most common abnormality in patients on haemodialysis, whereas the adynamic bone lesion is the most common finding in patients with peritoneal dialysis (Sherrard et al. 1993). The symptoms and signs of renal osteodystrophy are generally non-specific. Bone pain, often presenting as vague aches particularly in feet and legs is common. Muscular aches and muscle weakness are also very common complaints. Additional manifestations include joint pains, carpal tunnel syndrome, and occasional extraskeletal calcifications. Beta-2 microglobulin may accumulate in bones and joint ligaments and lead to carpal tunnel syndrome, destructive arthropathies, arthralgia, chronic joint swelling, and juxta-articular radiolucent cysts (Bardin and Fritz 1993). In uraemic patients, erosive azotaemic arthropathy occurs.

Hypoparathyroidism

Various forms of paravertebral ligamentous ossification (PVLO) were detected radiologically in 53 per cent of patients with hypoparathyroidism (Okazaki et al. 1984). A significant correlation was found between the period during which the patient was untreated and the incidence of ossification. Serum levels of calcium, phosphate, and their ionic product appeared not to influence the incidence. All the patients with PVLO exhibited evidence of ectopic calcification. Soft tissue calcification involving the paraspinal region, as well as the shoulders and hips, is found in patients with idiopathic hypoparathyroidism. Calcifications of muscles and tendons and paraspinal calcifications indistinguishable from diffuse idiopathic skeletal hyperostosis may occur. In patients with an ossifying diathesis, idiopathic hypoparathyroidism acts as a stimulant resulting in exuberant skeletal hyperostosis.

Diabetes mellitus

The late complications of diabetes mellitus are related to the two salvage pathways stimulated by chronic hyperglycaemia. Increased polyol pathway activity (aldose reductase) leads to accumulation of sorbitol and fructose. Excess of sorbitol in tissues causes damage most probably by an osmotic mechanism. Both hyperglycaemia and the activation of aldose reductase result in the overproduction of free oxygen radicals and in nitric oxide downregulation. The second pathway is a non-enzymatic protein glycation, which results in the accumulation of irreversible advanced glycation products (AGE) able to generate reactive oxygen intermediates and to interact with specific cellular receptors (RAGE) on different types of cells. AGE-modified proteins acquire different properties, such as increased resistance to enzymes, increased temperature stability and mechanical resistance, diminished solubility, and elasticity. This is particularly important for proteins forming the extracellular matrix, where collagen accumulates due to increased resistance to collagenases, reduced collagen turnover, and higher vessel wall rigidity. As a result, increased vascular resistance induces a decrease in tissue perfusion, leading to hypoxemia. The articular and neurological complications of diabetes mellitus are related to both vasculopathy and neuropathy on the one hand and the abnormal accumulation of proteins in soft tissues on the other.

Diabetic hand syndrome

Diabetic hand syndrome includes limited joint mobility (LJM), diabetic sclerodactyly, palmar flexor tendon synovitis, Dupuytren's contracture, and carpal tunnel syndrome.

LJM or cherioarthropathy involves mainly the small joints of the hand (Kapoor and Sibbit 1989). However, subtalar and metatarsophalangeal joints can be affected as well. LJM is most frequently found not only in juvenile diabetic patients, but also in adults with type I diabetes mellitus and even in some adults with type II diabetes mellitus. The prevalence varies from as low as 8.4 per cent to as high as 53 per cent depending on the report. Infante et al. (2001) compared the frequency of LJM between 1976–1978 and 1998 and found a more than fourfold reduction (31 versus 7 per cent), with a decrease in the proportion having moderate or severe LJM (35 versus 9 per cent). These findings confirm the hypothesis that the prevalence of LJM has decreased, most likely as the result of improved blood glucose control during the past two decades. LJM is characterized by thick, tight, waxy skin, joint restriction, and sclerosis of tendon sheaths reminiscent of scleroderma (Fig. 1). Contractures develop in the distal and proximal interphalangeal joints, metacarpophalangeal joints, and may extend to larger joints. Contractures can be demonstrated by having patient hold the palms of the hands together (prayer sign) or by attempting to flatten the fingers and palms against a flat surface (table-top test) (Fig. 2). Patients experience stiffness, weakness, clumsiness, and decreased job performance. LJM is associated with increased age, duration of diabetes mellitus, and microvascular complications of diabetes (defined as retinopathy, nephropathy, and neuropathy). Skin biopsy shows marked deposition of compact collagen fibres in the dermis and thickening of the basement membrane of the vessels. Electron microscopy reveals thickening and reduplication of the basement membrane. Aldose reductase inhibition by sorbinil led to sustained correction of limited joint mobility in severely compromised cases (Eaton et al. 1998).

Diabetic sclerodactyly is characterized by thickening of the skin closely resembling scleroderma. This condition is associated with, but not dependent on, the presence of LJM syndrome.

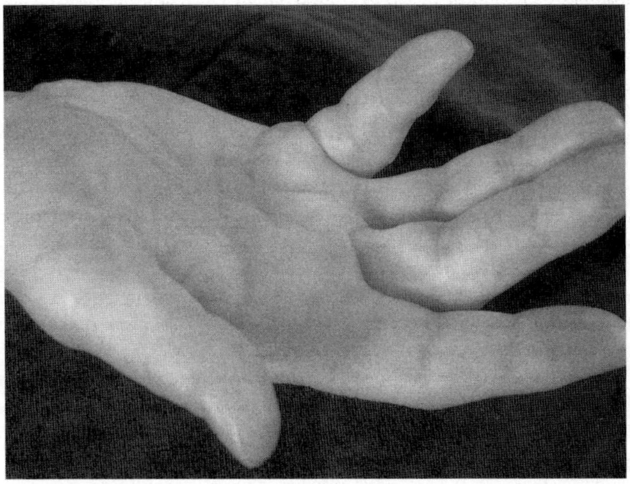

Fig. 1 A hand with thick, waxy, and scleroderma-like skin in a patient with a 30-year duration of type I diabetes. Mild flexion contractures in interphalangeal joints and incipient Dupuytren's contracture.

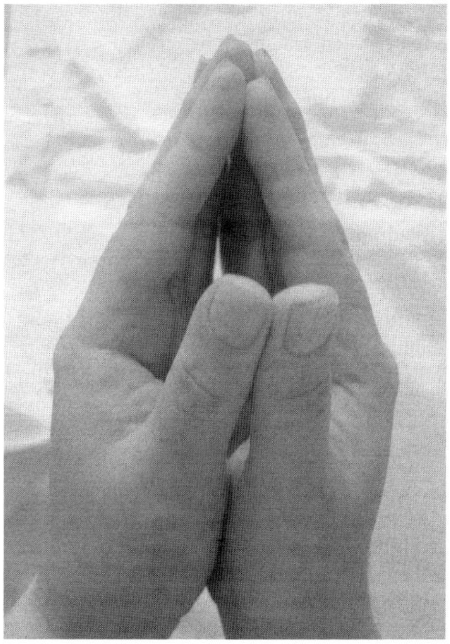

Fig. 2 Prayer sign in a patient with long-standing type II diabetes mellitus.

Multiple palmar *flexor tendon synovitis* causes 'trigger fingers' and can precede the onset of clinical diabetes. Excellent response to local corticosteroid injections in this condition as well as in limited joint mobility syndrome has been reported (Sibbit and Eaton 1997).

Dupuytren's contracture is a chronic nodular thickening of the palmar aponeurosis leading to various degrees of flexion deformity of the fingers. The reported prevalence in patients with diabetes varies from 2 to 63 per cent, depending on the patient's age and ethnic origin. Arkilla et al. (1996a) observed new development of Dupuytren's contracture in 17 out of 207 type I diabetic patients during 5-year follow-up (2 per cent per year). The prevalence is the same in types I and II diabetes and is dependent on the patient's age and disease duration. The disease is associated with macroalbuminuria in type II patients.

The prevalence of *carpal tunnel syndrome* ranges between 7 and 25 per cent in diabetic patients. Besides the compression of median nerve due to tissue infiltration, an ischaemia of the nerve secondary to microangiopathy of the vasa nervorum may be the cause. Nerve conduction measurements may distinguish carpal tunnel syndrome from diabetic polyneuropathy.

Periarthritis of the shoulder

Prevalence of *shoulder capsulitis* is 10.3 per cent in type I and 22.4 per cent in type II diabetic subjects (Arkkila et al. 1996b). It is associated with age in types I and II and with the duration of diabetes in type I patients. Independent associations exist between shoulder capsulitis and autonomic neuropathy in types I and II and with the history of myocardial infarction in type I diabetes. Bilateral involvement is more common (42 per cent) than in control subjects (5 per cent). There is a threefold increase in the prevalence of calcifications around shoulder joints in diabetics; 32 per cent of them are symptomatic.

Reflex sympathetic dystrophy of the hand may be a sequel of periarthritis of the shoulder.

Diabetic osteoarthropathy

Neuropathic arthropathy of the foot is a complication seen in about 0.15 per cent of diabetic population (Sinha et al. 1972). Diabetes is the most frequent cause of Charcot's joint. Neuropathic arthropathy can develop in both types I and II diabetes, usually after a long period of the disease, most often in patients with poor metabolic control. Changes are most frequently found in the age group 50–69 years. A very high frequency was noted by Cavanagh et al. (1994) with Charcot changes found in 16.7 per cent of diabetic neuropathy patients and with overall frequency of 6.5 per cent in diabetics. Seventy-five per cent of traumatic fractures found in these patients were previously unrecognized.

The metatarsophalangeal and tarsal joints are most often involved, while other joints affected, in decreasing order of frequency, include the ankle, knee, lumbar spine, but rarely, the upper extremity joints. The usual presenting complaint is unilateral foot swelling, accompanied with no or minimal pain, associated with skin ulcers under metatarsal heads. Patients report trauma, frequently trivial, prior to the onset of the condition. The clinical symptoms are much milder than would be expected on the basis of radiologic findings. They include swelling, warmth, redness, discomfort or pain, loosening of the articular capsule and ligaments, pathologic mobility of the joint, contractions, and development of deformities, such as 'rocker-bottom sole' due to the collapse of the arch of the foot. X-rays show initially circumscribed osteoporosis, followed by small, well-demarcated juxta-articular cortical defects. Subluxation and dislocation in the otherwise intact joints may develop. In the later stages, osteolysis, marked fragmentation, and fractures with or without dislocation occur. Within the soft tissue shards of bony debris may be observed. The changes result in bone 'whittling' and pencil deformities ('sucked candy' deformity). Typical is periosteal reaction, which in the advanced stages transforms into a thick periosteal ossification. The bone destruction can take place rapidly in weeks to months. Healing is characterized by degeneration of articular components, new bone formation, attempted repair by osteophytes, juxta-articular sclerosis, and possibly development of ankylosis.

Diabetic osteolysis is characterized by osteopenia, osteolysis, and resorption of the distal metatarsals and proximal phalanges. In contrast to neuroarthropathy, there is relative sparing of the joint.

The treatment of neuropathic arthropathy is conservative. The recommended measures are: immobilization of the affected joint, cessation of weight bearing, braces to correct subluxations. Surgical treatment is rarely indicated, arthrodesis is often unsuccessful, and joint replacement often results in loosening of the prosthesis. The most important task is to ensure good diabetic control. Usefulness of pamidronate has been reported in the treatment of Charcot arthropathy.

Differential diagnosis includes inflammatory, tumorous, degenerative processes, and neurogenic arthropathies, such as tabes dorsalis, syringomyelia, or leprosy.

Osteomyelitis is not uncommon in diabetes. It should be differentiated from extensive cellulitis that may affect the adjacent bone to give a picture of osteomyelitis. In this case, Indium-111-labelled leucocyte scanning is considered to be most accurate radionuclide study. Iodine-123-labelled murine monoclonal antigranulocyte antibodies may help differentiation between neuropathic joint and osteomyelitis.

Diffuse idiopathic skeletal hyperostosis

Diffuse idiopathic skeletal hyperostosis (DISH) is associated with diabetes, occurring in 13–49 per cent among diabetic patients (Fig. 3). Conversely, patients with ankylosing hyperostosis were found to have more frequently diabetes or impaired glucose tolerance. DISH is usually a radiographic diagnosis. It is more frequent in patients with type II diabetes and is associated with dyslipidaemia and/or hyperuricaemia in these patients (Vezyroglou et al. 1996). Hyperinsulinaemia and increased levels of growth hormone were implicated in the pathogenesis. There is no correlation between the degree of hyperglycaemia and the severity of DISH.

Other complications of diabetes

Diabetic femoral neuropathy (diabetic amyotrophy) is characterized by severe unilateral anterior thigh pain followed by wasting and weakness of the quadriceps muscle with loss of the knee jerk, becoming bilateral in approximately 50 per cent of patients (Coppack and Watkins 1991). The long-term outcome of this condition is good, with recovery apparent after 3 months and usually complete by 18 months, although some residual effects may persist. Diabetic amyotrophy may be a presenting symptom of the diabetes.

Diabetic muscle infarction is a rare cause of acute severe muscle pain in patients with diabetes mellitus (Silberstein et al. 2001). It is more frequent in type I diabetes and is usually found in patients with long-standing disease and extensive end-organ damage due to microvascular changes. The condition presents as an atraumatic tender swelling of the limb, commonly the thigh. The onset of pain is usually gradual, but can be sudden. It resolves within a few weeks, but frequently recurs. Muscle biopsy typically shows large confluent areas of muscle necrosis and oedema. The best imaging results are with T_2 weighted MRI scans, which have a fairly characteristic, but non-specific appearance showing the absence of a discrete mass and increased signal within the affected muscle. The differential diagnosis includes muscle tumour, localized abscess, haematoma, focal or systemic myositis, and deep venous thrombosis. The management should include bed rest, analgesia, tight metabolic control, and physiotherapy. Compartment syndrome, precipitated by small thrombotic/embolic syndrome, followed by ischaemia-reperfusion injury is considered to be implicated in the pathogenesis. Two cases of this condition associated with the presence of antiphospholipid antibodies have been described.

Diabetes mellitus is found slightly more frequently in patients with *chondrocalcinosis*. The prevalence of calcium pyrophosphate deposition disease in diabetes is reported to range from 8 to 73 per cent. Diabetics with chondrocalcinosis may be more susceptible to symptomatic pseudogout.

Several studies have suggested that *osteopaenia* can be observed in diabetes mellitus. While in type I diabetes the association has been confirmed in many reports, the issue is controversial in type II diabetes, where some studies also suggested increased bone mineral density in these patients. The bone turnover in diabetes is increased with lowered bone formation. No statistical difference in hip and Colles' fracture rate has been found between diabetic patients and reference group in one study (Melchior et al. 1994), and significantly fewer fractures in women with non-insulin-dependent diabetes mellitus in another report (van Daele et al. 1995).

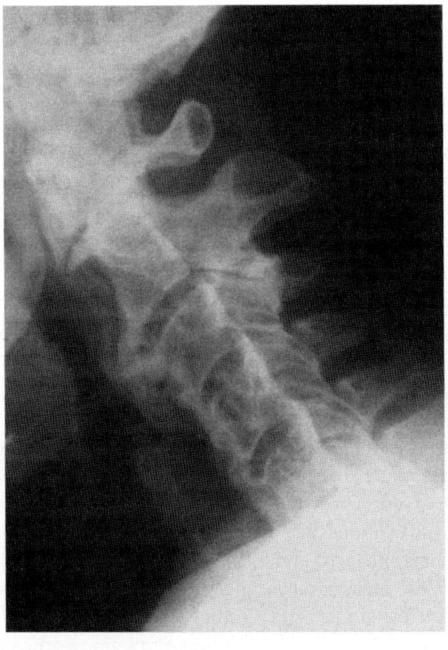

Fig. 3 Diffuse idiopathic skeletal hyperostosis in a 45-year-old diabetic man. Lateral view of the cervical spine demonstrates large osteophytes at C1, C2, and C3 and thick, flowing ossification along the anterior margins of the vertebral bodies below that level. Disc spaces are preserved.

Osteoarthritis

Evidence of an association between diabetes and osteoarthritis is inconsistent. Earlier studies, including a pathological study, suggested more severe and more prevalent osteoarthritis in subjects with diabetes mellitus. However, recent studies failed to confirm this association when controlled for age, sex, and obesity. In fact, osteophyte formation was significantly less common in patients with diabetes mellitus and, when present, tended to be less prominent than in those without diabetes.

Acromegaly

Acromegaly is usually caused by a benign tumour of the anterior pituitary gland with increased secretion of somatotropin or growth hormone after closure of the epiphyseal growth plates. Growth hormone stimulates the production of insulin-like growth factor-I (IGF-I, somatomedin C) by the liver. Both hormones have direct and indirect effects on bone cells, chondrocytes, fibroblasts, and muscle cells. IGF-I promotes DNA synthesis, cell replication, proteoglycan, and glycosaminoglycan synthesis in the articular chondrocytes.

Besides the dysmorphic syndrome, acromegalic patients frequently present with rheumatological complaints, which affect 10–17 per cent of patients at the time of onset of acromegaly and 50–70 per cent of patients with clearly identified disease (Detenbeck et al. 1973; Holt 1981; Dons et al. 1988). Musculoskeletal disorders in acromegaly are multiple and involve joint, spinal, neurological, and vascular abnormalities (Table 2).

Acromegalic arthropathy presents with a variety of symptoms. Patients start to complain usually after 10 years of onset of clinical acromegaly, but this delay decreases with patients' age. Acromegalic arthropathy affects both axial and peripheral sites and is generally non-inflammatory.

In *acromegalic limb arthropathy*, initially tightness of joints particularly in the hands is reported, which is probably secondary to thickening of the skin and subcutaneous tissue. Seventy-six per cent of patients complain of arthralgias. Typically large joints, knees, hips, and shoulders are symptomatically affected, though physical examination also shows abnormalities of the proximal and distal interphalangeal joints of the hands. Periarticular thickening is present involving both soft tissue and bone. Knee effusions are variable and usually small. Enlarged prepatellar, olecranon, and subacromial bursea contribute to joint enlargement. The typical finding is of

Table 2 Musculoskeletal disorders in acromegaly (modified from Lioté and Orcel 2000)

Peripheral joint involvement
Arthralgias
Acromegalic arthropathy
Cartilage hyperplasia
Bony proliferation
Synovial hyperplasia
Bursal hyperplasia
Premature osteoarthritis
Hypermobility
Spinal involvement
Cervical, thoracic, and particularly lumbar pain
Diffuse idiopathic skeletal hyperostosis
Neurologic involvement
Carpal tunnel syndrome
Nerve root compression
Myopathy
Peripheral neuropathy
Vascular involvement
Raynaud's phenomenon
Capillaroscopic abnormalities

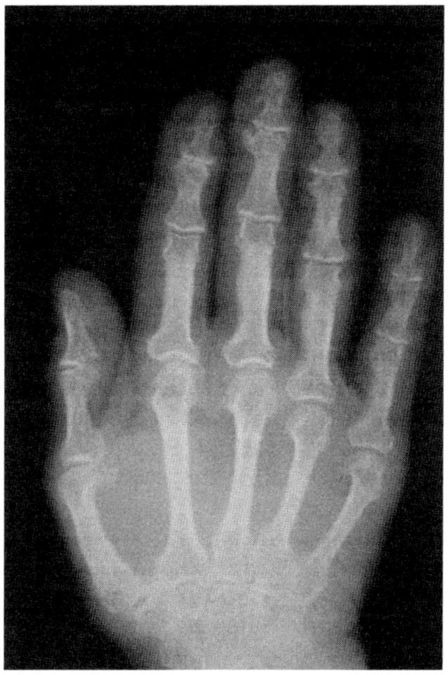

Fig. 4 Anteroposterior radiograph of the hand in a patient with acromegaly. The soft tissues are markedly thickened. The joint spaces are widened and the phalanges are squared. Tufting of the bones of the terminal phalanges is a characteristic finding.

coarse, continuous crepitus throughout movement, which is usually well maintained and only slightly painful. In late disease, increased pain and limitation of joint motion appear as a consequence of secondary osteoarthritis. Radiographic findings show thickening of soft tissues and broad metacarpals and phalanges in hands (Fig. 4). The distal tufts are prominent and spade-like. Cartilage hypertrophy leads to widened joint spaces, most marked at the metacarpophalangeal joints. The ends of the tubular bones of the hands and feet may be squared and exhibit small exostoses. An index over 40 of the medial sesamoid of the thumb strongly suggests acromegaly (longest diameter measured and multiplied by the diameter perpendicular to this line). In the feet, measurement of the thickness of the heel pad on a lateral film shows abnormal values—greater than 23 mm in males and 21.5 mm in females. The joint space in knees is widened, with hypertrophic spurring of the patella and the condyles of the femur and tibia. Later, a loss of joint space and advanced changes similar to severe degenerative osteoarthritis appear, frequently with angular deformity, especially varus. Similar changes are found in hips and shoulders, with large osteocartilaginous proliferation of the bone head, giving rise to a mushroom appearance (Detenbeck et al. 1973; Bland et al. 1979). Late changes in hips differ from classical osteoarthritis by the presence of excessive osteophytosis, moderate chronic lymphoplasmatic synovitis, an irregular pitting of the subchondral bone, and osteopaenia (Johanson et al. 1983).

Calcifications in the juxta-articular tissues occur and chondrocalcinosis may be found. Crystals of pyrophosphate or other joint debris may give rise to inflammatory episodes.

Analysis of the synovial fluid shows normal or increased viscosity, increased total protein concentration, normal to slightly elevated cell count, and sometimes an increase in hyaluronic acid concentration.

Spinal involvement includes kyphosis, non-radiating chronic low back pain (50 per cent), nerve root compression at cervical and lumbar sites, and spinal stenosis syndrome. Hypermobility, which may be seen in the peripheral joints as well, is especially noticeable in the spine. Radiographic abnormalities are characterized by new bone formation on the anterior surfaces of vertebrae and subsequent anteroposterior enlargement, increased intervertebral disc spaces, ligamentous calcification, and exaggeration of the posterior concavity, recognized as scalloping. These features are also frequently associated with degenerative spinal processes and with diffuse idiopathic skeletal hyperostosis. Palpable enlargement of the costochondral junctions (acromegalic rosary) is seen in almost all patients.

Acromegaly is associated with increased bone turnover. Increased bone mineral density was reported at the femoral neck in acromegalic patients. However, osteopaenia is also present (Johanson 1983). It may be related to a co-existent hypogonadism. Bone trabeculae are relatively thick, but widely spaced. Pathological fractures very seldom occur.

Carpal tunnel syndrome is a common complication of acromegaly seen in approximately 50 per cent of patients. It is usually bilateral and close correlation with disease activity has been demonstrated. Median nerve entrapment is often an early symptom of acromegaly.

Raynaud's phenomenon has been reported in up to 25 per cent of acromegalic patients. Morphological alterations of the peripheral microcirculation have been found by nailfold capillaroscopy with considerable increase in tortuosity of capillary loops and reduction in the density and length. This is associated with disease activity and reversible in some patients with non-active disease (Schiavon et al. 1999).

Myopathy manifests as proximal muscle weakness and decreased exercise tolerance. The weakness is insidious in onset and gradually progressive. Increased muscle size can be found, but it is not accompanied by corresponding increase in strength. Serum CK levels may be slightly elevated. Approximately 50 per cent of patients have myopathic changes on EMG. Histology is variable, both type II hypertrophy and atrophy, and type I hypertrophy have been described. The myopathy usually resolves when growth hormone levels return to normal.

Peripheral neuropathy is the result of thickening of peripheral nerves, which is associated with endoneural fibroblast overgrowth. It may take several forms: spontaneous pain, non-specific paresthesia, patchy sensory loss, or motor weakness, which may result in footdrop.

Treatment with somatostatin analogue has led to a substantial improvement in pain and functional ability. Decreased joint crepitus occurs. Symptoms of carpal tunnel syndrome usually quickly improve after lowering the growth hormone. Octreotide treatment has an immediate analgesic effect on headache associated with acromegaly. The only prospective study, in which ultrasonography to measure cartilage thickness was used, showed that after 6 months of octreotide treatment, a significant decrease in shoulder, wrist, and left knee articular cartilage was found (Colao et al. 1998). However, there is a general agreement that lowering of the growth hormone level by any form of currently available treatment does not arrest the evolution of the arthropathy once a significant build-up of abnormal cartilage has taken place (Dons 1988). Total arthroplasty in advanced cases is usually successful (Johanson 1983).

Adrenal disorders

Cushing's syndrome

Cushing's syndrome can be primary or iatrogenic, caused by long-term glucocorticoid therapy. Hypercorticism can induce osteoporosis, avascular bone necrosis, myopathy, tendinopathy, crystal-induced synovitis, and epidural lipomatosis.

Glucocorticoid induced *osteoporosis* is the most frequent form of secondary osteoporosis. It affects mainly trabecular bone and its loss starts soon after initiation of glucocorticoid therapy; peaks at 5–15 per cent loss within 6–10 months, and continues at a slower rate thereafter (Lioté and Orcel 2000). Bone resorption is enhanced and formation depressed. Glucocorticoids suppress serum levels of osteocalcin and osteoprotegerin. The prevalence of osteoporotic fractures in primary Cushing's syndrome is about 20 per cent and it is 30–50 per cent in patients on long-term glucocorticoid treatment. Young adult patients with progressive osteoporotic deformities should be inspected for endogenous production of cortico-steroids in Cushing's syndrome. Exogenous glucocorticoid induced bone loss is related to the dose and duration of treatment The highest-risk patients include elderly people, post-menopausal women, and those with prolonged immobilization. Each patient starting long-term (i.e. ≥3 months) therapy should be considered at risk. The minimal deleterious dose is still debated, but probably even as low as 5–7.5 mg of prednisolone has a negative impact on bone. However, in rheumatoid arthritis, dissecting out the relative contributions of the underlying inflammatory process, associated reduced mobility, and corticosteroids in the aetiology of bone loss has proved difficult. The issue in RA remains controversial, with some studies suggesting a possible protective effect by disease suppression. A qualitative defect contributes also to bone changes as vertebral fractures due to corticosteroids occur at a higher bone mineral density to that observed in other forms of osteoporosis. Steroid-induced bone loss is reversible. A recent controlled trial showed decreased incidence of fractures in alendronate treated patients receiving corticosteroids compared with placebo group (Adachi et al. 2001).

Avascular osteonecrosis is associated with Cushing's disease and particularly with glucocorticoid treatment. It may be multiple and bilateral. The femoral head is most commonly affected; less commonly the humeral head, distal femur, proximal tibia, and talus (Bland et al. 1979). The possible mechanism involves the induction of a hyperlipidaemic state, which increases the fat content in the femoral head, resulting in increased intracortical pressure that may lead to sinusoidal collapse and osteonecrosis. Statin therapy may reduce the risk of osteonecrosis in patients receiving steroids.

Myopathy develops in 50–80 per cent of patients with Cushing's disease, and in a majority of those with chronic glucocorticoid treatment (Kaminski and Ruff 1994). It manifests as a proximal muscle weakness and wasting, usually more prominent in the legs than in the arms. Myalgias may accompany the weakness. Ventilatory muscles may be affected. Patients usually have other stigmata of glucocorticoid excess. The fluorinated corticosteroids—tiamcinolone, bethametasone, and dexametasone—appear more likely to produce myopathy. Serum levels of muscle-associated enzymes are usually normal, but increased creatinine excretion is a classical feature. EMG findings are variable, motor unit potentials are of low amplitude and short duration. Histological studies show selective atrophy of type II muscle fibres. The muscle wasting in Cushing's disease reverses if the glucocorticoid levels are returned to the normal range. The treatment includes dose reduction to the lowest possible level, and exercise therapy.

Tendinopathy can develop as a consequence of long-term and high-dose glucocorticoid therapy. It manifests as tendinitis and tendon rupture. Involvement of Achilles' tendon is typical.

Acute synovitis induced by corticosteroid crystals may appear in about 2 per cent of patients treated with intraarticular injections, usually few hours after injection. Crystal size, low solubility in water, and phagocytosis by neutrophils initiates an inflammatory response in a manner identical to gout or pseudogout.

Epidural lipomatosis in patients receiving corticosteroid therapy is relatively common, whereas idiopathic forms are rare (Benamou et al. 1996). Epidural fat deposition excess can induce dural and cauda equina compression and cause nerve root pain, weakness of the lower limbs upon exertion, paraparesis, and bladder dysfunction. A prednisolone dose above 20 mg/day for at least 6 months or under 20 mg/day for at least 5 years' duration is a risk factor. The disease is best diagnosed by MRI. The treatment has usually been surgical with laminectomy and fatty tissue removal.

Addison's disease

Adrenocortical insufficiency is characterized by anorexia, weight loss, hypotension, and hyperpigmentation. Between 25 and 50 per cent of patients have severe generalized weakness, muscle cramping, and fatigue. Flexion contractures have been reported during an Addisonian crisis. Treatment with glucocorticoids provides rapid relief.

References

Adachi, J.D. et al. (2001). Two-year effects of alendronate on bone mineral density and vertebral fracture in patients receiving glucocorticoids: a randomized, double blind, placebo-controlled extension trial. *Arthritis and Rheumatism* **44** (1), 202–11.

Arkkila, P.E.T. et al. (1996a). Dupuytren's disease in type 1 diabetic patients: a five-year prospective study. *Clinical and Experimental Rheumatology* **14**, 59–65.

Arkkila, P.E.T. et al. (1996b). Shoulder capsulitis in type I and II diabetic patients: association with diabetic complications and related diseases. *Annals of the Rheumatic Diseases* **55**, 907–14.

Bardin, T. and Fritz, P. (1993). Rheumatological complication of dialysis. *Annals of Radiology* **36**, 74–80.

Benamou, P.-H. et al. (1996). Epidural lipomatosis not induced by corticosteroid therapy. Three cases including one in a patient with primary Cushing's disease. (Review of the literature). *Revue du Rhumatisme (English Edition)* **63**, 207–12.

Beutler, A. and Schumacher, H.R., Jr. (1994).Gout and pseudogout. When are arthritic symptoms caused by crystal deposition? *Postgraduate Medicine* **109**, 113–16.

Bhalla, A.K. (1986). Musculoskeletal manifestations of primary hyperparathyroidism. *Clinics in Rheumatic Diseases* **12**, 691–703.

Bland, J.H. et al. (1979). Rheumatic syndromes in endocrine disease. *Seminars in Arthritis and Rheumatism* **9**, 23–65.

Broulik, P.D., Štěpán, J.J., and Pacovský, V. (1987). Primary hyperparathyroidism and hyperuricaemia are associated but not correlated with indicators of bone turnover. *Clinica Chimica Acta* **170**, 195–200.

Cavanagh, P.R. et al. (1994). Radiographic abnormalities in the feet of patients with diabetic neuropathy. *Diabetes Care* **17**, 201–9.

Colao, A. et al. (1998). Reversibility of joint thickening in acromegalic patients: an ultrasonography study. *Journal of Clinical Endocrinology and Metabolism* **83**, 2121–5.

Coppack, S.W. and Watkins, P.J. (1991). The natural history of diabetic femoral neuropathy. *Quarterly Journal of Medicine* **288**, 307–13.

Detenbeck, L.C. et al. (1973). Peripheral joint manifestations of acromegaly. *Clinical Orthopaedics and Related Research* **91**, 119–27.

Dons, R.F. et al. (1988). Arthropathy in acromegalic patients before and after treatment: a long-term follow-up study. *Clinical Endocrinology* **28**, 515–24.

Dorwart, B.B. and Schumacher, H.R. (1975). Joint effusions, chondrocalcinosis, and other rheumatic manifestations of hypothyroidism. A clinicopathological study. *American Journal of Medicine* **59**, 780–90.

Duffin, A.C. et al. (1999). Limited joint mobility in the hands and feet of adolescents with type 1 diabetes mellitus. *Diabetic Medicine* **16**, 125–30.

Eaton, R.P. et al. (1998). A commentary on 10 years of aldosereductase inhibition for limited joint mobility in diabetes. *Journal of Diabetes Complications* **12**, 34–8.

Erickson, A.R. et al. (1994). The prevalence of hypothyroidism in gout. *The American Journal of Medicine* **97**, 231–4.

Frymoyer, J.W. and Bland, J.H. (1973). Carpal-tunnel syndrome in patients with myxedematous arthropathy. *Journal of Bone and Joint Surgery—American* **55**, 78–82.

Geelhoed, G.W. and Kelly, T.R. (1989). Pseudogout as a clue and complication in primary hyperparathyroidism. *Surgery* **106**, 1036–41.

Greenspan, S.L. and Greenspan, F.S. (1999). The effect of thyroid hormone on skeletal integrity. *Annals of Internal Medicine* **130**, 750–8.

Holt, P.J.L. (1981). Locomotor abnormalities in acromegaly. *Clinics in Rheumatic Diseases* **7**, 689–709.

Infante, J.R. et al. (2001). Changes in frequency and severity of limited joint mobility in children with type 1 diabetes mellitus between 1976–78 and 1998. *Journal of Pediatrics* **138**, 33–7.

Job-Deslandre, C. et al. (1993). Does hypothyroidism increase the prevalence of chondrocalcinosis. *British Journal of Rheumatology* **32**, 197–8.

Johanson, N.A. et al. (1983). Acromegalic arthropathy of the hip. *Clinical Orthopaedics and Related Research* **173**, 130–9.

Kaminski, H.J. and Ruff, R.L. (1994). Endocrine myopathies. In *Myology* (ed. A.G. Engel and C. Franzini-Armstrong), pp. 1726–53. New York: McGraw-Hill.

Kapoor, A. and Sibbit, W.L. (1989). Contractures in diabetes mellitus: the syndrome of limited joint mobility. *Seminars in Arthritis and Rheumatism* **18**, 168–80.

Kinsella, R.A., Jr. and Back, D.K. (1968). Thyroid acropachy. *Medical Clinics of North America* **52**, 393–8.

Klein, I. et al. (1981). Hypothyroidism presenting as muscle stiffness and pseudo-hypertrophy: Hoffman's syndrome. *American Journal of Medicine* **70**, 891–4.

Leriche, N.G.H. and Bell, D.A. (1984). Hashimoto's thyroiditis and polyarthritis: a possible subset of seronegative polyarthritis. *Annals of the Rheumatic Diseases* **43**, 594–8.

Lioté, F. and Orcel, P. (2000). Osteoarticular disorders of endocrine origin. *Baillières Clinical Rheumatology* **14**, 251–76.

McGill, P.E., Grange, A.T., and Royston, C.S. (1984). Chondrocalcinosis in primary hyperparathyroidism. Influence of parathyroid activity and age. *Scandinavian Journal of Rheumatology* **13**, 56–8.

Melchior, T.M., Sørensen, H., and Torp-Pedersen, C. (1994). Hip and distal fracture rates in peri- and postmenopausal insulin-treated diabetic females. *Journal of Internal Medicine* **236**, 203–8.

Nussbaum, A.J. and Doppman, J.L. (1982). Shoulder arthropathy in primary hyperparathyroidism. *Skeletal Radiology* **9**, 98–102.

Okazaki, T. et al. (1984). Ossification of the paravertebral ligaments: a frequent complication of hypoparathyroidism. *Metabolism* **33**, 710–13.

Punzi, L. et al. (1997). Clinical, laboratory and immunogenetic aspects of arthritis associated with chronic lymphocytic thyroiditis. *Clinical and Experimental Rheumatology* **15**, 373–80.

Resnick, D.L. (1974). Erosive arthritis of the hand and wrist in hyperparathyroidism. *Radiology* **110**, 263–8.

Sherrard, D.J. et al. (1993). The spectrum of bone disease in end-stage renal failure—an evolving disorder. *Kidney International* **43**, 436–42.

Schiavon, F. et al. (1999). Morphologic study of microcirculation in acromegaly by capillaroscopy. *Journal of Clinical Endocrinology and Metabolism* **84**, 3151–5.

Sibbit, W.L., Jr. and Eaton, R.P. (1997). Corticosteroid responsive tenosynovitis is a common pathway for limited joint mobility in the diabetic hand. *Journal of Rheumatology* **24**, 931–6.

Silberstein, L. et al. (2001). A unexpected cause of muscle pain in diabetes. *Annals of the Rheumatic Diseases* **60**, 310–12.

Silverberg, S.J. et al. (1999). Therapeutic controversies in primary hyperparathyroidism. *Journal of Clinical Endocrinology and Metabolism* **84**, 2275–82.

Sinha, S., Munichoodappa, C.S., and Kozak, G.P. (1972). Neuro-arthropathy (Charcot joints) in diabetes mellitus: clinical study in 101 patients. *Medicine (Baltimore)* **51**, 191–210.

van Daele, P.L. et al. (1995). Bone density in non-insulin-dependent diabetes mellitus. The Rotterdam Study. *Annals of Internal Medicine* **122**, 409–14.

Vezyroglou, G. et al. (1996). A metabolic syndrome in diffuse idiopathic skeletal hyperostosis. A controlled study. *Journal of Rheumatology* **23**, 672–6.

1.3.9 Links between malignant disease and musculoskeletal conditions

Deborah P.M. Symmons

Introduction

The links between malignant disease and musculoskeletal conditions seem to work in every possible direction. Both primary and secondary tumours may produce musculoskeletal symptoms, either because the musculoskeletal system is directly involved or as a paraneoplastic process. Malignancy may be a complication of a number of rheumatic diseases or their therapy. Finally, musculoskeletal conditions may develop as a side-effect of cancer chemotherapy. This chapter explores all these connections.

Malignant conditions presenting with musculoskeletal symptoms

Primary musculoskeletal tumours

Primary musculoskeletal tumours affecting either bone or soft tissue are relatively rare. Patients with suspected or confirmed primary malignant musculoskeletal tumours should be referred to specialist cancer centres for assessment and treatment.

Benign bone tumours

Osteoid osteomas are benign, slow-growing tumours which present most often in adolescents and young adults.

Malignant bone tumours

Osteosarcoma, chondrosarcoma, and Ewing's sarcoma together account for 75 per cent of malignant bone tumours. The incidence rates for bone tumours are generally higher for men than for women (Table 1).

Osteosarcoma is the most common primary malignant bone tumour. It has a bimodal distribution with peaks at age 10–19 and over 75. Seventy-five per cent of cases occur before the age of 30, mostly during the adolescent growth spurt. It has no gender or racial predilection. Upto 50 per cent of patients over the age of 60 with osteosarcoma have Paget's disease (Huvos 1986). Other risk factors for osteosarcoma are a previous hereditary retinoblastoma, the Li–Fraumeni syndrome (a germ-line mutation in the tumour-suppressor gene p53) (Arndt and Crist 1999), hereditary multiple exostoses, fibrous dysplasia, and prior exposure to ionizing radiation.

Osteosarcomas generally occur in the metaphyses of long tubular bones, especially the distal femur, proximal tibia, and proximal humerus. They present with constant bone pain which is unrelieved by rest. Later, a palpable mass may appear. They are rapidly progressive. Approximately 20 per cent of tumours have metastasized by the time of presentation, 90 per cent to the lungs and 10 per cent to bone (Kaste et al. 1999). MRI scanning is the best method of assessing the extent of the tumour and detecting skip metastases. Treatment is with pre- and post-operative chemotherapy and surgery. Osteosarcomas are relatively insensitive to radiotherapy.

Chondrosarcomas account for 10–13 per cent of malignant bone tumours. Incidence increases with age. Some cases occur as a complication of multiple enchondromatatosis. They usually present with pain and a firm swelling. They are relatively slow growing.

Ewing's sarcoma is an undifferentiated round-cell neoplasm. Around 95 per cent of patients have a t(11 : 22) or t(21 : 22) translocation (Denny 1996). Ewing's sarcoma is the second most common bone tumour in children and adolescents. Boys are affected slightly more often than girls (1.5 : 1). It is rare in Black or Asian children. It affects the metaphyses of long bones, the diaphyses of long bones, and flat bones with approximately equal frequency. It may also arise in soft tissue. It usually presents with pain and/or swelling in a bone or joint. The patient often has constitutional features such as fever and weight loss. Around 25 per cent of tumours have metastasized at the time of presentation: 50 per cent to lungs, 25 to bone, and 25 to bone marrow. Treatment is with multiagent chemotherapy and surgery. The tumours are radiosensitive but there is a high incidence of second cancers (10 per cent after 20 years).

Benign synovial and soft tissue tumours

Pigmented villonodular synovitis (PVNS) is a group of rare disorders characterized by localized or diffuse nodular thickening of the synovial membrane of joints, tendon sheaths, or bursae.

Synovial chondromatosis is a rare condition, characterized by the formation of multiple nodules of hyaline cartilage within the synovial membrane of joints, tendon sheaths, or bursae. If the nodules undergo endochondral ossification the condition is called synovial osteochondromatosis. It may be primary, or secondary to osteoarthritis or trauma. The condition is benign and predominantly affects one large joint.

Table 1 Age adjusted incidence and median survival rates for primary bone and connective tissue tumours by ethnic group and gender: United States 1973–1995

	Incidence (rate per million persons)				Median survival (months)			
	White		Black		White		Black	
	Male	Female	Male	Female	Male	Female	Male	Female
Bone	11.8	7.7	11.0	5.9	64	112	83	⩾120
Osteosarcoma	4.1	2.7	7.0	0.7	41	80	38	⩾120
Chondrosarcoma	3.5	2.1	0.0	3.2	⩾120	⩾120	⩾120	⩾120
Ewing's sarcoma	1.6	1.7	0.0	0.0	36	⩾120	⩾120	24
Soft tissue	29.7	20.9	28.8	20.8	77	95	73	113
Multiple myeloma	49.0	31.0	104.0	72.0	25	22	27	29

Source: Adapted from Praemer et al. (1999).

Malignant synovial and soft tissue tumours

Soft tissue sarcomas may arise from any of the mesodermal tissues of the limbs (50 per cent), trunk and retroperitoneum (40 per cent), or head and neck (10 per cent). Patients with neurofibromatosis, Gardner's syndrome (a rare autosomal dominant disorder characterized by multiple osteomas, polyposis coli leading to carcinoma and soft tissue sarcoma), Werner's syndrome (a rare autosomal-recessive disorder characterized by juvenile cataracts, scleroderma-like skin changes and accelerated aging), tuberous sclerosis, and Li–Fraumeni kindreds (p53 mutations) are at increased risk of soft tissue sarcomas.

Synovial sarcomas predominantly affect adolescents and adults aged under 50. The malignant cells probably arise from a primitive mesenchymal precursor cell and the term synovial sarcoma is a misnomer. In fact, less than 10 per cent of these tumours arise from the synovium. Around two-thirds of these tumours occur in the limbs near large joints. The popliteal fossa is the most frequently affected site. Symptoms have often been present for 2–4 years prior to diagnosis. Synovial sarcomas present as enlarging deep-seated soft tissue masses which are painful in around 50 per cent of cases. X-ray shows a well-circumscribed soft tissue mass which is invading adjacent bone in around 20 per cent of cases and shows stippled calcificaton in around 30 per cent of cases. MRI scans delineate the anatomic extent of disease. Cytogenetic techniques reveal the specific reciprocal chromosome translocation t(X : 18) (p11.2; q11.2). The tumour has a poor prognosis with a high rate of local recurrence followed by metastasis to regional lymph nodes, lung, and bone.

Rhabdomyosarcomas account for around 50 per cent of soft tissue sarcomas in children (Arndt and Crist 1999). Two-thirds occur before the age of 10. White children are affected more often than Black and Asian children. There are two histological types: embryonal (80 per cent) and alveolar (20 per cent). Rhabdomyosarcomas may occur in any muscle. Tumours affecting the orbit present with proptosis. They are mostly embryonal and have a high rate of cure. Limb tumours are usually alveolar and 50 per cent have already spread to the regional lymph nodes at the time of diagnosis. They have a less favourable outcome. Treatment is with chemotherapy and local resection. Metastases are treated with radiotherapy.

Secondary tumours

Skeletal metastases

Ninety-five per cent of malignant bone tumours are due to metastatic spread. The lumbar vertebrae, pelvis, femur, and ribs are most commonly affected. The tumours which most commonly metastasize to bone are carcinoma of the prostate, breast, kidney, and thyroid. On a tumour-by-tumour basis, lung cancer metastasizes less frequently but, as lung cancer is so common, it is actually second only to breast cancer as a source of bony secondary deposits.

Metastatic arthritis

Synovial metastasis without adjacent bone involvement is relatively uncommon. The knee, followed by the hip and shoulder, was the most frequently involved joint in a review of 47 cases of metastatic arthritis (Schwarzer et al. 1990). Arthritis was the initial manifestation of malignant disease in over 50 per cent of the cases. Carcinoma of the breast, gastrointestinal tumours, bronchogenic carcinoma, and melanoma are the most common malignancies to metastasize to synovium (Caldwell and McCallum 1986). The arthritis is usually asymmetrical. Metastatic deposits in the small joints of the hand are rare. Joint fluid is usually haemorrhagic and may contain malignant cells. Alternatively the diagnosis may be obtained from histological examination of a synovial biopsy. Radiographs show a destructive arthritis.

Leukaemic osteoarticular disease

Around 4 per cent of adults and 14–24 per cent of children with acute leukaemia develop an asymmetrical or migratory polyarthritis (Rennie and Auchterlonie 1991). In children, the arthritis may be the presenting feature. There are a number of possible underlying mechanisms including: leukaemic infiltration of the synovium, haemorrhage into the joint or surrounding structures, reactive synovitis adjacent to bony, periosteal or capsular lesions, and gout. The knee and ankle are most frequently affected. In chronic leukaemia, the arthritis tends to be a late manifestation and is frequently symmetrical.

Patients with leukaemic arthritis often have severe joint pain which is disproportionate to the degree of arthritis. The diagnosis is generally made from the peripheral blood film or bone marrow examination. Synovial fluid rarely contains leukaemic cells. The symptoms often resolve rapidly after chemotherapy has been commenced but may recur with relapse of the leukaemia.

In addition, leukaemic patients may complain of bone pain. In children, this appears to be sharp in quality and generally affects the limbs. In adults the pain is more dull and tends to affect the spine and ribs. The cause of the bone pain is unclear. X-ray may show osteolytic lesions, periosteal reaction, or metaphyseal rarefaction. Bone scan may be helpful but the changes are not specific. In addition patients with leukaemia may develop back pain due to meningeal involvement or osteoporotic fractures.

Lymphomatous osteoarticular disease

Bone involvement leading to bone pain is the most common osteoarticular feature of lymphomas and occurs in up to 25 per cent of patients with non-Hodgkin's lymphoma (NHL). In a review of the literature, McDonagh et al. (1994) found 10 cases of polyarthritis and seven of monoarthritis associated with NHL. They were predominantly T-cell lymphomas. The lymphoma can be diagnosed on synovial biopsy. Other osteoarticular features include hypertrophic osteoarthropathy and gout.

Paraneoplastic syndromes

Paraneoplastic syndromes are remote, non-metastatic effects of a tumour. They may precede the diagnosis of the underlying tumour (although seldom by more than 2 years), occur at the same time as the tumour becomes manifest, or develop when metastases appear. Paraneoplastic syndromes occur as a result of secretion of substances such as hormones, hormone-like peptides, or cytokines by the tumour; or as a result of autoimmmune phenomena. In some paraneoplastic syndromes the underlying mechanism is unknown.

Paraneoplastic syndromes due to hormones include Cushing's syndrome due to ectopic ACTH, and humoral hypercalcaemia due to parathyroid hormone-related protein.

Patients with malignant diseases (especially B-cell malignancies) may develop a wide range of autoantibodies including rheumatoid factor (RF), antinuclear antibodies (ANA), anti-DNA or antiphospholipid antibodies (aPL), or antibodies directed against histones, Ro, La, Sm, or RNP (Abu-Shakra et al. 2001). Raised levels of aPL may be associated with thrombosis in patients with cancer.

Patients with malignancy may develop autoantibodies directed against self-antigens expressed by the tumour cells as part of the antitumour immune response. These self antigens include oncoproteins, tumour suppressor proteins, proliferation-associated antigens, and onconeural antigens (Abu-Shakra et al. 2001). Screening for autoantibodies to p53, the most studied tumour suppressor protein, may be used to detect carcinoma in patients at high risk of developing malignancy. Oncoproteins play a part in the control of cell growth and differentiation. Antioncoprotein antibodies have been detected in patients with breast, lung, colon, and ovarian cancers. Their clinical significance is unclear.

Onconeural antigens are normally expressed only in the nervous system but, as a result of gene activation or depression, they can be expressed on tumours such as small cell lung cancer, breast cancer, Hodgkin's disease, and ovarian cancer. Anti-onconeural antibodies may be responsible for paraneoplastic neurological syndromes such as the Eaton–Lambert syndrome, cerebellar degeneration, or the stiff-person syndrome.

The major musculoskeletal paraneoplastic syndromes are shown in Table 2.

Paraneoplastic myopathies

Dermatomyositis

The association of cancer with dermatomyositis (DM) and polymyositis (PM) is discussed later. Zantos et al. (1994) performed a meta-analysis of four case control or cohort studies which included 565 cases of PM and 513 cases of DM. Cancer risk was increased both before and after the diagnosis of DM, but for PM cancer risk was only increased after the diagnosis of myositis. The finding of a high cancer rate before the diagnosis of DM suggests that DM is a paraneoplastic condition.

Table 2 Paraneoplastic rheumatic syndromes

Myopathies
Dermatomyositis
Eaton–Lambert myasthenic syndrome
Stiff-person syndrome
Arthropathies
Hypertrophic osteoarthropathy
Carcinomatous polyarthritis
Amyloid arthritis
Secondary gout
Vascular
Raynaud's phenomenon
Vasculitis
Erythromelalgia
Soft tissue
Fasciitis
Erythema nodosum
Panniculitis
Scleroderma
POEMS syndrome
Sweet's syndrome
Miscellaneous
Autoantibodies
Reflex sympathetic dystrophy
Oncogenic osteomalacia
Cryoglobulinaemia
Relapsing polychondritis

Eaton–Lambert myasthenic syndrome

The Eaton–Lambert syndrome is a rare disorder of neuromuscular transmission due to reduced release of acetyl choline from motor and cholinergic autonomic nerve terminals (Fam 2000). Many patients have auto-antibodies directed against voltage-gated calcium channel epitopes. The syndrome is characterized by myalgia and weakness (especially of the pelvic girdle and leg muscles), fatigability, and hyporeflexia. Patients often present with an abnormal gait. Autonomic symptoms include dry mouth, reduced sweating, postural hypotension, and impotence. There is an associated malignancy, usually a small-cell-lung carcinoma, in around 70 per cent of men and 25 per cent of women. Unlike myasthenia gravis, the Eaton–Lambert syndrome responds poorly to edrophonium and pyridostigmine. 4-Aminopyridine, which enhances release of acetylcholine, may be helpful. The syndrome may improve following eradication of the tumour.

Stiff-person syndrome

The stiff-person syndrome is a rare disorder of the central nervous system characterized by fluctuating but progressive muscle rigidity and spasms. Around 60 per cent of patients have autoantibodies to glutamic acid decarboxylase. In this group of patients, the stiff-person syndrome is usually associated with organ-specific autoimmune diseases, in particular insulin-dependent diabetes. Stiff-person syndrome has also been described in association with small-cell-lung cancer, breast cancer, Hodgkin's disease, and thymoma. These patients do not have antiglutamic acid decarboxylase antibodies. The paraneoplastic syndrome appears to be associated with autoantibodies directed against a neuronal protein on the synaptic terminal that binds the vesicle core protein adaptor AP2 and dynamin (Folli et al. 1993). Binding of this autoantibody prevents the release of neurotransmitters. The syndrome may respond to steroid therapy or removal of the tumour.

Paraneoplastic arthropathies

Hypertrophic osteoarthropathy (HOA)

HOA is characterized by clubbing of the fingers and toes, and periostitis of the distal ends of the tubular bones (Martinez-Lavin et al. 1993). Three incomplete forms are recognized: clubbing alone, periostosis without clubbing in the setting of any of the illnesses known to be associated with HOA (Fig. 1), and pachyderma associated with minor manifestations such as gynaecomastia, folliculitis, and hyperhydrosis.

Hereditary HOA (pachydermoperiostosis) affects male members of the family more commonly (in a ratio of 9 : 1). Isolated familial clubbing is more common and may represent an incomplete expression of the syndrome.

Clubbing may be asymptomatic or associated with a burning pain at the tips of the fingers. The bone changes of clubbing are seen first on X-rays of the feet. They include acro-osteolysis and tuftal overgrowth. Periostitis may cause periarticular pain or a deep-seated bone pain, which is aggravated by dependency. X-rays of affected long bones may show periosteal elevation as a sign of new bone formation. Isotope bone scans show increased uptake by the cortices of the shafts of affected bones (the so-called tramline sign). Some patients with HOA develop a symmetrical oligo- or polyarthritis. The knees, ankles, wrists, and MCPs are most frequently affected. Synovial fluid is non-inflammatory.

Ninety per cent of cases of HOA in the industrialized world are associated with non-small-cell carcinoma (adenocarcinoma) of the lung. Around 10 per cent of patients with this type of cancer have HOA. Proportionately, men are affected more often than women. HOA may precede the diagnosis of cancer by several months. HOA much less commonly accompanies

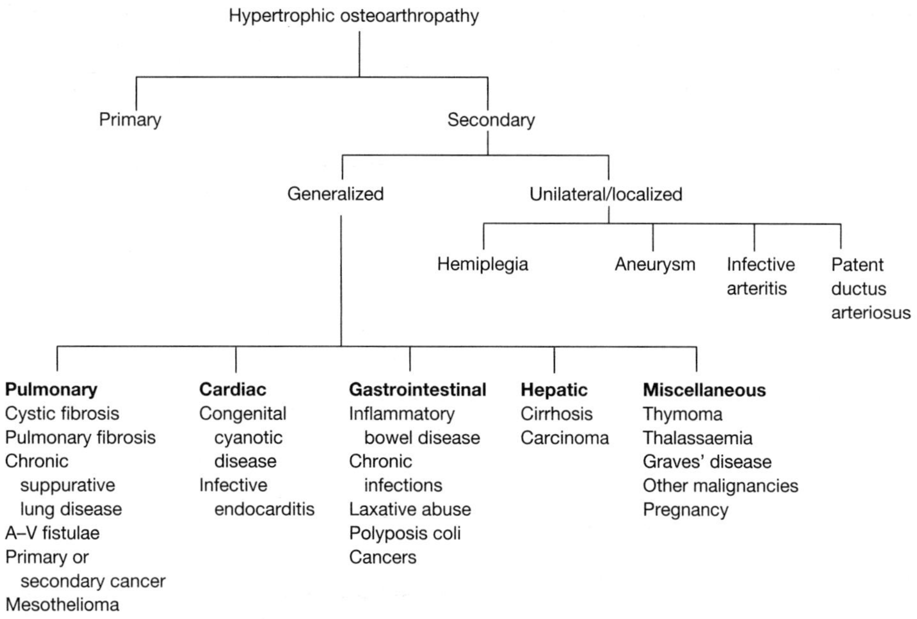

Fig. 1 Medical conditions known to be associated with HOA.

metastatic than primary lung cancer, and is more often associated with sarcomatous than carcinomatous metastases.

The symptoms of HOA may resolve rapidly after the treatment of the tumour. They may also resolve promptly after a peripheral vagotomy on the side of the tumour. The pathogenesis of the syndrome remains unclear.

Carcinomatous polyarthritis

Carcinomatous polyarthritis may be the presenting feature of a malignancy. It affects men and women with equal frequency. In 80 per cent of female patients, it is associated with breast cancer. In men, the primary tumour is most commonly in the lung. The most easily recognizable form of carcinomatous polyarthritis is characterized by an abrupt onset, patient aged over 60, predominant lower limb involvement with sparing of the hands and wrists (Caldwell and McCallum 1986). The mean time between the onset of arthritis and diagnosis of malignancy is 10 months. The arthritis is usually seronegative and non-erosive. Synovial fluid is mildly inflammatory and the ESR may be slightly elevated. In some patients, the arthritis more closely resembles RA with symmetric involvement of the MCP and PIP joints and may even be seropositive (Stummvoll et al. 2001). The favoured explanation is that there is cross reactivity of antigens shared by the neoplasm and synovium. The arthritis often (but not always) responds to NSAIDs and steroids. It resolves rapidly when the tumour is ablated.

Amyloid arthritis

Approximately 5 per cent of patients with multiple myeloma develop amyloid arthritis as a result of synovial deposition of monoclonal light chains (AL amyloid) secreted by the malignant plasma cells (Fam 2000).

Secondary gout

Hyperuricaemia and secondary gout may be associated with a number of myelo- and lymphoproliferative disorders including polycythaemia rubra vera, chronic myeloid leukaemia, lymphomas, and myelomas. It occasionally complicates carcinomas. Chemotherapy of these disorders can lead to severe hyperuricaemia as a result of destruction of large numbers of malignant cells. This can lead to acute renal failure as a result of urate crystal and stone formation. This can be prevented by prophylactic allopurinol and maintaining hydration.

Paraneoplastic vascular syndromes

Raynaud's phenomenon

Raynaud's phenomenon has been described as a presenting feature of a wide variety of malignancies including carcinomas of the oesophagus, stomach, ileum, pancreas, kidney, lung, breast, ovary, cervix, prostate, and maxillary antrum, as well as lymphoma, acute lymphocytic leukaemia, melanoma, and atrial myxoma. The onset is usually concurrent with the diagnosis of the tumour, although it may precede the diagnosis of malignancy by up to 2 years. The digital ischaemia may be unilateral and may progress to necrosis. In some cases, the Raynaud's phenomenon resolves following resection of the tumour. The pathogenesis is unknown. One case report described a carcinoma of the cervix which secreted interleukin-6 which was suspected to be the vasospastic stimulus (Murashima et al. 1992).

Paraneoplastic vasculitis

A wide variety of vasculitides has been described in association with malignancy. This includes small vessel (leucocytoclastic) vasculitis (LCV), Henoch–Schönlein purpura, polyarteritis nodosa, and temporal arteritis. Lymphoproliferative and haematopoietic malignancies (LHM) are associated with vasculitis more often than solid tumours. The solid tumours most commonly associated with vasculitis are non-small-cell lung cancer, prostate, breast, colon, and renal carcinoma (Kurzrock et al. 1994). The LHM most commonly associated with vasculitis are leukaemia (especially hairy cell leukaemia), multiple myeloma, and NHL (Greer et al. 1988).

A number of possible explanations have been put forward to explain the link between vasculitis and malignancy. These include: (i) vascular inflammation induced by immune complexes containing tumour-antigens, (ii) vasculitis associated with immune complexes from cryoglobulins in LHM, (iii) production of vascular lesions by antibodies which cross-react with tumour and endothelial cells, and (iv) a direct effect of malignant cells (e.g. hairy cells) on the blood vessel wall (Fam 2000).

Cutaneous vasculitis (LCV) is the most common form of paraneoplastic vasculitis (Sanchez-Guerrero et al. 1990). Crops of erythematous macules appear and may progress to palpable purpura. These most commonly affect the legs and follow a chronic relapsing course. Systemic manifestations include fever, arthralgia, respiratory, and gastrointestinal symptoms.

Henoch–Schönlein purpura has been described in patients with a number of malignancies including NHL, non-small-cell lung cancer, prostate cancer, and renal carcinoma. It occurs predominantly in men aged over 40 and presents with the classical triad of purpura, arthritis, and abdominal pain (Pertuiset et al. 2000).

A medium-sized vessel vasculitis resembling polyarteritis nodosa is seen in association with hairy cell leukaemia (Hasler et al. 1995). The vasculitis often occurs after the diagnosis of the hairy cell leukaemia, generally after splenectomy and infection. It is characterized histologically by perivascular and intramural leukaemic hairy cell infiltrates. Clinical features include fever, cutaneous vasculitis, myalgia, acute abdomen (due to mesenteric vasculitis), arthritis, coronary arteritis, and mononeuritis multiplex (Fam 2000). Hairy cell leukaemia may also be associated with LCV. Renal carcinoma may act as a trigger for Wegener's granulomatosis (Tatsis et al. 1999).

Temporal arteritis has been described in association with a number of malignancies. It is not clear whether this represents a true association as both conditions are common in the older age group.

The paraneoplastic vasculitides may respond to conventional treatment with steroids and immunosuppressants. However, the priority is to treat the underlying tumour. The vasculitis may recur when the tumour recurs.

Paraneoplastic erythromelalgia

Erythromelalgia is characterized by severe burning pain, erythema and warmth of the feet, and less commonly the hands. Heat, exercise, or dependency may provoke symptoms. Approximately 60 per cent of cases are idiopathic and 40 per cent secondary to other diseases (Fam 2000). About 20 per cent of patients with secondary erythromelalgia have an underlying myeloproliferative disorder such as polycythaemia rubra vera. The symptoms of erythromelalgia precede the diagnosis of the malignancy by a median of 2.5 years. The symptoms often respond to a single daily dose of 325–650 mg aspirin.

Paraneoplastic cutaneous and soft-tissue syndromes

Palmar fasciitis-arthritis syndrome

Palmar fasciitis is associated with rapidly progressive flexion contractures of both hands. The skin of the hands may be so taut as to be misdiagnosed as scleroderma. In addition patients have a symmetrical arthritis which most commonly involves the wrists, ankles, elbows, shoulders, and knees. Patients may also have plantar fasciitis. Most patients are women aged over 55, and about half are associated with ovarian adenocarcinoma (Pfinsgraff et al. 1986). The syndrome usually develops a few weeks before the tumour is diagnosed. In some cases, the syndrome has presented at the same time as the metastases. The pathogenesis is unknown. Treatment is difficult as the arthritis is often refractory to NSAIDs and steroids, and does not regress when the tumour is treated.

Paraneoplastic eosinophilic fasciitis

Eosinophilic fasciitis has been described in association with a number of LHM. In contrast to idiopathic eosinophilic fasciitis, cancer-associated fasciitis is more common in women. It is characterized by joint contractures, eosinophilia, and a raised ESR. The affected skin is thickened, taut, and tethered to the deep fascia. It usually affects the limbs but not the hands and feet. It often fails to respond to steroids but may improve when the underlying malignancy has been successfully treated.

Paraneoplastic erythema nodusum

Erythema nodusum has rarely been described in association with Hodgkin's disease, NHL, and leukaemia. It may precede diagnosis of the malignancy by several months or occur at the same time.

Sweet's syndrome

Acute febrile neutrophilic dermatosis (Sweet's syndrome) is associated with malignancy in 10–20 per cent of cases. The most common underlying malignancies are acute myeloid leukaemia, lymphomas, and multiple myeloma. Sweet's syndrome has also been described in association with genitourinary, breast, and gastrointestinal cancers and malignant melanoma. (Paydas et al. 2000). This skin disorder is characterized by tender, asymmetrical, erythematous plaques on the arms, head and neck, fever, arthralgia, anaemia, a raised ESR, and leucocytosis.

Panniculitis

The association of carcinoma of the pancreas and subcutaneous tender nodules and arthritis has been recognized since the early twentieth century. Both features are due to fat necrosis thought to be caused by blood borne pancreatic lipase. The nodules usually occur on the legs but may affect the trunk and buttocks. They may later break down giving a sterile yellow material containing globules of fat. The arthritis may be mono- or polyarticular. It often affects the ankles. Around half the patients also have an eosinophilia. The condition can be diagnosed on histology of a nodule. It responds poorly to treatment with steroids or NSAIDs.

Paraneoplastic scleroderma-like syndromes

Scleroderma-like skin changes may be a presenting feature of a number of malignancies including adenocarcinoma (usually of the breast, stomach, or lung) and carcinoid tumours. Women are affected three times as often as men. In patients with carcinoid syndrome, the tumour may secrete serotonin which may stimulate fibrous tissue proliferation.

POEMS syndrome (polyneuropathy, organomegaly, endocrinopathy, monoclonal protein, and skin changes suggestive of scleroderma) may occur in patients with IgA plasmacytoma.

Other paraneoplastic musculoskeletal syndromes

Paraneoplastic polymyalgia rheumatica and giant-cell arteritis

A syndrome resembling PMR may occasionally be the presenting feature of malignant disease. It has been seen in association with a variety of solid primary and metastatic tumours. Atypical features may include age younger than 50, asymmetry, ESR less than 40 or more than 100, and poor response to corticosteroids. Systemic features such as fever, night sweats, and malaise are common.

Oncogenic osteomalacia

Osteomalacia may occur in patients with benign tumours (such as fibromas or haemangiomas) or sarcomas. It is thought to be due to secretion of a hormone by the tumour which inhibits renal tubular re-absorption of phosphate. The onset is often insidious and patients complain of diffuse bone pain, proximal muscle weakness, and spontaneous fracture. Laboratory tests reveal hypophosphataemia, hyperphosphaturia, raised alkaline phosphatase, and low plasma 1,25-dihydroxyvitamin D_3 levels. Therapy with the latter agent is usually effective. The syndrome resolves if the tumour is completely resected.

Reflex sympathetic dystrophy (complex regional pain syndrome type II) has been described rarely in patients with carcinoma of the lung, colon, pancreas, and ovary, and in chronic myeloid leukaemia. Other musculoskeletal syndromes which appear rarely to be associated with malignancy include relapsing polychondritis, multicentric reticulohistiocytosis, and adult-onset Still's disease.

Musculoskeletal symptoms as a complication of cancer therapy

An increasing number of musculoskeletal complications of cancer therapy are being recognized. Raynaud's phenomenon (without associated autoantibody production) appears to be a common complication of bleomycin and vinblastine combination therapy (with or without cisplatin). It begins a median of 10 months after the start of chemotherapy and is persistent in around 50 per cent of cases (Vogelzang et al. 1981). Digital ischaemia and necrosis have been described after administration of 5-fluouracil. A scleroderma-like condition may develop as a complication of bleomycin therapy (Cohen et al. 1973).

Loprinzi et al. (1993) described a syndrome, which they called post-chemotherapy rheumatism, in eight women who had received adjuvant chemotherapy for breast cancer. The syndrome is characterized by symmetrical arthralgia, stiffness in the morning and after prolonged inactivity and, occasionally, mild swelling in both large and small peripheral joints. The same picture has since been described in a number of other malignancies in both men and women, and after a variety of chemotherapeutic regimes. All the regimes included cyclophosphamide. The symptoms respond poorly to NSAIDs or low-dose steroids, but do eventually resolve spontaneously.

Creamer et al. (1994) described three cases of acute inflammatory polyarthritis that developed 2 weeks, 9 weeks, and 1 year after tamoxifen had been started and resolved after tamoxifen was withdrawn. A persistent syndrome resembling fibromyalgia has also been described following adjuvant chemotherapy for breast cancer (Warner et al. 1997).

There are also descriptions of patients developing classical connective tissue disorders after combination chemotherapy but it is unclear whether this represents a true epidemiological association (Amft and D'Cruz 1996). There have been a number of reports of patients developing reactive arthritis after intravesical BCG therapy for bladder cancer (Goupille et al. 1994). There is an association between this complication and HLA-B27.

Malignancy as a complication of rheumatic disease

It is well recognized that patients with autoimmune diseases have an increased risk of lymphoproliferative and haematopoietic malignancies (LHM). This collective term includes Hodgkin's disease, NHL, leukaemia, and multiple myeloma. A number of other links between rheumatic disease and the subsequent development of malignancy at specific sites have been described.

Sjögren's syndrome and malignancy

The association of NHL and rheumatologic auto-immune disorders is strongest for Sjögren's syndrome. The risk of developing LHM in general, and NHL in particular is higher in patients with primary Sjögren's syndrome than those with secondary Sjögren's or RA alone (Table 3).

The first report of the association was published in 1951. Kassan et al. (1978) reported a 44-fold increased risk of developing NHL in 76 patients with primary Sjögren's syndrome. The risk was highest in those with an onset of Sjögren's syndrome before age 45. Other risk factors were parotid swelling, lymphadenopathy, splenomegaly, and irradiation of the parotid.

The evolution from a benign polyclonal lesion through an intermediate premalignant 'pseudolymphoma' stage to an overt monoclonal malignant B-cell NHL is gradual. The oncogene *bcl-2* has been identified in some follicular NHL seen in Sjögren's syndrome (Pisa et al. 1991). The reported latency between the onset of Sjögren's syndrome to the diagnosis of NHL ranges from 1.5 to 20 years or more. The NHL usually develops within lymphoepithelial lesions but may be extraglandular.

Rheumatoid arthritis and malignancy

The overall incidence of malignancy in RA is marginally increased. This equilibrium is achieved because some malignancies occur in excess while others are under-represented. The only cohorts of sufficient size to explore site-specific cancer morbidity in RA are derived either from national or regional databases of patients discharged from hospital with a diagnosis of RA, or of patients entitled to subsidized medication for RA. These records are then linked to the local cancer registry to investigate subsequent cancer incidence. The observed rates of malignancy are then compared to the expected rates for the local population (matched for age, sex, and follow-up period) to give a standardized incidence ratio (SIR). Four such studies have been published (Table 4). All have found an excess of LHM (especially Hodgkin's disease and NHL) and lung cancer. Smoking is a common risk factor for RA and lung cancer and this may account for the association between these two conditions. It is not clear whether the risk of lung cancer is increased in non-smokers with RA. All four studies found a significant reduction in the incidence of colorectal cancer and a non-significant reduction in stomach cancer. A large case–control study based in general practice found evidence of protection by aspirin and NSAIDs against oesophageal, gastric, and colorectal cancer (Langman et al. 2000).

In record linkage studies there is uncertainty about the accuracy of diagnosis of RA since standard classification criteria are not used. There is

Table 3 Standardized incidence ratios (SIR) for lymphoproliferative and haemopoietic malignancies (LHM) in patients with primary or secondary Sjögren's syndrome or rheumatoid arthritis. Data from record linkage of the Finnish Hospital Discharge Registry and the Finnish Cancer Registry 1970–1993 [adapted from Kauppi et al. (1997)]

	Diagnosis					
	Primary Sjögren's syndrome		**Secondary Sjögren's syndrome**		**Rheumatoid arthritis**	
Patients	676		709		9469	
Patient-years at risk	5336		4254		65391	
	SIR	(95% CI)	SIR	(95% CI)	SIR	(95% CI)
Malignancy						
All LHM	6.4	(3.8, 10.1)	3.1	(1.3, 6.4)	1.7	(1.3, 2.2)
All other malignancies	1.1	(0.8, 1.5)	0.7	(0.5, 1.1)	1.1	(1.0, 1.2)
Non-Hodgkin's lymphoma	8.7	(4.3, 15.5)	4.5	(1.5, 10.6)	2.2	(1.5, 3.1)
Hodgkin's disease	13.1	(1.6, 47.4)	—	—	2.2	(0.6, 5.7)
Leukaemia	3.6	(0.8, 10.8)	1.7	(0.0, 9.4)	1.3	(0.7, 2.2)
Myeloma	3.4	(0.4, 12.4)	2.2	(0.1, 12.1)	1.2	(0.5, 2.3)

Table 4 Prospective cohort studies which have explored the link between rheumatoid arthritis, based on hospital discharge diagnosis, and subsequent cancer incidence using record linkage

	Location							
	Finland		Sweden		Denmark		Scotland	
Reference	Isomaki et al. (1978)		Gridley et al. (1993)		Mellemkjaer et al. (1996)		Thomas et al. (2000)	
Person-years at risk	213 911		101 000		144 421		151 987	
	RR	(95% CI)	SIR	(95% CI)	SIR	(95% CI)	SIR	(95% CI)
All cancer	1.06	(1.0, 1.1)	0.95	(0.9, 10.0)	1.11	(1.1, 1.2)	1.01	(1.0, 1.0)
All LHM	2.18	(1.8, 2.6)	1.52	(1.2, 1.9)	1.71	(1.5, 2.0)	1.87	(1.6, 2.2)
Hodgkin's disease	2.79	(1.7, 4.4)	2.34	(1.2, 4.1)	3.40	(1.8, 5.6)	3.85	(2.2, 6.2)
NHL	2.68	(1.9, 4.7)	1.88	(1.3, 2.6)	2.40	(1.9, 2.9)	2.13	(1.7, 2.6)
Myeloma	2.20	(1.5, 3.2)	1.17	(0.7, 1.9)	1.10	(0.7, 1.7)	1.66	(1.2, 2.3)
Leukaemia	1.74	(1.3, 2.3)	1.43	(0.7, 2.6)	1.30	(0.9, 1.7)	1.38	(1.0, 1.8)
Colorectal	0.75	(0.6, 0.9)	0.66	(0.5, 0.8)	0.82	(0.7, 0.9)	0.75	(0.7, 0.9)
Lung	1.25[a]	(1.1, 1.4)	1.31	(1.0, 1.7)	1.50	(1.3, 1.7)	1.38	(1.3, 1.5)
Stomach	0.85	(0.7, 1.0)	0.63	(0.5, 0.9)	1.00	(0.8, 1.3)	0.83	(0.7, 1.0)

[a] All respiratory.

also little scope for exploring risk factors for the development of malignancy such as disease duration, treatment, and smoking status.

Rheumatology clinic based RA cohorts are inevitably much smaller but do offer greater diagnostic certainty and more patient details. The earliest, from the United Kingdom, showed a substantial increase in the incidence of LHM (RR 8.7; 95 per cent CI 4.3, 15.5) and of NHL in particular (RR 24.1; 95 per cent CI 9.7, 49.7) (Prior et al. 1984). The risk of NHL was strongly related to disease duration. None of the patients in the study had received immunosuppressive therapy. The most likely explanation of this association is that chronic stimulation of the immune system predisposes to malignant transformation. However, therapy (see 'Immunosuppressive therapy') and disease severity may also play a role in some cases. None of the record linkage or cohort studies has really been able to address the extent to which the association between RA and NHL may be explained by secondary Sjögren's syndrome. Even in the study of Kauppi et al. (1997) (Table 3) it remains possible that there were some cases of undiagnosed secondary Sjögren's syndrome amongst the patients labelled as 'RA alone'.

Gridley et al. (1994) found an SIR for NHL of 12.8 (95 per cent CI 7.7, 20.0) for male veterans with Felty's syndrome. They also found that, whereas 2 per cent of their total RA cohort had Felty's syndrome, 10 per cent of their RA patients with NHL had Felty's. Patients with Felty's syndrome may also develop T-cell chronic lymphocytic leukaemia as part of the large granular lymphocyte syndrome.

Although there does not appear to be an increased incidence of paraproteinaemia in patients with RA, there does appear to be a much higher risk of malignant transformation when paraproteinaemia and RA do occur together. The risk of myeloma is greatest in patients with a monoclonal IgA-paraprotein.

Systemic lupus erythematosus and malignancy

Four cohort studies have explored the link between systemic lupus erythematosus (SLE) and malignancy (Table 5). All showed an increased risk of NHL. A substantially increased risk of liver cancer has also been reported (RR 8.0; 95 per cent CI 2.6, 18.6) (Mellemkjaer et al. 1997). The authors postulated that patients with SLE are at increased risk of virus associated cancers. There was no evidence of an increased rate of exposure to immunosuppressant drugs in those patients who developed NHL. As with RA, it is possible that some of the cases of NHL may be related to secondary Sjögren's syndrome.

Although not conclusive, there is a suggestion of an increased risk of lung cancer in SLE. However, Mellemkjaer et al. reviewed the medical records and found that only 6 of the 15 cases of lung cancer satisfied the ACR criteria for SLE, and that a further two may have had SLE as a paraneoplastic syndrome.

Juvenile arthritis and malignancy

There is no evidence of a link between hospital admission with a diagnosis of juvenile arthritis and the development of malignancy in the next 10 years (Thomas et al. 2000).

Dermatomyositis/polymyositis and malignancy

An association between PM, DM, and malignancy was first described in 1916. A recent pooled analysis of published national data from Sweden, Denmark, and Finland found a three-fold increased risk of malignancy after the development of DM (SIR 3.0; 95 per cent CI 2.5, 3.6) and a 30 per cent increased risk after the development of PM (SIR 1.3; 95 per cent CI 1.0, 1.6) (Hill et al. 2001). DM was particularly associated with ovarian cancer (SIR 10.5; 95 per cent CI 6.1, 8.1), lung, pancreatic, stomach, and colorectal cancers and NHL (SIR 3.6; 95 per cent CI 1.2, 11.1). The increased risk of malignancy in patients with PM and DM is not related to immunosuppressant therapy (Airio et al. 1995).

Systemic sclerosis and malignancy

Patients with localized scleroderma confined to the skin (including those with morphoea or linear scleroderma) do not have an increased risk of malignancy (Rosenthal et al. 1995). An association between systemic sclerosis (SS) and malignancy was first seen in case reports. More recently two prospective cohort studies have demonstrated that patients with SS have an increased risk of malignancy compared to the general population (Table 6). The relative risk of malignancy is higher in men than women with SS. It is generally accepted that there is an increased incidence of breast cancer in the early years of follow-up in SS. Rosenthal et al. (1995) found 2.5 times the expected number of cases of breast cancer in the 12 months of follow-up after first hospital admission with SS. When cancers diagnosed in the first 12 months of follow-up were excluded (to reduce ascertainment bias) the risk of breast cancer was not increased.

Table 5 Prospective cohort studies which have explored the link between systemic lupus erythematosus and malignancy

	Location							
	Finland		USA		Canada		Denmark	
Reference	Pettersson et al. (1992)		Sweeney et al. (1995)		Abu-Shakra et al. (1996)		Mellemkjaer et al. (1997)	
Source of cases	Clinic attenders		Female clinic attenders		Clinic attenders		Hospital discharge diagnosis	
Method of cancer ascertainment	Record linkage—cancer registry		Postal questionnaire Record review		Record review		Record linkage—cancer registry	
Person-years at risk	2340		—		7233		10 807	
	RR	(95% CI)	SIR	(95% CI)	SIR	(95% CI)	RR	(95% CI)
All cancer	2.6	(1.5, 4.4)	1.4[a]	(0.5, 3.0)	1.1	(0.7, 1.6)	1.3	(1.1, 1.6)
All LHM	—		—		4.1	(1.5, 9.0)	3.5	(1.9,5.9)
NHL	44[a]	(11.9, 111)	10.0[a]	(0.3, 55.7)	5.4	(1.1, 15.7)	5.2	(2.2, 10.3)
Breast	2.7	(0.7, 6.8)	2.0	(0.4, 6.0)	0.7	(0.2, 1.8)	1.0	(0.5, 1.7)
Lung	—		—		1.5	(0.4, 3.9)	1.9	(1.1, 3.1)
Cervix	—		—		—		0.7	(0.1, 2.5)
Colon	—		4.3[a]	(0.1, 24.2)	2.0	(0.4, 6.0)	1.1	(0.5, 1.9)

[a] In women.

Note: RR, relative risk; SIR, standardized incidence ratio.

Table 6 Prospective cohort studies which have explored the link between scleroderma and malignancy

	Location			
	Canada		Sweden[a]	
Reference	Abu-Shakra et al. (1993)		Rosenthal et al. (1995)	
Source of cases	Clinic attenders		Hospital discharge diagnosis	
Method of cancer ascertainment	Record review		Record linkage—cancer registry	
Person-years at risk	2001		7403	
	SIR	(95% CI)	SIR	(95%CI)
All cancer	2.1	(1.2, 3.3)	1.5	(1.2, 1.9)
All LHM	—		2.3	(0.9, 4.8)
NHL	—		2.9	(0.8, 7.4)
Breast	6.1	(6.0, 6.2)	1.1	(0.5, 2.1)
Lung	8.3	(7.2, 9.6)	4.9	(2.8, 8.1)
Skin	—		4.2	(1.4, 9.8)

[a] Excludes malignancies occurring in the first year of follow-up.

Note: SIR, standardized incidence ratio.

While breast cancer is an early complication of SS, lung cancer is a late complication. Initial case reports suggested that alveolar cell carcinoma is the predominant type of lung cancer in SS. However, the prospective epidemiological studies found both squamous cell and adenocarcinomas.

The development of lung cancer in SS is related to pulmonary fibrosis rather than to smoking. Interestingly, an increased incidence of non-melanotic skin cancers has also been reported in SS (Rosenthal et al. 1995). Again this may be a complication of the fibrosing process.

Women who have developed SS in the last 5 years should be advised to undergo regular mammography. It has been suggested that patients with SS and pulmonary fibrosis should have periodic chest X-rays to screen for lung cancer (Bowles et al. 1999) although there is no evidence that mortality from lung cancer is reduced by regular screening.

Polymyalgia rheumatica and temporal arteritis

While polymyalgia rheumatica (PMR) may occur as a paraneoplastic syndrome (see earlier), there is no evidence that patients with idiopathic PMR have an increased risk of developing malignancy at a later date.

Paget's disease and malignancy

Paget reported sarcomas arising in five of the 23 patients he described with osteitis deformans. Osteosarcoma arising in pagetic bone remains one of the most serious complications of Paget's disease, affecting 0.7–5 per cent of patients. The majority of patients who develop osteosarcoma have polyostotic disease. In general, the sites of malignant transformation correspond to the distribution of Paget's disease. Around 20 per cent of these malignancies present as pathological fractures. It is thought that the two conditions may have a shared genetic basis and that the gene is located on chromosome 18 (Hansen et al. 1999).

Osteoarthritis and malignancy

A number of studies have found that patients who are hospitalized with osteoarthritis (OA) (Thomas et al. 2000) or undergo joint replacements for OA (Olsen et al. 1999) have a reduced subsequent risk of malignancy. The sites affected by this reduction were stomach, colon, rectum, and lung in both men and women; and gallbladder and bladder in women. It is unclear whether this reduction is due to a protective effect of OA, or whether patients admitted to hospital with OA (which would be predominantly for surgery) may be otherwise more healthy than their peers. The lower rate of colorectal cancer (which is also seen in RA) has been attributed to a protective effect of NSAIDs. The lower risk of lung cancer has been attributed to a negative association between smoking and OA (Felson et al. 1989). The incidence of prostate cancer was, however, increased in two studies (Nyren et al. 1995; Thomas et al. 2000). This may be a complication of NSAID therapy (Langman et al. 2000).

Malignancy as a complication of the treatment of rheumatic disease

Immunosuppressive therapy

The first evidence of an association between immunosuppressive drugs and malignancy came from a large UK–Australasian study of transplant and non-transplant patients published in 1979 (Kinlen et al. 1979). The transplanted patients showed a significant excess, compared to rates in the general population, of LHM. The non-transplant patient group, which included 623 patients with RA treated with immunosuppressants, showed a smaller excess of the same tumours. In the transplant field the association between immunosuppression and malignancy is most strong for LHM, skin cancer, and bladder cancer. In the rheumatic diseases, Silman et al. (1988) observed an increased risk of LHM in RA patients treated with azathioprine compared with non-azathioprine treated RA controls. Other studies observed an increased risk of bladder and skin cancer in RA patients treated with cyclophosphamide, and of leukaemia in patients with RA, SLE, and juvenile chronic arthritis treated with chlorambucil. The risk of bladder cancer persists for at least 17 years after stopping cyclophosphamide. There are case reports of LHM, some of them reversible, in patients with rheumatic diseases treated with methotrexate (Georgescu et al. 1997). Most of these tumours were Epstein–Barr virus positive.

In 1979, the European League Against Rheumatism (EULAR) established a registry of patients with rheumatic diseases who were enrolled when they first started on an immunosuppressive drug. They were followed annually for up to 10 years. Patients who received an immunosuppressive drug for 6 or more years had an adjusted incidence rate ratio of 3.74 (95 per cent CI 1.48, 9.47) of developing a LHM, skin or bladder cancer compared to those who received an immunosuppressive for less than 1 year (Asten et al. 1999). Thus, in addition to any increased risk of malignancy that may be conferred by individual rheumatic diseases (see 'Malignancy as a complication of rheumatic disease'), there is a further risk of specific types of malignancy that is related to the duration of exposure to immunosuppressive drugs. The attributable malignancy risk of azathioprine therapy in RA is around 5.7/1000 person-years of follow-up (Jones et al. 1996).

There are theoretical reasons for concern that treatment with the new tumour necrosis factor blocking drugs may be associated with an increased risk of malignancy. However, published data to date on long-term safety are reassuring (Moreland et al. 2001).

Irradiation

During the 1940s radiotherapy was used in the treatment of ankylosing spondylitis (AS). The link between leukaemia and radiotherapy in AS was established by the classic work of Court Brown and Doll (1965). They identified all AS patients ($N = 14\,554$) who had received treatment at one of the 87 UK radiotherapy centres between 1935 and 1954. Adequate follow-up data to January 1960 were obtained for 98 per cent of patients. This group had 29.4 times the expected rate of aplastic anaemia, 9.5 times the expected rate of leukaemia and 1.4 times the expected rate of cancer at other heavily irradiated sites. Follow-up has since been extended to January 1992 (Weiss et al. 1994). The SMR for cancer remained elevated at 1.3 (95 per cent CI 1.2, 1.4). The excess rate of lung cancer had disappeared by 35 years of follow-up but the RR for leukaemia and other neoplasms remained elevated, although less so than in the earlier period of follow-up. Studies from the United States and Canada have confirmed the increased mortality in AS patients who received radiotherapy.

The mortality rate from lymphoma in RA patients treated with total lymphoid irradiation is 5.9/1000 person years of follow-up (Uhrin et al. 2001).

References

Abu-Shakra, M., Guillemin, F., and Lee, P. (1993). Cancer in systemic sclerosis. *Arthritis and Rheumatism* **36**, 460–4.

Abu-Shakra, M., Gladman, D.D., and Urowitz, M.B. (1996). Malignancy in systemic lupus erythematosus. *Arthritis and Rheumatism* **39**, 1050–4.

Abu-Shakra, M. et al. (2001). Cancer and autoimmunity: autoimmune and rheumatic features in patients with malignancies. *Annals of the Rheumatic Diseases* **60**, 433–40.

Airio, A., Pukkala, E., and Isomaki, H. (1995). Elevated cancer incidence in patients with dermatomyositis, a population based study. *Journal of Rheumatology* **22**, 1300–3.

Amft, N. and D'Cruz, D. (1996). Postchemotherapy connective tissue diseases—more than just rheumatism? *Lupus* **5**, 255–6.

Arndt, C.A.S. and Crist, W.M. (1999). Common musculoskeletal tumours of childhood and adolescence. *New England Journal of Medicine* **341**, 342–52.

Asten, P., Barrett, J., and Symmons, D. (1999). Risk of developing certain malignancies is related to duration of immunosuppressive drug exposure in patients with rheumatic diseases. *Journal of Rheumatology* **26**, 1705–14.

Bowles, K.E., Wynne, C., and Baime, M.J. (1999). Screening for cancer in the patient with rheumatic disease. *Rheumatic Disease Clinics of North America* **25**, 719–44.

Caldwell, D.S. and McCallum, R.M. (1986). Rheumatologic manifestations of cancer. *Medical Clinics of North America* **70**, 385–417.

Cohen, I.S. et al. (1973). Cutaneous toxicity of bleomycin therapy. *Archives of Dermatology* **107**, 553–5.

Court Brown, W.M. and Doll, R. (1965). Mortality from cancer and other causes after radiotherapy for ankylosing spondylitis. *British Medical Journal* **2**, 1327–32.

Creamer, P. et al. (1994). Acute inflammatory polyarthritis in association with tamoxifen. *British Journal of Rheumatology* **33**, 583–5.

Denny, C.T. (1996). Gene re-arrangements in Ewing's sarcoma. *Cancer Investigation* **14**, 83–8.

Fam, A.G. (2000). Paraneoplastic rheumatic syndromes. *Baillières Clinical Rheumatology* **14**, 515–33.

Felson, D.T. et al. (1989). Does smoking protect against osteoarthritis? *Arthritis and Rheumatism* **32**, 166–72.

Folli, F. et al. (1993). Autoantibodies to a 128-kd synaptic protein in three women with the Stiff-man syndrome and breast cancer. *New England Journal of Medicine* **328**, 546–51.

Georgescu, L. et al. (1997). Lymphoma in patients with rheumatoid arthritis: association with the disease state or methotrexate treatment. *Seminars in Arthritis and Rheumatism* **26**, 794–804.

Goupille, P. et al. (1994). Three cases of arthritis after BCG therapy for bladder cancer. *Clinical and Experimental Rheumatology* **12**, 195–7.

Greer, J.M. et al. (1988). Vasculitis associated with malignancy. *Medicine (Baltimore)*, **67**, 220–30.

Gridley, G. et al. (1993). Incidence of cancer among patients with rheumatoid arthritis. *Journal of the National Cancer Institute* **85**, 307–11.

Gridley, G. et al. (1994). Incidence of cancer among men with Felty syndrome. *Annals of Internal Medicine* **120**, 35–9.

Hansen, M.F., Nellissery, M.J., and Bhatia, P. (1999). Common mechanism of osteosarcoma and Paget's disease. *Journal of Bone and Mineral Research* **14** (Suppl. 2), 39–44.

Hasler, P., Kistler, H., and Gerber, H. (1995). Vasculitides in hairy cell leukaemia. *Seminars in Arthritis and Rheumatism* **25**, 134–42.

Hill, C.L. et al. (2001). Frequency of specific cancer types in dermatomyositis and polymyositis: a population-based study. *Lancet* **357**, 96–100.

Huvos, A.G. (1986). Osteogenic sarcoma of bones and soft tissues in older persons. A clinicopathologic analysis of 117 patients older than 60 years. *Cancer* **57**, 1442–9.

Isomäki, H.A., Hakulinen, T., and Joutsenlahti, U. (1978). Excess risk of lymphomas, leukaemia and myeloma in patients with rheumatoid arthritis. *Journal of Chronic Diseases* **31**, 691–6.

Jones, M. et al. (1996). Does exposure to immunosuppressive therapy increase the 10 year malignancy and mortality risks in rheumatoid arthritis? A matched cohort study. *British Journal of Rheumatology* **35**, 738–45.

Kaste, S.C. et al. (1999). Metastases detected at the time of diagnosis of primary pediatric extremity osteosarcoma. *Cancer* **86**, 1602–8.

Kauppi, M., Pukkala, E., and Isomäki, H. (1997). Elevated incidence of haematologic malignancies in patients with Sjögren's syndrome compared to patients with rheumatoid arthritis (Finland). *Cancer Causes and Control* **8**, 201–4.

Kassan, S.S. et al. (1978). Increased risk of lymphoma in sicca syndrome. *Annals of Internal Medicine* **89**, 888–92.

Kinlen, L.J. et al. (1979). Collaborative United Kingdom—Australasian study of cancer in patients treated with immunosuppressive drugs. *British Medical Journal* **2**, 1461–6.

Kurzrock, R., Cohen, P.R., and Markowitz, A. (1994). Clinical manifestations of vasculitis in patients with solid tumours. *Archives of Internal Medicine* **154**, 334–40.

Langman, M. et al. (2000). Effect of anti-inflammatory drugs on overall risk of common cancer: case–control study in general practice. *British Medical Journal* **320**, 1642–6.

Loprinzi, C.L., Duffy, J., and Ingle, J.N. (1993). Postchemotherapy rheumatism. *Journal of Clinical Oncology* **11**, 678–70.

McDonagh, J.E. et al. (1994). Non-Hodgkin's lymphoma presenting as polyarthritis. *British Journal of Rheumatology* **33**, 79–84.

Martinez-Lavin, M. et al. (1993) Hypertrophic osteoarthropathy: consensus on its definition, classification, assessment and diagnostic criteria. *Journal of Rheumatology* **20**, 1386–7.

Mellemkjaer, L. et al. (1996). Rheumatoid arthritis and cancer. *European Journal of Cancer* **32** (A), 1753–7.

Mellemkjaer, L. et al. (1997). Non-Hodgkin's lymphoma and other cancers among a cohort of patients with systemic lupus erythematosus. *Arthritis and Rheumatism* **40**, 761–8.

Moreland, L.W. et al. (2001). Long-term safety and efficacy of etanercept in patients with rheumatoid arthritis. *Journal of Rheumatology* **28**, 1238–44.

Murasshima, A. et al. (1992). A case of Raynaud's disease with uterine cancer producing interleukin-6. *Clinical Rheumatology* **11**, 410–12.

Nyren, O. et al. (1995). Cancer risk after hip replacement with metal implants: a population-based cohort study in Sweden. *Journal of the National Cancer Institute* **87**, 28–33.

Olsen, J.H. et al. (1999). Hip and knee implantations among patients with osteoarthritis and risk of cancer: a record linkage study from Denmark. *International Journal of Cancer* **81**, 719–22.

Paydas, S., Sahin, B., and Zorludemir, S. (2000). Sweet's syndrome accompanying leukaemia: seven cases and review of the literature. *Leukaemia Research* **24**, 83–6.

Pertuiset, E. et al. (2000). Adult Henoch–Schönlein purpura associated with malignancy. *Seminars in Arthritis and Rheumatism* **29**, 360–7.

Pettersson, T. et al. (1992). Increased risk of cancer in patients with systemic lupus erythematosus. *Annals of the Rheumatic Diseases* **51**, 437–9.

Pfinsgraff, J. et al. (1986). Palmar fasciitis and arthritis with malignant neoplasms: a paraneoplastic syndrome. *Seminars in Arthritis and Rheumatism* **16**, 118–25.

Pisa, E.K. et al. (1991). High frequency of t(14 : 18) translocation in salivary gland lymphomas from Sjögren's syndrome patients. *Journal of Clinical Oncology* **174**, 1245–50.

Praemer, A., Furner, S., and Rice, D.P. *Musculoskeletal Conditions in the United States* 2nd edn. Rosemount IL: American Academy of Orthopaedic Surgeons, 1999.

Prior, P. et al. (1984). Cancer morbidity in rheumatoid arthritis. *Annals of the Rheumatic Diseases* **43**, 128–31.

Rennie, J.A.N. and Auchterlonie, I.A. (1991). Rheumatological manifestations of the leukaemias and graft versus host disease. *Baillières Clinical Rheumatology* **5**, 231–51.

Rosenthal, A.K. et al. (1995). Incidence of cancer among patients with systemic sclerosis. *Cancer* **76**, 910–14.

Sanchez-Guerrero, J. et al. (1990). Vasculitis as a paraneoplastic syndrome. Report of 11 cases and review of the literature. *Journal of Rheumatology* **17**, 1458–62.

Schwarzer, A.C. et al. (1990). Metastatic adeno squamous carcinoma presenting as an acute monoarthritis, with a review of the literature. *Journal of Orthopaedics and Rheumatology* **3**, 175–85.

Silman, A.J. et al. (1988). Lymphoproliferative cancer and other malignancy in patients with rheumatoid arthritis treated with azathioprine: a twenty year follow-up study. *Annals of the Rheumatic Diseases* **47**, 988–92.

Stummvoll, G.H. et al. (2001). Cancer polyarthritis resembling rheumatoid arthritis as a first sign of hidden neoplasms. *Scandinavian Journal of Rheumatology* **30**, 40–4.

Sweeney, D.M. et al. (1995). Risk of malignancy in women with systemic lupus erythematosus. *Journal of Rheumatology* **22**, 1478–82.

Tatsis, E. et al. (1999). Wegener's granulomatosis associated with renal cell carcinoma. *Arthritis and Rheumatism* **42**, 751–6.

Thomas, E. et al. (2000). Risk of malignancy among patients with rheumatic conditions. *International Journal of Cancer* **88**, 497–502.

Uhrin, Z. et al. (2001). Treatment of rheumatoid arthritis with total lymphoid irradiation. *Arthritis and Rheumatism* **44**, 1525–8.

Vogelzang, N.J. et al. (1981). Raynaud's phenomenon: a common toxicity after combination chemotherapy for testicular cancer. *Annals of Internal Medicine* **95**, 288–92.

Warner, E. et al. (1997). Rheumatic symptoms following adjuvant therapy for breast cancer. *American Journal of Oncology* **20**, 322–6.

Weiss, H.A., Darby, S.C., and Doll, R. (1994). Cancer mortality following X-ray treatment for ankylosing spondylitis. *International Journal of Cancer* **59**, 327–38.

Zantos, D., Zhang, Y., and Felson, D. (1994). The overall and temporal association of cancer with polymyositis and dermatomyositis. *Journal of Rheumatology* **21**, 1855–9.

Further reading

Miller, R.W., Boice, J.D., and Curtis, R.E. (1996). Bone cancer. In *Cancer Epidemiology and Prevention* 2nd edn. (ed. Schottenfield and Fraumeni). New York: Oxford University Press.

Schajowicz, F. *Tumors and Tumorlike Lesions of Bone* 2nd edn. Berlin: Springer-Verlag, 1994.

1.3.10 Haematology

Alexander Kai-Lik So

Introduction

Haematological changes are commonly present in systemic rheumatic diseases and in clinical practice, the full blood count is probably one of the most frequently requested laboratory investigations by rheumatologists. Haematological abnormalities may reflect the systemic nature of the disease in question, for example, systemic inflammation or autoimmunity. Occassionally, rheumatological symptoms may be a direct consequence of a primary disturbance of the haematological system, for example, primary AL amyloidosis and lymphomas. Of increasing importance is the haematological effects of the wide range of drugs used in treating rheumatic diseases that have toxic side-effects on haematopoiesis and gastrointestinal integrity. Rheumatic diseases and their treatments may also affect the pathways of coagulation and fibrinolysis. This chapter tries to cover some of the areas where haematological manifestations are frequently linked to rheumatic diseases.

Haematologic changes due to systemic inflammation

One of the most commonly encountered situations in rheumatology is the effect of systemic inflammation on haematological parameters. Our understanding of the mechanisms of acute and chronic inflammation has greatly increased due to progress in molecular and cellular biology, in particular in the elucidation of the roles of cytokines, chemokines, and prostaglandins on the cellular and humoral aspects of inflammation. Many of these same mediators have pleiotropic effects and can also act on blood cells and the bone marrow. The paradigm for inflammatory rheumatic disease in this setting is rheumatoid arthritis, though it has to be borne in mind that inflammatory mechanisms/mediators may differ in the different rheumatic diseases.

Table 1 Mechanisms of anaemia in chronic inflammation

Effect	Mechanism
Reduced RBC lifespan	Red cell membrane fragility
Impaired RBC formation	Direct inhibitory effect of inflammatory cytokines on erythropoiesis
	Reduced sensitivity to erythropoietin
	Reduced synthesis of erythropoietin
	Altered iron metabolism and iron trapping

Inflammation can affect all the blood cell lineages. The most frequently observed is on erythropoiesis, leading to anaemia of chronic disease (ACD). ACD is due to ineffective erythropoiesis in the presence of sufficient iron stores. This term is unsatisfactory as it does not indicate that inflammation is the main underlying cause, though it has the advantage of common usage. Similar pathophysiological mechanisms operate in the ACD encountered in malignancy, chronic infections, and chronic inflammation. In the rheumatological setting, it has been best studied in rheumatoid arthritis (RA). About 80 per cent of cases of anaemia in RA is attributable to systemic inflammation, with the other 20 per cent is due to other causes such as iron deficiency, drug toxicity, bone marrow disorders, etc. This form of anaemia presents typically as a mild normochromic, normocytic anaemia, and is characterized by decreased serum iron and total iron-binding capacity in the presence of normal or increased iron stores in the bone marrow. The aetiology of this form of anaemia is complex and is summarized in Table 1.

Both humoral and cellular factors inhibit erythropoiesis in chronic inflammation

Using *in vitro* cell culture techniques, an inhibitory effect by humoral factors and macrophages on erythropoiesis was demonstrated. With hindsight, it is likely that the macrophage effects are due to cytokines also. As for humoral factors, apart from cytokines, an immunoglobulin-like inhibitor may also be involved in some cases (Dainaiak et al. 1980).

Effects of inflammatory cytokines on erythropoiesis

Cytokines can act both directly and indirectly on erythropoiesis. *In vitro* studies have demonstrated that TNFα suppressed BFU-E formation directly, while inhibition of CFU-E was mediated by secretion of IFNβ from marrow stromal cells under the influence of TNF. IL-1 similarly had an indirect suppressive effect on CFU-E formation via IFNγ secreted by T-cells (Means et al. 1992).

The role of erythropoietin

Erythropoietin (EP) is a 166 amino acid, highly glycosylated hormone that is mainly synthesized by peritubular interstitial cells in the kidney (85–90 per cent) and is present in normal plasma at a range between 8 and 18 IU/l. Its circulating level is influenced by anaemia, hypoxia, and renal disease. EP acts by binding to erythropoietin receptors (EP-R) on early erythroid cells to stimulate haemoglobin synthesis, erythroid differentiation, and erythroid proliferation. In normal anaemic states, tissue hypoxia is detected in the kidney which stimulates renal EP production. This pathway provides a feedback loop which maintains red cell mass in a state of equilibrium.

During systemic inflammation, there is a reduced sensitivity of erythroid precursors to EP as well as a reduced production of EP. The serum levels of EP in anaemic RA patients are lower than that found in non-RA iron deficiency anaemia subjects. Furthermore, the slope of the curve between degree of anaemia and EP level is less steep in RA anaemia than in iron deficiency anaemia (Hochberg et al. 1998), indicating reduced tissue responsiveness to EP. At a cellular level, this can be accounted for by the direct inhibitory effect of cytokines such as IL1 and TNFα on renal cell EP production (Jelkmann et al. 1991) as well as a reduction of the erythroid response to EP. Finally, evidence for reduced sensitivitiy to EP in RA inflammatory anaemia is supported by the therapeutic effects of supra-physiological doses of EP when it is used to treat anaemia in RA.

Diagnosis of anaemia of chronic inflammation

Although bone marrow biopsy is the only way to establish conclusively that iron stores are adequate, in practice this can be inferred by indirect measurements. Low serum iron in the presence of reduced iron-binding capacity and a normal or raised ferritin level indicates that the problem is not a lack of available iron. Ferritin is an iron storage molecule which is synthesized as apoferritin in many organs, including the liver, spleen, heart, and macrophages. Generally, its serum level (normal ~100 ± 60 μg/l) accurately mirrors tissue iron stores, but during infection, inflammation and malignancy, its level can increase markedly due to increased cell death and the serum level therefore no longer reflects the state of iron storage. In RA, ferritin is only very reduced in the presence of true iron deficiency. Recently, the measurement of the serum level of the transferrin receptor (sTfR) has also been proposed as a diagnostic aid in differentiating anaemia of inflammation from other forms of anaemia. In iron deficiency anaemias and haemolytic anaemias, where there is increased red cell turnover, sTfR levels are increased from the norm (~5 mg/l), while in the anaemia of chronic disease, its level remains low or normal. In clinical practice, the identification of anaemia of chronic inflammation by the standard assays is usually straightforward, except when the clinical picture is complicated by other co-existing pathologies such as infection and malignancy or drug toxicity.

Effects of inflammation on other haematopoietic lineages

The effects on other lineages are much less marked. Thrombocytosis is often present in active RA, though generally at levels which do not exceed 1×10^9/l. In connective tissue diseases, thrombocytopaenia related to disease activity is explained by the specific immune processes implicated rather than inflammation per se. Although leucocytes play a key role in the pathogenesis of the inflammatory rheumatic diseases at a tissue level, their circulating levels do not betray their involvement, except for specific disorders such as eosinophilia syndromes. Specific analysis of leucocyte cell surface markers or of clonal expansion (of T- or B-cells) have not been useful in routine clinical practice and remains a research tool.

Haematological toxicity of antirheumatic drugs

Drug-related adverse effects are frequent in the treatment of rheumatic diseases. In a study of RA patients receiving DMARD and NSAID therapy, over 50 per cent developed an adverse event over a period of 3 years. Haematologic adverse events are the fourth most frequently affected organ system, preceded by skin, gastrointestinal, and renal side-effects. The polypharmacy often encountered in elderly patients increases the probability of developing interactions and increased drug toxicity. The toxic effects may be idiosyncratic or may be due to the intrinsic pharmacologic properties of the drug.

NSAIDs

The main haematological adverse effects of NSAIDs are summarized in Table 2. Phenylbutazone has been incriminated in agranulocytosis and aplastic anaemia for which its prescription has been strictly limited. However, these adverse effects have also been reported with many other NSAIDs at a reduced frequency. The mechanism of the bone marrow toxicity from NSAIDs is unknown, but is thought to be an idiosyncratic drug reaction to the drug with an increased susceptibility in the older patient. Although haematologic monitoring of NSAID therapy is not routinely

Table 2 Haematological adverse effects of NSAIDs

	Mechanism	Drugs implicated
Common		
Anaemia	Gastrointestinal bleeding	All NSAIDs except for COX-2 inhibitors
Uncommon		
Agranulocytosis	Not known. Idiosyncratic reaction most likely	Phenylbutazone, indomethacin, as well as other NSAIDs
Anaemia	Autoimmune haemolysis	Mefenamic acid and many other NSAIDs
Aplastic anaemia	Not known	Phenylbutazone and other NSAIDs
Eosinophilia	? Allergic	Naproxen, piroxicam
Leucopaenia	Not known	Many NSAIDs
Neutropaenia	Not known	Many NSAIDs
Thrombocytopaenia	Not known	Many NSAIDs

recommended, due to the rarity of most of these reactions, it is advisable to do so in the case of phenylbutazone therapy.

Table 3 Haematologic adverse effects of DMARDs

Drug	Adverse effect	Mechanism
Methotrexate	Macrocytosis and megaloblastic anaemia	Folate antagonism
	Agranulocytosis	Not known
	Thrombocytopaenia	Not known
	Lymphoma	Immunosuppression?
Gold (i.m. or oral)	Eosinophilia	Allergic
	Thrombocytopaenia	↑ Peripheral destruction or marrow suppression ? Autoimmune
	Aplastic anaemia	Not known
D-penicillamine	Thrombocytopaenia	Autoimmune?
Sulfasalazine	Haemolytic anaemia	Autoimmune, may be accompanied by a lupus-like syndrome
	Eosinophilia	Allergic
	Leucopaenia and neutropaenia	Not known
	Agranulocytosis	Not known

DMARDs

Treatment with DMARDs is frequently complicated by drug toxicity and haematological side-effects are common (Table 3). Haematological toxicity can present suddenly and with severe consequences. In my personal experience, severe reactions such as aplastic anaemia or agranulocytosis are often preceded by a period of a few weeks or months when the blood count declines gradually before the catastrophic presentation. This warning sign is frequently overlooked even though regular monitoring has been performed.

Low-dose methotrexate therapy inhibits dihydrofolate reductase (DHFR) activity and therefore may cause macrocytosis because of folate antagonism. Patients who already have low folic acid levels are likely to be more at risk to develop haematological toxicity, and co-administration of other folate inhibitors (e.g. trimethoprim) can augment toxicity. It is therefore advisable to supplement folic acid intake during methotrexate treatment, especially since it may also reduce the incidence of liver toxicity and offers protection against haematological toxicity (Griffith et al. 2001).

Haematological side-effects are well-recognized complications of gold and D-penicillamine treatment and blood monitoring is recommended at regular intervals. Thrombocytopaenia is probably the most commonly encountered side-effect that appears to be more frequent in patients who possess HLA-DR3 (Wooley et al. 1980).

Case reports of agranulocytosis secondary to sulfasalazine have been documented, though this complication is less frequent that leucopaenia, which has been reported to affect up to 5.6 per cent of RA patients treated with this drug. Haematologic reactions tend to occur early during treatment (less than 24 weeks). Sulfasalazine has also been linked to a lupus-like syndrome and can cause drug-induced lupus. Acute reactions of this type are thought to be immunologically mediated (Vyse and So 1992).

Immunosuppressive drugs

Alkylating agents act by inhibiting DNA synthesis. In rheumatic diseases, haematological toxicity with cyclophosphamide and chlorambucil have been clearly documented, and is explained by the pharmacology of these agents. Monitoring is therefore mandatory, and treatment should be suspended when major toxicity is detected. However, a degree of myelosuppression is often encountered with these agents and which can be managed by reducing the dosage (e.g. with cyclophosphamide in treatment of SLE and vasculitis). Oncogenesis related to alkylating agent treatment is also of concern, and is dealt with in a subsequent section.

Azathioprine and its metabolite 6-mercaptopurine are purine analogs which inhibit nucleic acid synthesis and therefore can interfere with haematopoeisis. In clinical practice, leucopaenia is the most commonly encountered problem, though thrombocytopaenia has also been reported. Megaloblastic anaemia or macrocytosis may be an early sign of bone marrow toxicity which is reversible if detected early. Adaptation of the dosage is often sufficient to avoid major toxicity. An interaction with allopurinol, which decreases the metabolism of 6-mercaptopurine, can increase azathioprine-related toxicity, and therefore the dose of azathioprine needs to be reduced if given in this setting.

Others

Of the other agents employed in antirheumatic therapies, dapsone is known to provoke haemolysis and methaemoglobinaemia and levamisole can induce granulocytopaenia.

Immune mediated haematological syndromes

Haemolytic anaemias

Immune-mediated haemolytic anaemias are mainly caused by the binding of warm-active IgG antibodies to erythrocytes. Antibody binding may be direct and detected by the direct Coombs test (see later), or due to alloantibodies or immune complexes that adhere to the red cell surface.

Among rheumatic diseases, two aetiologies dominate: the connective tissue diseases and drug-induced autoimmune haemolytic anaemias (AHAs). Although SLE is the most common cause, AHAs can also be found in patients suffering from RA, Sjögren's syndrome, and the primary antiphospholipid syndrome. In these conditions, production of antierythrocyte antibodies and the formation of circulating immune complexes are considered the main mechanisms of disease. The nature of the erythrocyte antigen remains incompletely elucidated; in some cases of AHAs, antibodies against the Rh antigens have been demonstrated (Barker et al. 1992). Although there is a correlation between the presence of antiphospholipid antibodies and AHA (Hazletine et al. 1988), it has not been shown that antiphospholipid antibodies are directly haemolytic but they can bind to the red cell membrane.

In drug-induced haemolysis, the drug may act as a hapten by binding to the red cell membrane to form a complex, which then becomes the target of immune destruction. Other mechanisms include drug-induced antibody formation or cross-reaction between antidrug antibodies with the erythrocyte. Among the commonly used antirheumatic drugs, haemolytic anaemias have been reported with gold, D-penicillamine, sulfasalazine, mefenamic acid, diclofenac, etodolac, sulindac, and other NSAIDs. In the case of mefenamic acid, drug sensitization can induce the production of a cross-reactive haemolytic antibody which has specificity for components of the Rh antigen complex, similar to methyldopa-induced haemolytic anaemia.

Mechanism of red cell destruction in AHA

IgG binding to erythrocytes may lead to red cell destruction either by complement-mediated intravascular haemolysis or receptor mediated clearance of 'opsonized' erythrocytes by the reticuloendothelial system. In most cases, it is the latter system which is responsible for anaemia, by trapping Ig-coated erythrocytes and facilitating their removal by erythrophagocytosis. Ig-coated red cells are cleared by the reticuloendothelial system via IgG Fc receptors, which are expressed at high concentrations (10^5 per cell) on macrophages and Kupffer cells in the sinuses of the liver and spleen. These receptors are surface glycoproteins which belong to the immunoglobulin superfamily and mediate specific binding to IgG, IgA, and IgE. Binding specificities for IgG and tissue distribution for the different receptors vary. Besides mediating an adherence function, FcR are also cell signalling molecules which transduce activation or inhibitory signals which modulate macrophage phagocytosis, neutrophil activation, or inhibition of B cell activation (van der Pol and van de Winkel 1998; Ravetch and Bolland 2001).

Animal studies confirm the importance of these receptors in the pathogenesis of AHAs (Shibata 1990). In an experimental murine model of AHA, IgG2a antierythrocyte antibodies provoked more severe anaemia than other IgG isotypes and is mediated by the low affinitiy receptor FcγRIII (23).

Although the complement system may also mediate red cell damage by activation of the lytic C5b-9 membrane attack complex, this pathway probably plays a minor role *in vivo* in haemolytic anaemias associated with the rheumatic diseases. Complement on red cells may, however, facilitate adhesion of red cells to the complement receptors CR1 (which binds to C3b) and CR3 (which binds to iC3b) and hence their clearance by the reticuloendothelial system.

Clinical presentation and diagnosis

Immune haemolytic anaemias secondary to SLE and other rheumatic diseases are usually chronic and mild. Occassionally, it may have an explosive onset, when the patient presents with symptoms of severe anaemia, mild jaundice, and hepatosplenomegaly. When severe, haemolysis may be accompanied by haemoglobinuria.

SLE and related connective tissue diseases account for up to 10 per cent of cases presenting with autoimmune haemolytic anaemia. In a small number of patients, HA may actually be the initial presentation of lupus. Evans' syndrome, which describes the clinical association of AHA and autoimmune thrombocytopenic purpura, overlaps with SLE and the antiphospholipid syndrome, and is present in 5–10 per cent of patients with these autoimmune diseases (Alarcon-Segovia et al. 1989).

Diagnosis of immune haemolytic anaemia depends on the demonstration of haemolysis and the presence of antibody or complement on the red cell surface. Conventional haematological tests will show anaemia and signs of increased erythropoiesis, such as a raised reticulocyte count or active erythropoiesis on bone marrow examination. The blood film will show polychromasia, anisocytosis, and spherocytosis. Indirect evidence of haemolysis include reduced serum haptoglobin concentration and increased bilirubin in the presence of normal liver function tests. However, direct evidence of immune haemolysis is the gold standard for diagnosis. In the direct Coombs' test, the patient's erythrocytes are first washed and are then probed with heterologous antibodies (of IgM class) to detect immunoglobulin or complement (C3) on the cell surface. A positive reaction produces red cell agglutination in the assay. In the indirect Coombs test, the patient's sera is used to coat normal compatible erythrocytes, which are then washed and probed with similar reagents as those used in the direct Coombs test. This test will detect antibodies which are capable of binding to red cells but which are not specific for red cell antigens. Not all patients who are Coombs' positive will have signs of active haemolysis.

Treatments for haemolysis

AHA encountered in SLE and the rheumatic diseases is usually mild and responds promptly to corticosteroids and/or the interruption of the provoking agent in the case of drug-induced haemolysis. The dose of corticosteroid used can be up to 100 mg of prednisone daily, which is then tapered after a clinical response develops. In steroid refractory cases, a trial of intravenous IgG is warranted (Flores et al. 1993) and may require infusion of large doses of immunoglobulin (from 0.5 g/kg/day upwards) given daily for five consecutive days followed by an intermittent treatment regime. Splenectomy and treatment with cytotoxic drugs (e.g. azathioprine, cyclosphosphamide) are kept in reserve for patients who have failed steroids and intravenous IgG.

Thrombocytopaenia

SLE occassionally presents as acute idiopathic thrombocytopaenic purpura (ITP) and low platelet count is a frequent finding in lupus patients and constitutes one of the clinical criteria for the classification of the disease. Indeed, chronic ITP share some of the clinical features of SLE, such as the predominant age of onset (20–40 years) and female predominance. Thrombocytopaenia is also a common clinical feature in the primary APS, where it may be found in 30–46 per cent of cases (Vincent and Mackworth-Young 2000). In other connective tissue and rheumtological diseases, thrombocytopaenia is more frequently related to the drug therapy, notable examples being gold and D-penicillamine therapy which probably has an immunological mechanism; and immunosuppressive drugs such as cyclophosphamide and chlorambucil.

Clinical manifestations of ITP

ITP may have an acute or chronic onset. Clinical manifestations include bruising and bleeding, particularly of mucosal surfaces and a history of spontaneous bruising and epistaxis. Splenomegaly may be a feature, particularly when ITP presents in the context of a connective tissue disease. When significant bruising is present, platelet counts are markedly reduced and if below 10 000/μl may be associated with severe and life-threatening bleeding. Diagnosis is based on the demonstration that platelet production is not impaired in the bone marrow, indicating that the problem is due to platelet consumption in the periphery. In severe ITP, marrow megakaryocytes are found in increased numbers but are less granular and more basophilic and platelet production may be increased up to eight-fold the normal rate.

ITP and autoantibodies

Peripheral consumption of platelets in ITP is explained by IgG and IgM binding to platelet surface antigens and the subsequent clearance of antibody coated platelets by the reticulo-endothelial system through Fc receptors. In chronic ITP, 95 per cent of patients possess platelet bound antibody, usually of the IgG class. A pathway for immunoglobulin mediated complement activation has also been demonstrated for platelet-bound IgM antibodies (Cines et al. 1985). The antigens recognized by these antibodies are in the main platelet glycoproteins, such as the GPIIb-IIIa complex, GpIb-IX, GpIa-IIa, etc. Patients with SLE and thrombocytopaenia have an increased frequency of antibodies against these antigens, as do patients with the primary APS syndrome with thrombocytopaenia (Macchi et al. 1997).

There has been particular interest in the association between antiphospholipid antibodies and thrombocytopaenia. As antiphospholipid anti-bodies are directed mainly against negatively charged membrane phospholipids, they were initally thought to be have a primary role in mediating thrombocytopaenia. However, patients with the primary antiphospholipid antibodies without thrombocytopaenia do not possess antiplatelet antibodies (Macchi et al. 1997), suggesting that there is no primary association between the APS and antiplatelet antibodies, and that the antigens which mediate platelet destruction in immune thrombocytopaenia are distinct from the antigens recognized by antiphospholipid antibodies. There is accumulating evidence that the antigens recognized by antibodies found in the antiphospholipid syndrome are in fact 'cofactor' proteins such as β_2-glycoprotein I, which interact with cell membrane phospholipids. Anti-β_2-glycoprotein I antibody binding to platelets that had been partially activated by ADP has been shown to be able to induce massive platelet activation *in vitro* (Arvieux et al. 1993), and may explain the thrombotic complications associated with antiphospholipid antibodies, but not the thrombocytopaenia.

Thrombotic thrombocytopaenic purpura (TTP)

TTP presents as a multisystem disorder with thrombocytopaenia, microangiopathic haemolytic anaemia, fluctuating neurologic symptoms, fever, and progressive renal failure. There is widespread subendothelial hyaline deposits and vascular microthrombi on pathologic examination which is due to massive deposition of platelet microthrombi in the circulation. The condition needs to be differentiated from disseminated intravascular coagulation and major thromboses in the setting of the antiphospholipid syndrome. The immunological mechanisms linking ITP to lupus are still unclear, but may involve a circulating inhibitor of von Willebrand factor (vWF)-cleaving protease. This leads to reduced protease activity and the presence of large multimers of vWF in the circulation (Furlan and Lammle 1998). In SLE, 40 cases of TTP have been reported in the literature, and the onset of TTP may occur simultaneously with the connective tissue disease (Musio et al. 1998). In paediatric cases of TTP, however, the link with SLE is stronger. In a retrospective analysis of 35 cases of TTP of childhood onset, nine (26 per cent) fulfilled four criteria or more of SLE, and the presence of proteinuria in this context is an important clinical pointer towards the presence of SLE (Brunner et al. 1999).

Leucopaenias including Felty's syndrome

The classical clinical manifestations of Felty's syndrome include neutropaenia and splenomegaly in a patient with RA. The RA is often long established, seropositive, and erosive. Other clinical features that may be present include skin ulcers, nodules, and vasculitis. The splenomegaly is variable, from mild to massive, while the neutropaenia may be cyclic, and may be associated with haemolytic anaemia and thrombocytopaenia. Among the mechanisms thought to be responsible for the clinical features are: (i) T cell mediated suppression of granulopoeisis in the spleen, (ii) hypersplenism, and (iii) antineutrophil antibodies. In support of the first mechanism is the demonstration of a suppressor T cell population which inhibits CFU-G formation and the reversal of neutropaenia when patients are treated with immunomodulatory drugs (e.g. D-penicillamine, leflunomide, cyclosporine A).

Recent interest has particularly focused on the relationship between Felty's and large granular lymphocyte (LGL) syndrome, a haematological disorder characterized by clonal proliferation of LGL, and which is considered a leukaemic condition. LGLs are CD3+, CD8+, and CD57+ and have natural killer (NK) activity. Clinical and immunogenetic studies show that there is an overlap between these two conditions; up to one-third of Felty's patients have clonal expansions of this subset of lymphocyte in their circulation (Bowman et al. 1995) and up to 25 per cent of patients with LGL syndrome turn out to have RA (Loughran and Starkebaum 1987). Immunogenetic studies also show a similarity in Felty's patients and LGL + RA patients, as 90 per cent possess HLA–DR4 (Starkebaum et al. 1997). Finally, LGLs from Felty's and normal subjects are capable of inhibiting CFU-GM development in an *in vitro* culture system, lending further support for a suppressive mechanism in the pathogenesis of neutropaenia (Coakley et al. 2000).

Haematological malignancies in rheumatic diseases (see Chapter 1.3.9)

A link between rheumatic diseases and neoplasia has long been noted. In clinical practice, this association presents most frequently in two settings: First, is the rheumatic disease a manifestation of an underlying malignancy? Second, is malignancy a result of the rheumatic disease or the treatment employed to treat the rheumatic disease ? I will confine my discussion to the haematological malignancies, which include the leukaemias, myeloproliferative disorders, lymphomas, and plasma cell disorders. In the first instance, we will address the question of whether there is a link between certain rheumatic diseases with these disorders, and secondly the recognized paraneoplastic manifestations of these disorders.

Epidemiology

In trying to establish if rheumatic diseases are associated with an increased risk of malignancy, investigators have relied on retrospective analysis of the causes of death or cancer incidence in cohort of patients and attempted to compare the rates with those found in the general population. The results are often expressed as relative risk or standardized incidence ratio (Table 4). The interpretation of these findings need to be considered, however, in the light of the size of the cohorts, and possible temporal trends in cancer incidence in the patient cohort, which may go back many years, with that of the comparator population, which is often taken at a single time point. Despite these reservations, there is a sizeable body of evidence on the major inflammatory rheumatic diseases, with most of the data coming from the Scandinavian countries where the health systems collect cancer statistics in a systematic manner.

Table 4 Epidemiological data of risks of haematological malignancies in rheumatic diseases

	No. of patients in study	**RR or SIR**
RA	9469[a]	
All haematologic malignancies		1.7 (1.3–2.2)
NHL		2.2 (1.5–3.1)
Hodgkin's		2.2 (0.6 –5.7)
Leukaemias		1.3 (0.7–2.2)
SLE		
Hodgkin's[b]	276	17.8 (0.45–99.23)
NHL[c]	205	44 (11.9–111)
NHL[d]	1585	5.2 (2.2–10.3)
Haematological[e]		4.1
Primary Sjögren's		
All haematological malignancies[a]	676	6.4 (3.8–10.1)
NHL[f]	110	13 (2.7–38)
NHL[g]	136	43.8
Scleroderma		
NHL[h]	233	9.6 (1.1–34.5)

[a] Kauppi et al. (1997).
[b] Sultan et al. (2000).
[c] Pettersson et al. (1992).
[d] Mellemkjaer et al. (1997).
[e] Abu-Shakra et al. (1996).
[f] Pertovaara et al. (2001).
[g] Kassan et al. (1978).
[h] Rosenthal et al. (1993).

Note: RR, relative risk; SIR, standardized incidence ratio with 95% CI; NHL, non-Hodgkin's lymphoma.

Rheumatoid arthritis

A slightly increased incidence of all types of cancer has been noted in RA, and it accounts for between 8 and 20 per cent of deaths in this population (Reilly et al. 1990). Since the 1960s, there was a suggestion that the incidence of lymphomas was elevated, and this was subsequently confirmed by Isomaki et al. (1978). However, more recent surveys showed only a slight increase (Kauppi et al. 1997) or no increase at all (Kvalvik et al. 2001). It has been suggested that the increased incidence of cancer, particularly non-Hodgkin's lymphoma, is linked to prior immunosuppressive treatment for RA, as has been found in the transplantation setting. Though of practical concern, this does not seem to be borne out by subsequent studies, except for the use of methotrexate and chlorambucil.

A clear role of an immunosuppressive agent in oncogenesis is the development of lymphomas in RA patients treated with methotrexate and which remits on stopping methotrexate (Georgescu et al. 1997). An additive role for EB virus has been proposed, and in a survey of 21 RA patients with lymphoma, 26 per cent of malignant lymph nodes from RA samples were positive when analysed by *in situ* hybridization, but no non-malignant nodes were positive (Dawson et al. 2001). These findings suggest that immunosuppressive drugs may play a permissive role in virus related oncogenesis, though there is insufficient data to determine if viral infection is a common cause for lymphomas developing while on other immunosuppressive agents.

SLE, Sjögren's, and scleroderma

While there seems to be an increased risk of malignancy in SLE patients overall, no excess in haematological malignancy was reported in studies by Manzi (1997) and Sultan (2000), while the studies of Canadian (Abu-Shakra et al. 1996), Danish (Mellemkjaer et al. 1997), and Finnish (Pertovaara et al. 2001) cohorts reported an excess of non-Hodgkin's lymphoma (RR 4, 5, and 44, respectively). In terms of mortality, cancer is not the major cause of death in SLE and trails behind SLE itself and infections. There is, in the literature, a handful of reports linking SLE with thymoma, which occurs more frequently than chance would suggest, suggesting that there is an aetiological link between the two diseases.

In primary Sjögren's syndrome, an increased incidence of haematological malignancies, especially non-Hodgkin's lymphoma is well documented. Initial reports cite an approximately 40-fold increased risk of developing lymphoma (Kassan et al. 1978). More recent studies suggest a lower risk, but there was still a significant association (Abu-Shakra et al. 1996). Clinical features at initial presentation of Sjögren's syndrome which should alert the clinician to an unfavourable outcome include non-exocrine organ involvement such as neuropathy, fever, and organomegaly. Laboratory features which are associated with development of lymphoma include mixed monoclonal cryoglobulinaemia and monoclonal rheumatoid factor. The lymphomas could involve the salivary glands themselves or present in other more typical sites such as the liver and spleen and lymph nodes.

In scleroderma, an increased incidence of lung and breast cancers has been reported by a number of groups (e.g. Jacobsen et al. 1998), and in a recent survey, an excess in haematological malignancies was also found (Rosenthal et al. 1993).

With few exceptions, the data presented does not separate out if the increased incidence in malignancies reported is due to the disease or to the treatment. There has been a sustained debate on the role of immunosuppressive treatments in the pathogenesis of malignancy, as they may suppress tumour immune surveillance or predispose the patient to other factors implicated in oncogenesis such as viral infections. While there may still be debate about the excess risk due to azathioprine or methotrexate, treatments such as radiotherapy in ankylosing spondylitis are known to be associated with an increase in leukaemias, most probably as a direct result of the treatment. In RA patients treated with chlorambucil, there is similarly an increased risk of haematological malignancies on long-term follow-up. However, any excess in cancer rate has also to be interpreted in the light of the data cited above, that is that some rheumatic diseases may, by itself, be associated with an increased rate of cancer.

Rheumatological presentations of haematological neoplasia

Rheumatological syndromes developing during the course of cancer are well known and recognized, and may be due to direct involvement of musculoskeletal system by the cancer or present as 'paraneoplastic' clinical manifestations. Among the haematological malignancies, a number of well described clinical associations are recognized, particularly in relation to myeloproliferative and lymphoproliferative diseases (Wooten and Jasin 1996). In childhood, acute leukaemia presenting as arthritis is well recognized; in adults, this may take the form of arthralgias or bone pains as the initial manifestations of haematological disease (Table 5). Occasionally, direct infiltration of synovial tissues by leukaemic cells in chronic leukaemias has been found.

Coagulation and thrombosis in rheumatic diseases

There is an increasing awareness that cardiovascular disorders and inflammatory rheumatic diseases may have much in common in terms of pathogenetic mechanisms and the growing body of data showing that there is an increased incidence of cardiovascular disease in patients with RA and SLE. Inflammation and immune mechanisms, similar to those implicated in the pathogenesis of inflammatory arthritis, also play a role in atherosclerosis (Ridker et al. 2000).

Vascular damage in RA and SLE

Cardiovascular complications can arise in both RA and SLE. In RA, vasculitis and cardiac disease are well-recognized extra-articular complications and support the notion that RA is not simply an articular disease, but a systemic disease with articular manifestations. In SLE, vasculitis, pericarditis, endocarditis are all recognized manisfestions. The presence of antiphospholipid antibodies in this condition is an additional marker for a range of vascular disorders which are dealt with elsewhere. However, beyond these classical complications is the realization that there is an increased prevalence of all types of cardiovascular disease (strokes, myocardial infarctions, thromboses, etc.) in association with these two diseases. The underlying mechanisms are likely to be multifactorial, and include persistent inflammation, treatments which predispose to vascular disease by changing lipid metabolism and immunological pathways that increase vascular injury.

Morbidity and mortality from cardiovascular disease

A number of different studies over the last three decades have documented that patients with RA have a higher mortality rate than the general population.

Table 5 Rheumatologic manifestations of haematological malignancies

Type	Rheumatological manifestation
Acute leukaemias	Arthralgias, gout, bone pains, septic arthritis
Chronic leukaemias	Arthralgias, arthritis, vasculitis
Hodgkin's	Erythema nodosum, arthralgias, arthritis
Non-Hodgkin's lymphoma	Arthralgias, arthritis, cryoglobulinaemia, vasculitis
Myeloma	Vasculitis, cryoglobulinaemia, amyloid
Polycythaemia rubra vera, essential thrombocythaemia	Gout, erythromelalgia
Hairy cell leukaemia	Cutaneous vasculitis
LGL syndrome	Arthritis

As cardiovascular disease is the most frequent cause of death in Western populations, it is not surprising that this is also the major cause of death in the RA group. However, when adjusted for the mortality rate of the reference population, there is a small and consistent increase of deaths due to cardiovascular disease in the studies undertaken to date. Male patients appear to be particularly at risk, and there may be an added risk related to rheumatoid factor positivity and the presence of extra-articular features of RA.

Although the data on SLE is not as extensive, there is also evidence that SLE patients have an increased risk of premature cardiovascular complications. SLE patients showed an increased rate of myocardial infarction and angina pectoris, especially if cardiovascular risk factors are present and if treated with corticosteroids for prolonged periods (Manzi et al. 1997). There is a suspicion that SLE itself may constitute a risk factor because of inflammation, antiphospholipid antibodies, and other mechanisms (Esdaile et al. 2001).

In practical terms, these studies highlight that in both RA and SLE, there is an increased risk of cardiovascular events related to accelerated atherosclerosis. Although the mechanisms underlying this increase remain to be elucidated, the clinician should be aware of this complication, and intervene promptly when cardiovascular risk factors are detected in this population. There is no current evidence to justify a preventive treatment.

Inflammation is linked to increased risk for atherosclerosis

Evidence from epidemiology and basic research show that inflammation plays a role in atherosclerosis. Population studies have found that even slightly raised levels of CRP are associated with an increased risk of cardiovascular events in men and women and is an independent risk factor for subsequent events (Ridker et al. 1997, 2000). From the pathological point of view, the mechanisms implicated in atherosclerosis share many common features of those implicated in chronic synovial inflammation (Ross 1999). In addition, immunological mechanisms such as endothelial damage and autoantibodies, which interact with LDL or cell membranes, may contribute to vascular injury and enhance development of atherosclerosis in patients with certain inflammatory rheumatic diseases.

Coagulation and fibrinolysis in rheumatic diseases

The coagulation cascade is made up of a series of proteolytic enzymes acting sequentially to regulate clot formation by amplifactory and inhibitory pathways. Although its main role is the formation of the fibrin clot, inflammation is also a potent trigger which can lead to extravascular fibrin deposition. Notable examples of this phenomenom include the synovium in rheumatoid arthritis, the kidney in glomerulonephritis and the lungs in alveolar inflammation. The formation of cross-linked fibrin results from the cleavage of fibrinogen by the serine protease thrombin, which in turn is generated by the conversion of prothrombin through the action of the 'prothrombinase complex' made up of Factors Xa and Va in the presence of phospholipid and Ca^{2+}. Tissue factor (TF), which is expressed on activated endothelium and activated macrophages, amplifies the conversion of X to Xa, in the presence of factor VIIa, and plays a critical role in initiating the coagulation cascade (see Fig. 1) (reviewed by Lutchman-Jones and Broze 1995). In RA, there is strong evidence that the coagulation pathway is active, as shown by the extensive fibrin deposits which are seen in the rheumatoid synovium and the raised levels of TAT (thrombin–antithrombin) complexes in the synovial fluid (Weinberg et al. 1991). In chronic rheumatoid effusions, fibrin aggregates in the form of rice bodies are often found and fibrin strands are seen attached to the synovial villi (Fig. 2). In addition to fibrin formation, activation of coagulation may also amplify inflammation by a number of receptor–ligand interactions, such as between Xa and its receptor EPR-1 (effector protease receptor), and thrombin with molecules in the protease-activated receptor (PAR) family (Coughlin 2001). These interactions are capable of inducing pro-inflammatory cellular proliferative responses in the synovium.

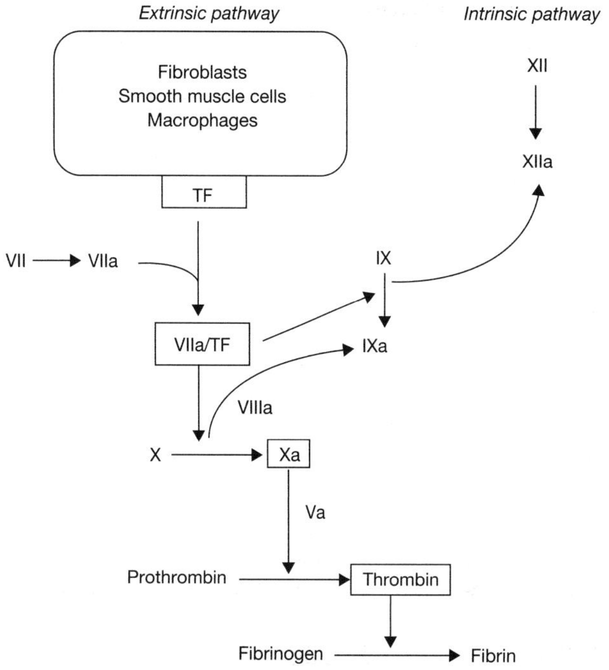

Fig. 1 Schematic representation of fibrin formation within the RA joint.

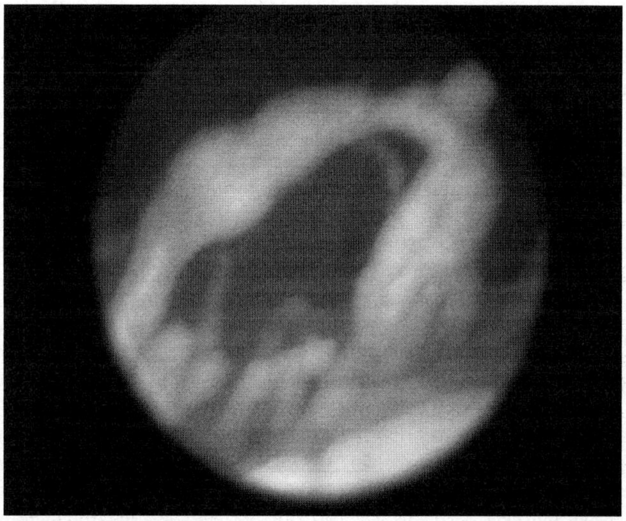

Fig. 2 Fibrin aggregates and fibrin strands seen attached to the synovial villi (as captured from video film).

The formation of fibrin in an inflammatory site or a clot is balanced by fibrinolytic pathways which serve to remove the deposited material. Plasmin is the main fibrinolytic enzyme which is generated from plasminogen in a process mediated by the two plasminogen activators: tPA (tissue plasminogen activator) or uPA (urokinase type plasminogen activator). In the RA synovium, there is an abundance of uPA which is produced by macrophages and synovial lining cells which may have both a beneficial role, by accelerating the clearance of fibrin or a more deleterious role by damaging cartilage and connective tissue within the joint (Busso and So 1997).

In prothrombotic states such as found in SLE and the antiphospholipid syndrome, besides the well-documented presence of antibodies that may react with membrane phospholipids and the endothelium, antiprothrombin antibodies have been demonstrated in a significant percentage of patients who are lupus anticoagulant positive (Bertolaccini et al. 2000). The pathological signficance of these antibodies remain to be clarified, but their presence appears to be correlated with thrombotic events in the SLE population. Increased TF levels have also been reported in patients with the antiphospholipid syndrome (Amengual et al. 1998) and may further contribute to the thrombotic predisposition.

References

Abu-Shakra, M., Gladman, D.D., and Urowitz, M.B. (1996). Malignancy in systemic lupus erythematosus. *Arthritis and Rheumatism* **39**, 1050–4.

Alarcon-Segovia, D. et al. (1989). Antiphospholipid antibodies and the antiphospholipid syndrome in systemic lupus erythematosus. A prospective analysis of 500 consecutive patients. *Medicine Baltimore* **68**, 353–65.

Amengual, O. et al. (1998). The role of the tissue factor pathway in the hypercoagulable state in patients with the antiphospholipid syndrome. *Thrombosis and Haemostasis* **79**, 276–81.

Arvieux, J. et al. (1993). Platelet activating properties of murine monoclonal antibodies to beta 2-glycoprotein I. *Thrombosis and Haemostasis* **70**, 336–41.

Barker, R.N. et al. (1992). Identification of autoantigens in autoimmune haemolytic anaemia by a non-radioisotope immunoprecipitation method. *British Journal of Haematology* **82**, 126–32.

Bertolaccini, M.L., Amengual, O., and Atsumi, T. (2000). Antiprothrombin antibodies. In *Hughes Syndrome* (ed M.A. Khamashta), pp. 245–52. London: Springer.

Bowman, S.J. et al. (1995). Hematologic and cytofluorographic analysis of patients with Felty's syndrome. A hypothesis that a discrete event leads to large granular lymphocyte expansions in this condition. *Arthritis and Rheumatism* **38**, 1252–9.

Brunner, H., Freeman, M., and Silverman, E.D. (1999). Close relationship between systemic lupus erythematosus and thrombotic thrombocytopenic purpura in childhood. *Arthritis and Rheumatism* **42**, 2346–55.

Busso, N. and So, A.K. (1997). Urokinase in rheumatoid arthritis: causal or coincidental? *Annals of the Rheumatic Diseases* **56**, 705–6.

Cines, D.B. et al. (1985). Platelet antibodies of the IgM class in immune thrombocytopenic purpura. *Journal of the Clinical Investigation* **75**, 1183–90.

Coakley, G. et al. (2000). CD8+, CD57+ T cells from healthy elderly subjects suppress neutrophil development in vitro: implications for the neutropenia of Felty's and large granular lymphocyte syndromes. *Arthritis and Rheumatism* **43**, 834–43.

Coughlin, S.R. (2001). Thrombin signalling and protease-activated receptors. *Nature* **407**, 258–64.

Dainaiak, N. et al. (1980). Humoral suppression of erythropoiesis in systemic lupus erythematosus (SLE) and rheumatoid arthritis. *American Journal of Medicine* **69**, 527–44.

Dawson, T.M. et al. (2001). Epstein–Barr virus, methotrexate, and lymphoma in patients with rheumatoid arthritis and primary Sjögren's syndrome: case series. *Journal of Rheumatology* **28**, 47–53.

Esdaile, J.M. et al. (2001). Traditional Framingham risk factors fail to fully account for accelerated atherosclerosis in systemic lupus erythematosus. *Arthritis and Rheumatism* **44**, 2331–7.

Flores, G. et al. (1993). Efficacy of intravenous immunoglobulin in the treatment of autoimmune hemolytic anemia: results in 73 patients. *American Journal of Hematology* **44**, 237–42.

Furlan, M. and Lammle, B. (1998). Deficiency of von Willebrand factor-cleaving protease in familial and acquired thrombotic thrombocytopenic purpura. *Ballière's Clinical Rheumatology* **11**, 509–14.

Georgescu, L. et al. (1997). Lymphoma in patients with rheumatoid arthritis: association with the disease state or methotrexate treatment. *Seminars in Arthritis and Rheumatism* **26**, 794–804.

Griffith, S.M. et al. (2001). Do patients with rheumatoid arthritis established on methotrexate and folic acid 5 mg daily need to continue folic acid supplements long term? *Rheumatology* **39**, 1102–9.

Hazletine, M. et al. (1988). Antiphospholipid antibodies in systemic lupus erythematosus: evidence of an association with positive Coombs' and hypocomplementemia. *Journal of Rheumatology* **15**, 80–6.

Hochberg, M.C. et al. (1998). Serum immunoreactive erythropoietin in rheumatoid arthritis: impaired response to anemia. *Arthritis and Rheumatism* **31**, 1310–18.

Isomaki, H., Hakulinen, T., and Joutsenlahti, U. (1978). Excess risk of lymphomas, leukemia and myeloma in patients with rheumatoid arthritis. *Journal of Chronic Diseases* **31**, 691–6.

Jacobsen, S., Halberg, P., and Ullman, S. (1998). Mortality and causes of death of 344 Danish patients with systemic sclerosis (scleroderma). *British Journal of Rheumatology* **37**, 750–5.

Jelkmann, W. et al. (1991). Monokines inhibiting erythropoietin production in human hepatoma cutlures and in isolated perfused rat kidneys. *Life Sciences* **50**, 300–1.

Kassan, S.S., Thomas, T.L., and Moutsopoulos, H.M. (1978). Increased risk of lymphoma in sicca syndrome. *Archives of Internal Medicine* **89**, 888–92.

Kauppi, M., Pukkala, E., and Isomaki, H. (1997). Elevated incidence of hematologic malignancies in patients with Sjögren's syndrome compared with patients with rheumatoid arthritis. *Cancer Causes and Control* **8**, 201–4.

Kvalvik, A.G., Jones, M.A., and Symmons, D.P. (2001). Mortality in a cohort of Norwegian patients with rheumatoid arthritis followed from 1977 to 1992. *Scandinavian Journal of Rheumatology* **29**, 29–37.

Loughran, T.P., Jr. and Starkebaum, G. (1987). Large granular lymphocyte leukemia. Report of 38 cases and review of the literature. *Medicine Baltimore* **66**, 397–405.

Luchtman-Jones, L. and Broze, G.J., Jr. (1995). The current status of coagulation. *Annals of Medicine* **27**, 47–52.

Macchi, L. et al. (1997). Anti-platelet antibodies in patients with systemic lupus erythematosus and the primary antiphospholipid antibody syndrome: their relationship with the observed thrombocytopaenia. *British Journal of Haematology* **98**, 336–41.

Manzi, S. et al. (1997). Age-specific incidence rates of myocardial infarction and angina in women with systemic lupus erythematosus: comparison with the Framingham Study. *American Journal of Epidemiology* **145**, 408–15.

Means, R.T., Dessypris, E.N., and Krantz, S.B. (1992). Inhibition of human erythroid colony-forming units by interleukin-1 is mediated by gamma interferon. *Journal of Cell Physiology* **150**, 50–9.

Mellemkjaer, L. et al. (1997). Non-Hodgkin's lymphoma and other cancers among a cohort of patients with systemic lupus erythematosus. *Arthritis and Rheumatism* **40**, 761–8.

Musio, F. et al. (1998). Review of thrombotic thrombocytopenic purpura in the setting of systemic lupus erythematosus. *Seminars in Arthritis and Rheumatism* **28**, 1–19.

Pettersson, T. et al. (1992). Increased risk of cancer in patients with systemic lupus erythematosus. *Annals of the Rheumatic Diseases* **51**, 437–9.

Pertovaara, M. et al. (2001). A longitudinal cohort study of Finnish patients with primary Sjögren's syndrome: clinical, immunological and epidemiological aspects. *Annals of the Rheumatic Diseases* **60**, 467–72.

Ramsey-Goldman, R. et al. (1998). Increased risk of malignancy in patients with systemic lupus erythematosus. *Journal of Investigation Medicine* **46**, 217–22.

Ravetch, J.V. and Bolland, S. (2001). IgG Fc receptors. *Annual Review of Immunology* **19**, 275–90.

Reilly, P.A. et al. (1990). Mortality and survival in rheumatoid arthritis: a 25 year prospective study of 100 patients. *Annals of the Rheumatic Diseases* **49**, 363–9.

Ridker, P.M. et al. (1997). Inflammation, aspirin, and the risk of cardiovascular disease in apparently healthy men. *New England Journal of Medicine* **336**, 973–9.

Ridker, P.M. et al. (2000). C-reactive protein and other markers of inflammation in the prediction of cardiovascular disease in women. *New England Journal of Medicine* **342**, 836–43.

Rosenthal, A.K. et al. (1993). Scleroderma and malignancy: an epidemiological study. *Annals of the Rheumatic Diseases* **52**, 531–3.

Ross, R. (1999). Atherosclerosis—an inflammatory disease. *New England Journal of Medicine* **340**, 115–26.

Shibata, T. et al. (1990). Monoclonal anti-erythrocyte autoantibodies derived from NZB mice cause autoimmune hemolytic anemia by two distinct pathogenic mechanisms. *International Immunology* **2**, 1133–41.

Starkebaum, G. et al. (1997). Immunogenetic similarities between patients with Felty's syndrome and those with clonal expansions of large granular lymphocytes in rheumatoid arthritis. *Arthritis and Rheumatism* **40**, 624–6.

Sultan, S.M., Ioannou, Y., and Isenberg, D.A. (2000). Is there an association of malignancy with systemic lupus erythematosus ? An analysis of 276 patients under long term review. *Rheumatology* **39**, 1147–52.

van der Pol, W.-L. and van de Winkel, J.G.J. (1998). IgG receptor polymorphisms: risk factors for disease. *Immunogenetics* **48**, 222–32.

Vincent, T. and Mackworth-Young, C. (2000). The primary antiphospholipid syndrome. In *Hughes Syndrome* (ed. M.A. Khamashta), pp. 111–26. London: Springer.

Vyse, T. and So, A.K. (1992). Sulphasalazine induced autoimmune syndrome. *British Journal of Rheumatology* **31**, 115–16.

Weinberg, J.B., Pippen, A.M., and Greenberg, C.S. (1991). Extravascular fibrin formation and dissolution in synovial tissue of patients with osteoarthritis and rheumatoid arthritis. *Arthritis and Rheumatism* **34**, 996–1005.

Wooley, P.H. et al. (1980). HLA–DR antigens and toxic reaction to sodium aurothiomalate and D-penicillamine in patients with rheumatoid arthritis. *New England Journal of Medicine* **303**, 300–2.

Wooten, M.D. and Jasin, H.E. (1996). Vasculitis and lymphoproliferative diseases. *Seminars in Arthritis and Rheumatism* **26**, 564–74.

1.3.11 An anaesthetic perspective

Allan I. Binder and Frances Dormon

Introduction

Rheumatic diseases have important implications in anaesthetic practice (Skues and Welchew 1993). Arthritis affecting the cervical spine, temporomandibular and cricoarytenoid joints, and involvement of the mouth, lips, nasopharynx, and oesophagus may result in increased risk and difficulty during intubation, maintenance, and recovery from general anaesthesia. Constitutional illness, anaemia, and the involvement of specific organs are common and may complicate anaesthetic management. Medication, in particular steroid and immunosuppressive agents may also be important. The sedentary life-style of many patients with rheumatic disease accelerates atherosclerotic vascular disease and increases the risk of infection postoperatively.

This chapter will concentrate on the problems from the anaesthetist's point of view, so that the rheumatologist can help by identifying problems in a particular patient in relation to the procedure involved. We include discussion of alternatives to general anaesthesia, such as regional and local blocks, with their relative advantages and disadvantages. Newer techniques to increase the safety of intubation and anaesthetic drugs with specific advantages are mentioned. Finally, the role of the pain clinic, usually run by anaesthetists, is examined.

Systemic factors in rheumatic disease and their relevance to routine pre-anaesthetic assessment and anaesthesia

Autoimmune diseases such as systemic lupus erythematosus (SLE), juvenile chronic arthritis, scleroderma, and rheumatoid arthritis are multisystem diseases. As the emphasis of clinical features varies greatly from patient to patient, with many patients showing features of more than one autoimmune disease, pre-anaesthetic investigation needs to be tailored specifically to the individual patient. In some circumstances, such as the pregnant patient with SLE, the anaesthetist needs to consider the risks of anaesthesia to both the mother and foetus (Davies 1991). In order that the risks of anaesthesia in patients with autoimmune disease may be anticipated and hence reduced, consideration will first be given to the impact of the disease on major organs, with appropriate pre-operative investigation.

Cardiac disease

Diseases

Patients with SLE, juvenile chronic arthritis, scleroderma, vasculitis, and rarely other autoimmune diseases can have serious cardiovascular pathology. Valvular vegetations may also develop in SLE patients, especially in association with anticardiolipin antibodies. Many patients with autoimmune disease have subclinical cardiac abnormalities, which are unlikely to affect anaesthetic management, provided that the procedure is uncomplicated. However, they can prove important if the anaesthetist experiences difficulties with intubation leading to inadvertent hypoxia. For this reason, careful pre-operative evaluation of the cardiovascular system should always be carried out.

Assessment

While clinical examination, electrocardiography, and chest radiographs will exclude major cardiac disease, echocardiography provides a non-invasive method of defining the extent of cardiac lesions. Although, exercise testing can be an excellent indicator of fitness for anaesthesia, many rheumatoid patients are not physically able to complete these tests. With a significant conduction defect, as occurs in some patients with spondarthropathies, the pre-operative insertion of a temporary pacing wire or facilities for pacing during surgery may be required. Patients with reduced cardiac reserve require more detailed monitoring of their central venous pressure, arterial pressure, and sometimes cardiac output. In all cases, the cardiac status should be optimized before surgery.

Anaesthesia

In patients with cardiac disease, general anaesthesia is often preferable to local anaesthesia as the blood pressure can usually be maintained with greater certainty. However, care is still necessary during induction and reversal of anaesthesia. If the patient awakes too rapidly or has excessive pain, an endogenous surge of adrenaline may destabilize the cardiac status.

If general anaesthesia is considered undesirable, local anaesthetic techniques can be considered. Limiting factors are the ability of patients to lie still for sufficiently long and the positioning required by the surgeon (Skues and Welchew 1993). A spinal block can cause a precipitous fall in the blood pressure due to rapid loss of sympathetic tone. Although, this can be treated with fluid and vasoconstrictors, epidural blockade is safer as it develops more slowly and the cardiovascular changes can be controlled more easily.

Patients with valvular abnormality, septal defect, or patent ductus arteriosus should be prescribed antibiotic prophylaxis, with the antibiotic being given 1 h pre-operatively if the oral or intramuscular route is used, or just prior to intubation if given intravenously.

Respiratory disease

Diseases

Pulmonary disease may be of several types. Pulmonary fibrosis is the most characteristic and important for anaesthesia as it causes a progressive reduction in lung compliance and vital capacity and the impairment of gas transfer can lead to pulmonary hypertension and respiratory failure.

In SLE, pleuropulmonary complications are common and often severe, especially when associated with vascular abnormalities as a result of antiphospholipid antibodies. Scleroderma also frequently has respiratory complications, resulting in complex abnormalities which include a restrictive ventilatory defect, airflow obstruction, and a reduced diffusing capacity for carbon monoxide. Pulmonary vascular disease and restriction of chest expansion may also coexist, increasing the risk of respiratory failure and pulmonary hypertension. The severity of lung involvement in scleroderma does not always correlate with the extent of extrapulmonary disease and can dominate the clinical picture.

Ankylosing spondylitis, and the seronegative spondarthropathies can reduce thoracic spine and costovertebral joint movement and seriously impair chest expansion. However, these patients maintain adequate ventilation, unless other factors such as bronchitis, pneumonia, or pneumothorax intervene. Reduction in chest expansion can also be found with severe kyphosis due to advanced osteoporotic collapse of thoracic vertebrae or weakness of the respiratory muscle as a result of dermatomyositis.

Assessment

Pre-operative assessment should identify significant respiratory disease. As a general rule, the ability to climb two flights of stairs without undue breathlessness suggests adequate respiratory reserve for general anaesthesia. If a problem is suspected, pulmonary function tests and baseline blood–gas analyses are necessary. The function tests should include transfer factor and a vitalograph, so the severity of restrictive and obstructive components of lung disease can be defined, and reversible elements treated. The baseline blood–gas analyses are especially helpful if respiratory failure develops in the postoperative period, and a knowledge of the pre-operative carbon dioxide level can assist in weaning the patient off the respirator.

Anaesthesia

The choice of anaesthetic technique usually depends upon the surgical requirements, with some consideration to the likely post-operative course. For major thoracic and abdominal surgery, the post-operative period can be complicated by respiratory insufficiency, owing to pain and the residual effect of the anaesthetic (Catley et al. 1985). Regional techniques are often preferred to general anaesthesia in patients with serious respiratory disease, although long operations and the supine position may be particularly unpleasant for breathless and disabled patients. If sedation is added to a regional technique, great care is necessary to avoid oversedation and dangerous respiratory depression. Adequate analgesia is just as important following regional as general anaesthesia, as respiratory failure may follow either technique if pain control is inadequate.

Renal disease

Diseases

Serious renal failure is a common finding in patients with SLE, but can occur in scleroderma and other autoimmune diseases. Subclinical renal dysfunction is common in rheumatoid and other connective tissue diseases, and can be exacerbated by non-steroidal anti-inflammatory drugs (NSAIDs) including COX-2-specific inhibitors, amyloidosis, or unrelated causes.

Assessment

With more serious renal failure, creatinine clearance and isotopic renography help to define the severity of the renal disease, although neither is accurate in advanced disease where expert nephrology advice should be sought.

Anaesthesia

Monitoring of the central venous pressure is usually needed to help maintain the fluid balance in patients with renal disease, especially during and after major surgery, where there may be large shifts of fluid complicating fluid balance. Whichever technique of anaesthesia is used in patients with autoimmune diseases, the plasma concentration of anaesthetic drugs may be affected by the degree to which they are protein-bound (Wood 1986) or by the degree of renal dysfunction. A mild reduction in renal function is not a problem to the anaesthetist, but if present should be noted so as to avoid prolonged perioperative fluid restriction combined with nephrotoxin agents such as gentamicin, NSAIDs, and frusemide.

Haemopoietic disease

Anaemia

This is a common feature of rheumatic diseases and can result from many causes. The 'anaemia of chronic disease', typical of inflammatory diseases such as rheumatoid arthritis, results from ineffective erythropoiesis, and rarely drops the haemoglobin to below 9 g/100 ml. Ideally, anaemia should be assessed, and where necessary treated before elective surgery. A haemoglobin of 8 g/100 ml is now considered adequate for general anaesthesia provided the anaemia is chronic and physiological adaptation has been achieved. Pre-operative oximetry is very helpful in the assessment of anaemic patients as it demonstrates the presence of desaturation without cyanosis. If transfusion is necessary, it should be completed at least 24 h before surgery to allow the transfused red cells to replenish the levels of 2,3-diphosphoglycerate and function in oxygen transfer. In an emergency, the blood should be given at the time of surgery to avoid fluid overload.

Neutropaenia

A low white-cell count as a result of SLE, Felty's syndrome, or rheumatic drugs increases the risk of post-operative sepsis without the expected white cell response. Antibiotic prophylaxis should be prescribed in susceptible patients.

Complex haematological abnormalities

These can develop as a result of SLE, Felty's syndrome, and occasionally, other rheumatic diseases or the drugs used in treatment. Full haematological assessment in these patients should include white blood count, platelet count, and a coagulation screen. Anticardiolipin antibodies and cryoglobulins may also be necessary. Anticardiolipin antibodies increase the risk of intravascular coagulation during surgery (Menon and Allt-Graham 1993) and paradoxically also occasionally cause excessive bleeding, especially when hypoprothrombinaemia and/or thrombocytopenia are also present (Shaulian et al. 1981). In these patients, fresh frozen plasma and platelet packs should be available for surgery. Expert haematological advice should be sought if complex abnormalities are found.

Prophylaxis against DVT

This is particularly important in patients undergoing major joint or abdominal surgery, where the risk of venous thrombosis and pulmonary embolism is increased (White 1985). Low molecular weight heparin, and pneumatic compression to the foot and calf reduce the risks of thromboembolism more effectively than low-dose warfarin following knee arthroplasty (Westrich et al. 2000; Brookenthal et al. 2001). Low molecular weight heparin and warfarin are effective following hip surgery, but the optimum duration of prophylaxis at both sites has yet to be determined.

Gastrointestinal disease

Oesophageal fibrosis and hypomotility are common in scleroderma and, even when not clinically apparent, markedly increase the risk of gastric reflux after anaesthesia (Orringer et al. 1976; Smith and Shribman 1984). Anaesthesia with a rapid sequence technique should be considered where there is risk of regurgitation. The laryngeal mask airway (see below) should only be used if the intubation risk is greater than that of regurgitation. Positioning and careful observation should be continued well into the post-operative period to avoid aspiration and identify cricoarytenoid joint inflammation (Funk and Raymon 1975), both of which could result in respiratory embarrassment after extubation. Extubation should also be delayed until the patient is able to maintain an independent airway.

Skin and joints

Particular care is necessary in the handling, positioning, and movement of patients with generalized arthropathy who undergo surgery, and corticosteroid therapy and rheumatoid nodules increase the risks of pressure-induced skin damage. Unusual parts of the body may also become weight bearing during surgery and will require additional padding and support. All patients with significant arthritis should be sent to theatre wearing a soft collar, to remind theatre staff to avoid excessive movement of the neck and to handle the patient with extreme care. Dry eyes need to be protected with regular methylcellulose eye drops and the application of petroleum jelly to the lips and nose will provide similar protection to oral and nasal mucosa.

Antirheumatic drugs

Corticosteroid therapy

Prolonged steroid use is associated with osteoporosis, deficient wound healing, reduced resistance to infection, and accelerated atherosclerosis. However, the suppressive effect on the hypothalamic–pituitary–adrenal axis is the most important complication to the anaesthetist, as it can persist for up to a year after corticosteroid therapy has ended. The levels of cortisol do not show whether the axis has recovered and other functional tests of the axis are complicated and unreliable. Steroid cover should therefore be given to these patients. Intravenous hydrocortisone is started with surgery, the doses being tapered over the next 2–4 days and returned to the maintenance levels within a week. For major surgery, 200 mg of intravenous hydrocortisone is given with anaesthetic induction. The dosage of hydrocortisone infused is then reduced by 25 per cent each day until the maintenance dose is reached. For lesser procedures, 100 mg of hydrocortisone, is adequate. The trend is to shorten the period of steroid cover, because of its adverse effect on wound healing and risk of infection.

The anaesthetist must minimize the risks of infection by maintaining scrupulous cleanliness of all equipment used. Bacterial filters should also be incorporated into the breathing circuits to reduce the risk of pulmonary infection. Antibiotic prophylaxis may be required and pre-operative dental hygiene should be considered for patients with severe scleroderma and Sjögren's syndrome.

Immunosuppressive drugs

Azathioprine, methotrexate, and other immunosuppressive agents are also associated with an increased risk of infection and similar precautions to those for steroids should be adopted. A reduction in the white blood count and platelet counts, and possible adverse effects on wound healing, may also be associated with these drugs. There is no evidence that stopping methotrexate, leflunomide, and biological agents reduces perioperative sepsis or other complications following elective orthopaedic surgery (Grennan et al. 2001). Where patients are on high dosage therapy or are particularly susceptible to infection, stopping immunosuppressive drugs for 1–2 weeks in the post-operative period might be prudent.

Intubation difficulties

Rheumatoid arthritis

Rheumatoid arthritis is by far the most common autoimmune rheumatic disease presenting to the anaesthetist. The advent of joint replacement has markedly increased planned surgical intervention, even in patients with advanced disease. Emergency operations are also frequently needed, especially for upper gastrointestinal bleeding induced by NSAIDs. Rheumatoid arthritis can affect any synovial joint and often affects the cervical spine (Crosby and Lui 1990) temporomandibular, and cricoarytenoid joints (Funk and Raymon 1975).

Cervical spine

Adequate extension at the cervical spine is important for direct laryngoscopy and endotracheal intubation, and can be compromised by rheumatoid neck involvement. Cervical subluxation, usually occurs at the atlantoaxial joint, but can affect any level. While subluxation can cause cervical myelopathy or radiculopathy, it is often asymptomatic. Atlantoaxial subluxation usually occurs anteriorly but can also occur posteriorly, as a result of odontoid peg erosion. Progressive subaxial cervical subluxation affecting multiple levels, the so-called 'stair-case spine', typically occurs in seropositive rheumatoid patients with severe deforming peripheral arthropathy. With progressive cervical disease, the neck becomes short and rigid, with superior migration of the dens, further complicating intubation. While neurological changes in rheumatoid patients usually results from subluxation, soft-tissue pannus formation can contribute to spinal cord compression.

Temporomandibular (TMJ) and cricoarytenoid (CAJ) joint involvement

TMJ disease limits mouth opening and can complicate direct laryngoscopy and intubation (Aiello and Metcalf 1992). A hoarse voice, a sense of fullness in the throat, dysphagia, exertional dyspnoea, and rarely stridor suggest CAJ involvement. Investigation by indirect laryngoscopy or fibre-optic examination of the cords may reveal rheumatoid nodules on the cords or cricoarytenoid joint involvement, with decreased cricoarytenoid movement, bowing of the cords during inspiration, fixed adduction of the cords, or glottic stenosis. In extreme cases, these findings indicate the need for elective tracheostomy or consideration of alternative methods of anaesthesia. The presence of such findings necessitates particular vigilance for signs of post-extubation stridor (Funk and Raymon 1975).

Pre-anaesthetic work-up

Two simple tests which may help to predict a difficult intubation are:

(i) an inability to visualize the soft palate or uvula when the mouth is fully opened and the tongue protruded (Mallampati et al. 1985); and

(ii) an inability of the patient to protrude the lower teeth beyond the upper incisors, suggesting reduced temporomandibular joint movement (Calder 1992).

These clinical tests should be carried out routinely in all patients, but even if normal, unexpected problems may arise and the anaesthetist needs to anticipate the possibility of a failed intubation (Wilson 1993).

In rheumatoid arthritis, radiographs of the cervical spine in flexion/extension with a through-mouth view of the odontoid peg are helpful in defining the presence and severity of any spinal instability, although the routine use of this investigation in asymptomatic rheumatoid arthritis patients has been questioned. Magnetic resonance imaging (MRI) is the investigation of choice in defining the presence and severity of subluxation and soft-tissue pannus affecting the cervical spine.

Having made a full assessment, the anaesthetist will choose to anaesthetize the patient in one of the ways listed in Table 1. The choice of anaesthetic approach is often based on individual preference and, with some of the techniques, the level of expertise. Intubation needs to be carried out with great care in patients with severe rheumatoid, as myelopathy may be precipitated by the procedure even in patients without symptomatic cervical involvement.

Juvenile idiopathic arthritis

Juvenile idiopathic arthritis, particularly of polyarticular or systemic onset, often results in serious and early involvement of the cervical spine

Table 1 Methods of airway maintenance during anaesthetic induction

No relaxant needed
Intravenous or inhalational induction
+/− Guedel airway or laryngeal mask airway
Relaxant needed
Intravenous or inhalational induction
delay relaxant until positive-pressure ventilation (PPV) is established with mask
intubate under (i) direct vision, or (ii) with introducer, or (iii) blind oral/nasal, or (iv) with a fibreoptic 'scope'
Awake intubation
using fibreoptic laryngoscope
Awake insertion of 'minitracheotomy'
ventilate through 'jet' for induction and intubation
Elective tracheostomy in the awake patient

(Hensinger et al. 1986). In addition to instability, growth abnormalities of the vertebral bodies, bony fusions, and sometimes torticollis add to the difficulties with intubation. Development of the temporomandibular joint and cricoarytenoid joints (Jacobs and Hui 1977) can be similarly affected with micrognathia and reduced mouth opening (Stabrun et al. 1988). MRI of the temporomandibular joints indicates the extent of disease.

The younger patient with potential for a difficult intubation presents the anaesthetist with a far greater problem (Smith 1990). There are fewer anaesthetic options in the child because techniques such as awake intubation are unsuitable and venous access may be difficult to achieve before induction of anaesthesia. The anatomy of the child is different from the adult, making visualization of the larynx more difficult. Sizes of the tracheal tube need to be scaled down according to age, and adult equipment cannot be used, increasing the hazards for anaesthetists unfamiliar with young patients. The physiological differences include a reduced respiratory reserve, which leads to more rapid onset of hypoxia if there is a delay in intubation or difficulty in maintaining the airway.

For all these reasons, young children with significant arthritis should be treated in specialist paediatric centres with expertise in difficult intubation techniques, although the options listed in Table 1 still generally apply. The laryngeal mask airway (see 'Techniques for difficult intubation'), can be used in all age groups, furthermore, intubation can be achieved using a smaller fibre-optic laryngoscope or a guide wire technique with the adult fibre-optic laryngoscope.

For certain procedures where intubation is unnecessary, ketamine can be used for anaesthesia (D'Arcy et al. 1976). This drug results in the maintenance of adequate respiration and a clear airway. However, it does not guarantee a safe airway and should not be used unless full intubation facilities and equipment for emergency tracheostomy are available. Ketamine is unsuitable for older children, who are more liable to suffer from troublesome hallucinations during the recovery phase.

Ankylosing spondylitis and seronegative spondarthropathies

Significant ankylosis of the cervical spine is common in ankylosing spondylitis, and can occur in any of the seronegative spondarthropathies. Disease of the cricoarytenoid joints can also be present. Ankylosis is rarely missed during the pre-anaesthetic assessment in patients with severe involvement, although these patients often generate more anxiety than is warranted. While difficult to intubate because of the rigidity of the neck, the airway is easy to maintain without intubation or manipulation. The laryngeal mask airway (Brain 1983) is easy to insert and, provided that the intercostal joints are not severely ankylosed, can be used to ventilate the patient. If intubation is considered essential, it should be achieved with minimal manipulation using the intubating laryngeal mask airway (Gabbott 2001), or the fibre-optic laryngoscope in the awake patient (Sinclair and Mason 1984). Care must be taken in these patients as atlantoaxial subluxation or vertebral fracture can occur from relatively minor trauma.

Sjögren's syndrome and scleroderma

These conditions, alone or in conjunction with other autoimmune states, can cause problems with intubation because of their specific effects on the mouth and nose.

Mouth and nose

In Sjögren's syndrome, xerostomia may result in reduced mouth opening, and dryness and friability of the oral mucosa, making it difficult to insert the laryngoscope. The poor dental state may result in loose teeth which could dislodge during intubation, or single-standing teeth which hamper laryngoscopy.

In scleroderma, the oral symptoms are often severe, and this combined with abnormalities of cervical and mandibular joints, makes intubation potentially hazardous. Poor dental hygiene is almost invariable in patients with severe scleroderma and patients need to be warned that if teeth are dislodged during anaesthesia, dentures may be impossible to fit. Whether the oral or nasal route is used for intubation, severe lacerations or bleeding from telangectasia may follow (Davidson-Lamb and Finlayson 1977).

Pulmonary

Pulmonary fibrosis is commonly found in patients with scleroderma, Sjögren's syndrome, and other autoimmune diseases. Progressive reduction in lung compliance and vital capacity can also result from sclerodermatous involvement of the chest wall.

Venous access

This is often difficult in scleroderma, limiting the choice for induction of anaesthesia (Smith and Shribman 1984). Vasospastic abnormalities are common and intravenous induction may provoke a painful cyanotic reaction, similar to that experienced by patients with Raynaud's phenomenon (Davidson-Lamb and Finlayson 1977). Vasodilatation may also cause significant cardiovascular instability after induction of anaesthesia (Eisele 1990), and fluids should be readily available to limit the fall in blood pressure, and should be warmed to prevent vasospastic irritability. Arterial lines, should only be used where absolutely necessary, as severe spasm could follow their introduction.

If local anaesthetic techniques are to be used, vasoconstrictors should be avoided, as the blood supply may be further compromised. Regional anaesthesia can also result in prolonged but reversible sensory blockade, which is useful as analgesia, but can be associated with prolonged vasospasm (Neill 1980).

Techniques for difficult intubation

Table 1 lists the range of techniques available to the anaesthetist. Not all patients require intubation, particularly for short procedures on the limbs, and local anaesthetic techniques may be more suitable in these cases. Repeated attempts at endotracheal intubation can increase the risk of neurological damage (Hastings and Kelley 1993) and also cause airway obstruction due to glottic trauma in the post-operative period.

Induction of general anaesthesia can be achieved smoothly with an intravenous or inhalational agent. If the airway is difficult to maintain, an oral or nasal airway may help. The laryngeal mask airway (Brain 1983; Gabbott 2001) passed orally, fits snugly over the larynx (Fig. 1), and is of proven value in the safer management of anaesthesia in arthritic patients. However, the airway is not protected from soiling by gastric contents and the laryngeal mask airway is not a replacement for intubation in all cases. Intubation is essential if the surgery requires muscle relaxation, the operation is longer, the patient needs to lie prone, or has pulmonary disease.

Despite careful assessment, it is not always possible to predict what will happen to the airway after induction (Wilson 1993). Obstruction can occur at any time and airway adjuncts may not help. Therefore, with all these patients, induction of anaesthesia is undertaken slowly, allowing repeated reassessment of the airway. Inhalational anaesthesia may be the safer option

(a)

(b)

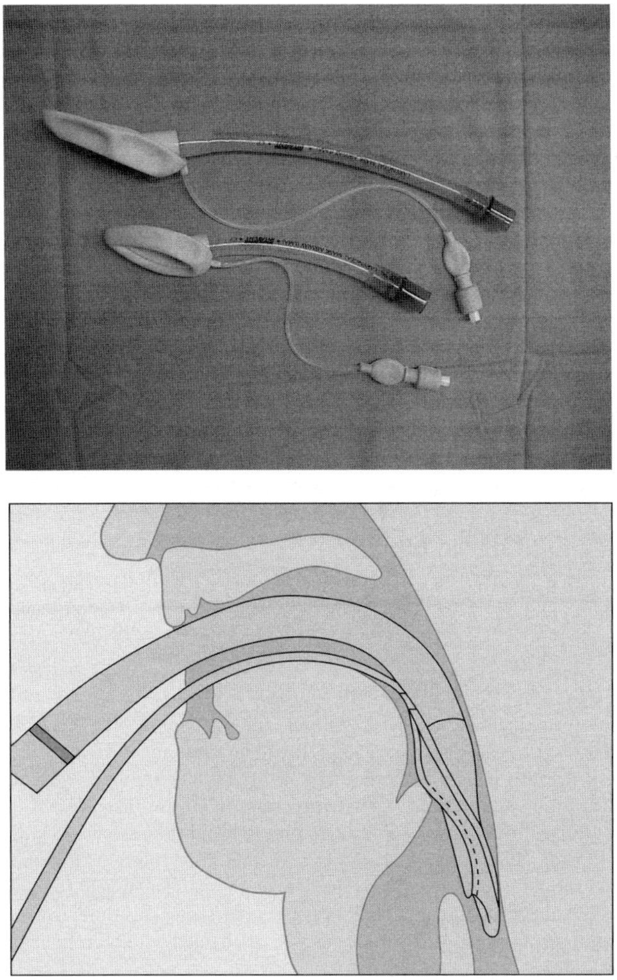

Fig. 1 (a) Laryngeal mask airway. (b) Diagram of a laryngeal mask airway in place.

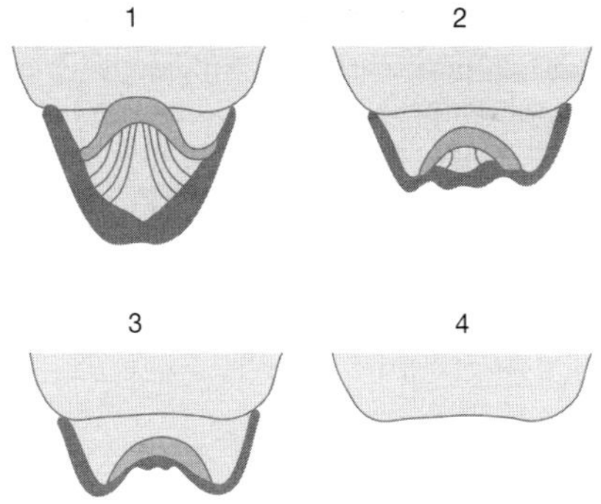

Fig. 2 Diagrammatic classification of the four grades of view of the larynx obtained at laryngoscopy. Grade 1, most of the glottis visible; grade 2, only epiglottis and posterior commissure seen; grade 3, only epiglottis seen; grade 4, not even the epiglottis can be exposed (Cormack and Lehane 1984).

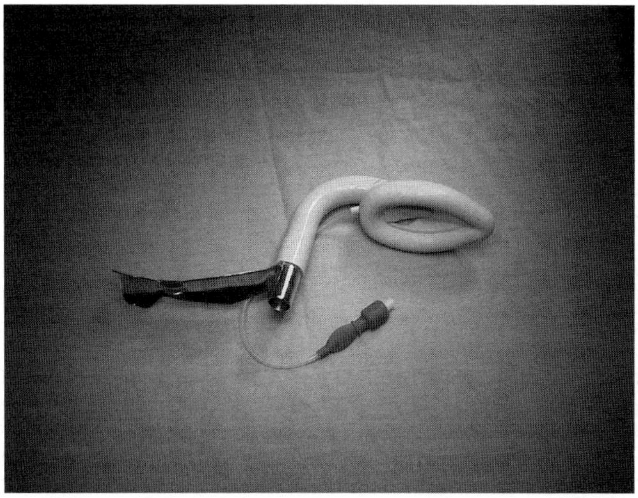

Fig. 3 Intubating laryngeal mask airway.

as the anaesthetic can be halted if the patient obstructs. Once the patient is asleep, and before muscle relaxants are given, the anaesthetist must ensure that it is possible to ventilate the patient manually with a bag, mask, and airway. Provided this is possible, there is sufficient time to try the several available techniques. If laryngoscopy is only moderately difficult and a grade 3 view of the larynx is obtained (Cormack and Lehane 1984) (Fig. 2), it is possible to intubate directly or use a soft bougie as an introducer over which the tracheal tube is passed. The McCoy laryngoscope, which is a modification of the mackintosh-bladed laryngoscope, has a hinged tip and improves the view to facilitate intubation. However, laryngoscopic intubation may still prove impossible. Some anaesthetists are sufficiently experienced with blind-nasal intubation, but the intubating laryngeal mask airway (Fig. 3) is now an accepted aid to intubation (Baskett et al. 1998). The intubating laryngeal mask airway is inserted and then used as a guide to blind insertion of a flexible endotracheal tube. In the most difficult cases, the fibreoptic intubating laryngoscope has radically altered the management of rheumatoid patients with cervical spine disease (King and Adams 1990). This device can be used when the patient is asleep but more commonly is used prior to anaesthesia where a difficult intubation is expected (Sinclair and Mason 1984; Sidhu et al. 1993).

A pre-operative explanation of the procedure will reassure the patient and the use of anticholinergic pre-medication will reduce secretions. However, anxiolytic agents should be used with care as respiratory depression may occur or the airway may become obstructed. Several methods have been described to achieve analgesia of the pharynx and upper trachea but care must be taken to avoid toxicity if a 4 per cent lignocaine spray is used.

Several other methods of airway management have been described. A 'minitracheotomy' (Matthews et al. 1986) can be made and a catheter passed through the larynx from below. The minitracheotomy can be used with a jet ventilator to maintain adequate ventilation while an alternative airway is secured. In other difficult situations the laryngeal mask airway may be inserted and elective tracheostomy performed either surgically or using a percutaneous dilatational kit. These kits are readily available and many intensivists have considerable expertise in their use (Bodenham 1993).

Emergency work-up for anaesthesia

Ideally there should be plenty of time for a full anaesthetic work-up to assess potential risks in patients with rheumatological disease (Skues and Welchew 1993) and this has been considered above. However, these patients often require emergency surgery, where a rapid bedside assessment must include:

- Cardiovascular—history (chest pain, paroxysmal nocturnal dyspnoea, palpitations), examination, and ECG.
- Respiratory—history (breathlessness, exercise tolerance, e.g. climbing stairs), examination.

- Drug history—cardiac drugs, NSAIDs, steroids, immunosuppressives.
- Airway and cervical spine assessment. With severe peripheral arthritis, assume cervical spine instability.
- Blood test—FBC, clotting, urea, and electrolytes.

If there is serious concern about the neck, awake intubation (Sinclair and Mason 1984), using the fibreoptic laryngoscope (Sidhu et al. 1993), should be considered. A soft collar to protect the vulnerable neck and careful handling have already been mentioned.

Post-operative care

Immediately following extubation, prolonged observation is necessary to ensure that airway obstruction does not develop, especially in patients with serious cricoarytenoid (Funk and Raymon 1975), temporomandibular, or cervical spine pathology. In some cases, post-operative ventilation may be necessary to ensure adequacy of the airway and oxygenation. Aspiration of gastric contents, which can lead to respiratory embarrassment, is a particular risk in scleroderma patients where gastro-oesophageal reflux is common (Orringer et al. 1976; Smith and Shribman 1984).

The main challenge facing the anaesthetist immediately following major surgery is the provision of effective analgesia without respiratory depression. Ventilatory insufficiency in the post-operative period can be precipitated by a number of causes such as restrictive lung disease, infection, obesity, diaphragmatic splinting due to pain, and the residual effect of the anaesthetic superimposed on pre-existing borderline respiratory function. If the carbon dioxide is significantly raised pre-operatively, then post-operative ventilation is usually necessary.

Early and regular chest physiotherapy, bronchodilators, and antibiotics are important in post-operative management. If the retention of sputum becomes a problem, a 'minitracheotomy' should be inserted to assist in the removal of secretions before the patient tires and develops respiratory failure.

Adjuvant epidural analgesia, cryotherapy to the intercostal nerves during thoracotomy, or patient-controlled intravenous opioid analgesia are all methods that optimize post-operative pain control and hence reduce the risk of respiratory failure. Patient-controlled analgesia systems may not be appropriate in rheumatoid patients with severe hand involvement (Jani and Trujillo 1994) and catheter techniques of regional blockade using local anaesthetic agents (see below) may be more effective.

Opioid drugs need to be used with particular care in rheumatoid patients as obstructive sleep apnoea may occur, especially in patients with temporomandibular joint involvement. NSAIDs given by the suppository, intramuscular, or buccal routes have particular value in post-operative pain control, by limiting the need for opioids that cause vomiting and respiratory depression.

After major abdominal or thoracic surgery, large shifts of fluid from the intravascular space may complicate fluid balance. As renal and cardiac abnormalities are so common in arthritic patients, cardiac or renal failure may result from minor variations in fluid balance. Continuous monitoring of the central venous pressure should therefore be extended well into the recovery period in these patients.

Careful positioning and additional padding and support to weight bearing parts of the body should also be maintained, with disabled patients being nursed on pressure relieving mattresses after surgery. Passive stretching and mobilization need to be started as early as possible to prevent joint contracture, pressure sores, and other post-operative complications in these patients. Rheumatoid therapy should also be reinstituted as soon as feasible and prophylaxis to prevent deep vein thrombosis, infection, and peptic ulceration should be continued in appropriate cases.

Alternatives to general anaesthesia

Local anaesthetic techniques, often combined with sedation, have gained increasing popularity in recent years. The improvement in education of the general public has contributed more to the increased usage than the introduction of new drugs or techniques. There are numerous techniques (Table 2) ranging in complexity from simple infiltration to blockade at the spinal level (Wildsmith and Armitage 1993).

Local infiltration

Careful explanation, with or without anxiolytic premedication, is all that is required before local infiltration. The appropriate use of sedative drugs also enables fairly complex operations to be undertaken. The combination of 1–2 mg of midazolam and 10–30 mg of propofol (see Table 3) provides sedation and amnesia with relative safety. Full monitoring and anaesthetic facilities should, however, be available, because of the rare (1–2 per cent) occurrence of respiratory depression in especially sensitive patients.

Peripheral nerve blocks

These blocks are suitable for many surgical procedures on the limbs, especially where a tourniquet is unnecessary (Wildsmith and Armitage 1993).

Regional nerve blocks

Regional nerve blocks are useful for many major procedures, and are sometimes combined with sedation or even light general anaesthesia without intubation.

Intravenous regional anaesthesia (Bier's block)

This form of anaesthesia is safe, simple, and useful for a wide range of procedures, given the necessary expertise. The local anaesthetic is injected intravenously into an arm or leg that has been isolated from the general circulation by a tourniquet. Care is necessary to ensure that the cuff is not inadvertently deflated for at least 20 min to avoid risks associated with the release of a bolus of local anaesthetic. Furthermore, full resuscitation facilities should be available. This type of anaesthesia is suitable for operations lasting about 40 min, as tourniquet pain occurs after this time. However, a major advantage is that patients can be discharged within an hour of the procedure.

Brachial plexus blocks

The brachial plexus can be approached by three distinct routes, each having some advantages and disadvantages.

The axillary approach

The axillary approach is the safest and therefore the most commonly used route, but has the disadvantages that the success rate is variable and supplementary peripheral nerve blocks are often required. The block of the radial nerve can also be patchy and, if a tourniquet is used, nerve blocks may be needed for the tourniquet area.

The subclavian approach

The subclavian approach is more reliable, particularly in the upper arm and tourniquet areas, but is associated with a greater risk of pneumothorax, making overnight observation in hospital desirable. A bilateral block should not be attempted because slow development of pneumothoraces may occur.

The interscalene approach

The interscalene approach is also reliable but the ulnar block may be patchy. It should be reserved for patients with emphysema or chronic obstructive airways disease, where the risk of pneumothorax is high, and for operations on the upper arm and shoulder.

Spinal anaesthesia

The use of narrow-gauge needles has reduced the incidence of spinal headache to under 5 per cent, and post-operative bed rest is unnecessary, making these blocks very popular. The block, which is established within 10 min, is more reliable and complete than an epidural block and lasts for up to 2 h. The time limit can be extended by the insertion of a fine-bore

Table 2 Newer drugs of value in anaesthesia

Drug	Function	Advantages and disadvantages
Rocuronium	Muscle relaxant	Very rapid onset, may avoid use of suxamethonium
Cisatracurium	Muscle relaxant	Non-enzymic elimination, especial value where renal and hepatic dysfunction co-exist
Propofol	Induction agent	Rapid metabolism allowing a quick and clear-headed recovery Major advance for anaesthesia for short procedures
Sevofluxane	Volatile anaesthetic agent	Rapid uptake and few side-effects Rapid elimination through the lungs Renal and hepatic damage unlikely Fast waking, hence ideal for day surgery
Midazolam	Benzodiazepine	Shortest-acting benzodiazepine (half-life 2 h compared with 36 h for diazepam) No active metabolites, so less mental impairment Favoured drug for intravenous sedation at doses of 2–7.5 mg (initial dose of 1 mg in elderly)
Flumazenil	Benzodiazepine antagonist	Useful for short-term reversal of sedation to assess the patient in the intensive care unit Avoid routine use to reverse sedation after minor surgery, as the half-life is short and resedation may occur
Alfentanyl	Opioid analgesic	Duration of action is 5–10 min, so useful in procedures of this duration High risk of respiratory depression
Remifentanyl	Opioid analgesic	Ultra short acting, given as infusion Rapidly metabolized by non specific blood and tissue esterases

Table 3 The approach of a 'pain clinic' and its therapeutic modalities

Multidisciplinary team	Anaesthetist, other physicians, social worker, physiotherapist, occupational therapist, psychologist, and/or psychiatrist
Drug therapy	Conventional analgesics, e.g. non-narcotic analgesics Narcotic analgesics as a last resort Centrally-acting, pain-modifying drugs: tricyclic antidepressants, antiepileptic agents
Nerve blocks	Local, regional, spinal blocks Autonomic blocks: stellate ganglion, coeliac plexus, and lumbar sympathectomy Facet joint injection or cryotherapy
Other	Guanethidine blocks Acupuncture Calcitonin injection therapy Clonidine injection Percutaneous cordotomy and other rare neuro-surgical techniques

catheter for continuous spinal anaesthesia, although the introduction of the combined spinal/epidural technique has reduced the use of spinal catheters. This type of block should be used with great care in patients with poor myocardial reserve, as its rapid onset can lead to peripheral vasodilatation and sudden hypotension (Malmqvist et al. 1987).

The use of a hyperbaric mixture of anaesthetic, such as bupivacaine in 4 per cent dextrose, allows the establishment of a unilateral block for surgery on one leg. For this type of block, the spinal needle is inserted with the patient lying on the side requiring surgery for at least 10 min while the block is established. The drop in blood pressure is far less with a unilateral block.

Epidural anaesthesia

This has gained wide usage even in the presence of extensive spinal disease. The wider-bore epidural needle allows a catheter to be inserted with ease for continuous infusion. The block takes longer to establish and may result in 'unblocked' segments, where nerve roots are left unaffected by the anaesthetic. Furthermore, if the needle is advanced too far, the dura may be pierced producing a CSF leak, resulting in severe headache and rarely complications such as arachnoiditis (Sklar et al. 1991).

Combined spinal and epidural anaesthesia

Using a special needle pack, the epidural space is identified and a long spinal needle is used to pierce the dura and perform a spinal block. The spinal needle is then removed and a catheter inserted into the epidural space. This combined technique offers the advantages of a rapid onset spinal block with the facility to administer 'top-ups' or a continuous infusion for longer operations or to provide post-operative analgesia.

Newer drugs of value in anaesthesia

A few agents recently introduced into anaesthetic practice have improved the safety and efficiency of anaesthesia for patients with multisystem disease. These drugs are shown in Table 2 with their relative advantages and disadvantages.

The pain clinic

Pain clinics are now established in most hospitals, where they are of value in the management of patients with intractable pain. Treatment is tailored to the individual needs of each patient and includes physical and psychological measures to reduce pain. Drugs and nerve blocks form the mainstay of treatment but in some cases other coping strategies enable patients to live with their pain. Pain clinics are usually run by anaesthetists, assisted by a multidisciplinary team. Detailed evaluation of these clinics is outside the scope of this chapter but the major treatment options are shown in Table 3. Although a large variety of conditions are referred to pain clinics, chronic mechanical backache, neck and shoulder pain, and reflex sympathetic dystrophy are the most commonly referred by rheumatologists.

Back pain unresponsive to conventional treatment may benefit from transcutaneous nerve stimulation, acupuncture, joint injections, epidurals, and other nerve blocks. Where these fail, antidepressants, behaviour modification, and other coping techniques can be successful.

Reflex sympathetic dystrophy (algodystrophy) is often intractable and when unresponsive to physiotherapy may benefit from guanethidine blocks, continuous epidural infusion, calcitonin injections, and chemical sympathectomy.

Patients with rheumatoid arthritis and inflammatory arthropathies form a very small proportion of referrals to pain clinics. However, there is increasing recognition of the value of pain specialists in the amelioration of pain from some sources. An example of this is the treatment of pain arising from the cervical spine, whether due to inflammatory or mechanical causes. Cervical epidural injection can be used to treat severe cervical pain without neurological deficit when unresponsive to physiotherapy. This treatment is particularly effective where muscle spasm and radicular pain are prominent features. Suprascapular blocks for intractable shoulder pain, and local injection around the hip, can have similar value. Moreover, the multidisciplinary approach of the pain clinic may help in the management of pain and development of coping mechanisms in patients with generalized inflammatory arthropathies whose pain is inadequately controlled despite optimal medical and surgical treatment. The true value of the pain clinics to rheumatology patients has not yet been fully explored.

Conclusions

This chapter has considered the systemic and joint abnormalities in patients with rheumatic disease from the perspective of the anaesthetist. The pre-anaesthetic assessment and techniques for general and regional anaesthesia have been described, with an insight into the difficulties often encountered and methods used for solving these problems. Finally, the role of the pain clinic has been considered.

References

Aiello, G. and Metcalf, I. (1992). Anaesthetic implications of temporomandibular disease. *Canadian Journal of Anaesthesia* **39**, 610–17.

Baskett, P.J.F., Parr, M.J., and Nolan, J.P. (1998). The intubating laryngeal mask. Results of a multicentre trial with experience of 500 cases. *Anaesthesia* **53**, 1174–9.

Bodenham, A.R. (1993). Percutaneous dilational tracheostomy. Completing the anaesthetists range of airway techniques. *Anaesthesia* **48**, 101–2 (editorial).

Brain, A.I. (1983). The laryngeal mask: a new concept in airway management. *British Journal of Anaesthesia* **55**, 801–5.

Brookenthal, K.R., Freedman, K.B., Lotke, P.A., Fitzgerald, R.H., and Lonner, J.H. (2001). A meta-analysis of thromboembolic prophylaxis in total knee arthroplasty. *Journal of Arthroplasty* **16**, 293–300.

Calder, I. (1992). Predicting difficult intubation. *Anaesthesia* **47**, 528–30.

Catley, D.M., Thornton, C., Jordan, C., Lehane, J.R., Royston, D., and Jones, J.G. (1985). Pronounced episodic oxygen desaturation in the postoperative period: its association with ventilatory pattern and analgesic regimen. *Anesthesiology* **63**, 20–8.

Cormack, R.S. and Lehane, J. (1984). Difficult tracheal intubation in obstetrics. *Anaesthesia* **39**, 1105–11.

Crosby, E.T. and Lui, A. (1990). The adult cervical spine: implications for airway management. *Canadian Journal of Anaesthesia* **37**, 77–93.

D'Arcy, E.J., Fell, R.H., Ansell, B.M., and Arden, G.P. (1976). Ketamine and juvenile chronic polyarthritis (Still's disease). Anaesthetic problems in Still's disease and allied disorders. *Anaesthesia* **31**, 624–32.

Davidson-Lamb, R.W. and Finlayson, M.C. (1977). Scleroderma. Complications encountered during dental anaesthesia. *Anaesthesia* **32**, 893–5.

Davies, S.R. (1991). Systemic lupus erythematosus and the obstetrical patient—implications for the anaesthetist. *Canadian Journal of Anaesthesia* **38**, 790–5.

Eisele, J.H. (1990). Connective tissue disease. In *Anaesthesia and Uncommon Diseases* 3rd edn. (ed. J. Katz, J.L. Benumof, and L.B. Kadis), pp. 645–67. Philadelphia PA: W.B. Saunders.

Funk, D. and Raymon, F. (1975). Rheumatoid arthritis of the cricoarytenoid joints: an airway hazard. *Anesthesia and Analgesia* **54**, 742–5.

Gabbott, D.A. (2001). Recent advances in airway technology. *British Journal of Anaesthesia/CEPD Reviews* **1**, 76–80.

Grennan, D.M., Gray, J., Loudon, J., and Fear, S. (2001). Methotrexate and early postoperative complications in patients with rheumatoid arthritis undergoing elective orthopaedic surgery. *Annals of the Rheumatic Diseases* **60**, 214–17.

Hastings, R.H. and Kelley, S.D. (1993). Neurological deterioration associated with airway management in a cervical spine-injured patient. *Anesthesiology* **78**, 580–3.

Hensinger, R.N., Devito, P.D., and Ragsdale, C.G. (1986). Changes in the cervical spine in juvenile rheumatoid arthritis. *Journal of Bone and Joint Surgery* **68**, 189–98.

Jacobs, J.C. and Hui, R.M. (1977). Cricoarytenoid arthritis and airway obstruction in juvenile rheumatoid arthritis. *Paediatrics* **59**, 292–4.

Jani, K. and Trujillo, M. (1994). Getting to grips with patient controlled analgesia—an evaluation of handgrip disability. *British Journal of Anaesthesia* **72** (Suppl. 1), 118.

King, T.A. and Adams, A.P. (1990). Failed tracheal intubation. *British Journal of Anaesthesia* **65**, 400–14.

Mallampati, S.R. et al. (1985). A clinical sign to predict difficult tracheal intubation: a prospective study. *Canadian Anaesthetic Society Journal* **32**, 429–34.

Malmqvist, L.A., Bengtsson, M., Bjornsson, G., Jorfeldt, L., and Lofstrom, J.B. (1987). Sympathetic activity and haemodynamic variables during spinal analgesia in man. *Acta Anaesthetica Scandinavica* **31**, 467–73.

Matthews, H.R., Fischer, B.J., Smith, B.E., and Hopkinson, R.B. (1986). Minitracheotomy: a new delivery system for jet ventilation. *Journal of Thoracic and Cardiovascular Surgery* **92**, 673–5.

Menon, G. and Allt-Graham, J. (1993). Anaesthetic implications of the anti-cardiolipin antibody syndrome. *British Journal of Anaesthesia* **70**, 587–90.

Neill, R.S. (1980). Progressive systemic sclerosis. Prolonged sensory blockade following regional anaesthesia in association with a reduced response to systemic analgesics. *British Journal of Anaesthesia* **52**, 623–5.

Orringer, M.B., Dabich, L., Zarafonetis, C.J., and Sloan, H. (1976). Gastro-oesaphogeal reflux in oesophogeal scleroderma: diagnosis and implications. *Annals of Thoracic Surgery* **295**, 120–30.

Shaulian, E., Shoenfeld, Y., Berliner, S., Shaklai, M., and Pinkhas, J. (1981). Surgery in patients with circulating lupus anticoagulant. *International Surgery* **66**, 157–9.

Sidhu, V.S., Whitehead, E.M., Ainsworth, Q.P., Smith, M., and Calder, I. (1993). A technique of awake fibreoptic intubation. Experience in patients with cervical spine disease. *Anaesthesia* **48**, 910–13.

Sinclair, J.R. and Mason, R.A. (1984). Ankylosing spondylitis. The case for awake intubation. *Anaesthesia* **39**, 3–11.

Sklar, E.M., Quencer, R.M., Green, B.A., Montalvo, B.M., and Post, M.J. (1991). Complications of epidural anaesthesia: MR appearance of abnormalities. *Radiology* **181**, 549–54.

Skues, M.A. and Welchew, E.A. (1993). Anaesthesia and rheumatoid arthritis. *Anaesthesia* **48**, 989–97.

Smith, B. (1990). Anesthesia in pediatric rheumatology. In *Pediatric Rheumatology Update* (ed. P. Woo, P.H. White, and B.M. Ansell), pp. 124–30. New York: Oxford University Press.

Smith, G.B. and Shribman, A.J. (1984). Anaesthesia and severe skin disease. *Anaesthesia* **39**, 443–55.

Stabrun, A.E., Larheim, T.A., Hoyeraal, H.M., and Rosler, M. (1988). Reduced mandibular dimensions and asymmetry in juvenile rheumatoid arthritis. Pathogenetic factors. *Arthritis and Rheumatism* **31**, 602–11.

Westrich, G.H., Haas, S.B., Mosca, P., and Peterson, M. (2000). Meta-analysis of thromboembolic prophylaxis after total knee arthroplasty. *Journal of Bone and Joint Surgery of Britain* **82**, 795–800.

White, R.H. (1985). Preoperative evaluation of patients with rheumatoid arthritis. *Seminars of Arthritis and Rheumatism* **14**, 287–99.

Wildsmith, J.A.W. and Armitage, E.N., ed. (1993). *Principles and Practice of Regional Anaesthesia* 2nd edn. Edinburgh: Churchill Livingstone.

Wilson, M.E. (1993). Predicting difficult intubation. *British Journal of Anaesthesia* **71**, 333–4.

Wood, M. (1986). Plasma drug binding: implications for anesthesiologists. *Anesthesia and Analgesia* **65**, 786–804.

1.3.12 The eye

Elizabeth M. Graham and Alison M. Leak

Introduction

The ophthalmologist has many roles in the management of patients with rheumatological problems. Most rheumatological diseases have ocular complications, many of which are specific to the disease, and consequently the ophthalmologist has an important diagnostic role. Many ophthalmic complications require specific therapy and in some cases may actually dictate the systemic therapy for the disease, giving the ophthalmologist a therapeutic role (Box 1). Rheumatological diseases require a wide range of drugs and several of these have important ocular side-effects; the ophthalmologist therefore has a guardian's role in monitoring the eye and preventing complications.

Most rheumatological diseases affect either the uvea, sclera, retina, or optic nerve, and produce symptoms and signs that confirm both their nature and aetiology. Involvement of the uvea or sclera usually produces painful red eyes with preserved vision, whereas involvement of the retina or optic nerve causes profound visual loss without pain or redness. Fortunately, with the particular exception of juvenile idiopathic arthritis, most of the ocular complications that can affect the sight are symptomatic, so that the rheumatologist can at once alert the patient to the possibility of future eye disease and then await events.

The ocular examination

All patients referred to the ophthalmologist undergo the same routine examination, whether or not they are symptomatic. Visual function is assessed by testing visual acuity via a pinhole to obtain the effects of refractive error. The visual field is assessed using a red pin, as red is the most sensitive colour for elucidating disease of the optic nerve. Colour vision, changes in which may indicate early disease of the optic nerve or severe macular disease, is tested with Ishihara colour plates.

The eyes are examined in detail for evidence of redness or squint, and then with a slit lamp to observe any medial opacity (e.g. uveitis, cataract) and to measure the intraocular pressure. Pupillary reactions and eye movements are tested before the pupils are dilated for examination of the fundi.

Box 1 Important key points for ophthalmologists to remember

1. Examine all children suspected of juvenile rheumatoid arthritis as soon as possible. It takes seconds!
2. Visual loss due to ischaemic optic neuropathy with cotton wool spots and/or minor retinal arteriolar occlusion is due to systemic vasculitis.
3. Uveitis associated with choroidal or pigment epithelial disease suggests sarcoidosis.
4. Uveitis and retinal infiltrates or retinal vein occlusions suggests Behçet's disease.
5. Scleritis associated with peripheral corneal ulceration indicates systemic vasculitis, particualrly Wegener's granulomatosis or polyarteritis nodosa.

Eye symptoms and signs

The more common eye symptoms encountered in patients with rheumatological diseases are dry, gritty eyes, photophobia, watering, redness, pain, floaters, and, most importantly, blurring or actual loss of vision. The differential diagnosis of the painful red eye and of sudden loss of vision is outlined in Tables 1 and 2.

The combination of symptoms with ocular signs indicates the site of the eye disease, and this may reflect both the nature and severity of the joint disease.

Common eye disorders encountered in rheumatological disease

Conjunctivitis

Bacterial conjunctivitis commonly presents as sore, red, sticky eyes with a purulent discharge. Patients complain of being unable to open their eyes in the morning and of blurred vision. Viral conjunctivitis is very common. It presents with red, watering, irritable eyes, and only minimal discharge, but often excessive photophobia as the cornea may become secondarily infected.

Dry eyes

Patients with dry eyes may complain of a foreign-body sensation, dryness, redness, grittiness, and excessive secretion of mucus. Their symptoms are aggravated by hot, dry, polluted atmospheres. Dry eyes may be due to local eye disease, particularly blepharitis and allergic eye disease, or keratoconjunctivitis sicca, which is associated with systemic disease. Keratoconjunctivitis sicca occurs when secretion of the lacrimal gland is of insufficient quality or quantity to maintain the tear film and ocular surface. It may be caused by reduction of tear secretion, destruction of the lacrimal glands, or scarring of the ducts. The systemic diseases associated with dry eyes are primarily autoimmune diseases, for example, primary Sjögren's syndrome, systemic lupus erythematosus, rheumatoid arthritis, and systemic sclerosis, and also include infiltrative disorders including lymphoma, sarcoidosis, or amyloidosis.

Slit-lamp examination is the essential investigation for patients with dry eyes. Offending local ocular disease can be diagnosed. The tear film is examined, particularly the break-up time of a fluorescent dye and the integrity of the cornea, which indicates adequacy of lubrication. In the absence of a slit lamp, Schirmer's test will identify patients with bone dry eyes but is otherwise not helpful. Rose Bengal stain denotes areas with an incomplete tear film. In early cases of keratoconjunctivitis sicca, the stain is limited to the conjunctiva and in severe cases can be seen all over the cornea.

Treatment of dry eyes requires patience from the sufferer and the physician. Frequent regular tear supplements are the mainstay and these range from viscous preparations to normal saline. Temporary or permanent canalicular ablation is rarely required. Modern treatments which are under investigation are epidermal growth factor, aldose reductase inhibitors, or cyclosporin eye drops (Tsubota 1994).

Episcleritis

The episclera is the thin layer of transparent tissue lying between the conjunctiva and the white sclera. It has its own blood supply and is incompletely

Table 1 The differential diagnosis of painful red eye

Ocular pathology	Vision	Pain	Distribution of redness	Extra signs	Likely systemic disease
Conjunctivitis	Good	Mild	Diffuse	Purulent sticky exudate	Reiter's syndrome
Dry eyes	Good	Gritty	Mild diffuse	Schirmer test Reduced tears Rose Bengal stain	Rheumatoid arthritis Systemic vasculitis Sjögren's syndrome (primary and secondary)
Episcleritis	Good	Irritation	Diffuse or nodular	Mobile nodules	Rheumatoid arthritis Systemic vasculitis
Scleritis	May be reduced	Very severe	Diffuse or nodular	Keratitis	Rheumatoid arthritis
Anterior uveitis	Reduced	Mild to severe	Circumcorneal	Keratic precipitates Small pupil Abnormal intraocular pressure Swollen optic disc	Seronegative spondyloarthropathy Sarcoidosis Behçet's disease Whipple's disease

Table 2 The differential diagnosis of sudden loss of central vision

Cause of visual loss	History	Field	Pupil reaction	Media	Fundus	Likely systemic disease
Vitreous haemorrhage	Sudden	Generalized constriction	Normal	Hazy (blood)	Not seen or new vessels Retinal vascular occlusion	Systemic vasculitis Behçet's disease
Macular oedema	Gradual, with distortion	Small, relatively central scotoma	Normal	Hazy Cells in anterior chamber and vitreous	Swollen disc	Behçet's disease Sarcoidosis Seronegative arthropathy
Central retinal artery occlusion	Sudden	Dense, large, central scotoma	Afferent pupillary defect	Clear	Normal or pale optic disc Cloudy swelling of the retina Cherry-red spot at macula Dark blood in arterioles	Systemic vasculitis, especially giant-cell arteritis Polyarteritis nodosa
Ischaemic optic neuropathy	Sudden	Dense altitudinal defect	Afferent pupillary defect	Clear	Pale, swollen, optic disc	Giant-cell arteritis Systemic vasculitis
Inflammatory optic neuropathy	Progressive	Central scotoma	Afferent pupillary defect	Clear or hazy	Optic disc oedema Optic atrophy	Sarcoidosis Wegener's granulomatosis

Note: All these are painless and occur in white eyes, except occasionally inflammatory optic neuropathy.

fixed to the underlying sclera. This is in contrast to the conjunctiva, which is freely mobile over the episclera. Episcleritis is a benign, self-limiting condition that is usually unilateral and often nodular, involving only a small segment of the eye's surface. Patients complain of irritation and redness rather than pain, although the nodules may be tender to the touch. The affected episcleral vessels are dilated, within a swollen episclera. The condition subsides spontaneously within 4–6 weeks. It is only rarely associated with systemic disease (Akpek et al. 1999).

Scleritis

Scleritis is a serious, potentially sight-threatening condition, which in contrast to episcleritis is painful and does not subside spontaneously. Pain is the most constant feature and may be excruciating. The inflamed area is red and may produce a nodular, diffuse, or necrotizing pattern. If adjacent tissues are involved in the inflammatory process, additional signs and symptoms develop: spread to the cornea produces peripheral ulceration, keratitis, and photophobia, whereas involvement of the posterior sclera causes proptosis, serous retinal detachment, a swollen optic disc, and, rarely, angle-closure glaucoma.

An unusual variant of scleritis is scleromalacia perforans, which occurs in elderly women with severe rheumatoid arthritis (see also below). This is characteristically painless and the affected sclera becomes dead white because the underlying lesion is arteritic infarction (Watson and Hazleman 1976). Eventually the sclera becomes atrophic and the blue, underlying choroid can be seen bulging through it. Actual perforation of the globe is very rare, despite the name. All forms of scleritis are very important to recognize for both the ophthalmologist and rheumatologist because they often herald activity of the systemic disease and may require systemic immunosuppression to prevent permanent ocular damage and blindness.

Acute anterior uveitis

Anterior uveitis is inflammation within the anterior chamber of the eye. The patient complains of an acutely painful, red eye with photophobia, sometimes associated with blurred vision. The pain is exacerbated by close work because the inflamed iris is stretched when the pupil constricts. The condition is generally unilateral and frequently recurrent. The ophthalmological signs, easily seen with the slit lamp, consist of circumcorneal redness and keratic precipitates on the endothelial surface of the cornea with flare and cells in the anterior chamber, looking like a cinema projection beam with specks of dust. In severe cases the cells gravitate to form a fluid level called a hypopyon. The pupil is small and poorly reactive; the intraocular pressure is often low in the acute stage and high in the convalescent stage.

Retinal vasculitis and posterior uveitis

The pattern of retinal disease in systemic inflammatory disease frequently reflects the nature of the disease and consequently may have important diagnostic value (Sanders 1987; Graham et al. 1989). In patients with seronegative arthropathies, Behçet's disease, and sarcoidosis, there may be inflammation in the posterior chamber of the eye (cells in the vitreous); the patient complains of floaters and of blurred or distorted central vision if the macula is oedematous. In mild cases, fundoscopy reveals focal or diffuse white sheathing of the retinal veins; in severe cases there are also scattered haemorrhages. Actual occlusion of the retinal veins and new vessels on the optic disc or peripheral retina may develop. The new vessels, similar to those in diabetes mellitus, generally develop as a consequence of retinal ischaemia secondary to occlusion of retinal veins. Their walls are fragile and vitreous haemorrhage is an important cause of visual morbidity in these patients.

By contrast, patients with systemic vasculitis do not develop inflammation within the eye but the vasculitic process affects the retinal capillaries and arterioles to produce retinal ischaemia, sometimes resulting in new vessels and vitreous haemorrhage. The ophthalmoscopic features range from asymptomatic, cotton-wool spots (due to occlusion of the retinal capillaries) to complete occlusion of the retinal artery causing blindness.

Optic neuropathy

Disease of the optic nerve invariably causes profound visual loss. Symptoms range from vague, blurred central vision and difficulty in differentiating colours to complete blindness. The cardinal ophthalmological signs of optic nerve disease are reduced visual acuity, impaired or absent colour vision, a central scotoma, and an afferent pupillary defect. The optic disc may look swollen, pale, or even normal. The pattern of visual loss varies from sudden, complete blindness, as experienced by patients with giant-cell arteritis in whom the optic nerve undergoes infarction, to a slowly progressive loss in patients with granulomatous disorders when the optic nerve becomes compressed by abnormal tissue. All patients who develop disease of the optic nerve require urgent investigation and treatment.

Specific ocular manifestations of systemic inflammatory diseases

The ocular manifestations of systemic inflammatory disease vary according to the size and type of vessel predominantly affected by the disease process. As a general rule, diseases that affect arterioles involve the cornea, episclera, sclera, and retinal arterioles, whereas those affecting the venules produce uveitis (intraocular inflammation), macular oedema, and retinal venous disease.

Giant-cell arteritis

Giant-cell arteritis is an ophthalmic emergency and an important cause of preventable blindness in elderly people. Twenty-five per cent of patients develop ocular disease and the majority experience sudden loss of vision in one eye, with a dense, inferior, altitudinal field defect (Ross Russell 1959, 1986). The cause of the blindness is usually infarction of the optic nerve (ischaemic optic neuropathy) (Plate 28), and occlusion of the central retinal artery in a minority of cases. Treatment is immediate, high-dose systemic steroids (e.g. prednisolone 1–2 mg/kg daily) to produce symptomatic relief of headache and, most importantly, to prevent blindness in the other eye, as recovery of vision is very unusual. If the patient has experienced symptoms of fluctuating vision in the good eye, treatment with intravenous steroids, heparin, and plasma expanders is indicated. Fluorescein angiography may show extremely delayed filling of both retinal and choroidal circulation and is an important diagnostic tool in difficult cases.

Unusual neurophthalmological complications of giant-cell arteritis include oculomotor palsies, ischaemic orbit with proptosis, and ophthalmoplegia. Horner's syndrome, cortical blindness (due to embolization from affected vertebral arteries), internuclear ophthalmoplegia, and visual hallucinations (Cullen and Coleiro 1976).

Systemic lupus erythematosus

Eye symptoms are very common in patients with systemic lupus erythematosus and range from minor, external problems (Frith et al. 1990) to severe retinopathy. Five per cent of patients will develop scleritis some time during the course of their disease, and this is occasionally seen at presentation (Plate 29). As usual, active scleritis indicates active systemic disease and may require adjustment of systemic therapy. Uveitis is very rare in systemic lupus and only occurs in association with severe scleritis.

The most important ophthalmic manifestation is the retinopathy described by Maumenee (1940). The hallmark of this is the cytoid body, which is the descriptive term used in systemic lupus for cotton-wool spot. A flurry of cotton wool spots may herald imminent fatal vasculitis and overall carry a poor prognosis. Retinal haemorrhages and occlusions of central and branch retinal arteries may also occur; these are due to deposition of immune complexes rather than vasculitis (Graham et al. 1985). Occlusions of branch retinal veins are usually secondary to hypertension. Serous detachment of the retina and choroidal infarcts (Plate 30) are seen in patients with active disease due to vasculitis of the choroidal vessels (Eckstein et al. 1993). The presence of anticardiolipin antibodies may be a marker for the development of retinal vascular occlusion (Levine et al. 1988) (Plate 31).

The primary antiphospholipid syndrome

The primary antiphospholipid syndrome is characterized by recurrent thrombosis and pregnancy loss, thrombocytopaenia, and the presence of lupus anticoagulant or antiphospholipid antibodies, leading to thrombophilia. The commonest visual symptom is transient monocular blindness experienced by 50 per cent of patients. Vaso-occlusive retinopathy is reported in 10 per cent patients, sometimes complicated by neovascularization and vitreous haemorrhage. Anterior ischaemic optic neuropathy and choroidal occipital infarcts are other complications of this thrombotic state. Ocular inflammatory disease including scleritis, episcleritis, and retinal vasculitis may occur (Gelfand et al. 1999).

Polyarteritis nodosa

This disease has similar ophthalmic manifestations to those of systemic lupus. However, necrotizing scleritis with peripheral corneal ulceration is relatively common. The retinopathy is usually secondary to accelerated hypertension and therefore characterized by arteriovenous nipping, cotton-wool spots, and flame-shaped haemorrhages. The appearance of isolated cotton-wool spots or branch-artery occlusion is unusual; sudden visual loss, due to either ischaemic optic neuropathy or occlusion of the central retinal artery, rarely occurs. The development of scleritis or retinal vascular disease in the absence of hypertension warrants investigation of the systemic disease.

Wegener's granulomatosis

Eye problems develop in about half of patients with Wegener's granulomatosis, particularly those with limited disease (Spalton et al. 1981). This is the only systemic inflammatory disease that commonly presents with orbital disease, which is due to infiltration of the orbit with granulomatous tissue (Fig. 1). The patient complains of proptosis, which is caused by the orbital mass, red eyes from the scleritis, and loss of vision from compression of the optic nerve by the granulomatous tissue, often accompanied by oedema of the optic disc and choroidal folds.

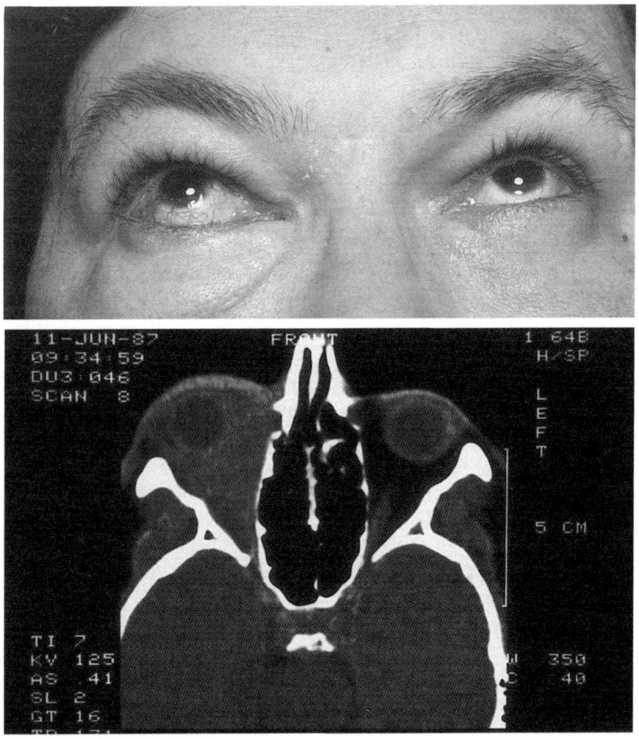

Fig. 1 Wegener's granulomatosis. A 32-year-old man presented with fever, malaise, sore red right eye, and blurred vision. The right eye was proptosed with dilated scleral vessels and an incidental finding of extensive xanthelasmas (top). A CT scan revealed a 'dirty' right orbit where the muscles and optic nerve could not be identified due to extensive granulomatous tissue.

Systemic sclerosis

The most common eye complaint is dryness. A minority develop retinopathy similar to that seen in the other systemic vasculitides, with cotton-wool spots, haemorrhages, and occlusion of retinal arteries and also with choroidal infarction (Grennan and Forrester 1977).

Rheumatoid arthritis

One-third of patients suffer with dry eyes and in 10 per cent this is combined with a dry mouth (Sjögren's syndrome). Five per cent of patients presenting with episcleritis and 30 per cent presenting with isolated scleritis have rheumatoid arthritis (Watson and Hazleman 1976). Patients with scleritis associated with rheumatoid arthritis more commonly have bilateral scleritis than patients with scleritis due to other systemic immune disease (Sainz de la Meza et al. 1994). The scleritis is associated with an occlusive vasculitis; this may be very severe and cause corneal melt and occasionally perforation requiring surgical repair. Scleromalacia perforans affects elderly women predominantly (Plate 32). Advancing scleral disease in these patients almost always heralds a flare-up of the systemic disease, particularly the vasculitic complications. Uveitis is not a feature of rheumatoid arthritis and involvement of the retinal vessels is very unusual.

Ankylosing spondylitis and the seronegative arthropathies

Acute anterior uveitis is the most important ocular disease in this group of patients. It occurs in 25 per cent of patients with ankylosing spondylitis and in 10–15 per cent of patients with other causes of seronegative arthropathy. The clinical symptoms and signs are identical, regardless of the accompanying disease. Attacks are usually unilateral but both eyes become affected during the course of the disease (Rothova et al. 1987). In severe cases, slit-lamp examination reveals a sticky, fibrinoid aqueous in the anterior chamber; posterior synechiae (adhesions between the iris and the lens) are common and raised intraocular pressure occurs. Patients who are HLA-B27 positive tend to be younger at the time of the first attack, have more severe ocular inflammation, and a longer duration of the acute attack than those who are HLA-B27 negative, in whom uveitis may be milder but sometimes more chronic (Linssen 1990). Conjunctivitis occurs in one-third of patients with Reiter's disease but there is no increased incidence in the other groups (Plate 33).

Interestingly, the posterior segment of the eye is rarely affected in seronegative arthropathies: only 10 per cent of patients develop cells in the vitreous from retinal vasculitis affecting predominantly the capillaries and the post-capillary venules, but the consequence of this may be cystoid macular oedema and oedema of the optic disc. In very severe cases, serous retinal detachment ensues (Rodriguez et al. 1994).

Sarcoidosis

Eye involvement occurs in 30–40 per cent of patients with systemic sarcoidosis (Jabs and Johns 1986; Karma et al. 1988). The most common ocular manifestation is acute or chronic, relapsing uveitis, often in the absence of active pulmonary disease. The anterior uveitis is characterized by granulomatous, 'mutton fat', keratic precipitates, and nodules on the iris (Plate 34). Patients may complain of dry eyes from involvement of the lacrimal glands, which can be very dramatic, particularly in patients of African ethnicity. Asymptomatic conjunctival and scleral nodules may develop and are of diagnostic use.

Twenty-five per cent of patients with ocular sarcoidosis develop posterior uveitis with cells in the vitreous, and retinal vasculitis. The diagnostic retinal features of sarcoidosis are periphlebitis, focal cuffing of the retinal veins, new vessels on the optic disc or in the peripheral retina (often in the absence of retinal ischaemia), choroidal nodules (Plate 35), and pigment epithelial lesions (Spalton and Sanders 1981).

Five per cent of patients develop granulomatous optic neuropathy with profound visual loss (Graham et al. 1986). This may mimic acute demyelinating optic neuritis, with pain and rapid visual loss, or it may produce progressive visual loss owing to a granuloma compressing the optic nerve (Plate 36). Both types may be acutely steroid-sensitive and therefore it is important to make the diagnosis rapidly.

Behçet's disease

Ocular manifestations in Behçet's disease occur in 70 per cent of patients and are very important as 25 per cent of patients will go blind (Michelson and Chisari 1982). Together with orogenital ulceration and thrombophlebitis, uveitis forms the major triad described in 1937 by Hulusi Behçet.

Severe anterior uveitis, often in a white eye, is common, with hypopyon formation in extreme cases. The anterior uveitis is typically recurrent but can resolve spontaneously. The high incidence of blindness in patients with Behçet's disease is due to the severity of the retinal changes. The pathognomonic features are sequential occlusions of branch retinal veins (Plate 37) and retinal infiltrates. The recurrent nature of the venous occlusions results in progressive retinal ischaemia and eventually the entire retinal vasculature becomes obliterated and the optic disc atrophic (Atmaca 1989). Retinal infiltrates, which are due to collections of polymorphs in the superficial retinal layers, are pathologically similar to a hypopyon and will resolve spontaneously over the course of a week. HLA-B51 and the presence of prothrombotic factor V Leiden mutation are risk factors for ocular involvement (Verity 1999).

Ocular involvement in rheumatic conditions of childhood

Introduction

Uveitis occurring before the age of 16 years is approximately four times less common than uveitis in the general population (Perkins 1966). In two reviews of uveitis in childhood, systemic illnesses such as sarcoidosis, Behçet's disease, and vasculitis accounted for less than 8 per cent of patients (Perkins 1966; Kanski and Shun-Shin 1984). The most common associated disorder in Kanski's series was seronegative juvenile chronic arthritis. Ocular complications of rheumatic diseases in childhood were reviewed by Petty (1990).

Juvenile idiopathic arthritis (JIA)

The chronic anterior uveitis that occurs in association with JIA deserves special mention, particularly as it does not occur in adults. Affected children are mostly girls, and are usually young at onset of arthritis (mean age, 3 years). Joint involvement is usually oligoarticular, although may become polyarticular. The presence of uveitis does not influence the longterm articular prognosis in oligoarticular onset JIA (Cimaz and Fink 1996). Most patients have associated antinuclear antibodies.

Arthritis generally pre-dates the eye involvement by 1–3 years or sometimes much longer, but 5–10 per cent of cases present with uveitis which may already be severe. If eye involvement has not developed within 5 years of onset of arthritis, the risk is much less, unlike the acute anterior uveitis in ankylosing spondylitis, which may occur for the first time very many years later than the first rheumatic symptoms. The ophthalmologist should consider asking for a paediatric rheumatological opinion in any young child presenting with chronic anterior uveitis. The rheumatologist must ask the ophthalmologist to not only arrange a slit-lamp examination on all Children with JIA, but also arrange appropriate follow-up screening at regular intervals (Leak 1992).

The non-granulomatous iridocyclitis runs an uncomplicated course in only one-third of affected children (Petty 1987), and many children develop complications of band keratopathy, posterior synechiae, cataracts, or glaucoma. Earlier papers reported 10–20 per cent blindness (Rosenberg 1987; Wolf et al. 1987), but more recent studies suggest that the severity of uveitis is decreasing. However, the worst prognosis is still often associated with the early cases, either symptomatic before onset of arthritis, or picked up at the first screening (Wolf et al. 1987; Kotaniemi et al. 1999; Edelsten et al. 2001).

Treatment of the uveitis is by topical corticosteroid drops and if necessary injections, with mydriatics, but many patients still need cataract extraction or vitrectomy. Several anecdotal reports have appeared of the benefits of low dose methotrexate for corticosteroid chronic uveitis (Singsen and Goldbach-Mansky 1997; Weiss et al. 1998), and in such cases close collaboration between the rheumatologist and ophthalmologist is advisable.

Spondyloarthropathies

As many as 8.6 per cent of patients with ankylosing spondylitis have their onset before the age of 16 years (Bennet and Wood 1968), frequently in an adolescent boy with pauciarticular arthritis of the legs, or enthesitis. Acute anterior uveitis probably occurs as frequently in juvenile-onset spondylitis as in adult ankylosing spondylitis, and over long follow-up up to 27 per cent of such children develop episodes of uveitis.

Bilateral, painless conjunctivitis is common in Reiter's syndrome but, in addition, acute anterior uveitis and keratitis with corneal ulcers have been described in children. Chronic anterior uveitis is only described in occasional children with juvenile spondylitis or Reiter's disease and always requires reconsideration of the diagnosis.

Although juvenile psoriatic arthritis is often grouped with the spondarthropathies, acute uveitis is uncommon and ocular involvement is usually chronic and clinically indistinguishable from that which occurs in association with early-onset juvenile chronic arthritis.

Multisystem systemic illness

Many systemic rheumatic diseases with ocular involvement in adults have counterparts in childhood, including systemic lupus erythematosus, Sjögren's syndrome, and systemic sclerosis (Leak and Isenberg 1989). Behçet's disease is rarely diagnosed before adolescence, although a history of oral ulcers may predate the appearance of other major manifestations by more than 8 years (Kim et al. 1994).

Sarcoidosis beginning under the age of 6 years with rash and arthropathy may be associated with chronic anterior uveitis (Hoover et al. 1986; Sahn et al. 1990). Features distinguishing this from juvenile chronic arthritis include the iris nodules, posterior eye involvement, and rather painless, non-evasive, boggy tenosynovitis. Blau syndrome is a familial form of granulomatous arthritis, uveitis, and rash with similar features to sarcoidosis in childhood (Blau 1985).

In childhood, classical polyarteritis nodosa and Kawasaki disease are the most common forms of systemic vasculitis. Bilateral, non-suppurative, bulbar, conjunctival injection is a recognized diagnostic criterion in Kawasaki disease, occurring in virtually all cases in the early stages of the illness; acute, bilateral uveitis is also very common (Ohno et al. 1982; Smith et al. 1989).

Differential diagnosis of coexistent ocular and arthritic problems in childhood includes infections such as Lyme disease, infantile-onset, multisystem inflammatory disease (Dollfus et al. 2000), and lysosomal storage diseases (Cassidy and Petty 1990).

Infective arthropathies and eye disease

Secondary syphilis may be accompanied by an acute panuveitis with an active anterior uveitis, cells in the vitreous, and retinal changes involving predominantly the capillaries, which produce oedema of the macula and optic disc, and also subretinal fluid in the inferotemporal quadrant, leading to a characteristic pale appearance.

Other infectious diseases that must be considered in undiagnosed patients presenting with arthritis and ocular inflammation include those involving Epstein–Barr virus, Lyme disease, Whipple's disease, brucellosis, and human immunodeficiency virus (Nussenblatt and Palestine 1989).

Temporal relationship of ocular involvement with other disease manifestations in specific conditions

The chronic anterior uveitis associated with juvenile chronic arthritis usually runs an intermittent course that is not associated with the current activity of the arthritis, although it is common for their onset to be within 1–2 years of each other. The severity of ocular and joint involvement is also independent such that blindness may occur in a child with minimal arthritis and no residual deformity. By contrast, in adult rheumatoid arthritis, scleritis indicates generalized, active disease.

The acute attacks of unilateral anterior uveitis that characterize the seronegative spondarthropathies occur randomly, whereas ocular involvement in Reiter's syndrome occurs as part of a symptom complex, usually within the first 2–3 years (Lee et al. 1986).

In Behçet's disease and sarcoidosis, uveitis is frequently found with other systemic manifestations at presentation, but subsequent flare-ups frequently occur in isolation such that eye and joint disease are not significantly associated.

In Kawasaki disease, eye involvement occurs as part of the acute inflammatory process, and Ohno et al. (1982) found a strong statistical correlation between the activity of uveitis, as measured by the numbers of inflammatory cells in the anterior chamber, and the erythrocyte sedimentation rate (ESR) and C-reactive protein.

Diagnostic and laboratory tests

The initial history and examination will provide the diagnosis in the majority of patients. The use of radiological or laboratory tests in the assessment of a patient with eye disease is limited. A useful screen for a patient with uveitis would be a full blood count, ESR, chest radiographs, and serology for syphilis. Further tests such as HLA-B27, angiotensin-converting enzyme, and antinuclear antibodies would be indicated by clinical evidence of disease elsewhere. In a prospective study of 865 patients, intensive investigation established a specific diagnosis in 628 patients (73 per cent) but an associated systemic disease was found in only 220 patients (26 per cent) (Rothova et al. 1992).

Evidence of an acute-phase response, for example, a raised ESR or C-reactive protein, suggests a generalized systemic illness with active ocular involvement. However, in diseases in which the activity of eye and joint disease do not run in parallel, active uveitis alone is usually not associated with a raised ESR.

Autoantibodies

Rheumatic diseases such as rheumatoid arthritis and systemic lupus erythematosus are often associated with serum autoantibodies but in this situation the antibodies are not of diagnostic use as the systemic disease would usually be obvious clinically.

Amongst a mixed group of patients with uveitis, antibodies to tissue antigens do not occur more frequently than in controls, except in children with juvenile chronic arthritis in which 80 per cent or more have antinuclear antibodies (Murray 1986). Patients with retinal vasculitis may have circulating immune complexes and/or antiretinal antibodies. The presence of antibodies alone may be associated with more severe disease (Kasp et al. 1986). Antineutrophil cytoplasmic antibodies have been found in 'fit' patients with severe necrotizing scleritis and may indicate an underlying systemic vasculitis that requires persistent vigilance by the ophthalmologist (Talks et al. 1994).

Immunogenetics

Determination of HLA-B27 in patients with acute anterior uveitis is valuable because B27-positive patients are more likely to have an associated spondarthropathy and should be referred for a rheumatological opinion (Feltkamp 1990).

Treatment of the ocular complications of systemic inflammatory disease

Mild, anterior-segment complications such as conjunctivitis, dry eyes, and episcleritis will invariably respond to local treatment.

Treatment of scleritis, anterior uveitis, retinal vasculitis, and optic neuropathy depends firstly on the severity of the eye disease and its effect on vision, and secondly on the activity of the systemic disease. In general, systemic therapy is dictated by the eye disease if the vision is reduced or potentially threatened by inflammation.

Scleritis

Scleritis is an indication for systemic therapy. Adequate doses of non-steroidal, anti-inflammatory drugs may suffice (e.g. flurbiprofen, 50 mg, three times a day), but if corneal or retinal involvement develops or the inflammation is uncontrolled, systemic steroids are indicated. In rare instances it is necessary to supplement the steroids by pulse cyclophosphamide (Meyer et al. 1987) or cyclosporin (Wakefield and McCluskey 1989). If the scleritis coincides with activity of the systemic disease, adjusting the treatment for the latter is usually sufficient.

Uveitis

The treatment of uveitis depends primarily on the visual acuity and the site of the inflammatory process. The rationale of treatment of uveitis is set out in Table 3. In the majority of cases, anterior uveitis can be treated topically with steroid eye drops (prednisolone betamethasone/dexamethasone) and a dilating agent (tropicamide/cyclopentolate/atropine), occasionally supplemented by a subconjunctival injection. A trial of systemic steroids may be necessary in selected patients with frequent persistent relapses of anterior uveitis. If the inflammation involves the posterior segment and the visual acuity drops below 6/12 (0.5), due either to cystoid macular oedema or vitreous cells, a subtenons injection of steroid or systemic steroids are indicated. If the vision drops because of occlusion of the retinal vessels or involvement of the optic nerve, systemic immunosuppression is immediately indicated. Corticosteroids and cyclosporin are effective (Towler et al. 1990; Howe et al. 1994), but these may be used in conjunction with azathioprine (Lightman 1991) or methotrexate (Shah et al. 1992; Samson et al. 2001) or Mofetil Mycophenolate (Jabs et al. 2000).

The most difficult management problem is Behçet's disease because of the severity and frequency of the attacks of uveitis, which almost invariably affect the retinal vessels. A combination of prednisolone, cyclosporin, azathioprine, and colchicine appears to be most effective in refractory patients. However, there are no controlled trials of these drugs in Behçet's uveitis and therefore the perplexing problem of benefits of treatment versus side-effects must be continuously evaluated. The management of Behçet's disease is discussed in Chapter 6.10.8.

Antirheumatic therapy with ocular side-effects

Most antirheumatic drug therapies cause no significant ocular side-effects but attention is drawn to toxicity of antimalarial drugs prescribed for rheumatoid arthritis, systemic lupus erythematosus, and related disorders, and to corticosteroids, widely used in many rheumatic conditions.

Table 3 Changing course of systemic steroids for patients with posterior uveitis

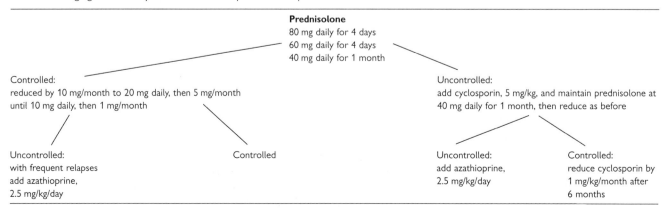

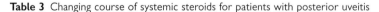

Prednisolone
80 mg daily for 4 days
60 mg daily for 4 days
40 mg daily for 1 month

Controlled:
reduced by 10 mg/month to 20 mg daily, then 5 mg/month until 10 mg daily, then 1 mg/month

- Uncontrolled:
with frequent relapses
add azathioprine,
2.5 mg/kg/day
- Controlled

Uncontrolled:
add cyclosporin, 5 mg/kg, and maintain prednisolone at 40 mg daily for 1 month, then reduce as before

- Uncontrolled:
add azathioprine,
2.5 mg/kg/day
- Controlled:
reduce cyclosporin by
1 mg/kg/month after
6 months

Antimalarial drugs

Use of these compounds in patients with rheumatic diseases has increased in recent years, both in combination with other DMARDs in RA, and also in SLE. Although there are still fears about retinal toxicity, reports of retinal toxicity are few. Non-retinal eye disease, for example, corneal deposits are minor and reversible.

Chloroquine has a high affinity for the melanin-containing tissue of the eye, including the retinal pigment epithelium (Maksymowych and Russell 1987). The pathophysiology of the retinal damage is related to malfunction of the phagolysosomes, resulting in faulty clearance of ageing photoreceptor membranes. The build-up of lamellar myelin bodies disturbs the metabolism of the retinal pigment epithelium.

In the advanced stage with an absolute scotoma and loss of visual acuity, there is granular pigmentation of the macula surrounded by a 'bull's eye' of rings of depigmentation and pigmentation. However, in the early stages, fundoscopy and other standard optic screening tests are normal despite the presence of a scotoma on a red Amsler grid (Plate 38). Identification at this stage is the goal of screening programmes, as cessation of treatment will usually prevent progression. To fully evaluate reports on retinal toxicity, data must be available on baseline screening, daily dose regime, renal function, other medication, and length of treatment.

All reviewers are agreed that the risk of toxicity is very small and initially related to the daily dosage, 3.5 mg/kg for chloroquine and 5.5 mg/kg for hydroxychloroquine (refs). In practical terms for a patient of 65 kg, 400 mg of OHCHL is safe, but only 225, not 250 mg of CHL. Current opinion favours OHCHL as having a better safety record than CHL, but there are occasional reports of toxicity, for example, after 6.5 and 8 years of OHCHL treatment at recommended dosages in 2 out of 58 Greek patients (Mavrikakis 1996), although none in a series of 1207 patients on OHCHL, when the dosage had been less than 6.5 mg/kg day (Levy et al. 1997). The cumulative dose has always been thought to have some importance.

Guidelines for screening have been produced by the Royal College of Ophthalmologists, in association with the British Society of Rheumatologists and British Association of Dermatologists (Fielder et al. 1998). Baseline screening when considering antimalarials should include renal and liver function, an enquiry about visual impairment, and a record of near visual acuity. Various colour vision tests can be employed to detect retinopathy. A study of six tests in patients with and without CHL retinopathy suggested that Standard Pseudoisochromatic Plates Part 2 (SPP-2) and American Optical Hardy Rand Rittler (AOHRR) are the most sensitive at detecting toxicity, whereas all tests were similarly specific (Vu et al. 1999). Follow up of patients on antimalarials should include enquiry about visual problems, re-assessment of visual acuity, and Amsler grid. Opinion is still divided as to whether regular colour vision testing is needed in low risk patients, but patients on treatment for 10 years should be followed more carefully, for example, at annual intervals (Spalton 1996; Levy et al. 1997).

Self-evaluation by the patient with an Amsler grid at regular intervals is an inexpensive and reproducible test that is both simple and sensitive (Easterbrook 1988; Lozier and Friedlander 1989), but not in widespread use. Detection of faded or distorted areas with the grid should prompt early evaluation with field testing by the ophthalmologist.

Evaluation of published reports on retinal toxicity is difficult because of the differences in dosage over variable periods of time and the exact criteria used to define retinopathy, as well as lack of baseline data in some patients.

The total dose of drug used before development of retinopathy is very variable whereas the daily dosage in relation to the patient's weight now seems to be the important factor. At daily doses of 250 mg for chloroquine or 400 mg for hydroxychloroquine, there are few cases of mild, reversible retinopathy. Reports of progressive retinopathy at 250 mg/day of chloroquine contain insufficient information on patients' weight.

Several reviewers are agreed that the risk of toxicity is very small at the recommended daily dosages: chloroquine 3.5 mg/kg; hydroxychloroquine 6.5 mg/kg (Maksymowych and Russell 1987; Rynes 1987; Easterbrook 1988; Lozier and Friedlaender 1989). In practical terms, for a patient of 65 kg, 400 mg of hydroxychloroquine are safe, or 225 mg of chloroquine (not 250 mg). However, smaller patients must take a reduced dose, as should those with renal or hepatic impairment. Current opinion favours hydroxychloroquine as having the best safety record (Bernstein 1991; Easterbrook 1993; Spalton et al. 1993).

An adequate, baseline ophthalmological examination is the ideal and should include visual acuity (corrected for distance and near), colour vision, red Amsler chart, and fundoscopy. Detection of coexistent eye disease such as age-related macular pigmentation will necessitate regular follow-up at 6-monthly intervals. In the absence of ocular abnormalities, opinion is divided as to the necessity and frequency of repeat tests. Some suggest no other ophthalmological review is necessary (Morsman et al. 1990), although the prescribing physician may wish to recheck the Amsler grid test every 6 months (Bernstein 1991). By contrast, Easterbrook (1993) still recommends annual ophthalmological assessment, whereas Spalton et al. (1993) feel this is only necessary after 5 years on antimalarial therapy. Self-testing by the patient with an Amsler grid at 2-weekly intervals is an inexpensive and reproducible test that is both simple and sensitive (Easterbrook 1988; Lozier and Friedlaender 1989). Detection of faded or distorted areas should prompt early evaluation with field testing by the ophthalmologist.

Corticosteroids

Both oral and topical corticosteroids may cause a variety of ophthalmic side-effects:

(i) Corneal and scleral thinning can occur with topical steroids and lead to perforation.

(ii) Cataracts are common, especially after higher doses of systemic steroids. Their development in chronic uveitis is partly related to the treatment but the advantages of topical therapy, in particular, far outweigh the side-effects.

(iii) Raised intraocular pressure is another common side-effect of steroids. Five per cent of the population are termed 'steroid reactors' because of a significant but asymptomatic increase in pressure. The frequency, duration, and type of topical or oral steroid all influence this effect, and use of an alternative steroid should be considered, for example from dexamethasone to fluorometholone.

(iv) Infectious problems: herpes simplex can cause an acute, unilateral anterior uveitis, and topical steroids risk exacerbating such eye infections; topical steroids should not be used indiscriminately on an undiagnosed red eye.

Immunosuppressives

Patients on long-term systemic immunosuppression may develop viral retinitis (herpes simplex, herpes zoster, cytomegalovirus) causing retinal necrosis and eventual blindness (Plate 39). Early symptoms include red eyes, floaters, and field defect, and require an urgent ophthalmological opinion.

References

Akpek, E.K., Uy, H.S., Gardal, C., and Foster, C.S. (1999). Severity of episcleritis and disease association. *Ophthalmology* **106**, 729–31.

Atmaca, L.S. (1989). Fundus changes in Behçet's disease. *Graefe's Archives of Clinical and Experimental Ophthalmology* **227**, 340–4.

Bennett, P.A. and Wood, P.H.N., ed. *Population Studies of the Rheumatic Diseases. Excerpta Medica International Congress series, No. 148*. Amsterdam: Excerpta Medica, 1968.

Bernstein, H.N. (1991). Ocular safety of hydroxychloroquine. *Annals of Ophthalmology* **23**, 292–6.

Blau, E.B. (1985). Familial granulomatous arthritis, iritis and rash. *Journal of Paediatrics* **5**, 689–93.

Cassidy, J.T. and Petty, R.E., ed. (1990). Storage diseases. In *Textbook of Pediatric Rheumatology* 2nd edn., pp. 555–7. New York: Churchill Livingstone.

Cullen, J.E. and Coleiro, J.A. (1976). Ophthalmic complications of giant cell arteritis. *Surveys of Ophthalmology* **20**, 247–60.

Dollfus, H. et al. (2000). Chronic infantile neurological cutaneous and articular/neonatal onset multisystem inflammatory disease syndrome. Ocular manifestations in a recently recognized chronic inflammatory disease of childhood. *Archives of Ophthalmology* **118**, 1386–92.

Easterbrook, M.E. (1988). Ocular effects and safety of antimalarial agents. *American Journal of Medicine* **85** (Suppl. 4A), 23–9.

Easterbrook, M.E. (1993). The ocular safety of hydroxychloroquine. *Seminars in Arthritis and Rheumatism* **23** (Suppl. 1), 62–7.

Eckstein, M.B., Spalton, D.J., and Holder G. (1993). Visual loss from central serous retinopathy. *British Journal of Ophthalmology* **77**, 263–4.

Feltkamp, T.E.W. (1990). Ophthalmological significance of HLA associated uveitis. *Eye* **4**, 839–44.

Fielder, A. et al. (1998). Royal College of Ophthalmologists guidelines—ocular toxicity and hydroxychloroquine. *Eye* **12**, 907–9.

Frith, P., Burge, S.M., Millard, P.R., and Wojnarowski, F. (1990). External ocular findings in lupus erythematosus; a clinical and immunopathological study. *British Journal of Ophthalmology* **74**, 163–7.

Gelfand, Y.A., Dovi, D., Miller, B., and Brennen, B. (1999). Visual disturbances and pathologic ocular findings in primary antiphospholipid syndrome. *Ophthalmology* **106**, 1537–40.

Graham, E.M., Spalton, D.J., Barnard, R.O., Garner, A., and Ross Russell, R.W. (1985). Cerebral and retinal changes in systemic lupus erythematosus. *Ophthalmology* **92**, 444–8.

Graham, E.M., Ellis, C.J.K., Sanders, M.D., and Macdonald, W.I. (1986). Optic neuropathy in sarcoidosis. *Journal of Neurology, Neurosurgery, and Psychiatry* **49**, 756–63.

Graham, E.M., Stanford, M.R., Sanders, M.D., Kasp, E., and Dumonde, D.C. (1989). A point prevalence study of 150 patients with idiopathic retinal vasculitis. 1. Diagnostic value of ophthalmological features. *British Journal of Ophthalmology* **73**, 714–21.

Grennan, D.M. and Forrester, J. (1977). Involvement of the eye in SLE and scleroderma. *Annals of the Rheumatic Diseases* **36**, 152–6.

Hoover, D.L., Khan, J.A., and Giangiacoma, J. (1986). Pediatric ocular sarcoidosis. *Surveys of Ophthalmology* **30**, 215–28.

Howe, L.J., Stanford, M.R., Edelsten, C., and Graham, E.M. (1994). The efficacy of systemic corticosteroids in sight threatening retinal vasculitis. *Eye* **8**, 443–7.

Jabs, D.A. and Johns, C.J. (1986). Ocular involvement in chronic sarcoidosis. *American Journal of Ophthalmology* **102**, 297–301.

Jabs, D.A. et al. (2000). Guidelines for the use of immunosuppressive drugs in patients with ocular inflammatory disorders: Recommendations of an expert panel. *American Journal of Ophthalmology* **130**, 492–513.

Kanski, J.J. and Shun-Shin, A. (1984). Systemic uveitis syndromes in childhood: an analysis of 340 cases. *Ophthalmology* **91**, 1247–52.

Karma, A., Huhti, E., and Poukkla, A. (1988). Course and outcome of ocular sarcoidosis. *American Journal of Ophthalmology* **106**, 467–72.

Kasp, E., Graham, E.M., Stanford, M.R., Sanders, M.D., and Dumonde, D.C. (1986). A point prevalence study of 150 patients with idiopathic retinal vasculitis. 2. Clinical relevance of antiretinal autoimmunity and circulating immune complexes. *British Journal of Ophthalmology* **73**, 722–30.

Kim, D.-K., Chang, S.N., Bang, D., Lee, E.-S., and Lee, S. (1994). Clinical analysis of 40 cases of childhood-onset Behçet's disease. *Paediatric Dermatology* **11**, 95–101.

Leak, A.M. (1992). Ophthalmological screening in seronegative juvenile chronic arthritis: a personal view. *British Journal of Rheumatology* **31**, 631–2.

Leak, A.M. and Isenberg, D.A. (1989). Autoimmune rheumatic disorders in childhood—a comparison with adult onset disease. *Quarterly Journal of Medicine* **73**, 875–93.

Lee, D.A., Barker, S.M., Su, W.P.D., Allen, G.L., Liesegant, T.J., and Illustrup, D.M. (1986). The clinical diagnosis of Reiter's syndrome, ophthalmic and non-ophthalmic aspects. *Journal of Ophthalmology* **93**, 350–6.

Levine, S.R., Crofts, J.W., Lesser, G.R., Floberg, J., and Welch, K.M.A. (1988). Visual symptoms associated with the presence of lupus anticoagulant. *Ophthalmology* **95**, 686–92.

Lightman, S. (1991). Use of steroids and immunosuppressive drugs in the management of posterior uveitis. *Eye* **5**, 294–8.

Linssen, A. (1990). B27+ disease versus B27− disease. *Scandinavian Journal of Rheumatology* **87** (Suppl.), 111–19.

Lozier, J.R. and Friedlaender, M.H. (1989). Complications of antimalarial therapy. *International Ophthalmology Clinics* **29**, 172–8.

Maksymowych, W. and Russell, A.S. (1987). Antimalarials in rheumatology: efficacy and safety. *Seminars in Arthritis and Rheumatism* **16**, 206–21.

Maumenee, A.E. (1940). Retinal lesions in lupus erythematosus. *American Journal of Ophthalmology* **23**, 971–81.

Meyer, A.R., Watson, P.G., and Franks, W. (1987). Pulsed immunosuppressive therapy in the treatment of immunologically advanced corneal and scleral disease. *Eye* **1**, 487–95.

Michelson, J.B. and Chisari, F.V. (1982). Behçet's disease. *Surveys in Ophthalmology* **26**, 190–203.

Morsman, C.D.G., Livesey, S.J., Richards, I.M., Jessop, J.D., and Mills, P.V. (1990). Screening for hydroxychloroquine retinal toxicity: is it necessary? *Eye* **4**, 572–6.

Murray, P. (1986). Serum autoantibodies and uveitis. *British Journal of Ophthalmology* **70**, 266–8.

Nussenblatt, R.B. and Palestine, A.G. *Uveitis: Fundamentals and Clinical Practice.* Chicago IL: Year Book Medical Publishers, 1989.

Ohno, S. et al. (1982). Ocular manifestations of Kawasaki's disease (mucocutaneous lymph node syndrome). *American Journal of Ophthalmology* **93**, 713–17.

Perkins, E.S. (1966). Pattern of uveitis in childhood. *British Journal of Ophthalmology* **50**, 169–85.

Petty, R.E. (1987). Current knowledge of the etiology and pathogenesis of chronic uveitis accompanying juvenile rheumatoid arthritis. *Rheumatic Disease Clinics of North America* **13**, 19–36.

Petty, R.E. (1990). Ocular complications of rheumatic diseases of childhood. *Clinical Orthopaedics and Related Research* **259**, 51–9.

Rodriguez, A., Akova, Y.A., Pedroza-Seres, M., and Foster, C.S. (1994). Posterior segment ocular manifestations in patients with HLA-B27-associated uveitis. *Ophthalmology* **101**, 1267–74.

Rosenberg, A.M. (1987). Uveitis associated with juvenile rheumatoid arthritis. *Seminars in Arthritis and Rheumatism* **16**, 158–73.

Ross Russell, R.V. (1959). Giant cell arteritis: a review of 35 cases. *Quarterly Journal of Medicine* **112**, 471–89.

Ross Russell, R.W. (1986). Giant cell (cranial) arteritis. In *Handbook of Clinical Neurology* Vol. 4 (ed. C. Rose), pp. 309–28. Amsterdam: Elsevier.

Rothova, A., van Veenendaal, W.G., Linssen, A., Glasius, E., Kjilstra, A., and de Jong, P.T.V.H. (1987). Clinical features of acute anterior uveitis. *American Journal of Ophthalmology* **103**, 137–45.

Rothova, A. et al. (1992). Uveitis and systemic disease. *British Journal of Ophthalmology* **76**, 137–41.

Rynes, R.I. (1987). Side effects of antimalarial therapy. *British Journal of Clinical Practice* **52** (Suppl.), 42–5.

Sahn, E.E., Hampton, M.T., Garen, P.D., Warnick J., Smith, D., and Silver R.M. (1990). Preschool sarcoidosis masquerading as juvenile rheumatoid arthritis: two case reports and a review of the literature. *Paediatric Dermatology* **7**, 208–13.

Sainz de la Maza, M., Foster, C.-S., and Jabbur, N.S. (1994). Scleritis associated with rheumatoid arthritis and with other systemic immune diseases. *Ophthalmology* **101**, 1281–8.

Samson, C.M., Waheed, N., Balatzis, S., and Foster, C.S. (2001). Methotrexate therapy for chronic manifestations uveitis. *Ophthalmology* **108**, 1134–9.

Sanders, M.D. (1987). Retinal arteritis, retinal vasculitis and autoimmune retinal vasculitis. *Eye* **1**, 441–65.

Shah, S.S. et al. (1992). Low dose methotrexate therapy for ocular inflammatory disease. *Ophthalmology* **99**, 1419–23.

Smith, L.B.H., Newburger, J.W., and Burns, J.C. (1989). Kawasaki syndrome and the eye. *Pediatric Infectious Disease Journal* **8**, 116–18.

Spalton, D.J. and Sanders, M.D. (1981). Fundus changes in histologically confirmed sarcoidosis. *British Journal of Ophthalmology* **65**, 348–58.

Spalton, D.J., Graham, E.M., Page, N.G.R., and Sanders, M.D. (1981). Ocular changes in limited forms of Wegener's granulomatosis. *British Journal of Ophthalmology* **65**, 553–63.

Spalton, D.J., Verdon Roe, G.M., and Hughes, G.R.V. (1993). Hydroxychloroquine, dosage, parameters and retinopathy. *Lupus* **2**, 355–8.

Talks, S.J., Luqmani, R.A., and McDonell, P.J. (1994). A severe antineutrophil cytoplasmic antibody associated anterior segment vasculitis. *Eye* **8**, 698–700 (letter).

Towler, H.M.A., Whiting, P.H., and Forrester, J.V. (1990). Combination low dose cyclosporin A and steroid therapy in chronic intraocular inflammation. *Eye* **4**, 514–20.

Tsubota, K. (1994). New approaches to dry eye therapy. In *Dry Eye. International Ophthalmic Clinics* Vol. 34 (ed. G. Smolin and M. Friedlaender), pp. 115–28. Boston MA: Little Brown.

Verity, D.H., Vaughan, R.W., Madanat, W., Kondeatis, E., Zureikat, H., Fayyad, F., Kanawati, C.A., Ayesh, I., Stanford, M.R., and Wallace, G.R. (1999). Factor V Leiden mutation is associated with ocular involvement in Behçet's disease. *American Journal of Ophthalmology* **128**, 352–6.

Wakefield, D. and McCluskey, P. (1989). Cyclosporin therapy for severe scleritis. *British Journal of Ophthalmology* **73**, 743–6.

Watson, P.G. and Hazleman, B.L. *The Sclera and Systemic Disorders*. London: Saunders, 1976.

Wolf, M.D., Lichter, P.R., and Ragsdale, C.G. (1987). Prognostic factors in the uveitis of juvenile rheumatoid arthritis. *Ophthalmology* **94**, 1242–8.

1.3.13 The kidney

Andrew S. O'Connor, Carolyn P. Cacho, and Gary M. Kammer

Introduction

Renal involvement is often the most catastrophic and potentially lethal complication of systemic rheumatic diseases. As such, it is vital for the rheumatologist to be familiar with the pathophysiology and clinical manifestations of renal disease. Many renal diseases are rapidly progressive and, therefore, the rheumatologist should recognize the early symptoms and signs, and have a framework for determining when consultation with a nephrologist is indicated. In many cases, urinary abnormalities, such as haematuria and proteinuria, will predate the onset of renal insufficiency, giving the rheumatologist an opportunity to determine the nature and severity of the renal lesion in consultation with the nephrologist. Similarly, the acute onset or worsening of hypertension may indicate renal involvement, warranting collaboration with the nephrologist to establish both diagnostic and therapeutic strategies.

Several rheumatic disorders have a relatively high incidence of renal involvement (Table 1). It is appropriate for patients with these illnesses to undergo a thorough initial assessment of renal function as well as frequent reassessments of renal parameters, even when the initial nephrological examination is negative. Renal involvement in the systemic rheumatic diseases is often variable and unpredictable. For example, systemic lupus erythematosus may present with isolated proteinuria, that is, the presence of proteinuria without hypertension or abnormalities of renal function. This proteinuria may or may not be an early indicator of renal lesions which progress to renal failure over time. At the other extreme, lupus nephritis may present as a rapidly progressive glomerulonephritis, characterized by haematuria, proteinuria, severe hypertension, and advanced renal insufficiency. Other rheumatic diseases with a relatively high incidence of renal involvement also show marked variability of symptoms and signs of kidney disease (Table 1). Furthermore, it is often difficult to differentiate rheumatic diseases either on the clinical or pathological basis of renal involvement. In many instances, the presentation of the renal disease and even the findings from renal biopsy may be identical. Thus, diagnoses of rheumatic disorders are defined on the basis of the clinical range of extrarenal findings and on serological analyses.

Table 1 Rheumatic disorders with a relatively high incidence of renal involvement

Systemic lupus erythematosus	60–70
Mixed connective tissue disease	6–47
Henoch–Schönlein purpura	30–70
Sjögren's syndrome	40–50
Systemic sclerosis	45
Wegener's granulomatosis	50
Classic polyarteritis	30–60
Microscopic polyarteritis	60–70

Note: Numbers are in percentages.

The overlap of rheumatic and renal diseases underscores the advantages of close collaboration between the nephrologist and the rheumatologist in the evaluation, diagnosis, and treatment of these disorders. The following sections seek to provide a broad perspective of the interaction between nephrologist and rheumatologist in the evaluation and management of renal complications in systemic rheumatic diseases by focusing on proteinuria, haematuria, acute renal failure, and hypertension. An exhaustive review of the most current treatment modalities for these diseases is, however, beyond the scope of this text.

Proteinuria

Definitions

The upper limit of protein excretion in healthy adults is approximately 150 mg/day. Functional proteinuria describes proteinuria without intrinsic renal disease. Such protein excretion is usually less than 500 mg/day and may be associated with high fever, strenuous exercise, or exposure to cold. Although proteinuria up to 1–2 g daily has been reported without clinical renal disease, proteinuria greater than 500 mg daily is strongly suggestive of intrinsic renal disease. Abnormal protein excretion of less than 3–5 g/day can occur in both glomerular and tubular interstitial diseases; however, more than 2 g of protein daily suggests a glomerular origin. The quantity of proteinuria as a result of glomerular disease does not always correlate with the nature or severity of the glomerular lesion. Proteinuria of greater than 20 g daily may be associated with minimal histological changes on renal biopsy and may be exquisitely sensitive to treatment with corticosteroids. By contrast, 3–5 g of proteinuria daily can be found in the presence of active lesions that are poorly responsive to therapy.

The prolonged presence of nephrotic-range proteinuria often leads to progressive renal insufficiency. While persistent proteinuria does not invariably progress to chronic renal failure, patients with a partial (<1 g daily) or complete (<150 mg daily) resolution of proteinuria in response to therapy have a lower rate of progression to end stage renal disease. Although remission of proteinuria is a favourable prognostic sign, rheumatic diseases do have periodic exacerbations and remissions, and there is a risk for recurrence of proteinuria and activation of the renal lesion. The presence of protein within the renal tubule has been implicated as an independent factor in the progression of a number of renal diseases (Remuzzi 1999). Therefore urinary protein excretion should be followed in order to assess the response to therapy and to determine the prognosis for renal survival. Patients with complete resolution of proteinuria also should have close follow-up by urinalysis approximately three to four times per year.

Diagnostic studies in the patient with proteinuria

The onset of proteinuria in a rheumatic disease does not necessarily implicate renal involvement from the systemic illness. Nonetheless, in the setting of a systemic rheumatic illness with a high incidence of renal involvement, the finding of proteinuria warrants a well-conceived and thorough diagnostic evaluation. Moreover, there are many patients under the care of the rheumatologist in whom the diagnosis of a systemic illness has not yet been established. With this in mind, the onset of proteinuria should trigger a more complete diagnostic evaluation. This should include quantification of urinary protein excretion and a careful microscopic examination of the urine sediment to exclude the presence of concomitant haematuria. The presentation of combined proteinuria and haematuria often indicates a more aggressive glomerular lesion with the potential to lead to a rapidly progressive loss of renal function. With such a presentation, active inflammatory lesions of the renal parenchyma and the possibility of diseases involving the glomerular and systemic vasculature should be investigated. This initial investigation should include a complete serologic workup, including antibodies directed against antineutrophil cytoplasmic antibodies. In select clinical scenarios, this workup may also potentially include a renal biopsy as the 'gold standard' for determination of the anatomic cause for proteinuria and haematuria (For additional comment, the reader is directed to the discussions of haematuria and the role of renal biopsy below.). Additional diagnostic studies for the new onset of proteinuria should include antinuclear antibodies, serum complement levels (C3 and C4), hepatitis B surface antigen, and anti-HCV antibodies. Because long-standing diabetes remains one of the most common causes of secondary nephrotic syndrome, an evaluation of proteinuria should include measurement of serum glucose and/or glycohaemoglobin. The increasing prevalence of human immunodeficiency virus (HIV) infection in the general population and the association of this infection with focal segmental glomerulosclerosis and heavy proteinuria warrants an anti-HIV antibody determination. Finally, paraproteinaemia is a significant cause of nephrotic syndrome due to glomerular amyloidosis and 'light chain nephropathy', a glomerular and tubular interstitial disorder. Therefore, a serum protein electrophoresis as well as immunofixation of abnormal protein fractions for the presence of Bence-Jones proteins should be done in patients with unexplained proteinuria.

When patients present with an extrarenal exacerbation of a rheumatic disorder, screening for proteinuria, examination of the urinary sediment, and measurement of renal function should be undertaken. Monitoring certain serological factors may also yield useful information that suggests an exacerbation of renal disease and, potentially, allows for early intervention by adjustment of immunosuppressive therapies. For example, in lupus nephritis an increase in the concentration of anti-native DNA antibody and a decrease in C3 and/or C4 complement levels have been shown to have an 80–90 per cent correlation with subsequent renal exacerbations within the following 10 weeks (ter Borg et al. 1990). However, because the serum C3 and C4 may or may not be chronically decreased, an isolated low complement level is not necessarily predictive of active disease. In this circumstance, both the blood pressure and renal function must be closely monitored.

Differential diagnosis of proteinuria in systemic rheumatic disease

The main causes of heavy proteinuria in rheumatic illnesses are divisible into two groups. The first group presents with isolated proteinuria with or without renal insufficiency. Systemic lupus erythematosus commonly presents in this manner and, indeed, presentation with the nephrotic syndrome may precede the diagnosis of lupus. The renal biopsy generally shows a non-inflammatory form of lupus nephritis, characterized either by (a) membranous nephropathy (WHO classification type V) with thickening of the glomerular basement membrane and subepithelial deposition of immune complexes; or (b) mesangial proliferative disease (WHO classification type II) with increased mesangial cellularity and matrix, but without significant proliferation of glomerular endothelial or epithelial cells and inflammatory infiltration. Patients with mesangial proliferation will generally have extensive deposition of immune complexes within the mesangial matrix, which may be accompanied by an increase in the number of cells in the mesangial matrix.

Secondary amyloidosis (AA type), although an overall rare condition, occurs in up to 15 per cent of patients with rheumatoid arthritis (RA) and may also complicate cases of psoriatic arthritis, ankylosing spondylitis, and long-standing systemic lupus erythematosus. In cases of RA-associated secondary amyloidosis, renal manifestations, specifically proteinuria and renal insufficiency, have been documented in up to 91 per cent of cases (Gertz and Kyle 1991). The diagnosis of renal involvement by amyloid is often inferred by the demonstration of amyloid A fibrils in a biopsy from an extrarenal site, such as the rectum, gingiva, or abdominal fat pad. However, in some cases, renal biopsy is required for the diagnosis. Renal amyloidosis often presents with massive proteinuria, hypoalbuminemia and is associated with high mortality.

Several therapeutic agents frequently used for connective tissue diseases have been associated with the development of heavy proteinuria. Traditional non-steroidal anti-inflammatory drugs (NSAIDs) have been associated with the development of heavy proteinuria, acute renal failure, and electrolyte disorders in up to 5 per cent of patients who take them (Whelton 1999). Although this overall rate may appear low, given the number of patients who use these medications and their availability, the number of patients at risk for this complication is significant. Proteinuria is variable, but may be as high as 20 g/day. Renal biopsy, when done, has usually revealed minimal-change glomerular disease and acute interstitial nephritis. Immunofluorescence staining is negative. Recent studies have indicated that 75–80 per cent of the mononuclear interstitial infiltrate is composed of T lymphocytes. It has been speculated that inhibition of cyclooxygenase by NSAIDs shunts arachidonic acid to the lipoxygenase pathway, with subsequent production of mediators of inflammation, such as the leukotrienes. The production of these mediators in turn leads to infiltration of T lymphocytes with subsequent damage to the glomeruli and the renal interstitium. The development of heavy proteinuria with or without renal insufficiency in a patient treated with these drugs should prompt discontinuation. In most cases, the proteinuria and renal insufficiency often resolve after elimination of the offending drug.

Approximately 3–4 per cent of patients treated with gold for RA develop proteinuria; however, only one-fourth of these show the nephrotic syndrome. Renal biopsy of these individuals has generally revealed a classic membranous glomerulopathy, a non-inflammatory lesion characterized by thickening of the glomerular basement membrane presumably resulting from *in situ* immune-complex deposition. The development of increasing proteinuria or nephrotic syndrome during gold therapy should prompt discontinuation of the drug. In over 80 per cent of patients, the proteinuria resolves within 1 year, and steroid therapy does not appear to be warranted.

Administration of penicillamine is associated with proteinuria in about 10 per cent of cases. There is no clear relationship between the development of proteinuria and either the daily or cumulative dose of the drug, suggesting an idiosyncratic reaction. As with gold therapy, renal biopsy in patients with penicillamine-associated proteinuria generally reveals a membranous glomerulopathy. Although the pathogenesis is unknown, the renal lesion usually resolves after discontinuation of the drug, but the proteinuria may persist for as long as 2 years. Renal insufficiency rarely develops, even when complicated by heavy proteinuria.

The second type of presentation is that of proteinuria of variable quantity accompanied by haematuria and possibly renal insufficiency, which can have a rapidly progressive course. Systemic rheumatic illnesses that can present in this manner include polyarteritis nodosa, Wegener's granulomatosis and cryoglobulinaemia. Systemic lupus erythematosus may also fall into this category, especially when it is associated with a focal or diffuse proliferative glomerular lesion (WHO classification type III to IV). Cryoglobulinaemia, also an immune-complex disease, is characterized by deposition of circulating immune complexes within the glomerulus and a proliferative glomerular lesion not unlike that seen in the more severe cases of lupus nephritis. In recent years it has been discovered that many cases of systemic cryoglobulinaemia, which had been previously labeled as essential or idiopathic, are in fact linked to infection with hepatitis C. Polyarteritis nodosa is associated with two relatively distinct renal syndromes. In classical polyarteritis nodosa, there is a vasculitis involving the large- and medium-sized vessels of the kidney, and this results in hypertension as the primary presenting symptom. When present, glomerular lesions are the result of ischaemia, not inflammation, and manifest primarily as haematuria, not proteinuria. In microscopic polyarteritis, rapidly progressive glomerulonephritis is characterized by red blood cell casts, proteinuria, acute renal failure, hypertension, and a necrotizing small vessel vasculitis. Wegener's granulomatosis, also associated with inflammation of the small vessels of the kidney including the glomeruli, presents with a similar clinical picture. Although the antiserine proteinase 3 directed c-ANCA (antineutrophil cytoplasmic autoantibody; see below) has a disease specificity of up to 98 per cent with active, untreated systemic Wegener's granulomatosis, the only definitive way to distinguish these various forms of acute necrotizing glomerulonephritis is to perform a renal biopsy (Jeannette and Falk 1997; Yi and Colby 2001).

Haematuria

Definitions

Haematuria is defined as the presence of red blood cells in the urine. The normal urine should be negative for haem pigment on dipstick examination and should reveal less than three red blood cells per high-power field on examination of the sediment. Significant bleeding from the lower portions of the urinary tract, such as the bladder or urethra, usually produces a red discoloration of the urine. Bleeding from the kidney, on the other hand, and especially from glomeruli, results in denaturation of haem proteins as the red blood cells traverse the urinary tract; this produces a 'tea' or 'cola' coloured urine. The dipstick haem test is not specific for intact red blood cells and will register positive if any haem pigment, including haemoglobin or myoglobin, is present in the urine. Free haemoglobin may be present in the urine as a result of massive intravascular haemolysis due to an immune mechanism in patients with severe systemic lupus or a non-immune mechanism in severe microangiopathies. Myoglobin may be present in the urine as the result of lysis of skeletal muscle. This is usually seen in traumatic or non-traumatic rhabdomyolysis, but rarely can be seen with chronic inflammatory muscle diseases in exacerbation, such as dermatomyositis and polymyositis. Myoglobinuria has also been associated with a number of different drug exposures.

Anatomical sources of haematuria in a patient with systemic rheumatic disease

Subjects with rheumatic disease may develop bleeding at various sites along the urinary tract either as a result of the underlying systemic disease or as a result of therapy for the rheumatic disorder. Lower urinary tract (bladder and urethra) bleeding most commonly results from urinary tract infection. Chronic immunosuppressive therapy and underlying renal insufficiency predispose to urinary tract infections, which can also present with either painless or painful microscopic or gross haematuria. The presence of white blood cells, leucocyte esterase, or nitrates on urinalysis is suggestive but not diagnostic for infection. Therefore, a urine culture should be included in the evaluation of unexplained haematuria. In addition, cyclophosphamide (Cytoxan), an immunosuppressive agent used in the therapy of several rheumatic diseases, can induce haemorrhagic cystitis, and has been associated with both transitional cell tumours of the uroepithelium and squamous cell carcinoma of the bladder. Haemorrhagic cystitis can present as painless microscopic or painful gross haematuria. This side-effect may be prevented by hydration and the use of mesna (2-mercaptoethane sulfonate). However, due to the increased risk of malignancy associated with the use of cyclophosphamide, it is extremely important for patients who have been treated with this cytotoxic agent to be closely monitored for the appearance of nonglomerular haematuria and appropriately screened for the presence of cystitis and malignancy (Talar-Williams et al. 1996).

Bleeding from the upper urinary tract (ureters and urinary collecting system) is often associated with long-term ingestion of non-narcotic analgesic agents. Renal papillary necrosis may occur with the accumulation of large doses of analgesic agents containing a combination of aspirin and phenacetin or with the sustained use of NSAIDs. The process can present with either painless microscopic or gross haematuria. Acute papillary necrosis can also induce renal colic, owing to ureteral spasm as the sloughed papilla passes down the ureter to the bladder. Occasionally, the diagnosis can be made by detecting the passage of gross tissue into the urine or from the presence of fragments of the sloughed papilla in the microscopic examination of the urine sediment. More commonly, the diagnosis is made from radiographic studies. The complications of renal papillary necrosis are pain and the potential for urinary tract obstruction. Recently, chronic heavy use of over-the-counter analgesics, including NSAIDs and acetaminofen, but not aspirin, has been associated with the development of endstage renal disease (Whelton 1999). Whether this association is due to analgesic nephropathy or to the increased prevalence of analgesic ingestion among patients with diseases which predispose them to endstage renal disease remains unclear. Occasionally, microscopic haematuria can complicate interstitial nephritis. A special case of this phenomenon may occur in the interstitial nephropathy associated with Sjögren's syndrome. In this entity, the haematuria may be secondary to nephrocalcinosis resulting from the distal renal tubular acidosis not infrequently encountered in patients with this disease .

Aside from the presence of a malignancy, the greatest concern in the patient with haematuria associated with systemic rheumatic illness is the development of glomerulonephritis. Glomerular haematuria, as opposed to isolated proteinuria, generally reflects an inflammatory process of the glomerulus, often resulting from immune-mediated injury, the deposition of circulating immune complexes or antiglomerular basement membrane (anti-GBM) antibody. Rheumatic disorders associated with this entity include systemic lupus erythematosus, Henoch–Schönlein purpura, Wegener's granulomatosis, and cryoglobulinaemia. Non-nephrotic or nephrotic-range proteinuria, cellular casts in the urinary sediment, and a deterioration of renal function may be present. The immediate danger from acute glomerulonephritis is deterioration of renal function.

Vascular diseases of the kidney can lead to haematuria by induction of ischaemic glomerular damage. Such injury causes destruction of the glomerular filtration barrier and leakage of red blood cells into Bowman's space. This mechanism occurs in both classical and microscopic polyarteritis as well as the microangiopathic syndromes, such as systemic sclerosis, malignant hypertension, thrombotic thrombocytopenic purpura, and haemolytic uraemic syndrome. Finally, renal vein thrombosis, which may occur in the nephrotic syndrome, may also lead to gross or microscopic haematuria.

Diagnostic studies

One of the greatest concerns with new onset haematuria, in the presence or absence of rheumatic disease, is the possibility of a tumour of the urinary tract. Therefore, in contrast to the evaluation of isolated proteinuria, the workup of haematuria should prompt both a urological and a nephrological evaluation. Normal urinary tract imaging with intravenous pyelography or renal ultrasonography and cystoscopy essentially rule out the bladder, ureters, and collecting system as the source of bleeding. On the other hand, the coexistence of haematuria and significant proteinuria or the presence of red blood cell casts in the urine sediment offer reasonable security that the haematuria is of glomerular origin and not due to neoplasm. Baseline renal function and protein excretion should be quantitated with a 24-h collection of urine. Once non-glomerular sources of the haematuria have been excluded, the exact nature of the glomerular disorder may be determined from the results of the serological tests and laboratory examination as previously described for the proteinuric patient. In addition, given the presentation of alteration in renal function in the presence of an 'active' urinary sediment, the antineutrophil cytoplasmic antibody (ANCA) along with measurement of antibodies directed against serine proteinase 3 (PR3) and to neutrophil myeloperoxidase (MPO) may be useful in the diagnosis of a systemic vasculitis. Alternatively, in the patient with an established vasculitis, measurements of titers of these antibodies may distinguish between vasculitic disease activity and complications of cytotoxic therapy, although there are conflicting data regarding the utility of serially monitoring ANCA titres as a marker of prognosis (Boomsma et al. 2000; Nowack et al. 2001). A renal biopsy may be indicated to establish the diagnosis or to ascertain the nature, activity, or chronicity of the glomerular lesion. These may be important in determining prognosis as well as potential response to therapy (Bajema et al. 1999).

Role of renal biopsy in the evaluation of proteinuria and haematuria

The role of renal biopsy in the evaluation of proteinuria and haematuria has been controversial. The decision to perform a renal biopsy in a specific clinical setting varies with the practice style of the nephrologist involved. Inferences can be made about the nature and activity of the renal lesion on the basis of renal functional abnormalities, the activity of the urine sediment, and the presence or severity of hypertension. Often, a diagnosis can be established from the extrarenal manifestations of the disease and its serological abnormalities. A therapeutic decision can then be made from this clinical information. The response of the renal lesion to therapeutic intervention can be assessed by changes in renal function, reduced cast excretion in the urine sediment, diminished quantity of proteinuria, and improvement in serological abnormalities. Such an approach can certainly be defended in the patient who may be at higher than usual risk for renal biopsy because of obesity, coagulation abnormalities, or the presence of a solitary kidney.

On the other hand, there are clinical circumstances in which a renal biopsy may be essential to establish a diagnosis. Neither serological studies nor the pattern of extrarenal involvement are specific for a particular renal pathology and, therefore, renal biopsy is a fundamental diagnostic procedure. Although the presence of the c-ANCA strongly supports the diagnosis of Wegener's granulomatosis, the identification of immune deposits on a renal biopsy specimen in a patient with rapidly progressive glomerulonephritis is still the 'gold standard' and an important determinant of whether corticosteroids, immunosuppressive agents, and/or plasmapheresis are the most appropriate course of therapy. In addition, the number of unaffected glomeruli found on a renal biopsy can have significance as a predictor for long-term renal outcomes in patients with ANCA-associated systemic vasculitis (Bajema et al. 1999).

An intermediate circumstance occurs when the diagnosis of systemic disease is established and a renal biopsy is being considered to ascertain the nature and severity of a glomerular lesion. The most typical case would be that of lupus nephritis, in which some nephrologists might recommend renal biopsy because of the prognostic implications of certain renal lesions. In addition to classifying patients with lupus nephritis according to the pattern of glomerular involvement (minimal, mesangial, focal proliferative, diffuse proliferative, and membranous), renal pathologists make note of the extent of activity (inflammatory, potentially reversible changes) and chronicity (sclerosing, irreversible changes) within the kidney (Balow and Austin 1988; Esdaile et al. 1989). Thus, given a patient with moderate renal failure, the presence of a high chronicity index may be considered a relative contraindication for intensive corticosteroid or immunosuppressive therapy because the likelihood of a therapeutic response would be outweighed by the potential toxicity. By contrast, a high activity index may prompt the nephrologist to institute aggressive treatment because of the potential for reversal of the underlying pathology (Boumpas et al. 1995).

The more conservative nephrologist might defer renal biopsy, attempt a limited trial of corticosteroid or immunosuppressive therapy, and then, if the renal disease fails to respond, consider renal biopsy at a later date to investigate a pathological explanation for the lack of response. Both approaches can be justified, and in fact, decision-analysis studies of this issue have failed to reveal any clearly favourable approach. The rheumatologist may, therefore, wish to choose a nephrology consultant on the basis of compatibility of their practice styles in this context.

An additional clinical scenario in which the role for renal biopsy is somewhat clouded is in the case of lupus nephritis, either during the course of therapy with cytotoxic agents or after the conclusion of therapy. Occasionally, patients will have a 'partial' response to therapy, have no response to therapy, or potentially have a relapse of haematuria/proteinuria after completing a course of directed therapy. In such patients, a case can be made for rebiopsying in order to determine if the patient has had a change in their glomerular pathology (a 'class switch' in the case of lupus nephritis), or potentially has a change in the pattern of glomerular/interstial involvement. During the course of therapy, patients occasionally will present with a decrease in overall renal function. In such cases the potential of an alteration in therapy, or potentially discontinuing potentially toxic medications based on the results of a repeated biopsy would justify a repeat biopsy (Moroni et al. 1999).

Acute renal failure

Definitions

Acute renal failure is defined as a sudden decline in renal function, usually measured by an increase in serum creatinine and blood urea nitrogen (BUN) or a decrease in glomerular filtration rate. The serum creatinine is a reliable marker of changes in the glomerular filtration rate if its limitations are understood. The BUN is a less reliable marker of changes in renal function, primarily because it may be elevated in several conditions where renal function is stable, such as gastrointestinal bleeding and steroid administration. As a result, rises in the BUN are best interpreted in relation to changes in the serum creatinine. Approximately 20 per cent of urinary creatinine excretion under physiological conditions is due to tubular secretion. Therefore, as glomerular filtration declines and tubular secretion of creatinine contributes a greater fraction of creatinine excretion, increases in the serum creatinine and a fall in the creatinine clearance tend to underestimate the true decrease in glomerular filtration rate that has occurred. Furthermore, therapeutic agents, such as cimetidine and trimethoprim, may competitively inhibit tubular creatinine secretion, leading to increases in the serum creatinine in the absence of any changes in glomerular filtration rate. Finally, because the serum creatinine is roughly inversely proportional to creatinine clearance or glomerular filtration rate, at relatively normal levels of renal function, changes in the serum creatinine tend to be relatively insensitive. For instance, an increase in the serum creatinine from 1 to 2 mg/dl would represent a halving (50 per cent decline) of the glomerular filtration rate. Once such a change has occurred, substantial renal function has been lost, despite what appears to be only a modest increase in the serum creatinine. An increase in the serum creatinine from 1.0 to 1.1 mg/dl, if real, represents a 9 per cent decline in glomerular filtration rate, also rather significant. However, the standard laboratory assay for serum creatinine has a variation of plus 10 per cent, meaning that any change of 0.1 mg/dl in the serum creatinine could correctly or incorrectly be attributed to laboratory variation. Therefore, it is important that even seemingly small changes in the serum creatinine should not be discounted and, if a more reliable indicator of renal function is required, creatinine clearance or radionuclide studies (such as iothalamate clearance) should be considered.

In the nephrotic syndrome, hypoalbuminaemia results in transudation of fluid from the vasculature into the interstitial space. Baroreceptors in the renal vasculature then 'sense' a decreased circulating volume. Sodium and water reabsorption increase and the volume of urine declines. Similarly in congestive heart failure, as may complicate systemic lupus erythematosus, low cardiac output is 'sensed' by the kidneys and a low urine output state develops. Acute changes in renal function, which are associated with such declines in either true or 'effective' circulating volume, are termed 'pre-renal' azotemia. NSAIDs, as well as a new class of anti-inflammatory medications, COX-2 inhibitors, by inhibiting renal vasodilatory prostaglandins, may also produce adverse haemodynamic changes and a decline in renal function independent of their potential to produce interstitial nephritis or proteinuria (Dunn 2000; Perazella 2000). It has been reported that sulindac has a 'renal sparing' effect because the enzyme that converts sulindac to its active form is not present in the kidney. However, the sparing effect of sulindac appears to be lost at daily dosages now in common use. Volume depletion, hepatic disease, and lupus nephritis predispose to the adverse renal haemodynamic changes associated with the NSAIDs. The alterations in renal function are reversed upon discontinuation of the offending drug. The angiotensin-converting enzyme (ACE) inhibitors and a related class of medications, the angiotensin receptor blockers, can induce decreased renal perfusion and an acute decline in renal function through dilation of intrarenal efferent arterioles. Such alterations in renal function are enhanced when there is underlying volume depletion, renal vascular disease, or pre-existing glomerular disease. In addition to being the preferred treatment for proteinuria, these antihypertensives have been particularly efficacious in the treatment of malignant hypertension associated with scleroderma renal crisis and the microangiopathies. When using these medications, renal function and serum electrolytes must be monitored closely because of the risk of acute renal failure and electrolyte abnormalities, such as hyperkalemia, due to a relative reduction of aldosterone.

Post-renal failure is oliguria caused by an intrarenal or extrarenal obstruction to urine flow. Intrarenal obstruction may be due to crystallization of a substance within the renal tubules. This might be endogenous, such as uric acid or a calcium salt, or exogenous, such as crystals of methotrexate or a sulphonamide. Clinically apparent extrarenal obstruction to urinary flow most commonly involves the lower urinary tract because the obstruction of only one of two functioning kidneys will allow the non-affected kidney to continue to make urine, so oliguria and renal failure will not result. Severe haemorrhagic cystitis complicating cyclophosphamide therapy may produce enough blood clot within the bladder to obstruct the flow of urine and acute oliguric renal failure develops. Bilateral papillary necrosis could lead to obstruction of the upper urinary tract through occlusion of both ureters, but this would be a most unusual event. Post-renal failure can be reversed if the site of obstruction is identified, and the obstruction is relieved before onset of renal parenchymal damage. Post-renal failure is characterized by low-to-absent urine output. Urinary sodium concentration and urine osmolarity are variable. In the acute phase, the urine electrolytes and osmolarity may mimic a pre-renal picture with a low urine sodium concentration and high urine osmolarity, however, as the obstruction becomes chronic, increasing tubular dysfunction is reflected by a high urine sodium concentration and low urine osmolarity. Obstruction is best diagnosed by renal ultrasound, which may reveal hydronephrosis, and cystoscopy, which could identify the presence of clots or tissue in the bladder.

Of most concern in the patient with acute renal failure is renal parenchymal disease, because this is most likely to lead to irreversible renal damage if appropriate diagnostic and therapeutic procedures are not undertaken. Acute renal failure due to renal parenchymal disease may be oliguric, that is, resulting in a urine volume of less than 500 ml/day, or non-oliguric (i.e. urine volumes >500 ml/day). The latter term implies that, despite an apparently normal daily volume of urine, solute clearance continues to decline as measured by serum creatinine or clearance techniques. The presence of normal urinary volumes may make patient management somewhat easier. Fluid and sodium restrictions may not have to be as severe, and not as much fluid may have to be removed on dialysis should this procedure become necessary. However, non-oliguric renal failure may be just as ominous as oliguric renal failure with regard to prognosis and potential response to therapy. Therefore, attention only to urinary volume without consideration to changes in the serum creatinine or creatinine clearance is misguided, because severe, progressive renal insufficiency may develop without an oliguric phase. Serial tests of the serum creatinine must be done in the unstable patient to adequately assess any changes in renal function. An estimation of creatinine clearance using the Modification of Diet in Renal Disease (MDRD) equation can then be made in order to adjust medication dosing. Urine collections of 24-hour duration for creatinine clearance are less helpful in the setting of acute renal failure due to the often cumbersome nature of timed collections and the potential for large changes in serum creatinine over relatively short periods of time, which may render the test inaccurate. The MDRD formula for the estimation of endogenous creatinine clearance is calculated as follows (Manjunath et al. 2001):

$$\mathrm{GFR} = 186.3 \times (P_{cr})^{-1-154}\,(\text{age in years})^{-0.203} \times 1.212\,(\text{if black race}) \times 0.742\,(\text{if female})$$

Anatomical sources of acute renal failure in the patient with systemic rheumatic disease

Acute renal failure has several pathophysiological mechanisms in systemic rheumatic diseases.

A. Pre-renal:
  1. True decreased circulating volume
     (a) overdiuresis
     (b) dehydration
  2. 'Effective' decreased circulating volume
     (a) nephrotic syndrome
     (b) congestive heart failure
     (c) non-steroidal anti-inflammatory drugs
     (d) cyclosporin
     (e) angiotensin-converting enzyme inhibitors
     (f) liver disease/cirrhosis

B. Intrinsic renal:
  1. Acute interstitial nephritis
     (a) non-steroidal anti-inflammatory agents
     (b) Sjögren's syndrome
  2. Acute tubular necrosis
     (a) sepsis
     (b) pigment
        (i) haemoglobin
        (ii) myoglobin
     (c) toxins/drugs
        (i) antibiotics
        (ii) radiocontrast media
  3. Rapid progressive glomerulonephritis
     (a) immune complex disease
        (i) systemic lupus erythematosus
        (ii) Henoch–Schönlein purpura
        (iii) cryoglobulinaemia
     (b) anti-GBM disease
     (c) pauci-immune
        (i) polyarteritis
        (ii) Wegener's granulomatosis
  4. Microangiopathic
     (a) scleroderma
     (b) thrombotic thrombocytopaenic purpura/haemolytic uraemic syndrome
     (c) cyclosporin

C. Post-renal/obstructive:
  1. Extrarenal
     (a) cyclophosphamide-induced haemorrhagic cystitis
     (b) bilateral papillary necrosis
  2. Intrarenal
     (a) Methotrexate-induced intratubular crystallization

The NSAIDs, as previously mentioned, may be associated with the development of heavy proteinuria, chronic renal insufficiency as well as acute renal failure. Approximately 10 per cent of cases have only nephrotic syndrome, about 15 per cent have only renal failure, and the remainder develop both. Wright's or Hansel's stain of the urinary sediment may rarely reveal eosinophiluria. Renal biopsy reveals an inflammatory infiltrate in the interstitial or tubular portion of the kidney parenchyma, which is termed interstitial nephritis. Interstitial nephritis induced by NSAIDs appears to be unique among the drug-induced tubular interstitial nephritides in its association with heavy proteinuria. Tubular interstitial nephritis generally occurs after prolonged exposure (mean, 5–6 months) to the offending agent, although acute hemodynamically associated changes in glomerular filtration rate can be associated with much shorter use of these medications. The propionic acid derivatives—fenoprofen, ibuprofen, and naproxen—have accounted for three-fourths of the cases reported, with fenoprofen alone accounting for over one-half of the incidence of tubular interstitial disease induced by NSAIDs. The lesions have also been found after the self-administration of over-the-counter ibuprofen and may recur after exposure to different NSAIDs of the same group or upon re-exposure to the same agent. The onset of nephrotic syndrome generally precedes that of renal failure. Supportive dialysis becomes necessary in about one-third of patients. An improvement in renal function occurs within days of discontinuing the offending agent, although proteinuria may persist for weeks to months. There appear to be no definite predisposing factors that identify subjects prone to developing nephritis induced by these drugs. Alternative agents infrequently associated with nephrotoxicity include meclofenamate and sulindac.

Sjögren's syndrome is associated with a chronic inflammatory infiltrate of the renal interstitium that may lead to a progressive deterioration in renal function. More common renal manifestations are those related to tubular dysfunction, including distal renal tubular acidosis and nephrogenic diabetes insipidus. Glomerular obsolescence with sclerosis may occur in association with severely damaged tubules; heavy proteinuria is uncommon. Renal involvement is generally inferred from a rising creatinine and tubular dysfunction, which may present with metabolic acidosis, hypokalaemia, hypophosphataemia, hypouricaemia, aminoaciduria, or polyuria. However, renal involvement is generally not a limiting factor in Sjögren's syndrome. A specific medical therapy for the renal lesion is not available.

Acute tubular necrosis has several potential pathophysiological mechanisms in systemic rheumatic diseases. Perhaps the most common is sepsis complicating chronic immunosuppression. Sepsis with endotoxaemia may lead to substantial renal dysfunction, even in the absence of overt septic shock, because local release of vasoactive substances in the kidney produces vasoconstriction and shunts blood flow away from the kidneys. While early acute renal failure of sepsis may resemble pre-renal azotaemia and may be characterized by a low urinary sodium and a high urinary osmolarity, it is more often associated with high urinary sodium and a low urinary osmolarity. Aggressive hydration often fails to reverse the oliguria and rising serum creatinine, which indicates that the defect is not merely a function of decreased renal perfusion. Sepsis-associated renal failure may respond to the renal vasodilator dopamine, although this form of therapy remains very controversial. Nonetheless, the treatment of choice is eradication of the infection with appropriate antibiotic therapy.

Large loads of haem pigment can result in renal tubular toxicity and acute renal failure with acute tubular necrosis. Severe intravascular haemolysis, which can occur in systemic lupus and the microangiopathic diseases, can result in the formation of haemoglobin casts within the tubules, intratubular obstruction, and direct tubular toxicity. There is considerable experimental evidence that red cell stroma contributes to the nephrotoxicity of acute haemolysis by inducing vasoconstrictive changes within the kidney. Such alterations in vascular tone promote tubular reabsorption of fluid, thereby further concentrating and enhancing the precipitation of haemoglobin within the tubular lumens. Polymyositis and dermatomyositis are rarely associated with myoglobinuric acute renal failure, because these diseases tend to be chronic rather than acute diseases of muscle.

The clinical course of pigment-induced nephropathy is similar to that of other forms of acute tubular necrosis with oliguria and (because of cell breakdown) significant hyperkalaemia. Mannitol may be useful in the early stages of the renal failure to increase urine flow, thereby washing out obstructing tubular casts, producing direct renal vasodilatation, and possibly preventing swelling of glomerular cells. Once renal failure due to pigment nephropathy becomes established, management is similar to that of other forms of acute renal failure. The electrolyte disorders, such as hyperkalaemia, that may be associated with cell lysis may necessitate early dialysis.

Rapidly progressive glomerulonephritis is a catastrophic form of inflammatory renal disease that sometimes complicates systemic rheumatic disease. It is a syndrome characterized by hypertension, proteinuria, haematuria with red blood cell casts, and a rapid decline in renal function. The pathological correlate of rapidly progressive glomerulonephritis is the formation of epithelial cell crescents in Bowman's space, often accompanied by a necrotizing vasculitis of the arterioles and glomerular capillaries. There are a number of systemic rheumatic diseases that can be associated with this type of glomerulonephritis, including systemic lupus erythematosus, polyarteritis nodosa, Wegener's granulomatosis, and cryoglobulinaemia. If the diagnosis can be established on the basis of the extrarenal manifestations of these diseases, then the cause of a rapidly progressive glomerulonephritis should be apparent. At times, the extrarenal manifestations are not sufficiently specific to allow for a diagnosis and glomerulonephritis can be the initial manifestation of disease. In such circumstances, the immunopathology of the renal lesion has traditionally been the basis for classifying the various forms of the rapidly progressive disease. The detection of deposits within the glomerular capillaries by immunofluorescence microscopy, or of subepithelial or subendothelial deposits by electron microscopy, suggests an immune-complex pathogenesis that is characteristic of lupus nephritis, post-infectious glomerulonephritis, or cryoglobulinaemic nephritis. The presence of linear immunofluorescence along the glomerular basement membrane is diagnostic for glomerulonephritis mediated by anti-GBM antibody which, in the presence of pulmonary haemorrhage, is termed Goodpasture's syndrome.

Much less well defined, however, are the forms of rapidly progressive glomerulonephritis that are not associated with immune-complex deposits or anti-GBM binding within the glomerulus, which have been termed pauci-immune glomerulonephritis. The diagnosis usually depends upon the pattern of extrarenal manifestations and includes polyarteritis nodosa in the presence of systemic necrotizing arteritis, Wegener's granulomatosis in the presence of pulmonary necrotizing granulomas, and idiopathic crescentic glomerulonephritis when no extrarenal disease is present. A scheme for the differential diagnosis of rapidly progressive glomerulonephritis is summarized in Table 2.

It has now been demonstrated that idiopathic, rapidly progressive glomerulonephritis and vasculitis-associated glomerulonephritis may share a common serological marker, ANCA. However, the ANCA test has also been associated with other systemic disorders in which renal disease may be absent, particularly inflammatory bowel disease. The ANCA test produces three patterns of indirect immunofluorescent staining: fine granular cytoplasmic (c-ANCA), perinuclear (p-ANCA), and a diffuse, atypical ANCA (a-ANCA) (Choi et al. 2001; Wiik 2001) (see Chapter 5.4). The autoantigen(s) stimulating the a-ANCA response have not been identified. PR3 and MPO are the most commonly identified autoantigens triggering the c-ANCA and p-ANCA responses, respectively, and therefore the terms PR3-ANCA and MPO-ANCA are coming into more common usage.

c-ANCA reflects an autoantibody response against a 29-kDa serine protease, known as proteinase 3 (PR3), which is localized within the azurophilic granules of quiescent neutrophils as well as on the cell surface of activated neutrophils . Localized in lysosomes, PR3 is a bifunctional protein with both enzymatic and antimicrobial functions. Acting as a proteinase, it hydrolyses naphthol-ASD-chloracetate. PR3-ANCA (c-ANCA) is a sensitive and specific autoantibody for active Wegener's granulomatosis. Although the frequency of this autoantibody in all patients with Wegener's granulomatosis approximates 90–95 per cent (Yi and Colby, 2001), the

Table 2 Differential diagnosis of rapidly progressive glomerulonephritis

Group	Glomerular immuno-fluorescence	Serological markers	Extrarenal manifestations	Diagnosis
Immune complex	Granular	Antinuclear antibodies	Skin, joints, haematological	Systemic lupus
		Cryoglobulins	Skin, joints	Cryoglobulinaemic glomerulonephritis
		Antistreptococcal antibodies	None	Poststreptococcal glomerulonephritis
		HBsAg	Skin, joints	Hepatitis-associated glomerulonephritis
		Increased IgA	Skin, joints, abdominal pain	Henoch–Schönlein purpura
Anti-GBM[a]	Linear	Anti-GBM antibodies	Lung haemorrhage	Goodpasture's syndrome
			None	Anti-GBM glomerulonephritis
Pauci-immune	None	Mostly c-ANCA[b]	Lungs, sinuses, joints	Wegener's granulomatosis
		c-ANCA or p-ANCA[c]	Skin, joints, lungs, nerves	Polyarteritis nodosa
		Mostly p-ANCA	None	Idiopathic crescentic glomerulonephritis

[a] Antiglomerular basement membrane.

[b] Cytoplasmic antineutrophil cytoplasmic autoantibodies.

[c] Perinuclear antineutrophil cytoplasmic autoantibodies.

overall sensitivity is estimated to be 66 per cent and the overall specificity is 98 per cent (Hewins et al. 2000). During active disease, the pooled sensitivity increases to 91 per cent and the pooled specificity rises to 99 per cent. Whether titres of ANCA correlate directly with disease activity remains controversial (Boomsma 2000; Nowack 2001). Based on an estimated 5 per cent prevalence of Wegener's granulomatosis, 37 per cent of patients with a positive c-ANCA may have a false-positive test result. These data underscore the importance of employing the c-ANCA test as corroborating evidence for the diagnosis of Wegener's granulomatosis in patients with the appropriate clinical stigmata and disease activity. In cases where such evidence is lacking, a renal biopsy should be considered prior to the initiation of cytotoxic therapies.

Although several azurophilic granule enzymes can drive the p-ANCA response, the principal autoantigen is myeloperoxidase (MPO) (Wiik et al. 1995). MPO is a 140-kDa cationic protein of azurophilic granules of neutrophils and certain granules of monocytes that generates chlorinated oxygen species upon activation of the cell by a microbe. The p-ANCA is most commonly associated with microscopic polyangiitis, Churg–Strauss syndrome, and pauci-immune glomerulonephritis. These disorders tend to be associated with MPO-ANCA. The p-ANCA pattern occurs in less than 5 per cent of subjects with Wegener's granulomatosis and classic polyarteritis nodosa.

At a recent consensus conference, the idiopathic vasculitides were reclassified into large, medium, and small vessel vasculitis (Jennette et al. 1994). Although Wegener's granulomatosis, microscopic polyangiitis, and Churg–Strauss syndrome were the small vessel vasculitic disorders predominantly associated with a positive ANCA test, it is also known that other non-renal and non-vasculitic processes, including ulcerative colitis and primary sclerosing cholangitis, are often associated with a positive p-ANCA.

Perhaps the most malignant form of renal involvement in the systemic rheumatic diseases is the microangiopathy that may be seen in systemic sclerosis, the thrombotic thrombocytopaenic purpura/haemolytic uraemia syndrome, and with the use of cyclosporin. The presence of microscopic renal lesions in patients with systemic sclerosis may be as high as 80 per cent, although only 40–50 per cent will present with clinical renal involvement, including hypertension, proteinuria, or azotaemia. Hypertension is very ominous in patients with systemic sclerosis. The death rate among hypertensive patients is about 2.5 times greater than among those with normal blood pressure. There are two distinct forms of hypertension seen in patients with systemic sclerosis. Mild to moderate hypertension associated with some degree of proteinuria may lead to the slow development of renal failure, and the extrarenal manifestations of systemic sclerosis usually dominate the clinical picture. However, in 15–20 per cent of patients who develop hypertension in the setting of systemic sclerosis, the onset is abrupt with severe elevation of blood pressure to greater than 130 mmHg diastolic, usually associated with cardiac failure and rapid deterioration of renal function (Steen et al. 2000). In some patients, severe hypertension may be the presenting feature of systemic sclerosis, with little involvement of skin, peripheral vessels, or joints. Classically, the small arterioles of the kidney in patients with the malignant form of hypertension in systemic sclerosis show extensive fibrinoid necrosis and microthrombus formation. Glomerular changes are variable and show varying degrees of thrombosis and necrosis secondary to ischaemia. Obviously, the accelerated hypertension and rapidly progressive renal failure of systemic sclerosis are life threatening and demand prompt, intensive intervention. The initial priority is to bring the blood pressure under control, and the ACE inhibitors have been the mainstay of therapy in this regard (Steen and Medsger 2000). Even if oliguria and progressive renal failure supervene despite control of blood pressure, antihypertensive therapy should be continued because it will protect other organs from the damaging effects of severe hypertension and renal function may return after months of dialysis support.

Thrombotic thrombocytopaenic purpura and haemolytic uraemic syndrome are classical examples of microangiopathic haemolytic anaemia and have many features in common, including anaemia, thrombocytopaenia, and renal involvement. The two syndromes are similar in most of their clinical and laboratory findings, differing primarily in age of onset and extent of renal involvement. An abnormal urinalysis characterized by haematuria, haemoglobinuria, proteinuria, and hyaline and granular casts is seen in the vast majority of patients with either disease, but those with haemolytic uraemic syndrome have a 90 per cent incidence of associated renal function abnormalities compared with a 50 per cent incidence in patients with thrombotic thrombocytopaenic purpura. The classical pathological finding in the kidney in both syndromes is occlusive lesions of arterioles and glomerular capillaries with fibrin, platelets, and red blood cells. Glomerular capillaries also show hyaline thrombosis with areas of infarction. The pathogenesis of these diseases is not completely understood, but it appears that some form of endothelial injury may be the underlying insult. Patients with systemic lupus erythematosus have been known to progress to thrombotic thrombocytopaenic purpura, and it is also seen in the setting of severe disseminated intravascular coagulation, sepsis, and other vasculitides, including polyarteritis nodosa and Wegener's granulomatosis. Plasma exchange has become the mainstay of therapy in thrombotic thrombocytopaenic purpura and haemolytic uraemic syndrome. Renal failure with its associated complications remains the most common cause of death (Hollenbeck et al. 1998).

Principles of treatment

Several general principles of evaluation and management of acute renal dysfunction in systemic rheumatic diseases should be emphasized. The prognosis of acute renal failure is determined both by the underlying disease and by the quality of medical management. Subjects with renal dysfunction complicating a rheumatic disorder should be followed-up jointly by a rheumatologist and nephrologist. Early consultation with a nephrologist is advisable in order to rapidly diagnose the underlying etiology of acute deterioration of renal function. In many situations, prompt resolution of the inciting factors can lead to a rapid return of renal function. In cases where deterioration cannot be halted, nephrologic support by means of renal replacement therapy can be initiated in a timely manner.

The chief cause of complications in the setting of acute renal failure is not azotaemia, but associated fluid and electrolyte abnormalities. The rheumatologist should manage these abnormalities with the nephrologist. In the acutely ill, highly catabolic patient with systemic illness, early and frequent dialysis may be required. Fluid overload may compound hypertension, leading to further renal injury, and should be managed intensively with high-dose diuretics. The rheumatologist and nephrologist should review the prescribed medications critically as soon as acute renal insufficiency is recognized. The dosage schedule for potentially nephrotoxic agents such as NSAIDs, aminoglycoside antibiotics, and amphotericin B should be adjusted for the level of renal failure or discontinued if possible. Intravascular radiocontrast procedures should be avoided during acute renal insufficiency. If it is necessary to use a diagnostic procedure requiring contrast, a minimal dose should be employed and the patient intensively hydrated before, during, and after the procedure to promote excretion of the radiocontrast. The presence of a highly catabolic state caused by corticosteroid therapy, gastrointestinal bleeding, parenteral nutrition, or septicaemia can induce a rise in the blood urea nitrogen by as much as 50 mg/dl per day in the setting of acute renal failure. Such levels of azotaemia are clearly detrimental to platelet and neutrophil function, and may potentiate a bleeding diathesis or further compromise host defenses. Therefore, intensive daily or continuous dialysis may be warranted.

Hypertension

Introduction

Hypertension is a very common finding in the adult population, affecting as many as 20–30 per cent of individuals over the age of 40. Raised blood pressure may be an incidental finding in the patient with systemic rheumatic illness and does not necessarily represent renal involvement from their disease. However, the onset of acute hypertension in a patient who was previously normotensive or whose blood pressure was well controlled may suggest renal involvement and may predate the onset of haematuria, proteinuria, or renal insufficiency. Anyone with a rheumatic disease who develops severe hypertension should be intensively investigated for the cause, and referral to a nephrologist should be considered. Intensive control of the blood pressure is important to minimize the renal and extrarenal complications of the severe hypertension, and a nephrologist may be best equipped to choose appropriate antihypertensive therapy in this setting. If incompletely treated, hypertension will further compound the renal injury by producing more intrarenal vascular damage. Therefore, intensive control of blood pressure is imperative. Malignant hypertension associated with renal vasculitis, systemic sclerosis, or microangiopathic disease results from extremely high concentrations of renin and angiotensin, released in response to focal areas of renal ischaemia. The ACE inhibitors, therefore, may be the only oral agents effective in the sustained reduction of blood pressure. Severe hypertension complicated by stroke, hypertensive encephalopathy, coronary ischaemia, pulmonary oedema, or aortic dissection requires concentrated intervention with confinement to an intensive care unit and use of a rapidly acting, parenteral, antihypertensive agent. There may be a further decline in renal function after hypertension has come under control, because of decreased renal perfusion pressure in the setting of high renal vascular resistance. However, once renal autoregulatory processes have stabilized, gradual return of renal function to physiological levels takes place after the successful control of blood pressure.

Specific diseases

Classical polyarteritis may produce hypertension through involvement of medium-sized arteries within the kidney, leading to distal areas of decreased perfusion and the release of potent vasoconstrictor substances. The glomeruli may not be directly affected in polyarteritis and, therefore, the presence of minimal haematuria, proteinuria, or other abnormal urinary sediment findings may presage abnormal results from renal function tests. Severe hypertension is, in fact, the most common renal manifestation of classical polyarteritis, affecting as many as 35 per cent of subjects with no other clinical renal manifestations of the disease. The diagnosis of classical polyarteritis in this setting is generally made from the extrarenal manifestations, most commonly mesenteric vasculitis with abdominal pain, abnormal liver function, and mononeuritis multiplex. Up to one-third will have a positive serology for hepatitis B surface antigen. In the absence of proteinuria or haematuria suggesting active glomerular involvement, renal biopsy is not helpful in the confirmation of the diagnosis. However, even without hypertension, polyarteritis nodosa is often found to involve medium-sized arteries on renal arteriography, characterized by segmental narrowing and aneurysmal dilatation.

Rapidly progressive glomerulonephritis can be associated with severe hypertension in the setting of acute glomerular injury. Intensive control of the blood pressure should be the objective, even before a specific diagnosis of the glomerular disease has been established. Inflammation is often compounded by ischaemia and, therefore, the hypertension will often prove refractory. High doses of multiple antihypertensive agents may be required for its control. A further decline in renal function may be anticipated as blood pressure control is achieved, because profound abnormalities in autoregulation of renal blood flow can occur, impairing the ability of the glomeruli to adapt to a fall in renal perfusion pressure. Nonetheless, a rise in the serum creatinine does not obviate the necessity to reduce the diastolic pressure to between 90 and 100 mmHg.

Summary and conclusions

The purpose of this chapter has been to provide the rheumatologist with a survey of the most important renal manifestations of systemic rheumatic illnesses, grouped according to the presentation most likely to be encountered in clinical practice. Table 3 is a list of important points to remember. Proteinuria, haematuria, acute renal failure, and hypertension can be ominous signs of direct renal involvement in systemic rheumatic diseases. However, they may also represent indirect involvement by complications of the primary disorder or its treatment, in which case the prognosis tends to be more favourable. The role of the rheumatologist here is to be familiar with the diseases most likely to affect the kidney and their renal manifestations, and to obtain the appropriate screening tests so that renal involvement can be identified promptly and appropriate intervention initiated without delay. When the patient does develop urinary abnormalities, decreasing renal function, or severe hypertension, the nephrologist should be involved early to assist the rheumatologist in the diagnosis and treatment of the renal disorder. Renal biopsy is a useful tool in many of these settings, but it should be understood that the information gained from it is more likely to be helpful in establishing the pathophysiological background, extent of activity, and chronicity of the renal lesion than it is to provide a specific diagnosis. The diagnosis of most of these systemic diseases is more likely to be established from the nature and pattern of extrarenal manifestations, and from serological abnormalities. Findings on renal biopsy can be helpful in choosing therapy in certain individuals, based on the confirmation of a suspected diagnosis, the activity compared with the chronicity of

Table 3 Important points to remember

1. Rheumatic disorders are frequently associated with renal disease. It is appropriate to initiate a thorough assessment of renal function when a rheumatic disease is diagnosed and periodically to reassess renal function, even when the initial nephrological examination is normal
2. The overlap of rheumatic and renal diseases underscores the advantages of close collaboration between the rheumatologist and the nephrologist in their evaluation, diagnosis, and treatment
3. Proteinuria, haematuria, acute renal failure, and hypertension; are four integral components of renal disease often associated with various rheumatic disorders
4. Proteinuria is a common manifestation of renal disease associated with rheumatic disorders. However, the quantity of proteinuria resulting from glomerular disease does not correlate with the nature or severity of the glomerular lesion. Although persistent proteinuria does not invariably progress to chronic renal failure, prolonged nephrotic-range proteinuria does often lead to progressive renal insufficiency
5. Renal vein thrombosis is not a cause of heavy proteinuria but, rather, a consequence of it
6. The evaluation of haematuria should prompt both a urological and a nephrological evaluation. Normal urinary tract imaging with intravenous pyelography or renal ultrasonography and cytoscopy essentially exclude the bladder, ureters, and collecting system as the source of bleeding, while the coexistence of haematuria and significant proteinuria offer reasonable security that the haematuria is of glomerular origin
7. Idiopathic, rapidly progressive glomerulonephritis and vasculitis-associated glomerulonephritis may share a common serological marker, the antineutrophil cytoplasmic autoantibody (ANCA)
8. New-onset hypertension in a patient who was previously normotensive or whose blood pressure has been well controlled may suggest renal involvement and may pre-date the onset of haematuria, proteinuria, or renal insufficiency. Any patient with a rheumatic disease who develops severe hypertension should be intensively investigated for the cause, and referral to a nephrologist should be considered

the lesion, the likelihood of responsiveness to therapy, and occasionally, an unexpected finding such as drug nephrotoxicity or amyloidosis.

Many deaths associated with systemic rheumatic disease are due to renal involvement. The improvement in diagnosis and treatment as well as the widespread availability of dialysis for chronic conditions have significantly reduced fatality for many of these illnesses. Nonetheless, the presence of renal involvement remains an ominous prognostic sign in many of these diseases and should be treated seriously. Relatively recent discoveries concerning the immunopathogenesis of the renal involvement in some of these illnesses are promising but also reminds much that yet remains unknown about these disorders.

References

Bajema, I.M. et al. (1999). Kidney biopsy as a predictor for renal outcome in ANCA-associated necrotizing glomerulonephritis. *Kidney International* **56**, 1751–8.

Balow, J.E. and Austin, H.A. (1988). Renal disease in systemic lupus erythematosus. *Rheumatic Disease Clinics of North America* **14**, 117–33.

Boomsma, M.M., Stegeman, C.A., Van der Leij, M.J., Vost, W., Hermans, J., Kallenberg, C.G.M., Limburg, P.C., and Cohen Tervaert, J.W. (2000). Prediction of relapses in Wegener's granulomatosis by measurement of antineutrophil cytoplasmic antibody levels: a prospective study. *Arthritis and Rheumatism* **43**, 2025–33.

Boumpas, D.T. et al. (1995). Systemic lupus erythematosus: emerging concepts Part 1: renal, neuropsychiatric, cardiovascular, pulmonary and hematologic disease. *Annals of Internal Medicine* **122**, 940–50.

ter Borg, E.J., Horst, G., Hummel, E.J., Limburg, P.C., and Kallenberg, C.G. (1990). Measurements of increases in anti-double-stranded DNA antibody levels as a predictor of disease exacerbation in systemic lupus erythematosus. A long-term, prospective study. *Arthritis and Rheumatism* **33** (5), 634–43.

Choi, H.K., Lin, S., Merkel, P.A., Colditz, G.A., and Niles, J.L. (2001). Diagnostic performance of antineutrophil cytoplasmic antibody tests for idiopathic vasculitides: metaanalysis with a focus on antimyeloperoxidase antibodies. *Journal of Rheumatology* **28**, 1584–90.

Dunn, M.J. (2000). Are COX-2 selective inhibitors nephrotoxic? *American Journal of Kidney Diseases* **35**, 976–7 (editorial).

Eras, J. and Perazella, M.A. (2001). NSAIDs and the kidney revisited: are selective cyclooxygenase-2 inhibitors safe? *American Journal of Medical Science* **321**, 181–90.

Esdaile, J.M. et al. (1989). The clinical and renal biopsy predictors of long-term outcome in lupus nephritis: a study of 87 patients and review of the literature. *Quarterly Journal of Medicine* **72**, 779–833.

Feutren, G. et al. (1992). Risk factors for cyclosporine induced nephropathy in patients with autoimmune diseases. *New England Journal of Medicine* **326**, 1654–60.

Gertz, M.A. and Kyle, R.A. (1991). Secondary systemic amyloidosis: response and survival in 64 patients. *Medicine* **70**, 246–56.

Hewins, P., Tervaert, J.W.C., Savage, C.O.S., and Kallenberg, C.G.M. (2000). Is Wegener's granulomatosis an autoimmune disease? *Current Opinion in Rheumatology* **12**, 3–10.

Hollenbeck, M., Katkahn, B., Aul, C., Leschke, M., Willers, R., and Grabensee, B. (1998). Haemolytic–uraemic syndrome and thrombotic–thrombocytopenic purpura in adults: clinical findings, and prognostic factors for death and end-stage renal disease. *Nephrology Dialysis and Transplantation* **13**, 76–81.

Jennette, J.C. and Falk, R.J. (1995). Clinical and pathological classification of ANCA-associated vasculitis: what are the controversies? *Clinical and Experimental Immunology* **101** (Suppl.), 18–22.

Jennette, J.C. et al. (1994). Nomenclature of systemic vasculitides: proposal of an international conference. *Arthritis and Rheumatism* **37**, 187–92.

Manjunath, G., Sarnak, M.J., and Levey, A.S. (2001). Prediction equation to estimate glomerular filtration rate: an update. *Current Opinions in Nephrological Hypertension* **10**, 785–92.

Moroni, G. et al. (1999). Clinical and prognostic value of serial renal biopsies in lupus nephritis. *American Journal of Kidney Diseases* **34**, 530–9.

Nowack, R., Grab, I., Flores-Suarez, L.-F., Schnüle, P., Yard, B., and van der Woude, F.J. (2001). ANCA titres, even of IgG subclasses, and soluble CD14 fail to predict relapses in patients with ANCA-associated vasculitis. *Nephrology Dialysis and Transplantation* **16**, 1631–7.

Perazella, M. and Eras, J. (2000). Are selective COX-2 inhibitors nephrotoxic? *American Journal of Kidney Diseases* **35**, 937–40.

Remuzzi, G. (1999) Nephropathic nature of proteinuria. *Current Opinion in Nephrology and Hypertension* **8** (6), 655–63.

Steen, V.D. and Medsger, T.A., Jr. (2000). Long-term outcomes of scleroderma renal crisis. *Annals of Internal Medicine* **133**, 600–3.

Talar-Williams, C. et al. (1996) Cyclophosphamide-induced cystitis and bladder cancer in patients with Wegener granulomatosis. *Annals of Internal Medicine* **124**, 477–84.

Whelton, A. (1999) Nephrotoxicity of nonsteroidal anti-inflammatory drugs: physiologic foundations and clinical implications. *The American Journal of Medicine* **106** (5b), 13s–24s.

Wiik, A. et al. (1995). The diversity of perinuclear antineutrophil cytoplasmic antibodies (pANCA) antigens. *Clinical and Experimental Immunology* **101** (Suppl.), 15–17.

Wiik, A. (2001). Laboratory diagnostics in vasculitis patients. *Israel Medical Association Journal* **3**, 275–7.

Yi, E.S. and Colby, T.V. (2001). Wegener's granulomatosis. *Seminars in Diagnostic Pathology* **18**, 34–46.

Yocum, D.E. et al. (1988). Cyclosporin A in severe, treated-refractory rheumatoid arthritis. *Annals of Internal Medicine* **109**, 863–9.

1.3.14 Psychiatric issues in rheumatology

Simon M. Helfgott and Malcolm P. Rogers

Introduction

The practice of rheumatology is not unlike the practice of psychiatry. Relationships with patients tend to be long term, most of the diseases are chronic and unpredictable in course, and the treatments available seldom cure but often are effective in increasing function and controlling the underlying disease. Function is an important focus of both specialties. The two disciplines have avoided a high-technology, disease-orientated approach in favour of a more comprehensive view of the patient's illness, open to relevant psychological and social data. Interestingly, a study by the Rand Corporation on the effects of six chronic disorders, including major depression and rheumatoid arthritis, showed that both had a similarly adverse affect on quality of life (Stewart et al. 1989). The number of days of missed work and time spent in bed at home were roughly equivalent for both disorders.

Stress and psychoneuroimmunology

While most of this chapter will concentrate on the recognition and treatment of the psychiatric complaints and disorders that occur frequently among patients with rheumatic disease, it is worthwhile first briefly discussing the topic of psychoneuroimmunology. There is an extensive literature on the possible effects of psychological stress and other emotional states on the onset and the course of rheumatic disease, particularly rheumatoid arthritis and systemic lupus erythematosus (Rimon 1989). For years, experienced clinicians and patients frequently connected flare-ups of disease with stressful life events. It is fair to say that the issue is not fully settled from a scientific point of view, despite many years of effort. The principal difficulty has been the practical necessity of relying on retrospective analyses. Some of the more imaginative approaches have included studies of identical twins discordant for rheumatoid arthritis, and attempted quantitation of the amount of life stress during the 6 months immediately before a flare-up of disease. They have have provided some suggestive evidence for a link between stress and illness but there have been negative results as well. These questions helped to stimulate what has now become the new and evolving field of psychoneuroimmunology (Kiecolt-Glaser and Glaser 1989). George Solomon was one of the first to ask whether psychological stress might influence rheumatoid arthritis by its effect on the immune system (Solomon 1969). Using an animal model of inflammatory arthritis he demonstrated that stress could indeed alter parts of the immune response. Subsequent studies with the model of arthritis induced by type II collagen in rodents have shown that various kinds of psychological stress have important but often conflicting effects on inflammation in joints, apparently without directly affecting antibody or cellular immune responses (Rogers et al. 1980).

Psychoneuroimmunology has also explored the effects of bereavement, depression, and relaxation on immunity in a variety of clinical states (Ader 1991). In simple terms, experimental and naturally occurring stress has been associated with altered measures of both cellular and humoral immunity. However, there is no clear demonstration as yet that these altered measures are biologically significant in the sense that they cause or adversely affect human disease. Certain forms of psychological intervention in cancer, for example, have been shown positively to affect the incidence of illness and death. Whether the psychological mechanism responsible for this clinical benefit acts through an immunological pathway remains unanswered.

Psychiatric manifestations of rheumatic diseases

The psychiatric manifestations of rheumatic diseases fall into three basic categories: (i) organic diseases caused by central nervous involvement of the underlying condition (primary disorders); (ii) psychiatric disturbances that are psychological 'reactions' to the impairments of rheumatic disease (secondary disorders); (iii) drug-induced psychiatric disorders (tertiary disorders). Each group is outlined in Tables 1 and 2. The difficult task for the rheumatologist or psychiatrist is to define which of the three groups best describes the underlying cause of the psychiatric impairment or whether there is an independent, primary psychiatric disorder. This chapter will attempt to outline an approach to the evaluation of psychiatric illness in the patient with rheumatic disease.

Rheumatic disease with primary psychiatric involvement (Table 1)

Organic mental syndromes occur frequently in this category. They include dementia, delirium, cognitive impairment, and sometimes more subtle changes of personality and affect. A disturbance of orientation, memory, language, or attention (and obviously specific motor and sensory symptoms) all strongly suggest organic disease of the central nervous system, and therefore help to identify primary psychiatric involvement.

Table 1 Rheumatic diseases with (a) primary and (b) secondary psychiatric involvement

	Psychiatric manifestations
(a) Rheumatic diseases with primary psychiatric involvement	
Systemic lupus erythematosus	Affective disorders Psychosis Organic mental disorder
Primary Sjögren's syndrome	Affective disorders Paranoid ideation Personality changes
Rheumatoid arthritis	Organic mental disorder (rare)
Giant cell arteritis/polymyalgia rheumatica	Organic mental disorder Depression
Granulomatous angiitis of the central nervous system	Organic mental disorder
Systemic necrotizing vasculitis—polyarteritis nodosa/Wegener's granulomatosis	Organic mental disorder Seizures
Cogan's syndrome	Seizures
Whipple's disease	Organic mental disorder Hypersomnia
Behçet's syndrome	Organic mental disorder Seizures
Sarcoidosis	Organic mental disorder Psychosis Affective disorder, hypersomnolence Confusion
Lyme disease	Organic mental disorder Cognitive impairment Sleep disturbance
Amyloidosis	Organic mental disorder
(b) Rheumatic diseases with secondary psychiatric involvement	
Rheumatoid arthritis	Mood disturbance (from endogenous depression to grief)
Juvenile idiopathic arthritis	
Spondyloarthropathies	
Osteoarthritis	
Polymyalgia rheumatica	
Systemic sclerosis	
Systemic lupus erythematosus	
Primary Sjögren's syndrome	
Myositis	

Systemic lupus erythematosus (SLE)

Systemic lupus can have major effects on the central nervous system, producing a variety of neuropsychiatric symptoms (see Chapter 6.6.1) *(editor's note: consensus is that Osler was not describing SLE)*. Daly (1942) was the first to emphasize the varied psychiatric presentations seen with systemic lupus, reporting 'toxic delirium' with confusion and disorientation as well as psychoses with paranoid features. Other psychiatric features include affective disorders, dementia, phobias, and autistic behaviour (Adelman et al. 1986). The true incidence of psychiatric symptoms is difficult to ascertain; most large series report an incidence of 15–20 per cent (Hay et al. 1992).

Clinical features

The psychiatric manifestations can sometimes pre-date the other clinical manifestations of systemic lupus. Most patients show some 'organic' symptoms suggestive of an organic mental disorder. However, a schizophrenic-like picture with hallucinations and paranoia and a grossly clear sensorium is sometimes found. Autistic behaviour has been seen, but infrequently. About half of the psychiatric episodes in the Johns Hopkins' study were accompanied by neurological signs or symptoms, with seizures being significantly associated (Feinglass et al. 1976). One-third of patients had no neurological features at any point in the course of the disease.

A 10-year prospective study of patients with neuropsychiatric lupus erythematosis noted three broad forms of presentation (West et al. 1995).

(i) A diffuse presentation characterized by an organic brain syndrome, depression, psychosis, generalized seizures, or coma.

(ii) Focal presentation with stroke, focal seizures, chorea, transverse myelitis, or migraine headaches.

(iii) Complex presentation usually manifested as an organic brain syndrome or other psychiatric disorder with stroke, seizure, or transverse myelitis.

Using standardized neuropsychological tests, a number of investigators noted significantly more cognitive impairment in patients with systemic lupus than in those with rheumatoid arthritis and in controls (e.g. Denburg et al. 1993). Neuropsychological testing has the advantage of being more directly relevant to the functional and behavioural capacity of the patient. Easily administered tests include the Bender Gestalt (with immediate and delayed recall), trail making, verbal fluency, and the Wechsler Adult Intelligence Scale—Revised. The American College of Rheumatology (ACR) Ad Hoc Committee on neuropsychiatric lupus nomenclature has recommended a short battery of tests, which takes approximately 1 h to complete. (It is available on the ACR World Wide Web site at http://www.rheumatology.org/ar/ar.html.)

Psychiatric assessment

Psychiatric assessment consists of a careful history, including the history of pre-existing psychiatric disorders or substance abuse. It is very useful to ascertain the patient's usual baseline of psychological functioning, including educational background, coping mechanisms, and view of their current illness. Particular investigation should focus on possible somatoform symptoms, such as conversion reactions, hypochondriasis, and frequent procedures or surgical interventions without evidence for organic disease. In addition, mental status should be carefully examined, with particular attention to orientation, memory (both remote and short-term), attention, language, reasoning, and visuospatial disturbance. Tests should include memory for remote events, such as names of political figures and the detail of historical events, as well as for repetition and retention of new information, such as four random words. Attention can be tested by having the patient repeat digits backward and forward, by naming the days of the week in reverse, or by subtracting serial 3s or 7s. Brief tests of naming objects in the room, reading, repeating a phrase, and writing a sentence should be given. Having the person copy a simple geometric figure or drawing a clock and putting in the time are effective screening techniques for visuospatial deficits. The best way to elicit symptoms of psychosis is to inquire about any unusual occurrences, unusual perceptions, the hearing or seeing of things that seem strange or unreal, or of possible fears that others are trying to hurt them.

Patients who show clear difficulties with such 'bedside' screening tests are most probably experiencing some organic brain disturbance. Others who do well on such tests yet still report prominent subjective difficulties may be suffering from more subtle organic disturbances. Both should have more detailed neuropsychological tests from experienced neuropsychologists.

The psychiatric disturbances may be due to failure of other organs. For example, uraemic encephalopathy may ensue, and renal failure or vasculitis with secondary severe hypertension can also result in hypertensive encephalopathy with the development of headaches, disorientation, coma, and seizures. Occult central nervous infections, especially in the immunocompromised patient, can lead to an organic mental syndrome. As mentioned later, high doses of corticosteroids, the mainstay of therapy for systemic lupus, can directly cause psychiatric disturbances.

Establishing the diagnosis of neuropsychiatric systemic lupus erythematosus

This remains a difficult task, even for the most astute clinician. The diagnosis should be considered in a young woman presenting with psychotic features, even if no other clinical or laboratory features of systemic lupus are present, as these psychiatric signs and symptoms may well be the initial presentation. In a study of 296 patients admitted to an acute psychiatric ward in Nottingham, United Kingdom, approximately 1 per cent of the patients met criteria for the diagnosis of systemic lupus (Hopkinson and Powell 1990). There is no consensus on the association between systemic and psychiatric lupus; most series have failed to document any relation between the two.

A number of immunological tests have been proposed as useful in the evaluation of neuropsychiatric systemic lupus. In a series of 70 female patients (Hanly et al. 1993), antineuronal antibodies were detected in 34 per cent, lymphocytotoxic antibodies in 47 per cent, anti-P antibodies in 17 per cent, and anticardiolipin antibodies in 24 per cent. However, there was no significant difference in the prevalence of any of these antibodies in patients with and without cognitive impairment. On the other hand, work by Denburg et al. (1994) has suggested a relation between specific cognitive deficits, namely visuospatial dysfunction, and the presence of lymphocytotoxic antibodies.

A Japanese study (Isshi and Hirohata 1998) comparing SLE patients with psychosis, non-psychotic central nervous system (CNS) lupus, and non-CNS SLE found that serum levels of antibody to ribosomal P protein (anti-P) were significantly elevated in patients with lupus psychosis compared with those with non-CNS SLE or those with non-psychotic CNS lupus. Cerebrospinal fluid (CSF) levels of anti-neuromal antibodies (anti-N) were significantly elevated in patients with lupus psychosis compared to the other groups. CSF antibodies to ribosomal P protein were not detected in most patients. These authors suggest that anti-P in the systemic circulation and anti-N in the CSF compartment might be important in the pathogenesis of CNS lupus.

Neuropsychiatric lupus may be seen in the context of antiphospholipid (aPL) antibodies, and/or in the presence of the antiphospholipid syndrome (APS). The syndrome includes many clinical manifestations of SLE and others that are more characteristic of APS such as pregnancy loss, vascular thrombosis, and livedo reticularis (see Chapter 6.6.4). A multicenter study of SLE patients identified APS as an independent predictor of CNS involvement (Karassa et al. 2000). A low serum C_4 complement level was another independent risk factor, whereas arthralgias, arthritis and a discoid rash were independent protective factors. Nearly 30 per cent of patients developed psychiatric features, primarily acute confusional states and psychosis.

Concentrations of interferon-α were increased in the cerebrospinal fluid in five of six patients with lupus psychosis (Shiozawa et al. 1992); these decreased when the psychosis subsided and they did not rise following seizures alone. These limited findings suggest that interferon-α, possibly synthesized in the brain, may play some part in the pathogenesis of psychosis in systemic lupus.

One study measured a variety of cytokines, prostaglandins, and autoantibodies in the CSF of patients with systemic lupus and infection (Tsai et al. 1994). The results suggested that high levels of interleukin (IL-6) and prostaglandin E_2 in the CSF favoured a diagnosis of infection of the CNS while modestly elevated IL-6, high IgG, and autoantibodies against calf thymus antigens in the CSF suggested a diagnosis of neuropsychiatric systemic lupus.

The autopsy findings in lupus of the CNS have recently been reviewed. Ellison et al. (1993) described small-vessel hyalinization and thickening, with fragments of platelet membrane found in the wails of small cortical and meningeal vessels. Concurrent thrombus formation, possibly related to antiphospholipid antibody formation, may facilitate the incorporation of platelet fragments into small-vessel walls, with resultant thickening and irregularity of the vessels. In another series of seven patients with confirmed neuropsychiatric systemic lupus (Hanly et al. 1992), four were found at autopsy to have multifocal cerebral cortical microinfarcts associated with microvascular injury. These studies suggest a vascular basis for neuropsychiatric systemic lupus in many, but not all patients.

Electroencephalography

The electroencephalogram may help to confirm the presence of an abnormal seizure focus that manifests as episodic changes in behaviour and mentation (e.g. temporal lobe epilepsy). It may help to distinguish delirium from a primary mental disorder with cognitive dysfunction such as acute mania. Clinically, delirium is characterized by diminished attention and sometimes diminished level of consciousness, associated with disorientation, agitation, reversal of the sleep–wakefulness cycle, perceptual distortions and misinterpretations, and impairment of short-term memory. Most patients with delirium have diffuse slowing of the background electroencephalogram, unlike in most primary mental disorders. Ritchlin et al. (1992) found that using neurometric quantitative electroencephalography as an indicator of cerebral dysfunction in patients with systemic lupus produced a diagnostic sensitivity of 87 per cent and specificity of 75 per cent.

Brain imaging

Advances in technology have resulted in four imaging techniques that may be helpful in evaluating neuropsychiatric systemic lupus; these four are outlined next.

Computed tomography (CT)

This technique initially described the presence of steroid-induced cortical atrophy and calcification of the paraventricular areas seen in systemic lupus. For the most part, CT has been supplanted by MRI. However, CT scans continue to serve an important diagnostic role in identifying emergent haemorrhage or cerebral infarction. They are also considerably less expensive than magnetic resonance imaging (MRI).

Magnetic resonance imaging

MRI is far more sensitive than CT for detecting disease of the CNS, and can demonstrate the reversal of some of the brain lesions in lupus. Three different patterns of disease can be demonstrated by MRI: cerebral infarction, multiple small areas of increased signal intensity secondary to microinfarctions, and focal areas of increased intensity in the cerebral grey matter (Bell et al. 1991).

A recent study (Baum et al. 1993) highlights the possibilities and difficulties in interpreting the MRI in neuropsychiatric systemic lupus. Twenty-one consecutive outpatients with systemic lupus were studied: 12 had focal lesions, primarily in the frontal lobes. Patients with focal neurological signs were more likely to have lesions on MRI. Ten patients had paraventricular hyperintensities, a finding noted in several other series as well. Yet, seven patients with abnormal MRI had no neuropsychiatric symptoms, and eleven had neuropsychiatric symptoms and signs that did not correlate with MRI findings.

To summarize, MRI may fail to detect abnormalities in diffuse, nonfocal, or mild lupus of the CNS. It is sensitive to focal lesions that are large enough to produce clear-cut localizing signs on neurological or cognitive examination.

Single photon-emission CT (SPECT)

SPECT appears to have limited value in the evaluation of neuropsychiatric systemic lupus. Rogers et al. (1992) noted abnormal findings in eight of 18 patients with subtle cognitive and affective changes, including a diffuse bilateral temporal–parietal pattern previously noted only in Alzheimer's disease. Another study (Rubbert et al. 1993) found normal SPECT scans in 90 per cent of those with overt neurological signs. SPECT may have a useful role in patients with diffuse symptoms, such as cognitive dysfunction and psychosis, in which MRI may be insensitive.

Positron-emission tomography (PET)

PET assesses cerebral blood flow and glucose metabolism. Carbotte et al. (1992) described an intensive longitudinal study of three women with neuropsychiatric systemic lupus. Fluorodeoxyglucose uptake indicated abnormalities in all three that had not been identified on plain CT, yet corresponded well with localizable cognitive deficits. Changes in each patient's cognitive profile on reassessment paralleled changes on PET. The high cost and limited availability of the necessary equipment has precluded more widespread use of PET.

Magnetization transfer imaging (MTI) is an MRI technique that is more sensitive to structural brain damage than conventional MRI and it permits easy quantification of such damage (Van Buchem et al. 1997). A study of SLE patients with and without neuropsychiatric disease revealed that volumetric MTI analysis can detect cerebral changes in the active phase of neuropsychiatric SLE (Bosma et al. 2000). These values differed from those obtained in patients in the chronic phase of disease, possibly reflecting the presence (or absence) of inflammation. The abnormalities in the brain parenchyma in patients with chronic neuropsychiatric SLE produced MTI valves that were similar to those observed in patients with inactive multiple sclerosis.

Treatment of the psychiatric symptoms

The usual treatments, ranging from antidepressants to antipsychotic medications and psychotherapy, have an important role. However, one must treat the underlying biological cause, the systemic lupus, as well. If the patient develops a frank psychosis on corticosteroids, the first task would be to define the aetiology of the change in mental status; is this drug-induced or a manifestation of the lupus or, less commonly, due to an occult infection of the central nervous system in an immunocompromised host? Generally, doses of prednisone in the range of 1–1.5 mg/kg per day have been given orally or systemically with variable results. Although steroid-induced psychosis can occur, the neuropsychiatric manifestations in patients taking corticosteroids are much more likely to be due to the disease than to the drug.

Patients who fail to respond to corticosteroids have been treated with cyclophosphamide: one study from the National Institutes of Health suggests the use of monthly pulse administrations of 0.75–1.0 g/m^2 of cyclophosphamide (Boumpas et al. 1991). The sample in most of these studies of treatment is too small for any meaningful extrapolation. In a retrospective study of 31 patients (Neuwelt et al. 1995) with severe neuropsychiatric systemic lupus refractory to corticosteroids and other oral immunosuppressive agents, intravenous cyclophosphamide was associated with substantial improvement in 18 patients, and stabilization of the condition in nine others. Patients with an organic brain syndrome or a large number of neuropsychiatric manifestations had a poorer outcome. The treatment of anticardiolipin-related thrombotic events remains controversial; recent studies suggest that warfarin appears to be superior to low dose aspirin in the management of this condition (see Chapter 6.6.4).

Sjögren's syndrome

One study found a high incidence of psychopathology in a group of patients with primary Sjögren's syndrome, in particular, high levels of hostility and paranoid ideation (Angelopoulos et al. 1988). Other studies have identified an increased incidence of affective disorders, cognitive impairment (in attention and concentration), and a correlation between neurological and psychiatric symptoms suggestive of an organic mental disorder. An increased incidence of neuropsychiatric symptoms may also accompany secondary Sjögren's syndrome.

Rheumatoid arthritis

The only primary neuropsychiatric syndrome in rheumatoid arthritis, described in two cases, is an organic mental disorder caused by rheumatoid nodules in the choroid plexus. Rarely, rheumatoid cranial vasculitis also appears as an organic mental disorder.

The vasculitides

The vasculitides associated with neuropsychiatric factors are listed in Table 1. Granulomatous angiitis of the CNS is a rare condition that presents with non-specific signs and symptoms including acute or subacute onset of confusion, headache, personality change, paresis, cranial neuropathy, or loss of consciousness. An elevated erythrocyte sedimentation rate may be the only abnormal laboratory finding. Cerebral angiography may reveal changes including vascular beading or aneurysms, but a definite diagnosis can only be made by brain or leptomeningeal biopsy. Pathological changes include an inflammatory process involving small arteries, with intimal proliferation, fibrosis, and multinucleated giant cells (Sigal 1987). A few cases have followed herpes zoster ophthalmicus.

Systemic vasculitides such as polyarteritis nodosa or Wegener's granulomatosis can involve the CNS. Psychiatric disturbances are rarely seen without neurological signs or symptoms. Depression and changes in mental status are not uncommon presentations for giant-cell arteritis. Helpful clinical clues for establishing this diagnosis include the presence of jaw claudication, new onset of headaches, visual changes, and proximal myalgias. An elevated erythrocyte sedimentation rate is generally found. Biopsy of the temporal artery is recommended for the patient with a new onset of depression and any of the aforementioned features. Improvement is noted after treatment with corticosteroids.

Behçet's syndrome

The central nervous manifestations of Behçet's syndrome consist of subacute, haemorrhagic, and necrotizing meningoencephalitis, most typically affecting the brainstem and hypothalamus. In addition to the focal neurological symptoms associated with these lesions, organic mental disorders, disorders of consciousness, and seizures have all been described (Bousser et al. 1988).

Whipple's disease

Behavioural changes, hypersomnia, memory disturbance, and dementia, which may antedate its usual gastrointestinal or joint manifestations, characterize some of the central nervous manifestations of Whipple's disease. There is one report of dementia partially reversed by antibiotic therapy.

Sarcoidosis

Involvement of the CNS occurs in 5 per cent of patients with sarcoidosis. Delirium, dementia, personality change, hypersomnolence, depression, and psychosis have all been described. Steroids have reversed at least some of these neuropsychiatric manifestations.

Lyme disease

The neuropsychiatric sequelae of untreated Lyme disease include a wide variety of symptoms, ranging from depression, mania, panic, dementia, anorexia nervosa, and obsessive-compulsive disorder to an acute schizophrenia-like psychosis that, if treated early enough, can be reversible (Fallon et al. 1994). Disseminated Lyme disease has been associated with long-term musculoskeletal, neurological, or cognitive impairment, especially memory, in a substantial percentage of individuals, particularly those who received delayed treatment (see Chapter 6.2.4).

Lyme disease has been associated with retrieval deficits and with impaired verbal memory, mental flexibility, verbal associative functions, and articulation (Benke et al. 1995). The degree of memory impairment does not appear to correlate with the level of anti-*B. burgdorferi* antibody titres in either serum or CSF; nor does it correlate with the MRI findings or the magnitude of mood disturbance.

Logigian et al. (1990) studied 27 patients with signs of earlier Lyme disease, current evidence of immunity to *B. burgdorferi*, and chronic neurological symptoms with no other identifiable cause. Twenty-four of them had a mild encephalopathy, which had begun 1 month to 14 years after the onset of the disease and was characterized by memory loss, mood changes, or sleep disturbance. Fourteen had memory impairment on neuropsychological testing and 18 had increased protein in cerebrospinal fluid, evidence of intrathecal production of antibody to *B. burgdorferi*, or both. Associated symptoms included fatigue, headaches, arthritis, and hearing loss. After a 2-week course of intravenous ceftriaxone, two-thirds of the patients had improved, one other had improved and then relapsed, and the remainder had no change in their condition.

A long-term follow-up (mean of 6 years) of a cohort of patients revealed significantly more verbal memory deficits in patients with higher IgG Lyme antibody titres who received treatment later (mean of 3 years) (Shadick et al. 1994). Similarly, Krupp et al. (1991) noted more memory impairment on formal testing of Lyme patients than healthy controls.

Untreated neuroborreliosis appears to have a course similar to that of neurosyphilis, leading to permanent and irreversible neurological disability. The differential diagnosis of new-onset psychosis may, therefore, need to include Lyme disease with the same emphasis as is given to syphilis, particularly in regions of the country where it is endemic.

There are medical challenges associated with 'pseudo-Lyme' disease. Subjective complaints such as chronic fatigue, headaches, or memory deficits may be incorrectly attributed to Lyme disease. It is of utmost importance that the diagnosis of Lyme disease be made using accepted serological techniques. The entity of 'seronegative' neuropsychiatric Lyme disease is probably quite rare.

A recent review of experience with Lyme disease in children (Adams et al. 1994) found no differences between disease and control groups for a number of neuropsychological measures. These data contrast with a number of case reports in the literature suggesting the existence of Lyme-related psychiatric disease, including paranoia, dementia, schizophrenia, bipolar disorder, panic attacks, major depression, anorexia nervosa, and obsessive–compulsive disorder (Fallon and Nields 1994).

Amyloidosis

Some of the types of primary amyloidosis may involve the blood vessels of the central nervous system. Cerebral amyloid angiopathy can produce a variety of organic mental disorders including dementia, a fact of increasing interest because of the isolation of B-amyloid protein in both plaques and skin in patients with Alzheimer's disease. It is unclear whether secondary amyloidosis may also be associated with brain pathology.

Rheumatological disease with secondary psychiatric involvement (Table 1)

Depression in rheumatoid arthritis

Estimates of the incidence of depression in rheumatoid arthritis have varied widely, from 30 per cent (more typically) to as high as 70 per cent. The variability has resulted from differences in the definition of depression as well as differences among the populations studied. Some studies have found that the prevalence of depression is no higher in rheumatoid arthritis than in other chronically ill medical patients (Walker et al. 1997).

Frank et al. (1988a) made one of the few studies using current operational criteria for depression in the context of rheumatoid arthritis. By using a structured diagnostic interview of predominantly male patients, they found a prevalence of major depressive disorder of 17 per cent. A much larger number, 41 per cent, met the criteria for dysthymic disorder, a less severe but more chronic form of depression in which symptoms must be present for at least 2 years and for more than half of the time. These diagnostic categories are not mutually exclusive: almost all of the patients with major depressive disorder met criteria for dysthymic disorder, so-called double depression. Overall, 41 per cent of this sample of 137 outpatients with rheumatoid arthritis were found to be depressed, with either of the two major depressive disorders or both. No correlation was found between the presence of a history of depression and higher levels of reported pain, as has been found in other studies.

Contrary to intuition, most studies have not found a significant correlation between depression and measures of disease activity, but rather with socio-economic factors, such as decreased social support and economic deprivation. One of the most comprehensive investigations of the origins of depression in rheumatoid arthritis found that a wide range of factors, including disability measures, duration of disease, social isolation, and economic deprivation, all made significant contributions to the explanation of depressed mood, together accounting for 44 per cent of the variation in depressed mood. Others have confirmed the complexity of determinants for depression in rheumatoid arthritis (Blalock and DeVellis 1992), indicating that loss of valued activities (Katz and Velin 1995) and social relationships (Crotty et al. 1994) may be as important as disease activity or functional status.

While most studies have found an increased incidence of depression in patients with rheumatoid arthritis, a few reports have not borne this out (Cassileth et al. 1984). Cassileth measured, on psychological rating scales, the psychological health of patients with a variety of chronic medical disease including rheumatoid arthritis. They showed that these persons were overall indistinguishable from the general population and significantly healthier mentally than a population of psychiatric outpatients (Cassileth et al. 1984). However, they did not use the standard, operationalized definitions of clinical depression.

Table 2 Drug-induced psychiatric manifestations

Medication	Psychiatric manifestations
Corticosteroids	Mania, depression, organic mental disorders, insomnia
Hydroxychloroquine	Psychosis, organic mental disorders, personality change, insomnia
Cyclosporin	Mania, depression, lethargy, organic mental disorders
Non-steroidal anti-inflammatory drugs	Depression, organic mental disorders
Methotrexate Azathioprine Gold salts D-Penicillamine	Mood changes, headaches
Monoclonal antibodies (e.g. anti-TNF, anti-IL-2)	Fatigue, headaches

Note: IL, interleukin; TNF, tumour necrosis factor.

Systemic lupus erythematosus

Because of the potential life-threatening nature of systemic lupus and the alteration in appearance, both from the underlying disease and from use of corticosteroids, the psychological toll can be enormous (Omdal et al. 1995). Given the younger age of onset and the female predominance, issues related to family planning and pregnancy are of foremost concern to both patient and physician. Most observers have found an increase in clinical depression and anxiety. Providing patients with information relating to their disease and its management may increase their knowledge base but does not affect their psychological response. Peer support groups for systemic lupus may have a beneficial role to play.

Juvenile idiopathic arthritis

Measurement of pain behaviours may be especially useful in studies of treatment outcome because these behaviours are relatively independent of depression (Jaworski et al. 1995). One recent survey found no correlation between scores on psychological testing and measures of functional status (Baildam et al. 1995), whereas another found that the proportion of patients demonstrating an anxious preoccupation with their disease increased with the degree of disability (David et al. 1994).

Miscellaneous disorders including systemic sclerosis, inflammatory myositis, spondylitis, severe osteoarthritis

The main connecting link in these conditions is the impairment in function due to joint and muscle problems and changes in appearance. These changes produce sadness, grief reactions, social isolation, and economic hardships. Some patients emphasize the positive, character-building aspects of these diseases and their potential for strengthening marital and family relationships.

Drug-induced psychiatric manifestations (Table 2)

Corticosteroids

Major psychiatric side-effects have been well described, occurring in approximately 6 per cent of all patients on steroids. These include: depression (40 per cent), mania (27 per cent), psychosis (14 per cent), delirium (10 per cent), and mixed depression and mania (8 per cent).

Female sex appears to be an important risk factor. Starting treatment with corticosteroids often results in euphoria. This may be due to a direct central nervous effect of the drug, or may relate to the psychological sense of well being from the beneficial effects of treatment on the disease process. Occasionally, steroids can induce a depressive state, especially with doses exceeding 0.5 mg/day or when rapidly tapered off after prolonged use. Wolkowitz et al. (1990) found that healthy volunteers given either a single, 1-mg dose of dexamethasone or 80 mg/day of prednisone for 5 days made significantly more errors of commission in verbal memory tasks, suggesting the possibility of specific, corticosteroid-related, cognitive impairments. Psychiatric symptoms are generally reversible when the drug is reduced or stopped. One prospective study found a good response to prophylactic treatment with lithium carbonate (Falk et al. 1979).

Cyclosporin

Cyclosporin produces its anti-inflammatory activity by binding to the interleukin-2 receptor on T cells. The observed psychiatric side-effects have included mania, depression, and lethargy. With the higher doses (5–15 mg/day) given after organ transplantation, irreversible dementia, encephalopathy, and fatal progressive neurological deterioration have been seen (Bertoli et al. 1988). Cyclosporin can attenuate the opiate withdrawal syndrome precipitated by naloxone in morphine-dependent animals and this effect can be adoptively transferred by splenic mononuclear cells (Dougherty and Dafny 1987). The drug can also alter the electrophysiological properties of discrete brain nuclei (Dougherty et al. 1987).

Antimalarials

Chloroquine and to a lesser extent hydroxychloroquine have associated toxic psychiatric reactions including personality change, depression, depersonalization, neurotic symptoms, confusional states, psychosis, and suicide (Good and Shader 1982). Chloroquine is concentrated in brain and spinal cord. The psychiatric effects may be related to acetylcholinesterase inhibitory activity.

Others

Gold salts, D-penicillamine, and azathioprine are not associated with any psychiatric findings (Rogers 1985). Methotrexate, given orally or parenterally in low weekly doses (i.e. 20 mg or less) for rheumatic diseases can be associated with headache, light-headedness, and mood swings.

Non-steroidal anti-inflammatory drugs

These are a class of agents distinguished by their ability to inhibit cyclooxygenase and thereby impair prostaglandin biosynthesis. Prostaglandins are synthesized in the brain and can modulate the effect of various neurotransmitters. In addition, these non-steroidal agents can cross the blood–brain barrier, which may explain their analgesic and antipyretic effects. These might be mediated by a direct effect on hypothalamic structures.

Indomethacin is the most potent inhibitor of cyclooxygenase among the non-steroidal anti-inflammatory drugs: it caused central nervous disturbances, including headache, light-headedness, dizziness, and vertigo, in almost one-half of the patients studied. These manifestations of toxicity can also occur, to a lesser extent, with virtually any of these drugs. More profound changes, including depression, confusional states, visual hallucinations, and suicides are reported with indomethacin. Interestingly, indomethacin contains an indole moiety similar to that in serotonin, which may explain its frequent psychiatric manifestations. Sulindac, structurally related to indomethacin, has been linked, in case reports, to delirium and paranoid psychosis. Tolmetin reportedly induced mania in a patient with a prior history of psychiatric disturbances. We speculate that its pyrrole moiety, also found in porphobilinogen, which is excreted in acute porphyria, a condition associated with intermittent psychosis, may be responsible.

Propionic acids such as ibuprofen, naproxen, and fenoprofen have been associated with depression and cognitive dysfunction, especially in elderly people (Goodwin and Regan 1982). Insomnia and nightmares have been described with several of the non-steroidal anti-inflammatory drugs.

Salicylates and salsalate in the therapeutic range have been associated with visual hallucinations, and confusion, especially in elderly individuals, in whom these can be misinterpreted as signs of Alzheimer's disease (Vivian and Goldberg 1982). Tinnitus and impaired hearing have also been encountered, even with subtherapeutic blood concentrations of salicylates.

Treatment

When should a patient with rheumatological disease be referred to a psychiatrist or other mental health professional? When functional impairment seems out of proportion to the underlying medical disorders, when there are cognitive changes, hallucinations, delusions, bizarre behaviour, confusional states, or when there are questions about the use of psychotropic medications as in patients with depression or significant anxiety states, referral to a psychiatrist should be considered. It becomes more urgent when the possibility of suicide or psychosis arises.

Support groups should be considered for patients who are more isolated as a result of their disorders and seeking more information than can reasonably be provided by the rheumatologist, or more social support than that currently available.

Managing depression

The word depression, to the confusion of some, has been used to describe conditions ranging from grief and adjustment reactions to the more serious and potentially life-threatening major depressive disorder (unipolar depression). In general, antidepressants are indicated for treatment of the more severe depressions.

By current consensus as defined in the *Diagnostic and Statistical Manual of Mental Disorders IV* (American Psychiatric Association 1995), a major depressive syndrome consists of at least a 2-week period during which at least five of the following nine symptoms will have consistently occurred, representing a change from a previous level of functioning:

(i) depressed mood;

(ii) markedly diminished interest or pleasure;

(iii) significant weight loss or gain;

(iv) insomnia or hypersomnia;

(v) agitation or psychomotor retardation;

(vi) fatigue;

(vii) feelings of worthlessness or excessive guilt;

(viii) diminished ability to think or concentrate; and

(ix) suicidal ideation.

A further stipulation is that one of the five symptoms is either (i) depressed mood or (ii) loss of interest or pleasure.

A contemporary epidemiological study has found that the lifetime prevalence of major depressive disorder in the normal population is 4.4 per cent. If treated with antidepressant medications, approximately 60–70 per cent of patients will respond with resolution of the episodes within a few weeks. If untreated, it is estimated that a typical episode of major depression will last from 6 to 12 months and then usually resolve spontaneously. However, depression may persist and present as a chronic depressive disorder in 20 per cent of individuals.

Accurate diagnosis of depression in medically ill patients is confounded by the overlap between symptoms of the medical disorder and symptoms of depression, particularly the neurovegetative symptoms. For example, fatigue, insomnia, and anorexia may all be directly related to medical conditions such as rheumatoid arthritis. For this reason, some investigators have suggested substituting the more cognitive/affective symptoms, such as guilt and low self-esteem, for the neurovegetative ones when diagnosing depression in patients with medical illness.

Psychological interventions and the course of rheumatic diseases

The belief that one can manage and control a specific stressful situation (so-called self-efficacy) is probably an effective antidote to the helplessness so often found at the core of depression in chronically ill patients. In a longitudinal study, Parker et al. (1988) demonstrated that increases in self-efficacy could be taught to patients with rheumatoid arthritis, in turn leading to improvements in pain, and in psychological and health status. Using a self-management course for patients with arthritis that emphasizes cognitive, behavioural, and stress management skills, together with mutual support groups, Strauss et al. (1986) demonstrated improvements in health status and specifically in measures of arthritis activity.

Muller et al. (1987) made a meta-analysis of 15 studies on the effects of psychoeducational interventions on disability, pain, and depression in individuals with rheumatoid arthritis or osteoarthritis. The results indicate that patient education and group psychotherapeutic support can improve the health status of patients with chronic arthritis.

The participation of patients with lupus in a specifically designed self-help course correlated with subsequent lower levels of depression, and greater enabling skills and use of relaxation and exercise (Braden et al. 1993).

Psychotropic medications

Mood stabilizers

Lithium is the mainstay of treatment for manic depressive or bipolar affective disorder. It is helpful as an adjunct in treatment-resistant depression and as a prophylaxis against corticosteroid-induced mania. Alternative drugs recently introduced for treatment of acute mania, such as carbamazepine and valproic acid, may also prove useful in this disorder.

Electroconvulsant therapy

This remains an effective treatment for major depression but is indicated only if the antidepressants are unsuccessful or not tolerated, or if there is an acute risk of suicide that necessitates immediate treatment.

Antidepressants

The four major categories of antidepressants include the serotonin-specific reuptake inhibitors (SSRIs), tricyclics, monamine oxidase inhibitors, and others. In general, the therapeutic response rate for all of the antidepressants is similar—approximately 70 per cent in major depression.

SSRIs

Over the past decade or so a number of new antidepressant agents have been introduced. The most important and widely used of these groups are the SSRIs. They are generally now the first-line agents used in the treatment of depression, primarily because they are better tolerated. Fluoxetine (Prozac) was introduced first, in 1987. It has received the most attention and controversy. Others in the same class, sertraline (Zoloft) and paroxetine (Paxil), fluvoxamine (Luvox) and, more recently, citalopram (Celexa) have been added to the list. The SSRIs have been so widely used and accepted because of their relatively limited side-effects. They have a highly specific action on serotonin reuptake and, as such, lack the anticholinergic side-effects, sedation, orthostatic hypotension, and cardiotoxicity that can be problematical with other antidepressants. Because of their potentially stimulating properties, they are the only antidepressants given in a single dose in the morning (Table 3). Fluvoxamine is almost always more sedating and therefore typically taken at bedtime. Nausea, jitteriness, insomnia, and headache are among the more common side-effects. Approximately 30 per cent of men will experience sexual dysfunction in the form of delayed ejaculation. All of the SSRIs have long half-lives, with fluoxetine the longest because of the activity of its metabolite. For this reason, medically ill patients should probably be treated with a non-fluoxetine SSRI. Once it has been effective, the antidepressant medication should be continued for about one year, at the same therapeutic level, and then gradually tapered off. However, if the patient has a history of recurrent depression, the medication is generally continued over a much longer period.

As with virtually all of the other antidepressants, there is an approximately 2- to 6-week lag time at therapeutic dosage before the antidepressants begin to exert their maximum effect on depression.

Tricyclics

Tricyclic antidepressants (Table 3) have been used in clinical practice for over 30 years. There is no evidence that one is more effective than another. The tertiary amines imipramine, amitriptyline, and doxepin are converted to their demethylated secondary amine metabolites desipramine, nortriptyline, and protriptyline, respectively, which retain pharmacological effectiveness and are used clinically as separate agents.

The tricyclics, and for that matter all of the antidepressants, are thought to exert their antidepressant effects through modulation of the availability of biogenic amines at receptor sites in the brain, particularly serotonin and noradrenaline, and through their effect on the responsiveness of adrenergic and serotonergic receptors. The side-effects of these medications also arise from receptor blockade. For example, sedation stems from antihistaminic effects, postural hypotension from α-adrenergic receptor blockade, and blurred vision, dry mouth, and constipation from the anticholinergic effects. The demethylated secondary amines, desipramine and nortriptyline, have been increasingly used, especially in elderly patients, because of their relatively low anticholinergic side-effects as well as less sedation and orthostatic hypotension.

Table 3 Serotonin-specific reuptake inhibitors and tricyclic antidepressants with usual dosage ranges

Agent	Daily dosage range (mg)
Serotonin-specific reuptake inhibitors	
Fluoxetine (Prozac)	10–40
Sertraline (Zoloft)	50–100
Paroxetine (Paxil)	20–40
Fluvoxamine (Luvox)	20–40
Tricyclic antidepressants	
Tertiary amines	
Imipramine	100–200
Amytriptyline	100–200
Doxepin	100–200
Trimipramine	100–200
Clomipramine	100–225
Demethylated secondary amines	
Desipramine	75–150
Nortriptyline	75–150
Protriptyline	15–40

A clinical advantage of the tricyclics is the ready availability of methods for measuring their plasma concentration, which can be used to determine compliance and to titrate the dosage for maximum therapeutic effect.

It is useful to start at a low dosage, generally between 10 and 25 mg, about an hour before bedtime, and then to increase gradually (approximately every 3 days) by the same amount, working up to a total dosage range of 50 mg/day. The 10-mg dosage increment is usually prudent in geriatric practice, while an increment of 25–50 mg is usually tolerated in the patient under 60 years of age. Once having gradually worked up to 50 mg it is usually easier to increase the dosage the rest of the way up to 150 mg/day or higher.

Patients respond to tricyclics at different dosages. This is probably due to individual biological variability and the rate at which the individual metabolizes the antidepressant. If a lower dosage does not result in remission or results in subtherapeutic blood concentrations, the dosage may need to be increased to 200–300 mg. Many patients with chronic rheumatic diseases may benefit from lower doses from the sedative and analgesic effects of the tricyclics.

Other antidepressants

Bupropion (Wellbutrin), a structurally unique compound, has minimal anticholinergic and antihistaminic properties. Its major contraindication has been in patients with seizure disorder. On the plus side, unlike the SSRIs, it does not disrupt ejaculation and other sexual function. In fact, it is sometimes added to an SSRI as an antidote to sexual side-effects. Maprotiline (Ludiomil) and trazodone (Desyrel) have side-effects similar to the tricyclic antidepressants. Venlafaxine (Effexor) is a relatively new addition that has been promoted on the basis of its combined serotonin and norepinephrine reuptake blockade (Feighner 1994). This can be associated with sustained increases in blood pressure in approximately 5 per cent of cases when dosages were maintained above 200 mg/day.

Other approved antidepressants areis nefazodone (Serzone) and mirtazapine (Remeron). Both tend to be more sedating and, given at bedtime, may help to promote sleep. Table 4 shows the dosage range and side-effects of the other antidepressants.

Monoamine oxidase inhibitors

The monoamine oxidase inhibitors (imipramine, desipramine tranylcypromine, phenelzine) were the first effective antidepressant drugs but because of tyramine-induced hypertensive episodes their use was limited. These drugs appear to have a special role in the treatment of atypical depressions characterized by hypersomnia, hyperphagia, and a reversed diurnal variation with symptoms typically worse at night than in the morning. They can often be effective in tricyclic-resistant patients and for the treatment of panic disorders. Concomitant ingestion of tyramine-containing foods, sympathomimetic agents, and meperidine (Demerol) must be avoided.

Treatment strategies

The choice of an antidepressant is often determined by its side-effects. Currently SSRIs are likely to be the first drug of choice because of their relatively

Table 4 Other antidepressants

Generic	Brand name	Side-effects
Bupropion	Wellbutrin	Jitteriness Seizures—avoid in patients with seizures
Venlafaxine	Effexor	SSRI—like side-effects
Nefazodone	Serzone	Sedation
Mirtazapine	Remeron	Weight gain, sedation
Trazodone	Desyrel	Priapism

Table 5 Antidepressant plasma concentrations

Drug	Therapeutic plasma concentration (mg)
Amitriptyline	150–250[a]
Doxepin	100–250[a]
Imipramine	200–300[a]
Trimipramine	200–300
Amoxapine	150–500
Desipramine	150–300
Maprotiline	100–300
Nortriptyline	50–150
Protriptyline	100–250
Bupropion	50–100
Fluxoetine	100–300
Sertraline	100–300
Paroxetine	100–300
Trazodone	800–1600

[a] Drug and metabolite.

benign side-effects. The most frequent reason for failure to respond to antidepressant treatment is inadequate dosage, so monitoring of the plasma concentration is an important step in guiding the clinician (Table 5).

After a satisfactory response has been obtained, the patient is generally continued on the medication for another 9 months before the dose is gradually tapered off. It is now clear that patients who have had a history of two or more depressions in the past should be kept on a maintenance dosage equal to the initial therapeutic dosage.

How does one proceed with the 10–40 per cent of patients who fail an initial trial of the medication? The main causes of a poor response are inadequate dosage, non-compliance, often associated with inability to tolerate side-effects, and inadequate duration of treatment. There are no precise guidelines in determining how to proceed after an initial full trial of an SSRI or tricyclic fails. It is important to allow an adequate trial of 4–6 weeks. Most clinicians choose another agent with a different pattern of side-effects or biochemical profile, for example, in a non-responder to an inhibitor of serotonin reuptake. If the second trial of an antidepressant fails, then the usual choice is between a newer agent, a combination of agents such as an SSRI boosted by a lower dosage of a tricyclic, or with a booster effect from lithium, or a monoamine oxidase inhibitor. For unclear reasons, individual patients may respond to one but not another of these agents. The addition of lithium is an adjunct may be effective in a subgroup of patients, especially those with a family history of bipolar illness.

Analgesic effects of antidepressants

Since their introduction over 30 years ago, tricyclics and, to a lesser extent, monoamine oxide inhibitors have found a role in the treatment of chronic pain syndromes, particularly for neuropathic pain, but also in the treatment of headaches, arthritis, low back, and facial pain. Approximately 50–60 per cent of patients with a chronic pain syndrome will benefit from the adjunctive analgesic effects of the antidepressants (Blackwell 1987). The analgesic action of the antidepressants cannot be entirely explained as a placebo effect, nor can it be indirectly related to the drug's effect on depression. In a review of 28 placebo-controlled studies, Magni (1991) concludes that antidepressants are helpful in a wide range of chronic pain syndromes, including fibromyalgia and rheumatoid arthritis, in addition to neuropathic pain, headache, migraine, and facial pain. Several studies of the use of antidepressants in chronic pain have shown pain relief in the absence of measurable changes in depression. Furthermore, structural congeners of imipramine such as carbamazepine and phenothiazine, which are not antidepressants, also have analgesic properties. Animal studies using antidepressants have also demonstrated some reduction in pain behaviour (Butler et al. 1985). Although the mechanisms of analgesia of the antidepressants remain unknown, their regulatory effects on serotonin and other biogenic amines, and their potential effect on opiate receptors, provide a theoretical basis.

Most of the antidepressants appear to have these analgesic effects. One must weigh the side-effects of the particular drug against the clinical setting. A patient with chronic pain and insomnia, for example, could benefit from a sedating antidepressant such as amitriptyline or trimipramine. These are generally described once daily, an hour or two before bedtime, and generally at a dose that is half of that used for the treatment of depression. It is wise to start with a low dose, either 10 or 25 mg, and gradually increase, similar to the approach in depression.

Antidepressants in rheumatoid arthritis

In the early 1960s, both anecdotal reports and uncontrolled studies suggested that antidepressants might have a role in providing pain relief to patients with rheumatoid arthritis. In the first controlled study of antidepressants in chronic pain, McDonald Scott (1969) demonstrated a significant improvement in rheumatoid arthritis with the use of imipramine. At a dosage of 75 mg daily, imipramine was compared to placebo in a double-blind, cross-over study of 22 patients with arthritis. Patients with a history of depression or other psychiatric disturbance were excluded. A significantly higher proportion of patients receiving imipramine improved both in subjective ratings of pain and in grip strength, and decreasing morning stiffness in 55 per cent of patients with various chronic arthritides.

Subsequent studies in patients with arthritis have suggested that not all antidepressants have similar analgesic properties. For example, Ganvir et al. (1980) failed to demonstrate a significant analgesic effect with 25 mg of clomipramine daily as compared to placebo, although they subsequently questioned whether the dosage was adequate. More recently, Frank et al. (1988b) compared amitriptyline, desipramine, trazodone, and placebo in a 32-week, double-blind, cross-over trial in 47 patient with rheumatoid arthritis. Although all of these drug regimens, including placebo, produced significant changes in pain measures, only amitriptyline was associated with a significant reduction in the number of painful and tender joints. Intriguingly, a study of the effects of amitriptyline or imipramine in rats with adjuvant-induced arthritis has suggested that the tricyclic antidepressants may have direct anti-inflammatory effects because of a reduction in the physical signs of inflammation (Butler et al. 1985).

Managing anxiety disorders

Anxiety disorders are common in the general population and may be more frequent in patients with rheumatic disorders. Acute anxiety reactions may benefit from short-term use of benzodiazepines if they do not interfere with balance or cognitive function. It is important to be alert to more specific kinds of anxiety disorder, such as panic disorder with agoraphobia, obsessive–compulsive disorder, and social phobia. Panic disorder with agoraphobia may benefit from a benzodiazepine, such as aiprazolam or clonazepam, or a tricyclic with antipanic effects, such as imipramine or desipramine. Pharmacotherapy should be given in conjunction with cognitive and behavioural approaches to the phobias. Obsessive–compulsive disorder specifically benefits from clomipramine (Anafranil) and the SSRIs. Patients with social phobia seem to do best with either imipramine or monoamine oxidase inhibitors. All of these disorders are significant problems in their own right and should be differentiated from the more non-specific and transient adjustment reactions seen with anxiety.

Patients needing 'anxiolytic' medications such as benzodiazepines who have a history of alcohol or substance abuse generally are better treated with buspirone (Buspar), which is non-addicting.

Managing sleep disturbances

These are common, particularly in patients with systemic lupus, rheumatoid arthritis, and fibromyalgia (see Chapter 6.13.1). Some patients with lupus may develop insomnia secondary to the use of prednisone. When

Box 1 Important points to remember

1. Neuopsychiatric illness is a common manifestation of many rheumatic diseases, particularly systemic lupus, where it may be associated with multiorgan involvement or as an isolated condition.
2. The neuropsychiatric manifestations of patients with systemic lupus on corticosteroids are much more likely to be due to the disease than to the steroids.
3. End-organ failure, e.g. renal or hepatic, and occult infection in the immunocompromised host should be excluded as causes for organic mental syndromes.
4. Consider potential drug toxicities, especially corticosteroids, as a cause of organic brain syndromes.
5. Depression complicating chronic rheumatic disease should be identified and when appropriate treated with antidepressant drugs.

prednisone is producing manic or hypomanic symptoms associated with loss of sleep, a mood stabilizer such as lithium should be considered. The pain and inflammation of rheumatoid arthritis may be associated with more frequent night-time awakenings. Anti-inflammatory medication is probably more helpful than sedative hypnotic medication at night.

Summary

Finally, some essential clinical guidelines that may be helpful when evaluating rheumatological patients for psychiatric illness are given in Box 1.

References

ACR Ad Hoc Committee on Neuropsychiatric Lupus Nomenclature (1999). *The American College of Rheumatology Nomenclature and Case Definitions for Neuropsychiatric Lupus Syndromes* **42**, 599–608.

Adams, W.R., Rose, C.D., Eppes, S.C., and Klein, J.D. (1994). Cognitive effects of Lyme disease in children. *Pediatrics* **94**, 185–9.

Adelman, D.C., Salteil, E., and Klinenberg, J.R. (1986). The neuropsychiatric manifestations of SLE: an overview. *Seminars in Arthritis and Rheumatology* **15**, 185–99.

Ader, R. *Psychoneuroimmunology* 2nd edn. New York: Academic Press, 1991.

American Psychiatric Association. *Diagnostic and Statistical Manual of Mental Disorders IV.* Washington DC: American Psychiatric Press, 1995.

Angelopoulos, N., Drosos, A.A., Kostouitsag, E., and Liskos, A. (1988). Personality and psychopathology in patients with primary Sjögren's syndrome. *Terapevticheskii Arkhiv* **60**, 49–52.

Baildam, E.M., Holt, P.J., Conway, S.C., and Morton, M.J. (1995). The association between physical function and psychological problems in children with juvenile chronic arthritis. *British Journal of Rheumatology* **34**, 470–7.

Baum, K.A., Hopf, U., and Nehrig, C. (1993). Systemic lupus erythematosus: neuropsychiatric signs and symptoms related to cerebral MRI findings. *Clinical Neurology and Neurosurgery* **95**, 29–34.

Bell, C.L. et al. (1991). Magnetic resonance imaging of central nervous system lesions in patients with lupus erythematosus. Correlation with clinical remission and antineurofilament and anticardiolipin antibody titers. *Arthritis and Rheumatism* **34**, 432–41.

Benke, T., Gasse, T., Hittmair-Delazer, M., and Schmutzhard, E. (1995). Lyme encephalopathy: long-term neuropsychological deficits eyars after acute neuroborreliosis. *Archives of Neurology* **48**, 1125–9.

Bertoli, M., Romagnoli, G.F., and Margreiter, R. (1988). Irreversible dementia following cyclosporin therapy in a renal transplant patient. *Nephron* **49**, 333–4.

Blackwell, B. (1987). Antidepressants as adjuncts in chronic idiopathic pain management. *International Drug Therapy Newsletter* **22**, 1–4.

Blalock, S.J. and DeVellis, R.F. (1992). Rheumatoid arthritis and depression: an overview. *Bulletin of Rheumatic Diseases* **41**, 6–8.

Bosma, G.P.T., Rood, M.J., Huizinga, T.W.J., deJong, B.A., Bollen, E.L.E.M., and VonBuchem, M.A. (2000). Detection of cerebral involvement in patients with active neuropsychiatric systemic lupus erythematosus by the use of volumetric magnetization transfer imaging. *Arthritis and Rheumatism* **43** (11), 2428–36.

Boumpas, D.T. et al. (1991). Pulse cyclophosphamide for severe neuropsychiatric lupus. *Quarterly Journal of Medicine* **81**, 975–84.

Bousser, M.G., Rougement, D., Youl, B.D., and Wechsler, B. (1988). Neurological manifestations of Behçet's disease. *Journal of Vascular Malformations* **13**, 231–4.

Braden, C.J., McGlone, K., and Pennington, F. (1993). Specific psychosocial and behavioral outcomes from the systemic lupus erythematosus self-help course. *Health Education Quarterly* **20**, 29–41.

Brooks, W.M., Jung, R.E., Ford, C.C., Grienel, E.J., and Sibbitt, W.L., Jr. (1999). Relationship between neurometabolite derangement and neurocognitive dysfunction in systemic lupus erythematosus. *Journal of Rheumatology* **26**, 81–5.

Butler, S.H., Weil-Fugazza, J., Godefray, F., and Besson, J. (1985). Reduction of arthritis and pain behavior following chronic administration of amitriptyline or imipramine in rats with adjuvant-induced arthritis. *Pain* **23**, 159–75.

Carbotte, S.M. et al. (1992). Fluctuating cognitive abnormalities and cerebral glucose metabolism in neuropsychiatric systemic lupus erythematosus. *Journal of Neurology and Neurosurgery* **55**, 1054–9.

Cassileth, B.R. et al. (1984). Psychological status in chronic illness: a comparative analysis of six diagnostic groups. *New England Journal of Medicine* **311**, 506–11.

Crotty, M., McFarlane, A.C., and Brooks, P.M. (1994). Psychosocial and clinical status of younger women with early rheumatoid arthritis: a longitudinal study with frequent measures. *British Journal of Rheumatology* **33**, 754–60.

Daly, D. (1942). Central nervous system in acute disseminated lupus erythematosus. *Journal of Nervous and Mental Disease* **102**, 461–3.

David, J. et al. (1994). The functional and psychological outcomes of juvenile chronic arthritis in young adulthood. *British Journal of Rheumatology* **33**, 876–81.

Denburg, S.D., Behmann, S.A., Carbotte, R.M., and Denburg, J.A. (1994). Lymphocyte antigens in neuropsychiatric systemic lupus erythematosus. *Arthritis and Rheumatism* **37**, 369–75.

Dougherty, P.M. and Dafny, N. (1988). Cyclosporine affects central nervous system opioid activity via direct and indirect means. *Brain and Behavioral Immunology* **2** (3), 242–53.

Dougherty, P.M., Aronowski, J., Drath, D., and Dafny, N. (1987). Evidence of neuro-immunologic interactions: cyclosporine modifies opiate withdrawal by effects on the brain and immune components. *Neuroimmunology* **13** (3), 331–42.

Ellison, D., Gatter, K., Heryet, A., and Esiri, M. (1993). Intramural platelet deposition in cerebral vasculopathy of systemic lupus erythematosus. *Journal of Clinical Pathology* **46**, 37–40.

Falk, W.E., Mahnke, M.W., and Poskanzer, D.C. (1979). Lithium prophylaxis of corticotrophin-induced psychosis. *Journal of the American Medical Association* **241**, 1011–12.

Fallon, B.A. and Nields, J.A. (1994). Lyme disease: a neuropsychiatric illness. *American Journal of Psychiatry* **151**, 1571–83.

Feighner, J.P. (1994). The role of venlafaxine in rational antidepressant therapy. *Journal of Clinical Psychiatry* **55** (Suppl. A), 62–8.

Feinglass, E.F., Arnett, F.C., Dorsch, C.A., Zizic, T.M., and Stevens, M.B. (1976). Neuropsychiatric manifestations of systemic lupus erythematosus: diagnosis, clinical spectrum, and the relationship to other features of the disease. *Medicine* **55**, 323–39.

Frank, R.G. et al. (1988a). Depression in rheumatoid arthritis. *Journal of Rheumatology* **15**, 920–5.

Frank, R.G. et al. (1988b). Antidepressant analgesia in rheumatoid arthritis. *Journal of Rheumatology* **15**, 1632–8.

Ganvir, P., Beammont, G., and Seldrup, J. (1980). A comparative trial of clomipramine and placebo as a adjunctive therapy in arthralgia. *Journal of International Medical Research* **8** (Suppl. 3), 60–6.

Good, M.I. and Shader, R.I. (1982). Lethality and behavioral side effects of chloroquine. *Journal of Clinical Psychopharmacology* **2**, 40–7.

Hanly, J.G., Walsh, N.M., and Sangalang, V. (1992). Brain pathology in systemic lupus erythematosus. *Journal of Rheumatology* **19**, 732–41.

Hanly, J.G. et al. (1993). Cognitive impairment and autoantibodies in systemic erythematosus. *British Journal of Rheumatology* **32**, 291–6.

Hay, E.M. et al. (1992). Psychiatric disorder and cognitive impairment in systemic lupus erythematosus. *Arthritis and Rheumatism* **35**, 411–16.

Hopkinson, N. and Powell, R. (1990). 'Occult' SLE amongst patients admitted to acute psychiatric wards (Abstract). *Arthritis and Rheumatism* **33**, S102.

Isshi, K. and Hirohata, S. (1998). Differential roles of the antiribosomal P antibody and antineuromal antibody in the pathogenesis of central nervous system involvement in systemic lupus erythematosis. *Arthritis and Rheumatism* **41**, 1819–27.

Jaworski, T.M., Bradley, L.A., Heck, L.W., Roca, A., and Alarion, G.S. (1995). Development of an observation method for assessing pain behaviors in children with juvenile rheumatoid arthritis. *Arthritis and Rheumatism* **38**, 1142–51.

Karassa, F.B., Ioannidis, J.P.A., Touloumi, G., Boki, K.A., and Moutsopoulos, H.M. (2000). Risk factors for central nervous system involvement in systemic lupus erythematosus. *Quarterly Journal of Medicine* **93** (3), 169–74.

Katz, P.P. and Velin, E.H. (1995). The development of depressive symptoms among women with rheumatoid arthritis. The role of function. *Arthritis and Rheumatism* **38**, 49–56.

Kiecolt-Glaser, J.K. and Glaser, R. (1989). Psychoneuroimmunology: past, present, and future. *Health Psychology* **8**, 677–82.

Krupp, L.B. et al. (1991). Cognitive functioning in Lyme borreliosis. *Archives of Neurology* **48**, 1125–9.

Logigian, E.L., Kaplan, R.F., and Steere, A.C. (1990). Chronic neurologic manifestations of Lyme disease. *New England Journal of Medicine* **323**, 1438–44.

McDonald Scott, N.A. (1969). The relief of pain with an antidepressant in arthritis. *Practitioner* **202**, 802.

Magni, G. (1991). The use of antidepressants in the treatment of chronic pain. A review of the current evidence. *Drugs* **42**, 730–48.

Muller, P.D., Laville, E.A., Biddle, A.K., and Lorig, K. (1987). Efficacy of psychoeducational interventions on pain, depression and disability in people with arthritis: a meta-analysis. *Journal of Rheumatology* **15**, 33–9.

Neuwelt, C.M., Lack, S., Kaye, B.R., Ellman, J.B., and Borenstein, D.G. (1995). Role of intravenous cyclophosphamide in the treatment of severe neuropsychiatric systemic lupus erythematosus. *American Journal of Medicine* **98**, 32–41.

Omdal, R., Husby, G., and Mellgren, S.I. (1995). Mental health status in systemic lupus erythematosus. *Scandinavian Journal of Rheumatology* **24**, 142–5.

Parker, J.C. et al. (1988). Pain management in rheumatoid arthritis patients: a cognitive behavioral approach. *Arthritis and Rheumatism* **31**, 593–601.

Rimon, R.H. (1989). Connective tissue diseases. In *Psychosomatic Medicine: Theory, Physiology, and Practice* Vol. 2 (ed. S. Cheren), pp. 565–609. Madison CT: International Universities Press.

Ritchlin, C.T. et al. (1992). Quantitative electroencephalography. A new approach to the diagnosis of cerebral dysfunction in systemic lupus erythematosus. *Arthritis and Rheumatism* **35**, 1330–42.

Rogers, M.P. (1985). Rheumatoid arthritis: psychiatric aspects and use of psychotropics. *Psychosomatics* **26**, 915–25.

Rogers, M.P. et al. (1980). Effect of psychological stress on the induction of arthritis in rats. *Arthritis and Rheumatism* **23**, 1337–42.

Rogers, M.P. et al. (1992). I-123 iodoamphetamine SPECT scan in systemic lupus erythematosus patients with cognitive and other minor neuropsychiatric symptoms. A pilot study. *Lupus* **1**, 215–19.

Rubbert, A. et al. (1993). Single photon emission computed tomography analysis of cerebral blood flow in the evaluation of central nervous system involvement in patients with systemic erythematosus. *Arthritis and Rheumatism* **36**, 1253–62.

Shadick, N.A. et al. (1994). The long-term clinical outcomes of Lyme disease. A population-based retrospective cohort study. *Annals of Internal Medicine* **121**, 560–7.

Shiowaza, S., Kuroki, Y., Kim, M., Hipohata, S., and Ogino, T. (1992). Interferon-alpha in lupus psychosis. *Arthritis and Rheumatism* **35**, 417–22.

Sigal, L.H. (1993). Lyme disease: testing and treatment: who should be tested and treated for Lyme disease and how? *Rheumatic Disease Clinics of North America* **19**, 79–93.

Smyth, J.M., Stone, A.A., Hurewitz, A., and Kaell, A. (1999). Effects of writing about stressful experiences on symptom reduction in patients with asthma or rheumatoid arthritis: a randomized trial. *Journal of the American Medical Association* **281**, 1304–9.

Solomon, G.F. (1969). Stress and antibody response in rats. *International Archives of Allergy* **35**, 97–104.

Stewart, A.I. et al. (1989). Functional status and well-being of patients with chronic conditions: results from the medical outcomes study. *Journal of the American Medical Association* **262**, 907–13.

Strauss, G.D. et al. (1986). Group therapies for rheumatoid arthritis: a controlled study of two approaches. *Arthritis and Rheumatism* **29**, 1203–9.

Thornton, T.L. (1980). Delirium associated with sulindac (Letter). *Journal of the American Medical Association* **243**, 1630–3.

Toubi, E., Khamashta, M.A., Panarra, A., and Hughes, G.R.V. (1995). Association of antiphospholipid antibodies with central nervous system disease in systemic lupus erythematosus. *American Journal of Medicine* **99**, 395–401.

Tsai, C.Y. et al. (1994). Cerebrospinal fluid interleukin-6, prostaglandin E_2 and autoantibodies in patients with neuropsychiatric systemic lupus erythematosus and central nervous system infections. *Scandinavian Journal of Rheumatology* **23** (2), 57–63.

VanBuchem, M.A. et al. (1997). Global volumetric estimation of disease border in multiple sclerosis based on magnetization transfer imaging. *American Journal of Neuroradiology* **18**, 1287–90.

Vivian, A.S. and Goldberg, I.B. (1982). Recognizing chronic salicylate intoxication in the elderly. *Geriatrics* **37**, 91–7.

West, S.G., Emlen, W., Wener, M.H., and Kotzin, B.L. (1995). Neuropsychiatric lupus erythematosis: a 10-year prospective study on the value of diagnostic tests. *American Journal of Medicine* **99** (2), 153–63.

Wilde, M.I., Plasker, G.L., and Benfield, P. (1993). Fluvoxamine. An updated review of its pharmacology and therapeutic use in depressive illness. *Drugs* **46**, 895–924.

Wolkowitz, O.M. et al. (1990). Cognitive effects of corticosteroids. *American Journal of Psychiatry* **147**, 1297–303.

2

Outcomes and issues in delivering rheumatological care

2 Outcomes and issues in delivering rheumatological care

2.1 Outcome assessment in rheumatology

Thomas Stoll and Gerold Stucki

Introduction

Rheumatic disorders vary in their clinical expression, yet each has a major effect on function and health status. The major goal in the management of patients with rheumatic disorders is to control or cure the disease and to preserve and control function and health status. To measure treatments' efficacy standardized assessment of organ morphology, function, and of health status are required. Health care professionals are accustomed to the measurement of organ pathology but if effective treatment is to improve, the standardized assessment of health status is critical. It can be done by: (i) the judgement of a physician or another health professional, (ii) performing standardized activities by the patient, and (iii) self-report of patients to standardized questionnaires.

In 1949, the American Rheumatism Association (now the American College of Rheumatology) Functional Classes were developed (Steinbrocker et al. 1949). Since then, hundreds of ad hoc, non-standardized, assessments of activities of daily living using one of the three approaches have been used. Beginning in the early 1980s, sophisticated, validated, and reproducible questionnaires to measure health status became available.

The literature on the psychometrics and properties of these instruments and their application to clinical trials is now commonplace, whereas their use in clinical practice is not established and the reasons why under study (Deyo 1989; Deyo and Carter 1992; Golden 1992).

This chapter reviews the patient-outcomes measurement of function, health status, and quality of life in the rheumatic and musculoskeletal diseases, conceptual limitations to their use, and guidelines for the selection of measures for specific applications. As assessments based upon the judgement of the physician are part of the disease-specific chapter (e.g. SLE activity indices and SLICC/ACR damage index are described under the chapter SLE) this chapter focuses on the self-report of patients to standardized questionnaire, and in children on performing standardized activities.

Definitions and conceptual framework

The terms which describe the impact of rheumatic conditions on the individual are defined according to ICF (WHO 2001):

'Impairment' means a problem in body function or structure, such as a significant deviation or loss. Body functions are the physiological functions of body systems including psychological functions. Body structures are anatomical parts of the body such as organs, limbs, and their components. Impairment may be reversible, for instance in synovitis the actual inflammatory state of the joint may resolve completely, or irreversible, that is, permanent damage.

'Disability' serves as an umbrella term for impairments, 'activity limitations' and 'participation restrictions'. It is perceived by an individual when there is a discrepancy between one's capacity and a higher actually perceived need for a specific function. The patient's expectations and limitations, psychosocial factors, and the actual demands are critical determinants of this perception. 'Activity' means the execution of a task or an action by an individual. In addition 'participation' includes a societal perspective and is defined as involvement in life situations.

'Functioning' is used as an umbrella term and refers to body functions, activities, and participation. Function changes over the course of people's development. In children and adolescents, maturation of physical, cognitive, behavioural, emotional, and psychological function are the rule, whereas in adult life, those capacities are stable but life circumstances are changing and physical abilities may be declining gradually in older age.

Environmental (extrinsic influences) or personal factors (intrinsic influences) may interact with all the components of 'functioning' or 'disability'.

'Health status' or 'quality of life' embodies the dimensions of physical, social, and emotional function. If these concepts are attributed to health, the term health-related quality of life is used. However, there is considerable variation in the terminology and interpretation of this concept. Most citations correspond to the World Health Organization definition of health as a state of 'complete physical, mental and social well-being' (WHO 1958). Health status instruments usually include the dimensions of physical function, social function, emotional function, pain, and perception of well being.

Characteristics of a health status measure

The attributes of any quantitative measure are validity, reliability, responsiveness, and practical usefulness (Liang and Jette 1981).

'Validity' refers to whether an instrument measures what it is supposed to measure. Ideally, one would compare a measure with a gold standard, for example, comparing a suspicious nodule on a chest radiograph with a biopsy showing cancer (criterion validity). For health status no reference or gold standard exists to judge the validity of a particular instrument. Instead one assesses the extent to which a measure is consistent with a theoretical concept (construct) concerning the phenomenon of interest (construct validity). Face validity (it 'looks like' it measures what it intends to measure) or content validity (it represents the domain of interest) are other techniques to strengthen the validity of a measure.

'Reliability' is the extent to which a measurement yields the same result on repeated administration of the questionnaire under the same circumstances (reproducibility). If scores of a health status instrument have little random error, they are considered reliable.

Validity and reliability are minimal criteria when one wants to differentiate individuals at one point in time. However, when used to evaluate changes over time, an instrument needs to be able to capture clinically meaningful changes. 'Sensitivity' denotes the capacity of a measure to show any change whether it is meaningful or not. This can be done by statistical techniques such as the standardized response mean (Liang et al. 1985), the effect size (Kazis et al. 1989), or Guyatt's responsiveness statistic (Guyatt et al. 1987). 'Responsiveness', on the other hand, is the capacity to show a change that is clinically meaningful to the patient and/or the physician. Responsiveness of a measure is the criterion which ultimately determines the usefulness of any outcome measure in the evaluation of chronic conditions but is the measurement criterion least established for health status instruments.

Finally, one needs to assess 'the practical utility' of a health status instrument for a given setting. In practice and research applications, the time needed to complete a questionnaire should be no more than 10–15 min to ensure compliance. In general, self-administered questionnaires are more practical than instruments requiring a trained interviewer. However, in multicultural populations or where literacy levels are variable, a standardized interview might be preferable.

In the following we describe commonly used instruments which have been evaluated for their metric properties.

Health status and quality of life measurement

The instruments for measuring health status or quality of life cover a variety of dimensions of health, including physical, social, and emotional functioning. Some instruments are general health status measures which have been applied to rheumatic disorders. Others are measures developed for rheumatoid arthritis, osteoarthritis, the spondyloarthropathies, and low back pain. Two rheumatoid arthritis instruments assess patient satisfaction with their function (Pincus et al. 1983; Meenan et al. 1992) and only one is an individualized measure of health status in rheumatoid arthritis (Tugwell et al. 1987). General health status instruments are suitable for the comparison of health status across multiple diseases or for examination of competing clinical programmes. Generic health status instruments are useful in the evaluation of subjects with multiple chronic conditions since they can detect changes arising from different diseases. This is also of interest when interventions can have effects or adverse effects on several organ systems.

Disease-specific instruments are useful for measuring clinically important changes in response to treatments (Patrick and Deyo 1989). Since these instruments include the elements most relevant to a particular disease, they are usually more sensitive to subtle improvements in health status than general health status instruments. Disease-specific instruments are as reliable as traditional measures of improvement in clinical status, such as anthropometric approaches (25-m walk time) or laboratory tests (erythrocyte sedimentation rate).

Health status instruments are interchangeable in their ability to measure major clinically significant improvement, but have varying ability to demonstrate changes in sub-dimensions such as social and global function (Liang et al. 1985; Bombardier et al. 1986). Measures of function or health status predict mortality and utilization of health services (McNevitt et al. 1986; Mitchell et al. 1986). A functional questionnaire is an economical and efficient technique for finding subjects with rheumatic and musculoskeletal diseases and has been applied in developing countries for evaluating community burden (Liang et al. 1981).

Generic health status measures

The Sickness Impact Profile (SIP) (Bergner et al. 1976) is a widely used general health status instrument containing 136 items that have true or false answers. Scores use pre-determined weights based on rater panel estimates of relative severity of the dysfunction. The categories of ambulation, body care (including continence), and mobility are aggregated into a physical dimension, and four categories (emotional behaviour, social interaction, alertness behaviour, and communication) into a psychosocial dimension. The remaining categories are work, sleep and rest, eating, home management, and recreation and pastimes. The SIP is available as a self-administered questionnaire or interview. It takes 30 min to complete as an interview. The instrument demonstrates change in groups of arthritis patients, but is relatively insensitive to changes in individual patients (Deyo and Inui 1984; Liang et al. 1985; Stucki et al. 1995).

The Quality of Well-Being Index (QWB) and an earlier version, the Index of Well-Being (Kaplan et al. 1976), assess mobility, physical activity, and social activity, but not pain. A trained interviewer asks what the patient did because of illness during the last 6 days. Scoring for particular functions is based on preference weights derived from the normal population. These have been validated in patients with rheumatoid arthritis (Balaban et al. 1986). The interview takes about 20 min. The instrument was valid, but not as sensitive to change as other measures in a clinical trial in rheumatoid arthritis (Bombardier et al. 1986). However, it has the advantage of being a ratio scale with a true zero point which, though not often relevant in rheumatic disease, allows for the calculation of quality-adjusted life years in cost–benefit studies. Major limitations are the complexity of the instrument and the requirement of a specially trained interviewer.

The McMaster Health Index Questionnaire (MHIQ) (Chambers et al. 1982) evaluates the quality of life in patients with rheumatoid diseases but has had limited application. A physical function index covers physical activities, self-care activities, mobility, communication, and global physical activity. A social index combines general well being, work performance, material welfare, support, participation with friends and family, and global social function. The emotional index measures feelings about personal relationships, self-esteem, the future, critical life events, and global emotional function. The MHIQ has 59 self-administered questions and takes 15–20 min to complete.

Short forms

One disadvantage of the instruments described above is that most require at least 15–20 min to complete (Table 1). This becomes burdensome if general health status is measured along with disease-specific measures. Shorter measures appear to retain the psychometric properties of the longer instruments.

The Medical Outcome Study Short Form 36 (SF-36) (Ware and Sherbourne 1992) comes from a larger battery of questions administered in the Medical Outcomes Study. The SF-36 includes eight multi-item scales containing 2–10 items each and a single item to assess health transition. The scales cover the dimensions of physical health, mental health, social functioning, role functioning, general health, pain, and vitality. Forms cover a week or a month. The use of sub-scales is encouraged and the questionnaire can be self-administered or interviewer administered. The SF-36 is the most widely used general health status instrument and has been translated into many languages. The instrument is suitable for subjects aged 14 years and older and takes approximately 10 min to complete. Studies show excellent psychometric properties and there seems to be good sensitivity to change in patients with rheumatic conditions compared with longer instruments (Katz et al. 1990b).

The SF-36 allows scoring of the eight sub-scales and the construction of two summary scales, the physical component summary (PCS) and the mental component summary (MCS) scales. Futher evaluation of these summary scales provided the foundation for the construction of an instrument that is much shorter than the SF-36 (Ware et al. 1995). This new short form, the SF-12, uses 12 items from the SF-36, and demonstrates satisfactory reproducibility of the PCS and MCS with correlation coefficients of 0.93–0.97 on cross validation with the whole instrument. The new short form is likely to perform well enough for monitoring general populations; however, it does not allow scoring of individual SF-36 sub-scales such as bodily pain or social functioning. While the SF-36 and SF-12 are commonplace in clinical and health services research, a previous version, the SF-20 (Stewart et al. 1988), is losing importance.

The Nottingham Health Profile (NHP) (McDowell et al. 1978) assesses perceived physical, social, and emotional health with 38 items answered

Table 1 Generic health status measures (including short forms)

Instrument	Dimensions covered	Mode of administration	Time to complete (min)
Sickness Impact Profile (SIP) (Bergner et al. 1976)	Physical function, psychosocial, work, sleep and rest, eating, home management, recreation and pastimes	Self-administered or interview	~30
Quality of Well-Being (QWB) (Balaban et al. 1986)	Mobility, physical activity, social activity	Interview	~20
McMaster Health Index Questionnaire (MHIQ) (Chambers et al. 1982)	Physical function, social function, emotional function	Self-administered	~15–20
Medical Outcome Study Short Form 36 (SF-36) (Ware and Sherbourne 1992)	Physical health, mental health, social functioning, role functioning, general health, vitality, pain	Self-administered or interview or telephone interview	~10
Nottingham Health Profile (NHP) (McDowell et al. 1978)	Physical mobility, pain, emotional reaction, energy level, sleep, social interaction	Self-administered	~10
European Quality of Life Instrument (EQ5D) (see Wells et al. 1999)	Mobility, self-care, usual activities, pain/discomfort, anxiety/depression	Self-administered	~5

yes or no. It uses weighted scores from panels' judgement about the severity of individual items. The NHP covers physical mobility, pain, emotional reaction, energy level, sleep, and social isolation and can provide dimension-specific scores. The NHP is designed to represent rather severe problems, giving individuals with minor difficulties little room to improve. The NHP's reliability and validity have been assessed in rheumatoid arthritis, osteoarthritis, and in patients undergoing hip replacement. The instrument is self-administered and takes 10 min to complete.

The European Quality of Life Instrument (EQ5D) is a self-administered questionnaire that describes health states in 5 dimensions: mobility, self-care, usual activities, pain/discomfort, and anxiety/depression (see Wells et al. 1999). Each dimension is divided into 3 levels which, when taken together, define a total of 243 (3^5) unique health states. In addition there is a VAS that measures the overall perception of health on a 0–100 scale. EQ5D is valid. It is recommended for use with other more generic measures such as SF-36.

WHO Disability Assessment Schedule (WHODAS II) is a new promising 36 item instrument, which has been developed to assess the activity limitations and participation restrictions in six domains (understanding and communicating, getting around, self care, getting along with people, life activities, participation in society) (http://www.who.int/ICIDH/whodas). Its reliability and validity await to be investigated.

Condition-specific measures

Rheumatoid arthritis

Rheumatoid disability is affected not only by the disease itself, but also by the person's age and social role. In middle age, rheumatoid arthritis may affect career development, raising a family, family relationships, or return to work when children are grown up. Rheumatoid arthritis in older persons accentuates the ageing process and accelerates physical dependency. Functional disability is the major consequence of rheumatoid arthritis. Relevant outcomes include the evaluation of physical function, pain, treatment side-effects, quality of life, and cost-effectiveness (Table 2).

The Health Assessment Questionnaire (HAQ) (Fries et al. 1980) asks questions about physical and psychological disability, pain, global severity, employment, income, cost of medical care, and drug-related side-effects. The portion about disability and pain is composed of 24 questions on activities of daily living and mobility including a single pain scale. The HAQ takes approximately 5 min to complete. The short form yields a summated index between 0 and 3 on a continuous scale. The HAQ is probably the most widely used health status instrument in rheumatoid arthritis and has been tested extensively for validity and reliability and captures clinically meaningful changes over time but may be insensitive to early or advanced disability. The HAQ may be used in other rheumatic diseases, for example, fibromyalgia (Wolfe et al. 2000).

The Arthritis Impact Measurement Scales (AIMS), a health status or quality of life instrument developed for rheumatoid arthritis, has 48 multiple-choice questions with nine sub-scales measuring mobility, physical activity, dexterity, social role functioning, social activity, activities of daily living, depression, anxiety, and pain (Meenan et al. 1980). The possible range of scores on each sub-scale is 0–10; sub-scale results are averaged to obtain a global score. The questionnaire is self-administered and takes 15–20 min to complete. AIMS 2 (Meenan et al. 1992) is an improved and expanded version which has additional scales measuring arm function, work, and support from family and friends, and a problem attribution section with yes/no questions. The scales also include three new questions to assess satisfaction with current level of functioning, specific impact of arthritis on an individual's health status, and prioritization of three areas where patients would most likely achieve improvement. Reliability, internal validity, and sensitivity to change of the AIMS 2 have been demonstrated.

Wallston et al. (1989) have shortened the original AIMS from 48 to 18 items by selecting two questions for each of the nine sub-scales. The abbreviated AIMS is slightly less reliable but has comparable validity to the whole instrument.

The Modified Health Assessment Questionnaire (MHAQ) (Pincus et al. 1983) reduces the HAQ disability sub-scales to eight questions. However, while it is shorter it may have a ceiling effect and thus may be less sensitive to change than the HAQ (Stucki et al. 1995).

The McMaster Toronto Arthritis Patient Preference Disability Questionnaire (MACTAR) (Tugwell et al. 1987) asks patients in a semi-structured interview to specify their own key functional activities. The five activities that rank highest are evaluated. On reassessment, patients are asked if their previously indicated limitations have improved, worsened, or remained the same. The MACTAR takes about 10 min to complete.

The Functional Status Index (FSI) (Jette 1980) measures pain, limitations, and dependence in performing 18 activities of daily living grouped as hand activities, gross mobility, personal care, home chores, and interpersonal activities. Studies on patients with rheumatoid arthritis show validity and a high degree of interobserver reliability. However, the FSI has had little usage as judged by publications.

The Toronto Functional Capacity Questionnaire (TFCQ) (Helewa et al. 1982) assesses function in personal care, activities using the upper extremities, mobility, and leisure activities. The TFCQ takes approximately 20 min to complete and requires an interviewer. Scoring includes weighting based on panels of occupational and physical therapists and rheumatologists. The instrument is valid and responsive in clinical trials (Bombardier et al. 1986).

Table 2 Arthritis-specific measures—polyarthritis

Instrument	Dimensions covered	Mode of administration (age)	Time to complete (min)
Adults			
Health Assessment Questionnaire (HAQ) (Fries et al. 1980)	Physical disability (dressing and grooming, arising, eating, walking, hygiene, grip, activities), pain	Self-administered	<10
Arthritis Impact Measurement Scales (AIMS) (Meenan et al. 1980)	Mobility, physical activity, dexterity, social role functioning, social activity, activities of daily living, depression, anxiety, pain	Self-administered	~20
McMaster Toronto Arthritis Patient Preference Disability Questionnaire (MACTAR) (Tugwell et al. 1987)	Open-ended self-identified functional priorities, closed-ended physical activities	Interview	~10
Functional Status Index (FSI) (Jette 1980)	Activities of daily living (hand activities, gross mobility, personal care, home chores, interpersonal acitvities)	Interview	20–30
Toronto Functional Capacity Questionnaire (TFCQ) (Helewa et al. 1982)	Function in personal care, activities of upper extremities, mobility, leisure activities	Interview	~20
Keitel Index (Keitel et al. 1971)	Mobility, ambulation, self-care tasks	Clinician observation	~15
Lee Functional Status Index (Lee et al. 1973)	Physical function	Self-administered or interview	<10
Convery Polyarticular Disability Index (Convery et al. 1977)	Mobility, acitivies of daily living	Self-administered	~15
Rheumatoid Arthritis Disease Activity Index (RADAI) (Fransen et al. 2001)	Previous global disease activity, today's disease activity, today's arthritis, pain, today's morning stiffness, today's amount of pain in each of several joint areas	Self-administered	5–10
Rheumatoid Arthritis Quality of Life (RAQOL)	30 questions with yes/no response derived from qualitative interviews with RA patients	Self-administered	~6
Children: development			
Hoskins and Squires Test for Gross Motor and Reflex Development (Hoskins and Squires 1973)	Gross motor, reflexes	Clinician observation (0–5 years)	30–60
Denver Development and Screening Test (DDST) (Frankenburg et al. 1970, 1971)	Personal–social, fine motor adaptive and gross motor skills, language	Clinician observation (1 month–6 years)	15–30
Newington Children's Hospital Juvenile Rheumatoid Arthritis Evaluation (Rhodes et al. 1988)	Motor tasks	Clinician observation (1–6 years)	30–60
Children: function			
Adapted Arthritis Impact Measurement Scales for Children (CHAIMS) (Coulton et al. 1987)	Physical disability (dressing and grooming, arising, eating, walking, hygiene, grip, activities), pain	Self-administered (parent or child) (all age)	<10
Juvenile Arthritis Functional Assessment Scale (JAFAS) (Lovell et al. 1989)	Physical activities	Clinician observation (7–18 years)	~10
Juvenile Arthritis Functional Assessment Report for Children (JAFAR-C) and parents (JAFAR-P) (Howe et al. 1991)	Physical activities	Self-administered (child or parent) (7–18 years)	~10
Rand Health Insurance Study Scale (HIS) (Eisen et al. 1980)	Mobility, physical activity, role functioning, self-care	Interview and parent report (0–13 years)	
Juvenile Arthritis Self Report Index (JASI) (see Duffy et al. 2000)	Self-care, domestic, mobility, school, extracurricular	Self-administered (>8 years)	30–50
Juvenile Arthritis Quality of Life Questionnaire (JAQQ) (see Duffy et al. 2000)	Gross motor function, fine motor function, psychosocial function, general symptoms	Parent-administered (<9 years) Patient-administered (≥9 years)	20

The Convery Polyarticular Disability Index (Convery et al. 1977) uses 16 items to rate functional impairment in polyarticular arthritis. The index is based on 9 mobility items and 7 activities of daily living. The questionnaire requires approximately 15 min to complete and is reliable and valid. There are no studies on its responsiveness.

The American College of Rheumatology (ACR) Revised Criteria for Classification of Global Functional Status in Rheumatoid Arthritis (Hochberg et al. 1992) rates patients from complete independence to limited abilities in performing usual self-care, vocational, and avocational activities. The criteria expand the original Rheumatoid Arthritis Classification of Functional Capacity (Steinbrocker et al. 1949). As an ordinal scale it is useful for stratifying or describing patients but less useful for showing change.

Unlike the questionnaires above, the Keitel Index (Keitel et al. 1971) consists of 24 standardized tasks which are rated by a trained examiner. The index tests motions of axial and peripheral joints focusing on mobility, ambulation, and self-care tasks. The complete test takes approximately 15 min to complete. Validity and reliability of the instrument, and the responsiveness in a clinical trial have been demonstrated.

The Lee Functional Status Index (Lee et al. 1973) includes 17 activities to assess the functional ability of the upper and lower extremities and the axial joints. The instrument has good psychometric properties and can be self-administered or interviewer based and takes less than 10 min to complete.

The RADAI (RA Disease Activity Index) is a 5 item questionnaire. Previous global disease activity, today's disease activity in terms of swollen and tender joints, today's arthritis pain, today's morning stiffness, and today's amount of pain in each of several joint areas are assessed by the patient. Validity and reliability of the instrument and its responsiveness have been demonstrated (Fransen et al. 2001).

The Rheumatoid Arthritis Quality of Life (RAQOL) (see Wells et al. 1999) has 30 items with a yes/no response format and takes about 6 min to complete. It is reliable and valid.

Childhood arthritis

In children, polyarthritis affects musculoskeletal, psychological, and social growth and development. It may interfere with the attainment of educational goals. In adolescence and young adulthood it may interfere with the acquisition of job skills, with emancipation from parents, achieving economic independence, interacting with peers, self-esteem, body image, and finding a partner.

The evaluation of physical function and health status in young patients requires measures different than those used to assess health status of adults with rheumatic diseases. Health status in children is conceptualized as achieving normal development and participating fully in developmentally appropriate physical, psychological, and social activities. Moreover, pain reporting is different in children than adults with a tendency to report less pain. Self-report is not considered reliable in children whose developmental or chronological age is below 4 years and necessitates a proxy or performance testing.

In children with juvenile rheumatoid arthritis, research has focused on the assessment of gross and fine motor skills and the evaluation of disability and pain (Table 2).

Measures of developmental status

The Hoskins and Squires Test for Gross Motor and Reflex Development (Hoskins and Squires 1973) asks an infant to perform 60 voluntary physical tasks that are rated by a clinician on a scale from 1 to 4. The 'motor age' is calculated by finding the highest level where the subject can perform at least 50 per cent of the required voluntary skills. The assessment covers children from birth to 5 years with normal values derived from the literature. The instrument has been tested for interrater reliability and validity.

The Denver Development and Screening Test (DDST) (Frankenburg et al. 1970, 1971) consists of a questionnaire to parents and a simple observational screening test for children. The test covers personal–social, fine motor-adaptive, language, and gross motor skills and is applicable to children aged between 1 month and 6 years. Test scores are used to assess whether a child has achieved age standardized milestones.

The Newington Children's Hospital Juvenile Rheumatoid Arthritis Evaluation (Rhodes et al. 1988) measures quality of motor performance against chronological age at which the task is typically mastered on a scale of 0–4. The index assumes that central nervous system development is normal and that tasks are sequentially learned. Fifty-eight motor tasks are evaluated. The instrument is designed to assess children aged from 1 to 6 years.

Health status measures

The Adapted Arthritis Impact Measurement Scales for Children (CHAIMS) (see Duffy et al. 2000) apply components of the AIMS to children with juvenile arthritis. The pain scale is most reliable in children with active and inactive arthritis, and the physical activity and dexterity scales have reasonable reliability. The AIMS for children is administered by a health professional to the parents of an affected child.

The Childhood Health Assessment Questionnaire (CHAQ) (see Duffy et al. 2000) is based on the adult HAQ (Fries et al. 1980). The questionnaire is either parent or self-administered and can be used for all age groups. The CHAQ covers two domains, pain and disability. The CHAQ has been tested for validity and reliability and can be completed in less than 10 min.

The Juvenile Arthritis Functional Assessment Scale (JAFAS) (Lovell et al. 1989) is a series of timed tests using items from the AIMS, HAQ, and MHIQ and a consensus process among paediatric occupational and physical therapists experienced with patients with juvenile rheumatoid arthritis. The test is administered by a health professional, takes approximately 10 min to complete, and requires special equipment. The Juvenile Arthritis Functional Assessment Report (JAFAR) is a self-reported version of the JAFAS (see Duffy et al. 2000). The JAFAR-C is administered to children, the JAFAR-P to their parents. Patient and parent reports correlate highly with each other and with objective assessment by a physical/occupational therapist. Questionnaire scores were independent of the child's age. JAFAS and JAFAR are reliable and valid, but there is no published data on their sensitivity. JAFAS and JAFAR cannot be administered to children under 6 years of age.

The Rand Health Insurance Study Scale (HIS) (Eisen et al. 1980) assesses health status in children from birth to 13 years. It is administered by an interviewer who asks the parents questions. It has good metric properties (McCormick et al. 1986).

The Juvenile Arthritis Self Report Index (JASI) consists of 100 questions covering five dimensions (self-care, domestic, mobility, school, and extracurricular). The questions use a 7-point Likert scale. The instrument is reliable and valid. There are two drawbacks: it takes 30–50 min to complete and it is recommended for use only in children over 7 years (see Duffy et al. 2000).

The Juvenile Arthritis Quality of Life Questionnaire (JAQQ) contains 74 items which are part of four domains (gross motor function, fine motor function, psychosocial function, and general symptoms). In each dimension the average score of 5 items (with a Likert scale from 1 to 7) selected by the questioned person is calculated. For children younger than 9 years it is completed by the parents. It takes 20 min. There are no published data on its reliability, but it has been shown to be valid and sensitive to change (see Duffy et al. 2000).

A further measure, the Childhood Arthritis Health Profile (CAHP) has only been published as abstract (see Duffy et al. 2000).

Osteoarthritis

Osteoarthritis disability unfolds slowly, paralleling the ageing process. Its impact on function occurs at a time when expectations and physical demands are less. Several studies have shown that the radiographic appearance of osteoarthritis does not correspond with symptoms (Lawrence et al. 1966).

Patient-centred measures of osteoarthritis have concentrated on a careful assessment of pain and functional status. These include measures for evaluating specific interventions such as surgery, osteoarthritis-specific measures, and measures of generic health status.

Generic health status instruments (Table 1) covering dimensions of social function, emotional function, role function, pain, and physical function assess relevant domains to patients with chronic osteoarthritis.

Measures to evaluate osteoarthritis-specific interventions

Since the advent of total joint arthroplasty surgery, rating schemes have been used to evaluate the success of surgery (Larson 1963; Harris 1969) but until recently were unstandardized, untested for validity and reliability, and based solely on the surgeons assessment or anthropometric criteria, disregarding the patient's judgement.

It is not surprising, therefore, that whether a surgical intervention is judged as a success is dependent on the rating scale employed (Andersson 1972). In recognition of these limitations orthopaedic societies have led the way in developing psychometrically sound, standardized instruments in shifting over to groups of related joints and to the evaluation of all interventions rather than only joint arthroplasty (Liang et al. 1991; Johanson et al. 1992; Katz et al. 1995).

The Hip Rating Questionnaire (Johanson et al. 1992) is a standardized instrument to assess the outcome of total hip replacement. The questionnaire is one of the very few rating scales in orthopaedic surgery that has been tested for validity, reliability, and sensitivity to change. The domains of global impact of arthritic pain, walking, and function are represented in the self-administered questionnaire that can be completed in about 10 min.

Osteoarthritis-specific measures

The WOMAC (Table 3) is a 24-item questionnaire focusing on the domains of pain, stiffness, and physical disability. The items were selected from the AIMS and HAQ and supplemented by questions felt to be important by 100 patients with hip and knee osteoarthritis. The WOMAC is tested for validity, reliability, and sensitivity to change, and has been used as the principal outcome measure in studies of surgical, physiotherapy, and pharmacological interventions. The instrument is self-administered and takes approximately 10 min to complete. Two versions of the WOMAC are available, a version utilizing 5 point Likert response categories and a version scoring responses on a 10 cm visual analogue scale. Both scales produce comparable results.

The Lequesne Index (Lequesne et al. 1987) contains two scales, one for the hip and one for the knee. Each scale covers pain and discomfort, activities of daily living, and maximum walking distance. The hip scale includes a question on sexual function. The Lequesne Index has been widely used in clinical and epidemiological studies of osteoarthritis and is tested for validity and reliability. It can be completed in less than 10 min. A time period covered by the items is not defined and may affect its sensitivity.

Both scales have been widely used in clinical studies. However the psychometric properties and sensitivity of the WOMAC may be superior (Stucki et al. 1998).

The AIMS (Meenan et al. 1980) and the Stanford HAQ (Fries et al. 1980) have been applied as outcome measures in pharmacological, surgical, and rehabilitative interventions in osteoarthritis too.

Spondyloarthropathies

Besides involvement of the axial skeleton, joints, and entesopathy spondylitis in young adults may affect self-esteem, body image, and leisure (Table 3).

Measurements used to evaluate the efficacy of treatments in ankylosing spondylitis include spinal and chest movement, duration and severity of morning stiffness, and quality of sleep. Health status indices such as the HAQ or AIMS are not readily applicable to ankylosing spondylitis since the items which might be affected by spinal mobility and symptoms are sparse.

Daltroy et al. (1988) developed a functional status measure (S-HAQ) for patients with spondylitis by adding five items to the HAQ, to cover the activities identified to be most problematic in a survey of 300 British patients with ankylosing spondylitis. The instrument is valid, reliable, and sensitive to change.

Dougados et al. (1988) developed a 20 item functional index for the assessment of ankylosing spondylitis (Dougados Functional Index = DFI). An item inventory was derived from a consensus of three rheumatologists and this was reduced by statistical procedures. The Dougados Index is valid and reliable and shows sufficient responsiveness (Dougados et al. 1990).

S-HAQ appears at least as sensitive to change as the Dougados Index (Kuzis and Ward 1999).

The Leeds Disability Questionnaire (Abbott et al. 1994) assesses disability in ankylosing spondylitis, inquiring about four areas of function: mobility, bending down, reaching up and neck movements, and postures. The 16 item self-administered questionnaire is valid, reliable, and sensitive to change.

The Bath Ankylosing Spondylitis Functional Index (BASFI) (Calin et al. 1995) is a 10 item self-administered questionnaire to assess function and activities of daily living in patients with ankylosing spondylitis. The questionnaire takes less than 10 min to complete and has been tested for validity, reliability, and sensitivity to change.

Low back pain and other miscellaneous measures

A number of questionnaires have been specifically designed for people with back pain of mechanical or structural origin. Probably, the most widely used are the Oswestry Low Back Pain Disability Questionnaire (Fairbank et al. 1980), the Roland Disability Questionnaire derived from the Sickness Impact Profile (Roland and Morris 1983), and the Million Visual Analogue Scale (Million et al. 1982). Other measures have been reported (Mooney et al. 1976; Lankhorst et al. 1982; Lehmann et al. 1983; Evans and Kagan 1986; Lawlis et al. 1989; Coste et al. 1993; for LBOS, NASS, ABPS, RADL, and QBPDS see Kopec 2000).

The dimensions measured in all these instruments include pain, function, and pain-limited activities. The instruments whose indicators of

Table 3 Arthritis-specific measures—osteoarthritis and spondyloarthropathy

Instrument	Dimensions covered	Mode of administration	Time to complete (min)
Osteoarthritis			
Western Ontario McMaster University (WOMAC) Osteoarthritis Index[a] (Bellamy et al. 1988)	Physical disability, pain, stiffness	Self-administered	~10
Lequesne Index[a] (Lequesne et al. 1987)	Pain, discomfort, activities of daily living, walking distance (separate scale for hip and knee joint)	Interview	~10
Hip Rating Questionnaire (Johanson et al. 1992)	Pain, function, walking	Self-administered	~10
Hip Arthroplasty Outcome Evaluation Questionnaire (Katz et al. 1995)	Pain, function	Self-administered	~10
Spondyloarthropathy			
Health Assessment Questionnaire for the Spondyloarthropathies (S-HAQ) (Daltroy et al. 1988)	Physical disability (dressing and grooming, arising, eating, walking, hygiene, grip, activities), pain	Self-administered	~10
Dougados Functional Index[a] (Dougados et al. 1988)	Physical function	Self-administered	~10
Leeds Disability Questionnaire (Abbott et al. 1994)	Pain, mobility, bending, reaching, neck movement, posture	Self-administered	~10
Bath Ankylosing Spondylitis Functional Index[a] (Calin et al. 1995)	Physical function, activities of daily living	Self-administered	<10

[a] Recommended by OMERACT III and IV for clinical trials.

reliability and validity have been reported include the Roland Disability Questionnaire (Roland and Morris 1983), Oswestry Low Back Pain Disability Questionnaire (Fairbank et al. 1980), Million Visual Analogue Scale (Million et al. 1982), Dallas Pain Questionnaire (Lawlis et al. 1989), North American Spine Society (NASS) Lumbar Spine Outcome Assessment Instrument (Daltroy et al. 1996), Quebec Back Pain Disability Scale (QBPDS) (see Kopec 2000), Low Back Outcome Scale (LBOS) (see Kopec 2000), Aberdeen Back Pain Scale (ABPS) (see Kopec 2000), Resumption of Activities of Daily Living scale (RADL) (see Kopec 2000), and EIFEL Questionnaire (Coste et al. 1993). The responsiveness of the Roland Disability Questionnaire was at least as good as that of the full SIP (Deyo 1986). Sensitivity to change has been demonstrated for the Oswestry, Million, NASS, LBOS, RADL, and ABPS instruments.

Other outcome questionnaires have been developed for carpal tunnel syndrome (Levine et al. 1993; Katz et al. 1994a), shoulder pain (Roach et al. 1991), disability of arm, shoulder, and hand (DASH) (Navsarikar et al. 1999), fibromyalgia (Burckhardt et al. 1991), and to assess fatigue in systemic lupus erythematosus (Krupp et al. 1989).

Limitations of outcomes measures

Multidimensional instruments or sub-scales of these instruments have floors or ceilings in their capacity to detect change and this relates to the subject's baseline score and the number of items or gradations of change that address one end or the other of the continuum of the function observed (Stucki et al. 1996).

Psychometrically sound instruments assume that function can be measured in all patients with the same instrument. Function is relative and, therefore, a small change in an individual's function may make a lot of difference. A small change may be totally adequate for the person's needs, yet may not be statistically significant or captured by a questionnaire. Individualized quality of life and functional measures have been developed to capture patient priorities better, but whether the greater resources required to administer these measures results in sufficiently improved validity or responsiveness remains largely unexplored. Moreover, from a clinical perspective, not all activities of daily living are equal for a given patient, and the technology of eliciting preference weights is far from perfect (Thompson et al. 1982, 1984; Katz et al. 1994b). Additionally, preferences of the sick and anxious do not remain constant during the vicissitudes of rheumatic illnesses, which are characterized by chronicity and an unpredictable waxing and waning course. Values change also with time because people learn, adjust, or accommodate over the course of illness.

The measurement of specific functions in questionnaires may be too coarse for monitoring patients closely. For example, function of hand and fingers may be assessed by a question on difficulty with fastening buttons or doing zippers. More subtle change would be assessed more appropriately by impairment measures such as pinch strength and standardized dexterity measures.

Self-reported symptoms and function do not necessarily correlate with objective impairments (Spiegel et al. 1985; Katz et al. 1990a; Liang et al. 1991; Davis et al. 1992) underscoring the fact that self-reported information complements measures of impairment and vice versa.

Selection of appropriate measures

For research applications, one should only use instruments with demonstrated psychometric properties which have been published. See Box 1 for the selection of appropriate measures.

Published instruments are frequently revised and improved, and it is important to get the latest version.

The validity and reliability of an instrument are characteristics of the instrument for a specific population and a reevaluation in a new population may be desirable. The scale should cover the range of severity and the magnitude of the changes expected. A small pilot on individuals that are

Box 1 Selection of appropriate health status measures

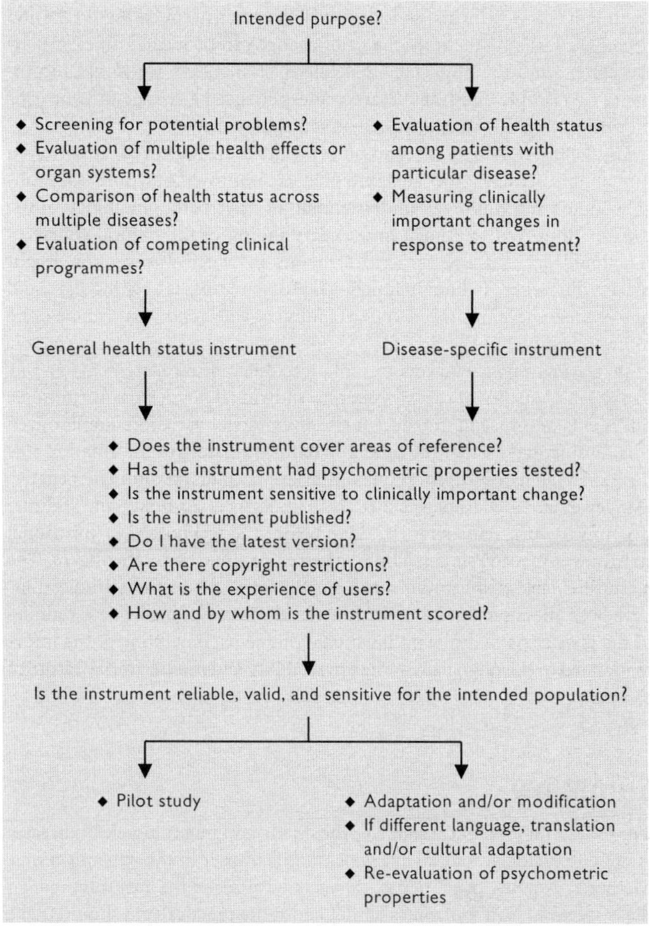

representative of the ones to be studied can be extremely informative. When a functional or health status measure is used in circumstances where language or cultural setting of the original instrument is different, a comprehensive procedure must be used to ensure its reliability and validity (Guillemin et al. 1994).

In selecting measures for clinical trials in rheumatic conditions one needs an understanding of the range of benefits and adverse effect that might be expected to get the best measure for each of the positive and negative consequences. It is also important to know how long it will take to the expected improvement. Traditional anthropometric measures should be supplemented by self-reported measures of physical function and health status. The battery should include a general health status measure if the results are to be used in health policy. If available, a disease-specific health status measure should also be used.

To the degree that psychosocial dysfunction results from the rheumatic condition, one would expect improvement of these parameters. However, prolonged psychological symptoms or innate traits are not likely to be helped by attention to for instance synovitis alone. In fact, a discrepancy between one's perceived function and objective signs of disease is often a clue that there is something else going on which needs attention.

General health status measures are needed in studies used in health policy in which decision makers must allocate resources to different conditions. The use of such scales in a clinical trial can help the investigator relate the findings to other diseases and the policy maker to understand the trade-offs in resource allocation. The use of a general health status measure may not capture the specific outcomes seen in a disorder. Disease-specific scales usually provide better coverage of dimensions of health thought to be important for that condition.

The evaluation should include a measure of whether or not a change has occurred and if the change was important to the patient, and whether the treatment was worthwhile considering all the positive effects on disease and negative effects. As the importance of change can be judged differently by the patient and the physician (Redelmeier et al. 1993), we would recommend two simple questions: 'Have you experienced a change in your condition?' (and, if so) 'Has this been an important change?'

Ultimately, if patient care and outcome are to be improved, attention to function must be incorporated into practice. Improved outcome will probably come from improved understanding of basic pathophysiology of the disease, improved treatment and understanding of the natural course of functional decline, and the critical points in which intervention might make a difference. To know a functional problem exists is only the start, and one needs to have improved understanding of when and what can be done to improve function.

Increasingly, policy makers are looking to outcome measurement as a way to assess the quality of care delivered by individual physicians, institutions, or systems of care, and to reduce ineffective practice variation. Randomized trials evaluating whether the collection of functional status information aids decision-making or improves outcomes have been disappointingly negative (McVey et al. 1989; Rubenstein et al. 1989; Kazis et al. 1990), and indicate that much work remains to be done before the technology of functional status assessment is successfully transferred to improved patient care. The reason for lack of improvement in functional status in these studies may have been the insensitivity of the functional measures, inadequate training of the physicians to deal with functional problems, the timing of the information fed to the physician, or the intractability and multifactorial nature of disability.

Summary

The evaluation of clinical status in rheumatic and musculoskeletal diseases is not complete without an assessment of its impact in the patient's terms. Measures evolving over the last 20 years have made the measurement of these so-called 'soft' outcomes harder and more practical and should make research and patient care more relevant to patient's concerns.

Acknowledgement

The authors would like to acknowledge Oliver Sangha (in memoriam), who was an author of this chapter in the previous edition.

References

Abbott, C.A., Helliwell, P.S., and Chamberlain, M.A. (1994). Functional assessment in ankylosing spondylitis: evaluation of a new self-administered questionnaire and correlation with anthropometric variables. *British Journal of Rheumatology* **33**, 1060–6.

Andersson, G. (1972). Hip assessment: comparison of nine different methods. *Journal of Bone and Joint Diseases* **54B**, 621–5.

Balaban, D.J., Sagi, P.C., Goldfarb, N.L., and Nettler, S. (1986). Weights for scoring the quality of well-being (QWB) instrument among rheumatoid arthritis: a comparison to general population weights. *Medical Care* **24**, 973–80.

Bellamy, N., Buchanan, W.W., Goldsmith, C.H., Campbell, J.J., and Stitt, L. (1988). Validation study of WOMAC: a health status instrument for measuring clinically important patient relevant outcomes to antirheumatic drug therapy in patients with osteoarthritis of the hip or knee. *Journal of Rheumatology* **15**, 1833–40.

Bergner, M., Babbitt, R.A., Pollard, W.E., Martin, D.P., and Gilson, B.S. (1976). The Sickness Impact Profile: validation of a health status measure. *Medical Care* **14**, 57–67.

Bombardier, C., Ware, J., Russell, I.J., Larson, M., Chalmers, A., Read, J.L., and the Auranofin Cooperating Group (1986). Auranofin therapy and quality of life in patients with rheumatoid arthritis: results of a multicenter trial. *American Journal of Medicine* **81**, 565–78.

Burckhardt, C.S., Clark, S.R., and Bennett, R.M. (1991). The fibromyalgia impact questionnaire: development and validation. *Journal of Rheumatology* **18**, 728–33.

Calin, A., Garrett, S., Whitelock, H., Kennedy, L.G., O'Hea, J., Mallorie, P., and Jenkinson, T. (1995). A new approach to defining functional ability in ankylosing spondylitis: the development of the Bath Ankylosing Spondylitis Functional Index. *Journal of Rheumatology* **21**, 2281–5.

Chambers, L.W., MacDonald, L.A., Tugwell, P., Buchanan, W.W., and Kraag, G. (1982). The McMaster Health Index Questionnaire as a measure of quality of life for patients with rheumatoid disease. *Journal of Rheumatology* **9**, 780–4.

Convery, F.R., Minteer, M.A., Amiel, D., and Connett, K.L. (1977). Polyarticular disability: a functional assessment. *Archives of Physical Medicine and Rehabilitation* **58**, 494–9.

Coste, J., LeParc, J.M., Berge, E., Delecouillerie, G., and Paolaggi, J.B. (1993). Adaptation and validation in French of a Disability Rating Scale for Low Back Pain Patients (The EIFEL Questionnaire). *Revue Rheumatism* (*English Edition*) **60**, 295–301.

Coulton, C.J., Zbarowsky, E., Lipton, J., and Newman, A.J. (1987). Assessment of the reliability and validity of the Arthritis Impact Measurement Scales for children with juvenile arthritis. *Arthritis and Rheumatism* **30**, 819–24.

Daltroy, L.H., Larson, M.G., Roberts, W.N., and Liang, M.H. (1988). A modification of the Health Assessment Questionnaire for the spondylarthropathies. *Journal of Rheumatology* **17**, 946–50.

Daltroy, L.H., Cats-Baril, W.L., Katz, J.N., Fossel, A.H., and Liang, H.H. (1996). The North American Spine Society outcome assessment instruments: reliability and validity tests. *Spine* **21**, 741–9.

Davis, M.A., Ettinger, W.H., Neuhaus, J.M., Barclay, J.D., and Segal, M.R. (1992). Correlates of knee pain among US adults with and without radiographic knee osteoarthritis. *Journal of Rheumatology* **19**, 1943–9.

Deyo, R.A. (1986). Comparative validity of the Sickness Impact Profile and shorter scales for functional assessment in low-back pain. *Spine* **11**, 951–4.

Deyo, R.A. and Carter, W.B. (1992). Strategies for improving and expanding the application of health status measures in clinical settings: a researcher–developer viewpoint. *Medical Care* **30** (Suppl.), MS176–86.

Deyo, R.A. and Inui, T.S. (1984). Towards clinical applications of health status measures: sensitivity of scales to clinical important changes. *Health Services Research* **19**, 275–89.

Deyo, R.A. and Patrick, D.L. (1989). Barriers to the use of health status measures in clinical investigation, patient care, and policy research. *Medical Care* **27**, S254–68.

Duffy, C.M., Tucker, L., and Burgos-Vargas, R. (2000). Update on functional assessment tools. *Journal of Rheumatology* **27**, 11–14.

Dougados, M., Gueguen, A., Nakache, J.-P., Nguyen, M., Mery, C., and Amor, B. (1988). Evaluation of a functional index and an articular index in ankylosing spondylitis. *Journal of Rheumatology* **15**, 302–7.

Dougados, M., Gueguen, A., Nakache, J.P., Nguyen, M., and Amor, B. (1990). Evaluation of a functional index for patients with ankylosing spondylitis. *Journal of Rheumatology* **17**, 1254–5.

Eisen, M., Donald, C.A., Ware, J.E., Jr, and Brook, R.H. *Conceptualization and Measurement of Health for Children in the Health Insurance Study.* Report Number R-2313-HEW. Santa Monica CA: Rand Corporation, 1980.

Evans, J.H. and Kagan, A. (1986). The development of a functional rating scale to measure the treatment outcome in chronic spinal patients. *Spine* **11**, 277–81.

Fairbank, J.C.T., Mbaot, J.C., Davies, J.B., and O'Brien, J.P. (1980). The Oswestry Low Back Pain Disability Questionnaire. *Physiotherapy* **66**, 271–3.

Frankenburg, W.K., Dodds, J., and Fandal, A. *The Denver Developmental Screening Test Manual.* Denver CO: Denver University Colorado Press, 1970.

Frankenburg, W.K., Camp, B.W., and Van Natta, P.A. (1971). Validity of the DDST. *Child Development* **42**, 475–85.

Fransen, J., Häuselmann, H., Michel, B.A., Caravatti, M., and Stucki, G. (2001). Responsiveness of the self-assessed rheumatoid arthritis disease activity index to a flare of disease activity. *Arthritis and Rheumatism* **44**, 53–60.

Fries, J.F., Spitz, P., Kraines, R.G., and Holman, H.R. (1980). Measurement of patient outcome in arthritis. *Arthritis and Rheumatism* **23**, 137–45.

Golden, W.E. (1992). Health status measurement. Implementation strategies. *Medical Care* **30** (Suppl.), MS187–95.

Guillemin, F., Bombardier, C., and Beaton, D. (1993). Cross-cultural adaptation of health-related quality of life measures: literature review and proposed guidelines. *Journal of Clinical Epidemiology* **46**, 1417–32.

Guyatt, G., Walter, S., and Norman, G. (1987). Measuring change over time: assessing the usefulness of evaluative instruments. *Journal of Chronic Diseases* **40**, 171–8.

Harris, W.H. (1969). Traumatic arthritis of the hip after dislocation and acetabular fractures: treatment by mold arthroplasty. An end-result study using a new method of result evaluation. *Journal of Bone and Joint Surgery* **51A**, 737–55.

Helewa, A., Goldsmith, C.H., and Smyth, H.A. (1982). Independent measurement of functional capacity in rheumatoid arthritis. *Journal of Rheumatology* **9**, 794–7.

Hochberg, M.C., Chang, R.W., Dwosh, I., Lindsey, S., Pincus, T., and Wolfe, F. (1992). The American College of Rheumatology 1991 revised criteria for the classification of global functional status in rheumatoid arthritis. *Arthritis and Rheumatism* **35**, 498–502.

Hoskins, T.A. and Squires, J.E. (1973). Developmental assessment: a test for gross motor and reflex development. *Physical Therapy* **53**, 117–25.

Howe, S., Levinson, J., Shear, E., Hanner, S., McGirr, G., Schulte, M., and Lovell, D. (1991). Development of a disability measurement tool for juvenile rheumatoid arthritis. *Arthritis and Rheumatism* **34**, 873–80.

Jette, A.M. (1980). Functional Status Index: reliability of a chronic disease evaluation instrument. *Archives of Physical Medicine and Rehabilitation* **61**, 395–401.

Johanson, M.A., Charlson, M.E., Szatrowski, T.P., and Ranawat, C.S. (1992). A self-administered hip rating questionnaire for assessment of outcome after total hip replacement. *Journal of Bone and Joint Surgery* **74A**, 587–97.

Kaplan, R.M., Bush, J.W., and Berry, C.C. (1976). Health status: types of validity for an index of well-being. *Health Services Research* **11**, 478–507.

Katz, J.N. et al. (1990a). Carpal tunnel syndrome: diagnostic utility of the history and physical examination findings. *Annals of Internal Medicine* **27**, 1495–8.

Katz, J.N., Larson, M.G., Phillips, C.B., Fossel, A.H., and Liang, M.H. (1990b). Comparative measurement sensitivity of short and longer health status measures. *Medical Care* **28**, 632–42.

Katz, J.N., Gelberman, R.H., Wright, E.A., Lew, R.A., and Liang, M.H. (1994a). Responsiveness of self-reported and objective measures of disease severity in carpal tunnel syndrome. *Medical Care* **32**, 1127–33.

Katz, J.N., Wright, E.A., Liang, M.H., and Cleary, P.D. (1994b). Differences between men and women undergoing orthopedic surgery for osteoarthritis. *Arthritis and Rheumatism* **37**, 687–94.

Katz, J.N. et al. (1995). The validity and reliability of a total hip arthroplasty outcome evaluation questionnaire. *Journal of Bone and Joint Surgery* **77A**, 1528–34.

Kazis, L.E., Anderson, J.J., and Meenan, R.F. (1989). Effect sizes for interpreting changes in health status. *Medical Care* **27**, 178–89.

Kazis, L.E., Callahan, L.F., Meenan, R.F., and Pincus, T. (1990). Health status reports in the care of patients with rheumatoid arthritis. *Journal of Clinical Epidemiology* **43**, 1243–53.

Keitel, W., Hoffman, H.L., and Weber, G. (1971). Ermittlung der prozentualen Funktionsminderung der Gelenke durch einen Bewegungsfunktionstest in der Rheumatologie. *Deutsches Gesundheitswesen* **26**, 1901–2.

Kopec, J.A. (2000). Measuring functional outcome in persons with back pain. *Spine* **25**, 3110–14.

Krupp, L.B., LaRocca, N.G., Muir-Nash, J., and Steinberg, A.D. (1989). The Fatigue Severity Scale: application to patients with multiple sclerosis and systemic lupus erythematosus. *Archives of Neurology* **46**, 1121–3.

Kuzis, S. and Ward, M.M. (1999). Validity and sensitivity to change of spondylitis-specific measures of functional disability. *Journal of Rheumatology* **26**, 121–7.

Lankhorst, G.J., Van de Stadt, R.J., Vogelaar, T.W., Van der Korst, J.K., and Prevo, A.J.H. (1982). Objectivity and repeatability of measurements in low back pain. *Scandinavian Journal of Rehabilitative Medicine* **14**, 21–6.

Larson, C.B. (1963). Rating scale for hip disabilities. *Clinical Orthopedics and Related Research* **31**, 85–93.

Lawlis, G.F., Cuencas, R., Selby, D., and McCoy, C.E. (1989). The development of the Dallas Pain Questionnaire. An assessment of the impact of spinal pain on behavior. *Spine* **14**, 511–16.

Lawrence, J.S., Breamer, J.M., and Brier, F. (1966). Osteoarthrosis: prevalence in the population and relationship between symptoms and X-ray changes. *Annals of the Rheumatic Diseases* **25**, 1–23.

Lee, P., Jasani, M.K., Dick, W.C., and Buchanan, W.W. (1973). Evaluation of a functional index in rheumatoid arthritis. *Scandinavian Journal of Rheumatology* **2**, 71–7.

Lehmann, T.R., Brand, R.A., and Gorman, T.W.O. (1983). A low back rating scale. *Spine* **8**, 308–15.

Lequesne, M.G., Mery, C., Samson, M., and Gerard, P. (1987). Indexes of severity for OA of the hip and knee. *Scandinavian Journal of Rheumatology* **65** (Suppl.), 85–9.

Levine, D.W. et al. (1993). Development and validation of symptom severity and functional status scales for carpal tunnel syndrome. *Journal of Bone and Joint Surgery* **75A**, 1585–92.

Liang, M.H. and Jette, A.M. (1981). Measuring functional ability in chronic arthritis: a critical review. *Arthritis and Rheumatism* **24**, 80–6.

Liang, M.H. et al. (1981). Evaluation of a pilot program for rheumatic disability in an urban community. *Arthritis and Rheumatism* **24**, 937–43.

Liang, M.H., Larson, M.G., Cullen, K.E., and Schwartz, J.A. (1985). Comparative measurement efficiency and sensitivity of five health status instruments for arthritis research. *Arthritis and Rheumatism* **28**, 542–7.

Liang, M.H., Katz, J.N., Phillips, C.B., Sledge, C.B., and Cats-Baril, W. (1991). The total hip arthroplasty outcome form of the American Academy of Orthopedic Surgeons. Results of a nominal group process. The American Academy of Orthopedic Surgeons Task Force on Outcomes Studies. *Journal of Bone and Joint Surgery* **73A**, 639–46.

Lovell, D.H. et al. (1989). Development of a disability measurement tool for juvenile rheumatoid arthritis. *Arthritis and Rheumatism* **32**, 1390–5.

McCormick, M.C., Stemmler, M.M., and Athreya, B.H. (1986). The impact of childhood rheumatic diseases on the family. *Arthritis and Rheumatism* **29**, 872–9.

McDowell, I.M., Martini, C.J.M., and Waugh, W. (1978). A method for self-assessment of disability before and after hip replacement operations. *British Medical Journal* **2**, 857–9.

McNevitt, M.C., Yelin, E.H., Henke, C.J., and Epstein, W.V. (1986). Risk factors for hospitalization and surgery for rheumatoid arthritis: implications for capitated medical payments. *Annals of Internal Medicine* **105**, 421–8.

McVey, L.J., Becker, P.M., Saltz, C.G., Feussner, J.R., and Cohen, H.J. (1989). Effect of a geriatric consultation on functional status of elderly hospitalized patients, a randomized, controlled trial. *Annals of Internal Medicine* **110**, 79–84.

Meenan, R.F., Gertman, P.M., and Mason, J.H. (1980). Measuring health status in arthritis: the Arthritis Impact Measurement Scales. *Arthritis and Rheumatism* **23**, 146–52.

Meenan, R.F., Mason, J.H., Anderson, J.J., Guccione, A.A., and Kazis, L.E. (1992). AIMS 2. *Arthritis and Rheumatism* **35**, 1–10.

Million, R., Hall, W., Nilsen, K.H., Baker, R.D., and Jayson, M.I.V. (1982). Assessment of the progress of the back-pain patient. *Spine* **7**, 204–12.

Mitchell, D.M., Spitz, P.W., Young, D.Y., Bloch, D.A., McShane, D.J., and Fries, J.F. (1986). Survival, prognosis, and causes of death in rheumatoid arthritis. *Arthritis and Rheumatism* **29**, 706–14.

Mooney, V., Cairns, D., and Robertson, J. (1976). A system for evaluating and treating chronic back disability. *Western Journal of Medicine* **124**, 370–6.

Navsarikar, A., Gladman, D.D., Husted, J.A., and Cook, R.J. (1999). Validity of the disabilities of arm, shoulder and hand questionnaire (DASH) for patients with psoriatic arthritis. *Journal of Rheumatology* **26**, 2191–4.

Patrick, D.L. and Deyo, R.A. (1989). Generic and disease-specific measures in assessing health status and quality of life. *Medical Care* **27**, S217–32.

Pincus, T., Summey, J.A., Soraci, S.A., Jr, Wallston, K.A., and Hummon, N.P. (1983). Assessment of patient satisfaction in activities of daily living using a modified Stanford Health Assessment Questionnaire. *Arthritis and Rheumatism* **26**, 1346–53.

Redelmeier, D.A., Rozin, P., and Kahneman, D. (1993). Understanding patient's decisions and emotional decisions. *Journal of the American Medical Association* **270**, 72–6.

Rhodes, V.J., Pumphrey, K.F., and Zemel, L. (1988). Development of a functional assessment tool for children with juvenile rheumatoid arthritis. *Arthritis and Rheumatism* **31** (Suppl. 4), S151.

Roach, K.E., Budiman-Mak, E., Songsiridej, N., and Lertratanakul, Y. (1991). Development of a shoulder pain and disability index. *Arthritis Care and Research* **4**, 143–9.

Roland, M. and Morris, R. (1983). A study of the natural history of back pain. Part I: Development of a reliable and sensitive measure of disability in low back pain. *Spine* **8**, 141–4.

Rubenstein, L.V., Calkins, D.R., and Young, R.T. (1989). Improving patient function: a randomized trial of functional disability screening. *Annals of Internal Medicine* **111**, 836–42.

Spiegel, J.S., Hirshfield, M.S., and Spiegel, T.M. (1985). Evaluating self-care activities: comparison of a self-reported questionnaire with an occupational therapist interview. *British Journal of Rheumatology* **24**, 357–61.

Steinbrocker, O., Traeger, C.H., and Battman, R.C. (1949). Therapeutic criteria in rheumatoid arthritis. *Journal of the American Medical Association* **140**, 659–62.

Stewart, A.L., Hays, R.D., and Ware, J.E. (1988). The MOS short-form general health survey. *Medical Care* **26**, 724–35.

Stucki, G., Stucki, S., Brühlmann, P., and Michel, B.A. (1995). Ceiling effects of the health assessment questionnaire and its modified version in some ambulatory rheumatoid arthritis patients. *Annals of the Rheumatic Diseases* **54**, 461–5.

Stucki, G., Daltroy, L.H., Katz, J.N., Johannesson, M., and Liang, M.H. (1996). Interpretation of change scores in ordinal clinical scales and health status measures. *Journal of Clinical Epidemiology* **49**, 711–17.

Stucki, G., Sangha, O., Stucki, S., Michel, B.A., Tyndall, A., Dick, W., Theiler, R. (1998). Comparison of the WOMAC (Western Ontario and McMaster Universities) Osteoarthritis Index and a Self Report Format of the Lequesne-Algofunctional Index in Patients with Knee and Hip Osteoarthritis. *Osteoarthritis Cart* **6**, 79–86.

Thompson, M.S., Read, J.L., and Liang, M.H. (1982). Willingness-to-pay concepts for societal diseases in health. In *Values and Long Term Care* (ed. R.L. Kane and R.A. Kane), pp. 103–5. Lexington MA: DC Health.

Thompson, M.S., Read, J.L., and Liang, M.H. (1984). Feasibility of willingness-to-pay measurement in chronic arthritis. *Medical Decision Making* **4**, 195–215.

Tugwell, P., Bombardier, C., Buchanan, W.W., Goldsmith, C.H., and Grace, E. (1987). The MACTAR Questionnaire—an individualized functional priority approach for assessing improvement in physical disability in clinical trials in rheumatoid arthritis. *Journal of Rheumatology* **14**, 446–51.

Wallston, K.A., Brown, G.K., Stein, M.J., and Dobbins, C.J. (1989). Comparing the short and long versions of the Arthritis Impact Measurement Scales. *Journal of Rheumatology* **16**, 1105–9.

Ware, J.E., Jr and Sherbourne, C.D. (1992). The MOS 36-item short-form health survey (SF-36). A. Conceptual framework and item selection. *Medical Care* **30**, 473–83.

Ware, J.E., Kosinski, M., and Keller, S.D. *SF-12. How to Score the SF-12 Physical and Mental Health Summary Scales.* Boston MA: The Health Institute, New England Medical Center, 1995.

Wells, G. et al. (1999) : Sensitivity to change of generic quality of life instruments in patients with rheumatoid arthritis. *Journal of Rheumatology* **26**, 217–21.

WHO (1958). Annex 1. Constitution of the World Health Organization. In *The First Ten Years of the World Health Organization*, p. 459. Geneva: WHO.

WHO. *International Classification of Functioning, Disability and Health* 1st edn. Geneva: WHO, 2001.

Wolfe, F., Hawley, D.J., Goldenberg, D.L., Russell, I.J., Buskila, D., and Neumann, L. (2000). *Journal of Rheumatology* **27**, 1989–99.

2.2 Rehabilitation of adults

Richard Haigh

Introduction

Rehabilitation is a process by which people disabled with injury or disease are able to regain their former abilities or, if full recovery is impossible, achieve their optimum potential (World Health Organization 1980). The rehabilitation approach aims to reduce disability and restore choice to individuals by concentrating on the consequence of disease, rather than the disease process and pathology itself. These definitions and statements serve to focus our approach to the disabled (or potentially disabled) patient with musculoskeletal disease and encourage, in the words of the World Health Organization (WHO), the use of 'all means' to achieve these goals.

Impairment, disability, and handicap

The WHO has developed a conceptual scheme for the assessment of the consequences of disease. Impairment, disability, and handicap distinguish between the anatomical and physiological results of disease and the psychosocial consequences such as the functional status of the individual.

- Impairment: Problems in body function or structure such as a significant alteration or loss.
- Disability: Any restriction or lack of ability to perform an activity.
- Handicap: The disadvantage suffered by the individual resulting from an inability to fulfil a role (depending on social and cultural factors).

This classification framework can be used to predict, guide, and plan the various needs of an individual. The WHO has released a new version of the International Classification of Functioning and Disability (Beta-2 version of ICIDH-2). ICIDH-2 organizes information according to three dimensions: body level, individual level, and society level (Table 1). Environmental factors form part of the classification. These have an impact on all three dimensions and are organized from the individual's most immediate environment to the general environment.

The biopyschosocial model

The classical medical approach emphasises diagnosis and treatment of a pathological process or disease. This Biomedical Model may neglect the secondary effects of disease and tends to polarise biological and psychological aspects of illness. Conversely, the Biopsychosocial Model addresses both the cause and the secondary effects of illness and injury, and acknowledges both the biological and psychosocial domains (Ferrari 2000). A rehabilitation approach formulates a patient centred action plan, setting goals in collaboration with a multidisciplinary team. These goals or outcomes are designed to increase the individual's potential, and are monitored throughout the rehabilitation process.

The rehabilitation process

Assessment

The assessment process should encompass a full evaluation of all the abilities of the patient and include the functional implications of each relevant symptom. It may be useful if the functional assessment is described in terms of the ICIDH framework (Table 1).

The following are important components of the rehabilitation assessment process:

- Assessment of disease activity/severity or stage of disease.
- Examine for and note: range of joint motion, muscle balance, strength and endurance, pain, cardiorespiratory, and neurological status.
- Evaluate the functional impact of impairments.

Table 1 An overview of ICIDH-2

	Part 1: Functioning and disability		Part 2: Contextual factors	
	Body functions and structures	**Activities and participation**	**Environmental factors**	**Personal factors**
Domains	Body functions Body parts	*Life areas* (task, actions)	*External* influences on functioning	*Internal* influences on functioning
Constructs	Change in body *function* (physiological) Change in body *structure* (anatomical)	*Capacity* executing tasks in a standard environment *Performance* executing tasks in the current environment	Facilitating or hindering impact of features of the physical, social, and attitudinal world	The impact of attributes of the person
Positive aspect	*Functional and structural integrity*	*Activity participation*	*Facilitators*	Not applicable
Negative aspect	*Impairment*	*Activity* limitation *Participation* restriction	*Barriers/hindrances*	Not applicable

Note: The Body dimension comprises two classifications, one for functions of body systems, and one for the body structure. *The Activities* dimension covers the complete range of activities performed by an individual. *The Participation* dimension classifies areas of life in which an individual is involved, has access to, and/or for which there are societal opportunities or barriers.

- Establish the impact on capacity and performance in personal, social, and vocational life areas.
- Determine the contextual factors such as physical environment.
- Development and implementation of a rehabilitation plan with patient and relevant team members.

The measurement of outcomes in rehabilitation

Outcomes have a high profile in health care practice. There is a need to clarify the desired outcome from an intervention, identify which interventions work and their utility in routine practice. These needs are important when dealing with individual patients as well as determining the needs of special groups.

Instruments designed to measure disability, handicap, and quality of life form a continuum with measures of impairment such as disease activity and radiology scores. The measures of handicap and quality of life give a broader perspective to the assessment of disease and its impact. Health care personnel tend to develop measures to assess what they think they can alter, and this is often reflected in what doctors, therapists, and family members regard as a treatment 'success'. However, recently there has been a re-emphasis on the notion that patients can report their perceptions of health impairment more effectively than doctors and health professionals.

There are several types of measure of disability and handicap, and many scores and questionnaires have been developed. These can be global, generic, disease specific, or dimension specific. The two most common instruments purporting to measure functional status in arthritis are the Health Assessment Questionnaire (HAQ) and the Arthritis Impact Measurement Scale (AIMS-2) (Fries et al. 1982; Meenan et al. 1992). The AIMS is a complex instrument comprising several dimensions including physical and social function, activities of daily living (ADL), and level of activity, as well as pain, mood, and anxiety. The HAQ can be viewed as a measure of self-perceived handicap, which takes account of the use of devices and aids. The physical disability scale of the HAQ is most often used. By using all the information gained from its 20 questions, rather than using scores from the eight categories, more useful information may be obtained. Also, the technique of Rasch Analysis can be employed to convert its ordinal scale to a linear scale to develop a hierarchical model that demonstrates the variation in difficulty of the various items. In comparison to other health status measures, the HAQ appears less sensitive to changes in mobility and pain, whilst AIMS is less sensitive to changes in social function. There does not seem to be a single instrument that is sensitive to change in all domains, which can be used as a generic health status measure.

Health status instruments attempt to measure a combination of disability, handicap, and quality of life. There is a considerable overlap with regard to the meaning of the terms handicap, disease impact, quality of life, and general health status, and overlap in the instruments that attempt to measure these subjective multidimensional constructs. Most of these measures are questionnaires that contain a series of questions or items in domains that include physical, psychological, emotional, and social well being. Alternatively, some require an independent observer. Table 2 contains examples of a series of instruments used to measure outcome, using RA and lower back pain as examples.

Table 2 Examples of outcome measures for rheumatoid arthritis and lower back pain

Modality measured	Rheumatoid arthritis	Lower back pain
Disease activity	Joint count[1]	
Pain	Visual Analogue Scale McGill Pain Questionnaire[2]	
Impairment	Joint deformity Radiology Score	Spinal range of motion
Disability/function	*RA specific:* AIMS-2[3] *General:* HAQ[4]	Oswestry LBP Disability Questionnaire[5]
Handicap and general health status	Short Form-36[6]	
Quality of life	EuroQoL Thermometer[7] Nottingham Health Profile[8]	
Psychological impact/ coping	*RA specific:* Coping with Rheumatic Stressors[9]	Coping Strategies Questionnaire[10]
	RA specific: Arthritis Self-Efficacy Scale[11]	General Self-Efficacy Scale[12]
	Beck Depression Inventory[13]	

1, Fuchs (1989); 2, Melzack (1975); 3, Meenan (1992); 4, Fries (1982); 5, Fairbank (1980); 6, Garratt (1993); 7, Euroquol group (1990); 8, Hunt et al. (1981); 9, van Lankveld et al. (1994); 10, Rosenstiel and Keefe (1983); 11, Lorig (1989); 12, Barlow (1996); 13, Beck (1961).

Multidisciplinary teamwork

Successful teamwork will lead to a better chance of resolving the patient's problem to their satisfaction. Ideally, members of the multidisciplinary team (MDT) will separately assess the patient, and then bring their discipline-specific goals to contribute to a management plan. To maximize the efficiency of MDT working, certain 'Ground Rules' have to be acknowledged:

- Team members have clearly defined roles.
- Clear lines of communication identified.
- Defined method of documenting decisions.
- Defined problem solving process by which decisions are made.
- An efficient, consistent, and evidence based decision making procedure.

The value of specialized services for rheumatology patients is taken for granted, though the evidence is not as convincing as many health care professionals might assume. Nevertheless, a meta-analysis concluded that MDT programmes for rheumatoid arthritis (RA) patients deliver better outcomes when compared with routine hospital outpatient follow-up (Vliet Vlieland and Hazes 1997). Self-management strategies have a positive effect on outcome in rheumatoid arthritis (RA), osteoarthritis, and chronic pain syndromes (see below).

Practical rehabilitation interventions in musculoskeletal disease

It is often difficult to tease out which part of a complex intervention or rehabilitation process is producing change, and in this respect it is difficult to produce strong evidence in support of many 'rehabilitation' interventions (Clarke 1999). The literature is full of studies that do not help decision making about effectiveness because of poor study design. These limitations include small numbers and lack of power, poor definition of case or diversity of condition, non-conformity of intervention, and differing non-standard outcome measures. Nonetheless, the lack of quality evidence for an intervention does not mean that the intervention is worthless or ineffective.

The prescription of exercise

Exercise is useful to humans, and there are many physiological and psychological benefits derived from habitual physical activity.

These include:

- General
  - endurance
  - reduces obesity
  - reduces platelet aggregation
- Cardiovascular/respiratory
  - increase in maximal oxygen uptake and cardiac output/stroke volume and reduced heart rate at given oxygen uptake
  - reduced blood pressure
  - increased efficiency of myocardium and vascularization
  - reduced cardiac morbidity and mortality
- Muscle
  - increased muscle strength
  - increased vascular supply
  - increased aerobic activity of muscle enzymes
- Joint
  - increases and maintains joint range of motion
  - increases co-ordination
  - improved biomechanical joint function
- Bone
  - can increase bone density and prevent/reduce osteoporosis
- Endocrine
  - beneficial effect on glucose tolerance and lipoprotein profile
- Psychological
  - enhanced perception of well being
  - reduced perception of exertion at a given work rate

Patients with RA have reduced muscle bulk, muscle strength, endurance, and aerobic capacity. There is a vicious cycle of pain, joint destruction, immobility, and reflex muscle inhibition leading to reduced joint protection, further mechanical stressors and ultimately, joint failure. Reduced muscle bulk and function also has an effect on balance and gait, and may predispose the individual to falls.

Range of motion, flexibility, and muscle imbalance

There is no increase in muscle strength gained from range of motion (ROM) exercises, though it is essential for immobile patients to have a daily regime of ROM exercises to maintain mobility of the joint. These exercises can prevent fixed deformity and contracture, and may have a role in maintaining normal joint physiology. ROM exercises can be active, assisted, or passive. Patients unable to perform active ROM exercise can be aided by a therapist or in certain situations, use continuous passive motion machines. ROM exercises can also enhance venous return in immobilized patients. Care must be taken not to provoke pain and damage to the joint with full range of motion exercises.

There are many techniques to increase flexibility, which can reduce the chance of injury and post-exercise pain, especially in myofascial pain syndromes. Muscle imbalance is a common finding in back pain and soft tissue problems, as well as in inflammatory and degenerative arthropathy. Exercises directed towards strengthening specific muscle groups may help restore muscle balance.

Active exercise

There are three types of contraction of a muscle or muscle group that can be used in an exercise programme—isometric, concentric, and eccentric. In isometric contractions there is no joint motion, and the muscle is exercised against a rigid object or with the aid of a therapist. Many patients can identify pain free postures and positions, enabling isometric exercises to be attempted, even when a joint is inflamed. However, the gain in strength is made at the joint angle of the exercises. It is not clear whether this gain can be generalized to other ranges of joint motion. Isometric exercises are able to increase muscle strength, but concentric contractions are probably more effective at increasing the bulk (cross sectional area) of the muscle. Concentric contractions are those in which the muscle shortens during contraction, and the force developed is in the direction of the movement. During eccentric contractions, the muscle is lengthened and pulled in the opposite direction during contraction by gravity, antagonist muscles, or devices. Dynamometer studies show, counter intuitively, that the greatest peak forces are in action during eccentric contractions, rather than with concentric contractions.

Dynamic exercise

Dynamic exercise therapy (i.e. exercises of low to moderate aerobic intensity) is used to increase aerobic capacity and muscle strength. Dynamic exercise therapy is a useful tool to reduce impairement in RA, though there is no strong evidence for a positive effect on function and disability (Van den Ende et al. 2000). One possible explanation for the lack of effect on disability is that outcome measures, such as the HAQ, do not reflect fatigue, levels of activity, and work ability. Improvement in these dimensions may be hidden. There have been suggestions that exercise may have a positive effect on swollen joint counts and on radiological progression, though these are not general findings. The anecdotal charge that exercise is detrimental to RA joints, however, can be challenged with confidence. There is no evidence that dynamic exercise therapy will exacerbate RA, nor any suspicion that it will promote radiological joint damage.

Aerobic exercise

Patients with arthritis have a reduced aerobic conditioning compared with age–sex matched controls. An aerobic training programme (e.g. aiming at 30–40 min of aerobic exercise reaching a target heart rate, three to four times a week), can increase aerobic capacity, walk times, and have psychological benefits. Low impact exercise, such as walking or swimming, is generally recommended. However, high resistance muscle strengthening programmes in patients with advanced OA can be undertaken with a low probability of further joint damage.

Wherever possible, exercise should be put in a social context, taking advantage of local leisure facilities that patients can have access to outside the hospital environment. In addition, advice on appropriate footwear for exercise is an essential part of the programme. Generally speaking, the residual benefit of an exercise programme drops off rapidly if exercises are not maintained, and especially if there is no supervision or arrangements made for review during the 'home exercise' period (Chamberlain et al. 1982).

Hydrotherapy

Water allows the almost wholly immersed body to have the benefit of buoyancy, which can nearly overcome the effect of gravity, thereby supporting body weight. Subsequently, the load through joints is reduced and the muscular effort required to move a joint or body part is minimized. Few studies have demonstrated the benefit of hydrotherapy over land based exercises, but there is no doubt that it has a place in the battery of physical therapy and exercise modalities, and is popular with patients. For example, patients unable to fully weight bear on land, often after major joint reconstruction surgery may benefit. Spa therapy or balneotherapy implies lying or soaking in hot spa water. It is important to recognize the physiological consequences of being immersed in warm water (renal, cardiovascular, respiratory effects and that there are contraindications to its use, e.g. ischaemic heart disease and skin ulceration).

Exercise in special situations

Idiopathic inflammatory myopathy

The underlying mechanisms responsible for the biochemical muscle abnormalities and loss of muscle function have not been defined in myosites. The disease process produces muscle weakness, pain, and fatigue resulting in disuse and inactivity. Cardiorespiratory involvement may also reduce activity and aerobic capacity. However, a training programme for patients with chronic muscle disease can be instituted without adversely affecting disease activity. For example, a programme including stationary cycling and step aerobics resulted in improvements in strength, oxygen uptake, activities of daily living (ADL) score, and well being (Wiesinger et al. 1998). Theoretically, concentric and isometric exercises should be employed because of possible ultrastructural damage to muscle with eccentric exercise. In active disease, ROM exercises are recommended, as contractures can develop quickly (often associated with muscle and sub-cutaneous calcification in children).

Ankylosing spondylitis

A regular programme of exercise should include ROM, stretching and strengthening, spinal extension, and aerobic exercise. The exercise programme should be carried out regularly by the individual, but can also be reinforced by group exercise. The optimum frequency and duration has not been determined. Patients with ankylosing spondylitis (AS) frequently complain of exercise intolerance and experience a decrease in aerobic capacity largely due to peripheral muscle function, deconditioning, and subjective fatigue rather than limitation of chest wall movements. Other useful approaches includes posture and sleep advice (sleep on firm mattress, thin pillow, regular periods of prone lying—approximately 20 min twice a day). Simple ergonomic measures include the use of an upright chair, an eye-level VDU screen, and a reading stand. All these measures are intended to prevent excessive spinal flexion.

Lower back pain

Exercise programmes are commonly used in the management of acute lower back pain (LBP), often in combination with other treatment modalities. Exercise programmes often involve flexion and extension exercises, isometric exercises (especially for abdominal and trunk muscles) and general aerobic fitness. Exercise regimes (general fitness or back specific) do not improve pain or functional status in acute LBP (van Tulder et al. 2000). In chronic LBP however, exercise therapy is more useful, but ineffective in providing long-term benefit or prevention of relapse. A generalized progressive exercise regimen aiming at global fitness, rather than back specific fitness, may be a more appropriate approach to reduce disability (Klaber Moffett et al. 1999). In general, the effects of exercise are largely short rather than long term and too few studies address the issue of 'return to work'.

Joint protection

Joint protection regimens aim to reduce pain, conserve energy, and help patients use strategies to reduce strain on their joints. Theoretically, less mechanical loading of a joint will lead to a reduction of local joint inflammation and pain.

Joint protection programmes include an educational component addressing posture, positioning and alignment, energy conservation, exercises, use of assistive devices, and adaptation of tasks and work patterns. Educational material is often provided such as leaflets and videotapes. Aids and appliances may be tried or demonstrated. There may be behavioural elements to some programmes (discussed below). Occupational therapists or physiotherapists usually deliver these programmes, but other MDT members may contribute. Joint protection can be taught on an individual basis, though it also lends itself to working with groups. These interventions have a well-defined short-term positive effect on pain and functional status, but the long-term benefits are not clear. However, a recent report described a comparison of an educational–behavioural programme with a standard joint protection programme, producing benefits in pain, function and disease activity measures that became more apparent at 1 year follow-up (Hammond and Freeman 2001).

Physical modalities

Therapeutic heat and cold

Heat and cold are amongst the most common modalities used to treat arthritis. Most studies on heat and cold show some beneficial effect on pain, joint ROM, grip strength, stiffness and function, though the supporting evidence is certainly not robust. Therapeutic heat and cold can be delivered in a number of ways (Table 3).

Therapeutic heat can reduce muscle tension and spasm, and increase the extensibility of connective tissue. Thus, heat can be applied prior to stretching and range of motion exercises. However, heat can exacerbate oedema and swelling, and due to the increase in enzymatic activity associated with an increase in temperature induced by deep heat, it can also theoretically promote joint damage and pain in active inflammatory joint disease. Therefore, superficial heat is generally used in arthritic joints. Cold can

Table 3 The delivery of therapeutic heat and cold

Heat		Cold
Infrared Liquid paraffin Hot packs Heating pad or mitten Heated pool/spa	Superficial heat (~1 cm below surface)	Ice packs Ice water Vapocoolant Baths
Short/medium wave diathermy Ultrasound	Deep heat (3–6 cm below surface)	

increase local pain threshold, reduce swelling and oedema, and also reduce muscle spasm. Nevertheless, some patients cannot tolerate ice packs at all.

Transcutaneous electrical nerve stimulation

Transcutaneous electrical nerve stimulation (TENS) is widely used for the treatment of arthritis and spinal pain. TENS is delivered by electrodes attached to the skin, connected to a small stimulator unit, which can be carried on a belt or in a pocket. The frequency, intensity and nature (pulsed or continuous, above or below sensory threshold) of applied stimulation, the position and size of the electrodes, and the duration of treatment can all be varied. Some patients have difficulty attaching the electrodes and operating the small dials and buttons on the stimulator box. TENS is used most widely for myofascial pain syndromes and spinal pain, and appears to be of most use in the chronic pain setting. TENS worn adjacent to certain joints (e.g. wrist and knee) may reduce pain and improve function. The inadequacy of control treatments and a strong placebo effect hinders an objective assessment of its efficacy. However, it is non-invasive, cheap and has few side effects.

Acupuncture

This ancient form of anaesthetic and treatment modality can be delivered by two distinct methods—Eastern Chinese and Western; each has its own theoretical basis. Whilst many patients with arthritis and spinal pain utilize complimentary therapies such as acupuncture principally for the relief of pain, the results of good quality trials do not support its use. In OA, the most rigorous studies suggest that both acupuncture and sham needling reduce the pain of OA to roughly the same degree (Ernst 1997). Systematic reviews of randomized controlled trials of acupuncture for neck pain and back pain provide similar conclusions.

Manipulation, mobilization, and massage techniques

Manipulation and mobilization techniques use 'a skilled passive movement to a joint (or spinal motion segment) either within or beyond its active range of motion' to treat arthritis and pain syndromes. The exact mechanism of pain relief is unclear, but may be due to raising the pain threshold, easing of muscle spasm, local circulatory effects, reduction in disc protrusion, changes in joint range of motion and psychological effects.

Spinal manipulation is a popular form of treatment, especially for both acute and chronic lower back pain, and is prescribed by many rheumatologists, yet debate about its clinical efficacy rages. The published evidence lends some weight towards supporting the use of manipulation, but poor methodology has complicated the assessment of many published trials. Sham-controlled, double blind, randomized clinical trials suggest that spinal manipulation is not associated with clinically relevant specific therapeutic effects (Ernst and Harkness 2001). It is important to note that manipulation may be associated with neurological complications, especially cervical spine manipulation. Interestingly, in a study comparing costs, chiropractors were shown to be the most expensive health care providers for patients with back pain with more visits to the chiropractor per LBP episode and higher outpatient costs (Shekelle et al. 1995).

There are various massage techniques involving stroking, kneading, friction, and percussion. Massage may have some potential as a therapy for LBP and for the treatment of muscle soreness after unaccustomed exercise.

Traction as treatment for spinal pain has been described since ancient times. By pulling, hanging, or motorized traction the vertebrae are said to be distracted and the presumed protruded disc is reduced. It would seem logical that acute LBP due to disc prolapse may benefit from traction though the published evidence is inconclusive.

Immobilization techniques

A formalized period of bed rest can be used to treat a flare of inflammatory arthritis, though this must be short-lived (less than 2 weeks) and could be combined with a simple exercise programme to maintain joint range of motion. Selective rest or splinting of a particular joint will result in reduction of inflammation. The negative effects of prolonged bed rest must be considered such as stiffening of periarticular structures, joint contracture, muscular weakness, and osteoporosis. It is rare for contracture to develop within 2–4 weeks of bed rest.

Taping or the application of devices that restrict their action can alter the forces developed by muscles. For example, medial taping of the patella can reduce pain in anterior knee pain syndrome or osteoarthritis of the knee. Taping can also be applied about the shoulder to aid control of posture and exercises restoring muscle balance. An epicondylitis clasp or brace can restrict the function of the forearm extensor apparatus, thus easing the pain of lateral epicondylitis.

Orthotics, aids and appliances, and environmental adaptation

Orthotics

An orthosis is a device worn outside the body that aids function, protects, or prevents pain. Orthoses may be custom-made or provided 'off the shelf'. An increasing variety of materials are being used to construct orthoses. Thermoplastics and alloys are superseding leather and steel, and Velcro™ and plastic loops are replacing straps and hooks.

Certain factors must be considered prior to the supply of an orthosis, for example, stability, alignment and integrity of the joint and surrounding muscle and ligament. Also, an assessment of cutaneous sensation and proprioception, vascular status, and skin integrity are mandatory and will greatly influence prescription. A trained orthotist or an experienced physician should review the prescription, preferably several weeks after supply.

Walking aids

The choice of a walking aid for an arthritis patient must take into account the extent of involvement of lower and upper limbs, and the terrain to be negotiated. A patient may require a variety of walking aids to use under different circumstances. Any walking aid that is prescribed should be fitted and checked by an experienced physiotherapist, who will be able to instruct the patient in its use and ensure that it is both correctly adjusted and in safe working order.

Crutches are often not appropriate for the RA patient. For example, elbow crutches cannot be used if a patient has over 40° fixed flexion of the elbow. In this situation, gutter type crutches with forearm supports may be required so a greater area of upper limb can take the load. However, these crutches are heavier and not as stable as axillary or elbow crutches.

If a walking stick is required it is held in the hand opposite the affected leg, increasing the size of the patient's base and taking some weight through the limb holding the stick. Some patients only need a walking stick outside the home, especially on uneven ground. Patients with RA may need a walking stick with a broad handle such as a Fischer stick.

It is necessary to make the simple but important point that a patient's mobility in the home is often improved or falls prevented by adequate lighting, reducing obstacles (often furniture), the removal of loose rugs, and fixing carpets.

Aids and appliances

In general, aids and appliances help to treat disability. Any functional limitation must be carefully defined, working with the patient, to provide an appropriate aid. Devices may compensate for either pain, weakness or for lack of joint range. Articles must be lightweight, strong and reliable, cheap, and acceptable to the patient and family. Patients must have adequate opportunity to trial these items before supply or purchase.

Devices used to compensate for poor handgrip function include large handles and knobs, key-holders, Velcro™ fasteners for garments, and jar and tin lid-opening aids. Aids such as trays, trolleys, and carts can get around difficulties with carrying objects. Problems with balance and rising from a sitting position make bathing difficult. Raised seats and bath-seats and lifts can be installed. The requirement to bend down whilst sitting or standing can be reduced by using long handled aids such as shoehorns, reaching aids, and cleaning implements, which can extend effective reach.

Environmental control

For a severely disabled patient, life may become a series of near impossible tasks that an able-bodied person can perform without thought, special attention or effort. Effective Environmental Control Systems (ECS) can improve the lives of many patients with severe disability by carrying out some of these tasks with the aid of technology, restoring the individual's independence and dignity. Following a comprehensive rehabilitation needs assessment, members of both the hospital and community based teams can consider an appropriate package which may include intervention with mobility aids, communication devices and ECS (British Society for Rehabilitation Medicine 1994).

ECS equipment is comprised of three components—a selection unit, an input from the user and various controlled appliances (Fig. 1). A lack of dexterity or a degree of cognitive impairement is no contraindication to ECS use. Using scanning software and an appropriate on–off switch, almost any movement that is under reliable voluntary control may be used to operate an environmental control unit. An assortment of switches are used for user input, and these can be mounted on a wheelchair, bedside, or can be completely portable. Switches come in many shapes and forms and may be a joystick, lever, keyboard, pressure pad, or suck/blow. ECS can control home security (personal alarms, door entry systems), communication aids, and appliances (home entertainment equipment and computers). Control of wheelchairs, voice control systems, synthetic speech output equipment, and the use of robotics are being developed for use in conjunction with ECS.

Wheelchairs

Some individuals consider the use of a wheelchair as an admission of defeat, but it may actually increase access and opportunity, especially in those patients that have limited outdoor mobility. It may also allow conservation of energy for more productive use. Attendant-operated chairs have small wheels that can be difficult to negotiate over kerbs. Self-propelling wheelchairs have larger wheels that make them easier to push. Many patients with arthritis will be unable to self-propel over any distance because of upper limb impairment, especially at the shoulder. Armrest position and seat height are important in determining how easy it is to get in and out of the chair. Special adaptations may have to be made to wheelchairs for patients with arthritis. For example, leg rests can accommodate lower limb deformity. Patients who spend much of their time in a wheelchair are at risk of pressure sores. They may require an appropriate pressure-relieving cushion as part of a special seating package, which should be dealt with by a specialist clinic. If there is difficulty propelling a wheelchair, consideration should

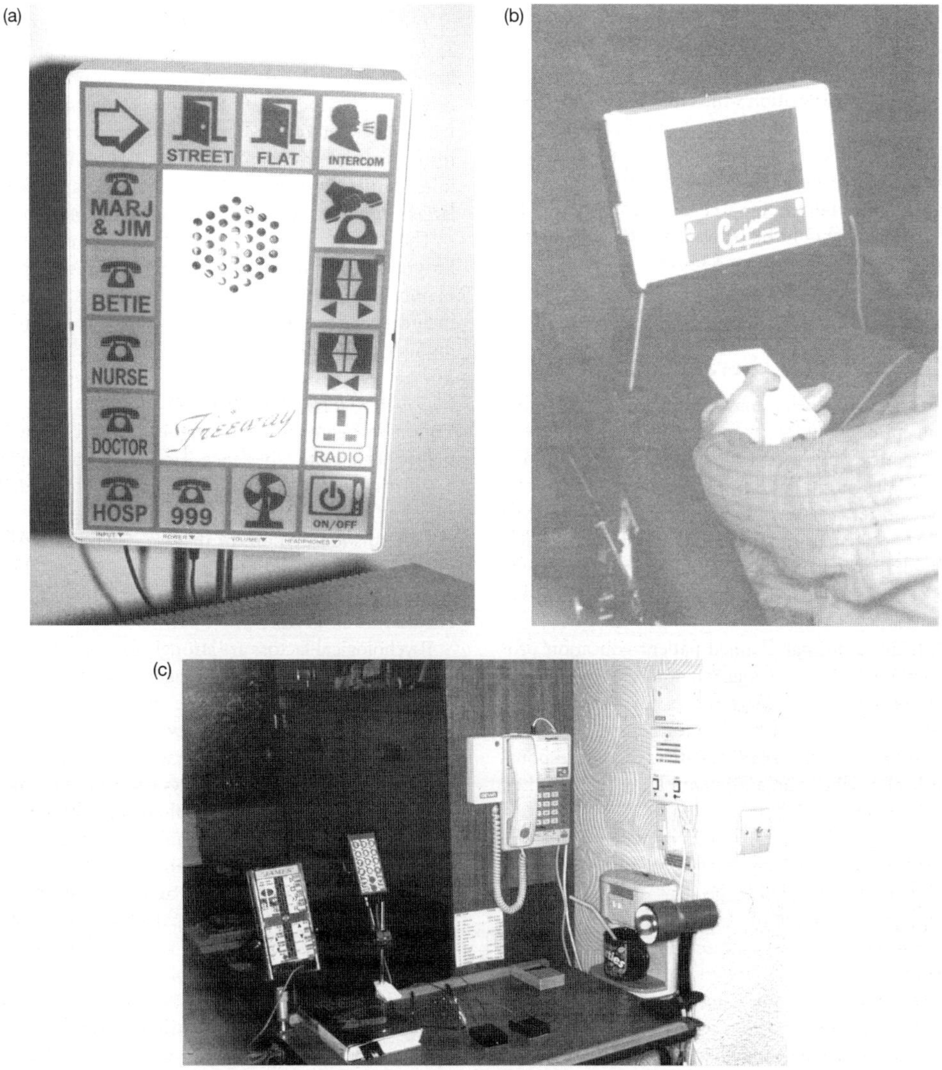

Fig. 1 Environmental control systems. (a) Control unit, (b) the input switch and control unit being used, and (c) a typical 'workstation' with ECS mounted onto desk.

be given to the prescription of an electric chair. The shape and position of the control may need to be modified for an arthritic patient.

If a wheelchair is contemplated, other factors in and around the home must be considered. Ramps may be needed, internal doorframes must be wide enough to pass through without trapping fingers, and there has to be room to manoeuvre. Patients may require equipment such as grab rails or a sliding board.

Driving

In most countries, if an individual develops arthritis that affects driving ability, the licensing authority must be informed. If severely affected, they may be required to undertake another driving test or assessment, which may be provided at a specialist centre. Patients unable to walk more than 100 m may be entitled to a disabled parking permit to facilitate convenient parking, obtained through the local government authority. Minor adjustments may make driving safer and more comfortable and include:

- steering wheel adaptation (padded cover or knobs)
- extra side-mirrors and additions to rear view mirror
- power steering and an automatic gearbox
- swivelling seats
- wheelchair hoists

Disability legislation

In many countries, disability legislation [such as The Disability Discrimination Act (UK) and The Americans with Disabilities Act (USA)] has been introduced to end the discrimination which many disabled people face. For example, attempts to protect disabled people in the areas of employment, access to goods, facilities, and services, and the management, buying or renting of land or property have been made. Requirements are also made of schools, colleges, and universities to provide information for disabled people. These measures should help to dismantle the barriers facing an individual, and facilitate participation in society.

Self-management strategies: patient education programmes and behavioural therapy

For an individual, the burden of arthritis may be immense. The future seems congested with pain episodes, disability, and the unravelling of social support networks. Not all patients can accept the uncertainties about diagnosis, drug treatments, and prognosis, and some have unrealistic expectations. Patients may often seek alternative methods of dealing with their chronic disease, which may not be part of a traditional Western approach. Moreover, non-medical factors, such as beliefs, attributions, behaviours, and perceived needs, play a major role in determining the consequence of chronic musculoskeletal disease.

In the face of such difficulties, formal planned patient education programmes have a fundamental role in the management of chronic musculoskeletal disease. The development of programmes for patients with arthritis, autoimmune diseases, and pain syndromes concord with the Biopsychosocial Model approach described earlier. Patients accept responsibility for changing their health behaviour, and obtain knowledge of their disease and its treatment (Edworthy 2000).

Certain concepts underpin the behavioural aspects of patient education programmes. Self-efficacy describes the confidence to undertake goal directed behaviour and it is task or behaviour specific—a patient may be confident to effect change in one aspect of their life, but not another. Appropriate levels of knowledge and realistic expectations are required to compliment confidence or self-efficacy, so that decisions can be made and goals achieved. Patient education programmes aim to teach not only new skills, but also the confidence to put them into practice in everyday life. The concept of 'learned helplessness'—the sense that external events control one's destiny is also relevant. Patients with arthritis often feel like 'an innocent bystander' with an unpredictable disease in amongst a complicated health care and social system. Again, self-management techniques aim to transfer the feeling of 'external' controlling factors, to a state where the individual has an increased sense of self-determination.

The contents of education and behavioural programmes can be very varied, though most include:

- *Educational elements*—disease specific anatomy and physiology, drugs, joint protection, nutrition, health and social systems
- *Cognitive elements*—cognitive restructuring, planning and problem solving, attention diversion, assertiveness and communication, recognizing depression and anxiety
- *Behavioural*—pacing exercise and activity, relaxation, rehearsal and practice of skills

The methods of delivery and location (community, primary care, hospital setting) of these programmes is also variable. Clinically meaningful improvements in pain, disability, fatigue, and depression have been demonstrated in a number of settings following arthritis patient education programmes. The benefits are estimated to be greater than or equal to prescription of NSAID, and are low cost. The evidence documenting these is strong (Lorig 1995), and though follow-up is usually limited to 1 year, some report benefits detectable for up to 5 years (Lindroth et al. 1995). The issue now is not whether arthritis education programmes improve the symptoms of patients with arthritis, but which elements of these programmes are most important and how can delivery be improved.

The utility of combined educational and exercise interventions, such as 'Back Schools' (BS) in spinal pain is less clear (Koes et al. 1994). The BS approach is mainly an education and skills programme with an exercise regimen, but may include a collection of processes such as posture advice and management, a formal exercise programme, biomechanical, and ergonomic instruction and sometimes cognitive–behavioural elements. There are definite short-term benefits of this intensive approach, which unfortunately, largely disappear within months after the intervention is completed.

There is now considerable overlap between arthritis patient education programmes and cognitive–behavioural therapy (CBT) interventions, mainly because pure educational learning is not as effective as learning that includes a behavioural element. Cognitive–behavioural interventions are discussed separately below.

Cognitive–behavioural therapy programmes

Cognitive–behavioural therapy is a process in which patients reconceptualize their pain experience, are taught pain coping skills, and are given opportunities for behavioural rehearsal and guided practice. The knowledge and skills obtained through the CBT process are then applied during a pain episode or flare of disease. CBT has been used in a number of musculoskeletal conditions with some success, both complimenting and adding to the improvements obtained with standard care (Superio-Cabuslay et al. 1996).

Psychological factors are strongly associated with disability and outcome in RA, and in fact may be stronger predictors of long-term outcome than any other biological or disease measure (McFarlane and Brooks 1988). Similar statements regarding psychosocial predictors of disability can also be made for patients presenting with back pain and fibromyalgia. Distress, coping strategies, and self-efficacy are important mediators between mood, physical impairment, and resultant disability in arthritis. Psychological therapies, either alone or combined with patient education or exercise regimes, are beneficial in managing pain and disability in RA, OA, fibromyalgia, and back pain. In addition, CBT has been effective in reducing psychological disturbance, pain, disability, and certain disease activity variables (such as acute phase reactants) in early arthritis (Sharpe et al. 2001). This approach is complimentary to the emphasis on aggressive medical management in early RA. Since a passive coping style predicts disability in RA, it would seem sensible to provide patients with RA (or other significantly disabling chronic musculoskeletal condition) the tools to focus on coping with relapse and maintenance of disease control. Addressing unhelpful coping styles such as avoidance and catastrophization early on in the experiences of an arthritis or back pain patient is likely to have a long-term effect.

There are several issues that need to be settled before the role of CBT in rheumatological practice can be adequately defined. These include whether the most important components of CBT can be identified and tested, developing strategies for matching CBT interventions to patients' readiness for behaviour change, testing the efficacy of different therapy formats (e.g. individual versus group, hospital versus primary care settings), and broadening the scope of CBT to address issues other than pain (Keefe et al. 1996).

Musculoskeletal problems in rehabilitation patients

Osteoporosis

Osteoporosis is common in neurological disorders causing paralysis and immobility. Fragility fractures occur more frequently in neuromuscular disorders in childhood, hemiplegia, Parkinson's disease, and spinal cord injury (SCI).

In SCI, sub-lesional osteoporosis is an important problem. This rapid onset and severe osteoporosis is due to a marked increase in bone resorption and reduced bone formation (Takata and Yasui 2001). This situation dramatically increases the risk of fragility fractures. For example, patients with SCI have a marked increase (at age 50: RR = 100) of pathological fracture in the long bones of the lower limb (Frisbie 1997). Sub-lesional bone may also undergo micro-structural changes following SCI, which alter its mechanical properties, and further increase the risk of fragility fractures. Imaging can demonstrate a coarse trabecular pattern and thinning of cortical bones. Measurement of femoral neck bone mineral density (BMD) can be used to quantify fracture risk in SCI patients. Heterotopic ossification (HO) (see below) around the hip can 'falsely' elevate BMD, leading to underestimation of fracture risk. Bone metabolism markers can indicate a high bone turnover state, and identify those who may require antiresorptive therapy. Strategies such as bed positioning, therapeutic standing and exercise, and possibly electrical stimulation, are used to provide an appropriate level of mechanical stress to the atrophied bone during rehabilitation. However, many cases of 'disuse osteoporosis' require a long time for bone to recover mineral density and strength.

Patients who have had a stroke have up to a 4-fold increase risk of hip fracture compared to control (Ramnemark et al. 2000). This is attributed to loss of bone mass in the paretic side and a high incidence of falls. Other risk factors include age, severity of stroke, and functional impairement. Stroke patients also experience a poorer outcome post-fracture in terms of higher mortality and a reduced chance of home discharge. It would seem sensible to preferentially target patients with stroke for treatment.

Heterotopic ossification

Heterotopic ossification is very familiar to orthopaedic surgeons; it is most often seen following hip replacement on X-rays (in the pericapsular region) within the first few months post-operatively. This condition is also commonly seen in patients with neuromuscular disorders, especially SCI and traumatic brain injury (TBI). It may mimic joint or soft tissue sepsis, inflammation, or tumour, and is therefore of relevance to the rheumatologist. HO occurs below the neurological level of the injury, usually at major joints. The incidence may be as high as 50 per cent in patients with SCI and TBI, though it is less common in stroke. It usually presents within 2–4 months following the neurological insult, though again in up to 50 per cent of cases, the lesion may be an incidental radiological finding. HO lesions can be massive and cause severe restriction to joint motion or ankylosis. However, the usual presentation is reduced range of joint motion, pain, and signs of local inflammation.

Investigation may reveal high levels of alkaline phosphatase activity, an acute phase response, increased bone turnover markers, and increased

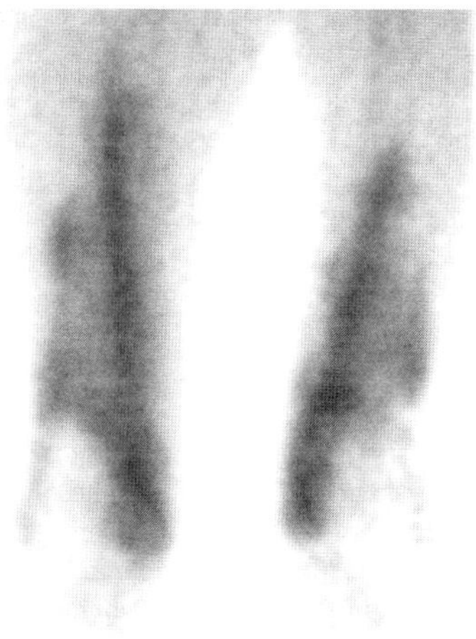

Fig. 2 Late phase isotope bone scan. Heterotopic ossification in tissues about the femur and knee in a patient with traumatic brain injury.

periarticular activity on the late (bone) phase of an isotope bone scan (Fig. 2). Bone scans may identify HO in patients without symptoms, and also multiple sites of involvement, which are clinically silent. The pathophysiology of HO is not understood, though neurohumeral mechanisms have been proposed along with an HLA-B27 associated predisposition. Certainly, the osteogenic response in patients with neuromuscular disorders is abnormal as evidenced by the high incidence of malunion, delayed union, or non-union of fractures in SCI and TBI patients. HO is associated with a poorer functional outcome in SCI and TBI, however, it is not clear whether this is a causal relationship or that HO is one of the many indicators of severity of neurological insult.

Careful non-traumatic exercise, such as range of motion exercises started early and maintained through the rehabilitation programme may prevent HO formation. Otherwise, treatment options are similar to those for post-surgical HO and include biphosphonates, indomethacin, radiation, and surgical excision. The timing of surgical excision differs according to aetiology as it is thought that lesions 'mature' and recur at a differing rates (Garland 1988). Traumatic HO may be resected at 6 months; SCI HO can be excised at 1 year; and TBI HO is removed after 18 months have elapsed. Patients with good neuromuscular control have the best functional result from surgery. The use of a continuous-passive-motion machine post-operatively may reduce the recurrence of HO.

Shoulder problems

The 'weightbearing shoulder'

Shoulder pain and dysfunction are common problems among patients with SCI. Shoulder pain and pain on transfer are reported in approximately 70 per cent of patients, with many experiencing regular pain within 6 months of injury (Daylan et al. 1999). Paraplegic patients rely almost exclusively on their upper limbs for weight-bearing activities such as transfers and wheelchair propulsion. Hence, the aetiology of shoulder pain in SCI patients has been attributed to overuse, with problems being more prevalent as the time since injury elapses (irrespective of age at injury). Rotator cuff lesions are important in the development and perpetuation of shoulder problems in wheelchair dependent SCI patients (Gellman et al. 1988). In cross sectional studies, rotator cuff lesions are present in 70 per cent of SCI patients. Shoulder muscle imbalance, with comparative weakness of the humeral head depressors (rotators and adductors) may lead to impingement. The 'depression transfer' may also stress shoulder girdle muscles and the glenohumeral joint, leading to pain. Other common causes of shoulder pain and weakness must also be considered. Unusually, osteonecrosis of the humeral head may occasionally present in this group.

Surgical reconstruction of a rotator cuff tear in a paraplegic patient is a thorny problem, as many of the post-operative restrictions that need to be observed pose Herculean difficulties for such an individual. Conservative management includes weight loss, review of transfer technique by an experienced SCI physiotherapist, analgesia, NSAIDs, stretching and strengthening exercise programmes designed to restore muscle balance (Pentland and Twomey 1994). The posterior shoulder musculature should be strengthened. The anterior muscle group, which is often very strong and shortened, need to be stretched for the balance to be restored.

Hemiplegic shoulder pain

The majority of stroke survivors suffer from shoulder pain. Its prevalence increases in the first weeks after discharge from hospital, and affects up to 70 per cent of patients (Walsh 2001). It causes considerable distress, functional impairment and can markedly hinder rehabilitation. There are many factors implicated in the aetiology of hemiplegic shoulder pain. They include:

- abnormalities of tone
    - spasticity (irritation of internal rotator/adductor muscle groups)
    - flaccidity (predispose to subluxation)
- glenohumeral subluxation
- rotator cuff pathology
- adhesive capulitis
- shoulder-hand syndrome (complex regional pain syndrome)
- central pain syndrome
- mechanical stress: manual handling/lifting; lack of upper limb support
- cold arm
- prior shoulder problems

A conservative management programme for hemiplegic shoulder pain could include measures to support the affected upper limb when the patient is seated and careful positioning in bed. In addition, a regime of daily static positional stretches, motor retraining, and strapping of the scapula to maintain postural tone and symmetry should be instituted (Bender and McKenna 2001). For prevention to be effective, it must begin immediately after the stroke. If shoulder pain persists, despite conservative measures and simple analgesia, further intensive treatment could include TENS and/or functional electrical stimulation, which may influence glenohumeral sub`luxation and reduce pain. Intra-articular or intra-lesional steroid and suprascapular nerve blocks also have a role in resistant cases.

Vocational rehabilitation

Patients disadvantaged by musculoskeletal disease may be unable to work. Vocational rehabilitation aims to enable individuals to access, return to, or remain in employment (British Society for Rehabilitation Medicine 2000). The roots of vocational rehabilitation lie in the period following the First World War, when interest in rehabilitation and retraining of disabled ex-servicemen began. In the United Kingdom, services dedicated to the delivery of vocational rehabilitation have been largely ignored. Nevertheless, vocational rehabilitation programmes have the potential to produce a significant return on costs by reducing payment of social benefits, increasing tax revenue, and reducing absence and retirement. Work disability is common in RA, and accounts for a significant portion of its costs to society. It is not restricted to those with severe established disease—it occurs in 50 per cent of patients with early RA working at the time of diagnosis.

Persistent abnormalities of ESR, HAQ disability, and pain, which may be detected in longitudinal follow-up, can predict work loss, though many other factors are related to work disability in RA (Table 4). For example, demographic variables, occupation, and level of education, as well as functional status in ADL, appear to identify work status more effectively than physiological variables. Work factors such as physical nature of work, control over the intensity of work, and job satisfaction are just as significant. Return to work depends on educational status, access, and work history. Work disability in OA has not been studied in such detail, but reports suggest that hours of work and employment are reduced in those with OA.

The negative effects of unemployment on the individual's physical and mental health are well known. The costs of work absence, both direct and indirect, are enormous. In certain settings, prolonged 'certification of sickness' can paradoxically hinder a return to work and curtail the promotion of healthy behaviour. The 'all or none' social welfare system does not encourage workers to seek rehabilitation or a graded return to work. The changing social and economic climate in industrialized western society has changed the working environment for many and brings new challenges to the working population.

The rheumatologist should include an employment history as part of the general assessment process. A more formal assessment of work disability may then be required, undertaken by other MDT members if necessary. Communication with employers, employment advisors, and social services will be necessary to implement job modifications and access to the workplace. Intensive rehabilitation can facilitate a return to work, if not commenced too late. The opportunities for vocational rehabilitation are also limited, and access often requires advice from a health professional with a detailed knowledge of the health and social care systems, and the plethora of voluntary sector agencies.

There have been many attempts to reduce work loss due to back pain. This is because of profound bio-psychosocial consequences and the huge cost to society of the 'back pain epidemic'. The chance of returning to work following absence due to back pain falls exponentially with time. Early intervention consisting of information, education, prompt access to physical therapy, and attention to manual handling and ergonomic issues can reduce work absences and promote return to work in a number of settings (Carter and Birrel 2000). Rather than concentrate on symptom control, intensive rehabilitation interventions emphasize health and well being promotion, in common with many rehabilitation programmes. Vocational rehabilitation in back pain is both beneficial and cost effective.

Vocational rehabilitation programmes may be delivered locally through community rehabilitation teams, day care facilities, sports and leisure centres, or at the place of work. Important elements of such programmes will include:

- physical therapy: fitness at home and work
- psychosocial interventions
- pain education

Table 4 Factors associated with work disability in rheumatoid arthritis

Disease parameters	Demographic	Disability	Vocational/educational	Psychosocial
Disease severity	Age	Functional impairment	Low socio-economic status	Depression
Disease duration	Female sex	High HAQ score	Low educational attainment	Emotional distress
Radiological damage		Pain	Physically demanding job	Behavioural coping styles
Diagnostic criteria				

- problem solving
- vocational education and skills retraining
- workplace/ergonomic assessment

Rehabilitation interventions in regional musculoskeletal problems

Cervical spine

Pain and limitation of cervical movements are common in arthritis and regional pain syndromes and can result in significant functional impairment. Impaired cervical flexion can lead to difficulty in eating and drinking, impaired extension can interfere with looking straight ahead and restrictions to rotation and lateral flexion can prevent safe driving. Compensatory strategies for cervical spine impairments include drinking straws and adapted cups and driving mirror extensions.

Cervical spine disease in RA

In RA, cervical spine involvement is almost universal; pain and functional impairment are common. An active conservative management programme for patients with atlanto-axial subluxation can educate and motivate patients to take active care of their neck and to relieve their chronic neck pain significantly (Kauppi et al. 1998). The effect on atlanto-axial instability has yet to be defined. In significant cervical spine instability at the atlanto-axial level, a rigid cervical orthosis ('hard collar') can be used to restrict excessive flexion in the A–P plane, and this can be confirmed using lateral cervical spine views (Fig. 3). The rigid cervical orthosis is worn when a passenger is in a motor vehicle or using public transport, and on transferring or hoisting if unsteady, to avoid cervical cord impingement with sudden jarring movements. In practice, rigid cervical orthoses are not well tolerated if worn continually. Soft collars can be used to support the neck relieving painful muscle spasm, especially at night.

(a) (b)

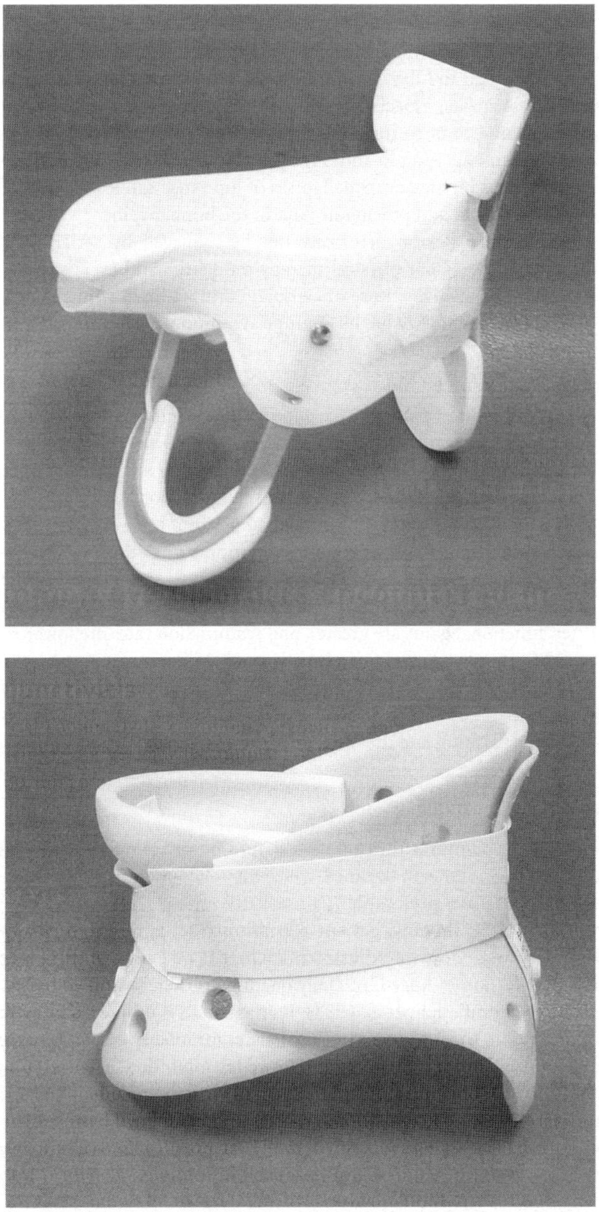

Fig. 3 Cervical orthoses ('hard collars'): (a) Combi and (b) Philadelphia. The 'Combi' is better tolerated by patients with RA and has the added advantage of a removable posterior component.

Shoulder

Lesions of the rotator cuff apparatus in the shoulder complex are common. Exercises (such as pendulum exercises with the patient bent forward, with the arm dependent, swinging to and fro) should be taught and continued regularly at home. Attention to posture is important, as a 'hunched' position will allow impingement of the rotator cuff apparatus. If possible, advice should be given to reduce or eliminate activities that aggravate pain, combined with suggestions of other methods of carrying loads, such as a trolley. A therapist may be able to provide aids and appliances that preserve independence and dignity such as long handled combs, dressing sticks, washing aids, and toilet aids.

Elbow

The elbow positions and stabilizes the hand for both fine and power tasks. With both elbows restricted to a 45° fixed flexion deformity, tasks such as driving, eating, drinking, and reaching the perineum become very difficult. Disability can be reduced by provision of aids, but regular exercise and prompt treatment of flares of inflammatory disease of the elbow can prevent the development of this impairment.

Hand

The power grip and pincer grip are important positions for hand function. The forces involved in pinch grip may encourage the development of MCP and IP joint subluxation. Aids that use a large grip or lever to reduce the force required for certain tasks could alleviate these problems.

Hand exercises often combined with a waxbath regime can reduce pain, increase grip and pincer strength, and improve finger flexor and extensor function. Debate continues whether hand exercises, promote or prevent deformity. Wrist and hand orthoses have a role in preventing deformity and improving function, providing analgesia, stability, and increased grip strength without causing muscle atrophy. Futura wrist splints stabilize the wrist in approximately 30° extension. The extensor bar is malleable and can be adjusted to ensure a good fit and improve position. Orthoses such as paddle splints are effective for pain relief, especially in a disease flare and hold the joint or limb in an optimal position, for example, the maintenance of finger extension. Because they render the hand functionally useless, they are usually worn at night. Thumb base pain in OA, especially on activity, is common. A rigid thumb post splint can be useful, holding the thumb in an abducted position, though many patients find these orthoses too restrictive.

Hip

Patients with arthritis of the hip should attempt a full set of range of motion exercises through the day. Swimming allows a wide range of joint movement (breast stroke, especially). Advice should be given to attempt prone rest or sleeping to encourage hip and knee extension. Raised chairs can address difficulty getting in and out of chairs; this will also help to prevent full or excessive hip flexion. Small losses of hip range can lead to secondary problems with gait and precipitate pain in the lumbar spine.

Hip and knee flexion deformity can be managed by serial splinting underpinned by regular physical therapy modalities and exercise. Surgical approaches can involve release of capsular contracture in younger patients but hip replacement may be the appropriate option.

Rehabilitation after hip fracture

The rehabilitation of patients after hip fracture is important in view of the number of patients involved and the significant mortality, morbidity, and functional disability following such an event. Of those who survive, only 25–50 per cent regain their pre-morbid level of function. Mortality rates are reported up to 30 per cent at 1 year and 40 per cent at 2 years. For patients receiving co-ordinated inpatient rehabilitation rather than routine inpatient care, outcome (e.g. death or institutional care) is better (Cameron et al. 2002). Other studies have shown that duration of inpatient stay is shorter, functional gains are greater, and readmission rates are lower in the groups of patients referred to an inpatient rehabilitation facility. Moreover, this intensive rehabilitation approach is associated with cost savings (Ruchlin et al. 2001). Overall, the goal orientated focus of attention on transferring, bathing and dressing, and pain management pays dividends.

Knee

Patients with painful arthritic knees should be discouraged from resting with a pillow underneath the knee, which may encourage flexion deformity; resting splints are preferable. Conservative management of knee OA involves exercise therapy, patient education (including an emphasis on weight loss) and footwear adjustments. There is no evidence that exercises cause progression of knee OA. Daily quadriceps exercises reduce pain and disability (Chamberlain et al. 1982). If an effusion is drained and the knee joint injected, a window of opportunity arises for intensive quadriceps exercise, with the muscle now released from reflex inhibition. Medial taping of the patella can also be effective. Orthoses can influence the loading and angulation of the knee. Knee braces may have an effect on proprioception in mild to moderate knee osteoarthritis and have a biomechanical function in more advanced cases, with a significant valgus deformity.

Foot and ankle

Problems with the foot and ankle are often relegated to the end of the consultation and may be overlooked by rheumatologists, though they may be responsible for one of our patients' main complaints—lack of mobility.

Many problems in the foot are related to abnormal alignment. The subtalar triplanar joint motions of supination and pronation (Fig. 4) result in the positions of valgus and varus being reached. Imbalance of the pronator or supinator muscle groups, weakness of ligaments, and joint destruction will all influence these motions. These structural variations result in predictable compensations, which can lead to pain and dysfunction.

Appropriate footwear is important for comfort, mobility, and stability. It must have adequate width and height to accommodate the toes, preferably a soft rubber sole and padded insole to provide shock absorption for the metatarsal heads, and an arch-support insole and strong medial side (or float) to the shoe to prevent valgus deformity of the ankle. Training shoes can provide some of these features, and because of the wide variety of styles, may be acceptable to many patients, both young and old.

A functional foot orthosis (FFO) can improve comfort and gait parameters, support the deformity, and eliminate the need to compensate for the abnormal alignment (Hodge et al. 1999). However, the evidence for a preventative role in early arthritis is lacking. The following section lists conservative interventions, with an emphasis on footwear and orthoses, in a number of common foot problems (Figs 5–7).

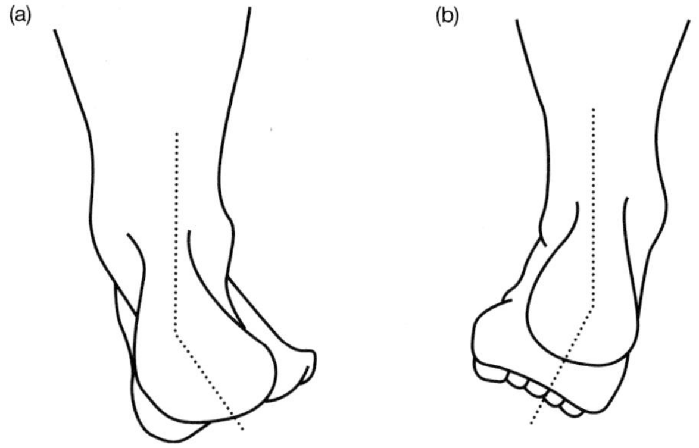

Fig. 4 Foot alignment: coordinated triplanar motion of the foot. (a) Pronation (abduction, eversion, and dorsiflexion) and (b) supination (adduction, inversion, and plantar flexion).

Hallux valgus

- accommodate deformity (broad fitting shoes)
- control excessive pronation (FFO)
- surgical intervention

Hallux rigidus

- restrict plantar flexion (sole stiffener)
- shift ground reaction force posteriorly, reducing the extension forces on MTP (rocker bottom sole)
- surgical intervention (fusion in a degree of dorsiflexion to facilitate toe off)

Metatarsalgia

- shift weight bearing load on MT heads proximally (FFO, MT cushion pads, dome or bar)
- treat callosities

Toe deformities (hammer, mallet, and claw toes)

- shift loading more proximally behind the MT heads and place pressure on toe flexor tendons (bar or dome)
- toe supports or props
- accommodate deformity (bespoke shoes)

Morton's neuroma

- replacing tight fitting footwear
- reduce the traction or mechanical pressure on intermetatarsal nerves/ligaments (FFO)

Midfoot and longitudinal arch pain

- Osteoarthritis and bony exostoses
  - reduce (painful) movement inside shoe/correct excessive pronation (FFO)
  - accommodate deformity in bespoke shoes

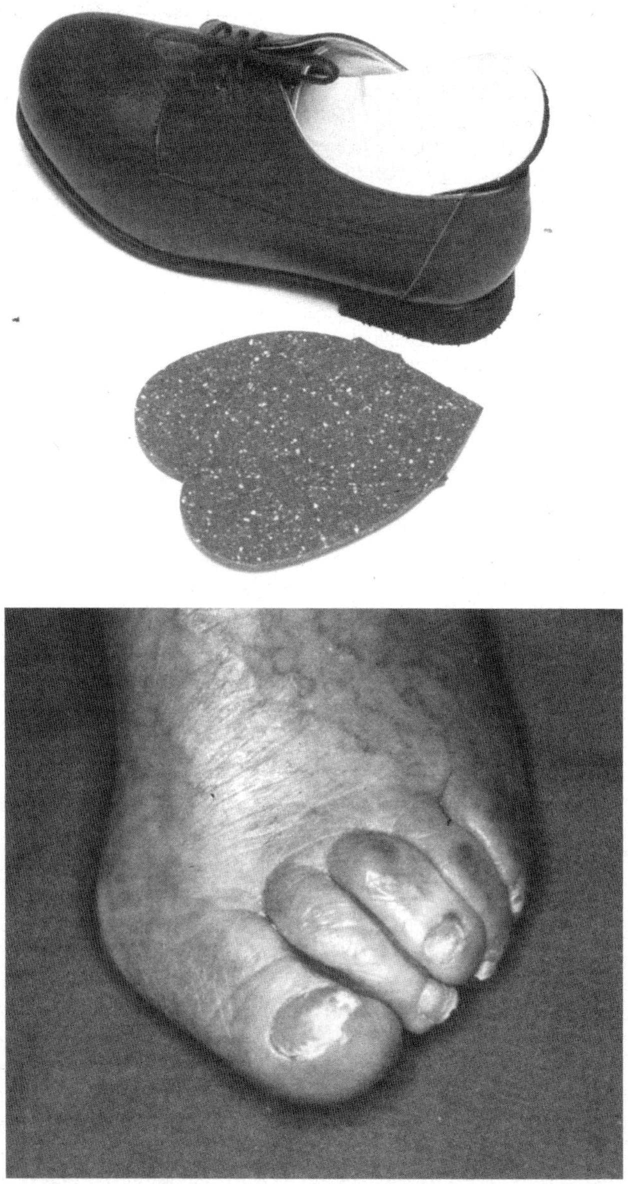

Fig. 5 Typical rheumatoid forefoot requiring bespoke shoe with functional foot orthosis and padding.

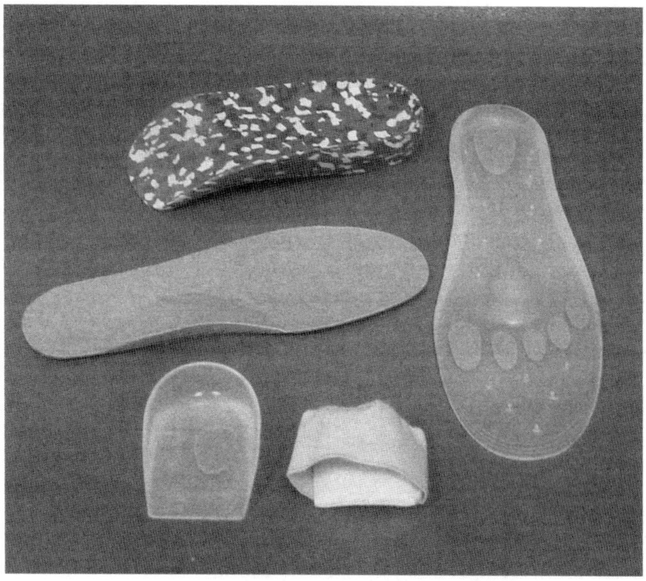

Fig. 6 Selection of orthotic devices. (Clockwise from top) 2/3 length functional foot orthosis with medial arch support and correction of hindfoot; off-the-shelf visco-elastic insole; metatarsal dome with 'garter'; visco-elastic heel insert; off-the-shelf insole with medial arch support.

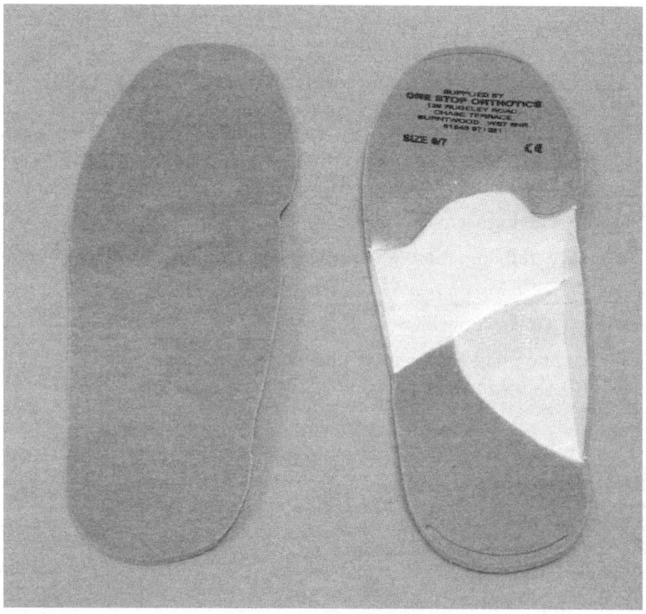

Fig. 7 Typical insole, turned upside down on right to display position of undersole with arch support and metatarsal bar.

- Tibialis posterior syndrome
  - support and maintain medial arch (footwear, FFO)
  - immobilize to reduce inflammation (ankle foot orthosis, cast)
  - surgical intervention (fusion of the talonavicular joint or 'triple fusion')

Ankle and hindfoot problems

- Ankle ligament injury
  - improve proprioceptive function and co-ordination (physical therapy regimes)
  - modified footwear ('high top shoes')
  - stabilize joint (orthoses Fig. 8/lateral ligament splints, ankle taping)
- Hindfoot in RA
  - reduce excessive strain on subtalar joint (FFO)
  - surgical options (fusion)
- Plantar fasciitis
  - correct the underlying biomechanical deformity (commonly excessive pronation, less commonly supination) FFO
  - prevent restriction of ankle dorsiflexion (stretching exercises to a short or tight tendo-achilles)
  - reducing impact (cushioned heel or heel insert)
  - reduce loading on heel during stance phase (medial arch support insole)

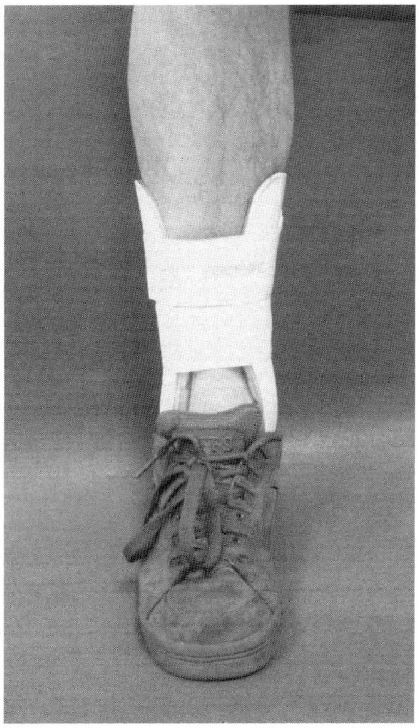

Fig. 8 Aircast ankle brace.

- Achilles tendonopathy
  - correct biomechanical predisposition—pronated or equinus foot (FFO)
  - relieve mechanical stresses to the tendon and its insertion (heel raises and FFO)
- Tarsal tunnel syndrome
  - reduce abnormal movement of the foot in the gait cycle (FFO)
  - reduce inflammation of surrounding structures (corticosteroid injection)
- Stress fractures in the lower limb
  - prevention and treatment of underlying biomechanical abnormality (FFO, shock absorbing insoles)

References

Barlow, J.H., Williams, B., and Wright, C. (1996). The generalized self-efficacy scale in people with arthritis. *Arthritis Care and Research* **9**, 189–196.

Beck, A.T. (1961). An inventory for measuring depression. *Archives of General Psychiatry* **4**, 561–71.

Bender, L. and McKenna, K. (2001). Hemiplegic shoulder pain: defining the problem and its management. *Disability and Rehabilitation* **23** (16), 698–705.

British Society for Rehabilitation Medicine. *Prescription for Independence: A Working Party Report of the BSRM Environmental Control Special Interest Group.* London: British Society for Rehabilitation Medicine, 1994.

British Society for Rehabilitation Medicine. *Vocational Rehabilitation—The Way Forward: Report of a Working Party (Chair: Frank AO).* London: British Society for Rehabilitation Medicine, 2000.

Cameron, I.D., Handoll, H.H., Finnegan, T.P., Madhok, R., and Langhorne, P. (2001). Co-ordinated multidisciplinary approaches for inpatient rehabilitation of older patients with proximal femoral fractures. *Cochrane Library* CD000106. Oxford: Update Software.

Carter, J. and Birrel, L. *Occupational Health Guidelines for the Management of Low Back Pain at Work: Evidence Review and Recommendations.* Faculty of Occupational Medicine: London, 2000.

Chamberlain, M.A., Care, G., and Harfield, B. (1982). Physiotherapy in osteoarthrosis of the knees. A controlled trial of hospital versus home exercises. *International Rehabilitation Medicine* **4**, 101–6.

Clarke, A.K. (1999). Effectiveness of rehabilitation for arthritis. *Clinical Rehabilitation* **13** (Suppl. 1), 51–62.

Dalyan, M., Cardenas, D.D., and Gerard, B. (1999). Upper extremity pain after spinal cord injury. *Spinal Cord* **37**, 191–5.

Edworthy, S.M. (2000). How important is patient self-management? *Baillière's Clinical Rheumatology* **14**, 705–14.

Ernst, E. (1997). Acupuncture as a symptomatic treatment of osteoarthritis. A systematic review. *Scandinavian Journal of Rheumatology* **26**, 444–7.

Ernst, E. and Harkness, E. (2001). Spinal manipulation: a systematic review of sham-controlled, double-blind, randomized clinical trials. *Journal of Pain and Symptom Management* **22**, 879–89.

EuroQuol Group (1990). EuroQuol—a new facility for the measurement of health-related quality of life. *Health Policy* **16**, 199–208.

Fairbank, J.C., Couper, J., Davies, J.B., and O'Brien, J.P. (1980). The Oswestry low back pain disability questionnaire. *Physiotherapy* **66**, 271–3.

Ferrari, R. (2000). The biopsychosocial model—a tool for rheumatologists. *Baillière's Clinical Rheumatology* **14** , 787–95.

Fries, J.F., Spitz, P., and Young, D. (1982). The dimensions of health outcomes: the Health Assessment Questionnaire disability and pain scales. *Journal of Rheumatology* **9**, 789–93.

Frisbie, J.H. (1997). Fractures after myelopathy: the risk quantified. *Journal of Spinal Cord Medicine* **20**, 66–9.

Fuchs, H.A., Brooks, R.H., Callahan, L.F., and Pincus, T. (1989). A simplified twenty-eight-joint quantitative articular index in rheumatoid arthritis. *Arthritis and Rheumatism* **32**, 531–7.

Garland, D.E. (1988). Clinical observations on fractures and heterotopic ossification in the spinal cord and traumatic brain injured populations. *Clinical Orthopedics* **233**, 86–101.

Garratt, A.M., Ruta, D.A., Abdalla, M.I., Buckingham, J.K., and Russell, I.T. (1993). The SF36 health survey questionnaire: an outcome measure suitable for routine use within the NHS? *British Medical Journal* **306**, 1440–4.

Gellman, H., Sie, I., and Waters, R.L. (1988). Late complications of the weight-bearing upper extremity in the paraplegic patient. *Clinical Orthopedics* **233**, 132–5.

Hammond, A. and Freeman, K. (2001). One year outcomes of a randomised controlled trial of an educational–behavioural joint protection programme for people with rheumatoid arthritis. *Rheumatology* **40**, 1044–51.

Hodge, M.C., Bach, T.M., and Carter, M.G. (1999). Novel Award First Prize Paper. Orthotic management of plantar pressure and pain in rheumatoid arthritis. *Clinical Biomechanics* **14**, 567–75.

Hunt, S.M., McEwan, J., and McKenna, S.P. *Measuring Health Status.* Beckenham: Croom Helm, 1986.

Kauppi, M., Leppanen, L., Heikkila, S., Lahtinen, T., and Kautiainen, H. (1998). Active conservative treatment of atlantoaxial subluxation in rheumatoid arthritis. *British Journal of Rheumatology* **3**, 417–20.

Keefe, F.J., Kashikar-Zuck, S., Opiteck, J., Hage, E., Dalrymple, L., and Blumenthal, J.A. (1996). Pain in arthritis and musculoskeletal disorders: the role of coping skills training and exercise interventions. *Journal of Orthopedics, Sports and Physical Therapy* **4**, 279–90.

Klaber Moffett, J. et al. (1999). Randomised control trial of exercise for low back pain: clinical outcomes, costs, and preferences. *British Medical Journal* **319**, 279–83.

Koes, B.W., van Tulder, M.W., van der Windt, D.A.W.M., and Bouter, L.M. (1994). The efficacy of back schools: a review of randomised clinical trials. *Journal of Clinical Epidemiology* **47**, 851–62.

Lindroth, Y., Bauman, A., Brooks, P.M., and Priestley, D. (1995). A 5-year follow-up of a controlled trial of an arthritis education programme. *British Journal of Rheumatology* **34**, 647–52.

Lorig, K., Chastain, R.L., Ung, E., Shoor, S., and Holman, H.R. (1989). Development and evaluation of a scale to measure perceived self-efficacy in people with arthritis. *Arthritis and Rheumatism* **32**, 37–44.

Lorig, K. (1995). Patient education: treatment or nice extra. *British Journal of Rheumatology* **34**, 703–6.

McFarlane, A. and Brooks, P. (1988). The determinants of disability in rheumatoid arthritis. *British Journal of Rheumatology* **27**, 7–14.

Meenan, R.F., Mason, J.H., Anderson, J.J., Kazis, L.E., and Guccione, A.A. (1992). AIMS2: the content and properties of a revised and expanded AIMS. *Arthritis and Rheumatism* **35**, 1–10.

Melzack, R. (1975). The McGill Pain Questionnaire: major properties and scoring methods. *Pain* **1**, 277–99.

Pentland, W.E. and Twomey, L.T. (1994). Upper limb function in persons with long term paraplegia and implications for independence: Part II. *Paraplegia* **32** (4), 219–24.

Ramnemark, A., Nilsson, M., Borssen, B., and Gustafson, Y. (2000). Stroke, a major and increasing risk factor for femoral neck fracture. *Stroke* **31**, 1572–7.

Rosenstiel, A.K. and Keefe, F.J. (1983). The use of coping strategies in chronic low back pain patients: relationship to patient characteristics and current adjustment. *Pain* **17**, 33–44.

Ruchlin, H.S., Elkin, E.B., and Allegrante, J.P. (2001). The economic impact of a multifactorial intervention to improve postoperative rehabilitation of hip fracture patients. *Arthritis and Rheumatism* **45**, 446–52.

Sharpe, L., Sensky, T., Timberlake, N., Ryan, B., Brewin, C.R., and Allard, S. (2001). A blind, randomised, controlled trial of cognitive-behavioural intervention for patients with recent onset rheumatoid arthritis: preventing psychological and physical disability. *Pain* **89**, 275–89.

Shekelle, P.G., Markovich, M., and Louie, R. (1995). Comparing the costs between provider types of episodes of back pain care. *Spine* **20**, 221–7.

Superio-Cabuslay, E., Ward, M.M., and Lorig, K.R. (1996). Patient education interventions in osteoarthritis and rheumatoid arthritis: a meta-analytic comparison with nonsteroidal anti-inflammatory drug treatment. *Arthritis Care in Research* **9** (4), 292–301.

Takata, S. and Yasui, N. (2001). Disuse osteoporosis. *Journal of Medical Investigation* **48** (3–4), 147–56.

Van den Ende, C.H.M., Vliet Vlieland, T.P.M., Munneke, M., and Hazes, J.M.W. (2000). Dynamic exercise therapy for rheumatoid arthritis (Cochrane Review). In *The Cochrane Library* Issue 2. Oxford: Update Software.

van Lankveld, W., van't Pad, B.P., van de, P.L., Naring, G., and van der, S.C. (1994). Disease-specific stressors in rheumatoid arthritis: coping and well-being. *British Journal of Rheumatology* **33** 1067–73.

van Tulder, M. et al. (2000). Exercise therapy for low back pain (Cochrane Review). In *The Cochrane Library*. Oxford: Update Software.

Vliet Vlieland, T.P. and Hazes, J.M. (1997). Efficacy of multidisciplinary team care programmes in rheumatoid arthritis. *Seminars on Arthritis and Rheumalotogy* **27**, 110–22.

Walsh, K. (2001). Management of shoulder pain in patients with stroke. *Postgraduate Medical Journal* **77**, 645–9.

Wiesinger, G.F. et al. (1998). Benefit of 6 months long-term physical training in polymyositis/dermatomyositis patients. *British Journal of Rheumatology* **37**, 1338–42.

World Health Organization. *The International Classification of Impairments, Disabilities and Handicaps (ICIDH).* Geneva: WHO, 1980.

2.3 Rehabilitation of children

Renate Häfner and Marianne Spamer

Introduction

Inflammatory arthritis is the most commonly seen feature in rheumatic disorders of children and adolescents. It occurs most often as idiopathic arthritis with different sub-types but may also be a symptom of an underlying disease such as systemic lupus erythematosus, sarcoidosis, or vasculitis. Rehabilitation follows the same principles as for all arthritic disorders. The therapy offered must give careful consideration to the child's age and developmental status, the pattern of joint involvement, and the individual disease course.

Aims of rehabilitation—a multidisciplinary team approach

The different aspects of rehabilitation require the cooperation of several health care professionals who work together to improve the child's function, independence, and self-esteem. This includes caring for the whole family and overseeing integration into the community. The team is guided and coordinated by a paediatric rheumatologist.

The physiotherapist works together with the occupational therapist to improve function of individual joints as well as general mobility.

The child's rheumatic disease always has an impact on the whole family, financial hardship is common. The social worker gives advice on financial entitlements and assists with individual social problems. A psychologist can be helpful to handle conflict situations.

A very important aspect of rehabilitation involves integrating the child into school life. To achieve this, it is necessary for several health care professionals to coordinate contact with teachers and other school staff to highlight the child's needs and help organize school life with the minimum of disruption for all concerned.

Perhaps the team's most important role is psychological—to create the highest possible level of integration so that children cease to see themselves as sick and different and acquire a sense of belonging.

Rehabilitation of joint function

Management of arthritis in children requires a wide-ranging knowledge of how functional impairment and deformities develop in individuals. The therapist must always keep in mind the progress of deformity and try to thwart this vicious circle as early as possible. It is much more beneficial to prevent deformities than to treat them.

Development of joint deformities

Pain in children with arthritis is often neglected as small children in particular rarely complain of painful joints. It is therefore important to note non-verbal expressions of pain (Scott et al. 1977; Melvin 1989; Truckenbrodt 1993; Spamer et al. 2001). Unfortunately, children rapidly adapt to painful arthritis with a reflex pain-relieving positioning of the affected joint. This is always a malposition which in turn produces a muscular imbalance. Those muscles which draw the joint into the pain-relieving position become hypertonic, and the antagonists become weak (Truckenbrodt 1993; Spamer et al. 2001). If caught at an early stage the deformity can still be corrected passively. If inflammation and pain persist the incorrect position becomes permanent and a normal part of daily activities.

Principles of physiotherapy

It is the aim of all therapeutic approaches to keep or restore joint function and alignment as much as possible and achieve a normal pattern of mobility (Jarvis 1980; Erlandson 1989; Melvin 1989; Spamer et al. 2001). Even slight restrictions of joint function must be taken seriously and treated. In this regard it is important to appreciate that children have a greater joint mobility than adults. Joint function which is normal in adults may already be impaired in a child and must be treated accordingly.

As a precondition for effective physiotherapy the child must relax during treatment, as fear and pain increase muscle tone and intensify the reflex

Table 1 Principles of physiotherapy in JIA. Garmisch therapy concept

1. Pain relief and relaxation —Physical modalities —Slow passive moving
2. Improvement of joint mobility —Passive or active assisted moving —Stretching of shortened muscles —Activation of hypotonic muscles
3. Training of muscular coordination

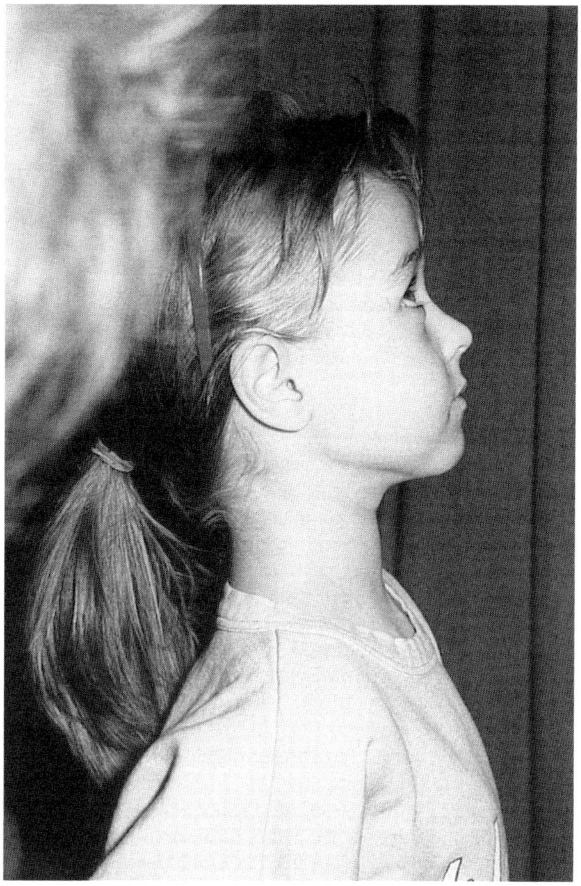

Fig. 1 Child with systemic onset disease and involvement of the cervical spine. Impaired extension is compensated by upward movement of the eyes.

pain-relieving position. A relationship of trust between child and therapist is of the utmost importance in achieving the most beneficial environment and results.

Effective physiotherapy requires a programme that is built on successive treatment steps (Spamer et al. 2001) (Table 1). The first step comprises methods for pain relief and relaxation. Cold packs, electrotherapy as well as weight release are helpful. Slow passive moving of the joints reduces pain. Even acutely inflamed and painful joints can be treated and protected from functional impairment.

Passive or active assisted moving is also the first part of joint mobilization. Next the hypertonic and shortened muscle groups, which keep the joint in its incorrect position, must be stretched. This procedure requires a relief positioning, and joint protection must be considered. Small children are treated with passive stretching alone, while older children can cooperate in active stretching procedures. At the end of each stretching the child is asked to hold the achieved joint function against a mild resistance. This procedure already introduces the next step: activation of hypotonic muscles.

The child must learn to tense those muscle groups which counteract the deformity. In a first step the therapist corrects the malposition and mobilizes the joint into the impaired direction, asking the child to hold the final position. When the child can tense the weak muscles isometrically he or she is ready to start with active movements of the joint. The child is encouraged to move the joint from the position of comfort all the way into the impaired direction. The therapist must correct immediately compensatory movements of neighbouring joints.

Finally, the restored mobility must be integrated into daily life, overcoming the pathological patterns of movement. Frequent repetition of simple actions helps to integrate these into daily activities. In the beginning the therapist will need to support and correct the joint movements. Later, more complex and faster movements can be achieved unaided. It is important, however, to adapt the training to the child's abilities.

Some therapists recommend strengthening of the weak muscles as a first step to overcome weakness and joint deformities (Jarvis 1980; Erlandson 1989; Melvin 1989). In our experience, however, this is ineffective as long as inflammation persists, joint alignment has not been regained adequately, and the child is still accustomed to a pathological pattern of motion. If, however, all these conditions have been restored, training of muscle coordination will simultaneously increase muscular power (Spamer et al. 2001).

The cervical spine

Cervical spine involvement is easily detected when the child is asked to look up or around. Extensive eye movements compensate for the restricted extension and rotation (Fig. 1). The typical pain-relieving position is mild flexion with restricted extension. Neck pain can be especially severe in children with systemic disease. It is induced by playing, writing, or working in a sitting position with the head slightly flexed. The cervical spine tends to early ankylosis in juvenile arthritis. Atlantoaxial subluxation is rare in children (Ansell and Kent 1977).

Therapy

Treatment of the cervical spine requires extreme caution and should be carried out in a relaxed position, preferably with the child lying on his or her back. Careful passive movement in all directions with slight traction can relieve pain and improve function. The dorsolateral neck muscles can be stretched by moving the shoulder girdle while the cervical spine remains in a fixed position. However, if spinal ankylosis has already developed no manipulation should be attempted.

A soft collar relieves pain and muscular tension of the cervical spine. It should be worn during long sedentary periods and as soon as pain starts. Children with severe neck problems may need to wear a collar all day. To aid comfortable sleep, pillows with a neck pad are helpful (Jarvis 1980; Erlandson 1989; Melvin 1989).

The temporomandibular joints

When temporomandibular joints become affected in early life significant growth disturbance of the mandible can occur (Bache 1964; Stabrun et al. 1988; Melvin 1989; Pedersen et al. 1995; Spamer et al. 2001). This micrognathia creates malocclusion and disturbs the facial appearance. Restricted mouth opening together with impaired extension of the cervical spine can cause problems if intubation becomes necessary.

Movement of the temporomandibular joint comprises a caudal and ventral gliding of the mandibular condyle to permit mouth opening. Arthritis leads to pain and restriction of both movements. Opening the mouth, especially the ventral protrusion, as well as lateral displacement of the jaw become impaired (Bache 1964; Melvin 1989; Spamer et al. 2001) (Fig. 2).

Therapy

Cautious traction with the therapist's thumbs on the lower dorsal dental rows can mobilize the caudal–ventral motion of the mandibula (Fig. 3).

(a)
(b)

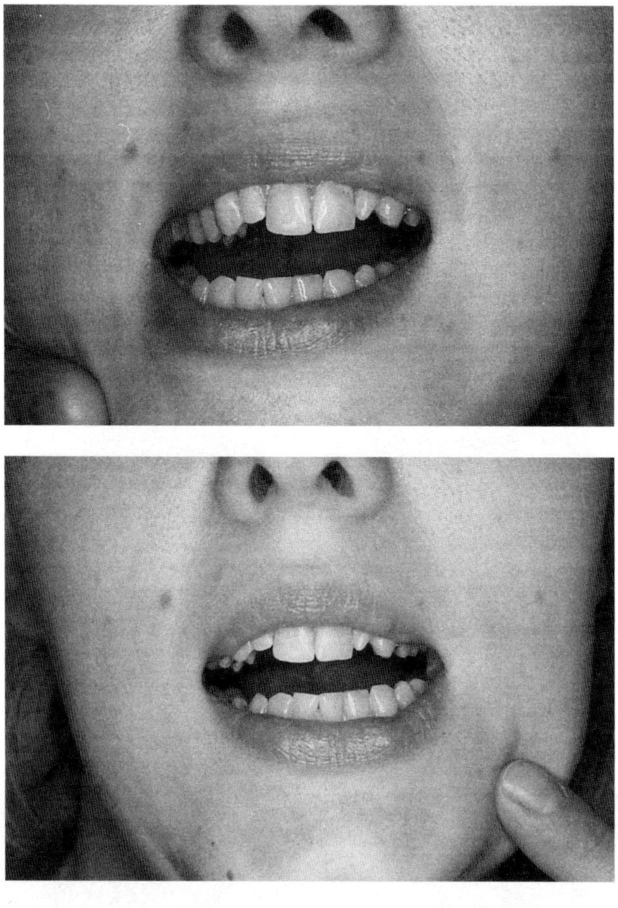

Fig. 2 Asymmetric involvement of the left temporomandibular joint. Lateral movement of the jaw is normal to the right (a) but markedly impaired to the left side (b).

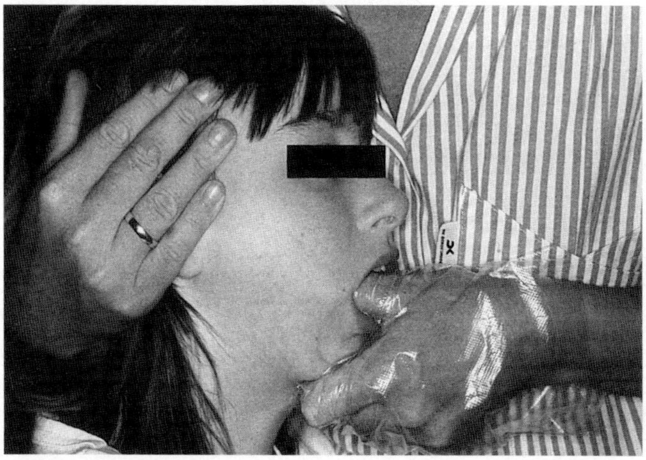

Fig. 3 Mobilization of the caudal–ventral motion of the jaw.

Active stretching of the hypertone masseter muscle can occur by inhibition of antagonists or the hold-relax technique. Finally, the weak musculus pterigoideus lateralis, which is responsible for protrusion of the mandible, must be activated (Spamer et al. 2001).

Temporomandibular joint involvement requires close collaboration with the dentist and orthodontist since dental or jaw regulation may be required to improve function and occlusion. Early treatment with a distraction splint is indicated. This splint initiates an anterior rotation of the mandible which unloads the joint and contributes to pain relief. When the active phase of arthritis has subsided an activator which generates a gradual protrusion of the mandible can be inserted (Pedersen et al. 1995).

The shoulder

Shoulder involvement impairs flexion and abduction. These movements involve a caudal gliding of the humeral head which is restricted in arthritis. Early cooperation of the shoulder blade during elevation and abduction compensates for impaired range of motion. The pain-relieving position tends towards abduction and protraction of the shoulder girdle. The scapula moves towards a cranial position (Spamer et al. 2001).

Therapy

First of all, the scapula must be mobilized towards its physiologic position caudo-lateral. Then mobilization of the glenohumeral joint into flexion, and abduction can follow. Careful manipulation of the caudal gliding of the humeral head is important (Melvin 1989). When adequate shoulder mobility has been achieved, muscular activation becomes possible which concentrates on the rotator cuff, the abductors, and the weak scapular muscles (Spamer et al. 2001).

The elbow

Synovitis of the elbow joint first impairs extension. A flexion contracture up to 30° may develop unnoticed since it hardly interferes with normal activities. Further contracture, however, significantly reduces arm length and can eventually lead to functional impairments.

Forearm rotation favours pronation as a position of comfort while supination is usually restricted. Severely impaired supination interferes with a lot of important daily activities and may become a very disabling condition.

Therapy

Mobilization is directed towards the restricted function, usually extension and supination. Since synovial tissue tends to fill the fossa olecrani, moving the elbow may be very painful. Manual traction vertical to the forearm can relieve pain and improve extension. Stretching of the flexor and pronator muscles is important to restore function.

The hand

Wrist involvement is easily detected while watching the child's activities. Hand prop is strictly avoided (Fig. 4). The typical pain-relieving position of the wrist in children is flexion and ulnar deviation (Erlandson 1989; Melvin 1989; Spamer et al. 2001). The extensors weaken while the flexor carpi ulnaris muscle becomes hypertonic. First active and later also passive dorsal wrist extension is limited. Secondary hyperextension of the metacarpophalangeal joints may occur (Fig. 5). To compensate for ulnar wrist deviation the metacarpophalangeal joints often drift radially even when they are not affected (Fig. 6), in contrast to adult hand deformity with radial deviation of the wrist and ulnar drift of the fingers. Occasionally an adult-type hand deformity can develop.

Involvement of finger joints can lead to swan-neck or boutonnière deformities. Swan-neck deformity develops mainly in index and middle fingers, boutonnière deformity in the fourth and fifth finger. The thumb tends towards opposition and adduction in its saddle joint and flexion deformity in the metacarpophalangeal joint. A compensatory hyperextension often develops in the interphalangeal joint (Fig. 7).

Flexotenosynovitis of the fingers is a common feature in juvenile arthritis. It can be very painful and may result in the adoption of a pain-relieving position with all three finger joints in flexion. Due to impaired tendon gliding, active flexion and extension are often reduced although passive movement is still possible (Fig. 8). Finally, shortening of the finger flexors develops with a significant impairment of hand function.

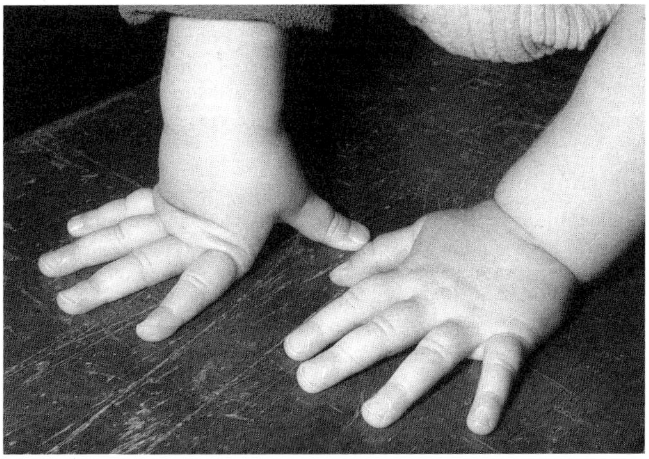

Fig. 4 A child with arthritis of the right wrist avoids hand prop when crawling.

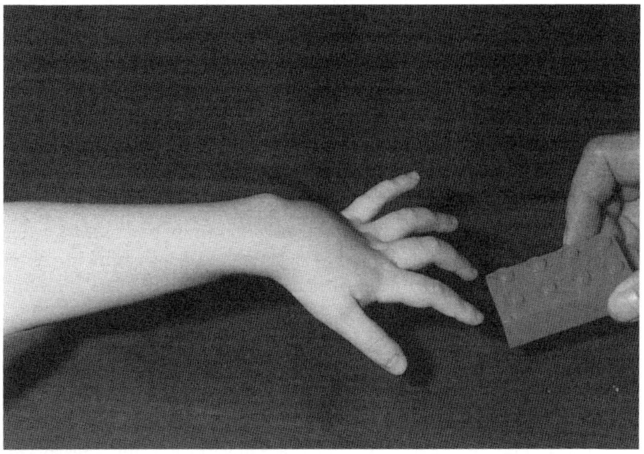

Fig. 5 Arthritis of the wrist joint with a typical malposition in flexion. Impaired extension is compensated by hyperextension in the metacarpophalangeal joints.

Therapy

Treatment of the wrist must include restoration of passive and later active dorsal extension as well as radial abduction. The therapist's grip during passive or active assisted movement should support the carpus and correct the hand axis (Fig. 9). When joint inflammation has subsided, activation of the extensor muscles becomes part of the programme. Since abduction of the thumb counteracts ulnar wrist deviation it is important to relearn and practise spreading the thumb. The therapist's assistance must correct inappropriate movements such as hyperextension of the fingers or flexion of the elbow that compensate for impaired dorsal extension.

In swan-neck deformity, it is important to mobilize impaired extension of the metacarpophalangeal joints and then continue with flexion of the proximal interphalangeal joints (Fig. 10). Muscular coordination of the extensor digitorum longus with the flexor digitorum superficialis muscle must be trained to achieve a physiological grip. In boutonnière deformity the often hyperextended metacarpophalangeal joints must be mobilized towards flexion. In a further step, stretching of the flexor digitorum superficialis muscle improves proximal interphalangeal flexion contracture.

In treatment of flexotenosynovitis, both passive and active movements are necessary to prevent adhesion of the tendons. To reduce pain, cold applications prior to physiotherapy are helpful.

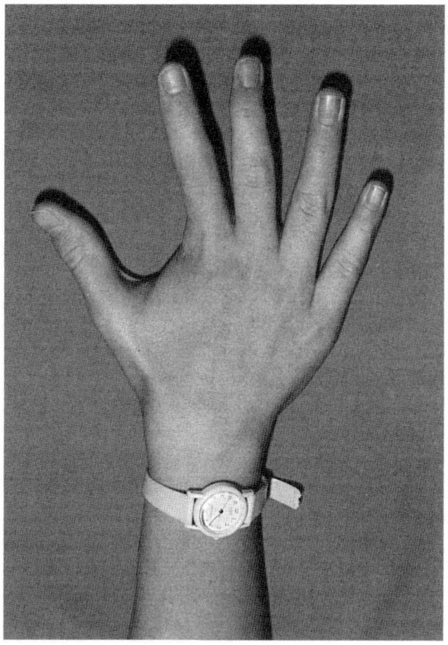

Fig. 6 Juvenile hand scoliosis with ulnar deviation of the wrist and compensatory radial drift of the fingers.

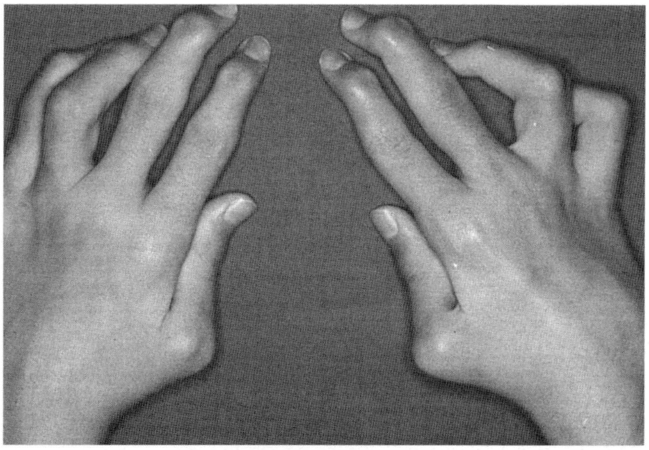

Fig. 7 Multiple finger deformities in a patient with juvenile polyarthritis: subluxation and abduction of the thumb at the metacarpophalangeal joint with hyperextension of the interphalangeal joint; swan-neck deformity of the index and middle fingers; and boutonnière deformity of the fourth and fifth fingers.

Hand orthoses

Therapy of wrist and finger deformities benefits from individual orthoses. The wrist joint can be stabilized by a short supporting splint to prevent or correct flexion position, ulnar (or radial) drift, and carpal subluxation (Jarvis 1980; Erlandson 1989; Melvin 1989; Spamer et al. 2001) (Fig. 11). These splints should be worn especially during manual activities since all active work with the hand increases the deviation. Stabilization of the carpus will improve power transfer in the finger–hand area and will also protect the inflamed joint structures from over- and misloading. Resting splints are indicated for finger deformities. They should be worn for several hours during the night and contribute to a careful passive stretching of shortened muscles and joint structures.

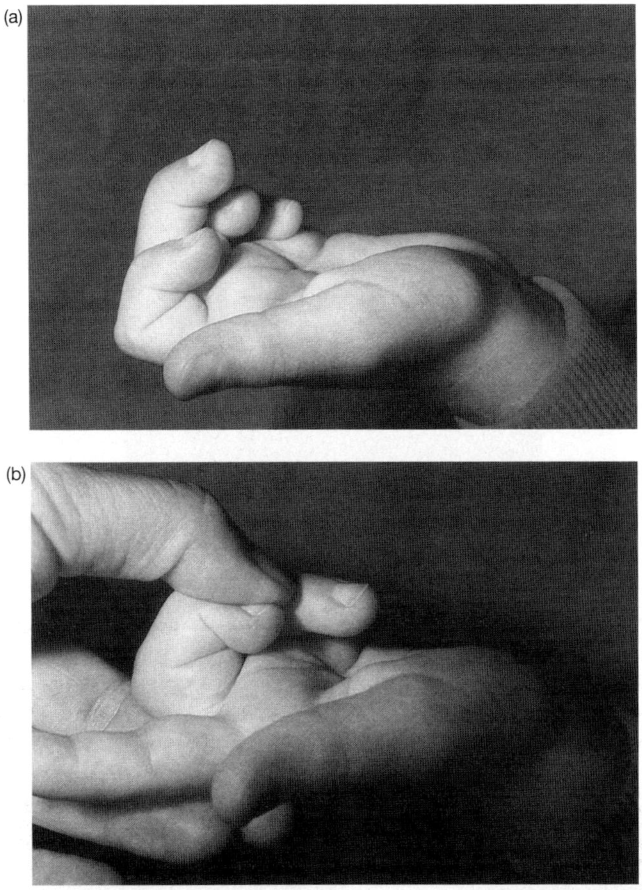

Fig. 8 Flexotenosynovitis of the middle finger. Active flexion is markedly impaired (a) while passive flexion is still complete (b).

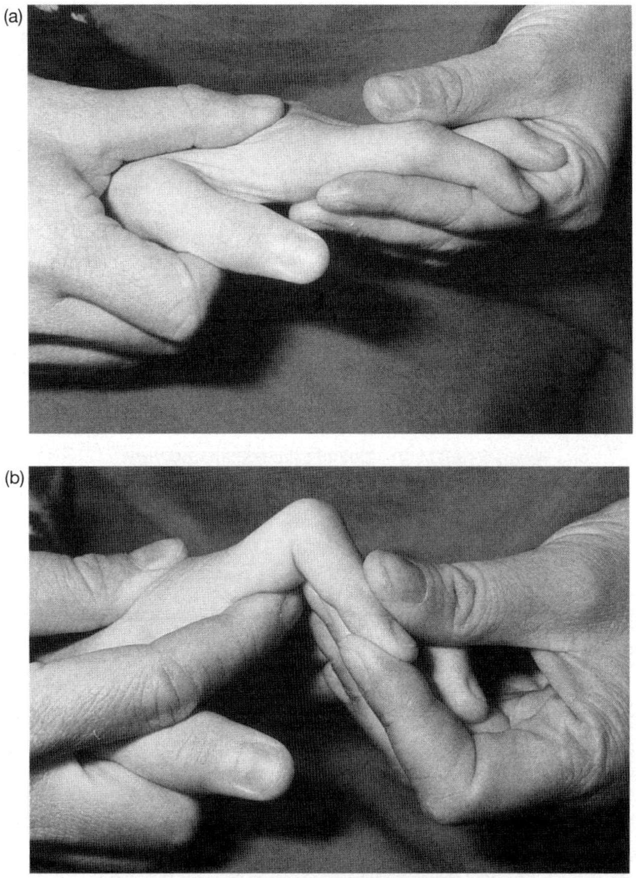

Fig. 10 Treatment of swan-neck deformity. Mobilization of extension at the metacarpophalangeal joint (a) is followed by flexion at the proximal interphalangeal joint (b).

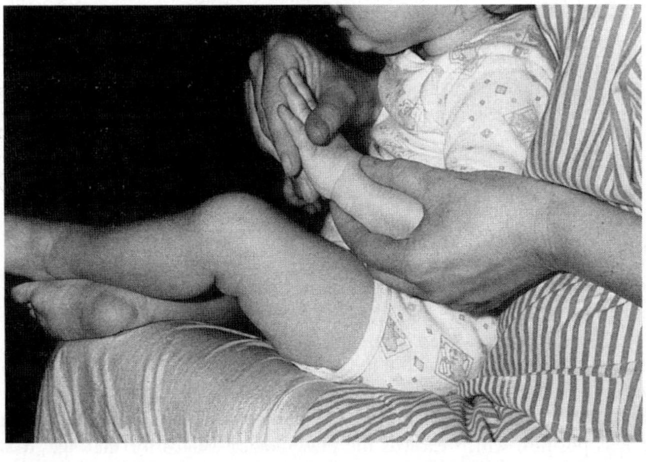

Fig. 9 Cautious passive moving of the wrist in a small child with polyarthritis.

The hip

Hip mobility in children exceeds that of adults. Young children with a free hip function can bend their hips until the knee reaches the belly and external rotation may reach 90°.

The first sign of hip involvement is pain during full range flexion with adduction. Later full extension, flexion, and internal rotation become painful. When the children stand or walk they usually deviate into abduction and internal rotation. Severe hip involvement is characterized by flexion, abduction, and internal rotation contractures. In such patients flexion position is compensated for by an increased lumbar lordosis as well as knee flexion (Swann 1978a; Erlandson 1989; Melvin 1989).

Therapy

In acute stages, only careful passive movement and mild traction are tolerated. This, however, should be done as often as possible to prevent contractures.

When pain subsides stretching should be done, concentrating on mainly the flexors. Later on, active exercises of extensor, abductor, and external rotator muscles is important to improve the range of movement of the joint (Spamer 1997).

Weight-bearing exercises for children with hip arthritis is controversial. Some therapists encourage ambulation to restore the joint structures and support joint congruity (Bernstein et al. 1977; Ansell 1978; Melvin 1989; Lloyd and Aldrich 1993; Hayem et al. 1994). Absence of weight bearing may interfere with a normal development of the femur and acetabulum in young children. Valgus deformity and lateralization of the femoral head and acetabular underdevelopment are often seen in children with onset of hip disease at an early age (Bernstein et al. 1977; Ansell 1978; Häfner 1997).

Conversely weight bearing may promote hip destruction. Therefore, partial weight bearing is a compromise for children with hip arthritis (Rombouts and Rombouts-Lindemans 1971; Ansell 1978; Jarvis 1980; Garcia-Morteo et al. 1981; Spamer 1997; Spamer et al. 2001). Depending on the child's age and the situation of the other joints, crutches, bicycles,

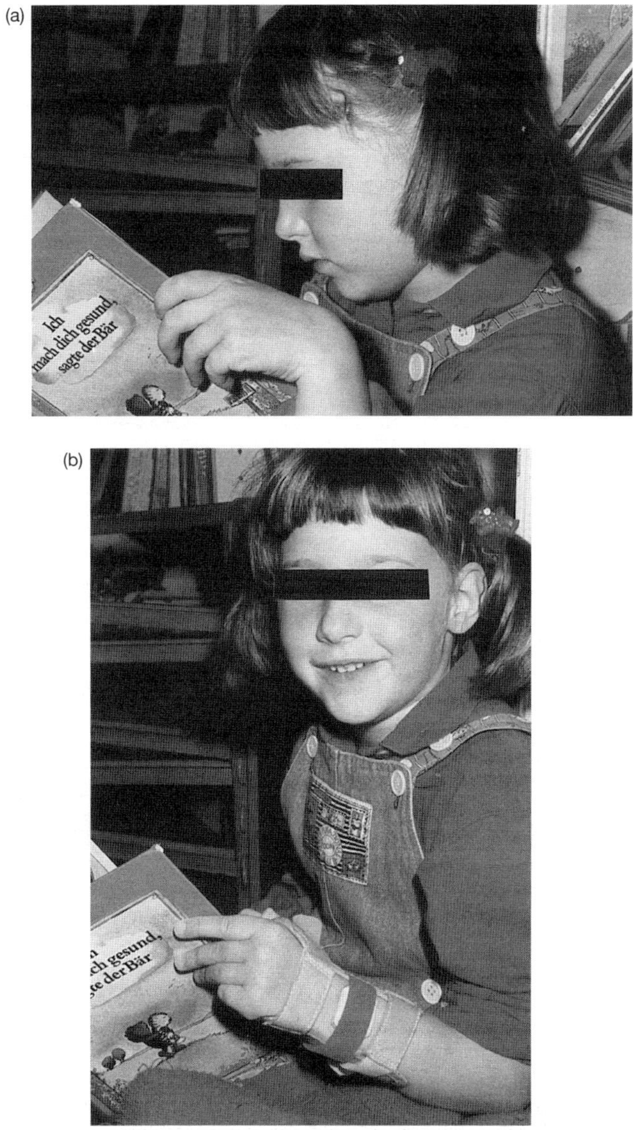

Fig. 11 Benefit of short supporting splints. The malposition in flexion and ulnar deviation (a) is corrected with a stabilizing splint (b).

tricycles, or scooters with a saddle are recommended (Fig. 12) for mobility. Wheelchair use is to be avoided since sitting increases flexion contractures of hips and knees (Ansell 1978; Swann 1978a; Melvin 1989).

Children have a good potential for restoration of joint cartilage and bone (Rombouts and Rombouts-Lindemans 1971; Bernstein et al. 1977; Melvin 1989; Häfner 1997) (Fig. 13). We therefore prefer partial weight bearing and regular, continuous moving of the hips in a relaxed position. The children benefit from using a sling suspension at home for daily exercises (Fig. 14).

The knee

The typical pain-relieving position is flexion of the knee joint which is stabilized by an increased tension of the hamstring muscles. The quadriceps muscle becomes hypotonic. Knee flexion contractures can develop into a very severe problem in young children. Each surgical procedure, even a small biopsy or arthroscopy, produces deterioration and should therefore be avoided in young children.

Predominant activity of the biceps femoris muscle in childhood arthritis results in an external rotation of the lower leg that is often compensated for by internal rotation of the hip joint, which then gives the impression of a valgus position of the knee but is really a pseudovalgus deformity (Spamer et al. 2001) (Fig. 15). Small children are particularly prone to develop a true valgus position which exceeds the physiological valgus for that age. It is caused by increased tension of the iliotibial band with ensuing instability of capsule and ligaments. Permanent knee flexion with dominant activity of the hamstring muscles favours dorsal subluxation of the tibia.

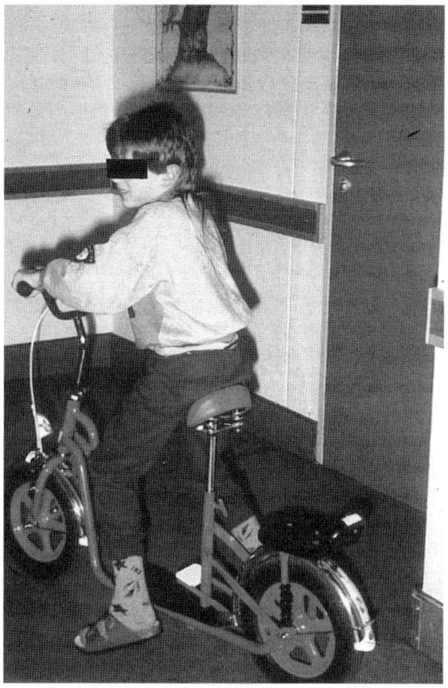

Fig. 12 Special vehicle for children with involvement of the lower limbs to avoid weight bearing.

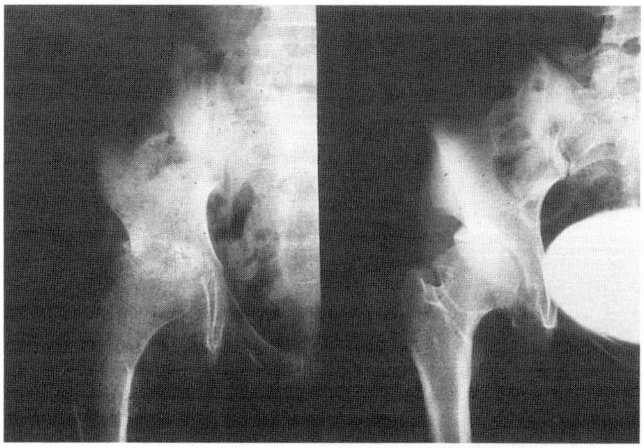

Fig. 13 Remodelling of hip joint destruction in a child with RF-negative polyarthritis.

Asymmetric knee involvement often results in a discrepancy in leg length due to increased growth at the affected knee joint.

Therapy

The first step in treatment of the knee should be to consider how to achieve full extension. When treating a knee flexion contracture it is especially important that the therapist is careful to respect the pain threshold, for only if the child is totally relaxed does it become possible to stretch the hypertonic hamstrings, in particular the biceps femoris muscle.

Once there is improvement of passive extension the quadriceps muscle can be activated.

Fast muscular coordination is best trained by letting the child kick including in water. However, the therapist must watch how far the full active extension is integrated in the course of movement.

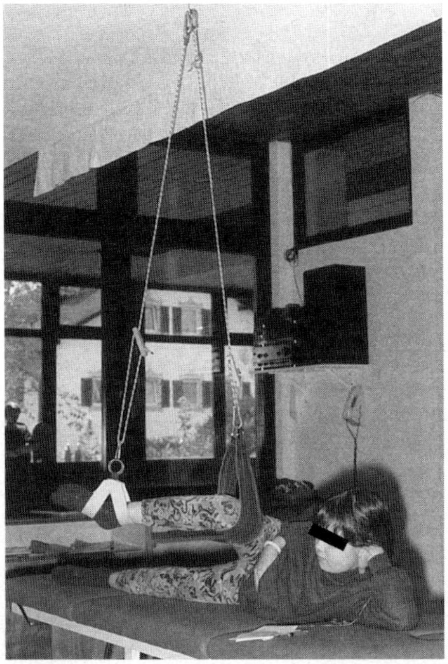

Fig. 14 Sling suspension for home exercises.

Additional aids

Stretching of the hamstring muscles can be supported by splints. They are put in place after physiotherapy in the position of maximum extension.

Arthritis of the knee benefits from partial weight bearing (Swann 1978a; Jarvis 1980; Melvin 1989; Spamer et al. 2001). It reduces stress to the joint, enables relaxation of the hypertonic muscles, and helps to avoid the wrong pattern of motion during walking.

A leg length discrepancy must be corrected by a combined sole and heel lift, otherwise pelvic tilting and scoliosis of the spine can develop. The increased leg length also promotes fixed knee flexion of the affected knee.

The foot

The numerous foot joints and variety in the pattern of joint involvement usually lead to a combination of different axial deformities. In most patients the gait becomes impaired. A neutral position or mild dorsal extension is the typical position of comfort when the ankle or talonavicular joint is inflamed (Melvin 1989; Spamer et al. 2001) (Fig. 16). The muscular imbalance includes a hypertonic tibialis anterior and a weak triceps surae and peroneus longus muscle. A rheumatic heel foot can develop. Plantar flexion and especially cranial movement of the heel become impaired. This is compensated by an increased flexion of the first metatarsophalangeal joint. The ball of the big toe, normally a major weight-bearing area, is spared and atrophies. During walking, body weight is transferred from the heel over the lateral rim to the distal phalanx of the big toe (Truckenbrodt et al. 1994; Spamer et al. 2001) (Fig. 17).

Young children in particular have a physiological tendency towards pes valgoplanus (Swann 1978b; Melvin 1989; Truckenbrodt et al. 1994; Spamer et al. 2001). During walking, impaired mobility is compensated by an outward turning of the leg and rolling over the medial rim (Fig. 18). This incorrect weight distribution increases the valgus deviation and flattening of the longitudinal arch. The forefoot seems to stand in pronation. However, if the heel is corrected into neutral position a supination of the forefoot becomes obvious (Fig. 19). Pronation is always impaired.

A rheumatic pes cavus develops less often and is seen mainly in older children with involvement of the distal intertarsal joints. These patients react with a reflex tension of the plantar muscles for pain relief (Fig. 20).

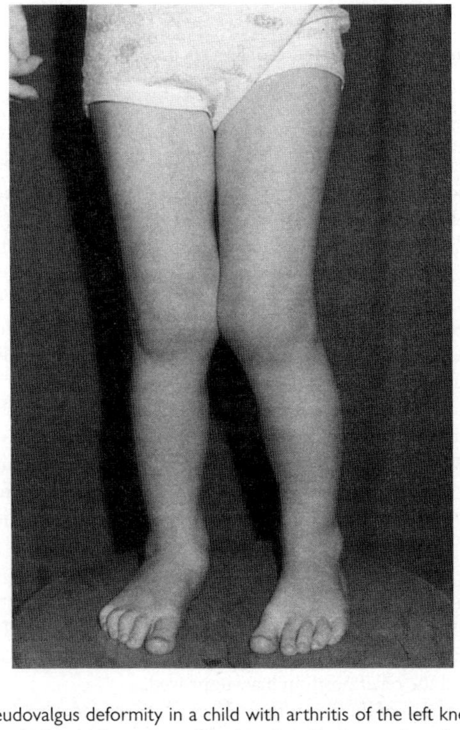

Fig. 15 Pseudovalgus deformity in a child with arthritis of the left knee. Flexion contracture with internal rotation of the leg gives the impression of a valgus position.

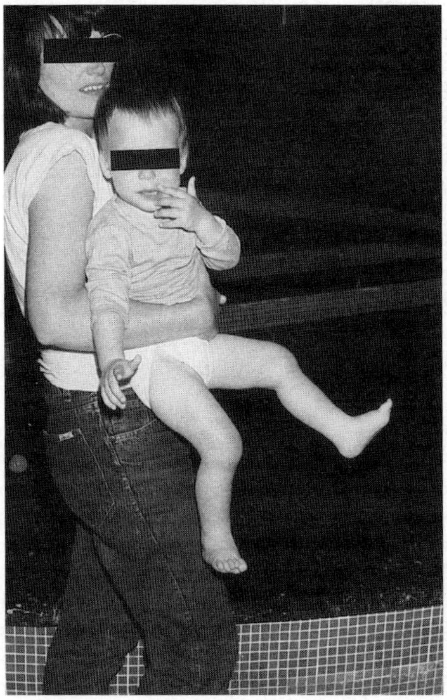

Fig. 16 Pain-relieving position with the feet in neutral position in a child with arthritis of both ankles.

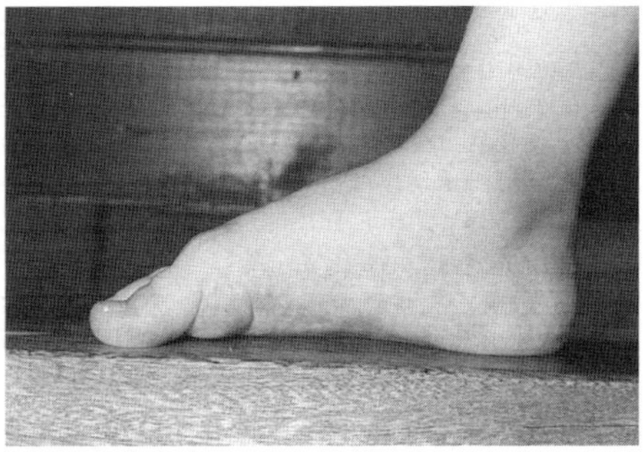

Fig. 17 Loading phase of a heel foot: the weight is shifted from the heel over the lateral rim to the distal phalanx of the big toe; the ball area is spared.

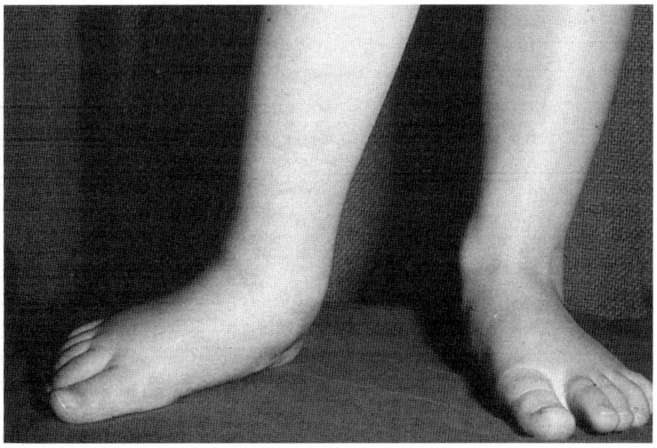

Fig. 18 Pes valgoplanus with external rotation of the leg and rolling over the medial rim.

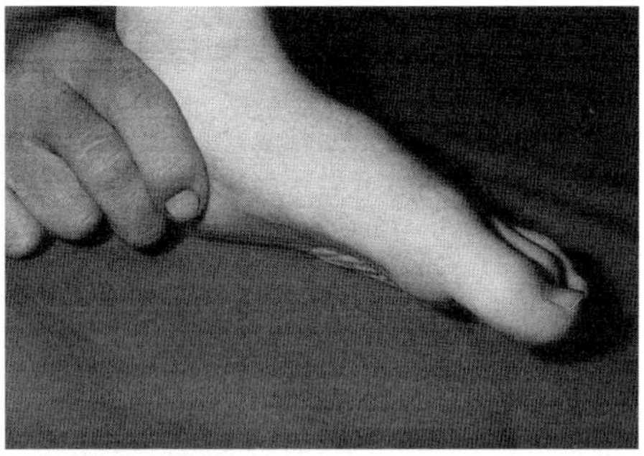

Fig. 19 Pes valgoplanus with erecting of the heel into neutral position. The forefoot stands in supination.

Heightening of the longitudinal arch occurs together with an increased loading of the ball area. This often induces flattening of the transversal arch and claw toes. When medial intertarsal joints are especially painful, the weight is shifted to the outer rim and the heel glides into a varus position (Swann 1978b; Melvin 1989; Truckenbrodt et al. 1994; Spamer et al. 2001).

Other foot deformities concern the forefoot and toes. Arthritis of the first metatarsophalangeal joint often results in a hallux flexus to relieve the painful area of the big toe ball. This deviation resembles the heel foot where a secondary hallux flexus can develop. A compensatory hyperextension of the interphalangeal joint may occur. A hallux valgus is seen mainly in children with polyarthritis and involvement of the metatarsophalangeal joints. These patients also tend to develop claw or hammer toes (Melvin 1989; Spamer et al. 2001).

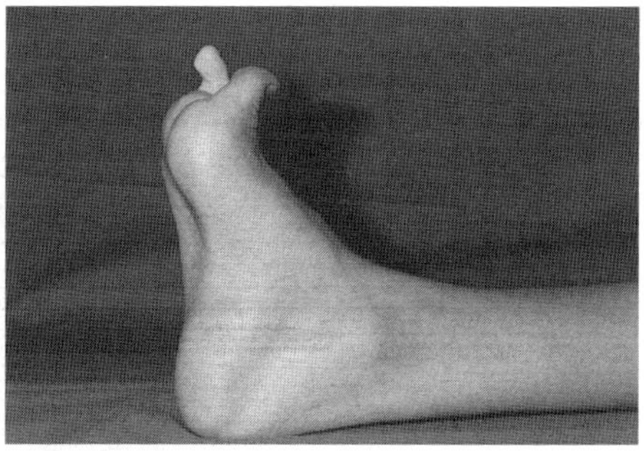

Fig. 20 Rheumatic pes cavus with tension of the plantar muscles.

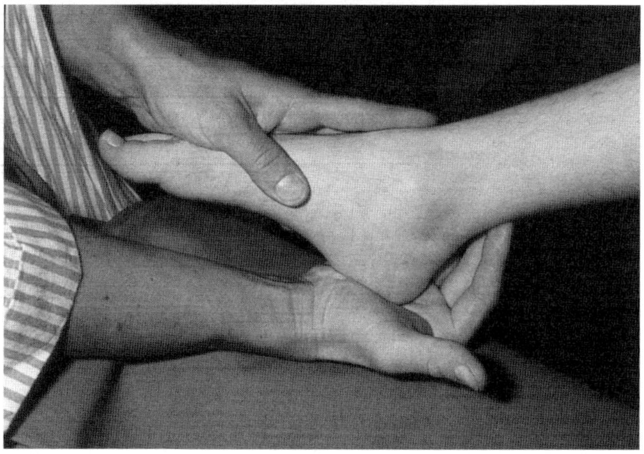

Fig. 21 Mobilization of plantar flexion with cranial moving of the calcaneus.

An equinus position of the foot is very rare in children with chronic arthritis.

Therapy

The first step should be to obtain mobility of each of the affected foot and toe joints. To achieve better plantar flexion in the ankle joint the therapist must concentrate in particular on cranial movement of the calcaneus (Fig. 21). Mobilizing forefoot pronation provides a strong fixation of the heel. It is also important to restore extension of the first metatarsophalangeal joint, which is necessary for the physiological loading of the big toe ball. To regain muscular balance the tibialis anterior muscle must be stretched and the triceps surae and peroneus longus muscles activated.

In a further procedure, the combined movement of forefoot pronation with extension of the big toe is exercised (Fig. 22).

To remedy the effects of foot involvement, intensive gait training is always necessary. The push-off with plantar flexion of the ankle and extension of the toes is very important. The therapist must correct wrong patterns and assist the re-education of each phase of a normal gait (Fig. 23).

Additional aids

Soft insoles should correct the deviation as long as they are adjustable without pain under full weight-bearing. Otherwise the insoles must primarily relieve the inflamed joints. It may even be necesssary to support a deviation until pain and the relief position have improved.

For stabilization of the upper foot, shoes which extend over the ankle are useful. Soft soles lower the transfer of concussions during walking. Severe foot deformities may require custom-made orthopaedic footwear. Partial weight-bearing is also recommended for children with inflamed foot joints.

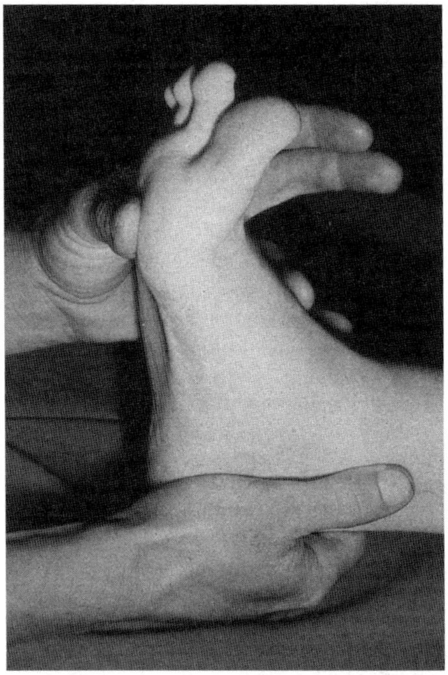

Fig. 22 Training of active toe extension together with forefoot pronation. The child is asked to push against the therapist's thumb.

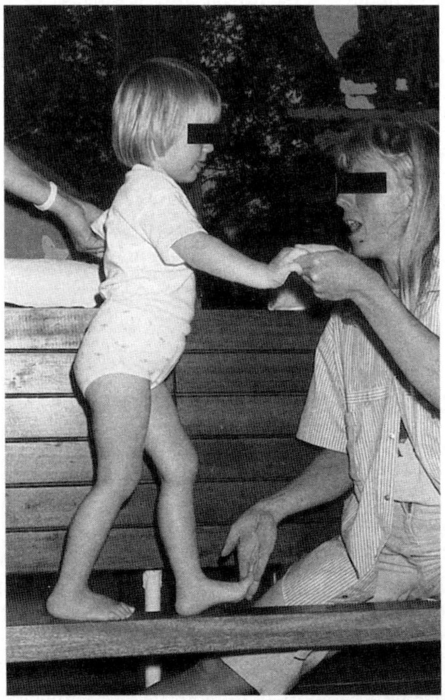

Fig. 23 Gait training with assistance to relearn each single phase of the gait cycle.

Joint protection and adapted devices

Joint protection training is an important task in the therapeutic regimen. The child with arthritis must learn how to reduce stress to the joints in daily activities. Effective joint protection relieves pain and can improve the inflammatory process. Principles of joint protection include:

1. proper positioning of joints to avoid deformities;
2. use of multiple instead of single joints;

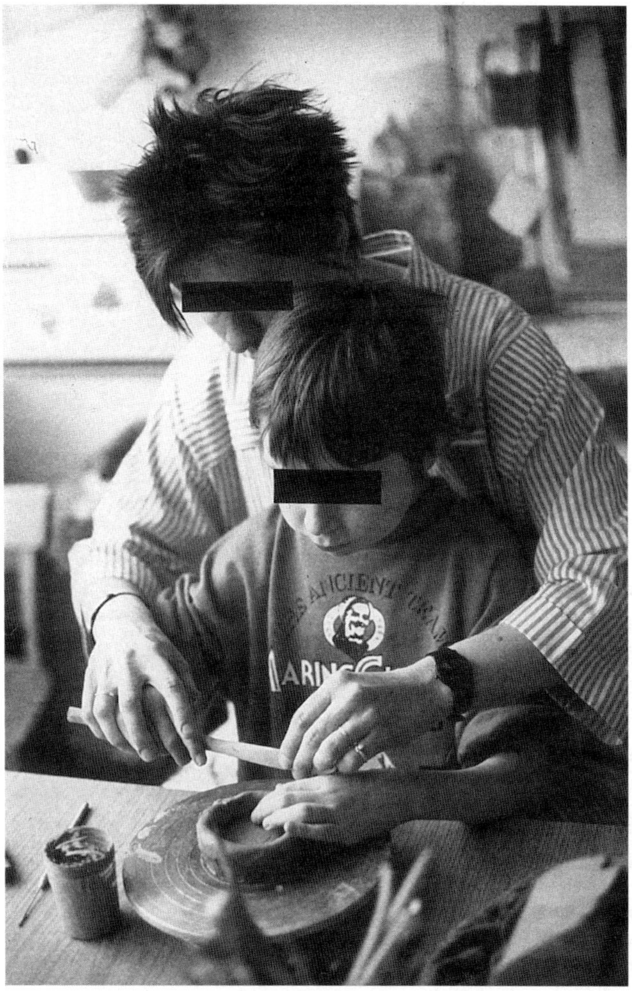

Fig. 24 The occupational therapist corrects a child's hand position during clay crafting.

3. transfer of a load from small to large joints or from involved to unaffected areas;
4. avoiding prolonged activity or positioning;
5. planning of rest breaks.

The child will assimilate these principles best if they are demonstrated during work or play (Fig. 24).

Joint protection may be supported by use of adapted devices. They help to reduce pain, preserve the proper joint position, minimize joint stress in daily activities, and increase the child's independence. In practice, such equipment is prescribed less often for children since they feel embarrassed to use such devices with their peers and prefer to use alternative techniques to perform a task or even to ask for help. Aid appliances, however, may become important for handicapped adolescents who wish to become independent.

Self-care equipment should be restricted to severely handicapped patients since most children with arthritis can learn to perform daily tasks without special equipment.

Integration into school

Most children with rheumatic diseases can and should be integrated into mainstream schools (Ansell and Chamberlain 1998). Classes for the physically handicapped are not the solution since they only serve to increase the child's sense of being abnormal.

(a)

(b)

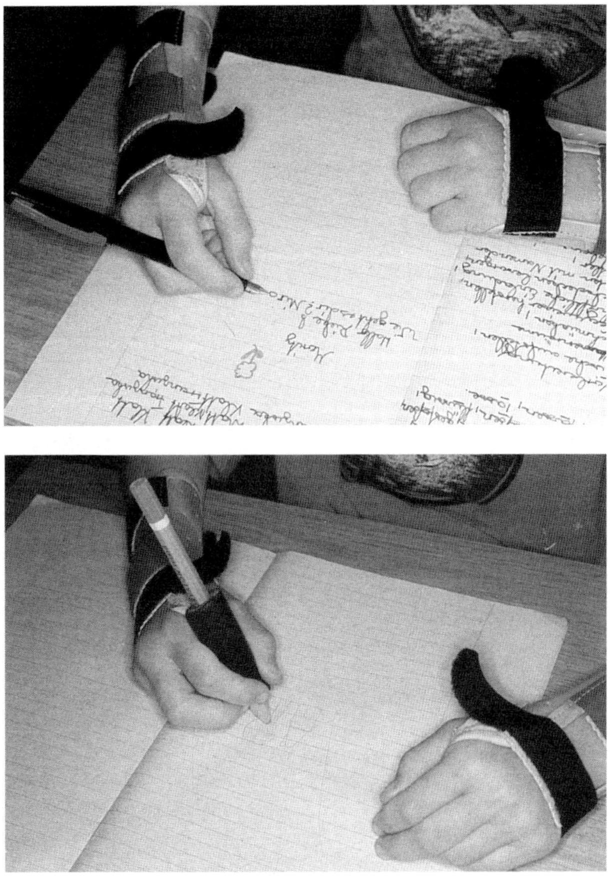

Fig. 25 Relief to finger joint pressure during writing occurs with an altered writing position (a) or a thickened pen handle (b).

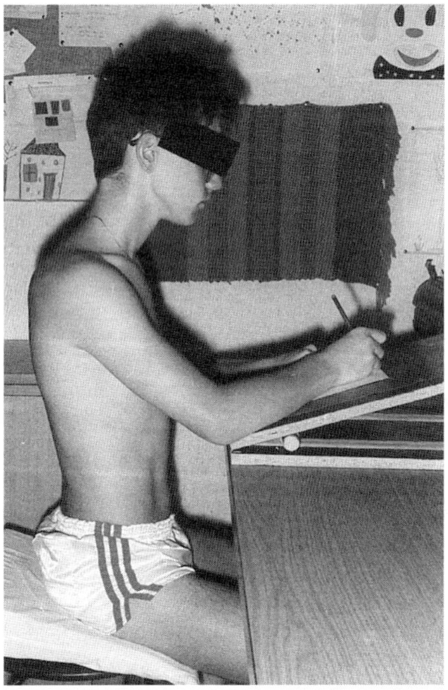

Fig. 26 Proper positioning during school or homework with an inclined bookstand and a slanting cushion.

Doctors, social workers, and therapists must communicate with educators and school nurses to find appropriate solutions and compromises for a practicable school life.

Keeping an extra set of books at home will save the child from having to carry heavy school bags. For necessary items backpacks should be preferred.

Children with arthritis of the hands may have a major problem with writing. Writing with splints is desirable to avoid ulnar deviation of the wrist but the changed position requires extra training. Pressure to the finger joints can be avoided if children learn to write holding the pen between index and middle finger and with the thumb in the opposed position. A thickened pencil also relieves joint stress (Fig. 25).

Despite all these aids, extended periods of writing may become painful and the child should receive extra time for class work to include rest periods. It is also helpful if the child is allowed to use a computer or dictaphone whenever possible.

Proper positioning during class and whilst doing homework is of the utmost importance, especially for children with back or neck problems. The solution consists of a chair adapted to the child's size, an inclined writing board or bookstand to avoid neck and back flexion, and a slanting cushion to tilt the pelvis and keep the spine erect (Fig. 26).

Parental involvement

For children with chronic progressive disease a regular, often daily, therapy programme is necessary. The best way to guarantee effective treatment at home is to integrate parents into the therapy programme. With adequate training most parents are able to undertake the task of daily exercises at home.

Problems with home therapy usually arise if progressive disease means treatment must be maintained over a prolonged period. In particular where patients suffer frequent relapse or continuous deterioration, general pessimism tends to reduce motivation. Parents and child may feel so discouraged that they abandon therapy. It is important to give them positive encouragement.

Parental education should also include advice on appropriate leisure activities. Sport is an important part of leisure activities in most families. It may be helpful if parents learn to give priority to sports which increase mobility without joint stress such as swimming or cycling. Depending on joint involvement and disease activity less aggressive sports may be acceptable (Häfner et al. 1998).

Guidance for the whole family

Arthritis in a child always has an impact on the whole family. Time-consuming demands, financial loss, and restriction of common activities alter the family's lifestyle; family members become resentful of their personal limitations and added responsibilities.

This situation requires guidance of the whole family, a task which all the team members may have to help resolve. Diagnosis of a chronic illness is usually devastating and adjustment to the new situation takes time, so it is vital that the health care team helps the families adapt to the altered situation. In the beginning, thorough information together with hope for a favourable outcome are important to motivate each family member.

Overprotection of the ill child and neglect of siblings is a common and understandable parental reaction, but should be avoided by early intervention. The ill child must learn to cope with frustrations and healthy siblings need support for their problems too.

On the other hand a child with chronic arthritis does need special attention. Pain and physical limitations often exceed what can be tolerated for appropriate social interaction. Regression, aggression, or other behavioural disturbances can result.

Cooperation within the family facilitates a positive adjustment and parents should be encouraged to share responsibility for all disease-related activities. Siblings may become involved in caring for the ill child. If they receive appropriate recognition for this extra demand they can develop a strong feeling of self-esteem.

Parents should be encouraged to join in family support groups as exchange of views among families with similar problems can be most helpful (Ansell and Chamberlain 1998). The health care team must, however, be aware of negative influences and uncertainty among the group. This situation can best be avoided if health professionals become regularly involved in support group meetings.

Helping children cope with their disease

Chronic diseases elicit different emotions in different children. Young children usually feel most disturbed by restrictions on their physical activity. In this age group normal motor activity is strongly related to psycho-social development, a process which is endangered in children with rheumatic diseases.

For older children and adolescents the disease has most impact on their social life, as this age group is strongly influenced by peer pressure. The rheumatic disease with its restrictions and special demands does not fit into the life concept of the peer group. Youngsters therefore tend to deny the illness and its consequences (Pelkonen 1997).

The health care team together with family, school staff, and friends must encourage positive adjustment. While treatment discipline is necessary, it should always leave enough time for play and hobbies. Friends and peers should be integrated into leisure activities. Healthy competition, which is important for the child's development, must be directed towards activities within the child's capabilities. Success at school or competence in music, crafts, games, etc. promote the child's self-esteem.

During the last years, we have gathered positive experience with patient education in small groups. Older children and adolescents share meetings with an expert who discusses a special aspect of the disease and its treatment. Topics are the characteristics of juvenile arthritis, drug therapy, principles of physiotherapy and occupational therapy as well as social aspects. The sessions have become very popular among our patients. They not only learn about their disease, but also benefit from the konwledge and personal experience of their co-patients.

Children who suffered from a long-standing rheumatic disease often learned to overcome obstacles which their friends could not even dream of. That can be a source for more self-reliance and positive self-esteem. The adolescent may be earlier and better qualified for an independent life despite some physical limitations. Parents and health care team members must recognize the child's struggle for freedom and facilitate appropriate self-determination and self-support.

References

Ansell, B.M. (1978). Rehabilitation. In *Surgical Management of Juvenile Chronic Polyarthritis* (ed. G.P. Arden and B.M. Ansell), pp. 201–15. New York: Grune & Stratten.

Ansell, B.M. and Kent, P.A. (1977). Radiological changes in juvenile chronic polyarthritis. *Skeletal Radiology* **1**, 129–44.

Ansell, B.M. and Chamberlain, M.A. (1998). Children with chronic arthritis: the management of transition to adulthood. *Baillière's Clinical Rheumatology* **12**, 363–74.

Bache, C. (1964). Mandibular growth and dental occlusion in juvenile rheumatoid arthritis. *Acta Rheumatica Scandinavica* **10**, 142–53.

Bernstein, B., Forrester, D., Singsen, B., Koster King, K., Kornreich, H., and Hanson, V. (1977). Hip joint restoration in juvenile rheumatoid arthritis. *Arthritis and Rheumatism* **20**, 1099–104.

Erlandson, D.M. (1989). Juvenile rheumatoid arthritis. In *Pediatric Rehabilitation. A Team Approach for Therapists* (ed. M.K. Logigian and J.D. Ward). Boston MA: Little, Brown and Company.

Garcia-Morteo, O., Babini, J.C., Maldonado-Cocco, J.A., Gagliardi, S., and Yabkowski, J. (1981). Remodeling of the hip joint in juvenile rheumatoid arthriris. *Arthritis and Rheumatism* **24**, 1570–4.

Häfner, R. (1997). Influence of inflammation and muscular imbalance on growth and form of the hip in juvenile chronic arthritis. *Revue du Rhumatisme (English Edition)* **64** (Suppl. 10), 169–72.

Häfner, R., Truckenbrodt, H., and Spamer, M. (1998). Rehabilitation in children with juvenile chronic arthritis. *Baillière's Clinical Rheumatology* **12**, 329–61.

Hayem, F., Calède, C., Hayem, G., and Kahn, M.F. (1994). Involvement of the hip in systemic-onset forms of juvenile chronic arthritis. A retrospective study of twenty-eight cases. *Revue du Rhumatisme (English Edition)* **61**, 516–22.

Jarvis, R.E. (1980). Treatment of arthritis in children. In *Physiotherapy in Rheumatology* (ed. S.A. Hyde). Oxford: Blackwell Scientific Publications.

Lloyd, S. and Aldrich, S. (1993). Paediatric rheumatology: meeting report. Second workshop of physiotherapy in JCA (Garmisch–Partenkirchen). *British Journal of Rheumatology* **32**, 425.

Melvin, J.L. *Rheumatic Disease in the Adult and Child: Occupational Therapy and Rehabilitation.* Philadelphia PA: F.A. Davis Company, 1989.

Pedersen, T.K. et al. (1995). Condylar condition and mandibular growth during early functional treatment of children with juvenile chronic arthritis. *European Journal of Orthodontics* **17**, 385–94.

Pelkonen, P.M. (1997). Impact of arthritis and its consequences on the psychological development of adolescents. *Revue du Rhumatisme (English Edition)* **64** (Suppl. 10), 191–3.

Rombouts, J.J. and Rombouts-Lindemans, C. (1971). Involvement of the hip in juvenile rheumatoid arthritis. A radiological study with special reference to growth disturbances. *Acta Rheumatica Scandinavica* **17**, 248–67.

Scott, P.J., Ansell, B.M., and Huskinsson, E.C. (1977). Measurement of pain in juvenile chronic polyarthritis. *Annals of the Rheumatic Diseases* **36**, 186.

Spamer, M. (1997). Conservative treatment of the hip in juvenile chronic arthritis. *Revue du Rhumatisme (English Edition)* **64** (Suppl. 10), 179–182.

Spamer, M., Häfner, R., and Truckenbrodt, H., ed. *Physiotherapie in der Kinderrheumatologie.* München: Pflaum Verlag, 2001.

Stabrun, A.E., Larheim, T.A., Hoyeraal, H.M., and Rösler, M. (1988). Reduced mandibular dimensions and asymmetry in juvenile rheumatoid arthritis. *Arthritis and Rheumatism* **31**, 602–11.

Swann, M. (1978a). Management of lower limb deformities. In *Surgical Management of Juvenile Chronic Polyarthritis* (ed. G.P. Arden and B.M. Ansell), pp. 97–115. New York: Grune & Stratton.

Swann, M. (1978b). The foot. In *Surgical Management of Juvenile Chronic Polyarthritis* (ed. G.P. Arden and B.M. Ansell), pp. 185–99. New York: Grune & Stratton.

Truckenbrodt, H. (1993). Pain in juvenile chronic arthritis: consequences for the musculo-skeletal system. *Clinical and Experimental Rheumatology* **11** (Suppl. 9), 59–63.

Truckenbrodt, H., Häfner, R., and von Altenbockum, C. (1994). Functional joint analysis of the foot in juvenile chronic arthritis. *Clinical and Experimental Rheumatology* **12** (Suppl. 10), 91–6.

2.4 Rheumatic disease and sexuality

David M. Siegel and John Baum

Introduction

Sexuality is a fundamental aspect of life for men and women. When one has a rheumatic disease both sexual desire and function are affected by the physical and psychological consequences of the illness. Although human sexual development is a lifelong process commencing *in utero*, many important aspects of the development of adult sexuality come to the fore during adolescence, and rheumatic illnesses are certainly present in the teenage population. Therefore, this chapter begins with a description of the psychosocial transitions that take place during adolescence leading toward the establishment of mature sexuality. Contributions to the literature describing the specific impact of rheumatological illness on sexuality and sexual function are reviewed and the chapter concludes with practical strategies for enhancing sexual satisfaction among those affected by rheumatic disease.

Adolescent sexuality

During childhood young boys and girls undergo similar sexual exploration through fantasy, play, and masturbation as they become aware of their bodies and gender differences (Zuengler and Neubeck 1983; Perrin and Gerrity 1984). In most societies it is during adolescence, however, that the sexual behaviours of males and females begin to differentiate. This is influenced by both the neuroendocrine changes of puberty and the sociocultural context in which the individual resides. In order to understand the potential impact of rheumatic disease on sexuality it is first necessary to recognize what is considered normal development for adolescents and young adults (Perrin and Gerrity 1984; McAnarney 1985; Strax 1988).

Adolescence is divided into early (11–15 years), middle (15–17 years), and late (17 years–early 20's) phases and significant developmental tasks challenge young people at each of these stages leading toward adulthood (Hamberg 1998). Pre-eminent in this process is a consolidation of identity including a capacity for intimacy that is made up, in part, by sexuality. For early adolescents, puberty arises with concomitant body changes representing concrete manifestations of the physical dimension of sexuality. These young people are powerfully preoccupied with both the adequacy and attractiveness of these changes and to varying degrees such focus on visible physical attributes persists through adulthood often reinforced by societal emphasis on stereotypic perceptions of beauty. Those teenagers who mature early or late may experience additional distress as their bodies seem to differ from their contemporaries. At the same time, social skills necessary for successful peer interaction begin to develop, and undergo repeated practice and rehearsal with family and friends, in school, and in other group settings. Toward the conclusion of middle adolescence most young people experience a slowing and completion of the bodily transformations whereas a more sophisticated repertoire of social and cognitive abilities continue to be established. It is during this period that overt sexual activity becomes increasingly incorporated into the individual's behaviour such that in the United States, for example, by age 19, over half will have experienced sexual intercourse. There is, in fact, a significant range of sexual experience as a function of age, gender, personality, and socio-cultural background (Netting 1992; Rodgers 1998).

Goals of adolescent psychosocial development that facilitate healthy adult sexuality have been articulated by Sarrel and Sarrel as 'sexual unfolding' (Sarrel and Sarrel 1981). Based on their work involving thousands of middle and upper middle class American college students, they have identified nine characteristics and tasks that culminate in a fully evolved, personally incorporated, and gratifying adult sexuality (Table 1). These general principles provide a useful paradigm with which to view the psychology of sexuality, albeit from a Western, industrialized socio-cultural perspective. It is also important to note that *mastery* of each of these points is not expected or necessarily predominant, but rather a gradual (and lifelong) striving for incorporation of these attributes into one's behaviour and relationships. Obviously, the full accomplishment of these goals does not occur during adolescence but personal development and experiences during the second decade of life lay the groundwork for one's eventual adult sexual adaptation and adjustment be it heterosexual, homosexual, or bisexual. Onset of rheumatic disease during adolescence and young adulthood can substantially disrupt the evolution of a number of these processes.

The presence of a rheumatic (or other chronic) disease during adolescence can adversely affect evolving sexuality through a variety of mechanisms

Table 1 Nine processes of sexual unfolding

1. Evolving sense of the body that is gender specific and free of body image distortion
2. Overcome guilt, shame, fear, and childhood inhibitions associated with sexual thoughts and behaviour
3. Loosening of emotional ties to parent and family
4. Learning to recognize what is erotically pleasing and displeasing and being able to communicate this to a partner
5. Resolution of sexual orientation
6. Absence of sexual dysfunction or compulsion
7. Awareness of being a sexual person and the place and value of sex in one's life, including the option of celibacy
8. Becoming responsible regarding sexuality (e.g. contraception, barriers, not use sex as a means of exploitation)
9. Increasing ability to experience eroticism as one aspect of intimacy with another person

Adapted from: Sarrel, L.J. and Sarrel, P.M. (1981). Sexual unfolding. *Journal of Adolescent Health Care* **2**, 93–9.

(Frauman and Sypert 1979; Perrin and Gerrity 1984; McAnarney 1985; Woodhead and Murph 1985; Strax 1988; Selekman and McIlvain-Simpson 1991). Confirmation of one's maleness or femaleness is centrally invested in the expected physical attributes that identify gender. The development of these characteristics during puberty are carefully monitored by the body-preoccupied early and middle adolescent as he/she searches for signs of those changes observed or reported by peers. The adolescent with persistent rheumatic disease is often faced with a significant delay in growth and appearance of secondary sex characteristics creating fear, uncertainty, and decreased self-esteem. This growth delay and suppression is a striking manifestation of juvenile arthritis as a consequence of both ongoing disease activity as well as from corticosteroid therapy (Stoeber 1976). Not only is there concern by the adolescent about whether adult features will *ever* manifest, but attractiveness and appeal are also questioned. These young people can be resentful and distressed about their slowed (or absent) development, but they may also be convinced that peers will judge them negatively as a consequence. The overwhelming importance placed by children in early and middle adolescence on peer perception and acceptance as a physically and sexually attractive individual explains the immediacy of this fear. As teenagers aspire to accept themselves, they typically display intolerance for those who appear and/or act differently. Thus, peer groups or cliques emerge, organized around patterns of speech, dress, attitude, etc. Adolescents with rheumatic illness can find themselves readily excluded from this social organization, at least in part because of their visible differences if not also due to their actual physical limitations. They may be unable to keep up with sports activities and often have only intermittent contact with their peers due to hospitalizations and frequent medical absences.

Impairments and abnormalities suffered as a result of rheumatic diseases such as juvenile arthritis, systemic lupus erythematosus, dermatomyositis, etc. affect the individual not only among their peers, but at home as well. While adolescence is a time during which increased autonomy and independence are appropriate goals, such illnesses can present serious obstacles to attainment of these developmental milestones. Initial diagnosis and management of diseases in adolescents is usually undertaken by parent(s). It is the adults (or adult) in the home who are expected to understand and take primary responsibility for the medical, psychosocial, and therapeutic dimensions of the illness while including the adolescent patient in the informational and decision-making processes. Soon, however, the teenager is faced with the developmental and logistic need to take on increasing self-care, a transition that can conflict with parental resistance to disrupting the status quo. Further, depending on the magnitude of care taking requirements, it may not be entirely possible for the patient with a rheumatic disease to adequately address the bulk of his/her needs.

These impediments to individual development, independence, and separation from family bear directly on sexuality. As cited by Sarrel and Sarrel

(1981), part of the maturation process necessary for the establishment of adult intimacy and sexuality includes a loosening of the primary bonds to family in order to make way for the next phase of relationships. While not an easy transition for any individual, the forced dependency imposed by rheumatic disease renders this step a particular challenge for the handicapped or disabled teenager. The obvious difficulty in accomplishing this shift from family bonding further exacerbates the potential problem regarding peer acceptance. That is, as the adolescent patient needs to explore ways of expressing and learning about his/her sexuality through interactions with others, these potential partners may be reluctant to pair with one who is unable to distance from parent(s). Furthermore just being exposed to a peer who cannot begin to separate from his/her family can be threatening and create anxiety in the healthy adolescent. In addition to holding on to primary caretaking for their maturing son or daughter for fear that he/she will otherwise lack for proper attention, parents confronted with their child's persistent physical immaturity (and dependence) are left without the usual visual and behavioural cues prodding them to recognize the coming of late adolescence and adulthood. This is particularly salient for sexuality when one considers the reluctance with which parents address the topic of sexuality even with their healthy children (Zuengler and Neubeck 1983). Thus, the adolescent with chronic rheumatic disease can be dually burdened by problems in moving *away* from his/her concerned and tenacious family of origin, as well as impaired steps *toward* the progressively more autonomous, but reluctantly accepting or inviting peer group.

Despite the intimidating potential for dysfunction among chronically ill teenagers, there are some reassuring data. In a comparison of patients with oncologic, cardiac, diabetic, rheumatic, or cystic fibrosis disease to healthy controls, overall measures of self-esteem and trait anxiety were similar in diseased and healthy groups (Kellerman et al. 1980; Zeltzer et al. 1980). Since self-esteem strongly influences sexuality this finding is positive and important. Conversely, in a report of 270 chronically ill children (of whom 24, or 9 per cent had juvenile arthritis) maternal responses to a behaviour check list indicated behavioural and social competence problems at rates higher than those standardized for healthy children. In the specific scale of 'externalizing behavior problems', however, children with arthritis scored lower (i.e. were described as having fewer of these problems) than the other disease groups (diabetes, spina bifida, haemophilia, chronic obesity, and cerebral palsy) (Wallander et al. 1988).

In a study of 363 children and young adults with juvenile arthritis, average scores on measures of self-concept revealed no differences with a normative sample of Australian children. When analysed separately, high school students who scored lower on the self-concept scale were, in fact, more socially isolated (defined, in part, as having fewer close friends and experiencing less dating). There was also a direct relationship between increased disease severity and decreased psychosocial functioning and adjustment (Ungerer et al. 1988). For all of these young people, during periods of illness exacerbation and increased disability one can anticipate even greater than normal levels of anxiety, depression, and dysfunction. Interestingly, in one study children with juvenile arthritis whose disability was less visually apparent reported greater psychosocial disruption than those with more noticeable impairment (McAnarney et al. 1974). Nevertheless, chronically ill adolescents do become sexually active, some (with milder impairments) at rates comparable to healthy teenagers (Choquet et al. 1997).

Interaction of rheumatic disease and sexuality

Having described these important aspects of sexuality and adolescent development, a further review of what is present in the literature regarding sexuality in teenagers and adults with rheumatic disease follows. It is notable that virtually all of the referenced papers describe patients with arthritis (juvenile or rheumatoid), and more recent articles are relatively few in number. Seeking to assess the degree to which adolescents with juvenile arthritis are concerned about sexuality, Wilkinson (1981) chose to examine the more severe range of the disease continuum by questioning a population of 27 adolescents with severe juvenile arthritis who were inpatients. Seventy per cent of this group were significantly socially isolated, and anxieties about lack of sexual contact, as a consequence of the isolation, were prominent.

Some 20 years later, Britto et al. (2000) identified as a problem the lack of questioning about sexual issues by paediatric rheumatologists during medical encounters with rheumatic disease patients (at one major US teaching children's hospital). Among 178 subjects with a mean age of 18.1 years (67 per cent female, 88 per cent white, 69 per cent with juvenile arthritis) screening for sexual activity was documented in the medical record for only 12.4 per cent of the visits. The authors designed and implemented an intervention consisting of three educational sessions for the (all male) rheumatologists in which these physicians were instructed on how to incorporate sexuality screening into their clinical routine. One year post-intervention the rate of screening had increased but to only 36.2 per cent and was more likely to have occurred among older, female, and black patients. When asked about obstacles to screening the paediatric rheumatologists cited time constraints and a skepticism of the effectiveness of screening in subsequently altering sexual practice among the study population.

In a study of 58 individuals with juvenile arthritis, participants were asked at a mean of 14.5 years after disease onset about marital status, dating, masturbation, orgasm, coitus, and limitation of coitus by pain, position, or fatigue (Hill et al. 1976; Herstein et al. 1977). The study sample included 21 men and 37 women with an age range at the time of questioning of 19–37 years. Age distribution was skewed toward late adolescence and young adults, however, with 50 out of 58 patients less than 28 years old and 17 subjects 19 or 20 years old. Fifty-two of the subjects were interviewed by a gynaecologist experienced in sexual counselling lending validity to the information gathered. When asked about frequency of coitus, marital status was a powerful determinant with all of those who were married reporting regular coitus, but only 17 out of 31 of those unmarried giving the same response. The authors stratified the group by arthritis functional class (I to IV) and found that those with greater disability (classes III, IV) had a lower prevalence of 'regular coitus' than did those with milder impairment (I, II). Interestingly, achievement of orgasm among the women did not differ by disease severity (9 per 23 with mild, 4 per 10 with severe disease). Limitation of coital activity due to pain, position, or fatigue was a factor for all patients with functional class III or IV and 16 out of 28 of those who were in class I or II. Thirty-eight per cent of the group desired sexual counselling. The authors, as would be expected, concluded that juvenile arthritis has an impact on sexual activity, although some of the most severely affected (two individuals confined to wheelchairs) nevertheless reported regular coitus. Intercourse does not make up the totality of sexuality, but these data certainly provide some insight into the coital dimension of sexuality for patients with juvenile arthritis.

Consistently high prevalences of loss of sexual interest and decrease in sexual desire have been reported (Ferguson and Figley 1979; Yoshino and Uchida 1981). Elst et al. (1984) utilized a standardized questionnaire to compare sexual motivation and coital position preference among adults with rheumatoid arthritis (RA, $n = 122$) to those with ankylosing spondylitis (AS, $n = 66$). Mean ages of the two groups were early to mid 40s and those with AS displayed a normal tendency to want to engage in sexual interaction whereas those with RA were abnormally averse to sexual interaction. High joint activity indices correlated with low sexual motivation and RA patients scored lower on length of foreplay and sexual enjoyment and were more likely to express need for help and advice regarding coital positioning.

Targeting only patients with RA, investigators from the Netherlands explored the degree of intrusiveness on sexuality presented by rheumatoid arthritis (Kraaimaat et al. 1996). Specifically they were interested in clarifying the effect of physical disability, pain, depression, and criticism by spouse on patient rated intrusiveness of RA on sexuality. All subjects (118 women and 102 men) were living with a spouse, at least 21 years old (mean age of

57 for women, and 61 for men), and had a disease duration of at least 2 years (mean of 14.5 years for females and 12.5 years for males). In response to the statement 'In general, the rheumatic disease interferes with my sexuality' approximately one-third of the population answered in each category of 'never', 'sometimes', and 'almost always' with slightly (but not statistically significantly) more males than females in 'never' (37 versus 30 per cent) and more females than males in 'almost always' (36 versus 30 per cent). Other measures in the study demonstrated that whereas degree of mobility, self-care, pain, and depression were correlated with intrusiveness, criticism by a spouse when in pain was not. The authors speculated that the latter item did not probe deeper or more pervasive partner conflicts that might bear on the nature of the sexual relationship.

Blake et al. (1987) assembled an appropriate, healthy concurrent control group (n = 130) to compare to 169 patients (mean age = 57 years) diagnosed with RA, osteoarthritis, or ankylosing spondylitis. More similarities than differences were observed. Subjects were asked about the quality of their current sexual adjustment and 36 per cent of patients and 39 per cent of controls indicated that they were *not* satisfied, whereas 35 and 33 per cent, respectively, were satisfied. When asked to compare past (pre-arthritis for patients) with present status 42 per cent of controls but 58 per cent of those with arthritis described a decrease in sexual satisfaction over time, and loss of sexual pleasure was reported by 21 per cent of controls versus 38 per cent of patients. These findings did not differ based on marital status either within or between groups. Thus, although age was clearly a factor, living with arthritis makes an additional negative contribution. Symptoms and concerns that can negatively impact on sexual function for patients with arthritis were also recorded. Joint pain, joint stiffness, and fatigue were ranked highest by patients, though controls also reported fatigue as a problem. Loss of libido and loss of lubrication were issues identified by both groups, and it is notable that feeling unattractive was of no greater concern for patients than for controls. Finally, being receptive to sexual counselling regarding guidance on changes in coital position, mutual masturbation, masturbation, and (of least interest) oral sex was comparable in both groups (independent of level of sexual satisfaction) and ranged from one-fifth to one-third of the population.

Rather than using a control group of healthy subjects, Lipe et al. (1990) compared 29 married men (mean age of 58 years) with arthritis (rheumatoid, psoriatic, or osteoarthritis) to 41 married men with Parkinson's disease (mean age of 62 years) using a self-administered, 17 item sexual functioning questionnaire. Subjects also completed a depression scale, and their health care providers rated the severity of their illness (RA or PD). The sexual functioning instrument was divided into 4 sub-scales consisting of desire, arousal, orgasm, and satisfaction. There was no significant difference on any of these parameters between the two study populations. Monthly frequency of intercourse was also similar (mean of 4 for PD and 3 for arthritis) as was patient rated satisfaction of mate. Both increasing age and greater severity of disease were significantly related to decreased sexual function. The results of this study support the contention that there is a common and noncategorical impact of chronic illness on sexual functioning despite differences in diagnosis, type of physical impairment, medication, etc.

The relationship between sexual satisfaction and functional disability was examined in a mailed questionnaire comparison of 113 married couples in which one spouse had a rheumatic disease (79.6 per cent had RA, 73 per cent were female, 94 per cent were white) compared to 37 healthy couples (Majerovitz and Revenson 1994). The mean age of patients was 56.7 years and for controls 53.6 years and there were similarly no significant differences between the groups in education, ethnicity, or years married. Sexual dissatisfaction was assessed using a 5 item scale (possible score range of 5–25) that measured frequency and level of interest in sex, feelings of sexual attraction for the spouse, and changes in level of sexual enjoyment. Illness severity, pain, and functional disability class were also measured. The majority of patients reported moderate disability and moderate levels of pain. Patients and controls reported similar overall levels of dissatisfaction (mean scores of 13.1 and 13.1, respectively; higher scores indicated greater dissatisfaction) and women were more sexually dissatisfied than men (mean scores of 13.9 versus 10.8). Not surprisingly, a positive correlation between a higher level of disability and increased sexual dissatisfaction was found. This study again confirms that the level of functional disability clearly impacts on sexual dissatisfaction, but also demonstrates a consistent effect on *spousal* sexual satisfaction, as well.

In a study from Norway by Ostensen and her colleagues (2000), 126 adult women and 35 adult men with a history of juvenile arthritis were administered a questionnaire about reproductive behaviour and health. The part of the questionnaire directly relating to sexuality found only two males and five females who noted that their physical handicap and disease activity prevented sex. Another possible deterrent, although minor because of the frequent use of birth control, was that one-third of the females had been advised against having children. This advice came half the time from doctors and about a third of the time from family members. An additional factor that was reported to interfere with sexual activity was a significantly higher frequency of metrorrhagia and needed surgery for cystic ovaries in the patients when compared to control. Pelvic inflammatory disease was seen twice as often in patients versus the normal controls although this was not a statistically significant difference. Sexual activity per se was as frequently reported in the patients as the controls (77 per cent) even though remission of disease was present in only about 50 per cent of the patients. Male patients reported rarer and less frequent sexual activity than the control population.

Gutweniger et al. (1999) recognized body image as an important component of sexuality and with this in mind studied a group of 40 women with RA. Specifically, the subjects were administered a 52 item questionnaire that measured four constructs. They were: (i) attractiveness/self-confidence, (ii) accentuation of external appearance, (iii) worry about possible physical deficits, and (iv) problems regarding sexuality. RA disease activity was assessed using functional classification, radiographs, joint counts, erythrocyte sedimentation rate, rheumatoid factor, and duration of morning stiffness. The patients had a mean age of 45 years and 75 per cent were married. The authors found that half of the women rated themselves as having a minimal degree of morning stiffness and half with a high degree and these two groups did not differ on any clinical or sociodemographic characteristics. Those with greater morning stiffness, however, reported significantly more worries about possible physical deficits and problems about sexuality than did their less stiff counterparts. This study points out the importance of subjective symptom reports (e.g. morning stiffness) in assessing risk for sexual problems, independent of other clinical or laboratory parameters of disease activity. The importance of morning stiffness as an indicator of persistent inflammatory activity is well-recognized by rheumatologists.

Several papers have been published that examine changes in sexual functioning among patients who have undergone arthroplasty (primarily hip joint replacement) as treatment for rheumatoid or osteoarthritis. Older studies by Currey (1970) and Todd et al. (1973) found 67 and 52 per cent, respectively, of adult patients reported sexual function disruption and attributed it to the pain and stiffness in their hip joints. The intriguing finding in these studies was that despite successful resolution of pain and stiffness in over 90 per cent of subjects after surgery, in both populations sexual difficulties improved in only 45 per cent (Currey 1970) and 57 per cent, respectively, (Todd et al. 1973) of those who reported preoperative problems. These results certainly speak to the additional psychologic (and perhaps other) factors that contribute to sexual dysfunction in these patients even in the presence of their perception that the aetiology is primarily physical. In a different population of 28 married RA patients with sexual problems felt to be secondary to hip pain, after total hip replacement 10 of these patients continued to have sexuality related difficulties (Baldursson and Brattstrom 1979). This could be related to the age of the patients when hip replacement was performed. Ostensen (1993) has reported that about 6000 patients have total hip replacements (THR) per year in Norway. She surveyed orthopaedists and obstetricians as well as reviewing the pertinent literature. Her synthesis of this material indicated that with advice to restrict sexual activity for 3 months following the procedure, uncomplicated THRs should result in no interference with sexual activity. Patients with joint replacement due to inflammatory arthritis with multiple joints and muscle involvement need more specific counselling regarding resumption of sexual activity.

Although this literature is not vast, there is ample evidence demonstrating problematic aspects of sexual function and sexuality in the lives of patients with rheumatic disease. More has been described about adult populations, but adolescents soon become adults [a transition with significant health care implications (Rettig and Athreya 1991)] and are at risk for similar outcomes, complicated by the additional complexity of chronic illness during their early physical and psychologic development (as discussed previously).

The importance and prevalence of this morbidity mandate that assessment of sexual function in patients with rheumatic disease be assigned a prominent place on the list of other physical and psychological parameters routinely inventoried during the health care encounter. A systematic review of the literature to identify valid, reliable, and generalizable instruments that assess sexual function of patients with specific rheumatic diseases was recently undertaken (Quaresma et al. 1997). Utilizing a comprehensive yet rigorous selection procedure, only 10 suitable articles were identified for critical appraisal. They addressed sexual function among those with systemic lupus erythematosus (3 studies), rheumatoid arthritis (2), osteoarthritis (1), chronic arthritis (3), and one paper compared patients with systemic sclerosis, SLE, and RA. The authors were discouraged to report that 'No article satisfied the quality criteria (for inclusion in the review), either because the study did not describe important issues of the instrument construction or because the properties (i.e. reliability, validity, responsiveness) of the instrument used were not tested (Quaresma et al. 1997)'. They went on to conclude that adequate questionnaire and scale development is urgently needed to evaluate sexual function in these patients. In a review of what had been written as of 1980 concerning sexuality and arthritis Richards (1980) noted the relative paucity of rigorous studies and also stressed the importance of asking patients with arthritis about the quality of their sex life and their perception of the contribution of joint disease to the latter. Again, valid and reliable questionnaires or instruments would greatly facilitate both research and patient care in this realm. Now, more than 20 years later quality and quantity of these studies is still lacking.

Strategies for improving sexual function and satisfaction in patients with rheumatic disease

The clinician participating in the care of patients with rheumatic disease can incorporate numerous strategies to better understand and potentially improve their sexuality experience. In the case of adolescents it is additionally necessary to forge a healthy compromise between the normal developmental needs of the patient and the demands of the chronic illness (Frauman and Sypert 1979; Woodhead and Murph 1985; Selekman and McIlvain-Simpson 1991). To begin, one cannot address sexuality without introducing the topic during the patient encounter. In working with the teenage population asking questions and soliciting information about sexuality should ideally begin just prior to early adolescence, in anticipation of puberty onset. For those with rheumatic illness, puberty onset can be delayed due to disease activity and/or medication (e.g. corticosteroids), but as 11- and-12-year olds begin to see their peers enter puberty, they will start to consider the changes in store for themselves and need the opportunity to talk about their own maturation even if it is to be later than normal. Deviations from normal physical and psychologic progression (as consequences of the disease) can be explained by the provider. This is also an important time for the clinician to start offering adolescents private, one-to-one time during the visit. This allows the teenager to speak confidentially and is also much more likely to result in accurate and complete information for the provider inquiring explicitly about sexuality. Interviewing the adolescent is different from interacting with adults. Assurances of confidentiality and a nonjudgmental approach are essential in soliciting sexuality related information (Deisher and Remafedi 1989). Some patients are reluctant to bring up the topic but almost certainly have questions and concerns to express.

In Britto's recently published Cincinnati study (Britto et al. 2000) of risk behaviours among adolescents and young adults with juvenile arthritis, the focus was on alcohol use and sexual activity. Although the authors made an important point about checking alcohol use in patients taking methotrexate, there is no indication that alcohol use or sexual activity was different from their healthy peers. The need to establish the proper use of birth control and barriers against the passage of sexually transmitted diseases underscores the importance of soliciting information from these patients regarding sexual activity. These individuals also warrant attention when they are *not* sexually active in order to find out why and provide appropriate guidance. There can be prohibitive religious or social mores for some, but if not, it behooves the physician to explore whether disease activity or physical disability are the problems and if so, these features should be addressed. Alcohol and cannabis use among adolescents is associated with initiation of sexual activity (Graves and Leigh 1995; Staton et al. 1999), and therefore these behaviours should be openly addressed as well.

As middle adolescence is reached, further discussion should take place around an evolving capacity for intimacy and specifically regarding sexuality. It is important at this point to remain nonjudgmental and particularly to avoid heterosexual stereotyping (e.g. asking males only about girlfriends and females only about boyfriends). It is common for physicians to unwittingly discourage rapport with gay adolescents by assuming that their patient's partner curiosity is heterosexual. Specific recommendations for soliciting information and communicating with adolescents are available to the reader elsewhere (Siegel and Baum 1999).

Problems in achieving autonomy can become more acute for the 15- to 17-year-old with a rheumatic (or other chronic) disease particularly if overt milestones such as obtaining a driver's license (Orr et al. 1984) or securing a part time job are prevented or delayed by the illness. Similarly, the limitations imposed on sexual experimentation by the rheumatic disease deserve attention. It is important to remember that unlike adults who develop a rheumatic illness after having already established their sexual attitudes, expectations, and behaviours, adolescents do not have a premorbid sexual status with which to compare. An inability to orchestrate one's own dating activities because of disability presents an opportunity for the patient, physician, and family to work out ways to allow this important psychosocial step to take place.

The reader is referred to Neumann's personal and insightful account of one juvenile arthritis patient's transition to sexual activity (Neumann 1988). In addition to encouraging young people to assume increasing responsibility for the management of their rheumatic disease, older adolescents should be pushed to consider their sexuality in a responsible way. Specifically, they need to think about the implications of becoming sexually active and whether the timing is appropriate for either them or their partner. If they have decided to engage in sexual intercourse then considerations of contraception, sexually transmitted diseases, and mechanical adjustments to allow for sexual activity must be taken into account. Some of these issues vary depending on the disease, as described below.

Regularly and clearly asking patients (and spouses or partners) about sexual functioning and satisfaction cannot be stressed enough. Not only does this provide important information that is typically not spontaneously volunteered by the patient, but it also transmits the message to the patient that the health care provider is interested in, and receptive to discussion about sexuality. In addition to encouraging patients to describe their global assessment of sexual functioning and level of satisfaction, it is important to take into consideration the mechanics of physical intimacy and therefore pay attention to the quantity and quality of joint involvement in the context of sexuality. Pain, stiffness, and tenderness of the hands and upper extremities can make touching, stroking, and caressing uncomfortable, thereby interfering with tactile pleasure and arousal, including during masturbation (Malek and Brower 1984). Coital positioning can be very important in determining whether intercourse is painful for one or both partners, let alone enjoyable. For example, in a woman with hip disease and limitations of abduction and rotation, the traditional heterosexual, frontal ('missionary') position may be quite uncomfortable if not impossible (Buckwalter et al. 1982).

The approach to these more physical limitations involves both awareness and communication of preferences and capabilities between partners as well as education by health professionals about adaptive techniques. Many patients with rheumatic diseases find it very difficult to express needs and choices about sexuality to their partner thus it is helpful for the physician or nurse to bring up the subject and support open communication, as well as the methodology to achieve sexual satisfaction (Hamilton and Hawkins 1977). More formal mental health consultation can often be helpful for individuals and couples struggling with the complexity of sexuality in the presence of illness. Low self-esteem, depression, anger, etc. are all expected concomitants and can result in decreased libido or insecurity about one's ability to satisfy a sexual partner.

In addition to talking with one's partner about what works best for sexual gratification, manipulation of medication and timing of intercourse can also facilitate more pleasurable physical intimacy. Knowing that fatigue is a significant factor in decreased sexual satisfaction and enjoyment, the patient with a rheumatic disease may need to plan for sex and carefully pace the balance of the day's activities. For some couples limiting the duration of foreplay can be helpful in reaching arousal and orgasm before pain and fatigue begin to set in for the affected partner. Furthermore, the pain and stiffness associated with arthritis can be temporarily addressed through 'pre-treatment' with heat, range of motion and anti-inflammatory and analgesic medication prior to physical closeness, stimulation, and intercourse. The application of heat and gentle range of motion can even become part of initial foreplay for the more mature, and less self-conscious patient. Obviously, what is recommended above precludes spontaneous, unplanned sexual activity, which is more typical among adolescents. The clinician caring for younger patients must be aware of this and acknowledge to the teenager that this may feel like yet another way in which the disease has complicated the emergence of their sexuality. On the other hand, without such strategies, sexual activity, including masturbation, may remain unpleasant, painful, and frustrating.

Rheumatic disease manifestations other than arthritis can also adversely affect sexuality (Table 2). Oral mucous membrane lesions in patients with SLE can make kissing and/or oral–genital contact painful. Patient's with Reiter's syndrome who have urethritis, cervicitis, or balanitis can find genital contact uncomfortable as can those with the ulcerative genital lesions and balanitis of Behçet's disease. Sjögren's syndrome complicated by xerostomia and atrophic vaginitis can result in pain with either oral or genital contact. The use of condoms and lubricants can help to alleviate some of the above problems (Lim 1995).

As described, the judicious use of pain-reducing medication can be useful in facilitating pleasurable sexual activity, but drugs can also interfere. Corticosteroids may cause difficulty in attaining penile erection, but when discontinued this problem should resolve. Numerous antihypertensives, often necessary in treating patients with renal disease, can also cause impotence, ejaculatory abnormalities, and loss of libido. Though uncommonly necessary in the management of rheumatic disease related pain, narcotic analgesics might contribute to fatigue, impotence, and loss of libido. Nonsteroidal anti-inflammatory drugs are not known to interfere with sexual desire or function. Hair loss secondary to immunosuppressive drugs (e.g. cyclophosphamide) might result in feelings of unattractiveness but sexual function is not directly affected. These cytotoxic therapies can also cause mouth and genital ulcers as can gold compounds. Medication considerations are also relevant in choosing a method of contraception. Patients with antiphospholipid antibodies (such as in SLE or the antiphospholipid antibody syndrome) are at increased risk for thromboembolic disease and should therefore not be given oral contraceptive preparations. General principles of 'safer sex' apply to everyone, including those with rheumatic disease, especially in the setting of oral and/or genital ulcers that can increase the efficiency of infection transmission (i.e. gonorrhoea, chlamydia, syphilis, human papillomavirus, HIV), in which cases spermicidal lubricated condoms are a must.

There are developmental, psychological, and physical aspects to sexuality in younger and older individuals with rheumatic disease. As an integral part of comprehensive care of these patients sexuality must be included. While it is incumbent on physicians to consistently inquire about this it is valuable to note that individuals may respond differently to various members of the health care team. This can be related to a desire to discuss sexuality with a professional of the same gender, or other aspects of what allows the patient to feel most comfortable and relaxed. It is particularly important to be sensitive to this consideration in working with adolescents (Conine and Quastel 1983). Nurses, occupational and physical therapists, social workers, psychologists, and physicians are *all* potential resources. While more research would lead to a broader, and perhaps more current understanding of sexuality issues for patients with rheumatic disease, sufficient knowledge and experience already exist to support an assertive approach in this important area of clinical rheumatology.

Table 2 Rheumatic diseases and interference with sexual function

Disease	Sexuality related impairment
Arthritis	Joint limitation of motion Hips—genital intercourse Hands and wrists—stroking, caressing, masturbation, hygiene
Systemic lupus erythematosus	Mucous membrane lesions
Reiter's	Urethritis, cervicitis, balanitis
Behçet's	Genital ulcers, balanitis
Sjögren's	Xerostomia, atrophic vaginitis
All diseases	Pain Stiffness Fatigue Depression Feeling unattractive Medication side effects

References

Baldursson, H. and Brattstrom, H. (1979). Sexual difficulties and total hip replacement in rheumatoid arthritis. *Scandinavian Journal of Rheumatology* **8** (4), 214–16.

Blake, D.J., Maisiak, R., Alarcon, G.S., Holley, H.L., and Brown S. (1987). Sexual quality-of-life of patients with arthritis compared to arthritis-free controls. *Journal of Rheumatism* **14**, 570–6.

Britto, M.T., Rosenthal, S.L., Taylor, J., and Passo, M.H. (2000). Improving rheumatologists' screening for alcohol use and sexual activity. *Archives of Pediatric and Adolescent Medicine* **154**, 478–83.

Buckwalter, K.C., Wernimont, T., and Buckwalter, J.A. (1982). Musculoskeletal conditions and sexuality (part II). *Sexuality and Disability* **5**, 195–207.

Choquet, M., Fediaevsky, L.D.P., and Manfredi, R. (1997). Sexual behavior among adolescents reporting chronic conditions: a French national survey. *Journal of Adolescent Health* **20**, 62–7.

Conine, T.A. and Quastel, L.N. (1983). Occupational therapists' roles and attitudes toward sexual rehabilitation of chronically ill and disabled children. *Canadian Journal of Occupational Therapy* **50**, 81–6.

Currey, H.L. (1970). Osteoarthrosis of the hip joint and sexual activity. *Annals of Rheumatic Diseases* **29**, 488–93.

Deisher, R. and Remafedi, G. (1989). Adolescent sexuality. In *Adolescent Medicine* (ed. A. Hofmann and D. Greydanus), pp. 337–46. New Jersey: Prentice Hall.

Elst, P., Sybesma, T., van der Stadt, R.J., Prins, A.P.A., Muller, W.H., and den Butter, A. (1984). Sexual problems in rheumatoid arthritis and ankylosing spondylitis. *Arthritis and Rheumatism* **27**, 217–20.

Ferguson, K. and Figley, B. (1979). Sexuality and rheumatic disease: a prospective study. *Sexuality and Disability* **2**, 130–8.

Frauman, A.C. and Sypert, N.S. (1979). Sexuality in adolescents with chronic illness. *Maternal and Child Nursing* **4**, 371–5.

Graves, K.L. and Leigh, B.C. (1995). The relationship of substance use to sexual activity among young adults in the United States. *Family Planning Perspectives* **27** (1), 18–22, 33.

Gutweniger, S., Kopp, M., Mur, E., and Günther, V. (1999). Body image of women with rheumatoid arthritis. *Clinical and Experimental Rheumatology* **17**, 413–17.

Hamberg, B.A. (1998). Psychosocial development. In *Comprehensive Adolescent Health Care* (ed. S.B. Friedman, M.M. Fisher, S.K. Schonberg, and E.M. Alderman), pp. 38–49. St Louis MO: Mosby.

Hamilton, A. and Hawkins, C. (1977). Sex and arthritis. In *Reports on Rheumatic Diseases* (ed. C. Hawkins and H.L.F. Currey), pp. 144–7. London: The Arthritis and Rheumatism Council for Research.

Herstein, A., Hill, R.H., and Walters, K. (1977). Adult sexuality and juvenile rheumatoid arthritis. *Journal of Rheumatism* **4**, 35–9.

Hill, R.H., Herstein, A., and Walters, K. (1976). Juvenile rheumatoid arthritis: follow-up into adulthood-medical, sexual and social status. *Canadian Medical Association Journal* **114**, 790–6.

Kellerman, J. et al. (1980). Psychological effects of illness in adolescence. I. Anxiety, self-esteem, and perception of control. *Journal of Pediatrics* **97**, 126–31.

Kraaimaat, F.W., Bakker, A.H., Janssen, E., and Bijlsma, J.W.J. (1996). Intrusiveness of rheumatoid arthritis on sexuality in male and female patients living with a spouse. *Arthritic Care and Research* **9**, 120–5.

Lim, P.A.C. (1995). Sexuality in patients with musculoskeletal diseases. *Physical Medicine and Rehabilitation: State of the Art Review* **9**, 401–15.

Lipe, H., Longstreth, W.T., Jr., Bird, T.D., and Linde, M. (1990). Sexual function in married men with Parkinson's disease compared to married men with arthritis. *Neurology* **40**, 1347–9.

Majerovitz, S.D. and Revenson, T.A. (1994). Sexuality and rheumatoid disease: the significance of gender. *Arthritic Care and Research* **7**, 29–34.

Malek, C.J. and Brower, S.A. (1984). Rheumatoid arthritis: how does it influence sexuality? *Rehabilitational Nursing* **Nov–Dec**, 26–8.

McAnarney, E.R. (1985). Social maturation: a challenge for handicapped and chronically ill adolescents. *Journal of Adolescent Health Care* **6**, 90–101.

McAnarney, E.R. et al. (1974). Psychological problems of children with chronic juvenile arthritis. *Pediatrics* **53**, 523–8.

Netting, N.S. (1992). Sexuality in youth culture: identity and change. *Adolescence* **27**, 961–76.

Neumann, R.J. (1988). Personal statement: experiencing sexuality as an adolescent with rheumatoid arthritis. In *Family Interventions Throughout Chronic Illness and Disability* (ed. P.W. Powers, A. Dell Orto, and M. Gibbons), pp. 156–63. New York: Springer.

Orr, D.P. et al. (1984). Psychosocial implications of chronic illness in adolescence. *Journal of Pediatrics* **104**, 152–7.

Ostensen, M. (1993). Hip prostheses in women of fertile age. Consequences for sexuality and reproduction. *Tidsskrift for Den Norske Laegeforening* **113** (12), 1483–5.

Ostensen, M., Almberg, K., and Koksvik, H.S. (2000). Sex, reproduction and gynecological disease in young adults with a history of juvenile chronic arthritis. *Journal of Rheumatism* **27** (7), 1783–7.

Perrin, E.C. and Gerrity, P.S. (1984). Development of children with a chronic illness. *Pediatric Clinics of North America* **31**, 19–31.

Quaresma, M.R., Goldsmith, C.H., Lamont, J., and Ferraz, M.B. (1997). Assessment of sexual function in patients with rheumatic disorders: a critical appraisal. *Journal of Rheumatism* **24**, 1673–6.

Rettig, P. and Athreya, B.H. (1991). Adolescents with chronic disease: transition to adult care. *Arthritic Care and Research* **4**, 174–80.

Richards, J.S. (1980). Sex and arthritis. *Sexuality and Disability* **3**, 97–104.

Rodgers, J.L. (1998). Development of sexual behavior. In *Comprehensive Adolescent Health Care* (ed. S.B. Friedman), pp. 49–54. St Louis MO: Mosby.

Sarrel, L.J. and Sarrel, P.M. (1981). Sexual unfolding. *Journal of Adolescent Health Care* **2**, 93–9.

Selekman, J. and McIlvain-Simpson, G. (1991). Sex and sexuality for the adolescent with a chronic condition. *Pediatric Nursing* **17**, 535–8.

Siegel, D.M. and Baum, J. (1999). Adolescent rheumatic disease and sexuality. In *Adolescent Rheumatology* (ed. D.A. Isenberg and J.J. Miller), pp. 291–9. London: Martin Dunitz.

Staton, M., Leukefeld, C., Logan, T.K., Zimmerman, R., Lynam, D., Milich, R., Martin, C., McClanahan, K., and Clayton, R. (1999). Risky sex behavior and substance use among young adults. *Health & Social Work* **24** (2), 147–54.

Stoeber, E. (1976). Corticosteroid treatment of juvenile chronic polyarthritis over 22 years. *European Journal of Pediatrics* **121**, 141–7.

Strax, T.E. (1988). Psychological problems of disabled adolescents and young adults. *Pediatry Annals* **17**, 756–61.

Todd, R.C., Lightowler, C.D.R., and Harris, J. (1973). Low friction arthroplasty of the hip joint and sexual activity. *Acta Orthopaedica Scandinavia* **44**, 690–3.

Ungerer, J.A. et al. (1988). Psychosocial functioning in children and young adults with juvenile arthritis. *Pediatrics* **81**, 195–202.

Wallander, J.L. et al. (1988). Children with chronic physical disorders: maternal reports of their psychological adjustment. *Journal of Pediatric Psychology* **13**, 197–212.

Wilkinson, V.A. (1981). Juvenile chronic arthritis in adolescence: facing the reality. *International Rehabilitational Medicine* **3**, 11–17.

Woodhead, J.C. and Murph, J.R. (1985). Influence of chronic illness and disability on adolescent sexual development. *Seminars in Adolescent Medicine* **1**, 171–6.

Yoshino, S. and Uchida, S. (1981). Sexual problems of women with rheumatoid arthritis. *Archives of Physical and Medical Rehabilitation* **62**, 122–3.

Zeltzer, L., Kellerman, J., Ellenberg, L., Dash, J., and Rigler, D. (1980). Psychological effects of illness in adolescence. II. Impact of illness in adolescents—crucial issues and coping styles. *Journal of Pediatrics* **97**, 132–8.

Zuengler, K.L. and Neubeck, G. (1983). Sexuality: developing togetherness. In *Stress and the Family* (ed. H. McCubben), pp. 41–53. New York: Bruner/Mazel.

2.5 The economics of the musculoskeletal diseases

Bruno Fautrel, John R. Penrod, and Ann E. Clarke

This chapter has two main objectives. The first is to describe the most common types of economic evaluations of diseases and medical interventions. This objective includes: providing some background motivating health economic studies; describing each type of study and how it can be used to support decision-making; and describing the general principles for carrying out such studies. The second objective is to review the literature specifically treating the economics of musculoskeletal diseases.

Economic evaluation

Background

In the industrialized countries, health care expenses have been steadily rising, both in absolute terms and as a proportion of national income. For example, in Canada, national health expenditures were 7.1 per cent of national income in 1975; by 1994 these expenses represented nearly 10 per cent of GDP (Anonymous 1996). After many years of deficit spending in many countries, the pressure for governments to balance budgets has focused attention on the fundamental economic problem: the use of society's scarce resources. Faced with unlimited possibilities for improving health and doing good, how should our limited resources be allocated? To this end, a rather large literature on the economic evaluation of medical interventions has developed. Recently, expert panels from various countries have published consensus guidelines for the methodological approach to these studies (Gold et al. 1996; Canadian Coordinating Office for Health Technology Assessment 1997).

Types of health economic studies

The five most common types of health economic evaluation studies are: cost of illness (COI) (burden of illness), cost minimization (CM) (cost identification), cost-effectiveness (C–E), cost-utility (C–U), and cost–benefit analyses (CBA) (Drummond et al. 1987).

Cost of illness

COI studies aim to describe the impact or burden of a disease on society in monetary terms. In their most common form, COI studies describe this monetary value as the sum of the direct and indirect costs imposed by the disease. The direct costs reflect the opportunity costs of resources employed to care for individuals. These resources have economic value whether they are compensated (e.g. nurses, physicians) or uncompensated (e.g. family caregivers). Indirect costs represent the value of productivity losses associated with morbidity and premature mortality. In practice, these losses are typically calculated by an application of the human capital method (Jackson 1992).

The uses of COI data have been discussed by several authors (Hodgson and Meiners 1982; Scitovsky 1982; Rice 1994; Moore et al. 1997). COI studies can be either prevalence-based or incidence-based. Prevalence studies may be useful for short- to medium-term resource planning in the health care system or for setting priorities for health research budgets across disease groups. However, because of changing patterns of treatment and health behaviours, incidence-based estimates such as those by Gabriel (Gabriel et al. 1999) for rheumatoid arthritis (RA) are needed.

Finally, the traditional COI studies based on the sum of direct and indirect costs have been criticized for theoretical shortcomings (O'Brien and Gafni 1996). For example, these estimates do not include intangible costs, such as pain and suffering, when they are not associated with productivity losses. Also, these studies focus on individuals with active disease. However, the presence of a disease in the population may impact healthy individuals, either through their concerns about their own future health or through altruistic sentiments. In principle, the willingness-to-pay (WTP) methodology could capture these valuations by surveying both affected and unaffected individuals on their WTP for a programme providing a hypothetical cure for the disease (O'Brien and Gafni 1996).

Cost minimization

CM studies simply describe the costs associated with competing interventions assumed to be clinically equivalent. Thus, the intervention with the lowest cost is judged to be superior.

Cost-effectiveness

C–E studies also compare alternative treatments for a given condition. C–E ratios are calculated by dividing the *incremental* cost of a particular therapy by its *incremental* effect on health outcomes. Examples of effectiveness measures would be years of life saved, Lequesne index scores, or hip fractures avoided. The C–E ratio is evaluated using the following formula:

$$\frac{\text{Cost}}{\text{Effectiveness}} = \frac{(\text{Cost}_{\text{treatment}} - \text{Cost}_{\text{control}})}{(\text{Effectiveness}_{\text{treatment}} - \text{Effectiveness}_{\text{control}})},$$

where the cost and outcome differences are evaluated over the relevant period of interest. In contrast to COI studies, it should be noted that current recommendations (Gold et al. 1996) advise excluding indirect costs associated with morbidity or mortality from the numerator of the C–E ratio, arguing that indirect costs are already counted in the effectiveness measure. Only indirect costs associated with the time costs of the interventions themselves should be counted in the numerator of the incremental C–E ratio.

Interventions that are less effective but more expensive are said to be 'dominated' and are automatically eliminated from consideration. In most cases, however, more effective interventions are also more expensive and the C–E ratio must be calculated and interpreted. This C–E ratio then can be compared to the C–E ratios for other interventions where the same measure of effectiveness was studied. This reveals one of the weaknesses of C–E analysis—comparisons can be made only across studies that use the same measure of effectiveness. Another weakness is that for multidimensional outcomes, the various disease-specific or general health-related quality of life measures weigh the importance of these dimensions arbitrarily and not according to patient preferences. Patient preferences for different health states are incorporated in C–U analyses, which allow comparison of interventions across different disease groups.

Cost-utility

The standard gamble and time-tradeoff methods are two ways of implementing preference weighting of multi-attribute health states (Gold et al. 1996). The standard gamble, which is explicitly based on expected-utility theory, asks individuals to trade off a given 'certain' health state with a lottery resulting in either perfect health (a utility of 1) or death (a utility of 0). In practice, a careful description of the health state of interest is provided, and the respondent is asked to choose between two hypothetical options: (i) to live for the rest of her/his life in that health state; or (ii) to undergo an intervention that would result in perfect health with probability p and death with probability $1 - p$. The probability is then varied until the respondent is indifferent between the two options (the certain health state or the lottery), and the utility is given by the probability of perfect health where the respondent is indifferent between the two options. The time-tradeoff method asks individuals to trade off a given health state with a smaller number of years of perfect health. The duration of life in perfect health is varied until the respondent is indifferent to living this duration in perfect health and some longer duration in the given health state of interest. The utility is computed by dividing the length of life in perfect health at this indifference point by the length of life in the health state of interest. Both standard gamble and time tradeoff methods can be used to develop measures of quality-adjusted life years (QALYs). Recently, utility measurement techniques have been applied in representative adult populations to the health states described by health-related quality of life surveys such as the Health Utilities Index (HUI) and the EuroQol instrument (Gold et al. 1996). Thus, as an alternative to the standard gamble or time tradeoff, it is now possible to derive utility scores from HUI or EuroQol questionnaire responses.

As in the case with C–E ratios, an incremental C–U ratio can be compared with incremental C–U ratios for commonly funded interventions and those of interventions that have not been funded to develop a sense of whether the evidence shows that the intervention is in the fundable range. Laupacis (Laupacis et al. 1992) suggests an incremental C–U of less than $20 000 per QALY is compelling evidence for adoption, while an incremental C–U of $100 000 per QALY or higher is weak evidence for adoption. However, both Laupacis (Laupacis et al. 1992) and Gold (Gold et al. 1996) stress that ethical and political considerations must also be factored into technology adoption decisions and they cannot recommend a fixed C–E threshold for generalized use.

Cost-benefit

In CBA, the benefits as well as the costs are valued in monetary terms. Thus, spending on a health care programme can be incorporated into a broader set of comparisons outside of health care. The benefits of a programme correspond to the public's WTP for it. The current principles for implementing WTP in medical care programmes are described in O'Brien and Gafni (1996). Since health care is mainly paid for through public or private insurance, they recommend that survey instruments measure the WTP for insurance coverage for a given service rather than the WTP for the service itself. Also, such surveys should be administered to the general population and not just affected individuals, since unaffected individuals may be WTP because of altruistic motives or concerns about their own future health. Although much has been learned about applying WTP to health care questions, the method presents many challenges, including the difficulty of measuring complex health outcomes in monetary terms, and the ethical considerations associated with a measure favouring programmes affecting those with a greater ability to pay. Given its inherent advantages, as these difficulties are addressed by researchers, CBA will increase in importance in health economic evaluation.

Implementation of economic evaluations

Direct costs

The first step in estimating direct costs is to exhaustively record the consumption of health care resources—either medical or non-medical (transport, etc.)—associated with the treatment of the illness over the relevant period. This involves the description of the therapeutic pathway containing all relevant downstream events. Treatment and effects may last until the end of life, so there will be a need to employ decision analytic techniques to model outcomes and resource use for the period after a randomized control trial has ended (Gold et al. 1996; Buxton et al. 1997). The second step in estimating the direct costs is to pair the resource utilization data with data on the opportunity costs of these resources. Finkler (1982) cautions that charges for services such as hospitalizations are probably poor estimates of opportunity costs, especially in systems such as that of the United States, where there is significant cross-subsidization between generous payers and less generous payers and the uninsured.

Indirect costs

Indirect costs reflect the reductions in productivity in market and household work due to morbidity and time seeking health care. For COI studies, this includes all time lost due to morbidity or seeking medical care, and for C–E or C–U analyses, this includes only the time seeking medical care. Since there are ethical considerations related to the valuation of hours lost, a sensitivity analysis employing replacement cost and opportunity cost versions of the human capital method should be carried out (Jackson 1992; Gold et al. 1996; Clarke et al. 2000).

Perspective

Since economic evaluations are carried out to aid in social decision making, it is recommended that the analysis adopt the social perspective (Gold et al. 1996; Canadian Coordinating Office for Health Technology Assessment 1997). However, the guidelines also specify that the analysis should be broken down into the various relevant viewpoints (health care system, patients, etc.).

Discounting future costs and outcomes

Since many interventions will have lasting effects, there is a need to discount future costs *and* effectiveness to the present. The need for discounting is not to adjust for inflation (all monetary amounts should already be inflation-adjusted to a constant given base year) but to reflect time preferences, which are society's preference to receive benefits earlier rather than later. Guidelines specify a 3–5 per cent base case discount rate (Gold et al. 1996; Canadian Coordinating Office for Health Technology Assessment 1997).

The economic burden of musculoskeletal diseases

Over the past few decades, several studies, using both population-based surveys and administrative databases, have provided national estimates of the economic burden of musculoskeletal diseases in the United States (Felts and Yelin 1989; Yelin et al. 1995), Canada (Badley 1995; Moore et al. 1997; Coyte et al. 1998), and Sweden (Jonsson and Husberg 2000). In the United States, in 1980, the total cost of musculoskeletal diseases was 0.8 per cent of GDP (Felts and Yelin 1989), 38 per cent due to indirect costs. In 1992, musculoskeletal conditions were estimated to cost $149 billion or approximately 2.5 per cent of the GDP, 52 per cent due to lost wages (Yelin et al. 1995). In Canada, in 1986, the cost of these conditions was estimated at $8.2 billion, representing 1.7 per cent of GDP, 78 per cent due to indirect costs (Badley 1995). In 1994, these costs had risen to $25.6 billion or 3.4 per cent of GDP, 71 per cent due to indirect costs (Coyte et al. 1998). It is estimated that musculoskeletal conditions account for 4.9 per cent of hospital expenditures, 6.5 per cent of medical expenditures, 6.8 per cent of medication expenditure, and for 35.2 per cent and 10.0 per cent of all lost income due to chronic and short-term disability, respectively (Moore et al. 1997). Although these studies are not directly comparable because of differences in methodology and health care structure and financing, it can be concluded that the economic burden of the musculoskeletal diseases has risen substantially in the past 20 years and likely will continue to do so in parallel with the ageing of the population and the rapid emergence of many novel, yet expensive therapies.

The economic burden of specific musculoskeletal diseases

To generate cost estimates for specific musculoskeletal diseases, clinic or community-based, rather than population-based samples, are often used. Each approach has limitations (Lubeck 1995; Gordon and Clarke 1999). Research involving national samples or community cohorts includes a more representative patient population. However, for uncommon diseases, such cohorts are difficult to assemble. In population surveys, disease diagnosis depends on self-reported illness and in community-based cohorts and managed care organizations, on administrative data and/or medical notes review. The reliance on self-reporting or diagnosis by a non-specialist may lead to aggregation of inflammatory and non-inflammatory rheumatic conditions. Given that resource use and disability can vary considerably between these conditions, national survey and administrative data can result in less precise cost estimates than clinic-based samples. Furthermore, clinic populations can potentially provide more detailed and longitudinal data.

For clinic-based populations, resource use is usually evaluated through a self-report questionnaire and/or review of medical notes or medical claims data; productivity impairment is usually assessed through self-report. Although self-report questionnaires are subject to recall bias, they elicit information on usage of non-physician health care professionals, non-prescription medications, and complementary and alternative medicine, which is not possible through other sources. The numerous cost assessment instruments that have been used were recently reviewed (Ruof et al. 2001). Medical notes review is feasible if the patient seeks care primarily from a single provider, but can become prohibitive if numerous providers and institutions are involved. Review of medical claims data is also feasible in settings where care is primarily financed through a single payer, such as in Canada, the United Kingdom, and in managed care organizations in the United States.

The remainder of this chapter will discuss studies, both population and community and clinic-based, which estimate the economic burden of specific musculoskeletal conditions, including (i) RA, (ii) osteoarthritis (OA), (iii) systemic lupus erythematosus (SLE), (iv) back pain (BP), (v) osteoporosis, (vi) fibromyalgia, and (vii) other autoimmune and inflammatory rheumatic diseases. We will attempt to focus primarily on studies which incorporate the elements of a comprehensive economic analysis as outlined earlier in this chapter.

Rheumatoid arthritis

Burden of illness

More COI studies have been conducted for RA than for any other arthritic condition at both the population, community, and clinic-based levels (Yelin 1994; Lubeck 1995; Rothfuss et al. 1997; Callahan 1998; Ruof et al. 1999; Cooper 2000a). C–E analyses conducted in RA are also summarized elsewhere (Bosi-Ferraz et al. 1997; Ruchlin et al. 1997).

Population studies

At the population level, both Yelin et al. and Coyte et al. who, as discussed above, have provided estimates for the cost of musculoskeletal diseases in the aggregate, have also provided estimates for more specific conditions. Coyte estimated costs for 'arthritis and rheumatism' at $5.9 billion, 64 per cent due to indirect costs (Coyte et al. 1998). Yelin used national survey data to develop cost estimates for persons with RA versus those without and calculated direct costs at $4.8 billion and indirect at $4.0 billion (1994 US $) for those with RA (Yelin 1996); the cost increment experienced by those with RA versus those without was $3.1 billion, 80 per cent of this increment being indirect costs. In England, in 1992, using several national data sources, McIntosh estimated the total economic impact of RA was £1256 billion with indirect costs responsible for 52 per cent of this total (McIntosh 1996). In Sweden, in 1994, Jonsson et al. (2000) estimated that of all the rheumatic diseases, RA was responsible for 5.5 per cent of expenditure with BP and OA responsible for 48 and 14 per cent, respectively. Of the total expenditure on RA, indirect costs accounted for 67 per cent of the total.

Clinic and community studies: methodologic issues

Clinic (Meenan et al. 1978; Liang et al. 1984; Lubeck et al. 1986; Yelin et al. 1987; Reisine et al. 1989; Allaire et al. 1991; Clarke et al. 1997; Albers et al. 1999; Kobelt et al. 1999; Barrett et al. 2000; Newhall-Perry et al. 2000; Cooper et al. 2000b; Merkesdal et al. 2001) and community-based (Jacobs et al. 1988; Pincus et al. 1989; Jonsson et al. 1992; Yelin 1996; Lanes et al. 1997; Gabriel et al. 1997a,b; Van Jaarsveld et al. 1998; Yelin and Wanke 1999) studies are more numerous than those conducted at the population level. Most express costs from a social perspective; a single one adopted an employer perspective (Birnbaum et al. 2000). Of these studies, almost all are prevalence-based; only two incidence-based studies have been published (Stone 1984; Gabriel et al. 1999). Most studies have used the human capital method; only two WTP studies have been conducted (Thompson 1986; Slothuus and Brooks 2000). Many of the human capital based studies consider direct and indirect costs; only the incidence-based studies considered mortality costs. Few conduct sensitivity analyses surrounding their most uncertain assumptions (Clarke et al. 1997).

Stone et al. published the first incidence-based study on the cost of RA. She estimated that for a cohort with initial onset of RA in 1977, the per capita lifetime costs were $20 412 (1977 US $), with indirect costs representing almost 80 per cent of this total. Gabriel et al. conducted the only other incidence-based study. She estimated total costs incurred in the 25 years after the incidence diagnosis, but, in contrast to the work of Stone et al., she compared her RA cohort with non-arthritic controls, enabling her to calculate the excess costs due to RA, rather than the total costs incurred by those with RA. She estimated the median lifetime incremental costs of RA at approximately $60 000 (1995 US $).

Using decision-analytic modelling, Thompson et al. published the first WTP study in RA. Although conceptually, the WTP methodology is anticipated to provide a more comprehensive valuation of the impact of RA than the human capital approach, the estimates generated by these studies were similar to those generated using the human capital approach. However, Thompson measured the WTP only among patients living with RA. Therefore, the valuations of unaffected individuals, which may arise from altruistic motives or concern about future help, were excluded from the analysis.

Over the past 20 years, of the prevalence-based studies on the cost of RA that have been published, most are from the United States (Meenan et al. 1978; Liang et al. 1984; Lubeck et al. 1986; Jacobs et al. 1988; Yelin 1996; Lanes et al. 1997; Gabriel et al. 1997a,b; Yelin and Wanke 1999; Newhall-Perry et al. 2000), but there is also work from Canada (Clarke et al. 1997, 1999b), the United Kingdom (Barrett et al. 2000; Cooper et al. 2000b), Sweden (Jonsson et al. 1992; Kobelt et al. 1999), the Netherlands (Van Jaarsveld et al. 1998; Albers et al. 1999), and Germany (Merkesdal et al. 2001). Costs differ across countries, but certain trends are evident. In most, inpatient costs were the largest component of total direct costs, averaging at least 50 per cent of the total (Meenan et al. 1978; Jacobs et al. 1988; Clarke et al. 1997; Gabriel et al. 1997a; Kobelt et al. 1999; Yelin and Wanke 1999; Newhall-Perry et al. 2000; Cooper et al. 2000b).

Direct costs attributable to RA

RA-attributed cost can be determined by either comparing an RA with a non-RA cohort (Gabriel et al. 1997a) or by estimating the total costs incurred and then assigning attribution (Yelin and Wanke 1999). Gabriel et al. compared a community-based cohort of persons with RA to a similar cohort from the same community who had never had a diagnosis of arthritis. They reported that the direct medical charges for the RA cohort exceeded the non-arthritic cohort by almost three-fold. In one of the most recent and comprehensive studies on the direct medical costs incurred by patients with RA, Yelin et al. reported on health service use both related and unrelated to RA. Annual direct medical costs for RA averaged $5919 (1996 US $) and $2582 for non-RA reasons. Although less than 10 per cent of the cohort were hospitalized in a year, hospitalization costs were responsible for 52 per cent of the total; admissions for total joint replacement surgery accounted for greater than 25 per cent of the RA direct cost total. Medications, physician visits, and laboratory/imaging studies comprised 26, 9, and 5 per cent, respectively, of total direct RA costs.

Long versus short disease duration

Some of the more recent studies have focused on costs incurred early in the disease course (Van Jaarsveld et al. 1998; Kobelt et al. 1999; Newhall-Perry et al. 2000; Cooper et al. 2000b; Merkesdal et al. 2001). In contrast to patients with long-standing RA, patients with RA of less than 1 year duration incur lower costs, primarily due to lower hospitalization costs which represented only 3.5 per cent of total direct costs (Newhall-Perry et al. 2000). Patients with longer disease duration are more likely to require hospitalization for joint replacement and complications of the disease and its therapy.

Indirect costs

Despite some of the population (Badley 1995; Yelin et al. 1995; Coyte et al. 1998) and clinic-based (Meenan et al. 1978; Kobelt et al. 1999; Newhall-Perry et al. 2000) and Stone's incidence-based work (Stone 1984) reporting that indirect costs exceed direct costs, some of the prevalence-based studies report that direct exceed indirect (Jonsson et al. 1992; Clarke et al. 1997). Indirect cost estimates are sensitive to the method of valuation. In studies where the population is predominantly elderly and no longer engaged in work-force activities, if diminished productivity is valued as lost employment income, then indirect cost estimates will be low.

Several clinic (Yelin et al. 1987; Reisine et al. 1989; Barrett et al. 2000; Merkesdal et al. 2001) and one community-based study (Pincus et al. 1989) describe the extent of work disability; the impact of RA on household work performance of women (Allaire 1991) and leisure time has also been described (Albers et al. 1999). At least 50 per cent of those with a history of paid employment had stopped working within a decade of diagnosis; 10 per cent leave within the first year and only 10 per cent remain employed until the usual age of retirement. Work disability is influenced by the patient's degree of functional impairment as well as the work characteristics (Yelin et al. 1987).

As she did for direct costs, Gabriel et al. (Yelin 1994; Gabriel et al. 1997b) compared the indirect and non-medical costs incurred by patients with RA to those from the same community not having RA, in an effort to determine the indirect costs attributable to RA. The annual indirect and non-medical costs incurred by those with RA exceeded that incurred by non-RA patients by over 2.5-fold ($2269 in 1992 US $ versus $816). Thirty-three per cent of those with RA reported a reduction in family income whereas 11.9 per cent of those without RA reported such reduction.

Osteoarthritis

Burden of illness

OA is the most frequent joint disease in the world (Tugwell 1996; March and Bachmeier 1997). Despite this high prevalence, few economic studies focus specifically on OA (Levy et al. 1993; Gabriel et al. 1995, 1997b; Lanes et al. 1997; Levy 1997; MacLean et al. 1998). Several reasons may explain this. First, OA has not been considered a major public health priority, since it was often perceived as an unavoidable consequence of increasing age (which is untrue), associated with no excess mortality. Second, comprehensive and accurate epidemiological data are difficult to obtain, since the identification of OA patients, manifesting different forms of the disease, is hampered because there is no unique definition of OA, and because the patients are often cared for by a variety of providers.

However, the available data show that the economic burden of OA is substantial. The high prevalence of OA is the main explanation; the majority of OA patients induce only minimal costs at the individual level compared to other diseases, but the large number of patients incurring such costs leads to high costs at the population level (Lanes et al. 1997). The economic burden of OA is often included in the global burden of musculoskeletal diseases, and information at a country level is scarce. In France, OA is responsible for 1 per cent of the national health insurance expenditure (Levy et al. 1993; Levy 1997). No such data have been published in other countries at the national level, but information from an American health maintenance organization (HMO) estimated that OA was responsible for 4.9 per cent of all medical expenditures (MacLean et al. 1998). This substantial difference may be explained by the differences in health care system organization, as well as the socio-economic characteristics of patients enrolled by HMOs (often fewer young people, upper socio-economic classes, and higher requirement for health services). At the individual level, similar differences are seen across studies (Gabriel et al. 1995, 1997b; Lanes et al. 1997; MacLean et al. 1998).

The main source of direct costs are hospital care and other facilities related to surgery (total joint replacement) or rehabilitation for the most disabling forms of OA. Other costs, that is, physician visits and drugs, are less substantial. Direct costs exceed indirect costs; since 80–90 per cent of OA patients are retired or not engaged in labour market activities (Gabriel et al. 1997b), calculated indirect costs are low since non-market work losses have not been valued.

Pharmacoeconomics of OA: the new NSAID dilemma

The pharmacoeconomics of OA has mainly focused on NSAIDs. At the patient level, NSAIDs are not very costly; however, because these drugs are widely used, they represent a substantial cost for the society (McCabe et al. 1998; Hunsche et al. 2001). Also, NSAIDs are able to induce considerable side effects because of gastrointestinal (GI) toxicity, which may have a significant impact on costs. The frequency of GI side effects is variable; GI discomfort is present in up to 50 per cent of NSAID users (van Dieten et al. 2000; Hunsche et al. 2001), 5.4 per cent of them developing a more serious event requiring hospitalization (van Dieten et al. 2000). Overall, the direct annual medical costs of NSAID-related GI complications has been estimated at 3.9 billion US dollars, which increases the cost of OA therapy approximately 1.5-fold (De Pouvourville 1995). An international comparison was conducted in 10 European countries and Australia to determine the total direct cost per GI event (Chevat et al. 2001).

The economic debate has intensified with the advent of the new NSAIDs (Cox-2 preferential or Cox-2 specific), which, despite being more costly, have lower GI toxicity. The central question is to determine if the higher price of these new drugs is compensated by a reduction in costs from fewer side effects. In the majority of economic evaluations, Cox-2 specific NSAIDs are cost saving compared with Cox-2 non-specific NSAIDs alone or associated with gastroprotective agents (Pettitt et al. 2000). This places Cox-2 specific NSAIDs in a 'dominant' position, meaning that these drugs are able to improve health at a reduced cost compared with the alternative. However, it remains to be clarified if cost savings result for all patients or for only a specific subset of patients with a high risk of GI side effects.

Systemic lupus erythematosus

Burden of illness

In contrast to RA, there are few economic studies on patients with SLE. Of those that have been conducted, all have evaluated the costs for clinic-based SLE populations (Clarke et al. 1993; Gironimi et al. 1996; Clarke et al. 1999a, 2000; Sutcliffe et al. 2001). Given the relative rarity of SLE compared to OA and RA, it is not surprising that economic evaluations based on a national survey have not been conducted. The costs incurred by SLE patients in Canada, the United Kingdom, and the United States have been estimated in separate studies (Clarke et al. 1993; Gironimi et al. 1996; Sutcliffe et al. 2001) and, in contrast to most other economic studies which evaluate patients in a single country, a cross-country comparison of expenditure involving SLE patients from Canada, the United Kingdom, and the United States has also been conducted (Clarke et al. 1999a). Although prices of health services vary across countries, consideration of natural units, that is, the number of resources utilized, makes it feasible to aggregate data across multiple sites. Clarke et al. (1999a) have shown that despite different patterns of resource utilization across countries, overall resource utilization was similar among this cohort of 700 patients. Mean annual direct costs were approximately $5000 (1997 Canadian $). Within each resource category, differences were observed. Canadians saw more specialists than the British, the British more generalists. Canadians and Americans were more frequent users of the emergency room; Americans of laboratory/imaging procedures. Canadians had greater hospital usage than Americans.

As with the other rheumatic diseases, indirect cost estimation in SLE is challenging. In RA and OA, many patients are elderly and not involved in labour market activities; in SLE, patients are almost exclusively women and, similarly, are less likely to be engaged in labour market activities. There is no consensus on valuing diminished non-labour market activity for which a wage is not received. Using the lupus cohort assembled from three countries as described above, Clarke et al. estimated the indirect costs incurred by these women with SLE under a variety of assumptions for the value of labour market and non-labour market activities (Clarke et al. 2000).

Six hundred and forty-eight women with SLE reported on employment status and time lost by themselves and their caregivers from labour market and non-labour market activities over a 6-month period. Depending on the value assigned to labour market and non-labour market activity, average annual indirect costs ranged from $1400 to $23 000 (1997 Canadian $). This work demonstrates that indirect cost estimates that do not incorporate long-term absenteeism in the market place and diminished non-labour market activity and that do not use gender neutral wages may lead to underestimates of the economic burden of women's diseases.

Back pain

Burden of illness

Back pain is, with OA, one of the main musculoskeletal problems affecting adults (Deyo et al. 1991; de Girolamo 1991; Linton 1998), involving annually up to 20 per cent of the population (Frymoyer and Cats-Baril 1991). However, the economic characteristics of BP contrast with those of OA in two ways. First, the majority of BP costs are due to a small number of patients: 10–20 per cent of the patients are responsible for 70–90 per cent of BP costs (Spengler et al. 1986; Abenhaim and Suissa 1987; Webster and Snook 1990; Engel et al. 1996; Hashemi et al. 1998) in contrast to OA, where the proportion of patients affected directly correlates with the proportion of total OA costs. These high cost patients are mainly those with chronic BP, their costs being directly related to the persistence of pain and the duration of disability (Engel et al. 1996). Second, since BP does not primarily affect the elderly and since a substantial portion results from work-related activities or injuries, indirect costs, representing productivity losses, exceed direct medical costs by a factor of 4–10 (van Tulder et al. 1995; Hutubessy et al. 1999; Maniadakis and Gray 2000).

Physiotherapy and other manual therapies and hospitalizations are the two major components of direct costs, the drug component being rather inexpensive compared to other diseases (Frymoyer and Cats-Baril 1991; van Tulder et al. 1995; Hutubessy et al. 1999; Maniadakis and Gray 2000). Indirect cost estimates vary, depending on the methodology used (Hutubessy et al. 1999; Maniadakis and Gray 2000); the 'friction cost' method provides low estimates, since only the first three months of absenteeism are included and the economic impact of the remaining absenteeism and long-term disability are completely ignored. The human capital method, which tries to integrate disability for the duration of the illness, provides higher estimates. Whatever the method used, the global economic burden of BP is substantial; because of the frequency of the disease and the impact on work ability, BP is in the 'Top 2' of health expenditures, with cardiovascular diseases (Deyo et al. 1991; van Tulder et al. 1995; Linton 1998; Maniadakis and Gray 2000). Moreover, its costs doubled between 1984 and 1991 (Frymoyer 1991). It represented 17 per cent of total health expenditure in the Netherlands in 1991 (Hutubessy et al. 1999).

Economic evaluation of back pain treatment

Two ways of reducing BP burden have been investigated. First, since BP is so prevalent, especially among some categories of workers, programmes have been developed to prevent BP occurrence. A controlled study conducted between 1986 and 1991 among 4000 US postal workers investigated an educational programme to prevent low back injuries (Daltroy et al. 1997). After 5.5 years, although the workers' knowledge about safe behaviour increased, there was no statistical difference in the prevalence of low back injuries and the number of lost workdays between the intervention and control group. This C–E evaluation provided sufficient information not to develop such programmes on a large scale. This result is not very surprising, since several studies demonstrated that the high economic burden is mainly linked to a small subset of patients with long-term disease (Spengler et al. 1986; Abenhaim and Suissa 1987; Webster and Snook 1990; Engel et al. 1996; Hashemi et al. 1998). Thus, some studies have been performed in patients with chronic BP or at risk of developing such BP.

A Norwegian controlled study compared the potential benefits of two supervised exercise programmes to self-exercise in 208 patients with BP of between 8 and 52 weeks duration (Torstensen et al. 1998). Those enrolled in the two supervised programmes experienced more improvement in pain and function than those enrolled in self-exercise. A CBA demonstrated that the supervised programmes were cost saving compared with the control self-exercise group (Torstensen et al. 1998).

Osteoporosis

Burden of illness

Osteoporosis is the most common metabolic disease of bone, responsible for fractures in elderly people, mainly of the wrist, vertebral body, and hip. During the past 10 years, it has become a substantial public health concern in many developed countries, since hip fracture is a main cause of death in the elderly (5–20 per cent of patients with femoral neck fracture are dead 1 year after the fracture) (Whittington and Faulds 1994; Walker-Bone et al. 2001). The fractures are also responsible for autonomy loss and dependence in the elderly, resulting in long-term stays in hospitals, admissions to nursing homes, or the need for home care facilities; 50 per cent of patients with hip fractures will require these services (Whittington and Faulds 1994; Johnell 1997; Zethraeus and Gerdtham 1998; Reginster 1999; Walker-Bone et al. 2001). This constitutes the main part of the economic burden of osteoporosis (Dolan and Torgerson 1998; Reginster et al. 1999; Ben Sedrine et al. 2001). Economic studies to date have focused mainly on direct costs. Estimates are quite variable, depending on the methodology and the definition of osteoporosis used (Levy 1989; Treves et al. 1989; French et al. 1995; Baudoin et al. 1996; Baudoin 1997; Ray et al. 1997; Dolan and Torgenson 1998; Hoerger et al. 1999; Reginster et al. 1999). However, the proportion of health care expenditure devoted to osteoporosis seems stable across countries and has been estimated between 0.5 and 2.4 per cent in France and the United States (Levy 1989; Treves et al. 1989; Baudoin et al. 1996; Ray et al. 1997; Hoerger et al. 1999). The average for each site of fracture is quite variable, which mainly reflects the differences between medical practices and health care system organization (Whittington and Faulds 1994; Johnell 1997; Ray et al. 1997; Reginster 1999). Hip fractures logically induce the main part of these expenditures: 40–60 per cent of acute hospital costs resulting from osteoporotic fractures are due to hip fractures (Ray et al. 1997; Zethraeus et al. 1997; Dolan and Torgenson 1998), and they are responsible for a higher percentage of non-acute care costs (Johnell 1997). Vertebral body and wrist fractures induce less disability and are thus less costly.

Economic evaluation of osteoporosis treatment

The treatment of osteoporosis is very heterogeneous. From a public health perspective, the main goal of such treatment is the prevention of hip and, to a lesser extent, vertebral fractures, which are the most important in terms of mortality and morbidity. However, several therapeutic protocols have been proposed, from primary prevention in post-menopausal women to curative treatment in people who have already experienced an osteoporotic fracture. Several factors influence the results of economic analyses: the target population, the potential side effects of therapy, compliance, and other risk factors for osteoporosis not influenced by therapy (Whittington and Faulds 1994). A recent paper reviewed all the economic evaluations published in this domain (Cranney et al. 1999). There are substantial discrepancies between these studies, which reflect the differences in drugs used and in the population treated. This may also partially explain the discrepancies which exist worldwide in the guidelines and public health recommendations about osteoporosis.

Fibromyalgia

Fibromyalgia (FM) is an increasing musculoskeletal problem in developed countries. The lack of very effective treatments often leads patients to consult several physicians, undergo multiple investigations, and experiment with numerous treatments (Wolfe et al. 1997). This high utilization of all sorts of health system resources results in high direct medical costs, estimated by an American multicentre study at 2274 US dollars per patient per year, with a trend to increase with disease duration (Wolfe et al. 1997). The main sources of expenses were hospitalization and drugs (Wolfe et al. 1997). In a smaller study conducted in Canada, the direct costs were less, which can reflect differences in the behaviour of FM patients as well as differences in the health care system (organization and available resources) (White et al. 1999). Important variations have been noted between patients and it seems that a substantial part of the costs are related to only a fraction of patients with high rates of health resource use (Wolfe et al. 1997).

Miscellaneous autoimmune and inflammatory diseases

There is less economic information on the less common rheumatic diseases. A multicentre study has been conducted in the United States in scleroderma patients; direct and indirect costs totaled approximately $1.5 billion in 1994, corresponding to 1–3 per cent of the economic burden of musculoskeletal diseases (Wilson 1997). For vasculitis (i.e. Wegener granulomatosis, periarteritis nodosa, giant cell arteritis), hospital costs have been studied in New York State and the results extrapolated to the whole American population; giant cell arteritis induced the greatest costs, probably because of its frequency (Cotch 2000). However, these results are incomplete, limited to a single cost component (acute hospital direct costs).

Conclusion

The costs of musculoskeletal diseases represent a significant proportion of health care spending, and the ageing of the population and the availability of new treatments will put yet additional pressure on health care budgets in coming years. Faced with unlimited possibilities for improving health, how should our limited resources be allocated? To make allocation choices that do the most good with the resources available, the tradeoffs between one use of resources and the best potential alternative uses must be understood. In this chapter, we have presented the most common types of economic studies used to aid decision makers and have described results from such studies carried out in the musculoskeletal disease area to date. We hope that this summary has provided a useful reference to readers looking for guidance in the interpretation and conduct of economic evaluations.

References

Abenhaim, L. and Suissa, S. (1987). Importance and economic burden of occupational back pain: a study of 2500 cases representative of Quebec. *Journal of Occupational Medicine* **29**, 670–4.

Albers, J.M. et al. (1999). Socio-economic consequences of rheumatoid arthritis in the first years of the disease. *Rheumatology (Oxford)* **38**, 423–30.

Allaire, S.H., Meenan, R.F., and Anderson, J.J. (1991). The impact of rheumatoid arthritis on the household work performance of women. *Arthritis and Rheumatism* **34**, 669–78.

Anonymous. *National Health Expenditures in Canada, 1974–1994. H21-99/1994.* Ottawa: Health Canada, 1996.

Badley, E.M. (1995). The economic burden of musculoskeletal disorders in Canada is similar to that for cancer, and may be higher (editorial). *Journal of Rheumatology* **22**, 204–6.

Barrett, E.M. et al. (2000). The impact of rheumatoid arthritis on employment status in the early years of disease: a UK community-based study. *Rheumatology (Oxford)* **39**, 1403–9.

Baudoin, C. (1997). The cost of osteoporosis in France. *Reviews in Rheumatology (English Edition)* **64**, 441–2.

Baudoin, C. et al. (1996). Hip fractures in France: the magnitude and perspective of the problem. *Osteoporosis International* **6**, 1–10.

Ben Sedrine, W., Radican, L., and Reginster, J.Y. (2001). On conducting burden-of-osteoporosis studies: a review of the core concepts and practical issues. A study carried out under the auspices of a WHO Collaborating Center. *Rheumatology (Oxford)* **40**, 7–14.

Birnbaum, H.G. et al. (2000). Direct and indirect costs of rheumatoid arthritis to an employer. *Journal of Occupational and Environmental Medicine* **42**, 588–96.

Bosi-Ferraz, M.B., Maetzel, A., and Bombardier, C. (1997). A summary of economic evaluations published in the field of rheumatology and related disciplines. *Arthritis and Rheumatism* **40**, 1587–93.

Buxton, M.J. et al. (1997). Modelling in economic evaluation: an unavoidable fact of life. *Health Economics* **6**, 217–27.

Callahan, L.F. (1998). The burden of rheumatoid arthritis: facts and figures. *Journal of Rheumatology Supplement* **53**, 8–12.

Canadian Coordinating Office for Health Technology Assessment. *Guidelines for Economic Evaluation of Pharmaceuticals* 2nd edn., Ottawa: Canadian Coordinating Office for Health Technology Assessment, 1997, pp. 1–85.

Chevat, C. et al. (2001). Healthcare resource utilisation and costs of treating NSAID-associated gastrointestinal toxicity. A multinational perspective. *Pharmacoeconomics* **19**, 17–32.

Clarke, A.E. et al. (1993). A Canadian study of the total medical costs for patients with systemic lupus erythematosus and the predictors of costs. *Arthritis and Rheumatism* **36**, 1548–59.

Clarke, A.E. et al. (1997). Direct and indirect medical costs incurred by Canadian patients with rheumatoid arthritis: a twelve year study. *Journal of Rheumatology* **24**, 1051–60.

Clarke, A.E. et al. (1999a). An international perspective on the well-being and health care costs for patients with systemic lupus erythematosus. *Journal of Rheumatology* **26**, 1500–11.

Clarke, A.E. et al. (1999b). Predicting the short term direct medical costs incurred by patients with rheumatoid arthritis. *Journal of Rheumatology* **26**, 1068–75.

Clarke, A.E. et al. (2000). Underestimating the value of women: assessing the indirect costs of women with systemic lupus erythematosus. *Journal of Rheumatology* **27**, 2597–604.

Cooper, N.J. (2000a). Economic burden of rheumatoid arthritis: a systematic review. *Rheumatology (Oxford)* **39**, 28–33.

Cooper, N.J. et al. (2000b). Secondary health service care and second line drug costs of early inflammatory polyarthritis in Norfolk UK. *Journal of Rheumatology* **27**, 2115–22.

Cotch, M.F. (2000). The socioeconomic impact of vasculitis. *Current Opinion in Rheumatology* **12**, 20–3.

Coyte, P.C. et al. (1998). The economic cost of musculoskeletal disorders in Canada. *Arthritis Care and Research* **11**, 315–25.

Cranney, A. et al. (1999). A review of economic evaluation in osteoporosis. *Arthritis Care and Research* **12**, 425–34.

Daltroy, L.H. et al. (1997). A controlled trial of an educational program to prevent low back injuries. *New England Journal of Medicine* **337**, 322–8.

de Girolamo, G. (1991). Epidemiology and social costs of low back pain and fibromyalgia. *The Clinical Journal of Pain* **7** (Suppl. 1), 1–7.

De Pouvourville, G. (1995). The iatrogenic cost of non-steroidal anti-inflammatory drug therapy. *British Journal of Rheumatology* **34**, 19–24.

Deyo, R.A. et al. (1991). Cost, controversy, crisis: low back pain and the health of the public. *Annual Review of Public Health* **12**, 141–56.

van Dieten, H.E. et al. (2000). Systematic review of the cost effectiveness of prophylactic treatments in the prevention of gastropathy in patients with rheumatoid arthritis or osteoarthritis taking non-steroidal anti-inflammatory drugs. *Annals of Rheumatic Diseases* **59**, 753–9.

Dolan, P. and Torgerson, D.J. (1998). The cost of treating osteoporotic fractures in the United Kingdom female population. *Osteoporosis International* **8**, 611–17.

Drummond, M.F., Stoddart, G.L., and Torrance, G.W. *Methods for the Economic Evaluation of Health Care Programmes.* Oxford: Oxford University Press, 1987.

Engel, C.C., von Korff, M., and Katon, W.J. (1996). Back pain in primary care: predictors of high health-care costs. *Pain* **65**, 197–204.

Felts, W. and Yelin, E. (1989). The economic impact of the rheumatic diseases in the United States. *Journal of Rheumatology* **16**, 867–84.

Finkler, S.A. (1982). The distinction between costs and charges. *Annals of Internal Medicine* **96**, 102–9.

French, F.H., Torgerson, D.J., and Porter, R.W. (1995). Cost analysis of fracture of the neck of femur. *Age and Ageing* **24**, 185–9.

Frymoyer, J.W. and Cats-Baril, W.L. (1991). An overview of the incidences and costs of low back pain. *Orthopedic Clinics of North America* **22**, 263–71.

Gabriel, S.E., Crowson, C.S., and O'Fallon, W.M. (1995). Costs of osteoarthritis: estimates from a geographically defined population. *Journal of Rheumatology Supplement* **43**, 23–5.

Gabriel, S.E. et al. (1997a). Direct medical costs unique to people with arthritis. *Journal of Rheumatology* **24**, 719–25.

Gabriel, S.E. et al. (1997b). Indirect and nonmedical costs among people with rheumatoid arthritis and osteoarthritis compared with nonarthritic controls. *Journal of Rheumatology* **24**, 43–8.

Gabriel, S.E. et al. (1999). Modeling the lifetime costs of rheumatoid arthritis. *Journal of Rheumatology* **26**, 1269–74.

Gironimi, G. et al. (1996). Why health care costs more in the US: comparing health care expenditures between systemic lupus erythematosus patients in Stanford and Montreal. *Arthritis and Rheumatism* **39**, 979–87.

Gold, M.R., Siegel, J.E., Russell, L.B., and Weinstein, M.C. *Cost-Effectiveness in Health and Medicine.* New York: Oxford University Press, 1996.

Gordon, C. and Clarke, A.E. (1999). Quality of life and economic evaluation in SLE clinical trials. *Lupus* **8**, 645–54.

allele into the structure of another allele causes functional changes with consequences for disease (Colbert et al. 1993).

Linkage disequilibrium

The evolution of the genome by recombination, gene conversion and gene duplication results in the concept of linkage disequilibrium, an understanding of which is central to pinpointing disease-related genes especially in complex traits. Linkage disequilibrium is the nonrandom occurrence of alleles of genes located close together. Again the MHC has well-documented examples with specific alleles of neighbouring loci consistently occurring together. These groups of alleles (haplotypes) may extend over 2000–3000 kilobases with several recombination hot spots breaking them up. Some 25 per cent of MHC haplotypes have this marked linkage disequilibrium often spoken of as extended or ancestral (Degli-Esposti et al. 1992). Many other HLA haplotypes exhibit small areas of linkage disequilibrium. The haplotype originally defined serologically by the HLA-A1, HLA-B8, HLA–DR3 alleles and often associated with autoimmunity is a well-documented and excellent example. The phenomenon of linkage disequilibrium radically impacts the ability to identify a gene directly involved in disease pathogenesis from within a chromosome region which has been shown in linkage studies to be related to disease (Goldstein 2001). Such chromosome regions typically may contain 50–150 genes, only a very small proportion of which will be involved in a specific disease. In this regard, investigators using murine systems, where extensive inbreeding allows separation of such genes within a cluster, have an advantage, although the number of matings involved to generate the required recombinants are substantial! A recent example is the documentation of a cluster of 3–4 genes involved in murine lupus located on chromosome 1 and recently identified as SLE 1a, 1b, 1c, 1d by Edward Wakeland and colleagues (2001).

Functional genomics

Functional genomics describes the study of gene expression at either the RNA or protein level. When a genome is studied from the RNA point of view then it is spoken of as the transcriptome, and from proteins as the proteome. Approaches used to study the expression of individual genes may include RNase protection, Northern blotting, and light cycle (quantitative) PCR and at the protein level include flow cytometry, Western blotting, or immunohistochemistry. These methods are now being complemented by microarrays in which the expression profiles of functionally related genes or even all genes can be tested at once. Labeled RNA from any source and, even RNA from a limited number of cells, if amplified first, can be selectively hybridized to genechips containing oligonucleotide probe sets or glass slides with spotted cDNAs. Specialized microarrays are being used to document expression of immunologically related genes and is a notable example of the application of the new technology (Shaffer et al. 2001). While issues of standardization of arrays are legion, the ability to look comprehensively at given biological pathway provides an outstanding tool for the investigator. Data gathered by expression arrays requires supporting studies using other techniques with protein-based methodologies, such as mass spectrometry and two-dimensional protein electrophoresis, providing additional confirmation in addition to the methodologies mentioned above.

Genome maps

Comprehensive maps of the genome are a necessary and important asset in the investigation of disease. Broadly speaking maps are either genetic or physical in nature. While both types provide the likely order of items along a chromosome, only physical maps provide an estimate of true distance in base pairs. Genome maps bring together data obtained by a variety of methods and are the current resources used to establish the chromosomal location of disease related genes. Information from the human genome project is maintained in databases available from www.ncbi.nlm.nih.gov while the assembled genome can be found at http://genome.ucsc.edu/.

Cytogenetic maps

Although a low resolution process, cytochemistry has allowed the identification of individual chromosomes and the mapping of genes to these chromosomes. The technique traditionally applied is known as fluorescent in situ hybridization (FISH). The number of genes so mapped is in the thousands, but the resolution is not better than 2–5 million base pairs (2–5 megabases) distance apart.

Genetic map

The classical genetic approach to mapping traits within families by co-inheritance of linked genes leads to a genetic map applying a statistical analysis known as logarithm of the odds or lod score, a score of greater than 3 is indicative of linkage between any particular genes. As previously discussed, two such closely linked genes may exhibit linkage disequilibrium if allelic variants of the genes occur together more often than expected on a chance basis. The greater the degree of linkage disequilibrium, that is, the lower the recombination rate, the more readily such linkage can be detected and the likelihood that one will establish close linkage between two particular traits or phenotypes. In this context, linkage disequilibrium can be an asset but when identifying genes in a specific chromosome region it can be a confounding variable when fine mapping. The map distances so defined from linkage groups is reported in centimorgans and there are approximately 3500 such centimorgans in the human genome although because of variable linkage disequilibrium the physical distance between traits so mapped may differ from the genetic map distance.

Physical map

In the past 10 years, genome centers all over the world have generated the raw sequence information by determining the sequence of the DNA subunits (bases) of small fragments of human DNA. This has resulted in a 'working draft' because there are still gaps where DNA sequence is missing, either due to lack of raw sequence data, or ambiguities in the positions of the fragments. The human genome project's ultimate goal producing a 'finished sequence' with few gaps and 99.99 per cent accuracy is well on its way to completion although issues still have to be resolved in terms of the ordering of genes within select overlapping components or contigs (Katsanis et al. 2001). Genes may be on the same segment of DNA but the correlation of that region of DNA with respect to its neighbours may not be clear. Interim maps based on two types of polymorphisms are also available. These polymorphic elements, which include SNPs and microsatellites or very numerous tandem repeats (VNTRs) are interspersed throughout the genome and have been extraordinarily helpful in looking for disease linkage.

Very numerous tandem repeat

These polymorphisms are present throughout the genome and there are approximately 10 000 in current VNTR maps, they are fairly randomly distributed and their utility depends on the extent to which they are individually polymorphic and their closeness to the disease related gene(s) of interest. High throughput genotyping of VNTRs is possible with a capacity of several thousand markers or greater per day. Genome-wide screens carried out in many diseases have to date utilized VNTRs (Todd et al. 1989; Todd 2001). The recent publication of a map constructed in the Icelandic population with some 5000 VNTRs used to plot recombinants provided substantially improved resolution over early VNTR genetic maps (Kong et al. 2002; Weber 2002).

Single nucleotide polymorphisms

In contrast, SNPs although less polymorphic in that they are biallelic, are much more numerous, with SNP maps of several millions now possible (Syvanen 2001). Such SNPs can also be detected by high throughput sequencing which will make an enormous contribution to the physical map and its application in understanding disease. SNPs, in contrast to microsatellites, are the main source of functional, that is, allelic variability, in genes. When they are present in the exons and alter the amino acid composition, they may alter the function of the protein, and when they are in the regulatory region, they could affect the gene expression. Such changes are likely to have an impact on the pathogenesis or severity of disease. The comprehensive physical maps will include nonfunctioning genes.

Functional map

The matching of expression data with the physical map will allow a determination of genes with functional status to be identified and mapped and will thus provide investigators with comprehensive knowledge of all genes linked to rheumatic disease. Such a map is still some way off at present, and will not be complete until a complete physical map is obtained.

The genome and disease

It is becoming increasingly understood that many, if not all, diseases have some genetic element, a contrast with the traditional monogenic view of genetic disease. These diseases have a single gene with a mode of inheritance recognized as dominant, recessive, sex-linked, or some variant of these. Diseases in which there is a polygenic involvement are also known as complex genetic traits. It is likely that such diseases, although they do not usually have a family history, nevertheless have an important but complicated genetic basis and account for many of the common rheumatic diseases (Risch and Merikangas 1996).

Monogenic disease

Monogenic diseases in rheumatology are not numerically important in the context of a standard rheumatology clinic although on an individual basis some of the gene defects provide insights into mechanisms of disease. Some monogenic diseases seen in rheumatology are described in chapters describing collagen mutations, and mutations leading to periodic fevers (see Chapters 3.2, 6.1, 6.3, 6.12.2, 6.12.3). Even common diseases may on occasions have a monogenic basis as suggested by several extensive kindreds with a dominant inheritance of early onset osteoarthritis. The recent documentation of linkage between a locus on chromosome 16p in an Icelandic osteoarthritic family is an excellent example of the value of such multiplex kindreds (Ingvarsson et al. 2001). That autoimmunity may on occasion be primarily monogenic can best be illustrated with the Fas and Fas ligand defects resulting in autoimmune disease in mice. The human equivalent of this defect (Adachi et al. 1993) is autoimmune lymphoproliferative syndrome, with some 500 patients reported (Fisher et al. 1995). The patients who present in childhood have massive lymphadenopathy and other autoimmune features including haemolytic anaemias.

Complex genetic traits

The characteristic features of a complex genetic trait, that is, one involving multiple genes, include many of the autoimmune diseases as well as other nonautoimmune conditions such as hypertension. Musculoskeletal diseases like rheumatoid arthritis, the spondyloarthropathies [including ankylosing spondylitis (AS)], systemic lupus erythematosus (SLE), and juvenile idiopathic arthritis (JIA) are all likely to be complex traits. The degree of family history is variable for these diseases, sometimes infrequent as in rheumatoid arthritis or more extensive as in SLE (Gregersen 1999; Wakeland et al. 2001). The lack of large multiplex kindreds means that association studies of disease phenotypes with polymorphic candidate genes have been the initial methods used to assess genetic influences in most rheumatic diseases. Genetic studies in autoimmunity have generally utilized case control methodology, the best documented of which are HLA associations. While many reports of HLA associations, particularly those with lower odds ratios, under 2, may well be founder effects due to population stratification, those with stronger genetic effects have been shown to be due to linkage to HLA (see Chapter 4.3).

In populations which are not homogeneous the issues of stratification are such that the much preferred methodologies involve family studies. At the association level, rather than linkage, pools of parental (or familial) nonproband genes can be compared with those from the disease probands, as described by Thomson (1995). For linkage, large multiplex kindreds, if available, would be the preferred approach—but an alternative for use in simplex families is the transmission disequilibrium test (TDT). TDT compares transmission of a given disease associated gene (or haplotype) from parents to affected individuals with the transmission of allelic variants that are not disease associated (Spielman et al. 1993, 1994). Comparison can also be made between affected and nonaffected in a sibship. Allele sharing is an alternative approach to linkage in families with disease limited to affected sib pairs (Todd et al. 1989).

The application of genome-wide polymorphic elements, particularly VNTRs, has led to the identification of other non-HLA chromosome regions likely to be involved in disease justifying the appellation, complex genetic trait (Todd et al. 1989). This does not identify the individual genes within those regions but suggests the complex nature of their genetic background.

Specific diseases

Systemic lupus erythematosus (also see Chapter 6.6.1)

This disease has similar clinical manifestations in all age groups. There is often a clear family pedigree and therefore a strong genetic component has been inferred. Linkage analysis can be applied and is being pursued in several centers (Gaffney et al. 1998; Moser et al. 1998). There are a number of extensive family databases, and linkage analysis has shown linkage of the disease to several regions on chromosome 1, and slightly less robust evidence to chromosome 4 and 6. The 'strong candidates' from murine models of disease have been proposed to be the HLA class II complex, the complement genes, and the immunoglobulin γ receptors IIIa (Wakeland et al. 2001).

SLE can be further subdivided into the syndromes that are due to complement deficiencies. These are examples of monogenic diseases in that the mutation of one gene leads to the phenotype, chiefly one of an inability to clear immune complexes as shown by splenic immune complex clearance studies. This applies to C2, C4, and rarely C67 deficiencies. C1q deficiency is particularly well studied in man and in animal models. In the C1q deficient mice, the nephritis is apparently due to the accumulation of apoptotic cells in the absence of C1q, revealing a novel role for C1q.

Rheumatoid arthritis (RA) (also see Chapter 6.3.1)

This is an example of a complex trait where there is a great deal of discussion as to whether genetic or environmental influences are most important in the pathogenesis of the disease. In a sense the discussion is not helpful as one needs to know about both. For RA, linkage to HLA has been observed in all major genome-wide screens employing microsatellite markers in multiplex families (Cornelius et al. 1998; Jawaheer et al. 2001, 2003; MacKay et al. 2002).

In addition to this relatively strong HLA component ($p < 0.00005$), several significant non-HLA loci have been reported ($p < 0.005$) which are in common between the genome-wide screens. (Jawaheer et al. 2001; MacKay et al. 2002). Of interest are overlaps in findings for other autoimmune diseases, SLE, IBD, AS, and MS. These findings are consistent with a meta-analysis of the genome-wide screens of autoimmune diseases (Becker et al. 1998), where the hypothesis that there are common autoimmune susceptibility loci was proposed.

The HLA association with DRB1 alleles and DQ alleles are described in detail in Chapters 4.3 and 6.3.1. Of interest is the finding of 'protective' DRB1 alleles containing the amino acid sequence DERAA, and the fact that

DQA3 and 5 can confer susceptibility to RA in the absence of DRB1*0401. The latter remains the strongest association with severe disease.

Ankylosing spondylitis

This disease is a good example of complex trait with a dominant genetic influence from the MHC locus. Family pedigrees are plentiful in AS, which has a more homogeneous phenotype than SLE. HLA-B27 has been implicated for over two decades, but it was clear that other factors are involved since only a small percentage of HLA-B27 individuals have AS. HLA-B27 transgenic rats are susceptible to a disease with features of AS, psoriatic arthritis, and IBD, but only when housed in a microbial environment (Hammer et al. 1990). A recent whole-genome screen performed in 185 families with 255 sibling pairs showed multiple areas of 'suggestive' or stronger linkage with the disease (Wordsworth 1998). The MHC locus has an overall LOD score of 15.6, and has the strongest linkage, followed by a region on chromosome 16q with a LOD score of 4.7, and areas on 1p, 2q, 9q, 10q, 19q (Laval et al. 2001). The transgenic model favours a role for B27 peptide presentation to T cells in arthritis. Recent work suggests that the misfolding of the peptide groove of the class I molecule is associated with aberrant formation of disulfide bonds, and so may influence peptide binding and therefore aberrant antigen presentation (Mear et al. 1999; Dangoria et al. 2002). Genes from the other regions could have a synergistic or modifying influence on the B27 effect. For example, the published case control studies showing association with transporter genes and the cytokines TNF and IL-10, could mean that the proteins of these genetic variants are involved in character of the final signal presented to activate the cytotoxic T cells (Reveille et al. 2001).

Juvenile idiopathic arthritis

This group of diseases are good examples of the importance of good phenotypic descriptions to allow dissection of genetic influence. They also represent complex traits without a major dominant gene locus as in AS.

The clinical classification of sub-types of JIA according to their clinical presentation and disease course has resulted in the identification of different genetic associations with different phenotypes. Family pedigrees are very rare, suggesting either a lack of genetic influence or that the disease is particularly a complex trait. Sibling pairs occur mainly in the oligoarticular group, particularly with onset at 5 years old or younger (Moroldo et al. 1997). Previous studies using the EULAR and ACR nomenclature, HLA class I and II genes are significantly associated with rheumatoid factor negative chronic arthritides in children except for the systemic group (Glass and Giannini 1999). A recent UK study using the ILAR classification confirm previous results showing disease association with HLA–DRB1*0801 (Thomson et al. in press). Furthermore this is increased in all children with an early age of onset (Murray et al. 1999), and linkage to disease was shown by TDT and by allele sharing in affected sib pairs (Prahalad et al. 2000). These studies suggest that genetic influence is age related, especially when the genes are immune response genes.

Based on the hypothesis that genes that regulate inflammation such as cytokine genes may cause persistent imbalance in the immune/inflammatory response, a number of candidate genes have been found to be associated with JIA in case control studies and await further confirmation. These include IL-10 and extended oligoarticular JIA, MIF, and IRF with JIA (without sub-grouping) (Crawley et al. 2001; Donn et al. 2001; Donn et al. in press). The association of TNFα SNP alleles and oligoarthritis was recently found in a TDT of simplex families in the United Kingdom (Zeggini et al. 2002), which does not include the −308 genetic variant, confirming negative association results with this allele in a case control study of Turkish and Czech patients (Ozen et al. 2002). The report of an association of a high expression allele of IL-6 with systemic JIA in a case control study (Fishman et al. 1998) was recently confirmed by a multinational TDT (Oglvie et al. 2003). Given that there are very few sibling pairs with systemic onset JRA, the disease could be the net consequence of a combination of alleles/mutations of proinflammatory and anti-inflammatory genes.

References

Adachi, M., Watanabe-Fukunaga, R., and Nagata, S. (1993). Aberrant transcription caused by the insertion of an early transposable element in an intron of the Fas antigen gene of lpr mice. *Proceedings of the National Academy of the Sciences of the United States of America* **90**, 1756–60.

Becker, K.G. et al. (1998). Clustering of non-major histocompatibility complex susceptibility candidate loci in human autoimmune diseases. *Proceedings of the National Academy of the Sciences of the United States of America* **95**, 9979–84.

Bork, P. and Copley, R. (2001). The draft sequences. Filling in the gaps. *Nature* **409**, 818–20.

Colbert, R.A. et al. (1993). Allele-specific B pocket transplant in class I major histocompatibility complex protein changes requirement for anchor residue at P2 of peptide. *Proceedings of the National Academy of Sciences of the United States of America* **90**, 6879–83.

Cornelius, F. et al. (1998). New susceptibility locus for rheumatoid arthritis suggested by a genome-wide linkage study. *Proceedings of the National Academy of the Sciences of the United States of America* **95**, 10746–50.

Crawley, E., Kon, S., and Woo, P. (2001). Hereditary predisposition to low interleukin 10 production in chldren wih extended oligiarticular juvenile idiopathic arthritis. *Rheumatology* **40**, 574–8.

Dangoria, N.S. et al. (2002). HLA-B27 misfolding is associated with aberrant intermolecular disulfide bond formation (Dimerization) in the endoplasmic reticulum. *Journal of Biological Chemistry* **277**, 23459–68.

Degli-Esposti, M.A. et al. (1992). Ancestral haplotypes: conserved population MHC haplotypes. *Human Immunology* **34** , 242–52.

Donn, R.P. et al. (2001). Cytokine gene polymorphisms and susceptibility to juvenile idiopathic arthritis. British Paediatric Rheumatology Study Group. *Arthritis and Rheumatism* **44**, 802–10.

Donn, R.P. et al. Mutational screening of the macrophage migration inhibitory factor (MIF) gene: positive association of a functional polymorphism of MIF with juvenile idiopathic arthritis. *Arthritis and Rheumatism* (in press).

Fisher, G.H. et al. (1995). Dominant interfering Fas gene mutations impair apoptosis in a human autoimmune lymphoproliferative syndrome. *Cell* **81**, 935–46.

Fishman, D. et al. (1998). The effect of novel polymorphisms in the interleukin-6 (IL-6) gene on IL-6 transcription and plasma IL-6 levels, and an association with systemic-onset juvenile chronic arthritis. *Journal of Clinical Investigation* **102**, 1369–76.

Flajnik, M.F. and Kasahara, M. (2001). Comparative genomics of the MHC: glimpses into the evolution of the adaptive immune system. *Immunity* **15**, 351–62.

Gaffney, P.M. et al. (1998). A genome-wide search for susceptibility genes in human systemic lupus erythematosus sib-pair families. *Proceedings of the National Academy of the Sciences of the United States of America* **95**, 14875–9.

Galas, D.J. (2001). Sequence interpretation. Making sense of the sequence. *Science* **291**, 1257–60.

Glass, D.N. and Giannini, E.H. (1999). Juvenile rheumatoid arthritis as a complex genetic trait. *Arthritis and Rheumatism* **42**, 2261–8.

Goldstein, D.B. (2001). Islands of linkage disequilibrium. *Nature Genetics* **29**, 109–11.

Gregersen, P.K. (1999). Genetics of rheumatoid arthritis: confronting complexity. *Arthritis Research* **1**, 37–44.

Hammer, R.E. et al. (1990). Spontaneous inflammatory disease in transgenic rats expressing HLA-B27 and human B2 m: an animal model of HLA-B27-associate human disorders. *Cell* **63**, 1099–112.

Hershey, G.K. et al. (1997). The association of atopy with a gain-of-function mutation in the alpha subunit of the interleukin-4 receptor. *New England Journal of Medicine* **337**, 1720–5.

Ingvarsson, T. et al. (2001). A large Icelandic family with early osteoarthritis of the hip associated with a susceptibility locus on chromosome 16p. *Arthritis and Rheumatism* **44**, 2548–55.

Jawaheer, D. et al. (2001). A genome wide screen in multiplex rheumatoid arthritis families suggests genetic overlap with other autoimmune diseases. *American Journal of Human Genetics* **68**, 927–36.

Jawaheer, D. et al. (2003). Screening the genome for rheumatoid arthritis susceptibility genes: a replication study and combined analysis of 512 multicase families. *Arthritis and Rheumatism* **48**, 906–16.

Katsanis, N., Worley, K.C., and Lupski, J.R. (2001). An evaluation of the draft human genome sequence. *Nature Genetics* **29**, 88–91.

Kong, A. et al. (2002). A high-resolution recombination map of the human genome. *Nature Genetics* **31**, 241–7.

Lander, E.S. et al. (2001). Initial sequencing and analysis of the human genome. *Nature* **409**, 860–921.

Laval, S.H. et al. (2001). Whole-genome screening in ankylosing spondylitis: evidence of non-MHC genetic-susceptibility loci. *American Journal of Human Genetics* **68**, 918–26.

MacKay, K. et al. (2002). Whole-genome linkage analysis of rheumatoid arthritis susceptibility loci in 252 affected sibling pairs in the United Kingdom. *Arthritis and Rheumatism* **46**, 632–9.

Martinez, F.D. et al. (1997). Association between genetic polymorphisms of the beta2-adrenoceptor and response to albuterol in children with and without a history of wheezing. *Journal of Clinical Investigation* **100**, 3184–8.

Mear, J.P. et al. (1999). Misfolding of HLA-B27 as a result of its B pocket suggests a novel mechanism for its role in susceptibility to spondyloarthropathies. *Journal of Immunology* **163**, 6665–70.

Moroldo, M.B. et al. (1997). Juvenile rheumatoid arthritis in affected sibpairs. *Arthritis and Rheumatism* **40**, 1962–6.

Moser, K.L. et al. (1998). Genome scan of human systemic lupus erythematosus: Evidence for linkage on chromosome 1q in African-American pedigrees. *Proceedings of the National Academy of the Sciences of the United States of America* **95**, 14869–74.

Murray, K.J. et al. (1999). Age-specific effects of juvenile rheumatoid arthritis-associated HLA alleles. *Arthritis and Rheumatism* **42**, 1843–53.

Ogilvie, E.M. et al. A multi-centre study using Simplex and Multiplex (JIA/JRA) families demonstrates that the -174G allele of the interleukin-6 gene confers susceptibility to systemic arthritis in children. *Arthritis and Rheumatism* (in press).

Ozen, S. et al. (2002). Tumour necrosis factor αG $\rightarrow$ A–238 and G $\rightarrow$ A–308 polymorphisms in juvenile idiopathic arthrits. *Rheumatology* **41**, 223–7.

Prahalad, S. et al. (2000). Juvenile rheumatoid arthritis: linkage to HLA demonstrated by allele sharing in affected sibpairs. *Arthritis and Rheumatism* **43**, 2335–8.

Reveille, J.D., Ball, E.J., and Khan, M.A. (2001). HLA-B27 and genetic predistposing factors in spondyloarthropathies. *Current Opinions in Rheumatology* **13**, 265–72.

Risch, N. and Merikangas, K. (1996). The future of genetic studies of complex human diseases. *Science* **273**, 1516–17.

Samonte, R.V. and Eichler, E.E. (2002). Segmental duplications and the evolution of the primate genome. *Nature Review Genetics* **3**, 65–72.

Shaffer, A.L. et al. (2001). Signatures of the immune response. *Immunity* **15**, 375–85.

Spielman, R.S., McGinnis, R.E., and Ewens, W.J. (1993). Transmission test for linkage disequilibrium: the insulin gene region and insulin-dependent diabetes mellitus (IDDM). *American Journal of Human Genetics* **52**, 506–16.

Spielman, R.S., McGinnis, R.E., and Ewens, W.J. (1994). The transmission/disequilibrium test detects cosegregation and linkage. *American Journal of Human Genetics* **54**, 559–60 (Discussion 560–3).

Syvanen, A.C. (2001). Accessing genetic variation: genotyping single nucleotide polymorphisms. *Nature Review Genetics* **2**, 930–42.

Thomson, G. (1995). Mapping disease genes: family-based association studies. *American Journal Human Genetics* **57**, 487–98.

Thomson, W. et al. (2002). Juvenile idiopathic arthritis (JIA) classified by the ILAR criteria: HLA associations in UK patients. *Rheumatology* **41**, 1183–9.

Todd, J.A. (2001). Human genetics. Tackling common disease. *Nature* **411**, 537–9.

Todd, J.A. et al. (1989). Identification of susceptibility loci for insulin-dependent diabetes mellitus by trans-racial gene mapping. *Nature* **338**, 587–9.

Venter, J.C. et al. (2001). The sequence of the human genome. *Science* **291**, 1304–51.

Wakeland, E.K. et al. (2001). Delineating the genetic basis of systemic lupus erythematosus. *Immunity* **15**, 397–408.

Weber, J.L. (2002). The Iceland map. *Nature Genetics* **31**, 225–6.

Wordsworth, P. (1998). Genes in the spondyloarthropathies. *Rheumatic Disease Clinics of North America* **24**, 843–62.

Zeggini, E. et al. (2002). Linkage and association studies of single-nucleotide polymorphism-tagged tumour necrosis factor haplotypes in juvenile oligoarthritis. *Arthritis and Rheumatism* **46**, 3304–11.

3.2 Molecular abnormalities of collagen and connective tissue

F. Michael Pope

Introduction

Collagen is a major connective-tissue protein family with certain important mechanical and scaffolding functions. Other important components of the extracellular matrix have tissue-regulating properties, including BMP 1, which is also the C collagen propeptidase. They are widespread in bone, cartilage, muscle sheaths, ligaments, joint capsules, skin, vascular structures, lungs, pleuroperitoneal linings, intestinal walls, hernial sacs, and glomeruli. Each can react with other proteins and bind to a variety of cellular components. Complex interactions between type V collagen and other fibrillar collagens (I and III) regulate fibril diameters in skin, ligaments, and arteries, whilst types V and XI collagens regulate the size of type II fibrils in cartilage and vitreous. Other collagens, such as types IX, XII, and XIV (the FACIT family), decorate compound fibres and bind to other matrix molecules. These interactions regulate embryonic foetal and later morphogenesis. Deformities result from errors in these interactions.

There are currently 19 collagen proteins with 32 genes. The first mutations were discovered as proteins in the mid-1970s and as genes in the early 1980s. Thus, *COL1A1* and *COL1A2* mutations of type I collagen cause either osteogenesis imperfecta (OI) or Ehlers–Danlos syndrome (EDS) type VII (Byers 1990). Collagen type II (*COL2A1*) mutations clearly cause certain chondrodysplasias (Horton 1995) and Stickler syndrome. Type III collagen (*COL3A1*) mutations usually cause the arterial form of EDS type IV, or types I or III. An X-linked, α5(IV) collagen basement-membrane protein coded by the *COL4A5* gene is implicated in X-linked Alport syndrome (Barker et al. 1990). In other cases, *COL4A1*, *-4A2*, *-4A3*, and *-4A4* genes have been implicated in autosomal-dominant and -recessive Alport syndrome. Collagen V (*COL5A1*) has recently been implicated in EDS types I and II, which are most probably allelic, whilst abnormalities of the *COL11A1* and *-11A2* genes have been implicated in the Stickler syndrome (Snead 1994; Li et al. 1995; Nicholls et al. 1996). There is also biochemical overlap between the Stickler syndrome and multiple epiphyseal dysplasia (Vikkula et al. 1995), with the clinical phenotype dictated largely by mutational type and position. *COL11A1* and *-11A2* have also been implicated in multiple epiphyseal dysplasia. Defects of type X collagen cause Schmid-type metaphyseal chondrodysplasia (Wallis et al. 1996).

Nevertheless, mutant mice null for *COL10A1* show normal growth and development of long bones, suggesting that *COL10A1* mutations act as dominant negatives (Rosati et al. 1994). Type VII collagen mutations cause dystrophic epidermolysis bullosa (Dunnill et al. 1994b). Unexpected collagens include the bullous pemphigoid antigen gene (*BPAG2/COL17A1*), which has both membrane bound and typical helical collagen domains, causing generalized atrophic benign epidermolysis bullosa (McGrath et al. 1995a). Another compound collagen is MARCO, which is a scavenger receptor protein. This has a large intracellular collagenous domain, but is also membrane-bound. Diseases caused by similar genes are highly probable. Other important players include those for collagen VI, present in skin, blood vessels, and fibrocartilage, and for type VIII, which is an endothelial collagen. Collagens IX, X, XI, and XII are important components of cartilage and bone, whilst type XIII collagen is keratinocyte-associated. Subsets of common disorders, such as osteoporosis, osteoarthritis, and congenital berry aneurysm are sometimes caused by mutations of collagen types I, II, and III, and resemble those of OI, certain chondrodystrophies, and vascular EDS (Ala-Kokko et al. 1990; Pope et al. 1991). Other diseases likely to be implicated include, EDS types I, II, and III (the benign hypermobility syndrome) and EDS VIII. Dystrophic epidermolysis bullosa is caused by *COL7A1* mutations. Other bone/cartilage abnormalities are caused by defects in matrix-regulatory proteins, collagen 2 and A, and sulfation abnormalities (the epiphyseal dysplasias). Pseudoxanthoma elasticum (PXE) is caused by a faulty ion transporter gene, which misassembles elastic fibres. In the same year as it was linked to chromosome 15, the fibrillin-5 and -15 genes were cloned. Subsequently, numerous mutations have been detected and the genomic organization of fibrillin 15 established (Corson et al. 1993; Nijbroek et al. 1995). In contrast, the fibrillin gene on chromosome 5 causes a slightly different disorder (congenital contractual arachnodactyly).

Structural mutations in the elastin gene cause certain types of autosomal dominant cutis laxa and supravalvular aortic stenosis. The clinical range is wide and includes various inherited single-gene diseases causing significant morbidity and mortality. Similar gene defects may also participate in other common abnormalities, such as varicose veins, inguinal and femoral hernias, and common forms of familial joint hypermobility syndromes.

The molecular analysis of human genetic disease proceeds in one of two ways. Most often a faulty candidate gene is suspected from structural (histological) finding or the protein chemistry, is subsequently cloned, sequenced, and then analysed for mutations. This approach has been impressively successful in inherited abnormalities of collagens I, II, and III. In other cases all obvious candidate genes have been excluded, leaving the cause completely unknown. Modern advances in sequencing the human genome provide not only a comprehensive catalogue of human genes, but also a collection of variable markers, such as single nucleotide polymorphisms or sequence-tagged sites (SNPs or STSs). Consequently, locating genes is now relatively simple and identifying new connective tissue gene markers is now possible. The recent location of the PXE and EDS VIII genes are good examples of this approach.

Modern recombinant DNA technology

The revolution in recombinant DNA technology includes methods for cutting DNA into fragments suitable for insertion into transmissible, extrachromosomal DNA elements (plasmids) easily grown in bacteria, facilitating the purification and amplification of any desired DNA fragment. Progressively larger DNA fragments have been amplified, whilst vectors have increased the length of clonable DNA from tens to hundreds of kilobases (gene sequencing). The preferential amplification of any DNA segment by the polymerase chain reaction (PCR) has revolutionized human molecular genetics (see Chapter 3.1).

Two approaches have been used for collagen gene defects and association with disease. Reverse genetics identifies the gene locus and then works backwards from gene sequencing to protein structure and function. The Marfan syndrome (MFS), which was only mapped to chromosome 15 in 1990 (Kainulainen et al. 1990), is an excellent example in the genetics of connective tissues. In the alternative approach, a candidate protein is identified in various ways and the gene subsequently cloned, followed by mRNA, cDNA, or genomic analysis. The coordinated efforts to sequence the human GENOME successfully culminating in the draft Human sequence, which began 15 years ago and ended in the assembly and analysis of the Human gene sequence in February 2001, has coincided with sequencing the worm (Caenorhabditis), fly (Drosophila), and mustard-cress (Arabidopsis) genomes. This, integrated comparative DNA, protein databases, and Human disease catalogues (OMIN), provide the means to locate, sequence, and dissect any human gene disorder. We can expect the localization on numerous gene errors to particular human diseases in the next 10 years, providing the potential for custom-made therapies, diagnosis, and identification in all fields of medicine, as well as connective tissue biology.

Collagen genes

The gene analysis of collagen and other connective tissue proteins is amenable to both approaches. In the classical approach, the candidate collagen protein is identified and cloned from cDNA or genomic libraries. Alternatively, a suitable autosomal-dominant disease can be tested for linkage to *COL1A1* or *-1A2* gene markers, or other restriction fragment length polymorphisms (RFLP) nearby.

The conventional approach has defined at least 30 genes coding for some 20 collagen (compound) proteins. In humans these are rather widely distributed, lying on chromosomes 1, 2, 6, 7, 10, 12, 13, 17, 21, and the X chromosome. There are multiple genes on chromosomes 2 (three), 6, 13, and 21 (two on each) (Vuorio and de Crombrugghe 1990). All code for extended triple helices of Gly–XY polymers (where X and Y are often proline or hydroxyproline). Collagen types I, II, III, V, and XI, the interstitial collagens, have *N*- and *C*-globular extensions with uninterrupted Gly–XY triple helices coded by 52 exons. All other collagens have either globular *N*-and/or *C*-terminal extensions, with varyingly large globular interruptions of the triple helix. Bending of the rigid helix at such globular interruptions may be important in different tissues and probably allows interaction with other associated macromolecular and cellular components. Cartilage also contains conventional, cross-striated, interstitial type II collagen fibres.

Historically, the genes for collagens I, II, III, and V were identified in numerical order of discovery (the numbering system originally arose from protein analysis 20 years earlier). These vertebrate proteins have well-defined *N*- and *C*-terminal extensions, essential for fibril alignment and formation and the central triple helices are coded by regular GlyXY subunits in cassettes of exon (coding) sequences, which are always multiples of 9 bp (Prockop and Kivirikko 1984). Such base-pair combinations suggest that there is duplication of the original 9-bp multiples in various combinations and permutations (Vuorio and de Crombrugghe 1990). Alternatively, an ancestral 54-bp exon with surrounding introns could produce 108 and 162 bp by intron loss and 45 and 99 bp by recombination.

Type I collagen is a heteropolymer of two distinct α-chains that spontaneously self-assemble in a 2 : 1 ratio to form $\alpha1(I)_2\alpha2$ triple helices. Rarely, there may be $\alpha1(I)_3$ trimers in skin, $\alpha2$ trimers cannot assemble and are thermodynamically unstable. Types II and III collagens form homotrimers: $\alpha1(II)_3$ and $\alpha1(III)_3$, respectively. The latter has two cysteine bonds in the α-helix, as well as the normal inter- and intrachain disulfide bonds within the *C*-propeptides found in other interstitial collagens. Type II collagen is confined to cartilage and the vitreous humour of the eye. Type III collagen is widely distributed in skin, ligaments, tendons, pleuroperitoneal linings, the intestinal wall, and blood vessels. It plays an important part in arterial strength and stability. These four collagens all have a central helix of $(GlyXY)_{333}$, with proline or hydroxyproline (10 per cent) and lysine or hydoxylysine (4 per cent) in the second and third positions (Prockop and Kirivikko 1984). The Gly–XY cassettes are crucial to the normal biophysical properties and correct winding of the collagen triple helix. The 3′ end of the gene codes for a *C*-terminus of between 243 and 247 amino acids (depending upon collagen type). It has a short telopeptide sequence, but is mostly globular with a highly conserved exon structure for all interstitial collagens (Vuorio and de Crombrugghe 1990). It is coded by exons 49–52; exons 49 and 50 vary in size and exons 51 and 52 are constant for the various interstitial genes. In most of the interstitial families, exon 49 codes for between 45 and 63 bp but in, α2XI it has reduced to only 15 bp.

The *N*-propeptides are more divergent, with substantial differences. *COL1A1*, *-1A2*, *-2A1*, and *-3A1* genes have cysteine-rich regions missing in *COL1A2*. The triple helical region of the *N*-propeptide also varies, being most complex in the *COL2A1* gene, where there are several extra exons. Other similarities at the 5′ and 3′ ends of the gene include regulatory sequences upstream of the gene. There are multiple binding sites for proteins upstream of this site and a highly conserved enhancer sequence within the first intron of *COL1A1*, *COL1A2*, and *COL3A1* collagens, sited between +418 and +1524 of *COL1A2* and +820 and +1602 of *COL1A1*. Deletion of certain promoter sequences causes positive or negative effects. There may also be enhancer sequences analogous to those β-globins downstream of the 3′-coding sequences. The genes for non-interstitial collagens, whilst somewhat different, also have family resemblances to the interstitial collagens. The *COL4* genes (*4A1*, *4A2*, *4A3*, *4A4*, and *4A5*), which all contain several globular interruptions within the triple helix, are highly homologous to each other, all possessing long, *C*-terminal, globular domains (NC1), with smaller *N*-terminal globular domains (NC2). Electron-microscopic and biochemical evidence shows that *N*- and *C*-terminal interactions between adjacent type IV molecules produce a chicken-wire model (Vuorio and de Crombrugghe 1990). There are more than 20 globular interruptions to the Gly–XY triple-helical repeat, 12 of which are single amino-acid deletions, whilst others are globular inserts of up to 24 amino acids depending upon the particular chain type. Nevertheless, exon sizes conform reasonably well to the 9-bp model. The *COL4A1* and *COL4A2* genes run in opposite orientation and direction from head-to-tail contiguous promoter sequences.

Type VI collagen is highly disulfide-linked and has a short triple helix with globular ends forming microfibrils of antiparallel dimers that are laterally associated. Three distinct genes *COL6A1*, *-6A2*, and *-6A3* code for α1, α2, and α3(VI) collagens. They are situated, respectively, on chromosomes 2 (*6A1* and *6A2*) and 21 (*6A3*). The helical exons are multiples of 9 bp. Type VII collagen (*COL7A1*) has globular *N*- and *C*-terminal extensions with a central helix of 320-kDa monomers packed as antiparallel fibrils. The *C*-terminus forms almost half of the molecule. Collagen VIII is an endothelial protein, collagens IX, X, and XI are all components of cartilaginous matrix, whilst the vitreous humour of the eye contains collagens II, V, and XI. In the Stickler syndrome, abnormalities of the vitreous structure and function are combined with myopia and osteoarthritis caused by mutations of the *COL2A1* or *COL11A1* and *-A2* genes. Fibrillin 15 and collagen VI have also been identified in the vitreous humour. Other important interactions include the decoration of collagen I/III by collagen V. There are strong hints that disturbances of such ordered structures produce distinct abnormalities. A good example is the cauliflower fibrils that occur in the skin of patients with EDS I or II. In other cases, certain molecular components that might fit into the gaps between the quarter-staggered fibrils include calcium (collagen I), collagen V (collagens I and III), proteoglycans, glycosaminoglycans, and other compound fibres. Similar constraints also apply to the NC1 (*N*-propeptide) of collagen IX. Site-directed mutagenesis of this region impairs chain registration, selection, or helical stability. The function of the *C*- and *N*-propeptide in those collagens with significant non-helical interruptions is clear, as evidenced by the fibrillogenesis of collagens IV, VI, VII, VIII, and X.

Collagens IX, X, and XI also contribute to cartilaginous matrix. Disorders of the vitreous, for example, Stickler syndrome, are caused by either homogeneous or heterogeneous anomalies of fibrillar collagens II, V, and XI. Errors in any of these components, either as homo or hetero-trimers, induce vitreous misassembly and disorder from faulty fibrillogenesis and distortion of the normal vitreous properties. The latter usually occurs in combination with myopia or osteoarthritis. Furthermore, other unexpected components have also been identified in the vitreous and defects of both fibrillin 15 (an essential component of lens suspensary ligament) and collagen VI genes are potentially pertinent to eye disorders. Compound heterozygosity of collagen types I and III and *COL1A1*, *-1A2*, and *-3A1* mutations and collagen I/II and III genetic compounds *COL1A1*, *-1A2*, *-3A1*, and *-2A1* could also produce clinical disease, though no convincing examples have so far been observed. Enzyme deficiencies of lysylhydroxylase (Wenstrup et al. 1989) and lysyloxidase (Byers et al. 1980) have been described, though the procollagen peptidase deficiency in humans originally postulated by Lichtenstein et al. (1973) was only identified in 1992 (Nusgens et al. 1992).

The molecular analysis of *COL2A1* mutations lagged initially, because of the difficulty culturing chondrocytes and obtaining cartilage samples from which the mutant proteins could be isolated. Errors closely resembled type I and III mutants, both in the pattern of the protein changes (Murray et al. 1989) and gene sequence (Lee et al. 1989). They are usually helical glycine substitutions or deletions. Collagen type II defects cause a variety of inherited disorders (Knowlton et al. 1990).

Type IX and XII collagens and FACIT collagens decorate the exterior of collagen type II, whilst the analagous collagen type XIII is secreted by keratinocytes, but also occurs in skin, bone, intestine, and muscle. Collagens IV, VI, IX, X, XII, and XIII have all been cloned and sequenced, but types VIII and XIII still await more detailed analysis. Interesting supramolecular interactions of collagen types have been observed at the fibrillar level. Collagens I and III and I and V form compound fibrils, whilst collagens II and XI coassociate with collagen IX, which coats the surface of type II and collagen XII decorates the surface of type I collagen. Collagens XIV to XVII include both FACIT and membrane-bound collagens. Errors of the latter, bullous pemphigoid-associated antigen type II, or BP180, cause a mild variant of dystrophic epidermolysis bullosa, the so-called generalized atrophic benign variant or GABEB. The gene specifies an intracellular globular domain, a transmembrane segment and 15 extracellular (GlyXY) sequences.

Collagen folding and self-assembly

The collagen triple helix contains multiple repeating polymers of $(\text{GlyXY})_n$. The flexible lysine bonds are interspersed with inflexible proline, or hydroxyproline, to confer a specific helical conformation, as defined by hydrogen bonding and water bridges linking individual α-chains to each other. For proper triple-helix formation, each of the three α-chains must be in correct register as redundant loops and mismatches could seriously impair the processing of the procollagen extensions. When the triple helix is correctly wound it is incorporated into mature collagen fibrils. Errors occur at any of several biosynthetic steps, for example, in the disulphide bonds between the α-chains. It is also essential that each component of the triple helix be properly aligned if proper superhelical winding is to take place. Helical winding next propagates towards the *N*-terminal end, twisting the three chains into a tightly wound, rod-like structure (Byers 1990).

There are also several important post-translational modifications, such as changing of GlyXPro to GlyXhydroxyproline by the enzyme prolyl-4-hydroxylase (Kivirikko and Myllyla 1982). This stabilizes the collagen helix at ambient body temperature, delaying crystallization of the 'in-register', *C*-propeptide-associated (potential) triple helix. Other important steps include limited lysyl hydroxylation, some of which have galactose, or glucosylgalactose, residues added. Hydroxylysine stabilizes the cross-links between collagen monomers. The chains cannot be efficiently folded without hydroxylation, but as the act of folding inhibits this modification the process is self-regulatory. After optimal winding, various cleavage enzymes (Byers 1990) dramatically alter the solubility of the precursor molecule. Spontaneous polymerization of individual triple-helical collagen α-helices into fibrils then follows. The self-assembly of collagen fibrils is probably affected by other constituents of the extracellular matrix.

The information above especially applies to the interstitial collagen types I [α1(I) and α2(I)], II [$\alpha 1(\text{II})_3$], and III [$\alpha 1(\text{III})_3$] proteins. Very probably, similar considerations and constraints apply to other interstitial collagens, such as collagen V (α1- and α2-chains) and collagen XI (α1- and α2-chains). It is also now apparent that defects of *COL5A1*, *-5A2*, *-11A1*, and *-11A2* also produce clinically detectable disease. More recently the *COL5A1* gene has been linked to EDS type I /II (Loughlin et al. 1995; Burrows et al. 1996). At least three other cartilage collagen genes, apart from collagen II, have the potential to produce cartilage-related inherited diseases. Furthermore, molecules such as tenascin, thrombospondin, the BMP family, and matrix-regulatory proteins and a wide repertoire of stimulatory molecules, play crucial roles in the immunomodulation of inflammation.

Mutations of collagen genes and proteins

Mutations of the genes coding for interstitial collagen types I, II, and III are extremely diverse and private to each family, with rare exceptions. Amino acid substitutions are disruptive when altering triple-helical glycines, but location and type of substitution are important. Very few second- or third-position (X + Y) mutations have been detected and their effects are not completely clear. Splice-junction point mutations are important mechanisms for collagen deletions, analogous to haemoglobin and other splice mutations. All dramatically affect protein structure or secretion, although overmodified secreted products are, in general, common in type I defects (Bonadio and Byers 1985), whilst overmodified retained protein is common in *COL3A1* mutations (Pope et al. 1996). Generally, the clinical phenotype is much more variable in mutations of collagen type I, ranging from virtual normality with mild osteoporosis, to congenital fractures with lethal disease in babies (Sillence et al. 1979). Defects of collagen type III rarely exhibit their lethal effects before adolescence with arterial rupture postponed until middle-age (Pope et al. 1996). Beighton et al. (1992), have attempted to correlate clinical chemical and molecular phenotypes.

Except for EDS type VII, all of which have exon-6 splicing defects of either $\alpha 1$(I) or $\alpha 2$(I), most families with mutations of collagen type I and III have private mutations (Pepin et al. 2000). To date, nearly all type I mutations have been observed in OI/EDS VII, only 5 per cent are recurrent between families. Many *COL3A1* mutants are unique, with noteable exceptions, such as exon 24 skips. The molecular analysis of *COL2A1*, which (as outlined above) previously lagged behind the others, but has recently advanced spectacularly with more than 50 recorded mutations (Horton 1995). Again, private mutations are the norm. As in collagen type I and III mutants, many are glycine substitutions or deletions, with similarly disturbed protein patterns (Murray et al. 1989) and gene-sequencing data (Lee et al. 1989). There is also impressive evidence that associates *COL2A1* mutations to various inherited disorders (Knowlton et al. 1990).

There have been equally spectacular advances in the analysis of Alport syndrome. These are in the linked *COL4A5* gene and the autosomal *COL4A3* and *COL4A4* genes. Gene linkage and mutational analysis of *COL7A1* mutants have also rapidly advanced, with linkage of the gene to both the autosomal-dominant and -recessive epidermolysis bullosa dystrophica and *COL7A1* mutations in both variants. Studies include combinations of cDNA and genomic sequencing of amplified gene fragments (Christiano et al. 1996). Usually cDNA is amplified as four or five fragments, whilst the 118 *COL7A1* genomic exon sequences are amplified with 70 pairs of separate primers, followed by a combination of HDE, SSCP, DGGE, or protein truncation analyses. Various null alleles, usually stop-codon mutants, but relatively few glycine helical substitutions, or splice junction deletions, have been detected. Null alleles are associated with both autosomal dominant and recessive DDB. In some double heterozygote parents they are clinically silent, in marked contrast to errors of fibrillar collagens I, II, or III.

There has also been rapid progress in the analysis of collagen IX and X mutants, which cause disorders such as spondylometaphyseal and Schmid-type chondrodysplasias. Other important advances include the identification of a collagen Vα1 and -α2 error in mice and man (*COL5A1* and *COL5A2* mutants), each of which produces specific connective-tissue diseases (Andrikopoulos et al. 1995; Nicholls et al. 1996). The original *COL5A1* mutant has been confirmed by linkage (Loughlin et al. 1995; Burrows et al. 1996) as well as exon skips, glycine substitutions, deletions, and null alleles (Burrows et al. 1998). Furthermore, EDS types I and II are allelic (Burrows et al. 1996).

Type I collagen mutations

Type I collagen is widespread in bones, particularly the metaphyses and diaphyses of long bones where it is the major matrix protein. It also occurs in tendons, joint capsules, the dermis, and blood vessels. Clinical abnormalities include weakened bones with variably diminished bone matrix proportional to the severity of the OI (Plate 40), ranging from mild, barely detectable familial osteoporosis, to lethal, short-limbed dwarfism. Sometimes, ligaments, joint capsules, scleral thickness, dentine, heart valves, and dermal thickness are affected, as judged by joint laxity, blue sclerae, dentinogenesis imperfecta (DI) and prolapsed, or incompetent, heart valves. Very severe joint laxity, with or without skin fragility, though usually without osteoporosis, is more typical of EDS VII, accompanied by short stature. In heterozygotes, mutations outside the main collagen helix produce either mild OI, or osteoporosis, but may be very severe in homozygotes (Byers 1990). One unusual patient with MFS, with an abnormal $\alpha 2$(I) collagen protein, had a second-position mutation affecting her father and herself. It is unclear whether the father in the former family is a true Marfan or a mosaic (Phillips et al. 1991). Furthermore, the general relevance is unclear as no other Marfan family has been linked to the *COL1A2*, or any other collagen gene and, with only one exception, all MFS families so far are linked to fibrillin 1 (Kainulainen et al. 1994; Dietz et al. 1995; Nijbroek et al. 1995). The one exception, a very large French family, is linked to 3p24.2–p25 (Collod et al. 1995). Whether or not this fulfills the MFS clinical criteria is controversial and hotly debated. Regularly updated MFS databases are available in Nucleic Acids Research, or on the web as OMIM number 154700 for MFS and 134797 for the gene, FBN1. There are similar databases for collagen type I and III mutations in OI and EDS.

Clinical features of OI

The clinical and pathological changes are those of inherited osteoporosis and, in severe disease, the bone matrix is severely disorganized and depleted (Plate 40). Here the periosteum persists normally, but there is often minor distortion and disorganization of the epiphyseal plates. Radiological changes range from mild osteoporosis with occasional fractures, to a widespread and severe skeletal abnormality with absent skull calcification, multiple rib fractures, platyspondyly with spinal collapse and distorted, multiply fractured bones either modelled, or unmodelled, depending upon clinical severity (Fig. 1).

The clinical phenotypes vary from normal-looking children with occasional fractures beginning in infancy, to severely crippled, short-limbed dwarves (dying either *in utero* or perinatally). Their variability is recognized by the Sillence classification (Sillence et al. 1979), which separates two mild and autosomal-dominant disorders (types I and IV) from two lethal or severely crippling disorders (types II and III) (Plate 41). Both autosomal-dominant and -recessive inheritance occurs.

Types I and IV OI

Both are mild disorders presenting in infancy or childhood with occasional fractures. Although the defect can present at birth, childhood fractures that improve at puberty are more usual. Type I OI differs from type IV only by the deep blue sclerae, which in patients with type IV are pale grey, or white. Common features include autosomal-dominant inheritance, multiple affected generations with transmission through either sex, variably short stature, and childhood fractures, improving at adolescence, but recurring after menopause. There are occasional variants where fractures are more common in females, but rare in males. Rather than improving in number in adolescence, they continue unabated throughout adulthood. Many different mutations have now been observed (Plate 42). Deafness or DI segregate separately, sparing some families, whilst being rampant in others. In families with DI, the primary dentition is uniformly opalescent (slate or brownish coloured), whilst the changes in the secondary dentition are usually patchy with lower incisors and first permanent premolars particularly prone. Dental radiographs characteristically show short, tapering roots and

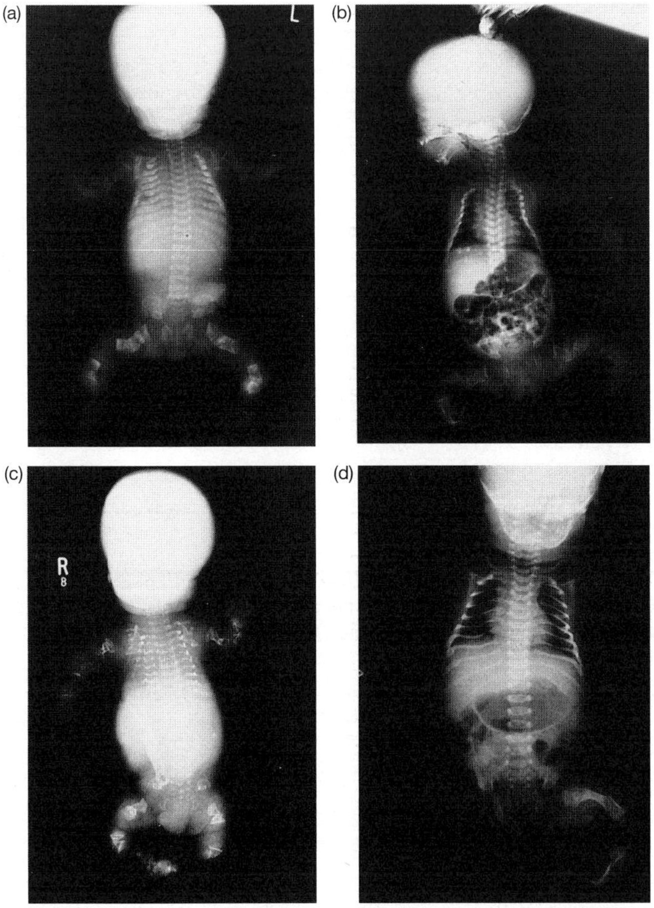

Fig. 1 Radiological phenotype of babies affected by OI ranging from (a) lethally affected, generalized involvement of ribs and unmodelled long bones (Sillence type IIa), to various combinations of unmodelled long bones and nodular or unbroken ribs (b–d). The least severe phenotype (sometimes called Sillence type IIc or III) has gracile, generally unfractured bones, but considerable distortion and fractures of the lower limbs (d).

expanded crowns. Histologically, there are sparse or agglomerated dentinal tubules, both by light and electron microscopy (Plate 43). The DI/OI disorder is separate from isolated DI, which affects the primary and secondary dentition equally. More rarely it is associated with minor joint laxity similar to EDS III (Komorowska et al. 1989) and is probably a connective tissue disorder. The gene lies on chromosome 4.

Sillence type II OI is a severely crippling and often lethal disease [Fig. 1(a) and (b) and Plate 41(d–f)]. Affected babies die *in utero* or perinatally from a variety of causes. The majority who die early do so from chest infections and pulmonary restriction, which complicate the widespread fractures. Sillence described three main types, IIa, IIb, and IId, of which the first two have unmodelled, rectangular limb bones, especially the femurs and humeri. OI type IIa has characteristically widened and multiple fractured ribs, which have a generalized, feathered appearance. OI type I, in contrast, shows either nodules (from callus formation) or unbroken, but thinned and slightly misshapen, ribs. This type [Fig. 1(a) and (b)], was called OI type III rather than Sillence type IIc by Thompson et al. (1987). It describes babies with very much more severely twisted, sometimes modelled, limb bones, distinct from OI IIa and IIb. Similarly, the ribs are thinned, nodular, or sometimes contain multiple fractures, but are always thinner and more distorted than those of IIa and IIb. With the thin-boned infantile variant, OI type III, most will survive to adulthood. Here there are slightly distorted ribs that are gracile rather than widened, whilst there are well-modelled limb bones, often with angulated, U-shaped tibiae [Plate 41(a)]. This subset might be better named Sillence IId OI in babies, but OI type III in surviving adults. OI type IIa is invariably lethal, as are many forms of IIb and IIc, so there are insufficient data to classify adult survivors. Probably OI type III would be an appropriate designation for most of them. In practice, the Sillence IIa–c classification is a useful guide for what is actually a continuous spectrum of clinical changes with broad-boned lethal OI and thin-boned OI. Inheritance is usually autosomal-dominant, and most affected babies have arisen from sporadic new mutations, 10 per cent of which have parents with somatic gonadal mosaics. Multiple reoccurrences in this circumstance simulate autosomal-recessive inheritance (Byers 1990). Authentic autosomal-recessive inheritance is also well documented but distinguishable from mosaicism only by sequencing. Occasional OI IId phenotypes are unlinked to both *COL1A1* and *COL1A2*. Proteins other than type I collagen must therefore participate.

Collagen type I mutations in OI

Bone matrix protein is made largely of type I collagen, with small amounts of type V and smaller traces of type III, coming from vascular structures. Over 200 mutations of type I collagen have been published, including point mutations, deletions, insertions, and a number of splicing mutations, as outlined below (Dalgleish 2001) [see Plate 42(a) and (b)]. The Sillence classification roughly correlates with the molecular pathology. Milder, Sillence type I and IV OI is caused by silent alleles, point mutations, or exon skipping of *COL1A1*, or *-1A2*, in relatively harmless parts of the molecule. Lethal and severely crippling OI mostly arises from glycine substitutions of *COL1A1* or *-1A2*, genes. These severely disrupt the collagen helix by producing homozygous, *C*-terminal mutations, or forming disruptive helical substitutions that consequently impair helical conformation, or even produce kinking distant to the substitution site. A good example is Gly–Cys748 of *COL1A1* in which processing of the distant *N*-propeptide is subsequently severely compromised (Vogel et al. 1988). Glycine substitutions are often position-specific, either interfering with helical folding, as measured by proteinase susceptibility, or impairing protein crystallization with normal folding. Mutations also produce the so-called *protein suicide* effect, in which the presence of one or more abnormal proα chains within triple helices causes both normal and abnormal products to be intracellularly degraded (Prockop 1990). Either one or two mutant molecules in a heterotrimer of wild-type and mutant products, destroy their companion normal components too. Only wild-type $\alpha1(I)2\alpha2$ heterotrimers survive to be successfully secreted.

Point mutations

Gly–Cys substitutions clearly illustrate how mutational location affects clinical phenotype [Plate 42(a)]. Two similar Gly–Cys substitutions, both within the *C*-terminal, CNBr fragment *α1(I)CB6*, cause widely disparate clinical phenotypes. One causes very mild, autosomal-dominant Sillence type I, whilst the other causes lethal, Sillence type II OI. The effect of the two errors correlates with their location. Both produce a novel, higher molecular-weight, disulfide-linked dimer, running above normal collagen $\alpha1(I)$ chains. Both individual peptide maps showed a pattern derived from collagen $\alpha1(I)$ chains, with *α1(I)CB6* running as a dimer. After reduction, the dimer disappeared, whilst *α1(I)CB6* reappeared (Steinmann et al. 1984) (Fig. 2). The lethal $\alpha1(I)$ dimer melted at 38°C, whereas, the dimer from the mild OI melted normally at 41°C (Fig. 3). This indicated disturbed helicity in the lethal but not mild mutation. At the time the location of both mutations to *CB6* belied their very different clinical phenotypes. Even though both mutations changed glycine (GCG) to cysteine (TCG) and were separated by only 10 amino acids, their effects were positional. The mild mutation substituted the first glycine outside the collagen triple helix with unimportant biophysical effects, whilst the 988 mutation changed the tenth glycine from the *C*-terminus of the $\alpha1(I)$ helix and is consequently lethal. The 988 substitution produced a protease-susceptible collagen that melted at 2°C lower than normal, the 1017 mutation produced an $\alpha1(I)$ collagen protein that melted normally [Fig. 3(a) and (b)]. Subsequently, many other

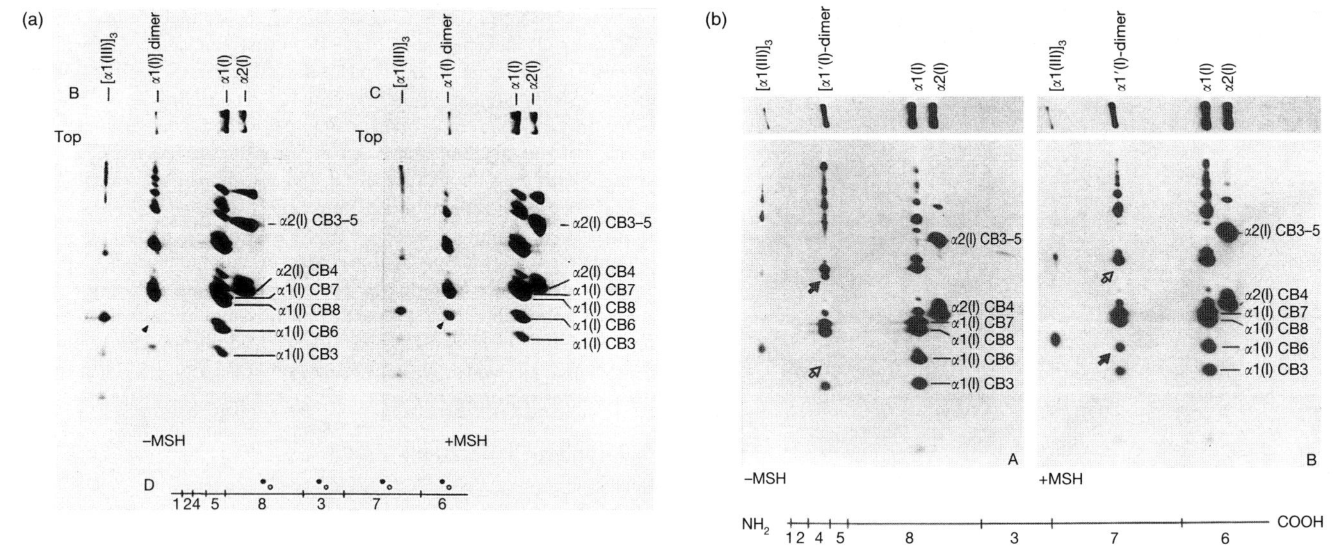

Fig. 2 Two-dimensional gel electrophoresis of radiolabelled collagens from (a) a lethally affected patient described by Steinmann et al. (1984) and (b) a mildly affected patient described by Steinmann et al. (1986). The lethally affected individual has tilted 'smiling' of all CNBr peptides and the mildly affected has horizontal, 'non-smiling' gels, yet both have mutations localized to *α1(I)CB6* and produce an additional, higher molecular-weight dimer running heavier than the α1(I) chains. This is obvious when the gels are compared before (−MSH) and after (+MSH) reduction with mercaptoethanol. The order of peptides from *N*- to *C*-termini is shown diagrammatically.

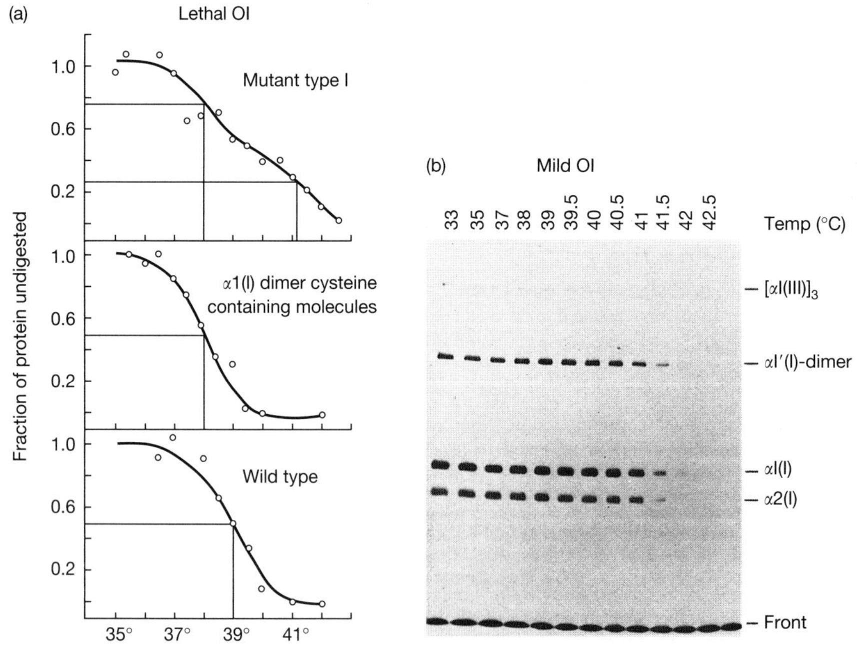

Fig. 3 Comparison of the melting profiles of the lethal and mild OI (from Steinmann et al. 1984). The lethally affected patient has differing melting curves for the cysteine-containing and normal α1(I) chains (shown as a graph). (a) The cysteine-containing α1(I) chain melts at 2°C earlier than its wild-type equivalent. In contrast, the cysteine-containing chain from the mildly affected individual melts identically to the wild-type α1 and α2(I) chains. The position of the mutated cysteine, therefore, influences the proteinase susceptibility of the two mutant collagen trimers. Whereas the melting curve is plotted as a ratio in (a), similar data are shown at each time point in (b) by gel electrophoresis.

cysteine substitutions have been identified at scattered locations ranging from near the *N*-terminus to as far 3′ as from the *C*-terminus [see Plate 42(a)]. Substitutions at the *C*-terminus of amino acid 690 to the end of the helix have been lethal, with those between amino acids 391 and 559 severely crippling. *N*-terminal 'left-hand' mutations between 94 and 223 have been uniformly mild (Cole and Dalgleish 1995). This is consistent with two other mutations, the one at residue 19 close to the *N*-terminus producing premature osteoporosis, the other at amino acid 415 producing a mixed Sillence type III/IV phenotype. Cysteine substitutions of α2(I) collagen produce less predictable phenotypes. One at position 259 had an OI type III phenotype, whilst at position 472 there was a genetic lethal and at position 646, a severe type IV phenotype (Byers 1990). Such differences are partly due to ascertainment bias. Whether severe crippling affects survivors or premature lethality kills younger babies is partly determined by randomly encountered respiratory pathogens or other systemic complications.

Other substitutions

There are over 200 mutations of type I collagen $\alpha 1$ or $\alpha 2$ genes (*COL1A1* and *COL1A2*), including those already discussed [Plate 42(a) and (b)]. The same broad generalizations apply to other *COL1A1* and *COL1A2* mutations, that is, errors closest to the *C*-terminus are the most disruptive (Dalgleish 2001). With the exception of glycine to alanine, all possible glycine substitutions have affected both the *COL1A1* and *COL1A2* genes. Severity varies with the position and type of substitution [Plate 42(a)]. The geometry of the triple helix is such that only hydrogen is small enough to project inwards between the triple chains. All other alternatives are very much larger and very disruptive to helical stability. Gly–Val , Gly–Asp substitutions are lethal wherever they occur. No Gly–Glu substitutions have been recorded for either type I gene, but several affect *COL3A1* (see below). Clinical severity reflects helical position, substitution size, with bigger amino acids being worse than smaller ones and local domain interactions with neighbouring molecules (Byers 1990). Less obvious mechanisms include Gly–Cys748, which not only locally disturbs the central triple helix, but has more puzzling distant effects upon the *N*-terminus, which is 500 residues away (Vogel et al. 1988).

Splitting the triple helix into collagenase A and B fragments shows micro-unfolding between 637 and 775 of collagen $\alpha 1$(I). Two nearby Gly–Ser substitutions in positions 598 and 631 show an adjacent region between amino acids 500 and 631 (Westerhausen et al. 1990). Other localized instabilities probably occur elsewhere in the collagen helix.

Exon-skipping deletions

Most vertebrate structural genes, including those for collagen types I and III, are interrupted by non-coding introns between 80 and 10 000 bp. Collagen introns lie at the lower end of this scale. The primary mRNA sequence is transcribed from genomic DNA. It is precisely cut and pasted as 52 consecutive exons. These include the 42 triple-helical exons, the four *C*-terminal exons, and the six exons of the *N*-propeptide. The 5′ and 3′ ends of each intron have invariant splice-junction donor and acceptor sites. The donor site at the 3′ end of the 5′-most exon is usually GT, whilst the acceptor sites at the 5′ end of the 3′-most exon is usually AG. Single nucleotide changes can destroy a normal splice site, or activate hidden alternatives. If the 3′ polyadenylation sequence is missing, translation continues to the next downstream 3′ equivalent. Such variability promotes evolutionary change.

The gradient of collagen exon-skipping deletions [Plate 42(b)] is similar to point mutations. Several *C*-terminal *COL1A1* mutations have been lethal (exons 43 and 44), whilst mid-gene defects are severe or lethal (exons 27 and 30). In contrast, *N*-terminal skipping can be either mild (17), or lethal (14) and similar considerations apply to the *COL1A2* exon skips. There are 36 *COL1A1* and *COL1A2* exon skips. *N*-terminal OI exon skips have phenotypical overlap with EDS VII and the closer to the *N*-terminus, the milder the OI. An atypical OI family with mild OI and marked joint laxity, with mis-spliced exon 9 of the COL1A2 gene producing a shortened $\alpha 2$(I) protein have been described. There was an 11 bp insertion spanning the exon–intron junction, which shortened the $\alpha 2$ collagen chain by 18 amino acids. Null alleles commonly cause Sillence type I OI (Dalgleish 2001).

Mutations with milder phenotypes that are neither deletions nor caused by exon skipping

Many Sillence type I OI patients produce less type I collagen than normal, detectable by polyacrylamide gel electrophoresis as a relatively higher abundance of type III collagen protein. Type I collagen is normally secreted not overmodified and has no structural abnormalities. Theoretically, mutations affecting gene expression, translational efficiency, stability of pro-α chains, and molecular assembly could all lower type I collagen protein. Steady-state cytoplasmic mRNA is either low or normal (Byers 1990). There is linkage to the *COL1A1* or *COL1A2* genes in 95 per cent of OI families (Sykes et al. 1990). Point mutations occur (as in our Gly–Cys family). Willing et al. (1990) described a collagen chain elongation mutant, caused by a stop codon deletion. Null mutants are distinguishable from wild-type genes by reverse transcriptase-PCR of allele-specific, intragenic cDNA polymorphisms. This allows confident discrimination between expressed or non-expressed alleles. Certain structural mutations cause identical protein profiles (Fig. 4), but different clinical phenotypes. Measurement of protein migration is insufficient to predict clinical severity, although the most crippling phenotypes usually show very obvious chemical changes.

COL1A2 mutations, which reduce $\alpha 2$(I) protein synthesis are detectable by altered $\alpha 1/\alpha 2$ ratios, increasing the expected 2/1 ratio, but also increasing III/I collagen ratios. In contrast, $\alpha 1$(I) depletion will lower $\alpha 1/\alpha 2$ ratios closer to 1 to 1. Those α chains not incorporated into heterotrimers could either form $\alpha 1$(I) trimers [$\alpha 1$(I) chains], or self-degrade ($\alpha 2$ chains). Chains with apparent $\alpha 2$ dimers can form anomalously. It is unclear whether these are stabilized by inter- or intramolecular cross-links, but the clinical phenotype is not OI.

A unique, 4-bp deletion in *COL1A2* was clinically silent in the heterozygote male, whilst the carrier female manifested premature osteoporosis. In contrast, the homozygous affected child had severe, Sillence type III OI. Both heterozygous parents also showed increased joint laxity and slightly thin bones (Nicholls et al. 1984). The 4-bp deletion produced a frameshift, with a nonsense downstream sequence, resulting in a defective sequence of the last 31 amino acids. It is possible that deletions at $\alpha 2$ might cause entirely different clinical phenotypes. There are strong hints that aortic dilatation, aortic incompetence and aortic arterial aneurysms can complicate certain *COL1A2* mutations, strongly implying a role for type I collagen $\alpha 2$ chains in maintaining aortic stability.

Gonadal mosaicism

Single *COL1A1*, or *COL1A2*, mutations often cause lethal OI. These are sporadic, new, autosomal-dominant mutations with negligible risks for recurrence. There are extraordinary families with four or more affected children, but normal parents, suggesting the possibility of germ-line mosaicism (Byers 1990). In the past, inheritance was usually interpreted as homozygous, or double heterozygous autosomal recessive, as in Sillence OI types IIb or IIc. Most are gonadal mosaics, as judged by the clinical expression of a milder (non-lethal) phenotype in the carrier parent, the properties

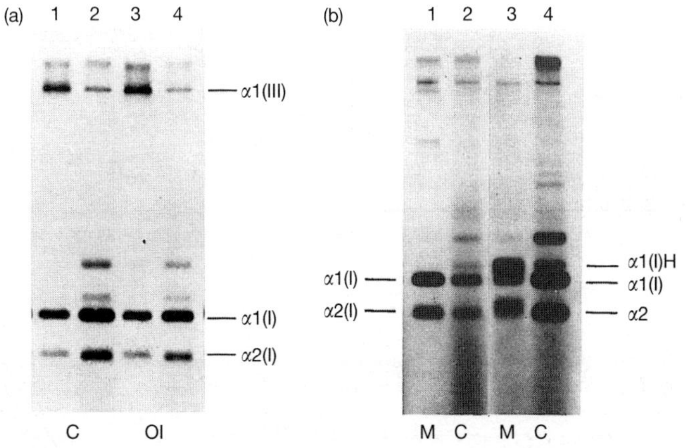

Fig. 4 Radiolabelled collagen profiles. (a) Low type I collagen-producing mild OI pattern. The intensity of the unreduced $\alpha 1$(III) band distinguishes affected individuals [relatively more type III collagen secreted into the medium (track 3) from unaffected (track 1)]. There is no difference in the cell-layer collagens (tracks 2 and 4). C, control. OI, osteogenesis imperfecta. This is typical of haploinsufficiency. (b) Double $\alpha 1$(I) components [one $\alpha 1$(I)H, of higher molecular weight] that occur in some rare, mild OI families. Here a double $\alpha 1$(I) band is secreted into the medium (M), whereas in the cell layer (C) mainly $\alpha 1$(I) is retained (tracks 3 and 4). The equivalent band retained in the cell layer of the control (track 2) is type V collagen.

of the mutant protein and expression of the mutant gene in fibroblasts, hair bulbs, saliva, lymphocytes, seminal fluid, or ovarian biopsies. A good example is Gly–Cys at position 472 of the *COL1A2* gene. Here a man with clinically mild OI fathered separately affected children with two different mothers. The mutant gene occurred in 33 per cent of sperm, 67 per cent of lymphocytes, and 100 per cent of dermal fibroblasts.

OI caused by neither *COL1A1* nor *COL1A2* mutations

We have studied several examples, some with Sillence type IId OI. One osteoporotic, but otherwise normal, mother partially expressed a doublet of normal and overmodified mutant $\alpha 1(\mathrm{I})$ chains. She has had three children lethally or severely affected by OI. In a second OI family, two clinically normal parents have produced six consecutively affected children with type IId. Both an overmodified and a normal protein are produced. Cyanogen bromide mapping suggests a defect at the 3′ end of either the *COL1A1* or *COL1A2* gene and the protein overmodification was sufficiently distinctive for prenatal diagnosis [Fig. 5(a)]. In the absence of such changes, ultrasonographic monitoring of limb length can be very useful [Fig. 5(b)]. Both compound heterozygosity and autosomal-recessive inheritance are unlikely (4096/1 against) and cloning and sequencing of the *α1(CB6)* region and the homologous region of *COL1A2* followed by allele-specific hybridization of parental tissues showed no collagen type I errors, suggesting mutations of genes other than *COL1A1* or *COL1A2*.

OI with normal collagen type I protein

Some OI patients have normal $\alpha 1(\mathrm{I})$ or $\alpha 2(\mathrm{I})$ collagen proteins, but still have abnormal *COL1A1* and *-1A2* genes. Genetic linkage studies are a valuable alternative in suitable families and will often pinpoint the mutant gene. Numerous RFLPs include *Msp*I and two *Rsa*I sites for *COL1A1* and *Eco*RI, *Msp*I, *Stu*I, and *Rsa*I for the *COL1A2*. All can be PCR'd (Sykes et al. 1990) with over 90 per cent of families linked to either *COL1A1* or *COL1A2* markers. Most Sillence type IV pedigrees segregate with *COL1A2* markers, whilst families with Sillence type I OI are three times more likely to be linked to *COL1A1* than *COL1A2*. Recently, the range and variety include 15 *COL1A1* and 37 *COL1A2* polymorphisms (Dalgleish 2001).

Linkage in autosomal-recessive OI

Such linkage data have been consistent for autosomal-dominant families but not for autosomal-recessive inheritance. We studied an unusual Irish 'traveller' family with three children lethally affected by type IId OI. Linkage data suggested that neither the *COL1A1* nor the *COL1A2* gene was to blame, yet the protein mapping data showed clear overmodification of collagen type I peptides. The latter usually indicates C-terminal mutations of either the *COL1A1* or *COL1A2* gene. To date this paradox remains unresolved. We have also observed at least three similar Asian Indian or Middle European families. Possible explanations include unusual somatic mosaicism, compound heterozygosity, or the involvement of unidentified matrix genes other than *COL1A1* or *COL1A2*.

EDS type VII

Whether collagen type I (*COL1A1/COL1A2*) mutations cause OI or EDS type VII depends entirely upon the location of the error. Type VII is a distinct subset of EDS, typified by extreme early joint laxity, increased skin fragility (similar to EDS I/II) and misshapen collagen fibrils by transmission electron microscopy [Plate 44(b)]. EDS VII overlaps clinically with OI mutations caused by *N*-terminal helical mutants, but patients with EDS VII rarely break bones, whilst OI lacks skin fragility. There are distinct genetic subsets of EDS VII. One group with structural abnormalities of type I collagen (*COL1A1* and *COL1A2*) and another with a faulty enzymes responsible for peptide cleavage (the *N*- and *C*-propeptidases). The former group usually has errors in exon 6 of either the *COL1A1* or *COL1A2* genes [Plate 44(a)]. The latter group has specific errors in the *N*-terminal propeptidase that cleaves the *N*-propeptide from both pro-$\alpha 1(\mathrm{I})$ and pro-$\alpha 2(\mathrm{I})$ chains. Intraexonic mutations of exon 6 and other more complex deletions of this region can probably produce similar disorders (see below). Here the subtleties of the protein chemistry will depend upon whether the *N*-proteinase or pepsin/trypsin cleavage sites, or lysine hydroxylation sequences are omitted [Plate 44(c)].

In EDS type VIIC, failure to remove any precursor *N*-propeptides causes lethal or severe skin fragility (Nusgens et al. 1992). Other notable features of EDS VIIC patients include identical biochemical changes, with disordered removal of the faulty *N*-propeptides and various novel clinical features including premature, generalized cutis laxa with severe blepharochalasis,

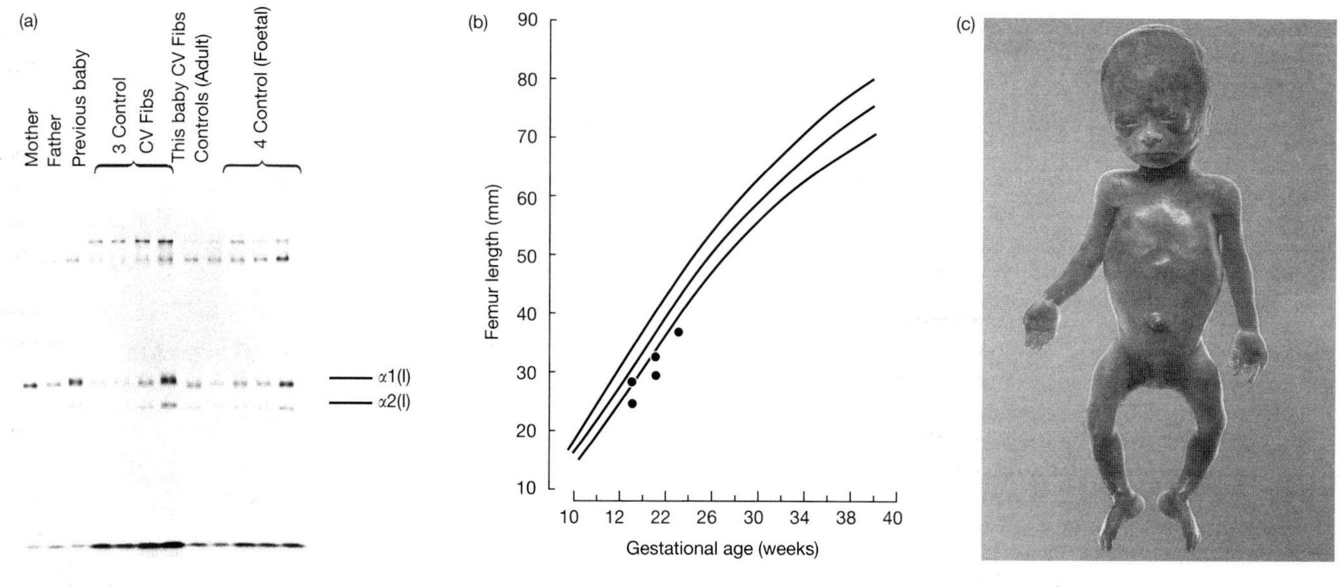

Fig. 5 (a) Patterns of overmodified $\alpha 1(\mathrm{I})$ and $\alpha 2(\mathrm{I})$ collagen profiles in two consecutively affected siblings. The seriously previously affected baby is compared with the current pregnancy in various parental normal and foetal controls. (b) The ultrasound calculation of femoral length was used as a back up. It consistently fell near or below the third percentile. (c) The terminated foetus had obvious deformities of his lower limbs.

severe joint dislocation particularly of the hips, and unusually wrinkled skin of the dorsum of the hands and feet as well as the palms and soles.

Types VIIA and B are possibly the most individual EDS phenotypes. Biochemically the molecular defect is remarkably consistent and so far, in published families, has involved a splicing failure of exon 6 of either the *COL1A1* or *COL1A2* collagen [Dalgleish 2001; Plate 44(a)]. This deletes the peptidase cleavage site from one or two of the three α-chain components of collagen type I heterotrimers, with consequent slippage and disruption of collagen helical packing and faulty formation of fibrils, visible as highly irregular, angulated fibrillar patterns [Plate 44(b)]. At the protein level, inefficient processing of procollagen to collagen causes persistence of pNα1 or pNα2 molecules after pepsinization [Plate 44(c)].

The clinical features include extreme, persistent joint laxity, presenting as congenital dislocation of the hips in infancy and joint laxity in childhood [Plate 44(d–f)], short stature, scarring of the knees [Plate 44(g)], forehead, and shins as severe, or even worse than in EDS I, with a typical criss-cross patterning of the palms. Inheritance is autosomal dominant. Surprisingly, fractures and osteoporosis are rare, although they commonly accompany nearby *N*-terminal helical, *COL1A1* or *-1A2* point mutations in severely loose-jointed variants of OI with osteoporosis and short stature [see Plate 42(a)]. Mutated sequences 5′ of exon 6 might also cause phenocopies of EDS VII. As mentioned earlier, more subtle mutations within exon 6 might produce similar phenotypes, especially if highly conserved residues are changed. Theoretically, errors in adjacent exons (3, 4, and 5) may produce similar structural or fibrillar phenotypes and we have studied an EDS VII patient deleting exons 3–6. Mutations of the first few helical exons of the *COL1A1*, *-1A2*, or *-3A1* genes regularly produce the expected skeletal or arterial phenotypes of OI and EDS IV, which are distinct from EDS VII. Mutations of the *N*-terminal propeptidase of *COL3A1* could still produce hieroglyphic fibrils, but with vascular, rather than predominantly ligamentous, pathology (Karl Kadler, personal communication).

Chondrodystrophies and chondrodysplasias

Until recently the mechanisms of the chondrodystrophies have been obscure (Maroteaux 1970; Beighton 1995). Since 1990, major advances have clarified their molecular pathology. Bone and cartilage matrix contain numerous structural proteins, collagen, proteoglycans, and the Gla proteins. *COL2A1* (cartilage collagen II protein) mutations are found in achondrogenesis, Kniest dysplasia, certain spondyloepiphyseal dysplasias, and Stickler syndrome (Ahmad et al. 1990). Other participating genes include *HOX*, *PAX*, and *SOX*, and certain regulatory proteins (e.g. bone morphogenetic protein BMP 5), *FGFR* receptor family and their ligands, glycosaminoglycan sulfation proteins, and the sulfate transport proteins (see below). More recently, studies of the cross-talk between osteoblasts and osteoclasts have clarified the role of proteins such as RANK, RANK-ligand, osteoprotogerin, and interferon B (Alliston and Derynck 2002). Additional conventional structural matrix collagens, for example, COL9 types 1–3 (type IX) and COL10A1 (collagen X), respectively, cause MED and Schmid metaphyseal dysplasia (Table 1). The Stickler phenotype and mutational spectrum shows great allelic, locus and phenotypical heterogeneity in mice and men. Stickler's original description included progressive premature myopia, retinal detachment with blindness, and premature osteoarthrosis. Stickler types I–III have been described and *COL2A1*, *-11A1*, and *-11A2* genes implicated. Human spondyloepiphyseal dysplasia (SED), osteoarthritis and deafness, without ophthalmic changes osteomegaepiphyseal dysplasia, is caused by homozygous *COL11A1* helical glycine substitutions. The clinical phenotype also includes severe degenerative OA of hips, knees and elbows, with mid-facial hypoplasia and sensory-neural deafness. Families unlinked to *COL11A2* have been linked to *COL11A1*, in which vitreo-retinal detachment without mid-facial hypoplasia predominates, (Snead and Yates 1999;

Table 1 Collagen gene mutations and their skeletal manifestations[a]

Gene	Chromosome	Type of protein	Disease	Genetics
COL2A1	12q13.11	ECM	Achondrogenesis type II Hypochondrogenesis SED congenita Kniest dysplasia Late-onset SED Stickler syndrome	D D D D D D
COL5A1	9q34	ECM	EDS I/II/Stickler overlap	D
COL9A2	1p33-p32.3	ECM	MED	D
COL10A1	bp21-q22.3	ECM	Schmid metaphyseal chondrodysplasia	D
COL11A1	1p32	ECM	Stickler syndrome	D
COL11A2	6p21.3	ECM	Stickler dysplasia-like	D R
COMP	19p13.1	ECM	Pseudoachondroplasia MED Fairbanks	D D
DTDST	5q31-q34	Sulfate transporter	Diastrophic dysplasia Achondrogenesis type 1B	R R
FGFR3	4p16.3	Tyrosine kinase transmembrane receptor	Thanatophoric dysplasia Achondroplasia Hypochondroplasia	D D D
PTHrPR	3p21-p11	G-protein transmembrane receptor	Jansen metaphyseal chondrodysplasia	D
SOX9	17q24.1-q25.1	Transcription factor	Campomelic dysplasia	D
ARS	Xp22.3	Enzyme	Chondrodysplasia punctata	SLR

[a] D, autosomal-dominant; R, autosomal-recessive; SLR, sex-linked recessive; ECM, extracellular matrix protein; EDS, Ehlers–Danlos syndrome; MED, multiple epiphyseal dysplasia; SED, spondyloepimetaphyseal dysplasia.

Richards et al. 2000). Snead has demonstrated, by slit-lamp examination, distinctive vitreoretinal morphology. He separates distinctive Stickler type 1 and 2 phenotypes, which he describes as 'membranous' and 'beaded' subtypes, respectively. The original Snead type 2 variant had a Gly–Val 97 substitution of *COL11A1*. The *COL2A1* mutational spectrum has continued to consolidate and expand. In addition to Stickler type I disease, a variety of errors have been described in Kniest syndrome and certain SED's. Human, autosomal-dominant negative, glycine substitutions in *COL10A1* cause Schmid metaphyseal dysplasia, another example in which a faulty collagen chain is very much more disruptive than a missing component. Other obvious examples of types I or III collagen cause severe OI and lethal EDS IV. Unexpected participants are the thrombospondin gene family; such as COMP 5 on chromosome 19, causing a variant of multiple epiphyseal dysplasia (MED) (Briggs and Chapman 2002).

Further examples of faulty molecules include the gene for chondrocalcinosis with OA on chromosome 8 and faulty proteoglycan sulfation in both diastrophic dwarfism and achondrogenesis type IB. The latter is caused by various homozygous or doubly heterozygous mutations of the DTDST gene. Founder mutations occur in Turkey, Japan, and Finland. The latter, especially, is an example of genetic drift, in an isolated founder population (Hastbacka et al. 1999; Superti-Furga et al. 1999). As with other chondrodysplasias, these mutations also cause other phenotypes. Studies of mutations of the FGFR family have clarified the molecular pathology of the craniofacial dysplasias, as well as achondroplasia, hypochondroplasia, pseudoachondroplasia, and thanataphoric dwarfism, all of which are allelic.

Chondrodysplasias caused by collagen mutations

The majority of cartilage and vitreous protein is collagen type II, coded by the *COL2A1* gene. Cartilage also contains IX, X, and XI, as well as the cartilage-specific matrix thrombospondin matrillin. Cartilage is phylogenetically ancient and, unlike skin or ligament matrix, rich in cells dispersed in a clear matrix, but is much less fibrous. In foetal life, the protoskeleton is cartilaginous with little or no bone. The latter progressively increases from infancy to adolescence, except for the articular surfaces. Even so, cartilaginous elements persist in the ears, nose, ribs, articular surfaces respiratory tracts, and other unexpected sites, such as the vitreous humour. Since it adheres closely to the retina, abnormalities and fibrous contractions result in retinal detachment and blindness.

Cartiliginous variants include hyaline and fibrocartilage, the latter with two varieties, collagen-rich fibrocartilage and elastin-rich yellow elastic cartilage. Articular hyaline cartilage lines the articular ends of bones within synovial cavities. Here it provides a robust and stable surface lubricated by synovial fluid. Collagen bundles align tangentially near the articular surface, but thicken if running vertically, or more deeply. Chondrocytes tend to be flattened superficially, but form distinctive vertical columns as they approach the bony metaphyses. Chondrocytes are firmly embedded in the cartilaginous matrix containing several collagenous proteins. Whole genes have been cloned and sequenced. Various other cartilage components include collagens types V and VI, fibrillin, matrillin, and other proteoglycans, most of which have been cloned and sequenced. Mutations of more than 12 genes have been identified in the past 10 years (Table 1).

Abnormalities of other components combine to produce the range of chondrodysplasias. COMP5 is a five-armed cartilage specific protein resembling thrombospondin mutations causing both SED and MED, similar to those caused by *COL9A1* and *-9A2* mutations. This implies common structural interactions between the two protein families.

FGFR receptor genes also have a role by binding fibroblast growth factors that orchestrate the expression and differentiation of numerous other mesenchymal growth factors. Their receptors are diverse but homologous, and include FGFR-1, -2, and -3. All have extracellular, immunoglobulin-like binding regions, with transmembranous tyrosine kinase-like domains and intracellular sequences that transmit certain cytoplasmic signals. Mutations of either the IgG or transmembranous regions of FGFR-1, -2, and -3 have been implicated in achondroplasia (FGFR-3), Crouzon, Apert, Pfeiffer, and Jackson–Weiss syndromes (FGFR-1 and -2), amongst other disorders. Mutations interfere with the orchestration and three-dimensional outcomes of skeletal morphology. They act upstream of those abnormalities caused by faulty structural components illustrating how disturbances in the hierarchical control of skeletal development produce varied, subtle disturbances of morphogenesis, as judged by size, shape, and three-dimensional organization. The 3 years to 1996 produced a revolution in the molecular pathology of skeletal dysplasia, in which a whole hierarchy of faulty products clearly participates including defects of pattern, structural, organizational and mechanical errors, or changes in structural elements with scaffolding functions.

Hyaline cartilage is translucent but opaque and scatters transmitted light. Polarized light shows a fibrillar organization with 10–20 nm fibres, detectable by electron microscopy. The *COL2A1* gene specifies a typical fibrillar collagen with a perfect *GlyXY* central helix, a variable *N*-terminus, and a conserved *C*-terminus. The latter is coded by exons 49–52. The *N*-terminus has unique triple-helical and two alternatively spliced exons, 4B and 5B, which are tissue specific. As in other fibrillar collagens, the central triple helix is coded by exons 7–48. The gene of 28 kbp maps to chromosome 12.

COL2A1 polymorphisms

These include *Hind*III and *Pvu*II variants, detectable with the 9.2 kb *Eco*R1 genomic fragment (Francomano et al. 1988; Wordsworth et al. 1988). The *Hind*III fragment links to familial OA, whilst the *Bam*H1 RFLP associates with common OA in caucasians. In other populations *COL2A1* is unassociated. The *Eco*R1/*Bam*H1 variable region in the 4.3 kb flanking region is also highly variable (in 30 bp multiples) and a 5′ *Hinf* RFLP segregates with SED Congenita (Anderson et al. 1990).

The recent efforts in mapping and sequencing the human genome have transformed the mapping of candidate genes in affected families. The combination of SNPs and STSs and the ordered genomic sequences of contiguous chromosomal sequences contained in cosmid, PAC, or BAC packaging vectors, displayed as gridded filters, allows the very rapid location of any inherited disease. A good recent example is the unexpected identification of the *COMP5* locus on chromosome 19 in MED (Briggs and Chapman 2002). Here, two separate lines of research converged. One had located the megaepiphyseal dysplasia locus, whilst the other pursued the basic structure, function, and biology of the *COMP5* gene and protein. We can confidently expect the identification of the gene for every known chondrodysplasia in the forseeable future.

Human diseases

Both McKusick and Spranger have emphasized the specificity and variability of the chondrodysplasias (McKusick et al. 1990; Beighton 1995). Mutations are identified by a combination of family studies, histology, and/or biochemistry of cartilage samples and DNA sequencing of the mutant genes. By means of chondrocyte culture (Benya and Shaffer 1982; Horton 1988) mutant collagen proteins can be purified and dissected, just as in OI or EDS patients with collagen types I, III, or V errors (Eyre et al. 1986; Nicholls et al. 1996; Pope et al. 1996). The illegitimate transcription of *COL2A1* mRNA by non-cartilaginous cells is also technically feasible (Cole et al. 1993). Other minority cartilage components are more widely expressed and can be tested by conventional skin fibroblast culture. Evidently, many lethal or severe *COL2A1* mutants secrete the faulty product and cannot incorporate mutant or even wild-type protein into their hyaline cartilage, instead retaining, or degrading, the faulty/wild-type heterotrimers intracellularly.

COL2A1 mutations in the chondrodystrophies

Wordsworth et al. (1988) first excluded *COL2A1* in achondroplasia, pseudoachondroplasia, multiple epiphyseal dysplasia, autosomal-recessive spondyloepiphyseal dysplasia tarda, diaphyseal aclasis, and the trichorhinophalangeal syndrome. Contrastingly, those chondrodysplasias with distorted hyaline cartilage, epiphyseal dysplasia, premature osteoarthritis, vitreoretinal detachment, or myopia frequently have *COL2A1* mutations.

The latter form two related groups. Firstly, the Stickler/Wagner group is autosomal-dominant. Clinical signs include vitreoretinal degeneration, myopia, cataracts, and retinal detachment with premature osteoarthritis, epiphyseal dysplasia, and facial abnormalities. These disorders are heterogeneous, some patients being marfanoid, whilst others are short though joint laxity is abnormal in both groups [see Fig. 6(a–d)]. The Kniest syndrome is also part of the Wagner/Stickler phenotypical complex. There are at least two types of Kniest syndrome. One relatively mild and autosomal-dominant, or sporadic, the other genetically lethal and sporadic. The milder overlaps with metatrophic dysplasia also show disproportionate short stature, prominent eyes, and mid-facial hypoplasia. Radiographs show epiphyseal irregularity, metaphyseal flaring, late ossification of the femoral heads, and platyspondyly. Histologically, the cartilage resembles Swiss cheese (McKusick et al. 1990).

Early evidence showed clear linkage to certain *COL2A1* RFLPs, whilst other evidence showed no linkage to *COL2A1* in the Wagner syndrome (Schwarz 1989). Subsequently, our own efforts show two distinct types of Stickler vitreous. Type I, linked to *COL2A1*, whilst type II segregates with *CO11A1*. Vitreous humour contains complex mixtures of collagens II, Vα 1, 2, and 3, XIα1, or XIα2, chains. Collagen 11alpha1 proteins are interchangeable in compound heterotrimers with collagen type II, whilst its companion, α2(XI), is not. Distinctive Stickler variants reflect this molecular complexity (Vikkula et al. 1995).

Autosomal dominant SED congenita is also linked to *COL2A1* [Fig. 6(d)]. It is clinically benign, causing odontoid hypoplasia, ovoid vertebrae, kyphoscoliosis, lumbar lordosis, chest deformities, poorly calcified epiphyses, and femoral heads and myopia. SED contrasts sharply with achondrogenesis, which is a severe short-limbed dwarfism with badly disorganized cartilage matrix, lethal either *in utero*, or perinatally. Affected infants are born prematurely with large heads, a short trunk, and severe micromelia (Plate 45).

Achondrogenesis types I and II (Langer–Saldino; Parente–Fraccaro) are distinguished by rather subtle radiological features that are separated into types IA, IB, and II by subtle differences in rib and limb morphology and fracture pattern. Generally, types IA and IB have stubby ribs and distorted limbs, whilst babies with type II have straighter limbs and ribs. Affected bone shows abnormal chondrocytes, with dilated endoplasmic reticulum and distorted growth plates [Plate 45(c,d)]. All these features suggest errors of collagen type II protein, whilst Superti-Furga et al. (1996, 1999) first

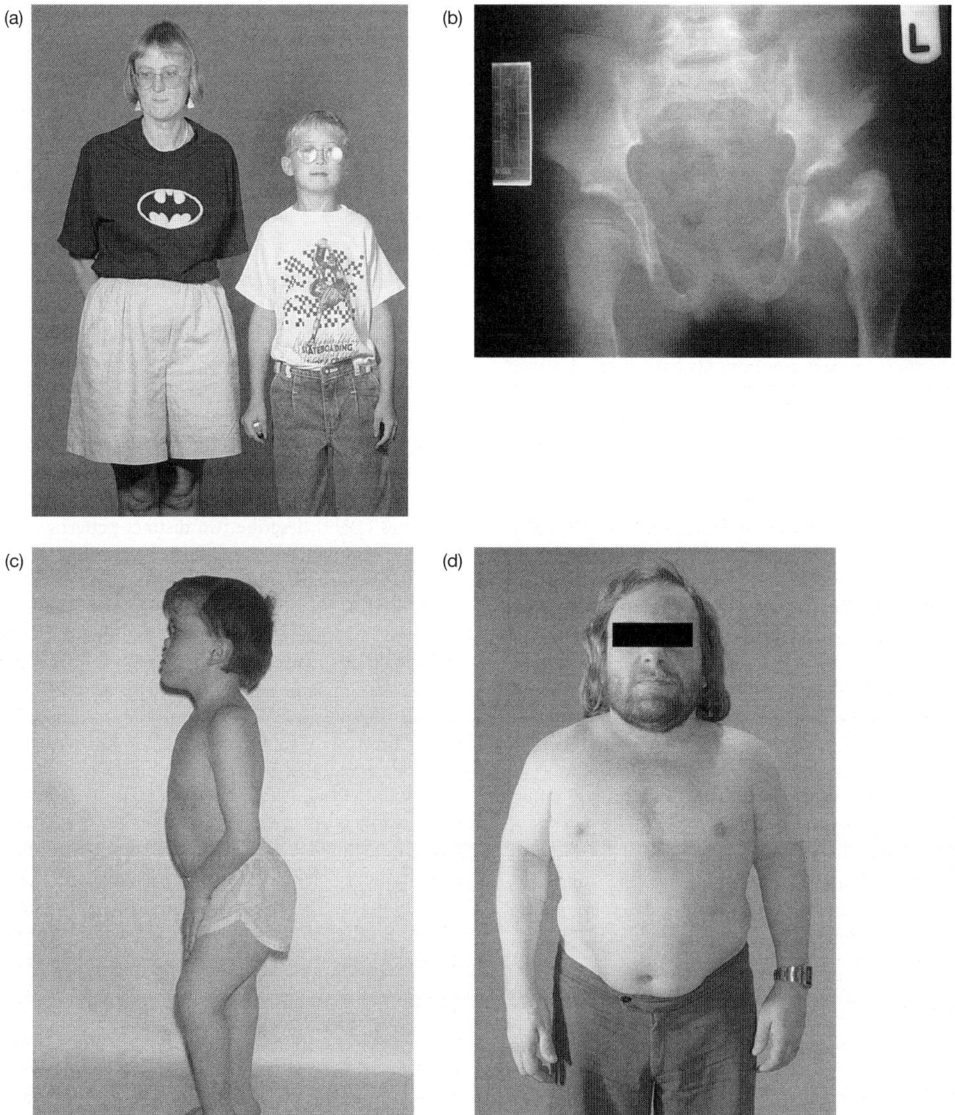

Fig. 6 Collagen II associated mutations. (a) Affected mother and son with *COL2A1*-linked Stickler syndrome. Note the high myopia. (b) Premature degenerative joint disease in similar patient. (c) Another Stickler variant. Note the lumbar lordosis and mid-facial hypoplasia. (d) Spondyloepiphyseal dysplasia with rhizomelic shortening of the upper segments of the upper limbs.

identified a sulfation abnormality in achondrogenesis type IB, as well as diastrophic dysplasia and MED.

The earliest evidence to implicate *COL2A1* in osteoarthritis was in three exceptional OA families with inherited OA without chondrodysplasia, (Knowlton et al. 1990). Knowlton's family had Heberden's nodes with conventional OA of hips, shoulders, wrists, and hands, but flattened metatarsal heads and vertebral end-plates consistent with mild chondrodysplasia. Naquamaland hip dysplasia, another mild chondrodysplasia with premature OA was also linked to *COL2A1* (Sher et al. 1991), but has subsequently been excluded as the candidate for Beukes familial OA (Beighton et al. 1994). The overall extrapolation to OA differs in UK, US, and South African data. These various OA syndromes (Dieppe 1987) are clearly genetically heterogeneous, with all cartilaginous structural gene being valid candidates.

Collagen protein analysis in the chondrodysplasias

Type II collagen protein analysis has been hampered by difficulties in obtaining cartilage samples and intricacies of chondrocyte culture. Primary chondrocyte culture is tricky (Benya and Shaffer 1982; Horton 1988) although agarose bead culture or the PCR amplification of 'illegitimate' *COL2A1* mRNA from skin fibroblasts, or purified lymphocytes, has lessened the technical difficulties. When available, cartilage biopsies can be analysed by conventional protein analysis (Eyre et al. 1986; Murray et al. 1989). As in OI and EDS protein analysis, mutant collagens are often overhydroxylated, or tilted, when analysed as CNBr peptides (by 2D electrophoresis) (Fig. 7). Overhydroxylation is least at the *N*-terminus and greatest with mutations at the *C*-terminus.

Molecular analysis of the chondrodysplasias (see Table 1)

Several *COL2A1* mutations have occurred in SED, achondrogenesis, and familial OA (Plate 46). Generally, mutational patterns resemble those of OI and EDS IV. Subsequently, mutations of other genes such as *COL9A1*, *-9A2*, *-11A1*, *-11A2*, *-5A2* and other cartilage components have been observed in a variety of disorders.

The first mutation was a 400-bp deletion, detected by the hypervariable *Eco*R1 3′ *COL2A1* genomic fragment (Lee et al. 1989). The genomic deletion extended from the middle of intron 47, to the 5′ splice-site of intron 48 deleting the 36 amino acids of triple helical residues 964–999, coded by the 108 bp exon 48. Collagen protein suicide follows (Prockop and Kivirikko 1984), with intracellular retention of mutant protein. Only one-eighth of collagen type II homotrimers are wild-type and correctly secreted. Shortly afterwords, Tiller et al. (1990) described a 45-bp duplication of exon 48 producing an elongated collagen type II protein, with an extra 155 amino acids.

Subsequent mutations are summarized in Plate 46 and include numerous glycine substitutions and a variety of deleted, or duplicated, segments. Unlike *COL1A1*, *-1A2*, and *-3A1* mutants, the clinical/mutational correlations have shallower and less clearly defined gradients. The three published examples included Gly–Val292, Gly–Cys709, and Gly–Cys302, all of which have convincingly abnormal collagen $\alpha1$(II) α-chains and abnormal CNBr peptides (Figs 7 and 8) (Tiller et al. 1995). Spondyloepiphyseal dysplasia has also been caused by *COL11A2* mutations. Tiller's patients were unusual in having *COL2A1* Gly–Cys substitutions. Transgenic mice heterozygous for *COL2A1* Gly85–Cys have a lethal chondrodysplasia (Garofalo et al. 1991).

Achondrogenesis

Achondrogenesis, hypochondrogenesis, and Kniest dysplasia form one disease spectrum. Clinical changes range from lethal asphyxiating chondrodystrophy, with very short limbs and multiple fractures (type IA achondrogenesis), to a milder disorder, with disproportionate short stature, cleft palate, mid-facial hypoplasia and a flattened nasal bridge (Kneist dysplasia). Infants with achondrogenesis usually die *in utero* or perinatally, whilst Kniest dysplasia, although deforming, is more benign.

Godfrey and Hollister (1988) accurately located a protein abnormality to the *C*-terminus (Fig. 7). Screening of a size-fractionated cosmid library showed two heterozygous *Hind*III *COL2A1* fragments. Amplification of exons 51 and 52 a Gly–Ser (GGC–AGC) at position 943, analogous to similar *COL1A1* OI lethal Gly–Ser mutations, 913–1003. The *C*-terminal position delays triple-helical winding, detectable as overmodified collagens. Shortly afterwards, Bogaert et al. (1992) detected a Gly–Glu 853 substitution in hypochondrogenesis. The field has rapidly advanced by the combination of conventional protein analysis, peptide mapping, reverse-phase high-performance liquid chromatography and genomic and cDNA PCR amplification (Tiller et al. 1995).

Since the first description of Gly–Ser *COL2A1* substitution (Vissing et al. 1989), numerous others have followed (see Plate 46). Although less position-specific than collagen type I, or type III, this implies much domain-related variability in the collagen II triple helix. The clinical phenotype of matrix cartilage disorganization correlates poorly with mutational position or type. Thus, Gly–Ser574 is as damaging as two similar changes at positions 943. Contrastingly, serine substitutions of position 493 cause non-lethal and relatively mild SED. The phenotype/genotype correlations in achondrogenesis/SED are more blurred than equivalent *COL1A1* mutations of OI. General, smaller substitutions have clearer gradients of severity, worse at the *C*-terminus and mildest at the *N*-terminus.

In Kniest dysplasia there is a cluster of deletions close to the *N*-terminus, deletions of 94–108, 102–108, 124–141, 142–156, 274–279, and 361–378. The same phenotype is caused by changes at positions 1007–1112 at the other end of the molecule. On the other hand, Gly103–D is much more severe than its *N*-terminal location would suggest. Shortening of the collagen triple helix is severely disruptive wherever it occurs and, whilst deletions are rare in *COL1A1*, *-1A2*, and *-3A1*, they are common in *COL2A1*.

Stickler syndrome

Stickler syndrome (STL) is both clinically heterogeneous and distinctive [Fig. 6(a–c)]. It combines premature myopia with retinal detachment and early joint degeneration. Joint hypermobility varies. Early myopia is typical of STL type I, whilst in other subtypes it is non-progressive, or absent. There is also overlap with the Wagner syndrome, which has similar retinal, facial, and skeletal abnormalities. The Pierre Robin anomaly, with mandibular hypoplasia and cleft palate, also overlaps with Stickler syndrome. Snead and Yates (1999) describe two distinct patterns of vitreoretinal fibrosis by slit-lamp examination. Furthermore, type I segregates with *COL2A1*, whilst type II sometimes segregates with *COL11A1* markers.

Classical STL1 includes progressive myopia from the first decade, with retinal detachment and potential blindness, combined with epiphyseal abnormalities and premature OA. The Wagner phenotype is narrower, lacking the skeletal pathology, but may also be linked to *COL2A1*. In STL2, the myopia is also early, but stable and the vitreous is beaded rather than generally fibrous. This subtype is often, but not exclusively, linked to *COL11A1*. Annunen et al. (1999) have shown both *COL2A1* and *COL11A1* mutations in the Marshall syndrome, whilst Martin et al. 1999 have shown that STL2 is never linked to *COL2A1*, often links to *COL11A1*, but in other cases is linked to neither gene, nor to other plausible candidates. The *non-COL2A1* phenotype also includes mid-facial hypoplasia, tall or short stature, and Marfanoid features. Other collagens form compound fibrils, whilst collagen VI and fibrillin 15 have also been deleted in the vitreous. Genes for all of these elements are, therefore, potential candidates for STL and related disorders. *COL11A2* mutations have been described in both autosomal-dominant and -recessive osteochondrodystrophies with STL (Vikkula et al. 1995). The corresponding homozygous mutation caused severe SED and sensorineural deafness, without vitreous changes [otospondylomegaepiphyseal dysplasia (OSMED) syndrome]. There was a homozygous glycine substitution of *COL11A2*. Although none of the *11A2* families had myopia or vitreoretinal degeneration, there was severe degenerative joint disease of the hips, knees, elbows and shoulders, and mid-facial hypoplasia, with a depressed nasal bridge. Homozygous stop-codon mutations in residue

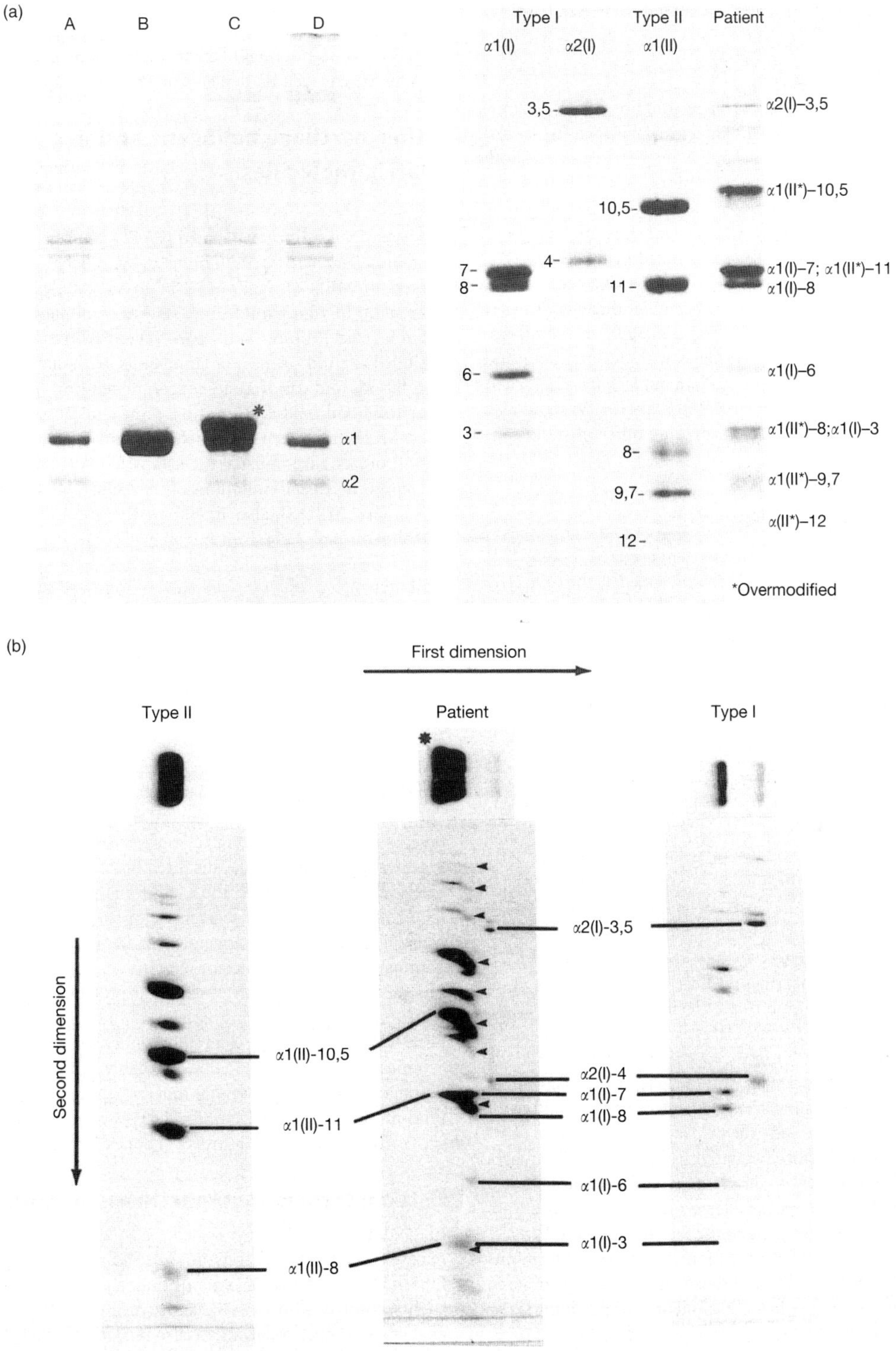

Fig. 7 (a) Collagen $\alpha 1$(II) chains from an achondrogenesis patient (track C), compared with control patterns (track B). The mutant produces normal and overmodified (*) forms. Similarly (right panel) all $\alpha 1$(II) cyanogen bromide fragments are overmodified (Godfrey and Hollister 1988). (b) The 2D peptide maps of forms excised from the collagen type II track showed typical 'smiling' of all cyanogen bromide peptides in an affected patient. These are analogous to the *α1(I)CB6* mutations causing OI, as illustrated in Fig. 3(b) and normal and overmodified species together form a diagonal 'smile'.

570 of the mouse *COL11A1* gene have been produced, and the equivalent human heterozygotes show Stickler syndrome with vitreoretinal degeneration (Snead et al. 1994). In other Stickler families, stop-codon mutations are common and the first three-generation family with retinal and joint degeneration linked to *COL2A1* and every other published Stickler (*COL2A1*) mutant has stop-codon defects. These include several Arg–STOP abnormalities and others created by unexpected 1-bp deletions (Vikkula et al. 1994). Our own studies have shown numerous exon 2 *COL2A1*

mutations in Stickler families with type I vitreoretinal degeneration (Richards et al. 2000).

Mutations of other collagens causing STS

In addition to collagen $\alpha1$(II) chains, cartilage contains $\alpha1$(V), $\alpha2$(V), $\alpha1$(XI), and $\alpha2$(XI) collagen chains. All are interstitial collagens with similarly organized triple helices and variably large *N*- and *C*-termini. In both the vitreous and articular cartilage, certain components are interchangeable. Collagen V $\alpha2$ chains can substitute for collagen XI $\alpha2$ in collagen XI trimers and collagens II, V, and XI are very important structural components of cartilage, which also contains collagen IX coded by the *-9A1*, *-9A2*, and *-9A3* genes, respectively. Hypertrophic cartilage is rich in collagen X. Mutations of such minority components have been identified in diseases, such as multiple epiphyseal dysplasia and Schmid metaphyseal dysplasia. Similarly, vitreous is as heterogeneous as cartilage, with permutations and hybrid combinations of $\alpha1$(II), $\alpha1$(XI), and $\alpha1$(V), but lacking $\alpha2$(XI) and $\alpha2$(V), which can form hybrid heterotrimers in other tissues. Vitreous also contains collagen type VI and fibrillin 15, providing other possible candidates for unlinked STS families.

Collagen XI mutations

Like types I and III collagen, type II fibrils are quarter-staggered. Type XI collagen is also fibrillar, containing $\alpha1$ and 2(XI) chains, coded by the *COL11A1* and *A2* genes, located on chromosomes 1p21 and 6p21.2, respectively. The $\alpha3$(XI) chain is an alternatively spliced variant of the *COL2A1* gene. Both the $\alpha1$(XI) and $\alpha1$(V) collagen genes regulate the thickness of compound collagen fibrils, most probably type II collagen fibres, by the former, and type I/III compound fibres, by the latter. Both collagens have prominent *N*-termini. Collagen $\alpha2$(XI) is expressed in cartilage, but not tendon, skin, or vitreous. Given the differential tissue distribution of the two type XI collagens, although both cause STS variants, they differ in the presence, or absence, of vitreous pathology and fibrosis. *COL11A2* links to autosomal-dominant STL without ophthalmic changes. The facial changes closely resemble those in Stickler's original descriptions, but segregated irregularly with cleft palate and early arthropathy. The mutation changes GT to AG at the donor splice site, causing an exon skip. A second homozygous Gly–Arg mutation in *COL11A2* was demonstrated in a more severe, autosomal-recessive chondrodysplasia, characterized by severe degenerative joint disease, facial hypoplasia, and sensorineural hearing loss (Vikkula et al. 1995). Identified errors include an exon-skip (Vikkula et al. 1995), a 27-bp deletion with hearing loss, bifid uvula, and cleft palate (Sirkko-Osadia et al. 1995) and a homozygous Gly–Arg175 in the OSMED syndrome (Vikkula et al. 1995). Heterozygous mutations in *COL11A2* cause isolated autosomal dominant *non-syndromic* sensorineural deafness. Collagen XI may influence fibril formation, cartilage cohesion, and growth-plate organization.

STL1 always has an associated congenital vitreous abnormality, with premature medium to high myopia (8–18 dioptres), whilst STL2 has a lesser non-congenital myopia of later onset. Stickler syndrome type I is always linked to *COL2A1*, whilst the type II never is. Snead's linked *COL11A1* STL2 family had inherited a Gly–Val substitution close to the *N*-terminus of collagen type XI $\alpha1$ (Richards et al. 1996). The clinical phenotype included medium to low myopia, retinal detachment, variable joint laxity regressing with age, minor skeletal disproportion, and cleft palate.

Collagen V $\alpha1$, which substitutes for collagen XI $\alpha1$ chains in heterotypic fibrils of the vitreous, is also a possible candidate. Recently, a *COL11A2* mouse knock-out model has been described (Andrikopoulos et al. 1995). Affected homozygotes had severe kyphoscoliosis, without limb shortening. Both skin and cornea showed fibril disorganization. In this context, *COL11A2* is linked to EDS II (Loughlin et al. 1995) and an exonic deletion of *COL11A2* has been identified in a patient with EDS II with corneal flattening. Other possible candidates include other cartilage-specific collagens, such as the *-5A1*, *-5A2*, *-9A1*, *-9A2*, and *-9A3* genes, although so far causing only EDS-like disorders. Snead (1994) considers that Wagner and Stickler syndromes cannot be distinguished by the type or location of the *COL2A1* mutation. He suggests that the vestigial vitreous of the STL1-linked group is caused by dominant negative disruption of the collagen triple helix, by either exonic deletions, or nonsense Gly substitutions of *COL2A1*. The latter might be analogous to the collagen I-depleted bones in OI and the collagen III-depleted arteries and skin of EDS IV.

Other cartilage collagens and extracellular matrix molecules

Collagen IX

Collagen IX is a fibril-associated (FACIT) collagen that decorates the surface of collagen II fibrils. The *COL-9A2* locus on chromosome 1p32 is linked to MED (Briggs and Chapman 2002). This is an autosomal-dominant, in which mild short stature combines with early-onset OA. It includes the Ribbing and more severe Fairbank subtypes. Symptoms include pain and stiffness of large joints, with onset varying between early childhood and mid-adolescence, depending upon clinical severity. Pseudoachondroplasia, part of the same clinical spectrum and overlapping with MED, has much shorter hands and very stubby fingers. Cartilage chondrocytes have unusual inclusions. Pseudoachondroplasia is linked to chromosome 19 and mutations of the *COMP5* gene have been identified at this locus. MED is also linked to the second chromosome 19 locus (Oehlmann et al. 1994; Kuivaniemi et al. 1997; Briggs and Chapman 2002).

Collagen X

Collagen X is a 'short chain' collagen, with a helical centre and large, globular, non-collagenous regions at the *N*- and *C*-termini. The *COL10A1* gene codes for two exons, a short one coding for the *N*-terminus and signal sequence, whilst the remaining 2940 bp codes for the entire triple helix and *C*-terminus. It is co-expressed along with collagen type II, but only in hypertrophic chondrocytes. The protein assembles into novel hexagonal structures and, probably, co-associates with collagen type II. Its actual function is unclear, possibilities include a role in vascularization or matrix mineralization. *COL10A1* with Schmid-type metaphyseal chondrodysplastic mutants have been described. The phenotype includes short stature, normal spines and hands, together with coxa vara and distorted distal femoral metaphyses. The 13-bp deletion, which disrupted the *C*-terminal propeptide, is analagous to the *COL1A2* homozygote in severely deforming OI. The *COL10A1* mutation causes a frameshift rearrangement of the 60 terminal amino acids of the *C*-propeptide, also truncated by nine amino acids. Schmid metaphyseal chondrodysplasias are invariably caused by *C*-propeptide mutations and 17 different *C*-propeptide mutations have been published. *COL10A1* mutations have been observed with non-Schmid phenotypes. The range of *C*-propeptide Schmid errors include alterations of highly conserved sequences, premature termination codons and several different glycine substitutions. Thus, mutations of the fibrillar collagens, FACIT collagens, and network forming collagens cause a spectrum of disorders in bone cartilage and blood vessels.

Osteoarthrosis (osteoarthritis or OA)

In 1990, Knowlton et al. reported a non-glycine, second position, autosomal dominant Arg–Cys mutation of *COL2A1* in an American family with inherited generalized OA and a minor chondrodysplasia. The validity of such second-position GlyXY substitutions is uncertain, but numerous analogues in other collagens are also recognized, such as types I (OI), IX, X and II (certain chondrodysplasias). All showed subtle changes of clinical phenotype, rather than the more conventional mutations caused by glycine substitutions or exon-skips, in other cases of typical OI, MED, Schmid type dysplasia and STL subtypes. Usually highly conserved or charged residues are altered to other residues. Knowlton's report confirmed other linkage, or association data (Hull and Pope 1989) of OA with *COL2A1*, although this association was very much weaker with the Heberdelon's node phenotype (Wordsworth et al. 1988). OA is certainly heterogeneous and, given the complexity of cartilage composition, genes such as *COL2A1*, *11A1*, *11A2*, *5A1*, *5A2*, *9A1–9A3*, *COMP5*, matrillin and fibrillin, are all plausible canditates in its aetiology. The segregation of late-onset OA, with the benign hypermobility syndrome, fits with this theory.

Type III collagen (*COL3A1*) mutations

Type III collagen clinical phenotypes reflect the distribution and functions of this protein. Skin, blood vessels, especially arteries, pleuroperitoneum, ligaments, tendons, and the walls of gastrointestinal tracts, are abnormally fragile and life-threatening if damaged (Pope et al. 1996). Tissues with abundant collagen III are very delicate. Arterial fragility is potentially lethal since small, medium, or even larger arteries are very easily torn. In practice, such catastrophes are most common in middle age, though not unknown even in adolescence. The collagen-depleted vessels are delicate and intolerant of sudden changes in arterial pressure. Isometric activities, such as weightlifting and sprinting, are potentially hazardous and should be forbidden. Pregnancy is also potentially hazardous. Rupture of the ascending or descending aorta with mediastinal bleeding can occur at any age, whilst medium-sized arteries, such as renal, splenic, iliac, axillary, femoral, popliteal, and anterior and posterior tibial, are also fragile, especially after the age of 30 years [Fig. 8(a)]. Unexpected or atypical abdominal pain should always be regarded with deep suspicion, but cautiously investigated, preferably non-invasively. The internal carotid artery and intracranial arteries are commonly prone to dissection and ectasia, whilst multiple premature intracranial aneurysms are also recorded. Rupture of the internal carotid artery within the cavernous sinus is well documented [Fig. 8(b)] (Pope et al. 1991).

Cerebral aneurysms occasionally occur in infancy and may be sporadic, or familial. Early bruising in infancy, or childhood is also typical, though non-specific. The phenotype varies from classical, acrogeric EDS IV, with typical facial features and short stature, to non-specific changes, indistinguishable from BHS/EDS III (Fig. 9). The latter is very heterogeneous. One particular subset, with lumbosacral striae, mitral-valve prolapse and, occasionally, aortic rupture, resembles the MFS, but is distinguished by normal lenses and bodily proportions.

EDS IV skin is thin and translucent, with prominent capillaries, especially over the anterior upper chest, shoulders, and upper back [Fig. 9(a)]. The dorsal skin of the hands and feet is unusually thin, haemosiderotic and prematurely aged, reminiscent of steroid atrophy. In younger women, the features include large, attractive eyes, little sub-cutaneous fat, lobeless, or small-lobed, ears and thin, straight nose and lips and can often be diagnosed in family photographs (Pope et al. 1996) [Fig. 9(c) and (d)]. Similar facial phenocopies segregate with EDS I/II, but merge with the normal population. Talipes can occur *in utero* and, although usually improving in childhood, can persist into adulthood. Lax joints are less obvious, except for the terminal phalanges of the fingers. Acrosteolysis of the finger tips is also common in acrogeric EDS IV [Fig. 9(e)] and congenital hip dislocations, with low birth weight, clinically overlap with EDS VI, VII, or the Larsen syndrome. Generalized laxity of joints is less obvious in EDS IV than other EDS subtypes. Skin histology shows abnormal dermal thinning, collagen depletion and elastic proliferation compared with normal [Fig. 9(b) and (c)], though similar lesser changes occur in EDS types I and II. Transmission electron microscopy of both skin and arteries shows variably sized, or misshapen, collagen fibrils [Fig. 9(e,f)]. This implies a role for type III collagen in regulating collagen fibril shape and diameter and varies with relative proportions of collagens I, III, and V, and other unspecified components. Collagen V deficiency causes EDS I/II collagen fibrils splay or fuse to form cauliflowers.

Biochemical and genetic changes

Collagen III can be extracted and rapidly analysed hours from 4 mm punch biopsies of skin. More usually radiolabelled, alcohol-precipitated protein synthesized by cultured skin fibroblasts is studied, but takes 4–6 weeks to produce and purify. The fastest screening method measures either radiolabelled type III procollagen, or pepsinized collagen in the medium and cell layers. Although 2D electrophoresis is an option, only the two most *C*-terminal cyanogen bromide peptides [α1(III)CB5 and CB9] are testable. They co-migrate after S–S reduction, before which CB9 is an S–S dimer, whilst CB5 runs as a monomer. The smaller peptides CB3, 4, 6, and 8 are less easily resolved. Vertebrate collagenase, which cuts collagen type III into *N*-terminal three-fourth and *C*-terminal one-fourth fragments, is also useful for molecular mapping.

Collagen III deficiency is typical of acrogeric EDS IV. Collagen secretion is impaired (Plate 47) and an abnormal overhydroxylated product is retained intracellularly [Plate 47(a), track 3]. Otherwise, either there is haploinsufficiency [Plate 47(b), track 1] or the mutant overmodified and normal wild-type products are secreted [Plate 47(b), track 2]. The degree of hydroxylation varies, depending upon the exonic location of the mutation and is greatest nearest the *C*-terminus [Plate 47(c), cell-layer tracks 2 and 3]. Two-dimensional electophoresis is technically tricky and less discriminating than for *COL1A1* mutants. It does separate the two large *C*-terminal peptides CB 5 and 9, but generally misses *N*-terminal errors [Plate 47(d); Nicholls et al. 1988; Pope et al. 1991, 1996].

Single-base substitutions, gene deletions, and splicing abnormalities are common, whilst other mechanisms, such as base insertions, are less frequent. Null alleles, many with premature chain termination, may also be expected. Mutational position and type correlate with clinical severity. Various splice-junction mutations have been described (Pepin et al. 2000). Protein screening is the optimal method of distinguishing acrogeric and

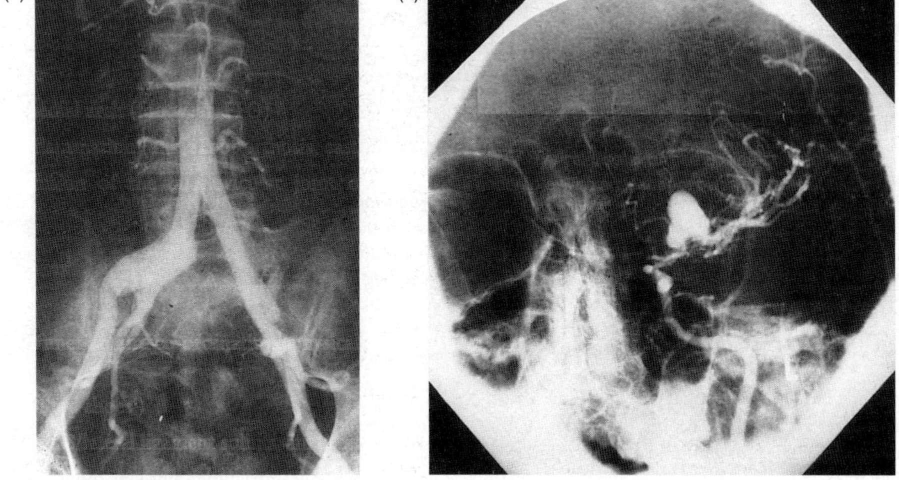

Fig. 8 (a) Aortogram showing fusiform right femoral aneurysm. (b) Large middle-cerebral aneurysm from two unrelated EDS IV patients.

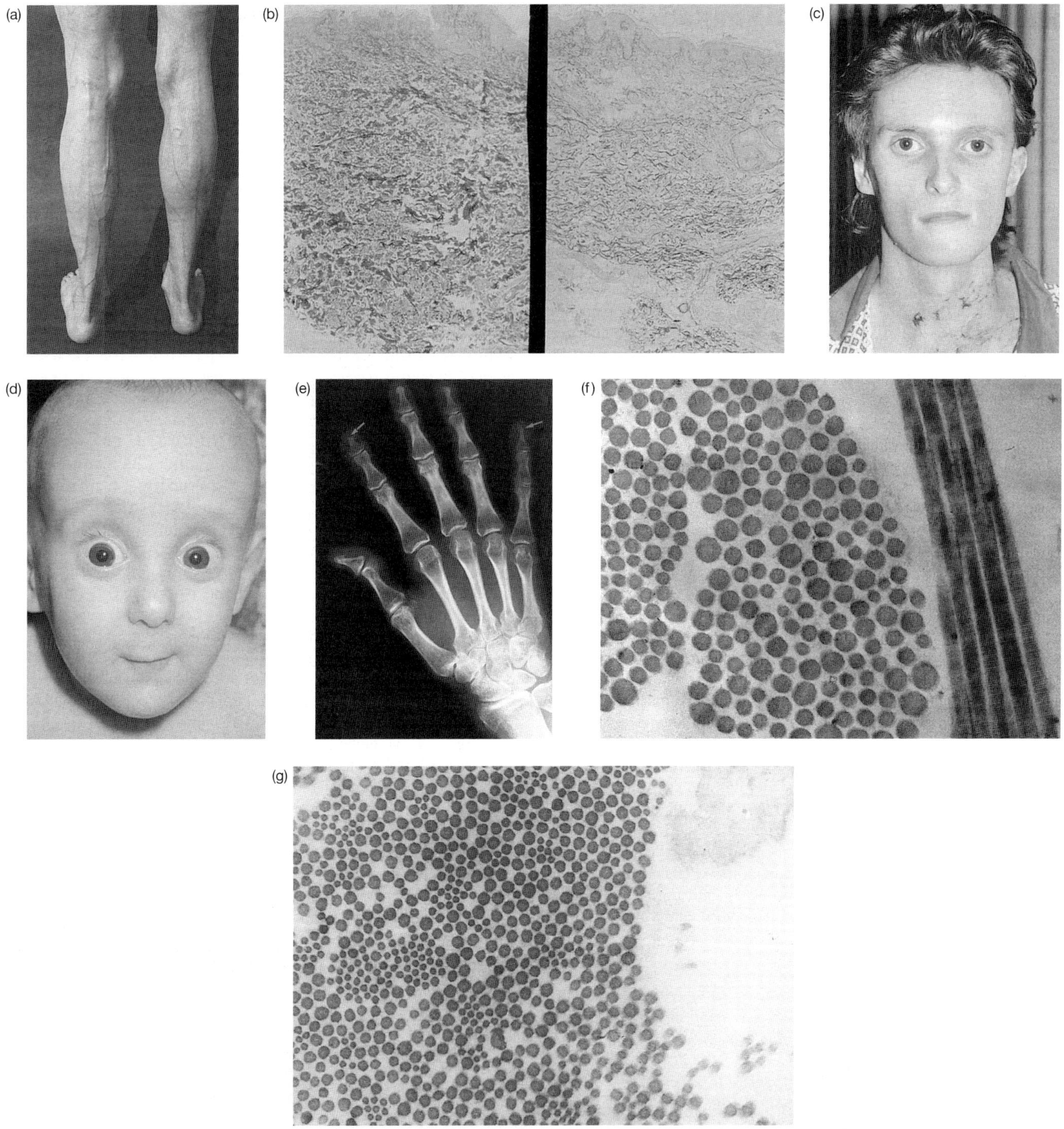

Fig. 9 (a) Typically thin skin of EDS IV, showing prominent capillary and venous pattern with some venous varicosity. (b) Histology of the thinned skin (R) shows collagen depletion and elastin proliferation, compared with the control (L). (c,d) The facial phenotype is especially characteristic with large eyes, thin lips, and lobeless ears in the acrogeric arterial type. This is equally easily recognized in adults (c) and babies (d). (e) Hand radiographs often show a subtle acro-osteolysis (arrowed). (f,g) Transmission electron micrographs showing irregularity of a collagen fibril diameters in (f) skin and (g) arterial walls.

haploinsufficient variants. Subtle reductions of collagen type III are distinguishable with difficulty and other approaches become necessary, such as osmium or hydroxylamine cleavage, cDNA or genomic amplification, with or without heteroduplex detection strategies. Automated direct sequencing is the most efficient of all.

Most mutations are unique. The future lies in detailed exonic screening from the detection of all theoretical variants, by microarray. For the present, cDNA or genomic amplification, followed by Wave detection of mutant heterodimers is efficient. Chip technology should detect any possible mutation in minutes, rather than weeks or months. Current best practice combines careful clinical classification, protein electrophoresis, electron microscopy, cDNA, and/or genomic sequencing.

The current situation

The *COL3A1* database maintained by Dr Raymond Dalgleish at the University of Leicester (http://www.le.ac.uk/genetics/collagen/col3a1.html), lists the following mutations: 106 glycine substitutions, of which 11 were recurrent at positions 82, 415, 499, 599, 736, 821, 1003, 1018, and 1021. Glycine to serine recurred seven times, whilst the others varied between two and three recurrences. Forty exon skips ranging from the first helical exon, number 7, to exon 47, the last helical exon before the *C*-propeptide. Exon 24 was exceptional in clustering 10 independent identical mutations, whilst exons 7, 8, 37, 41, 43, and 45 recurred two to three times. Other mutations include 3 frameshift terminations, from the *N*-propeptide to residue 77, pro18 to residue 48 and Asn 444 to residue 445, from four small exon deletions as well as four large deletions of 2.3, 3, 7.5, and 9 kb generally produce EDS IV phenotypes, although the 2 kb phenotype was unspecified and the 7.5 kb deletion was clinically mild. The overall effect is 40-exon skips and all the deletions. For other deletions see Pope et al. (1996) and Pepin et al. (2000). See also Fig. 10(b).

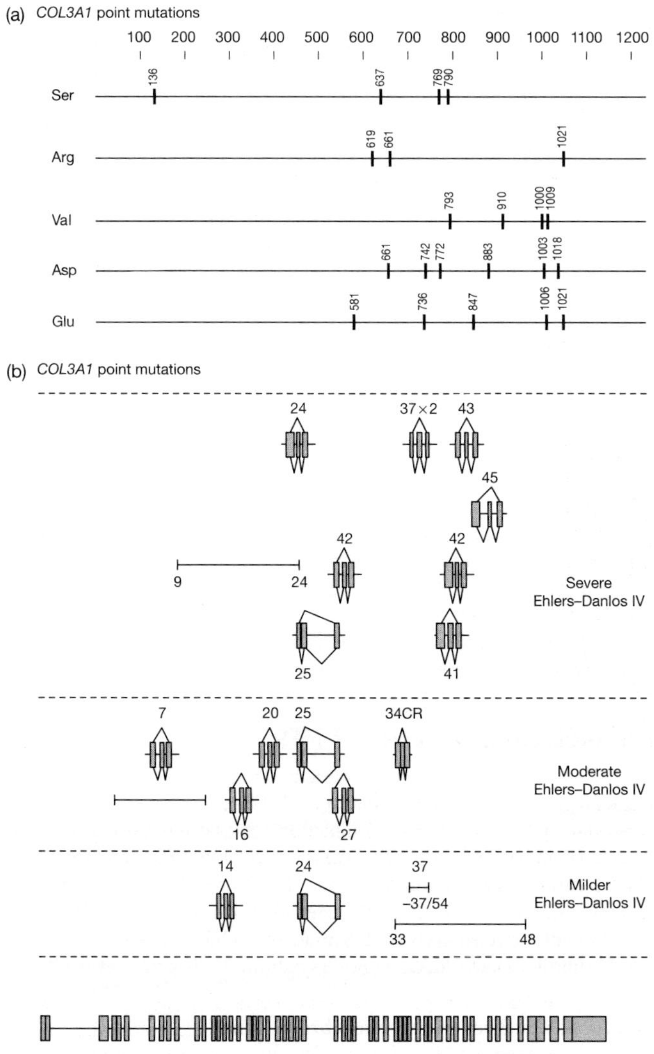

Fig. 10 Diagrams of the distribution of published *COL3A1* mutations (Pepin et al. 2000). (a) Point mutations. (b) Splicing and deletion mutations.

Our research programme identified many mutants at the *C*-terminal end of *COL3A1*, where mutational detection was technically easiest. EDS IV phenotypes vary by mutational position, acrogeria is commonest at the *C*-terminus. *COL3A1* mutants are highly dangerous at any location, thus a chemical gradient remains, with *C*-terminal mutants the most disruptive and most liable to arterial rupture. The acrogeric *COL3A1* EDS IV gradient contains anomalous benign mutants, such as *Gly–Glu*625, in which the phenotype includes mild generalized OA with Heberdens nodes, but without arterial fragility.

Mutations identified to date

Genetics of EDS

EDS is characterized by cutaneous fragility, with variable permutations of skin thinning, ligamentous laxity, short stature, spinal deformity, vascular fragility, or retinal detachment. There are at least nine distinct genetic subsets. Types IV, V, VI, and VII have specific biochemical abnormalities. Types I and II have mutations of collagen type V. Faulty collagen proteins cause types I, II, IV, VIIA, and VIIB, whilst enzyme errors cause types VIA, VIIC, and IX. EDS VII is caused by structural or enzyme abnormalities, whilst the causes of most EDS III's are still unknown. EDS VIII has at least two variants, one of which has been recently mapped to chromosome 12p13 whilst only two families with sex-linked EDS V have been reported. Lysyloxidase would be a strong candidate, but causes cutis laxa with bladder diverticulae, or Menkes syndrome.

There are many examples of *COL3A1* mutations in vascular EDS IV, whilst EDS VII A and B are caused by *N*-terminal collagen type I mutations in exon 6 of *COL1A1* or *COL1A2*. The phenotypes of EDS VIIA and B and EDS I and II overlap clinically, but are distinguished by transmission EM, which in EDS I and II shows cauliflower fibrils, whilst in EDS VIIA and B shows angulated collagen fibres in transverse section. In general, EDS VII patients are smaller, with mild generalized cutis laxa and earlier, more severe, joint laxity than EDS I and II probands, including late scoliosis and early congenital hip dislocations in types VIIA and B. Collagen V abnormalities cause both EDS types I and II, but other candidates for this phenotype include the *11A1*, *11A2*, and tenascin. Cutaneous fragility is the norm in EDS I, but can be as marked in VIIA and B [Plate 48(a–f)]. Other possibilities include compound, non-allelic, heterozygosity for collagens I, III, V, or XI as well as elastin, fibrillin, lysyloxidase, lysylhydroxylase, or other components of extracellular matrix, although, unlike globin mutations, none have been reported.

EDS VI is caused by specific enzymatic abnormalities, especially lysylhydroxylase deficiency. It differs from other subtypes of EDS by its inheritance, which is either autosomal-recessive or compound. There is severe infantile, or adolescent, scoliosis and spectacular generalized joint laxity. The lysylhydroxylase gene lies on chromosome 1p36 (Hautala et al. 1992). Known mutations include homozygous termination-codon duplication rearrangements and complex and single exon skips. EDS VIIC is more severe than VIIA or B and severely disturbs collagen fibrillogenesis with hieroglyphic fibrils in transversely sectioned electron micrographs. Both pNα1 and pNα2 propeptide extensions remain uncleaved so that the entire triple helix is faulty. All mutant molecules then misassemble to form flanged fibres appearing in transverse sections as hieroglyphs. The clinical phenotype includes spectacular cutis laxa, joint laxity, and short stature in adults, differing only slightly from the types VIIA and B phenotypes in which pNα1 or pNα2 chains are faulty. Faulty trimers incorporate one or two abnormal chains. Lysyloxidase deficiency can potentially cause several OI disorders, but it is unclear whether those families with apparent X-linked EDS V were actually lysyloxidase-deficient, which causes cutis laxa and extreme joint laxity, with bladder diverticula, a hydronephrosis, and chronic renal failure (Khakoo et al. 1997). Deficiency of procollagen peptidase produces autosomal-recessive EDS VIIC. Transmission electron microscopy shows angulated irregularities of collagen fibril shape in EDS VII, with size irregularities in *COL3A1* deficiency.

Collagen type V mutants

The evidence that faulty collagen V causes EDS I and II includes gene linkage, protein analysis, and gene sequencing data. The gene has 66 exons spanning 750 kb. Protein analysis is usually unhelpful, because of haplo-insufficiency, although we detected the first EDS I/II mutant by protein electrophoresis [Plate 49(c)]. Linkage studies of *COL5A1*, confirmed these data in other British families (Loughlin et al. 1995; Burrows et al. 1996) and a translocation deletion causing both EDS and hypomelanosis of Ito confirmed these data (Torriello et al. 1996). Subsequent progress has been swift, and has shown the expected range of fibrillar collagen mutations, such as glycine substitutions, exon skips and larger deletions. Haplo-insufficiency causing protein-dosage mutants are commonplace, making protein screening generally uninformative. Errors of *COL5A2* have also been identified (Burrows et al. 1998), as have unexpected homozygous mutations of tenascin, which causes a milder EDS III/BHS clinical phenotype (Schalkwijk et al. 2001). In other autosomal dominant EDS I and II families, both *COL5A1* and *COL5A2* have been eliminated, whilst other obvious candidate genes include *COL11A1* and *COL11A2*.

Collagen type IV mutations

The molecular genetics of *COL4A1–6* mutations has very rapidly advanced since X-linked Alport syndrome, with haematuria, glomerular basement-membrane thinning, and deafness was first linked to the *COL4A5* gene at Xq21.3–22.2 by Hostikka et al. (1990). The disorder OMIM 120070, 120131, 104200, 203780, 30150, 303630, is very heterogeneous, as is reflected by the various *COL4A1–4* homologues, which cause Alport variants. X-linked Alport disorders are caused by *COL4A5* mutations, whilst alterations of the autosomal equivalents, cause the remainder. These include six other types of Alport syndrome. All share a symptom complex of deafness, haematuria, and thickening, or splitting, of the glomerular basement membrane through the lamina densa, except for type III caused by autosomal genes. A common renal disease with an overall frequency of 1 per 5000, although less frequent than polycystic kidneys.

The first *COL4A5* mutation showed a 15-kb genomic deletion of exons 5–10 (Zhou et al. 1990). Autosomal-dominant Alport syndrome have been attributed mostly to *COL4A3* and *COL4A4* mutations. Goodpastures syndrome is caused by autoantibodies binding and damaging the *N*-terminal end of the *COL4A3* gene product α3(IV) chains of the lung and glomerular basement membrane collagen. Depending on the HLA susceptibility genotypes, the production of alveolar and/or glomerulus specific antibodies occurs, followed by renal failure, with or without interstitial pulmonary fibrosis.

Collagen type VI mutations

There are three collagen type VI genes coding for the *COL6A1, A2,* and *A3* genes on chromosomes 2q37 and 21q22.3. Mutations in two cause premature congenital myopathy with prominenet finger contractures (Bethlem myopathy). The three genes *COL6A1, -6A2,* and *-6A3* have been cloned and sequenced (Jobsis et al. 1996a, b) and typical glycine substitutions observed in Bethlem patients. *COL6A1* and *-6A2* are transcribed nose to tail on chromosome 21q22.3, whilst the *COL6A3* gene lies close to *COL3A1* and *COL5A2* on chromosome 2q37.

Collagen type VII mutations

Collagen VII is a basement membrane protein confined to stratified squamous epithelium, where it attaches epidermis to underlying dermal matrix at the level of the lamina densa of stratified squamous epithelial basement membrane. Faulty adhesion causes painful sub-epidermal blisters of skin, nails, buccal, oesophageal, and genitourinary epithelia. Collagen type VII protein has a central imperfect collagen helix with large *C*- and *N*-terminal globular ends. Unlike the fibrillar collagens, which are packed quarter staggered, collagen type VII assembles end to end at the *C*-termini to form antiparallel cross-striated anchoring fibrils.

Clinical phenotypes

Mutations of *COL7A1* cause certain inherited cutaneous blistering disorders, all of which scar. These are either autosomal dominant, or recessive, disorders of epidermal adhesion, with haemorrhagic blistering and scarring of the knees, shins and elbows, reminiscent of EDS I and II [Plate 50(a)]. The more severe recessive forms produce widespread generalized scarring [Plate 50(b–d)]. *COL7A1*, is a compact 32 kb with 118 exons and has an interrupted, imperfect collagen triple helix. The NC-1 domain contains both fibronectin III and von Willebrand (VWB) cassettes, as well as cartilage matrix protein (CMP) domains. Complex structural interactions are implicated between the anchoring fibrils and their various matrix associates (Parente et al. 1991; Christiano et al. 1994).

Mutations of *COL7A1*

As with other collagen gene mutations, linkage analysis is very important. It strongly implicates *COL7A1* in autosomal dominant EB (Ryynanen et al. 1991; Gruis et al. 1992). Single mutations cause mild autosomal dominant EB, whilst homozygous or heterozygous double hits cause the more severe autosomal recessive phenotypes. Errors are widely distributed throughout the NC1, helical and NC2 domains. Several important differences from *COL1A1, -1A2,* and *-3A1* patterns have emerged:

(i) Helical glycine substitutions can be clinically silent or apparent. For example, in some severely affected autosomal recessive double heterozygotes, clinically normal parents carry silent glycine substitutions of *COL7A1*, causing overt OI, or EDS IV, if similarly located in *COL1A1, -1A2,* or *-3A1*. In other examples, similar *COL7A1* glycine substitutions cause overt, but mild, dystrophic EB.

(ii) The mutational gradient is reversed for *COL1A1,-1A2,* and*-3A1*, this is normally greatest at the *C*-terminus and the fibrillar collagens wind from *C*- to *N*-termini, so winding is most severely impaired with *C*-terminal errors. Contrastingly, the *COL7A1* gradient is opposite, so the most severe autosomal recessive EB errors occur at the NC1 domain. Current UK strategy is to expand the mutational map, until genotype and phenotype correlations are nearly perfect. Mutational catalogues are available on line from OMIM, 12020, 131750, 22660, 226500. An updated classification has been published by Fine et al. (2000).

Marfan syndrome

MFS is characterized by arachnodactyly tall stature, pectusexcavatum, abnormalities such as dislocated lenses, myopia, high-arched palate, and mandibular hypoplasia [Plate 51(a–f)]. There is also a distressingly common predisposition to sudden aortic rupture, particularly in middle adulthood [Plate 51(g) and (h)] (Marfan 1896). Mitral-valve prolapse, joint laxity, and cutaneous striations are also common. None of these physical features are individually specific, it is their combination that makes the disorder recognizable. Beighton et al. (1988) published clear major and minor diagnostic criteria, which were updated by De Paepe et al. (1996). This modified the old requirement that at least one skeletal feature should combine with other major organ involvement, to attaching equal weighting to skeletal, cardiovascular, and ophthalmic clinical signs.

MFS is a clear autosomal-dominant [Weve 1931; Plate 51], with complete penetrance and a prevalence of approximately 1 per 25 000.

The molecular genetics of MFS

The MFS gene was mapped to chromosome 15 and, with the exception of a single atypical French family (Boileau et al. 1995; Dietz et al. 1995) which mapped to 3p21, every other MFS mutation has located to the MFS locus at D15S45 (Kainulainen et al. 1991). Maslen et al. (1991) first discovered fibrillin on chromosome 15, whilst Lee et al. (1991), described a second fibrillin gene on chromosome 5. Given the coincident locus of MFS, Dietz et al. (1991) rapidly detected the first MFS mutations, whilst the gene on chromosome 5 (fibrillin 2), was linked to Beal's syndrome by Tsipouras et al. (1992).

Molecular structure of the two fibrillin genes

Maslen et al. (1991) isolated a novel fibrillin sequence containing both 6- and 8-cysteine repeat motifs from a placental cDNA library. These fibrillin sequences were analagous to both vertebrate epidermal growth factor (EGF) and drosophila *Notch* protein. The 8-cysteine motif has homologies

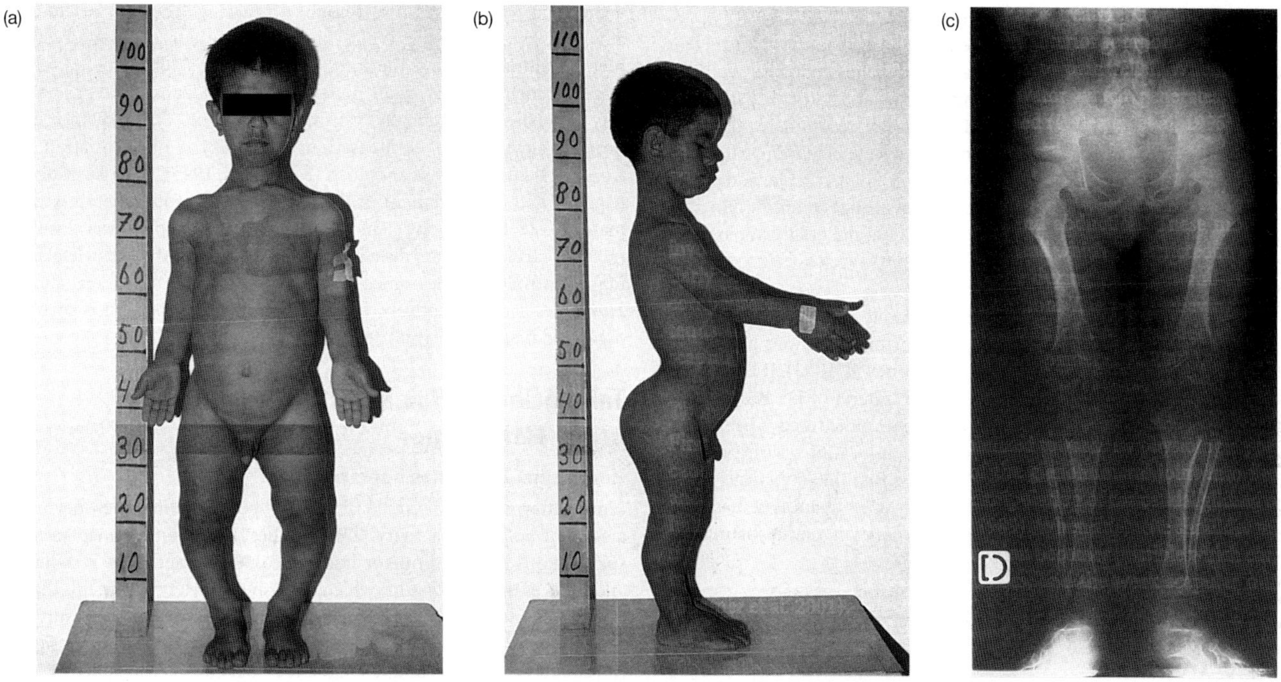

Fig. 11 A typical patient with achondroplasia. (a,b) Phenotypical features. (c) Radiographic features. The resemblance to Fig. 12 is obvious and both defects are caused by abnormalities of the same gene.

to TGF beta, as well as EGF. In contrast, Lee et al. (1991) had used monoclonal antibodies to identify fibrillin peptides, from which antisense sequences could be devised which hybridized to fibrillin cDNA sequences. In this way, they located fibrillin genomic sequences both on chromosome 15 (fibrillin 1) and 5 (fibrillin 2).

Other fibrillin cassettes

The complete genomic cDNA organization of the fibrillin 11 gene has a 11-kb coding region of 65 exons in a 110-kb genomic sequence (Pereira et al. 1993). There are numerous independent cassettes with distinctive *C*- and *N*-termini, 43 EGF-like calcium-binding motifs, four EGF-like non-calcium-binding regions, seven TGF-β_1-like binding regions, and two hybrid motifs. The EGF regions form two subsets, mostly 8-Cys and others with 6-Cys repeats. Calcium binding depends heavily upon highly conserved cysteines at residues 6, 7, 8, 17, 19, and 20, whilst residues 8 to 19 form the β-hydroxylase consensus sequence. Similarly, residue 10 is a β-hydroxylated Asp, whilst 15 is an aromatic Tyr. Calcium-binding cysteines of EGF bridge between residues 6/8, 7/17, and 19/20 and mutations at any of these highly conserved sites are pathological. A quadruple-loop secondary structure results, forming a double 'S' shape, upon which calcium binding depends. Various other residues are also strongly conserved, particularly the β-hydroxylase consensus sequence between residues 8 and 19. Other cassettes form TGF-β-like binding-protein domains (Lee et al. 1991; Corson et al. 1993; Pereira et al. 1993) interspersed with calcium-binding regions. Combinations of such domains regulate interchain disulfide bonds, whilst the calcium-binding cysteines form intrachain disulfide bonds (Dietz et al. 1995). At intervals between the *N*- and *C*-termini, TGF-β-like cassettes are occasionally coded by two exons, but more usually, by a single exon. The *N*- and *C*-termini are coded by two exons. There are 58 cassettes, coded by 61 exons. TGF-β domains are coded by cassettes 7, 14, 10, 33, 36, 44, and 50, with calcium regions of EGF in between (Corson et al. 1993; Pereira et al. 1993; Nijbroek et al. 1995).

Fibrillin mutations in MFS and congenital contractural arachnodactyly

Early mutational linkage studies linked fibrillin 15 to MFS and excluded important clinical overlaps, such as familial aortic dissection, annulo-aortic ectasia, the Marfanoid hypermobility syndrome, and congenital contractural arachnodactyly (Dietz et al. 1991; Lee et al. 1991; Maslen et al. 1991).

FIB 1 (fibrillin 1) mutations

Early mutational work quickly proved that adult MFS, isolated ectopia lentis, and MFS with aortic dilatation were allelic. By 1996, numerous mutational errors had been identified. The following general rules apply to phenotype–genotype correlations:

(i) A regularly up-dated MFS database is available online and is also published in *Nucleic Acids Research*, Collod-Beroud et al. (1998).

(ii) Forty three of the 65 *FIB 1* exons specify calcium-binding EGF cassettes, in which muations of conserved cysteines cause variable MFS phenotypes.

(iii) Whilst MFS phenotype and genotype are only loosely correlated, cysteine substitutions of exons 59–65 cause either mild MFS without aortic dilatation, or isolated ectopia lentis, without MFS.

(iv) A variety of errors form several distinct subsets, including missense cysteine substitutions, premature termination errors, in-frame deletions, insertions, or exon-skips.

(v) Infantile mutations, with a severe clinical phenotype, cluster in the middle of the gene, whilst premature termination mutations are generally mild.

(vi) Just as in the fibrillar collagens *COL1A1*, *-1A2*, and *3A1*, in which mutational type and position correlate with protein misassembly, *FIB 1* errors have similar dominant-negative effects, whereby a shortened or twisted mutant protein is very much more biologically disruptive than an absent protein.

(vii) Most mutations with clinical effects adversely alter sites, which are highly conserved between mice, bovines, and humans.

(viii) There is significant clustering of MFS mutations between exons 25, 27, and 28, of which 70 per cent are missense and 75 per cent cysteine substitutions.

(ix) Fibrillins assemble as beaded microfilaments, visible by either electron microscopy, or rotary shadowed preparations.

Fibrillin 2 (FIB 2) mutations

Analagous strategies apply to *FIB 2* mutations on chromosome 5q 23–31. Here the skeletal features closely resemble MFS, with dolichostenomelia, scoliosis, and adolescent striae. Contrastingly, the ophthalmic and aortic dilatation are missing, whilst crumpled ears and contracted fingers predominate (although may be absent). Tall stature is generally more variable, than in MFS, whilst the fibrillin 2 protein predominates in perichondrium, joint capsule, and vertebrae, producing more rheumatological orientated changes than fibrillin 1 in MFS, which more commonly presents to cardiologists and ophthalmologists.

Other pertinent genes for MFS

As mentioned earlier, a very large French MFS family with aortic dilatation, ectopia lentis, arachnodactyly, and pectus deformities showed linkage to 3p21, rather than the *FIB 1* locus at 15q21 (Collod et al. 1995). It is unclear, whether the phenotype truly fits the new MFS criteria of De Paepe et al. (1996). To date the mutant gene on 3p21, remains unidentified. The second exception is an affected MFS female without lens dislocations, with a second position GlyXY mutation of arginine 618 to glutamine substitution of *COL1A2* (Phillips et al. 1991). No other similar MFS phenotype has ever been linked to *COL1A1*, or *1A2* genes and the association may be fortuitous.

Chondrodysplasias

Introduction

With over 150 distinctive chondrodysplasias (Spranger 1992) inherited in autosomal-dominant, autosomal-recessive, or X-linked recessive patterns, the clinical heterogeneity of these disorders is bewildering. Advances in the biology of embryogenesis, pattern formation, and segmentation have impinged upon the molecular basis of these diseases. The regulation of three-dimensional shape in complex tissues have all been illuminated by these advances.

Mechanistically, there are two classes of mutant molecules: those in which structural components are faulty and those in which upstream regulatory substances are disturbed. Generally, structural components share phenotypical territories according to their site of distribution. This may be as single entities, or as interactive clusters of components able to assemble into cooperative macromolecules. Regulatory or orchestrational macromolecules have less specific effects in the local anatomical or structural sense and will affect general developmental timing and 3D shape, as is the case in the *HOX* or *FGFR* mutations. Collagen type IX interacts with COMP5, matrillin 3, and the diastrophic dysplasia sulfate transporter genes in the various manifestations of MED. Similarly, the diastrophic dysplasia spectrum includes lethal achondrogenesis, severe ateleosteogenesis type 2, and diastrophic dysplasias. Collagen X errors, on the other hand, cause variants of Schmid type metaphyseal chondrodysplasia, OMIM 156500 (Wallis et al. 1996).

The regulatory genes, such as *HOX, spiny hedgehog*, the *FGF* and *FGFR* genes, *BMP 1–5*, and the *GMP* genes have more generalized effects (Takahara et al. 1996). Horton (1995) has tabulated various examples of regulatory protein mutations.

Hierarchical development and skeletal patterning

Skeletal development, from embryo to foetus and afterwards, requires precise, temporally orchestrated growth and remodelling, morphogenesis is the final outcome of numerous interctions between the expression and degradation of complex matrix constituents in an ordered pattern (Erlebacher et al. 1995). It follows a defined sequence and pattern that determines overall growth and morphology and subtle variations in shape or location of particular components. These complicated symmetrical structures require precise regulation.

Skeletal patterning

Vertebrate skeletons have three major components, the head and neck (craniofacial region), the spine, ribs and pelvis (axial), and the limbs (appendicular skeleton). The craniofacial component derives from the embryonic branchial arches, which themselves arise from the neural crest. The axial skeleton originates from the sclerotomes, whilst the lateral mesoderm dictates which elements eventually become the limbs. Except for the skull and pelvis, which are largely of membranous origin, most of the remainder originates as cartilaginous templates that gradually transmute into bone. This sequence includes ordered mesenchymal condensation, chondrocytic differentiation, hypertrophic calcification, and apoptosis (Kraus et al. 1993). Vascularization is the trigger for the replacement of the cartilaginous protoskeleton with more mature, osteoblastic bony elements. Eventually, after epiphyseal closure, only traces of cartilage remain distally upon the articular surfaces. Skeletal patterning is controlled by the homeo-box family of transcriptional regualtors. The *Hox* genes act consecutively, from head to tail. The pattern is segmentally organized neuroectodermal development.

Tabulation of *Hox A2, A13, Pax 3, 6,* and other *MSX2* genes

How homeobox genes operate

Limb patterning signals are located in the posterior limb mesoderm, where a zone of polarizing activity (ZPA) resides. Embryonic transplantation of such regions induces a mirror-image second limb bud. ZPA is switched on and induces the *FGFR4* gene, which unleashes a variety of proteins that regulate the development of the embryo. Such a sequence is the result of *Hox* gene induction. The ZPA liberates a morphogen, which induces signalling molecules similar to segmental regulators that embryos produce for normal developmental tempero-spatial components. In Drosophila, genes, such as *armadillo, gooseberry*, and *wingless*, are essential for normal embryonic timetabling. *Hedgehog*, which is a concentration-dependent morphogen, is 78 per cent identical in chicks and flies, implying a very fundamental role in embryogenesis, extending over widely disparate animal phyla.

Control of bone shape

As far as connective tissue development is concerned, the *Hox* genes specify segmental patterns secondarily mediated by certain *TGF-β* family members. In turn, they control the distribution and patterning of connective tissue components with which they co-associate. In skeletal development, such substances orchestrate and timetable the development and three-dimensional patterning of precartilaginous mesenchyme. Similarly, the complexities of endochondral ossification necessitate the coordinated and orderly expression of epiphyseal, metaphyseal, and diaphyseal components.

FGF proteins and their receptor (*FGFR*) families

The *FGF* superfamily specifies proteins that bind to transmembrane *FGF* receptors (*FGF1–4*) (Givol and Yagon 1992). The latter (*FGFR*), which bind the former (*FGFR*), have proved to be extraordinarily disruptive of facial shape, sutural closure, and general craniofacial patterning. Others also regulate cutaneous proliferation.

In general, *FGFR1* and *FGFR2* mutations cause various craniosynostoses, such as Apert, Crouzon, Jackson–Weiss, or Pfeiffer syndromes. *FGFR3* errors affect cartilage, including achondroplasia, hypochondroplasia, and the thanatophoric dwarfisms. An excellent updated mutational catalogue has been published by Passos-Bueno et al. (1999).

FGFR mutations

The molecular pathology of certain apparently unrelated chondrodysplasias or craniofacial anomalies have all implicated the *FGFR1, FGFR2*, or *FGFR3* genes in a manner that is both domain and position related. Achondroplasia is caused by an *FGFR1* mutation, as are Crouzon, Apert, Pfeiffer, and Jackson–Weiss syndromes (Passos-Bueno et al. 1999).

Achondroplasia

Most achondroplastic mutations [Fig. 11(a–c)] change GGG–AGG in codon 380 of *FGFR3*. Occasionally there are GGG to CGG 380 variants and,

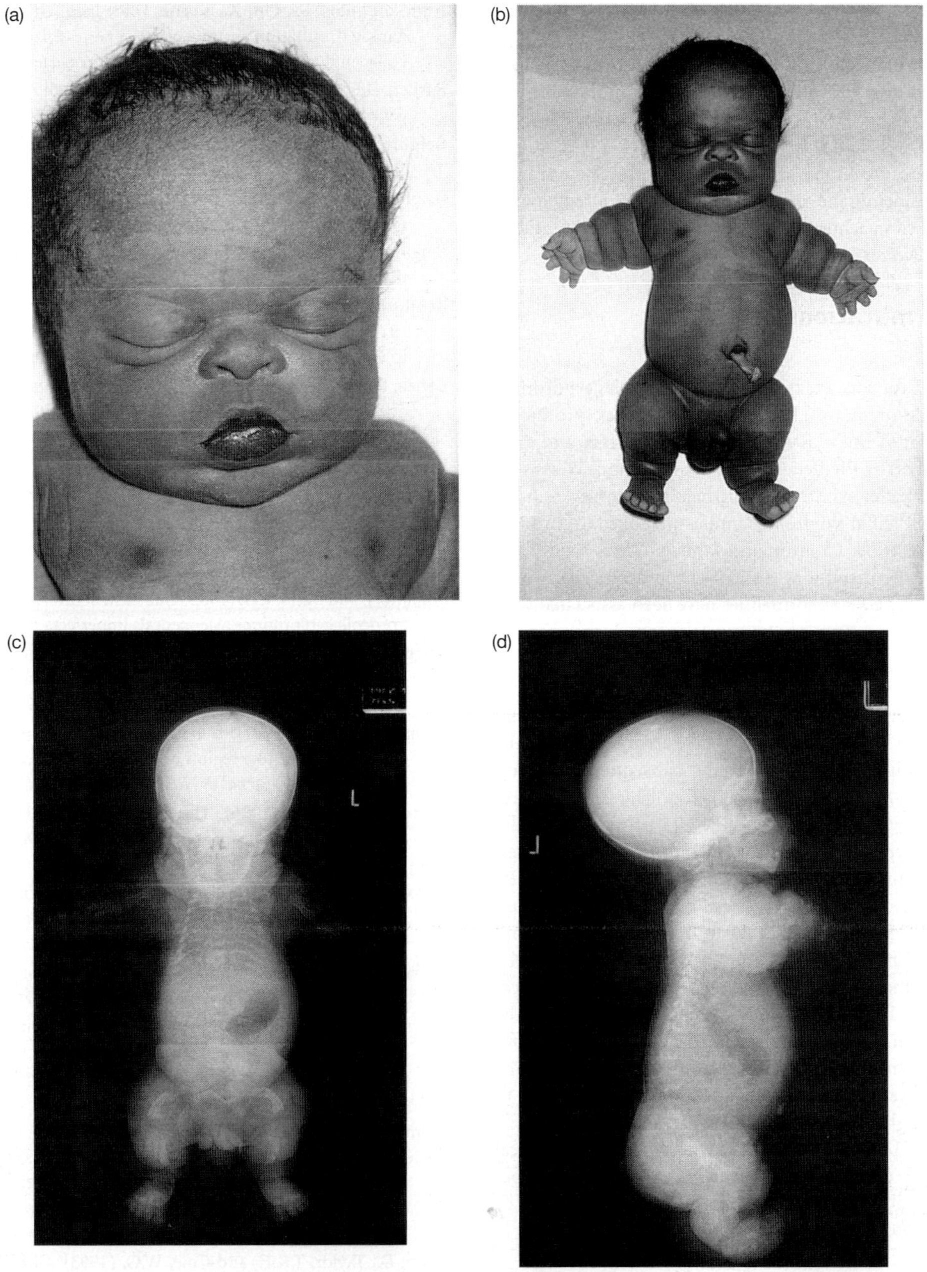

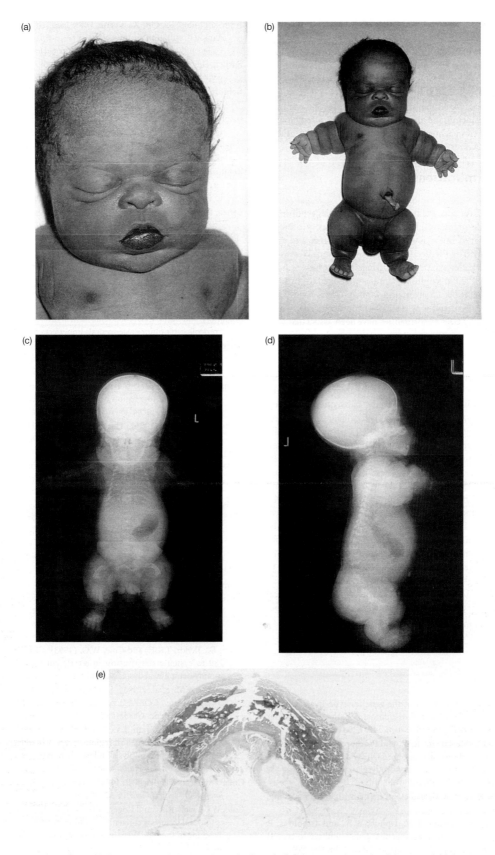

Fig. 12 (a,b) Facial and full-body phenotype of affected baby with thanatophoric dysplasia. (c,d) Babygram radiographs of the same child showing severe thoracic dysplasia, telephone-receiver femurs, and a dysplastic skeleton. (e) Histological appearance of section of femur showing a disturbed diaphysis and disorganized cartilage ×1.5.

exceptionally, there are unknown variants. Other allelic *FGFR3* mutations cause hypochondroplasia, or thanatophoric phenotypes (Fig. 12). Nucleotide 1138 is the mutational hot-spot for achondroplasia, whilst residue 1620 changes in at least half of hypochondroplasia mutations. The 1620 C–A transversion changes asparagine 540 to lysine. Both variants of thanatophoric dysplasia, types I and II, are also caused by *FGFR3* mutations.

Other *FGFR3* mutations cause entirely different phenotypes. These amino-acids lie within the transmembrane domain of *FGFR3* and radiological overlaps have been described in achondroplasia and the Crouzon-Acanthosis nigricans syndromes (Schwietzer et al. 2000).

FGFR1 and *FGFR2* mutations

Craniosynostoses

These include the Apert, Crouzon, Pfeiffer, and Jackson–Weiss syndromes. Common features include premature fusion of skull sutures, producing skull distortion, widely spaced, bulbous eyes with hyperteleorism, and mid-facial (Muenke et al. 1994). The Pfeiffer, Crouzon, and Jackson–Weiss syndromes overlap, but the Pfeiffer syndrome is distinguished by severe hand and foot anomalies. Some Pfeiffer syndrome families are linked to chromosome 8 with *FGFR1*, but not all. Crouzon and Jackson–Weiss syndromes were initially mapped to the distal long arm of chromosome 10, where *FGFR2* also lies and various *FGFR* abnormalities have been associated with these clinical phenotypes.

Examples

A highly specific Pro252–Arg substitution was detected in the extracellular domain of five families with Pfeiffer syndrome. There are mutations in the IgIIIc region of *FGFR2*, whereas the original and subsequent Crouzon mutations included IgIII Tyr328–Cys and Ser347–Cys. The tissue expression and distribution of *FGF1*, *FGFR2*, and *FGFR3* proteins partially explains the clinical phenotypes of Crouzon and Jackson–Weiss syndromes. Thus, whilst *FGFR1* is expressed throughout active limb bud, *FGFR2* expression at the equivalent stage of embryogenesis is confined to limb-bud ectoderm. *FGFR1* mutants might be expected to have more severe limb deformities. Those *FGFR2* mutations that cause Crouzon/Jackson–Weiss syndrome lie in exon 7, which codes for IgIII. These particular sequences are preferentially expressed in skull *FGFR* proteins and interfere with the timing of skull suture fusion. The Pro252–Arg *FGFR1* mutation in Pfeiffer syndrome lies in an exon shared by several isoforms of *FGFR1* protein. The clinical phenotype is, therefore, less specific. Mutations are located to sequences normally very highly conserved in both man and chickens.

Apert syndrome can also be allelic to Crouzon syndrome. Thus, identical mutations of the *FGFR1* gene can cause either Pfeiffer or Crouzon phenotypes (Rutland et al. 1995). Several Apert mutations mutate either Ser253–Trp or Pro253–Arg (Wilkie et al. 1995).

References

Ahmad, N.N. et al. (1990). A stop codon in the gene for type II procollagen *COL2A1* causes one variant of arthro-ophthalmopathy (the Stickler syndrome). *American Journal of Human Genetics* **47**, A206.

Ala-Kokko, L., Baldwin, C.T., Moskowitz, R.W., and Prockop, D.J. (1990). Single base mutation in the type II procollagen gene *COL2A1* as a cause of primary osteoarthritis associated with a mild chondrodysplasia. *Proceedings of the National Academy of Sciences USA* **87**, 6565–8.

Alliston, T. and Derynck, R. (2002). Medicine: interfering with bone modelling. *Nature* **416**, 686–7.

Anderson, I.J., Goldberg, R.B., Marion, R.W., Upholt, W.B., and Tsipouras, P. (1990). Spondyloepiphyseal dysplasia congenita: genetic linkage to type II collagen (*COL2A1*). *American Journal of Human Genetics* **46**, 896–901.

Annunen, S. et al. (1999). Splicing mutations of the 54 bp exons in the *COL11A1* gene cause Marshall Syndrome, but other mutations cause overlapping Stickler/Marshall phenotypes. *American Journal of Human Genetics* **65**, 974–83.

Andrikopoulos, K., Liu, X., Keene, D.R., Jaenisch, R., and Ramirez, F. (1995). Targeted mutation in the *col5a2* gene reveals a regulatory role for type V collagen during matrix assembly. *Nature Genetics* **9**, 31–6.

Barker, D.F. et al. (1990). Identification of mutations in the *COL4A5* collagen gene in Alport syndrome. *Science* **248**, 1224–7.

Beighton, P. *McKusick's Heritable Disorders of Connective Tissue 5th edn.* St Louis MO: Mosby, 1995.

Beighton, P. et al. (1988). International nosology of heritable disorders of connective tissue, Berlin, 1986. *American Journal of Medical Genetics* **29**, 581–94.

Beighton, P. et al. (1992). Molecular nosology of heritable disorders of connective tissue. *American Journal of Human Genetics* **42**, 431–48.

Beighton, P., Cilliers, H.J., and Ramesar, R. (1994). Autosomal dominant (Benkes) premature degenerative osteoarthropathy of the hip joint unlinked to *COL2A1*. *American Journal of Medical Genetics* **53**, 348–51.

Benya, P.D. and Shaffer, J.D. (1982). Dedifferentiated chondrocytes reexpress the differentiated collagen phenotype when cultured in agarose gels. *Cell* **30**, 215–24.

Bogaert, R. et al. (1992). An amino acid substitution (Gly853 → Glu) in the collagen $\alpha1$(II) chain produces hypochondrogenesis. *Journal of Biological Chemistry* **267**, 22522–6.

Boileau, C. et al. (1995). The question of heterogeneity in Marfan syndrome. *Nature Genetics* **9**, 230–1.

Bonadio, J. and Byers, P.H. (1985). Subtle structural alterations in the chains of type I procollagen produce osteogenesis imperfecta type II. *Nature* **316**, 363–6.

Briggs, M.D. and Chapman, K.L. (2002). Pseudoachondroplasia and multiple epiphyseal dysplasia; mutation review, molecular interactions, and genotype to phenotype correlations. *Human Mutation* **19**, 465–78.

Briggs, M.D. et al. (1994). Genetic mapping of a locus for multiple epiphyseal dysplasia EDM2 to a region of chromosome 1 containing a type IX collagen gene. *American Journal of Human Genetics* **55**, 678–84.

Burrows, N.P. et al. (1996). The gene encoding $\alpha1$(V) (COL5A1) is linked to Ehlers–Danlos syndrome type I/III. *Journal of Investigative Dermatology* **106**, 1273–6.

Burrows, N.P. et al. (1998). A point mutation in an intronic branch site results in aberrant splicing of *COL5A1* and in Ehlers–Danlos syndrome type II in two British families. *American Journal of Human Genetics* **63**, 390–8.

Byers, P.H. (1990). Brittle bones–fragile molecules: disorders of collagen gene structure and expression. *Trends in Genetics* **6**, 293–300.

Byers, P.H., Siegel, R.C., Holbrook, K.A., Narayanan, A.S., Bornstein, P., and Hall, J.P. (1980). X-linked cutis laxa: defective cross-link formation in collagen due to decreased lysyl oxidase activity. *New England Journal of Medicine* **303**, 61–5.

Chan, D. and Cole, W.G. (1991). Low basal transcription of genes for tissue-specific collagens by fibroblasts and lymphoblastoid cells. Application to the charcterization of a glycine 997 to serine substitution in alpha 1(II) collagen chains of a patient with spondyloepiphyseal dysplasia. *Journal of Biological Chemistry* **266**, 12487–94.

Chan, D., Taylor, T.K.F., and Cole, W.G. (1993). Characterisation of an arginine 789 to cysteine substitution in $\alpha1$(II) collagen chains of a patient with spondyloepiphyseal dysplasia. *Journal of Biological Chemistry* **268**, 15238–45.

Christiano, A.M. et al. (1994). Structural organisation of the human type VII collagen gene (*COL7A1*) comprised of more exons than any previously characterised gene. *Genomics* **21**, 169–79.

Christiano, A.M., McGrath, J.A., Tan, K.C., and Uitto, J. (1996). Glycine substitutions in the triple-helical region of type VII collagen result in a spectrum of dystrophic epidermolysis bullosa phenotypes and patterns of inheritance. *American Journal of Human Genetics* **58**, 671–81.

Cole, W.G. and Dalgleish, R. (1995). Perinatal lethal osteogenesis imperfecta. *Journal of Medical Genetics* **32**, 284–9.

Cole, W.G., Hall, R.K., and Rogers, J.G. (1993). The clinical features of spondylo-epiphyseal dysplasia congenita resulting from the substitution of glycine 997 by serine in the $\alpha1$(II) chain of type II collagen. *Journal of Medical Genetics* **30**, 27–35.

Collod, G. et al. (1995). A second locus for Marfan syndrome maps to chromosome 3p24.2-p25. *Nature Genetics* **8**, 264–8.

Collod-Beroud, G. et al. (1998). Marfan database (third edition): new mutations and new routines for the software. *Nucleic Acids Research* **26**, 229–33.

Corson, G.M., Chalberg, S.C., Dietz, H.C., Charbonneau, N.L., and Saiki, L.Y. (1993). Fibrillin binds calcium and is coded by cDNAs that reveal a multidomain, structural and alternatively spliced exons at the 5′ end. *Genomics* **17**, 476–84.

Dalgleish, R. (2001). Collagen type I and III databases at: http://www.le.ac.uk/genetics/collagen.

De Paepe, A., Devereux, R.B., Dietz, R.B., Hennekam, R.C., and Pyeritz, R.E. (1996). Revised diagnostic crtiteria for the Marfan Syndrome. *American Journal of Medical Genetics* **62**, 417–26.

De Paepe, A., Nuytinck, L., Hausser, I., Anton-Lamprecht, I., and Naeyaert, J.M. (1997). Mutations in the *COL5A1* gene are causal in Ehlers–Danlos syndromes I and II. *American Journal of Human Genetics* **60**, 547–54.

Dieppe, P. (1987). Osteoarthritis and related disorders. In *Oxford Textbook of Medicine* Vol. 2 (ed. D.J. Weatherall, J.G.G. Ledingham, and D.A. Warrell), pp. 16, 76–84. Oxford: Oxford University Press.

Dietz, H.C. et al. (1991). Marfan syndrome caused by a recurrent *de novo* missense mutation in the fibrillin gene. *Nature* **352**, 337–9.

Dietz, H.C. et al. (1995). The question of heterogeneity in Marfan syndrome. *Nature Genetics* **9**, 228–31.

Dunnill, M.G., Richards, A.J., Milana, G., Mollica, F., Eady, R.A., and Pope, F.M. (1994). A novel homozygous point mutation in the collagen VII gene (*COL7A1*) in two cousins with recessive dystrophic epidermolysis bullosa. *Human Molecular Genetics* **3**, 1693–4.

Erlebacher, A., Filvaroff, E.H., Gitelman, S.E., and Derynck, R. (1995). Toward a molecular understanding of skeletal development. *Cell* **80**, 371–8.

Eyre, D.R., Upton, M.P., Shapiro, F.D., Wilkinson, R.H., and Vawter, G.F. (1986). Nonexpression of cartilage type II collagen in a case of Langer–Saldino achondrogenesis. *American Journal of Human Genetics* **39**, 52–67.

Fine, J.D. et al. (2000). Revised classification for inherited epidermolysis bullosa. Report of the Second International Consensus Meeting on diagnosis and classification of epidermolysis bullosa. *Journal of American Academy of Dermatology* **42**, 1051–66.

Francomano, C.A. et al. (1988). The Stickler and Wagner syndromes: evidence for genetic heterogeneity. *American Journal of Human Genetics* **43**, A83.

Fryer, A.E. et al. (1990). Exclusion of *COL2A1* as the candidate gene in a family with Wagner–Stickler's syndrome. *Journal of Medical Genetics* **27**, 91–3.

Garofalo, S. et al. (1991). Reduced amounts of cartilage collagen fibrils and growth plate anomalies in transgenic mice harbouring a glycine-to-cysteine mutation in the mouse type II procollagen α1-chain gene. *Proceedings of the National Academy of Sciences USA* **88**, 9648–52.

Godfrey, M. and Hollister, D.W. (1988). Type II achondrogenesis-hypochondrogenesis: identification of abnormal type II collagen. *American Journal of Human Genetics* **43**, 904–13.

Givol, D. and Yagon, A. (1992). Complexity of FGF receptors: genetic basis for structural diversity and functional specificity. *FASEB Journal* **6**, 3362–9.

Gruis, N.A. et al. (1992). Genetic linkage between the collagen VII gene (*COL7A1*) and the autosomal dominant form of dystrophic epidermolysis bullosa in two Dutch kindreds. *Journal of Investigative Dermatology* **99**, 528–30.

Hastbacka, J. et al. (1999). Identification of the Finnish founder mutation for diastrophic dysplasia (DTD). *European Journal of Human Genetics* **7**, 664–70.

Hautala, T., Byers, M.G., Eddy, R.L., Shows, T.B., Kivirikko, K.I., and Myllyla, R. (1992). Cloning of human lysyl hydroxylase: complete cDNA derived amino acid sequence and assignment of the gene (*PLOD*) to chromosome 1p36.3–36.2. *Genomics* **13**, 62–9.

Horton, W.A. (1988). Approaches to investigating growth plate cartilage in the human chondrodysplasias. *Pathology and Immunopathological Research* **7**, 85–9.

Horton, W.A. (1995). Molecular genetics of the human chondrodysplasias—1995. *European Journal of Human Genetics* **3**, 357–73.

Hostikka, S.L., Eddy, R.L., Byers, M.G., Hoyhtya, M., Shows, T.B., and Tryggvarson, K. (1990). Identification of a distinct type IV collagen α chain with restricted kidney distribution and assignment of its gene to the locus of X chromosome-linked Alport syndrome. *Proceedings of the National Academy of Sciences USA* **87**, 1606–10.

Hull, R.G. and Pope, F.M. (1989). Osteoarthritis and cartilage collagen genes. *Lancet* **1**, 1337–8.

Jobsis, G.J. et al. (1996a). Type VI collagen mutations in Bethlem Myopathy, an autosomal dominant myopathy with contractures. *Nature Genetics* **14**, 113–15.

Jobsis, G.J. et al. (1996b). Genetic localization of Bethlem Myopathy. *Neurology* **46**, 779–82.

Kainulainen, K., Pulkkinen, L., Savolainen, A., Kaitila, I., and Peltonen, L. (1990). Location on chromosome 15 of the gene defect causing Marfan syndrome. *New England Journal of Medicine* **323**, 935–9.

Kainulainen, K. et al. (1991). Marfan syndrome: no evidence for heterogeneity in different populations, and more precise mapping of the gene. *American Journal of Human Genetics* **49**, 662–7.

Kainulainen, K., Karttunen, L., Puhakka, L., Saiki, L., and Peltonen, L. (1994). Mutations in the fibrillin gene responsible for dominant ectopia lentis and neonatal Marfan syndrome. *Nature Genetics* **6**, 64–9.

Khakoo, A., Thomas, R., Trompeter, R., Doffy, P., Price, R., and Pope, F.M. (1997). Congenital cutis laxa and lysyl oxidase deficiency. *Clinical Genetics* **51**, 109–14.

Kivirikko, K.I. and Myllyla, R. (1982). Post-translational enzymes in the biosynthesis of collagen: intracellular enzymes. In *Methods in Enzymology Extracellular Matrix: Structural and Contractile Proteins* Vol. 82, Part A (ed. L.W. Cunningham, and M. Frederiksen), pp. 245–304. New York: Academic Press.

Knowlton, R.G. et al. (1990). Genetic linkage of a polymorphism in the type II procollagen gene (*COL2A1*) to primary osteoarthritis associated with mild chondrodysplasia. *New England Journal of Medicine* **322**, 526–30.

Komorowska, A. et al. (1989). A Polish variant of isolated dentinogenesis imperfecta with a generalised connective tissue defect. *British Dental Journal* **167**, 239–43.

Krauss, S., Concordet, J.P., and Ingham, P.W. (1993). A functionally conserved homolog of the *Drosophila* segment polarity gene *hh* is expressed in tissues with polarizing activity in Zebrafish embryos. *Cell* **75**, 1431–44.

Kuivaniemi, H., Tromp, G., and Prockop, D.J. (1997). Mutations in fibrillar collagens (types I, II, III and XI), fibril-associated collagen (type IX), and network-forming collagen (type X) cause a spectrum of diseases in bone, cartilage and blood vessels. *Human Mutation* **9**, 300–15.

Lee, B., Vissing, H., Ramirez, F., Rogers, D., and Rimoin, D. (1989). Identification of the molecular defect in a family with spondyloepiphyseal dysplasia. *Science* **244**, 978–82.

Lee, B. et al. (1991). Linkage of Marfan syndrome and a phenotypically related disorder to two different fibrillin genes. *Nature* **352**, 330–4.

Li, Y. et al. (1995). A fibrillar collagen gene, *Col11a1*, is essential for skeletal morphogenesis. *Cell* **80**, 423–30.

Lichtenstein, J.R., Martin, G.R, Kohn, L.D., Byers, P.H., and McKusick, V.A. (1973). Defect in conversion of procollagen to collagen in a form of Ehlers–Danlos syndrome. *Science* **182**, 298–300.

Loughlin, J. et al. (1995). Linkage of the gene that encodes the α1 chain of type V collagen (*COL5A1*) to type II Ehlers–Danlos syndrome (EDS II). *Human Molecular Genetics* **4**, 1649–51.

Marfan, A.B. (1896). Un cas de déformation congénitale des quartre members, plus prononcée aux extrémités charactérisée par l'allongement des os avec un certain degré d'amincissement. *Bulletins et Memoires de la Societé Medical des Hopitaux de Paris* **13**, 220–6.

Maroteaux, P. (1970). Nomenclature internationale des maladies osseuses constitutionnelles. *Annals of Radiology* **13**, 455.

Martin, S., Richards, A.J., Yates, J.R., Scott, J.D., Pope, M., and Snead, M.P. (1999). Stickler syndrome: further mutations in *COL11A1* and evidence for additional locus heterogeneity. *European Journal of Human Genetics* **7**, 807–14.

Maslen, C.L., Corson, G.M., Maddox, B.K., Glanville, R.W., and Saiki, L.Y. (1991). Partial sequence of a candidate gene for the Marfan syndrome. *Nature* **352**, 334–7.

McGrath, J.A., Pulkkinen, L., Cristiano, A.M., Leigh, I.M., Eady, R.A.J., and Uitto, J. (1995). Altered laminin 5 expression due to mutation on the β_3 chain gene (*LAMB3*). *Journal of Investigative Dermatology* **104**, 467–74.

McGrath, J.A. et al. (1995a). Mutations in the 180 Kd bullous pemphigoid antigen (BPAG2), a hemidesmosomal transmembrane collagen in generalised atrophic benign epidermolysis bullosa. *Nature Genetics* **11**, 83–6.

McGrath, J.A. et al. (1995b). A homozygous nonsense mutation in the α3 chain of laminin 5 (*LAMA3*) in Herlitz junctional epidermolysis bullosa: prenatal diagnosis exclusion in a fetus at risk. *Genomics* **29**, 282–4.

McGrath, J.A. et al. (1995c). First trimester DNA-based exclusion of recessive dystrophic epidermolysis bullosa from chorionic villus sampling. *British Journal of Dermatology* **134**, 734–7.

McGrath, J.A. et al. (1999). Moderation of phenotype severity in dystrophic and junctional forms of epidermolysisa bullosa. In frame skipping at exons containing nonsense or frameshift mutations. *Journal of Investigative Dermatology* **113**, 314–321.

McKusick, V.A., Francomano, C.A., and Antonarakis, S.E. *Mendelian Inheritance in Man: Catalogs of Autosomal Dominant, Autosomal Recessive and X-linked Phenotypes* 9th edn. Baltimore MD: Johns Hopkins University Press, 1990.

Muenke, M. et al. (1994). A common mutation in the fibroblast growth factor receptor 1 gene in Pfeiffer syndrome. *Nature Genetics* **8**, 269–74.

Murray, L.W., Bautista, J., James, P.L., and Rimoin, D.L. (1989). Type II collagen defects in the chondrodysplasias. I. Spondyloepiphyseal dysplasias. *American Journal of Human Genetics* **45**, 5–15.

Nicholls, A.C. et al. (1984). The clinical features of homozygous $\alpha 2$(I) collagen deficient osteogenesis imperfecta. *Journal of Medical Genetics* **21**, 257–62.

Nicholls, A.C. et al. (1988). Linkage of a polymorphic marker for the type III collagen gene (*COL3A1*) to atypical autosomal dominant Ehlers–Danlos syndrome type IV in a large Belgian pedigree. *Human Genetics* **79**, 276–81.

Nicholls, A.C., Oliver, J.E., McCarron, S., Harrison, J.B., Greenspan, D.S., and Pope, F.M. (1996). An exon skipping mutation of a type V collagen gene (COL5A1) in Ehlers–Danlos syndrome. *Journal of Medical Genetics* **33**, 940–6.

Nijbroek, G. et al. (1995). Fifteen novel *FBN1* mutations causing Marfan syndrome detected by heteroduplex analysis of genomic amplicons. *American Journal of Human Genetics* **57**, 8–21.

Nusgens, B.V. et al. (1992). Evidence for a relationship between Ehlers–Danlos type VII C in humans and bovine dermatosparaxis. *Nature Genetics* **1**, 214–17.

Oehlmann, R., Summerville, G.P., Yeh, G., Weaver, E.J., Jimenez, S.A., and Knowlton, R.G. (1994). Genetic linkage of multiple epiphyseal dysplasia to the pericentromeric region of chromosome 19. *American Journal of Human Genetics* **54**, 3–10.

Parente, M.G. et al. (1991). Human type VII collagen: cDNA cloning and chromosomal mapping of the gene. *Proceedings of the National Academy of Sciences USA* **88**, 6931–5.

Passos-Bueno, M.R., Wilcox, W.R., Jabs, E.W., Sertie, A.L., Alonso, L.G., and Kitoh, H. (1999). Clinical spectrum of fibroblast growth receptor mutations. *Human Mutation* **14**, 115–25.

Pepin, M., Schwarze, U., Superti-Furga, A., and Vyers, P.H. (2000). Clinical and genetic features of Ehlers–Danlos Syndrome type IV, the vascular type. *New England Journal of Medicine* **342**, 673–80.

Pereira, L. et al. (1993). Genomic organization of the sequence coding for fibrillin, the defective gene product in Marfan syndrome. *Human Molecular Genetics* **2**, 961–8.

Phillips, C.L., Shrago-Howe, A.W., Pinnell, S.R., and Wenstrup, R.J. (1991). A substitution at a non-glycine position in the triple-helical domain of pro$\alpha 2$(I) collagen chains present in an individual with a variant of the Marfan syndrome. *Journal of Clinical Investigation* **86**, 1723–8.

Pope, F.M. et al. (1991). Type III collagen mutations cause fragile cerebral arteries. *British Journal of Neurosurgery* **5**, 551–74.

Pope, F.M., Narcisi, P., Nicholls, A.C., Germaine, D., Pals, G., and Richards, A.J. (1996). *COL3A1* mutations cause variable clinical phenotypes including acrogeria and vascular rupture. *British Journal of Dermatology* **135**, 163–81.

Prockop, D.J. (1990). Mutations that alter the primary structure of type I collagen. The perils of a system for generating large structures by the principle of nucleated growth. *Journal of Biological Chemistry* **265**, 15349–52.

Prockop, D.J. and Kivirikko, K.I. (1984). Heritable diseases of collagen. *New England Journal of Medicine* **311**, 376–86.

Richards, A.J. et al. (1996). A family with Stickler syndrome has a mutation in the *COL11A1* gene resulting in the substitution of glycine 97 by valine in $\alpha 1$(XI) collagen. *Human Molecular Genetics* **5**, 1339–43.

Richards, A.J. et al. (2000). Variation in the vitreous phenotype of Stickler syndrome can be caused by different amino acid substitutions in the X position of the type II collagen Gly-X-Y triple helix. *American Journal of Human Genetics* **67**, 1083–94.

Rosati, R. et al. (1994). Normal long bone growth and development in type X collagen-null mice. *Nature Genetics* **8**, 129–35.

Rutland, P. et al. (1995). Identical mutations in the *FGFR2* gene cause both Pfeiffer and Crouzon syndrome phenotypes. *Nature Genetics* **9**, 173–6.

Ryynanen, M., Knowlton, R.G., Parente, M.G., Chung, L.C., Chu, M.L., and Uitto, J. (1991). Human type VII collagen: genetic linkage of the gene (*COL7A1*) on chromosome 3 to dominant dystrophic epidermolysis bullosa. *American Journal of Human Genetics* **49**, 797–803.

Schalkwijk, J. et al. (2001). A recessive form of the Ehlers–Danlos syndrome caused by tenascin-X deficiency. *New England Journal of Medicine* **345**, 1167–75.

Schwartz, R.C. et al. (1989). Non allelic heterogeneity in the vitreo-retinal degradations of Stickler and Wagner types and evidence for iatrogenic recombination at *COL2A1* locus. *American Journal of Human Genetics* **45**, A128.

Sher, C., Ramesar, T., Martell, R., Leam monti, J., Tsipouras, P., and Beighton, P. (1991). Mild spondyloepiphyseal dysplasia (Naquamaland type): genetic linkage to the type II collagen gene. *American Journal of Human Genetics* **48**, 518–24.

Sillence, D.O., Senn, A., and Danks, D.M. (1979). Genetic heterogeneity in osteogenesis imperfecta. *Journal of Medical Genetics* **16**, 101–16.

Sirko-Osada, D.A., Murray, M.A., Scott, J.A., Lavery, M.A., Warman, M.L., and Robin, N.H. (1998). Stickler syndrome without eye involvement is caused by mutation in *COL11A2*, the gene encoding the alpha 2 (XI) chain of type XI collagen. *Journal of Pediatrics* **132**, 368–71.

Snead, M.P. (1994). Stickler syndrome: correlation between vitreoretinal phenotypes and linkage to *COL2A1*. *Eyes* **8**, 609–14.

Snead, M.P. and Yates, J.R.W. (1999). Clinical and molecular genetics of Stickler syndrome. *Journal of Medical Genetics* **36**, 353–9.

Spranger, J. (1992). International classification of the osteochondrodysplasias. The International Group on Constitutional Diseases of Bone. *European Journal of Paediatrics* **151**, 407–15.

Steinmann, R., Rao, V.H., Vogel, A., Bruckner, P., Gitzelmann, R., and Byers, P.H. (1984). Cysteine in the triple-helical domain of one allelic product of the $\alpha 1$(I) gene of type I collagen produces a lethal form of osteogenesis imperfecta. *Journal of Biological Chemistry* **259**, 11129–38.

Steinmann, B., Nicholls, A.C., and Pope, F.M. (1986). Clinical variability of osteogenesis imperfecta reflecting molecular heterogeneity: cysteine substitutions IN the $\alpha 1$(I) collagen chain producing lethal and mild forms. *Journal of Biological Chemistry* **261**, 8958–64.

Superti-Furga, A. et al. (1996). Achondrogenesis type 1B is caused by mutations in the diastrophic dysplasia sulfate transporter gene. *Nature Genetics* **12**, 100–2.

Superti-Furga, A. et al. (1999). Recessively inherited multiple epiphyseal dysplasia with normal stature, club foot, and double layered patella caused by a DTDST mutation. *Journal of Medical Genetics* **36**, 621–4.

Sykes, B. et al. (1990). Consistent linkage of dominantly inherited osteogenesis imperfecta to the type I collagen loci: *COL1A1* and *COL1A2*. *American Journal of Human Genetics* **46**, 293–307.

Takahara, K., Brevard, R., Hoffman, G.G., Suzuki, N., and Greenspan, D.S. (1996). Characterization of novel gene product (mamalian tolloid-like) with high sequence similarity to mamalian tolloid/bone morphogenetic protein-1. *Genomics* **34**, 157–65.

Thompson, E.M., Young, I.D., Hall, C.M., and Pembrey, M.E. (1987). Recurrence risks and prognosis in severe sporadic osteogenesis imperfecta. *Journal of Medical Genetics* **24**, 390–405.

Tiller, G.E., Rimoin, D.L., Murray, L.W., and Cohn, D.H. (1990). Tandem duplication within a type II collagen gene (*COL2A1*) exon in an individual with spondyloepiphyseal dysplasia. *Proceedings of the National Academy of Sciences USA* **87**, 3889–93.

Tiller, G.E. et al. (1995). Dominant mutations in the type II collagen gene, *COL2A1*, produce spondyloepiphyseal dysplasia, Strudwick type. *Nature Genetics* **11**, 87–9.

Torriello, H.V. et al. (1996). A translocation interrupts the *COL5A1* gene in a patient with Ehlers–Danlos syndrome and hypomelanosis of Ito. *Nature Genetics* **13**, 361–5.

Tsipouras, P. et al. (1992). Genetic linkage of the Marfan syndrome, ectopia lentis, and congenital contractural arachnodactyly to the fibrillin genes on chromosomes 15 and 5. The International Marfan Syndrome Collaborative Study. *New England Journal of Medicine* **326**, 905–9.

Vikkula, M., Mestaranta, M., and Ala-Kokko, L. (1994). Type II collagen mutations in rare and common cartilage diseases. *Annals of Medicine* **26**, 107–14.

Vikkula, M. et al. (1995). Autosomal dominant and recessive osteochondrodysplasias associated with the *COL11A2* locus. *Cell* **80**, 431–7.

Vissing, H., d'Alessio, M., Lee, B., Ramirez, F., Godfrey, M., and Hollister, D.W. (1989). Glycine to serine substitution in the triple helical domain of the pro$\alpha 1$(II) collagen results in a lethal perinatal form of short-limbed dwarfism. *Journal of Biological Chemistry* **264**, 18265–7.

Vogel, B.E., Doelz, R., Kadler, K.E., Hojima, Y., Engel, J., and Prockop, D.J. (1988). A substitution of cysteine for glycine 748 of the α1 chain produces a kink at this site in the procollagen I molecule and an altered N proteinase cleavage site over 225 nm away. *Journal of Biological Chemistry* **263**, 19249–55.

Wallis, G.A. et al. (1996). Mutations within the gene encoding the α1(X) chain of type X collagen (COL10A1) cause metaphyseal chondrodysplasia type Schmid, but not several other forms of metaphyseal chondrodysplasia. *Journal of Medical Genetics* **33**, 450–7.

Wenstrup, R.J., Murad, S., and Pinnell, S.R. (1989). Ehlers–Danlos syndrome type VI: clinical manifestations of collagen lysyl hydroxylase deficiency. *Journal of Pediatrics* **115**, 405–9.

Westerhausen, A., Constantinou, C.D., and Prockop, D.J. (1990). A mutation that substitutes valine for glycine α1 637 in type I procollagen gene, *COL1A1*, and causes lethal OI. *American Journal of Human Genetics* **47**, A242.

Weve, H. (1931). Über Arachnodaktylie (dystrophia mesodermalis congenital Typus Marfan). *Archives Augenheilkd* **104**, 1–46.

Wilkie, A.O. et al. (1995). Apert syndrome results from localized mutations of FGFR2 and is allelic with Crouzon syndrome. *Nature Genetics* **9**, 165–72.

Willing, M.C., Cohn, D.H., and Byers, P.H. (1990). Frameshift mutation near the 3′ end of the *COL1A1* gene of type I collagen predicts an elongated proα1(I) chain and results in osteogenesis imperfecta type I. *Journal of Clinical Investigation* **85**, 282–90.

Wordsworth, P., Ogilivie, D., Priestly, L., Smith, R., Wynne-Davis, R., and Sykes, B. (1988). Structural and segregation analysis of the type II collagen gene (*COL2A1*) in some heritable chondrodysplasias. *Journal of Medical Genetics* **25**, 521–7.

Zhou, J. et al. (1990). Cloning of the human α5(IV) collagen gene and characterization of mutations in Alport syndrome. *American Journal of Human Genetics* **47**, A85.

3.3 Articular cartilage

Timothy E. Hardingham

Introduction

Articular cartilage is a unique and long-time enigmatic tissue that is now revealing many of its secrets. Just a few millimetres thick, cartilage is ingeniously fashioned so as to withstand the considerable biomechanical forces created by walking, running, and jumping, over many decades (Muir and Hardingham 1986). Even during gentle walking, the force acting at the hip joint is equivalent to four times the body weight. Articular cartilage (Fig. 1) is unique in that it is a tissue with few cells and no basement membrane, no innervation, and no direct blood supply, relying on diffusion for its nutritive requirements. It is increasingly being realized that cartilage failure as seen in diseases such as osteoarthritis is far from being the passive degenerative condition long assumed, but represents an imbalance between dynamic reparative and catabolic processes, which in health proceed in a harmonized and strictly regulated manner (Hardingham 1990; Hardingham and Bayliss 1990).

The load-bearing properties of the tissue depend on the structure and matrix. The integrity of the matrix is maintained by the activity of the chondrocytes (Stockwell and Meachim 1979). The matrix contains more than 70 per cent water but, because of the high proteoglycan content, there is free diffusion of only small molecules. Solutes of large molecular weight are excluded from proteoglycan domains and, therefore, the mobility of molecules in the matrix depends on their size. The articular cartilage is bound to the underlying bone through a narrow calcified zone of cartilage. The junction between the calcified and non-calcified zone of cartilage forms the tidemark, which is named for its strong histological staining.

The articular surface is formed by a dense collagen layer of low proteoglycan content, but which is otherwise a part of the cartilage rather than a separate boundary layer. The articular joint and its component structures surrounding the synovial compartment are not bound by any basement membrane. There are no epithelial or endothelial boundaries. All the structures are of mesodermal origin. The synovial membrane has a thickness of one or a few cells and forms the surface layer of the synovial tissue, but it is otherwise not distinct from it. The deeper synovial tissue is well supplied with blood vessels and contains many cells rich in fat deposits. The synovial tissue becomes a site of major inflammatory reaction in joint diseases such as rheumatoid arthritis.

In chronic rheumatoid arthritis the synovium undergoes massive hyperplasia and forms a complex villous structure extending into the synovial space with a thickened cell lining layer and heavy lymphocytic infiltration with lymphoid follicles. The articular cartilage, synovium, and ligaments thus share a common compartment, with the synovial fluid linking them together. The tissues are therefore exposed to all the components that come into synovial fluid. Inflammatory events in the synovium that lead to the release of inflammatory mediators and cytokines will have consequences on ligaments and on articular cartilage.

The function of the articular joint is to give movement and mobility to the otherwise rigid bony skeleton (Mow and Lai 1980). The joint transmits force from one bone element to another. Bones are linked by ligaments and muscle/tendon elements. The articular cartilage provides two opposing smooth surfaces of extremely low friction for easy articulation, and a deformable and elastic tissue that helps distribute the load more evenly on to the underlying bone.

The different components in the joint have complimentary mechanical functions. All these connective tissues respond to the mechanical forces placed upon them and, in general, extra use leads to hypertrophy and mechanical strengthening. This is evident from experimental studies which showed that moderate running exercise in dogs resulted in an increase in articular cartilage thickness and proteoglycan content, and a rise in compressive stiffness (Kiviranta et al. 1992). This contrasted with excessively strenuous running exercise, which led to a fall in proteoglycan content, a loss of compressive stiffness, and some remodelling of the sub-chondral bone; but even severe exercise did not cause degeneration of the articular surface or lead to degenerative joint disease (Arokoski et al. 1993). High loading of a healthy joint is thus unlikely alone to initiate joint disease.

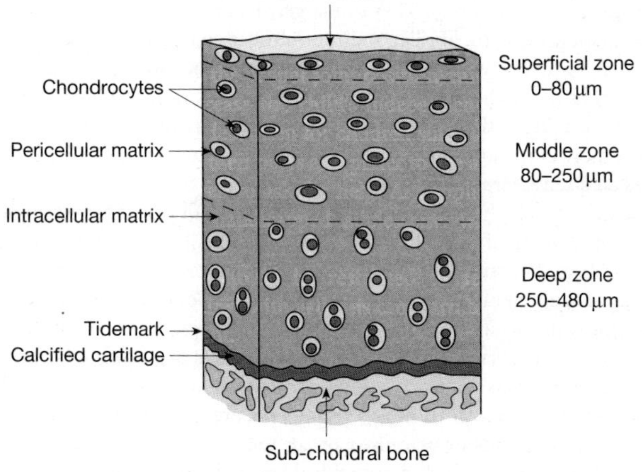

Fig. 1 Structure and organization of articular cartilage. Schematic drawing showing changes in organization from the articular surface to the sub-chondral bone.

Unlike exercise, disuse of the joint leads to atrophy of the articular cartilage (Buckwalter 1995). Even temporary immobilization of a joint can result in a fall in the synthesis and content of proteoglycan; more prolonged disuse can result in the degeneration of articular cartilage and its eventual complete loss and replacement of the joint space with fibro-fatty tissue. The healthy maintenance of the different tissues thus depends on their regular mechanical loading in normal use and this reflects a property of the cells within the tissue that controls the production and maintenance of the matrix. It is also clear that changes in the mechanical performance of any one joint tissue will have consequences on the loads experienced by other components causing further adaptive responses. This may be particularly prejudicial to articular cartilage integrity if it results in joint instability and greater impact loading. Therefore, the articular joint and its component tissues are far from being static structures and even in the mature animal they are in a constant dynamic state of adaptation and response. Many of the changes present in joints after many years of chronic joint disease may thus reflect adaptive responses to altered patterns of load distribution in the joint as well as direct effects of the disease processes themselves.

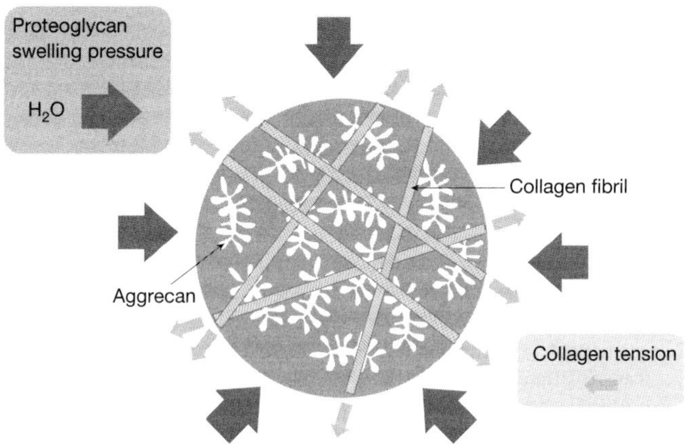

Fig. 2 The combined functions of collagen and proteoglycan in providing the compressive resilience of cartilage. The collagen fibres resist tension and provide the shape and form of the tissue. The proteoglycans (mainly aggrecan) are immobilized and create a large osmotic swelling pressure that extends the collagen network. The resulting tissue is tough, hard-wearing, and deforms elastically under load.

Cartilage

Cartilage occurs in various forms in the body and with different functions. In embryological development it is the important forerunner of long bone development and it persists in the growth plate as the major site of long bone growth. Cartilage is also formed in the body whenever there is a recapitulation of bone development, such as in fracture healing. Cartilage occurs in other sites of the body: it supports the air passageways as bronchial rings, in the larynx it supports the vocal chords, and it occurs as nasal cartilage. It is also found in considerable amounts as intercostal cartilages and at other sites it is in various ways reinforced by other connective tissue components. The cartilage supporting the external ear contains elastin fibres, and fibrocartilage, such as that found in the menisci of the knee, contains extra type I collagen reinforcement. The intervertebral discs also contain a radially reinforced collagen structure surrounding inner regions more similar to hyaline cartilage that resist compressive loading. A thin hyaline cartilage layer also forms an articular surface at the end plate of the vertebrae where they contact the intervertebral discs. In all these forms, the basic features of cartilage is that the cells within it produce a large expanded proteoglycan-rich matrix, which together with the fibrillar network make a stiff but elastically deformable tissue that is able to withstand repetitive compressive loading.

Physical properties of articular cartilage

The physical properties of articular cartilage depend on the structure and organization of the macromolecules in the extracellular matrix (Hardingham 1990, 1999). They can largely be understood in terms of the contribution made by fibrillar and non-fibrillar components (Fig. 2). The collagen fibrillar network is made up of fine fibres that have no preferred orientation in the mid-zone of the cartilage, although at the articular surface they are parallel to the surface with one preferred orientation, and they are rather more perpendicular to the surface in deeper zones. The collagen provides an essential framework to the tissue that gives it shape and form. The triple helical collagen molecules are organized into fibrils with overlapping and cross-linking of adjacent molecules, and fibrils laterally associate into longer fibres. The structure of collagen gives it impressive tensile properties and this is utilized in cartilage in a special way to produce a tissue that is not only strong in tension but also resistant to compression. This is achieved by filling the interfibrillar matrix with a very high content of proteoglycan, primarily aggrecan. The aggrecan at high concentration draws water into the tissue as it creates a large osmotic swelling pressure (Fig. 2).

The osmotic pressure is caused by all the negatively charged anionic groups on aggrecan, which carry with them mobile counter ions such as Na^+. This creates a large difference in the concentration of ions inside the cartilage compared with outside and also an imbalance amongst the freely diffusible anions and cations. Water is drawn into the tissue as a result of this osmotic imbalance and because aggrecan is too large and immobile to redistribute itself. The water thus swells and expands the aggrecan-rich environment. This places the collagen network under tension and an equilibrium is achieved when tension in the collagen network balances the swelling pressure, that is, when no more water enters the tissue because the force is insufficient to stretch the collagen network any further. At this equilibrium, with the tissue swollen with water, it has good compressive resilience as any new load on the tissue now places the collagen network under further tension. Another feature of the composite collagen/aggrecan organization is now important, as not only is aggrecan greatly restricted in its ability to move within the matrix and the collagen/aggrecan network is stiff and resists deformation, but aggrecan offers great resistance to any fluid flow and redistribution of water. The tissue thus behaves largely as a stiff elastic polymer to sudden impact loading, but shows some slow inelastic deformation with sustained loads. However, removal of all loads leads to a redistribution of water and a return to the preloading equilibrium position. The articular cartilage thus forms a tough but compliant load-bearing surface and these characteristics depend on the integrity of the collagen network and the retention within it of a high concentration of aggrecan.

Collagens

The collagens are a family of secreted matrix proteins that contain elements of a unique triple-helical peptide structure with a repeating motif, with glycine as every third amino acid and a high frequency of proline, 40–50 per cent of which is hydroxylated. The presence of hydroxyproline is essential for the stability of the collagen triple helix and hydroxylation of proline is an early post-translational step in synthesis. The collagen gene family is now known to be quite large, but its members fall into two main groups, those that contain long, uninterrupted, triple-helical 'collagenous' domains that form the main fibrillar collagens, types I, II, III, V, and XI, and those that contain shorter, non-fibrillar-forming collagenous domains that form a variety of beaded filament and network structures (Vuorio and de Crombrugge 1990). A further subgroup has been identified as the fibril-associated collagens with interrupted triple-helical domains, such as types IX, XII, and XIV (Olsen 1995). All the fibrillar collagens pack into fibres with a characteristic overlap between adjacent triple helices that gives a staggered array, which facilitates the formation of a cohesive cross-linked fibre, and accounts for the 67 nm banding pattern visible in electron micrographs of collagen fibres.

The most common collagen in the body is the type I fibrillar collagen that occurs as the main structural element in bone, skin, ligaments, and tendons, often occurring together with type III collagen. In contrast, articular cartilage contains collagens of a more restricted distribution that are specifically associated with cartilage (see Table 1). The major collagen of cartilage is type II, which forms 80–90 per cent of the total content. It is a long-chain fibrillar collagen and forms the major fibre network of the tissue. Type II collagen differs from type I in containing three identical chains, whereas type I contains two α_1 (I)-chains and one α_2 (I)-chain. Type II also contains more hydroxylysine than type I and is generally more glycosylated, with a higher content of galactose–glucose disaccharides attached to the hydroxylysine residues. Type II collagen has a very limited distribution in other tissues; apart from in cartilage and the intervertebral discs, it only occurs in the vitreous chamber of the eye. It forms a long-chain, fibrillar, triple helix that is 285 nm long and has large *N*- and *C*-terminal propeptides that are removed enzymatically by specific *N*- and *C*-propeptidases prior to fibril formation. The fibres it forms are generally of a smaller diameter than those formed by type I collagen and they are cross-linked at specific segments of the *N*- and *C*-terminal regions. These bonds are of a stabilized Schiff base that forms a pyridinolone. It is therefore a permanent covalent linkage and mature collagen fibres cross-linked in this way can only be solubilized and resorbed by extensive proteolytic action to excise the cross-linked segments (Eyre and Wu 1995).

Two more distinct collagens also occur in cartilage, these are types IX and XI (see Fig. 3). The latter is another long-chain fibrillar collagen comparable with type II. It can account for up to 10 per cent of the total collagen content of cartilage, but is typically about 3 per cent in adult articular cartilage. It is even more glycosylated than type II and is resistant to collagenase. There are two distinct type XI α-chains, but these show structural similarity to type V collagen α-chains, which are also expressed at a low level in cartilage and can be incorporated in hybrid type XI/V molecules. Type XI collagen in cartilage therefore contains a varying proportion of type V α-chains, which is reported to increase with development (Eyre and Wu 1995). Studies on the cross-links that join different peptides have shown that frequently type XI molecules are joined to each other, but some results show that linkages between type XI and type II chains are also present. Some of the collagen fibres in cartilage may therefore be cofibres of type II and type XI, and in these cases type XI may form the core elements, although analysis shows that some type XI collagen retains its *N*-propeptides in the tissue and this may be more compatible with a fibril surface role for these molecules.

Type IX collagen has a special structure with an interrupted collagenous sequence. It has three collagenous segments and four non-collagenous domains, and electron micrographs of the isolated molecule show it to be an elongated molecule with a kink towards one end. Type IX collagen contains three different α-chains and it has been shown that one of the α-chains (α_2 IX) has an attachment site for a chondroitin sulfate chain in the third non-collagenous domain. In fact the α_2-chain is slightly longer at this site than the α_1- or α_3-chains and this extension coincides with the kink in the electron micrograph image.

Localization of type IX collagen shows that it is found on the outside of type II fibrils and imaging has shown globular domains extending away from the surface of type II collagen fibrils at the end of short stalks, which would correspond with the fourth non-collagenous domain and the third collagenous segment lying at an angle with the axis of the first and second collagenous segments. Cross-links have been identified between the third non-collagenous domain and the *N*-terminal telopeptide region of type II collagen, and also between the second collagenous domain of type IX and the *C*-terminal region of type II collagen (Wu et al. 1992). The cross-linked fragments isolated show that type IX lies antiparallel to type II collagen in the fibres. Cross-links are also formed between type IX molecules. Type IX collagen therefore has the capacity to mediate covalent links between separate type II collagen fibrils. As stromelysin is able to cleave type IX collagen at the second non-collagenous domain and to cleave the telopeptides from type II collagen, it has the capacity to degrade these interfibrillar links (Eyre and Wu 1995). This would have major consequences on the collagen network and could provide a mechanism to facilitate matrix remodelling without great damage to major elements of the type II collagen fibrillar

Table 1 Collagens found in articular cartilage (modified from Eyre et al. 1991)

	Type	Molecular composition	Tissue distribution
Class 1 fibril forming	Type II	$[\alpha_1(\text{II})_3]$	Throughout tissue, major constituent
300 nm, triple helix	Type XI	$[\alpha_1(\text{XI})\ \alpha_2(\text{XI})\ \alpha_3(\text{XI})]$	Throughout tissue (possible core for type II fibrils)
Class 3, short helix molecules	Type VI	$[\alpha_1(\text{VI})\ \alpha_2(\text{VI})\ \alpha_3(\text{VI})]$	Concentrated pericellularly
	Type IX	$[\alpha_1(\text{IX})\ \alpha_2(\text{IX})\ \alpha_3(\text{IX})]$	Linked to type II on the outside of fibrils, some pericellular enrichment
	Type X	$[\alpha_1(\text{X})_3]$	Deep calcified zone only (abundant in growth plate cartilage)

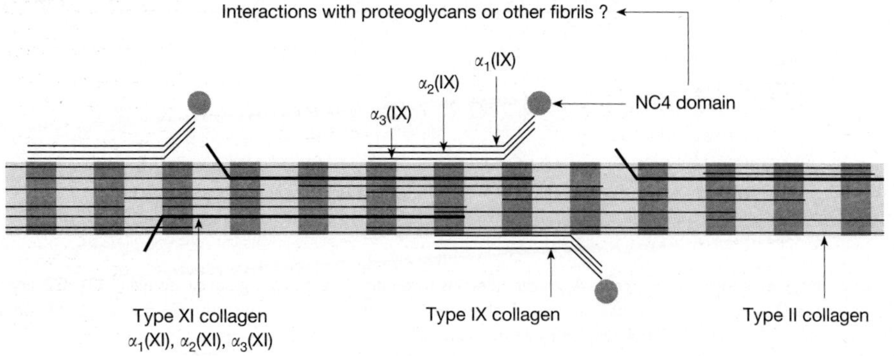

Fig. 3 Schematic showing collagen fibrils in cartilage formed from type II, type IX, and type XI collagen (from Jacenko and Olsen 1995).

network. Linkage analysis has identified defects in the genes of the fibrillar cartilage collagens II, IX, and XI as being responsible for some inherited diseases affecting the joints, including early-onset osteoarthritis, Stickler's syndrome, and various chondrodysplasias (Jacenko and Olsen 1995).

As with type II collagen, type IX is also expressed in the eye. In studies on avian eyes, it has been shown that its expression used a different gene promoter from that used in cartilage and the protein expressed has an additional peptide within its sequence that enlarges the fourth non-collagenous domain (Nishimura et al. 1989). It has also been shown in chickens that the chondroitin sulfate chain synthesized on the third non-collagenous domain in the vitreous chamber is almost 10 times longer than that synthesized in cartilage (Yada et al. 1990). The structure of type IX is thus strongly influenced by the tissue in which it is being expressed.

Type VI collagen is found in a number of different tissues in the body. It contains three different α-chains and forms a short, triple-helical segment only 100 nm long. There are large, disulfide-bonded, non-helical extensions that are not removed as propeptides, and fibril formation appears to involve the packing of antiparallel molecules in tetrameric units that form microfibrillar structures lacking the characteristic 67 nm banding of the main fibrillar collagens. Type VI collagen lacks the tight structure and extensive cross-linking of the fibrillar collagen and is easily extracted from the tissue in denaturing solvents. The distribution of type VI collagen in most tissues suggests a pericellular role, particularly associated with cell–matrix interactions. There is some evidence in cartilage that it is distributed principally in the pericellular region surrounding the chondrocyte, forming a lacuna bound by a dense meshwork of fine collagen fibrils that forms a basket or chondron. Type VI collagen contains several peptide sequences (RGD) that form possible sites for binding to cell receptors. It also shows properties of interaction with hyaluronan. Type VI collagen may thus participate in cell–matrix organization in a number of different ways.

Type X collagen is a short-chain collagen consisting of three identical α-chains that form a triple-helical segment of 150 nm in length. It occurs primarily in calcifying cartilage produced by hypertrophic chondrocytes in the growth plate. It has been proposed that type X collagen may have some function associated with calcification, but transgenic mice deficient in type X collagen were found to develop normally and endochondral ossification was not greatly affected. It may therefore have more of a temporary structural role in the growth plate during the transition from cartilage to bone. It is also present in a limited amount in the calcified zone at the junction of articular cartilage with the bone and its expression in articular cartilage appears to be increased in osteoarthritis.

Proteoglycans

The major proteoglycan of cartilage is aggrecan, which is of high molecular mass. Aggrecan contains a large core protein (molecular mass: approximately 250 kDa) but most of its mass is provided by the polysaccharide chains attached to it (see Fig. 2). There are about 100 chondroitin sulfate chains (molecular mass: 10–25 kDa each) and up to 50 keratan sulfate chains (molecular mass: 15 kDa each) on each aggrecan molecule and also some *O*-linked oligosaccharides and a few *N*-linked oligosaccharides. Each aggrecan molecule thus has a total molecular mass of 1.5×10^6 to 2.5×10^6 kDa and contains about 10 per cent protein and 90 per cent carbohydrate. The carbohydrate chains are all synthesized on the aggrecan core protein during post-translational glycosylation within the chondrocyte prior to its secretion into the matrix (Hardingham 1986). Proteoglycans follow pathways of synthesis in common with other secreted glycoproteins and the site of major glycosaminoglycan synthesis lies in the vesicular compartments of the medial/trans-Golgi. The mechanisms of biosynthesis are highly efficient and the time taken for protein synthesis in the rough endoplasmic reticulum to glycosaminoglycan chain synthesis and secretion from the chondrocyte is about 20–30 min.

The protein core of aggrecan is a single polypeptide chain with several subdomains of different function (Fig. 4) (Hardingham and Fosang 1992; Hardingham et al. 1992). At the *N*-terminal of the protein core there are two globular domains, G1 and G2, separated by a short extended segment (21 nm long). The G1 domain provides the site for aggregation, and has specific properties of binding to hyaluronan and a separate globular link protein. Aggregates are composed of aggrecan molecules bound to hyaluronan via their G1 domains and each hyaluronan chain can have up to a hundred or more aggrecans bound to it. The interaction of link protein with the G1 domain stabilizes its binding to hyaluronan and essentially 'locks' the aggrecan into the aggregate form. The protein structures of the G1 domain and link protein are interesting as they are closely related to each other and contain three structural motifs, one is an immunoglobulin-fold and the other two are a pair of link-modules, each of which is related to a C-lectin motif, which is found in a broad family of other proteins.

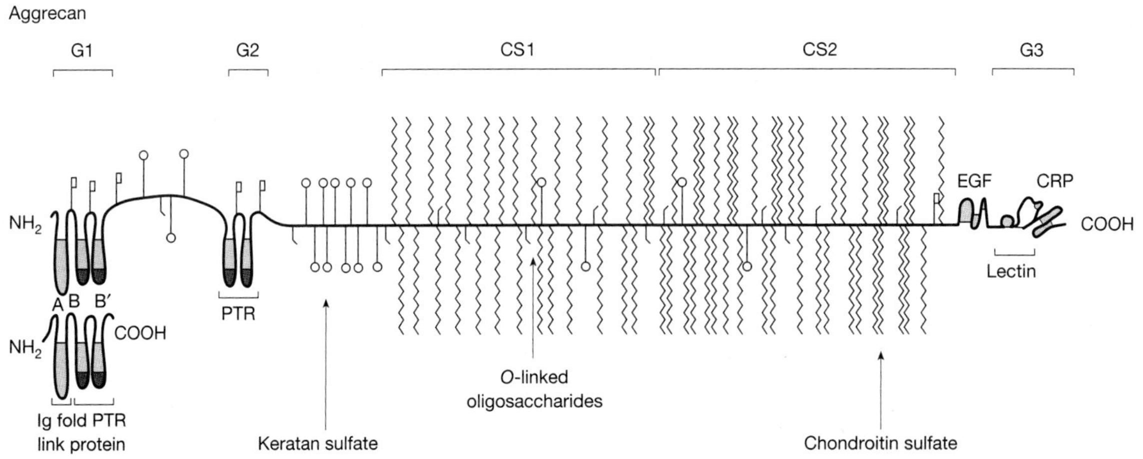

Fig. 4 The structure of the major cartilage proteoglycan, aggrecan. Aggrecan contains three disulfide-bonded globular domains, G1, G2, and G3, and has attached to it chondroitin sulfate, keratan sulfate, and *O*-, and *N*-linked oligosaccharides. Link protein is of similar structure to the G1 domain; both contain an immunoglobulin fold (Ig fold) and two link modules. Aggregation involves G1 binding to hyaluronan and this is stabilized by link protein, which binds to G1 and also to hyaluronan. G2 contains a further link module. G3 contains up to three protein motifs: an epidermal growth factor-like sequence (EGF), a mammalian type C-lectin sequence (lectin), and a complement regulatory protein sequence (CRP) (see Hardingham and Fosang 1992).

The tandemly repeated link modules in the G1 domain form the site of binding to hyaluronan and has specificity for a decasaccharide unit (hyaluronan HA10). The binding to HA is independent of calcium, in contrast with many other C-lectin interactions. The association between the G1 domain and link protein is by interaction of the immunoglobulin folds. The protein sequences of link protein are highly conserved amongst different species such that link protein from the cartilage of one species will bind and stabilize aggregate formation by aggrecan from another species. The formation of aggregates is an extracellular process. Aggrecan and link protein are synthesized and secreted together by chondrocytes, but hyaluronan is made separately at the chondrocyte cell surface. Aggregation can thus only occur after aggrecan has entered the matrix and it provides a mechanism for immobilizing it within the cartilage matrix.

The second globular domain also contains a link module similar to those tandemly repeated in the G1 domain and link protein, but it does not show any hyaluronan-binding activity (Fosang and Hardingham 1989). The main glycosaminoglycan attachment region of the proteoglycan is a long, extended protein sequence between the G2 domain and the *C*-terminal G3 domain. It is subdivided into three regions. Close to the G2 domain is a region rich in keratan sulfate, which contains a repeating sequence that varies in number in different animal species. The remaining major chondroitin sulfate attachment sequence involves two further patterns of sequence repeats. The attachment of chondroitin sulfate at serine–glycine sequences is restricted in aggrecan to these particular regions. Keratan sulfate has a wider distribution than chondroitin sulfate as it also occurs in the chondroitin sulfate-rich region and close to the G1 and G2 domains, and at some sites chains are *N*-linked rather than *O*-linked.

The globular *C*-terminal G3 domain contains sequences related to other protein families. One part is related to the mammalian type C-lectin family and is thus also distantly related to the link modules in the G1 domain. However, the G3 domain shows no HA binding properties, but interacts in a calcium dependant way with other matrix proteins. Two other epidermal growth factor-like repeat sequences may be variably expressed in the human aggrecan gene: and there is also a complement regulatory binding protein sequence. The incidence of these variations in aggrecan structure and their functional significance have yet to be determined. There are other proteoglycans structurally related to aggrecan in other tissues, which together form a family of hyaluronan-binding proteoglycans. These include versican in dermis, loose connective tissue, and smooth muscle, and neurocan and brevican in brain tissue. They all contain structurally related G1 and G3 domains although their glycosaminoglycan attachment regions are unrelated.

Aggrecan present in cartilage contains a heterogeneous population of molecules differing in size and composition. This has two main causes: first, variations in glycosylation and chain synthesis during biosynthesis result in a polydisperse product with a considerable range of sizes, and second and more importantly, the aggrecan molecules in the cartilage matrix are subject to some proteolytic attack (Hardingham 1986). As the lifetime of each aggrecan in the matrix is quite long (months, or years in mature cartilage), the composition of molecules extracted at any one time represents a cross-section of the population from newly synthesized to the oldest molecules present. The proteolytic action results in a selective loss of *C*-terminal structures such as G3 and preferential retention of the *N*-terminal structures. This arises because the *N*-terminal G1 domain provides the binding to hyaluronan and the mechanism of anchoring aggrecan in the matrix, and it follows that cleavage of the molecule results in the shortened forms containing intact G1 domains being retained in the tissue, whereas the *C*-terminal fragments are able to diffuse out of the matrix and become lost from the tissue.

The average turnover time of aggrecan appears to become longer with age and its size distribution also becomes steadily biased towards a population containing more partially cleaved molecules. Even in young cartilage there appears to be only a proportion (perhaps 50 per cent) of aggrecan molecules with an intact G3 domain and this appears to be lower in mature tissue. There is also a marked accumulation in older tissue of fragments of low molecular weight comprising only the G1 domain.

In addition to aggrecan, articular cartilage contains two chondroitin sulfate/dermatan sulfate proteoglycans of low molecular weight, decorin and biglycan (Heinegard and Oldberg 1989; Hardingham and Venn 1993). These small proteoglycans account for only about 5 per cent of the total glycosaminoglycans in the tissue, but as they are of small size they are present in molar amounts comparable with aggrecan. In human cartilage decorin is reported to increase in abundance with age whereas biglycan decreases. Both decorin and biglycan are also broadly distributed in other connective tissues besides cartilage. They have similar-sized core proteins and are structurally related, but appear to have quite different properties and presumably different functions. Decorin and biglycan form part of a family of leucine-rich proteoglycans, which contain a common sequence repeat rich in leucine (Iozzo and Murdoch 1996). Other members of this family include fibromodulin, which also occurs in cartilage, and lumican, a keratan sulfate proteoglycan, which is in the cornea. Whereas decorin and biglycan have chondroitin/dermatan sulfate chains attached towards the *N*-terminus (one chain for decorin, two for biglycan), fibromodulin has no chondroitin sulfate but has some sulfated tyrosines in the corresponding location, and also some molecules have keratan sulfate attached to *N*-linked oligosaccharide sites within the central leucine-rich repeats. Both decorin and fibromodulin have type II collagen-binding properties and *in vitro* they delay fibrillogenesis and cause the formation of thinner fibres. *In vivo* decorin has been localized at the d and e bands of type I collagen fibres, whereas fibromodulin binds to the a and c bands (Scott 1995) and these properties are functions of the protein cores. Biglycan in contrast does not have any collagen-binding properties and appears to be distributed close to a cell surface environment (Bianco et al. 1990). Experimental production of a decorin knockout-mouse showed a fragile skin phenotype with abnormal collagen fibres, but there was no cartilage pathology (Danielson et al. 1997).

A further interesting property of decorin is its ability to bind transforming growth factor-β (Ruoslahti and Yamaguchi 1991). It may thus function as a matrix repository for this growth factor that might be released as a result of proteinase action fragmenting the decorin protein core. Transforming growth factor-β has also been shown to stimulate selectively the synthesis of decorin and biglycan and modulate the synthesis of the attached chondroitin sulfate/dermatan sulfate chains. The ability of decorin to bind transforming growth factor-β and thereby block this action may thus form part of a feedback control of decorin synthesis and control of other actions of this growth factor. The binding of transforming growth factor-β in the matrix could also provide a store of growth factor that might be released through the action of proteolytic enzymes that attack the matrix following inflammation or tissue injury.

Aggrecan turnover

Proteoglycans in the cartilage matrix are constantly turned over even in mature non-growing tissue. There is a constant slow rate of aggrecan degradation and loss, and its replacement by new synthesis. The mechanisms of turnover, involving biosynthesis by the chondrocytes and degradation in the extracellular matrix, must therefore be co-ordinated so that the tissue content of aggrecan is maintained at a constant level. The chondrocytes are responsible for controlling these events and appear to be sensitive to the aggrecan content of the matrix surrounding them, and some feedback mechanisms enable synthesis and degradation to be coregulated (Morales and Hascall 1989).

The normal turnover of aggrecan in healthy cartilage appears to involve their proteolytic cleavage in the region close to the G1 domain. This is a most important site of attack as it releases a large glycosaminoglycan-bearing fragment and separates it from its site for aggregation. This is thus an efficient mechanism for mobilizing aggrecan as it involves the minimum of enzyme action. It is important that turnover is an essentially conservative process as cleavage and release of only a small fraction of the tissue content is required at any one time so that the overall tissue content is conserved and the biomechanical properties are sustained.

Several studies of cartilage from different sources have established that a major product of normal turnover is a large aggrecan fragment that has lost its G1 domain and is thereby able to diffuse slowly out of the matrix. Investigation of the released fragments from *in vitro* experiments and those released from tissue *in vivo* into synovial fluid has identified cleavage within the interglobular domain at a single predominant site (Sandy et al. 1991; Lohmander et al. 1993). Two aggrecanase enzymes have now been cloned and shown to belong to a family of ADAM-TS proteinases (Tortorella et al. 1999, 2001). These enzymes ADAM-TS4 and ADAM-TS5 are metalloproteinases and the former is induced in chondrocytes by inflammatory cytokines, such as interleukin (IL)-1 and tumour necrosis factor (TNF) α. Matrix metalloproteinases (MMPs) are also up-regulated by these cytokines and may be involved in the degradative process, particularly in the later stages of collagen degradation. Investigation of the actions of cytokines such as IL-1 or TNFα have shown that they not only stimulate chondrocytes to degrade their matrix, but also cause an inhibition of protein synthesis. They thus have a double action in depleting articular cartilage of its aggrecan content. In the presence of IL-1 or TNFα, the aggrecan fragments released from cartilage are more extensively degraded than those released in normal turnover. The rate of aggrecan release is greatly increased and this results from a large increase in matrix proteolysis with cleavage at several additional sites within the chondroitin sulfate attachment region of aggrecan. This is by the action of the same aggrecanase enzymes that cleave within the interglobular domain. The loss of aggrecan usually precedes the damage and loss of the fibrillar collagen matrix. Other inflammatory cytokines such as oncostatin M and IL-17 have a similar action to IL-1 and TNFα and may also act synergistically with these cytokines.

The neutral MMPs are a family of enzymes that are likely to be involved in many aspects of extracellular matrix breakdown and turnover (see Table 2) (Woessner 1991; Murphy 1995). There is now a large family of cloned enzymes, including collagenases, stromelysins, and gelatinases, which together have a range of complementary actions that enable them to attack and degrade all the major matrix macromolecules, but they clearly act in conjunction with related proteinase families of membrane associated metalloproteinases MT-MMPs and the ADAM and ADAM-TS families. The main MMPs are all secreted by cells in an inactive latent form that requires activation in the extracellular matrix. The process of activation involves a structural rearrangement and proteolytic cleavage with a reduction in molecular weight to give an active enzyme. Activation can be achieved *in vitro* with trypsin, which converts the proenzyme to active enzyme directly, or with APMA (aminophenyl mercuric acetate), which catalyzes a protein rearrangement that leads to an autocatalytic cleavage and self-activation. The physiological mechanism of activation has not been fully established, but could involve one metalloproteinase activating others, as in the proposal that gelatinase is the major activator of procollagenase. Other types of proteinase such as plasminogen activator may also catalyze metalloproteinase activation. In addition to activation, control of enzyme activity is also provided by a family of natural enzyme inhibitors tissue inhibitor of metalloproteinases (TIMP)1–4, which bind to active enzymes and irreversibly inactivates them. There is normally an excess of TIMPs in the extracellular matrix so that any activated enzymes are quickly inhibited. TIMPs are produced by the cells that secrete the proenzymes and they have selective action, for example, TIMP-3 effectively inhibit aggrecanases (ADAM-TS4 and 5), which are not inhibited by other TIMPs. The extent of proteinase activity in the matrix is thus under tight control and can be regulated in several ways. First, the production of latent proenzymes is varied; second, the production and availability of various activators of the proenzymes can be varied; and third, the production of specific inhibitors can be varied. The different metalloproteinase families are also inhibited by the general proteinase inhibitors in serum, such as α_2-macroglobulin. There are thus mechanisms to prevent proteinases causing more widespread tissue damage should they escape from local control.

Growth plate

The cartilage forming the growth plate provides the site for the major longitudinal growth of the long bones of the skeleton (Iannotti 1990; Poole 1991). In macromolecular terms, it has all the attributes of cartilage, containing a dense network of predominantly type II collagen fibres and an aggrecan-rich matrix, but its cells are very different. The growth plate chondrocytes, which are produced by the continuous division of progenitor cells, progress through a rapid programme of differentiation, matrix expansion, hypertrophy, matrix calcification, and further differentiation, or cell death, which is quite unlike other chondrocytes. This process results in endochondral bone formation. In addition to being responsible for long bone growth it is a process that also occurs in fracture healing and in osteophyte formation. It therefore has an important role in the growth of the skeleton and many inherited diseases affecting skeletal development are caused by mutations in genes that are active in the growth plate.

Cartilage formation begins during embryonic development as early as 6 weeks, with the condensation and differentiation of mesenchymal cells into chondrocytes to form the main elements of the skeleton. Soon after its formation, the central portion of each cartilage rudiment calcifies and is vascularized, which leads to the formation of a bony diaphysis capped at each end by a cartilaginous epiphysis. Later in development, a secondary centre of ossification develops in each epiphysis, which segregates the region of major cartilage growth from the cartilage that will be retained as the articular surface of the joint (Fig. 5). The transverse plate of cartilage which is sandwiched between the diaphysis and epiphysis remains as the site of growth throughout development, but finally calcifies and closes at skeletal maturity, typically between the ages of 14 and 18 years. The growth plate has a polarized and stratified structure (Fig. 5) that reflects the

Table 2 The neutral metalloproteinases

Enzyme	MMP family	Matrix substrates
Collagenase 1, 2, 3	MMP-1, -8, -13	Native collagen types I, II, III, VII, and X; also aggrecan and other non-collagenous proteins
Stromelysin 1	MMP-3	Aggrecan, link protein, fibronectin, laminin, gelatins, collagens III, IV, V, and IX, procollagen peptides
Gelatinases, 72 kDa, 92 kDa	MMP-2, -9	Gelatins, collagens IV, V, VII, and X; fibronectin, elastin
Range of activity		pH 5–9
Activation		Secreted latent enzymes require activation by other proteinases
Natural inhibitors		TIMP, TIMP-2, TIMP-3
Major plasma inhibitor		α_2-macroglobulin
Chemical inhibitors		EDTA, 1:10 phenanthroline

TIMP, tissue inhibitor of metalloproteinase; EDTA, ethylenediamine tetraacetic acid.

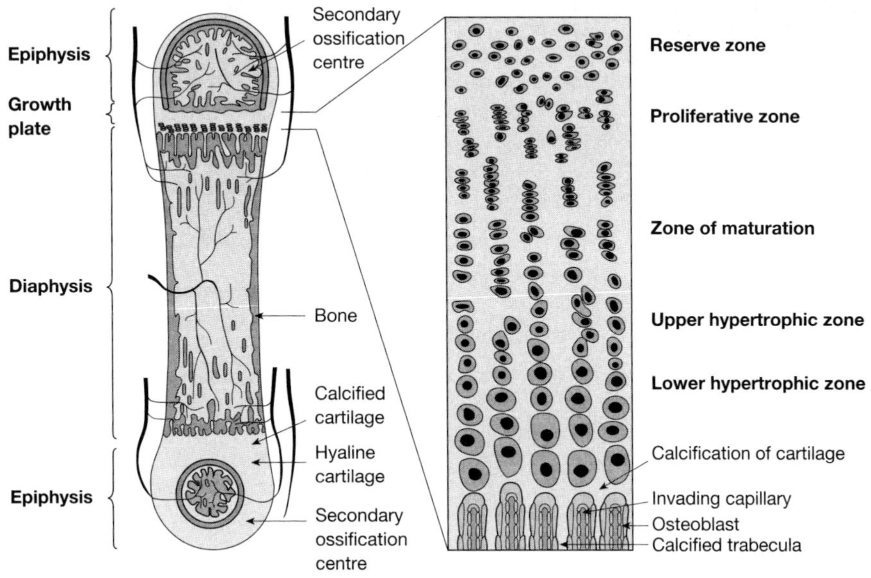

Fig. 5 The growth plate and cartilage development in a long bone at the late embryonic stage. The bone rudiment on the left shows the secondary centres of ossification that separate the growth plate cartilage from the articular cartilage. The expanded growth plate on the right shows the histologically distinct zones of the growth plate cartilage. Blood vessels penetrate the reserve zone of cartilage and the lower calcified zone, but the proliferative and hypertrophic zones are avascular. (Redrawn from Wallis 1993, with permission.)

processes that occur within it. These primarily include a sequence of cell division, matrix expansion, cell hypertrophy, matrix calcification, vascularization, resorption, and replacement by bone and this continues throughout its life. It is thus a dynamic structure, which proliferates chondrocytes at its leading edge and deposits bone at its trailing edge.

The cartilage of the growth plate has three histologically and functionally distinct zones (Fig. 5) (Iannotti 1990; Poole 1991; Cancedda et al. 1995). At the leading edge of the growth plate is the reserve zone of cartilage. It contains a sparse population of chondrocytes that are only slowly dividing and they reside in a collagen-rich matrix. This is a stable non-dynamic structure that forms the interface between the growth plate and the bone of the epiphysis. Blood vessels penetrate the reserve zone, but do not enter the adjacent proliferative zone. The progenitor cells mark the boundary between the reserve zone and the proliferative zone. These are the stem cells that generate the continuous supply of cells for cartilage growth. Columns of chondrocytes extend away from the stem cells and they deposit and expand the matrix surrounding them, thus providing the major mechanism to elongate the bone.

This highly active phase of chondrocyte maturation and matrix deposition is followed by cell hypertrophy. This is very evident histologically as the hypertrophic zone (Fig. 5), in which the cells become 5 to 10 times larger and the matrix is diminished prior to its calcification. The rate of cell division is again low in the hypertrophic zone and there is a much lower rate of synthesis of matrix macromolecules than in the proliferative zone. However, there is increased synthesis of some characteristic components of hypertrophic chondrocytes, such as alkaline phosphatase and type X collagen, and there is increased accumulation of intracellular calcium. Matrix vesicles, which are membrane-bound structures of 100–150 nm in diameter, are found in the interterritorial matrix of the hypertrophic zone. They are rich in calcium and their abundance increases towards the zone of calcification. It is undoubtedly the function of the chondrocytes in the hypertrophic zone to prepare the matrix for calcification, but the exact sequence of events and the mechanisms involved are a source of considerable debate. It is clear that hypertrophic chondrocytes accumulate calcium and produce matrix vesicles that are rich in calcium. They also produce alkaline phosphatase which can release inorganic phosphate, but what changes occur in the matrix to induce calcification are less clear. The unique expression of type X collagen in this region leads to the expectation that it may have a role in calcification; however, the development of transgenic mice that lack type X collagen but have apparently normal growth plate function suggested that it was not essential for calcification. The lowest calcified region of the hypertrophic zone forms the boundary for the penetration of blood vessels from the diaphyseal side of the growth plate and this forms an advancing front of cartilage matrix resorption and of new bone formation.

The fate of the chondrocytes in the calcified zone of the growth plate as the cartilage matrix is resorbed and bone takes its place is not completely clear (Cancedda et al. 1995). There is evidence of cell death amongst the hypertrophic chondrocytes in this region and in one model the resorption of the cartilage matrix and its replacement by bone could be caused by cells brought in by the blood vessels that penetrate into this region. However, there is also evidence that hypertrophic chondrocytes in culture can show some osteogenic potential and express matrix molecules, such as osteonectin, osteopontin, and switch from type II and type X collagen synthesis to type I, and deposit extracellular mineral. It therefore appears entirely feasible that some hypertrophic chondrocytes may survive and become osteoblasts and participate in the deposition of the growing bone. It may be that both these processes occur and that some hypertrophic chondrocytes undergo programmed cell death by apoptosis and are eliminated from the calcified zone as the matrix resorption and blood vessel invasion advances, whereas others may survive and proceed to participate in the generation of the new bone as osteoblasts. It may also be that the proportion of cells following either route varies from one site of endochondral ossification to another.

The chondrocytes in the growth plate are very sensitive to a range of growth factors including those of the insulin-like growth factor (IGF) family, the transforming growth factor (TGF)-β family (including bone morphogenic proteins), the fibroblast growth factor family, and vitamin D metabolites (Poole 1991; Cancedda et al. 1995). Some of these, such as the TGF-β family (and bone morphogenic proteins) are most active in promoting chondrocyte differentiation, whereas others, such as the fibroblast growth factors are most active in stimulating cell division, and these have little effect on fully differentiated cells. In contrast, the IGFs are very effective in stimulating the synthesis of matrix macromolecules and also suppressing matrix degradation and they thus have a very positive anabolic effect. The main effect of growth hormone on cartilage is the stimulation of local production of IGFs. The most rapid phase of growth is associated with sexual maturation at puberty and is driven by the hormonal changes and the accompanying increase in systemic growth factor production. Chondrocytes of the growth plate differ from other chondrocytes in that they are sensitive to vitamin D metabolites. These are essential for normal mineralization, and vitamin D deficiency, which causes rickets, is characterized by a slowing down of mineralization and an expansion of the hypertrophic zone of the growth plate. At the cellular level, the chondrocytes fail to accumulate calcium and there is poor production of matrix vesicles. The failure of calcification and bone formation causes widening of the growth plate, which leads to instability and deformed growth.

Investigation of many families that show inherited skeletal abnormalities, such as chondrodysplasias, has now identified a range of single gene defects that are responsible (Wallis 1993; Cancedda et al. 1995; Olsen 1995). Many of these are in the type II collagen gene in families with Kniest dysplasia, some forms of Stickler's syndrome, with spondyloepiphyseal dysplasia, and with hypochondrogenesis. Others have been identified in type IX collagen, type XI collagen, and in metaphyseal chondrodysplasia type Schmid in type X collagen. The sites of mutations in these various genetic diseases involve substitutions, deletions, and frame shifts and each family group contains a different form. The range of phenotype is also very variable from mild to severe and there is no clear pattern of correlation between the site of the mutation, or its form, and the phenotype that results. Several forms of multiple epiphyseal dysplasia and pseudoachondrodysplasia have also been linked to the cartilage oligomeric matrix protein gene (Deere et al. 1999); this produces a thrombospondin-like protein in cartilage matrix and changes in its structure may disrupt its calcium dependant collagen interactions (Holden et al. 2001). Some forms of hypochondrodysplasia are linked to polymorphisms in the IGF-1 gene. There are therefore a range of defects in genes that form part of the matrix or are involved in the processes that lead to the development of the matrix that can result in inherited skeletal abnormalities and with current techniques of molecular biology many more of these will be identified.

The basic process of chondrocyte differentiation, matrix expansion, matrix calcification, and its replacement by bone is not exclusive to the growth plate. A similar process occurs in fracture healing where the initial union in the fractured bone is made by chondrogenic development at the site of periosteal damage, which expands and forms the fracture callous, before it is eventually resorbed as cortical bone and healing becomes complete. The formation of osteophytes in synovial joints close to the articular surface also proceeds through an initial chondrophytic stage, often beginning at the site of the cartilage–bone junction. The differentiation of chondrocytes at this site forms a cartilage growth or chondrophyte, which then calcifies and becomes remodelled into a bone. It is only subsequently that the osteophyte fuses with the main cortical bone. Osteophytes therefore form not as direct outgrowths of the bone, but from separate, small, osteogenic centres that produce through a cartilage-mediated process, similar to that of the growth plate, a bony buttress joined with the main bone shaft.

Age-related change in articular cartilage

Age-related changes in articular cartilage are distinct from those characteristic of osteoarthritis, but give clues to the increasing susceptibility of cartilage to damage in old age. Age determines both the composition of the extracellular matrix as well as the distribution of chondrocytes and their response to external factors such as cytokines (see Table 3) (Hardingham and Bayliss 1990). Zonal changes in the distribution of chondrocytes are seen with ageing although the total number of chondrocytes shows little variation. Chondrocytes in the superficial cells mostly disappear with some increase in the cellular content of the deeper layers. Numerous changes in the extracellular matrix with ageing may compromise function. With old age there is a decrease in hydration of the matrix with a corresponding increase in compressive stiffness. This may have implications for the remarkable property of cartilage to undergo reversible deformation upon loading and may result in increased transmission of forces to sub-chondral structures. Loss of hydration is probably secondary to changes in the matrix components. Proteoglycan aggregation is adversely affected by proteolytic damage to link protein and a decrease in the available binding sites on hyaluronan; the latter is the result of binding of the free binding region domains that represent the limited digestion product of proteolysis of the glycosaminoglycan attachment region of core protein. Aggregation may also affect pore size distribution and solute permeability. Other changes observed include increasing proteoglycan heterogeneity with a general reduction in proteoglycan size accompanied by an increased ratio of keratan sulfate to chondroitin sulfate. Although the concentration of hyaluronan rises with age, this results from the gradual accumulation of partially degraded hyaluronan, rather than from a higher rate of synthesis. Age-related changes in the response of human cartilage to cytokines, especially to IL-1, have been documented with maturation, but little consistent change in response in old age has been noted. However, the reality is liable to be a complex interaction of endogenous anabolic and catabolic factors that are acting in articular cartilage in any age and considerable difficulties confront the investigator attempting to study their action *in vitro*.

Table 3 Age-related changes in articular cartilage following skeletal maturation

Chondrocytes	Loss of most superficial chondrocytes, some increase in the number of deeper cells
Extracellular matrix	Decreased hydration with greater compressive stiffness of the matrix; increase in stable collagen cross-links
Proteoglycans	Aggrecan of smaller average size and higher keratan sulfate/chondroitin sulfate ratio, increased content of free hyaluronan binding region domain (G1); content of decorin may increase and biglycan decrease
Hyaluronan and link protein	Increased hyaluronan content, but hyaluronan chains of shorter length, increased proteolytic damage of link protein

Cartilage response to cytokines and growth factors

IL-1 and TNFα have generally been shown to have major effects on articular cartilage, including the inhibition of proteoglycan synthesis and the stimulation of matrix proteoglycan degradation (Fig. 6). Studies with human cartilage have found only weak effects on matrix degradation, which is in contrast to results obtained using immature animal cartilages (Hardingham et al. 1992). Human cartilage studied *in vitro* has been found to respond typically with no significant increase in the release of proteoglycan over several days in culture, or by showing a delayed response with increased release after about 6 days in culture. This may correspond to a low level of activation of the catabolic process, rather than no activation at all. Aggrecan biosynthesis is much more sensitive to cytokine action than aggrecan catabolism and the effects are much more consistent amongst cartilages from human and animal sources. Human IL-1 causes a dose-dependent reduction in proteoglycan synthesis in animal and human cartilage and human TNFα is also effective. The sensitivity of human articular cartilage to IL-1 and TNFα declines with age. The effects on aggrecan synthesis show that there is no lack of penetration of the cytokines to the chondrocytes in human cartilage, but that some steps in the response of the chondrocytes that lead to increased matrix degradation are less stimulated in human cartilage than that from many animal sources. This might involve the production of less proenzyme, or of less activator of the proenzymes, or an increase

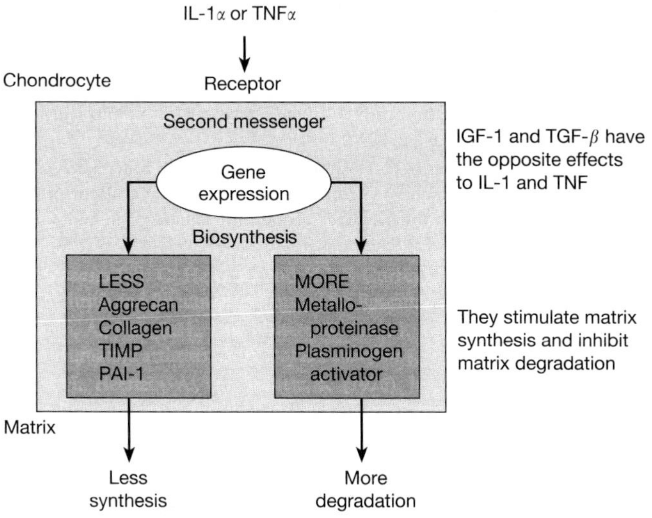

Fig. 6 Effects of cytokines and growth factors on articular chondrocytes.

in the inhibitors of the enzymes. Any of these effects may suppress the extent of proteolytic action and hence the rate of proteoglycan degradation and release from the matrix. This may be compounded by the dense collagenous network in human cartilage, which is less permeable to aggrecan fragments than in young animal cartilages and therefore requires more catabolism to give a significant increase in aggrecan release. The effects of IL-1 and TNFα are also mimicked and enhanced by IL-17, oncostatin M (IL-6 family member), and fibronectin fragments, but the actions are inhibited by anti-inflammatory cytokines, IL-4 and IL-13 (Cleaver et al. 2001). It has been speculated that the effects of cytokines on human articular cartilage in joint disease, which is typically slow and progressive may result primarily from shutting off aggrecan synthesis, rather than from any increase in matrix degradation.

Of the growth factors, IGF-1 is considered to be the major mediator of cartilage growth. As well as stimulating synthesis of proteoglycans, it may also reduce the rate of proteoglycan catabolism (Fig. 3), although human articular chondrocytes show a decrease in responsiveness to IGF-1 with increasing age. Other growth factors such as epidermal growth factor, fibroblast growth factor, and TGF-β have been shown to potentiate the effect of IGF-1 on proteoglycan synthesis. IGF-1 also inhibits the effects of the inflammatory cytokines, such as IL-1 and TNFα on chondrocytes.

TGF-β has been shown to enhance the synthesis of small proteoglycans (decorin or biglycan) relative to the large aggrecan proteoglycan. In explant cultures of cartilage from dogs that have undergone cruciate ligament transection, there was selectively more synthesis and a higher content of small proteoglycans, suggesting that TGF-β may be responsible in part for the increased activation of chondrocytes in experimental osteoarthritis (Venn et al. 1995).

In chronic rheumatoid arthritis TNFα has been successfully identified as a therapeutic target (Elliot et al. 1994). Neutralizing, humanized, monoclonal antibody to TNFα delivered to patients was effective in relieving clinical and laboratory parameters of disease activity, and the benefit was sustained over 1–3 months, after which there was a relapse. This suggested that TNFα was an important cytokine in driving the chronic arthritic process and also that IL-1 production in the joint was largely caused by TNFα, rather than vice versa and treatment with neutralizing TNFα antibodies has been shown to have great benefit to patients. In animal models of arthritis the treatment was shown to suppress inflammatory cell infiltration into the joint and reduce joint swelling, but it is not yet clear how far it can protect articular cartilage or reverse the damage. IL-1 receptor antagonist is a natural inhibitor of IL-1 and forms part of a biological mechanism controlling IL-1 action. Blocking IL-1 action with injections of recombinant IL-1 receptor antagonist has also been investigated in experimental arthritis, but very high doses are required to achieve any effect (Lewthwaite et al. 1995). One way in which the action of TNFα is controlled locally in tissues is by the release from the cell surface of the binding domains of TNFα receptors. The released domains not only no longer function as receptors, but also act as soluble ligands that bind and inactivate the available TNFα. The release of such receptors appears to be under the control of a cell surface metalloproteinase. The action of TNFα and IL-1 on articular chondrocytes is thus likely to be controlled, not merely by their local abundance, but also by a network of interactions, involving changes in the expression of receptors, the release from cells of soluble receptors and IL-1 receptor antagonist. Their actions are also modulated by the competing effects of local anti-inflammatory cytokines and local and circulating growth factors.

References

Arakoski, J., Kivaranta, I., Jurvelin, J., Tammi, M., and Helminen, H. (1993). Long distance running causes site dependent decrease of cartilage glycosaminoglycan content in the knee joint of beagle dogs. *Arthritis and Rheumatism* **36**, 1451–9.

Bianco, P., Fisher, L.W., Young, M.F., Termine, T.D., and Robey, P.G. (1990). Expression and localization of the two small proteoglycans decorin and biglycan in developing human skeletal and non skeletal tissues. *Journal of Histochemistry and Cytochemistry* **38**, 1549–63.

Buckwalter, J.A. (1995). Osteoarthritis and articular cartilage use, disuse and abuse: experimental studies. *Journal of Rheumatology* **22** (Suppl. 43), 13–15.

Cancedda, R., Cancedda, F.D., and Castagnola, P. (1995). Chondrocyte differentiation. *International Review of Cytology* **159**, 265–359.

Cleaver, C.S., Rowan, A.D., and Cawston, T.E. (2001). Interleukin-13 blocks the release of collagen from bovine nasal cartilage treated with proinflammatory cytokines. *Annals of the Rheumatic Diseases* **60**, 150–7.

Danielson, K.G., Baribault, H., Holmes, D.F., Graham, H., Kadler, K.E., and Lozzo, R.V. (1997). Targeted disruption of decorin leads to abnormal collagen morphology and skin fragility. *Journal of Cell Biology* **136**, 729–43.

Deere, M., Sandford, T., Francomano, C.A., Daniels, K., and Hecht, J.T. (1999). Identification of nine novel mutations in cartilage oligomeric matrix protein in patients with pseudoachondroplasia and multiple epiphyseal dysplasia. *American Journal of Medical Genetics* **85**, 486–90.

Elliot, M.J. et al. (1994). Randomised double-blind comparison of chimaeric monoclonal antibody to tumour necrosis factor (cA2) versus placebo in rheumatoid arthritis. *Lancet* **344**, 1105–10.

Eyre, D.R. and Wu, J.-J. (1995). Collagen structure and cartilage matrix integrity. *Journal of Rheumatology* **22** (Suppl. 43), 82–5.

Eyre, D.R., Wu, J.J., Woods, P.E., and Weis, M.A. (1991). The cartilage collagens and joint degeneration. *British Journal of Rheumatology* **30** (Suppl. 1), 10–15.

Fosang, A.J. and Hardingham, T. (1989). Isolation of the *N*-terminal globular domains from cartilage proteoglycans. *Biochemistry Journal* **261**, 801–9.

Hardingham, T. (1986). Structure and biosynthesis of proteoglycans. *Rheumatology* **10**, 143–83.

Hardingham, T. (1990). Degenerative joint disease. In *The Metabolic and Molecular Basis of Acquired Disease* (ed. R.D. Cohen, B. Lewis, K.G. Albert, and A.M. Denman), pp. 1851–69. London: Baillière Tindall.

Hardingham, T. and Bayliss, M. (1990). Proteoglycans of articular cartilage: changes in aging and in joint disease. *Seminars in Arthritis and Rheumatism* **20**, 12–33.

Hardingham, T. and Fosang, A.J. (1992). Proteoglycans: many forms, many functions. *FASEB Journal* **6**, 861–70.

Hardingham, T., Heng, B.C., and Gribbon, P. (1999). New approaches to the investigation of hyaluronan networks. *Biochemical Society Transactions* **27**, 124–7.

Hardingham, T.E. and Venn, G. (1993). Chondroitin sulfate/dermatan sulfate proteoglycans from cartilage: aggrecan, decorin and biglycan. In *Dermatan Sulfate Proteoglycans: Chemistry, Biology, Chemical Pathology* (ed. J.E. Scott), pp. 207–17. London: Portland Press.

Hardingham, T.E., Bayliss, M.T., Rayan, V., and Noble, D.P. (1992). Effects of growth factors and cytokines on proteoglycan turnover in articular cartilage. *British Journal of Rheumatology* **31** (Suppl. 1), 1–6.

Heinegard, D. and Oldberg, A. (1989). Structure and biology of cartilage and bone matrix noncollagenous macromolecules. *FASEB Journal* **3**, 2042–51.

Holden, P., Meadows, R.S., Chapman, K.L., Grant, M.E., Kadler, K.E., and Briggs, M.D. (2001). Cartilage oligomeric matrix protein interacts with type IX collagen and disruptions to these interactions identify a pathogenetic mechanism in a bone dysplasia family. *Journal of Biological Chemistry* **276**, 6046–55.

Iannotti, J.P. (1990). Bone disease. *Orthopedic Clinics of North America* **21**, 1–17.

Iozzo, R.V. and Murdoch, A.D. (1996). Proteoglycans of the extracellular environment: clues from the gene and protein side offer novel perspectives in molecular diversity and function. *FASEB Journal* **10**, 598–614.

Jacenko, O. and Olsen, B.R. (1995). Transgenic mouse models in studies of skeletal disorders. *Journal of Rheumatology* **22** (Suppl. 43), 39–41.

Kiviranta, I., Tammi, M., Jurvelin, J., Arakoski, J., Saamanen, A.-M., and Helminen, H.J. (1992). Articular cartilage thickness and glycosaminoglycan distribution in the canine knee joint after strenuous running exercise. *Clinical Orthopedics* **283**, 302–5.

Lewthwaite, J. et al. (1995). The role of TNFα in the induction of antigen-induced arthritis in the rabbit and the anti-arthritic effect of species-specific TNFα neutralising monoclonal antibodies. *Annals of the Rheumatic Diseases* **54**, 366–74.

Lohmander, L.S., Neame, P.J., and Sandy, J.D. (1993). The structure of aggrecan fragments in human synovial fluid: evidence that aggrecanase mediates cartilage degradation in inflammatory joint disease, joint injury and osteoarthritis. *Arthritis and Rheumatism* **36**, 1214–22.

Morales, T.I. and Hascall, V.C. (1989). Factors involved in the regulation of proteoglycan metabolism in articular cartilage. *Arthritis and Rheumatism* **32**, 1197–201.

Mow, V.C. and Lai, W.M. (1980). Recent developments in synovial fluid biomechanics. *Society for Industrial and Applied Mathematics Review* **22**, 275–317.

Muir, H. and Hardingham, T.E. (1986). Biochemistry of connective tissue. In *Copeman's Textbook of Rheumatic Diseases* (ed. J.T. Scott), pp. 177–98. Edinburgh: Churchill Livingstone.

Murphy, G. (1995). Matrix metalloproteinases and their inhibitors. *Acta Orthopaedica Scandinavica* **66** (Suppl. 26), 55–60.

Nishimura, I., Muragaki, Y., and Olsen, B.R. (1989). Tissue-specific forms of type IX collagen-proteoglycan arise from the use of two widely separated promotors. *Journal of Biological Chemistry* **264**, 20033–41.

Olsen, B.R. (1995). New insights into the function of the collagens from genetic analysis. *Current Biology* **7**, 720–7.

Poole, A.R. (1991). Cartilage assembly and mineralization. In *Cartilage: Molecular Aspects* (ed. B. Hall and S. Newman), pp. 179–211. Boca Raton FL: CRC Press.

Ruoslahti, E. and Yamaguchi, Y. (1991). Proteoglycans as modulators of growth factor activities. *Cell* **64**, 867–9.

Sandy, J.D., Neame, P.J., Boynton, R.E., and Flannery, C.R. (1991). Catabolism of aggrecan in cartilage explants: identification of a major cleavage site within the interglobular domain. *Journal of Biological Chemistry* **266**, 8683–5.

Scott, J.E. (1995). Extracellular matrix, supramolecular organisation and shape. *Journal of Anatomy* **187**, 259–69.

Stockwell, R.A. and Meachim, G. (1979). The chondrocytes. In *Adult Articular Cartilage* (ed. M.A.R. Freeman), pp. 115–22. London: Pitman Medical.

Tortorella, M.D. et al. (1999). Purification and cloning of aggrecanase-1: a member of the ADAM-TS family. *Science* **284**, 1664–6.

Tortorella, M.D., Malfait, A.-M., Deccico, C., and Arner, E. (2001). The role of ADAM-TS4 (aggrecanase-1) and ADAM-TS5 (aggrecanase-2) in a model of cartilage degradation. *Osteoarthritic Cartilage* **9**, 539–52.

Venn, G., Billingham, M.E.J., and Hardingham, T.E. (1995). Increased proteoglycan synthesis in cartilage in experimental canine osteoarthritis does not reflect a permanent change in chondrocyte phenotype. *Arthritis and Rheumatism* **38**, 525–31.

Vuorio, E. and de Crombrugge, B. (1990). The family of collagenases. *Annual Review of Biochemistry* **59**, 837–72.

Wallis, G.A. (1993). Here today, bone tomorrow. *Current Biology* **3**, 687–9.

Woessner, J.F. (1991). Matrix metalloproteinases and their inhibitors in connective tissue remodelling. *FASEB Journal* **5**, 2145–54.

Wu, J.-J., Woods, P.E., and Eyre, D.R. (1992). Identification of the cross-linking sites in bovine cartilage type IX collagen reveals an anti-parallel type II–type IX molecule relationship and type IX–type XI bonding. *Journal of Biological Chemistry* **267**, 23007–14.

Yada, T., Suzuki, S., Kobayashi, K., Hoshino, T., Horie, K., and Kimata, K. (1990). Occurrence in chick embryo vitreous humour of a type IX collagen proteoglycan with an extraordinarily large chondroitin sulfate chain and a short α1 polypeptide. *Journal of Biological Chemistry* **265**, 6992–9.

3.4 Bone in health and disease

Roger Smith

Bone is a metabolically active tissue that is formed, removed, and replaced throughout life. These processes depend on bone cells, whose activities are determined by many factors. They include genetic, mechanical, nutritional, and hormonal influences and a host of short-acting cellular messages, including growth factors, collectively termed cytokines. This chapter deals with the normal physiology of bone and outlines the changes in specific skeletal disorders. All aspects of bone physiology are dealt with by Bilezikian et al. (1996). Avioli and Krane (1998) and Favus (1999) give comprehensive accounts of metabolic bone disease. Advances in molecular and genetic knowledge have recently been reviewed by Econs (2000).

Bone in health

Structure

Bone consists of cells and an extracellular mineralized matrix (35 per cent organic and 65 per cent inorganic). About 90 per cent of the organic component is type I collagen. The remainder includes many non-collagen products of the osteoblast, such as osteocalcin, osteonectin, and proteoglycans. The mineral is present mainly as a complex mixture of calcium and phosphate in the form of hydroxyapatite.

Two anatomical types of bone may be defined: trabecular (cancellous) and cortical. The proportion of these in bones normally differs: for instance the vertebral bodies are predominantly trabecular and the shafts of the long bones are cortical.

This distribution is relevant both to the functions of the bone and to skeletal disorders such as osteoporosis. In trabecular bone, there are more metabolically active surfaces in a given volume than in cortical bone. The basic multicellular units (see below) act on the surfaces of trabecular bone and through resorbing channels (cutting cones) in cortical bones. The fine structure of bone is described by Boyde (1972).

Bone is often thought to be inert because of its structural rigidity and persistence after death, and also to be composed entirely of chalk because it contains 99 per cent of the body's calcium. Although both assumptions are superficially reasonable, neither is correct.

Bone cells

Conventional histological sections of bone demonstrate three types of bone cell, which are clearly different (Plates 52 and 53): osteoblasts, which may

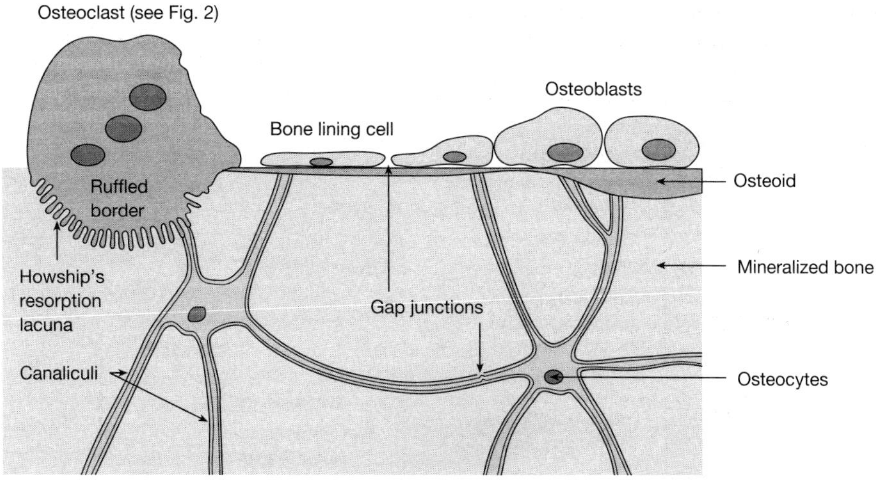

Fig. 1 A diagram of bone structure to show the relationship of different cell types.

be plump and apparently active, or flat and apparently inactive (otherwise called bone-lining cells); multinucleated osteoclasts, which most often occupy areas of resorption; and osteocytes within their lacunas in the mineralized bone, apparently in contact with other osteocytes and bone cells through their extensions in the canaliculi (Plate 53 and Fig. 1). All these cells may be seen together in one microscopic field. They are often in close contact with cells of the bone marrow, which contain their precursors and also bring them into close relationship with the immune system. These cells and the mineralized organic matrix have almost infinite possibilities for exchange of information. It is the complexity of bone that provides both the challenge and the fascination for those interested in its disorders. Histological techniques have been developed to study the sequential events enacted by teams of bone cells in so-called basic multicellular units (Eriksen et al. 1989). The techniques of cell biology are used to study the origin and functions of different types of cells and the communications between them. These approaches provide different information: the histology tells us about the temporal events in bone as a tissue whereas the cell biology provides clues about the activities of the different cells, albeit in artificial culture systems.

The cells of bone occupy a central position in its physiology. Osteoblasts are one particular cell form derived from the mesenchymal stromal cell system; fibroblasts and adipocytes are others. Osteoclasts are haemopoietic in origin. The marrow contains precursor cells for the stromal and haematopoietic system; currently these are referred to as fibroblast colony forming units and granulocyte–macrophage colony forming units, respectively (see below). The osteocytes that are imbedded in the mineralized bone are derived from osteoblasts, as are the bone-lining cells. All bone cells communicate with each other and control bone modelling during growth and remodelling throughout life. The constant processes of osteoclastic bone resorption and osteoblastic bone formation are closely linked and take place in basic multicellular units. The cellular cycle of such a unit (Fig. 2a) begins with activation of multinucleate osteoclasts from their macrophage-like mononuclear precursors; osteoclasts produce resorption (Howship's) lacunas (Fig. 1) on the surface of trabecular bone, or cutting cones in cortical bone. These are similar processes. In cancellous (trabecular) bone, the basic multicellular unit may be looked upon as a cortical multicellular unit sectioned through the middle. Resorption is followed by a reversal phase, during which a cement line is deposited, and then the formation by osteoblasts of new bone matrix, which is subsequently mineralized. In the young adult, when the bone mass is constant, the amount of new bone formed equals that resorbed; in childhood more bone is formed than resorbed; and in later years there is an imbalance between these two processes in favour of resorption, leading to osteoporosis. The timescale of the remodelling cycle is approximately established, although estimates differ (Fig. 2b).

Eriksen et al. (1989) give details of histomorphometrical findings in normal subjects and in those with metabolic bone disease. They point out that bone is one of the few tissues in which a time marker may be incorporated, and that histomorphometry can separate alteration in cellular activity from changes in cell number. The turnover of bone at the tissue level is determined by the activation frequency of basic multicellular units and the functional rates of individual cells. The mechanism of bone loss is different in different disorders. There are many unsolved mysteries about basic multicellular units. One is what factors lead to activation of the osteoclasts to initiate the resorbing cycle. Another is how cells communicate with each other (see later). However, it is becoming clear that many activities of the osteoclast depend on those of the osteoblast, which is a dominant cell in the skeletal scene.

Osteoblasts, osteocytes, and bone-lining cells

Osteoblasts (Plate 52) have many important functions (Fig. 3). It is possible that the functions are divided between them. They respond to endocrine factors, both systemic and local (cytokines), and to mechanical forces. They synthesize the organic bone matrix (mainly collagen) and non-collagen proteins, and they control bone mineralization. Importantly, they also appear to direct the activity of other cell types, particularly the osteoclasts. In this respect they may also activate the bone-resorbing cycle.

Osteocytes (Plate 53) occupy lacunas within the mineralized bone. They communicate with each other by gap junctions via processes within the canaliculi and probably have an important function in the detection of, and response to, mechanical forces within mineralized bone. Bone-lining cells, a form of flattened, inactive osteoblast, cover endosteal surfaces and bone trabeculas, being separated from each other by gap junctions. They may also isolate bone fluid (if this exists) from the general extracellular-fluid compartment.

Osteoclasts

These multinucleated cells are derived from precursors in the haemopoietic system (granulocyte–macrophage colony forming units). They resorb bone by attaching themselves to its surfaces and forming a seal to isolate their area of activity (Fig. 4). Within this sealed zone they produce a very acid environment, with the aid of a proton pump linked to the enzyme carbonic anhydrase II, within which digestion of whole bone by lysosomal enzymes occurs. Absence of carbonic anhydrase II is linked to a rare form of osteopetrosis (see later). Osteoclasts have receptors to calcitonin, which directly suppresses their activity, and also possibly to oestrogens, but not, so far as is known, to any other hormone. However, they do respond to prostaglandins. The resorptive effects of parathyroid hormone and of

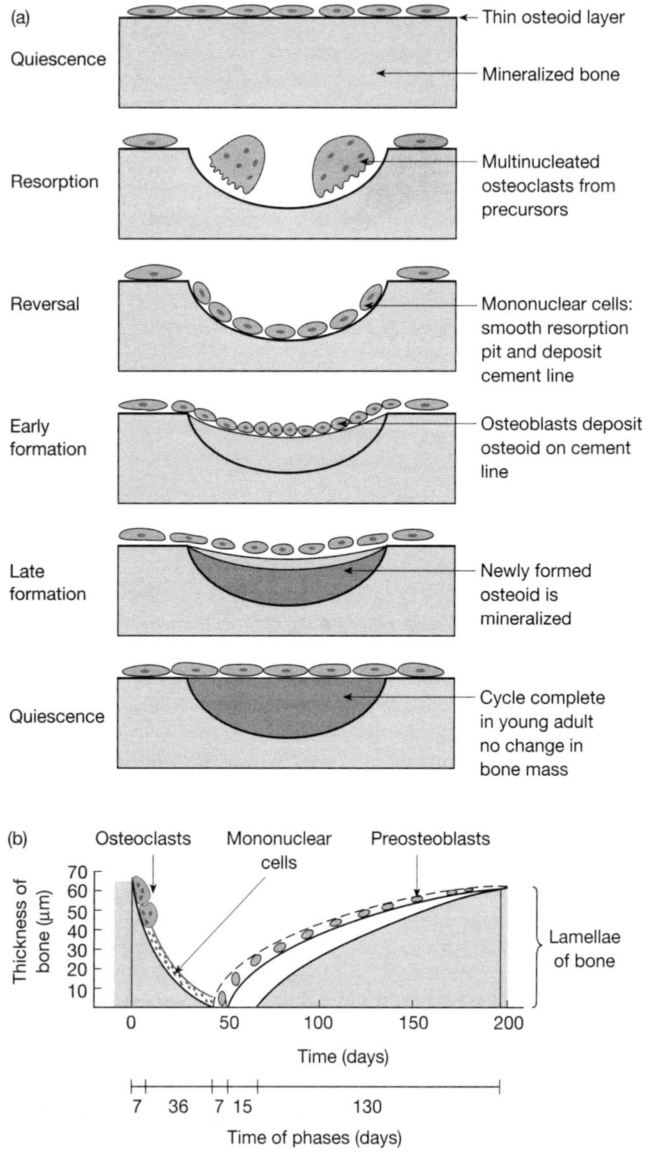

Fig. 2 (a) The remodelling events on the surface of bone during a bone multicellular-unit sequence. (b) The time sequences of these events from 20 young normal individuals [modified from Eriksen et al. (1989)].

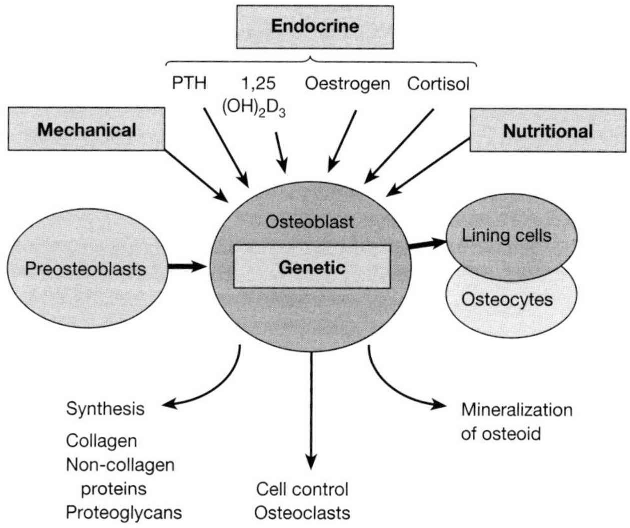

Fig. 3 The central position of the osteoblast in bone physiology. Broad arrows show the origin of osteoblasts from preosteoblasts, themselves derived from stromal cell (fibroblast colony forming unit) lineage, and of the lining cells and osteocytes.

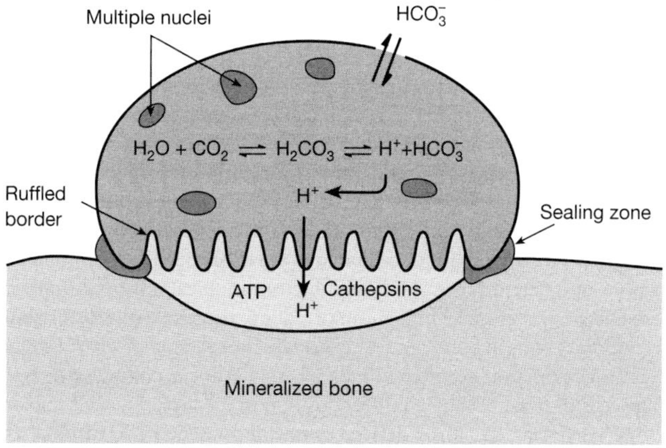

Fig. 4 A diagram of the main features and functions of the osteoclast.

1,25-dihydroxycholecalciferol (1,25$(OH)_2D_3$) are probably mediated through the osteoblast.

Bone formation

The factors that control bone formation are complex and not fully understood, but must work largely through the osteoblast. Osteoprogenitor cells, the precursors of osteoblasts, are found in the periosteum and the endosteal surfaces close to the bone marrow. The local remodelling stimulus for new bone formation comes from some aspect of bone resorption, which could, for instance, be polypeptide growth factors or morphogenetic proteins liberated by this process. The differentiation of a mesenchymal stromal cell into an osteoblast is particularly dependent on a specific transcription factor CBFAI.

The activities of bone cells are influenced by cytokines. A cytokine may be defined as a peptide, produced by a cell, that acts as an autocrine, paracrine, or endocrine mediator. In this sense, the definition includes a large number of substances of which many can be shown to have effects on bone and cartilage metabolism. Such effects have been demonstrated principally in experimental (and artificial) conditions and their physiological role is largely unknown. Many cytokines have alternative names and multiple actions, with synergism and antagonism; Table 1 provides examples of cytokines identified in bone matrix and produced by bone cells.

The local factors that control osteoblastic activity are of considerable importance. Only some of these have been identified. The osteoblastic activity that follows on osteoclastic bone resorption is thought by some to be stimulated by the production of local factors, either from the osteoclast itself or from the bone it has resorbed. It is now recognized that such bone contains many stimulating polypeptides and important morphogenetic proteins (see later). The situation is complex, as for example, transforming growth factor-β appears to belong to a family of multifunctional regulatory peptides, and bone is probably its most abundant source. Not only do osteoblasts synthesize this factor but they also have high-affinity receptors for it, and are mitogenically stimulated by it. Growth factors may be defined as polypeptides with mitogenic activity, although they also affect

Table 1 Cytokines, growth factors, and other mediators with effects on bone and those demonstrated in bone matrix and/or produced by bone cells

(a) Effective on bone
Interleukins (ILs)
Tumour necrosis factors (TNFs)
Interferons (IFN)
Growth factors (GF)
Haemopoietic and colony stimulating factors (CSFs)
Granulocyte (G-CSF)
Macrophage (M-CSF)
Granulocyte–macrophage (GM-CSF)
Osteoclast controlling factors
Osteoprotegerin (OPG/OCIF)[a]
Osteoclast differentiation factor (ODF; RANK-L)[a]
Others
(b) In bone matrix and/or produced by bone cells
Interleukins IL-1, IL-6, IL-8
Tumour necrosis factors
TNFα (cachectin)
TNFβ (lymphotoxin)
Platelet derived growth factors
Insulin-like growth factors (somatomedins) (IGF)
Fibroblast growth factors (FGF)
Transforming growth factors (TGF) α and β
Bone morphogenetic proteins (BMP)
Epidermal growth factor (EGF)
M-CSF
GM-CSF
OPG
ODF (RANK-L)
Parathyroid hormone related protein (PTHrP)

[a] For synonyms see text.

Table 2 Factors regulating osteoclast activity

Factor	Effect
Systemic hormones	
Calcitonin	Direct temporary inhibition
Parathyroid hormone and PTHrP	Indirect stimulation of differentiation and activity, via osteoblasts
1,25(OH)$_2$D	Stimulates differentiation and activity Probably indirect via osteoblasts
Oestrogens	Complex effects
Thyroid hormones	Increase bone resorption
Local hormones (cytokines)	
Interleukin 1 (IL-1)	Potent stimulator at all phases of osteoclast formation
Interleukin 6 (IL-6)	Osteoclast main source of IL-6 IL-6 also weakly stimulate osteoclast formation
Lymphotoxin and tumour necrosis factor (TNF)	Functionally related to IL-1
Colony stimulating factors (CSF and M-CSF)	Required for normal osteoclast formation
ODF (OPGL; RANK-L)[a]	Stimulates osteoclast bone resorption; acts on cells of osteoclast lineage
Osteoprotegerin (OPG)	Inhibits osteoclast differentiation and activity
Interferon γ (IFNγ)	Inhibits osteoclast formation
Transforming growth factor-β (TGF-β)	Complex species specific effects In most systems inhibits osteoclast formation and differentiation
Other factors	
Retinoids	Direct stimulation of osteoclasts
Transforming growth factor-α (TGF-α)	Powerful stimulation of osteoclasts
Prostaglandins	Complex effects species specific
Glucocorticoids	Variable effects on osteoclast-mediated bone resorption

[a] For synonyms see text.

the function of differentiated cells. They are produced by cells and, therefore, they may also be included under the general heading of cytokines. Important growth factors in bone matrix that have originated from cells within bone (Table 1) include platelet-derived growth factors, fibroblast growth factors, insulin-like growth factors (or somatomedins), transforming growth factors, and other osteoinductive factors.

Bone resorption

Osteoclasts are controlled by systemic and local hormones but there is no direct evidence that they are influenced by mechanical stress. Calcitonin directly inhibits the osteoclast, temporarily abolishes the active, ruffled border, and suppresses the generation of new osteoclasts. Bone resorption is increased by parathyroid hormone and 1,25(OH)$_2$D$_3$. As the osteoclast does not contain receptors to either of these hormones it is proposed that the resorbing activity is mediated via the osteoblast. Again, the messages that the osteoblasts use to turn on the resorbing activity of the osteoclast are largely unknown. The number and activity of the osteoclasts is increased by a variety of cytokines produced by lymphocytes or monocytes (lymphokines and monokines, respectively) and by peptide growth factors (epidermal growth factors, transforming growth factors). They are also stimulated by a group of factors previously called osteoclast-activating factors (see below) (Table 2).

Communication between bone cells

Although many bone hormones and cytokines regulate the differentiation and activity of the osteoclasts, it now seems that the two most important final effectors are osteoclast differentiation factor (ODF, RANK-L) and macrophage colony stimulating factor, M-CSF. The osteoclast possesses a receptor known as RANK which binds to ODF produced by the osteoblast: ODF is thus referred to as RANK ligand (RANK-L). This binding produces rapid differentiation of osteoclast precursor cells, increased functional activity and reduced apoptosis of mature osteoclasts. Osteoblast lineage cells also produce a decoy receptor known as osteoprotegerin (OPG), another member of the TNF receptor superfamily. This also binds to ODF, which is then also called OPGL. Osteoclast formation and activity is importantly determined by the ratio of OPG to OPGL. Figure 5 suggests how osteoclast stromal cells may regulate osteoclast differentiation and function (Yasuda et al. 1999).

Bone mass

The eventual size and density of the skeleton and its development during the early years of life is influenced by important genetic factors. This genetic background is modified by mechanical stress, nutrition, the systemic effects of hormones, and by local factors produced by the bone cells themselves (Fig. 6). The relative contributions of these may vary with age (Fig. 7). Recent investigations suggest that the rate of bone loss as well as peak bone mass may be genetically determined, that adequate calcium intake conserves bone mass at all ages, and that mechanical loading of the skeleton is also important at any age.

Genetic factors

Pocock et al. (1987) confirmed the heritability of bone mass in monozygotic twins and Seeman et al. (1989) provided evidence that the bone mass of daughters of osteoporotic women is less than that of daughters of non-osteoporotic women. Australian observations on mono- and dizygotic twins

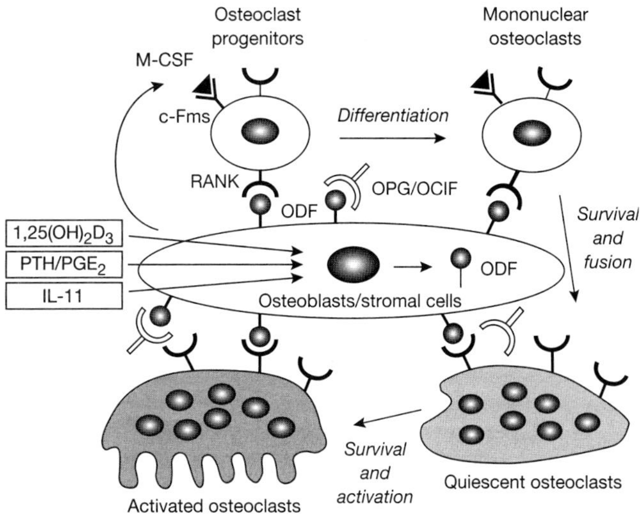

Fig. 5 A model illustrating a mechanism by which osteoblasts/stromal cells regulate osteoclast differentiation and function [from Yasuda et al. (1999), with permission].

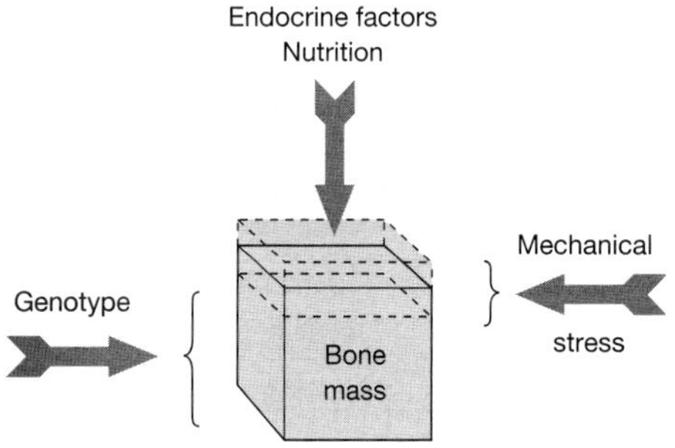

Fig. 6 A diagram of the main factors which influence bone mass [from Heaney (1986), with permission].

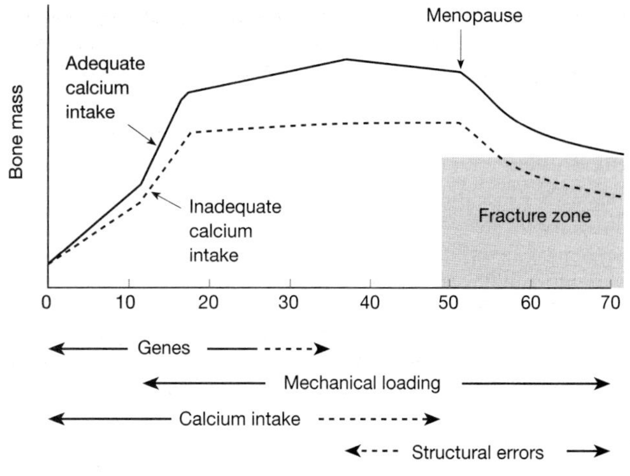

Fig. 7 The relative importance of factors contributing to bone mass with age [from Riggs and Melton (1988), with permission]. The post-menopausal rate of bone loss is also influenced by genetic factors and calcium intake.

and post-menopausal women have showed that bone mass in the populations studied is partly related to particular polymorphisms in the vitamin D receptor gene (Morrison et al. 1994), but this has not been widely confirmed. In a disorder such as osteogenesis imperfecta, where there is clear evidence of gene mutations, the heritable component of bone mass is very important (see below). Work on this syndrome has illuminated important genetic mechanisms that account for apparently non-Mendelian forms of inheritance, particularly somatic and germ-line mosaicism (Bernards and Gusella 1994). No mutations have been found in the helical region of collagen in osteoporosis; however, polymorphisms in the regulatory region of collagen appear to be related to bone mineral density and to fracture rate (Econs 2000).

Nutrition

It seems common sense that both the size and density of the skeleton should be related to nutrition, particularly of calcium, protein, and energy, but this has been difficult to prove. Twin studies have demonstrated a significantly greater increase in radial and vertebral bone density in those pre-pubertal twins on calcium supplements (Johnston et al. 1992) but this may not be sustained. Current evidence supports the notion that additional calcium is good for the skeleton at all ages (Marcus et al. 1996).

Mechanical factors

The main function of the skeleton is mechanical and it has long been known that within the skeleton bone is laid down along the lines of stress. Thus, at any age, stress-induced changes in bone mineral density are site-specific (Heinonen et al. 1993). *In vitro* experiments show that osteoblasts in culture can respond to mechanical stress by an increase in cAMP and phosphoinositol, partly mediated by prostaglandins. Since the osteocyte may be the primary sensor of mechanical loading, attempts are being made *in vivo* to identify the candidate gene in this cellular response.

Systemic hormones

Sex hormones, testosterone and oestrogen, encourage new bone formation. Growth hormone is an important anabolic skeletal agent during the early years of life, both directly and through the local production of insulin-like growth factors. A number of hormones primarily thought of as resorptive may also have anabolic actions on the osteoblasts. These include parathyroid hormone, which has a long-term anabolic effect increasing the proliferation of osteoblast precursors, and $1,25(OH)_2D_3$.

Bone matrix

The osteoblast synthesizes a large variety of substances that together form the organic bone matrix. These may be divided into collagen and non-collagen proteins, and the proteoglycans.

Collagen

Collagen is the major extracellular protein in the body and more than half is within the skeleton (Myllyharju and Kivirikko 2001). There are many different molecular types, with different functions, different structures and different genes (Chapter 3.2) (Table 3). The main fibrillar collagens are types I, II, and III; types V and XI are minor fibrillar collagens; types IX, XII, and XIV collagens are associated with fibrils. Collagen in bone is type I. This is a heteropolymer composed of two α_1-chains and one α_2-chain. The general structure of an α chain is $(GlyXY)_{338}$. The α-chains are synthesized as precursors within the osteoblasts and undergo a number of synthetic steps that include post-translational hydroxylation of proline and lysine residues; certain hydroxylysine residues are further modified into aldehydes and also glycosylated. After removal of their extensions the triple helical molecules form an exact structure with a quarter-stagger overlap, which is subsequently cross-linked (Fig. 8). In type I collagen, the so-called hole zones within this structure provide a template for early mineralization. The supramolecular assembly (Fig. 9) of the collagen molecules differ according to their tissue function. Mutations in the collagen genes and defects in posttranslational

Table 3 The vertebrate collagens

Type	α-Chains	Most common molecular form	Tissue distribution
I	α_1(I), α_2(I)	$[\alpha_1(I)]_2\ \alpha_2(I)$	Most connective tissues, e.g., bone, tendon, skin, lung, cornea, sclera, vascular system
II	α_1(II)	$[\alpha_1(II)]_3$	Cartilage, vitreous humour, embryonic cornea
III	α_1(III)	$[\alpha_1(III)]_3$	Extensible connective tissues, e.g., skin, lung, vascular system
IV	α_1(IV), α_2(IV), α_3(IV), α_4((IV), α_5(IV)	$[\alpha_1(IV)]_2\ \alpha_2(IV)$	Basement membranes
V	α_1(V), α_2(V), α_3(V)	$[\alpha_1(V)]_2\ \alpha_2(V)$	Tissues containing collagen I, quantitatively minor component
VI	α_1(VI), α_2(VI), α_3(VI)	$\alpha_1(VI)\ \alpha_2(VI)\ \alpha_3(VI)$	Most connective tissues, including cartilage
VII	α_1(VII)	$[\alpha_1(VII)]_3$	Basement-membrane-associated anchoring fibrils
VIII	α_1(VIII), α_2(VIII)	$[\alpha_1(VIII)]_2\ \alpha_2(VIII)$?	Product of endothelial and various tumour cell lines
IX	α_1(IX), α_2(IX), α_3(IX)	$\alpha_1(IX)\ \alpha_2(IX)\ \alpha_3(IX)$	Tissues containing collagen II, quantitatively minor component
X	α_1(X)	$[\alpha_1(X)]_3$	Hypertrophic zone of cartilage
XI	α_1(XI), α_2(XI), α_3(XI)[a]	$\alpha_1(XI)\ \alpha_2(XI)\ \alpha_3(XI)$	Tissues containing collagen II, quantitatively minor component
XII	α_1(XII)	$[\alpha_1(XII)]_3$	Tissues containing collagen I, quantitatively minor component
XIII	α_1(XIII)	$[\alpha_1(XIII)]_3$?	Quantitatively minor collagen, found, e.g., in skin, intestine
XIV	α_1(XIV)	$[\alpha_1(XIV)]_3$?	Tissues containing collagen I, quantitatively minor component

[a] Closely related to α1(II).

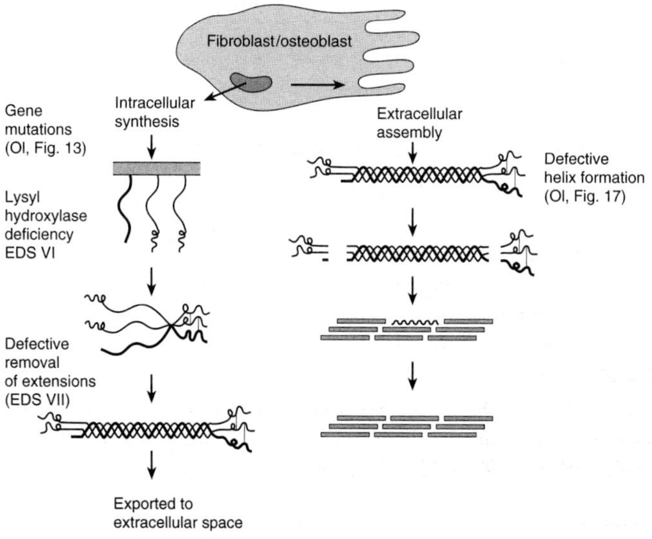

Fig. 8 Diagrammatic representation of the main synthetic pathways of collagen and the effects of some mutations. Type I collagen mutations which cause osteogenesis imperfecta are mirrored by similar mutations in type II collagen causing chondrodysplasias, and defects in minor collagens (type IX and X) [based on Prockop and Kivirikko (1984), with permission].

modification cause many inherited disorders of connective tissue, of which osteogenesis imperfecta is the main example. Recent work has demonstrated the causal importance of mutations in other collagens particularly those that cause chondrodysplasias (types II, IX, and X; see below).

Non-collagen proteins

Many proteins may be extracted from bone, which differ according to the starting material and the methods used (see Table 4). These include osteocalcin (Gla protein), sialoproteins, and various phosphoproteins such as osteonectin and osteopontin. Within the group of non-collagen proteins it is convenient also to include the bone proteoglycans and, importantly, the bone morphogenetic proteins. Osteoblasts are primarily responsible for the biosynthesis of all of these substances. However, other sources include substances selectively absorbed from the plasma, the products of monocytes, lymphocytes, and other cells within the bone marrow, the capillary network with its associated endothelial cells and basement membranes, and substances derived from the cartilage during endochondral ossification.

Many alternative names have been used for these substances. No unambiguous function has been determined for any bone matrix protein to date. Few, if any, are unique to bone, and bone matrix proteins can be expressed (at least transiently) in many tissues.

Osteonectin

This is the most abundant non-collagen protein produced by human osteoblasts. It binds strongly to calcium ions, utilizing high and low affinity binding sites, hydroxyapatite, and native collagen. It is not limited to mineralizing tissue, being also found in human platelets. Although osteonectin mRNA is widely distributed in developing tissues, osteonectin is most abundant in bone.

Bone sialoproteins

Two types of these are now recognized. Their relative abundance varies with species studied. Thus, sialoprotein I is a minor component of human bone, but a major contributor to total sialoprotein in rat bone. The protein contains a Arg–Gly–Asp cell-attachment sequence and is therefore called osteopontin. The major human bone sialoprotein is type II, similar to the substance originally described by Herring [for references see Favus (1999)].

Bone Gla-containing proteins

There are two of these, osteocalcin bone Gla protein and matrix Gla protein. The term Gla refers to the γ-carboxylated glutamic acid residues, formed by vitamin K-modulated, post-translational carboxylation of peptide-bound glutamic acid. These proteins have some sequence homology

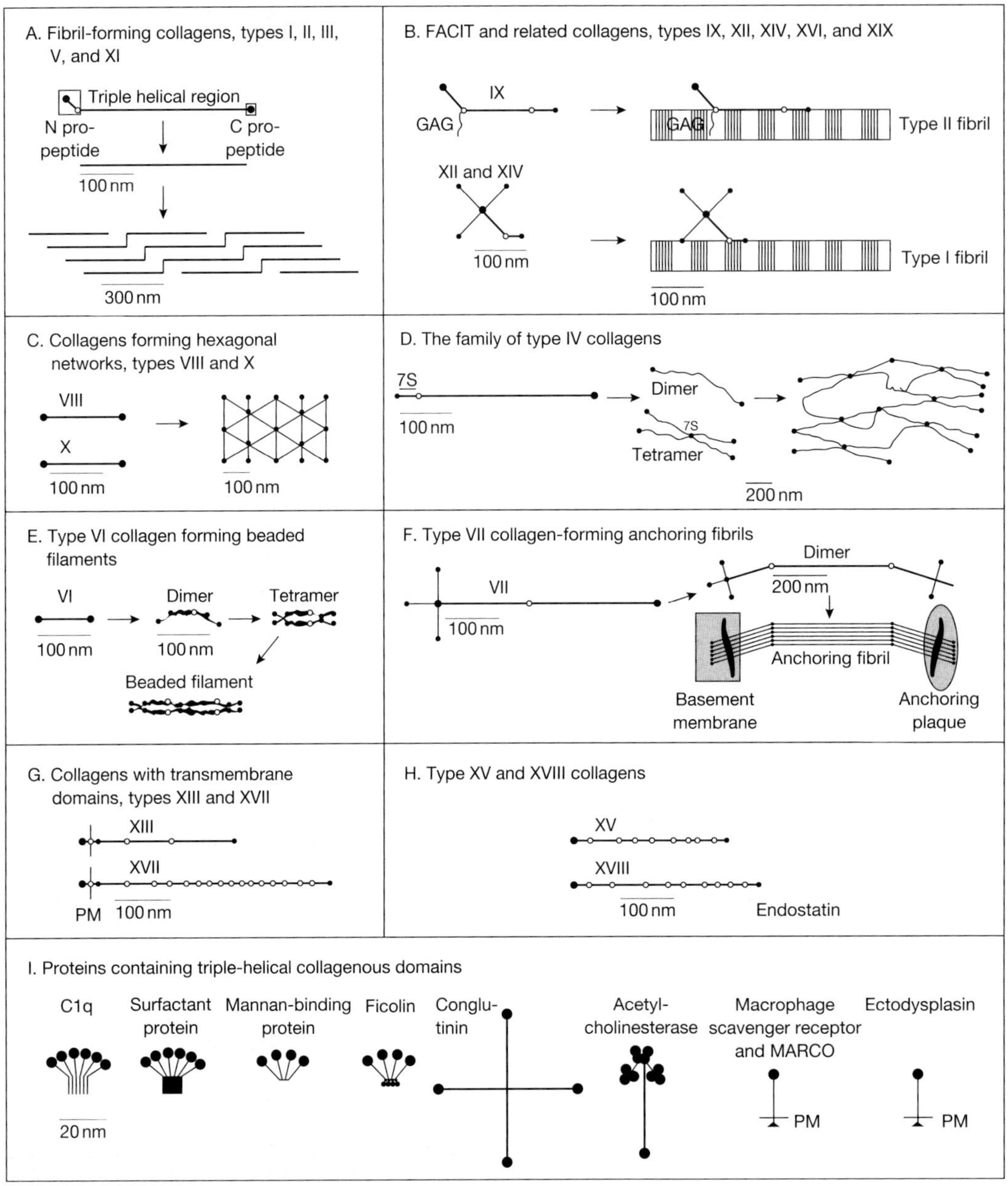

Fig. 9 Schematic representation of various members of the collagen superfamily and their known supramolecular assemblies [from Myllyharju and Kivirriko (2001), with permission].

but are products of different genes. Matrix Gla protein is also a cartilage protein, and is found at an earlier developmental stage than osteocalcin. Despite extensive research on osteocalcin, its function is unknown. Warfarin-treated animals do not show abnormal mineralization. Biosynthesis of osteocalcin is regulated by $1,25(OH)_2D_3$ (and no other hormone), which enhances its nuclear transcription and eventual secretion from bone cells. Plasma osteocalcin has been linked to the rate of bone formation or, less specifically, bone turnover.

Bone proteoglycans

Proteoglycans from cartilage have been studied more extensively than those from bone. Bone matrix proteoglycans differ in their small overall size, relatively larger amounts of protein, and longer chondroitin sulfate chains. The two proteoglycans of foetal bone (I and II) are different gene products. Small proteoglycans such as decorin and biglycan are thought to interact with growing collagen fibrils in a precise manner and to regulate their growth, maturation, and interactions.

Bone morphogenetic proteins

It has been known for many years that demineralized bone matrix contains substances capable of inducing ectopic bone formation. These substances are present in such small amounts that their extraction and isolation has presented great difficulties. A large number of bone morphogenetic proteins exist, many of which belong to the transforming growth factor-β family. The bone morphogenetic proteins act as differentiation factors concerned with the induction and expression of multiple phenotypes derived from mesenchymal cells. Investigation of recombinant bone morphogenetic proteins has shown that individually and together they are involved in chondrogenesis and osteogenesis. Additionally members of the family are involved in the patterning and development of the human skeleton

Table 4 Major non-collagen protein products of bone cells

Names	Properties
Alkaline phosphatase (bone-liver-kidney isoenzyme)	Gene on chromosome 1 Tissue specific post-translational modification Hydrolyses pyrophosphates
Osteonectin (SPARC)	Most abundant NCP Gene on chromosome 5 Binds to both collagen and hydroxyapatite Transiently synthesized by many cells. Found in platelets
Osteopontin (BSP I)	Expressed in different bone cells and in numerous other tissues including renal tubules and neuronal cells Has an RGD attachment sequence
Bone sialoprotein (BSP II)	Gene on chromosome 4 (same as osteopontin) Virtually specific to bone tissue
Osteocalcin (bone gla protein, BGP)	Gene on chromosome 1: found in young osteoblasts and odontoblasts. BGP deficient mice have dense bones
Matrix gla protein (MGP)	Not unique to bone; mRNA earlier than that for BGP in development MGP-deficient mice develop extraskeletal calcification. Gene on chromosome 12
Proteoglycan I (PG-I, byglycan)	Two separate species; share single heterogeneous core protein
Proteoglycan II (PG-II, decorin)	Involved in collagen fibrillogenesis
Bone morphogenetic proteins (BMPs)	Part of large TGF-β family

(Tickle 1994). It is becoming clear that recombinant bone morphogenetic proteins have clinical potential in the repair of bony defects.

Bone mineral and mineralization

Mineralization occurs against the background of the organic bone matrix. The ways in which mineralization happens continue to be debated (Boskey 1994) but there is good evidence that, in most mineralized tissues, calcifying vesicles derived from chondrocytes or osteoblasts provide a focus for mineralization. These vesicles are particularly demonstrable in cartilage, but their function in the organized matrix of bone is controversial. The precipitation of calcium within these vesicles may be controlled by the action of a pyrophosphatase, which locally destroys pyrophosphate, itself an inhibitor of mineralization. Alkaline phosphatase is one such pyrophosphatase and is readily demonstrable both in osteoblasts and in mineralizing vesicles.

It is possible, for the purposes of clarity, to consider two types of mineralization—homogeneous nucleation, which occurs in the lumen of the matrix vesicles from amorphous calcium phosphate to form crystalline hydroxyapatite, and heterogeneous nucleation, which is collagen-mediated and may partly rely on absorbed non-collagen proteins as nucleators. After this first phase (mediated either by vesicles or collagen) there is a second phase of rapid spread of mineralization, initially in the hole zones and later the overlap regions of the collagen matrix.

Calcium and phosphorus balance

Calcium is essential for innumerable functions such as reproduction, neurotransmission, hormone action, cellular growth, and enzyme action. The central position of calcium as an ionic messenger continues to be explored. There have been considerable advances in our understanding of the messengers which control cellular processes by generating internal calcium signals. Chief amongst these is inositol triphosphate, which is generated via G-protein and tyrosine kinase-linked receptors (Berridge 1993). Much has been written about external calcium balance and the main hormones that control it. Phosphate balance is less well understood. The circulating concentration of plasma calcium is determined by the amount of calcium absorbed by the intestine, the amount excreted by the kidney, and the exchange of mineral with the skeleton. The relative importance of these exchanges differs during growth and in different disorders. Total plasma calcium is closely maintained between 2.25 and 2.60 mmol/l, of which nearly half is in the ionized form (47 per cent ionized, 46 per cent protein bound, and the remainder complexed). The skeleton contains approximately 1 kg (25 000 mmol) of calcium. The main daily fluxes of calcium in the adult are shown in Fig. 10.

Parathyroid hormone

The gene for parathyroid hormone is on chromosome 11. The hormone is synthesized as a large precursor for export and its secretion is stimulated by a reduction in the plasma concentration of ionized calcium and reduced by an increase in $1,25(OH)_2D_3$. The way in which the parathyroid cells respond to very small changes in the extracellular concentration of calcium has been illuminated by the cloning and characterization of a calcium-sensing receptor from parathyroid-derived cells (Brown et al. 1993) (Fig. 11). Mutations within this receptor cause both hypercalcaemia and hypocalcaemia. An increase in parathyroid hormone secretion leads to an increase in calcium absorption through the gut, an increase in calcium reabsorption through the kidney, and an increase in bone resorption. Intestinal calcium absorption is mediated by $1,25(OH)_2D_3$ and 1α-hydroxylation is stimulated by parathyroid hormone, so that the effect of parathyroid hormone on intestinal calcium absorption is indirect and mediated by $1,25(OH)_2D_3$. In contrast, the renal effect of parathyroid hormone on calcium reabsorption is direct. The cellular effects of parathyroid hormone are mediated through specific G-protein-coupled receptors in kidney and bone and utilize more than one system. Parathyroid hormone encourages osteoclastic bone resorption by its effect on the osteoblast as previously described.

Vitamin D

Vitamin D (Fraser 1995; Favus 1999) is synthesized either as vitamin D_3 (cholecalciferol) within the skin from its precursor 7-dehydrocholesterol under the influence of ultraviolet light (usually as sunlight), or taken in with food, either as vitamin D_3 or D_2 (ergocalciferol). It is subsequently transported to the liver by a binding protein where it undergoes 25-hydroxylation; 25-hydroxyvitamin D ($25(OH)D_3$) is then hydroxylated in the 1 position by the renal 1α-hydroxylase, $1,25(OH)_2D_3$ is the active metabolite of vitamin D, and it has widespread effects (Fig. 12). Its classic effects are on calcium metabolism, where it promotes the synthesis of a calcium-transporting protein within the cells of the small intestine. Its effects are mediated through a widely distributed vitamin D receptor which contains DNA and hormone-binding components. This receptor combines with retinoid X-receptors and vitamin D response elements to produce its effect on target tissues. It is now realized that $1,25(OH)_2D_3$ has many effects outside mineral metabolism, concerned with the immune system and the growth and differentiation of a wide variety of cells. Measurement of plasma 25-OHD has proved to be a useful indicator of vitamin D status, and work on $1,25(OH)_2D_3$ and its receptors have illuminated the cause of the rarer forms of inherited rickets (see below). Although the kidney is the main sources of $1,25(OH)_2D_3$, it is now clear that this metabolite can be synthesized by a variety of granulomata, providing a partial explanation for the hypercalcaemia of sarcoidosis and (occasionally) lymphomas.

Calcitonin

Calcitonin (CT), a 32-amino-acid peptide, is one product of the calcitonin gene which also encodes the calcitonin gene-related peptide (CGRP).

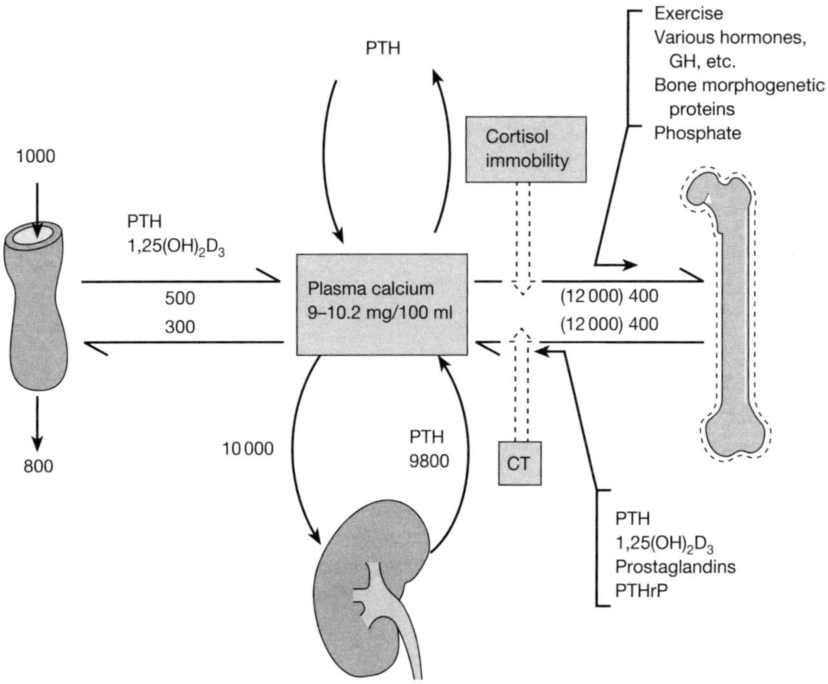

Fig. 10 Factors that control calcium balance; units are in mg per day (to convert to mmol divide by 40), and refer to an adult. The figures in parentheses are an estimate of exchange through the cellular barrier of bone. CT, calcitonin; GH, growth hormone; PTH, parathyroid hormone; PTHrP, parathyroid hormone-related peptide.

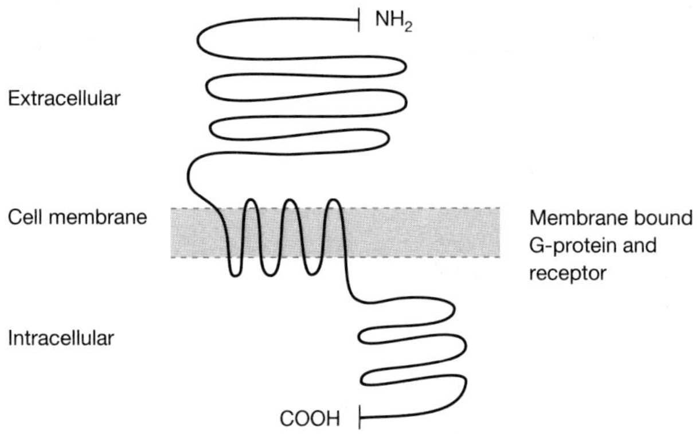

Fig. 11 A simplified diagram of the extracellular Ca^{2+}-sensing receptor from bovine parathyroid [redrawn from Brown et al. (1993)].

Experimentally its secretion (by the C cells of the thyroid) is increased by an increase in plasma calcium. The main effect of administered calcitonin is to reduce bone resorption by direct and reversible suppression of the osteoclast via a receptor closely related to the parathyroid hormone receptor. The physiological role of calcitonin is uncertain, although it is thought to protect the skeleton during physiological stresses such as growth and pregnancy.

Parathyroid hormone-related protein (PTHrP)

This hormone was discovered by studies on patients with non-metastatic hypercalcaemia of malignancy (see below). It has close sequence homology to parathyroid hormone at the amino-terminal end of the molecule and has very similar effects (Table 5). Its gene is located on the short arm of chromosome 12, which is thought to have arisen by a duplication of chromosome 11, which carries the human parathyroid hormone gene. It has been detected in a number of tumours, particularly of the lung. There is also evidence that it may have a role in foetal physiology, controlling the calcium gradient across the placenta, and maintaining the relatively higher concentrations in the foetal circulation. The recent observation that targeted disruption of the PTHrP gene leads to a lethal dysplasia has widened our knowledge of its possible functions (Karaplis et al. 1994).

Other hormones

Apart from the recognized calciotropic hormones, the skeleton is influenced by corticosteroids, the sex hormones, thyroxine, and growth hormone. The main effect of excess corticosteroids (either therapeutic or in Cushing's disease) is to suppress osteoblastic new bone formation. Both androgens and oestrogens promote and maintain skeletal mass. Osteoblasts have receptors for oestrogen, although they are not abundant. Two forms of oestrogen receptor exist, α and β, with different functions. Early postmenopausal bone loss is largely due to oestrogen deficiency but the mechanisms are not clear. In men oestrogen may also be skeletally important and osteoporosis occurs where the oestrogen receptor is ineffective or where the normal conversion of androgen to oestrogenic molecules is blocked. Thyroxine increases bone turnover and increases resorption in excess of formation; thyrotoxicosis thus leads to bone loss. Excess growth hormone leads to gigantism and acromegaly (according to the age of onset), with enlargement of the bones. Absence of growth hormone will lead to proportional short stature; where there is a wider pituitary failure the reduction in gonadotrophins will cause bone loss.

Biochemical measures of bone turnover

Knowledge of bone physiology allows interpretation of biochemical measures of bone turnover. These include the plasma bone-derived alkaline phosphatase and osteocalcin, and urinary total hydroxyproline and cross-linked, collagen-derived peptides. The first two of these are closely related to osteoblast function, and the second two to bone resorption. As formation and resorption are closely coupled, such measurements are usually closely related to each other, and to overall bone turnover.

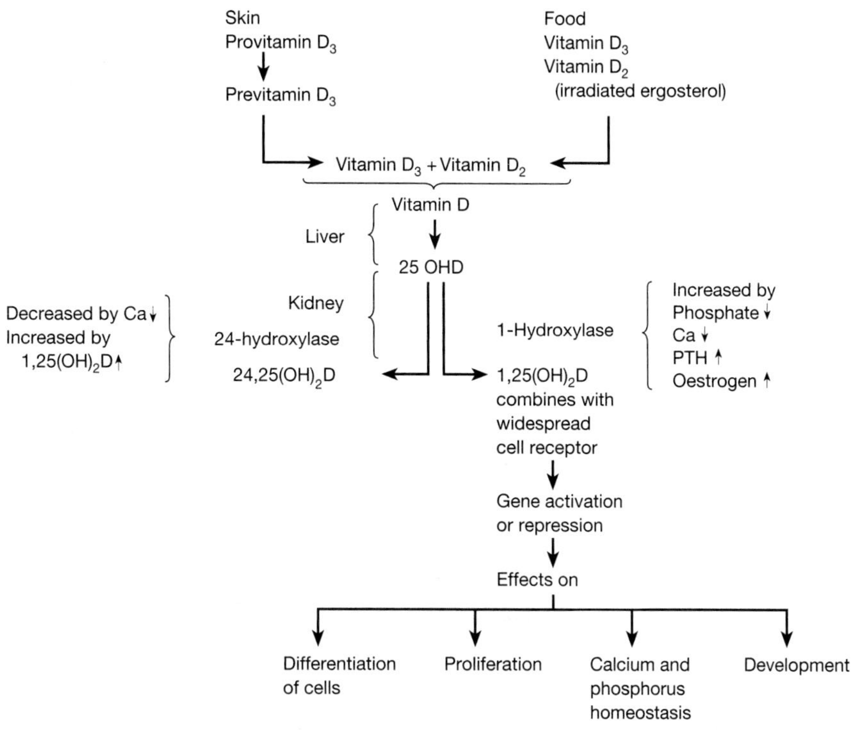

Fig. 12 The synthetic pathways and molecular and cellular effects of $1,25(OH)_2D$.

Table 5 Parathyroid hormone (PTH) and parathyroid-hormone related peptide (PTHrP) compared

	PTH	**PTHrP**
Source	Parathyroid glands	Non-metastatic solid tumours Many non-malignant tissues
Function	Control of Ca and P metabolism	Control of Ca and P metabolism Control of maternal/foetal calcium gradient
Gene locus	Chromosome 11	Chromosome 12
Structure	84 amino acids	3 isoforms, 8 of first 13 amino-terminal amino acids identical to PTH
Receptor	PTH/PTHrP PTH2	PTH/PTHrP
Biological activity	Amino terminal fragment	Many biologically active fragments
Primary hyperparathyroidism	PTH ↑	PTHrP undetectable
HHM	PTH ↓	PTHrP ↑
Biochemistry	In primary hyperparathyroidism Ca ↑ P ↓ Nephrogenous cAMP ↑ $1,25(OH)_2D$ ↑ Metabolic acidosis	HHM As for primary hyperparathyroidism except $1,25(OH)_2D$ not increased Metabolic alkalosis

Plasma alkaline phosphatase (largely derived from osteoblasts) provides a crude but readily accessible index of bone formation, being increased during periods of rapid growth and particularly where bone turnover is greatly increased, as in Paget's disease. Where more skeletal specificity is required measurement of bone-derived alkaline phosphatase can be useful. Early measurements of serum osteocalcin (bone Gla protein) were widely variable and depended on the origin, sensitivity, and stability of the antibodies used. Total urinary hydroxyproline excretion is influenced by dietary collagen (gelatin) and reflects both resorption and new collagen synthesis. The recent development of methods for the measurement of urinary collagen-derived pyridinium cross-links gives a reliable indication of bone resorption, unrelated to new collagen formation and uninfluenced by diet. The nomenclature of these degradation products has become unnecessarily complex. The cross-links of collagen fibres are formed via aldehydes derived from lysyl and hydroxylysyl residues. When collagen is degraded fragments containing these cross-links, referred to as pyridinium cross-links, are excreted in the urine. The cross-linked peptides are not further metabolized and the amount excreted is unaffected by dietary collagen (often in the form of gelatin). Pyridinoline (formed from hydroxylysyl cross-links) and deoxypyridinoline (from lysyl cross-links) derived from bone collagen are excreted in the same ratio as they exist in bone. Pyridinoline also comes from other tissues, especially tendon and cartilage. Since bone is metabolically more active than cartilage the main source of urinary pyridinium cross-linked, collagen-derived peptides is the skeleton. There is a diurnal variation in the amount excreted and according to the method used but significant increases are described in pre-adolescent growth and also in high turnover bone disease, particularly Paget's disease.

New immunoassay methods are being developed which are likely to supersede the original high-performance liquid chromatography (HPLC) procedure. Methods which measure other aspects of collagen turnover, such as the circulating concentration of carboxyl- and amino-terminal fragments of the molecule, have yet to establish themselves in practice. Eastell et al. (2001) have recently reviewed these so-called bone 'markers'.

Bone in disease

The causes of many bone diseases may now be explained by our increased understanding of skeletal physiology. These diseases may be acquired or inherited, and provide examples of disorders of bone formation and resorption, of mineralization, of matrix synthesis, of enzyme function, and of abnormal cell biology. Many conditions previously thought of as skeletal curiosities are now known to have a biochemical basis. Table 6 lists the identified molecular defects in a number of disorders affecting the skeleton. Further details are given by Favus (1999).

Osteoporosis

In osteoporosis, imbalance between resorption and formation leads to a reduction in the amount of bone per unit volume without a change in its composition. This reduction leads to microarchitectural deterioration, increased fragility, and increased fracture risk. Although osteoporosis is most frequent with increasing years, especially in post-menopausal women, there are a number of other recognizable causes that reduce the density of the younger skeleton (Table 7). These include anorexia nervosa, and excessive exercise in females associated with pre-menopausal oestrogen lack. The latter provides a striking example of the opposing effects of mechanical stress and hormone deficiency on the skeleton. A topical cause of osteoporosis is cardiac transplantation.

Immobilization causes both osteoblastic failure and osteoclast excess. Cushing's syndrome and excessive therapeutic corticosteroids suppress osteoblastic activity.

Table 6 Some molecular defects in bone and mineral disorders

Genetic disorder	Affected gene
Achondrogenesis	Collagen-2-A1 or diastrophic dysplasia sulfate transporter
Achondroplasia	Fibroblast growth factor receptor-3
Albright osteodystrophy (pseudohypoparathyroidism)	G-Protein, α subunit
Apert syndrome	Fibroblast growth factor receptor-2
Autosomal dominant hypocalcaemia	Calcium-sensing receptor
Campomelic dysplasia	SRY box-related-9 (SOX9)
Chrondrosarcoma	Exostosis-1
Cleidocranial dysplasia syndrome	CBFAI
Crouzon syndrome	Fibroblast growth factor receptor-2
Diaphyseal dysplasia (Camurati–Engelmann)	TGF β1
Diastrophic dysplasia	Diastrophic dysplasia sulfate transporter
Epiphyseal dysplasia	Cartilage oligomeric matrix protein-1 or COL-9-A1, 2, 3
Familial expansile osteolysis	TNFRSFIIA
Familial hypocalciuric hypercalcaemia	Calcium-sensing receptor
Familial hypoparathyroidism	Calcium-sensing receptor
Hereditary multiple exostoses	Exostosis-1 or -2
Hydrochondroplasia	Fibroblast growth factor receptor-3
Hypophosphataemic osteomalacia, dominantly inherited	Fibroblast growth factor 23 (FGF 23)
Hypophosphataemic rickets, X-linked	PHEX endopeptidase
Hypophosphatasia	Alkaline phosphatase
Jackson–Weiss syndrome	Fibroblast growth factor receptor-2
Kniest dysplasia	Collagen-2-A1
Marfan's syndrome	Fibrillin-1
McCune–Albright syndrome	G-protein, α subunit
Metaphyseal chondrodysplasia	Collagen-10-A1 or parathyroid hormone receptor
Multiple endocrine neoplasia, type 1	MEN1
Multiple endocrine neoplasia, type 2	RET protooncogene
Nephrolithiasis, X-linked, Dent disease	Renal-specific chloride channel
Neonatal hyperparathyroidism	Calcium-sensing receptor
Osteogenesis imperfecta	Collagen-1-A1, collagen-2-A1
Osteopetrosis with renal tubular acidosis	Carbonic anhydrase II
Osteoporosis–pseudoglioma syndrome	LRP5
Pseudoachondroplasia	Cartilage oligomeric matrix protein-1
Pycnodysostosis	Cathepsin-K
Sclerosteosis	SOST
Spondyloepiphyseal dysplasia	Collagen-2-A1
Stickler syndrome	Collagen-2-A1, collagen-11-A1
Thanatophoric dysplasia	Fibroblast growth factor receptor-3
Vitamin D–dependent rickets, type II	Vitamin D receptor
Williams syndrome	Elastin

Table 7 Causes of osteoporosis

Common
Increasing age
Menopause
Immobility
Less common
Cushing's syndrome
Hypogonadism
Coeliac disease
Rare
Generalized mastocytosis
Osteogenesis imperfecta
Turner's syndrome
Topical
Oestrogen deficient
Anorexia nervosa
Obsessional exercise
Satellite travel
Unknown
Idiopathic osteoporosis
Juvenile
Pregnancy-associated
In young people

Table 8 Some causes of rickets and osteomalacia

Nutritional
Immigrants from India to the United Kingdom
Housebound elderly people
Malabsorption
Coeliac disease
Small bowel resection
Renal
Renal glomerular failure
Renal tubular disorders
Inherited X-linked hypophosphataemia
Multiple renal tubular defects
Rare
Vitamin D dependent (type I; type II)
Oncogeneous (hypophosphataemic)

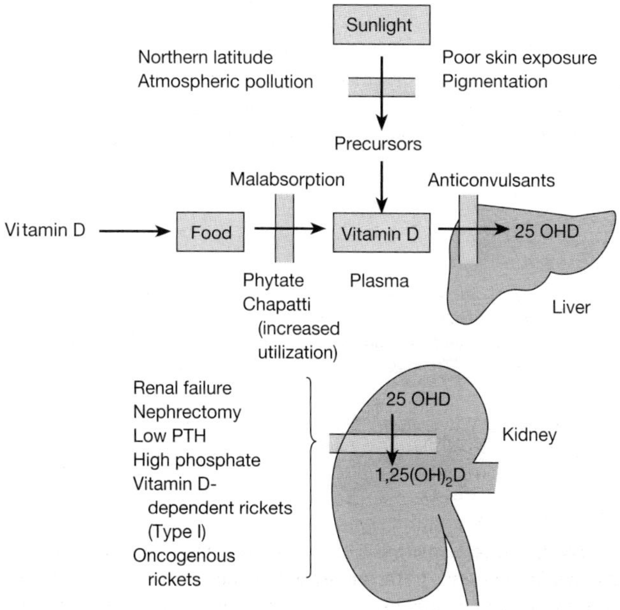

Fig. 13 The sources and metabolism of vitamin D and causes of rickets and osteomalacia.

The amount of bone in the adult depends on the peak bone mass and the subsequent rate of loss. As already stated, peak bone mass depends on genetic, nutritional, mechanical, and endocrine interactions. The rate of bone loss varies considerably between individuals and may also be genetically determined. It is also accelerated by certain so-called risk factors, such as immobility, excessive thinness, alcoholism, cigarette smoking, low calcium intake, prolonged periods of amenorrhoea, and early menopause. There is a relationship between reduced bone mass and fractures, but it is not a close one, as fractures depend as much on injury, including falls (especially in later life), as on loss of bone. How much excessive cytokine activity, especially of IL-6, contributes to post-menopausal bone loss is controversial. No differences have been found in circulating levels of this cytokine between normal and osteoporotic women (Khosla et al. 1994) but this is not unexpected since the action of IL-6 is likely to be very localized.

Osteomalacia and rickets

These conditions are distinguishable only by age. There is defective mineralization of the organic bone matrix due to vitamin D deficiency or a disturbance of its metabolism. The causes (Table 8) are best understood against the known metabolic pathways of vitamin D (Fig. 13). They include vitamin D deficiency, often in immigrants to the United Kingdom from the Indian sub-continent where an increased utilization of vitamin D (related to chapatti consumption) combines with lack of sunlight and lack of vitamin D in the diet, malabsorption (particularly coeliac disease), and renal disease. The causes of rickets from renal glomerular failure (renal glomerular osteodystrophy) are quite different from those due to renal tubular disease (Fig. 14), and may be modified by aluminium intoxication in those on dialysis. The most frequent cause of renal tubular rickets is inherited hypophosphataemia, but there are many others. The causal mutations on the PHEX gene have been identified in X-linked hypophosphataemia. Mutations in the chloride channel and fibroblast growth factor 23 genes have also been discovered in rare renal tubular forms of rickets (Dixon et al. 1998; ADHR Consortium 2000). Fibroblast growth factor 23 is also expressed in mesenchymal tumours associated with osteomalacia (Shimada et al. 2001). Investigation of one of the rarer forms of rickets, so-called vitamin D-dependent rickets, has shown that it may be due to defective 1α-hydroxylation of $25(OH)D_3$ (type I) or to end-organ resistance to $1,25(OH)_2D_3$ (type II). The molecular basis of the latter has been shown to be a number of mutations at either end of the 1,25-receptor (Fig. 15) (Hewison and O'Riordan 1994; Econs 2000).

Parathyroid bone disease

Most patients with primary hyperparathyroidism do not have clinically manifest bone disease (osteitis fibrosa cystica), although in the majority, the histological appearances are abnormal and improve after removal of the parathyroid tumour. Osteitis fibrosa cystica is characterized by an excess of fibrous tissue and osteoclasts within lesions that may become cystic (brown tumours). The most common cause of primary hyperparathyroidism is a parathyroid adenoma, and it is now recognized that a number of these are monoclonal in origin. Parathyroid overactivity also occurs in the multiple endocrine neoplasia syndromes (Thakker 1998; Econs 2000).

Parathyroid overactivity can result from prolonged hypocalcaemia (secondary hyperparathyroidism). Rarely, the parathyroids may become autonomous with hypercalcaemia (tertiary hyperparathyroidism). Finally

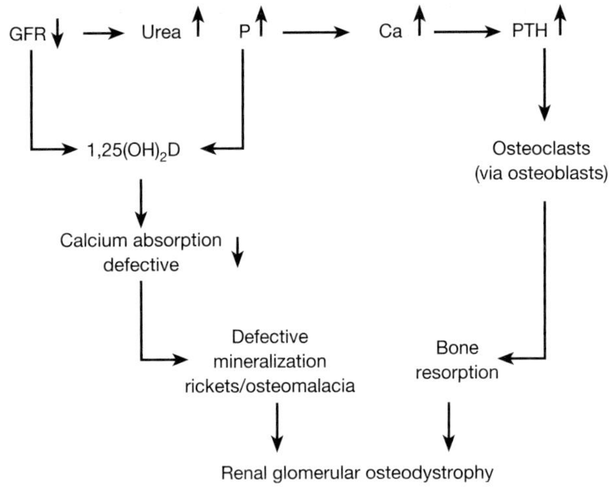

Fig. 14 The effects of renal glomerular failure on the skeleton.

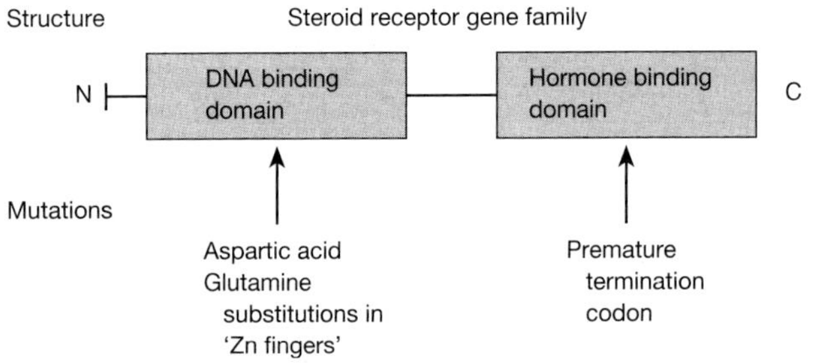

Fig. 15 Some molecular changes identified in type II vitamin D-dependent rickets.

familial hypocalciuric hypercalcaemia and familial hypocalcaemia can result from mutations in the parathyroid calcium-sensing receptor (Brown et al. 1993; Marx 2000).

Parathyroid insufficiency can result from inadvertent surgical removal of the parathyroids or may be idiopathic (Thakker 2001). The condition of pseudohypoparathyroidism is characterized by the presence of short fourth and fifth metacarpals, ectopic ossification calcification in the skin, and mental simplicity (Breslau 1989). It has now been shown that in a number of such patients there are loss of function mutations in the genes controlling the G-protein system that links parathyroid hormone to its effector tissue (Spiegel 1990; Lefkowitz 1995). This provides an explanation of the resistance to parathyroid hormone in this condition (Fig. 16). Interestingly there are activating G-protein mutations in polyostotic fibrous dysplasia (Econs 2000).

Paget's disease

In this disorder, the main skeletal abnormality appears to be overactivity of large multinucleated osteoclasts. At first this leads to excessive bone resorption but, because of the linkage between osteoclastic and osteoblastic activity, excessive new bone formation follows. Normally, this linkage is sufficiently close to prevent hypercalcaemia, however rapid the bone turnover, but this may occur if patients with Paget's disease are immobilized, in which case the osteoblasts become less active whilst resorption continues. It is currently considered that Paget's disease may be related to a viral infection of the osteoclasts, possibly with the respiratory syncytial virus, but current attempts to identify the viral nucleic acid continues to give

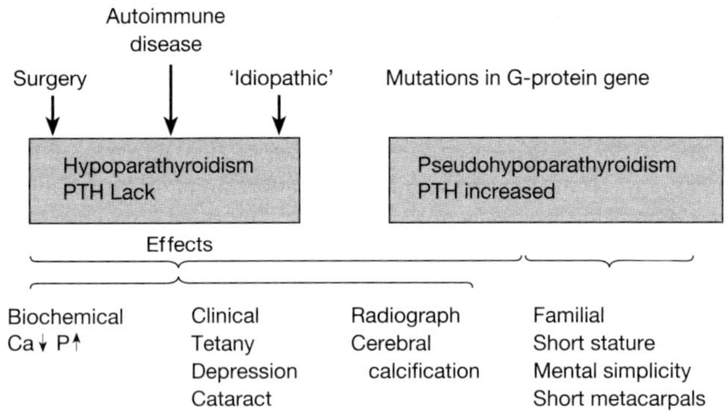

Fig. 16 The causes and effects of parathyroid hormone insufficiency or resistance. Mutations in the Ca^{2+}-sensing receptor may also mimic parathyroid resistance.

conflicting results. Linkage of Paget's disease to chromosome 18 has been described in some families; in a similar disorder, familial expansile osteolysis, mutations have been identified in the gene for the osteoclast receptor RANK (Hughes et al. 2000).

Disorders of bone matrix

Classically, these disorders have not been regarded as metabolic disorders of bone but it is now clear that mutations, especially in the collagen genes, can produce a wide variety of skeletal disorders (Table 9 and Chapter 3.2) (Royce and Steinmann 1993).

Osteogenesis imperfecta

Four clinical types are recognized, although many patients with this disorder cannot be accurately classified (Rowe and Shapiro 1998; Primorac et al. 2001). In the first, type I, the disorder is dominantly inherited and often appears to be due to a non-functional allele for type I collagen. The main result is that osteoblasts (and fibroblasts) make half as much type I collagen as they ought to, causing an inherited form of osteoporosis and affecting other tissues containing type I collagen (teeth, sclera, heart valves). Type II osteogenesis imperfecta is the lethal form of the disease; this is most often due to a single-base mutation in one of the type I collagen genes leading to an amino-acid substitution for one of the glycine residues normally present in every third position in the amino-acid chain. The importance of glycine is that it has no side-chain and can therefore fit into the interior of the helix (Sykes 1990). Replacement of such a 'core' glycine by an amino acid with a side-chain disturbs helix formation. The effect depends on the size of the side-chain and on the position of the replacement amino acid relative to the carboxyl-terminal end of the collagen molecule, where helix formation begins. The most lethal effects appear to be produced by large substitutions near to the carboxyl-terminal end of the molecule (Fig. 17).

Type III osteogenesis imperfecta is a progressively disabling disease. Infants survive but the skeleton becomes more and more deformed. The chemistry of this condition is not so well known as in other forms but again it is probably frequently related to a disturbance of helix formation by glycine substitutions. Type IV is rare and is a dominantly inherited disease. Extensive linkage studies have demonstrated that dominantly inherited (type I and IV) osteogenesis imperfecta is linked to mutations in either the α_1- or α_2-chain of type I collagen (Sykes et al. 1990). A detailed study on the variable expression of the mutant osteogenesis imperfecta gene demonstrates the importance of somatic mosaicism (Wallis et al. 1990). The relationship between genotype and phenotype is still complex (Smith 1994).

Other forms of inherited disorders of connective tissue

These include Marfan's syndrome, Ehlers–Danlos syndrome, and the skeletal dysplasias. It is clear that in most cases Marfan's syndrome is due to mutations in the fibrillin gene (Pyeritz 1993) on chromosome 15, although linkage to chromosome 3 has also been described (Collod et al. 1994). Since fibrillin is the major component of the suspensory ligament of the lens and of the elastin-associated microfibrillar system, mutations in its genes provide a neat explanation for the combination of lens dislocation and aortic dissection found in this disorder.

There are many different types of the Ehlers–Danlos syndrome. The most common (classic) forms (1 and 2) are often due to mutations in type V collagen, which is a minor collagen associated with type I collagen. Mutations in the gene for the non-collagen component tenascin-X have rarely been described in type 3 Ehlers–Danlos syndrome (Mao and Bristow 2001). In type 4 the major complication is rupture of the middle-sized blood vessels resulting from a variety of mutations in the gene for type III collagen. In type 6 Ehlers–Danlos syndrome, whose main features are ocular fragility and scoliosis, there is evidence of hydroxylysine deficiency. Another type of Ehlers–Danlos syndrome (type 7, with excessive joint mobility) results from defective removal of the procollagen extensions from the precursor molecule due to mutations at the peptidase site.

Table 9 a) Collagen gene mutations and disorders of bone matrix. b) Non-collagen gene mutations and disorders of bone matrix

Mutant gene	Disease family
(a) Collagen	
COL1A1 and COL1A2	Osteogenesis imperfecta and Ehlers–Danlos syndrome (EDS) type 7
COL2A1	Achondrogenesis type II
	Spondyloepiphyseal dysplasia (SED)
	Kniest dysplasia
	Stickler syndrome
COL3A1	EDS type 4
COL5A1	EDS types 1 and 2
COL9A1, A2, or A3	Multiple epiphyseal dysplasia
COL10A1	Metaphyseal chondroplasia (type Schmid)
COL11A2	Stickler syndrome (without ocular manifestations)
(b) Non-collagen	
COMP	Pseudoachondroplasia
	Multiple epiphyseal dysplasia
DTDST	Diastrophic dysplasia
	Atelosteogenesis type II
	Achondrogenesis type IB
PTH-PTHrP receptor	Jansen metaphyseal chondrodysplasia
SOX 9	Campomelic dysplasia
Arysulfatase E	Chondrodysplasia punctata
FGFR 3	Achondroplasia
	Thanatophoric dysplasia
	Hypochondroplasia
	Crouzon syndrome with acanthosis nigricans
FGFR 2	Crouzon syndrome
	Apert syndrome
	Jackson–Weiss syndrome
	Pfeiffer syndrome
FGFR 1	Pfeiffer syndrome
CBFA-1	Cleidocranial dysostoses
Cathepsin K	Pyknodyostosis
Tumour suppressor genes	Multiple hereditary exostoses
Sedlin gene	Spondyloepiphyseal dysplasia tarda (X-linked)

Skeletal dysplasias

These conditions (Wynne-Davies et al. 1985) which include achondroplasia, spondyloepiphyseal dysplasia, and achondrogenesis, were long thought of as orthopaedic curiosities. However, numerous mutations have now been described (Table 9). To begin with, exon deletions were described in the type II collagen gene in patients with spondyloepiphyseal dysplasia (Lee et al. 1989), and single-base mutations in the same gene in infants with achondrogenesis type II (Vissing et al. 1989). There was also evidence of genetic linkage of spondyloepiphyseal dysplasia congenita to type II collagen (Anderson et al. 1990). It seemed possible that mutations in type II collagen, which is the major collagen of cartilage, would be increasingly described as a cause of those disorders characterized by abnormal cartilage formation, although a number were excluded (Spranger et al. 1994; Winterpacht et al. 1994). Multiple epiphyseal dysplasia was linked to mutations in type IX collagen (a minor fibre-associated collagen). Mutations in type X collagen were also described in the Schmid type of metaphyseal dysplasia. Type X collagen is specifically produced by hypertrophic chondrocytes (McIntosh et al. 1994; Wallis et al. 1994). Most interesting of all mutations are those in the type 3 fibroblast growth-factor receptor (FGFR3) which has been identified as the cause of achondroplasia (Editorial 1994; Le Merrer et al. 1994; Rousseau et al. 1994; Shiang et al. 1994). The reason why such mutations should lead to specific changes in the skeleton is not yet understood. Mutations in a similar receptor, FGFR2, appear to cause Crouzon's syndrome (Reardon et al. 1994). Another (activating) mutation, this time in the PTH/PTHrP receptor, has recently been identified as a cause of the Jansen type of metaphyseal dysplasia (Schipani et al. 1996). Current

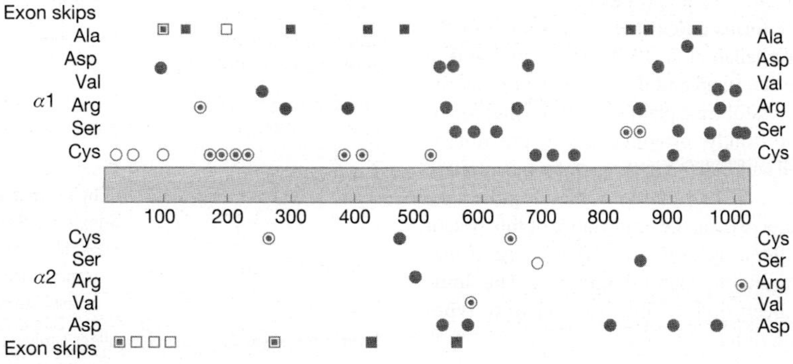

Fig. 17 Mutations in the collagen genes known to cause osteogenesis imperfecta [from Sykes (1990), with permission]. Axial glycine (circles) and exon skip (squares) mutations in the genes for the α_1- (upper) and α_2- (lower) subunits of type I collagen. The scale indicates the osteogenesis imperfecta phenotype from lethal (solid) through severe (dot) to mild (open). Note that the collagen triple helix winds up from the carboxyl (right) to the amino (left) terminal and that the least severe phenotypes are often associated with mutations near the amino terminus. Ala, Asp, etc., refer to the amino acid replacing the axial glycine.

information on the genetic causes of most skeletal dysplasias is summarized in Table 9 and reviewed by Vajo et al. (2000) and Cohn (2001).

Enzyme disorders

Some disorders that affect the skeleton result from abnormal enzyme function. These include hypophosphatasia, homocystinuria, and alkaptonuria.

Hypophosphatasia

In hypophosphatasia there are variable abnormalities in the skeleton associated with differing phenotypes. A common biochemical feature is an abnormally low plasma alkaline phosphatase associated with an excess of phosphoethanolamine in the urine. The disorder may be lethal, or it may cause hypercalcaemia in infants and early fusion of the cranial sutures. By contrast the disease can be mild in adults, although pathological fractures of the long bones may occur. Many mutations in the gene for the tissue non-specific alkaline phosphatase have been described (Mornet et al. 1998). Family studies linked the defect to chromosome 1 (Greenberg et al. 1990). Zurutuza et al. (1999) described the relationship between phenotype and genotype.

Homocystinuria

This condition, which mimics Marfan's syndrome, is due to a defect in cystathionine synthase, a pyridoxine-dependent enzyme. Accumulation of homocysteine behind the metabolic block leads to homocystinuria. Skeletal features of this disease are very similar to those of Marfan's syndrome with arachnodactyly and scoliosis. There is also dislocation of the lenses.

Alkaptonuria

In this disorder there is a deficiency of homogentisic acid oxidase; the accumulation of homogentisic acid is associated with the features of ochronosis, with pigmentation of articular cartilage, early osteoarthritis, and calcification of the intervertebral discs.

Disorders of cell biology

In two rare conditions, osteopetrosis and myositis ossificans progressiva, there is evidence that the disorder is primarily due to abnormalities in the bone cells.

Osteopetrosis

There are a number of inherited disorders in which there is an excessive amount of bone within the skeleton. The most well recognized is marble bone disease (Albers–Schönberg disease). This condition may be severe and recessively inherited, occurring in infancy, or it may be mild with dominant inheritance. There are intermediate forms and a rare form is due to deficiency of carbonic anhydrase II (Fathallah et al. 1994). In animals and in man, varying osteoclast defects are described and there is evidence that the infantile form may be cured by successful transplantation of normal osteoclasts (Fischer et al. 1986). Interestingly, osteopetrosis in the microophthalmic *op/op* mouse is associated with a defect in the gene for macrophage colony-stimulating factor (Yoshida et al. 1990) and mice lacking the c-*fos* oncogene develop osteopetrosis, emphasizing the importance of this system in bone physiology (Wang et al. 1992). Jackson et al. (1994) suggest that osteoblasts may also be defective in mammalian osteopetrosis. The dominantly inherited form has now been divided into two separate types (Benichoiu et al. 2000) possibly with different causes.

Fibrodysplasia (myositis) ossificans progressiva

In this disorder progressive ossification of the major striated muscles is associated with characteristic skeletal abnormalities from birth (Connor and Evans 1984; Cohen et al. 1993). The cause is unknown but it seems that the fibroblasts or mesenchymal cells within muscle behave as if they are osteoblasts to produce cartilage and true bone within muscles. This may be due to an inherited cellular abnormality; alternatively it could represent, for instance, an excess of one of the morphogenetic proteins. The combination of skeletal abnormalities and ectopic ossification, which often occurs in a specific order, would seem to implicate proteins involved in skeletal patterning as well as bone morphogenesis (Storm et al. 1994). The condition is fully described by Shore et al. (2000).

The skeleton in malignant disease

The skeleton is often affected in malignant disease, which is the most frequent cause of hypercalcaemia in hospital patients. This hypercalcaemia results from excessive bone resorption and increased renal tubular reabsorption of calcium. The relative importance of these depend on the type and distribution of the cancer. Bone resorption in cancer is due to an increase in osteoclastic activity (either as a direct response to hormonal factors or indirectly via other cells) and direct resorption of bone by the malignant cells themselves. The complexity of the mechanisms involved illustrates the multiple effects of cytokines and hormones on the skeleton (Avioli and Krane 1998).

Neoplastic hypercalcaemia may occur in three clinical settings—haematological malignancy, solid tumours with metastases, and solid tumours without. In the first of these the hypercalcaemia is usually due to the release of osteoclast-activating factors by the malignant cells (occasionally, as in lymphoma, the plasma calcium is increased because of excessive formation of $1{,}25(OH)_2D_3$ by the lymphomatous tissue); in the case of myeloma this activating factor is a lymphokine called lymphotoxin. Osteoclast-activating factors have been divided into those from T cells, B cells, and monocytes.

In solid tumours with lytic metastases, predominantly from the breast, lung, and kidney, a major contribution to hypercalcaemia is direct destruction of bone. However, where there are few or no detectable metastases, other mechanisms must be involved. Chief amongst these is the production of parathyroid hormone-related peptide by the tumour itself (Martin 1990; Strewler 2000). This hormone may also be relevant in metastatic and haematological malignancies. Parathyroid hormone-related peptide has been detected mainly in lung tumours, but also occurs in those from the breast (the mRNA for parathyroid hormone-related peptide is present in lactating mammary tissue) (Heath et al. 1990). The main biochemical effect of parathyroid hormone-related peptide is to produce changes similar to those of parathyroid hormone. These are hypercalcaemia and hypophosphataemia,

Table 10 Factors involved in the humoral hypercalcaemia of malignancy

Factor	Actions
Parathyroid hormone-related peptide (PTHrP)	See Table 5
Transforming growth factor-α (TGF-α)	Stimulates osteoclastic bone resorption Produced by same tumours as PTHrP
Tumour necrosis factor (TNF)	Powerful bone-resorbing cytokine; synthesized by normal activated macrophages Stimulates formation and activity of osteoclasts Probably produced by host cells under action of tumour-produced granulocyte-macrophage colony-stimulating factor
Interleukin 1 (IL-1)	Effect similar to TNF; associated with solid tumours Acts synergistically on bone resorption with TNF, parathyroid hormone, PTHrP, and TGF-α
Prostaglandins	Unlikely as a mediator for the humoral hypercalcaemia of malignancy

which has led in the past to terms like 'pseudohyperparathyroidism' and 'ectopic parathyroid hormone syndrome'. It is now clear that the concentrations of parathyroid hormone are low, although nephrogenous cAMP is increased. Increases in circulating parathyroid hormone-like protein have been recorded in such patients (Budayr et al. 1989). Finally, although the increase in parathyroid hormone-related peptide provides a neat explanation for hypercalcaemia in the absence of metastases, it may be only part of the story because the peptide may act in concert with other factors locally on bone. These have already been dealt with and include transforming growth factors-α and -β, prostaglandins, and interleukins (Table 10).

Conclusions

The skeleton fulfils many functions whose requirements are often in opposition. Bone is a very complex structure, which is continually being dismantled and replaced. This complexity leads to its fascination for investigators and provides many opportunities for a wide variety of bone diseases. Recent examples of rare diseases are provided by the discovery of mutations in the G-protein and Ca^{2+}-sensing receptor systems, in the minor collagens, and in the fibroblast growth factor receptors. Much more work is required before we fully understand the causes of the common polygenic disorders such as osteoporosis.

References

ADHR Consortium (2000). Autosomal dominant hypophosphateamic rickets is associated with mutations in FGF23. *Nature Genetics* **26**, 345–8.

Anderson, I.J., Goldberg, R.B., Marion, R.W., Upholt, W.B., and Tsipouras, P. (1990). Spondyloepiphyseal dysplasia congenita: genetic linkage to type II collagen (COL2A1). *American Journal of Human Genetics* **46**, 896–901.

Avioli, L.V. and Krane, S.M. *Metabolic Bone Disease and Clinically Related Disorders* 3rd edn. San Diego CA: Academic Press, 1998.

Benichou, O.D., Laredo, J.D., and de Vernejoul, M.C. (2000). Type II autosomal dominant osteopetrosis (Albers-Schonberg disease) Clinical and radiological manifestations in 42 patients. *Bone* **26**, 87–93.

Bernards, A. and Gusella, J.F. (1994). The importance of genetic mosaicism in human disease. *New England Journal of Medicine* **331**, 1447–9.

Berridge, M.J. (1993). Inositol trisphophate and calcium signalling. *Nature* **361**, 315–25.

Bilezikian, J.P., Raisz, L.H., and Rodan, G.A. *Principles of Bone Biology.* San Diego CA: Academic Press, 1996.

Boskey, A. (1994). Bone and cartilage mineralization. In *Bone Formation and Repair* 1st edn. (ed. C.T. Brighton, G. Friedlaender, and J.M. Lane), pp. 23–48. Rosemount IL: American Academy of Orthopedic Surgeons.

Boyde, A. (1972). Scanning electron microscope studies of bone. In *The Biochemistry and Physiology of Bone* Vol. 1, 2nd edn. (ed. G.H. Bourne), pp. 259–310. New York: Academic Press.

Breslau, N.A. (1989). Pseudohypoparathyroidism: current concepts. *American Journal of the Medical Sciences* **298**, 131–40.

Brown, E.M. et al. (1993). Cloning and characterization of an extracellular Ca^{2+}-sensing receptor from bovine parathyroid. *Nature* **366**, 575–80.

Budayr, A.A. et al. (1989). Increased serum levels of a parathyroid hormone-like protein in malignancy-associated hypercalcaemia. *Annals of Internal Medicine* **111**, 807–12.

Cohen, R.B. et al. (1993). The natural history of ectopic ossification in patients who have fibrodysplasia ossificans progressiva. A study of forty-four patients. *Journal of Bone and Joint Surgery* **75A**, 215–19.

Cohn, D.H. (2001). Defects in extracellular matrix structural proteins in the osteochondrodysplasias. In *The Molecular Basis of Skeletogenes is, Novartis Foundation Symposium* Vol. 232, pp. 195–212. Chichester: Wiley.

Collod, G. et al. (1994). A second locus for Marfan syndrome maps to chromosome 3 p24.2–p25. *Nature Genetics* **8**, 264–8.

Connor, J.M. and Evans, D.A. (1984). Fibrodysplasia ossificans progressiva. The clinical features and natural history of 34 patients. *Journal of Bone and Joint Surgery* **64B**, 76–83.

Dixon, P.H. et al. (1998). Mutational analysis of PHEX gene in X-linked hypophosphataemia. *Journal of Clinical Endocrinology and Metabolism* **83**, 3615–23.

Eastell, R., Baumann, M., Hoyle, N.R., and Wieczorek, L. *Bone Markers: Biochemical and Clinical Perspectives.* London: Martin Dunitz, 2001.

Econs, M.J. *The Genetics of Osteoporosis and Metabolic Bone Disease.* Totowa NJ: Humana Press, 2000.

Editorial (1994). Fingering fibroblast growth factor receptors. *Nature Genetics* **8**, 1–2.

Eriksen, E.F., Steiniche, T., Mosekilde, L., and Melsen, F. (1989). Histomorphometric analysis of bone in metabolic bone disease. *Endocrinology and Metabolism Clinics of North America* **18**, 919–54.

Fathallah, D.M., Bejaoui, M., Sly, W.S., Lakhoua, R., and Dellagi, K. (1994). A unique mutation underlying carbonic anhydrase II deficiency syndrome in patients of Arab descent. *Human Genetics* **94**, 581–2.

Favus, M.J. *Primer on the Metabolic Bone Diseases and Disorders of Mineral Metabolism* 4th edn. Philadelphia PA: Lippincott Williams and Wilkins, 1999.

Fischer, A. et al. (1986). Bone marrow transplantation for immunodeficiencies and osteopetrosis: European survey 1968–1985. *Lancet* **ii**, 1080–3.

Fraser, D.R. (1995). Vitamin D. *Lancet* **345**, 104–7.

Greenberg, C.R. et al. (1990). Infantile hypophosphatasia: localisation within chromosome region 1p36.1–34 and prenatal diagnosis using linked DNA markers. *American Journal of Human Genetics* **46**, 286–92.

Heaney, R.P. (1986). Calcium, bone health and osteoporosis. *Bone and Mineral Research* **4**, 255–301.

Heath, D.A., Senior, P.V., Varley, J.M., and Beck, F. (1990). Parathyroid hormone-related protein in tumours associated with hypercalcaemia. *Lancet* **335**, 66–9.

Heinonen, A., Pekka, O., Kannus, P., Sievanen, H., Mantari, A., and Vuori, I. (1993). Bone mineral density of female athletes in different sports. *Bone and Mineral* **23**, 1–14.

Hewison, M. and O'Riordan, J.L.H. (1994). Vitamin D resistance. *Baillière's Clinical Endocrinology and Metabolism* **8**, 305–15.

Hughes, A.E. et al. (2000). Mutations in TNFRSF 11A, affecting the signal peptide of RANK, causing familial expansile osteolysis. *Nature Genetics* **24**, 45–8.

Jackson, M.E., Shalloub, V., Lian, J.B., Stein, G.S., and Marks, S.C., Jr. (1994). Abberant gene expression in cultured mammalian bone cells demonstrates an osteoblast defect in osteopetrosis. *Journal of Cellular Biochemistry* **55**, 366–72.

Johnston, C.C. et al. (1992). Calcium supplementation and increases in bone mineral density in children. *New England Journal of Medicine* **327**, 82–7.

Karaplis, A.C. et al. (1994). Lethal skeletal dysplasia from targeted disruption of the parathyroid hormone-related peptide gene. *Genes and Development* **8**, 277–89.

Khosla, S., Peterson, J.M., Egan, K., Jones, J.D., and Riggs, B.L. (1994). Circulating cytokine levels in osteoporotic and normal women. *Journal of Endocrinology and Metabolism* **79**, 707–11.

Lee, B., Vissing, H., Ramirez, F., Rogers, D., and Rimoin, D. (1989). Indentification of the molecular defect in a family with spondyloepiphyseal dysplasia. *Science* **244**, 978–80.

Lefkowitz, R.J. (1995). G proteins in medicine. *New England Journal of Medicine* **332**, 186–7.

Le Merrer, M. et al. (1994). A gene for achondroplasia–hypochondroplasia maps to chromosome 4p. *Nature Genetics* **6**, 318–21.

Mao, J.R. and Bristow, J. (2001). The Ehlers–Danlos syndrome: on beyond c allogens. *Journal of Clinical Investigation* **107**, 1063–9.

Marcus, R., Feldman, D., and Kelsey, K. *Osteoporosis.* San Diego CA: Academic Press, 1996.

Martin, T.J. (1990). Properties of parathyroid hormone-related protein and its role in malignant hypercalcaemia. *Quarterly Journal of Medicine* **76**, 771–86.

Marx, S.J. (2000). Hyperparathyroid and hypoparathyroid disorders. *New England Journal of Medicine* **343**, 1863–5.

McIntosh, I., Abbott, M.H., Warman, M.L., Olsen, B.R., and Francomano, C.A. (1994). Additional mutations of type X collagen confirm COL10A1 as the Schmid metaphyseal chondrodysplasia locus. *Human Molecular Genetics* **3**, 303–7.

Mornet, E. et al. (1998). Identification of fifteen novel mutations in the tissue-non specific alkaline phosphatase (TNASLP) gene in European patients with severe hypophosphatasia. *European Journal of Human Genetics* **6**, 308–14.

Morrison, N.A. et al. (1994). Prediction of bone density from vitamin D receptor alleles. *Nature* 367, 284–7.

Myllyharju, J. and Kivirikko, K.I. (2001). Collagens and collagen-related diseases. *Annals of Medicine* 33, 7–21.

Pocock, N.A., Elsman, J.A., and Hopper, J.L. (1987). Genetic determinants of bone mass in adults: a twin study. *Journal of Clinical Investigation* 80, 706–10.

Primorac, D. et al. (2001). Osteogenesis imperfecta at the beginning of the bone and joint decade. *Croatian Medical Journal* 42, 392–414.

Prockop, D.J. and Kivirikko, K.I. (1984). Heritable diseases of collagen. *New England Journal of Medicine* 311, 376–86.

Pyeritz, R.E. (1993). The Marfan syndrome. In *Connective Tissue and its Heritable Disorders* 1st edn. (ed. P.M. Royce and B. Steinmann), pp. 437–68. New York: Wiley-Liss.

Reardon, W., Winter, R.M., Rutland, P., Pulleyn, L.J., Jones, B.M., and Malcolm, S. (1994). Mutations in the fibroblast growth factor receptor 2 gene cause Crouzon syndrome. *Nature Genetics* 8, 98–103.

Riggs, B.L. and Melton, L.J. *Osteoporosis. Etiology, Diagnosis and Management.* New York: Raven Press, 1988.

Rousseau, F. et al. (1994). Mutations in the gene encoding fibroblast growth factor receptor-3 in achondroplasia. *Nature* 371, 252–4.

Rowe, D.W. and Shapiro, J.R. (1998). Osteogenesis imperfecta. In *Metabolic Bone Disease and Clinically Related Disorders* 3rd edn. (ed. L.V. Avioli and S.M. Krane), pp. 651–95. San Diego CA: Academic Press.

Royce, P.M. and Steinmann, B. *Connective Tissue and its Heritable Disorders* 1st edn. New York: Wiley-Liss, 1993.

Schipani, E. et al. (1996). Constitutively activated receptors for parathyroid hormone and parathyroid-hormone related peptide in Jansens metaphyseal chondrodysplasia. *New England Journal of Medicine* 335, 708–14.

Seeman, E., Hopper, J.L., and Bach, L.A. (1989). Reduced bone mass in daughters of women with osteoporosis. *New England Journal of Medicine* 320, 554–8.

Shiang, R. et al. (1994). Mutations in the transmembrane domain of FGFR3 cause the most common genetic form of dwarfism, achondroplasia. *Cell* 78, 335–43.

Shimada, T. et al. (2001). Cloning and characterisation of FGF23 as a causative factor of tumor-induced osteomalacia. *Proceedings of the National Academy of Sciences USA* 98, 6500–5.

Shore, E.M. et al. (2000). Fibrodysplasia ossificans progressiva. In *The Genetics of Osteoporosis and Metabolic Bone Disease* (ed. M.J. Econs), pp. 211–36. Totowa NJ: Humana Press.

Smith, R. (1994). Osteogenesis imperfecta: from phenotype to genotype and back again. *International Journal of Experimental Pathology* 75, 233–41.

Spiegel, A.M. (1990). Albright's hereditary osteodystrophy and defective G proteins. *New England Journal of Medicine* 322, 1461–2.

Spranger, J., Winterpacht, A., and Zabel, B. (1994). The type II collagenopathies: a spectrum of chondrodysplasias. *European Journal of Paediatrics* 153, 56–65.

Storm, E.E., Huynth, T.V., Copeland, N.G., Jenkins, N.A., Kingsley, D.M., and Lee, S.-J. (1994). Limb alteration in brachypodism mice due to mutations in a new member of the TGFβ-superfamily. *Nature* 368, 639–42.

Strewler, G.L. (2000), The physiology of parathyroid hormone related protein. *New England Journal of Medicine* 342, 177–85.

Sykes, B. (1990). Bone disease cracks genetics. *Nature* 348, 18–20.

Sykes, B. et al. (1990). Consistent linkage of dominantly inherited osteogenesis imperfecta to the type I collagen loci COL1A1 and COL1A2. *American Journal of Human Genetics* 46, 293–307.

Thakker, R.V. (1998). Multiple endocrine neoplasia-syndromes of the twentieth century. *Journal of Clinical Endocrinology and Metabolism* 83, 2617–20.

Thakker, R.V. (2001). Genetic developments in hypoparathyroidism. *Lancet* 357, 974–6.

Tickle, C. (1994). On making a skeleton. *Nature* 368, 587–8.

Vajo, Z., Francomano, C.A., and Wilkin, D.J., (2000). The molecular and genetic basis of fibroblast growth factor receptor 3 disorders: the achondroplasia family of skeletal dysplasias. Muenke craniosynostosis, and Crouzon syndrome with acanthosis nigricans. *Endocrine Reviews* 21, 23–39.

Vissing, H., D'Alessio, M., Lee, B., Ramirez, F., Godfrey, M., and Hollister, D.W. (1989). Glycine to serine substitution in the triple helical domain of Pro α1(II) collagen results in a lethal perinatal form of short-limbed dwarfism. *Journal of Biological Chemistry* 264, 18265–7.

Wallis, G.A., Starman, B.J., Zinn, A.B., and Byers, P.H. (1990). Variable expression of osteogenesis imperfecta in a nuclear family is explained by somatic mosaicism for a lethal point mutation in the α1(I) gene (COL1A1) of type I collagen in a parent. *American Journal of Human Genetics* 46, 1034–40.

Wallis, G.A. et al. (1994). Amino acid substitutions of conserved residues in the carboxyl-terminal domain of the α1(X) chain of type X collagen occur in two unrelated families with metaphyseal chondrodysplasia type Schmid. *American Journal of Human Genetics* 54, 169–78.

Wang, Z.-Q. et al. (1992). Bone and haematopoietic defects in mice lacking *c-fos*. *Nature* 360, 741–5.

Winterpacht, A., Hilber, M., Schwarze, U., Mundlos, S., Spranger, J., and Zabel, B. (1994). Autosomal dominant spondylarthropathy due to a type II procollagen gene (COL2A1) point mutation. *Human Mutation* 4, 257–62.

Wynne-Davies, R., Hall, C.M., and Apley, A.G. *Atlas of Skeletal Dysplasias* 1st edn. Edinburgh: Churchill Livingstone, 1985.

Yasuda, H. et al. (1999). A novel molecular mechanism modulating osteoclast differentiation and function. *Bone* 25, 109–13.

Yoshida, H. et al. (1990). The murine mutation osteopetrosis is in the coding region of the macrophage colony stimulating factor gene. *Nature* 345, 442–3.

Zurutuza, L. et al. (1999). Correlations of genotype and phenotype in hypophosphatasia. *Human Molecular Genetics* 8, 1039–46.

3.5 The physiology of the joint and its disturbance in inflammation

David Blake, Paul Mapp, and Cliff R. Stevens

> No part of the physiology of bones abounds more in hypotheses and less in discoveries than the history of the synovial system.
>
> Many discussions and few facts; a long series of assumed principles; a brief assemblage of proofs; this is the analysis of all the hitherto known works on the subject. The notions already received throw but little light on those yet to be acquired.
>
> Marie-Francois-Xavier Bichat (1771–1802).

This chapter covers selected aspects of the physiology of the joint in health and disease. The normal synovium and synovial fluid will be described. Other areas of the joint such as the cartilage have been covered in previous chapters. Further, we will characterize the structural changes to the synovium and chemical changes in the fluid that occur in chronic inflammation and address the physiological implications of these changes. Finally, we will evaluate possible mechanisms by which these changes may lead to joint damage.

The synovium

The normal human body contains 187 synovial joints. In this chapter, the term synovium will be used to describe the connective tissue bound by the fibrous joint capsule on one side and by the joint space on the other.

One of the most striking histological features of the normal synovium is a lack of cellularity, apart from a discontinuous layer of cells, the synovial intimal cells, on the internal surfaces of the joint. Although variously described as synoviocytes, lining cells, or surface cells, here they will be referred to as intimal cells.

Intimal cells form a thin discontinuous layer lining the joint space and separate it from the fibro-fatty tissue and capsule that surrounds the whole joint. The intimal cells line all surfaces of the joint other than the cartilage and menisci. Synovial intimal cells, in common with other connective tissues, are derived in the embryo from the mesenchyme (O'Rhailly and Gardner 1978). What are apparently intimal cells may also be generated under certain other circumstances in connective tissue, as in the case of a pseudoarthrosis and as regenerated synovium covering the joint capsule connective tissue following synovectomy. Similar cells can be created in animal models when air is injected into loose connective tissue. The whole synovium is bathed in synovial fluid since there is no true basement membrane beneath the intimal cells. Since there is neither a continuous layer of cells nor any basement underneath them, the term synovial membrane is, strictly speaking, a misnomer.

Histology and ultrastructure of the normal synovium

Cellular morphology

By routine light microscopy the intimal cell layer appears as a homogeneous population of varying thickness. In some areas the cells may lie three or four layers deep whilst in others places there are gaps where no intimal cells are seen and the underlying stroma is apparently in direct contact with the joint fluid. The underlying tissue, however, may show markedly different appearances and this has led some authors to classify synovia on this basis. Divisions into areolar, fibrous, and fatty synovia have been applied to the synovium, although other researchers have recognized intermediate types such as fibroareolar synovium. In general, the normal synovium appears as a quiescent connective tissue containing some macrophages and fibroblasts with a thin layer of cells opposing the joint space. The particular nature of the underlying connective tissue is unlikely to be of significance.

Ultrastructural examination of the synovium has yielded much data but little agreement with regard to the predominant intimal cell type or their function. Intimal cells were first described by Barland et al. (1962) and divided into types A and B on a purely morphological basis. Other authors have made similar distinctions but have included an intermediate cell type postulating that this is a precursor of the two intimal cell types. The type A cell is characterized morphologically by a prominent Golgi apparatus, numerous vesicles and vacuoles, many filopodia, and mitochondria. This description is typical of a tissue macrophage. Type B cells, in contrast, contain large amounts of endoplasmic reticulum and a few large vacuoles, correlating well with ultrastructural descriptions of fibroblasts at other sites. The weight of scientific evidence suggests that the type A cell is a bone-marrow-derived macrophage and the type B cell is a mesenchymal fibroblast. The reader is particularly directed to the work of Edwards and Willoughby (1982), which demonstrates the arrival in the synovium of bone-marrow-derived macrophages using intracellular granules as a genetic marker.

Vascular system

Capillaries occur within the synovium and also the underlying tissues (fat, skeletal muscle, etc.). The synovium is considerably more vascular than the structures supporting the joint such as the capsule, ligaments, and tendons.

The first description of the vasculature within joints was made by Hunter (1743) who described the *circulus articuli vasculosus* as 'All around the neck of the bone there is a greater number of arteries and veins which ramify into smaller branches and communicate with one another by frequent anastomoses like those of the mesentery. This might be called the *circulus articuli vasculosus*, the vascular border of the joint'.

At the margins of articular cartilage the synovium forms villi and folds into which the plexus sends arcades of capillaries. The circulus articuli vasculosus anastomoses with deeper perichondrial vessels that communicate with the bone marrow vasculature. There are anastomosing plexuses in the deeper layers of areolar lining tissue, with decreasing vascular calibre towards the surface. A plexus of arterioles and venules also forms a quadrilateral array close to the surface of the synovium. This plexus yields capillary loops that pass through the cells or immediately below the layer of synovial intimal cells. The surface of the tissue carries a much denser capillary bed than the deeper tissue layers. The dimensions of the mesh of the arteriolar/venous plexus are between 0.9 and 1.5 mm.

Arteriovenous anastomoses (AVA) have been demonstrated to occur commonly in the joints of humans and animals. The pattern of the AVA suggests an important role in the regulation of the articular and, perhaps, the epiphysial blood flow, possibly by a shunt mechanism redistributing the blood flow between certain vascular beds. The AVA between muscle, capsule, and bone help to explain the production of endosseous blood stasis during rest or muscular inactivity and suggests that the AVA are related to regional haemodynamic regulation.

The vascularity of normal synovium appears to depend considerably on the type of underlying tissue. Capillary density is greatest where the substructure is areolar or adipose tissue and is virtually zero over fibrous areas. Away from the margins of articular cartilage the synovium is flatter, and the synovial capillaries form a flat loose polyhedral network supplied by several articular arteries. The capillaries are sinuous, which may reduce wall stress during motion, and are occasionally so coiled as to resemble glomerular capillaries.

Morphometry of normal human knee synovia has provided data on the spatial distribution of these vessels. The density of the capillaries is 240 mm^{-2} of synovial lining and their modal depth is 35 μm from the intimal cell/joint space boundary. The mean intercapillary distance is 17 μm (Stevens et al. 1991). Similar data have been obtained in rabbit synovia (Knight and Levick 1983). From these data, the functionally optimal range of vascular parameters for the synovium can be extrapolated. From this blood supply the bulk of the constituents of the synovial fluid is derived.

Nerve supply

Joints are supplied by both primary and accessory nerves. Primary nerves are branches of peripheral nerves passing near the joint whilst accessory nerves are branches of intramuscular nerves crossing the joint capsule. Some joints such as the knee and ankle also receive a nerve supply from cutaneous nerves in the overlying skin. The nerves to any one particular joint always arise from more than one level in the spinal cord. About 50 per cent of the axons that comprise articular nerves are less than 5 μm in diameter, those that are less than 2 μm in diameter are unmyelinated. These fibres carry nociceptive information with a slow conduction velocity. The nerve supply to the synovium was, until relatively recently, thought to be sparse. However, it is now known that the synovium contains a good supply of unmyelinated nerve fibres (Mapp et al. 1990). These are of two types: the post-ganglionic sympathetic adrenergic fibres located around the larger blood vessels are responsible for the control of articular blood flow and the unmyelinated C fibres, on the other hand, are responsible for pain transmission. The latter group of fibres are not normally active and are thought only to fire during tissue damage, either mechanical or chemical.

The unmyelinated fibres arise from cell bodies that are located in the dorsal root ganglion, close to the spinal cord. In addition to its peripheral projection the cell body also has a central projection to the spinal cord. The fine diameter nerve fibres terminate in the superficial layers of the spinal cord, laminae I and II of the dorsal horn, from where they synapse with ascending fibres in the spinal cord. The cell bodies are the site of manufacture of neuropeptides that are transported both centrally and peripherally along the nerve axons. The functions of these peptides are not clearly understood in the central nervous system but some, for instance substance P, are thought to be involved in pain transmission. Peripherally where the effects of these peptides are much easier to investigate they are clearly involved in the inflammatory process, both in its induction and in its modulation. They have the capacity individually or in synergism with other neuropeptides or mediators to modulate, mediate, or prime for an inflammatory response. In addition, they have an effect on vascular tone.

Having examined the structure of the synovium we turn to the fluid which is derived from it and which bathes the whole joint cavity.

Synovial fluid

The study of normal synovial fluid is difficult since the aspiratable volume of fluid is very small, in the range of 0–4 ml. The fluid is regarded as an ultrafiltrate of the plasma but in addition components secreted by the synovial cells are also present. The most important of these is hyaluronate. Hyaluronate is a linear repeating disaccharide, beta-D-glucuronyl-beta-D-*N*-acetyl-glucosamine, of high molecular weight (upwards of 10 000 000 Da). Hyaluronate forms the central axis of the proteoglycan aggregates necessary for the functional integrity of articular cartilage and other extracellular matrices. It comprises the major macro-molecular species of the synovial fluid and is responsible for the unique visco-elastic properties of the synovial fluid. More recently another component of human synovial fluid has been identified, lubricin, which as its name implies is thought to be involved in the lubrication of the joint (Swann et al. 1985). Lubricin is a protein with oligosaccharide side chains and has a molecular weight of 166 000 Da. *In vitro* its lubricating activity is concentration dependent and at concentrations thought to be present in the joint it acts as a highly efficient lubricant. A similar molecule has been isolated from bovine synovial fluid. As well as acting as a lubricant synovial fluid is also the source of nutrition for the articular cartilage.

The mechanism of formation of the synovial fluid is thought to be similar to that of interstitial fluid in any other body cavity. The flow across the capillary wall is driven by the difference between the pressure in the capillary and the joint fluid. This is opposed by both the osmotic and colloid pressure gradients, the Starling hypothesis (1896). Small physiological molecules of molecular weight less than 10 000 Da are in full equilibrium with the plasma. A graphic plot of the diffusion coefficient of a molecule (which takes into account mass and size) against the synovial permeability yields a broadly linear curve. Larger molecules such as proteins have only restricted access to the normal synovial fluid. The total protein content of the synovial fluid is 13 mg/l (as compared to the serum concentration of 65–80 mg/l), most of this protein being albumin. Proteins of higher molecular weight, such as fibrinogen, are excluded. Whilst proteins arrive in the joint at rates inversely proportional to their molecular size their rates of egress are similar. This is a reflection of the fact that protein is cleared from the synovial fluid by bulk flow through the lymphatic system that is not dependent on the size of the molecule.

Intra-articular pressure

The overall pressure within the normal joint is sub-atmospheric, pressures of −3 to −6 cmH_2O are typically recorded both at rest and during movement (Blake et al. 1989). This is true both in relaxation and during weight bearing. The 'joint space' is, therefore, only an apparent space since atmospheric pressure pressing on the soft tissues around the joint will cause the synovium to be in close opposition to the articular cartilage surface. This has the effect of optimizing the transfer of nutrients from the superficial blood vessels in the synovium to the avascular cartilage.

The intraarticular pressure is to be distinguished from the pressure that arises between the two cartilage surfaces, when under load.

Inflammatory disease

Histology of the inflamed synovium

Examination of the synovium in chronic inflammation reveals a wide variety of morphological changes, many of which may alter the physiology of the joint. The intimal cell layer becomes thickened, both by an increase in cell number and by an increase in cell size; hyperplasia and hypertrophy, respectively. The intimal cell layer is 6–8 cells deep. Underlying the intimal layer, changes typical of chronic inflammation are seen. There is a large increase in the number of cells, comprising mainly macrophages and lymphocytes. The lymphocytes accumulate perivascularly around the post-capillary venules and may organize into foci resembling lymphoid follicles: plasma cells are seen at the margins of the follicles. Large numbers of macrophages are also seen scattered widely throughout the tissue, these are thought to be migrating to the intimal cell layer replacing the turnover in type A cells.

Vasculature

The dominating vascular feature of chronic inflammatory disease is a vasculitis localized to the venules and capillaries, although it has been demonstrated that arterioles also become involved to a lesser degree. Using vital microscopy to study the rheumatoid synovium it has been found that venular dilatation of varying calibre, resulting in uneven outline and slow, almost stagnated corpuscular flow, is also a feature. In severe cases, focal and segmental venular-capillary necrosis and thrombosis are found in association with connective tissue necrosis. However, in less severe disease, vascular derangement is largely reversible and manifested by excessive venular-capillary dilatation, leakage, and occasionally by focal, partial, or temporary microvasculature obstruction.

Of particular relevance to the physiology of the joint are the changes seen in the synovial vasculature. Assuming that the data on capillary density and depth determined in normal joints represent the optimal situation, there is a significant reduction in vascularity in the functionally important superficial region of the synovium. The capillary number density in rheumatoid arthritis (RA) is reduced to about one-third of the normal value, from 240 to 80 capillaries per mm^2; mean intercapillary distance increased from 17 to 37 μm, reflecting not only an increase in spatial distribution of the vasculature but also a thickened synovial lining. The average capillary distance from the joint cavity is increased from 32.5 to 93.3 μm (Stevens et al. 1991). This apparent burial of the vasculature is due to the thickening of the synovial lining layer that would appear to proceed at a greater pace than angiogenesis (Fig. 1). In addition to these changes multilamination of the basement membranes (Matsubara et al. 1983) surrounding the blood vessel is also seen due to stimulation of endothelial cells (by unknown mediators) to produce excessive cellular components of basement membrane, this represents a further barrier to nutrient exchange. This is compounded by the deposition of fibrin that is often seen on the surface of the inflamed synovium.

The height of endothelium in small vessels is increased in chronic synovitis, with an increase in the number of vessels with histochemical features of the so-called high endothelial venules in tissue from rheumatoid patients. These vessels are thought to be the main site of lymphocyte traffic in lymph

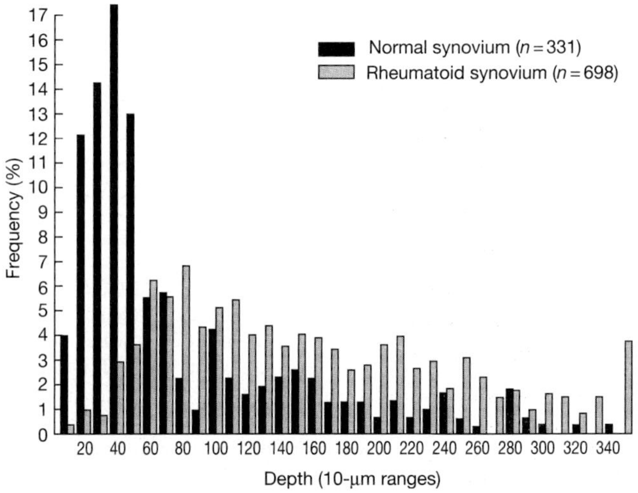

Fig. 1 Histogram showing the distribution of blood vessels in normal and rheumatoid synovia. The figures referred to relate to the distance of the vessels from the intimal cell surface.

and could represent a facilitated pathway for lymphocyte entry in pathological circumstances. One of the most frequent histologic findings affecting small vessels in chronic inflammation is that of perivascular cuffing by lymphocytes.

Nerve supply

In common with the vasculature, the nerve supply which normally extends to the synovial/joint space interface, is buried deeper within the rheumatoid synovium. It is probable that this is due to proliferation of the synovium but may be due to release of factors that are inhibitory to nerve proliferation or the inactivation of peptides that promote neuronal outgrowth, such as protease nexin 1 (Meier et al. 1990). The blood vessels that are in the superficial layers of the synovium, up to 150 μm from the joint space, appear not to be innervated by post-ganglionic sympathetic nerve fibres. This would imply that there is poor control over the superficial vascular supply. Free nerve fibres, assumed to be sensory in nature, are also absent from this area.

Nerve fibres, both free and perivascular, are, however, present in the deeper inflamed tissues (Fig. 2). These fibres appear to contain reduced amounts of neuropeptide, as determined by immunocytochemistry. The probable explanation for this is that the stored peptide is being released into the joint cavity.

In summary, the inflamed joint shows the following characteristics:

(i) Infiltration with numerous inflammatory cells.

(ii) The intimal layer becomes hypertrophic and hyperplastic.

(iii) The vasculature is buried deeper within the synovium rendering the tissue relatively hypoxic.

(a)

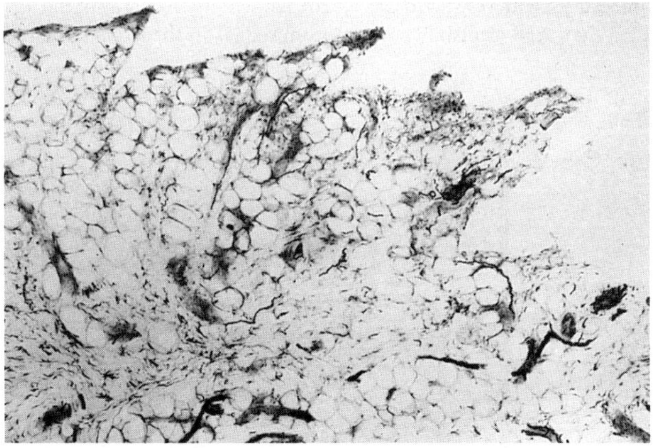

(b)

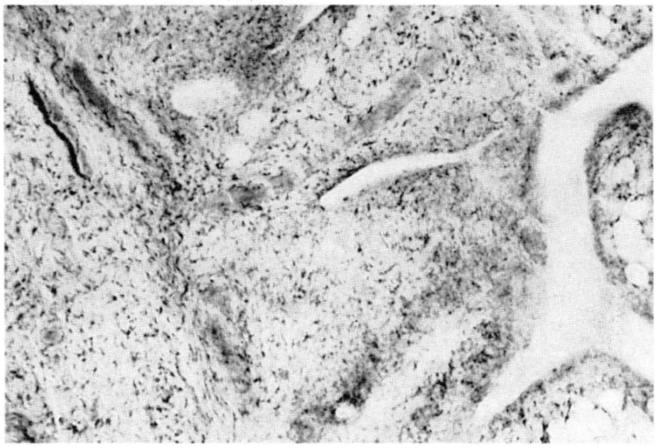

Fig. 2 Photomicrographs of normal (a) and rheumatoid (b) synovia. The specimens have been stained by immunocytochemistry to show all nerve fibres. Note the rich innervation of the normal specimen compared to the paucity of nerve fibres in the disease state.

(iv) The nervous supply is also buried deeper in the synovium perhaps releasing cells from normal neuronal regulation.

(v) The synovial fluid markedly increases in volume and changes in composition.

We now discuss how some of these basic changes induced by inflammation in turn influence the inflammatory process.

Ischaemia and hypoxia

The presence of a large cellular infiltrate in the inflamed synovium would lead one to think that there is an increased utilization of oxygen, often referred to as increased oxygen demand. This increased demand is not readily quantifiable. A working definition of ischaemia is that the steady-state rate of energy production, that is, ATP synthesis, cannot be supported by the existing blood flow. Since the necessary levels of energy production cannot be maintained this stimulates anaerobic metabolism, which, in turn, gives rise to lactic acid production and a fall in venous oxygen tension.

In order to determine whether the joint is ischaemic, attempts have been made to measure the blood flow in the synovium. Some studies, using the xenon (^{153}Xe) clearance technique have reported an increased perfusion in chronically inflamed synovia (Dick et al. 1970). The validity of such studies is in question because they fail to take account of the possibility of A–V shunting which would give rise to the impression of perfusion but would result in ischaemic, non-perfused synovial pockets. Other studies using ^{123}I or tritiated water appear to show that perfusion in chronic synovitis is markedly reduced (Simkin and Pizzorno 1979). The stage of the disease at which the perfusion is measured may be the all important factor here. In the early stages of RA, the temperature of the joint is raised relative to normal whereas in late stage disease their joint is cooler than normal. The implication of this is that in the early stages of the disease blood flow increases but in the later stages it decreases, the most affected joints being the ones with the least blood flow. Microvessel plugging by inflammatory cells also serves to reroute blood from the peripheral capillary beds. This is associated to a varying degree with microthrombi and extravascular aggregates of platelets.

Synovial fluid oxygen tension is more easily quantifiable than synovial ischaemia. The oxygen tension (pO_2) within the inflamed joint cavity (Lund-Oleson 1970) has been shown to be lower (27 mmHg) than in traumatic effusions (63 mmHg) or osteoarthritic knee fluids (43 mmHg). These results were confirmed by independent studies. In addition to a low pO_2, many studies have shown alterations in rheumatoid synovial fluid physiology, which would be anticipated in a hypoxic state, namely, raised carbon dioxide tension (pCO_2—upto 150 mmHg), raised lactate (upto 10 mM), lowered glucose and acidosis (pH as low as 6.6). The most comprehensive study summarizing these changes is by Falchuk et al. (1970) who showed that joints with the lowest pO_2 (as low as 9 mmHg) also exhibited large increases in pCO_2 and lactate: the same joints showed severe microvascular obliteration in the synovial membrane.

In summary, the inflamed joints are hypoxic because of increased metabolic demand of the inflamed synovium, and the inadequate oxygen delivery due to poor perfusion of the inflamed joint. It is important to note that physiological measurements in synovial fluid can vary with the patient's mobility. This observation has particular relevance to the concept of joint 'ischaemia-reperfusion' injury (Blake et al. 1989).

Synovial metabolism

The oxygen consumption of the rheumatoid synovial membrane per gram of excised tissue is approximately 20 times that of normal synovial membrane (Dingle and Page-Thomas 1956). This work also demonstrated that the activity of the glycolytic (Embden–Meyerhof) pathway for ATP production was markedly increased in rheumatoid compared to normal synovium. The raised metabolic rate of the rheumatoid synovium concomitantly raises the demand for ATP. The intracellular production of this molecule can be achieved by either the aerobic or anaerobic oxidation of glucose via the tricarboxylic acid (TCA) cycle or the glycolytic pathway, respectively. The oxygen-dependent TCA cycle is a much more efficient producer of ATP than the anaerobic system and so is generally favoured in normoxic tissues. The fact that the rheumatoid synovium favours the anaerobic glycolytic pathway indicates its hypoxic nature. In support of this, synovial intimal cells in rheumatoid arthritis contain significantly more glyceraldehyde-3-phosphate and lactate dehydrogenase activity than those of normal tissue. These are major enzymes of the glycolytic pathway. Their increase is more reasonably explained by a response to tissue hypoxia than by elevated metabolic activity as mitochondrial oxidation in the synovium is not similarly enhanced.

The terminal end-product of the anaerobic oxidation of glucose is lactate. The ratio of lactate to glucose, therefore, should give an indication of oxygen status in the synovium. This is indeed the case, as it has been shown that lowered glucose and raised lactate levels correlate well with falls in pO_2 and pH. Proton nuclear magnetic resonance (NMR) spectroscopy confirms the peculiar anaerobic environment in the inflamed joint. Comparison of paired synovial fluids and sera show that the concentrations of lactate, 3-D-hydroxybutarate and acetoacetate are all much higher in the synovial fluid than the serum pair. Additionally, high levels of ketone bodies are also found. The hypoxic conditions prevailing in the inflamed joint lead to an increase in fatty acid oxidation. However, the unavailability of NAD^+ results in an inability of the citric acid cycle to fully oxidize acetyl coenzyme A. This process leads to a build-up of unoxidizable metabolites, ketone bodies, recently demonstrated by NMR spectroscopy and illustrated in Fig. 3.

Acute exacerbation of chronic hypoxia

A distinguishing property of the joint is its ability to move. The inflamed joint of a mobile patient is unavoidably subjected to movement. This situation has profound significance in joint pathogenesis through the effects of hypoxic-reperfusion injury (Woodruff et al. 1986).

The environment for hypoxia and reperfusion in rheumatoid synovitis is created by the unique topography of the component parts of a joint that predisposes the synovium to pressure-induced fluctuations in blood supply. The synovium is the innermost confine of the joint space and its fluid. This moveable and compressible stroma is backed by the more rigid confines of the musculature and ligaments. It might be anticipated, therefore, that centripetal thickening and increasing fluid volume generates a pressurized system. This is indeed the case. We have confirmed (Blake et al. 1989) that the resting intra-articular pressure (IAP) in chronically inflamed joints is slightly above atmospheric pressure (+5 to 10 mmHg) compared with that of normal joints, which is sub-atmospheric (−5 mmHg). When normal joint are exercised, the pressure falls further, whereas in chronically inflamed joints IAP rises, sometimes as high as 300 mmHg and always above the capillary perfusion pressure in inflammation of 30–60 mmHg; this is illustrated in Fig. 4. It is, therefore, suggested that in chronically inflamed joints, the IAP rises during exercise above a critical level sufficient to occlude parts of the capillary bed thus inducing acute ischaemia in an already hypoxic environment. In rabbit knees IAPs as low as 19 mmHg cause synovial capillaries to assume a more flattened, elliptical profile.

In mobile patients who may be subjecting their joints to pressure induced ischaemia, subsequent rest allows reperfusion of blood and reoxygenation of the synovium, albeit to an inadequate degree. This eventuality has pathological repercussions consequent on the generation of reactive oxygen metabolites which accompanies post-ischaemic reperfusion.

Biochemical consequences of synovial hypoxia

There are a number of biochemical consequences of hypoxia; calcium imbalance is arguably the most influential of these events. Intracellular homeostasis, with respect to Ca^{2+}, is dependent upon energy in the form of ATP. When ATP availability is compromised, as in the hypoxic synovium,

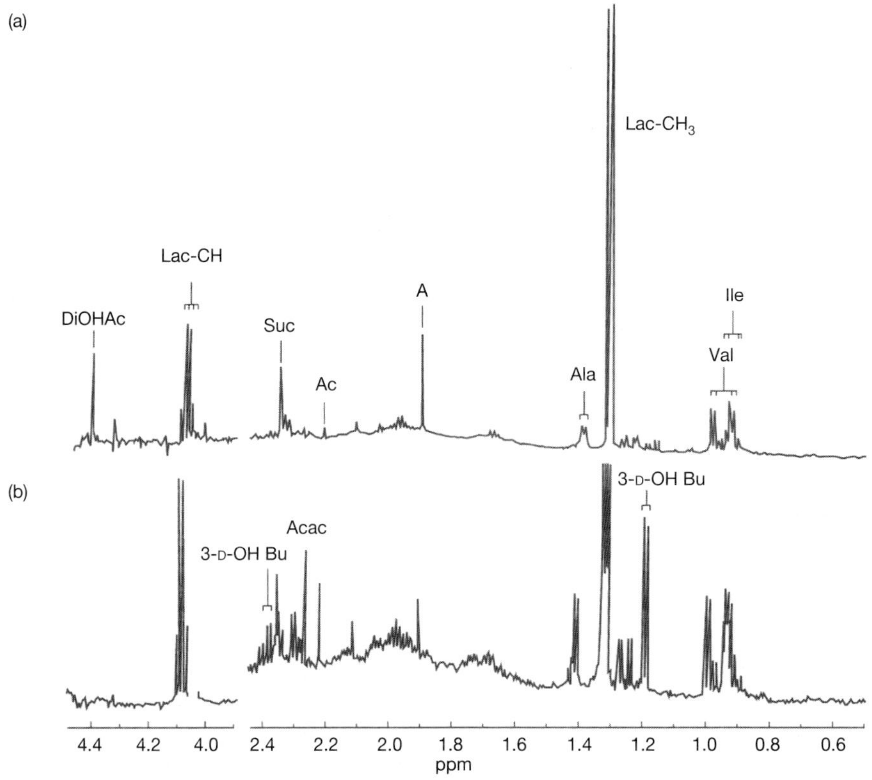

Fig. 3 600 MHz proton nuclear magnetic resonance spectra of low molecular mass, non-protein bound components of isolates from osteoarthritic (a) and rheumatoid (b) synovial fluids. DiOHAc, dihydroxyacetone; Lac, lactate; Suc, Succinate; Ac, acetone; A, acetate; Ala, alanine; Val, valine; Ile, isoleucine; 3-D-OH Bu, 3-D-hydroxybutarate; Acac, acetoacetate. (Samples were run in a Varian 600 MHz machine operating at 600 MHz at ambient temperature.)

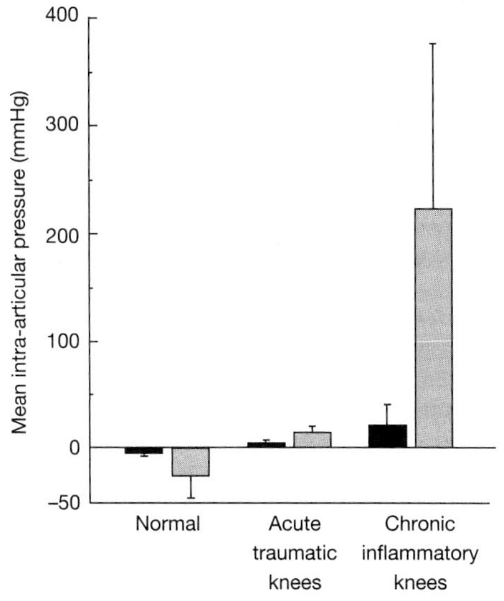

Fig. 4 Pressure changes on exercise. Black bars, rest; Grey bars, exercise.

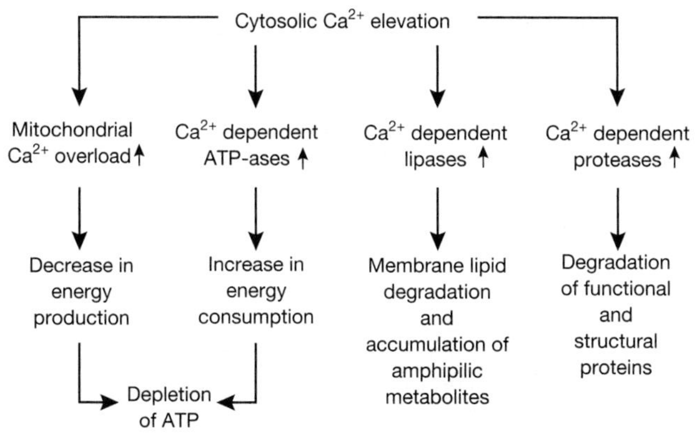

Fig. 5 Role of elevated cytosolic calcium in tissue injury.

cytosolic Ca^{2+} levels rise. Mitochondria are avid accumulators of Ca^{2+}, and when overloaded with Ca^{2+} their function is impaired, resulting in the further depletion of ATP levels and the maintenance of a calcium influx. Many important cellular functions and control mechanisms are Ca^{2+} dependent. The consequences of hypoxia-derived Ca^{2+} imbalance must be considered as possible contributing factors in the pathogenesis of rheumatoid arthritis (Fig. 5). The mechanism for increased vascular permeability for instance, which is associated with interendothelial gap formation, is thought to involve changes in the actin cytoskeleton of the endothelial cell. These changes can be elicited by calcium imbalance since actin binding proteins that regulate the endothelial cytoskeleton are calcium dependent. The failure of cellular phosphorylation mechanisms also leads to accumulation of adenosine and of its breakdown products, including hypoxanthine and xanthine, which are the substrates for the xanthine oxidase enzyme system, vide infra. The outcome of these events in the hypoxic synovium confers the facility for the inappropriate generation of reactive oxygen metabolites upon reperfusion of blood. There is much evidence to show that post-ischaemic reperfusion of the synovium evokes the generation of reactive oxygen metabolites, despite the underlying hypoxic environment that is not conducive to most conventional radical generating systems. One proposed mechanism that can achieve this is dependent on the enzyme xanthine oxidase, which is present within the capillaries of the synovium (Allen et al. 1987). The non-pathological dehydrogenase form of this enzyme oxidizes hypoxanthine and xanthine to uric acid using NAD^+ as an electron acceptor. Under ischaemic conditions, however, this enzyme can be converted to an NAD^+ independent form that catalyzes the same reaction using molecular oxygen as an electron acceptor and results in superoxide anion generation. The inappropriate production of superoxide in a biological system can have catastrophic repercussions particularly when the system facilitates the redox environment required for consequent hydroxyl radical ($^{\bullet}OH$) formation. The synovium is such a system enabling the spontaneous or enzymatic conversion of superoxide to hydrogen peroxide, which can then fuel a Fenton-type reaction catalyzed by decompartmentalized iron (Morris et al. 1986) forming the cytotoxic $^{\bullet}OH$ radical:

$$H_2O_2 + Fe^{2+} \rightarrow {}^{\bullet}OH + OH^- + Fe^{3+}$$

Iron is decompartmentalized as a consequence of hypoxia and can be detected bound to citrate in the synovial fluid. In such a form it may promote hydroxyl radical formation.

Biological consequences of reactive oxygen metabolites

Biochemical analysis of synovial fluid reveals the effects of radical damage to endogenous biomolecules in rheumatoid arthritis.

Lipids

The cell membrane, composed primarily of polyunsaturated fatty acids, is a well studied target for radical attack, and the resultant process of lipid peroxidation causes cell membrane damage. Polyunsaturated lipids undergoing the process of peroxidation give rise to the formation of lipid breakdown products such as lipid hydroperoxides, endoperoxides, aldehydes, and alkanes. These can be measured and correlate well with the clinical severity of the disease.

Proteins

Exposure of proteins to free radicals will lead to denaturation, cross-linking, aggregation, and fragmentation. There is much evidence of radical-mediated protein damage occurring in inflammatory synovitis. Immunoglobulin G (IgG) when exposed to free radicals *in vitro* develops a characteristic autofluoresence (excitation 360 nm, emission 454 nm) and forms both monomeric and aggregated complexes (Lunec et al. 1985). IgG with these characteristics is present in rheumatoid synovial fluid.

Additionally, the methionine residues on α-1-antitrypsin (the primary inhibitor of leucocyte elastase) are oxidized to sulfoxide adducts by free radicals, rendering the molecule biologically inactive. Such radical damaged α-1-antitrypsin is present in inflammatory synovial fluid.

Carbohydrates

Free radicals can also react with polysaccharides and induce fragmentation. The major macromolecule of the synovial fluid, which accounts for its viscosity, is the glycosaminoglycan hyaluronate. Loss of viscosity of the synovial fluid is thought to be due to the depolymerization of hyaluronate and an increase in the synovial concentration of dialyzable hyaluronan fragments and saccharide monomers. The alternative explanation for the reduction in the molecular weight of hyaluronan is defective synthesis with premature termination of the polysaccharide chain. Pulse-chase labelling experiments have supported the view that the presence of short-chain molecules of hyaluronan in the synovial fluid is due to post-synthetic degradation rather than defective synthesis. As neither normal nor inflammatory synovial fluids contain any measurable hyaluronidase activity it is inferred that the depolymerization of hyaluronan is the result of free radical attack. The degradation products have different biological properties from that of the native molecule. Low-molecular-mass fragments of hyaluronan are pro-angiogenic, whereas the high-molecular-mass hyaluronan has inhibitory effects on endothelial cell proliferation. Proliferation of both fibroblasts and mitogen-stimulated lymphocytes is similarly affected.

Effects on cells and cell viability

There are important effects of free radicals upon cells when considered as a whole. T lymphocytes in general have been shown to be susceptible to free radical attack. Free radicals are more toxic to T-cytotoxic/suppressor than to T-helper cells *in vitro* (Allan et al. 1986). These results support the speculation that free radical reactions, in addition to inducing the denaturation of proteins, can prevent immune suppressor/cytotoxic cells from controlling auto-immune reactions with subsequent immuno-pathological consequences. As well as the cytotoxic aspects of free radical attack on whole cells, which occurs at high concentrations, the data (Murrell et al. 1990) also suggest that at low concentrations free radicals can stimulate proliferation of cells. Under *in vitro* conditions fibroblasts were stimulated to proliferate by low concentrations of free radicals (the fibroblasts themselves release their own free radicals) and fibroblasts were inhibited from proliferation but were still viable when the endogenous free radicals were inhibited.

Many other examples of oxidative damage to the joint have been reported. Apart from these damaging or cytotoxic properties of free radicals, they also have the capacity to interfere subtly with finely controlled physiological mechanisms. One example of this occurs in the control of vascular tone by vasoactive substances.The activity of endothelium-derived relaxing factor (EDRF) has been ascribed to the nitrogen centred radical nitric oxide (NO) (Palmer et al. 1987) which is synthesized in endothelial cells by the Ca^{2+} dependent enzymatic conversion of L-arginine. It activates the cytosolic guanylyl cyclase of the adjacent smooth muscle cells increasing the levels of cGMP and resulting in relaxation of the cells and vasodilation. NO can interact with superoxide via peroxynitrite to produce the highly cytotoxic hydroxyl radical. *In vitro* this interaction abrogates the EDRF activity of NO. This is demonstrated by the ability of superoxide dismutase to enhance and prolong the relaxant effect of NO. NO is unstable and rapidly degrades to nitrate and nitrite, which are relatively stable in biological fluids. In inflammatory joints the synovial fluid levels of nitrite exceed those of the paired serum samples, thus indicating local production. The implication of this is that NO is also produced locally in the synovium. Vascular tone is controlled by the opposing actions of relaxing and contracting factors released from the endothelium in response to neurogenic stimuli or platelet products.

As mentioned above, NO can react with superoxide radicals leading to the formation of the potent oxidant peroxynitrite ($ONOO^-$). The attack of $ONOO^-$ upon aromatic amino acids leads to their nitration. One such reaction product, 3-nitrotyrosine (3-NT), is relatively stable, and its presence in tissues is strong evidence for the formation of $ONOO^-$ *in vivo*. We have examined rheumatoid arthritic and normal control synovia for the presence of 3-NT residues by immunohistochemistry. We found that 3-NT was present in the vascular smooth muscle of normal and diseased synovia (Mapp et al. 2001) (Fig. 6). The amount present in RA specimens was greatly increased as compared to normal material. It has been proposed that nitration of tyrosine residues is involved in the normal intracellular signalling process. However, it has also been demonstrated that exposure of rodent vascular smooth muscle *in vitro* brings about cellular energetic and contractile failure. We have, therefore, proposed that there is a physiologic role for $ONOO^-$ in modifying synovial vascular function.

Leucocyte chemotaxis and adhesion

The initiating factors of inflammatory cell infiltration are adherence to endothelium and chemotaxis. Synovial inflammatory cell infiltration is a major characteristic of RA as is the expression of membrane associated adhesion molecules. The contribution of hypoxia to this situation may have considerable significance particularly where oxygen free radicals are a consequence. Superoxide, hydrogen peroxide, or both can generate a chemoattractant for neutrophils from extracellular fluid (Perez et al. 1980; Petrone et al. 1980). The identity of the neutrophil chemotactic factor(s) generated in ischaemia is unknown. However, possible candidates are

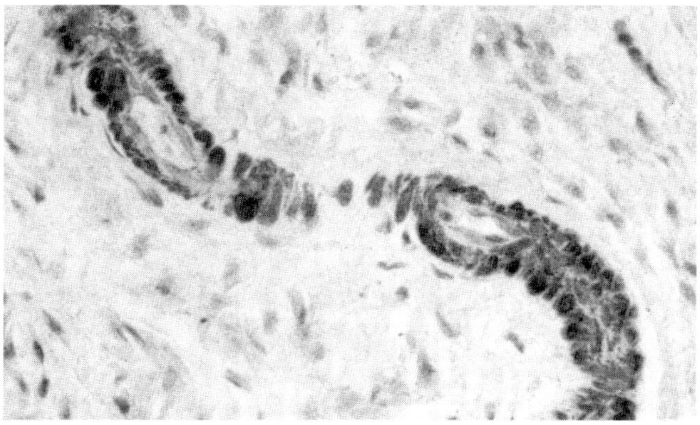

Fig. 6 Localization of 3-nitrotyrosine (dark area) in human rheumatoid synovium. Note that 3NT is present in the vascular smooth muscle of this resistance vessel but not in the endothelium.

cyclooxygenase and lipoxygenase metabolites of arachidonic acid, such as 12-hydroxyeicosatetraenoic acid, which is found to be raised in hypoxic states and is a neutrophil chemoattractant. In support of this, cultured endothelial cells are capable of responding to hypoxia by producing a neutrophil chemoattractant that is suppressible by lipoxygenase inhibitors.

The adhesion component of leucocyte infiltration can be facilitated by oxygen radicals (Suzuki et al. 1989) and by hypoxia alone. Interestingly, the adhesion of neutrophils to ischaemic arterial vasculature is associated with a loss of endothelium-dependent vasorelaxant activity.

Microvascular barrier function

In any inflammatory condition the manifestation of the inflammatory response is controlled by the permeability of the microvascular blood/tissue barrier. Increased transvascular exchange of macromolecules, emigration of leucocytes, and oedema formation are indicative of modified barrier function and are characteristic of synovial inflammation. The dynamics of barrier function, particularly solute exchange, are modulated physiologically by a complex assortment of mediators. During hypoxia, however, homeostasis is disrupted by, as yet, poorly understood mechanisms involving mediators of altered barrier function, such as PAF, complement, leukotrienes, and prostaglandins. Increased permeability during ischaemia or hypoxia has been reported in many vascular systems *in vitro* and *in vivo*, for example, heart (Armiger and Gavin 1975), lung (Lockhart and Saiag 1981), brain (Oleson 1986), and cultured bovine endothelium (Ogawa et al. 1990).

In addition to the effects of hypoxia alone, rheumatoid synovial microvascular function and permeability can be altered by the membrane damaging effects of oxygen free radicals. Measurement of von Willebrand factor (vWF) illustrates this. vWF, otherwise known as factor VIII-related antigen, is a large adhesive glycoprotein that is synthesized in endothelial cells and megakaryocytes and plays an important role in the adhesion of platelets to damaged vessel walls. Small sub-units of vWF are released constitutively by endothelial cells, accounting for normal circulating plasma levels. Larger multimers of vWF are stored in specific organelles called Weibel–Palade bodies within endothelial cells. Interestingly, these bodies are common in the synovium and have been implicated as a marker of angiogenesis in RA (Kumar et al. 1985). A variety of physiological stimuli can induce acute release of these multimers from the Weibel–Palade bodies *in vitro* including hypoxia, by a Ca^{2+} dependent process. Elevated levels of plasma vWF have been observed in various disease states including RA (Pottinger et al. 1989) where, in contrast to normal, levels increase with simple 'physiologic' exercise. This phenomenon has been assumed to indicate vascular damage (Greaves et al. 1987).

The attempts of the joint to limit the hypoxic damage

The immediate local response to tissue hypoxia is elicited by the vasculature, utilizing vasoactive substances that serve to enhance perfusion. It is clear that the facility for this response is impaired in rheumatoid synovitis. A longer term strategy for the re-establishment of adequate perfusion is neovascularization of hypoxic tissue. The facility for this, termed angiogenesis, most certainly exists in the rheumatoid synovium, to an extent which some believe to be pathological.

Under conditions of physiological stress, such as hypoxia, cell survival may become dependent on the expression of a specialized set of proteins, termed stress proteins.

Angiogenesis

The formation and growth of new blood vessels is under rigid control, so much so that in health angiogenesis only occurs in wound healing and during endometrial regeneration. Functional aberrations of the physiological regulation of new capillary growth such as seen in ischaemia and reperfusion are implicated in the pathogenesis (if not aetiology) of many neoplastic and non-neoplastic diseases.

The neovascularization of a wound progresses, logically, towards the centre where hypoxic macrophages are stimulated to produce angiogenic factors. The persistent synovitis characteristic of RA equates with persistent, though perhaps not fully effective, angiogenesis. The resulting fibroproliferative, inflammatory pannus invades and elicits the destruction of articular cartilage leading to joint deformation and loss of function. Clearly, there is angiogenesis in the rheumatoid synovium although morphometry suggests that this does not keep pace with synovial proliferation. This situation, as has been discussed earlier, promotes hypoxia in the peripheral region of the synovium that is rich in macrophages. The evidence that rheumatoid synovial tissue macrophages and hypoxic macrophages release a substance capable of inducing angiogenesis invites the hypothesis that hypoxia drives synovial angiogenesis. The macrophage-derived angiogenic factor is thought to be TNFα. TNFα has been localized histochemically to the synovial lining cells in RA but no prominent staining is seen in osteoarthritis non-inflammatory samples.

Stress proteins

Often inaccurately given the general term 'heat-shock proteins', these ubiquitous intracellular molecules form two groups. True heat-shock proteins (hsps) contain a specific consensus region within the promotor region of the gene while the second group, the glucose regulated proteins (grps), do not have this DNA sequence. Although the genes are normally quiescent or only partially active, stress protein mRNAs are actively transcribed following physiological stress, the proteins induced being dependent on the particular stressor; they are classified into families according to molecular weight.

Rheumatological interest in the hsps followed the implication of the 60 kDa family in the development of adjuvant-induced arthritis in rats; these observations have been extended to include other animal models of arthritis. Additionally, patients with rheumatoid arthritis have circulating isotype restricted antibodies to stress proteins and these same proteins are abundantly present in inflamed but not normal synovia; the high levels of the stress-inducible 72 kDa protein give a good indication of the physiological trauma of synoviocytes within the inflamed joint (Winrow et al. 1990).

It has been shown *in vitro* that grps are synthesized during hypoxia and hsps on reperfusion; similarly, animal experiments show that *de novo* intracellular synthesis occurs during exercise. Measurement of the 78 kDa grps synthesized during glucose deprivation is difficult to quantify in situ since the available antisera, which recognize this protein, also bind with other members of the 70 kDa family. The usual method of cell radiolabelling is impractical *in vivo*.

Natural defence mechanisms exist to limit damage from reactive oxygen metabolites. The 32 kDa heat-shock protein, now characterized as the enzyme haem oxygenase, is specifically induced by hydrogen peroxide, by heavy metals including iron, and by its substrate haem. Interestingly, it is also induced by the antirheumatic compound auranofin. Haem oxygenase, in the presence of NADPH and oxygen, cleaves haem to form biliverdin, which is then rapidly reduced to bilirubin, a radical scavenger. It has been suggested that increased production of this enzyme may be necessary to facilitate the turnover of haem-containing proteins like the mitochondrial cytochromes, which contribute to oxidative phosphorylation, by respiration-linked electron transfer. We have postulated that in the inflammatory joint, the production of this enzyme would be beneficial, decreasing the levels of haem whilst additionally increasing the levels of the antioxidant bilirubin and thus limiting damage by the haem iron catalyzed formation of hydroxyl radicals; the low pO_2 within the joint may limit activation of this enzyme. Auranofin and thiol reactive agents may act by helping to stimulate production of the 32 kDa protein and thus affect vascular changes; it is known that D-penicillamine suppresses neovascularization by generating low levels of hydrogen peroxide.

Reflex muscle inhibition

Exercise of the inflamed knee joints gives rise to elevated IAPs that is central to the mechanism of ischaemic reperfusion injury. However, this is not the case in all joints with effusions; there is a dramatic difference between a joint with an acute traumatic effusion and one with a chronic effusion. Measurement of the intra-articular pressure in the knee after quadriceps setting reveals that the acute traumatic patient is barely able to raise the intra-articular pressure at all (13 mmHg) whilst the chronic inflammatory patient is able to achieve pressures in excess of 250 mmHg. This phenomenon is explained by the fact that the acute traumatic patient has reflex muscular inhibition of the quadriceps whereas the chronic patient does not. This may be a defensive mechanism in the acute patient attempting to limit hypoxic-reperfusion injury. The mechanism behind this inhibition is not understood, neither is the manner by which it is overcome in the chronic inflammatory condition. However, it is reasonable to speculate that the depletion of the sensory nerve fibres in chronic arthritis (described earlier) is the cause. The transition from the acute to the chronic condition obviously involves the nervous system but again how this is regulated is not known. The nervous system also has other influences on the chronic inflammatory condition, some of which are only now being elucidated.

Nervous system

A number of clinical observations point to a neurogenic mechanism operative in chronic arthritis. The clearest example of this is provided by the synovitis that often accompanies reflexed sympathetic dystrophy. Sympathetic activity has also been implicated in the aetiology of the frozen shoulder (Maini et al. 1989). More controversial are the observations relating to hemiplegia and RA. In cases in which the RA develops after the hemiplegia the joints in the hemiplegic limbs are spared, but partially affected limbs were not always spared (Thompson and Bywaters 1962). In cases of patients paralysed by polio before the onset of the arthritis there is almost total sparing of the paralysed limbs (Glick 1967). While it is tempting to consider this as clear evidence for a neural component in RA other causal factors such a movement-induced hypoxic reperfusion injury (see earlier) need to be considered.

In animal model systems the available evidence is clearer. Experimental evidence for a neurogenic effect in acute arthritis is provided by the fact that antidromic (reversed) stimulation of the articular C fibres results in vasodilation and plasma extravasation within the joint. The intra-articular injection of capsaicin, a compound known to specifically stimulate C fibres gives similar results. Intra-articular infusion of 6-hydoxydopamine, a compound that stimulates post-ganglionic sympathetic nerves to release the contents of their peripheral terminals, can also produce a prolonged increase in synovial plasma extravasation. The acute vascular response to intra-articular injection of inflammatory compounds, such as carrageenan, can be significantly inhibited by prior joint denervation.

In human disease we have demonstrated that there is a change in the morphology of the nerve supply to the joint and have speculated on the release of neuropeptides in the inflamed joint. Neuropeptide-containing nerves are not found in the uppermost layers of the inflamed rheumatoid synovium. It is probable that synovial proliferation without concomitant fibre growth is the main cause of the reduced number of fibres observed (Buma et al. 2000).

Pain

One of the outstanding features of the inflamed joint is undoubtedly the pain that arises from it. As described earlier, the synovium contains unmyelinated C fibres that usually remain silent. However, in an inflammatory reaction the threshold of these fibres becomes lowered. This effect can be induced experimentally by agents such as prostaglandin E_1 and bradykinin (Konttinen et al. 1994). Both substances are found in inflammatory joint fluid. Not only can the nociceptive fibres alter their threshold but they may also alter their receptive field so as to widen it. Thus, movement in the normal range, which was once painless, now becomes painful.

Neurogenic inflammation

In addition to a nociceptive function, it is now widely accepted that neuropeptides contained within these nerve fibres play a role in the inflammatory response. The activation of the sensory nerves results not only in an impulse transmission to the spinal cord but also a antidromic transmission through the extensive branches in the peripheral C fibres. This is known as an axon reflex. This reversed transmission results in the release of neuropeptides, such as substance P, and stimulates an acute reaction—neurogenic inflammation (Foreman 1987). The major regulator of substance P gene expression in adult sensory nerves is nerve growth factor (NGF). NGF binds to a high affinity trkA receptor where it is internalized and retrogradely transported to the cell body. NGF has been found in the synovial fluid of patients with chronic arthritis. Systemic administration of anti-NGF neutralizing antibodies in an animal model of arthritis prevented the upregulation of neuropeptides and development of long-term changes in the spinal cord (Woolf et al. 1994). The changes that arise in the dorsal root ganglia in response to peripheral inflammation parallel changes seen in axotomy and chronic constriction injury, implying that the trophic support of NGF from the periphery has been lost. Over extended time periods, expression of proinflammatory peptides, such as SP and calcitonin gene-related peptide (CGRP), are downregulated and other peptides considered to be anti-inflammatory in nature are upregulated. The two peptides of current interest are galanin and vasoactive intestinal polypeptide (VIP). Galanin loss-of-function mutation mice show decreased peripheral nerve regeneration after a lesion (Holmes et al. 2000).

Adult sensory neurons from these animals show decreased axonal outgrowth *in vivo* and decreased neurite extension *in vitro* after axotomy compared to wild-type animals. The implied function for galanin must be the regeneration of peripheral nerves. Galanin has also been shown to be upregulated in the resolution phase on adjuvant arthritis (Calza et al. 2000) VIP has recently been shown to have potent anti-inflammatory effects in murine collagen-induced arthritis (Delgardo et al. 2001). It is proposed that VIP suppresses Th-1 type lymphocytes that produce proinflammatory mediators such as interferon-γ and IL-17. At the same time, Th-2 lymphocyte functions are activated producing anti-inflammatory cytokines such as IL4, IL10, and IL13. This latter discovery may hold therapeutic potential.

Degradation of peptides

The local activities of regulatory peptides, such as substance P and CGRP, depend on a combination of release and clearance from the vicinity of their receptors. Many peptides have short half-lives, rapid clearance being due to membrane-bound peptidases. These enzymes have characteristic regional distributions, and their activities may vary during inflammation. Understanding the local topography of membrane-bound peptidases and their relation to the sites of release and action of the peptides that may act as substrates is, therefore, essential to understanding peptidergic regulatory systems in the normal and diseased synovium.

NEP (EC 3.4.24.11) is responsible for the majority of the degradation of substance P in the human synovium. NEP is capable of the hydrolysis of many peptides including substance P. This enzyme is identical to the common acute lymphoblastic leukaemia antigen. Its activity has been shown in the synovium of patients with chronic arthritis. The activity of NEP was found to be higher in all patients with RA and in some patients with degenerative joint disease, when compared to traumatic arthritis controls. Our own data show the localization of this enzyme in human synovium, that fibroblasts are its source, and a restricted population of cells surrounding blood vessels are responsible for the majority of the activity (Mapp et al. 1992). These may represent a specialist sub-population of fibroblasts (Fig. 7). Since the function of NEP is probably the degradation of locally released regulatory peptides its presence around the blood vessels makes it ideally located to inactivate vasoactive peptides, such as substance P, which are released from perivascular nerve fibres.

In addition to NEP, several other peptide-degrading enzymes have been localized to the synovium including angiotensin-converting enzymes dipeptidyl peptidase IV and aminopeptidase M. The localization of these peptidases in the human synovium suggests not only a role limiting the duration of action of regulatory peptides but also in localizing activities to the vicinity of their release (Fig. 8). This functional compartmentalization of vascular and stromal regions in synovium is essential to the local regulatory function of peptides and is likely to influence responses to exogenous peptides administered into non-physiological compartments during experimental investigations.

(a)

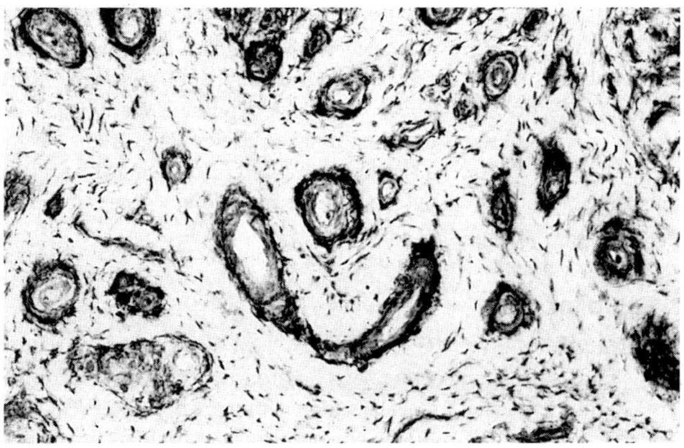

(b)

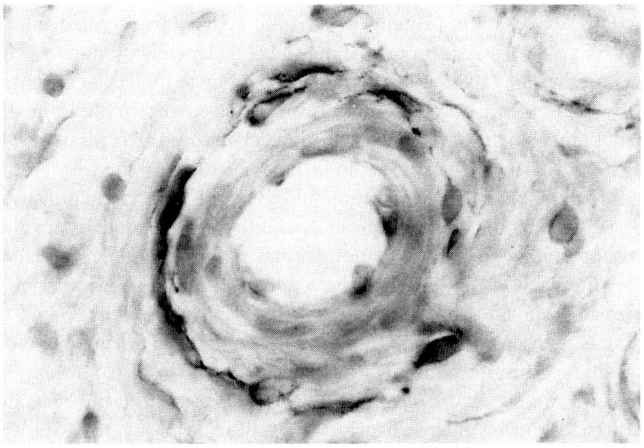

Fig. 7 Photomicrographs of rheumatoid synovia showing (a) the localization (black reaction product) of neutral endopeptidase, an enzyme that degrades neuropeptides, surrounding blood vessels and (b) at higher power, to a restricted population of cells surrounding those blood vessels.

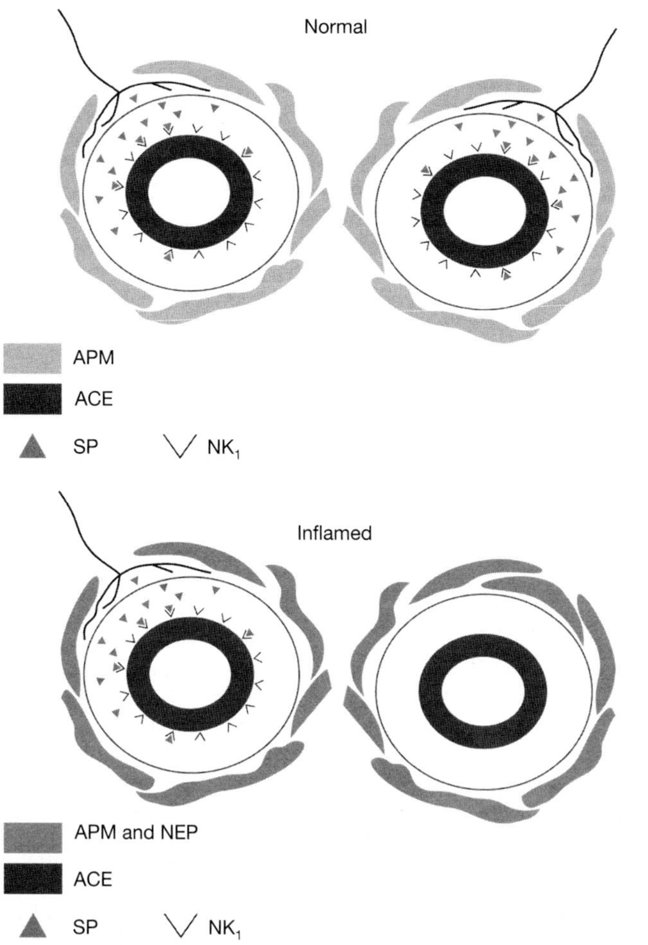

Fig. 8 Schematic diagram showing the distribution of enzymes, capable of degrading neuropeptides, in the normal and inflamed joints. Note how the neuropeptides are compartmentalized by the degrading enzymes.

Summary

In this chapter, we have shown how we believe the altered states of the synovium and synovial fluid arise in terms of the physiology of the joint. This is not intended to be a comprehensive review, since we have not attempted to address the involvement of the many other important mediator systems, to which separate chapters are devoted. The mechanisms that we have described are surely going on in parallel with several others. Previously, much attention was focused on mediators that promote inflammation. It is now realized that inhibitory mediators such as interferon-γ, and perhaps vasoactive intestinal peptide, are equally worthy of investigation.

References

Allan, I.M. et al. (1986). Reactive oxygen species (ROS) selectively deplete T-lymphocytes via a hydroxyl radical dependant mechanism. *Agents and Actions* **19**, 351–2.

Allen, R.E. et al. (1987). Xanthine oxido-reductase is present in human synovium. *Annals of the Rheumatic Diseases* **46**, 843–5.

Armiger, C. and Gavin, J.B. (1975). Changes in the microvasculature of ischaemic and infarcted myocardium. *Laboratory Investigation* **33**, 51–6.

Barland, P., Novikoff, A.B., and Hamerman, D. (1962). Electron microscopy of the human synovial membrane. *Journal of Cell Biology* **14**, 207–20.

Blake, D.R. et al. (1989). Hypoxic-reperfusion injury in the inflamed human joint. *Lancet* **1**, 289–93.

Buma, P. et al. (2000). Neurovascular plasticity in the knee joint of an arthritic mouse model. *The Anatomical Record* **260**, 51–61.

Calza, L. et al. (2000). Long-lasting regulation of galanin, opioid, and other peptides in dorsal root ganglia and spinal cord during experimental polyarthritis. *Experimental Neurology* **164**, 333–43.

Delgardo, M. et al. (2001). Vasoactive intestinal peptide prevents experimental arthritis by downregulating both autoimmune and inflammatory components of the disease. *Nature Medicine* **7**, 563–8.

Dick, W.C. et al. (1970). Derivation of knee joint synovial perfusion using the xenon (^{133}Xe) clearance technique. *Annals of the Rheumatic Diseases* **29**, 131–4.

Dingle, J.T.M. and Page-Thomas, D.P. (1956). *In vitro* studies on human synovial membrane. A metabolic comparison of normal and rheumatoid tissue. *British Journal of Experimental Pathology* **37**, 318–36.

Edwards, J.C.W. and Willoughby, D.A. (1982). Demonstration of bone marrow-derived cells in the synovial lining by means of giant intracellular granules as genetic markers. *Annals of the Rheumatic Diseases* **41**, 177–82.

Falchuk, K.H., Goetzl, E.J., and Kulka, J.P. (1970). Respiratory gases of synovial fluids. An approach to synovial tissue circulatory-metabolic imbalance in rheumatoid arthritis. *American Journal of Medicine* **49**, 223–31.

Foreman, J.C. (1987). Peptides and neurogenic inflammation. *British Medical Bulletin* **43**, 386–400.

Glick, E.N. (1967). Asymmetrical rheumatoid arthritis after poliomyelitis. *British Medical Journal* **3**, 26–9.

Greaves, M. et al. (1987). Changes in the factor VIII complex in diabetic ketoacidosis: evidence of endothelial damage? *Diabetologica* **30**, 160–5.

Holmes, F.E. et al. (2000). Targeted disruption of the galanin gene reduces the number of sensory neurons and their regenerative capacity. *Proceedings of the National Academy of Science USA* **97**, 11563–8.

Hunter, W. (1743). Of the structure and diseases of articulating cartilages. *Philosophical Transactions of the Royal Society of London Series B, Biological Sciences* **42**, 514–21.

Konttinen, Y.T. et al. (1994). Peripheral and spinal mechanisms in arthritis, with particular reference to treatment of pain and inflammation. *Arthritis and Rheumatism* **37**, 965–82.

Knight, A.D. and Levick, J.R. (1983). The density and distribution of capillaries around a synovial cavity. *Quarterly Journal of Experimental Physiology* **63**, 629–44.

Kumar, P. et al. (1985). Weibel–Palade bodies as a marker for neovascularization induced by tumour and rheumatoid angiogenesis factors. *Cancer Research* **45**, 4339–48.

Lockhart, A. and Saiag, B. (1981). Altitude and the human pulmonary circulation. *Clinical Science (London)* **60**, 599–605.

Lund-Oleson, K. (1970). Oxygen tensions in synovial fluids. *Arthritis and Rheumatism* **13**, 769–76.

Lunec, J. et al. (1985). Self perpetuating mechanisms of immunoglobulin G aggregation in rheumatoid inflammation. *Journal of Clinical Investigation* **76**, 2084–90.

Maini, R. et al. (1989). Use of laser doppler flowmetry and transcutaneous oxygen tension electrodes to assess local autonomic dysfunction in patients with frozen shoulder. *Journal of the Royal Society of Medicine* **82**, 536–8.

Mapp, P.I. et al. (1990). Substance P-, calcitonin gene-related peptide- and C flanking peptide of neuropeptide Y-immunoreactive fibres are present in normal synovium but depleted in patients with rheumatoid arthritis. *Neuroscience* **37**, 143–53.

Mapp, P.I. et al. (1992). Localisation of the enzyme neutral endopeptidase to the human synovium. *Journal of Rheumatology* **19**, 1838–44.

Mapp, P.I. et al. (2001). Localisation of 3-nitrotyrosine to rheumatoid and normal synovium. *Arthritis and Rheumatism* **44**, 1534–9.

Matsubara, T. et al. (1983). The thickening of basement membrane in synovial capillaries in rheumatoid arthritis. *Rheumatology International* **3**, 57–64.

Meier, R. et al. (1990). Induction of glia-derived nexin following peripheral nervelesion. *Nature* **342**, 548–50.

Morris, C.J. et al. (1986). Relationship between iron deposits and tissue damage in the synovium: an ultrastructural study. *Annals of the Rheumatic Diseases* **45**, 21–6.

Murrell, G.A.C., Francis, M.J.O., and Bromley, L. (1990). Modulation of fibroblast proliferation by oxygen free radicals. *Biochemical Journal* **265**, 659–65.

Ogawa, S. et al. (1990). Hypoxia modulates the barrier and coagulant function of cultured bovine endothelium. Increased monolayer permeability and induction of procoagulant properties. *Journal of Clinical Investigation* **85**, 1090–8.

Oleson, S.P. (1986). Rapid increase in blood–brain barrier permeability during severe hypoxia and metabolic inhibition. *Brain Research* **368**, 24–9.

O'Rhailly, R. and Gardner, E. (1978). The embryology of moveable joints. In *Joints and Synovial Fluid* (ed. L. Sokoloff), pp. 43–103. New York: Academic Press.

Palmer, R.M.J., Ferrige, A.G., and Moncada, S. (1987). Nitric oxide release accounts for the biological activity of endothelium derived relaxing factor. *Nature* **327**, 524–6.

Perez, H.D., Weksler, B.B., and Goldstein, I.M. (1980). Generation of a chemotactic lipid from arachidonic acid by exposure to a superoxide-generating system. *Inflammation* **4**, 313–28.

Petrone, W.F. et al. (1980). Free radicals and inflammation: superoxide-dependent activation of a neutrophil chemotactic factor in plasma. *Proceedings of the National Academy of Science USA* **77**, 1159–63.

Pottinger, B.E. et al. (1989). von Willebrand factor is an acute phase reactant in man. *Thrombosis Research* **53**, 9387–467.

Rodnan, G.P., Benedek, T.G., and Panatta, W.C. (1966). The early history of synovia (joint fluid). *Annals of Internal Medicine* **65**, 821–42.

Simkin, P.A. and Pizzorno, J.E. (1979). Synovial permeability in rheumatoid arthritis. *Arthritis and Rheumatism* **22**, 689–96.

Starling, E.H. (1896). On the absorbtion of fluids from connective tissue spaces. *Journal of Physiology* **19**, 312–26.

Stevens, C.R. et al. (1991). Hypoxia and inflammatory synovitis. *Annals of the Rheumatic Diseases* **50**, 124–32.

Suzuki, M. et al. (1989). Superoxide mediates reperfusion-induced leukocyte-endothelial cell interactions. *American Journal of Physiology* **257**, H1740–5.

Swann, D.A. et al. (1985). The molecular structure and lubricating activity of lubricin isolated from bovine and human synovial fluids. *Biochemical Journal* **225**, 195–201.

Thompson, M. and Bywaters, E.G. (1962). Unilateral rheumatoid arthritis following hemiplegia. *Annals of the Rheumatic Diseases* **21**, 370–7.

Winrow, V.R. et al. (1990). The heat shock response and its role in inflammatory disease. *Annals of the Rheumatic Diseases* **49**, 128–32.

Woodruff, T. et al. (1986). Is chronic synovitis an example of reperfusion injury? *Annals of the Rheumatic Diseases* **45**, 608–11.

Woolf, C.J. et al. (1994). Nerve growth factor contributes to the generation of inflammatory sensory hypersensitivity. *Neuroscience* **62**, 327–31.

3.6 Synovial pathology

Barry Bresnihan and Paul Peter Tak

Macroscopic appearances of synovitis in rheumatoid arthritis

The gross pathologic changes that are characteristic of rheumatoid arthritis (RA) result from chronic synovial inflammation (Tak and Bresnihan 2000). Typically, the surface of the synovium becomes hypertrophic and oedematous, with an intricate system of prominent villous fronds that expand into the joint cavity. The macroscopic appearances of synovitis may be readily quantified at arthroscopy (Veale et al. 1999), which provides easier access to human synovial tissue. This has produced new opportunities for those engaged in the study of arthritis (Bresnihan et al. 2000). Synovial tissue can now be selected from many sites within large and small joints, even in the earliest phases of disease, enhancing studies of aetiology, prognosis, and response to treatment (Bresnihan and Tak 1999). Contemporary imaging modalities, such as magnetic resonance imaging and ultrasonography, possess the capability of further characterizing and quantifying macroscopic synovial inflammation, joint effusion, cartilage integrity, and bone erosion (Backhaus et al. 2001; Peterfy 2001).

Microscopic appearances of synovitis in RA

The synovium in RA is hypertrophic and oedematous. There is marked hyperplasia of the lining layer, and accumulation of many cell populations, including T-cells, plasma cells, B-cells, macrophages, neutrophils, mast cells, natural killer (NK) cells, and dendritic cells in the sub-lining layer (Tak 2000) (Fig. 1).

The lining layer

The dominant cellular components of the lining layer are fibroblast-like synoviocytes (FLS) and macrophages. These cell populations release an array of proinflammatory cytokines and their inhibitors, which may promote further intraarticular perturbations. There is abundant production of matrix metalloproteinases (MMPs), cysteine proteases, and other tissue degrading mediators, which accumulate in the synovial fluid and augment joint damage by directly interacting with exposed cartilage matrix. These features are present very early in the disease course. Increased lining layer macrophage accumulation and perivascular mononuclear infiltration were prominent in tissue obtained days after the onset of symptoms (Schumacher and Kitridou 1972), and in the clinically uninvolved joints (Soden et al. 1989), of patients with RA. CD68+ macrophage accumulation in the synovium was more prominent in symptomatic joints (Pando et al. 2000), and the pre-clinical cellular infiltration of synovium, as well as tumour necrosis factor α (TNFα) and interleukin-1β (IL-1β) expression, observed in RA was similar in rhesus monkeys developing experimental arthritis (Kraan et al. 1998). Abundant protease gene expression has also

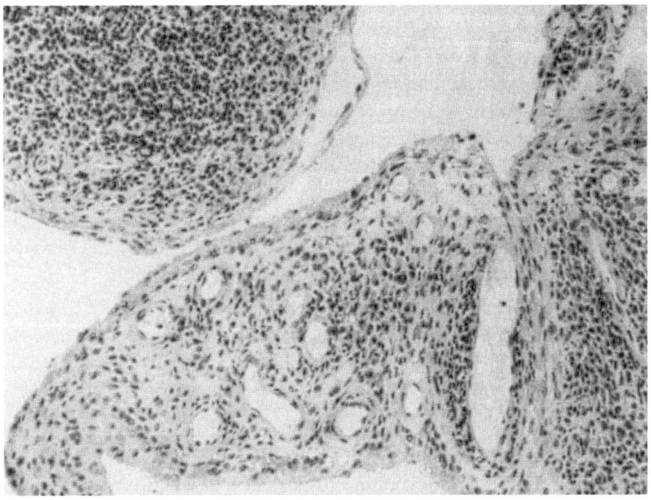

Fig. 1 Chronic inflammation in RA synovial membrane. Villous formation can be observed. Many blood vessels are seen, through which inflammatory cell populations have infiltrated the synovial sublining layer (haematoxylin and eosin; magnification ×100).

been observed in synovial tissue obtained only 2 weeks after the onset of symptoms, emphasizing the very early potential for joint destruction in RA (Cunnane et al. 1999). The intensity of some of these quantifiable immunohistologic features in the synovial lining layer may reflect the degree of joint damage (Yanni et al. 1994; Mulherin et al. 1996). This suggestion was highlighted in a recent study, which demonstrated that high levels of MMP-1 mRNA expression in the lining layer distinguished patients with more rapidly progressive erosive RA (Cunnane et al. 2001).

It remains to be clarified which factors account for the specific architecture of the lining layer and the interaction between FLS and intimal macrophages. The abundant expression of the transmembrane receptor CD97 on macrophages in the lining layer and the expression of its ligand, CD55, on FLS suggest that macrophages and FLS could interact functionally through CD97/CD55 binding (Hamann et al. 1999). Other molecules, including adhesion molecules and CD40 and its ligand CD40L may also be involved.

The sub-lining layer

T-cells and plasma cells are prominent in the synovial sub-lining layer. Lymphocyte aggregates are observed in 50–60 per cent of patients with RA. These aggregates can be surrounded by plasma cells. In addition, macrophages and lymphocytes infiltrate the areas between the lymphocyte aggregates. In some patients, areas with granulomatous necrobiosis are apparent (Klimiuk et al. 1997). These areas are characterized by regions with fibrinoid necrosis lined by a collar of epithelioid histiocytes and granulation tissue. Fibrin deposition and fibrosis can be observed. The macrophages often constitute the majority of inflammatory cells in the synovial sub-lining layer. Local disease activity is particularly associated with their number and with the expression of cytokines, such as TNFα and IL-6 (Tak et al. 1997; Kraan et al. 1998). The synovial sub-lining macrophages produce a variety of mediators of joint destruction (Konttinen et al. 1999; Onodera et al. 2000).

Large numbers of T-cells are also present in the synovial sub-lining. There are two basic patterns of T-cell infiltration (Firestein and Zvaifler 1990). First, perivascular lymphocyte aggregates can be found, which consist predominantly of CD4+ cells in association with B-cells, few CD8+ cells, and dendritic cells (Fig. 2). The second pattern of T cell infiltration is the diffuse infiltrate of T-cells scattered throughout the synovium. A subset of the CD4+ T-cells in synovial tissue is activated. A possible biologic effect of activated perivascular T-cells in the synovium is the activation of migrating macrophage populations through direct cell contact. This mechanism is known to stimulate macrophage production of cytokines and MMPs *in vitro* (Vey et al. 1992; Lacraz et al. 1994). A factor in human serum, identified as apolipoprotein A-1 (apo A-1), was recently shown to inhibit contact-mediated stimulation of monocytes by activated T-lymphocytes *in vitro* (Hyka et al. 2001). It was speculated that apo A-1 may play an important role in modulating T-lymphocyte-mediated effects in both acute and chronic inflammation. Many of the T-cells in synovial tissue are, on the other hand, in a state of hyporesponsiveness (Firestein and Zvaifler 1990; Maurice et al. 1997). Interdigitating dendritic cells, which are potent antigen presenting cells, are located in proximity to CD4+ T-cells in the lymphocyte aggregates and near the intimal lining layer (Duke et al. 1982; Thomas and Lipsky 1996; Pettit et al. 2000).

B-cells constitute a small proportion of the total amount of lymphocytes in the synovial sub-lining layer. However, numerous plasma cells may be present throughout the synovium, sometimes exceeding the number of infiltrating T-cells. A considerable number of the plasma cells synthesize and secrete rheumatoid factors and other autoantibodies (Hakoda et al. 1993; Otten et al. 1993). Follicular dendritic cells are observed in the same areas in proximity to proliferating B-cells. They are thought to play a crucial role in isotype switching and final differentiation of B-cells towards plasma cells or memory B-cells (Krenn et al. 1996; Schroder et al. 1996).

Granzyme positive NK cell and cytotoxic T-cells are present in both the synovial lining layer and in the synovial sub-lining. In line with the increased infiltration of granzyme positive cells in the synovium (Tak et al. 1994; Muller-Ladner et al. 1995; Smeets et al. 1998), there are markedly elevated levels of soluble granzymes in the synovial fluid and plasma of RA patients (Tak et al. 1999). Granzyme B could contribute to cartilage loss by degrading resident aggrecan (Froelich et al. 1993). Only few neutrophils are found in rheumatoid synovial tissue. However, large numbers of neutrophils traffic through the synovial lining layer into the synovial fluid. These cells are activated and contain a variety of proteinases and other enzymes, which might be of primary importance in destruction of the joint (Moore et al. 1999; van Meurs et al. 1999).

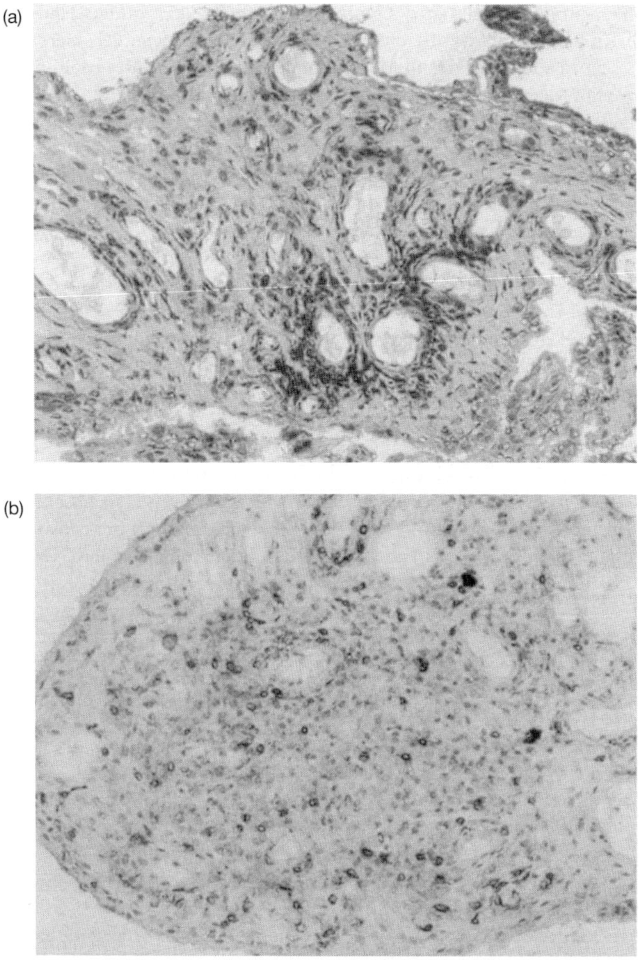

Fig. 2 Perivascular CD4+ T-cells in RA synovial membrane (a) CD8+ T-cells are scattered sparsely throughout the synovial sublining layer. (b) Immunoperoxidase; magnification ×100.

Mast cell sub-populations were found to expand in RA synovial tissue and an association between the intensity of infiltrating mast cells producing both tryptase and chymase, particularly in the superficial synovial layer, and inpairment of function have been described (Gotis-Graham and McNeil 1997). This observation is noteworthy as mast cells produce proteolytic factors, which can degrade proteoglycans. Synovial tissue from patients with relatively early RA was characterized by infiltrating mast cells producing tryptase only, suggesting that the synovial mast cell phenotype may alter as RA progresses (Gotis-Graham et al. 1998). However, the interpretation of this observation remains unclear, as it may be explained by differences in levels of disease activity.

TNFα and IL-1β production is prominent in the synovial lining layer and in some sub-lining layer cell populations at non-CPJ (CPJ stands for cartilage–pannus junction) sites (Tak and Bresnihan 2000). Using techniques that are highly specific for the detection of cytokine-producing cells,

TNFα-producing cells were prominent in the lining layer of most, but not all, RA tissue samples (Ulfgren et al. 1995). TNFα-producing cells were also present to a lesser degree in the sub-lining interaggregate areas and in the lymphoid aggregates. The impressive therapeutic effects of TNFα-blockade in RA may result from inhibition of the pathogenetic effects of TNFα produced by synovial tissue macrophages. Cells that are immunoreactive for IL-1 and IL-1Ra are also present in the lining and sub-lining layers (Deleuran et al. 1992a; Ulfgren et al. 1995) (Fig. 3). The distribution of IL-1Ra gene expression and protein production in RA differs from that in osteoarthritis, being notably less in the lining layer of RA synovium (Firestein et al. 1992). This observation is consistent with a relative deficiency of IL-1Ra production by RA synovial macrophages (Firestein et al. 1994). Taken together, studies of non-CPJ synovium from patients with late-stage RA suggest that TNFα, IL-1α, IL-1β, their inhibitors, and receptors are produced by most, but possibly not all, tissue samples. However, it is possible that the detection of cytokine production might depend on the site of biopsy. This was examined in multiple samples using reverse transcriptase PCR. TNFα was expressed in all samples from all biopsy sites, but at very low levels in the tissues of some. IL-1β was expressed in all samples from most sites (Kirkham et al. 1999). These observations are consistent with the findings at the CPJ and suggest that either synovial tissue TNFα or IL-1β production may be minimal or absent in some patients (Klimiuk et al. 1997; Tak et al. 1997). This is compatible with the heterogeneity of disease expression and response to treatment which is characteristic of RA.

IL-18 is a novel cytokine that is closely related to the IL-1 family in both structure and function (Okamura et al. 1998; Dinarello 1999). It induces both TNFα and IL-1β gene expression and protein synthesis, as well as MMP and iNOS gene expression by chondrocytes *in vitro*. It could, therefore, contribute to cartilage matrix degradation. IL-18 is produced by macrophages, chondrocytes, osteoblasts, and other cell populations. IL-18 mRNA and protein production have been described in RA synovial tissues (Gracie et al. 1999; Yamamura et al. 2001). It was predominantly expressed by synovial tissue macrophages within and adjacent to lymphocytic aggregates and, less prominently, by lining layer macrophages.

IL-15 in RA synovial tissue has been co-localized to macrophages, including lining layer macrophages, and sub-lining layer T-cells, and NK cells (McInnes et al. 1996; Thurkow et al. 1997). Inflamed synovial tissue also produces increased amounts of many other cytokines, colony stimulating factors and chemokines, which can modulate synovial cell functions (Dayer and Arend 1997). The role of many cytokines in the complex pathogenesis of joint degradation in RA remains to be clarified. The chemokines are a family of chemoattractant proteins which participate in the chemotaxis of cells to sites of inflammation. In RA, monocyte chemoattractant protein-1 (MCP-1), a member of the C–C sub-family, is constitutively expressed by lining layer macrophages and is upregulated in FLS by IL-1β or TNFα (Koch et al. 1992). Synovial MCP-1 production appears to be important in maintaining the accumulation of tissue macrophages.

There has been extensive analysis of proteolytic enzyme production by synovial tissue samples and primary synoviocyte cultures selected from non-CPJ sites in established RA (Tak and Bresnihan 2000). These studies have demonstrated MMP-1, MMP-3, and tissue inhibitor of metalloproteinase (TIMP) mRNA in the lining layer cells, including both macrophage and FLS populations, and in some sub-lining layer cell populations. Other MMPs, including MMP-9 (gelatinase B), have also been demonstrated in RA synovial tissue (Ahrens et al. 1996). The tissue distribution of MMP-9 was localized to sites of synovial inflammation, particularly the lining layer, endothelium, and tissue macrophages. MMP-13 has been cloned from RA synovial tissue (Wernicke et al. 1996). MMP-13 mRNA and protein was demonstrated in lining layer FLS and not in macrophages in most late-stage RA tissue samples. It seems likely that the degree of cartilage and bone degradation will depend on excessive MMP activity over the inhibitors in the synovium, especially within the pannus. In addition to MMPs, cathepsin B and cathepsin L production by synovial lining layer cells has also been demonstrated (Keyszer et al. 1995; Keyszer et al. 1998).

Synovial tissue is rich in blood vessels (Koch 1998; Walsh 1999) (Fig. 4). Angiogenesis is a complex process and a central feature in synovial inflammation and pannus formation. There are many regulators, including inhibitors, of angiogenesis that are produced and released by the human synovium. Angiogenic factors that have been demonstrated in RA synovium and implicated in the pathogenesis of progressive joint damage include VEGF, basic fibroblast growth factor, hepatocyte growth factor, IL-1, TNFα, IL-8, TGFα and TGFβ, angiogenin, and platelet-derived endothelial growth factor. Important inhibitors of angiogenesis produced by RA synovium include thrombospondin, TGFβ, TNFα, IFNγ, TIMP-1 and TIMP-2, and leukaemia inhibitory factor. In RA, evidence of angiogenesis and vascular regression may be observed in different microscopic foci of the same synovial samples. Angiogenesis may augment inflammation as newly formed blood vessels express increased levels of cell adhesion molecules such as E-selectin, which facilitate the migration of inflammatory cells. In turn, inflammatory cells generate angiogenic factors which further

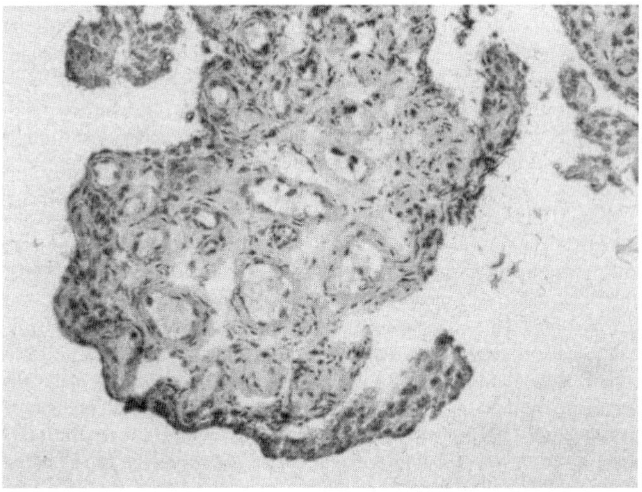

Fig. 3 Mononuclear cells producing interleukin-1β. Positively-stained cells (predominantly macrophages) accumulate in synovial lining layer and in the sub-lining layer (immunoperoxidase; magnification ×100).

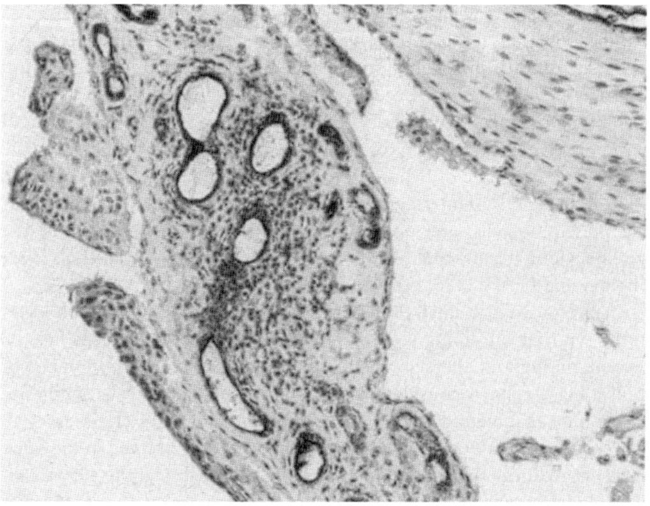

Fig. 4 Prominent proliferating blood vessels in the synovial sub-lining layer. Immunoreactive vascular endothelium is highlighted using an anti-factor VIII monoclonal antibody (immunoperoxidase; magification ×100).

increase angiogenesis. Angiogenesis permits continuing growth of the proliferating synovial pannus. Migrating endothelial cells produce proteases which may degrade adjacent cartilage and bone. However, the direct contribution of proliferating blood vessels to tissue destruction may be small compared to that of the FLS, macrophages, and other proteolytic enzyme-producing cells which accumulate at the CPJ.

The cartilage–pannus junction

The characteristic pattern of juxta-articular cartilage and bone erosion readily distinguishes RA from other forms of chronic arthritis (Resnick et al. 1997). Joint erosion results, at least in part, from the invasion of articular cartilage and adjacent sub-chondral bone by proliferating pannus (Fig. 1). However, joint erosion may also result more directly from bone-derived cells, particularly osteoclasts (Goldring and Gravallese 2000). The process of joint erosion is distinct from degradation or dissolution of the cartilage surface, which results from the direct effects of enzymes and other synovial cell products that accumulate in the synovial fluid.

In some patients with long-standing RA the CPJ tissue, examined at the time of surgery, may be relatively acellular (Kobayashi and Ziff 1975; Bromley and Woolley 1984). More typically, CPJ tissue contains several cell populations (Fig. 1) (Tak and Bresnihan 2000). FLS and macrophages are the dominant populations in the majority. Numerous clusters of macrophages and FLS are frequently observed at the leading edge where synovial tissue penetrates the degrading cartilage [Fig. 2(a)]. It is not known if these cells are pre-activated cells which continue to advance from the proliferative lining layer, cells which migrate through tissue channels from the bone marrow, or cells that are derived from the peripheral circulation. Synovial tissue adjacent to the CPJ in early RA demonstrates prominent cellular infiltration, with apparent preferential accumulation of macrophage populations compared to non-CPJ tissue (Youssef et al. 1998).

Both FLS and macrophages in the synovial lining layer and at the CPJ exhibit features which suggest a high level of activation (Firestein 1996; Burmester et al. 1997; Bresnihan and Youssef 2002). The functional properties of FLS in RA have been determined mostly from studies utilizing primary synoviocyte cultures or tissue samples selected from non-CPJ sites. Activated FLS exhibit many features of transformed cells and demonstrate increased cell adhesion molecule expression, proliferative and invasive activity, oncogene expression, and the release of proteolytic enzymes and cytokines (Firestein 1996). Activated synovial tissue macrophages demonstrate increased expression and transcription of IL-1β, TNFα, and C–C monokine chemoattractant protein-1 (MCP-1). Synovial tissue macrophages are multifunctional cells that incorporate biologic activities which may be destructive or protective (Firestein 1996; Burmester et al. 1997).

There is some evidence to suggest that the cell populations at the CPJ may undergo local functional modulation. Macrophages close to the CPJ were compared to those at sites distant from the CPJ with respect to the presence of myeloid-related proteins (MRP), which are myeloid differentiation markers on infiltrating tissue macrophages in inflammatory lesions (Youssef et al. 1999). Striking differences were observed. MRP8, MRP14, and the heterodimer MRP8/14 were expressed on lining layer macrophages adjacent to the CPJ but only in patients with active disease. Minimal or absent MRP staining was observed in sections from non-CPJ sites. These observations were consistent with altered macrophage differentiation at the site of maximal cartilage destruction during active phases of disease.

Other cell populations, including lymphocytes, plasma cells, and neutrophils may participate in the pathogenesis of joint destruction at the CPJ (Mohr and Menninger 1980; Kobayashi and Ziff 1975) (Fig. 1). Chondrocyte-derived cells are also known to appear in the proliferating pannus (Allard et al. 1987). Chondrocytes, when stimulated by TNFα or IL-1β, can produce proteolytic enzymes and cause cartilage matrix degradation (Borden et al. 1996). In addition, a morphologically distinct cell type that shares some of the characteristics of chondrocytes and FLS has been described at the CPJ (Zvaifler et al. 1997). It was suggested that this cell population, designated pannocytes, may represent an earlier stage of mesenchymal cell differentiation. Their role in joint destruction remains to be determined. A similar cell type, which expressed MMP-1, cathepsin B, and cathepsin L, has been cloned from an RA pannus lesion (Xue et al. 1997).

Mast cells have been identified at the site of cartilage erosion in RA (Bromley et al. 1984). Mast cell subsets can be defined according to their capacity to produce tryptase, or tryptase and chymase (Tetlow and Woolley 1995a). Local accumulations of mast cells were observed in approximately 50 per cent of late-stage RA synovial tissue samples selected from the CPJ (Tetlow and Woolley 1995b). Evidence of cell activation was present in most.

One mechanism implicating mast cells in joint damage may relate to the abundant production of vascular endothelial growth factor (VEGF), which enhances angiogenesis and could promote the growth of synovial pannus (Yamada et al. 1998). However, the exact role of mast cells in matrix degradation remains unknown and, in some experimental models, cartilage degradation and fibroblast invasion occurs in their absence (Geiler et al. 1994; Wang et al. 1997).

Osteoclasts at the CPJ also have a critical role in bone erosion (Goldring and Gravallese 2000). The calcitonin receptor (CTR) has been identified as a specific marker that distinguishes osteoclasts from other haematopoietic and bone cells (Chang et al. 1992; Ashton et al. 1993). Joint tissues obtained from the pannus–bone and pannus–cartilage interface in late-stage RA demonstrated strong osteoclast-specific CTR mRNA expression in multinucleated cells in the resorbtion lacunae of calcified cartilage and immediately adjacent sub-chondral bone (Gravallese et al. 1998). The multinucleated cells were also positive for tartrate-resistant alkaline phosphatase (TRAP) mRNA and TRAP enzyme activity. The important role of osteoclast precursors in the pathogenesis of joint erosion was further highlighted by the demonstration of osteoclast differentiation factor (ODF) (also known as osteoprotegerin ligand (OPG-L)) expression by both fibroblasts and activated T lymphocytes derived from the synovial tissues of patients with RA (Gravallese et al. 2000). The balance between osteoprotegerin and ODF/OPG-L production appears to be critical in the regulation of osteoclast activation (Lacey et al. 1998). Moreover, in murine adjuvant arthritis, it has been demonstrated that T-cell activation can lead to OPG-L production and subsequent bone loss (Kong et al. 1999).

TNFα and IL-1β are prominent in the pathogenesis of RA (Arend and Dayer 1995). Both are produced predominantly by macrophages, which accumulate maximally adjacent to the CPJ (Youssef et al. 1998; Youssef et al. 1999). Some TNFα-positive cells were identified adjacent to the CPJ in specimens from patients with long-standing erosive RA (Chu et al. 1991a, 1992). In contrast, in patients with relatively early RA (symptoms $<$18 months), all tissue samples from the CPJ demonstrated quantifiable TNFα-producing cells, suggesting that TNFα-producing macrophages accumulate at the CPJ early in the disease course and become less prominent for unknown reasons during the later phases. Both the p55 and p75 TNF receptors (TNF-R) are also present in abundance at the CPJ, especially by those cells invading cartilage (Deleuran et al. 1992a). Both receptors are expressed on a variety of cell types including fibroblasts, macrophages, and chondrocytes, supporting the view that a wide range of cells at the CPJ are potential targets for TNFα.

IL-1-producing macrophages have also been demonstrated at the CPJ in late-stage erosive RA (Chu et al. 1992). CPJ tissue from patients with long-standing disease (duration 6–29 years) demonstrated IL-1α- and IL-1β-producing cells in the majority, but not in all (Ulfgren et al. 2000). In patients with relatively early RA ($<$18 months), IL-1α- and IL-1β-producing cells were present at the CPJ in all, and measurements of the areas occupied by cytokine-producing cells suggested that considerably more IL-1α- and IL-1β-producing cells than TNFα-producing cells are present at the CPJ, especially in the earlier phases of RA. The apparent predominance of IL-1β-producing cells at the CPJ in these studies is consistent with quantitative analysis of gene expression in long-standing RA (Firestein et al. 1990). However, further study of this issue will need to apply strict criteria to the selection of biopsy material in relation to disease activity, medication, and other clinical parameters. The type I IL-1 receptor (IL-1RI) was also demonstrated in abundance on a variety of cell populations at the CPJ

(Deleuran et al. 1992b). As expected, cells producing IL-1 receptor antagonist (IL-1Ra) were less prominent at the CPJ than IL-1α-producing cells.

The production of several other cytokines and their inhibitors has also been demonstrated at the CPJ in advanced RA, including IL-6 (Chu et al. 1992b; Ulfgren et al. 2000), TGFβ (Chu et al. 1991b), IFN-γ, and GM-CSF (Chu et al. 1992). In contrast to the increased production of many cytokines at the CPJ, cells producing IL-8, a potent chemoattractant, were notably more prominent at non-CPJ sites (Deleuran et al. 1994). The relative influence of each of the pro- and anti-inflammatory mediators in matrix degradation at different disease stages is likely to be complex and requires considerable further analysis.

Cellular invasion and degradation of cartilage and sub-chondral bone is mediated in part by the secretion of proteolytic enzymes (Tak and Bresnihan 2000). Proteolytic mechanisms may be divided into extracellular pathways, which involve the MMPs and serine proteinases, active at neutral pH, and the intracellular pathways, which involve the cysteine and aspartate proteinases, active at a low pH (Nagase and Okada 1997). In RA synovial tissue, the MMPs and cysteine proteinases have been widely studied. The abundant production of MMP-1, which can digest collagen types I, II, III, VI, and X and gelatins, at sites of joint erosion was first demonstrated in late-stage RA using immunofluorescent techniques (Woolley et al. 1977). The large number of MMP-1-producing cells at the CPJ were subsequently identified as predominantly fibroblasts, although some chondrocytes close to the CPJ were also noted to express MMP-1 RNA and protein, confirming the capacity of chondrocytes to both degrade and synthesize cartilage matrix (Trabandt et al. 1992). The predominance of MMP-1 over MMP-13 production at sites of cartilage erosion by both synoviocytes and chondrocytes has also been demonstrated (Tetlow and Woolley 1998). MMP-13 gene expression in FLS at the CPJ was demonstrated and, in primary synoviocyte cultures, it was upregulated two- to four-fold following treatment with IL-1β or TNFα (Schulz Westhoff et al. 1999).

The cysteine proteases degrade major cartilage components including proteoglycans, collagen types I, II, IX, and XI and basement membrane components (Nagase and Okada 1997). In advanced RA, cathepsin B was demonstrated in most, but not all, synovial tissue samples selected from the CPJ and was localized to FLS at the invading front, and to the intimal and sub-intimal layers of adjacent tissue (Trabandt et al. 1991). Abundant macrophage cathepsin L expression was also observed at sites of cartilage erosion, suggesting a role in the pathogenesis of joint damage (Iwata et al. 1997). Cathepsin K has been implicated in osteoclast-mediated bone resorbtion (Inoaka et al. 1995; Drake et al. 1996) and cathepsin K mRNA was demonstrated at sites of articular destruction (Hummel et al. 1998). Not surprisingly, some of the cathepsin K positive cells were osteoclast precursors. However, cathepsin K mRNA, was also expressed in large numbers of FLS at the CPJ, and in areas adjacent to lymphocytic infiltration, strongly suggesting that it may not only contribute to matrix degradation but also facilitate the movement of mononuclear cells through perivascular interstitial tissue. Chondrocytes in RA cartilage also release the first component of complement C1s, which has collagenolytic activity and may participate in the degradation of cartilage matrix (Nakagawa et al. 1999).

Synovitis in other chronic inflammatory polyarthropathies

There are some similarities between RA and other categories of chronic polyarthritis, which are summarized below. Several categories of arthritis such as granulomatous diseases, crystal-related arthropathies, and infectious diseases, which are often mono- or pauci-articular and have specific inflammatory characteristics, are not considered in this chapter.

Ankylosing spondylitis

Synovial tissue from the sacroiliac joints of patients with ankylosing spondylitis (AS) demonstrate both mononuclear cell infiltration and islands of early ossification (Braun et al. 1995). Mononuclear cell infiltrates, which include lymphocytes, macrophages, and fibroblasts, are seen in synovium, and in adjacent cartilage and bone. Pannus formation similar to RA has been described. There is evidence to suggest that the primary site of inflammation is the enthesis, where ligament, tendon, or the joint capsule is inserted into bone. It is not clear how the inflammatory cell populations migrate to sacroiliac joint structures. It has been suggested that they may migrate from proliferating blood vessels, or directly from the bone marrow. Increased vascularity is seen in the early enthesitis lesion (McGonagle et al. 2002). Sacroiliitis is also characterized by TNFα, TGFβ2, IFN-γ, IL-4, and, IL-12 mRNA expression (Braun et al. 1998).

The manifestations of synovitis in the peripheral joints in AS are indistinguishable from RA in many respects. However, some quantitative differences have been described. Firstly, the cellularity of the lining layer appeared to be less in AS than in RA. Secondly, more intense mononuclear cell infiltration has been described in AS, but this observation has not been highlighted in all published studies (Kidd et al. 1989). Finally, large B-cell aggregates may be prominent in the peripheral joints of some patients with AS. Rheumatoid granulomas do not occur in AS. It has been suggested that the enthesis may be the primary site of inflammation in peripheral joints in AS (McGonagle et al. 1998).

Psoriatic arthritis

There are similarities between the manifestations of synovitis in psoriatic arthritis (PsA) and AS. In both, the cellularity of the lining layer is less than RA. Similarly, synovial tissue macrophages are more numerous in RA synovium than in PsA (Veale et al. 1993). Vascular changes are a dominant feature in PsA. For example, a comparison of synovial tissue obtained from patients with PsA and RA demonstrated that the number of blood vessels per square millimetre quantified microscopically in PsA tissue was almost double the number seen in RA. In addition, a distinct macroscopic pattern of blood vessel formation has been highlighted in PsA (Reece et al. 1999). Thus, under direct vision at arthroscopy, PsA and reactive arthritis synovium were characterized by the presence of tortuous, bushy vessels, and RA by straight, branching vessels.

Juvenile idiopathic arthritis

The synovial response to inflammation in children with juvenile idiopathic arthritis (JIA) is similar to adults with RA (Cassidy and Petty 1990). Macroscopically, villous formation is characteristic. Microscopically, there is increased cellularity of the synovial lining layer. In the sub-lining layer, vascular endothelial hyperplasia is prominent, associated with macrophage, lymphocyte, and plasma cell infiltration. Pannus formation is usual, leading to progressive erosion of adjacent cartilage and bone. The histopathologic manifestations of synovial inflammation in polyarticular and pauci-articular disease are indistinguishable.

Systemic lupus erythematosus

Synovitis in systemic lupus erythematosus is usually milder than RA. Vascular proliferation, perivascular mononuclear cell infiltration, and lining layer hypercellularity, consisting of both fibroblast-like synoviocytes and macrophages, are observed to varying degrees (Labowitz and Schumacher 1971). Deposition of fibrin-like material along the synovial surface and throughout the synovial membrane is characteristic. Features of synovial vasculitis, with infiltration of vessel walls and obliteration of the vascular lumen, is observed occasionally.

Osteoarthritis

Osteoarthritis (OA) is widely regarded as being primarily a degenerative disorder of articular cartilage. However, a considerable degree of synovial inflammation, often indistinguishable from RA, may be observed in many OA biopsy samples (Goldenberg et al. 1982; Kennedy et al. 1988). Well-developed lymphoid follicles and significant numbers of plasma cells are not seen in OA synovium.

References

Ahrens, D., Koch, A.E., Pope, R.M., Stein-Picarella, M., and Niedbala, M.J. (1996). Expression of matrix metalloproteinase 9 (96kd gelatinase B) in human rheumatoid arthritis. *Arthritis and Rheumatism* **39**, 1576–87.

Allard, S.A., Muirden, K.D., Campbelljohn, K.L., and Maini, R.N. (1987). Chondrocyte-derived cells and matrix at the rheumatoid cartilage–pannus junction identified with monoclonal antibodies. *Rheumatology International* **7**, 153–9.

Arend, W.P. and Dayer, J.-M. (1995). Inhibition of the production and effects of interleukin-1 and tumor necrosis factor α in rheumatoid arthritis. *Arhtritis and Rheumatism* **38**, 151–60.

Ashton, B.A., Ashton, I.K., Marshall, M.J., and Butler, R.C. (1993). Localisation of vitronectin receptor immunoreactivity and tartrate resistant acid phosphatase activity in synovium from patients with inflammatory or degenerative arthritis. *Annals of the Rheumatic Diseases* **52**, 133–7.

Backhaus, M., Burmester, G.-R., Gerber, T., Grassi, W., Machold, K.P., Swen, W.A., Wakefield, R.J., and Manger, B. (2001). Guidelines for musculoskeletal ultrasound in rheumatology. *Annals of the Rheumatic Diseases* **60**, 641–9.

Borden, P., Solymar, D., Sucharaczuk, A., Lindman, B., Cannon, P., and Heller, R.A. (1996). Cytokine control of interstitial collagenase and collagenase-3 gene expression in human chondrocytes. *Journal of Biological Chemistry* **271**, 23577–81.

Braun, J., Bollow, M., and Sieper, J. (1998). Radiologic diagnosis and pathology of the spondyloarthropathies. *Rheumatic Disease Clinics of North America* **24**, 697–735.

Braun, J. et al. (1995). Use of immunohistologic and in situ hybridization techniques in the examination of sacroiliac joint biopsy specimens from patients with ankylosing spondylitis. *Arthritis and Rheumatism* **37**, 499–505.

Bresnihan, B. and Tak, P.P. (1999). Synovial tissue analysis in rheumatoid arthritis. *Baillières Clinical Rheumatology* **13**, 645–59.

Bresnihan, B. and Youssef, P. (2002). Macrophages in rheumatoid arthritis. In *The Macrophage* (ed. B. Burke and C.E. Lewis), pp. 391–433. Oxford: Oxford University Press.

Bresnihan, B., Tak, P.P., Emery, P., Klareskog, L., and Breedveld, F. (2000). Synovial biopsy in arthritis research: five years of concerted Eurpean collaboration. *Annals of the Rheumatic Diseases* **59**, 506–10.

Bromley, M. and Woolley, D.E. (1984). Histopathology of the rheumatoid lesion. Identification of cell types at sites of cartilage erosion. *Arthritis and Rheumatism* **27**, 857–63.

Bromley, M., Fisher, W.D., and Woolley, D.E. (1984). Mast cells at the site of cartilage erosion in the rheumatoid joint. *Annals of the Rheumatic Diseases* **43**, 76–9.

Burmester, G.R., Stuhmuller, B., Keyszer, G., and Kinne, R.W. (1997). Mononuclear phagocytes and rheumatoid synovitis: mastermind or workhorse in arthritis? *Arthritis and Rheumatism* **40**, 5–18.

Cassidy, J.T. and Petty, R.E. (1990). Juvenile rheumatoid arthritis. In *Textbook of Pediatric Rheumatology* (ed. J.T. Cassidy and R.E. Petty), pp. 113–219. New York: Churchill Livingstone.

Chang, J.S. et al. (1992). Bone resorbtion by cells isolated from rheumatoid synovium. *Annals of the Rheumatic Diseases* **51**, 1223–9.

Chu, C.Q., Field, M., Feldmann, M., and Maini, R.N. (1991a). Localization of tumor necrosis factor a in synovial tissues and at the cartilage-pannus junction in patients with rheumatoid arthritis. *Arthritis and Rheumatism* **34**, 1125–32.

Chu, C.Q., Field, M., Abney, E., Zheng, R.Q., Allard, S., Feldmann, M., and Maini, R.N. (1991b). Transforming growth factor-beta 1 in rheumatoid synovial membrane and cartilage/pannus junction. *Clinical and Experimental Immunology* **86**, 380–6.

Chu, C.Q., Field, M., Allard, S., Abney, E., Feldmann, M., and Maini, R.M. (1992). Detection of cytokines at the cartilage/pannus junction in patients with rheumatoid arthritis: implications for the role of cytokines in joint destruction and repair. *British Journal of Rheumatology* **31**, 653–61.

Cunnane, G., FitzGerald, O., Hummel, K.M., Gay, R.E., Gay, S., and Bresnihan, B. (1999). Collagenase, cathepsin B and cathepsin L gene expression in the synovial membrane of patients with early inflammatory arthritis. *Rheumatology* **38**, 34–42.

Cunnane, G. et al. (2001). Synovial tissue protease gene expression and joint erosions in early rheumatoid arthritis. *Arthritis and Rheumatism* **44**, 1744–53.

Dayer, J.-M. and Arend, W.P. (1997). Cytokines and growth factors. In *Textbook of Rheumatology* (ed. W.N. Kelley, S. Ruddy, E.D. Harris, and C.B. Sledge), pp. 267–86. Philadelphia PA: W.B. Saunders.

Deleuran, B. et al. (1994). Localisation of interleukin 8 in the synovial membrane, cartilage–pannus junction and chondrocytes in rheumatoid arthritis. *Scandinavian Journal of Rheumatology* **23**, 2–7.

Deleuran, B.W. et al. (1992a). Localization of tumor necrosis receptors in the synovial tissue and cartilage–pannus junction in patients with rheumatoid arthritis. *Arthritis and Rheumatism* **35**, 1170–8.

Deleuran, B.W. et al. (1992b). Localisation of interleukin-1α, type 1 interleukin receptor and interleukin-1 receptor antagonist in the synovial membrane and cartilage/pannus junction in rheumatoid arthritis. *British Journal of Rheumatology* **31**, 801–9.

Dinarello, C.A. (1999). IL-18: a Th1-inducing, proinflammatory cytokine and new member of the IL-1 family. *Journal of Allergy in Clinical Immunology* **103**, 11–24.

Drake, F.H. et al. (1996). Cathepsin, K, but not cathepsin B, L, or S, is abundantly expressed in human osteoclasts. *Journal of Biological Chemistry* **271**, 12511–16.

Duke, O., Panayi, G.S., Janossy, G., and Poulter, L.W. (1982). An immunohistological analysis of lymphocyte subpopulations and their microenvironment in the synovial membranes of patients with rheumatoid arthritis using monoclonal antibodies. *Clinical and Experimental Immunology* **49**, 22–30.

Firestein, G.S. (1996). Invasive fibroblast-like synoviocytes in rheumatoid arthritis: passive responders or transformed aggressors? *Arthritis and Rheumatism* **39**, 1781–90.

Firestein, G.S. and Zvaifler, N.J. (1990). How important are T cells in chronic rheumatoid synovitis. *Arthritis and Rheumatism* **33**, 768–73.

Firestein, G.S., Alvaro-Garcia, J.M., and Maki, R. (1990). Quantitative analysis of cytokine gene expression in rheumatoid arthritis. *Journal of Immunology* **144**, 3347–53.

Firestein, G.S. et al. (1992). IL-1 receptor antagonist protein production and gene expression in rheumatoid arthritis and osteoarthritis synovium. *Journal of Immunology* **149**, 1054–62.

Firestein, G.S. et al. (1994). Synovial interleukin-1 receptor antagonist and interleukin-1 balance in rheumatoid arthritis. *Arthritis and Rheumatism* **37**, 644–52.

Froelich, C.J., Zhang, X., Turbov, J., Hudig, D., Winkler, U., and Hanna, W.L. (1993). Human granzyme B degrades aggrecan proteoglycan in matrix synthesized by chondrocytes. *Journal of Immunology* **151**, 7161–71.

Geiler, T., Kriegsmann, J., Keyszer, G.M., Gay, R.E., and Gay, S. (1994). A new model for rheumatoid arthritis generated by engraftment of rheumatoid synovial tissue and normal human cartilage into SCID mice. *Arthritis and Rheumatism* **37**, 1664–71.

Goldenberg, D.L., Egan, M.S., and Cohen, A.S. (1982). Inflammatory synovitis in inflammatory joint disease. *Journal of Rheumatology* **9**, 204–9.

Goldring, S.R. and Gravallese, E.M. (2000). Pathogenesis of bone erosions in rheumatoid arthritis. *Current Opinion in Rheumatology* **12**, 195–9.

Gotis-Graham, I. and McNeil, H.P. (1997). Mast cell responses in rheumatoid synovium: association of the MC TC subset with matrix turnover and clinical progression. *Arthritis and Rheumatism* **40**, 479–89.

Gotis-Graham, I., Smith, M.D., Parker, A., and McNeil, H.P. (1998). Synovial mast cell responses during clinical improvement in early rheumatoid arthritis. *Annals of the Rheumatic Diseases* **57**, 664–71.

Gracie, J.A. et al. (1999). A pro-inflammatory role for interleukin-18 in rheumatoid arthritis. *Journal of Clinical Investigation* **104**, 1393–401.

Gravallese, E.M., Harada, Y., Wang, J.-T., Gorn, A.H., Thornhill, T.S., and Goldring, S.R. (1998). Identification of cell types responsible for bone resorbtion in rheumatoid arthritis and juvenile rheumatoid arthritis. *American Journal of Pathology* **152**, 943–51.

Gravallese, E.M. et al. (2000). Synovial tissue in rheumatoid arthritis is a source of osteoclast differentiation factor. *Arthritis and Rheumatism* **43**, 250–8.

Hakoda, M., Ishimoto, T., Hayashimoto, S., Inoue, K., Taniguchi, A., Kamatani, N., and Kashiwazaki, S. (1993). Selective infiltration of B cells committed to the production of monoreactive rheumatoid factor in synovial tissue of patients with rheumatoid arthritis. *Clinical Immunology and Immunopathology* **69**, 16–22.

Hamann, J., Wishaupt, J.O., Van Lier, R.A.W., Smeets, T.J.M., Breedveld, F.C., and Tak, P.P. (1999). Expression of the activation antigen CD97 and its ligand CD55 in rheumatoid synovial tissue. *Arthritis and Rheumatism* **42**, 650–8.

Hummel, K.M. et al. (1998). Cysteine proteinase cathepsin K mRNA is expressed in synovium of patients with rheumatoid arthritis and is detected at sites of synovial bone destruction. *Journal of Rheumatology* **25**, 1887–94.

Hyka, N., Dayer, J.-M., Modoux, C., Kohno, T., Edwards, C.K, Roux-Lombard, P., and Burger, D. (2001). Apolipoprotein A-1 inhibits the production of interleukin-1β and tumor necrosis factor by blocking contact-mediated activation of monocytes by T lymphocytes. *Blood* **97**, 2381–9.

Inoaka, T., Bilbe, G., Ishibashi, O., Tezuka, K., Kumegawa, M., and Kokubo, T. (1995). Molecular cloning of human cDNA for cathepsin K: novel cysteine proteinase predominantly expressed in bone. *Biochemical and Biophysical Research Communication* **206**, 89–96.

Iwata, Y., Mort, J.S., Tateishi, H., and Lee, E.R. (1997). Macrophage cathepsin, L, a factor in the erosion of subchondral bone in rheumatoid arthritis. *Arthritis and Rheumatism* **40**, 499–509.

Kennedy, T.D., Plater-Zyberk, C., Partridge, T.A., Woodrow, D.F., and Maini, R.N. (1988). Morphometric comparison of synovium from patients with osteoarthritis and rheumatoid arthritis. *Journal of Clinical Pathology* **41**, 847–52.

Keyszer, G., Redlich, A., Haupl, T., Zacher, J., Sparmann, M., Ungethum, U., Gay, S., and Burmester, G.R. (1998). Differential expression of cathepsins B and L compared with matrix metalloproteinases and their respective inhibitors in rheumatoid arthritis and osteoarthritis: a parallel investigation by semiquantitative reverse transcriptase-polymerase chain reaction and immunohistochemistry. *Arthritis and Rheumatism* **41**, 1378–87.

Keyszer, G.M., Heer, A.H., Kriegsmann, J., Geiler, T., Trabandt, A., Keysser, M., Gay, R.E., and Gay, S. (1995). Comparative analysis of cathepsin L, cathepsin D, and collagenase gene expression in synovial tissues of patients with rheumatoid arthritis and osteoarthritis by in situ hybridization. *Arthritis and Rheumatism* **38**, 976–84.

Kidd, B.L., Moore, K., Walters, M.T., Smith, J.L., and Cawley, M.I.D. (1989). Immunohistological features of synovitis in ankylosing spondylitis: a comparison with rheumatoid arthrtis. *Annals of the Rheumatic Diseases* **48**, 92–8.

Kirkham, B., Portek, I., Lee, C.S., Stavros, B., Lenarczyk, L., Lassere, M., and Edmonds, J. (1999). Intraarticular variability of synovial membrane histology, immunohistology, and cytokine mRNA expression in patients with rheumatoid arthritis. *Journal of Rheumatology* **26**, 777–84.

Klimiuk, P.A., Goronzy, J.J, Bjornsson, J., Beckenbaugh, R.D., and Weyand, C.M. (1997). Tissue cytokine patterns distinguish variants of rheumatoid synovitis. *American Journal of Pathology* **151**, 1311–19.

Kobayashi, I. and Ziff, M. (1975). Electron microscopic studies of the cartilage–pannus junction in rheumatoid arthritis. *Arthritis and Rheumatism* **18**, 475–83.

Koch, A.E. (1998). Angiogenesis: Implications for rheumatoid arthritis. *Arthritis and Rheumatism* **41**, 951–62.

Koch, A.E., Kunkel, S.L., Harlow, L.A., Johnson, B., Evanoff, H.L., Haines, G.K., Burdick, M.D., Pope, R.M., and Strieter, R.M. (1992). Enhanced production of monocyte chemoattractant protein-1 in rheumatoid arthritis. *Journal of Clinical Investigation* **90**, 772–9.

Kong, Y.-Y. et al. (1999). Activated T-cells regulate bone loss and joint destruction in adjuvant arthritis through osteoprotegerin ligand. *Nature* **402**, 304–9.

Konttinen, Y.T., Salo, T., Hanemaaijer, R., Valleala, H., Sorsa, T., Sutinen, M., Ceponis, A., Xu, J.W., Santavirta, S., Teronen, O., and Lopezotin, C. (1999). Collagenase-3 (MMP-13) and its activators in rheumatoid arthritis: localization in the pannus-hard tissue junction and inhibition by alendronate. *Matrix Biology* **18**, 401–12.

Kraan, M.C., Versendaal, H., Jonker, M., Bresnihan, B., Post, W.J., 'tHart, B.A., Breedveld, F.C., and Tak, P.P. (1998). Asymptomatic synovitis precedes clinically manifest arthritis. *Arthritis and Rheumatism* **41**, 1481–8.

Krenn, V., Schalhorn, N., Greiner, A., Molitoris, R., Konig, A., Gohlke, F., and Mullerhermelink, H.K. (1996). Immunohistochemical analysis of proliferating and antigen-presenting cells in rheumatoid synovial tissue. *Rheumatology International* **15**, 239–47.

Labowitz, R. and Schumacher, H.R. (1971). Articular manifestations of systemic lupus erythematosus. *Annals of Internal Medicine* **74**, 911.

Lacey, D.L. et al. (1998). Osteoprotegerin ligand is a cytokine that regulates osteoclast differentiation and activation. *Cell* **93**, 165–76.

Lacraz, S., Isler, P., Vey, E., Welgus, H.G., and Dayer, J.-M. (1994). Direct contact between T lymphocytes and monocytes is a major pathway for induction of metalloproteinase expression. *Journal of Biological Chemistry* **269**, 22027–33.

Maurice, M.M., Nakamura, H., Van der Voort, E.A.M., Van Vliet, A.I., Staal, F.J.T., Tak, P.P., Breedveld, F.C., and Verweij, C.L. (1997). Evidence for the role of an altered redox state in hyporesponsiveness of synovial T-cells in rheumatoid arthritis. *Journal of Immunology* **158**, 1458–65.

McGonagle, D., Gibbon, W., O'Connor, P., Green, M., Pease, C., and Emery, P. (1998). Characteristic magnetic resonance imaging entheseal changes of knee synovitis in spondylarthropathy. *Arthritis and Rheumatism* **41**, 694–700.

McGonagle, Marzo-Ortega, H., O'Connor, P., Gibbon, W., Hawkey, P., Henshaw, K., and Emery, P. (2002). Histologic assessment of the early enthesitis lesion in spondyloarthropathy. *Annals of the Rheumatic Diseases* **61**, 534–7.

McInnes, I.B., Almughales, J., Field, M., Leung, B.P., Huang, F.P., Dixon, R., Sturrock, R.D., Wilkinson, P.C., and Liew, F.Y. (1996). The role of interleukin-15 in T-cell migration and activation in rheumatoid arthritis. *Nature Medicine* **2**, 175–82.

Mohr, W. and Menninger, H. (1980). Polymorphonuclear granulocytes at the pannus–cartilage joint in rheumatoid arthritis. *Arthritis and Rheumatism* **23**, 1413–14.

Moore, A.R., Appelboam, A., Kawabata, K., Da, S.J., D'Cruz, D., Gowland, G., and Willoughby, D.A. (1999). Destruction of articular cartilage by alpha 2 macroglobulin elastase complexes: role in rheumatoid arthritis. *Annals of the Rheumatic Diseases* **58**, 109–13.

Mulherin, D., FitzGerald, O., and Bresnihan, B. (1996). Synovial tissue macrophage populations and articular damage in rheumatoid arthritis. *Arthritis and Rheumatism* **39**, 115–24.

Muller-Ladner, U., Kriegsmann, J., Tschopp, J., Gay, R.E., and Gay, S. (1995). Demonstration of granzyme A and perforin messenger RNA in the synovium of patients with rheumatoid arthritis. *Arthritis and Rheumatism* **38**, 477–84.

Nagase, H. and Okada, Y. (1997). Proteinases and matrix degradation. In *Textbook of Rheumatology* (ed. W.N. Kelley, S. Ruddy, E.D. Harris, and C.B. Sledge), pp. 323–41. Philadelphia PA: W.B. Saunders.

Nakagawa, K., Sakiyama, H., Tsuchida, T., Yamaguchi, K., Toyoguchi, T., Masuda, R., and Moriya, H. (1999). Complement C1s activation in degenerating articular cartilage of rheumatoid arthritis patients: immunohistochemical studies with an active form specific antibody. *Annals of the Rheumatic Diseases* **58**, 175–81.

Okamura, H., Tsutsui, H., Kashiwamura, S.-I., Yoshimoto, T., and Nakanishi, K. (1998). Interleukin-18: a novel cytokine that augments both innate and acquired immunity. *Advances in Immunology* **70**, 281–312.

Onodera, S., Kaneda, K., Mizue, Y., Koyama, Y., Fujinaga, M., and Nishihira, J. (2000). Macrophage migration inhibitory factor up-regulates expression of matrix metalloproteinases in synovial fibroblasts of rheumatoid arthritis. *Journal of Biological Chemistry* **275**, 444–50.

Otten, H.G., Dolhain, R.J., de Rooij, H.H., and Breedveld, F.C. (1993). Rheumatoid factor production by mononuclear cells derived from different sites of patients with rheumatoid arthritis. *Clinical and Experimental Immunology* **94**, 236–40.

Pando, J.A., Duray, P., Yarboro, C., Gourley, M.F., Klippel, J.H., and Schumacher, H.R. (2000). Synovitis occurs in some clinically normal and asymptomatic joints in patients with early arthritis. *Journal of Rheumatology* **27**, 1848–54.

Peterfy, C.G. (2001). Magnetic resonance imaging in rheumatoid arthritis: current status and future directions. *Journal of Rheumatology* **28**, 1134–42.

Pettit, A.R., MacDonald, K.P.A., O'Sullivan, B., and Thomas, R. (2000). Differentiated dendritic cells expressing nuclear RelB are predominantly located in rheumatoid synovial tissue preivascular mononuclear cell aggregates. *Arthritis and Rheumatism* **43**, 791–800.

Reece, R., Canete, J.D., Parsons, W.J., Emery, P., and Veale, D.J. (1999). Distinct vascular patterns of early synovitis in psoriatic, reactive, and rheumatoid arthritis. *Arthritis and Rheumatism* **42**, 1481–4.

Resnick, D., Yu, J.S., and Sartoris, D. (1997). Imaging. In *Textbook of Rheumatology* (ed. W.N. Kelley, S. Ruddy, E.D. Harris, and C.B. Sledge), pp. 626–86. Philadelphia PA: W.B. Saunders.

Schroder, A.E., Greiner, A., Seyfert, C., and Berek, C. (1996). Differentiation of B cells in the nonlymphoid tissue of the synovial membrane of patients with rheumatoid arthritis. *Proceedings of the National Academy of Sciences USA* **93**, 221–5.

Schulz Westhoff, C., Freudiger, D., Petrow, P., Seyfert, C., Zacher, J., Kriegsmann, J., Pap, T., Gay, S., Stiehl, P., Gromnica-Ihle, E., and Wernicke, D. (1999). Characterization of collagenase 3 (matrix metalloproteinase 13) messenger RNA expression in the synovial membrane and synovial fibroblasts of patients with rheumatoid arthritis. *Arthritis and Rheumatism* **42**, 1517–27.

Schumacher, H.R. and Kitridou, R.C. (1972). Synovitis of recent onset. A clinicopathologic study during the first month of disease. *Arthritis and Rheumatism* **15**, 465–85.

Smeets, T.J.M., Dolhain, R.J.E.M., Breedveld, F.C., and Tak, P.P. (1998). Analysis of the cellular infiltrates and expression of cytokines in synovial tissue from patients with rheumatoid arthritis and reactive arthritis. *Journal of Pathology* **186**, 75–81.

Soden, M., Rooney, M., Cullen, A., Whelan, A., Feighery, C., and Bresnihan, B. (1989). Immunohistological features in the synovium obtained from clinically uninvolved knee joints of patients with rheumatoid arthritis. *British Journal of Rheumatology* **28**, 287–92.

Tak, P.P. (2000). Examination of the synovium and synovial fluid. In *Rheumatoid Arthritis. Frontiers in Pathogenesis and Treatment* (ed. G.S. Firestein, G.S. Panayi, and F.A. Wollheim), pp. 55–68. Oxford: Oxford University Press.

Tak, P.P. and Bresnihan, B. (2000). The pathogenesis and prevention of joint damage in rheumatoid arthritis. Advances from synovial biopsy and tissue analysis. *Arthritis and Rheumatism* **43**, 2619–33.

Tak, P.P., Kummer, J.A., Hack, C.E., Daha, M.R., Smeets, T.J.M., Erkelens, G.W., Meinders, A.E., Kluin, P.M., and Breedveld, F.C. (1994). Granzyme positive cytotoxic cells are specifically increased in early rheumatoid synovial tissue. *Arthritis and Rheumatism* **37**, 1735–43.

Tak, P.P., Smeets, T.J.M., Daha, M.R., Kluin, P.M., Meijers, K.A.E., Brand, R., Meinders, A.E., and Breedveld, F.C. (1997). Analysis of the synovial cellular infiltrate in early rheumatoid synovial tissue in relation to local disease activity. *Arthritis and Rheumatism* **40**, 217–25.

Tak, P.P., Spaeny-Dekking, L., Kraan, M.C., Breedveld, F.C., Froelich, C.J., and Hack, C.E. (1999). The levels of soluble granzyme A and B are elevated in plasma and synovial fluid of patients with rheumatoid arthritis (RA). *Clinical and Experimental Immunology* **116**, 366–70.

Tetlow, L.C. and Woolley, D.E. (1995a). Distribution, activation and tryptase/chymase phenotype of mast cells in the rheumatoid lesion. *Annals of the Rheumatic Diseases* **54**, 549–55.

Tetlow, L.C. and Woolley, D.E. (1995b). Mast cells, cytokines, and metalloproteinases at the rheumatoid lesion: dual immunolocalisation studies. *Annals of the Rheumatic Diseases* **54**, 896–903.

Tetlow, L.C. and Woolley, D.E. (1998). Comparative immunolocalisation studies of collagenase 1 and collagenase 3 production in the rheumatoid lesion, and by human chondrocytes and synoviocytes *in vitro*. *British Journal of Rheumatology* **37**, 64–70.

Thomas, R. and Lipsky, P.E. (1996). Presentation of self peptides by dendritic cells: possible implications for the pathogenesis of rheumatoid arthritis. *Arthritis and Rheumatism* **39**, 183–90.

Thurkow, E.W., Van der Heijden, I.M., Breedveld, F.C., Smeets, T.J.M., Daha, M.R., Kluin, P.M., Meinders, A.E., and Tak, P.P. (1997). Increased expression of IL-15 in the synovium of patients with rheumatoid arthritis compared to patients with Yersinia-induced arthritis and osteoarthritis. *Journal of Pathology* **181**, 444–50.

Trabandt, A., Gay, R.E., Fassbender, H.-G., and Gay, S. (1991). Cathepsin B in synovial cells at the site of joint destruction in rheumatoid arthritis. *Arthritis and Rheumatism* **34**, 1444–51.

Trabandt, A., Aicher, W.K., Gay, R.E., Sukhatme, V.P., Fassbender, H.-G., and Gay, S. (1992). Spontaneous expression of immediate-early response genes c-fos and egr-1 in collagenase-producing rheumatoid synovial fibroblasts. *Rheumatology International* **12**, 53–9.

Ulfgren, A.-K., Lindblad, S., Klareskog, L., Andersson, J., and Andersson, U. (1995). Detection of cytokine producing cells in the synovial membrane from patients with rheumatoid arthritis. *Annals of the Rheumatic Diseases* **54**, 654–61.

Ulfgren, A.-K., Grondal, L., Lindblad, S., Johnell, O., Klareskog, L., and Andersson, U. (2000). Interindividual and intra-articular variation of pro-inflammatory cytokines in rheumatoid arthritis patients: potential implications for treatment. *Annals of the Rheumatic Diseases* **59**, 439–47.

van Meurs, J., van Lent, P., Holthuysen, A., Lambrou, D., Bayne, E., Singer, I, and van den Berg, W. (1999). Active matrix metalloproteinases are present in cartilage during immune complex-mediated arthritis: a pivotal role for stromelysin-1 in cartilage destruction. *Journal of Immunology* **163**, 5633–9.

Veale, D., Yanni, G., Rogers, S., Barnes, L., Bresnihan, B., and FitzGerald, O. (1993). Reduced synovial membrane macrophage numbers, ELAM-1 expression, and lining layer hyperplasia in psoriatic arthritis as compared with rheumatoid arthritis. *Arthritis and Rheumatism* **36**, 893–900.

Veale, D.J., Reece, R.J., Parsons, W., Radjenovic, A., O'Connor, P.J., Orgles, C.S., Berry, E., Ridgway, J.P., Mason, U., Boylston, A.W., Gibbon, W., and Emery, P. (1999). Intra-articular primatised anti-CD4: efficacy in resistant rheumatoid knees. A study of combined arthroscopy, magnetic resonance imaging, and arthroscopy. *Annals of the Rheumatic Diseases* **58**, 342–9.

Vey, E., Zhang, J.H., and Dayer, J.-M. (1992). IFN-gamma and I,25(OH)2D3 induce on THP-1 cells distinct patterns of cell surface antigen expression, cytokine production, and responsiveness to contact with activated T cells. *Journal of Immunology* **149**, 2040–6.

Walsh, D.A. (1999). Angiogenesis and arthritis. *Rheumatology* **38**, 103–12.

Wang, A.Z., Wang, J.C., Fisher, G.W., and Diamond, H.S. (1997). Interleukin-1β-stimulated invasion of articular cartilage by rheumatoid synovial fibroblasts is inhibited by antibodies to specific integrin receptors and by collagenase inhibitors. *Arthritis and Rheumatism* **40**, 1298–307.

Wernicke, D., Seyfert, C., Hinzmann, B., and Gromnica-Ihle, E. (1996). Cloning of collagenase 3 from synovial membrane and its expression in rheumatoid arthritis and osteoarthritia. *Journal of Rheumatology* **23**, 590–5.

Woolley, D.E., Crossley, M.J., and Evanson, J.M. (1977). Collagenase at sites of cartilage erosion in the rheumatoid joint. *Arthritis and Rheumatism* **20**, 1231–9.

Xue, C., Takahashi, M., Hasunuma, T., Aono, H., Yamamoto, K., Yoshino, S., Sumida, T., and Nishioka, K. (1997). Characterisation of fibroblast-like cells in pannus lesions of patients with rheumatoid arthritis sharing properties of fibroblasts and chondrocytes. *Annals of the Rheumatic Diseases* **56**, 262–7.

Yamada, T., Sawatsubashi, M., Yakushiji, H., Itoh, Y., Edakuni, G., Mori, M., Robert, L., and Miyazaki, K. (1998). Localization of vascular growth factor in synovial membrane mast cells: examination with 'multi-labelling subtraction immunostaining'. *Virchows Archives* **433**, 567–70.

Yamamura, M., Kawashima, M., Taniai, M., Yamauchi, H., Tanimoto, T., Kurimoto, M., Morita, Y., Ohmoto, Y., and Makino, H. (2001). Interferon-γ-inducing activity of interleukin-18 in the joint with rheumatoid arthritis. *Arthritis and Rheumatism* **44**, 275–85.

Yanni, G., Whelan, A., Feighery, C., and Bresnihan, B. (1994). Synovial tissue macrophages and joint erosion in rheumatoid arthritis. *Annals of the Rheumatic Diseases* **53**, 39–44.

Youssef, P., Roth, J., Frosch, M., Costello, P., FitzGerald, O., Sorg, C., and Bresnihan, B. (1999). Expression of myeloid related proteins (MRP) 8 and 14 and the MRP8/14 heterodimer in rheumatoid arthritis synovial membrane. *Journal of Rheumatology* **26**, 2523–8.

Youssef, P.P., Kraan, M., Breedveld, F., Bresnihan, B., Cassidy, N., Cunnane, G., Emery, P., FitzGerald, O., Kane, D., Lindblad, S., Reece, R., Veale, D., and Tak, P.P. (1998). Quantitative microscopic analysis of inflammation in rheumatoid arthritis synovial membrane samples selected at arthroscopy compared with samples obtained blindly by needle biopsy. *Arthritis and Rheumatism* **41**, 663–9.

Zvaifler, N.J., Tsai, V., Alsalameh, S., von Kempis, J., Firestein, J.S., and Lotz, M. (1997). Pannocytes: distinctive cells found in rheumatoid arthritis articular cartilage erosions. *American Journal of Pathology* **150**, 1125–38.

3.7 Skeletal muscle physiology and damage

Joan M. Round and David A. Jones

Weakness and feelings of fatigue and myalgia are amongst the most common symptoms complained of by patients with a variety of disorders including muscle diseases of rheumatic and autoimmune origin. In evaluating these symptoms, it is important to have an understanding of the underlying physiology of normal skeletal muscle; how it grows, matures, and ages, the factors that determine its strength, the causes of fatigue and of pain and damage during normal activity.

Muscle structure and function

The major proteins of the contractile apparatus are actin and myosin. Actin and myosin are of great evolutionary antiquity being found in almost every living cell and are responsible for cytoplasmic streaming, the movement of organelles, and cell division in addition to generating force and movement in skeletal, cardiac, and smooth muscles. The fundamentals of muscle structure are dealt with in most textbooks (Jones and Round 1990).

Bundles of actin and myosin filaments form myofibrils which are separated from each other within the muscle fibre by sarcoplasmic reticulum, T tubules, and, frequently, mitochondria (Fig. 1).

Changes in myofibrillar size and number account for the alterations in the size of muscle during growth or atrophy. The number of myofibrils arranged in parallel defines the cross-sectional area of a muscle and is the major determinant of its strength. The main cause of weakness is loss of contractile material arranged in parallel, leading to a reduction in cross-sectional area, or muscle atrophy. In skeletal muscle the sarcomeres are held in an orderly array with the Z lines aligned at right angles to the long axis of the muscle fibre [Fig. 2(a)]. Any disruption of this structure, such as sarcomere streaming, indicates damage or disease Fig. 2(b).

There are a host of structural proteins that link the surface membrane and the basal membrane of a muscle cell to the underlying contractile proteins (Fig. 3). Whilst the precise function of these links remains unclear, the absence, or abnormality, of these proteins gives rise to a family of genetically determined diseases, the muscular dystrophies (see below).

Control of contraction

In mammalian skeletal muscle, the interaction of actin and myosin is controlled by the presence of the protein tropomyosin, which is closely associated with the actin filaments blocking the myosin binding sites. Three

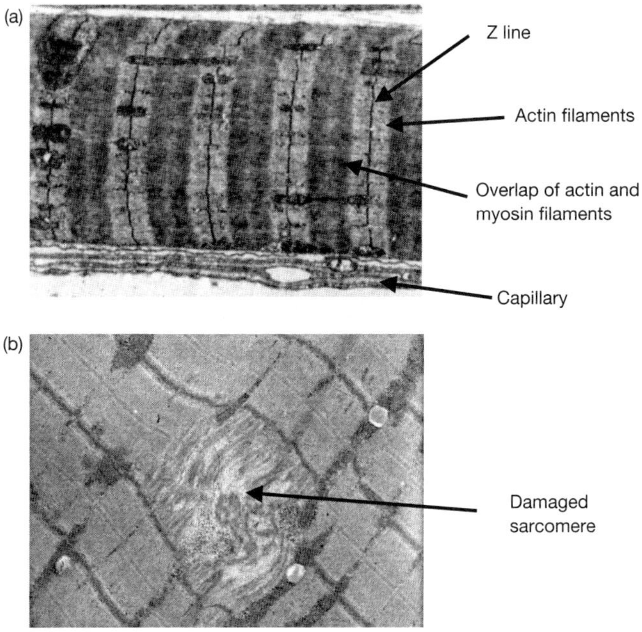

Fig. 2 Sarcomere structure in muscle fibres. (a) Normal muscle fibre showing the regular arrangement of sarcomeres. (b) Sarcomere damage caused by over extension during eccentric exercise.

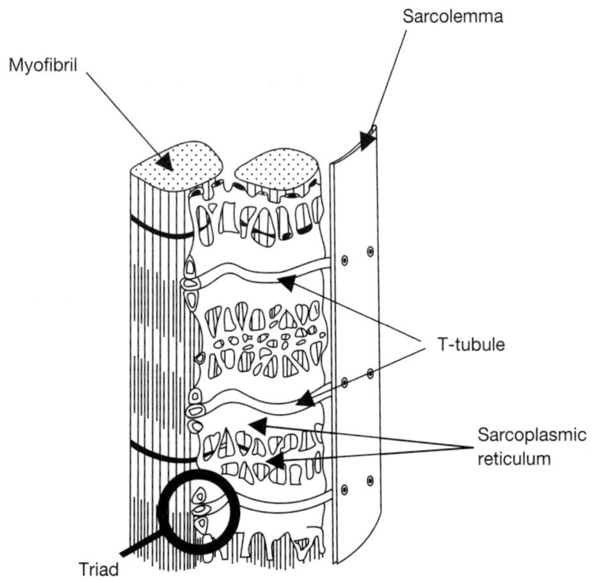

Fig. 1 T tubules, sarcoplasmic reticulum, and the myofibrils. Insert shows the structure of a triad.

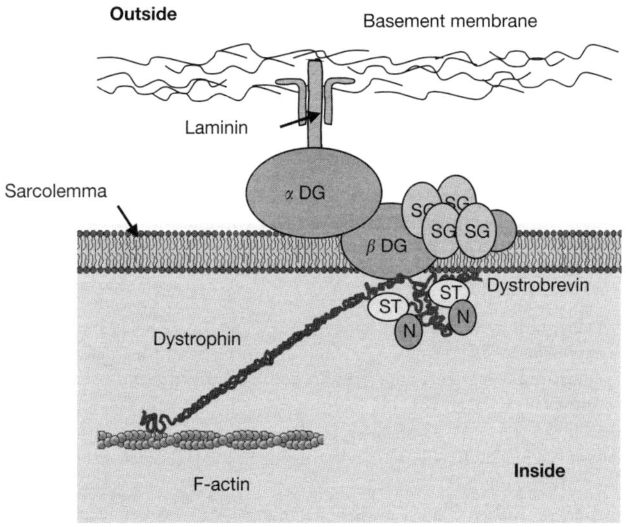

Fig. 3 Cytoskeletal proteins connecting the basement membrane and sarcolemma with the underlying contractile structures. DG, dystroglycan; SG, sarcoglycan, glycolsylated proteins in the surface membrane. N, nitric oxide synthase (NOS); ST, syntrophin which binds signalling molecules, such as NOS, to dystrophin and dystrobrevin.

other proteins associated with the tropomyosin occur at intervals along the actin filament. These are troponins I, T, and C. Troponin C binds calcium and this causes the tropomyosin molecule to move and expose the myosin binding sites on the actin filament. The actin and myosin can then combine and force is developed.

The calcium required for skeletal muscle contraction comes entirely from internal stores and is released from the membranous sarcoplasmic reticulum (SR) which encases the myofibrils. The SR acts as a store for the uptake and release of calcium in response to electrical activity in the surface membrane of the fibre. The SR also contains an active Ca^{2+} pump that can rapidly reduce intracellular calcium concentration, removing Ca^{2+} from troponin and causing the muscle to relax.

A complex branching T-tubular network runs through the whole fibre contacting every myofibril (Fig. 1) and is an extension of the surface membrane which conducts action potentials into the interior of the fibre. Where the T-tubular membrane comes into close proximity with the SR it forms the characteristic triad structure seen in EM sections. In this region the T-tubular membrane contains modified calcium channels (known as DHP receptors because they bind dihydropyridines such as verapamil), which act as voltage sensors and cause calcium channels in the SR membrane (known as ryanodine receptors) to open when an action potential passes along the T-tubule (Fig. 4). Calcium from the interior of the SR then rapidly diffuses to the myofibrils to initiate a contraction. The ryanodine receptors can also be opened by caffeine and halogenated anaesthetics such as halothane.

Muscle excitability

The electrophysiology of the muscle fibre is similar to that of nerve where the resting potential is largely determined by the K^+ gradient across the cell membrane. The passage of an action potential results in the movement of Na^+ into the cell and of K^+ outwards and during heavy exercise the flux of K^+ can be considerable giving rise to circulating K^+ concentrations as high as 6–7 mM which would normally be considered life-threatening. This danger is minimized by the fact that other resting muscles take up K^+ and, secondly, catecholamines, released during exercise stimulate this transport process. Since the pump is electrogenic ($3Na^+$ out to $2K^+$ in) this activity hyperpolarises both cardiac and skeletal muscles protecting against high circulating K^+ levels (McComas 1996).

Although muscle electrophysiology is basically the same as that of nerve, the T-tubular membrane complicates matters since action potentials pass from the surface of the fibre into the interior, along the T tubules, so the interior membranes may be depolarized when the surface is repolarizing. This voltage gradient could depolarize the surface membrane again and lead to repetitive firing. However, muscle membranes (unlike nerve) have a high chloride conductance which acts as a current leak, rendering the membrane less excitable and less prone to this problem.

The neuromuscular junction

A healthy adult muscle fibre has a single neuromuscular juntion (NMJ) situated about halfway along its length (the motor point).

The post-synaptic muscle fibre membrane of the NMJ is deeply convoluted with acetylcholine receptors situated at the crests of the folds close to the pre-synaptic (nerve) membrane. The membrane folds have a high density of sodium channels so that any depolarization as a result of acetylcholine binding to the receptor is amplified, ensuring reliable transmission from nerve to muscle. In foetal and denervated muscle, acetylcholine receptors are produced over the whole surface of the muscle fibres but when innervation, or re-innervation, occurs, contractile activity causes these extrajunctional receptors to disappear and acetylcholine receptors persist only at the NMJs. Although in normal circumstances the neuromuscular junction has considerable functional reserve, conditions which reduce the quantity of acetylcholine released or number of effective receptors on the post-synaptic membrane can lead to weakness and rapid fatigue.

The motor unit

Mature muscle fibres are innervated by a single branch of the axon from a motor neurone, the cell body of which is located in the ventral horn of the spinal cord (Fig. 5). Motor neurones vary in size and excitability, the smaller

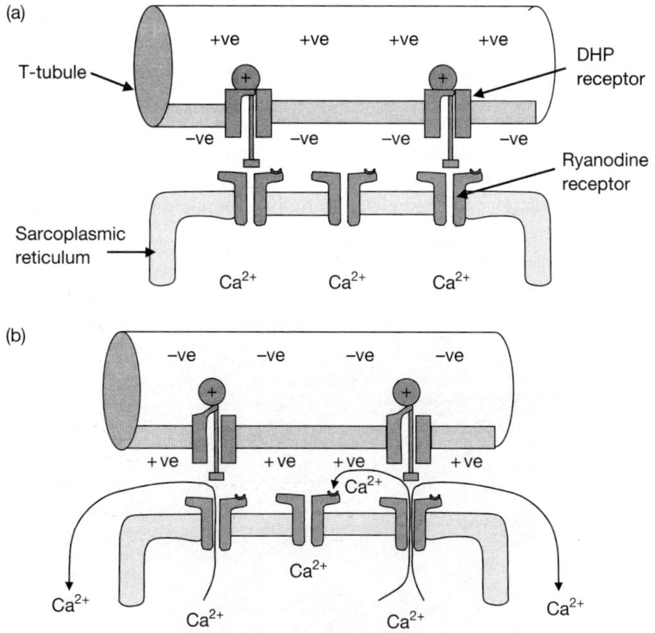

Fig. 4 Calcium channels and calcium release. (a) Resting muscle with the interior of the fibre negative relative to the interior of the T-tubule. DHP receptors act as voltage sensors closing the ryanodine receptors in the sarcoplasmic reticulum. (b) With the arrival of an action potential and depolarization of the T-tubular membrane, the DHP voltage sensor moves to open the ryanodine receptors and calcium diffuses out into the interior of the fibre. Released calcium also activates other ryanodine receptors (calcium-activated calcium release).

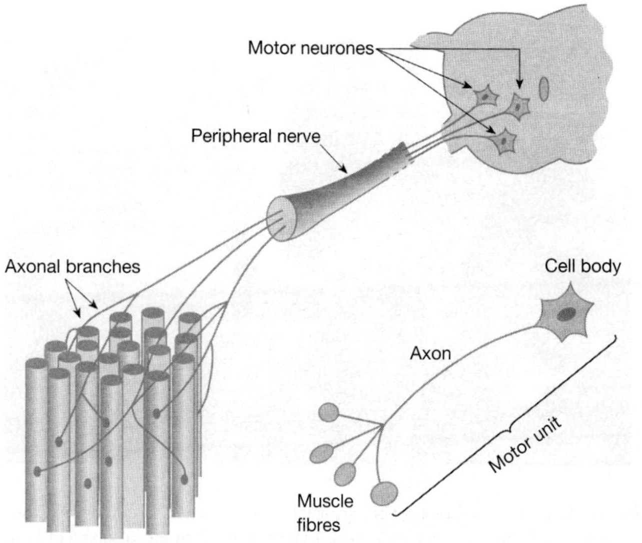

Fig. 5 The concept of the motor unit. A motor unit consists of the motor neurone and all the scattered muscle fibres which it innervates.

neurones being more excitable and most easily recruited. The number of axon branches that a motor neurone can sustain is a function of its size, the larger less excitable motor neurones having a large number of axon branches innervating a large number of muscle fibres. An action potential initiated by a motor neurone will pass down the axon in the motor nerve and along the axonal branches to initiate a simultaneous contraction in all the muscle fibres it innervates.

The motor neurone and the muscle fibres it innervates form a motor unit. The number of fibres in a motor unit varies widely from thousands in a large muscle, such as the quadriceps, down to tens in small muscles, such as those in the hand. The smaller, more excitable motor neurones are the first to be recruited when a muscle is required to contract and for most actions in every day life these are quite sufficient to provide the force required and are consequently used most frequently. The pattern of use has a major effect on the expression of proteins in the muscle fibres of a particular motor unit. Those units most frequently used express slow myosin isoforms, they contract relatively slowly, have less well developed T-tubular and SR systems and have a high mitochondrial content. Large motor units that are used relatively infrequently express fast myosin isoforms, have well-developed T-tubular and SR systems, a high content of glycolytic enzymes, and fewer mitochondria.

Human muscle fibres can be broadly classified into two groups: type 1, in the slow motor units, and type 2, in large fast units. In reality, there is a continuum between the two fibre types, and the type 2 fibre are often subdivided into 2A and 2B; type 2A having a higher oxidative capacity (more mitochondria) than type 2B and a slightly different content of myosin isoforms (Plate 54). Type 2C fibres, which contain embryonic myosins, are not normally seen in the adult unless the muscle is regenerating following damage or injury.

Patterns of imposed physical activity can have a considerable effect on the composition of a muscle, and interestingly the main effect has been found to be on the type 2A fibres. Enforced inactivity, as seen in patients with paraplegia, results in marked changes of muscle fibre type distribution with the inactive muscle consisting mainly of fast fibre types (Round et al. 1993). The implication is that the natural expression in muscle is of fast myosins while the expression of slow isoforms is a consequence of continual activity.

Although the pattern of imposed activity is a major determinant of fibre type, thyroid hormones also play an important role in this process. The muscles of hypothyroid patients have been found to have a marked predominance of slow fibres while type 2 fibres predominate in the muscles of hyperthyroid patients (Wiles et al. 1979).

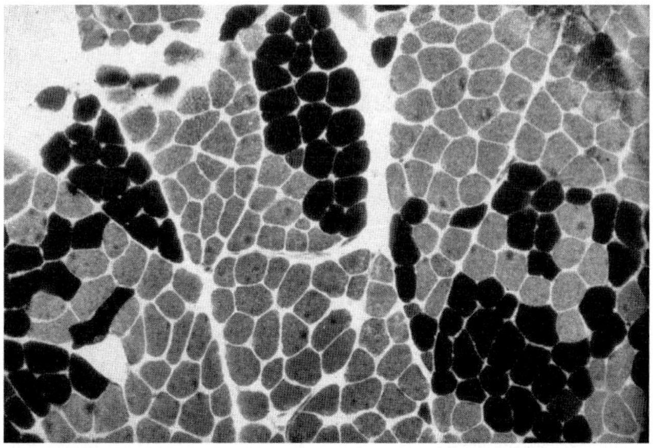

Fig. 6 Muscle biopsy showing fibre grouping. Biopsy stained for myosin ATPase, pH 9.4, type 2 fibres staining dark, type 1 fibres pale. Note the grouping of both fibre types compared to the random arrangement seen in normal muscle (Plate 54). The patient had suffered from a peripheral neuropathy due to heavy metal poisoning.

If a muscle fibre becomes denervated either by injury to the motor axon or by death of the motor neurone, nearby healthy axons will sprout and reinnervate the denervated fibres. Normally the fibres in fast and slow motor units are distributed fairly randomly within the muscle so that when muscle tissue is stained for different myosins a chequer board pattern of fibre types is seen (Plate 54). If, however, denervation is widespread whole areas of muscle can become innervated by axonal branches from a single motor neurone and will therefore express the same myosin isoforms, giving rise to fibre type grouping (Fig. 6).

Early development of muscle

Skeletal muscle is derived from the embryonic mesoderm. A myogenic fate is imposed on undifferentiated mesodermal cells in the somites by the action of a family of myogenic determining factors, the *myf* genes: *myf3 (MyoD)*, *myf4 (myogenin)*, *myf5*, and *myf6 (MRF4)* (mouse genes in parentheses; Buckingham 1992). These helix–loop–helix transcription factors continue to exert a controlling action on the genes encoding many muscle proteins and, together with thyroid hormone, they regulate the sequential development of muscle in the foetus. There is evidence that *myf* genes are also important in regulating gene expression in damaged and denervated adult muscle (Buckingham 1994).

At about the sixth week of gestation, mesodermal cells begin to divide and differentiate to form myoblasts. By weeks 7–9, the majority of myoblasts aggregate and fuse to form primary myotubes attached at their ends to tendons and the developing skeleton. Within a developing myotube a central chain of nuclei forms surrounded by basophilic cytoplasm rich in polyribosomes. By the ninth week of gestation the primordia of most muscle groups are well defined. At this time the synthesis of the contractile proteins, actin and myosin, occurs, the first signs of cross-striation are visible, and contractile activity begins (Fig. 7).

From 11 weeks of gestation onwards there is a proliferation of myofibrils leading to hypertrophy of the muscle fibres, which also grow in length by the addition of sarcomeres at the ends. Developing fibres express a number of different myosins including an embryonic form and an intermediate fast type often seen in regenerating adult muscle. Around 10 weeks of gestation, the nervous system makes contact with the developing muscle fibres and, in response to the patterns of contractile activity imposed by the motor nerves, the fibres differentiate so that, eventually, foetal myosins are no longer expressed. About 50 per cent of fibres contain adult slow myosin and 50 per cent fast myosin. This process, which is apparent by about 32 weeks of gestation, is not fully completed in human muscle until a few months after birth.

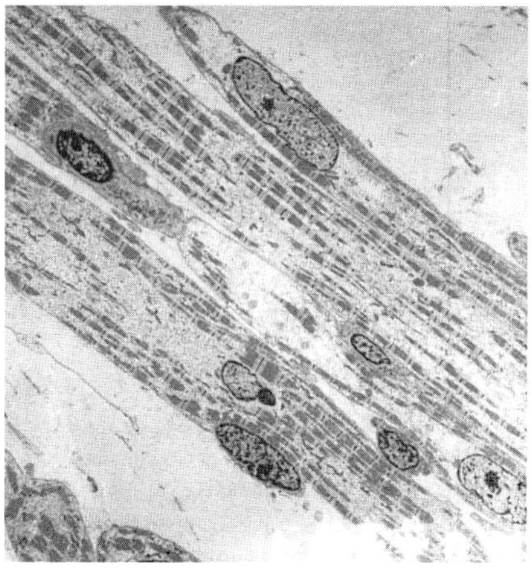

Fig. 7 Longitudinal section of developing myotubes showing the formation of myofibrils. Electron micrograph of tissue at 12 weeks of gestation.

Satellite cells

Muscle fibres are multinucleate structures and, in healthy fibres, the nuclei are situated at the periphery of the cell just under the surface membrane (sarcolemma). During development some of the mesodermal stem cells fail to fuse but remain closely associated with the developing myotubes. These undifferentiated cells are eventually enclosed by the basement membrane of the mature muscle fibres but remain outside the sarcolemma (Fig. 8). These are satellite cells, first described by Di Mauro (1961).

If the muscle fibre is damaged, the satellite cells enter the mitotic cycle, divide, and differentiate to form new myonuclei with which to repair or replace the damaged portions of the fibre. This process is tightly regulated by the *myf* genes and cyclin dependent kinases (Bornemann et al. 1999). The appearance of activated satellite cells is a good indication of perturbation, such as damage or rapid growth, occurring in a muscle. Successive cycles of damage lead eventually to a reduction in the numbers of satellite cells and in the efficiency of the remaining population (Endesfelder et al. 2000). This fact may provide an explanation for the decline in regenerative ability seen in the muscles of patients with advanced Duchenne muscular dystrophy (DMD) (Webster and Blau 1990).

Studies in mice suggest that satellite cells are a heterogeneous population, some being derived from progenitors in the embryonic vasculature. Putative stem cells isolated from skeletal muscle both reconstituted the haemopoetic compartment and participated in muscle regeneration while highly purified stem cells from bone marrow have been shown to participate in muscle regeneration (Seale et al. 2001). These observations suggest that tissue specific stem cells share a common embryonic origin, a finding which may lead to new therapies for degenerative muscle diseases such as muscular dystrophy.

Growth and maturation

Muscle fibre numbers in the rat do not change during life while the mean fibre cross-sectional area increases nearly 10-fold from the new-born to adult animal (Rowe and Goldspink 1969). The limited data available suggest that in human muscles there is also an increase in size without a change in fibre numbers as the muscles grow in size and strength (Plate 55). The final cross-sectional areas of adult muscle fibre are reached shortly after puberty. In an adult man about 40–45 per cent of the body weight is muscle and this figure is slightly lower for women.

Hypertrophy of muscle fibres occurs largely as a result of the activation and division of satellite cells which fuse with existing fibres and increase the amount of contractile material within the existing fibres. This process is controlled by a number of humoral factors including thyroid hormones, growth hormone, and adrenal androgens. During childhood there is little difference between the sexes and the increase in muscle bulk is in proportion to the general growth of the body. During puberty, there is a rapid increase in both height and weight influenced by the increasing levels of growth hormone and the sex hormones, oestrogen and testosterone (Round et al. 1999). For girls at this time, the relationship between strength and body weight remains similar to that seen during childhood. In boys, the increase in circulating testosterone leads to considerable muscle development which is particularly notable in the upper limb girdle where the final strength of the biceps is, on average, twice that found in mature girls (Fig. 9).

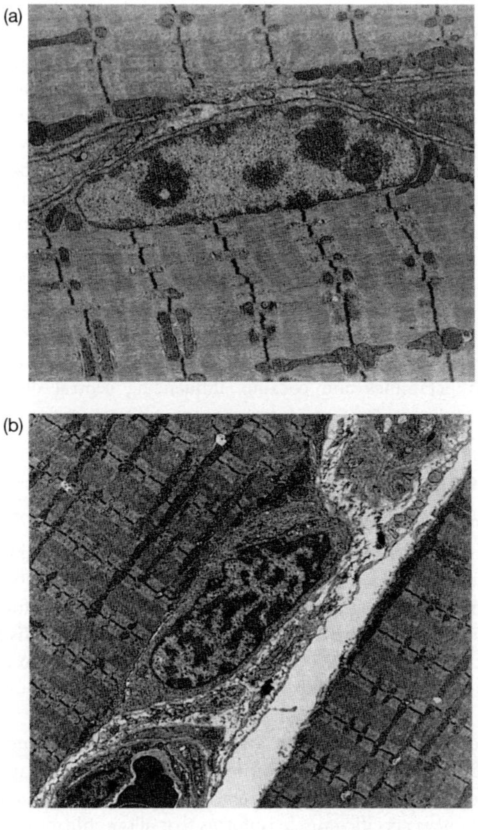

Fig. 8 Muscle fibre nucleus and satellite cell. (a) Muscle fibre nucleus lying just below the plasma membrane of the muscle cell. (b) Satellite cell lying outside the plasma membrane with a layer of cytoplasm around its nucleus.

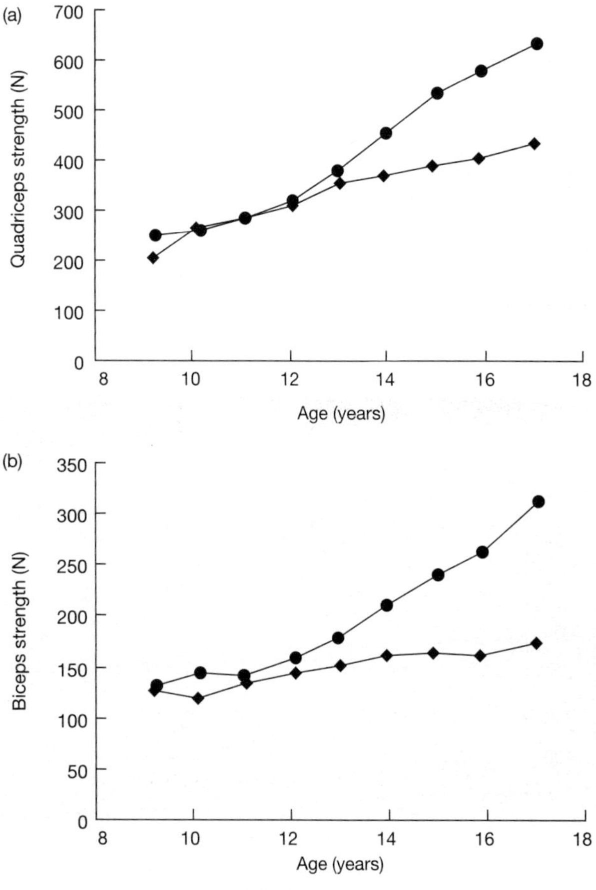

Fig. 9 Increases in muscle strength with growth and maturation: (a) quadriceps, (b) biceps. Girls' strength, diamonds, boys' strength, circles; mean isometric strength, longitudinal data. Note the divergence in strength at puberty.

Ageing

Ageing is characterized by a general reduction in mobility and an increased likelihood of damaging falls, partly due to loss of muscle bulk.

Peak muscle mass is reached early in the third decade after which muscle strength and bulk start to decline so that by the eighth decade muscle strength, which mirrors the reduction in bone density, may be reduced by about 40 per cent (Fig. 10). The loss of muscle fibre protein in elderly muscle is probably related to the reduction in circulating sex hormones and growth hormone which occurs with age (Rutherford and Jones 1992). Hormone replacement therapy in post-menopausal women is reported to increase both muscle strength and bone mineral density (Skelton et al. 1999).

The loss of muscle bulk with age is primarily due to a progressive atrophy of all skeletal muscle fibres but there is also a preferential loss of type 2 fibres, due to death of large, fast, motor neurones. Groups of type 1 fibres are not uncommon in muscle from otherwise healthy elderly subjects (Plate 56).

With increasing age, there is also a decrease in the number of satellite cells in muscle but the few reported studies of strength training in the elderly suggest that ageing muscles can be strengthened as efficiently as younger muscles (Frontera et al. 1988).

Loss of mobility is a serious problem for the elderly but whilst there must be a threshold strength required to rise from a chair or walk upstairs, it is not clear that these difficulties are entirely the result of reduced muscle strength. It is important not to overlook factors such as failing motor skills and eyesight, loss of balance, degenerative changes, and stiffness in the joints due to ageing of articular cartilage and rheumatic disease. Inflammation of joints causes muscle inhibition (Stokes and Young 1984) disrupting patterns of normal movement. In this situation, the problem with ageing is not primarily in the muscle but in the joints and failing senses. Muscle strengthening may have a role to play in maintaining mobility but therapy should also be directed towards mobilizing joints, assessing eyesight, and efforts to maintain or restore motor skills.

Skeletal muscle fatigue and damage

Fatigue and damage are features of many muscle diseases and it is important to understand these processes in normal muscle before considering pathological conditions.

Fatigue

Peripheral mechanisms

During high-intensity exercise, fatigue is primarily of a peripheral origin, that is, it can be attributed to failure within the muscle fibre or at the NMJ rather than to failure within the central nervous system (Jones 1999). The main features of this type of fatigue are a reduction in the force generating capacity of the muscle due to a decrease in calcium release and, secondly, a reduction in the velocity with which the muscle can shorten. Together, the deceased force and speed lead to a major loss of power (James et al. 1995; DeRuiter et al. 1999). The immediate cause is of metabolic origin, such as a decrease in ATP or accumulation of metabolites. It is clear, however, that the conventional view that lactic acid is the cause of fatigue is wrong, or at least a serious oversimplification since patients with McArdle's disease, who are unable to metabolize glycogen and produce lactate, suffer from very rapid fatigue (Cady et al. 1989a,b). During prolonged activity the situation is complex. When exercising at ~70 per cent VO_{2max} (marathon pace) most people can maintain a steady state, that is, a constant oxygen uptake and heart rate with blood lactate steady at between 2 and 4 mM. In theory, subjects should be able to exercise at this rate for about 90 min until muscle glycogen becomes depleted but, in practice, most are limited to between 20 and 60 min but show few signs of peripheral fatigue when they declare themselves exhausted. Evidence suggests that it is the ability to drive the muscles that is at fault in this situation. This is known as 'central fatigue'.

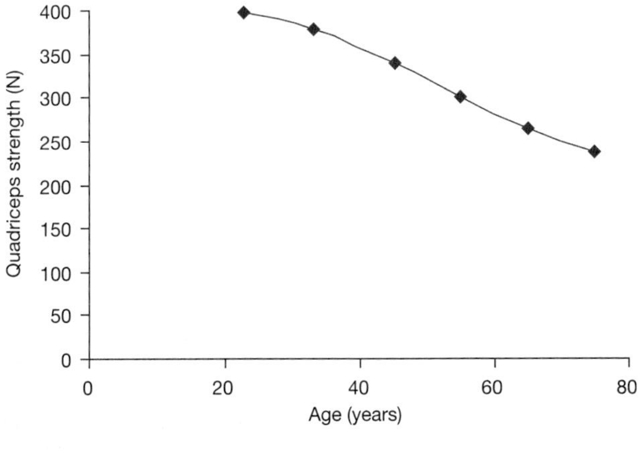

Fig. 10 Decline in strength with increasing age. Isometric quadriceps strength of healthy female subjects. Cross-sectional data.

Central fatigue

Very little is known of the mechanisms of central fatigue. Most work to date has centred on serotonergic pathways and, in animals, there is evidence that 5-HT agonists depress performance whereas antagonists enhance endurance times; there may also be a reciprocal relationship with dopamine (Bailey et al. 1993a,b). Exercise in warm and/or humid environments leads to a progressive rise in body temperature, which is associated with increasing feelings of discomfort and the secretion of pituitary hormones such as prolactin. Most subjects stop exercising when their core temperature reaches 39.5°C (Nielsen et al. 1993). Body temperature is probably only one of many afferent signals reaching the brain that contribute to inhibition of motor output. Chemo- and mechano-receptors in muscles, tendons, and joints have important projections into the brain stem involved in cardiovascular control and these may also influence motivation and motor pathways. In addition to direct neuronal input, it is likely that humoral factors affect mood and behaviour. There are clear links between the immune system and central processes regulating mood and perception and this has wide ranging implications for understanding the way disease modifies behaviour. For example, many cytokines induce changes in behaviour, mood, and cognition (Maier and Watkins 1998) and circulating cytokines can be increased by exercise, disease, and infection.

It is likely that individuals will vary in their tolerance of the various afferent signals associated with exercise and this tolerance may be improved with training or adversely affected by inactivity or disease. Tolerance can be altered pharmacologically with caffeine, which probably acts in a similar way to amphetamines and cocaine, influencing central dopaminergic pathways.

Muscle damage

Assessment of damage

The most common presentation of muscle damage is weakness often accompanied by myalgia. Simple functional tests, such as the ability to rise from a chair or squatting position, or stand on tiptoe, are useful guides to strength but more objective measures can be made using a relatively simple testing chair (Edwards et al. 1977). The technique is easy to apply and reliable measurements can be made even on children as young as 6 or 7 years.

Soluble constituents, such as creatine kinase (CK) and lactate dehydrogenase, will leak into the circulation from damaged skeletal muscle fibres and provide information about the extent and time course of damage. These two enzymes have specific muscle isoforms that allow effluxes from skeletal muscle to be distinguished from that coming from cardiac muscle or other tissues. Myoglobin can also be used as a marker but it provides little or no clinical advantage over the measurement of CK. A single laboratory report

(a)

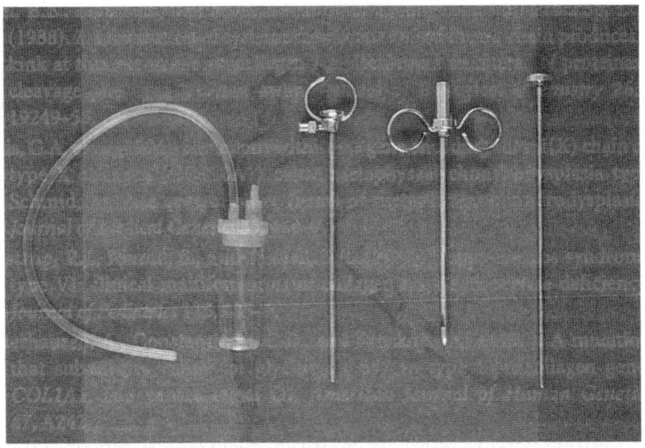

(b)

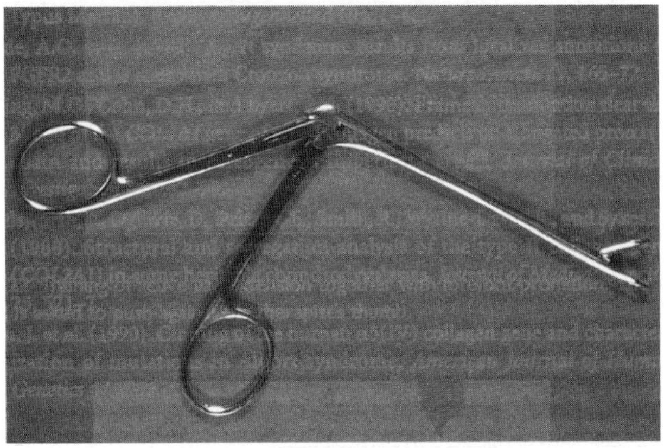

Fig. 11 (a) The University College Hospital (UCH) modification of Bergstrom's original percutaneous muscle biopsy needle. The cutting edge of the inner hollow cylinder is introduced within the outer pointed casing which contains a window at its lower end through which the muscle biopsy is taken. The sterile trap is attached to a suction mechanism which assists in pulling the muscle tissue into the outer window. The central solid portion of the instrument is used only to remove the specimen after the needle has been withdrawn. (b) Conchotome forceps for percutaneous muscle biopsy.

of an unexpectedly high CK value, particularly in an out-patient, should be checked by a repeat blood test about a week later and a history of any heavy or unaccustomed exercise should be sought.

Histological examination of a muscle biopsy specimen from large muscle groups such as the quadriceps or gastrocnemius, obtained either by the percutaneous needle or choncotome technique, can be valuable (Fig. 11). The presence of internalized muscle fibre nuclei is often a pointer to the fact that the muscle fibres have been damaged.

Damage due to physical trauma

Skeletal muscles are frequently subjected to physical trauma during everyday life and this risk is increased with participation in contact sports. It is probable that most of the painful sensations associated with bumps and bruises are due to inflammation of the skin, sub-cutaneous tissues, and the muscle fascia, with relatively little involvement of the muscle fibres. It is often said that procedures such as intramuscular injections or muscle biopsies lead to high circulating CK, but there is little evidence for this. Following orthopaedic surgery, in which large amounts of muscle were resected, circulating levels rose above 1000 IU/l only occasionally and values rapidly returned to normal 2–3 days after surgery (Jones et al. 1991).

Severe muscle fibre necrosis (rhabdomyolysis) can occur after crush injuries, or in cases where a patient has been found lying unconscious on a hard surface for some hours. The release of myoglobin into the circulation presents a serious risk of acute renal failure as myoglobin will precipitate in an acid environment and damage the proximal renal tubules. In these circumstances circulating myoglobin and CK are very high (>20 000 IU/l), reaching a peak about 24 h after circulation is restored to the damaged muscle. In these cases the damage is a result of reperfusion injury (see below).

For a tissue subjected to high mechanical stress and strain and a metabolic rate that fluctuates widely, skeletal muscle is remarkably resilient and resistant to damage. However, considerable damage can occur if untrained muscle is forcibly extended during what is often known as eccentric exercise or contractions.

Eccentric exercise

Many movements, such as sitting down, walking down stairs, running downhill, or lowering weights involve stretching movements, and following these types of exercise the muscle is weak and painful and the loss of force can persist for 2 or 3 weeks in severely damaged muscle.

The most intriguing feature of this type of muscle damage is the long delay (about 4–6 days) between the exercise and the leakage of soluble constituents from the muscle fibres. There is then an even longer delay (~10 days) before necrosis and regeneration are visible microscopically in biopsy samples of the affected muscle (Plate 57) (Newham et al. 1983; Jones et al. 1986).

Muscle pain after eccentric exercise

During eccentric exercise, there is no burning sensation such as produced by metabolically demanding high-intensity isometric or concentric activity. Typically the subject first notices pain the morning after the exercise. The major sensation is not of continuous pain but of discomfort, often described as stiffness or tenderness when the muscle is touched or stretched. Some degree of oedema is also often present (Newham et al. 1983). This pain is often referred to as 'delayed onset muscle soreness' or DOMS. Although severe muscle damage is associated with severe DOMS, all the indications are that DOMS is not a consequence of damage to muscle fibres but is part of an inflammatory reaction to damaged connective tissue elements in the muscle (Jones et al. 1987). It is notable that the nature and time course of DOMS is very similar to that experienced after a bruise or tendon sprain (involving connective tissue) while diseases such as muscular dystrophy and polymyositis, where there is major damage and destruction of muscle fibres, are largely pain free.

Muscle damage after reperfusion of an ischaemic limb

An unfortunate consequence of successful vascular surgery has been the occasional cases where the patient experiences severe rhabdomyolysis often accompanied by acute renal failure caused by myoglobin precipitating in the renal tubules. The huge rise in circulating CK and myoglobin does not occur immediately the circulation is restored but after a delay of 24–48 h. This suggests that the muscle damage is not the direct result of ischaemia but is due to some subsequent event occurring after oxygenated blood flow has been restored to the limb (Adiseshiah et al. 1992). Muscle specimens taken immediately after surgery show very little evidence of fibre damage, but biopsies obtained several days later show the characteristic picture of fibre necrosis, regeneration, and infiltration of the tissue by mononuclear cells (Plate 58).

Reperfusion injury as a consequence of free radicals generated by xanthine oxidase is a recognized and serious problem affecting tissues such as the brain and gut (McCord 1985; McArdle and Jackson 1994) and it is likely that similar mechanisms occur in skeletal muscle (Adiseshiah et al. 1992). Skeletal muscle is relatively resistant to this form of damage since the indications are that it requires 4–6 h of ischaemia before problems become apparent. Nevertheless, prophylactic treatment with an antioxidant, such as manitol, may help to reduce the muscle damage following vascular surgery, and maintaining alkaline urine with a bicarbonate infusion will help prevent renal failure following any rhabdomyolysis.

Muscle diseases

Figure 12 provides a classification of muscle disorders with a myopathic, as opposed to a neuropathic, origin.

The first division is between disorders where muscle bulk is relatively well maintained [Fig. 12(a)] and those where there is a loss of muscle bulk [Fig. 12(b)].

Disordered function, normal muscle bulk

This is a heterogeneous group of relatively rare muscle disorders where patients may present with abnormally rapid onset of fatigue, abnormally prolonged contractions, or episodes of flaccid paralysis [Fig. 12(a)].

The metabolic myopathies

Muscular activity places major demands on the energy metabolism, both anaerobic glycolysis and the oxidation of carbohydrates and fatty acids. All of these pathways are important in the secondary supply of energy to the muscles as the primary reserves of phosphocreatine become depleted. In general, patients with metabolic defects are of normal, or near-normal, strength when rested but are very limited in their exercise endurance.

The glycogenoses

Included in Table 1, are diseases where there are defects in the enzymes of the glycolytic pathway which affect skeletal muscle. In many of the glycogenoses, accumulation of abnormal glycogen damages the muscle fibre and an example of this is the type 2 condition, shown in Plate 59.

Muscle function has been most extensively studied in McArdle's disease (myophosphorylase deficiency, type 5) where the key clinical feature is of painful muscle fatigue, and sometimes contracture, in the absence of lactic acid. Muscles do not show any signs of damage or atrophy but an absence of phosphorylase on histochemical staining is diagnostic. In this condition, mild exercise such as walking slowly can be sustained by the oxidation of fatty acids and blood-borne glucose. Higher intensity exercise can be maintained for only a few seconds before the muscles begins to fatigue as the reserves of phosphocreatine are exhausted and muscle ATP levels are compromised (Cady et al. 1989a,b). If exercise continues, painful muscle contractures develop which are electrically silent (unlike muscle cramp in normal subjects, which is electrically active). These contractures which are extremely painful, resolve slowly, and can give rise to rhabdomyolysis when the blood supply eventually returns. Fortunately, patients are generally well aware of their limitations and take care to reduce the exercise level before any crisis can develop.

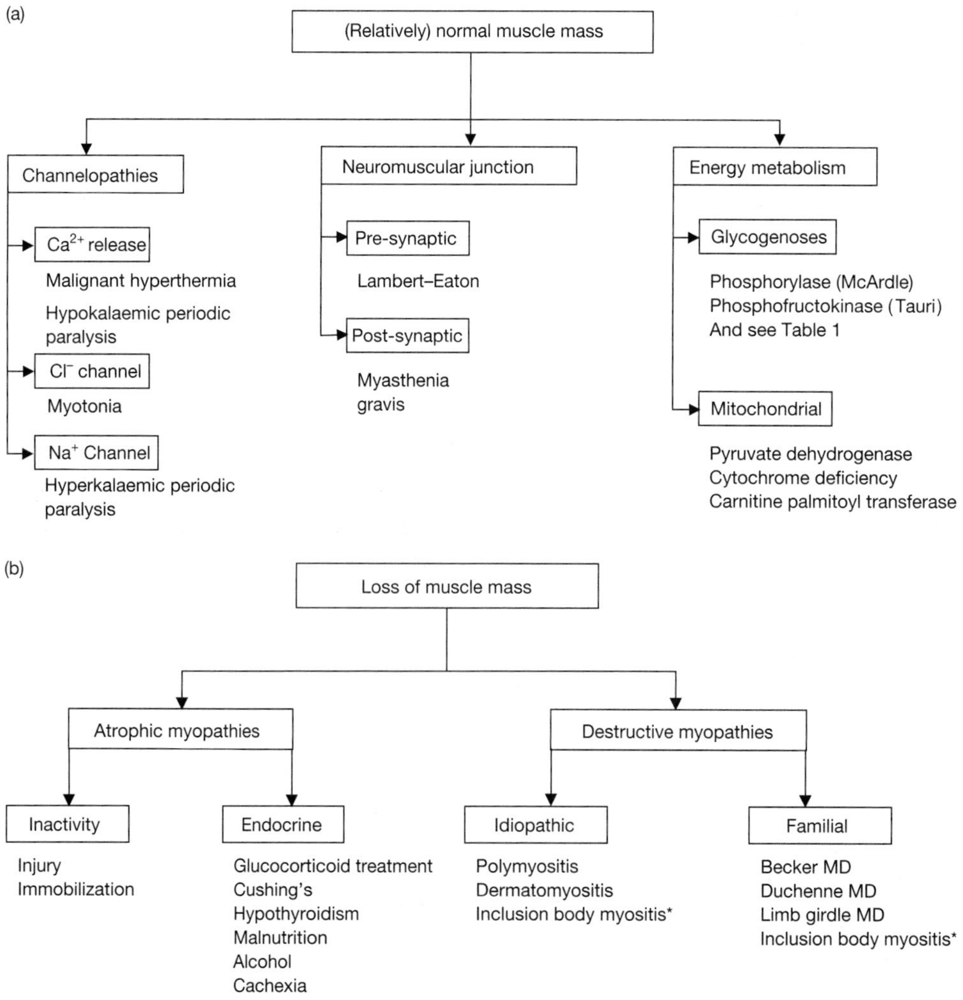

Fig. 12 Classification of muscle disorders. (a) Diseases in which muscle contractile material is relatively well preserved; the main problem being premature fatigue or episodes of flaccid paralysis. (b) Conditions where muscle tissue is lost and the main complaint is weakness. * Inclusion body myositis is included as being of both a familial and idiopathic origin since its autoimmune origin is uncertain.

Table 1 The glycogenoses. Only those conditions affecting skeletal muscle are listed

Type	Name	Deficiency	Affected organs/symptoms
1	Von Gierke's disease	Glucose-6-phosphatase	Hepatomegaly, growth retardation, hypoglycaemia, lacticacidosis
2	Pompe's disease	Lysosomal enzymes α-1,4 and α-1,6 glucosidase	Cardiomyopathy and severe weakness with large accumulations of glycogen in the muscle
3	Cori–Forbes disease	Absence of debrancher enzyme	Abnormal glycogen accumulates in the muscle. Clinical symptoms vary from severe muscle weakness in childhood to asymptomatic adult forms
5	McArdle's disease	Myo-phosphorylase deficiency	Cannot metabolise muscle glycogen. Severe exercise limitation in the absence of lactic acid accumulation
7	Tauri's disease	Phosphofructokinase deficiency	Enzyme missing in muscle and red cells. Similar to McArdle's, but more severe problems with exercise. Haemolytic anaemia may occur

McArdle's patients differ in the severity and onset of their symptoms and this may reflect the diverse genetic defects underlying the disease although no clear relationships have been demonstrated (Bartram et al. 1994). Some patients produce mRNA but no protein, others produce no mRNA or protein. This molecular heterogeneity implies the involvement of multiple mutations. The muscle glycogen phosphorylase gene is approximately 14 kb in size and has been assigned to the long arm of chromosome 11 (Lebo et al. 1984). A mutation in codon 50 (C to T) has been identified on at least one allele in all patients studied. McArdle's disease is usually considered as an autosomal recessive condition but heterozygotes expressing the disorder do occur, indicating that these patients must possess an additional mutation(s).

Mitochondrial myopathies

Patients with defective mitochondrial function have severely limited exercise capacity and even mild exercise is associated with breathlessness and severe metabolic acidosis, such as would be seen in a normal subject exercising at high intensity or under hypoxic conditions. Although severely limited in their exercise capacity, the normal glycolytic function in these patients must provide sufficient energy to prevent the development of the muscle contractures that are a feature of McArdle's disease. Histologically, patients show abnormal 'ragged red' fibres in muscle biopsy sections treated with trichrome stain, the periphery of the fibres being packed with numerous red-staining mitochondria (Plate 60). Scattered necrotic fibres are also seen. Both mitochondrial DNA and nuclear genes are necessary for the biogenesis of the respiratory chain and pathogenic mutations of both genomes are being identified. There are now many good correlations between genotype and phenotype in mitochondrial disorders (Larsson and Oldfors 2001; and see Smeitink et al. 2001 for review).

Disorders of fat metabolism

Patients with disorders of fatty acid metabolism have symptoms of weakness, exercise intolerance, muscle stiffness, and pain (sometimes accompanied by myoglobinuria). Symptoms are most evident at times when free fatty acids are the main substrates for energy metabolism, such as during prolonged sub-maximal exercise, particularly in the fasting state. The β-oxidation of fatty acids depends on the transport of free fatty acids into the mitochondria by a shuttle mechanism which involves carnitine and the carnitine palmitoyl transferase (CPT) enzymes. Low plasma carnitine and deficiencies of CPT have been described. Patients lacking carnitine are weak, whereas those lacking the CPT enzymes are of fairly normal strength at rest but after fasting or exercise they may show evidence of muscle damage, with a raised creatine kinase and occasionally myoglobinuria. Muscle biopsy may show large fat droplets in the muscle fibres.

Fatigue and disease states

Fatigue is one of the most common presenting symptoms and it is natural, when looking for explanations to think in terms of metabolic abnormalities as described above. In reality, problems such as McArdle's diseases are very rare and the majority of patients in whom the muscle bulk is relatively well preserved suffer from fatigue of a central nature rather than from peripheral metabolic problems in their muscles, vascular disease being an exception.

Fatigue is an almost universal experience of patients with chronic heart failure (CHF). Since the basic problem is a reduced central pump activity it would seem self evident that reduced blood supply to working muscles is the explanation of these feelings. However, there are many cases where limb blood flow is normal but exercise tolerance is reduced (Wilson et al. 1993) and there is little evidence of peripheral muscle abnormality (Buller et al. 1991). A survey of 52 ambulatory patients found no relationship between the feelings of fatigue and the severity of the cardiac impairment (Wilson et al. 1995) indicating a complex situation.

In cases of rheumatoid arthritis, osteoarthritis, and fibromyalgia, symptoms of fatigue are common but poorly related to the severity of the physical disease, with pain and sleep disturbance being the factors which most closely correlate with fatigue (Mahowald et al. 1989; Wolfe et al. 1996).

Patients with both hypothyroid and hyperthyroid disease complain of fatigue. Hypothyroid patients are especially interesting in the present context since, despite fatigue being one of their main complaints, their muscles, when tested objectively, prove to be more resistant to fatigue than normal (Wiles et al. 1981).

Basal ganglia

Feelings of fatigue are also a common complaint of patients suffering from arkinson's disease and there is growing interest in the possibility that dopaminergic and serotonergic pathways may mediate activity in the basal ganglia and the effort required to initiate movement (Chaudhuri and Behan 2000).

Chronic fatigue states

Chronic fatigue syndrome (CFS) is a complex condition which may arise from a number of precipitating events, including viral infections, and has a wide range of symptoms, but the one common factor is an abnormally low tolerance of whole body exercise (White 1990). Whilst there may well be alterations in cardiovascular and muscle function, evidence indicates that such changes are probably secondary to the decrease in activity and are not its underlying cause. Consequently much recent attention has turned to possible central nervous system changes, such as an increase in sensitivity to the sensations of exercise, and the role of the brain stem in regulating levels of attention and arousal. An increase in the sensitivity of brain 5-hydroxytryptamine receptor function is associated with chronic feelings of fatigue and exercise intolerance (Bakheit et al. 1992; Cleare et al. 1995) implicating pathways in the hypothalamus as possible sites where abnormalities may occur.

The ion channelopathies

Normal muscle physiology is dependent on the function of a variety of ion channels in the surface, T-tubular and SR membranes. A number of disorders due to mutations of cation channels have been identified (see Lehmann-Horn and Jurkat-Rott 1999, for review) these disorders give rise to a group of diseases designated as 'ion channelopathies'.

Malignant hyperthermia

This is an autosomal dominant disorder in which, during halothane anaesthesia, skeletal muscle responds with a prolonged contracture causing metabolic depletion of the muscle. The first signs of danger are muscle rigidity, a rise in the patient's temperature, and the release of potassium into the circulation, which brings with it the risk of cardiac arrest. If the patient survives this acute emergency, the skeletal muscles subsequently undergo rhabdomyolysis and there is the risk of acute renal failure. Rapid treatment with dantrolene (which inhibits Ca^{2+} release from the SR) and cooling has proved effective. This disorder is now known to be associated with a group of over 20 mutations in the ryanodine receptor (see Fig. 4) (Jurkat-Rott et al. 2000) which, in some families, are also associated with central core disease. *In vitro* tests for malignant hyperthermia (MH) are recommended for patients with central core disease and members of their families, if surgery is contemplated (Curran et al. 1999).

Myotonia congenita

In this condition there is a defect in the gene encoding the major skeletal muscle chloride channel (Lehmann and Jurkat-Rott 1999). Lack of a 'leak' conductance allows voltage gradients to build up between surface and deep T-tubular membranes leading to repetitive firing (see above) and an inability to relax a muscle particularly after a forceful movement. A characteristic EMG signal is seen with a rapid discharge which dies away after about 30 s.

Periodic paralyses

There are two forms of periodic paralysis, the hyper- and hypokalaemic varieties in which attacks of flaccid paralysis are provoked, respectively, by high or low plasma potassium concentrations (Jurkat-Rott et al. 2000). With hyperkalaemic periodic paralysis the defect is of a sodium channel that goes into an abnormal refractory state when the surface membrane is depolarised. The hypokalaemic variety is a defect in the calcium channels forming the DHP receptors that become inactive in the presence of low potassium concentrations and thus ineffective in linking electrical activity with release of calcium from the SR (Fig. 4). Restoring normal blood potassium reverses the paralysis in both cases but it is important to correctly diagnose the problem as giving potassium to a patient with the hyperkalaemic variety can only exacerbate the condition! High blood potassium can be reversed by giving glucose and/or insulin.

Diseases of the NMJ

Myasthenia gravis

This is an autoimmune disease in which antibodies are produced against post-synaptic acetylcholine receptors. The condition is more common in women often first affecting the eyes and tongue before spreading to other muscles and eventually threatening breathing and swallowing. Thymectomy in the early stages can be effective. At rest patients are of relatively normal strength but with use muscles fatigue rapidly as the quantity of acetylcholine released with each action potential decreases, leading to insufficient depolarization to activate the muscle fibre membrane. Anticholinesterase drugs such as edrophonium chloride provide dramatic short-term relief and can be used as a diagnostic test for this condition. Long-term treatment is with drugs to suppress the autoimmune activity and long acting anticholinesterase drugs such as atropine. Although muscle bulk is initially normal, inactivity eventually leads to muscle wasting. As with many autoimmune diseases the aetiology of this condition is obscure.

Lambert–Eaton syndrome

This is a myasthenia-like syndrome in which muscular weakness is the main problem. Unlike myasthenia gravis, where the problem gets worse as the muscle is used, with Lambert–Eaton syndrome, performance improves with activity. The differences can best be seen in response to a high frequency burst of stimulation where, with myasthenia gravis the evoked muscle action potentials decrease rapidly but with Lambert–Eaton syndrome they increase with time. The defect is thought to lie in the release of acetylcholine quanta and in particular with the voltage activated calcium channels in the motor nerve that are required to allow calcium entry and cause synaptic vesicles to fuse with the pre-synaptic membrane (McComas 1996). The syndrome is often associated with carcinoma, especially of the lung, and it is suggested that antibodies raised against calcium channels in the tumour also attack channels in the motor nerve terminals.

Diseases with a loss of muscle bulk

Muscle bulk may be lost as a result of the atrophy of individual muscle fibres while the number of fibres are relatively well maintained. In contrast, in the destructive myopathies muscle fibres are damaged, become necrotic and degenerate.

Atrophic myopathies

Patients frequently present with weakness which may be secondary to another diagnosis.

Fibre atrophy may occur after disuse. Extensive and rapid atrophy is seen if a limb is immobilized in plaster. This atrophy of the whole muscle is characterized by a reduction in muscle fibre size and a preferential loss of type 1 slow twitch fibres, occurring within a matter of weeks. Although apparent recovery of normal function may occur within 6 weeks after mobilization of the limb, residual muscle weakness may still be detectable several years after the injury unless specific strengthening exercises have been prescribed and followed (Rutherford et al. 1990).

Type 1 fibre atrophy, described above, is in marked contrast to the preferential atrophy of type 2 fibres which is commonly seen in a wide range of myopathies. These include starvation, cachexia, adrenal hyperplasia, hypothyroid disease, HIV positive patients, and often in patients receiving prolonged or intensive treatment with anti-inflammatory steroids (Fig. 13). Type 2 fibre atrophy is also seen with alcoholic myopathy, although this often includes a neurogenic component and may occasionally lead to severe rhabdomyolysis.

In general, it appears that type 2 fibre atrophy is a response to metabolic stress. Type 2 fibres are used for occasional rapid movement but their other role in the body is to constitute a store of protein. As a result of malnutrition or other stresses, this protein store is called upon to provide amino acids for the maintenance of other more vital organs and tissues. Type 2 fibre atrophy is a very common observation in muscle biopsy specimens and if the underlying problem can be diagnosed and treated, the atrophy will be corrected slowly and normal muscle fibre size and strength restored.

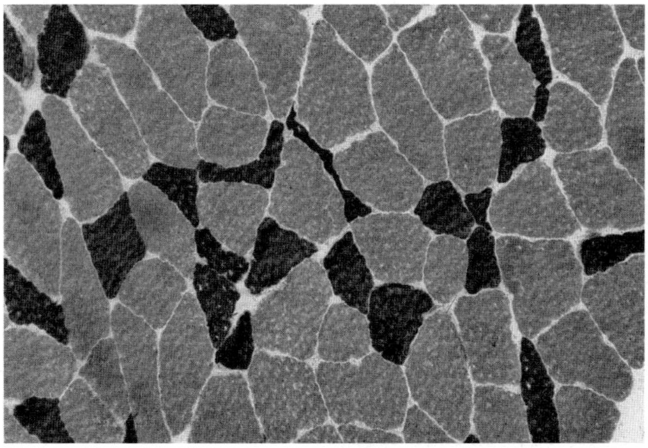

Fig. 13 Type 2 fibre atrophy in quadriceps muscle biopsy from a female patient on long term steroid therapy. ATPase stain at pH 9.4, type 2 fibres stain dark.

Destructive myopathies

This group includes the muscular dystrophies, where the defect is genetic, and the destructive myopathies of autoimmune origin, which are mainly idiopathic but may manifest a familial component influencing susceptibility.

The muscular dystrophies

The muscular dystrophies include all the familial progressive disorders of muscle which result in fibre destruction and the relentless replacement of muscle cells with fat and fibrous tissue. The most serious, though not the most common, type is DMD. It has a sex-linked recessive mode of inheritance, boys being affected and girls acting as carriers. If there is no family history the condition may not be noticed at first as there are few physical signs of the disease at birth, although the plasma CK may be as high as 10 000 IU/l. By about 4 years of age a delay in motor milestones becomes apparent and subsequently the child has increasing difficulty in standing and walking and is usually confined to a wheel chair by the start of the second decade. As the disease progresses, weakness of respiratory muscles, often complicated by scoliosis, becomes a problem and death usually occurs in or before the third decade.

Muscle biopsy in DMD shows the continuing destructive process, initially there is some increase in cellularity and some regeneration. As the condition progresses the increase in fat and fibrous tissue becomes more marked until virtually no contractile material remains. (Plate 61).

The defective gene in DMD was discovered by Kunkel et al. (1986) and assigned to position Xp21. This large gene of about 2000 kb codes for the structural protein dystrophin which provides a link between the surface membrane and the underlying contractile proteins (Fig. 3). Mutations of other proteins in this complex are implicated in other forms of muscular dystrophy; deletions in the sarcoglycans result in limb girdle dystrophy and congenital muscular dystrophy is the result of a defect in the gene determining laminin.

Dystrophin is absent in the muscle fibres of children with DMD due to deletions in the dystrophin gene which lead to either no, or nonsense, proteins. In the less severe Becker dystrophy an incomplete protein is produced with some residual function. Although relentless and tragic, the progression of Duchenne and Becker dystrophies is relatively slow and it appears that the loss of linkage between the surface membrane and the contractile apparatus leads to a cycle of continual damage and repair in which damage slowly predominates. Many attempts have been made to introduce the dystrophin gene into diseased muscle, most often in the form of implants of healthy myoblasts, but there has been limited success. Utrophin, a protein closely related to dystrophin, is ubiquitous in the body but in mature muscle is located only at the neuromuscular and myotendonous junctions; it is, however, found in all regenerating muscle fibres both in patients and in normal subjects. In the *mdx* mouse, a model for DMD, forced expression of full-length utrophin was found to prevent the development of dystrophy (Tinsley et al. 1998). Upregulation of the utrophin gene provides a plausible therapeutic approach in the treatment of DMD (Wakefield et al. 2000).

In clinical practice, the most likely form of dystrophy to be encountered in adults is myotonic dystrophy. This condition is dominantly inherited with variable gene penetration, and the gene maps on chromosome 19 in the q13.2–13.3 region. Weakness starts peripherally and only later are proximal muscle groups involved. Myotonia of the hands is often the initial symptom. This is a multisystem disease in which many organs, including brain, heart, endocrine organs, skin, and eyes are affected. Although giving its name to the disorder, myotonia itself is not the major problem.

Idiopathic destructive myopathies

Significant destruction of muscle fibres is seen in polymyositis and dermatomyositis with necrosis and regeneration being apparent, accompanied by invasion of the muscle by inflammatory cell infiltrates. Both diseases are the result of an autoimmune process and have a female to male preponderance of about 3 : 1. Plasma CK may be markedly elevated and a myopathic EMG is sometimes found. In severe acute polymyositis massive necrosis of muscle fibres with myoglobinuria has been reported with a consequent threat to renal function. In dermatomyositis, the skin is also affected with a patchy erythematous rash over the hands and sometimes the forearms.

The main pathological changes seen in muscle biopsies are muscle fibre necrosis with inflammatory infiltrates in perivascular, perimysial, and endomysial areas. Perifascicular atrophy is often a feature and fibres with abnormal architecture may be seen (Figs 14 and 15). Regenerating fibres are often present in acute cases but are less often seen in chronic polymyositis where the response to immunosuppressive drugs has been poor. In these cases atrophy of the remaining muscle cells, particularly of the type 2 fibres may occur due to the prolonged negative nitrogen balance produced by the anti-inflammatory steroid therapy.

For patients who respond well to steroid therapy and other immunosuppressive drugs, muscle strength will show good recovery, but because of the nitrogen losses caused by the high steroid doses, recovery may take many months. One of the dilemmas of treating polymyositis with high dose steroids is that the steroids themselves produce a negative nitrogen balance causing fibre atrophy and muscle weakness that may obscure recovery from the underlying disease. In this situation careful monitoring of muscle strength and CK can be most helpful in managing the withdrawal of immunosuppressive medication (Edwards et al. 1979).

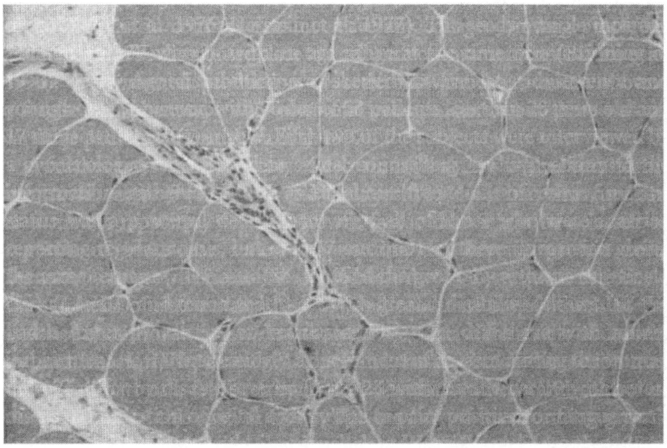

Fig. 14 Early polymyositis in a 38-year-old man. Inflammatory cells are seen in perimysial areas. Haematoxylin and eosin stain.

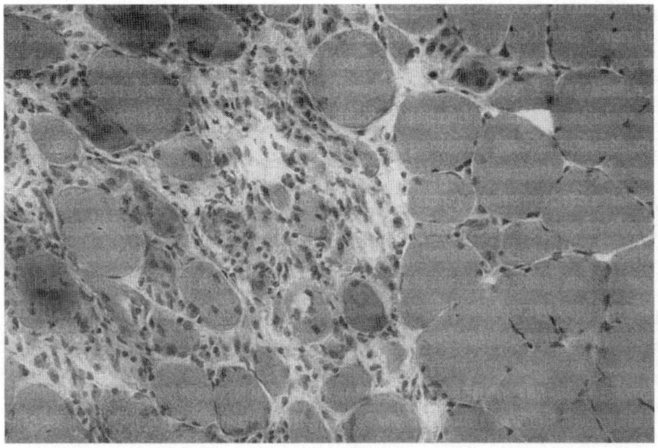

Fig. 15 Severe polymyositis in a 34-year-old woman. Necrotic and regenerating fibres are surrounded by inflammatory cells. One fascicle remains relatively normal showing the 'patchy' nature of the muscle damage. Haematoxylin and eosin stain.

Mechanisms of damage in autoimmune muscle disease

It is likely that autoimmune muscle disease develops as a result of some type of environmental exposure in genetically susceptible individuals. In dermatomyositis and polymyositis there may be an attack by the immune system on muscle fibres which have undergone some change in cell surface antigens, perhaps due to a virus infection, rendering them 'foreign' to the patient's immune system. Alternatively, muscle damage may be secondary to changes in the blood vessels and capillaries which are closely associated with muscle cells since immune reactions against the endothelial cells of small blood vessels can cause inflammation and necrosis. As a by-product of this inflammatory process, muscle fibres may become damaged leading to necrotic changes followed by invasion of the tissue by mononuclear cells.

Several genetic risk factors have been identified and in white Caucasians the HLA genes on chromosome 6, particularly HLA DRB1* 0301 and the linked allele DQA1* 0501, have the strongest association with all forms of autoimmune muscle disease. Different HLA alleles may confer risk in other ethnic, environmental, and serologic groups. Non-HLA genetic risk factors are also being identified (Shamim et al. 2000).

Inclusion body myositis (IBM)

In some cases diagnosed as polymyositis, the patient does not respond to steroids or other immunosuppressive drugs and the damage to muscle fibres becomes relentless, with a poor prognosis. Microscopic appearances resemble those seen in muscular dystrophy, with replacement of contractile material with fibrous connective tissue and fat. A characteristic finding in these cases is the presence of rimmed vacuoles in the muscle fibres.

It is now generally recognized that many of these cases represent a separate condition, designated inclusion body myositis. Unlike polymyositis the condition is most common in men over 55 years. Ninety per cent of patients possess the DR3 allele of the MHC complex, usually on a haplotype marked by HLA-B8 and have a deletion at the C4a (complement component) locus, or on a haplotype marked by HLA-B18 BfF1 with a deletion of C4b. Both these extended haplotypes have been associated with other autoimmune diseases such as myasthenia gravis, systemic lupus erythematosus, and autoimmune thyroid disease (Garlepp and Mastaglia 1996). Nevertheless, the autoimmune status of this disease is far from proven.

Most cases are sporadic but familial forms with variable genotypes also occur. In the latter cases, inflammatory infiltrates of T cells and macrophages are not usually seen and the CK may be normal. The recessive forms of IBM are currently linked to chromosome 9p1q1.

Muscle biopsies in sporadic cases reveal that the characteristic rimmed vacuoles seen in some fibres are filled with hyaline eosinophilic inclusions consisting of cytoplasmic twisted tubulofilaments, β-amyloid, ubiquitin, and an array of other proteins including prion proteins similar to those seen in the cerebral plaques in Alzheimer's disease. The latter finding has led to the intriguing suggestion that the degenerative process in inclusion body myositis may have something in common with the degenerative brain changes in Alzheimer's disease (Askanas et al. 1993). It has been postulated (Askanas and Engel 2001) that over expression of β-amyloid protein within the ageing muscle fibre in susceptible individuals is an early upstream event causing the subsequent pathogenic cascade.

If multisystem vasculitis occurs in association with autoimmune rheumatic diseases, the skeletal muscles may be affected and fibre damage may subsequently occur. Inflammatory vascular changes are associated with myositis in polyarteritis nodosa.

Sjögren's syndrome and rheumatoid arthritis

Although vasculitis can occur in rheumatoid arthritis, a more common cause of weakness is the atrophy of both type 1 and type 2 fibres, associated with loss of mobility owing to joint pain.

Muscle biopsy in systemic lupus erythematosus is seldom helpful since, although a broad spectrum of vascular abnormalities has been described (Weisman and Zvaifler 1980), the muscle usually appears relatively normal.

In scleroderma, the disordered collagen metabolism leads to excess collagen deposits which produce swelling and partial obstruction of the capillaries and small blood vessels in the muscles, which, in turn, leads to ischaemic changes and necrosis of the muscle cells, sometimes with the presence of inflammatory infiltrates. If the ischaemic damage is widespread, interstitial, and perivascular fibrosis is also seen.

References

Adiseshiah, M., Round, J.M., and Jones, D.A. (1992). Reperfusion injury in skeletal muscle a prospective study in patients with acute limb ischaemia and claudicants treated with revascularisation. *British Journal of Surgery* **79**, 1026–9.

Askanas, V. and Engel, W.K. (2001). Inclusion body myositis; newest concepts of pathogenesis and relation to ageing and Alzheimer disease. *Journal of Neuropathology and Experimental Neurology* **60**, 1–14.

Askanas, V., Masako, B., Engel, W.K., Alvarez, R.B., Tome, F., and Leclerc, A. (1993). Prion protein is accumulated in inclusion body myositis. *Clinical Neuroscience, Neuropathology: Neuroreport* **5**, 25–8.

Bailey, S.P., Davis, J.M., and Ahlborn, E.N. (1993a). Neuroendocrine and substrate responses to altered brain 5-HT activity during prolonged exercise to fatigue. *Journal of Applied Physiology* **74**, 3006–12.

Bailey, S.P., Davis, J.M., and Ahlborn, E.N. (1993b). Serotonergic agonists and antagonists affect endurance performance in the rat. *International Journal of Sports Medicine* **14**, 330–3.

Bakheit, A.M.O., Behan, P.O., Dinan, T.G., Gray, C.E., and O'Keane, V. (1992). Possible upregulation of hypothalamic 5-hydroxytryptamine receptors in patients with postviral fatigue syndrome. *British Medical Journal* **403**, 1010–12.

Bartram, C., Edwards, R.H.T., Clague. J., and Benyon, R.J. (1994). McArdle's disease a rare frameshift mutation of the glycogenphosphorylase gene. *Biochemica Biophysica Acta* **1226**, 341–3.

Bornemann, A., Maier, F., and Kuschel, R. (1999). Satellite cells as players and targets in normal and diseased muscle. *Neuropediatrics* **30**, 167–75.

Buckingham, M. (1992). Making muscle in mammals. *Trends in Genetics* **8**, 144–9.

Buckingham, M. (1994). Which myogenic factors make muscle? *Current Biology* **4**, 61–3.

Buller, N.P., Jones, D.A., and Poole-Wilson, P.A. (1991). Direct measurement of skeletal muscle fatigue in patients with chronic heart failure. *British Heart Journal* **65**, 20–34.

Cady, E.B., Elshove, H., Jones, D.A., and Moll, A. (1989a). The metabolic causes of slow relaxation in fatigued human skeletal muscle. *Journal of Physiology* **418**, 327–37.

Cady, E.B., Jones, D.A., Lynn, J., and Newham, D.J. (1989b). Changes in force and intracellular metabolites during fatigue of human skeletal muscle. *Journal of Physiology* **418**, 311–25.

Chaudhuri, A. and Behan, P.O. (2000). Fatigue and the basal ganglia. *Journal of the Neurological Sciences* **179**, 34–42.

Cleare, A.J., Bearn, J., Allain, T., McGregor, A., Wessely, S., Murray, R.M., and O' Keane, V. (1995). Contrasting neuroendocrine responses in depression and chronic fatigue syndrome. *Journal of Affective Disorders* **34**, 283–89.

Curran, J.L. et al. (1999). Segregation of malignant hyperthermia, central core disease and chromosome 19 markers. *British Journal of Anaesthesia* **83**, 217–22.

DeRuiter, C.J., Jones, D.A., Sargeant, A.J., and De Haan, A. (1999). Temperature effect on the rates of isometric force development and relaxation in the fresh and fatigued human adductor pollicis muscle. *Experimental Physiology* **84**, 1137–50.

Di Mauro, A. (1961). Satellite cells of skeletal muscle fibres. *Journal of Biophysics and Biochemical Cytology* **9**, 493–8.

Edwards, R.H.T., Young, A., Hosking, G.P., and Jones, D.A. (1977). Human skeletal muscle function: description of tests and normal values. *Clinical Science and Molecular Medicine* **52**, 283–90.

Edwards, R.H.T., Wiles, C.M., Round, J.M., Jackson, M.J., and Young, A. (1979). Muscle breakdown and repair in polymyositis: a case study. *Muscle and Nerve*, **2**, 223–8.

Endesfelder, S., Krahn, A., Kreuzer, K.A., Lass, U., Schmidt, C.A., Jahrmarkt, C., von Moers, A., and Speer, A. (2000). Elevated p21 mRNA level in skeletal muscle of DMD patients and mdx mice indicates either an exhausted satellite cell pool or a higher p21 expression in dystrophin-deficient cells per se. *Journal of Molecular Medicine* **78**, 569–74.

Frontera, W.R., Meredith, C.N., O'Reilly, K.P., Knuttgen, H.G., and Evans, W.J.J. (1988). Strength conditioning in older men: skeletal muscle hypertrophy and improved function. *Journal of Applied Physiology* **64**, 1038–44.

Garlepp, M.J. and Mastiglia, F.L. (1996). Inclusion body myositis. *Journal of Neurology, Neurosurgery and Psychiatry* **60**, 251–5.

James, C., Sacco, P., and Jones, D.A. (1995). Loss of power during fatigue of human leg muscles. *Journal of Physiology* **484**, 237–46.

Jones, D.A. (1999). Muscle fatigue during high intensity exercise. In *Limitations to Human Performance* (ed. B. Whipp and A.J. Sargeant), pp. 1–12. London: Portman Press.

Jones, D.A. and Round, J.M. *Skeletal Muscle in Health and Disease: A Textbook of Muscle Physiology.* Manchester: Manchester University Press, 1990.

Jones, D.A., Newham, D.J., Round, J.M., and Tolfree, S.E.J. (1986). Experimental human muscle damage: morphological changes in relation to other indices of damage. *Journal of Physiology* **375**, 435–48.

Jones, D.A., Newham, D.J., Obletter, G., and Giamberadino, M.A. (1987). Nature of exercise-induced muscle pain. *Advances in Pain Research* **10**, 207–18.

Jones, D.A., Round, J.M., and Carli, F. (1991). Plasma creatine kinase in patients following routine surgery: a comparison with experimental muscle damage. *Journal of Physiology* **43**, 173P.

Jurkat-Rott, K., McCarthey, T., and Lehmann-Horn, F. (2000). Genetics and pathogenesis of malignant hyperthermia. *Muscle and Nerve* **23**, 4–17.

Kunkel, L.M. et al. (1986). Analysis of deletions in DNA in patients with Becker and Duchenne muscular dystrophy. *Nature* **322**, 73–7.

Larsson, N.G. and Oldfors, A. (2001). Mitochondrial myopathies. *Acta Physiologica Scandinavica* **171**, 385–93.

Lehmann-Horn, F. and Jurkat-Rott, K. (1999). Voltage gated ion channels and hereditary disease. *Physiological Reviews* **79**, 1317–71.

Lebo, R.V., Gorin, F., Fletterick, R.J., Kao, F.T., Cheung, M.C., Bruce, B.D., and Kan, Y.W. (1984) High -resolution chromosome sorting and DNA spot-blot analysis assign McArdle's syndrome to chromosome 11. *Science* **225**, 57–9.

McComas A.J. *Skeletal Muscle Form and Function.* Leeds UK: Human Kinetics, 1996.

Mahowald, M.W., Mahowald, M.L., Bundlie, S.R., and Ytterberg, S.R. (1989). Sleep fragmentation in rheumatoid arthritis. *Arthritis and Rheumatology* **32**, 974–83.

Maier, S.F. and Watkins, L.R. (1998). Cytokines for psychologists: Implications of bi-directional immune-to-brain communication for understanding behaviour mood and cognition. *Psychological Review* **105**, 83–107.

McArdle, A. and Jackson, M.J. (1994). Intracellular mechanisms involved in damage to skeletal muscles. *Basic and Applied Myology* **4**, 43–51.

McCord, J.M. (1985). Oxygen derived free radicals in post ischaemic tissue injury. *New England Journal of Medicine* **312**, 159–63.

Nielsen, B., Hales, J.R.S., Strange, S., Christensen, N.J., Warberg, J., and Saltin, B. (1993). Human circulatory and thermoregulatory adaptations with heat acclimation and exercise in a hot, dry environment. *Journal of Physiology* **460**, 467–85.

Newham, D.J., Mills, K.R., Quigley, B.M., and Edwards, R.H.T. (1983). Pain and fatigue following concentric and eccentric muscle contractions *Clinical Science* **64**, 55–62.

Round, J.M., Barr, F.M.D., Moffat, B., and Jones, D.A. (1993). Fibre areas and histochemical fibre types in the quadriceps muscle of paraplegic subjects. *Journal of the Neurological Sciences* **116**, 207–11.

Round, J.M., Jones, D.A., Honour, J.W., and Nevill, A.M. (1999). Hormonal factors in the development of differences in strength between boys and girls during adolescence: a longitudinal study. *Annals of Human Biology* **26**, 49–62.

Rowe, R.W.D. and Goldspink, G. (1969). Muscle fibre growth in five different muscles in both sexes of mice:1 normal mice. *Journal of Anatomy* **104**, 519–30.

Rutherford, O.M. and Jones, D.A. (1992). The relationship of muscle and bone loss and activity levels with age in women. *Age and Ageing* **21**, 286–93.

Rutherford, O.M., Jones, D.A., and Round, J.M. (1990). Long lasting unilateral muscle wasting and weakness following injury and immobilisation. *Scandinavian Journal of Rehabilitation Medicine* **22**, 33–7.

Seale, P., Asakura, A., and Rudnicki, M.A. (2001). The potential of muscle stem cells. *Developmental Cell* **1**, 333–42.

Shamim, E.A., Rider, L.G., and Miller, F.W. (2000). Update on the genetics of the idiopathic inflammatory myopathies. *Current Opinions in Rheumatology* **12**, 482–91.

Skelton, D.A., Phillips, S.K., Bruce, S.A., Naylor, C.H., and Woledge, R.C. (1999). Hormone replacement therapy increases isometric strength of adductor pollicis in post-menopausal women. *Clinical Science* **96**, 357–64.

Smeitink, J., van den Heuvel, L., and DiMauro, S. (2001). The genetics and pathology of oxidative phosphorylation. *National Review of Genetics* **2**, 342–52.

Stokes, M. and Young, A. (1984). The contribution of reflex inhibition to arthrogenous muscle weakness. *Clinical Science* **67**, 7–14.

Tinsley, J., Deconinck, N., Fisher, R., Kahn, D., Phelps, S., Gillis, J.M., and Davies, K. (1998). Expression of full length eutrophin prevents muscular dystrophy in *mdx* mice. *Nature Medicine* **4**, 1441–4.

Wakefield, P.M., Tinsley, J.M., Wood, M.J., Gilbert, R., Karpati, G., and Davies, K.E. (2000). Prevention of the dystrophin phenotype in dystrophin/utrophin deficient muscle following adenovirus mediated transfer of a utrophin minigene. *Gene Therapy* **7**, 201–4.

Webster, C. and Blau, H.M. (1990). Accelerated age-related decline in replicative life span of Duchenne muscular dystrophy myoblasts: implications for cell and gene therapy. *Somatic Cell Molecular Genetics* **16**, 557–65.

Weisman, M.H. and Zvaifler, N.J. (1980). Vasculitis in connective tissue diseases. *Clinics in the Rheumatic Diseases* **6**, 351–72.

White, P. (1990). Fatigue and chronic fatigue syndromes. In *Somatization: Physical Symptoms and Psychological Illness* (ed. C. Bass), pp. 104–40. Oxford: Blackwell Scientific Publications.

Wiles, C.M., Jones, D.A., and Edwards, R.H.T. (1981). In *Human Muscle Fatigue: Physiological Mechanisms. Ciba Foundation Symposium* Vol. 82 (ed. R. Porter and J. Whelan), pp. 264–82. London: Pitman Medical Press.

Wiles, C.M., Young, A., Jones, D.A., and Edwards, R.H.T. (1979). Relaxation rate of constituent muscle-fibre types in human quadriceps. *Clinical Science* **56**, 47–52.

Wilson, J.R., Mancini, D.M., and Dunkman, W.B. (1993). Exertional fatigue due to skeletal muscle dysfunction in patients with heart disease. *Circulation* **87**, 470–75.

Wilson, J.R., Rayos, G., Gothard, P., and Bak, K. (1995). Dissociation between exertional symptoms and circulatory function in patients with heart failure. *Circulation* **92**, 47–53.

Wolfe, F., Hawley, D.J., and Wilson, K. (1996). The prevelance and meaning of fatigue in rheumatic disease. *Journal of Rheumatology* **23**, 1407–17.

3.8 Biomechanics of articulations and derangements in disease

Susan C. Scholes, Anthony M.J. Bull, Anthony Unsworth, and Andrew A. Amis

Introduction

Synovial joints are nature's bearings, and so large loads are transmitted while the frictional forces are kept to a minimum. This depends on the properties of cartilage and synovial fluid, which together maintain coefficients of friction of less than 0.02. This, at first sight, is surprising since cartilage surfaces are rough compared with engineering bearings, the transmitted loads are high, and the large range of sliding speeds found in human joints requires a range of lubrication mechanisms in order to maintain efficient articulation.

Typically, in the hip joint, loads of 3000 N are common, but an important feature of these loads is that they only have a duration of the order of 0.1 s. However, a lower limb might undergo up to 200 million impacts in a lifetime, often leading to some degree of failure. Osteoarthritis is a common disease that bears many of the typical signs of mechanical failure of the material, the first of which is the 'softening' of the cartilage, which reflects the change in the way it responds to loads. Fibrillation, or a breakdown in collagen structures of the surface layer, then leads to excessive wear of the cartilage that sometimes progresses to exposure of the underlying bone.

Mechanical factors alone cannot fully explain the aetiology of osteoarthritis but in this chapter we will discuss the synovial joint as a bearing and describe the mechanical factors that may contribute to failure. This includes the loading and how the cartilage responds by distributing it over the joint. The role of the menisci in the knee will be discussed and the consequences of damage to ligaments. The lubrication of joints and the mechanisms which have been identified as protecting joint surfaces from wear will lead on to a review of the breakdown of cartilage.

Mechanics of joints

Basic principles

Mechanics, when applied to human joints, can be studied under two main headings: statics or dynamics. Statics is the study of forces when there are no acceleration effects, and dynamics is the study of forces when accelerations are present. Both require knowledge of the loading on the joint and of the position or motion of the joint. In addition, the articular geometry and material properties need to be known in order to calculate the localized loading.

The loading on joints is due to forces, which tend to cause translational accelerations, and moments, which tend to cause rotational accelerations. For example, pushing a box along a surface is the application of a force that tends to cause translational acceleration of that box. Twisting a spinning top is the application of a moment that tends to cause rotational acceleration. There are generally two main sources of loading that cause compressive forces on the articular cartilage. These are: external forces to the joint (e.g. due to weightbearing) and internal forces (due to structures such as muscles and ligaments).

Although most joints have a large range of motion, not all positions are possible. For example, in a hip joint the femoral head rotates, but it generally does not translate relative to the acetabulum. These possible positions are related to the degrees of freedom (DOF) of the joint. In space, one body can move relative to another in translation (e.g. sliding) and rotation (e.g. rolling) in three dimensions. This means that this body has six DOF (three translations and three rotations). A synovial joint has a possible six DOF as it can be considered as one bone moving relative to another. Analysis of the mechanics of joints must take into account these DOF, although most joints effectively have fewer DOF. For example, the interphalangeal joints of the fingers can be considered as having one DOF—rotation in flexion/extension, with small out-of-plane effects.

Static force analysis of joints

The general principle, arising from Newton's laws, is that for a static analysis, all forces and moments are in equilibrium. If this were not the case, then the joint being analysed would be subjected to a resultant load or moment, causing it to accelerate. A dynamic analysis would then be needed. Statics does not mean that there is no movement, because movement can occur without accelerations. Therefore, for many slow activities, the joint can be considered as being in equilibrium. Static analysis requires knowledge of the positions as well as the magnitudes of the forces acting on the joints.

Static equilibrium uses the resolution of forces to account for translation effects, and the summation of the moments acting about a point to balance rotations. Although the body is a three-dimensional structure, it is often acceptable to simplify a situation into two dimensions. This applies to joints that have almost uniplanar motion. In this case, the general situation, which has six DOF, can be simplified to examine rotation about one axis, and then to two further components of force in order to calculate the joint load in the two-dimensional plane of motion.

The first step in this analysis is to measure the external load acting on the body. This is sometimes simple, such as when a weight is being supported in the hand. Walking is more complex, since the load can pass through a large area of foot-to-floor contact. Also, the loading may not be perpendicular to the floor, since there could be shearing actions (a tendency towards skidding), such as when the heel strikes the floor. In order to analyse complex situations, purpose-made load transducers are used, such as a 'force plate', which can give simultaneous output of all six DOF. Further, an array of force sensors (e.g. at each corner of a rectangular plate), can show the position and orientation of the resultant force, and thus where it acts on the sole of the foot. Further refinements include the study of pressures between the body and objects on which it acts using sheets of electroconductive rubber with electrodes painted on to each surface. These can give a 'contour map' of the foot-to-floor pressures.

The second step is to quantify the internal loads. Most of the loads acting on human joints arise from the muscles crossing the joints. These are much higher than the weight of the body or other external loads being supported, due to leverage effects. The tendons generally pass much closer to the axis of a joint than does the line of action of an external load, causing a considerable mechanical disadvantage. At the elbow, for example, the moment arm (the perpendicular distance from the line of action of the force to the axis of rotation) of the biceps tendon may be 35 mm, while that of a load in the hand may be 350 mm, in which case the tendon tension must be ten times the external load, if that were the only muscle acting. Because the muscles cause most of the load, it is important to identify which of them are active, and to obtain geometrical data, especially their moment arms about axes of rotation, and the directions in which they act.

The positions of the lines of action of muscles and tendons have been found by dissecting cadavers. If a range of joint positions is to be analysed, wires can be embedded in the tendons and three-dimensional data found by biplanar radiography (An et al. 1979), or by direct digitization of the structures *in vitro* (Amis et al. 1979). If the joint is surrounded by the fibre 'bellies' of muscles, such as at the hip, it is necessary to estimate the line of action within the muscle cross-section. These data can be obtained by digitizing photographs of sliced, frozen tissue, or from MRI scans of living subjects. Multiple slices can be obtained at a range of postures as a joint is flexed during a scanning procedure. Vertical access open configuration MR scanners now allow scans to be taken under weightbearing conditions (Bull and McGregor 2000).

Muscle activity is discerned by electromyography, using skin-mounted or needle electrodes. For analysis of a static situation there is much published electromyographic data (e.g. Basmajian 1967). For analysis of a moving subject, when different muscles will be switching on and off, subject-specific data must be obtained since the patterns of activitation vary between subjects. This applies particularly to antagonistic actions, which stabilize joints, causing great increases in the joint force. These data must be used to prepare a list of active muscles and then decide how they share the effort in order to reduce the number of unknown variables to solve a set of equations. Techniques used include minimizing the energy expended, or assigning the forces according to the physiological cross-sectional areas of the muscles (which allows for muscle fibre pennation geometry). This may be appropriate for strenuous isometric actions, when the muscles approach the limit of stress that they can create (Amis et al. 1980b).

With the muscle, geometrical, and external force data collected, a mathematical model of the joint is produced examining its equilibrium, placing the lines of action of the forces with the correct sharing of muscle tensions

Consider the finger tip pinch shown in Fig. 1. The moment is the product of the force times the moment arm. For moment equilibrium about the axis of flexion,

$$70\ \text{N} \times 15\ \text{mm} = T \times 5\ \text{mm}, \quad \text{so } T = 210\ \text{N}.$$

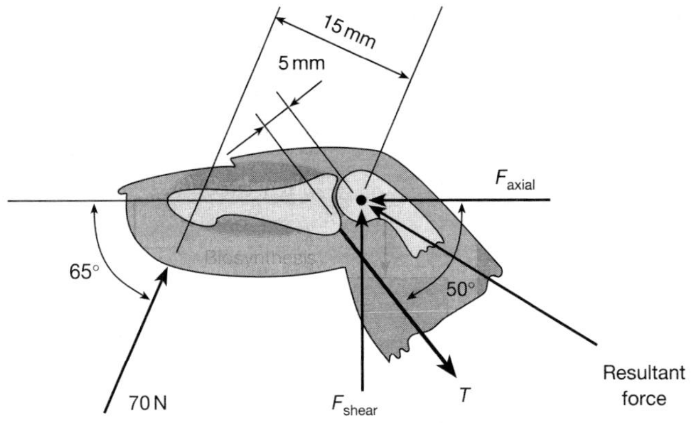

Fig. 1 Two-dimensional force analysis of finger tip pinch action. The flexor tendon tension $T = 210$ N, and the resultant joint force = 192 N at an angle of 31° to the axis of the distal phalanx.

For force equilibrium along the distal phalanx, it is necessary to use the components of each force that acts in this direction. Thus:

$$70 \cos 65° + T \cos 50° = F_{\text{axial}}, \quad \text{so } F_{\text{axial}} = 165 \text{ N}.$$

For force equilibrium across the distal phalanx,

$$F_{\text{shear}} + 70 \sin 65° = T \sin 50°, \quad \text{so } F_{\text{shear}} = 98 \text{ N}.$$

By the theorem of Pythagoras, the (resultant force)$^2 = F^2_{\text{axial}} + F^2_{\text{shear}}$, so the resultant force = 192 N and the angle of this force relative to the axis of the phalanx $= \tan^{-1}(F_{\text{shear}}/F_{\text{axial}}) = 31°$.

As noted above, this resultant force is much greater than the external pinch force.

Sometimes the analysis predicts a resultant joint force which is directed outside of the area of contact between the bones. This represents a potential instability, and ligament tensions may be invoked to regain equilibrium. For example, an analysis of pinching action showed that the axial force along the proximal phalanx, which would stabilize the metacarpal joint, was overcome by the shearing action of the flexor tendon tensions when the metacarpal joint was flexed. This would cause a palmar subluxation. Stability thus entailed tension in the collateral ligaments. In the rheumatoid hand, when the ligaments are slack because of loss of the joint surfaces, the shearing action causes palmar subluxation (Weightman and Amis 1982). This situation is at an extreme in the knee, where the tibiofemoral joint depends on the cruciate ligaments to resist the anterior–posterior actions of the muscles when walking (Morrison 1968).

The study of movement

Kinematics is the study of movement without reference to the forces involved. Kinematic studies provide data on the patterns of movements of the body, or the axes of rotation of individual joints that can be used when making static force analyses.

The main component of kinematic analysis is the capture of motion. A topic of debate in the nineteenth century was whether or not a trotting horse had all its limbs in the air. A photographer, E. Muybridge, set up a series of cameras, which were triggered as a horse galloped past. He showed that horses have a flight phase when galloping, and then he applied his techniques to the analysis of human motion (Ladin 1995). This has formed the basis for all types of video analysis of movement, although multiple viewing directions must be used for three-dimensional analyses. This allows details such as transverse rotations of the segments of the lower limb to be discerned. Techniques include video or multiple exposure radiographs with passive or active markers attached to the limb segments, electrical linkages fixed to body segments across joints, or electromagnetic devices. The drawbacks of such devices are that they can inhibit subject actions and move relative to the skeleton since they are usually fixed by adhesives. Invasive techniques have also been employed fixing markers, or devices, rigidly to the body segments using pins. Biplanar radiographic techniques using X-ray opaque markers fixed to anatomical landmarks are also used. These are very accurate for a small region of interest (Bull and Amis 1998).

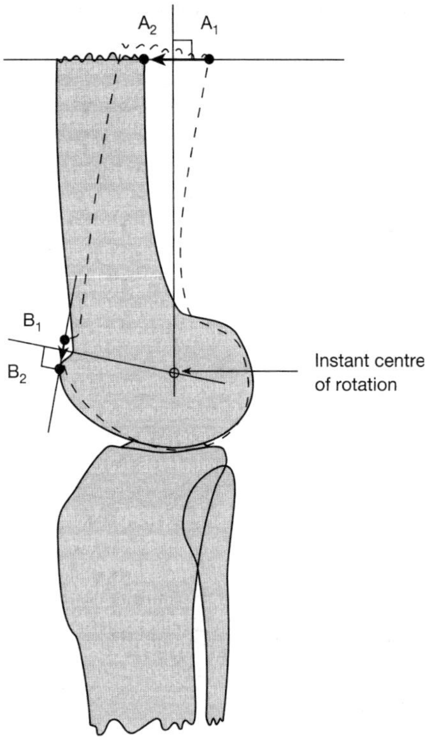

Fig. 2 Method to find 'instant centre of rotation' of a joint from double-exposure radiographs.

At any time, there will be an 'instant centre of rotation', about which all other points on a body are rotating. Since these points are all on arcs of circles centred at the axis, it is a simple geometrical calculation to identify the axis from the paths of several points (Fig. 2). This methodology has shown that the complexity of the carpus, for example, can be reduced to a simple uniaxial rotation about the proximal pole of the capitate during wrist flexion–extension and abduction–adduction (Youm et al. 1978), a finding used in the design of spherical geometries for the articular surfaces of wrist prostheses.

Dynamic analysis of joints

This approach is necessary when movements occur fast enough for inertial effects to be significant. Forces are required to accelerate the mass of limb segments to change their speed or direction of motion in translation or rotation. In the extreme, inertial effects limit the speed with which a joint can be moved, since active muscle tension capability diminishes as the speed of shortening increases (Elftman 1966), and large accelerations occur as the limb segment reaches the limits of motion. Accelerations of 20g during elbow flexion (Amis et al. 1980a) and 4g in the lower limb during walking (Paul 1974) have been reported.

To allow for these inertial effects requires data on the masses, locations of the centre of mass and inertial properties of the limb segments. This is available in the literature (e.g. Contini and Drillis 1966). However, such data are based on a small number of cadavers, which may not have the same mass distribution as a particular subject. It would be a major undertaking to gain such information from live subjects, and this is not normally attempted.

Joint forces during locomotion

The methods described above must all come together when a complex activity such as human locomotion is analysed, with simultaneous collection of spatial, electromyographic and force plate data. When the foot-to-floor forces are known, it is possible to estimate the joint forces. The external force action causes moments about the joints, which can have their equilibrium examined by means of 'static' methods that add in the inertial effects, which must themselves be calculated after analysing the accelerations of the limb segments. Although this has been facilitated by computers, the data collection still requires a well set-up and calibrated gait analysis facility.

Typical force predictions for walking have been approximately three, four, and four times body weight for the ankle, knee, and hip, with much higher loads anticipated in sporting activities.

Although gait analysis can find out the force distribution across a prosthetic knee when in use postoperatively, for example (Johnson et al. 1980), the amount of work required has meant that such analyses are not used regularly to monitor or correct force or motion patterns.

Direct measurement of joint forces

The many stages and assumptions needed to perform a dynamic analysis leading to joint force predictions lead to a large band of potential error in the results. Therefore, there have been attempts to measure the joint forces directly, mostly at the hip.

Hip prostheses have been implanted with the neck of the femoral component instrumented by strain gauges that respond to the deflections caused by loads applied to the joint. The early work by Rydell (1966) was hampered by the need to use transcutaneous wires, but Bergmann et al. (1993) transmitted a signal containing all components of load on the joint from within a sealed cavity in the prosthesis. This allowed the activities of patients to be followed for up to 2 years post-operatively, monitoring a return to relatively normal gait. Reassuringly, this work has largely confirmed the earlier force predictions, although this cannot be used to calculate localised loading on articular cartilage at the femoral head.

Lubrication of human joints

Having examined the loads passing through joints and seen how to measure these in clinical situations, we need to determine how the joints can respond to these with the minimum of damage. This leads us to look at the lubrication mechanisms in joints. Lubrication of human joints is important for two main reasons. A well lubricated joint has low friction and hence low energy loss, and if the lubrication mechanism separates the cartilage surfaces with a film of synovial fluid, this will minimize wear and may slow the process of osteoarthritic change (Unsworth 1984). A number of lubrication mechanisms have been identified for human joints under various conditions (Dowson 1967) some of which are better than others. Best of all is full-fluid film lubrication (FFL). Here, the two surfaces which are loaded together, are completely separated by a film of lubricant, albeit a very thin film (about 0.5 μm). This reduces both friction and wear. For the surfaces to be held apart by a film of fluid, the fluid must be pressurized in some way. One mechanism for this is 'hydrodynamic' lubrication (Reynolds 1886). Here the rolling and sliding motion between the surfaces generates pressure within the fluid. Thus motion and fluid viscosity are important. Another way is to pump the fluid between the surfaces using an external pump. This is called 'externally pressurized' or 'hydrostatic' lubrication.

If the load placed on the joint is not steady but varies such as when we jump in the air and land on the ground, pressure can be generated by 'squeeze film' mechanisms. This can be explained by imagining two surfaces separated by a film of fluid suddenly being squeezed together. This puts a high pressure on the fluid which therefore resists the applied force. With time this fluid film disappears unless it is re-charged by more fluid, but for dynamic loads and short loading times, as found in human joints, it is an important mechanism (Unsworth et al. 1975).

If these pressures are very high compared with the elastic properties of the solid boundaries (circa 2 MPa in the case of cartilage), then significant elastic deformation or 'squashing' of the surface will occur and this changes the geometry of the lubricating film. This then changes the pressures generated. This mechanism is called 'elastohydrodynamic lubrication' (EHL or EHD lubrication). Under FFL conditions, and all the above mechanisms are classified as FFL, the coefficient of friction is of the order of 0.01 or lower. However, under some conditions a fluid-film cannot be generated to separate the two surfaces. Here, intimate contact between the surfaces can be prevented by a boundary lubricant. A good boundary lubricant attaches itself to the solid surfaces by molecular forces and modifies the surfaces. This consequently reduces friction but not as much as FFL does (e.g. coefficient of friction 0.1–0.5). Coefficient of friction is also independent of speed of sliding or load in boundary lubrication whereas it is strongly dependent on both in FFL.

Many practical devices spend much of their working life running under a combination of fluid film and boundary lubrication known as 'mixed lubrication'. Here part of the load is carried by the fluid film and part by the solid to solid contact. Coefficients of friction tend to be between 0.1 and 0.05.

Most surfaces, cartilage included, are rough on the microscopic scale (Jones and Walker 1968; Sayles et al. 1979) so separation of the surfaces only occurs when the fluid film is so thick that the roughnesses on the surfaces do not touch each other (Fig. 3). Thus for complete separation and hence fluid film lubrication, the film thickness must be greater than the combined roughnesses of the two surfaces.

A brief history of studies of human joint lubrication

Because the subject of human joint lubrication has only recently become clear in scientific terms, a brief review of the history of the studies of human joint lubrication will be followed by a summary of the current thoughts on the subject.

The early texts suggested that human joints operated under FFL (Reynolds 1886; MacConaill 1932). Comparisons of anatomical features of the hip and knee with features of engineering bearings led to the belief that hydrodynamic lubrication was the principal mechanism. In order to have hydrodynamic lubrication, an entraining velocity and a physical wedge of fluid between the cartilage surfaces are necessary. This, according to MacConaill, came from the shape of the articulating surfaces.

Jones (1934) was the first to measure the coefficient of friction in a joint. A horse's stifle joint produced a coefficient of friction of 0.27 when dry and 0.02 when lubricated with synovial fluid. These experiments were carried out under unphysiological conditions of high constant load and low sliding speed so 2 years later he used a proximal interphalangeal joint of the finger as the fulcrum of a pendulum (Jones 1936). His results were consistent with FFL.

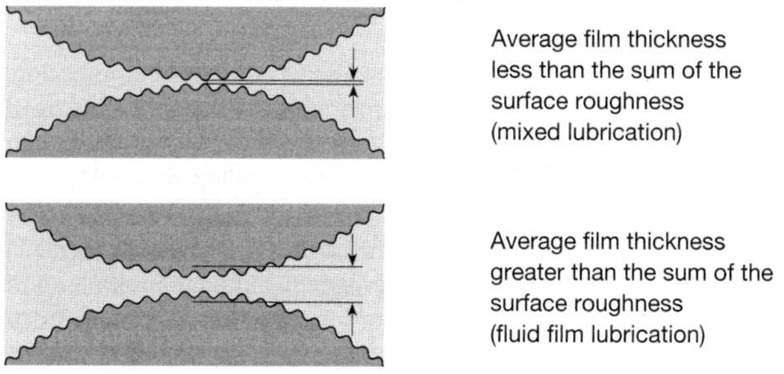

Fig. 3 Separation of surfaces.

Charnley (1959, 1960a,b) repeated Jones' experiments using a similar apparatus but found that the friction was the same whether synovial fluid was present or not and using a pendulum for human ankles found that the friction was independent of velocity of sliding and therefore boundary lubricated not fluid film. Charnley's measured values of friction were however very low for boundary lubrication (0.005–0.024).

Such low values of coefficient of friction at very low speeds of movement led McCutchen (1959) and Lewis and McCutchen (1959) to postulate a self-pressurizing hydrostatic lubrication mechanism which relied on pockets of liquid in the soft cartilage surface. Also because cartilage was porous, they believed that as the surface was loaded, the cartilage matrix compressed, pushing pressurized synovial fluid from its pores into the interface of the joint. This they called 'weeping lubrication'. Evidence of the pockets of liquid were supported by Unsworth et al. (1975) but the 'weeping' mechanism was shown by Maroudas (1967), to be controversial. She showed that the permeability of cartilage was so low as to be unrealistic as a method of replenishing fluid films between cartilage surfaces within the time scale of normal gait. However, this permeability was important to nutrition (Maroudas 1968).

Dintenfass (1963) discussed the importance of deformation of the low elastic modulus cartilage in human joint lubrication, thus highlighting the significance of EHL as a mechanism. This was supported by Tanner (1966) and later by Higginson and Unsworth (1981). However, squeeze film lubrication can act together with EHL and Fein (1966–67) showed that in human joints this combination can be an important feature of effective lubrication.

The importance of the type of loading can be seen from experiments carried out by Linn (1967, 1968) and Linn and Radin (1968). Using an 'arthrotripsometer' to measure the coefficient of friction in dog's ankle joints and under constant load, which is unphysiological and predisposes against FFL, they showed that mixed lubrication was present. In other words both hydrodynamic and boundary lubrication were acting together. The effects of boundary lubrication were examined by digesting synovial fluid with hyaluronidase and trypsin in turn. Trypsin, which removes the proteins, did not alter the synovial fluid's viscosity but doubled friction while hyaluronidase reduced viscosity but did not affect friction. This pointed to a protein component of synovial fluid acting as a boundary lubricant. It is important though to emphasize that these tests were carried out with a constantly loaded ankle joint whereas in real life such joints are dynamically loaded (loads from almost zero to five times body weight every second). O'Kelly et al. (1978) and Roberts et al. (1982) repeated Linn and Radin's work but using the dynamic walking cycles of Paul (1967) and English and Kilvington (1979), respectively, and found FFL throughout. An obvious conclusion is that under physiological loads (dynamic), FFL exists in human joints, while under static loads this reverts to 'mixed' lubrication, where boundary friction dominates. So what happens when we stand still under steady load for long periods? Under these conditions, McCutchen's theory of weeping lubrication may well be valid. In addition to this, 'boosted lubrication' was proposed by Walker et al. (1968) and can be thought of as the opposite of weeping lubrication. Here, the fluid flows from the trapped pools into the cartilage thereby concentrating the synovial fluid in the pools and increasing its viscosity and protein content to keep the surfaces apart. The same experimental evidence was often used by both sets of workers to justify the different conclusions. Ling (1974) produced a theoretical model of elastic porous discs on impervious substrata and showed that weeping and boosted were not mutually exclusive.

Further to this, work by Hills (2000) highlighted the boundary lubricating fraction of synovial fluid, surface active phospholipid (SAPL). Hills suggested that it is this part of the synovial fluid complex that is the vital ingredient, transported to the cartilage surface within the synovial fluid and then forming a lining on the articular surface. This lining provides boundary lubrication when the surfaces would normally be in contact. A comprehensive review paper by Batchelor and Stachowiak (1996) concluded that both gylcoproteins and phospholipids were important in synovial joint lubrication. Work by Murakami et al. (1998) and Forster and Fisher (1999) also supports the boundary lubricating ability of various constituents of synovial fluid including phospholipids.

Another important feature of human joints is their surface elasticity. Soft elastic layers are beneficial to lubrication and friction in pure-sliding (Bennett and Higginson 1970) and especially in squeeze film situations (Gaman et al. 1974). A combination of elasticity and porosity was not significantly better than elasticity alone (Higginson and Norman 1974) since the permeability of cartilage was far too low to affect lubrication.

A combination of dynamic loading (physiological) and soft elastic surfaces had a very great effect (Unsworth et al. 1987): the friction in a Charnley hip prosthesis could be reduced by a factor of 10 by adding a soft elastic layer. Thus the important features of healthy behaviour of human joints are high viscosity synovial fluid (>0.010 Pa s), dynamic loads and a soft elastic surface (hardness 4–8 N/mm^2).

Theoretical analyses

Using the experimental evidence already referred to, analytical and numerical studies have been carried out to help in the understanding of the lubrication mechanisms. A combined theoretical and numerical analysis of the movement of fluid in and out of cartilage during dynamic loading concluded that 'The natural lubrication process is neither the weeping mechanism nor the boosted mechanism', (Mansour and Mow 1977). In any analysis, simplifying assumptions are necessary and several workers have followed the advice of Higginson and Norman (1974) and neglected cartilage permeability. This is extremely convenient since EHL of soft impermeable layers is well documented in rolling/sliding situations for cylindrical contacts (Hooke and O'Donoghue 1972). This is probably sufficient for knee or ankle analysis though not for the hip. They give an equation for minimum fluid film thickness of $h_{min} \sim U^{0.6} W^{-0.2} R$, where $U = u\eta/ER$ and $W = w/ER$. R is the effective radius, η the viscosity of the lubricant, u is the rolling/sliding speed, E is the equivalent elastic modulus, and w is the load/unit length on a cylindrical contact. For a typical knee in normal walking this gives a film thickness of 1.4×10^{-7} m. Since cartilage is rough (10^{-6} m) this film thickness is unlikely to separate the cartilage surfaces unless the soft compliant surfaces are more tolerant of surface roughnesses than are metals. Higginson and Unsworth (1981) showed this to be the case and when account of this is taken, the film thickness is increased to about 6×10^{-7} m. This is still insufficient to separate the surfaces of cartilage. However, Dowson and Jin (1986) showed that using the ankle joint as a model the effect of high pressures generated on the roughnesses of the surfaces was to squash the high spots and produce a smoother surface. Adding squeeze film to the analysis increased film thicknesses to between 0.6 and 1.2 μm while the original surfaces had been smoothed to between 0.05 and 0.9 μm depending on the wavelength of the surface roughness. Thus for the first time theory had supported experiments on human joints.

This theory relates only to line contacts and so hips are not truly represented. Dowson and Yao (1990) analysed elliptical contacts and although the film thicknesses are smaller than for knees and ankles, Yao (1990) suggests that when combined with microelastohydrodynamic lubrication of Dowson and Jin (1986) fluid film lubrication is predicted theoretically.

The work of Dowson and Jin (1986) was taken further by Yao and Unsworth (1993) and while the basic mechanism of micro-elastohydrodynamic lubrication was still active, the predicted film thicknesses for realistic cartilage surfaces were very much smaller than the earlier predictions.

Summary of human joint lubrication

The important aspects of human joint lubrication are given in Fig. 4 which shows a hip joint at various stages in a walking cycle. During the lightly loaded swing phase, a relatively thick film of fluid can be entrained between the cartilage surfaces (Higginson and Unsworth 1981). When the heel strikes the ground, the load increases rapidly as the entraining velocity approaches zero. Here the thick film of fluid generated during the swing phase, begins to squeeze out and the fluid film thickness reduces. However

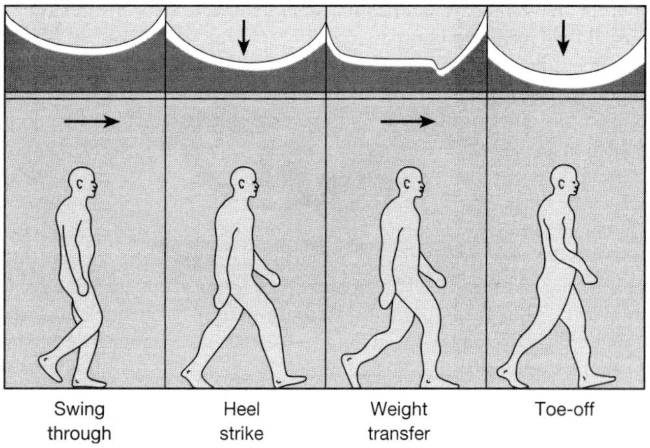

Fig. 4 A hip joint at various stages in a walking cycle.

since the load is only applied for a short time (circa 0.1 s), the film does not reduce too much at this stage. However, during the next phase of the walking cycle, the 'stance phase', the load reduces and the entraining velocity increases both of which help to generate elastohydrodynamic lubrication and so the fluid film separating the joint surfaces is maintained. Finally at 'toe off', the load is near to maximum and the entrainment velocity is low so 'squeeze film' lubrication is called upon to maintain the fluid-film and prevent surface to surface contact. With normal healthy tissue under physiological loads and motion, both theory and experiments show this to be true. During the time that the cartilage surfaces are completely separated by synovial fluid, little or no wear can take place. However, after resting, or standing motionless for long periods, we might expect our joints to squeeze all the fluid out from between the surfaces and therefore to have cartilage rubbing on cartilage (McCutchen 1959; Walker et al. 1968; Unsworth et al. 1975). When we start to move the joint again, the potential for wear is high except that a 'boundary lubricant' (Hills 2000) is present in the synovial fluid to keep friction low and help reduce wear. Once the motion has resumed, FFL takes over. Hence, FFL provides the lubrication mechanism wherever it can support the load but when needed, the ever present SAPL acts as a boundary lubricant.

Mechanical factors in the pathogenesis of osteoarthrosis

Although the initiation and progression of articular cartilage breakdown is not well understood, the process seems likely to include both 'mechanical' and 'biochemical' factors, which may interact. From the mechanical viewpoint, cartilage is a bearing material subjected to repetitive impulsive loads and movements. A normal engineering structure could accumulate microdamage that might lead to fatigue failure. This mechanism may explain the breakdown of articular cartilage, since it has limited regenerative capability. People typically take 2–3 million steps per annum, so cartilage must probably resist more than 100 million load cycles during a lifetime, which is effectively an infinite life in engineering design terms. In such a situation, a very small change in conditions can have a very large effect on the life of the structure. At 10^8 load cycles, a fatigue graph of cycles to failure versus stress is virtually flat even on a logarithmic scale, so a 5 per cent increase in stress can reduce the life to failure by a factor of 100.

Musculoskeletal tissues generally obey Wolff's law in that their form and structure are adapted to withstand the mechanical demands placed on them. Although this law was originally aimed at bone, it is accepted that articular cartilage also obeys it. The strength and stiffness of the articular surfaces increase with increased locally imposed stresses. Kempson et al. (1971) showed that the cartilage of the load-bearing area on the superior part of the femoral head had higher indentation stiffness than that from the inferior aspect. Swann and Seedhom (1985) found a correlation between compressive modulus and predicted compressive stress in the knee and ankle. Kempson (1979) also found a highly significant correlation with glycosaminoglycan content, and hypothesized that the loss of stiffness after early cartilage damage relates to damage to the collagenous framework that contains the glycosaminoglycans.

There is a significant loss of cartilage tensile strength (Kempson 1979) and fatigue strength (Weightman 1976) with advancing age. Since body weight does not fall greatly in most people with increasing age, the cartilage stresses will remain constant in normal activities, so there may be a convergence with the diminishing cartilage fatigue strength which would lead to failure when the repetitive load cycles exceed a damage threshold. A related hypothesis is that an increase in stress can result from changes in the underlying bone, either a localized irregularity in the contour of the subchondral plate or a more general stiffening of the bone (Radin and Paul 1970). Repetitive loading experiments on rabbit joints (Radin et al. 1984) showed that impacts caused trabecular microfractures, and that the healing response, with localized thickening of the damaged trabeculae, led to increased stiffness. These changes preceded cartilage damage. Trabecular hypertrophy is seen frequently as cartilage is lost from an osteoarthritic joint, and this is also part of a functional adaptation to the loss of the ability of the softened cartilage to support loads, which leads to localized areas of higher pressure. The growth of peripheral osteophytes is a further part of this adaptive process.

The studies above were careful to avoid testing damaged areas. With time, the early degenerative changes of softening and fibrillation (vertical fissures) seem to be found almost universally, but this is not the same as saying that fibrillation inevitably progresses to symptomatic osteoarthritis. In younger joints, fibrillation is found primarily in the non-loaded areas (Goodfellow and Bullough 1967; Byers et al. 1970; Waugh et al. 1980). These areas were different from those with 'progressive' lesions that led to full-thickness cartilage loss and which were associated with high stresses in use, such as the superior pole of the femoral head. It is interesting that there are differing frequencies with which the joints are affected by clinical degenerative changes. Beyond 70 years of age, most people have patellofemoral osteoarthritis, yet degeneration is rarely seen in the ankle. Part of the explanation comes from the pattern of movements, with 'linear' motion, such as in the ankle, appearing to be less damaging than a mixture of sliding and rotation, such as at the hip (Goodfellow and Bullough 1967). From a mechanical viewpoint, this appears to be related to the ability of the cartilage structure to adapt to resist the dominant loads. This can be visualized through the demonstration of surface 'split lines', which display the orientation of the collagen fibres in the articular surfaces. They are able to align themselves with the sliding of a hinge joint, but cannot do so for a sliding and rotating joint, when the shear forces might act across their orientation and 'separate' the fibre bundles.

It is usually accepted that the areas of fibrillation, which are areas of softening and are found in the majority of joints, do not lead directly to osteoarthritis. However, it must be a possibility that cartilage damage could spread from them into the areas that usually carry significant forces. A local area of cartilage softening will not carry its normal share of the joint force when the contact area covers it, thus, it is logical to expect elevated contact pressures in the adjacent cartilage. This phenomenon has been reported for chondromalacic lesions and for cartilage repairs that did not carry normal pressures when loaded (Shahgaldi et al. 1991). It is possible that large movements of joints that bring the loaded contact area over the softened zones at the normally unloaded aspect, can lead to expansion of the softened area until it is acted upon regularly, leading to breakdown in the heavily loaded area. This is similar to the hypothesis of Swann and Seedhom (1985) that damage relates to occasional overload of cartilage that is not adapted to high stresses, and may be the cause of progression of patellar changes from localized degeneration of the 'odd' medial articular facet, which only makes contact with the femur in full flexion (135°), across the full width of the patella.

Secondary arthritis

The discussion above concentrated on 'primary' osteoarthritis, where the cartilage changes have an insidious onset throughout a lifetime, and for which there is no obvious cause. There are, however, many cases where there is an obvious mechanical factor—'secondary' arthritis.

The principle underlying the concept of secondary arthritis is that there is a range of physiological stresses to which the articular surface is adapted, and that any sudden increase in loading, to a 'pathological' level, will initiate damage. This can arise from a range of problems, such as deformity of the joint surfaces due to malunion of articular fractures, depression of the subchondral plate due to trabecular crushing, or to deformity of the limb due to angulation of an extraarticular fracture. There is also a spectrum of disturbances arising from abnormal growth, muscle actions, etc. A typical situation would be an inaccuracy of alignment following a femoral supracondylar fracture, which might leave a valgus angulation. In such a case, the line of action of the body weight would be shifted laterally at the knee, and this would cause elevated stresses on the lateral tibiofemoral articulation. This can then cause a 'vicious circle', since lateral compartment cartilage loss will increase the valgus angulation on weight bearing, which will increase the load on the damaged articulation (that may now be devoid of cartilage). Total knee replacement can then act to restore the leg alignment, and balance the loads acting across the joint. For those whom joint replacement is not advisable (e.g. young patients) a realignment osteotomy, usually with some overcorrection, which allows the damaged area a respite, when reconstitution of a fibrocartilagenous surface and restoration of a healthy-looking joint space are sometimes observed (Maquet 1976).

Osteoarthritic changes can also be initiated by soft tissue damage. Knee joint kinematics are controlled largely by the cruciate ligaments, which stabilize the tibiofemoral articulation against the anterior–posterior actions of the muscles. Rupture of the anterior cruciate ligament is common in sport, and this allows abnormal tibiofemoral excursions. The resulting contact forces cause rapid articular damage in animals, and this has been a widespread animal model for osteoarthritis (Muir and Carney 1987). The changes in humans are less drastic, and often follow meniscal damage. Loss of stability allows abnormal bone excursions, which cause the menisci to be overridden by the femoral condyles, leading to damage. The menisci transmit much of the knee joint force (Seedhom and Hargreaves 1979), so meniscal damage in a ligament-deficient knee combines abnormal motion with abnormal stresses, causing degeneration. Knees in which a ruptured anterior cruciate ligament has not been reconstructed suffer increased rates of meniscal damage with time after the ligament injury, and this correlates directly with increasing areas of articular cartilage damage and loss (Murrell et al. 2001).

Failure of lubrication mechanism

Another factor in the development of osteoarthritis is a failure of the lubrication mechanism. This probably acts in conjunction with one of the other failure mechanisms already discussed.

Under normal conditions, human joints have the two articular cartilage surfaces separated by a full film of synovial fluid. This does two things to help limit the damage to articular cartilage. Firstly, by covering the rough surfaces of cartilage with a film of viscous fluid under pressure, the compressive stress transmitted to the cartilage is lower overall than if they were in direct contact. Rough, dry surfaces only contact at high spots, giving rise to very high stresses whereas the film of fluid spreads the load over a greater area and hence reduces the stress. The second method by which FFL protects cartilage is by reducing the shear stress due to friction acting on the surfaces of the articular cartilage. An effective boundary lubricating film also helps to limit damage. Although, in the case of boundary lubrication, the compressive stress transmitted to the cartilage will not be reduced, the friction and therefore shear stress will be reduced and this will increase the life of the joint further than that expected should direct cartilage contact occur. A reduction in compressive and shear stresses helps to avoid the failure of articular cartilage from fatigue stresses (Unsworth 1984). In other words, if FFL exists between the cartilage surfaces (along with boundary lubrication under the less forgiving conditions of prolonged standing, etc.), then they are likely to withstand a lifetime of use, whereas if they rub directly together, premature failure can be expected. The effects of this can be dramatic, reducing the life of 50-year-old cartilage to 4 years if lubrication fails (Unsworth 1984). This then raises another important feature of the way that the properties of synovial fluid and cartilage are affected by age, trauma, and disease. Anything that affects the joint's ability to produce a film of fluid can potentially cause damage to the cartilage surfaces and hence increase the effects of osteoarthritis.

Summary

It has been argued that cartilage is subjected to dynamic loading which can lead to a fatigue process causing damage to the surface layers of the joint. In addition, changes in the sub-chondral bone or in the stiffness of cartilage due to mechanical damage can also lead to accelerated mechanical failure of the articular surfaces. Changed kinematics in the joint, which might be due to the rupture of ligaments, can also increase the resultant contact force and cause premature failure, as can damage to menisci or a failure of the lubrication mechanisms which normally promote fluid film lubrication. All of these mechanisms effectively increase the resultant stress acting on the cartilage and this in turn will accelerate failure due to fatigue.

References

Amis, A.A., Dowson, D., and Wright, V. (1979). Muscle strengths and musculoskeletal geometry of the upper limb. *Engineering in Medicine* **8**, 41–8.

Amis, A.A., Dowson, D., and Wright, V. (1980a). Analysis of elbow joint forces due to high speed forearm movements. *Journal of Biomechanics* **13**, 825–31.

Amis, A.A., Dowson, D., and Wright, V. (1980b). Elbow joint force predictions for some strenuous isometric actions. *Journal of Biomechanics* **13**, 765–75.

An, K.-N., Chao, E.Y., Cooney, W.P., and Linscheid, R.L. (1979). Normative model of human hand for biomechanical analysis. *Journal of Biomechanics* **12**, 775–88.

Basmajian, J.V. *Muscles Alive* 2nd edn. Baltimore MD: Williams and Wilkins, 1967.

Batchelor, A.W. and Stachowiak, G.W. (1996). Arthritis and the interacting mechanisms of synovial joint lubrication. Part II: Joint lubrication and its relation to arthritis. *Journal of Orthopaedic Rheumatology* **9**, 11–21.

Bennett, A. and Higginson, G.R. (1970). Hydrodynamic lubrication of soft solids. *Journal of Mechanical Engineering Science* **12**, 218–22.

Bergman, G., Graichen, F., and Rohlmann, A. (1993). Hip joint measured in two patients. *Journal of Biomechanics* **26**, 969–90.

Bull, A.M.J. and Amis, A.A. (1998). Knee joint motion: description and measurement. *Proceedings of the Institution of Mechanical Engineers, Part H* **212**, 357–72.

Bull, A.M.J. and McGregor, A.H. (2000). Measuring spinal motion in rowers: the use of an electromagnetic device. *Clinical Biomechanics* **15**, 771–6.

Byers, P.D., Contempomi, C.A., and Farkas, T.A. (1970). A post mortem study of the hip joint. *Annals of the Rheumatic Diseases* **29**, 15–31.

Charnley, J. (1959). The lubrication of animal joints. *Institution of Mechanical Engineers Symposium on Biomechanics* **17**, 12–22.

Charnley, J. (1960a). The lubrication of animal joints in relation to surgical reconstruction by arthroplasty. *Annals of the Rheumatic Diseases* **19**, 10–19.

Charnley, J. (1960b). How our joints are lubricated. *Triangle* **4**, 175–80.

Contini, R. and Drillis, R.J. *Body Segment Mass Properties.* Technical report No. 1166.03, New York University, 1966.

Dintenfass, L. (1963). Lubrication in synovial joints: a theoretical analysis—a rheological approach to the problems of joint movements and joint lubrication. *Journal of Bone and Joint Surgery* **45A**, 1241.

Dowson, D. (1967). Modes of lubrication in human joints. *Proceedings of the Institution of Mechanical Engineers* **181**, 45–54.

Dowson, D. and Jin, Z.-M. (1986). Micro-elastohydrodynamic lubrication of synovial joints. *Engineering in Medicine* **15**, 63–5.

Dowson, D. and Yao, J.Q. (1990). A full solution to the problem of film thickness prediction in natural synovial joints. In *Mechanics of Coatings, Proceedings of 16th Leeds/Lyon Symposium on Tribology, Lyon 1989*, pp. 91–102. Amsterdam: Elsevier.

Elftman, H. (1966). Biomechanics of muscle. *Journal of Bone and Joint Surgery* **48A**, 363–77.

English, T.A. and Kilvington, M. (1979). *In vivo* records of hip loads using a femoral implant with telemetric output (a preliminary report). *Biomedical Engineering* **1**, 111–15.

Fein, R.S. (1966–67). Are synovial joints squeeze film lubricated? *Proceedings of the Institution of Mechanical Engineers* **181**, 125–8.

Foster, H. and Fisher, J. (1999). The influence of continuous sliding and subsequent surface wear on the friction of articular cartilage. *Proceedings of the Institution of Mechanical Engineers ar H* **213**, 329–45.

Gaman, I.D.C., Higginson, G.R., and Norman, R. (1974). Fluid entrapment by a soft surface layer. *Wear* **28**, 345–52.

Goodfellow, J.W. and Bullough, P.G. (1967). The pattern of ageing of the articular cartilage of the elbow joint. *Journal of Bone and Joint Surgery* **49B**, 175–81.

Higginson, G.R. and Norman, R. (1974). The lubrication of porous elastic solids with reference to the functioning of human joints. *Journal of Mechanical Engineering Science* **16**, 250–57.

Higginson, G.R. and Unsworth, A. (1981). The lubrication of natural joints. In *Tribology of Natural and Artificial Joints* (ed. J.H. Dumbleton), pp. 47–72. Amsterdam: Elsevier.

Hills, B.A. (2000). Boundary lubrication *in vivo*. *Proceedings of the Institution of Mechanical Engineers, Part* H **214**, 83–94.

Hooke, C.J. and O'Donoghue, J.P. (1972). Elastohydrodynamic lubrication of soft, highly deformed contacts. *Journal of Mechanical Engineering Science* **14**, 34.

Johnson, F., Leitl, S., and Waugh, W. (1980). The distribution of load across the knee: a comparison of static and dynamic measurements. *Journal of Bone and Joint Surgery* **62B**, 346–9.

Jones, F.S. (1934). Joint lubrication. *Lancet* **i**, 1426–7.

Jones, F.S. (1936). Joint lubrication. *Lancet* **i**, 1043.

Jones, H.P. and Walker, P.S. (1968). Casting techniques applied to the study of human joints. *Journal of the Institute of Science and Technology* **14**, 57–68.

Kempson, G.E. (1979). Mechanical properties of articular cartilage. In *Adult Articular Cartilage* 2nd edn. (ed. M.A.R. Freeman), pp. 333–414. Tunbridge Wells: Pitman Medical.

Kempson, G.E., Freeman, M.A.R., and Swanson, S.A.V. (1971). The determination of a creep modulus for articular cartilage from indentation tests on the human femoral head. *Journal of Biomechanics* **4**, 239–50.

Ladin, Z. (1995). Three-dimensional instrumentation. In *Three-Dimensional Analysis of Human Movement* (ed. P. Allard, I.A.F. Stokes, and J.-P. Blanchi), pp. 3–18. Leeds: Human Kinetics Europe Ltd.

Lewis, P.R. and McCutchen, C.W. (1959). Experimental evidence for weeping lubrication in animal joints. *Nature* **184**, 1285.

Ling, F.F. (1974). A new model of articular cartilage in human joints. *Transactions of the American Society of Mechanical Engineers, Journal of Lubrication Technology* **96**, 449–507.

Linn, F.C. (1967). Lubrication of animal joints: I—The arthrotripsometer. *Journal of Bone and Joint Surgery* **49A**, 1079–97.

Linn, F.C. (1968). Lubrication of animal joints: II—The mechanism. *Journal of Biomechanics* **1**, 193.

Linn, F.C. and Radin, E.L. (1968). Lubrication in animal joints III—The effect of certain chemical alteration of the cartilage and lubricant. *Arthritis and Rheumatism* **11**, 674–82.

MacConaill, M.A. (1932). Function of intra-articular fibrocartilages with special reference to the knee and inferior-radio-ulnar joints. *Journal of Anatomy* **66**, 210–27.

Mansour, J.M. and Mow, V.C. (1977). On the natural lubrication of synovial joints: normal and degenerative. *Transactions of the American Society of Mechanical Engineers, Journal of Lubrication Technology* **F99**, 163–73.

Maquet, P. *Biomechanics of the Knee*. Berlin: Springer-Verlag, 1976.

Maroudas, A. (1967). Hyaluronic acid films. *Proceedings of the Institution of Mechanical Engineers* **181**, 122–4.

Maroudas, A. (1968). Physiochemical properties of cartilage in the light of ion exchange theory. *Biophysics Journal* **8**, 575–95.

McCutchen, C.W. (1959). Sponge-hydrostatic and weeping bearings. *Nature* **184**, 1284–5.

Morrison, J.B. (1968). Bioengineering analysis of force actions transmitted by the knee joint. *Biomedical Engineering* **3**, 164–70.

Muir, H. and Carney, S.L. (1987). Pathological and biochemical changes in cartilage and other tissues of the canine knee resulting from induced joint instability. In *Joint Loading: Biology and Health of Articular Structures* (ed. H.J. Helminen et al.), pp. 47–63. Bristol: Wright.

Murakami, T. et al. (1998). Adaptive multimode lubrication in natural synovial joints and artificial joints. *Proceedings of the Institution of Mechanical Engineers ar H*, **212**, 23–35.

Murrell, G.A. et al. (2001). The effects of time course after anterior cruciate ligament injury in correlation with meniscal and cartilage loss. *American Journal of Sports Medicine* **29**, 9–14.

O'Kelly, J., Unsworth, A., Dowson, D., Hall, D.A., and Wright, V. (1978). A study of the role of synovial fluid and its constituents in the friction and lubrication of human hip joints. *Engineering in Medicine* **7**, 78–83.

Paul, J.P. (1967). Forces transmitted by joints in the human body. *Proceedings of the Institution of Mechanical Engineers, Part J* **181**, 1–15.

Paul, J.P. (1974). Force actions transmitted in the knee of normal subjects and by prosthetic joint replacements. *Proc. Symp. Total Knee Replacement*. London: IMECHE, pp. 126–31.

Radin, E.L. and Paul, I.L. (1970). Does cartilage compliance reduce skeletal impact loads? *Arthritis and Rheumatism* **13**, 139.

Radin, E.L., Martin, R.B., Burr, D.B., Caterson, B., Boyd, R.D., and Goodwin, C. (1984). Effects of mechanical loading on the tissues of the rabbit knee. *Journal of Orthopaedic Research* **2**, 221–34.

Reynolds, O. (1886). On the theory of lubrication and its application to Mr Beauchamp Towers' experiments. *Philosophical Transactions of the Royal Society of London* **177**, 157–235.

Roberts, B.J., Unsworth, A., and Mian, N. (1982). Modes of lubrication in human hip joints. *Annals of the Rheumatic Diseases* **41**, 217–24.

Rydell, N.W. (1966). Forces acting on the femoral head prosthesis in living persons. *Acta Orthopaedica Scandinavica* **37** (Suppl. 88), 1–132.

Sayles, R.S., Thomas, T.R., Anderson, J., Haslock, I., and Unsworth, A. (1979). Measurement of the surface microgeometry of articular cartilage. *Journal of Biomechanics* **12**, 257–67.

Seedhom, B.B. and Hargreaves, D.J. (1979). Transmission of load in the knee joint with special reference to the role of the menisci. *Engineering in Medicine* **8**, 220–8.

Shahgaldi, B.F., Amis, A.A., Heatley, F.W., McDowell, J., and Bentley, G. (1991). Repair of cartilage lesions using biological implants: a comparative histological and biomechanical study in goats. *Journal of Bone and Joint Surgery* **73B**, 57–64.

Swann, A.C. and Seedhom, B.B. (1985). The surveying of the stiffness of articular cartilage across total joint surfaces with reference to early stages of osteoarthritis. *British Journal of Rheumatology* **24**, 219.

Tanner, R.I. (1966). An alternative mechanism for the lubrication of synovial joints. *Physics in Medicine and Biology* **11**, 119.

Unsworth, A. (1984). Some biomechanical factors in osteoarthrosis. *British Journal of Rheumatology* **23**, 173–6.

Unsworth, A., Dowson, D., and Wright, V. (1975). The frictional behaviour of human synovial joints. Part 1: Natural Joints. *Trans. A.S.M.E. J. Lube. Tech.* **97**, 369–76.

Unsworth, A., Pearcy, M.J., and White, E.F.T. (1987). Soft layer lubrication of artificial hip joints. In *Proceedings of the Institution of Mechanical Engineers International Conference Volume on Tribology*, pp. 715–24. Bury St Edmunds: MEP.

Walker, P.S., Dowson, D., Longfield, M.D., and Wright, V. (1968). Boosted lubrication in synovial joints by fluid entrapment and enrichment. *Annals of the Rheumatic Diseases* **27**, 512–20.

Waugh, W., Newton, G., and Tew, M. (1980). Articular changes associated with a flexion deformity in rheumatoid and osteoarthritic knees. *Journal of Bone and Joint Surgery* **62B**, 180–3.

Weightman, B.O. (1976). Tensile fatigue of human articular cartilage. *Journal of Biomechanics* **9**, 193–200.

Weightman, B.O. and Amis, A.A. (1982). Finger joint force predictions related to the design of joint replacements. *Journal of Biomedical Engineering* **4**, 197–205.

Yao, J.Q. (1990). *A study of the deformation and lubrication of synovial joints.* Ph.D thesis. Leeds University.

Yao, J.Q. and Unsworth, A. (1993). Asperity lubrication in human joints. *Proceedings of the Institution of Mechanical Engineers, Part H* **207**, 245–54.

Youm,Y., McMurthy, R.Y., Flatt, A.E., and Gillespie, T.E. (1978). Kinematics of the wrist. *Journal of Bone and Joint Surgery* **60A**, 423–31.

3.9 The neurophysiology of pain

Hans-Georg Schaible

General pain physiology

Pain is the conscious sensation which is specifically evoked by potential or actual tissue-damaging (noxious) stimuli or by tissue injury (Table 1). The pain sensation has a sensory discriminative component (identification of the location, duration, intensity of the noxious stimulus) and an affective (emotional) component, the unpleasantness and aversion. Furthermore, noxious stimuli elicit motor reactions (e.g. withdrawal) and autonomic responses (e.g. changes in blood pressure, heart rate). Finally, pain sensations are evaluated and compared to pain in the past (cognitive component). The term *nociception* defines the neuronal events that occur in the peripheral and central nervous system when noxious stimuli are applied. Usually, pain is evoked when the *nociceptive system* is activated (Willis 1985; Schmidt 1989; Basbaum and Jessell 1999). However, during chronic pain the relationship between nociception and pain can be poor because chronic pain does not only depend on nociceptive processes but also on psychological and social factors (Turk 1997).

The nociceptive system is shown in Fig. 1. Nociceptive primary afferent neurons (*nociceptors*) convey nociceptive sensory information from the tissue to the spinal cord or to the brainstem (Fig. 1, left side). The axons of nociceptors are either unmyelinated (group IV or C-fibres, conduction velocities <2.5 m/s) or thinly myelinated (group III or Aδ-fibres, conduction velocities 2.5–30 m/s), and their sensory endings in the tissue are 'free nerve endings'. Most nociceptors are polymodal; they respond to noxious mechanical stimuli (e.g. painful pressure, squeezing the skin), noxious thermal stimuli (painful heat and/or cold), and chemical stimuli (Belmonte and Cervero 1996). Numerous nociceptors have also 'efferent functions'. They release neuropeptides from their sensory terminals into the innervated tissue thereby exerting effects on the vasculature and diverse non-neural cells (Lynn 1996). By contrast, non-nociceptive mechanoreceptors are nerve fibres that respond to innocuous mechanical stimuli such as touch or non-painful pressure. They have thick myelinated axons (group II or Aβ-fibres, conduction velocities >30 m/s) and corpuscular sensory endings. Smaller proportions of Aδ- and C-fibres are also non-nociceptive and respond to innocuous thermal (warmth, cold) or mechanical stimuli such as touch (Willis and Coggeshall 1991).

Table 1 Definitions

Aβ-fibre	Group II unit; afferent nerve fibre with a thick myelinated axon (conduction velocity >30 m/s) and a corpuscular sensory ending
Aδ-fibre	Group III unit; afferent nerve fibre with a thin myelinated axon (conduction velocity 2.5–30 m/s) and a free sensory nerve ending
Afferent nerve fibre	Primary afferent neurone; neurone that conveys information (action potentials) from the periphery to a neurone in the CNS
Algesic substance	Substance that causes pain
Allodynia	Sensation of pain evoked by gentle innocuous stimuli that do not cause pain under normal conditions
C-fibre	Group IV unit; afferent nerve fibre with an unmyelinated axon (conduction velocity <2.5 m/s) and a free sensory nerve ending
Chemosensitivity	Sensitivity of the sensory terminal of an afferent nerve fibre for chemical substances
Descending inhibition	Inhibition of spinal cord neurones by descending tracts (from brain stem)
Efferent function	Action evoked by action potentials that propagate from central to peripheral
Free nerve ending	Non-corpuscular sensory terminal of an afferent fibre
Hyperalgesia	Increased intensity of pain sensation evoked by noxious stimuli
Hyperexcitability	Enhanced sensitivity of a nerve cell to stimuli
Innocuous stimulus	Stimulus that does not threaten or damage the tissue
Mechanoinsensitive afferent	Silent nociceptor; primary afferent neurone that is not activated by mechanical stimuli under normal conditions
Mechanosensitivity	Sensitivity of the sensory ending of an afferent fibre to mechanical stimuli
Neurogenic inflammation	Vasodilatation and plasma extravasation in the tissue evoked by efferent (antidromic) activity of sensory afferent fibres
Nociception	Neuronal activity in the peripheral and central nervous system that is elicited by noxious stimuli
Nociceptive-specific neurone	Neurone that is activated by noxious but not by innocuous stimuli
Nociceptive system	System of neurones that process noxious stimuli
Nociceptor	Nociceptive primary afferent neurone; sensory neurone that is selectively activated by noxious stimuli
Noxious stimulus	Stimulus (mechanical, thermal, or chemical) that potentially or actually damages the tissue
Receptive field	Area of the tissue which when stimulated causes action potentials in a neurone
Polymodal nociceptor	Nociceptor that is excited by mechanical, thermal, and chemical noxious stimuli
Primary afferent neurone	Neurone in the peripheral nerve with sensory ending in the tissue
Sensitization	Generation of enhanced sensitivity of a nerve cell to stimuli
Sensory ending	Terminal site of a sensory afferent fibre in which mechanical, thermal or chemical stimuli are transduced into electrical potentials
Wide dynamic range neurone	Neurone that is activated by innocuous and noxious stimuli in a graded fashion

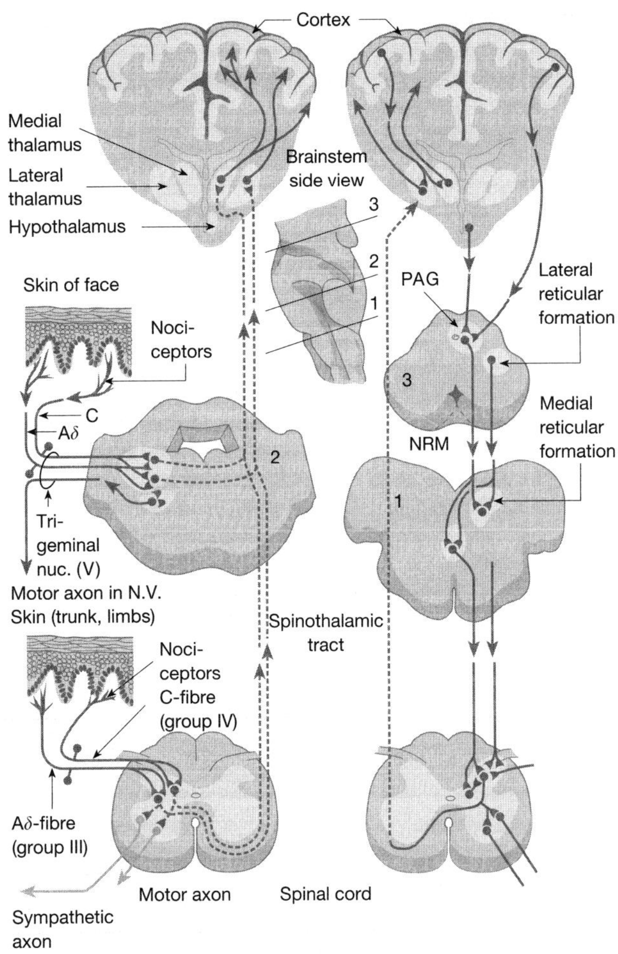

Fig. 1 The nociceptive system. The graph on the left shows a section through the spinal cord (bottom), of which the sensory neurones receive the afferent input from nociceptors supplying trunk and limbs. Sensory spinal cord neurones project to motor neurones and sympathetic neurones of the spinal cord (their axons leave the spinal cord in the ventral root) and to the brainstem and thalamus (top) via ascending tracts. The afferent input from the head is processed in the brainstem (above). Thalamic neurones project to the cerebral cortex. The graph on the right displays descending inhibitory systems which originate in the brainstem (two sections in the middle) and descend to the spinal cord. The brainstem is also influenced by pathways descending from the cortex. The central inset shows a side view of the brainstem with the three levels of the sections numbered 1–3. PAG, periaqueductal grey; NRM, nucleus raphe magnus. (Reproduced with permission from Schmidt 1989.)

The afferent sensory information is processed in the *spinal cord* (and in the *brainstem* for inputs from the head). Nociceptive-specific spinal cord neurones process only input from nociceptors, wide dynamic range neurons receive inputs from both non-nociceptive fibres and nociceptors. The latter neurones show weak responses to innocuous stimuli and stronger responses to noxious stimuli. Long ascending axons of spinal cord neurones project in the spinothalamic tract in the anterolateral quarter of the spinal cord to the thalamus, and in the spinoreticular tract to the brainstem. Spinal cord neurones also project, via interneurones, to motor neurones in the ventral horn and to sympathetic neurones in the lateral part of the grey matter. These pathways generate reflexes which are, however, controlled by descending systems (Willis 1985; Schmidt 1989; Jänig et al. 1996; Millan 1999).

In the brainstem, several nuclei (e.g. the periaqueductal grey, PAG; the nucleus raphe magnus, NRM) are interconnected and form pathways which descend mainly in the dorsolateral funiculus of the spinal cord (Fig. 1, right side). This *inhibitory descending system* partially suppresses the processing of nociceptive information in spinal cord neurones. The brainstem nuclei are activated via ascending tracts (thus forming a negative feed back system between spinal cord and brainstem) and from supraspinal sites (Willis 1985; Basbaum and Jessell 1999).

Activation of neurones in the *thalamus* and *cortex* is necessary to evoke the sensory, emotional, and cognitive components of the pain reaction. The pathway through the ventrobasal complex of the thalamus to the cortical areas SI and SII encodes the parameters of a noxious stimulus (intensity, localization, onset, and offset) and is thus sensory-discriminative. Other pathways run through the posterior and the intralaminar nuclei of the thalamus to the insula, the anterior cingulate cortex (ACC) and the prefrontal cortex. These and the connections to the hypothalamus and the limbic system are involved in the generation of affective aspects of pain (unpleasantness), in arousal reactions, and in pain memory (Basbaum and Jessell 1999; Treede et al. 1999).

The nervous system is not just a system of wires and switches which respond in a stereotyped manner to sensory stimuli. It rather shows considerable *plasticity*. Functional plasticity is an activity-dependent modification of the neuronal processing; it is observed, for example, during long-lasting noxious stimuli such as inflammation. Structural plasticity is characterized by anatomical changes such as sprouting of neurones, which is often seen after damage to the nervous system itself. Under both conditions a noxious stimulus will produce neuronal responses which are different to those seen under normal conditions. Changes in the nociceptive processing are thought to underly changes in the pain sensations such as allodynia and hyperalgesia (often present during inflammation, see below) or abnormal pain (often present after damage to the nervous system) (Coderre et al. 1993; McMahon et al. 1993; Schaible and Grubb 1993; Wall and Melzack 1994; Sandkühler et al. 2000).

Nociception in the joint—peripheral mechanisms

About one-fourth of nerve fibres in the joint nerve are sensory Aβ- and Aδ-fibres. Most fibres are sensory C-fibres or unmyelinated sympathetic efferent fibres. Non-nociceptive Aβ- (group II) fibres are equipped with corpuscular endings of the Ruffini, Golgi, and Pacini type which are located in the fibrous joint structures. By contrast, afferent Aδ- (group III) and C- (group IV) fibres, many of which are nociceptors, terminate as non-corpuscular or 'free nerve endings' in the fibrous capsule, the adipose tissue, the ligaments, the menisci, and the periosteum. In their ultrastructure the free nerve endings consist of a series of spindle-shaped thick segments connected by waist-like thin segments. These beads are not covered by Schwann cell processes and are assumed to be the sensory sites (Heppelmann et al. 1990). The innervation of the synovial layer (a major site of inflammatory foci in arthritic diseases) is still disputed since electron microscopy studies failed to identify nerve endings at these sites, whereas peptidergic structures in this layer are thought to represent afferent fibres (Schaible and Grubb 1993; Schmidt et al. 1994).

Most joint afferents are mechanosensitive; they respond to pressure applied to the joint and to movements of the joint. The receptive field of a sensory fibre is the area that causes the fibre to fire on palpation. At this site the sensory ending is located. Figure 2 displays the receptive fields of two joint afferents in the capsule (black spots). The non-nociceptive group III fibre in Fig. 2(a) is activated by innocuous extension (ext.) and inward rotation (pronation, IR) in the working range of the joint (normally non-painful movements). Non-nociceptive units serve probably proprioceptive functions such as movement and pressure sense. Although they exhibit higher discharge rates during noxious movements such as noxious inward rotation (n.IR) these units do not clearly discriminate innocuous from noxious stimuli in the whole range of movements.

By contrast, the C- (group IV) fibre displayed in Fig. 2(b) is a joint nociceptor. It does not respond to innocuous movements such as outward

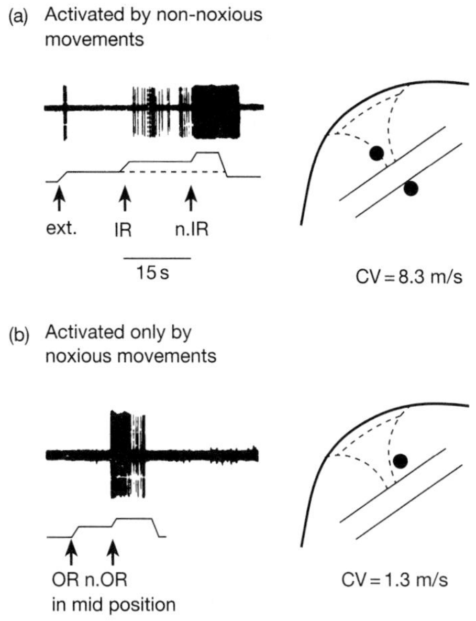

Fig. 2 (a) Response properties of a non-nociceptive unit with a low mechanical threshold in the innocuous range. The graph on the left shows the action potentials recorded from the axon during the application of the movements of the knee indicated by the traces underneath. Phasic response to extension of the knee, ext., and tonic response to inward rotation of the knee, IR, in extension (both movements in the working range of the knee joint); stronger response to noxious inward rotation of the knee, n.IR, in extension. The dots in the inset on the right show the location of two receptive fields of the unit in the capsule. (b) Nociceptive group IV unit with a high threshold. Same type of display as in (a). Strong response to noxious outward rotation, n.OR (and other noxious movements) but no response to outward rotation in the working range, OR, in mid-position (and any other movement in the working range). The dot shows the location of the receptive field in the capsule. CV, conduction velocity of the axon.

rotation in the working range (OR) but responds to noxious outward rotation against the resistance of the tissue (n.OR). Thus joint nociceptors have a high mechanical threshold and are only excited when painful pressure is applied to the joint and/or when movements are exceeding the working range of the joint. Most nociceptors also respond to chemical stimulation, for example, to algesic substances such as bradykinin, and are therefore polymodal. In awake humans, sensations of pain have been evoked when noxious mechanical, thermal, and chemical stimuli such as acids and hypertonic salt solutions were applied to the fibrous structures of the joint, the ligaments, and the fibrous capsule. By contrast, the application of mechanical and thermal stimuli to the cartilage did not evoke sensations and, interestingly, not much evidence was provided for sensations evoked by stimulation of the synovial layer (see Schaible and Grubb 1993). Muscle nerves contain nociceptors with similar response properties (Mense 1993).

A further group of afferents does not respond to innocuous or noxious mechanical stimuli; they are mechanoinsensitive afferents. These units do not have an apparent sensory function under normal conditions but they are important during inflammation of the joint (see below).

Nociception in the joint—mechanisms in the central nervous system

In the spinal cord, joint nociceptors activate second order neurones in the dorsal horn via synapses. Typically spinal cord neurones with input from the joint also receive inputs from adjacent deep tissues (muscles, other joints), and some neurones receive additional inputs from the skin. Figure 6(b) shows a spinal cord neurone with input from the knee. The total receptive field of this neurone (black area) includes the knee joint and adjacent muscles in thigh and lower limb. The receptive fields of spinal cord neurones are larger than the receptive fields of primary afferent neurones because many primary afferent neurones project to one and the same second order neurone. The convergence of nociceptive afferents to the spinal cord neurones provides some explanation for the diffuse and badly localized nature of joint pain.

Nociceptive-specific spinal cord neurones with joint input respond only to noxious compression of the joint and other structures of the hind limb(s) and/or to noxious movements of the knee. Wide dynamic range neurones show substantial responses to innocuous pressure applied to the knee and other structures and to movements in the working range of the knee but show more pronounced responses to stimuli of noxious intensity. Typically, most spinal cord neurones with joint input (and most other spinal cord neurones) are tonically inhibited by descending inhibitory systems; the interruption of descending inhibitory influences leads to enhanced sensitivity and enlargements of their receptive fields (Schaible and Grubb 1993).

Nociceptive spinal cord neurones project to supraspinal sites or to intraspinal neurones that mediate and control motor events (see Fig. 1). Stimulation of joint afferents by noxious hyperflexion, hyperextension, and hyperrotation can cause protective motor reflexes that counteract these movements. Under normal (innocuous) conditions joint afferents only exert weak effects on α-motoneurones (neurones that activate the muscles) but they evoke considerable reflex discharges in γ-motor neurones (γ-motor neurones adjust the length of muscle spindles thereby optimizing the gain of the reflexes which control the length of the muscle, for details see Schmidt 1989). Through this pathway, joint afferents may participate in the regulation of joint stiffness and joint stability during normal movement (Johansson et al. 1991).

The neurobiological response of the nociceptive system to joint inflammation

An inflammation in the joint evokes complex changes in the peripheral and central nervous system. These are summarized in Fig. 3. Briefly, the afferent inflow into the central nervous system is enhanced by activation and sensitization of afferent fibres supplying the inflamed joint (peripheral sensitization), and spinal cord neurones with input from the inflamed joint develop a state of hyperexcitability that significantly increases the gain of the processing of the afferent input (central sensitization). Output channels of the spinal cord (ascending axons, motoric and sympathetic pathways) are modified accordingly.

The inflammation-evoked changes in the nervous system are thought to be responsible for the allodynia (pain during application of innocuous stimuli such as gentle pressure and movements within the working range of the joint), hyperalgesia (enhanced pain during noxious stimulation), and persistent pain in the joint, which are typical symptoms of joint inflammation. Furthermore, the activation of the nociceptive system influences the inflammatory lesion through efferent mechanisms (see below). These changes in the spinal cord are produced by the increased or additional release of several transmitters/modulators and by the activation of receptors on postsynaptic neurones that are less activated, or not at all, under physiological conditions. They may be associated with an upregulation of the synthesis of transmitters and receptors in the long-term range.

Activation and sensitization of joint afferents—the peripheral neuronal basis of inflammatory pain in the joint

During joint inflammation, many joint afferents are sensitized. They exhibit ongoing discharges and respond stronger to mechanical stimuli applied to the joint. Many non-nociceptive Aβ-, Aδ-, and C-fibres show increased

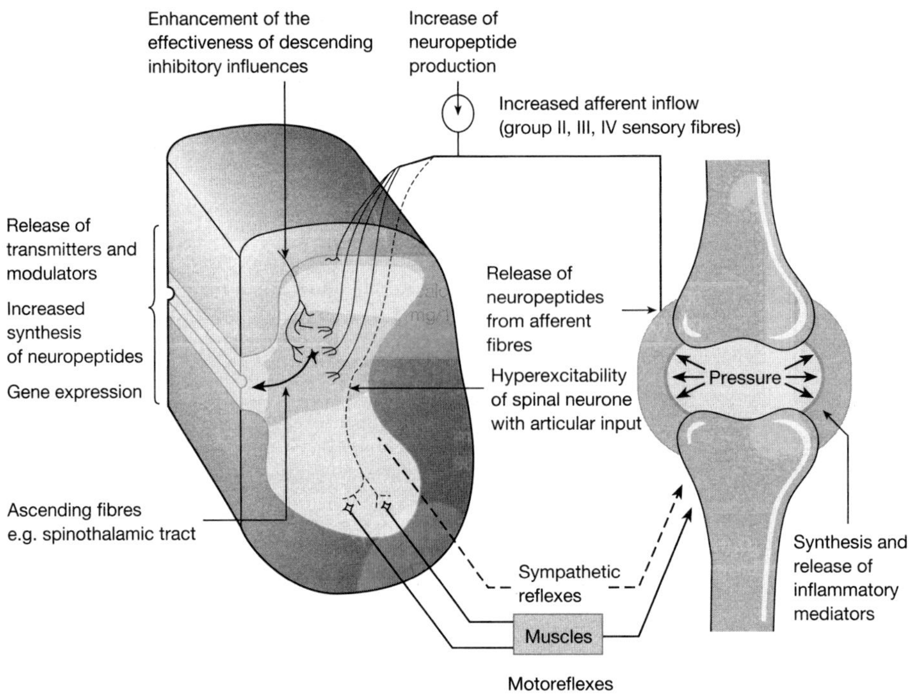

Fig. 3 Overview of neuronal events in the course of an inflammation in the joint. The graph displays the spinal cord with the afferent input from the joint via sensory fibres and the motor and sympathetic output pathways. [Reproduced from Schaible and Grubb (1993) with permission.]

responses to movements in the working range of the joints. This enhances the afferent input to the spinal cord quantitatively. Importantly, in most Aδ- and C-fibre nociceptors the activation threshold is lowered: they start to respond to normally innocuous stimuli such as movements within the working range of the joint and gentle pressure applied to the joint. Figure 4(a) shows the sensitization of an Aδ- (group III) nociceptor. Before inflammation the fibre responded only to noxious rotation of the joint, similar to the unit displayed in Fig. 2(b) but, during development of an acute inflammation, responses were also elicited by movements in the working range, for example, flexion of the knee [Fig. 4(a)]. This is a qualitative change of the sensory processing since sensitized nociceptors transmit their message 'noxious stimulus' to the spinal cord in response to an ordinarily innocuous stimulus and thus the central nociceptive system is already activated by normally non-painful stimuli (Schaible and Grubb 1993; Schmidt et al. 1994).

In addition, a proportion of mechanoinsensitive afferent fibres are rendered mechanosensitive during inflammation. Figure 4(b) displays a unit which was not excited even by noxious stimulation before inflammation (traces on the left: no response to movements, no receptive field identified by pressure). During development of inflammation, the fibre was activated even by innocuous movements and gentle pressure (see action potentials in the traces on the right and the dot on the knee joint showing the location of the receptive field identified during inflammation). Thus, these units are 'silent nociceptors', which play a role particularly under inflammatory conditions. By their activation these newly recruited nociceptive units increase the afferent drive of spinal neurones and contribute to spatial and temporal facilitation in the spinal cord (Schaible and Grubb 1993).

Mechanisms underlying the activation and sensitization of joint afferents

Many nociceptors are polymodal: they express sensor molecules for the transduction of mechanical, thermal as well as chemical stimuli into electrical potentials. Sensor molecules are either ion channels or receptor molecules in the membrane. Figure 5 shows the scheme of a sensory ending of a nociceptor with a variety of ion channels and receptors (Kress and Reeh 1996; Senba and Kashiba 1996; McCleskey and Gold 1999). Strictly speaking, the scheme is not entirely correct. Because the free nerve endings are extremely thin and embedded in the tissue it has not been possible to study ion channels and receptor activation at the free nerve endings in situ. However, ion channels and receptors are also expressed in the cell bodies in the dorsal root ganglia. These neurones can be isolated and cultured, and recordings can be made to study the properties of ion channels. The dorsal root ganglion neurone is therefore used as a model of the sensory ending.

It is likely that mechanoreception (depolarization of the ending by a mechanical stimulus) is due to the opening of cation channels. Changes in the mechanical conditions of inflamed joints (effusates, increase of intra-articular pressure, decrease in joint compliance) may open these channels more effectively than under normal conditions (Belmonte and Cervero 1996). Much progress has been made on heat-activated channels. Heat sensitivity is a characteristic feature of the recently cloned vanilloid 1 receptor (VR 1). This receptor is activated by capsaicin, the compound in the hot pepper that causes pain. Patch clamp recordings suggest that heat sensitivity is at least in part mediated by activation of the VR 1 receptor (Caterina et al. 1997). A proportion of joint nociceptors are capsaicin-sensitive suggesting that the VR 1 receptor also plays a role in joint nociception. Another important aspect is the proton sensitivity because many inflammatory exudates have a low pH. Protons may modulate the VR 1 receptor and other channels such as acid sensing ion channels (ASICs) (Kress and Reeh 1996). Concerning ion channels, the sodium channels became of interest because part of the sodium channels are tetrodotoxin (TTX) sensitive whereas others are TTX resistant. Interestingly, nociceptive neurones seem to express more TTX resistant sodium channels than thick myelinated neurones. Thus, selective antagonists at TTX resistant sodium channels could preferentially inhibit nociceptors. Sodium channels are expressed in the axon (conductance for the generation of action potentials) and probably also in the ending (McCleskey and Gold 1999).

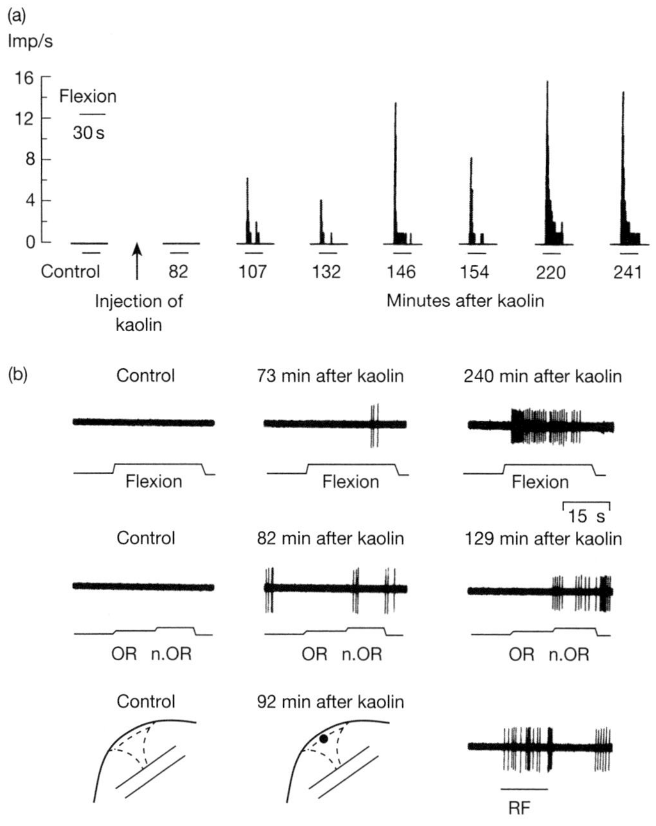

Fig. 4 (a) Sensitization of a nociceptive group III unit to mechanical stimulation of the joint during development of inflammation in the joint. The graph shows peristimulus time histograms indicating the number of action potentials elicted in this afferent fibre by flexion of the knee. No response to flexion of the normal joint. After the induction of inflammation by kaolin and carrageenan the previously high-threshold unit developed responses to flexion of the joint.
(b) Sensitization of a mechanoinsensitive group IV unit during development of inflammation of the knee joint. No responses to mechanical stimulation before inflammation (control, traces on the left), i.e. no response to flexion, outward rotation, OR, noxious outward rotation, n.OR, and palpation of the joint (no receptive field identified). After induction of inflammation by kaolin and carrageenan there was induction of mechanosensitivity (traces in the middle and on the right). At this stage responses were elicited by movements and by palpation of the joint (with identification of the receptive field, dot). RF, pressure applied to the receptive field; Imp, impulses. (Modified from Schaible and Schmidt 1988.)

Proportions of neurones exhibit receptors for the classical inflammatory mediators prostaglandins (mainly PGE_2 and PGI_2), bradykinin, serotonin, histamine, ATP, and acetylcholine (Fig. 5). These mediators are produced by inflammatory cells or released from plasma precursors. They not only produce the inflammatory response (Moncada et al. 1979; Salmon and Higgs 1987; Sedgwick and Willoughby 1989) but also exert significant effects on afferent fibres (Schaible and Grubb 1993; Kress and Reeh 1996). They either activate the neurone directly (the application of the mediator evokes action potentials) or they sensitize the neurone for other stimuli, for example, mechanical stimuli, temperature stimuli, or both. The identification of receptor subtypes on sensory endings is still in progress (Senba and Kashiba 1996). In addition, proportions of primary afferent neurones express receptors for neuropeptides such as substance P and somatostatin. When mediators bind to these receptors they activate second messenger systems such as phospholipase C and proteinkinase C (activated by bradykinin) and cAMP (activated by PGE_2). Through second messenger systems the mediators influence ion channels, for example, PGE_2 enhances the voltage-gated TTX-resistant sodium current and inhibits potassium currents. This enhances the excitability of the neuron, that is, the threshold for action potential firing is lower and more action potentials are elicited by suprathreshold stimuli (Bevan 1996).

Primary afferent neurones express receptors for neurotrophins and cytokines. Neurotrophins are survival factors during the development of the nervous system but they are also important for the adult nervous system. During inflammation of the tissue, the level of nerve growth factor (NGF) is substantially enhanced. By acting on tyrosine kinase A (trkA) receptors, NGF increases the synthesis of substance P and CGRP. Probably the synthesis of other molecules such as ion channels is also regulated by NGF. NGF may also act on mast cells and sensitize sensory endings by mast cell degranulation. The role of cytokines is currently being addressed.

It should be noted that DRG neurones are not homogenous, that is, not all of the primary afferent neurones express all the receptors and ion channels that are displayed in Fig. 5. Thus an antagonist or synthesis inhibitor applied for pain treatment may only affect proportions of neurons. However, some receptors (e.g. bradykinin receptors) are upregulated during inflammation, and then a greater proportion of neurones express this receptor (Segond von Banchet et al. 2000)

Activation of spinal cord neurones and generation of spinal hyperexcitability—a complex response of the central nervous system to peripheral inflammation

During the development of an inflammation in the joint, nociceptive spinal cord neurones show enhanced responses to noxious stimuli applied to the inflamed joint (central sensitization). Nociceptive-specific neurones exhibit a reduction in their mechanical threshold such that the application of innocuous stimuli to the inflamed joint is sufficient to excite the neurones. Before inflammation, the neurone in Fig. 6 had a high-threshold receptive field in the knee and the deep tissue of the thigh and lower leg [black area in Fig. 6(b)], that is, it responded to noxious pressure onto the knee and the adjacent structures but not to noxious pressure applied to the ankle and paw. After induction of inflammation (k/c), the neurone showed increase response to noxious pressure applied to the knee and it developed responses to noxious pressure applied to ankle and paw [Fig. 6(a)], that is the receptive field had expanded [Fig. 6(c), darker area]. At this stage innocuous pressure to all parts of the receptive field was sufficient to activate the neurone (Schaible and Grubb 1993).

The increased responses to stimuli applied to the inflamed joint most likely result from the enhanced discharge rate of the sensitized afferent units when the joint is stimulated. However, because the responses to mechanical stimuli applied to non-inflamed regions adjacent to and remote from the joint are also enhanced (although these areas are not inflamed) the spinal cord neurones obviously develop a state of hyperexcitability and responsiveness to inputs from both inflamed and non-inflamed areas is increased. This central sensitization can persist during chronic inflammation. It is thought to underly the pain, allodynia, and hyperalgesia in the inflamed joint, as well as adjacent and remote non-inflamed tissue. However, during inflammation segmental inhibitory influences on spinal neurones with input from inflamed areas and the effectiveness of the descending inhibition of spinal cord neurones (see Fig. 1) can also be increased. The balance between excitatory and inhibitory systems may determine the pain intensity (Schaible and Grubb 1993; Millan 1999).

It is thought that under certain circumstances the central sensitization can outlast the input from nociceptors, that is, the central nociceptive system remains in a sensitized state even after the disease process in the periphery has waned. Whether this is a proper explanation for pain syndromes in which patients suffer from pain in the absence of an obvious peripheral disease process needs to be clarified.

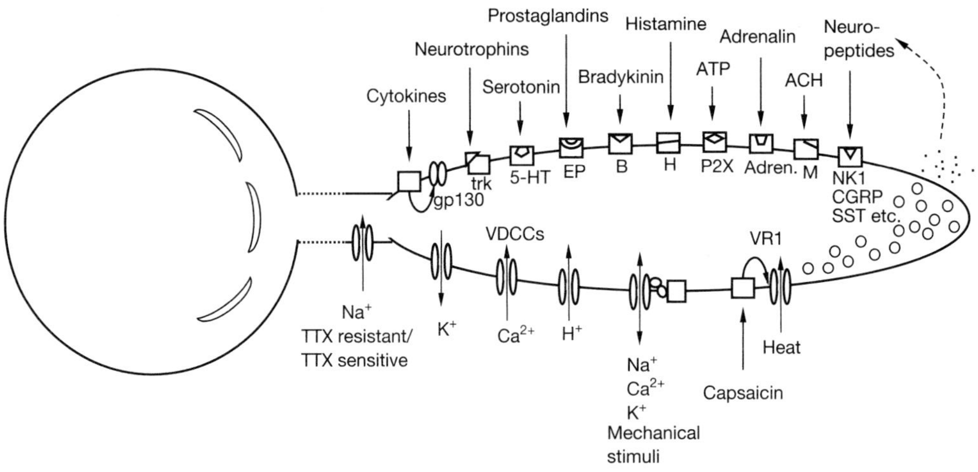

Fig. 5 Model of a nociceptive primary afferent neurone with its ion channels and receptors. The cell body of the neurone is shown on the left, the axon that conveys action potentials to the spinal cord is 'shortened', and the sensory ending where stimuli are transduced into local electrical potentials is 'enlarged'. The schema shows the expression of receptors for various compounds (top side) and ion channels (bottom side). The receptor subtypes are not specified in this figure. gp 130, glycoprotein 130; Trk, tyrosine kinase receptor; 5-HT, 5-hydroxytryptamine; EP, prostaglandin E receptor; B, bradykinin receptor; NK1, neurokinin 1 receptor for substance P; CGRP, calcitonin gene-related peptide receptor; SST, somatostatin receptor; P2X, purinergic receptor for ATP; H, histamine receptor; Adren, adrenergic receptor; M, muscarinergic receptor for acetylcholine, ACH; TTX, tetrodotoxin; VR1, vanilloid 1 receptor; VDCCs, voltage-dependent calcium channels. It should be noted that most nociceptors express only part of these receptors. Modified from Schaible, H.-G., Ebersberger, A., and Segond von Banchet, G. Mechanisms of pain in Arthritis. In *Neuroendocrine Immune Basis of the Rheumatic Diseases II* (ed. M. Cutulo, J.W.J. Bijlsma, R.G. Lahita, A.T. Masi, R.H. Straub, and H.L. Bradlow). *Annals of the New York Academy of Sciences*, Vol. 966, pp. 343–54 (2002).

Mechanisms underlying the synaptic activation of spinal cord neurones and the development of hyperexcitability

Neurones communicate via chemical transmission in synapses. Upon activation (propagation of action potentials into the axonal terminal) the presynaptic neurone releases excitatory or inhibitory transmitters which cross the synaptic cleft, bind to receptors, and then open ion channels on the post-synaptic neurones (Fig. 7). The sum of all excitatory and inhibitory synaptic potentials evoked in the post-synaptic neurone determines whether the neurone will fire. Importantly, many neurones do not only contain a classical transmitter (small molecules such as L-glutamate (Glu) or biogenic amines) but rather contain a classical transmitter and one or several neuropeptides (NP) such as substance P and CGRP in their presynaptic endings (principle of coexistence). These compounds can be coreleased when the neurone is adequately stimulated. Post-synaptic neurones contain a variety of receptors for classical transmitters and neuropeptides and other compounds (Willis and Coggeshall 1991; Millan 1999).

Figure 7 shows important aspects of the synaptic processing under normal and inflammatory conditions and it addresses the transmitters and receptors that have received most attention. Glu is the main excitatory transmitter in the central nervous system, and the most important transmitter of primary afferent neurones including the nociceptors (Fundytus 2001). Glu acts on three different receptors at postsynaptic neurones, namely on ionotropic α-amino-3-hydroxy-5-methylisoxazole-4-propionic acid (AMPA) receptors and ionotropic *N*-methyl-D-aspartate (NMDA) receptors (both ion channels have binding sites for Glu) and on metabotropic glutamate receptors. When innocuous, non-painful pressure is applied to the joint, non-nociceptive primary $A\beta$ afferents, but not the nociceptive $A\delta$- or C-fibres are activated. They release Glu and activate AMPA receptors in the post-synaptic neurone [Fig. 7(a)]. The opening of AMPA receptors allows the influx of sodium ions and the efflux of potassium ions, and by these ion fluxes the post-synaptic neurone is depolarized. For basal neuronal activity this is sufficient.

When noxious, painful pressure is applied to the healthy joint, non-nociceptive $A\beta$ as well as nociceptive $A\delta$- and C-fibres are activated and more Glu is released to the post-synaptic neurone [Fig. 7(b)]. This will open AMPA as well as NMDA receptors. The NMDA receptor is usually closed by a Mg^{2+} ion. However, when the neurone is strongly depolarized (e.g. when much Glu has been released) the magnesium ion is expelled and the channel allows the influx of both sodium and calcium ions. Importantly, calcium ions trigger numerous intracellular events that change excitability of the neurone. For this reason NMDA receptors are key receptors for many forms of neuroplasticity such as learning but they are also important in the development of hyperexcitability of spinal cord neurones (Sandkühler et al. 2000). The blockade of NMDA receptors prevents the generation of hyperexcitability during development of inflammation and even reduces the responses of the neurones to peripheral stimulation once hyperexcitability is established. Metabotropic glutamate receptors are not coupled to ion channels. When Glu binds to metabotropic receptors, G-proteins and intracellular second messengers are activated. These receptors also play a role in neuroplasticity (Neugebauer et al. 1993, 1994).

Proportions of primary afferent neurones, including nociceptors, synthesize and release NP such as substance P, neurokinin A, CGRP, from their spinal endings when they are adequately stimulated, and numerous spinal cord neurons express G-protein coupled receptors for these neuropeptides (NP-R). When the joint is normal, these peptides are only released in the spinal cord when noxious pressure is applied to the joint. However, during inflammation, when nociceptors are sensitized, innocuous pressure onto the joint is sufficient to elicit intraspinal release of these peptides (Schaible 1996). Thus, under inflammatory conditions a 'cocktail' of transmitters and/or modulators is released in the spinal cord which is quantitatively and qualitatively different to that released during noxious stimulation of normal tissue. Hence, more and different receptors on the post-synaptic neurones are activated [Fig. 7(c)]. In general, neuropeptides seem to amplify the glutamatergic synaptic transmission (Urban et al. 1994), and they also play a role in the generation (and maintenance) of hyperexcitability. When antagonists at the neuropeptide receptors are administered, development of inflammation-evoked hyperexcitability is attenuated but not abolished. Hence the analgesic potency of a single neuropeptide receptor antagonist is limited. In addition, the sensitivity of post-synaptic neurones is altered by intracellular processes that are induced by the synaptic activation (Schaible and Grubb 1993).

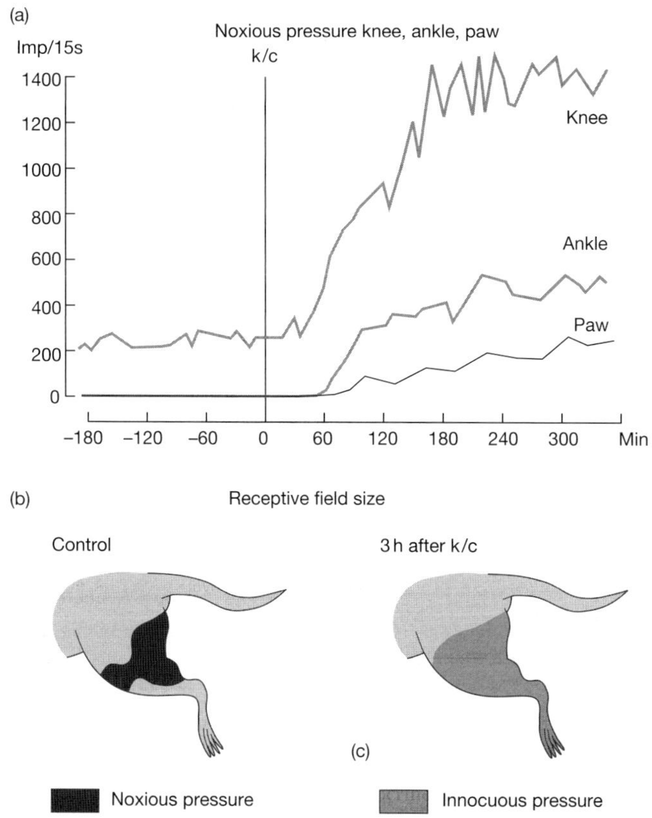

Fig. 6 Generation of hyperexcitability in a spinal cord neurone of the rat during development of inflammation in the knee joint. (a) Responses of the neurone (impulses /15 s) to noxious pressure applied to the knee, ankle, and paw before and after induction of inflammation in the knee joint. During development of inflammation in the knee the responses to noxious pressure applied to the knee were progressively enhanced and responses were also elicited by noxious pressure applied to the non-inflamed ankle and paw. (b) Receptive field of the neurone before inflammation. The neurone was only activated by noxious pressure applied to the knee and the adjacent muscles. (c) Expanded receptive field of the neurone 3 h after induction of inflammation. At this stage the neurone could be activated by gentle pressure applied to the whole leg. Imp, impulses; k/c, induction of inflammation. (Reproduced from Neugebauer et al. 1993 with permission.)

The role of other endogenous compounds in the synaptic processing and central sensitization is being explored. Neurotrophins, in particular brain derived neurotrophic factor (BDNF), and spinal prostaglandins can modify synaptic processing in the spinal cord (Vanegas and Schaible 2001). It should be noted that inhibitory compounds (endogenous opioids) are upregulated during inflammation, and this may set a new balance between excitatory drives and inhibitory mechanisms and thus control the degree of pain experienced (Dickenson 1994). However, one of the opioids, namely dynorphin, may have an antinociceptive role (by acting on κ-opioid receptors) as well as a pronociceptive role (by acting on different receptors).

The contribution of the nervous system to the inflammatory process in the joint

The nervous system is important for the sensation of pain. However, it may also contribute or influence the inflammatory process, by efferent functions of primary afferent fibres and by efferent sympathetic fibres. In addition, the hypothalamic–pituitary–adrenal/gonadal axis may influence the disease process. Thus, the nervous system with its neuronal and neuroendocrine functions is generally involved in the body reaction during chronic inflammation (Straub and Cutolo 2001).

As already mentioned, proportions of the joint afferents are peptidergic; they produce the NP substance P, neurokinin A, CGRP, and somatostatin. Peptides are transported from the perikarya in the dorsal root ganglia to the peripheral endings in the tissue. When peptidergic afferent fibres are stimulated they release substance P and CGRP from their sensory terminals. These peptides produce a 'neurogenic inflammation' characterized by vasodilation and plasma extravasation (Lynn 1996). They also stimulate white blood cells and synoviocytes to release and/or produce inflammatory compounds (Levine et al. 1987). Because the expression of acute and chronic inflammatory lesions is attenuated when afferent fibres have been destroyed by pretreatment with the neurotoxin capsaicin, neuropeptides are thought to contribute to the inflammatory process. Importantly, the synthesis of substance P and CGRP in the dorsal root ganglia is upregulated in segments supplying inflamed tissue (Schaible and Grubb 1993). Possibly, the efferent function of primary afferent fibres is also set in motion by neuronal processing in the spinal cord. In particular under inflammatoy conditions, action potentials may be elicited in the spinal terminals of afferent fibres. These action potentials propagate retrogradely to the periphery, invade the endings and presumably elicit peptide release (Willis 1999).

The joints are also supplied by efferent sympathetic nerve fibres that are vasoconstrictor neurones. As other sympathetic subsystems (e.g. the cardiac postganglionic sympathetic neurones) the sympathetic efferents to the joint show reflex discharges when noxious stimuli are applied (Jänig et al. 1996). In the polyarthritic rat, the sympathetic nervous system seems to contribute to the expression of the inflammatory lesions since the reduction of sympathetic activity and/or the blockade of the post-synaptic effects by antagonists at adrenergic receptors in the tissue partially reduced the severity of the lesions (Schaible and Grubb 1993). However, a reduction of sympathetic fibres has also been described during chronic inflammation, and the disturbed balance between afferent and efferent fibres may also support chronic inflammation (Straub and Cutolo 2001).

Principles of analgesic drug therapy

Pain can be treated either by reducing the excitation and sensitization of neurones and/or by activating inhibitory neurones. There are several targets sites to treat inflammatory pain. (i) Reduction of the inflammatory process and reduction of the activation and sensitization of sensory endings in NP. Any drug that reduces the inflammatory process will reduce the activation and sensitization of NP. Currently, this is best achieved by cyclooxygenase inhibitors (NSAIDs, see below) and TNFα inhibitors. Other compounds such as bradykinin receptor antagonists or ion channel blockers may be used in the future. (ii) Blockade of the conduction of action potentials in peripheral nerves by local anaesthetics. These compounds usually block the conduction of action potentials in nociceptive and in non-nociceptive afferent fibres, therefore, they cannot be used without general disturbance of the sensory system. Nevertheless, a low dose of systemic lidocaine can reduce pain without severe problems, probably because nociceptive neurones with thin axons are more sensitive to the effect of local anaesthetics. (iii) Reduction of excitatory synaptic transmission and of hyperexcitability in the central nociceptive system. This can be achieved by opioids and antagonists at receptors that are involved in the process of central sensitization, such as ketamine, an NMDA receptor antagonist. The central effects of NSAIDs (McCormack and Brune 1991) are being explored. (iv) Increase of inhibitory processes. Besides opioids, antidepressants (interfering with serotonin) and α-adrenergic agonists such as clonidine inhibit the nociceptive processing, mimicking, or potentiating the antinociceptive effects of descending inhibition (Allan and Zenz 1999; Schaible and Vanegas 2000).

The classical NSAIDs block both the cyclooxygenase-1 (COX-1) and the cyclooxygenase-2 (COX-2) while new selective drugs block only COX-2

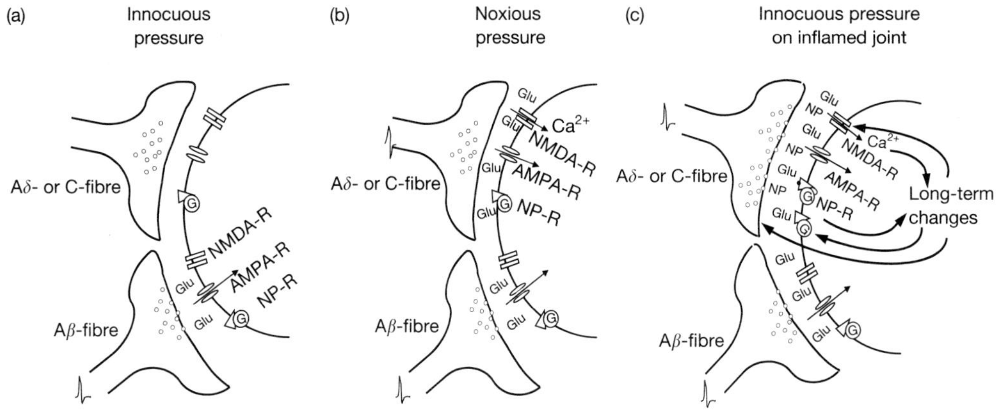

Fig. 7 Mechanisms involved in synaptic activation and generation, maintenance of inflammation-evoked hyperexcitability of spinal cord neurones. The graphs in (a), (b), and (c) show the central presynaptic ending of primary afferent fibres and the membrane of a post-synaptic neurone in the spinal cord with different receptors for transmitters, and the synaptic cleft between these neurones. (a) Synaptic activation of a spinal cord neurone by an innocuous stimulus (innocuous pressure) applied to the joint. L-glutamate (Glu) is released from non-nociceptive Aβ- fibres (it appears in the synaptic cleft) and activates only AMPA receptors (AMPA-R). (b) Synaptic activation of a neurone by noxious stimulation of the joint. L-glutamate is released from non-nociceptive Aβ- fibres and from nociceptive Aδ- and C-fibres, and it activates AMPA and NMDA receptors (NMDA-R). (c) Synaptic activity during joint inflammation. Upon pressure onto the joint, Aβ- fibres release L-glutamate, and Aδ- and C-fibres release L-glutamate and the neuropeptides substance P and calcitonin gene-related peptide (NP) and activate AMPA, NMDA, and neuropeptide receptors (NP-R). AMPA, (*R*,*S*)-α-amino-3-hydroxy-5-methylisoxazole-4-propionic acid, NMDA, *N*-methyl-D-aspartate. Modified from Schaible, H.-G., Ebersberger, A., and Segond von Banchet, G. Mechanisms of pain in Arthritis. In *Neuroendocrine Immune Basis of the Rheumatic Diseases II* (ed. M. Cutulo, J.W.J. Bijlsma, R.G. Lahita, A.T. Masi, R.H. Straub, and H.L. Bradlow). *Annals of the New York Academy of Sciences*, Vol. 966, pp. 343–54 (2002).

and thus in particular the production of prostaglandins in inflamed tissue. Inhibition of prostaglandin synthesis will reduce sensitization because both PGE_2 and PGI_2 act directly on nerve endings (see above). However, NSAIDs also effect the central nervous system. In the spinal cord both COX-1 and COX-2 are expressed, and thus the antinociceptive effect of NSAIDs and selective COX-2 inhibitors may result from peripheral and central effects (Vanegas and Schaible 2001). For further information see Chapter 4.5.1.

Opioids are strong analgesics. All opioids used for pain treatment are agonists at the μ-opioid receptor. Opioids inhibit the release of transmitters from primary afferent neurones by acting on presynaptic endings (thus attacking several transmitter systems) and they inhibit spinal cord neurones by hyperpolarization, that is, they also have post-synaptic actions (Stein 1999). Whether opioids should be given to treat inflammatory pain is under discussion because the views on the potential of opioids for inducing tolerance and addiction have changed. It is claimed that opioids do not necessarily induce tolerance to their analgesic effects and addiction (psychological dependence) when they are given in a strict application regime. However, opioids should only be given if non-opioidergic drugs are not sufficient to treat pain (Schaible and Vanegas 2000).

References

Allan, L. and Zenz, M. (1999). Chronic pain: a review. *Almere: Excerpta Medica Medical Communications* B.V.

Basbaum, A.I. and Jessell, T.M. (2000). The perception of pain. In *Principles of Neural Science* 4th edn. (ed. E.R. Kandel, J.H. Schwartz, and T.M. Jessell). pp. 472–91. New York: McGraw-Hill.

Belmonte, C. and Cervero, F., ed. *Neurobiology of Nociceptors.* Oxford: Oxford University Press, 1996.

Bevan, S. (1996). Signal transduction in nociceptive afferent neurons in inflammatory conditions. In *The Polymodal Receptor: A Gateway to Pathological Pain, Progress in Brain Research* Vol. 113 (ed. T. Kumazawa, L. Kruger, and K. Mizumura), pp. 201–13. Amsterdam: Elsevier Science B.V.

Caterina, M.J., Schumacher, M.A., Tominaga, M., Rosen, T.A., Levine, J.D., and Julius, D. (1997). The capsaicin receptor: a heat-activated ion channel in the pain pathway. *Nature* **389**, 816–24.

Coderre, T.J., Katz, J., Vaccarino, A.L., and Melzack, R. (1993). Contribution of central neuroplasticity to pathological pain: review of clinical and experimental evidence. *Pain* **52**, 259–85.

Dickenson, A.H. (1994). Where and how do opioids act? In *Proceedings of the 7th World Congress on Pain, Progress in Pain Research and Management* Vol. 2 (ed. G.F. Gebhart, D.L. Hammond, and T.S. Jensen), pp. 525–52. Seattle: IASP Press.

Fundytus, M.E. (2001). Glutamate receptors and nociception. *CNS Drugs* **15**, 29–58.

Heppelmann, B., Meßlinger, K., Neiss, W.F., and Schmidt, R.F. (1990). Ultrastructural three-dimensional reconstruction of group III and group IV sensory nerve endings ('free nerve endings') in the knee joint capsule of the cat: evidence for multiple receptive sites. *Journal of Comparative Neurology* **292**, 103–16.

Jänig, W., Levine, J.D., and Michaelis, M. (1996). Interactions of sympathetic and primary afferent neurons following nerve injury and tissue trauma. In *The Polymodal Receptor: A Gateway to Pathological Pain, Progress in Brain Research* Vol. 113 (ed. T. Kumazawa, L. Kruger, and K. Mizumura), pp. 161–84. Amsterdam: Elsevier Science B.V.

Johansson, H., Sjölander, P., and Sojka, P. (1991). Receptors in the knee joint ligaments and their role in the biomechanics of the joint. *CRC Critical Reviews in Biomedical Engineering* **18**, 341–68.

Kress, M. and Reeh, P.W. (1996). Chemical excitation and sensitization in nociceptors. In *Neurobiology of Nociceptors* (ed. C. Belmonte and F. Cervero), pp. 258–97. Oxford: Oxford University Press.

Levine, J.D., Goetzl, E.J., and Basbaum, A.I. (1987). Contribution of the nervous system to the pathophysiology of rheumatoid arthritis and other polyarthritides. *Rheumatic Disease Clinics of North America* **13**, 369–83.

Lynn, B. (1996). Efferent functions of nociceptors. In *Neurobiology of Nociceptors* (ed. C. Belmonte and F. Cervero), pp. 418–38. Oxford: Oxford University Press.

McCleskey, E.W. and Gold, M.S. (1999). Ion channels of nociception. *Annual Reviews of Physiology* **61**, 835–56.

McCormack, K. and Brune, K. (1991). Dissociation between the antinociceptive and anti-inflammatory effects of the nonsteroidal anti-inflammatory drugs. A survey of their analgesic efficacy. *Drugs* **41**, 533–47.

McMahon, S.B., Lewin, G.R., and Wall, P.D. (1993). Central hyperexcitability triggered by noxious inputs. *Current Opinion in Neurobiology* **3**, 602–10.

Millan, M.J. (1999). The induction of pain: an integrative review. *Progress in Neurobiology* **57**, 1–164.

Mense, S. (1993). Nociception from sceletal muscle in relation to clinical muscle pain. *Pain* **54**, 241–89.

Moncada, S., Ferreira, S.H., and Vane, J.R. (1979). Pain and inflammatory mediators. In *Handbook of Experimental Pharmacology, Part I: Inflammation* Vol. 50 (ed. J.R. Vane and S.H. Ferreira), pp. 588–616. Berlin: Springer.

Neugebauer, V., Lücke, T., and Schaible, H.-G. (1993). *N*-methyl-D-aspartate (NMDA) and non-NMDA receptor antagonists block the hyperexcitability of dorsal horn neurones during development of acute arthritis in rat's knee joint. *Journal of Neurophysiology* **70**, 1365–77.

Neugebauer, V., Lücke, T., and Schaible, H.-G. (1994). Requirement of metabotropic glutamate receptors for the generation of inflammation-evoked hyperexcitability in rat spinal cord neurones. *European Journal of Neuroscience* **6**, 1179–86.

Salmon, J.A. and Higgs, G.A. (1987). Prostaglandins and leukotrienes. In *Inflammation—Mediators and Mechanisms, British Medical Bulletin* Vol. 2 (ed. D.A. Willoughby), pp. 285–96. Edinburgh: Churchill Livingstone.

Sandkühler, J., Bromm, B., and Gebhart, G.F., ed. Nervous system plasticity and chronic pain. In *Progress in Brain Research* Vol. 129. Amsterdam: Elsevier Science B.V., 2000.

Schaible, H-G. (1996). On the role of tachykinins and calcitonin gene-related peptide in the spinal mechanisms of nociception and in the induction and maintenance of inflammation-evoked hyperexcitability in spinal cord neurons (with special reference to nociception in joints). In *The Polymodal Receptor: A Gateway to Pathological Pain, Progress in Brain Research* Vol. 113 (ed. T. Kumazawa, L. Kruger, and K. Mizumura), pp. 423–41. Amsterdam: Elsevier Science B.V.

Schaible, H.-G. and Grubb, B.D. (1993). Afferent and spinal mechanisms of joint pain. *Pain* **55**, 5–54.

Schaible, H.-G. and Schmidt, R.F. (1988). Time course of mechanosensitivity changes in articular afferents during a developing experimental arthritis. *Journal of Neurophysiology* **60**, 2180–95.

Schaible, H.-G. and Vanegas, H. (2000). How do we manage chronic pain? *Bailliere's Clinical Rheumatology* **14**, 797–811.

Schmidt, R.F. (1989). Nociception and pain. In *Human Physiology* 2nd edn. (ed. R.F. Schmidt and G. Thews), pp. 223–36. Heidelberg: Springer.

Schmidt, R.F., Schaible, H.-G., Meßlinger, K., Heppelmann, B., Hanesch, U., and Pawlak, M. (1994). Silent and active nociceptors: structure, functions, and clinical implications. In *Proceedings of the 7th World Congress on Pain, Progress in Pain Research and Management* Vol. 2 (ed. G.F. Gebhart, D.L. Hammond, and T.S. Jensen), pp. 213–50. Seattle: IASP Press.

Sedgwick, A.D. and Willoughby, D.A. (1989). Initiation of the inflammatory response and its prevention. In *Handbook of Inflammation. The Pharmocology of Inflammation* Vol. 5 (ed. I.L. Bonta, M.A. Bray, and M.J. Parnham), pp. 27–47. Amsterdam: Elsevier.

Segond von Banchet, G., Petrow, P.K., Bräuer, P., and Schaible, H.-G. (2000). Monoarticular antigen-induced arthritis leads to pronounced bilateral upregulation of the expression of neurokinin 1 and bradykinin 2 receptors in dorsal root ganglion neurons of rats. *Arthritis Research* **2**, 424–7.

Senba, E. and Kashiba, H. (1996). Sensory afferent processing in multi-responsive DRG neurons. In *The Polymodal Receptor: A Gateway to Pathological Pain, Progress in Brain Research* Vol. 113 (ed. T. Kumazawa, L. Kruger, and K. Mizumura) pp. 387–410. Amsterdam: Elsevier Science B.V.

Stein, C., ed. *Opioids in Pain Control. Basic and Clinical Aspects.* Cambridge: Cambridge University Press, 1999.

Straub, R.H. and Cutolo, M. (2001). Involvement of the hypothalamic-pituitary adrenal/gonadal axis and the peripheral nervous system in rheumatoid arthritis. *Arthritis and Rheumatism* **44**, 493–507.

Treede, R.-D., Kenshalo, D.R., Gracely, R.H., and Jones, A.K.P. (1999). The cortical representation of pain. *Pain* **79**, 105–11.

Turk, D.C. (1997). The role of demographic and psychosocial factors in transition from acute to chronic pain. In *Proceedings of the 8th World Congress on Pain. Progress in Pain Research and Management* Vol. 8 (ed. T.S. Jensen, J.A. Turner, and Z. Wiesenfeld-Hallin), pp. 185–213. Seattle: IASP Press.

Urban, L., Thompson, S.W.N., and Dray, A. (1994). Modulation of spinal excitability: cooperation between neurokinin and excitatory amino acid transmitters. *Trends in Neurosciences* **17**, 432–8.

Vanegas, H. and Schaible, H.-G. (2001). Prostaglandins and cyclooxygenases in the spinal cord. *Progress in Neurobiology* **64**, 327–63.

Wall, P.D. and Melzack, R., ed. *Textbook of Pain* 3rd edn. Edinburgh: Churchill Livingstone, 1999.

Willis, W.D. *The Pain System. The Neural Basis of Nociceptive Transmission in the Mammalian Nervous System.* Basel: Karger, 1985.

Willis, W.D. (1999). Dorsal root potentials and dorsal root reflexes: a double-edged sword. *Experimental Brain Research* **124**, 395–421.

Willis, W.D. and Coggeshall, R.E. *Sensory Mechanisms of the Spinal Cord* 2nd edn. New York: Plenum, 1991.

4

The process of inflammation

4 The process of inflammation

4.1 Cells, cytokines, and other mediators

Kevin A. Davies and Patricia Woo

Introduction

Inflammation is essential to protect organisms against external insults. Acute inflammation is short-lived and represents the process of removal of the external insult, and tissue repair. Disease results from failure of the regulatory process of inflammation, the persistence of a pro-inflammatory stimulus, an impairment of the mechanisms that halt inflammation, or a clonal disorder with pro-inflammatory consequences.

This chapter concentrates on the mechanisms involved in inflammation, how these mechanisms may be disrupted in rheumatic disease, the ways in which genetically determined differences in inflammation influences rheumatic disease, and how chronic and acute inflammations differs. Tissue specificity, pathways involved in inflammation, cytokines and matrix metalloproteinase enzymes (MMPs) will be summarized. Chemokines, now known as chemotactic cytokines, their receptors and functions are discussed in detail in Chapter 4.2.

Inflammation—an overview

In order to develop rational therapeutic strategies for chronic rheumatic disorders, a fuller understanding of acute, self-limiting, inflammatory processes is needed. Acute inflammation suggests an intact regulatory mechanism for inflammation. This involves recognition of the stimulus, followed by the orderly production of soluble mediators involved in the cellular process of inflammation, the acute phase response, and its resolution. Other mediator pathways involve proteins that work as stepwise activation cascades, for example, complement proteins, to opsonize and aid the removal of foreign antigens by effector cells.

An example of defects in the regulation of inflammation leading to chronic inflammation and disease is systemic lupus erythematosus (SLE) occurring in the context of complement deficiency. In this situation, a specific defect in host innate immunity results in abnormal clearance of immune complexes and apoptotic cells, resulting in tissue damage and possibly providing a stimulus for the development of autoimmunity.

Infection is the most common example of a foreign antigen persisting and causing chronic inflammation, for example, hepatitis C infection resulting in chronic hepatic damage and the subsequent development of cryoglobulinaemia. Among rheumatic diseases, tuberculosis, osteomyelitis, and HIV are typical examples.

Clonal disorders are much rarer, as in T cell neoplasms, for example, hypereosinophilic syndrome, or Castleman's disease, where cytokine production leads to persistent inflammation. Alternatively, clonal proliferations of B lymphocytes results in the production of an IgM rheumatoid factor, which complexes with IgG, resulting in cryoglobulinaemia, the clinical consequences of which are vasculitis, Raynauds, neuropathy, and glomerulonephritis (O'Shea et al. 1987; Callard and Turner 1990).

Genetic factors in inflammation

Complement genes

Figure 1 is a simplified diagram of the complement system. Inherited homozygous deficiencies of C1q, C1r, C1s, C4, or C2 are associated with SLE. There is a hierarchy of severity and susceptibility, according to the position of the missing protein within the classical pathway of complement activation. More than 90 per cent of patients with homozygous C1q deficiency develop SLE, typically at an early age. Disease is characterized by severe rashes, with a significant proportion of patients developing glomerulonephritis and/or cerebral lupus. A wide range of extractable nuclear antigen autoantibodies, incuding anti-Ro, anti-Sm, and anti-RNP, are found in these patients; anti-dsDNA antibodies are rarer. Approximately one-third of patients with C2 deficiency develop SLE and the autoantibody profile tends to be restricted to the presence of anti-Ro antibodies. The severity of disease is similar to that seen in lupus patients without homozygous complement deficiency. C3 deficiency is not usually associated with the development of full-blown SLE and up to one-third of C3-deficient patients develop a prominent rash in association with pyogenic infections.

Deficiency of two control proteins of the alternative complement activation pathway, Factor I and Factor H, is associated with severe secondary C3 deficiency due to a failure in regulating the alternative pathway of C3 cleavage. These patients show a similar phenotype to C3 deficiency and suffer from recurrent pyogenic infections and, occasionally, develop glomerulonephritis without autoantibody formation.

All four complement genes located in the Class III region of the major histocompatability complex (MHC) (C4A, C4B, C2, and Factor B) exhibit extensive genetic polymorphism. In the case of C4A and C4B this includes frequent 'null' alleles. The resultant partial deficiency of the C4 proteins has been found to be associated with SLE in different ethnic populations.

In patients with hereditary angioedema due to heterozygous C1 inhibitor deficiency, prolonged reduction in C4 and C2 levels occurs due to partially unregulated activity of C1r and C1s. Disordered regulation of both cell-mediated and humoral immunity has been described in these patients. Patients with prolonged, acquired C3 deficiency due to the presence of the autoantibody, C3 nephritic factor, develop SLE many years after presentation, in association with partial lipodystrophy. These associations lead to the hypothesis that the complement is key to the pathophysiology of these conditions and extensive surveys performed in normal populations showing that inherited homozygous complement deficiency in healthy individuals is extremely rare (Walport 1993).

Evidence for the role of complement and immune complexes in autoimmunity comes from animal models of complement deficiency. Dogs from a colony with C3 deficiency develop a very similar pattern of

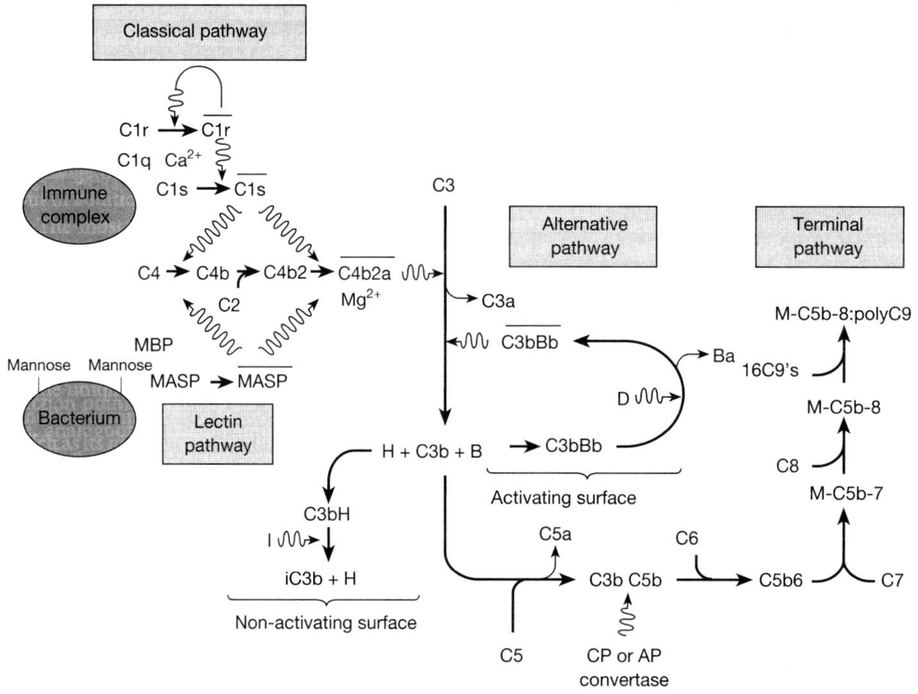

Fig. 1 Simplified diagram of the complement system. Complement may be activated by the classical pathway, the alternative pathway, or the newly characterized 'lectin' pathway, which is initiated by the binding of the collectin, mannose-binding protein, to bacterial surfaces rich in this carbohydrate. The 'amplification loop' of the alternative pathway on an activating surface can amplify C3 activation initiated by the other pathways, or by exogenous proteases from leucocytes, plasma (e.g. plasmin), or bacteria.

glomerulonephritis to that seen in C3-deficient humans (Botto and Walport 1993). Some pigs in Norway developed a severe, mesangiocapillary glomerulonephritis of early onset and were shown to have hereditary Factor H deficiency (Hogasen et al. 1997). C1q-deficient mice develop antinuclear antibodies and a significant proportion of the animals die with crescentic glomerulonephritis (Botto 1998).

Cytokine genes

Cytokines are key mediators of humoral and cellular inflammation. The best examples of polymorphic variation in cytokine genes resulting in susceptibility to rheumatic disease, or affecting the severity of the condition, are found in the tumour necrosis factor (TNF)α locus, the interleukin (IL)-1 gene cluster, and IL-6.

TNFα locus

TNFα is a key pro-inflammatory cytokine and is also responsible for apoptosis. Common TNF polymorphisms are illustrated in Fig. 2. The first polymorphic variant in the TNFα gene was described in the promoter region and consisted of an A–G nucleotide change 308 base pairs upstream of the transcription start site (Wilson et al. 1993). The rarer allele, −308A, occurred in approximately 20 per cent of populations in Western Europe and West Africa.

The −308 allele is part of the extended MHC haplotype commonly associated with autoimmunity, A1, B8, DR3, and DQ2. Many autoimmune diseases are associated with this haplotype, including insulin-dependent diabetes, SLE, coeliac disease, myaesthenia, and thyroiditis. Functional studies, using tranfection assays, demonstrate that the −308A allele is more efficient at directing transcription of a reporter gene than the more common −308G allele, but the results are still controversial. Nevertheless, these results led a number of investigators to explore the role of this polymorphic variant in a variety of infectious and autoimmune diseases, with the hypothesis that this allele might result in a more severe inflammatory

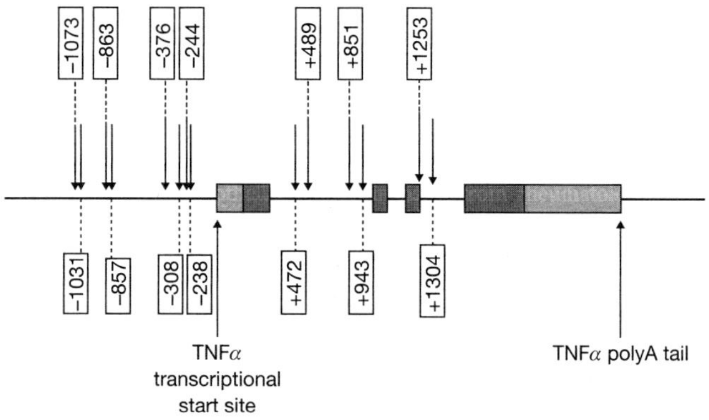

Fig. 2 A representative set of TNF SNPs and their location within the gene relative to the transcriptional start site (derived from GenBank sequence M16441). Dark grey boxes denote exons, while light grey boxes denote the 5′ and 3′ untranslated regions of the locus.

phenotype. An eightfold increased risk of death from cerebral malaria in a population in Gambia was subsequently found and the data appeared to support this view (McGuire et al. 1999).

The role of the TNFα locus has been studied in multiplex rheumatoid arthritis families. At least 14 single nucelotide polymorphisms (SNPs) have been found for the TNFα gene, eight being within the promoter region. In British Caucasians, two of the promoter polymorphisms are monomorphic (Zeggini et al. 2002). By transmission disequilibrium testing, the −308A and −857T alleles were found to be associated with rheumatoid arthritis in patients carrying the human leucocyte antigen (HLA)–DR shared epitope. Further stratification of data indicated that the −308A allele was significantly associated with susceptibility to rheumatoid arthritis in individuals heterozygous for the shared epitope, with a significance only occurring in patients carrying HLA–DR4, while the −857T allele was significant in individuals homozygous for the shared epitope (Waldron-Lynch et al. 2001).

More recently, investigators have explored the association between rheumatoid arthritis, TNF polymorphisms, and HLA alleles in non-caucasian populations. In Peruvian Mestizo patients, for example, it was observed that TNFα and HLA–DRB1*1402 independently conferred an increased risk of the disease (Castro et al. 2001).

The TNF locus has been found to be associated with juvenile idiopathic arthritis (JIA) also. A recent UK transmission disequilibrium testing of JIA has shown that −238G, +489A, and +851A alleles are significantly associated with persistent oligiarticular JIA. None of these SNPs are in linkage disequilibrium with HLA-A and DRB1 alleles associated with JIA (Zeggini et al. 2002). The −308A SNP has also been associated with juvenile dermatomyositis in the context of the autoimmune haplotype and −238A with anklylosing spondylitis in HLA-B27 negative individuals (Pachman et al. 2000; Gonzalez et al. 2001).

IL-1 and IL-1RN

IL-1 is an early response cytokine in inflammation. This, with its family members, is found in a cluster on chromosome 2q14-21. The genes found in this clusters are IL-1α, IL-β, IL-1 receptor antagonist (RA), IL-1 receptor type-1 (R1), and IL-18 receptor (R). A number of polymorphisms have been described across the region and specific genotypes defined by these DNA markers are over-represented in inflammatory diseases.

Several IL-1α polymorphisms have been described. The rarer variant, at position 889, was associated with an increase in JIA of the early onset pauciarticular type in Norwegian children, particularly in patients with a high ESR and chronic ocular inflammation, but this was not replicated in a larger UK population.

An association between psoriasis and a variant of IL-1α (exon 5 +3953) has been described, and early studies indicated that the rarer +3953 allele is related to the *in vitro* production of the cytokine (Cork et al. 1993). This is of interest as there is evidence that IL-1α is a key pro-inflammatory cytokine in immune-mediated skin disease of IL-1α transgenic mice (Groves et al. 1995). The most studied IL-RA genetic marker, in a clinical context, is found in intron 2, where there is a variable number of tandem repeats of an 86-bp sequence (Tarlow et al. 1993). More than five alleles are found in most human populations, but greater than 95 per cent of individuals have either four or two alleles. The frequency of IL-1RN2 is increased in a variety of conditions, including SLE, ulcerative colitis, alopecia areata, lichen sclerosis, and MS, but replication and family studies are needed to confirm association and linkage with disease. The frequency of different alleles in the IL-1β gene (at −511 and +3954), as well as the IL-1RA gene (at +2018), have been investigated in an association study involving 297 rheumatoid arthritis patients and 112 healthy controls from the same geographic area. Associations with rheumatoid arthritis susceptibility and severity as well as levels of IL-1RA and IL-1β were tested. The data suggest that the IL-1β (+3954) genetic variant is an important marker for the severity of joint destruction in rheumatoid arthritis and is associated with an imbalance in IL-1RA production. This genetic association was independent and additive to the risk of HLA–DR4/DR1 status, so it may be useful as a prognostic marker in early disease (Buchs et al. 2001).

IL-4 and IL-4R loci

IL-4 is a key cytokine in the polarization of T helper cells (Th) to type II phenotype. Variants of the IL-4 and IL-4R genes in patients with rheumatoid arthritis have recently been evaluated (Buchs et al. 2000). Allelic frequencies for polymorphisms in the IL-4 (variable number of tandem repeat polymorphism in intron 3) and IL-4Rα (transition at nucleotide 1902) genes were assessed in 335 rheumatoid arthritis patients and 104 controls. The frequency of the rare IL-4(2) allele was higher in patients with non-destructive rheumatoid arthritis (40 per cent) than in those with destructive rheumatoid arthritis and controls. Patients with this rare allele had significantly less joint destruction, assessed by the Larsen wrist index and a lower ESR. A significantly higher carriage rate of IL-4(2) was seen in HLA–DR4/DR1(−) patients with non-destructive rheumatoid arthritis, than in patients with destructive rheumatoid arthritis. This study suggested that the IL-4 allele may be a marker for good prognosis in rheumatoid arthritis. Like all single reports of association, confirmation from family or replicative studies is required.

IL-6

This cytokine is induced by multiple stimuli, including lipopolysaccharide (LPS), IL-1, and TNFα, and its production leads to further activation of pro-inflammatory molecules such as adhesion molecules and chemokines as well as inhibitors of IL-1 and TNF. In addition, it has effects on cells involved in the adaptive immune response, the hypothalamus and osteoblasts. There are three SNPs and a variable AT tract in the promoter (Fig. 3). All of these have been found to affect the rate of transcription of the gene. The −174G allele was found to be the most common, as well as most efficient, in gene expression (Fishman et al. 1998; Jeffery et al. 2003). The first disease association was with systemic JIA, and has recently been confirmed with a multicentre, multinational family study (Ogilvie et al. 2003). The −174G allele was significantly transmitted in excess and is consistent with the high serum levels of IL-6 found in this disease. The −174G allele has also been found to be associated, in case–control studies, with increased bone turnover in post-menopausal women, peak bone mass in adolescent men and pre-menopausal women with insulin, dependent diabetes (Ogilvie et al. 2003). Of interest is that the C allele is associated with an increased risk of coronary heart disease.

Fcg receptor genes

There are a number of reviews describing the relationship between polymorphisms of the genes encoding human Fc receptors and rheumatic disease (Salmon and Pricop 2001). FcγRIIα expressed on monocytes, platelets, and PMN is encoded by two co-dominantly expressed alleles (H and R131) bearing either a histidine or an arginine at amino acid position 131. The two variants differ in their capacity to bind immunoglobulin. The H131 variant binds IgG2 very efficiently, while R131 binds with low affinity. FcγRIIIα has two codominantly expressed allelic variants, F176 and V176, differing in one amino acid, phenylalanine or valine (Edberg et al. 1989; Kimberly et al. 1989). Homozygosity for V176 results in more avid binding of IgG1 and IgG3 than F176 homozygotes. Two common allelic variants of the neutrophil receptor FcγRIIIβ have also been described (NA1 and NA2), but IgG binding is not affected (Salmon et al. 1990). There is some evidence that FcγRIIIβ NA1/NA1 homozygous neutrophils have enhanced phagocytic responses compared with NA2/NA2 cells as a result of greater degranulation and oxidative burst responses in the former.

It has been suggested that FcγR genetic variants, encoding receptors that have an impaired capacity to ligate IgG in immune complexes, are likely to be susceptibility genes for SLE. This is supported by association studies suggesting FcγRIIα-R131 and FcγRIIIα-F176 are enriched in patients with

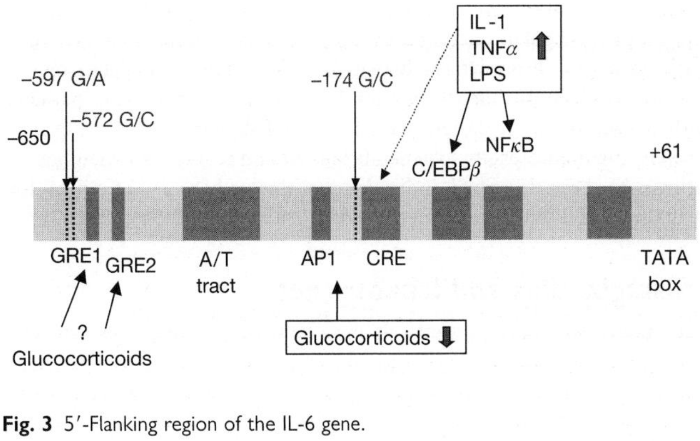

Fig. 3 5′-Flanking region of the IL-6 gene.

the disease (Duits et al. 1995; Salmon et al. 1996). More recent evidence from genome scanning in African-American SLE patients has also linked the FcγR gene cluster on chromosome 1q with lupus. However, this area remains controversial and associations between SLE and low-binding alleles have not been demonstrated in all populations studied (Botto et al. 1996). Current evidence would support an association between SLE and the FcγIIα-R131 allele in African-American patients, while in Caucasians the link with the FcγRIIIα-F176 variant appears more convincing. More specific associations with lupus nephritis, anti-C1q autoantibodies, and the FcγIIα-R131 variant have been described independently (Norsworthy et al. 1999). This suggests these genes have a role in dictating severity of disease, rather than acting as susceptibility factors.

FcγR allelic variants have been studied in Wegener's granulomatosis and rheumatoid arthritis. In rheumatoid arthritis, an increased frequency of FcγRIIIα-F176 homozygosity has been observed (Dijstelbloem et al. 1999). In Wegener's granulomatosis, the situation remains unresolved, but there is some evidence that a 'high'-binding variant of FcγRIIIβ on neutrophils predisposes to more severe disease, possibly as a consequence of facilitation of the binding of pathogenic ANCA to PMN.

Humoral mechanisms

A wide range of humoral mechanisms are involved in inflammation. These are enzyme cascades under tight regulatory control preventing autologous tissue damage. Overstimulation of the pathway, induced by an exogenous stimulus, or autoantibody and/or disruption of these regulatory mechanisms, can result in tissue injury and systemic upset. The main pathways that come into this category are the complement system, the coagulation and fibrinolysis systems, and the prostaglandin and leukotriene pathways.

Complement and immune complexes

The detailed biology of the complement system has been reviewed (Walport 2001a,b). Figure 1 illustrates the key pathways involved in complement activation. Activation of the complement, in the context of autoimmune disease, is mediated by the classical pathway. The resultant effects of complement activation are mediated by the insertion of the membrane attack complex into target cell membranes and ligation of specific receptors for complement split products on leucocytes.

Activation and cleavage of C3, C4, and C5 result in the production of anaphylotoxins, C3a and C5a, and opsonic molecules, C4b, C3b, C3dg, and iC3b. Receptors for these molecules are found on most leucocytes of both the mononuclear cell and granulocyte lineages. Chemotaxis and cellular activation result from the ligation of anaphylotoxin receptors. Opsonic receptor ligation also facilitates phagocytosis and cell activation, in addition to the activation via binding of the membrane attack complex at sub-lytic levels.

Fibrinolysis, coagulation, and kinin systems

These triggered enzyme cascades have an important role to play in diverse inflammatory sites. The mononuclear infiltrate in rheumatoid pannus produces procoagulant factors activating the coagulation system. There is also evidence for fibrinolytic activity in the inflamed joint and kallirein, and complement split products have been found in joint effusions in patients with active disease. A patient with factor XII deficiency (resulting in a severely impaired capacity to generate kinins) and co-incident rheumatoid arthritis has been described, indicating that this pathway is not critical for the pathological changes in rheumatoid arthritis (Donaldson et al. 1972).

Prostaglandins and leukotrienes

Eicosanoids play an important role in inflammation. Salicylates, conventional non-steroidal and the newly developed cyclooxygenase (COX)-2 inhibitors are all known to be highly effective anti-inflammatory agents in rheumatic disease. Figure 4 illustrates the metabolism of arachidonic acid.

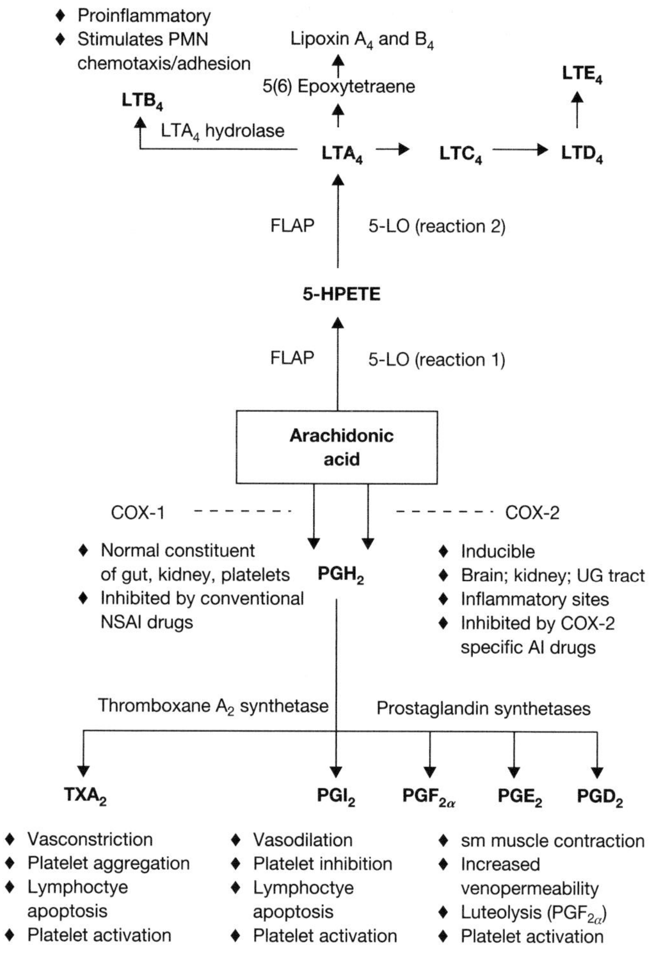

Fig. 4 The metabolism of arachidonic acid.

Cell types found in the inflamed joint can mobilize membrane arachidonic acid, metabolized to a range of pro-inflammatory mediators of the prostaglandin and leukotriene family (e.g. prostaglandin E_2, thromboxane A_2, leukotriene B_4, and prostacyclin). Certain of these mediators, including prostaglandin E_2 and prostacyclin, also have suppressive effects on inflammation (Funk 2001).

IL-1 and TNFα, amongst other cytokines, stimulate the activation of phospholipase A_2, releasing arachidonic acid from membrane phospholipids. This process may be inhibited by lipocortins, part of the anti-inflammatory effects produced by corticosteroids. Metabolism of arachidonate by lipoxygenase (primarily found in mammalian leucocytes) results in the production of leukotrienes. This pathway also has other substrates, such as eicosopentanoic acid, metabolized to the less potent pentaenoic leukotrienes. Metabolism of arachidonate by enzymes of the COX family results in prostaglandin production. These molecules have a range of pro-inflammatory effects, including local vasodilatation within the microcirculation, amplification of the effects of other mediators, causing oedema, and the stimulation of local pain receptors.

Leukotriene B_4 is a chemotactic agent for polymorphs and this group of mediators can have vasodilatory effects. Selective leukotriene B_4 inhibition has been shown to reduce severity of collagen-induced arthritis in mice (Griffiths et al. 1995) and there is increasing interest in the use of similar inhibitors in human inflammatory rheumatic disease. As with many biological systems, in the LT/PG system, there is a balance of pro- and anti-inflammatory effects. Prostaglandin E_2 can inhibit the synthesis of IL-1 and TNFα, but there is conflicting evidence in relation to its role in cartilage degradation and the interaction with these cytokines at a cellular level (Arsenis and McDonnell 1989; Stadler et al. 1991; Mohamed-Ali 1995; LeGrand et al. 2001).

Two forms of COX exist. COX-1 is constitutively expressed in many mammalian tissues and thought to have a major role in the synthesis of protaglandins within the GI tract mediating mucosal protection. COX-2 is an inducible form of the enzyme, primarily found at sites of inflammation and upregulated in response to pro-inflammatory stimuli. A wide range of drugs is now available specifically to inhibit COX-2 and evidence shows that these drugs have fewer adverse gastrointestinal side-effects than conventional non-steroidal anti-inflammatory drugs (NSAIDs) (see Chapter 4.5.1). However, the biology of COX inhibition remains far from fully elucidated and concerns remain in relation to the cardiovascular effects of COX-2 inhibition, bearing in mind that COX-2 is the main source of endothelial-derived prostacyclin (Verma et al. 2001). There is also experimental evidence that COX inhibitors may have a role in inhibiting T cell activation due to their ability to block transcription factors required for the expression of inducible response genes after T cell receptor (TCR) engagement. There is also evidence, from both epidemiologic and animal studies, that COX inhibition may have a role in cancer prevention. In both cases, the biological and clinical importance of these observations are unclear (Vainio 2001; Paccani et al. 2002).

Neuroendocrine factors in inflammation

Neural factors

Antidromic connections in sensory neurones are major contributors to the classical triple response (redness, flare, and weal) observed after injury to the skin. Synovium has a rich nerve supply and contains a network of small, unmyelinated afferent C fibres. These fibres release neuropeptides, including substance P. Synovial blood vessels also have an autonomic nerve supply, comprising primarily different noradrenergic synthetic fibres transmitting, among other mediators, neuropeptide Y (Kidd et al. 1990) (see also Chapter 3.5).

Triple response is mediated by substance P, causing vasodilatation and enhanced vascular mobility. Intrasynovial C fibres result in similar physiological effects. Synovial neuropeptides have a variety of potential pro- and anti-inflammatory actions (see Chapters 3.5 and 3.9). The most studied mediator is substance P which stimulates prostaglandin E2 synthesis, collagenase synthesis and cell division in the synoviocyte, and promotes neutrophil chemotaxis and degranulation. Substance P, also stimulates T cell proliferation, the synthesis of thromboxane-B2 by macrophage mast cell degranulation, leading to the release of histamine, and other inflammatory mediators.

Joint injury causes reflex inhibition of surrounding musculature, a factor in the muscle wasting around an inflamed joint and pain is a major stimulus of this phenomenon (see Chapter 3.9). While this response is physiologically appropriate after an acute injury, in the context of chronic inflammation it has adverse effects. The sympathetic nervous system has been explored in a number of animal models in the context of joint inflammation and has been shown to be more severe in animals with a higher basal sympathetic tone than in controls (Basbaum and Levine 1991).

Endocrine factors

There are associations between endocrine deficiency, or overactivity states, and rheumatic diseases, such as the arthropathy of acromegaly and Hoffman's syndrome. There is evidence to indicate that both sex hormones (e.g. the preponderance of the female sex in SLE and rheumatoid arthritis) and the hypothalamic–pituitary–adrenal axis are involved in the pathology of rheumatic diseases.

The hypothalamic–pituitary–adrenal axis

Evidence that the hyothalamic–pituitary–adrenal axis regulates inflammation comes from *in vitro* experimental observations, animal studies, and genetic studies of corticotrophin-releasing hormone (CRH). The production of CRH by the hypothalamus may be directly, or indirectly, influenced by a range of pro-inflammatory cytokines. The resultant downstream stimulation of adrenocorticotropic hormone (ACTH) and anti-inflammatory glucocorticoids may be an important mechanism in regulating inflammatory response. There is evidence that dysregulation of the control of these mechanisms influences the severity of inflammation. For example, there are differences in the severity of experimentally-induced arthritis observed in rats such as the Lewis rat, where CRH is blunted in response to stress, compared to the histocompatible Fischer rat. The latter are relatively resistant to adjuvant and streptococcal cell wall-induced arthritis and their susceptibility may be induced by hypophysectomy or adrenalectomy (Wilder 2002).

In man there are indications that the hypothalamic–pituitary axis is abnormal in patients with rheumatoid arthritis. Normal cortisol response to hip surgery was blunted in rheumatoid arthritis patients, compared with osteoarthritic controls (Chikanza et al. 1992) and studies suggest that diurnal variation of cortisol in rheumatoid arthritis is inappropriate to the level of inflammation observed (Neeck et al. 1990).

Peripheral expression of CRH is more complex (Karalis et al. 1991). CRH receptors are present on a variety of cells important to the arthritic immune response. CRH can be produced by peripheral blood mononuclear cells and this expression is increased at sites of inflammation. Association of the microsatellite marker, CRHRA1, is described in rheumatoid arthritis in 295 affected sibling pair families. Recently, positional cloning and sequence analyses have identified the genomic region linking the CRHRA1 marker and the CRH structural locus and a further marker, CRHRA2, was identified in strong linkage dysequilibrium with CRHRA1. The haplotypes CRHRA1*10 and CRHRA2*14 were found to be significantly overtransmitted in multiplex families with rheumatoid arthritis (Fife et al. 2002).

Sex hormones and arthritis

More females than males suffer from several rheumatic diseases, for example, SLE is nine times more common in adult females than males. Symptoms frequently develop around the time of puberty and improve post-menopausally. There is also evidence that the lupus is exacerbated by oestrogen-containing oral contraceptives, or when rapid changes in hormone levels occur, such as in the puerperium. Lupus patients are hyperoestrogenic, with reduced levels of testosterone (Lahita et al. 1993). There is an increased risk of rheumatoid arthritis in nulliparous females and evidence that the pill may be protective. There is increased susceptibility to rheumatoid arthritis during the first 3–4 months post-partum, with evidence that established disease improves during pregnancy (Silman 1994). The best example of the role of sex hormones in an animal model of rheumatic disease is in the NZB NZW F1 mouse. These animals develop a lupus-like syndrome and androgens clearly have a protective effect, while oestrogen exacerbates the severity of their disease.

A number of families are described with SLE occurring in multiple male members (Lahita 1983) and this has been regarded as the human counterpart of the BXSB mouse, another experimental model of lupus. In this animal, a variety of genes have been implicated in disease and a gene on the Y chromosome, the Yaa gene, has been shown to confer disease-enhanced susceptibility in a manner independent of sex hormone levels (Hogarth et al. 1998).

The other sex hormone extensively studied in rheumatoid arthritis is prolactin. Lymphocytes and cells of the mononuclear phagocytic system bear high affinity prolactin receptors and evidence shows excessive secretion of prolactin in patients with rheumatoid arthritis (Chikanza et al. 1993). There are a number of studies where drugs, such as bromocriptine, have been used for the experimental treatment of this condition, while hyperprolactaemia has been associated with exacerbation of lupus (McMurray et al. 1994) and collagen-induced arthritis (Mattsson et al. 1992). However, there is no clinical or experimental evidence that pharmacological interference with the prolactin system is of any therapeutic benefit in inflammatory arthritis or lupus.

Cytokines

Background

Cytokines are extracellular peptide mediators regulating cell growth, differentiation cellular activation, and interaction. Cytokines that are produced by leucocytes have a role in inflammation and immune responses and, in particular, linking innate and adaptive immune responses are called interleukins. There are 31 interleukins at the time of writing, but more are being discovered all the time. They can be grouped into families according to their structure or shared receptors (Table 1). TNFα is not named as an interleukin for historical reasons but exhibits a very similar range of biological activities. Characteristically, they have multiple functions that overlap with each other, largely due to their shared receptors and intracellular signalling pathways (Oppenheim et al. 2001).

The advent of specific immunoassays for cytokines was followed by the detection of these factors *in vivo* and identifying their relations to different indices of disease activity. The best correlations with systemic inflammatory disease have been obtained with IL-1β, IL-6, and TNFα. In situ hybridization studies have shown that the main source of IL-1β in rheumatoid joint synovium is the CD14+ macrophage (Wood et al. 1992). The stimuli for macrophage activation in rheumatoid arthritis are unknown, but the production of IL-1 by macrophages can be activated in an autocrine fashion by IL-1β, TNFα, other cytokines, and immune complexes.

The activity of a cytokine *in vivo* is the net effect of its concentration and the presence of inhibitory molecules. The shedding of cell-surface cytokine receptors has been found to occur widely and the shed receptors retain affinity for their ligands. They act as binding proteins competing with the cell-surface receptor for free ligands, thus acting as inhibitors (Symons et al. 1991). Some soluble receptors are stimulatory rather than inhibitory. For example, the complex formed between IL-6 and its soluble receptor stimulates the IL-6 signalling receptor gp130.

Other cytokine inhibitory molecules include IL-1RA, which has the same affinity to the two IL-1 surface receptors, but receptor occupancy does not transduce an activating signal. This molecule acts as a receptor antagonist and, along with inhibitory cytokines, such as naturally occurring antibodies to pro-inflammatory cytokines, IL-10 and transforming growth factor (TGF)β, has therapeutic potential.

Local and systemic inflammatory responses can often be explained by the actions of the major monocyte-derived cytokines IL-1α, IL-1β, IL-6, IL-8, and TNFα. The other major group of cytokines in the context of inflammation consist of immunomodulating interleukins, which are largely lymphocyte derived, includes TNFα amd IL-6.

Cytokine and cytokine receptor families

There are well over 100 molecules classified as cytokines, however, it is possible to identify large families of molecules based on sequence or structural homology of the DNA or proteins, or common usage of receptors (see Tables 1 and 2). Other important cytokines include the first described cytokine, macrophage inhibitory factor (MIF), which is pro-inflammatory, by stimulating other pro-inflammatory cytokines and suppressing the anti-inflammatory effects of glucocorticoids. There are viral homologues of a number of cytokines, such as IL-6, IL-10, vascular endothelial growth factor (VEGF), epidermal growth factor (EGF), and TGFα, and their interactions with host cells have yet to be explored in detail.

Regulation of cytokine gene expression is mainly at the transcriptional level, but regulation of the mRNA stability and, therefore, their usually short half-life, is an important factor in the overall control of inducible cytokines. Both mechanisms are dictated by common DNA sequences in the gene, serving as binding sites for transcription-enhancing factors, or mRNA, stabilizing or destabilizing proteins.

Cytokine receptor molecules are structurally dissimilar, but a major subgroup, called the haematopoietin receptor family, can be distinguished with shared structural features. It is possible to recognize homologous sequences in cytokine receptors representing an extended family, or similar receptors. These sequences have been found in vertebrates and invertebrates, suggesting important and highly conserved functions.

Table 1 Cytokines and chemotactic cytokines (chemokines) grouped by structural similarity of ligands and/or receptors

Haematopoietins	Interleukins 2, 3, 4, 5, 6, 7, 9, 11, 12 (p35), erythropoietin, leukaemia inhibitory factor, granulocyte-macrophage colony-stimulating factor, granulocyte colony-stimulating factor, oncostatin M, ciliary neurotropic factor, growth hormone, thrombopoietin, cardiotropin-1, leptin
TNF family	Tumour necrosis factor α, lymphotoxin α, β, CD40 ligand, CD30 ligand, CD27 ligand, Fas ligand, RANK ligand
IL-1 family	IL-1α, β, IL-1 receptor antagonist, IL-1 receptor I, IL-18 receptor, basic and acidic fibroblast growth factor, endothelial growth factor
α (CXC) family	IL-8, melanocyte growth-stimulating actor, neutrophil-activating protein, epithelial neutrophil-activating peptide, granulocyte chemotactic protein, platelet factor 4, connective tissue-activating peptide 3, monokine induced by IFNγ, IFNγ-inducible protein CX3C chemokine: fractalkine
β (CC) family	Monocyte chemoattractant proteins 1, 2, 3, macrophage inflammatory protein 1α, β, regulated upon activation, normal T cell expressed and secreted, I-309 C chemokine: lymphotactin
PDGF family	Platelet-derived growth factor A, B, macrophage colony-stimulating factor, stem cell factor
TGFβ family	Transforming growth factor β, inhibin β 2A, 2B, Activin 1 2A, 2B, 4, bone morphogenic protein
Interferon family	α and γ interferon, IL-10, 19, 20, 22, 28, 29

Table 2 Cytokine inhibitors

Inhibitors	Examples
Soluble, extracellular domain of cytokine receptors	Soluble TNFRs p55 and p75, soluble IL-1 receptors I and II, soluble IFNγ receptor, soluble gp130
Receptor antagonists and cytokine antibodies	IL-1 receptor antagonist, antibodies to IL-1, IL-6
Cytokines with mostly inhibitory properties	IL-4, IL-10, IL-13 for T helper 1 cells, IFNγ for T helper 2 cells, transforming growth factor β
Low affinity inhibitors	α_2-Macroglobulin
Glucocorticoids	

The tumour necrosis factor receptor superfamily

The tumour necrosis factor receptor (TNFR) superfamily is involved in lymphocyte signal transduction and the most important members of the TNFR superfamily are TNFR type 1 (TNFR1), TNFR type 2 (TNFR2), and Fas (CD95). TNFR1 and TNFR2 bind to TNFα and were the first members of the TNFR family to be identified. Studies performed in gene-targeted mice lacking expression of TNFR1 demonstrate that this receptor is involved in signalling, leading to inflammation and cell survival (Pfeffer et al. 1993). However, it has been observed that programmed cell death was impaired in TNFR1−/− mutants (Zheng et al. 1995). Therefore, TNFR1 mediates cell survival, inflammatory signalling, and proapoptotic signalling in response to a single ligand.

In response to TNFα binding, however, TNFR2 transduces signals principally for survival and inflammation (Yeh et al. 1999) and CD95 primarily mediates proapoptotic signals in response to the binding of its ligand FasL. Mice deficient in Fas, or FasL, show lymphoadenopathy and lymphocyte homeostasis is disrupted due to a lack of efficient programmed cell death.

TNFR superfamily members are categorized into two classes, based on the adaptor molecules recruited to their cytoplasmic domains. Class 1 receptors contain a death domain (DD) in the cytoplasmic tails and include TNFR1, Fas, death receptor (DR)3, DR4, DR5, and DR6 (Locksley et al. 2001). The DD in a receptor tail recruits intracellular adaptor proteins that also contain a DD. TNFR1's DD binds to the TNFα receptor-associated death domain protein (TRADD) and Fas contains a DD that binds to both Fas-associated death domain protein (FADD) and receptor-interacting protein (RIP) (Strasser et al. 2000; Baud and Karin 2001). Class 2 of TNFR superfamily receptors includes TNFR2, CD30, CD40, lymphotoxin receptor, the osteoprotegerin ligand (OPGL), receptor activator of NFκ-B (RANK), and B-lymphocyte activating factor (BAFF) receptors (Laabi et al. 2001; Locksley et al. 2001). The cytoplasmic tails of these receptors do not contain DDs, but have sequences permitting them to associate with a different set of intracellular adaptors called TNF receptor-associated factors (TRAFs) (Wajant et al. 2001). Six TRAF proteins have been identified to date (TRAF1–TRAF6), but only five (TRAF1, TRAF2, TRAF3, TRAF5, and TRAF6) actually bind to the cytoplasmic tails of the second class of TNFR superfamily receptors. Knock-out mice for signalling proteins downstream of these receptors have been generated and further insight into apoptotic mechanisms, amongst other consequences of TNFR ligation, could potentially provide new therapeutic targets.

Cytokines and T cell differentiation

Helper T cells (Th-CD4+) can be divided into two types depending on the function and range of the interleukins produced. Those that secrete IL-2, interferon-γ (IFNγ), IL-3, granulocyte-macrophage colony stimulating factor (GM-CSF), TNFα, and lymphotoxins are known as Th1 cells. These cells are involved in generating cell-mediated immunity targeted at intracellular pathogens, resulting in the delayed-type hypersensitivity response and are found in many chronic inflammatory diseases. Th2 cells secrete B-cell growth and differentiation factors IL-4, IL-5, IL-6, IL-10, IL-3, GM-CSF, and TNFα, inducing a predominantly humoral immune response that, generates antibodies. These two major pathways of T cell differentiation are mutually antagonistic and usually one type predominates in response to an antigenic challenge. In chronic inflammatory diseases with a cellular immune component, it may be possible to suppress inflammation with Th2 cytokines, such as IL-10, effective in abrogating collagen-induced arthritis in murine gene-transfer studies (Quattrocchi et al. 2001).

A coordinated programme of molecular events, initiated at the outset of T cell differentiation, leads to the generation of CD4+ Th effector cells and the outcome of this process dictates the host response to an exogenous stimulus. T-regulatory cells are also generated to maintain homeostasis. Three main stages are thought to be required for the acquisition of effector competence in T cells. These are often sub-divided into an initiation phase, a commitment phase, and a phase of acute gene transcription. In the initiation phase, naive T cells are engaged through their TCRs, by MHC/peptide complexes expressed on the surface of dendritic cells (DCs), followed by engagement of accessory surface molecules. Cytokines produced by DCs and T cells may lead to further differentiation. IL-12 and IL-18 are important for differentiation into Th1 cells. Evidence indicates that this initial engagement phase lasts from hours to days and usually results in the production of IL-2 and entry of the T cell into cell cycling. IL-1, IL-6, and TNFα contribute to the upregulation of the IL-2 receptor on the T cells. The commitment phase is characterized by the induction and recruitment of Th-subset-specific transcription factors, including GATA-3 and c-Maf for Th2 cells (Ho et al. 1996; Ouyang et al. 1998) and T-bet and ERM for Th1 cells (Ouyang et al. 1999; Szabo et al. 2000). Concommitant IL-4 signalling can affect this process. At this stage, differentiation is stabilized even in the absence of further TCR activation. Acute gene transcription is determined by secondary contact with antigen and necessitates the recruitment, to the transcription complex, of the nuclear factor of activated T cells (NFAT), together with subset-specific transcription factors. Finally, the initiation of lymphocyte proliferation is influenced by IL-15.

Cytokines in rheumatoid arthritis (also see Chapter 6.3.1)

Reports of IL-1 in rheumatoid arthritis exudates coincided with the demonstration that IL-1 was produced by mononuclear cells *in vitro* with potentially arthritogenic stimuli. *In vitro* synovial cells from rheumatoid arthritis joints were found to release IL-1 and concentrations of IL-1β in the blood of patients with rheumatoid arthritis was correlated with markers of disease activity (Eastgate et al. 1988). The main source of IL-1 in rheumatoid arthritis is the CD14+ synovial macrophage (Wood et al. 1992). The role of IL-1 in rheumatoid arthritis is evident from the success of therapeutic agents, such as IL-1 receptor anatagonist (Gabay 2002).

The other major cytokine implicated in rheumatoid arthritis is TNFα. In addition to its own pro-inflammatory activities, TNFα is also a potent inducer of IL-1. Spontaneous production of IL-1, by explanted synovial cells from rheumatoid joints, is inhibited by a TNFα antibody (Brennan et al. 1989). This demonstrates that the suppression of a wider cytokine cascade is achievable through the inhibition of a single cytokine. Clinical trials of a humanized antibody to TNFα in patients with rheumatoid arthritis were followed and sustained improvements in laboratory markers of inflammation and the clinical condition of the patients were reported (Elliott et al. 1993), leading to the development of new drugs.

Synovial mononuclear-cell infiltrates, including T cells, are chronically exposed to TNFα *in vivo* and a number of model systems have been devised to explore the consequences of this phenomenon. TCR variable signalling is impaired by TNFα. When recombinant TNFα was added repeatedly to T cell cultures, mimicking the sustained TNFα signalling believed to exist in inflamed joints, T cell activation was suppressed (Cope et al. 1994). Another study suggests that TNFα is costimulatory and a growth factor for T cells (Yokota et al. 1988). Peripheral blood T cell responses of patients with rheumatoid arthritis were rapidly restored after treatment with anti-TNFα (Cope et al. 1994). There is also a relationship between these parameters and clinical improvement (Elliott et al. 1994).

Angiogenesis and inflammation in the joints

Angiogenesis is critical to the pathogenesis of rheumatoid arthritis, as the development of new vessels is one of the earliest changes in rheumatoid synovium (Koch 1998, 2000). This neovascularization permits the delivery of cells, pro-inflammatory molecules and nutrients to the developing pannus. Proangiogenic cytokines have been identified in the rheumatoid joint, including VEGF, TNFα, basic fibroblast growth factor, TGFβ, and chemokines such as IL-8 (Koch et al. 1994; Feldmann 1996). VEGF is stimulated by hypoxia, as are pro-inflammatory cytokines. It induces endothelial cell proliferation, chemotaxis, and changes in vascular permeability (Paleolog et al. 1992). There is also a correlation with the degree of joint destruction in arthritis (Ballara et al. 1999). More information on this can be found in Chapters 3.5 and 3.6.

Angiogenesis is a target for novel anti-inflammatory therapies, but the complex nature of the angiogenic process provides such a plethora of potential targets that further work is required to identify the most effective sites for intervention. Work in rodents highlights the potential in this approach, with significant inhibition of collagen-induced arthritis by the angiogenic inhibitor AGM-1470 (Peacock et al. 1992; Oliver et al. 1994) and inhibition of $\alpha V\beta 3$ (Storgard et al. 1999) and VEGF. Many conventional antirheumatic drugs, including methotrexate and thalidomide, have angiostatic properties (Colville-Nash and Scott 1992; D'Amato et al. 1994) and the anti-TNFα monoclonal antibody, infliximab, is associated with a fall in serum VEGF concentrations (Paleolog et al. 1998).

Cellular component of inflammation and rheumatic disease

The endothelial cell

The endothelium, the interface between circulation and synovium, controls cell migration from the vascular space to tissues. The molecules on the cell surface also dictate the way in which humoral processes are initiated (e.g. the fibrinolysis or coagulation system). Activation of the endothelium mediated by cytokines, for example, results in the upregulation of adhesion molecules of the selectin and integrin families (see Chapter 4.2).

A number of clinical syndromes are described in association with deficiency of adhesion molecules. Patients with Type I leucocyte adhesion deficiency have a defect in the synthesis of the β chain, common to the three molecules LFA1, CR3, and CR4. Severely affected patients die in infancy from severe infections, partly as a result of ineffective killing of bacteria and partly because of failure of migration of leucocytes from the vascular space to the inflammatory sites.

Endothelial cells at different sites may affect the inflammatory mechanisms involved. While intracellular adhesion molecule (ICAM)-1 is upregulated by TNFα or IL-1 on all endothelial cells lining. The microvasculature, E-selectin and vascular cell adhesion molecule (VCAM)-1 are normally confined to endothelial cells of the post-capillary venule, the site of leucocyte rolling and margination (Petzelbauer et al. 1993). In certain pathological situations, however, capillaries express these molecules and the pattern of leucocyte diapedesis is altered to match that of the adhesion molecules. This occurs, for example, in psoriasis (Petzelbauer et al. 1994).

The time course for upregulation of adhesion molecules and chemokine expression is also critical. E-selectin expression, associated with neutrophil extravasation, peaks early after TNFα addition (around 24 h), coinciding with neutrophil recruitment. VCAM-1, which is associated with mononuclear cell binding, peaks at 12–24 h after TNFα addition, corresponding with T cell recruitment (Briscoe et al. 1992). T cell-induced cytokines also modify endothelial response. IFNγ prolongs the expression of E-selectin (Doukas and Pober 1990), while IL-4 stimulates the production of VCAM-1 (Thornhill et al. 1991), suppressing the expression of E-selectin and prohibiting Type 1 responses.

Human umbilical vein endothelial cells (HUVECs) bear very little TNFR1 on their surface, the main surface receptor being TNFR2 (Bradley et al. 1995; Gaeta et al. 2000). TNFR2 directly binds the signalling molecules TRAF2 and TRAF1, but does not activate the expression of adhesion molecules in these cells under physiological conditions (Slowik et al. 1993). TNFR2 increases cell sensitivity to TNFα, however, possibly by recruiting it to the other TNFR (Tartaglia et al. 1993). After TNFα binds to endothelial cells, it is rapidly internalized by association with caveolin 1, ending up in endosomal or lysosomal compartments (Bradley et al. 1995). A significant fraction of internalized TNFα molecules become associated with mitochondria and a third TNFα-binding protein (of approximately 60 kDa) has been identified in the inner membrane of this organelle (Ledgerwood et al. 1998). In cultured HUVECs, a significant proportion of TNFR1 molecules are located within the Golgi apparatus, retained there through an undefined interaction involving the DD (Al Lamki et al. 2001). Subsequent to the exposure of HUVEC to stimuli, TNFR1 is cleaved from the cell surface (Madge et al. 1999) and the soluble receptor becomes an inhibitor of TNFα. Receptor loss both desensitizes HUVECs to TNFα and serves as a source for the soluble receptor, a natural inhibitor of TNFα function. This is an important homeostatic mechanism, since the defective shedding of TNFR1 due to a mutation in the molecule leads to TRAPS, previously known as Familial Hibernian Fever (see Chapter 6.12.3).

Neutrophils

The primary role of neutrophils is in host defence against bacteria and parasites. They also provide a mechanism to remove debris from inflammatory sites. This role is illustrated by genetically determined or acquired neutropaenia, potentially resulting in life-threatening infections with Gram positive and negative bacteria, or fungi. Neutrophils are derived from colony forming unit-granulocyte/erythrocyte/macrophage/megakaryocytes (CFU-GEMMs) derived from CD34+ stem cells. The first morphogenically distinct member of the PMN lineage is the myeloblast, which differentiates into a promyelocyte, a band neutrophil and then a mature cell. This development takes around 2 weeks and a mature cell survives in circulation for 5–7 days. Growth factors or cytokines interact with these precursor cells at several stages. IL-1, IL-3, IL-6, and stem cell factor/c-*kit* ligand act on the early progenitors, either indirectly or directly. IL-1 induces the production of GM-CSF and G-CSF inflammatory mediators, affecting their growth. G-CSF, a 19 kDa glycoprotein, produced by macrophages, fibroblasts and endothelial cells, is specific for the neutrophil lineage. It binds to a single class of high affinity receptors on neutrophil precursors, leukaemic blasts and neutrophils, resulting in expansion of the myeloblast compartment with an increase in numbers and shorter maturation time (Nicola 1990). The signal transduction pathways involved include the protein tyrosine kinase families JAK, Src, and Akt. GM-CSF (22 kDa) is secreted by activated T cells, epithelial cells, macrophages, and fibroblasts (Baldwin 1992). It enhances the survival of macrophage and neutrophil precursors, in addition to acting directly on neutrophils via two types of receptor (Cannistra et al. 1990).

Mature neutrophils respond to a range of extracellular signals, translated into intracellular messages that cause changes in motility, adherence reactions, degranulation, the production of superoxide and phagocytosis. The cells respond to chemoattractant agents, with directed movements along concentration gradients, including fMLF, C5a, LTB_4, and PAF. Neutrophils recognize a number of other chemotactic peptides, including IL-8, neutrophilactivating peptide 2 (NAP-2), GRO-α, and MIP-1α and MIP-1β. The effects of these mediators are dictated by a family of receptors with guanine nucleotide binding sites and relative ligand-specific GTP-ase activity (known collectively as the seven transmembrane receptors). Signals from these receptors release calcium and result in respiratory burst and the release of oxygen as a free radical. Several receptors are also found on neutrophils responding specifically to chemokines (e.g. CXCR1 and CXCR2) that are receptors for IL-8, and CCR1 that binds MIP-1α, RANTES, MCP-2, and MCP-3. These cells produce a variety of inflammatory mediators (see Chapter 4.2).

Phagocytosis is an important function of neutrophils. The exogenous material is isolated in an intracellular phagosome, which fuses with cytoplasmic granules in order to facilitate the destruction of the pathogen. FcR family receptors that bind the Fc portion of immunoglobulin and the leucocyte integrin CR3 are involved. The two major antimicrobial pathways of neutrophils are classified as oxygen dependent and oxygen independent. The former involves the effect known as the respiratory burst, where oxygen is reduced to superoxide, then hydrogen peroxide and other toxic metabolites. Defects in this process result in chronic granulomatous disease. Part of the oxygen-dependent pathway is the peroxidase–peroxide–halide system where myeloperoxidase, a target for autoimmunity, converts hydrogen peroxide into chloramines and hypochlorous acid/chlorine (Winterbourn et al. 2000). Oxygen-independent antimicrobial activity is mediated by a number of specific proteins, some of which are autoimmune targets. These are found in the different neutrophil granules. The main mediators involved are lysozyme, lactoferrin, and cationic proteins and defensins, also functioning as monocyte and T cell chemoattractrants (Chertov et al. 1996).

Monocytes and macrophages

Monocytes and macrophages are similar to neutrophils in that one of their main functions is phagocytosis. However, they live longer and there is tremendous phenotypic variation depending on age, location, attachment, state of differentiation, and cytokine milieu. The circulating precursor pool is smaller than that of neutrophils and localization and recruitment of macrophages in inflammation is slower, due to this fact and the different adhesion molecules involved. The synovium contains resident macrophages as type-A lining cells and the liver and spleen contain specialized macrophages involved in antigen and immune complex processing. The activation of monocytes and macrophages is complex and many different genes are involved. The production of TNFα, IL-1, IL-6, IL-8, IL-10, and IL-12 by cells of the monocyte and macrophage lineage is a key driver of both local and systemic inflammatory responses. Immune complexes, endotoxin, IgG-, and C3-opsonized particles can all activate macrophages and receptors for immunoglobulin and LPS and complement products are implicated. IFNγ is an inducer of monocyte production of IL-1β and TNFα. T cells are the first infiltrating cells in most models of chronic inflammation, but macrophages soon follow. Pro-inflammatory synergistic interactions between these two cell types may help us to understand the pathogenesis of chronic inflammation in rheumatic diseases. T cell cytokines and TGF-β are predominantly anti-inflammatory, suggesting that soluble factors produced by T cells are not the primary mediators of inflammation. T cells might exert a pathological effect through direct cellular contact with monocyte or macrophages and a number of lines of evidence support this hypothesis. In some model systems, contact-mediated activation of monocytes, by stimulated T lymphocytes, is as effective as optimal doses of LPS at inducing IL-1 and TNFα in monocytes and cells of the monocytic lineage. Many T cell types, including T cell clones, freshly isolated T lymphocytes, and T cell lines also induce IL-1 and TNFα in macrophages (Vey et al. 1992; Isler et al. 1993; Li et al. 1995; Burger 2000). A number of stimuli induce T lymphocytes to activate monocytes by direct cellular contact (Chizzolini et al. 1997; Majewska et al. 1997; Parry et al. 1997). Depending on the type of T cell and stimulus, direct contact with stimulated T lymphocytes can induce different patterns of products secreted by macrophages. Brennan et al. (2002) showed that T cells can be cytokine-activated T cells (Tck), or TCR activated cells. Dysequilibrium between the production of anti- and pro-inflammatory cytokines has been observed where Type 1 T cell clones induce IL-1 rather than IL-1RA, while cytokine-stimulated T cells induce TNFα, but not the anti-inflammatory IL-10 (Chizzolini et al. 1997; Sebbag et al. 1997). Subsequent to contact with stimulated T cells, the balance between IL-1 and IL-1RA production in monocytes is dictated, in part, by Ser/Thr phosphatases (Vey et al. 1997). Contact-activated THP-1 cells express membrane-associated proteases, neutralizing TNFα activity by degrading the latter cytokine and cleaving its receptors at the cell surface (Vey et al. 1996). These data indicate that multiple ligands are involved in the contact-mediated activation of macrophages.

Mechanisms of tissue injury induced by cells

Matrix metalloproteinases and their inhibitors (TIMPs) (see Chapter 3.3)

Cartilage and bone destruction are major components of immune-mediated joint disease and osteoarthritis. Collagen, one of the major components of the extracellular matrix (ECM), is resistant to the activity of proteolytic enzymes as a result of its robust triple helical structure. However, a specific group of enzymes, MMPs, are vitally important in the normal homeostasis and modelling of the ECM and are involved in joint destruction. These molecules' TIMPs constitute exciting potential therapeutic targets in rheumatic disease and are reviewed in Nagase and Woessner (1999).

MMPs can degrade all the components of the ECM and are active at physiological values of pH. Most MMPs can be classified into five groups according to their primary structure, nature of their substrate, and cellular localization. These are the collagenases, gelatinases, stromelysins, matrilysins, and the membrane-type matrix metalloproteinases (MT-MMPs). Some MMPs, such as macrophage elastase (MMP-12), do not fall clearly into any of these categories, while some enzymes may be classified into more than one group.

There is evidence for the overexpression of MMPs in the joints of arthritic patients. Cell cultures derived from rheumatoid synovium secrete a collagenolytic activity into the medium (Dayer et al. 1976). Stromelysin-1 (Sirum and Brinckerhoff 1989) and collagenase-1 can be demonstrated at sites of cartilage erosion in rheumatoid joints by immunolocalization. TIMP-1 as well as these two enzymes have been immunolocalized in synovial samples from both rheumatoid arthritis and osteoarthritis patients (Hembry et al. 1995). It has also been demonstrated that collagenase-1, gelatinase A, and matrilysin have a role in the synovitis associated with rheumatoid arthritis, but the role of these enzymes in osteoarthritic joints is less well defined. Stromelysin-1 and collagenase-1 have been detected in the synovial fluids from rheumatoid and osteoarthritic knee joints (Ishiguro et al. 2001). Gelatinase B has been detected as both mRNA and protein in osteoarthritic cartilage, but not in normal tissue and is detectable in the synovial fluid from rheumatoid joints (Mohtai et al. 1993). Collagenase-2 and collagenase-3 have also been identified in arthritic cartilage (Tetlow et al. 2001). The expression of 16 MMPs at the mRNA level in rheumatoid arthritis and the following trauma has been analysed. Some MMPs (e.g. collagenase-3 and the MT2-MMP) were found to be exclusively present in rheumatoid tissue (Konttinen et al. 1999), though the biological significance of this observation is unclear.

The MMP family is not the only family of proteinases implicated in cartilage destruction and there has been considerable debate concerning their role in the degradation of cartilage proteoglycans relative to that of the related family of a disintegrin, a metalloproteinase, and thrombospondin aggrecanase (ADAM-TS) (Fosang et al. 1993; Bottomley et al. 1998). There is evidence from a model system of collagen degradation that stromelysin-1, collagenase-2, and collagenase-3 are unlikely to contribute to proteoglycan degradation, but collagenases and gelatinase have major roles in type II collagen breakdown (Kozaci et al. 1998). The specific collagenase responsible for cartilage collagen loss is the subject of detailed investigation and there is evidence that specific MMP-13 inhibitors can block IL-1-induced collagen loss, and an enhanced cleavage of type II collagen in osteoarthritic cartilage has been correlated with MMP-13 activity (Billinghurst et al. 1997). Studies on the role of TNFα in mediating the induction of MMPs in rheumatoid arthritis have shown that MT1-MMP is expressed and regulated by rheumatoid synovial fibroblasts (Migita et al. 1996).

In osteoarthritis, alterations in sub-chondral bone structure appear to precede changes in deep cartilage, with subsequent fibrillation of the articular surface. In rheumatoid arthritis, early changes appear in the surface layers with the majority of cartilage collagen destruction occurring at the cartilage–pannus junction.

MMP activity in the tissue is regulated by TIMPs (Brew et al. 2000). Four TIMPs (TIMP-1 to TIMP-4) are described in humans and it is the homologous *N*-terminal domains of TIMPs (N-TIMPs) that are primarily responsible for the inhibition of MMPs (Murphy et al. 1991), while *C*-terminal domains influence their binding affinity. The balance between the MMPs and TIMPs is critical for the homeostasis of the ECM structure. TIMP-1, -2, and -3 are demonstrable in joint tissue and raised levels of TIMP-1 have been reported both in synovial fluid and serum from rheumatoid arthritis patients, but not in the serum of patients with osteoarthritis. Overexpression of TIMP-1 using systemic adenovirus-based gene delivery has been shown to reduce joint destruction in TNFα transgenic mice (Schett et al. 2001), but did not prevent osteochondral injury in a murine model of collagen-induced arthritis (Apparailly et al. 2001).

A number of powerful MMP inhibitors have been developed and some have been clinically evaluated for the treatment of arthritis or cancer, but none were efficacious as recently reviewed (Zucker et al. 2000). There are a number of possible explanations for this failure and these drugs may also have unwanted side-effects. Marima-stat (British Biotech Pharmaceuticals, Oxford, UK), used in cancer patients, caused a range of musculoskeletal symptoms, including tendonitis, stiffness, arthralgia, and reduced mobility. These studies show that our current understanding of the biology and likely clinical importance of MMPs and TIMPs is at a relatively early stage.

References

Al Lamki, R.S., Wang, J., Skepper, J.N., Thiru, S., Pober, J.S., and Bradley, J.R. (2001). Expression of tumor necrosis factor receptors in normal kidney and rejecting renal transplants. *Laboratory Investigations* **81**, 1503–15.

Apparailly, F., Noel, D., Millet, V., Baker, A.H., Lisignoli, G., Jacquet, C., Kaiser, M.J., Sany, J., and Jorgensen, C. (2001). Paradoxical effects of tissue inhibitor of metalloproteinases 1 gene transfer in collagen-induced arthritis. *Arthritis and Rheumatism* **44**, 1444–54.

Arsenis, C. and McDonnell, J. (1989). Effects of antirheumatic drugs on the interleukin-1 alpha induced synthesis and activation of proteinases in articular cartilage explants in culture. *Agents and Actions* **27**, 261–4.

Baldwin, G.C. (1992). The biology of granulocyte-macrophage colony-stimulating factor: effects on hematopoietic and nonhematopoietic cells. *Developmental Biology* **151**, 352–67.

Ballara, S.C., Miotla, J.M., and Paleolog, E.M. (1999). New vessels, new approaches: angiogenesis as a therapeutic target in musculoskeletal disorders. *International Journal of Experimental Pathology* **80**, 235–50.

Basbaum, A.I. and Levine, J.D. (1991). The contribution of the nervous system to inflammation and inflammatory disease. *Canadian Journal of Physiology and Pharmacology* **69**, 647–51.

Baud, V. and Karin, M. (2001). Signal transduction by tumor necrosis factor and its relatives. *Trends in Cell Biology* **11**, 372–7.

Billinghurst, R.C., Dahlberg, L., Ionescu, M., Reiner, A., Bourne, R., Rorabeck, C., Mitchell, P., Hambor, J., Diekmann, O., Tschesche, H., Chen, J., Van Wart, H., and Poole, A.R. (1997). Enhanced cleavage of type II collagen by collagenases in osteoarthritic articular cartilage. *Journal of Clinical Investigations* **99**, 1534–45.

Botto, M. (1998). C1q knock-out mice for the study of complement deficiency in autoimmune disease. *Experimental and Clinical Immunogenetics* **15**, 231–4.

Botto, M. and Walport, M.J. (1993). Hereditary deficiency of C3 in animals and humans. *International Reviews in Immunology* **10**, 37–50.

Botto, M., Theodoridis, E., Thompson, E.M., Beynon, H.L., Briggs, D., Isenberg, D.A., Walport, M.J., and Davies, K.A. (1996). Fc gamma RIIa polymorphism in systemic lupus erythematosus (SLE): no association with disease. *Clinical and Experimental Immunology* **104**, 264–8.

Bottomley, K.M., Johnson, W.H., and Walter, D.S. (1998). Matrix metalloproteinase inhibitors in arthritis. *Journal of Enzyme Inhibitors* **13**, 79–101.

Bradley, J.R., Thiru, S., and Pober, J.S. (1995). Disparate localization of 55-kd and 75-kd tumor necrosis factor receptors in human endothelial cells. *American Journal of Pathology* **146**, 27–32.

Brennan, F.M., Chantry, D., Jackson, A., Maini, R., and Feldmann, M. (1989). Inhibitory effect of TNF alpha antibodies on synovial cell interleukin-1 production in rheumatoid arthritis. *Lancet* **2**, 244–7.

Brennan, F.M., Hayes, A.L., Ciesielski, C.J., Green, P., Foxwell, B.M., and Feldmann, M. (2002). Evidence that rheumatoid arthritis synovial T cells are similar to cytokine-activated T cells: involvement of phosphatidylinositol 3-kinase and nuclear factor kappaB pathways in tumor necrosis factor alpha production in rheumatoid arthritis. *Arthritis and Rheumatism* **46**, 31–41.

Brew, K., Dinakarpandian, D., and Nagase, H. (2000). Tissue inhibitors of metalloproteinases: evolution, structure and function. *Biochimica et Biophysica Acta* **1477**, 267–83.

Briscoe, D.M., Cotran, R.S., and Pober, J.S. (1992). Effects of tumor necrosis factor, lipopolysaccharide, and IL-4 on the expression of vascular cell adhesion molecule-1 *in vivo*. Correlation with CD3+ T cell infiltration. *Journal of Immunology* **149**, 2954–60.

Buchs, N., Silvestri, T., di Giovine, F.S., Chabaud, M., Vannier, E., Duff, G.W., and Miossec, P. (2000). IL-4 VNTR gene polymorphism in chronic polyarthritis. The rare allele is associated with protection against destruction. *Rheumatology (Oxford)* **39**, 1126–31.

Buchs, N., di Giovine, F.S., Silvestri, T., Vannier, E., Duff, G.W., and Miossec, P. (2001). IL-1B and IL-1Ra gene polymorphisms and disease severity in rheumatoid arthritis: interaction with their plasma levels. *Genes and Immunity* **2**, 222–8.

Burger, D. (2000). Cell contact interactions in rheumatology, The Kennedy Institute for Rheumatology, London, UK, 1–2 June (2000). *Arthritis Research* **2**, 472–6.

Callard, R.E. and Turner, M.W. (1990). Cytokines and Ig switching: evolutionary divergence between mice and humans. *Immunology Today* **11**, 200–3.

Cannistra, S.A., Koenigsmann, M., DiCarlo, J., Groshek, P., and Griffin, J.D. (1990). Differentiation-associated expression of two functionally distinct classes of granulocyte-macrophage colony-stimulating factor receptors by human myeloid cells. *Journal of Biological Chemistry* **265**, 12656–63.

Castro, F., Acevedo, E., Ciusani, E., Angulo, J.A., Wollheim, F.A., and Sandberg-Wollheim, M. (2001). Tumour necrosis factor microsatellites and HLA-DRB1*, HLA-DQA1*, and HLA-DQB1* alleles in Peruvian patients with rheumatoid arthritis. *Annals of Rheumatic Diseases* **60** (8), 791–5.

Chertov, O., Michiel, D.F., Xu, L., Wang, J.M., Tani, K., Murphy, W.J., Longo, D.L., Taub, D.D., and Oppenheim, J.J. (1996). Identification of defensin-1, defensin-2, and CAP37/azurocidin as T-cell chemoattractant proteins released from interleukin-8-stimulated neutrophils. *Journal of Biological Chemistry* **271**, 2935–40.

Chikanza, I.C., Petrou, P., Kingsley, G., Chrousos, G., and Panayi, G.S. (1992). Defective hypothalamic response to immune and inflammatory stimuli in patients with rheumatoid arthritis. *Arthritis and Rheumatism* **35**, 1281–8.

Chikanza, I.C., Petrou, P., Chrousos, G., Kingsley, G., and Panayi, G.S. (1993). Excessive and dysregulated secretion of prolactin in rheumatoid arthritis: immunopathogenetic and therapeutic implications. *British Journal of Rheumatology* **32**, 445–8.

Chizzolini, C., Chicheportiche, R., Burger, D., and Dayer, J.M. (1997). Human Th1 cells preferentially induce interleukin (IL)-1beta while Th2 cells induce IL-1 receptor antagonist production upon cell/cell contact with monocytes. *European Journal of Immunology* **27**, 171–7.

Colville-Nash, P.R. and Scott, D.L. (1992). Angiogenesis and rheumatoid arthritis: pathogenic and therapeutic implications. *Annals of Rheumatic Diseases* **51**, 919–25.

Cope, A.P., Londei, M., Chu, N.R., Cohen, S.B., Elliott, M.J., Brennan, F.M., Maini, R.N., and Feldmann, M. (1994). Chronic exposure to tumor necrosis factor (TNF) *in vitro* impairs the activation of T cells through the T cell receptor/CD3 complex; reversal *in vivo* by anti-TNF antibodies in patients with rheumatoid arthritis. *Journal of Clinical Investigations* **94**, 749–60.

Cork, M.J., Tarlow, J.K., Blakemore, A.I., Mee, J.B., Crane, A.M., Stierle, C., Bleehen, S.S., and Duff, G.W. (1993). Psoriasis and interleukin-1. A translation. *Journal of the Royal College of Physicians London* **27**, 366.

D'Amato, R.J., Loughnan, M.S., Flynn, E., and Folkman, J. (1994). Thalidomide is an inhibitor of angiogenesis. *Proceedings of the National Academy of Sciences USA* **91**, 4082–5.

Dayer, J.M., Krane, S.M., Russell, R.G., and Robinson, D.R. (1976). Production of collagenase and prostaglandins by isolated adherent rheumatoid synovial cells. *Proceedings of the National Academy of Sciences USA* **73**, 945–9.

Dijstelbloem, H.M., Scheepers, R.H., Oost, W.W., Stegeman, C.A., van der Pol, W.L., Sluiter, W.J., Kallenberg, C.G., van de Winkel, J.G., and Tervaert, J.W. (1999). Fcgamma receptor polymorphisms in Wegener's granulomatosis: risk factors for disease relapse. *Arthritis and Rheumatism* **42**, 1823–7.

Donaldson, V.H., Glueck, H.I., and Fleming, T. (1972). Brief recordings. Rheumatoid arthritis in a patient with Hageman trait. *New England Journal of Medicine* **286**, 528–30.

Doukas, J. and Pober, J.S. (1990). IFN-gamma enhances endothelial activation induced by tumor necrosis factor but not IL-1. *Journal of Immunology* **145**, 1727–33.

Duits, A.J., Bootsma, H., Derksen, R.H., Spronk, P.E., Kater, L., Kallenberg, C.G., Capel, P.J., Westerdaal, N.A., Spierenburg, G.T., and Gmelig-Meyling, F.H. (1995). Skewed distribution of IgG Fc receptor IIa (CD32) polymorphism is associated with renal disease in systemic lupus erythematosus patients. *Arthritis and Rheumatism* **38**, 1832–6.

Eastgate, J.A., Symons, J.A., Wood, N.C., Grinlinton, F.M., di Giovine, F.S., and Duff, G.W. (1988). Correlation of plasma interleukin 1 levels with disease activity in rheumatoid arthritis. *Lancet* **2**, 706–9.

Edberg, J.C., Redecha, P.B., Salmon, J.E., and Kimberly, R.P. (1989). Human Fc gamma RIII (CD16). Isoforms with distinct allelic expression, extracellular domains, and membrane linkages on polymorphonuclear and natural killer cells. *Journal of Immunology* **143**, 1642–9.

Elliott, M.J., Maini, R.N., Feldmann, M., Long-Fox, A., Charles, P., Katsikis, P., Brennan, F.M., Walker, J., Bijl, H., and Ghrayeb, J. (1993). Treatment of rheumatoid arthritis with chimeric monoclonal antibodies to tumor necrosis factor alpha. *Arthritis and Rheumatism* **36**, 1681–90.

Elliott, M.J., Maini, R.N., Feldmann, M., Kalden, J.R., Antoni, C., Smolen, J.S., Leeb, B., Breedveld, F.C., Macfarlane, J.D., and Bijl, H. (1994). Randomised double-blind comparison of chimeric monoclonal antibody to tumour necrosis factor alpha (cA2) versus placebo in rheumatoid arthritis. *Lancet* **344**, 1105–10.

Feldmann, M. (1996). The cytokine network in rheumatoid arthritis: definition of TNF alpha as a therapeutic target. *Journal of the Royal College of Physicians London* **30**, 560–70.

Fife, M., Steer, S., Fisher, S., Newton, J., McKay, K., Worthington, J., Shah, C., Polley, A., Rosenthal, A., Ollier, W., Lewis, C., Wordsworth, P., and Lanchbury, J. (2002). Association of familial and sporadic rheumatoid arthritis with a single corticotropin-releasing hormone genomic region (8q12.3) haplotype. *Arthritis and Rheumatism* **46**, 75–82.

Fishman, D., Faulds, G., Jeffery, R., Mohamed-Ali, V., Yudkin, J.S., Humphries, S., and Woo, P. (1998). The effect of novel polymorphisms in the interleukin-6 (IL-6) gene on IL-6 transcription and plasma IL-6 levels, and an association with systemic-onset juvenile chronic arthritis, *Journal of Clinical Investigations* **102**, 1369–76.

Fosang, A.J., Last, K., Knauper, V., Neame, P.J., Murphy, G., Hardingham, T.E., Tschesche, H., and Hamilton, J.A. (1993). Fibroblast and neutrophil collagenases cleave at two sites in the cartilage aggrecan interglobular domain. *Biochemical Journal* **295**, 273–6.

Funk, C.D. (2001). Prostaglandins and leukotrienes: advances in eicosanoid biology. *Science* **294**, 1871–5.

Gabay, C. (2002). Cytokine inhibitors in the treatment of rheumatoid arthritis. *Expert Opinions in Biological Therapy* **2**, 135–49.

Gaeta, M.L., Johnson, D.R., Kluger, M.S., and Pober, J.S. (2000). The death domain of tumor necrosis factor receptor 1 is necessary but not sufficient for Golgi retention of the receptor and mediates receptor desensitization. *Laboratory Investigations* **80**, 1185–94.

Gonzalez, S., Torre-Alonso, J.C., Martinez-Borra, J., Fernandez Sanchez, J.A., Lopez-Vazquez, A., Rodriguez, P.A., and Lopez-Larrea, C. (2001). TNF-238A promoter polymorphism contributes to susceptibility to ankylosing spondylitis in HLA-B27 negative patients. *Journal of Rheumatology* **28**, 1288–93.

Griffiths, R.J., Pettipher, E.R., Koch, K., Farrell, C.A., Breslow, R., Conklyn, M.J., Smith, M.A., Hackman, B.C., Wimberly, D.J., and Milici, A.J. (1995). Leukotriene B4 plays a critical role in the progression of collagen-induced arthritis. *Proceedings of the National Academy of Sciences USA* **92**, 517–21.

Groves, R.W., Mizutani, H., Kieffer, J.D., and Kupper, T.S. (1995). Inflammatory skin disease in transgenic mice that express high levels of interleukin 1 alpha in basal epidermis. *Proceedings of the National Academy of Sciences USA* **92**, 11874–8.

Hembry, R.M., Bagga, M.R., Reynolds, J.J., and Hamblen, D.L. (1995). Immunolocalisation studies on six matrix metalloproteinases and their inhibitors, TIMP-1 and TIMP-2, in synovia from patients with osteo- and rheumatoid arthritis. *Annals of the Rheumatic Diseases* **54**, 25–32.

Ho, I.C., Hodge, M.R., Rooney, J.W., and Glimcher, L.H. (1996). The proto-oncogene c-maf is responsible for tissue-specific expression of interleukin-4. *Cell* **85**, 973–83.

Hogarth, M.B., Slingsby, J.H., Allen, P.J., Thompson, E.M., Chandler, P., Davies, K.A., Simpson, E., Morley, B.J., and Walport, M.J. (1998). Multiple lupus susceptibility loci map to chromosome 1 in BXSB mice. *Journal of Immunology* **161**, 2753–61.

Hogasen, K., Jansen, J.H., and Harboe, M. (1997). Eradication of porcine factor H deficiency in Norway. *Veterinary Records* **140**, 392–5.

Ishiguro, N., Ito, T., Oguchi, T., Kojima, T., Iwata, H., Ionescu, M., and Poole, A.R. (2001). Relationships of matrix metalloproteinases and their inhibitors to cartilage proteoglycan and collagen turnover and inflammation as revealed by analyses of synovial fluids from patients with rheumatoid arthritis. *Arthritis and Rheumatism* **44**, 2503–11.

Isler, P., Vey, E., Zhang, J.H., and Dayer, J.M. (1993). Cell surface glycoproteins expressed on activated human T cells induce production of interleukin-1 beta by monocytic cells: a possible role of CD69. *European Cytokine Network* **4**, 15–23.

Jeffery, R., Fife, M., Le Luong, A., Ogilvie, E., MacFadyen, J., Humphries, S., and Woo, P. (2003). Differential binding of a transcription factor complex to the -174G/C varient of the interleukin-6 gene: rationale for disease susceptibility (in preparation).

Karalis, K., Sano, H., Redwine, J., Listwak, S., Wilder, R.L., and Chrousos, G.P. (1991). Autocrine or paracrine inflammatory actions of corticotropin-releasing hormone *in vivo*. *Science* **254**, 421–3.

Kidd, B.L., Mapp, P.I., Blake, D.R., Gibson, S.J., and Polak, J.M. (1990). Neurogenic influences in arthritis. *Annals of the Rheumatic Diseases* **49**, 649–52.

Kimberly, R.P., Salmon, J.E., Edberg, J.C., and Gibofsky, A. (1989). The role of Fc gamma receptors in mononuclear phagocyte system function. *Clinical and Experimental Rheumatology* **7** (Suppl. 3), S103–8.

Koch, A.E. (1998). Review: angiogenesis: implications for rheumatoid arthritis. *Arthritis and Rheumatism* **41**, 951–62.

Koch, A.E. (2000). The role of angiogenesis in rheumatoid arthritis: recent developments. *Annals of the Rheumatic Diseases* **59** (Suppl. 1), i65–71.

Koch, A.E., Harlow, L.A., Haines, G.K., Amento, E.P., Unemori, E.N., Wong, W.L., Pope, R.M., and Ferrara, N. (1994). Vascular endothelial growth factor. A cytokine modulating endothelial function in rheumatoid arthritis. *Journal of Immunology* **152**, 4149–56.

Konttinen, Y.T., Ainola, M., Valleala, H., Ma, J., Ida, H., Mandelin, J., Kinne, R.W., Santavirta, S., Sorsa, T., Lopez-Otin, C., and Takagi, M. (1999). Analysis of 16 different matrix metalloproteinases (MMP-1 to MMP-20) in the synovial membrane: different profiles in trauma and rheumatoid arthritis. *Annals of the Rheumatic Diseases* **58**, 691–7.

Kozaci, L.D., Brown, C.J., Adcocks, C., Galloway, A., Hollander, A.P., and Buttle, D.J. (1998). Stromelysin 1, neutrophil collagenase, and collagenase 3 do not play major roles in a model of chondrocyte mediated cartilage breakdown. *Molecular Pathology* **51**, 282–16.

Laabi, Y., Egle, A., and Strasser, A. (2001). TNF cytokine family: more BAFF-ling complexities. *Current Biology* **11**, R1013–16.

Lahita, R.G. (1993). Sex hormones as immunomodulators of disease. *Annals of the New York Academy of Sciences* **685**, 278–87.

Lahita, R.G., Chiorazzi, N., Gibofsky, A., Winchester, R.J., and Kunkel, H.G. (1983). Familial systemic lupus erythematosus in males. *Arthritis and Rheumatism* **26**, 39–44.

Ledgerwood, E.C., Prins, J.B., Bright, N.A., Johnson, D.R., Wolfreys, K., Pober, J.S., O'Rahilly, S., and Bradley, J.R. (1998). Tumor necrosis factor is delivered to mitochondria where a tumor necrosis factor-binding protein is localized. *Laboratory Investigations* **78**, 1583–9.

LeGrand, A., Fermor, B., Fink, C., Pisetsky, D.S., Weinberg, J.B., Vail, T.P., and Guilak, F. (2001). Interleukin-1, tumor necrosis factor alpha, and interleukin-17 synergistically up-regulate nitric oxide and prostaglandin E2 production in explants of human osteoarthritic knee menisci. *Arthritis and Rheumatism* **44**, 2078–83.

Li, J.M., Isler, P., Dayer, J.M., and Burger, D. (1995). Contact-dependent stimulation of monocytic cells and neutrophils by stimulated human T-cell clones. *Immunology* **84**, 571–6.

Locksley, R.M., Killeen, N., and Lenardo, M.J. (2001). The TNF and TNF receptor superfamilies: integrating mammalian biology. *Cell* **104**, 487–501.

Madge, L.A., Sierra-Honigmann, M.R., and Pober, J.S. (1999). Apoptosis-inducing agents cause rapid shedding of tumor necrosis factor receptor 1 (TNFR1). A nonpharmacological explanation for inhibition of TNF-mediated activation. *Journal of Biological Chemistry* **274**, 13643–9.

Majewska, E., Paleolog, E., Baj, Z., Kralisz, U., Feldmann, M., and Tchorzewski, H. (1997). Role of tyrosine kinase enzymes in TNF-alpha and IL-1 induced expression of ICAM-1 and VCAM-1 on human umbilical vein endothelial cells. *Scandinavian Journal of Immunology* **45**, 385–92.

Mattsson, R., Mattsson, A., Hansson, I., Holmdahl, R., Rook, G.A., and Whyte, A. (1992). Increased levels of prolactin during, but not after, the immunisation with rat collagen II enhances the course of arthritis in DBA/1 mice. *Autoimmunity* **11**, 163–70.

McGuire, W., Knight, J.C., Hill, A.V., Allsopp, C.E., Greenwood, B.M., and Kwiatkowski, D. (1999). Severe malarial anemia and cerebral malaria are associated with different tumor necrosis factor promoter alleles. *Journal of Infectious Diseases* **179**, 287–90.

McMurray, R., Keisler, D., Izui, S., and Walker, S.E. (1994). Hyperprolactinemia in male NZB/NZW (B/W) F1 mice: accelerated autoimmune disease with normal circulating testosterone. *Clinical Immunology and Immunopathology* **71**, 338–43.

Migita, K., Eguchi, K., Kawabe, Y., Ichinose, Y., Tsukada, T., Aoyagi, T., Nakamura, H., and Nagataki, S. (1996). TNF-alpha-mediated expression of membrane-type matrix metalloproteinase in rheumatoid synovial fibroblasts. *Immunology* **89**, 553–7.

Mohamed-Ali, H. (1995). Influence of interleukin-1 beta, tumour necrosis factor alpha and prostaglandin E2 on chondrogenesis and cartilage matrix breakdown *in vitro*. *Rheumatology International* **14**, 191–9.

Mohtai, M., Smith, R.L., Schurman, D.J., Tsuji, Y., Torti, F.M., Hutchinson, N.I., Stetler-Stevenson, W.G., and Goldberg, G.I. (1993). Expression of 92-kD type IV collagenase/gelatinase (gelatinase B) in osteoarthritic cartilage and its induction in normal human articular cartilage by interleukin 1. *Journal of Clinical Investigations* **92**, 179–85.

Murphy, G., Houbrechts, A., Cockett, M.I., Williamson, R.A., O'Shea, M., and Docherty, A.J. (1991). The N-terminal domain of tissue inhibitor of metalloproteinases retains metalloproteinase inhibitory activity. *Biochemistry* **30**, 8097–102.

Nagase, H. and Woessner, J.F., Jr. (1999). Matrix metalloproteinases. *Journal of Biological Chemistry* **274**, 21491–4.

Neeck, G., Federlin, K., Graef, V., Rusch, D., and Schmidt, K.L. (1990). Adrenal secretion of cortisol in patients with rheumatoid arthritis. *Journal of Rheumatology* **17**, 24–9.

Nicola, N.A. (1990). Characteristics of soluble and membrane-bound forms of haemopoietic growth factor receptors: relationships to biological function. *Ciba Foundation Symposium* **148**, 110–20.

Norsworthy, P., Theodoridis, E., Botto, M., Athanassiou, P., Beynon, H., Gordon, C., Isenberg, D., Walport, M.J., and Davies, K.A. (1999). Overrepresentation of the Fcgamma receptor type IIA R131/R131 genotype in caucasoid systemic lupus erythematosus patients with autoantibodies to C1q and glomerulonephritis. *Arthritis and Rheumatism* **42**, 1828–32.

Ogilvie, E.M., Fife, M.S., Thompson, S.D., Twine, N., Tsoras, M., Moroldo, M., Fisher, S.A., Lewis, C.M., Prieur, A.M., Glass, D.N., and Woo, P. (2003). The −174G allele of the interleukin-6 gene confers susceptibility to systemic arthritis in children: a multicenter study using simplex and multiplex juvenile idiopathic arthritis families. *Arthritis and Rheumatism* **48**, 3202–6.

Oliver, S.J., Banquerigo, M.L., and Brahn, E. (1994). Suppression of collagen-induced arthritis using an angiogenesis inhibitor, AGM-1470, and a microtubule stabilizer, taxol. *Cellular Immunology* **157**, 291–9.

Oppenheim, J.J. et al., ed. *Cytokine Reference.* London: Academic Press, 2001.

O'Shea, J.J., Jaffe, E.S., Lane, H.C., MacDermott, R.P., and Fauci, A.S. (1987). Peripheral T cell lymphoma presenting as hypereosinophilia with vasculitis. Clinical, pathologic, and immunologic features. *American Journal of Medicine* **82**, 539–45.

Ouyang, W., Ranganath, S.H., Weindel, K., Bhattacharya, D., Murphy, T.L., Sha, W.C., and Murphy, K.M. (1998). Inhibition of Th1 development mediated by GATA-3 through an IL-4-independent mechanism. *Immunity* **9**, 745–55.

Ouyang, W., Jacobson, N.G., Bhattacharya, D., Gorham, J.D., Fenoglio, D., Sha, W.C., Murphy, T.L., and Murphy, K.M. (1999). The Ets transcription factor ERM is Th1-specific and induced by IL-12 through a Stat4-dependent pathway. *Proceedings of the National Academy of Sciences USA* **96**, 3888–93.

Paccani, S.R., Boncristiano, M., Ulivieri, C., D'Elios, M.M., Del Prete, G., and Baldari, C.T. (2002). Nonsteroidal anti-inflammatory drugs suppress T-cell activation by inhibiting p38 MAPK induction. *Journal of Biological Chemistry* **277**, 1509–13.

Pachman, L.M., Liotta-Davis, M.R., Hong, D.K., Kinsella, T.R., Mendez, E.P., Kinder, J.M., and Chen, E.H. (2000). TNFalpha-308A allele in juvenile dermatomyositis: association with increased production of tumor necrosis factor alpha, disease duration, and pathologic calcifications. *Arthritis and Rheumatism* **43**, 2368–77.

Paleolog, E.M., Aluri, G.R., and Feldmann, M. (1992). Contrasting effects of interferon gamma and interleukin 4 on responses of human vascular endothelial cells to tumour necrosis factor alpha. *Cytokine* **4**, 470–8.

Paleolog, E.M., Young, S., Stark, A.C., McCloskey, R.V., Feldmann, M., and Maini, R.N. (1998). Modulation of angiogenic vascular endothelial growth factor by tumor necrosis factor alpha and interleukin-1 in rheumatoid arthritis. *Arthritis and Rheumatism* **41**, 1258–65.

Parry, S.L., Sebbag, M., Feldmann, M., and Brennan, F.M. (1997). Contact with T cells modulates monocyte IL-10 production: role of T cell membrane TNF-alpha. *Journal of Immunology* **158**, 3673–81.

Peacock, D.J., Banquerigo, M.L., and Brahn, E. (1992). Angiogenesis inhibition suppresses collagen arthritis. *Journal of Experimental Medicine* **175**, 1135–8.

Petzelbauer, P., Bender, J.R., Wilson, J., and Pober, J.S. (1993). Heterogeneity of dermal microvascular endothelial cell antigen expression and cytokine responsiveness in situ and in cell culture. *Journal of Immunology* **151**, 5062–72.

Petzelbauer, P., Pober, J.S., Keh, A., and Braverman, I.M. (1994). Inducibility and expression of microvascular endothelial adhesion molecules in lesional, perilesional, and uninvolved skin of psoriatic patients. *Journal of Investigative Dermatology* **103**, 300–5.

Pfeffer, K., Matsuyama, T., Kundig, T.M., Wakeham, A., Kishihara, K., Shahinian, A., Wiegmann, K., Ohashi, P.S., Kronke, M., and Mak, T.W. (1993). Mice deficient for the 55 kd tumor necrosis factor receptor are resistant to endotoxic shock, yet succumb to *L. monocytogenes* infection. *Cell* **73**, 457–67.

Quattrocchi, E., Dallman, M.J., Dhillon, A.P., Quaglia, A., Bagnato, G., and Feldmann, M. (2001). Murine IL-10 gene transfer inhibits established collagen-induced arthritis and reduces adenovirus-mediated inflammatory responses in mouse liver. *Journal of Immunology* **166**, 5970–8.

Salmon, J.E. and Pricop, L. (2001). Human receptors for immunoglobulin G: key elements in the pathogenesis of rheumatic disease. *Arthritis and Rheumatism* **44**, 739–50.

Salmon, J.E., Millard, S., Schachter, L.A., Arnett, F.C., Ginzler, E.M., Gourley, M.F., Ramsey-Goldman, R., Peterson, M.G., and Kimberly, R.P. (1996). Fc gamma RIIA alleles are heritable risk factors for lupus nephritis in African Americans. *Journal of Clinical Investigations* **97**, 1348–54.

Salmon, J.E., Edberg, J.C., and Kimberly, R.P. (1990). Fc gamma receptor III on human neutrophils. Allelic variants have functionally distinct capacities. *Journal of Clinical Investigations* **85**, 1287–95.

Schett, G., Hayer, S., Tohidast-Akrad, M., Schmid, B.J., Lang, S., Turk, B., Kainberger, F., Haralambous, S., Kollias, G., Newby, A.C., Xu, Q., Steiner, G., and Smolen, J. (2001). Adenovirus-based overexpression of tissue inhibitor of metalloproteinases 1 reduces tissue damage in the joints of tumor necrosis factor alpha transgenic mice. *Arthritis and Rheumatism* **44**, 2888–98.

Sebbag, M., Parry, S.L., Brennan, F.M., and Feldmann, M. (1997). Cytokine stimulation of T lymphocytes regulates their capacity to induce monocyte production of tumor necrosis factor-alpha, but not interleukin-10: possible relevance to pathophysiology of rheumatoid arthritis. *European Journal of Immunology* **27**, 624–32.

Silman, A.J. (1994). Epidemiology of rheumatoid arthritis. *Acta Pathologica, Microbiologica et Immunologica Scandinavica* **102**, 721–8.

Sirum, K.L. and Brinckerhoff, C.E. (1989). Cloning of the genes for human stromelysin and stromelysin 2: differential expression in rheumatoid synovial fibroblasts. *Biochemistry* **28**, 8691–8.

Slowik, M.R., De Luca, L.G., Fiers, W., and Pober, J.S. (1993). Tumor necrosis factor activates human endothelial cells through the p55 tumor necrosis factor receptor but the p75 receptor contributes to activation at low tumor necrosis factor concentration. *American Journal of Pathology* **143**, 1724–30.

Stadler, J., Stefanovic-Racic, M., Billiar, T.R., Curran, R.D., McIntyre, L.A., Georgescu, H.I., Simmons, R.L., and Evans, C.H. (1991). Articular chondrocytes synthesize nitric oxide in response to cytokines and lipopolysaccharide. *Journal of Immunology* **147**, 3915–20.

Storgard, C.M., Stupack, D.G., Jonczyk, A., Goodman, S.L., Fox, R.I., and Cheresh, D.A. (1999). Decreased angiogenesis and arthritic disease in rabbits treated with an alphavbeta3 antagonist. *Journal of Clinical Investigations* **103**, 47–54.

Strasser, A., O'Connor, L., and Dixit, V.M. (2000). Apoptosis signaling. *Annual Review of Biochemistry* **69**, 217–45.

Symons, J.A., Eastgate, J.A., and Duff, G.W. (1991). Purification and characterization of a novel soluble receptor for interleukin 1. *Journal of Experimental Medicine* **174**, 1251–4.

Szabo, S.J., Kim, S.T., Costa, G.L., Zhang, X., Fathman, C.G., and Glimcher, L.H. (2000). A novel transcription factor, T-bet, directs Th1 lineage commitment. *Cell* **100**, 655–69.

Tarlow, J.K., Blakemore, A.I., Lennard, A., Solari, R., Hughes, H.N., Steinkasserer, A., and Duff, G.W. (1993). Polymorphism in human IL-1 receptor antagonist gene intron 2 is caused by variable numbers of an 86-bp tandem repeat. *Human Genetics* **91**, 403–4.

Tartaglia, L.A., Pennica, D., and Goeddel, D.V. (1993). Ligand passing: the 75-kDa tumor necrosis factor (TNF) receptor recruits TNF for signaling by the 55-kDa TNF receptor. *Journal of Biological Chemistry* **268**, 18542–8.

Tetlow, L.C., Adlam, D.J., and Woolley, D.E. (2001). Matrix metalloproteinase and proinflammatory cytokine production by chondrocytes of human osteoarthritic cartilage: associations with degenerative changes. *Arthritis and Rheumatism* **44**, 585–94.

Thornhill, M.H., Wellicome, S.M., Mahiouz, D.L., Lanchbury, J.S., Kyan-Aung, U., and Haskard, D.O. (1991). Tumor necrosis factor combines with IL-4 or IFN-gamma to selectively enhance endothelial cell adhesiveness for T cells. The contribution of vascular cell adhesion molecule-1-dependent and -independent binding mechanisms. *Journal of Immunology* **146**, 592–8.

Vainio, H. (2001). Is COX-2 inhibition a panacea for cancer prevention? *International Journal of Cancer* **94**, 613–14.

Verma, S., Raj, S.R., Shewchuk, L., Mather, K.J., and Anderson, T.J. (2001). Cyclooxygenase-2 blockade does not impair endothelial vasodilator function in healthy volunteers: randomized evaluation of rofecoxib versus naproxen on endothelium-dependent vasodilatation. *Circulation* **104**, 2879–82.

Vey, E., Zhang, J.H., and Dayer, J.M. (1992). IFN-gamma and 1,25$(OH)_2D_3$ induce on THP-1 cells distinct patterns of cell surface antigen expression, cytokine production, and responsiveness to contact with activated T cells. *Journal of Immunology* **149**, 2040–6.

Vey, E., Burger, D., and Dayer, J.M. (1996). Expression and cleavage of tumor necrosis factor-alpha and tumor necrosis factor receptors by human monocytic cell lines upon direct contact with stimulated T cells. *European Journal of Immunology* **26**, 2404–9.

Vey, E., Dayer, J.M., and Burger, D. (1997). Direct contact with stimulated T cells induces the expression of IL-1beta and IL-1 receptor antagonist in human monocytes. Involvement of serine/threonine phosphatases in differential regulation. *Cytokine* **9**, 480–7.

Wajant, H., Henkler, F., and Scheurich, P. (2001). The TNF-receptor-associated factor family: scaffold molecules for cytokine receptors, kinases and their regulators. *Cell Signalling* **13**, 389–400.

Waldron-Lynch, F., Adams, C., Amos, C., Zhu, D.K., McDermott, M.F., Shanahan, F., Molloy, M.G., and O'Gara, F. (2001). Tumour necrosis factor 5′ promoter single nucleotide polymorphisms influence susceptibility to rheumatoid arthritis (RA) in immunogenetically defined multiplex RA families. *Genes and Immunity* **2**, 82–7.

Walport, M.J. (1993). Inherited complement deficiency—clues to the physiological activity of complement *in vivo*. *Quarterly Journal of Medicine* **86**, 355–8.

Walport, M.J. (2001a). Complement. First of two parts. *New England Journal of Medicine* **344**, 1058–66.

Walport, M.J. (2001b). Complement. Second of two parts. *New England Journal of Medicine* **344**, 1140–4.

Wilder, R.L. (2002). Neuroimmunoendocrinology of the rheumatic diseases: past, present, and future. *Annals of the New York Academy of Sciences* **966**, 13–19.

Wilson, A.G., de Vries, N., Pociot, F., di Giovine, F.S., van der Putte, L.B., and Duff, G.W. (1993). An allelic polymorphism within the human tumor necrosis factor alpha promoter region is strongly associated with HLA A1, B8, and DR3 alleles. *Journal of Experimental Medicine* **177**, 557–60.

Winterbourn, C.C., Vissers, M.C., and Kettle, A.J. (2000). Myeloperoxidase. *Current Opinions in Hematology* **7**, 53–8.

Wood, N.C., Dickens, E., Symons, J.A., and Duff, G.W. (1992). In situ hybridization of interleukin-1 in CD14-positive cells in rheumatoid arthritis. *Clinical Immunology and Immunopathology* **62**, 295–300.

Yeh, W.C., Hakem, R., Woo, M., and Mak, T.W. (1999). Gene targeting in the analysis of mammalian apoptosis and TNF receptor superfamily signaling. *Immunology Review* **169**, 283–302.

Yokota, S., Geppert, T.D., and Lipsky, P.E. (1988). Enhancement of antigen- and mitogen-induced human T lymphocyte proliferation by tumor necrosis factor-alpha. *Journal of Immunology* **140**, 531–6.

Zeggini, E., Thomson, W., Kwiatkowski, D., Richardson, A., Ollier, W., and Donn, R. (2002). Linkage and association studies of single-nucleotide polymorphism-tagged tumor necrosis factor haplotypes in juvenile oligoarthritis. *Arthritis and Rheumatism* **46**, 3304–11.

Zheng, L., Fisher, G., Miller, R.E., Peschon, J., Lynch, D.H., and Lenardo, M.J. (1995). Induction of apoptosis in mature T cells by tumour necrosis factor. *Nature* **377**, 348–51.

Zucker, S., Cao, J., and Chen, W.T. (2000). Critical appraisal of the use of matrix metalloproteinase inhibitors in cancer treatment. *Oncogene* **19**, 6642–50.

4.2 Leucocyte trafficking in inflammation

D.O. Haskard

Introduction

Whilst acute inflammation is dominated by a predominantly polymorphonuclear leucocyte infiltration of the tissues and by the exudation of fluid and plasma proteins, chronic inflammation is characterized by the presence of lymphocytes and monocyte/macrophages, and by the activation and proliferation of connective tissue. In some complex forms of inflammation such as rheumatoid synovitis, flares of acute inflammation may be periodically superimposed upon a background of chronic inflammation. The regulation of leucocyte trafficking into the tissues is critical to these processes.

Molecular basis of leucocyte trafficking

As long ago as the nineteenth century, Cohnheim postulated that a molecular change in the lining of the blood vessels in inflammation made them more adhesive for leucocytes. In recent years, monoclonal antibody (mAb) and DNA technology has led to the identification of a large number of adhesion molecules, chemoattractants, and chemoattractant receptors, which participate in leucocyte interactions with endothelial cells, and the migration and effector function of leucocytes within tissues (Springer 1995).

Adhesion molecules

Adhesion molecules concerned in leucocyte trafficking can be grouped into a number of families, based on similarities of structure and function (Springer 1995; Mojcik and Shevach 1997).

Selectins

The selectins are cell surface lectins that initiate intercellular interactions within flowing blood (Vestweber et al. 1999) (Table 1). The three members of the family are designated on the basis of the cell type on which the molecule was first characterized. Thus, L-selectin was first detected on leucocytes, P-selectin on platelets, and E-selectin on endothelial cells. Selectins have an extracellular *N*-terminal lectin domain, a proximal epidermal growth factor-like domain, a variable number of complement control protein (CCP) repeats (similar to those found in decay accelerating factor, e.g.), a transmembrane domain, and a short cytoplasmic domain. The lectin domains are highly conserved and are structurally similar to mammalian asialoglycoprotein receptors and mannose-binding proteins, with a functional dependence upon extracellular calcium ions. Each of the three molecules is encoded by genes that lie within 300 kb of each other on chromosome 1, suggesting that they are derived from duplications and mutations of a single gene. Whilst the primary function of selectins is adhesive, each of the selectins can perform cell signalling functions.

Consistent with their *N*-terminal lectin domains, the three selectins bind carbohydrate determinants (Varki 1997). However, high affinity selectin interactions depend on presentation of the glycan by appropriately modified glycoproteins. These are mostly sialomucins, which have a serine, threonine, proline-rich extracellular structure decorated with *O*-linked oligosaccharides. The best characterized selectin-binding carbohydrate is the sialylated, fucosylated terminal tetrasaccharide sialyl-3-fucosyl-*N*-acetyllactosamine (sialyl Lewis *x*), which can bind each of the selectins. For optimal L-selectin binding, the carbohydrate ligand is also sulfated (Galustian et al. 1999; Hemmerich et al. 2001). Cutaneous lymphocyte antigen (CLA) is an E-selectin ligand that marks a subset of memory T lymphocytes which traffic to skin. It is also expressed on neutrophils, eosinophils, monocytes, dendritic cells, and a subset of B cells. CLA is

Table 1 Selectins

	L-selectin	P-selectin	E-selectin
Synonyms	CD62L, LECAM-1, Leu-8, TQ1	CD62P, PADGEM, GMP-140	ELAM-1
Mol mass (kDa)	75–100	140	110–115
Complement control protein repeats	2	8/9	6
Distribution	Most leucocytes	Endothelial cells and platelets	Endothelial cells
Regulation	Constitutive expression	Translocation and transcription	Transcription
Cells bound	EC and leucocytes	Leucocytes, platelets	Leucocytes
Carbohydrate ligands	Sulfated, sialylated, and fucosylated	Sialyl Le^x	Sialyl Le^x, CLA
Protein ligands	GlyCAM-1, CD34, PSGL-1, MadCAM-1, others	PSGL-1	PSGL-1, others

a post-translational modification of P-selectin glycoprotein ligand-1 (PSGL-1, see below) and is related to sialyl Lewis *x* (Fuhlbrigge et al. 1997).

L-selectin was first identified by a monoclonal antibody (MEL-14), which inhibited the recruitment of lymphocytes to peripheral lymph nodes in mice, and was subsequently extensively characterized as a 'homing receptor' mediating the adhesion of lymphocytes to the endothelium of high endothelial venules (see below). However, L-selectin is expressed by most circulating leucocytes, apart from a subset of memory T lymphocytes, and also contributes to leucocyte–endothelial cell interactions in inflammation. Endothelial cell glycoproteins which can be modified to enable L-selectin binding include GlyCAM-1, CD34, podocalyxin, and MadCAM-1. Apart from its role in initiating leucocyte–endothelial cell adhesion, L-selectin also mediates the binding of leucocytes to PSGL-1 on leucocytes that are already adherent to endothelium, a process known as secondary capture (Walcheck et al. 1996). L-selectin tends to be enzymatically cleaved from the cell surface upon cell activation, explaining the reduced expression on tissue leucocytes.

P-selectin is the largest of the three selectins; in human having eight or nine CCP sequences, depending upon alternative mRNA splicing. It was first characterized as a platelet alpha granule antigen, appearing on the platelet surface after stimulation by thrombin. Subsequently, P-selectin was found to be synthesized also by endothelial cells and stored within intracellular granules known as Weibel–Palade bodies. Both platelet alpha granules and Weibel–Palade bodies can be mobilized to the plasma membrane within seconds of cellular activation, giving a very rapid mechanism for P-selectin expression. Additionally, endothelial cell P-selectin gene expression is upregulated by cytokines (see below). The principal counter-receptor for P-selectin is PSGL-1.

E-selectin expression is limited to activated endothelial cells (see below). Although E-selectin binds PSGL-1, there are other less well characterized E-selectin ligands. A number of candidates have been proposed, including L-selectin (Zollner et al. 1997), β_2 integrins (Kotovuori et al. 1993) and, in mouse, a 150 kDa (reduced) glycoprotein designated E-selectin ligand-1 (ESL-1) (Steegmaier et al. 1997).

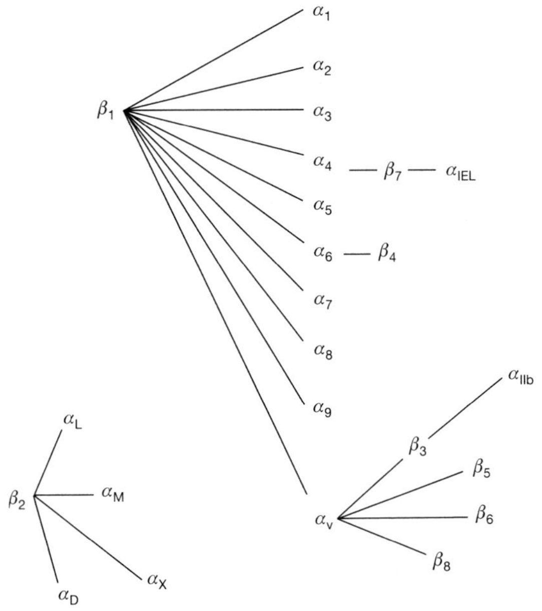

Fig. 1 The associations between integrin α and β sub-units, resulting in integrin sub-families.

Integrins

The integrins constitute a large family of non-covalently associated $\alpha\beta$ heterodimeric glycoproteins (sub-units of 95–200 kDa) that link the intracellular cytoskeleton with the extracellular environment (Hynes 1992). The importance of integrins is supported by their degree of species conservation, with similar molecules being found in the Drosophila fruit-fly and in the Xenopus toad. One or more integrin is found on most animal cell types.

At least 18 human α and 8 β chains have been defined, and the 22 recognized $\alpha\beta$ associations can be grouped into sub-families sharing a particular α or β chain. In general, there is considerable primary sequence similarity amongst the different α chains and also amongst the different β chains. However, despite the similarity between extracellular regions, there are substantial differences between the C-terminal cytoplasmic domains of different sub-units. Integrins that bind the same ligand may therefore differ markedly in their relationship with the cytoskeleton and in signalling functions.

While β sub-units complex with several different α sub-units, α sub-units themselves tend to combine with only one β sub-unit (with the exceptions of α_v, α_4, and α_6) (Fig. 1). Integrins expressed by leucocytes are shown in Table 2 (Shimizu et al. 1999; Harris et al. 2000). The ligand specificity of individual integrins depends not only on the particular $\alpha\beta$ combination but also on the cell type in which the integrin is expressed and upon the state of cellular activation.

The density of integrin expression by leucocytes is regulated by cellular activation. In the case of myeloid cells, $\alpha_M\beta_2$ and $\alpha_X\beta_2$ are translocated from intracellular granules, whereas changes in integrin expression on lymphocytes occur upon antigen stimulation. However, surface expression is not sufficient for ligand binding, which is regulated by rapid and reversible changes in integrin affinity and avidity. Changes in leucocyte integrin affinity are related to conformational alterations in the $\alpha\beta$ complex and are controlled in part by signals from within the cell ('inside-out signalling') and in part by initial contact with ligand ('ligand-induced adhesion'). Changes in integrin avidity occur upon integrin clustering in the cell membrane (van Kooyk and Figdor 2000). The reason for these complex mechanisms of regulating

Table 2 Leucocyte integrins[a]

Integrin	Synonyms	Distribution on leucocytes Blood cells	Ligands
$\alpha_L\beta_2$	LFA-1, CD11a/CD18	All	ICAM-1, -2, -3, -4, -5
$\alpha_m\beta_2$	Mac-1, CR3, CD11b/CD18	N, Bas, E, LGL, Mo, Mac, NK	ICAM-1, -4, iC3b, Factor X, Fb
$\alpha_x\beta_2$	p150,95, CD11c/CD18	N, Bas, DC, E, LGL, Mo, Mac, NK	Fb, iC3b
$\alpha_D\beta_2$	CD11d/CD18	Mo, Mac, E	VCAM-1, ICAM-3
$\alpha_1\beta_1$	VLA-1, CD49a/CD29	Mo, activated B and T	Collagen, Laminin
$\alpha_2\beta_1$	VLA-2, CD49b/CD29	Mo, activated T, B, P	Collagen, Laminin
$\alpha_3\beta_1$	VLA-3, CD49c/CD29	activated T, B	Collagen, Fn, Laminin
$\alpha_4\beta_1$	VLA-4, CD49d/CD29	Bas, E, Mo, NK, T, B	VCAM-1, Fn, ICAM-4
$\alpha_5\beta_1$	VLA-5, CD49e/CD29	M, T, B, P	Fn
$\alpha_6\beta_1$	VLA-6, CD49f/CD29	M, activated T, B	Laminin
$\alpha_4\beta_7$	LPAM-2	Bas, E, Mo, NK, sensitized T, B	MadCAM-1, VCAM-1, Fn
$\alpha_E\beta_7$	HML-1	Mucosa-associated T	E-cadherin
$\alpha_{IIa}\beta_3$	CD41a/CD61	P	Fb, Fn, TS, Vn, vWF
$\alpha_v\beta_3$	CD51/CD61	N, M, E, P	Vn, Fn, Ln, Tsp, Fb, vWF, ICAM-4

[a] B, B lymphocyte; Bas, basophil; DC, dendritic cells; E, eosinophil; EC, endothelial cell; Ep, epithelial cell; F, fibroblast; Fb, fibrinogen; Fn, fibronectin; LGL, large granular lymphocyte; LPAM, lymphocyte Peyer's patch adhesion molecule; Mac, macrophage; Mo, monocyte; N, neutrophils; NK, NK cell; P, platelet; T, T lymphocyte; TS, thrombospondin; vWF, von Willebrand Factor; Vn, vitronectin.

leucocyte integrin adhesiveness is most probably to maintain them in a relatively non-adhesive conformation while leucocytes are in the general circulation. Only under the control of specific cognate interactions, such as may be provided by chemokines at sites of inflammation (see below) do they convert to an adhesive state.

The ability of integrins to transduce signals into the cell is referred to as 'outside-in signalling' (Clark and Brugge 1995). Thus, integrin ligation may directly regulate cytoskeletal organization and activate the function of other integrins (Hogg and Leitinger 2001). Moreover, outside-in signalling through integrins can provide important costimulatory signals which influence leucocyte responsiveness to parallel stimuli. For example, several surface integrins, including $\alpha_L\beta_2$ and $\alpha_4\beta_1$, can act as costimulatory molecules for lymphocyte proliferation (Shimizu et al. 1990).

Immunoglobulin-like molecules

The immunoglobulin (Ig) supergene family consists of a large number of molecules that are structurally related to antibodies (Williams and Barclay 1988). Within this family falls a sub-group of single chain glycoprotein adhesion molecules (e.g. intercellular adhesion molecule (ICAM)-1-5, vascular cell adhesion molecule (VCAM)-1, mucosal addressin cell adhesion molecule (MadCAM)-1, platelet–endothelial cell adhesion molecule (PECAM)-1 and junctional adhesion molecules (JAM)-1-3, with many acting as ligands for integrins (Wang and Springer 1998) (Table 3). Other important lymphocyte surface molecules that are contained within the Ig superfamily are HLA Class I and II, CD4, CD8, CD2, and CD58 (lymphocyte function-associated antigen-3).

ICAM-1 has five C2-type extracellular Ig domains, with $\alpha_L\beta_2$ binding sites localized on the two domains nearest the *N*-terminal (van de Stope and van der Saag 2001). In contrast to their arrangement in antibodies, the Ig domains of ICAM-1 are unpaired and linear, with a potential bend between domains 2 and 3. ICAM-1 contains two recognized binding sites for integrins, one for $\alpha_L\beta_2$, localized to the outer domain one and the top of domain two, and one for $\alpha_M\beta_2$ on domain 3. The use of different binding sites on ICAM-1 by $\alpha_L\beta_2$ and $\alpha_M\beta_2$ suggests a mechanism for the strengthening of cellular adhesion to ICAM-1, which could be utilized by myeloid cells expressing both of these β_2 integrins.

ICAM-2 can be considered as a truncated form of ICAM-1, consisting of two Ig-like domains, which are similar to the two most *N*-terminal domains of ICAM-1. It is expressed on unstimulated endothelial cells with a density 10-fold greater than that of ICAM-1 and may therefore be the more important integrin $\alpha_L\beta_2$ ligand on endothelium in uninflamed tissues (De Fougerolles et al. 1991). However, ICAM-2 expression on endothelial cells is downregulated by proinflammatory stimuli, and consequently ICAM-1 may be the predominant $\alpha_L\beta_2$ ligand on endothelium in inflammation.

Although it is likely that ICAM-1 and ICAM-2 are the only ligands on endothelial cells which can bind integrin $\alpha_L\beta_2$, there is a third $\alpha_L\beta_2$ ligand in the form of ICAM-3. It is highly expressed on most resting leucocytes and may be particularly important for interactions between lymphocytes and dendritic cells. Consistent with this, ICAM-3 has been found to be an active signalling molecule. ICAM-4 is identical to the LW blood group protein and is expressed by erythroblasts (Spring et al. 2001). It is probably important for their adhesion and function in the bone marrow. ICAM-5 (telencephalin) is selectively expressed in the brain (Mizuno et al. 1997).

The VCAM-1 cDNA that was first sequenced predicted six C2-type Ig domains. However, the predominant form on endothelial cells has an additional domain, which is very similar in primary structure to the domain at the *N*-terminal and is situated between domains 3 and 4 of the 6-domain form. Whereas integrin $\alpha_4\beta_1$ binds domain one on both the 6- and 7-domain forms, $\alpha_4\beta_1$ binding can additionally occur to the homologous fourth domain of the 7-domain form, providing a mechanism for the strengthening of $\alpha_4\beta_1$-dependent adhesion. In general, α_4 integrins are expressed by eosinophils, monocytes, and lymphocytes and less so by neutrophils. VCAM-1 therefore makes an important contribution to the selective trafficking of eosinophils and mononuclear cells into inflamed tissues (Carter and Wicks 2001).

Human MadCAM-1 has two Ig domains which have structural similarities to ICAM-1 and VCAM-1, and which bind the integrin $\alpha_4\beta_7$. The membrane proximal portion of the molecule is occupied by a mucin region rich in *O*-linked sugars, which can act as an L-selectin ligand (Berg et al. 1993). MadCAM-1 is expressed by endothelial cells of post-capillary venules of Peyer's patches and mesenteric lymph nodes and also on blood vessels in lamina propria of the small intestine and in some forms of extramucosal inflammation (e.g. pancreas and CNS). It acts as a homing receptor ('vascular addressin') for lymphocyte trafficking to gut. Besides being expressed by gut endothelial cells, MadCAM-1 is also expressed by gut follicular dendritic cells, and may be involved in reprogramming naive T and

Table 3 Adhesion molecules within the immunoglobulin superfamily[a]

	CD	kDa	Ig domains	Expression	Ligands
ICAM-1	CD54	88–110	5	EC, Ep, F, DC, L, others	$\alpha_L\beta_2$, $\alpha_M\beta_2$
ICAM-2	CD102	55	2	EC, P, L	$\alpha_L\beta_2$, DC-SIGN
ICAM-3	CD50	124	5	L	$\alpha_L\beta_2$, $\alpha_D\beta_2$, DC-SIGN
ICAM-4	CD242	37–47	2	Erythroblasts	$\alpha_4\beta_1$, $\alpha_v\beta_1$, $\alpha_v\beta_3$, $\alpha_L\beta_2$, $\alpha_M\alpha_2$
ICAM-5		130	9	Neurons	$\alpha_L\beta_2$
VCAM	CD106	110	6/7	EC, Ep, DC, SB, other	$\alpha_4\beta_1$, $\alpha_D\beta_2$
MAdCAM		58–66	2	Gut-associated EC and FDC	$\alpha_4\beta_7$
PECAM	CD31	130	6	EC, L, P	$\alpha_v\beta_3$, PECAM, CD38
JAM-1		32–43	2	EC, Ep, P, L	JAM-1, $\alpha_L\beta_2$
JAM-2		48	2	EC	JAM-2, JAM-3
JAM-3		43	2	EC, L	JAM-2

[a] DC, dendritic cells; EC, endothelial cells; Ep, epithelial cells; F, fibroblasts; FDC, follicular dendritic cells; L, leucocytes; M, monocytes; P, platelets; SB, synovial type B cells.

B lymphocytes for gastrointestinal trafficking during their responses to antigen. Other cells that express MadCAM-1 include cells lining the marginal sinus of the spleen and choroid plexus epithelial cells. Notably, MdCAM-1 is not expressed in pulmonary, tonsillar, or oral mucosa, arguing that gastrointestinal trafficking of lymphocytes is not equivalent to mucosal trafficking.

PECAM-1 has six Ig domains, which self-associate in homotypic (i.e. PECAM-1–PECAM-1) interactions between cells. Another major structural feature of PECAM-1 is the presence in the cytoplasmic domain of an immunoreceptor tyrosine-based inhibitory motif, shared by molecules such as CTLA-4, CD22, and FcgRIIb (CD32) (Newman 1999). PECAM-1 is expressed by endothelial cells, platelets, neutrophils, monocytes, and a subset of T cells. On endothelium it is a major constituent of intercellular junctions, and contributes to contact inhibition of endothelial cell migration and proliferation. PECAM-1 is involved in modulating the function of surface integrins during the transmigration of leucocytes though endothelium into the tissues (Newman 1999).

JAM 1–3 are expressed at endothelial cell intercellular junctions and are involved in the regulation of paracellular permeability and in leucocyte transendothelial migration (Arrate et al. 2001; Aurrand-Lions et al. 2001). Recently JAM-1 has been found to act as a ligand for integrin $\alpha_L\beta_2$ (Ostermann et al. 2002).

P-selectin glycoprotein ligand-1

PSGL-1 is the principal leucocyte counter-receptor for P-selectin. It is also capable of binding L-selectin and is one of several possible counter-receptors for E-selectin (McEver and Cummings 1997). PSGL-1 is a 220 kDa sialylated homodimer with a disulfide bond situated extracellularly near the cell membrane. It is expressed in a functionally active form on most myeloid cells and on platelets (Frenette et al. 2000). Although it is widely expressed on lymphocytes, only a subset of memory T cells express PSGL-1 that is appropriately glycosylated for selectin-binding. PSGL-1 is similar to L-selectin in being shed upon leucocyte activation.

Vascular adhesion protein-1 (VAP-1)

VAP-1 is a 170–180 kDa homodimeric sialoglycoprotein that is surface expressed on a number of cells types, including endothelial cells and vascular smooth muscle cells (Salmi and Jalkanen 2001a). It is a semicarbazide-sensitive monoamine oxidase, and forms adhesions with an as yet unknown ligand(s) on leucocytes by catalysing the formation of transient covalent bonds. It plays a role in the primary capture of leucocytes to endothelium (see below).

CD44

CD44 (Pgp-1, HCAM, Hermes) is a highly polymorphic cell surface glycoprotein with similarity to cartilage link proteins (Pure and Cuff 2001). It has a wide cellular distribution, which includes lymphoid and myeloid cells, endothelial cells, epithelial cells, and fibroblasts. Heterogeneity of CD44 is partly attributable to alternative splicing of 10 exons lying in tandem within the extracellular portion of the CD44 gene and partly to differential glycosylation. Thus CD44 can be modified by *N*- and/or *O*-linked glysosylation and may also express chondroitin sulfate or heparan sulfate side-chains. CD44 acts as a receptor for several extracellular matrix components including hyaluronan and fibronectin. Furthermore, there is evidence that CD44 may support the adhesion of lymphocytes to endothelial cells. Apart from acting as an adhesion molecule, CD44 is also a signalling molecule capable of initiating integrin $\alpha_L\beta_2$ dependent adhesion and costimulating T lymphocyte proliferation. Variants of CD44 that express proteoglycan side-chains may bind cytokines and growth factors to the cell surface.

DC-SIGN

Dendritic cell specific-ICAM-grabbing non-integrin (DC-SIGN) is type 2 transmembrane mannose-binding C-type lectin that binds the second Ig domains of ICAM-2 and ICAM-3 and negatively regulates LFA-1 adhesion. It is involved in lymphocyte–dendritic cell interactions (Bleijs et al. 2001).

Chemoattractants

The directional movement of leucocytes in response to a soluble stimulus is known as 'chemotaxis'. A large number of leucocyte chemotactic factors have been described, including activated complement components (e.g. C5a), lipid metabolites (e.g. leukotrienes, platelet activating factor), and bacterial-derived peptides (e.g. F–Met–Leu–Phe). Amongst the cytokines, chemokines are 8–14 kDa proteins that play a key role in coordinating recruitment of leucocytes into and within tissues, during organogenesis, homeostatic lymphocyte recirculation, and inflammation (Rossi and Zlotnik 2000; Mackay 2001). Most chemokines have a basic charge, leading to the binding of sulfated proteins and proteoglycans. This feature is important for immobilization on the glycocalyx of endothelial cells and for establishing gradients of chemokine expression within tissues, along which leucocyte migration can take place.

Chemokines can be classified into CXC (α chemokines), CC (β chemokines), CX3C, and C sub-families, depending upon the number and spacing of cysteine residues at the amino terminal (Table 4). While equivalent chemokines can sometimes be identified in human and laboratory

Table 4 Chemokines

Classification	Synonym	Receptor
CXC chemokines		
CXCL1	Gro-α, MGSA-α	CXCR2 > CXCR1
CXCL2	Gro-β, MGSA-β	CXCR2
CXCL3	Gro-γ, MGSA-γ	CXCR2
CXCL4	PL4	?
CXCL5	ENA-78	CXCR2
CXCL6	GCP-2	CXCR1, 2
CXCL7	NAP-2	CXCR1, 2
CXCL8	IL-8	CXCR1, 2
CXCL9	Mig	CXCR3
CXCL10	IP-10	CXCR3
CXCL11	I-TAC	CXCR3
CXCL12	SDF-1α/β	CXCR4
CXCL13	BLC, BCA-1	CXCR5
CXCL14	BRAK, bolekine	?
CXCL15	Lungkine (as yet only mouse)	?
CXCL16		CXCR6
CC chemokines		
CCL1	I-309	CCR1, 8
CCL2	MCP-1, MCAF	CCR2
CCL3	MIP-1α, LD78α	CCR1, 5
CCL4	MIP-1β	CCR5
CCL5	RANTES	CCR1, 3, 5
CCL6	C10, MRP-1 (as yet mouse only)	?
CCL7	MCP-3	CCR1, 2, 3
CCL8	MCP-2	CCR3
CCL9/10	MRP-2, CCF18 (as yet mouse only)	?
CCL11	Eotaxin-1	CCR3
CCL12	MCP-5 (as yet mouse only)	CCR2
CCL13	MCP-4	CCR2, 3
CCL14	HCC-1	CCR1
CCL15	HCC-2, leukotactin, MIP-1δ	CCR1, 3
CCL16	HCC-4, LEC	CCR1
CCL17	TARC	CCR4
CCL18	DC-CK1, PARc, AMAC-1	?
CCL19	MIP-3β, ELC, exodus-3	CCR7, 11
CCL20	MIP-3α, LARK, exodus-1	CCR6
CCL21	6Ckine, SLC, exodus-2	CCR7, 11
CCL22	MDC, STCP-1	CCR4
CCL23	MPIF-1	CCR1
CCL24	MPIF-2, eotaxin-2	CCR3
CCL25	TECK	CCR9, 11
CCL26	Eotaxin-3	CCR3
CCL27	CTACK, ILC	CCR10
CCL28	MEC	CCR10
CX$_3$C chemokine		
CX3CL1	Fractalkine	CX3CR1
C chemokines		
XCL1	Lymphotactin, SCM-1α, ATAC	XCR1
XCL2	SCM-1β	XCR1

animals, this is not always the case. Thus no human equivalents have so far been discovered for mouse of CXCL15 and CCL6, 9, 10, and 12.

Some chemokines (e.g. SLC, ELC, BLC) are expressed by dendritic cells and lymphoid stromal cells and play a key role in homeostatic lymphocyte trafficking and sensitization (Cyster 1999). Expression of others, such as IL-8, MCP-1, and RANTES is induced by cytokines (e.g. IL-1, TNFα, IFNγ, IL-4) and other inflammatory mediators and stimulate leucocyte recruitment into inflamed tissues (Godessart and Kunkel 2001).

Fractalkine (CX3CL1) is unique amongst chemokines identified to date in being a membrane anchored molecule, with transmembrane and cytoplasmic domains (Bazan et al. 1997). Furthermore, fractalkine serves not only as a chemokine but also as an adhesion molecule (Haskell et al. 2000). The extracellular domain (about 95 kDa) has a long mucin stalk, which can be released from the membrane to give a soluble form with leucocyte chemotactic activity. Fractalkine is chemotactic for monocytes and lymphocytes but not neutrophils.

Chemoattractant receptors

As a general rule, chemoattractants stimulate leucocytes through receptors which span the membrane seven times ('serpentine receptors') and which activate cells through coupling to Gi-type heterotrimeric GTP-binding proteins (G proteins). Many chemokines bind with high affinity to several chemokine receptors, and conversely many chemokine receptors bind several different chemokines (Table 5) (Murphy et al. 2000). This apparent redundancy is probably more apparent than real, as receptor binding is not an accurate predictor of function. Chemokines acting through the same receptor may have distinct down-stream effects, be they agonistic, neutral, or antagonistic.

Leucocyte–endothelial cell interactions

Adhesion of leucocytes to the lumenal surface of vascular endothelial cells is the first step in their migration from the blood into the tissues. As such, leucocyte–endothelial cell interactions are of critical importance in determining the number and type of leucocytes recruited, both during constitutive lymphocyte trafficking and in inflammation. The term 'adhesion cascade' refers to the sequential participation of different adhesion molecules and chemoattractant receptors during the emigration process. Most studies have focused on events taking place in post-capillary venules, but important variations may exist in other tissues, such as in lung and liver, where leucocyte migration occurs via capillaries and sinusoids.

Tethering and rolling

Direct observation of leucocyte–endothelial cell interactions in post-capillary venules by intravital microscopy shows that leucocytes tether and then roll along the surface of endothelium before arresting on the vessel wall. As a result of rolling, the velocity with which leucocytes pass through the vessel drops from about 2000–3000 μm to approximately 10–25 μm, facilitating further interactions with the endothelial surface.

Leucocyte tethering and rolling are mediated in large part by selectins. Thus, both L- and P-selectin are effective at causing leucocyte tethering, perhaps since L-selectin and PSGL-1 are expressed on the tips of leucocyte microvillous processes. The role of E-selectin appears to be more involved in the stabilization of rolling rather than initial tethering (Jung and Ley 1999; Robinson et al. 1999). The bonds between selectins and their ligands have fast on–off kinetics and therefore form and break rapidly. Hence, they are well suited for initiating rather than maintaining leucocyte adhesion to endothelium. VAP-1 and CD44 may also be involved in leucocyte rolling under some circumstances.

Whereas neutrophils are highly dependent upon selectins for tethering and rolling, eosinophils, monocytes, and lymphocytes can also use α_4 integrins ($\alpha_4\beta_1$, $\alpha_4\beta_7$) for primary capture, through interactions with VCAM-1 or MAdCAM-1. This provides an important selectin-independent mechanism for initiating leucocyte–endothelial cell interactions with endothelium and may contribute to selective mononuclear recruitment.

Arrest of rolling cells

Whilst rolling, leucocytes are exposed to local factors that stimulate their arrest. The most important event mediating the conversion from rolling to arrest is the rapid stimulation of leucocyte integrin function (Lawrence and Springer 1991). This may be due to changes in either affinity or avidity of leucocyte integrins (Constantin et al. 2000). Stimuli leading to upregulated

Table 5 Chemokine receptors

Classification	Leucocyte distribution	Example of biological function
CXC chemokine receptors		
CXCR1	Neutrophils	Neutrophil recruitment
CXCR2	Neutrophils	Neutrophil recruitment
CXCR3	Th1 cells	Effector T cell responses
CXCR4	Most leucocytes	Lymphocyte migration in tissues
CXCR5	B cells, sensitized CD4 T cells	B cell follicle formation
CXCR6	Th1 cells, Tc1 cells	DC-T cell interactions
CC chemokine receptors		
CCR1	Eosinophils, monocytes	Antiviral responses
CCR2	Basophils, monocytes	Th1 cell responses
CCR3	Eosinophils, basophils, Th2 cells	Th2 responses
CCR4	Th2 cells, skin homing Th1 cells	Lymphocyte homing to skin
CCR5	Th1 cells, monocytes	Th1 cell responses
CCR6	Memory but not naive CD4 T cells, dendritic cells	DC homing to normal skin
CCR7	Naive and CD62L+ memory T cells, B cells, dendritic cells	Lymphoid tissue homing
CCR8	Th2 cells, monocytes	Th2 responses
CCR9	Gut-homing CD4 and CD8 T cells ($\alpha 4\beta 7$ integrin +)	Lymphocyte homing to gut
CCR10	? Memory T lymphocytes	Lymphocyte migration in skin
CCR11	Dendritic cells	?
CX_3C chemokine receptors		
CX3CR1	Monocytes, NK cells	Th1 cell responses

integrin function are usually associated with the endothelial surface, in the form of immobilized chemoattractants (Campbell et al. 1998; Tanaka et al. 1998). The correct presentation of chemokine is probably critical, as exposure of leucocytes to chemoattactants in solution may inhibit leucocyte emigration. The conversion from rolling to arrest is a critical selection point in the adhesion cascade, as many more cells may roll than will go on to arrest. For example, neutrophils roll in lymph node high endothelial venules but do not arrest unless the lymph node is inflamed.

Leucocyte transendothelial migration

The process by which leucocytes migrate through endothelium into the tissues is less well understood than the initial adhesion events (Imhof et al. 2001; Johnson-Léger et al. 2001). Although leucocytes usually emigrate through intercellular junctions, under some conditions they may actually pass through endothelial cells (Feng et al. 1998). The mechanisms guiding leucocytes through endothelium involve two-way signalling interactions between leucocytes and endothelial cells, which are modulated biomechanically by the shear forces of blood flow (Cinamon et al. 2001). The adhesion molecules involved in transmigration include similar integrin interactions with Ig-superfamily ligands to those supporting firm adhesion. In addition, other Ig-superfamily members (e.g. PECAM-1, JAM-1,2,3), which tend to be expressed selectively at endothelial cell junctions, are also involved. The mechanisms by which leucocytes penetrate the basal lamina, which is composed of types III, IV, and V collagen, heparan sulfate, laminin, and fibronectin, are not well understood but may involve the induced secretion or surface expression of degradative enzymes.

Zip-code model

The combination of adhesion and activation events necessary for successful leucocyte emigration provides a framework for understanding the diversity of leucocyte recruitment in different homeostatic and inflammatory settings (Butcher 1991; Springer 1995). The zip-code model proposes that adhesion molecules and chemokine/chemokine receptors guide leucocytes to their destination in a logical sequential fashion, as in the different codes of a long-distance telephone number. Thus adhesion or activation mechanisms with selective effects on particular leucocyte populations may have a major impact on the mix of leucocyte recruited.

Constitutive lymphocyte trafficking

Once myeloid cells are released from the bone marrow, their circulation tends to be confined to the vascular compartment. Lymphocytes on the other hand have a more complex distribution, which until the second half of the twentieth century was an enigma. Lymphocytes could be found in large numbers in thoracic duct lymph and these were thought to be the products of recent cell division within lymph nodes. Since lymphocytes that had been collected by thoracic duct drainage and reinjected intravenously were found to disappear from the circulation within an hour, it was assumed that lymphocytes were short-lived non-dividing cells. The classical experiments of Sir James Gowans in the rat provided a completely altered view of lymphocyte physiology. Gowans showed that blood lymphocytes rapidly enter lymph nodes on a recirculation pathway back to blood (Gowans and Knight 1964).

The life-span of lymphocytes

The demonstration of lymphocyte recirculation implied that small lymphocytes have much longer life-spans than had previously been realized. Studies on the longevity of chromosomal alterations in patients with ankylosing spondylitis who had undergone spinal irradiation showed that a population of small lymphocytes recirculates for years (Buckton et al. 1967), although a median survival time for lymphocytes in man is probably more like 2–3 weeks.

Function of lymphocyte trafficking

It is estimated that the human body has 10^{12} T lymphocytes, of which approximately two thirds are naive (unsensitized) cells. Since T cell receptor α and β chains can form approximately 2.5×10^7 combinations, the number of naive T cells expressing a particular $\alpha\beta$ T cell receptor may be as low as a few thousand (Arstila et al. 1999). The recirculation of lymphocytes therefore provides a mechanism that maximizes the chances of relatively small numbers of antigen-specific lymphocytes encountering cognate antigen associated with an antigen presenting cell (Von Andrian and Mackay 2000). In the case of naive cells, trafficking normally occurs predominantly through fixed lymphoid tissues, allowing access to antigen and antigen presenting cells transported via afferent lymphatics. Following sensitization and clonal expansion, lymphocytes develop the capacity to enter non-lymphoid tissues, particularly when these are inflamed.

Lymphocyte trafficking into lymph nodes

Recirculating lymphocytes enter lymph nodes by passing through post-capillary venules located primarily in the lymph node paracortex (Marchesi and Gowans 1964). These venules are referred to as high endothelial venules (HEV), because of their plump, columnar endothelial cells (Kraal and Mebius 1997). Their specialised properties require ongoing stimulation, since they are curtailed by ligation of afferent lymphatics. The recruitment of lymphocytes across HEV is highly efficient, with up to one in four lymphocytes that enter the venules passing into the lymphoid parenchyma (Young 1999).

The structure of HEV may provide a valve-like regulation of permeability to macromolecules, thereby minimizing the leak of plasma proteins that could occur with large scale constitutive lymphocyte trafficking. Furthermore, HEV are adapted for lymphocyte recruitment by expression of GlcNAc-6-sulfotransferase, an enzyme that enables the post-translational modification of molecules such as GlyCAM-1, CD34, and MadCAM-1 to become L-selectin ligands (Hemmerich et al. 2001). HEV also express chemokines on the endothelial lumenal surface, either synthesized within the endothelial cells or transported from within the lymph node parenchyma, or posted, via afferent lymphatics, from distant sites (Stein et al. 2000; Baekkevold et al. 2001).

Primary capture of leucocytes in lymph node HEV is mediated predominantly by L-selectin. T lymphocyte arrest is then selectively triggered by the chemokines CCL19 (ELC) and CCL21 (SLC) binding to their receptor CCR7 (Stein et al. 2000; Baekkevold et al. 2001), which in turn leads to $\alpha_L\beta_2$ integrin adhesion to ICAM-1/2. The arrest of B cells, which adhere to HEV in the vicinity to germinal centres, probably involves other chemokines (Campbell and Butcher 2000). Once lymphocytes have passed into the parenchyma of the node, their migration towards T cell zones is promoted by the chemokines ELC and SLC, whereas migration to B cell zones is promoted by BLC (Cyster 1999).

Effect of lymphocyte sensitization

The altered migration capacity of memory lymphocytes is attributable in large part to changes in expression of adhesion molecules and chemokine receptors that occur upon sensitization (Pitzalis et al. 1988; Sanders et al. 1988; Mackay et al. 1996). About 50 per cent of sensitized T cells retain L-selectin and CCR7, allowing their continued recirculation through secondary lymphoid tissues as central memory cells (Picker et al. 1993a; Sallusto et al. 1999). The other 50 per cent lose L-selectin and CCR7 expression and do not recirculate to lymph nodes following release into efferent lymphatics. Instead, they are capable of migrating into extralymphoid tissues, where they function as effector cells (Sallusto et al. 1999).

The changes in phenotype that occur upon lymphocyte differentiation in lymph nodes also confer on lymphocytes regional migration preferences (Butcher et al. 1999). For example, memory lymphocytes that home to skin express the E-selectin binding carbohydrate CLA (see above) and CCR4, which favour lymphocyte interactions with dermal endothelium (Picker et al. 1993b; Pitzalis et al. 1996; Campbell et al. 1999). While both $\alpha_4\beta_1$ and $\alpha_4\beta_7$ are upregulated upon sensitization of naive T cells, the α_4 integrin subunit associates with β_7 on lymphocytes sensitized in the gut immune system, and β_1 with in lymphocytes sensitized in peripheral lymph nodes. These pairings determine whether the cell selectively binds MAdCAM-1 in the gut or VCAM-1 in peripheral tissues (Rott et al. 1996). Whether or not there is a specific subset of lymphocytes that homes to inflamed synovium is still unclear. It is possible that the association between inflammatory bowel disease and arthritis relates in part to the ability of gut-homing lymphocytes to adhere to synovial endothelium (Salmi and Jalkanen 2001b).

Lymphocyte trafficking through spleen

Besides recirculating through lymph nodes, lymphocytes also circulate in large numbers through the spleen. Indeed, in the rat more lymphocytes circulate through spleen than through all the lymph nodes put together (Pabst 1988). Leucocytes are thought to pass freely through fenestrated arterial endothelium into splenic parenchyma, and, unlike in other tissues, endothelium is probably not a major control point for trafficking. Similar principles regulate the retention and distribution of lymphocytes in spleen as in lymph nodes (Cyster 1999).

Lymphocyte trafficking through liver

The liver contains large numbers of T lymphocytes and NK cells and is an important site for immunoregulation (Crispe et al. 1996). Lymphocytes can enter liver through vessels in the portal tracts, via the central veins or via the hepatic sinusoids. Adhesion molecules and chemokine receptors involved in entry of lymphocytes into liver include VAP-1, integrin $\alpha_L\beta_2$, CCR5, and CXCR3 (Grant et al. 2002).

Leucocyte trafficking into inflamed tissues

Entry of leucocytes into the tissues is a hall-mark of inflammation, and is promoted by the local induced expression of adhesion molecules and chemoattractants on the surface of vascular endothelium (Cines et al. 1998). Altered endothelial function is tightly regulated, allowing the interaction of leucocytes with endothelium to be one of the key control points determining the course of inflammatory responses.

Endothelial cell activation

Activation of endothelial cells occurs in response to changes in the extraluminal and lumenal microenvironment and may be classified according to the kinetics of the response.

Rapid activation

Endothelial cells are able to alter their expression of adhesion molecules and chemoattractants within seconds to minutes, through the translocation of intracellular storage granules, Weibel–Palade bodies, to the plasma membrane (Type 1 activation) (Wagner 1993). This results in the surface expression of P-selectin and the release of von Willebrand Factor and interleukin-8 (Utgaard et al. 1998; Wolff et al. 1998). Factors capable of stimulating Weibel–Palade body translocation include histamine, thrombin, and complement C5a and C5b-9.

Sub-acute activation

Injection of interleukin-1 (IL-1), tumour necrosis factor, or lipopolysaccharide *in vivo* stimulates a sub-acute inflammatory response associated with marked leucocyte emigration into the tissues. To a large extent this is attributable to an orchestrated induction of gene expression, de novo protein synthesis and surface expression of adhesion molecules and chemokines (Type 2 activation) (Mantovani et al. 1998). The transcriptional control of much of this response involves translocation to the nucleus of the transcription factor NFκB, which is autoregulated by the synthesis of the inhibitory protein IκBα (Read et al. 1994). Similar effects are induced by IL-18 or by ligation of endothelial cell CD40 (Karmann et al. 1995; Morel et al. 2001). Amongst the genes regulated in this way are adhesion molecules involved in the rolling and firm adhesion stages of leucocyte–endothelial cell interaction, including E-selectin, ICAM-1, VCAM-1, and MadCAM-1, as well as the synthesis and secretion of cytokines such as IL-1 and -6, colony stimulating factors (CSFs) G-CSF, GM-CSF, and M-CSF, platelet-derived growth factor, and a number of chemokines such as IL-8 and monocyte chemotactic protein-1. In general, increased protein expression is first detectable *in vitro* after 1–2 h and lasts for a variable time, depending upon the stimulus applied and the exact response measured.

Whilst IL-1 and tumour necrosis factor appear to be the dominant cytokines involved in the sub-acute phase of endothelial cell activation, their effects can be modulated by other cytokines, which in themselves may have little or no direct action on the expression of endothelial cell adhesion molecules and chemokines. For example, the effects of IL-1 and particularly tumour necrosis factor on the expression of ICAM-1 and VCAM-1 may be selectively upregulated by the actions of interferon-γ and IL-4 respectively, suggesting a possible differential control of endothelial cell activation during T-helper 1- and T-helper 2-type responses (Thornhill and Haskard 1990).

Although TNFα and IL-1 regulate P-selection in parallel with E-selectin in the mouse, P-selectin is not regulated by these cytokines in human. Instead, P-selectin expression is selectively upregulated by IL-4, IL-13, and oncostatin M (Yao et al. 1996).

Chronic activation

Understanding the nature of endothelial cell activation in chronic inflammation has been hampered by the limitations of endothelial cell cultures, which are difficult to prolong beyond a few days. Many endothelial cell responses are downregulated as the inflammatory process becomes chronic, either through the endogenous control of transcriptional mechanisms (Read et al. 1994) or through the downregulating actions of some cytokines and growth factors such as interferon-γ, IL-4, and transforming growth factor-β (Thornhill and Haskard 1990; Gamble et al. 1993; Melrose et al. 1998; Harari et al. 2001). On the other hand, chronic immune-mediated inflammation is characterized by lymphoid neogenesis (see below), in which post-capillary venules develop a HEV-like morphology (Freemont 1987) (Fig. 2). Endothelium of such vessels expresses the peripheral lymph node addressin, an antigen associated with L-selectin ligands in lymph nodes (Michie et al. 1993). It is likely, therefore, that lymphocyte trafficking into established chronic immune-mediated lesions becomes 'constitutive' as in lymph nodes.

Leucocyte migration within inflamed tissues

Leucocytes within tissues are in a dynamic state, governed by entry from the blood, retention, migration into afferent lymph or programmed cell death, and subsequent removal by phagocytosis (Akbar and Salmon 1997; Savill and Fadok 2000). Relatively small numbers of leucocytes actually proliferate in inflammatory lesions. Once leucocytes have passed through endothelium, they migrate towards afferent lymphatics, in part probably through passive convection with interstitial fluid (Seabrook et al. 1999). However, once within the tissues, leucocytes are stimulated sequentially by chemoattractants and contact with other cells and extracellular matrix components such as fibronectin, collagen, and hyaluronate, resulting in the promotion of their survival and accumulation (Foxman et al. 1999). For example, both T and B lymphocyte accumulation in synovium is enhanced by mechanisms involving SDF-1, a chemokine released by synovial fibroblasts (Buckley et al. 2000; Burger et al. 2001). Less is known about the molecular basis of active migration through tissues than is the case for leucocyte adhesion to and transmigration through endothelium, although it is likely that similar principles apply. Thus, interactions between leucocytes and extracellular matrix and stromal cells may be as important as selective leucocyte–endothelial cell interactions in determining the leucocytes populating an inflamed tissue.

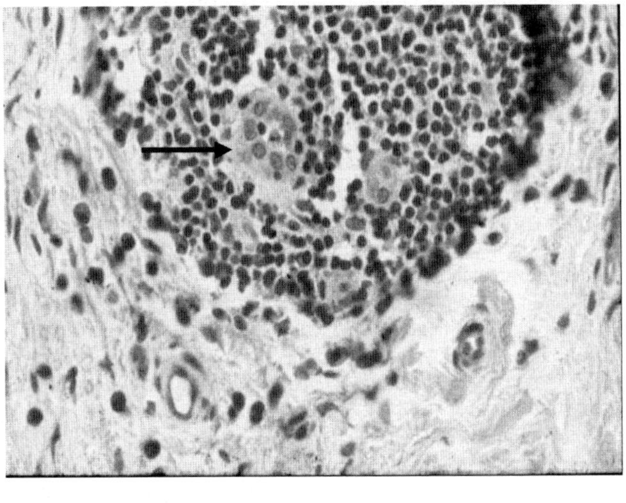

Fig. 2 Photomicrograph of rheumatoid synovium stained with haematoxylin and eosin. The arrow points to a 'high endothelial venule' within a lymphocyte aggregate.

Lymphoid neogenesis in inflammation

Lymphocytes not only migrate in increased numbers into inflamed tissues, but an increase also occurs in the number of lymphocytes present in the afferent lymph draining sites of inflammation, indicating an induced peripheral pathway of recirculation. Indeed, the number of lymphocytes in afferent lymphatics draining sites of chronic inflammation increases over days to weeks, eventually resembling that through lymph nodes (Smith et al. 1970). The ability of chronic inflammatory tissues to support the large scale recirculation of lymphocytes is associated with the development of HEV (see above) and germinal centres with B and T cells clustered around follicular dendritic cells (Hsi et al. 1998; Stott et al. 1998; Shi et al. 2001; Takemura et al. 2001a).

The molecular mechanisms responsible for this lymphoid neogenesis in inflammation are probably similar to those responsible for the development of lymph nodes during development (Ansel and Cyster 2001). Thus, ectopic lymphoid neogenesis can be induced in mice by overexpression of SLC (Fan et al. 2000) or BLC (Luther et al. 2000). Since BLC but not SLC is detectable in chronic synovitis, BLC may be the more important chemokine stimulating lymphoid neogenesis in the joint (Shi et al. 2001).

The consequence of lymphoid neogenesis in chronic inflammation is that inflamed tissues may adopt functions normally restricted to secondary lymphoid organs (Janossy et al. 1981). This might include the recruitment of lymphocyte phenotypes (i.e. naive T cells, B cells) that are less able to enter non-lymphoid tissues in acute inflammation. Furthermore, the lymphoid cytoarchitecture may allow the local sensitization of naive T cells, B cell–T cell interactions and the affinity maturation of antibodies (Takemura et al. 2001b).

The role of antigen in lymphocyte trafficking

A key event in lymphocyte trafficking is the encounter between the lymphocyte and an antigen-presenting cell, in which activation of the lymphocyte occurs via a focal area of adhesion known as the immunological synapse (Dustin 2002). At the onset of immune-mediated inflammation, the local activation of T lymphocytes sets up a cascade of events that results in the non-specific secondary recruitment of leucocytes, including more lymphocytes. The degree to which inflammation can be induced and amplified by this means is attested to by the ability to mount a delayed-type hypersensitivity response after passive transfer of a single T cell (Marchal et al. 1982). It is therefore likely that any oligoclonality of antigen specificity detected in populations of lymphocytes isolated from inflamed tissues is due predominantly to the selective retention, survival, and/or proliferation of cells activated within the tissues, rather than to the existence of a mechanism for the selective recruitment of antigen-specific lymphocytes.

Genetic abnormalities and polymorphisms affecting leucocyte trafficking

Although very rare, genetic abnormalities of leucocyte adhesion molecules provide important insights into molecular mechanisms of leucocyte trafficking and function in human.

Leucocyte adhesion deficiency types I and II

Striking evidence for the importance of adhesion molecules in leucocyte trafficking is found in leucocyte adhesion deficiency type (LAD) 1, which is due to failure to synthesize the β_2 integrin sub-unit (CD18) (Arnaout et al. 1990). Consequently, leucocytes have reduced or absent surface expression of all β_2 integrins. More recently, variants of LAD I have been described in which leucocytes have normal β_2 integrin expression but defective function (e.g. Hogg et al. 1999). Infants with LAD I often have delayed separation of the umbilical cord, reflecting the role of phagocytes in this process. The clinical course is characterized by recurrent pyogenic infections, in which affected tissues show a poverty of neutrophils. Typically patients have a high white cell count (sometimes as high as $150 \times 10^3/\text{mm}^3$), in part due to the inability of leucocytes to emigrate from the vascular compartment (Fig. 3). In spite of the abnormalities of leucocyte migration, problematic viral infections are rare and patients are able to mount satisfactory humoral and cell-mediated immune responses, probably because α_4 integrins and other adhesion molecules can compensate for the β_2 integrin deficiency.

In LAD II (also known as congenital disorder of glycosylation-IIc) there is an abnormality in fucosylation of glycoproteins, including selectin ligands (Etzioni and Tonetti 2000). Affected individuals have a spectrum of inflammatory manifestations, which overlap with those of leucocyte adhesion deficiency type I, and also show developmental abnormalities. The abnormal gene responsible for this condition is now known to be a GDP-fucose transporter.

Polymorphisms of adhesion molecules and chemokines

Genetic polymorphisms of adhesion molecules, chemokines, and their receptors may contribute to inter-individual differences in inflammatory responsiveness and disease expression, and may also provide insight into the potential of individual molecules as pharmacological targets (Marshall and Haskard 2002). While many of these associations may be due to linkage disequilibrium with other genes, in some cases adhesion molecule and chemokine polymorphisms have been shown to influence function or level of expression. Examples include E-selectin R128 E-selectin (gain in adhesive function), M29 ICAM-1 (ICAM-1^{kilifi}) (reduced adhesive function), I249 CX3CR1 (reduced expression) and Δ35 CCR5 (reduced expression). Furthermore, substitution of A for G at position −403 of the RANTES gene 5′ untranslated region leads to an augmentation of promoter activity.

Adhesion molecule expression in rheumatic diseases

Much of the new understanding of the mechanisms of leucocyte trafficking has been gained from investigations at the cellular and molecular level *in vitro*. Support for the relevance of *in vitro* work comes from a large number of immunocytochemical studies of synovium and other tissues, showing expression of adhesion molecules (Table 6). Owing to the constraints imposed by the availability of human tissue, there is also interest in measuring the soluble forms of the three selectins, ICAM-1, ICAM-3, and VCAM-1, as plasma or serum markers of cellular activation in tissues (Littler et al. 1997; Mojcik and Shevach 1997). In the case of E-selectin, synovial endothelial activation and E-selectin expression can be quantified and imaged non-invasively using intravenously injected, radiolabelled, monoclonal antibody (Fig. 4) (Jamar et al. 2002).

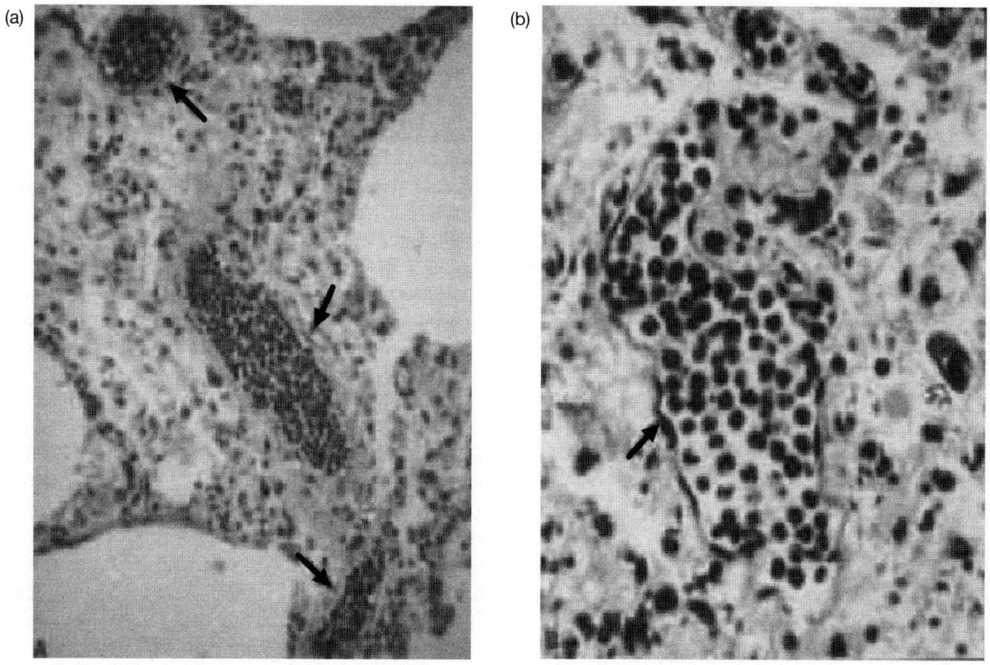

Fig. 3 Autopsy of infected lung tissue from a 19-year-old man with β_2-integrin deficiency, demonstrating the inability of neutrophils to extravasate into the tissues: (a) septal capillaries of the lung are filled with neutrophils (arrows) in contrast to the alveoli which contain macrophages and desquamated alveolar lining cells. Haematoxylin and eosin, magnification ×72; (b) the intravascular cells are mature and immature neutrophils. Haematoxylin and eosin, magnification ×220 (Davies et al. 1991, by courtesy of Blackwell Scientific Publications).

Table 6 Expression of adhesion molecules in arthritis

Molecule	Expression	Reference
L-selectin	Reduced on SM and SF leucocytes	Takahashi et al. (1992); Johnson et al. (1993)
P-selectin	Constitutive expression by SM EC	Grober et al. (1993); Johnson et al. (1993)
E-selectin	Minimal normally; increased on EC in synovitis	Koch et al. (1991); Fairburn et al. (1993)
Peripheral lymph node addressin	HEV in chronic synovitis	Michie et al. (1993)
β_2 and α_L integrin sub-units	All leucocytes	Hale et al. (1989); Takahashi et al. (1992)
α_M integrin sub-unit	Neutrophils and monocytes	Allen et al. (1989)
α_X Integrin sub-unit	SM macrophages	Allen et al. (1989); Koch et al. (1991)
β_1 and α_1, α_3, α_5, α_6 integrin sub-units	SM EC, type B synovial lining cells SM and SF lymphocytes	Takahashi et al. (1992); Nikkari et al. (1993) El-Gabalawy et al. (1993)
α_4 Integrin sub-unit	SM and SF monocytes and lymphocytes	Takahashi et al. (1992); Laffon et al. (1992)
ICAM-1	SM and SF MNC, EC and Fb	Hale et al. (1989); Szekanecz et al. (1994)
ICAM-2	SM and SF MNC, EC and lining cells	Takahashi et al. (1992); Szekanecz et al. (1994)
ICAM-3	SM and SF MNC and lining cells	El-Gabalawy et al. (1994); Szekanecz et al. (1994)
VCAM-1	Type B synovial lining cells, FDC and EC	Morales-Ducret et al. (1992); Wilkinson et al. (1993)
CD31	EC, macrophages (weak)	Johnson et al. (1993)
VAP-1	EC	Salmi and Jalkanen (1992)
CD44	SM and SF mononuclear cells, synoviocytes	Haynes et al. (1991); Johnson et al. (1993)
Fractalkine	Macrophages, DC, EC	Ruth et al. (2001)

DC, dendritic cells; EC, endothelial cells; Fb, fibroblasts; FDC, follicular dendritic cells; HEV, high endothelial venules; MNC, mononuclear cells; PB, peripheral blood; SF, synovial fluid; SM, synovial membrane.

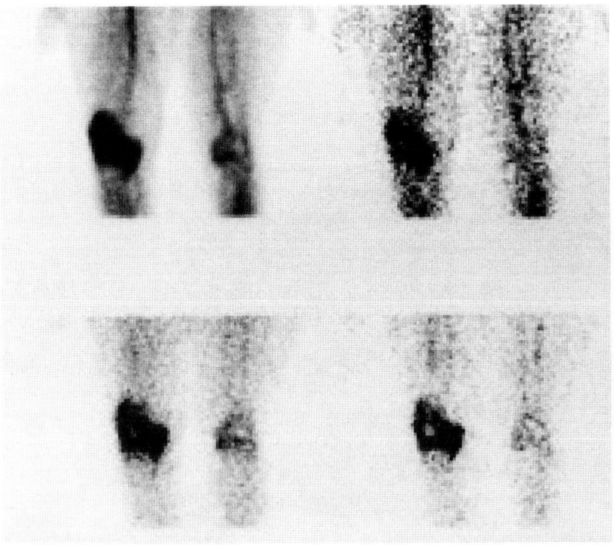

Fig. 4 Scintigraphic imaging of knees in rheumatoid arthritis with radiolabelled monoclonal antibody 1.2B6 (anti-E-selectin). Images were obtained four (top) and twenty (bottom) hours after injection of ^{99m}Tc-Fab (left) and ^{111}In-F(ab')$_2$ (bottom). E-selectin imaging is more prominent in the right knee (Jamar et al. 2002, by courtesy of Oxford University Press).

Functional evidence for the importance of different adhesion molecules for leucocyte trafficking can be gained from the Stamper and Woodruff technique, which measures leucocyte adhesion to blood vessels and other cells in tissue sections. Using this assay together with inhibitory monoclonal antibodies, a number of adhesion molecules have been implicated as mediating lymphocyte adhesion to synovial endothelial cells in situ, including α_L-, α_M-, β_2- and β_1-integrin sub-units, L-selectin, P-selectin, ICAM-1, VCAM-1, alternatively spliced fibronectin, CD44, and VAP-1 (Jalkanen et al. 1987; van Dinther-Janssen et al. 1991; Fischer et al. 1993; Grober et al. 1993; Elices et al. 1994; Salmi and Jalkanen 2001b). Studying trafficking into human tissues engrafted into immunodeficient mice is a useful approach for assessing the molecular mechanisms of leucocyte migration *in vivo* (Proudman et al. 1999).

Therapeutic possibilities

Reduced expression of cytokines, cell adhesion molecules, and leucocyte trafficking into tissues is to be expected as part of the successful suppression of synovial inflammation (Smith et al. 2001). However, some agents in routine use in rheumatological practice may directly affect leucocyte migration amongst other effects (Table 7).

Encouraging signs that deliberate manipulation of lymphocyte trafficking could have therapeutic effects have came form early studies using thoracic duct drainage or lymphocytaphoresis (Paulus et al. 1979; Karsh et al. 1981; Wahl et al. 1983). The development of antibodies against adhesion molecules has now allowed an analysis of the effects of inhibiting trafficking to be more precisely evaluated. In general, inhibiting selectins should only influence cellular interactions within the vasculature, while inhibiting integrin interactions may have widespread and lasting suppressive effects on the immune response (Isobe et al. 1992). Reduction in severity of animal models of arthritis has been demonstrated with anti-E-selectin (Issekutz et al. 2001), anti-ICAM-1 (Iigo et al. 1991), anti-β_2 integrin (Jasin et al. 1992), anti-α_1 and -α_2 integrins (De Fougerolles et al. 2000), and anti-α_4 integrin (Barbadillo et al. 1995). A limitation of studying chronic disease using antibodies is the generation of neutralizing antibodies with continued administration. The development of gene-targeted mice now allows the influence of individual adhesion molecules and chemokines to be more readily studied in models of arthritis and other forms of chronic inflammation. For example, mice deficient in CD44 show resistance to the development of collagen-induced arthritis (Stoop et al. 2001).

Table 7 Effect of drugs used in rheumatic diseases on leucocyte trafficking

Drug	Effect	References
Colchicine	Inhibition of leucocyte–EC interactions	Cronstein et al. (1995)
Corticosteroids	Inhibition of EC adhesion molecule expression	Cronstein et al. (1992)
Gold	Inhibition of EC adhesion molecule expression	Newman et al. (1994)
Methotrexate	Inhibits leucocyte function by stimulating adenosine release from fibroblasts and endothelial cells	Morabito et al. (1998)
Sulfasalazine	Inhibits TNFα-stimulated leucocyte integrin $\alpha_M\beta_2$ upregulation Inhibits leucocyte function by stimulating adenosine release from fibroblasts and endothelial cells	Greenfield et al. (1993) Morabito et al. (1998)

As yet there is relatively little clinical experience using antibodies or other agents to inhibit leucocyte trafficking in rheumatic disaeses, although results using anti-ICAM-1 and anti-β_2 integrin have been encouraging (Kavanaugh et al. 1994; Davis et al. 1995; Lockwood et al. 1999). However, the considerable pharmaceutical investment in this field has led to the development of a number of exciting new agents that will be evaluated over the next few years (Marshall and Haskard 2002).

References

Akbar, A.N. and Salmon, M. (1997). Cellular environments and apoptosis: tissue microenvironments control activated T cell death. *Immunology Today* **18**, 72–6.

Allen, C.A., Highton, J., and Palmer, D.G. (1989). Increased expression of p150,95 and CR3 leukocyte adhesion molecules by mononuclear phagocytes in rheumatoid synovial membranes. *Arthritis and Rheumatism* **32**, 947–54.

Ansel, K.M. and Cyster, J.G. (2001). Chemokines in lymphopoiesis and lymphoid organ development. *Current Opinion in Immunology* **13**, 172–9.

Arnaout, M.A. (1990). Leukocyte adhesion molecules deficiency: its structural basis, pathophysiology and implications for modulating the inflammatory response. *Immunological Reviews* **114**, 145–79.

Arrate, M.P. et al. (2001). Cloning of human junctional adhesion molecule 3 (JAM3) and its identification as the JAM2 counter-receptor. *Journal of Biological Chemistry* **276**, 45826–32.

Arstila, T.P. et al. (1999). A direct estimate of the human $\alpha\beta$ T cell receptor diversity. *Science* **286**, 958–61.

Aurrand-Lions, M. et al. (2001). Heterogeneity of endothelial junctions is reflected by differential expression and specific subcellular localization of the three JAM family members. *Blood* **98**, 3699–707.

Baekkevold, E.S. et al. (2001). The CCR7 ligand ELC (CCL19) is transcytosed in high endothelial venules and mediates T cell recruitment. *Journal of Experimental Medicine* **193**, 1105–12.

Barbadillo, C. et al. (1995). Anti-integrin immunotherapy in rheumatoid arthritis: protective effect of anti-a4 antibody in adjuvant arthritis. *Springer Seminars in Immunopathology* **16**, 427–36.

Bazan, J.F. et al. (1997). A new class of membrane-bound chemokine with a CX3C motif. *Nature* **385**, 640–4.

Berg, E.L. et al. (1993). L-selectin-mediated lymphocyte rolling on MadCAM-1. *Nature* **366**, 695–8.

Bleijs, D.A. et al. (2001). DC-SIGN and LFA-1: a battle for ligand. *Trends in Immunology* **22**, 457–63.

Buckley, C.D. et al. (2000). Persistant induction of the chemokine receptor CXCR4 by TGFβ1 on synovial T cells contributes to their accumulation within the rheumatoid synovium. *Journal of Immunology* **165**, 3423–9.

Buckton, K.E., Court Brown, W.M., and Smith, P.G. (1967). Lymphocyte survival in men treated with X-rays for ankylosing spondylitis. *Nature* **214**, 470–3.

Burger, J.A. et al. (2001). Fibroblast-like synoviocytes support B-cell pseudo-emperipolesis via a stromal cell-derived factor-1- and CD106 (VCAM-1)-dependent mechanism. *Journal of Clinical Investigation* **107**, 305–15.

Butcher, E.C. (1991). Leukocyte–endothelial cell recognition: three (or more) steps to specificity and diversity. *Cell* **67**, 1033–6.

Butcher, E.C. et al. (1999). Lymphocyte trafficking and regional immunity. *Advances in Immunology* **72**, 209–53.

Campbell, J.J. and Butcher, E.C. (2000). Chemokines in tissue-specific and microenvironment-specific lymphocyte homing. *Current Opinion in Immunology* **12**, 336–41.

Campbell, J.J. et al. (1998). Chemokines and the arrest of lymphocytes rolling under flow conditions. *Science* **279**, 381–4.

Campbell, J.J., Haraldsen, G., and Pan, J. (1999). The chemokine receptor CCR4 in vascular recognition by cutaneous but not intestinal memory T cells. *Nature* **400**, 776–80.

Carter, R.A. and Wicks, I.P. (2001). Vascular Cell Adhesion Molecule-1 (CD106): a multifaceted regulator of joint inflammation. *Arthritis and Rheumatism* **44**, 985–94.

Cinamon, G., Shinder, V., and Alon, R. (2001). Shear forces promote lymphocyte migration across vascular endothelium bearing apical chemokines. *Nature Immunology* **2**, 478–522.

Cines, D.B. et al. (1998). Endothelial cells in physiology and in the pathophysiology of vascular disorders. *Blood* **91**, 3527–61.

Clark, E.A. and Brugge, J.S. (1995). Integrins and signal transduction pathways: the road taken. *Science* **268**, 233–9.

Constantin, G. et al. (2000). Chemokines trigger immediate β_2 integrin affinity and mobility changes in lymphocyte arrest under flow. *Immunity* **13**, 759–69.

Crispe, I.N. and Mehal, W.Z. (1996). Strange brew: T cells in the liver. *Immunology Today* **17**, 522–25.

Cronstein, B.N. et al. (1992). A mechanism for the antiinflammatory effects of corticosteroids: The glucocorticoid receptor regulates leukocyte adhesion to endothelial cells and expression of endothelial–leukocyte adhesion molecule 1 and intercellular adhesion molecule 1. *Proceedings of the National Academy of Sciences USA* **89**, 9991–5.

Cronstein, B.N. et al. (1995). Colchicine alters the quantitative and qualitative display of selectins on endothelial cells and neutrophils. *Journal of Clinical Investigation* **96**, 994–1002.

Cyster, J.G. (1999). Chemokines and cell migration in secondary lymphoid organs. *Science* **286**, 2098–102.

Davies, K.A. et al. (1991). A 19-year-old man with leukocyte adhesion deficiency. *In vitro* and *in vivo* studies of leukocyte function. *Clinical and Experimental Immunology* **84**, 223–31.

Davis, L.S. et al. (1995). Induction by persistent T cell hyporesponsiveness *in vivo* by monoclonal antibody to ICAM-1 in patients with rheumatoid arthritis. *Journal of Immunology* **154**, 3525–37.

De Fougerolles, A.R. et al. (1991). Characterization of ICAM-2 and evidence for a third counter-receptor for LFA-1. *Journal of Experimental Medicine* **174**, 253–67.

De Fougerolles, A.R. et al. (2000). Regulation of inflammation by collagen-binding integrins $\alpha_1\beta_1$ and $\alpha_2\beta_1$ in models of hypersensitivity and arthritis. *Journal of Clinical Investigation* **105**, 721–9.

van Dinther-Janssen, A.C.H.M. et al. (1991). The VLA-4/VCAM-1 pathway is involved in lymphocyte adhesion to endothelium in rheumatoid synovium. *Journal of Immunology* **147**, 4207–10.

Dustin, M.L. (2002). Membrane domains and the immunological synapse: keeping T cells resting and ready. *Journal of Clinical Investigation* **109**, 155–60.

El-Gabalawy, H. and Wilkins, J. (1993). β_1 (CD29) integrin expression in rheumatoid synovial membranes: an immunohistologic study of distribution patterns. *Journal of Rheumatology* **20**, 231–7.

El-Gabalawy, H., Gallatin, M., Vazenx, R., Peterman, G., and Wilkins, J. (1994). Expression of ICAM-R (ICAM-3) a novel counter-receptor for LFA-1, in rheumatoid and non-rheumatoid synovium. *Arthritis and Rheumatism* **37**, 846–54.

Elices, M.J., Tsai, V., and Strahl, D. (1994). Expression and functional significance of alternatively spliced CS1 fibronectin in rheumatoid arthritis microvasculature. *Journal of Clinical Investigation* **93**, 405–16.

Etzioni, A. and Tonetti, M. (2000). Leukocyte adhesion deficiency II- from A to almost Z. *Immunology Reviews* **178**, 138–47.

Fairburn, K. et al. (1993). Intercellular adhesion molecules in normal synovium. *British Journal of Rheumatology* **32**, 302–6.

Fan, L. et al. (2000). Ectopic expression of chemokine TCA4/SLC is sufficient to trigger lymphoid neogenesis. *Journal of Immunology* **164**, 3955–9.

Feng, D. et al. (1998). Neutrophils emigrate from venules by a transendothelial cell pathway in response to FMLP. *Journal of Experimental Medicine* **187**, 903–15.

Fischer, C., Thiele, H.-G., and Hamann, A. (1993). Lymphocyte-endothelial interactions in inflamed synovia: involvement of several adhesion molecules and integrin epitopes. *Scandinavian Journal of Immunology* **38**, 158–66.

Foxman, E.F., Kunkel, E.J., and Butcher, E.C. (1999). Integrating conflicting chemotactic signals: the role of memory in leukocyte migration. *Journal of Cell Biology* **146**, 577–88.

Freemont, A.J. (1987). Molecules controlling lymphocyte-endothelial interactions in lymph nodes are produced in vessles of inflamed synovium. *Annals of the Rheumatic Diseases* **46**, 924–8.

Frenette, P.S. et al. (2000). P-Selectin glycoprotein ligand 1 (PSGL-1) is expressed on platelets and can mediate platelet-endothelial interactions *in vivo. Journal of Experimental Medicine* **191**, 1413–22.

Fuhlbrigge, R.C. et al. (1997). Cutaneous lymphocyte antigen is a specialized form of PSGL-1 expressed on skin-homing T cells. *Nature* **389**, 978–81.

Galustian, C. et al. (1999). L-selectin interactions with novel mono- and multi-sulfated Lewis x sequences in comparison with the potent ligand 3′-sulfated Lewis a. *Journal of Biological Chemistry* **274**, 18213–17.

Gamble, J.R., Khew-Goodall, Y., and Vadas, M.A. (1993). Transforming growth factor-β inhibits E-selectin expression on human endothelial cells. *Journal of Immunology* **150**, 4494–503.

Godessart, N. and Kunkel, S.L. (2001). Chemokines in autoimmune disease. *Current Opinion in Immunology* **13**, 670–5.

Gowans, J.L. and Knight, E.J. (1964). The route of recirculation of lymphocytes in the rat. *Proceedings of the Royal Society of London (Biology)* **159**, 257–82.

Grant, A.J. et al. (2002). Homing of mucosal lymphocytes to the liver in the pathogenesis of hepatic complications of inflammatory bowel disease. *Lancet* **359**, 150–7.

Greenfield, S.M. et al. (1993). Inhibition of leukocyte adhesion molecule upregulation by tumour necrosis factor α: a novel mechanism of action of sulphasalazine. *Gut* **34**, 252–6.

Grober, J.S. et al. (1993). Monocyte–endothelial adhesion in chronic rheumatoid arthritis. *In situ* detection of selectin and integrin-dependent interactions. *Journal of Clinical Investigation* **91**, 2609–19.

Hale, L.P. et al. (1989). Immunohistologic analysis of the distribution of cell adhesion molecules within the inflammatory synovial microenvironment. *Arthritis and Rheumatism* **32**, 22–30.

Harari, O. et al. (2001). Limited endothelial E- and P-selectin expression in MRL/lpr lupus-prone mice. *Rheumatology* **40**, 889–95.

Harris, E.S. et al. (2000). The leukocyte integrins. *Journal of Biological Chemistry* **275**, 23409–12.

Haskell, C.A., Cleary, M.D., and Charo, I.F. (2000). Unique role of the chemokine domain of fractalkine in cell capture. Kinetics of receptor dissociation correlate with cell adhesion. *Journal of Biological Chemistry* **275**, 34183–9.

Haynes, B.F. et al. (1991). Measurement of an adhesion molecule as an indicator of inflammatory disease activity: up-regulation of the receptor for hyaluronate (CD44) in rheumatoid arthritis. *Arthritis and Rheumatism* **34**, 1434–43.

Hemmerich, S. et al. (2001). Sulfation of L-selectin ligands by an HEV-restricted sulfotransferase regulates lymphocyte homing to lymph nodes. *Immunity* **15**, 237–47.

Hogg, N. and Leitinger, B. (2001). Shape and shift changes related to the function of leukocyte integrins LFA-1 and Mac-1. *Journal of Leukocyte Biology* **69**, 893–8.

Hogg, N. et al. (1999). A novel leukocyte adhesion deficiency caused by expressed but nonfunctional β2 integrins Mac-1 and LFA-1. *Journal of Clinical Investigation* **103**, 97–106.

Hsi, E.D. et al. (1998). Characterization of the lymphoid infiltrate in Hashimoto's thyroiditis by immunohistochemistry and polymerase chain reaction for immunoglobulin heavy chain rearrangement. *American Journal of Clinical Pathology* **110**, 327–33.

Hynes, R.O. (1992). Integrins: versatility, modulation, and signaling in cell adhesion. *Cell* **69**, 11–25.

Iigo, Y. et al. (1991). ICAM-1-dependent pathway is critically involved in the pathogenesis of adjuvant arthritis in rats. *Journal of Immunology* **147**, 4167–71.

Imhof, B.A., Engelhardt, B., and Vadas, M. (2001). Novel mechanisms of the transendothelial migration of leukocytes. *Trends in Immunology* **22**, 411–14.

Isobe, M., Yagita, H., Okumura, K., and Ihara, A. (1992). Specific acceptance of cardiac allograft after treatment with antibodies to ICAM-1 and LFA-1. *Science* **255**, 1125–7.

Issekutz, A.C. et al. (2001). E-selectin, but not P-selectin, is required for development of adjuvant-induced arthritis in the rat. *Arthritis and Rheumatism* **44**, 1428–37.

Jalkanen, S. et al. (1987). Lymphocyte recognition of high endothelium: antibodies to distinct epitopes of an 85–95 kDa glycoprotein antigen differentially inhibit lymphocyte binding to lymph node, mucosal, or synovial endothelial cells. *Journal of Cell Biology* **105**, 983–90.

Jamar, F. et al. (2002). Scintigraphy using a technetium 99m-labelled anti-E-selectin Fab fragment in rheumatoid arthritis. *Rheumatology (Oxford)* **41**, 53–61.

Janossy, G. et al. (1981). Rheumatoid arthritis: a disease of T-lymphocyte/macrophage immunoregulation. *Lancet* **ii**, 839–42.

Jasin, H.E. et al. (1992). Amelioration of antigen-induced arthritis in rabbits treated with monoclonal antibodies to leukocyte adhesion molecules. *Arthritis and Rheumatism* **35**, 541–9.

Johnson, B.A. et al. (1993). Adhesion molecule expression in human synovial tissue. *Arthritis and Rheumatism* **36**, 137–46.

Johnson-Léger, C., Aurrand-Lions, M., and Imhof, B.A. (2001). The parting of the endothelium: miracle, or simply a junctional affair? *Journal of Cell Science* **113**, 921–33.

Jung, U. and Ley, K. (1999). Mice lacking two or all three selectins demonstrate overlapping and distinct functions for each selectin. *Journal of Immunology* **162**, 6755–62.

Karmann, K. et al. (1995). CD40 on human endothelial cells: inducibility by cytokines and functional regulation of adhesion molecule expression. *Proceedings of the National Academy of Sciences USA* **92**, 4342–6.

Karsh, J. et al. (1981). Lymphapheresis in rheumatoid arthritis: a randomized trial. *Arthritis and Rheumatism* **24**, 867–73.

Kavanaugh, A.F. et al. (1994). Treatment of refractory rheumatoid arthritis with a monoclonal antibody to intercellular adhesion molecule-1. *Arthritis and Rheumatism* **37**, 992–9.

Koch, A.E. et al. (1991). Immunolocalization of endothelial and leukocyte adhesion molecules in human rheumatoid and osteoarthritic synovial tissues. *Laboratory Investigation* **64**, 313–20.

van Kooyk, Y. and Figdor, C.G. (2000). Avidity regulation of integrins: the driving force in leukocyte adhesion. *Current Opinion in Cell Biology* **12**, 542–7.

Kotovuori, P. et al. (1993). The vascular E-selectin binds to the leukocyte integrins CD11/CD18. *Glycobiology* **3**, 131–6.

Kraal, G. and Mebius, R.E. (1997). High endothelial venules: lymphocyte traffic control and controlled traffic. *Advances in Immunology* **65**, 347.

Laffon, A. et al. (1992). Upregulated expression and function of VLA-4 fibronectin receptors on human activated T cells in rheumatoid arthritis. *Journal of Clinical Investigation* **88**, 546–52.

Lawrence, M.B. and Springer, T.A. (1991). Leukocytes roll on a selectin at physiologic flow rates: distinction from and prerequisite for adhesion through integrins. *Cell* **65**, 859–73.

Littler, A.J. et al. (1997). A distinct profile of six soluble adhesion molecules (ICAM-1, ICAM-3, VCAM-1, E-selectin, L-selectin and P-selectin) in rheumatoid arthritis. *British Journal of Rheumatology* **36**, 164–9.

Lockwood, C.M. et al. (1999). Anti-adhesion molecule therapy as an interventional strategy for autoimmune inflammation. *Clinical Immunology* **93**, 93–106.

Luther, S.A. et al. (2000). BLC expression in pancreatic islets causes B cell recruitment and lymphotoxin-dependent lymphoid neogenesis. *Immunity* **12**, 471–81.

Mackay, C.R. et al. (1996). Phenotype, and migration properties of three major subsets of tissue homing T cells in sheep. *European Journal of Immunology* **26**, 2433.

Mantovani, A. et al. (1998). Regulation of endothelial cell function by pro- and anti-inflammatory cytokines. *Transplantation Proceedings* **30**, 4239–43.

Marchal, G. et al. (1982). Local adoptive transfer of skin delayed-type hypersensitivity initiated by a single T lymphocyte. *Journal of Immunology* **129**, 954–8.

Marchesi, V.T. and Gowans, J.L. (1964). The migration of lymphocytes through the endothelium of venules in lymph nodes: an electron microscope study. *Proceedings of the Royal Society of London (Biology)* **159**, 283–90.

Marshall, D. and Haskard, D.O. (2002). Clinical overview: where are we now? *Seminars in Immunology* **14**, 133–40.

McEver, R.P. and Cummings, R.D. (1997). Role of PSGL-1 binding to selectins in leukocyte recruitment. *Journal of Clinical Investigation* **100**, 485–92.

Melrose, J. et al. (1998). IFN-gamma inhibits activation-induced expression of E- and P-selectin on endothelial cells. *Journal of Immunology* **161**, 2457–64.

Michie, S.A. et al. (1993). The human peripheral lymph node vascular addressin: an inducible endothelial antigen involved in lymphocyte homing. *American Journal of Pathology* **143**, 1688–98.

Mizuno, T. et al. (1997). cDNA cloning and chromosomal localization of the human telencephalin and its distinctive interaction with lymphocyte function-associated antigen-1. *Journal of Biological Chemistry* **272**, 1156–63.

Mojcik, C.F. and Shevach, E.M. (1997). Adhesion molecules—a rheumatological perspective. *Arthritis and Rheumatism* **40**, 991–1004.

Morabito, L. et al. (1998). Methotrexate and sulfasalazine promote adenosine release by a mechanism that requires ecto-5′-nucleotidase-mediated conversion of adenine nucleotides. *Journal of Clinical Investigation* **101**, 295–300.

Morales-Ducret, J. et al. (1992). α_4/β_1 Integrin (VLA-4) ligands in arthritis: Vascular cell adhesion molecule-1 expression in synovium and on fibroblast-like synoviocytes. *Journal of Immunology* **149**, 1424–31.

Morel, J.C. et al. (2001). A novel role for interleukin-18 in adhesion molecule induction through NF kappa B and phosphatidylinositol (PI) 3-kinase-dependent signal transduction pathways. *Journal of Biological Chemistry* **276**, 37069–75.

Murphy, P.M. et al. (2000). International Union of Pharmacology. XXII. Nomenclature for chemokine receptors. *Pharmacological Reviews* **52**, 145–76. {14935}

Newman, P.J. (1999). Switched at birth: a new family for PECAM-1. *Journal of Clinical Investigation* **103**, 5–9.

Newman, P.M. et al. (1994). Effect of gold sodium thiomalate and its thiomalate component on the *in vitro* expression of endothelial cell adhesion molecules. *Journal of Clinical Investigation* **94**, 1864–71.

Nikkari, L. et al. (1993). Expression of integrin family of cell adhesion receptors in rheumatoid synovium. *American Journal of Pathology* **142**, 1019–27.

Ostermann, G. et al. (2002). JAM-1 is a ligand of the $\beta2$ integrin LFA-1 involved in transendothelial migration of leukocytes. *Nature Immunology* **3**, 151–8.

Paulus, H.E. et al. (1979). Prolonged thoracic duct drainage in rheumatoid arthritis and systemic lupus erythemmatosus. *Western Journal of Medicine* **130**, 309–24.

Picker, L.J. et al. (1993a). Control of lymphocyte recirculation in man: I. Differential regulation of the peripheral lymph node homing receptor L-selectin on T cells during the virgin to memory cell transition. *Journal of Immunology* **150**, 1105–21.

Picker, L.J. et al. (1993b). Control of lymphocyte recirculation in man: II. Differential regulation of the cutaneous lymphocyte-associated antigen, a tissue-selective homing receptor for skin-homing T cells. *Journal of Immunology* **150**, 1122–36.

Pabst, R. (1988). The spleen in lymphocyte migration. *Immunology Today* **9**, 43–5.

Pitzalis, C., Cauli, A., and Pipitone, N. (1996). Cutaneous lymphocyte antigen-positive T lymphocytes preferentially migrate to the skin but not to the joint in psoriatic arthritis. *Arthritis and Rheumatism* **39**, 137–45.

Pitzalis, C. et al. (1988). The preferential accumulation of helper-inducer T lymphocytes in inflammatory lesions: evidence for regulation by selective endothelial and homotypic adhesion. *European Journal of Immunology* **18**, 1397–404.

Proudman, S.M., Cleland, L.G., and Mayrhofer, G. (1999). Effects of tumor necrosis factor-α, interleukin 1β, and activated peripheral blood mononuclear cells on the expression of adhesion molecules and recruitment of leukocytes in rheumatoid synovial xenografts in SCID mice. *Journal of Rheumatology* **26**, 1877–89.

Pure, E. and Cuff, C.A. (2001). A crucial role for CD44 in inflammation. *Trends in Molecular Medicine* **7**, 213–21.

Read, M.A. et al. (1994). NFκB and IκBβ: an inducible regulatory system in endothelial activation. *Journal of Experimental Medicine* **179**, 503–12.

Robinson, S.D. et al. (1999). Multiple, targeted deficiencies in selectins reveal a predominant role for P-selectin in leukocyte recruitment. *Proceedings of the National Academy of Science U.S.A.* **96**, 11452–7.

Rossi, D. and Zlotnik, A. (2000). The biology of chemokines and their receptors. *Annual Review of Immunology* **18**, 217–42.

Rott, L.S. et al. (1996). A fundamental subdivision of circulating lymphocytes defined by adhesion to mucosal addressin cell adhesion molecule-1. Comparison with vascular cell adhesion molecule-1 and correlation with β_7 integrins and memory differentiation. *Journal of Immunology* **156**, 3727–36.

Ruth, J.H. et al. (2001). Fractalkine, a novel chemokine in rheumatoid arthritis and in rat adjuvant-induced arthritis. *Arthritis and Rheumatism* **44**, 1568–81.

Sallusto, F. et al. (1999). Two subsets of memory T lymphocytes with distinct homing potentials and effector functions. *Nature* **401**, 708–12.

Salmi, M. and Jalkanen, S. (1992). A 90-kilodalton endothelial cell molecule mediating lymphocyte binding in humans. *Science* **257**, 1407–9.

Salmi, M. and Jalkanen, S. (2001a). VAP-1: an adhesin and an enzyme. *Trends in Immunology* **22**, 211–16.

Salmi, M. and Jalkanen, S. (2001b). Human leukocyte subpopulations from inflamed gut bind to joint vasculature using distinct sets of adhesion molecules. *Journal of Immunology* **166**, 4650–7.

Sanders, M.E. et al. (1988). Human memory T lymphocytes express increased levels of three cell adhesion molecules (LFA-3, CD2, and LFA-1) and three other molecules (UCHL1, CDw29, and Pgp-1) and have enhanced IFNγ production. *Journal of Immunology* **140**, 1401–7.

Savill, J. and Fadok, V. (2000). Corpse clearance defines the meaning of cell death. *Nature* **407**, 784–8.

Seabrook, T. et al. (1999). The traffic of resting lymphocytes through delayed hypersensitivity and chronic inflammatory lesions: a dynamic equilibrium. *Seminars in Immunology* **11**, 115–23.

Shi, K. et al. (2001). Lymphoid chemokine B cell attracting chemokine-1 (CXCL13) is expressed in germinal center of ectopic lymphoid follicles within the synovium of chronic arthritis patients. *Journal of Immunology* **166**, 650–5.

Shimizu, Y. et al. (1990). Roles of adhesion molecules in T-cell recognition: fundamental similarities between four integrins on resting human T cells (LFA-1, VLA-4, VLA-5, VLA-6) in expression, binding, and co-stimulation. *Immunological Reviews* **114**, 110–43.

Shimizu, Y., Rose, D.M., and Ginsberg, M.H. (1999). Integrins in the immune system. *Advances in Immunology* **72**, 325–80.

Smith, J.B., McIntosh, G.H., and Morris, B. (1970). The migration of cells through chronically inflamed tissues. *Journal of Pathology* **100**, 21–9.

Smith, M.D. et al. (2001). Successful treatment of rheumatoid arthritis is associated with a reduction in synovial membrane cytokines and cell adhesion molecule expression. *Rheumatology (Oxford)* **40**, 965–77.

Spring, F.A. et al. (2001). Intercellular adhesion molecule-4 binds $\alpha_4\beta_1$ and α_V-family integrins through novel integrin binding mechanisms. *Blood* **98**, 458–66.

Springer, T.A. (1995). Traffic signals on endothelium for lymphocyte recirculation and leukocyte emigration. *Annual Review of Physiology* **57**, 827–72.

Stamper, H.B. and Woodruff, J.J. (1976). Lymphocyte homing into lymph nodes: *in vitro* demonstration of the selective affinity of recirculating lymphocytes for high-endothelial venules. *Journal of Experimental Medicine* **114**, 828–33.

Steegmaier, M. et al. (1997). The E-selectin-ligand ESL-1 is located in the golgi as well as on microvilli on the cell surface. *Journal of Cell Science* **110**, 687–94.

Stein, J.V. et al. (2000). The CC chemokine thymus-derived chemotactic agent 4 (TCA-4, secondary lymphoid tissue chemokine, 6Ckine, Exodus-2) triggers lymphocyte function-associated antigen-1-mediated arrest of rolling T lymphocytes in peripheral lymph node high endothelial venules. *Journal of Experimental Medicine* **191**, 61–75.

Stoop, R. et al. (2001). Increased resistance to collagen-induced arthritis in CD44-deficient DBA/1 mice. *Arthritis and Rheumatism* **44**, 2922–31.

van de Stope, A. and van der Saag, P.T. (2001). Intercellular adhesion molecule-1. *Journal of Molecular Medicine* **74**, 13.

Stott, D.I. et al. (1998). Antigen-driven clonal proliferation of B cells within the target tissue of an autoimmune disease: the salivary glands of patients with Sjögren's syndrome. *Journal of Clinical Investigation* **102**, 938–46.

Szekanecz, Z. et al. (1994). Differential distribution of intercellular adhesion molecules (ICAM-1, ICAM-2, and ICAM-3) and the MS-1 antigen in normal and diseased human synovia. *Arthritis and Rheumatism* **37**, 221–31.

Takahashi, H. et al. (1992). Integrins and other adhesion molecules on lymphocytes from synovial fluid and peripheral blood of rheumatoid arthritis patients. *European Journal of Immunology* **22**, 2879–85.

Takemura, S. et al. (2001a). Lymphoid neogenesis in rheumatoid synovitis. *Journal of Immunology* **167**, 1072–80.

Takemura, S. et al. (2001b). T cell activation in rheumatoid synovium is B cell dependent. *Journal of Immunology* **167**, 4710–18.

Tanaka, Y., Fujii, K., Hubscher, S., Aso, M., Takazawa, A., Saito, K., Ota, T., and Eto, S. (1998). Heparan sulfate proteoglycan on endothelium efficiently induces integrin-mediated T cell adhesion by immobilizing chemokines in patients with rheumatoid synovitis. *Arthritis and Rheumatism* **41**, 1365–77.

Thornhill, M.H. and Haskard, D.O. (1990). IL-4 regulates endothelial activation by IL-1, tumor necrosis factor or IFNγ. *Journal of Immunology* **145**, 865–72.

Utgaard, J.O. et al. (1998). Rapid secretion of prestored interleukin-8 from Weibel–Palade bodies of microvascular endothelial cells. *Journal of Experimental Medicine* **188**, 1751–6.

Varki, A. (1997). Selectin ligands: will the real ones please stand up? *Journal of Clinical Investigation* **99**, 158–62.

Vestweber, D. and Blanks, J.E. (1999). Mechanisms that regulate the function of selectins and their ligands. *Physiological Reviews* **79**, 181–213.

Von Andrian, U.H. and Mackay, C.R. (2000). T cell function and migration. *New England Journal of Medicine* **343**, 1020–34.

Wagner, D.D. (1993). The Weibel–Palade body: the storage granule for von Willebrand factor and P-selectin. *Thrombosis and Haemostasis* **70**, 105–10.

Wahl, S.M. et al. (1983). Leukapheresis in rheumatoid arthritis. *Arthritis and Rheumatism* **26**, 1076–84.

Walcheck, B. et al. (1996). Neutrophil-neutrophil interactions under hydrodynamic shear stress involve L-selectin and PSGL-1. *Journal of Clinical Investigation* **98**, 1081–7.

Wang, J. and Springer, T.A. (1998). Structural specializations of immunoglobulin superfamily members for adhesion to integrins and viruses. *Immunological Reviews* **163**, 197–215.

Wilkinson, L.S. et al. (1993). Expression of vascular cell adhesion molecule-1 (VCAM-1) in normal and inflamed synovium. *Laboratory Investigation* **68**, 82–8.

Williams, A.F. and Barclay, A.N. (1988). The immunoglobulin superfamily-domains for cell surface recognition. *Annual Review of Immunology* **6**, 381–405.

Wolff, B., Burns, A.R., and Middleton, J. (1998). Endothelial cell 'memory' of inflammatory stimulation: human venular endothelial cells store interleukin 8 in Weibel–Palade bodies. *Journal of Experimental Medicine* **188**, 1757–62.

Yao, L. et al. (1996). Interleukin 4 or oncostatin M induces a prolonged increase in P- selectin mRNA and protein in human endothelial cells. *Journal of Experimental Medicine* **184**, 81–92.

Young, A.J. (1999). The physiology of lymphocyte migration through the single lymph node *in vivo*. *Seminars in Immunology* **11**, 83–3.

Zollner, O. et al. (1997). L-selectin from human, but not from mouse neutrophils binds directly to E-selectin. *Journal of Cell Biology* **136**, 707–16.

4.3 Specific immune responses

Frances C. Hall and B.P. Wordsworth

The immune response has evolved as an orchestrated array of defence mechanisms, designed to neutralize the threat posed by a plethora of microbial pathogens. The response is typically initiated following recognition of a microbial invasion. Effector mechansims appropriate to the nature of the microbe are selected and many of these are amplified according to the site and scale of the challenge. Finally, when microbial eradication is complete, the effectors must be withdrawn or destroyed, in order that resolution may occur in the affected tissue. The immune system utilizes two broad strategies. The innate immune system forms the 'rapid response force', a network of circulating cells and molecules, which, together, recognize a few hundred different conserved microbial components and mount an immediate aggressive response. In contrast, the adaptive immune system can recognize, with high specificity, more than 10^{14} distinct molecules. This is achieved by virtue of the diversity of antigen receptors expressed by T and B lymphocytes. Activated T cells perform a myriad of functions, including direct killing of virally infected host cells, production of a range of cytokines, which determine the nature of the adaptive response, and the provision of help for B cells. Certain activated B cells mature into plasma cells, which produce antibodies. The diversity of antigen receptors on the surface of T and B cells maximizes the chance that every possible pathogen can be recognized. However, the frequency of T and B lymphocytes able to respond to a given specificity is low and amplification is critical for the success of the adaptive response. This problem is partially redressed by the generation of 'memory', which ensures that the adaptive immune response to rechallenge with the same microbe is more rapid than during the primary response. Although innate and adaptive strategies are often considered separately, they are, in fact, integrated at every stage of the immune response.

Immune effector mechanisms are intrinsically dangerous! An arsenal with sufficient potency to destroy invading organisms, and to efficiently clear swathes of foreign molecules from the circulation, necessarily results in some collateral damage. A fundamental property of an effective but safe immune system is the ability to discriminate self from foreign molecules. A single failure on this front can lead to the development of autoimmune disease. Further issues relate to the selection of appropriate effector mechanisms which eliminate the microbe with minimal host tissue damage, the localization of the response to the infected tissue, efficient but measured amplification of the response, and, finally, timely resolution, when the microbe has been eradicated. Failure to regulate any of these processes can lead to chronic inflammatory disease.

Innate immunity

The innate immune system consists of a battery of cells and molecules that circulate, in large numbers, usually in an inactive state. The innate response is triggered by recognition of a limited number of invariant features associated with microbes and the effector mechanisms are rapidly deployed (Medzhitov and Janeway 2000). The major strategies include: clearance of the microbe and conserved microbial products from the extracellular space, ingestion and intracellular destruction of the microbe by specialized phagocytes, neutralization of conserved microbial molecules, which may be essential to microbial function, and destruction of the microbes in the extracellular space.

The soluble mediators of the innate system include components of a number of molecular cascades, which are designed for rapid activation and amplification of proinflammatory chemicals. These include the complement cascade, the kinin system, which results in bradykinin release, and both clotting and fibrinolytic systems. Some of these cascade components are also acute phase reactants, which are rapidly released in response to infection and tissue injury. C-reactive protein is an acute phase reactant, which is involved both in the activation of complement and in the clearance of immune complexes. Cytokines are produced by cellular components of the immune system; they convey messages both locally and to distant sites, thereby coordinating both innate and adaptive arms of the immune response. Chemokines are a sub-group of chemoattractant cytokines, which selectively recruit and orchestrate cellular effectors in affected tissues.

The cellular components of innate immunity include macrophages and neutrophils, which are phagocytes specialized for intracellular killing of ingested bacteria. In contrast, eosinophils are only weakly phagocytic and specialize in attacking large multicellular parasites, by the release of cationic proteins and reactive oxygen species directly onto the microbial wall, in the extracellular space. Basophils and mast cells are responsible for releasing a variety of inflammatory mediators, which increase blood flow to the infected region and attract further cellular components in innate and adaptive immune responses. Mast cells and basophils exhibit further cooperation between the innate and adaptive systems, since they express high affinitiy receptors for IgE (FcϵR) and accumulate IgE antibodies on their surface. Natural killer cells destroy nucleated host cells that have ceased to express the normally ubiquitous MHC class I molecules; failure to express MHC class I molecules usually indicates that the affected host cells have undergone either malignant transformation or infection by viruses that 'hijack' the cellular synthetic machinery. Natural killer cells also destroy cells that are coated (opsonized) with IgG, a process called antibody-dependent cellular cytotoxicity, again illustrating the interdependence of innate and adaptive systems. Dendritic cells (DC) are phagocytic but, unlike macrophages and neutrophils, their primary purpose is not to 'ingest and destroy' but to fulfil the role of professional antigen-presenting cells (APC). DC become activated by 'danger signals', such as heat shock proteins, reactive oxygen intermediates, extracellular matrix breakdown products, or cytokines secreted by cellular components of the innate response. DC process complex microbial antigens and present them as peptide antigens bound to MHC class II molecules, for recognition by T lymphocytes. Activated DC also express costimulatory molecules that enable the activation of naive T lymphocytes and the initiation of the primary adaptive immune response.

It is important to appreciate that innate and adaptive immunity and, indeed the whole inflammatory process, operate as a completely integrated system. The adaptive immune response is only initiated after a pathogen has been recognized by the innate immune system. A primary adaptive response requires that the naive T cells receive at least two signals: one is recognition of a specific peptide/MHC complex, the second is usually provided by the expression of CD80 (B7.1) and CD86 (B7.2) molecules on the professional antigen-presenting cell. However, DC only express CD80 and CD86 in response to the 'danger signals' produced by the innate immune system. These, in turn, are produced, by the host, only on pattern recognition of conserved microbial components, a process that is mediated through Toll-like receptors (Akira et al. 2001).

Defects or variants in components of the innate immune response can contribute to autoimmune pathology. For example, rare deficiencies of early classical pathway complement components (C1q, C2, and C4) are strongly associated with the development of systemic lupus erythematosus (SLE) (Schur 1995). The inheritance of an extended human leucocyte antigen (HLA) haplotype bearing a C4A null allele is also associated with SLE. Although there have been several reports of HLA associations with susceptibility to SLE, the C4A null allele has been shown to be an independent susceptibility factor (Wakeland et al. 2001). Polymorphism in the complement component C5 may be involved in other inflammatory arthritides since it influences the severity of inflammatory arthritis in two murine models of disease, the collagen-induced arthritis (Johansson et al. 2001) and the recently defined K/B × N model (Ji et al. 2001). Natural killer cell function has recently been implicated in the pathogenesis of type I diabetes in the non-obese diabetic mouse model. Both numerical and functional deficiencies of natural killer cells have been demonstrated in this mouse strain and correction of the defect has been shown to prevent the onset of diabetes (Poulton et al. 2001).

Adaptive immunity

Adaptive or acquired immunity relies on recognition of microbial antigens by cells from two distinct lymphocyte lineages, B cells and T cells. Each of these lineages has the capacity to recognize in excess of 10^{14} different antigenic specificities. In contrast to the innate system, which can respond rapidly to the presence of a variety of conserved microbial products, the lymphocytes' response is relatively slow but ensures that every novel pathogen or pathogenic variant can be recognized. The adaptive immune response also displays 'memory', such that secondary exposure to a particular antigenic challenge will elicit a faster and more efficient response.

The essence of adaptive immunity resides in the nature of antigen receptors expressed by the B and T cells. The incredible diversity of B and T cell receptors is achieved by a process of gene rearrangement in the developing B and T cells. Neither the B cell receptor (BCR) nor the T cell receptor (TCR) is encoded exclusively in the germline. Instead the genes encoding the individual chains of these heterodimeric molecules are formed somatically by the splicing together of gene segments, which are selected from a pool of germline gene segments. Additional nucleotide diversity is generated at the junctions of these recombining segments by random addition of single nucleotides. This remarkable process provides the potential for at least 10^{14} different BCR and TCR in each individual. Since this process is somatic, even monozygotic twins will form different repertoires of BCR and TCR. A further essential characteristic shared by B and T lymphocytes is the phenomenon of clonality. Generally, each B cell or T cell expresses a single specificity of BCR or TCR. An important difference between B and T cells, however, lies in the ability of the BCR to undergo somatic mutation during the development of an immune response; this potentially increases the affinity of the antibody produced for its antigen (affinity maturation). TCRs do not undergo somatic mutation; presumably the potential for enhancing T cell autoreactivity poses too great a threat.

B and T lymphocytes also differ with respect to the nature of antigen recognized. BCR recognize antigens directly, usually in their native and functional form, for example, soluble or cell surface proteins. In contrast, TCR recognizes antigens in the form of a linear peptide, presented by an MHC molecule (discussed below). This difference reflects the fundamentally different roles played by B and T cells in the immune response.

T lymphocytes

It has become an immunological cliché to describe the T cell as the 'conductor of the immune orchestra'. While this is an oversimplification, a subset of T cells is certainly instrumental in initiating the antigen-specific response and for selectively activating appropriate adaptive effector mechanisms. There are, in fact, several categories of T cells. In the majority, the TCR is comprised of an $\alpha\beta$ heterodimer. This consists of a membrane-proximal constant region, including a transmembrane and a short cytoplasmic domain, and a membrane-distal variable region. The antigen-binding site is located at the distal end of the variable region; it is formed by six solvent-accessible loops, corresponding to three hypervariable regions from each of the two (α and β) chains. The TCRs are always membrane-bound. The $\alpha\beta$ TCRs recognize peptides presented by MHC class I or class II molecules (Davis et al. 1998). In contrast, many $\gamma\delta$ T cells recognize antigen directly, as do antibodies, whereas a few recognize lipid or glycolipid antigens presented by 'non-classical MHC' molecules, such as CD1 (Born et al. 1999). Hereafter, the T cells discussed will be the $\alpha\beta$ T cells. These can be further classified according to their expression of CD8 or CD4. Generally, CD8+ T cells recognize peptide antigen in the context of MHC class I molecules, whereas CD4+ T cells recognize antigen presented by MHC class II molecules.

T cells perform several functions. CD8+ T cells commonly differentiate into cytotoxic T cells. These kill virally infected cells by a combination of perforin, which literally perforates the target cell membrane, and by initiating Fas-mediated apoptosis in the target cell. All categories of T cells can produce cytokines. However, the most extensively studied group are the so-called 'helper' T cells (Th), which derive their name from their contribution to B cell activation and differentiation into plasma cells. Th cells can be classified according to the cytokine profile produced. Mosmann and Coffman proposed the Th1/Th2 dichotomy in 1989 (Mosmann and Coffman 1989). Typically, Th1 cells produce cytokines, IL-2 and IFNγ, which promote inflammation and activate macrophages, thereby enabling them to kill intracellular organisms. Th2 cells secrete IL-4, IL-5, IL-6, and IL-10, which together attract and activate eosinophils and which provide B cell help, thereby facilitating the production of antibody. The division of CD4+ T cells into two functional subsets is almost certainly an oversimplification (Mosmann and Sad 1996). Recently, a group of regulatory CD4+ T cells, which constitutively express the IL-2Rα chain (CD25) and CTLA-4, has been defined (Maloy and Powrie 2001). These cells appear to inhibit immune responses by cell contact with effector T cells, antigen-presenting cells, or possibly both. The role of cytokines in this regulatory process is controversial. In rodent models, depletion or deficiency of this regulatory subset leads to a variety of spontaneous autoimmune diseases.

Since CD4+ T cells initiate the adaptive immune response, safeguards are required to ensure that activation occurs only in appropriate circumstances and by T cell clones of appropriate specificity. These safeguards include the destruction of T cells with high autoaggressive potential in the thymus, the requirement of naive T cells for at least two activation signals, the absence of somatic mutation in the TCR, and a process of active inhibition of responses.

The requirement that the TCR specifically recognizes peptide/MHC complexes presents a fundamental paradox of adaptive immunity. The TCR must be able to recognize a linear peptide antigen, presented by a *self*-MHC molecule and yet activation by *self-peptide*/self-MHC molecules must be avoided, since this could lead to devastating autoimmunity. The process of thymic selection screens individual nascent T cells on the basis of the avidity of their TCR for a large panel of self-peptide/MHC complexes (Anderson et al. 1996). Failure of a TCR to recognize self-MHC results in apoptotic death, since this T cell would be essentially 'blind' and unlikely to recognize a foreign peptide/self-MHC complex. High avidity recognition of self-peptide/MHC complexes also results in T cell death; this negative selection removes the T cells with the highest autoaggressive potential. The remaining T cells, in which TCR recognition of self-peptide/MHC is of moderate avidity are postively selected; the sum of TCR selected in this way comprise the peripheral TCR repertoire. Aberrant selection of the TCR repertoire may cause susceptibility to autoimmune disease (Ridgway and Fathman 1999).

It is clear that some degree of affinity for self-proteins is necessary for a T cell to be selected for development. However, the vast majority of autoreactive T cells never become frankly autoaggressive and respond, instead, only to foreign peptide/MHC complexes. This can partly be explained by the requirement of a naive T cell for at least two activation signals, prior to activation. Here the integration of innate and adaptive immune systems plays a critical role. Ligation of the TCR by peptide/MHC complex provides signal 1. The strength of this signal is related to the avidity of the TCR for its ligand and a high-avidity interaction in the periphery is likely to arise from the recognition of foreign peptide/MHC complexes. However, this signal in isolation will lead to anergy (non-responsiveness) or apoptosis unless it is acccompanied by other signals. The classical signal 2 is provided by the binding of the T cell molecule CD28 to its ligand CD80 or CD86. These are induced on professional APCs by their recognition of conserved microbial components. T cell activation is therefore a consequence of both antigen recognition and detection of 'danger signals' provided by the innate immune system. It is now recognized that CD28 is one of many costimulatory molecules, which can mediate the supplementary signals required for activation. Others include receptor–ligand pairs CD40–CD154, ICOS–LICOS, PD1–PDL, CD27–CD70, and RANK–TRANCE (Kwon et al. 1999; Watts and DeBenedette 1999) and cytokines, including IL-1, IL-6, and TNFα (Joseph 1998 #1821). Each of these costimulatory pathways imparts a different signal, which influences T cell effector function. For example, expression of TRANCE (or OPGL) on activated T cells in the rheumatoid synovium is responsible for activating osteoclast progenitors, thereby contributing to the periarticular osteoporosis and bone erosion typical of this disease (Kong et al. 1999).

An additional safeguard against inappropriate T cell activation is the action of regulatory T cells, which have been identified in the CD4+ CD25+ constitutive subset. Their mechanism(s) of action remain to be resolved but they appear to be activated following recognition of peptide/MHC via their specific TCR. The inhibitory effect appears to be mediated by direct cell contact. However, their suppressive activity is local and antigen-non-specific (Shevach 2001). It is interesting that NOD mice, which spontaneously develop insulin-dependent diabetes mellitus, exhibit a deficiency of CD25+ CD4+ T cells (Salomon et al. 2000). CD25+ CD4+ regulatory T cells have recently been demonstrated in humans but their role in human autoimmunity is, as yet, unknown (Dieckmann et al. 2001; Jonuleit et al. 2001; Stephens et al. 2001).

B lymphocytes

B cells also express an antigen-specific receptor on their surface, the BCR and, like T cells, they exhibit clonality. The BCR is an immunoglobulin molecule, which is composed of two heavy chains and two light chains (either κ or λ). Together these are organized into a membrane-proximal constant region (the Fc region) and two membrane-distal variable regions (Fig. 1). The BCR is therefore bivalent, with an antigen binding site contained in each variable region. BCR recognizes epitopes on the surface of molecules; a single molecule usually has several B cell epitopes. The

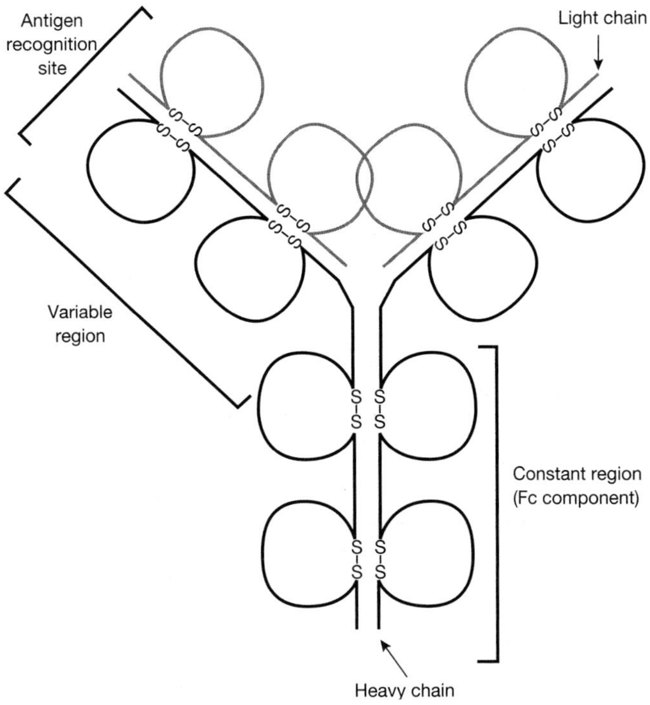

Fig. 1 Structure of immunoglobulin. An immunoglobulin molecule consists of two heavy chains and two light chains. Each immunoglobulin has two antigen-binding sites. These are formed from the variable regions of both heavy and light chains. The constant region of the heavy chain determines the class and sub-class of the immunoglobulin (IgM, IgA, IgE, IgG1, IgG2, IgG3, IgG4). The constant regions vary in the number and nature of immunoglobulin domains; these confer different properties, including complement fixation, affinity for Fc receptors, transplacental transport (different classes/sub-classes not illustrated).

diversity of the BCR repertoire is achieved by somatic gene rearrangement, as for the TCR repertoire. Gene segments are recombined in the developing B cell to generate the genes encoding the heavy chain and the light chain. In contrast to the TCR, the BCR can be secreted in soluble form (antibody) and different forms of the constant region are available, giving rise to IgD, IgM, IgG, IgE, and IgA isotypes. These antibodies have functionally distinct roles. IgM and IgG fix complement efficiently and activate the classical pathway of complement. IgG, IgA, and IgE bind to corresponding Fc receptors (FcγR, FcαR, FcϵR) on phagocytic cells. IgG and IgE can mediate antibody-dependent celluar cytotoxicity by opsonizing the target and binding to the requisite Fc receptors on natural killer cells, macrophages or neutrophils (IgG mediated) or eosinophils (IgE mediated). IgA is secreted in saliva and other fluids. Its Fc region enables it to be transported across the epithelium to protect mucosal surfaces. IgD is not secreted but operates as a surface BCR. The process of class-switching during B cell differentiation enables a B cell and its progeny to secrete antibody of a single specificity but of different isotypes according to the function required.

As for T cells, there are different categories of B cells. The B1 cells develop early during ontogeny and express CD5. They produce so-called 'natural' IgM antibodies, which recognize epitopes on common pathogens and autoantigens, for example, microbial polysaccharides. The specificities of these antibodies are determined by germ-line encoded gene segments and the antibodies exhibit relatively low affinity for their epitopes. B1 cells do not require T cell help in order to secrete antibody. With these characteristics, the B1 cells can be regarded as part of the innate immune system.

In contrast, the majority of B cells are B2 cells; they do not express CD5 and develop later in ontogeny. Antigen-naive B2 cells express IgM and IgD istotypes on the cell surface. B2 cells are dependent on CD4+ T cells for activation and maturation into antibody-secreting plasma cells. This critical interaction takes place in a specialized microenvironment called the germinal centre, which is located in lymph nodes and other lymphoid tissues (see below). In the germinal centre, B cells bind antigen via the cell surface BCR. This imparts an activation signal and the antigen is ingested, processed and presented on the B cell surface, as linear peptide fragments, in the context of MHC class II. The peptide/MHC class II complexes are then recognized by a panel of specific CD4+ Th cells, which are thereby stimulated to express CD40L. CD40L binds to its ligand CD40 on the surface of the B cell and triggers the processes of somatic hypermutation and isotype class switching within the B cell. Somatic mutation results in a series of sequence alterations in the variable region of the antibody produced by the B cells. Daughters of the original B cell thereby produce subtle variations on the parent antibody specificity. B cells that produce variants with higher affinity for the target antigen are favoured. The process of somatic hypermutation thereby results in affinity maturation of the antibodies produced and this 'experience' is retained in the immune system in the form of long-lived memory B cells, which encode high-affinity antibodies. In addition to signalling via CD40, the Th cell provides 'help' in the form of cytokines, such as IL-2, IL-4, and IL-5; these influence the selection of heavy chain isotype during the process of class switching. The result of this process in the germal centre is the maturation of a population of plasma cells, which produce high-affinity antibodies of an isotype appropriate to the nature of the challenge and a population of memory B cells, which enable this refined adaptive response to be produced rapidly, if the organism is rechallenged with the same antigen.

B cell overactivity is an important feature of several autoimmune diseases. SLE is characterized by hypergammaglobulinaemia and a panoply of autoantibodies, many of which are specific for antigens that appear on the surface of apoptotic cells in apoptotic blebs (Eguchi 2001). Many of these antigens are proteins involved in DNA structure or processing, thereby accounting for the frequency of the autoantibodies specific for these components.

Secondary lymphoid tissue

Since the frequency of T and B cells, which are specific for a particular epitope, is low, the success of adaptive immunity depends on a strategy that enables them to be efficiently brought into contact with the antigen and each other. This function is fulfilled for most tissues by their draining lymph nodes, for the bloodstream by the spleen, and for mucosal surfaces by the mucosal-associated lymphoid tissue (MALT). For the purpose of this overview, only the process lymphoid cell entry into a peripheral lymph node will be described in detail.

Lymph nodes receive afferent lymphatics, which drain extracellular fluid and migratory cells from the regional tissues. The lymph contains dendritic cells, which have phagocytosed soluble antigens and immune complexes in the tissues. If the innate immune response has been triggered in the tissues, the DC will have been exposed to local 'danger signals' and will have been activated. Whereas immature DC specialize in antigen ingestion, activated DC mature into efficient antigen-presenting cells, able to provide all the signals required for activation of a naive CD4+ T cell.

T cells enter the lymph node from the circulation via the high endothelial venules. Here, the specialized endothelial cells express peripheral node addressin (PNAd), which is recognized by L-selectin (CD62L) on the surface of naive T cells. This interaction mediates rolling of the T cell along the surface of the venule endothelium. The glycosaminoglycans covering the endothelial surface trap secondary lymphoid tissue chemokine (SLC), which is secreted by the endothelial cells. This binds to chemokine receptor 7 (CCR7) on the surface of the T cell and initiates a signalling cascade that results in the activation of the integrin $\alpha_L\beta_2$, on the surface of the T cell. This integrin binds with high affinity to intercellular adhesion molecules-(ICAM-)1 and 2 on the endothelial cell surface and halts the rolling process. The T cell will then diapedese across the endothelium and migrate along chemokine gradients to the T cell area in the paracortex, where it encounters the DC.

B cells expressing CXCR5 congregate in the lymph node follicles, to which they migrate along a chemotactic gradient of B lymphocyte chemokine (BLC). B cells stimulated by BLC secrete lymphotoxin-β, which is essential for the development of follicular dendritic cells (FDC), and the generation of a follicle. The FDCs collect and retain immune complexes as a source of antigen with which to stimulate the B cells. Activation of neighbouring CD4+ Th cells results in their expression of CD40L and the production of cytokines, which initiate the formation of a germinal centre within the follicle. This contains rapidly dividing B cells, which undergo somatic mutation and class-switching. The process results in the generation of mature plasma cells and memory B cells.

In several autoimmune diseases, for example, rheumatoid arthritis (RA), Hashimoto's thyroiditis, type I diabetes, and Sjögren's syndrome, lymphoid follicles and germinal centres may develop at extranodal sites. In RA synovium, this lymphoid neogenesis has been shown to involve the local production of BLC and lymphotoxin-β (Takemura et al. 2001). There may be an association between lymphoid neogenesis and erosive disease, since activated synovial T cells express OPGL (also known as RANKL or TRANCE). This molecule has been implicated both in lymphoid organogenesis and in the maturation of osteoclasts (Kong et al. 1999). BLC overproduction has also been implicated in producing lupus-like symptoms in (NZB $\times$ NZW)F1 mice (Ishikawa et al. 2001) by stimulating the production of autoantibodies by B1 cells.

Effector T cells express adhesion molecules that enable them to enter sites of inflammation, rather than recirulating through lymph nodes. Since the differentiation of naive CD4+ T cells into Th1 or Th2 sub-types is associated with the ability to produce different spectra of cytokines, it is important that the correct type of effector is recruited to the site of infection. For this reason, Th1 and Th2 cells express different chemokine receptors. Th1 cells express CCR5 and CXCR3, which bind inflammatory cytokines, whereas Th2 cells express CCR3, the eotaxin receptor, which is also expressed on eosinophils, basophils, and mast cells. CCR4, CCR8, and CXCR4 are also preferentially expressed on Th2 cells. This ensures that Th1 and Th2 cells congregate appropriately at sites requiring their respective effector functions. In RA, the majority of synovial T cells express CCR5 (Qin et al. 1998) and there is some evidence that individuals, who are homozygous for a disrupted CCR5 variant, are less susceptible to RA (Paxton and Kang 1998).

Antigen presentation and the trimolecular complex

The recognition of peptide MHC ligand by a specific TCR is pivotal both for the activation of naive T cells and the targetting of many T cell mediated effector functions. The efficiency and specificity of this interaction is critical. It determines the ability to initiate an adaptive response to foreign antigen, while maintaining neutrality to self. It enables the professional APC, which activate T cells, to be distinguished from virally infected cells that must be destroyed by T cells. How are these demands achieved?

Antigen is recognized by specific TCR in the form of a linear peptide presented by an MHC molecule. Two distinct classes of MHC molecule enable the responding T cell to distinguish between an antigen-presenting cell and a target for lysis. MHC class I molecules are expressed on all nucleated cells. They present peptides generated in the cytosol to CD8+ T cells. The primary purpose of this pathway is to indicate whether individual cells are infected with virus. In contrast, MHC class II molecules are usually expressed only by a subset of immune cells, the professional antigen-presenting cells. These molecules present peptides derived from endocytic pathways that sample the extracellular environment. This pathway is used to initiate an adaptive immune response by presenting fragments of microbes or microbial products to CD4+ T cells. The distinct pathways of antigen presentation in the context of MHC class I or class II molecules refelect their different functions (Parham 1999) (Fig. 2).

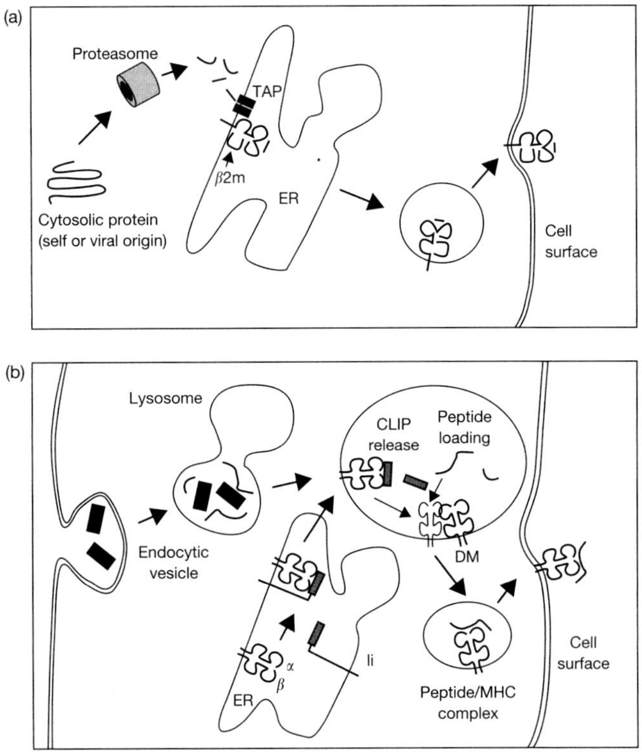

Fig. 2 (a) MHC class I pathway of antigen presentation. The nascent MHC class I heavy chain associates with β_2m in the endoplasmic reticulum (ER). Cytosolic protein, which may be of self or viral origin is degraded by the proteasome complex. Peptides are translocated to the lumen of the ER via an active transporter associated with antigen processing (TAP). The class I molecule folds around the short peptide and is transported to the cell surface. (b) MHC class II pathway of antigen presentation. The MHC class II molecule is formed by association of α and β chains. This heterodimer is chaperoned by the invariant chain (Ii). Exogenous proteins are ingested by phagocytosis or endocytosis and the resulting endosomes fuse with lysosomes, which contain degradative enzymes. In the mature endosomal compartment, the MHC class II/Ii complex encounters proteases, which degrade Ii leaving only the class II invariant peptide (CLIP) blocking the peptide binding groove. The atypical MHC class II molecule, HLA–DM (DM) catalyses the release of CLIP from the MHC class II antigen-binding groove, in exchange for a peptide derived from extracellular protein. The peptide/MHC class II complex translocates to the cell surface.

Classical MHC class I molecules consist of a polymorphic heavy chain, which includes the membrane-distal peptide-binding groove, a single membrane-proximal domain, transmembrane and cytoplasmic domains. This is non-covalently associated with β_2-microglobulin (Fig. 3). A linear peptide of approximately eight residues in length (8-mer) is incorporated into the MHC class I molecule as it folds in the endoplasmic reticulum (ER). The peptides presented are derived from the population of endogenous cytoplasmic proteins, that is, those that are synthesized within the cell. A cytoplasmic proteasome (large molecular weight proteolytic enzyme complex) is responsible for degradation of complex proteins and the resulting peptides are actively transported into the ER. In a healthy cell, the surface MHC class I molecules will present a panel of self peptides. These cells will not be targets for T cells. A subset of these normal peptide/MHC class I subsets will be recognized by killer inhibitory receptors (KIR) on natural killer cells. The resulting negative signal imparted to the natural killer cells prevents cytotoxic attack. However, in a malignant cell or virally infected cell, expression of MHC class I molecules may be absent or sub-normal. Such cells will not inhibit natural killer cell activation and will be killed by MHC-independent cytotoxicity. Cells expressing abnormal proteins, such as viral products, will present peptide fragments of these on the cell surface, in the context of MHC class I molecules and will activate CD8+ cytotoxic T lymphocytes. These will kill target cells by a combination of perforin and granzyme or by inducing Fas-mediated apoptosis.

In addition to the 'classical' MHC class I molecules, the so-called 'non-classical' MHC class I (class Ib) molecules also play important roles in antigen presentation, although usually to a limited subset of lymphocytes. For example, HLA-E presents leader peptides, derived from certain other classical MHC class I molecules, to natural killer cells; this delivers a negative signal via the NK cell CD94/NKG2 receptor (Braud et al. 1999). The MHC class Ib molecule CD1d presents lipids antigens to NK/T cells (natural killer cells with certain T cell markers). These cells can be considered as a component of the innate immune system, they exhibit a restricted TCR repertoire and secrete large quantities of IL-4, which influences the effector function of an emerging adaptive immune response (Elewaut and Kronenberg 2000). The stress-induced MHC class I related proteins MICA/B and ULBP do not present antigen but activate NK cells via the NKG2D receptor (Vivier et al. 2002). Similarly, non-classical MHC class I molecules T22 and T10 activate a subset of $\gamma\delta$ T cells, without presenting antigen (Chien and Hampl 2000). Other non-classical MHC class I molecules function as highly specific molecular transporters. Examples include nFcR, which mediates transmucosal and transplacental IgG transport and the HFE molecule, which is involved in iron metabolism (see below).

In contrast to classical MHC class I molecules, MHC class II molecules are normally expressed only by professional APC, including DC, B cells, macrophages, activated T cells, and thymic epithelial cells. A range of other cells can be induced to express MHC class II molecules, in the presence of IFNγ. A further key difference between the MHC class I and class II antigen-presentation pathways is that the peptides presented by MHC class II molecules are derived either from extracellular proteins or from proteins destined for cell surface expression or secretion [Fig. 2(b)]. Professional APC are equipped with a number of mechanisms for ingesting exogenous proteins, ranging from phagocytosis of whole opsonized microbes, to receptor-mediated endocytosis and pinocytosis of fluid-phase proteins. The endosomes formed by these processes fuse with lysosomes, which contain proteolytic enzymes. Here the exogenous proteins are degraded into linear peptides for presentation by MHC class II molecules.

The heterodimeric MHC class II molecules are synthesized in the ER and consist of non-covalently linked α and β chains. Unlike MHC class I molecules, class II molecules are not loaded with peptide in the ER but, instead, are chaperoned by the invariant chain (Ii). In this form they are transported to the mature endosomal compartment. Here the majority of the invariant chain is degraded, leaving only the Class II associated invariant peptide (CLIP) which blocks the peptide-binding groove. A non-classical MHC class II molecule, HLA–DM interacts with the CLIP/MHC class II complex and catalyses the release of CLIP, enabling the pool of exogenous peptides to gain access to the antigen-binding groove. The peptides bound by MHC class II molecules are often much longer than the MHC class I-bound nonamers and the *N*- and *C*-terminal ends of the peptide may project either side of the antigen-binding groove. The pool of MHC class II molecules, presenting a panel of endosomal peptides is translocated to the cell surface for recognition by CD4+ T cells.

The peptide/MHC class I and class II complexes present a rather flat surface to the TCR (Plate 62). Six solvent-accessible loops extend from the membrane-distal domains of the TCR (three from the α chain and three from the β chain). The TCR positions itself diagonally over the peptide lying in the antigen-binding groove with the CDR1 and CDR2 loops of the TCRα chain overlying the *N*-terminal portion of the peptide and surrounding MHC α-helices, while the CDR1 and CDR2 loops of the TCRβ chain contact the *C*-terminal peptide and enveloping MHC α-helices. The CDR3α and CDR3β loops mainly make contact with the peptide within the groove, while the less variable CDR1 and CDR2 loops primarily contact relatively conserved contacts on the MHC molecule. The CDR3 loops, therefore, contribute most to the specificity of peptide/MHC recognition by TCR, whereas the CDR1 and CDR2 loops are more responsible for the orientation of the interaction (reviewed by Garcia et al. 1999).

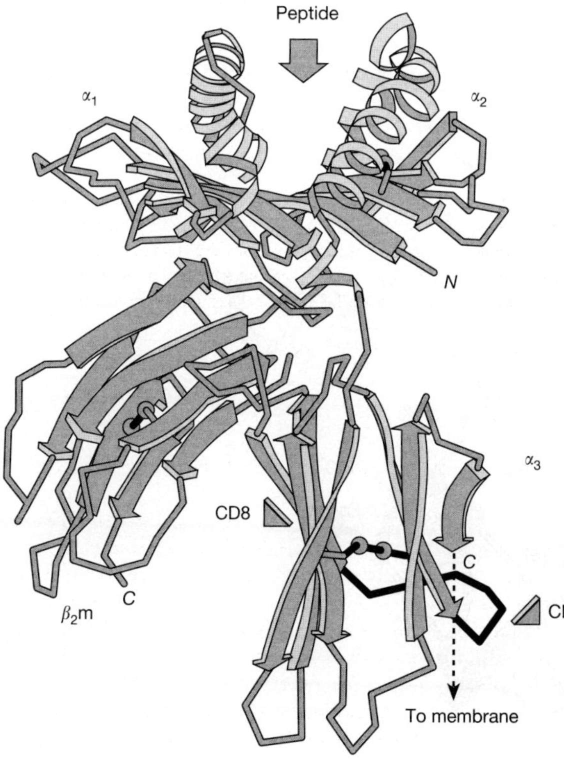

Fig. 3 Ribbon diagram of the HLA-A2 class I molecule, indicating the antigen-binding cleft. Polymorphic residues are concentrated around this structure pointing towards the peptide antigen from the floor and sides. The sites of interaction with the CD8 molecule and β_2-microglobulin are indicated.

Since the MHC class I pathway identifies cells that are infected, or altered by malignant tranformation, it is critical that these are recognized by the CD8+ cytolytic T cells. In contrast, the peptide/MHC class II complexes must be recognized by CD4+ T cells, which can initiate an adaptive immune response, if evidence of extracellular microbial invasion is to be detected. Surveillance by the appropriate class of T cell is achieved partly by the location in which antigen presentation occurs and partly by the coreceptors CD4 and CD8, which define the T cell subsets. CD8 and CD4 coreceptors directly recognize MHC class I and class II molecules, respectively.

MHC molecules and disease

Human MHC molecules are referred to as human leucocyte antigens. The HLA gene complex on chromosome 6p21.3 is a gene-dense region, which encodes both classical and non-classical MHC class I and class II molecules, MHC class I related chains, molecules concerned with loading peptides onto classical MHC class I molecules (TAP, LMP, tapaisin), complement components, inflammatory mediators (e.g. TNFα and LTα), heat shock proteins, and many other proteins, many with immunological functions (Trowsdale 2001) (Plate 63). The classical MHC class I sub-classes are HLA-A, HLA-B, and HLA-C, in each case, the α chain is encoded by a single locus in the MHC complex. The β chain (β2 microglobulin) is encoded on chromosome 15. The class II sub-classes, HLA–DR, HLA–DQ, and HLA–DP are each encoded by at least one α-chain and one β-chain locus (e.g. HLA–DRA1 and HLA–DRB1). Most of these loci are highly polymorphic, with more than 250 HLA-A alleles, more than 500 HLA-B alleles, more than 300 HLA–DRB1 alleles, 24 HLA–DQA alleles, more than 50 HLA–DQB, and more than 100 HLA–DPB alleles worldwide (Robinson et al. 2001). Each MHC molecule can bind a broad selection of peptides but the sequence differences between MHC molecules ensure that distinct panels of peptides are preferentially selected by different molecules. Since most MHC loci are highly polymorphic, most individuals are heterozygous at loci encoding MHC molecules. These loci are expressed co-dominantly ensuring that each individual expresses several MHC class I and class II molecules, thereby increasing the range of antigens that can be presented to the immune system.

Many HLA associations with disease have been demonstrated and the diseases discussed below represent a few illustrative examples (Tiwari and Terasaki 1985). Many hypotheses have been advanced to explain these associations; most assume that disease pathogenesis is related to the role of HLA molecules in antigen presentation (Table 1; reviewed in Hall and Bowness 1996). Most HLA-associated diseases are immunologically mediated and many are rheumatological. The association of ankylosing spondylitis with HLA-B27 has been recognized since 1973 (Brewerton et al. 1973). Approximately 94 per cent of patients with ankylosing spondylitis are HLA-B27 positive (Brown et al. 1996). HLA-B27 is associated, to a lesser degree, with arthritis in the context of inflammatory bowel disease

Table 1 Hypotheses advanced to explain HLA association with disease

Presentation of a pathogenic peptide by the associated HLA molecule
T cell receptor repertoire selection in the thymus in the presence of the associated HLA molecule
Presentation of a peptide fragment of the associated HLA molecule by other HLA molecules
Interaction of HLA (class II) molecules with superantigens
Chemical modification or expression of an aberrant form of the HLA molecule
Specific binding of microorganisms
Differential intereaction of HLA molecule with chaperone or other regulatory proteins
Linkage of the associated HLA locus with the disease locus

(30 per cent), reactive arthritis (50–80 per cent), psoriatic arthritis and uveitis (95 per cent). Studies in rodents expressing HLA-B27 transgenes directly implicate this MHC class I molecule in the pathogenesis of both arthritis and inflammatory bowel disease (Taurog et al. 1999). However, this is only evident in certain rodent strains, indicating that non-HLA genes also contribute to susceptibility. It has recently been demonstrated that HLA-B27 has a propensity for forming heavy chain homodimers. This aberrant molecule may present novel peptides to CD8 or NK cells and elicit abnormal inflammatory responses (Edwards et al. 2000).

Although the association of ankylosing spondylitis with HLA-B27 is strong, most HLA associations with autoimmune or chronic inflammatory disease are with MHC class II molecules. The association of RA with the HLA–DRB1 locus has been extensively studied. Careful analysis of the sequences of HLA–DRB1 alleles indicated that a conserved sequence, which translates into a region around pocket P4 of the peptide-binding groove, was more strongly associated with RA than any individual HLA–DRB1 allele. This has become known as the 'shared epitope' or 'consensus sequence' (Gregersen et al. 1987; Wordsworth et al. 1989). The significance of the shared epitope has been demonstrated elegantly by comparing the different associations of individual HLA–DRB1*04 alleles with RA. The RA-associated alleles, which contain the consensus sequence, include a series of basic residues in the third hypervariable region. In contrast, closely related HLA–DR4 alleles, for example, DRB1*0402, *0402, are not associated with RA; these alleles have non-conservative substitutions in the third hypervariable region. The positions of these influential residues are shown in Fig. 4 and the sequence of the third hypervariable region in a selection of RA-associated and non-associated alleles is presented in Table 2. The importance of the HLA–DRB1 locus in RA has been further supported by the finding that the combination of two RA-associated HLA–DRB1 alleles confers greater susceptibility to disease than the inheritance of either alone (Wordsworth et al. 1992). However, it is not known whether this reflects a direct synergistic effect between the two HLA–DR alleles are effects from other genes on these haplotypes.

An association has also been demonstrated between HLA haplotypes and SLE (Wakeland et al. 2001). HLA–DR2 and –DR3 have shown consistent associations with SLE in European–Caucasian populations, with a two- to three-fold increase in the frequency of these two alleles compared with controls but associations in non-Caucasian populations have been less impressive. SLE is a highly heterogeneous disease and particular clinical pictures are associated with the presence of certain autoantibodies. Interestingly, the MHC class II associations with the presence of individual autoantiobody specificities (e.g. HLA–DQ2 and anti-Ro antibodies) are stronger than the overall association with SLE (Schur 1995).

Several other autoimmune diseases are associated with MHC class II genes. Coeliac disease (CD) is associated with the HLA–DQ molecule encoded by HLA–DQA1*0501/HLA–DQB1*0201. Both the α and β chains of HLA–DQ are polymorphic and this particular HLA–DQ molecule may be expressed if both HLA–DQA1*0501 and DQB1*0201 are inherited on the same HLA haplotype (*cis*-encoded) or on different haplotypes (*trans*-encoded). This is thought to explain the lesser association of CD with allele DRB1*0301 (on a haplotype containing both HLA–DQA1*0502 and DQB1*0201) or with genotype DRB1*0501/DRB1*0701 (haplotypes DRB1*0501–DQA1*0501 and DRB1*0701–DQB1*0201) (Sollid 1998) (Fig. 5). Recent evidence supports the notion that CD4+ T cells promote a pathological inflammatory response to gluten in patients with CD. Gluten-reactive CD4+ T cells have been isolated from small intestinal biopsies of patients with CD; these are usually restricted by HLA–DQ molecules known to be associated with diesase but not by other MHC class II molecules expressed by the patients (Sollid 2000).

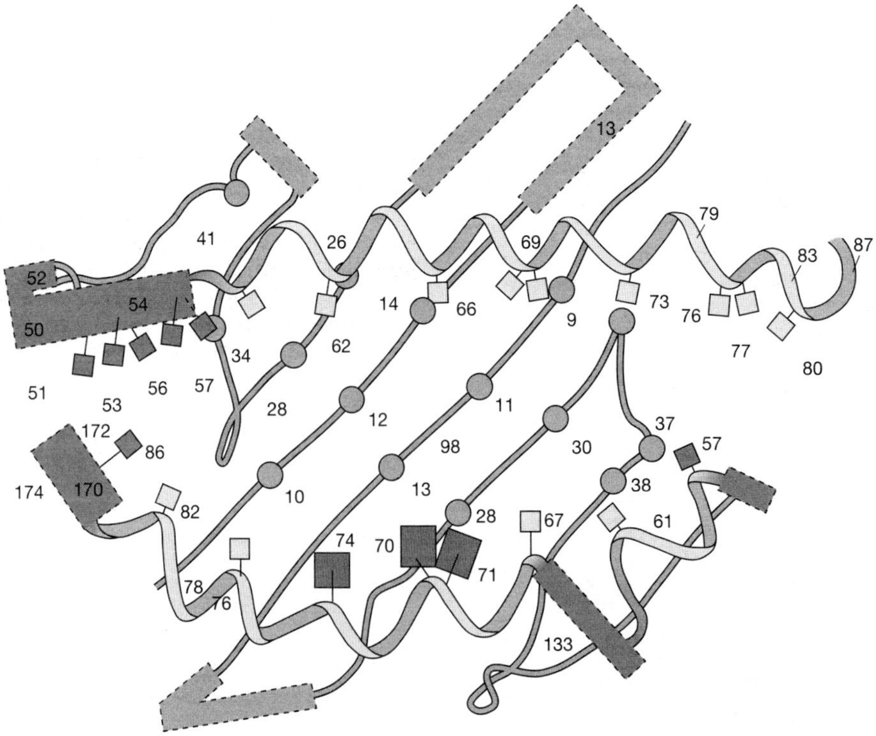

Fig. 4 Diagrammatic representation of the HLA–DR molecule, illustrating the peptide binding groove. Substitution of charged amino acids at positions (70, 71, 74) alter the susceptibility to rheumatoid arthritis (shown as solid symbols on the DR β-chain α-helix). The residues at these positions influence the nature of peptide that can bind in the groove and can also be directly contacted by the T cell receptor.

Table 2 Comparison of the amino acid sequences found in the third allelic hypervariable region of DR β-chains associated with susceptibility or non-susceptiblity to rheumatoid arthritis and those that are not

			67			70	71			74		
Susceptible	DR4	DRB1*0404/8	Asp	Leu	Leu	Glu	Glu	Arg	Arg	Ala	Ala	Val
Susceptible	DR4	DRB1*0405	—	—	—	—	—	—	—	—	—	—
Susceptible	DR4	DRB1*0401	—	—	—	—	—	Lys	—	—	—	—
Susceptible	DR1		—	—	—	—	—	—	—	—	—	—
Susceptible	DR10		—	—	—	—	Arg	—	—	—	—	—
Susceptible	DR6	DRB1*0402	—	—	—	—	—	—	—	—	—	—
Not susceptible	DR4	DRB1*0402	—	Ile	—	—	Asp	Glu	—	—	—	—
Not susceptible	DR4	DRB1*0403/7	—	—	—	—	—	—	—	—	Glu	—
Not susceptible	DR2		—	Phe	—	—	Asp	—	—	—	—	—

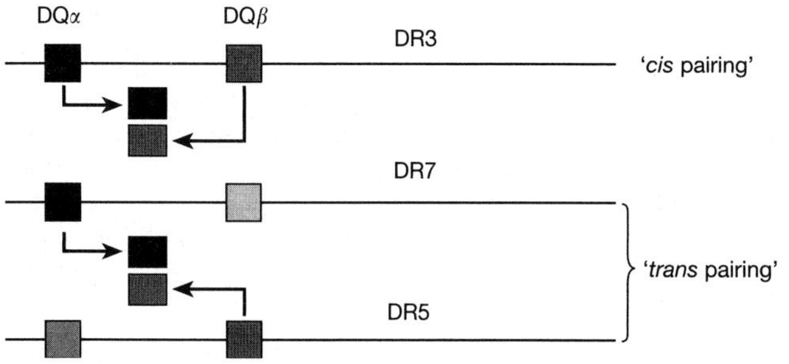

Fig. 5 The same DQ heterodimer may be assembled from the DQα and DQβ paired in *cis* formation from a single DR3 haplotype or from the DQα of a DR5 haplotype with the DQβ of a DR7 haplotype.

Several susceptibility loci, within and outside the HLA complex, have been demonstrated for type I diabetes mellitus. HLA haplotypes have been shown to confer both susceptibility and, unusually, dominant resistance to disease (Todd and Wicker 2001). In particular, HLA–DQβ chains with aspartic acid at position 57 in the binding groove confer resistance to disease. As for the HLA–DQ molecules in coeliac disease, MHC class II molecules have been shown to be involved in antigen presentation in the pancreatic lymph nodes and islets (Lee et al. 2001).

In addition to HLA associations with autoimmune disease, the host response to certain infectious agents is also influenced by the inheritance of particular HLA class I or class II alleles. An influence of HLA genes on a variety of infections, including leprosy, malaria, tuberculosis, AIDS, and hepatitis viruses have been demonstrated (Hill 1998). More surprising has been the association of HLA loci with metabolic or neurological disorders, such as hereditary haemochromotosis and narcolepsy. The original HLA association of haemochromotosis was with HLA-A3. It is now recognized that this is in linkage disequilibrium with the disease locus, HFE (Ehrlich and Lemonnier 2000). The HFE locus encodes a non-classical MHC class I molecule that is involved in iron metabolism. Patients with hereditary haemochromotosis have a mutated form of the HFE protein, typically a substitution of tyrosine for cysteine in the extracellular domain, which is unable to associate with β2m on the cell surface. It is hypothesized that this interferes with transferrin/iron transport. In contrast to hereditary haemochromotosis, the strongest HLA association with narcolepsy is with HLA–DQB1*0602 and no linked disease gene has been identfied (Mignot et al. 2001). The recent discovery of the hypocretin peptide system and its involvement in the physiology of sleep has restimulated interest in possibility that narcolepsy is an autoimmune condition which targets hypocretins and/or their receptors (Lin et al. 2001).

Summary

The immune system mirrors the central nervous system in complexity. The capacity to respond to microbial challenge with speed and efficacy relies upon the orchestration of the innate and adaptive arms of the immune system. The cellular and molecular agents of the innate response are marshalled rapidly following the pattern recognition of microbial components. This induces local inflammation and sets the scene for the generation of an adaptive response. This effector response is tailored to the nature of the challenge, in part by the behaviour of the innate system. Virtually any novel exogenous molecule can be recognized by the T cells and antibodies, which are fundamental to the adaptive immune response. Unlike innate defences, an effective primary response takes several days to develop. Once established, however, immunological 'memory' ensures that a second challenge with the same novel agent elicits a larger, faster secondary response. The flexibility and specificity of the adaptive response is based upon the B cell receptors (antibodies) and T cell receptors; the remarkable diversity of these receptors enables the recognition of virtually any antigen. The ability of the adaptive immune response to discriminate between endogenous and exogenous antigens is critical if self-tissues are to be protected from the harmful arsenal of immune effector mechanisms. Several levels of regulation appear to contribute to this 'self-tolerance', including thymic selection, the milieu created by the innate immune response and active regulation by T cells. The failure of such regulatory mechanisms may result in autoimmunity. The challenge is to understand how variations in immune function may predispose an individual to disease, what mechanisms serve to perpetuate the damaging inflammatory response and how this may be prevented or intercepted for therapeutic benefit.

References

Akira, S., Takeda, K., and Kaisho, T. (2001). Toll-like receptors: critical proteins linking innate and acquired immunity. *Nature Immunology* **2**, 675.

Anderson, G., Moore, N.C., Owen, J.J., and Jenkinson, E.J. (1996). Cellular interactions in thymocyte development. *Annual Review of Immunology* **14**, 73.

Born, W., Cady, C., Jones-Carson, J., Mukasa, A., Lahn, M., and O'Brien, R. (1999). Immunoregulatory functions of gamma delta T cells. *Advances in Immunology* **71**, 77.

Braud, V.M., Allan, D.S., and McMichael, A.J. (1999). Functions of nonclassical MHC and non-MHC-encoded class I molecules. *Current Opinion in Immunology* **11**, 100.

Brewerton, D.A., Caffrey, M., Hart, F.D., James, D.C.O., Nichols, A., and Sturrock, R.D. (1973). Ankylosing spondylitis and HL-A27. *Lancet* **i**, 904.

Brown, M.A. et al. (1996). HLA class I associations of ankylosing spondylitis in the white population in the United Kingdom. *Annals of the Rheumatic Diseases* **55**, 268.

Chien, Y.H. and Hampl, J. (2000). Antigen-recognition properties of murine gamma delta T cells. *Springer Seminars in Immunopathology* **22**, 239.

Davis, M.M. et al. (1998). Ligand recognition by alpha beta T cell receptors. *Annual Review of Immunology* **16**, 523.

Dieckmann, D., Plottner, H., Berchtold, S., Berger, T., and Schuler, G. (2001). *Ex vivo* isolation and characterization of CD4(+)CD25(+) T cells with regulatory properties from human blood. *Journal of Experimental Medicine* **193**, 1303.

Edwards, J.C., Bowness, P., and Archer, J.R. (2000). Jekyll and Hyde: the transformation of HLA-B27. *Immunology Today* **21**, 256.

Eguchi, K. (2001). Apoptosis in autoimmune diseases. *Internal Medicine* **40**, 275.

Ehrlich, R. and Lemonnier, F.A. (2000). HFE—a novel nonclassical class I molecule that is involved in iron metabolism. *Immunity* **13**, 585.

Elewaut, D. and Kronenberg, M. (2000). Molecular biology of NK T cell specificity and development. *Seminars in Immunology* **12**, 561.

Garcia, K.C. et al. (1996). An alphabeta T cell receptor structure at 2.5 A and its orientation in the TCR-MHC complex *Science* **274**, 209 (see comments).

Garcia, K.C., Teyton, L., and Wilson, I.A. (1999). Structural basis of T cell recognition. *Annual Review of Immunology* **17**, 369.

Gregersen, P.K., Silver, J., and Winchester, R.J. (1987). The shared epitope hypothesis. An approach to understanding the molecular genetics of susceptibility to rheumatoid arthritis. *Arthritis and Rheumatism* **30**, 1205.

Hall, F.C. and Bowness, P. (1996). HLA and disease: from molecular function to disease association? In *HLA and MHC Genes, Molecules and Function* (ed. M. Browning and A. McMichael), pp. 353–81. Oxford: BIOS Scientific Publishers Ltd.

Hill, A.V. (1998). The immunogenetics of human infectious diseases. *Annual Review of Immunology* **16**, 593.

Ishikawa, S. et al. (2001). Aberrant high expression of B lymphocyte chemokine (BLC/CXCL13) by C11b+CD11c+ dendritic cells in murine lupus and preferential chemotaxis of B1 cells towards BLC. *Journal of Experimental Medicine* **193**, 1393.

Ji, H. et al. (2001). Genetic influences on the end-stage effector phase of arthritis. *Journal of Experimental Medicine* **194**, 321.

Johansson, A.C. et al. (2001). Genetic control of collagen-induced arthritis in a cross with NOD and C57BL/10 mice is dependent on gene regions encoding complement factor 5 and FcgammaRIIb and is not associated with loci controlling diabetes. *European Journal of Immunology* **31**, 1847.

Jonuleit, H., Schmitt, E., Stassen, M., Tuettenberg, A., Knop, J., and Enk, A.H. (2001). Identification and functional characterization of human CD4(+) CD25(+) T cells with regulatory properties isolated from peripheral blood. *Journal of Experimental Medicine* **193**, 1285.

Joseph, S.B., Miner, K.T., and Croft, M. (1998). Augmentation of naive Th1 and Th2 effector CD4 responses by IL-6, IL-1 and TNF. *European Journal of Immunology* **28**, 277.

Kong, Y.Y. et al. (1999). Activated T cells regulate bone loss and joint destruction in adjuvant arthritis through osteoprotegerin ligand. *Nature* **402**, 304.

Kwon, B., Youn, B.-S., and Kwon, B. (1999). Functions of newly identified members of the tumor necrosis factor receptor/ligand superfamilies in lymphocytes. *Current Opinion in Immunology* **11**, 340.

Lee, K.H., Wucherpfennig, K.W., and Wiley, D.C. (2001). Structure of a human insulin peptide-HLA–DQ8 complex and susceptibility to type 1 diabetes. *Nature Immunology* **2**, 501.

Lin, L., Hungs, M., and Mignot, E. (2001). Narcolepsy and the HLA region. *Journal of Neuroimmunology* **117**, 9.

Medzhitov, R. and Janeway, C. (2000). Innate immunity. *New England Journal of Medicine* **343**, 338.

Mignot, E. et al. (2001). Complex HLA–DR and –DQ interactions confer risk of narcolepsy-cataplexy in three ethnic groups. *American Journal of Human Genetics* **68**, 686.

Maloy, K.J. and Powrie, F. (2001). Regulatory T cells in the control of immune pathology. *Nature Immunology* **2**, 816.

Mosmann, T.R. and Coffman, R.L. (1989). TH1 and TH2 cells: different patterns of lymphokine secretion lead to different functional properties. *Annual Review of Immunology* **7**, 145.

Mosmann, T.R. and Sad, S. (1996). The expanding universe of T-cell subsets: Th1, Th2 and more. *Immunology Today* **17**, 138.

Parham, P., ed. (1999). Pathways of antigen processing and presentation. *Immunological Reviews* **172** (whole edition).

Paxton, W.A. and Kang, S. (1998). Chemokine receptor allelic polymorphisms: relationships to HIV resistance and disease progression. *Seminars in Immunology* **10**, 187.

Poulton, L.D. et al. (2001). Cytometric and functional analyses of NK and NKT cell deficiencies in NOD mice. *International Immunology* **13**, 887.

Qin, S. et al. (1998). The chemokine receptors CXCR3 and CCR5 mark subsets of T cells associated with certain inflammatory reactions. *Journal of Clinical Investigation* **101**, 746.

Ridgway, W.M. and Fathman, C.G. (1999). MHC structure and autoimmune T cell repertoire development. *Current Opinion in Immunology* **11**, 638.

Robinson, J., Waller, M.J., Parham, P., Bodmer, J.G., and Marsh, S.G. (2001). IMGT/HLA Database—a sequence database for the human major histocompatibility complex. *Nucleic Acids Research* **29**, 210.

Salomon, B. et al. (2000). B7/CD28 costimulation is essential for the homeostasis of the CD4+CD25+ immunoregulatory T cells that control autoimmune diabetes. *Immunity* **12**, 431.

Schur, P.H. (1995). Genetics of systemic lupus erythematosus. *Lupus* **4**, 425.

Shevach, E.M. (2001). Certified professionals: CD4(+)CD25(+) suppressor T cells. *Journal of Experimental Medicine* **193**, F41.

Sollid, L.M. (1998). Genetics of the immune response to gluten in coeliac disease. *Digestive Diseases* **16**, 345.

Sollid, L.M. (2000). Molecular basis of celiac disease. *Annual Review of Immunology* **18**, 53.

Stephens, L.A., Mottet, C., Mason, D., and Powrie, F. (2001). Human CD4(+)CD25(+) thymocytes and peripheral T cells have immune suppressive activity *in vitro*. *European Journal of Immunology* **31**, 1247.

Takemura, S. et al. (2001). Lymphoid neogenesis in rheumatoid synovitis. *Journal of Immunology* **167**, 1072.

Taurog, J.D. et al. (1999). Inflammatory disease in HLA-B27 transgenic rats. *Immunology Reviews* **169**, 209.

Tiwari, J.L. and Terasaki, P.I. *HLA and Disease Associations* Vol. I. New York: Springer, 1985.

Todd, J.A. and Wicker, L.S. (2001). Genetic protection from the inflammatory disease type 1 diabetes in humans and animal models. *Immunity* **15**, 387.

Trowsdale, J. (2001). Genetic and functional relationships between MHC and NK receptor genes. *Immunity* **15**, 363.

Vivier, E., Tomasello, E., and Paul, P. (2002). Lymphocyte activation via NKG2D: towards a new paradigm in immune recognition? *Current Opinion in Immunology* **14**, 306.

Wakeland, E.K., Liu, K., Graham, R.R., and Behrens, T.W. (2001). Delineating the genetic basis of systemic lupus erythematosus. *Immunity* **15**, 397.

Watts, T.H. and DeBenedette, M.A. (1999). T cell co-stimulatory molecules other than CD28. *Current Opinion in Immunology* **11**, 286.

Wordsworth, B.P., Lanchbury, J.S., Sakkas, L.I., Welsh, K.I., Panayi, G.S., and Bell, J.I. (1989). HLA–DR4 subtype frequencies in rheumatoid arthritis indicate that DRB1 is the major susceptibility locus within the HLA class II region. *Proceedings of the National Academy of Sciences of the USA* **86**, 10049.

Wordsworth, B.P. et al. (1992). HLA heterozygosity contributes to susceptibility to rheumatoid arthritis. *American Journal of Human Genetics* **51**, 585.

4.4 Animal models of arthritis

Wim B. van den Berg

Introduction

A major research goal in the field of arthritis is to unravel the pathogenesis of chronic arthritis and the concomitant joint destruction. A second, more practical goal, is to discover a treatment that selectively inhibits the progression of destructive arthritis yet leaves the host defence mechanisms virtually intact. This requires a critical understanding of the cells and mediators involved in the destruction and in the initiation, maintenance, and remission of the arthritic process. Studies in human arthritis are hampered by the fact that the precise time of onset is unknown, whereas lesional tissue is often obtained from endstage disease at the moment of joint replacement. The latter holds in particular for cartilage specimens, since it is widely accepted that this tissue has a limited capacity for repair. In the past, synovial biopsies and synovial fluid were only taken from patients experiencing an exacerbation of symptoms that necessitated arthroscopy or the *aspiration* of an effusion, inherently representing extremes of the natural history of the disease. Moreover, specimens come from patients who have been receiving various drugs, and the shortage of control tissue is obvious. Numerous arthritis units have now started to run early arthritis clinics, in which early biopsies are *taken more often* and even the taking of small biopsies of articular cartilage surfaces from *affected* areas may be considered. Another way to circumvent the problems is to resort to the use of experimental models of arthritis.

Although not ideal in the eyes of many in terms of precise mimicry of human arthritic disease, experimental models of arthritis do reflect key aspects of their human counterparts. Their *established* time course, the easy access to tissue samples, and the *ease* of experimental therapeutic manipulation offer a useful approach to further understanding of the pathogenesis of arthritis. Models may also provide valuable insights into biological approaches to arthritis therapy, ranging from cytokines, cytokine inhibitors, and 'tolerizing' antigens to monoclonal antibodies against cellular receptors and vaccination directed against effector cells. Potential therapies need to be evaluated in the human diseases, indirectly approving the predictive value of findings in particular models. It *must be accepted* that no single animal model of arthritis truly represents the human disease. In fact, the wide variety of agents that can induce an experimental arthritis with clinical and histopathological features close to those of the human arthritides supports the hypothesis that rheumatoid arthritis may have a variety of causes and that the characteristic features reflect common end-points. Analysis of aspects peculiar to an individual model may be of limited value and the emphasis should be on general validity and common concepts in various models. In the following sections, the models most widely used in the study of rheumatoid arthritis will be summarized and their value will be illustrated with some recent research findings. Since the questions to be answered in models must arise from elements of the human disease, current concepts will be briefly addressed first.

Concepts and features of rheumatoid arthritis

Rheumatoid arthritis is characterized by chronic inflammation in the joints and progressive destruction of bone and cartilage. Its pathogenesis is unknown, but the disease is often considered as an autoimmune process. The articular cartilage is an intriguing tissue, since it may function both as the trigger as well as the victim of this disease. Two major events may underlie the chronic synovial inflammation: persistent stimulation of T and B cells by as yet unknown (auto-) antigens, or direct activation of the synovial cells by non-antigenic triggers. The latter may imply continuous stimulation by bacterial or viral triggers, but may also reflect deranged behaviour and tumour-like growth.

Table 1 Recent approaches in arthritis models

Application of MHC blockade
Manipulation of defined T-cell subsets
Selective T-cell receptor usage/blockade
Regulatory role of heat-shock proteins
Control by bacterial flora
Preventive induction of tolerance
Immunomodulation in established arthritis?
Induction of bystander suppression
Neutralization of key cytokines
Upregulation of cytokine inhibitors
Blockade of adhesion molecules
Identification of destructive cells/enzymes
Aberrant cell survival/apoptosis
Disease course in transgenic/knock-out mice

Plate 64 depicts potential cascades in the synovial inflammation and concomitant joint destruction. It illustrates the various levels of potential therapeutic interference, ranging from antigen presentation to T cells, control by regulatory T cells, production of antibodies, activation of synovial cells, and release of destructive mediators acting on the articular cartilage. It is, of course, attractive to target research in models at the level of the arthritogen. However, in the absence of an established antigen, to seek further understanding of effector mechanisms characteristic of joint inflammation and destruction seems at least as valuable. Recent research approaches in models are summarized in Table 1, which for obvious reasons cannot all be covered in detail. An overview of classic arthritis models by Wooley (1991) is recommended.

Characteristic histopathological features in the rheumatoid arthritic joint include immune complexes in the articular cartilage layers and variable amounts of macrophages and T cells in the synovium, often accompanied by fibrosis and synovial hyperplasia. The antigens in the immune complexes in the cartilage are still poorly defined and, although candidates for a role in the synovitis, may even reflect an epiphenomenon of immune-complex deposition and retention in damaged areas. Increasing attention is now focused on the role of cytokines, with tumour necrosis factor (TNF) and interleukin-1 (IL-1) being seen as master cytokines, orchestrating the synovial inflammation and concomitant tissue destruction. However, considerable variation is found in relative cytokine levels and immune elements between patients and at various stages in one patient, making it difficult or even impossible to define critical correlations in animal models. The latter can at best reflect *specific* aspects.

Models of arthritis

Historically, models of arthritis have been used to understand the stimuli provoking chronic arthritis and the mechanisms regulating chronicity and tissue destruction. When a model is established, the potential of a given stimulus is proven. The next step would be to obtain evidence that such reactions do occur in human arthritides, for instance, T-cell reactivity against a cartilage antigen. If this is the case, it has still to be proved that this reactivity is of pathogenetic importance and not an epiphenomenon, for example, by showing that antigen-specific immunomodulation really affects the course of the disease. Up to now, such research has not yielded

Table 2 Common models of arthritis

Model	Species	Immunization	Induction	Pers. Ag[a]	Auto Ag	T cells
Adjuvant arthritis	Rat	CFA		Bact?	?	+
Collagen-induced arthritis	Rat, mouse, primate	CII/CFA			Collagen II	+
Proteoglycan arthritis	BALB/c mouse	PG/CFA			Proteoglycan	+
Streptococcal cell-wall arthritis	Rat		i.p. SCW	SCW		+
Antigen-induced arthritis	Rabbit, rat, mouse	Ag/CFA	i.a. Ag	Antigen		+
Oil-induced arthritis	Rat, mouse	Oil			?	+
MRL-lpr/lpr	MRL mouse			Virus?		−
K/BxN arthritis	Mouse	Cross breeding	TCR	GPI	GPI	+

[a] Relates to persistent antigen in the joints.

Note: Ag, antigen; CFA, complete Freund's adjuvant; CII, collagen type II; PG, proteoglycan; SCW, streptococcal cell-wall; i.p., intraperitoneal; i.v., intravenous; TCR, T-cell receptor; GPI, glucose-6-phosphate isomerase.

a clue about the definitive trigger *for* rheumatoid arthritis and continuing investigations can be divided into those that attempt further understanding of principles in established models and those that are still looking for new, putative triggers, and novel models and concepts.

In line with the historical concepts in rheumatoid arthritis, the models most widely studied in the past decades are those of adjuvant arthritis, collagen-induced arthritis (CIA), antigen-induced arthritis, and streptococcal cell-wall arthritis. T cells play a dominant part in all of these models (Table 2). The second common principle is the presence of a chronic stimulus, either in the form of a persistent antigen or an autoantigen akin to joint structures. Persisting antigens are non-degradable bacterial cell walls in the synovial tissue, or antigen trapped in the collagenous reservoirs such as ligaments and articular cartilage (antigen-induced arthritis). Both conditions reflect escape from proper clearance by the phagocytic system. A second category of persistent stimuli is formed by autoantigens from the articular cartilage, such as collagen type II and proteoglycans. Other, yet unknown cartilage antigens probably fulfil a similar role. In adjuvant and streptococcal cell-wall arthritides the cartilage could as well function as an autoantigen, related to structural mimicry between bacterial peptidoglycans and cartilage proteoglycans. However, ultimate proof that these cross-reactive responses really contribute to the arthritis has still to be provided. Of interest, destructive forms of rheumatoid arthritis tend to decline at the moment that the cartilage is fully destroyed. Moreover, total joint replacement often results in a complete remission of the arthritis in that particular joint, without the need for concomitant synovectomy. These are possible arguments for a direct role of cartilage antigens in the pathogenesis or an indirect role of cartilage components in the maintenance of the inflammatory process in the joint. The latter receives recent attention, since it is shown that degraded fragments of cartilage components can directly stimulate synoviocytes to release inflammatory cytokines.

The third lesson from the models is that microbial components, particularly cell-wall fragments from enteric organisms, are potential causative agents in humans. Apart from their ability to induce arthritis by direct localization to joint tissues, they may induce arthritis remotely as a result of structural mimicry with joint structures. There is ample evidence from clinical observations that bacterial infections and development of arthritis may somehow be related.

It is almost a matter of taste whether persistent exogenous antigens or autoantigens should be considered as different entities or as reflecting integral parts of the body that need tight regulation of suppression and/or tolerance. Certainly, it is as yet unclear whether the regulation of these forms of immunity is similar or dissimilar.

In line with the increasing doubt in various research groups about the critical role of a T-cell-driven reaction to a defined (auto-) antigen, increasing attention is nowadays focused on less defined models, such as the spontaneous arthritis in MRL/lpr mice and the arthritis induced in susceptible strains with mineral oils. In addition, plain overexpression of cytokines IL-1 and TNF-α or H_2-c-*fos* in transgenic animals provides further evidence that the expression of chronic destructive arthritis may occur in the absence of a clear involvement of T cells. In addition, T cells may help in autoantibody production, but immune complex arthritis can persue on its own as long as antibody levels remain high. In the following sections, some of the commonly used models will be critically evaluated. Comparative information is given in Table 3. Technical details can be found in some overviews (Bliven and Otterness 1985; Hunneyball et al. 1989).

Table 3 Characteristic features of the arthritis models

	AA	CIA	SCW-A	AIA
Main site of expression	Ankle	Peripheral	Ankle	Knee[a]
Bone marrow inflammation	++	−	+	−
Local plasma cells	−	±	−	++
Immune complexes in cartilage	−	++	−	++
Cartilage destruction	±	+++	+	++
Effects of NSAIDs[b]	+	++	+	−
Dominant feature	Periostitis	Destructive	Fibrosis	Destructive

[a] To be chosen by intra-articular injection.

[b] Effect on ongoing destruction.

Note: AA, adjuvant arthritis; CIA, collagen-induced arthritis; SCW-A, streptococcal cell-wall arthritis; AIA, antigen-induced arthritis; NSAID, non-steroidal anti-inflammatory drug.

Adjuvant arthritis

This is the first and most extensively studied model of polyarthritis, which was discovered some 40 years ago by Stoerk in 1954 as an experimental accident. Whilst trying to produce immunity to spleen extracts emulsified in Freund's adjuvant, an arthritis developed in the immunized rats. Pearson (1956) demonstrated that the arthritis was due simply to the bacterial component. The model has since been extensively used for the screening of drugs to be used in rheumatoid arthritis.

Nowadays, the classical model is induced by intradermal injection of Freund's complete adjuvant containing heat-killed mycobacteria and the arthritis develops within 2 weeks in susceptible rat strains. In general, the model is induced in Lewis rats. The volume, type of oil, and composition of the suspension are critical variables that determine the incidence and severity of the arthritis. The active component in the bacteria is the cell-wall peptidoglycan and the disease can be induced with various bacteria.

The histopathological features of adjuvant arthritis mainly reflect a periarthritis, with marked periostitis instead of a synovitis, and massive inflammation in the bone marrow. Immune-complex deposition in the cartilage is not a characteristic feature and cartilage destruction is limited in early disease (Plate 65). Given the highly destructive attack on the cartilage as seen in the autoimmune collagen type-II arthritis, this argues against cross-reactivity with cartilaginous autoantigens in adjuvant arthritis as the driving principle.

Adjuvant arthritis is T-cell dependent and the strongest argument for an autoimmune process is the induction of arthritis by passive transfer of T cells from diseased animals. The joint inflammation may reflect the generation of a T-cell reaction to bacterial epitopes cross-reacting with endogenous bacterial fragments continuously present in synovial tissues or with cartilaginous antigens. It may also be based on non-specific immunomodulation, reflecting the adjuvant properties of the bacterium in oil preparations and the generation of a disregulated expression of autoimmunity to whatever autoimmune epitope. The fact that non-antigenic adjuvants, such as the oil preparation avridin (CP 20961) and other mineral oils, can induce an arthritis indistinguishable from adjuvant arthritis underlines the potential existence of such a pathway.

In classic adjuvant arthritis, a bacterium-specific pathogenesis remains most likely since conventionally bred rats are generally resistant to adjuvant arthritis, whereas germ-free Fisher or Wistar rats are susceptible (van de Langerijt et al. 1994, 1994a). The germ-free rats are lacking early contact with bacteria and are therefore not 'tolerized'; colonization with bacteria before the induction of adjuvant arthritis prevented susceptibility (Kohashi et al. 1986). Susceptibility is furthermore influenced by the level of the steroid feedback response. Lewis rats are generally susceptible to numerous autoimmune processes and are low steroid responders to a large range of stimuli. Steroid responsiveness of a rat strain or a particular individual is an element modulating the severity of the disease.

The most intriguing observation in the model of adjuvant arthritis is the occurrence of spontaneous remission and the lack of susceptibility to reinduction. This resistance is antigen-specific. T-cell lines and clones were isolated that can induce disease, but when attenuated can also induce protective responses (Holoshitz et al. 1983). It probably involves regulatory T cells that recognize antigen-specific receptors on the T cells driving the arthritis and which are able to block the activity of those cells.

Treatment with antibodies against CD4 induced suppression of adjuvant arthritis and tolerance to the initiating arthritogen (Billingham 1994). Subsequently, it was found that rats undergoing anti-CD4 treatment before the induction of arthritis with either streptococci or non-antigenic adjuvants (mineral oils, CP 20961) displayed a shared tolerance to the reinduction of both models, implying that there might be common bacterial epitopes in the regulation of adjuvant arthritides.

The identification of epitopes on bacterial heat-shock proteins and the recognition of cross-reactive, highly conserved, endogenous heat-shock proteins in eukaryotes, has implicated these proteins as the target antigen in adjuvant arthritis (van Eden 1991, 1999). However, subsequent research demonstrated a role for heat-shock proteins in other autoimmune models also, and a regulatory role in inflammation rather than as a critical antigen in arthritis seems more likely.

In industry, adjuvant arthritis is often the model of first choice for screening new therapeutic agents for antiarthritic efficacy. This is mainly based on its ease of induction and the simple macroscopic observation of arthritis in the paws. The fact that non-steroidal anti-inflammatory drugs are effective inhibitors of cartilage and bone destruction in this model, in clear contrast to observations in human rheumatoid arthritis, puts some doubt on its applicability.

Collagen-induced arthritis

The model of collagen arthritis in rats was first described in 1977 by Trentham and colleagues, again as a coincidental finding in protocols to induce antibodies to purified collagen preparations (Trentham et al. 1977). The initial observation indicated that arthritis was confined to sensitization with native collagen type II, a major component of articular cartilage. Denatured collagen type II or other collagen types were not arthritogenic. Minor collagen types from articular cartilage may also function as arthritogens, for instance collagen types IX and XI (Holmdahl et al. 1993).

The crucial element in this arthritis is the induction of immunity to foreign collagen type II, subsequently cross-reacting with homologous collagen type II. Plain immunization with homologous collagen type II can also be used, but then much stronger immunization regimens are needed to override natural tolerance. The disease can easily be induced in rats, with full-blown expression within 14 days, whereas expression in mice follows genetic restriction (Wooley et al. 1981). Moreover, disease expression in mice is more gradual, starting after 3–4 weeks in some, whereas a 100 per cent incidence commonly takes 8–10 weeks. Of interest, collagen arthritis can also be induced in non-human primates. Most rhesus monkeys were susceptible and instead of *a susceptibility gene*, linkage studies on the major histocompatibility complex (MHC) revealed the presence of a gene regulating resistance.

Unlike adjuvant arthritis, collagen arthritis is *less systemic as an illness, but involves mainly the* peripheral joints and spares the spine. However, the ears may be affected, and this feature is mainly found at late stages in rats. This may suggest a role for this type of reactivity in polychondritis. In murine CIA, marked expression was also found in knee joints, in addition to the paws, ankle, and wrist. Histopathology of collagen arthritis shows a distinct, acute synovitis with numerous granulocytes, and bone erosions as well as periosteal new bone formation. Involvement of the bone marrow is limited in early disease. A characteristic feature is the direct attack by granulocytes at the cartilage surface. In contrast to findings in other models, a complete loss of articular cartilage is often seen within 2 weeks (Plate 65) and the arthritis ends up in ankylosis, with limited inflammation. The lack of sustaining antigen is probably the main reason for the remission of the arthritis. In addition, regulating T cells have been demonstrated in late-phase disease, which demonstrates that one should be careful with anti-T-cell therapy in human arthritis, since, dependent of the phase, such treatment can either improve the condition or make it worse.

The mechanism of arthritis expression is based on two principles: the presence of anticollagen antibodies and the generation of anticollagen type II T-cell immunity. Although antibodies alone are able to induce arthritis after passive administration to naive recipient animals, high concentrations are needed and, at best, a transient arthritis occurs. Passive transfer with bulk T cells or clones also yielded poor disease expression. Probably, antibodies are needed to bind to the cartilage surface and to release further collagen epitopes upon complement fixation and the attraction of leucocytes, including granulocytes and lymphocytes. An influx of anticollagen type II (CII)-specific T cells will then further drive the arthritic process.

Expression can be enhanced by extra anticollagen type II antibodies, non-specific inflammatory stimuli such as lipopolysaccharide or yeast particles (zymosan), or the simple addition of single inflammatory mediators such as IL-1, TNF-α, or transforming growth factor-β (TGF-β) (Joosten et al. 1994). It proves an intriguing principle that quiescent autoimmune arthritis comes to a full expression with a combination of potentiating elements, which also include bacterial infections and IL-12 release. Recent studies not only implicate potentiating cytokines, but also the temporary control by modulators such as IL-4 and IL-10. This is further addressed under the heading 'Cytokines' below.

Much research has been focused on oral and nasal tolerance induction with collagen type II fragments. It is now accepted that the route of administration and the local cytokine milieu, rather than the existence of tolerizing or arthritogenic epitopes on fragments, determine the impact on arthritis (Brand et al. 2002). Collagen-induced arthritis, using a defined autoantigen, is also a suitable model for analysing the restricted usage of T-cell receptors (*TCR*) and the possibility of suppressing arthritis by blocking a particular receptor. Although challenging scientifically, therapeutic applicability of this principle in RA patients *remains a remote possibility*.

Significant T-cell reactivity to collagen type II cannot easily be detected in patients with rheumatoid arthritis, making it difficult to analyse efficacy of specific immunomodulation. Recent immunomodulation approaches include the principle of bystander suppression, where oral or nasal administration of a nonrelated antigen is used to generate the production of suppressive cytokines (IL-10, TGF-β). These mediators will then by way of bystander activity suppress anti-CII immunity and indirectly collagen arthritis (Miossec and van den Berg 1997; Joosten et al. 2000). If variable antigen usage is accepted as a likely condition reflecting heterogeneity in various rheumatoid arthritis patients, such a non-specific therapeutic approach might prove more useful.

A worrying finding in terms of comparison with human arthritis is the highly destructive character of collagen arthritis and the marked sensitivity to non-steroidal anti-inflammatory drugs. Indomethacin is a very potent suppressor of both the inflammation and the joint destruction; steroids are also highly effective. The latter complicates experimental studies, since stress influences can profoundly disturb the expression of the arthritis. In contrast to the female preponderance in rheumatoid arthritis, male rodents are more susceptible to collagen arthritis.

Proteoglycan arthritis

This is a logical extension of collagen arthritis, since both collagen type II and proteoglycan are major components of articular cartilage. Yet again the discovery of the model was coincidental, following the immunization of mice to prepare antibodies. Repeated boosting was needed to induce consistent arthritis after 8 weeks, implicating poor antigenicity or strong tolerance. Arthritis was noticed in inbred female Balb/c mice upon immunization with human foetal articular proteoglycan, stripped of chondroitin sulfate (Mikecz et al. 1990; Finnegan et al. 1999). The arthritogenic epitope resides in the core protein. The mechanism of induction of the arthritis is probably quite similar to that in CIA: the induction of immunity to foetal human proteoglycan, subsequently cross-reacting with murine proteoglycans.

The proteoglycan model shows a polyarthritis, with severe cartilage erosion and marked ankylosis. In addition, involvement of the lumbar spine and disc regions was found, making it a model for spondylitis also. Like collagen arthritis, the most severe expression of proteoglycan arthritis is found in the presence of both antibodies and antiproteoglycan T-cell immunity. Of interest, antiproteoglycan antibodies on their own were capable of causing marked loss of proteoglycan from the cartilage in the absence of distinct synovitis.

Screening for the occurrence of such antiproteoglycan immunity in patients with rheumatoid arthritis did not yield unequivocal data in support of a role in human arthritis sofar. Further characterization of proteoglycan subtypes and epitopes may provide more insight.

Streptococcal cell-wall arthritis

This model was originally described by Cromartie and Schwab (1977). It was induced in Lewis rats by the systemic injection of cell-wall fragments of group A streptococci, which are highly resistant to biodegradation. Later on a similar disease was induced with cell-wall fragments from other bacteria, such as *Lactobacillus casei* or *Eubacterium aerofaciens.* The common principle resides in the poor degradability of the fragments, thereby creating a persistent stimulus. The lactobacillus and eubacterial models are of particular interest for the human disease, since these bacteria are part of the normal gastrointestinal flora (Stimpson et al. 1986; Hazenberg et al. 1992), which implies that an enormous load of potential arthritogenic stimuli is continuously present in the normal gastrointestinal tract.

Within 24 h of the administration of cell-wall fragments, acute inflammation develops in peripheral joints, coincident with the dissemination of cell-wall fragments in the blood vessels of the synovium and in the subchondral bone marrow. This acute, complement-dependent inflammation subsides over the next week and is followed within 2 weeks by a chronic, erosive polyarthritis, which involves mainly peripheral joints. In contrast with the acute phase, the chronic joint inflammation develops in only a limited number of rat strains, with the highest incidence in Lewis rats. The chronic phase often shows waxing and waning of arthritis, which brings it close to human rheumatoid arthritis. Mice strains studied so far are not susceptible to this i.p. model of arthritis. In general, female rats show a more severe arthritis than males.

Although macrophages become stimulated by the persistent bacterial fragments, cogent evidence now exists that the chronic phase is dependent on T cells. The chronic phase was not inducible in nude Lewis rats (no T cells) and cyclosporin A effectively inhibited this phase. In addition, chronic arthritis can be prevented with antibodies against the $\alpha\beta$ TCR. Moreover, streptococcal cell wall-specific T-cell responses were found in arthritis-susceptible Lewis rats, whereas resistant Fisher rats did not mount this immune reaction. Finally, germ-free Fishers rats were susceptible and did show streptococcal cell wall-specific T-cell reactivity. This suggests that the chronic arthritis is driven by a streptococcal cell wall-specific T-cell reaction to persistent bacteria. Normal animals and most individuals are strongly tolerant of threatening arthritogenic reactions to bacterial cell walls, whereas Lewis rats and similar individuals display weak tolerance and easily lose tolerogenic control. Lewis rats display a disturbance in the hypothalamic–pituitary–adrenal axis, reflected in a low feedback response to endogenous corticosteroid. Such a defect is also noted in patients with rheumatoid arthritis, which is not attributable to chronic inflammation itself. The defect in the hypothalamic–pituitary–adrenal axis is probably not a *critical but more a regulatory effect.*

In addition to streptococcal cell wall-specific T-cell reactions, cross-reactive autoimmunity to cartilage proteoglycans may contribute to the chronic arthritis. However, it is unlikely that this is a major factor in its onset. In fact, early histopathological appearances are those of a strong, mononuclear synovitis, with a sparse exudate in the joint space and limited loss of proteoglycan from the articular cartilage (Plate 65). Only at later stages of the chronic arthritis were marked pannus formation and severe erosions of underlying cartilage and bone frequently observed.

In line with the involvement of growth factors and the tumour-like behaviour of synovial cells in patients with rheumatoid arthritis, similar characteristics have been found in synoviocytes from streptococcal cell-wall arthritic rats. Probably due to the persistent bacterial stimuli, synovial cells do show continued proliferation *ex vivo*, with apparent paracrine and autocrine regulation by growth factors (Lafyatis et al. 1989). This observation further delineates that macrophage–fibroblast activation may be a perpetuating principle, but it leaves unanswered why *in vivo* the observed T-cell dependence is still a critical, controlling factor.

The model has not been frequently used for drug studies, which is an omission. Cyclosporin A shows efficacy and it has been claimed that non-steroidal anti-inflammatory drugs and steroids are suppressive as well. Gold and penicillamine were without effect, whereas methotrexate showed moderate activity. The main reason for limited studies in this model is the difficulty of preparing proper arthritogenic *bacterial cell walls.*

CpG arthritis

As an extension of involvement of bacteria in arthritis it was recently identified that bacterial DNA could induce arthritis. In particular, the CpG motifs in bacterial DNA are arthritogenic and substantial amounts can be found in joint tissues (Deng and Tarkowski 2001). Macrophages play a major role in this arthritis through TNF production. However, in comparison to cell wall fragments, the cytokine inducing capacity is weak.

Antigen-induced arthritis

Since human rheumatoid arthritis was/is believed to be an immunologically mediated disease, albeit with an unknown inciting antigen, a model based on local antigenic challenge in a primed host appeared logical. Such a model was first developed by Dumonde and Glynn (1962) in rabbits. In principle, it can be induced in any species, provided that proper immunity to a particular antigen can be mounted, and extensions have since been developed in mice, rats, and guinea pigs. In contrast to the polyarthritis models described so far, this type of arthritis remains confined to the injected joint, enabling comparison with a contralateral control joint of the same animal.

Commonly used antigens were ovalbumin, bovine serum albumin, and fibrin. Pre-immunization is performed with antigen in complete Freund's adjuvant to induce strong humoral as well as cell-mediated immunity. Arthritis is usually induced 3 weeks later by a local injection in the knee joint of a large amount of antigen. Initially an Arthus type of reaction develops, followed by a T-cell-mediated chronic inflammation. In the rabbit, chronicity may last for years. The histopathological appearances are of a granulocyte-rich exudate in the joint space, thickening of the synovial lining layer, and, at later stages, a predominantly mononuclear infiltrate in the synovium, which later includes numerous T cells and clusters of plasma cells. Interestingly, a large proportion (50 per cent) of these plasma cells are still making antibodies to the inciting antigen, providing evidence that the retained antigen still is the driving force in the chronic arthritis. Intense immune-complex formation is seen in the superficial layers of the articular cartilage, which may contribute to the process of cartilage destruction. Early loss of proteoglycan, followed by pannus formation and cartilage and bone erosion, is a common finding. Of the models described so far these characteristics are the closest to those found in human rheumatoid arthritis.

Two important principles emerged from studies on antigen-induced arthritis: first, chronicity is only found in the presence of sufficient antigen retention in joint tissues, in combination with proper T-cell-mediated delayed hypersensitivity; second, joints contain numerous, non- or avascular collagenous tissues such as cartilage, ligaments, and tendons, which allow for prolonged antigen retention by antibody-mediated trapping and charge-mediated binding (Cooke et al. 1972; van den Berg et al. 1984) (Plate 66). A key finding was the observation that antigen injected in the skin produced transient inflammation, whereas a similar dose in the joints caused chronic arthritis. The chronicity of arthritis in the standard model is probably related to the generation of local hyper-reactivity. Antigen trapped in the collagenous tissues will be released in tiny amounts to sustain low-grade chronic arthritis. As a consequence the local T-cell infiltrate will gain specificity, since retention of specific T cells is enhanced by homologous antigen. This means that small amounts of antigen are sufficient to sustain arthritis, whereas relatively large amounts are needed to induce it. This is a pivotal finding and forms the basis for exacerbations of arthritis described below.

Cationic antigens are proper arthritogens in this model, owing to their ability to stick to the negatively charged collagenous structures of the joint. This led to a search for putative natural antigens with similar properties. Interestingly, cationic components of bacteria such as streptococci appeared to be *sufficient* stimuli in the model, but subsequent searches for such T-cell reactivities in human rheumatoid arthritis were negative. However, similar reactivity was demonstrated in reactive arthritis, and antigen-induced arthritis, using a cationic antigen, probably makes a good model for reactive arthritis.

The model of antigen-induced arthritis is most suited to studies into the mechanism of cartilage destruction, which are facilitated by knowledge of the exact time of onset, the accessibility of the knee joint (as compared with ankles), and the presence of a contralateral control joint. Moreover, the model can be adequately used to test the feasibility of approaches to therapeutic immunomodulation. Comparison with autoimmune models may provide insight into similarities or dissimilarities in regulation of immunity to chosen protein antigens or cartilage autoantigens.

Antigen-induced arthritis is insensitive to non-steroidal anti-inflammatory drugs (de Vries and van den Berg 1989; Hunneyball et al. 1989), like the human condition. Steroids are highly effective, cytotoxic drugs are potent suppressants, and gold compounds were shown to be effective in the rabbit model.

Flares of arthritis

In comparison to the chronic process of human rheumatoid arthritis, a general shortcoming of most models is the relatively short duration of a severe and rapidly destructive inflammation. In that respect, models of repeated flares of arthritis, with slower development of lesions, provide a valuable extension. An arthritic joint bearing a chronic T-cell infiltrate displays a state of local hyper-reactivity against retained antigens, contributing to chronicity. This is not restricted to retained antigen but also applies to new antigen entering the sensitized joint. Flares of smouldering arthritis could easily be induced with as little as 10 ng of antigen. This is a T-cell-dependent process and can be completely blocked by *in vivo* antibody treatment against MHC (Ia) or CD4 (Lens et al. 1984). Flares can be induced by local rechallenge, but also by intravenous or even oral antigen administration. Higher dosages are, of course, needed for intravenous or oral challenges, and access to the joint is dependent on systemic antibodies and the physicochemical properties of the antigen. A model of repeated flares is probably more akin to the human state than is a model showing severe inflammation for some weeks, followed by rapid waning of arthritis. In a considerable proportion of patients with rheumatoid arthritis the disease course is characterized by exacerbations and remissions.

An important extension of the flare model was found by comparative dosing of IL-1 to naive joints and joints bearing a chronic infiltrate. The infiltrated joint was much more sensitive to IL-1, and the reactivity seemed to reside in the macrophage infiltrate. Most importantly, the IL-1-induced flare was more destructive to the articular cartilage than the initial insult.

In addition to flare models based on protein antigen, similar models have been developed in rats and mice using bacterial cell-wall constituents. In contrast to small protein antigens, which are only inflammatory in the context of an immune response, bacterial fragments may function as an antigen as well as a phlogistic irritant in their own right, and ensuing reactions are a mixture of T-cell- and macrophage-driven processes. The generation of local hyper-reactivity asks for large, persistent bacterial peptidoglycan–polysaccharide components, but the recurrence may happen with a variety of components ranging from fragments, to lipopolysaccharide, to CpG motifs, to cytokines like IL-1. The strongest flares occur in the presence of T-cell immunity and a correlation was found between the potential of fragments to induce an exacerbation and to elicit cell wall-specific T-cell proliferation *in vitro* (van den Broek et al. 1988). One other important aspect of these flares with cell-wall fragments resides in the presence of considerable cross-reactivity between cell walls from different bacterial origins. Flares can be induced with homologous as well as heterologous fragments and this may even extend to cross-reactive autoantigens from the cartilage. These principles open up a wide range of putative stimuli involved in exacerbations, simultaneously complicating the search for the driving 'antigen' in humans.

Immune complex arthritis

Autoantibodies are a key feature of rheumatoid arthritis. In some of the models discussed above, such as collagen, proteoglycan and antigen induced arthritis, immune complex formation at joint tissues is a major element. Although there is no doubt that excessive immune complex formation can cause destructive arthritis, common observations indicate that chronicity is limited and in fact, only seen in the presence of T cells. The latter may be linked to the need of T cells to sustain antibody production, or points to the necessity of T-cell macrophage interaction in sustained joint pathology. Minute amounts of antigen suffice to stimulate T cells, whereas considerable amounts of ICs are needed to stimulate inflammatory mediator release from phagocytes. Anyway, immune complex models mimic part of the rheumatoid arthritis pathology.

There is growing interest in the use of the passive immune complex models, along with availability of a range of transgenic knockouts to identify crucial pathways of inflammation and tissue destruction. In general, the advantage of passive systems is the lower dependence of genetic background, herein avoiding excessive backcrossing to create the transgenics in suitable, susceptible mouse strains. Passive transfer of collagen arthritis can be done with a critical mixture of a number of anti-CII monoclonal antibodies, including complement binding IgG2a. Sets are now commercially available, routinely recommending DBA mice as sensitive recipients. Accepted concepts of inflammation include immune complex mediated complement and Fc-gamma receptor activation on phagocytes.

Proteoglycan antibodies from the proteoglycan arthritis model can induce transient arthritis upon transfer, with concomitant proteoglycan loss from the cartilage, but no erosive damage. IgG1 seems the critical subclass, but the limited destructive potential as compared to anti-CII, is yet unclear.

An intriguing, novel IC model emerged from the elegant series of experiments in transgenic mice, overexpressing a self-reactive TCR. The cross of K/BxN mice developed arthritis (Korganow et al. 1999) and it was found that the TCR recognized the ubiquitous self-antigen glucose-6-phosphate isomerase (GPI) and provoked through B cell differentiation and proliferation high levels of anti-GPI antibodies. The antibodies are directly pathogenic upon transfer and appear to recognize endogenous GPI, associated with the cartilage surface, which may explain the joint specificity. IgG1 antibodies are dominant and cause a sustained, erosive arthritis after continued transfer. Complement C5 is a regulatory element and might explain some of the variable susceptibility of various mouse strains (Ji et al. 2001; Maccioni et al. 2002).

A final model to be mentioned here is the passive transfer of rabbit anti-lysozyme antibodies to mice which are locally injected in one knee joint with Poly-L-lysine (PLL)-lysozyme. PLL coupled lysozyme is highly cationic and sufficiently large to be retained in the joint for prolonged periods of time. Both association with synovial tissue and heavy sticking to cartilage surfaces contributes to chronicity and cartilage destruction (van Lent et al. 1997). An intriguing observation was the more chronic and destructive nature of this arthritis in DBA/1j mice, which seems related to high sustained levels of activating Fc receptors on macrophages of this mouse strain (Blom et al. 2000). Further reading on activating and inhibitory Fcg receptors is recommended (Ravetch and Bolland 2001; van Lent et al. 2001).

Other models

In line with the trend of increasing concern about a particular T-cell-driven pathogenesis in rheumatoid arthritis, models not based on a specific antigenic trigger have received major attention in recent years. These include arthritis with various types of mineral oils, spontaneous models displaying arthritis amongst other changes, models based on superantigens or viral antigens exacerbating established models, and transgenic models based on overexpression of cytokines or mediators involved in cellular activation like *c-fos* or *c-jun*. These models reflect the hyper-reactivity of synovial cells or a general disturbance of the control of autoimmunity, either spontaneous or caused by compounds showing distinct adjuvant properties.

SCID mice

In addition, interest has been raised in the SCID (severe combined immunodeficiency disease) mouse. This immunocompromised animal allows for the *in vivo* study of the pathological potential of cells from animal models or patients with rheumatoid arthritis. For this purpose, cells or pieces of synovial tissue are transferred to the SCID mouse and behaviour and pathological changes analysed (Williams et al. 1992b). An interesting design is the combination of cells or tissue with cartilage as a target tissue, to obtain further insight into mechanisms of cartilage destruction (Muller-Ladner et al. 1996). Using the latter approach it was found that rheumatoid arthritis synovial fibroblasts, without the need of T cells can display invasive behaviour and cause cartilage destruction. This behaviour is promoted by IL-1.

Adjuvant oils and pristane

Adjuvant oils can induce a symmetrical, destructive polyarthritis when injected intradermally in DA rats (Kleinau et al. 1991). Expression of arthritis occurs between days 11 and 14, is found in 100 per cent of rats, and lasts for 6 weeks. As in classical adjuvant arthritis, readministration of oil to rats that had recovered from oil-induced arthritis fails to induce arthritis a second time. This points to an immunological background and indeed the arthritis could be transferred with concanavalin A-activated T cells from arthritic rats to irradiated recipients. A seemingly similar disease could be induced with adjuvant oil in certain strains of mice and was termed pristane arthritis (Wooley et al. 1989; Thompson and Elson 1993). The pristane disease, however, has proved difficult to characterize, due to late onset, variable penetrance, and difficulty of transfer. Moreover, in late disease numerous types of autoantibodies were noted, including rheumatoid factor, which may contribute to the expression of the arthritis and make this model less clearly T-cell driven. In clear contrast to findings in adjuvant and streptococcal cell-wall arthritides, pristane arthritis was suppressed in germ-free mice, implying a bacterium-specific pathogenesis. Interestingly, spontaneous arthritis may occur in DBA/1 mice, the strain that is highly susceptible to CIA. The spontaneous model seems to reflect aspects of the collagen arthritis since downregulation could be achieved with anti-idiotypic antibodies to anticollagen antibodies. This is in sharp contrast with adjuvant arthritis, which has been demonstrated to have a pathogenetic pathway different from that of collagen arthritis.

MRL/lpr mice

Spontaneous arthritis is also described in MRL–lpr/lpr mice (Hang et al. 1982; Koopman and Gay 1988). These animals develop a severe autoimmune disease, mainly characterized by massive lymphadenopathy, arteritis, immune complex-mediated glomerulonephritis, and chronic arthritis. The serological abnormalities in these animals include antibodies against native DNA, rheumatoid factors, and circulating immune complexes. This strain of mice may thus be regarded as a model of both systemic lupus erythematosus and rheumatoid arthritis. The presence of rheumatoid factors, which is lacking in most of the induced models, makes this model of potential interest. However, the incidence of arthritis is much lower than the incidence of the systemic lupus-like syndrome and is much more variable in presentation. Moreover, upon standard breeding it is often noted that the incidence of arthritis is further diminished, due to preferential breeding of the more healthy individuals. Arthritis is characterized by predominantly synovial and mesenchymal cell hyperplasia, late T-cell infiltration, and preceding cartilage destruction. The first signs are synovial cells with a transformed appearance and invasion of these cells into cartilage and bone, resulting in a rheumatoid arthritis-like pannus. Significant arthritis occurs only in aged mice, and signs are mild or absent before the age of 5 months. A viral cause has been suggested, but is it now established that these mice display prolonged cell survival due to defective Fas mediated apoptosis. Expression of arthritis can be enhanced with an injection of Freund's complete antigen or superantigen. In line with the autoimmune character, immunosuppressive drugs such as cyclophosphamide and leflunomide are effective in this model (Bartlett et al. 1988). In addition, chloroquine and gold were antiarthritic.

TNF and IL-1 transgenics

Transgenic mice expressing the human TNF transgene develop chronic polyarthritis with a 100 per cent incidence (Keffer et al. 1991). Hyperplasia of the synovium, inflammatory infiltrates in the joint space, pannus formation, and cartilage destruction were observed, and the model runs in RAG mice, in the absence of immune cells. Expression could be completely blocked with anti-TNF-α antibodies, but also with antibodies to the IL-1 receptor, identifying that the pathology runs through induction of IL-1. Uncoupling of the proinflammatory and immunosuppressive properties were identified at the p55 TNF receptor (Kassiotis and Kollias 2001). Subsequently, transgenic IL-1 overexpression was also shown to induce chronic, destructive arthritis (Niki et al. 2001). These models illustrate that systemic overexpression of TNF-α and IL-1 may lead to the precipitation of inflammatory processes in the joints, and are suitable for the screening of cytokine related downstream effects and therapeutic applicability of cytokine scavengers.

Others

The potential involvement of retroviral antigens in chronic arthritis was further underlined by the occurrence of arthritis after 2–3 months in mice transgenic for human T-cell leukaemia virus (Iwakura et al. 1991; Yamamoto et al. 1993). Transgenic mice overexpressing *c-fos* were used in combination with arthritis models. Plain overexpression of *c-fos* in synovial cells did not lead to arthritis. However, the eliciting of antigen-induced or collagen arthritides in these *c-fos* mice yielded more severe and more destructive arthritis. Remarkably, the cellular infiltrate in these mice contained hardly any lymphocytes, yet marked cartilage destruction was found, stressing the role of mesenchymal cells in that damage (Shiozawa et al. 1992). The expression of *c-fos* coincides with the enhanced expression of stromelysin and collagenase, enzymes involved in cartilage destruction.

Involvement of cytokines

The synovial inflammation in patients with rheumatoid arthritis is characterized by an abundance of macrophage- and fibroblast-derived mediators and a relative lack of the T-cell factors IL-2 and interferon-γ (Firestein 1991). It is encouraging to note that considerable hierarchy exists in the plethora of cytokines and growth factors, putting major emphasis on the cytokines TNF-α and IL-1. The relative absence of IL-2 and interferon-γ in rheumatoid synovia must not be overinterpreted, since minor amounts of activated T cells can be sufficient to drive arthritis. Moreover, the novel T cell cytokine IL-17 is clearly present, and can accelerate inflammation and tissue destruction in CIA, independent of IL-1 (Lubberts et al. 2001). In addition, the macrophage derived cytokines IL-12, IL-15, and IL-18 are abundant as well, can contribute to Th1 maturation and activation, and were shown to promote collagen arthritis (McInness and Liew 1998; Gracie et al. 1999). Detailed discussion goes beyond the scope of the present chapter, but upcoming clinical trials will certainly address these cytokines as novel therapeutic targets.

Animal model studies have greatly contributed to the identification of TNF and IL-1 as so-called master cytokines. Powerful approaches were the use of neutralizing antibodies, specific binding proteins or receptor antagonists (Henderson and Blake 1992) and more recently, the evaluation of arthritis models in cytokine deficient backgrounds. Major findings are summarized in Table 4. Instead of going through all the details in the common models, some general elements will be highlighted and some reviews are suggested for further reading (van den Berg and Bresnihan 1999; van den Berg 2000).

In murine collagen arthritis, anti-IL-1 and anti-TNF have been used before onset, shortly after onset, and in the established phase. TNF plays an important part in the onset of CIA, but is less dominant in late arthritis (Williams et al. 1992a; Wooley et al. 1993). In contrast, IL-1 is a pivotal mediator in both early and established CIA. The elimination of IL-1 greatly suppressed the arthritis and yielded marked protection against cartilage destruction (van den Berg et al. 1994). The protection could be demonstrated using either neutralizing antibodies or IL-1 receptor antagonist, provided that large amounts (1 mg/day per mouse) of the antagonist were continuously supplied in osmotic minipumps. Given the poor pharmacokinetics and the need for sustained receptor blocking, it must be stressed that any therapeutic application with IL-1Ra in patients with rheumatoid arthritis would need high dosages.

In immune complex arthritis models also a strong dependence of IL-1 was found (van Lent et al. 1995) which might imply that immune complex driven pathology is a dominant feature in early collagen arthritis. In the single flare model of streptococcal cell-wall arthritis in the rat both TNF-α and IL-1 appeared to be important (Schwab et al. 1991). An alike study in the mouse with continued flares after repeated injections of cell wall fragments in the knee joint showed that every flare was TNF dependent in terms of joint swelling, yet IL-1 appeared crucial in sustained cellular infiltration and cartilage destruction (van den Berg 2000).

In antigen-induced arthritis in the rabbit and the mouse, elimination of both TNF-α and IL-1 was not that effective in suppressing joint inflammation, pointing to substantial 'overkill' by other mediators (Lewthwaite et al. 1994). However, elimination of IL-1 did yield protection against cartilage destruction (van de Loo et al. 1992) and this was even more striking in the antigen-induced flare (van de Loo et al. 1995).

In rat adjuvant arthritis a marked synergy was noted when the combination of soluble TNF receptor and IL-1Ra was used (Bendele et al. 2000). The beneficial effect of the combination of TNF and IL-1 blocking, to eliminate both joint inflammation and tissue destruction, was also seen in murine SCW arthritis.

In conclusion, TNF is a major mediator in early stages of joint inflammation in every model. Although IL-1 is not a dominant inflammatory cytokine in all models, it is certainly the pivotal cytokine in the inhibition of chondrocyte proteoglycan synthesis in all models studied so far and the blocking of IL-1 has a great impact on net cartilage destruction. In line with this, a chronic destructive arthritis could not be induced in IL-1 deficient mice, using any of the models mentioned above. In contrast, TNF deficiency reduced incidence of arthritis expression, but once joints become afflicted full progression to erosive arthritis did occur (van den Berg 2000; Campbell et al. 2001).

Regulation of arthritis susceptibility

Apart from the cytokines TNF-α and IL-1, modulatory cytokines such as IL-4, IL-10, IL-12, and TGF-β, and specific endogenous inhibitors like shed receptors or IL-1 receptor antagonist are of prime importance. Although it has long been thought that susceptibility or resistance of a particular mouse strain to induction of collagen arthritis was mainly related to different epitope recognition, it becomes now clear that the cytokine milieu and the different production and sensitivity to regulatory cytokines has a major impact. In general, endogenous Th2 cytokines IL-4 and IL-10 are protective, enhanced incidence of models like CIA and proteoglycan arthritis is seen in IL-4- and IL-10-deficient mice, and treatment with IL-4/IL-10 suppresses arthritis (Joosten et al. 1997). In addition, IL-12 and IL-18 promote such diseases, through enhancement of Th1 reactivity, and strong immunization with high or repeated adjuvant exposure makes seemingly resistant animals susceptible. The enhanced expression of arthritis with a single lps injection shortly before expected onset is also dependent on IL-12 generation.

Table 4 Cytokine dependence in various murine arthritis models

Model	Acute inflammation		Chronic inflammation		Cartilage destruction	
	TNF-α	IL-1	TNF-α	IL-1	TNF-α	IL-1
CIA	++	+++	±	++	±	++
ICA	±	++			±	++
SCW-A	++	−	−	++	−	++
SCW-A-flare-up[a]	+	+	±	++	−	++
AIA	±	±	−	+	−	++
AIA-flare[b]	+	+			−	++

[a] SCW-A-flare-ups reflect the situation after three consecutive SCW flare-ups with a 7-day interval.

[b] AIA-flare is induced by antigen rechallenge at day 21.

Note: TNF-α, tumour necrosis factor-α; IL-1, interleukin-1; AIA, antigen-induced arthritis; CIA, collagen-induced arthritis; SCW-A, streptococcal cell-wall arthritis; ICA, passive immune complex arthritis.

An important remark to be made is that mediators like IL-10 and TGF-β are generally immunosuppressive when given systemically, yet they can display proinflammatory activity at local sites through upregulation of adhesion molecules and local cell activation.The latter also holds for IL-4. It implies that both Th1 and Th2 cytokines can play an arthritogenic role and various forms of human arthritis might be viewed as a result of dysregulated cytokine environment (Ortman and Shevach 2001). As an illustration, Balb/c mice deficient in IL-1Ra and lacking proper control of IL-1, develop spontaneous arthritis (Horai et al. 2000).

Uncoupling of joint destruction/joint inflammation

Apart from studies on the involvement of cytokines and on immunotherapeutic approaches, models of arthritis are valuable tools for further identifying subpopulations of infiltrating leucocytes or synovial cells involved in cartilage destruction. The damage observed in the different models ranged from a selective loss of matrix in cartilage underlying pannus tissue to an overall loss of proteoglycans and, later on, of collagen, or even to the killing of numerous chondrocytes and the complete loss of the superficial and middle cartilage layer. This underlines that arthritic processes can be more or less destructive, dependent on the underlying process and cytokine mixture (van den Berg 2001). Large variation in progressive destruction is also noted in populations of patients with rheumatoid arthritis, which may indicate separate pathogenetic pathways. Enhanced degradation of matrix and inhibited synthesis of proteoglycans by the chondrocyte are general findings in all models.

In antigen-induced arthritis, clear uncoupling of joint swelling from cartilage destruction is a common observation. Non-steroidal anti-inflammatory drugs are effective in reducing the swelling but leave the destructive process untouched. It is even suggested that most non-steroidal anti-inflammatory drugs are harmful, by inhibition of prostaglandin production. Prostaglandin E_2 is a potent feedback regulator of IL-1 production and concentrations of this cytokine are higher in the presence of non-steroidal anti-inflammatory drugs with cyclooxygenase inhibitory activity.

The contribution of neutrophils to cartilage destruction is still unclear. Although the enzymes from neutrophils, such as elastase, can be highly destructive *in vitro*, neutrophils also contain TGF-β and IL-1 receptor antagonist and can be protective as well. Normally, neutrophils do not attach to the cartilage surface and released enzymes will be scavenged by enzyme inhibitors of the synovial fluid. Depletion of neutrophils in antigen-induced arthritis did not influence cartilage destruction and damage was similar in elastase-deficient mice. However, in the presence of dense immune complexes in the superficial cartilage layers, marked sticking of neutrophils is found in antigen- and in collagen-induced arthritis in particular. This attachment is potentiated by immobilization of the joint. The ruffled cartilage surface under those conditions indicates direct destruction by the attached cells (van Lent et al. 1990).

Although neutrophils may be destructive under limited conditions, these cells are certainly not essential to the destruction and neither are lymphocytes. Observations in MRL–lpr/lpr mice and the H_2-c-*fos* transgenic mice indicate that macrophage-rich infiltrates can be highly destructive without the presence of neutrophils and lymphocytes. Similarly, macrophage but not lymphocyte numbers in rheumatoid synovial tissue correlate with the radiological progression of joint destruction (Bresnihan 1998). The critical enzymes involved in destruction in arthritis models and human rheumatoid arthritis are still far from understood. Detailed discussion of the various approaches to identify key enzymes in the models is beyond the scope of this chapter.

A general lesson that may be deduced from observations in most models is that continuing, irreversible destruction can occur under conditions that will be hardly considered as inflammatory. Symptomatic relief by anti-inflammatory therapy is promising but the main challenge remains to interrupt joint destruction. It is intriguing that combined, repeated injections of IL-1 and TGF-β give a much more profound synovitis than IL-1 alone, yet cartilage destruction is less. Similarly, local gene transfer with IL-4 did not suppress local inflammation, yet markedly reduced cartilage and bone destruction in CIA (Lubberts et al. 2000). It has recently been identified that RANKL is the crucial activating cytokine of the bone resorbing osteoclasts. In the absence of RANKL, immune complex driven joint inflammation continues, but bone erosion is prevented (Petit et al. 2001). These observations argue for carefull monitoring of both joint inflammation and destructive features in clinical trials.

References

Bartlett, R.R., Popovic, S., and Raiss, R.X. (1988). Development of autoimmunity in MRL/lpr mice and the effects of drugs on this murine disease. *Scandinavian Journal of Rheumatology* **75** (Suppl.), 290–9.

Bendele, A.M. et al. (2000). Combination benefit of treatment with the cytokine inhibitors IL-1ra and PEGylated soluble TNF receptor type I in animal models of RA. *Arthritis and Rheumatism* **43**, 2648–59.

Billingham, M.E.J. (1994). Monoclonal antibody therapy of experimental arthritis: comparison with cyclosporin A for elucidating cellular and molecular disease mechanisms. In *Immunopharmacology of Joints and Connective tissue* (ed. M.E. Davies and J.T. Dingle), pp. 65–86. New York: Academic Press.

Bliven, M. and Otterness, I. (1985). Laboratory models for testing nonsteroidal antiinflammatory drugs. In *Nonsteroidal Anti-inflammatory Drugs* (ed. J.G. Lombardino), pp. 111–252. New York: Wiley.

Blom, A.B., van Lent, P.L.E.M., van Vuuren, H., Holthuysen, A.E.M., van de Winkel, J.G., Jacobs, C., van de Putte, L.B.A., and van den Berg, W.B. (2000). FcgammaR expression on macrophages is related to severity and chronicity of synovial inflammation and cartilage destruction during experimental immune-complex-mediated arthritis (ICA). *Arthritis Research* **2**, 489–503.

Brand, D.D. et al. (2002). Detection of early changes in autoimmune T cell phenoptype and function following intravenous administration of type II collagen induced TCR-transgenic model. *Journal of Immunology* **168**, 490–8.

Bresnihan, B. (1999). Pathogenesis of joint damage in RA. *Journal of Rheumatology* **26**, 717–19.

Campbell, I.K., O'Donnell, K., Lawlor, K.E., and Wicks, I.P. (2001). Severe inflammatory arthritis and lymphadenopathy in the absence of TNF. *Journal of Clinical Investigation* **107**, 1519–27.

Cooke, T.D.V., Hird, E.R., Ziff, M., and Jasin, H.E. (1972). The pathogenesis of chronic inflammation in experimental antigen induced arthritis. *Journal of Experimental Medicine* **135**, 323–38.

Cromartie, W.L. and Schwab, J. (1977). Arthritis in rats after systemic injection of streptococcal cell walls. *Journal of Experimental Medicine* **146**, 1485–602.

Deng, G.M. and Tarkowski, A. (2001). Synovial cytokine mRNA expression during arthritis triggered by CpG motifs of bacterial DNA. *Arthritis Research* **3**, 48–53.

de Vries, B.J. and van den Berg, W.B. (1989). Impact of NSAIDs on murine antigen induced arthritis. I. An investigation of anti-inflammatory and chondroprotective effects. *Journal of Rheumatology* **18** (Suppl. 16), 10–18.

Dumonde, D.C. and Glynn, L.E. (1962). The production of arthritis in rabbits by an immunological reaction to fibrin. *British Journal of Experimental Pathology* **43**, 373–83.

Finnegan, A., Mikecz, K., Tao, P., and Glant, T.T. (1999). Proteoglycan (aggrecan)-induced arthritis in BALB/c mice is a Th1-type disease regulated by Th2 cytokines. *Journal of Immunology* **163**, 5383–90.

Firestein, G.S. (1991). The immunopathogenesis of rheumatoid arthritis. *Current Opinion in Rheumatology*, **3**, 398–406.

Gracie, J.A. et al. (1999). A proinflammatory role for IL-18 in rheumatoid arthritis. *Journal of Clinical Investigation* **104**, 1393–401.

Hang, L., Theofilopoulos, A.N., and Dixon, F.J. (1982). A spontaneous rheumatoid arthritis-like disease in MRL/1 mice. *Journal of Experimental Medicine* **155**, 1690–701.

Hazenberg, M.P., Klasen, I.S., Kool, J., Ruseler-van Embden, J.G.H., and Severijnen, A.J. (1992). Are intestinal bacteria involved in the etiology of rheumatoid arthritis? *Acta Pathologica, Microbiologica, et Immunologica Scandinavica* **100**, 1–9.

Henderson, B. and Blake, S. (1992). Therapeutic potential of cytokine manipulation. *Trends in Pharmacological Science* **13**, 145–52.

Holmdahl, R., Malmstrom, V., and Vuorio, E. (1993). Autoimmune recognition of cartilage collagens. *Annals of Medicine* **25**, 251–64.

Holoshitz, J., Naparstek, Y., Ben-Num, A., and Cohen, I.R. (1983). Lines of T lymphocytes induce or vaccinate against autoimmune arthritis. *Science* **219**, 56–8.

Horai, M. et al. (2000). Development of chronic inflammatory arthropathy resembling RA in IL-1ra-deficient mice. *Journal of Experimental Medicine* **191**, 313–20.

Hunneyball, I.M., Billingham, M.E.J., and Rainsford, K.D. (1989). Animal models of arthritic disease: influence of novel compared with classical antirheumatic agents. In *New Developments in Antirheumatic Therapy* (ed. K.D. Rainsford), pp. 93–132. Dordrecht: Kluwer.

Iwakura, Y. et al. (1991). Induction of inflammatory arthropathy resembling rheumatoid arthritis in mice transgenic for HTLV-I. *Science* **253**, 1026–8.

Ji, H. et al. (2001). Genetic influences on the end stage effector phase of arthritis. *Journal of Experimental Medicine* **194**, 321–30.

Joosten, L.A.B., Helsen, M.M.A., and van den Berg, W.B. (1994). Accelerated onset of collagen-induced arthritis by remote inflammation. *Clinical and Experimental Immunology* **97**, 204–11.

Joosten, L.A.B., Lubberts, E., Durez, P., Helsen, M.M.A., Jacobs, M.J.M., Goldman, M., and van den Berg, W.B. (1997). Role of IL-4 and IL-10 in murine collagen-induced arthritis: Protective effect of IL-4 and IL-10 treatment on cartilage destruction. *Arthritis and Rheumatism* **40**, 249–60.

Joosten, L.A.B., Coenen-de Roo, C.J.J., Helsen, M.M.A., Lubberts, E., Boots, A.M.H., van den Berg, W.B., and Miltenburg, A.M.M. (2000). Induction of tolerance with intranasal administration of human cartilage gp39 in DBA/1 mice. Amelioration of clinical, histologic, and radiologic signs of type II collagen-induced arthritis. *Arthritis and Rheumatism* **43**, 645–55.

Kassiotis, G. and Kollias, G. (2001). Uncoupling the proinflammatory from the immunosuppressive properties of TNF at the p55 TNF receptor level: implications for pathogenesis and therapy of autoimmune demyelination. *Journal of Experimental Medicine* **193**, 427–34.

Keffer, J. et al. (1991). Transgenic mice expressing human tumor necrosis factor: a predictive genetic model of arthritis. *EMBO Journal* **13**, 4025–31.

Kleinau, S., Erlandsson, H., Holmdahl, R., and Klareskog, L. (1991). Adjuvant oils induce arthritis in the DA rat. I. Characterization of the disease and evidence for an immunological involvement. *Journal of Autoimmunity* **4**, 871–80.

Kohashi, O., Kohashi, Y., Takahashi, T., Ozawa, A., and Shigematsu, N. (1986). Suppressive effect of *Escherichia coli* on adjuvant-induced arthritis in germ-free rats. *Arthritis and Rheumatism* **29**, 547–53.

Koopman, W.J. and Gay, S. (1988). The MRL–lpr/lpr mouse. A model for the study of rheumatoid arthritis. *Scandinavian Journal of Rheumatology* **75** (Suppl.), 284–9.

Korganow, A.S. et al. (1999). From systemic T cell self-reactivity to organ-specific autoimmune disease via immunoglobulins. *Immunity* **10**, 451–61.

Lafyatis, R. et al. (1989). Transforming growth factor-β production by synovial tissues from rheumatoid patients and streptococcal cell wall arthritic rats. *Journal of Immunology* **143**, 1142–8.

Lens, J.W., van den Berg, W.B., and van de Putte, L.B.A. (1984). Flare-up of antigen-induced arthritis in mice after challenge with intravenous antigen. Studies on the characteristics of and mechanisms involved in the reaction. *Clinical and Experimental Immunology* **55**, 287–94.

Lewthwaite, J., Blake, S.M., Hardingham, T.E., Warden, P.J., and Henderson, B. (1994). The effect of recombinant human IL-1 receptor antagonist on the induction phase of antigen induced arthritis in the rabbit. *Journal of Rheumatology* **21**, 467–72.

Lubberts, E., Joosten, L.A.B., Chabaud, M., van den Bersselaar, L., Oppers, B., Coenen-de Roo, C.J.J., Richards, C.D., Miossec, P., and van den Berg, W.B. (2000). IL-4 gene therapy for collagen arthritis suppresses synovial IL-17 and osteoprotegerin ligand and prevents bone erosion. *Journal of Clinical Investigation* **105**, 1697–710.

Lubberts, E., Joosten, L.A.B., Oppers, B., van den Bersselaar, L., Coenen-de Roo, C.J.J., Kolls, J.K., Schwarzenberger, P., van de Loo, F.A.J., and van den Berg, W.B. (2001). IL-1 independent role of IL-17 in synovial inflammation and joint destruction during collagen induced arthritis. *Journal of Immunology* **167**, 1004–13.

Maccioni, M. et al. (2002). Arthritogenic monoclonal antibodies from K/BxN mice. *Journal of Experimental Medicine* **195**, 1071–7.

McInnes, I.B. and Liew, F.Y. (1998). Interleukin-15: a proinflammatory role in rheumatoid arthritis synovitis. *Immunology Today* **19**, 75–9.

Mikecz, K., Glant, T.T., Buzas, E., and Poole, A.R. (1990). Proteoglycan induced polyarthritis and spondylitis adoptively transferred to naive BALB/C mice. *Arthritis and Rheumatism* **33**, 866–76.

Miossec, P. and van den Berg, W.B. (1997). Th1/Th2 cytokine balance in arthritis. *Arthritis and Rheumatism* **40**, 2105–15.

Müller-Ladner, U. et al. (1996). Synovial fibroblsts of patients with RA attach to and invade normal human cartilage when engrafted into SCID mice. *American Journal of Pathology* **149**, 1607–15.

Niki, Y. et al. (2001). Macrophage- and neutrophil-dominant arthritis in human IL-1 alpha transgenic mice. *Journal of Clinical Investigation* **107**, 1127–35.

Ortmann, R.A. and Shevach, E.M. (2001). Susceptibility to collagen-induced arthritis: cytokine-mediated regulation. *Clinical Immunology* **98**, 109–18.

Pearson, C.M. (1956). Development of arthritis, periarthritis and periostitis in rats given adjuvants. *Proceedings of the Society for Experimental Biology (New York)* **91**, 95–101.

Petit, A.R. et al. (2001). TRANCE/RANKL knockout mice are protected from bone erosion in a serum transfer model of arthritis. *American Journal of Pathology* **159**, 1689–99.

Ravetch, J.V. and Bolland, S. (2001). IgG Fc receptors. *Annual Review of Immunology* **19**, 275–90.

Schwab, J.H., Anderle, S.K., Brown, R.R., Dalldorf, F.G., and Thompson, R.C. (1991). Pro- and anti-inflammatory roles of interleukin-1 in recurrence of bacterial cell wall-induced arthritis in rats. *Infection and Immunity* **59**, 4436–42.

Shiozawa, S., Tanka, Y., Fujita, T., and Tokuhisa, T. (1992). Destructive arthritis without lymphocyte infiltration in H_2-c-*fos* transgenic mice. *Journal of Immunology* **148**, 3100–4.

Stimpson, S.A. et al. (1986). Arthropathic properties of peptidoglycan-polysaccharide polymers from normal flora bacteria. *Infection and Immunity* **51**, 240.

Thompson, S.J. and Elson, C.J. (1993). Susceptibility to pristane-induced arthritis is altered with changes in bowel flora. *Immunology Letters* **36**, 227–32.

Trentham, D.E., Townes, A.S., and Kang, A.H. (1977). Autoimmunity to type II collagen: an experimental model of arthritis. *Journal of Experimental Medicine* **146**, 857–68.

van de Langerijt, A.G.M., van Lent, P.L.E.M., Hermus, A.R.M.M., Sweep, C.G.J., Cools, A.R., and van den Berg, W.B. (1994). Susceptibility to adjuvant arthritis: relative importance of adrenal activity and bacterial flora. *Clinical and Experimental Immunology* **97**, 33–8.

van de Langerijt, A.G.M., Kingston, A.E., van Lent, P.L.E.M., Billingham, M.E.J., and van den Berg, W.B. (1994a). Cross-reactivity to proteoglycans in bacterial arthritis: lack of evidence for *in vivo* role in induction of disease. *Clinical Immunology and Immunopathology* **71**, 273–80.

van de Loo, A.A.J., Arntz, O.J., Otterness, I.G., and van den Berg, W.B. (1992). Protection against cartilage proteoglycan synthesis inhibition by anti-interleukin 1 antibodies in experimental arthritis. *Journal of Rheumatology* **19**, 348–56.

van de Loo, A.A.J., Arntz, O.J., Bakker, A.C., van Lent, P.L.E.M., Jacobs, M.J.M., and van den Berg, W.B. (1995). Role of interleukin-1 in antigen-induced exacerbations of murine arthritis. *American Journal of Pathology* **146**, 239–49.

van den Berg, W.B. (2000). What we learn from arthritis models to benefit arthritis patients. *Bailliere's Clinical Rheumatology* **14**, 599–616.

van den Berg, W.B. (2001). Uncoupling of inflammatory and destructive mechanisms in arthritis. *Seminars in Arthritis and Rheumatology* **30** (Suppl. 2), 7–16.

van den Berg, W.B. and Bresnihan, B. (1999). Pathogenesis of joint damage in RA: evidence of a dominant role for IL-1. *Bailliere's Clinical Rheumatology* **13**, 577–97.

van den Berg, W.B., van de Putte, L.B.A., Zwarts, W.A., and Joosten, L.A.B. (1984). Electrical charge of the antigen determines intraarticular antigen handling and chronicity of arthritis in mice. *Journal of Clinical Investigation* **74**, 1850–9.

van den Berg, W.B., Joosten, L.A.B., Helsen, M., and van de Loo, F.A.J. (1994). Amelioration of established murine collagen-induced arthritis with anti-IL-1 treatment. *Clinical and Experimental Immunology* **95**, 237–43.

van den Broek, M.F., van den Berg, W.B., van de Putte, L.B.A., and Severijnen, A.J. (1988). Streptococcal cell wall induced arthritis and flare-up reactions in mice induced by homologous and heterologous cell walls. *American Journal of Pathology* **133**, 139–49.

van Eden, W. (1991). Heatshock proteins as immunogenic bacterial antigens with the potential to induce and regulate autoimmune arthritis. *Immunology Reviews* **121**, 5.

van Eden, W. (1999). Heat shock proteins in rheumatoid arthritis. *Stress Proteins* **136**, 329–46.

van Lent, P.L.E.M., van den Bersselaar, L., van de Putte, L.B.A., and van den Berg, W.B. (1990). Immobilization aggravates cartilage damage during antigen-induced arthritis in mice. Attachment of polymorphonuclear leucocytes to articular cartilage. *American Journal of Pathology* **136**, 1407–16.

van Lent, P.L.E.M., van de Loo, F.A.J., Holthuysen, A.E.M., van den Bersselaar, L.A.M., Vermeer, H., and van den Berg, W.B. (1995). Major role for IL-1 but not for TNF in early cartilage damage in immune complex arthritis in mice. *Journal of Rheumatology* **22**, 2250–8.

van Lent, P.L.E.M., Blom, A., Holthuysen, A.E.M., Jacobs, C.W.M., van de Putte, L.B.A., and van den Berg, W.B. (1997). Monocytes/macrophages rather than PMN are involved in early cartilage degradation in cationic immune complex arthritis in mice. *Journal of Leucocyte Biology* **61**, 267–78.

van Lent, P.L.E.M., Nabbe, K., Blom, A.B., Holthuysen, A.E.M., Sloetjes, A., van de Putte, L.B.A., Verbeek, S., and van den Berg, W.B. (2001). Role of activatory Fcγ RI and Fcγ RIII and inhibitory Fcγ RII in inflammation and cartilage destruction during experimental antigen-induced arthritis. *American Journal of Pathology* **159**, 2309–20.

Williams, R.O., Feldmann, M., and Maini, R.N. (1992a). Anti-tumor necrosis factor ameliorates joint disease in murine collagen-induced arthritis. *Proceedings of the National Academy of Sciences (USA)* **89**, 9784–8.

Williams, R.O., Plater-Zyberk, C., Williams, D.G., and Maini, R.N. (1992b). Successful transfer of collagen-induced arthritis to severe combined immunodeficient (SCID) mice. *Clinical and Experimental Immunology* **88**, 455–60.

Wooley, P.H. (1991). Animal models of rheumatoid arthritis. *Current Opinion in Rheumatology* **3**, 407–20.

Wooley, P.H., Luthra, H.S., Stuart, J.M., and David, C.S. (1981). Type II collagen-induced arthritis in mice. I. MHC (I-region) linkage and antibody correlates. *Journal of Experimental Medicine* **154**, 688–700.

Wooley, P.H., Seibold, J.R., Whalen, J.D., and Chapdelaine, J.M. (1989). Pristane induced arthritis. The immunologic and genetic features of an experimental murine model of autoimmune disease. *Arthritis and Rheumatism* **32**, 1022–30.

Wooley, P.H., Dutcher, J., Widmer, M.B., and Gillis, S. (1993). Influence of a recombinant human soluble tumor necrosis factor receptor FC fusion protein on type II collagen-induced arthritis in mice. *Journal of Immunology* **151**, 6602–7.

Yamamoto, H., Sekiguchi, T., Itagaki, K., Saijo, S., and Iwakura, Y. (1993). Inflammatory polyarthritis in mice transgenic for human T cell leukemia virus type I. *Arthritis and Rheumatism* **36**, 1612–20.

4.5 Modification of inflammation

4.5.1 Non-steroidal anti-inflammatory drugs—old and new

Burkhard Hinz and Kay Brune

Mode of action of antipyretic analgesics

Inhibition of cyclooxygenase enzymes

In 1971, Vane showed that the anti-inflammatory action of non-steroidal anti-inflammatory drugs (NSAIDs) rests in their ability to inhibit the activity of the cyclooxygenase (COX) enzyme, which in turn results in a diminished synthesis of proinflammatory prostaglandins (Vane 1971). This action is considered to be not the sole but a major factor of the mode of action of NSAIDs. The pathway leading to the generation of prostaglandins has been elucidated in detail. Within this process, the COX enzyme (also referred to as prostaglandin H synthase) catalyzes the first step of the synthesis of prostanoids by converting arachidonic acid into prostaglandin H_2, which is the common substrate for specific prostaglandin synthases. The enzyme is bifunctional, with fatty-acid COX activity (catalyzing the conversion of arachidonic acid to prostaglandin G_2) and prostaglandin hydroperoxidase activity (catalyzing the conversion of prostaglandin G_2 to prostaglandin H_2) (Fig. 1).

In the early 1990s, COX was demonstrated to exist as two distinct isoforms (Masferrer et al. 1990; Xie et al. 1991). COX-1 is constitutively expressed as a 'housekeeping' enzyme in nearly all tissues, and mediates physiological responses (e.g. cytoprotection of the stomach, platelet aggregation). On the other hand, COX-2 expressed by cells that are involved in inflammation (e.g. macrophages, monocytes, synoviocytes) has emerged as the isoform that is primarily responsible for the synthesis of prostanoids involved in pathological processes, such as acute and chronic inflammatory states. COX-2-derived prostaglandins may cause inflammation by virtue of their chemotactic and oedema-promoting actions.

The expression of the COX-2 enzyme is regulated by a broad spectrum of other mediators involved in inflammation. Glucocorticoids and anti-inflammatory cytokines (interleukin-4, interleukin-10, interleukin-13) have been reported to inhibit the expression of the COX-2 isoenzyme (Masferrer et al. 1990; Onoe et al. 1996; Niiro et al. 1997). Moreover, products of the COX-2 pathway (i.e. prostaglandin E_2 by virtue of its second messenger cAMP) may exert a positive feedback action on the expression of its biosynthesizing enzyme in the inflamed tissue (Nantel et al. 1999a) as well as in numerous cell types (Hinz et al. 2000a,b; Maldve et al. 2000).

NSAIDs interfere with the enzymatic activity of COX-2. However, all conventional NSAIDs inhibit both COX-1 and COX-2 at therapeutic doses (Patrignani et al. 1997). Whereas many of the side-effects of NSAIDs (e.g. gastrointestinal ulceration and bleeding, platelet dysfunctions) are due to a suppression of COX-1-derived prostanoids, inhibition of COX-2-derived prostanoids facilitates the anti-inflammatory, analgesic, and antipyretic effects of NSAIDs. Consequently, the hypothesis that specific inhibition of COX-2 might have therapeutic actions similar to those of NSAIDs, but without causing the unwanted side-effects, was the rationale for the development of specific COX-2 inhibitors (see 'Specific COX-2 inhibitors').

However, the simple concept of COX-2 being an exclusively proinflammatory and inducible enzyme cannot be sustained in the height of more recent experimental findings. Recently, COX-2 has also been shown to be expressed under basal conditions in organs as the ovary, uterus, brain, spinal cord, kidney, cartilage, bone, and even the gut, suggesting that this isozyme may play a more complex physiological role than previously recognized

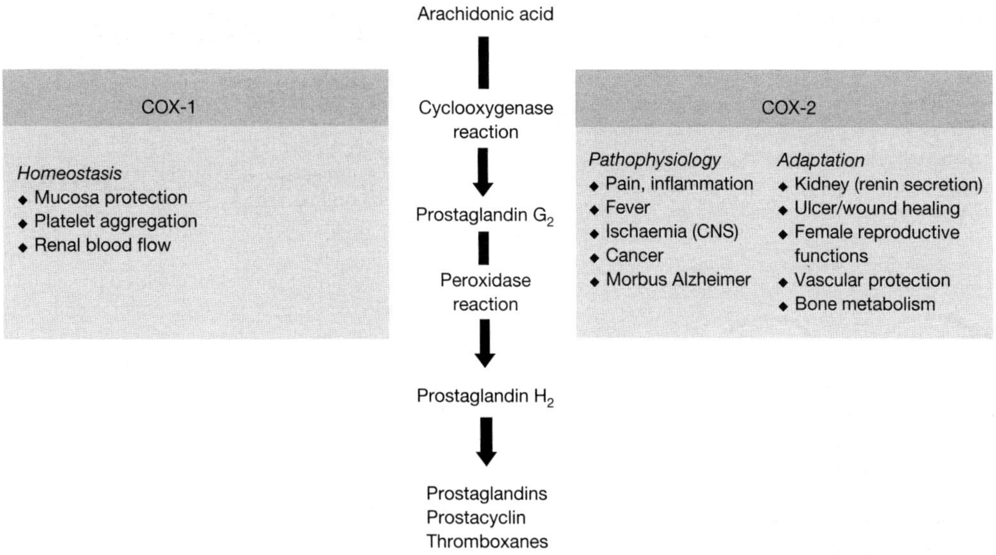

Fig. 1 Physiological and pathophysiological roles of COX-1 and COX-2. The COX-1 isozyme is expressed constitutively in most tissues and fulfills housekeeping functions by producing prostaglandins. The COX-2 isoform is an inducible enzyme, which becomes expressed in inflammatory cells (e.g. macrophages, synoviocytes) after exposure to endotoxin, mitogens, or proinflammatory cytokines. COX-2 has been implicated in the pathophysiology of various inflammatory and mitogenic disorders. However, in some tissues (e.g. genital tract, bone, kidney, endothelial cells) COX-2 is already significantly expressed even in the absence of inflammation and appears to fulfil various physiological functions.

(for review see Hinz and Brune 2000) (Fig. 1). Moreover, during past years, evidence has increased to suggest that a constitutively expressed COX-2 may play a role in physiological renal functions. In the human kidney, COX-2 immunoreactivity has been observed in the renal vasculature, medullary interstitial cells, and the macula densa, whereas COX-1 was detected in the collecting ducts, thin loops of Henle, and portions of the renal vasculature (Nantel et al. 1999b). In the rat kidney COX-2 is expressed constitutively, particularly in the macula densa (Harris et al. 1994) and becomes upregulated following salt restriction. COX-2 expression has also been observed in the uterine epithelium at different times during early pregnancy. Here, COX-2 may be involved in the implantation of the ovum, in the angiogenesis needed for the establishment of the placenta, and in the induction of labour (Gibb and Sun 1996). Furthermore, recent findings suggest that COX-2 may be involved in ovulation as female COX-2 knock-out mice are infertile (Lim et al. 1997).

Impact of biodistribution on pharmacological effects of antipyretic analgesics

Following the discovery that aspirin-like drugs exert their pharmacological action by suppressing the synthesis of prostaglandins (see COX enzymes above), the question was asked why aspirin and its pharmacological relatives, the (acidic) NSAIDs, exerted anti-inflammatory activity and analgesic effects whereas the non-acidic drugs phenazone and paracetamol were analgesic only (Brune 1974). It was speculated that all acidic anti-inflammatory analgesics, which are highly bound to plasma proteins and show a similar degree of acidity (pK_A values between 3.5 and 5.5), should lead to a specific drug distribution within the body of man or animals (Fig. 2). In fact, high concentrations of these compounds are reached in blood stream, liver, spleen, and bone marrow (due to high protein binding and an open endothelial layer of the vasculature), but also in body compartments with acidic extracellular pH values (Brune et al. 1976). The latter type of compartments includes the inflamed tissue, the wall of the upper gastrointestinal tract and the collecting ducts of the kidneys. By contrast, paracetamol and phenazone, compounds with almost neutral pK_A values and a scarce binding to plasma proteins, are distributed homogeneously and quickly throughout the body due to their ability to penetrate barriers such as the blood–brain barrier easily (Brune et al. 1980). It is evident that the degree of inhibiton of prostaglandin synthesis due to inhibition of the responsible cyclooxygenases depends on the potency of the drug and its local concentration.

Impact of biodistribution on side effects of antipyretic analgesics

Due to the accumulation of NSAIDs high drug concentrations may lead to an almost complete inhibition of the COX enzymes in some body compartments, for example, the inflamed tissue, blood stream, stomach wall, and the kidney, whereas uniform distribution throughout the body may lead to some inhibition throughout. These contrasting observations did explain the fact that only the acidic, antipyretic analgesics (NSAIDs) are anti-inflammatory and cause acute side-effects in the gastrointestinal tract (ulcerations), the blood stream (inhibition of platelet aggregation), and the kidney (fluid and sodium retention), while the non-acidic drugs paracetamol and phenazone as well as their derivatives are devoid of both anti-inflammatory activity, and gastric and (acute) renal toxicity. Finally, chronic inflammation of the upper respiratory tract (e.g. asthma, nasal polyps) leads to the accumulation of inflammatory prostaglandin-producing cells in the respiratory mucosa. Inhibition of COX appears to shift part of the metabolism of the prostaglandin precursor arachidonic acid to the production of leukotrienes that may induce pseudoallergic reactions (i.e. aspirin asthma). These patients comprise a well-defined risk group and should receive antipyretic analgesics, particularly acidic NSAIDs, only under the control of a physician.

Mechanisms of hyperalgesia

Inflammation causes an increased synthesis of COX-2-dependent prostaglandins, which sensitize peripheral nociceptor terminals and produce localized pain hypersensitivity. Recently, it has been shown that prostaglandins regulate the sensitivity of so-called polymodal nociceptors

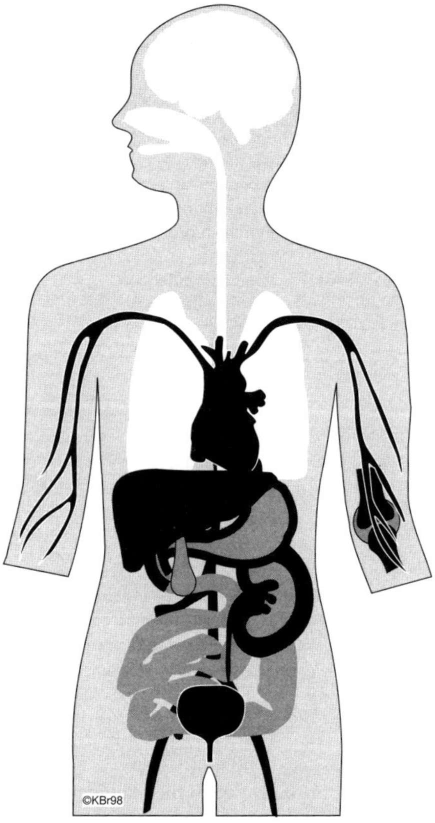

Fig. 2 Scheme of the distribution of acidic antipyretic analgesics in the human body (transposition of the data from animal experiments to human conditions). Dark areas indicate high concentrations of acidic antipyretic analgesics, that is, stomach and upper wall of the gastrointestinal tract, blood, liver, bone marrow, spleen (not shown), inflamed tissue (e.g. joints) as well as the kidney (cortex > medulla). Some acidic antipyretic analgesics are excreted in part unchanged in urine and achieve high concentration in this body fluid, others encounter enterohepatic circulation and are found in high concentrations as conjugates in the bile.

that are present in nearly all tissues. A significant portion of these nociceptors cannot be easily activated by physiological stimuli such as (mild) pressure or (some) increase of temperature (Schaible and Schmidt 1988). However, following tissue trauma and subsequent release of prostaglandins, 'silent' polymodal nociceptors become excitable to pressure, temperature changes, and tissue acidosis (Neugebauer et al. 1995). This process results in a phenomenon called hyperalgesia—in some instances, allodynia. Prostaglandin E_2 and other inflammatory mediators facilitate the activation of tetrodotoxin (TTX)-resistant Na^+ channels in dorsal root ganglion neurons. A certain type of TTX-resistant Na^+ channels has recently been cloned (Akopian et al. 1996) that appears to be selectively expressed in small- and medium-sized dorsal root ganglion neurons. Compelling evidence indicates that these small dorsal root ganglion neurons are the somata that give rise to thin and unmyelinated C- and Aδ-nerve fibres, both conducting nociceptive stimuli. Increased opening of these Na^+ channels involves activation of the adenylyl cyclase enzyme and increases in cyclic AMP possibly leading to protein kinase A-dependent phosphorylation of the channels. On the basis of this mechanism, prostaglandins produced during inflammatory states may significantly increase the excitability of nociceptive nerve fibres, thereby contributing to the activation of 'sleeping' nociceptors. As such, it appears reasonable that at least a part of the peripheral antinociceptive action of acidic antipyretic analgesics arises from prevention of this sensitization.

Apart from sensitizing peripheral nociceptors, prostaglandins may also act in the central nervous system to produce hyperalgesia. Experimental data suggest that COX inhibitors act primarily in the dorsal horn to cause analgesia. Here, nociceptor signals are transferred to secondary neurons, which propagate the signals to the higher centres of the central nervous system. COX-2 is expressed constitutively in the dorsal horn of the spinal cord, and becomes upregulated briefly after a trauma, such as damage to a limb, in the corresponding sensory segments of the spinal cord (Beiche et al. 1996). The induction of spinal cord COX-2 expression may facilitate transmission of the nociceptive input. In line with a role of COX-2 in central pain perception, Smith et al. (1998) reported that the specific COX-2 inhibitor celecoxib suppressed inflammation-induced prostaglandin levels in cerebrospinal fluid, whereas the selective COX-1 inhibitor SC-560 was inactive in this regard. These observations were substantiated by recent findings that show a widespread induction of COX-2 expression in spinal cord neurons and in other regions of the central nervous system following peripheral inflammation (Samad et al. 2001).

Moreover, it has been shown that the non-acidic antipyretic analgesics of the phenazone type exert their analgesic effects predominantly in the spinal cord that is easily accessible to these compounds due to their physicochemical characteristics allowing a fast passage through the blood–brain barrier (Neugebauer et al. 1995).

Acidic antipyretic analgesics

Based on the finding that aspirin at high doses (>3 g/day) not only inhibits fever and pain but also interferes with inflammation, Winter et al. (1962), in the United States, developed an assay to search for drugs with a similar profile of anti-inflammatory activity. Amazingly, all substances that survived the test of experimental pharmacology and clinical trials turned out to be acids with a high degree of lipophilic–hydrophilic polarity, similar pK_A values, and a high degree of plasma protein binding (for review see Brune and Lanz 1985; Hinz et al. 2000c). Suggestions for indications including treatment of rheumatoid diseases are listed in Table 1. Apart from aspirin, all of these compounds differ in their potency, that is, the single dose necessary to achieve a certain degree of effect ranges from a few milligrams (e.g. lornoxicam) to about 1 g (e.g. salicylic acid). They also differ in their pharmacokinetic characteristics, that is, the speed of absorption (time to peak, t_{max}) (which may also depend on the galenic formulation used), the maximal plasma concentrations (c_{max}), the elimination half-life ($t_{1/2}$), and the oral bioavailability. Interestingly, all traditional NSAIDs lack a relevant degree of so-called COX-2 selectivity (Patrignani et al. 1997). This is surprising since they have all been selected on the basis of high anti-inflammatory potency and low gastrotoxicity that depends on COX-1 inhibition. The key characteristics of the most important NSAIDs are compiled in Table 2 (most data are from Brune and Lanz 1985). This table also contains the data of aspirin which differs in many respects from the other NSAIDs and is therefore discussed at the end of this chapter in detail (see 'Compounds of special interest'). Otherwise, the drugs can be categorized in four different groups that are discussed in the following sections.

NSAIDs with low potency and short elimination half-life

The drugs of this group are particularly useful for blocking occasional mild inflammatory pain. The prototype of this type of compounds is ibuprofen. Depending on its galenic formulation, fast or slow absorption of ibuprofen may be achieved. A fast absorption of ibuprofen was observed following administration of the respective lysine salt (Geisslinger et al. 1993). The bioavailability of ibuprofen is close to 100 per cent and the elimination is always fast even in patients suffering from mild or severe impairment of liver (metabolism) or kidney function (Brune and Lanz 1985). Ibuprofen is used as single doses ranging from 200 mg to 1 g. A maximum dose of 3.2 g/day (United States) or 2.4 g (Europe) for rheumatoid arthritis

Table 1 Indications for antipyretic analgesics

Acute and chronic pain, produced by inflammation of different aetiologies	High dose	Middle dose	Low dose
Acidic antipyretic analgesics (anti-inflammatory antipyretic analgesics, NSAIDs)[a]			
Arthritis: chronic polyarthritis (rheumatoid arthritis), ankylosing spondilytis (Morbus Bechterew), acute gout (gout attack)	Diclofenac, indometacin, ibuprofen, piroxicam (phenylbutazone)[b]	Diclofenac, indometacin, ibuprofen, piroxicam (phenylbutazone)[b]	No
Cancer pain (e.g. bone metastatis)	(Indometacin[c]), diclofenac[c], ibuprofen[c], piroxicam[c]	(Indomethacin[c]), diclofenac[c], ibuprofen[c], piroxicam[c]	Aspirin[d], ibuprofen[c]
Active arthrosis (acute pain-inflammatory episodes)	No	Diclofenac, indometacin, ibuprofen piroxicam	Ibuprofen, ketoprofen
Myofascial pain syndromes (antipyretic analgesics are often prescribed but of limited value)	No	Diclofenac, ibuprofen, piroxicam	Ibuprofen, ketoprofen
Post-traumatic pain, swelling	No	(Indometacin), diclofenac, ibuprofen	Aspirin[d], ibuprofen[c]
Post-operative pain, swelling	No	(Indometacin), diclofenac, ibuprofen	Ibuprofen
Acute pain and fever	**Pyrazolinones (high dose)**	**Pyrazolinones (low dose)**	**Anilines (high dose is toxic)**
Non-acidic antipyretic analgesics			
Spastic pain (colics)	Yes	Yes	No
Conditions associated with high fever	Yes	Yes	No
Cancer pain	Yes	Yes	Yes
Headache, migraine	No	Yes	Yes[f]
General disturbances associated with viral infections	No	Yes[e]	Yes

[a] Dosage range of NSAIDs and example of monosubstances (but note dosage prescribed for each agent).

[b] Indicated only in gout attacks.

[c] Compare the sequence staged scheme of WHO for cancer pain.

[d] Blood coagulation and renal function must be normal.

[e] If other analgesics and antipyretics are contraindicated, for example, gastro-duodenal ulcer, blood coagulation disturbances, asthma.

[f] In particular patients.

is possible. At low doses ibuprofen appears particularly useful for the treatment of acute occasional inflammatory pain. High doses of ibuprofen may also be administered, although with less benefit, for the treatment of chronic rheumatic diseases. Remarkably, at high doses the otherwise harmless compound has been shown to result in an increased incidence of gastrointestinal side-effects (Kaufman et al. 1993; Silverstein et al. 2000). In some countries, ibuprofen is also administered as the pure *S*-enantiomer, which comprises the active entity of the racemic mixture in terms of COX inhibition. On the other hand, a substantial conversion of the less potent COX inhibitor *R*-ibuprofen (comprises 50 per cent of the usual racemic mixture) into the active *S*-enantiomer has been observed following administration of the racemic mixture (Rudy et al. 1991). Other drugs of this group are salicylates and mefenamic acid. The latter does not appear to offer major advantages; on the contrary, this compound and other fenamates are rather toxic at overdosage (central nervous system).

NSAIDs with high potency and short elimination half-life

These drugs are predominantly prescribed for the treatment of rheumatic (arthritic) pain. The most widely used compound of this group is diclofenac which appears to be less active on COX-1 as compared to COX-2 (Patrignani et al. 1997; Tegeder et al. 1999; Hinz et al. 2003). This is taken as a reason for the relatively low incidence of gastrointestinal side-effects of diclofenac (Henry et al. 1996). The limitations of diclofenac result from its usual formulation (monolythic acid-resistant coated dragee or tablet). In fact, retention of such formulations in the stomach for hours or even days may cause retarded absorption of the active ingredient (Brune and Lanz 1985). Moreover, diclofenac has a considerable first-pass metabolism that causes its limited (about 50 per cent) oral bioavailability. Consequently, a lack of therapeutic effect may require adaptation of the dosage or change of the drug. New formulations (microencapsulations, salts, etc.) remedy some of these deficits. The slightly higher incidence of liver toxicity associated with diclofenac may result from the high degree of first-pass metabolism, but other interpretations appear feasible. Recently, it has been demonstrated that pharmacologically relevant concentrations of diclofenac are generated through limited but sustained bioactivation following oral administration of aceclofenac (Hinz et al. 2003). As aceclofenac per se does not interfere with the COX enzymes, diclofenac seems to confer a major part of the pharmacological action of aceclofenac.

This group contains further important drugs such as lornoxicam, flurbiprofen, and indomethacin (very potent), but also ketoprofen and fenoprofen (less active). All of them show a high oral bioavailability and good effectiveness, but also a relative high risk of unwanted drug effects (Henry et al. 1996).

NSAIDs with intermediate potency and intermediate elimination half-life

The third group is intermediate in potency and speed of elimination and comprises drugs such as diflunisal and naproxen. Because of its slow absorption, diflunisal is rarely used anymore.

NSAIDs with high potency and long elimination half-life

The fourth group consists of the oxicams (meloxicam, piroxicam, and tenoxicam). These compounds are characterized by a high degree of

Table 2 Physicochemical and pharmacological data of acidic antipyretic analgesics

Pharmacokinetic/ chemical sub-classes	pK_A	Binding to plasma proteins (%)	Oral bioavailability (%)	t_{max}[a]	$t_{1/2}$[b]	Single dose (maximal daily dose) for adults
Low potency/ short elimination half-life						
Salicylates						
Aspirin	3.5	50–70	~50 Dose-dependent	~15 min	~15 min	0.05–1 g[c] (~6 g)
Salicylic acid	3.0	80–95 Dose-dependent	80–100	0.5–2 h	2.5–4.5 h Dose-dependent	0.5–1 g (6 g)
2-Arylpropionic acids						
Ibuprofen	4.4	99	100	0.5–2 h	2 h	200–800 mg (2.4 g)
Anthranilic acids						
Mefenamic acid	4.2	90	70	2–4 h	1–2 h	250–500 mg (1.5 g)
High potency/ short elimination half-life						
2-Arylpropionic acids						
Flurbiprofen	4.2	>99	No data	1.5–3 h	2.5–4(–8) h	50–100 mg (200 mg)
Ketoprofen	5.3	99	~90	1–2 h	2–4 h	25–100 mg (200 mg)
Aryl-/heteroarylacetic acids						
Diclofenac	3.9	99.7	~50 Dose-dependent	1–12 h[e] Very variable	1–2 h	25–75 mg (150 mg)
Indometacin	4.5	99	~100	0.5–2 h	2–3(–11 h)[d] Very variable	25–75 mg (200 mg)
Oxicams						
Lornoxicam	4.7	99	~100	0.5–2 h	4–10 h	4–12 mg (16 mg)
Intermediate potency/ intermediate elimination half-life						
Salicylates						
Diflunisal	3.3	98–99 Dose-dependent	80–100	2–3 h	8–12 h Dose-dependent	250–500 mg (1 g)
2-Arylpropionic acids						
Naproxen	4.2	99	90–100	2–4 h	12–15 h[d]	250–500 mg (1.25 g)
Arylacetic acids						
6-Methoxy-2-naphthyl-acetic acid (active metabolite of nabumetone)	4.2	99	20–50	3–6 h	20–24 h	0.5–1 g (1.5 g)
High potency/ long elimination half-life						
Oxicams						
Piroxicam	5.9	99	~100	3–5 h	14–160 h[d]	20–40 mg; initial: 40 mg
Tenoxicam	5.3	99	~100	0.5–2 h	25–175 h[d]	20–40 mg; initial: 40 mg
Meloxicam	4.08	99.5	89	7–8 h	20 h[e]	7.5–15 mg

[a] Time to reach maximum plasma concentration after oral administration.

[b] Terminal half-life of elimination.

[c] Single dose for inhibition of thrombocyte aggregation: 50–100 mg; single analgesic dose: 0.5–1 g.

[d] Enterohepatic circulation.

[e] Monolithic acid-resistant tablet or similar galanic form.

enterohepatic circulation, slow metabolism, and slow elimination (Brune and Lanz 1985). Because of their long half-lives (days), oxicams do not represent drugs of first choice for the treatment of acute pain with (probably) short duration. The main indication of the oxicams is inflammatory pain that likely persists for days, that is, pain resulting from cancer (bone metastases) or chronic polyarthritis. The high potency and long persistence in the body may be the reason for the somewhat higher incidence of serious adverse drug effects in the gastrointestinal tract and in the kidney observed in the presence of these drugs (Henry et al. 1996). Recently, it has been claimed that meloxicam is particularly well tolerated by the gastrointestinal tract because it inhibits predominantly the COX-2 isozyme. These results are not fully accepted. When tested in the human whole blood assay, the

COX-2 selectivity of meloxicam is not superior to that of diclofenac (Patrignani et al. 1997).

Compounds of special interest

Asprin, the prototype of NSAIDs, deserves special discussion. Aspirin irreversibly inactivates both COX-1 (highly effective) and COX-2 (less effective) by acetylating an active-site serine, this covalent modification interferes with the binding of arachidonic acid at the COX active site. Most cells compensate the enzyme loss due to acetylation by aspirin via de novo synthesis of this enzyme. However, as platelets are unable to generate fresh enzyme, a single dose of aspirin may suppress platelet COX-1-dependent thromboxane synthesis for whole life-time of thrombocytes (8–11 days) until new platelets are formed.

Following oral administration, aspirin is substantially cleaved before, during, and shortly after absorption, to yield salicylic acid. Consequently, the plasma half-life of aspirin is only about 15 min. Aspirin may be used as a solution (effervescent) or as a (lysine) salt allowing very fast absorption, distribution, and fast pain relief. Aspirin may cause bleeding from existing ulcers due to its long-lasting antiplatelet effect and topical irritation of the gastrointestinal mucosa. The inevitable irritation of the gastric mucosa may be acceptable in otherwise healthy patients. Aspirin should not be used in pregnant women (premature bleeding, closure of ductus arteriosus) or children before puberty (Reye's syndrome).

When low doses of aspirin (≤100 mg) are administered, aspirin acetylates the COX-1 isozyme of platelets presystemically in the portal circulation before aspirin is deacetylated to salicylate in the liver. By contrast, COX-2-dependent synthesis of vasodilatory and antithrombotic prostacyclin by vascular endothelial cells outside the gut is not altered by low-dose aspirin. The reason for this phenomenon lies in the rapid cleavage of aspirin leaving little if any unmetabolized aspirin after primary liver passage. Thus, low-dose aspirin has its only indication in the prevention of thrombotic and embolic events. An unresolved question concerns the use of low-dose aspirin together with other COX-2-selective or non-selective NSAIDs. Recently, it has been shown that the combination of low-dose aspirin with the COX-2-specific inhibitor celecoxib may abrogate the gastrointestinal-sparing effects of the latter (Silverstein et al. 2000) (see 'Specific COX-2 inhibitors').

Over the past three decades, the theory that suppression of prostaglandin biosynthesis accounts for the pharmacological actions of NSAIDs has been questioned by comparing the actions of salicylic acid and aspirin (for review see Weissmann 1993). Salicylate does not, unlike its acetylated derivative aspirin, inhibit COX-1 and COX-2 activity *in vitro*. On the other side, sodium salicylate has been demonstrated to be an effective inhibitor of prostaglandin formation *in vivo* at sites of inflammation and to be equally effective against arthritis as aspirin. From the data published by Kopp and Ghosh (1994) it appears that inhibition of the transcription factor NF-κB could be a mechanism by which salicylates exert their anti-inflammatory action. However, relatively high concentrations of sodium salicylate (i.e. higher than that obtained after therapeutic dosing) were required to provide inhibition of NF-κB activation. On the other hand, pharmacological concentrations of salicylates have been shown to inhibit COX-2 expression in human umbilical vein endothelial cells and foreskin fibroblasts (Xu et al. 1999) pointing towards a possible (cell-specific) target of salicylic acid upstream to COX-2 enzyme activity. Furthermore, metabolites of salicylic acid have recently been shown to inhibit the COX-2-dependent synthesis of prostaglandins (Hinz et al. 2000d), suggesting that bioactivation may confer, at least in part, the capacity of salicylic acid to interfere with prostaglandin formation *in vivo*.

Non-acidic antipyretic analgesics

Aniline derivatives

The main representative of this group is paracetamol (Table 3). Paracetamol is a poor inhibitor of the COX isozymes with, consequently, only weak anti-inflammatory activity. By contrast, induction of fever is clearly blocked by paracetamol in several species. The major advantage of paracetamol lies in its relative lack of (serious) side effects given that the dose limits are obeyed, although serious events can be observed with low doses although rarely so (Bridger et al. 1998). A small proportion of paracetamol is metabolized to the highly toxic nucleophilic *N*-acetyl-benzoquinoneimine that is usually inactivated by reaction with sulfydryl groups in glutathione. However, following ingestion of large doses of paracetamol hepatic glutathione is depleted, resulting in covalent binding of *N*-acetyl-benzoquinoneimine to DNA and structural proteins in parenchymal cells (e.g. in liver and kidney) (for review see Seef et al. 1986). Under these circumstances, dose-dependent, potentially fatal hepatic necrosis may occur. When detected early, overdosage can be antagonized within the first 12 h after intake of paracetamol by administration of *N*-acetylcysteine that regenerates detoxifying mechanisms by replenishing hepatic glutathione stores. Paracetamol should not be given

Table 3 Physicochemical and pharmacological data of paracetamol, pyrazolinone derivatives, and specific COX-2 inhibitors

Chemical/pharmacological class	Binding to plasma proteins	Oral bioavailability (%)	t_{max}[a] (h)	$t_{1/2}$[b] (h)	Single dose (maximal daily dose) for adults
Anilin derivatives					
Paracetamol (acetaminophen)	5–50 Dose-dependent	70–100 Dose-dependent	0.5–1.5	1.5–2.5	0.5–1 g (4 g)
Pyrazolinone derivatives					
Phenazone	< 10	~100 Dose-dependent	0.5–2	11–12	0.5–1 g (4 g)
Propyphenazone	~10	~100 Dose-dependent	0.5–1.5	1–2.5	0.5–1 g (4 g)
Metamizol-Na[c]	<20	—	—	—	0.5–1 g (4 g)
4-Methylaminophenazone[d]	58	~100	1–2	2–4	—
4-Aminophenazone[d]	48	—	—	4–5.5	—
Specific COX-2 inhibitors					
Celecoxib	94–98	60–80	2–4	11	100–200 mg (400 mg)
Rofecoxib	~98	~100	2–4	~17	12.5–25 mg (50 mg)

[a] Time to reach maximum plasma concentration after oral administration.

[b] Terminal half-life of elimination.

[c] Noraminopyrinemethansulfonate-Na.

[d] Metabolites of metamizol.

to patients with seriously impaired liver function. The predominant indication of paracetamol is fever and mild forms of pain occurring in the context of viral infections, but not in, for example, post-operative pain. In addition, many patients with recurrent headache benefit from paracetamol and its low toxicity. Paracetamol is also used in children, but despite its somewhat lower toxicity in juvenile patients, fatalities due to unvoluntary overdosage have been reported. It is presently unclear to what extent paracetamol in combination with aspirin and caffeine act synergistically (Laska et al. 1984). Moreover, the mechanism of the so-called analgesic nephropathy associated with such analgesic mixtures is still a matter of debate (Elseviers and De Broe 1996; Porter 1996). Also, claims that such combinations are more frequently abused than single-entity analgesics are supported only by (weak) epidemiological data. Acetanilide and phenacetine, the precursors of paracetamol, have definitely been banned because of their higher toxicity.

Pyrazolinone derivatives

Following the discovery of phenazone 120 years ago, the drug industry has tried to improve this compound in three ways: phenazone was chemically modified (i) to have a more potent compound, (ii) to yield a water-soluble derivative to be given parenterally, and (iii) to find a compound which is eliminated faster and more reliable than phenazone. The results of these attempts are the phenazone derivatives aminophenazone, dipyrone, and propyphenazone (Table 3). Aminophenazone is not in use anymore because it has been associated with formation of nitrosamines that may increase the risk of stomach cancer. The other two compounds differ from phenazone in their potency and elimination half-life, their water solubility (dipyrone is a water-soluble prodrug of methylaminophenazone), and their general toxicity (propyphenazone and dipyrone do not lead to the formation of nitrosamines in the acidic environment of the stomach). Phenazone, propyphenazone, and dipyrone are the predominantly used antipyretic analgesics in many countries (Latin America, many countries in Asia, Eastern and Central Europe). Dipyrone has been accused to cause agranulocytosis. Although there appears to be a statistically significant link, the incidence is extremely rare (1 case per million treatment periods) (The International Agranulocytosis and Aplastic Anemia Study 1986; Kaufman et al. 1991). Moreover, all antipyretic analgesics have also been claimed to cause Stevens–Johnson's syndrome and Lyell's syndrome as well as shock reactions. New data indicate that the incidence of these events is in the same order of magnitude as with, for example, penicillins (Roujeau et al. 1995; Mockenhaupt et al. 1996; The International Collaborative Study of Severe Anaphylaxis 1998). All non-acidic phenazone derivatives lack anti-inflammatory activity, and are devoid of gastrointestinal and (acute) renal toxicity. In contrast to paracetamol, dipyrone is safe even when given at overdosages. If one compares aspirin, paracetamol, and propyphenazone when used for the same indication (e.g. occasional headache), it is evident that aspirin is more dangerous than either propyphenazone or paracetamol.

Specific COX-2 inhibitors

Specific COX-2 inhibitors are expected to exert anti-inflammatory and analgesic effects without causing gastric ulcerogenic effects or platelet dysfunction. By definition, a substance may be regarded as a specific COX-2 inhibitor if it causes no clinically meaningful COX-1 inhibition (i.e. suppression of platelet thromboxane formation and gastric prostaglandin synthesis) at maximal therapeutic doses. Among the variety of available test systems, the *ex vivo* whole-blood assay has emerged as the best method to estimate COX-2 selectivity in humans. This assay provides a direct indication of the ability of a test substance to inhibit the enzymatic activities of COX-1 (i.e. thromboxane formation from platelets during blood clotting) and COX-2 (i.e. prostaglandin E_2 synthesis in lipopolysaccharide-stimulated monocytes). Using this assay, celecoxib and rofecoxib have been shown to cause no significant inhibition of COX-1-dependent thromboxane formation over the entire range of clinically used doses (Ehrich et al. 1999; Leese et al. 2000).

X-ray crystallography of the three-dimensional structures of COX-1 and COX-2 has provided more insights into how COX-2 specificity is achieved. Within the hydrophobic channel of the COX enzyme a single amino acid difference in position 523 (isoleucine in COX-1, valine in COX-2) has been detected that is critical for the COX-2 selectivity of several drugs. Accordingly, the smaller valin molecule in COX-2 gives access to a side pocket, which has been proposed to be the binding site of COX-2 selective substances (Luong et al. 1996). Thus, the increased NSAID-binding pocket of the COX-2 isozyme can bind bulky inhibitors more readily than the COX-1 isoform. Celecoxib and rofecoxib are novel specific COX-2 inhibitors of the diarylheterocyclic family. The 4-methylsulfonylphenyl and 4-sulfonamoylphenyl groups of these compounds interact with specific residues within the 'side pocket' of the COX-2 isozyme. Valdecoxib, parecoxib sodium (prodrug of valdecoxib that can be administered intramuscularly or intravenously) and the dipyridinyl compound etoricoxib are the latest developments belonging to this type of specific COX-2 inhibitors.

Celecoxib and rofecoxib have been shown to be effective analgesics in dental pain models and effective anti-inflammatory and analgesic substances in patients with rheumatoid arthritis and osteoarthritis. The analgesic potency is comparable to that of of traditional NSAIDs (Ehrich et al. 1999; Lefkowith 1999). Celecoxib was approved in December 1998 by the US Food and Drug Administration for relief of the signs and symptoms of osteoarthritis (recommended oral dose is 200 mg/day administered as a single dose or as 100 mg twice per day) and rheumatoid arthritis in adults (recommended oral dose is 100–200 mg twice per day). Rofecoxib became available in 1999 and is indicated for relief of the signs and symptoms of osteoarthritis (recommended starting dose is 12.5 mg/day, maximum recommended daily dose is 25 mg), for the management of acute pain in adults, and for the treatment of primary dysmenorrhoea (recommended initial doses are 50 mg once daily, use of rofecoxib at this dose for more than 5 days in the management of pain has not been studied). As compared with celecoxib, rofecoxib has a longer half-life and exhibits a higher potency and COX-2 selectivity (Table 3). However, their pharmacokinetic characteristics (slow absorption, slow elimination) make both drugs poor candidates for the treatment of acute pain of short duration. Whereas the metabolism of rofecoxib is primarily mediated through cytosolic enzymes, celecoxib is metabolized predominantly via cytochrome P4502C9 (CYP2C9). Thus, significant interactions may occur when celecoxib is administered together with drugs that inhibit CYP2C9 (e.g. fluconazole). As NSAIDs have been reported to elevate plasma lithium levels, patients receiving specific COX-2 inhibitors and lithium should be observed carefully for signs of lithium toxicity. Furthermore, specific COX-2 inhibitors may diminish the anti-hypertensive effect of angiotensin converting enzyme (ACE) inhibitors. In patients receiving warfarin, anticoagulant activity should be monitored particularly in the first few days after initiating therapy with specific COX-2 inhibitors.

Published clinical studies support the hypothesis that specific COX-2 inhibitors may provide a significantly improved risk–benefit ratio in terms of gastrointestinal safety as compared with conventional NSAIDs. Accordingly, the use of specific COX-2 inhibitors rather than traditional NSAIDs should be preferred in patients at increased risk of serious upper gastrointestinal complications. These patients include individuals older than 60 years, those with a history of peptic ulcer disease and those taking glucocorticoids (with a high-dose NSAID) and anticoagulants. In the Vioxx Gastrointestinal Outcomes Research (VIGOR) study (Bombardier et al. 2000), treatment with rofecoxib at twice the approved maximal dose for long-term use resulted in significantly lower rates of clinically important upper gastrointestinal events and complicated upper gastrointestinal events than did treatment with a standard dose of naproxen. Moreover, the incidence of complicated upper gastrointestinal bleeding and bleeding from beyond the duodenum was significantly lower among patients who received rofecoxib. In the Celecoxib Long-term Arthritis Safety Study (CLASS) (Silverstein et al. 2000), incidences of symptomatic ulcers and/or ulcer complications were not significantly different in patients taking celecoxib versus NSAIDs who were also taking concomitant low-dosage aspirin, indicating that the use of low-dose aspirin may abrogate the gastrointestinal-sparing effects of celecoxib. By contrast, analysis of non-aspirin users alone demonstrated that celecoxib, at a dosage two- to four-fold greater than the maximum therapeutic dosages, was associated with a significantly lower incidence of symptomatic ulcers and/or ulcer complications compared with NSAIDs.

Moreover, an interesting finding of the past years was the observation that COX-2 may influence ulcer healing and the associated angiogenesis. In accord with this concept, COX-2 has previously been shown to be induced in tissue on the edges of ulcers (Mizuno et al. 1997). In animal studies, selective COX-2 inhibitors have been demonstrated to retard ulcer healing (Schmassmann et al. 1998). As a consequence, it will be necessary to test whether effective ulcer healing occurs in patients with NSAID-associated ulcers switched to specific COX-2 inhibitors.

The involvement of COX-2 in human renal function is supported by clinical studies (Catella-Lawson et al. 1999; Whelton et al. 2000) that showed that specific COX-2 inhibitors, similar to other NSAIDs, may cause peripheral oedema, hypertension, and exacerbation of pre-existing hypertension by inhibiting water and salt excretion by the kidneys. Moreover, in healthy elderly volunteers, specific COX-2 inhibitors decreased renal prostacyclin production and led to a significant transient decline in urinary sodium excretion (Catella-Lawson et al. 1999). However, although decreases in sodium excretion were comparable between NSAIDs and specific COX-2 inhibitors, only NSAIDs were shown to reduce the glomerular filtration rate in volunteers with normal renal function (Catella-Lawson et al. 1999).

COX-2 localized in the endothelium has been suggested to confer vasoprotective and antiatherogenic actions by virtue of its major product, prostacyclin, which is a potent inhibitor of platelet aggregation, activation and adhesion of leucocytes, and accumulation of cholesterol in vascular cells. Upregulation of endothelial COX-2 has been shown to be induced by laminar shear stress (Topper et al. 1996) or lysophosphatidylcholine (a component of atherogenic lipoproteins) (Zembowicz et al. 1995), suggesting that COX-2 may provide an adaptive vascular protection. In clinical studies, specific COX-2 inhibitors have been reported to decrease systemic prostacyclin production in healthy volunteers (Catella-Lawson et al. 1999).

In this context, it is interesting to note that specific COX-2 inhibitors that do not inhibit platelet COX-1 might (at least in theory) unfavourably alter the thromboxane–prostacyclin balance by inhibiting COX-2-dependent synthesis of vasoprotective prostacyclin in endothelial cells. However, hitherto published clinical studies have yielded discrepant results in this regard. In the CLASS trial no difference was noted in the incidence of cardiovascular events (cerebrovascular accident, myocardial infarction, angina) between celecoxib and NSAIDs (ibuprofen, diclofenac) (Silverstein et al. 2000). On the other hand, in the VIGOR study, patients receiving rofecoxib had a significant four-fold increase in the incidence of myocardial infarctions, as compared with patients randomized to naproxen (Bombardier et al. 2000). However, as both compounds are known to cause a similar inhibition of systemic prostacyclin production without altering platelet-derived thromboxane synthesis, the apparent discrepancy of these studies in terms of cardiovascular outcome is most likely due to differences in the study protocols (e.g. eligibility criteria, study population, study duration) and the use of different NSAID comparators. It is noteworthy that 22 per cent of the patients included in the CLASS trial took aspirin as a cardioprotective agent, whereas the entry criteria for the VIGOR study precluded aspirin consumption. In addition, the VIGOR study was performed on patients with rheumatoid arthritis, a condition that has been associated with an enhanced rate of cardiovascular events. In contrast, the CLASS trial included patients with osteoarthritis who do not have increased risk of cardiovascular complications. As a consequence, a possible thrombogenicity of specific COX-2 inhibitors deserves further well-controlled studies.

On the other hand, the involvement of the COX-2 isozyme in other pathological states suggests that specific COX-2 inhibitors may have further indications in conditions such as colonic polyposis, colorectal cancer, and Alzheimer's disease (Thun et al. 1991; Giardiello et al. 1993; Tocco et al. 1997). Specific COX-2 inhibitors have been shown to possess a strong chemopreventive action against colon carcinogenesis in rats, inhibiting tumours to a greater degree than conventional NSAIDs (Kawamori et al. 1998). With regard to the functions of the COX isozymes, Tsujii et al. (1998) found that COX-2 may modulate the production of angiogenic factors by colon cancer cells, while COX-1 regulates angiogenesis in endothelial cells. Moreover, recent studies indicate that COX-2 overexpression is not necessarily unique to cancer of the colon, but may be a common feature of other epithelial cells. Accordingly, increased COX-2 levels have been identified in lung, breast, and gastric cancers. On the basis of these data, it is conceivable that specific COX-2 inhibitors might be used as adjuvants in the treatment of tumours as well as in cancer prevention.

References

Akopian, A.N., Sivilotti, L., and Wood, J.N. (1996). A tetrodotoxin-resistant voltage-gated sodium channel expressed by sensory neurons. *Nature* **379**, 257–62.

Beiche, F., Scheuerer, S., Brune, K., Geisslinger, G., and Goppelt-Struebe, M. (1996). Upregulation of cyclooxygenase-2 mRNA in the rat spinal cord following peripheral inflammation. *FEBS Letters* **390**, 165–9.

Bombardier, C., Laine, L., Reicin, A., Shapiro, D., Burgos-Vargas, R., Davis, B., Day, R., Ferraz, M.B., Hawkey, C.J., Hochberg, M.C., Kvien, T.K., and Schnitzer, T.J. (2000). Comparison of upper gastrointestinal toxicity of rofecoxib and naproxen in patients with rheumatoid arthritis. VIGOR Study Group. *New England Journal of Medicine* **343**, 1520–8.

Bridger, S., Henderson, K., Glucksman, E., Ellis, A.J., Henry, J.A., and Williams, R. (1998). Deaths from low dose paracetamol poisoning. *American Medical Journal* **316**, 1724–5.

Brune, K. (1974). How aspirin might work: a pharmacokinetic approach. *Agents and Actions* **4**, 230–2.

Brune, K. and Lanz, R. (1985). Pharmacokinetics of non-steroidal anti-inflammatory drugs. In *Handbook of Inflammation. The Pharmacology of Inflammation* Vol. 5 (ed. M.A. Bray, I.L. Bonta, and M.J. Parnham), pp. 413–49. Amsterdam: Elsevier Science Publishers.

Brune, K., Rainsford, K.D., and Schweitzer, A. (1980). Biodistribution of mild analgesics. *British Journal of Clinical Pharmacology* **10** (Suppl. 2), 279–84.

Brune, K., Glatt, M., and Graf, P. (1976). Mechanism of action of anti-inflammatory drugs. *General Pharmacology* **7**, 27–33.

Catella-Lawson, F., McAdam, B., Morrison, B.W., Kapoor, S., Kujubu, D., Antes, L., Lasseter, K.C., Quan, H., Gertz, B.J., and FitzGerald, G.A. (1999). Effects of specific inhibition of cyclooxygenase-2 on sodium balance, hemodynamics, and vasoactive eicosanoids. *Journal of Pharmacology and Experimental Therapeutics* **289**, 735–41.

Ehrich, E.W., Dallob, A., De Lepeleire, I., van Hecken, A., Riendeau, D., Yuan, W., Porras, A., Wittreich, J., Seibold, J.R., De Schepper, P., Mehlisch, D.R., and Gertz, B.J. (1999). Characterization of rofecoxib as a cyclooxygenase-2 isoform inhibitor and demonstration of analgesia in the dental pain model. *Clinical Pharmacology and Therapeutics* **65**, 336–47.

Elseviers, M.M. and De Broe, M.E. (1996). Combination analgesic involvement in the pathogenesis of analgesic nephropathy: the European perspective. *American Journal of Kidney Diseases* **28** (Suppl. 1), 48–55.

Geisslinger, G., Menzel, S., Wissel, K., and Brune, K. (1993). Single dose pharmacokinetics of different formulations of ibuprofen and aspirin. *Drug Investigations* **5**, 238–42.

Giardiello, F.M., Hamilton, S.R., Krush, A.J., Piantadosi, S., Hylind, L.M., Celano, P., Booker, S.V., Robinson, C.R., and Offerhaus, G.J. (1993). Treatment of colonic and rectal adenomas with sulindac in familial adenomatous polyposis. *New England Journal of Medicine* **328**, 1313–16.

Gibb, W. and Sun, M. (1996). Localization of prostaglandin H synthase type 2 protein and mRNA in term human fetal membranes and decidua. *Journal of Endocrinology* **150**, 497–503.

Harris, R.C., McKanna, J.A., Akai, Y., Jacobson, H.R., Dubois, R.N., and Breyer, M.D. (1994). Cyclooxygenase-2 is associated with the macula densa of rat kidney and increases with salt restriction. *Journal of Clinical Investigation* **94**, 2504–10.

Henry, D., Lim, L.L., Garcia Rodriguez, L.A., Perez Gutthann, S., Carson, J.L., Griffin, M., Savage, R., Logan, R., Moride, Y., Hawkey, C., Hill, S., and Fries, J.T. (1996). Variability in risk of gastrointestinal complications with individual non-steroidal anti-inflammatory drugs: results of a collaborative meta-analysis. *British Medical Journal* **312**, 1563–6.

Hinz, B. and Brune, K. (2000). New insights into physiological and pathophysiological functions of cyclooxygenase-2. *Current Opinion in Anaesthesiology* **13**, 585–90.

Hinz, B., Brune, K., and Pahl, A. (2000a). Cyclooxygenase-2 expression in lipopolysaccharide-stimulated human monocytes is modulated by cyclic AMP, prostaglandin E_2 and nonsteroidal anti-inflammatory drugs. *Biochemical and Biophysical Research Communications* **278**, 790–6.

Hinz, B., Brune, K., and Pahl, A. (2000b). Prostaglandin E_2 up-regulates cyclooxygenase-2 expression in lipopolysaccharide-stimulated RAW 264.7 macrophages. *Biochemical and Biophysical Research Communications* **272**, 744–8.

Hinz, B., Dorn, C.P., Shen, T.Y., and Brune, K. (2000c). Anti-inflammatory—antirheumatic drugs. In *Ullmann's Encyclopedia of Industrial Chemistry. 2000 Electronic Release* 6th edn. Weinheim: Wiley-VCH.

Hinz, B., Kraus, V., Pahl, A., and Brune, K. (2000d). Salicylate metabolites inhibit cyclooxygenase-2-dependent prostaglandin E_2 synthesis in murine macrophages. *Biochemical and Biophysical Research Communications* **274**, 197–202.

Hinz, B., Rau, T., Auge, D., Werner, U., Ramer, R., Rietbrock, S., and Brune, K. (2003). Aceclofenac spares cyclooxygenase 1 as a result of limited but sustained biotransformation to diclofenac. *Clinical Pharmacology and Therapeutics* **74**, 222–35.

Kaufman, D.W., Kelly, J.P., Levy, M., and Shapiro, S. (1991). The drug etiology of agranulocytosis and aplastic anemia. *Monographs in Epidemiology and Biostatistics* **18**. New York: Oxford University Press.

Kaufman, D.W., Kelly, J.P., Sheehan, J.E., Laszlo, A., Wiholm, B.-E., Alfredsson, L., Koff, R.S., and Shapiro, S. (1993). Nonsteroidal anti-inflammatory drug use in relation to major upper gastrointestinal bleeding. *Clinical Pharmacology and Therapeutics* **53**, 485–94.

Kawamori, T., Rao, C.V., Seibert, K., and Reddy, B.S. (1998). Chemopreventive activity of celecoxib, a specific cyclooxygenase-2 inhibitor, against colon carcinogenesis. *Cancer Research* **58**, 409–12.

Kopp, E. and Ghosh, S. (1994). Inhibition of NF-κB by sodium salicylate and aspirin. *Science* **265**, 956–9.

Laska, E.M., Sunshine, A., Mueller, F., Elvers, W.B., Siegel, C., and Rubin, A. (1984). Caffeine as an analgesic adjuvant. *Journal of the American Medical Association* **251**, 1711–18.

Leese, P.T., Hubbard, R.C., Karim, A., Isakson, P.C., Yu, S.S., and Geis, G.S. (2000). Effects of celecoxib, a novel cyclooxygenase-2 inhibitor, on platelet function in healthy adults: a randomized, controlled trial. *Journal of Clinical Pharmacology* **40**, 124–32.

Lefkowith, J.B. (1999). Cyclooxygenase-2 specificity and its clinical implications. *American Journal of Medicine* **106**, 43S–50S.

Lim, H., Paria, B.C., Das, S.K., Dinchuk, J.E., Langenbach, R., Trzaskos, J.M., and Dey, S.K. (1997). Multiple female reproductive failures in cyclooxygenase 2-deficient mice. *Cell* **91**, 197–208.

Luong, C., Miller, A., Barnett, J., Chow, J., Ramesha, C., and Browner, M.F. (1996). Flexibility of the NSAID binding site in the structure of human cyclooxygenase-2. *Nature Structural Biology* **3**, 927–33.

Maldve, R.E., Kim, Y., Muga, S.J., and Fischer, S.M. (2000). Prostaglandin E_2 regulation of cyclooxygenase expression in keratinocytes is mediated via cyclic nucleotide-linked prostaglandin receptors. *Journal of Lipid Research* **41**, 873–81.

Masferrer, J.L., Zweifel, B.S., Seibert, S., and Needleman, P. (1990). Selective regulation of cellular cyclooxygenase by dexamethasone and endotoxin in mice. *Journal of Clinical Investigation* **86**, 1375–9.

Mizuno, H., Sakamoto, C., Matsuda, K., Wada, K., Uchida, T., Noguchi, H., Akamatsu, T., and Kasuga, M. (1997). Induction of cyclooxygenase 2 in gastric mucosal lesions and its inhibition by the specific antagonist delays healing in mice. *Gastroenterology* **112**, 387–97.

Mockenhaupt, M., Schlingmann, J., Schroeder, W., and Schoepf, E. (1996). Evaluation of non-steroidal anti-inflammatory drugs (NSAIDs) and muscle relaxants as risk factors for Stevens-Johnson syndrome (SJS) and toxic epidermal necrolysis (TEN). *Pharmacoepidemiology and Drug Safety* **5**, 116.

Nantel, F., Denis, D., Gordon, R., Northey, A., Cirino, M., Metters, K.M., and Chan, C.C. (1999a). Distribution and regulation of cyclooxygenase-2 in carrageenan-induced inflammation. *British Journal of Pharmacology* **128**, 853–9.

Nantel, F., Meadows, E., Denis, D., Connolly, B., Metters, K.M., and Giaid, A. (1999b). Immunolocalization of cyclooxygenase-2 in the macula densa of human elderly. *FEBS Letters* **457**, 475–7.

Neugebauer, V., Geisslinger, G., Rümenapp, P., Weiretter, F., Szelenyi, I., Brune, K., and Schaible H.-G. (1995). Antinociceptive effects of R(−)- and S(+)-flurbiprofen on rat spinal dorsal horn neurons rendered hyperexcitable by an acute knee joint inflammation. *Journal of Pharmacology and Experimental Therapeutics* **275**, 618–28.

Niiro, H., Otsuka, T., Izuhara, K., Yamaoka, K., Ohshima, K., Tanabe, T., Hara, S., Nemoto, Y., Tanaka, Y., Nakashima, H., and Niho, Y. (1997). Regulation by interleukin-10 and interleukin-4 of cyclooxygenase-2 expression in human neutrophils. *Blood* **89**, 1621–8.

Onoe, Y., Miyaura, C., Kaminakayashiki, T., Nagai, Y., Noguchi, K., Chen, Q.R., Seo, H., Ohta, H., Nozawa, S., Kudo, I., and Suda, T. (1996). IL-13 and IL-4 inhibit bone resorption by suppressing cyclooxygenase-2-dependent prostaglandin synthesis in osteoblasts. *Journal of Immunology* **156**, 758–64.

Patrignani, P., Panara, M.R., Sciulli, M.G., Santini, G., Renda, G., and Patrono, C. (1997). Differential inhibition of human prostaglandin endoperoxide synthase-1 and -2 by nonsteroidal anti-inflammatory drugs. *Journal of Physiology and Pharmacology* **48**, 623–31.

Porter, G.A. (1996). Paracetamol/aspirin mixtures: experimental data. *American Journal of Kidney Diseases* **28** (Suppl. 1), 30–3.

Roujeau, J.C., Kelly, J.P., Naldi, L., Rzany, B., Stern, R.S., Anderson, T., Auquier, A., Bastuji-Garin, S., Correia, O., Locati, F., Mockenhaupt, M., Paoletti, C., Shapiro, S., Sheir, N., Schöpf, E., and Kaufman, D. (1995). Drug etiology of Stevens-Johnson syndrome and toxic epidemal necrolysis, first results from an international case–control study. *New England Journal of Medicine* **333**, 1600–9.

Rudy, A.C., Knight, P.M., Brater, D.C., and Hall, S.D. (1991). Stereoselective metabolism of ibuprofen in humans: administration of R-, S- and racemic ibuprofen. *Journal of Pharmacology and Experimental Therapeutics* **259**, 1133–9.

Samad, T.A., Moore, K.A., Sapirstein, A., Billet, S., Allchorne, A., Poole, S., Bonventre, J.V., and Woolf, C.J. (2001). Interleukin-1beta-mediated induction of Cox-2 in the CNS contributes to inflammatory pain hypersensitivity. *Nature* **410**, 471–5.

Schaible, H.G. and Schmidt, R.F. (1988). Time course of mechanosensitivity changes in articular afferents during a developing experimental arthritis. *Journal of Neurophysiology* **60**, 2180–95.

Schmassmann, A., Peskar, B.M., Stettler, C., Netzer, P., Stroff, T., Flogerzi, B., and Halter, F. (1998). Effects of inhibition of prostaglandin endoperoxide synthase-2 in chronic gastro-intestinal ulcer models in rats. *British Journal of Pharmacology* **123**, 795–804.

Seeff, L.B., Cuccherini, B.A., Zimmerman, H.J., Adler, E., and Benjamin, S.B. (1986). Paracetamol hepatotoxicity in alcoholics. *Annals of Internal Medicine* **104**, 399–404.

Silverstein, F.E., Faich, G., Goldstein, J.L., Simon, L.S., Pincus, T., Whelton, A., Makuch, R., Eisen, G., Agrawal, N.M., Stenson, W.F., Burr, A.M., Zhao, W.W., Kent, J.D., Lefkowith, J.B., Verburg, K.M., and Geis, G.S. (2000). Gastrointestinal toxicity with celecoxib vs nonsteroidal anti-inflammatory drugs for osteoarthritis and rheumatoid arthritis: the CLASS study: a randomized controlled trial. Celecoxib Long-term Arthritis Safety Study. *Journal of the American Medical Association* **284**, 1247–55.

Smith, C.J., Zhang, Y., Koboldt, C.M., Muhammad, J., Zweifel, B.S., Shaffer, A., Talley, J.J., Masferrer, J.L., Seibert, K., and Isakson, P.C. (1998). Pharmacological analysis of cyclooxygenase-1 in inflammation. *Proceedings of the National Academy of Sciences USA* **95**, 13313–18.

Tegeder, I., Lotsch, J., Krebs, S., Muth-Selbach, U., Brune, K., and Geisslinger, G. (1999). Comparison of inhibitory effects of meloxicam and diclofenac on human thromboxane biosynthesis after single doses and at steady state. *Clinical Pharmacology and Therapeutics* **65**, 533–44.

The International Agranulocytosis and Aplastic Anemia Study (1986). Risks of agranulocytosis and aplastic anemia: a first report of their relation to drug use with special reference to analgesics. *Journal of the American Medical Association* **256**, 1749–57.

The International Collaborative Study of Severe Anaphylaxis (1998). *Epidemiology* **9**, 141–6.

Thun, M.J., Namboodiri, M.M., and Heath, C.W., Jr. (1991). Aspirin use and reduced risk of fatal colon cancer. *New England Journal of Medicine* **325**, 1593–6.

Tocco, G., Freire-Moar, J., Schreiber, S.S., Sakhi, S.H., Aisen, P.S., and Pasinetti, G.M. (1997). Maturational regulation and regional induction of cyclooxygenase-2 in rat brain: implications for Alzheimer's disease. *Experimental Neurology* **144**, 339–49.

Topper, J.N., Cai, J., Falb, D., and Gimbrone, M.A., Jr. (1996). Identification of vascular endothelial genes differentially responsive to fluid mechanical stimuli: cyclooxygenase-2, manganese superoxide dismutase, and endothelial cell nitric oxide synthase are selectively up-regulated by steady laminar shear stress. *Proceedings of the National Academy of Sciences USA* **93**, 10417–22.

Tsujii, M., Kawano, S., Tsuji, S., Sawaoka, H., Hori, M., and DuBois, R.N. (1998). Cyclooxygenase regulates angiogenesis induced by colon cancer cells. *Cell* **93**, 705–16.

Vane, J.R. (1971). Inhibition of prostaglandin synthesis as a mechanism of action of aspirin-like drugs. *Nature New Biology* **231**, 232–5.

Weissmann, G. (1993). Prostaglandins as modulators rather than mediators of inflammation. *Journal of Lipid Mediators* **6**, 275–86.

Whelton, A., Maurath, C.J., Verburg, K.M., and Geis, G.S. (2000). Renal safety and tolerability of celecoxib, a novel cyclooxygenase-2 inhibitor. *American Journal of Therapeutics* **7**, 159–75.

Winter, C.A., Risley, E.A., and Nuss, G.W. (1962). Carrageenin-induced edema in hind paw of the rat as an assay for anti-inflammatory drugs. *Proceedings of the Society of Experimental Biology, New York* **111**, 544–52.

Xie, W., Chipman, J.G., Robertson, D.L., Erikson, R.L., and Simmons, D.L. (1991). Expression of a mitogen-responsive gene encoding prostaglandin synthase is regulated by mRNA splicing. *Proceedings of the National Academy of Sciences USA* **88**, 2692–6.

Xu, X.M., Sansores-Garcia, L., Chen, X.M., Matijevic-Aleksic, N., Du, M., and Wu, K.K. (1999). Suppression of inducible cyclooxygenase 2 gene transcription by aspirin and sodium salicylate. *Proceedings of the National Academy of Sciences USA* **96**, 5292–7.

Zembowicz, A., Jones, S.L., and Wu, K.K. (1995). Induction of cyclooxygenase-2 in human umbilical vein endothelial cells by lysophosphatidylcholine. *Journal of Clinical Investigation* **96**, 1688–92.

4.5.2 The place of glucocorticoids in the management of rheumatic disease

John R. Kirwan

Introduction

The history of glucocorticoid use is linked with some of the most important advances in medical science this century. Philip Hench and his colleagues, later awarded the Nobel Prize, used them in rheumatoid arthritis (RA) with dramatic results (Hench et al. 1949). The subsequent widespread use of glucocorticoids as anti-inflammatory agents made its mark in many conditions with an inflammatory or autoimmune basis.

This chapter will briefly consider the structure and function of glucocorticoids, then go on to review current practice in the use of glucocorticoids to treat polymyalgia rheumatica (PMR) and temporal arteritis (TA), vasculitic episodes typified by those in systemic lupus erythematosus (SLE), and chronic inflammatory arthritis typified by RA. In the latter, in particular, the evidence base of current practice will be carefully scrutinized. Adverse effects of glucocorticoids as used in rheumatology clinical practice will be considered, and weighed against the data available to support their use. Finally, some of the potential for further developments in glucocorticoid use in arthritis will be explored.

Brief overview of mechanisms and biology

The principal glucocorticoid hormone of the human adrenal cortex is cortisol (hydrocortisone), derived from hydroxylation of cortisone [Fig. 1(a)]. The 11β and 17α hydroxyl groups are important for glucocorticoid activity. The additional double bond in the synthetic analogue prednisolone enhances glucocorticoid activity without increasing mineralocorticoid activity, an effect that is increased by 6α methylation (methylprednisolone), 9α fluorination (triamcinolone), or both (dexamethasone) (Goulding and Fowler 2001). Prednisone is a synthetic metabolic precursor of prednisolone.

Plasma cortisol is normally maintained at a concentration of 5–25 ng/ml. Most (80 per cent) is bound to the α-globulin transcortin and some (10 per cent) to albumin (Baxter and Forssham 1972). The remaining 10 per cent provides biological activity. Based on recent experimental findings as well as clinical observations of the effects of glucocorticoids at different doses, current

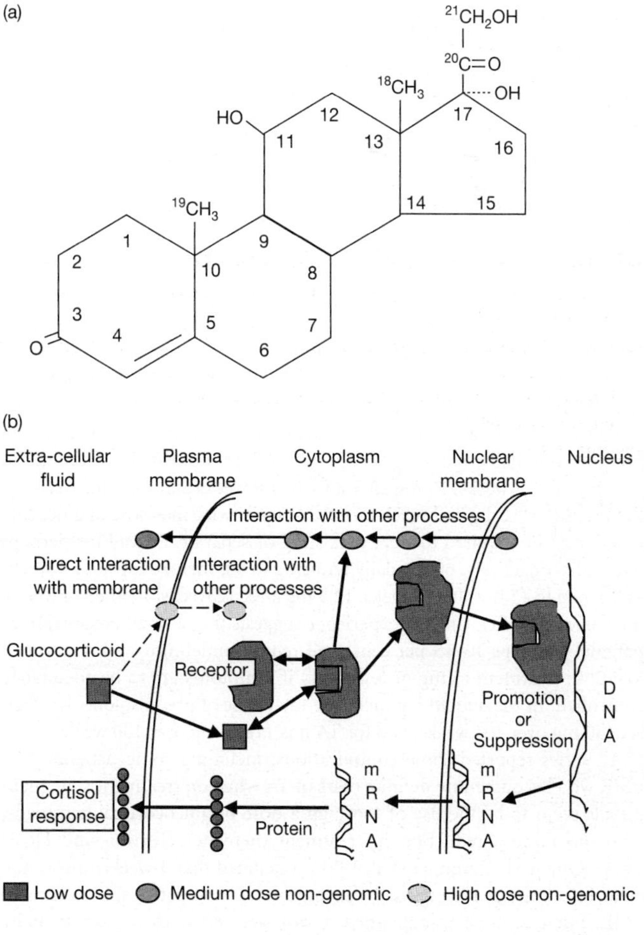

Fig. 1 (a) Chemical structure of hydrocortisone and (b) modes of action of glucocorticoids.

understanding suggests glucocorticoid actions are strongly dose-dependent not only in a quantitative, but also in a qualitative manner (Buttgereit et al. 1998, 2002). There are probably three principal mechanisms of action. The first is well known and involves the passage of glucocorticoid molecules through the plasma membrane to specific receptor proteins in the cytoplasm. The human glucocorticoid receptor is a 95 kDa phosphorylated protein with glucocorticoid binding, deoxyribonucleic acid (DNA) binding, and strongly antigenic regions, each of roughly equal size. The receptor gene has now been cloned and sequenced, confirming and extending the general description of this protein (Oakley and Cidlowski 2001).

The glucocorticoid and receptor form a complex that undergoes a conformational change, and moves to the nucleus, where it binds reversibly to specific DNA sites promoting (or suppressing) the production of messenger ribonucleic acid (mRNA), and the proteins that produce the hormonal effects. Most cellular responses can be detected within 2 h of glucocorticoid exposure and some within 10 min (Baxter and Forssham 1972). In general, a response is not observed if RNA synthesis is inhibited.

A second mechanism of action becomes increasingly important as the number of glucocorticoid and receptor complexes in the cytoplasm increases (i.e. with higher doses of glucocorticoid). These complexes are then able to interact with other metabolic pathways and induce effects that do not depend on interaction with the genes (non-genomic effects). When the plasma concentration of glucocorticoid is even higher, then glucocorticoid molecules interact directly with the cell membrane and influence a further set of cellular activities. These three modes of action are illustrated in Fig. 1(b) and help to explain the very complex dose–response effects of glucocorticoids observed in clinical practice.

Further complexity is introduced by the circadian variation in the natural production of hydrocortisone and by the hypothalamic pituitary adrenal (HPA) interaction that controls it. The negative feedback loop that suppresses the production of hypothalamic corticotrophin releasing hormone (CRH) and pituitary corticotrophin (ACTH) turns out to be more complicated than previously recognized (Cowell and Buckingham 2001) and is probably functioning abnormally and causing relative under-secretion of hydrocortisone in RA (Harbuz and Jessop 1999).

Glucocorticoids in PMR and TA

The signs and symptoms of PMR and TA overlap and can often be confused, but both are treated with glucocorticoids. There are no controlled trials to define the best treatment regimen, but four substantial cohorts of patients have been reported in the literature (Salvarini 1987; Delecoeuillerie et al. 1988; Kyle and Hazleman 1989; Lundberg and Hedfors 1990). The evidence points to a requirement to treat PMR initially with about 15 mg prednisolone daily, reducing slowly over 18–24 months, for example, to 12.5 mg after 8 weeks, 10 mg after a further 8 weeks and for a further year, then reduce by 1 mg daily each month. At least twice that dose of glucocorticoids will be required to treat coexisting or separate TA and for perhaps 6 months longer (e.g. 60 mg daily reducing to 40, then 20 mg after 4 weeks each, then to 15 mg after 4 weeks, 12.5 mg after 12 weeks, 10 after 14 weeks, then as with PMR). Clinical experience suggests that a small proportion of patients (perhaps 10–15 per cent) will require indefinite continuation of low dose treatment (5 mg or less daily) if symptoms are to be adequately controlled. In the quoted regimens the total dose of prednisolone for PMR is 6440 mg over 104 weeks, and for TA it is 11865 mg over 130 weeks.

All series reported some complications, including some patients with PMR who become more definite cases of TA while on treatment. The main pitfalls seem to be the use of too high a dose of glucocorticoids initially, with too rapid a reduction in treatment thereafter (Kirwan and Hosie 1994). One trial (Dasgupta et al. 1991) concluded that 3-weekly intramuscular injections of 120 mg methylprednisolone were better able to control PMR, but treatment was planned to last only 80 weeks, a substantially shorter period of treatment than recommended above. As a result only two-thirds of patients achieved remission, there were frequent relapses, and in more than half the patients glucocorticoids were still being taken at 96 weeks. The cause of symptoms in PMR does not seem to relate to signs of inflammation (Poutain and Hazleman 1995), so it is intriguing that glucocorticoids are so effective.

In a recent randomized, controlled trial in 42 patients with biopsy-proven, giant-cell arteritis, high initial doses of glucocorticoid were given, then tapered quickly, and withdrawn (Jover et al. 2001), while methotrexate or placebo was given weekly from the start for 24 months. The methotrexate reduced the high proportion of patients who relapsed (45 versus 84.2 per cent) but once again this study has a relatively high rate of relapse using a regimen that is clearly at substantially lower level of treatment (about 5000 mg prednisolone) than that recommended above.

High dose pulsed glucocorticoids in nephritis, vasculitis, and active RA

Pulse therapy involves the i.v. infusion of a large dose of glucocorticoid (usually 1 g of methylprednisolone) over a short time—perhaps 1–3 h. Current regimens use three pulses on alternate days, followed by a resting phase of around 6 weeks. Most also use immunosuppressive or cytotoxic agents such as azathioprine or cyclophosphamide. This treatment started in renal transplant recipients, but spread to other renal disorders, notably the nephritis of SLE (Rubinger et al. 1986). It is now used for severe vasculitis in any organ system associated with SLE, RA, or other vasculitides such as polyarteritis nodosa. There is a disappointing dearth of new clinical trials exploring the best regimens and measuring their true benefits. A few papers in the last 10 years deal with Wegener's granulomatosis (Guillevin et al. 1997), polyarteritis nodosa, Churg–Straus syndrome (Guillevin et al. 1995), and giant-cell arteritis (Chevalet et al. 2000). One regimen in current use follows:

Day 1: i.v. mesna 200 mg
i.v. cyclophosphamide 1000 mg in 500 ml normal saline over 1 h
i.v. methylprednisolone 1000 mg in 250 ml normal saline over 1 h
Oral mesna 400 mg 4 h after infusion
Oral mesna 400 mg 6 h after infusion
Day 3: i.v. methylprednisolone 1000 mg in 250 ml normal saline over 1 h
Day 5: i.v. methylprednisolone 1000 mg in 250 ml normal saline over 1 h
Continuing treatment.

But much more information from adequately controlled studies is required.

Pulsed methylprednisolone has also been used in severe RA to produce an early initial response, especially in patients commencing second-line agents, thus effectively bridging the gap between initiation and response with these agents. A review (Weusten et al. 1993) of the use of pulsed methylprednisolone stresses the impressive favourable risk–benefit ratio of this therapy with few or minor adverse effects. Most of the serious adverse effects—cardiovascular collapse, myocardial infarction, severe infection—have occurred in patients with compromised cardiovascular or immune systems as a result of their disease, or due to concomitant drug treatment. The minimal effective dose of methylprednisolone is uncertain at present. It has been reported that doses as low as 320 mg (Radia and Furst 1988), 250 mg (Vischer et al. 1986), or even 100 mg (Iglehart et al. 1990) may be as effective as 1 g, although others (Shipley et al. 1988) have concluded that using only 500 mg results in substantial loss of efficacy. If equivalent oral doses are as effective as i.v. treatment (Needs et al. 1988), this will allow pulsed treatment to become an outpatient procedure with reduced costs and less patient discomfort, although Choy et al. (1993) found that intramuscular methylprednisolone was superior to equivalent oral doses.

Reports of complications following pulse glucocorticoids therapy have usually arisen in renal transplant patients. Most important among these is sudden death, most probably arising as a result of ventricular dysrhythmia and consequent myocardial infarction. Nevertheless, the incidence appears to be extremely low, given that well over 10 000 renal transplant patients are likely to have been treated with pulse glucocorticoids. Other reported complications include transient arthralgias and synovitis, hyperglycaemia, pancreatitis, gastrointestinal bleeding, visual disturbance, acute psychosis, and severe infections.

Glucocorticoid treatment in moderate RA: reviewing the evidence

The management of RA concentrates on the control of joint inflammation, which is seen to be the cause of day-to-day symptoms and the gradually accumulating long-term joint damage that occurs in the majority of hospital patients with RA. Non-steroidal anti-inflammatory drugs (NSAIDs) provide the first line of treatment. Second line agents (also called specific, slow acting, or disease modifying antirheumatoid drugs) can reduce inflammation over weeks or months by unknown mechanism(s) of action.

The view clinicians take on the role of glucocorticoids in disease management is clouded by prejudice and failure to recognize current practice weaknesses. Initial euphoria at the success of glucocorticoid treatment in RA gave way to disillusionment as clinicians and the public became aware of the serious adverse effects that can occur with prolonged use of high doses. However, protests that glucocorticoid use should be limited were at odds with their actual widespread use (in up to 40 per cent of hospital outpatients with RA) (Criswell and Redfearn 1994).

The relatively short-term anti-inflammatory effect of glucocorticoids has recently been reviewed by Saag et al. (1996). It is clear that, over a few weeks, glucocorticoids have stronger anti-inflammatory effects than NSAIDs. These symptom-improving benefits wear off, however, an effect known since the earlier long-term clinical trials in RA (Joint Committee of the Medical Research Council and Nuffield Foundation 1954). However, of greater interest in a chronic condition such as RA are the medium- and long-term effects of treatment. The key to long term outcome must lie to some extent in the control of joint destruction, which accumulates over the years and is seen on radiographs as joint erosions. Much debate has focused on whether it is possible to sufficiently modify the natural history of RA to make a difference to long-term patient outcome (Scott et al. 1989). This is a difficult question but the clinical impression is that medical intervention does improve outcome measured by clinical, functional, and structural change. Whether and by how much joint damage can be prevented or reduced by glucocorticoids is an important question.

The immune dysfunction in RA is diffuse and glucocorticoids have the potential to influence it at various levels. It seems logical that an agent such as glucocorticoid, which has actions further 'upstream' in the pathological pathways than do NSAIDs, is more likely to prevent structural damage. In active inflammatory RA serum cortisol levels are reduced and the cortisol response during surgical stress is dampened compared with patients who have osteomyelitis, another chronic inflammatory condition (Chikanza et al. 1992). This raises the possibility that alterations in glucocorticoids action or control may play a more fundamental role in the development and progress of RA than previously thought.

Studies that address the progression of joint destruction have been few. In the early 1950s several attempts were made to define their role.

A study conducted by the Empire Rheumatism Council (1955) randomized 100 adult patients to receive cortisone (mean dose equivalent to 14 mg prednisolone) or aspirin (mean dose 4 g daily) for 2 years. On this occasion X-rays of the hands and feet were taken during the second half of the second year and showed a higher erosion score in the aspirin-treated patients (71 versus 49 per cent), although this did not reach statistical significance. There were no radiographs at entry so progression could not be estimated.

A third trial (Joint Committee of the Medical Research Council and Nuffield Foundation 1959) compared prednisolone with aspirin in 84 patients. The patients receiving prednisolone had a daily mean dose of 12 mg at the end of the first year and 10 mg at the end of the second year. Radiographs were obtained of the hands and feet initially and after 1 and 2 years of treatment, and radiographic progression was analysed by assessing a variety of rheumatoid changes including erosions. There were lower rates of progression in erosion scores in the prednisolone group as shown below:

	Prednisolone		Aspirin	
Time	Hands	Feet	Hands	Feet
1 year	17	12	49	44
2 years	41	10	72	71

During the third year, 5/26 (19 per cent) of patients in the analgesic group progressed but only 4/49 (8 per cent) in the prednisolone treated group did (Joint Committee of the Medical Research Council and Nuffield Foundation 1960). Four years later West (1967) was able to follow-up 74 of the original 77 patients who completed this study and reported that over 7 years only 9/39 (23 per cent) patients who had continued on prednisolone developed new erosions compared with 32/34 (94 per cent) patients who had continued on aspirin alone. Published in 1967, in a journal not readily accessible and with a title that did not indicate the nature of the findings, this paper went unnoticed until referenced by Masi (1983).

Meanwhile a variety of short term inconclusive studies were published which did not satisfactorily address the question of alteration in radiological progression (summarized in Table 1). Berntsen (Berntsen and Freyberg 1961) compared 183 RA patients on various glucocorticoids to patients already on gold ($n = 155$) or analgesics alone ($n = 50$). The period of follow-up was at least 5 years and radiological progression was present in both groups, leading the authors to conclude that glucocorticoids were no better than gold or analgesics. However, the formulations and doses of glucocorticoids varied widely, the control group(s) had not been randomized, and (in keeping with thinking at that time) glucocorticoids would have been used generally in more aggressive disease.

Three other randomized trials were published in 1981, 1983, and 1984 (Leibling et al. 1981; Harris et al. 1983; Million et al. 1984). The first showed no advantage for monthly intravenous methylprednisolone compared with placebo over a 6-month period. The second was a small study involving only 18 patients. The authors concluded that erosive progression was lesser in the prednisolone treated group compared with placebo over a 10-month period. The third study compared patients treated with prednisolone (mean dosage 10.3 mg daily) with those without prednisolone. This study included 103 patients followed up over a period of 120 months. The suggestion from this study was that the hand X-rays showed significantly lesser erosions in the prednisolone treated group. In a later study comparing pulse intravenous methylprednisolone with saline infusion, no long-term benefit was found in terms of clinical outcome or radiological progression (Hansen et al. 1990).

In 1986, Byron and Kirwan (1986) reviewed and re-analysed the results of both the 1959 MRC trial (Joint Committee of the Medical Research Council and Nuffield Foundation 1960) and the follow-up report by West (1967) and concluded that there was a good case for the potential of glucocorticoids therapy to reduce the rate of joint destruction. Subsequently, a multicentre trial (Kirwan and The ARC Low Dose Glucocorticoid Study Group 1995; Hickling et al. 1998) recruited 128 patients with RA of less than 2 years since diagnosis and compared placebo treatment with prednisolone 7.5 mg daily. Patients were allowed to continue on routine medication including second line agents. The patients treated with prednisolone had greater reductions than the placebo group in the number of inflamed joints (articular index) [Fig. 2(a)], pain, and disability during the first few months of the treatment, but were indistinguishable from them during the second year of treatment and after withdrawal of glucocorticoid therapy.

The development of erosions and radiological progression were assessed by changes in the Larsen score (Larsen et al. 1977). After 2 years the Larsen score had shown very little change in the prednisolone treated patients while the placebo group had substantial joint destruction ($P = 0.004$). This effect was lost during the 1 year blinded post-treatment follow-up [Fig. 2(b)]. In addition, the onset of erosions in non-erosive patients was

Table 1 Some randomized controlled trials of glucocorticoids in rheumatoid arthritis

Study	Year	Ref.	No. of patients	Treatment (mg/day)	Comparator	Duration (months)	Radiographic result	Comments
MRC	1954	Kirwan (1997)	61	Cortisone 80	Aspirin 4.5 g/d	12	Not assessed	Withdrawal flares
ERC	1955	Brook and Corbett (1977)	100	Cortisone 69	Aspirin 4 g/d	12	Non-significant but higher porosis and erosion scores in aspirin group	Erosion score could have been refined. If cut off taken at moderate to severe scores, cortisone did far better
MRC	1959	Wolfe et al. (1994) Saag et al. (1994)	77	Prednisolone 12 for year 1, 10 for year 2	Aspirin	36	Less after 1 and 2 years	Followed up for 3 years. Prednisolone probably held advantage into third year
Berntsen	1961	Laan et al. (1993)	183	Hydrocortisone 25–100	Analgesics, 50 I/M gold	>60	No difference (steroid group had better functional outcome)	Poorly matched, different doses and formulations, steroid group worse at start
West	1967	Fries et al. (1993)	74	Prednisolone <15	Aspirin	84	Less progression	10 mg better than 7.5 mg Publication not readily accessable
Liebling	1981	Sambrook et al. (1986)	10	Methyl-prednisolone 1 g/month	Placebo	6	No difference	Very few patients
Harris	1983	Adachi et al. (1994)	18	Prednisolone 5	Placebo and crossover at 24/52	10	Less progression in steroid group (and better functional outcome)	Very few patients
Million	1984	Klippel (2000)	103	Prednisolone 10.3	No steroids	120	Less erosions	Broad treatment comparison with contamination between groups
Hansen	1990	Breedveld et al. (2000)	97	Methyl-prednisolone 1 g i.v. monthly	IV saline	12	No difference in erosion scores	
ARC	1995	Byron and Kirwan (1986) Hickling et al. (1998)	128	Prednisolone 7.5	Placebo	24	Reduced erosive change	
COBRA	1997	Larsen et al. (1977)	155	Prednisolone, methotrexate, and sulfasalazine	Sulfasalazine	9, 11	Reduced erosive change	

reduced: 25.7 per cent on placebo versus 1.9 per cent on prednisolone. One can conclude that a fixed daily low dose of prednisolone (7.5 mg) can prevent radiological progression over 2 years in patients with early RA who are taking concomitant treatment with other second line agents.

In a study from the Netherlands [the COBRA study (Boers et al. 1997)], 76 test and 79 control patients received continuous sulfasalazine. Test subjects also took methotrexate for 40 weeks and prednisolone for 28 weeks. The daily prednisolone dose was 60 mg in week 1, 40 mg in week 2, 25 mg in week 3, 20 mg in week 4, 15 mg in week 5, 10 mg in week 6, and 7.5 mg thereafter. Both methotrexate and prednisolone were discontinued gradually. Erosive progression was prevented during the period of treatment with prednisolone and methotrexate, while patients on sulfasalazine alone more than doubled their erosion score. The benefits of the prednisolone seemed to persist for several weeks after treatment was discontinued, but erosive progression resumed between 56 and 80 weeks.

The report (Rau et al. 2000) of a double blind randomized controlled clinical trial by Rau and colleagues compared 5 mg of prednisolone with placebo in 196 patients with RA of only 2 years duration. All patients also received co-medication with auranofin or methotrexate. Using a modified Sharp method, erosions progressed three times faster in the control group compared to prednisolone.

With the exception of the very early ERC and MRC studies, all of the investigations reviewed above have been accompanied by the concomitant use of disease modifying antirheumatic agents. Thus, it has been difficult to discern the independent effects of glucocorticoids. The most recent randomized controlled trial, by van Everdingen and colleagues (2000), tested prednisolone (10 mg daily) without second line therapy for up to 2 years. This reduced the rate of radiological progression by half.

As most of the studies summarized here included patients of similar severity and disease duration, it is reasonable to directly compare their results. Fig. 3(a) shows such a comparison, based on the proportionate change from baseline. The cumulative magnitude and consistency of these findings supports a significant protective effect of glucocorticoids on joint destruction.

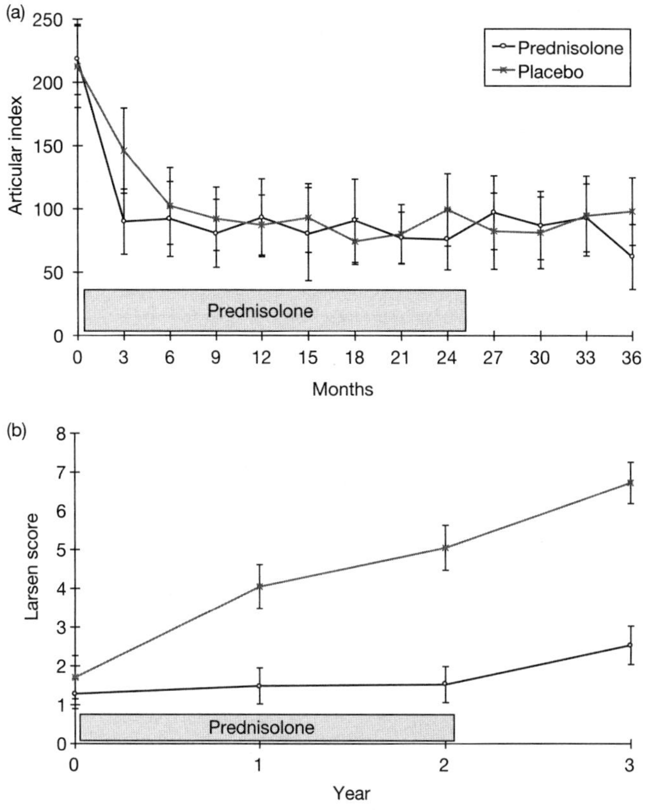

Fig. 2 (a) Mean (95% CI) articular index for 75 patients with radiographs at all time points. The difference between groups is significant at 3 months only. (b) Mean (95% CI) Larsen score after log transformation for 75 patients with radiographs at all time points. The difference between groups is significant at 1, 2, and 3 years.

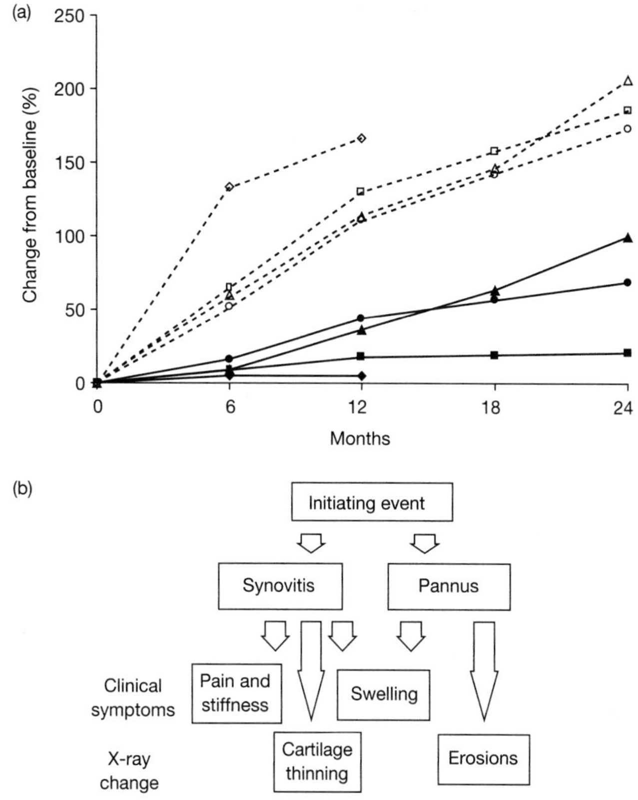

Fig. 3 (a) Proportion change in erosion scores in four trials of prednisolone in RA. Results are from Kirwan (1995) [■, □], Boers et al. (1997) [◆, ◇], van Everdingen et al. (2002) [▲, △], and Wassenberg (1999) [●, ○] [Broken line = placebo, solid line = prednisolone]. (b) A model of rheumatoid arthritis consistent with the currently available data.

Implications of long-term glucocorticoid treatment response for disease pathology

An important observation made in several of these studies is that, compared to the placebo group, any beneficial reduction in the symptoms of synovitis was evident only for 6–9 months. In contrast, control of radiological progression was evident for the whole period of treatment.

This observation does not fit well with the traditional model of RA in which erosive change is a direct consequence of synovitis. Evidence is now accumulating that the process of synovitis is T-cell driven while that of cartilage and bone destruction may be more macrophage mediated (Bresnihan et al. 1995). Thus, the causative link between synovitis and erosions is less convincing. A re-analysis of some of the data from the ARC study demonstrated (Kirwan et al. 1997) that the correlation between the ongoing presence of synovitis and erosive progression in individual joints of the hand was weak ($r = 0.248$) and explained only 6 per cent of the variance in measurements. These findings argue against there being a direct causal relationship between synovitis and erosions. A model of RA that can accommodate these observations is shown in Fig. 3(b). This model is open to a variety of tests, such as finding out whether synovial histological correlates with clinical progression, whether joint space narrowing and erosions are dissociated in clinical studies, whether other differential treatment effects can be demonstrated, and whether there are different risk factors and prognostic indicators for erosive and non-erosive disease.

Logical treatment strategies for glucocorticoids in RA

There are certain situations in which glucocorticoids may be the preferred treatment for symptom control. Owing to their relatively good safety profile glucocorticoids may be used during arthritic flares in pregnancy. Low-dose prednisolone may be a preferable alternative to NSAIDs in the elderly in order to avoid aggravation of renal or cardiac failure. The use of high-dose glucocorticoids in systemic and vasculitic crises is widely practised (see above). From the evidence reviewed above, there is a case for using 7.5 mg prednisolone to treat some patients with RA in the early years of their disease (Table 2). Treating non-erosive patients more than 3 years after diagnosis will result in no benefit, as such patients are extremely unlikely to develop radiological change (Brook and Corbett 1977). The published findings for radiological protection could reasonably be extrapolated into the fourth and fifth years of disease, but further extension of these findings would be difficult to justify without additional evidence of efficacy.

Adverse effects of glucocorticoid treatment in inflammatory arthritis

There are many well-documented adverse effects of glucocorticoids taken in moderate to high doses for many months or years (Table 3). Perhaps the main concern is the possible accumulation of adverse effects with low doses of

Table 2 Evidence based policy for selecting and treating patients with prednisolone 7.5 mg daily to reduce the progression of erosions in RA. Patients should have active inflammatory disease and all other treatment modalities should be used as clinically indicated. Discontinuation of therapy should be by rapid tapering off. One suitable regimen is alternate-day treatment for 2 weeks then every third day for 2 weeks, then stop (Kirwan et al. 1995; Hickling et al. 1998)

Radiographic findings at time of decision	Disease duration			
	<2 years	2–3 years	3–4 years	>4 years
Erosions	Treat with prednisolone 7.5 mg daily for approximately 4 years	Treat with prednisolone 7.5 mg daily for approximately 2 years	Treat with prednisolone 7.5 mg daily for approximately 2 years	Do not treat until more evidence is available
No erosions	Treat with prednisolone 7.5 mg daily for approximately 4 years	Treat with prednisolone 7.5 mg daily for approximately 2 years	Do not treat	Do not treat

Table 3 Adverse effects of systemic glucocorticoid therapy

Metabolic	Obesity Glucose/protein metabolism Electrolyte imbalance Enzyme induction
Predisposition to infection	
Musculoskeletal	Myopathy Osteoporosis Osteonecrosis Tendon rupture Glucocorticoid withdrawal syndrome
Gastrointestinal	Peptic ulcer disease Pancreatitis
Ophthalmic	Cataract Glaucoma
Central nervous system	Psychosis Depression Benign intracranial hypertension
Dermatologic	Acne Striae Alopecia Bruising Skin atrophy
Growth retardation	
Hypothalamic–pituitary–adrenal axis suppression	

glucocorticoids spread over many years, where the information available is far less clear in its implications. Because studies of glucocorticoid toxicity in RA tend to be retrospective and observational their ability to differentiate bad outcomes attributable to glucocorticoids from those occurring due to RA or other co-morbidities is limited. The picture is further complicated by the use of glucocorticoids at different times in the disease course, limited data defining the 'threshold' dose for particular adverse events and toxicity reports covering heterogeneous groups of diseases that may not extrapolate to RA.

Data from the Arthritis Rheumatism and Aging Medical Information System (ARAMIS) database, suggests a 1.5-fold increased risk of mortality for glucocorticoid-treated patients was seen when compared with controls (hazards ratio ranging from 1.3 to 1.6) (Wolfe et al. 1994). In a recent study, (Saag et al. 1994) even after statistical adjustment for significant disease severity factors such as the presence of rheumatoid nodules and bony erosions, average prednisone dose was the strongest predictor of a serious AE potentially attributable to glucocorticoid therapy [odds ratio (OR) = 4.5 for 5 to 10 mg, 95 per cent confidence interval (CI) 2.1–9.6 and OR = 32.3 for 10–15 mg, 95 per cent CI 4.6–220 per cent]. It seems reasonable to conclude that, over and above the reduced life expectancy due to RA alone, glucocorticoid toxicity probably does include an element of increased mortality in the long term. The confounding effects of patient selection, physician bias, and co-morbidity will continue to make it difficult to estimate the risk precisely.

However, compared with other antirheumatic agents, glucocorticoids have a low incidence of short-term symptomatic toxicity and patients uncommonly discontinue therapy for these reasons (Fries et al. 1993). There has been some debate about the potential for an exacerbation of disease following cessation of glucocorticoid treatment. However, in a blind randomized follow-up of withdrawal from 7.5 mg prednisolone daily for 2 years there was no evidence of any change in disease status (Hickling et al. 1998).

Many long-term, high-dose adverse effects have been identified and some of these may be relevant in the treatment of RA. Most immediate concern is centred on the emergence of adverse effects during medium- or long-term low-dose therapy, which fall broadly into four categories: infections, peptic ulceration, osteoporosis, and atherosclerosis (Saag and Kirwan 2001). For the first two, the evidence is probably against any major association, although glucocorticoids may exacerbate the ulcerogenic properties of NSAIDs. The evidence linking glucocorticoid therapy with atherosclerosis falls far short of proof, but if true, even a small effect would have considerable clinical significance. The bone loss associated with glucocorticoid therapy principally effects trabecular bone. Studies using photon absorptiometric measurement of bone mineral density have shown that bone loss is greater in the lumbar spine, less in the proximal femur, and least in the forearm. Studies of bone loss in patients treated with glucocorticoids do not clearly suggest a threshold dose below which osteoporosis can be avoided. Bone loss has been reported with prednisolone doses of 10 mg daily, reducing to zero over 20 weeks (Laan et al. 1993). Other studies suggest maintenance of bone stock on doses up to 7.5 mg daily (Sambrook et al. 1986). There appears to be a consistent relationship between doses above 7.5 mg daily and rate of bone loss.

RA patients on glucocorticoids tend to have more severe disease and as such are at greater risk of osteoporosis due to the disease itself and the associated functional disability. The improved function resulting from glucocorticoid treatment would reduce the rate of bone loss because of increased functional activity, which has a positive effect on bone density. Finally, even if low-dose glucocorticoid treatment does cause increased bone loss in RA it is not entirely clear how this translates into clinically important fractures. Treatment with bisphosphonates and/or hormone replacement therapy may retard bone loss with the potential to reduce the frequency of fractures (Adachi et al. 1994).

One reasonable approach allowing for bone and cardiovascular complications may be to avoid prescribing glucocorticoids in patients at high risk of serious adverse effects. These include: thin, frail, elderly women; patients with a history of serious cardiovascular disease (ischaemic heart disease, hypercholesterolaemia, and hypertension); and those with poorly controlled diabetes.

Research agenda and recent developments

The exciting clinical and scientific observations reviewed above provide evidence for clinical efficacy and raise issues related to disease pathology, how it responds to glucocorticoid therapy, and whether this response might be related to specific mechanisms of action in different diseases and at different glucocorticoid doses. A suggested research agenda (Saag and Kirwan 2001) includes: are there different mechanisms of action related to effects on inflammation and joint destruction? Can the mechanisms responsible for the beneficial effects of glucocorticoids be separated from those causing the adverse effects? Is there action in the central nervous system that explains the 'sense of well-being' induced in some patients? Will low-dose glucocorticoids reduce radiologic progression is patients with disease duration greater than 4 years? What is the most effective time in the circadian variation of RA to administer glucocorticoids? What dose reducing strategies will be most effective?

All these questions are open to direct investigation, and answering them will elucidate disease mechanisms as well as improve treatment strategies. The suppression of joint destruction as also been an aim of new 'biological' therapies (Klippel 2000), currently centred on inhibition of the effects of TNFα. Reports of rapid clinical responsiveness and delayed radiographic progression are strikingly similar to the findings with glucocorticoid therapy combined with traditional antirheumatoid treatments, such as methotrexate. The costs and potential adverse effects (Breedveld et al. 2000) of biological therapies are likely to be much greater than those for glucocorticoid treatment, and it will be of interest to discover which treatment strategies will be most cost-effective.

References

Adachi, J.D. et al. (1994). Intermittent cyclic therapy with etidronate in the prevention of glucocorticoid induced bone loss. *Journal of Rheumatology* **21** (10), 192.

Baxter, H.D. and Forssham, P.H. (1972). Tissue effects of glucocorticoids. *American Journal of Medicine* **53**, 573–89.

Berntsen, C.A. and Freyberg, R.H. (1961). Rheumatoid patients after five or more years of glucocorticoid treatment: a comparative analysis of 183 cases. *Annals of Internal Medicine* **54**, 938–53.

Boers, M. et al. (1997). Randomised comparison of combined step down prednisolone, methotrexate and sulphasalazine with sulphasalazine alone in early rheumatoid arthritis. *Lancet* **350**, 309–18.

Breedveld, F., Bresnihan, B., Maini, R., van Riel, P., and Symmons, D. (2000). Proposal to establish a register for the long term surveillance of adverse events in patients with rheumatic diseases exposed to biological agents. *Annals of the Rheumatic Diseases* **59**, 419–20.

Bresnihan, B., Mulherin, D., and FitzGerald, O. (1995). Synovial pathology and articular erosions in rheumatoid arthritis. *Rheumatology in Europe* **24** (Suppl. 2), 158–60.

Brook, A. and Corbett, M. (1977). Radiographic change in early rheumatoid disease. *Annals of the Rheumatic Diseases* **36**, 71–3.

Buttgereit, F., Wehling, M., and Burmester, G.R. (1998). A new hypothesis of modular glucocorticoid actions. Glucocorticoid treatment of rheumatic diseases revisited. *Arthritis and Rheumatism* **41**, 761–7.

Buttgerit, F., da Silva, J., Boers, M., Burmester, G., Cutolo, M., Jacobs, J., Kirwan, J., Köhler, L., van Riel, P., Vischer, J., and Bijlsma, J.W.J. (2002). Standardised nomenclature for glucocorticoid dosages and glucocorticoid treatment regimens: current questions and tentative answers in rheumatology. *Annals of the Rheumatic Diseases* **61**, 718–22.

Byron, M.A. and Kirwan, J.R. (1986). Corticosteroids in rheumatoid arthritis: is a trial of their 'disease modifying' potential feasible? *Annals of the Rheumatic Diseases* **46**, 171–3.

Chevalet, P., Barrier, J.H., Pottier, P., Magadur-Joly, G., Pottier, M.A., Hamidou, M., Planchon, B., El Kouri, D., Connan, L., Dupond, J.L., De Wazieres, B., Dien, G., Duhamel, E., Grosbois, B., Jego, P., Le Strat, A., Capdeville, J., Letellier, P., and Agron, L. (2000). A randomized, multicenter, controlled trial using intravenous pulses of methylprednisolone in the initial treatment of simple forms of giant cell arteritis: a one year followup study of 164 patients. *Journal of Rheumatology* **27**, 1484–91.

Chikanza, I.C., Petrou, P., Kingsley, G., Chrousos, G., and Panayi, G.S. (1992). Defective hypothalamic response to immune and inflammatory stimuli in patients with rheumatoid arthritis. *Arthritis and Rheumatism* **35**, 1281–8.

Choy, E.H.S., Kingsley, G., Corkhill, M.M., and Panayi, G.S. (1993). Intramuscular methylprednisolone is superior to pulse oral methylprednisolone during the induction phase of chrysotherapy. *British Journal of Rheumatology* **32**, 734–9.

Cowell, A.M. and Buckingham, J.C. (2001). Glucocorticoids and the HPA axis. In *Milestones in Drug Therapy: Glucocorticoids* (ed. N.G. Goulding and R.J. Flower), pp. 129–45. Basel: Birkhauser Verlag.

Criswell, L.A. and Redfearn, W.J. (1994). Variation among rheumatologists in the use of prednisolone and second-line agents for the treatment of rheumatoid arthritis. *Arthritis and Rheumatism* **37**, 476–80.

Dasgupta, B., Gray, J., Fernandes, L., and Olliff, C. (1991). Treatment of polymyalgia rheumatica with intramuscular injections of methylprednisolone. *Annals of the Rheumatic Diseases* **50**, 942–5.

Delecoeuillerie, G., Joly, P., de Lara, A.C., and Paolaggi, J.B. (1988). Polymyalgia rheumatica and temporal arteritis: a retrospective analysis of prognostic features and different corticosteroid regimens (11 year survey of 210 patients). *Annals of the Rheumatic Diseases* **47**, 733–9.

Empire Rheumatism Council (1955). Multi-centre controlled trial comparing cortisone acetate and acetyl salicylic acid in the long-term treatment of rheumatoid arthritis. *Annals of the Rheumatic Diseases* **14**, 353–67.

van Everdingen, A.A., Jacobs, J.W.G., van Reesema, D.R.S., and Bijlsma, W.J. (2002). Low-dose prednisone therapy for patients with early active rheumatoid arthritis: Clinical efficacy, disease-modifying properties, and side effects. *Annals of Internal Medicine* **136**, 1–12.

Fries, J.F. et al. (1993). The relative toxicity of disease-modifying antirheumatic drugs. *Arthritis and Rheumatism* **36**, 297–306.

Goulding, N.J. and Fowler, R.J. (2001). Glucocorticoid biology—a molecular maze and clinical challenge. In *Milestones in Drug Therapy: Glucocorticoids.* (ed. N.G. Goulding and R.J. Flower), pp. 3–16. Basel: Birkhauser Verlag.

Guillevin, L., Lhote, F., Cohen, P., Jarrousse, B., Lortholary, O., Genereau, T., Leon, A., and Bussel, A. (1995). Corticosteroids plus pulse cyclophosphamide and plasma exchanges versus corticosteroids plus pulse cyclophosphamide alone in the treatment of polyarteritis nodosa and Churg–Strauss syndrome patients with factors predicting poor prognosis. A prospective, randomized trial in sixty-two patients. *Arthritis and Rheumatism* **38**, 1638–45.

Guillevin, L., Cordier, J.F., Lhote, F., Cohen, P., Jarrousse, B., Royer, I., Lesavre, P., Jacquot, C., Bindi, P., Bielefeld, P., Desson, J.F., Detree, F., Dubois, A., Hachulla, E., Hoen, B., Jacomy, D., Seigneuric, C., Lauque, D., Stern, M., and Longy-Boursier, M. (1997). A prospective, multicenter, randomized trial comparing steroids and pulse cyclophosphamide versus steroids and oral cyclophosphamide in the treatment of generalized Wegener's granulomatosis. *Arthritis and Rheumatism* **40**, 2187–98.

Hansen, T.M., Kryger, P., Elling, H., Haar, D., Kreutzfeldt, M., IngemanNielsan, M.W., Olsson, A.T., Pedersen, C., Rahbek, A., Tvede, N., and Winge, J. (1990). Double blind placebo controlled trial of pulse treatment with methylprednisolone combined with disease modifying drugs in rheumatoid arthritis. *British Medical Journal* **301**, 268–70.

Hansen, M. et al. (1999). A randomised trial of differentiated prednisolone treatment in active rheumatoid arthritis: Clinical benefits and skeletal side effects. *Annals of the Rheumatic Diseases* **58**, 713–18.

Harbuz, M. and Jessop, D. (1999). Is there a defect in cortisol production in rheumatoid arthritis? *Rheumatology* **38**, 298–302.

Harris, E.D., Jr. et al. (1983). Low dose prednisolone therapy in rheumatoid arthritis: a double blind study. *Journal of Rheumatology* **10**, 713–21.

Hench, P.S. et al. (1949). Effects of a hormone of the adrenal cortex (17-hydroxy-11 dehydrocorticosterone: compound E) and of pituitary adrenocorticotrophic hormone on rheumatoid arthritis. Preliminary report. *Proceedings of Staff Meetings of Mayo Clinic* **24**, 181–97.

Hickling, P., Jacoby, R.K., Kirwan, J.R. and The Arthritis and Rheumatism Council Low-Dose Glucocorticoid Study Group (1998). Joint destruction after glucocorticoids are withdrawn in early rheumatoid arthritis. *British Journal of Rheumatology* **37**, 930–6.

Iglehart, I.W., III, Sutton, J.D., Bender, J.C., Shaw, R.A., Ziminski, C.M., Holt, P.A., Hochberg, M.C., Zizic, T.M., Engle, E.W., and Stevens, M.B. (1990). Intravenous pulsed steroids in rheumatoid arthritis: a comparative dose study. *Journal of Rheumatology* **17**, 159–62.

Joint Committee of the Medical Research Council and Nuffield Foundation (1954). A comparison of cortisone and aspirin in the treatment of early cases of rheumatoid arthritis. *British Medical Journal* **29**, 1223–7.

Joint Committee of the Medical Research Council and Nuffield Foundation (1959). A comparison of prednisolone with aspirin or other analgesics in the treatment of rheumatoid arthritis. *Annals of the Rheumatic Diseases* **18**, 173–87.

Joint Committee of the Medical Research Council and Nuffield Foundation (1960). A comparison of prednisolone with aspirin or other analgesics in the treatment of rheumatoid arthritis. *Annals of the Rheumatic Diseases* **19**, 331–7.

Jover, J.A., Hernandez-Garcia, C., Morado, I.C., Vargas, E., Banares, A., and Fernandez-Gutierrez, B. (2001). Combined treatment of giant-cell arteritis with methotrexate and prednisone. a randomized, double-blind, placebo-controlled trial. *Annals of Internal Medicine* **134**, 106–14.

Kirwan, J.R. (1997). The relationship between synovitis and erosions in rheumatoid arthritis. *British Journal of Rheumatology* **36**, 225–8.

Kirwan, J.R. and Hosie, G. (1994). Management policies for polymyalgia rheumatica. *British Journal of Rheumatology* **33**, 690–1.

Kirwan, J.R. and The ARC Low Dose Glucocorticoid Study Group (1995). The effect of glucocorticoids on joint destruction in rheumatoid arthritis. *New England Journal of Medicine* **333** (3), 142–6.

Klippel, J. (2000). Biologic therapy for rheumatoid arthritis. *New England Journal of Medicine* **343**, 1640–1.

Kyle, V. and Hazleman, B.L. (1989). Treatment of polymyalgia rheumatica and giant cell arteritis. II. Relation between steroid dose and steroid associated side effects. *Annals of the Rheumatic Diseases* **48**, 662–6.

Laan, R.F.J.M., Van Reil, P.L.C.M., van de Putte, L.B.A., van Erning, L.J.T.O., van't Hof, M.A., and Lemmens, J.A.M. (1993). Low dose prednisolone induces rapid reversible axial bone loss in patients with rheumatoid arthritis: a randomised controlled study. *Annals of Internal Medicine* **119**, 963–8.

Larsen, A., Dale, K., and Eek, M. (1977). Radiographic evaluation of rheumatoid arthritis and related conditions by standard reference films. *Acta Radiologica* **18**, 481–91.

Leibling, M.R., Leib, E., and McLaughlin K. (1981). Pulse methyl-prednisolone in rheumatoid arthritis. *Annals of Internal Medicine* **4**, 21–6.

Lundberg, I. and Hedfors, E. (1990). Restricted dose and duration of corticosteroid treatment in patients with polymyalgia rheumatica and temporal arteritis. *Journal of Rheumatology* **17**, 1340–5.

Masi, A.T. (1983). Low dose glucocorticoid therapy in rheumatoid arthritis. *Journal of Rheumatology* **10**, 675–8.

Million, R. et al. (1984). Long-term study of management of rheumatoid arthritis. *Lancet* **1**, 812–16.

Needs, C.J. et al. (1988). Comparison of methylprednisolone (1 gram IV) with prednisolone (1 gram orally) in rheumatoid arthritis: a pharmokinetic and clinical study. *Journal of Rheumatology* **15**, 224–8.

Oakley, R.H. and Cidlowski, J.A. (2001). The glucocorticoid receptor: expression, function, and regulation of glucocorticoid responsiveness. In *Milestones in Drug Therapy: Glucocorticoids* (ed. N.G. Goulding and R.J. Flower), pp. 55–80. Basel: Birkhauser Verlag.

Poutain, G. and Hazleman, B. (1995). ABC of Rheumatology: polymyalgia rheumatica and giant cell arteritis. *British Medical Journal* **310**, 1057–9.

Radia, M. and Furst, D.E. (1988). Comparison of three pulse methylprednisolone regimens in the treatment of rheumatoid arthritis. *Journal of Rheumatology* **15**, 242–56.

Rau, R., Wassenberg, S., Zeidler H., and LDPT-Study Group (2000). Low dose prednisolone therapy (LDPT) retards radiographically detectable destruction in early rheumatoid arthritis—preliminary results of a multicenter, randomized, parallel, double blind study. *Zeitschrift für Rheumatologie* **59** (Suppl. 2), II/90–6.

Rubinger, D., Drukker, A., Shvil, Y., Kopolovic, Y., Friedlaender, M.M., Shalit, M., and Popovtzer, M.M. (1986). Combined cyclophosphamide and corticosteroid-induced remission in severe glomerulopathy associated with systemic vasculitis. *American Journal of Nephrology* **6**, 346–52.

Saag, K.G. and Kirwan, J.R. (2001). Glucocorticoid therapy in rheumatoid arthritis. In *Modern Therapeutics of Rheumatoid Disease* (ed. G.C. Tsokos). New Jersey, USA: Humana Press.

Saag, K.G. et al. (1994). Low dose long-term corticosteroid therapy in rheumatoid arthritis: an analysis of serious adverse events. *American Journal of Medicine* **96**, 115–23.

Saag, K.G., Criswell, L.A., Sems, K.M., Nettleman, M.D., and Kolluri, S. (1996). Low-dose corticosteroids in rheumatoid arthritis. A meta-analysis of their moderate-term effectiveness. *Arthritis and Rheumatism* **39**, 1818–25.

Salvarini, C. et al. (1987). Polymyalgia rheumatica and giant cell arteritis: a 5-year rpidemiologic and clinical study in Reggio Emilia, Italy. *Clinical and Experimental Rheumatology* **5**, 205–15.

Sambroook, P.N., Eisman, J.A., Yeates, M.G., Pocock, N.A., Eberl, S., and Champion, G.D. (1986). Osteoporosis in rheumatoid arthritis: safety of low dose corticosteroids. *Annals of the Rheumatic Diseases* **45**, 950–3.

Scott, D.L., Spector, T.D., Pullar, T., and McConkey, B. (1989). What should we hope to achieve when treating rheumatoid arthritis? *Annals of the Rheumatic Diseases* **48**, 256–61.

Shipley, M.E., Bacon, P.A., Berry, H., Hazleman, B.L., Sturrock, R.D., Swinson, D.R., and Williams, I.A. (1988). Pulsed methylprednisolone in active early rheumatoid disease. A dose ranging study. *British Journal of Rheumatology* **15**, 211–14.

Vischer, T.L., Sinniger, M., Ott, H., and Gerster, J.C. (1986). A randomized, double-blind trial comparing a pulse of 1000 with 250 mg methylprednisolone in rheumatoid arthritis. *Clinical Rheumatololgy* **5**, 325–6.

Wassenberg, S., Rau, R., and Zeidler, H. (1999). Low dose prednisolone therapy (LDPT) retards radiographically detectable destruction in early rheumatoid arthritis. *Arthritis and Rheumatism* **42** (Suppl.), S243.

West, H.F. (1967). Rheumatoid arthritis. The relevance of clinical knowledge to research activities. *Abstracts of World Medicine* **41**, 401–17.

Wolfe, F. et al. (1994). The mortality of rheumatoid arthritis. *Arthritis and Rheumatism* **37**, 481–94.

Weusten, B.L.A.M., Jacobs, J.W.G., and Bijlsma, J.W.J. (1993). Corticosteroid pulse therapy in active rheumatoid arthritis. *Seminars in Arthritis and Rheumatism* **23**, 183–92.

4.5.3 Immunosuppressive and other drugs—monotherapy versus combination therapy

Ferdinand C. Breedveld and Edward C. Keystone

Introduction

The active search for new treatment modalities of established rheumatoid arthritis (RA) has created a dynamic period for rheumatology. Both innovative application of established disease-modifying antirheumatic drugs (DMARDs) and the availability of targeted interventions with products of the biotechnology industry have improved therapeutic results. Targeted therapies with novel small molecules are expected to further improve these results. Like all new therapeutic strategies much remains to be learned about their optimal use and possible limitations. Experience suggests that a complex disease like RA can be brought under control and that the knowledge about the pathogenetic pathways obtained with the targeted therapies will be a stimulus for further drug development.

The motivation to develop new treatments for RA may be explained, in part, by three developments over the last decade: accurate description of the natural history of RA; availability of improved DMARDs; and, above all, the recognition that partial control of inflammation with an effective DMARD does not prevent joint damage (Pincus et al. 1999). Most patients with RA and seen in clinical settings have persistent inflammatory symmetrical arthritis that has not responded adequately to traditional therapies. It is recognized that patients monitored upto the 1980s experienced poor long-term outcomes, including radiographic progression, joint deformity, functional declines, work disability, joint replacement surgery, high costs, extra-articular disease, and premature mortality (Pincus et al. 1994). Furthermore, it was realized that many patients develop irreversible radiographic joint damage in the first years of the disease, which emphasizes the need for preventive treatment strategies (Drossaers-Bakker et al. 1999).

Descriptions of the natural history of RA include the results of its therapy. Continuous treatment with DMARDs does ameliorate the course of RA, including retardation of radiographic progression, but rarely induces sustained remission. Furthermore, contemporary DMARDs such as methotrexate (MTX) and sulfasalazine have a considerable greater efficacy/toxicity ratio than traditional agents such as gold salts, penicillamine, and azathioprine. MTX emerged as an important DMARD during the 1990s with long-term effectiveness and acceptable toxicities compared to other treatments (Weinblatt et al. 1998). Nonetheless, sustained remission is unusual and, therefore, many physicians started to propose combination DMARD therapy.

The emphasis in RA clinical research has been directed towards the measurement of inflammatory activity such as joint scores and acute phase response. Control of inflammatory activity is regarded as an effective strategy to improve long-term outcome although few studies are available to assess how completely inflammation can be controlled. Several studies reported that some improvement in joint scores, global severity scores, and acute phase response can be paralleled by significant progression of functional disability (Mulherin et al. 1996). Taken together, these observations provide powerful arguments that new therapeutic principles have to be developed for RA, particularly in early disease when drug therapy might prevent long-term damage.

During the past decade much progress has also been made with regard to understanding mechanisms leading to tissue destruction in RA. Based on this increasing knowledge, therapeutic principles have been developed with novel biological agents that act more specifically by targeting immune processes considered to be essential in RA. Table 1 gives an overview of the biological therapies already investigated in patients with RA. The overall aetiology of RA cannot be described more precisely than that it is the interaction of a genetically susceptible host with an unidentified external inflammatory stimulus (Feldmann et al. 1996). Therefore, a disease-specific therapy is not at present realistic. Targeted therapies follow the most recent knowledge of the pathophysiology of a disease, which is dynamic given the rapid improvement in gaining knowledge in cell biology and inflammation. All interventions that were investigated in the clinic have shown efficacy in animal models of arthritis. Arthritis is mediated by a vast array of cells and soluble factors that recruit more cells at the site of inflammation. T-lymphocytes, particularly those with a memory CD4+ phenotype, accumulate. Typically, for an autoimmune reaction these cells show a T-helper 1 cytokine production profile (Dolhain et al. 1996). Such cytokines activate signalling pathways in target cells that lead to gene activation and effector functions. The end result is that resident synovial macrophages, mast cells, and endothelial cells, which together with blood derived cells such as B-lymphocytes and neutrophils, maintain a state of chronic inflammation.

Activated cells produce a wide array of mediators such as cytokines, chemokinase, and destructive enzymes that also contribute to the creation of typical hypertrophic and destructive synovial inflammation in RA. Observations of the presence of such components in the rheumatoid inflammation and insight into the biological significance motivated the development of new therapies.

Table 1 Biological interventions investigated in RA

Cell surface directed therapy
Anti-CD3 mAb, anti-CD4 mAb, anti-CD5 mAb, anti-CD7 mAb, anti-CD25 mAb, anti-CD52 mAb, anti-CD28 mAb, IL-2 fusion protein, anti-ICAM-1, CTLA4Ig (CD86 binding)
Cytokine targeted therapy
TNF antagonists (mAb, soluble TNF receptor)
IL-1-receptor antagonist
IL-6 antagonist (mAb against IL-6 or IL-6 receptor)
Administration of cytokines (IL-4, IL-10, IFN-gamma and -beta)
Tolerance induction
Application of antigens (collagen II, HCGP-39)
T cell or T cell receptor vaccination
Interference with T cell activation (CTLA-4-Iγ)
Inhibition of chemokines
Inhibition of complement activation
High-dose intravenous immunoglobulins
Plasmapheresis, immunoadsorption column
Autologous bone marrow transplantation

These developments were also made possible by the rapid developments in biotechnology. Monoclonal antibodies (mAbs) are produced by a single clone of B-cells, are monospecific, and thereby effective tools for therapies and diagnostics (Breedveld 2000). The conventional route to derive mAbs is to immunize mice and grow the selected hybridomas in laboratory animals. Now, various systems for *in vitro* mAb production are being developed that allow large-scale production for therapeutic use. The phage display technique now allows the selection and production at a high level without using animals as intermediates. Furthermore, recombinant engineering techniques have emerged that permit the construction of mAbs customized with respect to the binding site but with possible variations in size and effector function. This design flexibility resulted in the development of chimeric humanized and now fully human mAbs.

Tumour necrosis factor (TNF) and interleukin (IL)-1 with their broad spectrum of biological activities were, together with T cells, the first targets selected for biological therapy in RA (Arend and Dayer 1995; Feldmann et al. 1997; Breeveld 2000). Both cytokines are actively produced at the synovial site of inflammation in RA. Several biological activities of TNF overlap with those of IL-1. Both stimulate metalloproteinase (MTX) and PGE_2 production by synovial fibroblasts. This effect, together with the suppression of synthesis of matrix components by mesenchymal cells and the activation of osteoclasts, explains their capacity to promote cartilage and bone destruction. TNF and IL-1 are also potent activators of endothelial cells with the promotion of adhesion molecule expression and subsequent leucocyte transmigration into tissues. They also stimulate the production of other cytokines and chemokines, increase phagocytic function of leucocytes, and stimulate proliferation of fibroblasts and endothelial cells.

TNF, IL-1, and other proinflammatory cytokines exert their effect on many cells and their activity is controlled by many cells and molecules. At the time when the trials on TNF and IL-1 inhibition were designed there was fear that blockage of one molecule would not provide results of substantial biological effects. However, the results of a substantial number of clinical trials have now led to the conclusion that such fears were unjustified.

TNF antagonists in RA

Administration of a chimeric monoclonal antibody, infliximab (Remicade™), which binds to TNF specifically and neutralizes its activity, was found to be of substantial clinical benefit in RA. Infliximab is a chimeric mAb that consists of the variable regions of a murine mAb linked to a human IgG1 molecule. Infliximab has a high affinity for TNF and has been shown to inhibit both secreted and cell-associated TNF (Arend and Dayer 1995). Preliminary open-label studies in patients with refractory disease attending the Charing Cross Hospital in London showed a remarkable and direct clinical improvement and substantial improvement of biochemical and histological parameters of disease activity (Feldmann et al. 1997). In the first randomized trial a single infusion of 1 or 10 mg/kg infliximab was compared with placebo in 73 patients (Elliot et al. 1994). After 4 weeks, 8 per cent of the placebo recipients fulfilled the response criteria compared to 44 and 79 per cent of the patients treated with low and high doses respectively. The medium duration of the response in the high-dose group was 8 weeks, which could directly be related to the persistence of the circulating infliximab with its half-life of ±10 days. In a second controlled trial infliximab in combination with a fixed dose of MTX in RA patients with active disease showed enhanced degree and duration of efficacy (Maini et al. 1998). In the largest trial published till date 428 patients with active RA despite treatment with MTX were randomized to placebo or one of four regimens of infliximab given every 4 or 8 weeks intravenously in a background of a stable dose of MTX. At 30 weeks response criteria were achieved in 52–58 per cent of patients receiving infliximab compared with 20 per cent of patients receiving placebo plus MTX (Maini et al. 1999). The anti-inflammatory effect as well as the improvements in physical function and parameters of quality of life persisted when the patients were studied after 2 years (Lipsky et al. 2000a). Most remarkable was the analysis of joint X-rays taken after 1 year of treatment (Lipsky et al. 2000b). The median scores for joint space narrowing and bone erosion on X-rays of hands and feet progressed in the placebo and MTX-treated group, but was unchanged in the infliximab-treated group.

Three other TNF binding antibodies are under clinical development. CDP571 was studied in dosages upto 10 mg/kg in 36 patients with active RA (Rankin et al. 1995). The best effects were seen in patients receiving the highest dose. CDP870 is a pegylated humanized Fab fragment produced by *Escherichia coli*. With the addition of two PEG chains a half-life of 12–15 days is obtained. In a dose-finding randomized controlled trial 200 patients with severe RA were treated with subcutaneous (s.c.) injections of placebo, 50, 100, 200, or 400 mg per 4 weeks. After 12 weeks, the percentage of ACR 20 per cent responders was, respectively, 15, 21, 20, 34, and 60 per cent (Keystone et al. 2001a). Further studies are in progress.

Adalimumab is a human anti-TNF mAb produced by means of the phage display technique. After completion of several phase II and III studies that included over 2500 patients, the dossier for the registration for RA treatment is now under review. The antibody has a half-life of 2 weeks and can be administered s.c. every other week. A 24-week placebo controlled study was conducted in 271 patients with active RA and receiving stable concurrent doses of MTX. The patients were randomized to receive placebo or s.c. adalimumab at doses of 20, 40, or 80 mg every alternate week. After 24 weeks, 14 per cent of the placebo-treated individuals fulfilled an ACR 20 per cent response versus 65 per cent of the patients receiving 40 and 80 mg per 2 weeks (Keystone et al. 2001b). The results of phase III studies, which include studies on X-rays and function, will be presented in 2003.

Etanercept (Enbrel™) was developed by linking DNA encoding the extracellular portion of the p75 TNF receptor with DNA encoding the Fc portion of human IgG1 (Mohler et al. 1993). The resulting fusion protein is expressed in a hamster ovary cell line and binds both soluble TNF and lymphotoxin with higher affinity than the naturally occurring monomers of soluble TNF receptors. Etanercept was first evaluated in a double-blind, placebo controlled, dose evaluating study in patients with active refractory RA. Given the half-life of ±90 h, the drug was administered SC twice weekly in doses of 2, 4, or 16 mg/m^2 for 4 weeks following a single intravenous leading dose (Moreland et al. 1996). In every dose group three received the active drug and one the placebo. Over 50 per cent reduction in individual response variables such as joint counts and acute phase response was observed in the highest dose group. These results were confirmed in a study in which patients received placebo, 0.25, 2, or 16 mg/m^2 SC twice weekly for 3 months (Moreland et al. 1997). Of the patients receiving the highest dose 75 per cent fulfilled the ACR 20 per cent response criteria versus only 14 per cent of the placebo-treated patients. In another placebo-controlled trial in which patients (n = 234) were treated during 6 months with placebo, 10 or 25 mg of etanercept SC twice weekly, 51 and 59 per cent of the 10 and 25 mg treated groups fulfilled the ACR 20 per cent response criteria which was significantly higher than the 11 per cent of the placebo-treated patients (Moreland et al. 1999). To study whether the addition of etanercept to MTX would provide additional benefit to patients who had persistent active RA despite receiving MTX (15–25 mg), patients received either 25 mg etanercept or placebo injections while continuing MTX (Weinblatt et al. 1999). At 24 weeks 71 per cent of the patients receiving etanercept and 27 per cent of those receiving placebo met the ACR 20 per cent response criteria.

To study the effect of etanercept in patients in an early phase of the disease, 632 patients with a mean disease duration of 1 year received either twice weekly s.c. etanercept (10 or 25 mg) or weekly oral MTX (mean 19 mg/week) for 12 months (Bathon et al. 2000). At 12 months, 72 per cent of the patients in the group assigned to receive 25-mg of etanercept had an ACR 20 per cent response, as compared with 65 per cent of those in the MTX group. As also noted in previous studies the 25 mg dose was more effective than the 10-mg dose. Among patients who received the 25-mg dose of etanercept 72 per cent has no increase in the erosion score as compared with 60 per cent of the patients in the MTX group.

Interleukin-1 receptor antagonist in RA

The IL-1 gene family consists of IL-1α and β and their natural inhibitor, IL-1 receptor antagonist (IL-1Ra) (Rankin et al. 1995). IL-1α and β are antagonists that exert their function from the interaction between these molecules and a receptor on target cells. The effects of IL-1α and β are blocked by the interaction of the IL-1 receptor with IL-1Ra. The production of IL-1Ra has been found to be deficient relative to the total production of IL-1 in RA patients. This did lead to the hypothesis that administering IL-1Ra to patients with active RA might restore the IL-1Ra/IL-1 balance. Clinical studies with a recombinant IL-1Ra, anakinra (Kineret™), have substantiated this hypothesis. In a preliminary trial 15 patients with active RA received daily s.c. injections of anakinra for a total of 28 days. Major reductions in the joint counts and acute phase reactants were observed in 12 of 15 patients within 2 weeks of treatment. In a subsequent controlled trial 175 RA patients were randomized to receive 20, 70, or 200 mg of kineret with varying dosing intervals during 3 weeks (Campion et al. 1996). Daily dosing appeared most effective. Subsequently, a randomized placebo-controlled trial where 472 patients with relatively early and active RA were treated with daily injections of 30, 75, or 150 mg kineret or placebo for 24 weeks was organized (Bresnihan et al. 1998). The clinical responses in patients receiving 150 mg/day were greater than those in the other treatment groups. An ACR 20 per cent response was achieved in 43 per cent of the 150 mg/day group compared to 27 per cent of the patients in the placebo group after 24 weeks. Radiographic evaluations in this study found a statistically significant decrease in the rate of joint damage progression after treatment with kineret when compared to placebo (Jiang et al. 2000). All patients who completed the 24-week extension phase of the study were radiographically assessed after 1 year of treatment. It was reported that joint destruction was reduced even more in the second half-year of treatment.

The efficacy of anakinra plus MTX was evaluated in a 24-week randomized study on 419 patients who had active RA despite MTX treatment (12.5–25 mg/week for at least 6 months) (Cohen et al. 2002). Patients were randomized to daily s.c. injections of placebo, 0.04, 0.1, 1.0, or 2.0 mg/kg per day for up to 24 weeks. The ACR 20 per cent response at 24 weeks was seen in 42 per cent of patients who received 1 mg/kg and in 23 per cent of the patients in the placebo/ MTX group.

Adverse reactions to TNF and IL-1 inhibitors in RA

Data from clinical trials with TNF and IL-1 antagonists have reported relatively low levels of toxicity of these drugs and the incidence of adverse events during the first years of therapy seem to be acceptable low. The most common reactions in the infliximab clinical trial program in RA were headache, nausea, upper respiratory tract infections, and infusion related reactions (Hanauer 1999). The latter were mild necessitating withdrawal in less than 2 per cent of the patients. Serious adverse reactions occurred in 4.4 per cent of the infliximab recipients compared to 1.8 of the placebo recipients in a pooled analysis. These reactions included fever (0.9 per cent), pneumonia (0.9 per cent), dyspnoea (0.4 per cent), and rash (0.4 per cent). About 6 per cent of infliximab patients withdraw from treatment because of adverse events.

With etanercept, the withdrawal rates because of adverse events were also low and similar to placebo in randomized trials (Moreland et al. 1999; Weinblatt et al. 1999). The most common adverse events were injection site reactions, upper respiratory tract infections, and headache. Post-marketing studies confirm the relative safety of TNF antagonists. Of the 4794 patients enrolled in the etanercept studies and long-term open label studies there was no increase in the rate of serious infection, malignancy, or death. Data of infliximab follow-up programmes are also reassuring in this respect but recently an increased risk of exacerbations of latent tuberculosis appeared (Day 2002). The probability to unmask tuberculosis may be greater with antibody therapies against TNF than with soluble receptor therapies. These observations have led to warnings in the prescribing information and to recommendations for prevention.

Wider use of TNF antagonists in RA has led to reports, largely of individual cases of a range of serious adverse neurological, hematological, heart failure, and serious infectious complications. It is important to realize, however, that there may be an increased risk of such complications in RA independent of whatever treatment they have received. It is, therefore, fundamentally important not just to document the occurrence of these events in a treated cohort of patients but also to compare their occurrence with that of which might have occurred if such patients had remained on conventional therapy.

The most frequently documented side-effect of kineret therapy is injection site reaction. In controlled trials these were reported in 25 per cent of patients given placebo and ±75 per cent of patients given anakinra. This resulted in the premature withdrawal from the study in 5 per cent of anakinra-treated patients. Infections that required antibiotic therapy occurred in 12 per cent of the placebo-treated patients and 16 per cent of the kineret-treated patients.

Immunogenicity

Administration of large proteins can lead to the formation of antibodies against the treatment. In the case of mAb the formation of antiidiotypic antibodies is an integral element of immunoregulation. However, the exact clinical relevance of such antibodies is currently unknown. The frequency of antibody formation against infliximab is irreversibly related to the dose and is lower when MTX is given concomitantly. The formation of anti-infliximab antibodies during MTX occurred in 15.7 and 0 per cent, respectively, with 1.3 and 10 mg/kg infliximab (Maini et al. 1998). These antibodies neutralize the binding activity of infliximab to TNF. Etanercept also induces antibody formation which seems to be non-neutralizing for TNF binding activity. Antibody formation against anakinra has not been reported.

Both infliximab and etanercept lead to formation of autoantibodies against nuclear factors in clinical trials with RA patients. The percentage of patients was ±50 with infliximab and ±10 with etanercept. Less than 5 per cent of these patients also developed antibodies against double stranded DNA. Recently, there were some case reports of RA patients being treated with either infliximab or etanercept who developed drug-induced systemic lupus erythematosus (Debandt et al. 2001; Shakoor et al. 2002). Further studies are necessary to clarify its prevalence and pathogenesis.

Combination therapy in RA

Recently, the expectations of rheumatologists have been raised with regards to improved outcomes in RA patients. A substantial reduction in signs and symptoms, improvement in disability, and inhibition of radiographic progression are now key objectives. This concept arises from the significant improvement observed with TNF antagonists and the recent demonstration that aggressive early treatment has long-term radiographic benefit (Lard et al. 2001; Landewe et al. 2002). Early introduction of DMARDS has been associated with a better disease outcome (van Jaarsveld et al. 2000). Moreover, aggressive therapy in patients with recent onset RA has resulted in reduced, long-term radiographic progression. This is particularly important since over time disability becomes an increasing function of radiographic damage in addition to disease activity (Scott et al. 2000).

Combinations of DMARDs have recently been used with a view of achieving additional efficacy or synergy without increase in toxicity compared with the same agents used sequentially. In combining DMARDs, three strategies are utilized: step up, parallel, and step down (Verhoeven et al. 1998; Goekoop et al. 2001).

Step up strategies

Step up therapy involves the addition of a second DMARD to a DMARD to which the patient has an incomplete response:

(i) Cyclosporine A (CyA) added to MTX: In a trial of 6 months duration involving 148 patients (mean duration ~10 years), CyA (mean dose 2.0 mg/kg) was added to MTX (mean dose 10.2 mg/week) in patients with partial response to the MTX (Tugwell et al. 1995). At 6 months, the response rate (ACR 20 per cent) was higher with the combination (48 per cent) than with MTX alone (16 per cent). A mean improvement in tender joints (25 per cent) and swollen joints (25 per cent) was achieved with the combination. Side-effects were not substantially increased. The dropout rate was higher with the combination (25 per cent) versus MTX alone (16 per cent).

(ii) Hydroxychloroquine (HCQ) and/or salazopyrine (SSZ) added to MTX: In a trial of 2 years duration, HCQ (400 mg/day) and/or SSZ (1500 mg/day) were added to patients partially responsive to MTX (O'Dell et al. 1999). The response rates (ACR 20 per cent) were higher in the group to which both HCQ and SSZ were added to MTX compared with the addition of HCQ or SSZ alone. The combinations were well tolerated.

(iii) Leflunomide (LEF) added to MTX: In a trial of 6 months duration, LEF (100 mg/day for 2 days followed by 10 mg/day for 2 months) was added to MTX. Patients with an adequate response at 2 months could increase the dose to 20 mg/day (Kremer et al. 2000). By 24 weeks, response rates (ACR 20 per cent success) were higher in the combination group (46 per cent) than in the group receiving MTX alone (20 per cent). In this trial, AST and ALT elevations were seen in 17 and 31.5 per cent of the LEF-treated patients, respectively.

Parallel strategy

Parallel strategy involves a therapeutic regimen in which patients are started on a combination of new drugs simultaneously:

(i) Combination MTX, SSZ, and HCQ: In a trial of 2 years duration, involving 102 patients (mean disease duration 6–9 years), combination MTX (mean dose ~16 mg/week), SSZ (dose 1 g), and HCQ (dose 400 mg) were compared with HCQ plus SSZ and MTX alone (O'Dell et al. 1996). At 9 months, patients failing to achieve 50 per cent improvement (in three of the following: morning stiffness, joint tenderness, joint swelling, normal ESR) were considered non-responders. At 2 years, the 50 per cent improvement rate was higher in the triple combination group, 24/31 (77 per cent), compared with the double combination group, 14/35 (40 per cent) or the group treated with MTX alone, 12/36 (33 per cent). The combinations were well tolerated and no more toxic than the group receiving MTX alone. Confounders in the study included mild disease (MTX naive with ~8 years disease duration).

(ii) Combination MTX, SSZ, HCQ, and prednisolone: In an open randomized trial of 2 years duration, involving 199 patients (mean duration ~7.5 months), combination MTX (escalated as required up to 15 mg/week at 9 months; median dose 7.5 mg), HCQ (300 mg), SSZ (up to 3 g), and prednisolone (5 mg to a maximum of 10 mg) was compared with SSZ with or without prednisolone (Mottonen et al. 1999). If less than a 25 per cent clinical response was achieved at 6 months in the SSZ group, SSZ was replaced by MTX or azathioprine (2 mg/kg) or others if azathioprine failed. Radiological progression increased more in the combination therapy group than in the SSZ group. The frequency of adverse effects were similar in both groups. At 1 year of therapy, response rates (ACR 20 per cent) were higher in the combination group (75 per cent) than in the SSZ group (60 per cent). The 2-year rates were 71 and 58 per cent respectively. Confounders in the study include the open label design, switching to other DMARD (75 per cent) intra-articular injections as required.

(iii) Combination MTX, SSZ, and HCQ: In an open randomized study of 2 years duration involving 180 patients, triple combination of, MTX (7.5–15 mg), HCQ (200 mg), and SSZ (1–3 g) ($n = 60$) were compared with double combinations MTX/SSZ ($n = 30$) and MTX/HCQ ($n = 20$) (Calguneri et al. 1999). At 6 months, if 50 per cent improvement (Modified Paulus) was not achieved, patients in monotherapy and double therapy were switched to another drug or combination. At 2 years, response rates (50 per cent improvement) was greater in triple combination (87.9 per cent) compared with double combination (44.6 per cent) or single DMARD therapy (31.5 per cent). Radiological damage (Larsen score) significantly increased only with single DMARD therapy. No radiological progression was seen in triple therapy (68 per cent) versus double therapy (64.2 per cent), versus single therapy (24.5 per cent). Confounders in the study include open label design, use of Paulus criteria, mild disease at onset of study, and inadequate information regarding method of analysis.

Step down strategies

This involves sequential withdrawl of simultaneously started drugs after improvement with the initial combination regimen:

(i) Combination MTX, SSZ, and prednisolone: In a study of 2 years duration involving 155 patients (median disease duration, 4 months), combination therapy with MTX (7.5 per cent/week), SSZ (2 g), and prednisolone (initially 60 mg/day tapered in 6 weekly steps to 7.5 mg) was compared with SSZ alone (Boers et al. 1997). Prednisolone was stopped after 7 months and MTX after 10 months. At 7 months of therapy, the response rate (ACR 20 per cent) was higher with combination therapy (72 per cent) than SSZ alone (49 per cent). By 10 months, there was no difference between the two groups. Radiological damage (Sharp/Van der Heijde) was less with combination therapy compared to SSZ alone at 7 months, 1 year, and $1\frac{1}{2}$ years (80 weeks). Combination therapy immediately suppressed damage progression whereas SSZ did so with a lag of 6–12 months. Few dropouts were seen in the combination group (8 per cent) versus SSZ alone (23 per cent). At 5 years, radiological progression was still occurring at a faster rate in the SSZ group despite the option to switch to standard of care after 2 years in both groups (Chen et al. 1995).

Novel small molecule therapy

A clinical trial with TNF and IL-1 antagonists showed an unprecedented clinical efficacy in a therapy refractory patient population but the efficacy was never complete. Studies on synovial biopsies showed heterogeneous patterns of cytokine production in individual patients. This argues for the existence of different disease pathways between patients. Therefore, future treatment with antagonists of both cytokines as well as treatment of cell activation pathways downstream of the interaction of proinflammatory cytokines and cell surface receptors seem to be attractive. Cell activation and differentation is associated with gene transcription initiated by transcription factors binding to the promoter region of DNA. Several transcription factor families are involved in these processes in RA: (i) mitrogen-activated protein kinase (MAPK) and (ii) nuclear factor kB (NFkB) (Firestein and Manning 1999).

Mitogen-activated protein kinase (MAPK) inhibitors

MAPK inhibitors are part of a signalling cascade, that is, series of MAKP activation steps (through phosphorylation) leading to AP-1 activation (Marshall et al. 1994). There are three major MAPK signalling cascades, including ERK (extracellular signal-regulated kinase), JNK (Jun *N*-terminal kinase), and p38 MAPK. These MAPKs are activated by upstream kinases, MAPK kinases, which are further activated by MAPK kinase kinases. ERKs are activated by cytokines and growth factors while JNK and p38 kinase are activated in response to many proinflammatory cytokines, that is, TNF and IL-1 as well as cellular stress.

Activation of the MAPK cascade leads downstream to the phosphorylation of AP-1 which is the transcription factor binding DNA resulting in gene transcription of MMPs and cytokines.

All three MAPK families are expressed in RA FLS (Han et al. 1999). IL-1 induces rapid phosphorylation of ERK and p38 in RA FLS. Phosphorylated JNK is detected in RA synovial tissues but not in OA tissues. JNK-1 and JNK-2 knockout mice cause markedly diminished collagenase gene expression.

Immunohistochemical studies demonstrate AP-1 in RA synovium, mainly in fibroblast-like synoviocytes (FLS) in the initial lining layer (Kinne et al. 1995). Administration of AP-1 decoy oligonucleotides that interfere with binding of AP-1 at the promoter binding site *in vivo* suppresses IL-1, IL-6, TNFα, MMP-3, and MMP-9 in synovial tissues and inhibits murine collagen-induced arthritis (Shiozawa et al. 1997).

In vivo studies have confirmed the therapeutic potential for targeting MAPKs for the treatment of RA. Certain members of the pyridinyl imidazole class of compounds have been shown to be selective inhibitors of p38 MAPK. One such compound, an orally administered agent, SB 242235, resulted in significantly reduced signs of arthritis in adjuvant arthritis. (Badger et al. 2000) The compound exerted a protective effect on joint integrity suggesting disease modifying properties. A number of small molecule inhibitors of p38 MAPK are currently in development for use in RA. Phase II trials are underway with several inhibitors.

Nuclear factor kB inhibitors

NFkB is a ubiquitous transcription factor that plays an important role in inflammatory gene transcription (Baeuerle and Henkel 1994; Chen et al. 1995; Barnes and Karin 1997; Firestein and Manning 1999; Yamamoto and Gaynor 2001). NFkB exists as a dimer and the classic dimer consists of p50 (NFkB1) and p65 (Rel A). Other components of NFkB include p52 (NFkB2), Rel B, and c-Rel.

NFkB is activated by a large number of different signals including TNF, IL-1, lipopolysaccharide (LPS) and H_2O_2. NFkB resides in the cytoplasm in an inactive form, associated with inhibitory proteins referred to as inhibitor of NFkB (IkB). IkB family members include IkBα, IkBβ, and IkBε. NFkB activation occurs after extracellular stimulation causes degradation of the inhibitor IkB in the cytoplasm.

The degradation process is initiated by two IkB kinases, Ikk-1 (Ikkα) and Ikk-2 (Ikkβ), that phosphorylate IkB. The phosphorylated IkB is then ubiquinated and degraded by 26S proteosome. NFkB is subsequently translocated to the nucleus where it binds the DNA of its target genes to initiate transcription.

The therapeutic potential for targeting NFkB has been demonstrated in several animal models of arthritis.

NFkB proteins p50 and p65 are abundant in RA synovium in synovial lining cells, vascular endothelium, and CD14 positive macrophages

(Handel et al. 1995; Marok et al. 1996). Ikk-1 and Ikk-2 are constitutively expressed in cultured FLS and induced by IL-1 and TNF. Inhibition of Ikk2 prevents TNFα mediated cytokine production in FLS, whereas inhibition of Ikk1 does not. NFkB inhibition suppresses clinical arthritis in adjuvant arthritis (Pierce et al. 1997; Tsao et al. 1997) and streptococcal cell wall arthritis (Miagkov et al. 1998). Novel small molecules are currently in development as therapy for RA.

The oral use of proteosome inhibitors that block the degradation of IkB reduced the severity of peptidoglycan polysaccharide-induced arthritis in Lewis rats. An oral novel T cell specific NFkB inhibitor SP100030 used in established collagen induced severity with a trend towards improvement on histological evaluation (Gelay et al. 2000).

TNFα converting enzyme (TACE) inhibition

TNFα converting enzyme (TACE) is the MMP that processes the 26-kDa membrane-bound precursor of TNFα (pro-TNF) to the 17 kDa soluble component (Moss et al. 1998). A number of orally bioavailable, selective, and potent TACE inhibitors are currently in development and are currently in phase II studies in RA. These inhibitors effectively block TACE-mediated processing of pro-TNF in human monocytes and are capable of reducing TNF production in normal human subjects. TACE processing of pro-TNF has recently been shown to occur intracellularly. One issue raised as a consequence of intracellular processing is the fate of unprocessed pro-TNF since cell surface associated pro-TNF has potential biological activity. Recent studies demonstrate that more than 80 per cent of unprocessed pro-TNF is degraded intracellularly. The rest is transiently expressed on the cell surface.

In animal models of arthritis, oral TACE inhibitors are efficacious therapeutically in established collagen-induced arthritis. The efficacy is greater than the strategies used to neutralize soluble TNF, presumably due to greater tissue penetration.

Interleukin converting enzyme (ICE) inhibition

Another approach to decrease cytokine activity is to reduce its production by interfering with its processing and secretion. This approach can be used with IL-1 and IL-18. IL-1β and IL-18 are synthesized in the cytoplasm as inactive precursors (pro-IL-1β and pro-IL-18). In order for IL-1β and IL-18 to be secreted the pro-form of the cytokines are processed by interleukin converting enzyme (ICE), a cysteine protease that cleaves pro-IL-β and IL-18 to generate natural forms that can be secreted.

The therapeutic potential for targeting ICE has been demonstrated in animal models of arthritis. ICE knockout mice are not susceptible to collagen-induced arthritis. Treatment with an ICE inhibitor reduced the severity of established collagen-induced arthritis. Since inhibition of ICE potentially effects both IL-1 and IL-18, synergistic effects of inhibiting both T-cell and non-T-cell mediated processes may be particularly effective. Recent data have shown IL-18 to have a variety of proinflammatory effects on multiplicity of cells in the synovium. Since inhibition of ICE may prolong the life of cells, the potential for development of malignancies and autoimmune disease may exist. However, ICE knockout mice do not seem to develop these diseases.

Angiogenesis inhibition

Neovascularization is an important process in perpetuating immune cell migration, proinflammatory molecule generation, and pannus formation in RA (Koch 1998; Szekanecz and Koch 2001). Orally bioavailable agents (inhibiting angiogenesis) (e.g. Fumagillin derivative, AGM-1470) have been extensively studied in animal models of arthritis (Peacock et al. 1992). AGM-147O has been shown to have both anti-inflammatory as well as disease modifying effects such as preventing pannus formation and neovascularization. Another critical effector molecule for blood vessels undergoing angiogenesis (as well for differentiation of osteoclasts) is the integrin $\alpha V\beta 3$ (Storgand et al. 1999; Badger et al. 2001). Intra-articular administration of a cyclic peptide antagonist of $\alpha V\beta 3$ to rabbits with antigen induced arthritis early in disease resulted in inhibition of synovial angiogenesis, and reduced synovial infiltrate, pannus formation, and cartilage erosions (Storgand et al. 1999). When administered in chronic disease, the $\alpha V\beta 3$ antagonist effectively diminished the severity of arthritis. Recently, an orally bioavailable inhibitor of $\alpha V\beta 3$ (and $\alpha V\beta 5$) was shown to substantially inhibit clinical inflammation and prevent cartilage and bone destruction in an established adjuvant arthritis mouse model (Badger et al. 2001). In addition, taxol, an oral compound that induces endothelial cell apoptosis, has been shown to be effective in collagen-induced arthritis. Taxol is currently being evaluated in patients with RA.

Summary and conclusions

The concept of a targeted therapy that could affect one or more specific pathological processes in RA has enormous implications for the future. Heretofore all the available therapies have been truly non-specific, often borrowed from other disciplines (e.g. oncology, infectious diseases) and containing side-effect profiles that limit their usefulness. With the new biological agents new therapeutic perspectives come up but many questions need to be addressed to further clarify their role. These include (i) do these drugs maintain efficacy with treatments longer than 5 years; (ii) do these treatments maintain integrity of joint structures during long-term therapy; (iii) are they safe with long-term therapy; (iv) how to explain non-responders; (v) how to select patients for the different forms of targeted therapies; (vi) is it justified to use, due to restricted financial means, in health care for long-term RA treatment with biological agents?

Currently, the US Food and Drug Administration and the European Medical Agency for Drug Evaluation have approved etanercept, infliximab, and anakinra for patients who failed DMARD therapy. Whether this will change depends on more studies in early RA.

RA is a severe disease despite established treatment. The most promising therapies at present include those based on biotechnology. These therapies, which have become available for many rheumatologists, may certainly be seen as breakthroughs in the treatment of RA. The optimization of TNF and IL-1 blockade through increasing experience and extended careful surveillance of patients should ensure cytokine-targeted agents a pivotal place in the therapy for RA.

References

Arend, W.P. and Dayer, J.M. (1995). Inhibition of the production and effects of interleukin-1 and tumor necrosis factor alpha in rheumatoid arthritis. *Arthritis and Rheumatism* **38**, 151–60.

Badger, A.M. et al. (2000). Disease modifying activity of SB 242235, a selective inhibitor of P38 mitogen-activated protein kinase, in rat adjuvant-induced arthritis. *Arthritis and Rheumatism* **43**, 175.

Badger, A.M. et al. (2001). Disease modifying activity of SB 273005, an orally active non-peptide $\alpha v\beta 3$ (vitronectin receptor) antagonist in RAJ adjuvant-arthritis. *Arthritis and Rheumatism* **44**, 128–37.

Baeuerle, P.A. and Henkel, T. (1994). Function and activation of NFkB in the immune system. *Annual Review of Immunology* **12**, 141.

Barnes, P.J. and Karin, M. (1997). Nuclear factor-kappa B. A pivotal transcription factor in chronic inflammatory diseases. *New England Journal of Medicine* **336**, 1066.

Bathon, J.M. et al. (2000). A comparison of etanercept and methotrexate in patients with early rheumatoid arthritis. *New England Journal of Medicine* **343**, 1586–93.

Boers, M. et al. (1997). Randomized comparison of combined step-down prednisolone, methotrexate and sulphasalazine with sulphasalazine alone in early rheumatoid arthritis. *Lancet* **350**, 309–18.

Breedveld, F.C. (2000). Therapeutic monoclonal antibodies. *Lancet* **355**, 735–40.

Bresnihan, B. et al. (1998). Treatment of rheumatoid arthritis with recombinant human interleukin-1 receptor antagonist. *Arthritis and Rheumatism* **41**, 2196–204.

Calguneri, M. et al. (1999). Combination therapy versus monotherapy for the treatment of patients with rheumatoid arthritis. *Clinical and Experimental Rheumatology* **17**, 699–704.

Campion, G.V. et al. (1996). Dose-range and dose-frequency study of recombinant human interleukin-1 receptor antagonist in patients with rheumatoid arthritis. *Arthritis and Rheumatism* **39**, 1092–101.

Chen, C.C. et al. (1995). Selective inhibition of E-selectin, vascular cell adhesion molecule-1, and intercellular molecule-1 expression by inhibitors of 1 kappa B-alpha phophorylation. *Journal of Immunology* **155**, 3538.

Cohen, S. et al. (2002). Treatment of rheumatoid arthritis with anakinra, a recombinant human interleukin-1 receptor antagonist, in combination with methotrexate: results of a twenty-four-week, multicenter, randomized, double-blind, placebo-controlled trial. *Arthritis and Rheumatism* **46**, 574–8.

Day, R. (2002). Adverse reactions to TNF-α inhibitors in rheumatoid arthritis. *Lancet* **359**, 540–1.

DeBandt, M.J., Descamps, V., and Meyer, O. (2001). Two cases of etanercept-induced systemic lupus erythematosus in patients with rheumatoid arthritis. *Annals of the Rheumatic Diseases* **60**, 175.

Dolhain, R.J.E.M. et al. (1996). Shift toward T lymphocytes with a T helper 1 cytokine-secretion profile in the joints of patients with rheumatoid arthritis. *Arthritis and Rheumatism* **39**, 1961–9.

Drossaers-Bakker, K.W. et al. (1999). Long-term course and outcome of functional capacity in rheumatoid arthritis. *Arthritis and Rheumatism* **42**, 1854–60.

Elliott, M.J. et al. (1993). Treatment of rheumatoid arthritis with chimeric monoclonal antibodies to TNFα. *Arthritis and Rheumatism* **36**, 1681–90.

Elliot, M.J. et al. (1994). Randomised double-blind comparison of chimeric monoclonal antibody to tumour necrosis factor alpha (cA2) versus placebo in rheumatoid arthritis. *Lancet* **344**, 1105–10.

Feldmann, M., Brennan, F.M., and Maini, R.N. (1996). Rheumatoid arthritis. *Cell* **85**, 307–10.

Feldmann, M., Elliot, M.J., Woody, J.N., and Maini, R.N. (1997). Anti-tumor necrosis factor-alpha therapy of rheumatoid arthritis. *Advances in Immunology* **64**, 310–50.

Firestein, G.S. and Manning, A.M. (1999). Signal transduction and transcription factors in rheumatic disease. *Arthritis and Rheumatism* **42**, 609.

Gelay, D.M. et al. (2000). Effect of a T cell-specific NFkB inhibitor on *in vitro* cytokine production and collagen-induced arthritis. *Journal of Immunology* **165**, 1652–8.

Goekoop, Y.P.M., Allaart, C.F., Breedveld, F.C., and Dijkmans B.A.C. (2001). Combination therapy in rheumatoid arthritis. *Current Opinion in Rheumatology* **13**, 177–83.

Han, Z. et al. (1999). Jun *N*-terminal kinase in rheumatoid arthritis. *Journal of Pharmacology and Experimental Therapy* **291**, 124.

Hanauer, S.B. (1999). Safety of infliximab in clinical trials. *Alimentary Pharmacology & Therapeutics* **4** (Suppl. 4), 16–22.

Handel, M.L., McMorrow, L.B., and Gravellese, E.M. (1995). Nuclear factor-kappa B in rheumatoid synovium. Localization of p50 and p65. *Arthritis and Rheumatism* **38**, 1762.

Jiang, Y. et al. (2000). A multicenter, double-blind, dose-ranging, randomized and placebo controlled study of recombinant human interleukin-1 receptor antagonist in patients with rheumatoid arthritis: radiologic progression and correlation of Genant and Larsen scoring methods. *Arthritis and Rheumatism* **43**, 1001–9.

Keystone, E. et al. (2001a). CDP870, a novel, pegylated, humanised TNFα inhibitor, is effective in healing signs and symptoms of rheumatoid arthritis. Presented at the 2001 ACR Annual Scientific Meeting (late breaking abstracts).

Keystone, E. et al. (2001b). The fully human anti-TNF monoclonal antibody, adalimumab (D2E7), dose ranging study: the 24-week clinical results in patients with active RA on methotrexate therapy (the Armade trial). *Annals of the Rheumatic Diseases* **60**, 67 (abstract).

Kinne, R.W. et al. (1995). Synovial fibroblast-like cells strongly express jun-B and c-fosprote-oncogenes in rheumatoid and osteoarthritis. *Scandinavian Journal of Rheumatology* **101**(Suppl.), 121.

Koch, A.E. (1998). Angiogenesis, Implications for RA. *Arthritis and Rheumatism* **41**, 951–62.

Kremer, J.M. et al. (2000). The combination of leflunomide and methotrexate in patients with active rheumatoid arthritis who are failing on methotrexate alone: a double blind placebo controlled study. *Arthritis and Rheumatism* **43**, 5224 (abstract).

Landewe, R.B. et al. (2002). COBRA combination therapy in patients with early rheumatoid arthritis: long-term structural benefits of a brief intervention. *Arthritis and Rheumatism* **46**, 283–5.

Lard, L. et al. (2001). Early versus delayed treatment in patients with recent-onset rheumatoid arthritis: comparison of two cohorts with different treatment strategy during 2 years. *American Journal of Medicine* **111**, 446–51.

Lipsky, P. et al. (2000a). 102-Week clinical and radiological results from the ATTRACT trial: a 2 year, randomized, controlled, phase 3 trial of infliximab (Remicade®) in patients with active RA despite MTX. *Arthritis and Rheumatism* **43** (Suppl.), 269 (abstract).

Lipsky, P.E. et al. (2000b). Infliximab and methotrexate in the treatment of rheumatoid arthritis. Anti-tumor necrosis factor trial in rheumatoid arthritis with Concomitant Therapy Study Group. *New England Journal of Medicine* **343**, 1594–602.

Maini, R. et al. (1999). Infliximab (chimeric anti-tumour necrosis factor α monoclonal antibody) versus placebo in rheumatoid arthritis patients receiving concomitant methotrexate: a randomised phase III trial. *Lancet* **354**, 1932–9.

Maini, R.N. et al. (1998). Therapeutic efficacy of multiple intravenous infusions of anti-tumour necrosis factor α monoclonal antibody combined with low-dose weekly methotrexate in rheumatoid arthritis. *Arthritis and Rheumatism* **41**, 1552–63.

Marshall, C.J. (1994). MAP kinase kinase kinase, MAP kinase kinase, and MAP kinase. *Current Opinion in Genetics Development* **4**, 82.

Marok, R. et al. (1996). Activation of the transcription factor nuclear factor-kappa B in human inflamed synovial tissue. *Arthritis and Rheumatism* **39**, 583.

Miagkov, A.V. et al. (1998). NF-kappa B activation provides the potential link between inflammation and hyperplasia in the arthritis joint. *Proceedings of the National Academy of Science USA* **95**, 13859.

Mohler, K.M. et al. (1993). Soluble tumor necrosis factor (TNF) receptors are effective therapeutic agents in lethal endotoxemia and function simultaneously as both TNF carriers and TNF antagonists. *Journal of Immunology* **151**, 1548–61.

Moreland, L.W. et al. (1996). Recombinant soluble tumor necrosis factor receptor (p80) fusion protein: toxicity and dose finding trial in refractory rheumatoid arthritis. *Journal of Rheumatology* **23**, 1849–55.

Moreland, L.W. et al. (1997). Treatment of rheumatoid arthritis with recombinant human tumor necrosis factor receptor (p75)-Fc fusion protein. *New England Journal of Medicine* **337**, 141–7.

Moreland, L.W. et al. (1999). Etanercept therapy in rheumatoid arthritis: a randomized, controlled study. *Annals of Internal Medicine* **130**, 478–86.

Moss, M.L. et al. (2001). TACE and other ADAM proteases as targets for drug discovery. *Drug Discovery Today* **16**, 417–26.

Mottonen, T. et al. (1999). Comparison of combination therapy with single-drug therapy in early rheumatoid arthritis: a randomized trial Fin-RaCO trial group. *Lancet* **353**, 1568–73.

Mulherin, D., Fitzgerald, O., and Bresnihan, B. (1996). Clinical improvement and radiological deterioration in rheumatoid arthritis: evidence that pathogenesis of synovial inflammation and articular erosion may differ. *British Journal of Rheumatology* **35**, 1263–8.

O'Dell, J. et al. (1999). Methotrexate (M)—hydroxychloroquine (H)—sulfasalazine (S) versus M-H or M-S for rheumatoid arthritis (RA): results of a double-blind study. *Arthritis and Rheumatism* **42**, S117 (abstract).

O'Dell, J.R. et al. (1996). Treatment of rheumatoid arthritis with methotrexate alone, sulfasalazine and hydroxychloroquine or a combination of all three medications. *New England Journal of Medicine* **334**, 1287–9.

Peacock, D.J., Banduerigo, M.L., and Braker, E. (1992). Angiogenesis Inhibition suppresses collagen arthritis. *Journal of Experimental Medicine* **175**, 1135–8.

Pierce, J.W. et al. (1997). Novel inhibitors of cytokine-induced IkBα phosphorylation and endothelial cell adhesion molecule expression show anti-inflammatory effects *in vivo*. *Journal of Biological Chemistry* **272**, 21096–103.

Pincus, T., Breedveld, F.C., and Emery, P. (1999). Does partial control of inflammation prevent long-term joint damage? Clinical rationale for combination therapy with multiple disease-modifying antirheumatic drugs. *Clinical and Experimental Rheumatology* **17** (Suppl. 18), S2–7.

Pincus, T., Brooks, R.H., and Callahan, L.F. (1994). Prediction of long-term mortality in patients with rheumatoid arthritis according to simple questionnaire and joint count measures. *Annals of Internal Medicine* **120**, 26–34.

Rankin, E.C. et al. (1995). The therapeutic effect on an engineered human anti-tumor-necrosis factor alpha antibody (CDP571) in rheumatoid arthritis. *British Journal of Rheumatology* **34**, 334–42.

Scott, D.L. et al. (2000). The links between joint damage and disability in rheumatoid arthritis. *Rheumatology* **39**, 122–32.

Shakoor, N., Michalska, M., Harris, C.A., and Block, J.A. (2002). Drug-induced systemic lupus erythematosus associated with etanercept therapy. *Lancet* **359**, 579–80.

Shiozawa, S. et al. (1997). Studies on the contribution of c-fos/AP-1 to arthritic joint destruction. *Journal of Clinical Investigation* **99**, 1210.

Storgand, C.M. et al. (1999). Decreased angiogenesis and arthritic disease rabbits treated with an $\alpha v\beta 3$ antagonist. *Journal of Clinical Investigation* **103**, 47–54.

Szekanecz, Z. and Koch, A.E. (2001). Chemokines and angiogenesis. *Arthritis Research* **13**, 202–8.

Tsao, P.N. et al. (1997). The effect of dexamethasone on the expression of activated NF-kappa B in adjuvant arthritis. *Clinical Immunology and Immunopathology* **83**, 173.

Tugwell, P. et al. (1995). Combination therapy with cyclosporine and methotrexate in severe rheumatoid arthritis. *New England Journal of Medicine* **333**, 137–41.

van Jaarsveld, C.H.M., Jacobs, J.W.G., van der Veen, M.J. (2000). Aggressive treatment in early rheumatoid arthritis: a randomized controlled trial. *Annals of the Rheumatic Diseases* **59**, 468–47.

Verhoeven, A.C., Boers, M., and Tugwell, P. (1998). Combination therapy in rheumatoid arthritis: an updated systematic review. *Rheumatology* **37**, 612–19.

Weinblatt, M.E., Maier, A.L., Fraser, P.A., and Coblyn, J.S. (1998). Longterm prospective study of methotrexate in rheumatoid arthritis: conclusion after 132 months of therapy. *Journal of Rheumatology* **25**, 238–42.

Weinblatt, M.E. et al. (1999). A trial of Etanercept, a recombinant tumor necrosis factor receptor: Fc fusion protein, in patients with rheumatoid arthritis receiving methotrexate. *New England Journal of Medicine* **340**, 253–9.

Yamamoto, Y. and Gaynor, R.B. (2001). Therapeutic potential of inhibition of the NFkB pathway in the treatment of inflammation and cancer. *Journal of Clinical Investigation* **107**, 135–42.

4.5.4 Future targeted therapies

Gabriel S. Panayi

Why present targeted therapies are inadequate

The success of therapies directed against tumour necrosis factor (TNF)α and against interleukin (IL)-1 testifies to the strength of the paradigm that inhibition of cytokine activity will be of therapeutic benefit in rheumatoid arthritis (RA). On the basis of this success, one can draw up a whole list of cytokines, enzymes, and other molecules that are involved in the inflammatory and destructive processes within the rheumatoid joint and that can be targeted for therapy. Indeed, this is the approach being followed at present by the overwhelming majority of pharmaceutical companies. It may be concluded, however, that this approach will be of benefit to a patient only with continuous therapy. There is an additional and very important point. That is, despite the hypothesis that TNFα is at the apex of an inflammatory cascade, some 30 per cent of patients treated with TNFα blocking drugs have little or no response to them. The implication here is that other mechanisms may be involved at any particular time in individual patients or that the pathogenesis of RA is more complex than the current paradigms suggest. This chapter aims to explore the reasons why there is this failure of response by a significant number of patients given anticytokine therapy and to think of possible targeted therapies that will have a more fundamental effect on disease activity in RA, perhaps leading to permanent switch off of the inflammatory events. Whether this can be defined as 'cure' in a bacteriological sense is debatable. Such a cure, however, would depend on the induction and expansion of regulatory networks that could permanently control inflammation within the joint.

RA is a T cell driven disease

The primary hypothesis being proposed in this chapter is that RA is a disease that is triggered by unknown factor(s) but in which inflammation is maintained by the continued activation of T cells (Fig. 1). T cells are activated by unknown antigenic peptides presented in the groove of Class II MHC molecules (see below) on the surface of dendritic cells that are professional antigen presenting cells. T cells, with particular T cell receptors on their surface, recognize this molecular complex and, with the help of co-stimulatory molecules, are activated. Functional and phenotypic studies have shown that the activated T cells within the RA synovium are of the TH1 type (for review see Panayi et al. 2001).

The activation of T cells has many consequences for the pathogenesis of RA (Fig. 2). Activated T cells, either directly, by cell-to-cell contact, or indirectly, by the release of cytokines, stimulate macrophages to contribute to inflammation. T cells provide help so that B cells can undergo clonal expansion and somatic mutation to produce high affinity rheumatoid factors that

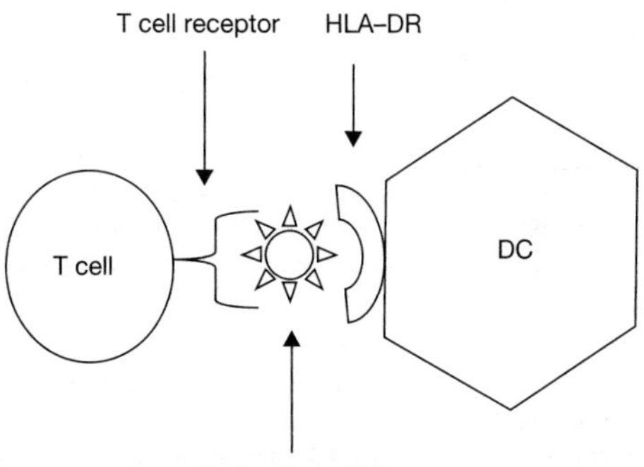

Fig. 1 T cell stimulation is brought about by the interaction of the T cell receptor (TCR) with the antigenic peptide held in the groove of the HLA–DR molecule on the surface of dendritic cells (DCs).

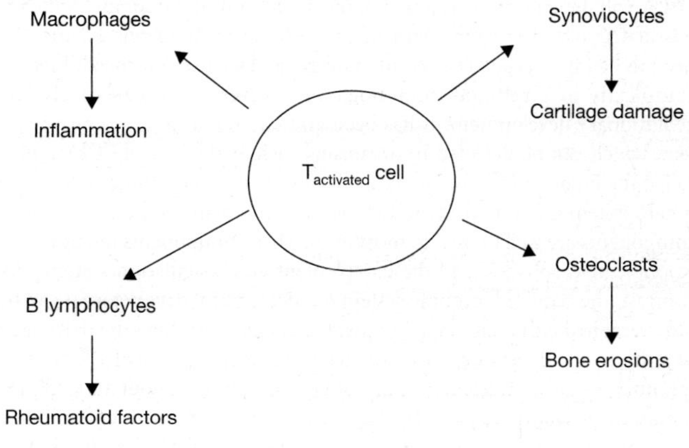

Fig. 2 The consequences of T cell activation in rheumatoid arthritis.

contribute to inflammation by the formation of immune complexes. T can activate directly or indirectly fibroblast-like synovial cells (synoviocytes) to cause cartilage damage by the release of matrix metalloproteinases. Finally, T cells can stimulate osteoclasts to cause bone erosions. They can do this indirectly, by the release of IL-17 or soluble RANK ligand (RANK L), and directly, by expressing RANK L on their surface. Cell-bound or soluble RANK L then engages RANK on the surface of osteoclast progenitors inducing their differentiation and activation into mature osteoclasts that cause bone erosion (Chabaud and Miossec 2001; Hofbauer and Heufelder 2001).

Control of T cell activation in RA could lead to prolonged disease remission

The secondary hypothesis being proposed is that the successful induction of regulatory circuits that suppress or down modulate the TH1 response within the rheumatoid synovium will lead to suppression of rheumatoid inflammation. Thus, the primary focus of this account of future targeted therapies will be on antigen presenting cells and T cells and the mechanisms of their mutual interactions and how these can be regulated to the clinical benefit of the patient.

What to target?

There are two major targets in the therapeutic sense. The first target is commonly thought of as the individual molecules, pathways, and cells involved in a particular process. Thus, in RA synovitis, we may focus our therapeutic efforts, for example, on cytokines, chemokines, and their receptors or on the cells producing them. The second target is the patient. Why do some patients respond to a drug whilst others do not? Why do some patients develop toxic side-effects to a drug while others do not? These differences obviously will depend on genetic factors. We already know that drug toxic side-effects are due to genetic differences between individuals. However, we have only just scratched the surface of this vast field. The same applies to differences in response to drugs. We know, for example, that the failure to respond to a drug may be due to genetic differences in its metabolism or pharmacokinetics. Both of these genetic variables, toxicity and response, are now being studied by genome scanning methods described under the generic term of pharmacogenomics. This will be, undoubtedly, an important future development in the delivery of targeted therapies that will focus on pathogenetic processes and on the genetic makeup of the individual.

The innate and acquired immune responses

Since the hypothesis being proposed is that effective long-term intervention in RA will depend on manipulating the T cell immune response, which is postulated to be driving the synovitis, some basic immunological principles need to be introduced. The acquired immune response, which exhibits the complexity of T cell and immunoglobulin diversity, is a relatively late evolutionary development. It has been grafted onto a more primitive system, which can be detected in organisms such as the fruit fly *Drosophila*, called the innate immune system. Unlike the acquired immune system, the innate system is always ready to function at a moment's notice. Some of its components are well known to most of us. These components include neutrophils, macrophages, and the complement and coagulation systems. By contrast, the acquired immune system requires several days before it can be fully recruited although, on subsequent challenge with the same pathogen or antigen, it will respond with the accelerated tempo typical of a secondary immune response. T cell activation cannot take place without antigen presentation by dendric cells (DCs) (Fig. 1). DCs are components of the innate immune system (Liu et al. 2001). Hence, the state of the DC at the time of antigen presentation will determine the nature of the ensuing immune response (see below). The situation can be best summarized by quoting Liu et al. (2001): 'The diverse functions of DCs in immune regulation are dictated by the instructions they receive during innate immune responses to different pathogens and from their evolutionary lineage heritage'. Hence, regulating or modifying DC function within the RA SM could downregulate the TH1 response within the joint.

Potential mechanisms available for the immunotherapy of RA

Since it is being proposed that RA is a disease of unknown aetiology being driven by TH1 T cell responses, then it follows that methods, which downregulate such responses, could be used for the immunotherapy of RA. A summary of these methods is shown in Fig. 3. Let us consider each one briefly before proceeding to a more detailed analysis of each one below. TH1 T cell responses can be downregulated by TH2 T cell responses and, although this is easier to do during the induction of an immune response, it can still be achieved with primed, memory T cells. A switch from a TH1 to a TH2 response can be achieved by the use of appropriate cytokines or by manipulating the function of DCs so that they induced TH2 rather than TH1 T cell responses. Regulatory or suppressor T cells are now recognized to exist despite decades of scepticism by most immunologists. One group of regulatory T cells have a very characteristic phenotype being CD4+CD25+. They can be isolated from human blood. Other regulatory cells can be induced by appropriate manipulations, such as mucosal delivery of antigen, or by gene transfer. The manipulation of the Class II MHC is an obvious target for immunotherapy as this is at the apex of the T cell stimulatory pathway (Fig. 1). Finally, a number of costimulatory molecules are involved in the activation of T cells. Inadequate costimulatory activity can lead to the development of T cell anergy or failure to respond to the inciting antigen. We shall now consider each of these mechanisms in turn.

The major caveat to the therapeutic approaches to be discussed in this section is whether it is possible to reset the TH1 immune response in RA, in which there are already primed memory T cells particularly in the synovial membrane. Such T cells are notorious for having a lower threshold for activation when compared to naive T cells. However, this goal may be achievable as the commitment of T cells to either the TH1 or the TH2 pathway could be influenced, even in established disease, by the exact cytokine field generated by the immune cells (Kourilsky and Truffa-Bachi 2001).

The manipulation of DCs and induction of a TH2 response

Manipulation of DCs

DCs are professional antigen presenting cells. They can be considered as the link between the innate and acquired immune systems (for a review

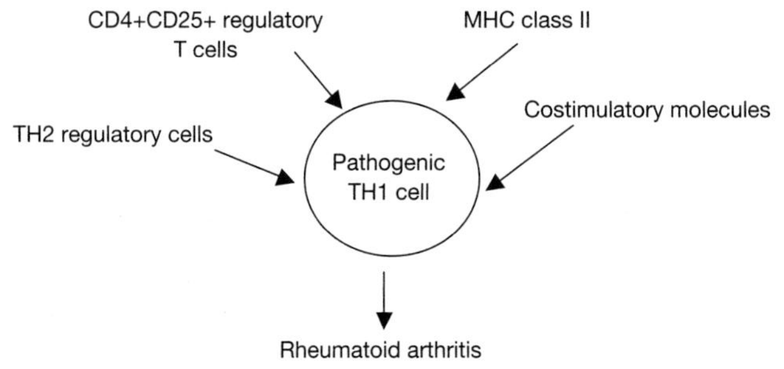

Fig. 3 Methods available to downregulate TH1 pathogenic T cell responses that could be used for the immunotherapy of rheumatoid arthritis.

see Banchereau and Steinman 2001). DCs are widely dispersed in both lymphoid and non-lymphoid tissues. The have two distinct functions. First, they sample self-antigens to maintain T cell self-tolerance. Second, immature DCs possess pattern-recognition receptors on their surface that can be triggered by adhesion of pathogens or their products. This interaction causes immature DCs to mature to immunogenic DCs. These DCs can initiate primary T cell-mediated responses since they express high amounts of cell surface MHC and costimulatory molecules. DCs can induce different types of T cell responses, such as TH1 or TH2, depending on their lineage, maturation stage, and activation signals.

In human blood, there are two types of DC precursors: myeloid monocytes (pre-DC1) and plasmacytoid (pre-DC2) DC precursors. DC1 cells produce large amounts of IL-12 and preferentially induce TH1 development. DC2 cells produce lower amounts of IL-12 and preferentially induce TH2 development. There is an element of functional plasticity during the course of DC development (Fig. 4). Thus, the presence of lipopolysaccharide and T cell signals such as CD40L and interferon (IFN)γ direct DC1 to induce TH1 differentiation. Conversely, a variety of signals stimulate DC to induce TH2 differentiation or to inhibit TH1 differentiation including IL-10, transforming growth factor (TGF)β, and glucocorticoids.

During the course of DC maturation, important functional changes take place. Immature DC specialize in capturing and processing antigens into antigenic peptides inserted into the groove of the MHC. By contrast, mature DC prime T cells for immune functions such as clonal expansion, interacting with other cells such as B cells (for antibody production), macrophages (for cytokine release), and target cells (for cytolysis). DC/T cell interactions are bidirectional with T cells enhancing DC survival, upregulation of the costimulatory molecules CD80 and CD86, secretion of IL-12, and release of chemokines such as IL-8, M1P-1α and β.

DC, in addition to their ability to induce immune responses in both T and B cells, are involved in tolerance induction. In the thymus, during the induction of central tolerance, they delete developing autoreactive T cells whilst in lymphoid organs, during the induction of peripheral tolerance, they induce anergy or deletion of mature T cells.

Induction of a Th2 response

IL-10 blocks maturation of DC. In humans, DC may be generated from peripheral blood monocytes by culture with GM-CSF and IL-4. It is of interest that endogenously produced IL-10 prevents the spontaneous maturation of DC (Coriniti et al. 2001). Thus, enhancing the concentration of IL-10 could be one strategy by which T cell functions could be regulated in RA. Parenteral administration of IL-10 has been ineffective and associated with toxic side-effects (van Roon et al. 2003). This outcome, though disappointing at first glance, suggests that in order for adequate levels of IL-10 to be present in lymph nodes, where the majority of T cell priming occurs, more direct targeting is necessary. This would reduce the amount of systemic IL-10 and hence the possibility of toxicity. There are several ways by which this could be achieved:

(i) The systemic gene delivery of IL-10. A proportion of the administered genes will reach the lymph nodes and IL-10 protein produced locally. Adenoviral vectors are commonly used for systemic gene delivery. This form of gene therapy is currently under a moratorium because of unwanted toxic side-effects and even death in patients.

(ii) The local delivery of genes into the joint may obviate some of the dangers of systemic gene delivery. We already know from the work of Evans and his colleagues that soluble IL-1 and TNFα receptor genes delivered to one joint also have a clinical effect in the contralateral joint (Ghivizzani et al. 1998; Lechman et al. 1999). It appears that the genes are transported by cells of the monocytic series. Thus, DC precursors, isolated from the blood or bone marrow, could be used as vehicles for genes coding for IL-10. Of course, this approach can be used for the delivery of other genes of interest.

(iii) The administration of plasmid DNA, coding for IL-10 or other relevant genes encapsulated in liposomes, systemically to patients either by parenteral injection or by mucosal administration, nasal or oral (Chun et al. 1999; Fellowes et al. 2000). DC or macrophages would take some of the DNA up and the contained IL-10 gene expressed as protein. By this means, high lymph node and synovial membrane IL-10 levels could be achieved without high systemic levels.

(iv) Glucocorticoids direct the maturation down the TH2 pathway (Fig. 4). The exact molecular mechanisms are not known but may be related to the inhibition of IL-12 production thus driving DC maturation in the direction of DC2. However, it may be possible to develop orally active drugs to exploit this particular property of glucocorticoids. Such drugs will probably not have the other associated side-effects of glucocorticoids. More recently, vasoactive intestinal peptide (VIP) has been shown to inhibit collagen induced arthritis in mice by three mechanisms: (i) by inhibiting the production of IFNγ and IL-17 from TH1 cells; (ii) by directly inhibiting macrophages and fibroblast-like synovial cells; (iii) by activating TH2 cells (Delgado et al. 2001). Thus, pharmacological regulation of TH1 responses is envisaged as playing an increasingly important role in our management of RA in the future.

(v) The final approach is related to the preceding. The signal transduction pathways leading to IL-10 production are beginning to be unravelled (Benkhart et al. 2000; Brightbill et al. 2000). Such pathways would be very attractive targets for the development of orally active drugs able to induce the production of IL-10. This would be another pharmacological, as opposed to a biological, approach to therapy.

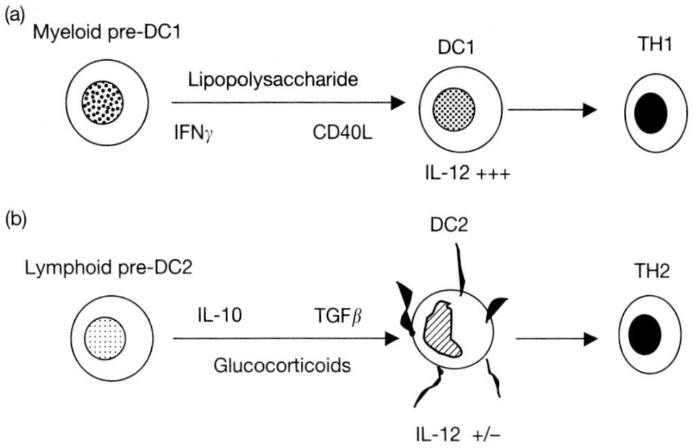

Fig. 4 The development of the two types of dendritic cells, DC1 and DC2, that direct the the induction of TH1 and TH2 T cells, respectively.

Regulatory T cells

Over the years, immunologists have been perplexed by observations that pointed to the existence of T cells with immunoregulatory functions. These cells were given different names including, that of 'suppressor' cells. However, since these cells could not be isolated or expanded, most immunologists denied that they existed. The situation today is dramatically different as the existence of these cells is now universally accepted. These cells are characterized by the phenotype CD4+CD25+ (for a review see Shevach 2001). These cells are found in and can be isolated from human peripheral blood (Dieckmann et al. 2001; Jonuleit et al. 2001). They can suppress naive and memory T cell proliferation (Levings et al. 2001) [Fig. 5(a)]. They express the immunoregulatory molecule CTLA4 on their surface. In mice, blockade of CTLA4 on CD4+CD25+ regulatory T cells leads to loss of function and the development of autoimmune disease in otherwise normal animals (Takahashi et al. 2000) [Fig. 5(b)].

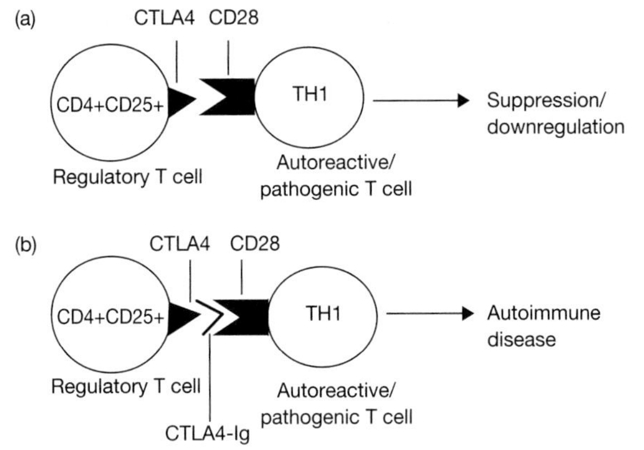

Fig. 5 (a) The infusion of CD4+CD25+ regulatory T cells leads to disease improvement via the downregulation of autoreactive/pathogenic T cells. (b) The administration of CTLA4-Ig, by blocking regulatory T cell function, could lead to the development of autoimmune disease.

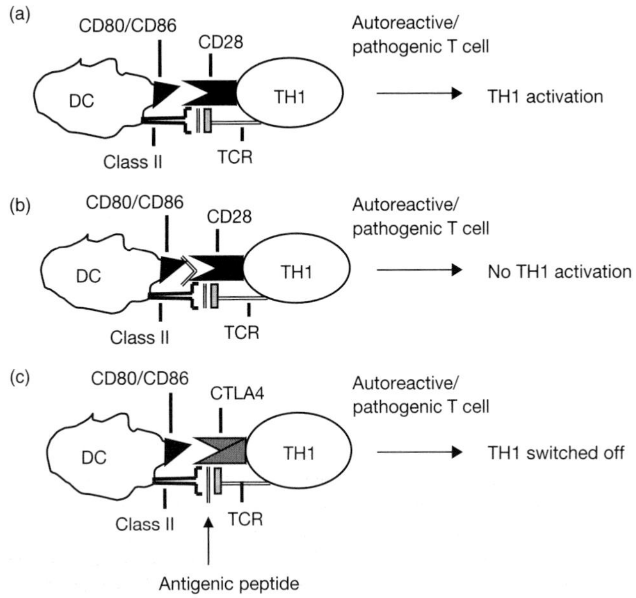

Fig. 6 Costimulation required for T cell activation. (a) Interaction of CD28 with CD80/CD86 leads to T cell activation. (b) Infusion of CTLA4-Ig (>) inhibits T cell activation. (c) The appearance of CTLA4 later in T cell activation leads to the T cell being switched off.

Thus, the therapeutic infusion of these cells into patients with RA is a very attractive proposition. However, there is a problem in the therapeutic use of these cells: they are difficult to expand although *in vitro* the combination of IL-2 and IL-15 is of some value. Despite this reservation, immunotherapy with *in vitro* expanded CD4+CD25+ regulatory T cells could be a feasible proposition [Fig. 5(a)]. This is particularly relevant because of their ability to suppress the function of memory T cells—cells notoriously difficult to suppress unlike naive T cells that are easily downregulated. There is at least one pharmaceutical company that is trialling CTLA4-Ig as an inhibitor of costimulatory activation of T cells because of the importance of costimulation for T cell activation [Fig. 6(a)]. DCs activate T cells via a 'two-signals' mechanism. The first signal is provided by the antigenic peptide presented in the groove of the MHC molecule. The second signal is provided by the costimulatory molecules CD80 and CD86 on the surface of DC interacting with CD28, which appears on the surface of the T cell early in activation. Later in activation CTLA4 appears on the surface of the T cell and engages CD80/CD86 with higher affinity than CD28. This interaction switches off T cell activation [Fig. 6(c)]. It can therefore be seen how infusing CTLA4-Ig could inhibit T cell activation [Fig. 6(b)]. This therapeutic approach needs to be viewed with caution since, if it leads to inhibition of the activity of CD4+CD25+ regulatory T cells [Fig. 5(b)], it may inadvertently produce unwanted immunological side-effects. It could also mean that there would be no clear, cut therapeutic benefit as any downregulation of costimulatory activity via the inhibition of CD28 would be counterbalanced by inhibition of the immunomodulatory role of the regulatory CD4+CD25+ T cells [Fig. 5(b) and Fig. 6(b)].

Manipulation of the MHC Class II activation system

There are at least two mechanisms by which the MHC Class II T cell activation pathway could potentially be manipulated in order to downregulate the immune response in RA. In some respects, these two approaches are based on a contradictory view of the exact role of MHC Class II antigens in the pathogenesis of RA.

The 'shared epitope' hypothesis

The shared epitope hypothesis (Nepom 2001) states that HLA–DRB chains that bear the QKRRA amino acid motif or motifs with conserved substitutions such as QRRAA or RRRAA present unknown antigenic peptides to T cells bearing particular T cell α and β receptor chains. These pathogenic T cells are activated thereby initiating the inflammatory cascade in the rheumatoid joint. The relevant disease causing DRB1 alleles are DRB1*0101, *0401, *0404, *0405, and *1001 [Fig. 7(a)].

On this model, the inflammatory cascade could be blocked if the DRB1 groove were occupied by 'therapeutic' peptides that were designed to bind and displace the 'RA-causing' peptides. This displacement would prevent the activation of disease causing T cells because the new MHC–peptide complex would not be recognized by their T cell receptors [Fig. 7(b)]. It should be noted that this therapy would not induce a general immunosuppression because of the heterogeneity of the MHC Class II system. Such therapeutic studies are presently under way by several companies utilizing this approach. Thus, Organon is using peptides derived from the HCgp39 protein whilst AstraZeneca is using peptides whose specificity has not been revealed. The outcome of these studies is awaited with great interest.

The RA protection hypothesis

The RA protection (RAP) hypothesis proposes that certain DQ, but not DR, alleles predispose to the development of RA (Zanelli et al. 1995) [Fig. 7(c)]. DR alleles modulate the effect of DQ by either enhancing or dominantly protecting against the disease-inducing propensity of DQ. The disease predisposing DQ alleles are DQ5 and the DQA*03-chain containing alleles (DQ4, DQ7, DQ8, and DQ9) (Snijders et al. 2001). Using the terminology of the shared epitope hypothesis, enhancing DRB1 alleles would be DRB1*0401, *0404, *0101, and *1001 whereas DRB1 alleles, which contain the motif DERAA in the HV3 region of the protein, such as DRB*1040, *1301, and *1302 are protective. The RAP hypothesis has not only received support from clinical studies (van der Horst-Bruinsma et al. 1999) but also from experiments in transgenic mice (Bradley et al. 1997). More recently the DRB1-derived peptide DERAA has been shown to be naturally processed by human antigen presenting cells (Snijders et al. 2001). Thus, the implications of the RAP hypothesis for the immunotherapy of RA are obvious [Fig. 7(c)]. 'RA-causing' peptides are presented in the context of

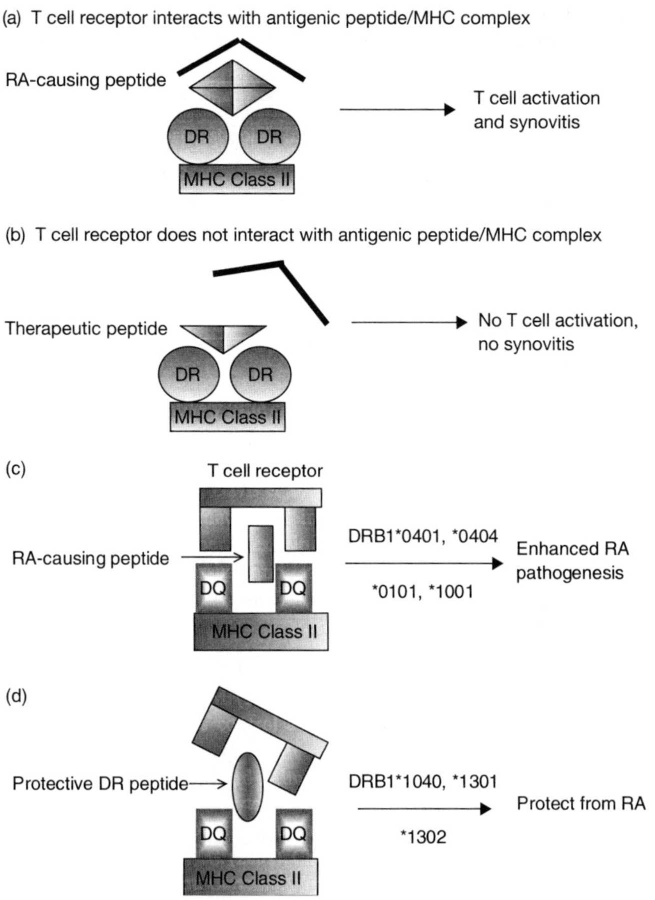

Fig. 7 Potential therapeutic intervention based on the MHC Class II association, the 'shared epitope', with rheumatoid arthritis. (a) A disease causing peptide being presented in the context of HLA–DR B1 molecule activating disease causing T cell via its T cell receptor. (b) A therapeutic peptide binds to HLA–DR, displacing the causing peptide, but unable to stimulate the T cell receptor. As a consequence, arthritis is suppressed. (c) HLA–DQ present disease causing peptides to T cells with appropriate T cell receptors. Disease severity is determined by the HLA–DR make-up of the individual. (d) Peptides derived from protective HLA–DR molecules displace the disease causing peptide, there is no T cell activation and thus protection from arthritis.

appropriate HLA–DQ molecules to T cells, which induce synovitis. The degree of synovitis can be enhanced by certain HLA–DR molecules and inhibited by others.

From the therapeutic point of view interruption of this pathway should downmodulate RA inflammation. It is postulated that 'protective' peptides would inhibit synovitis by displacing 'RA-causing' peptides from the groove of the DQ molecules and thereby preventing activation of T cells [Fig. 7(d)]. The recent demonstration that such protecting peptides can be generated by processing of appropriate HLA–DR molecules (Snijders et al. 2001) suggests that this may very well be a viable therapeutic proposition.

Summary and conclusions

There are undoubtedly many avenues to the induction of tolerance and/or the regulation of TH1 responses within the RA synovium. At first, many of these therapies will be based on biologics but they will eventually be based on xenobiotics—small molecular weight, orally active molecules. This will reduce cost and be more patient friendly. The major prediction of this review is that such therapies, singly or in combination, will lead to life long control of inflammation without the necessity for repeated treatments.

References

Banchereau, J. and Steinman, R.M. (1998). Dendritic cells and the control of immunity. *Nature* **392**, 245–52.

Benkhart, E.M. et al. (2000). Role of Stat3 in lipopolysaccharide-induced IL-10 gene expression. *Journal of Immunology* **165**, 1612–17.

Bradley, D.S. et al. (1997). HLA–DQB1 polymorphism determines incidence, onset, and severity of collagen-induced arthritis in transgenic mice. Implications in human rheumatoid arthritis. *Journal of Clinical Investigation* **100**, 2227–34.

Brightbill, H.D. et al. (2000). A prominent role for Sp1 during lipopolysaccharide-mediated induction of the IL-10 promoter in macrophages. *Journal of Immunology* **164**, 1940–51.

Cauli, A., Yanni, G., and Panayi, G.S. (1994). Endogenous avidin-binding activity in epithelial cells of the ducts of human salivary glands. *Clinical and Experimental Rheumatology* **12**, 45–7.

Chabaud, M. and Miossec, P. (2001). The combination of tumor necrosis factor alpha blockade with interleukin-1 and interleukin-17 blockade is more effective for controlling synovial inflammation and bone resorption in an *ex vivo* model. *Arthritis and Rheumatism* **44**, 1293–303.

Chun, S. et al. (1999). Distribution fate and mechanism of immune modulation following mucosal delivery of plasmid DNA encoding IL-10. *Journal of Immunology* **163**, 2393–402.

Corinti, S. et al. (2001). Regulatory activity of autocrine il-10 on dendritic cell functions. *Journal of Immunology* **166**, 4312–18.

Dieckmann, D. et al. (2001). *Ex vivo* isolation and characterization of CD4(+)CD25(+) T cells with regulatory properties from human blood. *Journal of Experimental Medicine* **193**, 1303–10.

Delgado, M. et al. (2001). Vasoactive intestinal peptide prevents experimental arthritis by downregulating both autoimmune and inflammatory components of the disease. *Nature Medicine* **7**, 563–8.

Fellowes, R. et al. (2000). Amelioration of established collagen induced arthritis by systemic IL-10 gene delivery. *Gene Therapy* **7**, 967–77.

Ghivizzani, S.C. et al. (1998). Direct adenovirus-mediated gene transfer of interleukin 1 and tumor necrosis factor alpha soluble receptors to rabbit knees with experimental arthritis has local and distal anti-arthritic effects. *Proceedings of the National Academy of Sciences USA* **95**, 4613–18.

Hofbauer, L.C. and Heufelder, A.E. (2001). The role of osteoprotegerin and receptor activator of nuclear factor kappaB ligand in the pathogenesis and treatment of rheumatoid arthritis. *Arthritis and Rheumatism* **44**, 253–9.

Jonuleit, H. et al. (2001). Identification and functional characterization of human CD4(+)CD25(+) T cells with regulatory properties isolated from peripheral blood. *Journal of Experimental Medicine* **193**, 1285–94.

Kourilsky, P. and Truffa-Bachi, P. (2001). Cytokine fields and the polarization of the immune response. *Trends in Immunology* **22**, 502–9.

Lechman, E.R. et al. (1999). Direct adenoviral gene transfer of viral IL-10 to rabbit knees with experimental arthritis ameliorates disease in both injected and contralateral control knees. *Journal of Immunology* **163**, 2202–8.

Levings, M.K., Sangregorio, R., and Roncarolo, M.G. (2001). Human CD25(+)CD4(+) T regulatory cells suppress naive and memory T cell proliferation and can be expanded *in vitro* without loss of function. *Journal of Experimental Medicine* **193**, 1295–302.

Liu, Y.J. et al. (2001). Dendritic cell lineage, plasticity and cross-regulation. *Nature Immunology* **2**, 585–9.

Nepom, G.T. (2001). The role of the DR4 shared epitope in selection and commitment of autoreactive T cells in rheumatoid arthritis. *Rheumatic Disease Clinics of North America* **27**, 305–15.

Panayi, G.S., Corrigall, V.M., and Pitzalis, C. (2001). Pathogenesis of rheumatoid arthritis. The role of T cells and other beasts. *Rheumatic Disease Clinics of North America* **27**, 317–34.

Shevach, E.M. (2001). Certified professionals: CD4(+)CD25(+) suppressor T cells. *Journal of Experimental Medicine* **193**, F41–6.

Snijders, A. et al. (2001). An HLA–DRB1-derived peptide associated with protection against rheumatoid arthritis is naturally processed by human APCs. *Journal of Immunology* **166**, 4987–93.

Takahashi, T. et al. (2000). Immunologic self-tolerance maintained by CD25(+)CD4(+) regulatory T cells constitutively expressing cytotoxic T lymphocyte-associated antigen 4. *Journal of Experimental Medicine* **192**, 303–10.

van der Horst-Bruinsma, I.E. et al. (1999). HLA–DQ-associated predisposition to and dominant HLA–DR-associated protection against rheumatoid arthritis. *Human Immunology* **60**, 152–8

van Roon, J., Wijngaarden, S., Lafeber, F.P., Damen, C., van de Winkel, J., and Bijlsma, J.W. (2003). Interleukin 10 treatment of patients with rheumatoid arthritis enhances Fc gamma receptor expression on monocytes and responsiveness to immune complex stimulation. *Journal of Rheumatology* **30** (4), 648–51.

Zanelli, E., Gonzalez-Gay, M.A., and David, C.S. (1995). Could HLA–DRB1 be the protective locus in rheumatoid arthritis? *Immunology Today* **16** (4), 274–8.

5

Investigation of the rheumatic diseases

5 Investigation of the rheumatic diseases

5.1 Acute phase response

Douglas Thompson and Howard A. Bird

What is the acute phase response and how is it assessed?

The acute phase response

The acute phase response is the term generally used to describe the concerted series of diverse systemic and local events which accompany inflammation resulting from tissue damage. Despite the term 'acute phase', the changes may be present in both acute and chronic inflammatory situations. These events are usually considered to be protective in nature, facilitating the inflammatory process and ultimately culminating in removal of tissue debris and foreign organisms, and tissue repair. They include fever, endocrine changes, leucocytosis, muscle proteolysis, and an increase in the synthesis of specific liver-derived proteins—the acute phase proteins. It is this latter event which is often used as an indicator of the presence and extent of the inflammatory process and indeed it is often used synonymously with the term 'acute phase response'. We will also follow this convention for the purposes of this chapter.

There are approximately 30 acute phase proteins. They fall into several different structural and functional categories of plasma proteins and fulfil various roles in inflammation such as inhibition of phagocyte-derived proteases, scavenging of cellular debris, and mediation and inhibition of the inflammatory process (Table 1) (reviewed by Mackiewicz et al. 1993; Gabay and Kushner 1999). The increase in serum concentration of these proteins (which by definition must be by at least 25 per cent in the first 7 days following tissue damage) probably serves to maintain their circulating and tissue levels, which may otherwise become depleted as a result of their consumption at the site of inflammation.

The increased synthesis of the acute phase proteins by the liver has been ascribed to several cytokines, including interleukin-1 (IL-1), tumour necrosis factor-α (TNF-α), and particularly interleukin-6 (IL-6). These cytokines are predominantly derived from activated macrophages at the site of injury although they can be produced by many other cell types such as fibroblasts and endothelial cells, and they have also been implicated in mediating other aspects of the acute response such as fever. It has become apparent that the regulation of the acute phase proteins is complex and that subsets of acute phase proteins are induced by different cytokines (reviewed by Baumann and Gauldie 1994). The IL-1 group of cytokines, IL-1α and β and TNF-α and -β, induce the production of so-called type-1 acute phase proteins which include α_1-acid glycoprotein, serum amyloid A protein, C-reactive protein, and complement component C3, whereas the IL-6 family of cytokines (IL-6, IL-11, leukaemia inhibitory factor, oncostatin M, and ciliary neurotrophic factor) induce the synthesis of type-2, IL-6 specific, acute phase proteins, fibrinogen, α_1-antitrypsin, α_1-antichymotrypsin, haptoglobin, haemopexin, and caeruloplasmin. In most cases IL-1 or TNF have no effect on the production of type-2 acute phase proteins but the IL-6 group of cytokines can induce type-1 acute phase proteins and synergistically enhance the IL-1 and TNF-mediated production of the type-1 acute phase proteins. However, to a certain extent these actions depend on the species and hepatocytes being examined. In addition, two groups of factors modulate cytokine-induced acute phase protein synthesis, namely the glucocorticoids and the growth factors such as insulin, insulin-like growth factor, hepatic growth factor, fibroblast growth factor, and transforming

Table 1 The positive acute phase proteins and their proposed functions

Protein	Proposed functions in inflammation
Inflammatory mediators	
Complement components	Opsonization, chemotaxis, mast cell degranulation
C-reactive protein	Phosphorylcholine binding, complement activation and opsonization, cytokine induction
Plasminogen	Activation of complement, clotting, fibrinolysis
α_1-Antitrypsin	Induction of IL-1ra
Kininogenase (kallikrein)	Vascular permeability and dilation
Inhibitors	
α_1-Antitrypsin	Serine protease inhibition, particularly elastase
α_1-Antichymotrypsin	Inhibition of cathepsin G
Thiol protease inhibitor	Cysteine protease inhibition
Haptoglobin	Inhibition of cathepsin B, H, L
Antithrombin III	
C1 1NH	Control of mediator pathways
Factor I, factor H	
C-reactive protein	Inhibition of cell surface expression of L-selectin
Scavengers	
Haptoglobin	Scavenges haemoglobin and free radicals
Serum amyloid A	Scavenger of cholesterol
C-reactive protein	Scavenger of DNA?
Caeruloplasmin	Free-radical scavengers
α_1-Antichymotrypsin	Free-radical scavengers
Cellular immune regulation	
C-reactive protein	B and T-cell interactions
α_1-Acid glycoprotein	Membrane protein of lymphocytes and monocytes
Repair and resolution	
α_1-Acid glycoprotein	Promotes fibroblast growth
α_1-Antitrypsin	Bonds to surface of new elastic fibres. Inhibition of tissue remodelling by leucocyte-derived proteinases?
α_1-Antichymotrypsin	
Fibrinogen	Endothelial cell adhesion, spreading, and proliferation
Haptoglobin	Stimulation of angiogenesis

growth factor-β (Baumann et al. 1987). The net result achieved is dependent on the overall interactions (Fig. 1).

Most of the changes in acute phase protein production are thought to be mediated at the transcriptional level, however, post-transcriptional modulation such as increases in stability of mRNA for positive acute phase proteins and altered glycosylation and hence possibly bioactivity/stability may also contribute to their regulation (reviewed by Steel and Whitehead 1994). Although the liver is generally accepted as being the site of acute phase protein synthesis, it is now recognized that extrahepatic tissues also have this capability. It has been shown, for example, that cells of the monocyte–macrophage lineage can produce several complement components and α_1-antitrypsin. The significance of this and the extent to which it normally occurs *in vivo*, particularly at the site of inflammation, is not known.

A small group of proteins including albumin, transthyretin, retinol-binding protein, and transferrin decrease in serum concentration during inflammation. These are often referred to as the 'negative acute phase proteins'. This decrease has been attributed to increased catabolism and vascular permeability although cytokines are capable of decreasing transcription of at least some of the negative acute phase protein genes.

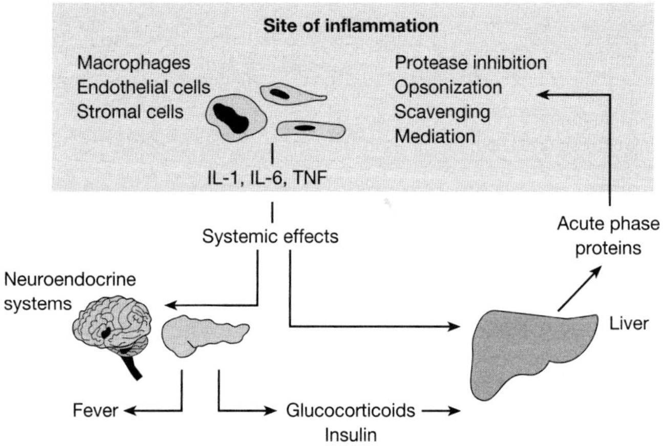

Fig. 1 The regulation of the acute phase protein response. The systemic acute phase protein response is mediated by cytokines such as IL-6, IL-1, and TNF-α released by activated macrophages, endothelial cells, and stromal cells at the site of inflammation. The systemic effects of these cytokines include muscle proteolysis, fever, and the production of acute phase proteins, which exert a range of function at the site of inflammation. The synthesis of acute phase proteins can also be modulated by hormones such as the glucocorticoids and insulin.

Kinetics of the acute phase response in disease

The rate and extent of the increase in plasma concentration of any acute phase protein depends on factors such as molecular size, volume of distribution, rate and sensitivity to induction, and the rate of catabolism. Considerable incremental and kinetic differences are therefore seen between the various proteins. In acute inflammation, the overall pattern of the response is relatively constant, provided that the magnitude of the response is sufficient to elicit a detectable change in all the proteins. The properties of the major acute phase proteins and typical magnitudes and time courses of response are shown in Table 2. It is important to appreciate the differences in kinetics of these changes, for example, while some proteins are elevated within 6–8 h of stimulus, there is no apparent change in others for appreciably longer. These relative changes in the acute phase proteins are exemplified in Plate 67 which shows the changes in positive acute phase proteins *in vivo* following administration of IL-6.

Generally, the magnitude of the response is related quantitatively to the activity or extent of inflammation in the acute situation. In bacterial infection, an extremely large response is seen, probably as a result of systemic endotoxin-induced release of cytokines such as IL-1, IL-6, and TNF from macrophages. However, particularly in chronic inflammation, differential increases in catabolic rate may also result in altered 'profiles' for several proteins. For example, when vasculitis is present, concentrations of α_1-antitrypsin are inappropriately low when compared with a group of other acute phase proteins, owing to its consumption by leucocyte enzymes. Similarly if intravascular coagulation is a complication, levels of fibrinogen may be lower than would otherwise be expected and haptoglobin is lower if haemolysis is occurring. Such differences in themselves may be useful in drawing attention to possible complications which may be present with the inflammatory process, but would contraindicate the effective use of that particular protein as an inflammatory marker in that particular situation. Often in chronic inflammation the magnitude of the overall response is lower than expected for the degree of inflammatory activity, possibly as a result of downregulation. As will be discussed later in this chapter, some diseases show little or no acute phase response even though acute inflammation is clinically apparent.

Laboratory measurements of the acute phase response

The main parameters usually measured to assess the acute phase response are the erythrocyte sedimentation rate (ESR), plasma viscosity (PV), and

Table 2 Properties of the major acute phase proteins

Protein	Response time (h)	Molecular weight	Adult reference ranges
Group I: <1× increase			
Caeruloplasmin	48–72	132 000	0.20–0.60 g/l (5th–95th centile)
Complement components C3	48–72	180 000	0.75–1.65 g/l (5th–95th centile)
C4	48–72	206 000	0.20–0.65 g/l (5th–95th centile)
Group II: 2–4× increase			
α_1-Acid glycoprotein	24	41 000	0.6–1.2 g/l (male); 0.4–1.0 g/l (female); 5 to 50 years of age
α_1-Antitrypsin	10	54 000	1.1–2.1 g/l (5th–95th centile)
α_1-Antichymotrypsin	10	68 000	0.3–0.6 g/l
Haptoglobin	24	86 000	0.5–2.0 g/l (male); 0.4–1.6 g/l (female)
Fibrinogen	24	340 000	2.0–4.0 g/l
Group III: up to 1000× increase			
C-reactive protein	6–10	110 000	0.068–8.0 mg/l
Serum amyloid A	6–10	180 000	

the plasma concentrations of the acute phase proteins (CRP in particular). General guidelines as to the relative merits of these tests have been drawn up by the International Committee for Standardization in Haematology (ICSH 1988). In view of the role of cytokines in the control of the acute phase response, it may be relevant in the future to include plasma levels of cytokines as an additional parameter to be used. Most of the identified cytokines can now be measured by immunoassay, but problems exist such as poor interlaboratory reproducibility and lack of standardization (reviewed by Banks 2000). It is now appreciated that it may be the ratio of pro- and anti-inflammatory cytokines that will give the most clinically relevant information.

ESR and PV

ESR is the oldest and probably still the most widely used index of the acute phase response. It is a laboratory measurement of the rate of sedimentation of erythrocytes that is dependent on their degree of aggregation and the packed cell volume (PCV). Aggregation is strongly influenced by the concentration of large asymmetric plasma proteins such as fibrinogen, α_2-macroglobulin, and immunoglobulins. The ESR is therefore a composite measurement reflecting changes in several slow changing proteins.

There are several disadvantages to this assay. It is influenced by red cell number and characteristics, abnormal immunoglobulins or complexes such as in myeloma or cryoglobulinaemia, age and sex, smoking, menstrual cycle, drugs, and dietary lipids therefore resulting in a circadian rhythm. In addition, the ESR in the acute phase is mainly influenced by fibrinogen, an acute phase protein that is slow to increase and persists long after the inflammation subsides because of its long half-life. Its reliance on fibrinogen levels means that the ESR is often insensitive and relates poorly to the time-course of the inflammation, and is influenced by complications that result in the consumption of fibrinogen, such as the presence of intravascular coagulation. Due to the relative instability of red blood cells in terms of their deformability and aggregation, stored samples cannot be used. Standardization and quality control are difficult although recent recommendations may improve this (ICSH 1993).

PV is increasingly being used in place of the ESR and has several advantages as a routine measurement. It is dependent on the concentrations of the same group of large-molecular-weight proteins but shows less inter-individual variation than the ESR. This is at least partly because the PV, unlike the ESR, is affected minimally by age, sex or pregnancy, and it is not affected by anaemia or red cell morphology. In addition it is a more rapid test to perform, easier to standardize and stored samples are suitable for use.

Despite the above reservations about the ESR and PV, these are technically simple and inexpensive assays to perform and may provide a better screening test for the detection of many diseases than the measurement of a single acute phase protein. For example, the ESR integrates the effects of anaemia, immune response, and acute phase response. These tests thus still play an important role in the detection and monitoring of chronic inflammation where the hyperproteinaemia is more complex than in the acute situation, involving changes in other pathologically important proteins such as immunoglobulins.

Acute phase proteins

Individual acute phase proteins are usually assayed using specific antisera, the precise immunochemical technique being dependent on the particular laboratory. The techniques most often used are, enzyme-linked immunosorbent assay (ELISA), turbidimetry, and nephelometry. Proposed functions of the acute phase proteins have been given in Table 1 and the properties of the major acute phase proteins together with their reference ranges are shown in Table 2. However, it must be emphasized that reference ranges vary between laboratories and clinicians should consult their own laboratories for appropriate figures. The relative merits of the major acute phase proteins as markers of inflammation are discussed below. Detailed reviews have been published, for example, Gabay and Kushner (1999).

C-reactive protein

CRP is a non-glycosylated protein composed of five identical 21 kDa non-covalently bound globular subunits, a member of the pentraxin family. It is the most useful index of the acute phase response being specific, sensitive, and rising rapidly within 6–10 h following the inflammatory event. This time lag represents the time for complete synthesis of the molecule as no hepatic store exists. Peak concentrations are reached by about 48 h and, because of its short half-life of approximately 19 h in man, declines rapidly following the decrease in inflammatory activity. It has been shown in humans that the catabolism of CRP is independent of its plasma concentration and is not affected by the presence of inflammatory illnesses such as rheumatoid arthritis, systemic lupus erythematosus, or infections. This, coupled with the fact that there is no significant tissue sequestration of CRP, indicates that the circulating concentration is determined solely by its rate of synthesis and hence inflammatory stimulus. However, the reference range for CRP is very wide, from 0.068 to 8.0 mg/l with a median value of 0.58 mg/l (Claus et al. 1976), and with many routine assay methods only having a lower limit of detection between 5 and 10 mg/l, it is apparent that CRP concentrations in some individuals could increase more than a 100-fold and still remain within normal limits. It is therefore an unsuitable protein for detecting very mild inflammation unless sensitive assays are used, serial determinations are made and the normal values are known for the individual. Typically, mild infections are associated with CRP levels of between 10 and 40 mg/l (Peltola 1982), acute inflammation and moderate bacterial infection with levels of between 40 and 200 mg/l, and severe bacterial infection can produce levels in excess of 300 mg/l (Morley and Kushner 1982). For detecting or monitoring chronic inflammation, an additional slower reacting acute phase protein such as α_1-antichymotrypsin or α_1-acid glycoprotein or the ESR should also be measured as CRP may be transiently normal during brief remission periods. A World Health Organization (WHO) international standard is available.

Serum amyloid A (SAA) protein

SAA proteins are a family of at least three different apolipoproteins with similar kinetics to CRP but possibly greater sensitivity (reviewed by Uhlar and Whitehead 1999). It is elevated even in relatively mild conditions such as the common cold. Higher levels of SAA have been reported in diseases that carry an increased risk of amyloidosis such as rheumatoid arthritis and systemic juvenile rheumatoid arthritis. However, since SAA is not routinely measured in most laboratories, even though most of the technical problems have been overcome, it will not be covered further here.

α_1-Antichymotrypsin (ACT)

ACT is a glycoprotein consisting of a single polypeptide chain, with oligosaccharide chains accounting for approximately 23 per cent of its molecular weight. Measurement of ACT is often available routinely and normal levels lie in the range of 0.3–0.6 g/l. It increases almost as rapidly as CRP and SAA following tissue injury, although normally only increasing two- to four-fold. It remains elevated for longer than CRP, is easy to measure, and does not suffer from genetic variation or differential catabolism. There is, however, an interlaboratory standardization problem as values obtained are dependent on the antibody and standard used.

Haptoglobin

Haptoglobin is a member of a family of polymers of α–β chains with the α-chain having two main genetic variants. It is much slower in response but can be measured routinely. It is generally unsuitable as an acute phase response indicator, however, because of its consumption associated with haemolysis, and genetic variations giving rise to phenotypic reference ranges.

α_1-Antitrypsin (AAT)

The glycoprotein AAT (α_1-proteinase inhibitor) can be routinely assayed and standardized with WHO preparations. It is generally unsuitable as an indicator of the acute phase response, however, as genetic variants give rise to decreased serum concentrations. Approximately 15 per cent of the Caucasian population are heterozygous and have lower normal concentrations than the 1.1–2.1 g/l found in the normal homozygous MM phenotype. In addition concentrations increase in pregnancy or with oestrogen treatment, and may be inappropriately lowered in vasculitis because of its consumption.

Fibrinogen

Fibrinogen is composed of three pairs of non-identical polypeptide chains, two of which are glycosylated. Fibrinogen is slow to exhibit changes in concentration during inflammation and is relatively insensitive. In routine laboratories, fibrinogen is usually measured by a functional assay of its clotting ability.

α_1-Acid glycoprotein (AGP)

AGP (orosomucoid), as its name suggests, is glycosylated with polysaccharide chains accounting for 45 per cent of the molecule. Genetic variants exist although these have no effect on normal serum ranges. AGP is not often measured routinely, being less sensitive than CRP or ACT. In addition, concentrations may be decreased in pregnancy or during oestrogen treatment and a disproportionate increase in AGP concentration may occur in chronic renal disease, resulting from a reduction in the glomerular filtration rate.

C3, C4, and caeruloplasmin

Complement components C3 and C4, and the copper-binding glycoprotein caeruloplasmin are very insensitive and too slow to increase to be of use as markers of the acute phase response, although low C3 or C4 concentrations, indicating their consumption may be of use for monitoring of immunologically based diseases.

Clinical use of the acute phase response

Although the presence of an acute phase response is associated unequivocally with inflammation, the reverse is not always true. Inflammation occurring with mild chronic tissue damage, localized disease, recurrent attacks, or certain diseases including ulcerative colitis and systemic lupus erythematosus is often found associated with a normal ESR or CRP level. The acute phase response by nature is a non-specific response in terms of the disease and therefore must be used in conjunction with other more specific tests for diagnostic purposes as it can be elevated in many pathological conditions and indeed some acute phase proteins such as AAT and caeruloplasmin also exhibit elevated concentrations in physiological circumstances such as pregnancy. Although the magnitude of the acute phase response is related generally to the mass or activity of inflammation, this is not always the case. As previously indicated, an extremely large acute phase response is seen in bacterial infections, for example, presumably as a result of the systemic endotoxin-induced release of IL-1, IL-6, and TNF from macrophages.

However, together with other clinical and laboratory measurements, the assessment of the acute phase response is generally used in three main ways to assist the rheumatologist:

(i) detection of organic disease;

(ii) assessment of extent or activity of the disease, monitoring of therapy, and indication of prognosis; and

(iii) detection of intercurrent infection.

There is no acute phase response in patients with soft tissue rheumatism or osteoporosis. The use of the acute phase response is given below for each of the main disease groups within the arthritides.

Crystal deposition diseases

The acute phase response may be only mild or absent in crystal deposition diseases unless accompanied by superimposed infection in the joints. In gout, however, an acute phase response is often seen and CRP levels may reach in excess of 100 mg/l, even in the absence of intercurrent infection (Roseff et al. 1987).

Osteoarthritis

Primary generalized or nodal osteoarthritis is not associated with an acute phase response, the ESR being normal or only mildly elevated in the majority of cases (reviewed by Altman and Gray 1985). This may be partly age related. No difference is seen between erosive and non-erosive osteoarthritis and there is no practical value in attempting to determine the severity of episodes of inflammation by the measurement of the acute phase response. PV, however, has been reported to be slightly elevated in more than 80 per cent of patients examined with non-erosive osteoarthritis.

Polymyalgia rheumatica and giant cell arteritis

Most studies report a raised ESR in 95–100 per cent of patients with polymyalgia rheumatica/giant cell arteritis at presentation, and indeed an ESR of greater than 50 mm/h is now included as one of five diagnostic criteria to be used in the classification of giant cell arteritis. This marked acute phase response is of use clinically to differentiate between polymyalgia rheumatica and other causes of myalgia such as depression, myositis, and thyroid disease, due to the lack of other abnormal biochemical findings in polymyaglia rheumatica. However, there are reports of patients with biopsy-proven giant cell arteritis in whom the ESR is normal and it has been suggested that at least in some cases this may be because of prior use of steroids. A significant correlation between PV and ESR has been reported, but in 30 out of the 112 paired readings, one parameter was abnormal in the presence of a normal value for the other. Acute phase proteins such as CRP, AGP, ACT, and haptoglobin are also elevated in the majority of untreated patients with polymyalgia rheumatica or giant cell arteritis (CRP may be in excess of 100 mg/l). However, the elevation of AGP by corticosteroids and the consumption of haptoglobin limit their potential usefulness in monitoring disease activity, and ACT does not decrease with clinical remission although lower concentrations during follow-up may be indicative of a reduced risk of subsequent relapse (Pountain et al. 1994). There is some controversy as to whether CRP or ESR is the better index of disease activity and both may remain normal during clinical relapse on treatment (Pountain et al. 1994). If clinical suspicion of the disease is strong yet the chosen parameter is not abnormal, it may be appropriate to measure the other. Measurement of either CRP or the ESR may be used together with clinical assessment to monitor the initial effectiveness of steroid therapy, thus minimizing the risk of arteritis, with the change in CRP more rapidly reflecting the clinical improvement and in most cases reaching normal levels within 7–14 days of the start of steroid administration. Neither CRP nor ESR levels can be used to predict a relapse, however.

A galaxy of other serum biological markers have been reported as raised in untreated polymyalgia rheumatica. These include IL-6 and IL-6 receptor antagonist, serum soluble intercellular adhesion molecule 1, IL-10, and vascular endothelial growth factor (VEGF). However, there is no evidence that these are useful in measuring response to therapy and these cytokines are, in any case, only available in certain laboratories and then only at considerable expense.

Autoimmune rheumatic disorders

The acute phase response is often moderate or absent in these disorders, even when clinically active, and if marked may suggest alternative pathology. However, in systemic lupus erythematosus the ESR is elevated in nearly all patients, often falling with a decline in disease activity, although it is of little use clinically. The use of CRP levels to discriminate between intercurrent infection (with or without fever) and disease exacerbation is controversial. Most studies report generally higher CRP levels in patients with infection compared with active disease (reviewed by Pepys et al. 1982). It has been proposed that a serum CRP level of greater than 60 mg/l is strongly indicative of infection, with CRP levels of less than 30 mg/l making it unlikely that severe infection is present. However, the discriminatory power of CRP levels is not absolute and must be viewed with caution as levels in excess of 60 mg/l have been reported in patients with systemic lupus erythematosus in the absence of infection, and patients with this disease and intercurrent infection may have normal or only moderately elevated levels of CRP. Recently it has been proposed that the discriminatory ability of CRP levels is only of value in the absence of serositis (Ter Borg et al. 1990). In addition, patients with Jaccoud's arthropathy or polyarthritis appear to have higher CRP concentrations (Spronk et al. 1992).

The reason for the relative lack of acute phase response in many of the autoimmune rheumatic disorders even in the presence of active inflammation is not clear, but the finding of identical clearance rates for CRP in patients with systemic lupus erythematosus compared with healthy controls make it unlikely that altered clearance mechanisms account for the apparent lack of response. It is also unlikely to be due to a straightforward lack of hepatic responsiveness as these patients can present such a response in the case of bacterial infection. However, with the complex regulation of the acute phase response by a network of cytokine interactions, it is possible that the response may be impaired by certain combinations of cytokines that are present in this disease, either at the level of the hepatocyte or because of cytokine inhibitors (reviewed by Gordon and Emery 1993).

Plasma fibrinogen has recently been advocated as an acute phase reactant of value in monitoring the progression severity of systemic lupus erythematosus, independent of the more modest age effect and more likely to be raised in the presence of thrombosis (Ames et al. 2000) but this is no substitute for the screening for antiphospholipid antibodies, dealt with elsewhere in the book.

Seronegative spondyloarthritides

Ankylosing spondylitis is variably associated with a raised ESR, PV, and CRP. Reports regarding correlation with disease activity are conflicting, possibly due at least in part to differences in study design and definitions of active disease. Generally, CRP levels are between 10 and 30 mg/l although levels in excess of 100 mg/l have been reported in active disease. CRP or PV have been advocated as being more sensitive markers of active disease than the ESR (Dixon et al. 1981) and significantly elevated CRP levels have been found in patients with active disease compared with inactive disease (Nashel et al. 1986). In other studies, although the ESR was found to correlate with levels of CRP and other acute phase proteins, none of these parameters correlated with disease activity (Laurent and Panayi 1983). More recently a significant correlation between disease activity and CRP levels was only shown in HLA-B27 positive patients.

CRP levels in patients with Behçet's syndrome do not usually exceed 20 mg/l. Most patients with psoriatic arthritis have an increased PV compared with controls. Both psoriatic arthritis and Reiter's syndrome are associated generally with normal or only mildly elevated levels of CRP, although levels as high as 40 mg/l have been reported in patients with active Reiter's syndrome (Nashel et al. 1986). The few reports concerning the use of CRP or ESR to monitor disease activity in these illnesses are contradictory and hence no conclusion can be drawn.

There is lack of unanimity about increased serum levels of creatine kinase in ankylosing spondylitis. A recent study has suggested that the serum biochemical markers of muscle origin (aldolase, creatinine, alanine aminotransferase, and aspartate aminotransferase) are low in patients with active ankylosing spondylitis, the first correlating with high CRP levels, implying specific protein degradation, predominantly in skeletal muscle, in this disease.

Early synovitis

With an increased acceptance that rheumatoid arthritis is a more serious disease than once thought and the realization that early treatment reduces later joint damage, early synovitis clinics in which patients are seen within 4–6 weeks of the onset of their joint symptoms have become an accepted and important part of rheumatological care. In turn, particularly if potent early treatment is to be encouraged, there has been increased interest in the first change in acute phase reactants (which are of assistance diagnostically in excluding patients who have milder conditions that mimic inflammatory arthritis) and which would be of value in monitoring and confirming the benefit of early drug intervention. In this respect the ESR and CRP are time-honoured and figure in conventional clinical assessments. The PV is sometimes substituted. In general, CRP has proved to be the most valuable standard first index of inflammation, the ESR too subject to variables other than inflammatory disease and PV a little slower to change. This mirrors the relative speed of change of these parameters in polymyalgia rheumatica. Once disease is established and abnormalities present, ESR, CRP, and PV have proved equally useful in calculating ACR 20 per cent response rate in patients with early active rheumatoid arthritis. Known aggressors have been suggested and published to allow interchange, since not all of these are measured in each unit (Paulus et al. 1999). However, not all have found CRP to be so reliable.

More complicated tests have sometimes been suggested. Serum amyloid A may be preferable to either ESR or CRP in patients with recent onset arthritis, very high levels claimed to have exclusive diagnostic reliability. Serum amyloid A protein also falls as the disease comes under control but this test is not yet universally available (Cunnane et al. 2000). Serum matrix metalloproteinase 3 (MMP-3) has also been advocated as a useful marker for predicting bone damage in the early stages of rheumatoid arthritis (Yamanaka et al. 2000).

Rheumatoid arthritis

Rheumatoid arthritis is associated generally with a marked acute phase response although fever is usually absent. PV, ESR, and CRP levels are nearly always elevated and in many cases, although not all, reflect disease activity (reviewed by Van Leeuwen and Van Rijswijk 1994). CRP levels are generally in the range of 30–40 mg/l in patients with moderate disease activity, and may reach in excess of 100 mg/l in severe disease, although in a small group of patients CRP levels lie within the normal range despite clinical evidence of active disease. CRP concentrations in excess of 150 mg/l may be indicative of an intercurrent bacterial infection. The question of which of these parameters is the best index of disease activity is open to debate. ACT has also been reported to reflect disease activity in rheumatoid arthritis, being elevated even in those patients in whom CRP levels are normal despite clinical evidence of active disease (Chard et al. 1988), and merits further investigation.

Studies examining the prognostic implications of the acute phase response in rheumatoid arthritis have recently been reviewed (Van Leeuwen and Van Rijswijk 1994). In general it appears that isolated measurements of the acute response are of little use in predicting outcome of the disease. However, persistently higher ESR and CRP measurements have been associated with a higher rate of radiological progression. More recently, time-integrated values of CRP and ESR have been found to correlate significantly with radiological progression both in patients with early disease and in those with long-standing disease (Hassell et al. 1993; Van Leeuwen et al. 1993, 1994). However, with the considerable interindividual variation in CRP values found, it would be inappropriate to attempt to use a single cut-off value for prognostic purposes but rather the longitudinal findings need to be interpreted for each individual patient.

Following an examination of the literature, the American College of Rheumatology have recommended that the ESR or CRP should be one of the core set of disease activity measures in clinical trials (Felson et al. 1993). The slow-acting disease-modifying drugs such as gold, sulfasalazine, D-penicillamine, and hydroxychloroquine are usually associated with a decline in the acute phase protein response (reviewed by Kvien and Husby 1992). An exception is cyclosporin which has no effect on the ESR. A recent European collaborative study found ESR to be a more useful measure of disease activity than CRP, with CRP presenting standardization problems between countries and laboratories. Although a vast majority of studies have failed to find any effect of non-steroidal anti-inflammatory drugs on the acute phase response, a study which differentiated between clinical 'responders' and 'non-responders' in their analysis, did suggest a decline in

ESR and CRP levels in the 'responders', correlating with improvement in clinical variables (Cush et al. 1990). However, the finding that CRP decreases even in some clinical 'non-responders' suggests that this decline in acute phase protein response may not be secondary to a suppression of joint inflammation and cytokine production by the drugs, but rather to some other mechanism. Obviously, under these circumstances, the use of the acute phase reactants to monitor drug efficacy would be inappropriate.

Conflicting reports exist regarding a possible association between AAT phenotype and rheumatoid arthritis but the evidence overall does not currently support any such association (Kahl et al. 1989). IgA-AAT levels in rheumatoid arthritis do not appear to be associated with inflammation per se, neither are they related to obvious bacterial stimulation.

Other markers have recently been studied. Serum 5′-nucleotidase, mainly from the liver, acts as a marker of general inflammation. 5′-Nucleotidase in the synovial fluid was mainly produced locally, possibly a valuable marker of joint inflammation (Johnson et al. 1999). Stromelysin-1 (MMP-3), one of several metalloproteinase raised in rheumatoid arthritis, proves not to be an independent marker of joint damage but correlates better with overall systemic inflammation (So et al. 1999). Serum ferritin is a valuable and accepted marker of disease activity in adult onset Still's disease. The percentage of glycosylated ferritin is low both in the active disease and in remission, though the specificity of this test is not yet sufficient to allow its use as a diagnostic marker, particularly when adult onset Still's disease has an atypical presentation.

Diagnostic confusion sometimes arises between normochromic normacytic anaemia of rheumatoid disease and officially anaemia, often consequent upon the use of non-steroidal anti-inflammatory drugs. Serum transferrin receptor (sTfR) may prove superior to serum ferritin in clarifying this, irrespective of the concurrent iron storage status.

References

Altman, R.D. and Gray, R. (1985). Inflammation in osteoarthritis. *Clinics in the Rheumatic Diseases* **11**, 353–65.

Ames, P.R.J. et al. (2000). Fibrinogen in systemic lupus erythematosus: more than an acute phase reactant? *Journal of Rheumatology* **27**, 1190–5.

Banks, R.E. (2000). Measurement of cytokines in clinical samples using immunoassays: problems and pitfalls. *Critical Reviews in Clinical Laboratory Sciences* **37**, 131–82.

Banks, R.E. et al. (1995). The acute phase protein response in patients receiving subcutaneous IL-6. *Clinical and Experimental Immunology* **102**, 217–23.

Baumann, H. and Gauldie, J. (1994). The acute phase response. *Immunology Today* **15**, 74–80.

Chard, M.D. et al. (1988). Serum α_1-antichymotrypsin concentration as a marker of disease activity in rheumatoid arthritis. *Annals of the Rheumatic Diseases* **47**, 665–71.

Claus, D.R., Osmand, A.P., and Gewurz, H. (1976). Radioimmunoassay of human C-reactive protein and levels in normal sera. *Journal of Clinical and Laboratory Medicine* **87**, 120–8.

Cunnane, G. et al. (2000). Serum amyloid A in the assessment of early inflammatory arthritis. *Journal of Rheumatology* **27**, 58–63.

Cush, J.J. et al. (1990). Correlation of serologic indicators of inflammation with effectiveness of non-steroidal anti-inflammatory drug therapy in rheumatoid arthritis. *Arthritis and Rheumatism* **33**, 19–28.

Dixon, J.S., Bird, H.A., and Wright, V. (1981). A comparison of serum biochemistry in ankylosing spondylitis, seronegative and seropositive rheumatoid arthritis. *Annals of the Rheumatic Diseases* **40**, 404–8.

Felson, D.T. et al. (1993). The American College of Rheumatology preliminary core set of disease activity measures for rheumatoid arthritis clinical trials. *Arthritis and Rheumatism* **36**, 729–40.

Gabay, C. and Kushner, I. (1999). Mechanisms of disease: acute phase proteins and other systemic responses to inflammation. *New England Journal of Medicine* **340**, 448–54.

Gordon, C. and Emery, P. (1993). Cytokines and the acute phase response in SLE. *Lupus* **2**, 345–7.

Hassell, A.B. et al. (1993). The relationship between serial measures of disease activity and outcome in rheumatoid arthritis. *Quarterly Journal of Medicine* **86**, 601–7.

ICSH (International Committee for Standardization in Haematology, Expert Panel on Blood Rheology) (1988). Guidelines on selection of laboratory tests for monitoring the acute phase response. *Journal of Clinical Pathology* **41**, 1203–12.

ICSH (International Committee for Standardization in Haematology, Expert Panel on Blood Rheology) (1993). ICSH recommendations for measurement of erythrocyte sedimentation rate. *Journal of Clinical Pathology* **46**, 198–203.

Johnson, S.M. et al. (1999). 5′Nucleotidase as a marker of both general and local inflammation in rheumatoid arthritis patients. *Rheumatology* **38**, 391–6.

Kahl, L.E. et al. (1989). Alpha-1-antitrypsin (Pl) and vitamin-D binding globulin (GC) phenotypes in rheumatoid arthritis: absence of an association. *Disease Markers* **7**, 71–8.

Kushner, I. (1982). The phenomenon of the acute phase response. *Annals of the New York Academy of Sciences* **389**, 39–48.

Kvien, T.K. and Husby, G. (1992). Disease modification in rheumatoid arthritis with special reference to cyclosporin A. *Scandinavian Journal of Rheumatology* **21** (Suppl. 95), 19–28.

Laurent, M.R. and Panayi, G.S. (1983). Acute phase proteins and serum immunoglobulins in ankylosing spondylitis. *Annals of the Rheumatic Diseases* **42**, 524–8.

Mackiewicz, A., Kushner, I., and Baumann, H., ed. *Acute Phase Proteins: Molecular Biology, Biochemistry and Clinical Applications.* London: CRC Press, 1993.

Morley, J.J. and Kushner, I. (1982). Serum C-reactive protein levels in disease. *Annals of the New York Academy of Sciences* **389**, 406–18.

Nashel, D.J. et al. (1986). C-reactive protein: a marker for disease activity in ankylosing spondylitis and Reiter's syndrome. *Journal of Rheumatology* **13**, 364–7.

Paulus, H.E. et al. (1999). Equivalence of the acute phase reactants, C-reactive protein, plasma viscosity, and Westergren erythrocyte sedimentation rate when used to calculate American College of Rheumatology 20 per cent improvement criteria or the disease activity score in patients with early rheumatoid arthritis. *Journal of Rheumatology* **26**, 2324–31.

Peltola, H.O. (1982). C-reactive protein for rapid monitoring of infections of the central nervous system. *Lancet* **i**, 980–3.

Pepys, M.B., Lanham, J.G., and De Beer, F.C. (1982). C-reactive protein in SLE. *Clinics in the Rheumatic Diseases* **8**, 91–103.

Pountain, G.D., Calvin, J., and Hazleman, B.L. (1994). α1-antichymotrypsin, C-reactive protein and erythrocyte sedimentation rate in polymyalgia rheumatica and giant cell arteritis. *British Journal of Rheumatology* **33**, 550–4.

Roseff, R. et al. (1987). The acute phase response in gout. *Journal of Rheumatology* **14**, 974–7.

So, A. et al. (1999). Serum MMP-3 in rheumatoid arthritis: correlation with systemic inflammation but not with erosive status. *Rheumatology* **38**, 407–10.

Spronk, P.E., Terborg, E.J., and Kallenberg, C.G.M. (1992). Patients with systemic lupus-erythematosus and Jaccoud's arthropathy—a clinical subset with an increased C-reactive protein response. *Annals of the Rheumatic Diseases* **51**, 358–61.

Steel, D.M. and Whitehead, A.S. (1994). The major acute phase reactants: C-reactive protein, serum amyloid P component and serum amyloid A protein. *Immunology Today* **15**, 81–8.

Ter Borg, E.J. et al. (1990). C-reactive protein levels during disease exacerbations and infections in systemic lupus erythematosus: a prospective longitudinal study. *Journal of Rheumatology* **17**, 1642–8.

Uhlar, C.M. and Whitehead, A.S. (1999). Serum amyloid A, the major vertebrate acute phase reactant. *European Journal of Biochemistry* **265**, 501–23.

Van Leeuwen, M.A. and Van Rijswijk, M.H. (1994). Acute phase proteins in the monitoring of inflammatory disorders. *Baillière's Clinical Rheumatology* **8** (3), 531–52.

Van Leeuwen, M.A. et al. (1993). The acute-phase response in relation to radiographic progression in early rheumatoid arthritis: a prospective study during the first three years of the disease. *British Journal of Rheumatology* **32** (Suppl. 3), 9–13.

Van Leeuwen, M.A. et al. (1994). Interrelationship of outcome measures and process variables in early rheumatoid arthritis. A comparison of radiologic damage, physical disability, joint counts, and acute phase reactants. *Journal of Rheumatology* **21**, 425–9.

Yamanaka, H. et al. (2000). Serum matrix metalloproteinase 3 as a predictor of the degree of joint destruction during the six months after measurement, in patients with early rheumatoid arthritis. *Arthritis and Rheumatism* **43**, 852–8.

5.2 Biochemistry

Douglas Thompson and Howard A. Bird

The rheumatologists' requirements of the clinical biochemistry laboratory vary according to the disease being managed. Automation of assays has led to a wider variety of biochemical estimations becoming more easily and inexpensively available. However, the contribution of the clinical biochemist to the diagnosis and management of the rheumatic illnesses is still relatively minor when compared with many other illnesses, possibly reflecting the relative chronicity and non-life-threatening nature of many of the rheumatic illnesses and the difficulty of devising new clinical laboratory tests when the aetiology of the disease is relatively uncertain. This chapter concentrates on those biochemical assays that are likely to be available in most hospitals for the routine management of patients with rheumatic disease.

The clinical problem in rheumatology

Rarely is a single biochemical laboratory test truly diagnostic (except in the case of inborn errors of metabolism); rather, they point to a pathological process or suggest damage or dysfunction of a particular organ, or they are used to monitor the course of a disease. As in most specialities, biochemical tests serve a number of well-defined purposes in rheumatology, which may be outlined as follows:

1. Indication of a pathological process and its intensity, for example, inflammation, immune response, haemolysis, malignancy.
2. Indication of damage or dysfunction of organs, for example, liver and kidney.

Tests may be used to:

1. Confirm or exclude a specific diagnosis. Several tests must be interpreted together with the clinical picture to create a probability of a diagnosis. Critical decisions are whether a particular organ or tissue is affected and what process (e.g. inflammation) is present.
2. Exclude other disorders that could (although deemed unlikely in the clinical context) give rise to the same symptoms. A panel of screening tests for other disorders is required, tailored to the clinical presentation, to ensure that different diagnoses are not overlooked. For example, malignant disease may be associated with myositis, myopathy, or generalized symptoms suggestive of soft tissue rheumatism. However, normal test results never completely exclude a condition.
3. Assess and monitor disease activity. Prognosis and choice of therapy may depend on disease activity at presentation and control of therapy may depend on monitoring disease activity. Examples include longitudinal measurements of acute-phase proteins to assess disease activity in rheumatic diseases and the use of serum uric acid levels to monitor the effectiveness of long-term prophylactic allopurinol therapy for gout.
4. Detect a complication of the disease. This usually means detecting damage to an organ, such as the kidney, either at the time of diagnosis or during the course of the disease. Rheumatic diseases particularly associated with such complications include systemic lupus erythematosus, polyarteritis nodosa, and gout.
5. Detect side-effects of therapy. Many of the drug therapies used in rheumatology can have unwanted side-effects, particularly in elderly people, often involving the liver or kidney. Sulfasalazine, azathioprine, and methotrexate are amongst this group of drugs.

The biochemical tests in rheumatology

Table 1 indicates the appropriate biochemical tests for assessing organ/tissue pathology and disease processes in rheumatic diseases. In the following section we will explain the use of these tests, suggest how they may be interpreted, and examine their clinical relevance in rheumatology. A guide to the use of these tests in the overall management of patients in rheumatology is provided in Table 2.

Organ or tissue pathology mimicking rheumatic disease or arising from it or from therapy

At presentation and during the course of the disease, the presence of various organ or tissue abnormalities, which may either be the cause of the symptoms or occur as a result of complications of the disease or therapy, needs to be excluded.

Renal function

The tests available for the assessment of renal function are described below (reviewed by Duarte and Preuss 1993; Lindeman 1993; Moore and Carome 1993).

Table 1 Biochemical tests for assessing organ/tissue pathology and pathological processes in rheumatic disease

Clinical problem	Laboratory test
Organ/tissue pathology mimicking rheumatic disease or arising from it or therapy	
Renal damage	
Glomerular	Plasma urea or creatinine, electrolytes
Tubular	Urinary β_2-microglobulin, α_2-microglobulin, *N*-acetyl glucosaminidase, electrolytes
Liver damage	Plasma AST/ALT, alkaline phosphatase, GGT, bilirubin, total protein, albumin
Bone metabolism	Plasma calcium, phosphate, alkaline phosphatase, albumin, osteocalcin, collagen crosslinks
Muscle disease	Plasma creatine kinase
Malignancy	
Myeloma	Serum and urine electrophoresis
Metastatic	Plasma alkaline phosphatase, prostate-specific antigen
Pathological processes occurring in rheumatic disease	
Inflammation	Acute-phase proteins
Immune response	IgG, IgA, IgM
Immune complex deposition	Immune complexes, C3, C4, and breakdown products
Crystal deposition	Uric acid

ALT, alanine transaminase; AST, aspartate transaminase; GGT, γ-glutamyl transpeptidase; Ig, immunoglobulin.

Table 2 Routine biochemical management of rheumatic patients

Disease	At diagnosis A	At diagnosis B	At follow-up
Soft-tissue rheumatism	N/A	Acute-phase response, full profile, creatine kinase	N/A
Gout	Uric acid, acute-phase response	N/A	Uric acid every 2 weeks during initial therapy, then every second year; lipids every 5 years; renal profile annually
Pyrophosphate deposition	N/A	Bone profile, uric acid	N/A
Polymyalgia rheumatica/ temporal arteritis	Acute-phase response	Creatine kinase, serum/urine electrophoresis	Acute-phase response every 2 months for 2 years, then monitor while decreasing steroids
Osteoarthritis	N/A	Acute-phase response, full profile	N/A
Rheumatoid arthritis	Acute-phase response, rheumatoid factor	Full profile	Diagnostic tests every 3–6 months, if disease-modifying antirheumatic drugs used, test more frequently; renal and hepatic profiles as appropriate and dipstick urinary protein monitoring
Psoriatic arthritis	Acute-phase response	Rheumatoid factor, full profile	Acute-phase response annually
Ankylosing spondylitis	Acute-phase response	Rheumatoid factor, full profile	Acute-phase response annually
Systemic lupus erythematosus	Acute-phase response, antinuclear antibodies	Rheumatoid factor, full profile	Acute-phase response, DNA binding, C3, C4, renal profile every 6 months; regular dipstick urinary protein monitoring
Polymyositis/dermatomyositis	Creatine kinase, acute-phase response	N/A	Repeat tests and renal profile annually
Systemic sclerosis	Acute-phase response	N/A	Repeat tests and renal profile annually

It is emphasized that this is a personal view and the actual practice will vary between hospitals and be dependent upon factors such as local laboratory resources and ease of attendance of patients. Tests at diagnosis are divided into (A), those which provide positive diagnostic information for the disease, and (B), those which are usually used to exclude other conditions or possible complications of the proposed diagnosis. 'Full profile' refers to the measurements usually available on multichannel analysers and consists of urea, creatinine, sodium, potassium, chloride, bicarbonate, calcium, phosphate, albumin, AST/ALT, bilirubin, alkaline phosphatase, and total protein. The terms we have used here are 'renal profile' to include urea, creatinine, sodium, and potassium; 'hepatic profile' to include AST/ALT, bilirubin alkaline phosphatase and albumin; and 'bone profile' to include calcium, alkaline phosphate, albumin, and phosphate. Acute-phase response indicates the use of plasma viscocity, erythrocyte sedimentation rate or acute-phase proteins, as available. N/A, not applicable.

Glomerular function

The two principal indicators of glomerular function are the permeability of the glomerular basement membrane and the glomerular filtration rate (GFR). The GFR can be assessed by measuring the clearance of substances that must fulfil the requirements of being freely filtered at the glomerulus, neither secreted nor reabsorbed by the renal tubule, be physiologically and metabolically inert, and have a constant concentration in the plasma throughout the period of urine collection. Although the fructose polymer inulin is an ideal substance, the requirement of administration by intravenous infusion precludes its use routinely. An alternative is ^{51}Cr-labelled EDTA, the clearance of which can be assessed from the plasma radioactivity at one time-point after a single intravenous dose rather than collecting timed urine samples. However, disadvantages include cost and unsuitability of use during pregnancy. Although clearance of inulin or radioisotopes are the most accurate methods of measuring GFR, they are used less frequently than the more inaccurate methods described below, largely because of the relative complexity and cost (Duarte and Preuss 1993).

The GFR is most often assessed by measuring the creatinine clearance. This is not ideal as creatinine is secreted actively by the renal tubules, the assay of plasma creatinine is subject to interference from non-creatinine chromogens, the reference range is age dependent, and plasma concentrations may increase after exercise or after the consumption of cooked meat during the period of urine collection (24 h). Although creatinine clearance provides a reasonably accurate assessment of GFR when renal function is normal, as glomerular function becomes impaired the GFR is increasingly overestimated. This partly results from increased tubular secretion of creatinine, together with the decreasing inaccuracy of the plasma creatinine measurement as the relative contribution from the non-creatinine chromogen falls. The overall imprecision of creatinine clearance measurements can be high [up to 70 per cent coefficient of variation (CV), Walser 1998] since it is calculated from three measurements, namely, plasma and urinary creatinine, and 24 h urine volume, each having its own imprecision. The main sources of error include incomplete and inaccurately timed urine collection, and bacterial degradation of urinary creatinine. It is recommended that clearance measurements should be discontinued (Walser 1998).

In view of the inaccuracy and imprecision of measurements of creatinine clearance, the concentration of plasma creatinine is viewed by many to be a more useful indicator of glomerular function. Measurements of plasma creatinine are less imprecise than those of urinary creatinine, and the adult reference range for plasma creatinine is not affected by age, although it is sex dependent and affected by pregnancy and muscle mass. The plasma creatinine may be elevated falsely by drugs that block tubular secretion (e.g. cimetidine and salicylates), ketone bodies and bilirubin (which may interfere in some assays), exercise, and the consumption of meat. It is a relatively insensitive indicator of renal impairment, with no appreciable change in plasma creatinine until the GFR is reduced by about half, after which point the creatinine rises exponentially with the decline in GFR. The reciprocal of the creatinine concentration at several time-points may provide a better indicator of declining GFR. As the reciprocal of the plasma creatinine decreases linearly with progressive renal failure, the rate of progression of renal impairment can be determined from the slope of the line. Additional adverse occurrences or effects of therapy are thus apparent from a change in the slope of the line (Fig. 1).

The decline in GFR that occurs with increasing age is not reflected in the serum creatinine, which remains within the 'normal' range. This is due to the coincidental reduction in lean body mass and resultant decrease in

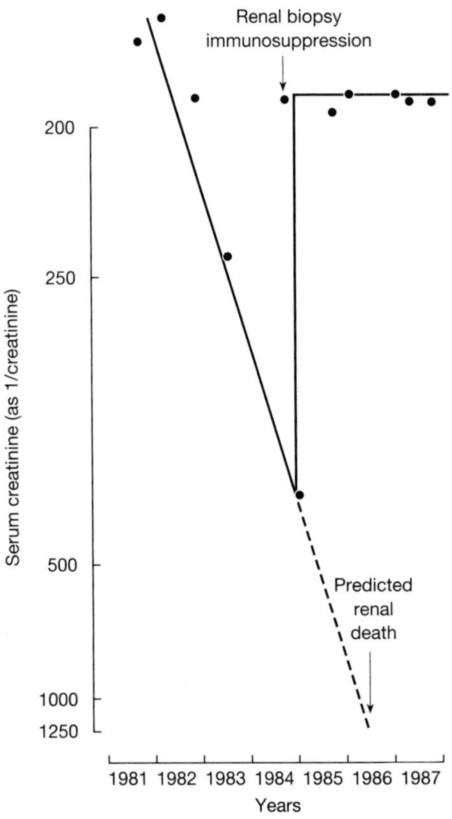

Fig. 1 The use of reciprocal plasma creatinine to monitor renal function. The reciprocal creatinine concentrations are shown for a female Caucasian (date of birth 18 August 1941) who developed arthralgia, photosensitive skin rash, and mildly positive serology for systemic lupus. Persistent proteinuria and a progressive rise in plasma creatinine were found. On nephrological referral 3 years later, a renal biopsy showed diffuse, proliferative glomerulonephritis with deposition of immunoglobulins and complement, and the patient was treated with prednisolone and cyclophosphamide. The graph illustrates the use of the reciprocal creatinine to monitor the progressive decline in renal function. With therapy, renal function improved and reached a new steady state, although it was permanently impaired.

endogenous creatinine production. When using the serum creatinine (S_{cr}) to predict the creatinine clearance (C_{cr}), there are several nomograms and formulae, such as the one below, which allow correction for effects of body weight and age (Cockroft and Gault 1976):

$$C_{cr} = \frac{(140 - \text{age}) \times \text{bodyweight (kg)}}{0.81 \times S_{cr}\ (\mu\text{mol/l})}$$

For an adult woman, the value obtained should be reduced by 15 per cent to allow for lower muscle mass. It must be emphasized that the analytical and pre-analytical variability of creatinine measurements are inherent in such formulae.

Plasma urea is a less sensitive measurement than plasma creatinine and is influenced by the rate of protein catabolism, diet, fluid balance, infection, and concomitant medication such as corticosteroids (Moore and Carome 1993). As the excretion of urea is very dependent on urine flow rate, dehydration leads to an elevated plasma urea, owing to increased reabsorption. In patients known to have chronic renal failure, intercurrent infection may drastically increase the rate of protein catabolism, with a deterioration of the biochemical abnormality and possible rapid clinical impairment. In this situation, plasma urea is a more rapid and sensitive indicator of the clinical state than is creatinine. If the patient with chronic renal failure is undergoing strict dietary control to reduce the rate of urea formation, measurement of creatinine is appropriate as the levels of urea may fall considerably as the result of the dietary measures alone. The urea : creatinine ratio can be used to indicate reductions in renal blood flow that occur as a result of either real or apparent hypovolaemia. A reduction of the normal ratio (approximately 1 : 20 SI units) indicates renal outflow obstruction, hypotension, increased protein intake, or dehydration.

Cystatin C is a low molecular weight protein that has many of the features of an ideal GFR marker. Indications are that plasma cystatin C concentrations are a good indicator of GFR throughout life and that it shows a better correlation with reference procedures than plasma creatinine (Price and Finney 2000).

Proteinuria can reflect either glomerular or tubular damage, and can be characterized as primarily glomerular, primarily tubular, or of mixed origin, based on the protein constituents of the urine (Moore and Carome 1993). Haematuria, together with proteinuria, usually localizes the cause of the proteinuria to a glomerular pathology. Glomerular proteinuria is often associated with larger amounts of urinary protein (>2.5 g/24 h) and the urine contains proteins of moderate and high molecular weight to a much greater extent than in primary tubular proteinuria (4.4 g/24 h compared with 0.4 g/24 h). Proteinuria may also result from strenuous exercise and the possibility of Bence-Jones proteinuria should not be overlooked.

Tubular function

The proximal tubule is the most common site of renal tubular damage and substances normally reabsorbed at this site appear in the urine in increased concentrations (e.g. glucose, amino acids, proteins, phosphate, and potassium). The most sensitive test of proximal tubular reabsorption is the measurement of low molecular weight proteins such as β_2-microglobulin (11.8 kDa), α_1-microglobulin (27 kDa), and retinol-binding protein (21 kDa), which are filtered normally by the glomeruli and almost totally reabsorbed in the proximal tubule. Increased plasma concentrations of these proteins, such as may occur with β_2-microglobulin in lymphoproliferative disorders or when the GFR falls excessively in chronic renal failure, may also result in low molecular weight proteinuria as the tubular reabsorptive capacity may be exceeded. In acid urine β_2-microglobulin is unstable, thus favouring measurement of retinol-binding protein or α_1-microglobulin.

Renal enzymes such as the lysosomal enzyme *N*-acetyl-D-glucosaminidase (NAG) and the brush-border enzyme alanine aminopeptidase are released during damage to tubular cells and are sensitive markers, usually preceding changes in urinary protein. Such enzymes are of most use for monitoring the acute rather than the chronic state, where protein assays may be superior.

Clinical relevance in rheumatic disease

Soft tissue rheumatism and osteoarthritis are usually associated with normal renal function tests but it is important to exclude serious coincidental renal pathology particularly since osteoarthritis patients are elderly. Similarly, renal function is virtually never impaired in the temporal arteritis–polymyalgia rheumatica syndrome (Sonnenblick et al. 1989). Apart from drug toxicity, the kidney is not often clinically involved in systemic juvenile chronic arthritis or adult rheumatoid arthritis, with abnormalities mainly occurring as a result of amyloid deposition or, less frequently, vasculitis. Most patients with amyloidosis present with a marked proteinuria, and the disease runs a variable but slow course towards end-stage renal failure that can be monitored by the reciprocal of serum creatinine. It has been suggested that in view of the many renal-associated deaths in rheumatoid arthritis, which are not amyloid-related, it remains sub-clinical during the course of the disease because of insensitive screening methods.

Between 10 and 20 per cent of patients with ankylosing spondylitis have some renal abnormality (reviewed by Youssef and Russell 1990). These may be coincidental, related to therapy with non-steroidal anti-inflammatory drugs (NSAIDs), the result of amyloid deposition that is associated with long-term ankylosing spondylitis, or alternatively due to IgA nephropathy.

Systemic lupus erythematosus, polyarteritis nodosa, and Sjögren's disease, which may complicate rheumatoid arthritis, all carry a much higher risk of renal involvement. Renal disorders, mainly mild interstitial nephritis with distal tubular acidosis, can occur in up to 30 per cent of patients with primary Sjögren's syndrome (reviewed by Boers 1990), although clinically overt renal disease is generally found in less than 5 per cent of patients. Vasculitis, which may be primary as in Wegener's granulomatosis and polyarteritis nodosa, or secondary to disorders such as rheumatoid arthritis and many of the autoimmune rheumatic disorders, may cause a glomerulonephritis with temporary or permanent glomerular dysfunction, a decrease in GFR, and ultimately renal failure.

Potentially serious renal disease may complicate systemic lupus (Cameron 2001) and regular renal assessment is essential. The onset may be insidious or abrupt, usually following a chronic course with remissions and exacerbations. The pathogenesis is complex and the renal disease may be glomerular, tubular, or vascular, with concomitant biochemical changes as described above, predominantly those of glomerulonephritis. Serial creatinine clearances have been reported to be of little use in patients with lupus nephropathy, as they do not accurately measure the direction or the magnitude of the change in GFR (Petri et al. 1988). Both plasma creatinine and qualitative urinary protein can predict mortality in systemic lupus (reviewed by Gladman 1990). However, there are patients with systemic lupus who have normal plasma creatinine concentrations and urinalysis but abnormal findings on renal biopsy.

Tests of renal function are essential in patients with gout, both at diagnosis and at regular intervals thereafter, in order to detect the important complication of renal damage, which may dictate the need for specific drug therapy with allopurinol. Approximately half of patients with chronic gout have proteinuria with normal plasma creatinine concentrations. The incidence of renal stones (predominantly uric acid) is in excess of 100-fold greater than in the general population. Hypertension and atherosclerosis may also result from renal damage, as well as being associated with gout.

Some drugs used in the treatment of rheumatic diseases may cause nephrotoxicitiy. NSAIDs are associated with a slight reduction of renal function, as measured by slight impairment of creatinine clearance, although this is normally reversible on discontinuing the drug (Bird et al. 1989). Greater caution should be used when NSAIDs are prescribed with ACE inhibitors and angiotensin 2 antagonists since risk of renal impairment is greater with a risk of hypercalcaemia. Diuretics also increase the risk of nephrotoxicity from NSAIDs. Amongst disease modifying drugs for rheumatoid arthritis, cyclosporin is most likely to be associated with an increase in serum creatinine and subsequently with renal impairment, additionally associated with hypertension, though the hypertension seen with leflunomide is less likely to cause renal damage.

If renal function is already compromised, the risk of nephrotoxicity may be greatly increased. In addition, with drugs that are excreted primarily by the kidneys, such as methotrexate, a decrease in renal function may lead to accumulation of the drug and increased toxicity, though in the low dose used for rheumatoid arthritis this is only occasionally a problem.

Liver function

The standard 'liver function tests (LFTs)', that is, serum or plasma bilirubin, aspartate aminotransferase (AST), alanine aminotransferase (ALT), alkaline phosphatase, γ-glutamyl transferase (GGT), and albumin, are used routinely to identify the presence of and monitor the course of liver disease, although they are generally poor at identifying the precise pathology (reviewed by Rosalki and Dooley 1994; Dufour et al. 2000).

Serum bilirubin

Bilirubin is excreted in the bile after conjugation with glucuronide in the liver. Although less than 500 mg of bilirubin is produced each day from breakdown of haem, the liver is capable of conjugating up to three times this amount. Hyperbilirubinaemia is therefore an insensitive indicator of parenchymal liver disease. Clinical jaundice may not be apparent until the bilirubin concentration is more than twice the upper limit of normal. The major causes of hyperbilirubinaemia include haemolysis (usually accompanied by normal LFTs), hepatitis, cirrhosis, gallstones, tumour infiltration, and drugs such as rifampicin that impair the handling of bilirubin.

Serum enzymes

The aminotransferases AST and ALT are released from damaged cells and are used as markers of hepatocellular integrity, although they are not liver specific, being released from other tissues such as skeletal muscle, heart muscle, and kidney. Very high activities ($>10\times$ the upper limit of normal) occur in acute hepatocellular disease, with even higher values ($>20\times$ the upper reference limit) strongly suggestive of acute hepatitis from drugs or viral infection. Very high values may also occur in shock, cardiac failure, or sepsis.

Total circulating alkaline phosphatase consists of several different forms (isoenzymes) with the main two in the healthy adult being derived from liver and bone. The liver isoenzyme is produced by hepatocytes adjacent to the biliary canaliculi and elevated plasma activities of alkaline phosphatase are found in extra- or intrahepatic bile-duct obstruction (cholestasis) as a result of increased synthesis. Normal or only mildly elevated levels are found in hepatitis. A high plasma alkaline phosphatase and low plasma aminotransferase indicate cholestatic jaundice, although cholestasis may be accompanied by hepatocellular damage and resultant increases in AST and ALT. Pregnancy also results in an elevated plasma alkaline phosphatase. If the elevation in alkaline phosphatase is unaccompanied by abnormalities of other LFTs, a non-hepatic source should be considered. For example, the most common rheumatological cause of an isolated rise in plasma alkaline phosphatase is due to an increase in the circulating bone isoenzyme in Paget's disease. A hepatic origin of the alkaline phosphatase is indicated by the finding of a simultaneous elevation of a liver-derived enzyme such as GGT, which does not occur in bone disease. This enzyme is sensitive but not tissue-specific and may be elevated either through hepatocellular damage or induction by drugs or alcohol. The finding of a normal GGT result does not necessarily imply a bone origin for the alkaline phosphatase, however, as an isolated increase in alkaline phosphatase is often the only abnormality in cases of liver metastases. A more specific approach is the actual determination of the alkaline phosphatase isoenzymes (reviewed by Moss 1987). Placental and intestinal alkaline phosphatases are 'true' isoenzymes, being encoded by individual structural genes. The kidney, liver, and bone isoenzymes are all encoded by the same gene but differ through tissue-specific glycosylation. Isoenzymes can be differentiated by their heat stability or more precisely through electrophoretic separation, which is not always routinely available. Specific immunoassays measuring the bone isoenzyme are now available.

Cirrhosis results in a modest increase of plasma AST and GGT, sometimes accompanied by alkaline phosphatase. Drug-induced hepatitis may be primarily hepatocellular (often without jaundice) or the result of intrahepatic cholestasis with jaundice. The AST, GGT, and alkaline phosphatase are usually raised, the last especially with cholestasis. Alkaline phosphatase is raised in many inflammatory conditions, primarily as part of the acute phase response. Sometimes inflammation elsewhere results in an inflammatory infiltration of the biliary tracts with modest jaundice and greater increases of alkaline phosphatase. The mechanism of this is not understood.

Clinical relevance in rheumatic disease

Systemic juvenile idiopathic arthritis may present with abnormal liver function, and abnormal transaminases are often found after salicylate therapy. In patients with rheumatoid arthritis, plasma transaminases are usually normal, although occasionally the AST may increase, suggesting low-level hepatitis. Between 7.5 and 50 per cent of patients with rheumatoid arthritis have an abnormal alkaline phosphatase level, an abnormality which has been proposed to be primarily of hepatic origin, based on the finding (although variable) of simultaneous elevations of GGT or 5′-nucleotidase, but it may reflect the acute-phase response rather than hepatobiliary dysfunction. However, other studies attribute this increase to the bone isoenzyme and it is a question that still remains unresolved, both in patients with rheumatoid arthritis and in those with ankylosing spondylitis. Patients with rheumatoid arthritis have also been found to have elevated GGT (less than 5–77 per cent of patients depending on the study). It has been suggested that a latent or sub-clinical hepatobiliary pathology may exist in patients with rheumatoid arthritis, with an association between this involvement and disease activity (Aida 1993). The possibility of sub-clinical hepatobiliary damage is supported by the non-specific histopathological changes of liver biopsies from patients with rheumatoid arthritis (reviewed by Aida 1993).

Serious hepatic pathology is not usually found in osteoarthritis, although a wider variation in results of LFTs may be expected than would be encountered in a younger population.

Elevated plasma alkaline phosphatase may be found in patients with the temporal arteritis–polymyalgia rheumatica syndrome (Sonnenblick et al. 1989), with abnormal aminotransferases being infrequent and elevated serum bilirubin extremely rare. Resolution of the biochemical abnormalities occurs after successful corticosteroid therapy. Of patients undergoing liver biopsy, 73 per cent overall had positive findings, although the pathogenesis of the liver involvement in this illness is not clear.

In patients with polymyositis and dermatomyositis, lactate dehydrogenase and AST may be elevated. An elevated serum alkaline phosphatase is a common finding in systemic sclerosis (approximately 25 per cent) and this condition is often seen in patients with chronic liver disease (reviewed by Weinblatt et al. 1982). Although most studies find little evidence of clinically significant hepatic disease in systemic lupus erythematosus (Weinblatt et al. 1982), liver disease as detected by altered LFTs and confirmed in most cases histologically has been reported in more than 20 per cent of patients studied (Runyon et al. 1980). This was unrelated to aspirin-induced hepatitis, which is recognized as a potential complication in patients with systemic lupus.

Several of the drugs used in the treatment of the rheumatic diseases may be hepatotoxic, particularly sulfasalazine, azathioprine, cyclophosphamide, and methotrexate. It is essential that hepatic function is assessed before commencing therapy and at regular intervals thereafter. A major practical problem is disentangling a rise in liver enzymes that act as acute-phase reactants (Chapter 5.1) from increases in enzymes because of hepatotoxicity particularly, as in the case of sulfasalazine there may be an autoimmune element. In general, a rise in alkaline phosphatase and a modest rise in GGT both accepted as acute-phase reactants, causes less concern than a rise in aminotransferases, which is more likely to be drug induced. The serial plotting of results is invaluable and liver enzymes are more likely to behave as acute-phase reactants in the presence of a raised rheumatoid factor and raised platelet count than in the absence of these. However, when drug toxicity is suspected or proven, serial change in GGT is the most sensitive indicator of improvement.

Calcium and bone

An elevated plasma alkaline phosphatase, particularly in the absence of other abnormal LFTs, may reflect an increase in the bone isoenzyme and hence indicate increased bone turnover. Appropriate measures can be used to identify the origin of the isoenzyme (as discussed previously).

Calcium is present in blood combined with plasma proteins (40 per cent, 1.0 mmol/l), complexed to anions such as citrate and phosphate (10 per cent, 0.25 mmol/l), or as the free ion (50 per cent, 1.2 mmol/l). The maintenance of the blood calcium is achieved by parathyroid hormone, which promotes calcium absorption from the gut and renal tubule and mobilization from bone, calcitonin, which has a less pronounced action tending to lower blood calcium, and vitamin D, which increases the blood calcium directly by acting on the gut and renal tubule and indirectly via a synergistic action with parathyroid hormone on bone (described in Chapter 2.4). As the secretion of parathyroid hormone is under direct feedback control by ionized calcium, it is this form of calcium that should ideally be measured. However, this is often not routinely available and total plasma calcium is usually assayed by one of a large number of available methods. Several preanalytical factors can affect the result (reviewed by Bourke and Delaney 1993), two of the most important of which are venous stasis and the posture of the patient at sample collection. Total plasma calcium should always be corrected for the plasma albumin concentration, as this corrected result shows a better correlation with ionized calcium. The simultaneous measurement of phosphate provides an indication of the pathology of any calcium abnormality, with calcium and phosphate concentrations usually changing in the same direction unless parathyroid hormone is inappropriately in excess or deficient, or unless renal failure is present.

Clinical relevance in rheumatic disease

Bone pains may be confused with pains of articular or soft-tissue origin. Bone pain in adults may be caused by osteomalacia, Paget's disease, bony metastases, myeloma, or very occasionally primary hyperparathyroidism. All these conditions, with the exception of myeloma, are associated with increased osteoblastic activity and a consequent raised plasma alkaline phosphatase due to an increase in the bone isoenzyme. A raised alkaline phosphatase of bone origin is most likely to be associated with Paget's disease. Myeloma is investigated easily by serum and urine protein electrophoresis, with the almost invariable finding of a paraprotein in the serum or Bence-Jones protein in the urine. Advanced osteomalacia may be associated with frank hypocalcaemia, while hypercalcaemia is invariably present in primary hyperparathyroidism, and often in myeloma and bony metastases.

Serial biochemical assessments are not useful in soft-tissue rheumatism but plasma alkaline phosphatase and serum calcium should be measured to exclude osteomalacia. Similarly, clinical biochemistry plays no part in the management of calcium pyrophosphate deposition disease, osteoarthritis, or osteoporosis with a normal calcium, phosphate, and alkaline phosphatase. Occasionally, osteoporosis may be secondary to metabolic disorders such as Cushing's syndrome. As previously discussed, there is controversy as to whether elevations in the hepatic or the bone isoenzyme account for the elevated total alkaline phosphatase often seen in diseases such as rheumatoid arthritis, and to the relationship of this elevation with disease activity.

Many assays are available for the measurement of bone and cartilage turnover but the use of these in the rheumatology field is still experimental. It remains to be decided which, if any, of the markers will give information that will be useful in the routine management of the patient (Young-Min et al. 2001).

Muscle disease

Muscle pains may be due to myositis, with damage to muscle fibres resulting in the release of various enzymes. The most clinically useful is creatine kinase (CK). This is composed of two monomers designated M and B and exists in human tissues as three isoenzymes. The isoenzymes CK-1 (CK-BB), CK-2 (CK-MB), and CK-3 (CK-MM) differ in electrophoretic mobility. Skeletal muscle contains predominantly CK-MM (98 per cent) whereas CK-BB is confined mainly to the brain and thyroid. Myocardium contains both CK-MM and CK-MB, with a much greater proportion of CK-MB than skeletal muscle (30 and 2 per cent, respectively). Myocardial infarction, myopathies including those induced by alcohol and drugs, severe exercise, intramuscular injection, surgery, or hypothyroidism can all cause an elevated total creatine kinase. Abnormal levels can occur in asymptomatic female carriers of Duchenne muscular dystrophy. Most serum creatine kinase is normally CK-MM, rising with damage to skeletal muscle. Increases in CK-MB as a percentage of total creatine kinase are indicative of myocardial infarction, whereas an increase of CK-BB indicates brain damage.

Plasma electrolytes should also be measured to exclude electrolyte imbalance, particularly hypocalcaemia, as a cause of muscle pain.

Clinical relevance in rheumatic disease

If soft-tissue rheumatism is suspected, measurement of CK may be required to exclude myositis, although this condition is usually obvious clinically. The myalgia accompanying polymyalgia rheumatica–giant-cell arteritis is not associated with abnormal serum activities of muscle enzymes. Other causes of myalgia, such as anxiety, depression, fibrositis, thyroid disease, and

Parkinson's disease, must be excluded. CK is the most reliable enzyme test in polymyositis and dermatomyositis, with plasma activity levels correlating with disease activity (Vignos and Goldwin 1972). Rarely, CK may be normal but an elevation usually distinguishes polymyositis from polymyalgia.

Several antirheumatic drugs including corticosteroids, D-penicillamine, aspirin, gold salts, and the non-steroidal anti-inflammatories, are known to cause myopathy (reviewed by Zuckner 1990).

Malignancy

Apart from metastatic malignancy of bone, malignant disease may cause myositis, myopathy, or generalized symptoms suggestive of soft-tissue rheumatism. Serum and urinary electrophoresis may be required to exclude myeloma, and plasma alkaline phosphatase and serum calcium analysis to exclude other neoplastic involvement. Prostate-specific antigen in conjunction with digital rectal examination can be used to check for carcinoma of the prostate. Pain caused by such conditions affecting bone is interpreted frequently by the patient as arising in adjacent soft tissues. Further clinical tests will be required to investigate this.

Pathological processes occurring in rheumatic disease

The division between clinical chemistry and immunology laboratories is becoming blurred, particularly with the automation of many assays. The measurements used to detect and monitor the following pathological processes may be carried out in laboratories of either discipline. For completeness, they are mentioned briefly here, being covered in greater detail elsewhere.

Inflammation

Inflammatory cells release cytokines that initiate local and systemic effects (see Chapter 4.1). Although assays are available for most of the known cytokines it is more usual to measure CRP as a surrogate marker of the inflammatory episode (see Chapter 5.1). Cytokines stimulate other cells to release enzymes (e.g. elastase) and reactive oxygen species (e.g. nitric oxide) which may damage surrounding extracellular elements. Although elastase measurement has been shown to be rather insensitive, the measurement of NO (as nitrite or nitrate) has shown much promise (Ralston 1997).

Immune response

Immune responses feature in many rheumatic diseases, being most notable early in the disease or during exacerbation. During a phase of immune stimulus, IgM is raised modestly, subsiding in 2–3 weeks to be replaced by IgG. Raised concentrations of IgG are found commonly, especially in the connective tissue diseases. Infiltration of the synovium with plasma cells results in IgA production. Thus the immunoglobulin profile is complex and is related insufficiently to disease process or activity to be useful for differential diagnosis or monitoring.

Immune complex diseases

Although the presence of immune complexes is usually not in itself a very helpful marker of clinical disease or its treatment and is difficult to assay, significant deposition of complexes in the vascular system results in activation of mediator systems, notably complement, which may be measured. Complement activation implies the occurrence of immune complex mediated damage, indicating the need for therapeutic intervention. Total C3 and C4 concentrations may be measured as they are consumed by the process of activation, although their consumption may be masked by their increased synthesis as part of the acute-phase response. Breakdown fragments of C3 or C4, for example, C3a, are a much more sensitive indicator of complement activation. Changes in C4 are frequently more sensitive than those in C3, particularly in the case of systemic lupus erythematosus, when used in conjunction with anti-DNA antibody measurements.

Crystal deposition

Biochemical tests are mainly useful in the case of gout. The relationship between hyperuricaemia and gout has been reviewed by Becker (1988). Uric acid, the end product of the metabolism of purines, is present normally as the urate ion at physiological pH and has a low solubility. Saturation and consequently precipitation of urate crystals can occur after only minor elevations of circulating concentrations. The serum urate concentration is governed by the rate of excretion (approximately two-thirds via the kidneys and the remainder via the gut) and the rate of formation, which is dependent on the balance between dietary intake, de novo synthesis, and degradation of nucleotides. Serum levels tend to be higher in males, rise with age, and reference ranges vary between ethnic groups.

Gout may be secondary to conditions that cause increased formation or decreased excretion of uric acid, such as hyperparathyroidism or myeloproliferative disorders. Dietary factors and alcohol often exacerbate hyperuricaemia. Such conditions need to be excluded before appropriate treatment can be commenced. Gout is more often primary or idiopathic, being found in patients who have an elevated rate of urate synthesis (10–15 per cent) or inappropriately low excretion (85–90 per cent). The exact nature of the defects is not known. Measurement of the urinary uric acid excretion aids in the differentiation of the two mechanisms. Although the risk of gout increases with a higher serum urate, hyperuricaemia does not necessarily imply the presence or the development of gout. Figure 2 shows clearly that while measurements of uric acid are useful, the relationship between the concentration of uric acid and clinical gout is not very clear. The definitive diagnosis of gout can only be made on the finding of crystals of monosodium urate in joint fluid. Gout may cause, or occur as a result of, renal failure, and assessment of renal function is essential in the interpretation of raised concentrations of uric acid. It is also prudent to screen at diagnosis for conditions sometimes associated, such as hypertension and hyperlipidaemia. Measurements of serum uric acid can be used to determine the efficacy of long-term prophylactic therapy with allopurinol or uricosuric agents. Hyperuricaemia has also been reported to occur in 10–20 per cent of patients with psoriatic arthritis (Lambert and Wright 1977), probably reflecting the increased breakdown of nucleoprotein with the rapid turnover of skin cells.

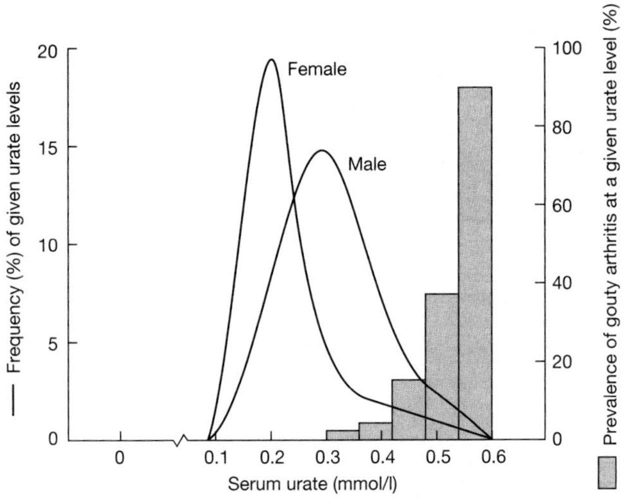

Fig. 2 Frequency distribution of serum uric acid values and the prevalence of gouty arthritis (adapted from Whicher et al. 1989). Serum urate concentrations are not normally distributed and the upper limit of the reference ranges (2 SD above the mean) are 0.42 and 0.36 mmol/l for males and females, respectively. Approximately 20% of subjects with urate concentrations within the reference range suffer from gout and a significant percentage of individuals with hyperuricaemia are not affected by gout.

Although relatively uncommon as causes of the deposition of calcium pyrophosphate, metabolic disorders such as hyperparathyroidism, hypomagnesaemia, or hypophosphatasia should be excluded in pseudogout, using appropriate tests.

References

Aida, A. (1993). Alkaline phosphatase isoenzyme activities in rheumatoid arthritis: hepatobiliary enzyme dissociation and relation to disease activity. *Annals of the Rheumatic Diseases* **52**, 511–16.

Becker, M.A. (1988). Clinical aspects of monosodium urate monohydrate crystal deposition disease (gout). *Rheumatic Disease Clinics of North America* **14**, 377–93.

Bird, H.A., Clarke, A.K., Fowler, P.D., Little, S., Podgorski, M.R., and Steiner, J. (1989). An assessment of tenoxicam, a nonsteroidal anti-inflammatory drug of long half-life, in patients with impaired renal function suffering from osteoarthritis or rheumatoid arthritis. *Clinical Rheumatology* **8**, 453–60.

Boers, M. (1990). Renal disorders in rheumatoid arthritis. *Seminars in Arthritis and Rheumatism* **20**, 57–68.

Bourke, E. and Delaney, V. (1993). Assessment of hypocalcemia and hypercalcemia. *Clinics in Laboratory Medicine* **13**, 157–81.

Cameron, J.S. (2001). Clinical manifestations of lupus nephritis. In *Rheumatology and the Kidney* (ed. D. Adu, P. Emery, and M. Medaio), pp. 17–22. Oxford: Oxford University Press.

Cockroft, D.W. and Gault, M.H. (1976). Prediction of creatinine clearance from serum creatinine. *Nephron* **16**, 31–41.

Duarte, C.G. and Preuss, H.G. (1993). Assessment of renal function—glomerular and tubular. *Clinics in Laboratory Medicine* **13**, 33–52.

Dufour, D.R., Lott, J.A., Nolte, F.S., Gretch, D.R., Koff, R.S., and Seeff, L.B. (2000). Diagnosis and monitoring of hepatic injury. II. Recommendations for use of laboratory tests in screening, diagnosis and monitoring. *Clinical Chemistry* **46**, 2050–68.

Gladman, D.D. (1990). Prognosis of systemic lupus erythematosus and factors that affect it. *Current Opinion in Rheumatology* **2**, 694–702.

Lambert, J.R. and Wright, V. (1977). Serum uric acid levels in psoriatic arthritis. *Annals of the Rheumatic Diseases* **36**, 264–7.

Lindeman, R.D. (1993). Assessment of renal function in the old. *Clinics in Laboratory Medicine* **13**, 269–77.

Moore, J., Jr. and Carome, M.A. (1993). Proteinuria. *Clinics in Laboratory Medicine* **13**, 21–31.

Moss, D.W. (1987). Diagnostic aspects of alkaline phosphatase and its isoenzymes. *Clinical Biochemistry* **20**, 225–30.

Petri, M. et al. (1988). Serial assessment of glomerular filtration rate in lupus nephropathy. *Kidney International* **34**, 832–9.

Price, C.P. and Finney, H. (2000). Developments in the assessment of glomerular filtration rate. *Clinica Chimica Acta* **297**, 55–66.

Ralston, S.H. (1997). Nitric oxide: what a gas! *British Journal of Rheumatology* **36**, 831–8.

Rosalki, S.B. and Dooley, J.S. (1994). Liver function profiles and their interpretation. *British Journal of Hospital Medicine* **51**, 181–6.

Runyon, B.A., LaBrecque, D.R., and Anuras, S. (1980). The spectrum of liver disease in systemic lupus erythematosus. Report of 33 histologically-proved cases and review of the literature. *American Journal of Medicine* **69**, 187–94.

Sonnenblick, M., Nesher, G., and Rosin, A. (1989). Nonclassical organ involvement in temporal arteritis. *Seminars in Arthritis and Rheumatism* **19**, 183–90.

Vignos, P.J. and Goldwin, J. (1972). Evaluation of laboratory tests in diagnosis and management of polymyositis. *American Journal of Medicine* **263**, 291–308.

Walser, M. (1998). Assessing renal function from creatinine measurements in adults with chronic renal failure. *American Journal of Kidney Diseases* **32**, 23–31.

Weinblatt, M.E., Tesser, J.R.P., and Gilliam, J.H., III (1982). The liver in rheumatic diseases. *Seminars in Arthritis and Rheumatism* **11**, 399–405.

Whicher, J., Walters, G., and Henley G. (1989). Using the biochemistry laboratory. *Medical Forum* **31**, 6–9.

Young-Min, S.A., Cawston T.E., and Griffiths I.D. (2001). Markers of joint destruction: principles, problems, and potential. *Annals of the Rheumatic Diseases* **60**, 545–7.

Youssef, W. and Russell, A.S. (1990). Cardiac, ocular, and renal manifestations of seronegative spondyloarthropathies. *Current Opinion in Rheumatology* **2**, 582–5.

Zuckner, J. (1990). Drug-induced myopathies. *Seminars in Arthritis and Rheumatism* **19**, 259–68.

5.3 Microbiology and diagnostic serology

Geoffrey Scott

Optimal use of the microbiology laboratory

The aim of the microbiologist is to help the clinician make a more tangible diagnosis if infection or reactive arthritis is suspected. The clinician can help the microbiologist by ensuring that appropriate specimens are taken, that they get to the laboratory quickly, and by communicating with the laboratory scientist or doctor so that all relevant tests can be done. The request form that accompanies a specimen is the principal method of communication but most are completed inadequately. In most hospitals, microbiologists will see patients on request, examine notes, advise on prescribing of antimicrobials, and may even impose restrictions on their use. In an acute or difficult clinical setting, direct communication helps to ensure that someone in the laboratory will take a special interest in the processing of a specimen. In most laboratories, some simple tests, such as examination for acid-fast bacilli, will be made only if specially requested by the clinician. Purists would say that all tests should be done on every specimen and that they should be examined for 'all' possibilities. In practice, this would be impossibly expensive and time wasting. The interpretative microbiologist requires some sense of what the clinician is searching for. The more relevant (concise) history that can be given, the better.

In clinical pathology, it is important to consider the likelihood that a result is actually a true representation. Computer-printed results sometimes suggest a degree of scientific precision that, particularly in microbiology, may be unfounded. A patient must not be made to fit an unlikely diagnosis suggested by test results, especially when they are preliminary (Stokes et al. 1993). The sensitivity of a test is the percentage of the infected group detected as positive by the test. The specificity indicates the percentage of the negative group detected as negative by the test. These values are in themselves meaningless unless put into the context of the total number of tests done, and the expected rates of positives and negatives in a population. The figures that can be calculated to express these data are the predictive values of positive (PVP) and negative (PVN) test results, respectively (Easmon 1990). The problem in trying to calculate these values is that one needs to know how many in the population actually do or do not have the infection. PVP and PVN can be calculated for a new test when compared with a 'gold standard' test assumed to be 100 per cent sensitive and specific. An example would be the comparison of a new enzyme immunoassay for chlamydial antigen against culture of the organism (the 'gold standard'), or against amplification of chlamydial DNA. The last will inevitably detect more positives than culture but it will be impossible to know whether they are truly positive for a variety of reasons, including difficulty in identifying specific DNA and the risk of contamination. When comparing two tests, it becomes obvious that one test can detect positives which the other cannot. Yet the more sensitive test will almost certainly have a higher rate of false positivity.

If a test gives a continuum of signals between positive and negative, a cut-off point has to be chosen to categorize its results. This is illustrated by the microbiology of urine specimens. The cut-off between positive and negative is chosen by examining large numbers of samples and selecting a point (10^5 CFU/ml) between the two peaks of the bimodal distribution of the concentration of bacteria present. Some of those with 'significant bacteriuria' will, by definition, have only 10^4–10^5 organisms per millilitre of urine. Rather than accepting this single result as meaningful, the microbiologist will hope to confirm or refute the suggestion of positivity by requesting a repeat test. In recently developed enzyme immunoassays, the cut-off between negative and positive is selected in exactly the same way. If the cut-off is selected at 20 units and the test has a result of 19 units, this should be reported as negative yet may well be positive. Only alternative, confirmatory tests can be of real help in these cases and the clinician must again avoid the temptation to make a patient fit a dubious result. False-positive immunoassays are common in some conditions (e.g. assays for antibody to human immunodeficiency virus), but repeated tests of different design and specificity will yield more reliable results.

Unless the sensitivity and specificity of a test are both 100 per cent, PVP and PVN will be markedly influenced by the prevalence of the disease in the population under study. Comparing likely isolation rates of chlamydia in patients attending a genitourinary medicine clinic (17 per cent) with those attending a rheumatology clinic (assumed 1 per cent), and using a test with sensitivity of 90 per cent (i.e. 1 in 10 positive patients give a negative result) and specificity of 95 per cent (1 in 20 tests are false positive), the PVPs in the two clinics would be 78 and 15 per cent, respectively. In the low-prevalence population this is of profound importance in trying to make a microbiological diagnosis in a patient with reactive arthritis.

Table 1 Outline of microbiology in investigations for rheumatology patients

Monoarthropathy with constitutional symptoms
Synovial fluid
It is essential to send fluid rather than a swab for microscopy and culture
Consider whether it is necessary to look for mycobacteria
Tests performed
Cell count
Giemsa: cell morphology
Gram, acridine orange, methylene blue: micro-organism morphology
Ziehl–Nielsen, auramine: acid-fast bacilli
Gas–liquid chromatography: anaerobes, *Pseudomonas*, etc.
Culture: chocolatized blood agar enriched CO_2: most bacteria
Enrichment in broth (e.g. Robertson's cooked meat)
Lowenstein Jensen (solid) or Middlebrook (broth): mycobacteria
Also
Serum to save
Blood culture
Polyarthropathy with constitutional symptoms
As above plus investigations to exclude rheumatic fever
Serum: process for antistreptolysin titre, etc.
Throat swab: culture for *Streptococcus pyogenes*
Seronegative arthritis
Post-hepatitis
Check liver function tests for persistent abnormalities
Serum for hepatitis A, B, C, and E
If negative, serum for hepatitis C RNA detection
Post-diarrhoea
Stool culture: *Salmonella* and *Yersinia*
Serum: *Yersinia* antibodies
Post-rash and constitutional illness
Serum: rubella and parvovirus antibodies
With rash and neurological symptoms
Serum: *Borrelia* spp. antibodies
Urethritis
Urethral swabs for *Chlamydia* and *Neisseria*

Tests and their limitations

The influence of antibiotics on culture

Microbiological culture studies are relatively insensitive and will be almost certainly negative when the patient is already on antimicrobial agents. Prophylactic antibiotics are often prescribed as a matter of routine for orthopaedic operations, but when infection is suspected and the operation is partly for diagnostic purposes, it is crucial that the administration of antimicrobials be delayed until after all the specimens have been taken. We advise that anaesthetists give the antimicrobials intraoperatively in infected cases.

Specimens

The rheumatologist will tend to send fluid or biopsies from joints or blood in order to diagnose bacterial infection, and special culture specimens from elsewhere (e.g. faeces, urethral fluid), or serum, to support the diagnosis of reactive arthritis. All specimens are treated in the laboratory as though there is a risk of infection to the staff. Contamination of the outside of a container is obviously a particular hazard, so all containers should be sent in a sealed, clear-plastic bag separate from the request form. Staples should not be used. Specimens that leak may be discarded in the laboratory because opening the bag poses a high risk to the staff. Unlabelled specimens and those accompanied by an inadequate request form should also be discarded.

An outline of microbiological investigations is shown in Table 1.

Synovial fluid (pus)

Specimens must be of the highest quality. Take specimens using aseptic precautions. Interpretation of the relevance of a culture containing avirulent skin commensals such as coagulase-negative staphylococci, *Acinetobacter* spp., or α-haemolytic streptococci is almost impossible. Furthermore, the inoculation of any of these organisms into a damaged joint may result in secondary infection.

Pus will be examined by Gram stain. Modified Giemsa is necessary to identify cell morphology. Methylene blue and acridine orange may reveal organisms that do not stain with Gram because they are damaged. Acridine orange will stain DNA and RNA, and will confirm the presence of micro-organisms, but will not reveal their classical morphology. When indicated, acid-fast bacilli are stained with auramine O and Ziehl–Nielsen.

The specimen is cultured under a range of conditions on non-selective media and, when a clue is given by the Gram stain, on selective media. It is quite common to see organisms in pus but for these not to grow, and this may reflect inhibition by host defences still present in the pus rather than insensitive culture conditions. Restoration of 'stressed' organisms is done very poorly in clinical laboratories. There is a move to apply special techniques used in food microbiology to clinical specimens. Essentially, the culture is enriched under optimal conditions for bacterial growth without any potentially suppressive selective pressure.

All fluids should be incubated alone and inoculated into enrichment broth or cooked-meat medium, then sub-cultured at 24 and 48 h. Dilution in broth may allow growth, even in the presence of antimicrobial agents.

It is better to send a good volume of fluid or pus rather than a swab of the pus. It is not worth looking for mycobacteria from a swab. If the specimen is aspirated with a syringe, send the capped syringe to the laboratory rather than decanting the pus into another container. Aeration of a specimen may reduce the yield of anaerobes. Anaerobes and moulds are usually found only after penetrating trauma. The pus can be subjected to gas–liquid chromatography to demonstrate volatile fatty acids, which are products of anaerobic metabolism. This is a rather more technical way of identifying anaerobes than simply smelling the offensive odour of a specimen. Specific gas–liquid chromatographic patterns may indicate a particular anaerobic genus, long before it has been cultured and identified.

Most fluids are cultured aerobically on enriched media (such as chocolatized blood agar), in an atmosphere of 5–10 per cent CO_2, and anaerobically because certain facultative anaerobes (e.g. *Streptococcus pyogenes*) show more characteristic colonial morphology under these conditions. Many true anaerobes require several days of incubation before they give visible growth.

If swabs of wounds are taken, they should be placed in transport medium supplied (e.g. Stuart or Amies). The best recovery that can be expected from a swab is less than 30 per cent of the organisms sampled. Swabs and pus from joints should in general not be refrigerated because of the risk of killing cold-sensitive organisms such as *Neisseria gonorrhoeae*.

Blood cultures

Blood cultures should be taken from any patient suspected of having pyogenic arthritis. Two sets taken by separate venepuncture at different times will increase the positive yield but it is not worth taking more. Disinfection of the skin twice with 70 per cent isopropyl alcohol allowed to dry is quite sufficient provided that the venepuncture is done deftly. Contamination of the culture with skin commensals nearly always follows poor technique or difficult venepuncture. Blood-culture bottles should be filled from a syringe before other sample containers because often these others are not sterile.

Handling the blood is dangerous. Needlestick injuries while changing needles and inoculating the bottles are very common, so extreme care must be taken. Some recommend not changing needles for this reason and because it has been shown not to reduce significantly the level of contamination. The bottles should not be overfilled with blood (easily done for bottles with a vacuum), because blood over a certain concentration is inhibitory to bacterial growth. Different style bottles require different sizes of inoculum. Most modern bottles have a cap over a sterile rubber membrane and it is important to read the label to find out whether the membrane should be swabbed with alcohol before inoculation of blood.

Three main types of automatic culture detection systems are in use: detection of $^{14}CO_2$ released from labelled carbohydrate; detection of CO_2 by infrared spectrophotometry or some patented indicator system; and detection of increased pressure of gas within a bottle by a simple cap indicator. These systems do away with the routine sub-cultures and accelerate the process of detection. It is not unusual for a blood culture taken during the night to cue positive in the morning with coliforms or *Streptococcus pneumoniae*, without visible signs of growth.

The blood-culture system routinely used in the local laboratory will have limitations. Do cultures regularly detect fastidious organisms such as neisseriae and brucellae? When in doubt, cultures should be specially subcultured on to rich medium after a week's incubation, but this will only be done by special request.

Antimicrobial sensitivity testing

In general, antibiotic tests are performed when an organism has been isolated in pure culture. However, direct sensitivities can be done by plating the specimen and using antibiotic discs, but this depends on having seen an organism with characteristic morphology. The inoculum is inaccurate so the preliminary results are suspect until confirmed using the isolated organism in pure culture.

Antimicrobial testing is done in most laboratories by one of two methods. The principle of the first is that antimicrobials diffuse from a small filter-paper disc into agar in such a way that exponential concentration is inversely proportional to the distance from the disc. A sensitive organism plated on to the agar is inhibited up to but not beyond the minimal inhibitory dilution of the antibiotic. The zone radius or diameter is then measured and recorded. In the United Kingdom, the practice is to compare the zone of inhibition of test organisms with a control of known sensitivity (Stokes method; Stokes and Ridgway 1987), but in the United States the size of the zone given by the unknown is compared with a database of known sensitive organisms (Kirby–Bauer or NCCLS method). A modification of NCCLS method (BSAC) is being introduced in many laboratories. A reduction in zone size indicates reduced sensitivity, which may be declared 'moderate' or 'resistant'. The advantages of the test are that the organism can be seen to have grown with characteristic morphology, that it is not contaminated, and that 'sensitivity' is a clear signal. The main limitations of the disc diffusion test are that it is standardized for fast-growing organisms and causes problems with difficult organisms (e.g. *Haemophilus* spp., *Neisseria* spp.). Some other specific problems are as follows:

1. Requirement for a special medium or culture conditions:
   (a) enriched for *Neisseria*, *Haemophilus* spp., etc.;
   (b) thymidine-free—testing folate antagonists (sulfonamide, etc.);
   (c) special supplements—pyridoxine for streptococci;
   (d) staphylococcal sensitivity to methicillin is temperature-dependent (best demonstrated at 30°C).
2. Poor diffusion of antibiotics (a small zone of inhibition is difficult to interpret) as with:
   (a) glycopeptides—vancomycin and teicoplanin;
   (b) polymyxin.
3. Inaccurate results:
   (a) inappropriate sensitivity of inactivating enzyme producers, for example:
      (i) *Enterobacter* spp. may appear sensitive to ampicillin yet almost always produce β-lactamase;
      (ii) penicillin-resistant *Staphylococcus aureus* often shows a good zone of inhibition to penicillin;
      (iii) penicillin-resistant pneumococci may show a zone to penicillin but not to oxacillin.
   (b) Organism shows heterogenous resistance (some clones more resistant than others):
      (i) *S. aureus* to methicillin/oxacillin.

The other method in common use involves the incorporation of antimicrobials into agar or broth at concentrations above and below the so-called breakpoint between sensitive and resistant. Unknown and control sensitive and resistant organisms are included in tests. Although this method gives more precise information about the minimal inhibitory dilution of an antibiotic against a certain organism, it also has flaws. If an organism does not grow, one cannot be certain that the organism was not dead when inoculated. Broth sensitivities may be automated (e.g. VITEK system).

The effect of penicillin against *N. gonorrhoeae* is a good example where there is a continuum of increasing resistance conferred by sequential changes in penicillin-binding proteins, permeability, and finally β-lactamase. It is difficult to know where to set the breakpoint between sensitive and resistant in this situation.

Sensitivity to antibiotics of slow growers such as mycobacteria is best done by a modified agar incorporation method that has been standardized. Mycobacterial sensitivities should be ready 3 weeks after primary isolation but rapid sensitivity tests employing radiocarbon release as $^{14}CO_2$ from a suitable broth can be done in specialized laboratories. Molecular methods are available for species identification (e.g. of *Mycobacterium tuberculosis*) and to detect important antibiotic resistance genes (e.g. *rpoB* gene for rifampicin resistance).

These examples illustrate the point that sensitivity testing of bacteria *in vitro* has problems whatever method is adopted. In addition, when large numbers of tests are done, there are likely to be transcriptional errors. When a patient does not appear to respond to recommended therapy, question first the appropriateness of the results of sensitivity tests, have them double-checked in the laboratory, and meanwhile consider the pharmacology of the antimicrobial selected.

The minimal inhibitory and the minimal bactericidal dilutions of an antimicrobial are tested in broth culture using highly accurate concentrations of antimicrobial. This is done for isolates causing infective endocarditis but may exceptionally be done also for a pyogenic arthritis that is failing to resolve. Antimicrobial activity can also be measured in synovial fluid as a check on pharmacokinetics. Experimentally, killing of organisms and the post-antibiotic effect (inhibition of growth even after the antibiotic has been removed) may be measured; such tests are part of the development, and may influence the use, of new antimicrobials.

Antibiotic choice

Antibiotics chosen empirically for joint infections should be appropriate to the isolate or most likely organism, but also need to penetrate well. Some agents, such as chloramphenicol, co-trimoxazole, tetracycline, clindamycin, rifampicin, or metronidazole, are well absorbed from the intestine and will probably be effective when given orally. Most β-lactam antimicrobials are poorly absorbed and penetrate into bone and joint tissue poorly, so the first phase of treatment for acute pyogenic infections should be given parenterally in high doses.

Antimicrobials that penetrate well into joint fluid include tetracycline (useful for brucellae), co-trimoxazole (active against coliforms and some *S. aureus*), rifampicin and fucidic acid (very active against *S. aureus*, but should not be given alone), and chloramphenicol. Ciprofloxacin in recommended doses may not achieve sufficiently high concentration to inhibit *Pseudomonas aeruginosa*. Although absorbed from the gut and suitable for pseudomonal urinary infection, the antimicrobial should probably be given parenterally to achieve sufficiently high concentrations in the synovium. *Stenotrophomonas maltophilia*, an emerging nosocomial pathogen in immunosuppressed patients, is usually resistant to carbapenems so may be selected by the widespread use of these drugs. Nosocomial enterococcal infections are also selected by using cephalosporins.

Newer antibiotics for resistant Gram-positive infections included quinupristin-dalfopristin, newer quinolones, and linezolid (von Eiff and Peters 1999). The latter is particularly useful for resistant staphylococci and enterococci in soft tissues and is orally active (Perry and Jarvis 2001).

Antigen detection

Tests for antigen detection have developed in two rather different directions. First, rapid tests, which usually depend on agglutination of latex particles, red cells, or staphylococci (binding Fc) coated with antibody, are sold in kit form to the routine laboratory for rapid detection or confirmation of common organisms found in certain specimens. An example would be *Haemophilus influenzae* type b in cerebrospinal fluid. Kits are designed so that a single test can be done economically, together with positive and negative controls.

The alternative tests for antigen are immunoassays [either radiometric or enzyme-linked (ELISA)], suitable for processing large numbers of specimens. These are often highly sensitive but may not be specific, so confirmatory tests of positives are required. Reference laboratories tend to develop and validate their own immunoassays. The classical application of successful immunodiagnosis of antigen is in the detection of hepatitis B virus surface antigen. Single-tube ELISA assays have been developed to process individual specimens.

Despite antigenic diversity, only a limited number of the antigenic shapes expressed on micro-organisms are useful for the detection of species. Monoclonal antibodies are preferred to polyclonal ones for their greater specificity, but polyclonals will usually include some antibody of greater avidity, which can significantly improve a test. Sandwich immunoassays using high-avidity antibody capture and one highly specific antibody seem to be the most reliable. The antigen recognized by the antibody chosen should be common to and expressed on all of the species and subspecies that are to be sought. Yet there should be no cross-reactivity with antigens on other species and this is unachievable. In an immunofluorescence test, where the antibody (directly or indirectly labelled) is applied to a clinical specimen and examined microscopically, it is possible for the experienced reader to detect alternative organisms or debris that appear to bind yet have a different shape from the organism under investigation. This indicates a serious problem with ELISA in which positives are detected simply by a graded colour change. It must be assumed that some of the results will be false-positive and that secondary confirmatory tests are required.

Specific DNA or RNA detection

Labelled, specific, single-stranded DNA probes will anneal with complementary DNA that has been cleaved into single strands at high temperature. The labelled complex is detected in the appropriate way (radioisotope detection or enzymatic colour change). This method appears to be specific (although it is often impossible to prove positives or negatives) but is not sensitive because it will detect only relatively large amounts of DNA. Labelled DNA probes can also be made to anneal with ribosomal RNA, which will be present at a higher copy number than the DNA.

DNA segments in the test sample may be amplified using flanking sequences that define a specific segment and a heat-stable polymerase to replicate the DNA repeatedly (polymerase chain reaction, PCR). The problems with DNA amplification are extreme sensitivity and false-positivity due to contamination: the test should be done away from laboratories where the organism being sought is routinely grown and handled. Recent advances in PCR technology include 'nesting', using two pairs of primers, the second internal to the first, which increases the sensitivity of the test some 100-fold and also the specificity. Second, viral and bacterial RNA can be amplified after it has been converted to complementary DNA by reverse transcription. Third, the amplification product can be annealed to a specific labelled probe to confirm the specificity of the product.

Good examples of the useful application of PCR are to be found in the study of viruses that cannot (easily) be grown (e.g. hepatitis C virus, human immunodeficiency virus).

New tests are experimental and are often used to detect rare diseases. When a new test is introduced, inevitably there is an exploratory period when the results are uninterpretable and unreliable.

Antibody detection

A single serum test for antibody rarely yields a definitive diagnosis. Even a confirmed positive antibody test for human immunodeficiency virus merely indicates exposure to, and latent infection with, the virus. It does not infer anything about the relation of the present symptoms and the stage of the disease.

Two specimens separated by at least 2 and preferably 4 weeks should be tested to make a diagnosis of a recent infection. Only the evolution of titre can indicate how recent an infection was and then only within wide confidence limits. Some infections (e.g. legionellosis) are associated with a delayed rise in antibody, up to 3 weeks after the onset of illness and some fail to stimulate any detectable antibody response at all. Antibody tests are the only way of making a non-invasive diagnosis in many infections that predispose to arthritis. Patients with polyclonal B-cell activation may show strong positivity in several tests and anamnestic responses are common.

The tests for antibody have developed enormous sophistication. Nevertheless, crude agglutination reactions are still made on dilutions of serum mixed with polyclonal antisera, usually as screening tests. This is the basis for screening tests for brucellae and enteric fever. Positive screening for *Brucella* agglutination in the routine laboratory is usually non-specific, cross reacts with *Bartonella* and cannot be confirmed in the reference laboratory by other immunoassays, and should not be taken automatically as indicating brucellosis.

With the high rate of false-positive tests in the first-generation enzyme immunoassays for human immunodeficiency virus, particularly in patients from Africa, it became conventional to confirm the specificity of antibodies by Western immunoblotting. The antigens of the organism under test are separated by chromatography and transferred to a membrane for reaction with the patient's serum. The patterns of reactivity are then compared with positive controls. Non-specific Western blot reactivity has been clearly shown not to indicate infection with human immunodeficiency virus. Western blotting may also be used to confirm the specificity of antibody in other conditions (e.g. Lyme disease) (Karlsson 1990). Enthusiasm for what was thought to be a very specific test has now waned because of difficulties in standardization and definition of a positive test.

Specific tests have been developed over the years for certain organisms. They include the dye test for *Toxoplasma gondii*. This is still used as the 'gold standard' in reference laboratories, but routine agglutination tests have been replaced by highly sensitive latex-particle agglutination and specific IgM kits, which can be applied in routine laboratories. Some IgM kits have been found to be oversensitive.

The antistreptolysin-O titre for antibodies to *S. pyogenes* remains the mainstay of laboratory diagnosis of recent infection. It uses the neutralization of a standard inoculum of streptolysin by dilutions of the patient's serum. The indicator is haemolysis of sheep or human erythrocytes but the test is not specific. Anti-DNAase B, streptokinase, and hyaluronidase are more useful additional tests.

The likelihood of accurate results from serological tests for antigen and antibody depend on how frequently the tests are done in the laboratory. Furthermore, commercial test kits are very expensive: hence the reliance on reference laboratories for support and verification. Inevitably, such test results are delayed.

Acute joint infections (Figs 1–2 and Plate 68)

Acute joint infections are a small part of rheumatology practice in Europe and America. In certain parts of the world, however, brucellosis and tuberculosis of joints are common. With increasing invasive health care, nosocomial bacteraemia, especially from intravenous-line infections, may contribute to some bone and joint infections.

Microbiological examination of fluid from an infected joint is only important because of the guidance the results ultimately give towards sensible chemotherapy. In the relatively few acutely inflamed joints that are infected, a very wide range of organisms is involved and, with very few exceptions, isolates have increasingly unpredictable sensitivity patterns to antimicrobials. Moreover, when positive, culture gives a firm diagnosis in a doubtful case.

Bacterial infections of healthy joints occur after bacteraemia with virulent organisms including *S. pneumoniae, S. pyogenes, S. aureus,* and *N. gonorrhoeae* but are much more likely to occur in joints damaged by other conditions such as osteoarthrosis or rheumatoid arthritis. Patients are often debilitated and on corticosteroids. In these patients, it is critical to make a positive diagnosis as soon as possible to prevent the inadvertent injection of steroids into an infected joint. Clinically, acute spontaneous pyogenic arthritis in a previously healthy individual is often restricted to one joint and is relatively easy to recognize, but may be much less evident when it supervenes on a chronic inflammatory polyarthropathy in a patient on steroids. To make a diagnosis, none of the surrogate markers of infection (e.g. white blood-cell count, ESR, and CRP) compares favourably with direct examination of synovial fluid from inflamed joints or blood for relevant micro-organisms. It may be sufficient to take blood cultures and treat with antimicrobials on the basis of the most probable organism, in expectation of a positive culture in due course. However, always consider sampling synovial fluid, which can also be examined for crystals and other important markers (see Chapter 5.5).

Routine cultures should readily yield *Brucella melitensis* within a week but less certainly *Brucella abortus*. Special cultures are needed for mycobacteria and negative results are not available for 8 or 12 weeks, depending on laboratory routine. Simple tests will distinguish *M. tuberculosis* from atypical species but the laboratory scientist will be reluctant to declare a species to the clinician until reference laboratory identification is completed.

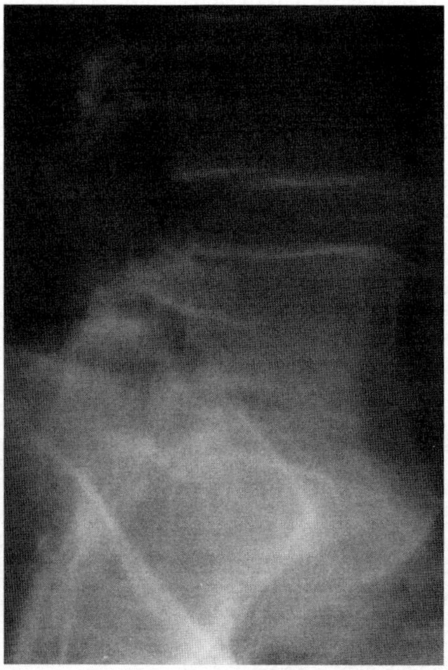

Fig. 1 Acute back pain with fever may be due to spinal osteomyelitis. Tuberculosis would be a common cause but in this case an aspirate of pus yielded *Brucella melitensis*. The patient came from Turkey.

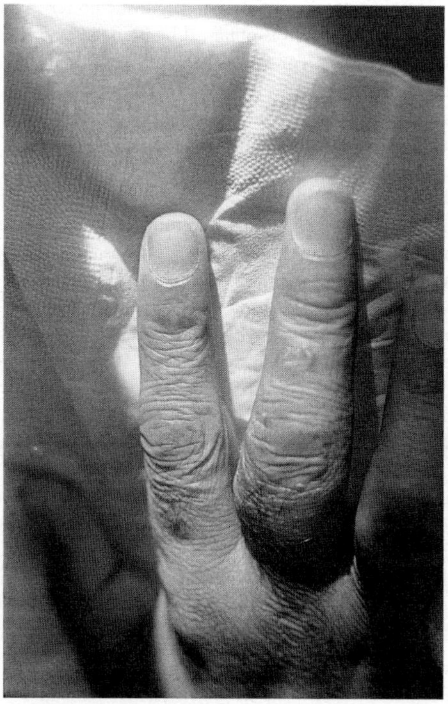

Fig. 2 A chronic discharging sinus from the back of the finger of this man with psoriatic arthropathy surprisingly yielded *Mycobacterium tuberculosis*.

The best way of monitoring the success of long-term therapy for deep *S. aureus* infections is to test serial sedimentation rates and CRP levels. Antibodies to staphylococcal α- and γ-lysins should not be used to make a diagnosis of deep staphylococcal infection because false-positives may occur. However, if the diagnosis has been made by conventional culture, then serial assays of sera taken every 1–2 months or so can be done in parallel to monitor progress.

Investigation of reactive arthritis

Many infections predispose to reactive arthritis. These arise because of immune reactivity to organisms infecting particularly the genitourinary and gastrointestinal tracts. It may be possible to elicit a very specific, temporally relevant history of a symptom complex that points to a diagnosis. Common syndromes preceding arthritis are 'febrile rash' illness, diarrhoea, urethritis (sometimes with uveitis), and influenza-like illness with and without jaundice. Unless there is a preceding illness or accompanying signs, searching for the cause is likely to be fruitless.

Urethritis

It is important to search for the cause. When urethritis or prostatitis precedes arthritis, then it should be presumed to have been sexually acquired. Patients should ideally be examined in a department of genitourinary medicine, where there are facilities to take the optimal specimens and direct liaison with the laboratory. Furthermore, staff there will arrange contact tracing and may obtain circumstantial evidence for infection of the proband, by detecting chlamydiae or *N. gonorrhoeae* in an asymptomatic carrier partner.

The quality of the specimens is of great importance. For chlamydia, separate special swabs must be used for immunodiagnosis (enzyme immunoassay), immunofluorescence, DNA detection, and culture. Special transport media containing 2-sucrose phosphate and preservation at −70°C are required if the swabs are not to be inoculated directly into tissue culture. Special tissue culture is labour-intensive and does not detect 1/10 positives (by all tests) but has the advantage of being highly specific. The antigen-detection tests by immunofluorescence or by enzyme immunoassays tend to yield false-positives for a variety of technical reasons. Optimal diagnostic power in patients with low risk of chlamydial infection is obtained by doing several tests (Ridgway and Taylor-Robinson 1991). For the patient with post-urethritis arthritis or Reiter's disease, diagnosis is important because eradicative antibiotic therapy is an important part of management even though the immunological disease is usually not affected by such treatment.

Experimental methods, such as direct probes to detect chlamydial DNA or RNA, or DNA amplification, are under development. The direct probes are not particularly sensitive, but DNA amplification is oversensitive, very prone to contamination, and may yield false-positive results. Antigen-detection tests alone and DNA amplification are not yet specific enough to be absolutely sure about the meaning of a positive result.

The chlamydiae, therefore, are typical examples of organisms that commonly cause disease and are detected by rapid, simple means other than conventional staining and culture, that is, enzyme immunoassay and immunofluorescence of antigen, with DNA or RNA hybridization proving a useful experimental tool. In contrast, detection of gonorrhoea should be by culture.

The likelihood of detecting these organisms diminishes progressively with time from the acute infection. Therefore, the tests may be negative in patients with reactive arthritis. Although antibody may be detected, this does not help with the diagnosis of recent infection. A very high titre of antibody to *Chlamydia trachomatis* would be a pointer to the diagnosis. The results of tests for antibody to *N. gonorrhoeae* are so totally unreliable that they should not be requested or performed.

Diarrhoea-associated reactive arthritis

When a patient gives a history of diarrhoea preceding the arthropathy then it is worth examining stools for continuing carriage of salmonellae, shigellae, and yersiniae, even though the acute illness may have occurred some time ago. All culture methods are selective, so lack sensitivity. Three separate stools should be examined to increase the value of a negative result. Intestinal biopsies may reveal organisms by immunofluorescence but this technique is very likely to be misleading because of cross-reactivity (de Koning et al. 1989). There is preliminary evidence that fluoroquinolones such as ciprofloxacin may be able to eradicate the carriage of certain organisms in the stool, but this action has not yet been shown to affect post-dysenteric arthropathy.

Yersinia enterocolitica causes a syndrome of prolonged diarrhoea with abdominal pain a particular feature (Cover and Aber 1989). Patients may have terminal ileitis and pseudoappendicitis. Five per cent of patients develop erythema nodosum or reactive arthritis or full-blown Reiter's disease. *Yersinia enterocolitica* serogroups O3 and O9 are particularly associated with postinfective arthritis in Scandinavia, in parallel with a high incidence of HLA-B27. Antibodies to *Yersinia*, particularly IgA, persist and can be measured in reference laboratories. Cross-reactivity between numerous O serogroups and other organisms (*Brucella, Morganella, Salmonella*) and thyroid tissue antigens is likely to make agglutination tests for antibodies unreliable, although experimental enzyme immunoassays are under evaluation (Gronberg et al. 1989).

Like *Yersinia* spp., infection with *Tropheryma whippelii* may present with musculoskeletal as well as neurological, cardiac, pulmonary, and skin manifestations may present without or before the classical intestinal features of Whipple disease. The isolation of the responsible organism (Raoult et al. 2000) and development of blood PCR as diagnostic tool (Razman et al. 1997) suggests that it should be soon possible to make a non-invasive diagnosis.

Non-specific illness

Short-lived, influenza-like illness predisposing to arthritis will probably not be diagnosed. From a survey of 10 microbiology laboratories, Waghorn (1995) discovered that the following serological tests might be performed on serum from a 30-year-old female with 'an influenza-like illness and arthralgia': (in order of frequency) rubella, parvovirus, *Mycoplasma*, influenza, *Chlamydia*, adenovirus, enterovirus, hepatitis B, Q-fever, Epstein–Barr virus, antistreptolysin titre, *Borrelia*, mumps, respiratory syncytial virus, *Yersinia*, *Legionella*, toxoplasmosis, syphilis, and cytomegalovirus.

More protracted illness would be a feature of glandular fever, toxoplasmosis, or viral hepatitis. It is worth checking particularly for evidence of recent anicteric hepatitis. Markers of recent infection with hepatitis B virus include IgM antihepatitis B core antibody. Serial sera will also reveal the evolution of an acute infection or chronic carrier state. Hepatitis A virus IgM is specific to recent infection within the last 6 months because the carrier state does not occur.

Positive hepatitis C virus antibody tests occurred particularly in rheumatoid arthritis, implying a causal link until it was discovered that this reactivity was non-specific. However, there have been a small number of case reports of reactive arthritis associated with this infection.

Rash illness

Common exanthematous infections such as rubella and parvovirus are associated with arthritis either during the latter stages of the acute infection, when the diagnosis is usually clear, or when the infection appears to have resolved. Serological tests are needed to make the diagnosis. Specific IgM tests are available for these organisms.

Lyme disease (see also Chapter 6.2.4)

The rheumatologist may be alerted to the possibility of Lyme disease as a cause of rheumatic symptoms during the secondary stage of the disease by concomitant rash, neurological signs, or myopericarditis. History of exposure, of known tick bite, and of the erythema chronicum migrans of the primary illness will also be useful. Large-joint arthritis is characteristic of the tertiary stage and there may or may not be skin and neurological manifestations.

Although the spirochaetes can sometimes be seen in biopsy material, realistically the diagnosis can only be made serologically and several methods of detecting antibody are available in kit form: indirect immunofluorescence (based on the fluorescent treponemal antibody test but using *Borrelia burgdorferi*), passive haemagglutination of red cells or latex beads coated with *B. burgdorferi*, various enzyme immunoassays, and a specific IgM capture test (Barbour 1988). Rheumatoid factor will give false-positives in the last. Many laboratories will do one of these as a screening test will rely on reference laboratories for confirmatory (Schwartz et al. 1989).

False-positives are common in all tests, probably because of exposure to commensal spirochaetes, and the most specific tests use a preliminary absorption step. Schwartz et al. (1989) found some discrepancies between test results from different laboratories. It is important that the screening test should be highly sensitive (and therefore gives some false-positives) so that positives are not missed. False-positives should be excluded by confirmatory tests but Western immunoblotting does not add much to the specificity of a good enzyme immunoassay (Karlsson 1990).

Rheumatic fever (see Chapter 6.2.12)

In the relatively rare condition of acute rheumatic fever, *S. pyogenes* may be obtained from the throat swab of the proband and family contacts several weeks after the acute infection. During an outbreak it is worth determining the serotype of any isolate. However, except in very unusual conditions, these are not consistently of one M-type (Kaplan et al. 1989). Certain M-types seem to be more commonly associated with rheumatic fever but this is probably an epiphenomenon and the diversity of types usually found suggests an epidemic cofactor, such as a coincident viral infection. No such cofactor has ever been identified. Isolation of *S. pyogenes* is a helpful indication but is not the mainstay of the diagnosis (Pope 1989). High titres, preferably with a demonstrated fourfold rise or fall in antistreptolysin-O and anti-DNAase B titres in serial samples, are the strongest supportive evidence for rheumatic fever. However, only 80 per cent of patients who fulfil the clinical criteria for acute rheumatic fever have a significantly raised antistreptolysin-O titre, and antibodies against other determinants may be more sensitive.

Conclusion

The rheumatologist can gain much information by using the diagnostic microbiology laboratory to the best advantage but can also expend much money and fruitless energy uncritically requesting irrelevant serology. Withholding antibiotics until all the relevant culture specimens have been taken and consultation over difficult cases may be helpful.

References

Barbour, A.G. (1988). Laboratory aspects of Lyme borreliosis. *Clinical Microbiology Reviews* **1**, 399–413.

Cover, T.L. and Aber, R.A. (1989). *Yersinia enterocolitica. New England Journal of Medicine* **321**, 16–24.

Easmon, C.S.F. (1990). Laboratory diagnosis of bacterial diseases. In *Principles of Bacteriology, Virology, and Immunity* Vol. 3 (ed. G.R. Smith and C.S.F. Easmon), pp. 1–9. London: Edward Arnold.

von Eiff, C. and Peters, G. (1999). Comparative *in-vitro* activities of moxifloxacin, trovafloxacin, quinupristin/dalfopristin and lionezolid against staphylococci. *Journal of Antimicrobial Chemotherapy* **43**, 569–73.

Gronberg, A., Fryden, A., and Kihlstrom, E. (1989). Humoral response to individual *Yersinia enterocolitica* antigens in patients with and without reactive arthritis. *Clinical and Experimental Immunology* **76**, 361–5.

Kaplan, E.L., Johnson, D.R., and Cleary, P.P. (1989). Group A streptococcal serotypes isolated from patients and sibling contacts during the resurgence of rheumatic fever in the United States in the mid-1980s. *Journal of Infectious Diseases* **159**, 101–3.

Karlsson, M. (1990). Western immunoblot and enzyme-linked immunosorbent assay for serodiagnosis of Lyme borreliosis. *Journal of Clinical Microbiology* **28**, 2148–50.

de Koning, J., Heeseman, J., Hoogkamp-Korstanje, J.A.A., Festen, J.J.M., Houtman, P.M., and Van Oijen, P.L.M. (1989). *Yersinia* from intestinal biopsy specimens from patients with seronegative spondyloarthropathy: correlation with specific IgA antibodies. *Journal of Infectious Diseases* **159**, 109–12.

Perry, C.M. and Jarvis, B. (2001). Linezolid: a review of its use in the management of serious Gram-positive infections. *Drugs* **61**, 525–51.

Pope, R.M. (1989). Rheumatic fever in the 1980s. *Bulletin on the Rheumatic Diseases* **38**, 1–8.

Raoult, D., Birg, M.L., La Scola, B., Fournier, P.E., Enea, M., Lepidi, H., Roux, V., Piette, J.C., Vandenesch, F., Vital-Durand, D., and Marrie, T.J. (2000). Cultivation of the bacillus of Whipple's disease. *New England Journal of Medicine* **342**, 620–5.

Razman, N.N., Loftus, E., Jr., Burgart, L.J., Rooney, M., Batts, K.P., Wiesner, R.H., Fredricks, D.N., Relamn, D.A., and Persing, D.H. (1997). Diagnosing and monitoring of Whipple disease by polymerase chain reaction. *Annals of Internal Medicine* **126**, 520–7.

Ridgway, G.L. and Taylor-Robinson, D. (1991). Current problems in microbiology. 1. Chlamydial infections: which laboratory test? *Journal of Clinical Pathology* **44**, 1–5.

Schwartz, B.S., Goldstein, M.D., Ribeiro, J.M.C., Schulze, T.L., and Shahied, S.I. (1989). Antibody testing in Lyme disease: a comparison of results in four laboratories. *Journal of the American Medical Association* **262**, 3431–4.

Stokes, E.J. and Ridgway, G.L. (1987). Antibiotic sensitivity tests. In *Clinical Microbiology*, pp. 204–33. London: Edward Arnold.

Stokes, E.J., Ridgway, G.L., and Wren M. (1993). The practice of clinical microbiology. In *Clinical Microbiology*, pp. 1–11. London: Edward Arnold.

Waghorn, D.J. (1995). Serological testing in a microbiology laboratory of specimens from patients with suspected infectious disease. *Journal of Clinical Pathology* **48**, 358–63.

5.4 Serological profile

Peter J. Maddison and Pearl Huey

Autoantibodies, typically found in autoimmune rheumatic diseases, have been the subject of intensive study to understand their origin and role in pathogenesis. Laboratory methods to detect certain of these antibodies have provided the clinician with valuable tools to assist in diagnosis and, to some extent, prognosis in patients with autoimmune rheumatic diseases. Serology is of particular value in situations where clinical expression of a disease such as systemic lupus erythematosus (SLE) is incomplete when the presence of a particular antinuclear antibody (ANA) profile can be diagnostic. However, autoantibodies can be found in a variety of clinical settings and their occurrence does not necessarily indicate the presence of disease. Therefore, it is imperative that serological tests are planned and the results are interpreted in the light of the clinical findings. Conversely, to be of most use to the clinician, the serology laboratory should have the facility to detect a wide range of relevant antibody specificities.

An important observation is that autoantibodies are directed to very characteristic autoantigen targets in patients with autoimmune rheumatic diseases. Furthermore, in the individual patient, the autoantibody profile is often quite restricted. It is now appreciated that certain profiles are associated with diagnostic categories of autoimmune rheumatic diseases and sometimes with particular patterns of clinical manifestations (Reichlin and Harley 1997). Therefore, for example, once ANA have been detected with a screening test, it is important to determine their specificity. This is now part of the standard operating procedures of serology laboratories but the process is greatly facilitated by the clinician providing adequate clinical information when serological testing is requested.

Methods of detecting autoantibodies

To obtain a complete serological profile, the laboratory will use a combination of different techniques (Miles et al. 1998).

Antinuclear antibodies

Indirect immunofluorescence (IMF) is used to detect a wide range of autoantibodies, both organ-specific and non-organ-specific (Box 1). The type of substrate used will depend on the suspected autoantibody specificity. For many years, rodent tissues were used to screen for almost all autoantibodies but these are being superseded by more specific and more sensitive substrates such as monkey tissue and cultured human cells.

IMF using whole cell preparations detects a wide range of ANA specificities and is the technique used by most serology laboratories as a primary screening test for ANA. ANA are a diverse group of antibodies, often directed to large cellular complexes containing protein and nucleic acid components. The most frequently occurring ANA react with components of DNA–protein or RNA–protein complexes. A large number of studies indicates that the production of these autoantibodies, which are generally high titre, high affinity IgG antibodies, is T-cell dependent and driven by the host autoantigen (Reichlin and Harley 1997).

Human cell lines, particularly HEp-2 epithelial cells, derived from a human laryngeal carcinoma, are now used in preference to cryostat sections of rodent tissues such as mouse or rat liver or kidney. This is because it is easier to visualize individual HEp-2 cells and their organelles and, more importantly, as rapidly dividing cells, they present antigens only expressed during certain stages of the cell cycle, which are either absent or occur only in small quantities in the resting nuclei of tissue sections. Also, ANA in autoimmune rheumatic diseases, such as anti-Ro antibodies, are directed primarily to the human antigen. Some commercial suppliers have transfected human genes into the cells so that they hyperexpress antigens such as Ro, making detection of corresponding antibodies a lot easier (Pollock and Toh 1999). Interpretation of this assay still depends on the skill of the technician, but with the advent of commercially available cell culture substrates, easily available positive standards and the requirement for laboratories to participate in quality assurance schemes, the IMF technique is generally reliable and reproducible.

Most patients with an autoimmune rheumatic disease will have a positive ANA. Therefore, if the ANA is negative, the differential diagnosis should be reviewed. As illustrated in Table 1, in addition to autoimmune rheumatic diseases, ANA are found in organ-specific autoimmune diseases and in other clinical settings such as infection and lymphoproliferative disorders. About 15 per cent of healthy adults and 8 per cent of children have detectable ANA, usually in low titre (Forslid et al. 1994). The frequency of ANA in normal people is higher in women and increases with age so that at least 30 per cent of women over the age of 60 years are positive. The frequency is also higher in healthy first degree relatives of patients with autoimmune rheumatic diseases (Maddison et al. 1993).

Both the ANA pattern and the titre will generally be reported. The pattern of immunofluorescence will give some hints to the principal ANA specificity in the serum and may influence the subsequent approach to determine the antibody specificity (Homburger 1995). Some staining patterns such as those corresponding to centromere and nucleolar antibodies are closely associated with a diagnosis of systemic sclerosis (SSc). Other patterns such as the peripheral nuclear pattern is almost exclusively seen in SLE. Although a low-titre ANA is not necessarily clinically insignificant, higher titres ($>1:160$) are more likely to indicate the presence of an autoimmune rheumatic disease (Tan et al. 1997). In some instances, the IMF ANA test gives a false negative result. This may occur if the antigen is located outside the nucleus (e.g. anti-Jo-1 and anti-ribosomal P, both frequently categorized under the umbrella term 'ANA') or if it is present in a form not recognized by a particular autoantibody (e.g. when anti-Ro is directed exclusively to determinants on the native Ro molecule not expressed in cultured HEp-2 cells) (Plate 69). In these situations, the clinical picture will dictate that specific assays need to be undertaken. The titre of ANA frequently fluctuates in individual patients but this does not correspond well to disease activity. The titre per se does not have a prognostic significance.

Automated enzyme-linked immunosorbent assay (ELISA) technology is now available for ANA detection. This potentially cuts hands-on testing time

Box 1 Use of IMF in detecting autoantibodies

In *indirect immunofluorescence*, the patient's diluted serum is incubated on the substrate to allow any antibodies present to bind to the corresponding antigens. After washing to remove unbound immunoglobulin, fluorescein-conjugated antihuman, class-specific antibody is added and allowed to react. After further washing, the slide is viewed under ultraviolet light. A positive reaction is indicated by bright fluorescence at the site of antigen–antibody binding. There are alternative visualization reagents that rely on a chemical reaction using an enzyme-linked conjugate to detect bound antibodies. Such methods are useful if a fluorescence microscope is unavailable. The titre and pattern of fluorescence will be reported.

Table 1 Antinuclear antibodies in various diseases detected by indirect immunofluorescence

Condition	Frequency of ANA (%)
Autoimmune rheumatic disease	
Drug-induced lupus	100
Systemic lupus erythematosus	98
Systemic sclerosis	98
Sjögren's syndrome	80
Pauciarticular juvenile idiopathic arthritis	70
Polymyositis/dermatomyositis	60
Rheumatoid arthritis	50
Organ-specific autoimmunity	
Primary autoimmune cholangitis	100
Autoimmune hepatitis	70
Myaesthenia gravis	50
Autoimmune thyroid disease	45
Other conditions	
Waldenstrom's macroglobulinaemia	20
Subacute bacterial endocarditis	20
Infectious mononucleosis	15
Leprosy	15
Normal population	
Children	8
Adults	15

and reduces the need for experience to interpret IMF results. These commercial assays employ various principles for preparing the substrate including whole cell extracts and specific mixtures of purified or recombinant autoantigens. However, there is considerable variability in their sensitivity and specificity (Emlen and O'Neill 1997) and they have not yet taken over from IMF which is still the gold standard.

Antibodies to DNA

Autoantibodies binding native, double-stranded DNA (nDNA) and/or denatured, single-stranded DNA (ssDNA) have a central place in the immunology of lupus. It is techniques to detect anti-nDNA antibodies, which are most specific for SLE, that are routinely used in the diagnostic laboratory. IMF using the haemoflagellate, *Crithidia luciliae*, is a frequently used technique for detecting anti-nDNA, combining high sensitivity with high disease specificity but is only semiquantitative. This microorganism contains a giant mitochondrion that consists of pure circular nDNA and it is the fluorescence of this which constitutes a positive test. The Farr assay is a fluid phase radioimmunoassay in which antibodies combined to ^{125}I-labelled DNA are precipitated by 50 per cent saturated ammonium sulfate (Smeenk et al. 1990). Modifications of this include the use of filters or an antihuman immunoglobulin serum. It is important that the substrate is impeccably pure, double-stranded DNA. The Farr assay detects high affinity antibody, is at least as specific as IMF using Crithidia and titres correlate best with disease activity. Increasingly, however, laboratories are turning for convenience to ELISA. The ELISA is more sensitive but generally less specific than the Farr and IMF assays because it detects low as well as high affinity antibody. Different commercial ELISA assay systems are not always comparable (Aviña-Zubieta et al. 1995) and are influenced by important factors such as characteristics of the DNA antigen, how the DNA is presented to antibody in the serum, and the reaction conditions.

Antihistone antibodies

Antibodies to histones are detected in idiopathic and drug-induced lupus, rheumatoid arthritis, and other conditions including scleroderma-related disorders. Histones are a set of basic proteins that organize chromosomal DNA in eukaryotes into nucleosomes, which are the repeating units of chromatin. The nucleosome consists of the histone octamer $(H2A–H2B–H3–H4)_2$, approximately 200 base pairs of DNA and H1. Antibodies are directed to a range of epitopes expressed on individual histones, histone–histone complexes, and histone–DNA complexes (Burlingame and Rubin 1990). They can be detected by IMF, typically producing an homogeneous nuclear pattern which can be abolished by acid treatment of the substrate (Fritzler and Tan 1978). These antibodies primarily react with the (H2A–H2B)–DNA complex which is exposed in chromatin. ELISA have also been developed (Burlingame and Rubin 1990) but can be affected by DNA contamination of the antigen preparation. Immunoblotting using commercial sources of extracted histones can be used to detect antibodies to all five histones, although only the reactivity to denatured individual histones is measured by this technique.

Recent studies have demonstrated that antibodies reacting specifically with native nucleosomes are important in idiopathic SLE. These antibodies, which can be measured by ELISA, occur early in the course of the disease and can precede classical anti-DNA antibodies. These assays may become more widely used in routine serology.

Nucleic acid-binding proteins

Many of the antibodies detected by IMF in patients with autoimmune rheumatic diseases are reactive with a group of highly conserved, nucleic acid-binding proteins, colloquially known as extractable nuclear antigens (ENA). Traditionally, these molecules have been extracted using either saline or acetone from rabbit and calf thymus or human spleen but other human tissues have also proved to be good sources of antigens. Increasingly, recombinant proteins have been made available for assays. The presence of antibodies to ENA is a very characteristic feature of autoimmune rheumatic diseases and certain profiles of these antibodies are associated with particular patterns of disease. A variety of methods are available to detect and classify these antibodies such as double immunodiffusion (Fig. 1), ELISA, Western blotting, and immunoprecipitation. In practice, the diagnostic laboratory uses a combination of techniques to detect and identify antibodies to ENA.

Traditionally, these antibodies, generally IgG and of high titre, have been detected by immunodiffusion using extracts of mammalian tissue as the antigen source. A range of prototype sera, available from the CDC, Atlanta, are used to identify a precipitin system.

Counter-current immunoelectrophoresis (CIE) (Kurata and Tan 1976) is quicker to complete and about 10-fold more sensitive than the Ouchterlony technique but is more demanding and capricious. The main drawbacks of the immunodiffusion methods include lack of sensitivity, variability of the substrate and operator error.

Increasingly, more sensitive methods of antibody detection are being used, such as immunoblotting, protein or RNA immunoprecipitation, and ELISA. The techniques of immunoblotting and immunoprecipitation are described elsewhere (Verheijen et al. 1993). They tend to be too labour intensive for the routine laboratory but are the principal ways of identifying many of the myositis- and scleroderma-associated antibodies. In Western immunoblotting, specific antibodies are recognized by binding to a profile of proteins of particular molecular weight which have been separated by electrophoresis of a cell extract and transferred to nitrocellulose sheets. It is not a suitable method to screen large numbers of sera and another disadvantage is that it only detects antibodies to epitopes on denatured proteins and, consequently, there are frequent false negatives with sera containing, for example, anti-Ro. However, methods using dot blots or line blots are gaining popularity in diagnostic laboratories. Here, purified native, recombinant or synthetic peptides are dotted on to nitrocellulose support or thin strips of antigen-impregnated nitrocellulose are placed on a slide. The patient's serum is then tested in a similar way to the Western

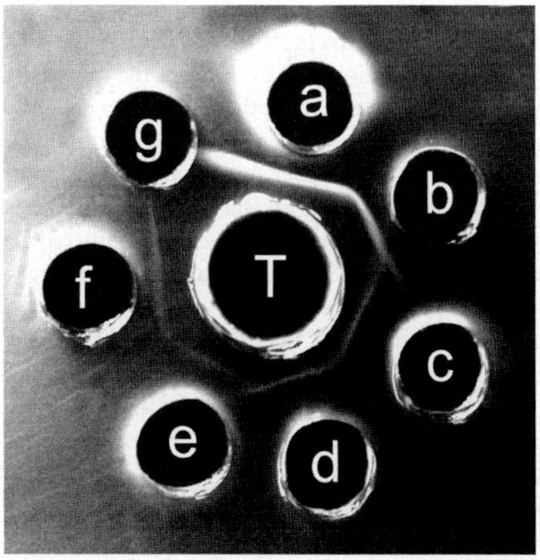

Fig. 1 The Ouchterlony technique of double immunodiffusion. In this procedure, the antigen and antibody are allowed to diffuse towards each other in an agarose gel medium and a line of precipitation forms where the two reactants meet. A sharp line is produced at the point of equivalence but is soluble in excess antibody or antigen. The position of the line is determined by the molecular weight of the reactants and the concentration of the antigen and antibody. Identification of the antibody is achieved by running prototype sera in wells adjacent to the positive unknown sera. Sera (a) and (b) are anti-Sm; sera (c) and (d) are anti-Ro; sera (e) and (f) are anti-topoisomerase-1.

Box 2 ELISAs using purified antigens for detecting antibodies

ELISA methods generally involve the use of plastic microtitre plates coated with antigen. Diluted patients' sera are incubated in the wells for a set time. After extensive washing to remove unbound immunoglobulin, in the second step the bound antibodies are detected with enzyme-conjugated antihuman antibodies. Bound antibodies are then visualized in a third step by the use of a chromagen substrate, which gives a visible coloured reaction in the test well. The intensity of the colour produced is quantified by measuring the optical density, which is proportional to the amount of antibody in the serum.

blot technique. These blots are much easier to interpret than Western blots, as there is usually only one antigen specificity in each dot.

ELISAs using purified antigens have been developed and provide a sensitive, quantitative way of detecting these antibodies (Box 2). Initially, immunoaffinity purified antigens were used but recombinant antigens are increasingly used as the substrate.

ELISA methods lend themselves to automation and eliminate many of the variables associated with IMF. They are rapid, sensitive and specific, however, there are marked variations between commercial ELISA kits (Tan et al. 1999). This is largely due to the quality, purity, structure, and concentration of antigen coated on to the plate. As with most other tests an increase in sensitivity often leads to loss of specificity and a decrease in positive and negative predictive values.

Antiphospholipid antibodies

The presence of antiphospholipid (APL) antibodies is the serological marker of the hypercoagulable disorder known as the antiphospholipid syndrome (APS) (Wilson et al. 1999). APL comprise a family of antibody specificities that need a combination of assays for detection. Previously, it was assumed that APL bound to cardiolipin or other negatively charged phospholipids such as phosphotidylinositol and phosphotidylserine. However, in contrast to APL induced by infection, antibodies associated with the APS primarily react with a number of phospholipid-binding proteins especially the 50 kDa plasma protein termed β2-glycoprotein I (β2GPI) (Roubey 1994). The anticardiolipin ELISA test is the most sensitive screening test for APS and is positive in more than 80–90 per cent of patients with the disorder. Generally, high levels of anticardiolipin antibodies are strongly suggestive of APS where as in other non-related disorders the antibody levels tend to be low. Similarly, IgG anticardiolipin antibodies are most frequently associated with clinical disease. The lupus anticoagulant (LAC) is less frequently positive in APS but is regarded as a more specific test. Since, about 10–20 per cent of patients with APS have a LAC but are anticardiolipin antibody-negative, the consensus at the present time is that a combination of an ELISA for anticardiolipin and a functional assay for the presence of LAC, for example, prolongation of the Russell's viper venom time, serves as a confirmatory screen for APS (Harris et al. 1998). However, some investigators feel that detection of anti-β2GPI by ELISA should replace assays for anticardiolipin antibodies since this is more specific for the diagnosis of APS (Koike and Matsuura 1996).

Antineutrophil cytoplasmic antibodies

The detection of antineutrophil cytoplasmic antibodies (ANCA), which react principally with myeloid-specific lysosomal enzymes, is well established as a tool for the diagnosis and assessment of certain forms of primary vasculitis (see Wiik 1995 for a review).

The standard method of screening for these antibodies is IMF using normal neutrophils, carefully separated and fixed in ethanol. Using this technique, different patterns of fluorescence indicate different antibody specificities (Plate 70).

All sera from suspected cases of vasculitis should be screened by IMF at a serum dilution of 1 : 20. As ANCA are usually of the IgG class it is recommended that a human IgG monospecific polyclonal IgG immunofluorescent conjugate is used as the secondary antibody. IgA class antibodies have been reported in Henoch–Schönlein purpura and IgM class antibodies in some cases of pulmonary haemorrhage. If such conditions are suspected, the laboratory needs to be informed so that an antihuman IgA or IgM fluorescent conjugate can be used. Considerable experience and great care are needed in the interpretation of results since there is such a wide variety of fluorescence patterns (Savige et al. 1998).

The ANCA specificity should be confirmed using ELISA specific, for example, for antiproteinase-3 (PR3) or antimyeloperoxidase (MPO). This will also provide a quantitative result which can be helpful in monitoring disease activity. However, up to 10 per cent of ANCA-positive sera from patients with Wegener's granulomatosis (WG) or microscopic polyangiitis (MPA) can only be demonstrated by IMF and are negative in MPO and PR3 ELISA tests. Conversely, about 5 per cent of ANCA-positive sera will only be detectable using ELISA. A recent development has been the Quickcard method of detecting antibodies to PR3, MPO, and glomerular basement membrane, using dot blot technology, which is simple and rapid and shows good specificity and sensitivity.

Rheumatoid factor

This is one of the most requested tests for rheumatic diseases. Rheumatoid factors (RF) are antibodies directed against antigenic determinants on the Fc fragment of IgG. Most methods detect the 19s pentameric IgM but IgA and IgG RF have also been detected although their clinical significance is less clear. In rheumatoid arthritis, RF is polyclonal and reacts with a wide range of determinants on both the CH2 and CH3 domains of IgG. It is detected in many laboratories by techniques employing agglutination or flocculation of IgG-coated cells or particles. An example is the rheumatoid arthritis latex test that uses latex beads coated with human IgG that are cross-linked by RF to produce visible flocculation. This detects primarily IgM RF because of its high valency. The RF latex test also detects antiallotypic antibodies resulting from transfusion or pregnancy; thus, to increase specificity, techniques such as the Rose–Waaler test have been used in which RF interacts with sheep cells coated with subagglutinating doses of rabbit IgG to cause haemagglutination. Since the presence of heterophile antibodies which react directly with sheep red cells can give rise to false-positive results, sera are usually tested in parallel with both coated and uncoated red cells and the difference in titres is expressed as the differential agglutination titre. Alternatively, the test serum is pre-incubated with uncoated sheep red cells (SCAT technique). Methods using rabbit IgG are less sensitive and give lower titres than the rheumatoid arthritis latex test because only a minor proportion of RF cross-react with rabbit IgG in rheumatoid arthritis. The presence of immune complexes or aggregated IgG can interfere with these techniques, sometimes to the extent that there is a false-negative result ('hidden rheumatoid factors'). Other methods for detecting RF include laser nephelometry, which is highly reproducible, and radioimmunoassays and ELISAs which are sensitive and quantitative and can be used to detect different isotypes of RF.

RF is non-specific, is found in many other clinical conditions (Table 2) and is present, usually in low titres in 1–5 per cent of the healthy population. In an unselected population the positive predictive value of the RF test for rheumatoid arthritis is low (20–30 per cent) but, in a selected population with polyarthritis, the positive predictive value increases to over 80 per cent with a negative predictive value of 95 per cent.

Antifilaggrin antibodies

Antibodies to filaggrin, a cytokeratin filament-binding protein involved in the differentiation of epithelial cells and keratinization, and its precursor, pro-filaggrin, are commonly found in rheumatoid arthritis. Initially, these antibodies were detected by IMF as 'antiperinuclear factor' (APF) (Nienhuis and Mandema 1964) characterized by a pattern of fluorescent perinuclear dots in epithelial cells from human buccal mucosa. Later, 'anti-keratin' antibodies (AKA) were frequently identified in APF-positive sera by Johnson et al. (1981) using IMF on rat oesophagus. Subsequent studies (Sebbag et al. 1995), strongly suggested that the targets of APF and AKA were pro-filaggrin and filaggrin, respectively. Neither of these IMF techniques is in common use due to the difficulty in obtaining consistently reliable substrate although, of the two, AKA, recognized by linear laminated labelling of the stratum corneum in the superficial layers of the epithelium of rat oesophagus, is the most reliable. ELISAs have been established using purified filaggrin preparations for clinical research (Paimela et al. 2001) but are not commercially available at the present time. Schellekens et al. (2000) have developed an ELISA to detect antibodies to a cyclic citrullinated peptide, based on the observation that citrulline residues are an important constituent of the antigenic regions reacting with antifilaggrin antibodies, in up to 70 per cent of the patients with rheumatoid arthritis with a specificity of over 95 per cent.

Table 2 Diseases commonly associated with rheumatoid factor

Rheumatoid arthritis	75%
Other rheumatic diseases	Systemic lupus erythematosus, systemic sclerosis, Sjögren's syndrome, mixed connective tissue disease
Acute viral infections	Mononucleosis, hepatitis, influenza, etc., after vaccination
Parasitic infections	Trypanosomiasis, malaria, schistosomiasis, etc.
Chronic inflammatory diseases	Tuberculosis, leprosy, syphilis, subacute bacterial endocarditis, etc.
Neoplasms	After irradiation or chemotherapy
Other hyperglobulinaemic states	Hyperglobulinaemic purpura, sarcoidosis, chronic liver disease, cryoglobulinaemia

Other autoantibodies

Table 3 summarizes the methods used to detect a number of other organ-specific and non-organ-specific antibodies of relevance to patients with rheumatic diseases.

Autoantibody profiles in autoimmune rheumatic diseases

Systemic lupus erythematosus

The use of HEp2 cells enhances the sensitivity of the ANA test in SLE so that ANAs can be detected in 95 per cent of active, untreated patients. The main

Table 3 Summary of methods used to detect organ-specific and non-organ-specific antibodies

Antibody specificity	Antigen	Assay	Disease association
Liver/kidney microsomal antibodies (LKM-1, LKM-2, LKM-3)	P-450 Other enzymes	IMF (rodent/monkey liver and kidney) ELISA	Anti-LKM-1 strongly associated with autoimmune hepatitis type II
Liver cytosol Type 1	LC1	IMF (rodent liver)	Type II autoimmune hepatitis
Liver soluble antigen	Glutathione S transferase	ELISA	Type II autoimmune hepatitis
Mitochondrial	Pyruvate dehydrogenase	IMF (rodent liver/kidney/stomach, HEp-2 cells) ELISA	Primary biliary cirrhosis
Parietal cell	Gastric pump	IMF (rodent/monkey fundus of stomach)	Autoimmune gastritis Pernicious anaemia Often associated with thyroid disease
Smooth muscle	F- or G-actin Desmin Vimentin	IMF (rodent/monkey stomach blood vessels)	Autoimmune hepatitis (associated with antibodies to F- or G-actin, whereas antibodies to other muscle filaments are more associated with viral hepatitis
Endomysial	Tissue transglutaminase	IMF (monkey oesophagus/human umbilical cord)	Coeliac disease (IgA antibodies) Sensitivity $>$ 90%; specificity $>$ 95%
Glomerular basement membrane	Alpha3 chain of Type IV collagen	IMF (monkey kidney) ELISA (best method to confirm)	Goodpasture's syndrome
Thyroid	Thyroglobulin Microsomal peroxidase	IMF (thyroid) ELISA	Autoimmune thyroid disease
GAD	Glutamic acid decarboxylase (GAD 65 kDa, 67 kDa)	IMF (pancreas) ELISA (preferred method)	Stiff man syndrome Diabetes mellitus

difference from using rodent substrates is the increased detection of patients with an immune response predominantly to Ro. The identification of this patient subset can be further enhanced by using HEp-2 cells transfected with human 60 kDa Ro antigen gene (Pollock and Toh 1999). Thus, in the situation where the clinician wishes to exclude the possibility of SLE, IMF is sufficient as a screening test for ANA and it is not cost-effective automatically to test for anti-DNA or other antibody specificities. However, a very small number of SLE patients are ANA-negative even using HEp2 cells and proceeding with other techniques to look for SLE-associated antibodies is indicated if the clinical picture dictates. Conversely, since the positive predictive value in an ANA test for SLE is low, as low as 11 per cent in some studies (Slater et al. 1996), once the ANA test is positive, then it is important to look for antibodies reacting with DNA or nucleic acid-binding proteins.

Approximately 70 per cent of untreated patients with active SLE have anti-nDNA detected by IMF or the Farr technique. In many patients, an increase in anti-DNA levels precedes a clinical exacerbation. In some a fall in these raised levels is observed just prior to the disease flare (ter Borg et al. 1990). Consequently, there is value in monitoring serial serum anti-DNA levels. In studies where the relative proportion of high and low avidity anti-DNA antibodies was measured, clinical exacerbation was often heralded by an increase in high avidity antibodies.

In SLE, antibodies react most frequently with four groups of RNA-binding proteins, namely Sm, U1RNP, Ro, and La (Reichlin and Harley 1997). The antigens have been well characterized at a molecular level. High titres of these antibodies, for example as detected by immunodiffusion, are found frequently and almost exclusively in the context of autoimmune rheumatic diseases. Anti-Sm has the greatest specificity for SLE but there is a marked ethnic variation in the presence of these antibodies, being more commonly found in Afro-Caribbeans than in northern European Caucasians (Arnett 1988). These antibodies identify distinctive serological subsets within the spectrum of SLE. Antibodies to Sm frequently occur in association with anti-U1RNP and antibodies to La are virtually always accompanied by anti-Ro. It is apparent that these serological subsets are associated with certain patterns of disease expression (Table 4) in which they may have a pathogenetic role.

These antibodies are usually present from the beginning of the clinical presentation and are detectable throughout the course of the disease. Using an ELISA, fluctuations in antibody titre can be detected but there is an inconsistent relationship between titre measured in longitudinal studies and disease activity. A variety of other antibody specificities, for example, anti-PCNA (cyclin) (Asero et al. 1987), SL (Ki) (Sakamoto et al. 1989), and ribosomal P protein (Elkon et al. 1994), can be detected in SLE. They occur in a small proportion of sera and although clinical associations have been reported these associations require confirmation in larger, prospective studies and the role of these antibodies in 'routine' SLE serology is not yet defined.

Antibodies to ribosomal P proteins are directed predominantly to a conserved region of the *C*-terminus, which is shared by the P proteins. They occur in approximately 10 per cent of patients with SLE but have been reported in a higher proportion with active disease with an association with diffuse neuropsychiatric manifestations (Elkon et al. 1994). However, this association is not apparent in all published studies (reviewed by Teh and Isenberg 1994). Reasons for discrepancies between reports include methodological differences for detecting antiribosomal P, a lack of uniform criteria for classifying patients with lupus involving the central nervous system, and demographic variation between the study populations.

Antihistone antibodies are a striking feature of the immune response in drug-induced lupus, occuring in over 90 per cent cases whereas, in contrast to idiopathic lupus, autoantibodies to nDNA and ENA are uncommon. Although they lack disease specificity, the presence of autoantibodies primarily to histones in the appropriate clinical setting strongly suggests a drug-induced syndrome (Thompson et al. 1993).

Table 4 ANA specificities in diagnosis and disease expression

Disease	Antibody	Frequency (%)	Clinical association
SLE	Anti-nDNA	70	Lupus nephritis
	Anti-Sm	10–25[a]	Vasculitis; CNS lupus
	Anti-U1RNP	30	Raynaud's, swollen fingers, arthritis, myositis, MCTD
	Anti-Ro	40	Photosensitive rash, SCLE[b], neonatal lupus, CHB, Sjögren's
	Anti-La	15	As for anti-Ro
	Anti-rRNP	15	CNS lupus (psychosis, depression)
Sjögren's syndrome	Anti-Ro	60–90[c]	Extraglandular disease, vasculitis, lymphoma
	Anti-La	35–85[c]	As for anti-Ro
Systemic sclerosis	Anticentromere	30	Limited cutaneous disease, micro/macrovascular disease, telangiectasia
	Anti-ThRNP	4	Limited cutaneous disease
	Anti-topoisomerase-1	25	Diffuse cutaneous disease, interstitial lung disease
	Anti-RNA-polymerases	20	Diffuse cutaneous disease, renal disease
	Anti-U3RNP	5	Diffuse cutaneous disease, pulmonary hypertension
	Anti-PM-Scl	5	Scleroderma/polymyositis overlap
	Anti-Ku	2	Scleroderma/polymyositis overlap
Dermato/polymyositis	Anti-Jo-1	30	Antisynthetase syndrome
	(antibodies to other tRNA synthetases)	(3)	
	Anti-SRP	4	Severe myositis
	Anti-Mi2	10	Dermatomyositis

[a] Higher frequency in Blacks and Asians.

[b] Subacute cutaneous lupus.

[c] Using sensitive ELISA assays.

Mixed connective tissue disease

The concept of mixed connective tissue disease was initially predicated upon the identification of autoantibodies to U1RNP. Whether or not mixed connective tissue disease is a distinctive autoimmune rheumatic disease is controversial (Maddison 2000). However, the serological profile of autoantibodies not only to U1RNP but also another splicosome-related constituent, HnRNP-A2 (RA33) is quite distinctive. The pattern of antibody binding to RA33 epitopes in MCTD, for example, appears to be different from other autoimmune rheumatic diseases such as SLE, SSc, and RA (Smolen and Steiner 1998).

Sjögren's syndrome

With sensitive techniques, antibodies to Ro and La can be detected in virtually all patients with Sjögren's (Harley et al. 1986). They are a marker for Sjögren's syndrome developing in SLE, SSc, and primary biliary cirrhosis. Several studies, including that of Pease et al. (1993), have shown that antibodies to Ro and La identify patients at greatest risk of developing extraglandular complications such as vasculitis. Sjögren's syndrome in rheumatoid arthritis is usually not associated with anti-Ro. However, the small proportion of rheumatoid arthritis patients with anti-Ro have a distinctive clinical picture (Tishler et al. 1994).

Systemic sclerosis

Antinuclear and/or antinucleolar antibodies are an almost universal feature of patients with SSc. Several of these antibodies are highly specific for the disease, are rarely found in other clinical settings and occur as an early feature so that their identification has an important role in in early diagnosis. Certain of these antibodies can be detected in the routine serology laboratory by observing a typical pattern of IMF (in the case of anti-centromere antibodies) or using immunodiffusion or a specific ELISA (in the case of anti-topoisomerase-1). However, many of these systems require techniques such as immunoprecipitation for their detection and it is recommended to have sera from SSc patients analysed by a specialized reference laboratory when possible. An important observation is that there is virtually no overlap between subsets of patients identified by a particular antibody profile and these subsets tend to be associated with certain patterns of clinical expression. Thus, anticentromere antibodies (Steen et al. 1988) and antibodies to the nucleolar constituent, ThRNP are almost exclusively found in patients with limited cutaneous SSc (Falkener et al. 1998) and identify patient at risk of micro- and macrovascular disease. By contrast, antibodies to topoisomerase-1, RNA polymerase I, II, and III and to U3RNP identify clinical subsets of SSc with severe disease involving extensive scleroderma and visceral organ involvement (Bunn et al. 1998).

Polymyositis/dermatomyositis

Multiple antibody systems are also found in polymyositis or dermatomyositis. These include a number of myositis-specific antibodies (see Chapter 6.8.1). Each specificity occurs in a small proportion of patients and is associated with a characteristic pattern of clinical expression.

About 30 per cent of patients have antibodies to tRNA synthetases. Most commonly these antibodies react with histidyl-tRNA synthetase (Jo-1), and much less commonly, other aminoacyl tRNA synthetases (including threonyl, alanyl, glycyl, and isoleucyl tRNA synthetase). These patients frequently develop additional clinical features such as interstitial lung disease, polyarthritis, Raynaud's phenomenon and 'mechanics fingers' (the 'antisynthetase syndrome').

Antibodies to signal recognition particle occur in about 5 per cent patients and appear to be associated with severe, treatment-resistant polymyositis. In contrast, antibodies to Mi-2 occur almost exclusively in patients with dermatomyositis. Antibodies to U1RNP, U2RNP, Ku, and the PM-Scl system identify overlap syndromes between myositis and other connective tissue diseases, often with features of scleroderma.

Anti-Jo-1 antibodies can be detected in the routine serology laboratory but other myositis-specific antibodies require the input of a specialized reference laboratory.

Primary vasculitis

ANCA serology has a well-established role in the diagnosis and assessment of primary vasculitis (Gross et al. 2000). In current classification schemes, WG, MPA, and Churg–Strauss vasculitis are grouped as 'ANCA-associated small vessel vasculitis'. The high specificity (>95 per cent) of cANCA for WG has been confirmed in several studies (Rao et al. 1995) particularly if the presence of antibodies to PR3 is confirmed by ELISA. Overall, sensitivity is 60–70 per cent for the disease depending on the patient population selected. cANCA are found in at least 90 per cent of patients with diffuse WG and renal involvement but less commonly in patients with more localized disease. The presence of cANCA is of especial value in systemically ill patients when positive serology should prompt treatment in the absence of histological confirmation. In many patients, but not all, the titre of cANCA relates to disease activity but rising titres per se should not be a reason for modifying treatment.

The presence of pANCA with confirmation of antibodies to MPO by ELISA is commonly found in MPA. However, pANCA, reactive with MPO or other lysosomal enzymes, is found in a variety of chronic inflammatory are inflammatory disorders including RA, SLE, drug-induced lupus, and inflammatory bowel disease (Gross et al. 1993).

Rheumatoid arthritis

For many years, RF has been the only widely used serological test for diagnosis and assessment of rheumatoid arthritis. Tests for RF have some value as screening tests for rheumatoid arthritis, since RF is present in at least 75 per cent of patients with rheumatoid arthritis using a cut-off level for positivity, which excludes 95 per cent of the normal population. However, the clinical setting for interpreting this test is all important and the chance finding of RF on routine screening of a disease unlikely to be rheumatoid arthritis is of little clinical significance. The presence of RF in rheumatoid arthritis indicates a poorer prognosis (Heliövaara et al. 1995) and a high frequency of systemic and extra-articular manifestations.

Recently, there has been renewed interest in the clinical relevance of other autoantibodies associated with this disease such as antifilaggrin antibodies, anti-RA33, and anti-Sa (Menard et al. 1998). Each of these specificities is found early in the course of rheumatoid arthritis and while each occurs only in 30–40 per cent of patients, they show a high specificity of the order of 85–95 per cent. Since these antibodies occur in rheumatoid arthritis patients negative for RF, their detection may have a role in early diagnosis. Anticyclic citrullinated peptide, present in up to 70 per cent of patients with RA, have been shown to predict radiographic joint damage (Meyer et al. 2003). There is a potential for these antibodies to identify patients at an early stage that require aggressive treatment. However, further studies are needed to confirm the role of these antibodies in routine clinical practice.

References

Arnett, F.C. (1988). Increased frequencies of Sm and nRNP autoantibodies in American blacks compared to whites with systemic lupus erythematosus. *Journal of Rheumatology* **15**, 1773–6.

Asero, R., Origgi, L., Crespi, S., Bertetti, E., D'Agostino, P., and Riboldi, P. (1987). Autoantibody to proliferating cell nuclear antigen (PCNA) in SLE: a clinical and serological study. *Clinical and Experimental Rheumatology* **5**, 241–6.

Aviña-Zubieta, J.A., Galindo-Rodriguez, G., Kwan-Yeung, L., Davis, P., and Russell, A.S. (1995). Clinical evaluation of various selected ELISA kits for the detection of anti-DNA antibodies. *Lupus* **4**, 370–4.

Bunn, C.C., Denton, C.P., Shi-Wen, X., Knight, C., and Black, C.M. (1998). Anti-RNA polymerases and other autoantibody specificities in systemic sclerosis. *British Journal of Rheumatology* **37**, 15–20.

Burlingame, R.W. and Rubin, R.L. (1990). Subnucleosome structures as substrates in enzyme-linked immunoabsorbent assays. *Journal of Immunological Methods* **134**, 187–99.

Elkon, K.B., Bonfa, E., Weissbach, H., and Brot, N. (1994). Antiribosomal antibodies in SLE, infection, and following deliberate immunisation. *Advances in Experimental Medicine and Biology* **347**, 81–92.

Emlen, W. and O'Neill, L.O. (1997). Clinical significance of antinuclear antibodies. Comparison of detection with immunofluorescence and enzyme-linked immunosorbent assays. *Arthritis and Rheumatism* **40**, 1612–18.

Falkener, D., Wilson, J., Medsger, T.A., Jr., and Morel, P.A. (1998). HLA and clinical associations in systemic sclerosis patients with anti-Th/To antibodies. *Arthritis and Rheumatism* **41**, 74–80.

Forslid, J., Heigl, Z., Jonsson, J., and Scheynius, A. (1994). The prevalence of antinuclear antibodies in healthy young persons and adults, comparing rat liver tissue sections with HEp-2 cells as antigen substrate. *Clinical and Experimental Rheumatology* **12**, 137–41.

Fritzler, M.J. and Tan, E.M. (1978). Antibodies to histones in drug-induced and idiopathic lupus erythematosus. *Journal of Clinical Investigation* **62**, 560–7.

Gross, W.L., Schmitt, W.H., and Csernok, E. (1993). ANCA and associated diseases: immunodiagnostic and pathogenetic aspects. *Clinical and Experimental Immunology* **91**, 1–12.

Gross, W.L., Trabandt, A., and Reinhold-Keller, E. (2000). Diagnosis and evaluation of vasculitis. *Rheumatology* **39**, 245–52.

Harley, J.B. et al. (1986). Anti-Ro (SSA) and anti-La (SSC) in patients with Sjögren's syndrome. *Arthritis and Rheumatism* **29**, 196–201.

Harris, E.N., Pierangeli, S.S., and Gharavi, A.E. (1998). Diagnosis of the antiphospholipid syndrome: a proposal for use of laboratory tests. *Lupus* **7** (Suppl. 2), 144–8.

Heliövaara, M., Aho, K., Knekt, P., Aromaa, A., Maatela, J., and Reunanen, A. (1995). Rheumatoid factor, chronic arthritis and mortality. *Annals of the Rheumatic Diseases* **54**, 811–14.

Homburger, H.A. (1995). Laboratory medicine and pathology: cascade testing for autoantibodies in connective tissue diseases. *Mayo Clinic Proceedings* **70**, 183–4.

Johnson, G.D., Carvalho, A., Holborrow, E.J., Goddard, D.H., and Russell, G. (1981). Antiperinuclear factor and keratin antibodies in rheumatoid arthritis. *Annals of the Rheumatic Diseases* **40**, 263–6.

Koike, T. and Matsuura, E. (1996). Anti-β2GP1 antibody: specificity and clinical significance. *Lupus* **5**, 378–80.

Kurata, N. and Tan, E.M. (1976). Identification of antibodies to nuclear acid antigens by counter immunoelectrophoresis. *Arthritis and Rheumatism* **19**, 574–9.

Maddison, P.J. et al. (1993). Connective tissue disease and autoantibodies in the kindreds of 63 patients with systemic sclerosis. *Medicine* **72**, 103–12.

Maddison, P.J. (2000). MCTD: overlap syndromes. *Clinical Rheumatology* **14**, 111–24.

Menard, H.A., el Amine, M., and Despres, N. (1998). Rheumatoid arthritis associated autoimmune systems. *Journal of Rheumatology* **25**, 835–7.

Meyer, O., Labarre, C., Dougados, M., Goupille, Ph., Cantagrel, A., Dubois, A., Nicaise-Roland, P., Sibilia, J., and Combe, B. (2003). Anticitrullinated protein/peptide antibody assays for predicting five year radiographic damage. *Annals of the Rheumatic Diseases* **62**, 120–6.

Miles, J., Charles, P., and Riches, P. (1998). A review of methods available for the identification of both organ-specific and non-organ-specific autoantibodies. *Annals of Clinical Biochemistry* **35**, 19–47.

Nienhuis, R.L.F. and Mandema, E. (1964). A new serum factor in patients with rheumatoid arthritis: the antiperinuclear factor. *Annals of the Rheumatic Diseases* **23**, 302–5.

Paimela, L., Palosuo, T., Aho, K., Lukka, M., Kurki, P., Leirisalo-Repo, M., and von Essen, R. (2001). Association of autoantibodies to filaggrin with an active disease in early rheumatoid arthritis. *Annals of the Rheumatic Diseases* **60**, 32–5.

Pease, C.T., Charles, P.J., Shackles, W., Markwick, J., and Maini, R.N. (1993). Serological and immunogenetic markers of extraglandular primary Sjögren's syndrome. *British Journal of Rheumatology* **32**, 574–7.

Pollock, W. and Toh, B.-H. (1999). Routine immunofluorescence detection of Ro/SS-A autoantibodies using Hep-2 cells transfected with human 60 kDa Ro/SS-A. *Journal of Clinical Pathology* **52**, 684–7.

Rao, J.K., Weinberger, M., Oddone, E.Z., Allen, N.B., Lansman, P., and Fuessner, J.R. (1995). The role of antineutrophil cytoplasmic antibody (cANCA) testing in the diagnosis of Wegener's granulomatosis. *Annals of Internal Medicine* **123**, 925–32.

Reichlin, M. and Harley, J.B. (1997). Antinuclear antibodies: an overview. In *Dubois' Lupus Erythematosus* 5th edn. (ed. D.J. Wallace and B.H. Hahn), pp. 397–405. Baltimore MD: Williams & Wilkins.

Roubey, R.A.S. (1994). Autoantibodies to phospholipid-binding plasma proteins: a new view of lupus anticoagulant and other 'antiphospholipid' autoantibodies. *Blood* **84**, 2854–67.

Sakamoto, M., Takasaki, Y., Yamanaka, K., Kodama, A., Hashimoto, H., and Hirose, S. (1989). Purification and characterization of Ki antigen and detection of anti-Ki antibody by enzyme-linked immunosorbent assay in patients with systemic lupus erythematosus. *Arthritis and Rheumatism* **32**, 1554–62.

Savige, J.A. et al. (1998). A review of immunofluorescent patterns associated with anti-neutrophil cytoplasmic antibodies (ANCA) and their differentiation from other antibodies. *Journal of Clinical Pathology* **51**, 568–75.

Schellekens, G., Visser, H., DeJong, B.A.W., van den Hoogen, F.H., Hazes, J.M.W., Breedveld, F.C., and van Venrooij, W.J. (2000). The diagnostic properties of rheumatoid arthritis antibodies recognizing a cyclic citrullinated peptide. *Arthritis and Rheumatism* **43**, 155–63.

Sebbag, M., Simon, M., Vincent, C., Masson-Bessierre, C., Girbal, E., Durieux, J.J., and Serre, G. (1995). The antiperinuclear factor and the so-called antikeratin antibodies are the same rheumatoid arthritis-specific autoantibodies. *Journal of Clinical Investigation* **95**, 2672–9.

Slater, C.A., Davis, R.B., and Shmerling, R.H. (1996). Antinuclear antibody testing: a study of clinical utility. *Archives of Internal Medicine* **156**, 1421–5.

Smeenk, R., Brinkman, K., Van den Brink, H., and Swaak, T. (1990). A comparison of assays used for the detection of antibodies to DNA. *Clinical Rheumatology* **9**, 63–73.

Smolen, J.S. and Steiner, G. (1998). Mixed connective tissue disease. To be or not to be? *Arthritis and Rheumatism* **41**, 768–77.

Steen, V.D., Powell, D.L., and Medsger, T.A., Jr. (1988). Clinical correlations and prognosis based on serum autoantibodies in patients with systemic sclerosis. *Arthritis and Rheumatism* **31**, 196–203.

Tan, E.M. et al. (1997). Range of antinuclear antibodies in 'healthy' individuals. *Arthritis and Rheumatism* **40**, 1601–11.

Tan, E.M. et al. (1999). A critical evaluation of enzyme immunoassays for detection of antinuclear autoantibodies of defined specificities I. Precision, sensitivity and specificity. *Arthritis and Rheumatism* **42**, 455–64.

Teh, L.S. and Isenberg, D.A. (1994). Antiribosomal P protein antibodies in systemic lupus erythematosus. A reappraisal. *Arthritis and Rheumatism* **37**, 307–15.

ter Borg, E.J., Horst, G., Hummel, E.J., Limburg, P.C., and Kallenberg, C.G. (1990). Measurement of increases in anti-double-stranded DNA antibody levels as a predictor of disease exacerbation in systemic lupus erythematosus. A long-term, prospective study. *Arthritis and Rheumatism* **33**, 634–43.

Thompson, D., Juby, A., and Davis, P. (1993). The clinical significance of autoantibody profiles in patients with systemic lupus erythematosus. *Lupus* **2**, 15–19.

Tishler, M., Golbrut, B., Shoenfeld, Y., and Yaron, M. (1994). Anti-Ro(SSA) antibodies in patients with rheumatoid arthritis—a possible marker for gold induced side effects. *Journal of Rheumatology* **21**, 1040–2.

Verheijen, R., Salden, M., and van Venrooij, W.J. (1993). Protein blotting. In *Manual of Biological Markers of Disease* Vol. A4 (ed. W.J. van Venrooij and R.N. Maini), pp. 1–25. Dordrecht, The Netherlands: Kluwer.

Wiik, A. (1995). Anti-neutrophil cytoplasmic antibodies in Wegener's granulomatosis. Some clinical and pathogenetic aspects. *Seminars in Clinical Immunology* **9**, 5–13.

Wilson, W.A. et al. (1999). International consensus statement on preliminary classification criteria for definite antiphospholipid syndrome. Report of an International Workshop. *Arthritis and Rheumatism* **42**, 1309–11.

5.5 Joint fluid

J. Lawrence Houk

Formation, composition, and function of joint fluid

Joint fluid acts as a lubricant for the lining of the joint cavity. It is particularly effective for decreasing the coefficient of resistance during low-impact joint loading and motion while its adhesiveness enhances joint stability and tracking. Joint fluid also is a vehicle providing nutrients to and removing metabolic products from the articular cartilage (Simkin 1991).

The fluid is composed of molecules filtered from plasma plus a glycoprotein, hyaluronate, produced by synovial cells. The composition and concentrations of synovial components are determined primarily by their molecular weights. Small molecules such as glucose, amino acids, uric acid, bilirubin, and several enzymes are freely filtered through the endothelium and synovial tissues. Consequently the concentrations of small molecules normally reflect those seen in plasma. The influx of larger molecules such as fibrinogen requires increased vascular permeability and is normally impeded by filtration through the synovial tissue meshwork of hyaluronate proteins. Accordingly, large molecules found in serum are not normally present in joint fluid. Molecules leave the joint fluid via lymphatics. This process is usually unaffected by joint disease. Inflammation can change the normal distribution of joint fluid molecules. The inflammatory response can increase vascular permeability, allowing larger molecules such as fibrinogen to enter. These molecules account for the clotting of synovial fluid samples in abnormal fluid. At the same time, inflammation decreases vascular perfusion, thus reducing the number of small molecules that are available for diffusion into the joint fluid.

Indications for joint fluid examination

Why should joint fluid be examined? Even when performed by an experienced physician, the procedure is time consuming. A busy outpatient practice does not allow for many delays, and consequently, joint fluid examination is often omitted from the evaluation of the patient with arthritis.

Nonetheless, the results of a carefully conducted joint fluid examination usually have important diagnostic value. In fact, it may be the only source of a conclusive diagnosis. For example, a diagnosis of gout or calcium pyrophosphate crystal deposition disease cannot be certain unless the appropriate intracellular crystals are observed. Information gained from analysing joint fluid often provides more important data than any combination of blood tests or radiological procedures. In one report, treatment plans were changed in 53 per cent of 180 patients after synovial fluid analysis (Eisenberg et al. 1984).

The coexistence of two or more arthropathies is common, and at times only joint fluid testing can distinguish the diseases. Rheumatoid arthritis and osteoarthritis frequently occur simultaneously. Although conventional radiography can demonstrate the osteoarthritis, joint fluid evaluation may be necessary to reveal concomitant rheumatoid inflammation and suggest the correct decisions regarding therapy. Similarly, the risk of septic arthritis is increased in joints affected by rheumatoid arthritis and other arthropathies. A culture of joint fluid is the most sensitive and specific test for the recognition of a septic arthritis. Any articular site that is markedly more inflamed than other areas must undergo arthrocentesis to rule out infection. Gout, particularly the polyarticular form, can involve the hands, and tophi can occur in the region of the distal interphalangeal joints commonly involved in osteoarthritis (see 'Gout'). Microscopic examination of joint fluid for tophaceous material may be necessary to reveal this association. Likewise, gout and calcium pyrophosphate crystal deposition disease can coexist (Dieppe et al. 1988).

When should joint fluid be obtained? Generally joint fluid should be aspirated whenever a diagnosis has not been established or if there is a new articular event. Objective findings in a previously uninvolved area or increased swelling, pain, or erythema in an already affected site are indications for joint fluid aspiration. There is no absolute contraindication to an arthrocentesis unless the needle insertion site is in a potentially infected area. Joint fluid analysis should be considered a mandatory procedure in any individual with an unexplained articular effusion (Cohen et al. 1975). Additionally, joint fluid should be removed when injecting a corticosteroid preparation. Weitoft et al. (2000) instilled 20 mg of triamcinolone hexacetonide into 191 inflamed knees of 147 patients with rheumatoid arthritis. The joint fluid was removed prior to injection in 95 knees but not aspirated in 96 knees. The relapse rate was 23 per cent in the knees from which fluid was removed and 47 per cent when the fluid was not aspirated.

Aspirate fluid whenever the diagnosis is not known or if there is an unexplained change in joint swelling.

When the examination of joint fluid is believed to be of diagnostic or therapeutic value it should be obtained without delay. In inflammatory disorders such as rheumatoid arthritis, simple rest can decrease inflammation; the joint effusion may resolve, and consequently, an opportunity for a diagnosis is lost. Monosodium urate, and hydroxyapatite crystals can decrease over a period of time occasionally in as little as 6 h (Kerolus et al. 1989). Thus, a delay in synovial fluid analysis may eliminate the only source of a diagnosis. Septic joints have to be diagnosed immediately. Postponement of fluid aspiration can result in delay of treatment, possibly resulting in joint destruction. On the other hand, antibiotics started before fluid aspiration can prohibit growth of the infecting organism in culture; the diagnosis may never be established with certainty, and the patient may be subjected to inappropriate treatment.

The arthrocentesis itself can be therapeutic. Joint capsule distention can produce pain, loss of motion, or both, particularly in the knee. Removal of fluid can rapidly reduce discomfort and allow restoration of movement. However, excess fluid should not be aspirated repeatedly just because it is present. The additional medical expense and even the small risk of arthrocentesis must be justified by the possibility of correcting the diagnosis or improving the patient's condition.

Sites accessible to obtaining joint fluid

Potentially, any diarthrodial joint or bursal space can be entered with a needle. However, some areas are easier than others and some sites usually are not aspirated in a medical office setting. The knee is generally the simplest

Krey, P.R. (1992a). Practical guide to the analysis of synovial fluid. In *Analysis of Synovial Fluid* (ed. P.R. Krey and D.M. Lazaro), pp. 74–86. Summit NJ: Ciba-Geigy Corp.

Krey P.R. (1992b). Arthrocentesis. In *Analysis of Synovial Fluid* (ed. P.R. Krey and D.M. Lazaro), pp. 74–86. Summit NJ: Ciba-Geigy Corp.

Krey, P.R. and Bailen, D.A. (1979). Synovial fluid leukocytosis: a study of extremes. *American Journal of Medicine* **67**, 436–42.

Krey, P.R. and Lazaro, D.M. (1992). Specific tests. In *Analysis of Synovial Fluid* (ed. P.R. Krey and D.M. Lazaro), pp. 28–52. Summit NJ: Ciba-Geigy Corp.

Lally, E.V., Zimmermann, B., Ho, G., and Kaplan, S.R. (1989). Urate-mediated inflammation in nodal osteoarthritis: clinical and roentgenographic correlations. *Arthritis and Rheumatism* **32**, 86–90.

Lawrence, C. and Seife, B. (1971). Bone marrow in joint fluid: a clue to fracture. *Annals of Internal Medicine* **74**, 740–2.

McCarty, D.J. (1975). Diagnostic mimicry in arthritis: patterns of joint involvement associated with calcium pyrophosphate dihydrate crystal deposits. *Bulletin on the Rheumatic Diseases* **25**, 804–9.

McCarty, D.J. (1976). Calcium pyrophosphate dihydrate crystal deposition disease—1975. *Arthritis and Rheumatism* **19**, 275–86.

McCarty, D.J., Kohn, N.N., and Faires, J.S. (1962). The significance of calcium phosphate crystals in the synovial fluid of arthritis patients: the 'pseudogout syndrome' I. Clinical aspects. *Annals of Internal Medicine* **56**, 711–37.

McKnight, K.M. and Agudelo, C. (1991). Comment on the article by Kerolus et al. *Arthritis and Rheumatism* **34**, 118.

Nordstrom, D., Konttinen, Y.T., Bergroth, V., and Leirisalo-Repo, M. (1985). Synovial fluid cells in Reiter's syndrome. *Annals of the Rheumatic Diseases* **44**, 852–6.

Owen D.S., Jr. (1978). Synovial fluid glucose. *Journal of the American Medical Association* **239**, 193.

Pascual, E. (1991). Persistence of monosodium urate crystals and low-grade inflammation in the synovial fluid of patients with untreated gout. *Arthritis and Rheumatism* **34**, 141–5.

Pekin, T.J., Malinin, T.I., and Zvaifler, N.J. (1967). Unusual synovial fluid findings in Reiter's syndrome. *Annals of Internal Medicine* **66**, 677–84.

Punzi, L., Ramonda, R., Glorioso, S., and Schiavon, F. (1992). Predictive value of synovial fluid analysis in juvenile chronic arthritis. *Annals of the Rheumatic Diseases* **51**, 522–4.

Reginato, A.J., Feldman, E., and Rabinowitz, J.I. (1985). Traumatic chylous knee effusion. *Annals of the Rheumatic Diseases* **44**, 793–7.

Reginato, A.J. et al. (1986). Arthropathy and cutaneous calcinosis in hemodialysis oxalosis. *Arthritis and Rheumatism* **29**, 1387–96.

Rodnan, G.P., Eisenbeis C.H., Jr., and Creighton, A.S. (1963). The occurrence of rheumatoid factor in synovial fluid. *American Journal of Medicine* **35**, 182–8.

Rouault, T., Caldwell, D.S., and Holmes, E.W. (1982). Aspiration of the asymptomatic metatarsalphalangeal joint in gout patients with hyperuricemic controls. *Arthritis and Rheumatism* **25**, 209–12.

Schumacher, H.R. (1986). Reproducibility of synovial fluid analysis. *Arthritis and Rheumatism* **29**, 770–4.

Shmerling, R.H., Delbanco, T.L., Tosteson, A.N., and Trentham, D.E. (1990). Synovial fluid tests, what should be ordered. *Journal of the American Medical Association* **264**, 1009–14.

Simkin, P.A. (1991). Physiology and pathophysiology. In *A Practical Handbook of Joint Fluid Analysis* 2nd edn. (ed. R.A. Gattar and H.R. Schumacher), pp. 8–23. Philadelphia: Lea and Febiger.

Simkin, P.A., Campbell, P.M., and Larson, E.B. (1983). Gout in Heberden's nodes. *Arthritis and Rheumatism* **26**, 94–7.

Talbot, J.H., Altman, R.D., and Yu, T. (1978). Gouty arthritis masquerading as rheumatoid arthritis or vice versa. *Seminars in Arthritis and Rheumatism* **8**, 77–113.

Thomas, R. and Carroll, G.J. (1993). Reduction of leukocyte and interleukin-1B concentrations in the synovial fluid of rheumatoid arthritis patients treated with methotrexate. *Arthritis and Rheumatism* **36**, 1244–52.

Wallace, S.L., Robinson, H., Masi, A.T., Decker, J.L., McCarty, D.J., and Yu, T. (1977). Preliminary criteria for the classification of the acute arthritis of primary gout. *Arthritis and Rheumatism* **20**, 895–900.

Ytterberg, S.R. (1993). Viral arthritis. In *Arthritis and Allied Conditions: A Textbook of Rheumatology* 12th edn. (ed. D.J. McCarty and W.J. Koopman), pp. 2047–65. Philadelphia: Lea and Febiger.

5.6 Imaging

5.6.1 Imaging in adults

Peter Renton and Philip G. Conaghan*

Introduction

This chapter provides a general overview of techniques currently available for the imaging of the musculoskeletal system. It also provides an overview of appropriate investigations for both specific anatomical sites and common musculoskeletal conditions. Details on individual diseases will be described in the appropriate sections.

Radiology has undergone a major technological revolution in the last 20 years and a wide range of imaging methods is now available. Rapid advances in hardware and software continue to change the applications of these tools. These technologies vary in terms of their usefulness, expense, and availability; optimal use of these investigations will result from radiologists and clinicians working together to tailor tests to individual patient needs.

Plain radiography

Conventional radiography is available generally and is usually the first imaging technique used. Changes in film and X-ray technology have occurred in recent years with faster films, rapid automatic processing, the use of rare earth screens, and ultimately the move away from analog to digital imaging. This has not necessarily meant an improvement in image quality but a lower radiation dose.

Plain film images of bones and joints are usually obtained in two planes. For many joints, for example, the knee, this will mean at least an anteroposterior and lateral radiograph; for some joints, however, an oblique view is necessary, for example, at the hip, as the lateral view of the pelvis superimposes the two hip joints.

Plain film imaging of soft tissues

Soft tissue swelling is an unfailing indicator of underlying musculoskeletal disease. It follows that images must be correctly exposed for both bone and soft tissue. Digital imaging allows operator control of these factors. Soft tissue swelling is seen as an increase in width over involved bones or joints, that is, over the ulnar styloid (Fig. 1) or over the 5th or 1st metatarsal head. The thickened soft tissues are also radiologically denser and, therefore, the involved area looks 'greyer' and the underlying bone detail is less well seen, as it is 'filtered' by the soft tissue thickening. Comparison can be made with an unaffected or normal joint.

Filling in of web spaces in between fingers, which become convex rather than concave, or similar soft tissue swelling over metatarsal heads projecting over basal phalanges may be seen. Fat planes overlie joints and separate muscle bundles. Displacement of fat planes is an indicator of muscle thickening,

* It is with regret that we must report the death of Peter Renton during the preparation of this Textbook.

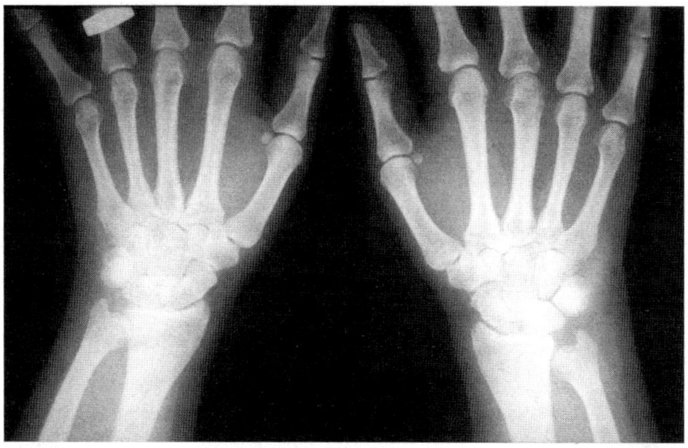

Fig. 1 Rheumatoid arthritis. Soft tissue swelling over the right ulnar styloid.

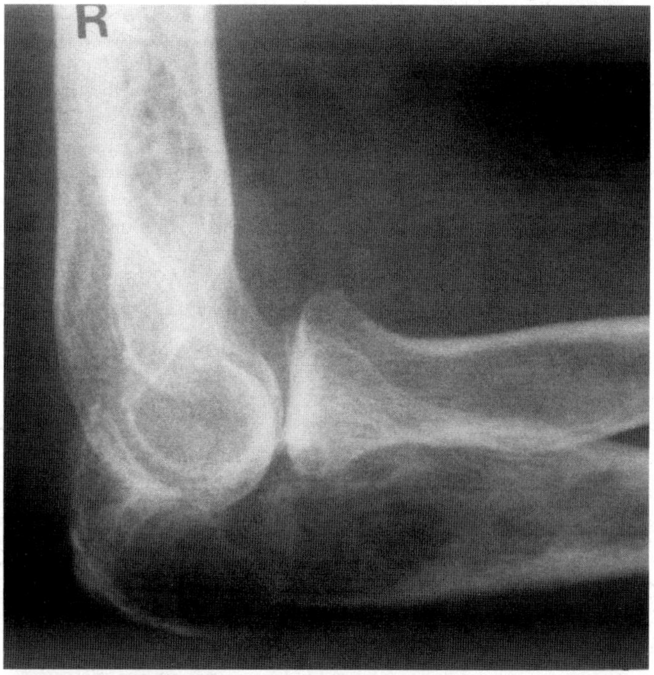

Fig. 2 Rheumatoid arthritis. Pathological fracture through a large cyst is associated with elevation of the anterior fat pad (sail sign).

oedema, or haemorrhage or, conversely, muscle atrophy. Joint effusions also displace overlying fat lines (Fig. 2).

Plain film changes with soft tissue thickening and fat plane displacement

Skull

These changes occur following trauma, over fractures, and at sites of foreign bodies. It may be found in the paranasal air sinuses with trauma, infection, or tumour.

Cervical spine

On a lateral view of the cervical spine, the retropharyngeal soft tissues are applied closely to the anterior aspect of the upper four cervical vertebral bodies. Below C4, the tracheal translucency is situated around 1 cm anterior to the cervical spine. Air is seen occasionally in the oesophagus, and an anterior cervical fat stripe may also be present. Soft tissue thickening following infection, trauma, or malignancy is demonstrated by displacement of the air shadows (Fig. 3).

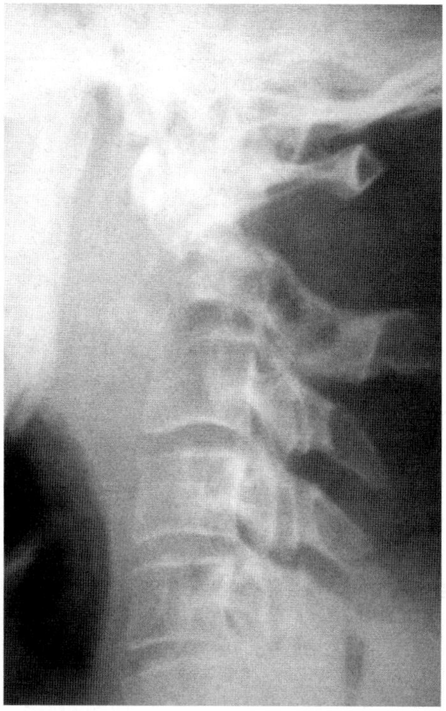

Fig. 3 Pathological collapse of the body of C2 with an associated large anterior soft tissue mass. The destructive lesion in this 27-year-old male was a chordoma.

Thoracic spine

In the thoracic region, soft tissues closely approximate to the vertebral bodies and are well demonstrated on a correctly exposed anteroposterior view. These are best seen on the left, are mainly pleural, and are separate from the descending aorta. These paraspinal lines are displaced by osteophytes and syndesmophytes but especially by bleeding in malignancy, trauma, infection, etc. Generally, the widest point of the soft tissue swelling lies at the site of maximal skeletal change (Fig. 4).

Lumbar spine

In the lumbar region the spine is not surrounded by air, but by soft tissues. Nonetheless, masses can still be assessed by inspection of the psoas and its overlying fat plane on an anteroposterior view, and by displacement of gut gas shadows on the lateral view. Similarly, sacral disease displaces the rectal gas shadow.

Shoulder

The axillary recess of the joint can be assessed on a plain radiograph and effusion diagnosed. Similarly, a large subdeltoid bursal effusion or, conversely, deltoid atrophy may also be assessed (Fig. 5).

Elbow

Anterior and posterior fat pads lie on the synovium and are usually just visible on the lateral radiograph. This is taken with the arm in the flexed position. Under these circumstances, the posterior fat pad is pressed inwards by the triceps tendon while the anterior capsule and fat pad are redundant. Effusions elevate the anterior fat pad more easily, therefore, than the posterior (Fig. 2). A 'sail' sign results, and is suggestive of a fracture

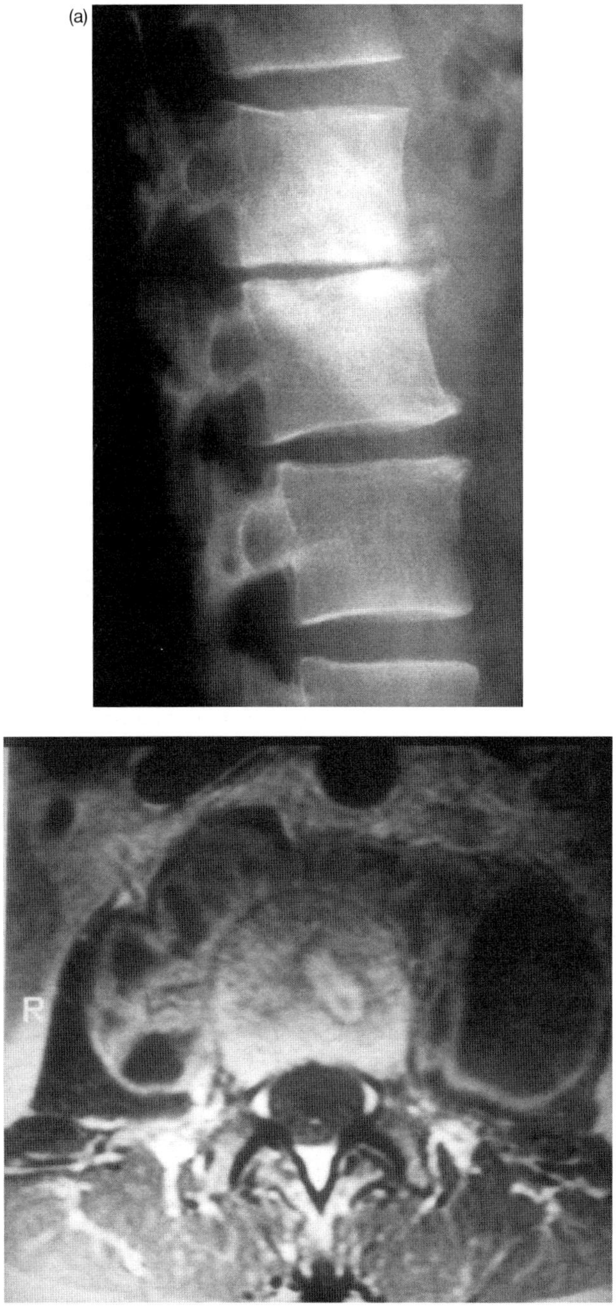

Fig. 4 Paraspinal soft tissue mass in spinal tuberculosis. (a) The radiograph demonstrates narrowing of an upper lumbar disc space with reversal of the curve. There is destruction of the adjacent end-plates with reactive new bone formation anteriorly, and a soft tissue mass is demonstrated anterior to the affected disc. (b) The axial MR images demonstrate not only the erosive destruction of the vertebral body but also psoas abscesses. The images are obtained after intravenous gadolinium and show both areas of enhancement and necrosis in the psoas muscles as well as anteriorly in the retroaortic tissues.

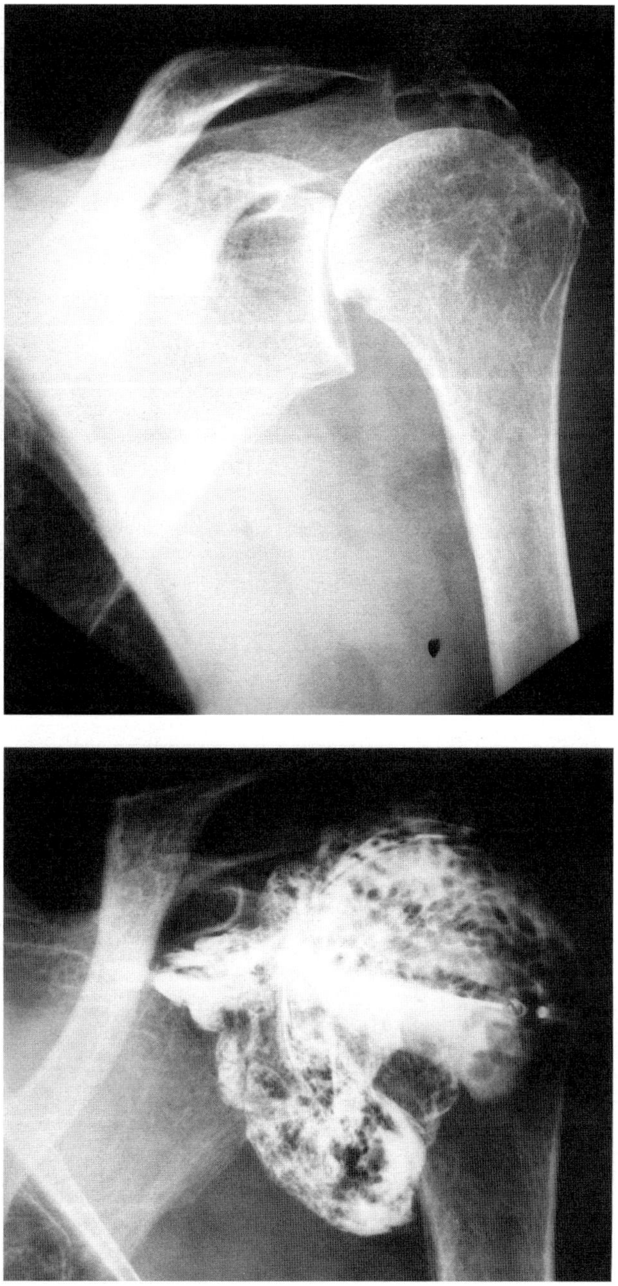

Fig. 5 Rheumatoid arthritis with a large effusion which can be seen on the plain film. (a) Upward subluxation of the humeral head is associated with marginal erosions, as well as erosion of the under surface of the acromion. The displaced fat plane beneath the glenoid and humeral head is seen on the subsequent arthrogram to represent the margin of the distended capsule. (b) A rotator cuff tear is demonstrated at arthrography with filling of the subacromial bursa. The distended joint capsule is demonstrated, especially inferiorly. Numerous loose bodies lie within the joint space. These may represent areas of synovial proliferation or osteochondral fragments but, in the main, represent fibrinous loose bodies.

given a history of trauma, especially if the posterior fat plane is elevated; this only happens with larger quantities of fluid.

Wrist

There are numerous bursae and tendons around the wrist and soft tissue swelling may occur at many sites (Fig. 1). These should be sought especially over the radial and ulnar styloids and laterally. Pronator quadratus muscle lies on the palmar aspect of the distal radius and ulna, and a fat plane lies on it. Trauma to the distal radius or ulna elevates this fat pad, which assumes an abnormal convex palmar appearance (Fig. 6). Similarly, soft tissue swelling may be seen over interphalangeal joints, and especially at distal interphalangeal joints in cases of osteoarthritis, and over the dorsum of the carpus.

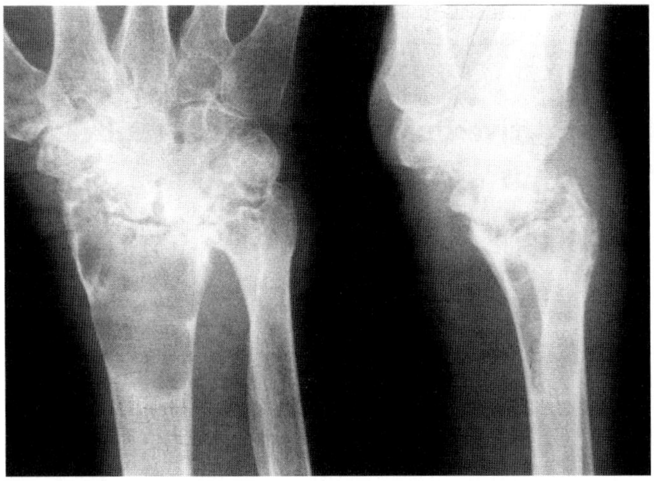

Fig. 6 Displacement of pronator quadratus. On the lateral view there is diffuse soft tissue swelling over the wrist in this patient with severe rheumatoid arthritis. The fat plane over pronator quadratus is displaced in a palmar direction over the large cyst in the distal radius.

Pelvis and hips

The acetabulum is difficult to visualize in a conventional anteroposterior film. For this reason, 45°-oblique views are needed to demonstrate the anterior and posterior pillars satisfactorily (Judet views). The obturator internus lies just inside the acetabulum and the fat line internal to it is seen as a thin stripe lying on, and parallel to, the iliopectineal line. Trauma to the acetabulum, malignant disease, or cortical bone destruction elevates the fat pad. Hip joint effusion also displaces two commonly seen fat pads round the medial and lateral aspects of the femoral neck.

Knee

The suprapatellar pouch is seen in the undistended state arising almost vertically from the patellofemoral joint space. It is a thin (2–3 mm) parallel-walled or rectangular structure surrounded by fat. With progressive distention, it enlarges to a lentiform shape of soft tissue density surrounded by fat.

Ankle

Both malleoli lie directly subcutaneously. Bony trauma causes soft tissue swelling more proximally than damage to the collateral ligaments, which is associated with swelling distally. Joint effusions are demonstrated on the lateral view. Anterior and posterior soft tissue masses project from the joint space and are seen as soft tissue densities, especially posteriorly where they project into the fatty triangle bounded by tendo-Achilles, calcaneus, and posterior tibia (Kager's triangle). Behind this triangle lies the Achilles tendon, which inserts into the posterior aspect of the calcaneus, some 2–3 mm beneath its upper angle. Between tendon and bone lies a small, normally non-visualized bursa. The tendon is some 6 mm thick at the insertion, and sharply defined anteriorly and posteriorly by overlying fat. In the presence of Achilles tendinitis or posterior calcaneal erosive disease, the distal tendon thickens and its insertion, being oedematous, becomes poorly defined. The retrocalcaneal bursa enlarges, first fills the space known as the retrocalcaneal recess, then further encroaches into Kager's triangle.

Foot

Changes at the metatarsal heads mirror those seen in the hands. Early on in an erosive arthritis, therefore, particular attention should be paid to the soft tissues over the metatarsal heads.

Arthrography

The injection of contrast into joints was in use for many years prior to the advent of image intensification. However, arthrography is now infrequently used alone due to the increasing use of magnetic resonance imaging (MRI). The major use of arthrography was in the knee, to demonstrate meniscal tears. In experienced hands, arthrography is as accurate as arthroscopy in the diagnosis of meniscal lesions and probably more accurate in the diagnosis of lesions of the posterior horn of the medial meniscus.

Arthrography has also been used for years in the shoulder: Lindblom (1939) performed shoulder arthrography using Myodil by a technique of direct injection. Arthrography is mainly used to diagnose rotator cuff tears and restrictive capsulitis—tasks for which the examination is admirably suited, being cheap, and quick (Fig. 5). Arthrography may also be used in the temporomandibular joint to display the meniscus and in the wrist to assess the triangular cartilage.

Computed tomography scanning

This technique uses X-rays to obtain axial images of the body in serial slices (tomography). As the attenuated beam, having passed through the patient is detected and analysed by computer, a much wider grey scale is available on the computer-based reconstructions than on X-ray film.

Axial tomography not only enables spatial relationships to be obtained in the sagittal and coronal planes simultaneously, but also allows densities to be assessed visually and also directly from the computer, measured in Hounsfield units. Enhancement with intravenous water-soluble iodine-based contrast media further opacifies vascular tissues, enhancing their intrinsic differences, especially vascular tumours and infections. Computed tomography (CT) can differentiate between fat (which shows low attenuation) serous fluid, and blood, and between muscle and cortical and medullary bone.

Radionuclide scanning

Until the advent of MRI, isotope scanning was the most accurate method of demonstrating the presence of pathological change in bones and joints (Fig. 7). Technetium-99m phosphate images demonstrate increased blood flow to inflamed synovium in the early or vascular phase of the scan and, on delayed images obtained 3 h after injection, increased uptake is demonstrated at sites of increased bone turnover due to isotope deposition on hydroxyapatite crystals.

Radioisotope scanning is an invasive technique with good sensitivity but poor specificity for individual diseases. Radioisotope scanning may be more sensitive than clinical examination for detecting inflamed joints. Early and persistently positive scans are a good prognosticator for subsequent erosive change, but chronic inactive erosions may often be negative at phosphate scanning (Rosenthall 1991). Spatial discrimination has been improved by use of single photon emission computed tomography (SPECT) imaging. The various arthropathies can only be distinguished by the distribution of the abnormal foci of increase in uptake.

An exciting new development aimed at increasing the specificity of radionuclide scanning in the diagnosis of inflammatory arthritis has been the linking of technetium-99m to a monoclonal antibody which reacts with the endothelial activation molecule E-selectin (Jamar et al. 2002). Such *radiolabelled monoclonal antibodies* may provide new tools for both diagnosis and assessment of disease severity.

Measurement of bone density

Screening for osteoporosis in post-menopausal women and inflammatory arthritis patients represents a huge task and requires non-invasive technology. Care must be taken in choosing techniques as the agreement between methods may be poor (Grampp et al. 1997). In general, imaging at a particular site

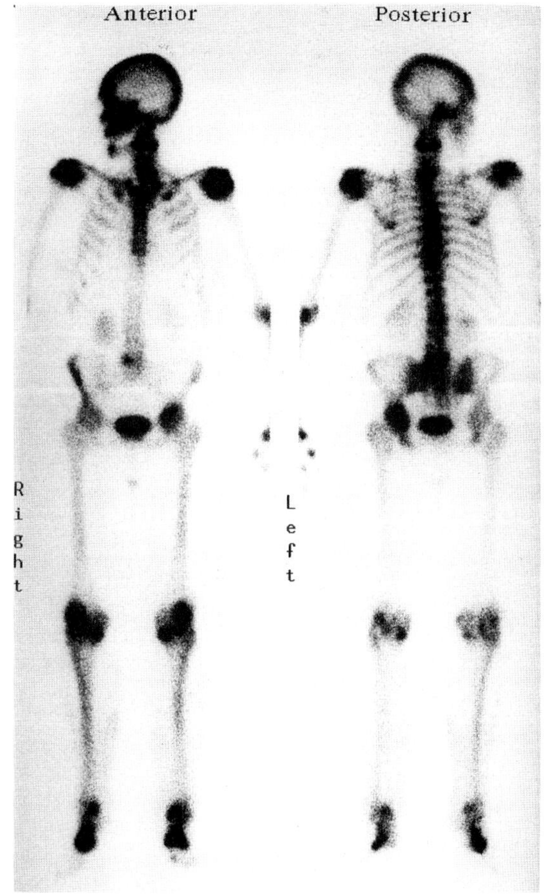

Fig. 7 Rheumatoid arthritis. Radioisotope bone scan showing increase in uptake in both shoulder joints, the left hip, both knees, and the hindfeet. (By courtesy of Dr A. Hilson, Royal Free Hospital.)

(e.g. spine) provides the best risk for fracture at that site. There may also be a poor correlation between bone mineralization in the axial and appendicular skeleton due to local factors such as osteoarthritis.

Up to 50 per cent of bone mineral in a given area must be lost before being radiologically visible on plain films. Subjectivity results in observer variation. Early methods for assessing bone density included photographic densitometry, an aluminium wedge being included on the film, or a cadaver metacarpal matched for age and sex. Images of the hand can also be used to measure cortical thickness in the metacarpal, and resorption of the cortex gives an indication of demineralization. Photon absorptiometry uses a single source of photon energy through the radius or calcaneus, and absorption of the isotope by bone is compared with that in adjacent soft tissues. Dual photon densitometry utilizes photons of two energies from a single isotope (gadolinium-153). The results are independent of thickness of local soft tissues (whereas single photon absorptiometry requires a uniform thickness of soft tissue over the bony part being investigated). Radiation dose is relatively low and double photon absorptiometry is particularly accurate, with only 2–3 per cent error. Double photon absorptiometry enables both central and peripheral bone to be assessed. These two techniques have now largely been superseded by dual energy X-ray absorptiometry (DEXA).

Quantitative CT scanning can be used to assess bone density, especially in the spine, by comparing attenuation of single or dual energy CT beams with attenuation by phantoms, which may be scanned simultaneously or separately. This technique distinguishes cortical and trabecular bone, can give three-dimensional estimates of mineralization but involves relatively more irradiation than DEXA.

Quantitative dual energy radiography (X-ray absorptiometry; DEXA)

This is now the technique of choice as it is precise, scanning time is short, and radiation dose low. It uses an X-ray tube rather than an isotope as the source, which results in greater resolution and speed of investigation (Sartoris and Resnick 1990). The X-ray source provides a beam alternating between two energies. The beam is finely collimated and also passes through a disc containing attenuating materials, used as a reference. A ratio of attenuation is given. Accurate measurements are usually taken from the lumbar spine and proximal femur and results are usually expressed in terms of the number of standard deviations above or below the mean of an age-related control population (*Z*-score) or of a young healthy adult population (*T*-score) (Fig. 8).

Other bone density screening tools

Some other screening tools for osteoporosis are worth mentioning. Quantitative ultrasonography utilizes the principles of ultrasound described below and reflects structural properties and bone density (Fuerst et al. 1995). It has been used for screening at peripheral sites such as the hand and calcaneus. The early use of measurements from a plain radiograph have been mentioned, but the advent of digital radiographs and computerized image analysis has re-awoken interest in radiogrammetry (Rosholm et al. 2001). Radiogrammetry techniques differ and may, for example, measure combined cortical thickness or a metacarpal cortical index. The development of these tools is awaited with interest.

Ultrasonography

Diagnostic ultrasound utilizes sound frequencies above those audible to the human ear, that is, 20 000 cycles/s (Hertz). Frequencies in use clinically range from 2 to 10 MHz.

Ultrasound waves are generated by a piezoelectric crystal in the usually hand-held transducer, which both transmits the sound waves and receives back the resultant echoes. The returning signal impinges upon the crystal which converts the attenuated sound waves into electronic impulses, processed via a computer.

Images are displayed on a screen, film, or paper using a grey scale, or colour to show venous/arterial flow, or a combination of both. Real-time imaging allows dynamic continuous scanning of body parts. Linear images can be obtained in any plane of the body (Van Holsbeeck and Introcaso 1991).

Images obtained depend on the following:

1. The frequency of the ultrasound. The higher the frequency, the better is the resolution of the images, but the penetration of the body by sound waves is limited.
2. The nature of the tissues into which the sound waves must pass. Bone is totally refractory to sound waves (as is air) and so deep structures in joints are inaccessible. At the knee, therefore, the superficial ligaments and tendons are well imaged, as are the superficial parts of the menisci, but not the deep structures.
3. The angle of incidence of the beam. Sound waves pass through matter and the speed of sound in a tissue varies with the nature of the tissue, materials of the greatest density transmitting sound at the highest velocity. Sound is also reflected at tissue interfaces, while the amount of reflected sound also depends on the angle of incidence of the beam, the least reflection occurs with a beam which is at right angles to the

(ai)

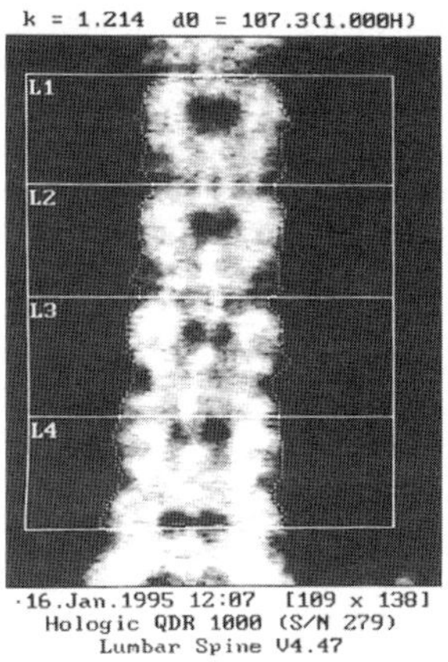

TOTAL BMD CV FOR L1-L4 1.0%

Region	Area (cm2)	BMC (gr)	BMD (g/cm)
C.F.	1.005	1.044	1.000
L1	13.06	12.46	0.954
L2	13.91	14.86	1.069
L3	15.86	17.12	1.079
L4	16.79	18.33	1.092
TOTAL	59.61	62.77	1.053

(bi)

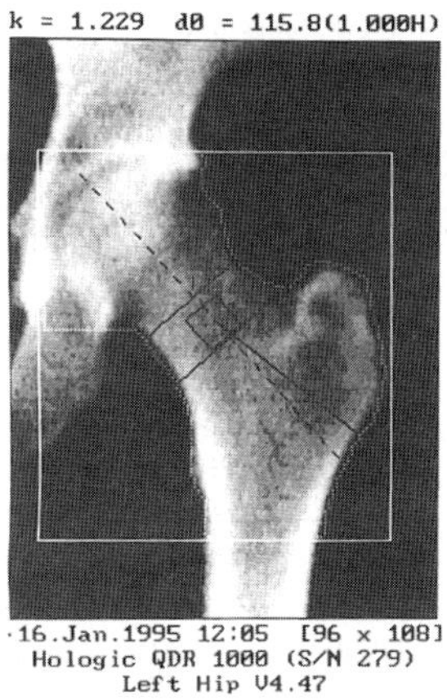

Region	Area (cm2)	BMC (gr)	BMD (g/cm2)
C.F.	1.005	1.044	1.000
Neck	5.53	3.95	0.715
Troch	12.62	8.86	0.702
Inter	17.36	18.05	1.040
TOTAL	35.51	30.86	0.869
Ward's	1.26	0.80	0.641

Midline (94,120)-(166, 40)
Neck -63 x 16 at [31, 9]
Troch 10 x 50 at [0, 0]
Ward's -11 x 11 at [5, 5]

(aii)

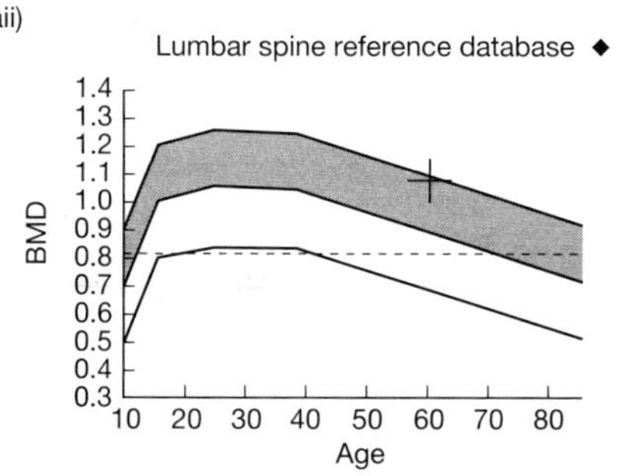

BMD (L1–L4) = 1.053 g/cm²

Region	BMD	*T*(30.0)		*Z*	
L1	0.954	+0.27	103%	+1.56	122%
L2	1.069	+0.37	104%	+1.81	123%
L3	1.079	−0.04	100%	−1.47	118%
L4	1.092	−0.22	98%	−1.35	116%
L1–L4	1.053	+0.05	101%	+1.52	119%

◆ Age and sex matched
T = peak bone mass
Z = age matched
BMD = bone mass density

(bii)

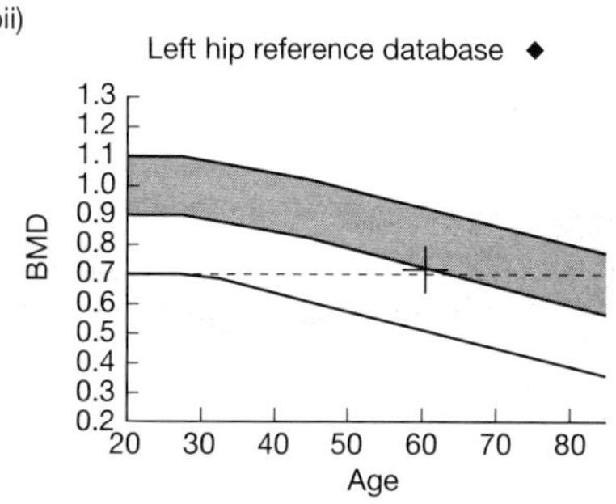

BMD (neck[L]) = 0.715 g/cm²

Region	BMD	*T*		*Z*	
Neck	0.715	−1.79 (22.0)	80%	−0.12	98%
Troch	0.702	−0.23 (30.0)	97%	+0.84	112%
Inter	1.040	−0.77 (29.0)	91%	+0.27	104%
Total	0.869	−0.88 (28.0)	89%	+0.22	103%
Ward's	0.641	−1.41 (20.0)	81%	+1.05	122%

◆ Age and sex matched
T = peak bone mass
Z = age matched
BMD = bone mass density

Fig. 8 DEXA scan of femur demonstrating that the patient's values lie on the predicted value for bone density at that age.

reflecting surface (Van Holsbeeck and Introcaso 1991). The returning pulses of sound characterize the tissues and tissue interfaces. A cyst is echo-free, calculi cast an acoustic shadow, and soft tissues show numerous interfaces, giving a complex but regular pattern if normal and a more irregular pattern in the presence of disease.

Ultrasound is thus used in:

1. joint disease to show effusions, intra-articular loose bodies or other structures, and the capsule and synovium;
2. surrounding ligaments and tendons;
3. muscle tears, haematomas, and tumours;
4. vascular lesions—arterial and venous flow using Doppler.

It is not primarily used in the diagnosis of bone disease although it can be used to visualize bone erosions in joints where it has access such as the metacarpophalangeal joints.

The shoulder region is thus much more amenable to ultrasound investigation than the knee, as the rotator cuff is more accessible to the ultrasonic waves (Plate 71).

Magnetic resonance imaging

MRI does not involve ionizing radiation, but utilizes the different biophysical properties of the various constituents of the body tissues, especially the number of hydrogen nuclei or protons in a given tissue. MR images reflect the distribution of these nuclei. Grey scale changes on film reflect the number of protons in a given tissue, and reflect their behaviour in the externally applied magnetic fields. These field strengths are generally between 0.5 and 1.5 T (Tesla), although newer magnets may have strengths up to 4 T. Such field strengths cause the hydrogen nuclei to precess or gyrate at frequencies in the range of radiowaves or radiofrequency (RF).

RF stimulation (i) excites protons and (ii) also brings them into phase with each other. Once the RF pulse is turned off, the system returns to normal. The protons return to a low energy state. A measure of the time taken for dephasing to occur is the T_2 (or transverse relaxation time) and the T_1 (or longitudinal relaxation time) is that taken for the protons to re-establish their equilibrium (Nixon 1987).

MRI has become the investigation of choice for the musculoskeletal system. It enables primary, not reformatted, images to be obtained in all planes and is non-invasive. Inherent differences in structure of the body tissues result in greater differences in grey-scale contrast than are obtainable by any other imaging technique.

In most cases, the sequences used are simple T_1- and T_2-weightings. In T_1-weighted images fat is bright, fluid is grey, and bone is black. With T_2-weighted images, fat is less bright, fluid is very bright, and bone is black. Signal is altered by disease, so that oedema, inflammation, or haemorrhage all cause local increase in signal. Cell death, however, decreases signal, as does calcification.

Fat suppression STIR (short tau inversion recovery) sequences cause the bright signal from fat to be suppressed completely. Muscle is therefore a more homogeneous grey (as the internal fat is black). Fat, and fatty marrow, is black. Fluid, however, remains very bright and so oedema, vascular tumours, fluid collections, and veins stand out clearly from the surrounding suppressed bone, muscle, and fat. Avascular and necrotic tissues are also black (i.e. of low signal) (Fig. 9).

MR scanning is not inevitably successful and may be stressful. The dark and noisy environment leads to a patient rejection rate of around 2 per cent and also to degradation of images due to patient movement. Modern scanners are more open in design, with small magnet peripheral scanners requiring only limb insertion and consequently better patient tolerance. Sedation is rarely necessary in adolescents and adults. Intravenous sedation needs to be performed in an environment where the patient can be monitored. Non-ferromagnetic anaesthetic and resuscitation equipment is not inevitably available.

Before scanning, the presence of ferromagnetic and electric implants should be excluded. Metallic implants cause artefacts due to signal void or, on occasion, marked hyperintensity. Ferromagnetic implants cause a greater artefact than non-ferromagnetic, and are seen as an irregular area of low signal in and around the implant. Non-ferromagnetic implants may be associated with signal void, which does not significantly impair image quality. Larger field strength magnets also cause a larger artefact. A low-signal artefact is due to both the presence of the metal itself and the surrounding effect on the magnetic field.

Pacemakers may be affected by the magnetic field and their presence creates image degradation. The pacemaker may move and pacemaker function may be interfered with. Current may be induced in leads sufficient to induce fibrillation or burns. Prosthetic heart valves are not generally a contraindication to MR scanning.

Ferromagnetic surgical clips can move in a magnetic field and their presence in a vulnerable situation, for example, at an aneurysm, is a contraindication to MR scanning. Similarly, cochlear implants may be ferromagnetic. Some cochlear implants are held in place by magnets; others may be electronically activated. MRI should not be performed on these patients. Copper IUCDs are not ferromagnetic and are safely included in a scan.

Skin and body temperature are not increased by MRI but conductive materials may be heated and currents induced in leads resulting in burns.

Patients should also be screened for the presence of metallic foreign bodies, such as shrapnel, pellets, or bullets. It is often not possible to say whether pellets, bullets, or shrapnel are ferromagnetic. Movement may cause damage to adjacent vital structures. Blindness may result if intraocular metal fragments are displaced by the magnetic field. Metal workers should have radiographs of the orbit performed prior to MRI (Berquist 1991).

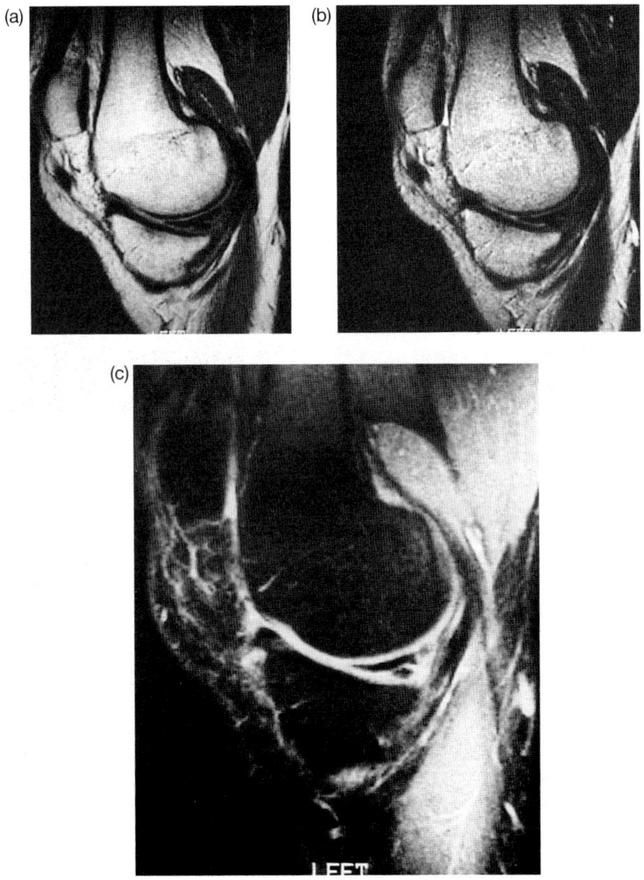

Fig. 9 Meniscal tears demonstrated with (a) T_1-, (b) T_2-, and (c) STIR weightings. The STIR weighting has the added advantage of graphically demonstrating cystic change or oedema in the adjacent bone much more clearly than the other modes.

Future imaging techniques

There are a number of new imaging techniques that remain research tools at present, but which may be used to image joint components especially the synovium. Scanning laser Doppler uses laser light in the near-infrared spectral range to generate a spatial perfusion map, and has been used to study inflammation in finger joints of rheumatoid arthritis (RA) patients (Ferrell et al. 2001). Positron emission tomography (PET) uses a radiotracer analogue of glucose, 18F-fluorodeoxyglucose, to detect those cells using an excess of glucose. Although PET scanning has largely been used to detect malignant tissues, there are preliminary reports on its ability to detect areas of inflammation in the hands of inflammatory arthritis patients (Yun et al. 2001). Information from such scans may be complimentary to the structural information gained from MRI scans.

Imaging the spine

Anatomy of the lumbar spine

The lumbar spine is lordotic, convex anteriorly. In part, this is because the lower lumbar vertebral bodies are greater in height anteriorly. At L5, the difference may be as much as 0.9 cm. At L1, however, the reverse is the case and the body of L1 may normally be wedged anteriorly. Similarly, the mid- and lower lumbar discs may be significantly thicker anteriorly (Farfan 1973).

Although it is often stated that the height of the L5/S1 disc is around 50 per cent of that at L4/5, in one small study 40 per cent of L5/S1 discs were thicker posteriorly that the L4/5 disc, and an even larger number showed the discs to be equal in height posteriorly.

With segmentation anomalies the intervening disc is rudimentary and diminished in height. Discs of smaller heights have diminished movement. The L5 disc may be high, that is, at or just below the level of the iliac crest, or deep, that is, much lower than the crest. Higher discs are said to be more vulnerable to degeneration. Disc degeneration in the lumbar spine has the highest incidence at the lumbosacral junction and the incidence decreases to be lowest at L1/2. If the lower lumbar disc is also sacralized, wholly or in part, that is, associated with large L5 transverse processes, that disc will be small, 'protected', and less likely to be diseased.

The transverse processes at L5 may be the bulkiest and unilaterally or bilaterally articulate with, or be totally or partially fused to, the sacrum in some 15–30 per cent. Large transverse processes at L5 thus protect the disc below, but seem to be associated with increased levels of degeneration at the level above, which is thus high, 'free', and potentially unstable.

The sacrum also contributes to the lordosis as its upper surface is angled distoanteriorly. The L3/4 disc is aligned horizontally. Loss of the lordosis is shown by reduction of the angle that the lumbosacral disc makes with the plane of the L3/4 disc. Also, in a normal spine, the anterior surfaces of the vertebral bodies are always tangential to each other, while in a spastic painful or degenerate and immobile segment, adjacent anterior vertebral surfaces are in alignment.

The transverse processes are seen on a lateral view of the spine along a line drawn from the L1 transverse process to the anterior surface of the femoral head. On the anteroposterior film, the transverse processes differ in size and shape. The transverse process at L3 is often the most lateral and its inferior surface often the lowest to be inclined horizontally.

The facet joints

The facet joints in the lumbar spine vary in their orientation. At L1, the facet joints have an almost vertical orientation but, passing inferiorly, change direction so that at L5/S1 the superior facet faces superiorly, medially, and posteriorly. Facets are generally symmetrically orientated. The angle of the facets to the midline is around 52° at the L5/S1 joint, and 10° less at L4/5. Facet asymmetry is also greatest at L5/S1. A high correlation has been reported between the side of increased facet rotation and disc protrusion with sciatica (Farfan 1973).

Facetal changes of osteoarthritis follow discal height loss. These changes are seen on plain films, especially with oblique views, and very well demonstrated at CT scanning, where bony hypertrophy and synovial thickening are seen to narrow the lateral recess and exit foramina (Fig. 10). Yellow ligament thickening is seen at axial imaging to indent the theca from behind, and posterolaterally.

Plain film demonstration of disc narrowing, facet slip and rotation, foraminal encroachment, and marginal new bone formation are all indicative of established discal degeneration.

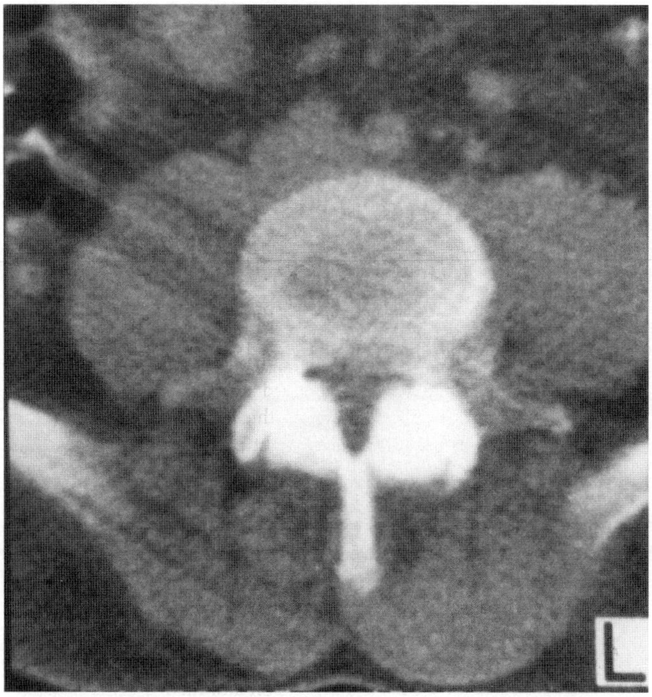

Fig. 10 A rather old scan, but a good example of facet hypertrophy causing lateral recess stenosis and a trefoil deformity.

Scoliosis associated with vertebral asymmetry is seen commonly on routine chest radiographs and occurs in up to 13 per cent of spines. It has been stated that these curves are due to primary vertebral asymmetry with a diminished body height on the concavity, as well as shorter pedicles and a flatter neural arch.

Pain sources in the spine

Pain may arise: (i) in the motion segment and surrounding structures, comprising the discal nucleus and annulus, vertebral end-plates, and the two local facet joints, as well as surrounding ligaments and muscles; (ii) in the superficial structures around the spinous processes; and (iii) referred from spinal nerves and the sympathetic chain. Pain may arise in isolation but, because all three areas are interdependent, a complex pain pattern may result (O'Brien 1984).

The disc is the largest structure in the motion segment. The nucleus and inner annulus have no innervation but the outer annulus has a rich multilevel sensory nerve supply. Similarly, the vertebral body has a rich sensory nerve supply.

The emerging nerve root occupies about 50 per cent of the exit foramen and so is compromised easily by changes in the local bone and soft tissue. The dura around the nerve is itself innervated anteriorly, but not posteriorly. The capsule of the facet joint (but not the synovium) has a three-level innervation. It is also likely that each anatomic level of the anterior and posterior longitudinal ligaments derive their innervation from the level above.

Patterns of spinal and referred pain are complicated because of the overlap of innervation (Plate 72). Pain fibres are also present in the sympathetic chain which lies in close contact with the spine, and they too are affected by local disease, bony osteophytes, and lesions of the annulus (Fig. 11).

At least 50 per cent of the population suffers from back pain at some time. Abnormal anatomy predisposes to abnormal stresses on the disc. Discal degeneration is an inevitable fact of life; no spine remains unaffected.

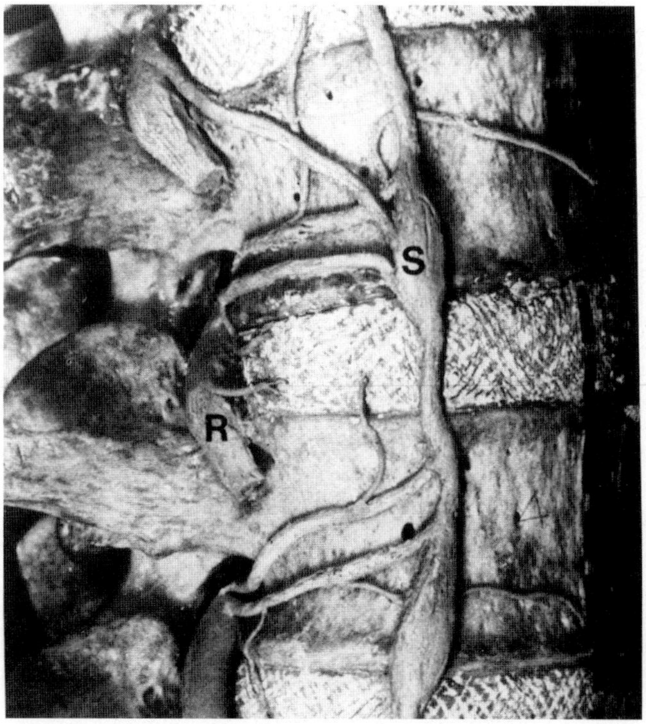

Fig. 11 Superficial view of lumbar spine demonstrating the nerve supply of the disc. Note the close proximity of the sympathetic chain to the disc and vertebral margin and also the communication between the nerve root and sympathetic chain just above the level of the disc. R, nerve root; S, sympathetic trunk. (Reproduced from *Textbook of Pain*, by courtesy of Mr J.P. O'Brien FRCS and Churchill Livingstone.)

Discal narrowing causes alteration of facet alignment and subsequent degeneration. Exit foraminal encroachment by soft tissue and osteophytes compromise the emerging nerve roots.

Pathology in the disc

Many disc protrusions regress spontaneously with time and conservative therapy (Cowan et al. 1992). Diagnosis of degeneration based solely on MR or CT criteria often does not address the cause of pain and, indeed, inappropriate surgery may worsen the patient's condition.

Posterior annular circumferential fissures start to form in the lower lumbar spine as early as puberty (Fig. 12). Subsequently, the nucleus starts to dehydrate and radial tears occur, perhaps related to the orientation of facets.

Forces acting on the nucleus can cause both nuclear protrusion and annular fissuring, as well as end-plate fractures (Fig. 13); not to be confused with Schmorl's nodes, which are nuclear herniations through corticated defects in the end-plates which had transmitted blood vessels in infancy (Fig. 14).

Osteophyte formation

Osteophytes are seen at vertebral marginal edges and so-called traction spurs are seen some 2–3 mm away from the vertebral margin. These are intimately related to, and are usually indicative of, local annular tears (Fig. 15). Traction spurs may be related to change in the more superficial layers of the annulus and adjacent anterior longitudinal ligament.

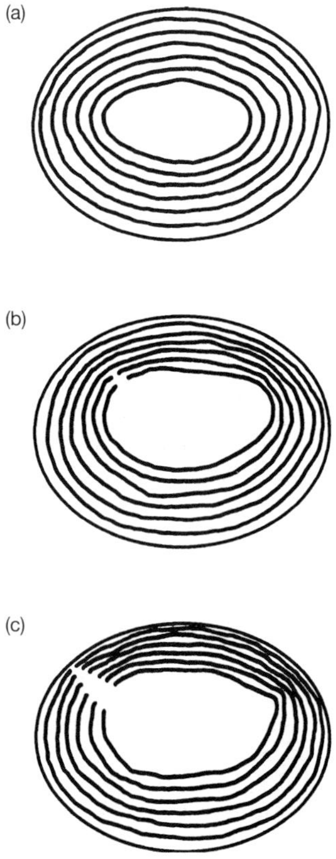

Fig. 12 Formation of radial fissure: (a) concentric laminae of equal number at all points around the circumference; (b) some of the inner lamellations become discontinuous and the clefts in the annulus become larger; and (c) the annular clefts and the tears of the minor annular layers continue to form a radial fissure. (Reproduced from Farfan, H.F. (1993), *Mechanical Disorders of the Low Back*, by courtesy of Lea and Febiger.)

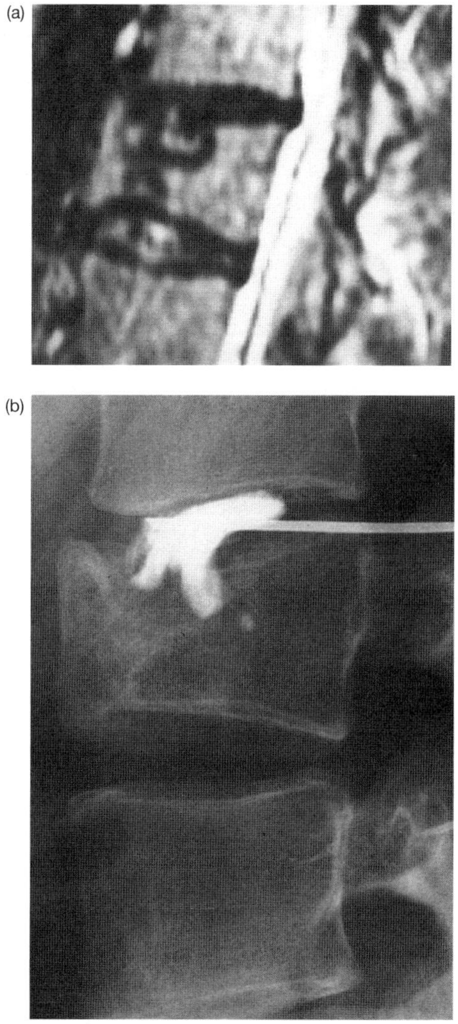

Fig. 13 End-plate fracture. (a) Defects are demonstrated on the upper surface of a lumbar vertebral body with depression of the cortex at MR scanning together with some loss of signal in the local disc. (b) At discography the defects are shown to fill with contrast injected into the nucleus.

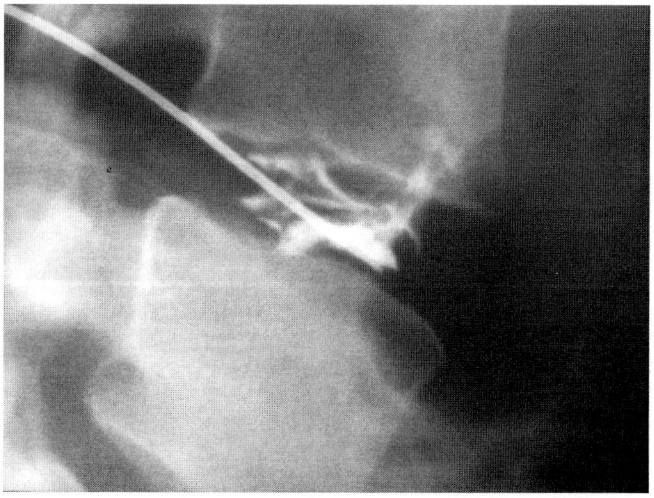

Fig. 14 Schmorl's node. At discography defects around the injected disc are demonstrated at the upper and lower end-plates.

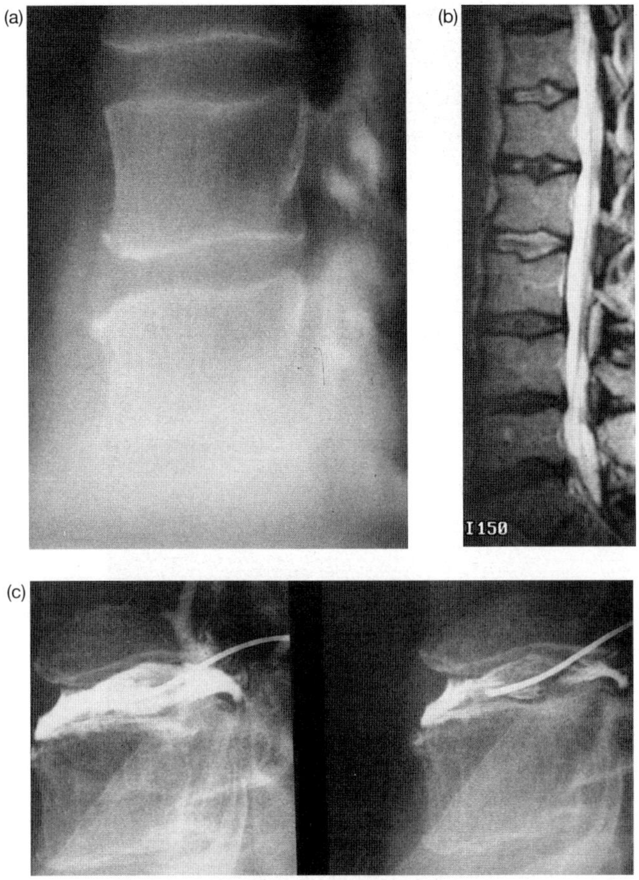

Fig. 15 Disc degeneration. (a) Plain tomography showing disc narrowing and anterior osteophytes. (b) MRI showing disc degeneration especially at L4/5. (c) Anterior and posterior annular tears at discography. Note vascular filling, presumably the result of superficial inflammation. Anteriorly, the contrast in the tear creeps over a traction spur on the superior surface of the lower end-plate at that disc level.

Radiological investigation of low back pain

Griffiths (1991) has recommended simple anteroposterior and lateral views as adequate for the first examination for the general practitioner or accident and emergency department, while the specialist may require further views. Lateral views in flexion can be used to demonstrate loss of movement in both the cervical and lumbar regions.

Plain radiography

The plain film of the spine is rapidly obtained and can provide information on alignment, disc height, disc pathology (indicated by erosions, osteophytes, or traction spurs). Rotational abnormalities can be assessed in both planes, together with an assessment of bony density. End-plate density is lost with infection and increased with degeneration and instability. However, up to 50 per cent of bone must be resorbed before foci of demineralization can be seen on the film. Marrow changes are thus better seen with isotope and MR scanning.

Myelography and radiculography

These procedures are rarely performed now with the increasing use of MRI. Intrathecal negative-contrast investigation of the spinal canal using air was first performed in 1921 and this was followed by the use of positive-contrast iodinated oil (Lipiodol/Myodil) in 1922. The bulging disc protrudes into the canal and causes a filling defect to be seen in the contrast. Oily media cause arachnoiditis and theoretically should have been removed after the study but, in practical terms, this was not always possible. Even though Myodil is very slowly absorbed naturally, remnants may be seen in the canal after many years. Using modern non-ionic media and fine non-bevelled needles, the incidence of meningism and other complications are lessened, but postlumbar-puncture headaches still occur, though these can be minimized if the patient is well hydrated and given prophylactic corticosteroids. Unfortunately, only the areas reached by contrast can be investigated, that is, the nerves are shown as far as the tip of the root sheaths.

CT scanning

Axial scanning using CT added a new dimension to the conventional water-soluble contrast study. Delayed CT scanning allows total mixing of the contrast with cerebrospinal fluid. CT on its own demonstrates bone detail well and, in the axial mode, the discs, facets, lateral recesses, and pedicles are all clearly seen together with their relationships to theca and roots, even in the absence of intravenous contrast, so that CT alone has been used as a screening test, as a non-invasive study with no side-effects (other than those of a cumulative irradiation dose). If sufficient fine contiguous slices are obtained, reformatting allows visualization in any plane.

The examination is limited in extent by time, cost, and radiation exposure, so that a standard examination of the lumbar spine is usually only of the L3/S1 motion segments, and plain films are still needed to show higher levels, but most significant degenerative disease of the spine is below L4. The combination of CT and radiculography may give better appreciation of the soft tissue interfaces, especially between disc, root, and theca, while at the same examination, the lateral recesses, facets, and yellow ligaments are better imaged than at radiculography.

MRI of the spine

MRI of the spine is non-invasive and tomographic and has now largely replaced CT and radiculography. Metal implants in the spine sometimes contraindicate MRI but this technique can still be used to assess change in discs above, for instance, a fused level. In the post-operative spine, enhancement by gadolinium occurs with recurrent disc protrusions, but fibrotic masses do not enhance as they are relatively water-free. It is important to correlate symptoms with pathology as disc protrusion imaged at a particular level may not be the cause of the patient's pain—many such discs are asymptomatic (Jensen et al. 1994).

In MR scanning, bony changes are not as well demonstrated as at CT, though the low signal of cortical bone is shown. The disc height may be diminished, and nuclear signal decreased on T_2-weighted images. Disc protrusions, both posterior and anterior, are seen, especially against bright cerebrospinal fluid on T_2-weighted images (Fig. 16), and the displaced low-signal posterior longitudinal ligament on T_1-weighting.

Sagittal slices through the pedicles demonstrate the emerging nerve roots in exit foramina and show them against bright fat when normal, or impinged upon by soft tissue or bony masses. Axial scans confirm these changes.

Discography

This procedure has again been largely superseded by MRI. Discography provides an image of disc anatomy and pathology. It may aid the diagnosis and demonstrate pathology not shown by any other method. Controversially, discal injection may also be used to reproduce the patient's pain or to exclude that disc level as a pain source. However, MRI demonstrates spinal anatomy and pathology more clearly, as (i) extradiscal structures are also displayed; (ii) the entire cervical, thoracic, or lumbar spine is imaged in one study; and (iii) the technique is non-invasive, and without the risks of discitis or anaphylaxis at discography.

A painful disc can be associated with a normal MRI scan. Radial or circumferential tears of the disc or end-plate fractures may all be associated with pain in the presence of normal plain films, radiculograms, CT, and

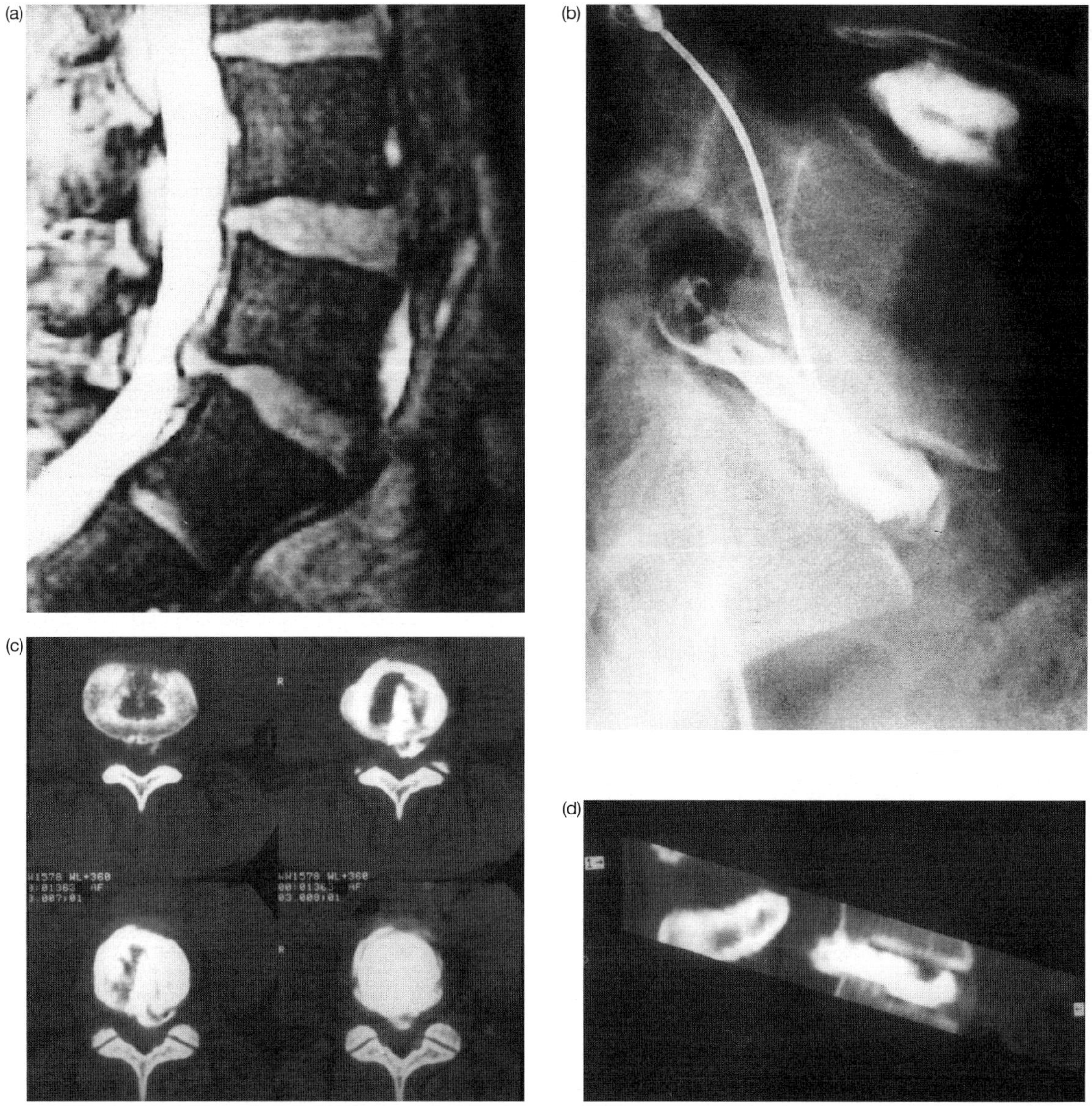

Fig. 16 Disc prolapse. (a) MR scan, T_2-weighted image. There is dorsal protrusion of a disc impinging upon the theca and narrowing the sagittal diameter of the canal. (b) The discogram demonstrates this lesion, showing a posterior annular tear with partial opacification of the bulge. A normal disc is demonstrated at the L4/5 level. (c) CT scanning following this study shows the degenerate disc with the central and left-sided protrusion. Sagittal reconstructions are also obtained (d).

MR scans (it will be remembered that the outer fibres of the annulus are innervated) (Collins et al. 1990). A partial radial tear need not be associated with MR change and this tear antedates rather than follows degenerative change. The normal and abnormal patterns demonstrated at discography are represented in Fig. 17. A plain film is an essential adjunct to discography. Experience with discography leads to the realization that even so-called minor abnormalities on the plain film may be associated with discal pathology and pain. Spurs in particular, however small, can be associated with painful radial tears and do indicate underlying disc disease, as does loss of lordosis and minor malalignment on a lateral view, especially even minimal retrolisthesis of L5 on S1 (Fig. 18).

Imaging and the spondyloarthritides

New bone formation around the spine occurs in ankylosing spondylitis as well as in the other seronegative spondyloarthritides. In ankylosing spondylitis, the changes may occur first at the thoracolumbar junction and spread in both directions. The new bone, or syndesmophyte, is usually vertically aligned in the annulus, gracile, and vertebromarginal (Fig. 19). This change follows the demonstration of vertebromarginal erosions which may be sclerotic and can give an impression of vertebral 'squaring' (Fig. 20). Non-marginal and floating syndesmophytes also occur in ankylosing spondylitis, but seem more common in the other seronegative spondyloarthropathies (Fig. 21).

In the cervical spine, change occurs from C2 down, in continuity, and cervical spondyloarthritis may be the presenting symptom in juvenile chronic arthritis and ankylosing spondylitis.

Ankylosing spondylitis

Paradiscal ossification in ankylosing spondylitis arises when the patient is relatively young, that is, before discal degeneration. Disc heights are often then well-preserved, even in the elderly. On the lateral view of the spine in ankylosing spondylitis, the disc shows increased density, partly because of

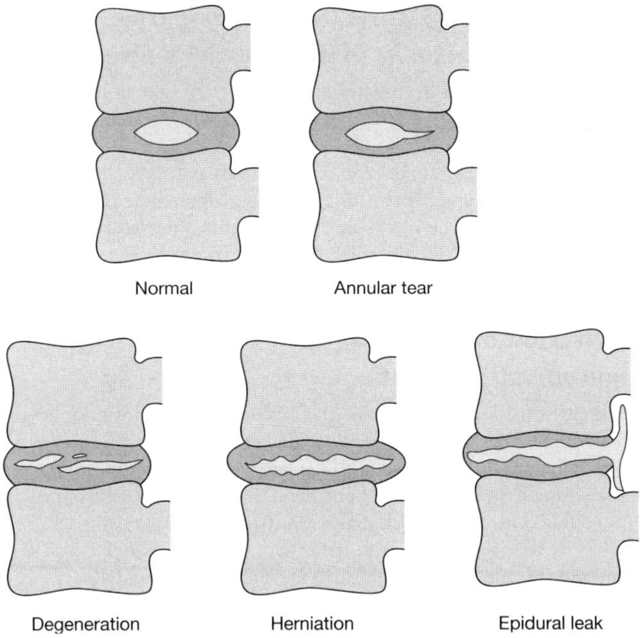

Fig. 17 Diagramatic representation of the progression of discal degeneration, starting with an annular tear.

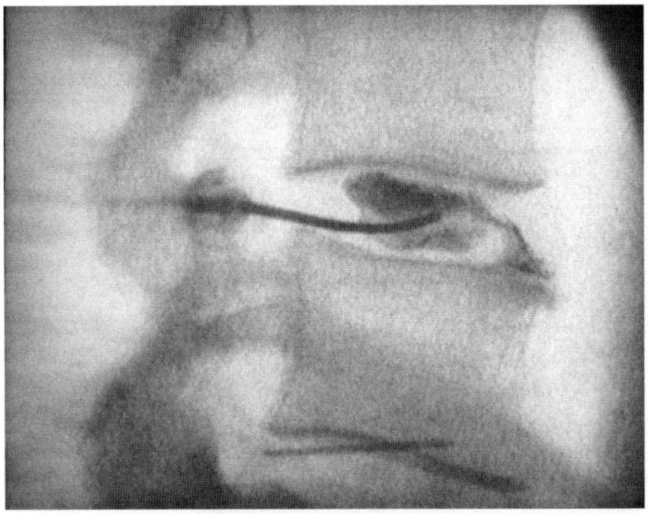

Fig. 18 An annular tear is associated with, and leads to, the spur on the subjacent end-plate anteriorly. The spur is the site of considerable reactive bone sclerosis. The disc is otherwise normal.

marginal new bone, but also because of discal nuclear calcification. This is seen as an added central density and occurs in other situations where there is bony fusion across discs (Fig. 22).

The earliest changes in the spine in this disease are best recognized with MRI. This demonstrates bone oedema (especially visible using T_2-weighted or fat-suppressed images) at the anterior corners of the vertebral bodies (Fig. 23). It seems likely that these changes precede bony erosion and vertebral 'squaring'. This bone oedema may be reversible with modern therapies (Brandt et al. 2000). Involvement of the sacroiliac joints in ankylosing spondylitis is discussed below.

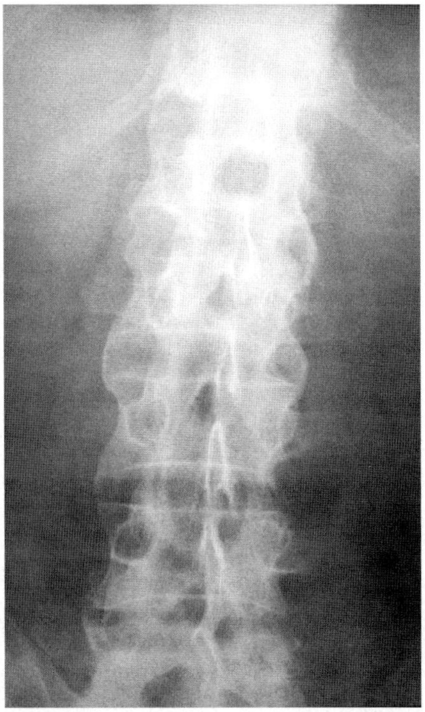

Fig. 19 Ankylosing spondylitis. Gracile, vertically orientated new bone runs between adjacent vertebral body margins.

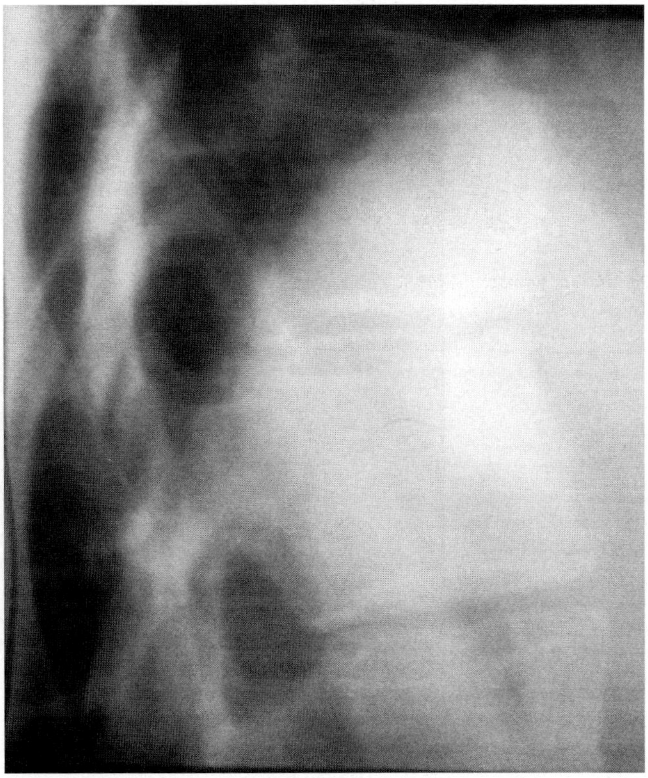

Fig. 20 Ankylosing spondylitis. Vertebral squaring results from margin erosion and also new bone laid down on the anterior concavity of the vertebral body.

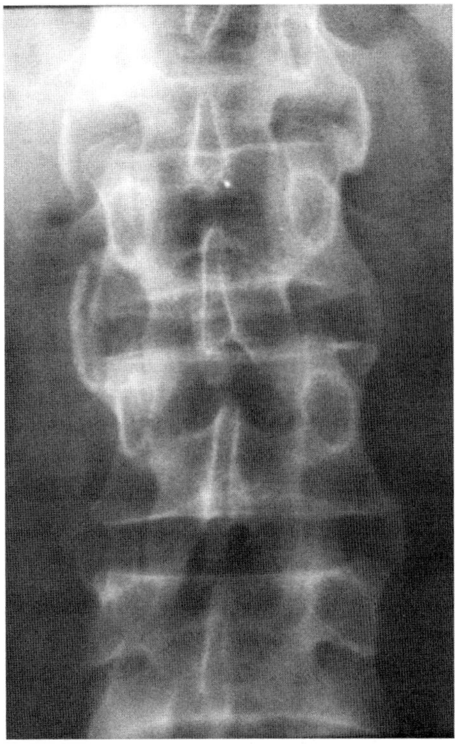

Fig. 21 Psoriatic spondylitis. The presence of non-marginal and also 'floating' (non-attached) syndesmophytes is demonstrated in this seronegative spondyloarthritis.

Ankylosing hyperostosis (diffuse idiopathic skeletal hyperostosis, DISH; Forestier's disease)

In ankylosing hyperostosis, the new bone is accreted later in life, is much more extensive, thicker, and florid, and is not necessarily seen in association with degeneration (Fig. 24).

Paraspinal new bone can be seen on plain films and, as expected, on CT scanning. In ankylosing hyperostosis, it is especially well demonstrated in the thoracic spine on the right side on CT scanning, the left being spared presumably because pulsation in the descending aorta prevents its formation (Jones et al. 1988).

Ossification of the posterior longitudinal ligament

New bone formation is also seen in the distribution of the posterior longitudinal ligament of the spine as an isolated phenomenon [ossification of the posterior longitudinal ligament (OPLL)], often in healthy Japanese, but also in ankylosing hyperostosis. The bone here, as elsewhere, is well shown on CT scanning (Fig. 25) (Resnick et al. 1978; Tsuyama 1984).

Where bone formation is gross, increase in uptake of isotope is also seen in the spine in ankylosing hyperostosis and ankylosing spondylitis.

Imaging of the sacroiliac joints

Erosive change at the sacroiliac joints is the pathognomonic feature in ankylosing spondylitis. In children, the sacroiliac joints are poorly defined as the cortex is not readily visualized and, as a result, the joint seems wider than in the adult. Also, at isotope scanning, the images of the adolescent sacroiliac joints are more prominent—'hotter' and wider than in the adult. The plain film diagnosis of erosive disease can be difficult to make in patients under 18 years of age.

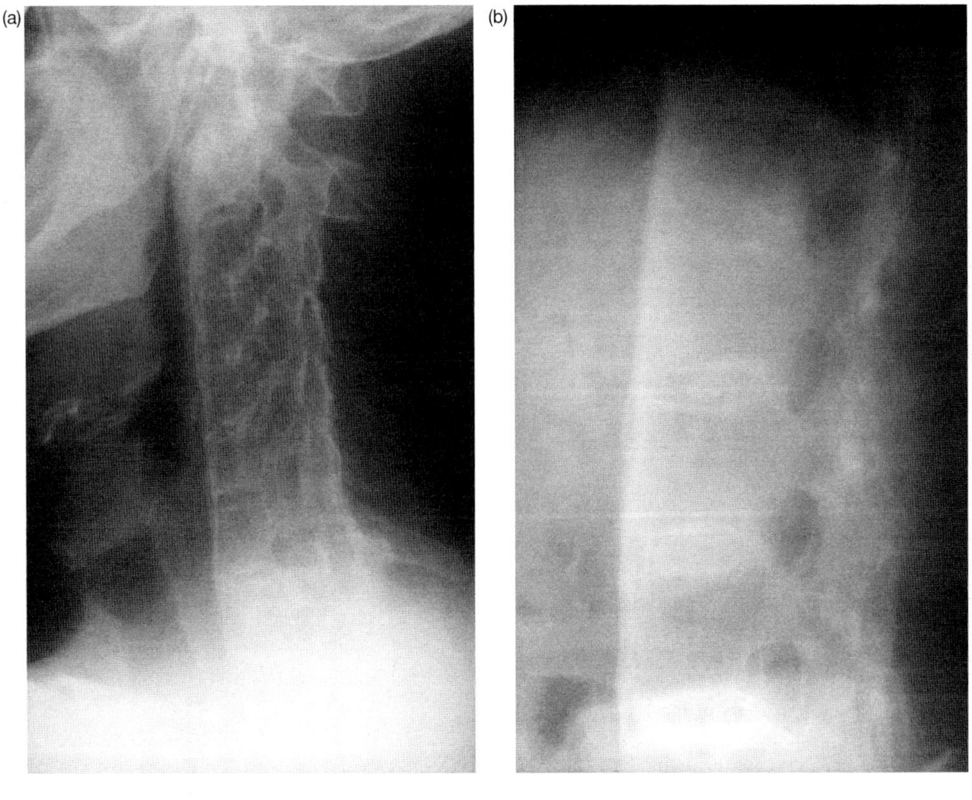

Fig. 22 Ankylosing spondylitis showing bony bridging with nuclear calcification.

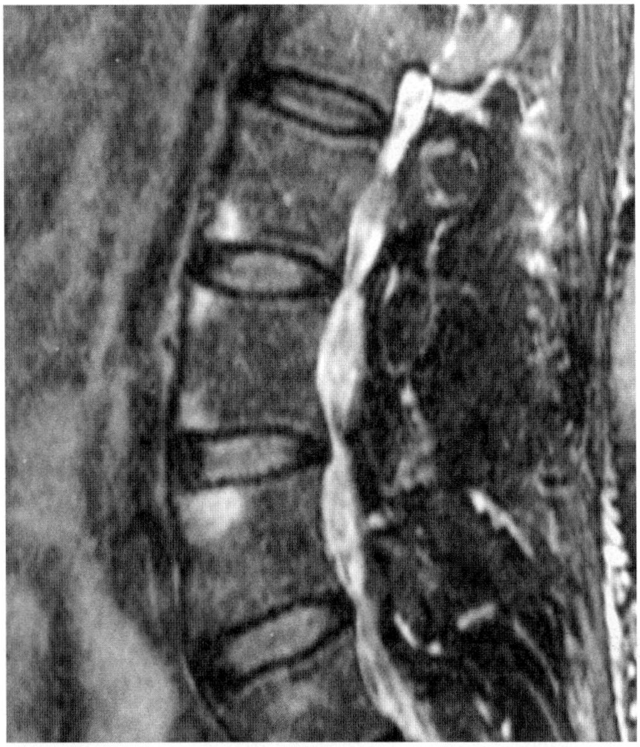

Fig. 23 MRI of the spine in ankylosing spondylitis demonstrating oedema of the anterior corners of the vertebral bodies. (By courtesy of Dr P. O'Connor, Leeds General Infirmary.)

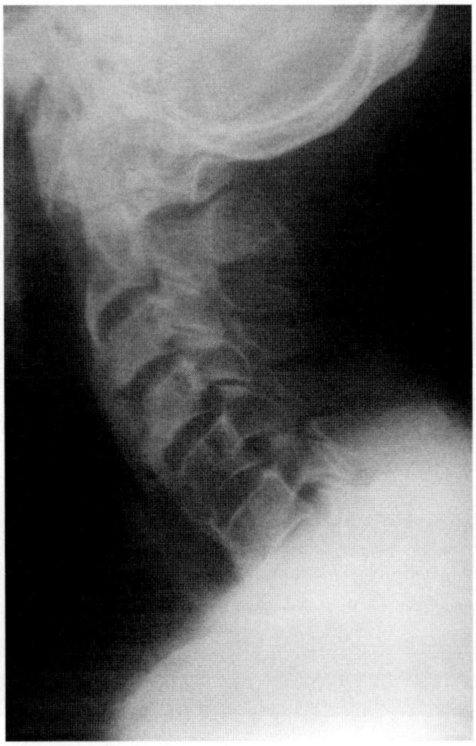

Fig. 24 Diffuse idiopathic skeletal hyperostosis. Preserved disc spaces are demonstrated in association with anterior ankylosis across many segments with a continuous bar of anterior new bone formation, which considerably increases the sagittal diameter of the vertebral body complex.

(a)

(b)

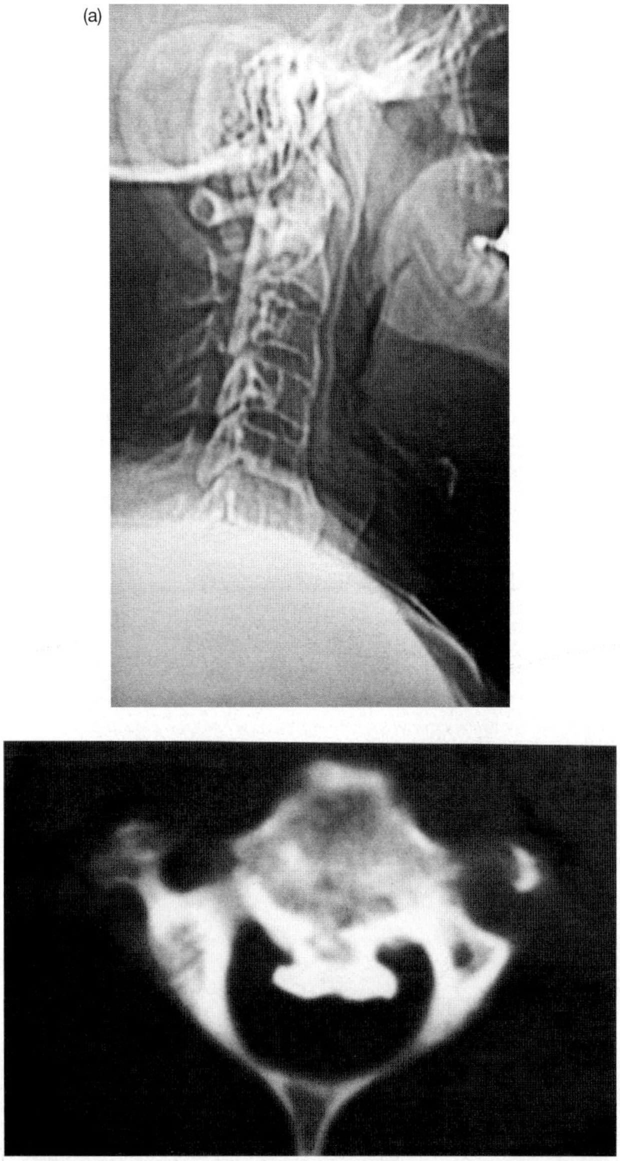

Fig. 25 Ossification of the posterior longitudinal ligament. To show the presence of new bone formation applied to the posterior aspect of the vertebral bodies of C2 and C3, considerably narrowing the sagittal diameter of the canal and indenting the theca.

In children and adults, infection of the sacroiliac joints is usually unilateral. Clinical onset of disease can antedate radiological change by up to 2 weeks. Gut gas, especially in sick children, may obscure the joint on plain radiographs.

Plain radiography

Conventional imaging is a simple anteroposterior radiograph centred on the sacrum (Fig. 26). This is probably the least effective means of imaging the joint as the beam diverges from, and the joint converges to, the midline. It is therefore more logical to image the sacroiliac joint prone, as the beam then passes down the joint space parallel to the articular surfaces. Oblique views and a 30° shoot-up anteroposterior image demonstrate the sacroiliac joint cortices much better than a single anteroposterior vertical beam.

CT scanning

CT scans are useful in assessing the sacroiliac joints as the images are free of overlying gut shadows and the articular cortices can be assessed for erosions and fusion and subcortical cysts. Detail is generally better with CT scans than with plain films or linear tomography and, by altering windows, small erosions can be visualized (Fig. 27). Only a few images need be taken of what is quite a long structure as excess irradiation is to be avoided.

Radionuclide bone scanning

Radioisotope scanning gives poor spatial resolution of sacroiliac joint disease but demonstrates pathology, albeit in a non-specific way by showing increase in uptake unilaterally or bilaterally. Unilateral sacroiliitis should be seen clearly because of asymmetric increase in uptake. Bilateral change can be more difficult to assess if uptake is symmetrically increased.

Fusion is a well-recognized sequel to endstage sacroiliitis—bilateral in ankylosing spondylitis but often unilateral in other seronegative spondyloarthritides and following tuberculosis and other infections. Fusions at the sacroiliac joints are also seen in the elderly in whom no other evidence of ankylosing spondylitis exists, often in elderly females who might not be expected to have had sacroiliitis. It is also seen in patients with ankylosing hyperostosis, due to ligamentous and osteophytic ankylosis in the absence of erosions (Fig. 28) (Durback et al. 1988), and in patients with Paget's disease, thalassaemia, and X-linked hypophosphataemic osteomalacia.

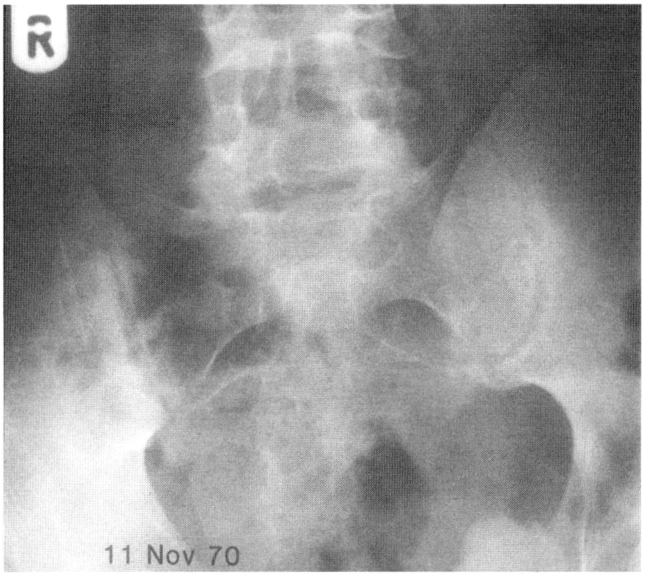

Fig. 26 Bilateral erosive sacroiliitis in ankylosing spondylitis.

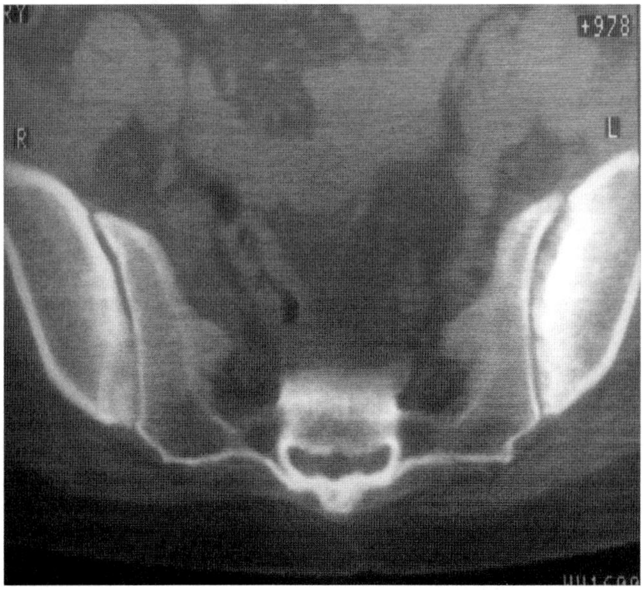

Fig. 27 Ankylosing spondylitis. Erosive sacroiliitis at CT scanning. There is narrowing of the sacroiliac joints bilaterally with erosive changes, initially confined to the lateral side of the joint. Reactive sclerosis is demonstrated in the underlying bone.

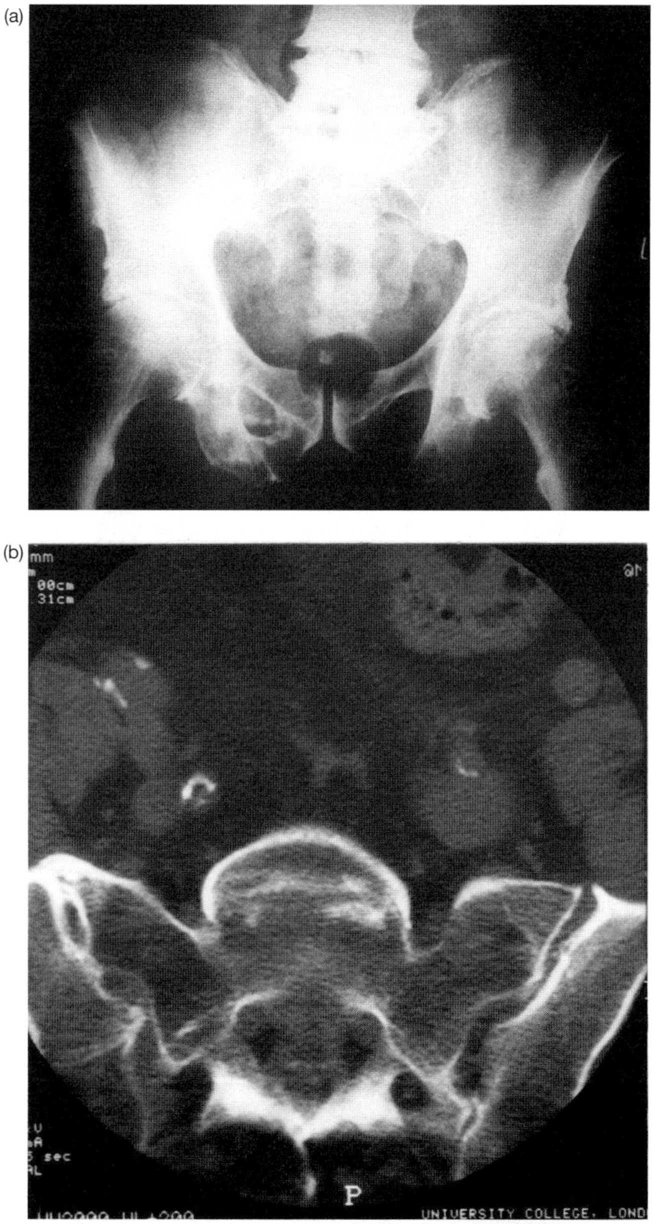

Fig. 28 Diffuse idiopathic skeletal hyperostosis. (a) There is new bone formation on the iliac crest and, in particular, superiorly at the sacroiliac joints, giving an impression of fusion across these. (b) CT scan to show new bone formation anteriorly across the sacroiliac joints in another patient with DISH. There are no erosions.

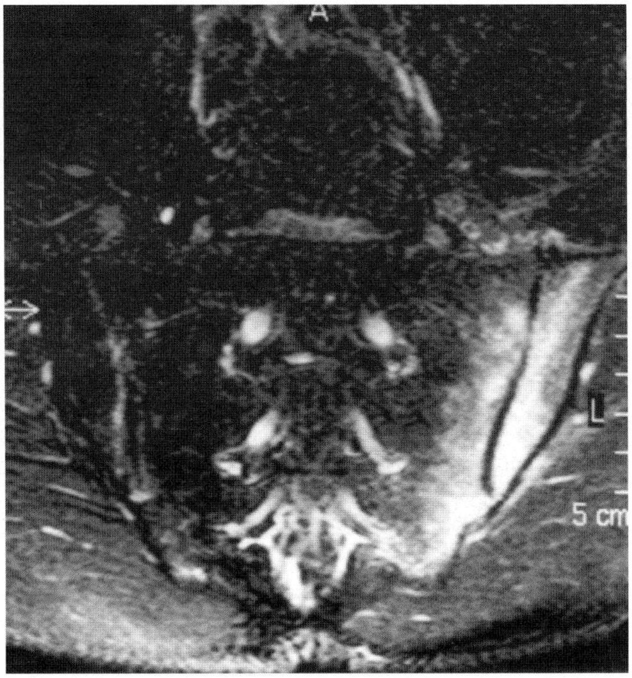

Fig. 29 Fat-suppressed MRI of sacroiliac joints demonstrating peri-joint oedema. (By courtesy of Dr H. Marzo-Ortega, Leeds General Infirmary.)

Magnetic resonance imaging

Whereas plain radiographs and CT scanning can identify established bony changes, they cannot localize bone oedema and inflammation. Scintigraphy lacks specificity, but MRI can assess the location and severity of these inflammatory changes at the sacroiliac joints (Fig. 29). It is therefore well placed to aid early diagnosis as well as staging of disease severity in the spondyloarthropathies (Braun et al. 2000). It can also help in the differential diagnosis of infection at the sacroiliac joint, where spread to adjacent muscles may be visualized.

Imaging the peripheral joints

The shoulder

Plain radiography and arthrography

The presence of an impinging subacromial osteophyte and upward subluxation of the humeral head can be seen on the plain film. In the evaluation of impingement, an elevated humeral head on the plain film is compatible with tendinous narrowing or total rupture. Using arthrography a rotator cuff tear is easily demonstrated (Figs 30 and 31), while restrictive capsulitis is shown by demonstration of the contracted capsular outline and volumetric assessment of capacity (Fig. 32) (Renton 1991).

MR imaging

This is said to have 100 per cent sensitivity and 95 per cent specificity in the diagnosis of complete tears, while in the differentiation of a normal tendon from one affected by tendinitis with impingement, the sensitivity and specificity are 93 and 87 per cent, respectively. For labral tears, these are also around 90 per cent (Iannotti et al. 1991). Changes of hypertrophy of bone and soft tissue at the acromioclavicular joint may cause compression of the underlying supraspinatus, often associated with tendon oedema (Fig. 33). The demonstration of a low-signal subacromial spur or osteophyte directs attention to the subjacent tendon, which may be thickened and oedematous, thinned, frayed, or frankly torn and distracted, allowing the humeral head to sublux upwards (Fig. 34).

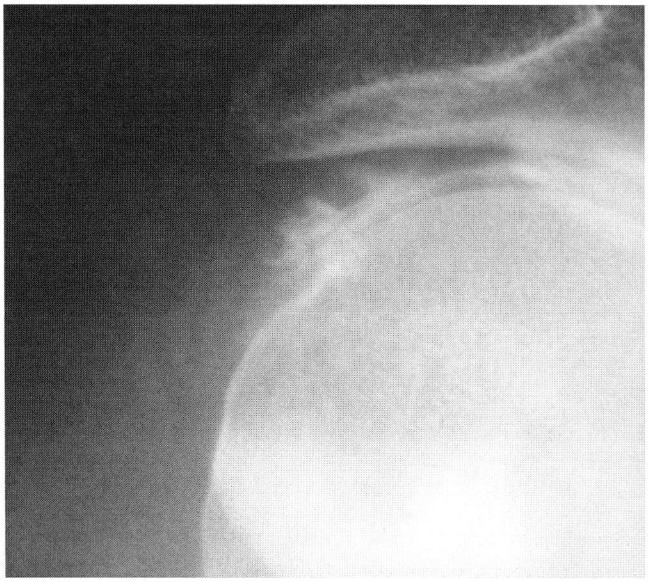

Fig. 30 Arthrogram of the shoulder showing partial tear of the rotator cuff. Irregularity of the inferior surface of the rotator cuff tendon is demonstrated. Contrast fills the tendon but does not reach the subacromial space.

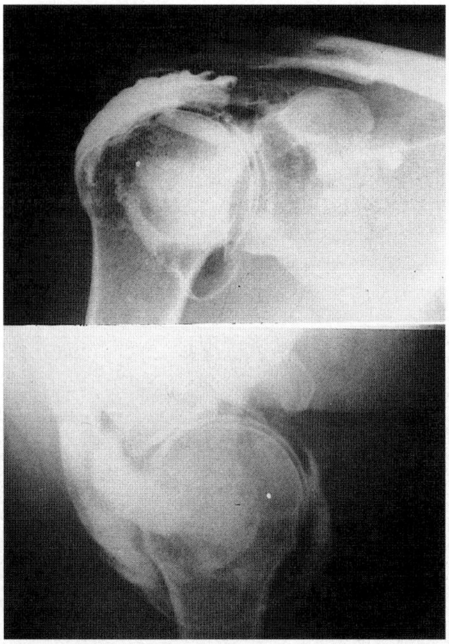

Fig. 31 Rotator cuff tear. Contrast medium now fills the subacromial bursa in continuity with the shoulder joint proper. On the axial view, the contrast medium in the subacromial bursa overlies that in the joint space proper.

Fluid is seen clearly on T_2-weighted or STIR sequences in the tendon, as well as in degenerative bone cysts at the greater tuberosity, and in the subacromial bursa. The deltoid may be atrophied. Axial scans show the long head of the biceps and its relationship to the bicipital groove, as well as the glenoid labrum.

CT arthrography

CT arthrography does demonstrate these findings but is invasive and has been largely superseded by MRI. Axial imaging by CT post-arthrography

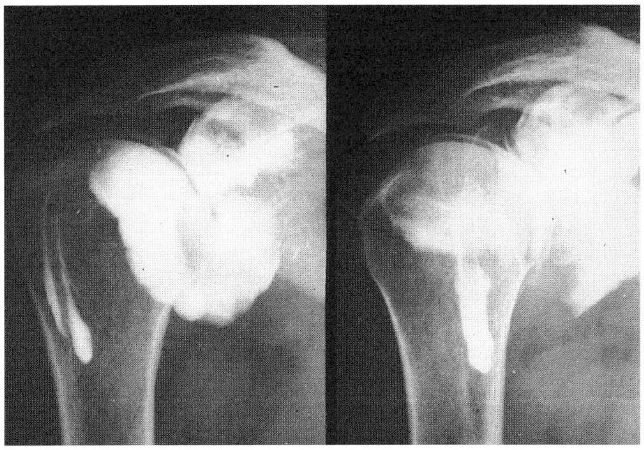

Fig. 32 Restrictive capsulitis. The capsule is reduced in size and is irregular. The long head of the biceps tendon sheath is filled as contrast medium seeks to escape from the tight shoulder joint capsule.

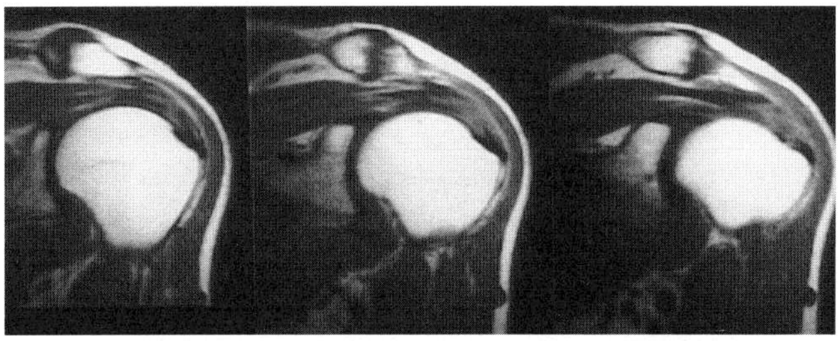

Fig. 33 MR scan of the shoulder. Hypertrophy of the acromioclavicular joint causes changes of oedema in the subjacent supraspinatus tendon. More distally there is a tear of the rotator cuff tendon shown as an area of increased signal replacing the normal low signal of the tendon.

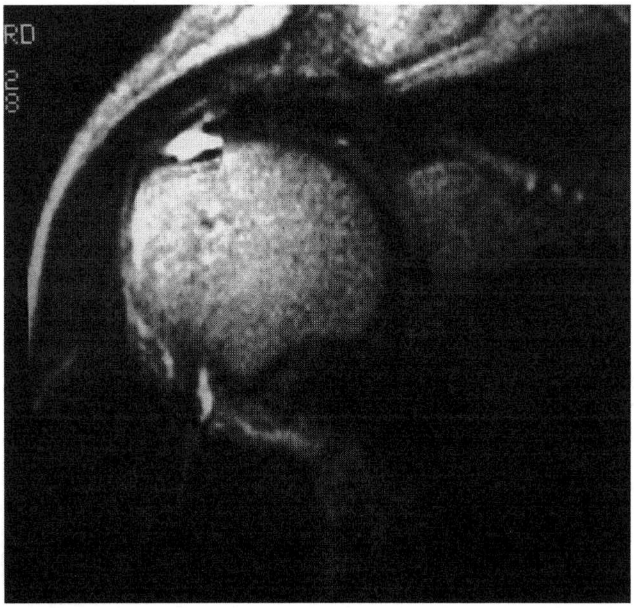

Fig. 34 MR scan of the shoulder. The tendon is seen to be retracted and fluid occupies the gap just proximal to the insertion into the greater tuberosity in a patient with a total rupture of the rotator cuff tendon.

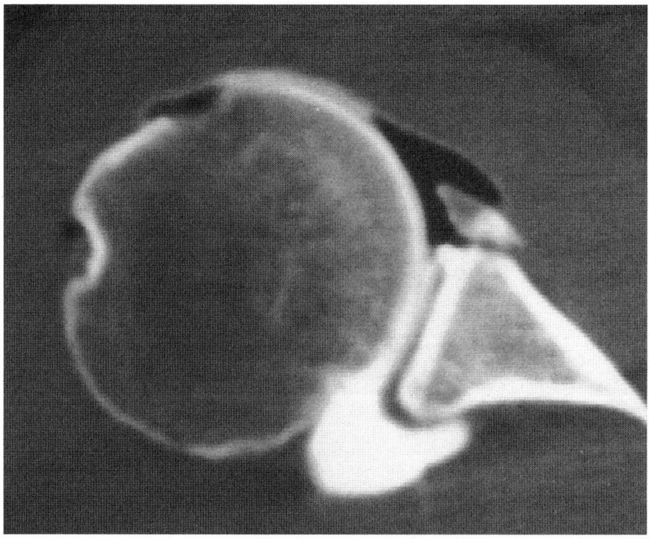

Fig. 35 CT arthrogram following trauma. There is avulsion of the anterior lip of the labrum and the underlying corner of the glenoid.

will show the long head of the biceps, the glenoid labra (Fig. 35), and a possible Hill–Sachs or hatchet defect after recurrent dislocation (Fig. 36) (all are also seen at MRI) (Kieft et al. 1988).

Ultrasonography

While ultrasound is operator dependent and the images maybe difficult to interpret, it is a quick and useful tool for assessing full thickness rotator cuff tears. A study comparing ultrasonography with arthrography demonstrated an accuracy of 84 per cent for ultrasonography and 94 per cent for arthrography (Paavolainen and Ahovuo 1994). Ultrasonography does have the added advantage of examining the patient in real time and can provide appropriately guided corticosteroid injection at the same time.

The elbow joint

Plain films have been discussed above. Arthrography of the elbow has always been of limited use. It was employed mainly for the diagnosis of loose bodies. Osteochondritis dissecans can also be shown. Unfortunately, the introduction of even the smallest of bubbles into a small joint makes the diagnosis of a loose body rather difficult. Opaque bodies in the joint are probably better demonstrated using CT.

MRI of the elbow joint represents a substantial advance in the diagnosis, not merely of abnormalities of bone, articular cartilage, synovium, and joint space, but also in showing the related structures around the elbow joint. Fat suppression studies, especially of the elbow, are useful in showing changes of a local tendinitis at the medial and lateral condyles and adjacent flexor and extensor origins. Changes within the elbow joint are well demonstrated.

The wrist

Plain films have been discussed above. Arthrography has been used at the wrist to demonstrate the integrity of the triangular cartilage. The radiocarpal joint is injected with contrast and a tear or defect in the triangular cartilage is then demonstrated by the passage of contrast medium into the distal radioulnar joint. Unfortunately, this tends to occur in around 15 per cent of normal patients and tends to increase with age. CT scanning of the wrist has some use in the demonstration of rheumatoid change.

MRI of the wrist is of great use in inflammatory arthritis for assessing soft tissue and bony changes and may also be used to demonstrate the integrity

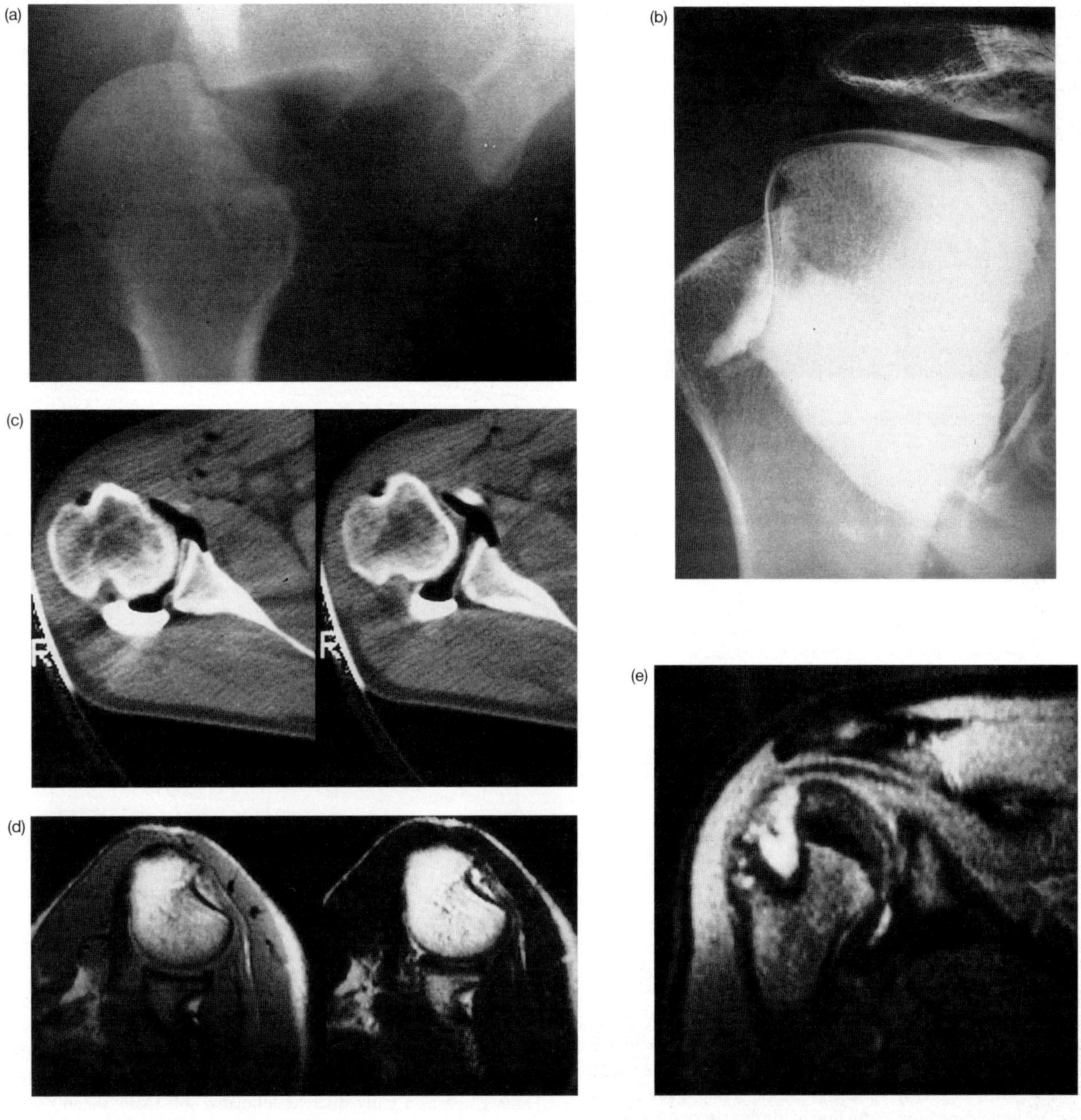

Fig. 36 Hill–Sachs or hatchet defect. Following anterior dislocation of the humeral head, especially if recurrent, a defect arises posteriorly following impingement upon the anterior lip of the glenoid. This may be demonstrated (a) on plain film, (b) at arthrography, (c) at CT, and (d, e) at MR scanning.

of the triangular cartilage. On coronal images the cartilage should be seen extending from the ulnar styloid to the radius, on the radial aspect of the distal radioulnar joint. Failure to do so may indicate avulsion. Bright signal on T_2 images, and especially on fat suppression studies, demonstrates either internal degeneration of the meniscus or a complete tear.

The hip joint

The presence of fluid in the joint can be seen on a plain radiograph. Ultrasound and MRI are more sensitive in diagnosing hip effusions and, using either fluoroscopy or ultrasound, the joint can be aspirated and contents analysed.

Arthrography may be used in the assessment of prosthetic loosening and infection. Again, the joint is aspirated, the specimen sent for microbiological investigation, then contrast injected. Loosening is shown by contrast filling the lucent gap between bone and cement or prosthesis. The width of this gap, if present at all, should be less than 1 mm.

Tumours of synovium are infrequent. Benign lesions are pigmented villonodular synovitis (Goldman and Dicarlo 1988) and synovial osteochondromatosis. In pigmented villonodular synovitis, a distended capsule is associated with synovial proliferation and bone scalloping (Fig. 37). The joint space is preserved initially as cartilaginous destruction is a later phenomenon. Aspiration may give a serosanguinous fluid. Synovial chondromatosis is associated with multiple (four or more) pearl-like chondral tumours, either floating loose or in the fronds of proliferating synovium. When these pearls ossify, they may be seen on a plain film.

With malignant synovioma, a patchily ossifying articular mass is associated with bone invasion.

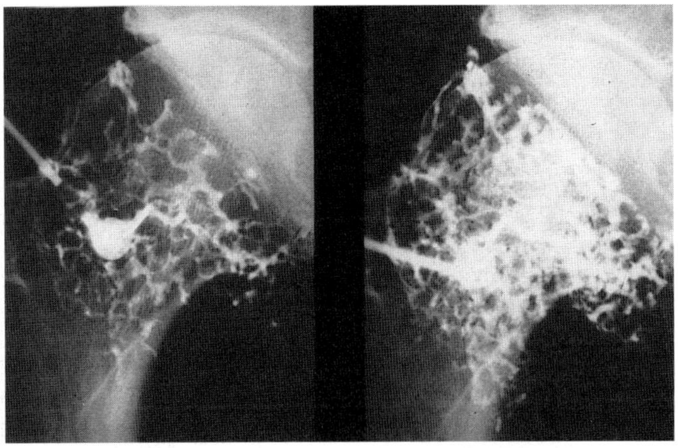

Fig. 37 Pigmented villonodular synovitis. At arthrography the frond-like proliferation of the synovium is demonstrated. This is associated with corticated erosion of the underlying bone.

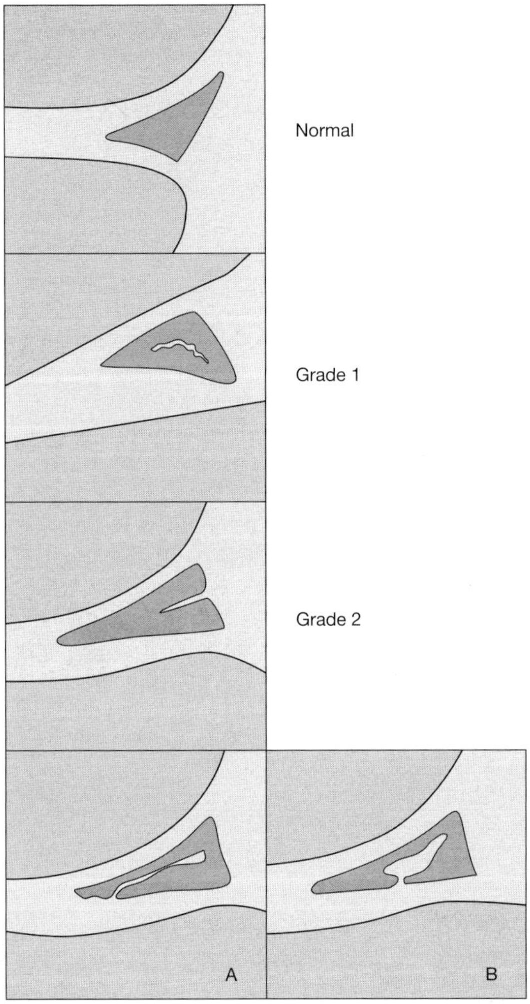

Fig. 38 Classification of meniscal change at MRI from normal to tear, according to Mink et al. (1993).

The knee joint

The tomographic nature of MRI and its ability to visualize soft tissue makes it ideal for studying the knee, where it can demonstrate all the key tissues: bone, cartilage, synovium, menisci, ligaments, and tendons.

Use of MRI

About 95 per cent of meniscal lesions can be diagnosed accurately, a similar accuracy rate to arthroscopy (Ireland et al. 1980). Fluid in the meniscus is shown as a band, or disc, of increased signal in the meniscus and may be graded accordingly (Fig. 38) (Mink and Deutsch 1990). Degree of extrusion can also be evaluated.

Areas of increased signal may be seen in adolescents and in older asymptomatic knees and are usually the result of myxoid degeneration (Stoller et al. 1987). Should the bright signal extend to the meniscal surface, a tear should be diagnosed and would be seen at arthroscopy. Equivocal or doubtful extension to the articular surface of the meniscus is responsible for false-positive diagnoses and, if in doubt, a tear should not be diagnosed (Kaplan et al. 1991).

Studies on American football players have shown progression from grade II to grade III lesions during the season, so that extension of intrameniscal degeneration to tear occurs (Reinig et al. 1991). Discoid lateral menisci and tears in them are also easily recognized (Fig. 39). Collateral ligament lesions in particular are well defined and disruption of the ligaments, local haemorrhage, and subsequent fibrosis may all be seen. The relationship between meniscal tears and degenerative changes in the underlying bone is clearly demonstrated (Fig. 40).

MRI is said not to be as accurate as arthroscopy in the diagnosis of stages I and II of chondromalacia patellae, but compares favourably for stages III and IV (Brown and Quinn 1993).

The accuracy of MRI in the diagnosis of cruciate ligament lesions approaches 100 per cent (Lee et al. 1988). The posterior ligament is better imaged as it is larger, while the anterior, besides being thinner, is also inclined at an angle to the midsaggital plane. It is thus necessary to image the anterior cruciate ligament with the limb in around 15° of external rotation. Tears, in the acute phase, may be partial or rupture of a cruciate ligament may be total and are associated with fluid seen with T_2-weighted or STIR sequences. The tear may be seen, or total retraction may occur, so that the ligament is no longer visible along its normal course (Fig. 41).

MRI is also useful for demonstrating adventitial cysts such as the Baker's cyst—an enlargement of the gastrocnemio–semimembranosus bursa which communicates with the posterior joint space. Baker's cysts are associated with meniscal tears and other forms of internal derangement, as well as inflammatory arthritis, presumably because of increased amounts of joint fluid and pressure in the joint. Such cysts can be seen on a plain lateral radiograph as a fairly discrete, lobulated soft tissue shadow posterior to the knee. Loose bodies may lie in it, or if multiple densities are present inferoposterior to the knee, the presence of local synovial osteochondromatosis can be inferred. Cyst rupture causes leak of synovial fluid into the calf, between skin and muscles, or between soleus and gastrocnemius. Rupture results in calf pain and swelling, mimicking a deep vein thrombosis. Ultrasound is the preferred examination as it confirms the presence of a cyst, the leak, and the absence of a deep vein thrombosis. MRI demonstrates the cyst, the effusion, and the leak as well as any associated meniscal abnormality (Fig. 42).

The ankle

Arthrography at the ankle has been used to demonstrate tears of the collateral ligaments, even acutely after injury. Tenosynovitis at the ankle tendons has been diagnosed by contrast injection of the tendon sheath, which is performed easily by direct puncture of the palpated tendon. MRI is good for evaluating structures at and around the ankle joint, including tendons and ligaments, as well as articular surfaces and the joint space (Fig. 43). Ultrasound may also be particularly useful in evaluating soft tissue changes at the ankle.

(a)

(b)

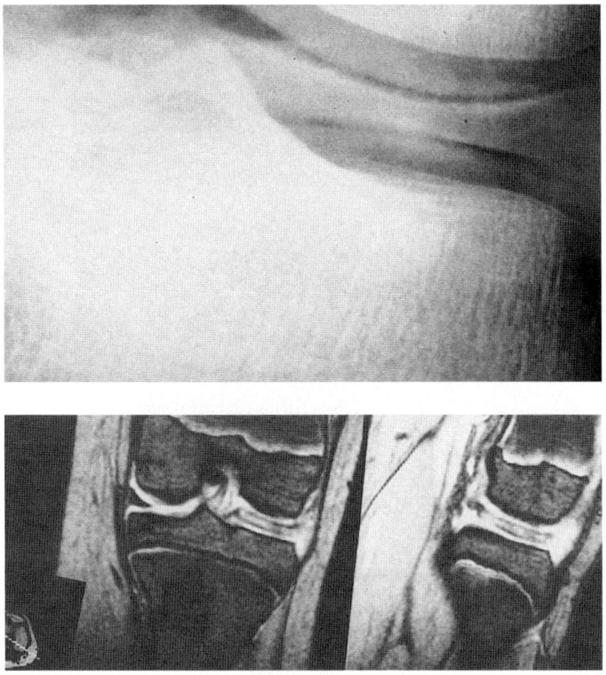

Fig. 39 Discoid meniscus. (a) On arthrography, instead of the normal triangular shape of the meniscus, its internal aspect is elongated and expanded. (b) The MR scan of a discoid meniscus shows the expansion of the meniscus, but also increased signal in it. This is extensive and presumably indicates widespread internal degeneration of the meniscus.

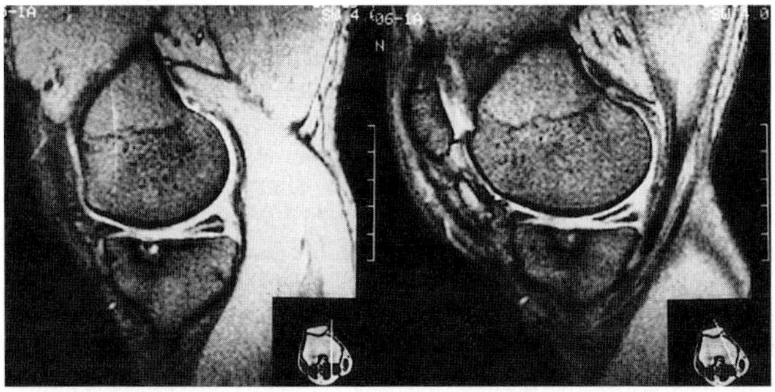

Fig. 40 MR scan of the knee showing a tear in the posterior horn of the medial meniscus and associated degenerative changes in the tibial plateau.

The hind foot

Radiographs may demonstrate erosions at various sites around the heel, at target areas for the various arthritides (Resnick et al. 1977). Erosions occur above, at, and below the Achilles tendon insertion on the posterior aspect of the calcaneus and will be associated with local increase in uptake on a radioisotope bone scan. Similarly, erosions form on the plantar surface of the calcaneus in the region of the origin of the plantar fascia in the seronegative arthritides. CT scanning demonstrates the bony erosions and can also show tendinous thickening, but the soft tissue changes are clearly demonstrated at MRI.

Twenty-two per cent of normal individuals have plantar spurs, which increase in incidence with age (Resnick et al. 1977). Normal spurs are 4 mm or less in size and smooth in outline. Rheumatoid patients may have benign-looking spurs which may be painless, but fluffy irregular spurs occur in seronegative patients, often associated with periostitis on the more distal inferior surface of the calcaneus, retrocalcaneal recess abnormalities, tendon thickening, and erosions. Benign spurs may become irregular with progression of disease and, similarly, irregular spurs may become smooth with remission of disease. Larger, denser, and fluffier plantar spurs are strongly suggestive of reactive arthritis (Fig. 44).

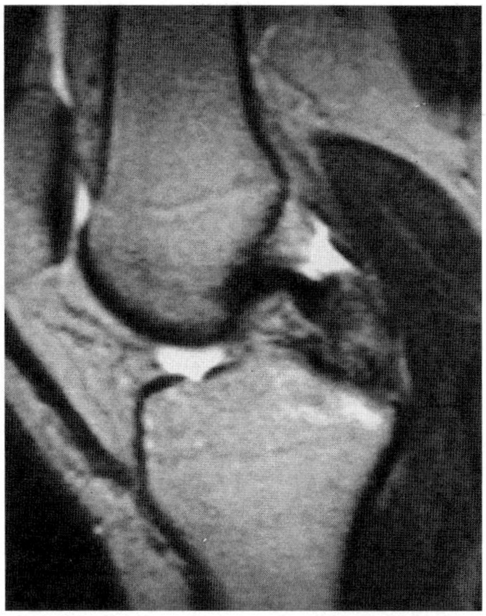

Fig. 41 MR scan of the knee. The posterior cruciate ligament is avulsed and has also taken the sub-adjacent cortical bone from the upper tibia with it. Note the oedema in the underlying tibial plateau.

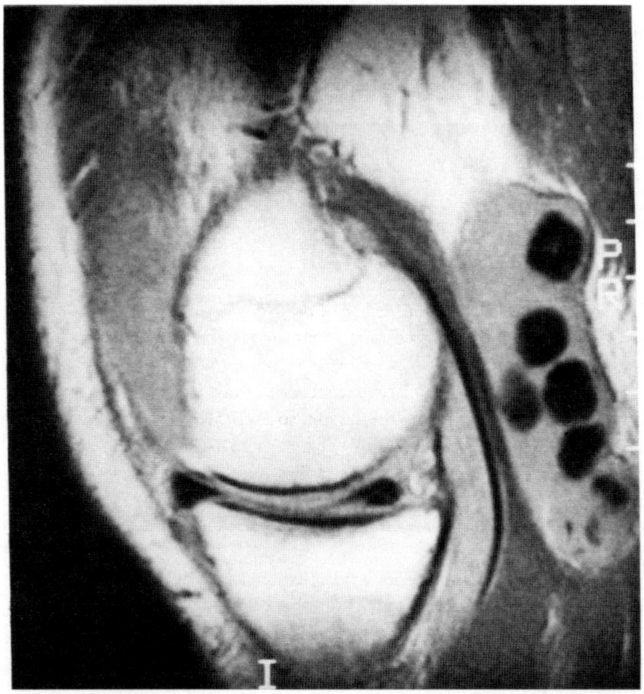

Fig. 42 Baker's cyst. MR scan of the knee demonstrating a large posterior cyst containing numerous loose bodies. This is associated with a tear of the posterior horn of the medial meniscus.

(a)

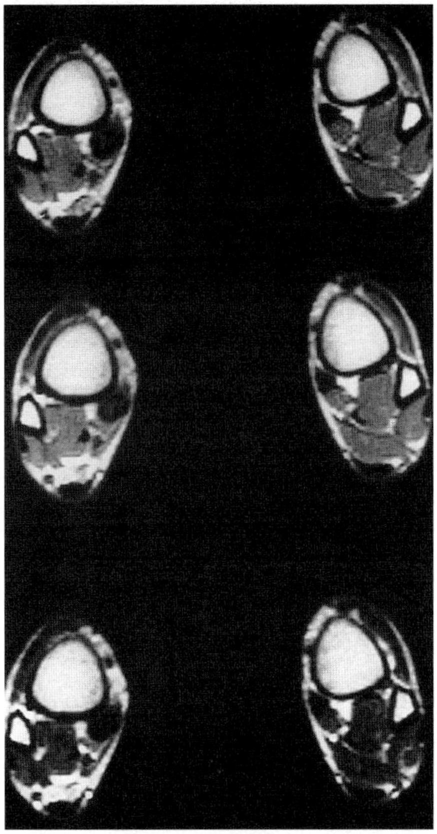

(b)

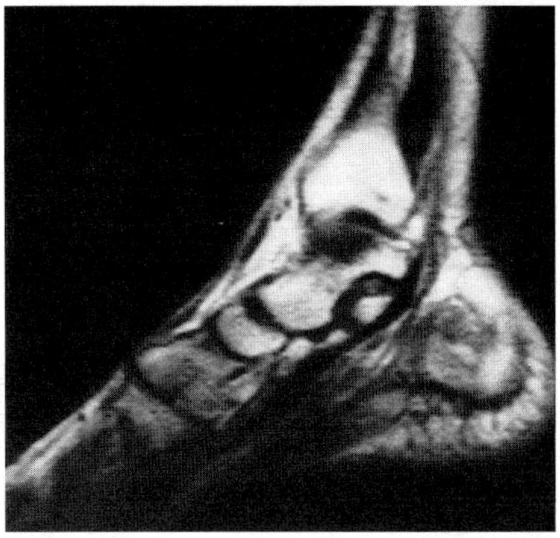

Fig. 43 Ruptured tibialis posterior tendon; sagittal and axial MR images. (a) The axial slices show both ankles. On the normal left side, the tendons behind the medial malleolus are well defined and compact. On the right, there is obvious thickening. This is due to retraction and the changes are easily identified then on the sagittal image (b).

The tendo-Achillis may be easily and quickly visualized with ultrasonography. Tears and tendinitis in the tendo-Achillis are especially well shown at MR scanning (Fig. 45).

Os trigonum

The os trigonum is seen in between 3 and 15 per cent of feet. It is almost certainly a tarsal accessory bone, rather than an old non-united fracture of the normal posterior process seen in 38 per cent of feet. The ossicle is demonstrated clearly on a lateral view of the foot. It may be the cause of symptoms of pain and tenderness due to impingement in plantar flexion

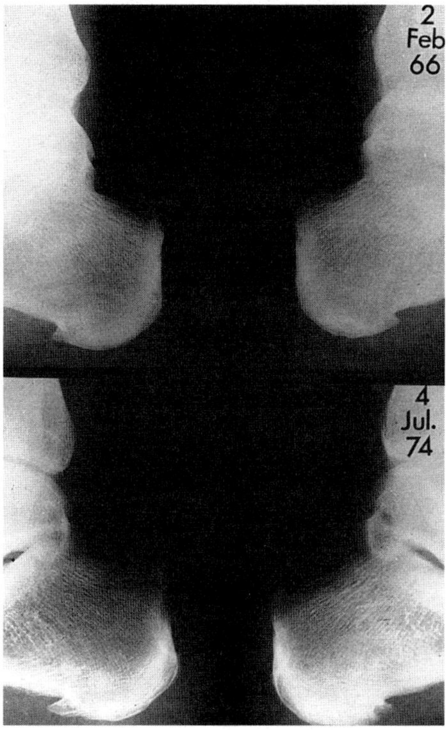

Fig. 44 Reactive arthritis. A large, fluffy plantar periostitis is shown.

in footballers or ballet dancers. The normal ossicle is smooth and well corticated, as indeed is the normal posterior tubercle, but with a normally lucent central medulla. With chronic impingement, central sclerosis and cortical irregularity with pitting and local soft-tissue oedema result. These changes can all be seen on a plain lateral radiograph. Changes of osteonecrosis and soft tissue swelling are also seen at MR scanning.

The subtalar joint

There are three compartments of the subtalar joint—posterior, middle, and anterior. The posterior and middle lie parallel to each other, inclined at around 35–40° to the weight-bearing plane. Imaging on plain films of these compartments is performed with a lateral view in the weight-bearing plane. Weight-bearing films are more easily reproducible between examinations and between patients and, though static, demonstrate the foot in a position of function. The axial view is taken with the X-ray beam projected along the line of the middle and posterior facets, that is, at 35–40° to the weight-bearing plane. These joints are clearly demonstrated at CT and MRI scanning.

The peroneal spastic flat foot syndrome

Tarsal coalition exists in many forms. It has been shown to exist *in utero* and is the result of failure of segmentation of the cartilaginous primordia. The most common form is talocalcaneal synostosis, usually at the middle facet and well demonstrated on the axial view. Calcaneonavicular fusion is the next most commonly seen type, easily seen on an oblique view of the foot. These lesions become clinically manifest when the cartilaginous bridge between the ossific nuclei matures, usually into a continuous bar of bone (Fig. 46), though formes frustes are also found. The resulting fusion causes hindfoot rigidity and a flattening of the longitudinal arch, resulting in stretching pain and spasm in the peroneus longus tendon. The syndrome was seen in 2 per cent of Canadian army recruits (Harris and Beath 1948). CT scanning and MRI demonstrate the fusion directly (Fig. 47).

Stress fracture in the foot

Stress fractures are caused by (i) regular, repeated submaximal stress on normal bone or (ii) normal stresses on abnormal, that is, Pagetic, osteomalacic,

(a)

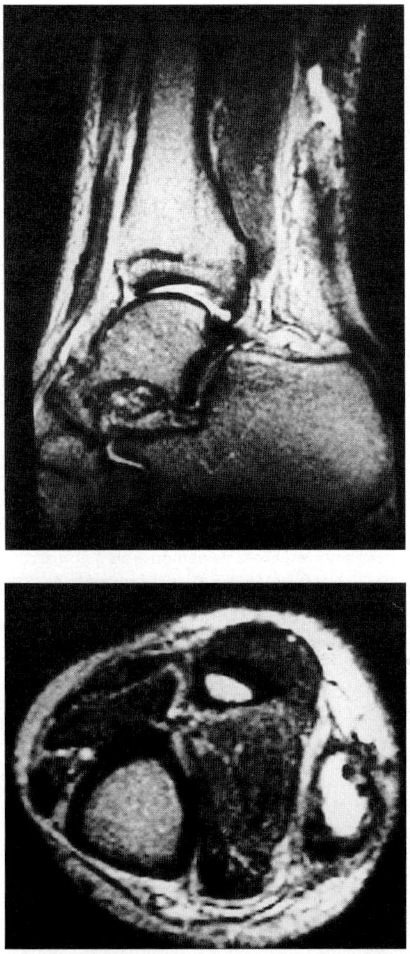

(b)

Fig. 45 MRI of the tendo-Achilles showing a degenerate and ruptured tendon. The capsule around the tendon seems intact but the space between the two frayed ends is filled with fluid.

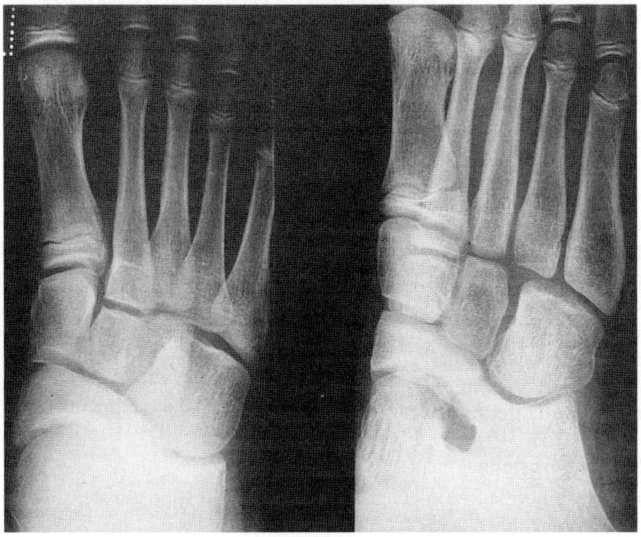

Fig. 46 Oblique radiograph of the foot demonstrates calcaneonavicular synostosis.

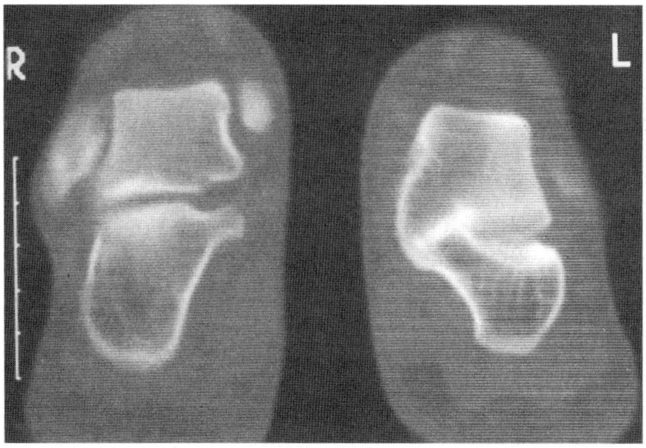

Fig. 47 Hindfoot fusion at the sustentaculotalar joint. Compare normal and abnormal sides.

(a)

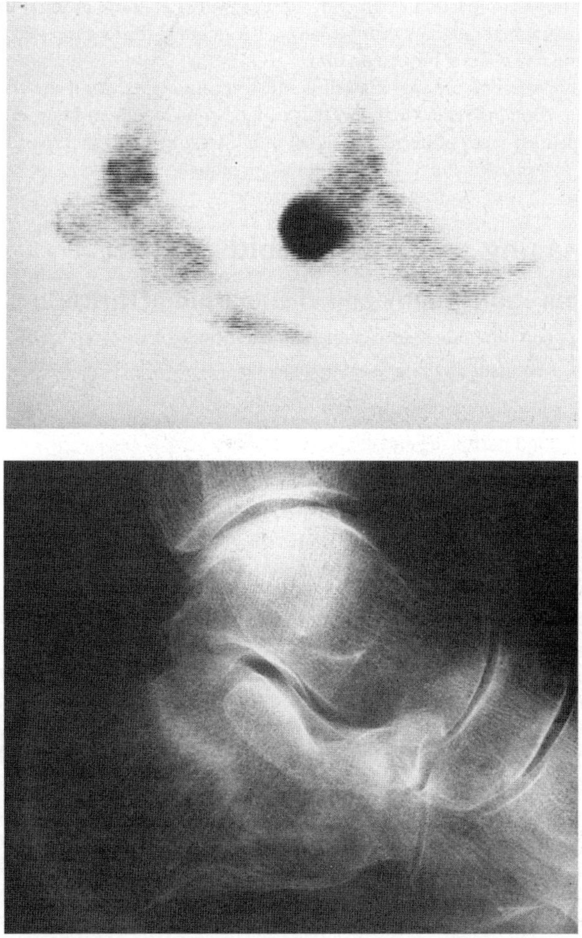

(b)

Fig. 48 Occult fracture of the calcaneum where initial radiograph showed no abnormality but a radioisotope bone scan (a) shows a gross increase in uptake in the calcaneum. (b) Another patient showing a stress or increment fracture in an osteoporotic calcaneum, seen as a serpiginous dense line extending to the upper cortex of the bone and reaching it at a right angle.

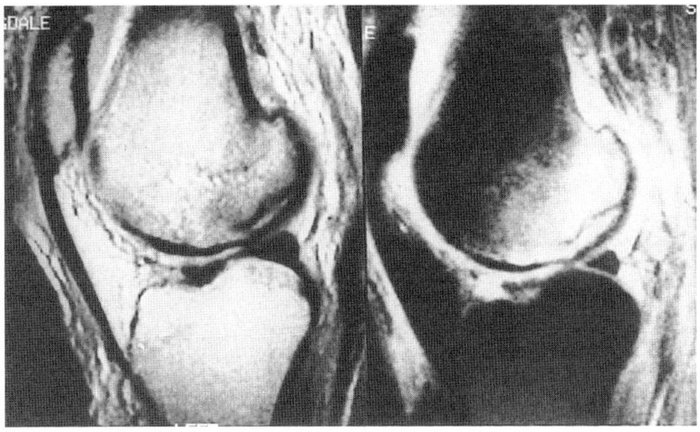

Fig. 49 Occult fracture of medial femoral condyle seen on a T_1-weighted image (a) as a serpiginous band of low signal extending to the posterior femoral cortex surrounded by some loss of the fatty bright signal. The bone oedema, however, is much better demonstrated on the STIR sequence (b).

or osteoporotic bone. Stress fractures in the tarsus are usually calcaneal. As with stress fractures elsewhere, the history may be typical but no abnormality may be present on the initial radiograph. Under these circumstances, a radioisotope bone scan will be positive (Fig. 48), and a dense line representing bone compaction or fracture healing will later show up on a lateral radiograph, tomograph or, especially, CT scan but, if the foot is rested, bony changes may never be seen on film.

Stress lesions are well imaged is MR scanning, especially if the affected bone contains yellow marrow, that is, fat. Stress lesions in bone show as ill-defined areas of decreased signal on T_1-weighted and increased signal on T_2-weighted and STIR fat-suppression sequences (Fig. 49).

Imaging and rheumatoid arthritis

Plain radiography and rheumatoid arthritis

The plain film radiological changes in RA include:

(i) soft tissue swelling, local or general;

(ii) alteration in bony density;

(iii) joint narrowing and alignment changes;

(iv) periostitis;

(v) surface irregularity, cortical loss, and erosions;

(vi) muscle wasting; and

(vii) calcification or ossification in surrounding soft tissues.

Erosions are often first seen in the feet rather than in the hands (Brook and Corbett 1977). Erosions are first described at the metatarsophalangeal joints, and most commonly at the 5th metatarsophalangeal joint. The metatarsal head is eroded before the adjacent phalangeal base. Approximately 30–50 per cent of patients with newly diagnosed RA will have erosions at presentation. Erosions have been studied extensively by Buckland-Wright and coworkers using macroradiography. This process uses a very small target and the object is placed close to the X-ray tube. The advantages of using such a fine X-ray tube focus are large magnification (up to ×10 or 20) and high spatial resolution (Dacre and Buckland-Wright 1992). Changes in RA have thus been reported as early as 2 weeks after onset of symptoms (Fig. 50). Buckland-Wright (1984) also demonstrated that erosions are symmetrical and bear no relation to hand dominance, though others do not agree. Erosions also vary in size, with the largest at the radiocarpal, medial carpometacarpal, and second and third metacarpophalangeal joints.

Martel et al. (1980) described 'bare areas' of bone between articular cartilage and synovium, and pointed out that pannus logically would erode bone at this site which was free of cartilage. Erosions therefore commence as small areas of juxta-articular radiolucency adjacent to the margin of the articular cartilage. These lucencies are due to trabecular loss and cortical thinning. Small defects (0.1–0.3 mm diameter) begin to be seen in the cortex at sites of ingrowth of pannus. With progression of these changes, visible classical erosions form. Migration of pannus below the articular cortex results in subchondral erosions and, with weakening of local bone, the articular cortex collapses (Fig. 51). Alternatively, direct invasion by pannus from above destroys articular cartilage and also causes subchondral invasion.

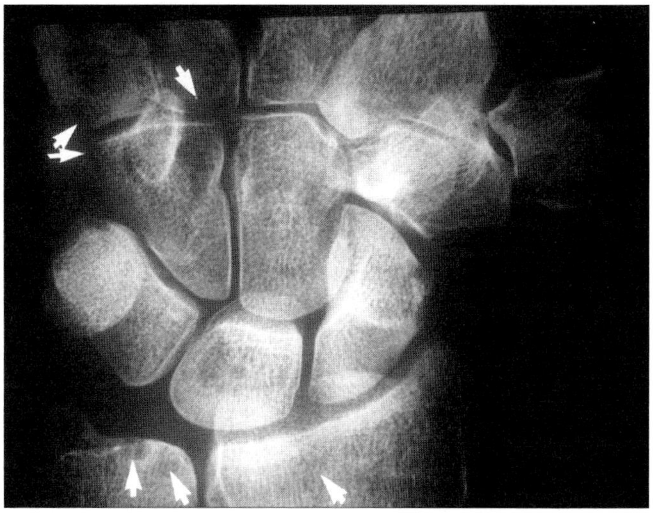

Fig. 50 Rheumatoid arthritis. Erosions demonstrated at macroradiography. (By courtesy of Dr F. Buckland-Wright, Guy's Hospital.)

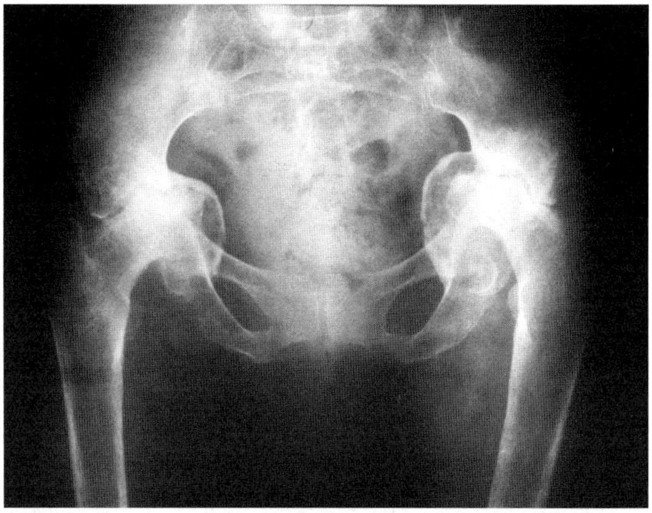

Fig. 51 Rheumatoid arthritis. Collapse of the femoral head associated with protrusio acetabuli.

Pressure erosions

Where two normally non-congruous bony surfaces approximate, and one moves on the other, well-corticated pressure erosions develop. With large rotator cuff tears, upward subluxation of the humeral head results in it eroding the undersurface of the acromion. Subsequently, the inferior glenoid lip erodes the adjacent humeral neck (Fig. 52).

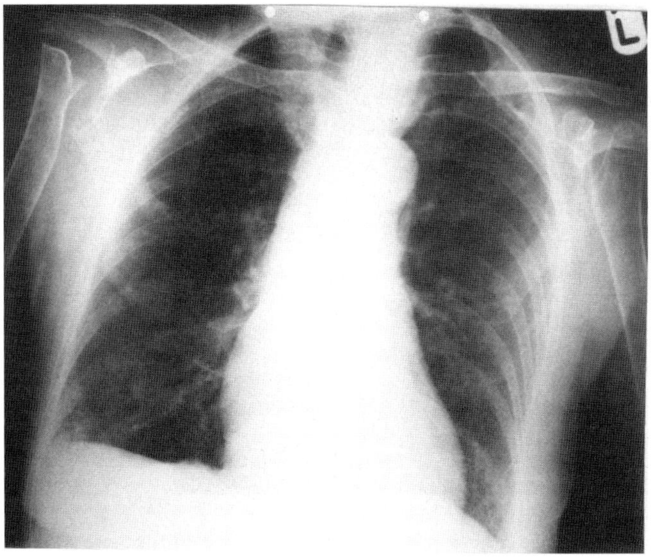

Fig. 52 Rheumatoid arthritis. Upward subluxation of the resorbed humeral head has eroded the inferior aspect of the acromion and clavicle. The neck of the humerus is eroded by the glenoid, and the superior aspects of the third and fourth ribs are also eroded superiorly.

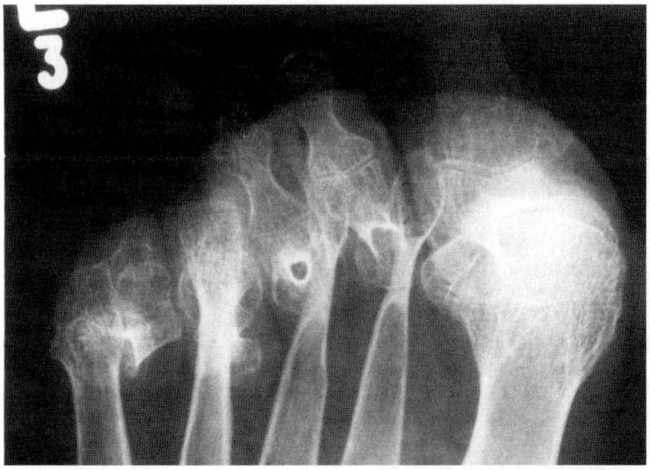

Fig. 53 Rheumatoid arthritis. Phalangeal subluxation causes pressure erosion of the metatarsal necks.

Proximal phalangeal subluxation in scleroderma and after Jaccoud's arthritis similarly allows the phalangeal base to erode the metacarpal neck (Fig. 53). In the foot, impinging malleoli cause defects on the adjacent talus.

The use of radiographs as outcome measures in RA has recently been reviewed (Boini and Guillemin 2001). Care should be taken when choosing views, scoring methods, and in reader training.

MRI in rheumatoid arthritis

As a result of the inherent contrast of MR images, the components of a joint, bone, and soft tissue are better defined than in any other modality. Synovial fluid, synovium, cartilage, ligaments, tendon, and bone can all be identified, and pathology seen in them (Fig. 54). This makes MRI an ideal tool for evaluation of RA which is primarily a synovial disease.

Erosions are the pathognomonic change in RA and it is important to conceptualize that MRI erosions represent different lesions to radiographic erosions—the former visualizes hydrogen proton content where latter represents calcified bone cortex. However, the MRI lesion is likely to precede the radiographic erosion. One study demonstrated approximately one in four of the MRI lesions progressed to radiographic erosions over 1 year (McQueen et al. 2001). This discrepancy in progression rate may in part be explained by the tomographic nature of MRI compared with plain films.

The MRI erosions are visualized as marginal low-signal defects on T_1-weighted images and they seem to be preceded by, and often accompanied, by bone marrow oedema (high signal on T_2-weighted images) (Conaghan et al. 1999). Such erosions are detected earlier in the disease process and with greater frequency on MRI scans than on plain films.

Synovial tissue shows on conventional images as an intermediate signal mass adjacent to the erosions. Effusions in joints or tendon sheaths are bright (brighter than pannus) on T_2-weighted views. The use of intravenous gadolinium with T_1-weighted sequences further distinguishes inflammatory from non-inflammatory fibrous synovial tissue by demonstration of synovial enhancement where synovial proliferation is hypervascular. Gadolinium-detected synovitis has been correlated with macroscopic and microscopic findings of synovitis (Conaghan et al. 1999). The degree of synovitis at baseline has also predicted subsequent development of MRI erosions (McQueen et al. 1998; Østergaard et al. 1999).

The sensitivity of MRI for detecting synovitis and erosions means it has the ability to diagnose RA earlier. The effects of adding MRI criteria to the classification criteria for RA has been favourably demonstrated (Sugimoto et al. 1996). MRI has also been used to assess outcomes in RA and in clinical trials has helped the evolution of its clinical applications in RA (Peterfy 2001). Efforts to develop semi-quantitative and automated scoring methods for quantifying synovitis are on-going. The technique of dynamic gadolinium-enhanced MRI (DEMRI) combined with computer-aided quantification has been used to demonstrate differences in therapy for RA, by analysing changes in signal intensity of multiple images taken immediately after gadolinium injection (Reece et al. 2002). Parameters such as the initial rate of enhancement and maximal enhancement of signal intensity are calculated.

Changes at the C1–C2 interface

Cervical spine involvement occurs in up to 86 per cent of patients with RA and atlantoaxial subluxation occurs in up to 40 per cent. Ligamentous laxity and rupture may be associated with erosive change around the peg due to local pannus. Instability may involve anterior displacement of C1 or posterior displacement of the peg. A conventional lateral radiograph taken in flexion should not result in a space between arch and peg of more than 2.5 mm in an adult. Superior and lateral displacement of the peg also occur.

Erosion of the lateral masses at C1–C2 allows the odontoid peg to shift upward. The distance from the anteroinferior surface of C2 to McGregor's line should be more than 34 mm in men and 29 mm in women (McGregor's line is a line drawn from the back of the hard palate to the lowest part of the occiput). These changes can be visualized by CT with radiculography, which was until the advent of MRI, the investigation of choice (Fig. 55).

MRI is now the investigation of choice for imaging the craniocervical region. Pannus, cerebrospinal fluid, bone, and cord are all shown (Fig. 56). Scans can also be obtained in flexion and extension, but there is probably no advantage to this over a single MR study with plain lateral flexion and extension views and tomography to show erosions. In addition, the status of the cord can be assessed at MRI for oedema, gliosis, or atrophy (Einig et al. 1990).

Ultrasonography in rheumatoid arthritis

With the advent of smaller, portable ultrasound machines with better image quality, there has been a growing use of this technique for the examination of peripheral joints in RA. As well as being non-invasive, ultrasonography can be performed in the clinic with multiple peripheral joints being evaluated at a single visit. There are, of course, important training issues in the use of this technique and access to joints may be limited by transducer size.

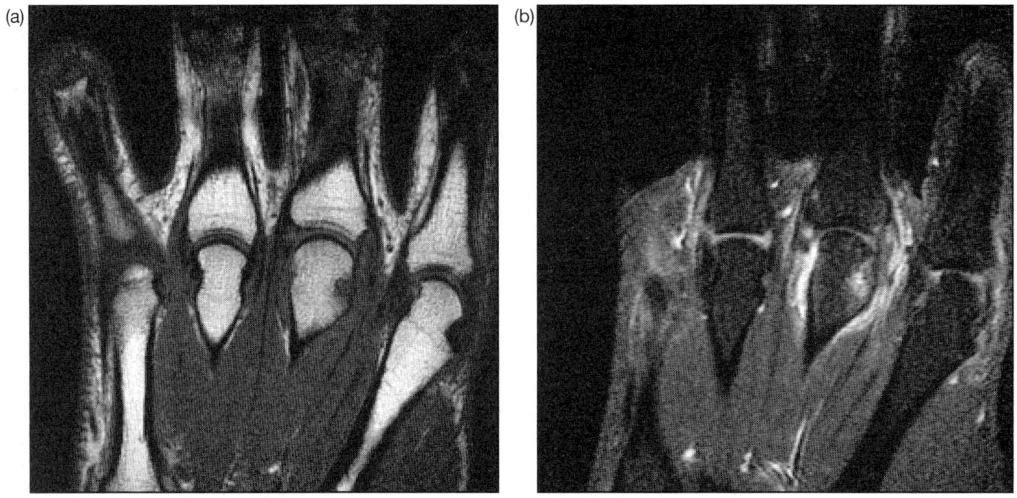

Fig. 54 Sagittal MRI scans of metacarpophalangeal joints of a rheumatoid arthritis hand. (a) T_1-weighted image demonstrating MRI erosions and (b) T_1 fat-suppressed post-gadolinium image demonstrating bone oedema. (By courtesy of Dr P. O'Connor, Leeds General Infirmary.)

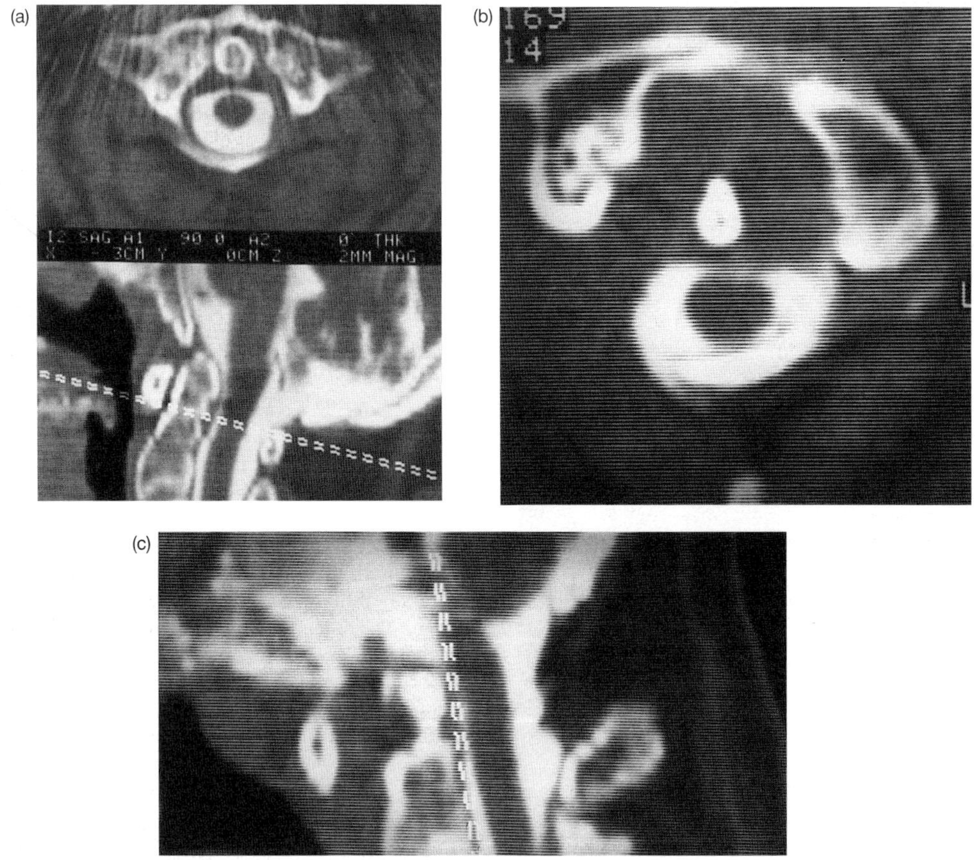

Fig. 55 CT radiculography. (a) Normal relationship of peg, arch of atlas, theca, and cord in the axial mode, together with sagittal reconstruction. (b) In this patient with rheumatoid arthritis, the odontoid peg is eroded (see lateral reconstruction) and no longer has an intimate relationship with the arch of atlas. There is a large soft-tissue mass interposed between the two. The cord is displaced posteriorly and the theca impressed upon. (By courtesy of Dr J. Steven, National Hospital, Queen Square.)

Ultrasonography may be useful for both early diagnosis and assessing outcome of disease in RA, by virtue of its abilities to detect synovitis more sensitively than clinical examination (Backhaus et al. 1999) and to detect bone erosions with greater sensitivity than plain radiographs (Fig. 57) (Wakefield et al. 2000).

Problems remain with the quantification of synovial tissue volumes but recent studies with power Doppler ultrasonography suggest it may aid quantification of inflammation (Walther et al. 2001). Ultrasound may be particularly useful in RA tendon and bursal disease where clinical examination alone is insensitive (Gibbon and Wakefield 1999).

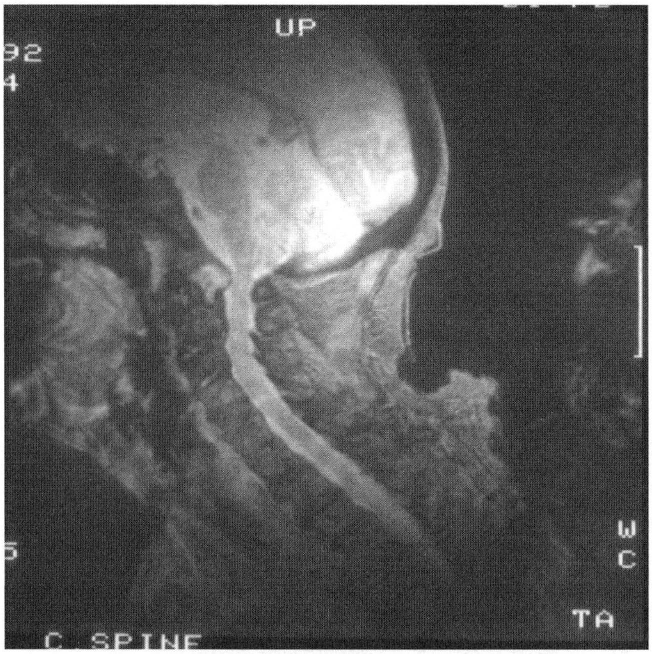

Fig. 56 Rheumatoid arthritis. MR sagittal T_2-weighted image shows erosion of the odontoid peg with pannus and compression of the cervical cord.

Another advantage of ultrasonography is to accurately guide local corticosteroid injection therapy. A recent study demonstrated that the planned site of injection was changed in many cases after ultrasonographic assessment (Karim et al. 2001).

(a)

(b)

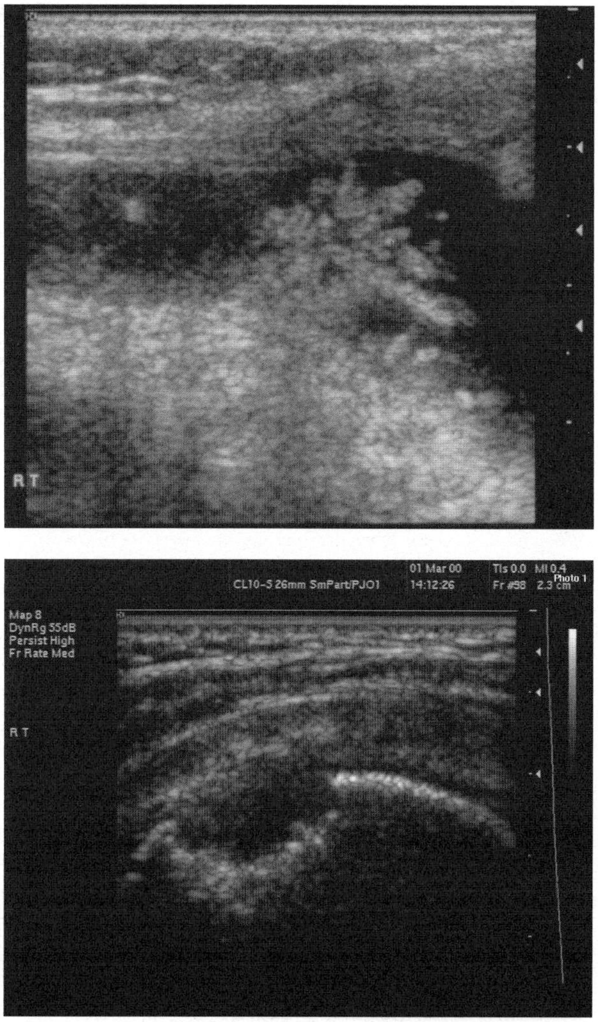

Fig. 57 Ultrasonography in rheumatoid arthritis. Ultrasound of (a) knee, demonstrating fronds of synovitis, and (b) shoulder, demonstrating an erosion (By courtesy of Dr P. O'Connor, Leeds General Infirmary.)

Imaging and osteoarthritis

Osteoarthritis typically affects the joints involved in weight-bearing, such as the hips, knees, and lumbar and cervical spine. In the hand, the first carpometacarpal and distal interphalangeal joints are commonly involved, the latter joint involvement frequently seen in older women. Plain films provide a cheap, quick, and simple method of imaging affected joints for diagnosis and long-term evaluation of structural progression. However, they have a poor correlation with symptoms. Plain radiographic changes include joint space narrowing due to cartilage and meniscal destruction, marginal osteophytes, cyst formation and articular collapse, reactive sclerosis, and malalignment. Many of these changes relate to cortical bone and may also be imaged with CT scanning (Fig. 58) or MRI (Fig. 59). Axial imaging demonstrates the joint spaces, osteophytes, cysts, and changes in bony density especially well. Loose bodies are also well seen. The images may be enhanced by the use of single or double contrast arthrography.

MRI has significant advantages in osteoarthritis imaging because it can visualize all the components now thought important in the disease process: the synovium, cartilage, subchondral bone, and ligaments. MRI is better at demonstrating cartilage loss than any other imaging modality (Chan et al. 1991), so that a joint which appears normal on plain films is shown to have cartilage loss on MRI. This technique is also better than conventional radiography in demonstration of osteophytes, though CT does this equally well. At present, MRI use is still limited by cost and availability—the advent of smaller scanners may change usage.

Most MRI work in osteoarthritis has involved developing semiautomated assessments of cartilage volume (Loeuille et al. 1998). Although still far from routine use, these techniques are demonstrating improved reliability and sensitivity to change. Newer MRI studies have focused on features of subchondral bone, such as trabecular bone and bone oedema

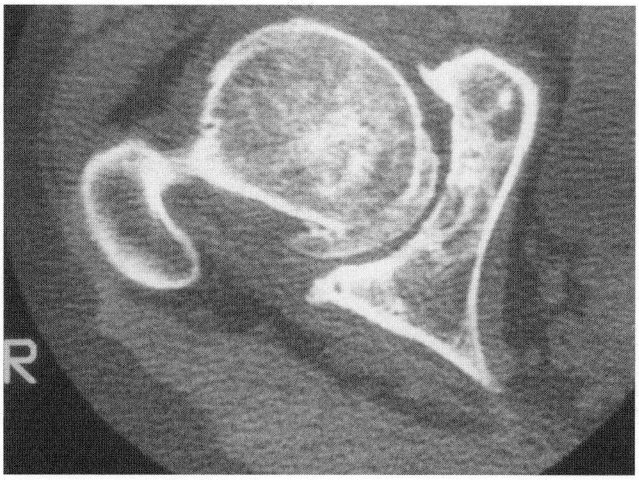

Fig. 58 Osteoarthritis demonstrated at CT scanning. New bone proliferation is seen around the articular surfaces and internally within the joint on the femoral head.

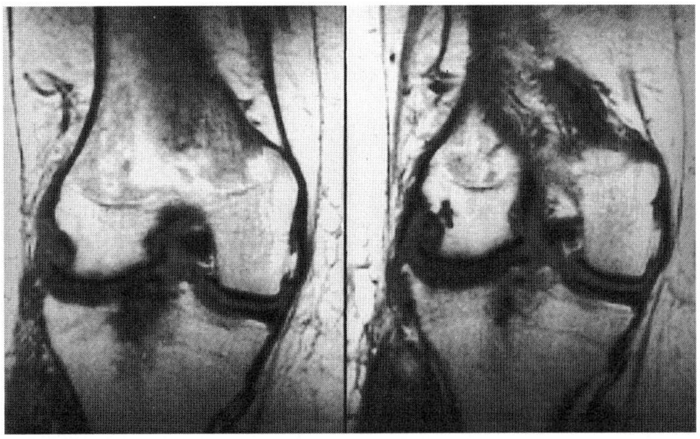

Fig. 59 Osteoarthritis demonstrated at MR scanning. Coronal images show irregular articular surfaces, marginal osteophytes, synovial proliferation and irregularity, or even loss of the adjacent meniscus.

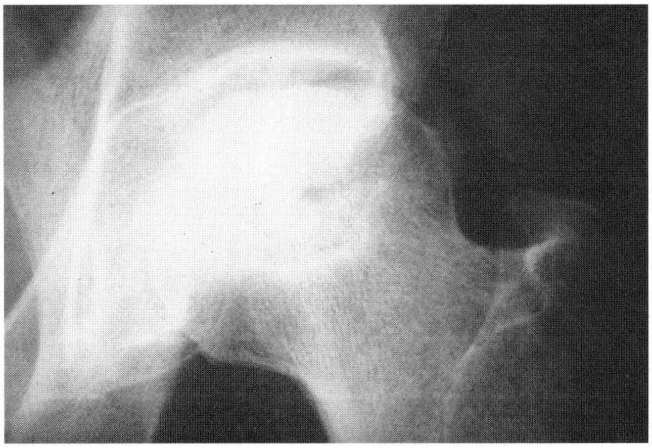

Fig. 60 Avascular necrosis. A sclerotic rim of creeping substitution is seen beneath an area of structural failure of the femoral head.

(Felson et al. 2001; Beuf et al. 2002). Recent studies of large MRI osteoarthritis cohorts have given new insights into the discrepancy between plain radiographs and symptoms: sites of patient pain have been correlated with sites of subchondral bone oedema and the degree of symptoms has been correlated with the degree of synovial hypertrophy (Felson et al. 2001; Hill et al. 2001). Improved imaging will doubtless lead to better understanding and management of this extremely common condition.

Transient regional osteoporosis

Transient regional osteoporosis is an uncommon, painful condition first described in pregnant women, but more commonly seen in middle-aged men. It is associated with marked demineralization of bone around the hip seen on a plain film associated with preservation of the joint space, a feature that makes septic arthritis perhaps less likely in the presence of severe osteoporosis. The disease is self-limiting and clinical and radiographic changes revert to normal, usually within 6 months. A radioisotope scan will show marked increase in uptake in the femoral head. The MR scan shows decreased marrow signal on T_1-weighted images, but generally increased signal on T_2-weighted studies—changes compatible with marked oedema (Bloem 1988)—and this may be seen, in the presence of a normal radiograph, early on in the disease.

Avascular necrosis

Deprivation of blood supply to cortex and medulla results in marrow cell death. No changes are seen on the plain film in the early phase, but this still has to be obtained to exclude other abnormalities and for a baseline study. The early isotope scan demonstrates photopaenia and subsequently, with repair, will show increased uptake around the abnormal devitalized area corresponding to healing at the zone of creeping substitution. Subsequent radiographs may demonstrate a subcortical crest of lucency which prognosticates structural failure and articular collapse (Fig. 60). The joint space remains intact until secondary osteoarthritis supervenes. The plain film may also subsequently show cyst formation and necrotic bone, which remains dense in the midst of demineralization and resorption.

At MRI, changes in ischaemia precede plain film change, and probably isotope scan changes too (Brower and Kransdorf 1990). Linear or confluent areas of low signal in epiphyses replace bright marrow signal on T_1-weighted images. The linear bands may be subcortical or deep in the bone. The position of the avascular areas can be assessed on axial, sagittal, and coronal slices (Fig. 61).

On T_2-weighted images, the low-signal band often has a parallel adjacent area of increase in signal representing oedema, or even neovascularity.

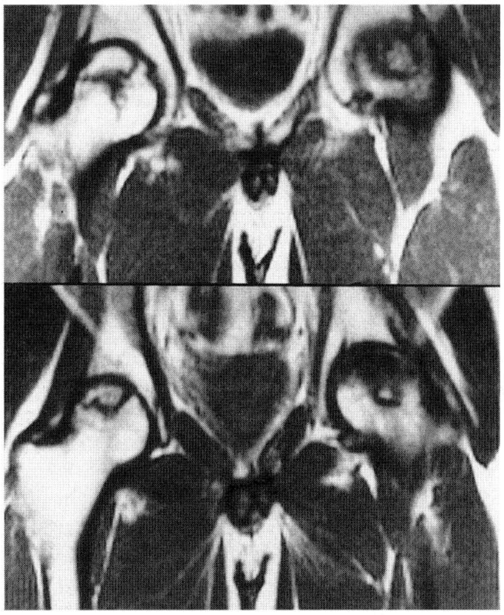

Fig. 61 Avascular necrosis of both femoral heads seen at MR scanning. The areas of low signal are avascular.

It should be noted that even a negative MR scan does not rule out avascular necrosis, as there is a temporal lag between the initial insult and subsequent cell death. Serial studies may be necessary (Mitchell et al. 1986; Beltran et al. 1988).

References

Backhaus, M. et al. (1999). Arthritis of the finger joints. *Arthritis and Rheumatism* **42**, 1232–45.

Beltran, J. et al. (1988). Femoral head avascular necrosis. MR imaging with clinical-pathologic and radionuclide correlation. *Radiology* **166**, 215–20.

Berquist, T.H. (1991). Magnetic resonance techniques in musculoskeletal disease. *Rheumatic Diseases Clinics of North America* **17**, 599–615.

Beuf, O. et al. (2002). Magnetic resonance imaging of normal and osteoarthritic trabecular bone structure in the human knee. *Arthritis and Rheumatism* **46**, 385–93.

Bloem, J.L. (1988). Transient osteoporosis of the hip. MR imaging. *Radiology* **167**, 753–5.

Boini, S. and Guillemin, F. (2001). Radiographic scoring methods as outcome measures in rheumatoid arthritis: properties and advantages. *Annals of the Rheumatic Diseases* **60**, 817–27.

Brandt, J. et al. (2000). Successful treatment of active ankylosing spondylitis with the anti-tumor necrosis factor alpha monoclonal antibody infliximab. *Arthritis and Rheumatism* **43**, 1346–52.

Braun, J., Sieper, J., and Bollow, M. (2000). Imaging of sacroiliitis. *Clinical Rheumatology* **19**, 51–7.

Brook, A. and Corbett, M. (1977). Radiographic changes in early rheumatoid disease. *Annals of the Rheumatic Diseases* **36**, 71–3.

Brower, A.C. and Kransdorf, M.J. (1990). Imaging of hip disorders. *Radiologic Clinics of North America* **28**, 955–74.

Brown, T.R. and Quinn, S.F. (1993). Evaluation of chondromalacia of the patellofemoral compartment with axial magnetic resonance imaging. *Skeletal Radiology* **22**, 325–8.

Buckland-Wright, J.C. (1984). Microfocal radiographic examination of erosions in the wrist and hand of patients with rheumatoid arthritis. *Annals of the Rheumatic Diseases* **43**, 160–71.

Chan, W.P. et al. (1991). Osteoarthritis of the knee. Comparison of radiography, CT and MR imaging to assess extent and severity. *American Journal of Radiology* **157**, 799–806.

Collins, C.D. et al. (1990). The role of discography in lumbar disc disease. Comparative study of magnetic resonance imaging and discography. *Clinical Radiology* **42**, 252–7.

Conaghan, P.G., McGonagle, D., Wakefield, R., and Emery, P. (1999). New approaches to imaging of early rheumatoid arthritis. *Clinical and Experimental Rheumatology* **17**, S37–42.

Cowan, N.C., Bush, K., Katz, D.E., and Gishen, P. (1992). The natural history of sciatica: a prospective radiological study. *Clinical Radiology* **46**, 7–12.

Dacre, J.E. and Buckland-Wright, J.C. (1992). Radiological measures of outcome. *Baillière's Clinical Rheumatology* **6**, 39–67.

Durback, M.A., Edelstein, G., and Schumacher, H.R. (1988). Abnormalities of the sacroiliac joints in diffuse idiopathic skeletal hyperostosis. Demonstration by computed tomography. *Journal of Rheumatology* **15**, 1506–10.

Einig, M., Higger, H.P., Meairs, S., Faust-Tinnefeldt, G., and Kapp, H. (1990). Magnetic resonance imaging of the craniocervical junction in rheumatoid arthritis: value, limitations, indications. *Skeletal Radiology* **19**, 341–6.

Farfan, H.F. *Mechanical Disorders of the Low Back*. Philadelphia PA: Lea and Febiger, 1973.

Felson, D.T. et al. (2001). The association of bone marrow lesions with pain in knee osteoarthritis. *Annals of Internal Medicine* **134**, 541–9.

Ferrell, W.R., Balint, P.V., Egan, C.G., Lockhart, J.C., and Sturrock, R.D. (2001). Metacarpophalangeal joints in rheumatoid arthritis: laser Doppler imaging—initial experience. *Radiology* **220**, 257–62.

Fuerst T., Gluer, C.C., and Genant, H.K. (1995). Quantitative ultrasound. *European Journal of Radiology* **20**, 188–92.

Gibbon, W.W. and Wakefield, R.J. (1999). Ultrasound in inflammatory disease. *Radiologic Clinics of North America* **37**, 633–51.

Goldman, A.B. and Dicarlo, E.F. (1988). Pigmented villonodular synovitis. Diagnosis and differential diagnosis. *Radiologic Clinics of North America* **26**, 1327–47.

Grampp, S. et al. (1997). Comparisons of non-invasive bone mineral measurements in assessing age-related loss, fracture discrimination, and diagnostic classification. *Journal of Bone and Mineral Research* **12**, 697–711.

Griffiths, H.J. *Imaging of the Lumbar Spine*. Gaitherburg MA: Aspen, 1991.

Harris, R.I. and Beath, T. (1948). Aetiology of peroneal spastic flat foot. *Journal of Bone and Joint Surgery* **30B**, 624–34.

Hill, C.L. et al. (2001). Knee effusions, popliteal cysts, and synovial thickening: association with knee pain in osteoarthritis. *Journal of Rheumatology* **28**, 1330–7.

Iannotti, J.P., Zlatkin, M.B., Esterhai, J.L., Kressel, H.Y., Dalinka, M.K., and Spindler, K.P. (1991). Magnetic resonance imaging of the shoulder. *Journal of Bone and Joint Surgery* **73A**, 17–28.

Ireland, J., Trickey, E.L., and Stoker, D.J. (1980). Arthroscopy and arthrography of the knee. *Journal of Bone and Joint Surgery* **62B**, 3–6.

Jamar, F. et al. (2002). Scintigraphy using a technetium 99m-labelled anti-E-selectin Fab fragment in rheumatoid arthritis. *Rheumatology* **41**, 53–61.

Jensen, M.C., Brant-Zawadzki, M.N., Obuchowski, N., Modic, M.T., Malkasian, D., and Ross, J.S. (1994). Magnetic resonance imaging of the lumbar spine in people without back pain. *New England Journal of Medicine* **331**, 69–73.

Jones, M.D., Pais, M.J., and Omiya, B. (1988). Bony overgrowths and abnormal calcifications about the spine. *Radiologic Clinics of North America* **26**, 1213–34.

Kaplan, P.A., Nelson, N.L., Garvin, K.L., and Brown, D.E. (1991). MR of the knee. The significance of high signal in the meniscus that does not clearly extend to the surface. *American Journal of Roentgenology* **156**, 333–6.

Karim, Z. et al. (2001). The impact of ultrasonography on diagnosis and management of patients with musculoskeletal conditions. *Arthritis and Rheumatism* **44**, 2932–5.

Kieft, G.J., Bloem, J.L., Rozing, P.M., and Obermann, W.R. (1988). MR imaging of recurrent anterior dislocation of the shoulder. Comparison with CT arthrography. *American Journal of Roentgenology* **150**, 1083–7.

Lee, J.K., Yao, L., Phelps, C.T., Wirth, C.R., Czajka, J., and Lozman, J. (1988). Anterior cruciate liagment tears. MR imaging compared with arthroscopy and clinical tests. *Radiology* **166**, 861–4.

Lindblom, K. (1939). Arthrography and roentgenography in ruptures of tendons of the shoulder joint. *Acta Radiologica* **20**, 548–62.

Loeuille, D., Olivier, P., Mainard, D., Gillet, P., Netter, P., and Blum, A. (1998). Magnetic resonance imaging of normal and osteoarthritic cartilage. *Arthritis and Rheumatism* **41**, 963–75.

Martel, W., Stuck, K.J., Dworin, A.M., and Hylland, R.G. (1980). Erosive osteoarthritis and psoriatic arthritis. *American Journal of Roentgenology* **134**, 125–35.

McQueen, F.M. et al. (1998). Magnetic resonance imaging of the wrist in early rheumatoid arthritis reveals a high prevalence of erosions at four months after symptom onset. *Annals of the Rheumatic Diseases* **57**, 350–6.

McQueen, F.M. et al. (2001). What is the fate of erosions in early rheumatoid arthritis? Tracking individual lesions using X-rays and magnetic resonance imaging over the first two years of disease. *Annals of the Rheumatic Diseases* **60**, 859–68.

Mink, J.H. and Deutsch, A.L. (1990). The knee. In *MRI of the Musculoskeletal System: A Teaching File* (ed. J.H. Mink and A.L. Deutsch), pp. 251–387. New York: Raven Press.

Mink, J.H., Reicher, M.A., and Crues, J.V. *MRI of the Knee* 2nd edn., pp. 100–3. New York: Raven Press, 1993.

Mitchell, M.D., Kundel, H.L., Steinberg, M.E., Kressel, H.Y., Alavi, A., and Axel, L. (1986). Avascular necrosis of the hip. Comparison of MR, CT and scintigraphy. *American Journal of Roentgenology* **147**, 67–71.

Nixon, J.R. (1987). Basic principles and terminology. In *Magnetic Resonance of the Musculoskeletal System* (ed. T.H. Berquist), pp. 1–12. New York: Raven Press.

O'Brien, J.P. (1984). Mechanisms of spinal pain. In *Textbook of Pain* (ed. P.D. Wall and R. Melzack), pp. 2–13. Edinburgh: Churchill Livingstone.

Østergaard, M. et al. (1999). Magnetic resonance imaging-determined synovial membrane volume as a marker of disease activity and a predictor of progressive joint destruction in the wrists of patients with rheumatoid arthritis. *Arthritis and Rheumatism* **42**, 918–29.

Paavolainen, P. and Ahovuo, J. (1994). Ultrasonography and arthrography in the diagnosis of tears of the rotator cuff. *Journal of Bone and Joint Surgery* **76A**, 335–40.

Peterfy, C.G. (2001). Magnetic resonance imaging of rheumatoid arthritis: the evolution of clinical applications through clinical trials. *Seminars in Arthritis and Rheumatism* **30**, 375–96.

Reece, R.J. et al. (2002). Comparative assessment of leflunomide and methotrexate for the treatment of rheumatoid arthritis, by dynamic enhanced magnetic resonance imaging. *Arthritis and Rheumatism* **46**, 366–72.

Reinig, J., McDevitt, E.R., and Ove, P.N. (1991). Progression of meniscal degenerative changes in college football players. Evaluation with MR imaging. *Radiology* **181**, 255–7.

Renton, P. (1991). Arthrography. In *Surgical Disorders of the Shoulder* (ed. M. Watson), pp. 97–117. Edinburgh: Churchill Livingstone.

Resnick, D., Feingold, M.L., Curd, J., Niwayama, G., and Goergen, T.G. (1977). Calcaneal abnormalities in articular disorders. *Radiology* **125**, 355–66.

Resnick, D., Guerra, J., Jr., Robinson, C.A., and Vint, V.C. (1978). Association of diffuse idiopathic skeletal hyperostosis and calcification and ossification of the posterior longitudinal ligament. *American Journal of Roentgenology* **131**, 1049–53.

Rosenthall, L. (1991). Nuclear medicine techniques in arthritis. *Rheumatic Diseases Clinics of North America* **17**, 585–97.

Rosholm, A., Hyldstrup, L., Bæksgaard. L., Grunkin, G. and Thodberg, H.H. (2001). Estimation of bone mineral density by digital X-ray radiogrammetry: theoretical background and clinical testing. *Osteoporosis International* **12**, 961–9.

Sartoris, D.J. and Resnick, D. (1990). Current and innovative methods for non-invasive bone densitometry. *Radiologic Clinics of North America* **28**, 257–8.

Stoller, D.W. et al. (1987). Meniscal tears. Pathologic correlation with MR imaging. *Radiology* **163**, 731–5.

Sugimoto, H., Takeda, A., Masuyama, J., and Furuse, M. (1996). Early-stage rheumatoid arthritis: diagnostic accuracy of MR imaging. *Radiology* **198**, 185–92.

Tsuyama, N. (1984). Ossification of the posterior longitudinal ligament of the spine. *Clinical Orthopaedics and Related Research* **184**, 71–83.

Van Holsbeeck, M. and Introcaso, J.H. *Musculoskeletal Ultrasound.* St Louis MO: Mosby Year Book, 1991.

Wakefield, R.J. et al. (2000). The value of sonography in the detection of bone erosions in patients with rheumatoid arthritis. *Arthritis and Rheumatism* **43**, 2762–70.

Walther, M., Harms, H., Krenn, V., Radke, S., Faehndrich, T., and Gohlke, F. (2001). Correlation of power Doppler sonography with vascularity of the synovial tissue of the knee joint in patients with osteoarthritis and rheumatoid arthritis. *Arthritis and Rheumatism* **44**, 331–8.

Yun, M., Kim, W., Adam, L.E., Alnafisi, N., Herman, C., and Alavi, A. (2001). F-18 FDG uptage in a patient with psoriatic arthritis: imaging correlation with patient symptoms. *Clinical Nuclear Medicine* **26**, 692–3.

Futher reading

Resnick, D. *Diagnosis of Bone and Joint Disorders* 3rd edn. Philadelphia PA: W.B. Saunders, 1995.

Resnick, D. and Niwayama, G. *Bone and Joint Imaging* 2nd edn. Philadelphia PA: W.B. Saunders, 1989.

Weissman, B.N., ed. (1991). Imaging of rheumatic diseases. *Rheumatic Diseases Clinics of North America* **17**, 457–816.

5.6.2 Imaging in children

G.H. Sebag, Tal Laor, and J.F. Quignodon

Introduction

The use of imaging in paediatric rheumatology reflects the old adage that a child is not a small adult. This chapter will illustrate the specificity of joint imaging in children. Successful imaging in children requires a thorough knowledge of the anatomical variants resulting from growth and development, knowledge of paediatric diseases and their manifestations, and finally the need for radiation protection. Furthermore, in this era of advancing imaging technology, knowledge of the relative values of available imaging techniques is necessary to optimize the management of children with arthritis. The theoretical basis of imaging techniques, including conventional radiography, radionuclide scanning, sonography, computed tomography (CT), and magnetic resonance imaging (MRI) are described in Chapter 5.6.1. Each is being used in paediatric radiology. Changes in individual diseases will be presented in the appropriate section. As in adult radiology, investigations have to be tailored to the individual need of the child, and radiologists and paediatricians must collaborate to ensure that the needs of all are best matched.

Practical considerations

High quality, diagnostic examinations of sick children can be obtained consistently with care, time, and patience. The child's cooperation usually requires an explanation of exactly what is going to happen in language that can be understood. It is also crucial to reassure the parents that the procedure will go smoothly and that they will be informed of the results.

Expertise in immobilizing and imaging children is essential to perform the examination quickly and efficiently. It is important that technologists are trained in the handling of neonates, small infants, and small children. A number of immobilization devices are available; the simplest ones are very efficient (Velcro straps, wooden immobilization boards, bags). Immobilization need not be traumatic to the child. It will allow better positioning for conventional radiography, fluoroscopy, CT, MRI, and radionuclide scanning and make motion much less likely. This will result in less radiation to the child as smaller fields of view can be used and the chance of repeat examinations is reduced. In some cases (especially children under the age of 6 years), it is necessary to use sedation of the child for imaging procedures such as CT and MRI. The choice of drug and route of administration must be made on an individual basis according to the type of examination, the child, the facility, and the experience of the radiologist and the support team (Egelhoff et al. 1997).

Musculoskeletal radiography

The conventional radiograph is almost always the initial imaging technique used in the evaluation of the musculoskeletal system. Its predominance in diagnosing, for example, fractures, bone tumours, congenital dysplasias, metabolic and inflammatory disorders, is confirmed by the fact that it is the only technique needed for most children. It is the most widely available modality and can be obtained more quickly and easily than any other type of imaging (Fig. 1). Conventional radiography plays an important role in localizing and defining the nature of a lesion, especially when the clinical history and physical examination are uncertain or not contributory. This property is especially true in infants and young children who do not localize pain accurately or effectively communicate symptoms to the physician. For example, conventional radiographs are invaluable in the diagnosis of the aetiology of acute or newly discovered limping for which a traumatic cause is not obvious (Blumhagen 1994) (Table 1).

As in adult radiology, conventional radiographs allow grouping of the various arthritides on the basis of the distribution and the pattern of joint space changes (Fig. 2). However, radiological findings, although very important are only one of the criteria by which arthritis is judged to be present and by which a specific diagnosis is established (Ansell 1990). Furthermore, assessment of disease progression (e.g. juvenile chronic arthritis) is made possible by repeating the conventional radiograph. In young children especially, radiographic changes (i.e. joint space narrowing indicative of cartilage loss) represent late and indirect signs of synovial disease.

Technical considerations

Radiation protection must be a priority in children. Proper coning of the X-ray beam, use of high-speed intensifying screens, and the use of gonadal shielding all help reduce exposure. In the assessment of scoliosis, the frontal film is taken from a posterior position in order to reduce breast irradiation, and lateral view radiographs should be kept to the minimum in follow-up evaluation. Other ways of reducing radiation to the patient include the use of digital radiography, if available. Electronic image manipulation permits viewing of segments of the image, adjustment of contrast, and measurement of curve or length. This reduces the need for repeat studies when the initial technique is unsatisfactory. Contrast manipulation allows the enhancement of soft tissue thickening and periarticular fat pad displacement. Evaluation of these structures is especially useful

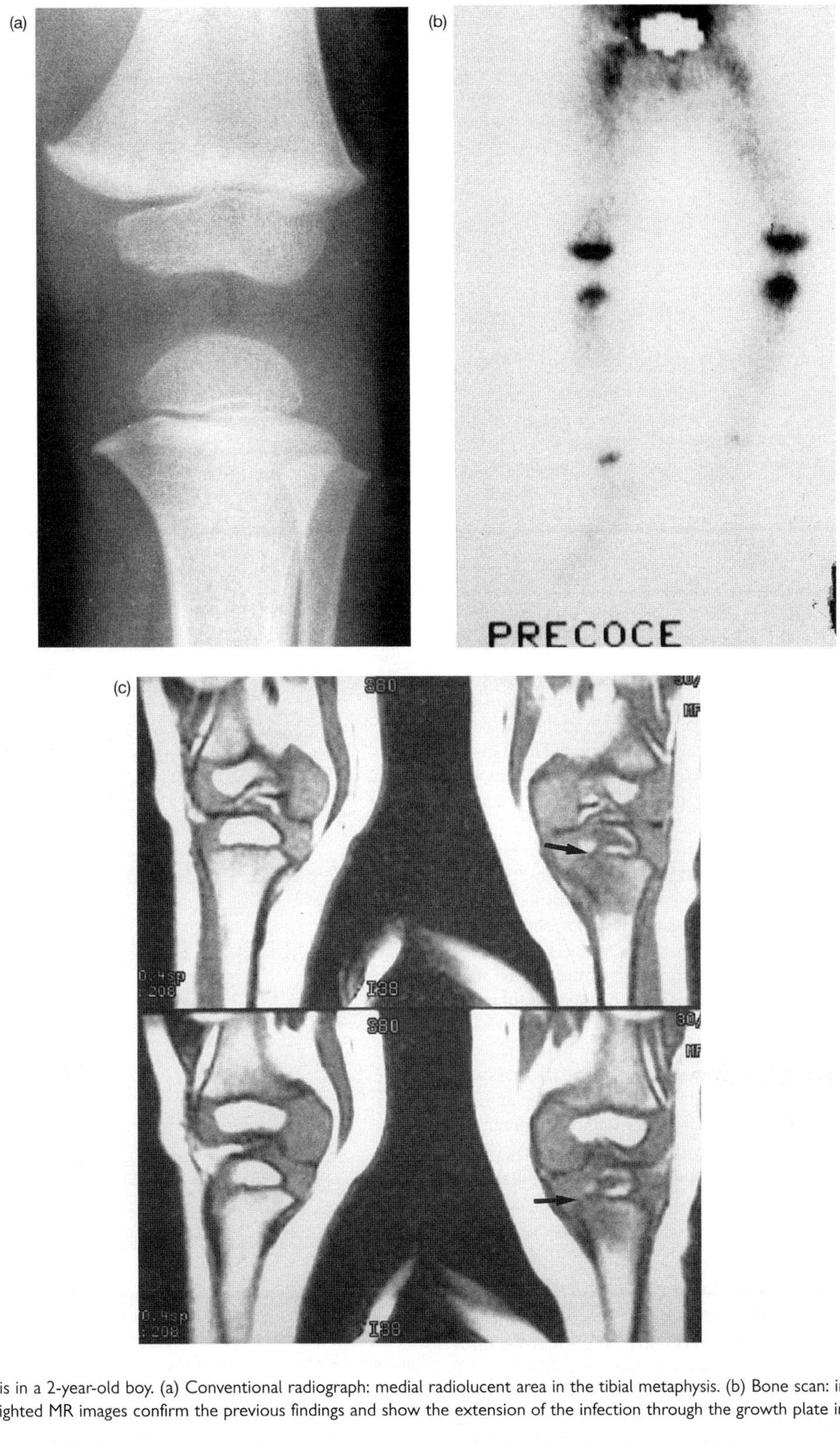

Fig. 1 Acute osteomyelitis in a 2-year-old boy. (a) Conventional radiograph: medial radiolucent area in the tibial metaphysis. (b) Bone scan: increased uptake in the upper left tibia. (c) T_1-weighted MR images confirm the previous findings and show the extension of the infection through the growth plate in the epiphysis (arrow).

in infants and young children. At least two views at right angles, a true frontal and a lateral projection, should be obtained of the involved joint or extremity.

Correct positioning is important for accurate interpretation. A variety of radiographic guidelines (drawing lines, measurements of angle and distance) have been suggested to detect any distortion of the anatomical relationship. Use of guidelines is highly dependent upon proper positioning. For instance, obliquity of the pelvis can result in false interpretation of hip malposition when evaluating an infant for developmental dysplasia of the hip (DDH) (Fig. 3).

Recognition of even minimal pelvic and femoral rotation is necessary to avoid the false-positive results of joint space widening, especially in

Table 1 Common causes of limping in children

Traumatic
Fractures
Stress fractures
Non-accidental trauma
Foreign body
Inflammatory
Transient synovitis
Osteomyelitis
Septic arthritis
Discitis
Soft tissue abscess
Congenital/developmental
Developmental dysplasia of the hip (DDH)
Club foot
Spinal dysraphism
Avascular necrosis and related conditions
Legg–Calve–Perthes' disease
Osteochondrosis
Osteochondritis dissecans
Slipped capital femoral epiphysis
Neoplastic

a painful hip that is held typically in abduction and external rotation (Fig. 4). Unrotated pelvic views show symmetry of obturator foramina and of the medial acetabula as well as alignment of the pubic symphysis with the sacral midline. Joint space widening secondary to the accumulation of fluid in the hip joint has been found to be a more reliable sign in young children and infants. In older children, detecting fluid in the hip joint is best accomplished with sonography.

Frog-leg lateral views (in addition to anteroposterior neutral views) of the hip are mandatory when Legg–Calve–Perthes' disease or a slipped capital femoral epiphysis is suspected. The abnormal anterior subchondral surface of Legg–Calve–Perthes' disease and early posterior slippage are demonstrated better on these views.

In addition, it is useful to obtain comparative views of the normal side, especially in cases where abnormal findings are subtle. It is very useful in the assessment of the shape and size of the ossification centres (normal variants, advanced maturation). However, comparative views are not systematically required, although occasionally these, oblique, or other special views will facilitate a diagnosis. When choosing the right views, one must keep in mind that symptoms in children can be very confusing. For instance, children with discitis can experience symptoms suggesting lower extremity disease (limp, failure to bear weight, referred hip pain) and in this case, a spinal view should be obtained.

Special views include:

- weight-bearing films, bending films,
- flexion views of the cervical spine (C1 to C2 dislocation).

These views are performed to determine whether a joint is stable or not. The C1 to dens distance is normally wider in children (as great as 4–5 mm) than in adults and flexion views are very useful to detect instability.

Growth abnormalities are an important issue in children with rheumatological disease. Epiphyseal overgrowth (caused by hyperaemia), epiphyseal deformities, accelerated ossification with premature fusion of growth plate, and compression fractures lead to malalignment and length discrepancy, especially in unilateral disease. Measurement is an important part in the evaluation of growth abnormalities. It includes estimation of valgus and varus angles, leg-length discrepancy, spinal curvature, femoral anteversion, and tibial torsion amongst others. Tables, charts, and graphs of standard measurements have been widely published and are referred to daily by practising orthopaedists and radiologists (Pettersson and Ringertz 1991; Ozonoff 1992). The use of these measurements correlated with the patient's skeletal age at each determination allows a prediction of future growth and effect and timing of surgery to be made (Pettersson and Ringertz 1991; Ozonoff 1992).

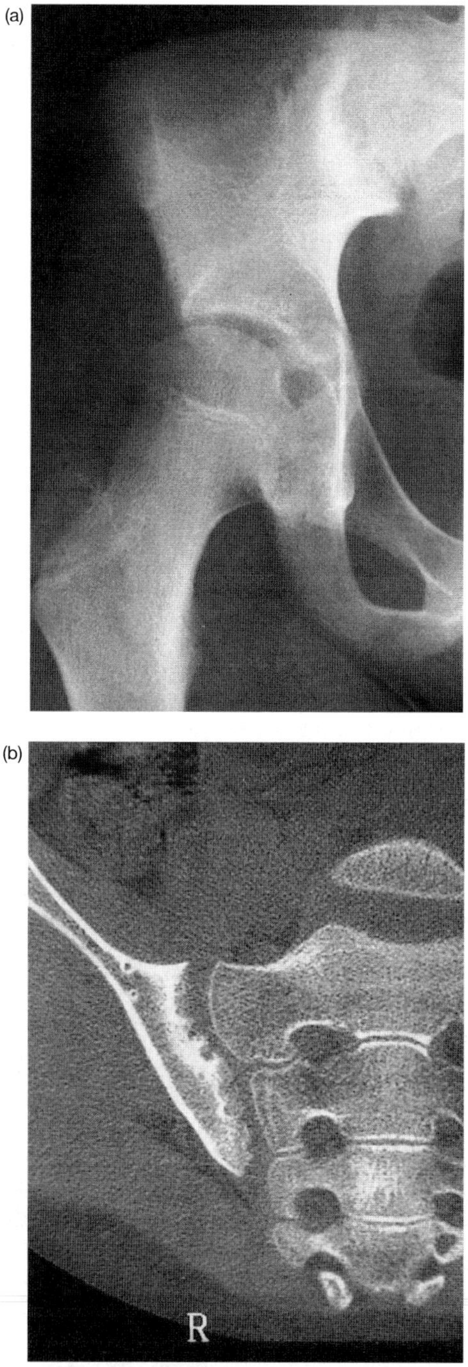

Fig. 2 Juvenile spondyloarthropathy in an 11-year-old boy. (a) Conventional radiograph: lateral subluxation of the femoral head with superolateral narrowing of the joint space. Sclerosis of the sacroiliac joint. (b) CT: sclerosis, irregularity, and erosion of the sacroiliac joint.

General growth abnormalities are influenced by the disease (type, onset, and duration), immobilization, and steroid therapy which lead to growth delay. Skeletal age assignment is the most common evaluation. After 1 year of age, the number, shape, and stage of development of the epiphyses in the left hand and wrist are compared with standards for various ages up to the time of epiphyseal fusion; the atlas of Greulich and Pyle (1959) is normally used. In addition, spinal growth in scoliosis can be estimated using Risser's method (Risser 1948) by assessing iliac crest development on the frontal view of the entire spine.

Osteoporosis, induced, for example, by immobilization and steroid therapy, can be assessed on conventional radiography both in the appendicular and axial skeleton. Measurement of the cortical thickness of tubular bones is commonly performed (in metacarpals and tibia for instance).

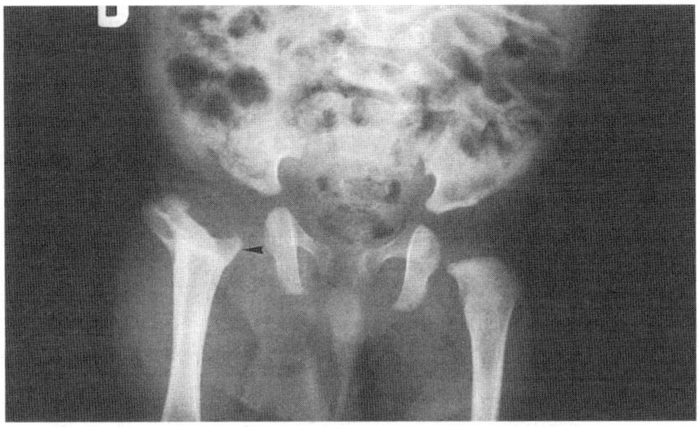

Fig. 3 Septic arthritis in a 4-month-old baby with dislocation of the left hip. Conventional radiograph shows lateral displacement of the femoral head and new bone formation.

(a)

(b)

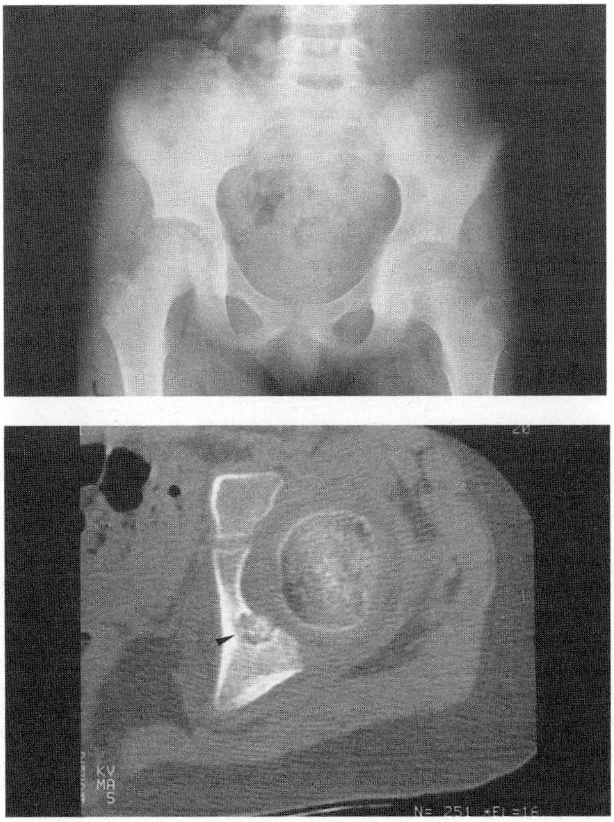

Fig. 4 Osteoid osteoma affecting the left hip in a 9-year-old boy. (a) Conventional radiograph: left hip effusion with severe osteoporosis. (b) CT scan: localizes the site of nidus in the acetabulum.

Evaluation of musculoskeletal changes on conventional radiography

Proper interpretation of conventional radiography is pivotal in directing further diagnostic evaluation that can be both complex and expensive in children. One should use a systemic approach to analyse conventional radiographs. For example:

- joint space (widening, narrowing, malalignment, ankyloses, calcification, gas) (Figs 1 and 4);
- soft tissues (obliterated or displaced fat pads, calcification, ossification opacities, thickening and reticulation, tendon width changes) (Figs 5 and 6);
- bone density (increased or decreased, generalized or localized);
- epiphysis (shape, size, subchondral bone, defect, erosion);
- metaphysis (transverse bands, widening, cupping, destruction);
- growth plate;
- diaphysis (cortical bone, periosteal reaction, tubulation).

By grouping the findings and using the complete range of the common causes of these findings, one can narrow the differential diagnosis (Swischuk et al. 1993) (Tables 2–9). This practical approach allows a proper interpretation of conventional radiography, especially for clinicians or radiologists who practise paediatric rheumatology only occasionally.

Finally, knowledge of the normal is a prerequisite for recognition of the abnormal. Familiarity with appearances at the various ages of development is learned by experience but considerable help may be gained from

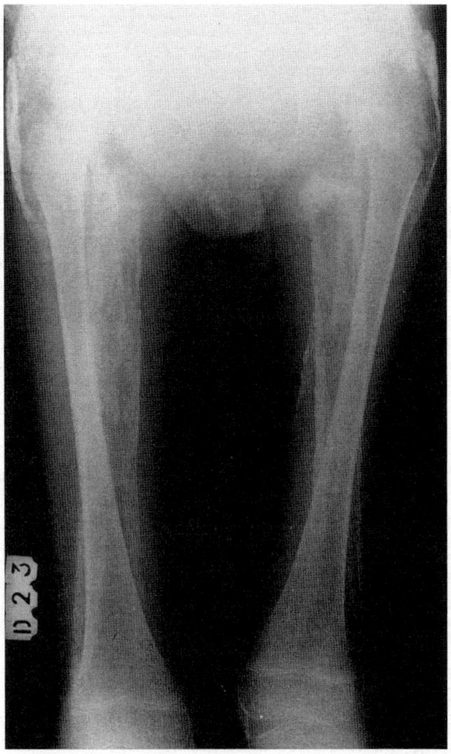

Fig. 5 Dermatomyositis in a 7-year-old girl. Conventional radiograph of extensive calcinosis in the subcutaneous tissue and in the muscles.

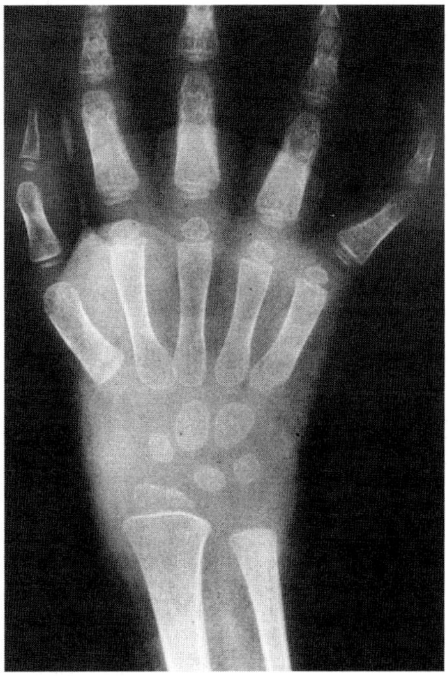

Fig. 6 Juvenile chronic arthritis in a 4-year-old boy at the early stage. Conventional radiograph of the wrist shows marked soft tissue swelling.

Table 2 Joint space widening

Traumatic effusion and/or dislocation
Septic arthritis (hip, shoulder)
Transient synovitis (hip)
Legg–Calve–Perthes' disease
Developmental dysplasia of the hip
Juvenile chronic arthritis
Bleeding disorders
Joint laxity (neuromuscular) (Larsen syndrome, Ehlers–Danlos syndrome)
Collagen vascular disease
Pigmented villonodular synovitis
Synovial tumour
Synovial osteochondromatosis
Winchester–Grossman syndrome

Table 3 Joint space narrowing

Septic arthritis
Juvenile chronic arthritis
Haemophilic arthropathy
Degenerative arthritis (long-term complication of Legg–Calve–Perthes' disease, avascular necrosis, trauma)
Slipped capital femoral epiphysis (post-operative)
Pigmented villonodular synovitis
Idiopathic chondrolysis

Table 4 Transverse radiolucent metaphyseal band

Prematurity
Severe illness, trauma
Leukaemia, lymphoma
Metastasis (neuroblastoma)
Neonatal infections (toxoplasmosis, syphilis, cytomegalovirus, rubella)
Scurvy
Hypermagnesaemia
Cushing's syndrome
Hypervitaminosis D
Osteogenesis imperfecta
Idiopathic juvenile osteoporosis

Table 5 Epiphyseal defect

Normal variants
Osteochondritis dissecans
Osteochondral avulsion
Juvenile chronic arthritis
Haemophilic arthritis
Septic arthritis (tuberculosis, fungus, pyogenic)
Epiphyseal osteomyelitis
Langerhans cell histiocytosis (LCH)
Tumours (synovial, chondroblastoma metastases)

Table 6 Periarticular calcifications

Collagen disease (dermatomyositis)
Trauma
Infection
Hypervitaminosis D and A
Hyperparathyroidism
Tumoural calcinosis

Table 7 Intra-articular calcifications

Traumatic avulsion
Osteochondritis dissecans
Idiopathic (in hips of infant after taps)
Synovial tumours
Synovial inflammation
Synovial chondromatosis
Oxalosis
Ochronosis

Table 8 Diffuse decreased bone density

Rickets (privational, vitamin D resistant)
Osteogenesis imperfecta
Mucopolysaccharidosis
Hypophosphatasia
Renal osteodystrophy
Malabsorption disorders
Disuse (immobilization, neuromuscular)
Haematological disorders (malignant, haemolytic anaemia)
Endocrinological disorders (Cushing's disease)
Steroid therapy

Table 9 Periosteal bone reaction

Fracture Trauma Pathological Battered child
Infection Osteomyelitis Neonatal infection (syphilis)
Infarction
Bleeding disorders
Caffey's disease
Metabolic Rickets Prematurity Scurvy Hypervitaminosis D and A Thyroid acropachy
Storage disease Gaucher's disease Mucolipidosis
Tumours Metastasis Leukaemia-lymphoma Primary malignant (sarcomas) Benign Langerhans cell histiocytosis Soft tissue tumour
Vascular malformation (soft tissue or intra-osseous)
Osteoarthropathy
Prostaglandin E treatment
Juvenile chronic arthritis

atlases both of normal variants and of normal development at different ages (Keats 1991; Swischuk et al. 1993). The following poiknts should be borne in mind:

1. the bone-within-bone appearance: most commonly seen in the spine in newborns and premature infants;
2. symmetrical periosteal new bone seen in normal neonates up to about 6 months of age, especially in the femoral diaphysis;
3. transverse sclerotic lines in the metaphysis (growth recovery lines);
4. irregular ossification centre seen especially in the medial aspect of the lower femoral epiphysis;
5. fibrous cortical defect occurring particularly around the knee and located in the superficial bony cortex;
6. gas in the joint: the 'vacuum' joint effect commonly seen in the shoulders and the hips of infants.

Role of conventional radiography in the management of children with musculoskeletal disease

Diagnostic study

Conventional radiographs provide crucial information in the early stages of diagnosing disease in children (Jacobs 1982; Swischuk 1994; Thomas et al. 1994) (Figs 1, 2, 4, and 7). For instance, in cases of non-specific clinical presentation (such as limp, failure to bear weight, joint pain, back pain) the findings of conventional radiography can be straightforward:

1. stress and pathological fractures (Figs 8–10);
2. transverse radiolucent metaphyseal band and osteolysis in metastatic neuroblastoma or leukaemia (Figs 11 and 12);
3. joint effusion, subluxation of the femoral head with or without bone destruction in infant with septic arthritis of the hip (Fig. 3);
4. posterior slippage of the femoral head indicative of slipped capital femoral epiphysis (Fig. 13);
5. disc narrowing with indistinct vertebral endplate indicative of spondylodiscitis;
6. small subchondral fragment within a defect in the medial femoral condyle indicative of osteochondritis dissecans of the knee;
7. small crescentic subchondral lucency of the femoral head on the frog-leg view indicative of Legg–Calve–Perthes' disease.

Furthermore, in the imaging evaluation of bone tumours or tumour-like disorders, conventional radiographs are pivotal in directing further investigations. Conventional radiographs are very often sufficient to separate lesions into two categories:

1. those that may be left alone, such as:
   (a) non-ossifying fibroma,
   (b) fibrous dysplasia,
   (c) chondroid lesions (Fig. 14),
   (d) myositis ossificans,
   (e) tumorous calcinosis,
   (f) bone cysts,
   (g) Langerhans cell histiocytosis (LCH) (Fig. 15);
2. those that require intervention such as biopsy:
   (a) malignant lesions (sarcoma),
   (b) complicated lesions,
   (c) undetermined lesions.

It is important that developmental variations and benign lesions are not mistaken for malignancy. It is equally important that the diagnosis of malignancy is not delayed.

A skeletal survey or bone sonography is often required to establish if the lesion is solitary or polyostotic (LCH, fibrous dysplasia, malignancy) and to guide an eventual biopsy to the optimal site (Figs 11, 12, and 15).

Chest films are often required in childhood rheumatic diseases. A frontal chest film is obtained most frequently. Pleural effusion and lymph node enlargement may be detected on a lateral film. Chest films are performed to rule out any pulmonary nodules, cavities or infiltrate, pleural effusion, mediastinal and/or hilar lymph node enlargement, and cardiomegaly

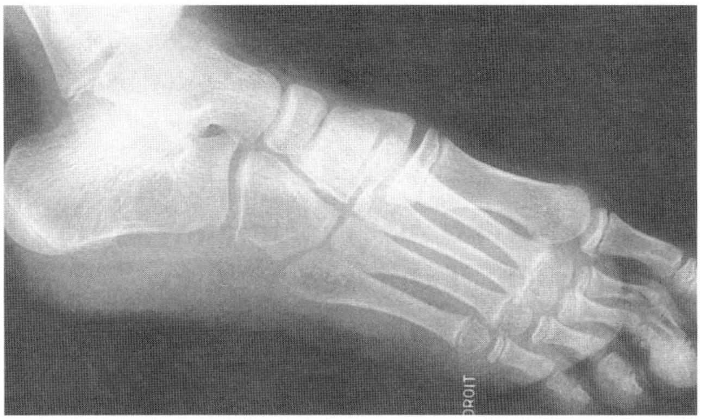

Fig. 7 Talocalcaneal coalition in a 10-year-old boy with foot pain.

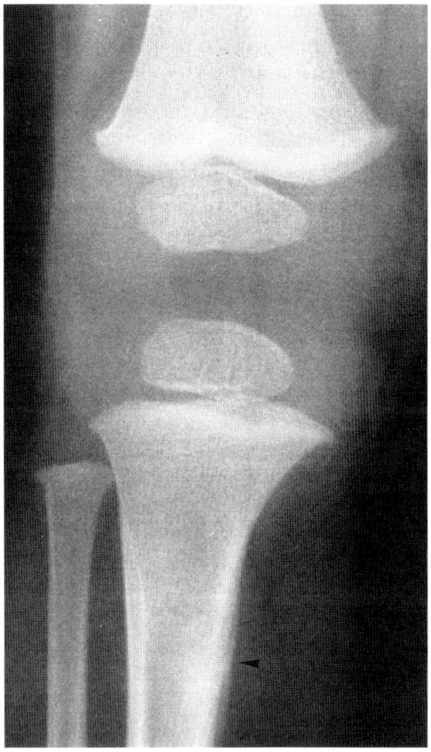

Fig. 8 Stress fracture in a 5-year-old boy. Area of increased sclerosis and periosteal bone deposition in the upper tibia.

(pericardial fluid, cardiac failure, myocarditis). Chest films are indicated especially in systemic juvenile chronic arthritis, systemic lupus erythematosus, scleroderma, dermatomyositis, Kawasaki disease, systemic vasculitis, sarcoidosis, rheumatic fever, the occurrence of a positive tuberculin test, or if otherwise clinically required.

Follow-up study

Conventional radiography is of major importance in evaluating disease progression and/or the effect of treatment in paediatric rheumatology in a reproducible and standardized manner (Jacobs 1982) (Figs 2, 6, and 16). In the literature, various methods of radiographic grading system have been proposed, especially in juvenile chronic arthritis and haemophilic arthritis

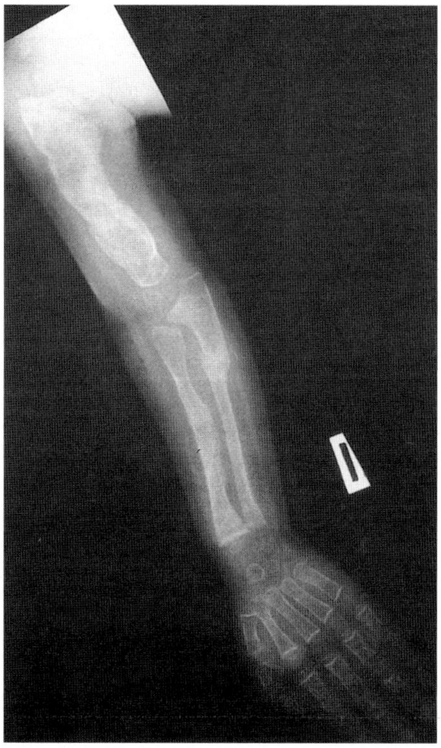

Fig. 9 Pathological fractures in a 2-year-old boy with osteogenesis imperfecta. Conventional radiograph shows multiple fractures, diffuse decreased bone density, and transverse radiolucent metaphyseal bands.

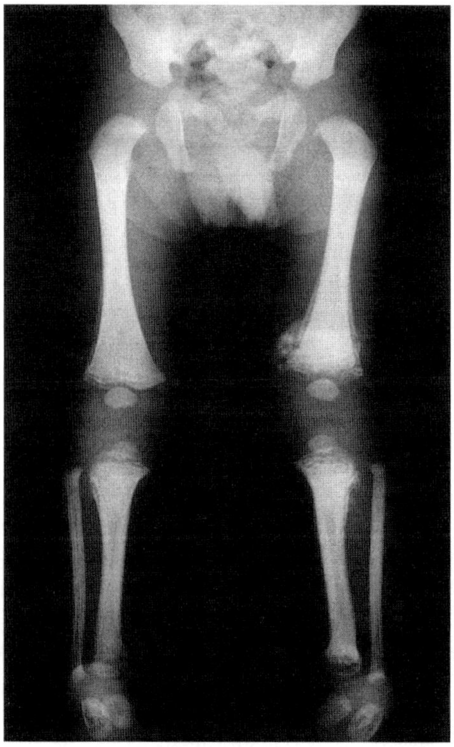

Fig. 10 Child abuse in a 4-month-old baby refusing to move his left limb. Conventional radiograph shows bilateral metaphyseal corner fractures at different stages of healing.

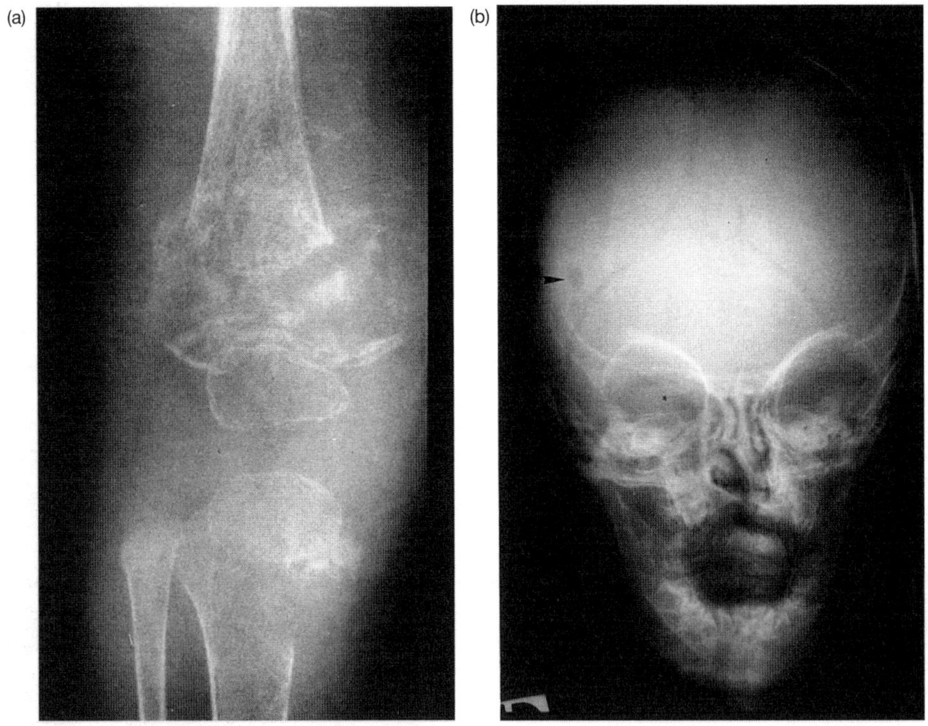

Fig. 11 Metastatic neuroblastoma in a 2-year-old boy with intense knee pain. (a) Radiograph of the knee. Extensive osteolysis and periosteal bone reaction. (b) Radiograph of the skull. Osteolytic area in the right parietal bone.

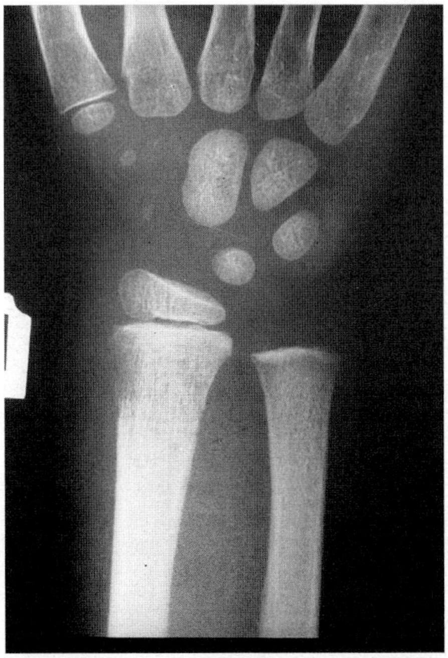

Fig. 12 Acute leukaemia in a 7-year-old-boy with wrist pain. Distal metaphyseal destruction of the cubitus on conventional radiography.

(Pettersson et al. 1980; Pettersson and Rydholm 1984). Grading systems in adult rheumatology (such as the Steinbrocker method of evaluation of rheumatoid arthritis) have not been adapted for paediatric rheumatology (Steinbrocker et al. 1949).

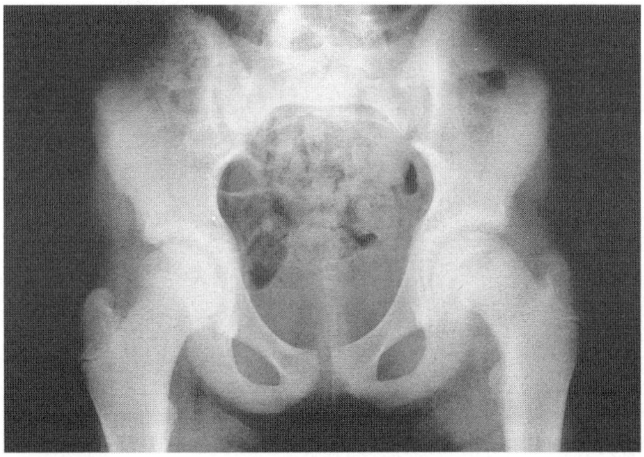

Fig. 13 Slipped capital femoral epiphysis in an 11-year-old boy.

In children, less attention is paid to the loss of joint space. The reason is that estimating the joint space in children (especially young) is difficult because of:

- the thickness of the epiphyseal cartilage,
- weight-bearing difficulties on the painful joint,
- projectional error associated with flexion and/or valgus deformity,
- joint space loss (often late and/or less prominent feature).

In children, scoring systems pay much attention to growth abnormality (Dale et al. 1994) (Table 10). In juvenile chronic arthritis, a radiographic

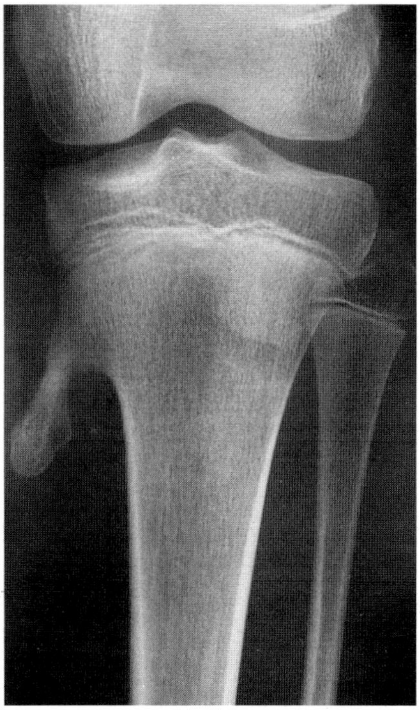

Fig. 14 Exostosis in a 13-year-old girl with a medial mass of the knee.

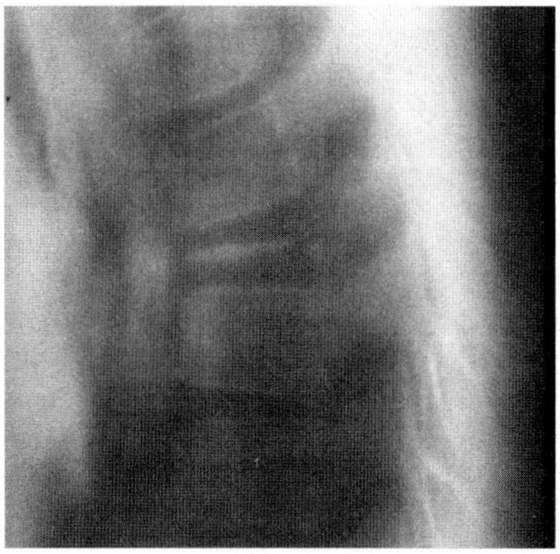

Fig. 15 LCH in a 7-year-old boy with typical vertebra plana.

classification system is often applied to the knee, which is the most commonly affected joint in childhood (Tables 10 and 11).

Pettersson and Rydholm (1984) proposed radiological scoring of the knee joint destruction in juvenile chronic arthritis by dividing the joint into three separate compartments (i.e. femur, tibia, and patella). Each of the bones participating in the articulation is examined for signs of osteoporosis, enlargement, erosions, subchondral cysts, and deformity of the joint surface. The presence or the absence of these parameters in the joint is allotted 1 or 0 points, respectively (Table 11). This scoring method has a very significant correlation with the clinical status. Unfortunately, radiographic findings are seen in later stages of disease activity.

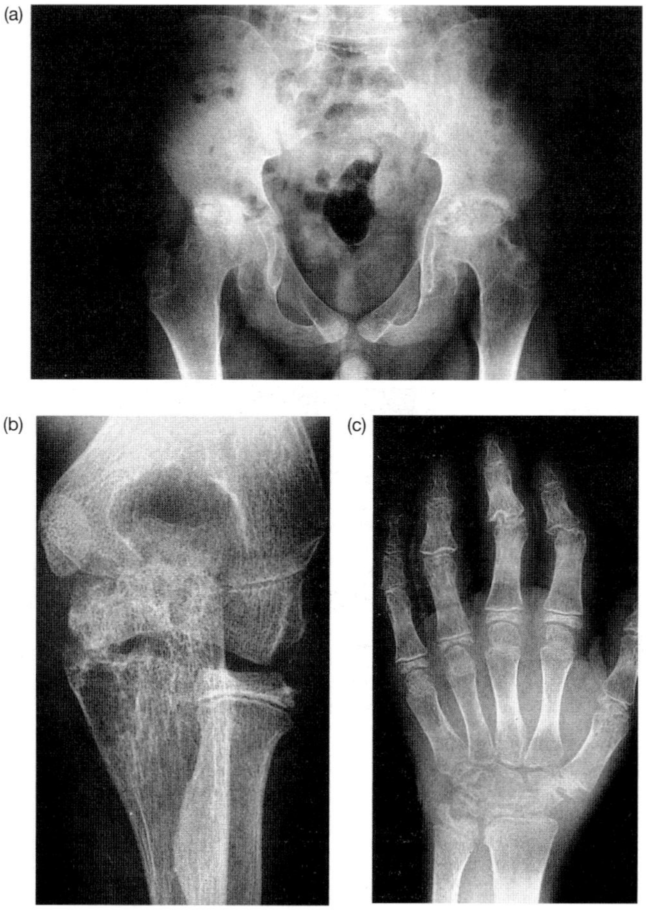

Fig. 16 Juvenile chronic arthritis in a 12-year-old girl with severe destructive abnormalities on the conventional radiography of the (a) hips, (b) elbow, and (c) wrist and hand.

Table 10 Radiological grading system applied to the knee in juvenile chronic arthritis (Dale et al. 1994)

Grade 0: normal condition
Grade I: slight abnormality Juxta-articular osteoporosis ± joint effusion
Grade II: growth abnormality Epiphyseal, patellar overgrowth
Grade III: destructive abnormality Overgrowth + marginal bony erosions ± malalignment
Grade IV: severe destructive abnormality Marginal bony erosions Epiphyseal deformations Malalignment
Grade V: mutilating abnormality Pronounced alignment changes and destruction Bony ankylosis

Finally, evaluation of complications of disease and treatment is commonly performed by looking for delayed bone age, decreased bone density, local growth abnormalities, compression fractures, avascular osteonecrosis, and instability of the cervical spine.

Table 11 Radiological scoring of knee destruction in juvenile chronic arthritis (Petterson and Rydholm 1984)

	Femur	Tibia	Patella
Osteoporosis	0–1	0–1	0–1
Enlargement of epiphysis or patella	0–1	0–1	0–1
Erosion	0–1	0–1	0–1
Subchondral cyst deformation	0–1	0–1	0–1
Deformed joint surfaces	0–1	0–1	0–1
Score	0–5	0–5	0–5
Total score		0–15	

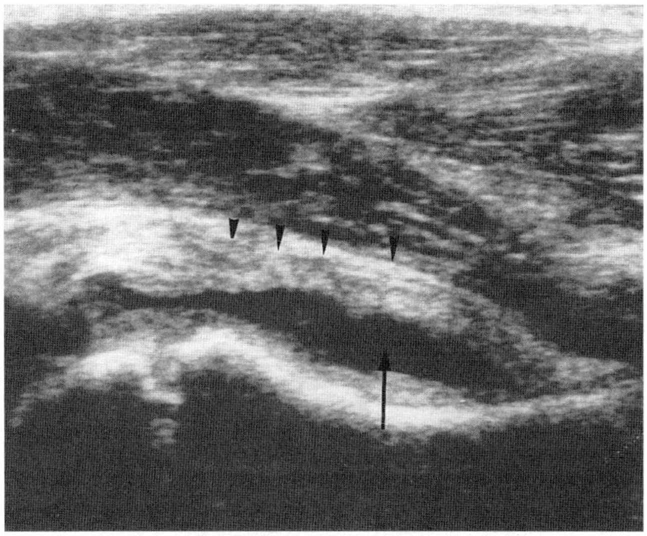

Fig. 17 Fluid in the hip joint. Sonography shows anterior accumulation of fluid (arrow) with distension of the joint capsule and synovial thickening (arrowhead).

Doppler sonography

Doppler sonography use has expanded greatly for the musculoskeletal system and has become a primary imaging tool for many aspects of paediatric rheumatology. In infants and young children, sonography shows the cartilaginous forms of bones that cannot be visualized with conventional radiography. Use of Doppler sonography continues to increase as resolution of the equipment improves and anatomic structures become more easily identified with high frequency transducers (5–13 MHz). Sonography is widely available, safe, non-ionizing, and non-invasive, easily accepted by children, and can be performed at the bedside, in intensive care, or in a neonatal unit. Sonography also allows dynamic stress examination of the hip joint.

Colour and pulsed Doppler facilitate identification of vascular anomalies. With the advent of power Doppler, visualization of femoral head vascularization is achievable consistently in newborns and shows promise in the detection of occlusion of feeding nutrient vessels (septic arthritis, congenital dislocation of the hip) (Plate 73). Therefore, in some particular conditions, sonography has become the primary imaging study performed, especially in the hip, replacing conventional radiography. The early detection of DDH or dislocation allows prompt treatment and is the key to successful management. By treating this condition at a young age, most of the sequelae that occur when DDH goes unrecognized can be avoided.

Clinical screening programmes have been instituted for all neonates. The use of imaging has been allied closely with programmes for detection and treatment. In the newborn period, conventional radiography are unreliable since the key structures of the hip are composed of cartilage.

On sonographic images the cartilaginous components of the acetabulum and femoral head can be distinguished from other soft tissue structures. Real-time sonography permits multiplanar evaluation that clearly defines femoral head dislocation in relation to the acetabulum. The ability to observe changes in hip position with movement is a further advantage of sonography. The benefits of using sonography in the diagnosis and management of DDH have been widely reported (Graf 1983; Harcke 1994; Harcke and Walter 1995; Grissom and Harcke 1999).

Variations in technique exist and, regardless of the method used, sufficient experience with both normal and abnormal hips should be gained. Initial assessment should be performed at approximately 4–6 weeks of age. In most cases, referral for initial assessment is a questionable or abnormal physical examination or presence of an increased risk factor (firstborns, breech position, oligohydramnios, family history, congenital torticollis, foot deformities). From a posterolateral approach, sonography can be used to assess hip position after application of an abduction splint.

Sonography is very useful in the detection of joint effusion especially in the hip, which is commonly evaluated in children. The common indications are the child with a limp who refuses to bear weight on the limb, and suspicion of septic arthritis in newborns or infants. Thus, the crucial question is whether or not the hip is involved and specifically whether there is fluid in the hip joint. The examination of the hip is quick and within minutes anterior accumulation of fluid with joint capsule distension can be detected (Fig. 17). It is more important to rely on the configuration and shape than on absolute measurements echotexture or Doppler tracing (Strouse et al. 1998). Furthermore, comparison with the opposite hip is always helpful unless bilateral effusions are present.

The use of sonography is simple and more sensitive than conventional radiography (reported sensitivity range: 88–100 per cent) (Marchal et al. 1987). However, the nature of a joint effusion cannot be assessed accurately. We do not attempt to distinguish the different types of fluid and defer to the clinicians for determination of which effusions should be tapped (Zawin et al. 1993).

In the knee, sonography can be used for evaluation of synovial hypertrophy, (Lamer and Sebag 2000) detection of cysts, and exclusion of popliteal thrombosis (Fig. 18) (Grobbelaar and Bouffard 2000). In contrast, conventional radiographs are not helpful in differentiating synovial effusions from synovial thickening. The distinction is easy with sonography where synovial thickening appears as an irregular echogenic area surrounding the effusion (Fig. 17). Unfortunately, in chronic arthritis (such as juvenile chronic arthritis), sonography does not permit a reliable detection of joint loculation, which might make intra-articular injection of steroid difficult.

Cartilage erosions and thinning can be detected (Sureda et al. 1994). However, the whole surface of cartilage cannot be assessed. Sonography does provide an objective method for observing disease course during therapy (Eich et al. 1994; Sureda et al. 1994).

Power Doppler also shows promise in evaluating the amount and the activity of pannus in juvenile chronic arthritis. Proliferative synovium, which is extremely vascular, shows high power Doppler signal (Plate 74).

Finally, in a child presenting with a swollen red extremity, Doppler sonography can be very useful by distinguishing:

- fluid collection (sub-periosteal, abscess, bursitis),
- thrombophlebitis (Plate 75),
- non-opaque foreign body,
- vascular malformation,

and guiding a needle for aspiration or catheter for drainage of fluid collection.

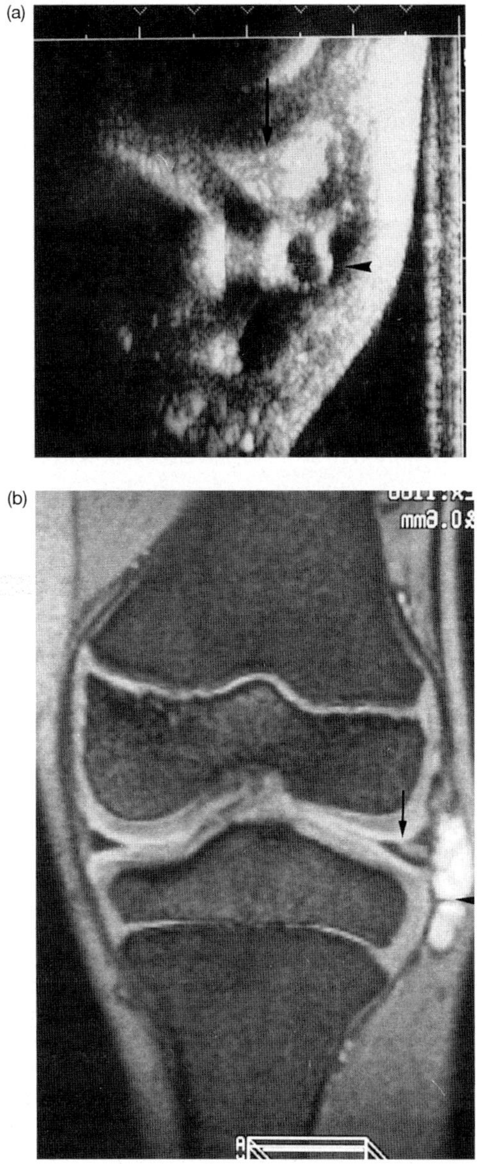

Fig. 18 Meniscal cyst in an 8-year-old boy with knee pain and medial mass. (a) Sonography shows a cystic mass (arrowhead) adjacent to the medial meniscus (arrow). (b) Frontal T_2-weighted MR image shows a torn medial meniscus (arrow) and a meniscal cyst (arrowhead).

Sonography can be employed easily in the initial evaluation and subsequent follow-up of soft tissue haemorrhage in trauma and bleeding disorders.

Abdominal sonography can demonstrate peritoneal, pleural, and pericardial effusion, and hepatosplenomegaly in systemic juvenile chronic arthritis.

Echocardiography can demonstrate coronary aneurysms in Kawasaki disease or cardiac involvement in rheumatic fever.

Pulsed and colour Doppler can be useful in systemic vasculitis (Plate 74).

Arthrography and myelography

The use of arthrography and CT arthrotomography has decreased dramatically over the past few years in most paediatric practices because of the increasing availability of MRI and of arthroscopy. Arthrography requires general anaesthesia in young children and sedation in older children. The advantage of arthrography over CT and MRI is that it provides a dynamic study and depicts joints as they move. Hip arthrography is still an important test for assessing femoral head containment and assessing incongruity between the femoral head and the acetabulum (DDH, Legg–Calve–Perthes' disease). It is an excellent tool in the operating room where it gives the surgeon an opportunity to visualize key relationships as the position of head is changed. It is a valuable aid for performing closed reduction in DDH and for guiding femoral or pelvic osteotomy in Legg–Calve–Perthes' disease. Finally, arthrography is performed occasionally in the detection of non-opaque loose bodies and the evaluation of articular surface irregularities.

Myelography has been widely replaced in children by CT and MRI, which are presently the first examinations to be performed. However, myelography is still very useful in the assessment of the cord in a few situations:

1. severe spinal deformities (spinal malformations, dysraphism, severe scoliosis) in which the interpretation of planar MRI or CT images is very difficult;
2. surgical metallic spinal fixation in which the hardware creates CT and MR artefacts;
3. spinal instability (spondylolisthesis, spondylolysis) in which erect or dynamic films are crucial.

Angiography

In children, angiography is used only occasionally because of its invasive aspect and the low incidence of collagen vascular disease. In its place, non-invasive, vascular imaging modalities such as pulsed and colour Doppler sonography, CT angiography, and magnetic resonance angiography are now widely available. Multiple modalities can be performed including arteriography, phlebography, and direct percutaneous injection. Highly selective studies are now possible in infants using digital subtraction angiography, low osmolar contrast, and small catheters. Arteriography infrequently is indicated in the planning of resection of musculoskeletal tumours and can demonstrate neovascularity, displacement, encasement, or occlusion of major vessels.

Pre-operative chemotherapy or embolization can be performed on children with sarcoma or an aneurysmal bone cyst. It also makes surgical procedure easier and less vascular. Therapeutic angiography can be particularly helpful in the management of synovial vascular malformation. Angiography cannot distinguish between malignant and benign disease. Cardiac angiography is indicated in Kawasaki disease to detect coronary aneurysms. Arteriography of the aorta and major arteries is useful in the evaluation of vasculitis, especially Takayasu's arteritis. However, MRI is now frequently performed.

Balloon dilatation can be an effective treatment of arterial stenosis in Takayasu's arteritis. Phlebocavography is also very effective in the detection of thrombophlebitis and collateral flow in children at risk (Behçet's syndrome, coagulation disorders, lupus).

Radionuclide studies

Imaging the skeleton with bone-seeking radionuclide tracers offers the major advantage of high sensitivity in the detection of early pathological osseous changes in the entire skeleton. In children, scintigraphy with bone-seeking and inflammatory agents, is the primary investigation to survey the skeleton for multifocal disease such as infection and malignancy (Fig. 1). Scintigraphy also provides critical information for the evaluation of musculoskeletal pain when conventional radiographs are unrevealing. Disadvantages of bone scintigraphy are the lack of specificity and the poor spatial resolution. Correlating the results of a radionuclide study with information from other imaging techniques helps to overcome the lack of specificity inherent with this technique. The amount of radiation exposure during bone scintigraphy depends upon the radionuclide used and the dose administered. Children receive a portion of the adult dose calculated on the basis of body weight. The total body exposure from a technetium-99m bone study is comparable with that from a radiographic skeletal survey. Target organs such as the bladder and growth plates receive increased exposure. For bone scanning, the most commonly used and practical radio-pharmaceutical in paediatrics is a phosphate compound labelled with technetium-99m.

The diagnostic accuracy of bone scintigraphy is closely related to the quality of the study. A technetium-99m bone scan is one of the most technically demanding nuclear imaging procedures. As with radiographs, meticulous attention should be given to positioning children for scintigraphic images. Positioning without rotation is essential. Homologous bones and joints must be shown with mirror-image positioning to allow careful comparison and detection of subtle asymmetry. Immobilization and/or sedation may be required. High-resolution techniques, using pinhole collimator views, are necessary to resolve small or subtle abnormalities that occur near the intense metabolic activity of the bone of the growing metaphyses of young children. Long scanning times from 10 to 15 min per pinhole collimator view are required to obtain sufficient count density.

In general, images of the entire skeleton should be obtained even when symptoms are localized to a single site. This rule allows the recognition of unsuspected asymptomatic skeletal lesions. Pinhole views are used to resolve adequately the metaphyses, the epiphyses, and regions of the skeleton that are of specific clinical or radiological interest. Most false-negative diagnoses are secondary to metaphyseal lesions (osteomyelitis, corner fractures, and metastases). Familiarity with the scintigraphic appearance of the normal growth zone is necessary to detect subtle abnormalities in this region. The shape of the area of increased activity of the growth zone varies with age. In children of less than 18 months, the growth zone has an ovoid or elliptical form. After the age of 2 years, the growth zone is represented by a transverse linear band of increased activity that is always flat or slighty convex in the direction of the diaphysis. Moderate or marked convexity of this margin is abnormal. At all ages, the demarcation of the growth zone activity from the diaphysis is sharp.

Recent advances in nuclear radiology have improved the scintigraphic evaluation of musculoskeletal disease in children. A new generation of single-photon emission computed tomography (SPECT) cameras can demonstrate subtle lesions that are undetectable by planar scintigraphy. State of the art SPECT systems feature multiple camera heads in a fixed ring design. More powerful post-processing has led to faster image reconstruction including sagittal, axial, and coronal planes and three-dimensional views. In paediatrics, SPECT has been particularly useful in the evaluation of the femoral heads for Legg–Calve–Perthes' disease, and in the evaluation of the lumbar spine for posterior element lesions (usually defects of the pars interarticularis). In a study of 162 young patients presenting with back pain, SPECT demonstrated posterior element stress injury in 44 per cent, from which planar scintigraphy was abnormal in 20 per cent (Bellah et al. 1991).

Demonstration of occult fractures and sports injuries has increased in children with the use of bone scanning. Scintigraphic abnormalities, particularly of the tarsus and calcaneus, thought to reflect occult stress fracture, have been found in pre-school children with unexplained lower extremity pain and normal radiographs (Englaro et al. 1992).

Bone scanning is useful in the evaluation of soft tissue and bone infection. Three phases bone scan is useful in the febrile infant or toddler when localization of infection can be difficult or in the older child with focal but non-specific complaints (Fig. 1). As in adults, scintigraphy helps to distinguish a purely soft tissue infection from infection with bone involvement and to differentiate acute bone infarcts from acute osteomyelitis in children with sickle cell anaemia.

Leucocyte scans, using autologous cells labelled with indium-111 or technetium-99m detect osteomyelitis with high sensitivity (Lawson et al. 1994). The use of leucocyte scans in paediatrics is more limited because of the moderately high radiation dose to the spleen. Leucocyte bone scans can be considered for children in whom the identification of a source of infection is critical and who can tolerate the removal of at least 20 ml of blood.

Other pharmaceuticals including polyclonal IgG, monoclonal antigranulocyte antibodies, and IgG fragments can be used to detect inflammation (Oyen et al. 1992). A major advantage of these agents is the ease of preparation compared with that required for leucocyte labelling.

Finally, one disadvantage of scintigraphy is its low spatial resolution (Fig. 1). Therefore, when a bone scan reveals a lesion that was not seen on conventional radiography, the site of the lesion should be studied with a high resolution anatomical technique such as CT or MRI.

Computed tomography

The use of CT has decreased dramatically over the past few years because of the superiority and increasing availability of MRI. However, CT is the better modality for imaging the mineralized portion of the bone, and is most effective when clinical evaluation, conventional radiography, or bone scan have targeted a definite area.

The radiation dose received by a child during a CT examination is similar to that of multiple conventional radiographs. The newer multidetector helical CT scanners allow for more rapid imaging that results in radiation dose reductions. Two- and three-dimensional reformations are readily performed. CT software programs permit the data acquired from serial slices to be reformatted into any plane (even a curved plane) and to be reconstructed. The three-dimensional programs allow 'disarticulation' of joints and 'removal' or 'isolation' of any bone which may obscure the visualization of the underlying pathology or anatomy. Thus, three-dimensional CT provides a demonstration of complex anatomy, which can be of value in the management of complex malformations or trauma in children (Fig. 19).

The maximum pre-operative information can be obtained by manipulating the data set in order to simulate the operative approach and the operation (osteotomy for instance). Reformations have proven to be valuable in a number of disorders such as neoplasms, malformation, or trauma affecting the pelvis, hip, feet, and spine.

CT techniques and software modifications have been developed so that quantitative measures of bone mineral can be performed. Evaluation of the lumbar spine for osteopaenia is the usual procedure and normal values for children are available (Pettersson and Rydholm 1984; Gilsanz et al. 1988; Thomas et al. 1991). CT offers an alternative to conventional radiography for determining:

- femoral and tibial torsion (Hernandez et al. 1981),
- leg-length (using the scout view).

With careful positioning, almost any bone end can be imaged in a direct coronal or sagittal projection. In tarsal coalition, CT has proved to be the modality of choice. It is also more cost-effective (Emery et al. 1998). CT is the preferred method of evaluation in suspected cases of talocalcaneal coalition. The direct sagittal section is particularly valuable in demonstrating the anterior talocalcaneal articulation or coalition. For depiction of a calcaneonavicular coalition with CT, sections of the feet are obtained with the plantar surfaces perpendicular to the table, or images reformatted from a coronal sequence can be used.

In sacroiliac arthritis, the orientation of sacroiliac joints and the ability to tilt the gantry to coincide with the plane of the joint make CT an excellent tool. The ability to demonstrate the joint completely with CT gives greater confidence in making a diagnosis of chronic sacroiliac disease when secondary bony changes such as erosions and sclerosis may be seen. Acute sacroilitis is better evaluated with MRI (Fig. 2).

CT remains the most satisfactory method for demonstrating sequestra in cases of chronic osteomyelitis (Hernandez 1985). CT is invaluable for definition of the osseous anatomy of lesions arising in bones that are difficult to image in two standard orthogonal planes, for example, pelvis or vertebra, and for guiding a biopsy of such lesions when necessary.

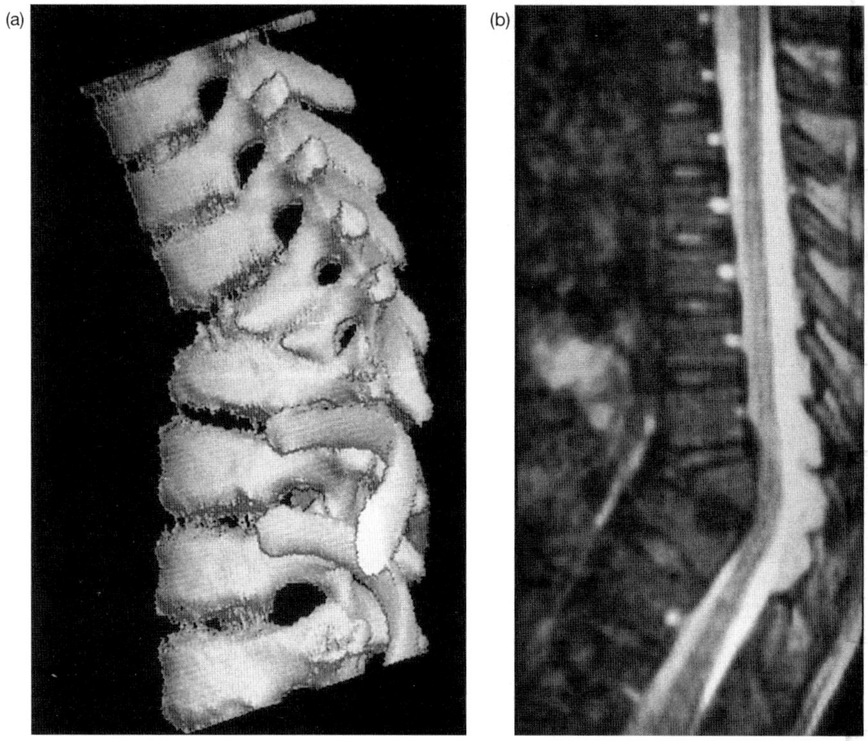

Fig. 19 Spondylodiscitis in a 12-year-old boy with dorsal kyphosis and vertebral block. (a) Three-dimensional CT shows the spinal deformity. (b) T_2-weighted MR image shows the cord compression.

CT has been an important adjunct to conventional radiography for the evaluation of the spine, however MRI has now challenged this role. CT offers the advantage of being more widely available especially in emergencies (trauma, spondylodiscitis). It is also the most sensitive modality for detecting calcifications and ossifications; this is invaluable for characterizing:

- calcifications in a chondroid matrix,
- phlebolithis in soft tissue or synovial venous malformations,
- ossification in early myositis ossificans.

CT is very effective in localizing precisely the site of the nidus of an osteoid osteoma (Fig. 4). Once the likely site of the osteoid osteoma has been determined with conventional radiographs and/or bone scan, a high resolution CT study is performed in that limited area, and can be used to guide a biopsy (Rosenthal 1997; Woertler et al. 2001). Attention should be directed to areas of high incidence of osteoid osteomas, such as the proximal femur where a reactive hip arthritis may be the revealing symptom (Fig. 4). Refinement of the technique has allowed percutaneous ablation of the nidus of osteoid osteoma.

Magnetic resonance imaging

MRI has revolutionized the diagnostic evaluation of paediatric musculoskeletal disorders, becoming the modality of choice in many indications. The paediatric musculoskeletal system is ideally suited for investigation by MRI since it is the only technique which can differentiate clearly the individual components of the normal joints from one another (articular cartilage and fibrocartilage, growth plate, synovial membrane, joint effusion, ligaments). MRI also allows identification of bone marrow, muscles, tendons, fascia, nerves, and vessels with high contrast between these structures.

However, one must not overlook the issue of clinical efficacy and cost-effectiveness. When deciding whether to use MRI, one should consider the financial cost, the time required, the potential need for sedation, and the operator dependency in comparison with good physical examination and conventional radiography. Therefore, physical examination must be performed and conventional radiography obtained prior to any decision to use MRI. Thus, cost-effectiveness is maximized and the diagnostic information of the MRI study optimized by choosing the best protocol for a specific indication.

Technical considerations

Without the use of ionizing radiation, MRI can safely produce high-contrast, high-resolution images of the paediatric musculoskeletal system in virtually any plane (Lawson et al. 1994). The success of MRI depends heavily upon multiple technical factors. The setting of the sequence needs to be adjusted for the individual examination. The magnetic field strengths and radiofrequencies currently employed with MRI produce no biological hazards. Immobilization is essential because of the intrinsic motion sensitivity of MRI. Unfortunately, the noise produced by the gradient coils of MRI scanners disturbs young infants and children, albeit to a variable degree.

Some form of sedation may be required in young children but general anaesthesia is exceptional. MR examinations generally require more scan time (on the average 30 min) than do other imaging modalities such as CT and sonography. Therefore, careful monitoring of children is essential (including heart rate, oxygen saturation). Newer magnet configuration designs such as small bore magnets for MRI of the extremities have recently been developed. 'Open' magnets, although better tolerated by children and offer the potential for unrestricted motion studies and weight-bearing position, have diminished signal, and require more imaging time. This can result in increased motion artefact (Lawson et al. 1994).

In children, the choice of the appropriate surface coil is crucial and is dependent on both the body part to be examined and the clinical question to be answered (Fig. 20). The smaller size of children may allow designated coils for adults to be used for a different body part of the child. In some

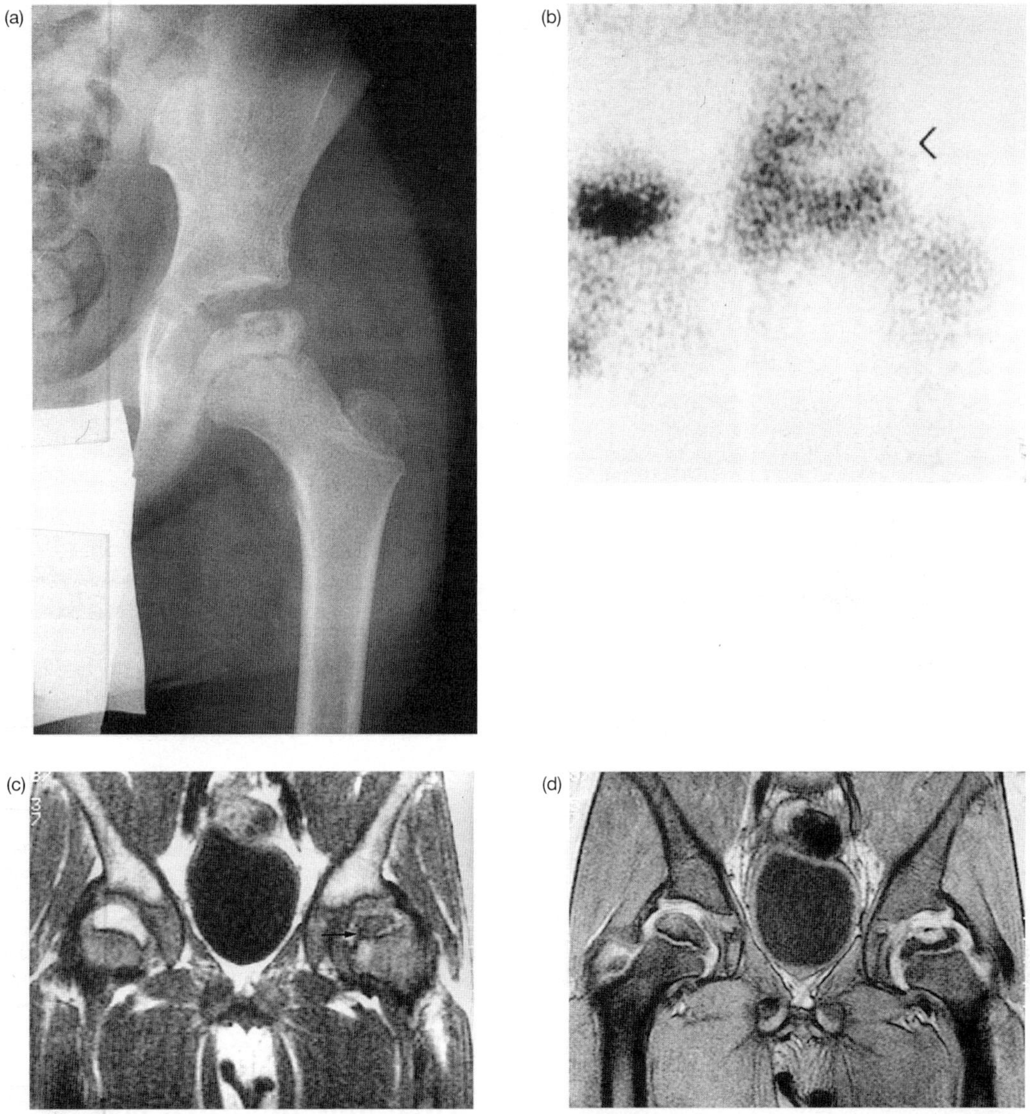

Fig. 20 Legg–Calve–Perthes' disease involving the left hip in an 8-year-old boy. (a) Conventional radiograph shows a typical fragmented appearance of the femoral head with lateral loss of containment. (b) Bone scan shows a decreased uptake in the necrotic bone. (c) T_1-weighted MR image shows the extent of necrosis (arrow). (d) Gradient-echo image shows the cartilaginous containment of the femoral head and the extent of the osteolytic area.

instances, a coil designed to image an adult's head may be effective for imaging simultaneously both hips of an infant or a small child (or an orbit or temporomandibular coil for imaging a single joint). In-plane spatial resolution of structures smaller than 1 mm with high signal and contrast-to-noise ratio is routinely achievable with this modality in children.

Pulse sequences

The appropriate choice of pulse sequences is critical to high-quality diagnostic MRI of the musculoskeletal system (Barnewolt and Chung 1998). The ideal combination of parameters depends on the anatomy being examined and the suspected abnormality in addition to the available hardware, time constraints, and local preferences. Each sequence has relative advantages and disadvantages (Jaramillo and Shapiro 1998). Spin-echo sequences are the mainstay of musculoskeletal MRI and are available on all MRI systems producing either T_1, spin-density or T_2-weighted sequences (Fig. 21) (Barnewolt et al. 1997). Following the administration of an intravenous contrast agent (usually gadolinium-based), T_1-weighted sequences are obtained (Fig. 21). The efficacy of spin-echo has been firmly established in various musculoskeletal applications in the paediatric literature and any new sequence should be compared with spin-echo before its routine clinical use. More rapid imaging sequences are currently available and are desired when imaging children.

Gradient-echo and fast spin-echo allow faster imaging than conventional spin-echo. The use of rapid gradient-echo with a three- or two-dimensional acquisition mode allows dynamic gadolinium-enhanced examinations studying musculoskeletal tissue vascularization and perfusion. This technique is maximized using post-processing software with pre- and post-contrast image subtraction (Fig. 22). The use of gradient-echo with a three-dimensional acquisition mode allows high spatial resolution. The acquisition of isotropic voxels allows reformatting in any plane and three-dimensional reconstruction.

The gradient-echo contrast can be advantageous for studying the trabecular bone structure and detecting haemorrhage (Sebag and Moore 1990) (Fig. 20). The use of the gradient-echo sequence is particularly useful in

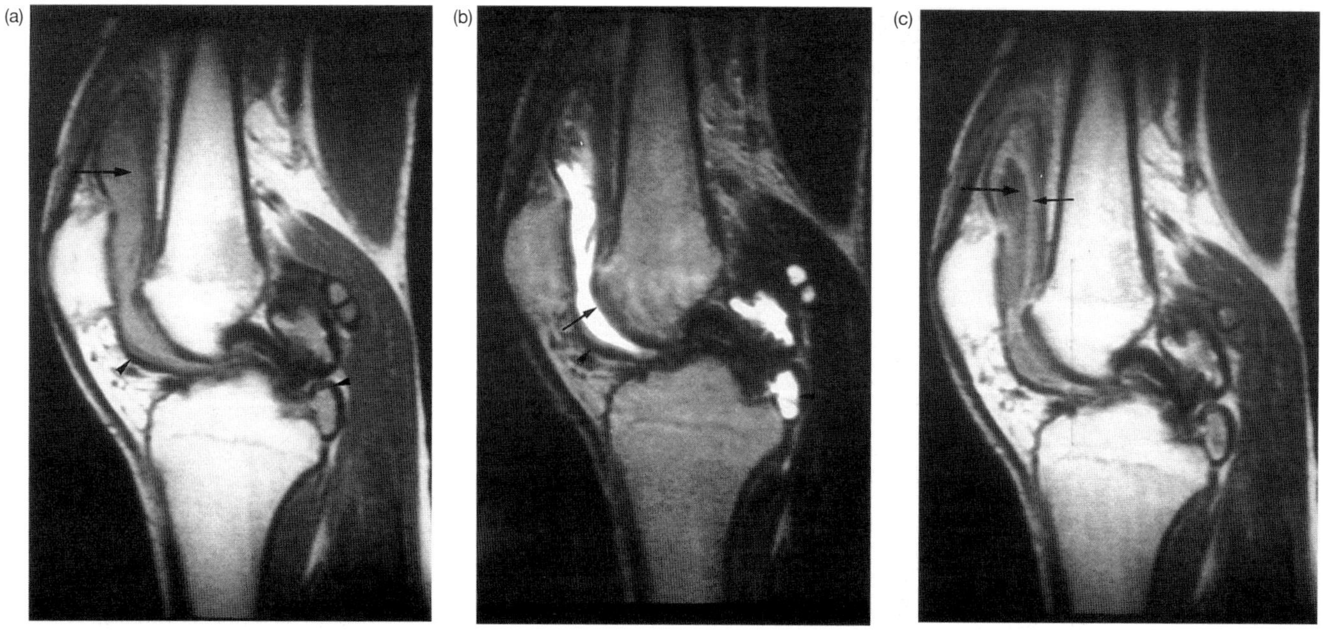

Fig. 21 Haemophilic arthropathy affecting the knee in a 14-year-old boy. (a) T_1-weighted MR image shows joint effusion (arrow) and synovial haemosiderin deposition (arrowhead). (b) T_2-weighted MR image shows articular surfaces with an arthrographic-like appearance (arrow). Haemosiderin deposition has a decreased signal (arrowhead). (c) Enhanced T_1-weighted MR image shows enhancement in the proliferative synovium (arrow) and allows a reliable distinction of active synovium from joint effusion (long arrow).

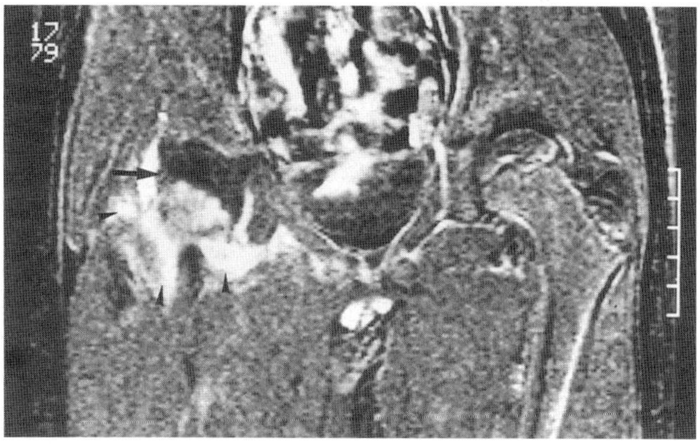

Fig. 22 Legg–Calve–Perthes' disease mimicking a right hip arthritis in an 8-year-old boy. Enhanced substraction MR image shows an avascular right femoral head (arrow) with enhancing reactional synovitis (arrowhead).

detecting osteolytic areas but can be problematic when identifying bone marrow oedema (Fig. 20). With certain gradient-echo parameters, epiphyseal, physeal, and articular cartilage appears brighter and better defined than it does on spin-echo images (Fig. 20). This contrast allows a very good demonstration of cartilage abnormalities in children. Fast spin-echo produces in a shorter time images with contrast similar to spin-echo. Fast spin-echo is especially advantageous for obtaining rapid, high resolution, heavily T_2-weighted images with a high signal-to-noise ratio. This is very useful for spinal studies with a myelographic effect (Fig. 19).

The transfer magnetization technique allows the contrast between joint fluid and articular cartilage to be increased, with an arthrogram-like effect (Wolf and Balaban 1994). The fat-suppression technique by decreasing or eliminating the signal from fat is also increasingly used in musculoskeletal MRI. It allows a good study of cartilage structures (which appear bright) and cartilaginous abnormalities, a better detection of gadolinium enhancement, and a better differentiation of sub-acute haemorrhage from fat (Barnewolt and Chung 1998). Finally, the short-TI inversion recovery (STIR) fat-suppressed sequence is a very sensitive screening method for detecting musculoskeletal disorders and especially marrow diseases in older children and teenagers (Fig. 23).

Normal and abnormal MRI musculoskeletal appearance in children

It is important when assessing a joint that the observer is familiar with the appearance of a normal MRI in the growing child. In the near-term foetus, the epiphyses are entirely cartilaginous. As ossified epiphyses develop with increasing age, there is gradual thinning of the epiphyseal cartilage. The ossification centres develop a bright signal representing the fatty marrow content (Jaramillo et al. 1991). Growth plates and epiphyseal cartilage have intermediate signal intensity on both T_1 and T_2 spin-echo sequences (Figs 20 and 21). They have a bright signal on T_2^* gradient-echo sequences and on fat-suppressed T_1 sequences (Fig. 20). Furthermore in children, the epiphyseal cartilage that surrounds the ossification centre, has a non-uniform signal pattern. A non-homogeneous hypointense zone is seen lying between the articular cartilage and the hemispherical growth zone of the ossification centre (Jaramillo and Hoffer 1992; Varich et al. 2000). This hypointense area is thought to represent a broad zone of poorly organized chondrocytes. With increasing age, the growth plate is reduced to a narrow zone between the epiphysis and the metaphysis, which shows an intermediate signal on T_1 and T_2 images and a high signal on T_2^* and fat-suppressed images (Jaramillo and Shapiro 1998) (Fig. 20).

In most long bones, physiological closure of the growth plate begins centrally. The distal tibial physis is an exception. Gadolinium-enhanced

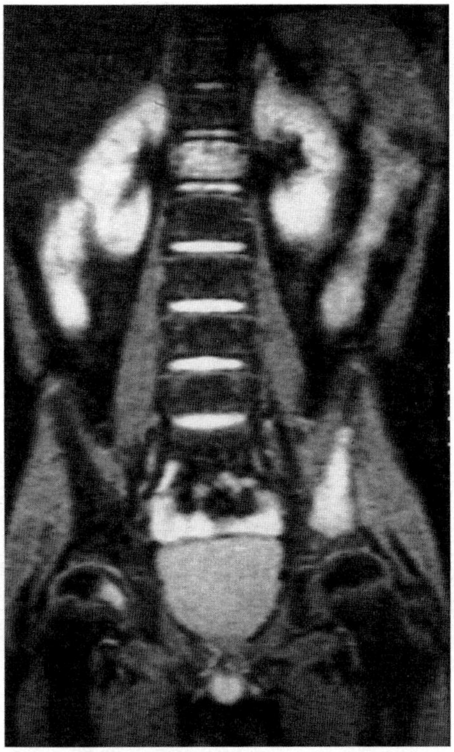

Fig. 23 Acute leukaemia relapsing in a 9-year-old boy with normal conventional radiographs. Frontal STIR image. Infiltration of the T12 vertebral body, of the right femoral head, and of left iliac wing.

subtraction MRI depicts the increased vascularization and perfusion of the metaphyseal growth zone (Dwek et al. 1997) (Fig. 22).

The distribution of fatty and haematopoietic marrow changes in the paediatric skeletal system from infancy to adulthood (Babyn et al. 1998). In a consistent pattern, the high fat content of fatty marrow results in an increased signal on T_1-weighted sequences and a lower signal on T_2-weighted sequences (Vogler and Murphy 1988; Zawin and Jaramillo 1993; Babyn et al. 1998). In contrast, the higher water and protein content of haematopoietic marrow results in a signal on T_1-weighted sequences that is low in neonates and slightly increased in the older child, together with a signal that is intermediate or increased on T_2-weighted sequence. After injection of contrast material, haematopoietic marrow shows a greater enhancement than fatty marrow, especially in small children and infants (Dwek et al. 1997).

Starting in infancy, the haematopoietic marrow is converted progressively to a fatty marrow. This begins in the distal appendicular skeleton and progresses to the axial skeleton. In an individual bone, the epiphysis converts to fatty marrow first, followed by the diaphysis and then the metaphysis, reaching the adult pattern by 25 years (Vogler and Murphy 1988; Jaramillo et al. 1991; Babyn et al. 1998). Knowledge of the type of marrow that is normally present in a given bone at a given age is essential to recognize any local or diffuse marrow abnormality in children. T_1-weighted spin-echo sequences are optimal for showing the status of marrow conversion, while STIR and T_2-weighted sequences are better at distinguishing an abnormal marrow (Fig. 23).

The articular surfaces are smooth and show up well on T_2 and gradient echo sequences, with an arthrographic-like appearance from bright joint fluid (Figs 20 and 21). The synovium is not seen in the normal joint when imaged without intravenous contrast. Without contrast enhancement, proliferative synovial tissue (i.e. pannus) has a variable signal and cannot be distinguished reliably from joint effusion and cartilage (Fig. 21). After injection of a paramagnetic agent (most often, gadolinium), proliferative synovium,

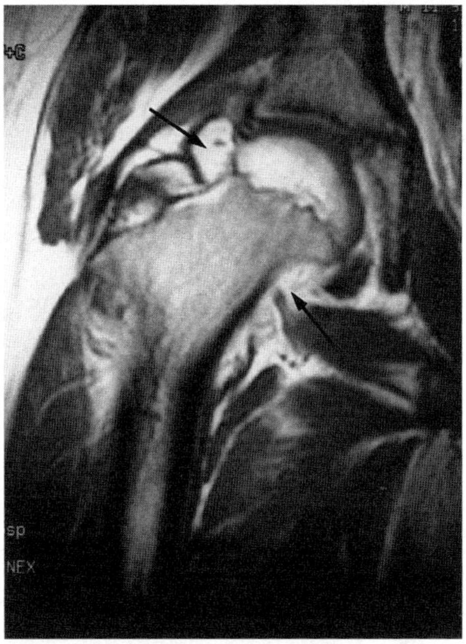

Fig. 24 Tuberculosis of the hip in an 11-year-old boy. Enhanced T_1-weighted MR image shows a non-specific intense enhancement of a dramatic synovial proliferation in the right hip (arrow).

which is extremely vascular, may be enhanced. Enhancement is indicative of disease activity and allows a precise assessment of pannus extension, joint effusion, and cartilage loss [Gylys-Morin 1998; Gylys-Morin et al. (in press)].

Contrast-enhanced MRI is the most sensitive modality to determine whether an arthritis is present, but rarely helps in establishing a specific diagnosis (Fig. 24).

In haemarthrosis and lipohaemarthosis, MRI can document the presence of haemorrhage owing to a predictable sequence in the chemical degradation of haemoglobin in extravasated blood (Fig. 21). Decreased signal intensity resulting from haemosiderin deposition can be demonstrated within an abnormal synovial proliferation (Fig. 21). Although this finding is suggestive, it is not specific and can be seen in haemophilia, bleeding disorders, pigmented villonodular synovitis, and intra-articular neoplasms such as a vascular malformation (Jelinek et al. 1989; Gaary et al. 1996) (Fig. 25).

Role of MRI in paediatric musculoskeletal system

MRI is an extremely sensitive modality for bone marrow imaging; however, the pattern of MR changes is non-specific and the diagnosis may be dependent on clinical information.

Joints are ideally suited for investigation by MRI in children (Gylys-Morin 1998). In most centres arthrography and CT arthrotomography have been replaced by MRI, which is currently used to evaluate congenital, traumatic, and inflammatory processes involving various joints. While the knees and hips are the joints most commonly examined with this modality, MRI of ankles, shoulders, wrist, elbow, and C1 to C2 are being performed with increasing frequency. Within the knee, MRI is ideal for determining internal derangement; discoid menisci and meniscal tears are easily visualized (Zobel et al. 1994) (Fig. 18). In osteochondritis dissecans, the extent of involvement can be evaluated as well as the status of the overlying cartilage.

In Legg–Calve–Perthes' disease, MRI allows the detection and definition of the extent of necrotic bone, which is essential for the diagnosis, prognosis,

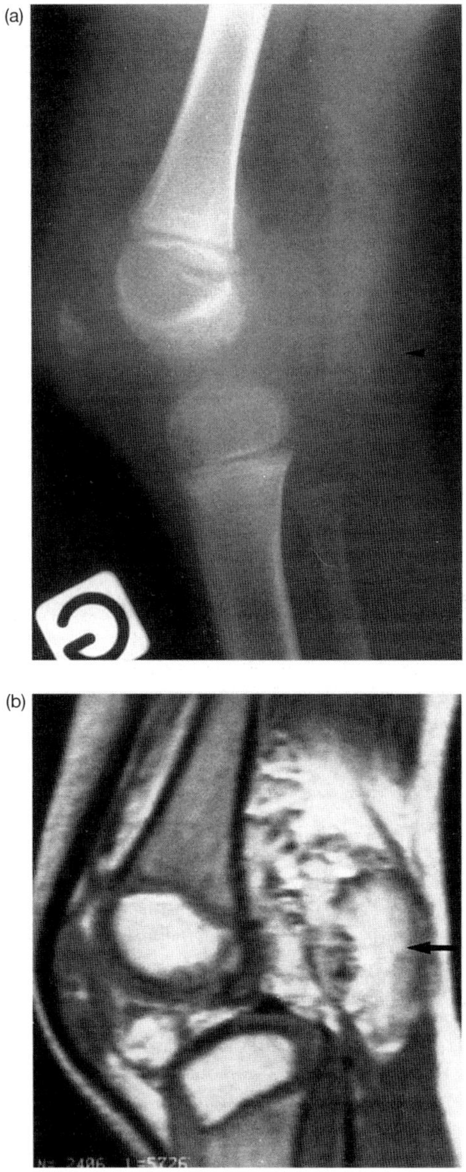

Fig. 25 Synovial vascular malformation affecting the knee in a 5-year-old boy. (a) Conventional radiograph demonstrates a phlebolith and a popliteal mass. (b) Enhanced T_1-weighted MR image shows the extension of the synovial vascular malformation.

and successful treatment of this condition (Ducou le Pointe et al. 1994) (Figs 20 and 22). Cartilage abnormalities also are depicted well (Jaramillo et al. 1995).

Within the hip, MRI allows detection of vascular changes and assessment of femoral head incongruity. It is useful to evaluate femoral head containment within the acetabulum even in abduction (Fig. 20) (Jaramillo et al. 1999). The role of MRI compared with that of scintigraphy is still under study (Conway 1993; Uno et al. 1995). MRI also allows early detection of osteonecrosis in children at risk and, especially, complications of steroid therapy (Mulliken et al. 1994). MRI is also useful in demonstrating late changes of DDH including deformity of the femoral head, acetabular dysplasia, infolding of the labrum, hypertrophy of the pulvinar, invagination of the iliopsoas tendon, and superimposed osteonecrosis (Johnson et al. 1988; Bos et al. 1991).

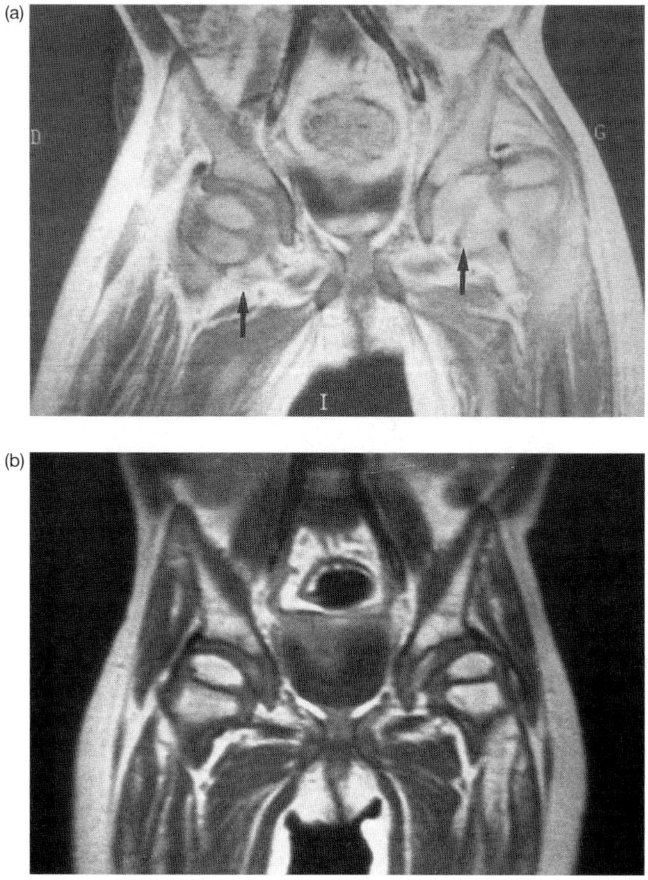

Fig. 26 Juvenile chronic arthritis. Systemic onset disease with hip involvement in a 3-year-old girl. Enhanced T_1-weighted MR image: (a) Prior to intra-articular injection of steroid: bilateral, active enhancing pannus is seen (arrow) with left hip dislocation. (b) After intra-articular injection of steroid: bilateral decrease in volume and enhancement of pannus with normal femoral head containment.

MRI is essential for pre-operative planning in congenital limb deficiency by showing the unossified structures and the hypoplastic or aplastic bones (Laor et al. 1996). MRI is the most satisfactory modality for diagnosing possible growth plate abnormalities prior to the osseous abnormality (Jaramillo 1992; Jaramillo and Shapiro 1998).

The early detection of any damage (most often acute or chronic trauma) is essential to avoid severe growth deformity and long-term sequella (Jaramillo and Shapiro 1998). MRI is very useful in the evaluation of sport injuries, showing occult fractures and trabecular bone impaction, which are seen increasingly in children and adolescent (Kapelov et al. 1993).

Inflammatory and synovial diseases in children are increasingly being studied by MRI (Harcke et al. 1997; Gylys-Morin 1998; Ramsey et al. 1999; Suenaga et al. 2000). In juvenile chronic arthritis, clinical evaluation of symptomatic joints is frequently supplemented with conventional radiographs; but radiographic changes represent late and indirect signs of synovial disease.

Contrast-enhanced MRI can be used to evaluate precisely the extension of synovial proliferation, the status of articular cartilage, joint effusion, and bone erosion in juvenile chronic arthritis [Gylys-Morin et al. (in press)] and haemophilic arthropathy (Fig. 26) (Gaary et al. 1996).

Cartilage loss is detected better on MRI than on conventional radiography, especially in young children with thick, growing cartilage and at the early stage of the disease [Gylys-Morin et al. (in press)].

Contrast-enhanced MRI is promising in the evaluation of the effectiveness of intra-articular therapy in juvenile chronic arthritis (Eich et al. 1994).

Enhanced MRI allows better evaluation of residual anatomic lesions after treatment. MRI may be used to predict subsequent therapeutic failure (fluid loculations) or early relapse (persistence of pannus enhancement) (Fig. 26). It is particularly valuable for hip appraisal in which clinical evaluation is difficult.

MRI is now the preferred approach for evaluating children for lesions of the spine and spinal cord (either congenital, traumatic, inflammatory, or neoplastic).

Finally, as in the adult, MRI has proved to be essential in the evaluation of:

- extent of soft tissue tumours and bone tumours (Jaramillo et al. 1996),
- evaluation of the response to treatment of musculoskeletal tumours (Debaert et al. 1992),
- musculoskeletal infection (acute and chronic osteomyelitis) (Gylys-Morin 1998).

In osteomyelitis, MRI should be performed in cases that may require surgical drainage including infections of the spine or pelvis, infections extending into the growth plates of long bones, and infections that fail to respond to antibiotics (Dangman et al. 1992; Jaramillo et al. 1995) (Fig. 1).

Conclusion

Selection of the appropriate sequence of imaging studies for a given child and a given diagnostic problem has become a complex undertaking. Investigations have to be tailored to the individual need of the child, and radiologists and paediatricians have to work together to ensure that the needs of all are best matched. Clinical examination and/or conventional radiography remain the initial investigations. The need for radiation protection must remain a priority in children. Finally, in this era of advancing imaging technology, a knowledge of the relative values of available imaging techniques is necessary to optimize the management of children with musculoskeletal disease.

References

Ansell, B.M. (1990). Classification and nomenclature. In *Update in Paediatric Rheumatology* (ed. P. Woo, P. White, and B.M. Ansell), pp. 3–5. Oxford: Oxford University Press.

Babyn, P., Ranson, M., and McCarvile, M.E. (1998). Normal bone marrow. Signal characteristics and fatty conversion. *Magnetic Resonance Imaging Clinics of North America* **6** (3), 473–95.

Barnewolt, C.E. and Chung, T. (1998). Techniques, coils, pulse sequences, and contrast enhancement in pediatric musculoskeletal MR imaging. *Magnetic Resonance Imaging Clinics of North America* **6** (3), 441–53.

Barnewolt, C.E., Shapiro, F., and Jaramillo, D. (1997). Normal gadolinium-enhanced MR images of the developing appendicular skeleton: Part I. Cartilaginous epiphysis and physis. *American Journal of Roentgenology* **169** (1), 183–9.

Bellah, R.D. et al. (1991). Low back pain in adolescent athletes: detection of stress injury to the pars interarticularis with SPECT. *Radiology* **180**, 509–12.

Blumhagen, J.D. (1994). The child with a limp. In *Practical Pediatric Radiology* (ed. S.W. Hilton, D.K. Edwards, and J.W. Hilton), pp. 391–442. Philadelphia PA: W.B. Saunders.

Bos, C., Bloem, J.L., and Verbout, A.J. (1991). Magnetic resonance imaging in acetabular residual dysplasia. *Clinical Orthopaedics* **265**, 207–17.

Conway, J.J. (1993). A scintigraphic classification of Legg–Calve–Perthes disease. *Seminars in Nuclear Medicine* **23** (4), 274–5.

Dale, K., Paus, A.C., and Laires, K. (1994). Radiographic classification system in juvenile rheumatoid arthritis applied to the knee. *European Radiology* **4**, 27–32.

Dangman, B.C. et al. (1992). Osteomyelitis in children: gadolinium-enhanced MR imaging. *Radiology* **182**, 743–7.

Debaert, T., Vanel, D., Shapeero, L.G., Charpentier, A., Terrier, P., and Di Paola, M. (1992). Osteosarcoma after chemotherapy: evaluation with contrast material-enhanced substraction MR imaging. *Radiology* **185**, 587–92.

Ducou Le Pointe, H., Haddad, S., Silberman, B., Filipe, G., Monroc, M., and Montagne, P. (1994). Legg–Calve–Perthes' disease: staging by MRI using gadolinium. *Pediatric Radiology* **24**, 888–91.

Dwek, J.R., Shapiro, F., Laor, T., Barnewolt, C.E., and Jaramillo, D. (1997). Normal gadolinium-enhanced MR images of the developing appendicular skeleton: Part 2. epiphyseal and metaphyseal marrow. *American Journal of Roentgenology* **169** (1), 191–6.

Egelhoff, J.C., Ball, W.S., Jr., Koch, B.L., and Parks, T.D. (1997). Safety and efficacy of sedation in children using a structured sedation program. *American Journal of Roentgenology* **168** (5), 1259–62.

Eich, G.F., Halle, F., Hodler, J., Seger, R., and Willi, U.V. (1994). Juvenile chronic arthritis: imaging of the knees and hips before and after intraarticular steroid infection. *Pediatric Radiology* **24**, 558–63.

Emery, K.H., Bisset, G.S., III, Johnson, N.D., and Nunan, P.J. (1998). Tarsal coalition: a blinded comparison of MRI and CT. *Pediatric Radiology* **28** (3), 612–16.

Englaro, E.E., Gelfand, M.J., and Paltiel, H.J. (1992). Bone scintigraphy in preschool children with lower extremity pain of unknown origin. *Journal of Nuclear Medicine* **33**, 351–4.

Gaary, E., Gorlin, J.B., and Jaramillo, D. (1996). Pseudotumor and arthropathy in the knees of a hemophiliac. *Skeletal Radiology* **25** (1), 85–7.

Gilsanz, V. et al. (1988). Vertebral bone density in children: effect of puberty. *Radiology* **166**, 847–50.

Graf, R. (1983). New possibilities for the diagnosis of congenital hip joint dislocation by ultrasonography. *Journal of Pediatric Orthopedics* **3** (3), 354–9.

Greulich, W.W. and Pyle, S.J. *Radiographic Atlas of Skeletal Development of the Hand and Wrist.* Stanford CA: Stanford University Press, 1959.

Grissom, L.E. and Harcke, H.T. (1999). Ultrasonography and developmental dysplasia of the infant hip. *Current Opinion in Pediatrics* **11** (1), 65–6.

Grobbelaar, N. and Bouffard, J.A. (2000). Sonography of the knee, a pictorial review. *Seminars in Ultrasound, CT, and MR* **21** (3), 231–74.

Gylys-Morin, V.M. (1988). MR imaging of pediatric musculoskeletal inflammatory and infectious disorders. *Magnetic Resonance Imaging Clinics of North America* **6** (3), 537–59.

Gylys-Morin, V.M., Graham, T.B., Blebea, J.S., Laor, T., Dardzinski, B.J., Johnson, N.D., Oestreich, A.E., and Passo, M.H. (2001). Knee in early juvenile rheumatoid arthritis: MR imaging findings. *Radiology* **220**, 696–706.

Harcke, H.T. (1994). Screening newborns for developmental dysplasia of the hip: the role of sonography. *American Journal of Roentgenology* **162** (2), 395–7.

Harcke, H.T. and Walter, R.S. (1995). Ultrasound screening for dysplasia of the hip. *Pediatrics* **95** (5), 799–800.

Harcke, H.T., Mandell, G.A., and Cassell, I.L. (1997). Imaging techniques in childhood arthritis. *Rheumatic Disease Clinics of North America* **23** (3), 523–44.

Hernandez, R.J. (1985). Visualization of small sequestra by computerized tomography: report of 6 cases. *Pediatric Radiology* **15**, 238–41.

Hernandez, R.J., Tachdjian, M.O., Poznanski, A.K., and Dias, L.S. (1981). CT determination of femoral torsion. *American Journal of Roentgenology* **137**, 97–101.

Jacobs, J.C. *Pediatric Rheumatology for the Practitioner* 2nd edn. Berlin: Springer-Verlag, 1982.

Jaramillo, D. and Hoffer, F.A. (1992). Cartilaginous epiphysis and growth plate: normal and abnormal MR imaging findings. *American Journal of Roentgenology* **158**, 1105–10.

Jaramillo, D. and Shapiro, F. (1998). Growth cartilage: normal appearance, variants and abnormalities. *Magnetic Resonance Imaging Clinics of North America* **6** (3), 455–71.

Jaramillo, D., Laor, T., Hoffer, F.A., Zaleske, D.J., Cleveland, R.H., Buchbinder, B.R., and Egglin, T.K. (1991). Epiphyseal marrow in infancy: MR imaging. *Radiology* **180** (3), 809–12.

Jaramillo, D., Kasser, J.R., Villegas-Medina, O.L., Gaary, E., and Zurakowski, D. (1995). Cartilaginous abnormalities and growth disturbances in Legg–Calve–Perthes disease: evaluation with MR imaging. *Radiology* **197** (3), 767–73.

Jaramillo, D., Treves, T.S., Kasser, J.R., Harper, M., Sundel, R., and Laor, T. (1995). Osteomyelitis and septic arthritis in children: appropriate use of imaging to guide treatment. *American Journal of Roentgenology* **165**, 399–403.

Jaramillo, D., Laor, T., and Gebhardt, M.C. (1996). Pediatric musculoskeletal neoplasms. Evaluation with MR imaging. *Magnetic Resonance Imaging Clinics of North America* **4** (4), 749–70.

Jaramillo, D., Galen, T.A., Winalski, C.S., DiCanzio, J., Zurakowski, D., Mulkern, R.V., McDougall, P.A., Villegas-Medina, O.L., Josesz, F.A., and Kasser, J.R. (1999). Legg–Calve–Perthes disease: MR imaging evaluation during manual positioning of the hip—comparison with conventional arthrography. *Radiology* **212** (2), 519–25.

Jelinek, J.S. et al. (1989). Imaging of pigmented villonodular synovitis with emphasis on MR imaging. *American Journal of Roentgenology* **152**, 337–42.

Johnson, N.D., Wood, B.P., and Jackman, K.V. (1988). Complex infantile and congenital hip dislocation: assessment with MR imaging. *Radiology* **168**, 151–6.

Kapelov, S.R. et al. (1993). Bone contusions of the knee: increased lesion detection with fast spin-echo MR imaging spectroscopic fat saturation. *Radiology* **189**, 901–4.

Keats, T.E. *An Atlas of Normal Variants that may Simulate Disease* 5th edn. Chicago IL: Year Book Medical Publishers, 1991.

Lamer, S. and Sebeg, G.H. (2000). MRI and ultrasound in children with juvenile chronic arthritis. *European Journal of Radiology* **33** (2), 85–93.

Laor, T., Jaramillo, D., Hoffer, F.A., and Kasser, J.R. (1996). MR imaging in congenital lower limb deformities. *Pediatric Radiology* **26** (6), 381–7.

Lawson, J.P., Keller, M.S., and Rattner, Z. (1994). Recent advances in pediatric musculoskeletal imaging. In *Advances in Musculoskeletal Imaging* Vol. 32, Issue 2 (ed. D.J. Sartoris), pp. 353–75. Philadelphia PA: W.B. Saunders.

Marchal, G.J. et al. (1987). Transient synovitis of the hip in children: role of US. *Radiology* **162**, 825–8.

Moore, S.G. and Sebag, G.H. (1990). Primary disorders of bone marrow. In *Magnetic Resonance Imaging of Children* (ed. M.D. Cohen and M.K. Edwards), pp. 824–65. Philadelphia PA: B.C. Decker.

Mulliken, B.D., Renfrew, D.L., Brand, R.A., and Whitten, C.G. (1994). Prevalence of previously undetected osteonecrosis of the femoral head in renal transplant recipients. *Radiology* **192**, 831–4.

Oyen, W.J. et al. (1992). Diagnosis of bone joint and joint prosthesis infections with in-111-labeled nonspecific human immunoglobulin G scintigraphy. *Radiology* **182**, 195–9.

Ozonoff, M.B., ed. (1992). Special radiologic techniques measurements and calculations. In *Pediatric Orthopedic Radiology* 2nd edn., pp. 765–85. Philadelphia PA: W.B. Saunders.

Pettersson, H. and Rydholm, V. (1984). Radiologic classification of knee joint destruction in juvenile chronic arthritis. *Pediatric Radiology* **14**, 419–21.

Pettersson, H. and Ringertz, H. (1991). *Measurements in Pediatric Radiology* pp. 20–98. London: Springer-Verlag.

Pettersson, H., Ahlberg, G.A., and Nilsson, I.M. (1980). A radiologic classification of hemophilic arthropathy. *Clinical Orthopaedics* **149**, 153–9.

Ramsey, S.E., Cairns, R.A., Cabral, D.A., Malleson, P.N., Bray, J.H., and Petty, R.E. (1999). Knee magnetic resonance imaging in childhood chronic monarthritis. *Journal of Rheumatology* **26** (10), 2238–43.

Risser, J.C. (1948). Important practical facts in the treatment of scoliosis. *American Academic Orthopedic Surgery* **5**, 248–60.

Rosenthal, D.I. (1997). Percutaneous radiofrequency treatment of osteoid osteomas. *Seminars in Musculoskeletal Radiology* **1** (2), 265–72.

Sebag, G.H. and Moore, S.G. (1990). Effect of trabecular bone on the appearance of marrow in gradient-echo imaging of the appendicular skeleton. *Radiology* **174**, 855–9.

Steinbrocker, O., Trager, G.H., and Butterman, R.C. (1949). Therapeutic criteria in rheumatoid arthritis. *Journal of the American Medical Association* **140**, 659–62.

Strouse, P.J., DiPietro, M.A., and Adler, R.S. (1998). Pediatric hip effusions: evaluation with power Doppler sonography. *Radiology* **206** (3), 731–5.

Suenaga, S., Ogura, T., Matsuda, T., and Noikura, T. (2000). Severity of synovium and bone marrow abnormalities of the temporomandibular joint in early rheumatoid arthritis: role of gadolinium-enhanced fat-suppressed T1-weighted spin echo MRI. *Journal of Computer Assisted Tomography* **24** (3), 461–5.

Sureda, D., Quiroga, S., Arnal, C., Boronat, M., Andreu, J., and Casas, L. (1994). Juvenile rheumatoid arthritis of the knee. Evaluation with US. *Radiology* **190**, 403–6.

Swischuk, L.E. (1994). The extremities. In *Emergency Imaging of the Acutely Ill or Injured Child* 3rd edn., pp. 361–567. Baltimore MD: Williams and Wilkins.

Swischuk, L.E. and John, S.D. (1995). Bones and soft tissues. In *Differential Diagnosis in Pediatric Radiology* 2nd edn., pp. 187–342. Baltimore MD: Williams and Wilkins.

Swischuk, L.E., Swischuk, P.N., and John, S.D. (1993). Wedging of C-3 in infants and children: usually a normal findings and not a fracture. *Radiology* **188**, 523–6.

Thomas, K.A., Cook, S.D., Bennet, J.T., Whitecloud, T.S., III, and Rice, J.C. (1991). Femoral neck and lumbar spine bone mineral densities in a normal population 3–20 years of age. *Journal of Pediatric Orthopedics* **11**, 48–58.

Thomas, P.S., Renton, P., Hall, C., Kalifa, G., Dubousset, J., and Lalande, G. (1994). The musculo skeletal system. In *Imaging Children* (ed. H. Carty, F. Brunelle, D. Shaw, and B. Kendall), pp. 845–1291. London: Churchill Livingstone.

Uno, A., Hattori, T., Noritake, K., and Suda, H. (1995). Legg–Calve–Perthes' disease in its evolutionary period: comparison of MRI with bone scintigraphy. *Journal of Pediatric Orthopedics* **15**, 362–7.

Varich, L.J., Laor, T., and Jaramillo, D. (2000). Normal maturation of the distal femoral epiphyseal cartilage: age-related changes at MR imaging. *Radiology* **214** (3), 705–9.

Vogler, J.B., III and Murphy, W.A. (1988). Bone marrow imaging. *Radiology* **168** (3), 679–93.

Woertler, K., Vestring, T., Boettner, F., Winkelmann, W., Heindel, W., and Lindner, N. (2001). Osteoid osteoma: CT-guided percutaneous radiofrequency ablation and follow-up in 47 patients. *Journal of Vascular and Interventional Radiology* **12** (6), 717–22.

Wolf, S.D. and Balaban, R.S. (1994). Magnetization transfer imaging: practical aspects and clinical applications. *Radiology* **192**, 593–9.

Zawin, J.K. and Jaramillo, D. (1993). Conversion of bone marrow in the humerus, sternum, and clavicle: changes with age of MR images. *Radiology* **188** (1), 159–64.

Zawin, J.K., Hoffer, F.A., Rand, F.F., and Teele, R.L. (1993). Joint effusion in children with an irritable hip: US diagnosis and aspiration. *Radiology* **187** (2), 459–63.

Zobel, M.S., Borrello, J.A., Siegel, M.J., and Stewart, N.R. (1994). Pediatric knee MR imaging: pattern of injuries in the immature skeleton. *Radiology* **190**, 397–401.

5.7 Histopathology

Patrick J. Gallagher and Janice R. Anderson

Most chronic rheumatological disorders affect multiple tissues and systems (Plates 76 and 77). This has the potential to generate a wide variety of histological biopsies, and the problems associated with processing and interpretation of some of these are considered in this section. The value of skin, gastrointestinal, renal, liver, pulmonary, marrow, and other biopsies have been considered in various chapters in Section 1.3.

Synovial biopsies

Methods of closed synovial biopsies were described many years ago and comprehensive accounts of the histological features in large clinical series were published before modern pathological methods were developed (Rosenberger et al. 1981). These detailed studies clarified exactly which alterations are most common in each disorder, but the precision with which diagnoses can be made in individual patients did not necessarily increase. In the 1980s and 1990s, the value of synovial biopsy was seriously questioned by rheumatologists and pathologists. It is, therefore, important that collaborative work between European rheumatologists and pathologists has now defined and confirmed the value of synovial biopsy, particularly in the assessment of the efficacy of new treatments (Tak and Bresnihan 2000).

Technical aspects

Most biopsies obtained by needle arthroscopy are 5–10 mm in dimension and ideally three or more fragments are required (Plate 78). Besides histology, biopsies can be used for RNA and DNA extraction, bacterial or lymphocyte culture, and cell isolation. It has been calculated that at least 2.5 mm^2 of synovial tissue is needed to reflect the variation in cellular density expected in rheumatoid synovium (Kennedy et al. 1998a,b). In a recent large series of needle biopsies, one group moved from a 1.8 to a 2.7 mm biopsy forceps and reported improved tissue retrieval (Baeten et al. 1999). Satisfactory histological specimens can be obtained from needle biopsy of metacarpophalangeal joints (Ostendorf et al. 1999). For diagnostic histology, no special processing techniques are required, but multiple levels should be examined. All of the monoclonal antibodies directed against the usual panel of leucocyte antigens now give good results in formalin-fixed tissue. If the biopsies are performed largely for investigative, rather than diagnostic, reasons the use of methyl methracylate as an embedding medium should be considered. The pattern of immunohistochemical staining with this medium is far superior and lends itself to more accurate quantification by image analysis.

Evaluation of biopsies

At least 10 per cent of biopsies are unsatisfactory, either because the material retrieved is too small for evaluation or only collagenous joint capsule has been biopsied. Until recently it was not known whether arthroscopic synovial biopsies, selected under direct vision, produced better histological information than closed needle biopsy specimens. When these two procedures were compared in the same joint, it was found that assessment of the microscopic features was not affected by the way in which the samples had been obtained. Furthermore, as the macroscopic features of inflammation seen at arthroscopy did not predict the microscopic change it is probably unnecessary to perform arthroscopy solely for the purposes of obtaining a biopsy (Youssef et al. 1998a).

There are only a limited range of pathological changes that occur in synovial biopsies (Table 1) and each of these should be carefully assessed. Most practising pathologists allocate abnormalities to one of three grades (e.g. mild, moderate, or severe; well, moderately, or poorly differentiated). Even such a simple system is far from reproducible and experienced pathologists can fail to agree over the grading of common biopsies such as the uterine cervix. However, the European Synovitis Study Group compared a semi-quantitative and quantitative method of analysing cellular infiltration in rheumatoid arthritis and showed a close relationship between the two methods (Youssef et al. 1998b). In investigative studies, however, quantitative methods of measuring synovial thickness and inflammatory cell infiltration are probably essential (Cunnane et al. 1999; Kraan et al. 2000).

It has often been stated that synovial fluid examination, rather than synovial biopsy, is the pathological investigation of choice in most joint disorders. This may no longer be true. Johnson and Freemont (2001) compared the information that was obtained when 103 patients had simultaneous synovial fluid aspiration and synovial biopsy. In many cases, both investigations produced the same amount of information, which were generally equally specific or non-specific. However, biopsy produced more information than the fluid in 29 per cent of cases and vice versa in 18 per cent. These experienced articular pathologists concluded that the diagnostic usefulness of a biopsy approximates to, and occasionally exceeds, that of fluid aspiration.

Table 1 Histopathological changes in synovial biopsies

Frequent changes, no specific diagnostic value
Hyperplasia of synovial lining cells
Villous synovial hyperplasia
Synovial ulceration and fibrin deposition
Acute and chronic inflammatory cell inflammation
Chronic inflammatory aggregates, with germinal centre formation
Less frequent changes, possible diagnostic value
Granulomatous lesions in joint capsule (rheumatoid arthritis) or synovium (sarcoidosis)
Dense acute inflammatory infiltration with micro-organisms (infective arthritis) or urate crystals (gout)
Subsynovial deposits of amyloid
Dense haemosiderin deposits (repeated haemorrhage, e.g. haemophilia)

Histological changes in individual disorders

Although histopathologists rarely make a definitive diagnosis on a synovial biopsy, there are some general features that suggest particular disorders and a few changes that indicate specific diseases.

Rheumatoid disease

The chief microscopic features in rheumatoid arthritis are (Plate 79):

- Marked thickening of the synovial membrane as a result of proliferation and reduced apoptosis of type B synovial lining cells and infiltration by CD68 positive macrophage like cells.
- Infiltration of the sub-synovial layer by aggregates of both CD4 positive T cells, some CD8 positive T cells, B lymphocytes, plasma cells, macrophages, and some antigen presenting cells.
- A substantial increase in vascularity as a result of vasodilatation and neovascularization.
- Synovial ulceration, fibrin deposition, and some scarring (Plates 80 and 81).

These histological alterations represent a primary pathological process, responsible for cartilagenous destruction, rather than a secondary effect of the joint destruction itself. Strong support for this concept has emerged from studies that have compared biopsies taken in early and late rheumatoid arthritis and which have related the histopathological changes to the degree of clinical joint disease (Baeten et al. 2000). When joints with effusions were compared to those without, the majority of the histopathological features summarized above were more marked in patients with effusions. There were increased numbers of plasma cells and both CD4 and CD8 positive lymphocytes. The maximum thickness of the synovial lining was greater in patients with long-standing disease (Plate 82) but other histopathological changes were related to the level of disease activity rather than its duration (Plate 83).

In practical terms, pathologists should be told what, if any, treatments patients have received, especially if disease modifying drugs have been used before the biopsy was taken. Although immunohistochemistry has no specific diagnostic role, it can easily be performed on synovial biopsy specimens. It readily allows the pathologist to identify CD68 positive cells within the synovium and to assess the density of CD4 positive T lymphocytic infiltration. If these features are confirmed, the suspicion of rheumatoid disease is enhanced.

Osteoarthritis

There can be substantial, and largely unexplained, inflammatory cell infiltration in some synovial biopsies from patients with undoubted osteoarthritis. In one classical study, 40 per cent of osteoarthritic samples could not be differentiated from rheumatoid biopsies and half of all osteoarthritic synovia had moderate or marked inflammation (Goldenberg et al. 1982). Quite understandably, the focus of recent research has been in the analysis of rheumatoid synovia and its response to new disease modifying drugs (Bresnihan et al. 2000). Some of these studies have included subsets of patients with osteoarthritis and have confirmed that the inflammatory changes are significantly greater in rheumatoid than in osteoarthritis (Fonesca et al. 2000). In addition, it has been shown that the mean and maximum thickness of the synovial lining, the numbers of CD68 positive cells in the sub-synovial zone and CD4 positive lymphocytes tend to be lower in patients with osteoarthritis as compared to rheumatoid disease. Nevertheless, there is overlap in these measurements, especially when patients with osteoarthritis and effusion are compared to rheumatoid joints with no effusion (Baeten et al. 2000). Synovial ulceration and markedly hyperplastic, hydropic, synovial villae are not, in our experience, common features of osteoarthritis. Pathologists should look carefully for small bony masses within the synovium (bone shards), a feature that is more suggestive of osteoarthritis than rheumatoid disease.

Other arthropathies

Inflammatory changes are seen in most of the less common forms of chronic joint disease such as psoriatic or enteropathic arthropathy, juvenile idiopathic arthritis, reactive arthritis, or ankylosing spondilitis. Predictably, there is no single histological feature that is in any way diagnostic of a particular disorder. Traditionally, it has been said that in both adults and children with the less common arthropathies the density of inflammatory infiltrates is usually less than in typical long-standing rheumatoid disease (Kidd et al. 1989). This has been convincingly confirmed in a recent study in which the numbers of CD20 positive B cells, and CD3 and CD4 positive T cells were reduced in patients with spondyloarthropathy and joint effusions in comparison to similar patients with rheumatoid disease (Baeten et al. 2000). There was also evidence of changes in the immunohistochemical staining for integrin molecules but these specialized staining methods are not in routine use in diagnostic laboratories.

Severe acute purulent *synovial membrane* inflammation strongly suggests infective arthropathy. Although polymorphs are often found in the synovial fluid in rheumatoid disease, and the movement of polymorphs in rheumatoid disease has been studied in detail (Youssef et al. 1996), polymorphs are only occasionally seen in the synovium itself, even in active rheumatoid disease. In unusual disorders, such as sarcoidosis or amyloidosis, a specific histological diagnosis is sometimes possible.

Prosthetic joints

An exuberant histological reaction may be seen in synovial biopsies taken during 're-do' joint replacement. The abraded material from these joints, particularly the polyethylene fragments, may stimulate a marked macrophage response and there may be a florid associated synovial hyperplasia. Most practising pathologists are now aware of these changes and biopsies of this nature rarely pose diagnostic problems.

Salivary gland biopsy

Inflammatory infiltration of the lacrymal and salivary glands may occur as an isolated event, or in association with a variety of autoimmune diseases. Chronic inflammation and the inevitable associated fibrosis and loss of glandular tissue leads to a reduction in the production of saliva and tears. This causes dryness of the mouth and eyes and may progress to a sicca syndrome with kerato-conjunctivitis.

The typical, well developed, lesions in major salivary glands in Sjögren's syndrome have been termed benign lymphoepithelial lesions or myoepithelial sialadenitis (MESA). Although much glandular tissue can be lost, the larger salivary ducts may be preserved. The subsequent proliferation of their lining epithelium and myoepithelial covering produces characteristic histological structures termed 'myoepithelial islands'. Patients with Sjögren's syndrome and MESA have an increased risk of developing malignant lymphoma, usually of the so-called mucosa-associated lymphoid tissue lymphoma (MALT) type. In addition, there is an increased incidence of lymphoproliferative abnormalities such as lymphocytic interstitial pneumonitis and unusual forms of atypical hyperplasia in lymph nodes.

Technical aspects

Malignant lymphoma should be suspected in any patient with an autoimmune rheumatic disease who presents with salivary gland enlargement or cervical lymphadenopathy. With modern immunohistochemical techniques, satisfactory staining reactions with almost all antibodies can be obtained in formalin-fixed, paraffin-processed tissue. However, fresh tissue is valuable for cytological and cytogenetic studies and the extraction of DNA.

In Sjögren's syndrome, both major and minor salivary glands are involved and the small glands on the inner aspect of the cheek and lower lip are easily biopsied (Plate 84). The lower lip is everted and a 15–20 mm incision is made under local anaesthesia, parallel to the vermilion border in the labial mucosa. In normal subjects, the procedure is relatively innocuous; occasionally, a feeling of numbness around the biopsy site remains. In patients with severe stomatitis, the biopsy site may become infected and ulcerate.

Evaluation of biopsies

Major salivary glands and cervical lymph nodes

In the majority of centres in the United Kingdom and North America, histopathological reporting is undertaken by teams of sub-specialists. Oncologists are seldom willing to treat patients until the histology has been reviewed formally by pathologists with whom they have a close working relationship. The classification of malignant lymphomas has evolved continually, over a period of at least 20 years and may progress further in the future. However, at present, all specialist lymphoreticular pathologists adhere to the World Health Organization classification that has been summarized in a recent comprehensive guide (Jaffe et al. 2001).

Early diagnosis of malignant lymphoma in the salivary or lacrymal glands requires careful cytological analysis of the lymphoid infiltrates and good quality immunohistochemical preparations. Virtually all of these lymphomas are derived from B cells and are most correctly known as extra nodal marginal zone B cell lymphomas of mucosa associated lymphoid tissue (MALT lymphomas). Although they make up only 7–8 per cent of all B cell lymphomas, they are the most common malignant lymphoma in sites such as the salivary gland, the orbit and eye, and the stomach. The tumour cells typically express IgM and less often IgA or IgG and only one form of immunoglobulin light chain. Immunoglobulin heavy and light chain genes are rearranged in the majority of cases. The outlook for MALT lymphomas in the head and neck region is good and they are slow to disseminate. Recurrences may involve other extra nodal sites but the tumours are sensitive to radiotherapy. Even the most experienced lymphoreticular pathologists have difficulties in distinguishing early MALT lymphomas from myoepithelial sialadenitis and general pathologists should refer these specimens for an expert opinion.

Minor salivary gland biopsies

Biopsies are most often taken in the investigation of patients with an obscure sicca syndrome (Plate 85). In a study of over 360 cases, Daniels demonstrated that multiple lymphoid aggregates (greater than 1 focus per 4 mm^2) in adequate biopsies of labial salivary glands were better indicators of Sjögren's syndrome than a reduced salivary flow from the parotid or subjective symptoms of a dry mouth (Daniels 1984). Subsequently, interest in salivary gland biopsies declined in many centres but there has been a recent resurgence in interest in this technique. For example, Lee and colleagues studied 121 patients with sicca symptoms, performing a detailed clinical evaluation, serology, and salivary gland biopsy. They concluded that labial salivary gland biopsy was most useful in patients who had only some of the established clinical criteria for a sicca syndrome but positive anti-Ro or anti-La antibodies. Where there was no reasonable clinical suspicion of salivary gland involvement, or where the diagnosis was clinically obvious, salivary gland biopsy was thought to add little useful clinical information (Lee et al. 1998).

Ideally, between four and eight small salivary glands should be sectioned in order to obtain the most reproducible result. Furthermore, multiple sections of each biopsy should be examined. It has been demonstrated that examination at multiple levels had an impact on the diagnosis of Sjögren's syndrome in approximately 60 per cent of biopsies (Al-Hashimi et al. 2001).

Another study used two different methods of grading the density of inflammatory infiltrates and compared the positive yield from both labial salivary gland (Plate 86) and lacrymal gland biopsy. Perhaps surprisingly the number of lymphocytic foci and myoepithelial islands in severe lymphocyte infiltration were greater in lacrymal than labial glands. The authors emphasize the value of performing both types of biopsies but this has not become a standard clinical practice (Xu et al. 1996). In all studies, females make up the majority of cases. This has been confirmed in a recent clinical and physiological study (Saito et al. 1999). Clear clinical indications are, therefore, necessary before biopsy is undertaken in male patients.

Despite the various technical reservations, labial salivary gland biopsy could be used more widely. Gene rearrangement and chromosomal translocation studies can easily be performed on material extracted from these fresh biopsies. In a study of 70 patients with Sjögren's syndrome, 13 had light chain restriction in labial gland biopsy. Four of these 13 patients later developed extra salivary lymphoma (Jordan et al. 1995).

Bone biopsy

In systemic bone disorders, such as osteomalacia, renal osteodystrophy, and hyperparathyroidism, bone biopsy can be a valuable aid in establishing a diagnosis and in assessing the severity of the disease process and the response to treatment (Malluche et al. 1999; Pecovnik Balon and Bren 2000). The role of biopsy in the common forms of osteoporosis is less clear but it certainly has a place in the investigation of patients less than about 50 years old and in those with associated abnormalities of calcium metabolism (Eriksen et al. 1994). Biopsies should only be referred to pathologists whose laboratories have the technical expertise to process and section undecalcified bone and who have sufficient experience to evaluate and quantify the histological changes.

Technical aspects

Eriksen and his colleagues have produced an excellent short guide to bone biopsy which is required reading for pathologists and rheumatologists with an interest in metabolic bone disease (Eriksen et al. 1994). The terminology can be confusing but an international group has attempted to standardize the nomenclature and specialist journals, such as *The Journal of Bone and Mineral Research*, give succinct guidelines in their instructions to authors. Virtually all biopsies are from the ilium, usually within 20–30 mm of the anterior superior iliac spine. The iliac crest should be avoided as the demarcation between cortical and trabecular bone can be indistinct (Vigorita 1984). A core should be taken in a horizontal place through the full thickness of the gluteal surface. An ideal biopsy should, therefore, include the inner and outer cortical plates and the full width of trabecular bone. A 5-mm Jamshidi needle produces a more than adequate biopsy. Cores of 10 mm are less likely to fragment but in our experience this advantage is offset by the added difficulties in processing and sectioning.

Tetracycline is a naturally fluorescent antibiotic that binds to immature bone at the 'calcification front'—the interface between osteoid and mineralizing bone. Tetracycline fluorescence can, therefore be used to estimate how much of the bone surface is undergoing mineralization. If two doses are given at a fixed interval the rate of bone calcification can also be calculated (Fallon and Teitelbaum 1982). Two separate 3-day courses of oxytetracycline are given (250 mg, four times a day) at least 10 days apart. The biopsy should be taken no less than 3 days after the end of the second course. The results are unpredictable, especially in severe osteomalacia, when it may be difficult to identify two clear lines of fluorescence. If there is strong clinical evidence of osteomalacia or renal bone disease, it is advisable to increase or prolong the doses of tetracycline and to extend the intervals between the two courses of antibiotic and between the second dose and the biopsy, as described below. When tetracycline has been given the biopsies should be fixed in 70 per cent alcohol rather than formalin.

Bone that has not been decalcified is difficult to section especially if it has been routinely processed into paraffin wax. Trabecular bone tends to tear and shatter during cutting and the alignment of marrow with the bony trabeculae can be lost. Bone biopsies can be dehydrated satisfactorily in modern tissue processors and we use a kit (JB4; Polysciences Inc.) to embed the samples in 2-hydroxyethylmethacrylate. Sections are then cut with glass knives at 3 μm. It is sometimes possible to distinguish osteoid from mineralized bone in haematoxylin and eosin stains but better definition is obtained with Goldner's trichome method or the Van Kossa stain for calcium phosphate.

Histopathological assessment

Although simple histological assessment can allow a confident diagnosis in florid cases of osteomalacia (Plate 87) and renal osteodystrophy, quantitative microscopy is required when osteoporosis is suspected or the changes of osteomalacia are more subtle. Almost all histological features can be measured with a suitable range of eye-piece graticules and highly reproducible results can be obtained by experienced observers. However, excellent low-power histological images can now be obtained from simple flat bed scanners. Most large laboratories have some form of image analysis system and even the simplest of these can be adapted for bone histomorphometry.

Most pathologists assume that the information obtained from a two-dimensional image is a reflection of the results that would be obtained from the full three-dimensional structure. This is not necessarily true and two respected reviews have outlined mathematical methods by which three-dimensional measurements can be estimated from a small number of sections taken at known intervals in a carefully defined plane (Cruz-Orive and Weibel 1990). These methods can be applied to bony tissue (Gundersen et al. 1988) and are especially useful for estimating trabecular bone volume.

Many different measurements can be made in bone biopsies (Melsen et al. 1978) but comparatively few of these are use in the diagnosis of osteoporosis and the various forms of osteomalacia (Table 2). The histological features of some variables such as trabecular bone volume, are clear cut, at least if the sections are free of artefactual tears or fissures. If the measurements are made from a scanned image at suitable magnification, even an inexperienced pathologist should obtain reproducible results. There is much more variation when subtle microscopic changes are evaluated. For example, trabecular resorptive surfaces are defined on the basis of the irregular or scalloped surfaces but the identification of these is highly subjective.

Osteoporosis

As there are no reliable, qualitative features that distinguish osteoporotic from normal bone, some form of quantitation is essential for diagnosis. The comprehensive approach used in experimental studies sets an ideal standard but is impractical in most routine laboratories (Storm et al. 1993). As a first step we measure trabecular bone volume and osteoid volume. Trabecular bone volume is defined as the percentage of the medullary cavity occupied by trabecular bone. In most studies of this volume there are differences between groups of patients with osteoporosis and healthy controls, but in elderly people there may be a considerable overlap. Furthermore, measurements of trabecular bone volume in biopsies taken from different sites in the same patient can vary by as much as 80 per cent (Chavassieux et al. 1985). Healthy young adults have trabecular bone volumes in the range 20–32 per cent but mean results in elderly subjects have been quoted as 11.9 and 19.9 per cent (normal) and 8.7, 9.6, and 13.3 per cent (osteoporotic patients). Patients with trabecular bone volumes of 20 per cent or greater are most unlikely to have osteoporosis, but volumes as low as 6 per cent can occasionally be recorded in elderly subjects with no clinical or pathological evidence of osteoporosis (Ashton-Key and Gallagher 1992).

Mean trabecular-plate thickness and mean trabecular-plate density can be derived from the trabecular bone volume using simple formulae (Parfitt et al. 1983). The plate thickness is an indication of the size and the density an index of the number of trabecular plates per unit area. By using these three measurements together it is possible to determine whether bone loss has resulted from loss of complete trabeculae, by thinning of trabeculae, or a combination of both. In non-osteoporotic controls there is an almost

Table 2 Histological measurements in bone biopsies

Parameter (abbreviation)	Definition	Approximate normal values	Comments
Trabecular bone volume (TBV)	Percentage of medullary cavity occupied by trabecular bone	20–32%, young adults 12–16%, elderly	Lower in osteoporotic patients than in age-matched controls, but considerable overlap. Note variation between adjacent sites in individual patients
Mean trabecular plate thickness (MTPT)	A mathematical index closely related to size of individual trabeculae[a]	~140 μm	No direct relationship with increasing age. Reduced in severe osteoporosis only
Mean trabecular plate density (MTPD)	A mathematical index closely related to the number of trabeculae per unit area[a]	1.4–1.8/mm	Reduced with increasing age in both sexes and in osteoporosis
Trabecular osteoid surface	Percentage of the trabecular surface which stains as osteoid	~20%	
Trabecular resorption surface	Percentage of trabecular bone with an irregular (scalloped) appearance	~5%	Objective variation between different pathologists
Osteoclastic resorption surface	Definition of percentage of the surface of trabecular bone lined by osteoclasts	Normal value less than 0.15%	May be increased in hyperpara thyroidism and renal osteodystrophy
Osteoclast number	The number of osteoclasts per mm^2 of trabecular bone	Normal value approximately $0.2/mm^2$	
Calcification rate	The distance between double tetracycline labelling lines divided by the number of days between tetracycline dosages	Normal values 0.15–1.0 μm/day	Several different areas should be measured if there is satisfactory fluorescence
Percentage tetracycline labelling	The percentage of the trabecular osteoid surface that labels with tetracycline (single or double lines acceptable)	~15%	Most easily measured from photographs: graticule examination is difficult

[a] See Parfitt et al. (1983).

linear decline in both trabecular bone volume and mean trabecular-plate density with increasing age, and this is accentuated in patients with vertebral fractures and in patients receiving corticosteroids (Hanyu et al. 1999). It is now accepted that the underlying cellular mechanisms in age-related and post-menopausal osteoporosis are different (Dempster and Lindsay 1993) (see also Chapter 6.16.1). In post-menopausal disease enhanced osteoclastic activity during the erosive phase of bone remodelling may cause deep perforations of trabeculae with a generalized loss of 'connectivity'. In contrast, in age-related osteoporosis there is a reduction in trabecular plate thickness but the trabeculae retain their 'connections' with each other. At least two methods have been described to assess that—the marrow star volume (Eriksen et al. 1994) and node-strut analysis. The value of these measurements is illustrated clearly in a study of hyperparathyroidism in post-menopausal women (Pariesen et al. 1995). In practice, these methods are not difficult to master (Shore et al. 2000), especially as low-power images can now be scanning slides directly.

There is no evidence that osteoid volume is increased in either the 'post-menopausal' or 'senile' form of osteoporosis. Furthermore, most reports indicate that osteoid volume is not affected by increasing age. If a high osteoid volume is recorded in an osteoporotic patient, an additional form of metabolic bone disease should be suspected.

Osteomalacia

The histological appearances of florid cases of osteomalacia are characteristic (Plate 87) and histopmorphometry is not strictly necessary for immediate diagnosis. Trabecular bone volume, osteoid volume, and osteoid surface should be measured in all cases, along with an index of hyperparathyroidism such as percentage trabecular or osteoclastic resorption surface. When tetracycline has been given it is usually possible to calculate the calcification rate and percentage tetracycline labelling. In practice, a perfect pattern of fluorescence is seldom obtained. If severe osteomalacia or renal osteodystrophy is suspected the interval between the two courses of antibiotic should be increased and the biopsy taken 1 or 2 weeks after the last dose. Even if this is possible the number of true double lines may be small and the real value of this technique may be doubtful. Nevertheless, we use tetracycline in all adults in whom there is a suspicion of osteomalacia or renal osteodystrophy. It should not, of course, be used in children. Confocal laser microscopy can produce excellent fluorescent images of tetracycline-labelled bone biopsies.

Biopsies from patients with renal bone disease or hyperparathyroidism should be handled in much the same way. Reabsorption surfaces should be measured. Some form of 'hard copy', such as an image from a digital camera, makes these measurements easier. Osteoblasts and osteoclasts should be counted when there is any suspicion of hyperparathyroidism. Their distribution is not random in these disorders, nor even in normal bone. Because of this a set of measurements made from a single section may be imprecise. Gundersen and his colleagues have described simple techniques that allow more accurate estimation of irregularly distributed histological features (Gundersen et al. 1988). By examining a comparatively small number of sections it is possible to estimate volumetrically, rather than in two-dimensional terms.

Vascular disorders

Introduction

Although the underlying causes of systemic vasculitis are imperfectly understood, there have been significant advances in the clinical and laboratory diagnosis of these disorders and their management (see Section 6.10). Because systemic vasculitis is a serious, but potentially treatable, disorder it is essential that surgical pathologists consider this diagnosis in biopsies from a wide variety of different sites. In some clinical settings, the diagnosis is obvious and rapidly confirms the clinical impression. For example, vasculitis is an obvious diagnosis to consider in any renal biopsy and is the diagnosis of exclusion in temporal artery specimens. Vasculitis has been reported in virtually every organ and system and may, therefore, produce many different clinical signs and symptoms. In contrast, there are only a restricted number of histological changes. A diagnosis of vasculitis must be considered in any unusual inflammatory lesion, especially in the lung or paranasal region and in skin and gastro-intestinal biopsies.

Although pathologists have access to an increasing range of immunological and molecular methods these are of limited value in the everyday diagnosis of vasculitis. The most practical advance has been the widespread use of a diagnostic classification based on the size of the vessels involved in different disorders (Jeanette and Falk 1997) (Table 3). In some inflammatory and reactive disorders, blood vessels show changes that are indistinguishable from true vasculitis. There is no simple answer to this problem and even the most experienced vascular pathologists find difficulties in this distinction. General guidelines are summarized in Table 4 but there are exceptions to most of the points that have been summarized. The single most important point is to consider vasculitis in any tissue in which unexplained infarction is detected. Undoubted histological features of vasculitis may be found incidentally in patients in whom there is no suspicion at all of systemic disease. This so-called 'isolated vasculitis' has a predilection for the cervix, uterus, spermatic chord, and testes. Some patients develop evidence of systemic disease but many do not (Burke and Virmani 2001).

The range of biopsy material clearly varies from centre to centre, largely dependent on the enthusiasms of physicians and rheumatologists. A recent report from a Danish centre (Table 5) has produced results that are very much in keeping with United Kingdom practice. The commonest type of vasculitis identified is self-limiting cutaneous leucocytoclastic angiitis. The overall instance of primary renal vasculitis is approximately 18 cases per million. The commonest underlying causes are Wegener's granulomatosis and microscopic polyangitis.

Table 3 Major types of vasculitis

Large-vessel vasculitis
Giant-cell arteritis
Takayasu's arteritis
Medium-sized-vessel vasculitis
Polyarteritis nodosa
Kawasaki's disease
Primary granulomatous central nervous system vasculitis
Small-vessel vasculitis
ANCA-associated small-vessel vasculitis
Microscopic polyangiitis
Wegener's granulomatosis
Churg–Strauss syndrome
Immunologically mediated small-vessel vasculitis
Henoch–Schönlein purpura
Lupus vasculitis
Rheumatoid vasculitis
Cutaneous leucocytoclastic vasculitis
Idiopathic or drug related
Vasculitis as part of the spectrum of systemic disease
Para-neoplastic vasculitis
In association with inflammatory bowel disease

Note: This is a simplification of the classification described by Jeanette and Falk (1995).

Small vessel vasculitis

Wegener's granulomatosis, microscopic polyangiitis, and Churg–Strauss syndrome have distinctive clinical patterns of disease but virtually indistinguishable histologically. All but a very few patients have circulating antibodies to neutrophil cytoplasmic antigens (ANCA) (see Chapter 5.4). In each disorder, small vessels, arterioles, capillaries, and venules are preferentially affected. Characteristically, there is no evidence of immune complex deposition in lesions. Necrotizing granulomas are frequently identified in paranasal and lung biopsies in Wegener's and Churg–Strauss syndrome.

Henoch–Schönlein purpura is the one form of small vessel vasculitis in which the pathologists can usually provide evidence of immune mediated abnormalities. Characteristically, IgA dominant immune complexes are identified in glomeruli or in vessels in the skin or gastrointestinal tract. There are case reports of Henoch–Schönlein purpura in unusual sites such as the heart and central nervous ststem. As the overall prognosis for this condition is excellent, supportive treatment is sufficient for the majority of patients. It is, therefore, essential that pathologists make an accurate diagnosis of this disorder. Patients with ANCA associated small vessel vasculitis and who present with skin rashes and abdominal pain should not be diagnosed as Henoch–Schönlein purpura. These patients do not have a good prognosis and require specific therapy.

Table 4 Histological features of systemic vasculitis in comparison to reactive changes in vessels

Systemic vasculitis	Inflammatory conditions with secondary involvement of blood vessels
Vessels of a specific size are preferentially involved in different disorders	Different vessels may be involved, including both arteries and veins
Inflammatory cells penetrate the full thickness of the vessel wall	Inflammatory cells surround vessels and are largely confined to the adventitia and the alter media
Vessel walls may show necrosis, often with fibrin deposition	Fibrinoid necrosis is uncommon, although exceptions do occur
Reactive intimal thickening is uncommon	Intimal thickening in small arteries (endarteritis obliterans) is often a feature
Vascular changes may induce localized areas of infarction	Cutaneous and mucosal ulceration are the characteristic secondary changes

Table 5 Vasculitis in a single hospital in 1993–1998

Diagnosis	Number of cases
Cutaneous leucocytoclastic vasculitis	37
Wegener's granulomatosis	22
Cranial arteritis	14
Microscopic polyangiitis	12
Churg–Strauss syndrome	2
Polyarteritis nodosa	2
Henoch–Schönlein purpura	2
Takayasu's arteritis	1

Small vessel vasculitis, which is confined to the skin, is termed cutaneous leucocytoclastic vasculitis. The characteristic vessel that is affected is the post-capillary venule in the skin. Histological features are no different from the more aggressive forms of systemic vasculitis, which have cutaneous involvement. In the acute stages there is an acute inflammatory reaction and associated vessel wall necrosis. However, most biopsies are taken from patients with persistent or unusual rashes and the appearances may be subtly different. The infiltrate may be a mixture of acute and chronic cells and vessel wall necrosis and endothelial necrosis will be less evident. Occasional cases are seen in which the infiltrate is composed only of chronic inflammatory cells. Most patients with cutaneous leucocytoclastic vasculitis have a single episode of disease that resolves spontaneously. Only 10 per cent have recurrent or persistent vasculitis. At least 10 per cent of cases are associated with recent administration of drugs such as penicillins and streptokinase, cytokines, and monoclonal antibodies. Cutaneous vasculitis may also be a para-neoplastic change, usually in patients with leukaemia or lymphoma (Paydas et al. 2000).

Vasculitis in muscular arteries

The three important forms of vasculitis that affect muscular arteries are:

- Polyarteritis nodosa
- Kawasaki's disease
- Granulomatous angiitis of the central nervous system

Kussmaul and Maier described a patient with nodular inflammatory lesions in medium-sized and small arteries throughout the body in 1866. They called this condition periarteritis nodosa but this has changed to polyarteritis nodosa. Until the recent concensus conference (Jeanette and Falk 1995), this diagnostic label was often applied to any patient with necrotizing arteritis. It is now essential that it is confined to the rather uncommon form of systemic vasculitis, which *chiefly* affects muscular arteries, tending to spare small vessels. If this definition is adhered to strictly, comparatively few patients will fall into this diagnostic grouping. The lesion is usually diagnosed in liver or muscle biopsies. There is florid inflammation with necrosis of the muscular wall and aneurysm formation. Glomerulonephritis is not a primary feature of this disorder and antineutrophil cytoplasmic antibodies may not be detected. The histological diagnosis is usually straightforward as there is dense mixed inflammatory cell infiltration and fibrinoid necrosis of the muscular wall.

The two other forms of vasculitis affecting muscular arteries are seldom important in rheumatological practice. Kawasaki's disease (mucocutaneous lymph node disorder) is an important disease in the Far East but is seen occasionally in paediatric practice in the West. The preferential involvement of coronary arteries is a puzzling feature of this disorder. Aneurysms may form in any part of the epicardial coronary artery tree and are often identified by echocardiography.

Granulomatous angiitis of the central nervous system affects small- and medium-sized arteries of the meninges and cerebrum. As in cranial arteritis giant cells may be prominent, but if anything, the inflammatory infiltrates are denser and there may be extensive necrosis of the muscular wall. Patients present with a variety of focal or diffuse neurological symptoms but visual symptoms are not especially common and the scalp vessels do not appear to be affected. If cerebral angiography is performed, a characteristic beaded appearance of vessels may be seen. Occasionally, the diagnosis has been confirmed by meningial biopsy. Some patients have responded to cyclophosphamide and corticosteroids. The cause of this disorder is unknown. There is an association with cerebral amyloid angiopathy, a form of vascular amyloid deposition distinct from the usual pattern seen in Alzheimer's disease. Several reports have described an association with previous Hodgkin's or non-Hodgkin's lymphoma. This is a puzzling association.

Vasculitis in large muscular arteries or the aorta

Temporal artery biopsy

Despite many clinical, pathological, and epidemiological studies, very little is known about the cause of cranial (giant cell or temporal arteritis). Although medium-sized arteries of the head and neck are most frequently involved, almost any area of the body, including the aorta, may be affected. It is disease of the ophthalmic artery and its small posterior cilary branches that leads to blindness but biopsies are usually taken from the superficial temporal branch of the external carotid or, occasionally, the terminal branches of the occipital artery.

Technical aspects

Many patients with the classical, clinical features of temporal arteritis have normal biopsies and this is the result of focal involvement of the artery by disease (Poller et al. 2000). To minimize these false-negative biopsies, samples for histological examination must be as long as possible and should be taken from areas that are tender. Although pathologists traditionally suggest a 20–30 mm length should be biopsied, this is rarely the end-result of surgery. Most biopsies are less than 15 mm in length and in general terms, these are satisfactory. All of the biopsies should be processed and there is some evidence that the whole of the wax block should be cut into serial sections (Chakarbarty and Franks 2000). Besides improving the chance of finding typical areas of inflammation, it will clarify the importance of unusual histological findings such as involvement of small branch vessels and adventitial lymphocytic infiltration. Some sections should be stained in order to demonstrate the elastic lamellae and the distribution of collagen. The elastic Van Gieson stain or one of the many trichrome methods is satisfactory for this.

Evaluation of biopsies

The microscopic features of acute and sub-acute cranial arteritis and the arterial changes associated with ageing are summarized in Table 6. The classical picture of granulomatous acute and chronic inflammation, with multi-nucleated giant cells in close relationship to an extensively fragmented internal elastic lamella, is seen in approximately 60 per cent of typical cases. Giant cells are not a prerequisite for diagnosis. However, there must be evidence of inflammation within the muscular wall. In some biopsies from patients with acute cranial arteritis, there is florid intimal oedema, and it may be the resolution of this that underlies a prompt response to anti-inflammatory drugs.

Surgical pathologists must be familiar with the full range of ageing changes that occur in the aorta and muscular arteries. These alterations can be misinterpreted and prompt an erroneous diagnosis of healed arteritis (Cox and Gilks 2001). Various clinico-pathological questions raised by rheumatologists and other physicians are summarized in Table 7. Two new problems in the histological diagnosis have been addressed in recent reports. A small proportion of biopsies show only adventitial lymphocytic infiltration (Corcoran et al. 2001). This can, of course, be a feature of common arterial diseases such as atherosclerosis but this is uncommon in the temporal artery. If this change is seen, biopsies should be serially sectioned for a significant proportion will then show more convincing evidence of arteritis. It has been appreciated for some time that the inflammation in temporal artery biopsies may be restricted to branching points or small arteries or arterioles in the adventitia. The majority of these patients have good clinical evidence of cranial arteritis and further sectioning may reveal disease in the main arterial stem which was biopsied. Nevertheless, a small proportion have evidence of a disseminated small vessel vasculitis and this possibility must be investigated clinically and immunologically.

Inflammatory disease of the aortic root and aorta

Most cardiovascular pathologists have experience of the range of changes that are seen in aortic biopsies in patients undergoing surgery for proximal aortic aneurysms or aortic incompetence. Most of these biopsies show degenerative changes in the elastic media which are the underlying cause of the aortic dilatation. In occasional patients with established rheumatological diseases, there will be considerable thickening of the wall with medial and adventitial inflammation, sometimes with associated changes in the aortic valve. These biopsies rarely present diagnostic difficulty. However, in occasional aortic biopsies, small inflammatory foci are seen within the

Table 6 Histological changes in temporal artery biopsies

'Ageing changes' (arteriosclerosis)	Active cranial arteritis	Sub-acute or healed cranial arteritis
Concentric intimal and inner medial fibrosis	Acute and chronic transmural inflammation, often in relationship to small branches	Focal aggregates of lymphocytes and macrophages in the media
Focal fragmentation and apparent reduplication of internal elastic lamella	Prominent giant cells in relation to destructed internal elastic lamella	Bizarre, irregularly arranged intimal fibrous tissue
Focal calcification, especially around elastic lamellae and adjacent media	Marked intimal fibrosis and oedema	Fragmentation of elastic lamella, usually involving more than one-quarter of the arterial circumference
Hyalinization of muscular media	Focal areas of intimal and medial necrosis; not extensive necrotizing change with fibrin deposition and luminal thrombus formation unusual	Medial scarring with ingrowth of new blood vessels (neo-vascularization)
Aggregates of lymphocytes and macrophages in adventitia, especially in association with atherosclerosis		

Table 7 Common clinico-pathological questions in cranial arteritis

I have a patient with tender temporal arteries, headache, an ESR of 95 mm/h and a raised C-reactive protein. What is the chance of a positive biopsy?
About 60%. This is the mean figure of a number of different studies. It is the result of patchy involvement of the superficial temporal artery
Well, why should I bother with a biopsy? I am going to start steroid treatment whatever you report
You, or another colleague, will be very grateful for objective evidence of the diagnosis in a year's time when your patient has steroid-induced problems!
My patient has been on steroids for almost a week. What is the chance of a positive biopsy?
Much less. Probably not more than 25%. It is still worth doing but the pathologist must look for changes such as intomal oedema and fibrosis in focal rather than diffuse inflammation
What is the relationship between polymyalgia rheumatica and giant cell arteritis pathologically?
About 50% of patients with giant cell arteritis have muscle pain. The arteritis is confined to vessels of the head and neck. Less than 10% of patients who present with polymyalgia rheumatica ultimately develop giant cell arteritis. Muscle biopsy and polymyalgia do not show vasculitis
Does involvement of small branch vessels matter if the main artery is normal?
Yes, this is uncommon but the changes are important and must not be disregarded. Most of these patients have cranial arteritis. About 10% will have systemic small vessel vasculitis and this possibility must be investigated
The surgical pathologist has reported adventitial lymphocytic only. What does this mean?
Again this must not be disregarded. Serial sectioning of these biopsies will reveal more specific histological evidence of cranial arteritis in 15% of cases

aortic media and there may be occasional clusters of giant cells. In our experience, only two such patients have had previous clinical evidence of cranial arteritis (Plate 88). These changes must, therefore, be interpreted with caution for steroids are strongly contraindicated in the post-operative period. Although a now historic study suggested that almost 20 per cent of patients with cranial arteritis had involvement in the aorta, the exact incidence of clinically important aortic disease is probably unknown.

Pathologist in most centres in Europe have very little direct experience of the histopathological changes of Takayasu's disease. The diagnosis is best made on clinical grounds, supplemented by newer methods of CT scanning. The detailed histological changes have been summarized by Lie (1995).

Muscle biopsy in the rheumatic disorders

Technique

Muscle biopsy, obtained by either needle or open biopsy, is a minor procedure that can be done under local anaesthesia in almost all patients. An open biopsy requires a small skin incision but has the advantage that a larger specimen is obtained. In comparison, a needle biopsy provides a smaller sample but several biopsies in different directions can be obtained through the same small incision, and it is much less likely to leave a scar. In addition, the patient is more likely to tolerate repeat biopsies. With either method, careful handling and freezing of the specimen is essential to obtain maximum histological information. It is best to orientate the specimen before freezing and then to snap-freeze in isopentane cooled in liquid nitrogen. This rapid freezing eliminates ice-crystal artefact, which can grossly distort the muscle fibres and obscure pathological changes. A simple technique for freezing biopsy specimens is illustrated (Fig. 1). It is important to keep the specimen completely frozen and to avoid contact with fingers or metal instruments at room temperature, as these may cause thawing at the periphery. For diagnostic purposes, transverse sections generally yield the most information. Fibre atrophy is one of the more common pathological changes in the rheumatic disorders and fibre size can be accurately assessed from fibre diameter, but only in genuine transverse sections (Fig. 2). If there is enough material, it is always sensible to store a small frozen sample for biochemical analysis and to put a tiny strip into glutaraldehyde for electron microscopy, lest either of these investigations prove necessary.

Site

A positive muscle biopsy is an important diagnostic criterion of polymyositis and dermatomyositis (see Chapter 6.8), where skeletal muscle is the main and often sole pathological target. In other systemic rheumatic disorders, muscle biopsy may assist in primary diagnosis, but more often is done to elucidate the cause of muscle symptoms, particularly to detect an active myositis. The site of biopsy is best determined by the clinical picture. A severely wasted muscle in a patient with a chronic disorder should be avoided. A tender muscle may yield a positive result in inflammatory disorders; electromyographic abnormalities on one side in symmetrical muscle disease may assist localization of an appropriate muscle to biopsy in the opposite limb.

Muscle fibre types and staining reactions

A wide variety of enzyme histochemical and tinctorial stains is available, but only a few are necessary for initial screening (Fig. 3). Differences in

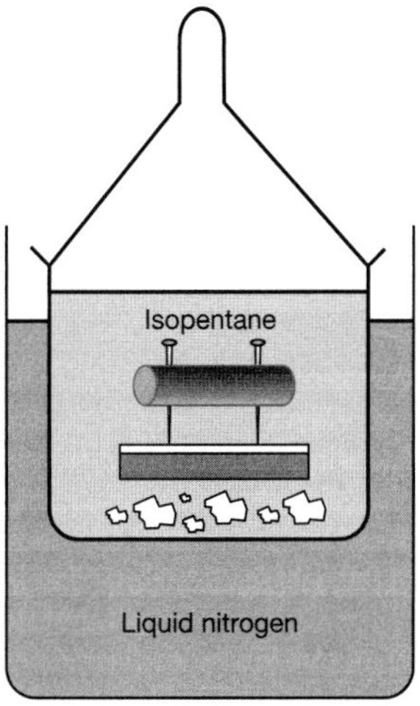

Fig. 1 A small cylinder of muscle under slight tension is pinned to a piece of rubber and prevented from sticking to it by a layer of plastic. When dropped into isopentane, cooled by liquid nitrogen until crystals appear on the bottom of the beaker, the specimen freezes instantly.

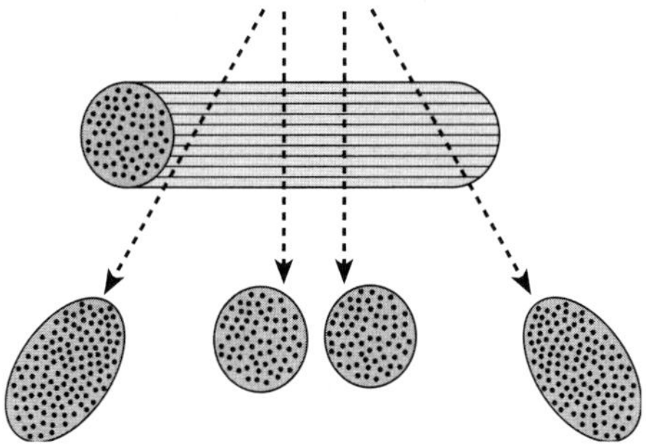

Fig. 2 Fibre size can be reliably assessed from fibre diameter or area, but only in true transvere sections. Poor orientation results in larger elliptical sections and erroneous measurements of fibre size.

Myosin ATPase*	Fibre typing
Oxidative enzymes* Gomori trichrome	Intermyofibrillar network Mitochondria
Acid phosphatase*	Lysosomes, macrophages
Periodic acid Schiff	Glycogen
Oil Red O	Lipid

* Histochemical reaction

Fig. 3 Basic panel of special stains for muscle biopsy interpretation.

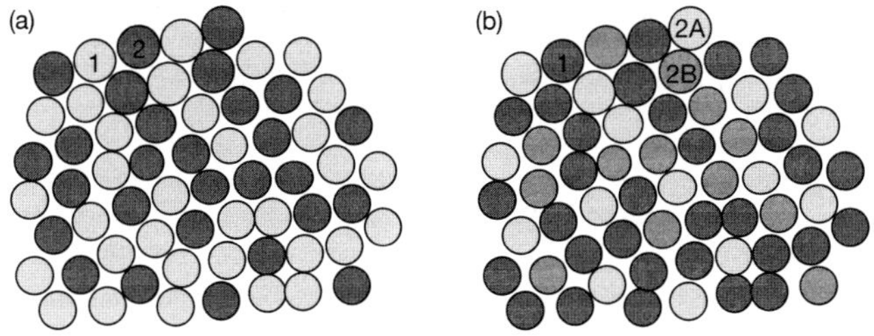

Fig. 4 Fibre types. (a) Myosin ATPase at pH 9.4 shows strong reactivity in type 2 fibres (dark), but enzyme activity is inhibited in type 1 fibres (pale). (b) At acid pH 4.6 there is a reversal of this pattern. The type 1 fibres are dark and the type 2 fibre sub-types are revealed, type 2A (pale) and 2B (intermediate). The intermingling of fibres of adjacent motor units creates the normal mosaic pattern.

physiological properties, that is, differences in twitch speed and fatiguability, correlate with differences in enzyme profile of individual muscle fibres. One fibre category may be selectively involved in disease; therefore identification of fibre types and their variation from the normal pattern are important diagnostic criteria. The myosin ATPase histochemical reaction is the best and most readily reproducible method, by which three types can be distinguished: slow-twitch, fatigue-resistant type-1, and fast-twitch type-2 fibres, which are sub-divided into 2A with intermediate fatiguability and 2B with rapid fatigue (Fig. 4). The muscle fibres within a motor unit are of uniform type but fibres from adjacent units are intermingled, creating a normal mosaic pattern in all normal human limb muscles. A fourth type, 2C fibres, are immature fibres found only in foetal, neonatal, or regenerating muscle. Other stains give additional information about sarcoplasmic contents, the arrangement of myofibrils, and other organelles. Immunocytochemistry may be used to identify and type infiltrating lymphocytes and macrophages in inflammatory disease. Electron microscopy has played an important research role in muscle disorders but has little diagnostic value in the rheumatic disorders.

Clinicopathological correlation

Histological abnormalities in a muscle biopsy are rarely pathognomonic of a single disorder. Rheumatic diseases and conditions with totally different pathogenesis, such as dystrophies or neurogenic atrophy, may not always be distinguished by histological features alone. Close clinicopathological correlation is essential to obtain the maximum diagnostic information from a muscle biopsy. For detailed descriptions of the pathology of neuromuscular disease and biopsy interpretation the reader is referred to elsewhere (Anderson 1985; Engel and Banker 1986; Emslie Smith and Engel 1990). However, a guide to the usual pattern of immunological injury is shown in Plate 89.

Peripheral nerve biopsy in the rheumatic disorders

Definition of the peripheral nervous system

The peripheral nerves include all the neural structures external to the pial sheath of the central nervous system, that is, the axons and sheaths of all cranial nerves except optic and olfactory, all spinal and autonomic nerves, and the dorsal root and autonomic ganglia.

Factors that influence the decision to biopsy

Peripheral nerve biopsy is not an investigation that should be undertaken lightly. Not only is it an invasive procedure, with inevitable scarring and not insignificant post-operative sensory disturbance, but the diagnostic yield is negligible unless there are specialist laboratory facilities for processing the nerve and a pathologist experienced in interpretation. Furthermore, only a tiny, possibly unrepresentative, section of an extensive network can be examined. There are no histological criteria that differentiate motor and sensory fibres, and patterns of degeneration are limited and stereotyped. Only rare disorders, such as leucodystrophies, exhibit disease-specific fine-structural changes. In most peripheral neuropathies, molecular pathogenetic mechanisms are unknown. Morphological clues may incriminate the axon or myelin sheath as the primary target but, inevitably, because of structural and metabolic interdependence, secondary changes will occur. In a single biopsy, the sequence of events is not always easy to reconstruct and diagnostic interpretation must be amplified by close correlation with clinical and electromyographic data.

Indications for biopsy

Biopsy is unnecessary in a large proportion of patients with a peripheral neuropathy because they have a known cause, such as diabetes, or a family history and recognized pattern of hereditary disease. Diseases that selectively involve motor neurones, namely motorneurone disease and hereditary motor neuropathies, manifest as muscle weakness. Muscle biopsy and electromyography, rather than nerve biopsy, are more appropriate methods of investigation.

Nerve biopsy is generally only applicable to peripheral neuropathies with a definite sensory component. In the rheumatoid and autoimmune rheumatic diseases, a diagnostic quest for vasculitis, which is not only the most common cause of peripheral neuropathy in these disorders but also potentially treatable, is the foremost indication for nerve biopsy. Entrapment neuropathies and neuropathy due to drug toxicity occur but are usually recognized without biopsy.

Site

Certain factors dictate the site of nerve biopsy:

1. It must be easily accessible through a small skin incision made under local anaesthetic, therefore superficial, but not subject to repetitive trauma in everyday life, as this alone will injure the nerve.
2. Biopsy must not give rise to unacceptable deficit; therefore cutaneous sensory nerve is preferable to a motor or mixed sensory–motor nerve.
3. The nerve selected must be involved and in most polyneuropathies, the lower legs are earliest and most severely affected.

Hence, the sural nerve, which is purely sensory and easily identified subcutaneously at the ankle, is most often appropriate, but the superficial peroneal and radial nerves are useful alternatives. After exposure the proximal end of the nerve should be incised first. The distal end can then be handled without the patient experiencing abnormal sensations. To minimize discomfort during and deficit after surgery, only partial transection of the nerve and excision of several fascicles is necessary (Plate 90) but, ideally, these should be at least 3 cm long. The success of biopsy relies heavily on careful surgical technique. Artefactual disruption of delicate axons and myelin sheaths is easily produced by stretching or pinching with forceps. The specimen is best transferred immediately, fresh and unfixed, to the laboratory where a skilled technician can sub-divide it for the most appropriate methods of study—generally resin-embedded transverse sections, teased fibre preparations, and electron microscopy. Quantitation of internodal length and nerve fibre diameter and density has an important role in the interpretation of the nerve biopsy (Plates 91 and 92).

Interpretation of the biopsy

Pathological changes are related to the neuronal components principally involved, with an attempt to explain resulting clinical and electrophysiological abnormalities. For a detailed guide to the pathological changes seen on nerve biopsy the reader is referred elsewhere (Thomas and Ochoa 1984; Said et al. 1988; Chaunu et al. 1989; Kissel et al. 1989).

References

Achkar, A.A., Lie, J.T., Hunder, G.G., O'Fallon, M., and Gabriel, S.E. (1994). How does previous corticosteroid treatment affect the biopsy findings in giant cell temporal arteritis? *Annals of Internal Medicine* **120**, 987–92.

Al-Hashimi, I., Wright, J.M., Cooley, C.A., and Nunn, M.E. (2001). Reproducibility of biopsy grade in Sjögren's syndrome. *Journal of Oral Pathology and Medicine* **30**, 408–12.

Allison, M.C. and Gallagher, P.J. (1984). Temporal artery biopsy and steroid treatment. *Annals of the Rheumatic Diseases* **43**, 416–17.

Allsop, C.J. and Gallagher, P.J. (1981). Temporal artery biopsy in giant cell arteritis: a reappraisal. *American Journal of Surgical Pathology* **5**, 317–23.

Anderson, J.R. *Atlas of Skeletal Muscle Pathology*. Lancaster: MTP Press, 1985.

Ashton-Key, M.R. and Gallagher, P.J. (1992). The value of simple morphometric techniques in the diagnosis of osteoporosis. *Pathology Research and Practice* **188**, 616–19.

Baeten, D. et al. (1999). Needle arthroscopy of the knee with synovial biopsy sampling: technical experience in 150 patients. *Clinical Rheumatology* **18**, 434–41.

Baeten, D. et al. (2000). Comparative study of the synovial histology in rheumatoid arthritis, spondyloarthropathy and osteoarthritis: influence of disease duration and activity. *Annals of the Rheumatic Diseases* **59**, 945–53.

Bresnihan, B., Tak, P.P., Emery, P., Klareskog, L., and Breedveldt, F. (2000). Synovial biopsy in arthritis research: five years of concerted European collaboration. *Annals of the Rheumatic Diseases* **59**, 506–10.

Burke, A.P. and Virmani, R. (2001) Localised vasculitis. *Seminars in Diagnostic Pathology* **18**, 59–66.

Chakarbarty, A. and Franks, A.J. (2000). Temporal artery biopsy: is there any value in examining biopsies at multiple levels. *Journal of Clinical Pathology* **53**, 131–6.

Chaunu, M.P. et al. (1989). The spectrum of changes on 20 nerve biopsies in patients with HIV infection. *Muscle and Nerve* **12**, 452–9.

Cox, M. and Gilks, B. (2001). Healed or quiescent arteritis versus senescent changes in temporal artery biopsy specimens. *Pathology* **33**, 163–6.

Corcoran, G.M., Prayson, R.A., and Herzog, K.M. (2001). The significance of perivascular inflammation in the absence of arteritis in temporal artery biopsy specimens. *American Journal of Clinical Pathology* **115**, 342–7.

Cruz-Orive, L.M. and Weibel, E.R. (1990). Recent stereological methods for cell biology: a brief survey. *American Journal of Physiology* **258**, L148–56.

Cunnane, G. et al. (1999). Quantitative analysis of synovial membrane inflammation: a comparison between automated and conventional microscopic measurements. *Annals of the Rheumatic Diseases* **58**, 493–9.

Dalakas, M.C., Isabel, I., Pezeshkpour, G.H., Laukaitis, J.P., Cohen, B., and Griffin, J.L. (1990). Mitochondrial myopathy caused by long term zidovudine therapy. *New England Journal of Medicine* **322**, 1098–105.

Daniels, T.E. (1984). Labial salivary gland biopsy in Sjögren's syndrome. Assessment as a diagnostic criterion in 362 suspected cases. *Arthritis and Rheumatism* **27**, 147–56.

Dempster, D.W. and Lindsay, R. (1993). Pathogenesis of osteoporosis. *Lancet* **341**, 979–801.

Dyck, P.J., Karne, J., Lais, A., and Clarke Stevens, J. (1984). Pathologic alterations of the peripheral nervous system of humans. In *Peripheral Neuropathy* Vol. 1, 2nd edn. (ed. P.J. Dyck, P.K. Thomas, E.H. Lambert, and R. Bunge), pp. 760–870. Philadelphia PA: W.B. Saunders.

Emslie-Smith, A.M. and Engel, A.G. (1990). Microvascular changes in early and advanced dermatomyositis. *Annals of Neurology* **27**, 343–56.

Engel, A.G. and Arahata, K. (1986). Mononuclear cells in myopathies. *Human Pathology* **17**, 704–21.

Engel, A.G. and Banker, B.Q. *Myology*. New York: McGraw-Hill, 1986.

Eriksen, E.G., Axelrod, D.W., and Melsen, F. *Bone Histomorphometry*. New York: Raven Press, 1994.

Fonesca, J.E. et al. (2000). Histology of the synovial tissue: value of semiquantitative analysis for the prediction of joint erosions in rheumatoid arthritis. *Clinical and Experimental Rheumatology* **18**, 559–64.

Gallagher, P.J. (1991). Blood vessels. In *Histology for Pathologists* (ed. S.S. Sternberg), pp. 195–213. New York: Raven Press.

Goldenberg, D.L., Egan, M.S., and Cohen, A.S. (1982). Inflammatory synovitis in inflammatory joint disease. *Journal of Rheumatology* **9**, 204–9.

Gundersen, J.J.G. et al. (1988). Some new, simple and efficient stereological methods and their use in pathological research and diagnosis. *Acta Pathologica Microbiologica et Immunologica Scandinavica* **96**, 379–94.

Hanyu, T., Arai, K., and Takahashi, H.E. (1999). Structural mechanisms of bone loss in iliac biopsies: comparison between rheumatoid arthritis and post menopausal osteoporosis. *Rheumatology International* **18**, 193–200.

Jeanette, J.C. and Falk R.J. (1995). Small vessel vasculitis. *New England Journal of Medicine* **337**, 1512–23.

Johnson, J.S. and Freemont, A.J. (2001). A 10 year retrospective comparison of the diagnostic usefulness of synovial fluid and synovial biopsy examination. *Journal of Clinical Pathology* **54**, 605–7.

Jordan, R.C.K., Pringle, J.G., and Speight, P.M. (1995). High frequency of light chain restriction in labial gland biopsies of Sjögren's syndrome detected by *in situ* hybridization. *Journal of Pathology* **177**, 35–40.

Kennedy, T.D., Plater-Zyberk, C., Partridge, T.A., Woodrow, D.R., and Maini, R.N. (1988a). Representative sample of rheumatoid synovium: a morphometric study. *Journal of Clinical Pathology* **41**, 841–6.

Kennedy, T.D., Plater-Zyberk, C., Partridge, T.A., Woodrow, D.F., and Maini, R.N. (1988b). Morphometric comparison of synovium from patients with osteoarthritis and rheumatoid arthritis. *Journal of Clinical Pathology* **41**, 847–52.

Kidd, B.L., Moore, K., Walters, M.T., Smith, J.L., and Crawley, M.I.D. (1989). Immunohistochemical features of synovitis and ankylosing spondylitis: a comparison with rheumatoid arthritis. *Annals of the Rheumatic Diseases* **48**, 92–8.

Kissel, J.R., Riethman, J.L., Omerza, J., Rammohan, K.W., and Mendell, J.R. (1989). Peripheral nerve vasculitis: immune characterisation of the vascular lesions. *Annals of Neurology* **25**, 291–7.

Leger, J.M. et al. (1989). The spectrum of polyneuropathies in patients affected with HIV. *Journal of Neurology, Neurosurgery and Psychiatry* **52**, 1369–74.

Lie, J.T. (1995). Systemic, pulmonary and cerebral vasculitis. In *Vascular Pathology* (ed. W.E. Stehbens and J.T. Lie), pp. 623–53. London: Chapman and Hall.

Malluche, H.H., Langub, M.C., and Monier-Faugere, M.C. (1999). The role of bone biopsy in clinical practice and research. *Kidney International* **73**, S20–5.

Mata, M., Kahn, S.N., and Fink, D.J. (1988). A direct electron microscopic immunocytochemical study of IgM paraproteinemic neuropathy. *Archives of Neurology* **45**, 693–7.

Nishino, J., Engel, A.G., and Rima, B.K. (1989). Inclusion body myositis. The mumps virus hypothesis. *Annals of Neurology* **25**, 260–4.

Ostendorf, B., Dann, P., and Wedekind, F. (1999). Miniarthroscopy of metacarpophalangeal joints in rheumatoid arthritis. Rating of diagnostic value in synovitis staging and efficiency of biopsy. *Journal of Rheumatology* **26**, 1901–8.

Pariesen, M. et al. (1995). Bone structure in postmenopausal hyperparathyroid, osteoporotic and normal women. *Journal of Bone and Mineral Research* **10**, 1393–9.

Paydas, S., Zorludemir, S., and Sahin, B. (2000). Vasculitis and leukaemia. *Lymphoma and Leukemia* **40**, 105–12.

Pecovnik Balon, B. and Bren, A. (2000). Bone histomorphometry is still the gold standard for diagnosing renal osteodystrophy. *Clinical Nephrology* **54**, 463–9.

Poller, D.N., van Wyk, Q., and Jeffrey, M.J. (2000). The importance of skip lesions in temporal arteritis. *Journal of Clinical Pathology* **53**, 2.

Ropert, A. and Metral, S. (1990). Conduction block in neuropathies with necrotizing vasculitis. *Muscle and Nerve* **13**, 102–5.

Rosenberger, J.L., Cooper, N.S., Soren, A., and McEwen, C. (1981). A statistical approach to the histopathologic diagnosis of synovitis. *Human Pathology* **12**, 329–37.

Said, G., Lacroix-Ciaudo, C., Fujimura, H., Blas, C., and Faux, N. (1988). The peripheral neuropathy of necrotizing arteritis: a clinicopathological study. *Annals of Neurology* **23**, 461–5.

Saito, T. et al. (1999). Low prevalence of clinicopathological and sialographic changes in salivary glands of men with Sjögren's syndrome. *Journal of Oral Pathology and Medicine* **28**, 12–16.

Shore, P.A., Shore, A.C., and Aaron, J.E. (2000). A three-dimensional histological method for direct determination of the number of trabecular termini in cancellous bone. *Biotechnic and Histochemistry* **75**, 183–92.

Silver, R.M., Heyes, M.P., Maize, J.C., Quearry, B., Vionnet-Fuasset, M., and Sternberg, E.M. (1990). Scleroderma, fasciitis and eosinophilia associated with the ingestion of tryptophan. *New England Journal of Medicine* **322**, 874–81.

Soren, A. *Histodiagnosis and Clinical Correlations of Rheumatoid and other Synovitis.* Stuttgart: Thieme, 1978.

Storm, T., Steiniche, T., Thamsborg, G., and Melsen, F. (1993). Changes in bone morphometry after long term treatment with intermittent, cyclic etridonate for post menopausal osteoporosis. *Journal of Bone and Mineral Research* **8**, 199–208.

Tak, P.P. and Bresnihan, B. (2000). The pathogenesis and prevention of joint damage in rheumatoid arthritis: advances from synovial biopsy and tissue analysis. *Arthritis and Rheumatism* **43**, 2619–33.

Thomas, P.K. and Ochoa, J. (1984). Microscopic anatomy of peripheral nerve fibres. In *Peripheral Neuropathy* Vol. 1, 2nd edn. (ed. P.J. Dyck, P.K. Thomas, E.H. Lambert, and R. Bunge), pp. 39–96. Philadelphia PA: W.B. Saunders.

Vital, C. et al. (1988). Peripheral neuropathy with essential mixed cryoglobulinemia: biopsies from 5 cases. *Acta Neuropathologica* **75**, 605–10.

Vital, A., Viral, C., Rigal, B., Decamps, A., Emeriau, J.P., and Galley, P. (1990). Morphological study of the ageing human peripheral nerve. *Clinical Neuropathology* **9**, 10–15.

Xu, K.P., Katagiri, S., Takeuchi, T., and Tsubota, K. (1996). Biopsy of labial salivary glands and lacrimal glands in the diagnosis of Sjögren's syndrome. *Journal of Rheumatology* **23**, 76–82.

Youssef, P.P. et al. (1996). Neutrophil trafficking into inflamed joints in patients with rheumatoid arthritis and the effect of methylprednisolone. *Arthritis and Rheumatism* **39**, 236–42.

Youssef, P.P. et al. (1998a). Quantitative analysis of inflammation in rheumatoid arthritis synovial membrane samples selectes at arthroscopy compared with samples obtained blindly by needle biopsy. *Arthritis and Rheumatism* **41**, 663–9.

Youssef, P.P. et al. (1998b). Microscopic measurement of cellular infiltration in the rheumatoid arthritis synovial membrane: a comparison of semiquantitative and quantitative analysis. *British Journal of Rheumatology* **37**, 1003–7.

5.8 Electrophysiology

Adam Young

Modern nerve conduction studies and electromyography provide unique quantitative information about the function of nerves and muscles. These investigations can be an invaluable aid to both the diagnosis and management of musculoskeletal and neuromuscular disorders. The general aims of electrical tests in these disorders are to:

(i) detect and distinguish between disorders of:
   (a) anterior horn cells,
   (b) nerve roots,
   (c) plexus,
   (d) peripheral nerves,
   (e) neuromuscular junction,
   (f) muscles;

(ii) define location, extent, and severity;

(iii) relate neurophysiological abnormalities to clinical features;

(iv) infer pathology if possible.

The principal application of electrical studies to rheumatic disease is in diagnostic and prognostic assessment of neurological and myopathic features which complicate inflammatory, autoimmune, rheumatic, and soft tissue disorders. Clinical features include muscle weakness or wasting, sensory symptoms, pain, deformity, or a combination of these, and often as the presenting complaint. The most frequently encountered indications,

Table 1 Indications for electrodiagnosis in rheumatic disorders

Clinical feature	Pathophysiology	Examples
Muscle weakness or wasting	Atrophic	Rheumatoid joint
	Myopathic	Polymyositis
	Neuropathic	Rheumatoid or entrapment neuropathy
Sensory symptoms	Peripheral neuropathy	Rheumatoid arthritis or vasculitis
	Entrapment neuropathy	Ulnar neuropathy
Pain	Entrapment neuropathy	Carpal tunnel syndrome
	Nerve injury	Causalgia
Deformity	Hereditary or rare neuromyopathies	Muscular dystrophy
	Entrapment neuropathy	Ulnar nerve claw hand

possible pathophysiological processes, and some examples for electrodiagnosis in rheumatological practice are shown in Table 1.

Several procedures are available and good clinical information is essential for planning an individual examination. The clinician should consider the following points when an electrical test is planned:

(i) The optimum diagnostic yield depends on thorough clinical evaluation of the patient's symptoms and signs, with the appropriate radiology and laboratory tests.

(ii) It only provides physiological information but will complement other studies of pathological (e.g. biopsy) or structural disturbances (e.g. radiology).

(iii) It is uncomfortable for the patient, but safe, and, except for needle sampling, non-invasive.

(iv) It requires specialized equipment and expertise.

(v) Biopsy and electromyography must not be done in the same muscle, and muscle enzymes (e.g. creatine phosphokinase) should be assayed either before or after 2 weeks of muscle sampling.

General principles and methods

Standard texts cover detailed descriptions and technical aspects of stimulation and recording methods (Ludin 1980; Brown and Bolton 1993).

Nerve conduction studies

Compound action potentials are measured in sensory, motor, or mixed nerve fibres by stimulating the nerve and recording the response with surface electrodes. The amplitude, duration, and shape of the evoked response are measured to obtain an estimate of the number of functioning axons contributing to that response. Nerve conduction velocity is obtained by delivering a supramaximal stimulus at two sites along the peripheral nerve and measuring the distance and time between the two [speed (m/s) = distance (cm)/time (ms)]. These findings are compared with the contralateral side and other peripheral nerves, and also to normal values available in standard tables (Ludin 1980) or developed by the user's own laboratory. Values vary from nerve to nerve, but faster velocities are generally seen in the upper (50–70 m/s) compared to the lower limb (40–50 m/s).

Motor nerve conduction

With the surface electrode over the appropriate muscle, the onset of the muscle response, the motor action potential, measured in millivolts, gives the distal motor latency in milliseconds. Figures 1 and 2 show the stimulation and recording sites and traces obtained in an evaluation of the ulnar nerve.

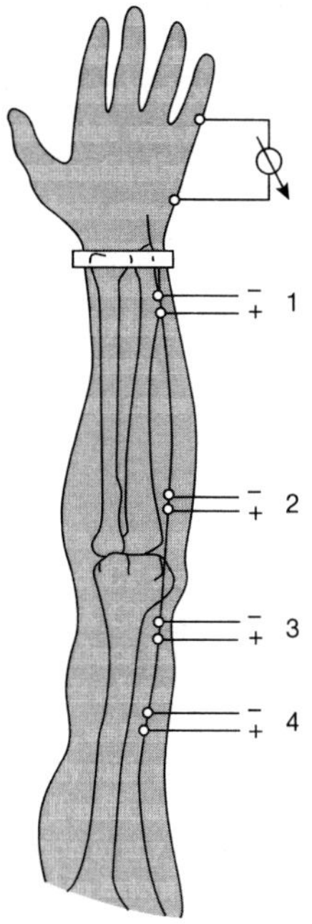

Fig. 1 Stimulation and recording sites of ulnar nerve. The stimulation points of the ulnar nerve are shown at the wrist, below and above the elbow, in the axilla, and at Erb's point in the supraclavicular fossa. A muscular response is recorded from adductor digiti minimi. The distance between the stimulation and recording sites is measured in centimetres, time in milliseconds, and velocities in metres per second. This examination will demonstrate any localized slowing of the ulnar nerve (e.g. compression by Osborne's band at the elbow). More generalized slowing suggests axonal or wallerian degeneration, and if widespread involving other nerves, may be part of a peripheral neuropathy.

Sensory and mixed nerve conduction

Sensory and mixed nerve action potentials can be recorded with skin electrodes placed distally (antidromic) or proximally (orthodromic) to the stimulation site, whichever is technically easier to do. The amplitudes recorded are much lower, in the order of microvolts, and because they are more difficult to elicit, may require averaging techniques. Results are expressed as either distal (to onset) or peak latencies (to peak response). An example of a median nerve sensory study is shown in Fig. 3. The amplitude and latency of the mixed nerve action potential of the median nerve are tested by stimulating in the median fossa, and recording at the wrist.

Reflex latencies

Conduction velocities in proximal segments of nerves are more difficult to measure, and other techniques are available. The most widely used is the *F* response. When a motor nerve is stimulated impulses travel proximally to the anterior horn cells followed by recurrent conduction back down the nerve where the small muscle response (the '*F* wave') can be detected over muscles of the appropriate root distribution. This latency is compared to the other side or height related normal values. They are sometimes technically difficult to elicit and their interpretation is controversial, but a delayed *F* wave in the presence of normal peripheral conduction implies slowing of proximal motor fibres at plexus or root level.

Specific involvement of nerve roots are indicated from conduction studies of the central segments of peripheral nerves by measuring latencies of limb reflexes. The 'H' reflex is mediated through the Ia fibres in the afferent arc of the reflex, most commonly elicited for the monosynaptic reflex arc of the first sacral (S1) root. Increased latencies in the presence of normal

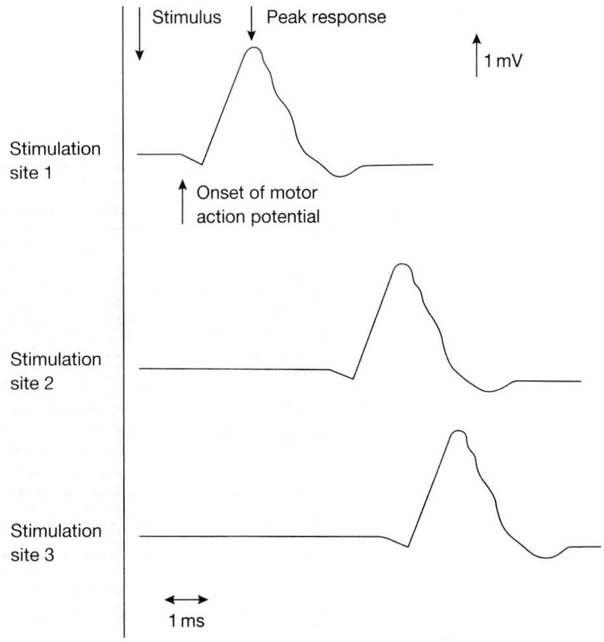

Fig. 2 Recordings of ulnar nerve study. Tracings of a patient with pain, numbness, and weakness in the right hand. Power of fifth finger adduction was reduced. The referring clinician suspected an ulnar nerve lesion and planned ulnar nerve exploration. Stimulation and recording sites were the first three shown in Fig. 1. Amplitudes are recorded in millivolts. The distal latency recorded following stimulation of the ulnar nerve at the wrist was 2.5 ms, and velocities below and above elbow were 59.3 and 58.1 m/s, respectively. These are normal results for ulnar nerve studies, and with the clinical abnormalities suggested a lesion other than in the ulnar nerve itself. This indicated proceeding to other electrical tests described in this chapter. In this example, all motor and sensory studies were normal, but electrical evidence of denervation in adductor digiti minimi was detected, highly suggestive of a pre-ganglionic lesion of the T1 nerve root or in the anterior horn cell.

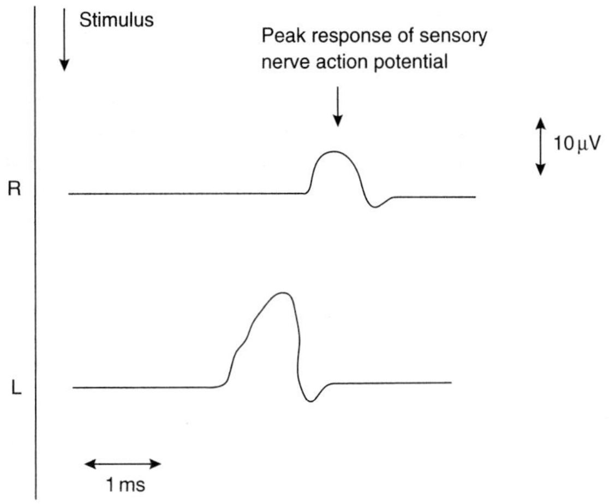

Fig. 3 Sensory nerve conduction study in median nerve. Tracings of a patient referred for suspected carpal tunnel syndrome, which had not responded to conservative measures. The recording electrodes are placed over the index finger as shown in Fig. 1 and median nerve stimulated at wrist. The amplitude is measured in microvolts (vertical scale) and peak latency in milliseconds (horizontal scale). The latency for the right median nerve is delayed compared to the normal reference range and to the left (asymptomatic) side. Although not shown here, right median nerve motor conduction was delayed at the wrist but normal in the forearm, thus confirming the clinician's diagnosis.

peripheral conduction imply dysfunction of this root. The posterior tibial nerve is stimulated at below threshold strength in the popliteal fossa and the motor response recorded in medial head of gastrocnemius muscle in the calf. A technique using an electronically triggered patella hammer has made reflex studies easier to perform and more comfortable for patients. The ankle jerk is elicited in the usual way, the latency (milliseconds) recorded with a surface electrode over gastrocnemius, and compared to the other side. Its absence or a delay of 2 ms or more is found in conditions that affect this reflex. For example, in a patient who presents with sciatica but no evidence of tension signs or abnormal neurology, a delayed ankle jerk latency in the presence of normal conduction of the peripheral segments of sciatic and peroneal nerves is suggestive of a S1 root lesion.

Neuromuscular function

Repetitive nerve stimulation and recordings of motor action potentials can reveal abnormalities of neuromuscular transmission. In myasthenia gravis, significant decrement occurs in about 60 per cent if one muscle is sampled but can be improved to 95 per cent if other muscle groups are included.

Electromyography

Electromyography is the recording and study of spontaneous and voluntary electrical activity of muscle. The first objective is to distinguish between primary muscle disease and the secondary changes due to neurogenic disorders. Then, the pattern of muscle involvement in conjunction with nerve conjunction studies helps distinguish between conditions of the anterior horn cell, nerve roots, plexus, or peripheral nerve.

A normal muscle at rest has no detectable electrical activity, apart from initial insertional activity or in the vicinity of the motor end plate. If a motor unit loses its nerve supply, sensitivity to acetylcholine increases and spontaneous discharges can be detected by the needle electrode, and amplified and displayed on a cathode ray oscilloscope as small spontaneous fibrillation potentials (less than 300 μV). They may be confused with normal 'motor end plate noise', an important distinction because spontaneous fibrillation is characteristic of denervation, as is the related positive sharp wave. The interpretation of these changes requires considerable skill and experience and is largely a matter of personal judgement.

Motor action potentials recorded during voluntary contraction are much larger and vary from 1 to 8 mV depending on the muscle. They are reduced if motor units are lost (e.g. primary myopathy) or muscle fibres cannot be activated (e.g. myasthenia gravis). In axonal degeneration, sprouting of surviving axons attempt to reinnervate nearby denervated muscle fibres and this can be detected electrically by the appearance of polyphasic and large amplitude motor action potentials ('giant units'). When the force of contraction is increased more units are activated, and these recruitment patterns vary with different conditions. Analysis of these interference patterns remains subjective.

Other features recognized include the complex repetitive discharges of polymyositis, fasciculation potentials characteristic of denervation, and the myotonic discharges of myotonia. Single fibre techniques can be useful in detailed examination of the motor unit particularly in the diagnosis of motor end plate disorders and re-innervation. This was initially a very time consuming refined method, but has been simplified to some extent by modern methods. The 'blanket technique' described by Payan (1978) bridges the gap between single-fibre and conventional electromyography.

Sensory evoked potentials

Very small potentials, evoked by repetitive percutaneous stimulation of peripheral nerves, can be detected by surface electrodes over the skin of spinal cord or scalp using averaging techniques. These somatosensory evoked potentials have been extensively used in the investigation of patients with multiple sclerosis, particularly in suspected cases and in revealing clinically silent lesions (Jones 1982). They have also been used to investigate peripheral neuropathies, and are particularly well suited to the investigation of proximal lesions of the brachial plexus and spinal nerve roots, which are so inaccessible to normal recording methods (Jones et al. 1981). Dermatotomal somatosensory evoked potentials found a place in the assessment of radicular symptoms in degenerative lumbar spinal disease (Katifi and Sedgwick 1987), but have now largely been replaced by modern and improved radiological imaging.

Clinical application

How can electrical methods assist the clinician in rheumatological practice? The answer to this depends on the nature, site and chronicity of the lesion, the clinical information available, and the knowledge of other features, which may affect the electrical findings, for example, the presence of neurological anomalies or dual pathology. This investigation can be crucial in decisions regarding surgery.

Three main pathological processes result in the electrical abnormalities of conduction studies:

- demyelination (e.g. hereditary neuropathies, diabetes mellitus)
- axonal degeneration (e.g. polio, motor neurone disease)
- metabolic effects (e.g. renal failure)

It is customary to use the term demyelination for neuropathies with a primary disorder of the myelin sheath. Prolonged distal latencies and conduction velocities are the characteristic electrical findings, the best-known examples being the hereditary neuropathies. The degree of slowing parallels the degree of demyelination, and conduction velocities are usually reduced by at least 30 per cent. Segmental demyelination is found localized to one segment of a nerve in the entrapment neuropathies at the site of compression. Conduction block refers to failure of conduction in an intact axon or nerve fibre, and is important to recognize because full recovery of muscle weakness or sensory loss is possible if the block is reversed (e.g. carpal tunnel syndrome).

More prolonged compression of a peripheral nerve results in further damage to the axons distal to the lesion causing wallerian degeneration (Levin 1993). Absent or reduced amplitudes of sensory, motor or mixed action potentials in the presence of normal or slightly reduced conduction velocities are characteristic of axonal degeneration. This is because, as in most peripheral neuropathies, the disease process affects fast conducting, large diameter fibres preferentially and the remaining smaller diameter fibres conduct at slightly slower rates. Motor conduction velocities of less than 40 m/s are unusual (McLeod et al. 1973). In rheumatological practice, axonal degeneration is typical of the vasculitides, for example, mononeuritis multiplex. Certain conditions result in a mixed pattern of electrical findings, for example, in diabetes mellitus and Guillain–Barre syndrome. The rapid improvement in conduction times after renal transplants has been explained on the basis of metabolic effects.

The degree and site of these changes (Table 2) indicate the presence of axonal degeneration or widespread or segmental demyelination, thus focusing the differential diagnosis. Electrical studies also help to distinguish the relative importance of the coexistence of these processes, for example, entrapment neuropathies in the presence of generalized neuropathies of rheumatoid arthritis. Timing of the investigation may be important, and serial studies may be helpful. For example, because the amplitude of the motor action potential reflects the number of surviving axons, the response in the thenar muscles on stimulating the median nerve at wrist is a useful prognostic indicator in the early stages of a polyradiculitis (Miller et al. 1988). Significant demyelination in the childhood and hereditary neuropathies can be a useful predictor of response to steroid treatment.

Table 2 Summary of electrical findings of conduction studies in neuropathy

Electrical features	Axonal degeneration	Segmental demyelination
Amplitude	Markedly reduced	Normal/slight reduction
Distal latency	Normal/slight delay	Marked delay
Velocity	Normal/slight delay	Marked delay
Examples	Vasculitis	Diabetes

Common clinical conditions

Acute nerve injury

The study of traumatic nerve lesions has contributed much to the understanding of nerve conduction, and has been successfully applied to other lesions of peripheral nerves. The basic principles of nerve damage, the differences between contusion (neuropraxia), trauma (neurontemesis), and nerve division (axontemesis), and detailed clinical descriptions can be found elsewhere (Smith 1998).

A surgical opinion should be sought early in these cases because the timing of surgery can be crucial to recovery. Planning rehabilitation can be helped by the prognostic information provided by electrical methods. Wallerian degeneration requires nerve regrowth and if present the time scale of recovery is inevitably longer and dependent on the length of nerve and degree of damage.

Acute compression neuropathies

Sudden but prolonged compression of a peripheral nerve leads to mild focal demyelination affecting large fibres preferentially. Nerve conduction studies reveal motor and sensory conduction block at the damaged site, but normal conduction studies distally because the nerve is electrically still intact (Ochoa et al. 1973). This is followed by gradual electrical and clinical recovery accompanied by wallerian degeneration, which may be detected by evidence of electromyographic features of denervation. The clinical syndromes most often seen in rheumatological practice are shown in Table 3.

The so-called 'tourniquet palsy' may in fact be due to prolonged pressure due to poor positioning of a limb during prolonged anaesthesia. Similar clinical and electrical features are sometimes seen following the reduction of difficult fractures and the removal of tight plaster casts. Bonney (1986) has reviewed iatrogenic nerve damage extensively. Post-surgical complications include traction of peripheral and cervical nerve roots during anaesthesia, damage to ulnar nerve (elbow arthroplasty), common peroneal nerve (knee surgery), sciatic nerve (total hip replacement), superficial radial nerve (De Quervain's tenosynovitis), digital nerve (Dupytren's contracture), and spinal accessory nerve (neck). The changes detected electrically depend critically on when they are performed after injury. Spontaneous fibrillation so characteristic of denervation does not appear for at least 10 days. The appearance of this or other electrical signs of axonal degeneration indicate a slow recovery.

Table 3 Acute nerve entrapment syndromes

Sign	Nerve	Condition
Wrist drop	Radial nerve palsy	Saturday night palsy Tourniquet palsy
Weak hand	Ulnar nerve	Tourniquet palsy
Foot drop	Common peroneal nerve	Crossed leg palsy Tight plaster cast Tourniquet palsy
	Sciatic nerve	Total hip replacement Haematoma in haemophilia or poor anticoagulation control

Chronic or subacute compressive (entrapment) neuropathies

Mononeuropathies developing after prolonged mechanical damage to a nerve at a site of anatomical constriction are common. The best known is the median nerve in the carpal tunnel. Following focal demyelination, segmental demyelination occurs and progresses to wallerian degeneration. Varying degrees of slowing of nerve conduction velocities are found and in early or mild cases sensory nerves studies are more sensitive (Buchtal and Rosenfalk 1971). Needle sampling may reveal denervation in the relevant muscles in more severe cases.

Electrical studies determine the exact site and severity of a lesion in these conditions, and may also help to assess prognosis and treatment response, depending on the nature and site of the lesion. However, correlation of clinical and electrical findings is not always straight forward. For diagnosis it is important to demonstrate that delay in conduction distal to the site of compression is disproportionate to any mild proximal slowing. Electrodiagnostic demonstration of an isolated motor nerve root lesion can be achieved by finding evidence of denervation in a group of muscles corresponding to the distribution of the spinal segment rather than the peripheral nerve. A pre-ganglionic root lesion will not affect the distal sensory action potential whereas a post-ganglionic lesion may do so because the integrity of the peripheral nerve fibre may be affected. This may be vital information in differentiating between a lesion of the anterior horn cell (e.g. motor neurone disease) and a localized post-ganglionic lesion (e.g. in the brachial plexus). Greater details of all the entrapment neuropathies can be found in surgical and neurology texts (Smith 1998; Dawson et al. 1999).

Median nerve

Carpal tunnel syndrome is the commonest chronic nerve entrapment. Although usually idiopathic, underlying causes have been well described and fortunately mild cases usually respond to conservative measures. Electrodiagnosis is generally indicated with atypical or progressive clinical presentations to exclude other conditions such as radiculopathies or proximal median nerve lesions:

1. Wasting or weakness of thenar muscle. In the presence of osteoarthritis of the CMC joint of the thumb, this may be difficult to determine clinically. If sensory symptoms are absent or minimal, or it progresses, motor neurone disease should be considered.
2. Dual pathology is suspected at cervical spine level and at wrist, the so-called double crush syndrome (Upton and McComus 1973). This information may affect treatment.
3. If surgical exploration and/or decompression is considered.
4. Recurrent symptoms following surgery for median nerve decompression may be due to inadequate surgery. This can be better demonstrated electrically in comparison with a pre-operative result.

The minimal diagnostic criterion is a prolonged median sensory conduction velocity at the wrist with a normal ulnar sensory velocity. The distal motor latency to abductor pollucis brevis is normally also determined. Using these criteria, Boniface et al. (1994) reported that nerve conduction studies excluded the clinical diagnosis of carpal tunnel syndrome in 36 per cent, and most of these patients (72 per cent) responded to conservative treatment. In this study, it was clear that decisions whether to perform decompressive surgery were greatly influenced by positive electrical findings, and the authors highlight the importance of the investigation as part of good clinical practice as well as health service costs. Although the decision to operate is essentially a clinical one, the absence of a sensory action potential or a distal motor latency of more than 5 ms in median nerve, or evidence of denervation in abductor pollucis muscle are strong indicators for surgery.

Post-operative electrical studies are difficult to interpret without pre-operative data. Goodman and Gilliat (1961) reported that electrical recovery depended on degree of delay of distal motor latencies recorded pre-operatively. Values greater than 10, 7–10, and 5–7 ms respectively, required up to 18, 8–12, and 6 months to recover. Surgeons still report patients with typical carpal tunnel symptoms who respond to decompressive surgery in the presence of normal electrical findings, which can be normal in 5–10 per cent (Wilcox and Bilbao 1993). Refinements of electrodiagnosis reported by Mills (1985) in which the median nerve is stimulated in the palm and recorded at the wrist improves sensitivity.

Ulnar nerve

The second most frequent entrapment neuropathy affects this nerve, mainly at the elbow in the cubital tunnel or medial epicondylar groove. Causes include injury, iatrogenic, arthropathies of the elbow, repeated pressure, but in the majority idiopathic. The common indications for ulnar nerve studies are:

(i) the degree and exact site of damage at the elbow;

(ii) whether the lesion is in the ulnar nerve or the 1st thoracic root;

(iii) whether an ulnar nerve lesion of the hand is proximal or distal to the bifurcation into deep muscle and superficial sensory branches;

(iv) part of work up for a peripheral neuropathy.

Conduction studies of ulnar nerve lesions at the elbow correlate well with clinical severity and localization is correct in 95 per cent (Payan 1969). Classification systems to guide treatment are based mainly on patient symptoms, and supported by clinical and electrical findings. Mild symptoms without objective signs can usually be best treated conservatively, and excellent results have been reported in 58 per cent for non-operative treatment of minimal lesions (Dellon 1989). Surgery should be considered in patients with moderate symptoms, pain, motor symptoms, or signs that progress, and in patients who fail to respond to non-operative treatment. Electrical tests are an important adjunct to this clinical assessment. A reduction of more than 25 per cent in the amplitude of the motor action potential from abductor digiti minimi muscle suggests conduction block. Ulnar nerve decompression without transposition is often all that is needed, especially in patients with a short history, mild weakness, and mild abnormalities of sensory nerve action potentials. Transposition of the ulnar nerve is still being performed purely on clinical grounds. It should be reserved for patients with objective evidence of ulnar nerve damage, because repair or mobilization of peripheral nerves can cause causalgia and become long term treatment problem (Wynn Parry 1988).

Radial nerve

Entrapment of this nerve is uncommon, but can be injured in the axilla (e.g. pressure from a crutch), in spiral groove (Saturday night palsy), or by fracture of humerus or radius. Thorough clinical examination is usually sufficient for initial diagnosis and monitoring recovery. As with the ulnar nerve it may occur post-operatively from faulty positioning or prolonged tourniquet pressure. If there is any dispute about the cause or timing of such a lesion, electrodiagnosis may be required for medicolegal reasons. Surgery is not often indicated.

Cervicothoracic nerve roots and brachial plexus

Radicular symptoms in the upper limb are common in rheumatology clinics. They are usually due to cervical disc or facet joint degeneration, and conservative measures are normally successful. Cervical ribs and bands in the thoracic outlet syndrome, tumours, and irradiation are uncommon. If further investigation is required, magnetic resonance imaging is the most productive. Electrical studies may contribute to diagnosis if a structural lesion has not been demonstrated radiologically, or this is not consistent with the clinical findings, or there is clinical progression, or surgery is considered. '*F*' waves and somatosensory evoked potentials can sometimes be helpful in the diagnosis of lesions of the proximal segments of these nerves. Electrical studies will exclude lesions of these nerves at more peripheral sites in patients with unusual presentations or poor response to treatment, and those with dual pathology. The latter includes carpal tunnel syndrome and cervical radiculopathy, rheumatoid involvement of both cervical spine (often silent) and hand or elbow, and multiple nerve entrapment syndromes. In neuralgic amyotrophy (brachial neuritis), when muscle weakness and wasting of shoulder or scapula muscles can be rapid and severe, needle sampling will show spontaneous fibrillation, typical of denervation. The diagnosis and planning of treatment for traction lesions of the brachial plexus has been shown to be greatly helped by expert electrical examination in special centres (Jones et al. 1981; Wynn Parry 1988).

Sciatic and common peroneal nerves

The sciatic nerve may be injured following traction during hip surgery. The common peroneal nerve is vulnerable to injury at the fibula head. Electrical studies are indicated when:

(i) recovery is poor,

(ii) decompressive surgery is considered, or

(iii) there is difficulty distinguishing between an isolated palsy or a 5th lumbar nerve root lesion.

If the diagnosis is uncertain or the lesion is complete and recovery is not apparent or appears very slow, decisions about planning physiotherapy, rehabilitation, and type of leg appliances all require prognostic information early. This can often only be obtained by electromyography. In distinguishing between a L5 root lesion and peroneal nerve palsy causing a foot drop, the weakness of foot eversion which is found in peroneal nerve palsies is not always easy to demonstrate. The posterior tibialis is one of the few muscles innervated by the L5 root and not via peroneal nerve and therefore an important muscle to examine to distinguish these two lesions. It is a difficult muscle to examine clinically but ideal for needle sampling. Sensory studies of sural and superficial peroneal nerves can be helpful.

Back pain and sciatica

Electrical studies do not have a place in the routine work up of acute or chronic mechanical back pain with or without sciatica. Over 95 per cent of prolapsed disc disorders are successfully diagnosed by careful clinical examination followed by radiological studies. Modern imaging methods of the lumbosacral spine have greatly improved the visualization of the spinal canal and its recesses. Electrical methods provide physiological information and can still be occasionally useful in the following circumstances (Young and Wynn Parry 1988):

(i) the problem of failed surgery,

(ii) clinical and radiological signs which do not correspond, or

(iii) isolating single nerve root involvement by epidural fibrosis in extensive arachnoiditis.

Electrical abnormalities can remain for more than a year post-operatively in paraspinal and peripheral muscles and must be interpreted carefully (Young et al. 1983).

Other less commonly affected nerves (Smith 1998)

Lesions in anterior and posterior interosseus nerves in forearm and deep branch of ulnar nerve within Guyon's canal of the hand can be confirmed with motor conduction studies and by finding abnormalities in the appropriate muscles on needle sampling. Conduction studies are difficult in the lateral cutaneous nerve of the thigh (meralgia paresthetica). This also applies for the facial nerve, for which needle sampling is uncomfortable, a problem to interpret, and prognostic information limited, but can determine whether loss of motor units is complete or not. The tarsal tunnel syndrome is uncommon, it is a painful area to examine electrically but denervation found on needle sampling proves reliable and treatment can be rewarding.

Peripheral neuropathies

Motor, sensory, and mixed conduction studies in both arms and legs are essential if a generalized neuropathy is suspected. Sensory investigations are more sensitive than motor studies, especially the sural sensory and peroneal mixed action potentials in sensory neuropathies. The differential diagnosis can be reduced by careful appraisal of the clinical features, the degree of slowing and magnitude of amplitude responses, and which sensory and/or motor nerves are affected. Differentiation between the numerous possible causes of peripheral neuropathies on the basis of electrical findings alone is possible in only a few cases. The common causes of peripheral neuropathy such as diabetes, drug and alcohol effects, and vitamin deficiencies can usually be diagnosed by means of full and detailed clinical, radiological, laboratory, and electrical investigations.

Two varieties of peripheral neuropathy are well-recognized features of rheumatoid disease (Pallis and Scott 1965). Low amplitudes and slowing of sensory conduction suggest segmental demyelination found in the more common mild distal sensory neuropathy which has a good prognosis. Reduced amplitudes with or without widespread denervation in the presence of relatively normal conduction suggest axonal degeneration found in the more severe sensorimotor neuropathy. This may start as an isolated neuropathy and progress as part of a vasculitic process as in mononeuritis multiplex. Electrical studies are clearly valuable in distinguishing the two and demonstrating the extent of involvement, which may not be apparent clinically because of joint deformity or synovitis.

It is not unusual to record normal electrical values in patients who present with features of a peripheral neuropathy. These cases can be explained on the basis of very early mild disease, involvement of small diameter fibres only, central lesions of the nerve root, or non-organic disorders (Payan 1985). Most series record that as many 50 per cent of cases remain undiagnosed, but in detailed studies inherited disorder accounted for 42 per cent, inflammatory demyelinating polyradiculopathies in 21 per cent, and 13 per cent had other acquired neuropathies (Dyke and Thomas 1993).

Myopathies

Primary myopathic disorders can affect muscle fibres (e.g. hereditary myopathies), nerve terminals (e.g. polymyositis), or the neuromuscular junction (e.g. myasthenia gravis). The electrophysiological diagnosis of many myopathies is based on needle sampling and generally conduction studies are normal. Electrodiagnosis is most rewarding in the acute phases of the inflammatory myopathies. The classic changes in polymyositis are those of myopathic degeneration and acute denervation. Fibrillation potentials have been reported in 74 per cent of polymyositis and 33 per cent of dermatomyositis patients (Bohan et al. 1977), but are not an essential prerequisite for the diagnosis of an inflammatory myopathy. Other changes include myopathic motor potentials (low amplitude short duration motor unit potentials) and polyphasic potentials. These changes allow successful diagnosis in about two-thirds of cases, including the other inflammatory arthropathies that can be complicated by myopathy, such as rheumatoid arthritis and systemic lupus erythematosus. The diagnosis depends on the typical clinical features, an elevated creatine phosphokinase, electromyographic abnormalities, and histological changes seen on muscle biopsy.

The most common drug-induced myopathy is steroid treatment, which is at least partially dose dependent, often sub-clinical, and frequently electromyography and biochemistry are normal. It may be difficult to distinguish between the changes of polymyositis and the myopathic changes seen in chronic steroid treatment (particularly fluoridized corticosteroids). However, florid spontaneous activity makes an inflammatory aetiology a high probability. A muscle biopsy is usually the only way to make the distinction safely. The other causes of myopathy, for example, metabolic myopathies and the muscular dystrophies, require other more detailed investigations in addition to electromyography for a definitive diagnosis. The assessment of treatment of the myopathies is mainly a clinical skill and although occasionally helpful in some instances, electrodiagnosis has not found a place in the routine management of these cases.

Multifocal pathology

This may be suspected clinically, for example, in mononeuritis multiplex, but more often is revealed by the appropriate electrical tests. Certain conditions characterized by mild generalized neuropathic changes, which are often sub-clinical, are also prone to localized entrapment neuropathies because of mechanical pressure as in diabetes, hypothyroidism, chronic alcoholism, inflammatory arthritis, and familial pressure palsies. Cervical and/or lumbar root pathology, although clinically mild, is not uncommon in the older patient and may be found during investigation for other conditions. In a series of patients with carpal tunnel syndrome reported by Murray-Leslie and Wright (1976), a third had other soft tissue lesions, at elbow, shoulder, or neck. Cervical spine dimensions were significantly smaller in this group. A full clinical summary is vital to explain unusual electrical findings due to dual pathology.

Safety issues and pitfalls in electrodiagnosis

The normal ranges for motor nerve conduction were first established by Hermann von Helmolz in the summer months of the early 1850s. Subsequent studies by him in the winter demonstrated the significant effect of temperature on nerve conduction and present day electromyographers are well aware of the necessity to provide standard temperatures (preferably warm ones) for this examination. The limbs of cold patients need to be warmed to obtain meaningful results. Age is another factor that can influence electrical readings, with peak conduction velocities seen in the teens. Full term neonates have half the normal adult ranges. There is a reduction of 0.5–1.8 m/s every 10 years after the age of 20. Amplitude decay increase with age. This may be clinically relevant, for example, in loss of sural nerve sensory action potentials in patients over 65. Anomalies of innervation can affect the interpretation of electrophysiological findings (Sonck et al. 1991). The most common is the Martin-Gruber anastomosis between ulnar and median nerves which occurs in 10–20 per cent of the population. Conventional electrical tests will be essentially normal in patients with upper motor neurone lesions or with non-organic signs. In the latter, when the hysteria-conversion reaction or malingering posture makes clinical examination so difficult, electrical testing can be extremely helpful in excluding severe organic disease, but occasionally reveals a genuine underlying pathological lesion. Safety precautions include patients with pacemakers, although modern versions protect against electrical stimulation, and needle sampling in patients with clotting disorders. Risk of bleeding is increased if the prothrombin time is double normal values or platelet counts are less than 50 000/cm^3. Transmission of infectious disease (e.g. hepatitis B or C, and HIV) is negligible using disposable needle electrodes.

References

Bohan, A., Peter, J.B., Bowman, R.L., and Pearson, C.M. (1977). A computerised assisted analysis of 153 patients with polymyositis and dermatomyositis. *Medicine* **56**, 255–86.

Boniface, S.J., Morris, I. M., and Macleod, A. (1994). How does neurophysiological assessment influence the management and outcome of patients with carpal tunnel syndrome? *British Journal of Rheumatology* **33**, 1169–70.

Bonney, G. (1986). Iatrogenic injury of nerves. *Journal of Bone and Joint Surgery* **68B**, 9–13.

Brown, W. and Bolton, C. *Clinical Electromyography* 2nd edn. Boston MA: Butterworth Heinmann, 1993.

Buchtal, F. and Rosenfalck, A. (1971). Sensory potentials in neuropathy. *Brain* **94**, 241–62.

Dawson, D.M., Hallet, M., and Wilbourn, A.J. *Entrapment Neuropathies.* Lippincott-Raven, 1999.

Dellon, A.L. (1989). Review of treatment results for ulnar nerve entrapment at the elbow. *Journal of Hand Surgery* **14**, 688–99.

Dyke, P.J. and Thomas, P.K. *Peripheral Neuropathy.* Philadelphia PA: W.B. Saunders, 1993.

Dyck, P., Oviatt, K.F., and Lambert, E.H. (1981). Intensive evaluation of referred unclassified neuropathies yields improved diagnosis. *Annals of Neurology* **10**, 222–6.

Goodman, H.V. and Gilliat, R.J. (1961). The effect of treatment of median nerve conduction in patients with carpal tunnel syndrome. *Annals of Physical Medicine* **6**, 137.

Jones, S.J. (1982). Clinical applications of short latency somatosensory evoked potentials. *Annals of the New York Academy of Sciences* **388**, 369–87.

Jones, S.J., Wynn Parry, C.B., and Landi, A. (1981). Diagnosis of brachial plexus traction lesions by sensory nerve action potentials. *Injury* **12**, 376–82.

Katifi, H.A. and Sedgwick, E.M. (1987). Evaluation of the dermatomal somatosensory evoked potentials in the diagnosis of lumbo-sacral root compression. *Journal of Neurology, Neurosurgery and Psychiatry* **50** (9), 1204–10.

Levin, K.G. (1993). Common focal mononeuropathies and their electrodiagnosis. *Clinical Neurophysiology* **10**, 181–9.

Ludin, H.P. *Electromyography in Practice.* New York: Georg Thieme Verlag Thieme–Stratton, 1980.

McLeod, J.G., Prineas, J.W., and Walsh, J.C. (1973). The relationship of conduction velocity to pathology in peripheral nerves. In *New Developments in EMG and Clinical Neurophysiology* Vol. 2 (ed. J.E. Desmedt). Basel: Karger.

Miller, R.G., Petersen, G.W., Daube, J.R., and Albers, J.W. (1988). Prognostic value of electrodiagnosis in Guillain–Barre syndrome. *Muscle and Nerve* **11**, 769–74.

Mills, K.R. (1985). Orthodromic sensory action potentials from palmar stimulation in the diagnosis of carpal tunnel syndrome. *Journal of Neurology, Neurosurgery and Psychiatry* **48**, 250–5.

Murray-Leslie, M. and Wright, V. (1976). Carpal tunnel syndrome, humeral epicondylitis and the cervical spine: a study of clinical and dimensional relations. *British Medical Journal* **1**, 1439–42.

Ochoa, J., Fowler, T.J., and Gilliatt, R.W. (1973). Changes produced by a pneumatic tourniquet. In *New Developments in EMG and Clinical Neurophysiology* Vol. 2 (ed. J.E. Desmedt). Basel: Karger.

Pallis, C.A. and Scott, J.T. (1965). Peripheral neuropathy in rheumatoid arthritis. *British Medical Journal* **1**, 1141.

Payan, P. (1969). Electrophysiological localisation of ulnar nerve lesions. *Journal of Neurology, Neurosurgery and Psychiatry* **32**, 208–20.

Payan, P. (1978). The Blanket principle: a technical note. *Muscle and Nerve* **1**, 423–6.

Payan, P. (1985). Peripheral neuropathy. In *Contemporary Neurology* (ed. M. Harrison), pp. 225–33. London: Butterworths.

Smith, S.J.M. (1998). Electrodiagnosis. In *Surgical Disorders of the Peripheral Nerves* (ed. R. Birch, G. Bonney, and C.B. Wynn Parry), pp. 467–90. Edinburgh: Churchill Livingstone.

Sonck, W.H., Francx, M.H., and Engels, H.L. (1991). Innervation anomolies in upper and lower extremities: potential clinical implications. *Electromyography and Clinical Neurophysiology* **31** (2), 67–80.

Upton, A.R.M. and McComus, A.J. (1973). The double crush in nerve entrapment syndromes. *Lancet* **ii**, 359–62.

Wilcox and Bilbao (1993). Sensitivity of electrophysiological studies and carpal tunnel syndrome. *Muscle and Nerve* **16**, 1265–6.

Wynn Parry, C.B. (1988). Update on peripheral nerve injuries. *International Disability Studies* **10**, 11–20.

Young, A., Getty, J., Jackson, A., Kirwan, E., Sullivan, M., and Wynn Parry, C.B. (1983). Variations in the pattern of muscle innervation by L5 and S1 nerve roots. *Spine* **8**, 616–24.

Young, A. and Wynn Parry, C.B. (1988). The assessment and management of the failed back. *International Disability Studies* **10**, 21–5.

6

The scope of rheumatic disease

6 The scope of rheumatic disease

6.1 Epidemiology

6.1.1 Epidemiology and the rheumatic diseases

Karen Walker-Bone and Cyrus Cooper

Introduction

Derived from the Greek words, *epi-* (among) and *demos* (the people), epidemiology is the scientific study of the distribution and determinants of disease among human populations. The geographical distribution of a disease, the variations in its frequency at different times, and the special characteristics of people affected by it, are part of the basic description by means of which it is defined and recognized. Historically, when medical practice was overshadowed by epidemics of infectious diseases, doctors were inevitably concerned with disease distributions, leading to early successes such as that with cholera, whereby study of the distribution led to identification of causes and thence to prevention (Box 1).

During the twentieth century, however, the discipline of epidemiology has evolved and attention has expanded from acute infectious and dietary diseases to the study of chronic degenerative diseases (such as arthritis and osteoporosis), that are now among the leading causes of morbidity in the developed world.

The principles of epidemiology

Three closely interrelated components—frequency, distribution, and determinants—encompass all epidemiological principles and methods (Fig. 1).

Box 1

In London, during the mid-nineteenth century, drinking water was supplied to residents by several water companies. John Snow, a British physician, compared the cholera mortality rates for residents using water from two of the major water companies: the Southwark and Vauxhall Company, which used sewage contaminated water from the Thames and the Lambeth Water Company, which obtained its water from a source free of London sewage. Within the area supplied by both companies, John Snow walked from house to house and collected information about the water supply for every household from which a cholera death occurred. Snow demonstrated that the cholera outbreak could be traced back to water supplied by the Southwark and Lambeth Water Company (Snow 1860).

Measurement of the frequency of disease involves quantification of the existence or occurrence of a disease. The distribution of disease considers such issues as who is getting the disease within a population and when and where a disease is occurring. Such issues may be studied in different populations at the same time, in the same population at different times, or between sub-groups of the population. The third component, the determinants of disease, derives from the first two, since epidemiological hypotheses are formulated and tested from knowledge of the frequency and distribution of disease (see Box 2).

The frequency of the rheumatic diseases

Measures of disease frequency are tools used to describe how common an illness is with reference to the size of the population 'at risk'. The most basic measure is a simple count of affected individuals, which provides information for public health planners and administrators who wish to determine the allocation of health care resources in a particular community (Table 1). In City A, 4200 people have rheumatoid arthritis, while in City B, there are 2060 people with the disease. This information allows health care administrators to allocate resources in the two cities in order to care for the affected individuals. However, count data alone are of limited utility for epidemiologists.

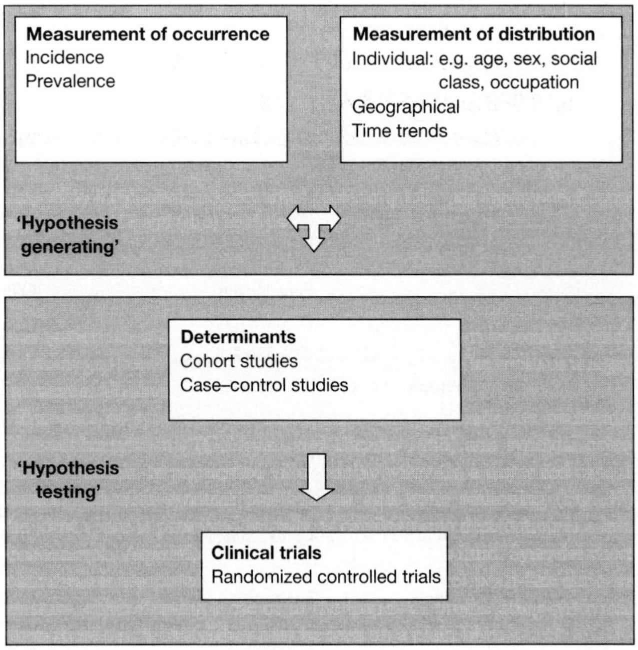

Fig. 1 The epidemiological principles.

Box 2

During the first half of the last century, researchers documented a dramatic increase in the frequency of cases of bronchial carcinoma, associated with a similar trend in the number of deaths. Epidemiologists initiated studies of the distribution of lung cancer, several of which suggested that cigarette smoking might be an important factor. It was then that two seminal case control studies were carried out, in the United Kingdom and in the United States, both of which demonstrated a strong association between cigarette smoking and carcinoma of the lung (Doll and Hill 1950; Wynder and Graham 1950). Thus, from surveys of frequency and distribution, combined with formal hypothesis testing, strong epidemiological evidence was generated to link smoking and lung cancer within just 15 years. Armed with the epidemiological evidence, public health physicians have been able to implement changes in policy and experimental scientists have gone on to develop an understanding of the toxic effects of the components of tobacco smoke on the lung parenchyma.

Table 1 Hypothetical data on the frequency of rheumatoid arthritis

Location	No. of people with rheumatoid arthritis	Total population	Prevalence (%)
City A	4200	211 718	2
City B	2060	103 078	2

Table 2 Measures of disease frequency

Prevalence	Number of existing cases of a disease (at a given point in time) *as against* Total population
Incidence	Number of new cases of a disease during a given period of time *as against* Total population at risk

To investigate distributions and determinants of disease, the size of the 'at risk' population must be known, and the time period over which data were collected. The use of such measures allows direct comparisons of disease frequencies in two or more groups of individuals.

Prevalence

The *prevalence* of a disease describes the proportion of existing cases in a population. In Table 1, the prevalence of rheumatoid arthritis in Cities A and B was 2 per cent, that is, the number of people affected by the disease divided by the total 'at risk' population at a given point in time (Table 2). Prevalence estimates for some of the commoner rheumatic diseases are summarized in Table 3. Prevalence normally refers to *point prevalence,* that is, the number of cases existing at a notional point in time. However, with some conditions, for example, soft tissue disorders of the neck or back, which relapse and remit frequently, it may be more appropriate to measure the *period prevalence,* that is, the number experiencing the disorder during a stated time period. Duration is conventionally measured over 1 week, 1 month, 1 year, or a lifetime.

Incidence

The *incidence* of a disease describes the number of new cases of a disease arising in the 'at risk' population over a specified time period (Table 2). Conventionally, incidence rates are usually measured over 1 year, that is, *annual incidence rates.* However, incidence can be applied more broadly. For incidence rates to be measured correctly, precise definition of the denominator is essential. The incidence rates should only include the population 'at risk' and those who cannot develop the disease for any reason should be excluded from the denominator. For example, osteoporosis is rare in those aged less than 50 years. By convention therefore, the incidence rates of osteoporotic fractures are measured as the rate at which fractures occur in those aged 50 years and over (Cooper and Melton 1996).

Incidence or prevalence?

Frequently, only one of the measures is appropriate. Obviously, these two measures are related: prevalence = incidence × duration; as suggested by this equation, prevalence increases with duration. Thus, treatments that prolong life, for example, renal transplantation for patients with chronic renal failure from systemic lupus erythematosus will increase the prevalence of the disease without any change in the incidence rates. For these reasons,

Table 3 Prevalence of the major rheumatic diseases

Disease	Population	Reference	Prevalence (%)		
			Males	Females	All
Rheumatoid arthritis	North American	Cathcart and O'Sullivan (1970)	—	—	0.9
	European	Lawrence (1961)	0.5	0.6	1.1
	Asian	Lau et al. (1993)	—	—	0.3
	Pima Indians	O'Brien et al. (1967)	0.6	2.5	1.3
Ankylosing spondylitis	United States	Carter et al. (1979)	—	—	0.13
	Pima Indians	Gofton et al. (1972)	—	—	0.54
Psoriatic arthritis	Scandinavian	Hellgren (1969)	0.02	0.02	—
Osteoarthritis	United States (25–74 years)	Lawrence et al. (1989)	—	—	Hands 32.5 Feet 22.2 Knees 3.8
Gout	European (>45 years)	Gardner et al. (1982)	4.3	—	—
	United States	National Center for Health Statistics (1987)	—	—	0.9
Systemic lupus erythematosus	England	Hochberg (1987)	—	0.01	—
	Japan	Nakae et al. (1987)	—	—	0.02
	US Whites	Fessel (1974)	0.007	0.07	—
	US Blacks	Fessel (1974)	0.05	0.28	—

the prevalence rate of a disease is seldom of direct interest in aetiological studies, since it reflects the incidence rate and the probability of surviving with disease. In the example above, renal transplantation may be positively associated with the prevalence of systemic lupus and so be misconstrued as a cause. However, prevalence is extremely useful in the study of chronic diseases with no clear moment of onset, for example, osteoarthritis.

In order to measure incidence, the timing of onset of a disorder must be known. For conditions such as acute neck pain, which is frequent, mild, and usually self-limiting, it is difficult to measure true incidence rates unless elaborate methods of self-reporting are employed. Alternative strategies are to measure *cumulative incidence*, that is, 'ever' had acute neck pain, or *episode incidence*, that is, 'first ever' episodes, or 'all episodes', of acute neck pain over a defined period.

Approaches to measurement of the frequency of the rheumatic diseases

Although there are several approaches to measuring occurrence (Table 4), the appropriate method is usually predicated by the frequency and severity of disease.

Cross-sectional surveys in the general population

It is virtually impossible to derive incidence data from a cross-sectional survey, since a single survey will miss cases that died or went into remission. However, such surveys are essential in the study of the prevalence of common conditions such as osteoarthritis or soft tissue rheumatic disorders, capturing a representative picture of the occurrence and distribution of disease at a notional point in time (Table 3). However, many of the rheumatic diseases, in particular the connective tissue disorders, are rare with estimated prevalence of less than 80/100 000 population (Safavi et al. 1990). Because they are so infrequently observed, very large populations must be studied in order to estimate reliably the prevalence of such conditions. Generally, such large-scale population surveys are impractical and prohibitively expensive.

Surveys of health care use

Another approach is to estimate occurrence by health care use. Clearly, it would not be appropriate to ascertain back pain by review of hospital attendances as many of those affected will not seek medical attention. However, for rarer and more severe diseases, it is reasonable to assume that the majority of those affected will seek medical care. For example, the prevalence of systemic lupus erythematosus was estimated in Birmingham, England, using data from four sources: notification by rheumatologists and primary care physicians, laboratory search for positive DNA binding, and data on hospital admissions (Johnson et al. 1995). Additionally, the investigators maximized ascertainment by contacting the local branch of the lupus patient support group. Even using multiple sources, however, there is evidence that such surveys tend to underestimate the true prevalence, with a magnitude of underascertainment of the order of 10 per cent (Hochberg 1985).

Population-based information systems

Certain very large population based data sets are available and have been exploited to study the epidemiology of uncommon conditions. The *Rochester Epidemiology Project* (REP) is perhaps the most extensively used information system (Kurland 1984). The Mayo Clinic in Rochester, Minnesota, together with the Olmstead Medical Practice, provides apparently the only source of medical care to the local population of approximately 100 000. The Mayo Clinic system maintains a single medical record (dossier) for all contacts with any individual. These dossiers have been indexed by diagnoses (inpatient or outpatient), operations, and histology since 1910 and can be retrieved with remarkable accuracy. This database has been used in the study of many rheumatic diseases.

In the United Kingdom, where health care delivery is centred around general practitioners, a large database has been constructed, owned by the UK Department of Health and managed by the Medicines Control Agency, known as the *General Practice Research Database* (GPRD). The database incorporates computerized records from 683 general practices in the United Kingdom, comprising approximately 6.5 per cent of the total population of England and Wales. The demographic characteristics are representative of the whole UK population. Within the database, comprehensive information as to demography, prescriptions, clinical events, preventive care, referrals to specialist care, and hospital admissions together with the major outcomes, are recorded (Hall 1992). Several independent validation studies have suggested that the database has a high level of completeness and accuracy (Van Staa et al. 2000). This database has provided

Table 4 Approaches to the measurement of disease occurrence

Approach	Measure	Rheumatic disease	Reference
Cross-sectional population survey	Prevalence	Osteoarthritis	Kellgren and Lawrence (1958)
		Rheumatoid arthritis	Lawrence (1961)
		Vertebral osteoporosis	O'Neill et al. (1996)
		Fibromyalgia syndrome	Wolfe et al. (1995)
		Low back pain	Reigo et al. (1999)
Surveys of health care use	Incidence and prevalence	Systemic lupus erythematosus	Johnson et al. (1995)
		Scleroderma	Maricq et al. (1989)
Population-based information systems	Incidence and prevalence	Rochester epidemiology project	
		Rheumatoid arthritis	Linos et al. (1980)
		Ankylosing spondylitis	Carbone et al. (1992)
		Reiter's syndrome	Michet et al. (1988)
		Temporal arteritis	Chuang et al. (1982)
		Systemic lupus erythematosus	Michet et al. (1985)
		Juvenile rheumatoid arthritis	Towner et al. (1983)
		GPRD	
		Corticosteroid induced osteoporosis	Van Staa et al. (2000)
Disease-specific registries	Incidence and prevalence	NOAR	
		Rheumatoid arthritis	Symmons and Harrison (2000)
			Harrison and Symmons (2000)
		ARAMIS	
		Systemic lupus erythematosus	Fries (1990)

Table 5 Examples of rheumatic disease classification criteria

Rheumatic disease	Study group	Reference
Rheumatoid arthritis	American Rheumatism Association	Arnett et al. (1988)
Osteoarthritis		
Knee	American Rheumatism Association	Altman et al. (1986)
Hip	American College of Rheumatology	Altman et al. (1991)
Hand	American College of Rheumatology	Altman et al. (1990)
Scleroderma	American Rheumatism Association	ARA Subcommittee (1980)
Fibromyalgia	American College of Rheumatology	Wolfe et al. (1990)
Sjögren's syndrome	European Community Sjögren's Study Group	Vitali et al. (1993)
Behçet's disease	International Study Group for Behçet's disease	International Study Group (1992)
Ankylosing spondylitis	European Spondyloarthropathy Study Group	Dougados et al. (1991)
Upper limb soft tissue disorders	Health and Safety Executive, UK	Harrington et al. (1998)

a rich resource for the study of many diseases, in particular the pharmacoepidemiology of the rheumatic diseases.

Disease-specific registries

Although initially developed for cancer surveillance, there are specific features of design and operation that make a registry useful for studying the descriptive epidemiology of the rheumatic diseases. In order to be useful, however, a registry must cover a sufficiently large population to have significant numbers of cases of the condition of interest, the population must be well-defined so that cases that are not from the population may be excluded, and the population must be well characterized in terms of size and composition (World Health Organization Working Group 1988). Clearly, such a scheme is logistically difficult and expensive, but results from such a scheme in Norfolk, England, for the monitoring of rheumatoid arthritis, suggest that it can be remarkably successful (Harrison and Symmons 2000; Symmons and Harrison 2000).

What is a 'case'?

Accurate estimates of occurrence rely upon a clear differentiation of 'caseness'. There are particular challenges to classification of the rheumatic disorders, which comprise in excess of 100 heterogeneous conditions, acute and chronic, some with multisystem involvement and others affecting musculoskeletal regions. Many of the rheumatic diseases are syndromes with overlapping and variable clinical features that lack diagnostic laboratory tests. Furthermore, the aetiology and pathogenesis of many of these conditions is incompletely understood. Consequently, classification of rheumatic conditions is non-uniform, including various types of information, such as clinical and laboratory features, tests of specific pathogenic mechanisms (e.g. autoantibodies), anatomical abnormalities, organ system involvement, genetic risk factors (e.g. HLA B27), or aetiological agents.

Why is classification important?

The purpose of classification criteria is to separate patients with a disease both from those without the disease and from normal subjects (Fries et al. 1994). Classification criteria are tools in the construction of a uniform language; where identical criteria have been employed in different populations, direct comparisons might be drawn. Thus, uniformity of language facilitates our understanding of the epidemiology of rheumatic diseases. However, the choice of criteria will vary, depending upon the specific objectives of the study. In clinical trials of drug treatments, for example, considerable stringency is required, that is, only patients with clearly established disease are eligible for study, to prevent dilution of an effect. By contrast, if the aim is the investigation of familial clustering, even mild disease in affected probands is of importance.

The appropriateness of a diagnostic criterion for a particular study may be determined from knowledge of its *sensitivity* and *specificity* in the setting in question. A very specific test will have no false positives and would be appropriate for use in randomized controlled trials of a drug in a group of patients. A very sensitive test will have no false negatives and would be more appropriate in the investigation of familial clustering. Although there are an increasing collection of published classification criteria in the field of rheumatology (Table 5), the majority are derived by comparing groups of patients with a disease with groups of patients with similar, though distinct, diseases. Consequently, the available criteria will not always be appropriate for the desired application.

The distribution of rheumatic diseases

As in the earlier examples (see Boxes 1 and 2), differences in the distribution of disease provide useful starting points for the investigation of disease causation. Conceptually, distribution of disease can be examined between individuals, between geographical or geopolitical divisions, or over time (Fig. 2).

Individual factors

Genetic factors

There are several approaches that may be used to assess the genetic contribution to disease.

Comparison between different ethnic groups

Genetic influences may be studied by comparing ethnic groups. However, it can be difficult to dissociate genetic from environmental influences in these types of studies.

Family studies

The second approach involves examining the occurrence of disease in relatives. A major advantage of these studies is that family members are generally enthusiastic participants and high response rates can be achieved. However, families share environments as well as genes, which may confound the results. In addition, it can be difficult to categorize the relatives of the probands as 'affected' or 'not affected', for several reasons. First, some of the rheumatic diseases may be manifest in a mild form. For example, the relatives of probands with ankylosing spondylitis frequently have either clinical or radiographic evidence of sacroiliitis, but not both. Another difficulty is that many of the rheumatic diseases present late in life so that misclassification of subjects yet to develop a disease may easily occur. In contrast, relatives might be misclassified if they have had disease in the past, but it has gone into remission by the time of the survey. Another potential

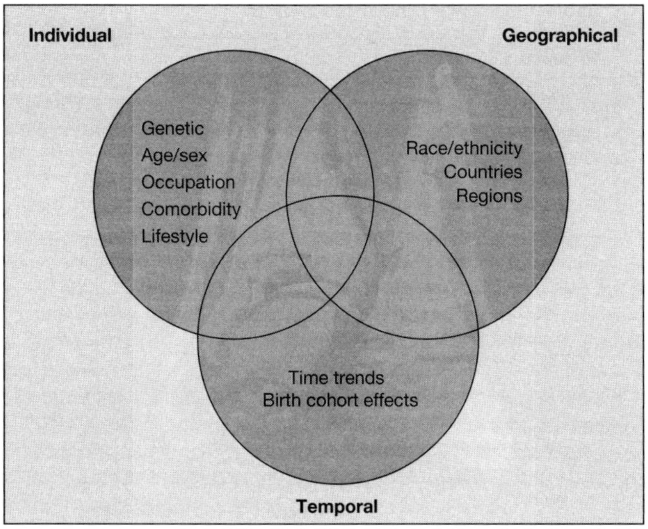

Fig. 2 The distribution of disease.

source of bias arises when subjects are selected for family studies from among hospital patients; it is well recognized that hospital subjects are more likely to have affected relatives than population-derived subjects. It might be that individuals are selected for referral to hospital clinics more easily when there is a family history, perhaps because the individual and their physician have a greater awareness of the disease.

Twin studies

A unique way of exploring genetic influences is to compare disease concordance between identical and non-identical twins. A major advantage of twin studies is the excellent matching for environmental factors. However, it is virtually impossible to perform twin studies of sufficient number in the rarer rheumatic diseases.

Genetic markers

Studies of genetic markers are performed in population samples where a proportion of the population has the diseases in question. This approach assumes that the candidate gene is involved in the pathogenesis of the disease, so that genetic markers will be over-represented in patients with the disease. The advantage of this technique is that it gives information on the possible role of a candidate gene in the population context. However, demonstration of an association does not mean that the candidate gene is a cause of the disease.

Linkage studies

In this technique, the disease is followed through a multicase family, aiming to establish linkage between the disease and polymorphic genetic markers throughout the genome. This is a powerful technique, but limited by the availability of suitable families. One drawback is that results from multicase families may not necessarily be important in the general population.

The genetic associations of the rheumatic diseases

Among others, osteoporosis, osteoarthritis, rheumatoid arthritis, ankylosing spondylitis, systemic lupus erythematosus, scleroderma, and juvenile chronic arthritis show evidence of familial clustering. Studies in monozygotic twins have shown a concordance as high as 50 per cent in ankylosing spondylitis and 40 per cent in osteoarthritis and juvenile chronic arthritis and around 25 per cent in systemic lupus erythematosus. The concordance rate for rheumatoid arthritis is of the order of 12 per cent.

Age

There are striking differences in the age distribution of many of the rheumatic diseases. For example, systemic lupus erythematosus frequently presents in women of childbearing age, osteoarthritis is increasingly common with age, but ankylosing spondylitis rarely occurs after aged 65 years.

Table 6 Age- and sex-specific prevalence of vertebral deformity in Europe (adapted from O'Neill et al. 1996)

Age (years)	Prevalence (%)	
	Males	Females
50–54	16.5	11.5
55–59	18.5	14.6
60–64	21.0	16.8
65–69	20.9	23.5
70–74	20.7	27.2
75–79	29.1	34.8

Sex

With the particular exceptions of ankylosing spondylitis and gout, which are commoner in men, the majority of the rheumatic disorders are more frequent among women. The proportion of female predominance is variable between different diseases; for example, osteoarthritis is twice as common in women as men, rheumatoid arthritis is three times more frequent in women, and systemic lupus erythematosus is up to nine times more common. This distribution raises particular aetiological hypotheses, including a potential role for hormonal and reproductive factors in some of these diseases (Silman and Black 1988).

As a result of these striking age- and sex-effects, it is impossible to compare the results from different studies without considering the demographic characteristics of the populations in question. Crude estimates of occurrence (i.e. all age and sex combined) may well be explained simply by differences in the proportion of men and women or in the age structures of the populations. There are two approaches to overcoming this problem. First, data may be presented separately for each age and sex group (e.g. Table 6). For many of the less common rheumatic diseases, however, the number of cases will be very small in each age and sex band, resulting in less precise estimates. Another approach is to adjust the crude rates to a 'standard population', producing a *standardized rate.* This latter approach is effective, providing that the results of different investigations are standardized to the *same population* before they are compared.

Anthropometry

Obesity is a contributory factor in the development of osteoarthritis of the knee (Cooper et al. 1994) and hip (Cooper et al. 1998), carpal tunnel syndrome (Lam and Thurston 1998), and gout (Hall et al. 1967). Conversely, low body mass index is a risk factor for low bone mineral density and osteoporotic fractures (Johnell et al. 1995). Tallness may be a risk factor for the development of low back pain.

Hormonal/reproductive factors

As already discussed, many of the rheumatic disorders show a marked female preponderance, suggesting a role for hormonal or reproductive factors in their aetiology. In polyarticular osteoarthritis, for example, the condition increases in prevalence after the menopause and is associated with previous hysterectomy. Furthermore, there is some evidence that post-menopausal hormone replacement therapy may retard the development of knee disease (Hannan et al. 1990). Rheumatoid arthritis is associated with early menarcheal age and nulliparity and frequently presents in the early post-partum period. Osteoporosis is associated with late menarcheal age, early menopause, and short number of fertile years. Systemic lupus erythematosus usually presents in women during their fertile years and may be precipitated at the time of pregnancy. Having demonstrated such associations, no assumptions can be made about a causative role of these factors, but such factors might be useful in explaining sex differences in occurrence.

Lifestyle

Cigarette smoking

There is contradictory evidence to suggest that cigarette smoking is (Heliovaara et al. 1993) and is not (Vessey et al. 1987) a risk factor for rheumatoid arthritis. In population surveys, smoking is associated with reporting musculoskeletal pain at all sites (Brage and Bjekedal 1996) and with osteoporosis (Law and Hackshaw 1997). Some, but not all, population studies have suggested that cigarette smoking has a protective effect against the development of osteoarthritis, even after adjusting for body mass index, a potential confounder.

Alcohol

Excessive intake of alcohol is associated with hyperuricaemia and possibly acute gout (Glynn et al. 1983). Whilst moderate levels of alcohol intake may have a positive effect on bone mass, excessive intake substantially increases the risk of osteoporotic fracture (Bikle et al. 1986).

Diet

Patients with rheumatic diseases frequently consider that diet plays a role in their disease. Although much has been written about this subject (Mansfield 1995), scientifically validated studies are scant and often inconclusive. The influence of diet on rheumatic diseases is difficult to study, because accurate recall is difficult, particularly over years and individuals vary their diet considerably. A recent ecological study suggested a possible association between dietary intake of meat and offal and inflammation in rheumatoid arthritis (Grant 2000), but more research is required.

Occupation

Occupation has been implicated as a risk factor for the development of several of the rheumatic diseases. For example, associations have been demonstrated between occupations that involve lifting and osteoarthritis of the hip among men (Coggon et al. 1996) and between occupational squatting and kneeling and osteoarthritis of the knee among men and women (Cooper et al. 1994). Soft tissue rheumatic disorders of the shoulder are more common among workers who perform prolonged overhead or repetitive work (Bernard 1997). Hand transmitted vibration has been linked with Raynaud's phenomenon (Palmer et al. 2000). A number of toxic exposures have been linked to the development of scleroderma, including silica dust (coal miners, stonemasons), organic chemicals (toluene, benzene, xylene, white spirit, vinyl chloride), toxic oils, epoxy resins, biogenic amines, and urea (formaldehyde foam insulations). It remains unclear as to whether silicone breast implants play a role in the development of this and other, connective tissue diseases (Cooper and Dennison 1998).

Comorbidity

Diseases

A number of rheumatic diseases occur secondary to another underlying pathology (e.g. Table 7). Overall however, the proportion of each of these diseases which is found to have a primary cause is generally extremely small, so that the comorbidity is of limited relevance for the disease in general. Of greater relevance are the rheumatic disorders that are seen to occur in association with other pathology, although the latter does not 'cause' the former (e.g. Table 8).

Drugs

Pharmaceutical agents have been linked with a number of rheumatic diseases (e.g. Table 9). Drug-induced systemic lupus erythematosus is thought to occur in those who are genetically slow acetylators, not as a result of direct drug toxicity. There is epidemiological evidence to suggest that the oral contraceptive pill either protects against the development of rheumatoid arthritis, or postpones its progression, although the mechanism is obscure (Silman and Vandenbroucke 1989; Spector and Hochberg 1990).

Table 7 Secondary rheumatic diseases

Rheumatic disease	Primary pathology
Adhesive capsulitis	Stroke Diabetes mellitus
Gout	Polycythaemia rubra vera Chronic renal failure Psoriasis
Osteoporosis	Anorexia nervosa Hyperthyroidism Malabsorption (e.g. coeliac disease) Transplantation
Chondrocalcinosis	Haemachromatosis Ochronosis Osteoarthritis Wilson's disease Hyperparathyroidism Hypomagnesaemia Acromegaly Diabetes mellitus Gout
Carpal tunnel syndrome	Acromegaly Hypothyroidism Diabetes mellitus

Table 8 Associations between rheumatic disorders and other pathology

Rheumatic disease	Associated pathology
Chronic regional pain syndromes	Anxiety and depression
Fibromyalgia syndrome	Irritable bowel syndrome
Rheumatoid arthritis	Autoimmune thyroid disease
Osteoarthritis	Diabetes mellitus Hypertension Hyperuricaemia
Stiff man syndrome	Diabetes mellitus
Dermato- and polymyositis	Malignancy
Polymyalgia rheumatica	Autoimmune thyroid disease
Giant cell arteritis	Autoimmune thyroid disease
Gout	Hypertension Ischaemic heart disease
Ankylosing spondylitis	Acute anterior uveitis Multiple sclerosis Inflammatory bowel disease

Table 9 Drugs and the rheumatic diseases

Rheumatic disease	Drug
Systemic lupus erythematosus	Tetracyclines Hydralazine Procainamide Isoniazid
Eosinophilia myalgia syndrome	L-Tryptophan
Osteoporosis	Corticosteroids Anticonvulsants
Acute gout	Thiazide diuretics Allopurinol

Geographical factors

Geographical distribution of disease may be compared between countries or within countries to the level of a small area (e.g. see Box 3).

Race and ethnicity

Variations in the occurrence of rheumatic diseases by racial group are of considerable interest, although they are inevitably difficult to interpret. Apparent differences may occur as a result of differences in symptom reporting, physician consultation and bias in physician diagnosis. Ethnic groups share genes and environments, so different patterns of disease might be explained by any combination of these influences. One useful approach therefore, is to compare disease occurrence in migrant populations (e.g. see Box 4).

Temporal factors

Time trends in disease occurrence may also be very revealing. Clusters of incident cases in a particular season of the year or sporadic clusters of cases at one particular time or place suggest a common aetiological agent. Thus, it was the clustering of cases of arthritis in one place over a short time that led to the establishment of the causative agent in Lyme disease (see Box 5).

Changes in the occurrence of a disease over time may reflect patterns of change in exposure to putative risk factors, leading to potentially important aetiological clues. However, changes in the prevalence of diseases are potentially difficult to interpret, since they may reflect either change in exposure to causative agents, or in the pattern of survival from the disease. Changes in incidence rates of a disease are less subject to confounding, but unfortunately, long-term data on incidence are currently available for few of the rheumatic diseases, with the notable exception of rheumatoid arthritis. Between 1950 and 1975, the epidemiologists in Rochester, Minnesota, documented a decline in the incidence of rheumatoid arthritis among women, but not among men. Several hypotheses were put forward to explain this decline, one of which was that it coincided with increasing use of the oral contraceptive pill. There is some evidence to suggest that these two phenomena may be linked (Spector and Hochberg 1990).

Birth cohort effects

As time advances, individuals grow older, they are diagnosed more recently and individuals born more recently can be compared. These three separate but interrelated factors may be studied in birth cohort analyses. The aim is to separate the way in which these factors contribute to the pattern of disease occurrence over time. If the presumed environmental trigger of a disease occurs early in life (e.g. health of parents, number of siblings, early

Box 3

Rheumatoid arthritis

The prevalence of rheumatoid arthritis has been studied in more geographical locations than any other rheumatic disease (Table 10). There are methodological differences in the studies and many were too small to reliably detect a disease with a prevalence of less than 1%. However, the striking feature is that the prevalence is very consistently between 0.5 and 1% across all five continents, suggesting that the causative factors (genetic and/or environmental) are ubiquitous.

Osteoporosis

In contrast, the incidence of osteoporotic fractures shows striking geographical variation (Table 11) (Lau 1996). Some of the differences are accounted for by ethnic and racial differences in bone mass and hip axis length. However, across Europe there is a sevenfold difference in the incidence of hip fracture, which is not explained by racial and ethnic factors (Johnell et al. 1992). Although these differences are not fully understood, factors such as latitude, socio-economic deprivation, proportion of agricultural land, reduced sunlight, and fluoridated water may be contributory.

Table 10 Geographical variation in prevalence of rheumatoid arthritis

Population	*N*	Prevalence of definite rheumatoid arthritis at age 15+ years (%)
Europe		
Leigh and Wensleydale, UK	2234	1.1
Sofia, Bulgaria	4318	0.9
Rotterdam, Netherlands	19647	0.9
Sweden	39418	0.9
Samso, Denmark	4557	0.8
Heinola, Finland	8000	2.0
Asia		
Shizouko, Japan	3006	0.8
Kinmet, China	5629	0.3
Java, Indonesia	4683	0.2
Africa		
Phokeng, South Africa	801	0.12
Soweto, South Africa	964	0.9
Venda, South Africa	543	Nil
America		
Kingston, Jamaica	530	1.9
Sudbury, MA, USA	4552	0.9
Chippewa Indians, USA	205	6.8
Inuit, Canada	2055	0.6
Puerto Rico	3883	0.3
Oceania		
New Zealand	432	1.0
Maori, New Zealand	175	3.9

Table 11 Age-adjusted incidence rates per 100 000 person-years for hip fractures in different populations (Walker-Bone et al. 2001)

Population	Rate per 100 000	
	Women	Men
Norway (1983–1984)	1290	550
Stockholm (1972–1981)	620	290
California Whites (1983–1984)	560	210
Rochester, MN (1965–1974)	510	170
Hong Kong (1965–1967)	150	100
Hong Kong (1985)	350	180
Singapore (1955–1962)	80	100
California Asians (1983–1984)	340	100
California Blacks (1983–1984)	220	140
California Hispanics (1983–1984)	200	90
Beijing, China (1990–1992)	90	100
Canada (1993–1994)	480	190
Kuwait (1992–1995)	295	200
Japan (1986–1988)	115	41
Japan (1992–1994)	145	60

Incidence rates age-standardized to US population.

Box 4

Systemic lupus erythematosus

It has been consistently demonstrated that African populations resident in the United States and the United Kingdom develop systemic lupus erythematosus three to four times as commonly as Caucasians. Furthermore, the Africans develop more severe disease, with higher morbidity at a younger mean age. Some, but not all, studies among Asian populations have also suggested an excess compared with Caucasians (Samanta et al. 1991).

Osteoarthritis

Hand involvement appears to be over-represented among the Pima and Blackfoot Indian populations of North America (Cooper 1998). African-American women have a higher age-adjusted prevalence of knee osteoarthritis than Caucasians, but are less likely to have Heberden's nodes on physical examination. Heberden's nodes are also seen less frequently among African Blacks in Nigeria, Liberia, and Jamaica. Osteoarthritis of the hip is infrequently seen in African Blacks, Asian Indians, Hong Kong Chinese, and Japanese populations.

Gout

Filipino and Polynesian populations such as the Maoris have shown the largest excess population risk. Studies among migrants from these populations who migrate to Western countries suggest that these populations have an inherited tendency to clear uric acid poorly, but become susceptible to gout only when exposed to the Western diet (high purine levels and alcohol) (Silman and Hochberg 1993).

Box 5

In November 1975, a resident of Old Lyme, Connecticut, informed the State Health Department that 12 children from the local rural community of 5000 residents had been diagnosed recently with juvenile rheumatoid arthritis. Almost concurrently, a second mother from Old Lyme informed physicians at Yale that she, her husband, two of their children, and several neighbours had all developed arthritis (Steere et al. 1977). In all, 39 children and 12 adults in three local rural communities had developed arthritis over a 4-year period. In most, the onset was June–September and the presenting symptoms were of intermittent pain and swelling in one or more large joints, sometimes associated with a prior skin lesion. One person recalled being bitten by a tick prior to the onset of the skin lesion. Epidemiological studies pointed to an ixodid tick in the region where the cases were occurring. Subsequent serological testing linked the spirochaete, *Borrelia burgdorferi* with this tick and with skin lesions, blood tests, and CSF fluid from Lyme disease patients.

diet, etc.), this will be highlighted by analyses of morbidity by period of birth (e.g. Box 6).

The determinants of disease

As described in Fig. 1, the ultimate aim of the epidemiologist is to use the available information on frequency and distribution in order to generate aetiological hypotheses that may be tested in formal analytical studies. There are two major observational analytical epidemiological study designs: the *case-control study* and the *cohort study*. The essential difference between these designs is one of *sampling* (Fig. 3).

Box 6

The Pima Indians have one of the highest incidences of rheumatoid arthritis, but observation of secular trends suggests that the incidence is declining. Potentially, this could be explained by changes in environmental factors, either acting in early life, or in later adult life. To explore these influences further, Silman et al. analysed the trends in rheumatoid factor over 30 years among Pima Indians, taking into account age, calendar year and birth cohort (Silman et al. 2000). A strong birth cohort trend was evident with an almost linear 10-fold reduction in the presence of rheumatoid factor from those born between 1896 and 1905 to those born between 1966 and 1975. The presence of such a strong association with period of birth suggests that environmental influences, which operated early in the lives of these individuals, have contributed to the subsequent development of rheumatoid factor and that these factors (whatever they are) are changing over time.

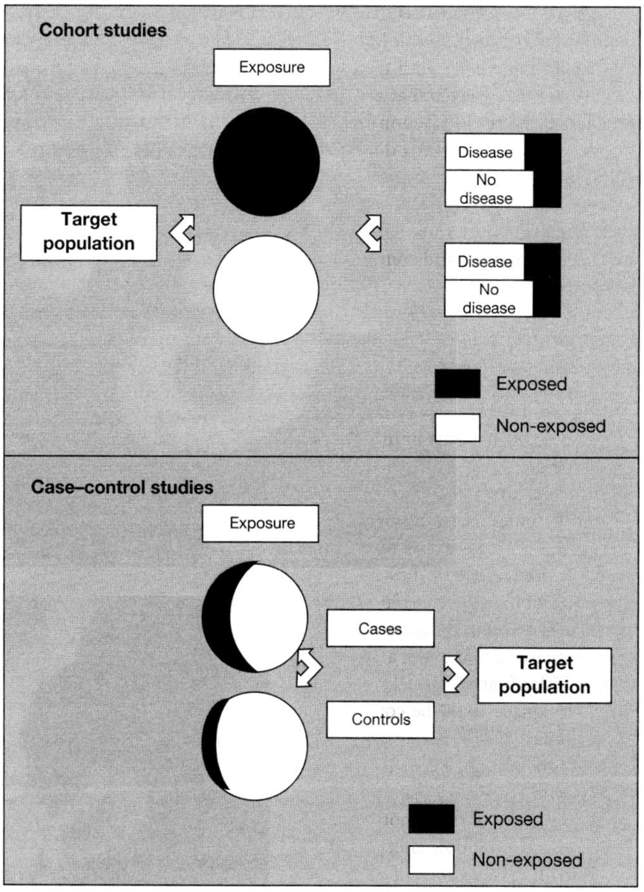

Fig. 3 Observational analytical epidemiology studies.

Case–control studies

In case–control studies, the sampling is on the basis of whether individuals do (cases) or do not (controls) have the disease in question. The groups are then compared with respect to the proportion having a history of an exposure or characteristic of interest (e.g. Box 7).

The main advantage is in studying chronic rheumatic diseases with potentially long latency periods; epidemiologists take a group of affected

Box 7

Cooper and colleagues explored the risk factors for the development of osteoarthritis of the hip in a population-based case–control study (Cooper et al. 1998). They studied 611 patients listed for hip replacement over an 18-month period in two health districts of the United Kingdom. Each case was individually matched with a control, selected by age, sex, and general practitioner. All cases and controls were interviewed about suspected risk factors using a standardized questionnaire, and were examined. The investigators found that the hip osteoarthritis cases were more likely to be obese, to have experienced a previous hip injury and to have Heberden's nodes. The male controls were more likely to be cigarette smokers.

Box 8

Between 1968 and 1974, the Oxford Family Planning Association (United Kingdom), incepted a large cohort of 17 032 women, then aged 25–39 years, attending one of 17 local family planning associations. The aim of the study was to investigate the long-term effects of exposure to oral contraceptives. These women have been followed-up for periods up to 26 years and information has been collected about illnesses requiring hospital inpatient or outpatient care. From this cohort, considerable information has been published about many medical disorders. Among the rheumatic disorders, the incidence of carpal tunnel syndrome (Vessey et al. 1990), rheumatoid arthritis (Vessey et al. 1987), and back pain requiring hospital referral (Vessey et al. 1999), among women exposed to oral contraceptives have all been studied.

individuals and assess exposure retrospectively, rather than studying those with an exposure over a very prolonged period of time until disease intervenes. Case–control studies also provide a means of studying the rarer rheumatic diseases, since cases are selected on the basis of their disease status. In a disease like scleroderma, for example, a vast population would need to be studied over a considerable length of time in order to accumulate sufficient numbers of individuals with the outcome of interest. Another advantage of the case–control study is that a large number of different exposures may be considered, and the interaction between them, which can be particularly useful when knowledge about a disease is in its early stage of development.

The major disadvantage of the case–control study is that both the disease and the exposure have occurred at the time of the subject entering the study. This can lead to a susceptibility to the introduction of bias, either in the selection of cases and controls, or differential reporting or recording of exposures.

Cohort studies

In cohort studies, sampling is based upon exposure. Groups are defined according to the presence or absence of exposure to a suspected risk factor for a disease. At the time of inception of the cohort, all individuals must be free of the disease in question and the cohort are then followed forward to assess the occurrence of the outcome (e.g. Box 8).

Cohort studies have a number of advantages for evaluating the influence of exposure on disease. For one thing, since participants are disease-free at inception, and exposure has already occurred, the temporal sequence of exposure and disease occurrence is more readily defined. Cohort studies are particularly useful in the situation where an exposure is rare. For example, if it is hypothesized that use of a particular hand-held vibrating tool leads to an elevated risk of carpal tunnel syndrome, subjects who regularly use this tool in the workplace could be compared with other subjects in the workplace doing similar jobs, but not using the particular tool of interest. Otherwise, the proportions of individuals with exposure to this tool among a group of subjects with carpal tunnel syndrome would be far too small to allow a meaningful assessment of risk. Another advantage of a cohort design, as illustrated in Box 5, is that multiple effects of a single exposure may be studied.

The main disadvantage of cohort studies is that they usually involve the follow-up of a large group of individuals over a long period of time, which is generally time-consuming and expensive. Because of the resources involved, the cohort study is inefficient for the study of rarer diseases, particularly if the exposure is followed by a prolonged latent period prior to disease onset. Clearly, huge numbers of young women would need to be followed-up over many years if sufficient numbers of them were to develop a connective tissue disease in relation to a particular exposure. Inevitably, the longer a period of follow-up that is attempted, the higher the rates of dropout will become. This may introduce bias, since loss to follow-up may not be a random process. One particularly attractive research design is to use a historical cohort. It is cheaper and quicker than having to incept a new cohort, and might be the only realistic option if the follow-up period is decades later.

Randomized clinical trials

The intervention study, or clinical trial, is an epidemiological study that artificially creates a controlled experiment resembling those performed by basic scientists. As with cohort studies, subjects are recruited on the basis of their exposure status, but the investigator allocates the exposure (intervention). If the intervention is allocated randomly in sufficiently large numbers of subjects, the results of well-conducted intervention trials may be expected to have some assurance of validity to the degree that observational study design cannot provide.

Increasingly, health care decision-making is guided by evidence from valid, applicable studies. Randomized clinical trials are rightfully regarded as the best tools for gathering evidence on the effectiveness of health care interventions and they are given the greatest weight in grading levels of evidence for/against an intervention (Agency for Health Care Policy and Research 1992). However, the maturity of randomized trials, now over 50 years old, is not always reflected in the rigour in which they are conducted or the transparency with which they are reported (Bossuyt 2001). It is an obligation of the investigators that they report the results, not just their opinions and that the reader may judge the potential for bias in the design, conduct, analysis, and interpretation of studies, together with the generalizability of the findings. Towards this end, guidelines have been developed, and recently revized (Moher et al. 2001) by the CONSORT (Consolidated Standards of Reporting Trials) group. The use of such guidelines should enable readers to understand a trial's conduct and assess the validity of its results.

References

Agency for Health Care Policy and Research. *Guidelines for Clinical Practice* (ed. M.J. Field and K.N. Lohr). Washington DC: National Academic Press, 1992.

Altman, R. et al. (1986). Development of criteria for the classification and reporting of osteoarthritis of the knee. *Arthritis and Rheumatism* **29,** 1039–49.

Altman, R. et al. (1990). The American College of Rheumatology criteria for the classification and reporting of osteoarthritis of the hand. *Arthritis and Rheumatism* **33,** 1601–10.

Altman, R. et al. (1991). The American College of Rheumatology criteria for the classification and reporting of osteoarthritis of the hip. *Arthritis and Rheumatism* **34,** 505–14.

ARA Subcommittee for Scleroderma Criteria of the American Rheumatism Association Diagnostic and Therapeutic Criteria Committee (1980). Preliminary criteria for the classification of systemic sclerosis (scleroderma). *Arthritis and Rheumatism* **23,** 581–90.

Arnett, F.C. et al. (1988). The American Rheumatism Association 1987 Revised criteria for the classification of rheumatoid arthritis. *Arthritis and Rheumatism* **31,** 315–24.

Arnett, F.C. et al. (1990). Connective tissue disease in south east Georgia. A community based study of immunogenetic markers and autoantibodies. *Journal of Rheumatology* **17,** 1029–35.

Bernard, B.P. *Musculoskeletal Disorders (MSDs) and Workplace Factors.* Cincinnati OH: US Department of Health and Human Services, 1997.

Bikle, D.D. et al. (1986). Bone disease in alcohol abuse. *Annals of Internal Medicine* **103,** 42–8.

Bossuyt, P.M.M. (2001). Better standards for better reporting of RCTs. *British Medical Journal* **322,** 1317–18.

Brage, S. and Bjekedal, T. (1996). Musculoskeletal pain and smoking in Norway. *Journal of Epidemiology and Community Health* **50,** 166–9.

Carbone, LD. et al. (1992). Ankylosing spondylitis in Rochester, Minnesota 1935–1989. Is the epidemiology changing? *Arthritis and Rheumatism* **35,** 1476–82.

Carter, E.T. et al. (1979). Epidemiology of ankylosing spondylitis in Rochester, Minnesota, 1935–73. *Arthritis and Rheumatism* **22,** 365–70.

Cathcart, E.S. and O'Sullivan, J.B. (1970). Rheumatoid arthritis in a New England town. *New England Journal of Medicine* **282,** 421–4.

Chuang, T.Y. et al. (1982). Polymyalgia rheumatica. *Annals of Internal Medicine* **97,** 672–80.

Coggon, D. et al. (1996). Osteoarthritis of the hip and occupational lifting. *American Journal of Epidemiology* **147,** 523–8.

Cooper, C. (1998). Epidemiology of osteoarthritis. In *Rheumatology* (ed. J.H. Klippel and P.A. Dieppe), pp. 8.2.1–8.2.8. London: Mosby.

Cooper, C. and Coggon, D. (1999). Physical activity and knee osteoarthritis. *Lancet* **353,** 217–78.

Cooper, C. and Dennison, E. (1998). Do silicone breast implants cause connective tissue disease? *British Medical Journal* **316,** 403–4.

Cooper, C. and Melton, L.J. (1996). Magnitude and impact of osteoporosis and fractures. In *Osteoporosis* (ed. R. Marcus, D., Feldman, and J. Kelsey), pp. 419–34. San Diego CA: Academic Press Inc.

Cooper, C. et al. (1994). Occupational activity and osteoarthritis of the knee. *Annals of the rheumatic diseases* **53,** 90–3.

Cooper, C. et al. (1998). Individual risk factors for hip osteoarthritis: obesity, hip injury, and physical activity. *American Journal of Epidemiology* **147,** 516–22.

Doll, R. and Hill, A.B. (1950). Smoking and carcinoma of the lung: preliminary report. *British Medical Journal* 739–48.

Dougados, M. et al. (1991). The European Spondyloarthropathy Study Group preliminary criteria for the classification of spondyloarthropathy. *Arthritis and Rheumatism* **34,** 1218–27.

Fessel, W.J. (1974). Systemic lupus erythematosus in the community: incidence, prevalence, outcome, and first symptoms; the high prevalence in women. *Archives of Internal Medicine* **134,** 1027.

Fries, J.F. (1990). The epidemiology of systemic lupus erythematosus—1950–1990. Conceptual advances and the ARAMIS databanks. *Clinical Rheumatology* **9,** 5–9.

Fries, J.F. et al. (1994). Criteria for rheumatic disease. *Arthritis and Rheumatism* **37,** 454–62.

Gardner, M.J. et al. (1982). The prevalence of gout in three English towns. *International Journal of Epidemiology* **11,** 71–5.

Glynn, R.J., Campion, E.W., and Silbert, J.E. (1983). Trends in serum uric acid levels. 1961–80. *Arthritis and Rheumatism* **26,** 87–93.

Gofton, J.P. et al. (1972). Sacroiliitis and ankylosing spondylitis in North American Indians. *Annals of the Rheumatic Diseases* **31,** 474–81.

Grant, W.B. (2000). The role of meat in the expression of rheumatoid arthritis. *British Journal of Nutrition* **84,** 589–95.

Hall, A.P. et al. (1967). Epidemiology of gout and hyperuricaemia. *American Journal of Medicine* **42,** 27–37.

Hall, G. (1992). Pharmacoepidemiology using a UK database of primary care records. *Pharmacoepidemiological Drug Safety* **1,** 33–7.

Hannan, M.T. et al. (1990). Estrogen use and radiographic osteoarthritis of the knee in women. *Arthritis and Rheumatism* **33,** 525–32.

Harrington, J.M. et al. (1998). Surveillance case definitions for work related upper limb pain syndromes. *Occupational and Environmental Medicine* **55,** 264–71.

Harrison, B. and Symmons, D. (2000). Early inflammatory polyarthritis: results from the Norfolk Arthritis Register with a review of the literature. II. Outcome at three years. *Rheumatology* **39,** 939–49.

Heliovaara, M. et al. (1993). Smoking and the risk of rheumatoid arthritis. *Journal of Rheumatology* **20,** 1830–5.

Hellgren, L. (1969). Association between rheumatoid arthritis and psoriasis in total populations. *Acta Rheumatologica Scandinavica* **15,** 316–26.

Hochberg, M.C. (1985). The incidence of systemic lupus erythematosus in Baltimore, Maryland, 1970–1977. *Arthritis and Rheumatism* **28,** 80–6.

Hochberg, M.C. (1987). Prevalence of systemic lupus erythematosus in England and Wales, 1981–2. *Annals of the Rheumatic Diseases* **46,** 664.

International Study Group for Behçet's Disease (1992). Evaluation of diagnostic ('classification') criteria in Behçet's disease—towards internationally agreed criteria. *British Journal of Rheumatology* **31,** 299–308.

Johnell, O. et al. (1992). The apparent incidence of hip fracture in Europe: a study of national register sources. MEDOS Study Group. *Osteoporosis International* **2,** 298–302.

Johnell, O. et al. (1995). Risk factors for hip fractures in European women: the MEDOS study. *Journal of Bone Mineral Research* **10,** 1802–15.

Johnson, A.E. et al. (1995). The prevalence and incidence of systemic lupus erythematosus in Birmingham, England. *Arthritis and Rheumatism* **38,** 551–8.

Kellgren, J.H. and Lawrence, J.S. (1958). Osteoarthritis and disc degeneration in an urban population. *Annals of the Rheumatic Diseases* **17,** 388–97.

Kurland, L.T. (1984). The Rochester epidemiology program project. *Epidemiology of the Rheumatic Diseases, Proceedings of the Fourth International Conference.* New York: Gower.

Lam, N. and Thurston, A. (1998). Association of obesity, gender, age and occupation with carpal tunnel syndrome. *Australia and New Zealand Journal of Surgery* **68,** 190–3.

Lau, E. et al. (1993). Low prevalence of rheumatoid arthritis in the urbanized Chinese of Hong Kong. *Journal of Rheumatology* **20,** 1133–7.

Lau, E.M. (1996). The epidemiology of hip fracture in Asia: an update. *Osteoporosis International* **6** (Suppl. 3), 19–23.

Law, M.R. and Hackshaw, A.K. (1997). A meta-analysis of cigarette smoking, bone mineral density and risk of hip fracture: recognition of a major effect. *British Medical Journal* **315,** 493–503.

Lawrence, J.S. (1961). Prevalence of rheumatoid arthritis. *Annals of the Rheumatic Diseases* **20,** 11–17.

Lawrence, R.C. et al. (1989). Estimates of the prevalence of selected arthritis and musculoskeletal disorders in the United States. *Journal of Rheumatology* **16,** 427–41.

Linos, A. et al. (1980). The epidemiology of rheumatoid arthritis in Rochester, Minnesota: a study of incidence, prevalence, and mortality. *American Journal of Epidemiology* **111,** 86–98.

Mansfield, J. *Arthritis: Allergy, Nutrition and the Environment.* London: Thorsons, 1995.

Maricq, H.R. et al. (1989). Prevalence of scleroderma spectrum disorders in the general population of South Carolina. *Arthritis and Rheumatism* **32,** 998–1006.

Michet, C.J. et al. (1985). Epidemiology of systemic lupus erythematosus and other connective tissue diseases in Rochester, Minnesota, 1950 through 1979. *Mayo Clinic Proceedings* **60,** 105–13.

Michet, C.J. et al. (1988). Epidemiology of Reiter's syndrome in Rochester, Minnesota: 1950–1980. *Arthritis and Rheumatism* **31,** 428–31.

Moher, D., Schulz, K.F., and Altman, D.G., for the CONSORT Group (2001). The CONSORT statement: revised recommendations for improving the quality of reports of parallel-group randomised trials. *Lancet* **357,** 1191–4.

Nakae, K. et al. (1987). A nationwide epidemiological survey on diffuse collagen diseases: estimation of prevalence rate in Japan. In *Mixed Connective Tissue Disease and Anti-Nuclear Antibodies* (ed. R. Kasukawa and G.C. Sharp), p. 9. Amsterdam: Elsevier.

National Center for Health Statistics (1987). Current Estimates from the National Health Interview Survey, United States, 1986. *Vital and Health Statistics.* Series 10, No. 164. DHHS Pub. No. (PHS) 87–1592. Public Health Service. Washington DC: US Government Printing Office.

O'Brien, W.M. et al. (1967). A genetic study of rheumatoid arthritis and rheumatoid factor in Blackfeet and Pima Indians. *Arthritis and Rheumatism* **10,** 163–79.

O'Neill, T.W. et al. (1996). The prevalence of vertebral deformity in European men and women: The European Vertebral Osteoporosis Study. *Journal of Bone Mineral Research* **11,** 1010–18.

Palmer, K.T. et al. (2000). Prevalence of Raynaud's phenomenon in Great Britain and its relation to hand transmitted vibration: a national postal survey. *Occupational and Environmental Medicine* **57**, 448–52.

Reigo, T., Timpka, T., and Tropp, T. (1999). The epidemiology of back pain in vocational age groups. *Scandinavian Journal of Primary Health Care* **17**, 17–21.

Safavi, K.H., Heyse, S.P., and Hochberg, M.C. (1990). Estimating the incidence and prevalence of rare rheumatologic diseases: a review of methodology and available data sources. *Journal of Rheumatology* **17**, 990–3.

Samanta, A. et al. (1991). The prevalence of diagnosed systemic lupus erythematosus in Whites and Indian Asian immigrants in Leicester City, UK. *British Journal of Rheumatology* **30** (Suppl. 1), 21.

Silman, A.J. and Black, C. (1988). Increased incidence of spontaneous abortion infertility in women with scleroderma before disease onset. *British Journal of Rheumatology* **47**, 441–4.

Silman, A.J. and Hochberg, M.C. (1993). Gout. In *Epidemiology of the Rheumatic Diseases* (ed. A.J. Silman and M.C. Hochberg), pp. 2891–314. Oxford: Oxford University Press.

Silman, A.J. and Vandenbroucke, J.P. (1989). Female sex hormones and rheumatoid arthritis. *British Journal of Rheumatology* **28** (Suppl. 1), 1–73.

Silman, A.J. et al. (2000). Strong influence of period of birth on the occurrence of rheumatoid factor: results from a 30 year follow-up study on Pima Indians. *Arthritis and Rheumatism* **43** (Suppl.), 605.

Snow, J. *On the Mode of Communication of Cholera.* London: John Churchill, 1860.

Spector, T.D. and Hochberg, M.C. (1990). The protective effect of the oral contraceptive pill on rheumatoid arthritis. *Journal of Clinical Epidemiology* **43**, 1221–30.

Steere, A.C. et al. (1977). An epidemic of oligoarticular arthritis in children and adults in three Connecticut communities. *Arthritis and Rheumatism* **20**, 7–17.

Symmons, D. and Harrison, B. (2000). Early inflammatory polyarthritis: results from the Norfolk Arthritis Register with a review of the literature. I. Risk factors for the development of inflammatory polyarthritis and rheumatoid arthritis. *Rheumatology* **39**, 835–43.

Towner, S.R. et al. (1983). The epidemiology of juvenile arthritis in Rochester, Minnesota, 1960–1979. *Arthritis and Rheumatism* **26**, 1208–13.

Van Staa, T.P. et al. (2000). The use of a large pharmacoepidemiological database to study exposure to oral corticosteroids and risk of fractures: validation of study population and results. *Pharmacoepidemiological Drug Safety* **9**, 359–66.

Vessey, M., Painter, R., and Mant, J. (1999). Oral contraception and other factors in relation to back disorders in women: findings in a large cohort study. *Contraception* **60**, 331–5.

Vessey, M.P., Villard-Mackintosh, L., and Yeates, D. (1987). Oral contraceptives, cigarette smoking, and other factors in relation to arthritis. *Contraception* **35**, 457–65.

Vessey, M.P., Villard-Mackintosh, L., and Yeates, D. (1990). Epidemiology of carpal tunnel syndrome in women of childbearing age. Findings in a large cohort study. *International Journal of Epidemiology* **19**, 655–9.

Vitali, C. et al. (1993). Preliminary criteria for the classification of Sjögren's syndrome: results of a prospective concerted action supported by the European Community. *Arthritis and Rheumatism* **36**, 340–7.

Walker-Bone, K., Dennison, E., and Cooper, C. (2001). Osteoporosis. In *The Epidemiology of the Rheumatic Diseases* (ed. A.J. Silman and M.C. Hochberg), pp. 259–92. Oxford: Oxford University Press.

Wolfe, F. et al. (1990). The American College of Rheumatology 1990 criteria for the classification of fibromyalgia: report of the multicenter criteria committee. *Arthritis and Rheumatism* **33**, 160–72.

Wolfe, F. et al. (1995). The prevalence and characteristics of fibromyalgia in the general population. *Arthritis and Rheumatism* **38**, 19–28.

World Health Organization Working Group (1988). The use of registers in the epidemiologic study of rheumatic diseases including planning. *Scandinavian Journal of Rheumatology* **71** (Suppl.), 3–16.

Wynder, E.L. and Graham, E.A. (1950). Tobacco smoking as a possible etiologic factor in bronchiogenic carcinoma: a study of six hundred and eighty-four proved cases. *Journal of the American Medical Association* **143**, 329–36.

6.1.2 Epidemiology of rheumatic diseases in selected non-European populations

Patricia A. Fraser

The primary focus of this chapter is the variation in frequencies of rheumatic diseases among several racial and ethnic groups. The study of race and ethnicity-specific disease expression may provide clues to aetiological factors for rheumatic diseases. Observed variations in incidence, prevalence, and clinical and laboratory manifestations of systemic rheumatic diseases between racial and ethnic groups may result from genetic and environmental factors, or complex interactions between genes and the environment (Bae et al. 1998). Inherited factors contribute to susceptibility to rheumatic diseases. These genetic factors may be linked to, or regulated by, multiple loci throughout the human genome (e.g. Jawaheer et al. 2001). If the genes of interest are polymorphic, their allelic frequencies may vary between ethnic groups. Such genetic variation may be the basis for ethnic differences in susceptibility and disease expression. Infectious agents in our environment may contribute to susceptibility to rheumatic diseases. The association between Epstein–Barr virus infection and systemic lupus erythematosus (SLE) (James et al. 2001) and the correlation between exposure to *Mycoplasma pneumoniae* respiratory infections and cyclic variation in incidence of juvenile rheumatoid arthritis in one Canadian province (Oen et al. 1995) are consistent with a role for microbial exposures in the modulation of predisposition to rheumatic and connective tissue diseases. Chemicals in our environment may also trigger connective tissue diseases. This is exemplified by the observations that occupational exposures to silica and organic solvents are risk factors for lupus, scleroderma, and undifferentiated connective tissue diseases (Cooper et al. 1999, 2002; Lacey et al. 1999; Povey et al. 2001). The investigation of gene–environment interactions in the rheumatic and connective tissue diseases is a relatively new discipline. Such gene–environment interactions are hypothesized to account for the high prevalence of scleroderma (systemic sclerosis) among Choctaw Native Americans residing in Oklahoma in the United States (Michet 1998) and have been shown to explain scleroderma risk among some individuals who have been exposed to organic solvents (Povey et al. 2001).

Survival is one important prognostic feature of disease expression. Ethnic differences in disease mortality may be multifactorial. Studies of the prognosis for SLE in African Americans emphasize the importance of modifiable risk factors related to socio-demographic, behavioural, and psychosocial variables (Alarcon et al. 2001a,b). Future epidemiological studies of the rheumatic diseases should be designed to obtain data on multiple variables such as genetic markers at multiple loci, climate, microbial exposures, social, cultural, and behavioural factors (e.g. dietary habits, tobacco, and alcohol use) (Adebajo 1995).

Interethnic comparisons of the epidemiology of rheumatic diseases are hampered by the lack of uniform sampling and disease definitions, and also by limited or missing data on many ethnic groups. Clinical case series have been included for several ethnic groups when formal epidemiological studies of prevalence or incidence are not available. These data are not equivalent in their scientific rigor to formal epidemiological studies. They are presented for the purpose of completeness of information on rheumatic diseases worldwide.

Juvenile arthritis

Definition

Descriptive terms and definitions of chronic inflammatory arthritis in childhood are numerous (see Chapter 1.1.2 and Section 6.5).

Occurrence

Juvenile arthritis (JA) is the most common, childhood, chronic systemic rheumatic disease in the United States. This statistic reflects the frequency of juvenile arthritis in the largest ethnic group, Caucasians, and in Native Americans. Data on the occurrence of juvenile arthritis in Africa, Australia, and Asia are sparse.

Several survey methods have been used to estimate the occurrence of juvenile arthritis and other rheumatic diseases (Gewanter et al. 1983). The field population survey is the most accurate method because it includes actual physical examination of the population under study by trained observers. It is also the most costly. Estimates are also based on the number of cases presenting to a central clinic. The size of the source population must be known and it is assumed that all cases from this population base would present to this centre. The review of a medical records database for the diagnoses of interest has been used extensively. This approach also assumes the database captures virtually all of the source population. The practitioner survey interviews practitioners by questionnaire, which may be a preferable method in a population with a decentralized health care system and has been used effectively to estimate frequencies for childhood rheumatic diseases in the United States (Gewanter et al. 1983).

Juvenile arthritis is twice as common among Native Americans than among Caucasians in western Canada. Susceptibility to juvenile arthritis also varies between Native American tribal groups. In this analysis, data from Eskimo ethnic groups are compared to those from other Native American tribal groups. The two-fold difference in the prevalence of juvenile arthritis between Native Americans in Manitoba and British Columbia (Rosenberg et al. 1982) may be due to the high prevalence of juvenile-onset spondyloarthropathy among the Native Americans of Manitoba (Hochberg 1984). Similarly designed studies reveal a variable prevalence for juvenile arthritis in several samples of Eskimos and Alaskan Native Americans (Oen et al. 1986; Boyer et al. 1988, 1990, 1991). The Inuit and Native Americans from the southeast coast of Alaska have the two highest reported prevalence rates for juvenile arthritis (126/100 000 and 83/100 000, respectively) (Oen et al. 1986; Boyer et al. 1991). Figure 1 includes estimates of the period prevalence of juvenile arthritis in Native Americans, Eskimos (Rosenberg et al. 1982; Oen et al. 1986; Boyer et al. 1988, 1990, 1991), and African-Americans in Baltimore (Hochberg et al. 1983), and the frequency of juvenile arthritis in Caucasians in the United States (Lawrence et al. 1989) and Arabs in Kuwait, another Caucasian population (Khuffash and Majeed 1988).

Cases of juvenile arthritis have been observed in Chinese in Hawaii (Hicks 1977) and California (Hanson et al. 1977), but a formal estimate of the incidence of juvenile arthritis in British Columbia indicates that it is rare in North American Chinese (Hill 1976; Kelsey 1982). The incidence of juvenile arthritis in African Americans approximates that observed in Caucasians in the United States (Lawrence et al. 1989). Differences in method may account for the disparity in incidence estimates between US and Canadian Caucasians. Incidence rates by race and ethnicity are listed in Table 1.

Gender differences and laboratory manifestations

The distribution of the different onset types of juvenile arthritis varies by race, ethnicity, and region. For example, onset types varied among three predominantly Caucasian samples in the United States (Hanson et al. 1977; Jacobs 1982; Aaron et al. 1985). In view of the strong genetic component in predisposition to juvenile arthritis and the known variation in the frequency of genetic markers within an ethnic group, the observed difference in the distribution of onset types in US Caucasians may reflect the particular ethnic composition (e.g. ratio of individuals of northern versus southern European origin) in these samples. Smaller samples of individuals with juvenile arthritis in other ethnic groups also demonstrate variability in the distribution of onset types. Polyarticular-onset juvenile arthritis was twice as common among Canadian Native Americans as Canadian Caucasians (Rosenberg et al. 1982). Comparison of three samples of patients with juvenile arthritis among Black Africans revealed different proportions of onset types and no evidence for a regional trend (Kanyerezi and Mbidde 1980; Gupta et al. 1981; Haffejee et al. 1984). The studies of juvenile arthritis among Kuwaiti Arabs (Khuffash and Majeed 1988), Ugandans (Kanyerezi and Mbidde 1980), Zambians (Gupta et al. 1981), Black and Indian South Africans (Haffejee et al. 1984), Costa Ricans (Oen and Cheang 1996), and Mexicans (Martinez-Cairo Cueto et al. 1978) are presented in Table 2.

Equal sex ratios among Black and Indian South African (Haffejee et al. 1984) and Mexican individuals with juvenile arthritis (Martinez-Cairo Cueto et al. 1978) contrast with the female predominance in samples of Native American and North American Caucasians with juvenile arthritis (Rosenberg et al. 1982; Aaron et al. 1985) (Table 3). With the exception of two studies on sex ratios (Hanson et al. 1977; Aaron et al. 1985), data were not analysed to demonstrate the age dependence of sex ratios in pauci-articular juvenile arthritis (i.e. girls more often affected than boys in early onset, boys more than girls in late onset).

Case series must be utilized when we consider comparisons of rheumatoid factor positivity. With the exception of Black Ugandans, rheumatoid factor-positive juvenile arthritis is three-fold greater in the non-European populations included, although the proportion of polyarticular-onset juvenile arthritis is not significantly different among these populations. The disparity between the proportions of polyarticular-onset juvenile arthritis and seropositivity may indicate the presence of other stimuli for rheumatoid factor production such as malaria or other recurrent parasitic infections and tuberculosis (Haffejee et al. 1984). Estimates of the seroprevalence of rheumatoid factor in juvenile arthritis are presented in Table 4.

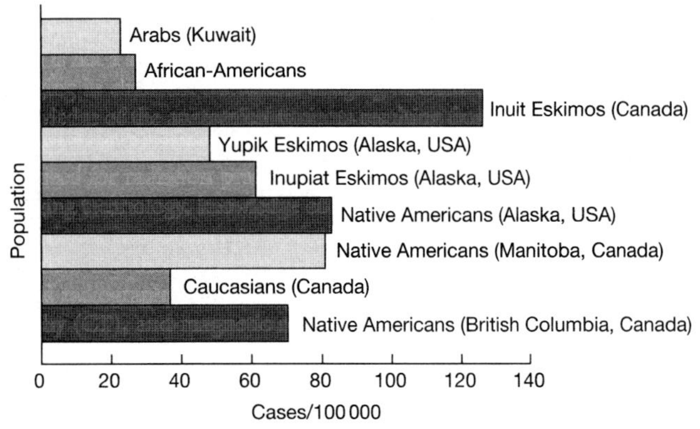

Fig. 1 Prevalence of juvenile arthritis.

Table 1 Annual incidence rate per 100 000 of juvenile arthritis

Population	Rate
Chinese (Canada)	0.00
Caucasian (British Columbia, Canada)	2.20
Native American (British Columbia)	7.20
Native Americans (S.E. Alaska, USA)	38.6
Inupiat Eskimo (Alaska, USA)	28.0
Yupik Eskimo (Alaska, USA)	42.5
Inuit Eskimos (Canada)	23.6
African-American	6.20
Caucasian (USA)	9.20
Costa Rican	5.0

Table 2 Juvenile arthritis onset types by author, race, or ethnicity

Race/ethnicity/ (author and/or locale)	Number	Systemic (%)	Polyarticular (%)	Pauci-articular (%)
Caucasians[a] (USA, Jacobs)	260	9	1675	
Caucasians[a] (USA, Hanson et al.)	563	43	2334	
Caucasians[a] (USA, Aaron et al.)	327	15	2758	
Native Americans	34	11.8	58.8	29.4
Arabs (Kuwait)	41	39	3922	
Blacks (Uganda)	41	54	379	
Blacks (Zambia)	8	37.5	37.5	25
Blacks (S. Afr.)	42	15	5035	
Indians (S. Afr.)	18	16.6	44.4	39
Mexicans	46	28.3	45.6	26.1
Asians (India)[b]	—	—	41–87	—
Japanese[b]	—	—	53	—
Thai[b]	—	—	77	—
Costa Rican[b]	—	—	—	75
African-Caribbean[b]	—	—	—	64

[a] Sample composition is more than 95% US Caucasian.

[b] Summarized by Oen and Cheang (1996).

Table 3 Female : male ratio by onset type or all juvenile arthritis (JA)

Race or ethnicity	Systemic	Polyarticular	Pauci-articular	All JA
Native Americans (British Columbia)	—	—	—	4.6 : 1
Caucasians (British Columbia)	—	—	—	5.8 : 1
Blacks/Indians (S. Afr.)	1.25 : 1	1.1 : 1	0.83 : 1	1 : 1
Mexicans	0.63 : 1	2 : 1	0.7 : 1	1.1 : 1
Arabs	2.2 : 1	33 : 1	8 : 1	1.3 : 1
US Caucasians (Hanson et al.)	1.1 : 1	3.8 : 1	3.2 : 1	2 : 1
US Caucasians (Aaron et al.)	1.6 : 1	5.3 : 1	2 : 1	2.4 : 1
Inuit				1 : 1

Juvenile spondyloarthropathies

Juvenile-onset seronegative spondyloarthropathies, which include ankylosing spondylitis, Reiter's syndrome, and seronegative enthesopathy and arthropathy syndrome (Rosenberg and Petty 1982), account for at least half of the arthritides of childhood in native North American populations. Specific criteria for childhood-onset ankylosing spondylitis are necessary since the application of adult criteria have limited value (Singsen 1990) and may result in underestimation of this condition. The demographic, clinical, and laboratory features of juvenile-onset spondyloarthropathies (Rosenberg et al. 1982; Oen et al. 1986; Boyer et al. 1988, 1990, 1991) are summarized in Table 5.

Table 4 Frequency (%) of rheumatoid factor by race, or ethnicity by onset sub-type or unclassified juvenile arthritis (JA)

Race or ethnicity	Systemic	Polyarticular	Pauci-articular	JA
Native Americans (Alaska)	—	—	—	32
Native Americans (British Columbia)	—	—	—	36
Caucasians (British Columbia)	—	—	—	9.1
Black (S. Afr.)	—	—	—	38
Indian (S. Afr.)	—	—	—	33
Mexican	30.7	42.8	16.6	33
Black (Uganda)	—	—	—	10

Rheumatoid arthritis

Definition

The case definition of rheumatoid arthritis (RA) varies between studies. This non-uniform disease definition resulted from the evolution of disease criteria for rheumatoid arthritis over time—the Manchester grading system, the 1958 and 1962 American Rheumatism Association criteria, the New York criteria, 1987 revised, for rheumatoid arthritis (see Chapter 6.3.2). The earliest prevalence estimates to be presented in this section, from New Zealand Maoris (Rose and Prior 1963), rural Japan (Shichikawa et al. 1981), Jamaica (Lawrence et al. 1966), Puerto Rico (Mendez-Bryan et al. 1964), Liberia and Nigeria (Muller 1970), and among the South African Bantu (Beighton et al. 1975; Solomon et al. 1975), included probable and definite cases of rheumatoid arthritis. In later studies, prevalence rates were based on classical and definite cases of rheumatoid arthritis.

Occurrence

Rheumatoid arthritis does not occur at the same frequency at all ages. Its age distribution may vary between populations. Crude estimates of prevalence in populations with a younger age structure will be lower than age-adjusted prevalence rates since rheumatoid arthritis is a disease of middle age. This potential source of bias is one explanation offered for the very low prevalence of rheumatoid arthritis in several studies from different Asian and African, and African-derived population samples (Mijiyawa 1995).

Rheumatoid arthritis occurs in India, Pakistan, Oman, and Iraq at frequencies (0.75–1.98 per cent) similar to that observed in the United Kingdom and the United States (Al-Rawi et al. 1978; Pountain 1991; Malaviya et al. 1993a; Hameed et al. 1995). The common methods used to estimate the occurrence of rheumatoid arthritis among samples of Native American facilitate the comparison of prevalence estimates among these groups. It is noteworthy that rheumatoid arthritis was confined to women in an Inuit sample, although records of both sexes were reviewed (Oen et al. 1986). In contrast, a field population survey among the Yakima was limited to women (Beasley et al. 1973). Within this ethnic group, we observe variability between tribal groups and by locale. The majority (76 per cent) of those with rheumatoid arthritis among south-eastern Alaskan Native Americans were of Tlingit ancestry (Boyer et al. 1991). The prevalence of rheumatoid arthritis varied among the groups of Native Americans studied (Chippewa, Haida, Nootka and Pima, Yupik, and Inupiat Eskimos) from 0.6 to 7.1 per cent, with the highest rates among the Chippewa and the Pima (7.1 and 5.3 per cent, respectively) (Gofton et al. 1964; Harvey et al. 1983; Atkins et al. 1988; Del Puente et al. 1989; Boyer et al. 1990; Boyer et al. 1991).

Rheumatoid arthritis occurs at a lower frequency in populations of African ancestry when compared to Caucasians. This is best exemplified in a study in Manchester, England, where the age-adjusted prevalence

Table 5 Juvenile spondyloarthropathies (SPA): prevalence (cases/100 000), incidence (cases/100 000/year), ratio of SPA : juvenile arthritis (JA), and frequency of HLA-B27 (%)

Population	Dx	Number of cases	Prevalence	Incidence	SPA : JA	HLA-B27
Native Americans (British Columbia)	All SPA	14	29.4		0.82:1	70
	SEA	5				
	AS	3				
	RS	4				
Native Americans (Alaska)	All SPA	9			3.75:1	
	SEA	7				
	RS	2				
Yupik Eskimos	All SPA	21			7:1	
	SEA	17				
	RS/AS	4				
Inupiat Eskimos	All SPA	5		47.4	5:1	
	SEA	2				
	RS	2				
	AS	1				
Inuit	All SPA	11	367		105.6	4.5:1

of rheumatoid arthritis was significantly lower in Afro-Caribbeans (Afro-Caribbean:Caucasian 0.36:1) (MacGregor et al. 1994), and in a study that failed to detect any cases of rheumatoid arthritis among 2000 rural Nigerians (Silman et al. 1993).

Comparison of the prevalence rates of rheumatoid arthritis among populations of Sub-Saharan African descent is more problematical and necessitates review of the raw data. This is necessary because several disease definitions were used in the studies of interest. Intercontinental differences in population age structure may also contribute to the observed differences in the prevalence of rheumatoid arthritis. For example, the age distribution in the United States is significantly older than that in most Sub-Saharan African nations (Hall 1991). Since rheumatoid arthritis occurs most frequently in young and middle-aged adults, a country such as the United States may have a higher prevalence of rheumatoid arthritis on the basis of the age distribution of its population. The combined prevalence of definite and classical rheumatoid arthritis has been estimated for African-Americans (Lawrence et al. 1989), while prevalence data for probable and definite rheumatoid arthritis are available from Jamaica and several Black African samples. We observe variability if we compare the prevalence of definite rheumatoid arthritis among samples of Sub-Saharan African descent. Although the prevalence of definite rheumatoid arthritis is similar for African-Americans, rural Jamaicans, and urban South African Bantu (Lawrence et al. 1966; Solomon et al. 1975; Lawrence et al. 1989), estimates from rural Africa are significantly lower (Beighton et al. 1975; Moolenburgh et al. 1984; Brighton et al. 1988). With the exception of the Jamaican sample, there is a striking difference between urban and rural black populations. This is best illustrated in southern Africa, where rural and urban estimates among the Tswana reveal a more than threefold difference in the prevalence of rheumatoid arthritis (Beighton et al. 1975; Solomon et al. 1975). It is difficult to draw any conclusions about ethnic differences in predisposition in Sub-Saharan African populations. A study of 39 patients with rheumatoid arthritis admitted to a central hospital in Uganda did not show any ethnic predisposition among the Baganda, Banyarwanda, and Banyankole, the major tribal groups in that region (Kanyerezi 1969). A similar investigation in western Nigeria also failed to show heightened susceptibility in any ethnic group (Greenwood 1969).

Table 6 lists 45 prevalence estimates for rheumatoid arthritis.

Comparative analyses of seropositivity in rheumatoid and non-rheumatoid arthritis show rates of seropositivity in non-rheumatoid from 2 to 20 per cent and between 9 and 94 per cent in rheumatoid (Table 7). It is interesting that two studies from Nigeria made more than 20 years apart provide very different estimates of the seroprevalence of rheumatoid factor (Greenwood 1969; Adebajo et al. 1993). A longitudinal study of rheumatoid factor and rheumatoid arthritis in the Pima indicated that the titre of rheumatoid factor predicts the risk of developing rheumatoid arthritis in this population (Del Puente et al. 1988). This observation may also explain the high prevalence rates of rheumatoid arthritis and of seropositive rheumatoid arthritis (78–94 per cent) among other Native American groups.

Systemic lupus erythematosus

Definition

The analysis of Jamaicans with systemic lupus erythematosus (SLE) (Wilson and Hughes 1979) utilized 1971 criteria to define the disease (Cohen et al. 1971). The remainder of the studies used the 1982 revised criteria (Tan et al. 1982).

Occurrence

Although there is little evidence for geographic clustering of SLE (Wallace and Quismorio 1995), there are abundant data to support the concept of differential susceptibility to lupus associated with ethnicity. The prevalence of SLE among African-Americans is more than threefold greater than among Caucasians in the same regions (Siegel and Lee 1973; Fessel 1974). The available rates for systemic lupus in African-Americans are stratified by sex and age, with peak prevalence between 15 and 64 years. United States incidence data are two- to three-fold greater in African-American than Caucasian women (McCarty et al. 1995). The same trends are seen in data from African-Caribbeans in Birmingham, United Kingdom (Johnson et al. 1995). These statistics contrast sharply with the very low prevalence of lupus in Sub-Saharan Africans. This prevalence gradient of low lupus risk in resident Sub-Saharan Africans and high risk in migrant populations of Sub-Saharan African ancestry residing outside continental Africa is unexplained. Genetic admixture (Symmons 1995) and environmental factors (Bae et al. 1998) are hypothesized to account for this variation. The only study to address admixture in systemic lupus found no difference in its level (approximately 28 per cent) between African-American patients in Baltimore and local controls (Bias et al. 1992). In several samples, age of onset in African-Americans and Afro-Caribbeans is significantly younger

Table 6 Prevalence rates of rheumatoid arthritis

Population	Type of estimate	Criteria for Dx	Prevalence (cases/100)	
			Females	Total
Inuit Eskimos	Database	1958[a]		1.82
Yupik Eskimos	Database	1958	1.0	0.6
Inupiat Eskimos	Database	1958	1.1	0.7
Native Americans (Alaska)	Database	1958	3.5	2.4
Haida Native Americans (Canada)	Population	1958, 1962 Manchester[b]	1.5	1.0
Nootka Native Americans (Canada)	Population	1958		1.4
Pima Native Americans (USA)	Population	1962[c]	6.95	5.3
Yakima Native Americans (USA)	Population	NewYork[d]	3.4	
Chippewa Native Americans (USA)	Population	1958		5.3
Wayakama, Japan (rural)	Population	1962		0.5
Hiroshima + Nagasaki, Japan (urban)	Population	1958	0.64	0.47
African-Americans	Population	1958		0.9[e]
Jamaica	Population	1958	6.0/1.6[e]	4.3/1.1[e]
Black Caribbean (Manchester, UK)	Population	1987		0.29
Liberia	Population	1962 + Manchester	2.1	2.3
Igbo-Oro (Nigeria)	Population	1962 + Manchester	0	1.0
Isheri (Nigeria)	Population	1962 + Manchester	3.7	3.1
Igbo-Oro (Nigeria)	Population	1987	0	0
Bantu (S. Afr.—urban)	Population	1962	3.7/1.4[e]	3.3/0.9[e]
Tswana (S. Afr.—rural)	Population	1962	0.4	0.87/0.12[e]
Basutho (Lesotho—rural)	Central	1962	0.19	0.23/0.20[e]
Venda (S. Afr.—rural)	Population	1962		0.0026[e]
Xhosa (S. Afr.—rural)	Population	1962		2.2/0.68[e]
Puerto Rico	Population	1958	1.2	0.93
Maoris, New Zealand	Population	1962		3.3
Kinmen, China (rural)	Population	1962	0.4	0.3[e]
Hong Kong (urban)	Population	1958, 1962, 1987		0.35
Han (North China, rural)	Population	?		0.34
Han (South China, rural)	Population	?		0.32
Taiwan (rural)	Population	1958		0.26
Taiwan (suburban)	Population	1958		0.78
Taiwan (urban)	Population	1958		0.93
India (rural)	Population	1987		0.75
Pakistan (urban, poor)	Population	1987		0.9
Pakistan (urban, affluent)	Population	1987		1.98
Indonesia (rural)	Population	1958		0.2
Indonesia (urban)	Population	1958		0.3
Oman	Population	1987		0.84
Iraq	Population	1958		1.0
Santiago, Chile	Central	1962		0.1[e]
Monterrey, Mexico	Central	1987		0.68
El Salvador	Not specified	1987		0.86

[a] Ropes et al. (1958).
[b] Lawrence (1961).
[c] Kellgren (1962).
[d] Lawrence and Wood (1963).
[e] Computed from definite or definite + classical RA cases only.

Table 7 Frequency (%) of rheumatoid factor seropositivity in selected normal and rheumatoid arthritis (RA) samples

Population/locale	Type of sample	Total	non-RA	RA
USA	Population		2.6	32
Uganda	Hospitalized			51.3[a]
Western Nigeria	Hospitalized		11.4	13.0[b]
Ibadan, Nigeria	Central clinic		4	47[c]
Jamaica	Population	1.6		20.0
Tswana (rural S. Afr.)	Central clinic			8.90[d]
Tswana (urban S. Afr.)	Central clinic			12.1[d]
Xhosa (rural S. Afr.)	Central clinic			17.0[d]
Cape Town (S. Afr.)	Central clinic			85.0[e]
Xhosa (rural S. Afr.)	Population	17	14.7	50.0[f]
Basutho (Lesotho)	Population		12–19	54.8[g]
Chippewa (USA)	Population		10	92
Yakima (USA)	Population		3	94
Haida (Canada)	Population	3.5	2	50
Yupik (Alaska)	Population			78
Inuit (Canada)	Population			83
Japan (urban)	Population	8.9	7.4	75
China (rural)	Population		1.7	28

[a] Kanyerezi (1969); [b] Greenwood (1969); [c] Adebajo (1993); [d] Meyers et al. (1983); [e] Mody et al. (1989); [f] Meyers et al. (1977); [g] Moolenburgh et al. (1984).

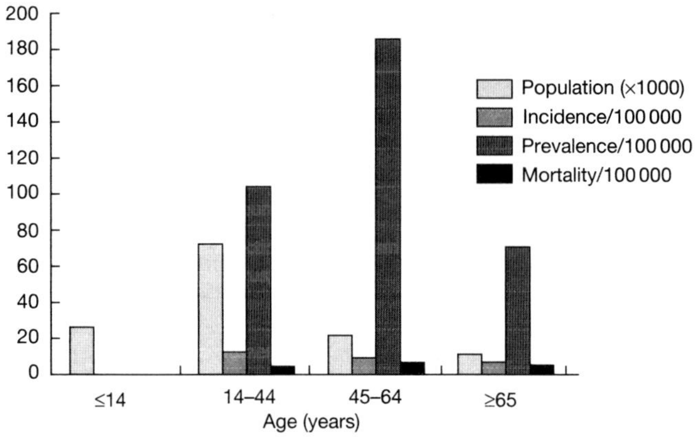

Fig. 2 Age-specific population, prevalence, incidence, and mortality in Curacao.

than locale-matched Caucasian lupus patients (Johnson et al. 1995; McCarty et al. 1995). Estimates of SLE occurrence in Curacao, a Caribbean island largely populated by descendants of enslaved Africans, differ slightly from other samples of African ancestry. Although the peak incidence occurs among women 45–65 years exceeds that for the 15–44 age group (186.6 versus 102.9/100 000) (Nossent 1992). The minor discordance between these two rates is not due to differences in mortality rates. Figure 2 summarizes age-specific population, prevalence, incidence, and mortality data for the Curacao sample.

Among Native American women in Alaska aged 15–64 years, the prevalence of SLE is 280/100 000, which is intermediate between estimates for US Caucasians and African-Americans (140/100 000 and 410/100 000, respectively) (Boyer et al. 1991). The Nootka Native Americans in British Colombia have the highest reported prevalence of systemic lupus (500 cases/100 000 population) (Atkins et al. 1988), while the Sioux, Crow, and Arapaho exhibited the highest incidence rates of systemic lupus in a survey of 75 Native American peoples (Morton et al. 1976). The estimates for the Nootka, Crow, and Arapaho were derived from small populations (2000–3000) and it is likely that the incidence estimate for the Sioux is the most accurate (Hochberg 1990) because they were the most numerous group studied (population = 30 000).

Black South Africans were over-represented among inpatients with SLE in Cape Town (Fessel 1988). Since admission to hospital with systemic lupus is highly correlated with disease severity, the disproportionate number of Blacks may reflect more severe disease rather than excess risk of lupus. Studies of Pacific rim, southeast Asian and New Zealand populations provide prevalence rates of SLE for India (Malaviya et al. 1993b), Chinese, Japanese, and Filipinos in Hawaii, and Polynesians in New Zealand (Serdula and Rhoads 1979; Hart et al. 1983; Catalano and Hoffmeier 1989). An overall prevalence estimate from Malaysia, which includes lupus cases of Chinese, Asian Indian, and Malay ancestry is also available (Wang et al. 1997.) Comparisons among these rates are difficult because of the variability in methods. Table 8 summarizes the data on lupus occurrence.

Clinical and laboratory manifestations

The ratio of females to males with SLE in the Unites States is 8–10 : 1 (Siegel and Lee 1973; Fessel 1974) and approaches 12 : 1 in Venezuela (Abadi and Gonzalez 1990). Case series in Latin America may indicate higher female to male ratios than among US Caucasians (Alarcon 1986). Populations of Black African descent in Jamaica and the United States demonstrate an earlier age of onset than Caucasians (Wilson and Hughes 1979; Hochberg et al. 1985; Ward and Studenski 1990), more frequent and more severe renal involvement, and greater mortality (Harris et al. 1989; Williams et al. 1990). Earlier age of onset is associated with HLA–DR8 in African-Americans (Reveille et al. 1989). Among African-Americans, discoid lupus (Hochberg et al. 1985; Ward and Studenski 1990), lupus pneumonitis, serositis, nephritis, hypocomplementaemia, hyperglobulinaemia (Hochberg et al. 1985), and anti-Sm and antiribonucleoprotein (Ward and Studenski 1990) are significantly more common than among US Caucasians, while photosensitivity is significantly less frequent (Hochberg et al. 1985; Ward and Studenski 1990). Photosensitivity occurs with a similar frequency among African-Americans residing in a temperate climate and Jamaicans who are exposed to a subtropical climate. Interestingly, photosensitivity is twice as common in Black South Africans who also reside in a temperate zone as among African-Americans. The LUMINA study in the United States is a longitudinal study of three lupus cohorts—Caucasian, African-American, and Mexican-American in the southeastern region of the United States. This study shows that disease activity, disability, and organ damage are significantly worse for African-Americans and Mexican-Americans when compared to (Alarcon et al. 2001a,b). The frequencies of clinical and laboratory features of SLE in African-American, Jamaican, and Black South African, and Zimbabwean samples are listed in Table 9 (Wilson and Hughes 1979; Hochberg et al. 1985; Taylor and Stein 1986; Dessein et al. 1988; Ward and Studenski 1990; Nossent 1993).

Seronegative spondyloarthropathies

Definition

The seronegative spondyloarthropathies are a group of chronic rheumatic diseases characterized by variable combinations of asymmetrical peripheral arthritis, enthesopathy, involvement of the axial skeleton, mucocutaneous symptoms, higher than expected frequencies of the *HLA-B27* allele, and the absence of rheumatoid factor. Ankylosing spondylitis, Reiter's syndrome/'reactive arthritis', psoriatic arthritis/spondylitis, and inflammatory bowel disease-associated spondylitis are included within the spondyloarthropathy category. The term undifferentiated spond(ylo)arthropathy has been designated for these conditions (Boyer et al. 1988).

Table 8 Prevalence (cases/100 000) and incidence (new cases/100 000 year) of systemic lupus

Population (locale)	Type of sample	Prevalence		Incidence
		All	15–64 years	
African-American female	Not specified	283[a]	410[a]	8.1[b], 11.4[c]
African-American male[d]	Not specified	53		
African-American female	Population-based registry			9.2[e]
African-American male	Population-based registry			0.7[e]
Afro-Caribbean female (UK)	Multisource registry	197.2[f]		
Curacao female	Hospital			7.9[g]
Curacao male	Hospital			1.1[g]
Venezuela female	Inpatient	9.27		
Venezuela male	Inpatient	0.8[h]		
Native American-female[i] (Alaska)	Population		280	
Eskimo (Alaska)[j]	Population		11.4	
Sioux Native American[j]	Inpatient			16.6
Caucasian female (USA)[d]	Not specified	71	140	3.9
Caucasian (New Zealand)[k]	Composite[l]	14.6		
Polynesian (New Zealand)[k]	Composite	51	99	
Japanese (Japan)[m]	Not specified	21		
Japanese (Hawaii)[n]	Not specified	27.5		
Chinese (China)[o]	Population		40–70	
Chinese (Hawaii)[n]	Not specified	33.5		
Caucasian (Hawaii)[p]	Not specified	10.3		
Caucasian (S. Afr.)[p]	Central clinic	23.9		1.95
Black (S. Afr.)[p]	Central clinic	12.2		1.03
Coloured (S. Afr.)[p]	Central clinic	20.7		1.6
Asian Indian (S. Afr.)[p]	Central clinic	69.3		6.33
Malaysia[q]	Central clinic	43		
India[r]	Population		3.2	

[a] Fessel (1974), data from Hochberg (1990), table 4; [b] Siegel and Lee (1973), data from Hochberg (1990), table 3; [c] Data from Hochberg (1990), table 3; [d] Fessel (1974); [e] McCarty et al. (1995); [f] Johnson et al. (1995); [g] Nossent (1992); [h] Abadi and Gonzalez (1990); [i] Boyer et al. (1991); [j] Morton et al. (1976); [k] Hart et al. (1983); [l] Hospital disch data and practitioner survey; [m] Nakae et al. (1987), from Hochberg (1990), table 2; [n] Catalano and Hoffmeier (1989), from Hochberg (1990), table 5; [o] Nai-Zheng (1989), from Hochberg (1990); [p] Morrison et al. (1990); [q] Wang et al. (1997); [r] Malaviya et al. (1993).

The Rome criteria and the New York criteria (see Chapter 6.4.1) have been developed to assess the frequency of ankylosing spondylitis in populations. The Rome criteria are more suited to field studies since they do not require radiographs to make the diagnosis of definite ankylosing spondylitis. The criteria for Reiter's syndrome (see Chapter 6.4.5) and the undifferentiated spondyloarthropathies have not been used as extensively as those for ankylosing spondylitis. Also problematical is the relation of sacroiliitis to the groups of spondyloarthropathy. Is asymptomatic sacroiliitis distinct from clinical spondyloarthropathy or does it represent one end of the spectrum of spondarthropathic disease expression?

Occurrence

Prevalence estimates for spondyloarthropathies for several Native American and Eskimo groups and the Chinese (Morse et al. 1980; Beasley et al. 1983; Oen et al. 1986; Boyer et al. 1988, 1990, 1991) appear in Table 10. HLA-B27 and spondyloarthropathies occur at higher frequencies in several Native American groups than in Caucasians, with the highest recorded rates among the Haida in Canada.

In sharp contrast to the Native American groups, spondyloarthropathy is diagnosed infrequently in African-Americans and Sub-Saharan Africans (Baum and Ziff 1971). The frequency of spondyloarthropathies in African-Americans is not known. The ratio of Caucasians to African-Americans with ankylosing spondylitis (range 20:1–6.5:1) admitted to US Veterans' hospitals serves as an indirect estimate of the prevalence of ankylosing spondylitis in African-Americans (Baum and Ziff 1971). The rarity of spondyloarthropathies in West Africans, who are racially heterogeneous and are one of the source populations for African-Americans, has been attributed to the low frequency of HLA-B27. For example, the *HLA-B*2703* allele has been found in Gambians but ankylosing spondylitis has not been observed (Hill et al. 1991). Because of the low overall frequency of HLA-B27 (2.6 per cent) in Gambians, it is possible that one might not see cases of ankylosing spondylitis since only a proportion of HLA-B27-positive individuals develop ankylosing spondylitis. Alternatively, the absence of ankylosing spondylitis in a population with HLA-B27 may indicate the absence of environmental factors that interact with HLA-B27 to trigger spondyloarthropathies, or that the HLA-B27 molecules in the population do not confer susceptibility to spondyloarthropathies (Hill et al. 1991).

Table 9 Frequency (%) of clinical and laboratory manifestations of systemic lupus erythematosus in selected samples

Feature	US		Jamaica	Curacao	Southern Africa		
	Ward[a]	Hochberg[b]	Wilson[c]	Nossent	Morrison[d]	Taylor[e]	Dessein[f,i,ii,iii]
Oral/nasal ulcers	21.4	—	—	19	—	19	23
Photosensitivity	15.5	11	12	25	32/8/27	16	13
Discoid rash	16.0	35	—	—	—	19	27
Renal	51.9	49	40	78	83/66/100	71	60
All CNS	—	—	58	—	—	13	20
Seizures	14.4	—	—	—	—	6	10
Psychosis	13.4	—	—	3	—	6	—
Anti-DNA	63.6	30	—	97	48/100/86	100	81
Anti-Sm	17.1	24	—	4	—	—	—
Anti-RNP	26.2	41	—	—	—	—	—
Hypocomplementaemia	61	81	—	—	—	—	—

[a] Ward and Studenski (1990), tables 2 and 3; [b] Hochberg et al. (1985), table 3; [c] Wilson and Hughes (1979), tables 6 and 8; [d] Morrison et al. (1990); [e] Taylor and Stein (1986), table 1; [f] Dessein et al. (1988), tables 1 and 2; [i] Frequency in South African Blacks; [ii] Frequency in Coloureds; [iii] Frequency in Indians.

Table 10 Prevalence of seronegative spondyloarthropathies (SPA)

Population (locale)	Disease	Criteria	Rate (cases/100)
Haida Native Americans (Canada)	AS	New York	6.7
Haida Native Americans (Alaska)	AS	New York	0.8
Other Native Americans (Alaska)	All SPA	Composite[a]	1.1
Yupik Eskimos (Alaska)	AS	Rome	0.2
Yupik Eskimos (Alaska)	RS	A.R.A., 1981	0.23
Inupiat Eskimos (Alaska)	AS	Rome	0.1
Inupiat Eskimos (Alaska)	RS	A.R.A., 1981	0.6
Inuit (Alaska)	AS	New York	0.34
Inuit Eskimos (Alaska)	RS	—	0.63
Inuit (Greenland)	RS	A.R.A., 1981	1.08/0.34[b]
Navajo Native Americans (USA)	RS	—	0.3[c]
Chinese (Kinmen Island)	AS	—	0.3[d]

[a] Boyer et al. (1991) used New York criteria for AS, A.R.A. (1981) criteria for RS and working criteria for USPA.

[b] Estimates from Greenland Community's A and B, respectively, from table 3, Boyer et al. (1990).

[c] Morse et al. (1981).

[d] Beasley et al. (1983).

Table 11 Relative frequencies (%) of spondyloarthropathy (SPA) subsets and sex ratios in several populations

Population (locale)	SPA	Frequency	Male : female ratio
Native American (Alaska, USA)	AS	32.8	5.3:1
	RS	32.8	0.58:1
	USPA	34.4	0.33:1
Inuit (Alaska, USA)	AS	11.8	
	RS	41.2	
	PSA/S	5.9	
	USPA	41.1	
	All SPA		3.3:1
Yupik Eskimo (Alaska, USA)	AS	22.4	6.5:1
	RS	28.4[a]	
	USPA	32.8[b]	1.6:1
	PSA/S	1.4[a]	
	All SPA		5:1
Navajo Native American (USA)	RS	100	
Caucasian (England)	AS	85	2.4:1
Shona (Zimbabwe)	AS	47.4	8:1
	RS	52.6	4:1

[a] No females were observed with this diagnosis.

[b] Includes cases of USPA and overlap SPA syndromes.

In support of this latter theory, *HLA-B*2703* differs from other *B27* alleles at amino acid position 59 in the α_1-domain. This observation may explain the results of experiments with alloreactive T-cell clones with this allele (Calvo et al. 1990) and may indicate that peptide binding for *HLA-B*2703* is different from other B27 subtypes (Woodrow 1991).

Distribution of spondyloarthropathy subsets and sex ratios

The relative frequencies of the spondyloarthropathy subtypes vary within and between racial groups. As shown in Table 11, ankylosing spondylitis is the predominant spondyloarthropathy in Caucasians of Northern European descent (Edmunds et al. 1991). Equal frequencies of ankylosing spondylitis and Reiter's syndrome are seen in Alaskan Native Americans and Eskimos (Boyer et al. 1990, 1991) and the Shona cultural group in Zimbabwe (Stein et al. 1990). Cases of ankylosing spondylitis comprise only 11 per cent of spondyloarthropathies among the Alaskan Inuit, where the frequencies of Reiter's syndrome and undifferentiated spondyloarthropathy are equal. With the exception of Native Americans in Alaska (Reiter's syndrome and undifferentiated spondyloarthropathies are more common in females), males outnumber females with spondyloarthropathies (Table 11).

References

Aaron, S. et al. (1985). Sex ratio and sibship in juvenile rheumatoid arthritis kindreds. *Arthritis and Rheumatism* **28**, 753–8.

Abadi, I. and Gonzalez, N. (1990). Epidemiologia de lupus eritematosos sistemico en Venezuela. Sindrome clinico e immunologico. In *Ediciones Anno Acta Medica Colombiana* (ed. M. Sanchez, M. Diaz, F. Rondon, and G. Ucros), pp. 17–22.

Adebajo, A.O. (1995). Tropical rheumatology. Epidemiology and community studies: Africa. *Baillières Clinical Rheumatology* **9**, 21–30.

Adebajo, A.O., Charles, P.J., Hazleman, B.L., and Maini, R.N. (1993). Serological profile of rheumatoid arthritis in West Africa. *Rheumatology International* **12**, 235–8.

Alarcon, G.S. (1986). Epidemiologia de las enfermedades reumaticas en America Latina. *Bol Oficina Sanit Panam* **101**, 309–27.

Alarcon, G.S., McGwin, G., Jr., Bartolucci, A.A., Roseman, J., Lisse, J., Fessler, B.J., Bastian, H.M., Friedman, A.W., and Reveille, J.D., and LUMINA Study Group (2001a). Lupus in minority populations, nature versus nurture. Systemic lupus erythematosus in three ethnic groups. IX. Differences in damage accrual. *Arthritis and Rheumatism* **44** (12), 2797–806.

Alarcon, G.S., McGwin, G., Jr., Bastian, H.M., Roseman, J., Lisse, J., Fessler, B.J., Friedman, A.W., and Reveille, J.D. (2001b). Systemic lupus erythematosus in three ethnic groups. VII (correction of VIII). Predictors of early mortality in the LUMINA cohort. LUMINA Study Group. *Arthritis and Rheumatism* **45** (2), 191–202.

Al-Rawi, Z.S., Alazzawi, A.J., Alajili, F.M., and Alwakil, R. (1978). Rheumatoid arthritis in population samples in Iraq. *Annals of the Rheumatic Diseases* **37**, 73–5.

Atkins, C. et al. (1988). Rheumatic disease in the Nuu-Chah-Nulth native Indians of the Pacific Northwest. *Journal of Rheumatology* **15**, 684–90.

Bae, S.C., Fraser, P.A., and Liang, M. (1998). The epidemiology of systemic lupus erythematosus in populations of african ancestry: a critical review of the 'Prevalence Gradient Hypothesis'. *Arthritis and Rheumatism* **41**, 2091–9.

Baum, J. and Ziff, M. (1971). The rarity of ankylosing spondylitis in the black race. *Arthritis and Rheumatism* **14**, 12–18.

Beasley, R.P., Willkens, R.F., and Bennett, P.H. (1973). High prevalence of rheumatoid arthritis in Yakima Indians. *Arthritis and Rheumatism* **16**, 743–8.

Beasley, R.P., Bennett, P.H., and Lin, C.C. (1983). Low prevalence of rheumatoid arthritis in Chinese. *Journal of Rheumatology* **10** (Suppl.), 11–15.

Beighton, P., Solomon, L., and Valkenburg, H.A. (1975). Rheumatoid arthritis in a rural South African Negro population. *Annals of the Rheumatic Diseases* **34**, 136–41.

Bias, W.B., Hochberg, M.C., McLean, R.H., and Machan, C. (1992). Systemic lupus erythematosus joint report. In *HLA 1991: Proceedings of the Eleventh International Histocompatibility Workshop and Conference* Vol. 1 (ed. K. Tsuji, M. Aizawa, and T. Sasazuki), pp. 740–5. Oxford: Oxford University Press.

Boyer, G.S., Lanier, A.P., and Templin, D.W. (1988). Prevalence rates of spondyloarthropathies, rheumatoid arthritis, and other rheumatic diseases in an Alaskan Inupiat Eskimo population. *Journal of Rheumatology* **15**, 678–83.

Boyer, G.S. et al. (1990). Spondyloarthropathy and rheumatoid arthritis in Alaskan Yupik Eskimos. *Journal of Rheumatology* **17**, 489–96.

Boyer, G.S., Templin, D.W., and Lanier, A.P. (1991). Rheumatic diseases in Alaskan Indians of the southeast coast: high prevalence of rheumatoid arthritis and systemic lupus erythematosus. *Journal of Rheumatology* **18**, 1477–84.

Brighton, S.W. et al. (1988). The prevalence of rheumatoid arthritis in a rural African population. *Journal of Rheumatology* **15**, 405–8.

Calvo, V. et al. (1990). Structure and diversity of HLA-B27-specific T-cell epitopes: analysis with site-directed mutants mimicking HLA-B27 subtype polymorphism. *Journal of Immunology* **144**, 4038–45.

Catalano, M.A. and Hoffmeier, M. (1989). Frequency of systemic lupus erythematosus (SLE) among ethnic groups of Hawaii. *Arthritis and Rheumatism* **32** (Suppl. 4), S30.

Cohen, A.S. et al. (1971). Preliminary criteria for the classification of SLE. *Bulletin on the Rheumatic Diseases* **21**, 643–8.

Cooper, G.S., Germolec, D., Heindel, J., and Selgrade, M. (1999). Linking environmental agents and autoimmune diseases. *Environmental Health Perspectives* **107** (Suppl. 5), 659–60.

Cooper, G.S., Miller, F.W., and Germolec, D.R. (2002). Occupational exposures and autoimmune diseases. *International Immunopharmacology* **2** (2–3), 303–13.

Del Puente, A. et al. (1988). The incidence of rheumatoid arthritis is predicted by rheumatoid factor titer in a longitudinal population study. *Arthritis and Rheumatism* **31**, 1239–44.

Del Puente, A. et al. (1989). High incidence and prevalence of rheumatoid arthritis in Pima Indians. *American Journal of Epidemiology* **129**, 1170–8.

Dessein, P.H.M.C., Gledhill, R.F., and Rossouw, D.S. (1988). Systemic lupus erythematosus in black South Africans. *South Africa Medical Journal* **74**, 387–9.

Edmunds, J.E., Kennedy, L.G., and Calin, A. (1991). Primary ankylosing spondylitis, psoriatic and enteropathic spondyloarthropathy: a controlled analysis. *Journal of Rheumatology* **18**, 696–8.

Fessel, W.J. (1974). Systemic lupus erythematosus in the community incidence, prevalence, outcome and first symptoms: the high prevalence in black women. *Archives of Internal Medicine* **134**, 1027–35.

Fessel, W.J. (1988). Epidemiology of systemic lupus erythematosus. *Rheumatic Disease Clinics of North America* **14**, 15–23.

Gewanter, H.L., Roghman, K.J., and Baum, J. (1983). The prevalence of juvenile arthritis. *Arthritis and Rheumatism* **26**, 599–601.

Gofton, J.P., Robinson, H.S., and Price, G.E. (1964). A study of rheumatic disease in a Canadian Indian population. II. Rheumatoid arthritis in the Haida Indians. *Annals of the Rheumatic Diseases* **23**, 364–71.

Greenwood, B.M. (1969). Polyarthritis in Western Nigeria. *Annals of the Rheumatic Diseases* **28**, 489–96.

Gupta, K., Chintu, C., and Raghu, M.B. (1981). Juvenile rheumatoid arthritis in Zambian children. *East Africa Medical Journal* **58**, 344–5.

Haffejee, I.E., Raga, J., and Coovadia, H.M. (1984). Juvenile chronic arthritis in Black and Indian South African children. *South Africa Medical Journal* **65**, 510–14.

Hall, P. (1991). Rheumatoid arthritis in sub-Saharan Africa. *Proceedings First AFLAR Congress of Rheumatology* (Abstract 17).

Hameed, K., Gibson, T., Kadir, M., Sultana, S., Fatima, Z., and Syed, A. (1995). The prevalence of rheumatoid arthritis in affluent and poor urban communities of Pakistan. *British Journal of Rheumatology* **34**, 252–6.

Hanson, V. et al. (1977). Three subtypes of juvenile rheumatoid arthritis. *Arthritis and Rheumatism* **20** (Suppl.), 184–6.

Harris, E.N., Williams, E., Shah, D.J., and De Ceular, K. (1989). Mortality of Jamaican patients with systemic lupus erythematosus. *British Journal of Rheumatology* **28**, 113–17.

Hart, H.H., Grigor, R.R., and Caughey, D.E. (1983). Ethnic difference in the prevalence of systemic lupus erythematosus. *Annals of the Rheumatic Diseases* **42**, 529–32.

Harvey, J. et al. (1983). Rheumatoid arthritis in a Chippewa band. II. Field study with clinical serologic and HLA-D correlations. *Journal of Rheumatology* **10**, 28–32.

Hill, R. (1976). Juvenile arthritis in various racial groups in British Columbia. *Arthritis and Rheumatism* **20** (Suppl.), 162–4.

Hill, A.S.V. et al. (1991). HLA class I typing by PCR: HLA-B27 and an African HLA-B27 subtype. *Lancet* **337**, 640–2.

Hochberg, M.C. (1984). The epidemiology of juvenile rheumatoid arthritis: review of current status and approaches for future research. In *Epidemiology of the Rheumatic Diseases. Proceedings of the Fourth International Conference, National Institutes of Health* (ed. R.C. Lawrence and L.E. Shulman), pp. 220–30. London: Gower Medical.

Hochberg, M.C. (1990). Systemic lupus erythematosus. *Rheumatic Disease Clinics of North America* **16**, 617–39.

Hochberg, M.C., Linet, M.S., and Sills, E.M. (1983). The prevalence and incidence of juvenile rheumatoid arthritis in an urban black population. *American Journal of Public Health* **73**, 1202–3.

Hochberg, M.C. et al. (1985). Systemic lupus erythematosus: a review of clinicolaboratory features and immunogenetic markers in 150 patients with emphasis on demographic subsets. *Medicine* **64**, 285–95.

Jacobs, J.C. *Pediatric Rheumatology for the Practitioner.* New York: Springer-Verlag, 1982.

James, J.A., Neas, B.R., Moser, K.L., Hall, T., Bruner, G.R., Sestak, A.L., and Harley, J.B. (2001). Systemic lupus erythematosus in adults is associated with previous Epstein-Barr virus exposure. *Arthritis and Rheumatism* **44** (5), 1122–6.

Jawaheer, D., Seldin, M.F., Amos, C.I., Chen, W.V., Shigeta, R., Monteiro, J., Kern, M., Criswell, L.A., Albani, S., Nelson, J.L., Clegg, D.O., Pope, R., Schroeder, H.W., Jr., Bridges, S.L., Jr., Pisetsky, D.S., Ward, R., Kastner, D.L., Wilder, R.L., Pincus, T., Callahan, L.F., Flemming, D., Wener, M.H., and Gregersen, P.K. (2001). A genomewide screen in multiplex rheumatoid arthritis families suggests genetic overlap with other autoimmune diseases. *American Journal of Human Genetics* **68** (4), 927–36.

Johnson, A.E., Gordon, C., Palmer, R.G., and Bacon, P.A. (1995). The prevalence and incidence of systemic lupus erythematosus in Birmingham, England. *Arthritis and Rheumatism* **38**, 551–8.

Kanyerezi, B.R. (1969). Rheumatoid arthritis in Uganda. *East Africa Medical Journal* **46**, 71–5.

Kanyerezi, B.R. and Mbidde, E. (1980). Juvenile chronic polyarthritis in Ugandan African children. *East Africa Medical Journal* **57**, 484–9.

Kelsey, K.L. (1982). Juvenile rheumatoid arthritis. In *Epidemiology of Musculoskeletal Disorders,* pp. 94–7. Oxford: Oxford University Press.

Khuffash, F.A. and Majeed, H.A. (1988). Juvenile rheumatoid arthritis among Arab children. *Scandinavian Journal of Rheumatology* **17**, 393–5.

Lacey, J.V., Jr., Garabrant, D.H., Laing, T.J., Gillespie, B.W., Mayes, M.D., Cooper, B.C., and Schottenfeld, D. (1999). Petroleum distillate solvents as risk factors for undifferentiated connective tissue disease (UCTD). *American Journal of Epidemiology* **149** (8), 761–70.

Lawrence, J.S. et al. (1966). Rheumatoid arthritis in a subtropical population. *Annals of the Rheumatic Diseases* **25**, 59–66.

Lawrence, R.C. et al. (1989). Estimates of the prevalence of selected arthritic and musculoskeletal disease in the United States. *Journal of Rheumatology* **16**, 427–41.

McCarty, D.J., Thomas, S.M., Medsger, T.A., Ramsey-Goldman, R., LaPorte, R.E., and Kentworth, C. (1995). Incidence of systemic lupus erythematosus. *Arthritis and Rheumatism* **38**, 1260–70.

MacGregor, A.J., Riste, L.K., Hazes, J.M., and Silman, A.J. (1994). Low prevalence of rheumatoid arthritis in black-Caribbeans compared with whites in inner city Manchester. *Annals of the Rheumatic Diseases* **53**, 293–7.

Malaviya, A.N., Kapoor, S.K., Singh, R.R., Kumar, A., and Pande, I. (1993a). Prevalence of rheumatoid arthritis in the adult Indian population. *Rheumatology International* **13**, 131–4.

Malaviya, A.N., Singh, R.R., Singh, Y.N., Kapoor, S.K., and Kumar, A. (1993b). Prevalence of systemic lupus erythematosus in India. *Lupus* **2** (2), 115–18.

Martinez-Cairo, C.S., Antonio, O.D., and Frati, A. (1978). Arthritis reumatoide juvenil. Estudio de 46 casos. *Boletin Medico del Hospital Infantil de Mexico* **35**, 711–17.

Mendez-Bryan, R., Gonzalez-Alcover, R., and Roger, L. (1964). Rheumatoid arthritis: prevalence in a tropical area. *Arthritis and Rheumatism* **7**, 171–6.

Mijiyawa, M. (1995). Epidemiology and semiology of rheumatoid arthritis in third world countries. *Expansion Scientifique Francaise* **62**, 121–6.

Moolenburgh, J.D., Moore, S., Valkenburg, H.A., and Erasmus, M.G. (1984). Rheumatoid arthritis in Lesotho. *Annals of the Rheumatic Diseases* **43**, 40–3.

Morse, H.G. et al. (1980). High frequency of HLA-B27 and Reiter's syndrome in Navajo Indians. *Journal of Rheumatology* **7**, 900–2.

Morton, R.O. et al. (1976). The incidence of systemic lupus erythematosus in North American Indians. *Journal of Rheumatology* **3**, 186–9.

Muller, A.S. *Population Studies on the Prevalence of Rheumatic Diseases in Liberia and Nigeria.* Unpublished doctoral thesis, University of Leiden, 1970.

Nossent, J.C. (1992). Systemic lupus erythematosus in the Caribbean island of Curacao: an epidemiological investigation. *Annals of the Rheumatic Diseases* **51**, 1197–201.

Nossent, J.C. (1993). Course and prognostic value of systemic lupus erythematosus disease activity index in Black Caribbean patients. *Seminars in Arthritis and Rheumatism* **23**, 16–21.

Oen, K.G. and Cheang, M. (1996). Epidemiology of chronic arthritis in childhood. *Seminars in Arthritis and Rheumatism* **26** (3), 575–91.

Oen, K. et al. (1986). Rheumatic disease in an Inuit population. *Arthritis and Rheumatism* **29**, 65–74.

Oen, K., Fast, M., and Postl, B. (1995). Epidemiology of juvenile rheumatoid arthritis in Manitoba, Canada, 1975–92: cycles in incidence. *Journal of Rheumatology* **22**, 745–50.

Pountain, G. (1991). The prevalence of rheumatoid arthritis in the Sultanate of Oman. *British Journal of Rheumatology* **30**, 24–8.

Povey, A., Guppy, M.J., Wood, M., Knight, C., Black, C.M., and Silman, A.J. (2001). Cytochrome P2 polymorphisms and susceptibility to scleroderma following exposure to organic solvents. *Arthritis and Rheumatism* **44** (3), 662–5.

Reveille, J.D. et al. (1989). DNA analysis of HLA–DR and DQ genes in American blacks with systemic lupus erythematosus. *Arthritis and Rheumatism* **32**, 1243–51.

Rose, B.S. and Prior, I.A.M. (1963). A survey of rheumatism in a rural New Zealand Maori community. *Annals of the Rheumatic Diseases* **22**, 410–15.

Rosenberg, A.M. and Petty, R.E. (1982). A syndrome of seronegative enthesopathy and arthropathy (SEA syndrome). *Arthritis and Rheumatism* **25**, 1041–7.

Rosenberg, A.M. et al. (1982). Rheumatic diseases in Western Canadian Indian children. *Journal of Rheumatology* **9**, 589–92.

Serdula, M.K. and Rhoads, G.G. (1979). Frequency of systemic lupus erythematosus in different ethnic groups in Hawaii. *Arthritis and Rheumatism* **22**, 328–33.

Shichikawa, K. et al. (1981). A longitudinal population survey of rheumatoid arthritis in a rural district in Wakayama. *The Ryumachi* **21** (Suppl.), 35–43.

Siegel, M. and Lee, S.L. (1973). The epidemiology of systemic lupus erythematosus. *Seminars in Arthritis and Rheumatism* **3**, 1–54.

Silman, A.J. et al. (1993). Absence of rheumatoid arthritis in a rural Nigerian population. *Journal of Rheumatology* **20**, 618–22.

Singsen, B.H. (1990). Rheumatic disease of childhood. *Rheumatic Disease Clinics of North America* **16**, 581–99.

Solomon, L., Robin, G., and Valkenburg, H.A. (1975). Rheumatoid arthritis in an urban South African Negro population. *Annals of the Rheumatic Diseases* **34**, 128–35.

Stein, M. et al. (1990). The spondyloarthropathies in Zimbabwe: a clinical and immunogenetic profile. *Journal of Rheumatology* **17**, 1337–9.

Symmons, D.P.M. (1995). Occasional series: lupus around the world; frequency of lupus in people of African origin. *Lupus* **4**, 176–8.

Tan, E.M. et al. (1982). The 1982 revised criteria for the classification of systemic lupus erythematosus. *Arthritis and Rheumatism* **25**, 1271–7.

Taylor, H.G. and Stein, C.M. (1986). Systemic lupus erythematosus in Zimbabwe. *Annals of the Rheumatic Diseases* **45**, 645–8.

Wallace, D.G. and Quismorio, F.P., Jr. (1995). The elusive search for geographic clusters of systemic lupus erythematosus. *Arthritis and Rheumatism* **38**, 1564–7.

Wang, F., Wang, C.L., Tan, C.T., and Manivasagar, M. (1997). Systemic lupus erythematosus in Malaysia: a study of 539 patients and comparison of prevalence and disease expression in different racial and gender groups. *Lupus* **6** (3), 248–53.

Ward, M.M. and Studenski, S. (1990). Clinical manifestations of systemic lupus erythematosus. *Archives of Internal Medicine* **150**, 849–53.

Williams, W. and Shah, D. (1990). Lupus nephritis at the University Hospital of the West Indies, Kingston, Jamaica: a 10-year experience. *Renal Failure* **12**, 25–33.

Wilson, W.A. and Hughes, G.R.V. (1979). Rheumatic disease in Jamaica. *Annals of the Rheumatic Diseases* **38**, 320–5.

Woodrow, J. (1991). Genetics of the spondyloarthropathies. *Current Science* **3**, 586–91.

6.2 Infections

6.2.1 Pyogenic arthritis in adults

Marc L. Miller

Septic arthritis caused by pyogenic bacteria is a true medical emergency. Prompt recognition of an infected joint and an immediate start to proper treatment are essential for a good outcome. Despite advances in antimicrobial therapy and surgical approaches, the death rate in several large series has ranged up to 10 per cent (Dubost et al. 1993; Kaandorp et al. 1997a), and up to one-third of cases are affected by residual functional impairment, persistent pain, or other complications (Cooper and Cawley 1986; Kaandorp et al. 1997a; Weston et al. 1999). In several series, the incidence of pyogenic arthritis has been less than 10 cases per 100 000 population (Cooper and Cawley 1986; Kaandorp et al. 1997b; Weitoft and Makitalo 1999), with a frequency as high as 29.1 cases per 100 000 in selected populations (Morgan et al. 1996).

This chapter will discuss pyogenic bacterial infections in adults only. Paediatric infections will be addressed in Chapter 6.2.2.

Pathophysiology

Bacteria can reach the joint by one of three routes:

(i) by haematogenous spread from a distant infected site;

(ii) by direct penetration through the skin to the joint space;

(iii) by direct spread from a contiguous infected site.

Haematogenous seeding is by far the most common route. The synovium is a highly vascular tissue without a limiting basement membrane to block bacterial access to the synovial fluid. The presence of synovitis, effusion, granulation tissue, or foreign material increases the likelihood of bacterial colonization of the joint. Therefore, joints affected by chronic arthritis, particularly rheumatoid arthritis, and prosthetic joints are at increased risk (Goldenberg and Reed 1985).

Altered host immunity also increases the risk of joint infection. This may be due to inherited immunodeficiency states or to acquired immunodeficiency due to immunosuppressive therapy or diseases such as cancer, diabetes, chronic liver disease, or human immunodeficiency virus infection (Saraux et al. 1997).

Characteristics of the infecting organisms help to explain why some bacteria that are frequent causes of bacteraemia are rare causes of joint infections. Those organisms that most commonly cause pyogenic arthritis, staphylococci and *Neisseria gonorrhoeae*, have an enhanced ability to adhere to synovial tissue or produce toxins that facilitate colonization (Switalski et al. 1993). These organisms are able to infect normal joints in normal hosts. Those organisms with low virulence for joint infection, such as Gram-negative bacilli, typically cause infections only in individuals with risk factors.

Direct entry of bacteria into the joint space can occur as the result of penetrating trauma or iatrogenic causes including arthrocentesis, arthroscopy, and arthroplasty. Infection following arthrocentesis and intra-articular steroid injection is very rare, occurring in less than 1 in 10 000 injections (Weitoft and Makitalo 1999). Persistent drainage from surgical portals should always raise the suspicion of post-arthroscopic infection.

Direct spread from an adjacent focus of infection occurs in several clinical settings. Pyogenic arthritis may result from an adjacent osteomyelitis in adults, although this complication is rare, owing to the infrequency of untreated osteomyelitis in the antibiotic era. In adults, but not in children, there is an anastomosis between the metaphyseal and synovial vascular beds allowing direct entry of bacteria from an osseous focus of infection into the joint. Direct extension of an enteric fistula in inflammatory bowel disease, of a psoas abscess, or of a gluteal abscess in a paraplegic can result in pyogenic arthritis of the hip.

Once infection is established bacteria multiply and spread throughout the synovium and eventually into the synovial fluid. Organisms are phagocytosed by polymorphonuclear leucocytes and a classic inflammatory reaction develops. Cytokines and proteinases are released from phagocytic cells leading to degradation of cartilage. In animal models, the proteoglycan content of cartilage is reduced by 40 per cent within 48 h of the induction of joint infection. Significant loss of collagen develops within 2–3 weeks. This rapid destruction underscores the importance of prompt detection and initiation of treatment, including draining bacterial and leucocyte degradation products from the joint. Chronic inflammatory tissue that resembles rheumatoid pannus may develop in untreated infections and further erode cartilage and subchondral bone.

Non-gonococcal arthritis

Clinical manifestations

The clinical manifestations, epidemiology, and natural history of gonococcal and non-gonococcal arthritis are sufficiently distinct (Table 1) that infections due to *Neisseria* spp. will be discussed separately.

The typical patient with non-gonococcal bacterial arthritis presents with acute onset of pain, swelling, erythema, warmth, and tenderness of the infected joint. There may be a tense effusion. The patient usually guards the joint against any movement. The severity of pain, tenderness, and swelling is generally greater than in other causes of joint inflammation and should immediately raise the suspicion of infection. Very rarely, patients present with a sub-acute or even chronic course and a paucity of inflammatory signs. This presentation is more commonly associated with less virulent organisms.

In deep-seated joints, localization of pain and tenderness may be difficult, and erythema, warmth, and swelling are not detectable. Hip infections produce pain deep in the buttock, in the anterior thigh, or even in the knee, while pain from the sacroiliac joint may be referred to the buttock or posterior thigh and may mimic sciatica.

Fever is commonly, but not invariably, present in cases of septic arthritis. The patient may also show signs and symptoms of an infection at a distant site from the joint, such as the skin, respiratory tract, or urinary tract.

The knee accounts for more than half of cases and the hip another 20 per cent. The remainder of cases is divided largely among the shoulder, wrist,

Table 1 Distinguishing features of gonococcal and non-gonococcal arthritis

Gonococcal	Non-gonococcal
Most often affects healthy, sexually active, young adults	Most often affects the very young or very old. Underlying joint or other medical conditions
Females more often than males	Males more often than females
Hip uncommonly affected	Hips involved in 20%
Migratory polyarthralgias common	Polyarthralgias uncommon
Rash, tenosynovitis common	Extra-articular manifestations common
Synovial fluid Gram's stain positive, 25% Culture positive, 50% Lactate not elevated	Synovial fluid Gram's stain positive, 50–65% Culture positive, 90% Lactate elevated
Rapid response to therapy	Response often slow; may require surgical drainage
Full recovery in most cases	10% mortality; one-third with residual joint damage

elbow, and ankle (Cooper and Cawley 1986). Involvement of the small joints of the fingers and toes or of the axial joints (sacroiliac, sternoclavicular, sternomanubrial, or pubic symphysis) is rare. Typically, pyogenic infections cause monarticular arthritis, but in approximately 20 per cent of cases bacteraemia can lead to polyarticular involvement (Epstein et al. 1986; Dubost et al. 1993). A polyarticular presentation should not deter a search for infection in a patient with acute onset of illness, signs of toxicity, or a distant site of infection.

Bacteriology

Table 2 shows the frequency of infecting organisms in non-gonococcal pyogenic arthritis.The bacteriology of pyogenic arthritis has changed very little over the past three decades (Goldenberg and Cohen 1976; Goldenberg and Reed 1985; Cooper and Cawley 1986; Ryan et al. 1997; Weston et al. 1999). Staphylococcal and streptococcal species remain the most commonly isolated organisms. *Staphylococcus aureus* accounts for more than 80 per cent of staphylococcal infections. Gram-negative organisms occur third most commonly. The incidence of *Streptococcus pneumoniae* infections has fallen in the antibiotic and vaccine era.. Case reports have documented the infrequent occurrence of arthritis due to *Listeria monocytogenes, Streptobacillus moniliformis,* and *Pasteurella multocida.* While *Staph. aureus* is the most common cause of both monarticular and polyarticular infections, streptococci, and *Haemophilus influenzae* are more frequently associated with polyarticular presentations than would be expected based on the overall incidence of joint infections with these organisms (Epstein et al. 1986; Dubost et al. 1993).

A variety of streptococcal species, most commonly group A β-haemolytic, but also group B, group C, group G, enterococcus, *Streptococcus milleri* and *Strep. viridans* have been found in infected joints. Associated conditions and risk factors are present in most infected patients, and mortality and residual joint damage have been significant (Schattner and Vosti 1998).

H. influenzae is an encapsulated organism requiring opsonizing antibody and an effective reticuloendothelial system for optimal clearance. Patients with *H. influenzae* arthritis therefore often have predisposing conditions such as alcoholism, hypogammaglobulinaemia, multiple myeloma, systemic lupus erythematosus, or asplenia. Almost half of reported cases have been polyarticular (Borenstein and Simon 1986).

Advanced age and intravenous drug abuse are risk factors for Gram-negative joint infections. Elderly patients often have underlying joint disease and multiple medical problems. The presentation in the elderly is usually abrupt, with frequent fevers and rigors. The most common organism is *Escherichia coli* (Newman et al. 1988). Also reported with some frequency are *Pseudomonas aeruginosa, Proteus mirabilis, Serratia marcesens,* and *Klebsiella 'pneumoniae'.* Scattered case reports document rare joint infections with a number of Gram-negative organisms including *Aeromonas hydrophila, Acinetobacter* spp., *Arizona hinshawii, Burkholderia pseudomallei, Eikenella corrodens, Enterobacter* spp., and *Kingella kingae*; these reports indicate the importance of bacteriological identification by culture in patients with suspected Gram-negative infections.

Table 2 Infecting organisms in non-gonococcal arthritis in adults

Organism	Percentage of cases
Staphylococcus	
aureus	40–50
epidermis	10–15
Streptococcal species	20
Gram-negative bacteria	15
S. pneumoniae	2
H. influenzae	2
Anaerobes	5

Intravenous drug abusers tend to be younger and have no pre-existing joint disease. Their presentation is often more insidious with a longer duration of illness before diagnosis (Bayer et al. 1977; Chandrasekar and Narula 1986). There is a predilection for the axial joints, and periarticular soft-tissue abscess or osteomyelitis are frequently encountered. *P. aeruginosa* and *S. 'marcesens'* have been reported in increased frequency in some but not all series from large urban centres.

Salmonellal arthritis is a rare complication of salmonellosis. *Salmonella typhimurium* is the most common serotype cultured from joints, followed by *S. choleraesuis.* Patients with systemic lupus erythematosus or sickle-cell anaemia are at increased risk because the chronic salmonellal carrier state is more common in these conditions. This is the result of impaired clearance by the reticuloendothelial system, owing to inhibition of Fc receptors by circulating immune complexes in systemic lupus and to the functional hyposplenism that can accompany either condition. The presentation is usually monarticular, but polyarticular cases have been reported. In many cases there is no history of a preceding diarrhoeal illness. The diagnosis of salmonellal arthritis may not be suspected after arthrocentesis because the synovial fluid is often non-purulent, and described as turbid, serosanguinous, or straw-coloured, despite a positive culture from it (Cohen et al. 1987; Medina et al. 1989).

Rat-bite fever caused by *Streptobacillus moniliformis,* a pleomorphic Gram-negative organism, presents as an acute illness with fever, rash, vomiting, and arthritis that is usually polyarticular. The infection is acquired from bites or close contact with infected rodents or from ingestion of contaminated food or beverages. When articular symptoms are prominent the clinical presentation may be confused with rheumatoid arthritis, adult Still's disease, systemic lupus, or gonococcaemia. Joint effusions can be either sterile and inflammatory or purulent with positive synovial fluid cultures. Identification and isolation of the organism are difficult due to its variable staining characteristics and specific growth requirements (Holroyd et al. 1988).

Past. multocida is a small, Gram-negative coccobacillus that causes joint infections after animal bites, most commonly from cats or dogs. In approximately one-third of patients there is no history of a bite. Arthritis with this organism has been reported in both normal hosts and in patients with rheumatoid arthritis, chronic liver disease, or immunosuppression (Weber et al. 1984).

L. monocytogenes infections in general have been increasing in recent years, owing to the increased survival of immunocompromised patients. The few case reports of *L. monocytogenes* infections of the joints suggest that these occur in immunocompromised patients or in those with previous joint disease (Kurosh and Perednia 1989).

In recent years, there has been increasing recognition of the role of anaerobic organisms in pyogenic arthritis, although the incidence of anaerobic bacterial arthritis is still quite low. Anaerobic joint infections typically occur after joint surgery, after penetrating trauma, or in patients with underlying diseases. In the setting of surgery or trauma, bacteria are introduced directly from the skin or from soil contaminated with faecal organisms. Peptococcal and clostridial species, and *Propionibacterium acnes* predominate. In the setting of underlying disease the anaerobic Gram-negative organisms, particularly *Bacteroides fragilis,* predominate. The route of infection can be haematogenous from a distant site such as the bowel or direct extension from an adjacent site such as a deep sacral decubitus. A single organism will be cultured in about half of cases, while half will be polymicrobial, usually mixed aerobic and anaerobic organisms (Brook and Frazier 1993).

Anaerobic joint infections are probably underdiagnosed. There are no specific diagnostic signs and therefore synovial fluid must be cultured specifically for anaerobic organisms whenever the clinical setting suggests the possibility of anaerobic infection. Anaerobic cultures should also be obtained in any patient with suspected joint infection in whom initial aerobic cultures of synovial fluid are negative. Any anaerobic organisms isolated from synovial fluid should not be dismissed merely as contaminants if the clinical setting suggests infection.

Diagnosis

Pyogenic joint infection should be suspected in any patient with acute onset of monarticular or polyarticular joint pain and swelling. The presence of fever, extra-articular bacterial infection, and risk factors for infection should heighten the suspicion of joint infection. Risk factors include underlying joint disease, advanced age, diabetes mellitus, treatment with immunosuppressive medications, immunosuppressive disease states, and intravenous drug abuse. Joint infection should also be suspected in painful prosthetic joints and in chronically inflamed joints in which no other diagnosis has been established, again particularly in the setting of underlying risk factors (Goldenberg 1998).

Laboratory studies

The critical test in the evaluation of a patient with suspected pyogenic arthritis is the analysis of synovial fluid. The aspiration of frank pus immediately suggests bacterial infection, although chylous effusions associated with long-standing rheumatoid arthritis and effusions due to gout or pseudogout may at times appear grossly purulent.

The leucocyte count in synovial fluid is greater than 50 000/mm^3 in most cases and often exceeds 100 000/mm^3. The differential count will show greater than 90 per cent and often 100 per cent polymorphonuclear leucocytes. However, when the infection has been partially treated with antibiotics before aspiration, the count may never exceed 50 000/mm^3. Synovial fluid glucose is decreased in about half of cases, but cannot distinguish infected from rheumatoid effusions. A markedly elevated synovial fluid lactic acid is associated with non-gonococcal pyogenic arthritis but not with non-infectious inflammatory effusions (Riordan et al. 1982). The concentration of lactic acid may be of diagnostic help before cultures of synovial fluid are available or in cases of partially treated infections in which synovial fluid cultures remain negative.

Gram's stain of synovial fluid is positive in 50–65 per cent of all cases of non-gonococcal arthritis, approaching 75 per cent in staphylococcal infections but only about 50 per cent in infections caused by Gram-negative bacilli (Goldenberg and Cohen 1976). Bacteria can be cultured from synovial fluid in nearly all cases of non-gonococcal arthritis. The occasional negative results can be attributed to preceding antibiotic therapy, poor handling of specimens, failure to culture for anaerobic organisms, or theoretically to the localization of organisms to the synovium rather than the fluid during the very early stage of infection.

The erythrocye sedimentation rate and C-reactive protein are almost universally elevated in pyogenic joint infections and are good markers of response to treatment. The peripheral white blood cell count is elevated in about one-half and blood cultures are positive in about one-third of cases.

Imaging studies

Plain radiographs will generally show only periarticular soft-tissue swelling or joint effusion in uncomplicated pyogenic arthritis. However, plain radiographs may aid in differential diagnosis by demonstrating a fracture, chondrocalcinosis, gouty erosions, or avascular necrosis, and are useful in assessing pre-existing joint disease, the extent of joint damage and cartilage loss in cases in which diagnosis and treatment have been delayed, and the presence of accompanying osteomyelitis.

Except in a few clinical situations, radionuclide scanning also has limited value in the assessment of the suspected infected joint. While pyogenic arthritis of peripheral joints is readily detectable on physical examination, infections of the axial joints are often difficult to localize from the patient's description or by physical examination. In these cases, a technetium-99m bone scan can demonstrate increased activity that suggests involvement of a deep-seated joint (Vyskocil et al. 1991). For example, in the evaluation of the patient with signs of infection and complaining of diffuse low back or buttock pain, the technetium scan may identify involvement of the sacroiliac joint. This may help to differentiate joint sepsis from intra-abdominal or retroperitoneal abscess, or from osteomyelitis of the pelvis. The technetium bone scan, however, does not differentiate between infectious and non-infectious inflammatory arthritis and therefore cannot distinguish an infected sacroiliac joint from sacroiliitis due to reactive arthritis, or an infected from an uninfected but actively inflamed peripheral joint in rheumatoid arthritis.

The accuracy of detecting joint infections with radionuclide scanning can be improved by scanning with either gallium-67- or indium-111-labelled leucocytes. Gallium scans used in sequence after a positive technetium scan may increase the specificity of technetium scanning. The gallium scan may become positive earlier than the technetium in poorly vascularized joints such as the sacroiliac or sternoclavicular, making it a useful test to consider even when the technetium scan is negative (Lopez-Longo et al. 1987). False-positive gallium scans have been reported in rheumatoid arthritis, thereby limiting the usefulness of this technique in evaluating the possibility of joint sepsis in that condition. Gallium and indium scans are of most value in suspected infection of a prosthetic joint, where they may distinguish an infected from an uninfected, painful, loose prosthesis. Although indium scanning does require the additional steps of removing, labelling, and then reinfusing the patient's leucocytes, it is more sensitive and specific than sequential technetium/gallium scanning and results are available at 24 h rather than 72 h as with gallium scanning (Molina-Murphy et al. 1999).

Conventional fluoroscopy or computed tomographic scanning can be of value in guiding aspiration of deep-seated joints such as the hip, sternoclavicular, or sacroiliac joint. While computed tomography and magnetic resonance imaging are seldom necessary in the evaluation of pyogenic arthritis, these imaging techniques can be of great value when an infected joint fails to respond as expected to appropriate treatment because of adjacent osteomyelitis or abscess formation around an axial joint (Wohlgethan et al. 1988). Magnetic resonance imaging's precision in specifically locating an abnormality to soft tissue, bone or joint may be very helpful in the early evaluation of a patient with a suspected infection in an extremity (Forrester and Feske 1996).

Differential diagnosis

The differential diagnosis of pyogenic joint infection includes:

- *Crystal-induced arthritis:* both gout and pseudogout typically present with acute monarticular or polyarticular arthritis that may suggest pyogenic arthritis. Previous history of gout or pseudogout attacks, presence of gouty tophi, involvement of the the first MTP joint, presence of risk factors such as diuretic therapy, alcohol abuse, or renal insufficiency suggest but do not prove crystal-induced arthritis. The diagnosis of crystal-induced arthritis is proven by the identification of crystals in the synovial fluid by polarizing microscopy. Rarely infection and crystal-induced arthritis occur concurrently. If this is suspected, appropriate Gram's stain and culture must also be performed.
- *Lyme disease:* Lyme arthritis is a late manifestation of Lyme disease that presents as an acute, often recurrent, monarthritis most commonly affecting the knee joint. Fever may be present. Diagnostic clues include the history of previous similar episodes, history of tick exposure and rash, and residence in an endemic area. Synovial fluid leucocyte count may be markedly elevated but bacterial cultures will be negative and the diagnosis is confirmed by serologic testing.
- *Rheumatoid arthritis:* the difficulty in distinguishing a flare-up of rheumatoid arthritis from an infected joint is discussed in the next section.
- *Reactive arthritis:* acute monarticular or polyarticular arthritis occurring 2–3 weeks after an infection, particularly a dysenteric infection, is termed reactive arthritis. Associated manifestations include eye or genitourinary inflammation, and oral ulcers. Synovial fluid leucocyte count may exceed 100 000/mm^3.
- *Adult Still's disease:* the triad of 'rheumatoid' rash, arthritis and high-spiking fever is characteristic of this condition. The quotidian or double quotidian fever pattern typical of adult Still's disease would be unusual in pyogenic joint infection.

- *Neuropathic joint:* in this condition, rapidly destructive joint changes may suggest an infectious process. The presence of peripheral neuropathy with sensory deficit and marked fragmentation of periarticular bone in the setting of relatively little joint effusion helps distinguish this from an infectious process.
- *Haemarthrosis:* often occurring after trauma, acute haemarthrosis presents as an acutely painful joint effusion that may be distinguishable from pyogenic arthritis only by diagnostic arthrocentesis. Patients with chronic haemophiliac arthritis may present with recurrent haemarthrosis and in addition are at increased risk for superimposed pyogenic joint infections.

Joint infections and rheumatoid arthritis

Patients with rheumatoid arthritis are at increased risk of pyogenic arthritis. While the precise prevalence of joint infections in rheumatoid arthritis is not known, approximately 10 per cent of all cases of non-gonococcal arthritis in several large series occurred in patients with that condition (Goldenberg and Cohen 1976; Cooper and Cawley 1986).

Staph. aureus is the infecting organism in 70 per cent of reported cases, followed by streptococci in 9 per cent, Gram-negative bacilli in 8 per cent, pneumococci in 7 per cent, and anaerobes in 3 per cent. Blood cultures are positive in 20–25 per cent of cases. The knee is involved in about half the cases. The hip, shoulder, elbow, wrist, and ankle are each involved in about 10 per cent of cases, while infections in the smaller joints of the hands and feet are unusual. Polyarticular infections are reported in about 30 per cent of cases. The source of infection can be identified in half of these patients. The skin is the most common site of distant infection, followed by the lungs, and the urinary and gastrointestinal tracts (Gardner and Weisman 1990).

Identifying joint infections in the patient with rheumatoid arthritis can be difficult. Fewer than one-half of rheumatoid patients with joint infections present with fever and even fewer develop a leucocytosis (Gardner and Weisman 1990). The erythrocyte sedimentation rate is of limited value in distinguishing infection from disease flare. Both infection and exacerbation of the rheumatoid condition can be monarticular or polyarticular. This difficulty in distinguishing between the two often leads to delay in diagnosis. Joint infection should be suspected in those patients whose disease activity changes abruptly from its normal pattern, particularly if only one or a few joints are involved; in those with systemic signs of toxicity; in those with a remote site of active or recent infection; or in patients on immunosuppressive therapy with long-standing, deforming disease or with accompanying, debilitating illnesses. Whenever one of these clinical states is present, synovial fluid should be obtained, Gram stained, and cultured before considering any treatment (such as an intra-articular steroid injection or systemic anti-inflammatory medication) for a flare-up of rheumatoid disease (Goldenberg 1989).

Distinguishing infection from disease exacerbation is further complicated in the occasional patient who develops a 'pseudoseptic' arthritis. In these cases there is an abrupt onset of usually monarticular joint pain and effusion accompanied by fever. The synovial fluid is purulent, with the leucocyte count usually greater than 100 000/mm^3. Gram's stain and culture of the synovial fluid are negative, and the process quickly resolves within a few days without antibiotics (Call et al. 1985). These episodes may be recurrent and identical in presentation in an individual patient, in which case antibiotics may be withheld pending the results of synovial fluid culture. In most instances, however, empirical antibiotic therapy should be started as soon as infection is suspected and cultures obtained. If adequate cultures are negative, then 'pseudoseptic' arthritis should be considered and antibiotics discontinued.

Joint infections in rheumatoid patients tend to have a poorer outcome than in other groups with pyogenic arthritis. The death rate in reported series is about 20 per cent, more than doubling in patients with polyarticular involvement (Gardner and Weisman 1990). Only about one-third will recover without any worsening of basic joint function. Osteomyelitis or draining cutaneous fistulas will develop in some cases.

Prosthetic joint infection

Although assessment and treatment of pre-operative infections, improved surgical technique, and perioperative prophylactic antibiotics, has reduced the incidence of infection after hip or knee arthroplasty to less than 1 per cent of cases, infection remains a major cause of failed joint replacement surgery. The incidence of infection for prosthetic joint revisions is about 5–10 times that of primary procedures (Wymenga et al. 1992).

Prosthetic joint infections should be suspected in cases of new or increasing prosthetic joint pain, even in the absence of clinical signs of infection. Cultures should be obtained at all revision operations for presumed aseptic loosening, as infection cannot be completely excluded pre-operatively (Tsukayama et al. 1996). Over 90 per cent of all prosthetic joint infections present with joint pain; fever, and erythema and swelling of the joint occur in less than half of cases. Leucocytosis is unusual while an elevated erythrocyte sedimentation rate or C-reactive protein is almost always present.

About one-quarter of infections are detected in the first 3 months after surgery (Inman et al. 1984). These early cases are usually the result of bacteria introduced at the time of surgery or are due to wound infections. A large proportion of these patients will have or have had wounds complicated by haematoma, stitch abscess, dehiscence, or infection. These patients usually have an acute illness with fever, pain, and local signs of infection, including persistent drainage from the joint, but infection should also be suspected in the patient with no local signs of infection who has fever, leucocytosis, or an elevated erythrocyte sedimentation rate that fails to drop with time after surgery.

The prosthetic joint remains at risk for infection indefinitely. Infections diagnosed more than one year after surgery are usually the result of haematogenous seeding from a distant site. The onset of pain is usually insidious, and local and systemic signs of joint infection are absent. There is often a delay of months from onset of pain to diagnosis. Occasionally, late infections present with draining sinus tracts.

Diagnosis of prosthetic joint infection is often difficult. In the early period, infection of the actual joint space must be distinguished from adjacent wound and soft tissue infection. In later infections presenting with only joint pain, the infected prosthesis must be distinguished from the uninfected but painful, loose prosthesis. Plain radiographs are usually normal in early infections. Loosening is defined as greater than 2 mm of lucency at the bone–cement or bone–metal (in cementless prostheses) interface, or any lucency at the metal–cement interface. Other findings in late infections include progressive cortical bone loss around the prosthesis, fractured cement, or a periosteal reaction when the infection has spread through the thickness of cortical bone.

Radionuclide scans are useful in the evaluation of prosthetic joint loosening. A negative technetium-99m bone scan is strong evidence against infection, and sequential technetium-99m and gallium-67 scanning can help to distinguish infected from non-infected loosening. Similarly, indium-111 uptake favours diagnosis of infection.

Joint aspiration is necessary when infection is suspected on a clinical basis or if imaging studies are suggestive of infection or are equivocal. Culturing for anaerobic organisms is imperative. Frozen section histology of specimens removed at revision surgery has a high predictive value for infection, and culture of the removed material provides the definitive bacteriological diagnosis in many cases (Atkins et al. 1998).

Staphylococcal species account for 50–60 per cent of prosthetic joint infections. *Staph. epidermis* is a more common cause of prosthetic than native joint infections. Various streptococcal species and Gram-negative bacilli each account for 15–20 per cent and anaerobes 5–10 per cent of cases. Mixed organisms are cultured in 10–20 per cent of cases, particularly those occurring in the early post-operative period (Inman et al. 1984). Organisms of low virulence that are seldom considered pathogens, such as diphtheroids, propionibacteria, and lactobacilli, are occasional causes of prosthetic joint infections and must not be dismissed as contaminants if cultured from synovial fluid or biopsy material.

Neisserial arthritis

Gonococcal arthritis

Disseminated gonococcal infection complicates approximately 0.1–0.3 per cent of localized infections. Seventy-five per cent of cases of disseminated gonococcal infection result from asymptomatic local infections (Eisenstein and Masi 1981). This makes effective preventive measures difficult. In the past, gonococcal infection has been considered the most common cause of joint infection in adolescents and young adults, but in the past two decades disseminated gonococcal infection has almost disappeared in industrialized countries. This is likely the result of a decrease in the prevalence of those strains associated with disseminated disease and to a decline in the overall incidence of gonococcal infections in these countries (Rompalo et al. 1987). However, in the past few years there has been an increase in genitourinary gonococcal infections reported from several industrialized countries reversing the trend of the previous 10 years (Martin and Ison 2000). It remains to be seen if this will lead to an increase in disseminated cases. Gonococcal arthritis remains a significant problem in developing countries and urban centers throughout the world where the largest reservoirs of localized gonococcal infection exist.

Individuals with inherited deficiencies of the terminal complement components, C5–C9, have an increased risk of neisserial infection (Ross and Densen 1984). Complement deficiencies should be searched for in individuals with recurrent gonococcal or meningococcal infections. Women are affected three to five times more often than men.

Those strains of *N. gonorrhoeae* associated with disseminated disease differ biologically from those strains associated with symptomatic, localized disease (O'Brien et al. 1983). The strains that disseminate are more likely to be resistant to killing by normal human serum, have specific nutritional requirements when grown in culture, have specific cell-surface proteins, and tend to be more sensitive to antibiotics. These characteristics are also shared by those strains that cause asymptomatic localized infections. These strains do not provoke a local inflammatory reaction and thus the organism is not limited to the mucosa, allowing seeding of the bloodstream.

About two-thirds of patients with disseminated gonococcal infection present with an acute illness of 3–4 days' duration, consisting of fever, rash, tenosynovitis, and migratory polyarthralgias or polyarthritis with non-purulent effusions. The rash, present in 60–90 per cent of this group, is a diffuse, maculopapular eruption or a more limited number of vesiculopustular lesions on an erythematous base of approximately 5 mm in diameter. Less commonly the lesions appear as haemorrhagic pustules or bullae. The rash generally spares the face and scalp but can appear anywhere on the trunk and extremities. The lesions may be painful. When effusions are present they are small and cultures of synovial fluid are negative.

Another group of patients presents with a purulent arthritis that resembles non-gonococcal arthritis. Typically, these patients present with an acute illness of 4–5 days' duration. Most have a monarticular arthritis, with the knee most commonly involved, followed by the ankle, wrist, and elbow. Involvement of the hip, shoulder, temporomandibular, and axial joints is rare, as is polyarticular involvement. About one-third of these patients will also have rash or tenosynovitis and about two-thirds will give a history of polyarthralgia preceding the development of monarthritis.

Leucocyte counts in the synovial fluid of patients with purulent arthritis range from about 30 000/mm^3 to greater than 200 000/mm^3. This range overlaps with that in non-gonococcal arthritis, although counts tend to be slightly lower in gonococcal infections. Gram's stain is positive in about one-quarter of cases. *N. gonorrhoeae* is difficult to culture due to its fastidious growth requirements and can be successfully cultured from only about half of purulent effusions (Scopelitis and Martinez-Osuna 1993). Some effusions with negative cultures may be due to the presence of bacteria cell wall constituents such as lipopolysaccharide that remain behind after the phagocytosis and successful clearance of intact organisms. In animal studies, both killed gonococci and purified lipopolysaccharide can induce a purulent synovitis after injection into the joint space (Goldenberg et al. 1984).

There is a strong negative correlation between positive blood cultures and the presence of purulent joint effusions. This suggests that there is a bacteraemic phase of disseminated infection in which patients may present with rash, tenosynovitis and arthralgias and a joint localization phase in which purulent arthritis follows bacteraemia.

As positive cultures of synovial fluid are obtained in only a minority of patients, the diagnosis of disseminated gonococcal infection usually must be presumed from a suggestive clinical presentation, together with isolation of *N. gonorrhoeae* from a site other than the joint. Positive cultures can be obtained from the cervix in 80–90 per cent of women, the urethra in 50–75 per cent of men, and the blood in 25 per cent. The pharynx and the rectum will be positive in a smaller number of cases (Scopelitis and Martinez-Osuna 1993). To culture *N. gonorrhoeae* from the joint, synovial fluid should be immediately spread on a pre-warmed, chocolate-agar plate and incubated in an atmosphere enriched with carbon dioxide, or sent to the laboratory on transport media. Antibiotic-enriched culture media such as Thayer–Martin are used for isolating *N. gonorrhoeae* from sites that have a native bacterial flora, such as the pharynx, cervix, urethra, and rectum, but are not necessary and in fact may inhibit growth when culturing synovial fluid.

The differential diagnosis of disseminated gonococcal infection is broad. Reactive arthritis and disseminated gonococcal infection both commonly affect young, sexually active individuals. Urethritis, rashes, and inflammatory monarthritis or oligoarthritis occur in both. Table 1 lists the features that help distinguish non-gonococcal arthritis from monarticular purulent gonococcal infection. Other infectious illnesses may present with fever, rash, and polyarthralgias or polyarthritis, such as the prodrome of hepatitis B, sub-acute bacterial endocarditis, and bacterial arthritis due to *N. meningitidis*, group A streptococcus, *H. influenzae*, or *Streptobac. moniliformis*. Acute rheumatic fever may present with fever and migratory arthritis distinguishable from disseminated gonococcal infection by evidence of a recent streptococcal infection, accompanying chorea or typical rash. Systemic lupus erythematosus, hypersensitivity vasculitis, and adult Still's disease may all present with fever, rash, and arthritis that at times might be confused with disseminated gonococcal infection, although the nature of the rash and the involvement of other organ systems should help to distinguish most cases.

The course of the disseminated infection is variable. In the preantibiotic era, some cases underwent spontaneous remission, while in others there was progression to destructive joint changes. In general the progression to irreversible damage in the cartilage and joint is not as rapid as with staphylococci, streptococci, or Gram-negative bacilli. Rash, tenosynovitis, and polyarthralgias respond very promptly to antibiotics, while purulent effusions respond somewhat more slowly.

Meningococcal arthritis

Arthritis due to *N. meningitidis* follows one of several clinical patterns and may be confused with disseminated gonococcal infection (Fam et al. 1979; Schaad 1980). Joint manifestations complicate about 2–10 per cent of cases of acute meningococcaemia and may follow one of three clinical patterns. In the first, patients develop polyarthralgias, polyarthritis, or tenosynovitis during the acute phase of their meningococcal infection. They are acutely ill with fever, meningitis, and/or a diffuse, erythematous, macular rash or diffuse haemorrhagic skin lesions typical of acute meningococcaemia. When effusions occur in this group they are small and non-purulent. Synovial cultures are negative but *N. meningitidis* can be recovered from blood or cerebrospinal fluid. The articular manifestations respond rapidly to antibiotic therapy.

The second group of patients develops purulent joint effusions that are most commonly monarticular or oligoarticular during the acute phase of meningococcaemia. Cultures of synovial fluid can be positive or negative.

In some cases, these effusions may be slow to resolve, even after appropriate antibiotics are given and the synovial fluid cultures are sterile.

A small number of patients with acute meningococcaemia will develop articular manifestations only after the acute stage of infection has responded to antibiotics and the patient is clearly improving (Jarrett et al. 1980). In these cases, monarticular, oligoarticular, or polyarticular effusions develop 1–2 weeks after the onset of the acute illness. Cultures of synovial fluid are negative but immune complexes are detectable in blood and synovial fluid, suggesting an immunological basis for the synovitis, which eventually resolves without further antibiotic therapy.

Patients with purulent arthritis, usually monoarticular, but without signs of acute meningococcaemia are classified as primary meningococcal arthritis (Andersson and Krook 1987). The knee and ankle are most commonly involved. Cultures of synovial fluid are positive in 90 per cent of cases. Despite prompt and appropriate therapy these patients are at risk for joint damage and at times may require open drainage. Blood cultures are negative in this group.

Finally, joint manifestations may occur in the setting of chronic meningococcaemia, a condition marked by chronic rash and positive blood cultures. These patients generally present with polyarthralgias rather than frank arthritis. When effusions are present, cultures are negative, suggesting an immune-mediated mechanism.

Management

The three basic principles of management of pyogenic joint infections are: (i) prompt diagnosis and institution of therapy; (ii) appropriate antibiotics; and (iii) adequate drainage of the infected joint.

The most important factors in determining outcome are the length of time before beginning treatment and the length of time to sterilization of synovial fluid cultures. There should be no delay in aspirating any joint about which there is a suspicion of infection. The synovial fluid should be analysed for total and differential cell count and crystals, Gram stained, and cultured. Blood cultures should be obtained and a search for a distant focus of infection should be undertaken as appropriate for the individual patient.

If Gram's stain is positive or the analysis is otherwise suggestive of pyogenic infection, treatment should begin immediately. The patient should be admitted to hospital and given intravenous antibiotics as soon as all cultures have been obtained. Intra-articular antibiotics should be avoided because adequate concentrations in synovial fluid can be achieved via the parenteral route and because there is a risk of chemical synovitis with the intra-articular route. The concentration of antibiotics in synovial fluid parallels that in serum, and adequate levels can be achieved with standard parenteral doses. Although they may achieve bactericidal levels in synovial fluid, aminoglycosides are sometimes less effective than other agents, possibly due to inhibition by the reduced pH of infected synovial fluid. Aminoglycosides are therefore inadequate for primary treatment of pyogenic arthritis. Most often the initial choice of antibiotics is empirically guided by the results of Gram's stain when positive, or by the clinical features when Gram's stain is negative. In choosing antibiotics, one must consider the age of the patient, any underlying disease, and the presence of extra-articular infection. Table 3 provides a guide to the empirical choice of antibiotics. Antibiotic coverage can then be changed to the most appropriate agent when sensitivity results are reported.

In recent years, methicillin-resistant strains of *Staph. aureus* have become more prevalent in both hospital- and community-acquired infections. Vancomycin should be the initial drug of choice for suspected *Staph. aureus* infection in those communities and hospitals where resistant strains exist.

Although those strains of *N. gonorrhoeae* that cause disseminated gonococcal infection are more likely to be antibiotic sensitive than those causing localized infections, strains that have chromosomally-mediated resistance to penicillin or are resistant because they produce plasmid-mediated penicillinase have become more common and widespread, and have been reported in disseminated infection (Wise et al. 1994). Therefore, in communities with resistant strains, a third-generation cephalosporin should replace penicillin G until antibiotic sensitivities are reported.

The duration of antibiotic therapy must be tailored to the individual presentation and response to therapy and to the infecting organism. In general,

Table 3 Guidelines for initial antibiotic therapy of bacterial arthritis based on Gram's stain

Gram's stain result	Probable pathogen	Antibiotic choice
Gram-positive cocci		
Clusters	*Staph. aureus*	Nafcillin (2 g every 4 h)
	(methicillin resistance suspected)	Vancomycin (1 g every 12 h)
	Staph. epidermis	Vancomycin (1 g every 12 h)
Pairs and chains	Streptococci (enterococcal)	Penicillin G (2.5 million U every 4 h)
(urinary, biliary, bowel)	Enterococci	Penicillin G (2.5 million U every 4 h) and gentamycin (1 mg/kg every 8 h)
Gram-negative cocci	*N. gonorrhoeae*	Ceftriaxone (1–2 g every 12 h)
(haemorrhagic rash, meningitis)	*N. meningitidis*	Penicillin G (2.5–5 million U every 6 h)
Gram-negative coccobacilli	*H. influenzae*	Ampicillin (2 g every 6 h)
	(ampicillin resistance suspected)	Cefotaxime (1 g every 8 h)
Gram-negative bacilli	Enterobacteriaceae	Cefotaxime (2 g every 8 h)
	Pseudomonas spp.	Ceftazidime (2 g every 8 h)
No organisms seen		
(healthy young adult)	*N. gonorrhoeae*	Ceftriaxone (1–2 g every 12 h)
(older adult, underlying disease)	Staphylococci Streptococci Enterobacteriaceae	Vancomycin and cefotaxime
(intravenous drug abuser)	Staphylococci *Pseudomonas* spp. Enterobacteriaceae	Vancomycin and ceftazidime

Source: Reprinted with modification from Parker, R.H. (1988). Acute bacterial arthritis. In *Orthopedic Infections* (ed. D. Schlossberg), p. 74. New York: Springer-Verlag.

intravenous antibiotics should be continued until signs of joint inflammation have resolved, joint effusions have resolved or significantly decreased, and synovial cultures are sterile. Oral antibiotics can then be used to complete the course of treatment, which is usually about 2 weeks in uncomplicated cases but should be extended to 4 weeks or more where there was a significant delay in starting treatment, or a slow response, where infection was with virulent organisms such as *Staph. aureus* or Gram-negative bacilli, and in immunosuppressed patients (Syrogiannopoulos and Nelson 1988). The development of ambulatory intravenous antibiotic delivery systems has allowed earlier hospital discharge in appropriate patients (Williams et al. 1989).

The duration of parenteral antibiotic therapy for disseminated gonococcal infection is generally shorter than for non-gonococcal arthritis. In most patients with gonococcal arthritis with a good response to therapy, parenteral antibiotics can be substituted by oral after about 3 days of intravenous therapy to complete a 2-week course. Patients who have dermatitis/tenosynovitis only, without purulent arthritis, can be treated as outpatients, provided they are compliant and closely followed.

Occasional patients with purulent gonococcal effusions will develop a persistent inflammatory effusion lasting weeks after sterilization of synovial fluid with antibiotics. These effusions eventually resolve without further antibiotics. Recovery may be speeded by giving non-steroidal anti-inflammatory drugs.

Infected joints can be drained by closed needle aspiration, tidal irrigation (Ike 1993), arthroscopy, or arthrotomy. Each procedure has its appropriate place in the treatment of septic arthritis depending on the clinical situation. Which modality is chosen is probably not as critical to the ultimate outcome as the duration of time from onset of infection to adequate drainage and sterilization of the joint fluid (Goldenberg et al. 1975; Lane et al. 1990; Ho 1993).

Initial treatment with serial, closed-needle aspiration avoids the expense and surgical morbidity and mortality of the more invasive procedures and is a satisfactory approach as long as the joint can be completely drained and there is clear evidence of improvement as indicated by resolution of systemic signs of toxicity, serial decrease in synovial fluid white blood-cell count and sterilization of the synovial fluid culture within 48–72 h (Broy and Schmid 1986).

The presence of risk factors for a poor outcome include delayed diagnosis, virulent organism, polyarticular involvement, or underlying disease, such as rheumatoid arthritis, and should prompt the early use of a more invasive procedure. Arthroscopy has the advantage of good visualization of the joint space and articular cartilage combined with effective drainage and irrigation, while avoiding the post-operative joint stiffness and slow functional improvement sometimes associated with arthrotomy (Thiery 1989). Arthroscopy is best suited for drainage of the knee joint, although, depending on the skill of the arthroscopist, it can be applied to other smaller joints.

Septic arthritis of the hip should be treated primarily by arthrotomy because of the difficulty and uncertainty of achieving adequate joint drainage by closed aspiration. Infection of the deep axial joints complicated by abscess formation requires open drainage.

Regardless of the mode of drainage, early mobilization of the infected joint is important in regaining maximal function. Most often the infected joint will be too painful to allow mobilization during the first few days of therapy. However, passive, range-of-motion exercises should be instituted as soon as pain permits. Both animal and human studies have demonstrated the advantages of a continuous, passive-motion device soon after surgical drainage of the knee. Isometric exercises to restore strength to the limb muscles and progressive ambulation to prevent the complications of prolonged bed-rest should also be implemented (Mikhail and Alarcon 1993).

In general, management of infected prosthetic joints requires removal of the prosthesis. Exceptions include some very early post-operative infections in which the joint can be effectively drained and irrigated or the polypropylene component of a knee prosthesis can be exchanged. Another exception is the patient who is not considered a candidate for surgery because of poor medical status and who is infected with an organism of low virulence. In this case, chronic suppression of infection by antibiotics has at times been successful in salvaging the prosthesis and preventing further infectious complications.

In nearly all other instances, the prosthesis, cement, and all necrotic bone and soft tissue should be removed as soon as infection is detected or strongly suspected. Appropriate antibiotics should be started, as outlined in Table 3, keeping in mind the increased frequency of *Staph. epidermis*, Gram-negative bacilli, and anaerobic infections. After 6 weeks of intravenous antibiotics a prosthesis can be reimplanted with a greater than 90 per cent chance of success and with a better functional outcome and greater patient satisfaction than with arthrodesis of the knee or excision arthroplasty (Girdlestone procedure) of the hip, which should be reserved for those patients unable or unwilling to tolerate a second surgical procedure (Brandt et al. 1999). Others have reported success with a one-step procedure in which a new prosthesis is implanted at the time of removal of the infected prosthesis (Goksan and Freeman 1992).

Pyogenic bursitis

The many bursae found throughout the body are lined with a synovial membrane identical to that found in synovial joints. Bursitis may result from trauma, inflammatory conditions such as rheumatoid arthritis or gout, or from infection. Bacteria enter the bursa directly from the skin as a result of trauma, unlike pyogenic arthritis in which the route of infection is most commonly haematogenous seeding. Immunosuppression, diabetes, alcoholism, and chronic bursitis due to rheumatoid arthritis or gout increase the risk of infection (Canoso and Barza 1993).

Nearly all cases of pyogenic bursitis involve the olecranon or prepatellar bursae. Presentation is usually acute, with sudden onset of bursal pain, tenderness, swelling, and erythema. Less commonly, presentation may be subacute or chronic with minimal localized signs and symptoms present for weeks to months before the diagnosis is established. Involvement of the bursa is readily distinguishable from joint infection by the presence of very superficial, often tense, distension of the bursal sac with preservation of movement in the underlying joint and no joint effusion. Fever is a common but not universal finding. Regional lymphadenopathy and adjacent cellulitis of the forearm or peripatellar skin are frequently present. Desquamation of the skin overlying the infected bursa and spontaneous drainage of the bursa through the skin may occur. Osteomyelitis of the underlying bone may occasionally complicate chronic cases.

The characteristics of synovial fluid from an infected bursa are variable. The gross appearance ranges from clear to frankly purulent. The leucocyte count may range from less than 2000 to greater than 100 000 cells/mm^3, with the proportion of polymorphs ranging from 50 to nearly 100 per cent. In contrast to pyogenic arthritis, the leucocyte count in infected bursal fluid is often less than 10 000/mm^3, so that relatively low counts should not deter one from pursuing the diagnosis of infection in the appropriate clinical setting (Ho et al. 1978; Canoso and Barza 1993).

In the absence of previous antibiotic therapy, culture of bursal synovial fluid will be positive in every case. Gram's stain is positive in about two-thirds of cases. *Staph. aureus* is the infecting organism in more than 90 per cent of cases. Sporadic cases are due to *Staph. epidermis* or group A streptococci.

Uncomplicated septic bursitis can be treated effectively with serial, closed-needle aspiration and oral antibiotics. Patients with underlying bursal disease, immunosuppressed patients, or those who fail to respond promptly to treatment as outpatients with oral antibiotics should be admitted to hospital and treated with intravenous antibiotics (Ho and Su 1981; Canoso and Barza 1993). Incision and drainage or excision of the infected bursa may be necessary in those cases with extensive involvement or failure to respond to closed drainage. Empirical antibiotic treatment should be with a semisynthetic, penicillinase-resistant penicillin or vancomycin, if methicillin-resistant *Staph. aureus* is a concern.

References

Andersson, S. and Krook, A. (1987). Primary meningococcal arthritis. *Scandinavian Journal of Infectious Disease* **19**, 51–4.

Atkins, B.L., Athanasou, N., Deeks, J.J., Crook, D.W.M., Simpson, H., Peto, T.E.A., McLardy-Smith, P., Berendt, A.R., and the OSIRIS Collaborative Study Group (1998). Prospective evaluation of criteria for microbiological diagnosis of prosthetic-joint infection at revision arthroplasty. *Journal of Clinical Microbiology* **36**, 2932–9.

Bayer, A.S., Chow, A.W., Louie, J.S., Nies, K.M., and Guze, L.B. (1977). Gram-negative bacillary septic arthritis: clinical, radiographic, therapeutic, and prognostic features. *Seminars in Arthritis and Rheumatism* **7**, 123–32.

Borenstein, D.G. and Simon, G.L. (1986). *Hemophilus influenzae* septic arthritis in adults. *Medicine* **65**, 191–201.

Brandt, C.M., Duffy, M.C.t., Berbari, E.F., Hanssen, A.D., Steckelberg, J.D., and Osmon, D.R. (1999). *Staphylococcus aureus* prosthetic joint infection treated with prosthesis removal and delayed reimplantation arthroplasty. *Mayo Clinic Proceedings* **74**, 553–8.

Brook, I. and Frazier, E.H. (1993). Anaerobic osteomyelitis and arthritis in a military hospital: a 10-year experience. *American Journal of Medicine* **94**, 21–8.

Broy, S.B. and Schmid, F.R. (1986). A comparison of medical drainage (needle aspiration) and surgical drainage (arthrotomy or arthroscopy) in the initial treatment of infected joints. *Clinics in the Rheumatic Diseases* **12**, 501–22.

Call, R.S., Ward, J.R., and Samuelson, C.O. (1985). Pseudoseptic arthritis in patients with rheumatoid arthritis. *The Western Journal of Medicine* **143**, 471–3

Canoso, J.J. and Barza, M. (1993). Soft tissue infections. *Rheumatic Disease Clinics of North America* **19**, 293–309.

Chandrasekar, P.H. and Narula, A.P. (1986). Bone and joint infections in intravenous drug abusers. *Reviews of Infectious Diseases* **8**, 904–11.

Cohen, J.I., Bartlett, J.A., and Corey, G.R. (1987). Extra-intestinal manifestations of salmonella infections. *Medicine* **66**, 349–88.

Cooper, C. and Cawley, M.I.D. (1986). Bacterial arthritis in an English health district: a 10 year review. *Annals of the Rheumatic Diseases* **45**, 458–63.

Dubost, J. et al. (1993). Polyarticular septic arthritis. *Medicine* **72**, 296–310.

Eisenstein, B.I. and Masi, A.T. (1981). Disseminated gonococcal infection (DGI) and gonococcal arthritis (GCA): I. Bacteriology, epidemiology, host factors, pathologic factors and pathology. *Seminars in Arthritis and Rheumatism* **10**, 155–72.

Epstein, J.H., Zimmermann, B., III, and Ho, G., Jr. (1986). Polyarticular septic arthritis. *Journal of Rheumatology* **13**, 1105–7.

Fam, E.G., Tenenbaum, J., and Stein, J.L. (1979). Clinical forms of meningococcal arthritis. A study of 5 cases. *Journal of Rheumatology* **6**, 567–73.

Forrester, D.M. and Feske, W.I. (1996). Imaging of infectious arthritis. *Seminars in Roentgenology* **31**, 239–49.

Gardner, G.C. and Weisman, M.H. (1990). Pyarthrosis in patients with rheumatoid arthritis: a report of 13 cases and a review of the literature from the past 40 years. *American Journal of Medicine* **88**, 503–11.

Goksan, S.B. and Freeman, M.A.R. (1992). One-stage reimplantation for infected total knee arthroplasty. *Journal of Bone and Joint Surgery* **74B**, 78–82.

Goldenberg, D.L. (1989). Infectious arthritis complicating rheumatoid arthritis and other chronic rheumatic diseases. *Arthritis and Rheumatism* **32**, 496–502.

Goldenberg, D.L. (1998). Septic arthritis. *Lancet* **351**, 197–202.

Goldenberg, D.L. and Cohen, A.S. (1976). Acute infectious arthritis. *American Journal of Medicine* **60**, 369–77.

Goldenberg, D.L. and Reed, J.I. (1985). Bacterial arthritis. *New England Journal of Medicine* **312**, 764–71.

Goldenberg, D.L., Reed, J.I., and Rice, P.A. (1984). Arthritis in rabbits induced by killed *Neisseria gonorrhoeae* and gonococcal lipopolysccharide. *Journal of Rheumatology* **11**, 3–8.

Goldenberg, D.L., Brandt, K.D., Cohen, A.S., and Carthcart, E.S. (1975). Treatment of septic arthritis—comparison of needle aspiration and surgery as initial modes of joint drainage. *Arthritis and Rheumatism* **18**, 83–90.

Ho, G., Jr. (1993). How best to drain an infected joint. Will we ever know? *Journal of Rheumatology* **20**, 2001–3.

Ho, G., Jr. and Su, E.Y. (1981). Antibiotic therapy of septic bursitis: it's implications in the treatment of septic arthritis. *Arthritis and Rheumatism* **24**, 905–11.

Ho, G., Jr., Tice, A.D., and Kaplan, S.R. (1978). Septic bursitis in the prepatellar and olecranon bursae. *Annals of Internal Medicine* **89**, 21–7.

Holroyd, K.J., Reiner, A.P., and Dick, J.D. (1988). *Streptobacillus moniliformis* polyarthritis mimicking rheumatoid arthritis: an urban case of rat bite fever. *American Journal of Medicine* **85**, 711–14.

Ike, R.W. (1993). Tidal irrigation in septic arthritis of the knee: A potential alternative to surgical drainage. *Journal of Rheumatology* **20**, 2104–11.

Inman, R.D., Gallegos, K.V., Brause, B.D., Redecha, P.B., and Christian, C.L. (1984). Clinical and microbial features of prosthetic joint infection. *American Journal of Medicine* **77**, 47–53.

Jarrett, M.P., Moses, S., Barland, P., and Miller, M.H. (1980). Articular complications of meningococcal meningitis. An immune complex disorder. *Archives of Internal Medicine* **140**, 1656–66.

Kaandorp, C.J.E., Krijnen, P., Moens, H.J.B., Habbema, J.D.F., and van Schaardenburg, D. (1997a). The outcome of bacterial arthritis. *Arthritis and Rheumatism* **40**, 884–92.

Kaandorp, C.J.E., Dinant, H.J., van de Laar, M.A.F.J., Moens, H.J.B., Prins, A.P.A., and Dijkmans, B.A.C. (1997b). Incidence and sources of native and prosthetic joint infection: a community based prospective survey. *Annals of the Rheumatic Diseases* **56**, 470–5.

Kurosh, N.A. and Perednia, D.A. (1989). *Listeria monocytogenes* septic arthritis. *Archives of Internal Medicine* **149**, 1207–8.

Lane, J.G., Falahee, M.H., Wojtys, E.M., Hankin, F.M., and Kaufer, H. (1990). Pyarthrosis of the knee. Treatment considerations. *Clinical Orthropedics and Related Research* **252**, 198–204.

Lopez-Longo, F.-J., Menard, H.-A., Carreno, L., Cosin, J., Ballesteros, R., and Monteagudo, I. (1987). Primary septic arthritis in heroin users: early diagnosis by radioisotopic imaging and geographic variations in the causative agents. *Journal of Rheumatology* **14**, 991–4.

Martin, I.M.C. and Ison, C.A. (2000). Rise in gonorrhoea in London, UK. *Lancet* **355**, 623.

Medina, F., Fraga, A., and Lavalle, C. (1989). Salmonella septic arthritis in systemic lupus erythematosus. The importance of the chronic carrier state. *Journal of Rheumatology* **16**, 203–8.

Mikhail, I.S. and Alarcon, G.S. (1993). Nongonococcal bacterial arthritis. *Rheumatic Disease Clinics of North America* **19**, 311–31.

Molina-Murphy, I.L., Palmer, E.L., Scott, J.A., Prince, M.R., and Strauss, H.W. (1999). Polyclonal, nonspecific 111In-IgG scintigraphy in the evaluation of complicated osteomyelitis and septic arthritis. *Quarterly Journal of Nuclear Medicine* **43**, 29–37.

Morgan, D.S., Fisher, D., Merianos, A., and Currie, B.J. (1996). An 18 year clinical review of septic arthritis from tropical Australia. *Epidemiology and Infections* **117**, 423–8.

Newman, E.D., Davis, D.E., and Harrington, T.M. (1988). Septic arthritis due to Gram negative bacilli: older patients with good outcome. *Journal of Rheumatology* **15**, 659–62.

O'Brien, J.P., Goldenberg, D.L., and Rice, P.A. (1983). Disseminated gonococcal infection: a prospective analysis of 49 patients and a review of pathophysiology and immune mechanisms. *Medicine* **62**, 395–406.

Riordan, T., Doyle, D., and Tabaqchali, S. (1982). Synovial fluid lactic acid measurement in the diagnosis and management of septic arthritis. *Journal of Clinical Pathology* **35**, 390–4.

Rompalo, A.M., Hook, E.W., III, Roberts, P.L., Ramsey, P.G., Handsfield, H., and Holmes, K.K. (1987). The acute arthritis-dermatitis syndrome: the changing importance of *Neisseria gonorrhoeae* and *Neisseria meningitides*. *Archives of Internal Medicine* **147**, 281–3.

Ross, S.C. and Densen, P. (1984). Complement deficiency states and infections: epidemilogy, pathogenesis and consequences of neisserial and other infections in an immune deficiency. *Medicine* **63**, 243–73.

Ryan, M.J., Karnaugh, R., Wall, P.G., and Hazleman, B.J. (1997). Bacterial joint infection in England and Wales: analysis of bacterial isolates over a four year period. *British Journal of Rheumatology* **36**, 370–3.

Saraux, A., Taelman, H., Bbblanche, P. Batungwanayo, J., Clerinx, J., Kagame, A., Kabagabo, L., Ladner, J., Van de Perre, P., Le Goff, P., and Bogaerts, J.

(1997). HIV infection as a risk factor for septic arthritis. *British Journal of Rheumatology* **36**, 333–7.

Schaad, U.B. (1980). Arthritis in disease due to *Neisseria meningitidis*. *Reviews of Infectious Disease* **2**, 880–8.

Scopelitis, E. and Martinez-Osuna, P. (1993). Gonococcal arthritis. *Rheumatic Disease Clinics of North America* **19**, 363–77.

Schattner, A. and Vosti, K.L. (1998). Bacterial arthritis due to beta-hemolytic streptococci of serogroups A, B, C, F, and G. *Medicine* **77**, 122–39.

Singleton, J.D., West, S.G., and Nordstrom, D.M. (1991). 'Pseudoseptic' arthritis complicating rheumatoid arthritis: a report of six cases. *Journal of Rheumatology* **18**, 1319–22.

Switalski, L.M., Patti, J.M., Butcher, W., Gristina, A.G., Speziale, P., and Hook, M. (1993). A collagen receptor on *Staphylococcus aureus* strains isolated from patients with septic arthritis mediates adhesion to cartilage. *Molecular Microbiology* **7**, 99–107.

Syrogiannopoulos, G.A. and Nelson, J.D. (1988). Duration of anti-microbial therapy for acute suppurative osteoarticular infections. *Lancet* **i**, 37–40.

Thiery, J.A. (1989). Arthroscopic drainage in septic arthritis of the knee: a multicenter study. *Arthroscopy* **5**, 65–9.

Tsukayama, D.T., Estrada, R., and Gustilo, R.B. (1996). Infection after total hip arthroplasty. *Journal of Bone and Joint Surgery* **78-A**, 512–23.

Vyskocil, J.J., McIroy, M.A., Brennan, T.A., and Wilson, F.M. (1991). Pyogenic infection of the sacroiliac joint. *Medicine* **70**, 188–97.

Weber, D.J., Wolfson, J.S., Swartz, M.N., and Hooper, D.C. (1984). *Pasteurella multocida* infections. Report of 34 cases and review of the literature. *Medicine* **63**, 133–54.

Weston, V.C., Jones, A.C., Bradbury, N., Fawthorp, F., and Doherty, M. (1999). Clinical features and outcome of septic arthritis in a single UK health district 1982–1991. *Annals of the Rheumatic Diseases* **58**, 214–19.

Weitoft, T. and Makitalo, S. (1999). Bacterial arthritis in a Swedish health district. *Scandinavian Journal of Infectious Diseases* **31**, 559–61.

Williams, D.N., Gibson, J.A., and Bosch, D. (1989). Home intravenous antibiotic therapy using a programmable infusion pump. *Archives of Internal Medicine* **149**, 1157–60.

Wise, C.M., Morris, C.R., Wasilauskas, B.L., and Salzer, W.L. (1994). Gonococcal arthritis in an era of increasing penicillin resistance. *Archives of Internal Medicine* **154**, 2690–5.

Wohlgethan, J.R., Newberg, A.H., and Reed, J.I. (1988). The risk of abscess from sterno-clavicular septic arthritis. *Journal of Rheumatology* **15**, 1302–6.

Wymenga, A.B., van Horne, J.R., Theeuwes, A., Muytjens, H.L., and Slooff, T.J.J.H. (1992). Perioperative factors associated with septic arthritis after arthroplasty. *Acta Orthopaedica Scandinavia* **63**, 665–71.

6.2.2 Pyogenic arthritis in children

Douglas S. Swanson and Mary Anne Jackson

Introduction

The terms septic arthritis, suppurative arthritis, pyogenic arthritis, and infectious arthritis are all used interchangeably to denote purulence in the joint space, usually due to microbial infection. A successful outcome to suppurative arthritis in infancy and childhood is contingent upon early recognition and timely antimicrobial and surgical therapy. Despite the advent of newer antimicrobials that penetrate readily into infected joints, complications and permanent changes still arise in some cases of septic arthritis. This chapter reviews the epidemiology and pathogenesis of joint infection, and outlines the approach to diagnosis and management. Changes in the spectrum of childhood skeletal infection in the era of the *Haemophilus influenzae* type b (Hib) vaccine are highlighted. The emergence of resistant pneumococci and staphylococci as well as the occurrence of *Kingella kingae* disease in younger infants provides new therapeutic challenges to the clinician.

Epidemiology

Acute septic arthritis is a relatively uncommon infection. It is estimated that two of every 1000 admissions to general hospitals are for septic arthritis. In a 30-year study of paediatric skeletal infection reported by Nelson, 682 cases of suppurative arthritis were described with an occurrence of 25 cases among 10 000 annual admissions (Nelson 1991). Our institution serves a large, urban population in the American Midwest where approximately 10 000 children are admitted to the hospital each year. During the most recent 1 year evaluation there were 34 admissions for septic arthritis.

Suppurative joint infection is an important disease of young children, with more than half of the cases occurring in children less than 3 years of age (Table 1). Although boys are reported to be affected twice as often as girls, in our series this predominance is seen most in the child older than 5 years; in the younger patient, the sex distribution tends to be more equal.

A history of non-penetrating trauma can be elicited in many children with septic arthritis; however, most investigators have questioned its role in the pathogenesis of the infection. In one study (Welkon et al. 1986), patients with septic arthritis and sterile cultures more frequently reported a history of trauma than those with culture-confirmed pyarthrosis.

An antecedent infection of the upper respiratory tract frequently precedes septic arthritis due to *H. influenzae* type b and *K. kingae* compared with pyarthrosis due to *S. aureus* (Yagupsky et al. 1993).

Pathogenesis

In most cases, bacteria enter the joint space haematogenously. Less often, direct inoculation of bacteria into the joint space occurs during an episode of penetrating trauma. Contiguous extension of disease from infected soft tissues is felt to be rare in paediatric practice, and occurs most often in the adult diabetic.

Concomitant osteoarticular infection frequently occurs in the neonate and occasionally in the older infant because transphyseal blood vessels, which connect the vasular supply of the epiphysis and metaphysis, facilitate the spread of infection from the metaphysis across the growth plate to the epiphysis and adjacent joint space (Ogden 1979). By 18 months of age, the transphyseal vessels are interrupted and the blood supply between the metaphysis and epiphysis is separated.

In children, there are four areas where the bony metaphysis is intracapsular: the proximal femur, proximal humerus, proximal radius, and distal lateral tibia. Rupture of a metaphyseal abscess through the periosteum in these locations permits bacterial invasion into the joint space, resulting in a clinical presentation similar to that of isolated joint infection. Data from our institution suggest this type of skeletal infection may occur in up to 20 per cent of cases. In these cases, longer treatment with antibiotics is

Table 1 Suppurative joint infection. The Children's Mercy Hospital Kansas City

Age	Total	%
≤2 months	11	8
3–23 months	58	42
2–5 years	36	26
6–11 years	19	14
>11 years	14	10

needed than in primary joint infection. More importantly, these patients have a greater frequency of permanent disability (Jackson et al. 1992).

Clinical manifestations

Monoarticular infection of weight-bearing joints is characteristic, with involvement of the knee, hip, or ankle accounting for 70 per cent of cases. Usually the child with pyogenic joint infection presents acutely with fever and an exquisitely painful, swollen joint. In some cases, it may be difficult to localize the involved joint, especially in a febrile, irritable infant. A careful examination after giving a short-acting sedative may be needed to locate the affected joint. The typical distribution of involved joints I suppurative arthritis in order of decreasing frequency are: knees, hip, ankles, elbows, shoulders, joints of the hands and feet, and sacroiliac joints.

Diagnostic evaluation should be pursued promptly, especially in cases of septic arthritis of the hip where compromise of the vascular supply to the femoral head may result in destruction of the capital epiphysis and growth plate. An evaluation would include a complete blood count, erythrocyte sedimentation rate (ESR), C-reactive protein (CRP), and radiographs of the joint, as well as culture of blood and synovial fluid. In most cases, leucocytosis and elevation of the ESR in the range of 50–90 mm/h will be found; however, the diagnosis should not be excluded even if both of these are normal. Klein et al. (1997) found the ESR to be a much more sensitive predictor of septic hip arthritis than either temperature or leucocyte count. Radiographs may reveal periarticular, soft tissue swelling and joint effusion but also may be non-diagnostic.

Radioisotope bone scanning is helpful in occasional cases where localization of the diseased joint is difficult. An increase or decrease in uptake on either side of the joint line with limitation to the joint capsule is seen in suppurative arthritis (Tuson et al. 1994). Magnetic resonance imaging has been shown to be a sensitive tool in the diagnosis of septic sacroiliitis (Sandrasegaran et al. 1994). In the child whose hip is painful on examination but plain radiographs are unrevealing, ultrasonography of the hip is useful in identifying fluid and in guiding arthrocentesis (Zawin et al. 1993).

Aspiration of the joint is imperative to confirm the diagnosis. The fluid is usually frankly purulent and low glucose concentrations may be found. In most cases, the white blood cell count in the synovial fluid is greater than 50 000 and a differential count reveals more than 90 per cent polymorphonuclear leucocytes. A Gram-stained smear of the joint fluid will provide a presumptive identification of the causative agent in approximately one-third of cases. Culture of the joint fluid will reveal the precise organism in 50–60 per cent of cases. Inoculation of joint fluid aspirates into blood culture bottles may improve the recovery of fastidious pathogens. In 10 per cent blood culture will demonstrate the causative agent when cultures of the joint fluid are sterile. Despite careful culture of blood, joint fluid, and other appropriate sites, a microbiological diagnosis will not be obtained in 25–30 per cent of cases. If the clinical diagnosis is deemed to be septic arthritis, lack of a defined pathogen should not change the management of the patient.

General aetiology

The most commonly identified causative bacteria of suppurative arthritis are presented in Table 2. Although *H. influenzae* type b has historically caused the majority of cases of suppurative arthritis in infants less than 2 years of age, since the implementation of Hib vaccine in the United States in 1985, this organism has virtually disappeared as a cause of septic arthritis and other invasive diseases (Bowerman et al. 1997; Howard et al. 1999). Currently, *S. aureus* and streptococci account for close to 70 per cent of culture-confirmed cases of suppurative arthritis. Most streptococcal infections in neonates are caused by group B (*Streptococcus agalactiae*), in children less than 2 years old by pneumococci, and in children greater than 2 years old by group A (*S. pyogenes*) (Gutierrez 1997). In teenagers with multiple joint involvement, gonococci are the most common pathogens. Primary meningococcal arthritis is a rare form of meningococcal disease characterized by polyarticular infection, no involvement of other organs, and excellent prognosis. *Pseudomonas aeruginosa* may cause infection in cases of puncture wound to the foot; other Gram-negative organisms cause infection infrequently. Occasionally, salmonella arthritis occurs in the setting of salmonellosis or in the sickleaemic patient (Mallouh and Talab 1985). Anaerobes including *Bacteroides* spp., *Fusobacterium* spp., and *Eikenella corrodens* are most commonly involved in joint infection following a human bite (Resnick et al. 1985). *K. kingae* has become a more commonly recognized cause of bone and joint infections in young children (Yagupsky and Dagan 1997; Lundy and Kehl 1998). Recovery of this fastidious organism is enhanced by inoculating the synovial fluid into blood culture bottles (Yagupsky et al. 1992).

Table 2 Aetiology of the most common pathogens causing suppurative arthritis according to age

Age	Sterile	*S. aureus*	Hib[a]	Cocci[b]	GC[c]	Other[d]
<2 months	9	36	0	36	0	18
2–6 months	40	0	0	60	0	0
7–12 months	26	11	41	15	0	7
13–23 months	36	25	32	0	0	7
24–36 months	29	7	14	36	0	14
3–5 years	35	30	5	20	0	10
6–11 years	35	30	10	10	0	30
>11 years	13	33	0	0	27	20

[a] *H. influenzae* type 6.
[b] Streptococci including enterococci, group A and B streptococci, viridans streptococci, pneumococci.
[c] Gonococcal.
[d] *P. aeruginosa*, acinetobacter, enterobacter, klebsiella, coagulase-negative staphylococci, *Eikenella corrodens*, salmonella, *Brucella* spp.

Septic arthritis of specific joints

Hip

When the hip is involved in septic arthritis, the child will assume a position of comfort with the hip flexed, externally rotated, and abducted. Asymmetry of the skin folds of the buttocks and thighs may be apparent, and significant limitation of passive hip abduction and extension is typical. Pathological subluxation of the hip may occur, and was found in 8 per cent of children with septic arthritis of the hip at our institution.

There is much potential for permanent disability in cases of septic arthritis of the hip. The femoral capital epiphysis is entirely intra-articular and capsular distension may interfere with the vascular supply to the femoral head. Therefore, in all cases where septic arthritis of the hip is suspected, the diagnosis should be promptly confirmed by aspiration of the joint under ultrasound guidance or fluoroscopy. If purulent material is found, immediate drainage of the hip should be performed.

Sacroiliac joint

Infection of the sacroiliac joint is relatively unusual, accounting for 1–2 per cent of cases of septic arthritis. These children tend to be older (mean age, 10 years) and usually do not appear systemically ill. Most have acute onset of fever, with pain in the buttocks, groin, hip, or abdomen. Often the patient has an antalgic gait but pain is poorly localized. The duration of symptoms before diagnosis averaged 7 days in one study (Patterson 1970), but chronic symptoms of up to 1 month have been reported (Schaad et al. 1980). The most common physical finding in patients with sacroiliac arthritis is a positive Fabere sign (pain with flexion, abduction, and external rotation of the hip while stressing the sacroiliac joint by placing pressure on the flexed ipsilateral knee).

As in many cases of septic arthritis, plain radiographs are often normal. A bone scan may localize the involved sacroiliac joint; however, a computed tomographic or magnetic resonance imaging scan is more sensitive and specific.

S. aureus is the most commonly recognized pathogen and a positive blood culture is often found. Antistaphylococcal therapy usually results in a prompt clinical response and drainage of the sacroiliac joint is usually unnecessary. *Brucella* spp. have a predilection for sacroiliac involvement and should be considered in individuals who were born or have travelled to endemic areas or have ingested raw milk. Diagnosis of brucella sacroiliitis may be confirmed by culture or serology and therapy should usually include trimethoprim sulfamethoxazole or doxycycline (for patients over 9 years of age) possibly with the addition of rifampicin.

Septic arthritis in specific hosts

Neonates

Although suppurative skeletal infection in a newborn infant often reflects systemic infection with *Staphylococcus aureus, Candida albicans*, or group B streptococci, systemic symptoms and signs are generally not apparent. Non-specific symptoms such as irritability, lethargy, or poor feeding may occur. However, a non-toxic appearance and absence of fever is found in more than one-half of cases, and a normal white cell count and ESR are generally found (Fox and Sprunt 1978). Local swelling of an extremity with overlying inflammation and/or flexion contracture are the most common clinical findings. Occasionally, a newborn with hip pyarthrosis may present with abdominal distension secondary to rupture into the abdomen of intra-articular pus.

A high index of suspicion is necessary and aspiration of all suspected joints is absolutely essential to confirm the diagnosis. Permanent sequelae are frequent in this age group. Hallel and Salvati (1975) found deformities of the femoral head in 70 per cent of neonates followed up for suppurative arthritis of the hip. Complications from skeletal infection in the neonate can be minimized by a high index of suspicion, detailed evaluation with a careful musculoskeletal examination in any baby with suspected sepsis, and early surgical drainage and antibiotic therapy.

Adolescents

Suppurative arthritis due to *Neisseria gonorrhoeae* is one of the manifestations of the disseminated gonococcaemia syndrome and must be considered in sexually active adolescents. In more than one-half of cases, polyarticular disease is found, with joints of the arm, especially wrists and fingers, most frequently involved. A history of migratory polyarthralgia in a febrile adolescent with arthritis of the wrist is so clinically distinct that a presumptive diagnosis can be made and appropriate therapy begun. Although analysis and culture of joint fluid is mandatory in all patients, the organism is found in joint fluid in less than one-half of cases. It is essential to culture from the pharynx, rectum, and vagina/urethra in all patients with a suspected diagnosis of gonococcal arthritis.

Septic arthritis in chronic joint disease

The diagnosis of suppurative joint infection may be particularly difficult in the patient with underlying chronic disease of the joints, such as those with haemophilia or systemic juvenile chronic arthritis. Although there is no hallmark for differentiating chronic, active disease from acute suppurative infection of the joint, most infected patients are febrile, have a more toxic appearance, and have marked local manifestations.

In haemophiliacs, septic arthritis has been considered a rare complication of haemarthrosis. Severe joint pain and systemic toxicity that persist despite giving coagulation factors should be considered an indication for needle aspiration of the affected joint. Pneumococci (which have a predilection for diseased joints) and staphylococci, are the most common pathogens of septic arthritis in haemophiliacs (Scott et al. 1985). Generally, a single joint, usually the knee, is involved and diagnosis may be delayed when a septic joint is superimposed on haemarthrosis. Recently, septic arthritis complicating pneumococcal, staphylococcal, or salmonella bacteraemia has been reported in haemophiliacs infected with human immunodeficiency virus. Polyarticular disease with significant destruction occurred despite appropriate therapy (Ragni and Hawley 1989). However, a more favourable outcome has been reported in four recent cases where non-operative management with prompt antimicrobial therapy was advocated (Merchan et al. 1992).

Joint infection during rheumatoid arthritis is more common in adults than children. Usually, worsening of pain of an isolated joint occurs during a flare-up of the underlying disease; however, there is polyarticular involvement in almost 40 per cent of cases (Kaufman et al. 1976). As in other cases where septic arthritis complicates underlying chronic disease of the joint, a high index of suspicion is necessary to avoid a delay in diagnosis and poor subsequent outcome.

Septic arthritis in patients with sickle haemoglobinopathy

Septic arthritis is uncommon in children with sickle haemoglobinopathy. Localized joint pain and fever are usually found, and symptoms and signs tend to persist for 4 days or longer (Syrogiannopoulos et al. 1986). Encapsulated bacteria typically cause infection in the patient with sickle haemoglobinopathy. Pneumococci are the most commonly recognized pathogens in such children with septic arthritis, although occasional disease secondary to *H. influenzae* type b is reported (Mallouh and Talab 1985). Salmonella have a predilection for bone in sicklaemic patients and may be found in cases of suppurative arthritis in association with an adjacent osteomyelitis.

Penetrating injuries and arthritis

Suppurative arthritis following a penetrating injury to a joint is well described, although when first reported was most commonly associated with sewing-needle injury to the knee. The knee is still the joint usually involved, but sewing needles have rarely been implicated as the agent of trauma in the last two decades. The clinical presentation is similar to other cases of pyarthrosis. In our series, 8 per cent of cases of suppurative arthritis followed a penetrating injury (Table 3). All cases were boys, with a mean age of 6 years. A wide variety of pathogens was found; however, *P. aeruginosa* arthritis of the metatarsal joint following nail puncture through a tennis shoe occurred most frequently.

Reactive or so-called traumatic arthritis follows an injury, usually a thorn or splinter puncture, and may be severe and difficult to distinguish from acute suppurative infection. In most cases, symptoms have been present for longer than a week and although there is pain on moving the joint, it is usually not as severe as that associated with a pyarthrosis (Green and Edwards 1987). Exploration of the joint to exclude a foreign body should be considered in cases where traumatic synovitis persists.

Management

The essentials of management of suppurative arthritis in childhood include the combination of an appropriately selected antimicrobial agent and adequate drainage of the pyarthrosis (see Box 1). Simple needle aspiration of the affected joint may be sufficient in some cases. However, emergency surgical drainage of the joint is mandatory in pyarthrosis of the hip and probably shoulder infection. Arthrotomy and drainage should also be considered in cases where the pus is thick, or when significant symptoms and signs persist despite initial needle aspiration of pus from the affected joint. Aggressive surgical management of Pseudomonas osteochondritis and septic arthritis following a nail puncture wound to the foot permits shortened antimicrobial therapy of only 7–10 days (Jacobs et al. 1989). An aminoglycoside plus ceftazidime are often used as initial therapy until susceptibility test results are available.

Table 3 Suppurative arthritis following puncture wound

Age (years)	Sex	Joint	Trauma	Pathogen
2	M	Knee	Toothpick	Viridans streptococci
3	M	Knee	Plastic	Group A streptococci
3	M	Knee	Dog bite	Unknown
1	M	Knee	Human bite	*Eikenella corrodens*
4	M	Metatarsal	Nail	*Pseudomonas aeruginosa*
12	M	Knee	Nail	Gram-negative rods
4	M	Metatarsal	Nail	*Pseudomonas aeruginosa*
9	M	Metatarsal	Unknown	*Escherichia coli, Enterobacter cloacae*
7	M	Metatarsal	Nail	*Pseudomonas aeruginosa*
9	M	Metatarsal	Nail	*Pseudomonas aeruginosa*
10	M	Metatarsal	Nail	*Pseudomonas aeruginosa*

When a presumptive diagnosis of septic arthritis is made, parenteral antibiotics should be begun promptly. The choice of antimicrobial agents in the healthy child without a puncture wound should be based on the age of the child and the suspected pathogen. Infants under 3 months of age should be treated initially with antimicrobial agents active against *S. aureus*, Gram-negative enteric organisms, and group B streptococcus. Children 3 months to 2 years of age should receive therapy active against *S. aureus*, *S. pneumoniae* (including penicillin-resistant strains), and *K. kingae*. Cefuroxime is appropriate initial coverage as long as concomitant meningitis is not present. Alternatively, a combination of an antistaphylococcal penicillin with a third-generation cephalosporin (usually cefotaxime or ceftriaxone) until the results of culture are known is reasonable. Use of an expanded spectrum agent such as meropenem, imipenem/cilastatin, or cefepime is another option; however, concerns over developing antimicrobial resistance precludes the routine prescribing of these drugs. In older children, an antistaphylococcal penicillin or cephalosporin is the drug of choice. Parenteral antimicrobial agents readily penetrate into infected joints, so intra-articular installation of antibiotics is not necessary.

Drug resistance

Community-aquired methicillin-resistant *S. aureus* (MRSA) infections in children are becoming an increasing concern (Herold et al. 1998; Centers for Disease Control and Prevention 1999). Clinical infection caused by such

Box 1 Management of suspected pyogenic arthritis in the child

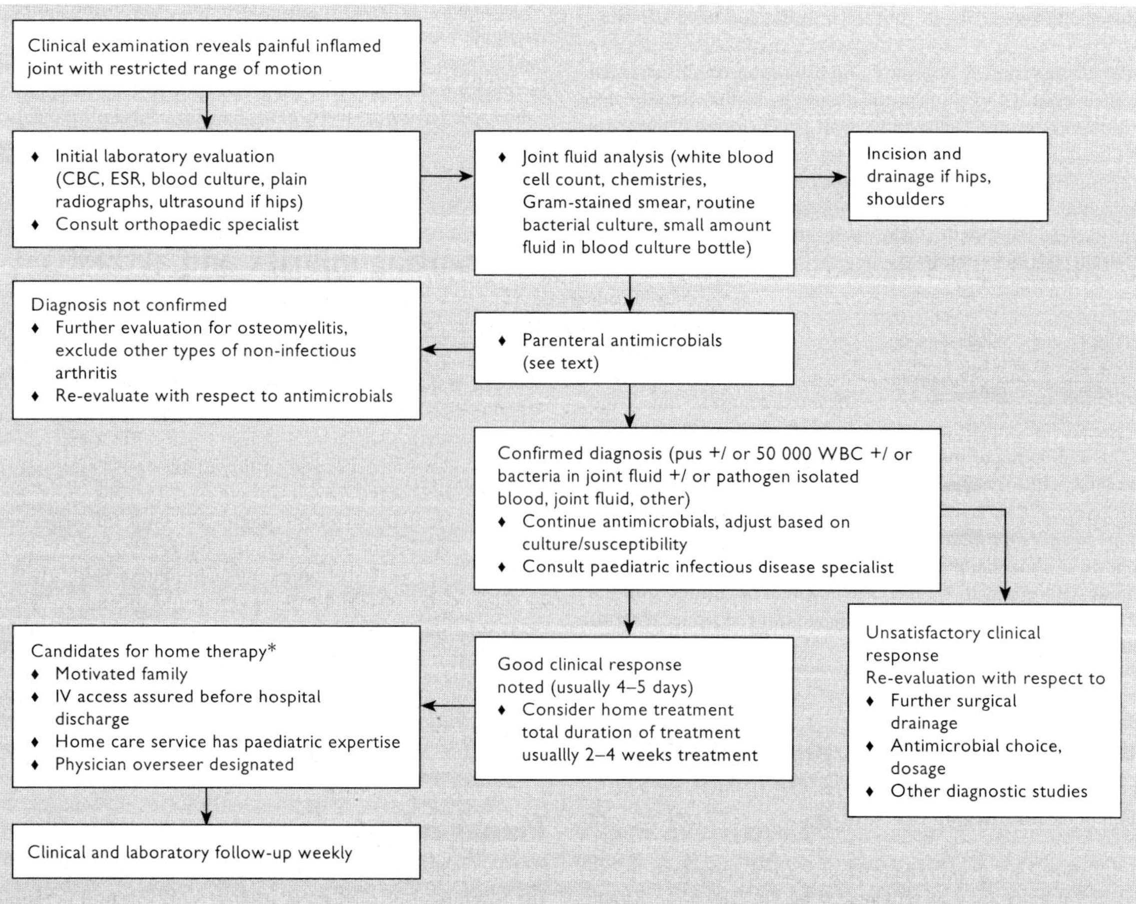

* Some patients are not candidates for home therapy. The decision may be based on clinical or microbiological features of diseases. There may be situations where therapy cannot be provided in a technically satisfactory manner.

strains are similar to those caused by methicillin-susceptible *S. aureus.* In contrast to hospital-acquired MRSA, community-acquired isolates are more likely to be susceptible to clindamycin which effectively penetrates bone and joint. The prevalence of community-acquired MRSA infection increased from 10/100 000 admissions to 208/100 000 admissions over the last decade. Established risk factors for MRSA infection were absent in one-half of such patients identified at a large Mid western urban facility. If rates continue to increase, clindamycin may be the first line agent for skeletal infections in the paediatric population (Hussain et al. 2000).

Worldwide, *S. pneumoniae* isolates that are resistant to penicillin and cephalosporins have been increasingly recovered from patients with both systemic infections and infections of the upper respiratory tract. Risk factors for infection with a drug-resistant strain include daycare attendance and prior beta-lactam antibiotic therapy. Empiric therapy for septic arthritis due to suspected drug-resistant pneumococcus includes cefotaxime, ceftriaxone, clindamycin, or vancomycin. If vancomycin is administered, it should be discontinued as soon as antimicrobial susceptibility test results identify effective alternative agents (American Academy of Pediatrics 2000). Recently, conjugated pneumococcal vaccine was approved for infants beginning at two months of age. As use of this vaccine becomes more routine, the incidence of pneumococcal septic arthritis is expected to diminish significantly.

Sequential intravenous–oral regimens

The efficacy of a sequential intravenous–oral antimicrobial regimen has been demonstrated by numerous prospective studies (e.g. Feigin et al. 1975; Jackson and Nelson 1982). Usually, intravenous therapy is given for 5–7 days. Because the CRP rapidly decreases with appropriate treatment of bacterial arthritis, it is a useful test to monitor the initial response to therapy. If the CRP remains high or increases again during treatment, it may indicate increased inflammation due to inadequate therapy or the need for surgical drainage of the joint (Kallio et al. 1997). After all surgical procedures and when there is definite clinical improvement, a patient may be considered for an oral regimen if (i) an appropriate oral antimicrobial is available, (ii) the patient is able to take and retain oral medication, and (iii) reliable follow-up is guaranteed. The need to test for bactericidal activity of serum samples is controversial and many experts do not use this assessment in the child who has a good clinical and laboratory response to treatment (Nelson 1997; Peltola et al. 1997).

The oral dosage of the selected antibiotic is two to three times that used for otitis media or skin and soft tissue infection. A peak serum bactericidal titre is sometimes used to monitor oral therapy. A serum specimen for blood levels is obtained 1 h after the oral dose is given (after the drug has reached steady-state concentrations) and adequate bactericidal activity should be confirmed. A serum bactericidal activity of at least 1 : 8 is considered adequate except in cases of streptococcal infection where a titre of 1 : 32 is needed. Adjustment of the antimicrobial dosage is usually required in 15 per cent of cases. In less than 5 per cent of cases, satisfactory bactericidal activity cannot be achieved and a total parenteral regimen must be used for the duration of therapy (Prober and Yeager 1979). Oral antibiotic regimens should not be used outside the hospital setting in a child unless adherence to therapy can be assured.

The optimum duration of antimicrobial therapy for children with suppurative arthritis is dependent upon the duration of symptoms before diagnosis of the pathogen, the response to medical and surgical treatment, and whether or not there is concomitant bone infection. Generally, if the patient's clinical response is good and the ESR returns to normal, 3 weeks of therapy is adequate for staphylococcal and Gram-negative bacillary infection (Syrogiannopoulos and Nelson 1978). Shorter courses have been successful for streptococcal and haemophilus infection, in which a total of 10–14 days of therapy may be adequate. In all cases where an oral regimen is used, ESR should be monitored weekly until therapy is considered complete.

The risk of relapse or recurrent disease is quite small in cases of primary joint infection; however, for the child with pyarthrosis and concomitant bone infection, the potential for relapse or sequelae is significant. Therefore, if adherence cannot be guaranteed, an oral regimen is not appropriate for such patients. Delayed diagnosis, delay in surgical drainage, slow clinical response, and undocumented compliance are all risk factors for chronic disease (Hallel and Salvati 1975).

Prognosis

In the child over 1 month of age, the prognosis for primary septic arthritis of the knee is good and more than 90 per cent have a satisfactory outcome. However, poor outcome has been estimated to occur in approximately 40 per cent of hip, 20 per cent of ankle, and 30 per cent of shoulder infections, particularly if there is an adjacent osteomyelitis (Welkon et al. 1986). There should be careful orthopaedic follow-up for at least 6–12 months in all children with suppurative joint infection.

References

American Academy of Pediatrics (2000). Pneumococcal infections. In *2000 Red Book: Report of the Committee on Infectious Diseases* 25th edn. (ed. L.K. Pickering), pp. 452–60. Elk Grove Village IL: American Academy of Pediatrics.

Bowerman, S.G., Green, N.E., and Mencio, G.A. (1997). Decline of bone and joint infections attributable to *Haemophilus influenzae* type 6. *Clinical Orthopaedics and Related Research* **341**, 128–33.

Centers for Disease Control and Prevention (1999). Four pediatric deaths from community-acquired methicillin-resistant *Staphylococcus aureus*–Minnesota and North Dakota, 1997–1999. *Journal of the American Medical Association* **282**, 1123–5.

Feigin, R.D., Pickering, L.K., Anderson, B., Kooney, R.D., and Shackleford, P.G. (1975). Clindamycin treatment of osteomyelitis and septic arthritis in children. *Pediatrics* **55**, 213–23.

Fox, L. and Sprunt, K. (1978). Neonatal osteomyelitis. *Pediatrics* **62**, 535–42.

Green, N.E. and Edwards, K. (1987). Bone and joint infections in children. *Orthopedic Clinics of North America* **18**, 555–76.

Gutierrez, K.M. (1997). Infectious and Inflammatory Arthritis. In *Principles and Practice of Pediatric Infectious Diseases* (ed. S.S. Long, L.K. Pickering, and C.G. Prober), pp. 537–48. New York: Churchill Livingston.

Hallel, T. and Salvati, E.A. (1975). Septic arthritis of the hip in infancy. End result study. *Clinical Orthopaedics* **132**, 115–28.

Herold, B.C. et al. (1998) Community-acquired methicillin-resistant *Staphylococcus aureus* in children with no identified predisposing risk. *Journal of the American Medical Association* **279**, 593–8.

Howard, A.W., Viskontas, D., and Sabbagh, C. (1999). Reduction in osteomyelitis and septic arthritis related to *Haemophilus influenzae* type b vaccination. *Journal of Pediatric Orthopaedics* **19**, 705–9.

Hussain, F.M., Boyle-Vavra, S., Bethel, C.D., and Daum, R.S. (2000). Current trends in community-acquired methicillin-resistant *Staphylococcus aureus* at a tertiary care pediatric facility. *Pediatric Infectious Disease Journal* **19**, 1163–6.

Jackson, M.A. and Nelson, J.D. (1982). Etiology and medical management of acute suppurative bone and joint infections in pediatric patients. *Journal of Pediatric Orthopaedics* **2**, 313–23.

Jackson, M.A., Burry, V.F., and Olson, L.C. (1992). Pyogenic arthritis associated with adjacent osteomyelitis: identification of the sequelae-prone child. *Pediatric Infectious Disease Journal* **11**, 9–13.

Jacobs, R.F., McCarthy, R.E., and Elser, J.M. (1989). Pseudomonas osteochondritis complicating puncture wounds of the foot in children: a 10-year evaluation. *Journal of Infectious Diseases* **160**, 657–61.

Kallio, M.J.T., Unkila-Kallio, L., Aalto, K., and Peltola, H. (1997). Serum C-reactive protein, erythrocyte sedimentation rate and white blood cell count in septic arthritis of children. *Pediatric Infectious Disease Journal* **16**, 411–13.

Kaufman, C.A., Watanakunakorn, C., and Phair, J.P. (1976). Pneumococcal arthritis. *Journal of Rheumatology* **3**, 409–19.

Klein, D.M., Barbera, C., Gray, S.T., Spero, C.R., Perrier, G., and Teicher, J.L. (1997). Sensitivity of objective parameters in the diagnosis of pediatric septic hips. *Clinical Orthopaedics and Related Research* **338**, 153–9.

Lundy, D.W. and Kehl, D.K. (1998). Increasing prevalence of *Kingella kingae* in osteoarticular infections in young children. *Journal of Pediatric Orthopedics* **18**, 262–7.

Mallouh, A. and Talab, Y. (1985). Bone and joint infection in patients with sickle cell disease. *Journal of Pediatric Orthopedics* **5**, 158–62.

Merchan, E.C.R., Magallon, M., Mauso, F., and Martin-Billar, J. (1992). Septic arthritis in HIV positive haemophiliacs. *International Orthopaedics* **16**, 302–6.

Nelson, J.D. (1991). Skeletal infections in children. In *Advances in Pediatric Infectious Diseases* Vol. 6 (ed. S.C. Aronoff, W.T. Hughes, S. Kohn, W.T. Speck, and E.R. Wald), pp. 59–76. St Louis MO: Mosby Year Book.

Nelson, J.D. (1997). Toward simple but safe management of osteomyelitis. *Pediatrics* **99**, 883–4.

Ogden, J.A. (1979). Pediatric osteomyelitis and septic arthritis: the pathology of neonatal disease. *Yale Journal of Biological Medicine* **52**, 423–48.

Patterson, D.C. (1970). Acute suppurative arthritis in infancy and childhood. *Journal of Bone and Joint Surgery* **52B**, 414–82.

Peltola, H. et al. (1997). Simplified treatment of acute Staphylococcal osteomyelitis of childhood. *Pediatrics* **99**, 846–50.

Prober, C.G. and Yeager, A.S. (1979). Use of serum bactericidal titer to assess the adequacy of oral antibiotic therapy in treatment of acute hematogenous osteomyelitis. *Journal of Pediatrics* **95**, 131–55.

Ragni, M.V. and Hawley, E.N. (1989). Septic arthritis in hemophiliac patients and infection with human immunodeficiency virus. *Annals of Internal Medicine* **110**, 168–9.

Resnick, D., Pineda, C.J., Weisman, M.H., and Kerr, R. (1985). Osteomyelitis and septic arthritis of the hand following human bites. *Skeletal Radiology* **14**, 263–6.

Sandrasegaran, K., Saifuddin, M.B., Coral, A., and Butt, W.P. (1994). Magnetic resonance imaging of septic sacroiliitis. *Skeletal Radiology* **23**, 289–92.

Schaad, V.B., McCracken, G.H., and Nelson, J.D. (1980). Pyogenic arthritis of the sacroiliac joint in pediatric patients. *Pediatrics* **66**, 375–9.

Scott, J.P., Maurer, H.S., and Dias, L. (1985). Septic arthritis in two teenaged hemophiliacs. *Journal of Pediatrics* **107**, 748–51.

Syrogiannopoulos, G.A. and Nelson, J.D. (1978). Duration of antimicrobial therapy for acute suppurative osteoarticular infections. *Lancet* **i**, 37–40.

Syrogiannopoulos, G.A., McCracken, G.H., and Nelson, J.D. (1986). Osteoarticular infections in children with sickle cell disease. *Pediatrics* **78**, 1090–6.

Tuson, C.E., Hoffman, E.B., and Mann, M.D. (1994). Osotope bone scanning for acute osteomyelitis and septic arthritis in children. *Journal of Bone and Joint Surgery* **76B**, 306–10.

Welkon, C.J., Long, S.S., Fisher, M.C., and Alburger, P.D. (1986). Pyogenic arthritis in infants and children: a review of 95 cases. *Pediatric Infectious Disease Journal* **5**, 669–76.

Yagupsky, P. and Dagan, R. (1997). *Kingella kingae*: an emerging cause of invasive infections in young children. *Clinical Infectious Diseases* **24**, 860–6.

Yagupsky, P., Dagan, R., Howard, C.W., Einhorn, M., Kassis, I., and Simu, A. (1992). High prevalence of *Kingella kingae* in joint fluid from children with septic arthritis revealed by the BACTEC blood culture system. *Journal of Clinical Microbiology* **30**, 1278–81.

Yagupsky, P., Dagan, R., Howard, C.W., Einhorn, M., Kassis, I., and Simu, A. (1993). Clinical features and epidemiology of invasive *Kingella kingae* infections in Southern Israel. *Pediatrics* **92**, 800–4.

Zawin, J.K., Hoffer, F.A., Rand, F.F., and Teele, R.L. (1993). Joint effusion in children with an irritable hip: US diagnosis and aspiration. *Radiology* **187**, 459–63.

6.2.3 Osteomyelitis and associated conditions

Emilio Bouza and Patricia Munoz

Introduction

The term osteomyelitis used to describe any infection involving the bone and the marrow. Important developments in the field of osteomyelitis include newer diagnostic techniques, the use of aggressive surgery in infection associated with implantation of new prosthetic devices, and antibiotic releasing bead implants. The availability of non-toxic, highly efficacious, oral antimicrobial agents frequently permits a long-term approach to these difficult-to-treat infections during which the patient remains ambulatory. The increasing number of immunosuppressed patients (particularly those with HIV/AIDS and those on immunosuppressive therapy) at risk of osteomyelitis, and the emergence of antimicrobial resistance, pose serious problems for clinical management of osteomyelitis.

Classification

A universally applied classification system for stratifying osteomyelitis and prosthetic joint infection is required to provide a framework to evaluate the efficacy of medical and surgical treatments in different institutions. To date, there is no single classification system that is satisfactory. Osteomyelitis can be classified on the basis of several characteristics (Table 1):

1. The age of the patient must always be considered, since pathogenesis and aetiology are usually different in neonates, children, or adults. Haematogenous osteomyelitis is far more frequent in children. *Staphylococcus aureus*, *Enterobacteriaceae*, and group A and B β-haemolytic streptococci are the most common aetiological agents in neonates. In children under 4 years of age, *Haemophilus influenzae* is the most important pathogen, followed by streptococci and *S. aureus*. In children older than 4 years *S. aureus*, streptococci, and *H. influenzae* predominate.
2. The affected bone is also an important factor. Long bones, particularly those of the lower limbs, are more susceptible to infection because their blood supply is poorer than in short bones. Also, they bear more weight and have worse venous return. Pelvic and cranial bones are infrequently involved.
3. Host factors are important in susceptibility to osteomyelitis. In patients with HIV/AIDS and intravenous drug abusers, atypical locations are more frequently encountered (pubic bones, clavicle, or vertebra) and,

Table 1 Classification criteria for osteomyelitis

Criteria	Classification
1. Age	Children–adults
2. Affected bone	Long–short
3. Host factors	HIV/AIDS, immunosuppressed–immunocompetant
4. Aetiology	Bacterial–non-bacterial
5. Pathogenesis	Haematogenous–contiguous
6. Existence of fracture	Consolidated–non-unions
7. Risk factors	With–without prosthetic material
8. Blood supply	Adequate–inadequate
9. Evolution	Acute–chronic

besides staphylococci and streptococci, several unusual bacterial and fungal infections cause disease. Patients with haemoglobinopathies, such as sickle-cell disease, have a higher incidence of infections caused by encapsulated bacteria such as *S. pneumoniae, H. influenzae*, or *Salmonella* spp. Chronic haemodialysis is also a risk factor for osteomyelitis and the ribs and thoracic spine are commonly involved.

4. A range of microorganisms cause osteomyelitis. While Gram-positive bacteria (*S. aureus* or *Staphylococcus epidermidis*) predominate, up to one-third of cases can be due to Gram-negative bacteria. They are frequently found in post-traumatic and post-surgical osteomyelitis. Anaerobic and mixed infections should also be considered in osteomyelitis associated with poor vascular supply such as in diabetics. Mycobacteria, and particularly *Mycobacterium tuberculosis*, are an increasing cause of osteomyelitis in HIV-endemic areas. Fungal infections of the bone have been described in all agents responsible for systemic mycosis in both the normal and the immunocompromised host.
5. Osteomyelitis can be classified according to the route by which the infection reaches bone: (a) haematogenous, (b) secondary to a contiguous focus of infection, and (c) direct inoculation. Acute haematogenous osteomyelitis is more common in children and is discussed later. In adults, haematogenous osteomyelitis frequently involves the spine. This constitutes a diagnostic challenge since clinical and radiological manifestations may be non-specific and rapid evolution may produce significant neurological sequelae. HIV-related adult haematogenous osteomyelitis is a relatively new disease in Africa. *Staphylococcus* spp., *Salmonella* spp., or other gut flora are common aetiological agents. Mixed infections are also common. Despite vigorous treatment with rest, elevation, antibiotics, surgical drainage, and sequestrectomies, effective cure is rarely possible.
6. The existence of an underlying fracture, sometimes with non-union (pseudoarthrosis), will influence the surgical approach.
7. The presence of any kind of prosthetic material near the infection site must be carefully sought, since it facilitates persistence of infection, increases the pathogenicity of microorganisms such as *S. epidermidis*, and hinders the efficacy of antimicrobial treatment. Although the withdrawal of prosthetic materials is regularly recommended, it is not always necessary, or possible.
8. Osteomyelitis can also be classified according to the integrity of the bone's vascular supply. Neuropathic and vascular changes characteristic of diabetes, leprosy, and other neuropathies, put patients at risk of developing chronic foot damage after minor trauma and subsequent bone infection.
9. The disease activity in osteomyelitis can be classified as acute or chronic. Osteomyelitis is considered acute when the appearance of symptoms is recent, and when there has been no previous therapy. This usually occurs in children who present with excruciating pain, high fever, and are toxic and irritable. On the other hand, osteomyelitis is chronic when symptoms have been present for 4–6 weeks or previous therapy has been given. This classification is important, since therapy and prognosis will be very different. At the present time, less than 6 per cent of haematogenous osteomyelitis becomes chronic but practically all post-traumatic infections are chronic.

Previous classifications have considered these important aspects, the most essential being the presence of vascular compromise, the presence of prosthetic material, and the rate of evolution.

Cierny and Mader (1984) proposed a classification for adult chronic osteomyelitis that takes into account the anatomical status of the bone lesion, the involvement of soft tissues, and the expected host response to infection. Accordingly, each case of adult chronic osteomyelitis must be classified with a number and a letter. Nevertheless, the system is imprecise and has not been broadly accepted or generally incorporated into clinical practice. Details of the classification are as follows.

Table 2 Local and systemic factors that affect the immunological, metabolic, and vascular response to osteomyelitis

Systemic	Local
Malnutrition	Chronic lymphoedema
HIV/AIDS	Venous stasis
Immunodeficiency/ immunosuppressive therapy	Large/small vessel disease
Diabetes mellitus	Arteritis
Renal and/or hepatic failure	Neuropathy
Malignancy	Scars
Extremes of age	Post-radiation fibrosis
Drug abuse	
Smoking	
Chronic hypoxia	

Anatomical classification

Type I: Intramedullary infection or infected (but consolidated) fractures with an intramedullary rod. Surgical treatment is simple and will not result in bone instability.

Type II: Cortical bone infection (pressure sore). Bone excision is easy, although soft-tissue coverage may be more complicated.

Type III: Osteomyelitis affecting cortical bone and marrow, but not including the whole bone circumference (sequestrum). Surgical debridement is complicated, although does not necessarily result in instability.

Type IV: Osteomyelitis affecting the whole bone circumference. The surgical approach usually requires ablation of a bone segment and may result in bone instability. Includes infected non-unions and infected articular prostheses.

Type IV physiological classification

Class A: Patients and tissues with normal response to infection and surgery.

Class B: Patients with local or systemic immune deficiencies, which may predispose to infection (Table 2).

Class C: Patients not considered to be suitable surgical candidates, for whom the morbidity of treatment is greater than the risk of disease or exceeds the expected benefit.

Microbial aetiology of osteomyelitis

A wide range of microorganisms (bacteria, viruses, fungi, spirochaetes, mycoplasma) can be isolated from patients with osteomyelitis (Bouza and Muñoz 1999).

Gram-positive bacterial infections

Gram-positive bacteria are the most common causative agents of osteomyelitis. *S. aureus* is, undoubtedly, the most common aetiological agent of osteomyelitis of any kind (Guerrero 1987). In recent years, the emergence of methicillin-resistant strains (MRSA) (strains resistant to all β-lactam drugs) has been described in many hospitals worldwide. *S. epidermidis* is one of the most common agents of bone and joint infection in patients with prosthetic materials, and a high proportion of these infections are resistant to methicillin. The aetiological role of *S. epidermidis* should only be fully accepted when the isolate is obtained from a usually sterile body fluid or tissue, and skin contamination can be reasonably ruled out. *S. epidermidis* infection is extremely rare without the presence of underlying prosthetic material.

Although streptococci are of great importance in skin and soft tissue infections, they are not frequent causes of osteomyelitis. Group B β-haemolytic streptococcus (*Streptococcus agalactiae*) is exceptional as a cause of osteomyelitis. It is most commonly described in children, the elderly, or immunosuppressed patients (Garcia Leuchuz et al. 1999). *S. pneumoniae* osteomyelitis is also extremely uncommon in adults and may occur as a single focus of infection in normal children (Jacobs 1991). *Enterococcus* spp. is very rarely implicated in osteomyelitis. In a well-designed study of biopsy confirmed, non-prosthetic osteomyelitis, *Enterococcus* spp. accounted for 3 per cent of the cases (Gentry and Rodríguez-Gomez 1991). Vancomycin-resistant *E. faecium* osteomyelitis has also been described. Other Gram-positive microorganisms such as *Listeria* spp. or *Bacillus* spp. have only rarely been implicated in osteoarticular infections.

Gram-negative bacterial infections

Among the Gram-negative bacteria, *Pseudomonas* is one of the most commonly involved in bone infections. It is usually found in osteomyelitis following open fractures or surgical procedures. It is the most frequent cause of calcaneus osteomyelitis following infected puncture wounds of the foot (Lavery et al. 1994). *Salmonella* osteomyelitis occurs either as a complication of typhoid fever or in patients with various underlying diseases, including immunosuppressed patients and those with sickle-cell disease (Anand and Glatt 1994). Other Enterobacteriaceae have also been described, particularly in infections following open fractures or as a consequence of haematogenous bone involvement in patients with bacteraemia of another origin (Voss et al. 1992). *Brucella* spp. osteomyelitis, especially affecting the vertebrae, is common in brucellosis-endemic countries.

Anaerobic bacterial infections

Conditions predisposing to anaerobic bone infections are vascular disease, human and animal bites, a contiguous focus of infection, peripheral neuropathy, haematogenous spread, and trauma. Anaerobes are more frequently detected in osteomyelitis under pressure sores, or in bone infections of the diabetic foot (Hudson 1993). Pigmented *Prevotella* and *Porphyromonas* spp. were mostly isolated in infections of the skull and following bites. Members of the *Bacteroides fragilis* group have been detected in cases of hand and foot infection, and *Fusobacterium* spp. in skull, bite wounds, and haematogenous long-bone infections.

Mycobacterium tuberculosis (see Chapter 6.2.7)

Mycobacterium tuberculosis is a common cause of osteomyelitis in tuberculous-endemic areas (both in normal and immunocompromised hosts) (Jellis et al. 1995; Jellis 2002). Tuberculosis has been declared a global emergency by the World Health Organization and the epidemic affects all parts of the globe. Thus, all cases of chronic osteomyelitis of any bone must be screened for *M. tuberculosis*.

Viruses

In the tropics, hepatitis B and the arboviruses (e.g. sindbis, chikungunya, dengue, mayaro, and yellow fever) can cause arthritis.

Fungal infections

Fungal osteomyelitis is found in both normal and immunocompromised hosts. *Candida* spp., *Cryptococcus* spp., *Coccidioides immitis, Histoplasma duboisii*, and other fungi can cause osteomyelitis (Miller and Mejicano 2001; Wang and Lee 2001). Mucormycosis of long bones can also occur (Holtom et al. 2000).

Diagnostic procedures

The diagnosis of osteomyelitis and prosthetic joint infections is usually made on the basis of clinical, laboratory, and imaging techniques. A complete clinical history and examination must be performed. Information on the presence of any kind of prosthetic material, previous surgical and medical therapy, duration of previous antimicrobial courses, and the response must be carefully recorded. Physical examination should focus on the integrity of involved bone and surrounding tissues, and on evidence of inflammatory signs, pain, bone instability, sinus tracts, or neurovascular changes. The nutritional status of the patient should also be considered. The detection of a sinus tract with suppurative drainage will establish the diagnosis in an appropriate clinical setting. Further diagnostic techniques will be required to confirm the diagnosis, if necessary, and to establish the aetiology.

Laboratory investigations

Laboratory data are not essential for the diagnosis of osteoarticular infections. The erythrocyte sedimentation rate is usually high with active infections and tends to fall after effective therapy. Its accuracy in infected prostheses is variable. In our experience, the erythrocyte sedimentation rate is not useful as an index of either activity or resolution in osteomyelitis. C-reactive protein is also usually increased, although its measurement is less widely used (Unkila-Kallio et al. 1994). Only one-third of patients have leucocytosis at the time of admission. No single laboratory measure is reliable enough to be used routinely for the diagnosis of osteomyelitis.

Imaging techniques

Imaging plays an important part in establishing the diagnosis and directing the treatment of osteomyelitis (Griffith et al. 2002). A variety of imaging methods are available:

1. plain radiography,
2. radionuclide imaging,
3. computerized tomography (CT),
4. magnetic resonance imaging (MRI).

Decisions on the best method can be challenging and should reflect the location of the suspected infection and associated underlying systemic or bone disorder. Once the microorganism reaches the bone, a suppurative reaction is produced, followed by a marrow oedema, which can only be readily detected by MRI. The next step consists of vascular congestion, thrombosis, and ischaemia. At this time, soft tissue changes may be detected by CT but not by plain radiology. Finally (after at least 2–3 weeks), bone reaction begins, with the production of new periosteal bone, sequestrum, decalcification, and new bone formation, which can be detected even with plain films.

Plain X-ray films

The detection of *acute* osteomyelitis on a plain film requires at least a 35 per cent loss of calcium content in the bone lesion. This usually takes a minimum of 15 days. This is not the issue in *chronic* osteomyelitis, in which the dilemma is to establish whether radiological changes correspond to active infection, surgical sequelae, or just trauma.

The detection of a sequestrum (a clearly defined, isolated necrotic area of bone surrounded by a osteopenic zone), an involucrum (a hyperdense zone of bone under an elevated periosteum), a Brodie's abscess is considered pathognomonic of osteomyelitis. Other signs that should suggest the presence of active infection are the detection of poorly delineated osteolytic areas, periosteal hyperplasia, or irregular periosteal bone extending into adjacent soft tissue (Gómez 1987).

The presence of periprosthetic bone reabsorption or new periosteal bone formation is highly suggestive of infection in the appropriate clinical setting. Considering their simplicity and low price, conventional radiographs should always be obtained if osteoarticular infection is suspected.

Isotope bone scanning

In most cases of chronic osteomyelitis, clinical and radiological data permit an easy diagnosis. However, sometimes bone changes from other causes and soft-tissue infection make laboratory and radiographic signs unreliable as indicators of osteomyelitis. This happens regularly in acute haematogenous osteomyelitis. In this situation, scintigraphic methods can be helpful (Alazraki 1993; Kothari et al. 2001). Since it provides physiological data, scintigraphy is also useful in the evaluating therapeutic response. However, anatomical definition is inferior to that of CT or MRI.

$^{99}Tc^{m}$ *methylene diphosphonate*

$^{99}Tc^{m}$ methylene diphosphonate (MDP) is taken up in areas of increased blood flow or osteoblastic activity. A three-phase bone MDP scan (vascular, pool, and late or bone phase) increases specificity, and is the first-line diagnostic imaging technique after a plain radiograph in evaluating suspected osteomyelitis.

Image quality is fairly good, the dose of irradiation is small, the cost is reasonable, and the technique is available in most centres. Preparation is simple, and the technique provides an earlier and more sensitive diagnosis than plain radiography. However, specificity is poor and the negative predictive value of this technique is more reliable than positive prediction. False-positives may be due to neoplasm, fractures, heterotopic ossification, arthritis, neuropathic osteopathy, trauma, or arthrosis. It is not very useful in children or following recent surgery to bone.

67-Gallium citrate

^{67}Ga is taken up in areas where leucocytes or bacteria accumulate and provides quantitative information about inflammatory activity. Gallium scans become positive earlier than MDP and are sensitive in detecting active bone/joint lesions. A normal gallium scan virtually excludes the presence of an inflammatory process. False-positive gallium scans in ununited fractures or after recent surgery are common. Images are less precise than MDP scans. Adult patients with previous bone disorders and possible osteomyelitis or patients with dubious results from MDP scanning should have a gallium scan. Gallium may also be the preferred technique for following response to therapy.

111-Indium or 99-Tc autologous leucocyte scintigraphy

If the other bone scans are inconclusive, ^{111}In-labelled leucocyte scintigraphy is the next line to take, particularly in adults with other bone disorders. Patient's leucocytes are obtained and labelled. Afterwards, they are re-infused into the patient and accumulate in the focus of infection where they can be detected. Indium scans have higher specificity than the previous techniques for the diagnosis of infection, particularly in previously traumatized bone. They provide very good results in osteomyelitis of the diabetic foot, infections associated with delayed or non-union, and prosthetic infections.

Indium scans have higher sensitivity in acute osteomyelitis than in chronic cases (60 versus 100 per cent), probably due to the massive presence of leucocytes in the former (Schauwecker et al. 1984). False-positives may occur after trauma, tumours, and other osseous disorders. The quality of the image is inferior to that of Tc scintigraphy and it is not very accurate for the axial skeleton. Preparation is complex and long, and the major concerns about this technique are the hazards associated with the handling of blood, and the need to delay imaging for 18–24 h, which precludes a rapid result. Potential alternative agents for ^{111}In-labelled leucocytes include labelled immunoglobulin and labelled antigranulocyte antibody reagents. Indium scans should be reserved for patients with a suspicion of osteomyelitis of the lower extremities not diagnosed with the previous techniques.

None of the types of scintigraphy can differentiate between septic and non-septic inflammatory processes with sufficient accuracy. For this reason, other techniques are sometimes required.

Computed tomography

CT scanning accurately detects increased medullary density (typical of the early stages of osteomyelitis), as well as subsequent changes in soft tissues and cortical bone. Its principal advantage is excellent definition of cortical bone, including zones of necrosis, sclerosis, demineralization, periosteal changes, and adjacent soft-tissue swelling. CT does not provide information about the activity of the process and there may be image interference caused by the presence of prosthetic material. Radiation exposure is rather high and it is an expensive technique. CT is especially recommended in chronic osteomyelitis before surgery. It may help to delineate the presence of abscesses, a sinus tract or sequestrum. It may also be useful for evaluation of infected joint prostheses and osteomyelitis of the spine, pelvis, and sternum.

Magnetic resonance imaging

MRI readily detects the oedema of bone marrow that characterizes the earlier phases of bone infection. Typical features of osteomyelitis on MRI include a low-intensity area in T_1 (less fat) and a hyperintense area in T_2. Bone reaction to fracture or surgery would appear as low marrow intensity in T_1 and normal signal in T_2. Sinus tract and cellulitis would appear as hyperintense areas in T_2. MRI has proved to be as sensitive as bone scintigraphy in the early detection of osteomyelitis, and, with its superior spatial resolution, it is often more specific than planar scintigraphy in differentiating bone from soft-tissue infection and in separating arthritis, cellulitis, and soft-tissue abscesses from osteomyelitis. In several comparative studies, MRI has been more accurate in detecting the presence and determining the extent of osteomyelitis than scintigraphy, CT scan, and conventional radiography. MRI may facilitate differentiation of acute from chronic osteomyelitis and may help to detect foci of active infection in the presence of chronic inflammation or post-traumatic lesions (Spaeth et al. 1991). The patient is not irradiated and newer techniques such as fat-suppressed, contrast-enhanced MRI are significantly more sensitive than scintigraphy, and more specific than non-enhanced MRI or scintigraphy (Hopkins et al. 1995).

MRI has some drawbacks. It does not provide very precise images of cortical bone and its usefulness decreases in the presence of metallic materials. False-positive results may be obtained in the presence of neoplasm, or intra-/extramedullary inflammation. Experience with MRI is as yet limited and the cost is high. A major indication for MRI is in osteomyelitis of the vertebrae and the foot, and when diagnosis is still not established after using the previously described techniques.

Microbiological diagnosis

The aetiological diagnosis usually relies on microbiological analysis of local samples (biopsy tissue, exudates/discharge, sinus swabs). In acute haematogenous osteomyelitis, blood cultures and/or locally obtained aspirates are the procedures of choice. It is important to note that only in a small proportion of cases do microorganisms recovered from sinus tracts reflect the real causative agent present in the bone. Consequently, bone biopsy culture is now the standard method for determining specific antimicrobial therapy (sensitivity and specificity of 87 and 93 per cent, respectively) (Howard et al. 1994). Bone biopsy should be taken, using local anaesthesia and imaging control, from the most painful site. The specimen must be transported to the laboratory immediately where it is processed systematically:

1. Microscopy after Gram stain and acid-fast stain.
2. Culture and identification of most common pathogens, including aerobes, anaerobes, fungi, and mycobacteria. Quantitative bone cultures have not been effective in differentiating osteomyelitis from infection or colonization of adjacent soft tissue.
3. Molecular analysis for detecting pathogen-specific DNA. Recent developments in molecular methods utilizing polymerase chain reaction (PCR) or ligase chain reaction (LCR) using appropriate organism-specific primers for detecting microbial DNA in tissues may be useful in identification of the organism.

Histological diagnosis

Histological diagnosis of osteomyelitis is particularly necessary in cases where there is reasonable doubt about the reliability of cultures. It is required in patients already receiving antimicrobial drugs, in osteomyelitis potentially caused by pathogens that are difficult to grow, and in patients where bone

environmental microorganisms and 10-fold reduction in the incidence of infection. Some orthopaedic surgeons recommend prophylactic antimicrobial agents for prevention of infection in patients with prosthetic joints undergoing certain invasive procedures. Particular attention should be paid to bacteriuria, the implantation of intravascular devices, drainage, and dental manipulations, for which a prophylactic approach similar to that for endocarditis is recommended.

Chronic post-traumatic osteomyelitis

Most information to date comes from experience with chronic post-traumatic osteomyelitis. The risk of infection after an open fracture varies widely with the site, size, and nature of an open fracture. Chronic osteomyelitis is usually a local disease that only rarely produces systemic manifestations. The most common symptoms are pain and suppurative discharge. As mentioned previously, the infection is characteristically recurrent and resistant to short courses of antibiotic therapy (Ciampolini and Harding 2000). Fever is more common in acute infections or in the presence of soft-tissue abscesses. The presence of an open draining fistula is always a marker of clinical activity of osteomyelitis.

The main principle of management of infection in non-consolidated bone fractures is to retain fracture fixation whenever possible. When infection becomes apparent, ultrasonography may determine the presence or absence of collections requiring drainage. In the absence of a collection or a wound discharge, only antimicrobial treatment should be provided. If discharge or collections are present, surgical drainage and debridement are necessary, the organisms present must be identified, and antimicrobial treatment prescribed. Implants should be retained unless fracture has occurred, in which case repeated debridement with removal of all devitalized bone and soft tissue is required. After this, either exchange implants or external fixation are undertaken.

Osteomyelitis in decubitus ulcers

The incidence of osteomyelitis under decubitus ulcers ranges from 28 to 70 per cent (Bruck et al. 1991). Most patients with osteomyelitis have radiological changes but to confirm its activity and aetiology requires needle or surgical bone sampling. Antibiotics are indicated only if osteomyelitis is present. After surgical debridement, soft-tissue coverage is essential. Myocutaneous flaps are superior to skin flaps in securing skin cover.

Acute haematogenous osteomyelitis in children

Bacteria are carried by the blood to the metaphysis of long bones (tibia, femur, humerus) where they produce inflammatory changes, with consequential rise in intraosseous pressure, which in turn occludes the endosteal circulation and produces a septic necrosis (Vazquez 2002). The infection spreads to the diaphysis along the medullary cavity. Pus eventually breaches the cortex lifting the periostium. The dead cortex becomes a sequestrum.

Haematogenous osteomyelitis may appear as an acute onset of bone pain or limited motion of an extremity, regardless of the presence or absence of signs of infection such as fever, local tenderness, redness, swelling, or heat (Bonhoeffer et al. 2001). Acute haematogenous osteomyelitis in children was becoming infrequent until the advent of the HIV/AIDS epidemic. In most children with acute haematogenous osteomyelitis no obvious predisposing factors are apparent apart from HIV/AIDS and sickle-cell anaemia where it is associated with a higher risk of haematogenous osteomyelitis, particularly due to and *Staphylococcus*. It is often difficult to distinguish acute osteomyelitis from bony infarction in sickle-cell disease (Wong et al. 2001).

Pain, pseudoparalysis (voluntary limitation of movement of one extremity), and fever are the most common clinical manifestations. Initially, local inflammatory signs are rarely present. Plain radiographs are frequently negative and isotope bone scanning is required. The disease is almost always monostotic and long-bone metaphyses are the sites most frequently involved. In experienced hands the diagnosis of acute pyogenic osteomyelitis is often made clinically. Diagnostic confirmation requires needle aspiration or surgical debridement. Early surgical decompression prevents the sequelae of chronic osteomyelitis and therefore can be a surgical emergency. Blood cultures are, in contrast to chronic osteomyelitis, frequently positive (in at least one-third of the episodes). Both blood and local samples should be always be obtained because, not uncommonly, only one of the samples is positive. *S. aureus* is responsible for at least 50 per cent of the cases. The remaining cases are caused by different microorganisms, among them *Streptococcus* and *Haemophilus* spp.

When pain is severe, needle or surgical decompression should be undertaken. If the infection opens into the synovial cavity, repeated needle aspiration may be sufficient. When no pain or large collection of pus is present, antimicrobial treatment alone may be enough. Sequential treatment (intravenous drugs followed by oral antimicrobial agents) may be adequate. A total of 10–14 days of intravenous antibiotics is followed by 2–6 additional weeks of oral agents. These should have an acceptable flavour, good oral absorption, low toxicity profile, and be active against Gram-positives and *Haemophilus*. Nowadays, the prognosis of acute haematogenous osteomyelitis in childhood is much better than in the past. Death from this cause in HIV-negative patients is almost non-existent and evolution to chronicity occurs in less than 5 per cent of cases.

Vertebral osteomyelitis

The spinal column is the most common site of haematogenous osteomyelitis in adults, probably due to vertebrae having abundant red marrow and a slow and tortuous blood flow.

Aetiology

Bacteria reach the vertebral bodies preferentially by the arteries but occasionally also through the venous plexus. More than 50 per cent of the episodes of vertebral osteomyelitis are due to *S. aureus*, approximately 30 per cent to Enterobacteriaceae, and the remaining 10–20 per cent to other microorganisms such as *Brucella* spp., *M. tuberculosis*, *Listeria monocytogenes*, and fungi (Khan et al. 2001). These figures will vary according to the endemicity of certain organisms. *Brucella* osteomyelitis is a major health problem in South America, the Middle East, and the Mediterranean (Kubler and Klestov 2001). Osteomyelitis due to *M. tuberculosis* is now increasing in frequency in HIV-positive patients in Sub-Saharan Africa, reflecting the growing tuberculosis epidemic. Tuberculosis can affect any bone in the body (Kutty et al. 2002). Pott's disease (tuberculosis of the bone) is common in tropical countries and with the rise in the number of cases of tuberculosis in the United Kingdom, a high index of suspicion is warranted. Tuberculous osteomyelitis occurs most commonly in the thoracic spine leading to vertebral collapse and kyphosis. The spinal cord may be affected and associated neurological features occur. Spinal tuberculosis can be treated with standard quadruple antituberculosis chemotherapy and a few cases may require anterior decompression and fusion. Osteomyelitis due to fungal infections such as *Candida* have been described (Wang 2001).

Clinical presentation

Backache and pain that increases with spinal movement is the most common clinical manifestation of any vertebral osteomyelitis. Lump on the affected area may be the first clinical sign. Other symptoms depend on the site of involvement. In patients with cervical osteomyelitis and prevertebral abscesses, odinophagia and dysphagia may be present. Fever and/or an increased white blood-cell count is absent in up to half of the cases. An increased erythrocyte sedimentation rate has traditionally been considered to be a very sensitive marker for the presence of active vertebral infection.

In our experience this is not the case and the diagnosis of vertebral osteomyelitis should not be rejected in patients with a normal erythrocyte sedimentation rate. Overall, the lumbar spine is the most frequent location and is involved in more than 50 per cent of episodes of vertebral osteomyelitis, followed by 35 per cent in the dorsal spine, and the remaining 15 per cent in the cervical spine.

Lumbar osteomyelitis occurs occasionally as a septic metastasis of infections of the pelvis and genitourinary tract; cervical bone infection is frequently a complication of parenteral drug abuse.

X-ray changes

Most cases of vertebral osteomyelitis have abnormalities on plain radiographs when first seen but in very acute presentations, the plain film may be normal. Erosive, irregular images in the vertebral bodies and the adjacent intervertebral disc are common. Pre- and paravertebral abscesses and vertebral collapse are common complications.

Isotope imaging

Isotope imaging is diagnostically very sensitive in patients with normal or equivocal plain films. Both CT and MRI offer early and well-defined images that are very useful for directing aspiration or surgery.

Microbiological investigations

Microbiological confirmation requires culture of vertebral material and blood cultures. Only one-fourth of the episodes are documented with blood cultures and consequently bone aspiration should be undertaken whenever possible and subject to intense microbiological workup as described previously.

Management

Most cases of vertebral osteomyelitis recover on appropriate antibiotic therapy and do not require surgical debridement. Surgery should be reserved for patients with spinal instability, neurological impairment, a large, progressive abscess impossible to drain by guided needle aspiration, or cases of unknown aetiology not responding rapidly to appropriate antimicrobial therapy. Considerations governing antimicrobial therapy described previously also apply to vertebral involvement. Immobilization in bed is only required for patients with pain or vertebral instability and casts are not necessary in most cases.

Infected prosthesis (see Chapter 6.2.1)

Infections related to joint prostheses have been divided into those presenting in the first 3 months after surgery (type I), those presenting between 3 months and 1 year post-operatively (type II), and those occurring after 1 year post-surgery (type III). Type I infections are almost exclusively acquired during surgery and may be divided into superficial (involving soft tissues but not the prosthesis) and deep (involving the prosthesis). In group II, most infections are surgically acquired and practically all of them involve the prosthesis. Finally, group III infections are of haematogenous origin and involve the prosthesis. At least 70 per cent of prosthetic joint infections are monomicrobial and the remaining 20–30 per cent are either polymicrobial or not documented (Buchholz et al. 1984; Munoz and Bouza 1999). Among the responsible microorganisms, *S. epidermidis* and *S. aureus* are far ahead of other bacteria, followed by Gram-negative rods and anaerobes.

Chronic infection of articular prostheses usually begins as continuous pain, frequently without obvious drainage through a sinus tract, prosthetic dysfunction, or complete loosening (Fig. 1). Infections associated with prosthetic material are extremely difficult to treat and often require surgical removal of foreign bodies, which may be very radical when artificial joints are involved. Attempts to implant a new prosthesis are usually made after prolonged courses of antimicrobial therapy, leaving the patient with major incapacity for a long time.

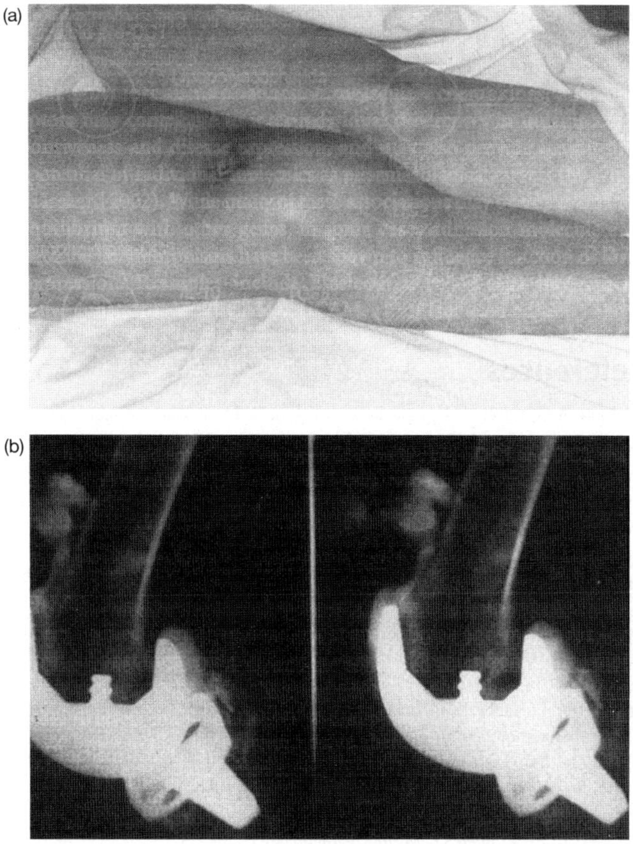

Fig. 1 Infected knee prosthesis: (a) fistulous tract; (b) fistulography.

Type I infections with superficial involvement and no evidence of prosthetic dysfunction should be treated with antimicrobial agents, removal of blood or collections, soft-tissue debridement, and irrigation. A high proportion of these cases (approximately 70 per cent) do not require future prosthetic replacement (Buchholz et al. 1984). Even in cases with deep infections, antimicrobial therapy and early debridement and irrigation save at least 50 per cent of the prostheses.

In HIV-infected patients with a significant degree of immunosuppression (CD4+ lymphocyte counts <200/mcl) prosthesis and implants can become foci of infection many years after their initial insertion (Jellis et al. 1995).

In patients with type II and III infections the final objective is to preserve a functional, pain-free prosthesis. In patients with no prosthetic dysfunction and with no or minimal pain, a trial of antimicrobial therapy without surgical replacement of the prosthesis can be attempted. We use, whenever possible, oral antimicrobial agents, usually including rifampin in a combination regimen. Treatment is continued for a 6- to 12-month period, provided an adequate response was rapidly obtained. In case of a late relapse, the treatment is individualized depending on many variables such as the age of the patient, functional status, and the risk for surgical replacement. In patients with pain, prosthetic dysfunction, or loosening, surgical replacement is necessary. It may be performed in two stages or in a single step, with a low rate of reinfection.

Other musculoskeletal infections

Infective polymyositis

Pyomyositis is an acute inflammation of skeletal muscle which is mainly found in the tropics (Adebajo 2002). It can occur at any age but is frequently found in children and young adults. It is now also common in HIV-infected adults. *Staphylococcus pyogenes* is the usual aetiology. Trauma, HIV/AIDS, malnutrition, viral and parasitic infections are common predisposing factors. Any muscle group can be affected and clinical features are those of a localized abscess with systemic features. Untreated the condition progresses to extensive muscle destruction. The more acute presentation and the peripheral site distribution makes the diagnosis difficult to differentiate from haematogenous osteomyelitis. Treatment involves adequate doses of appropriate antibiotics active against penicclinase-resistant organisms, given parenterally initially. Surgical drainage of fluctuant abscesses should be carried out.

References

Adebajo, A.O. (2002). Musculoskeletal disorders. In *Manson's Tropical Diseases* 21st edn., Chapter 22 (ed. G.C. Cook and A. Zumla). Edinburgh: Saunders.

Alazraki, N.P. (1993). Radionuclide imaging in the evaluation of infections and inflammatory disease. *Radiologic Clinics of North America* **31**, 783–94.

Anand, A.J. and Glatt, A.E. (1994). *Salmonella* osteomyelitis and arthritis in sickle cell disease. *Seminars in Arthritis and Rheumatism* **24**, 211–21.

Bamberger, D.M. (1993). Osteomyelitis. A commonsense approach to antibiotic and surgical treatment. *Postgraduate Medicine* **94**, 177–84.

Berman, S. and Jensen, J. (1990). Cytomegalovirus-induced osteomyelitis in a patient with the acquired immunodeficiency syndrome. *Southern Medical Journal* **83**, 1231–2.

Bonhoeffer, J., Haeberle, B., Schaad, U.B., and Heininger, U. (2001). Diagnosis of acute haematogenous osteomyelitis and septic arthritis: 20 years experience at the University Children's Hospital Basel. *Swiss Medical Weekly* **131**, 575–81.

Bouza, E. and Muñoz, P. (1999). Microorganisms responsible for osteoarticular infections. *Bailliere's Clinical Rheumatology* **13**, 21–36.

Bouza, E. et al. (1992). Eficacia del cotrimoxazol en el tratgamiento de infecciones estafilocócicas graves. Abs 217 (Proceedings) V Congreso de la Sociedad Española de Enfermedades Infecciosas y Microbiología Clínica (SEIMC). Barcelona.

Brook, I. and Frazier, E.H. (1993). Anaerobic osteomyelitis and arthritis in a military hospital: a 10-year experience. *American Journal of Medicine* **94**, 21–8.

Bruck, J.C., Buttemeyer, R., Grabosch, A., and Gruhl, L. (1991). More arguments in favour of myocutaneous flaps for the treatment of pelvic pressure sores. *Annals of Plastic Surgery* **26**, 85–8.

Buchholz, H.W. et al. (1981). Management of deep infection of total hip replacement. *Journal of Bone and Joint Surgery (B)* **63**, 342.

Buchholz, H.W., von Foerster, G., and Heinert, K. (1984). Management of infected prostheses. *Orthopedics* **7**, 1620.

Cattaneo, R., Catagni, M., and Johnson, E.E. (1992). The treatment of infected nonunions and segmental defects of the tibia by the methods of Ilizarov. *Clinical Orthopedics* **280**, 143–52.

Ciampolini, J. and Harding, K.G. (2000). Pathophysiology of chronic bacterial osteomyelitis. Why do antibiotics fail so often? *Postgraduate Medical Journal* **898**, 479–83.

Cierny, G. and Mader, J.T. (1984). Adult chronic osteomyelitis. *Orthopedics* **7**, 1557.

Cierny, G. and Mader, J.T. (1989). Adult chronic osteomyelitis: an overview. In *Orthopaedic Infections* (ed. R.D. D'Ambrosia and R.L. Marier), pp. 31–47. Thorofare NJ: SLACK International.

Dunkle, L.M. and Brock, N. (1982). Long-term follow-up of ambulatory management of osteomyelitis. *Clinical Pediatrics* **21**, 650.

García Leuchuz, J., Bachiller, P., Vasalo, F.J., Muñoz, P., Padilla, B., amd Bouza, E. (1999). Group B streptococcal osteomyelitis in adults. *Medicine (Baltimore)* **78**, 191–9.

Gentry, L.O. and Rodríguez-Gomez, G. (1991). Ofloxacin versus parenteral therapy for chronic osteomyelitis. *Antimicrobial Agents and Chemotherapy* **35**, 538–41.

Griffith, J.F., Kumta, S.M., Leung, P.C., Cheng, J.C., Chow, I.T., and Metrewell, C. (2002). Imaging of musculoskeletal tuberculosis: a new look at old disease. *Clinical Orthopaedics* **398**, 32–9.

Guerrero, A. (1987). Estudio etiológico de las osteomielitis bacterianas. *Enfermedades Infecciosas Microbiología Clínica* **5**, 517–20.

Guerrero, A. (1989). Infecciones del aparato locomotor. In *Monografía en Comentarios a la Literatura en Enfermedades Infecciosas* Vol. 5 (2) (ed. E. Bouza), pp. 9–88. Madrid: CIMSA.

Holtom, P.D., Obuch, A.B., Ahlmann, E.R., Sheperd, L.E., and Patzakis, M.J. (2000). Mucormycosis of the tibia: a case report and review of the literature. *Clinical Orthopaedics* **381**, 222–8.

Hopkins, K.L., Li, K.C., and Bergman, G. (1995). Gadolinium-DTPA-enhanced magnetic resonance imaging of musculoskeletal infectious processes. *Skeletal Radiology* **24**, 325–30.

Howard, C.B., Einhorn, M., Dagan, R., and Yagupski, P. (1994). Fine-needle bone biopsy to diagnose osteomyelitis. *Journal of Bone and Joint Surgery (B)* **76**, 311.

Hudson, J.W. (1993). Osteomyelitis of the jaws: a 50-year perspective. *Journal of Oral and Maxillofacial Surgery* **51**, 1294–301.

Jellis, J. (2002). Surgery in the Tropics. In *Manson's Tropical Diseases* 21st edn., Chapter 24 (ed. G.C. Cook and A. Zumla). Edinburgh: Saunders.

Jellis, J., Mulla, Y., McSweeney, L., Forster, A., Youbo, C., and Mouritzen, L. (1995). Bone and joint tuberculosis and HIV disease. *East and Central African Journal of Surgery* **1** (2), 90–91.

Khan, K.M., Pao, W., and Kendler, J. (2001). Epidural abscess and vertebral osteomyelitis caused by *Listeria monocytogenes*: case report and literature review. *Scandinavian Journal of Infectious Diseases* **33**, 714–16.

Kothari, N.A., Pelchovitz, D.J., and Meyer, J.S. (2001). Imaging of musculoskeletal infections. *Radiological Clinics of North America* **39**, 619–51.

Kubler, P.A. and Klestov, A.C. (2001). Osteoarticular brucellosis with long latent period. *Clinical Rheumatology* **20**, 444–6.

Kutty, S., Bennett, D., Devitt, A., and Dowling, F.E. (2002). Tuberculous osteomyelitis of the sternum in an infant: a case report and review of the literature. *Paediatrics International* **44**, 186–8.

Mader, J.T., Shirtliff, M., and Calhoun, J.H. (1999). The host and the skeletal infection: classification and pathogenesis of acute bacterial and joint sepsis. *Baillieres Best Practice Research in Clinical Rheumatology* **1**, 1–20.

Miller, D.J. and Mejicano, G.C. (2001). Vertebral osteomyelitis due to *Candida* species: case report and literature review. *Clinical Infectious Diseases* **33**, 523–30.

Munoz, P. and Bouza, E. (1999). Acute and chronic adult osteomyelitis and prosthesis related infections. *Baillieres Best Practice Research in Clinical Rheumatology* **1**, 129–47.

Nepola, J.V., Seabold, J.E., Marsh, J.L., Kirchner, P.T., and el-Khoury, G.Y. (1993). Diagnosis of infection in ununited fractures. Combined imaging with indium-111-labeled leukocytes and technetium-^{99}m methylene diphosphonate. *Journal of Bone and Joint Surgery (A)* **75**, 1816–22.

Newman, L.G. et al. (1992). Leukocyte scanning with ^{111}In is superior to magnetic resonance imaging in diagnosis of clinically unsuspected osteomyelitis in diabetic foot ulcers. *Diabetes Care* **15**, 1527–30.

Spaeth, H.J. et al. (1991). Magnetic resonance imaging detection of early experimental periostitis. Comparison of magnetic resonance imaging, computed tomography, and plain radiography with histopathologic correlation. *Investigative Radiology* **26**, 304–8.

Stengel, D., Bauwens, K., Sehouli, J., Ekkernkamp, A., and Porzsolt, F. (2001). Systematic review and meta-analysis of antibiotic therapy for bone and joint infections. *Lancet Infectious Diseases* **3**, 175–88.

Unkila-Kallio, L., Kallio, M.J., Eskola, J., and Peltola, H. (1994). Serum C-reactive protein, erythrocyte sedimentation rate, and white blood cell count in acute hematogenous osteomyelitis of children. *Pediatrics* **93**, 59–62.

Vazquez, M. (2002). Osteomyelitis in children. *Current Opinion in Paediatrics* **14**, 112–15.

Voss, L.M., Rhodes, K.H., and Johnson, K.A. (1992). Musculoskeletal and soft tissue *Aeromonas* infection: an environmental disease. *Mayo Clinic Proceedings* **67**, 422–7.

Wang, Y.C. and Lee, S.T. (2001). Candida vertebral osteomyelitis: a case report and review of the literature. *Chang Gung Medical Journal* **12**, 810–15.

Wong, A.L., Sakamoto, K.M., and Johnson, E.E. (2001). Differentiating osteomyelitis from bone infarction in sickle cell disease. *Paediatric Emergency Care* **17**, 60–3.

6.2.4 Lyme disease

Gerd-Rüdiger Burmester, Thomas Kamradt, and Andreas Krause

Introduction

Lyme disease or Lyme borreliosis is a multisystem infectious disease that is endemic in large parts of Europe, North America, and Asia. The disease is caused by at least three species of the tick-borne spirochaete *Borrelia burgdorferi* sensu lato, namely *B. burgdorferi* sensu stricto, *B. garinii*, and *B. afzelii*. Lyme disease was first recognized as a clinical entity about 25 years ago because of a clustering of children with arthritis in the three contiguous communities of Lyme, Old Lyme, and East Haddam, Connecticut. It was soon realized that arthritis was only one manifestation of this systemic infection and that many of the clinical manifestations of Lyme disease had already been described in Europe in the first half of the twentieth century. Lyme borreliosis primarily affects the skin, the nervous system, and the joints, but many other organs may also be affected. There are some differences in the clinical presentation between Europe and the United States which may in part be explained by the local distribution and different organotropisms of the pathogenic *B. burgdorferi* species. Lyme disease is usually cured by antibiotic treatment in any disease stage. Therapy is easier and more successful the earlier it is started.

Epidemiology

Approximately 15 000 cases of Lyme disease are reported every year in the United States (Anonymous 2001). The distribution pattern of Lyme disease is highly focal with over 90 per cent of the cases reported from eight states along the Atlantic Coast and from Wisconsin. In these regions, the annual reported incidence may exceed 100 cases per 100 000 inhabitants. In some areas, such as Old Lyme, the incidence reaches 1000 cases per 100 000 inhabitants. The incidence in children aged 5–10 years is approximately twice as high as in adults (Anonymous 2001).

In Europe, the disease is most prevalent in Scandinavia and Central Europe. In southern Sweden, a population-based, prospective survey revealed an annual incidence of 69 cases per 100 000 population. In some areas of endimicity the annual incidence reached 160 per 100 000 (Berglund et al. 1995). A similar study in southern Germany found an annual incidence of 111 per 100 000 (Huppertz et al. 1999). In both European studies, the incidence in children was higher than in adults.

Aetiology

Lyme disease is caused by *B. burgdorferi* sensu lato, a gram-negative spirochaete. *B. burgdorferi* undergoes enzootic cycles between ixoid ticks—*Ixodes ricinus* in Europe and *I. scapularis* and *I. pacificus* in the United States—and small mammal reservoirs. The ixoid ticks may carry other pathogens such as Babesia, viruses (e.g. the FSME virus), or the agent of human granulocytic ehrlichiosis in addition to *B. burgdorferi*.

At least three species are human pathogens: *B. burgdorferi* sensu stricto, *B. garinii*, and *B. afzelii* (reviewed in Wang et al. 1999). The somewhat different clinical manifestations of Lyme disease in Europe and North America may be explained by the fact that only *B. burgdorferi* sensu stricto occurs in the United States whereas all three species occur in Europe. Furthermore, *B. garinii* or *B. afzelii* are more frequently isolated from European ticks than *B. burgdorferi* sensu stricto. The late dermatologic manifestation acrodermatitis chronica atrophicans (ACA) which is observed in Europe but rarely, if ever, in the United States was found to be mostly but not exclusively associated with *B. afzelii*. Neuroborreliosis is frequently caused by *B. garinii*. All three species can cause Lyme arthritis, which occurs both in Europe and North America (Lunemann et al. 2001; Steere 2001; Kamradt 2002).

The *B. burgdorferi* (strain B31) genome has been sequenced. A linear chromosome of approximately 920 000 base pairs (bp) contains 853 genes. In addition there are at least 17 linear and circular plasmids with another approximately 530 000 bp (Fraser et al. 1997). *B. burgdorferi* does not possess the enzymes necessary to synthesize LPS. Instead *B. burgdorferi* has approximately 130 genes coding for lipoproteins (Fraser et al. 1997). These proteins, which are anchored to *B. burgdorferi's* outer membrane via their lipid moieties are called outer surface proteins (Osps). The Osps are important for *B. burgdorferi's* lifecycle and pathogenicity because they are differentially expressed in different hosts. Environmental clues regulate the switch from OspA-expression to OspC-expression which seems to be important for the migration of *B. burgdorferi* from the tick's midgut to the salivary gland and for the subsequent invasion of the mammalian host.

Pathogenesis

Early infection and immune response

Upon transmission by an infected ixodes tick to a susceptible host, *B. burgdorferi* locally spreads in the skin. Within a few days, the spirochaetes disseminate via the blood stream and invade multiple organs, especially the central nervous system. Local spreading and dissemination is facilitated by a number of mechanisms including the activation of degrading host enzymes and the adhesion to various host extracellular-matrix proteins, glycosaminoglycans, and integrins. In addition, the recently detected induction of an array of matrix-metalloproteinases may contribute to both the invasion and destruction of host tissues by the spirochaetes (Steere 2001). Inflammation is primarily caused by the activation of monocytes and other cells of the innate immune system. This activation is caused chiefly by the binding of the spirochaetes' Osps to the Toll-like receptor (TLR)-2 on host cells such as macrophages resulting in the induction of proinflammatory cytokines and chemokines (Medzhitov and Janeway 2000). The adaptive immune response evolves more slowly and specific antiborrelial antibodies may not be detected in sera from patients with Lyme disease before 3–4 weeks after the infection. Lytic antibodies are critical for eradicating the spirochaetes. There is only limited cross-reactivity of antibodies between different species of *B. burgdorferi*. Therefore, the humoral immune response may not be protective and re-infections do occur even in patients with high antibody titres. Moreover, *B. burgdorferi* may evade the host's immune response and can cause chronic infections. It has been isolated from an ACA lesion more than 10 years after the initial symptoms (Steere 2001).

Lyme arthritis

The pathogenesis of Lyme arthritis is associated with the presence of spirochaetes in the affected joints except, perhaps, for the rare cases of treatment-resistant arthritides (see below). *B. burgdorferi* strongly activates not only infiltrating inflammatory cell such as monocytes and lymphocytes, but also resident fibroblasts are induced to produce various cytokines, chemokines, matrix-metalloproteinases, and adhesion molecules. This results in a strong local inflammatory reaction with proliferation and dense infiltration of the synovial membrane.

Although *B. burgdorferi* can only very rarely be isolated or cultured from joints, *B. burgdorferi* DNA may be detected by polymerase chain reaction (PCR) in synovial fluids and synovial tissues in more than 80 per cent of untreated patients with Lyme arthritis. It is of note that after successful antibiotic therapy, PCR for *B. burgdorferi* in synovial fluids rapidly becomes negative even in patients with ongoing arthritis after treatment. However, recent studies demonstrated *B. burgdorferi* DNA in synovial tissue of these patients, suggesting that intra-articular bacterial persistence plays an important pathogenetic role in chronic Lyme arthritis (Nocton et al. 1994; Priem et al. 1998; Carlson et al. 1999). Ultrastructural studies suggest that the spirochaetes may not only be found extracellularly, but may also persist within the cytoplasm of synovial cells (Steere 2001; Kamradt 2002).

Treatment-resistant Lyme arthritis

Most patients with Lyme arthritis respond to antibiotic therapy; however, in about 10 per cent of patients with Lyme arthritis the inflammation persists despite antibiotic therapy (Steere 2001). The synovial lesion in treatment-resistant Lyme arthritis resembles that of other chronic arthritides such as rheumatoid arthritis, including the formation of germinal centre like structures within the inflamed synovium (Steere 2001). Whereas children have a higher incidence of Lyme disease than adults, the incidence of treatment-resistant Lyme arthritis is lower in children than in adults. In Europe, both *B. burgdorferi* sensu stricto and *B. garinii* can cause treatment-resistant Lyme arthritis (Kamradt 2002).

Most patients with treatment-resistant Lyme arthritis yield consistently negative PCR results in synovial fluid and synovial tissue after antibiotic treatment (Nocton et al. 1994; Priem et al. 1998; Carlson et al. 1999). Therefore, host factors may be crucial for the pathogenesis of treatment-resistant Lyme arthritis (Steere 2001; Kamradt 2002). HLA–DR4 and the presence of antibodies or a T-cell response against OspA have been associated with a lack of response to antibiotic therapy. Therefore, the HLA–DR4-restricted response to *B. burgdorferi* OspA has been suspected to trigger chronic synovitis. Immunological cross-reactivity between OspA and a self-antigen has been suggested and refuted as cause of treatment-resistant Lyme arthritis (Steere 2001; Kamradt 2002). It has become clear that the idea that cross-reactivity between one particular microbial peptide and one particular self-peptide is indicative of pathogenicity is most likely too simple (Kamradt and Mitchison 2001).

An alternative explanation for the development of treatment-resistant Lyme arthritis would be hypersensitivity that develops to traces of persistent antigen. Cytokines such as IL-1β, IL-6, IL-10, IL-11, or IL-12 that are produced by cells of the innate immune system have been implicated in the regulation of arthritis severity in patients or animal models (Kamradt 2002). *B. burgdorferi* lipoproteins such as OspA strongly activate cells of the innate immune system via their binding of TLR-2. Thus, *B. burgdorferi* induces in host cells the production of IL-1β, IL-6, IL-10, IL-12, and TNF-α. *B. burgdorferi*-OspA via its activation of the innate immune system both in mice and in humans also induces the differentiation of Th cells that produce IL-17 (Infante-Duarte et al. 2000). IL-17, in turn induces the production of IL-6 and other proinflammatory mediators. This reciprocal enhancement of IL-17 and IL-6 could therefore fuel chronic synovitis. Alltogether, it is likely that antigen-non-specific mechanisms mediate, perhaps in synergy with antigen-specific mechanisms, the immunopathology that finally leads to treatment-resistant Lyme arthritis in susceptible patients (Steere 2001; Kamradt 2002).

Clinical manifestations

The clinical manifestations of Lyme disease have been reviewed in a recent series of excellent reviews (Nadelman and Wormser 1998; Sigal 1998; Shapiro and Gerber 2000; Steere 2001).

Lyme disease is traditionally grouped into three stages (localized, stage 1; early disseminated, stage 2; late or chronic, stage 3) (Table 1). However, the illness does not necessarily develop in stages. It may manifest in any of these stages and earlier stages may be skipped, missed by the patients, or coincide with later states. In our experience, only one-third of patients with Lyme arthritis remembers a tick bite and less have experienced an erythema migrans, the initial lesion. This appears to be especially true in European patients. Moreover, the differentiation into localized and disseminated infection is questionable since even in patients with a single localized erythema migrans the borreliae may already have spread haematologically. Therefore, from a pragmatic standpoint it is more useful to discriminate between patients with early (erythema migrans), acute extracutaneous (neurological, non-neurological, especially carditis, early arthritis) and late forms or chronic disease (arthritis, acrodermatitis). Even though only Lyme arthritis lies within the medical domain of rheumatologists, frequently this specialty is also confronted with the other manifestations of Lyme borreliosis. This can happen either in retrospect to search for initial symptoms or because the rheumatologist dealing with Lyme disease is visited by potential Lyme patients, especially those suffering from neurological symptoms or for the differential diagnosis of fibromyalgia and chronic fatigue syndrome. Therefore, rheumatologists are confronted with all manifestations of Lyme disease.

The clinical manifestations of Lyme borreliosis are similar worldwide and will be described in detail below. However, there are some regional variations in frequency and appearance of certain symptoms between Europe/Eurasia and America that are summarized in a simplified form in Table 1.

Early Lyme borreliosis

Early Lyme disease has two typical features: firstly, the characteristic erythema migrans, and, secondly, systemic constitutional signs with low-grade fever, constitutional symptoms, arthralgias, malaise, headaches, and paraesthesias which may accompany erythema migrans or occur without a recognized skin lesion. Headaches and paraesthesias may reflect early neurological dissemination. These constitutional signs may vary from day to day, and symptoms such as fatigue and lethargy may recur for months, independent of the initial skin lesion. Since these features are non-characteristic and many patients have not recognized a tick bite or experienced an erythema migrans, the diagnosis of early Lyme disease is frequently missed or can only be assumed in retrospect.

Erythema migrans starts as a red macule or papule at the site of the tick bite. After an incubation period of a few days up to 8 weeks, the lesions gradually expands—sometimes reaching a size so large that the margins of an erythema originating at the abdomen may meet in the back of the patient. However, sometimes the lesion is small in diameter, and in these cases it is difficult to discriminate it from a hyperergicic 'insect' bite lesion. The typical lesion is flat, red or bluish-red, and non-scaling. In Europe, less often in America, lesions lasting for a longer period will clear in the central part leaving a demarcated ring and a small red spot inside where the initial tick bite had taken place [Plate 93(a) and (b)]. The centre may be flat, sometimes indurated, vesicular, or necrotic. However, erythema migrans may also manifest as a faint diffuse reddening, which can only be recognized upon application of heat such as after a warm bath. Except for an occasional itching or burning, there are usually no further symptoms which alert the patient so that the lesion may go unrecognized, especially if the redness is not very marked or the skin manifestation occurs at the back or at hairy sites. The typical site of the erythema are those locations, where the ticks have been stopped by mechanical barriers such as the belt region, the posterior thigh, popliteal fossa, or hairy areas such as the groin, axilla, or hair on the head, especially in children. Even without antibiotic treatment, erythema migrans will resolve within 4–12 weeks; however, in many cases bacteria will persist at other sites and will cause subsequent Lyme manifestations.

Half of the American patients develop multiple secondary erythema skin lesions within days of the tick bite, which is rather rare in Europe. An additional dermatological manifestation in the early phase is the lymphocytoma cutis, especially in Europe, usually presenting as a purplish nodule at the ear lobe, the nose, the forehead or at the nipple [Plate 93(c)]. In the latter case it may be mixed up with gynaecomasty in male patients. Histologically, this lesion is characterized by germinal centers surrounded by lymphohistiocytic cells. Interestingly, European investigators had shown in the 1960s that both the erythema migrans and the lymphocytoma contain infectious organisms by transfer experiments to normal volunteers.

The differential diagnosis of the erythema migrans includes all other erythematous skin diseases such as erythema gyratum repens, erythema anulare, and the erythema necrolyticum migrans. There are usually no laboratory abnormalities in early Lyme disease except for rare elevations of the ESR, mild anaemia, leucocytosis, and slight elevations of liver enzymes. At this stage of the disease, only 50 per cent of patients develop serological signs of a *B. burgdorferi* infection (see later).

Table 1 Clinical manifestations of Lyme borreliosis in Eurasia and North America [Modified after Steere (2001) and Gray et al. (2002)]

Organ system	Clinical feature	Europe/Eurasia (*B. afzelii, B. garinii, B. burgdorferi* ss)	North America (*B. burgdorferi* ss)
Skin			
Acute phase	Erythema migrans	Slower spreading, less intensely inflamed, and of longer duration; less frequent haematogeneous dissemination, but possible regional or contiguous spread to other sites	Central clearing <35%; systemic symptoms common; frequent, possibly widespread haematogeneous dissemination
	Borrelial lymphocytoma	Rarely and predominantly seen in children and scarcely in adults	None reported
Chronic phase	Acrodermatitis chronica atrophicans	Caused primarily by *B. afzelii*	Rarely reported
	Circumscribed scleroderma and Lichen sclerosus et atrophicus	Reports about the isolation of *B. afzelii* from lesional skin and improvement after antibiotic therapy in single cases	None reported
Nervous system			
Acute phase	Meningopolyradiculoneuritis (Bannwarth) Cranial nerve palsy	Severe radicular pain, meningitis more severe in children, intrathecal pleocytosis and antibody production, caused primarily by *B. garinii*	Meningitis, less prominent radiculoneuritis
Chronic phase	Encephalitis Encephalomyelitis Cerebral vasculitis Peripheral neuropathy	Subtle sensory neuropathy within areas affected by acrodermatitis Severe encephalomyelitis, spasticity, cognitive abnormalities, marked intrathecal antibody production	Subtle sensory polyneuropathy without acrodermatitis Subtle encephalopathy, cognitive disturbance, slight intrathecal antibody production
Heart			
Acute phase	Carditis	Atrioventricular block and subtle myocarditis	Atrioventricular block and subtle myocarditis
Chronic phase	Dilated cardiomyopathy	Isolation of *B. burgdorferi* s.l. from endomyocardial biopsies in only a few cases	None reported
Musculoskeletal			
Acute phase	Arthritis	Less frequent oligoarticular arthritis, less intense joint inflammation	More frequent oligoarticular arthritis, more intense joint inflammation
Chronic phase	Arthritis Myositis Bursitis	Persistent arthritis less frequent	Treatment-resistant arthritis in about 10% of patients, probably due to immunopathologic mechanism
Antibody response		Expansion of response to fewer borrelial antigens	Expansion of response to many borrelial antigens

Acute extracutaneous and chronic Lyme disease

Neurological manifestations

In a minority of patients (about 15 per cent), typical neurological symptoms develop within weeks or months after the tick bite: cranial neuropathy (most commonly involving the facial nerve), meningitis, especially in children, and radiculoneuropathy alone or in combination. The rare manifestations of chronic neurological Lyme disease occurring months to years after infection include demyelinating encephalopathy or myelopathy, chronic encephalopathy, cerebral vasculitis, peripheral polyneuropathy, and transverse myelitis.

The earlier neurological manifestations are characterized by two major entities: the radiculoneuropathy (if accompanied by meningitis termed Bannwarth's syndrome) and facial palsy or other cranial nerve lesions. Radiculoneuropathy is usually a very painful acute condition frequently with a significant increase of pain at night. It may affect any dermatome or several contiguous dermatomes and is frequently mixed up with a 'slipped disc' even prompting surgery. Further symptoms include paraesthesia, sensory deficits and motor weakness.

Facial palsy may even be bilateral, especially in children. It may occur when the erythema migrans is still present or subsequently after a few weeks. A relationship to Lyme disease in endemic areas should especially be considered in children and in tick exposed individuals such as forest workers, housewives working in the garden, farmers, and hunters. Even in these risk groups, however, idiopathic facial palsy is more prevalent than Lyme-associated neuropathy; clinically, however, a distinction is not possible. Other manifestations include the paresis of the abducent nerve (5 per cent). Lyme meningitis is usually found in children and is characterized by initial headaches, additional signs of mild encephalopathy and neck stiffness, while overt meningism is rare. All acute manifestations may eventually remit without treatment, however, in a significant number of patients mild symptoms may last for years in non-treated patients.

In rare cases, chronic varieties of neuroborreliosis occur. These include distal symmetric polyneuropathy (often associated with acrodermatitis), mononeuritis multiplex, stroke-like disorders, chronic encephalitis, encephalomyelitis, or meningoencephalomyelitis. The latter are characterized by slowly progressive courses with increasing spastic para-, tetraparesis or hemiparesis. Other manifestations include cognitive defects, memory loss, and concentration deficits. The diagnosis has to be made with great caution and under strict criteriae since especially the latter symptoms are difficult to discriminate from neuropsychiatric or neurotic diseases, and particularly in the latter cases patients consult rheumatologists for the treatment of self-diagnosed 'chronic lyme disease'.

In all suspected cases of neuroborreliosis, cerebrospinal fluid analysis is necessary to establish the diagnosis. This is characterized by a lymphocytic pleocytosis with a cell number up to 1000/μl, elevated protein levels (1–2 g/l) and an intrathecal Ig production. This immune response is directed against *B. burgdorferi* as shown by a relatively increased Ig production compared to blood values. However, in early cases of neuroborreliosis, spinal fluid findings may still be negative, and in cases of chronic disease only mild elevations of protein may persist. Especially in these circumstances, detection of *B. burgdorferi* DNA by PCR may be important to establish the diagnosis.

Ocular manifestations of Lyme disease

Ophthalmological changes can occur in all disease stages. These include a conjunctivitis in early disease and upon dissemination all varieties of a uveitis (anterior, intermedia and posterior and panuveitis) are possible. Meningitis may lead to a papillar oedema. In the chronic stage uveitis, keratitis and episcleritis may evolve. Therefore, in endemic areas, infection with *B. burgdorferi* must be considered in these cases. Moreover, upon routine eye examination in rheumatological cases ocular manifestations may be an incidental finding, especially monocular chorioiditis with no apparent symptoms. The recognition of Lyme borreliosis as a cause of ocular conditions is important since a causative treatment with antibiotics usually results in the resolution of the disease.

Carditis

Lyme carditis is a rather rare entity occurring in about 5 per cent of patients. It frequently develops after a preceding erythema migrans. Many patients also have neurological symptoms and arthralgias. Typical manifestations are conduction abnormalities with varying degrees of atrioventricular block, right or left bundle block, atrial fibrillations or tachycardias. Lyme carditis should be particularly suspected in younger individuals without apparent other risk factors. Rare incidences of a chronic Lyme carditis have been described in Europe only resulting in cardiomyopathy even with a fatal course. However, usually cardiac involvement subsides spontaneously within a few weeks and does not recur. Histologically, Lyme carditis is characterized by transmural lymphoplasmacellular infiltrates, interstitial fibrosis, occasional necrosis, and fibrinous pericarditis. Spirochaetes have been successfully cultured out of cardiac biopsies. Therapy is symptomatic plus antibiotic treatment which usually results in a prompt resolution, in the case of conduction abnormalities steroids have been added.

Articular manifestations

In America, arthritis is the predominat manifestation of disseminated *B. burgdorferi* infection with about 60 per cent of untreated patients developing joint manifestations usually weeks to years after the initial infection. In Europe, a lesser proportion of patients experience arthritis which may either occur in early disseminated disease or, more typically, in late disease stages. Nevertheless, the onset of arthritis is acute making the differential diagnosis to other acutely occurring arthritides difficult. In our experience, only a minority of patients will remember a tick bite, and in Europe only few individuals have had an erythema migrans. Moreover, other manifestations of disseminated infection are usually missing, and arthritis may be the sole presentation of Lyme disease. Therefore, the diagnosis of Lyme arthritis is one of the most challenging in rheumatology.

The clinical course is usually intermittent with acute attacks with transient seeming 'remissions' and left untreated may go on for months and years. In most cases, there is a mono- or oligoarticular course predominantly affecting the knees, ankles, and sometimes ellbows usually with massive effusions. In some cases, there is no overt arthritis, and the disease is characterized by non-specific arthralgias, myalgias, and periarticular pain making the differential diagnosis difficult with regard to functional syndromes and fibromyalgia, especially in seropositive individuals living in endemic areas.

Clinical manifestations of frank arthritis are usually non-specific with effusions, pain, and movement restriction. Popliteal (Baker's) cysts are common, and—if present—dactylitis and Achilles tendon involvement can be helpful as diagnostic signs, if reactive arthritis, psoriatic arthritis, or spondyloarthropathies have been ruled out. Involvement of the sacroiliac joints or the spine do not occur in Lyme borreliosis and therefore are most valuable to differentiate Lyme arthritis from the latter arthritides. Otherwise, Lyme arthritis cannot be distinguished from reactive arthritis or other acutely presenting oligoarticular diseases on clinical grounds alone. Joint fluid analysis usually shows non-specific inflammatory changes with a cell count of about 25 000 cells/mm^3, predominantly granulocytes. Histological investigations of the synovial membrane have concentrated on chronic cases and have documented rheumatoid arthritis like changes with a hyperplasia of the lining and lymphocytic infiltration. While it is generally not possible to culture *B. burgdorferi* from intra-articular sites, PCR analysis of the joint fluid and synovial biopsies have shown the presence of spirochaetes. Therefore, PCR investigations may be helpful in unclear cases (see below).

The prognosis of the disease is usually good. Joint destruction even in long-standing cases is rare. After adequate therapy, more than 80 per cent of patients are cured already after a single course of antibiotic therapy. In some patients repeated therapy is necessary. The success of antibiotic treatment often cannot be evaluated before several weeks after completion of treatment since symptoms usually fade slowly and complete recovery may take several months.

However, there is a small proportion of patients who do not respond even to repeated courses of antibiotic treatment. In our (European) experience, these therapy-resistant courses are rare while in America a proportion of 10 per cent has been described. The incidence is lower in children than in adults. Treatment with steroids, especially given intra-articularly, before adequate antibiotic treatment significantly increases the risk of developing treatment-resistant Lyme arthritis. While some of these cases may be driven by intra-articular persistence of *B. burgdorferi*, there is some evidence that others are maintained by infection-induced immunopathology including autoimmune mechanisms.

Differential diagnosis

A remarkable finding in Lyme arthritis is the frequent absence of systemic inflammatory signs. Thus, despite massive effusions ESR and CRP-values are usually normal with the exception of occasional patients. Therefore, if, for example, a knee swelling is the initial symptom especially in a younger athletic person, acute meniscopathy may be a wrong diagnosis if Lyme arthritis is not considered. On the other hand, reactive arthritis is normally characterized by significant elevations of the ESR and CRP. In contrast to spondyloarthropathies, Lyme arthritis is not associated with HLA-B27 and axial involvement is missing. In severe cases of Lyme arthritis, rheumatoid factor and antinuclear antibodies may be positive making the differential diagnosis of Lyme diseases difficult, especially in rare cases of a polyarticular or erosive disease course. An important disease to consider is Loefgren's syndrome frequently presenting with an acute arthritis of the lower extremeties. The erythema nodosum and bihilar lymphadenopathy will help to distinguish this condition from Lyme arthritis.

Extra-articular manifestations in the musculoskeletal system

Compared to arthritis, other rheumatological manifestations are much rarer. These consist of tenosynovitis and bursitis. Despite frequent myalgias, overt myositis or dermatomyositis have been described only in rare cases; they could, however, be confirmed by a positive culture out of a muscle biopsy. Also three cases of a polymyalgia like disease have been reported after an erythema migrans with a good reponse to antibiotic therapy. In contrast to these rare cases, fibromyalgia developing after Lyme disease has been the focus of many investigations. Thorough studies have now demonstrated that there is no evidence of a persistent infection, and even prolonged antibiotic therapy does not help to resolve this disorder. Moreover, the generalized pain, trigger points, fatigue, sleep disturbances, and other constitutional symptoms are clearly different from the arthritic pain in Lyme disease. Therefore, a previous infection with *B. burgdorferi* does not appear to rarely cause chronic unspecific symptoms leading to the so-called post-Lyme syndrome or to be just one of many triggers causing fibromyalgia, and does not affect the course or the therapeutic options in this condition. However, misdiagnosis of fibromyalgia as Lyme borreliosis has led to an extensive overdiagnosis of Lyme disease and antibiotic overtreatment, especially in America. The controversies about fibromyalgia, chronic fatigue syndrome, and Lyme disease clearly point out the diagnostic difficulties in endemic areas where more than 10 per cent of the normal population are seropositive and patients with difficult to treat conditions seek alternative explanations for the course of the disease.

Acrodermatitis chronica atrophicans

Chronic borreliosis of the skin is a rare event in America, but quite common in untreated European patients. ACA (see section on 'Aetiology') occurs after more than 12 months after the initial infection and is characterized by a unilateral extended distal atrophic skin lesion frequently preceded by an oedematous violaceous stage. Typical is the cigarette paper like appearance with a wrinkled violet thin skin without hairs and with translucent veins [Plate 93(d)]. Frequently, it is associated with pain in the joints underneath the skin lesion (usually the PIP joints or toes) and is, therefore, sometimes called 'arthrodermatitis'. Other symptoms are paraesthesias indicating an underlying vasculitis of the vasa nervorum and juxta-articular nodules, especially at the knees, ellbows and along the ulna. Rare complication of ACA include squamous cell carcinoma and B cell lymphoma of the skin. Diagnosis is quite easy due to the typical skin manifestation and usually an extremely marked immune response upon serology. If recognized early, treatment results in a resolution of the skin lesion, however, in prolonged cases atrophic changes may remain.

Diagnosis

A typical erythema migrans may be diagnosed only by appearance. In all other cases the diagnosis of Lyme borreliosis is based on clinical grounds and supported by laboratory analyses, especially Lyme serology. A history of tick exposure or a tick bite in an area that is endemic for Lyme disease, symptoms characteristic for, or at least compatible with, Lyme disease and the detection of specific antibodies against *B. burgdorferi* are the most important diagnostic hallmarks. In Lyme neuroborreliosis, the diagnosis may be confirmed by the detection of CNS pleocytosis and of an intrathecal antibody production against borrelial antigens. In contrast, in Lyme arthritis it is difficult to establish the diagnosis. Patients usually present with unspecific symptoms and often do not remember having had specific early Lyme manifestations. The direct detection of the spirochaete is still difficult, and therefore it is only possible to give the likely diagnosis of Lyme arthritis after having ruled out other forms of arthritis.

The European Concerted Action Against Lyme Borreliosis (EUCALB) and the Centers for Disease Control (CDC) have published case definitions for Lyme disease, which combine clinical and laboratory data (URL: http://www.dis.strath.ac.uk/vie/LymeEU/) (Anonymous 1990; Smith et al. 1998). These may be used for public health surveillance and studies on Lyme disease.

Serology

Serology is usually performed when Lyme disease is suspected. The standard procedure is to start with an ELISA and use Western blotting for the confirmation of positive ELISA results (Anonymous 1990; Sigal 1998; Steere 2001). IgM antibodies against *B. burgdorferi* first become detectable 3–4 weeks after the infection, peak after 6–8 weeks, and decline subsequently. IgG antibodies appear 6–8 weeks after the infection and remain detectable for many years (Steere 2001). For diagnostic purposes it is important to keep in mind that both IgG and IgM responses can persist for over 10 years even after successful antibiotic treatment (Steere 2001).

The sensitivity, specificity, and reproducibility of the currently available commercial tests are poor. The CDC have published guidelines for test performance and interpretation for the serologic diagnosis of Lyme disease (CDC 1995) and the American College of Physicians has issued recommendations for the cost-effective use of serological testing (Nichol et al. 1998). Serological testing is not clinically useful if the pretest probability of Lyme disease is less than 0.20 or greater than 0.80.

Whereas Lyme disease is uniformly caused by *B. burgdorferi* sensu stricto in the United States, three different species of *B. burgdorferi* sensu lato cause Lyme disease in Europe. This more diverse microbiological aetiology results not only in different clinical manifestations but also in very different serologic response to *B. burgdorferi*. Therfore, there are currently no generally accepted diagnostic criteria for Lyme disease in Europe.

Asymptomatic infection

In areas endemic for Lyme disease, many inhabitants are seropositive yet lack any history or symptoms of Lyme disease (Steere 2001). The frequency of asymptomatic infection may be considerable and further complicates the interpretation of serological data. During the 2-year observation period of the clinical trial of the Lyme vaccine, 137 of the placebo recipients seroconverted on Western blotting. Twenty-eight of those (20 per cent) did not show any clinical symptoms of Lyme disease (Steere et al. 1998). A retrospective Swedish study even found that more than half of the people who were seropositive by ELISA could not recall any symptoms suggestive of Lyme disease (Gustafson et al. 1990).

Culture, DNA detection

The culture of *B. burgdorferi* from patient specimens would prove the diagnosis of Lyme disease. Unfortunately, it is extremely difficult to perform and rarely attempted for diagnostic purposes, except for unclear skin manifestations of Lyme borreliosis (Steere 2001). *B. burgdorferi* DNA can be detected by PCR in synovial fluid (Nocton et al. 1994) or synovial tissue (Priem et al. 1998) from patients with Lyme arthritis, and in the CSF from patients with early CNS manifestations of Lyme disease (Nocton et al. 1996). However, PCR-detection of *B. burgdorferi* DNA is currently not considered a routine method, partly because there is considerable interlaboratory variation in the results (Steere 2001).

Prevention and treatment

Exposure prophylaxis

Prophylactic measures to avoid tick bites include simple physical measures such as wearing long sleeves and long pants that are tucked into the socks, the complete avoidance of wooded areas, and drastic measures such as area application of insecticides. One popular recommendation is the use of tick and insect repellents. However, to maintain effectiveness, DEET (*N,N*-diethylmetatoluamide)-containing repellents need to be applied every 1–2 h. Moreover, their use may result in severe complications, including encephalopathy, seizures, coma, and death in children (Kamradt 2002). Permethrin kills ticks and can be sprayed on clothing but skin exposure should be avoided due to its possible carcinogenicity. In infested areas, daily careful screening for tick bites seems to be the most realistic and useful prophylactic measure (Steere 2001). Experimental and observational data indicate that transmission of *B. burgdorferi* occurs only after ticks have been attached to the host for at least 24–50 h (Kamradt 2002). Persons who have been bitten by a tick should be informed about early Lyme disease manifestations and advised to seek immediate treatment in case of the development of respective symptoms.

Immunization

Immunization with several different *B. burgdorferi* proteins including OspA can induce protective antibody responses in experimental animals. The protection induced by immunization with OspA has a unique mode of action. When a tick feeds on an immunized host the serum antibodies against OspA kill the spirochaetes in the tick's midgut (Fikrig et al. 1992). A vaccine consisting of recombinant lipidated OspA was found to be safe and effective in a large clinical trial involving more than 10 000 participants aged 15–70 years who lived in areas of the United States where Lyme disease is endemic (Steere et al. 1998). This vaccine has since been approved by the FDA for use in persons older than 16 years. However, the manufacturing company discontinued producing the vaccine in February 2002 because of non-medical reasons.

Clinical and experimental studies gave rise to concerns that an immune response against OspA might be detrimental and could perhaps trigger autoimmune synovitis (Steere 2001; Kamradt 2002). In two clinical trials there was no significant increases in the frequency of arthritis in vaccinees (Sigal et al. 1998; Steere et al. 1998). The recent experience with a rotavirus vaccine illustrates that very rare side-effects of any vaccine cannot be detected even in careful clinical studies (Anonymous 1999). However, approximately 1.5 million doses of the OspA vaccine have been administered to date and there was no post-licensure discovery of a serious adverse effect. Thus, there is currently no indication that the vaccine might provoke arthritis.

The OspA vaccine is not licensed in Europe. In contrast to the United States where Lyme disease is exclusively caused by *B. burgdorferi* sensu stricto, *B. burgdorferi* sensu stricto, *B. garinii*, and *B. afzelii* all cause Lyme disease in Europe. The OspA-sequence heterogeneity among European isolates prevents the effectiveness of the OspA vaccine which is based on one single sequence from *B. burgdorferi* sensu stricto. Currently, there is no vaccine against Lyme borreliosis available in Europe.

Secondary prevention

The risk of acquiring *B. burgdorferi* infection through a tick bite is low and varies between 1.2 and 3.2 per cent. It increases, however, to greater than 25 per cent when someone has been bitten by an infected tick (Maiwald et al. 1998). Transmissions hardly occur within the first 24 h of the tick bite and can only take place when the tick had at least partially become engorged with blood. Weighing the low risk and the possible side-effects of doxycycline treatment, the Infectious Diseases Society of America has published a recommendation that antibiotic treatment should not routinely be administered to tick-bitten persons (Wormser et al. 2000). In a study, which was performed in Westchester County, NY, where the incidence of Lyme disease is probably the highest in the world, one dose of 200 mg doxycycline p.o. administered within 72 h after a tick bite was 87 per cent effective in preventing Lyme disease (Nadelman et al. 2001). Importantly, of the placebo recipients in this study, only 3 per cent developed Lyme disease. Forty doses of doxycycline had to be administered to prevent one case of Lyme disease. This number would be higher in areas with a lower incidence of Lyme disease. The efficacy of prophylactic doxycycline administration is further reduced by the fact that most cases of Lyme disease result from unrecognized tick bites. However, the observation period in that study was only 6 weeks and the first symtoms of Lyme disease may occur much later after a tick bite. Taken together, routine antibiotic prophylaxis is not recommended. Individuals with tick bites should be stratified according to their risk to be infected by borreliae. Only in those rare patients who have really been bitten by a tick and not, for example, by an insect, and with high infection risk (i.e. nymphal tick from an endemic area, long duration of tick attachment, ticks at least partially engorged) antibiotic prophylaxis may be considered.

Treatment

There is no need to treat persons with positive Lyme serology but without any symptoms of Lyme disease. Treatment decisions should always be based on clinical signs. All manifestations of Lyme borreliosis should be treated antibiotically so as to shorten the clinical course and prevent the progression of the disease. Detailed and essentially comparable recommendations have been issued by EUCALB (URL: http://www.dis.strath.ac.uk/vie/LymeEU/) and by the Infectious Disease Society of America (Wormser et al. 2000). Therapeutic decisions depend on duration, stage, and symptoms of the disease. Amoxicillin, doxycycline, and third-generation cephalosporins are the drugs of choice (Nadelman and Wormser 1998; Sigal 1998; Shapiro and Gerber 2000; Steere 2001). Doxycycline has the advantage of being also effective against the agent of human granulocytic ehrlichiosis, which may be co-transmitted by ticks. In early infections, azithromycin and oral cephalosporines are also effective and may serve as alternatives if the first line drugs are contraindicated. However, their efficacy has not been proven in later disease stages. Penicillin G is also recommended for disseminated infections but has the disadvantage of short dosage intervals. Erythromycin is less effective than the recommended compounds and therefore regarded as the last choice. Treatment duration ranges from 2 to 4 weeks. Details are given in Table 2.

Uncomplicated Lyme arthritis, that is, without neurologic or any other organ manifestations, may be treated orally with amoxicillin or doxycycline. However, one study found the subsequent development of neuroborreliosis in patients treated with doxycycline but not in those primarily treated with ceftriaxone. If the oral regimen was not effective, which may occur in some 20 per cent of patients, or in cases with symptoms of neurologic or other organ involvement, parenteral therapy with ceftriaxone or cefotaxime should be given. In patients with persistent symptoms, a second parenteral antibiotic therapy should be given, again following the evaluated approaches for parenteral treatment. There is no need to change the drug since borreliae do not become resistant to any of the recommended antibiotics. Likewise, other therapeutic regimens like high-dose pulse therapy or long-term antibiotic treatment are neither necessary nor evaluated and may be associated with a substantial risk of serious side-effects.

Using the recommended therapeutic approach the prognosis of Lyme disease is excellent. Almost all early infections are rapidly cured without sequelae. In later disease stages, especially in Lyme arthritis, symptoms often wane slowly and clinical improvement is observed only several weeks after therapy. It should be kept in mind that there are several potential reasons for treatment failures or incomplete responses to therapy including misdiagnosis and irreversable tissue damage caused by the infection. However, about 10 per cent of patients with Lyme arthritis in the United States and probably a smaller percentage of European patients do not respond sufficiently even to repeated courses of antibiotic treatment. The pathogenesis of this so-called treatment-resistant Lyme arthritis has not been fully elucidated yet but there is some evidence that infection-induced immunopathology plays a major role in most of these cases. Since no controlled therapeutic studies, for example, with disease modifying antirheumatic drugs, have been performed yet, symptomatic treatment with anti-inflammatory agents should be given. In patients with persistent monarthritis, especially with proliferative synovitis, synovectomy can be beneficial.

Clinical problems arise in a small percentage of patients who have been appropriately treated for Lyme disease but still complain about multiple, mostly unspecific symptoms including fatigue, myalgias, arthralgias, and cognitive impairement. This so-called 'post-Lyme disease syndrome' may be severely disabling with a substantially reduced health-related quality of life and has many features in common with the chronic fatigue syndrome and fibromyalgia. The frequency, pathogenesis, diagnosis, and treatment of this syndrome have been a highly contentious issue for more than a decade.

Table 2 Treatment of Lyme borreliosis

Condition	Drug	Dose/day (dosages for children[a])	Duration
Early infection	Doxycycline	1 × 200 mg or 2 × 100 mg orally	14 days
	Amoxicillin	3 × 500–750 mg or 2 × 1000 mg orally (50 mg/kg)	14 days
	Azithromycin[b]	2 × 500 mg orally	1st day
		500 mg	2nd to 5th day
	Cefuroxime acetyl[b]	2 × 500 mg orally	14 days
Acute neuroborreliosis[c]	Ceftriaxone	1 × 2 g i.v. (50 mg/kg)	14–21 days
	Cefotaxime	3 × 2 g i.v. (100 mg/kg)	14–21 days
	Penicillin G	4 × 5 MioU i.v. (500 000 U/kg)	14–21 days
	Doxycycline[d]	1 × 200 mg or 2 × 100 mg orally	14–21 days
Carditis[e]	Ceftriaxone	1 × 2 g i.v.	14 days
	Cefotaxime	3 × 2 g i.v.	14 days
	Penicillin G	4 × 5 MioU i.v.	14 days
Arthritis Acrodermatitis	Doxycycline	1 × 200 mg or 2 × 100 mg orally	30 (–40) days
	Amoxicillin	3 × 500–750 mg or 2 × 1000 mg orally	30 (–40) days
	Ceftriaxone	1 × 2 g i.v.	14–21 days
	Cefotaxime	3 × 2 g i.v.	14–21 days
Lyme borreliosis during pregnancy	Amoxicillin	3 × 500–750 mg or 2 × 1000 mg orally	14–21 days
	Penicillin G	4 × 5 MioU i.v.	14–21 days
	Ceftriaxone[f]	1 × 2 g i.v.	14 days
	Cefotaxime[f]	3 × 2 g i.v.	14 days

[a] Dosages for adults are the maximum dosages.

[b] Only in cases of doxycyclin and amoxicillin allergy or contraindications.

[c] In chronic neuroborreliosis i.v. therapy only for 14–28 days.

[d] Only in cases with facial palsy alone.

[e] In patients with first degree atrioventricular block oral therapy for 14–21 days may be sufficient.

[f] Should be used with caution in the first trimester because of lack of data on safety.

However, a number of recently published studies demonstrated that the risk of developing a post-Lyme syndrome is low. When persons who had had Lyme disease were compared to an age-matched group of persons who had not had this infection the general health status was good in both groups and patients reported about an array of chronic complains with comparable frequency. Only patients with early nervous system involvement and without or delayed antibiotic treatment appear to more often have residual neurologic deficits and pain. Moreover, patients who had had Lyme arthritis more frequently reported about knee pain than the control subjects (Kalish et al. 2001).

There are no diagnostic criteria for the post-Lyme disease syndrome yet. This diagnostic uncertainty together with a widespread irrational anxiety about the risk of chronic sequelae from Lyme disease often lead to an overdiagnosis of chronic Lyme borreliosis or the post-Lyme syndrome in patients with unspecific symptoms. Even worse, certain physicians' and patients' groups have stirred up the fear, and published by various media including the Internet, a number of unsubstantiated therapeutic recommendations mostly consisting of long-term antibiotic regimens, sometimes even with combination therapies. Two recently published studies tested the effect of a long-term therapy in patients with well documented Lyme disease and who had various persisting symptoms despite an average of three previous antibiotic courses. Patients received either 2 g ceftriaxone daily for 30 days followed by 200 mg doxycycline daily for another 60 days or placebo. The study was stopped prematurely after the first 107 patients had been evaluated because there was no difference between the treatment group and the placebo group and therefore it was highly unlikely that even this massive antibiotic therapy was of any benefit. Taken together, especially in patients with late stages of Lyme disease it may be necessary to give two or sometimes even three antibiotic courses with the antibiotics, dosages, and durations recommended above (Klempner et al. 2001). Despite this therapy, there is a small group of patients with ongoing, so-called treatment-resistant arthritis or various, sometimes disabling symptoms of the post-Lyme syndrome. While we do not know the optimum treatment for these patients yet it is obvious that prolonged antibiotic treatment should be avoided since it is not only ineffective, but also expensive and burdened with a number of severe and sometimes lethal side-effects.

References

Anonymous (1990). Case definitions for public health surveillance. Lyme disease. *Morbidity and Mortality Weekly Reports* **39 (RR-13)**, 19–21.

Anonymous (1999). Intussusception among recipients of rotavirus vaccine—United States, 1998–1999. *Morbidity and Mortality Weekly Reports* **48**, 577–81.

Anonymous (2001). Lyme disease—United States, 1999. *Morbidity and Mortality Weekly Reports* **50**, 181–5.

Berglund, J. et al. (1995). An epidemiologic study of Lyme disease in southern Sweden. *New England Journal of Medicine* **333**, 1319–27.

Carlson, D. et al. (1999). Lack of *Borrelia burgdorferi* DNA in synovial samples from patients with antibiotic treatment-resistant Lyme arthritis. *Arthritis and Rheumatism* **42**, 2705–9.

CDC (1995). Recommendations for test performance and interpretation from the Second National Conference on Serologic Diagnosis of Lyme Disease. *MMWR Morbidity and Mortality Weekly Reports* **44**, 590–1.

Fikrig, E. et al. (1992). Elimination of *Borrelia burgdorferi* from vector ticks feeding on OspA-immunized mice. *Proceedings of the National Academy of Sciences USA* **89**, 5418–21.

Fraser, C. et al. (1997). Genomic sequence of a Lyme disease spirochaete, *Borrelia burgdorferi*. *Nature* **390**, 580–6.

Gray, J.S. et al. *Lyme Borreliosis: Biology, Epidemiology and Control*. Wallingford: CABI Publishing, 2002.

Gustafson, R. et al. (1990). Prevalence of tick-borne encephalitis and Lyme borreliosis in a defined Swedish population. *Scandinavian Journal of Infectious Diseases* **22**, 297–306.

Huppertz, H.I. et al. (1999). Incidence of Lyme borreliosis in the Wurzburg region of Germany. *European Journal of Clinical Microbiology of Infectious Diseases* **18**, 697–703.

Infante-Duarte, C. et al. (2000). Microbial lipopeptides induce the production of IL-17 in T helper (Th) cells. *Journal of Immunology* **165**, 6107–15.

Kalish, R.A. et al. (2001). Evaluation of study patients with Lyme disease, 10–20-year follow-up. *Journal of Infectious Diseases* **183**, 453–60.

Kamradt, T. (2002). Lyme disease and current aspects of immunization. *Arthritis Research* **4**, 20–9.

Kamradt, T. and Mitchison, N.A. (2001). Advances in immunology: tolerance and autoimmunity. *New England Journal of Medicine* **344**, 655–64.

Klempner, M.S. et al. (2001). Two controlled trials of antibiotic treatment in patients with persistent symptoms and a history of Lyme disease. *New England Journal of Medicine* **345**, 85–92.

Lunemann, J.D. et al. (2001). Rapid typing of *Borrelia burgdorferi* sensu lato species in specimens from patients with different manifestations of Lyme borreliosis. *Journal of Clinical Microbiology* **39**, 1130–3.

Maiwald, M. et al. (1998). Transmission risk of *Borrelia burgdorferi* sensu lato from *Ixodes ricinus* ticks to humans in southwest Germany. *Epidemiology and Infection* **121**, 103–8.

Medzhitov, R. and Janeway, C., Jr. (2000). Innate immunity. *New England Journal of Medicine* **343**, 338–44.

Nadelman, R.B. et al. (2001). Prophylaxis with single-dose doxycycline for the prevention of Lyme disease after an *Ixodes scapularis* tick bite. *New England Journal of Medicine* **345**, 79–84.

Nadelman, R.B. and Wormser, G.P. (1998). Lyme borreliosis. *Lancet* **352**, 557–65.

Nichol, G. et al. (1998). Test-treatment strategies for patients suspected of having Lyme disease: a cost-effectiveness analysis. *Annals of Internal Medicine* **128**, 37–48.

Nocton, J.J. et al. (1994). Detection of *Borrelia burgdorferi* DNA by polymerase chain reaction in synovial fluid in Lyme arthritis. *New England Journal of Medicine* **330**, 229–34.

Nocton, J.J. et al. (1996). Detection of *Borrelia burgdorferi* DNA by polymerase chain reaction in cerebrospinal fluid in Lyme neuroborreliosis. *Journal of Infectious Diseases* **174**, 623–7.

Priem, S. et al. (1998). Detection of *Borrelia burgdorferi* by polymerase chain reaction in synovial membrane, but not in synovial fluid from patients with persisting Lyme arthritis after antibiotic therapy. *Annals of the Rheumatic Diseases* **57**, 118–21.

Shapiro, E.D. and Gerber, M.A. (2000). Lyme disease. *Clinical Infectious Diseases* **31**, 533–42.

Sigal, L.H. (1998). Musculoskeletal manifestations of Lyme arthritis. *Rheumatic Disease Clinics of North America* **24**, 323–51.

Sigal, L.H. et al. (1998). A vaccine consisting of recombinant *Borrelia burgdorferi* outer-surface protein A to prevent Lyme disease. *New England Journal of Medicine* **339**, 216–22.

Smith, M. et al. (1998). The European Union Concerted Action World Wide Web site for Lyme borreliosis. *Zentralblatt für Bakteriologie* **287**, 266–9.

Steere, A.C. (2001). Lyme disease. *New England Journal of Medicine* **345**, 115–25.

Steere, A.C. et al. (1998). Vaccination against Lyme disease with recombinant *Borrelia burgdorferi* outer-surface lipoprotein A with adjuvant. *New England Journal of Medicine* **339**, 209–15.

Wang, G. et al. (1999). Molecular typing of *Borrelia burgdorferi* sensu lato: taxonomic, epidemiological, and clinical implications. *Clinical Microbiology Reviews* **12**, 633–53.

Wormser, G.P. et al. (2000). Practice guidelines for the treatment of Lyme disease. The Infectious Diseases Society of America. *Clinical Infectious Diseases* **31**, (Suppl. 1), 1–14.

6.2.5 Viral arthritis

Stanley J. Naides

Viruses may affect the joints by a number of mechanisms. The mechanisms employed vary with the infecting virus based on mode of tissue entry, tissue tropism, mechanisms of replication, direct viral effects on cellular functions, the ability to establish persistent infection, local immune response, expression of host-like antigens, ability to alter host antigens, host age and genetic makeup, and the infection history of the host. Several viruses directly infect the cells of the synovium. The mechanism of injury may be through lysis of target cells. The target cells may die by one of three mechanisms. First, viral infection may result in classic cell necrosis with karyorrhexis. Second, the virus may initiate the cellular machinery for programmed cell death, or apoptosis. Third, the virus may express virally encoded antigens on the cell surface that elicit an immune response that, in turn, targets killing of virally infected cells.

Direct infection may also result in non-lytic mechanisms of viral arthritis pathogenesis. Viral gene products may transactivate host cell genes. Immune activation may result from cell surface expression of normally sequestered autoantigens, viral antigens or virally encoded cytokines. The infected cell would become a target for immune attack or the focus of recruitment of cytokine responsive cells. Viral infection leading to expression of viral antigens on the cell surface may serve as a novel foreign antigen and elicit an immune response. Alternatively, molecular mimicry of host autoantigens may break immune tolerance resulting in generation of an autoimmune response. Immune complex disease may result when the humoral response generates sufficient antibody to cause deposition of immune complexes either locally, at the site of viral infection, or systemically with deposition of circulating immune complex in synovium.

Parvovirus B19

Human parvovirus B19 was first discovered serendipitously in 1975. It is a member of the family Parvoviridae, consisting of the smallest known DNA viruses, and the genus Erythrovirus, consisting of parvoviruses autonomously replicating in erythroid precursors. Numerous autonomous parvoviruses are known to infect mammalian animal species. However, these viruses are extremely species specific and are not known to cross species barriers. B19 is a non-enveloped, single-stranded DNA virus measuring approximately 23 nm in diameter. Although infection of other tissue types may occur, viral replication is usually not as brisk in cells other than erythroid progenitors.

Epidemiology

B19 infection is common and geographically widespread. Seroepidemiological studies of community outbreaks of B19 infection demonstrate that a large proportion of B19 infections remain asymptomatic or present as undiagnosed non-specific viral illnesses. Approximately 50 per cent of the general adult population has serological evidence of past B19 infection. Outbreaks of B19 infection occur in late winter and spring, although epidemics have also been reported in summer and fall. Within a community, B19 outbreaks tend to cycle every 3–5 years, representing the period of time for a fresh cohort of susceptible children to enter the school system. Since the seroprevalence of anti-B19 IgG antibodies is only approximately 50 per cent in adults, these periodic outbreaks often involve susceptible adults as well. The risk of infection in susceptible adults may be as high as 50 per cent with multiple exposures (Gillespie et al. 1990). Workers in occupations with increased exposure to children, such as school teachers, day care workers, and hospital personnel, have increased risk of infection. Sporadic cases occur between outbreaks. Transmission is via nasopharyngeal secretions.

The incubation period between infection and onset of symptoms is 7–18 days. In human volunteer studies, introduction of B19 nasally was followed in 7 days by a flu-like illness associated with viraemia, viral shedding in nasal secretions, and areticulocytosis. At approximately 11 days post-infection, an incipient anti-B19 IgM antibody response was associated with clearing of viraemia, cessation of nasal shedding of virus, and a second phase of clinical illness characterized by rash, arthralgia, and arthritis. Onset of the anti-B19 IgG antibody response occurred almost concurrently with the IgM response (Anderson et al. 1985). In natural infections, the temporal separation between the two phases of clinical illness is often blurred.

Clinical features

Since 1981, well-defined clinical syndromes have been attributed to B19 infection. B19 is the cause of transient aplastic crisis in the setting of chronic haemolytic anaemias such as sickle cell disease, hereditary spherocytosis, α- and β-thalassaemias, pyruvate kinase deficiency, glucose-6-phosphate dehydrogenase deficiency, pyrimidine 5′-nucleotidase deficiency, hereditary stomatocytosis, autoimmune haemolytic anaemia, and HEMPAS [hereditary erythrocytic multinuclearity associated with a positive acidified (HAMS) test] (Naides 2000). B19 is the aetiologic agent of erythema infectiosum, or fifth disease, a common rash illness of children characterized by bright red 'slapped cheeks' and a macular, maculopapular, and occasionally vesicular or haemorrhagic eruption on the torso and extremities (see Plate 94). While infection in children may be asymptomatic, when symptoms do occur they tend to be mild and include sore throat, headache, fever, cough, anorexia, vomiting, diarrhoea, and arthralgia. Erythema infectiosum may also be seen in adults not previously infected. In adults, the rash tends to be subtler and the bright red 'slapped cheeks' absent. A number of uncommon dermatologic manifestations of B19 infection have been reported including a vesiculopustular eruption, purpura with or without thrombocytopaenia, Henoch–Schönlein purpura, and a gloves and socks erythema.

B19 infection may be associated with paraesthesias in the fingers. Rarely, progressive arm weakness has occurred as has numbness of the toes. In such instances, nerve conduction studies show mild slowing of nerve conduction velocities and decreased amplitudes of motor and sensory potentials.

B19 may cross the placenta to infect the foetus. Clinically affected foetuses develop hydrops foetalis either on the basis of B19-induced anaemia resulting in a high output cardiac failure, or on the basis of viral cardiomyopathy. B19 has been reported to less commonly cause pancytopaenia, isolated anaemia, thrombocytopaenia, leucopaenia, myocarditis, neuropathy, hepatitis, or vasculitis (Karetnyi et al. 1999; Naides 2000). Patients with congenital or acquired immune deficiencies, including prior chemotherapy for lymphoproliferative disorders, immunosuppressive therapy for transplantation, or human acquired immune deficiency syndrome (AIDS) may fail to clear B19 infection. Such individuals may have chronic or recurrent anaemia, thrombocytopaenia, or leucopaenia. B19 infection is the leading cause of pure red cell aplasia in AIDS patients (Frickhofen et al. 1994).

Among B19 infected immune competent children under 10 years of age, arthralgia may occur in about 5 per cent and joint swelling in only approximately 3 per cent. In adolescents, joint pain and swelling occur in about 12 per cent and 5 per cent, respectively. However, joint pain occurs in about 77 per cent and joint swelling in 60 per cent of adults 20 years of age or older. In adults, B19 infection may be associated with a severe flu-like illness in which polyarthralgia and joint swelling are prominent. The distribution of involved joints is rheumatoid-like with prominent symmetric involvement of the metacarpophalangeal, proximal interphalangeal, wrist, knee, and ankle joints. Patients usually experience sudden onset polyarthralgia or polyarthritis. Onset of joint symptoms may or may not be preceded by a viral prodrome consisting of fever, malaise, chills, and myalgias. Most adults present with acute, moderately severe, symmetric polyarthritis that usually starts in the hands or knees and within 24–48 h spreads to include the wrists, ankles, feet, elbows, and shoulders. Spinal involvement is uncommon. Joint symptoms in adults are usually self-limited, but a minority of adults may have symptoms for prolonged periods of time. Chronic symptoms fall into one of two patterns. Approximately two-thirds of patients have continuous symptoms of morning stiffness and arthralgis with intermittent flares. The remaining one-third of patients are symptom-free between flares. Morning stiffness is prominent. Approximately one-half of adult arthropathy patients meet diagnostic criteria for rheumatoid arthritis. Rheumatoid factor may be present in low to moderate titre during the acute phase of infection but usually resolves. Anti-DNA, antilymphocyte, antinuclear antibodies, and antiphospholipid antibodies may also be found acutely. Joint erosions and rheumatoid nodules have not been reported. Chronic B19 arthropathy may last for up to 8 years, the longest follow-up to date. Several weeks after the initial infection, symptoms of acute synovitis tend to resolve. Joint pain and stiffness remain prominent features in patients who continue to have symptoms. Approximately 12 per cent of patients presenting with 'early synovitis' have B19-induced rheumatoid-like arthropathy, the majority of whom are women (Naides 2000). Adults usually lack the classic slapped-cheek rash seen in children.

The distribution of joint involvement in B19 arthropathy and its symmetry may suggest a diagnosis of a rheumatoid arthritis. About half of all patients with chronic B19 arthropathy meet the criteria of the American Rheumatism Association for a diagnosis of rheumatoid arthritis: morning stiffness which may last for more than an hour, symmetric involvement, involvement of at least three joints, and involvement of the hand joints. Joint erosions and rheumatoid nodules are absent. While an initial report suggested that chronic B19 arthropathy may be associated with HLA–DR4 as is seen in classic erosive rheumatoid arthritis, subsequent studies by the same group have demonstrated no increased association with DR4. The absence of rheumatoid nodules or joint destruction aids in the differential diagnosis of B19 arthropathy from classic, erosive rheumatoid arthritis (Naides et al. 1990).

Diagnosis

Diagnosis is based on laboratory confirmation in the appropriate clinical setting. A number of approaches and methodologies have been used in the laboratory to confirm B19 infection. Immune electron microscopy, detection of B19 DNA during viraemia, and detection of anti-B19 IgM antibody may be used. However, the most useful modality in the Rheumatology Clinic is the IgM serology because patients usually have anti-B19 IgM antibodies and have begun to clear viraemia at the time of presentation with polyarthralgia/polyarthritis. Both radioimmunoassays (RIA) and enzyme-linked immunoabsorbent assays (ELISA) have been used to detect B19 antigen and specific antibody to B19 capsid. A number of laboratories developed recombinant B19 antigens for B19 diagnostics in response to the difficulty in obtaining B19 viraemic serum to use as an antigen source. Commercial diagnostic kits are now available.

The anti-B19 IgM antibody response is usually positive for at least 2 months following onset of joint symptoms, but may wane shortly thereafter. However, the IgM antibody may be detectable in occasional patients for 6 months or longer. Because of the high seroprevalence of anti-B19 IgG in the adult population, detection of anti-B19 IgG antibody shortly after presentation of acute onset joint symptoms in a patient, in the absence of anti-B19 IgM, suggests past B19 infection and other diagnoses should be pursued. Failure to obtain B19 serologic testing at presentation may leave the diagnostic IgM antibody response undetected, leading to failure to diagnose B19 arthropathy in those patients in whom joint symptoms persist. Testing for B19 DNA at the time of arthropathy presentation is unlikely to be useful. At that time, antibody response has cleared viraemia or reduced serum virus load. Finding B19 DNA in synovium in chronic arthropathy is of questionable diagnostic value given the finding of B19 DNA in synovium by sensitive polymerase chain reaction (PCR) techniques in half of healthy military recruits undergoing arthroscopy for injury (Soderlund-Venermo et al. 2002).

Pathogenesis

Anti-B19 IgM antibody and acute-phase IgG antibody (less than 1 week post-inoculation) recognize determinants on the major capsid protein,

VP2. In convalescent serum, anti-B19 IgG antibody recognizes determinants on the minor capsid protein VP1 structural protein (Kurtzman et al. 1989). Since B19 VP1 and VP2 are products of alternate transcription of the same open reading frame, VP1 contains an additional 227 *N*-terminal amino-acids not present in VP2. VP1, therefore, contains unique determinants not present in the truncated form represented by VP2; these determinants may be in the unique non-overlapping *N*-terminal region or, alternatively, represent conformational differences in the sequences shared between the two proteins. Western blot analysis of serum from individuals with congenital immune deficiency, prior chemotherapy, or AIDS, demonstrated the absence of convalescent anti-B19 IgG antibodies directed against VP1. These sera were unable to neutralize B19 virus in experimental bone marrow culture systems (Kurtzman et al. 1989). In the absence of neutralizing antibodies to B19, B19 persists in the bone marrow and may cause chronic or intermittent suppression of one or more haematopoietic lineages.

Management

There is no specific vaccine or treatment for B19 infection at this time. Neutralizing activity to B19 is found in commercially available pooled immunoglobulin because the seroprevalence of anti-B19 IgG antibodies in the adult population is approximately 50 per cent. Intravenous immunoglobulin has been successful in the treatment of bone marrow suppression and B19 persistence in immunocompromised patients. However, this may not be applicable to chronic arthropathy patients. Treatment is symptomatic with non-steroidal anti-inflammatory agents (Naides et al. 1990).

Rubella virus

Rubella virus is the sole member of the genus rubivirus in the *Togaviridae* family of enveloped RNA viruses. The spherical rubella virion measures 50–70 nm in diameter with a 30 nm dense core. An envelope is acquired by budding at vesicles or the cell surface. Spike-like projections on the envelope measuring 5–6 nm contain haemagglutinin activity detected by agglutination of erythrocytes from a variety of animal species.

Epidemiology

Rubella host range is restricted to humans. Like B19 infection, transmission is by nasopharyngeal secretions with peak incidence in late winter and spring. Widespread rubella vaccination altered the epidemiology of rubella infection, which had previously occurred in 6–9-year cycles with most cases in children. Now, the age profile has shifted towards young adults whose risk of infection of 10–20 per cent is comparable to that during the pre-vaccine era. More recent rubella outbreaks in college students and in adults underscores the public health need for maintaining vaccination programmes.

Incubation time from infection to onset of rash is 14–21 days. Viraemia occurs 6–7 days before skin eruption, peaks immediately prior to eruption, and clears within 48 h of rash. Virus shedding in nasopharyngeal secretions may be detected from 7 days before and until 14 days after skin eruption, but is maximal just before onset of rash until 5–6 days post-eruption (Chantler et al. 2001).

Clinical features

The spectrum of clinical disease in children and adults ranges from asymptomatic infection to a classic syndrome of low-grade fever, rash, coryza, malaise, and prominent posterior cervical, post-auricular, and occipital lymphadenopathy. Constitutional symptoms may precede the skin eruption by 5 days. The eruption may vary during a brief 2–3 day period, starting as a morbilliform facial eruption before spreading to the torso, and upper then lower extremities. The eruption may coalesce on the face and clear as the extremities become involved. Alternatively, the eruption may be limited to a transient blush.

Joint complaints are common in adult infection, especially in women. Joint symptoms may occur 1 week before or after onset of the rash. Joint involvement is usually symmetric and may be migratory, resolving over a few days to 2 weeks. Arthralgias are more common than frank arthritis. Stiffness is prominent. The metacarpophalangeal and proximal interphalangeal joints of the hands, the knees, wrists, ankles, and elbows are most frequently involved. Periarthritis, tenosynovitis, and carpal tunnel syndrome may be seen. In some patients, symptoms may persist for several months or years.

Live attenuated vaccines have been employed in rubella vaccination with a high frequency of post-vaccination arthralgia, myalgia, arthritis, and paraesthesias. The HPV77/DK12 strain was the most arthritogenic of the vaccine strains made available. The pattern of joint involvement was similar to natural infection. Arthritis usually occurred 2 weeks post-inoculation and lasted less than a week. However, symptoms may have persisted in some patients for more than a year. The currently used vaccine RA27/3 may likewise cause post-vaccination joint symptoms. While it had been considered safer than HPV77/DK12 and Cendehill vaccine strains, studies following a vaccination campaign in response to a rubella outbreak in Canada led to recognition that as many as 15 per cent or more of recipients of RA27/3 vaccine strain may develop arthropathy (Howson and Fineberg 1992; Mitchell et al. 1993).

In children, two syndromes of rheumatologic interest may occur. In the 'arm syndrome', a brachial radiculoneuropathy causes arm and hand pain, and dysaesthesias that are worse at night. The 'catcher's crouch' syndrome is a lumbar radiculoneuropathy characterized by popliteal fossa pain on arising in the morning. Those affected assume a 'catcher's crouch' position. The pain gradually decreases through the day. Both syndromes occur 1–2 months post-vaccination. The initial episode may last up to 2 months, but recurrences are usually shorter in duration. Episodes of 'arm syndrome' and 'catcher crouch syndrome' may recur for up to 1 year, but there is no permanent damage.

Diagnosis

Rubella is readily cultured from tissues and body fluids including throat swabs. Virus is detected in either direct assays of cytopathic effects in tissue culture or in an indirect assay of interference of enterovirus growth in primary African green monkey kidney cell culture. Detection of antirubella IgM antibody or anti-IgG antibody seroconversion is diagnostic of rubella infection. Antirubella IgM and IgG are usually present at onset of joint symptoms. IgM antibody peaks 8–21 days after symptoms then decreases over the next 4–5 weeks to undetectable levels in most patients. Therefore, detection of antirubella IgM indicates recent infection, usually in the last 1–2 months. Since antirubella IgG rises rapidly over a period of 7–21 days after onset symptoms, a diagnosis of rubella infection based on IgG serology can only be made with paired acute and convalescent sera. The presence of IgG in a single serum sample only documents immunity.

Pathogenesis

Failure to mount an adequate immune response to specific epitopes may allow rubella virus to persist in patients with rubella arthritis. Virus may be detected in synovial fluid during arthritis flares and in lymphocytes years after symptom resolution. Onset of rash and arthritis is coincident with the appearance of antibodies, including neutralizing antibodies to whole virus suggesting a role for antibody or immune complexes in the synovitis (Chantler et al. 2001).

Management

Non-steroidal anti-inflammatory agents may be used for symptom control. Low to moderate doses of steroids have been used to control symptoms and viraemia (Mitchell et al. 1993).

Hepatitis B virus

Hepatitis B virus (HBV) is a member of the family Hepadnaviridae, genus orthohepadnavirus. HBV is an enveloped double-stranded DNA icosahedral virus measuring 42 nm in diameter (Hollinger and Liang 2001).

Epidemiology

HBV is transmitted by parenteral and sexual routes. HBV infection occurs worldwide, but prevalence of hepatitis B surface antigen (Australian antigen) is higher in Asia, the Middle East, and Sub-Saharan Africa. The prevalence in China may be as high as 10 per cent compared to 0.01 per cent in the United States. There is no known seasonality to primary HBV infections. Most acute infections in endemic regions occur at an early age with many acquired perinatally from infected mothers and is usually asymptomatic; incidence of infection in children may be as high as 5 per cent annually, with gradual decline of carriage rates and specific antibody with advanced age. In the West, most infections are acquired in adulthood during sexual or needle exposures. Adult infection is more often associated with acute hepatitis; 5–10 per cent of those with hepatitis develop persistent infection. In endemic regions, HBV is a common cause of chronic liver disease and a leading cause of hepatocellular carcinoma (Robinson 1994).

Clinical features

The incubation period from infection to hepatitis is usually 45–120 days. A pre-icteric prodromal period lasting several days to a month and may be associated with fever, myalgia, malaise, anorexia, nausea, and vomiting. HBV infection may cause an immune complex mediated arthritis during this period. Significant viraemia occurs early in infection; soluble immune complexes with circulating HBsAg are formed as antihepatitis B surface antigen antibodies (HBsAb) are produced. Arthritis onset is usually sudden and often severe. Joint involvement is usually symmetric with simultaneous involvement of several joints at onset, but arthritis may be migratory or additive. The joints of the hand and knee are most often affected, but wrists, ankles, elbows, shoulders, and other large joints may be involved as well. Fusiform swelling may be seen in the small joints of the hand. Morning stiffness is common. Arthritis and urticaria may precede jaundice by days to weeks and may persist several weeks after jaundice. However, arthritis and rash usually subsides soon after onset of clinical jaundice. While arthritis is usually limited to the pre-icteric prodrome, those patients who develop chronic active hepatitis or chronic HBV viraemia may have recurrent arthralgias or arthritis. Polyarteritis nodosa (PAN) is frequently associated with chronic hepatitis B viraemia (Guillevin et al. 1995).

Diagnosis

Urticaria in the presence of polyarthritis should raise the possibility of HBV infection. Acute hepatitis may be asymptomatic, but elevated bilirubin and transaminases are usually present when the arthritis appears. Joint fluid examination is not diagnostic. At the time of arthritis onset, peak levels of serum HBsAg are detectable. Virions, viral DNA, polymerase, and hepatitis B antigen may be detectable in serum. Antihepatitis B core antigen IgM antibodies are present and indicate acute HBV infection as opposed to past or chronic infection.

Pathogenesis

HBV arthritis is thought to be mediated by immune complex deposition in synovium. Immune complexes containing HBsAg, antibody, and complement components may be detected.

Management

Management is limited to supportive measures including non-steroidal anti-inflammatory agents.

Hepatitis C virus

HCV is a member of the family Flaviviridae. HCV is an enveloped single-stranded RNA spherical virus measuring 38–50 nm in diameter (Purcell 1994).

Epidemiology

HCV is distributed world-wide. Using current diagnostic tools, seroprevalence is less than 1 per cent in developed western countries but is higher in Africa and Asia where it may cause one-fourth of acute and chronic hepatitis. In Japan, this figure may reach 50 per cent. HCV is transmitted by the parenteral route; sexual transmission is considered rare. HCV is responsible for 95 per cent of post-transfusion hepatitis in countries routinely screening donated blood for HBV. More than half of all cases of non-A, non-B hepatitis are attributable to HCV infection (Bhandari and Wright 1995). HCV genotypic variants have been described and these differ in their pathogenicity including severity of disease and response to α interferon. HCV has six major genotypes groups or clades and over 50 genotypic sub-types (Bhandari and Wright 1995).

Clinical features

Acute HCV infection is usually benign. Up to 80 per cent of post-transfusion infections are anicteric and asymptomatic. Prior to cirrhosis, liver enzymes are usually minimally elevated to normal. Community acquired cases present because of more symptomatic illness in which significant enzyme elevations occur; however, fulminant HCV hepatitis is rare. HCV is strongly associated with HBV negative hepatocellular carcinoma, especially in Africa and Japan.

Acute onset polyarthritis in a rheumatoid distribution, including the small joints of the hand, wrists, shoulders, knees, and hips, may occur in acute HCV infection. HCV is often associated with type II cryoglobulinaemia in established infection. It may present as essential mixed cryoglobulinaemia, a triad of arthritis, palpable purpura, and cryoglobulinaemia. Indeed, a majority of patients originally described as having essential mixed cryoglobulinaemia were eventually discovered to have HCV infection. HCV infection is also seen in non-essential secondary cryoglobulinaemia although less commonly. The presence of anti-HCV antibodies in essential mixed cryoglobulinaemia is associated with more severe cutaneous involvement, for example, Raynaud's phenomena, purpura, livedo, distal ulcers, and gangrene. HCV RNA may be found in 75 per cent of cryoprecipitates from patients with essential mixed cryoglobulinaemia and anti-HCV antibodies (Munoz-Fernandez et al. 1994).

Diagnosis

Serological tests utilize an array of antigens in an enzyme immunoassay while a recombinant strip immunoblot assay (RIBA) is confirmatory. A minority of patients may have HCV RNA detectable by PCR amplification methods in the absence of a positive serology.

Pathogenesis

Chronic HCV infection leads to cirrhosis, end-stage liver failure, and hepatocellular carcinoma but the frequency of these sequelae and the mechanisms by which they occur are not known. HCV infection persists despite vigorous antibody response to an array of viral epitopes. A high rate of mutation in the envelope protein is responsible for emergence of neutralization escape mutants and quasispecies (Shimizu et al. 1994). HCV is suspected to elicit cryoglobulins because HCV envelope glycoprotein has antibody Fc receptor properties that allow epitope spreading from HCV to bound immunoglobulin Fc (Wunschmann et al. 2000).

Management

Interferon α has been shown to be efficacious in the treatment of chronic HCV hepatitis and HCV-associated cryoglobulinaemia. Interferon α2b at a dose of 3 million units thrice weekly for 6 months suppresses viral titres and ameliorates clinical disease in about half of patients (Jenkins et al. 1996). Ribavarin in combination with interferon α2b, or higher doses of interferon α2b alone when tolerated, has improved response rates. Relapse after completion of the initial course of therapy is common. Those with cryoglobulinaemic vasculitis failing interferon therapy may require immunosuppressive therapy. There is controversy whether interferon therapy precipitates autoimmune disease such as autoimmune thyroiditis.

Retroviruses (see Chapter 6.2.6)

Human immune deficiency virus (HIV)

Several musculoskeletal syndromes have been described in HIV-infected patients. Whether reactive arthritis, and psoriatic arthritis are more prevalent in HIV-infected populations remains somewhat controversial. The incidence and prevalence of these rheumatic diseases may vary between populations studied and may depend on geography, mode of HIV transmission, exposure to different infectious agents, racial and ethnic makeup, risk behaviours, and patient ascertainment (Reveille 2000). Reactive arthritis may have a prevalence as high as 11 per cent in some HIV-infected populations. These patients differ from 'idiopathic' reactive arthritis patients in that they do not have sacroiliitis or anterior uveitis, nor do they present with the classic triad of arthritis, urethritis, and uveitis. The prevalence of HLA-B27 positivity appears to be lower in the HIV-infected patients compared to non-HIV-associated reactive arthritis. In Africa, where the route of HIV transmission is predominantly heterosexual, approximately 40 per cent of HIV patients with joint symptoms in Zimbabwe have reactive arthritis, and another 40 per cent have a pauciarticular presentation without extra-articular features. In the United States, psoriatic arthritis limited to a pattern of asymmetric oligoarthritis may be seen in as many as a third of HIV-infected patients with psoriasis, but the overall incidence of psoriasis does not appear to be significantly increased. Whether the different patterns of rheumatic disease expression are attributable to HIV infection itself or co-infection with other agents remains controversial (Cuellar and Espinoza 2000). The caprine arthritis-encephalitis virus, a goat retrovirus, causes an inflammatory destructive arthritis and lends support to the notion that HIV infection alone may have musculoskeletal manifestations.

Initial HIV infection may be associated with a transient flu-like illness with arthralgias. Later, three pain syndromes not associated with synovitis may be seen. The concurrence of rheumatoid arthritis and HIV is thought to be very rare. An acute symmetric polyarthritis involving the small joints of the hands and the wrists have been described but it was associated with periosteal new bone formation about the involved joints, a feature not seen in rheumatoid arthritis. A sub-acute oligoarticular arthritis primarily of the knees and ankles may cause severe arthralgia and disability but is transient, peaks in intensity within 1–6 weeks, and responds to non-steroidal anti-inflammatory agents. The synovial fluid is non-inflammatory. Mononuclear cell infiltrates may be seen in the synovium of the involved joints. As many as 10 per cent of HIV-infected patients may experience 'painful articular syndrome' characterized by intermittent severe joint pain predominantly of the shoulders, elbows, and knees that lasts about a day. The pain may be incapacitating and require short-term narcotic analgesics. Fibromyalgia has been reported in HIV-infected patients with prevalence as high as 29 per cent in one series. The role of HIV and other potential agents in these pain syndromes remains to be clarified. In addition to arthritis, disseminated interstitial lymphocytosis syndrome (DILS) may be seen in AIDS patients. In effected patients, a CD8 positive lymphocyte infiltrate of salivary glands causes parotid swelling. This entity needs to be differentiated from classic Sjögren's syndrome (Reveille 2000).

Human T lymphocyte leukaemia virus 1

Human T lymphocyte leukaemia virus 1 (HTLV-1) is endemic in Japan where it has been observed to be associated with oligoarthritis and a nodular rash. The patients have positive serology for anti-HTLV-1 antibodies. Type C viral particles are seen in skin lesions. The presence of atypical synovial cells with lobulated nuclei and T cell synovial infiltrates suggests direct involvement of the synovial tissue by the leukaemic process (Nishioka et al. 1993). Patients with HTLV-1 infection may also have sicca symptoms (Merle et al. 1999).

Alphaviruses

Chikungunya virus

Chikungunya virus was originally isolated during an epidemic of febrile arthritis in Tanzania in 1952–1953. The local tribal word, Chikungunya, 'that which twists or bends up', was applied to the virus and the disease. Retrospectively, it is likely that similar epidemics occurred in Indonesia, Africa, India, Asia, and possibly the southern United States from 1779 to 1828 (Griffin 2001). Humans are the major reservoir for Chikungunya virus which is transmitted by *Aedes* mosquitoes. The reinfestation of *Aedes aegypti* and the introduction of *Aedes albopictus* into the western hemisphere raises the spectre of an expanded geographic distribution. Indeed, the emergence of West Nile virus in the United States underscores the potential for alphaviruses to spread to new geographic ranges.

Epidemiology

Chikungunya virus is transmitted from its reservoir hosts (baboons, monkeys, and in Senegal, *Scotophilus* bat species) to man by *Aedes* mosquitoes in south and west Central Africa, Thailand, Vietnam, and India. *Mansonia africana* and mosquitoes from other genera may also act as a vector. In a 1964 epidemic in Bangkok, Thailand, an estimated 40 000 patients out of an urban area of 2 million were infected (Halstead et al. 1969). Thirty-one per cent of the prospectively studied cohort seroconverted to Chikungunya virus antibody positivity. Communities, particularly urban centres, where Chikungunya fever has not been encountered either endemically or epidemically for a prolonged period have a cohort of school age children without herd immunity. Therefore, those communities are at risk for significant infections. Globalization may also contribute to increasing risk of spread. An outbreak in Malaysia in 1998–1999 was attributed to migrant workers from endemic areas (Lam et al. 2001).

Clinical features

Chikungunya fever has explosive onset associated with fever and severe arthralgia. Constitutional symptoms and rash follow an illness that lasts from 1 to 7 days. The incubation period is usually 2–3 days but ranges over 1–12 days. Fever elevations occur quickly reaching 39–40°C and are accompanied by rigours. The acute illness may last 2–3 days with a range of 1–7 days. Following the acute illness, fever may resolve for 1–2 days before recrudescence. Polyarthralgia is migratory and predominantly affects the small joints of the hands, wrists, feet, and ankles with less prominent involvement of the large joints. Previously injured joints may be more severely affected. Stiffness and swelling may occur but large effusions are uncommon. In severe cases, symptoms may persist for months. Approximately 10 per cent of patients have joint symptoms 1 year post-infection. Generalized myalgia, and back and shoulder pain are common. Skin eruption is characterized by facial and neck flushing followed by macular or maculopapular eruption beginning 1–10 days after illness onset. Typically, a rash occurs on days 2–5 and is associated with defervescence. The rash may last 1–5 days and may recur with fever. It is located on the torso, extremities and occasionally the face, palms, and soles. It may be pruritic. In some patients, involved skin desquamates.

Isolated petechiae and mucosal bleeding may occur, usually without significant haemorrhage. Suffusion of the conjunctiva is prominent. Sore throat, pharyngitis, headache, photophobia, retro-orbital pain, anorexia, nausea, vomiting, and abdominal pain may accompany the acute illness. Lymphadenopathy may be tender but is usually not massive. Symptoms in children tend to be milder (Halstead et al. 1969). In symptomatic children, nausea and vomiting, pharyngitis, and facial flushing are prominent features. Arthralgia, arthritis, and rash are uncommon. Children may present with mild dengue-like haemorrhagic fever, headache, pharyngeal injection, vomiting, abdominal pain, constipation, diarrhoea, cough, or lymphadenopathy. Arthralgia and arthritis in children are milder and briefer in duration. A destructive arthropathy may occur in a few adult patients with chronic symptoms. Low titre rheumatoid factor may be found in those with long-standing symptoms.

The pathogenesis of this infection has not been studied intensively. As noted above, few patients may have chronic symptoms of arthralgia. Case reports would suggest that a few patients go on to have destructive lesions resulting from chronic disease manifestations.

Diagnosis

Chikungunya fever should be considered in any febrile patient resident in or returning from endemic areas. A history of epidemic occurrence should be sought. Mayaro virus, Ross River virus, rubella virus, parvovirus B19, and HBV virus infections may present similarly. Synovial fluid shows decreased viscosity with poor mucin clot, 2000–5000 white cells/mm^3. Therefore, the diagnosis depends on laboratory confirmation.

Virus may be isolated during days 2–4 post-infection. In some patients, viral antigen may be detected in acute sera by haemagglutination assay due to the intensity of the viraemia. Haemagglutination inhibition antibodies develop as viraemia is cleared. Complement fixation antibodies are positive by the third week and slowly decrease over the subsequent year. Neutralizing antibody production parallels haemagglutination inhibition activity. Chikungunya virus specific IgM antibodies may be found for 6 months or longer. Reverse transcriptase polymerase chain reaction (RT-PCR) methods offers an approach to more rapid diagnosis than viral culture or antibody testing (Hasebe et al. 2002).

Pathogenesis

Following mosquito bite, intense viraemia occurs within 48 h. Viraemia begins to wane around day 3. The appearance of haemagglutination inhibition activity in neutralizing antibodies clears the viraemia. Involved skin shows erythrocyte extravasation from superficial capillaries and perivascular cuffing. The virus absorbs to human platelets causing aggregation, suggesting a mechanism for bleeding. Synovitis in Chikungunya fever probably results from direct viral infection of synovium.

Management

Management for the patient is supportive. During the acute attack, range of motion exercises ameliorates stiffness. Non-steroidal anti-inflammatory agents are useful. However, chloroquine phosphate (250 mg/day) has been used when non-steroidal anti-inflammatory agents failed (Brighton 1984).

O'nyong-nyong virus

This virus is closely related to Chikungunya virus. O'nyong-nyong virus was first described in the Acholi province of northwestern Uganda in February 1959. Within 2 years, it had spread through Uganda and the surrounding region, affecting 2 million people. Serologically determined attack rates ranged from 50–60 per cent with 9–78 per cent of infected individuals becoming symptomatic. Disease spread at a rate of 2–3 km daily. After the epidemic, the virus was not detected again until it was isolated from *Anopheles funestus* mosquitoes in Kenya in 1978. *Anopheles gambiae* also serves as a vector. Serological surveys indicate that O'nyong-nyong virus is endogenous. The non-human vertebrate reservoir for O'nyong-nyong virus is not known. In 1996–1997, O'nyong-nyong virus again appeared during an outbreak in southcentral Uganda (Lanciotti et al. 1998).

Clinical features

O'nyong-nyong fever is clinically similar to Chikungunya infection. The name derives from the Acholi word meaning 'joint breaker'. The incubation period lasts at least 8 days and is followed by sudden onset polyarthralgia/polyarthritis. Four days later, appearance of skin eruptions are typically associated with improvement in joint symptoms. The eruption is uniform in nature and lasts 4–7 days before fading. The fever is less prominent but post-cervical lymphadenopathy may be marked. Although residual joint pain often persists, there appears to be no long-term sequelae.

Diagnosis

Viral isolation by intracerebral injection into suckling mice produces runting, rash, and alopecia (Williams et al. 1962). Haemagglutination inhibition or complement fixation tests identify the virus. The differential diagnosis is similar to that of Chikungunya fever. Mouse antisera raised against Chikungunya virus or O'nyong-nyong virus react equally well with O'nyong-nyong virus, but O'nyong-nyong antisera does not react well with Chikungunya virus. The mechanisms of O'nyong-nyong virus pathogenesis are unknown.

Management

Management is symptomatic. Patients recover without sequelae.

Igbo Ora virus

Igbo Ora virus is serologically similar to Chikungunya and O'nyong-nyong viruses (Moore et al. 1975). A single patient with fever, sore throat, and arthritis was identified. In 1984, an epidemic of fever, myalgias, arthralgias, and skin eruption occurred in four villages in the Ivory Coast. Igbo Ora was coined as 'the disease that breaks your wings'. The virus was isolated from *A. funestus* and *A. gambiae* mosquitoes, and from affected individuals.

Ross River virus (epidemic polyarthritis)

Epidemics of fever and rash have been observed in Australia since 1928. Epidemics occurred among soldiers stationed in Australia during the Second World War. Isolation of Ross River virus from mosquitoes, its serological association with epidemic polyarthritis, and the isolation of the virus from epidemic polyarthritis patients in Australia confirmed Ross River virus as the aetiologic agent of epidemic polyarthritis (Aaskov et al. 1985). Antibodies to Ross River virus have been observed in the sera of endogenous populations in Papua New Guinea, West New Guinea, the Bismarck Archipelago, Rossel Island, and the Solomon Islands (Scrimgoeur et al. 1987). From 1979 to 1980, a major epidemic of febrile polyarthritis occurred in the Fiji Islands, affecting over 40 000 individuals (Bennett et al. 1980). Serological surveys suggested that a low level of Ross River virus infection was present throughout the Fiji Islands before 1979 but that following the epidemic, up to 90 per cent of the residents of some communities had antibody. A similar epidemic occurred in the Cook Islands early in 1980. Weber's line is a hypothetical line separating the Australian geographic zone from the Asiatic zone. West of Weber's line, antibodies to Ross River virus are not found.

In Australia, both endemic cases and epidemics occur in tropical and temperate regions. Significant numbers of cases are reported in Queensland and New South Wales, although cases and outbreaks are described in other regions as well. Seroprevalence may reach only 6–15 per cent in temperate coastal zones but is 27–39 per cent in the plains of the Murray Valley river system (Boughton et al. 1984). High rainfall usually precedes epidemic periods due to increased mosquito populations. Cases occur from the spring through the fall (Woodruff et al. 2002).

Aedes vigilax is the major vector on the eastern coast of Australia where the mosquito breeds in salt marshes. *Aedes camptorhynchus* similarly breeds in salt marshes of southern Australia. *Culex annulirostris* is a fresh-water breeding vector. Other Australian *Aedes* species and *Mansonia uniformus* may also serve as vectors. Several mammalian species may serve as intermediate hosts, including domestic animals, rodents, and marsupials. In the Pacific islands outbreaks, *Aedes polynesiensis, A. aegypti, A. vigilax,* and *C. annulirostris* may have contributed as well.

In Queensland, annual rates of disease range from 31.5 to 288.3 per 100 000 person years (Kelly-Hope et al. 2002). During epidemics in Fiji and New South Wales, the majority of those infected were symptomatic (Hawkes et al. 1985). While male and female infection rates were similar, there was a predominance of women in presenting cases. The children have a case to infection ratio lower than adults.

Clinical features

Arthralgias occur abruptly after a 7–11 day incubation period (Fraser 1986). A macular, papular, or maculopapular skin eruption, that may be pruritic, typically follows onset of arthralgia by 1–2 days; in some patients, rash may precede or follow joint symptoms by 11 or 15 days, respectively. Occasionally, vesicles, papules, or petechiae are seen. The trunk and extremities are typically involved although involvement of the palms, soles, and face may occur. The rash resolves by fading to a brownish discoloration or by desquamation. Despite its name, half of patients have no fever, and in those who do, modest fevers may last only 1–3 days. Headache, nausea, and myalgia are common. Mild photophobia, respiratory symptoms, and lymphadenopathy may occur.

A majority of patients have severe, incapacitating arthralgia. Joint distribution is often asymmetric and migratory, commonly involving the metacarpophalangeal and finger interphalangeal joints, wrists, knees, and ankles. Shoulders, elbows, and toes may also be involved. Axial, hip, and temporomandibular involvement occasionally occurs. Arthralgias are worse in the morning and after periods of inactivity. Mild exercise tends to improve joint symptoms. One-third will have frank synovitis. Polyarticular swelling and tenosynovitis are common. As many as one-third have paraesthesias, or palm or sole pain. Some patients have classic carpal tunnel syndrome. Half of all patients are able to resume their activities of daily living within 4 weeks although residual polyarthralgia may be present. Joint symptoms recur but episodes of relapse gradually resolve. A few patients will continue to have joint symptoms for up to 3 years (Fraser 1986).

Diagnosis

The diagnosis of Ross River virus infection should be considered in anyone with a febrile arthritis in the appropriate geographic setting. Acute rubella arthritis may present in a similar fashion although the signs and symptoms of an upper respiratory are more prominent in rubella. Patients may present without a rash. The differential diagnosis then would include early seronegative rheumatoid arthritis, systemic lupus erythematosus, parvovirus B19 infection, HBV infection, HCV infection, other alphavirus infections, Henoch–Schönlein purpura, and drug hypersensitivities. In those individuals who develop vesicles, differential from varicella or the occasional parvovirus B19 infection would need to be considered.

Synovial fluid cell counts range from 1500 to 13 800 cells/mm^3. Monocytes and vacuolated macrophages dominate with few neutrophils. Virus has been isolated only from antibody negative sera. In the Australian epidemics prior to 1979, patients were antibody positive at the time of presentation. However, in the Pacific Island epidemics of 1979–1980, patients remained viraemic and serologically negative for up to a week following onset of symptoms (Aaskov et al. 1981). Ross River virus antigen is detectable by fluorescent antibody staining of C6/36 cells inoculated with acute patient serum. Virus in serum is stable for up to a month at 0 to -10°C.

Pathogenesis

Ross River viral antigen may be detected by specific immunofluorescence in monocytes and macrophages early but intact virus is not identifiable by electron microscopy or cell culture. The dermis shows mild perivascular mononuclear cell, mostly T lymphocytic, infiltrate in both erythematous and purpuric eruptions. The purpuric form of eruption also shows extravasation of erythrocytes. Synovium demonstrates synovial lining layer hypertrophy, vascular proliferation, and mononuclear cell infiltration. Viral RNA can be found by RT-PCR (Soden et al. 2000). Ross River virus antigen may be found in epithelial cells in the erythematous or purpuric skin lesions, and in the perivascular zone in the erythematous lesion. However, viral antigens have not been found in the perivascular zone of the purpuric lesions (Fraser et al. 1983).

Management

Management of the acute infection is symptomatic. Aspirin or non-steroidal anti-inflammatory drugs provide relief for joint pain. Occasional patients may develop more persistent joint symptoms, but full recovery is usual.

Barmah Forest virus

Barmah Forest virus may present in a fashion similar to epidemic febrile polyarthritis (Doggett et al. 1999).

Sindbis virus

Sindbis virus is the prototype alphavirus used for molecular virology studies. It was isolated from *Culex* mosquitoes in the Egyptian village of the same name in 1952.

Epidemiology

Sindbis virus infection occurs in Sweden, Finland, and the neighbouring Karelian isthmus of Russia where it is known locally as Okelbo disease, Pogosta disease, or Karelian fever, respectively. *Aedes, Culex*, and *Culiseta* species transmit the virus to humans. Birds are an intermediate host. Cases are confined to predominately forested areas. Individuals involved in outdoor activities or occupations are at risk. Sindbis virus infection has also been reported as sporadic cases and small outbreaks in Uganda, South Africa, Zimbabwe, Central Africa, and Australia (Griffin 2001).

Clinical features

Skin eruption and arthralgia are the initial symptoms although one may precede the other by a few days. Fever may be present although it is not high. Constitutional symptoms including headache, fatigue, malaise, nausea, vomiting, pharyngitis, and paraesthesias may be present but are usually not severe. Macular skin eruptions typically begin on the torso, spreading to the arms legs, palms, soles, and occasionally head. The macules may evolve to papules that have a tendency to vesiculate. Vesiculation is particularly prominent on pressure points including the palms and soles. As the eruption fades, a brownish discoloration is left. Vesicles on the palms and soles may become haemorrhagic. The rash may recur during convalescence.

Arthralgia and arthritis involves the small joints of the hands and feet, wrists, elbows, ankles, and knees. Occasionally, the axial skeleton becomes involved. Tendonitis is common, often involving the extensor tendons of the hand and the Achilles tendon. Non-erosive chronic arthropathy is common in both Swedish and Finnish reports, with up to half of patients having symptoms 2.5 years after onset. A smaller number have symptoms as long as 5–6 years post-infection (Laine et al. 2000).

Diagnosis

Haemagglutination inhibition and complement fixation tests may establish the diagnosis. Antibodies appear during the first week of illness.

Pathogenesis

Little is known about the pathogenesis of Sindbis virus disease. Virus has been isolated from a skin vesicle in the absence of viraemia. Skin lesions show perivascular oedema, haemorrhage, lymphocytic infiltrates, and areas of necrosis. Antiviral IgM may persist for years raising the possibility that Sindbis virus arthritis is associated with viral persistence and direct viral effect on the synovium (Niklasson et al. 1988).

Management

Management is supportive.

Mayaro virus

Was first recognized in Trinidad in 1954 and has caused epidemics in Bolivia and Brazil. Mayaro virus has a monkey reservoir and is transmitted to man by *Haemogogus* mosquitoes feeding in the South American tropical rain forest. Mayaro virus was responsible for an outbreak in Belterra, Brazil, in 1988 with 800 out of 4000 exposed latex gatherers becoming infected. The clinical attack rate was 80 per cent. Illness was characterized by sudden onset of fever, headache, dizziness, chills, and arthralgias in the wrists, fingers, ankles, and toes. About 20 per cent had joint swelling. Unilateral inguinal lymphadenopathy was seen in some patients. Leucopaenia was common. Viraemia was present during the first 1–2 days of illness. After 2–5 days, fever resolved but a maculopapular rash on the trunk and extremities appeared. The rash lasted about 3 days. Recovery was complete, although some patients had persistent arthralgias at 2 month follow-up. Several cases of imported Mayaro virus infection have presented in the United States after travel from an endemic area in the Brazil–Bolivia–Peru inter-border region (Tesh et al. 1999). Of interest, Mayaro virus has been isolated from a bird in Louisiana (Calisher et al. 1974), raising the spector of emergence of Mayaro virus in the North American hemisphere.

Other viruses

Apart from specific viral infections noted above in which arthralgia and/or arthritis is typically a prominent feature, there are a host of commonly encountered viral syndromes in which joint involvement is occasionally seen. Children with varicella have been reported rarely to develop brief monoarticular or pauciatricular arthritis that is thought to be viral in origin. Adults who develop mumps occasionally develop small or large joint synovitis lasting up to several weeks. Arthritis may precede or follow parotitis by up to 4 weeks.

Infection with adenovirus and coxsackieviruses A9, B2, B3, B4, and B6 have been associated with recurrent episodes of polyarthritis, pleuritis, myalgia, rash, pharyngitis, myocarditis, and leucocytosis. Epstein–Barr virus associated mononucleosis is frequently accompanied by polyarthralgia, but occasional monoarticular knee arthritis occurs. Polyarthritis, fever, and myalgias due to echovirus 9 infection has been reported in a few cases. Arthritis associated with herpes simplex virus or cytomegalovirus infections are likewise rare. Herpes hominis occasionally causes arthritis of the knee known as herpes gladiatorum because it is seen in wrestlers. Vaccinia virus has been associated with post-vaccination knee arthritis in only two reported cases.

References

Aaskov, J.G., Mataika, J.U., Lawrence, G.W., Rabukawaqa, V., Tucker, M.M., Miles, J.A., and Dalglish, D.A. (1981). An epidemic of Ross River virus infection in Fiji, 1979. *American Journal of Tropical Medicine and Hygiene* **30**, 1053–9.

Aaskov, J.G., Ross, P.V., Harper, J.J., and Donaldson, M.D. (1985). Isolation of Ross River virus from epidemic polyarthritis patients in Australia. *Australian Journal of Experimental Biology and Medical Science* **63**, 587–97.

Anderson, M.J., Higgins, P.G., Davis, L.R., Willman, J.S., Jones, S.E., Kidd, I.M., Pattison, J.R., and Tyrrell, D.A. (1985). Experimental parvoviral infection in humans. *Journal of Infectious Diseases* **152**, 257–65.

Bennett, N.M., Cunningham, A.L., Fraser, J.R., and Speed, B.R. (1980). Epidemic polyarthritis acquired in Fiji. *Medical Journal of Australia* **1**, 316–17.

Bhandari, B.N. and Wright, T.L. (1995). Hepatitis C: an overview. *Annual Reviews in Medicine* **46**, 309–17.

Boughton, C.R., Hawkes, R.A., Naim, H.M., Wild, J., and Chapman, B. (1984). Arbovirus infections in humans in New South Wales. Seroepidemiology of the alphavirus group of togaviruses. *Medical Journal of Australia* **141**, 700–4.

Brighton, S.W. (1984). Chloroquine phosphate treatment of chronic Chikungunya arthritis. An open pilot study. *South African Medical Journal* **66** (6), 217–18.

Calisher, C.H., Gutierrez, E., Maness, K.S., and Lord, R.D. (1974). Isolation of Mayaro virus from a migrating bird captured in Louisiana in 1967. *Bulletin of the Pan American Health Organization* **8**, 243–8.

Chantler, J., Wolinsky, J.S., and Tingle, A. (2001). Rubella virus. In *Fields Virology* 4th edn. (ed. D.M. Knipe et al.), pp. 815–38. Philadelphia PA: Lippincott Williams & Wilkins.

Cuellar, M.L. and Espinoza, L.R. (2000). Rheumatic manifestations of HIV-AIDS. *Bailliere's Best Practice and Research in Clinical Rheumatology* **14**, 579–93.

Doggett, S.L., Russell, R.C., Clancey, J., Haniotis, J., and Cloonan, M.J. (1999). Barmah Forest virus epidemic on the south coast of New South Wales, Australia, 1994–1995: viruses, vectors, human cases, and environmental factors. *Journal of Medical Entomology* **36**, 861–8.

Feder, H.M. (1994). Fifth disease. *New England Journal of Medicine* **331**, 1062.

Fraser, J.R.E. (1986). Epidemic polyarthritis and Ross River virus disease. *Clinics in the Rheumatic Diseases* **12**, 369–88.

Fraser, J.R., Ratnamohan, V.M., Dowling, J.P., Becker, G.J., and Varigos, G.A. (1983). The exanthem of Ross River virus infection: histology, location of virus antigen and nature of inflammatory infiltrate. *Journal of Clinical Pathology* **36**, 1256–63.

Frickhofen, N., Chen, Z.J., Young, N.S., Cohen, B.J., Heimpel, H., and Abkowitz, J.L. (1994). Parvovirus B19 as a cause of acquired chronic pure red cell aplasia. *British Journal of Haematology* **87**, 818–24.

Gillespie, S.M., Cartter, M.L., Asch, S., Rokos, J.B., Gary, G.W., Tsou, C.J., Hall, D.B., Anderson, L.J., and Hurwitz, E.S. (1990). Occupational risk of human parvovirus B19 infection for school and day-care personnel during an outbreak of erythema infectiosum. *Journal of the American Medical Association* **263**, 2061–5.

Griffin, D.E. (2001). Alphaviruses. In *Fields Virology* 4th edn. (ed. D.M. Knipe et al.), pp. 917–62. Philadelphia PA: Lippincott Williams & Wilkins.

Guillevin, L., Lhote, F., Cohen, P., Sauvaget, F., Jarrousse, B., Lortholary, O., Noël, L.H., and Trépo, C. (1995). Polyarteritis nodosa related to hepatitis B virus—a prospective study with long-term observation of 41 patients. *Medicine (Baltimore)* **74**, 238–53.

Halstead, S.B., Nimmannitya, S., and Margiotta, M.R. (1969). Dengue and chikungunya virus infection in man in Thailand, 1962–1964. II. Observations on disease in outpatients. *American Journal of Tropical Medicine and Hygiene* **18**, 972–83.

Hasebe, F., Parquet, M.C., Pandy, B.D., Mathenge, E.G., Morita, K., Balasubramaniam, V., Saat, Z., Yusop, A., Sinniah, M., Natkunam, S., and Igarashi, A. (2002). Combined detection and genotyping of Chikungunya virus by a specific reverse transcription-polymerase chain reaction. *Journal of Medical Virology* **67**, 370–4.

Hawkes, R.A., Boughton, C.R., Naim, H.M., and Stallman, N.D. (1985). A major outbreak of epidemic polyarthritis in New South Wales during the summer of 1983/1984. *Medical Journal of Australia* **143**, 330–3.

Hollinger, F.B. and Liang, T.J. (2001). Hepatitis B virus. In *Fields Virology* 4th edn. (ed. D.M. Knipe et al.), pp. 2971–3036. Philadelphia PA: Lippincott Williams & Wilkins.

Howson, C.P. and Fineberg, H.V. (1992). Adverse events following pertussis and rubella vaccines. Summary of a report to the Institute of Medicine. *Journal of the American Medical Association* **267**, 392–6.

Jenkins, P.J., Cromie, S.L., Bowden, D.S., Finch, C.F., and Dudley, F.J. (1996). Chronic hepatitis C and interferon alfa therapy: predictors of long term response. *Medical Journal of Australia* **164**, 150–2.

Karetnyi, Y.V., Beck, P.R., Langnas, A.N., and Naides, S.J. (1999). Human parvovirus B19 infection in acute fulminant liver failure. *Archives of Virology* **144**, 1713–24.

Kelly-Hope, L.A., Kay, B.H., Purdies, D.M., and Williams, G.M. (2002). The risk of Ross River and Barmah Forest virus disease in Queensland: implications for New Zealand. *Australian and New Zealand Journal of Public Health* **26**, 69–77.

Kurtzman, G.J., Cohen, B.J., Field, A.M., Oseas, R., Blaese, R.M., and Young, N.S. (1989). Immune response to B19 parvovirus and an antibody defect in persistent viral infection. *Journal of Clinical Investigation* **84**, 1114–23.

Laine, M., Luukkainen, R., Jalava, J., Ilonen, J., Kuusisto, P., and Toivanen, A. (2000). Prolonged arthritis associated with sindbis-related (Pogosta) virus infection. *Rheumatology* **39**, 1272–4.

Lam, S.K., Chua, K.B., Hooi, P.S., Rahimah, M.A., Kumari, S., Tharmaratnam, M., Chuah, S.K., Smith, D.W., and Sampson, I.A. (2001). Chikungunya infection—an emerging disease in Malaysia. *Southeast Asian Journal of Tropical Medicine and Public Health* **32**, 447–51.

Lanciotti, R.S., Ludwig, M.L., Rwaguma, E.B., Lutwama, J.J., Kram, T.M., Karabatsos, N., Cropp, B.C., and Miller, B.R. (1998). Emergence of epidemic O'nyong-nyong fever in Uganda after a 35-year absence: genetic, characterization of the virus. *Virology* **252**, 258–68.

Merle, H., Cabre, P., Smadja, D., Josset, P., Landau, M., and Vernant, J.C. (1999). Sicca syndrome and HTLV-1-associated myelopathy/tropical spastic paraparesis. *Japanese Journal of Ophthalmology* **43**, 509–12.

Mitchell, L.A., Tingle, A.J., Shukin, R., Sangeorzan, J.A., McCune, J., and Braun, D.K. (1993). Chronic rubella vaccine-associated arthropathy. *Archives of Internal Medicine* **153**, 2268–74.

Moore, D.L., Causey, O.R., Carey, D.E., Reddy, S., Cooke, A.R., Akinkugbe, F.M., David-West, T.S., and Kemp, G.E. (1975). Arthropod-borne viral infections of man in Nigeria, 1964–1970. *Annals of Tropical Medicine and Parasitology* **69**, 49–64.

Munoz-Fernandez, S., Barbado, F.J., Martin Mola, E., Gijon-Banos, J., Martinez Zapico, R., Quevedo, E., Arribas, J.R., Gonzalez Anglada, I., and Vazquez, J.J. (1994). Evidence of hepatitis C virus antibodies in the cryoprecipitate of patients with mixed cryoglobulinemia (Review). *Journal of Rheumatology* **21**, 229–33.

Naides, S.J. (2000). Parvoviruses. In *Clinical Virology Manual* 3rd edn. (ed. S. Specter, R.L. Hodinka, and S.A. Young), pp. 487–500. New York: Elsevier Science Publishers.

Naides, S.J., Scharosch, L.L., Foto, F., and Howard, E.J. (1990). Rheumatologic manifestations of human parvovirus B19 infection in adults. Initial two-year clinical experience. *Arthritis and Rheumatism* **33**, 1297–309.

Niklasson, B., Espmark, A., and Lundstrom, J. (1988). Occurrence of arthralgia and specific IgM antibodies three to four years after Ockelbo disease. *Journal of Infectious Diseases* **157**, 832–5.

Nishioka, K., Nakajima, T., Hasunuma, T., and Sato, K. (1993). Rheumatic manifestation of human leukemia virus infection. *Rheumatic Disease Clinics of North America* **19**, 489–503.

Purcell, R.H. (1994). Hepatitis C virus. In *Encyclopedia of Virology* (ed. R.G. Webster and A. Granoff), pp. 569–74. San Diego CA: Academic Press.

Reveille, J.D. (2000). The changing spectrum of rheumatic disease in human immunodeficiency virus infection. *Seminars in Arthritis and Rheumatism* **30**, 147–66.

Robinson, W.S. (1994). Hepatitis B viruses. In *Encyclopedia of Virology* (ed. R.G. Webster and A. Granoff), pp. 554–9. San Diego CA: Academic Press.

Scrimgoeur, E.M., Aaskov, J.G., and Matz, L.R. (1987). Ross River virus arthritis in Papua New Guinea. *Transactions of the Royal Society of Tropical Medicine and Hygiene* **81**, 833–4.

Shimizu, Y.K., Hijikata, M., Iwamoto, A., Alter, H.J., Purcell, R.H., and Yoshikura, H. (1994). Neutralizing antibodies against hepatitis C virus and the emergence of neutralization escape mutant viruses. *Journal of Virology* **68**, 1494–500.

Soden, M., Vasudevan, H., Roberts, B., Coelen, R., Hamlin, G., Vasudevan, S., and La Brooy, J. (2000). Detection of viral ribonucleic acid and histologic analysis of inflamed synovium in Ross River virus infection. *Arthritis and Rheumatism* **43**, 365–9.

Soderlund-Venermo, M., Hokynar, K., Nieminen, J., Rautakorpi, H., and Hedman, K. (2002). Persistence of human parvovirus B19 in human tissues. *Pathologie-Biologie (Paris)* **50**, 307–16.

Tesh, R.B., Watts, D.M., Russell, K.L., Damodaran, C., Calampa, C., Cabezas, C., Ramirez, G., Vasquez, B., Hayes, C.G., Rossi, C.A., Powers, A.M., Hice, C.L., Chandler, L.J., Cropp, B.C., Karabatsos, N., Roehrig, J.T., and Gubler, D.J. (1999). Mayaro virus disease: an emerging mosquito-borne zoonosis in tropical South America. *Clinical Infectious Diseases* **28**, 67–73.

Williams, M.C., Woodall, J.P., and Porterfield, J.S. (1962). O'nyong-nyong fever: an epidemic virus disease in East Africa. *Transactions of the Royal Society of Tropical Medicine and Hygiene* **56**, 166–72.

Woodruff, R.E., Guest, C.S., Garner, M.G., Becker, N., Lindesay, J., Carvan, T., and Ebi, K. (2002). Predicting Ross River virus epidemics from regional weather data. *Epidemiology* **13**, 384–93.

Wunschmann, S., Medh, J.D., Klinzmann, D., Schmidt, W.N., and Stapleton, J.T. (2000). Characterization of hepatitis C virus (HCV) and HCV E2 interactions with CD81 and the low-density lipoprotein receptor. *Journal of Virology* **74**, 10055–62.

6.2.6 HIV and other retroviruses

Patrick Venables

The human retroviruses

Introduction

Retroviral infection in humans is almost synonymous with human immunodeficiency virus (HIV). The current global pandemic is estimated to involve over 36 million people. Because HIV infection is frequently associated with rheumatic complaints, the virus is becoming increasingly prominent in the practice of rheumatology. Besides HIV, there are at least three exogenous retroviruses known to infect humans: HIV-2, HTLV-I, and HTLV-II. Of these HTLV-I, estimated to infect 10–20 million people worldwide, is also associated with autoimmune phenomena, many of which have only recently been described. The diseases associated with each of these viruses are summarized in Table 1. In addition, both HIV and HTLV-I cause a number of serological abnormalities which may prompt rheumatological referral. Besides the known retroviruses, there may be others, perhaps not yet described, which have a role in rheumatic disease. The human genome is also a graveyard for a large number of endogenous retroviral sequences. These are the remnants of previous retroviral infections that have become incorporated into germ line DNA during evolution. Although most are disabled by mutations, many are transcriptionally active and may play a role in immune modulation. Thus, retroviruses represent a small but significant part of clinical practice and research in autoimmune rheumatic disease.

Biology of retroviruses

Retroviruses are a large family of enveloped animal viruses with single-stranded, ribonucleic acid (RNA) genomes. Following infection of a target cell, the viral RNA is converted to DNA, termed proviral DNA, which becomes integrated permanently into the chromosomal DNA of the host. It is the reverse transcription (RNA to DNA) that gives the family its name. The DNA provirus directs the synthesis of viral proteins using the host cell mechanisms, resulting in the production of new viral particles that are capable of infecting other cells.

Retroviral virions are 80–130 nm in diameter and are composed of a nucleoprotein core surrounded by a phospholipid envelope. The core of the retroviral virion contains two molecules of RNA (of 8–13 kilobase, kb) closely associated with many copies of a nucleocapsid protein and a transfer RNA (tRNA) molecule, which is required for initiation of reverse transcription. The basic retroviral genome organization (Plate 95) consists of *gag* (*g*roup specific *a*ntigens), *pol* (*pol*ymerase), and *env* (*env*elope) genes. At each end there is the long terminal repeat (LTR), which regulates viral

Table 1 Disease associations of human retroviruses

Retrovirus	Disease associations
HIV-1	Acquired immunodeficiency syndrome (AIDS) Malignancies: lymphomas and sarcomas Autoimmune-like conditions Diffuse infiltrative lymphocytosis syndrome (DILS), arthritis, myositis, vasculitis, neuropathies
HIV-2	AIDS
HTLV-I	Adult T-cell leukaemia/lymphoma (ATL) Tropical spastic paraparesis (TSP) Autoimmune-like conditions Uveitis, Sjögren's syndrome, arthritis, polymyositis, TSP
HTLV-II	Chronic neurological disease/TSP-like syndrome

transcription. In complex retroviruses, there are additional regulatory genes including a transcriptional activator (e.g. *tat* in HIV, *tax* in HTLV), and a regulator of messenger RNA (mRNA) splicing (e.g. *rev* in HIV, *rex* in HTLV).

The replication cycle of infectious retroviruses is outlined in Plate 96. An intact retroviral virion binds to specific cell surface molecules which act as receptors. Fusion between the retroviral envelope and the cell membrane then occurs, with the resultant release of the viral capsid into the cell cytoplasm. The principal cell surface receptor for HIV-1 and HIV-2 is the cell differentiation antigen CD4 and this is reflected in the primary tropism of these viruses for helper T-lymphocytes, monocytes, and macrophages. Recently, a number of co-receptors for HIV have been identified, such as the chemokine receptor CCR5, which facilitates fusion of the virion envelope and the macrophage cell membrane. Polymorphisms in the gene for CCR5 have been described which confer resistance to HIV infection and influence disease progression in infected individuals.

Reverse transcription and integration

In the cell cytoplasm, the retroviral virion undergoes a process of uncoating to expose the viral nucleoprotein complex. This complex is transported to the nucleus where the viral RNA is reverse transcribed by reverse transcriptase (RT) into a linear, double-stranded DNA. The DNA becomes integrated into the host cell DNA, mediated by the retroviral enzyme integrase.

Transcription and translation

Once integrated, retroviral genes are transcribed by the host cell's own mechanisms. Retroviral proteins are translated as larger polyprotein precursors which are subsequently cleaved by protease into their mature forms upon budding. Protranslational modification of the proteins also occurs, including glycosylation of the envelope proteins.

Particle assembly and budding

The assembly of progeny virions involves a complex series of interactions between viral proteins, viral RNA, and a specific host cell tRNA (reviewed by Wills and Craven 1991). Virions exit from the cell by budding from the plasma membrane and undergo maturation after release.

Transmission

All infectious human retroviruses have similar modes of transmission, horizontal via sexual or parenteral transmission and vertical perinatal transmission, which may occur *in utero*, during birth, or postnatally via infected breast milk. Retroviruses may also be transmitted from parent to child as a provirus in the germ line DNA and, as such, become endogenous retroviruses.

Human immunodeficiency viruses

A human lentivirus was first isolated from a homosexual patient with lymphadenopathy and was designated lymphadenopathy associated virus (LAV). Other isolates were independently reported, named HTLV-III and acquired immunodeficiency syndrome (AIDS) related virus (ARV). The virus was renamed HIV in 1986. In the same year, a separate human immunodeficiency virus HIV-2, was isolated from two West African patients with clinical features of AIDS who were seronegative for HIV-1. HIV-1 and HIV-2 are both very recent infections of humans in terms of evolution. The earliest confirmed case of HIV/AIDS was in an African in 1959 (Zhu et al. 1998) and it was suggested that its introduction into humans was as a zoonosis from chimpanzees, an event which occurred only a few decades before.

Both HIV-1 and HIV-2 have *gag*, *pol*, and *env* genes characteristic of retroviruses. In addition, there are several regulatory genes in the 3′ region of the genome which encode proteins that are translated from multiple spliced mRNAs and are essential for viral replication. The *tat* gene encodes a 14 kDa protein essential for initiation and elongation of viral transcripts. The *rev* gene encodes a 19 kDa protein involved in regulation of viral RNA splicing. Other regulatory genes have been described which are not essential for viral replication in cultured cells and have been termed 'accessory' genes (reviewed by Frankel and Young 1998).

The host reponse to HIV infection

Primary infection with sexually transmitted HIV usually occurs via CD4 positive macrophages in mucosal surfaces. When it is transmitted by blood products or intravenous drug abuse HIV can bypass this early phase and directly infect the recipients lymphocytes. The initial illness is characterized by a syndrome very similar to infectious mononucleosis with fever, lymphadenopathy, and fatigue, which usually resolves over weeks. During this phase, the immune response to HIV is similar to any other virus, with high levels of virus detectable in the circulation and a vigorous antiviral immune response. After the initial or 'seroconversion' illness has passed, the virus goes into a so-called latent phase with macrophages still being the main reservoir of virus. During this period, the effects of the virus are more in the direction of immune activation rather than suppression. Peripheral blood lymphocyte counts are normal or raised, monocytes are activated with the widespread production of cytokines. B cells are activated with the production of autoantibodies and hypergammaglobulinaemia. It is mainly during this phase of infection that most of the autoimmune phenomena occur and the first group or 'inflammatory' rheumatic diseases may occur. The illness can then proceed along one or both of two paths. The virus gradually mutates to become more tropic to CD4 T cells and immunodeficiency associated with CD4 lymphopaenia begins to supervene. When the CD4 count falls below 400 cells/ml, the patient becomes increasingly susceptible to opportunistic infections. Many of these can include infections of the musculoskeletal system. In some patients, the CD4 count does not fall and in these persistent B cell activation leading to the development of non-Hodgkin's lymphomas dominates the clinical picture.

Inflammatory rheumatic diseases associated with HIV-1 infection

HIV-1 infection and the diffuse infiltrative lymphocytosis syndrome

A Sjögren's-like syndrome, termed diffuse infiltrative lymphocytosis syndrome (DILS) is now a well-established manifestation of HIV infection that may present to the rheumatologist. These patients have sicca symptoms, swelling of the parotid and submandibular salivary glands, reduced tear and reduced saliva production. Biopsies of minor salivary glands show lymphocytic infiltration with a preponderance of $CD8^+$ T-cells. The frequency of DILS in HIV positive subjects is reported as being between 3 and 8 per cent though using histological criteria alone in African patients a frequency as high as 48 per cent was reported (McArthur et al. 2000). The frequency of DILS amongst patients referred to rheumatologists as Sjögren's syndrome is unknown. The author has seen three cases amongst a population of over 300 Sjögren's syndrome, patients (Venables, unpublished observations) suggesting that in London, at least, DILS may comprise approximately 1 per cent of patients referred to a Sjögren's clinic. None of the three was previously known to be HIV positive, indicating the importance of clinicians being aware of this disease.

The largest series (35 patients) of DILS was described by Kazi et al. (1996) where all had bilateral parotid gland enlargement and 94 per cent had sicca symptoms. This high frequency is not surprising because sicca symptoms are one of the defining features of the disease. Pulmonary involvement, manifest as lymphocytic interstitial pneumonitis was the most common extraglandular feature (31 per cent). An additional feature recognized in this study was clinical and pathological evidence of myositis in 26 per cent of patients (drug-induced myopathy with zidovudine had

Table 2 Comparison of clinical features between Sjögren's syndrome and HIV-associated 'diffuse infiltrative lymphocytosis syndrome'

Clinical features common to both Sjögren's syndrome and DILS
Sicca symptoms
Salivary gland swelling (often massive in DILS)
Extraglandular involvement, e.g. hepatitis, renal tubular acidosis
Lymphocytic infiltration on salivary gland biopsy
Neutropaenia and/or lymphopaenia in peripheral blood
Polyclonal hypergammaglobulinaemia

Clinical features which differ between Sjögren's syndrome and DILS

	Sjögren's syndrome	DILS
Sex	90% female	90% male[a]
Lymphadenopathy	Common	Massive
Extraglandular involvement	Uncommon	Common
Autoantibodies	Anti-Ro, anti-La	Multiple, low titre
HLA–DR association	HLA–DR2, DR3	HLA–DR5, DR6
Infiltrating lymphocyte type	Mainly $CD4^+$	Mainly $CD8^+$

[a] The male preponderance of DILS probably reflects the male preponderance of HIV infection in western populations. It is likely as heterosexual spread of HIV increases, the male : female ratio of DILS will decline. There have been no studies on the prevalence of DILS in populations from areas with high female HIV infection e.g. East Africa.

Sources: Itescu et al. (1989); Kazi et al. (1996).

been excluded). Apart from these similarities between DILS and idiopathic Sjögren's syndrome, there are also differences (Table 2). The autoantibodies (anti-Ro and anti-La) characteristic of Sjögren's syndrome are rarely found, although antibodies to the cytoplasm of a salivary gland epithelial cell line have been reported (Atkinson et al. 1993). The predominant cell infiltrate in salivary glands from DILS patients is $CD8^+$ lymphocytes, compared to $CD4^+$ lymphocytes in Sjögren's syndrome. Finally, the HLA associations of DILS (DR-5 and DR-6) differ from the HLA association (DR-3) of primary Sjögren's syndrome.

Diagnosis

The diagnosis of DILS is simply based on the clinical features of Sjögren's syndrome in association with HIV infection. If HIV serology has not been done, DILS may be suspected, the patient being male, in a high-risk group and with very prominent systemic features. The diagnosis may be missed because most of these patients do not have AIDS, and may well have a lymphocytosis rather than a lymphopaenia. Furthermore high immunoglobulin levels, low titre ANA and antiphospholipid antibodies may mislead the clinician into believing that they are dealing with a primary autoimmune disease rather than a retroviral infection. The only way to be sure of making a diagnosis is to think of DILS in every patient with Sjögren's syndrome and arrange for appropriate serology if HIV infection is suspected.

Treatment

There is no evidence-base for any specific treatment of DILS. Steroids have been used though there is always concern that, in high doses at least, they might increase the viral load. Maintenance doses equivalent to prednisolone less than 10 mg daily have been recommended with careful monitoring of the viral load. Since low-dose steroids have become more frequent in the routine management of HIV-infected patients (McComsey et al. 2001), most clinicians feel reassured about the relative safety of prednisolone in the management of DILS. Calabrese (1998) has also indicated that patients with DILS also respond particularly well to treatment with zidovudine. There is also a limited experience of the use of hydroxychloroquine in doses ranging from 200 to 600 mg/day. The clinician can feel reassured that hydroxycholoroquine has been reported to have a weak anti-retroviral effect of its own (Boelaert et al. 1999) and therefore it is unlikely to do any harm.

HIV-1 and arthritis

The association of HIV-1 with arthritis is controversial. Rynes et al. (1988) described an HIV-associated arthritis in four patients characterized by an asymmetrical oligoarthritis affecting the knees and ankles. Synovial biopsies from affected joints showed mild chronic synovitis and the symptoms responded rapidly to intra-articular corticosteroids. Stein and Davis (1996) described a similar large joint arthritis in association with HIV infection in 26 patients. Arthritis associated with HIV infection has been reported to improve with treatment with sulfasalazine and intramuscular gold. Solinger and Hess (1993) prospectively examined 1100 HIV seropositive patients for arthritis and found nine patients with 'non-specific' arthralgias, four with psoriatic arthritis, and one with Reiter's syndrome, but none with an oligoarthritis that would correspond to the HIV-associated arthritis previously described. They concluded that there was little evidence to associate HIV with a specific virally induced arthritis.

The association between Reiter's syndrome and HIV is also controversial. Winchester et al. (1987) reported 13 HIV seropositive patients with Reiter's syndrome. Subsequent studies (Stein and Davis 1996) reported a reactive arthritis in HIV seropositive patients with prevalence rates of up to 10 per cent. Davis et al. (1989) observed an increased frequency of Reiter's syndrome in association with HIV infection in Zimbabwe, where Reiter's syndrome was previously rarely seen. Over a period of 6 months, the authors saw 20 cases of Reiter's syndrome, 14 of which were subsequently found to be seropositive for HIV (Davis et al. 1989). In contrast, Clark et al. (1992) reviewed three large cohort studies of American homosexuals with and without HIV-1 infection and showed a similar prevalence of Reiter's syndrome (<1 per cent) between the two groups. A large Spanish study of 556 HIV seropositive patients identified a prevalence of Reiter's syndrome of 0.5 per cent (Munoz-Fernandez et al. 1991). The main risk factor for the development of Reiter's syndrome was not HIV infection, but a previous history of bacterial enteritis (*Shigella*, *Salmonella*, or *Campylobacter*) or non-gonococcal urethritis, suggesting that it was these organisms rather than HIV that were the underlying cause.

HIV infection can precipitate or worsen pre-existing psoriasis and the de novo appearance of psoriasis during the course of infection is now a well-recognized cutaneous manifestation of HIV. The clinical and histological appearances of the skin lesions in HIV-associated psoriasis is similar to that of idiopathic disease but is often much more severe. Seborrhoeic dermatitis occurs in up to 20 per cent of patients with HIV infection and its overlap with psoriasis (so-called seborrhoeic psoriasis) is an uncommon but highly characteristic manifestation of HIV infection (Fig. 1). In contrast to the debate about the frequency of reactive arthritis, psoriatic arthritis is definitely more common in HIV seropositive individuals (Solinger and Hess 1993). As with reactive arthritis psoriatic arthritis is often much more severe and sometimes associated with quite spectacular nail dystrophies (Plate 97).

Treatment

Psoriatic arthritis and other seronegative spondyloarthropathies can be rapidly progressive and extremely destructive in the context of HIV infection. Treatment is similar to idiopathic disease though methotrexate should be used only with extreme caution as it has been shown to precipitate AIDS. Nevertheless, the risks of methotrexate are justified in selected cases given how incapacitating these forms of arthritis can be.

HIV-1 infection and myositis

An inflammatory myositis indistinguishable from polymyositis was described in patients infected with HIV-1 (reviewed by Calabrese 1998). As in idiopathic polymyositis, the presenting symptoms are generally proximal muscle weakness involving both the arms and legs, but predominating in the legs. The serum creatine kinase (CK) is usually elevated and histology of affected muscle shows an infiltration with predominantly $CD8^+$ T-cells. Patients with HIV-associated myositis do not have the characteristic autoantibodies associated with idiopathic inflammatory myositis.

Treatment

Treatment with corticosteroids have been shown to improve symptoms and patients usually respond to a lower dose (prednisolone 0.5 mg/kg) than that traditionally used in idiopathic inflammatory myositis (Calabrese 1998). Myositis in association with HIV infection may also occur due to treatment with zidovudine that can cause a toxic mitochondrial myopathy that usually improves on withdrawal of the drug (Dalakas et al. 1990). Myositis has been reported as a prominent feature in patients with DILS, occurring in over one-fourth of the patients (Kazi et al. 1996).

HIV infection and vasculitis

A number of patterns of vasculitis are now recognized to occur in patients with HIV infection (reviewed by Gheradi et al. 1993). Small vessel involvement is the most common and may present with peripheral neuropathy, often misdiagnosed as drug toxicity. Large vessel involvement may present as giant cell arteritis (Solinger and Hess 1993) and medium vessel involvement as polyarteritis nodosa (Gheradi et al. 1993). Henoch–Schönlein purpura has also been reported (Gheradi et al. 1993). The vasculitides associated with HIV are usually not life-threatening and present as a single flare rather than a relapsing illness. Although antibodies to neutrophil cytoplasmic antigens (ANCA) have been described in HIV seropositive patients, these antibodies do not appear to be associated with the HIV-associated vasculitides. Histopathological examination of HIV-associated vasculitic lesions showed perivascular infiltration by $CD8^+$ T-cells (Gheradi et al. 1993), histologically similar to the infiltration observed in tissues from patients with DILS. In addition, IgM and complement were demonstrated in vessel walls consistent with immune complex deposition (Gheradi et al. 1993) suggesting that immune complexes may be playing a pathogenic role in HIV-associated vasculitis.

Neurological manifestations of HIV infection

An MS-like syndrome, encephalitis and subacute and chronic idiopathic demyelinating polyneuropathies have been described in association with HIV infection (reviewed by Price 1996). These neuropathies usually occur in the early and mid phases of HIV infection and may therefore often present before the diagnosis of HIV infection is made. Though normally the province of neurologists, neurological manifestations may present to the rheumatologist as encephalopathies or neuropathies associated with connective tissue diseases, such as CNS lupus, particularly as some of the serological features of HIV infection may mimic SLE or Sjögren's syndrome.

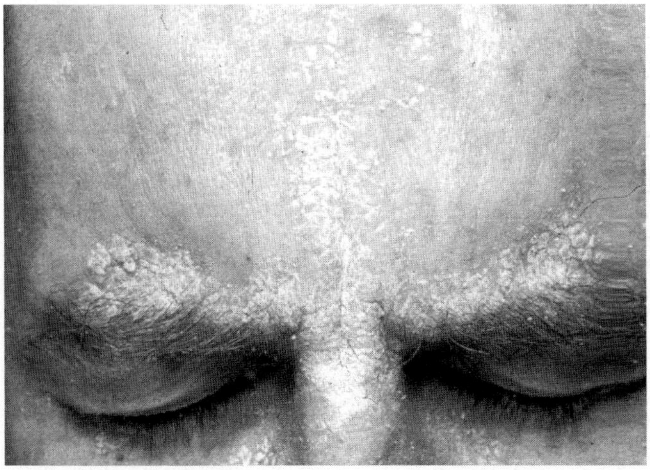

Fig. 1 Sebopsoriasis in an HIV positive patient. Sebopsoriasis (psoriasis with a similar distribution and character to seborrhoeic dermatitis) is a highly characteristic feature of psoriasis in HIV positive patients. Such lesions occurring de novo should always give rise to suspicion of underlying HIV infection (kindly donated by Dr Eleanor Mallon).

Serological manifestations of HIV infection

Rheumatologists are being increasingly referred patients because of abnormal blood tests. Traditionally one of these has been 'raised ESR query cause'. HIV can cause a raised ESR as well as a plethora of other haematological and serological abnormalities. To appreciate some of these, it is important to understand that HIV, in spite of its name, is not really an immunosuppressive virus, at least not early in infection. In early disease HIV predominantly infects macrophages, with an increased production of proinflammatory cytokines, lymphocyte proliferation, and activation of B cells to produce hypergammaglobulinaemia and autoantibodies. These are listed in Table 3. Most prominent amongst these are antiphospholipid antibodies, which may be of both IgG and IgM class. They are not associated with antibodies to B1 glycoprotein nor are they associated with the thrombotic phenomena seen in primary antiphospholipid syndrome or lupus. Antinuclear antibodies are seen in 10–30 per cent of patients but in general are not directed against native DNA or nuclear ribonucleoproteins such as U1 RNP, Sm Ro, and La. Thus, most of these antibodies are indicators of B cell activation rather than involvement in pathogenesis. The few autoantibodies that are pathogenic include antiplatelet and erythrocyte antibodies, which cause immune thrombocytopaenic purpura and haemolytic anaemia in a minority of patients. Antibodies reactive with CD4 or class II have also been described by some units. Whether these have any pathogenic significance *in vivo* remains to be established.

Musculoskeletal manifestations of AIDS

The musculoskeletal manifestations described above are attributable to activation of the immune system via infected monocytes. As the virus becomes more lymphotropic, the CD4 count begins to fall and coinfection with other organisms tends to dominate the clinical picture. Features of such infections are summarized in Table 4. It is estimated that musculoskeletal infection, predominantly septic arthritis, osteomyelitis and pyomyositis occur in 0.3–3.5 per cent of HIV-infected individuals (Vassilopoulos et al. 1997). The commonest organisms are those which also occur in musculoskeletal sepsis in the absence of HIV infection. These include *Staphylococcus aureus* and *Streptococcus pneumoniae.* In addition to these familiar organisms, opportunistic infections can occur when the CD4 count falls below 100. Typically, these are organisms which are normally targeted by cell-mediated immunity. They include intracellular bacteria such as mycobacteria and fungi and often include species that are not associated with infection in individuals with a normal immune system.

Table 3 Autoantibodies occurring in association with HIV-1 infection

Antibody	Frequency (%)	Reference
Blood components		
Antierythrocyte	a	Telen et al. (1990)
Anti-CD4 lymphocyte	60	Muller et al. (1994)
Antiplatelet	a	Dominguez et al. (1994)
RF (anti-IgG)	10–41	Montero et al. (1998)
		Munoz-Fernandez et al. (1991)
Antiprotein S	56	Lafeuillade et al. (1994)
Anticardiolipin	23–76	Solinger et al. (1991)
		Calabrese (1998)
Intracellular antigens		
Antinuclear	Up to 30	Calabrese (1998)
ANCA	10	Klaassen et al. (1992)

a Frequency not specified.

Table 4 Effect of AIDS on musculoskeletal sepsis

Frequency	Probably increased (0.3–3.5%)
Site of infection	More commonly multifocal, often unusual, e.g. sacroiliac, sternoclavicular joints, pyomyositis
Organisms	
Acute	Similar organisms to HIV negative: Staphylococcus, Pneumococus
Chronic	Atypical mycobacteria, e.g. *Mycobacterium kansasii* and M. avium Fungi
Symptoms/signs	Signs of inflammation may be less marked in some patients
Treatment	May be more prolonged, success rate similar to HIV negative

Septic arthritis

Septic arthritis may be the first manifestation of AIDS and as such represents another situation when the rheumatologist may be the first physician to make the diagnosis of HIV infection. In most case series (Hughes et al. 1992; Adebajo and Davis 1994; Vassilopoulos et al. 1997), *S. aureus* is the commonest organism (30–60 per cent) with streptococcal species coming a close second. Standard risk factors such as previous needling of the joint, psoriasis or pustular infection elsewhere apply as they do to idiopathic septic arthritis. However, most HIV positive individuals are not otherwise at risk from septic arthritis unless the CD4 count has fallen significantly. The exception may be individuals who have acquired HIV from intravenous drug abuse. In these patients it has been suggested that the frequency of septic arthritis is no more frequent in HIV positive compared to HIV negative individuals. These patients are also particularly susceptible to *Pseudomonas* infections, such that should it occur, attention should be directed to the possibility of parenteral drug abuse (Munoz-Fernandez et al. 1991). In Africa, where HIV is usually acquired by sexual promiscuity, gonococcal arthritis is the most common musculoskeletal infection. Septic arthritis complicating HIV infection usually presents as an acutely swollen, painful, erythematous process in one or several joints, accompanied by systemic symptoms of bacteraemia. Staphylococcal infections may be particularly widespread, causing septic bursitis, tendonitis and juxta-articular osteomyelitis. It has been suggested that, even with pyogenic organisms, immunosupression by HIV may modify the immune response such that inflammation and fever may be less prominent (Hughes et al. 1992).

The joint may also be a site for true opportunistic infections with organisms normally controlled by a cell-mediated immune response. These characteristically include Mycobacteria, with *Mycobacterium tuberculosis* being common, as it is in patients who are not immunocompromised. Infection with atypical mycobacteria rarely occurs unless there is profound immunosupression. Relatively prominent amongst these is *Mycobacterium kansasii*, which has been described in at least 50 cases in the world literature (Bernard et al. 1999). *Mycobacterium avium intracellulare* is one of the most frequent atypical mycobacterial species associated with pulmonary infection in AIDS but there are only isolated reports of its causing septic arthritis. Non-mycobacterial isolates include *Candida, Cryptococci*, and *Histoplasma* species. The literature also contains individual case reports of bizarre infective agents, too numerous to list, and emphasize the need for close collaboration between rheumatologists and infectious disease experts when investigating opportunistic infections of the joint. Furthermore, infection with these relatively low virulence organisms, together with an impaired immune response by the host, may be accompanied by minimal signs of inflammation. These rather bland clinical findings, together with an acellular synovial fluid, could therefore suggest a seronegative oligoarthritis. This emphasizes the need to examine the synovial fluid of every HIV positive patient with arthritis for the possibility of an opportunistic infection.

Osteomyelitis and pyomyositis

Osteomyelitis may also affect patients with AIDS. This may be juxta-articular osteomyelitis, usually caused by *S. aureus*, which in some cases can lead to multidigit dactylitis. Other organisms causing osteomyelitis in HIV-infected individuals include the same species which can lead to septic arthritis including *C. albicans*.

Pyomyositis of the thigh is regarded as a particular complication of AIDS infection and usually occurs when the CD4 count falls below 50/cumm. Presentation is with an acute onset of unilateral thigh pain associated with soft-tissue swelling, erythema, and woody induration of the distal thigh. Diagnosis is made by imaging techniques, including ultrasound, CT, and MRI scans and confirmed by microscopy and culture of aspirated pus.

Treatment

The treatment of musculoskeletal sepsis in HIV positive patients is similar to that of HIV negative patients. It is likely, though not proven, that therapy needs to be prolonged beyond that normally seen in HIV negative patients because of the inability of the immune system to 'mop up' any remaining viable organisms. In the case of most opportunistic infections, treatment is usually continued for life. In spite of profound immunosuppression, the mortality rate of septic arthritis in AIDS is surprisingly low at 20 per cent and in the case of pyomyositis 10 per cent (Vassilopoulos et al. 1997). This apparently better prognosis compared to HIV negative cases may reflect the relative absence of pre-existing distortion of joint architecture (by RA or joint surgery) seen in at least half of idiopathic musculoskeletal infections.

Human T-cell lymphotropic viruses

HTLV-I was first isolated from a cell line established from a patient with a cutaneous T-cell lymphoma. A retrovirus with 60 per cent sequence identity to HTLV-I was subsequently isolated from a patient with a benign T-cell variant of hairy cell leukaemia and designated HTLV-II. Both HTLV-I and HTLV-II possess a number of regulatory genes at the 3′ end of the genome, initially referred to as the X region due to its unknown function. Two important genes have been identified within the X region, the *tax* (*transactivating*) gene which encodes a 40 kDa protein (Tax) and a second gene *rex*, which encodes proteins of 21 and 27 kDa. The Tax protein is a potent activator of the provirus LTR and activates certain host cellular genes including some of those encoding pro-inflammatory cytokines and some oncogenes by binding to host transcription factors, such as nuclear factor-κB (NF-κB). Tax is considered to be responsible for many of the pro-inflammatory and oncogenic transforming properties of HTLV-I.

HTLV-I is endemic in southwestern Japan, the Caribbean, and western Africa. Infection is rare in Europe (Taylor 1996) with a prevalence of one in 20 000 blood donations in London (Brennan et al. 1993) although the prevalence is higher in immigrants from endemic areas (Murphy et al. 1993).

Diseases associated with HTLV-I infection

HTLV-I infection differs from that of HIV in that most individuals remain asymptomatic carriers, but are capable of transmitting the virus. About 5 per cent of infections are associated with two major classes of disease: adult T-cell leukaemia/lymphoma (ATL), and a myelopathy termed tropical spastic paraparesis (TSP) in Western countries and HTLV-I associated myelopathy (HAM) in Japan.

ATL is an aggressive malignancy of $CD4^+$ T-cells, which is characterized by the presence of leukaemia cells with polymorphic nuclei ('flower' cells) in the peripheral blood and lymph nodes. ATL is resistant to chemotherapy and patients have a mean survival time of only a few months. Epidemiological studies have shown that for HTLV-I seropositive subjects, the lifetime risk of developing ATL is approximately 1 per cent. The mechanism by which HTLV-I causes ATL probably involves transactivation of cellular genes by Tax. It is likely that the resulting cell proliferation leads to an accumulation of chromosomal abnormalities which ultimately result in malignant transformation and ATL.

TSP was first described in Jamaican patients in 1964 (Montgomery et al. 1964) and was linked with HTLV-I infection by serological studies in 1985 (Gessain et al. 1985). It is a chronic progressive demyelinating disease characterized by low back pain, weakness and pain in the legs, impaired bladder control and mild peripheral sensory loss. It is more common in females and usually the onset of symptoms occurs between the third and sixth decades of life. In contrast to typical multiple sclerosis (MS), TSP does not result in acute relapsing and remitting disease. Patients with TSP respond well to corticosteroid treatment indicating a possible role of autoimmunity in this condition (Oger and Dekaban 1995).

For HTLV-I seropositive subjects, the lifetime risk of developing TSP is approximately 2 per cent. Although TSP is often thought of as a neurological disease, such patients may be referred to a rheumatologist as a possible transverse myelitis, or a myelopathy due to disc disease. The importance of considering HTLV-I infection lies in the simplicity of making a positive diagnosis by a single serological test.

HTLV-I associated Sjögren's syndrome

The association between HTLV-I infection and Sjögren's syndrome was first described in 1988 by Vernant et al. who documented five patients from the West Indies, with HTLV-I associated TSP and lymphocytic alveolitis, with abnormal Schirmer's test and positive salivary gland biopsies (Vernant et al. 1988). Like patients with DILS due to HIV, these patients were anti-Ro/La negative, but in other respects tended to mimic idiopathic Sjögren's syndrome. Four years later, Eguchi et al. (1992) showed that Japanese patients with Sjögren's syndrome, in an area endemic for HTLV-I, had a high prevalence of HTLV-I infection. Since then several studies have shown that in endemic areas, the frequency of antibodies to HTLV-I is increased above controls. For example, in Nagasaki, 23 per cent of patients with Sjögren's syndrome were seropositive compared to 3 per cent of blood donors (Terada et al. 1994). The histological appearance of salivary gland biopsies between patients with and without HTLV-I infection is identical though using in situ hybridization, HTLV-I proviral DNA was found in infiltrating lymphocytes rather than salivary gland epithelial cells.

It can therefore be concluded that like HIV, HTLV-I can cause a sialadenitis similar to idiopathic Sjögren's syndrome. In non-endemic areas this is rare, but may be found occasionally in a multicultural society. For example, out of over 300 patients documented at our unit we have three with HTLV-I associated Sjögren's syndrome. Therefore, even in a clinical setting in Europe, HTLV-I infection is worth considering in patients with atypical Sjögren's syndrome.

HTLV-I associated arthropathy

Sato et al. (1991) described 10 patients from Japan with an HTLV-I associated arthropathy, characterized by a chronic non-erosive oligoarthritis predominantly involving the large joints, such as shoulders and knees. These observations do not prove that HTLV-I causes arthritis. An unexplained synovitis of the knees is a common problem facing rheumatologists and HTLV-I is a common infection in endemic areas. Thus a causal relationship between the virus and the arthritis remains to be established. Nevertheless some investigators are sufficiently convinced that the arthritis caused by HTLV-I does exist as an entity and is now listed as HTLV-I associated arthropathy or 'HAAP' as one of the increasing number of diseases caused by the virus.

There is also some evidence of a role for HTLV-I in idiopathic RA in endemic areas. The frequency of HTLV-I among female patients with RA in Japan (20.4 per cent) was significantly higher than among normal female blood donors (4.2 per cent) (Eguchi et al. 1996). There were no apparent clinical or laboratory differences between HTLV-I infected patients with RA and those without HTLV-I infection and it was concluded that HTLV-I infection increases the risk of developing RA.

Polymyositis

Morgan et al. (1989) first suggested that HTLV-I infection may cause polymyositis based on the observation that 85 per cent of a group of Jamaican patients with polymyositis were seropositive for HTLV-I (compared to a seroprevalence of 7.5 per cent in a control group). Further reports of polymyositis in association with HTLV-I infection have subsequently been published (e.g. Sowa 1992). Bowness et al. (1991) did not detect antibodies to HTLV-I in sera from 36 European patients with polymyositis suggesting that although HTLV-I is a recognized cause of polymyositis in endemic areas, the virus is not associated with polymyositis in non-endemic areas. Uveitis and vasculitis have been described in association with HTLV-I infection, though many of these are isolated case reports or small series and the evidence for a pathogenic role for the virus is not compelling.

HTLV-I infection: conclusion

Autoimmune manifestations of HTLV-I infection are not a large part of rheumatological practice, but clearly it can be easily missed, based on the assumption that the virus is rare in many parts of the world. However, it must be remembered that HTLV-I is most frequently transmitted vertically and many patients may not have the risk factors associated with HIV infection. Therefore, in an increasingly multiracial society, HTLV-I infection should be part of the differential diagnosis, particularly in patients presenting with symptoms of myelopathy or Sjögren's syndrome.

Diseases associated with HTLV-II infection

Although HTLV-II was originally isolated from patients with an atypical (T-cell) hairy cell leukaemia, a causal association has not yet been firmly established. Recent reports have linked HTLV-II with neurological diseases including TSP/HAM, spinocerebellar atrophy and ataxia with cognitive impairment. In addition, an increase in soft tissue infections and pneumonias have been observed in HTLV-II seropositive subjects, chiefly in intravenous drug users (Modahl et al. 1997), however, further studies are required to prove a causal role for HTLV-II in these conditions.

Endogenous retroviruses

It has been known for over 20 years that the human germ line DNA contains multiple sequences corresponding to human endogenous retroviruses (HERVs). Most of these sequences appear to have been acquired at least 10 million and possibly up to a 100 million years ago and may constitute up to 5 per cent of our germ-line DNA (Prak and Kazazian 2000). Larsson et al. (1989) proposed a unified nomenclature whereby HERV are named according to the type of tRNA primer binding site contained in the leader region located between the HERV 5′ LTR and the *gag* region. For example, HERV-K is named by the presence of a primer binding site complementary to lysine tRNA (K being the single letter amino acid code for lysine). HERV-K is the large family of human endogenous retroviruses with at least 30 copies per haploid genome. Other important HERVs include HERV-W, HERV-R (also known as ERV3), and HERV-H. Other HERVs, which have largely escaped this classification system, include ERV3 (still used in preference to HERV-R) ERV9 and HRES-1.

Over time, the vast majority of HERV loci have mutated and are no longer able to encode full length proteins. However, some HERV loci encode open reading frames and may produce viral particles. Some of these open reading frames express proteins which are differentially expressed in certain cell types. Whole virus particle production has been described in the placenta which contain HERV-K derived sequences and carry detectable levels of RT activity (Simpson et al. 1996). Given that some of these HERV proteins have the capacity to modulate the immune system as well as being antigenic in their own right, it is possible that they could have a role in autoimmune rheumatic disease.

Retroviruses and idiopathic rheumatic disease

The occurrence of autoimmune syndromes in association with human retroviral infections supports the hypothesis that idiopathic autoimmune disease could be caused by an unknown exogenous retrovirus infection or conceivably by an expressed endogenous retroviral sequence. However, there is no direct evidence that retroviruses cause any rheumatic disease in humans beyond what is seen in HIV-1 and HTLV-I infection. However, there are retroviruses which can cause clinical or laboratory phenomena suggesting that they have the necessary properties to cause rheumatic disease. Such suggestive phenomena can be summarized as follows:

1. Rheumatic disease occurring in patients with known retroviral infections.
2. Animal models of retrovirus infection.
3. Retroviral products may suppress or activate the immune system.
4. Retroviral proteins may function as autoantigens.
5. Molecular mimicry between retroviral and host proteins may occur.
6. Random insertion of proviral DNA may activate or disrupt immune genes.
7. Retroviruses can induce or inhibit apoptosis.

Rheumatic disease in patients with known retroviral infections

Amongst the plethora of autoimmune manifestations, particularly noteworthy are of features of Sjögren's syndrome and polymyositis in both HIV and HTLV-I infection. Also notable is the relative rarity of these syndromes in patients infected with either retrovirus; occurring in less than 5 per cent of seropositive individuals. This suggests that, if idiopathic disease were caused by an unknown retrovirus, it is likely to be an uncommon reaction to infection in predisposed individuals. A difficulty with the retroviral hypothesis is that most patients with idiopathic rheumatic disease are not exposed to risk factors normally associated with retroviral transmission such as promiscuity, drug abuse, etc. Counter to this argument might be that the infection could be ubiquitous and that the main means of transmission is vertical rather than via blood products or bodily fluids.

Animal models of retrovirus infection

Perhaps the most compelling animal model of retrovirus induced autoimmune rheumatic disease is the caprine arthritis encephalitis virus (CAEV). Goats infected with CAEV may develop a chronic large joint arthritis clinically and histopathologically similar to RA (Narayan et al. 1993). Synovial hyperplasia and cartilage erosion by synovial fibroblasts also occurs and the cytokine profile in affected joints was similar to that seen in RA (Lechner et al. 1997).

HTLV-I transgenic mice may also develop rheumatic disease: either Sjögren's syndrome or arthritis. The first model was described by Green et al. (1989) in which mice transgenic for *tax* and *env* developed a sialadenitis similar to that of Sjögren's syndrome. Apart from the characteristic histological features the expression of mRNA for *tax* was maximal in salivary gland suggesting that the Tax protein itself was directly responsible for the inflammation. Another model was later described in which *tax* mRNA was strongly expressed in the joints. A number of pro-inflammatory cytokines including interleukin (IL)-1α, IL-1β, IL-6, and tumour necrosis factor (TNF)-α, were increased in the synovium (Iwakura et al. 1995) supporting a direct role for Tax in inflammation.

Retroviral products may activate or suppress the immune system

As demonstrated in the transgenic mice, HTLV-I Tax protein activates a number of genes, including some of the pro-inflammatory cytokines. The development of a chronic arthritis in mice transgenic for HTLV-I *tax* may be due to the Tax-induced production of pro-inflammatory cytokines. This is a relatively novel concept where inflammatory disease can occur as a direct result of retroviral infection without the need to invoke the breakdown of tolerance as a central mechanism.

Retroviral proteins may also activate the immune system as superantigens. Superantigens are proteins of microbial origin that bind to major histocompatability complex (MHC) class II molecules and stimulate T-cells via interaction with the Vβ domain of the T cell receptor. Examples include the retrovirus mouse mammary tumour virus which encodes a superantigen in its 3′ LTR (reviewed by Acha-Orbea and MacDonald 1995). Based on the preferential expansion of an autoreactive T-cell repertoire in humans with insulin dependent diabetes (IDDM), Conrad et al. (1997) suggested that a member of the HERV-K family encoded a superantigen, which triggered T-cell mediated destruction of the pancreatic beta cells. The superantigen activity of this sequence was not confirmed in a more recent report (Lapatschek et al. 2000).

In vivo infection with HIV-1 or HTLV-I results in polyclonal activation of B-cells and hypergammaglobulinaemia. In the case of HIV infection it may be due to upregulation of co-infection with other B-cell activators such as Epstein–Barr virus or it may be due to one of the accessory proteins of the virus itself. In the case of HTLV-1, the role of Tax is particularly compelling as it can upregulate most of the B cell stimulatory cytokines such as IL-6 and IL-10.

There is evidence in animals that ERV encoded proteins may have immunosuppressive properties. Immunosuppressive sequences include the transmembrane envelope proteins (p15E) of murine and feline leukaemia viruses (reviewed by Haraguchi et al. 1995). The TM glycoproteins of some HERV elements share significant amino acid similarity with p15E. If immunosuppressive properties of expressed HERV proteins could be demonstrated *in vivo*, it is possible that defects in the proteins themselves or in their regulation could be of aetiological importance in autoimmunity. At the present time it is quite clear that such a hypothesis is long way from being proven.

Retroviral proteins may act as autoantigens

Over 25 years ago, the increased expression of a murine ERV-encoded Env protein ($gp70^{env}$) was associated with the development of glomerulonephritis in lupus-prone strains of mice (Yoshiki et al. 1974). Immune complexes of $gp70^{env}$–anti-$gp70^{env}$ were thought to be responsible (Izui et al. 1979). This was the first study to investigate an association between expression of retroviral antigens and autoimmunity. Since then, little work has been published in pursuit of the involvement of gp70 in murine lupus and the original observations remain unconfirmed.

Endogenous retroviral proteins are by definition self-antigens and a number of studies have detected antibodies to HERV proteins in healthy individuals, pregnant women, and in patients with malignancies and autoimmune diseases. A recent study from our own group has shown that antibodies to HERV-K10 envelope proteins occur in as many as 30 per cent of healthy individuals (Herve et al. 2002). This and other studies demonstrates that ERV proteins may act as autoantigens though it is difficult to establish which of many expressed proteins are driving the immune response because antibodies to Gag proteins cross-react with several retroviral sequences (Brookes et al. 1992). Moreover, the pathogenic roles of these autoantibodies are not clear.

Molecular mimicry between retroviral and host proteins may occur

If a viral antigen is similar in conformation or sequence to a host cellular component, an antiviral response may result in autoantibodies or autoreactive T-cells, a process known as 'molecular mimicry'. Retroviral proteins have partial homology to more than 15 different self-antigens (reviewed by Krieg et al. 1992), a number of which are frequent targets of autoantibodies characteristically associated with Sjögren's syndrome, SLE, mixed connective tissue disease (MCTD), or systemic sclerosis. Such cross-reactivity may explain the observation that patients with Sjögren's syndrome and SLE produce antibodies to retroviral proteins.

Integration of a retrovirus may disrupt the structure or regulation of host genes

The integration of a retroviral provirus into the host cell genome allows potential for activation or disruption of host genes. Retroviral LTRs may activate neighbouring genes, which if involved in the immune response or apoptosis could potentially result in autoimmunity. In the MRL-*lpr/lpr* strain of mouse, the integration of an endogenous retroviral element within the *fas* apoptosis gene results in abnormal splicing of *fas* transcripts and lymphocyte maturation defects, with the subsequent development of a lymphoproliferative and lupus-like autoimmune disease (Wu et al. 1993). Mutations in the *fas* gene in humans are associated with a rare autoimmune lymphoproliferative syndrome (also named Canali Smith syndrome, Fisher et al. 1995), however, the defect in *fas* is not due to a retroviral integration.

Although, in theory, the site of integration by a retrovirus is random, studies have shown that ERV integrations are found in higher frequency at specific sites, particularly areas rich in the nucleotides guanidine and cytidine. Up to 23 per cent of the human MHC class II region consists of retroelements, in contrast to a much smaller proportion of the remainder of the genome. It was suggested that retroelements in the HLA–DR genes contribute to the polymorphisms observed. Solitary ERV LTRs have been detected in some HLA–DQ haplotypes and one study has associated such an integration (a HERV-K LTR) with susceptibility to IDDM (Badenhoop et al. 1996).

Given the associations between complement deficiencies and autoimmune disease (e.g. SLE, reviewed by Atkinson, 1989), it is possible that if an ERV integration in the human complement genes resulted in complement deficiencies, autoimmunity could occur. The integration of HERV-K elements is responsible for some of the polymorphisms observed in the human C2 (Zhu et al. 1992) and C4 complement genes (Tassabehji et al. 1994) but there is currently no evidence to implicate these integrations with autoimmune disease.

Retroviruses may alter the homeostasis of apoptotic pathways

A lack of balance between cell division and apoptosis (programmed cell death) may have a role of apoptosis in the pathogenesis of autoimmunity. Failure of apoptosis of autoreactive cells, increased apoptosis of cells in target organs and the release of immunogenic antigens by apoptotic cells, have been suggested as possible mechanisms of autoimmunity in the rheumatic diseases (reviewed by Vaishnaw et al. 1997). Retroviruses (including HIV-1 and HTLV-I) have been shown to both prevent *and* induce apoptosis (reviewed by Kaplan and Sieg 1998; Chen et al. 1997). Increased apoptosis was demonstrated in the peripheral blood lymphocytes of patients with SLE (Emlen et al. 1994) and Sjögren's syndrome and in the salivary gland epithelial cells of patients with Sjögren's syndrome (Kong et al. 1997). Nakamura and colleagues examined salivary gland biopsies from patients with Sjögren's syndrome with and without HTLV-I infection for evidence of apoptosis and found no difference between the two groups, suggesting that the glandular destruction in HTLV-I induced Sjögren's syndrome was not specifically mediated by retrovirus-induced apoptosis (Nakamura et al. 1998). Conversely, in the *tax* transgenic mouse, inhibition of apoptosis using an anti-Fas monoclonal antibody (Fujisawa et al. 1996) resulted in an improvement of the arthropathy, suggesting that in this case the *tax*-induced arthropathy may be driven by apoptosis. Further studies are required to elucidate the influence of retroviruses on apoptosis in the retrovirus associated autoimmune conditions.

Retroviral infection and rheumatic disease: conclusion

Retroviral infection is therefore a rare diagnostic challenge for the rheumatologist but an important one because the correct diagnosis can fundamentally affect management. In the future, as HIV infection becomes more frequent and, with racial migration and integration, the epidemiology of HTLV-I more widespread, the rheumatologist will see increasing numbers of patients with rheumatic symptoms attributable to retrovirus infection. Although these are never likely to be common, recognition is important, as specific antiretroviral treatments become available. It is still an open question whether unknown retroviruses could cause what is currently regarded as idiopathic autoimmune rheumatic disease. Although much of the research to date has been inconclusive, the striking similarity between rheumatic disease and rheumatic syndromes caused by retroviruses in humans and animals provides a major stimulus for continuing research in this area.

References

Acha-Orbea, H. and MacDonald, H.M. (1995). Superantigens of mouse mammary tumour virus. *Annual Review of Immunology* **13**, 459–86.

Adebajo, A. and Davis, P. (1994). Rheumatic diseases in African blacks. *Seminars in Arthritis and Rheumatism* **24**, 139–53.

Atkinson, J.P. (1989). Complement deficiency: predisposing factor to autoimmune syndromes. *Clinical and Experimental Rheumatology* **7**, S95–101.

Atkinson, J.C., Schiodt, M., Robataille, S., Greenspan, D., Greenspan, J., and Fox, P.C. (1993). Salivary autoantibodies in HIV-associated salivary gland disease. *Journal of Oral Pathology & Medicine* **22**, 203–6.

Badenhoop, K., Tonjes, R.R., Rau, H., Donner, H., Rieker, W., Braun, J., Herwig, J., Mytilineos, J., Kurth, R., and Usadel, K.H. (1996). Endogenous retroviral long terminal repeats of the HLA–DQ region are associated with susceptibility to insulin-dependent diabetes mellitus. *Human Immunology* **50**, 103–10.

Bernard, L., Vincent, V., Lortholary, O., Raskine, L., Vettier, C., Colaitis, D., Mechali, D., Bricaire, F., Bouvet, E., Sadr, F.B., Lalande, V., and Perronne, C. (1999). *Mycobacterium kansasii* septic arthritis: French retrospective study of 5 years and review. *Clinical Infectious Diseases* **29**, 1455–60 (review).

Boelaert, J.R., Sperber, K., and Piette, J. (1999). Chloroquine exerts an additive *in vitro* anti-HIV type 1 effect when associated with didanosine and hydroxyurea. *AIDS Research and Human Retroviruses* **15**, 1241–7.

Bowness, P., Davies, K.A.A., Tosswill, J., Bunn, C.C., MacAlpine, L., Weber, J.N., and Walport, M.J. (1991). Autoimmune disease and HTLV-1 infection. *British Journal of Rheumatology* **30**, 141–3.

Brennan, M., Runganga, J., Barbara, J.A.J., Contreras, M., Tedder, R.S., Garson, J.A., Tuke, P.W., Mortimer, P.P., McAlpine, L., and Tosswill, J.H.C. (1993). Prevalence of antibodies to human T cell leukaemia/lymphoma virus in blood donors in north London. *British Medical Journal* **307**, 1235–9.

Brookes, S.M., Pandolfino, Y.A., Mitchell, T.J., Venables, P.J., Shattles, W.G., Clark, D.A., Entwistle, A., and Maini, R.N. (1992). The immune response to and expression of cross-reactive retroviral gag sequences in autoimmune disease. *British Journal of Rheumatology* **31**, 735–42.

Calabrese, L.H. (1998). Rheumatic aspects of human immunodeficiency virus infection and other immunodeficient states. In *Rheumatology* 2nd edn., 6.7.1–12. London: Mosby.

Chen, X., Zachar, V., Zdravkovic, M., Guo, M., Ebbesen, P., and Liu, X. (1997). Role of the Fas/Fas ligand pathway in apoptotic cell death induced by the human T cell lymphotropic virus type I Tax transactivator. *Journal of General Virology* **78**, 3277–85.

Clark, M.R., Solinger, A.M., and Hochberg, M.C. (1992). Human immunodeficiency virus infection is not associated with Reiter's syndrome. Data from three large cohort studies. *Rheumatic Diseases Clinics of North America* **18**, 267–76.

Conrad, B., Weissmahr, R.N., Boni, J., Arcari, R., Schupbach, J., and Mach, B. (1997). A human endogenous retroviral superantigen as candidate autoimmune gene in type I diabetes. *Cell* **90**, 303–13.

Dalakas, M.C., Illa, I., Pezeshkpour, G.H., Laukaitis, J.P., Cohen, B., and Griffin, J.L. (1990). Mitochondrial myopathy caused by long-term zidovudine therapy. *New England Journal of Medicine* **322**, 1098–105.

Davis, P., Stein, M., Latif, A., and Emmanuel, J. (1989). Acute arthritis in Zimbabwean patients: possible relationship to human immunodeficiency virus infection. *Journal of Rheumatology* **16**, 346–8.

Dominguez, A., Gamallo, G., Garcia, R., Lopez-Pastor, A., Pena, J.M., and Vazquez, J.J. (1994). Pathophysiology of HIV related thrombocytopenia: an analysis of 41 patients. *Journal of Clinical Pathology* **47**, 999–1003.

Eguchi, K., Matsuoka, N., Ida, H., Nakashima, M., Sakai, M., Sakito, S., Kawakami, A., Terada, K., Shimada, H., Kawabe, Y., Fukuda, T., Sawada, T., and Nagataki, S. (1992). Primary Sjögren's syndrome with antibodies to HTLV-I: clinical and laboratory features. *Annals of the Rheumatic Diseases* **51**, 769–76.

Eguchi, K., Origuchi, T., Takashima, H., Iwata, K., Katamine, S., and Nagataki, S. (1996). High seroprevalence of anti-HTLV-I antibody in rheumatoid arthritis. *Arthritis and Rheumatism* **39**, 463–6.

Emlen, W., Niebur, J., and Kadera, R. (1994). Accelerated *in vitro* apoptosis of lymphocytes from patients with systemic lupus erythematosus. *Journal of Immunology* **152**, 3685–92.

Fisher, G., Rosenberg, F., Straus, S., Dale, J., Middleton, L., Lin, A., Strober, W., Lenardo, M., and Puck, J. (1995). Dominant interfering *fas* gene mutations impair apoptosis in a human autoimmune lymphoproliferative syndrome. *Cell* **81**, 935–46.

Frankel, A.D. and Young, J.A. (1998). HIV-1: fifteen proteins and an RNA. *Annual Review of Biochemistry* **67**, 1–25.

Fujisawa, K., Asahara, H., Okamoto, K., Aono, H., Hasunuma, T., Kobata, T., Iwakura, Y., Yonehara, S., Sumida, T., and Nishioka, K. (1996). Therapeutic effect of the anti-Fas antibody on arthritis in HTLV-1 tax transgenic mice. *Journal of Clinical Investigation* **98**, 271–8.

Gessain, A., Barin, F., and Vernant, J.C. (1985). Antibodies to human T-lymphotropic virus type-1 in patients with tropical spastic paraparesis. *Lancet* **2** (8452), 407–10.

Gheradi, R., Belec, L., Mhiri, C., Gray, F., Lescs, M., Sobel, A., Guillevin, L., and Wechsler, J. (1993). The spectrum of vasculitis in human immunodeficiency virus-infected patients. *Arthritis and Rheumatism* **36**, 1164–74.

Green, J.E., Hinrichs, S.H., Vogel, J., and Jay, G. (1989). Exocrinopathy resembling Sjögren's syndrome in HTLV-I *tax* transgenic mice. *Nature* **341**, 72–4.

Haraguchi, S., Good, R.A., and Day, N.K. (1995). Immunosuppressive retroviral peptides: cAMP and cytokine patterns. *Immunology Today* **16**, 595–603.

Herve, C.A., Lugli, E.B., Brand, A., Griffiths, D.J., and Venables, P.J. (2002). Autoantibodies to human endogenous retrovirus-K are frequently detected in health and disease and react with multiple epitopes. *Clinical and Experimental Immunology* **128**, 75–82.

Hughes, R.A., Rowe, I.F., Shanson, D., and Keat, A.C. (1992). Septic bone, joint and muscle lesions associated with human immunodeficiency virus infection. *British Journal of Rheumatology* **31**, 381–8 (review).

Itescu, S., Brancato, L.J., and Winchester, R. (1989). A sicca syndrome in HIV infection: association with HLA-DR5 and CD8 lymphocytosis. *Lancet* **2** (8661), 466–8.

Iwakura, Y., Saijo, S., Kioka, Y., Nakayama-Yamada, J., Itagaki, K., Tosu, M., Asano, M., Kanai, Y., and Kakimoto, K. (1995). Autoimmunity induction by human T cell leukaemia virus type I in transgenic mice that develop chronic inflammatory arthropathy resembling rheumatoid arthritis in humans. *Journal of Immunology* **155**, 1588–98.

Izui, S., McConahey, P.J., Theofilopoulos, A.N., and Dixon, F.J. (1979). Association of circulating retroviral gp70–anti-gp70 immune complexes with murine systemic lupus erythematosus. *Journal of Experimental Medicine* **149**, 1099–116.

Kaplan, D. and Sieg, S. (1998). Role of the Fas/Fas ligand apoptotic pathway in human immunodeficiency virus type 1 disease. *Journal of Virology* **72**, 6279–82.

Kazi, S., Cohen, P.R., Williams, F., Schempp, R., and Reveille, J.D. (1996). The diffuse infiltrative lymphocytosis syndrome: clinical and immunogenetic features in 35 patients. *AIDS* **10**, 385–91.

Klaassen, R.J.L., Goldschmeding, R., Dolman, K.M., Vlekke, A.B.J., Weigel, H.M., Eeftinck Schattenkerk, J.K.M., Mulder, J.W., Westedt, M.L., and Von Dem Borne, A.E.G.K. (1992). Anti-neutrophil cytoplasmic antibodies in patients with symptomatic HIV infection. *Clinical and Experimental Immunology* **87**, 24–30.

Kong, L., Ogawa, N., Nakabayashi, T., Liu, G.T., D'Souza, E., McGuff, H.S., Guerrero, D., Talal, N., and Dang, H. (1997). Fas and Fas ligand expression in the salivary glands of patients with primary Sjögren's syndrome. *Arthritis and Rheumatism* **40**, 87–97.

Krieg, A.M., Gourley, M.F., and Perl, A. (1992). Endogenous retroviruses: potential etiologic agents in autoimmunity. *FASEB Journal* **6**, 2537–44 (review).

Lapatschek, M., Durr, S., Lower, R., Magin, C., Wagner, H., and Miethke, T. (2000). Functional analysis of the env open reading frame in human endogenous retrovirus IDDMK (1,2)22 encoding superantigen activity. *Journal of Virology* **74**, 6386–93.

Larsson, E., Kato, N., and Cohen, M. (1989). Human endogenous proviruses. *Current Topics in Microbiology and Immunology* **148**, 115–32.

Lechner, F., Vogt, H.R., Seow, H.F., Bertoni, G., Cheevers, W.P., von Bodungen, U., Zurbriggen, A., and Peterhans, E. (1997). Expression of cytokine mRNA in lentivirus-induced arthritis. *American Journal of Pathology* **151**, 1053–65.

McArthur, C.P., Subtil-DeOliveira, A., Palmer, D., Fiorella, R.M., Gustafson, S., Tira, D., and Miranda, R.N. (2000). Characteristics of salivary diffuse infiltrative lymphocytosis syndrome in West Africa. *Archives of Pathology & Laboratory Medicine* **12**, 1773–9.

McComsey, G.A., Whalen, C.C., Mawhorter, S.D., Asaad, R., Valdez, H., Patki, A.H., Klaumunzner, J., Gopalakrishna, K.V., Calabrese, L.H., and Lederman, M.M. (2001). Placebo-controlled trial of prednisone in advanced HIV-1 infection. *AIDS* **15**, 321–7.

Modahl, L.E., Young, K.C., Varney, K.F., Khayam-Bashi, H., and Murphy, E.L. (1997). Are HTLV-II-seropositive injection drug users at increased risk of bacterial pneumonia, abscess and lymphadenopathy? *Journal of Acquired Immune Deficiency Syndromes and Human Retrovirology* **16**, 169–75.

Montero, A., Giovannoni, A.G., Fernandez, M.A., Pons-Estel, B., and Sen, L. (1998). Autoantibodies in human immunodeficiency virus-infected patients with and without concurrent hepatitis C infection. *Arthritis and Rheumatism* **41**, 2077–9.

Montgomery, R., Cruickshank, E., Robertson, W., and McMenemy, W. (1964). Clinical and pathological observations in Jamaican neuropathy. A report of 206 cases. *Brain* **87**, 425–62.

Morgan, O.S., Rodgers-Johnson, P., Mora, C., and Char, G. (1989). HTLV-1 and polymyositis in Jamaica. *Lancet* **2**, 1184–7.

Muller, C., Kukel, S., Schneweis, K.E., and Bauer, R. (1994). Anti-lymphocyte antibodies in plasma of HIV-1-infected patients preferentially react with MHC class II-negative T cells and are linked to antibodies against gp41. *Clinical and Experimental Immunology* 97, 367–72.

Munoz-Fernandez, S., Cardenal, A., Balsa, A., Quiralte, J., del Arco, A., Pena, J.M., Barbado, F.J., Vazquez, J.J., and Gijon, J. (1991). Rheumatic manifestations in 556 patients with human immunodeficiency virus infection. *Seminars in Arthritis and Rheumatism* 21, 30–9.

Murphy, E.L., Varney, K.F., Miyasaki, N.T., Moore, R.J., Umekubo, J.I., Watanabe, A.N., and Khayam-Bashi, H. (1993). Human T-lymphotropic virus type I seroprevalence among Japanese americans. *The Western Journal of Medicine* 158, 480–3.

Nakamura, H., Koji, T., Tominaga, M., Kawakami, A., Migita, K., Kawabe, Y., Nakamura, T., Shirabe, S., and Eguchi, K. (1998). Apoptosis in labial salivary glands from Sjögren's syndrome (SS) patients: comparison with human T lymphotropic virus-I (HTLV-I)-seronegative and -seropositive SS patients. *Clinical and Experimental Immunology* 114, 106–12.

Narayan, O., Zink, M.C., Gorrell, M., Crane, S., Huso, D., Jolly, P., Saltarelli, M., Adams, R.J., and Clements, J.E. (1993). The lentiviruses of sheep and goats. In *The Retroviridae*, pp. 229–55. New York: Plenum Press.

Oger, J. and Dekaban, G. (1995). HTLV-I associated myelopathy: a case of viral-induced auto-immunity. *Autoimmunity* 21, 151–9.

Prak, E.T. and Kazazian, H.H. (2000). Mobile elements and the human genome. *Nature Reviews. Genetics* 1, 134–44.

Price, R.W. (1996). Neurological complications of HIV infection. *Lancet* 348, 445–52.

Rynes, R.I., Goldenberg, D.L., DiGiacomo, R., Olson, R., Hussain, M., and Veazey, J. (1988). Acquired immunodeficiency syndrome-associated arthritis. *American Journal of Medicine* 84, 810–16.

Sato, K., Maruyama, I., Maruyama, Y., Kitajima, I., Nakajima, Y., Higaki, M., Yamamoto, K., Miyasaka, N., Osame, M., and Nishioka, K. (1991). Arthritis in patients infected with human T lymphotropic virus type I. *Arthritis and Rheumatism* 34, 714–21.

Simpson, G.R., Patience, C., Lower, R., Tonjes, R.R., Moore, H.D., Weiss, R.A., and Boyd, M.T. (1996). Endogenous D-type (HERV-K) related sequences are packaged into retroviral particles in the placenta and possess open reading frames for reverse transcriptase. *Virology* 222, 451–6.

Solinger, A.M. and Hess, E.V. (1991). Induction of autoantibodies by human immunodeficiency virus infection and their significance. *Rheumatic Diseases Clinics of North America* 17, 157–76 (Review).

Solinger, A.M. and Hess, E.V. (1993). Rheumatic diseases and AIDS-is the association real? *Journal of Rheumatology* 20, 678–83.

Sowa, J.M. (1992). Human T lymphotropic virus 1, myelopathy, polymyositis and synovitis: an expanding rheumatic spectrum. *Journal of Rheumatology* 19, 316–18.

Stein, C.M. and Davis, P. (1996). Arthritis associated with HIV infection in Zimbabwe. *Journal of Rheumatology* 23, 506–11.

Tassabehji, M., Strachan, T., Anderson, M., Duncan Campbell, R., Collier, S., and Lako, M. (1994). Identification of a novel family of human endogenous retroviruses and characterisation of one family member, HERV-K (C4), located in the complement C4 gene cluster. *Nucleic Acids Research* 22, 5211–17.

Taylor, G.P. (1996). The epidemiology of HTLV-I in Europe. *Journal of Acquired Immune Deficiency Syndromes and Human Retrovirology* 13 (Suppl. 1), s8–14.

Telen, M.J., Roberts, K.B., and Bartlett, J.A. (1990). HIV-associated autoimmune hemolytic anemia: report of a case and review of the literature. *AIDS* 3, 933–7 (Review).

Terada, K., Katamine, S., Eguchi, K., Moriuchi, R., Kita, M., Shimada, H., Yamashita, I., Iwata, K., Tsuji, Y., Nagataki, S., and Miyamoto, T. (1994). Prevalence of serum and salivary antibodies to HTLV-1 in Sjögren's syndrome. *Lancet* 344, 1116–19.

Vaishnaw, A.K., McNally, J.D., and Elkon, K.B. (1997). Apoptosis in the rheumatic diseases. *Arthritis and Rheumatism* 40, 1917–27.

Vassilopoulos, D., Chalasani, P., Jurado, R.L., Workowski, K., and Agudelo, C.A. (1997). Musculoskeletal infections in patients with human immunodeficiency virus infection. *Medicine (Baltimore)* 4, 284–94 (review).

Vernant, J.C., Buisson, G., Magdeleine, J., de Thore, J., Jouannelle, A., Neisson-Vernant, C., and Monplaisir, N. (1988). T-lymphocyte alveolitis, tropical spastic paresis and Sjögren's syndrome. *Lancet* 1, 177 (letter).

Wills, J.W. and Craven, R.C. (1991). Form, function and use of retroviral gag proteins. *AIDS* 5, 639–54 (editorial).

Winchester, R., Bernstein, D.H., Fischer, H.D., Enlow, R., and Solomon, G. (1987). The co-occurrence of Reiter's syndrome and acquired immunodeficiency. *Annals of Internal Medicine* 106, 19–26.

Wu, J., Zhou, T., He, J., and Mountz, J. (1993). Autoimmune disease in mice due to an integration of an endogenous retrovirus in an apoptosis gene. *Journal of Experimental Medicine* 178, 461–8.

Yoshiki, T., Mellors, R.C., Strand, M., and August, J.T. (1974). The viral envelope glycoprotein of murine leukemia virus and the pathogenesis of immune complex glomerulonephritis of New Zealand mice. *Journal of Experimental Medicine* 140, 1011–27.

Zhu, Z.B., Hsieh, S., Bentley, D.R., Duncan Campbell, R., and Volanakis, J.E. (1992). A variable number of tandem repeats locus within the human complement C2 gene is associated with a retroposon derived from a human endogenous retrovirus. *Journal of Experimental Medicine* 175, 1783–7.

Zhu, T., Korber, B.T., Nahmias, A.J., Hooper, E., Sharp, P.M., and Ho, D.D. (1998). An African HIV-1 sequence from 1959 and implications for the origin of the epidemic. *Nature* 391, 594–7.

6.2.7 Mycobacterial diseases

Sanjiv N. Amin

Tuberculosis and leprosy are infectious diseases characterized by chronic inflammation. Tuberculosis is caused chiefly by the organism *Mycobacterium tuberculosis* and much less commonly by *M. bovis* and atypical mycobacteria (*M. avium, intercellulare, scrofulaceum, gordonae, marium*, etc.). Leprosy is caused by *M. leprae*. Most of these infections are readily amenable to modern medical and surgical treatment, which almost always cures the infection.

Tuberculosis

Epidemiology and immunopathogenesis

The World Health Organization (WHO) estimated over 8 million new tuberculosis patients in 1999, and has suggested that till 2005 the annual rate of increase in tuberculosis incidence is 3 per cent globally, 7 per cent in Eastern Europe, and over 10 per cent in African countries that are most affected by HIV/AIDS. Tuberculosis kills about 2 million people every year. Between 1 and 5 per cent of all tuberculosis patients have bone or joint infection (Pertuiset et al. 1997).

In the majority of instances, *M. tuberculosis* is transmitted from person to person via the respiratory route. Infection of a host occurs when a few bacilli are inhaled. These are sufficiently small to reach the pulmonary alveoli and are phagocytosed by alveolar macrophages. The *M. tuberculosis* multiply slowly, dividing approximately every 10–24 h, and rupture the alveolar macrophage. Growth and multiplication of the organism are essentially unimpeded, until a specific cell-mediated immune response develops after 4–8 weeks, and only if a threshold number of *M. tuberculosis* organisms is reached. Cellular immunity mediated by interferon-γ-secreting CD4+ is the major protective immune response, and of recent there is increasing evidence that a major role exists for MHC class-1 restricted CD8+ T cells. The CD8+ T cells have been shown to produce cytokines, become cytolytic and possess direct antimycobacterial activity (Flynn and Ernst 2000; Smith and Dockrell 2000). However, their protective function remains unclear.

In most infected persons, the immune response elucidated is adequate to control the infection. However, in few individuals the disease may appear within a few weeks of primary infection, and in others the bacilli may remain dormant within the macrophages for many years before entering a phase of exponential multiplication to cause the disease. The bacilli reach the bloodstream either by being carried in the lymph to the draining lymph nodes and thence to the thoracic duct, or by erosion of blood vessels in the walls of developing tuberculous lesions in the lungs. Skeletal infection can develop either by hematogenous or lymphatic spread from chronic pulmonary or lymph node foci, or by reactivation of latent mycobacteriae at sites seeded in the primary infection.

Clinical manifestations

Skeletal tuberculosis typically is a chronic and insidious infection that seldom affects more than one site. Pre-existing arthritis or old trauma, alcoholism, prolonged use of corticosteroids, and immunodeficiency diseases are significant predisposing factors. Localized pain is the commonest manifestation, usually accompanied by swelling and function impairment. The spine is affected in almost half the patients, whereas large joints—hip, knee, elbow, wrist, and shoulder are less common sites. Small joints, metaphysis of long and short bones, tendon sheaths of hands and feet, bursae, muscle and deep fasciae are rarely affected. Systemic symptoms such as fever, night sweats, body weight loss, and malaise may or may not accompany. Poncet described symmetric polyarthritis of hands and feet in 12 patients with recent and concomitant visceral tuberculosis in 1887. The concept of a reactive arthritis to tuberculosis has remained debatable and occasionally reported (Southwood et al. 1988; Dall and Long 1989).

Other, less frequently seen clinical features of tuberculosis include necrotic skin ulcers of erythema nodosum, shoulder–hand syndrome, parotid gland swelling, and red eye caused by uveitis and chorioretinitis. Secondary amyloidosis may appear many years after the tuberculous infection.

Spine tuberculosis

Tuberculosis can affect any part of the spine, although dorsal and lumbar regions are most common sites. The infection may begin in and remain confined to a vertebral body, eventually leading to its collapse and kyphotic deformity or gibbus at that site, or begin with end-plate of the vertebral body with early involvement of the adjacent disc and the next vertebral end-plate. Anterior lesions develop under the anterior spinal ligament to involve several vertebrae. The transverse or spinous processes are infrequently involved (Lindahl et al. 1996), but pedicles and laminae are affected more commonly. The formation of a paravertebral abscess is usual, and it may remain localized at the same site or track along tissue planes and neurovascular bundles to cause symptoms at a remote site. In the lumbar spine, the abscess may track along the psoas muscle to present as a swelling in groin or thigh; from thoracic vertebrae it may follow the course of a rib and present anteriorly on the chest wall. The local symptoms are pain, muscle spasm, and limited movement. The pain is characteristically worse during sleep, which perhaps is due to relaxation of the protective muscle spasm. In the occasional patient, pain may not be the predominant symptom, and kyphosis or a cold abscess is the first manifestation.

Tuberculosis involving the first and second cervical vertebrae may begin in the retropharyngeal space with secondary involvement of the bone, or more rarely in the bone itself (Lifeso 1987) (Fig. 1). With progression there is increasing ligamentous involvement, with minimal osteolytic erosions, into the odontoid or the arch of the first cervical vertebra. This would allow anterior subluxation of C1 on C2, increasing rotatory subluxation, and proximal translocation of the odontoid. In a final stage of the disease, bone destruction increases, with complete loss of the C1 arch or fracture through the base of the odontoid, leading to a grossly unstable articulation between the occiput and C2. The diagnosis is suspected if an individual with prolonged neck pain has restriction in all ranges of movement.

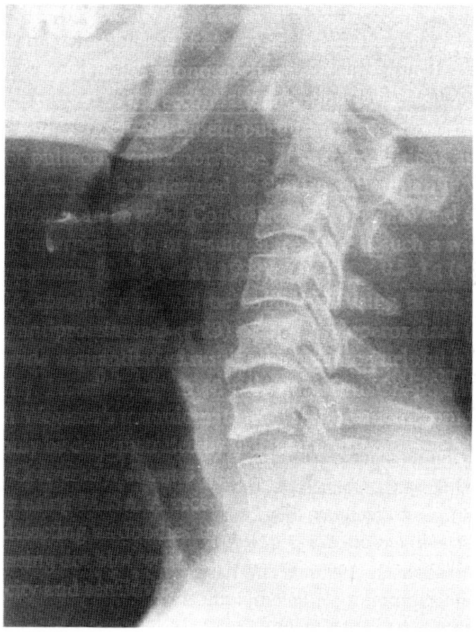

Fig. 1 Tuberculosis of C1 and C2 with a large retropharyngeal abscess.

The most serious complication of spinal tuberculosis is involvement of the spinal cord causing a neurological deficit. This may occur incompletely and slowly, with the patient complaining of difficulty in walking, or it can appear more dramatically, with complete spastic paraplegia or quadriplegia and loss of sphincter control. The neurological deficit may be secondary to medullary and radicular inflammation, cord compression by an abscess, tuberculoma, or subluxation of a vertebral body, and rarely by inflammatory vasculitis and thrombosis of spinal blood vessels.

Limb joint tuberculosis

Tuberculous arthritis is usually monoarticular, though occasionally three or more joints may be simultaneously affected, particularly in immunocompromised patients (Linares et al. 1991). Weight-bearing joints are more frequently affected, and microtrauma to cartilage is thought to predispose to the infection (Figs 2–4). The joints commonly involved are the hip, knee, ankle, sacroiliac, wrist, and shoulder, in that order (Garrido et al. 1988). Mycobacteriae from the bloodstream may directly seed the synovium or the adjacent epiphyseal bone may develop a focus of osteomyelitis that erodes through the articular surface into the joint space. The synovium gets inflamed and accumulates granulation tissue and forms a pannus that erodes the cartilage and overlying capsule and tendons. Rarely, a sinus may form from within the joint.

The infected individual usually has a long history of mild or moderate joint or bone pain along with a swelling or large effusion. On examination, there is synovial thickening and mild warmth. There is always significant muscle atrophy around the joint. If a sinus track has formed, there may be signs of superimposed pyogenic infection. Even in the early stages, there is limitation in the range of motion by effusion and synovial thickening. As infection progresses, flexion contractures and joint deformity develop. The end-result may be fibrous or bony ankylosis (Kramer and Rosenstein 1997).

Investigations and diagnosis

Laboratory tests

Tuberculosis is diagnosed if the clinical pattern is suggestive and acid-fast bacilli are demonstrated in the lesions. A smear from the infected site such

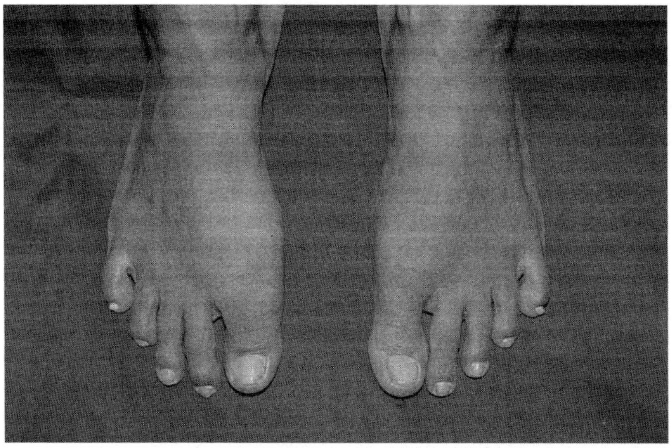

Fig. 2 The base of the right great toe was painful and swollen for 5 years in a 40-year-old pre-menopausal female; this was an indolent and slowly progressive lesion of tuberculosis.

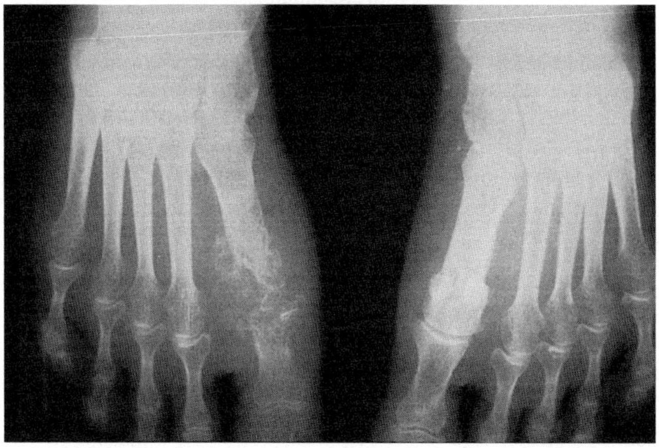

Fig. 3 Radiograph of the feet of the patient in Fig. 2 at 5 years after the onset of pain, revealing remarkable destruction of the bones and joints by tuberculous infection.

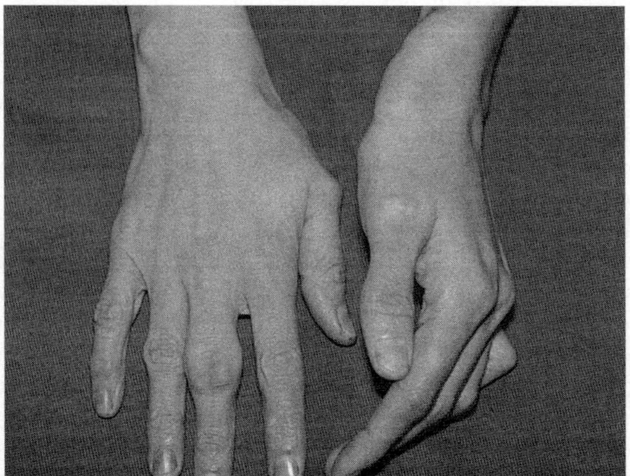

Fig. 4 Tuberculous inflammation of the right middle proximal interphalangeal joint and left abductor pollicis longus tendon sheath in a 36-year-old woman.

as a paraspinal abscess usually provides the required evidence and typical histological feature is a tuberculous granuloma with partial or complete caseation necrosis. However, typical granulomas are not always seen (particularly in the synovium) and only a tuberculoid infiltrate may be visible. In this infiltrate are seen irregular accumulations of epitheloid cells among mononuclear cells, with or without necrosis and giant cells (Levy et al. 1986).

Tuberculin or purified protein derivative (PPD) has been used for the past 50 years to support diagnosis of tuberculosis. The greatest limitation is the fact that most protein components in this substance are shared between mycobacterial species or with unrelated bacteriae. The specificity of the test is poor because patients sensitized by prior exposure to non-tuberculosis mycobacteria or vaccinated with BCG respond immunologically to PPD prepared from *M. tuberculosis* in many cases as well or better than individuals infected with *M. tuberculosis* itself. PPD replaced by specific antigens of *M. tuberculosis* have been tested for *in vitro* detection of specific interferon-γ-secreting lymphocytes sensitized by mycobacterial antigens. The assay is done as a lymphocyte stimulation with specific antigens of *M. tuberculosis*, most conveniently directly in whole blood for 24 h, followed by ELISA detection of interferon-γ produced after stimulation. The status of research in this field suggests that tuberculosis-specific antigens for *in vitro* immune-based diagnosis are likely to become a reality (Anderson et al. 2000).

In endemic tuberculosis regions, patients suspected to have bone or joint tuberculosis could be prescribed treatment without culture confirmation of the diagnosis because of lack of adequate facilities. However, in developed countries where tuberculosis is an uncommon disease, culture of a specimen or histopathology confirmation is desired before initiation of treatment (Watts and Lifeso 1996).

To culture tubercle bacilli on the Lowenstein–Jensen medium requires 4–8 weeks to detect growth. Substantial improvement in the time taken for detection and total number of positive cultures can be gained by using a carbon-14 broth based growth system such as BACTEC 460 TB (Becton Dickinson Diagnostic Instrument Systems). Mycobacterial growth metabolizes carbon-14 liberating CO_2 that can be detected by the BACTEC 460 TB instrument in about 4–14 days (Morgan et al. 1983). Conventional methods of species identification using biochemical test reactions to niacin, nitrate reduction, catalase, and several others take on average 10 days for full confirmation. The introduction of nucleic acid probes for detection of *M. tuberculosis* and other pathogenic species has gained acceptance for their excellent sensitivity and specificity, and shortened the time required to less than 4 h. In one such assay, a labelled DNA probe is reacted with the target rRNA, forming a DNA–RNA hybrid. In a chemiluminescent assay hybridized acridium ester is detected by a luminometer (Evans et al. 1992). In practice, more than half mycobacteriae isolates detected in public health laboratories of developed nations are mycobacteriae other than tuberculosis.

Advances in molecular genetics have resulted in impressive DNA hybridization probes that are non-radioactive to directly test body fluids. Several kits have become available that are based on target amplification system wherein a characteristic component of the organism is amplified to a detectable level (Woods 2001). Some of the methods available include polymerase chain reaction (PCR) amplification, RNA amplification, strand displacement amplification, and ligase chain reaction (LCR) amplification. However, these assays are expensive, not validated for non-respiratory specimens, and should be interpreted in conjunction with patient's clinical data. These techniques are extremely useful in identifying mutations responsible for drug resistance, for example, rifampicin resistance by the PCR amplified *rpoB* gene (Gamboa et al. 1998; Traore et al. 2000).

Enzyme linked immunoassays to detect antibodies against mycobacterial antigens in either serum or body fluids in patients with bone and joint tuberculosis do appear to hold great potential; however, these tests at the current state of development cannot be accepted as alternative to conventional methods due to their sub-optimal sensitivity and poor ability to distinguish between active and latent infection and between infection of *M. tuberculosis* and mycobacterium other than tuberculosis (Chan et al. 2000).

Imaging studies

Plain radiographs of the skeleton will have features suggestive of tuberculous infection though none described are diagnostic. Osteoporosis is the first sign of active infection. If long bones are affected (osteomyelitis), small zones of clearly defined radiolucency indicate granular foci. Diffuse demineralization surrounds these osteolytic areas. As caseation takes place, the osteolytic foci become more evident. When the healing process begins, the perifocal bone becomes sclerotic. If the central demineralized area is merely exudative, healing results in reossification with eventual return of the normal trabecular pattern. If central caseation occurs during the active phase of infection, with calcium deposition, then the dense image of a sequestrum is surrounded by an osteolytic ring representing the fibrous wall beyond which the bone is demineralized. In tuberculous dactylitis the soft tissue swelling is obvious and there may be mild or exuberant periostitis of phalanges, metacarpals, or metatarsals (Bush and Schneider 1984). Expansion of the bone accompanied by cystic change is termed spina ventosa. In involvement of a peripheral joint the synovial shadow may be clearly visible in a slightly underexposed radiograph. If the arthritis is destructive, then the joint space narrows due to erosion of cartilage, and the subchondral cortex of bone becomes ragged and osteoporotic. Vague, irregular densities seen in the surrounding soft tissues may signify abscess formation.

The radiographic appearance of spinal tuberculosis depends on the extent of infection. Destructive changes occasionally confined to a vertebral body or part of two posterior elements of the vertebral complex such as the lamina or pars, but these are uncommon and easily confused with malignant disease. More typically seen is reduction of the disc space, with irregularity of adjacent end-plates, surrounded by a soft tissue swelling due to a paravertebral abscess. Later, more extensive destruction and increased abscess formation are evident. Kyphotic or scoliotic deformity develops as vertebral destruction progresses. In children, secondary changes, such as an increase in vertebral height, may develop in uninvolved adjacent vertebrae to produce a compensatory lordosis above and below the kyphotic deformity. A severe kyphotic deformity may increase with time, even after healing has occurred, because of the gravitational effect on the deformed spine.

Radiological evidence of healing after successful drug treatment is usually observed late on routine radiographs, both in limb bones or joints and the spine. Sclerosis is a feature of healing, and appears variably from onset to within 5 months of starting drug treatment. The change from sclerosis to normal bone density takes 5 years or much longer. Paravertebral soft-tissue masses may also take as long as 15 months to resolve. Involvement of adjacent vertebrae is often associated with the reduction in disc space, fusion of the vertebrae, and the formation of syndesmophyte-like bone bridges.

Computed tomography (CT) is provenly superior to conventional radiographs in detecting and monitoring paravertebral abscesses and particularly to target the biopsy site (Watts and Lifeso 1996). The CT findings indicative of an abscess include an abnormal mass of low attenuation number, displacement of surrounding structures, obliteration of normal fascial planes, and macroscopic calcifications. However, none of these features is specific for and differential diagnoses include other pyogenic infections, usually of the more chronic nature such as brucellosis and nocardiosis. Magnetic resonance imaging (MRI) is a useful modality because it can discriminate between abcesses and granulation tissue, delineate soft tissue masses, and identify the amount of bone destruction (Kim et al. 1994). Nuclear medicine imaging can detect a small focus of bone infection as a hot spot in the initial stages of vertebral tuberculosis. However, if bone destruction has occurred, scans with technetium-99, gallium-67, and indium-111 are often negative (Watts and Lifeso 1996).

Treatment

The cornerstone of the treatment of musculoskeletal tuberculosis is a good regimen of antituberculous drugs, with surgical intervention in selected cases. Drug susceptibility testing is recommended on all *M. tuberculosis* isolates. The available drugs are listed in Table 1. Isoniazid is recommended in conjunction with other drugs for the entire duration of therapy, and in absence of drug resistance, a regimen of isoniazid and rifampicin for 9 months is curative. The antituberculosis agents have excellent tissue penetration and hence the treatment of bone and joint tuberculosis should be no more difficult than pulmonary tuberculosis. However, due to paucity of controlled trials in patients with extra-pulmonary tuberculosis, at least 12 months duration therapy is recommended for all ages (Bass et al. 1994). Some of the regimens for bone and joint tuberculosis are:

1. rifampicin, isoniazid, and pyrazinamide daily for initial 2 months, followed by rifampicin and isoniazid daily or two times a week or three times a week for 10 months;
2. rifampicin, isoniazid, pyrazinamide daily for the first 2 weeks, followed by
   (a) rifampicin, isoniazid, pyrazinamide two times a week for 6 weeks, followed by,
   (b) rifampicin and isoniazid daily or two times a week or three times a week for 10 months, with ethambutol added if the patient is from or in an endemic region of tuberculosis;
3. rifampicin, isoniazid, pyrazinamide, streptomycin, or ethambutol, three times a week for 6 months, followed by isoniazid and ethambutol for 6 months.

The treatment differs for persons infected with drug resistant strains. In adults, baseline estimate of liver enzymes, bilirubin and creatinine, and complete blood count should be organized. If pyrazinamide is prescribed, the uric acid levels must be estimated and for ethambutol the visual acuity and red–green colour perception should be tested. During treatment, all patients should be clinically reviewed at least once in 2 or 3 months and monitored for adverse effects. The duration of treatment must be extended if clinical features have failed to improve during the initial 12 months. Most relapses are likely to occur within 12 months after omission of treatment. Multidrug-resistant tuberculosis (defined as resistance to at least isoniazid and rifampicin) is usually curable and extended regimens for 12, 18, or 24 months should be planned according to the drug susceptibility results if available and must include at least 4 or 6 drugs, for example, ciprofloxacin or ofloxacin, ethambutol, kanamycin or amikacin, ethionamide or pyrazinamide, aminosalicylic acid, and cycloserine (Iseman 1993; Fujiwara et al. 2000).

HIV-infected patients do not have increased risk of treatment failure or relapse, if they adhere to standard treatment regimes, though the treatment should be extended if clinical response is slow or less than anticipated (Zumla et al. 2000). Rifampicin reduces the blood levels of concomitantly ingested antiretroviral agents, particularly the protease inhibitors and non-nucleoside reverse-transcriptase inhibitors. In these patients, Rifabutin is preferred as it has fewer interactions with the protease inhibitors and non-nucleoside reverse-transcriptase inhibitors, except ritonavir and delavirdine, respectively (Center for Disease Control and Prevention 1998).

Indications for adjunctive surgical procedures include presence of large abcesses, in case of vertebral tuberculosis the development of neurologic deficits (acute deterioration, paraparesis, paraplegia) and/or spinal instability or deformity of more than 5°. The posterior (laminectomy), posterolateral (costotransverseectomy), or anterior approach would be planned depending on the pattern of affection and experience of the surgeon. External bracing for 6–12 months is recommended for patients with spine tuberculosis (Rezai et al. 1996). Surgery is not indicated for tuberculous limb joint arthritis if the infection is limited to the synovium (or bursa), with little or no radiographic involvement of the adjacent bone. If the synovium is affected and adjacent bone and cartilage are partially eroded but without gross instability of the joint, there is an argument for synovectomy together

Table 1 Drugs for tuberculosis

Drug, route	Dose			Adverse effects	Recommended regular monitoring	Comments
	Daily	Twice weekly	Thrice weekly			
First-line agents						
Isoniazid, oral	Child, 10 mg/kg Adults, 300 mg (maximum 300 mg)	Child, 20–70 mg/kg Adults, 15 mg/kg (maximum 900 mg)	Adults, 15 mg/kg (maximum 900 mg)	Hepatitis, peripheral neuritis, CNS effects	Serum liver enzymes (if baseline value abnormal)	Overdose may be fatal; aluminium containing antacids reduce absorption and pyridoxine hydrochloride may reduce neurologic effects
Rifampicin, oral	Child, 10–20 mg/kg Adults, 600 mg (maximum 600 mg)	Child, 10–20 mg/kg Adults, 600 mg	Adults, 600 mg	Hepatitis, fever and flu-like syndrome, thrombocytopaenia, renal failure	Serum liver enzymes, creatinine	Body fluids orange discoloration, single dose on empty stomach preferred
Pyrazinamide, oral	Child, 20–30 mg/kg Adults, 1.5–2.5 g	Child, 40–50 mg/kg Adults, 2.5–3.5 gm	Adults, 2.0–3.0 g	GI disturbance, rash, hyperuricaemia, arthralgia	Serum liver enzymes (if baseline value abnormal)	Treat increased uric acid only if symptomatic; interaction with oral hypoglycaemics
Ethambutol, oral	Child and adults, 15–25 mg/kg, (maximum 2.5 g)	Child, 30–50 mg/kg Adults, 50 mg/kg	Adults, 30 mg/kg	Diminished red–green discrimination and visual acuity, rash	Monthly colour vision and acuity	Optic toxicity may be unilateral; to to be avoided in children unable to comprehend vision testing
Streptomycin, intramuscular	Child, 20–30 mg/kg Adults, 15 mg/kg			Vestibular and auditory effects, renal insufficiency, eosinophilia, hypokalaemia and hypomagnesaemia	Audiometry, serum creatinine, potassium and magnesium	
Second-line agents						
Capreomycin, intramuscular	Child, 15–30 mg/kg Adults 15 mg/kg			Vestibular and auditory effects, renal insufficiency, eosinophilia, hypokalaemia and hypomagnesaemia	Audiometry, serum creatinine, potassium and magnesium	
Ciprofloxacin, oral	Adults, 750–1500 mg			GI disturbance, insomnia, tremulousness, headache		Variable absorption
Clofazimine, oral	Child, 50–200 mg Adults, 100–300 mg			GI disturbance		Efficacy not proved, orange-brown skin discoloration
Cycloserine, oral	Child, 15–20 mg/kg Adults, 500–1000 mg (in three or four divided doses)			Seizures, depression, psychosis, rash	Mental status assessment	Increase dose gradually, pyridoxine hydrochloroide 50 mg with each 250 mg cycloserine will reduce CNS effects
Ethionamide, oral	Child, 15–20 mg/kg Adults, 500–1000 mg (in three or four divided doses)			GI disturbance, metallic taste, hepatitis, hypothyroidism	Serum liver enzymes and thyroid hormones	Increase dose gradually and as tolerated, concomitant antiemetic may be necessary
Kanamycin and amikacin, intramuscular	Child, 15–30 mg/kg Adults, 15 mg/kg			Vestibular and auditory effects, renal insufficiency, hypokalaemia and hypomagnesaemia	Audiometry, serum creatinine, potassium and magnesium	
Ofloxacin, oral	Adults, 600–800 mg			GI disturbance, insomnia, tremulousness, headache		Variable absorption
Levofloxacin, oral	Adults, 500–1000 mg			GI disturbance, insomnia, tremulousness, headache		Variable absorption
Aminosalicylic acid, oral	Child, 150 mg/kg			GI disturbance, hypersensitivity, hepatotoxicity, hypothyroidism	Serum thyroid hormones	Contraindicated in G6PD deficient patients, increase dose gradually and as tolerated
Rifabutin, oral	Child, 10–20 mg/kg Adults, 5 mg/kg (maximum 300 mg)	Child, 10–20 mg/kg Adults, 5 mg/kg (maximum 300 mg)		Rash, hepatitis, neutropaenia and thrombocytopaenia	CBC monthly, serum liver enzymes (if baseline value abnormal)	Body fluids orange discoloration, interaction with concomitant protease inhibitors or non-nucleoside reverse-transcriptase inhibitor
Rifapentine		Adults, 600 mg once or twice a week		GI disturbance, hepatitis, hyperuricaemia, dizziness	Serum liver enzymes, bilirubin, CBC	Cross-resistance with rifampicin, body fluids orange discoloration

with antituberculous drugs to reduce the time needed for convalescence and reduce limitation in the range of joint movement. For advanced joint destruction (complete loss of cartilage and disorganization of the bones), the appropriate surgery is synovectomy, debridement, and fusion of the involved joint. Total arthroplasty is contraindicated in the presence of active tuberculosis. After the infection has been controlled, arthroplasty may be planned for weight-bearing joints (Kim 1988).

Skeletal non-tuberculous mycobacterial infection

Immunocompromised patients, for example, suffering from AIDS or malignancy or taking corticosteroids are more susceptible to atypical mycobacterial infections. Common sites of infection are small long bones (phalanges), tendon sheaths, bursae or synovium on wrist, knee, and ankles. Local pain and swelling would be the manifestation associated with increased systemic symptoms such as low grade fever and weight loss. Mycobacterial diseases in HIV patients usually occurs in advanced stages and after CD4+ count is lower than 100 cells/mm^3. Multiple site affection, concomitant skin infection, and dissemination of infection occurs frequently (Hirsch et al. 1996). The most common isolated bacteriae are *Mycobacterium avium intercellulare, M. chelonei, M. fortuitum, M. haemophilum*, and *M. kansasii. M. avium intracellulare* is usually resistant to isoniazid and pyrazinamide, hence the combination therapy must include a new macrolide (clarithromycin or azithromycin), ethambutol, and a third drug—rifampicin, ciprofloxacillin, amikacin, and clofazimine (Benson 1994). *M. chelonei* and *M. fortuitum* infections too are usually resistant to all conventional antituberculosis drugs, therefore alternative agents such as amikacin, with clarithromycin or cefoxitin, ciproflaxacillin, or a tetracycline are prescribed (French et al. 1997). *M. haemophilum* appears to be an emerging pathogen against which rifampicin, amikacin, and ciproflaxacillin seem to be effective (Straus et al. 1994), whereas *M. kansasii* responds well to rifampicin, isoniazid, and ethambutol combination for extended duration of 18 months (Witzig et al. 1995).

Summary of management

The diagnosis of tuberculosis is suspected from the clinical features and appropriate imaging. The final diagnosis is by smear of the aspirate for acid-fast bacilli or from histopathological examination of excised tissue. Appropriate specimens must be obtained before treatment is begun. The material is cultured whenever possible, chiefly to ascertain sensitivity to antituberculous drugs.

The initial drug treatment is with rifampicin, isoniazid, and pyrazinamide for the first 2 months, followed by rifampicin, isoniazid (and ethambutol in endemic regions) for 10 months. Drug resistance is suspected if there is worsening of clinical signs and symptoms after the first 3 or 4 months of treatment and imaging reveals increased tissue destruction. If reports on culture and antituberculous drug sensitivity are available, then at least four of the appropriate drugs are selected, of which two or three must be bactericidal. In the absence of drug sensitivity reports, the treatment must be changed to kanamycin, isoniazid, ethionamide, cycloserine, and ofloxacin or ciprofloxacin. The duration of treatment is then extended to 18 or 24 months. Majority of atypical mycobacteriae are resistant to the conventional antituberculosis drugs and they respond to longer duration (12–24 months) combinations of aminoglycosides, macrolides, fluroquinolones, or tetracycline.

Surgical intervention is most often necessary to obtain a specimen for diagnosis and sometimes as adjunctive to drugs treatment. Immobilization of the affected region is desired, at least for spinal tuberculosis. Joint infection seldom necessitates synovectomy, except for the occasional patient in whom the diagnosis was delayed and there is a discharging sinus. Most patients not requiring synovectomy can remain ambulatory; if a leg joint is affected, partial weight bearing is recommended for the first 3 or 4 months. This is followed by physiotherapy to build lost muscle mass and tone. Surveillance for 1 year after the end of drug treatment is recommended.

Leprosy

Leprosy is a chronic infectious disease caused by *M. leprae*, an acid fast, rod-shaped bacillus that mainly affects skin, peripheral nerves, mucosa of upper respiratory tract and occasionally the eyes, bones, and joints. G.A. Hansen discovered *M. leprae* in 1873.

The WHO estimate of leprosy patients worldwide at the beginning of 2000 was about 640 000, as reported by 91 countries, of which 70 per cent are in India, Myanmar, and Nepal. Africa is the next most affected area, followed by Brazil. It is impossible to estimate the number of unreported patients. Leprosy can affect an individual at any age, but cases in infants of less than 1 year old are extremely rare. No major interaction between HIV infection and leprosy is documented (Gebre et al. 2000).

Mycobacterium leprae is virtually non-toxic and all persons who get infected do not suffer the disease. Genetic factors are considered to play a role in the clinical expression of the diseases after infection. Leprosy is acquired by direct person-to-person transmission (Reich 1987). The possibility of transmission of leprosy through the respiratory route is gaining increasing attention, although spread by insects has also been suspected. The incubation period is difficult to measure, and estimates vary from 6 months to a few decades.

Although the usual course of leprosy is indolent, occasional interruption by 'reactional states' is observed in patients who are either untreated or already receiving antileprosy drugs. Tender sub-cutaneous nodules develop and the associated features are low-grade fever, lymphadenopathy, and arthritis.

The earliest histopathological events in leprosy are not known. Perhaps the majority of infections are overcome at the site of entry (possibly the mucosa of the respiratory tract) and the bacilli destroyed. The Schwann cells of the nerves in the upper respiratory tract may be the first to harbour the bacilli and haematogenous spread occurs thereafter. The skin is probably involved via the endothelial cells of small vessels. Bacilli are seen in superficial nerve plexuses and perivascular macrophages in the skin in early lesions, with mild local lymphocytic infiltration. In majority of infected persons, these lesions resolve spontaneously with eradication of bacilli. If the bacilli do persist and multiply in skin and/or nerves, the inflammatory reactions are amplified and lesions of leprosy appear. These lesions range from organized epithelioid-cell granulomas containing giant cells with few or no bacilli, through intermediate stages with less-organized epithelioid cells containing more bacilli, to containing mainly macrophages and abundant bacilli. In the reactional states, there is increased inflammation in the lesions with activation of epithelioid cells, oedema, polymorphonuclear leucocyte infiltration, and often a necrotizing vasculitis.

The intraosseous lesions of leprosy are characterized by granulomatous tissue reactions that lead to trabecular destruction. The lesions are evident in the epiphysis and metaphyses of tubular bones, and direct involvement of the medullary canal can also occur.

Clinical manifestations

The first signs of leprosy are usually cutaneous. Single or multiple, hypopigmented macules or plaques may appear. Fully developed skin lesions are densely anaesthetic and have lost sweat glands and hair follicles. Their distribution is not symmetrical. Nerve involvement occurs early and the superficial nerve leading from lesion is enlarged. The supraorbital, facial, greater auricular, ulnar, median, radial cutaneous, common peroneal, sural, anterior, or posterior tibial nerves may be grossly enlarged and easily palpated. There may be severe paraesthesias initially, followed by muscle atrophy. If the disease progresses and the hands and feet are affected, then contractures develop. In a more advanced stage, osteolysis of the terminal phalanges occurs. In lepromatous leprosy, the skin lesions are macules, nodules, papules, or plaques with predilection for the face, wrists, elbows, buttocks, and knees. Involvement of major nerve trunks in common and leads to glove-and-stocking paraesthesias in the extremities.

The incidence of direct involvement of the skeleton in leprosy is probably under-reported. Symmetrical, peripheral, inflammatory polyarthritis of insidious onset with a pattern of exacerbation and remission is observed in some patients (Atkin et al. 1989; Gibson et al. 1994), which is different from the joint involvement of erythema nodosum leprosum. Affected joints can include the wrist, knees, and hands and feet. Morning stiffness is variable from 30 min to 1 h. Symptomatic improvement is observed within a few weeks of starting multidrug treatment.

A different pattern of involvement is with changes that are usually confined to the small bones of the face, the hands, and feet (Atkin et al. 1989). At the fingers and toes it may appear as a dactylitis. The osseous involvement is probably due to extension of infection from overlying dermal or mucosal areas. The periosteum is initially contaminated (leprous periostitis) and subsequently the cortex and marrow are infected (leprous osteitis and osteomyelitis). In an occasional patient, haematogenous spread of infection can occur, leading to other intramedullary foci in the tubular long bones and the ribs. Overall, the progression of the lesions is very slow.

Neuroarthropathy is a progressive, degenerative joint change due to lesions of peripheral nerves and the skeletal changes may follow the involvement of nerves by two or three decades. The bones of the hands and feet are most susceptible. In the feet the changes usually start in the medial arch and later involve the lateral arch, talus, and calcaneus (Horibe et al. 1988). In extreme cases, dissolution of the mid-foot results in separation of the forefoot and the hind foot, and the tibia is driven downwards to become weight-bearing. Infection and bone injury, which can occur separately as sequelae to neuropathy and trophic ulcers, tend to accelerate the skeletal changes, leading to disintegration of the affected bones and joints.

The acute and chronic arthritis associated with the reactional state of erythema nodosum leprosum is common (Karat et al. 1966). The development of synovitis and/or dactylitis coincides closely with the appearance of fulminant skin lesions (Plate 98), and the patient is febrile and toxic.

Diagnosis, classification, and investigations

The principal criteria for the diagnosis of leprosy are:

1. skin lesion consistent with leprosy and with definite sensory loss, with or without thickened nerves,
2. positive skin smears.

Two indices that depend on observation of *M. leprae* in smears from skin or nasal smears are useful in assessing the amount of infection, and the viability of the organisms and also the progress of the patient under treatment. They are the bacteriological index and the morphological index.

The bacteriological index (BI) is an expression of the bacterial loads that is calculated by counting six to eight stained smears under the 100× oil immersion lens. The smear is made by nicking the skin with a sharp scalpel and scraping it; the fluid and tissue obtained are spread fairly thickly on a slide and stained by the Ziehl–Neelsen method and decolourized (but not completely) with 1 per cent acid alcohol.

The results are expressed on a logarithmic scale.

1+ At least 1 bacillus in every 100 fields.

2+ At least 1 bacillus in every 10 fields.

3+ At least 1 bacillus in every field.

4+ At least 10 bacilli in every field.

5+ At least 100 bacilli in every field.

6+ At least 1000 bacilli in every field.

The bacteriological index is affected by the depth of the skin incision, the thoroughness of the scrape, and the thickness of the film.

The morphological index (MI) is calculated by counting the numbers of solid-staining acid-fast rods. Only the solid-staining bacilli are viable. Solid-staining *M. leprae* may reappear for short periods in patients being successfully treated with drugs and measurement of MI is liable for observer variations and therefore not always reliable.

Leprosy can be classified on the basis of clinical manifestations and skin smear results. In the classification based on skin smears, patients showing negative smears at all sites are grouped as paucibacillary (PB) leprosy, while those showing positive smears at any site are grouped as having multibacillary (MB) leprosy. However, in practice, clinical criteria are used for classifying and deciding the appropriate treatment regimen for individual patients, particularly in view of the non-availability or non-dependability of the skin-smear services. The clinical system of classification for the purpose of treatment includes the use of number of skin lesions and nerves involved as the basis for grouping leprosy patients into MB and PB leprosy.

Patients with MB leprosy frequently have mild anaemia, an elevated erythrocyte sedimentation rate, and hypergammaglobulinaemia; 10–20 per cent of patients show a false-positive reaction to antiphospholipid antigens (Elbeialy et al. 2000), rheumatoid factor, and antinuclear antibodies (Garcia-de la Torre 1993).

Mycobacterium leprae is an acid-fast bacillus morphologically and biochemically similar to *M. tuberculosis.* It does not grow in artificial media or tissue cultures but is consistently propagated in the footpads of mice and nine-banded armadillos for the purpose of epidemiological studies and drug evaluation. The bacillus is slow to multiply and the doubling time is around 12 days in optimal conditions in murine footpads. The technique is expensive and time-consuming, and it takes at least 10 months for the organism to grow.

The radiographic features of leprous osteitis are enlarged nutrient foramina, osteoporosis, endosteal thinning, and cyst-like lesions that are best appreciated in the phalanges. Bone sclerosis, which signifies the healing process, may also be seen. In the face, nasal destruction is characteristic. Destruction of the alveolar process and the anterior nasal spine of the maxilla appear to be related to primary involvement of the bone as well as to secondary infection. In patients with neuroarthropathy the typical changes begin with erosion of the terminal tufts of the phalanges and in the more advanced cases the entire length of terminal group of phalanges may be resorbed. A rare but specific radiographic finding is calcification of a large peripheral nerve such as the radial or ulnar.

Treatment

The current multidrug therapy recommended by the WHO for leprosy in adults is, for MB disease (BI, >2+), rifampicin, 600 mg orally once monthly, dapsone 100 mg orally daily, and clofazimine, 300 mg orally once monthly and additionally 50 mg daily. The duration of treatment is at least 1 year and until negative skin tests are obtained, which occasionally extends to beyond 5 years. For PB disease (BI, 2+) the regimen is rifampicin, 600 mg orally once monthly, and dapsone, 100 mg orally daily. The duration of treatment is 6 months. All drugs are prescribed in full doses from the beginning of treatment and continued without interruption, even during the reactional states.

Evidence of clinical improvement should appear after 8–12 weeks from the beginning of treatment. The clinical response to adequate therapy may be confused by reactional states. Mild lepra reactions are controlled by non-steroidal anti-inflammatory drugs such as aspirin or indomethacin. In severe cases, prednisolone (60–100 mg/daily) may be required. For the reactional state of erythema nodosum leprosum, clofazimine 100 mg orally three times a day for 2 or 3 weeks followed by tapering off to a lower dose may be helpful. An alternative, effective drug is thalidomide, especially for those patients who later take a chronic course with erythema nodosum leprosum. The usual dose of thalidomide is 200 mg orally twice daily, which is then gradually tapered off to a maintenance dose of 50–100 mg daily. Thalidomide is absolutely contraindicated in pregnancy.

Non-steroidal anti-inflammatory drugs usually fail to alleviate the symptoms of the polyarthritis, and they regress within a few weeks after starting antibiotic treatment. Those who present with neuroarthropathy are far more difficult to treat, particularly when the feet are involved (Warren 1973). Absolute rest for the affected limbs and control of superimposed infection are mainstays of treatment. Immobilization in plaster until all ulcerative lesions of the skin have healed may be necessary. Regular exercises are required to maintain the flexibility of the other joints until the ulcers heal. Thereafter, graded weight bearing is permitted. Amputation may be indicated if advanced disintegration of bones and joints has occurred, as the patient would be better off with a prosthesis. Advanced deformities of the hands, associated with tendon rupture, can be functionally improved by appropriate tendon-transfer surgery.

Summary of management

The diagnosis is usually evident from the clinical examination of the skin, and tender nerves are palpable at the elbows, wrists, and near the head of the fibula. Polyarthritis and enthesitis are sometimes observed in all stages of the disease. Multidrug treatment is the mainstay of therapy, and the duration largely depends on the extent of dermal involvement. The bacillary count on the slit-skin smear enables one to judge if the patient has PB or MB disease. Dapsone and rifampicin are given for 6 or 12 months to patients with PB disease. Those with MB disease are given dapsone, rifampicin, and clofazimine for 2 years, and if the slit-skin smears remain positive the treatment may be extended to 5 years. The symptoms of arthritis and enthesitis regress within 3 or 4 months of the start of treatment. In late stages, some patients develop a neuropathic foot and subluxation of joints that require surgical rehabilitation. Reactive states are occasionally observed in the first year of treatment and the patient is then given aspirin or low-dose prednisolone for 6–8 weeks to alleviate the symptoms, while the multidrug therapy is continued.

References

Anderson, P. et al. (2000). Specific immune-based diagnosis of tuberculosis. *Lancet* **356**, 1099–104.

Atkin, S.L. et al. (1989). Clinical and laboratory studies of arthritis in leprosy. *British Medical Journal* **298**, 1423–5.

Bass, J.B. et al. (1994). Treatment of tuberculosis and tuberculosis infection in adults and children. *American Journal of Respiratory Critical Care in Medicine* **149**, 1359–74.

Benson, C.A. (1994). Treatment of disseminated disease due to the *Mycobacterium avium* complex in patients with AIDS. *Clinical Infectious Diseases* **18** (Suppl. 3), S237–42.

Bush, D.C. and Schneider, L.H. (1984). Tuberculosis of the hand and wrist. *Journal of Hand Surgery* **9A**, 391–8.

Center for Disease Control and Prevention (1998). Prevention and treatment of tuberculosis among patients infected with human immunodeficiency virus: principles of therapy and revised recommendations. *Morbidity and Mortality Weekly Report* **47** (RR-20), 1–58.

Chan, E.D., Heifets, L., and Iseman, M.D. (2000). Immunologic diagnosis of tuberculosis: a review. *Tubercle and Lung Disease* **80** (3), 131–40.

Dall, L. and Long, L. (1989). Stanford Poncet's disease: tuberculous rheumatism. *Review of Infectious Diseases* **11**, 105–7.

Elbeialy, A. et al. (2000). Antiphospholipid antibodies in leprotic patients: a correlation with disease manifestations. *Clinical and Experimental Rheumatology* **18** (4), 492–4.

Evans, K.D. et al. (1992). Identification of *Mycobacterium tuberculosis* and *Mycobacterium avium-intercellulare* directly from primary BACTEC cultures using acridine-ester-labelled DNA probes. *Journal of Clinical Microbiology* **30**, 2427–31.

Flynn, J.L. and Ernst, J.D. (2000). Immune responses in tuberculosis. *Current Opinion in Immunology* **12**, 432–6.

French, A.L., Benator, D.A., and Gordin, F.M. (1997). Nontuberculous mycobacterial infections. *Medical Clinics of North America* **81**, 361–79.

Fujiwara, P.I., Simone, P.M., and Munsiff, S.S. (2000). The treatment of tuberculosis. In *Tuberculosis: A Comprehensive International Approach* 2nd edn. (ed. L.B. Reichman and E.S. Hershfield), pp. 401–46. New York: Marcel Dekker.

Gamboa, F. et al. (1998). Evaluation of a commercial probe asay for detection of rifampicin resistance in *Mycobacterium tuberculosis* directly from respiratory and non-respiratory clinical specimens. *European Journal of Clinical Microbiology of Infectious Diseases* **17**, 189–92.

Garcia-de la Torre, I. (1993). Autoimmune phenomenon in leprosy, particularly antinuclear antibodies and rheumatoid factor. *Journal of Rheumatology* **20**, 900–3.

Garrido, G. et al. (1988). A review of peripheral tuberculous arthritis. *Seminars in Arthritis and Rheumatism* **18**, 142–9.

Gebre, S. et al. (2000). The effect of HIV status on the clinical picture of leprosy: a prospective study in Ethopia. *Leprosy Review* **71** (3), 338–43.

Gibson, T., Ahsan, Q., and Hussein, K. (1994). Arthritis of leprosy. *British Journal of Rheumatology* **33**, 963–6.

Hirsch, R. et al. (1996). Human immunodeficiency virus-associated atypical mycobacterial skeletal infections. *Seminars in Arthritis and Rheumatism* **25**, 347–56.

Horibe, S. et al. (1988). Neuroarthropathy of the foot in leprosy. *Journal of Bone and Joint Surgery* **70**, 481–5.

Iseman, M.D. (1993). Treatment of multidrug-resistant tuberculosis. *New England Journal of Medicine* **329**, 784–91.

Karat, A.B. et al. (1966). Acute exudative arthritis in leprosy: rheumatoid arthritis like syndrome in association with erythema nodosum leprosum. *British Medical Journal* **ii**, 770–3.

Kim, Y.H. (1988). Total knee, arthroplasty for tuberculous arthritis. *Journal of Bone and Joint Surgery* **70A**, 1322–30.

Kim, N.H., Lee, H.M., and Suh, J.S. (1994). Magnetic Resonance Imaging for the diagnosis of tuberculous spondylitis. *Spine* **19**, 95–103.

Kramer, N. and Rosenstein, E.D. (1997). Rheumatologic manifestations of tuberculosis. *Bulletin on the Rheumatic Diseases* **46**, 5–8.

Levy, A. et al. (1986). Early recognition of tuberculous arthritis assisted by CT scan and closed needle synovial biopsy. *Clinical Rheumatology* **5**, 523–6.

Linares, L.F. et al. (1991). Tuberculous arthritis with multiple joint involvement. *Journal of Rheumatology* **18**, 635–6.

Lindahl, S. et al. (1996). Imaging of tuberculosis. IV: spinal manifestations in 63 patients. *Acta Radiologica* **37**, 506–11.

Lifeso, R.M. (1987). Atlanto axial tuberculosis in adults. *Journal of Bone and Joint Surgery* **69B**, 183–7.

Morgan, M.A. et al. (1983). Comparison of a radiometric method (BACTEC) and conventional culture media for recovery of mycobacteria from smear negative specimens. *Journal of Clinical Microbiology* **18**, 384–8.

Pertuiset, E. et al. (1997). Aspects epidemiologiques de la tuberculose osteo-articulaire de l'adulte. *Presse Medicale* **26**, 311–15.

Reich, C.V. (1987). Leprosy: cause, transmission and a new theory of pathogenesis. *Review of Infectious Diseases* **9**, 590–4.

Rezai, A.R., Lee, M., and Cooper, P.R. (1996). Pott's disease. In *Tuberculosis* (ed. W.N. Rom and S. Garay), pp. 623–33. Boston MA: Little Brown.

Smith, S.M. and Dockrell, H.M. (2000). Role of CD8+ cells in mycobacterial infections. *Immunology and Cell Biology* **78**, 325–33.

Southwood, T.R. et al. (1988). Tuberculous rheumatism (Poncet's disease) in a child. *Arthritis and Rheumatism* **31**, 1311–13.

Straus, W.L. et al. (1994). Clinical and epidemiologic characteristics of *Mycobacterium haemophilum*, an emerging pathogen in immunocompromised patients. *Annals of Internal Medicine* **120**, 118–25.

Traore, H. et al. (2000). Detection of rifampicin resistance in *Mycobacterium tuberculosis* isolates from diverse countries by a commercial line probe assay as an initial indicator of multidrug resistance. *International Journal of Tuberculosis and Lung Diseases* **4**, 481–4.

Warren, G. (1973). The management of tarsal disintegration. *Leprosy Review* **43**, 137–47.

Watts, H.G. and Lifeso, R.M. (1996). Tuberculosis of bone and joints. *Journal of Bone and Joint Surgery of America* **78** (2), 288–98.

Witzig, R.S. et al. (1995). Clinical manifestations and implications of coinfection with *Mycobacterium kansasii* and human immunodeficiency virus type 1. *Clinical Infectious Disease* **15**, 1–12.

Woods, G.L. (2001). Molecular techniques in mycobacterial detection. *Archives of Pathology and Laboratory Medicine* **25**, 122–6.

Zumla, A. et al. (2000). Impact of HIV infection on tuberculosis. *Postgraduate Medical Journal* **76**, 259–68.

6.2.8 Brucellar arthritis

Eliseo Pascual

Introduction

Infection of the joints is the most frequent localized complication of Brucellosis, and a common cause of infectious arthritis in the countries where the disease is endemic.

Epidemiology

Brucellosis occurs naturally in domesticated animals. It constitutes an important economic problem and a serious health hazard in many countries, specially in the Mediterranean basin, Arabic peninsula, Indian subcontinent, Mexico, and parts of Central and South America. Of the six recognized species of *Brucella*, only four are known to be human pathogens (Young 1995) the most virulent *B. melitensis*, which causes disease in goats, sheep, and camels, *B. abortus* in cattle, *B. suis* in pigs, and *B. canis* in dogs; multiple viobars have been identified in *B. melitensis*. Localization of brucellae in the male and female reproductive organs accounts for the major clinical manifestation—abortion. Human infection is contracted from infected animals, and is closely linked to poor methods of animal husbandry, feeding habits, and hygiene standards. Handling of infected animals or viscera make the disease common in some professions, where the organism is acquired either through breaches in the skin or by infectious aerosol reaching the conjunctiva or the airways. Ingestion of unpasteurized dairy products is the most common cause of infection due to *B. melitensis*. Because its high infectiveness, brucellae are a common cause of accidental infection in laboratory workers (Young 1995).

Infection acquired during foreign travel, often through consumption of infected illegally marketed dairy products, is the cause of imported disease. The possibility of illegal import of such products should be borne in mind.

General characteristics of the organism

Brucellae are small, aerobic, non-motile gram-negative coccobacilli which grow well at 37°C, in any high-quality peptone-based media enriched with blood or serum. Their growth requires a much longer incubation period than pyogenic organisms. Many strains of *B. abortus* and *B. suis* require supplementary CO_2 (Young 1995). Characterization of the molecular genetics of Brucellae have shown that the genus is highly homogeneous with all members showing over 95 per cent homology in DNA–DNA pairing studies, thus classifying *Brucella* as a monospecific genus (Verger 1985).

The host defence

Experiments in rats have shown that after entering the blood-stream, brucellae are phagocytosed by polymorphonuclear leucocytes. Within hours, phagocytosed organisms can be seen in the mononuclear-phagocytic cells of the liver sinusoids, lymph nodes, spleen, and bone marrow and probably in other organs rich in mononuclear-phagocytic cells, where they reproduce (Spink 1964). The frequent isolation of brucellae from bone marrow cultures in diseased humans (Gotuzzo et al. 1987) as well as from liver biopsies (Spink 1964) indicates a similar distribution in humans. The permanence and reproduction of the organisms inside the cells, may be important to the understanding of some of the characteristics of the disease.

The tissue response in established disease, is a non-specific granulomatous lesion, very similar to sarcoidosis. Brucellae cannot be identified in these tissues, but can be cultured from them (Spink 1964). Localized areas of suppuration or caseation may occur, most frequently in *B. suis* (Spink 1964) and in *B. melitensis* (Rotés-Querol 1957).

General characteristics of the disease

The manifestations of brucellosis are non-specific, and no combination of signs or symptoms can be considered to be characteristic. *B. melitensis* causes more severe disease than *B. abortus* and *B. suis*, probably because of its greater ability to avoid the host's defenses. *B. suis* has higher tendency to suppurative complications. The large published series relate mainly to *B. melitensis*, and generalization to disease caused by the other brucellae may be inaccurate.

Brucellosis is more common in men than in women both in the Middle East and Mediterranean countries (Andonopoulos et al. 1986; Colmenero et al. 1986; Ariza 1988; Mousa et al. 1988; Batlle et al. 1989). In the same areas, the disease occurs with equal frequency in children of both sexes (Gomez-Reino et al. 1986; Lubani et al. 1986; Al-Eissa et al. 1990), as happens with adults in Perú (Gotuzzo et al. 1987). It may be that where brucellosis is contracted as a professional hazard, more males are affected. Ingestion of milk, which is the usual cause of the disease in children and in Peruvian adults (Gotuzzo et al. 1987), would result in equal incidence in both sexes.

The incubation period may be as short as 1 week, but usually lasts from 2 to 8 weeks (Young 1995). The disease usually presents with fever—often without an undulant pattern—sweats, which may be drenching, and a general feeling of malaise. Weakness, anorexia, myalgia, and arthralgia are common. Patients often recall possibly infected animals or their unpasteurized products, but this evidence may be missing. Physical examination may show lymphadenopathy, and hepatosplenomegaly. Localized infections, especially skeletal, are common. Other manifestations include neurobrucellosis, endocarditis, hepatitis, and epididimo-orchitis.

Sub-clinical disease occurs, and may heal spontaneously. Patients may present with relapses following previous sub-clinical disease, or with late, localized complications, simulating a very long incubation period.

The concept of chronic brucellosis was coined before the antibiotic era, to refer to a group of patients who complained of ill health after having suffered from brucellosis, generally due to *B. abortus*. A careful study showed that some of these patients had a bacteriologically proven relapse, or localized disease; in others, no explanation was found for the symptoms, and it was felt that they were related to an unstable emotional state. It is unclear whether chronic brucellosis in the absence of infection exists, and such diagnosis must be handled with care.

Brucellar arthritis

Arthralgia is more common in brucellosis than in other febrile illnesses. It has been recorded in 65 per cent (Colmenero et al. 1986; Ariza 1988) of adult patients studied prospectively, and in 74 per cent (Al-Eissa et al. 1990) of the children thus studied; its presence may be a clue to the disease. Bone scanning of patients with brucellosis and musculoskeletal symptoms has been reported as being very frequently abnormal, often in multiple sites (el Desouki 1991). Perhaps some of the minor musculoskeletal symptoms of these patients are due to localized infection. Since the treatment of brucellar arthritis and that of uncomplicated brucellosis is the same, once brucellosis is diagnosed, it is not worthwhile searching for arthritis to explain minor or unclear musculoskeletal symptoms.

Infection in the joints is the most common form of localized disease in brucellosis. It appears in 25 per cent (Colmenero et al. 1991), 29 per cent (Ariza 1988), 24 per cent (Gotuzzo et al. 1987), and 22 per cent (Andonopoulos et al. 1986) of adult patients studied prospectively, and in 38 per cent (Al-Eissa et al. 1990) of children. In areas where brucellosis is endemic, brucellar arthritis may outnumber tuberculous arthritis. All the above series refer to *B. melitensis*.

The general clinical characteristics of brucellar arthritis are similar to those of infectious arthritis due to other organisms. The disease is generally monoarticular, but in 18 per cent of our patients more than one joint was affected (Batlle et al. 1989). The large peripheral joints, sacroiliacs, and the

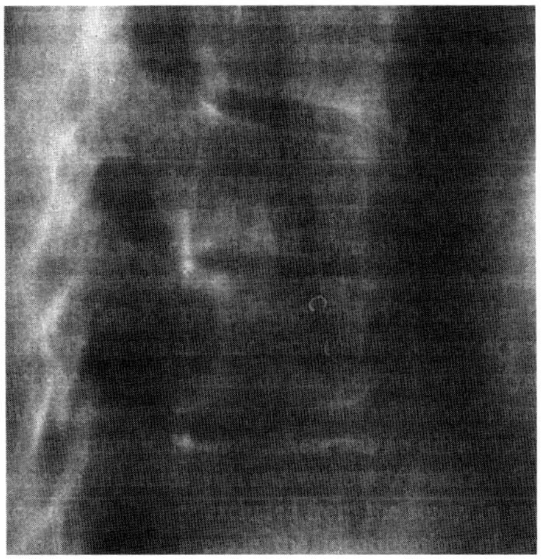

Fig. 3 Lateral tomography of the dorsal spine, showing diminished disc space height and vertebral end-plate erosions in a patient with brucellar spondylitis.

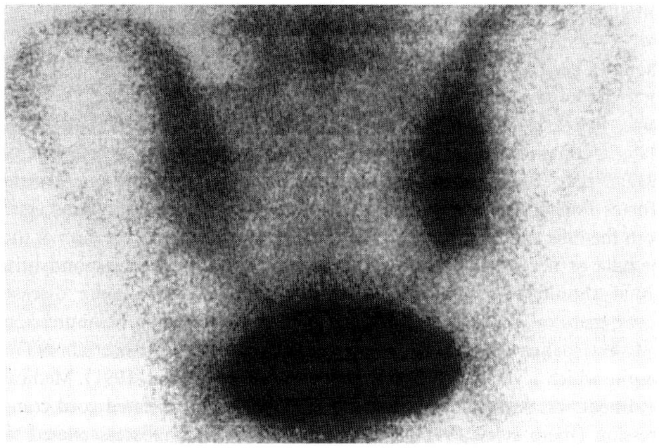

Fig. 4 Bone scan of the posterior pelvis of a patient with left brucellar sacroiliitis of short duration and normal radiograph.

a prospective study showed abnormalities in signal intensity of the vertebral body marrow at the lession site; subchondral areas of the vertebra were most commonly affected. Most patients had unifocal disease, but multifocal involvement was also seen. Small soft tissue masses seen early in the disease, some of them epidural, which regressed with medical treatment were also noted in this series, as well as narrowing of the disc space as a later feature.

Bone scan frequently shows increased uptake at the level of the affected disc-space, even when radiologically normal (Bahar et al. 1988; Madkour et al. 1988; Sharif et al. 1989) (Fig. 4). On the other hand, in a prospective study of brucellar spondylitis, bone scans were normal in some patients during the first 3 months of the disease, and later, at times, only slightly abnormal (Ariza et al. 1985).

Osteomyelitis

Osteomyelitis is an unusual feature of brucellosis, which may present as local pain and tenderness. *Brucella melitensis* has predilection for the ribs and epiphyses of long bones, but may occur in other locations (Rotés-Querol 1957; Serre et al. 1981; Mousa et al. 1988). *Brucella suis* seems to prefer the long bones (Kelly et al. 1960).

Reactive arthritis

Although a report (Hodinka et al. 1978) of higher frequency of HLA B27 in patients with brucellar spondylitis raised the possibility of brucellar reactive arthritis, other studies have failed to find such association (Alarcón et al. 1981, 1985; Al-Rawi et al. 1987). My own experience with 86 prospectively followed patients with brucellar arthritis is that in none of them has any type of chronic arthritis remaining after antimicrobial treatment. As a rule, the symptoms clearly improve after appropriate treatment, in both peripheral and axial arthritides. Reactive brucellar arthritis therefore appears an unlikely possibility, and this diagnosis should be made cautiously.

Other musculoskeletal manifestations

Acute brucellosis may present as a leucocytoclastic vasculitis. Patients with brucellosis may also show lesions resembling panniculitis from which brucella can be grown. Soft tissue abscesses have been reported.

General laboratory features

With the exception of serological and bacteriological data, the laboratory features of brucellosis are non-specific. The erythrocyte sedimentation rate generally shows some elevation: it was below 44 mm in 70 per cent of the patients with brucellar arthritis (Mousa et al. 1988) and normal in 16 per cent in another series (Rotés-Querol 1957). Frequent slight elevations or normal values have been found by others, in both adults (Colmenero et al. 1986; Al-Rawi et al. 1987) and children (Gómez-Reino et al. 1986; Al-Eissa et al. 1990). Similar pattern is seen with *B. abortus* and *B. suis* (Kelly et al. 1960). Normal values are not unusual in late, localized forms, as is spondylitis (Serre et al. 1981). A normal or low leucocyte count, associated with lymphocytosis is usual (Colmenero et al. 1986; Mousa et al. 1988). Lymphopaenia may be associated with more severe clinical manifestations. Leucocytosis is unusual, but may occur. Thrombocytopaenia, anaemia, and pancytopaenia, all may occur.

Abnormal liver function tests are a common feature of the disease, especially in the early phases.

Synovial fluid analysis

Published data of synovial fluid analysis in brucellar arthritis are scarce. Cell counts have been found to be lower than 50 000/mm^3, (Gotuzzo and Carrillo 1988), or even lower, 4460–8800 (Andonopoulos et al. 1986) and 6000–18 000/mm^3 (Mousa et al. 1988). Glucose levels were within normal limits in the above series. Lactic acid levels have also been found to be normal. *Brucella melitensis* has been isolated from some of the above synovial fluids. Our own unpublished data from 18 prospectively studied patients showed different results. The cell counts were 3200–90 000/mm^3; glucose was low in some of the fluids (0–100 mg/dl, mean 47 ± 33 SD), and lactic acid was also high in some occasions (13–138 mg/dl, mean 74 ± 36 SD). *Brucella melitensis* was recovered from 73 per cent of those fluids, many of them with characteristics suggestive of non-infectious, inflammatory synovial fluid.

Diagnostic investigations

Importance of the clinical features

The clinical features of brucellosis are non-specific. The manifestations of brucellar joint disease are similar to those of other infectious peripheral or axial arthritides, and may also resemble some inflammatory arthritides. Nevertheless, in the following circumstances, appropriate testing for brucellosis should always be done: (a) in all undiagnosed arthritides, with features fitting those of brucellosis, occurring in areas where the disease is endemic, or in patients with a history of possible exposure to the disease; (b) in all cases of undiagnosed acute unilateral sacroiliitis; (c) in all cases of undiagnosed disc-space infection, specially those with radiological evidence of localized vertebral angle infection, or infection of multiple levels.

About 25 per cent do not recall exposure to possibly infected animals or unpasteurized dairy products.

Bacteriological diagnosis

Isolation of brucellae from blood, synovial fluid, or other sources, should always be attempted when the disease is suspected. It provides a definitive diagnosis, and the possibility of differentiating *B. melitensis*, *B. abortus*, and *B. suis*, which cannot be done with the usual serological tests. When brucellosis is suspected, the laboratory should always be warned, since: (a) brucellae are slow growing organisms, and most cultures will be negative if not kept long enough, ideally up to 6 weeks (Rodríguez Torres 1988). In a series of 262 positive blood cultures, the growth was apparent in 8 per cent of the samples during the first week, 36 during the second, 31 during the third, 17 during the fourth, 6 during the fifth, and 2 during the sixth. The culture was not pursued further (Ariza 1988); (b) brucellae are a common cause of acquired infection in the laboratory, and such personnel should take special precautions. Any high-quality peptone-based enriched with blood or serum, are suitable for growing brucellae (Young 1995); a 10 per cent CO_2 atmosphere increases the yield, and is necessary for most strains of *B. abortus*; culture systems with a solid phase are easier and less risky to handle in the laboratory (Rodríguez Torres 1988). Of practical importance, blood cultures processed by the lysis-centrifugation system allows isolation of Brucellae in a shorter period of time (Navas et al. 1993). Using this system, 15 of 22 blood cultures were detected positive for *B. melitensis* after 72 h incubation (Yagupsky 1999).

Blood cultures are often positive in disease due to *B. melitensis*. The organism was isolated in 78 per cent (Ariza 1988), 62 per cent (Colmenero et al. 1986), and 72 per cent (Colmenero et al. 1991) of series of unselected adults, and in 75 per cent (Al-Eissa et al. 1990) of children. In patients with brucellar arthritis, blood cultures were positive in 58 per cent (Rotés-Querol 1957), 41 per cent (Batlle et al. 1989), and 41 per cent (Al-Rawi et al. 1989), 70 per cent (Lubani et al. 1986), and 33 per cent (Gómez-Reino et al. 1986) of children also had positive blood cultures. Patients with relapsing disease have the same rate of positive blood cultures as new patients (Ariza 1988).

Although blood cultures should be obtained when patients are febrile, in 30 per cent (Ariza 1988) and 31 per cent (Rodríguez Torres 1988) of afebrile patients the organism grew. Isolation of *B. melitensis* from blood cultures is less frequent in late, localized disease, such as spondylitis (Serre et al. 1981; Gotuzzo and Carrillo 1988; Colmenero et al. 1991). Differences in disease characteristics or laboratory procedures probably account for the wide differences found between series: a 7 per cent positivity was found in a large series in which blood cultures were frequently kept less than 10 days (Mousa et al. 1987). The isolation rate of *B. abortus* and *B. suis* is lower than that of *B. melitensis*.

Synovial fluid should always be cultured. *B. melitensis* grew in 73 per cent of the synovial fluids inoculated in blood culture flasks (Carro et al. 1988). Other series have obtained a 62 per cent (Gotuzzo and Carrillo 1988), 60 per cent (Andonopoulos et al. 1986), and 27 per cent (Gotuzzo et al. 1982) growth in the cultured samples. *B. abortus* has been cultured from synovial fluid (Al-Rawi et al. 1989), as well as *B. canis* (Young 1995). Material obtained by needle puncture from infected disc spaces or surgically from the sacroiliac joint, may also grow brucellae. *Brucella abortus* or *B. suis* may grow in samples obtained from bone, bursa, tendons, and joints (Kelly et al. 1960).

Serological diagnosis

Attempts to isolate brucellae from blood or other sources are not always successful; moreover, cultures when positive, require a long incubation period. Under these circumstances, the possibility of serological diagnosis offers great advantages. Serological tests allow the detection of antibodies produced against the lipopolysaccharide of the bacterial cell wall, which is common to *B. melitensis*, *B. abortus*, and *B. suis*, but not *B. canis*, which needs a specific antigenic suspension (Polt et al. 1982; Devi et al. 1987).

The standard tube agglutination test (STA) is the most widely used test. The antigen used in it is generally obtained from *B. abortus*; it reacts against *B. abortus*, *B. melitensis*, and *B. suis*, not allowing differentiation between them (Rodríguez Torres 1988; Young 1995). A positive STA is indicative of contact with brucellae. Although high titres are indicative of current infection, the presence of any positive titre, if the clinical features are compatible, must be investigated further. As in other serological investigations, individual response, antigen preparations, and laboratory procedures influence the final titre (Rodríguez Torres 1988).

Blocking antibodies may result in negative STA at low dilutions, while a positive test is obtained with further serum dilution. This phenomenon occurs mainly in late, localized brucellosis (Rodríguez Torres 1988). The brucellar Coomb's test detects these blocking antibodies, and allows the diagnosis. The brucellar Coomb's test always gives higher titres than the STA (Rodríguez Torres 1988). A combination of the STA and the brucellar Coomb's test allows detection of the large majority of infections, and seem adequate for routine clinical practice (Ariza 1988; Rodríguez Torres 1988). If simple agglutination methods or the Rose Bengal slide agglutination test (Rodríguez Torres 1988) are used for screening, standard tests must be performed in the positive sera for definite serological diagnosis.

The pattern of the antigenic response may be measured with an ELISA test. IgM antibodies appear first, and may disappear within a mean time of 9 months. IgG peaks at about 2 months, but significant titres persist after 18 months or more (Ariza 1988). In a large group of serially followed patients, STA and IgM antibodies had a parallel decline, as did the Coomb's test and IgG antibodies (Ariza 1988; Ariza et al. 1992a). The measurement of specific antibodies allows the detection of occasional patients not discovered by other serological tests (Ariza et al. 1992a). Detection of an elevation of the IgG antibody during the follow-up is a very useful serological sign for the diagnosis of relapses (Pellicer et al. 1988; Ariza et al. 1992a). The definitive diagnosis of a relapse requires either bacteriological or clinical evidence of the disease.

Occupationally exposed workers may have low abnormal serological tests in the absence of disease. Due to similitude in the cell wall components, serological test for brucellosis may be positive in infections due to *P. tularensis*, *Y. enterocolitica* 0 : 9, *V. cholera* and *E. coli* 0 : 157; when positivity is due to cross-reaction, titres tend to be lower against the cross-reacting antigenic suspension.

Several brucella-specific genes have now been cloned, including the BP26 and BCS P31. Detection of the later by polymerase chain reaction in peripheral blood allowed the diagnosis of the disease in 50 cases of brucellosis; 60 healthy subjects were used as controls. The sensitivity and specificity found for this test was 100 and 98.3 per cent, respectively (Queipo-Ortuño et al. 1997). These rapid PCR essays have diagnostic potential.

Treatment

The treatment of brucellar arthritis is similar to that of uncomplicated brucellosis. The regimen presently recommended by the World Health Organization (1986) includes a combination of rifampicin 900 mg combined with doxycycline at 200 mg, both given once a day during a period of 6 weeks; a relapse rate of about 5 per cent is seen with this regimen. Doxycycline, 100 mg every 12 h and rifampin 15 mg/kg per day in a single morning dose for 45 days showed a similar efficacy than a combination of doxycycline for 45 days plus streptomycin, 1 g/day for 15 days, although the doxycycline–rifampin combination was less effective in patients with spondylitis (Ariza et al. 1992b). A meta-analysis of six published randomized trials comparing the relative efficacy of rifampicin and doxycycline versus streptomycin and doxycycline or another tetracycline concluded that the treatment of rifampicin and doxycycline presents a greater number of recurrences and lower number of cures than the classical treatment with streptomycin and tetracycline (Solera et al. 1994). Probably a regimen including streptomycin and a tetracycline should be preferred for patients with more severe disease, such as spondylitis associated with epidural abscesses.

Brucellae isolated from patients with relapses show similar drug sensitivities to the pre-treatment isolates of the same patients (Ariza et al. 1986), showing that the relapses are not due to drug resistance. A second course of treatment is generally effective in these patients.

A therapeutic study conducted on 1100 children with early disease, showed that very few relapses were seen after oral monotherapy combined with either streptomycin or gentamicin. These combinations fared better than other regimens. It was concluded that children of 8 years or younger should receive trimethoprim–sulfamethoxazole, 10–50 mg/kg/day, given b.i.d., for 3 weeks with gentamicin, 5 mg/kg/day im, b.i.d. given the first 5 days. Children of 9 years or older, should receive doxycycline 5 mg/kg/day b.i.d., for 3 weeks, combined with gentamicin, 5 mg/kg/day im, b.i.d. the initial 5 days (Lubani et al. 1989). Monotherapy with trimethoprim–sulfamethoxazole (Gómez-Reino et al. 1986; Lubani et al. 1989), or with rifampin (Lubani et al. 1989) results in a higher relapse rate. Combination of 10–12 mg/kg trimethoprim, 50–60 mg/kg sulfamethoxazole, and rifampin 15–20 mg/kg in two divided doses for 6 weeks of 113 children resulted in only four relapses, and offers a convenient oral therapy for children (Khuri Bulos et al. 1993).

Apart from antibiotics, patients with peripheral arthritis do not require periodical evacuation of the joint, as is necessary in pyogenic arthritides. Rarely large paravertebral abscesses have been drained, though the need for this is not determined. Epidural abscesses with cord compression may need surgery, though a reported patient was medically treated with good results (Ibero et al. 1997) and it is not established if the more aggressive approach offers advantages over medical treatment alone.

References

Adam, A., MacDonald, A., and MacKenzie, I.G. (1967). Monoarticular brucellar arthritis in children. *The Journal of Bone and Joint Surgery* **49B**, 652–7.

Agarwal, S., Kadhi, S.K., and Rooney, R.J. (1991). Brucellosis complicating bilateral total knee arthroplasty. *Clinical Orthopedics and Related Research* **267**, 179–81.

Alarcón, G.S., Bocanegra, T.S., Gotuzzo, E., Hinostroza, S., Carrillo, C., Vasey, F.B., Germain, B.F., and Espinoza, L.R. (1981). Reactive arthritis associated with brucellosis: HLA studies. *Journal of Rheumatology* **8**, 621–5.

Alarcón, G.S., Gotuzzo, E., Hinostroza, S.A., Carrillo, C., Bocanegra, T.S., and Espinoza, L.R. (1985). HLA studies in brucellar spondylitis. *Clinical Rheumatology* **4**, 312–14.

Al-Eissa, Y.A., Kambal, A.M., al-Nasser, M.N., al-Habib, S.A., al-Fawaz, I.M., and al-Zamil F.A. (1990). Childhood brucellosis: a study of 102 cases. *Pediatric Infectious Diseases Journal* **9**, 74–9.

Al-Rawi, Z.S., Al-Khateeb, N., and Khalifa, S.J. (1987). Brucella arthritis among Iraqi patients. *British Journal of Rheumatology* **26**, 24–7.

Al-Rawi, T.I., Thewaini, A.J., Shawket, A.R., and Ahmed, G.M. (1989). Skeletal brucellosis in Iraqi patients. *Annals of the Rheumatic Diseases* **48**, 77–9.

Andonopoulos, A.P., Asimakopoulos, G., Anastasiou, E., and Bassaris, H.P. (1986). Brucella arthritis. *Scandinavian Journal of Rheumatology* **15**, 377–80.

Ariza, J., Gudiol, F., Valverde, J., Pallarés, R., Fernández Viladrich, P., Rufí, G., Espadaler, L., and Fernández Nogués, F. (1985). Brucellar spondylitis: a detailed analysis based on current findings. *Reviews of Infectious Diseases* **7**, 656–64.

Ariza, J., Bosch, J., Gudiol, F., Liñares, J., Fernández-Viladrich, P., and Martín, R. (1986). Relavance of *in vitro* antimicrobial susceptibility of *Brucella melitensis* to relapse rate in human brucellosis. *Antimicrobial Agents and Chemotherapy* **30**, 958–60.

Ariza, J. *Brucelosis: perspectiva actual de la enfermedad. Perfil de las inmunoglobulinas específicas en el curso de su evolución.* Tesis Doctoral. Universidad de Barcelona, 1988.

Ariza, J., Pellicer, T.-Pallares, R., Foz, A., and Gudiol, F. (1992a). Specific antibody profile in human brucellosis. *Clinics in Infectious Diseases* **14**, 131–40.

Ariza, J., Gudiol, F., Pallares, R., Viladrich, P.F., Rufi, G., Corredoira, J., and Miravitlles, M.R. (1992b). Treatment of human brucellosis with doxycycline plus rifampin or doxycycline plus streptomycin. A randomized, double-blind study. *Annals of Internal Medicine* **117**, 25–30.

Ariza, J., Valverde, J., Nolla, J.M., Rufi, G., Viladrich P.F., Corredoira. J.M., and Gudiol, F. (1993). *Brucellar sacroiliitis*: findings in 63 episodes and current relevance. *Clinics in Infectious Diseases* **16**, 761–5.

Bahar, R.H., Al-Suhaili, A.R., Mousa, A.M., Nawaz, M.K., Kaddah, N., and Abdel-Dayem, H.M. (1988). Brucellosis: appearance on skeletal imaging. *Clinical Nuclear Medicine* **13**, 102–6.

Batlle, E., Pascual, E., Salas, E., Plazas, J., Román, J., and Vela, P. (1989). Brucellar arthritis: an study of 86 prospectively collected patients (abstract). *British Journal of Rheumatology* **28** (Suppl. 2), 25.

Benjamin, B. and Khan, M.R. (1994). Hip involvement in childhood brucellosis. *Journal of Bone and Joint Surgery (British)* **76**, 544–7.

Benjamin, B., Annobil, S.H., and Khan, M.R. (1992). Osteoarticular complications of childhood brucellosis: a study of 57 cases in Saudi Arabia. *Journal of Pediatric Orthopedics* **12**, 801–5.

Berrocal, A., Gotuzzo, E., Calvo, A., Carrillo, C., Castañeda, O., and Alarcon, G.S. (1993). Sternoclavicular brucellar arthritis: a report of 7 cases and a review of the literature. *Journal of Rheumatology* **20**, 1184–6.

Carro, A., Batlle, E., Pascual, E., Castellano, J.A., and Plazas, J. (1988). Blood culture flasks for synovial fluid culture: a more sensitive method for the isolation of bacteria from synovial fluid, particularly *Brucella melitensis* (abstract). *British Journal of Rheumatology* **27** (Suppl. 2), 33.

Colmenero, D.J., Porras, J.J., Valdivieso, P., Porras J.A., de Ramón, E., Cause, M., and Juárez, C. (1986). Brucelosis: estudio prospectivo de 100 casos. *Medicina Clínica (Barcelona)* **86**, 43–8.

Colmenero, J.D., Reguera, J.M., Fernandez-Nebro, A., and Cabrera-Franquelo, F. (1991). Osteoarticular complications of brucellosis. *Annals of the Rheumatic Diseases* **50**, 23–6.

Colmenero, J.D., Cisneros, J.M., Orjuela, D.L., Pachon, J., Garcia-Portales, R., Rodriguez-Sampedro, F., and Juarez, C. (1992). Clinical course and prognosis of Brucella spondylitis. *Infection* **20**, 38–42.

Colmenero, D.J., Jiménez Mejías, M.E., Sánchez Lora, F.J., Reguera, J.M., Palomino Nicás, J., Martos, F., García de las Heras, J., and Pachón, J. (1997). Pyoginic, tuberculous, and brucellar vertebral osteomyelitis: a descriptive and comparative study of 219 cases. *Annals of the Rheumatic Diseases* **56**, 709–15.

Cordero Sánchez, M., Alvarez Ruiz, S., López Ochoa, J., and García Talavera, J.R. (1990). Scintigraphic evaluation of lumbosacral pain in brucellosis. *Arthritis and Rheumatism* **33**, 1052–5.

el Desouki, M. (1991). Skeletal brucellosis: assessment with bone scintigraphy. *Radiology* **181**, 415–18.

Devi, S.J.N., Polt, S.S., Boctor, F.N., and Peter, J.B. (1987). Serological evaluation of brucellosis: importance of species in antigen preparation. *The Journal of Infectious Diseases* **156**, 658–61.

Gómez-Reino, F.J., Mateo, I., Fuertes, A., and Gómez-Reino, J.J. (1986). Brucellar arthritis in children and its successful treatment with trimethoprim-sulphamethoxazole. *Annals of the Rheumatic Diseases* **45**, 256–8.

Gotuzzo, E., Alarcón, G.S., Bocanegra, T.S., Carrillo, C., Guerra J.C., Rolando, I., and Espinoza, L.R. (1982). Articular involvement in human brucellosis: a retrospective analysis of 304 cases. *Seminars in Arthritis and Rheumatism* **12**, 245–55.

Gotuzzo, E., Seas, C., Guerra, J.G., Carrillo, C., Bocanegra, T.S., Calvo, A., Castañeda, O., and Alarcón, G.S. (1987). Brucellar arthritis: a study of 39 Peruvian families. *Annals of the Rheumatic Diseases* **46**, 506–9.

Gotuzzo, E. and Carrillo, C. (1988). Brucella arthritis. In *Infections in the Rheumatic Diseases* (ed. L. Espinoza, D. Goldenberg, F. Arnett, and G. Alarcón), pp. 31–41. Orlando FL: Grune & Stratton.

Hodinka, L., Gomor, B., Meretey, K., Zahumenszky, Z., Geher, P., Telegdy, L., and Bozsoky, S. (1978). HLA-B27-associated spondylarthritis in chronic brucellosis (letter). *Lancet* **i**, 499.

Ibero, I., Vela, P., and Pascual, E. (1997). Arthritis of the shoulder and spinal cord compression due to brucella dysc infection. *British Journal of Rheumatology* **36**, 377–81.

Joint FAO/WHO expert committee on brucellosis. Geneva: WHO, 1986.

Kelly, P.J., Martin, W.J., Shirger, A., and Weed, L.A. (1960). Brucellosis of the bones and joints. *The Journal of the American Medical Association* **174**, 347–53.

Khuri Bulos, N.A., Daoud, A.H., and Azab, S.M. (1993). Treatment of childhood brucellosis: results of a prospective trial on 113 children. *Pediatric Infectious Disease Journal* **12**, 377–81.

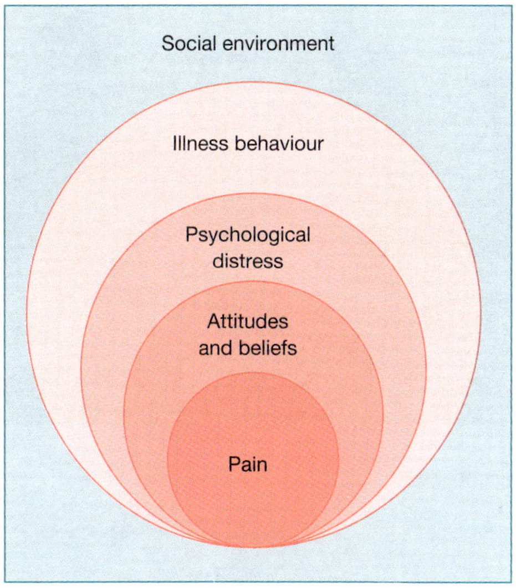

Plate 1 A biopsychosocial model of low-back-pain disability. From Clinical Standards Advisory Group, 1994.

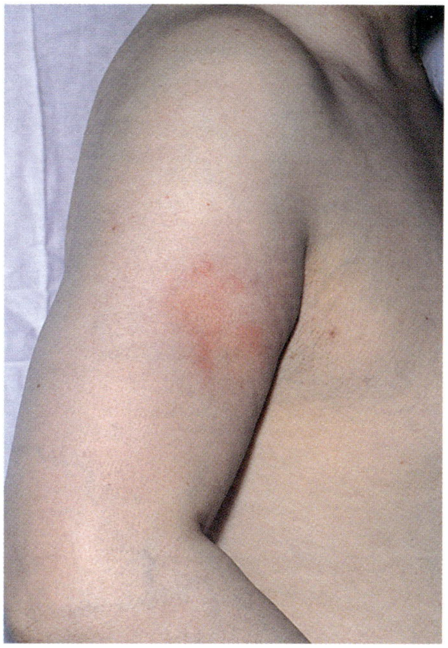

Plate 2 Man who presented with fever, marked raised erythrocyte sedimentation rate (>100), and right upper arm pain due to a septic arthritis of the right shoulder tracking down the long head of the biceps to present as swelling in the right upper arm.

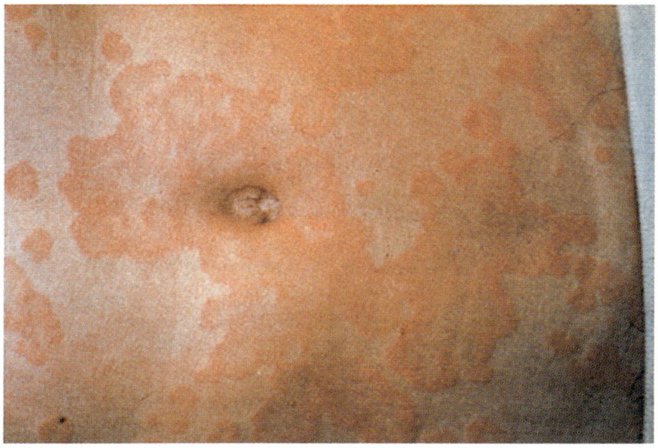

Plate 3 Erythema marginatum in rheumatic fever: reddish annular lesions may expand rapidly to form large figurate patches; the eruption is typically evanescent, lasting 2–3 days at most (photograph by courtesy of Dr E. Pascual).

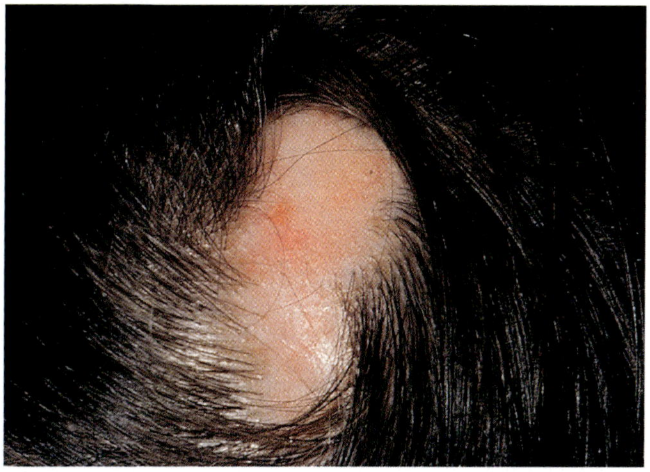

Plate 4 Scarring alopecia of the scalp in discoid lupus erythematosus.

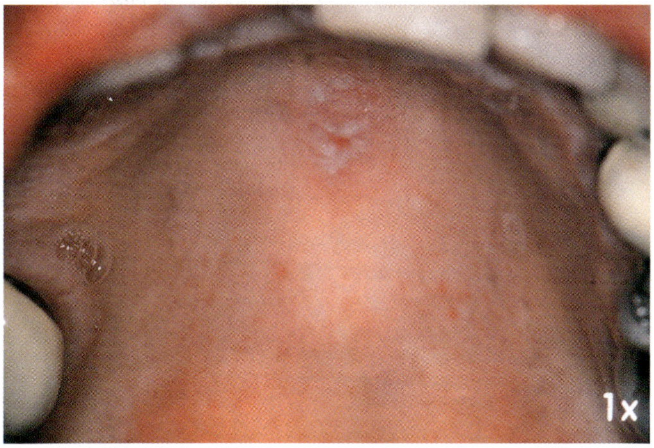

Plate 5 Involvement of hard palate in subacute lupus erythematosus.

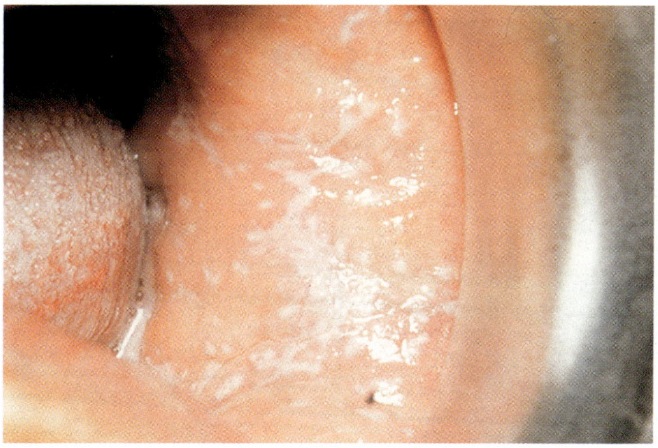

Plate 6 Oral lichen planus—white streaks on buccal mucosa.

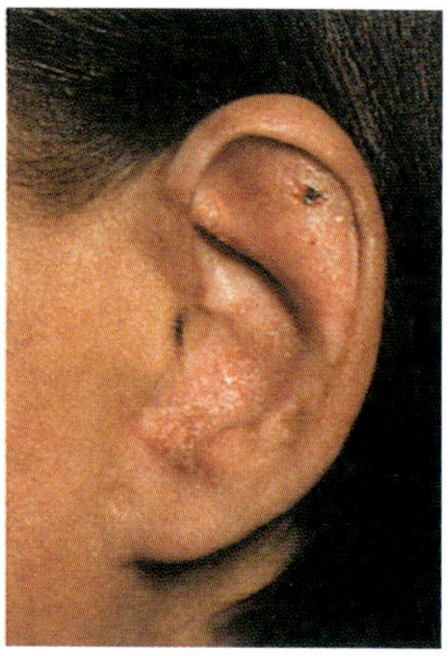

Plate 7 Discoid lupus erythematosus affecting the external ear.

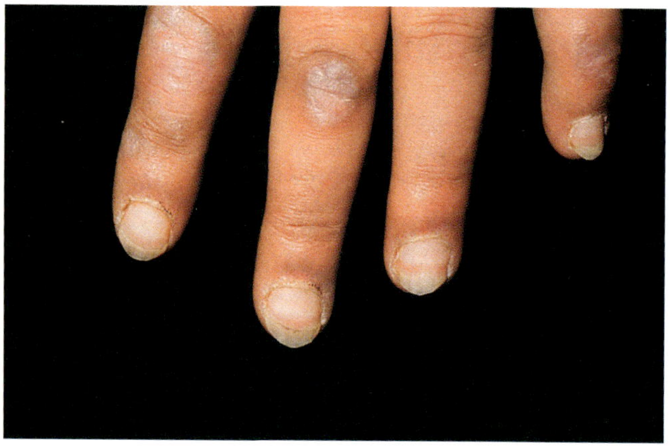

Plate 8 Plaques of discoid lupus erythematosus on the fingers.

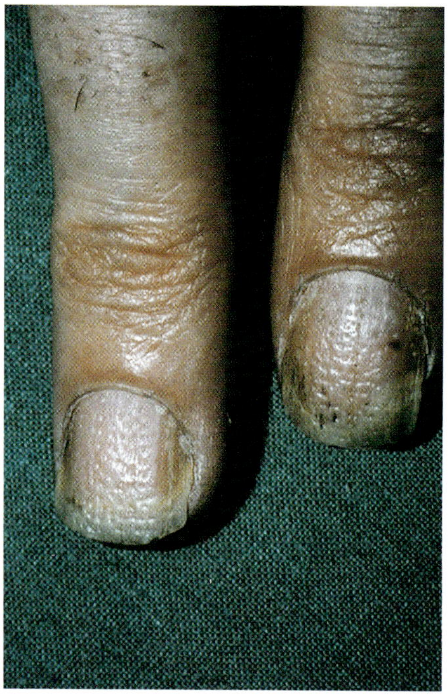

Plate 9 Psoriasis: nail pits with early onycholysis.

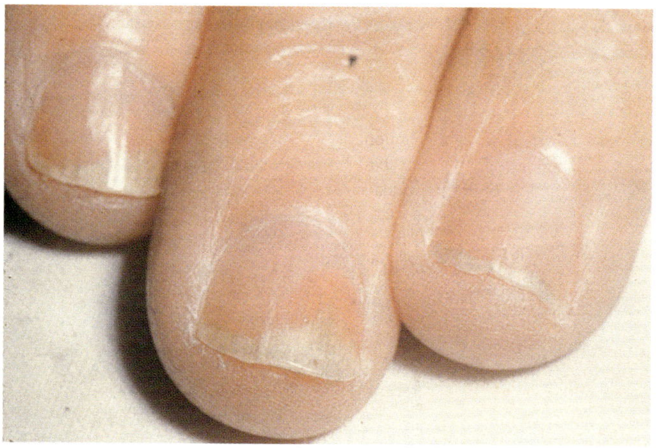

Plate 10 Psoriasis: onycholysis with 'salmon patch'.

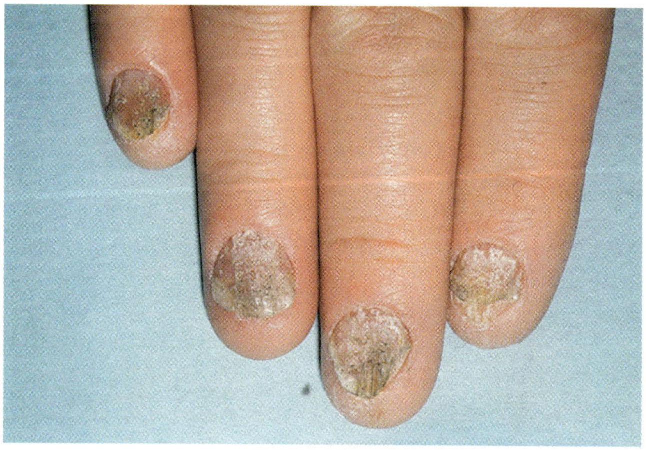

Plate 11 Psoriasis: onycholysis, gross pitting, and nail deformity.

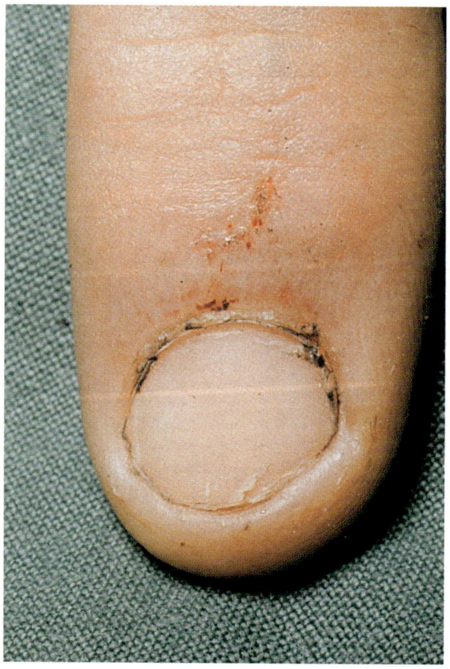

Plate 12 Dermatomyositis: nailfold vasculopathy (photograph by courtesy of Dr R.S.-H. Tan).

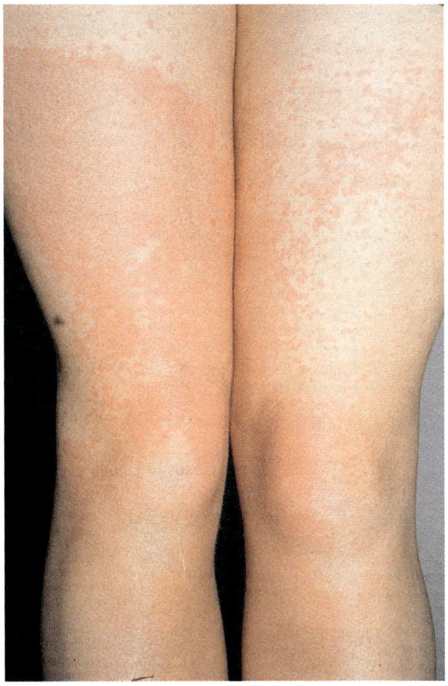

Plate 13 Polymorphic light eruption: itchy maculopapular lesions occur within hours of sun exposure to sites habitually covered (in this patient the eruption extends to the line of her Bermuda shorts).

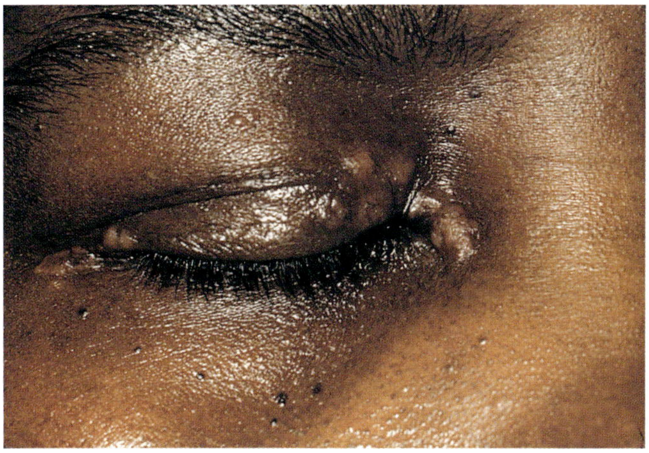

Plate 14 Cutaneous sarcoid in an Afro-Caribbean patient: yellowish papules around the eyelids.

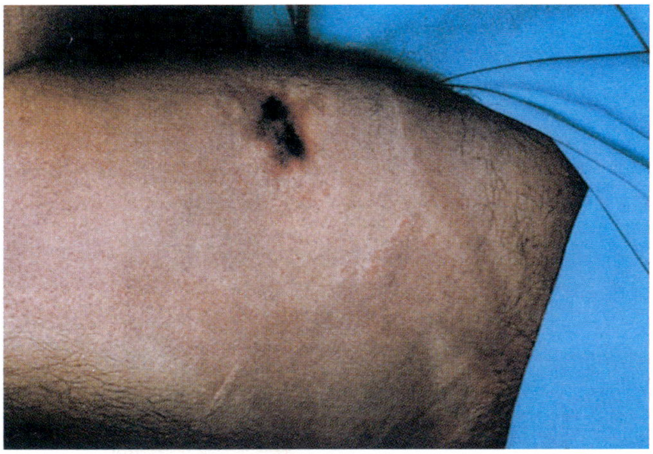

Plate 15 Erythema chronicum migrans: annular erythema is developing around the site of the tick bite on the thigh (photograph by courtesy of Dr E. Pascual).

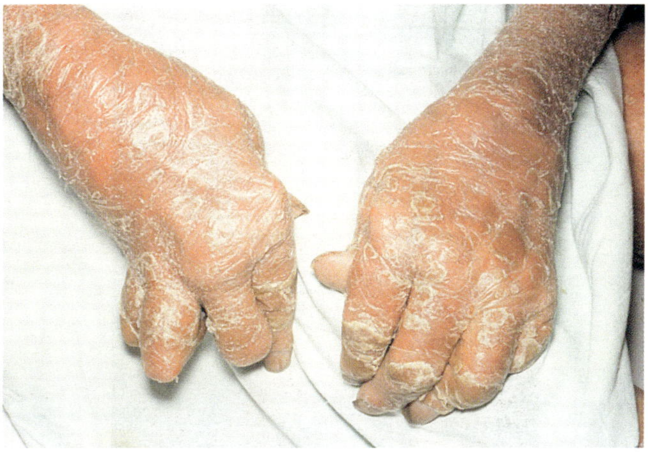

Plate 16 Erythrodermic psoriasis involving the hands in an elderly man with psoriatic arthritis.

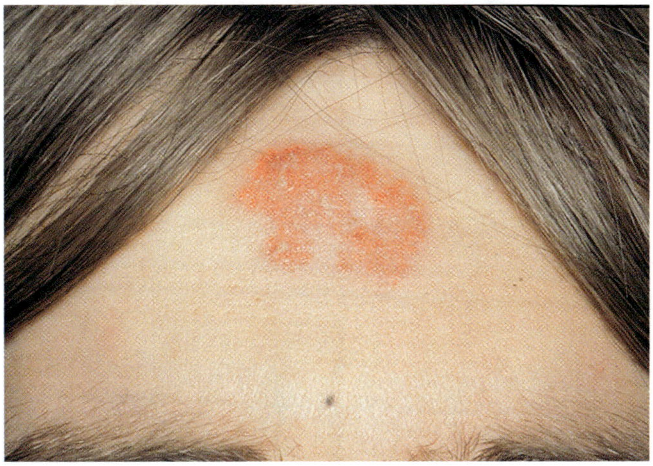

Plate 17 Scaling plaque of discoid lupus erythematosus on a light-exposed area of forehead.

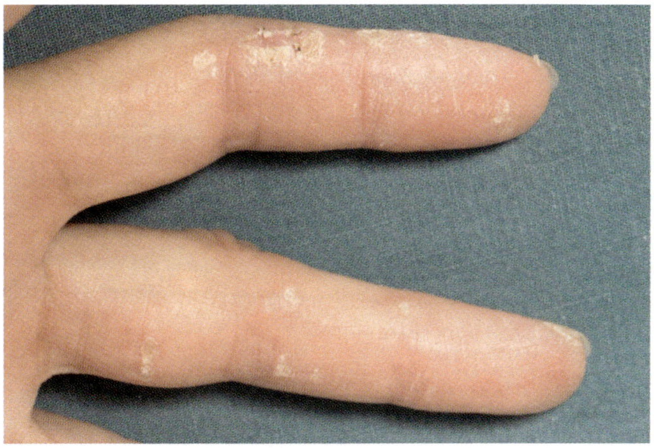

Plate 18 Discrete hyperkeratotic lesions on radial aspect of fingers ('mechanic's hands').

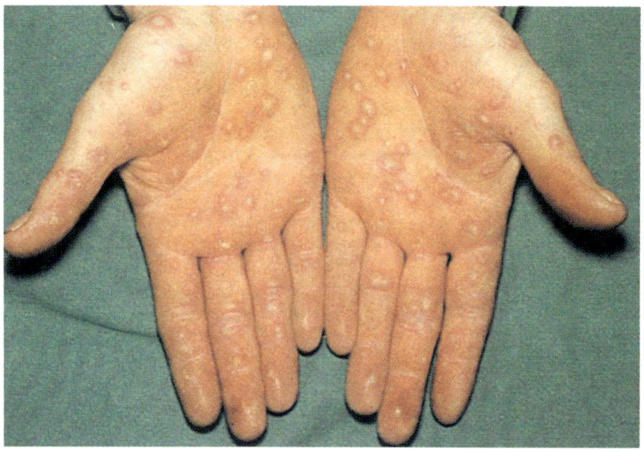

Plate 19 Erythema multiforme: characteristic 'target lesions' on the palms.

(a)

(b)

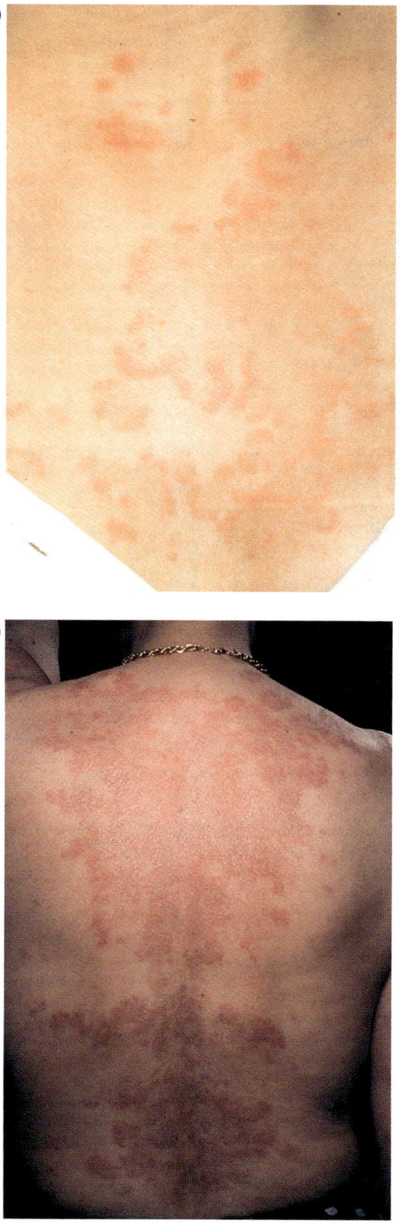

Plate 21 Osteopoikilosis: note stippling of bone, especially adjacent to joint (photograph by courtesy of Dr G. Evison).

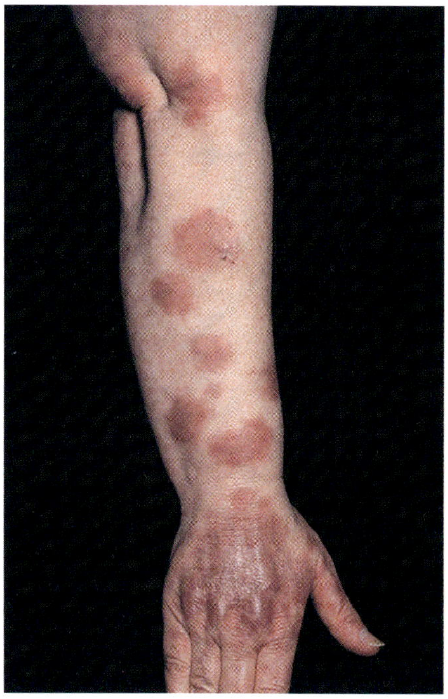

Plate 20 Sweet's syndrome: plum-coloured plaques on forearm and hand.

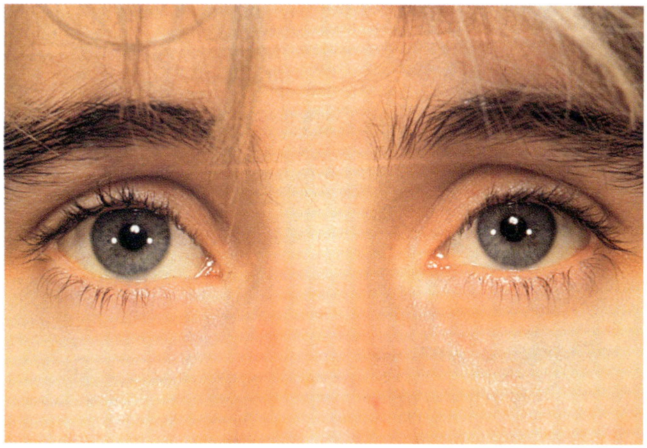

Plate 22 Yellow pigmentation of the skin and sclerae due to mepacrine.

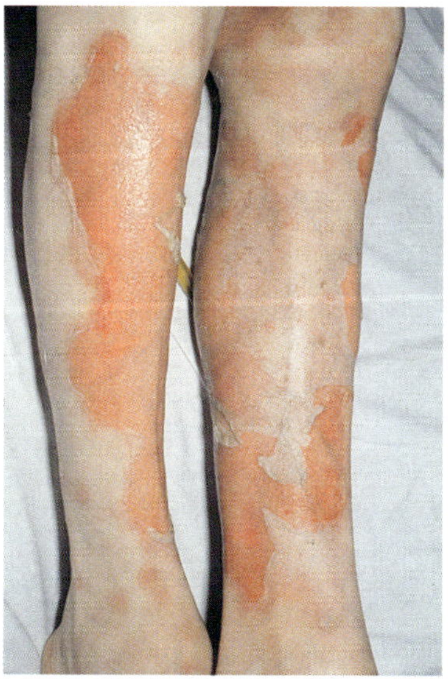

Plate 23 Toxic epidermal necrolysis.

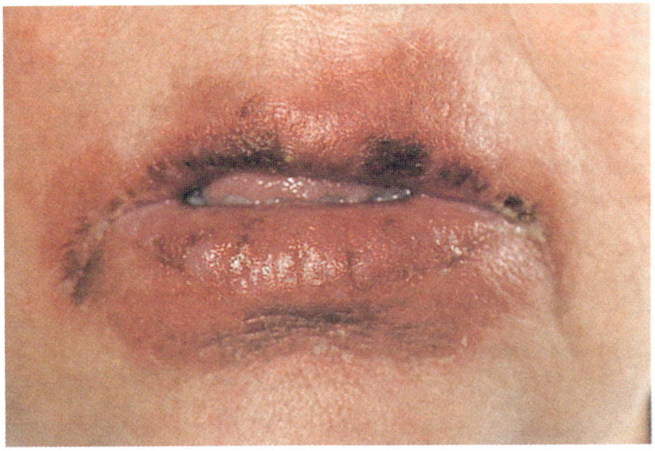

Plate 24 Fixed drug eruption. A well-demarcated, often ovoid, dusky area of erythema, later followed by slatey hyperpigmentation.

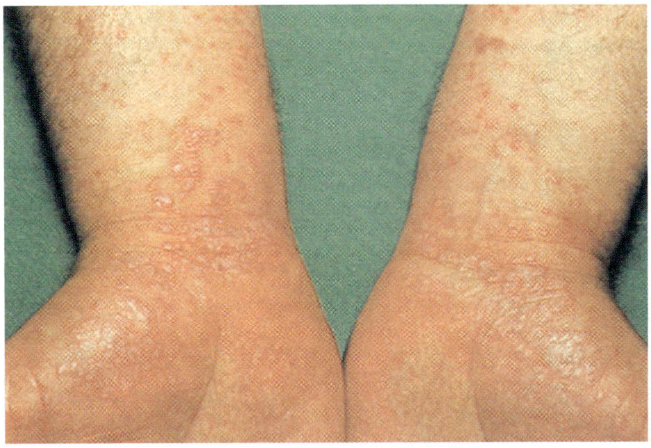

Plate 25 Lichen planus: typical violaceous papules. Drug-induced lichen planus may be indistinguishable from the idiopathic form or may also exhibit eczematous features.

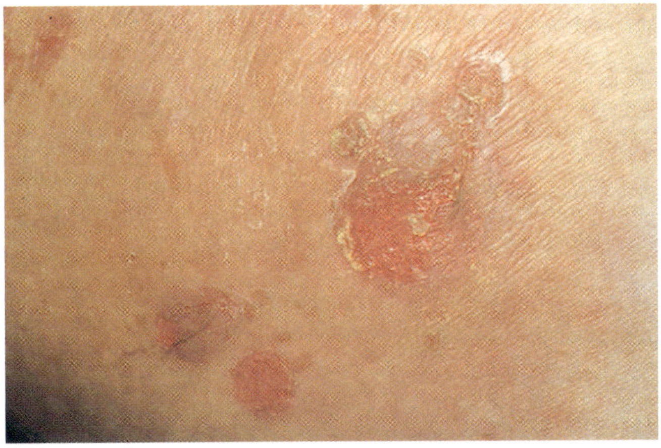

Plate 26 Pemphigus foliaceus of the trunk, induced by D-penicillamine. The superficial, eroded eruption can be confused with eczema.

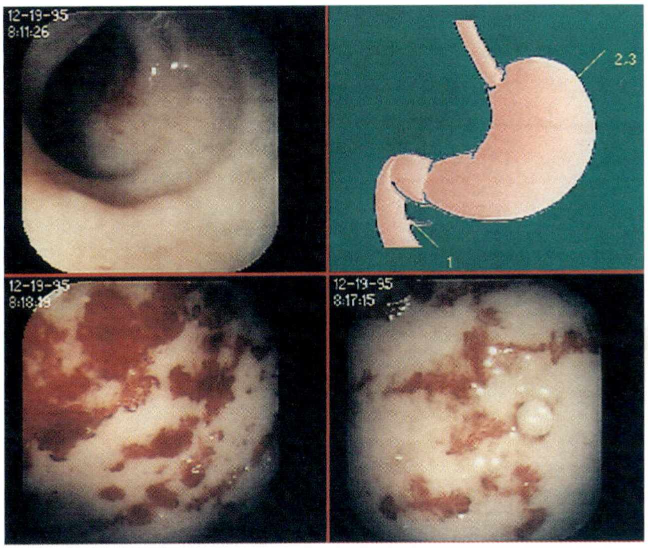

Plate 27 Gastric lesions in a patient taking non-steroidal anti-inflammatory drugs (NSAIDs).

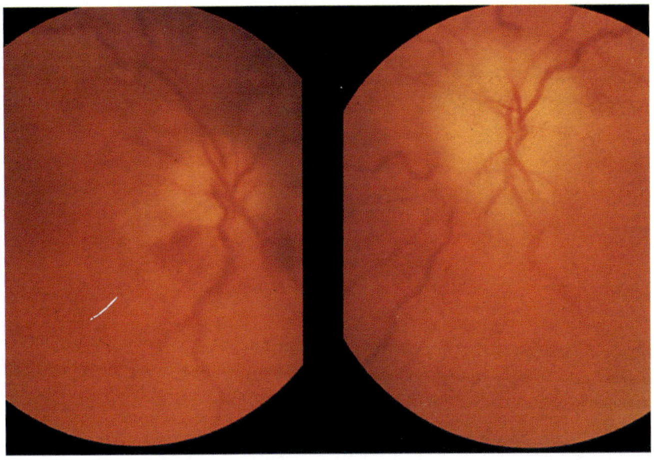

Plate 28 Giant-cell arteritis. An 81-year-old woman with severe scalp tenderness woke up blind in her left eye, followed 3 days later by blindness in her right eye. The right fundus (left) has a swollen optic disc with peripapillary haemorrhages. The left optic disc (right) is swollen and pale, typical of ischaemic optic neuropathy.

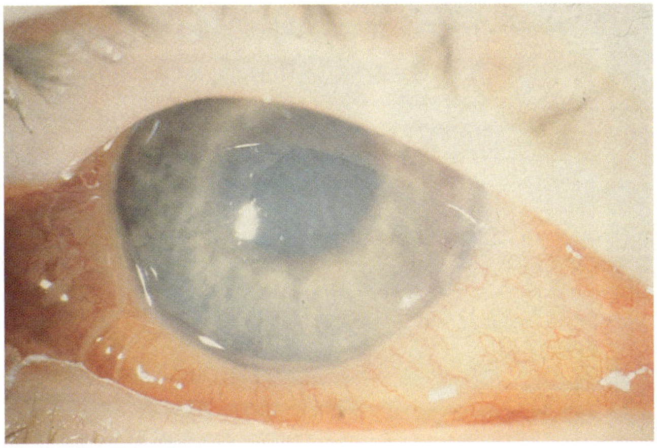

Plate 29 Scleritis. A 32-year-old Caucasian woman presents with a 3-week history of general malaise and fever and a 1-week history of loss of vision associated with severe pain. The eye is red, the sclera is inflamed, the conjunctiva is chemosed. The cornea appears hazy because of corneal folds caused by hypotension in the eye secondary to severe ischaemia. Investigations confirmed acute, fulminant systemic lupus erythematosus.

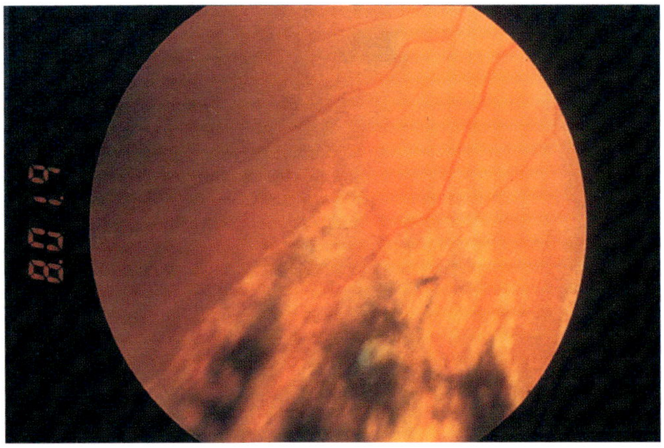

Plate 30 Choroidal infarcts in systemic lupus erythematosus. A 22-year-old woman presents with headaches and confusional state. Systemic lupus is diagnosed. Ten years later she has further thrombotic events when antiphospholipid antibodies were identified and these infarcts observed. They are asymptomatic.

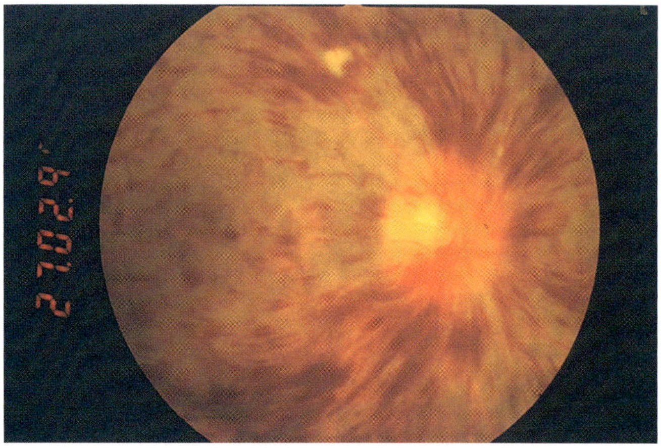

Plate 31 Retinal vein occlusion in a woman who suffers with systemic lupus erythematosus and has antiphospholipid antibodies.

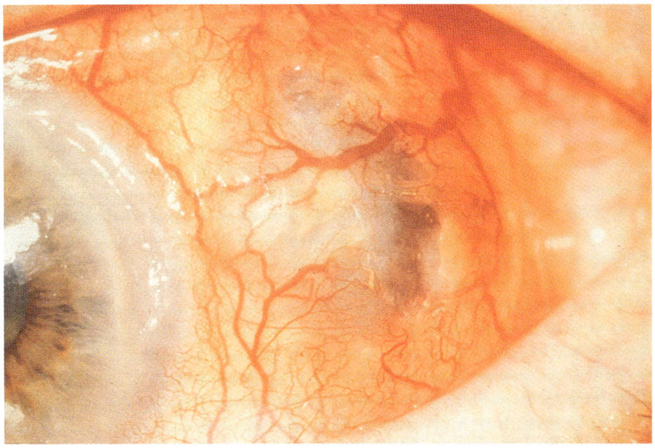

Plate 32 Scleromalacia perforans. A 75-year-old man has suffered with severe rheumatoid arthritis and scleritis for many years. He now has an area of very thin sclera due to ischaemia and ulceration of the adjacent peripheral cornea.

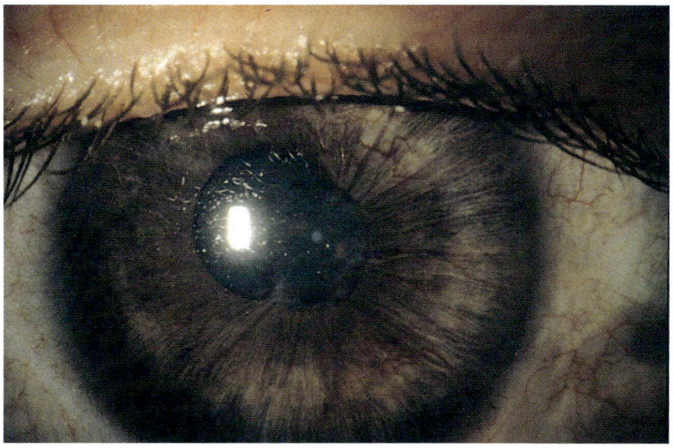

Plate 33 Uveitis associated with ankylosing spondylitis. A 24-year-old man is blind from chronic anterior uveitis. The eye is white but the pupil is irregular due to posterior synechiae and abnormal new vessels are present on the iris.

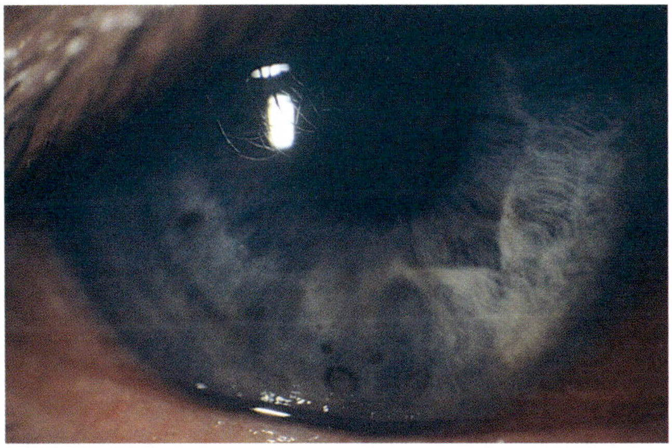

Plate 34 Granulomatous anterior uveitis. A 58-year-old man presents with episodes of breathlessness and red eyes, due to sarcoidosis. The conjunctiva is infected; large, grey, keratic precipitates are seen inferiorly on the corneal endothelium.

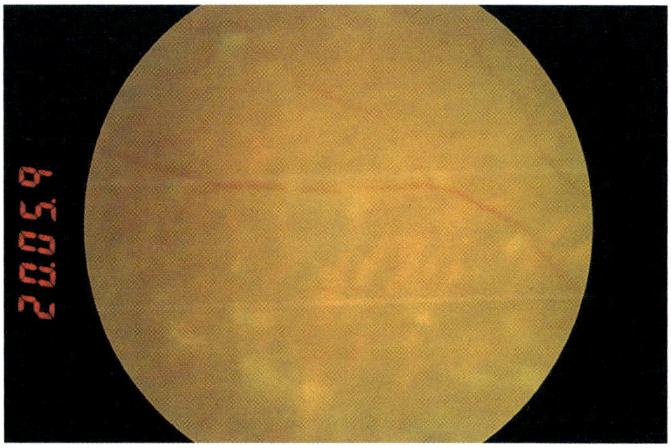

Plate 35 Sarcoidosis. A 40-year-old Asian man has suffered with uveitis and sarcoidosis for 15 years. He has sheathing of his retinal veins and multiple pale areas in the pigment epithelium and choroid, which probably represent granulomas.

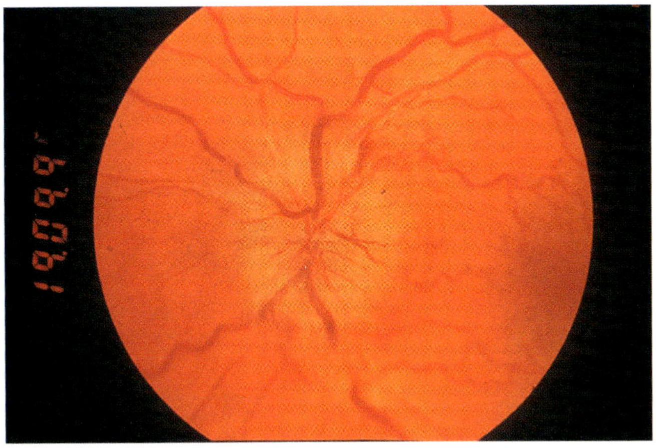

Plate 36 Optic nerve infiltration by sarcoidosis. A 24-year-old Caucasian man presents with sudden loss of vision associated with pain in the left eye. Investigations reveal a lymphopaenia, a high angiotensin-converting enzyme, raised protein, and 11.0 million lymphocytes in the cerebrospinal fluid.

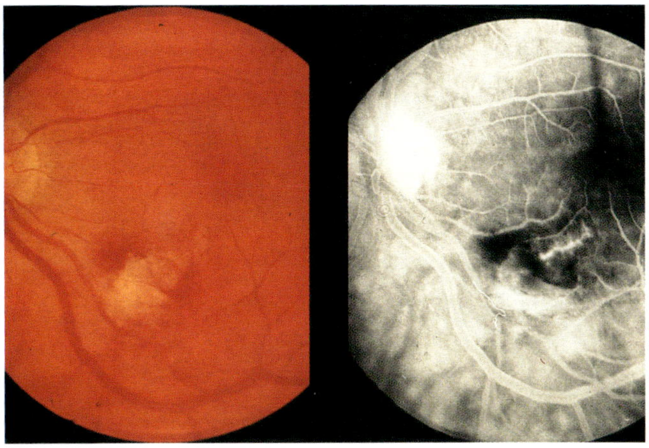

Plate 37 Behçet's disease. A 24-year-old woman with a history of severe orogenital ulceration and thrombophlebitis suddenly developed blurred central vision in her left eye. An area of haemorrhage and infiltrate was present inferior to the macula (left) and a fluorescein angiogram (right) revealed occlusion of a small retinal vein.

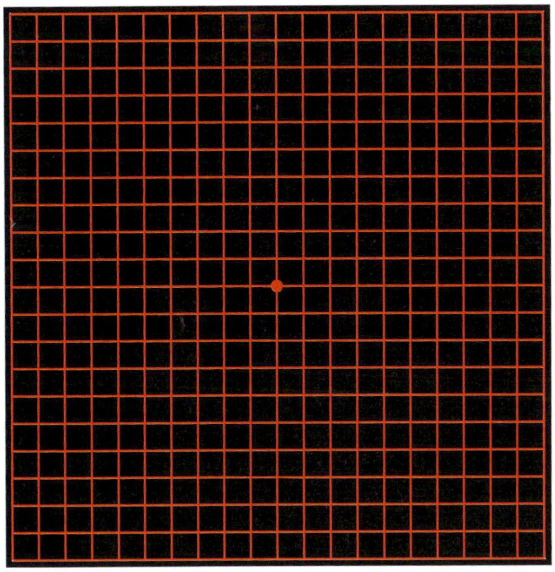

Plate 38 The red Amsler grid.

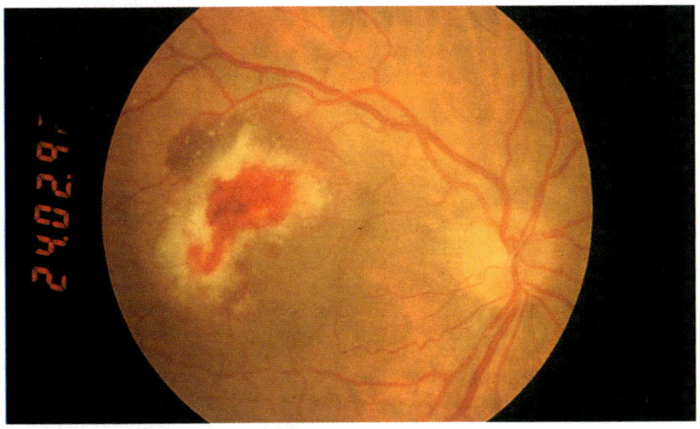

Plate 39 Cytomegalovirus retinitis. A middle-aged man has Wegener's granulomatosis controlled with prednisolone and azathioprine. After 12 months' treatment he develops blurred vision. The area of retinal necrosis with haemorrhage and satellite lesions is typical of cytomegalovirus retinitis. The retinitis resolved with ganciclovir and reduction of immunosuppressive therapy.

(a)

(b)

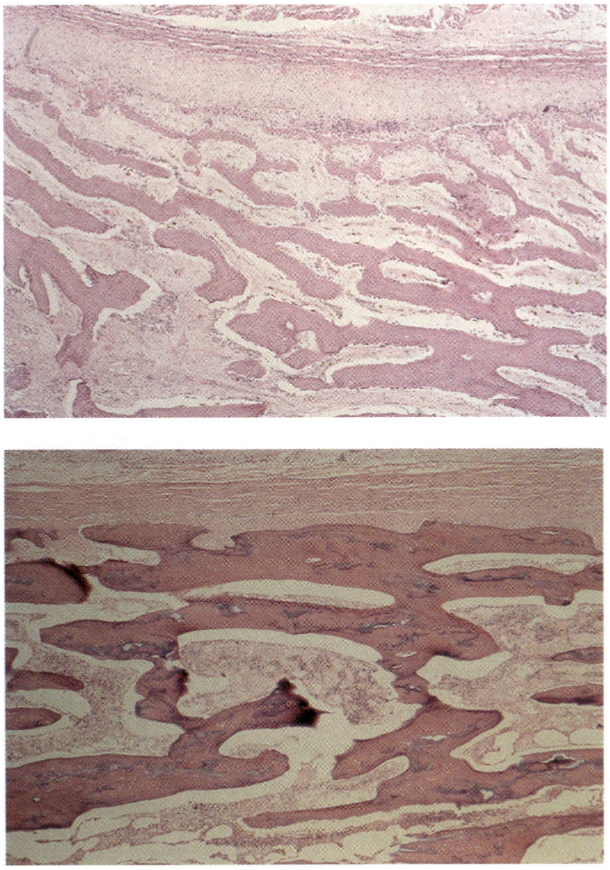

Plate 40 Histological features of foetal bone in mild osteogenesis imperfecta (OI) (a) compared with normal control; (b) at 24 weeks' gestation. The trabecular bone is obviously thinner in the OI sample. Original magnification ×4.

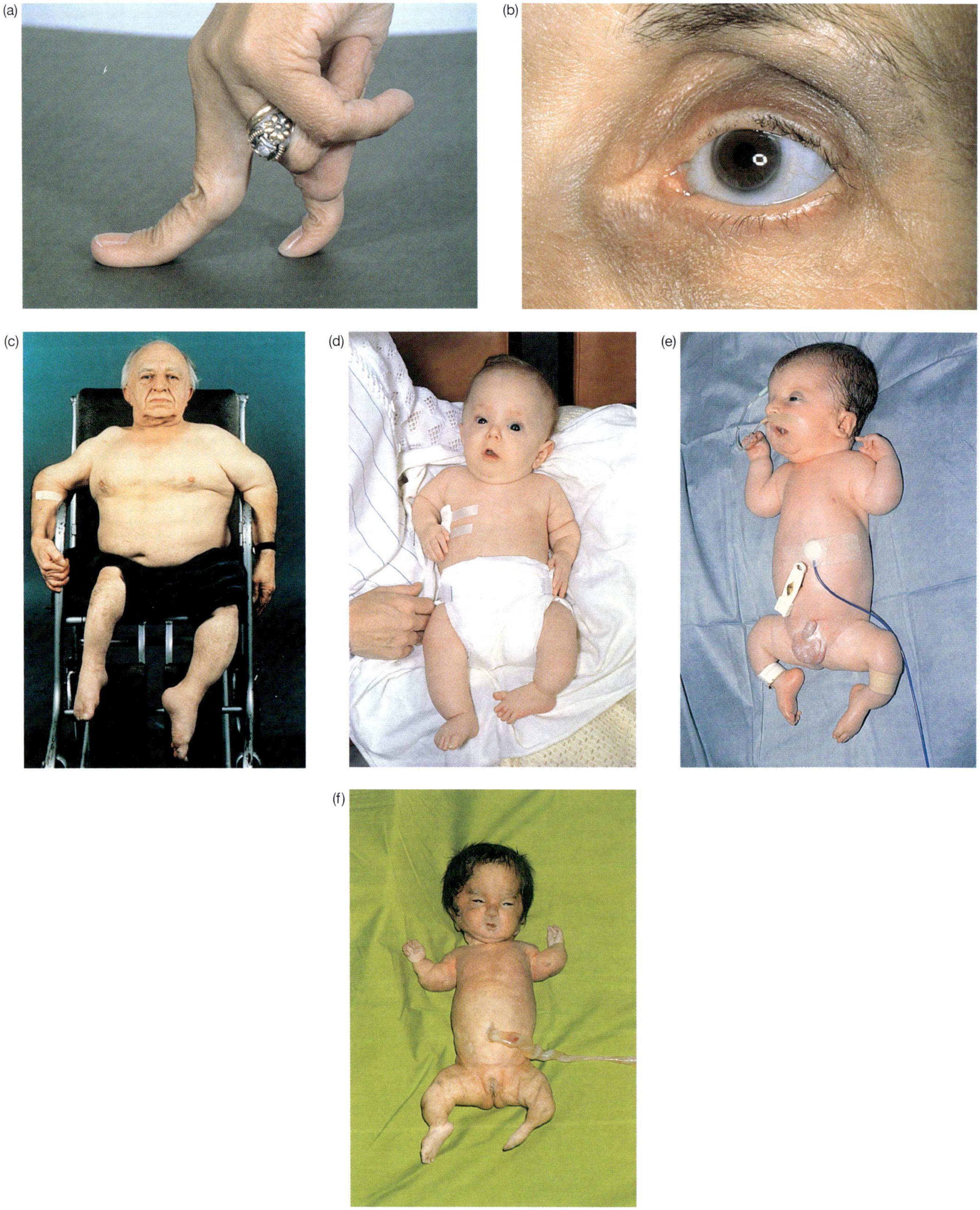

Plate 41 (a) Many patients with Sillence type I osteogenesis imperfecta (OI) have generalized joint laxity (shown here at finger tips). (b) Here, this was associated with premature corneal arcus caused by the OI. (c) Severely crippling Sillence type II OI. This patient has a relatively normal face, shortened upper-limb segments, a broadened and distorted chest, and convex, distorted lower limbs. He had a Gly–Cys mutation at position 415 of the collagen a1(I) chain. (d) Severely affected patient with Sillence type IIb OI. (e) Lethally affected patient with Sillence type IIa OI. (f) Lethally affected OI baby with OI type IIb.

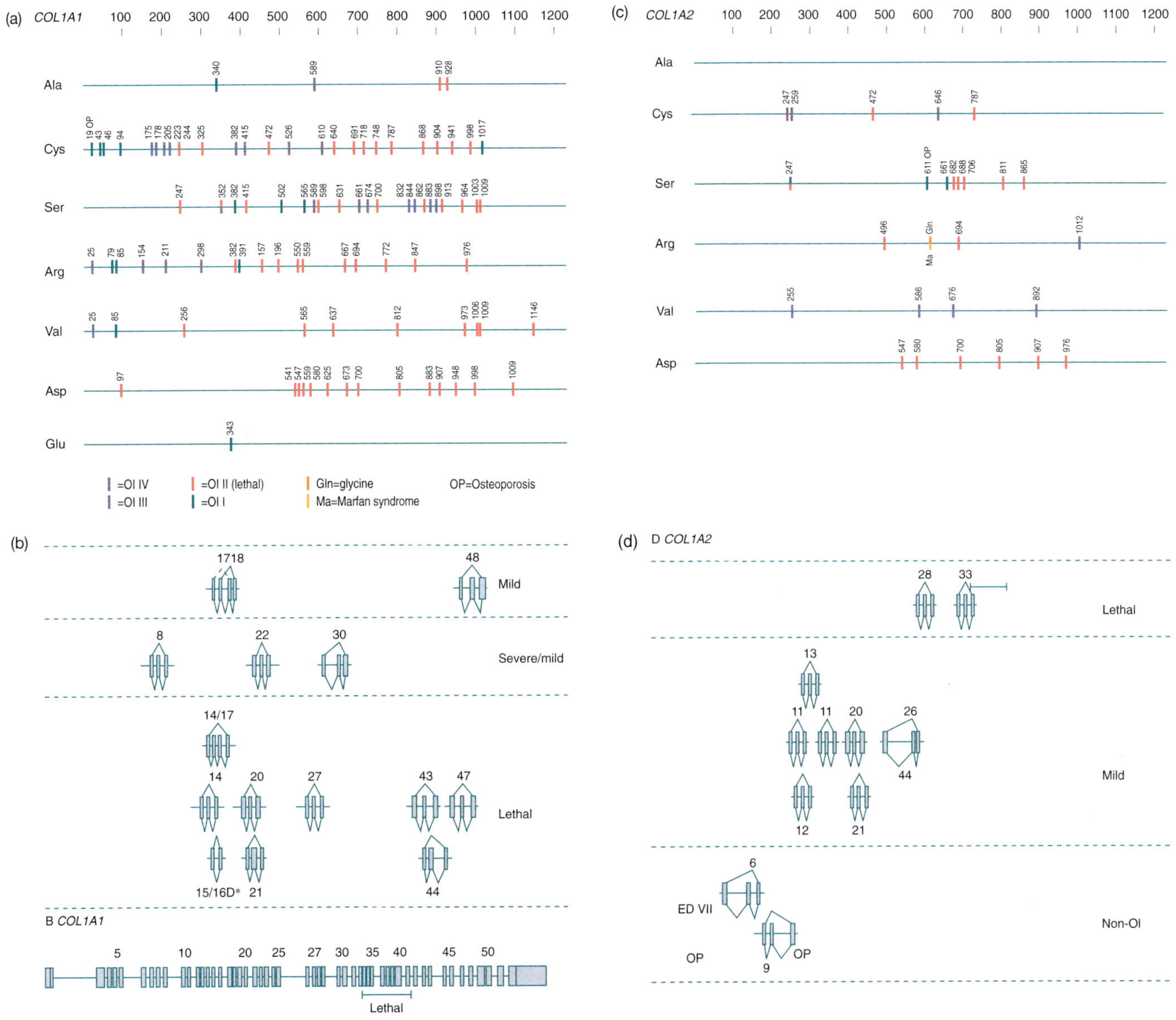

Plate 42 Distribution of type I collagen mutations arranged by glycine substitutions for *COL1A1* and *COL1A2* (a and b) and by exon skips (c and d). Updated from information by Byers (1990), Cole and Dalgleish (1995), and Dalgleish (2001). Different colours indicate the severity of OI and exon skips are denoted by superscripts. OI = osteogenesis imperfecta, EDS = Ehlers–Danlos syndrome, OP = osteoporosis.

(a)

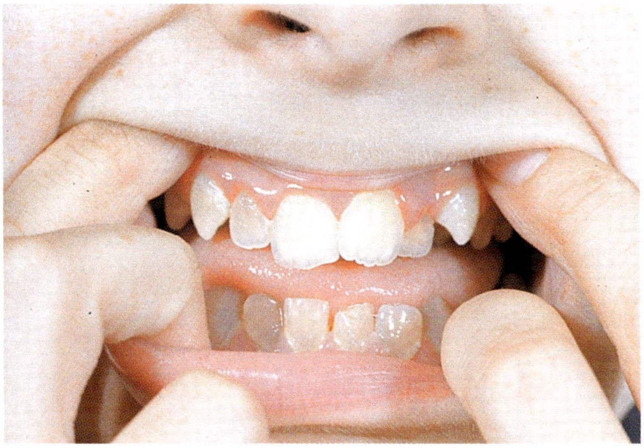

(b)

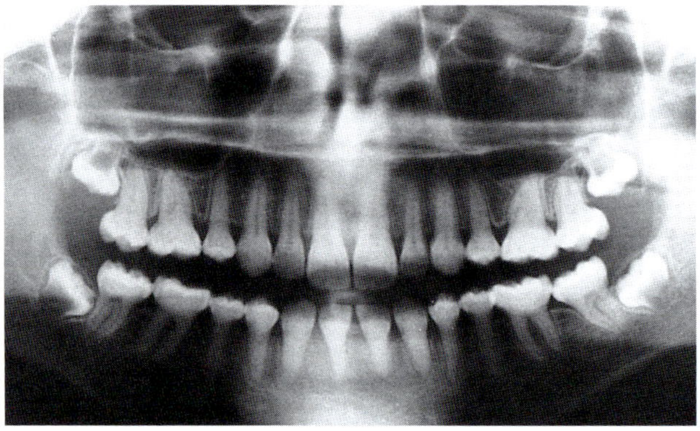

(c)

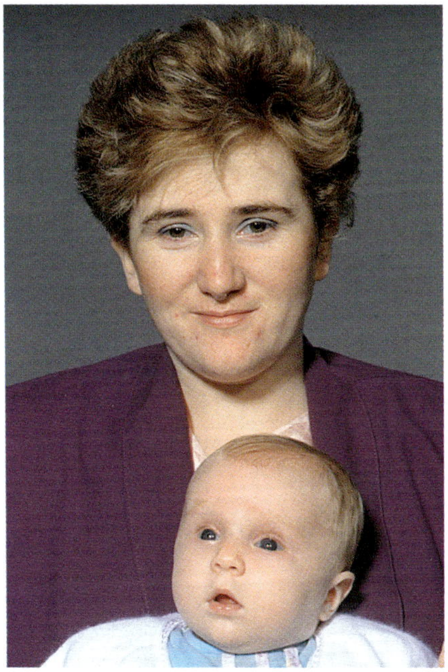

Plate 43 (a) Typically patchy distribution of dentinogenesis imperfecta in adolescent teeth of mild Sillence type I OI. The lower incisors and premolars are particularly affected. (b) Dental radiographs in typical osteogenesis imperfecta (OI) showing shortened, tapering roots, obliterated pulp cavities, and tulip-like crowns. (c) This mother and baby both have mild Sillence type I OI. Note mother's triangular-shaped head. Both individuals have blue sclerae.

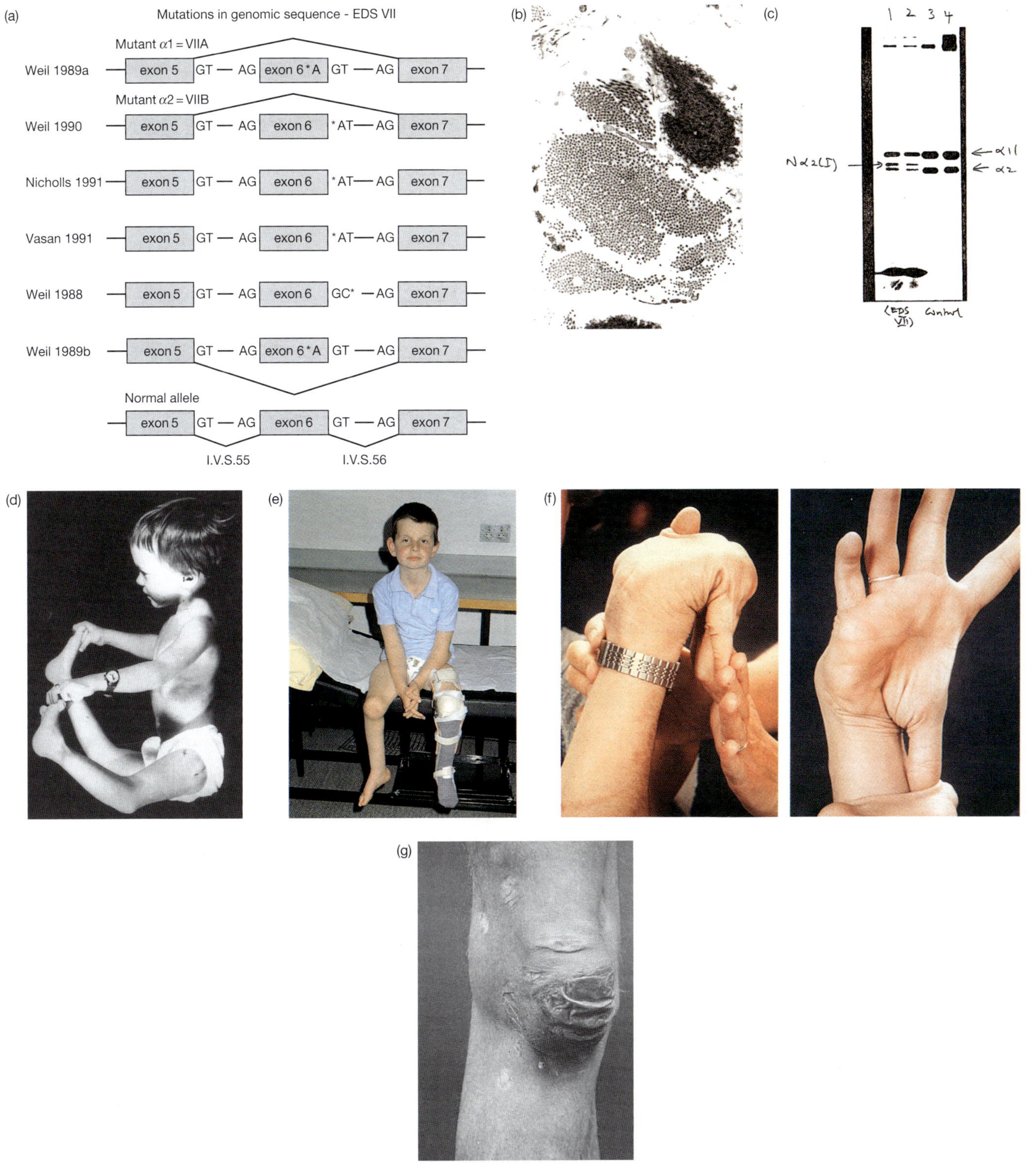

Plate 44 (a) Diagrammatic representation of certain published mutations in Ehlers–Danlos syndrome (EDS) VII affecting the splicing of exon 6 of either the *COL1A1* or *COL1A2* genes. (b) Collagen fibril patterns in our Dutch patient (Pope et al. 1991). (c) Radiolabelled collagen profiles from EDS VII patients (tracks 1 and 2) compared with normal control (tracks 3 and 4) with persistent pNα2 chains after pepsinization. (d) Affected patient with EDS VII (Beighton 1995). Note extreme rotation of hips and knees. (e) British patient with *COL1A1* splice-junction mutation. Note early premature cutis laxa and joint laxity sufficiently severe to require bracing of the unstable knees. (f) Laxity of finger joints. (g) Abnormal scarring of knees and shins from the Dutch patient whose fibres are shown in (b) and (c). These changes resemble EDS I/II (see also Plates 48 and 49).

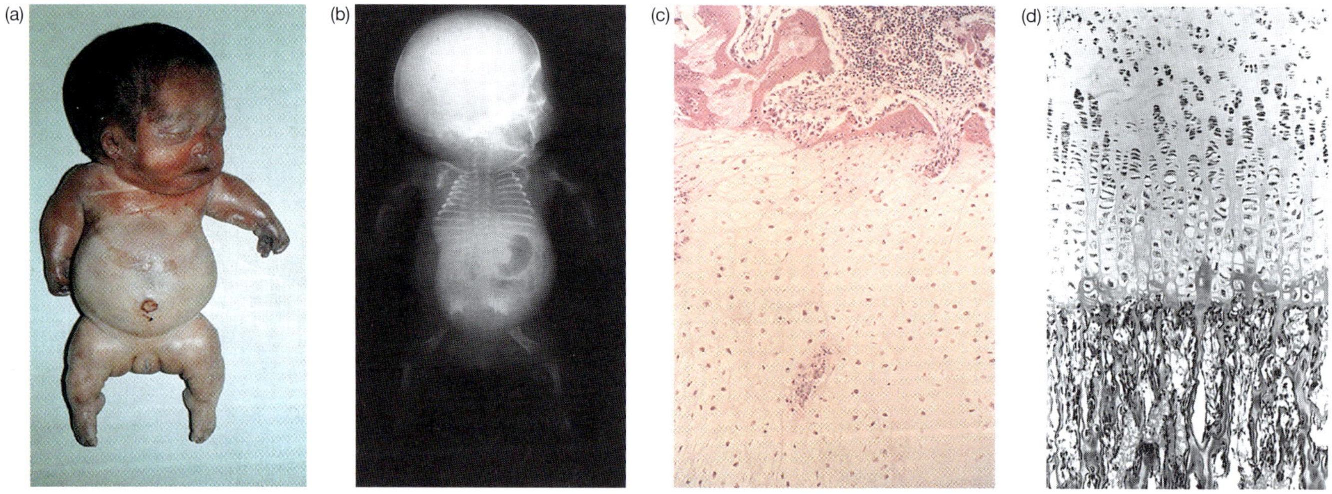

Plate 45 (a) Typical clinical appearance of patient with lethal achondrogenesis II. Note the rhizomelia and abdominal distension with the constricted small chest. (b) The radiographs show shortened ribs, metaphyseal flaring, and shortened long bones. (c) The histological appearance of the femur shows bulbous hyperplasia of the epiphyses and disorganization of cartilage columns, including a fibroblastic inclusion at the epiphyseal plate, compared with the normal control. (d) The bony trabeculae are also disorganized in the achondrogenesis bone. Original magnification ×157.

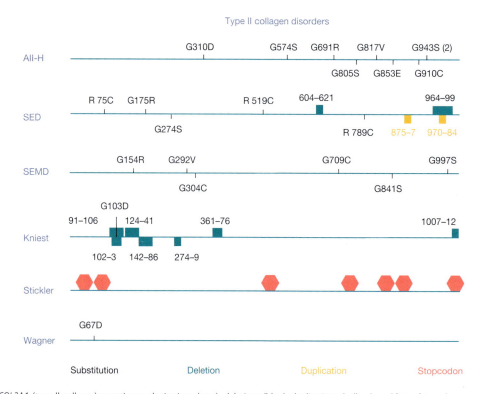

Plate 46 Diagram of *COL2A1* (type II collagen) mutations, substitutions (grey), deletions (blue), duplications (yellow), and 'stops' in red.

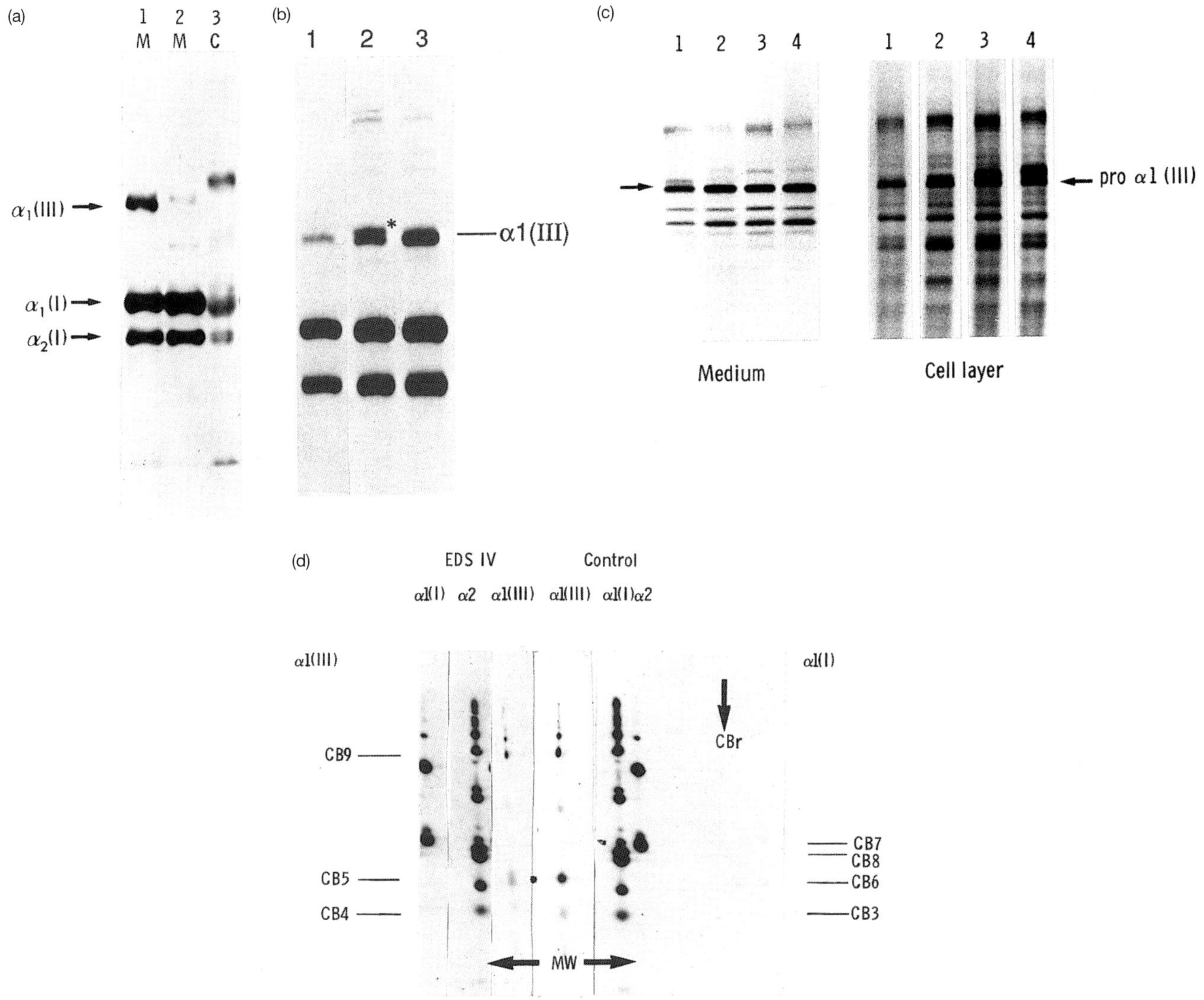

Plate 47 (a) Typically, poor secretion and intracellular retention of pepsinized collagen α1(III) chains in an Ehlers–Danlos syndrome IV mutant. Here the medium collagens (track 1) are diminished and an overmodified form is retained within the cell layer, compared with the normal control (track 3). (b) The mutant form is secreted as an α1(III) doublet (track 2) in which the secreted mutant product is starred. Otherwise, a normal and a shortened form of the protein are simultaneously secreted (not shown). (c) Overmodification of retained, cell layer, pro-α1(III) chains is variable (cell layer, tracks 2, 3, and 4) according to the helical position of the mutation, the nearer the C terminus the greater the overmodification and the more retarded the band. The effect on collagen secretion is similar (medium, tracks 2, 3, and 4). (d) Two-dimensional electrophoresis of collagen α1(III) chains. In this instance there is an α1(III) CB5 doublet in the mutant, left hand a1(III) track, compared with the normal, right hand, sample. α1(I) and α2(I) tracks are identical.

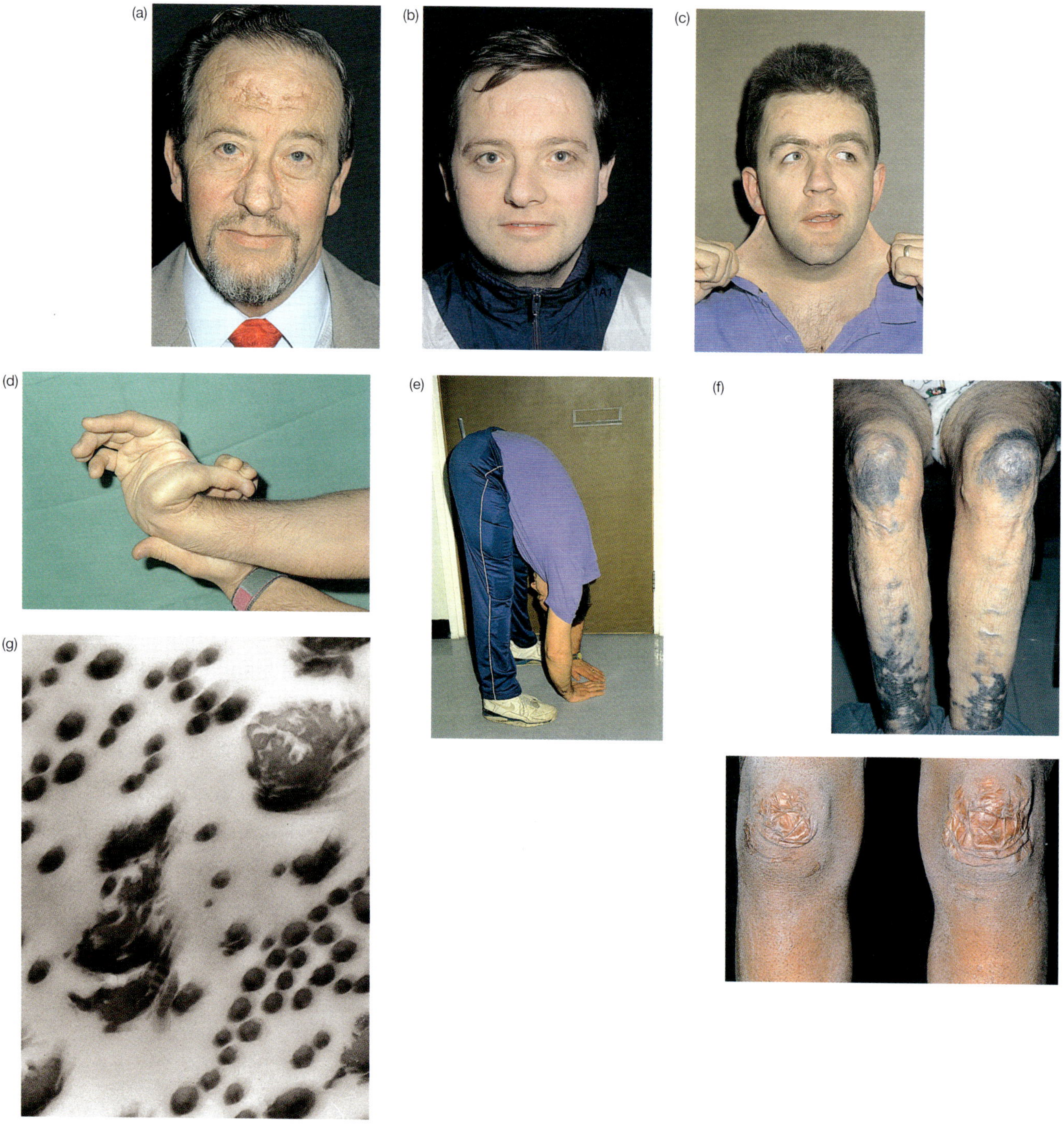

Plate 48 (a, b) Faces of affected father and son with Ehlers–Danlos syndrome (EDS) I, both showing typical scarring. (c) There is also abnormal cutaneous extensibility or epicanthic folds. (d, e) Joint laxity is both widespread and commonplace. (f) Scarring of the shins and knees is also usual, closely resembling that of certain patients with EDS VI [see Plate 44(e)]. (g) Cauliflower fibrils are typical (as viewed by transmission electron microscopy $\times$62 500).

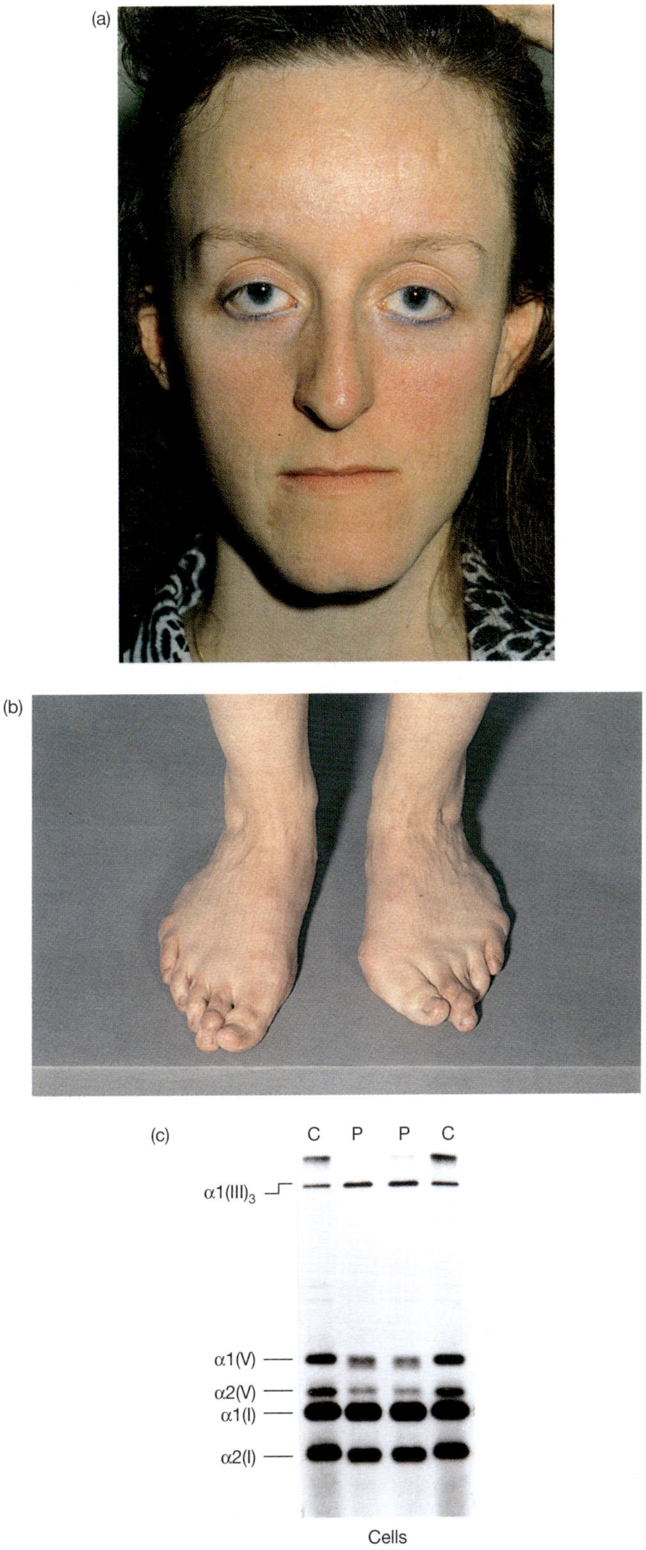

Plate 49 (a, b) Face and feet of the first Ehlers–Danlos syndrome patient with a *COL5A1* mutation. The eyes have flattened corneas, but the general physical features resembled those shown in Plates 44 and 48. (c) Gel electrophoresis of cell layer collagens from affected patient showing normal (upper) and shortened (lower) collagen α1 (V) chains in the patient (tracks PP); as compared with the controls (tracks CC), which show only normal (upper) patterns.

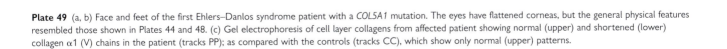

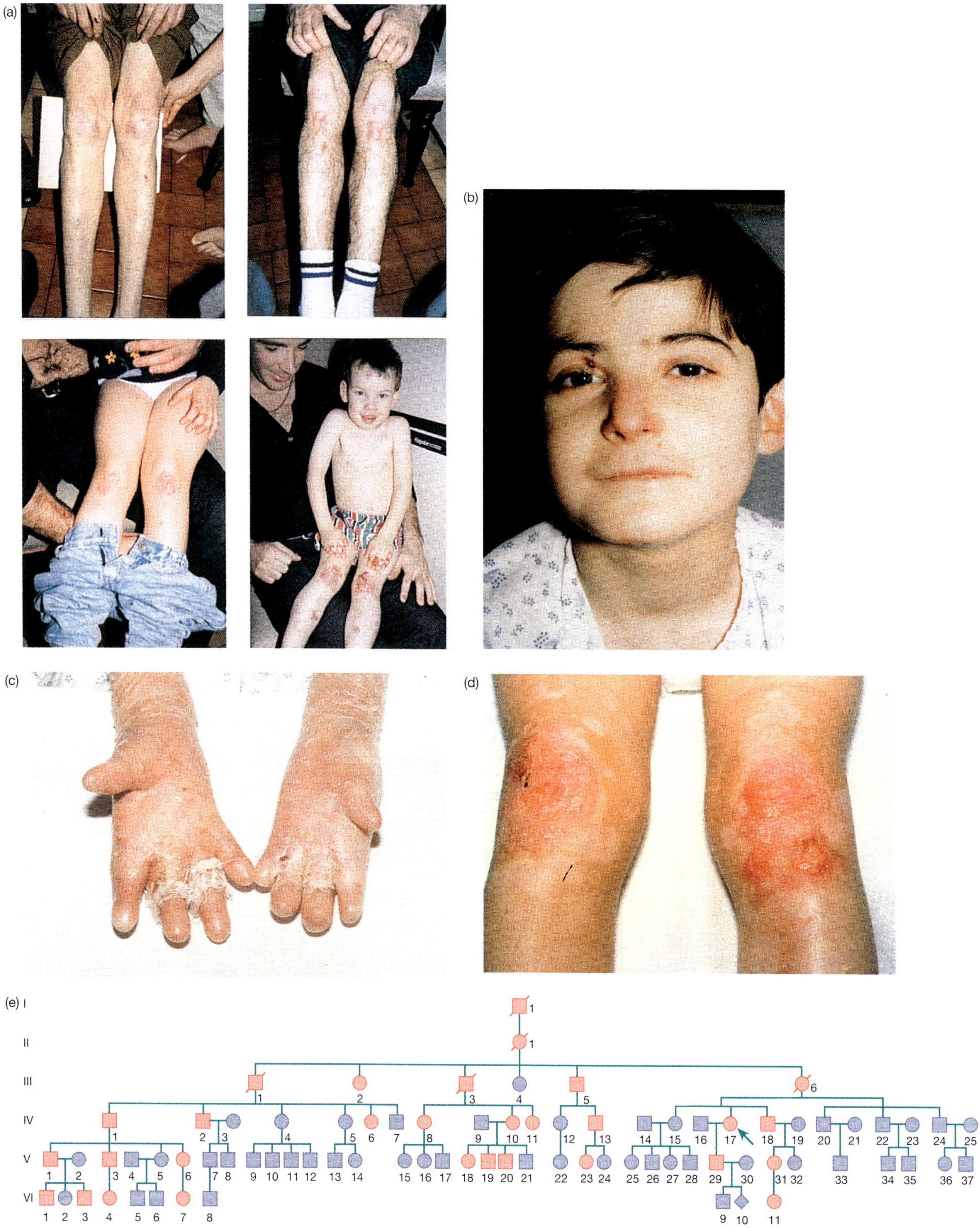

Plate 50 (a) Montage of family with autosomal-dominant dystrophic epidermolysis bullosa (DEB) showing typical scarring and blistering of knees, shins, and the hands. (b, c, d) Severe recessive (R) DEB. (b) Facial scars. (c) Mittening of the hands. (d) Scarring of the knees. (e) Typical multigenerational pedigree of autosomal-dominant DEB.

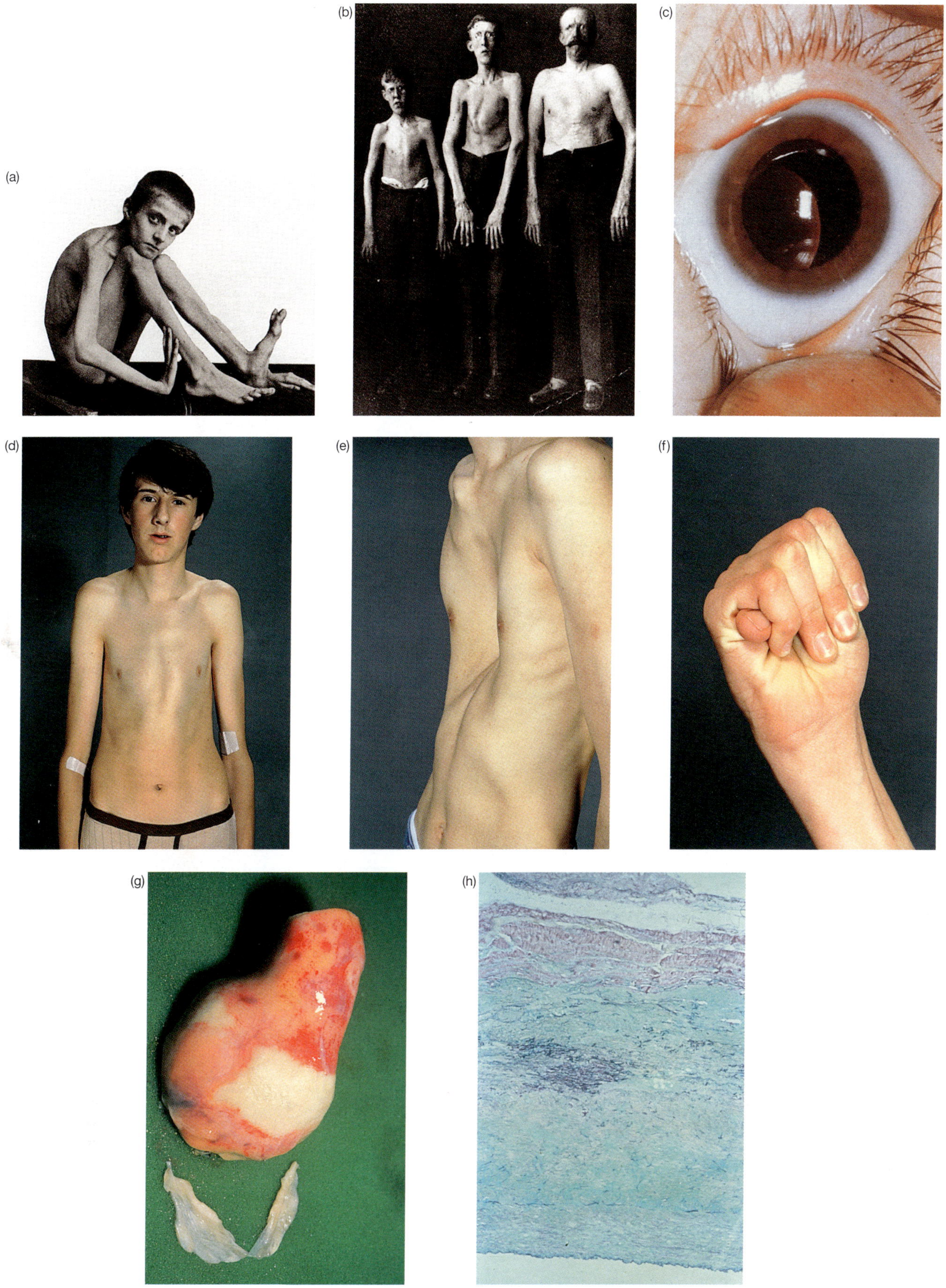

Plate 51 Marfan syndrome (MFS) clinical phenotypes. (a) Marfan's original patient. (b) Original family described by Weve (1931). Note chest deformities and elongated fingers and arms. (c) Typical dislocated lens from individual with classical MFS. (d, e) Pectus excavatum and carinatum from two different patients with MFS. (f) Positive thumb sign (the grasped thumb protrudes beyond the width of the palm). (g) Dilated aortic root from typical MFS patients. (h) Medial elastic degeneration of MFS.

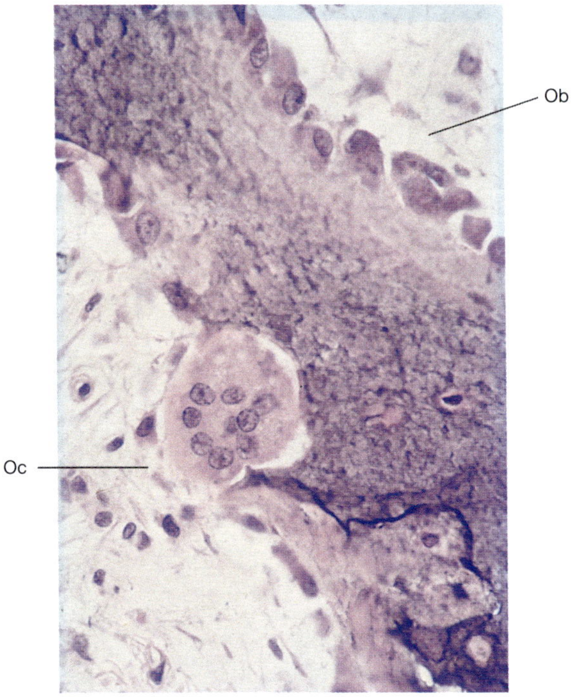

Plate 52 A multinucleated osteoclast (centre: ↔, Oc) is present in a Howship's resorption lacuna along one edge of a bone trabecula; a row of plump mononuclear osteoblasts lie along the opposite edge (right: →, Ob). Haematoxylin and eosin, magnification ×4000.

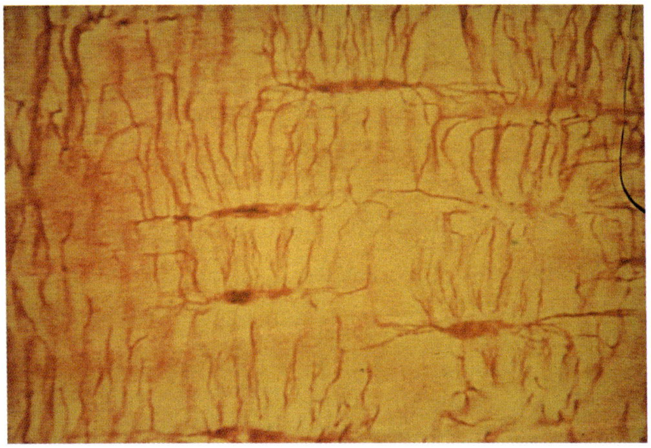

Plate 53 A ground bone section showing osteocytes with numerous canaliculi, magnification ×400.

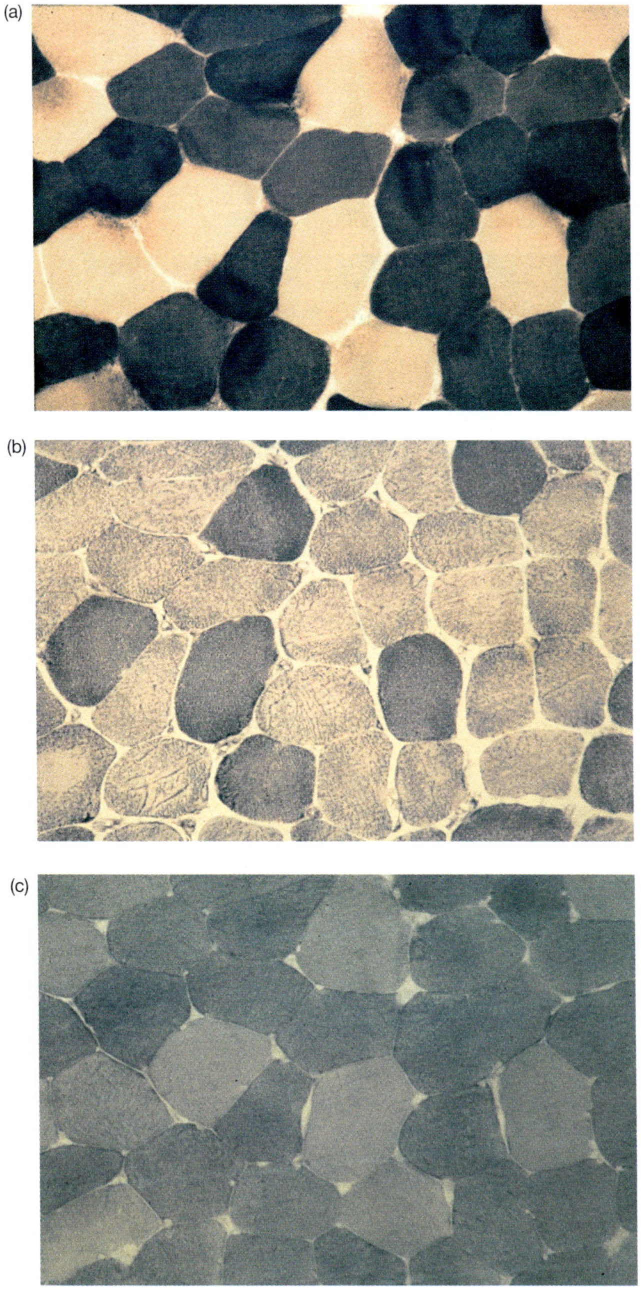

Plate 54 Serial transverse sections of human quadriceps muscle stained with (a) ATPase at pH 9.4; (b) NADH tetrazolium reductase for mitochondrial activity; and (c) for phosphorylase. Fibres high in phosphorylase are low in mitochondrial activity and stain darkly (type 2) with ATPase at pH 9.4.

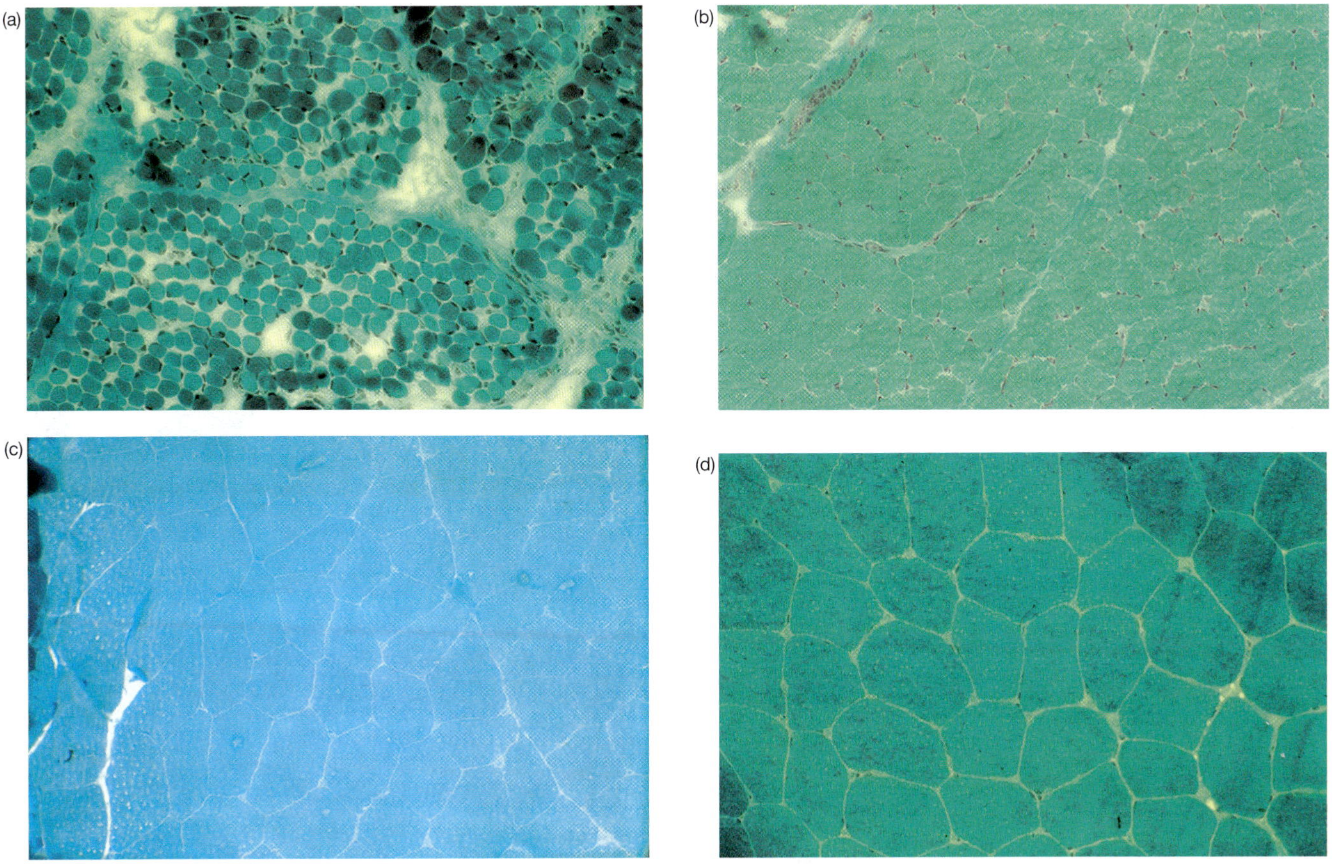

Plate 55 Growth of muscle fibre size in the human quadriceps. (a) In a baby aged 8 months, (b) in a child of 5 years, (c) in a boy aged 14 years, and (d) in an adult male. All at the same magnification.

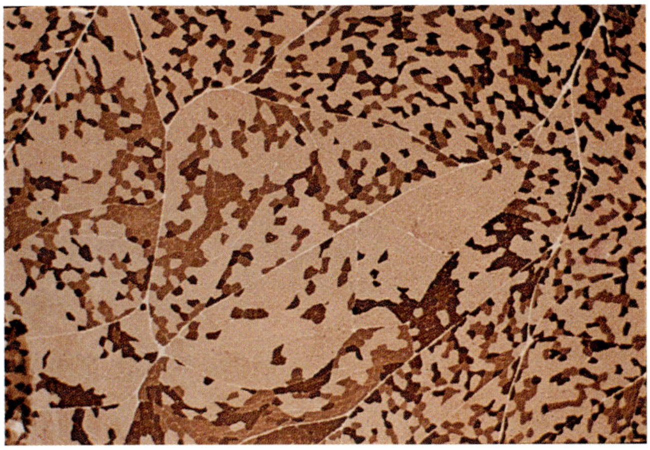

Plate 56 Adductor pollicis muscle of the hand from an 80-year-old woman with no clinical or neurological signs. Transverse section of an autopsy sample, several fascicles consist largely of only type 1 fibres indicating reinnervation. ATPase stain at pH 9.4.

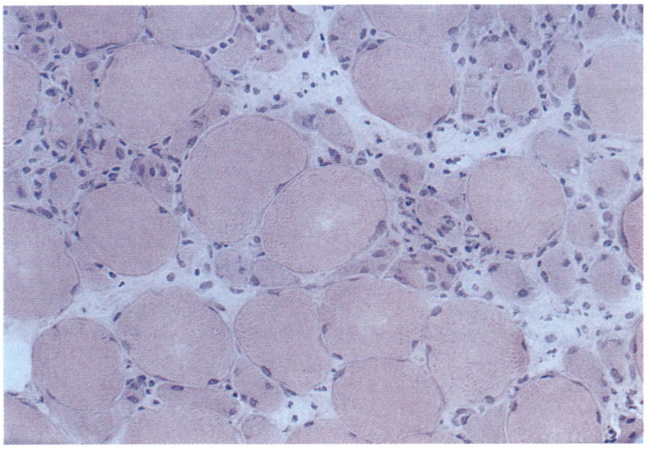

Plate 57 Haematoxylin and eosin stains of transverse section of quadriceps muscle, 12 days after eccentric exercise.

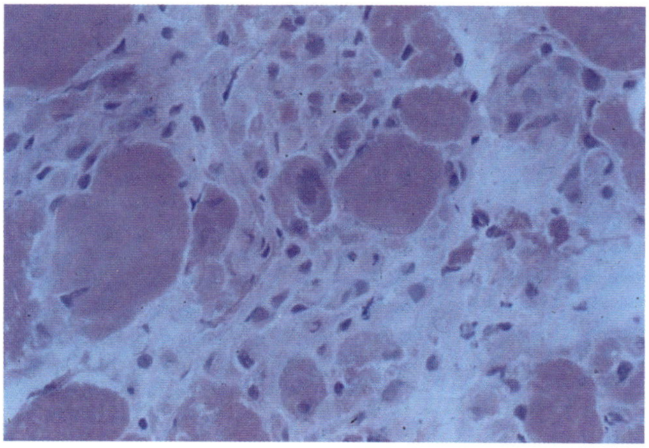

Plate 58 Muscle damage due to ischaemia and reperfusion. Histological appearance of a biopsy from anterior tibialis muscle 10 days after surgical revascularization of the limb. Haematoxylin and eosin stain.

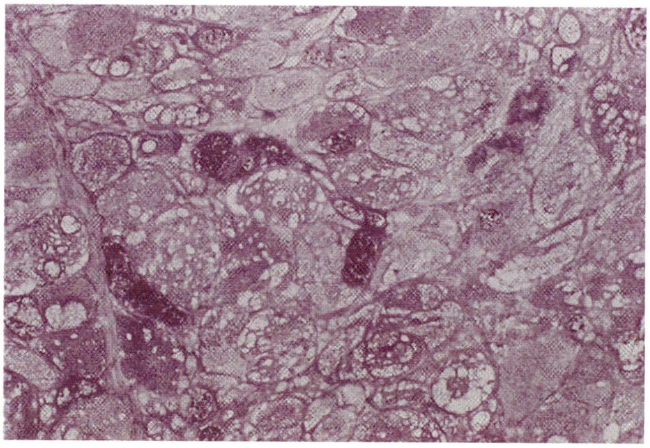

Plate 59 Muscle biopsy of a patient with acid maltase deficiency (type 2 glycogenosis). Note the severe vacuolar myopathy with fibres packed with glycogen. Periodic acid–Schiff stain.

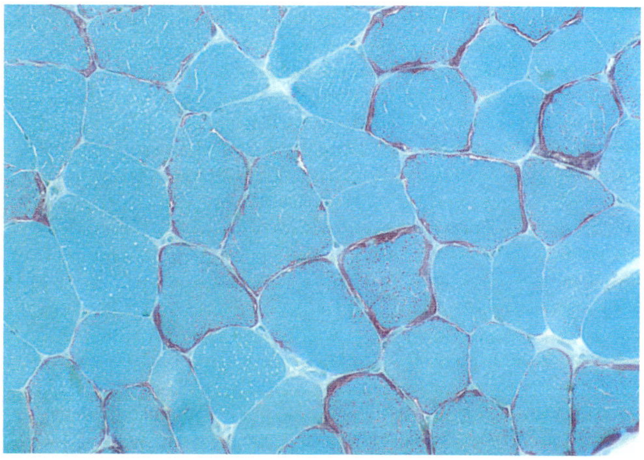

Plate 60 Ragged red fibres in a transverse section of quadriceps muscle from a 19-year-old boy with a mitochondrial myopathy. Dark red staining at the periphery of the fibres is caused by aggregations of mitochondria. Trichrome stain.

(a)

(b)

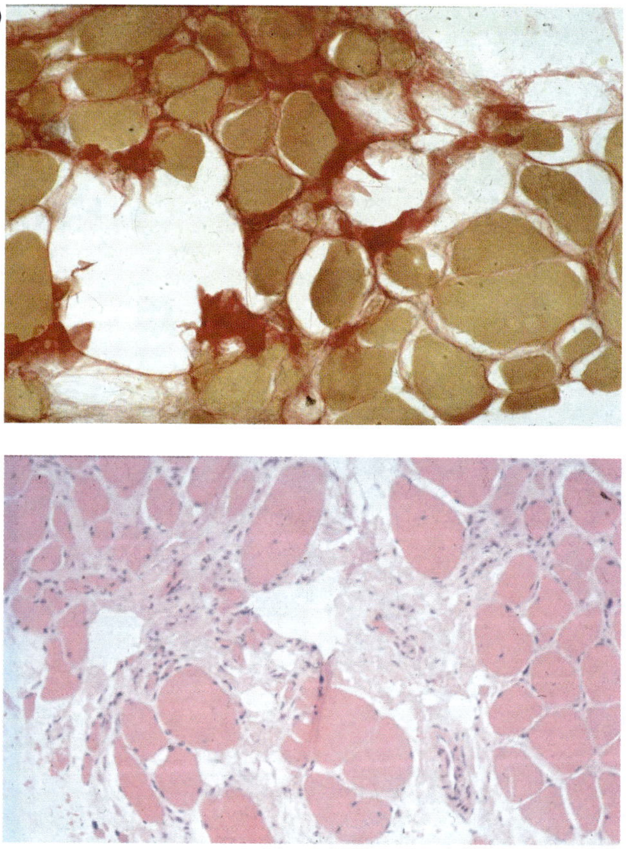

Plate 61 (a) Transverse section of quadriceps muscle from a 15-year-old boy with Duchenne muscular dystrophy showing replacement of muscle fibres by fibrous connective tissue. Van Geison stain; fibrous tissue stained red, muscle fibres stained yellow. (b) Transverse section of calf muscle from the same boy showing replacement of muscle by fibrous tissue and fat, the fat has dissolved during processing and appears as spaces in the section.

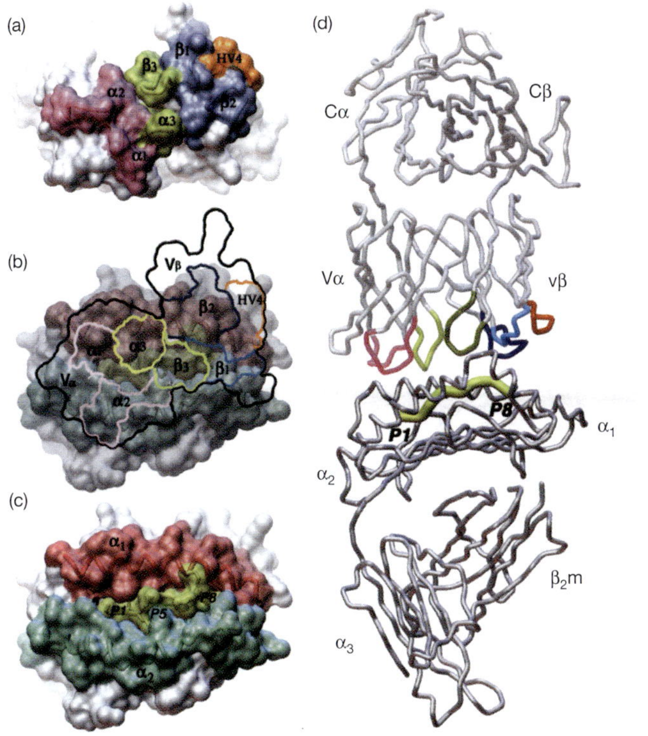

Plate 62 TCR/peptide/MHC triple complex. This figure is derived from crystallographic analysis of the murine $\alpha\beta$ TCR (2C) bound to the MHC class I molecule (H-2K^b) presenting a peptide (dEV8). (a) View of the antigen-binding site of the TCR, showing the six CDR loops (α1, α2, α3, β1, β2, β3). (b) View of the surface of the peptide/MHC complex, indicating the position of the CDR loops when the TCR docks with the peptide/MHC. (c) View of the surface of the peptide/MHC complex depicting the two α-helices (α1 and α2) of the MHC class I heavy chain and the peptide (yellow), showing the positions of residues P1, P5, and P8. (d) Representation of the relationship between the TCR (top) and peptide/MHC (below). (From Garcia et al. 1996.)

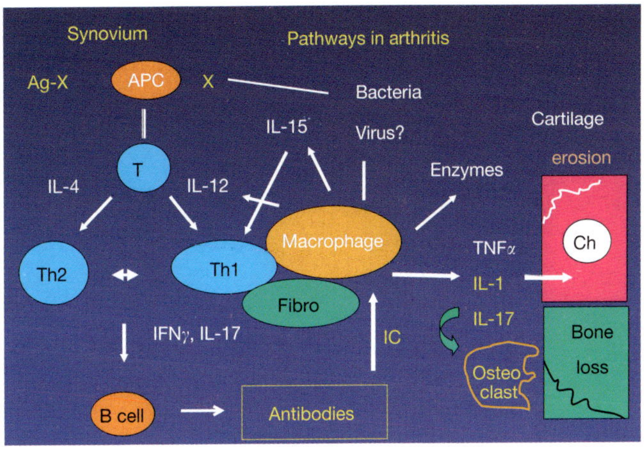

Plate 64 Pathways in arthritis.

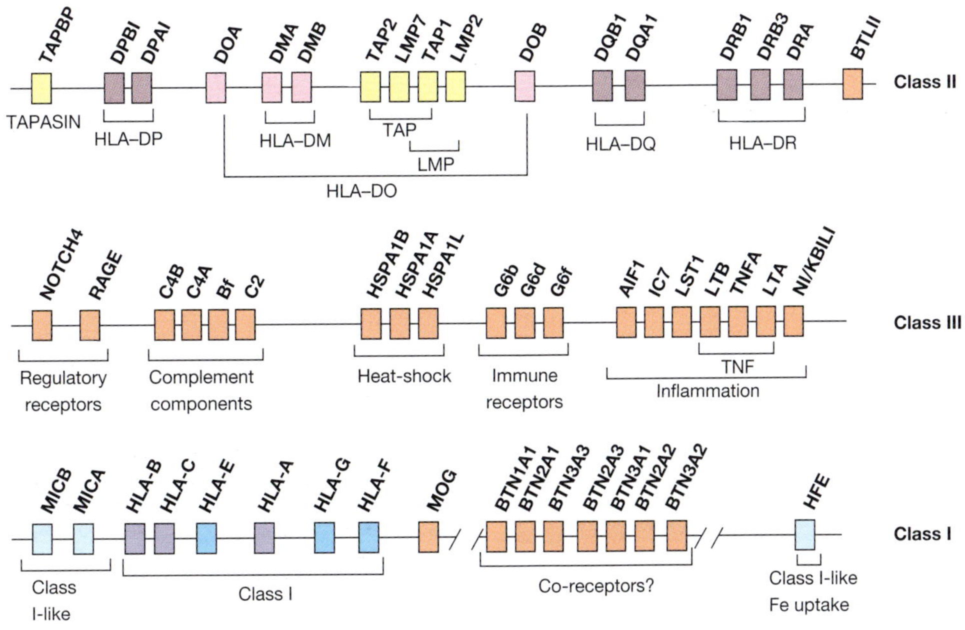

Plate 63 Main genes in the MHC locus. Classical class II genes are purple and non-classical are pink. Classical class I are dark blue, non-classical are blue, and others are pale blue. (From Trowsdale 2001.)

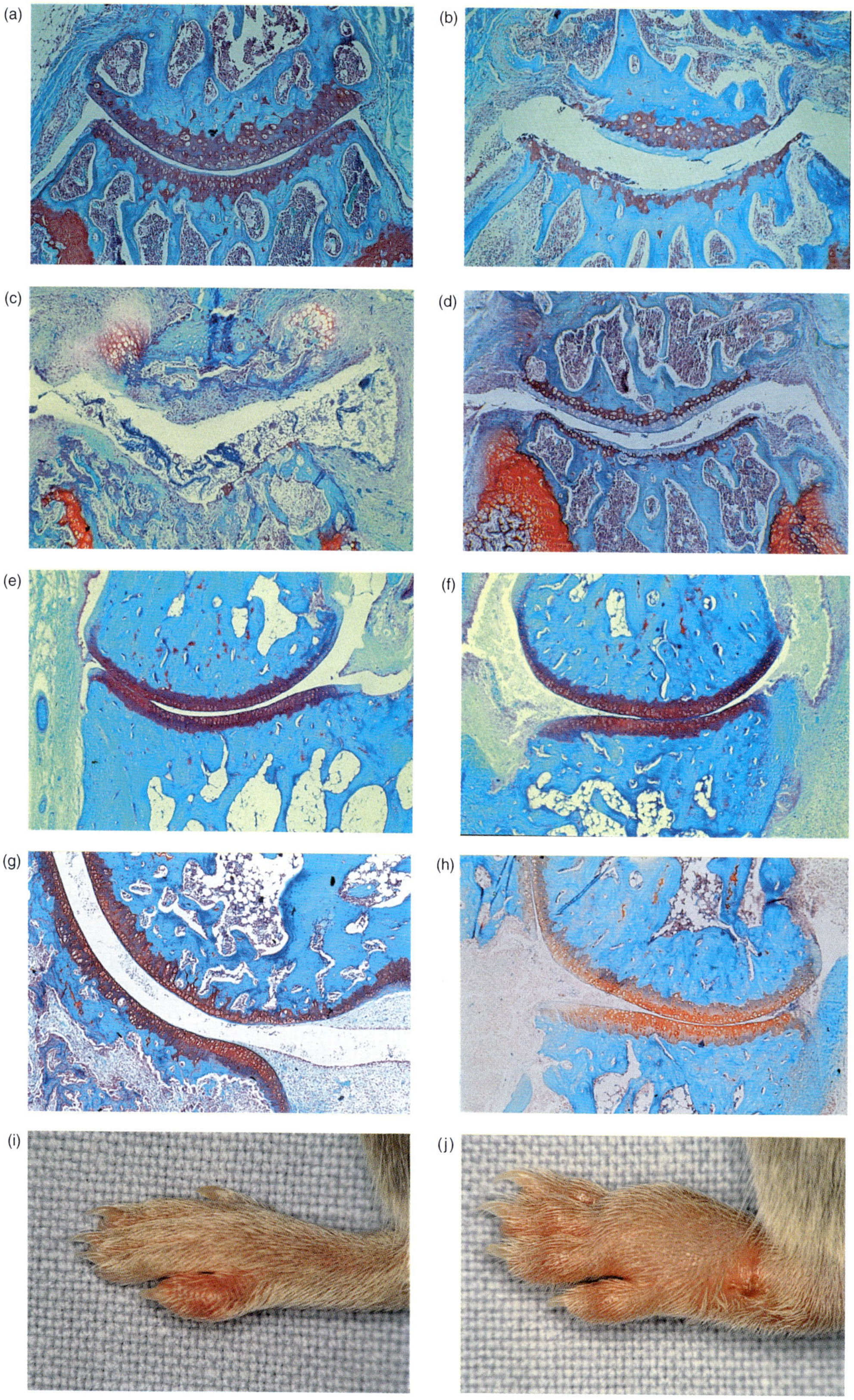

Plate 65 Light-microscopic analysis of cartilage proteoglycan (PG) depletion in safranin O-stained knee (a–d) and ankle (e–h) joints. (a) Normal knee joint; (b) destructive collagen arthritis (CIA), day 28 after onset; (c) complete destruction in CIA, day 28; (d) antigen-induced arthritis, day 28, showing superficial loss of PG and bone erosion as well as outgrowth at the edges; (e) normal ankle; (f) adjuvant arthritis, day 17; (g) adjuvant arthritis, day 28; (h) streptococcal cell-wall, arthritis, day 17, macroscopic appearance of collagen arthritis; (i) first onset in one toe; and (j) full-blown expression.

(a)

(b)

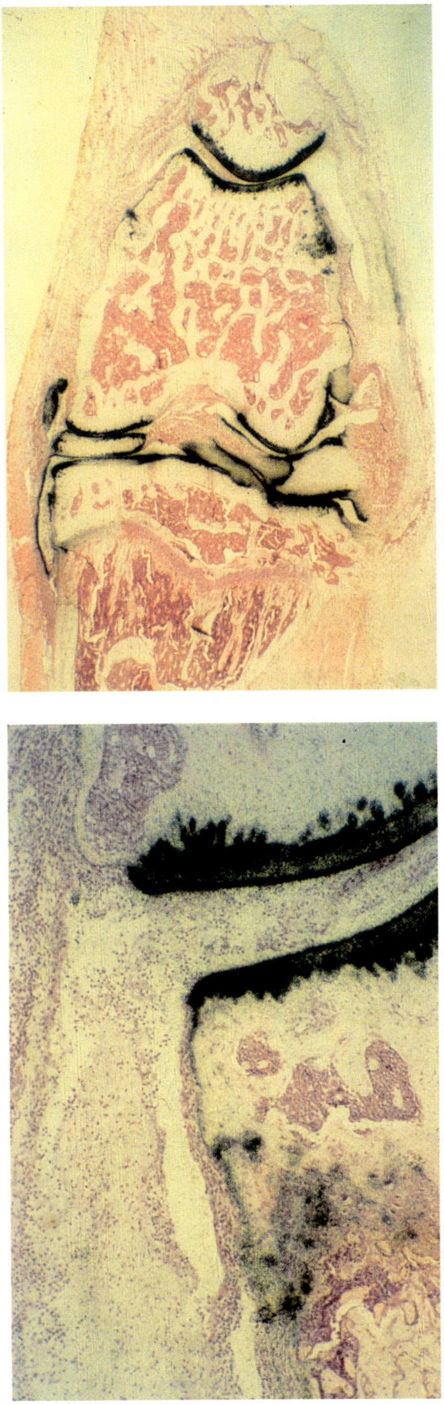

Plate 66 Autoradiograph at day 2 after intra-articular injection of [^{125}I]-labelled bovine serum albumin (BSA) in BSA/Freund's complete adjuvant immunized mice: (a) whole knee joint, and (b) detail of patella and femur; note the deep penetration of antigen in cartilaginous structures.

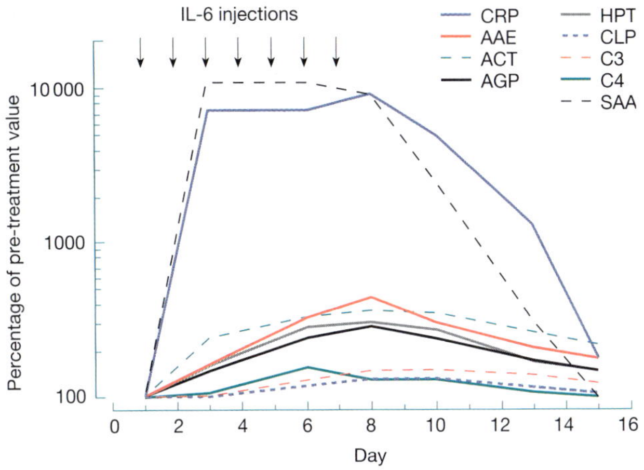

Plate 67 Profile of the relative changes in the positive acute phase proteins following IL-6 treatment in a patient with cancer. IL-6 was administered subcutaneously once daily for 7 days (arrows) at a dose of 10 mg/kg per day (reproduced from Banks et al. 1995, with permission).

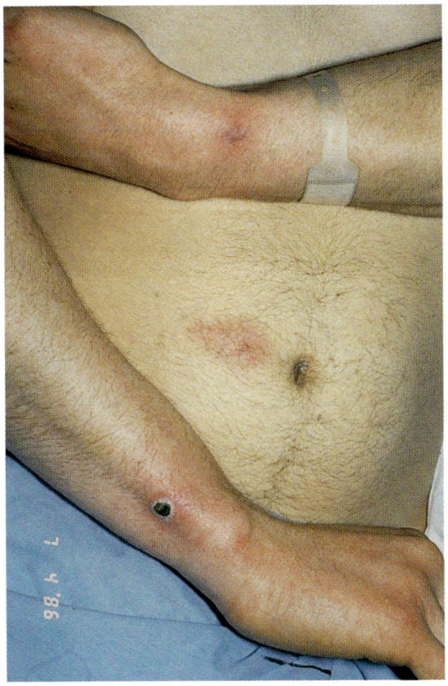

Plate 68 This patient has acute arthritis of one knee and these skin lesions indicate bacteraemia particularly with *Neisseria gonorrhoeae*.

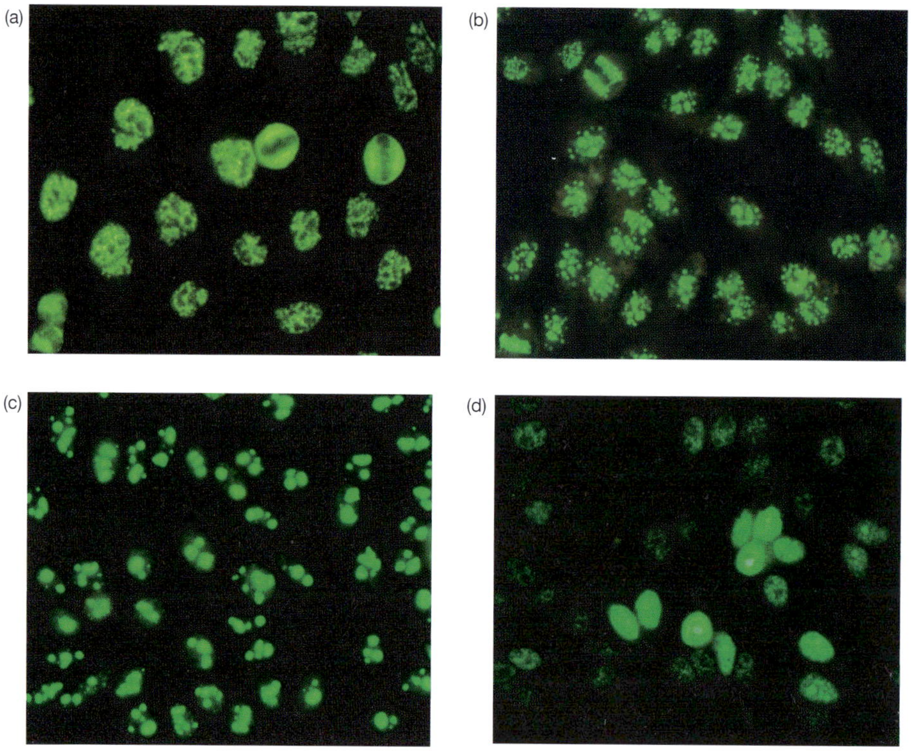

Plate 69 Patterns of immunofluorescence using Hep-2 cells: (a) speckled (pattern typical of anti-U1RNP); (b) centromere: characterized by discrete speckles in interphase nuclei which segregate on to the metaphase plate during cell division; (c) nucleolar; (d) a serum containing predominantly anti-Ro produces characteristic speckled fluorescence of the nucleus, nucleolus and, sometimes, the cytoplasm in the Hep-2 cells transfected with the 60kDa human Ro gene that hyperexpress Ro antigen.

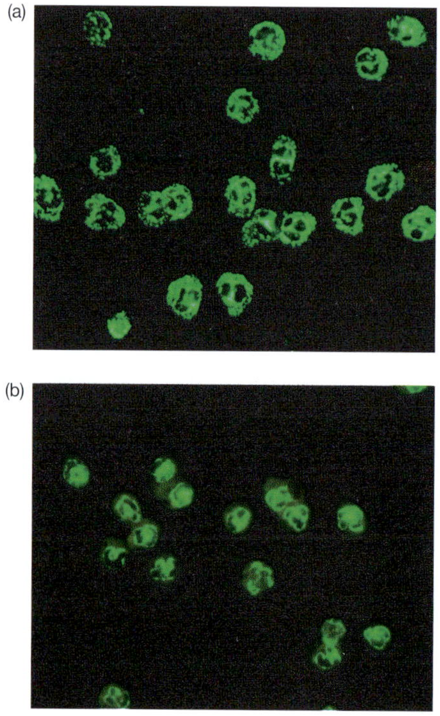

Plate 70 Detection of ANCA using normal human polymorphonuclear leucocytes fixed in ethanol. (a) cANCA corresponding to antibodies to proteinase 3 showing coarse granular staining of the cytoplasm with central accentuation. (b) pANCA corresponding to antibodies directed to a variety of constituents, often myeloperoxidase but sometimes elastase, lactoferrin, cathepsin G, and other lysosomal enzymes. This pattern is artefactual and is due to the release of highly charged components of the primary granules on fixation of the cells, which are attracted to DNA.

(a)

(b)

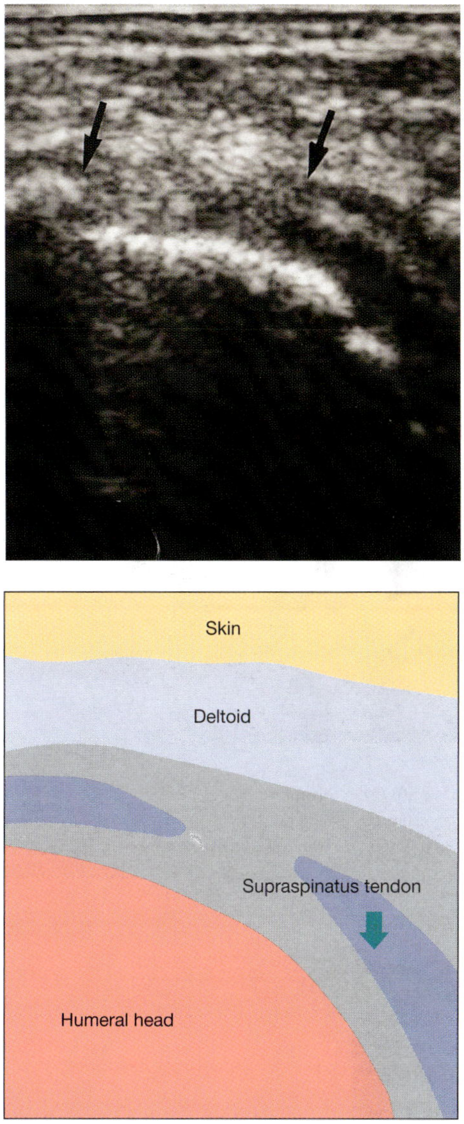

Plate 71 Rotator cuff tear in a 56-year-old woman who fell off her horse. The free ends of the supraspinatus tendon (arrows) are seen deep to the deltoid. (By courtesy of Dr S. Burnett, St Mary's Hospital.)

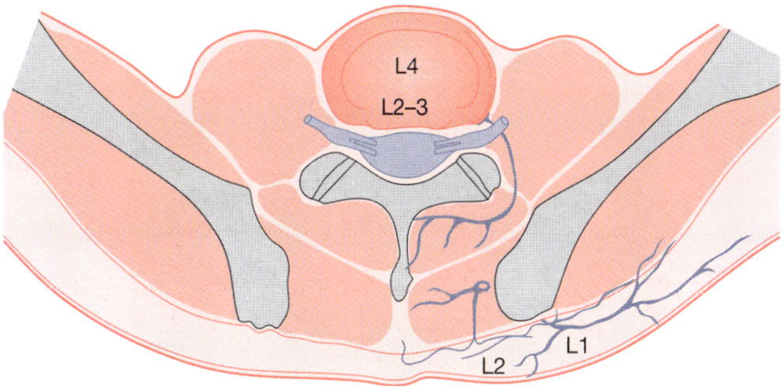

Plate 72 Transverse section of the spine and associated structures at L4 to illustrate the different innervations of structures at the same anatomical level. (Reproduced from *Textbook of Pain*, by courtesy of Mr J.P. O'Brien FRCS and Churchill Livingstone.)

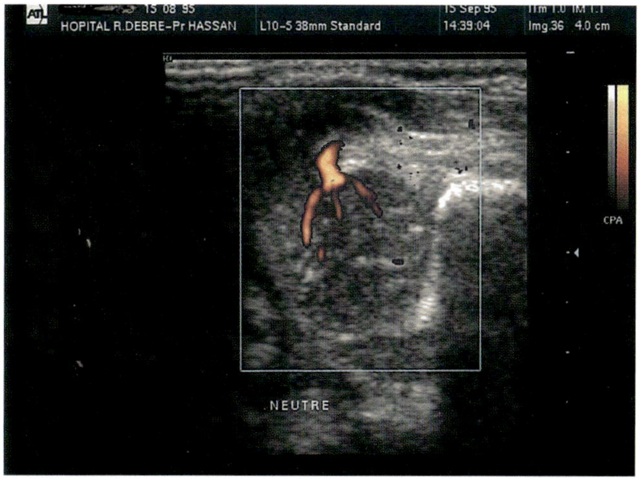

Plate 73 Femoral head vascularization in a newborn. Power Doppler visualizes the branches of the circumflex arteries.

(a)

(b)

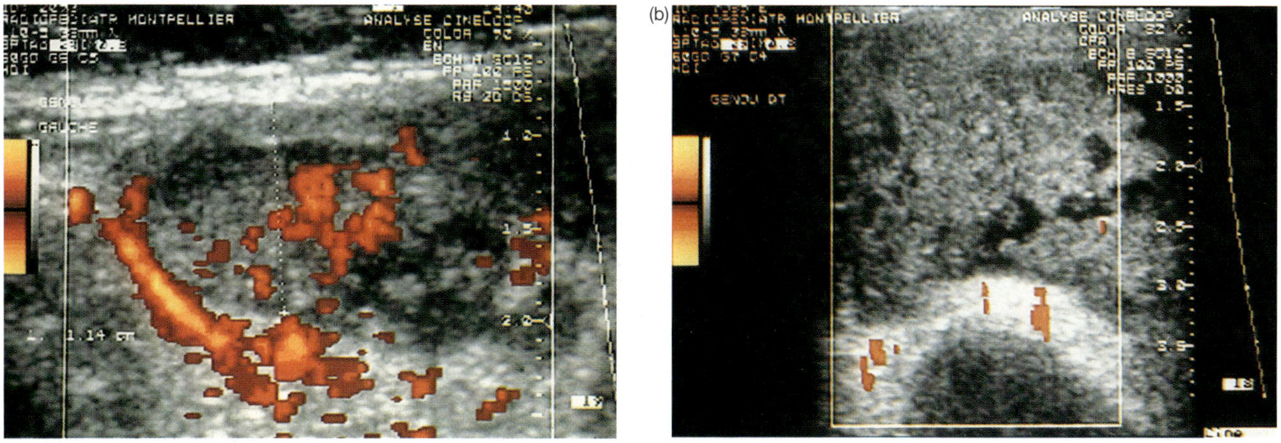

Plate 74 Juvenile chronic arthritis affecting the knee in a 5-year-old girl (by courtesy of Dr A. Couture, Montpellier, France). (a) Power Doppler shows hypervascularization of the active pannus. (b) After intra-articular injection of steroid, there is a decrease of power Doppler signal within the pannus.

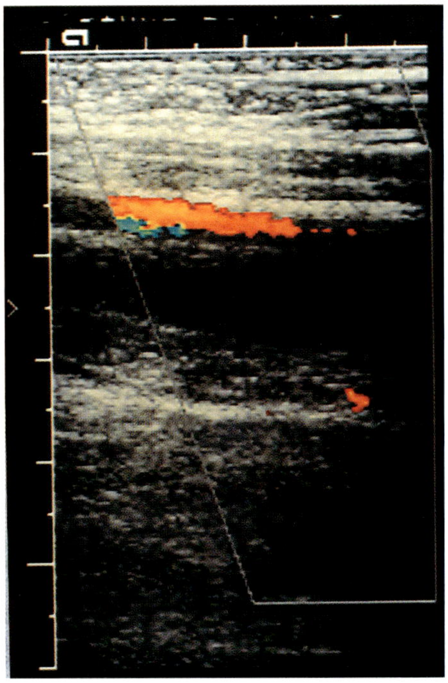

Plate 75 Thrombophlebitis in a 15-year-old girl with Behçet's disease. Colour Doppler shows a thrombosis of the superficial femoral vein.

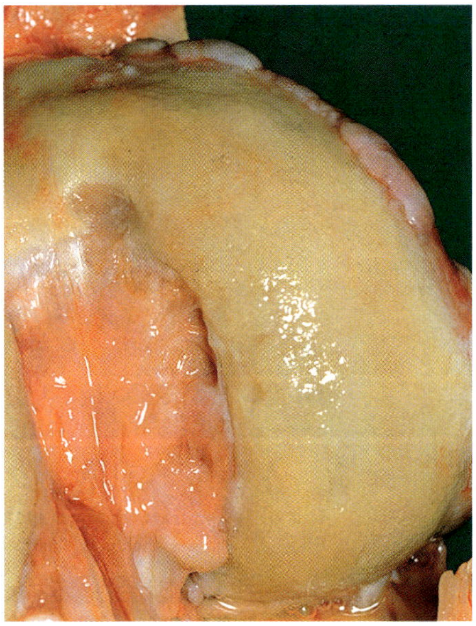

Plate 76 Early rheumatoid disease. There is synovial hyperplasia in the intertrochanteric area and a small erosion on the median aspect of the condyle.

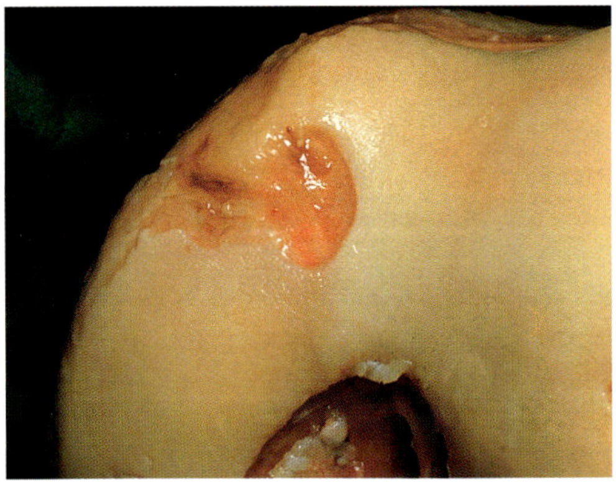

Plate 77 Rheumatoid disease. An erosive lesion with a base of pannus.

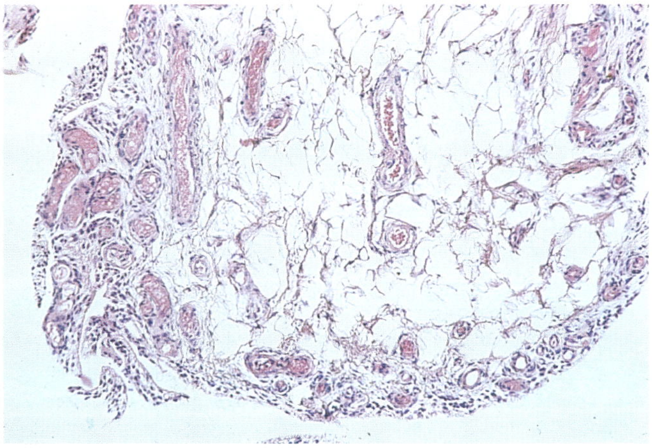

Plate 78 A normal synovial biopsy. The bulk of the biopsy is loose fibroadipose tissue. Blood vessels are prominent but the appearances are within normal limits.

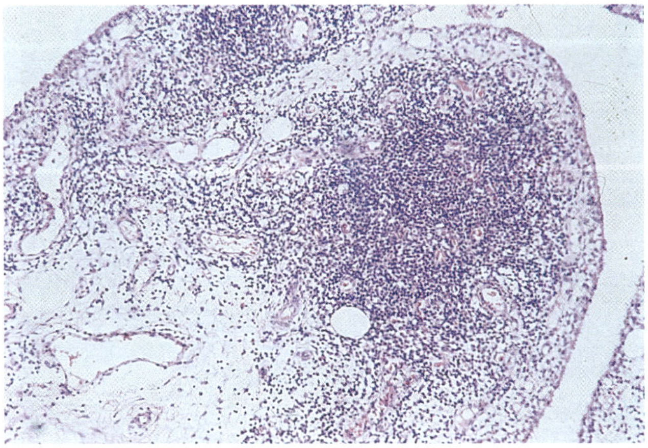

Plate 79 Chronic rheumatoid arthritis. The synovium shows villous hypertrophy and there is a prominent lymphoid aggregate.

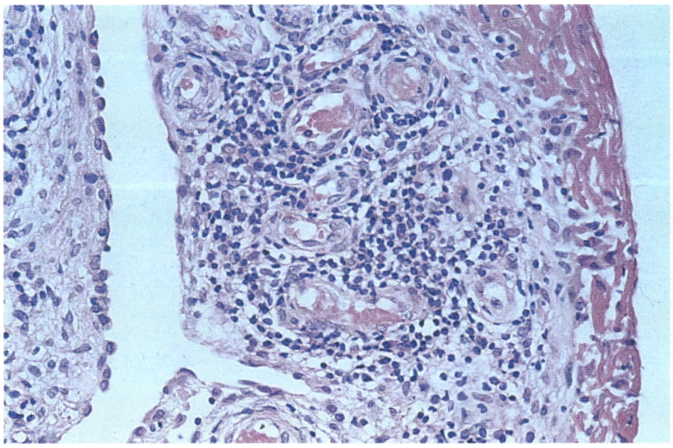

Plate 80 Chronic rheumatoid arthritis. There is diffuse lymphocytic infiltration, the synovial membrane is ulcerated, and there is a superficial layer of fibrin (right hand side).

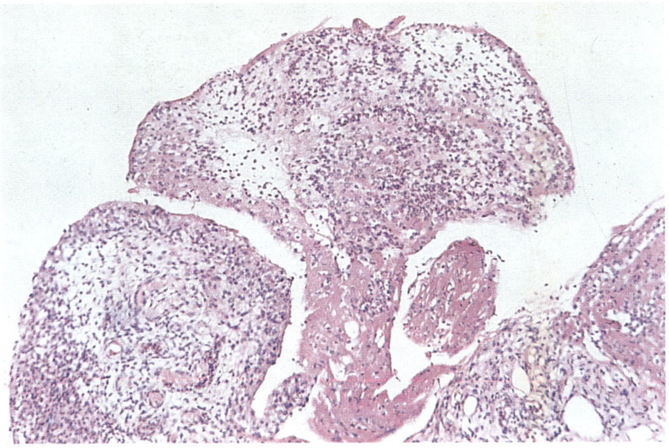

Plate 81 Early rheumatoid arthritis. There is a mass of fibrin in the centre and the underlying synovium is infiltrated with acute and chronic inflammatory cells.

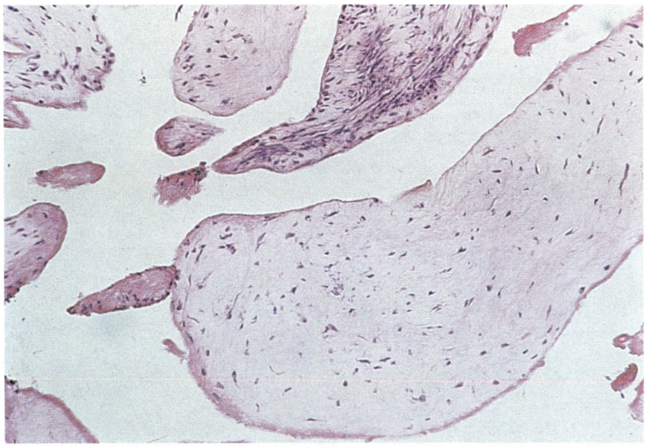

Plate 82 Villous synovial hyperplasia in long-standing rheumatoid arthritis. In this field there is no associated inflammation.

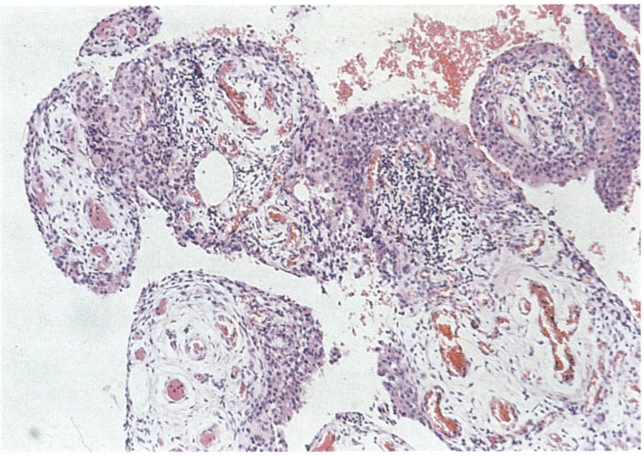

Plate 83 Villous synovial hyperplasia and moderate associated chronic inflammation in osteoarthritis. Inflammation of this degree is not uncommon.

(a)

(b)

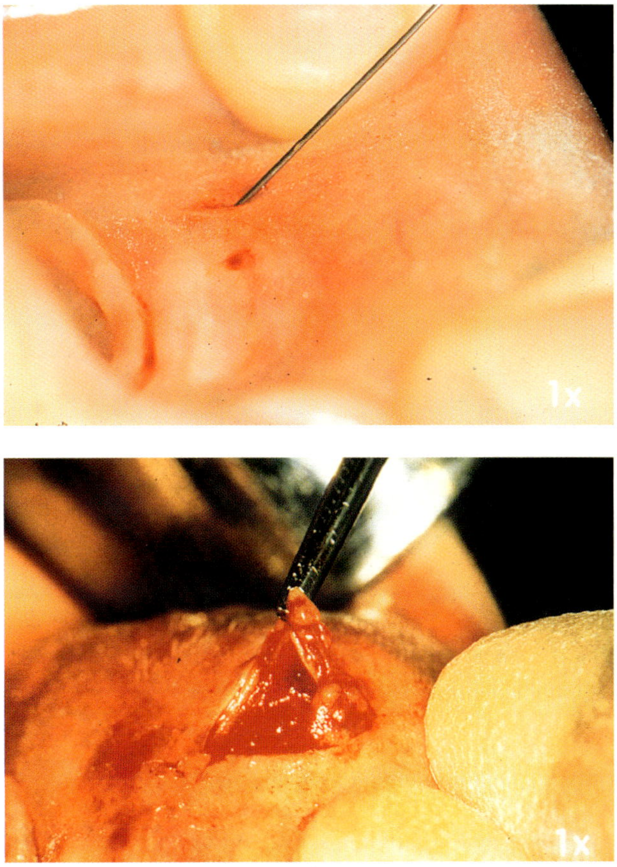

Plate 84 Biopsy of a minor salivary gland on the inner aspect of the lower lip.

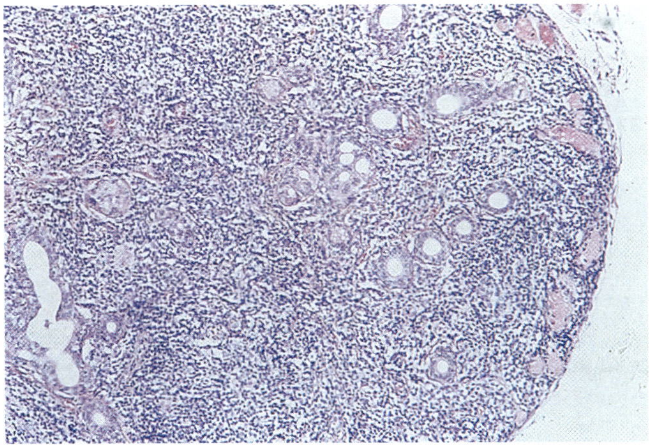

Plate 85 Labial salivary gland biopsy in a patient with sicca syndrome. The normal architecture of the gland has been effaced by a diffuse lymphocytic infiltrate.

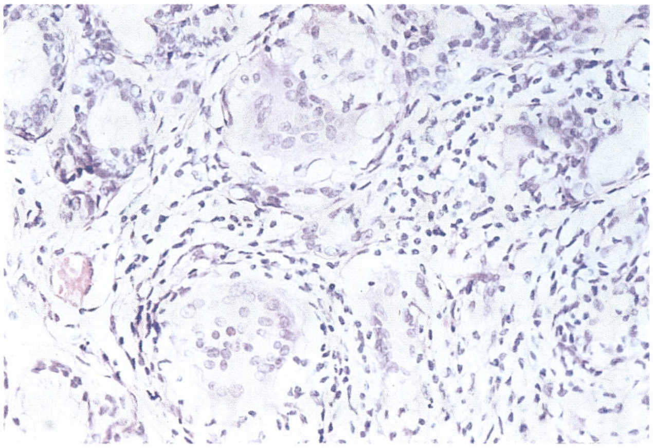

Plate 86 A non-caseating granuloma, with prominent giant cells, in the labial salivary gland of a patient with sarcoidosis.

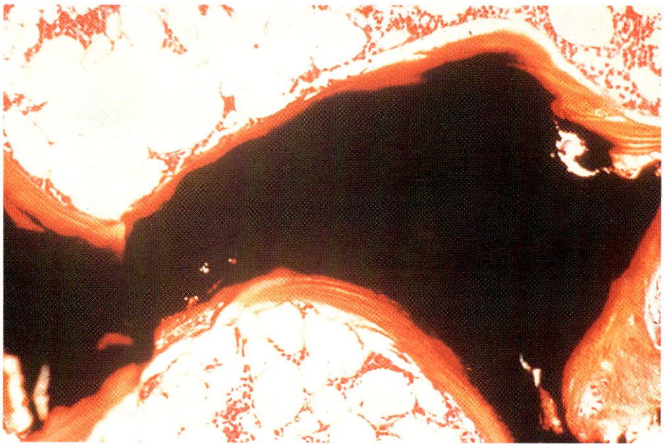

Plate 87 Bone biopsy from a patient with osteomalacia. The material was not decalcified and was stained by the von Kossa method. An abnormally thick rim of non-calcified osteoid (orange-yellow colour) surrounds the mineralized trabeculum (black).

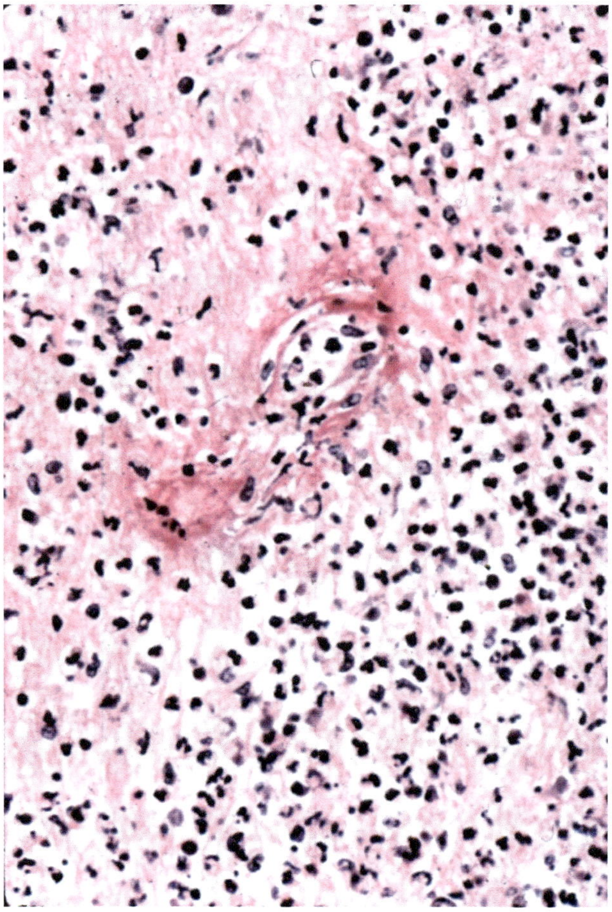

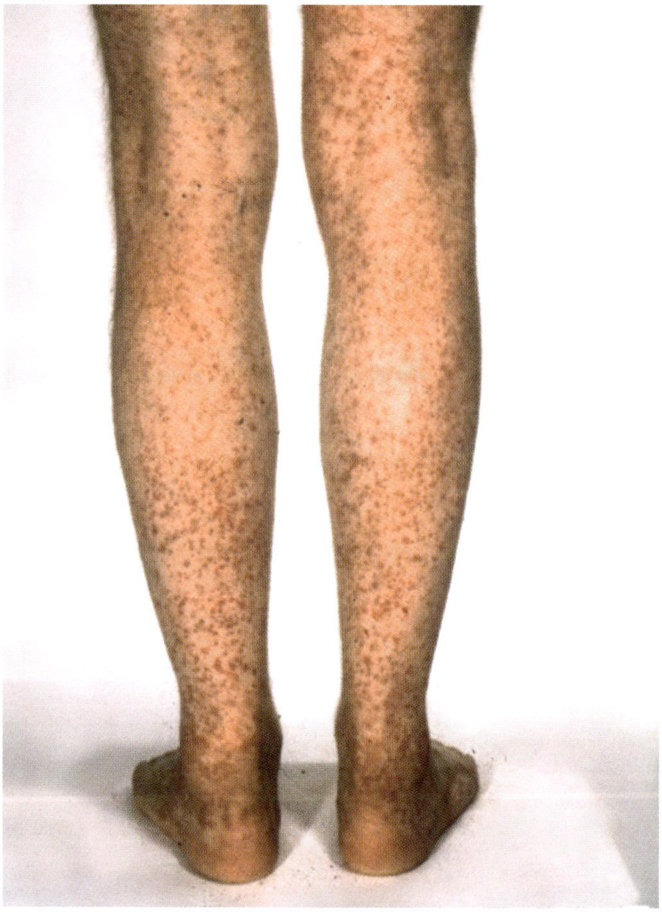

Plate 88 Leucocytoclastic vasculitis. The biopsy taken from this patient shows an acute and chronic inflammatory reaction centred around small capillaries. Some cases of persistent cutaneous vasculitis show only chronic inflammatory changes.

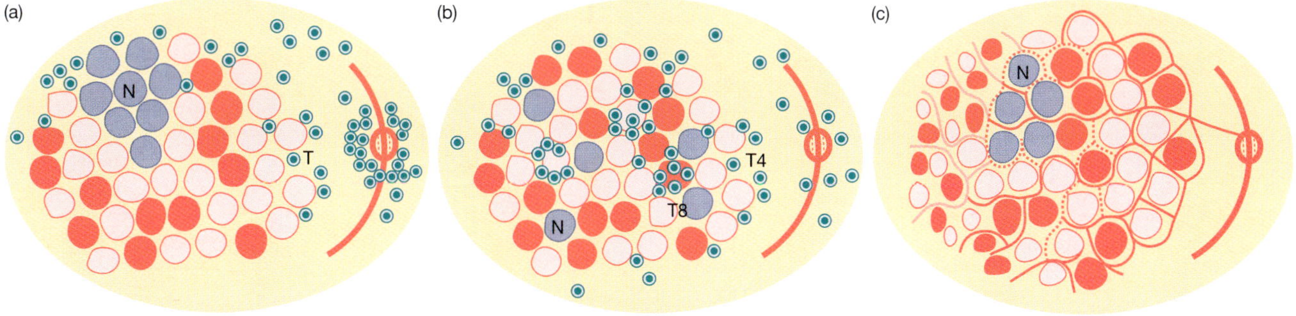

Plate 89 Immunological injury. (a) Pattern of lymphocytic (T and B cell) infiltration in dermatomyositis. Necrotic fibres (N) in small groups suggesting microinfarcts. (b) Pattern of lymphocytic infiltration in polymyositis. Invasion of non-necrotic fibres by cytotoxic T cells (T8) and spotty fibre necrosis (N). (c) Membrane attack complex (MAC) deposition of capillaries (dotted line) precedes capillary loss. Reduction of flow in capillary bed causes microinfarcts (N) and atrophy of fibres at periphery of vascular field.

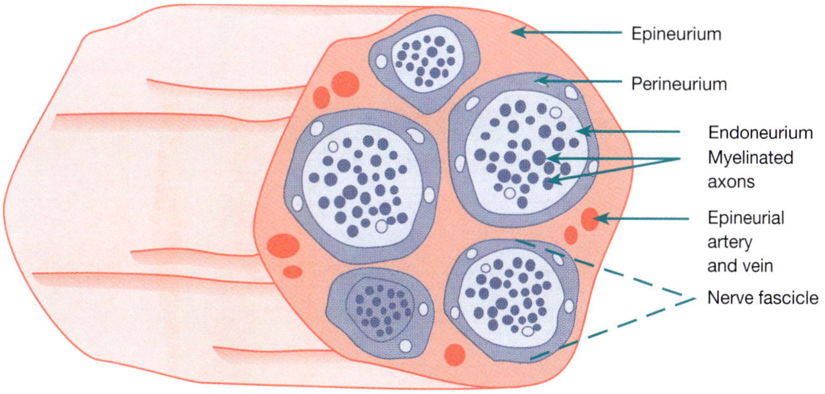

Plate 90 Diagram of transected nerve to show the arrangement of fascicles bounded by connective tissue sheaths. The sural nerve at the ankle contains five or six fascicles and thus partial transection may be adequate. Full thickness is preferable for detection of vasculitis because arteries, most often involved, lie within the epineurium.

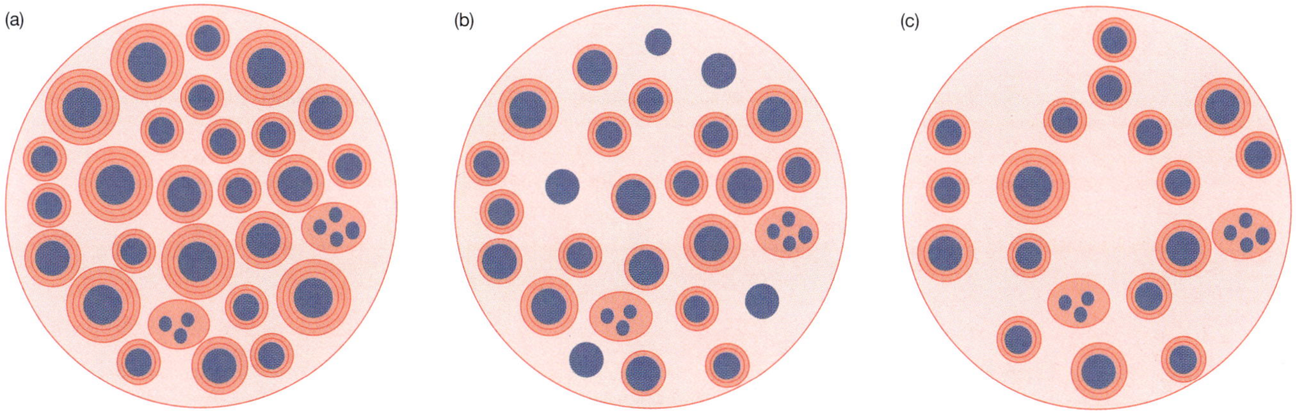

Plate 91 Transverse sections are required for measurement of nerve fibre density and fibre diameters. (a) The normal nerve has three major populations; (i) large myelinated fibres; (ii) small myelinated fibres; (iii) unmyelinated axons—the smallest fibres. (b) Demyelination and remyelination. No axonal loss. Large fibres with abnormally thin myelin sheaths indicate remyelination. (c) Axonal loss. Decreased fibre density, chiefly due to loss of large diameter fibres.

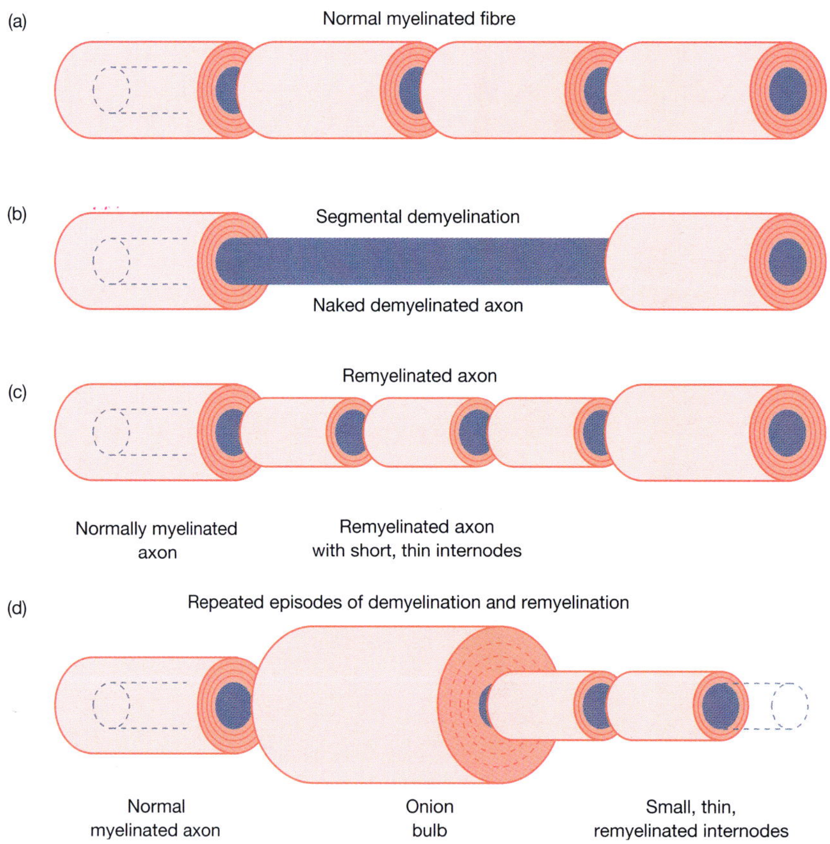

Plate 92 Teased fibre preparations permit examination of the thickness of several consecutive internodes and are particularly valuable for recognition of demyelination and remyelination: (a) normal myelinated fibre, (b) segmental demyelination, (c) remyelinated axon, (d) repeated episodes of demyelination and remyelination.

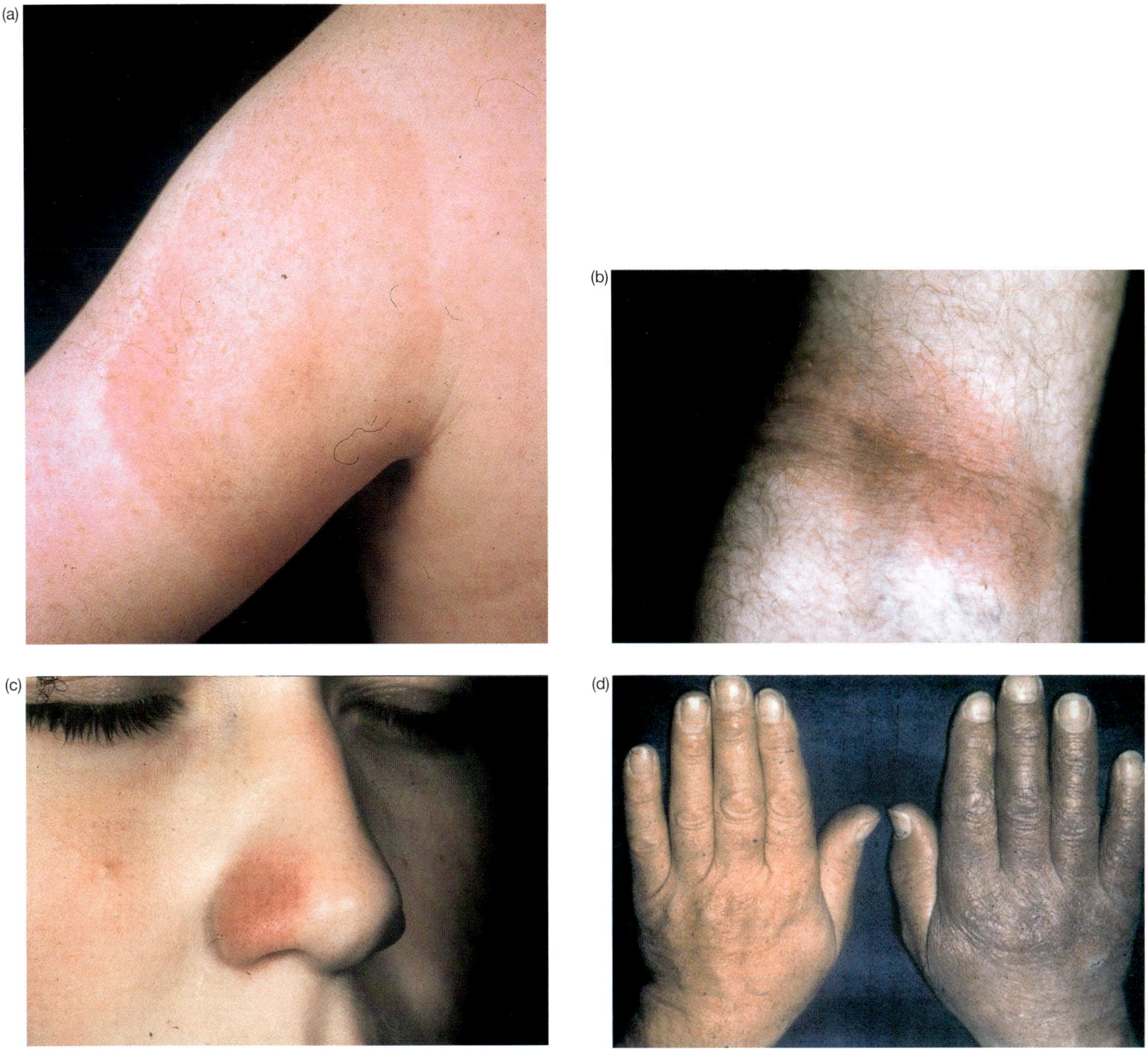

Plate 93 (a, b) Erythema migrans. The lesions starts as a red macule or papule at the site of the tick-bite and then slowly expands. Central clearance may or may not be present. (c) Borrelial lymphozytoma, typically presenting as a painless bluish-red nodule (by courtesy of Prof. W. Sterry, Department of Dermatology, Charité University Hospital, Berlin, Germany). (d) Acrodermatitis chronica atrophicans. Starting with a bluish-red discoloration, usually on the extensor surface of the extremities, the affected skin slowly becomes atrophic.

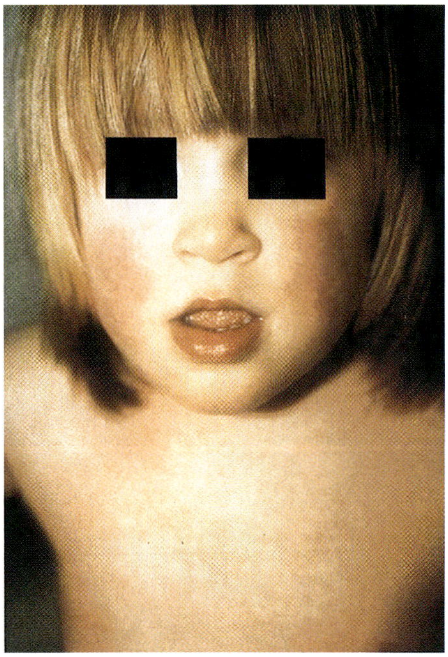

Plate 94 Classic 'slapped cheeks' of a child with erythema infectiosum, or fifth disease, caused by parvovirus B19. A lacy macular erythematous eruption is also present on the trunk but not in focus. (With permission from H.M. Feder, Jr. (1994). Fifth disease. *New England Journal of Medicine* **331**, 1062.)

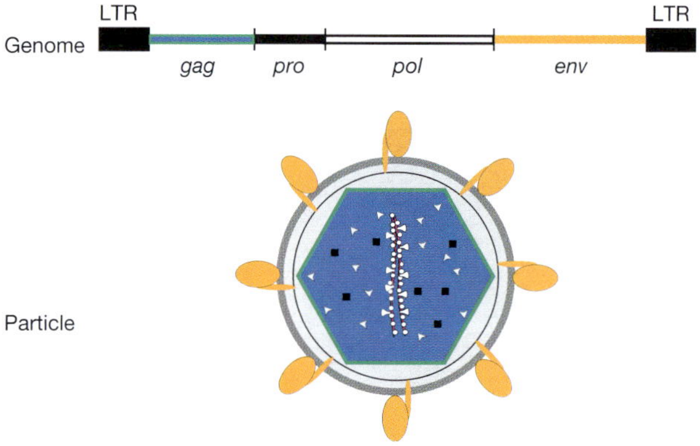

Plate 95 Genomic organization and structure of a typical retrovirus. The long terminal repeats (LTR) are shown at each end of the genome with the core proteins or group specific antigens (*gag*) in blue, protease (*pro*) in black, the enzymes encoded by the polymerase gene (*pol*) in white, and the envelope glycoproteins (*env*) in orange.

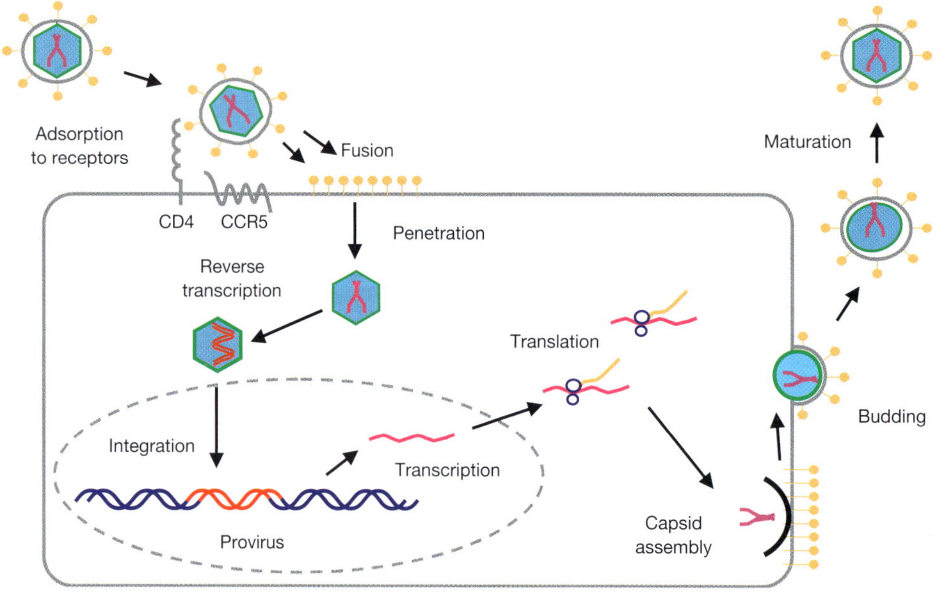

Plate 96 Life cycle and replication of HIV. Following binding of the virus to its receptors (in the case of HIV this is CD4 and CCR5) the core of the virus enters the cell where its RNA is reverse-transcribed to DNA which becomes incorporated in the genome as proviral DNA. Upon activation of the cell, proviral DNA is transcribed by the host cell machinery to produce viral genomic RNA and the capsid that surrounds it. The capsid then buds through the host cell membrane containing the envelope glycoproteins to form new virus particles.

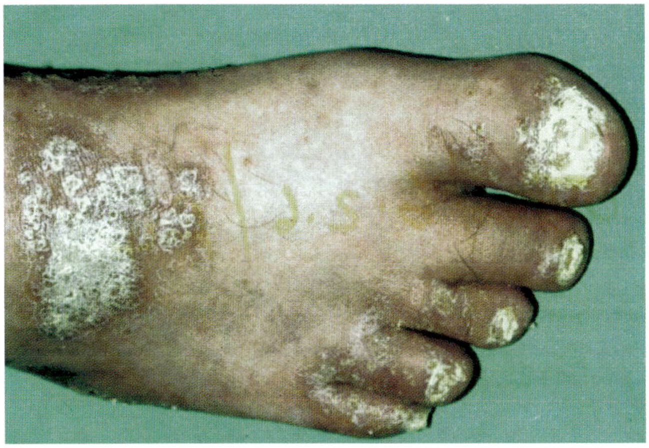

Plate 97 Severe nail dystrophies with associated psoriasis in an HIV positive patient with psoriatic arthritis (kindly donated by Dr Eleanor Mallon).

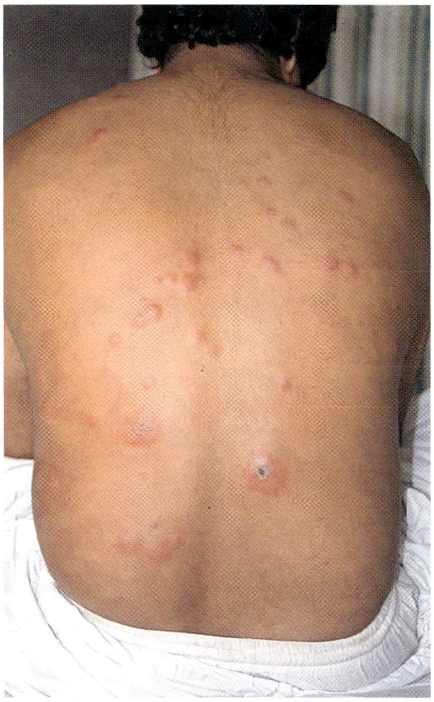

Plate 98 Erythema nodosum lesions in the lepra reaction.

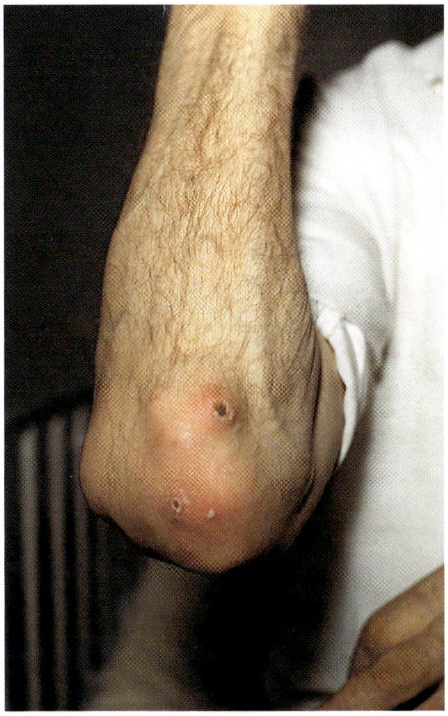

Plate 99 Subcutaneous nodule over elbow with ulceration in a patient who developed necrotizing vasculitis and gangrene of toes.

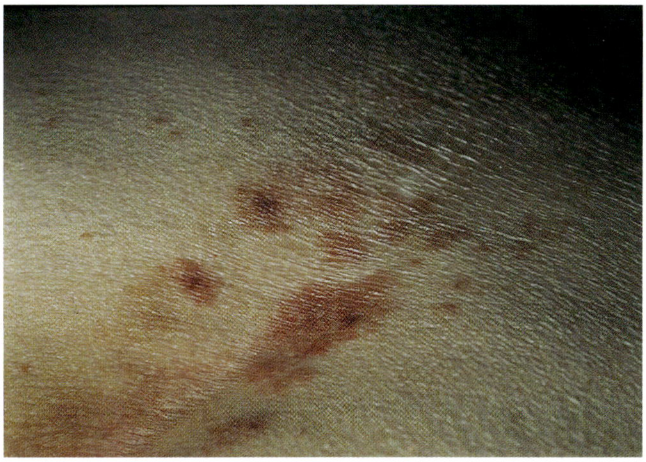

Plate 100 Palpable purpura in a case of rheumatoid arthritis, where healing occurred without immunosuppressive therapy.

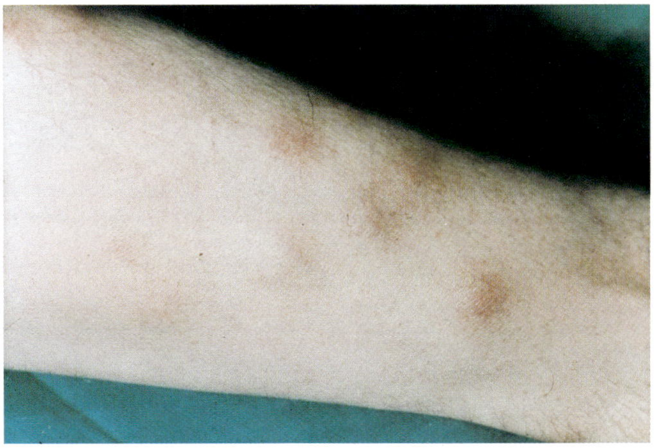

Plate 101 Erythema nodosum at the forearm.

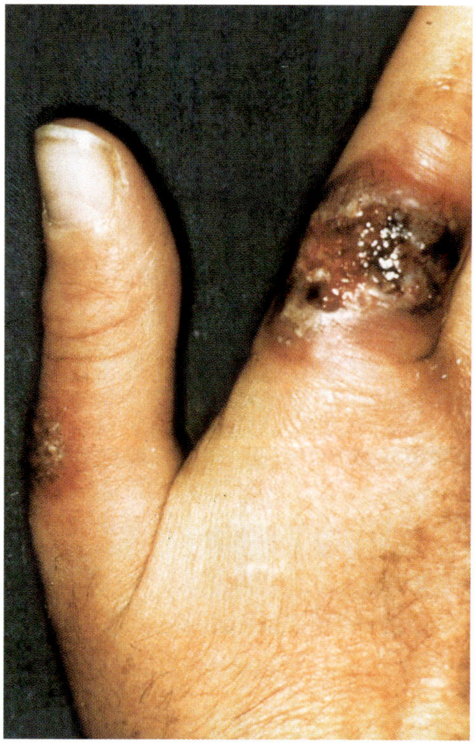

Plate 102 Pyoderma gangrenosum at a finger.

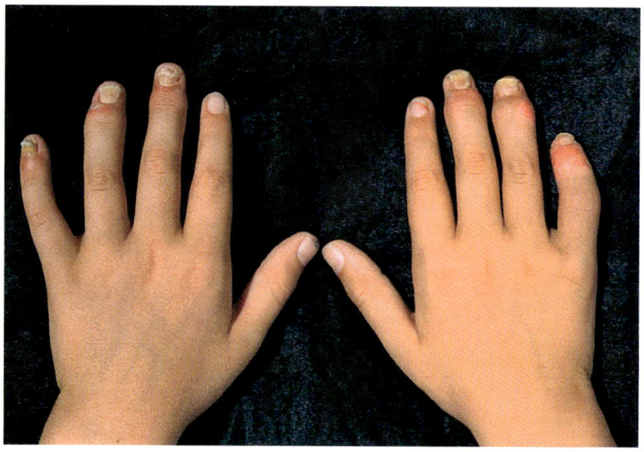

Plate 103 The hands of an 8-year-old boy with severe psoriatic nail changes. They show arthritis of distal interphalangeal joints, dactylitis of the right fifth digit, and diffuse metacarpophalangeal involvement.

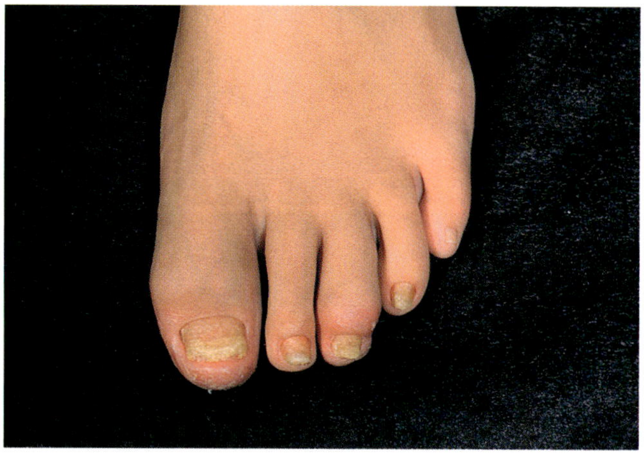

Plate 104 The foot of the boy whose hands are depicted in Plate 103, showing arthritis of the interphalangeal joint of the great toe and dactylitis of the third toe, as well as classical psoriatic nail changes.

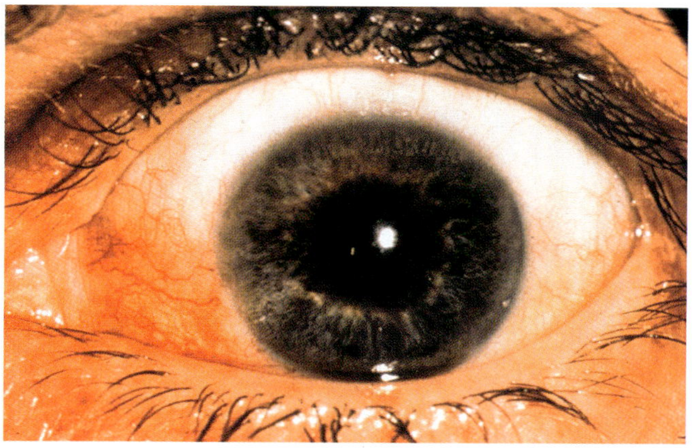

Plate 105 An example of severe recurrent iritis with both active change and evidence of old damage.

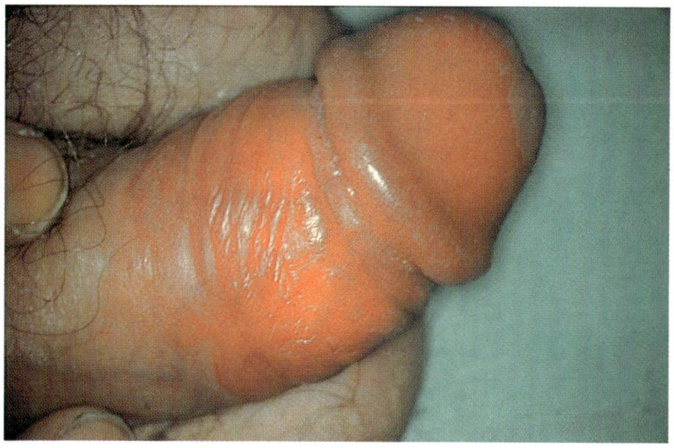

Plate 106 Balanitis.

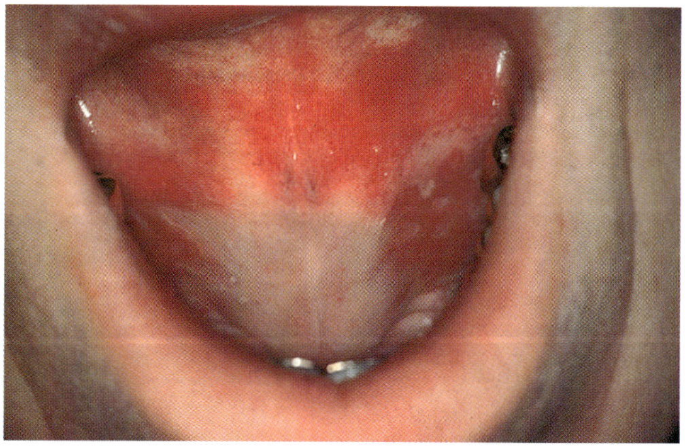

Plate 107 An erythematous, painless, palatal mucosal lesion.

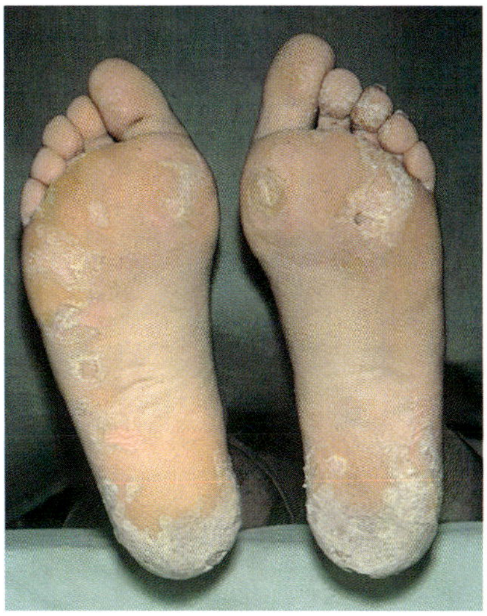

Plate 108 Keratoderma blennorrhagica.

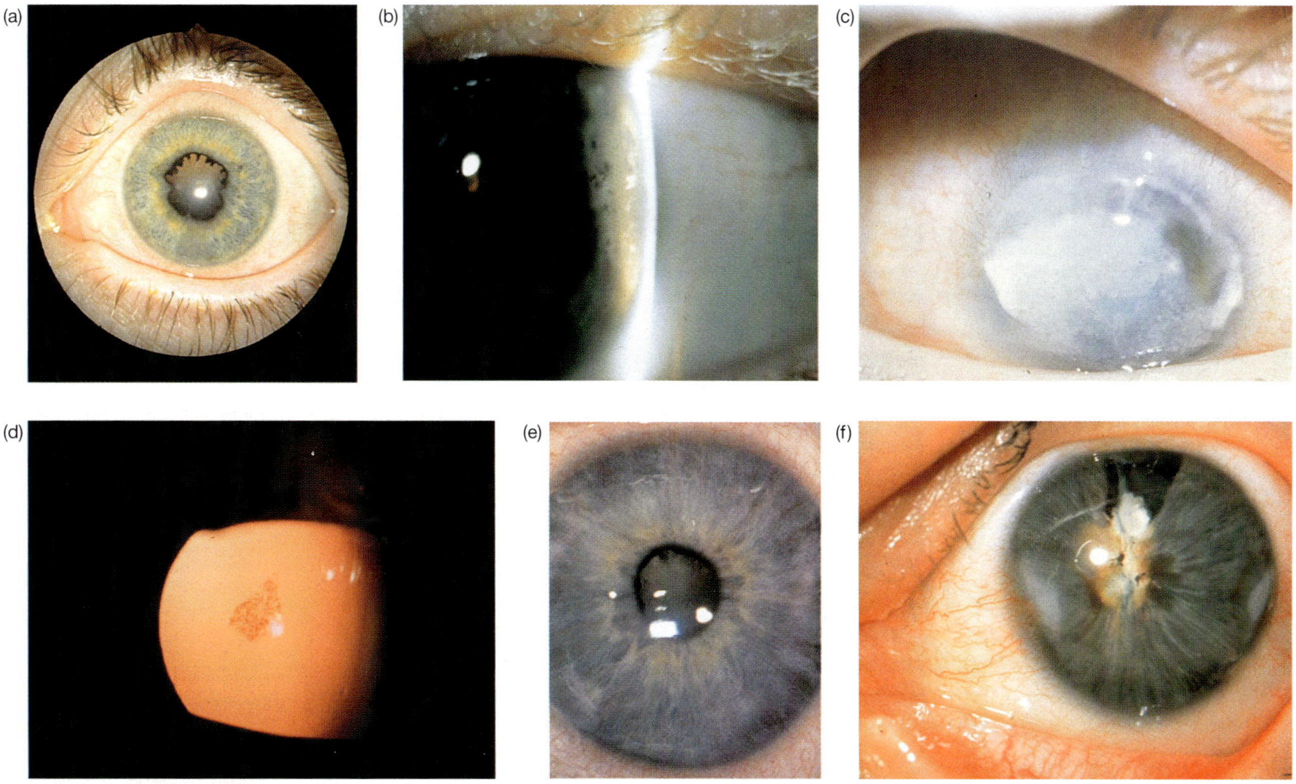

Plate 109 Ocular involvement in JIA. (a) Signs of uveitis visible on clinical examination. This eye has developed pupillary irregularities from synechiae, which adhere the iris to the lens capsule. The dilation of the pupil reveals numerous areas of adhesion. The clouding of the pupillary reflex is caused by keratitic precipitates, which are clumps of inflammatory cells on the posterior surface of the cornea. (b) The white lacy area represents paralimbal band keratopathy, caused by deposition of calcium in Bowman's layer. (c) Extremely severe, untreated band keratopathy. (d) Small posterior subcapsular cataract, seen by retroillumination. Cataract formation may result from either steroid therapy or disease. (e) Chronic iritis with more advanced, complicated cataract. Posterior synechiae are also visible and can induce secondary glaucoma. (f) Ocular findings after surgical intervention for complicated cataract. The pupil has been secondarily scarred down, after removal of cataract membrane. Ocular inflammation predisposes to this degree of scarring, which severely compromises vision. Current surgical techniques attempt to avoid these complications. Note the horseshoe iridectomy, performed for glaucoma, as well as the paralimbal band keratopathy at 3 and 9 o'clock.

(a)
(b)
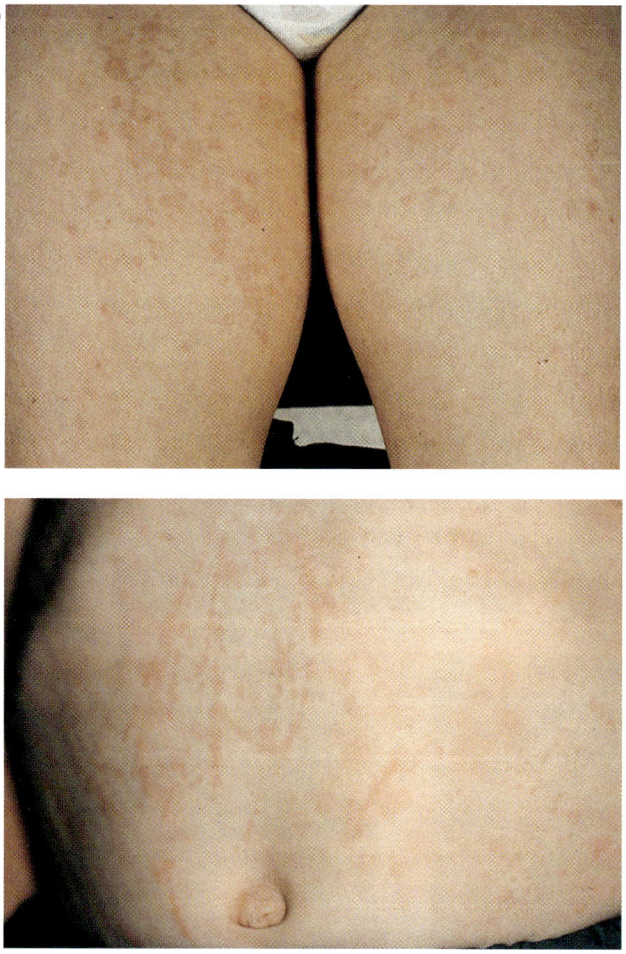

Plate 110 (a) Rash of systemic arthritis showing characteristic salmon-pink macular eruptions with central clearing. (b) Koebner phenomenon (appearance of exaggeration of rash in areas of minor trauma).

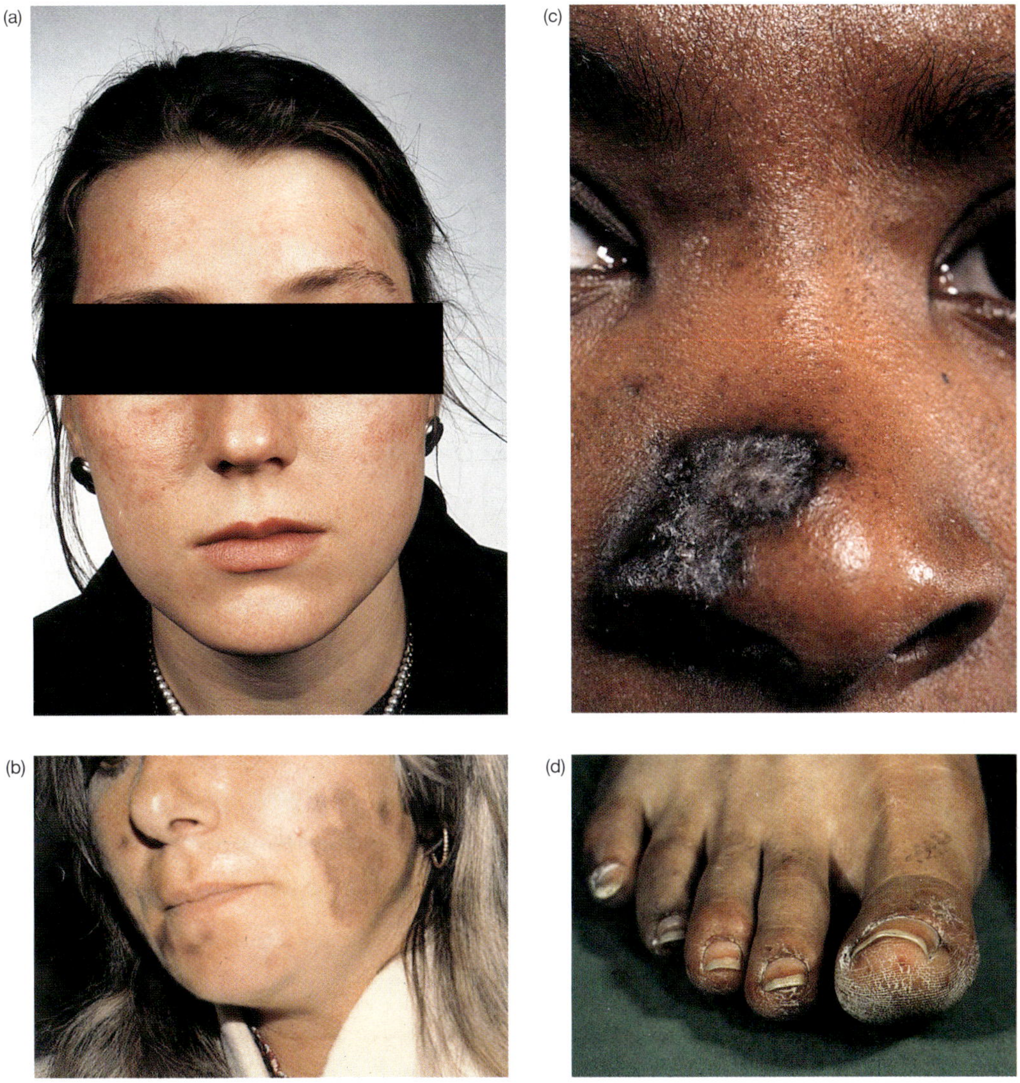

Plate 111 (a) Butterfly rash; (b) a discoid lupus rash; (c) nasal ulceration; (d) vasculitis affecting the toes, with associated hyperkeratosis.

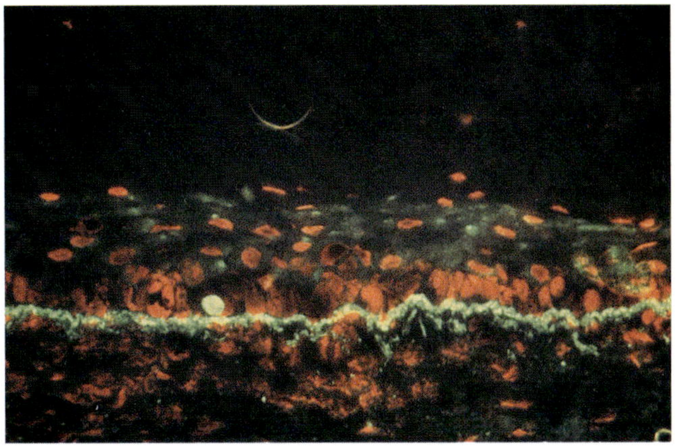

Plate 112 Lupus band tests—the linear green staining is due to the deposition of IgM identified by a fluoresceinated antihuman antibody; the red counterstain is propidium iodide.

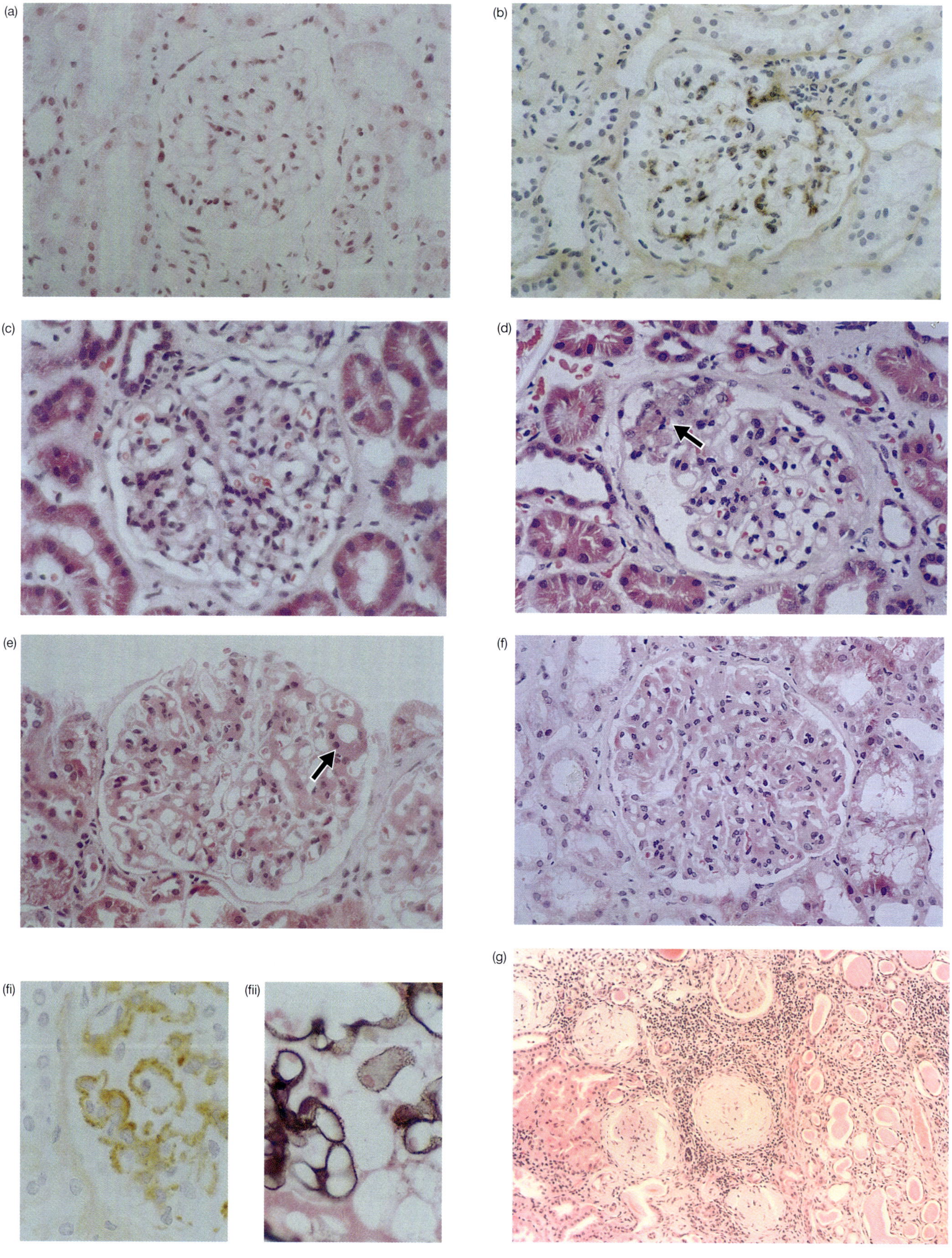

Plate 113 Continued.

(h)

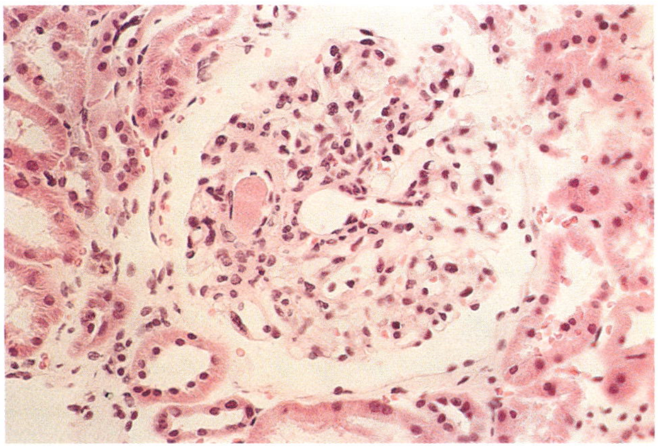

Plate 113 Renal lupus (by courtesy of Dr M.H. Griffiths). (a) Systemic lupus erythematosus, no renal lesions, WHO class I. In addition to the mesangial immune deposit there is a mesangial cell proliferation and the glomerulus appears hypercellular (haematoxylin and eosin). (b) Mesangial lupus nephritis, WHO class IIA. Immune complexes are demonstrable in the mesangium, seen here as granular brown deposits (immunoperoxidase technique for IgG). (c) Mesangial lupus nephritis, WHO class IIB. In addition to mesangial immune deposit there is mesangial cell proliferation and the glomerulus appears hypercellular (haematoxylin and eosin). (d) Focal proliferative lupus nephritis, WHO class III. Segmental proliferation (arrow) is seen in this glomerulus (haematoxylin and eosin). (e) Diffuse proliferative lupus nephritis, WHO class IV. The glomerular capillary walls are irregularly thickened forming, in places, classical 'wire loops' (arrow). There is variable cellular proliferation (haematoxylin and eosin). (f) Membranous lupus nephritis, WHO class V. There is diffuse capillary-wall thickening produced by abundant immune deposits in and on the basement membrane, seen in (i) as granular brown staining (immunoperoxidase technique for IgG). The basement membrane extends out between and around the deposits to produce a series of spikes and circles shown with silver staining in (ii) (hexamine silver technique). (g) Endstage renal disease showing completely sclerosed, non-functional glomeruli. (h) Hyaline thrombus in the glomerulus of a patient with systemic lupus and a high titre of antiphospholipid antibodies.

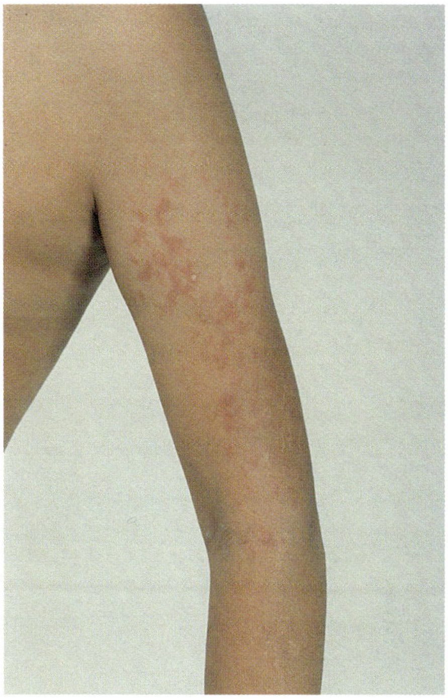

Plate 114 A patient with known systematic lupus erythematosus developed a severe, vasculitic rash on arms and legs following sun exposure.

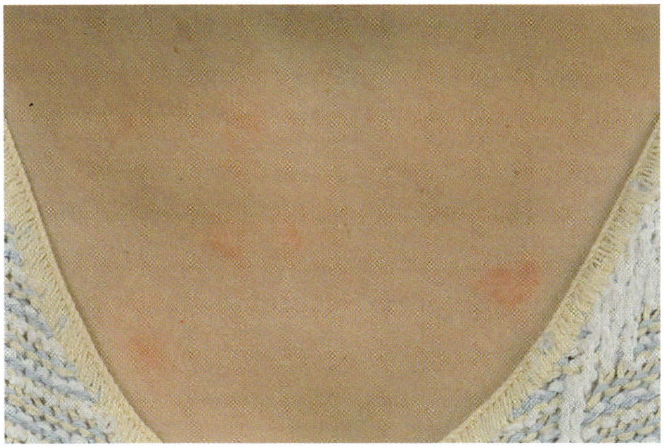

Plate 115 Annular erythema on the neck of a systematic lupus erythematosus patient with anti-Ro and anti-La antibodies.

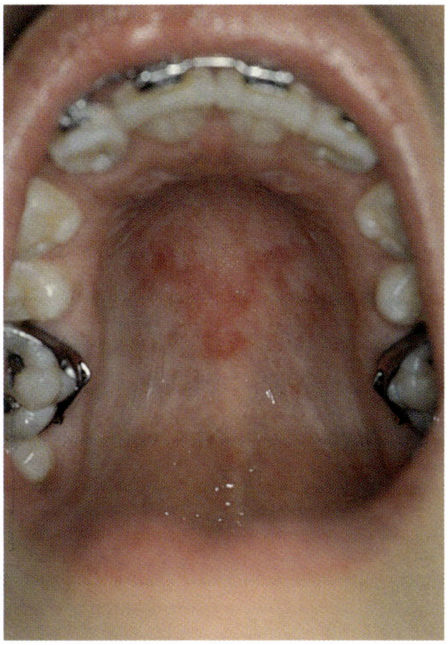

Plate 116 Hyperaemia and petechiae on hard palate secondary to vasculitis.

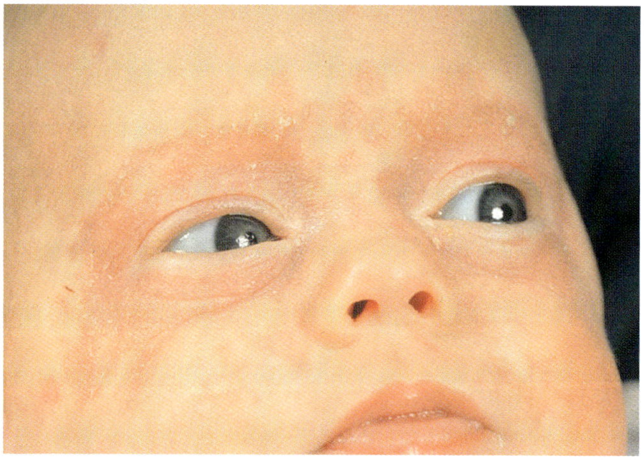

Plate 117 The face of a 3-month-old baby delivered to a healthy mother with anti-Ro and anti-La antibodies. Note the scaly erythematosus areas around the eyes. This rash healed without scarring following the use of topical steroid cream.

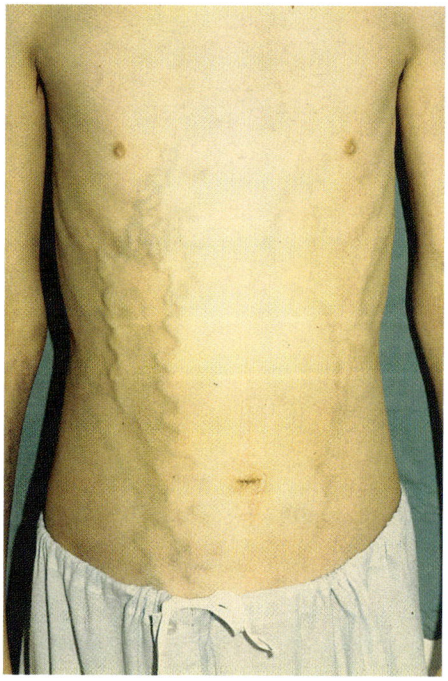

Plate 118 Budd–Chiari syndrome in a 20-year-old patient with primary antiphospholipid syndrome (by courtesy of Dr L. Pallares, Servicio de Medicina Internal, Hospital Son Dureta, Palma de Mallorca, Spain).

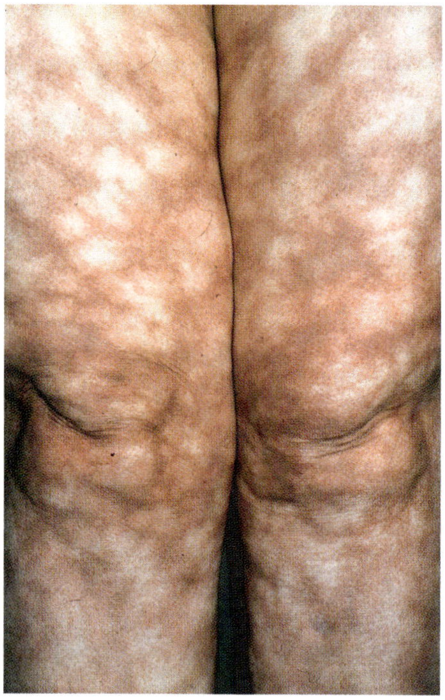

Plate 119 Extensive livedo reticularis in a patient with primary antiphospholipid syndrome.

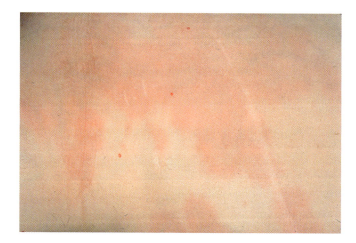

Plate 120 Localized morphoea showing discrete lesions with central depigmentation and circumferential inflammation.

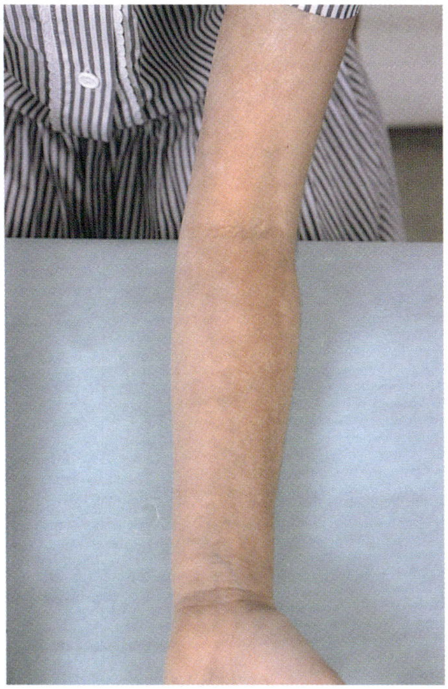

Plate 121 Linear scleroderma occurring in childhood. Defective growth of the involved limb is a major clinical problem in childhood-onset disease.

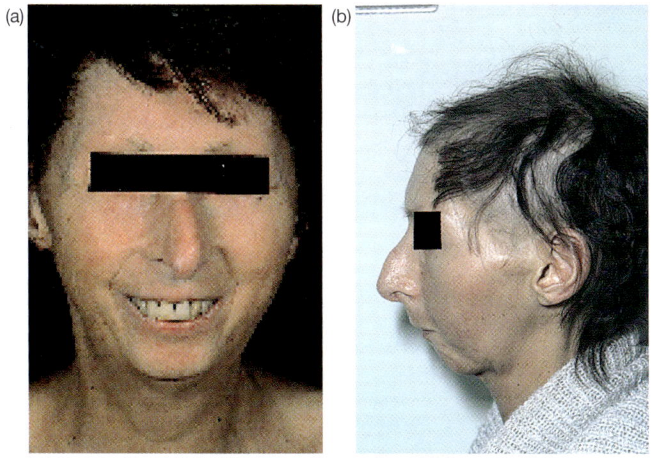

Plate 122 (a, b) Typical facial appearance of diffuse cutaneous systemic sclerosis, with tight shiny skin, contrasting with the widespread facial telangiectasis often present in advanced, limited cutaneous systemic sclerosis.

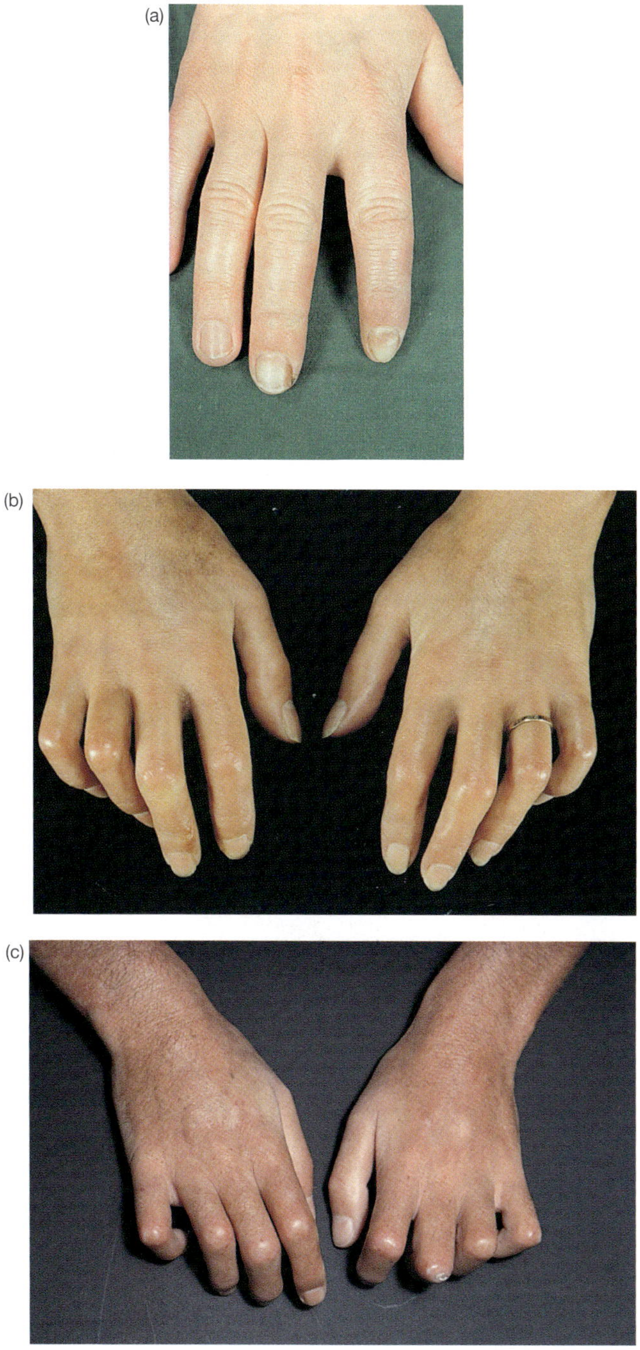

Plate 123 The three phases of skin involvement in the hands of a patient with systemic sclerosis: (a) initial puffiness of the skin; (b) tight shiny skin with induration, loss of finger pulp, and contractures; (c) late changes of contractures with atrophic skin and ulceration.

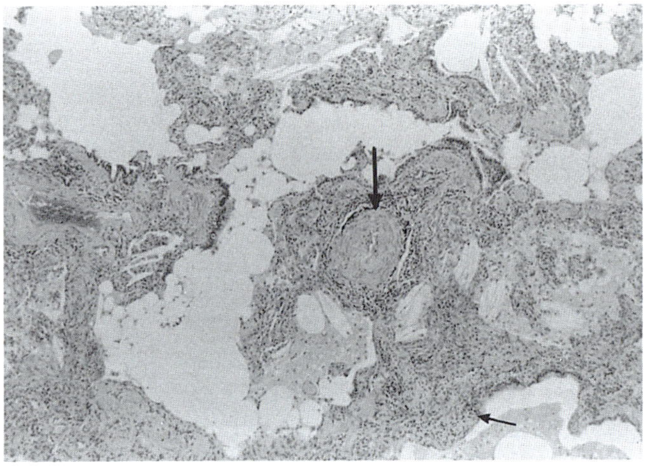

Plate 124 Open lung biopsy of patient with systemic sclerosis showing interstitial chronic inflammation and fibrosis (small arrow) and thick-walled arteriole showing intimal fibrosis (large arrow). Haematoxylin and eosin, × 300. (Courtesy of Dr Mary N. Sheppard, Department of Lung Pathology, Royal Brompton Hospital, London.)

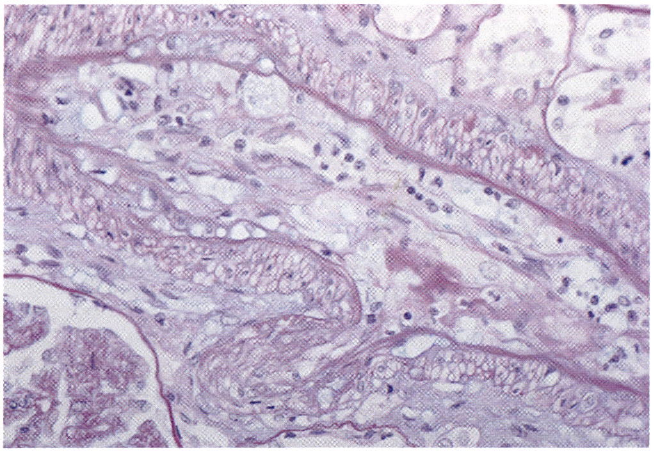

Plate 125 An artery in the corticomedullary region. This section has been stained by the Alcian-blue/diastase-periodic acid–Schiff method. The lumen of the blood vessel has been entirely effaced by proliferation and swelling of the intima. Intimal cells can be seen to have developed an unusual bubbly, blue (mucoid) cytoplasm that is characteristic of scleroderma-related acute renal arteriopathy. There is a scattered small-lymphocytic infiltrate as well. (By courtesy of Dr A.P. Dhillon, Department of Histopathology, Royal Free Hospital Medical School, London.)

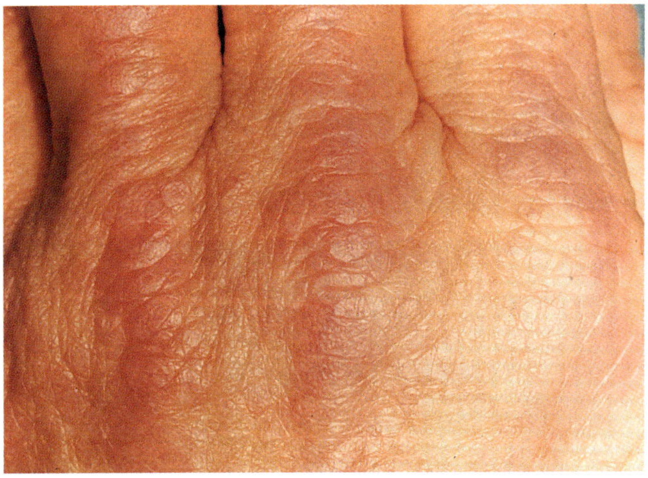

Plate 126 Skin over the metacarpophalangeal (MCP) joints of a patient with dermatomyositis showing characteristic erythematous lesions of Gottron's sign. (Courtesy of Department of Dermatology, University of Oklahoma Health Sciences Center.)

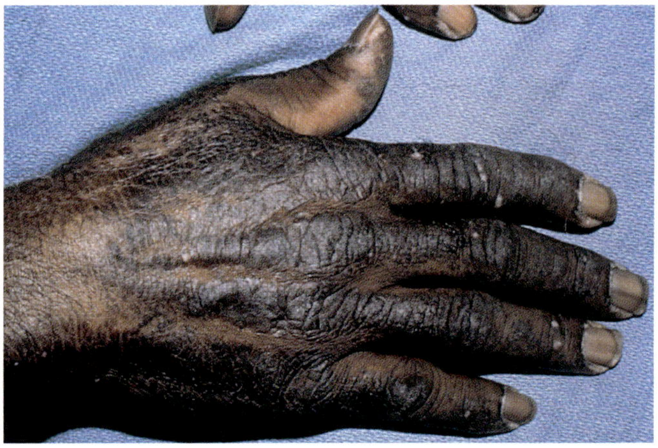

Plate 127 Hand of a patient with dermatomyositis. Gottron's papules over the PIP and MCP joints, with marked linear extensor erythema extending from the joints along the tendons. In Black patients, the lesions may appear hyperpigmented. (Courtesy of Dr Frank C. Arnett, University of Texas at Houston HSC.)

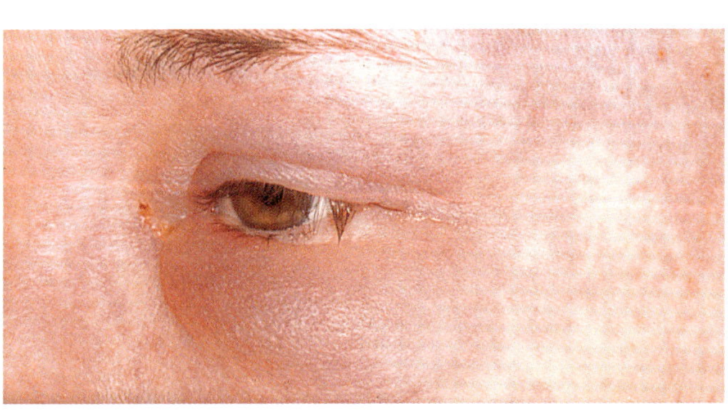

Plate 128 A severe heliotrope rash of dermatomyositis, with the characteristic lilac color and accompanying periorbitaloedema. (Courtesy of Department of Dermatology, University of Oklahoma Health Sciences Center.)

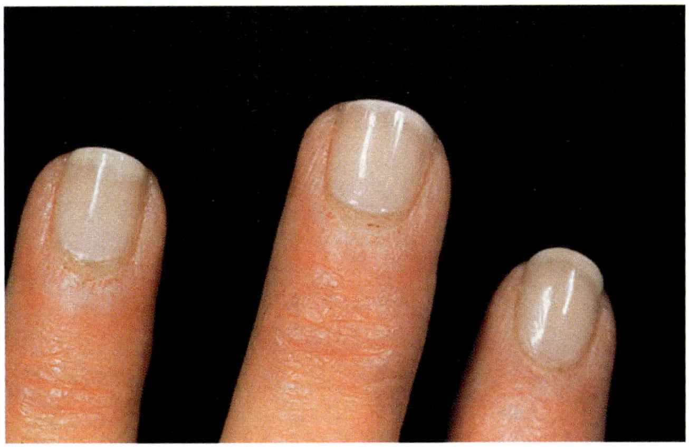

Plate 129 Nailfold vascular changes in a patient with amyopathic dermatomyositis for 4 years. Dilatation, dropout, and haemorrhage are evident without microscopy. Gottron's papules are present over the proximal interphalangeal joints of the index and middle fingers, and the suggestive lesions over the distal interphalangeal joints. (Courtesy of Dr Lela Lee, Department of Dermatology, University of Oklahoma Health Sciences Center.)

(a) (b)

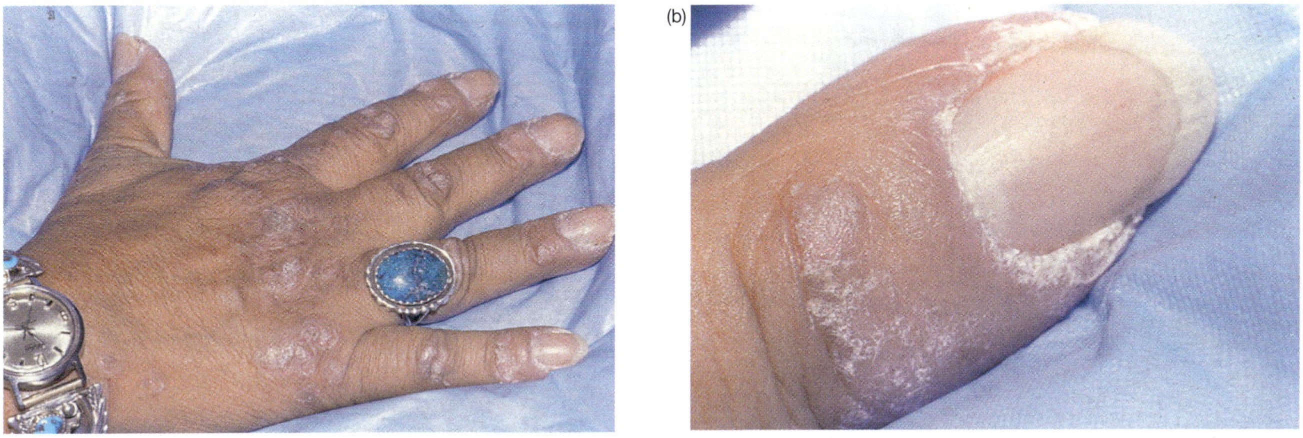

Plate 130 (a) Hand of a patient with anti-Mi-2 positive dermatomyositis with severe weakness of 2 months duration. Typical Gottron's papules are seen over the MCPs, PIPs, and DIPs, with more scale than in Plate 131. There is cuticular hyperkeratosis around many nails, and mechanic's hand change on the thumb. (Courtesy of Dr E. Taylor-Albert, University of Oklahoma Health Sciences Center.) (b) Thumb of the patient in (a). Cuticular changes are evident. A Gottron's papule is over the IP joint.

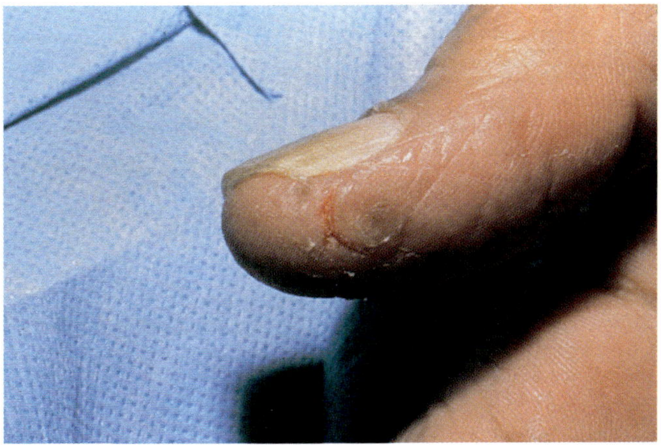

Plate 131 Thumb of a patient with anti-Jo-1 positive polymyositis. The edge of the thumb shows fissuring and some hyperkeratosis as in mechanic's hands. (Courtesy of Dr Frank C. Arnett, University of Texas at Houston Health Sciences Center.)

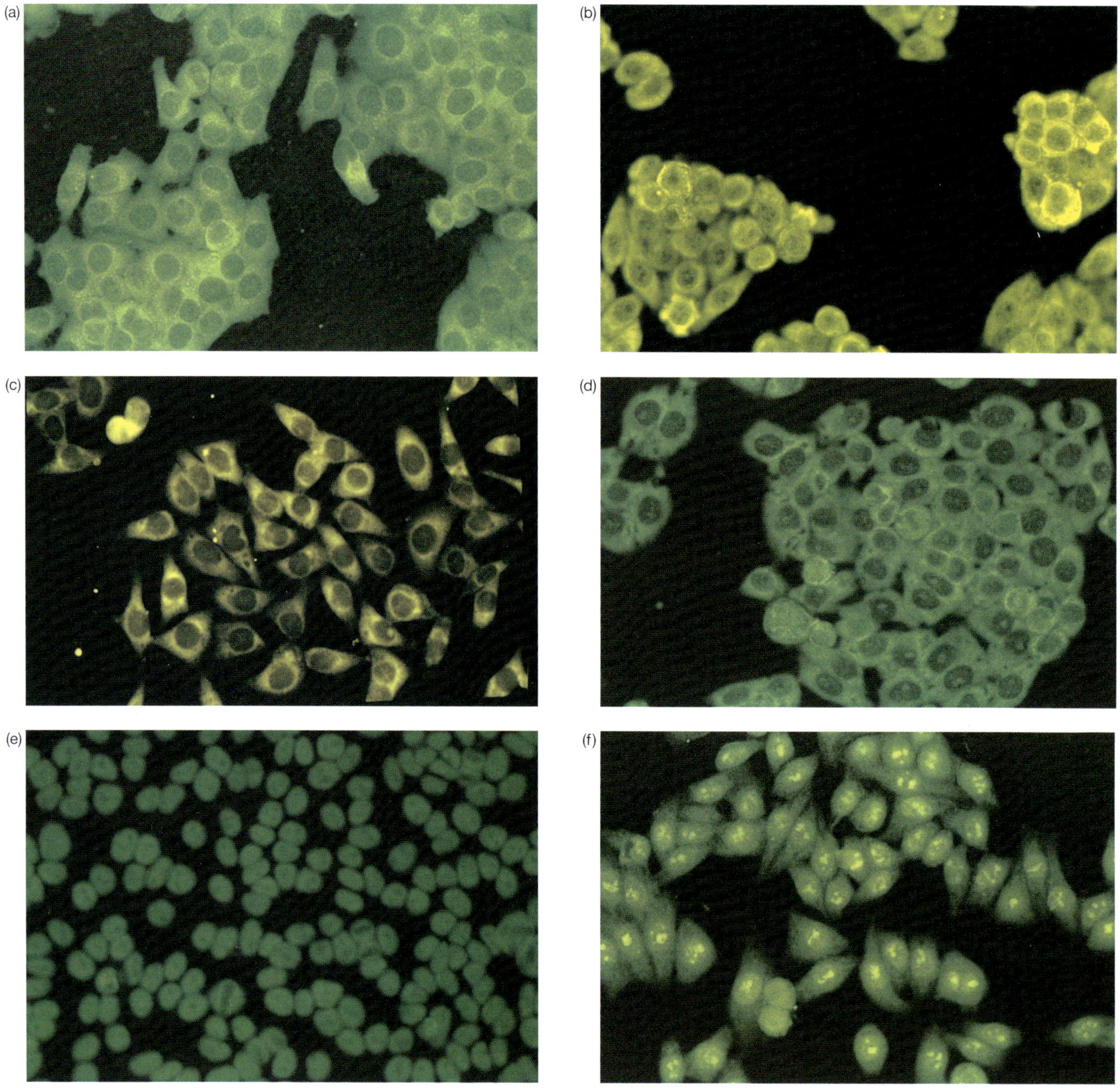

Plate 132 Indirect immunofluorescence on HEp-2 cells using sera with myositis-associated autoantibodies. (a) Anti-Jo-1 autoantibodies (reacting with histidyl-tRNA synthetase): finely speckled cytoplasmic pattern of fluorescence. (b) Anti-PL-7 autoantibodies (antithreonyl-tRNA synthetase): cytoplasmic pattern (more homogeneous at higher concentration). (c) Anti-SRP autoantibodies (antisignal recognition particle): cytoplasmic pattern. (d) Anti-KJ autoantibodies (reacting with a translation factor): cytoplasmic pattern with slight nucleolar staining. (e) Anti-Mi-2 autoantibodies (reacting with an unidentified nuclear protein): nuclear pattern, sparing nucleoli, without cytoplasmic staining. (f) Anti-PM-Scl autoantibodies (reacting with a complex of 11 proteins): intense nucleolar staining with significant nuclear staining.

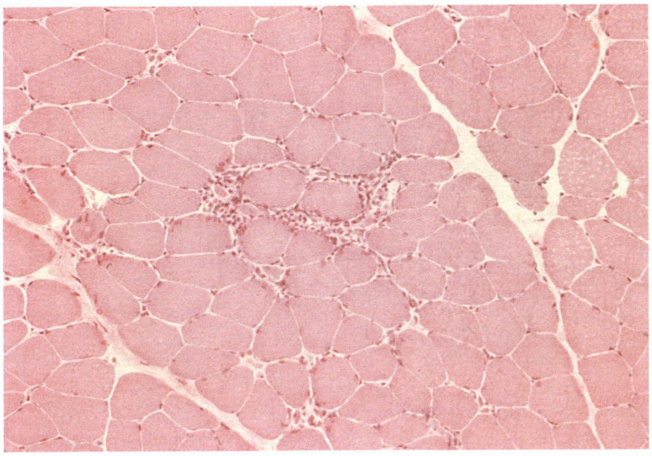

Plate 133 Muscle biopsy (haematoxylin and eosin stain) from a patient with polymyositis. Endomysial inflammation (infiltration with mononuclear cells between fibers within the fascicle) is seen, a pattern characteristic of biopsies from patients with polymyositis.

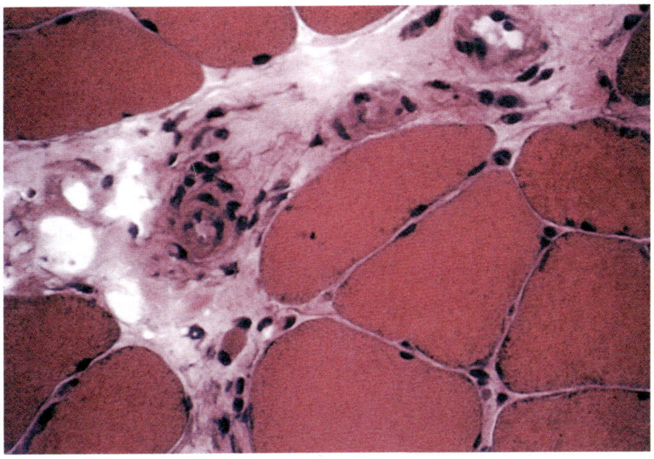

Plate 134 Muscle biopsy from a patient with severe myositis associated with Sjögren's syndrome, showing inflammation surrounding small vessels.

(a)

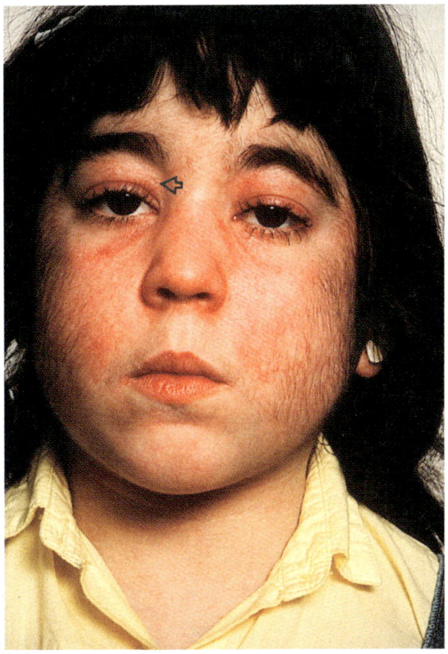

(b)

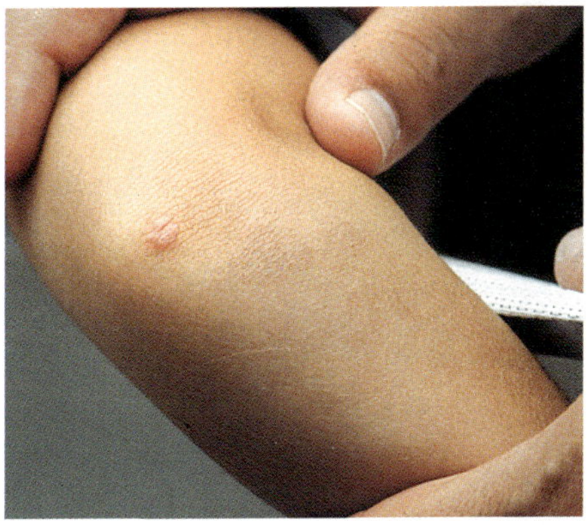

Plate 135 (a) This young girl has the typical rash of juvenile dermatomyositis (JDM). Erythema and oedema involving the eyelids are seen, with healed microinfarcts at the medial aspect of the right upper eyelid (open arrow). The rash crosses the bridge of the nose. (b) Gottron's papules on the elbow of a 4-year-old child with recurrent JDM.

(a)

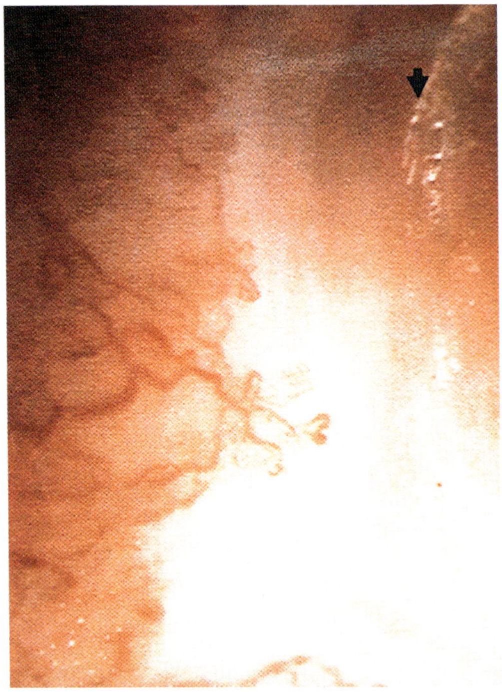

(b)

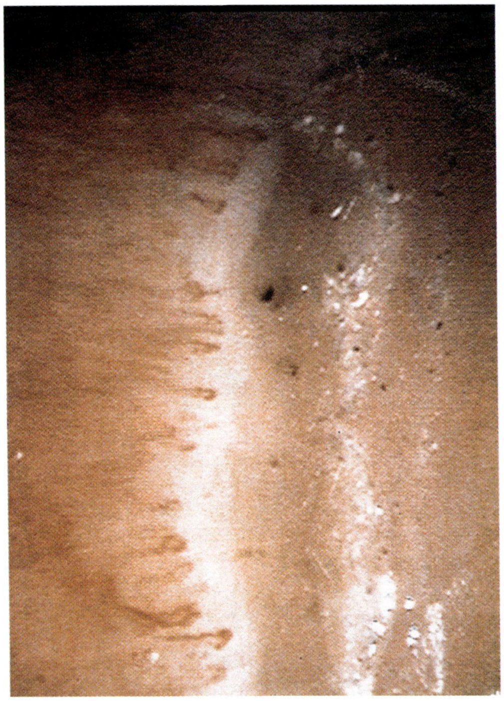

Plate 136 (a) Nailfold capillary studies of a child with dermatomyositis of 2-year duration with severe active disease. Her nailfolds display a prominent subcapillary venous plexus and marked avascularity with decreased numbers of end capillary loops. The few end capillaries that are present are tortuous and show terminal bushing characteristic of this disease. The black arrow indicated the edge of the nail. (b) The same nailfold 2 years and 4 months later: the child is now walking, but still requires intensive therapy. The prominent subcapillary venous plexus has been aided by new capillary formation.

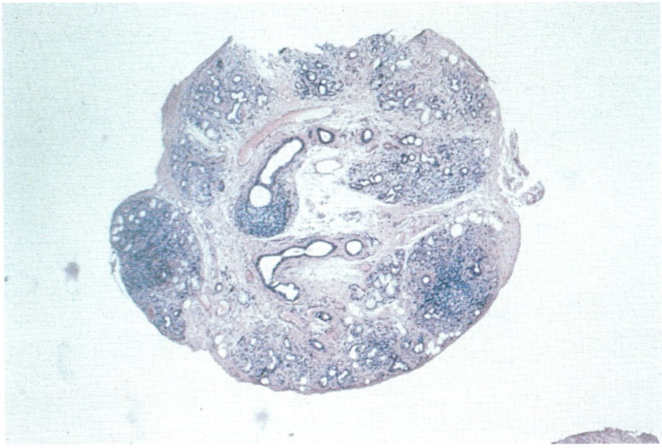

Plate 137 Minor salivary gland biopsy of a patient with Sjögren's syndrome, showing moderate and large focal lymphocytic infiltrates around the acini and ducts.

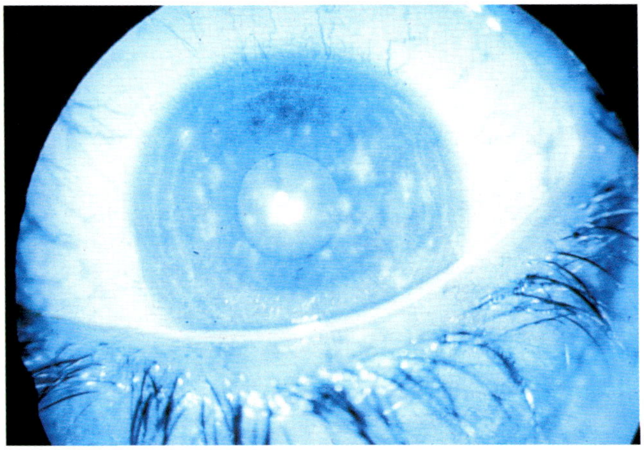

Plate 138 Slit-lamp examination of the eye of a patient with Sjögren's syndrome after rose bengal staining. The retention of the stain in the corneal conjunctiva shows damaged epithelium and filaments, which are diagnostic of keratoconjunctivitis sicca.

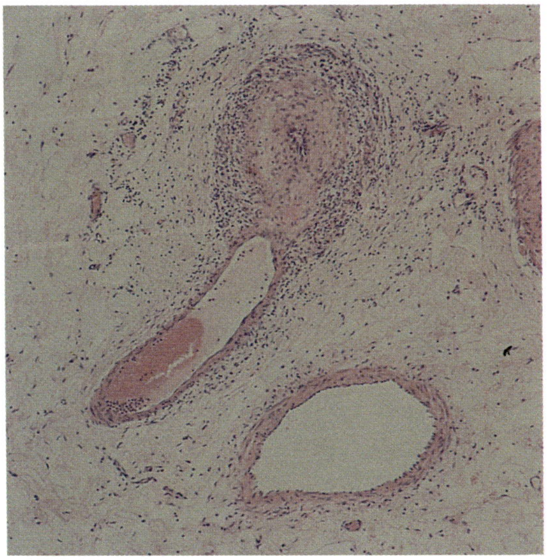

Plate 139 Histology showing typical necrotizing vasculitis.

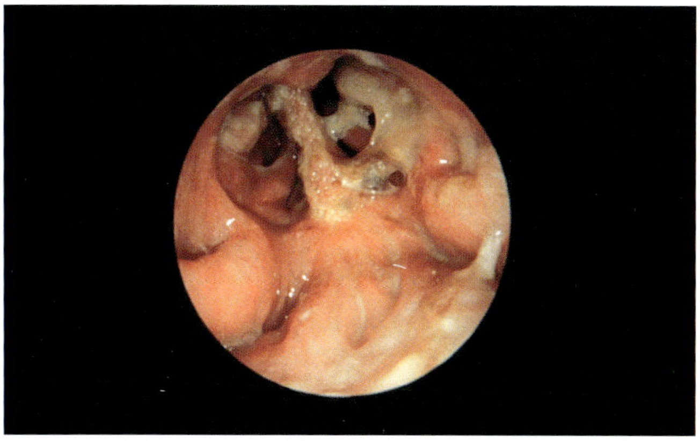

Plate 140 Intranasal bilateral and septal mucosal disease with granulations and crusts leading to permanent serosanguineous discharge.

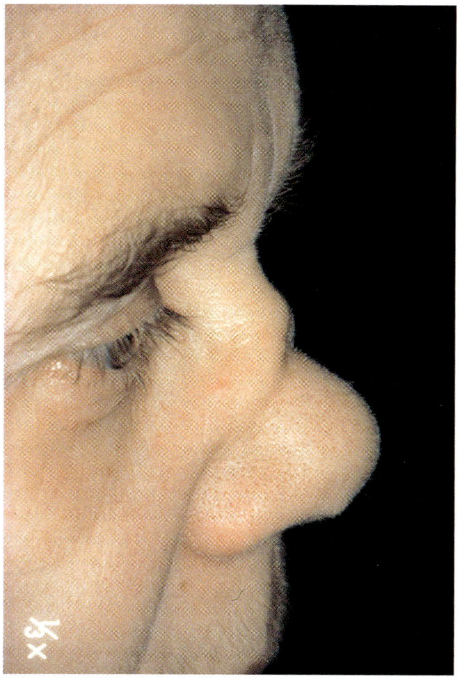

Plate 141 Saddling of the nose due to destruction of the septal cartilage is a common finding in Wegener's granulomatosis.

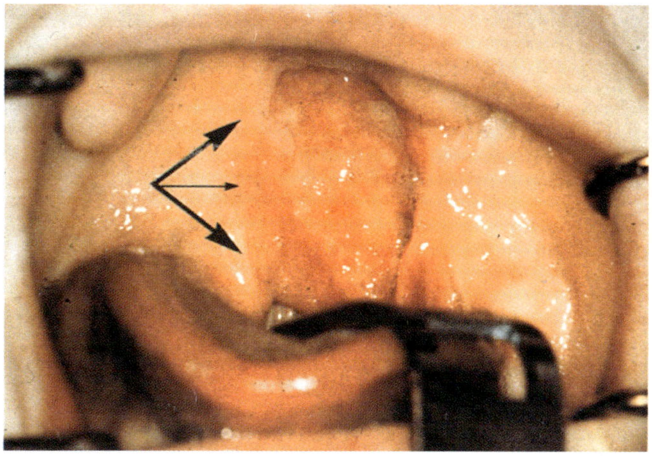

Plate 142 Ulceration of the palate—an unusual site of Wegener's granulomatosis (WG) manifestation—whose characteristic histology led to the diagnosis of WG in a patient with cavitating round nodules of the lung.

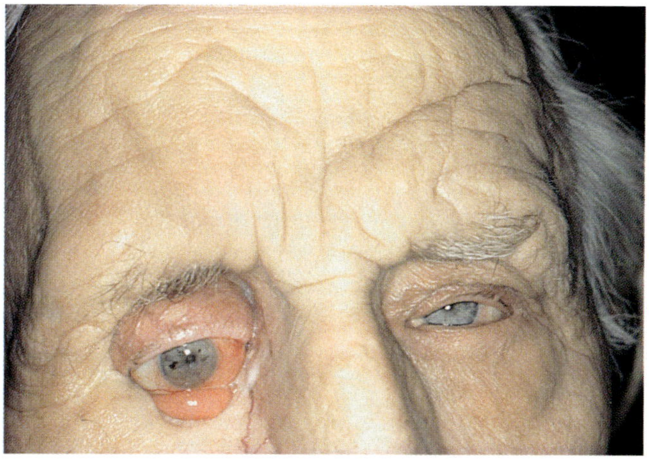

Plate 143 Eye disease in Wegener's granulomatosis usually manifests itself in one of two ways: retro-orbital granuloma masses leading to proptosis (etc.), and small vessel vasculitis leading to 'red eye'.

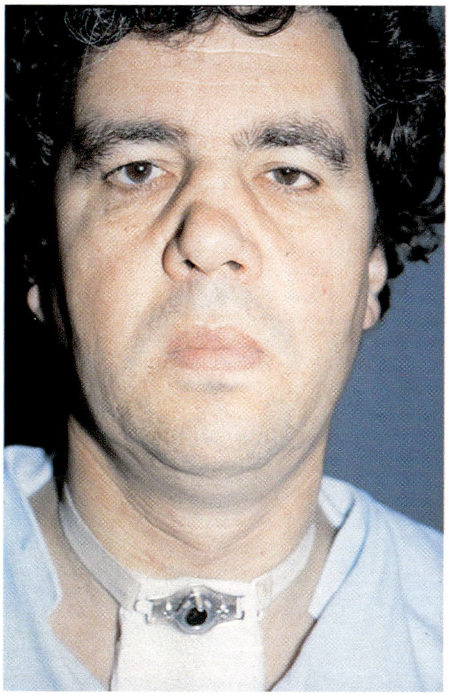

Plate 144 Laryngeal involvement: the circumferential narrowing just below the cords led to subglottic stenoses requiring tracheostomy (see also: saddle nose deformity).

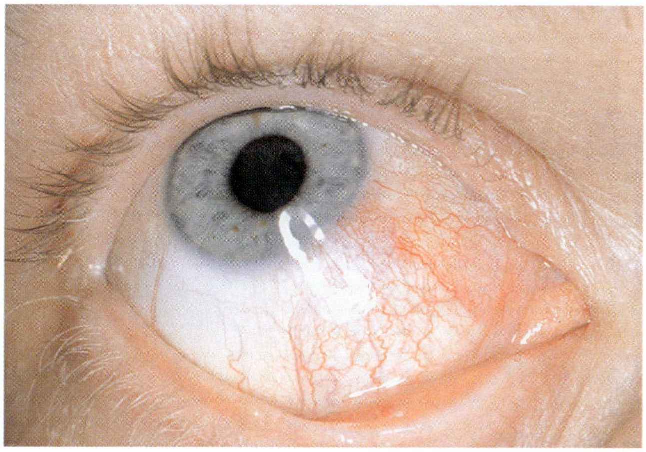

Plate 145 Episcleritis as a characteristic clinical sign of active generalized Wegener's granulomatosis.

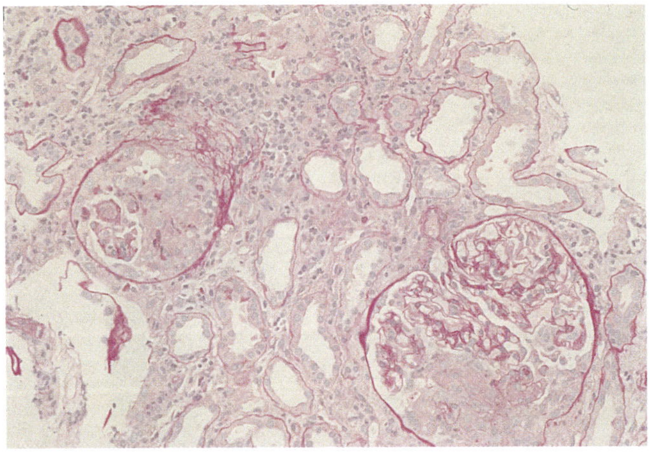

Plate 146 Histopathology of a necrotizing and crescentic glomerulonephritis from a patient with rapidly progressive glomerulonephritis in Wegener's granulomatosis.

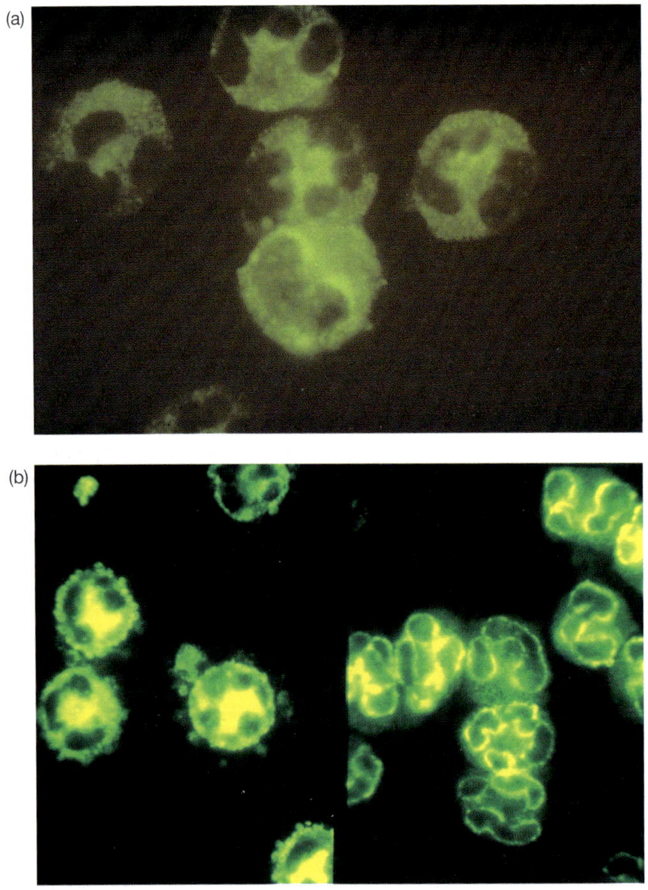

Plate 148 Antineutrophil cytoplasmic autoantibodies: (a) cANCA and (b) pANCA-fluorescence pattern.

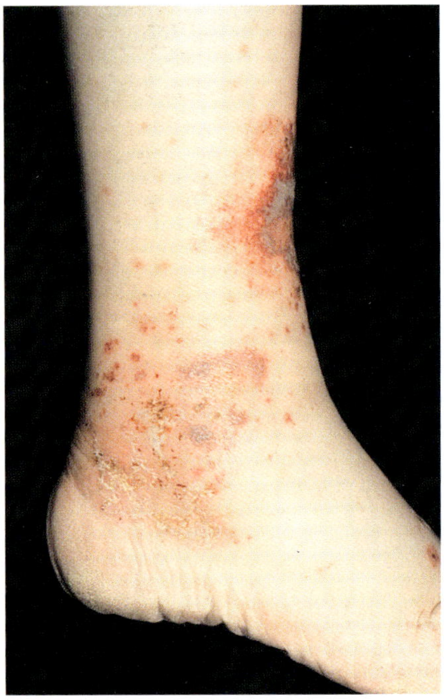

Plate 147 Palpable purpura in a patient with fulminant Wegener's granulomatosis.

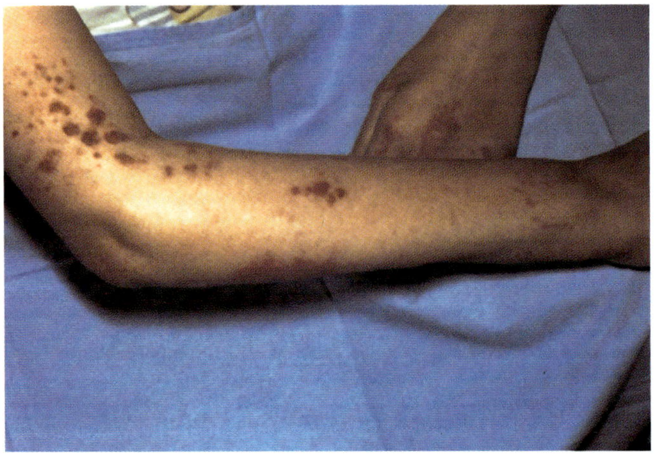

Plate 149 Vasculitic rash in a patient with metastatic adenocarcinoma of unknown origin.

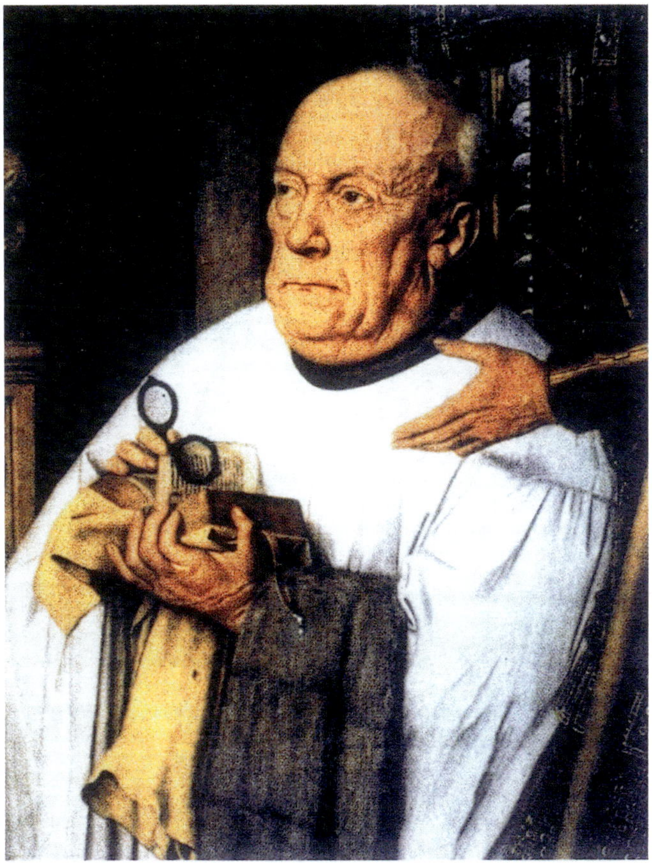

Plate 150 'The Holy Virgin with Canon Van der Paele', by Flemish painter Jan van Eyck, 1436. The prominent temporal arteries along with a scar formation and loss of hair in the left temporal region, have been considered to be caused by GCA. (The municipal museum of Bruges.)

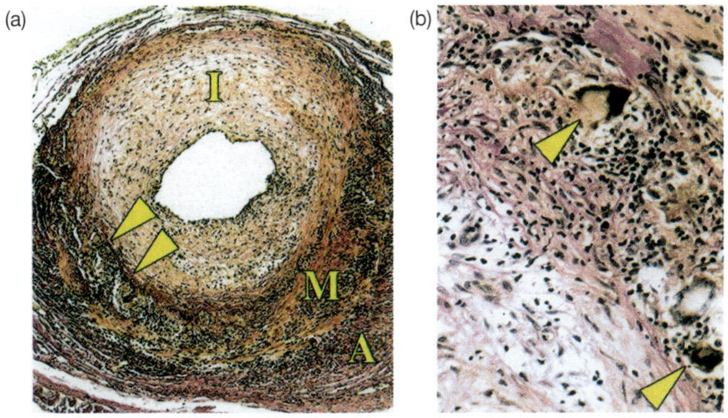

Plate 151 GCA. (a) Cross-sectioned temporal artery with severe chronic inflammation in the adventitia (A), media (M), and intima (I). Note the pronounced thickening of the intima. Arrowheads: giant cells at the media–intima border. (b) Larger magnification, showing multinucleated giant cells at the media–intima border (arrowheads) (van Gieson).

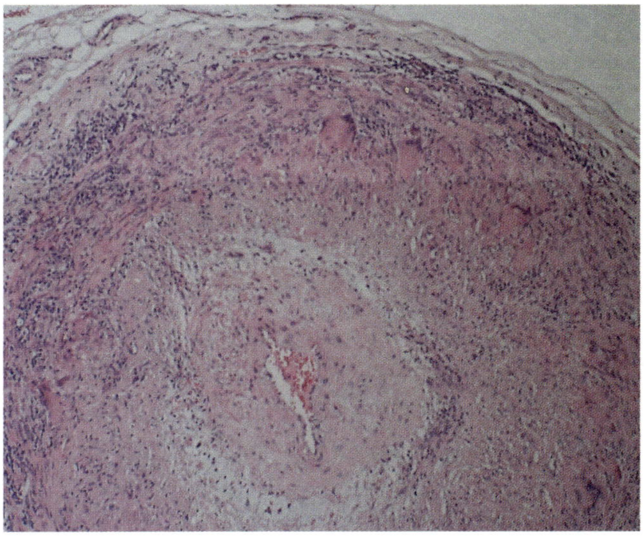

Plate 152 Temporal artery biopsy showing intimal thickening, panarteritis, and giant cells. (Courtesy: Dr Wolfe—Southend General Hospital, United Kingdom.)

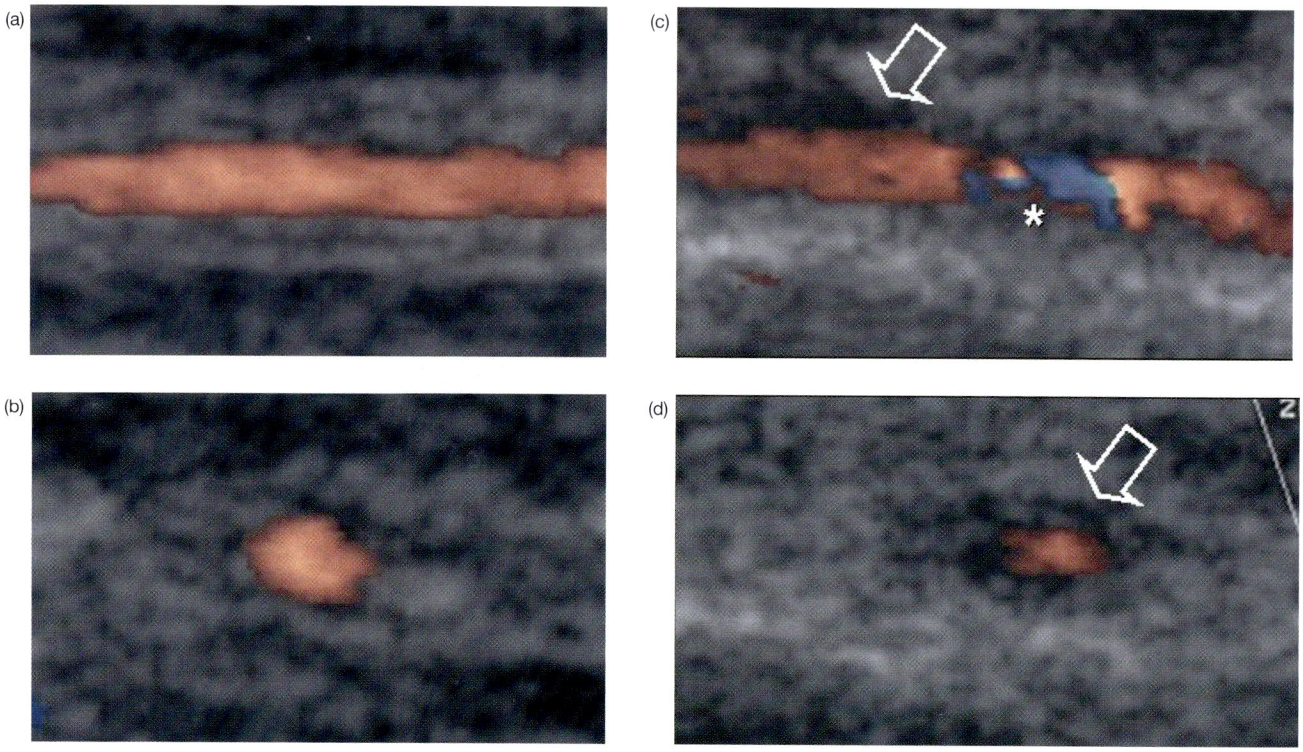

Plate 153 Showing frontal ramus of the right common superficial temporal artery in a longitudinal (a, c) and a transverse plane (b, d). (a, b) Normal temporal artery; (c, d) temporal artery of a 64-year-old female with acute temporal arteritis. The arrows show the inflammatory wall thickening (halo), the asterisk is located at a stenosis with turbulent blood flow. (Courtesy: Dr Schmidt—Medical Centre for Rheumatology, Berlin-Buch.)

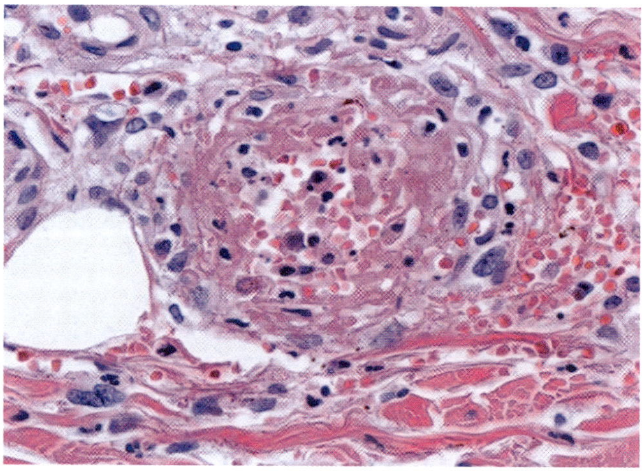

Plate 154 Small artery with wall vessel destruction, fibrinoid necrosis, and leucocytoclasia (HE).

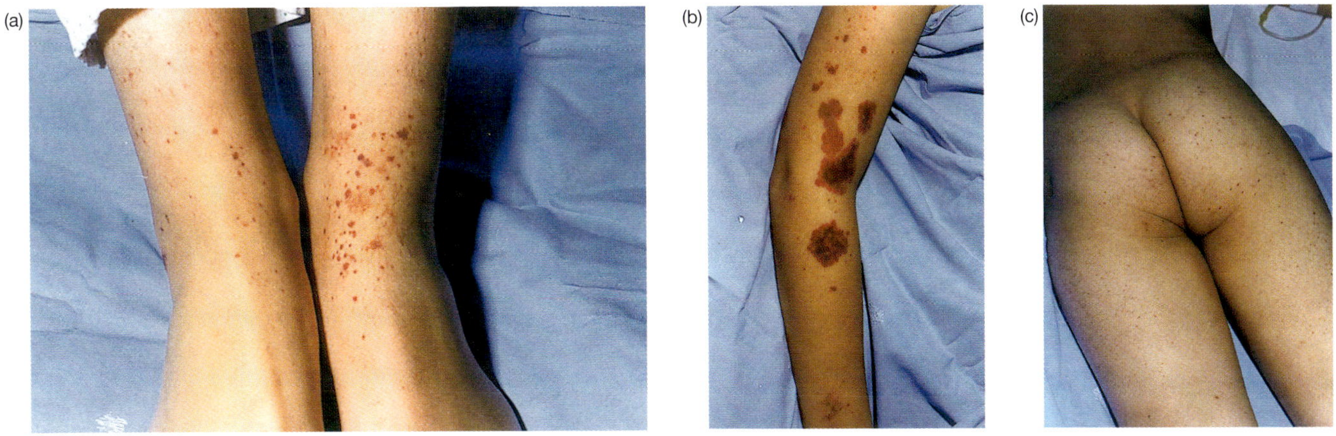

Plate 155 (a) Symmetrical palpable purpura in a patient with small vessel vasculitis. (b) Combination of different lesions in a boy with biopsy proven small-sized blood vessel vasculitis. (c) Henoch–Schönlein purpura. Petechial and purpuric rash in buttocks as expression of a dependent and pressure-bearing area.

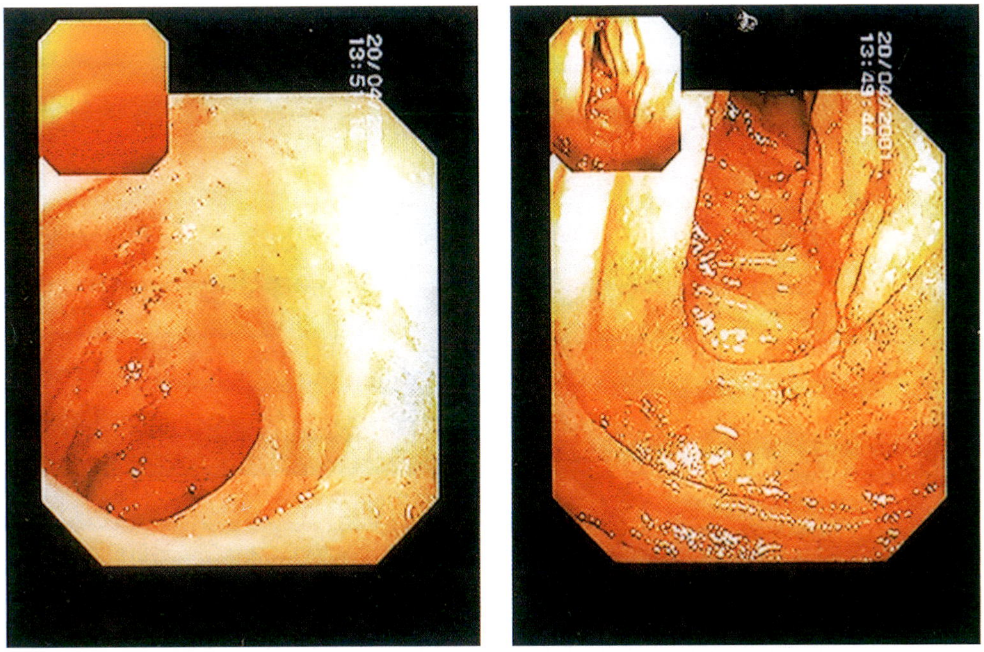

Plate 156 Erythema, oedema, petechial lesions, and superficial erosions of the duodenal mucosa in a boy with Henoch–Schönlein purpura.

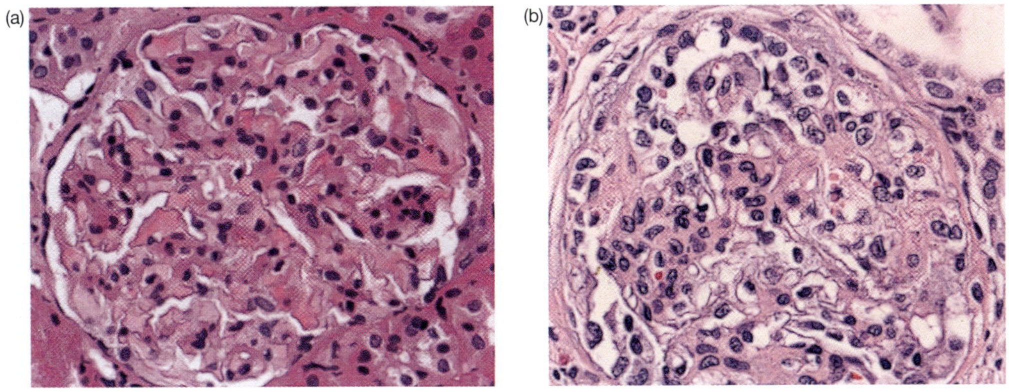

Plate 157 (a) Glomerulus of a patient with Henoch–Schönlein purpura and mesangial IgA glomerulonephritis showing increased mesangial matrix and mesangial hypercellularity (HE). (b) Glomerulus with epithelial capsular proliferation in an adult with Henoch–Schönlein purpura and rapidly progressive crescentic glomerulonephritis (HE).

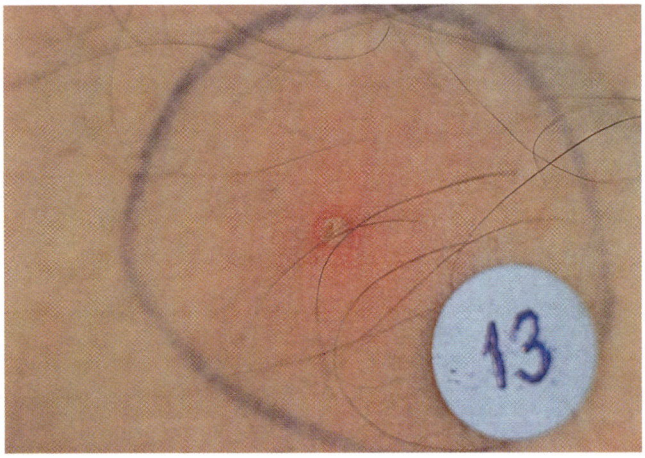

Plate 158 The pathergy reaction in the form of a pustule.

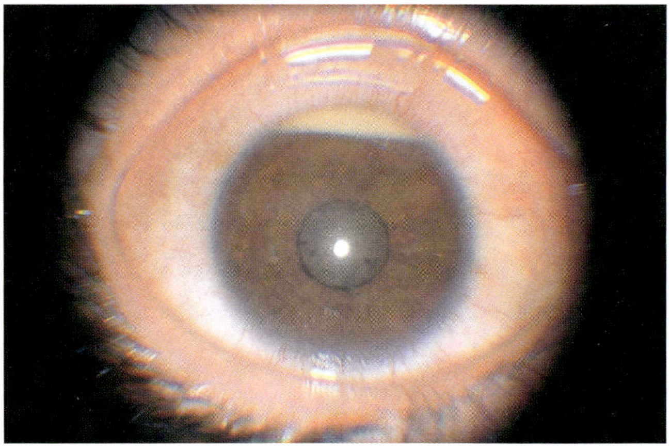

Plate 159 Hypopyon uveitis.

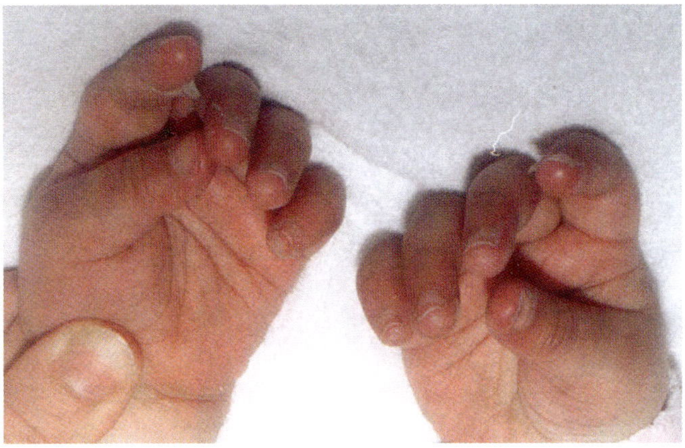

Plate 160 Kawasaki disease showing desquamation of the skin in the convalescent phase.

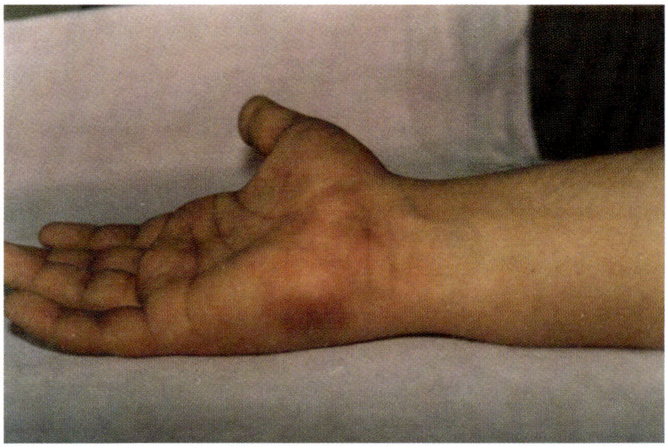

Plate 161 Painful nodule of systemic PAN, the 'nodose' of the disease.

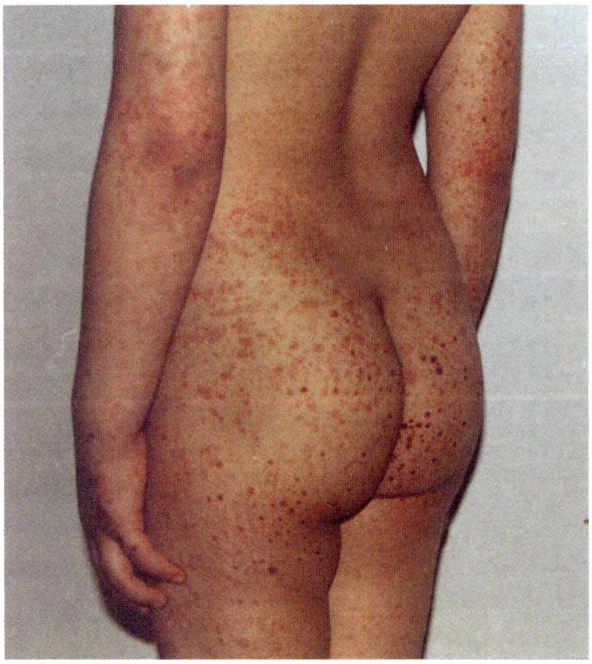

Plate 162 Typical purpura of Henoch–Schönlein purpura.

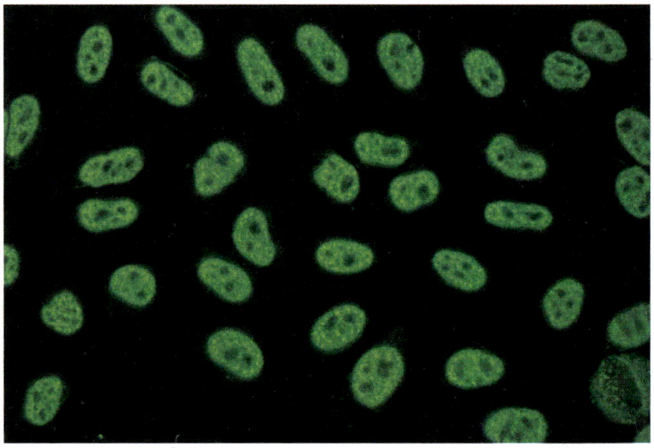

Plate 163 Typical coarse speckled pattern of ANA detected by indirect immunofluorescence in serum from a patient with mixed connective tissue disease. Note the relative sparing of staining of the nucleolus within the cell nucleus.

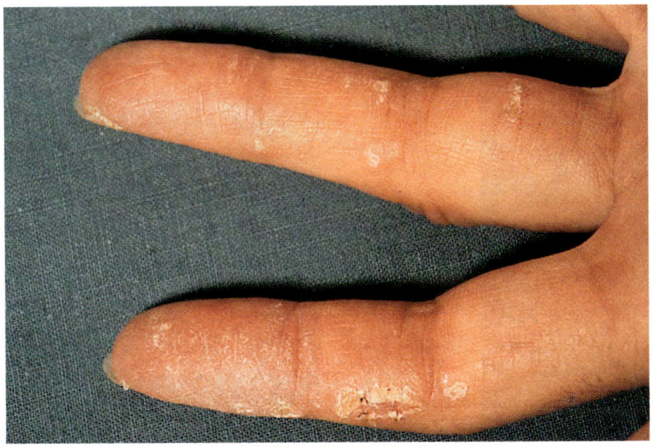

Plate 164 Mechanic's finger.

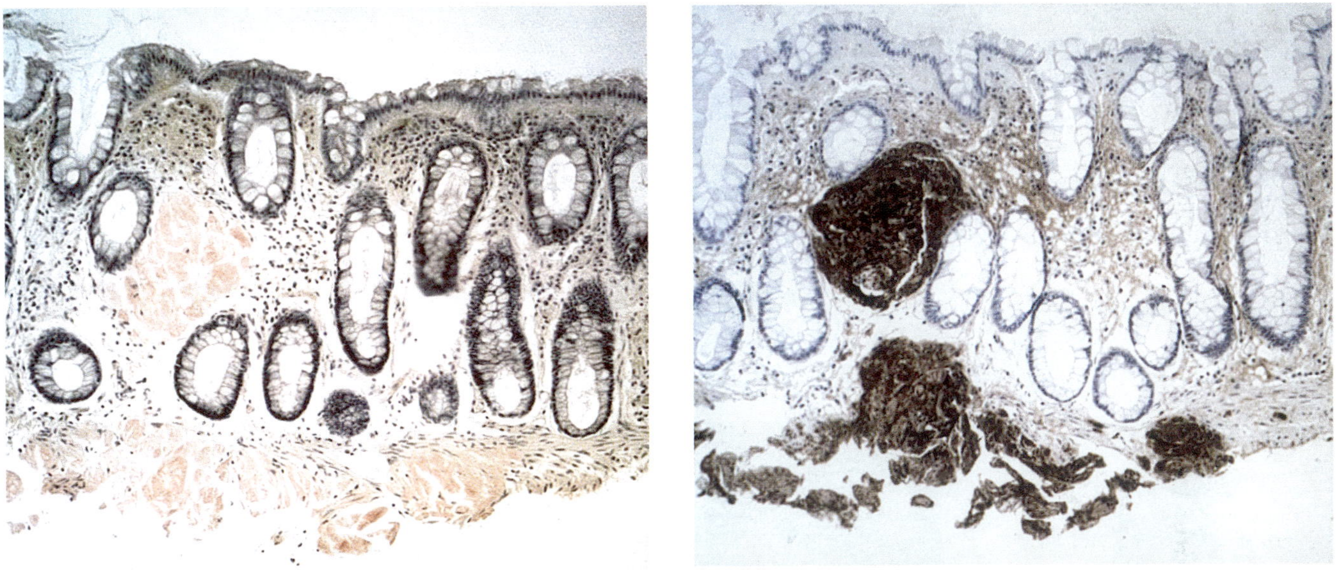

Plate 165 Rectal biopsy sections treated with Congo red (left) and with antibodies to transthyretin (right), staining amyloid deposits pink and brown staining respectively, confirming the presence of transthyretin amyloidosis.

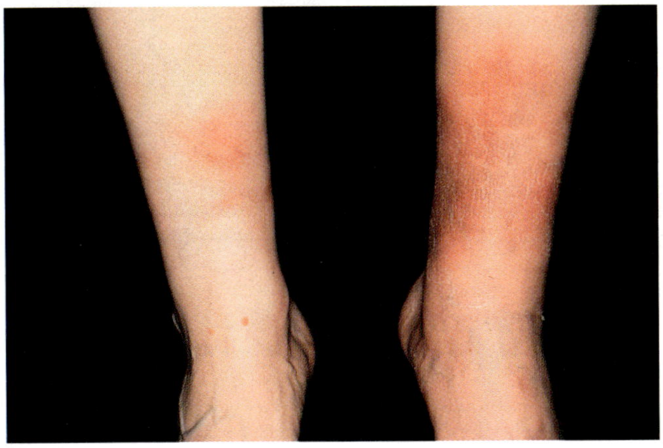

Plate 166 Erythema nodosum—multiple tender subcutaneous erythematous nodules.

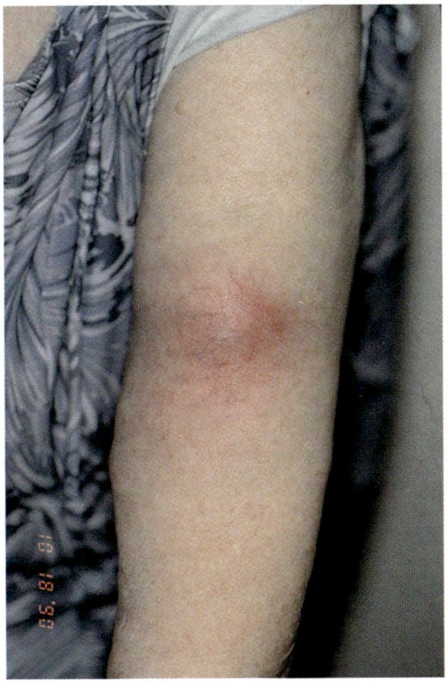

Plate 167 Weber–Christian disease—this patient developed multiple recurrent subcutaneous lesions with accompanying fever and arthritis.

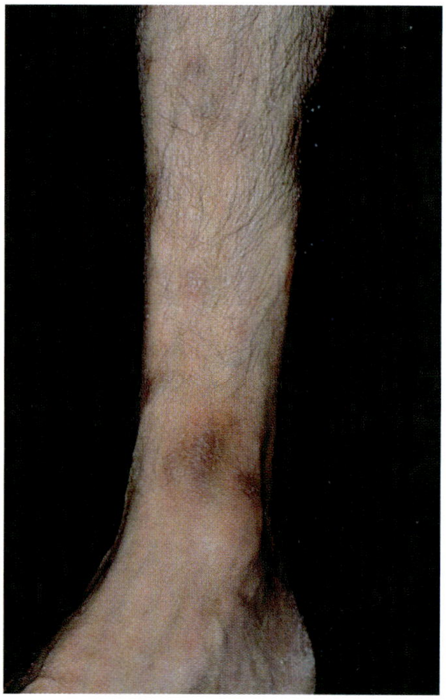

Plate 168 Pancreatic panniculitis. Tender, erythematous subcutaneous nodules in a patient with pancreatitis (by courtesy of Robert Schosser, MD, Lexington KY, USA).

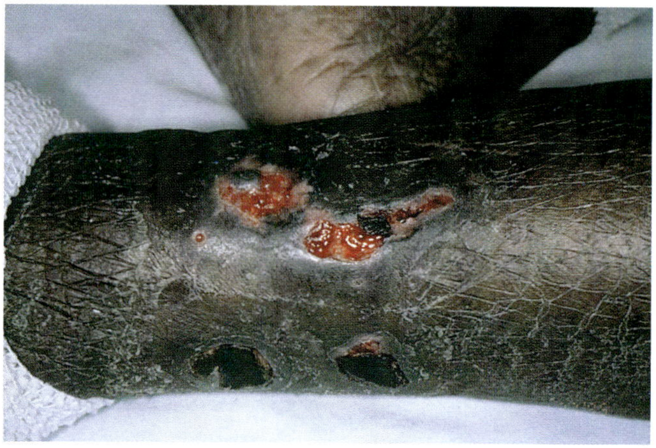

Plate 169 Calcifying panniculitis (calciphylaxis) in this patient with renal failure. The reaction has resulted in necrosis and ulceration of the nodular lesions on the lower extremity.

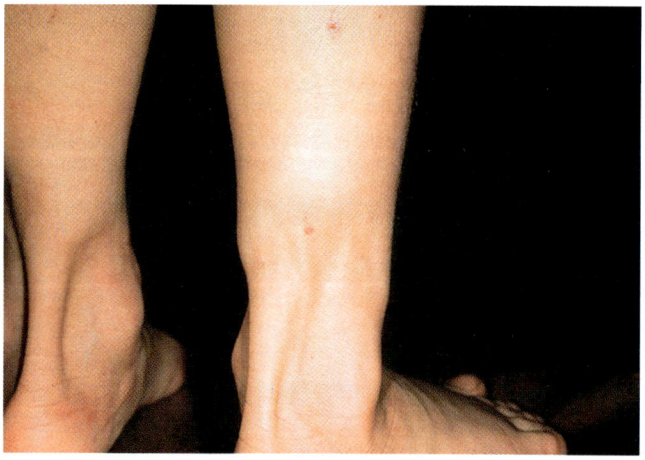

Plate 170 Lipoatrophy following an active panniculitis of unknown cause in this child.

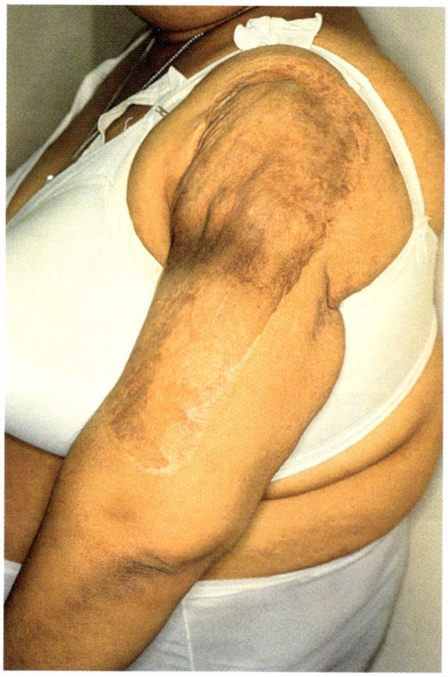

Plate 171 Factitial panniculitis—this patient developed multiple lesions, which were surgically drained or excised; only after careful inspection of several specimens by polarized microscopy was refractile material found.

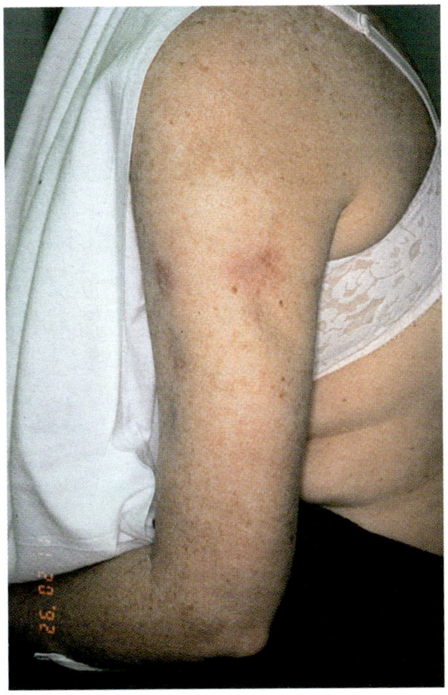

Plate 172 Lupus erythematosus panniculitis. Erythematous to violaceous nodules with resultant atrophy of the subcutaneous tissue.

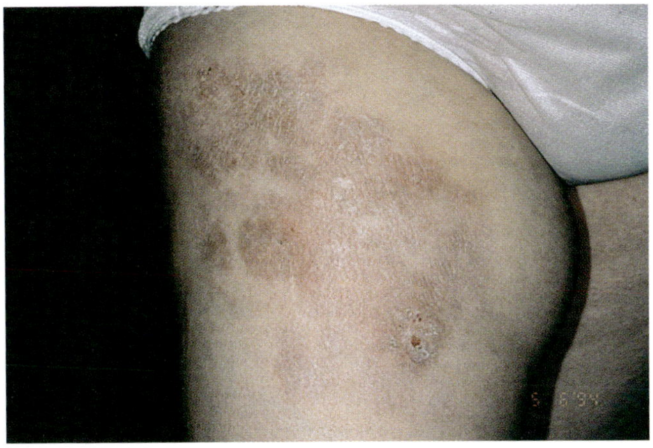

Plate 173 Calcified subcutaneous nodules of lupus erythematosus.

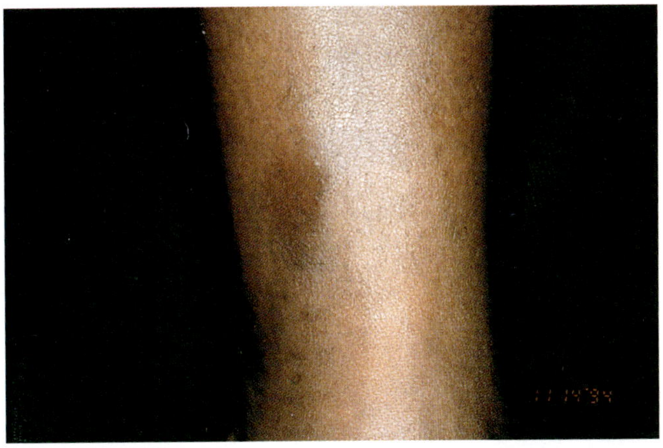

Plate 174 Sclerosing panniculitis. Tender, subcutaneous nodule in a patient with peripheral oedema.

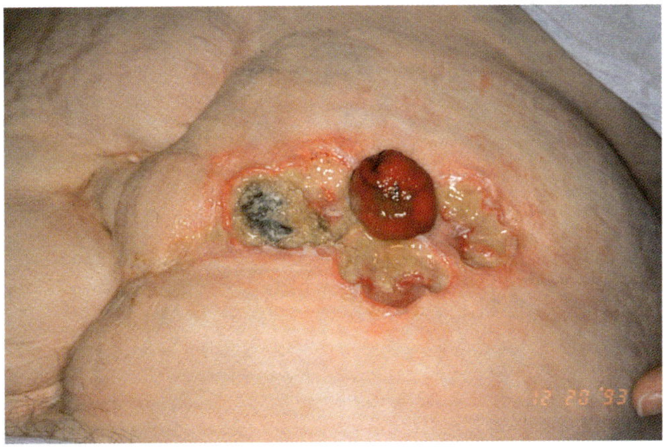

Plate 175 Peristomal pyoderma gangrenosum in a patient with an ileostomy after bowel surgery for ulcerative colitis.

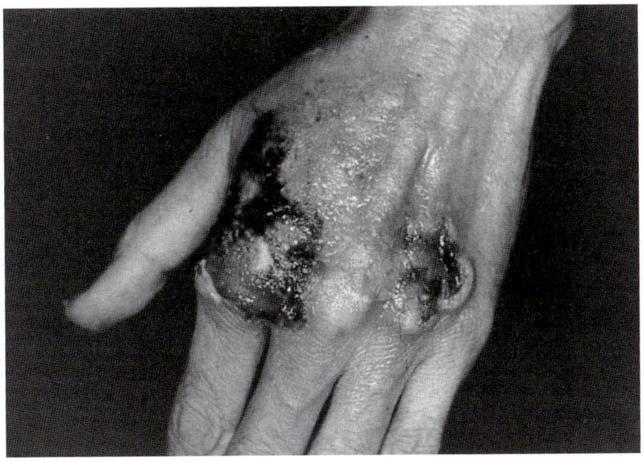

Plate 176 Atypical pyoderma gangrenosum in a patient with a pre-leukaemic state. The lesion is a shallow ulcer with a bullous, blue-grey border.

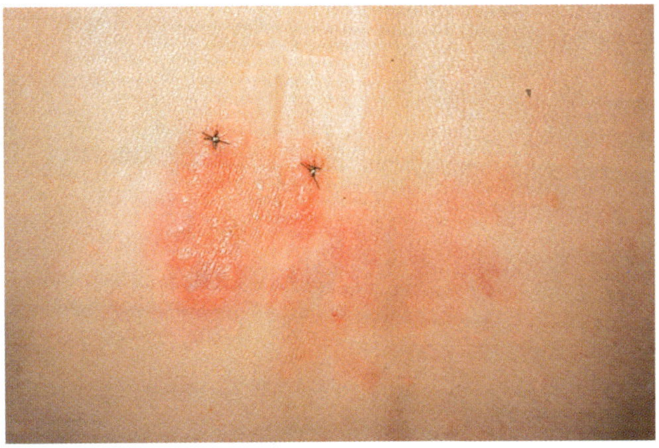

Plate 177 Vesiculopustular eruption in a patient with previous ulcer surgery (Billroth II) and a blind loop—the so-called 'bowel bypass syndrome without a bowel bypass'.

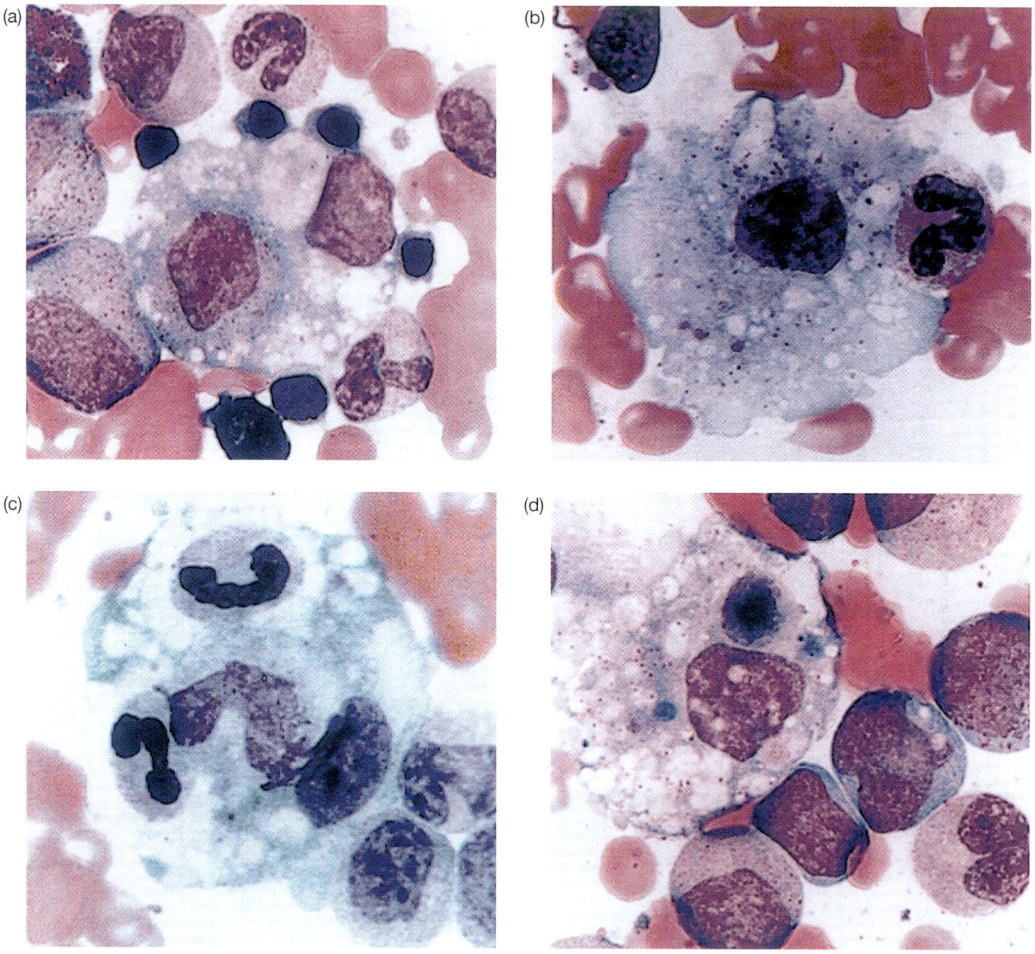

Plate 178 Bone marrow aspirate specimens from a patient with macrophage activation syndrome revealing histologically benign actively phagocytic macrophages (haematoxylin and eosin stain). (a) Myelocyte within activated macrophage. In addition, there are multiple adherent red blood cell and myeloid precursors. (b) Activated macrophage engulfing a neutrophilic band form. (c) Neutrophilic band forms and metamyelocyte within an activated macrophage. Nuclei of band forms appear condensed. (d) Activated macrophage with haemosiderin deposits and a degenerating phagocytosed nucleated cell. (Reproduced with permission from Prahalad et al. (2001). *Journal of Rheumatology* **28**, 2120–4.)

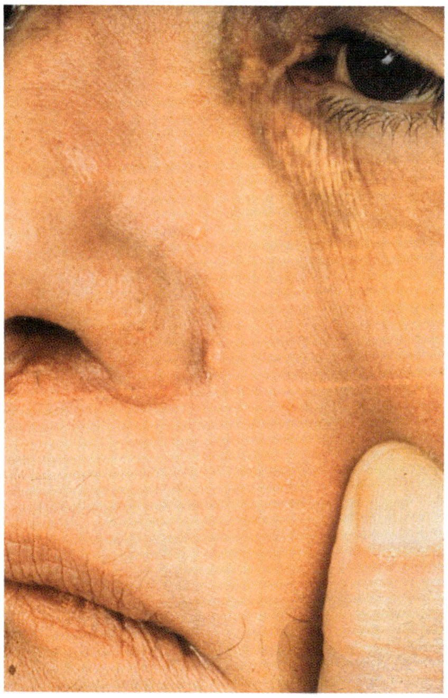

Plate 179 Multicentric reticulohistiocytosis: involvement of the face.

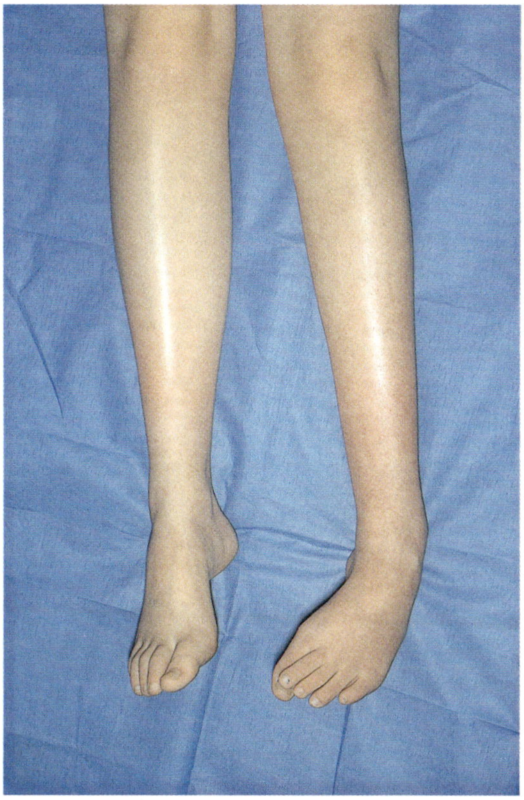

Plate 180 Lower limbs of a 13-year-old girl with a 12 month history of severe reflex sympathetic dystrophy of the right foot unresponsive to multiple procedures prior to referral. For 3 months she had been experiencing similar features in the left leg leading to complete loss of mobility. A pre-existing mild spastic diplegia was noted from early childhood which had only minimally affected her gait previously.

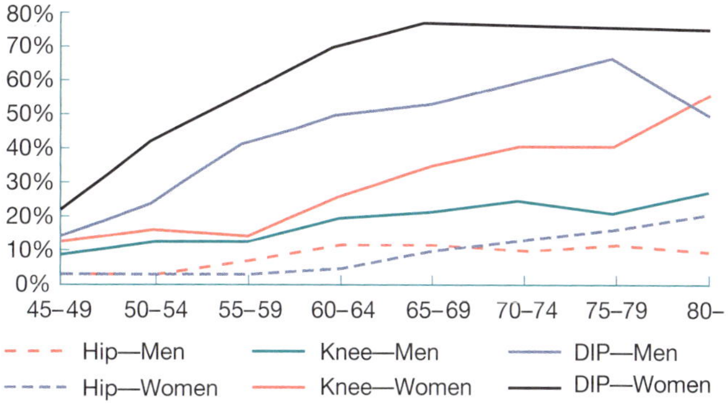

Plate 181 Prevalence of radiological osteoarthritis by age group and gender in a Netherlands community population. Derived from van Saase et al. (1989).

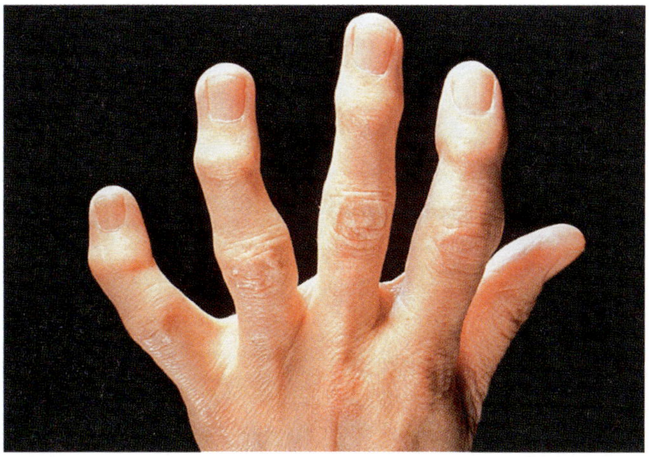

Plate 182 Typical appearance of multiple Heberden's and Bouchard's nodes in nodal generalized osteoarthritis.

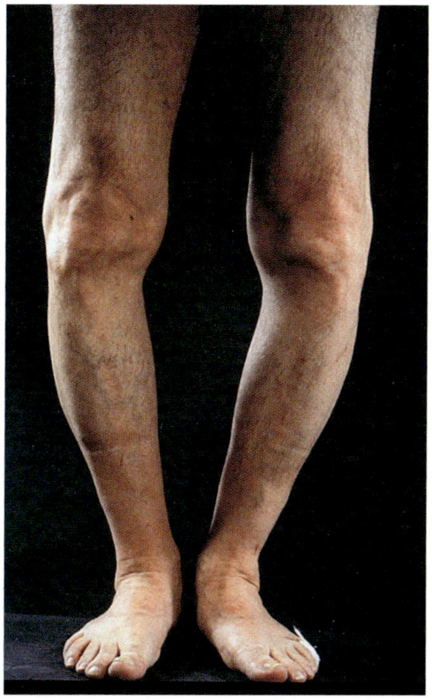

Plate 183 Typical varus deformity of knee osteoarthritis.

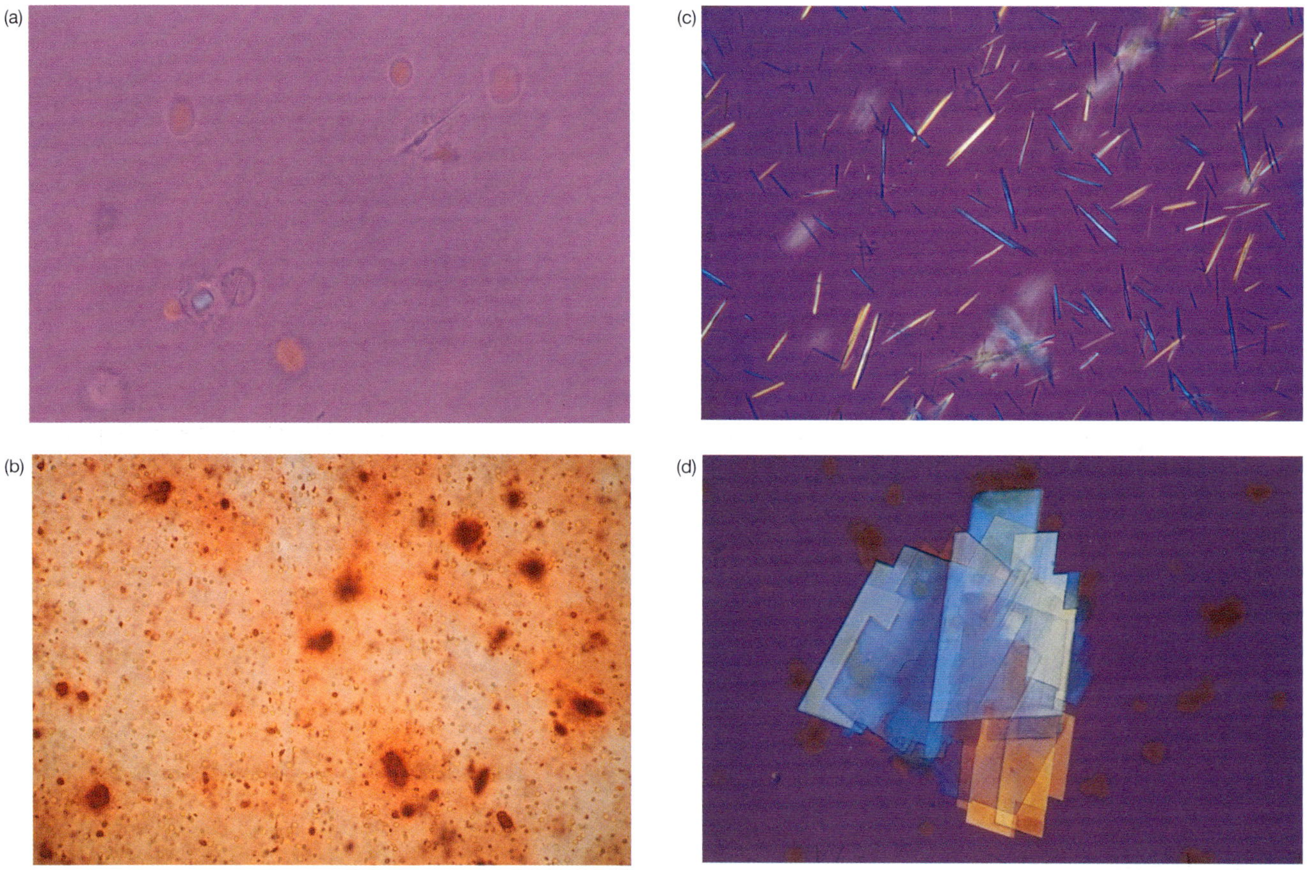

Plate 184 (a) Calcium pyrophosphate dehydrate; (b) monosodium urate monohydrate; (c) apatite; and (d) cholesterol crystals.

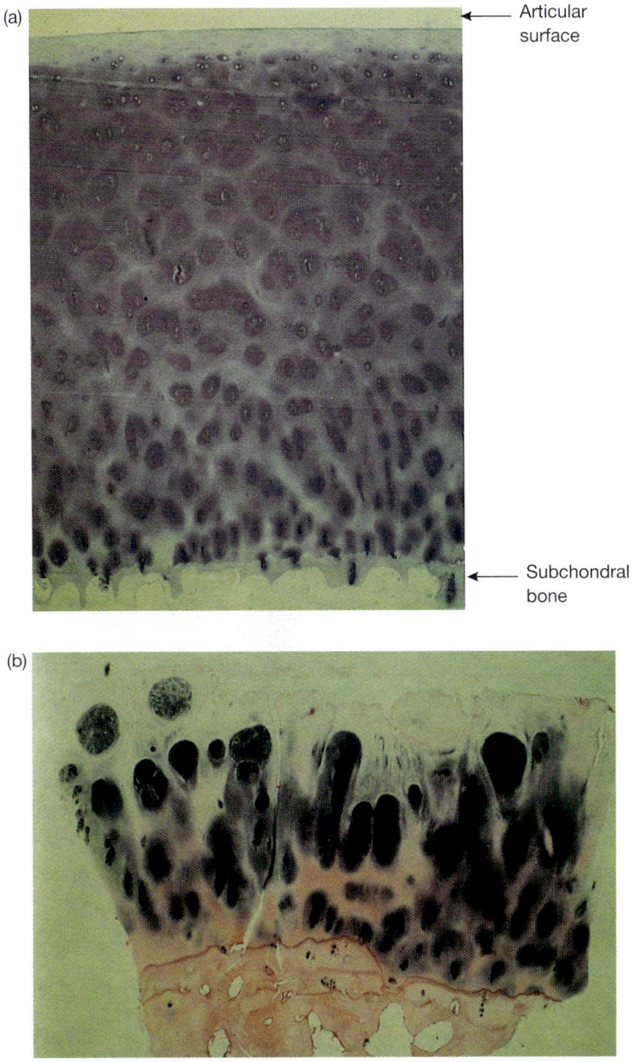

Plate 185 (a) Normal and (b) osteoarthritic human articular cartilage (toluidine blue). Note the extensive cell clustering, loss of metachromatic staining, fissuring of the tissue, and duplication of the 'tide-mark' in the osteoarthritis specimen.

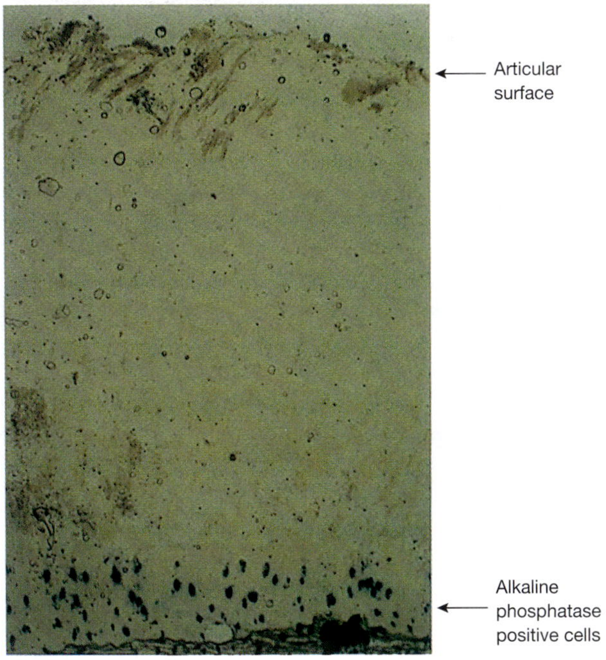

Plate 186 Localization of alkaline phosphatase in human osteoarthritic cartilage (55-year-old patient).

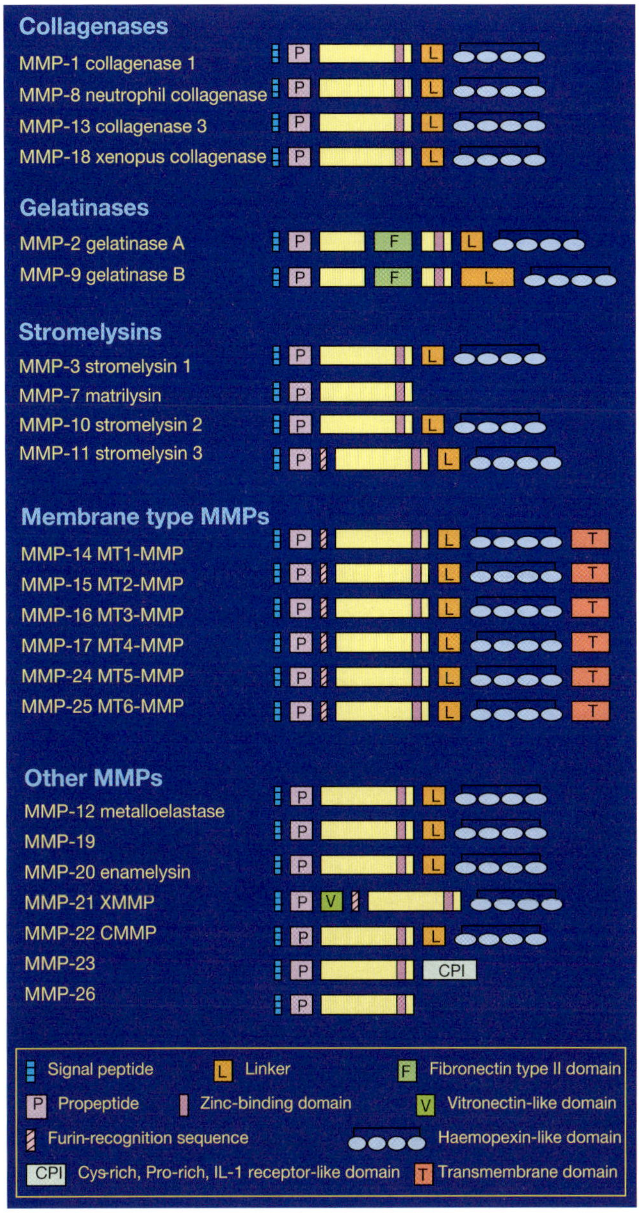

Plate 187 Metalloproteinase domain structure.

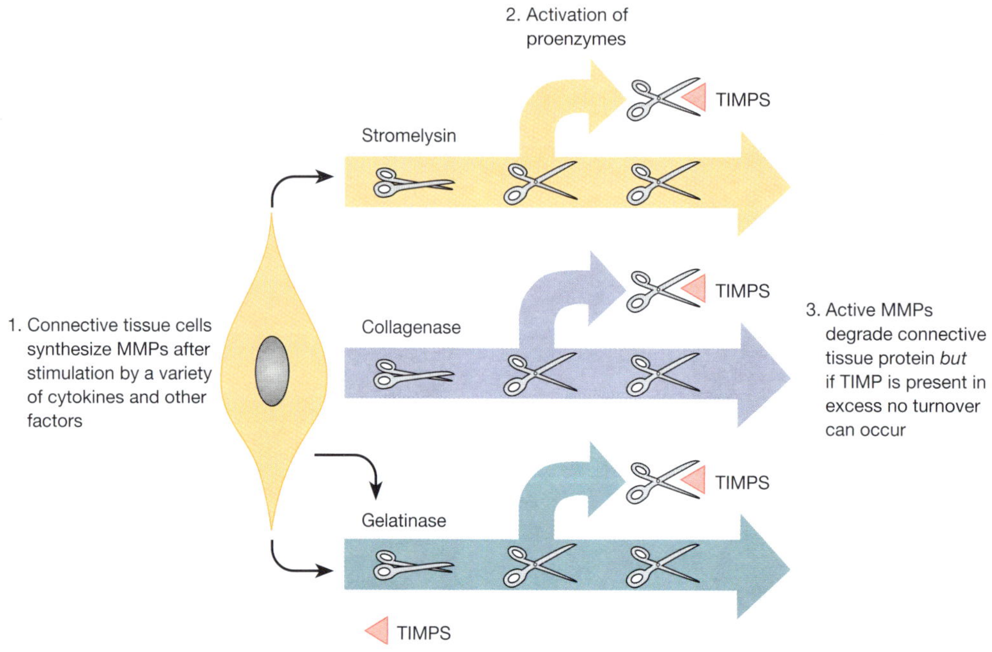

Plate 188 Control of metalloproteinase activity.

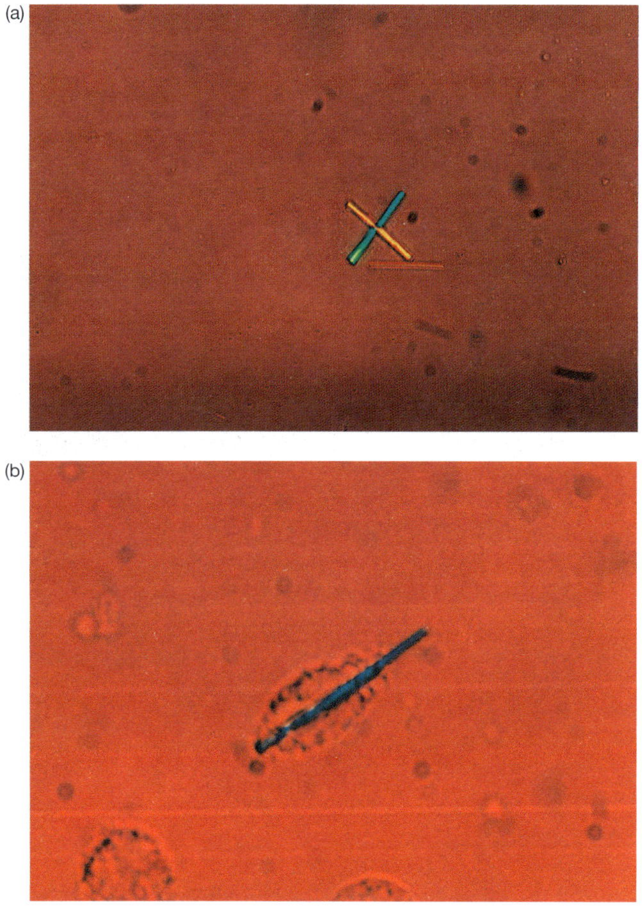

Plate 189 Typical, needle-shaped, negatively birefringent crystals are seen under polarizing light microscopy in the synovial fluid of patients with gouty arthritis. These crystals may be (a) extracellular or (b) intracellular.

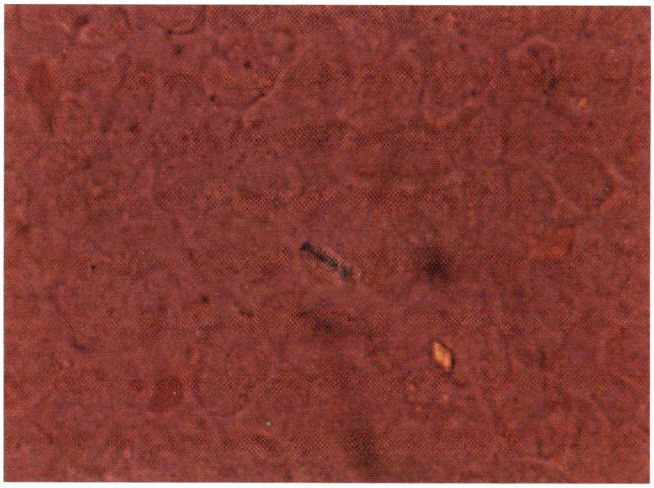

Plate 190 Typical, positively birefringent crystals of calcium pyrophosphate dihydrate are seen here. Note the rhomboid shape and the weak birefringence.

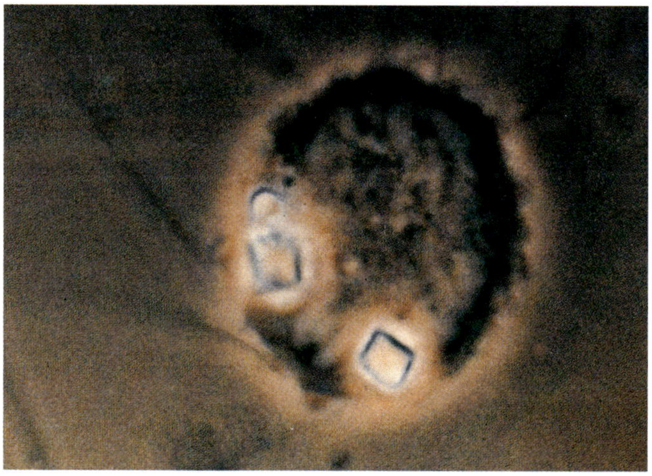

Plate 191 The typical bipyramidal crystals of calcium oxalate dihydrate are seen here inside a cell.

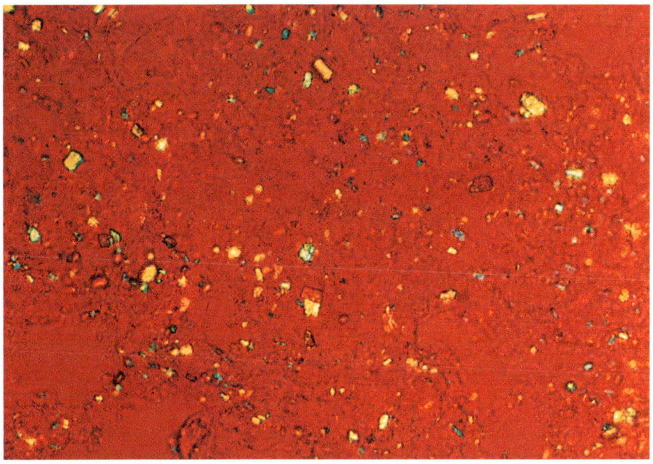

Plate 192 Steroid crystals can be seen in synovial fluids after intra-articular corticosteroid injections.

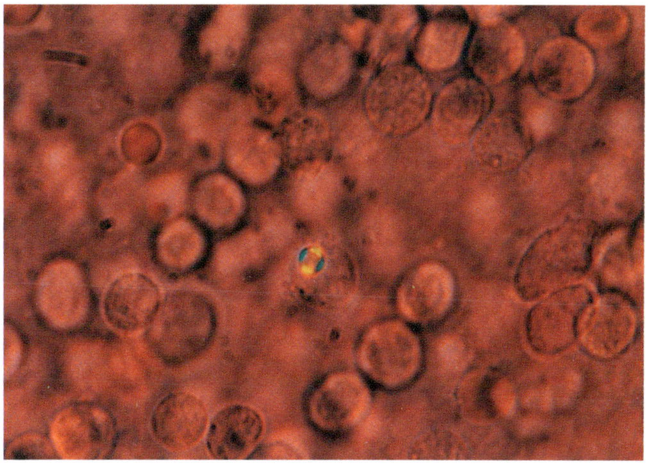

Plate 193 The typical appearance of lipid crystals in synovial fluid.

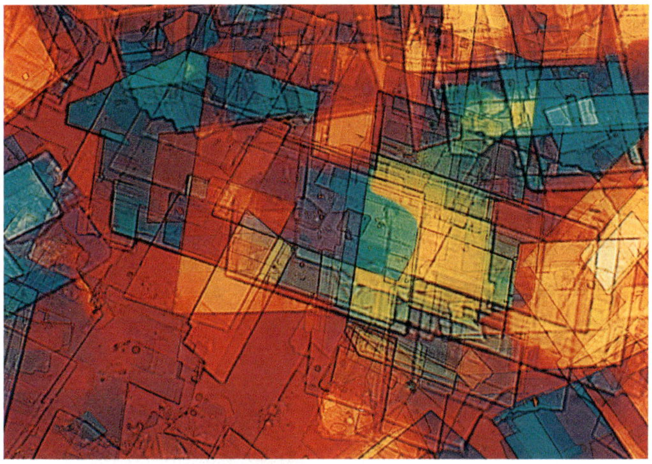

Plate 194 The typical appearance of cholesterol crystals in synovial fluid.

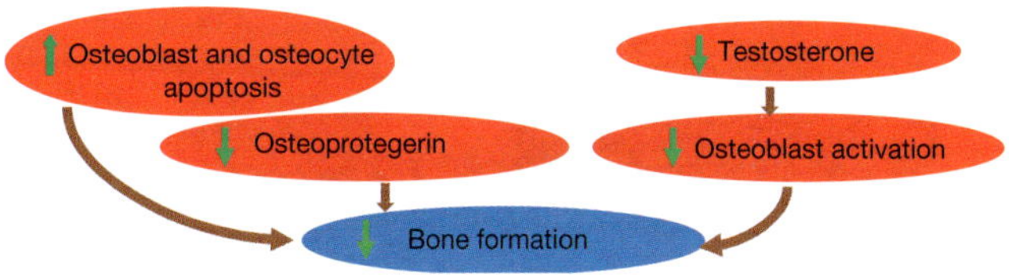

Plate 195 Effects of excess corticosteroids on bone formation.

(a)

(b)

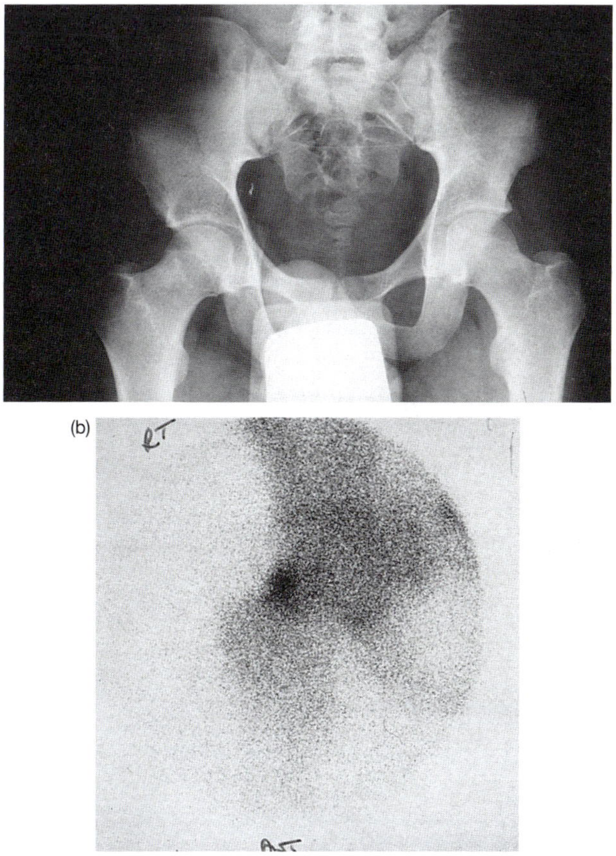

Plate 196 (a) Plain pelvic radiograph showing an osteoid osteoma of the femoral neck in an 18-year-old male who presented with a 3-month history of progressively worsening pain. (b) Radionuclide bone scan showing increased uptake of isotope by the lesion.

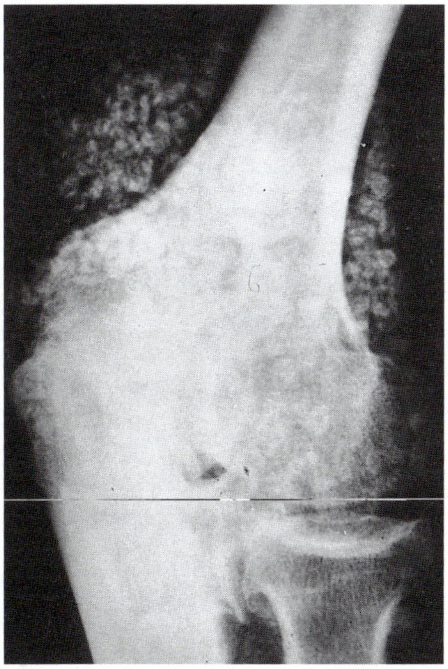

Plate 197 Anteroposterior view of the elbow demonstrating multiple osteochondral bodies, regularly shaped and uniform in size. This is typical of synovial chondromatosis. (By courtesy of Dr P. Renton, University College, London.)

(a)
(b)
(c)
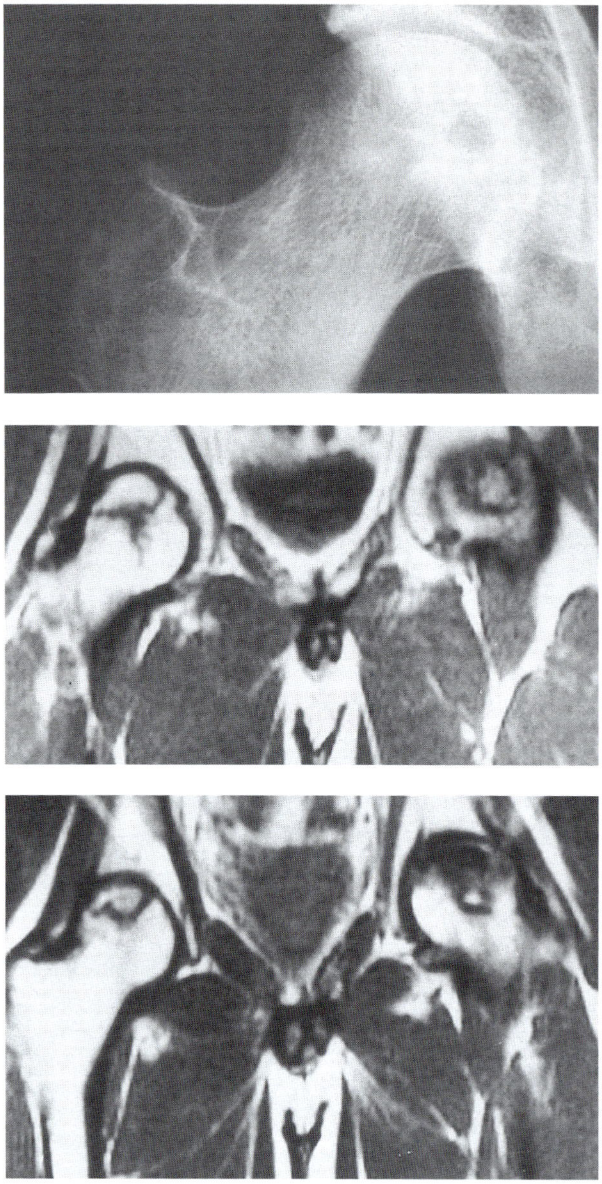

Plate 198 (a) Early changes of osteonecrosis of the femoral head shown on plain radiograph (Arlet and Ficat stage II). (b) MRI clearly detects osteonecrosis at an early stage in T_1-weighted and (c) T_2-weighted images. (By courtesy of Dr P. Renton, University College, London.)

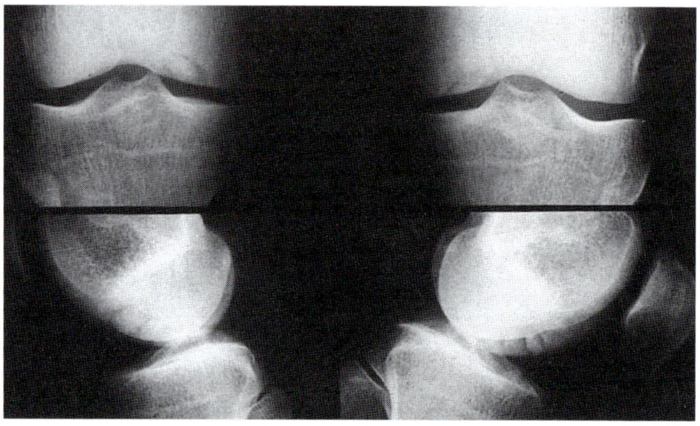

Plate 199 Anteroposterior and lateral views showing typical lesions of osteochondritis dissecans in both medial femoral condyles. A radiolucent line separates the oval-shaped, in situ body from the femoral condyle. (By courtesy of Dr P. Renton, University College, London.)

(a) (b)
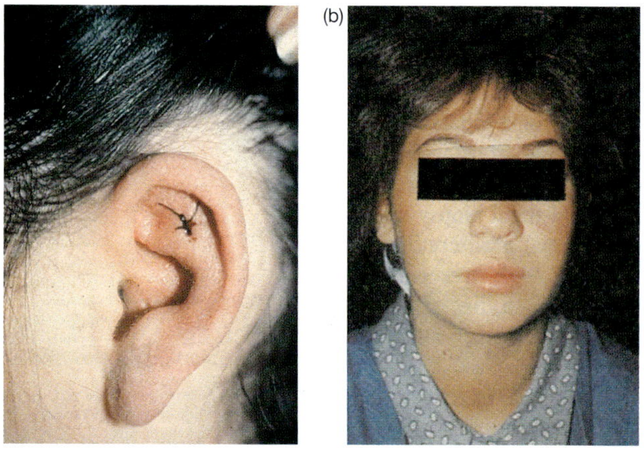

Plate 200 Clinical features of relapsing polychondritis. (a) Acute inflammation of the external ear. (b) Saddle nose deformity. (By courtesy of Dr A. Balsa, La Paz Hospital, Madrid.)

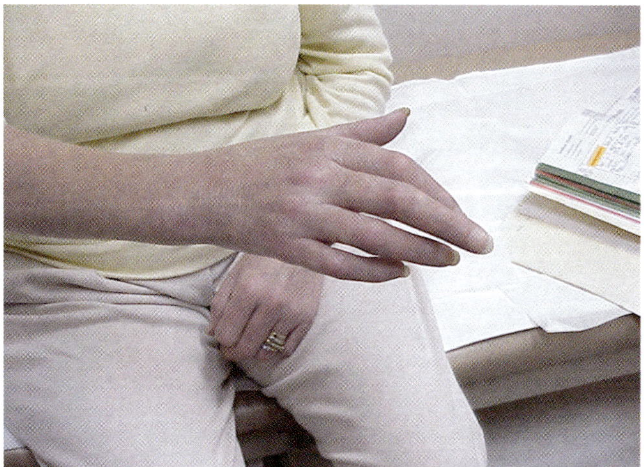

Plate 201 Tightened joints and soft-tissue dystrophic changes in right hand of a 43-year-old woman 18 months after injury.

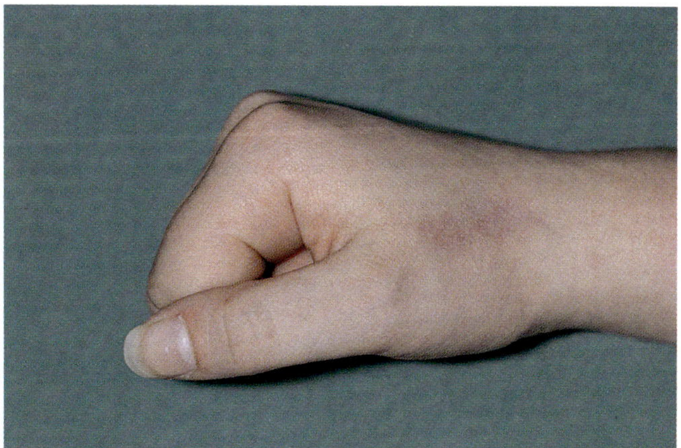

Plate 202 Subcutaneous tissue atrophy following steroid injection of De Quervain's tenosynovitis lesion.

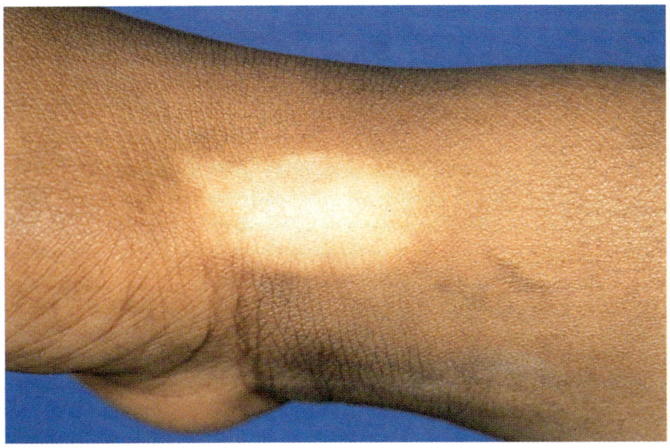

Plate 203 Depigmentation following steroid injection of De Quervain's tenosynovitis lesion.

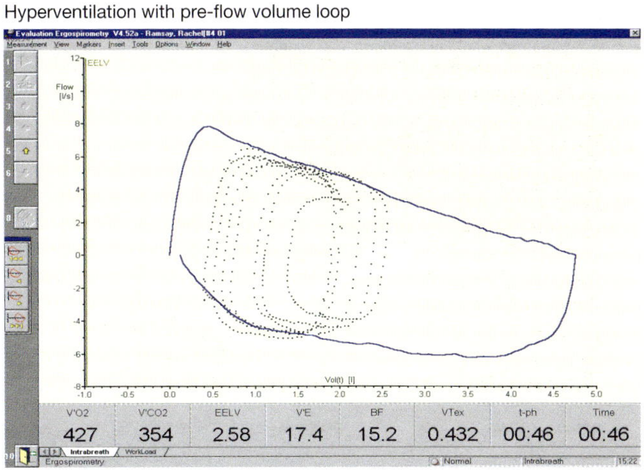

Plate 204 During exercise, breath circles are contained within the envelope of the maximum effort flow loop. The harder the exercise, the larger the breath circles, which must move to the left, closer to full inspiration, where the airways are widest.

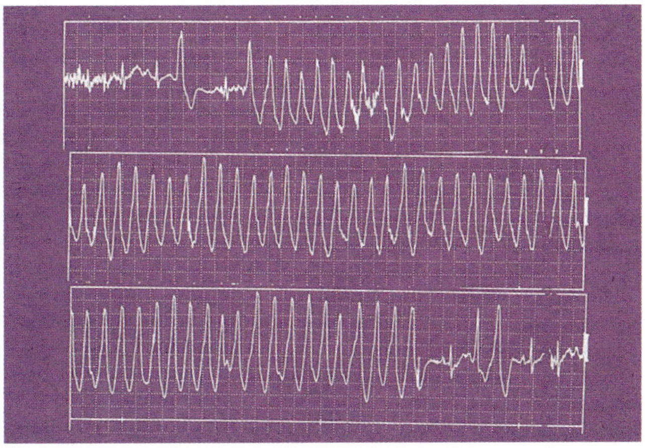

Plate 205 Ventricular tachycardia running for 3 min precipitated occurring during exercise in a female rower.

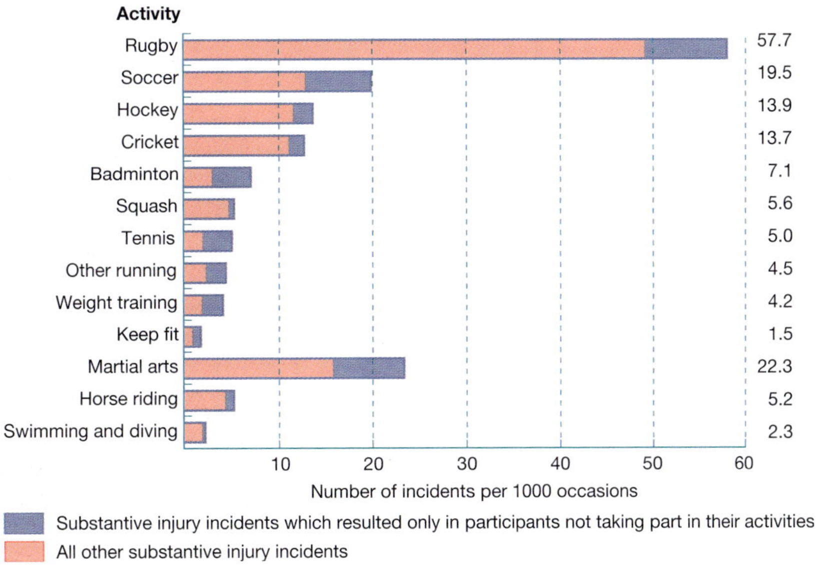

Plate 206 New substantive injury incident rates by activity in a random sample of 17 564 people aged between 16 and 45 in England and Wales (Nicholl et al. 1991).

Lifeso, R.M., Harder, E., and McCorkell, S.J. (1985). Spinal brucellosis. *The Journal of Bone and Joint Surgery* **67 B**, 345–51.

Lubani, M.M., Sharda, D.C., and Helin, I. (1986). Brucella arthritis in children. *Infection* **14**, 233–6.

Lubani, M.M, Dudin, K.I., Sharda, D.C., Mana Ndhar, D.S., Araj, G.F., Hafed, H.A., Al-Saleh, Q.A., Helin, I., and Salhi, M.M. (1989). A multicenter therapeutic study of 1100 children with brucellosis. *Pediatric Infectious Diseases Journal* **8**, 75–8.

Madkour, M.M., Sharif, H.S., Abed, M.Y., and Al-Fayez, M.A. (1988). Osteoarticular brucellosis: results of bone scintigraphy in 140 patients. *American Journal of Radiology* **150**, 1101–5.

Mousa, A.R., Elhag, K.M., Khogali, M., and Marafie, A.A. (1988). The nature of human brucellosis in Kuwait: study of 379 cases. *Reviews of Infectious Diseases* **10**, 211–17.

Navas, E., Guerrero, A., Cobo, J., and Loza, E. (1993). Faster isolation of Brucella spp. from blood by isolator compared with BACTEC NR. *Diagnostic Microbiology and Infectious Disease* **16**, 79–81.

Pellicer, T., Ariza, J., and Foz, A. (1988). Specific antibodies detected during relapse of human brucellosis. *The Journal of Infectious Diseases* **157**, 918–24.

Polt, S.S., Dismukes, W.E., Flint, A., and Schaefer, J. (1982). Human brucellosis caused by *Brucella canis*: clinical features and immune response. *Annals of Internal Medicine* **97**, 717–19.

Queipo-Ortuño, M.I. et al. (1997). Rapid diagnosis of human brucellosis by peripheral blood PCR essay. *Journal of Clinical Microbiolology* **35**, 2927–30.

Rodríguez Torres, A. (1988). Diagnóstico de la brucelosis humana. *Revista Española de Reumatología* **15**, 204–14.

Rotés Querol, J. (1957). Osteo-articular sites of brucellosis. *Annals of the Rheumatic Diseases* **16**, 63–8.

Serre, H., Kalea, G., Brousson, A., Sany, J., Bertrand, A., and Simon, L. (1981). Manifestations ostéo-articulaires de la brucellose. *Revue du Rhumatisme et des Maladies Ostéoarticulaires* **47**, 143–8.

Sharif, H.S., Aideyan, O.A., Clark, D.C., Madkour, M.M., Aabed, M.Y., Mattsson, T.A., al-Deeb, S.M., and Moutaery, K.R. (1989). Brucellar and tuberculous spondylitis: comparative imaging features. *Radiology* **171**, 419–25.

Solera, J., Martínez-Alfaro, E., and Saez, L. (1994). Metaanalisis sobre la eficacia de la combinacion de rifampicina y doxiciclina en al tratamiento de la brucelosis humana. *Medicina Clinica (Barcelona)* **102**, 731–8.

Spink, W.W. (1964). Host–parasite relationship in brucellosis. *Lancet* **ii**, 161–4.

Torres Rojas, J., Taddonio, R.F., and Sanders, C.V. (1979). Spondylitis caused by *Brucella abortus*. *Southern Medical Journal* **72**, 1166–9.

Verger, J.M., Grimont, F., Grimont, P.A.D., and Grayon, M. (1985). Brucella: a monospecific genus as shown by deoxyribonucleic acid hybridization. *International Journal of Systematic Bacteriology* **35**, 292–5.

Yagupsky, P. (1999). Detection of Brucellae in blood cultures. *Journal of Clinical Microbiology* **37**, 3437–42.

Young, E.J. (1995). Brucella species. In *Principles and Practice of Infectious Diseases* (ed. G.L. Mandell, J.E. Bennett, and R. Dolin), pp. 2053–60. New York: Churchill Livingstone.

6.2.9 Parasitic involvement

Yusuf I. Patel

Parasitism defines the relationship between two organisms, where the host provides both habitat and nourishment to the parasite. In order to establish itself within the environment of the host, the parasite must develop the ability to evade or tolerate the immune response of the host (Dogiel 1964; Zelmer 1998). Pathogenicity depends on a variety of factors including host fitness and parasitic virulence (Beverley 1996; Poulin and Combes 1999).

Immunity to parasites

Host immune responses to parasites are geared to eliminate the foreign organism, and include both innate and specific immune responses. Innate responses involve complement-mediated lysis and macrophage/neutrophil phagocytosis and killing. Some parasites evade complement-mediated lysis by altering surface molecules that bind complement or by acquiring host proteins that inhibit complement pathways (e.g. CD55, decay accelerating factor). The tegument of helminths makes them resistant to neutrophil and macrophage cytocidal mechanims.

Specific immune responses appear to segregate into two groups. Cellular immunity against protozoa mediated through $CD4^+$-driven macrophage activation or CTL (cytotoxic T-lymphocyte) responses, and antibody (IgE) or eosinophil (major basic protein) mediated defence against helminthic infections.

Immune responses against parasites may in fact produce some of the damage seen in the host. Examples include the fibrosis and granuloma formation in schistosomiasis, immune complex deposition in malaria and schistosomiasis, autoimmune myocarditis, and neuropathy in Chaga's disease caused by *Trypanosoma cruzi* (Abbas et al. 1997). Autoimmune disease in chronic parasitic infections may be associated with molecular mimicry (Abu-Shakra et al. 1999).

Parasites use a number of mechanisms to evade the host immune system. These are crucial adaptations in ensuring the survival of the species from the point of view of the parasite, but equally may contribute significantly to the pathology seen in the host.

The immune evasive mechanisms include:

Anatomic sequestration

- intracellular replication (malaria, toxoplasma),
- cyst formation (entamoeba),
- residence within the intestinal lumen (helminths).

Antigen masking

- parasite acquires surface coat of host proteins (schistosomiasis).

Antigenic variation

- antigenic shift with stages of parasitaemia (malaria),
- continuous variation of surface antigens (African trypanosomiasis).

Antigen shedding

- loss of surface antigen spontaneously or after antibody binding (*E. histolytica*, trypanosomes, schistosome larvae).

Resistance to host immune effector mechanisms

- development of tegument (resistant to antibodies, complement, or CTL attack),
- inhibition of complement (various mechanisms),
- resistance to phagocytosis (various mechanisms),
- resistance to antibody (production of ectoenzymes).

Parasitic infections are a particular problem in developing countries. In developed countries, they usually occur in isolated outbreaks or in people travelling to endemic areas (Weller 1992). An increased incidence of parasitic disease is found throughout the world amongst patients infected with human immunodeficiency virus (HIV) (Mannheimer and Sloave 1994).

Even in endemic areas, direct parasitic involvement of the musculoskeletal system is relatively rare. Systematic epidemiologic studies are lacking and therefore the true prevalence of rheumatic manifestations in parasitic infections remains unknown. No specific manifestations or rheumatic syndromes have been identified in association with parasitic infection. Diagnostic criteria for 'parastic rheumatism' have been suggested (Doury 1981, 1994), but due to a relatively low prevalence, together with other problems related to conducting epidemiologic studies in developing countries, there has not been a rigorous study of 'parasitic rheumatism' and its diagnostic criteria. Where data is available, the musculoskeletal manifestations are varied and the outcome usually very good either with or without therapy (Ferraccioli et al. 1988).

Parasitic infection as a cause of rheumatic disease is not frequently considered in the primary differential diagnosis. Factors that must alert the clinician to a parasitic association include:

- patients from endemic areas,
- travellers to endemic areas,
- elevation of eosinophil count,
- failure to respond to anti-inflammatory therapy.
- coincidental identification of parasitic infection in index patient.

Initiation of relevant investigations for parasitic infection depends on the clinician having a heightened level of awareness for the association of parasitic infection and musculoskeletal disease. An appropriate search for parasites and/or their immune phenomena may assist in making a diagnosis. This includes a search in blood, urine, and stool, and where appropriate, tissue for histological analysis (Garcia et al. 1995).

Direct identification of parasitic material in muscle, synovium, and bone has highlighted the role of parasitic infections in causing musculoskeletal disease. However, it is rare to find parasites at the site of pathology and this depends on the type of parasite involved. Parasitic material has been identified at the site of musculoskeletal pathology in cases with cysticercosis, gnathostomiasis, filariasis, Guinea worm infestation, hydatid disease, malaria, schistosomiasis, strongyloidiasis, toxocariasis, toxoplasmosis, trichinella infections, and trypanosomiasis. With the advent of molecular methods of identification of parasites, including specific polymerase chain reaction (PCR) techniques, the percentage of cases with identifiable 'parasitic material' may increase in future (Weiss 1995).

More often, rheumatic syndromes are associated as a remote manifestation accompanying a parasitic infection elsewhere in a given individual. In this case, parasitic material may be identified at a site remote from the musculoskeletal system, or immune phenomena may indicate the possibility of a parasitic infection. These include elevated blood eosinophils (usually with nematode infections), infiltration of eosinophils into tissue, specific antiparasitic antibodies, deposition of immune complexes, and signs of immune damage such as granuloma formation or fibrosis.

Parasites are broadly classified into two groups, protozoa and helminths. A wide variety of parasites from both groups have been associated with rheumatic manifestations (Tables 1 and 2). These include oligoarthritis, polyarthritis resembling rheumatoid arthritis, enthesitis, myositis and myopathic syndromes, and vasculitis either localized or systemic. However, no specific 'parasitic syndrome' has been identified, and the pathogenesis remains uncertain. Evidence exists for both direct parasitic involvement of musculoskeletal tissue as well as possible reactive arthritis or immune-mediated mechanisms causing the rheumatic manifestations.

The response to therapy is variable. Whilst some patients only require NSAID therapy to keep symptoms under control, others may need specific antiparasitic drugs or surgical removal of parasites (Tables 1 and 2). Complete resolution of symptoms and signs have been demonstrated with antiparasitic therapy, particularly where strong evidence of infection has been found. However, no systematic study has been performed to assess the need for antiparasitic therapy in all patients. As many of the antiparasitic drugs are relatively toxic, a trial of therapy in 'suspected cases' should not be undertaken lightly. However, where clinical suspicion is high, and if evidence exists for parasitic infestation, a trial of therapy should be undertaken under close supervision. Typically, therapeutic responses to antiparasitic therapy occurs where standard anti-inflammatory therapy and/or steroids have previously failed (Doury 1994). There are no long-term outcome studies to indicate the benefit of antiparasitic therapy for musculoskeletal manifestations of parasitic infections.

Table 1 Protozoa have been associated with a variety of musculoskeletal manifestations. Therapeutic choices and references of case reports or case series are indicated

Protozoa	Musculoskeletal manifestations	Therapy	Reference
Blastocystis hominis	Arthritis	Metronidazole, iodoquinol	Lee et al. (1990); Lakhanpal et al. (1991)
Cryptosporidium	Arthritis	Paromomycin	Hay et al. (1987)
Entamoeba histolytica	Arthralgia, arthritis, focal vasculitis	Metronidazole	Rappaport et al. (1951); Desphande et al. (1992)
Giardia lamblia	Arthritis, vasculitis	Metronidazole, tinidazole	Goobar (1977); Woo and Panayi (1984)
Isospora belli	Arthritis, myositis, vasculitis	Trimethoprim–sulfamethoxazole	McGill (1957); Jeffrey (1974); Gonzalez-Dominguez et al. (1994)
Microsporidia spp.	Myositis	Albendazole	Ledford et al. (1985)
Plasmodium spp.	Muscle necrosis, vasculitis	Chloroquine, quinine, others	De Silva et al. (1988); Swash and Scwartz (1993)
Toxoplasma gondii	Arthritis, myositis, vasculitis	Pyrimethamine and sulfadiazine	McNicholl and Underhill (1970); Antezana (1979); Topi et al. (1979); Balleari et al. (1991); Carmeni et al. (1991)
Trypanosoma spp. American—*cruzi* African—*rhodesiense, gambiense*	Myositis	Suramin, eflornithine, nifurtimox	Cossermelli et al. (1978)

Table 2 Helminth infections causing musculoskeletal manifestations are summarized, with therapeutic choices and selected references indicated

Helminth	Musculoskeletal manifestations	Therapy	References
Ancylostoma (*A. duodenale*)	Arthritis	Mebendazole	Bissonnette and Beaudet (1983)
Ascaris (*A. lumbricoides*)	Arthritis, vasculitis	Mebendazole	Treusch et al. (1981); Grcevska and Polenakovic (1993)
Coeneurosis (*Taenia multiceps*)	Nodules in subcutaneous tissue and muscle	Surgical excision	Templeton (1968)
Cysticercus (*Taenia solium*)	Arthralgia, myopathy, localized vasculitis	Albendazole, mebendazole	Serre et al. (1970); Estañol et al. (1986); Gupta et al. (1994)
Dirofilaria (*D. immitis, D. tenuis*)	Arthritis	Self-limiting	Corman (1987)
Dracunculus (*D. medinensis*)	Arthralgia, arthritis, myalgia	Metronidazole	McLaughlin et al. (1984); Garf (1985)
Filariae (*W. bancrofti, Loa Loa, O. volvulus*)	Arthralgia, arthritis, myalgia, vasculitis	Diethylcarbamazine, ivermectin	Alhadeff (1955); Carme et al. (1989)
Gnathostoma (*G. spinigerum*)	Soft tissue masses, nodular panniculitis	Albendazole, surgical excision	Rusnak and Lucey (1993); Stevens and Bryson (1994)
Hydatid (*Echinococcus* spp.)	Arthralgia, arthritis, myalgia, vasculitis, bone lesions	Albendazole, surgical excision	Fyfe et al. (1990); Buskila et al. (1992); Bakkaloglu et al. (1994)
Schistosoma (*Schistosome* spp.)	Arthralgia, arthritis, enthesitis, myopathy	Praziquantel	Bassiouni and Kamel (1984); Atkin et al. (1986)
Sparganosis (*Spirometra* spp.)	Soft tissue mass in muscle or subcutaneous tissue	Surgical excision	Cho and Patel (1978)
Strongyloides (*S. stercoralis*)	Arthralgia, arthritis, vasculitis	Thiabendazole	Bocanegra et al. (1981); Akoglu et al. (1984) Forzy et al. (1988)
Taenia (*T. saginata*)	Arthritis	Praziquantel	Bocanegra et al. (1981)
Toxocariasis (*T. canis, T. catis*)	Arthralgia, arthritis, panniculitis, myositis	Diethylcarbamazine, mebendazole	William and Roy (1981); Walsh et al. (1988)
Trichinosis (*Trichinella* spp.)	Myalgia, myositis, vasculitis	Mebendazole, albendazole	Frayha (1981); MacLean et al. (1989); Durán-Ortiz et al. (1992)
Trichuris (*T. trichiura*)	Arthritis	Mebendazole	Treusch et al. (1981)

In addition to uncertainty related to outcome measures, there is the possibility of exacerbating musculoskeletal symptoms on initiation of antiparasitic therapy. This is more of a problem when treating tissue invasive parasites, and varies with type of parasite, parasite load, and the drug used (Bocanegra 1998). 'Start low and go slow' should help avoid most major complications of therapy but there may be a need for concomitant steroids particularly in the Mazzotti reaction described in the treatment of filariasis with diethylcarbazine or ivermectin (Ottesen 1987; Kumaraswami et al. 1988).

References

Abbas, A.K., Lichtman, A.H., and Pober, J.S. *Cellular and Molecular Immunology* 3rd edn. Philadelphia PA: W.B. Saunders Company, 1997.

Abu-Shakra, M., Buskila, D., and Shoenfeld, Y. (1999). Molecular mimicry between host and pathogen: examples from parasites and implication. *Immunology Letters* **67**, 147–52.

Akoglu, T. et al. (1984). Parasitic arthritis induced by *Strongyloides stercoralis*. *Annals of the Rheumatic Diseases* **43**, 523–5.

Alhadeff, R. (1955). Clinical aspects of filariasis. *Journal of Tropical Medicine and Hygiene* **58**, 173–9.

Antezana, E. (1979). Polytenosynovitis caused by *Toxoplasma gondii*. *South African Medical Journal* **56**, 746.

Atkin, S.L. et al. (1986). Schistosomiasis and inflammatory polyarthritis: a clinical, radiological and laboratory study of 96 patients infected by *S. mansoni* with particular reference to the diarthrodial joint. *Quarterly Journal of Medicine* **59**, 479–87.

Bakkaloglu, A. et al. (1994). A possible relationship between polyarteritis nodosa and hydatid disease. *European Journal of Paediatrics* **153**, 469.

Balleari, E., Cutolo, M., and Accardo, S. (1991). Adult-onset Still's disease associated with *Toxoplasma gondii* infection. *Clinical Rheumatology* **10**, 326–7.

Bassiouni, M. and Kamel, M. (1984). Bilharzial arthropathy. *Annals of the Rheumatic Diseases* **43**, 806–9.

Beverley, S.M. (1996). Hijacking the cell: parasites in the driver's seat. *Cell* **87**, 787–9.

Bissonnette, B. and Beaudet, F. (1983). Reactive arthritis with eosinophilic synovial infiltrations. *Annals of the Rheumatic Diseases* **42**, 466–8.

Bocanegra, T.S. et al. (1981). Reactive arthritis induced by parasitic infestation. *Annals of Internal Medicine* **94**, 207–9.

Bocanegra, T.S. (1998). Parasitic involvement. In *Oxford Textbook of Rheumatology* 2nd edn. (ed. P.J. Maddison et al.), pp. 945–54. Oxford: Oxford University Press.

Buskila, D. et al. (1992). Polyarthritis associated with hydatid disease (echinococcosis) of the liver. *Clinical Rheumatology* **11**, 286–7.

Carme, B. et al. (1989). Clinical and biological study of Loa-Loa filariasis in Congolese. *American Journal of Tropical Medicine and Hygiene* **41**, 331–7.

Carmeni, G. et al. (1991). Vascular involvement and toxoplasma infection. *British Journal of Dermatology* **124**, 14.

Cho, C. and Patel, S.P. (1978). Human Sparganosis in northern United States. *New York State Journal of Medicine* **78**, 1456–8.

Corman, L.C. (1987). Acute arthritis occurring in association with subcutaneous *Dirofilaria tenuis* infection. *Arthritis and Rheumatism* **30**, 1431–4.

Cossermelli, W. et al. (1978). Polymyositis in Chaga's disease. *Annals of the Rheumatic Diseases* **37**, 277–80.

De Silva, H.J. et al. (1988). Skeletal muscle necrosis in severe falciparum malaria. *British Medical Journal* **296**, 1039.

Desphande, R.B. et al. (1992). Necrotising arteritis in amoebic colitis. *Journal of Postgraduate Medicine* **38**, 151–2.

Dogiel, V.A. *General Parasitology*. London: Oliver and Boyd, 1964.

Doury, P. (1981). Parasitic rheumatism (letter). *Arthritis and Rheumatism* **24**, 638–9.

Doury, P. (1994). Parasitic arthritis and parasitic rheumatism. *Semaine des Hospitaux Paris* **7**, 522–8.

Durán-Ortiz, J.S. et al. (1992). Trichinosis with severe myopathic involvement mimicking polymyositis. Report of a family outbreak. *Journal of Rheumatology* **19**, 310–12.

Estañol, B., Corona, T., and Abad, P. (1986). A prognostic classification of cerebral cysticercosis: therapeutic implications. *Journal of Neurology, Neurosurgery and Psychiatry* **49**, 1131–4.

Ferraccioli, G.F. et al. (1988). Prospective rheumatological study of muscle and joint symptoms during *Trichinella nelsoni* infection. *Quarterly Journal of Medicine* **69**, 973–84.

Forzy, G. et al. (1988). Reactive arthritis and strongyloides. *Journal of the American Medical Association* **259**, 2546–7.

Frayha, R.A. (1981). Trichinosis related polyarteritis nodosa. *American Journal of Medicine* **71**, 307–12.

Fyfe, B. et al. (1990). Intra-osseous echinococcosis: a rare manifestation of echinococcal disease. *Southern Medical Journal* **83**, 66–8.

Garcia, L.S. et al. (1995). Diagnosis of parasitic infections: collection, processing and examination of specimens. In *Manual of Clinical Microbiology* 6th edn. (ed. P.R. Murray et al.), pp. 1145–58. Washington DC: ASM Press.

Garf, A.E. (1985). Parasitic rheumatism: rheumatic manifestations associated with calcified Guinea worm. *Journal of Rheumatology* **12**, 976–9.

Gonzalez-Dominguez, J. et al. (1994). *Isospora belli* reactive arthritis in a patient with AIDS. *Annals of the Rheumatic Diseases* **53**, 618–19.

Goobar, J.P. (1977). Joint symptoms in Giardiasis. *Lancet* **i**, 1010–11.

Grcevska, L. and Polenakovic, M. (1993). Renal vasculitis associated with ascaridiasis and good prognosis. *Nephron* **64**, 327–8.

Gupta, P.K. et al. (1994). Unusual clinical manifestations of cysticercosis. *Journal of the Association of Physicians of India* **42**, 411–12.

Hay, E.M., Windfield, J., and McKendrick, M.W. (1987). Reactive arthritis associated with cryptosporidium enteritis. *British Medical Journal* **295**, 248.

Jeffrey, H.C. (1974). Sarcosporidiosis in man. *Transactions of the Royal Society for Tropical Medicine and Hygiene* **68**, 17–29.

Kumaraswami, V. et al. (1988). Ivermectin for the treatment of *Wuchereria bancrofti* filariasis: efficacy and adverse reactions. *Journal of the American Medical Association* **259**, 3150–3.

Lakhanpal, S., Cohen, S.B., and Fleischmann, R.M. (1991). Reactive arthritis from *Blastocystis hominis*. *Arthritis and Rheumatism* **34**, 251–3.

Ledford, D.K. et al. (1985). Microsporidiosis myositis in a patient with the acquired immunodeficiency syndrome. *Annals of Internal Medicine* **102**, 628–30.

Lee, M.G. et al. (1990). Infective arthritis due to *Blastocystis hominis*. *Annals of the Rheumatic Diseases* **49**, 192–3.

MacLean, J.D. et al. (1989). Trichinosis in the Canadian arctic: report of five outbreaks and a new clinical syndrome. *Journal of Infectious Diseases* **160**, 513–20.

Mannheimer, S.B. and Sloave, R. (1994). Protozoal infections in patients with AIDS. Cryptosporidiosis, isosporiasis, cyclosporiasis, and microsporidiosis. *Infectious Disease Clinics of North America* **8**, 483.

McGill, R.J. (1957). Sarcosporidiosis in a man with polyarteritis nodosa. *British Medical Journal* **2**, 333–4.

McLaughlin, G.E. et al. (1984). Rheumatic syndromes secondary to Guinea worm infestation. *Arthritis and Rheumatism* **27**, 694–7.

McNicholl, B. and Underhill, D. (1970). Toxoplasmic polymyositis. *Irish Journal of Medical Science* **3**, 525–7.

Ottesen, E.A. (1987). Description of mechanisms and control of reactions to treatment in the human filariases. *Ciba Foundation Symposium* **127**, 265–83.

Poulin, R. and Combes, C. (1999). The concept of virulence: interpretations and implications. *Parasitology Today* **15** (12), 474–5.

Rappaport, E.M., Rossien, A., and Roseblum, L. (1951). Arthritis due to intestinal amoebiasis. *Annals of Internal Medicine* **34**, 1224–31.

Rusnak, J.M. and Lucey, D.R. (1993). Clinical gnathostomiasis: a case report and review of the English language literature. *Clinics in Infectious Diseases* **16**, 33–50.

Serre, H. et al. (1970). Muscular manifestations of human cysticercosis. *Rheumatologie* **22**, 537–63.

Stevens, C.O. and Bryson, A.D. (1994). Gnathostomiasis as a cause of soft tissue swellings. *British Journal of Rheumatology* **33** (Suppl. 65), 36.

Swash, M. and Scwartz, M.S. (1993). Malaria myositis. *Journal of Neurology, Neurosurgery and Psychiatry* **56**, 1238.

Templeton, A.C. (1968). Human coeneurosis: a report of 14 cases from Uganda. *Transactions of the Royal Society for Tropical Medicine and Hygiene* **62**, 251–5.

Topi, G.C. et al. (1979). Dermatomyositis-like syndrome due to toxoplasma. *British Journal of Dermatology* **101**, 589–91.

Treusch, P.J., Swatnam, R.E., and Woelke, B.J. (1981). Eosinophilic joint effusion and intestinal nematodiasis. *Annals of Emergency Medicine* **10**, 614–15.

Walsh, S.S., Robson, W.J., and Hart, C.A. (1988). Acute transient myositis due to Toxocara. *Archives of Diseases in Childhood* **63**, 1087–8.

Weiss, J.B. (1995). DNA probes and PCR for diagnosis of parasitic infections. *Clinical Microbiology Reviews* **8**, 113.

Weller, P.F. (1992). Eosinophilia in travelers. *Medical Clinics of North America* **76**, 1413.

William, D. and Roy, S. (1981). Arthritis and arthralgia associated with Toxocaral infestation. *British Medical Journal* **283**, 192.

Woo, P. and Panayi, G.S. (1984). Reactive arthritis due to infestation with *Giardia lamblia*. *Journal of Rheumatology* **11**, 719.

Zelmer, D.A. (1998). An evolutionary definition of parasitism. *International Journal for Parasitology* **28**, 531–3.

6.2.10 Fungal arthritis

Carol A. Kemper and Stanley C. Deresinski

Introduction

Fungal infection of joints is an uncommon but challenging clinical problem whose recognition and management is often belated. The initial challenge to the clinician is in making the distinction between these infrequently encountered cases of fungal joint infection and other infections or inflammatory processes. A high degree of suspicion for fungal infection must be maintained in the face of persistent monoarticular or, less commonly, asymmetric polyarticular, arthritis, especially in an immune suppressed host. Fungal joint infection most often results from the haematogenous dissemination of the pathogen from a primary portal of infection (usually pulmonary) directly to the synovial tissue or occurs as the result of infection of para-articular bone with subsequent rupture into a joint space. Less commonly, such infection occurs as the result of direct inoculation of the organism into the joint space or synovial tissue. An inflammatory, aseptic arthritis may also occur in association with certain fungal infections (e.g. coccidioidomycosis, histoplasmosis) as a consequence of the immune response to the organism, rather than a result of infection of the joint space itself.

Epidemiology

Only a handful of fungi, perhaps five or six species at most, are responsible for most human mycotic musculoskeletal infections (Bradsher 1988; Fader and McGinnis 1988; Cuellar et al. 1992, 1993) (Table 1), but virtually all of the approximately 100 fungi pathogenic in man have been reported, at one time or another, to cause infection of bones and/or joints. The frequency with which fungal arthritis occurs, its clinical presentation, and its outcome varies depending on the specific pathogen as well as upon host variables. For example, fungal arthritis due to the endemic dimorphic fungi, such as *Histoplasmosis capsulatum*, *Blastomycosis dermatiditis*, and *Coccidioides immitis*, is often seen in patients without overt immunodeficiency. In contrast, infection due to *Candida* species is usually found in association with intravascular infection in individuals with readily apparent host factors, such as those with indwelling central venous catheters (often in association with the administration of long-term antibiotic therapy and/or parenteral nutrition), or those undergoing haemodialysis, or in intravenous drug users. Defects in cellular immunity are critical to the dissemination of certain fungi from their initial portal of infection and the secondary infection of joint spaces. Patients with haematologic malignancy, haematopoietic and organ transplant recipients, and those receiving long-term corticosteroids and immunosuppressive therapy are especially at risk for fungal arthritis due to *Candida*. On the other hand, persons with advanced HIV infection are especially vulnerable to disseminated infection, with occasional complicating fungal arthritis, due to *Cryptococcus neoformans* and *C. immitis*, whereas candidal joint space infection is rare in these patients.

Rarely, joint infection occurs secondary to direct inoculation of the organism into the joint during aspiration or injection, trauma, or surgical intervention. Human-to-human transmission of these mycoses does not, for all practical purposes, occur.

Unlike the other fungi, infection with *C. albicans* and related yeasts is ordinarily the consequence of host invasion by endogenous colonizing organisms. In contrast, exposure to *B. dermatiditis*, *C. immitis*, *H. capsulatum*, or *Paracoccidioides brasiliensis* primarily occurs because of exposure within an endemic area (see Table 1). *C. immitis* is limited to endemic zones in North, Central, and South America, while *H. capsulatum* is found in areas of both hemispheres, often in association with avian and chiropteran habitats. *B. dermatiditis* is most often acquired in the United States. *P. brasiliensis* is found in Central and South America, although rare cases have been described in North America. For each of these four dimorphic fungi, inhalation of conidia or arthroconidia released by the mycelial phase of the organism results in a primary pulmonary infection that is either sub-acute or acute, and typically self-limited, or that, in some cases, becomes chronic. Secondary dissemination of each of these infections during the acute or chronic phase of pulmonary infection results, with a varying frequency, in clinical joint space infection. Two of the more common fungi found in joint space infections, *C. neoformans* and *Sporothrix schenckii*, have a worldwide distribution.

Clinical picture

The clinical presentation of joint infection is generally indolent, although the onset of some infections, such as those due to *B. dermatiditis*, *Candida* species, and, occasionally, other fungi, may be acute, with hot, erythematous, and tender joints and accompanying fever. The presentation may thus resemble an acute bacterial septic arthritis. Most cases, however, present with the usual findings of monoarticular (or, occasionally, asymmetric

Table 1 Risk factors for infection and the clinical setting of fungal joint infection

Organism	Endemicity	Host risk factors	Mode of infection	Joint Involvement
Candida spp.	Normal human commensal	Haematological malignancy, immunodeficiency, neonates, indwelling catheters, central catheters, long-term antibiotic use, exogenous steroids	Haematogenous, rarely direct inoculation from trauma or injections	Monoarticular; predominately large joints (knee 70%)
Coccidioides immitis	Arizona, New Mexico, California	Usually immunocompetent host	Haematogenous	Monoarticular (>90%); predominately knee and ankle
Blastomyces dermatitidis	Ohio, Missouri, Mississippi river valley, south-eastern United States, Africa, Middle East	Usually immunocompetent host (>90%)	Haematogenous, rarely direct inoculation	Monoarticular (>90%); knee, ankle, elbow, and wrist
Sporothrix schenkii	Worldwide	Alcoholic, diabetic, rarely severely immunocompromised	Haematogenous, may be direct inoculation	Monoarticular (50%), polyarticular (50%); knee, ankle, wrist, small joints of the hand
Histoplasma capsulatum	Ohio, Missouri, Mississippi river valleys, Central and South America	Both normal and immuno-deficient hosts (e.g. AIDS)	Haematogenous	Monoarticular; knee, wrist, small joints of the hand
Cryptococcus neoformans	Worldwide	Organ transplant, AIDS haematological malignancy, diabetes, exogenous steroids	Haematogenous	Monoarticular (65%), polyarticular (35%); knee (60%), ankle, wrist, sterno/acromial-clavicular
Paracoccidioides brasiliensis	Central and South America	Immunocompetent host	Haematogenous	

polyarticular) arthritis with decreased range of motion, tenderness, and swelling. There is often evidence of joint effusion; but in some cases of chronic infection due to *C. immitis*, joint swelling may be due to synovial proliferation rather than the accumulation of fluid. The initial list of differential diagnoses may therefore be quite broad, and includes septic arthritis, rheumatoid arthritis, mycobacterial infection, brucellosis, and pigmented villonodular synovitis. While fungal arthritis may present in the setting of widespread fungal infection, in many instances there is little clinical evidence of extra-articular infection. Large weight-bearing joints, particularly the knee, are the usual targets.

Roentgenographic examination generally reveals evidence of joint effusion. Other findings that may be seen with varied frequency, depending upon the aetiology, host factors, and the chronicity of the infection, include erosion of juxta-articular cortex, osteoporosis, and associated para-articular osteomyelitis. These radiographic findings are also common to those found in tuberculosis, rheumatoid arthritis, sarcoidosis, metastatic neoplasm, eosinophilic granuloma, and pigmented villonodular synovitis.

Clinically important information about joint integrity and the presence of otherwise unapparent para-articular osteomyelitis may be provided by magnetic resonance imaging that has greater sensitivity and resolution than other conventional techniques (see Chapter 5.6.1). However, the role of this modality in the clinical evaluation and management of fungal arthritis has not been critically evaluated. Nuclear medicine techniques, such as scanning after injection of technetium pyrophosphate, may serve to confirm clinical evidence of joint inflammation [see Fig. 1(a)].

Synovial fluid examination reveals an elevated white blood cell count. Although candidal and blastomycotic joint infections typically present with frankly purulent synovial fluid with a predominance of polymorphonuclear leucocytes, the other fungi often cause lesser degrees of inflammation with lower cell counts and variable predominance of either polymorphonuclear leucocytes or lymphocytes. The protein concentration is usually in excess of 3.0 gm/dl while the glucose concentration is low to normal. Routine direct examination (e.g. Gram stain) usually does not reveal the organism, but cytologic preparations are useful in the diagnosis of blastomycosis,

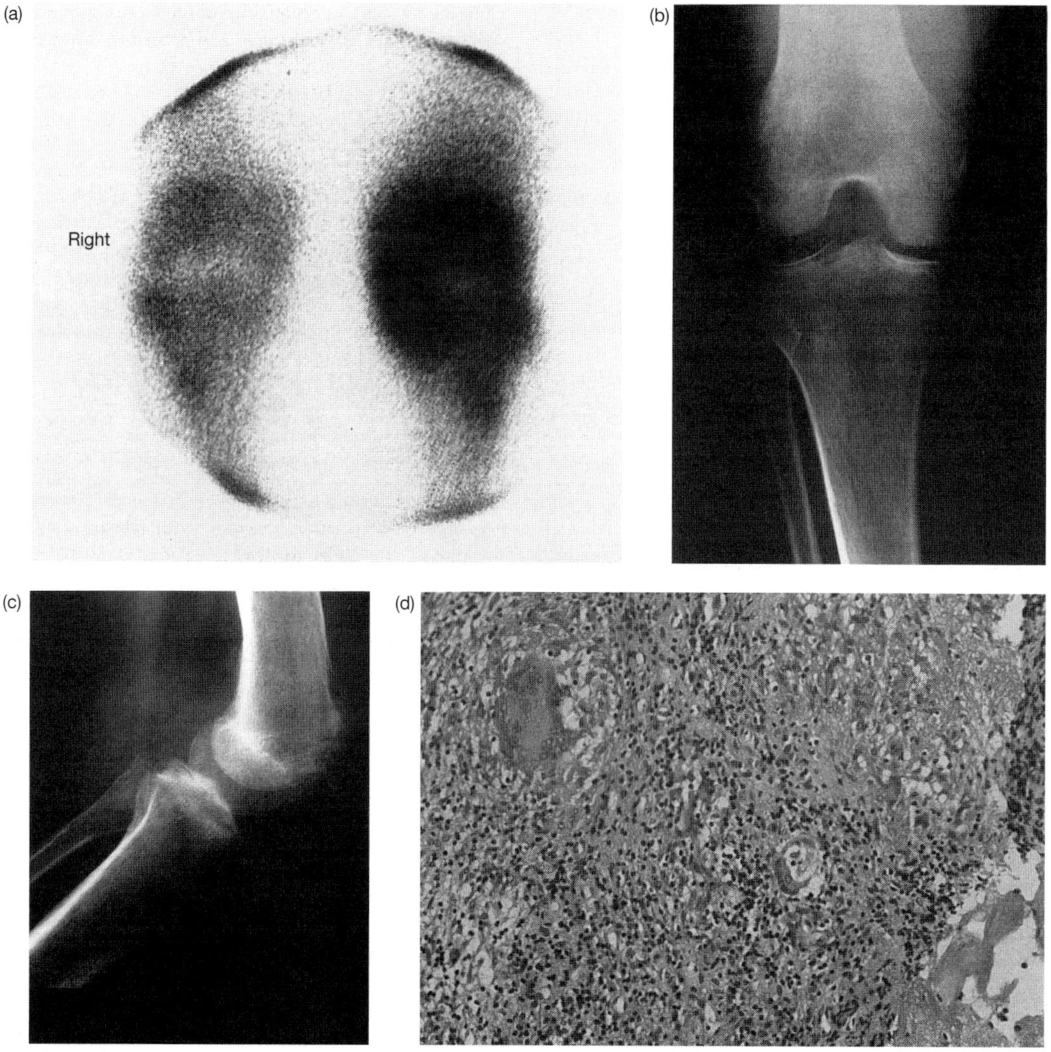

Fig. 1 (a) Bone scintigraphy, using technetium-99M, demonstrating intense uptake of the radionuclide in the left knee of a patient with synovitis due to *Sporothrix schenckii*. (b) and (c) Roentgenographs of the left knee demonstrating only patchy osteopaenia of the distal femur and proximal tibia from the same patient. (d) Granulomatous reaction with typical giant cells of synovium obtained from the same patient. Organisms were not visualized with this stain or with Gomori-methamine silver or PAS stains and the diagnosis was made by recovery of the organism in culture from the synovial tissue. Haematoxylin and eosin, original magnification ×200 (courtesy of Jesse Hofflin).

cryptococcus, and, to a lesser degree, coccidioidomycosis. Culture of synovial fluid or synovial tissue usually yields the organism. Synovial tissue histopathology is variable and often non-specific, such as in infection due to *S. schenckii* in which the organisms are few and difficult to visualize. A granulomatous reaction is most commonly observed and the resulting differential diagnosis that must be considered includes fungal infection, brucellosis, mycobacterial infection, syphilis, protothecosis, rheumatoid arthritis, pigmented villonodular synovitis, sarcoidosis, Crohn's disease, foreign body reaction, gout, pseudogout, and oxalosis.

The use of additional diagnostic procedures, such as blood cultures, bone marrow examination and culture, antibody tests, or tests for the detection of fungal antigen in serum or other body fluids, depend upon the clinical setting and the suspected aetiology. Tests of delayed dermal hypersensitivity to fungal antigens are generally not useful for diagnostic purposes.

Some infections may cause tenosynovitis in the absence of osteomyelitis or arthritis. Tenosynovitis may occur as the result of haematogenous dissemination or of direct inoculation, and is most often associated with *S. schenkii* infection, as well as, to lesser degrees, with infections due to *C. immitis* and *C. neoformans*.

During the primary pulmonary infection with *C. immitis*, an acute self-limited arthritis or periarthritis, commonly referred to as 'desert rheumatism', may be seen in association with erythema nodosum, erythema multiforme, and occasionally hilar adenopathy. Thus, the clinical picture may resemble sarcoidosis. An immunologic process, probably immune complex deposition, is thought to be aetiologic. Acute aseptic inflammatory arthritis may also be seen in histoplasmosis, as well as in acute blastomycosis.

Management

Amphotericin B remains the initial therapeutic agent of choice for many serious fungal infections, especially for those who are severely immune suppressed, have life-threatening or central nervous system disease, or who have failed azole therapy. Lipid-associated or -complexed formulations of amphotericin allow the administration of higher dosages of drug with less toxicity than the conventional formulation, although the relative efficacy of these agents in fungal skeletal infection is unproven. The triazoles, fluconazole and itraconazole, have greatly added to our ability to treat fungal infections, especially in the outpatient setting, with similar efficacy but reduced toxicity and morbidity than that of Amphotericin B. A newer azole, voriconazole, was recently introduced. In addition, the first of a series of echinocandin antifungal agents, caspofungin, may prove to have a role in the treatment of selected infections. Despite this expanded armamentarium, some infections remain recalcitrant to therapy.

Amphotericin B, administered intravenously, penetrates into synovial fluid to some extent. While some authors have advocated directly injecting or irrigating the joint space with Amphotericin B, the necessity for this mode of therapy is unproven, and there is concern that a chemical synovitis and articular damage may result. The toxicities of amphotericin are well known and include fever, chills, nausea, vomiting, hypotension, renal dysfunction, hypokalaemia, and hypomagnesaemia. The renal toxicity is frequently dose limiting.

Fluorocytosine (5-FC) enters susceptible fungal cells through a specific permease system and is then converted to 5-fluorouracil. It has a narrow spectrum of activity that includes most *Candida* species as well as *C. neoformans*. In most instances, 5-FC is not administered as a single agent because of the possibility of the development of drug resistance during therapy. The drug penetrates well into all body fluids, including synovial fluid, and is renally excreted. The major toxicity, bone marrow suppression and resultant cytopaenias, is directly related to serum concentrations in excess of 100 μg/ml. Serum concentrations of 5-FC should be closely monitored during administration, and dose adjustments must be made in the presence of changing renal function.

The azoles, such as fluconazole, itraconazole, ketoconazole, and miconazole, inhibit the C-14 demethylation of lanosterol, thus impairing fungal cell membrane assembly. They have variable pharmacokinetic, toxicity, and antifungal profiles. The intravenous form of miconazole has limited utility because of toxicity, and unfavourable pharmacokinetics; its use is now limited (on an emergency basis) for severe infections due to *Pseudoallescheria boydii*.

Fluconazole is a water-soluble bis-triazole with a high degree of oral bioavailability and the ability to penetrate into body fluids, including synovial fluid, where it achieves concentrations similar to those in serum (O'Meeghan et al. 1990). It has efficacy in a variety of fungal infections including those due to most *Candida* species (*C. krusei* is always resistant), *H. capsulatum*, *B. dermatiditis*, *C. neoformans*, and *C. immitis*. Both oral and parenteral formulations are available. Dose adjustment is required in the presence of renal insufficiency. Drug interactions occur with phenytoin, rifampicin, and rifabutin, as well as with astemizole and terfenadine. Hepatic toxicity is rare; steroid hormone synthesis is not affected.

Another bis-triazole, itraconazole, has a broader spectrum of activity than either fluconazole or ketoconazole. It is approved by the US Food and Drug Administration (FDA) for use in both blastomycosis and histoplasmosis, and is also very active against *S. schenkii* and most *Aspergillus* species, as well as *Candida* species, Trichophyton, and the *dematiaceous* fungi. Itraconazole is variably absorbed after oral administration, and elimination is non-renal. Body fluid penetration is less than that of fluconazole. Cortisol synthesis is not impaired by itraconazole. Pharmacokinetic interaction with cyclosporin occurs, as well as with a number of other drugs metabolized by the hepatic cytochrome P450 system; the same precautions regarding drug interactions should be observed with itraconazole as with ketoconazole. Gastrointestinal side-effects are common. Although there is some disagreement whether or not serum concentrations of itraconazole correlate with therapeutic outcome, itraconazole, which requires stomach acid for absorption, should not be administered to patients who are receiving antacids, H-2 blockers, or those who have achlorhydria, unless adequate serum levels can be demonstrated. The newer formulation as an oral suspension overcomes these barriers to some extent, providing better absorption. A parenteral formulation of the drug is also now available.

Ketoconazole was the first of the azoles available for oral administration, although fluconazole and itraconazole have largely replaced its use. Its spectrum of activity is similar to that of fluconazole but has less favourable pharmacokinetics and more frequent drug interactions. Similar to itraconzole, absorption is impaired in the absence of gastric acid.

One of the newer azoles, voriconazole, which has a spectrum of activity similar to that of itraconazole, is available in both oral and parenteral formulations. Similar to itraconazole, voriconazole is solubilized for i.v. administration by use of a cyclodextran base. Caspofungin, the first of the echinocandins (drugs that inhibit 1,3-β-D-glucan synthase), has received FDA approval for salvage therapy for *Aspergillus*. It is thus far available only in parenteral form. Combinations of antifungal agents may be effective in certain infections. For example, *in vitro* studies suggest that combinations of terbenafine with azoles may be beneficial in treating certain infections, such as *Aspergillus*. Similarly, caspofungin and Amphotericin B may be synergistic against some fungi. Finally, adjunctive therapy with immune modulators, such as granulocyte-macrophage colony-stimulating factor or interferon-γ, may be useful in certain patients with more severe disease or immune deficiency.

Individual mycoses

Aspergillus

Various species of *Aspergillus* have rarely resulted in joint space infection, often associated with contiguous osteomyelitis (Denning and Stevens 1990). Severely immune suppressed hosts, such as those with haematopoetic and organ transplants, as well as those with chronic granulomatous disease, are at greatest risk for *Aspergillus* infection. Clinically apparent pulmonary infection is present in two-thirds of subjects with disseminated aspergillus, although a recent report described two patients suffering from graft versus host disease with aspergillus knee joint involvement, one of which was largely asymptomatic and not associated with other signs of systemic infection (Panigrahi et al. 2001). Haematogenous dissemination of the organism is implicated in most cases, although introduction of the organism into the joint space has occurred during surgical or arthroscopic procedures, or as a result of trauma.

While Amphotericin B remains the treatment of choice for life-threatening invasive *Aspergillus* infection, itraconazole, voriconazole, or caspofungin may be useful alternatives in certain cases.

Blastomycosis

Blastomycosis is an uncommonly encountered mycotic infection primarily endemic to parts of the Midwestern, Southeastern, and Appalachian areas of the United States (see Table 1). *B. dermatiditis* is a thermal dimorph whose mycelial phase is thought to reside in soil. Conversion to the yeast phase occurs after inhalation of spores. Primary pulmonary infection may be acute, sub-acute, or sub-clinical, but is usually self-limited; chronic infections are unusual. Haematogenous dissemination is relatively frequent during the initial phase of the disease, leading to infection at almost any body site. While skin and bones are the most frequent sites of dissemination (25–60 per cent), only 2.5–8 per cent of patients develop joint infection (McDonald et al. 1990). Those patients with particularly severe pulmonary disease, miliary involvement, or those who are immune compromised are at the greatest risk for dissemination (Sarosi and Davies 1981; Recht et al. 1982). Endogenous reactivation, which usually occurs within the first 2–3 years of the initial pulmonary infection, is rare. Very rarely, joint infection is the result of direct inoculation secondary to trauma.

While many patients with progressive or disseminated disease due to *B. dermatiditis* suffer from potentially predisposing conditions, such as diabetes, alcoholism, renal failure, and malignancy, this organism is not generally considered an opportunistic pathogen. Recht and colleagues described 78 patients with blastomycosis, six (13 per cent) of whom were immune compromised, none, however, due to T-lymphocyte dysfunction (Recht et al. 1982). Those six patients had a similar clinical presentation and therapeutic response as the remaining patients who were not immune suppressed. Nevertheless, rapidly progressive and unusually severe disease has been reported in patients with profoundly impaired immunity, such as transplant recipients and those with AIDS (Davies and Sarosi 1991).

Myalgias and arthralgias are common during the acute pulmonary phase of the disease, but erythema nodosum is not. A reactive arthritis, similar to that seen with coccidioidomycosis, has been reported (Berger and Kraman 1981).

The arthritis is monoarticular in more than 95 per cent of cases with the knee most commonly involved, followed by the ankle, elbow, and wrist (see Table 2). Infrequent reports describe patients with initial monoarticular infection with the subsequent development of polyarthritic disease (Abril et al. 1998). Joint pain is often acute in onset and patients usually appear toxic. In contrast to coccidioidal arthritis, active pulmonary disease is present in more than 90 per cent of patients with joint involvement, and more than 70 per cent have evidence of additional dissemination to cutaneous or subcutaneous sites. In contrast to those with candidal or sporotrichal arthritis, less than one-third of patients have roentgenographic evidence of juxta-articular osteomyelitis.

Synovial fluid findings are similar to those seen in candida arthritis. The fluid is usually cloudy or frankly purulent with white blood cell counts that may exceed 100 000/mm^3 and with a predominance of polymorphonuclear leucocytes. The concentration of protein in the synovial fluid exceeds 3.0 g/dl while the glucose is low to normal. Cytologic examination of synovial fluid may be more sensitive in detecting the organism than is culture. The organism may also be recovered in culture or visualized on histopathology from synovial biopsy specimens. Histopathological examination of infected synovium reveals prominent polymorphonuclear leucocytes, often with microabscesses and occasional granulomata.

While most patients with acute self-limited pulmonary blastomycosis have demonstrable delayed dermal hypersensitivity to blastomycin, this reactivity wanes over time and is not of diagnostic value. Available serologic tests have been disappointing with both false negative and positive results commonly seen.

Amphotericin B remains the drug of choice for many patients, particularly those who are critically ill, have central nervous system disease, who are immunosuppressed, or who are experiencing progressive disease despite appropriate azole therapy (Bradsher 1988). The total dose required is usually 1.0–2.0 g. Limited data suggest that lipid-complexed Amphotericin B may

Table 2 Clinical and laboratory data helpful in the diagnosis of fungal joint infection

Organism	Serology	Synovial fluid white blood cell count	Synovial glucose	Synovial fluid examination	Cultures
Candida spp.	Not useful	Frankly purulent, <100 000/mm^3	Variable, low to normal	20% positive	Blood and/or synovial fluid, >95% positive
Coccidioides immitis	Complement fixation, immunodiffusion diagnostic	<50 000/mm^3, mononuclear cells	Low	Rarely positive	Synovial fluid, >95% positive
Blastomyces dermatitidis	Low sensitivity, low specificity	Frankly purulent, < 100 000/mm^3 polymorphonuclear	Variable, low to normal	By cytological preparation, 88% positive	Synovial fluid, 50% positive
Sporothrix schenkii	Not available	2000–60 000/mm^3 lymphocytes and polymorphonuclear	Variable, low to normal	Rarely positive	Synovial tissue more often positive than synovial fluid
Histoplasma capsulatum	Complement fixation, immunodiffusion diagnostic			Not helpful	Blood and/or synovial fluid, 20–25% positive
Cryptococcus neoformans	Cryptococcal antigen diagnostic	200–5000/mm^3, no particular cellular predominance	Variable, usually normal	India ink very helpful	Blood and/or synovial fluid, >80% positive
Paracoccidioides brasiliensis	Serum antibody			Not helpful	Usually positive, slow growth (longer than 4 weeks)

be useful. In patients with joint infection and otherwise stable disease, itraconazole is recommended (approximate 90 per cent response rate) (Chapman et al. 2000). The usual starting dose is 200 mg once daily, increasing to 400 mg daily as necessary. Therapy should be continued for approximately 6 months.

Ketoconazole also has some efficacy in patients without meningeal disease who are not severely immunocompromised (Bradsher 1988). Fluconazole does not appear to be nearly as effective as itraconazole in the treatment of blastomycosis.

Candida species

Candida albicans is a normal commensal of man and endogenous colonization is the source of most infections by *Candida* species. *Candida* species that have been implicated in septic arthritis include *C. albicans, Candida tropicalis, Candida parapsilosis, Torulopsis* (*Candida*) *glabrata*, and, less commonly, *Candida guilliermondii, Candida krusei*, and *Candida zeylanoides*. Deep tissue infection generally occurs after amplification of colonization during an intervening immunodeficient state or during administration of broad-spectrum antibacterial therapy coupled with breaches in integumentary and mucosal barriers. *Candida* infection of joints is typically the consequence of haematogenous dissemination (often from indwelling intravenous catheters in predisposed immunodeficient hosts or in intravenous drug users) (Marina et al. 1991). Joints previously afflicted by rheumatoid arthritis appear to be at increased risk of infection with candidal organisms. Less commonly, joint infection occurs secondary to direct inoculation of the organism into the joint during aspiration or injection of corticosteroids, trauma, or surgical intervention (including simple arthrotomy) (see Table 1). Immunocompromise due to HIV infection does not appear to predispose to disseminated candidiasis or to candida arthritis, except in those who use parenteral drugs (Munoz-Fernandez et al. 1991).

In contrast to many of the other fungal joint infections discussed here, the onset of disease due to *Candida* species is acute in approximately two-thirds of cases. The remaining patients present with less acute disease, except for those few remarkably indolent presentations. The large joints are most commonly affected.

Synovial fluid examination demonstrates a markedly elevated white blood cell count (15 000–100 000 cells/mm^3) with a predominance of polymorphonuclear leucocytes (see Table 2). The protein concentration is elevated while that of glucose is either low or normal. Histologic examination of synovium reveals mononuclear cell infiltration but usually an absence of granulomata. The organism is visualized in only 20 per cent of cases on direct examination of synovial fluid by Gram stain or other methods. Synovial fluid or tissue consistently yield the organism in culture. Recovery of the organism from blood cultures may provide an important clue to the aetiology of the joint process.

The cornerstone of management consists of systemic antifungal chemotherapy. Intravenously administered Amphotericin B, with or without 5-FC, remains the standard of treatment for immediately life-threatening infection. However, increasing evidence suggests that fluconazole may be as effective against susceptible strains, at least in non-neutropaenic hosts (Weers-Pothoff et al. 1997). Certain yeasts (e.g. *C. krusei, T. glabrata*) often exhibit decreased susceptibility to fluconazole and itraconazole (although they may remain susceptible to voriconazole and caspofungin), resulting in treatment failure to these agents (Zmierczak et al. 1999). Fungal susceptibility studies, performed by a reliable laboratory, may help to guide therapy in more complicated cases. Caspofungin may also prove efficacious. The potential role of lipid-associated or -complexed Amphotericin B in the treatment of joint infection is unknown. Intra-articular Amphotericin B has been utilized but the necessity or desirability of this method of treatment is questionable. Repeated joint aspiration is usually indicated. Surgical debridement, both to confirm the diagnosis and to remove infected tissues, is often necessary (in addition to antifungal chemotherapy), particularly in cases of hip joint infection.

Neonatal candida arthritis

Candida species are aetiologic in almost one-fifth of cases of nosocomial septic arthritis in neonates (Dan 1983), occurring frequently in high-risk infants receiving antibiotic therapy and total parenteral nutrition. Other risk factors include prematurity, low birth weight, abdominal surgery, umbilical cord and central venous line catheterization, and administration of corticosteroids.

In most neonatal cases, candida arthritis presents as just one facet of a systemic disease process and the organism may be recovered from a variety of extra-articular sites including blood, urine, and spinal fluid. In an examination of the frequency of end-organ involvement in 86 neonates with candidemia from 1989 to 1999, Noyola and colleagues found that nearly half of the infants (46.5 per cent) had *Candida* isolated from sites other than blood, but only one (1.2 per cent) had fungal arthritis (Noyola et al. 2001). Most of the bloodstream isolates in this study were either *C. albicans* (63 per cent) or *C. parapsilosis* (30 per cent), although neonates receiving fluconazole for pre-emptive therapy are more likely to be infected with non-albicans *Candida* species (Kaufman et al. 2001).

In the largest reported series of neonatal *Candida* arthritis, one or both knees were involved in 71 per cent of cases; polyarticular infection was seen in one-third (Dan 1983). The synovial fluid white blood cell count was as high as 100 000/mm^3 with a predominance of polymorphonuclear leucocytes. The synovial membrane was hyperemic and purulent with erosion of cartilage. Roentgenographic evidence of adjacent osteomyelitis was observed in almost 90 per cent of joints, suggesting that infection of the metaphysis is frequently the original site of haematogenous dissemination with subsequent rupture into the articular cavity. Other radiographic findings included peri-articular soft tissue swelling and joint effusion and, in the case of hip joint infection, subluxation of the femoral head. Major orthopaedic sequelae are uncommon.

Neonates with septic arthritis due to *Candida* species usually receive parenterally administered Amphotericin B for a minimum of 4 weeks, at least until their infection is adequately controlled. Fluconazole has been effective in some cases. Candida arthritis may occur up to 1 year following apparently successful treatment of initial fungemia.

Prosthetic joint infection

Fungal infection of total joint arthroplasties is rare (Brooks and Pupparo 1998). Infection is likely the result of implantation of skin microflora at the time of the original surgery. The infections are clinically low-grade, indolent, and present late following reconstructive arthroplasty ($\geq$6 months). Pain, decreased range of motion, and peri-articular swelling are common. Sinus tracts may be seen. Roentgenographic examination shows evidence of loosening and adjacent areas of osteolysis indicative of osteomyelitis.

Technetium pyrophosphate and gallium nitrate scans are not useful, since they are often positive in the presence of a loosened prosthesis, regardless of the presence of infection. The value of indium-111 white blood cell scanning is unknown. Consistent with a more sub-acute presentation, synovial fluid white blood cell counts were less inflammatory than that typically seen in native joint infections (4000–15 000/mm^3); polymorphonuclear leucocytes were predominant.

Amphotericin B, with or without 5-FC, in combination with removal of the prosthesis and other foreign material, and debridement of affected tissue is the initial treatment of choice. Fluconazole, itraconazole, and ketoconazole may have a role in long-term 'maintenance' therapy of such cases. Two reports describe the successful salvage of total knee arthroplasties infected with *Candida* species (Fukasawa and Shirakura 1997; Brooks and Pupparo 1998), and reimplantation has been reported in one patient 10 months after resection arthroplasty (Younkin et al. 1984).

Coccidioidomycosis

Coccidioides immitis is endemic to the soils of certain areas of the Lower Sonoran Life Zone of the Western Hemisphere, with most cases resulting from exposure to airborne arthroconidia in Arizona and the central valley of California (see Table 1) (cases also occur in New Mexico, Northern Mexico, and, recently, the first cases were reported from Utah). Upon reaching the alveoli of the infected host, the organism, a tissue dimorph, converts to the spherule-endospore phase. Approximately one-half of infected patients become symptomatic and, in the vast majority of these, the infection is self-limited with influenza-like symptoms. Transient arthralgias or aseptic inflammatory arthritis, which probably represents an immunologically mediated inflammatory process similar to erythema nodosum (which is also often seen), occur in 3–5 per cent of patients with primary pulmonary coccidioidomycosis. Treatment consists of the administration of non-steroidal anti-inflammatory agents.

Clinically important extrapulmonary dissemination occurs in fewer than 0.5 per cent of cases, although woman who are pregnant (especially the third trimester) or in the immediate post-partum state, and Filipinos, African Americans, and Latinos are at greater risk for dissemination. While many patients with disseminated disease have no impairment in immune function, approximately one-half are immunocompromised by HIV-infection, corticosteroids, diabetes, renal failure, or other immunosuppressive therapy. Most cases that occur outside of the endemic area are the result of travel, especially older folks who frequent the southwestern US during the winter months and who have no pre-existent immunity.

Joint space infection occurs in up to 25–30 per cent of patients with disseminated disease, with occasional extension into adjacent bony areas (Deresinski 1980). Monoarticular arthritis occurs in more than 90 per cent of cases, with large weight bearing joints, particularly the knee and ankle, being most frequently affected. While the larger joints are more commonly involved in adults, the small joints of the hand appear to be more commonly affected in children. At the time of presentation with joint disease, occult sites of dissemination are present in up to 25 per cent of cases. Extrapulmonary sites of infection, including meningeal, bone and joint infection, should, therefore, be avidly sought for in any patient with disseminated coccidioidomycosis.

While some patients may initially present with an acutely inflamed joint, most infections are indolent with progressive effusion and synovial thickening. The diagnosis of joint infection is often delayed, and chronic infection frequently results in significant articular and bony destruction with resultant loss of joint function [see Fig. 2(a)]. Occasionally, chronic arthrocutaneous fistulas develop with drainage of synovial fluid [see Fig. 2(b)]. Baker's cysts may occur as a consequence of knee involvement. Roentgenographic examination may be unremarkable during the initial phase of infection, effusion, and erosion of articular cortex and adjacent osteoporosis are commonly seen as the infection progresses (Bayer and Guze 1979). Technetium pyrophosphate radioisotope scans usually localize to the affected joints.

Synovial fluid is inflammatory with total white blood cell counts as high as 50 000/mm^3 (see Table 2). Mononuclear cells usually, but not always, predominate. Protein is greater than 3.0 gm/dl, glucose is low, and mucin clot is poor (Deresinski and Stevens 1974). Culture of synovial fluid yields the organism in approximately 50 per cent of cases, usually within 3–6 days. Greater yield is seen with culture and histologic examination of synovial tissue. The affected proliferative synovium, which often invades cartilage and articular surfaces, exhibits granulomatous villonodular inflammatory changes with the characteristic endosporulating spherules visible on microscopic examination. Most importantly, if coccidioidomycosis infection is suspected, the microbiology laboratory must be notified because of the significant biohazard represented by this organism in culture.

Serum complement fixing antibody to coccidioidin is almost universally present with the height of the titre reflecting the extent of dissemination, as in other manifestations of disseminated infection with this organism (Deresinski 1980). Delayed dermal hypersensitivity to coccidioidin may be absent. Magnetic resonance imaging in adults with coccidioidal arthritis frequently reveals synovitis, sub-articular bone loss, and loss of cartilage, but less frequent marrow involvement.

Among the endemic fungal infections, coccidioidomycosis is the most recalcitrant to therapy. Patient prognosis depends upon the extent of dissemination to other sites, particularly the central nervous system. Treatment consists of systemic administration of antifungal agents, and Amphotericin B remains the treatment of choice in many cases, especially for those with life-threatening disease, central nervous system involvement, immune suppression, as well as those who have failed appropriate azole therapy. Patients with disseminated disease often receive a total of 1.0–2.5 g

(a)

(b)

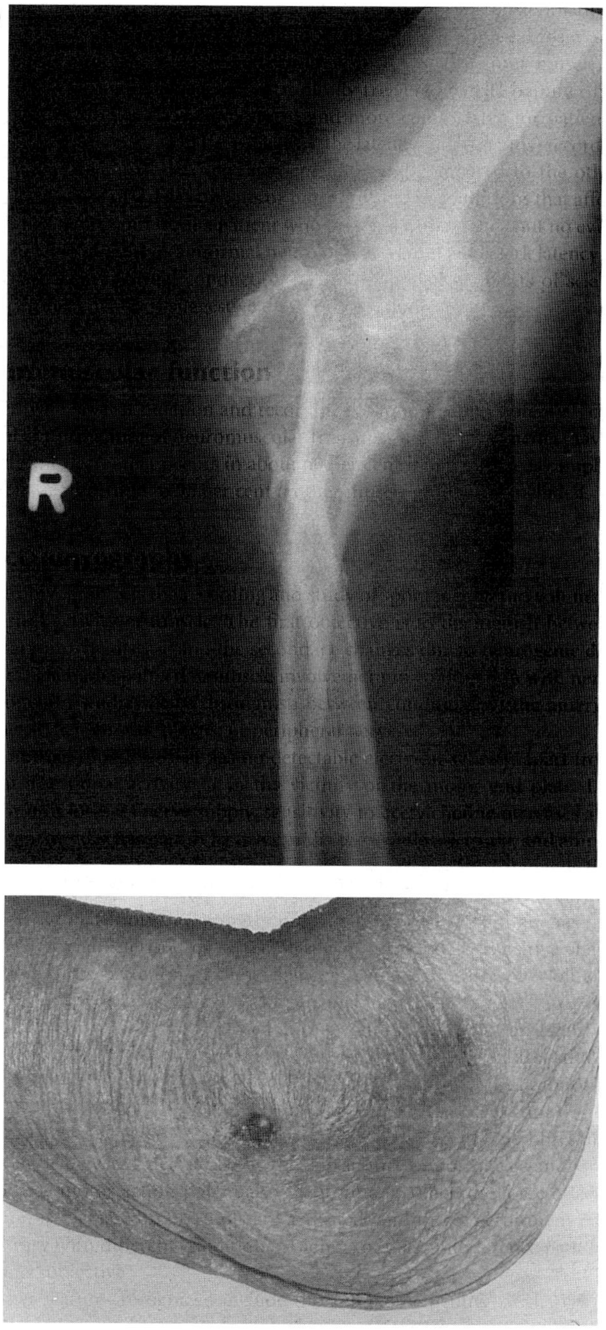

Fig. 2 (a) Roentgenograph of the right elbow demonstrating destruction of the articular cortex and osteomyelitis of contiguous bone of an elderly women with chronic coccidioidal arthritis of many years duration despite multiple courses of antifungal therapy. (b) Chronic coccidiodal arthritis of the same patient as in (a) demonstrating the right elbow joint fixed in flexion. The sinus tracts intermittently drain material from which *Coccidioides immitis* is recoverable in culture (courtesy of John S. Hostetler).

of Amphotericin B. Continued therapy is indicated until remission has been achieved, as defined by objective clinical measures, and improvement in serological and radiographic data. Life-long therapy for disseminated infection is often necessary.

Guidelines for the management of patients infected with *C. immitis*, recently published by the Infectious Disease Society of America, recommend that patients with life-threatening, non-meningeal disseminated disease receive Amphotericin B 0.6–1.0 mg/kg daily, or orally administered fluconazole (≥400 mg daily) or itraconazole (≥200 mg twice daily) for a minimum of 1 year (Galgiani et al. 2000a). Patients with stable or slowly progressive disease may receive either fluconazole or itraconazole. Patients with skeletal infection may do better in response to itraconazole than fluconazole (Galgiani et al. 2000b). Given the favourable pharmacologic and toxicity profiles for both fluconazole and itraconazole, many clinicians initiate treatment at higher dosages (fluconazole 800–1000 mg daily or itraconazole 400–600 mg daily). Even higher dosages have been used in patients who have failed to respond or who are intolerant of Amphotericin B. Ketoconazole (400–800 mg/day) also has some efficacy in skeletal disease, but the relapse rate is high (approximately 30 per cent), depending on the severity of disease.

The need for synovectomy and debridement of infected bone and tissue remain controversial. Despite appropriate medical and surgical intervention, the joint infection often remains progressive and disabling. In one study, seven of 14 patients who received amphotericin alone failed therapy, whereas none of the 14 patients who were treated with a combination of medical and surgical approaches relapsed (Bried and Galgiani 1986). In another similar study, seven of nine patients who received Amphotericin B and who underwent surgical debridement remained disease-free at least 4 years later (Bisla and Taber 1976). The two remaining patients developed recurrent disease, despite having received more than 3.0 g of Amphotericin B each. Patients with complement fixation titres greater than or equal to 1 : 128 were most likely to fail in response to medical therapy alone (Bried and Galgiani 1986). Amphotericin B has also been administered intra-articularly, but the therapeutic necessity or advisability of this is uncertain. Arthrodesis is generally effective, but not desirable.

An unusual case of prosthetic hip joint infection due to *C. immitis* responded to long-term therapy with fluconazole (Nomura and Ruskin 1994).

Cryptococcosis

Cryptococcus neoformans is worldwide in distribution. Skin test surveys suggest that sub-clinical infection is quite common in normal hosts. Clinical disease occurs predominantly, but not exclusively, in individuals with defects in cellular immunity (see Table 1). Patients with renal failure and HIV infection are especially vulnerable to infection with this encapsulated yeast. The primary portal of entry for the organism is believed to be the respiratory tract, although clinical recognizable pulmonary infection is infrequent. Haematogenous dissemination leads to varying organ involvement, although the organism has a particular predilection for the brain and meninges. Cryptococcal arthritis, frequently associated with areas of contiguous osteomyelitis and osteomyelitis occurs in up to 10 per cent of patients with systemic disease (Stead et al. 1988). Most, but not all, patients have severe deficits in cellular immunity, such as those with AIDS, sarcoidosis, diabetes, and renal allograft recipients (Bosch et al. 1994). Both gout and calcium pyrophosphate disease appear to increase the risk of cryptococcal infection in affected joints.

Although soft-tissue swelling, inflammation, and frank cellulitis have been reported in cases of cryptococcal joint infection, most cases are indolent in presentation. The knee is involved in approximately 60 per cent of reported cases, followed by an equal number of cases in the sternoclavicular and acromial-clavicular joints, elbow, wrist, and ankle (see Table 2). Approximately one-third of the cases are polyarticular. Roentgenograms demonstrate an erosive arthritis and juxta-articular osteomyelitis, and computed tomographic scans often show evidence of surrounding soft-tissue inflammation. Examination of the synovial fluid reveals a white blood cell count of 200–20 000/mm^3, with a predominance of mononuclear cells. The peripheral white blood cell count and erythrocyte sedimentation rate is often normal.

Amphotericin B may be administered as initial therapy in most cases of life-threatening, disseminated infection. Many experts advocate the concomitant administration of 5-FC for approximately 4 weeks for more severe infection. Once the systemic disease is under control and the joint disease is improving, consideration can be given to completing treatment with fluconazole (400–800 mg/day). Itraconazole may also be effective, but the data are limited. Patients with advanced HIV infection should remain on life-long suppressive maintenance therapy, as long as severe immunocompromise persists. Debridement may be useful, especially in cases with significant synovial thickening and peri-articular extension of infection.

Histoplasmosis

Histoplasmosis capsulatum is endemic to many areas within the temperate zones of the world, but is most heavily concentrated in the Ohio, Mississippi, and Missouri River valleys of the United States (see Table 1). The organism is a thermal dimorph with the mycelial phase existing in soil, generally in association with bird and bat guano. Large outbreaks occur in urban endemic areas. Speleologists throughout the world may be at risk. An African form, due to *H. capsulatum* v. *duboisii*, also occurs.

Upon inhalation by the human or animal host, microconidia reach the alveoli where they convert to the yeast phase. While greater than 95 per cent of infections are sub-clinical, a flu-like respiratory illness may result from infection. Haematogenous dissemination is rare and occurs most commonly in patients with impaired cellular immunity. Persons with HIV infection who travel to or have previously lived in an endemic area are at risk for reactivation disease.

Immunologically mediated arthralgias and aseptic inflammatory arthritis, similar to that reported for coccidioidomycosis, are common in primary histoplasmosis (Rosenthal et al. 1983). Erythema nodosum and erythema multiforme may also occur. During a single outbreak of acute histoplasmosis in 381 symptomatic patients, 16 (4.1 per cent) developed arthralgias and six (1.6 per cent) developed aseptic arthritis (Rosenthal et al. 1983). The knees, ankles, wrists, and small joints of the hands were the most common sites of involvement; approximately 50 per cent of the cases were polyarticular. The joint involvement may be additive or migratory, and is often symmetric. Synovial fluid is inflammatory. This clinical problem is self-limited and is treated with non-steroidal anti-inflammatory agents.

In contrast to candidiasis and coccidioidomycosis, infection of the synovium or joint space by *H. capsulatum* is exceedingly rare (Weinberg et al. 2001). Juxta-articular osteomyelitis is often present. Joint involvement is usually monoarticular and has been reported in both apparently immunologically normal and compromised hosts.

The diagnosis of histoplasmosis can be made by culture of both blood and infected sites, including synovial fluid, and histologic demonstration of the infecting organism. The organism is readily cultivated on a variety of media. The lysis–centrifugation technique hastens recovery from the blood of patients with active dissemination, although weeks may still be required. Detection of histoplasma antigen in serum or urine is highly useful in the diagnosis of disseminated histoplasmosis (Wheat et al. 1986). Although both falsely positive and negative results occur, antibody tests may be useful. Histoplasmin skin testing is useful only for epidemiological purposes.

Amphotericin B remains the initial treatment of choice for severe, life-threatening forms of histoplasmosis. Itraconazole, which has largely replaced ketoconazole in the treatment of non-life-threatening, non-central nervous system forms of disease, is now recommended for use in the treatment of histoplasmosis. In a non-comparative treatment trial, itraconazole (200–400 mg/day) was effective in 81 per cent of patients with histoplasmosis (Sharkey-Mathis et al. 1993). Itraconazole is also the preferred agent for maintenance therapy in AIDS patients, for which use it is clearly superior to fluconazole.

Paracoccidioidomycosis

Paracoccidioidomycosis is endemic only to areas of Central and South America where it is the most commonly encountered respiratory mycotic infection. *P. brasiliensis* is thermally dimorphic, and as is true for the other dimorphic fungi, conidia released by the mycelial phase of the fungus are inhaled and convert to the yeast phase in the alveoli. Acute, self-limited pulmonary infection may occur, although most patients present with chronic pulmonary disease and evidence of chronic haematogenous dissemination, including painful granulomata of the skin, lymphadenopathy, and ulceration of mucous membranes. Skeletal disease occurs but is rare (see Table 1) (Castaneda et al. 1985). Typical budding yeast forms were seen on examination of the synovial fluid and cultures were positive. The diagnosis is usually made on the basis of visualization of the organisms in synovial fluid or tissues, or by culture. Serological tests have been utilized with varying success. Skin tests are useful only for epidemiologic surveys.

Although the disease is rarely encountered outside endemic areas, the diagnosis should be suspected in any individual at epidemiological risk. Paracoccidioidomycosis primarily occurs in persons without evidence of immune dysfunction, but cases of severe disseminated disease have been described in immunosuppressed patients (Sugar et al. 1984).

Amphotericin B is effective in the treatment of disseminated paracoccidioidomycosis, although itraconazole (and ketoconazole) appear as effective in the treatment of less severe cases (Kwon-Chung and Bennett 1992). Relapses after treatment are common, and chronic suppressive therapy with one of the azoles or a sulfonamide is, therefore, recommended.

Sporotrichosis

Sporothrix schenckii, a tissue dimorph, is commonly found on decaying vegetation and in soil in many areas of both hemispheres. Infections are both sporadic and epidemic. In contrast to the other soil fungi discussed here, cutaneous disease occurs secondary to the inoculation of the organism as a result of trauma to the skin. The lymphocutaneous form, with the development of an ulcer at the site of cutaneous inoculation and proximal nodules in the area of lymphatic drainage, is the most common manifestation of infection (Belknap 1989). Persons at particular risk for this infection include rose cultivators and those who handle soil and spagnum moss.

While arthralgias occur in approximately 2 per cent of those with acute cutaneous or lymphocutaneous disease, infection of the joint space with *S. schenkii* is rare, having occurred in only one of 3300 patients (0.03 per cent) in a large outbreak of sporotrichosis (Lurie 1963). Arthritis may occur in the presence of widespread dissemination to other sites, but is much more common as an isolated finding (Bayer et al. 1979a). Bayer and colleagues described 44 cases of sporotrichal joint infection, 20 per cent of which were associated with systemic and pulmonary disease (Bayer et al. 1979a). Most cases of sporotrichal arthritis are, therefore, believed to be due to haematogenous dissemination of the organism, although some cases may be the result of articular extension of infection from an adjacent site of osteomyelitis or skin infection or, occasionally, from direct inoculation of the organism into the joint. The majority of patients with systemic infection have predisposing underlying disease, including myeloproliferative disorders, malignancy, chronic corticosteroid use, and alcoholism.

Sporotrichal arthritis is an indolent and slowly progressive infectious process that predominantly affects the knee and other large weight-bearing joints, although the small joints of the hand and wrist are also commonly affected (Bayer et al. 1979a). Calhoun and colleagues described 11 cases of systemic sporotrichosis; eight involved the skeletal system with a total of 12 joints being affected, including the wrist (63 per cent), knee (38 per cent), ankle (25 per cent), and elbow and phalanx (13 per cent each) (Calhoun et al. 1991). Monoarticular and polyarticular involvement occurs with equal frequency. Most cases present as a slowly progressive synovitis or tenosynovitis with pain, warmth, swelling, and restricted range of motion (Bayer et al. 1979a; Chang et al. 1984).

Radiographic abnormalities are seen in more than 90 per cent of cases, possibly reflecting the chronicity of infection prior to diagnosis. Osteoporosis of contiguous bone is the most common roentgenographic finding, followed by soft tissue swelling with effusion, 'punched out' osteolytic lesions, articular cartilage erosion, and joint space narrowing (Bayer et al. 1979a; Jones 1999) [see Figs 1(b) and (c)].

Synovial fluid white blood cell count is reported to range from 2800 to 60 000/mm^3. Both lymphocytes and polymorphonuclear leucocytes may be seen (see Table 2). The protein concentration is high while that of glucose is low to normal. The diagnosis may be delayed because of the isolated nature of the infection, the rarity of visualizing the organism on smears of synovial fluid, the often non-specific nature of synovial histopathology (which may resemble that of rheumatoid or tuberculous arthritis), and the paucity of organisms in tissue [see Fig. 1(d)]. Asteroid bodies, often said to be pathognomonic of sporotrichosis, may, in fact, be seen in other infections. Isolation of the organism in culture is the cornerstone of diagnosis. Synovial tissue is more likely to yield the organism (usually within 5 days) than is synovial fluid. Skin tests are only useful for epidemiologic surveys. A variety of serologic tests have been utilized with varying results.

While Amphotericin B had been recommended for the treatment of skeletal sporotrichosis, more recent data indicate that itraconazole is also very effective. In a National Institute of Allergies and Infectious Diseases non-comparative clinical treatment trial of 30 patients with both lymphocutaneous and systemic sporotrichosis, one-half of whom had osseous or articular infection, itraconazole (100–600 mg daily for 3–18 months) was effective in 83 per cent, although several cases relapsed later (Sharkey-Mathis et al. 1993).

Despite reasonably effective penetration by the drug into synovial fluid, ketoconazole has effected responses in only approximately two-thirds of patients with systemic sporotrichosis, including patients with joint infection (Calhoun et al. 1991). Fluconazole has been similarly disappointing in lymphocutaneous infection. Potassium iodide, which is effective in the lymphocutaneous form of the disease, has no role in the treatment of deep tissue infection, such as arthritis.

Intra-articular administration of Amphotericin B has also been utilized, but this is unlikely to be necessary. Surgical debridement may also be necessary on occasion, but should be reserved for persistent culture positivity and in cases of tenosynovitis.

Miscellaneous mycoses

A variety of additional fungi have been implicated in joint infections. Skeletal infections due to *Alternaria* species and *Bipolaris hawaiiensis, Acremonium* species, *Cunninghamella bertholletiae, Exiophiala jeanselmei, Exiophila spinifera, Fusarium solan, Madurella mycetomi, Phialophora parasitica, Saccharomyces* species, *P. boydii, and Trichosporon beigeli* are among those that have been reported (Cuellar et al. 1993).

References

Abril, A., Campbell, M.D., Cotten, V.R., Jr., Steckleberg, J.M., El-Azhary, R.A., and O'Duffy, J.D. (1998). Polyarticular blastomycotic arthritis. *Journal of Rheumatology* **25**, 1019–21.

Bayer, A.S., Scott, V.J., and Guze, L.B. (1979a). Fungal arthritis. III. Sporothrichal arthritis. *Seminars in Arthritis and Rheumatism* **9**, 66–74.

Bayer, A.S., Scott, V.J., and Guze, L.B. (1979b). Fungal arthritis. IV. Blastomycotic arthritis. *Seminars in Arthritis and Rheumatism* **9**, 145–51.

Belknap, B.S. (1989). Sporotrichosis. *Dermatologic Clinics* **7**, 193–202.

Berger, R. and Kraman, S. (1981). Acute miliary blastomycosis after 'short-course' corticosteroid treatment. *Archives of Internal Medicine* **141**, 1223–5.

Bisla, R.S. and Taber, T.H. (1976). Coccidioidomycosis of bone and joints. *Journal of Clinical Orthopedic Related Research* **121**, 196–204.

Bosch, X., Roman, R., Font, J., Alemany, S., and Coca, A. (1994). Bilateral cryptococcosis of the hip. *Journal of Bone and Joint Surgery* **76A**, 1234–8.

Bradsher, R.W. (1988). Blastomycosis. *Infectious Disease Clinics of North America* **1**, 877–98.

Bried, J.M. and Galgiani, J.N. (1986). *Coccidioides immitis* infections of bones and joints. *Clinical Orthopedics* **211**, 235–43.

Brooks, D.H. and Pupparo, F. (1998). Successful salvage of a primary total knee arthroplasty infected with *Candida parapsilosis*. *Journal of Arthroplasty* **13**, 707–12.

Calhoun, D.L., Waskin, H., White, M.P., Bonner, J.R., Mulholland, J.H., Rumans, L.W., Stevens, D.A., and Galgiani, J.N. (1991). Treatment of systemic sporotrichosis with ketoconazole. *Journal of Infectious Diseases* **13**, 47–51.

Castaneda, O.J., Alarcon, G.S., Garcia, M.T., and Lumbreras, H. (1985). *Paracoccidioides brasiliensis* arthritis. Report of a case and review of the literature. *Journal of Rheumatology* **12**, 356–8.

Chang, A.C., Destouet, J.M., and Murphy, W.A. (1984). Musculoskeletal sporotrichosis. *Skeletal Radiology* **12**, 23–8.

Chapman, S.W., Bradsher, R.W., Jr., Campbell, G.D., Jr., Pappas, P.G., and Kauffman, C.A. (2000). Practice guidelines for the management of patients with blastomycosis. Infectious Disease Society of America. *Clinical Infectious Diseases* **30**, 679–83.

Cuellar, M.L., Silveira, L.H., and Espinoza, L.R. (1992). Fungal arthritis. *Annals of the Rheumatic Diseases* **51**, 690–7.

Cuellar, M.L., Silveira, L.H., Citera, G., Cabrera, G.E., and Valle, R. (1993). Other fungal arthritides. *Rheumatic Disease Clinics of North America* **19**, 439–55.

Dan, M. (1983). Neonatal septic arthritis. *Israel Journal of Medical Science* **19**, 967–71.

Davies, S.F. and Sarosi, G.A. (1991). Clinical manifestations and management of blastomycosis in the compromised patient. In *Fungal Infection in the Compromised Patient* 2nd edn. (ed. D.W. Warnock and M.D. Richardson), pp. 215–29. Chichester: John Wiley & Sons, Ltd.

Denning, D.W. and Stevens, D.A. (1990). Antifungal and surgical treatment of invasive aspergillosis: review of 2121 published cases. *Review of Infectious Diseases* **12**, 1147–201.

Deresinski, S.C. (1980). Coccidioidomycosis of the musculoskeletal system. In *Coccidioidomycosis* (ed. D.A. Stevens), pp. 195–212. New York: Plenum Press.

Deresinski, S.C. and Stevens, S.C. (1974). Coccidioidomycosis in compromised hosts. *Medicine* **54**, 377–95.

Fader, R.C. and McGinnis, M.R. (1988). Infections causes by dermatiaceous fungi: chromoblastomycosis and phaeohyphomycosis. *Infectious Disease Clinics of North America* **1**, 925–38.

Fukasawa, N. and Shirakura, K. (1997). Candida arthritis after total knee arthroplasty—a case of successful treatment without prosthesis removal. *Acta Orthopaedica Scandinavica* **68**, 306–7.

Galgiani, J., Ampel, N.H., Catanzaro, A., Johnson, R.H., Stevens, D.A., and Williams, P.L. (2000a). Practice guidelines for the treatment of coccidioidomycosis. *Clinical Infectious Diseases* **30**, 658–61.

Galgiani, J.N., Catanzaro, A., Cloud, G.A., Johnson, R.H., Williams, P.L., Mirels, L.F., Nassar, F., Lutz, J.E., Stevens, D.A., Sharkey, P.K., Singh, V.R., Larsen, R.A., Delgado, K.L., Flanigan, C., and Rinaldi, M.G. (2000b). Comparison of oral fluconazole and itraconazole for progressive, non-meningeal coccidiodomycosis: a randomized, double-blind trial. *Annals of Internal Medicine* **133**, 676–86.

Jones, N. (1999). Photo quiz. Osteoarticular sporothrichosis. *Clinical Infectious Diseases* **29**, 202–3.

Kaufman, D., Boyle, R., Hazen, K.C., Patrie, J.T., Robinson, M., and Donowitz, L.G. (2001). Fluconazole prophylaxis against fungal colonization and infection in preterm infants. *New England Journal of Medicine* **345**, 1660–6.

Kwon-Chung, K.J. and Bennett, J.E. (1992). Paracoccidioidomycosis. In *Medical Mycology* (ed. K.J. Kwon-Chung and J.E. Bennett), pp. 594–619. Philadelphia PA: Lea & Febiger.

Lurie, H.I. (1963). Five unusual cases of sporotrichosis from South Africa showing lesions in muscles, bone and viscera. *British Journal of Surgery* **50**, 585–91.

Marina, N., Flynn, P., Rivera, G., and Hughes, W. (1991). *Candida tropicalis* and *Candida albicans* fungemia in children with leukemia. *Cancer* **68**, 594–9.

McDonald, P.B., Black, G.B., and MacKenzie, R. (1990). Orthopaedic manifestations of blastomycosis. *Journal of Bone and Joint Surgery* **72A**, 860–4.

Munoz-Fernandez, S. et al. (1991). Rheumatic manifestations in 556 patients with human immunodeficiency virus infection. *Seminars in Arthritis and Rheumatism* **21**, 30–9.

Nomura, J. and Ruskin, J. The prosthetic joint and disseminated coccidioidomycosis (abstract 32). *Centennial Conference on Coccidioidomycosis, Stanford, CA*, (1994).

Noyola, D.E., Fernandez, M., Moylett, E.H., and Baker, C.J. (2001). Ophthalmologic, visceral, and cardiac involvement in neonates with candidemia. *Clinical Infectious Diseases* **32**, 1018–23.

O'Meeghan, T., Varcoe, R., Thomas, M., and Ellis-Preger, R. (1990). Fluconazole concentration in joint fluid during successful treatment of *Candida albicans* arthritis. *Journal of Antimicrobial Chemotherapy* **26**, 601–2.

Panigrahi, S., Nagler, A., Or, R., Wolf, D.G., Slavin, S., and Shapira, M.Y. (2001). Indolent aspergillus arthritis complicating fludarabine-based non-myeloablative stem cell transplantation. *Bone Marrow Transplant* **27**, 659–61.

Recht, A.D., Davies, S.F., and Eckman, M.R. (1982). Blastomycosis in immunosuppressed patients. *American Review of Respiratory Diseases* **125**, 359–62.

Rosenthal, J., Brandt, K.D., Wheat, J.L., and Slama, T.G. (1983). Rheumatologic manifestations of histoplasmosis in the recent Indianapolis epidemic. *Arthritis and Rheumatism* **26**, 1065–70.

Sharkey, P.K. et al. (1990). Itraconazole treatment of phaeohyphomycosis. *Journal of American Academy of Dermatology* **23**, 577–86.

Stead, K.J., Klugman, K.P., Painter, M.L., and Koornhof, H.J. (1988). Septic arthritis due to *Cryptococcus neoformans*. *Journal of Infection* **17**, 139–45.

Sugar, A.M., Restrepo, A.A., and Stevens, D.A. (1984). Paracoccidioidomycosis in the immunosuppressed host: report of a case and review of the literature. *American Review of Respiratory Diseases* **129**, 340–2.

Tunkel, A.R., Thomas, C.Y., and Wispelwey, B. (1993). *Candida* prosthetic arthritis: report of a case treated with fluconazole and review of the literature. *American Journal of Medicine* **94**, 100–3.

Weers-Pothoff, G., Havermans, J.F., Kamphuis, J., Sinnige, H.A., and Meis, J.F. (1997). *Candida tropicalis* arthritis in a patient with acute myeloid leukemia successfully treated with fluconazole: case report and review of the literature. *Infection* **25**, 109–11.

Weinberg, J.M., Ali, R., Badve, S., and Pelker, R.R. (2001). Musculoskeletal histoplasmosis. A case report and review of the literature. *Journal of Bone and Joint Surgery of America* **83A**, 1718–22.

Wheat, L.J., Kohler, R.B., and Tewari, R.P. (1986). Diagnosis of disseminated histoplasmosis by detection of *Histoplasmosis capsulatum* antigen in serum and urine specimens. *New England Journal of Medicine* **314**, 83–8.

Younkin, S., Evarts, C.M., and Steigbigel, R.T. (1984). *Candida parapsilosis* infection of a total hip-joint replacement: successful reimplantation after treatment with amphotericin B and 5-fluorocytosine. A case report. *Journal of Bone and Joint Surgery of America* **66A**, 142–3.

Zmierczak, H., Goemaere, S., Mielants, H., Verbruggen, G., and Veys, E.M. (1999). *Candida glabrata* arthritis: case report and review of the literature of *Candida* arthritis **18**, 406–9.

6.2.11 Immunodeficiency

A.D.B. Webster

Introduction

There has been a rapid advance over the past decade in our understanding of the molecular mechanisms for most of the inherited 'primary' immunodeficiencies (PIDs). Joint disease is an uncommon but important complication of PID, and affected patients are often referred to rheumatologists for advice on diagnosis and management. Patients with PID usually complain initially of recurrent respiratory infection, although the average time in

Table 1 Classification of immunodeficiency (based on IUIS Report 1999)

Primary
Antibody deficiency
X-linked agammaglobulinaemia (XLA)
Common variable immunodeficiency (CVID)
Hyper IgM syndromes (HIM) (X-linked or autosomal recessive)
Autosomal recessive agammaglobulinaemia
Selective IgA deficiency (IgAD)
Selective IgG subclass deficiency
Thymoma with hypogammaglobulinaemia
Transient hypogammaglobulinaemia of infancy
Functional antibody deficiency
Severe T-cell deficiency (often with partial antibody deficiency)
Thymic aplasia (Di George syndrome)
Purine nucleoside phosphorylase deficiency
CD3 complex defects (γ or ϵ chain)
Mixed T- and B-cell defects
Severe combined immunodeficiency (SCID)
Myeloid dysgenesis
X-linked γc chain defect
Adenosine deaminase (ADA) deficiency
Defects in:
Recombinase activating gene 1 and 2
Artemis gene
Janus kinase-3 (JAK-3)
HLA Class 11 transcription factor (C11TA, RFX complex)
Zeta chain associated protein (ZAP-70) defect
$P56^{lck}$ kinase
Interleukin-7 receptor α chain
CD 45
Moderate mixed immunodeficiency
Ataxia telangiectasia (A-T)
Nijmegen breakage syndrome (NBS)
Ligase 1 defect
Wiskott–Aldrich syndrome (WAS)
Transporter for antigen presentation (TAP-2) defect
X-linked lymphoproliferative syndrome (XLPS)
Interferon-γ/interleukin-12 circuit defects
Defects in:
IL-12p40 subunit
IL-12 receptor β1 subunit
Interferon-γ receptor (chain 12)
STAT-1
Complement deficiencies
Neutrophil defects
Neutropaenia
Chronic granulomatous disease (CGD)
Leucocyte adhesion disorder (LAD)
Secondary
Involving lymphocytes
Lympho-reticular malignancy
Chronic lymphatic leukaemia[a]
Myeloma[a]
Viruses
HIV[b]
Rubella[a]
Metabolic and vitamin deficiencies
Vitamin A[a]
Zinc[b]
Selenium[b]
Renal and liver failure[a,b]
Trauma[a,b]
Burns[a]

Table 1 Continued

Hypercatabolism or increased loss of immunoglobulin
Nephrotic syndrome
Protein-losing enteropathy:
1° and 2° lymphangiectasia
Inflammatory bowel disease
Dystrophia myotonica
Therapeutic agents
Corticosteroids[b]
Cyclophosphamide [a,b]
Azathioprine[b]
Methotrexate[b]
Vincristine[a,b]
Cyclosporin[b]
Anti-T-cell antibodies[b]
Anti-B cell antibodies[a]
Sulfasalazine[a]
Gold[a,c]
Penicillamine[a,c]
Chloroquine[a,c]
Fenclofenac[a,c]
Valproate[a,c]
Phenytoin[a]
Carbamazepine[a]
Captopril[a,c]
Thyroxine[c,d]
Ibuprofen[c,d]
Salicylic acid[c,d]
Levamisole[d]
Involving neutrophils
Drug induced
Autoimmune neutropaenia

[a] Predominant effect on antibody production.

[b] Predominant effect on cellular immunity.

[c] Only IgA deficiency reported.

[d] Needs independent confirmation.

the United Kingdom before the diagnosis is confirmed is about 5 years; therefore, patients with joint disease may present to rheumatologists in ignorance of their underlying diagnosis. In these circumstances, some patients have been diagnosed as having a 'connective tissue' disorder, and inappropriately treated. These mistakes can be easily avoided by routinely measuring the levels of serum immunoglobulins to exclude the most common types of PID. Rheumatological complications are rare in patients with 'secondary' immunodeficiency caused by lymphoid malignancy, drugs, or viruses.

It is useful to sub-classify the causes of immunodeficiency into groups depending on whether the defect compromises mainly humoral or cellular immunity, or both (combined immunodeficiency) (see Table 1).

Diagnosis

The history will usually reveal a predisposition to infection; unexplained infections in family members suggests PID. The initial screening tests are cheap and rapid (i.e. full blood count, serum immunoglobulins and (in adults) immunoelectrophoresis for paraproteins) and will identify over 90 per cent of patients with suspected immunodeficiency, who should then be referred to an immunologist for further investigation.

It is important to remember that the normal ranges for serum immunoglobulins and blood lymphocyte counts in children are different from adults. Most patients with severe combined immunodeficiency have a very low blood lymphocyte count. Secondary immunodeficiency associated with other diseases is usually obvious, except when the patient has been treated with potentially immunosuppressive drugs for a rheumatic or autoimmune disorder (Table 1).

Primary immunodeficiency

Antibody deficiency (PAD)

The principal diseases of the joints that are associated with PAD are shown in Table 2. Mycoplasma infection is the most common cause, and investigations should be initially focused on this likely diagnosis.

Mycoplasma arthritis

Mycoplasmas are prokaryotic organisms which frequently infect mammals but which also occur in fish and reptiles (Taylor-Robinson and Bradbury 1998). Infection is a major problem in veterinary practice, causing arthritis in pigs, sheep, and cattle. Many different species are found in humans, the majority colonizing mucosal surfaces and, in general, behaving as commensals. However, *Mycoplasma pneumoniae* is a recognized human pathogen causing pneumonia, and ureaplasmas can cause 'non-specific' urethritis in otherwise healthy men. Mycoplasmas will activate the first component of complement in the absence of antibody, facilitating uptake into the phagocytic vacuoles of neutrophils, and probably macrophages (Webster et al. 1988); these cells are then probably responsible for disseminating the infection to joints where the organism thrives in the synovial fluid. Only about 10 per cent of PAD patients are prone to mycoplasma joint disease, so there must be additional predisposing factors other than the absence of specific antibodies. Recently, a low plasma level of mannose binding lectin (MBL), which occurs in about 40 per cent of the general population, has been identified as one cofactor; MBL probably inhibits growth of mycoplasmas by binding to mannose residues on the surface of the organism (Hamvas et al. unpublished).

This type of joint disease in similar PAD patients had previously been diagnosed as 'rheumatoid arthritis', supporting the view in the 1950s that PID patients were prone to autoimmune and connective tissue disorders (Good et al. 1957). However, there is now a consensus that mycoplasmas are the direct cause of the joint disease and not merely 'passengers' in an immunocompromised host.

Origin of infection

Ureaplasmas are commonly present in the vagina of pregnant women, neonates often being colonized in the respiratory tract shortly after birth, although the organisms then disappear by mechanisms that are not understood (Taylor-Robinson and Bradbury 1998). Bacterial vaginosis favours colonization with *Mycoplasma hominis*. In later life, colonization of the urinary tract may occur from sexual intercourse; since about one-third of healthy women are persistently colonized, most men are exposed to these organisms. Colonization is usually transient and asymptomatic, although a minority of men will develop ureaplasmal urethritis. In contrast, both men and women with hypogammaglobulinaemia are prone to symptomatic ureaplasma urethritis, which may progress to chronic cystitis, fibrosis with contraction of the bladder, and occasionally pyelonephritis (Webster et al. 1981). The lungs may be another source of infection with some species (e.g. *M. pneumoniae*). Trauma to a joint, which may be minor, can trigger septic mycoplasmal arthritis, suggesting that the organisms are present in small numbers in the circulation and become established at an inflammatory focus within the joint. Once one joint has been infected, there is a tendency for other joints to follow if the infection is not eliminated with appropriate antibiotics.

M. hominis, M. pneumoniae, and *Ureaplasma urealyticum* are the mycoplasma species most likely to be isolated from the joints of PAD patients (Franz et al. 1997). *Mycoplasma salivarium*, presumably originating from the upper respiratory tract where it is found in the saliva of about 80 per cent of healthy individuals, is a rare cause of arthritis (So et al. 1982). Other mycoplasma species, normally found in animals, have rarely caused extra-articular disease in PAD patients (e.g. meningitis, deep abscesses).

Table 2 Joint disease in primary hypogammaglobulinaemia

Disease	Comments
Mycoplasma arthritis	Mainly large joints, occurs before and after immunoglobulin therapy
Tenosynovitis/arthralgia	Usually hands and feet, responds rapidly to immunoglobulin therapy Arthralgia may be due to quinolones
Enterovirus disease	Flexion contractures of elbows and knees Oedema/rash on limbs Mild arthritis
Monoarthritis of knee	Mainly in children, improves slowly after immunoglobulin therapy
Rheumatoid arthritis (seronegative)	Rare, may be difficult to distinguish from secondary hypogammaglobulinaemia caused by drugs for RA

Clinical features

Large joints are usually affected, particularly the knees, although the ankles, hips, shoulders, and wrists (including carpal bones) are frequently involved in persistent infections. The fingers and toes are rarely affected, and when this does occur it usually involves a single inter-phalangeal joint. The initial symptoms are swelling and stiffness of the affected joint, usually with an obvious effusion when the knee is involved. Nodules may occur on the elbows that have the same histological features as classical rheumatoid nodules. Systemic symptoms are rare and there is usually no fever or blood leucocytosis. Joint pain increases over a few weeks or months, and if the infection persists the synovium will gradually deteriorate through chronic inflammation, leading eventually to fibrosis and fixation of the joint (Fig. 1). This sequence usually takes months, or sometimes years to reach a conclusion if inappropriate or no treatment is offered.

Some patients may enter a severe phase, presumably reflecting high levels of circulating organisms. Subcutaneous abscesses may then occur, sometimes at sites of minor trauma (e.g. injection sites), but more often in communication with a joint; the skin then breaks down leaving a chronically discharging sinus. Even at this relatively late stage, the patient may have minimal systemic effects.

Diagnosis

Organisms can be cultured from the synovial fluid in specialized laboratories. There are also PCR techniques that focus on sequences in the 16S ribosomal RNA gene, an initial PCR often being used to identify a common sequence to all known human mycoplasmas, followed by a second amplification to identify individual species. Although this is a useful screening test to establish the diagnosis, culture of the organism is required to provide antibiotic sensitivities which may take up to 6 weeks to complete.

It should be remembered that a serological diagnosis, often used to confirm *M. pneumoniae* lung infection in general medical practice, is of no use in antibody deficient patients. Synovial fluid should always be sent for the routine culture of common pathogens, such as staphylococci and *Haemophilus influenzae*, which may rarely cause arthritis in patients with hypogammaglobulinaemia. The fluid is usually yellow and/or turbid in active mycoplasma infection, and contains many neutrophils. If the routine culture is negative, then the working diagnosis should be mycoplasma arthritis until proved otherwise.

Management

Patients should be given doxycycline as soon as synovial fluid has been aspirated. This should preferably be given intravenously (Pfizer) at a dose of 200 mg daily for 7 days, followed by 100 mg/day until there is improvement in joint swelling and the level of serum C-reactive protein (CRP) is normal, the CRP being a useful marker of disease activity. Since the tetracyclines are

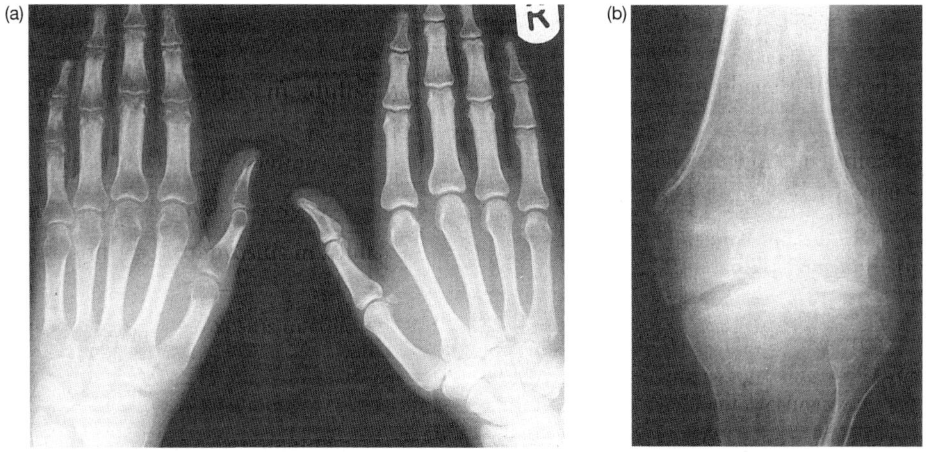

Fig. 1 (a) Chronic infection with *Ureaplasma urealyticum* of the wrist in a 30-year-old man with X-linked agammaglobulinaemia, showing destruction of the left distal ulna, the medial radius, and lunate, with osteoporosis of all joint levels related to disuse. (b) The left knee of the same patient showing destruction of the cartilage, obliteration of the joint space, and disorganization of the joint.

only static for mycoplasmas, treatment should continue with oral doxycycline (100 mg/day) for at least 3 months. Fortunately, most mycoplasma strains are sensitive to doxycycline and there will be obvious improvement in the joint symptoms within a few days. However, it is useful to arrange sensitivity tests against a range of antibiotics as soon as possible in case of resistance. Sensitivity testing should routinely include macrolides (e.g. erythromycin, clindamycin, and azithromycin) and doxycycline. In our experience, patients who are infected with a doxycycline-resistant strain are difficult to manage and usually progress to multi-joint involvement despite various combinations of antibiotics (Franz et al. 1997). Recently, a pleuromutilin antibiotic used in veterinary practice (Econor) has been made available on a compassionate basis for human disease. Most mycoplasmas are sensitive to Econor (Heilmann et al. 2001), but to reduce the chance of emerging resistance our policy is to use at least two antibiotics (i.e. Econor and clindamycin) in patients with tetracycline resistant organisms.

Surgical interference of the joint should be kept to a minimum; arthroscopy and lavage is unhelpful, although drainage under vacuum of a very tense effusion for 24 h may rarely be necessary. Trauma from surgical interference appears to increase the growth of mycoplasmas, as well as increasing the risk of sinus formation. The joint should be immobilized until there is no longer any swelling; if there is damage to ligaments the joint must be stabilized by splinting. Provided the diagnosis is made early and the mycoplasmas are sensitive to tetracyclines, there is usually full recovery.

It may be necessary to resort to immunotherapy in patients with multi-antibiotic resistant organisms who continue to deteriorate. Unfortunately, standard intravenous human immunoglobulin (IVIG) replacement therapy will not control mycoplasma infection because it contains inadequate levels of specific antibody. For those with established mycoplasma disease, it is reasonable to give high-dose IVIG (i.e. 2 g/kg/week for 8 weeks), hoping that this will provide enough specific antibody to help eradicate the organism. Patients with PAD can be treated with regular hyperimmune animal serum because they do not develop serum sickness. We have successfully treated two patients with goat hyperimmune serum taken from animals immunized with the patient's own isolate (Taylor-Robinson et al. 1985). Finally, monoclonal antibodies to mycoplasmas are not commercially available, and would have to be 'tailor-made' for the particular strain involved. Nevertheless, this may be an option for the future as technology develops to produce such antibodies faster and cheaper.

Bacterial septic arthritis

Patients with hypogammaglobulinaemia are prone to septicaemia and pneumonia caused by pneumococci, non-typeable *H. influenzae*, and staphylococci, any of which can occasionally cause septic arthritis (Asherson and Webster 1980). However, in contrast to mycoplasma arthritis, bacterial arthritis is usually more acute and painful, and is very rare in patients already established on replacement immunoglobulin therapy. There may be difficulty in making a diagnosis when nothing is cultured from joint fluid in patients already treated with antibiotics, although PCR tests for mycoplasmas should remain positive.

Rheumatoid arthritis

Although the literature prior to 1980 emphasized the high incidence of 'rheumatic' disease in PAD, it is now conceded that the majority of affected patients were suffering from mycoplasma arthritis. However, rheumatoid arthritis (RA) does occur in about 1 per cent of patients with common variable immunodeficiency (CVID). It is often difficult to ascertain whether the arthritis precedes or follows the onset of hypogammaglobulinaemia, and there is the added complication that a number of drugs used to treat rheumatoid arthritis (Table 1) are known to cause hypogammaglobulinaemia (see below). Nevertheless, there are rare patients in whom the hypogammaglobulinaemia clearly precedes the onset of classical RA, with the typical involvement of small joints of the hand, rheumatoid nodules, and gradual destruction of small and large joints (Hermaszewski et al. 1993). These patients are seronegative for rheumatoid factor and other relevant autoantibodies. However, an exhaustive search for mycoplasmas, using modern PCR and culturing techniques, should be undertaken before accepting the diagnosis. It is interesting that these classical features of RA have never been reported in patients with X-linked agammaglobulinaemia (XLA) who lack mature B-lymphocytes, particularly in view of recent claims that clearance of B-lymphocytes with monoclonal antibodies induces remission of RA (see Chapter 6.3.1). Since CVID patients retain mature B-lymphocytes, the presence of B-cells in the synovial membrane may be critical for the development of RA perhaps through their antigen presenting capacity or cytokine profiles, rather than through production of autoantibodies.

Miscellaneous arthritides associated with hypogammaglobulinaemia

Chronic synovial effusion of the knee

Children with hypogammaglobulinaemia, particularly those with XLA, are prone to a chronic insidious arthritis of the knee which is usually unilateral. There is a chronic effusion with little or no pain, which may persist for many years, sometimes with hypertrophy of the epiphysial cartilage (Fig. 2).

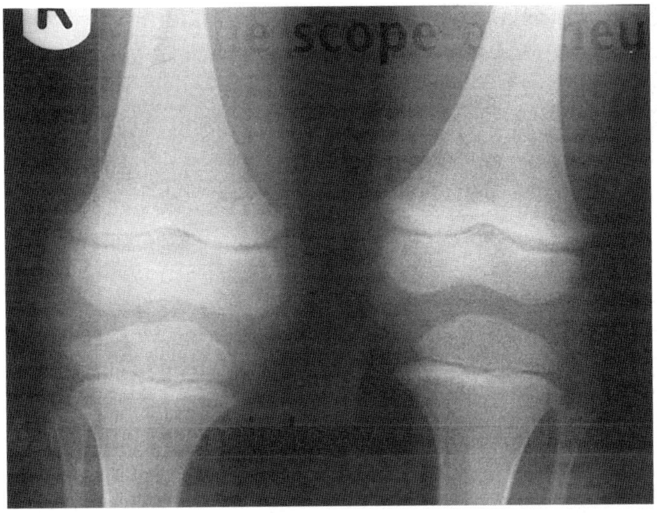

Fig. 2 Epiphyseal hypertrophy in the right knee of a 3-year-old boy with X-linked agammaglobulinaemia. There was a sterile effusion; the knee subsequently improved spontaneously.

The condition usually recovers spontaneously after a few months or years, leaving very little permanent damage apart from the unsightly appearance of enlarged condyles. Damage to the cartilage may necessitate menisectomy in later years.

The synovial fluid is colourless and contains mainly lymphocytes; it is sterile when cultured for bacteria, viruses, and mycoplasmas. Nevertheless, there is still a possibility that this is a low-grade mycoplasma infection, although antimycoplasma drugs such as doxycycline or erythromycin have no effect. Anti-inflammatory drugs are often useful.

This complication is now very rare, probably because children with PID are diagnosed earlier and treated with higher doses of IVIG therapy; in one of our cases the effusion disappeared after IVIG.

Chronic tenosynovitis/arthralgia

This condition was relatively common in British patients with hypogammaglobulinaemia in the 1970s but is now very rare (Webster et al. 1976). It usually occurred in adult patients with CVID as one of the presenting features of the disease. The usual pattern was of a patient suffering from recurrent respiratory infections for many years, who then developed stiffness in the wrists, elbows, and ankles with swelling of the tendon sheaths on the dorsal aspects of the wrist, hands, and feet. This sometimes led to tendon tethering with cystic swellings that required surgery; any associated arthritis was usually mild and fluctuating.

The condition can be confused with the early manifestations of RA, but there are no bony erosions. Furthermore, there is rapid improvement following immunoglobulin replacement therapy, even with the 'low dose' intramuscular immunoglobulin that was given routinely before the early 1980s. Possible causes are inflammation caused by IgM immune complexes (CVID patients can often make IgM antibodies) in response to chronic bacterial antigenaemia, or viruses which could be rapidly neutralized by immunogloulin therapy; since this condition has not been reported in XLA patients, who make no IgM, the former is more likely.

More recently, mild arthropathy, and occasionally tendonitis, has occurred in PID patients on immunoglobulin therapy who are taking quinolones as prophylaxis against *H. influenzae* bronchitis. About 10 per cent of PID patients on quinolone prophylaxis in the clinic at The Royal Free Hospital, London, have developed mild pain and stiffness in joints, without swelling; all have improved within a few weeks of discontinuing the drug.

Enteroviral disease

Patients with PID are prone to chronic enteroviral infection of the central nervous system and muscles, particularly with echo and coxsackie viruses (McKinney et al. 1987); a recent survey of published cases shows that arthritis is a rare feature, occurring in only 2 per cent of affected patients (Halliday et al. 2003). This is a 'slow' virus disease that mainly affects small vessels in the meninges, subcutaneous tissues, and muscles, which in the latter causes fibrosis with a 'woody' sensation on palpation. The arms and legs are predominantly affected, and the muscle fibrosis can lead to flexion contractures at the knees and elbows, sometimes producing a characteristic stooped posture (Webster 1984). An erythematous rash may occur transiently, which together with the subcutaneous oedema led clinicians before the mid-1970s to call this 'dermatomyositis'. At the time this provided further evidence that PID patients were predisposed to autoimmune and 'connective tissue' disorders.

Until the late 1980s, enteroviruses could usually be cultured from the cerebral spinal fluid (CSF) of affected patients, even when there were minimal or no central nervous system features. However, with the increasing use of higher dose IVIG therapy, the disease now often presents more insidiously with a wide range of neurological symptoms, sometimes being mistaken for a psychiatric disorder. Although IVIG prophylaxis may not protect against enteroviral infection, the small amounts of specific antibody present in these preparations is probably enough to partially neutralize these viruses and prevent culture from the CSF. In this situation the diagnosis depends upon a positive PCR identification of viral RNA, although this technique cannot yet identify the specific enteroviral species (Rotbart et al. 1997).

Dermatomyositic features are still being described in PID patients in eastern Europe and Russia where many receive inadequate replacement immunoglobulin therapy. Enteroviruses can be cultured directly from a muscle biopsy in this situation, although the CSF is also usually positive. Muscle histology characteristically shows a perivascular lymphocytic infiltration with foci of fibrosis. Plasma levels of creatine kinase are a poor indicator of disease activity. These extra-CNS features are now very rare in the Western world, probably because adequate immunoglobulin therapy is given before the virus can produce chronic muscle changes. Following diagnosis, it is useful to give high-dose IVIG therapy (2 g/kg/week for 8 weeks); there have been a few apparent cures from CNS disease with regular injection of immunoglobulin into the CSF via an Ommaya reservoir.

The recent availability of Pleconaril (Viropharma Inc., USA), a novel compound which prevents uncoating of the enteroviral capsid, has improved the outlook for affected patients, most of whom previously died within 5 years (Rotbart et al. 2001). Pleconaril, given orally, should be started as soon as the diagnosis is confirmed, in combination with standard or high-dose immunoglobulin therapy. Fortunately, most enteroviruses are sensitive to the drug.

Enteroviral disease occurs in only about 5 per cent of PID patients, particularly in children with XLA, with about 20 per cent of these developing dermatomyositic features; there are no clues to the additional susceptibility factor(s) which must be present in these patients. Early diagnosis of XLA is therefore important, and meticulous attention should be paid to keeping the trough serum IgG level above 7 g/l with immunoglobulin prophylaxis. There is a strong clinical impression in the major PID centres in Europe that this has reduced the incidence of enteroviral disease.

Severe T-cell and combined immunodeficiency

There are a variety of inherited single gene disorders causing T-lymphocyte dysfunction, often in combination with antibody deficiency (Table 1). Survival for most of these patients depends on a successful bone marrow graft. These disorders generally present in early childhood, and rheumatological problems are rare. Nevertheless, paediatricians should be aware of the possibility of mycoplasma or enteroviral disease, particularly in infants and children with severe combined immunodeficiency (SCID). Rare defects in either the production of γ-interferon by lymphocytes, or the activation of macrophages by this cytokine, causes a selective susceptibility to multisystem mycobacterial disease.

Inherited complement deficiencies

Defects in the early components of the classical complement pathway are associated with vasculitis and immune complex disease, including systemic lupus erythematosis (see Chapter 6.6.3). Pneumococcal, meningococcal, and gonococcal septicaemia, occasionally with septic arthritis, may occur in patients with genetically determined homozygous complement deficiencies involving C2 and subsequent components in the cascade which ultimately leads to lysis of bacteria. Combinations of these defects, particularly homozygous C2 deficiency which occurs in about 1 in 10 000 of the population, with mild antibody deficiency may together predispose to susceptibility to a wider range of organisms, including *H. influenzae.* Patients with defects in the late complement components (C3–C9) are prone to meningococcal septicaemia, as are those with inherited defects in the alternate pathway (e.g. properdin, Factor B or I deficiency). Classical (CH50) and alternate complement (AP50) pathway activity should be tested in all patients with gonococcal and meningococcal arthritis, particularly if they have had a previous neisserial infection.

Inherited neutrophil defects

Primary neutropaenia predisposes to septic arthritis and osteomyelitis, particularly caused by staphylococci. However, septicaemia and superficial or deep abscesses are usually the main focus of clinical management; if patients fail to benefit from treatment with granulocyte stimulating factors, bone marrow transplantation is usually required. Inherited functional defects either lead to a failure of neutrophils to adhere to vessel walls and migrate towards infection (mutations in β integrins) or to a failure to digest catalase negative bacteria and fungi (chronic granulomatous disease—CGD). Integrin defects are not associated with joint disease. CGD predisposes to chronic infection with salmonella, staphylococci, *Burkholderia cepacia*, candida and *Aspergillus* species, as well as other less common fungi (Mouy et al. 1989). Involvement of the joints is rare, but osteomyelitis is a well-known feature. Once the organism has been identified, antibiotics which will penetrate the phagocytic vacuole should be used (e.g. rifampicin, itraconazole).

Secondary immunodeficiency

Chronic lymphatic leukaemia (CLL) is often associated with hypogammaglobulinaemia, although it is rare for this to be as severe as that in PAD. Septic arthritis is not a recognized complication of CLL, but this should be considered in patients presenting with a swollen joint. Myeloma is also associated with antibody deficiency which recovers during remission. Occasionally patients with myeloma present with amyloid involvement of joints, the underlying diagnosis being mistaken for PAD. For this reason, laboratories measuring serum immunoglobulins in adults should routinely screen the first sample received for paraproteins to help exclude myeloma.

Premature neonates are also prone to systemic mycoplasma infection, which rarely may involve joints, probably because of inadequate amounts of protective antibody passing through the placenta. There have been anecdotal reports of mycoplasma involvement of joints and osteomyelitis in severely ill patients following trauma or major surgery. Most of these patients were not investigated from an immunological perspective, but it is likely that they were severely immunocompromised.

Many types of therapy in Western hospitals induce partial defects in cellular immunity (e.g. cytotoxic/immunosuppressive drugs for organ transplantation, autoimmune disease, and cancer). Antibody production is not usually severely compromised in these patients, who are more likely to develop disease due to reactivation of latent viruses (e.g. EBV associated lymphoma, CMV hepatitis). Joint infection is rare.

Drug-associated hypogammaglobulinaemia

A variety of antirheumatic and anticonvulsant drugs are associated with hypogammaglobulinaemia (Hammarstrom and Smith 1999) (Table 1), which partly explains the raised incidence of selective IgA deficiency in Still's disease (Barclay et al. 1979). The immunoglobulin levels usually return to normal after withdrawal of the drug although this may take many months or years. There is no obvious common molecular mechanism for the effect of these drugs on the immune system. Sulfasalazine inhibits NF-κB-dependent transcription and could affect immunoglobulin class switching, while lysosomotropic agents like chloroquine can interfere with antigen processing (reviewed by Truedsson et al. 1995). Since some of the genes predisposing to CVID and selective IgA deficiency are relatively common in the general Caucasian population, it is possible that drugs may 'trigger' these immunodeficiencies in genetically susceptible patients.

References

Asherson, G.L. and Webster, A.D.B. *Diagnosis and Treatment of Immunodeficiency Diseases.* Oxford: Blackwell, 1980.

Barclay, D., Ansell, B., Howard, A., Hohermuth, H., and Webster, A.D.B. (1979). IgA deficiency in juvenile chronic polyarthritis. *Journal of Rheumatology* **6**, 219–24.

Franz, A., Webster, A.D.B., Furr, P.M., and Taylor-Robinson, D. (1997). Mycoplasmal arthritis in patients with primary immunoglobulin deficiency: clinical features and outcome in 18 patients. *British Journal of Rheumatology* **36**, 661–8.

Good, R.A., Rotstein, J., and Mazzitello, W.F. (1957). The simultaneous occurrence of rheumatoid arthritis and agammaglobulinaemia. *Journal of Laboratory and Clinical Medicine* **49**, 343–57.

Hammarstrom, L. and Smith, C.I.E. (1999). Genetic approach to common variable immunodeficiency and IgA deficiency. In *Primary Immunodeficiency Diseases. A Molecular and Genetic Approach* (ed. H.D. Ochs, C.I.E. Smith, and J.M. Puck), pp. 250–62. Oxford UK: Oxford University Press.

Halliday, E., Winkelstein, J., and Webster, A.D.B. (2003). Enteroviral infections in primary immunodeficiency (PID): a survey of morbidity and mortality. *Journal of Infection* **46**, 1–8.

Heilmann, C., Jensen, L., Jensen, J.S., Lundstrom, K., Windsor, D., Windsor, H., and Webster, A.D. (2001). Treatment of resistant mycoplasma infection in immunocompromised patients with a new pleuromutilin antibiotic. *Journal of Infection* **43**, 234–8.

Hermaszewski, R., Ratnavel, R., Webster, A.D.B., and Denman, A.M. (1993). Rheumatoid arthritis in a patient with primary hypogammaglobulinaemia. *British Journal of Rheumatology* **32**, 636–9.

McKinney, R.E., Jr., Katz, S.L., and Wilfert, C.M. (1987). Chronic enteroviral meningoencephalitis in agammaglobulinaemic patients. *Review of Infectious Diseases* **9**, 334–56.

Mouy, R., Fischer, A., Vilmer, E., Seger, R., and Griscelli, C. (1989). Incidence, severity, and prevention of infections in chronic granulomatous disease. *Journal of Pedatrics* **114**, 555–60.

Primary Immunodeficiency Diseases. Report of an IUIS Scientific Committee. *Clinical and Experimental Immunology* **118** (Suppl. 1), Oct. 1999.

Rotbart, H.A., Ahmed, A., Hickey, S., Dagan, R., Mc Cracken, G.H., Jr., Whitle, R.I., Modlin, J.F., Cascino, M., O'Connell, J.F., Menegus, M.A., and Blum, D. (1997). Diagnosis of enterovirus infection by polymerase chain reaction of multiple specimen types. *Pediatric Infectious Disease Journal* 409–11.

Rotbart, H.A. and Webster, A.D.B. for the Pleconaril Treatment Registry Group (2001). Treatment of potentially life threatening enterovirus infection with Pleconaril. *Clinical Infectious Diseases* **32**, 228–35.

So, A.K.L., Furr, P.M., Taylor-Robinson, D., and Webster, A.D.B. (1982). Arthritis caused by *Mycoplasma salivarium* in hypogammaglobulinaemia. *British Medical Journal* **286**, 762–3.

Taylor-Robinson, D. and Bradbury, J. (1998). Mycoplasma diseases. In *Topley and Wilson's Microbiology and Microbial Infections* 9th edn. *Bacterial Infections* (ed. W.J. Hausler and M. Sussman), pp. 1013–37. London: Arnold.

Taylor-Robinson, D., Furr, P.M., and Webster, A.D.B. (1985). *Ureaplasma urealyticum* causing persistent urethritis in a patient with hypogammaglobulinaemia. *Genitourinary Medicine* **61**, 404–8.

Truedsson, L., Baskin, B., Pan, Q., Rabbani, H., Vorechovsky, I., Smith, C.I.E., and Hammarstrom, L. (1995). Genetics of IgA deficiency. *Acta Pathologica, Microbiologica et Immunologica Scandinavica* **103**, 833–42.

Webster, A.D.B. (1984). Echovirus disease in hypogammaglobulinaemic patients. *Clinics in Rheumatology* **10**, 189–203.

Webster, A.D.B., Loewi, G., Dourmsahkin, R.D., Golding, D.N., Ward, D.J., and Asherson, G.L. (1976). Polyarthritis in adults with hypogammaglobulinaemia and its rapid response to immunoglobulin treatment. *British Medical Journal* **1**, 1314–16.

Webster, A.D.B., Taylor-Robinson, D., Furr, P.M., and Asherson, G.L. (1981). Chronic cystitis and urethritis associated with ureaplasmal and mycoplasmal infection in primary hypogammaglobulinaemia. *British Journal of Urology* **54**, 287–91.

Webster, A.D.B., Furr, P.M., Hughes-Jones, N.C., Gorick, B.D., and Taylor-Robinson, D. (1988). Critical dependence on antibody for defence against mycoplasmas. *Clinical and Experimental Immunology* **71**, 383–7.

Further reading

Hans, D., Ochs, C.I., Smith, E., and Puck, J.M., ed. *Primary Immunodeficiency Diseases. A Molecular and Genetic Approach.* Oxford: Oxford University Press, 1999.

Webster, A.D.B. (1997). Secondary immunodeficiency. In *Encyclopaedia of Immunology* (ed. I.M. Roitt and P.J. Delves). London: Saunders Scientific Publications.

6.2.12 Rheumatic fever

Allan Gibofsky and John B. Zabriskie

Introduction

Acute rheumatic fever is a delayed, non-suppurative sequel to a pharyngeal infection with the group A streptococcus. Following the initial streptococcal pharyngitis, there is a latent period of 2–3 weeks. The onset of disease is usually characterized by an acute febrile illness, which may show itself in one of three classical ways: (i) the patient may present with migratory arthritis predominantly involving the large joints; (ii) there may be concomitant clinical and laboratory signs of carditis and valvulitis; and (iii) there may be involvement of the central nervous system, manifesting itself as Sydenham's chorea. The clinical episodes are self-limiting but damage to the valves may be chronic and progressive, resulting in cardiac decompensation and death.

Although there has been a dramatic decline in both the severity and fatality of the disease since the turn of the century, there are recent reports of its resurgence in the United States (Veasy et al. 1987) and in many military installations in the world, reminding us that it remains a public health problem even in developed countries. In addition, the disease continues essentially unabated in many of the developing countries: estimates suggest there will be 10–20 million new cases per year in those countries where two-thirds of the world population lives.

Epidemiology

The incidence of rheumatic fever actually began to decline long before the introduction of antibiotics into clinical practice, decreasing, for example, from 250 to 100 patients/100 000 population from 1862 to 1962 in Denmark (Gordis 1985). The introduction of antibiotics in 1950 caused a rapid acceleration of this decline, until in 1980 the incidence ranged from 0.23 to 1.88 patients per 100 000, primarily children and teenagers. A notable exception has been in the Hawaii and Maori populations (both of Polynesian ancestry), where the rate continues to be 13.4/100 000 children admitted to hospital per year (Pope 1989).

Table 1 Positive throat cultures—group A β-haemolytic streptococci (Rockefeller University Hospital, rheumatic fever patients; $n = 78$)

M type	RHD	No RHD	Total
Non-typable	1	5	6
1	1	1	2
2	0	1	1
5	1	1	2
6	1	1	2
12	0	2	2
18	2	2	4
19	2	2	4
28	1	0	1
Total	9	14	23

Note: RHD, patients with rheumatic heart disease; no RHD, patients without rheumatic heart disease.

As reviewed by Markowitz (1987), only a few M-streptococcal serotypes (types 5, 14, 18, 24) have been implicated in outbreaks of rheumatic fever, suggesting there could be a particular 'rheumatogenic' potential of certain strains of group A streptococci. However, in Trinidad, types 41 and 11 have been the most common strains isolated from rheumatics. In our own series, gathered over 20 years (see Table 1), a large number of different M serotypes were isolated, including six strains that were not typable. Kaplan et al. (1989) found that several different M types were isolated from the patients seen during an outbreak of rheumatic fever, and that these strains were both mucoid and non-mucoid in character. Whether or not certain strains are more 'rheumatogenic' than others remains unresolved. What is true, however, is that a streptococcal strain capable of causing a well-documented pharyngitis is almost always potentially capable of causing rheumatic fever, although some notable exceptions have been recorded (reviewed by Whitnack and Bisno 1980).

Pathogenesis

There is little evidence for the direct involvement of group A streptococci in the affected tissues of patients with acute rheumatic fever, but there is a large body of epidemiological and immunological evidence indirectly implicating the group A streptococcus in the initiation of the disease process. For example: (i) it is well known that outbreaks of rheumatic fever closely follow epidemics of either streptococcal sore throats or scarlet fever (Whitnack and Bisno 1980); (ii) adequate treatment of a documented streptococcal pharyngitis markedly reduces the incidence of subsequent rheumatic fever; (iii) approximate antimicrobial prophylaxis prevents recurrences of the disease in patients known to have had acute rheumatic fever, and (iv) if one tests the serum of the majority of patients with acute rheumatic fever for three antistreptococcal antibodies (streptolysin O, hyaluronidase, and streptokinase), the vast majority of samples (whether or not the patients recall an antecedent streptococcal sore throat) will have elevated antibody titres to these antigens.

A note of caution is necessary concerning the documentation (either clinical or microbiological) of an antecedent streptococcal infection. The rate of isolation of group A streptococci from the oropharynx is extremely low, even in populations who generally do not have access to microbial antibiotics. Further, there appears to be an age-related discrepancy in the clinical documentation of an antecedent sore throat. In older children and young adults, the recollection of a streptococcal sore throat approaches 70 per cent; in younger children, it approaches only 20 per cent (Veasy et al. 1987). Thus, it is important to have a high index of suspicion of acute rheumatic fever in children or young adults presenting with signs of arthritis and/or carditis, even in the absence of a clinically documented sore throat.

Another intriguing, and as yet unexplained, observation has been the invariable association of rheumatic fever only with streptococcal pharyngitis rather than other streptococcal lesions. While there have been many outbreaks of impetigo, rheumatic fever almost never follows infection with these impetigo strains. Furthermore, as Potter et al. (1978) have pointed out, in Trinidad, where both impetigo and rheumatic fever are concomitant infections, the strains colonizing the skin are different from those associated with rheumatic fever, and did not influence the incidence of acute rheumatic fever.

These observations remain inexplicable. It is clear that group A streptococci fall into two main classes based on differences in the C-repeat regions of the M protein (Bessen et al. 1989). One class is clearly associated with streptococcal pharyngeal infection, the other (with some exceptions) belongs to strains commonly associated with impetigo. Thus, the particular strain of streptococcus may be crucial in initiating the disease process. The pharyngeal site of infection, with its large repository of lymphoid tissue, may also be important in the initiation of the abnormal humoral response by the host to those antigens cross-reactive with target organs (see below). Finally, while impetigo strains do colonize the pharynx, they do not appear to elicit as strong an immunological response to the M-protein moiety as do the pharyngeal strains. This may prove to be an important factor, especially in light of the known cross-reactions between various streptococcal structures and mammalian proteins.

Group A streptococcus

Figure 1 is a schematic cross-section of the group A streptococcus. The capsule is composed of equimolar concentrations of *N*-acetyl glucosamine and glucuronic acid, and is structurally identical to hyaluronic acid of mammalian tissues.

Numerous past attempts to demonstrate antibodies to this capsule were unsuccessful. More recently, Fillit et al. (1986) successfully demonstrated high titres to hyaluronic acid, using techniques designed to detect non-precipitating antibodies in the serum of animals. Similar antibodies have been found in man (Faarber et al. 1984). Almost no published data implicate this capsule as important in human infections, although Stollerman (1975) commented on the presence of a large mucoid capsule as one of the more important characteristics of certain 'rheumatogenic' strains.

Investigations by Dr Rebecca Lancefield and others, spanning almost 70 years (reviewed by Fischetti 1989), have established that the M-protein molecule (at least 80 distinct serological types) is perhaps the most important virulence factor in human group A streptococcal infections. The protein is a helical, coiled-coil structure; it has striking structural homology with the cardiac cytoskeletal proteins tropomyosin and myosin, as well as with many other coil-coiled structures like keratin, DNA, lamin, and vimentin.

Once the amino acid sequence of a number of M proteins became known, it was possible to localize specifically those cross-reactive areas. The studies of Dale and Beachey (1985) showed that the part of the M protein involved in the opsonic reaction also cross-reacted with human sarcolemmal antigens. Sargent et al. (1987) more precisely localized this cross-reaction to the M-protein amino acid residues 164–197.

The evidence implicating these cross-reactions in the pathogenesis of acute rheumatic fever remains scant. Antibodies to myosin have been detected in the serum of patients with acute rheumatic fever, but they are also present in a large percentage of sera obtained from individuals who have had a streptococcal infection but did not subsequently develop acute

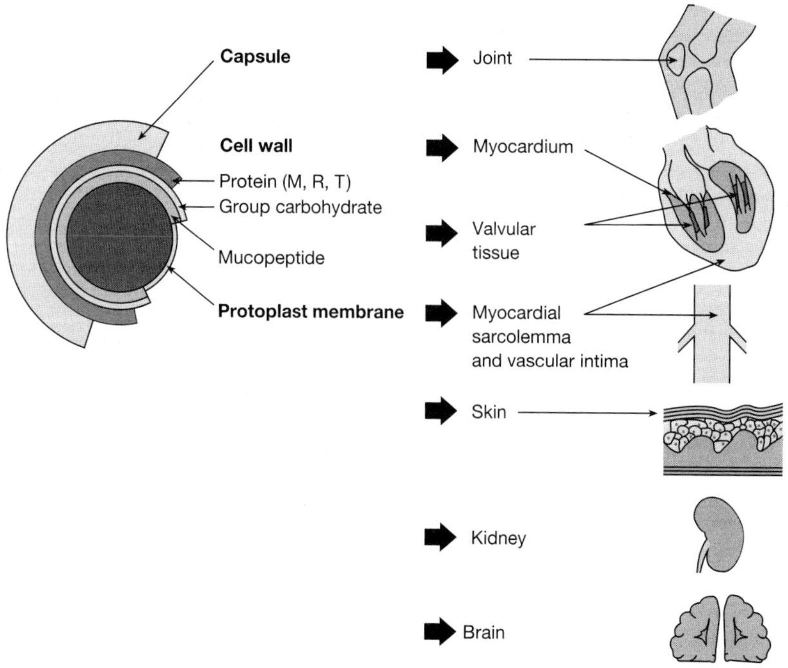

Fig. 1 Schematic representation of the various structures of the group A streptococcus. Note the wide variety of cross-reactions between its antigens and mammalian tissues.

rheumatic fever (Cunningham et al. 1988). The significance of this observation is unclear, since myosin is an internal protein of cardiac muscle cells and therefore not easily exposed to M-protein cross-reacting antibodies.

The group-specific carbohydrate of the streptococcus is a polysaccharide chain consisting of repeating units of rhamnose capped by *N*-acetyl glucosamine molecules. The *N*-acetyl glucosamine is immunodominant and gives rise to the serological group specificity of group A streptococci. The cross-reaction between group A carbohydrate and valvular glycoproteins was first described by Goldstein et al. (1968), and the reactivity was related to the *N*-acetyl glucosamine moiety present in both structures. Goldstein and Caravano (1967) noted that serum from patients with rheumatic fever reacted with the heart-valve glycoprotein. More recently, H.M. Fillit (personal communication) has observed strong reactivity of such sera with purified proteoglycan material. Thus, these cross-reactions could involve the sugar moiety present in both the proteoglycan portion of the glycoprotein and the carbohydrate.

It has always been assumed that group A anticarbohydrate antibodies did not play a part in the phagocytosis of group A streptococci. However, the studies of Salvadori et al. (1995) have demonstrated that human serum containing high titres of anti-group A carbohydrate antibody were opsonophagocytic for a number of different M-protein-specific strains, and that the opsonophagocytic properties were directed to the *N*-acetyl glucosamine moiety of the group A carbohydrate.

The mucopeptide portion of the cell wall is the 'backbone' of the organism and thus rather rigid in structure. It is composed of repeating units of muramic acid and *N*-acetyl glucosamine, cross-linked by peptide bridges. It is particularly difficult to degrade and induces a wide variety of lesions when injected into various species, including arthritis in rats and myocardial granulomas in mice that resemble (but are not identical to) lesions in rheumatic fever.

The connection between cell-wall mucopeptides and the pathogenesis of rheumatic fever remains obscure. Elevated titres of antimucopeptide antibody have been detected in the serum of patients with acute rheumatic fever, and also in the serum of patients with rheumatoid and juvenile rheumatoid arthritis (Heymer et al. 1976), but their pathogenetic relation to the clinical disease has been difficult to establish. There is no evidence that cell-wall antigens are present either in the Aschoff lesion or in the myocardial tissue obtained from patients with rheumatic fever.

Perhaps the most significant cross-reactions lie in the streptococcal membrane structure. We have shown (Zabriskie 1985) that immunization with membrane material elicited antibodies that bound to sections of heart in a pattern similar to that observed with serum from acute rheumatic fever.

Kingston and Glynn (1971) were the first to show that animals immunized with streptococcal antigens develop serum antibodies that stain astrocytes. Husby et al. (1976) demonstrated that serum from patients with acute rheumatic fever with chorea contains antibodies that were specific for caudate cells. Absorption of the serum with streptococcal membrane antigens eliminated the reactivity with caudate cells.

Numerous other cross-reactions between streptococcal membranes and other organs have also been reported, for example, renal basement membranes, basement membrane proteoglycans, and skin, particularly keratin. Here, space does not permit an exhaustive discussion of these cross-reactions, and the reader is referred to our recent review (Froude et al. 1989) for more detail. Whether or not these cross-reactions (especially those seen with basement membranes and skin) play a part in the disease awaits further study.

Genetics

The concept that rheumatic fever might be the result of a host genetic predisposition has intrigued investigators for over a century. It has been variously suggested that the disease gene is transmitted in an autosomal-dominant fashion, an autosomal-recessive fashion with limited penetrance, or that it is possibly related to the genes conferring blood-group secretor status.

Renewed interest in the genetics of rheumatic fever came with the recognition that gene products of the human major histocompatibility complex (MHC) were associated with certain clinical disease states. Using an alloserum from a multiparous donor, an increased frequency of a B-cell alloantigen was reported in several genetically distinct and ethnically diverse populations of individuals with rheumatic fever, and was not MHC-related (Patarroyo et al. 1979).

Most recently, studies were accomplished with a monoclonal antibody (D8/17) prepared by immunizing mice with B cells from a patient with rheumatic fever (Khanna et al. 1989). This B-cell antigen was expressed on increased numbers of B cells in 100 per cent of rheumatics of diverse ethnic origin, and only in 10 per cent of normal individuals. The antigen defined by this monoclonal antibody showed no association with, or linkage to, any of the known MHC haplotypes, nor did it appear to be related to B-cell activation antigens.

These findings are in contrast to reports of an increased frequency of HLA–DR4 and HLA–DR2 in white and black patients with rheumatic heart disease (Ayoub et al. 1986). Other studies have implicated HLA–DR1 and –DRW6 as susceptibility factors in Black South African patients with rheumatic heart disease (Maharaj et al. 1987). Most recently, Guilherme et al. (1991) have noted a close association of HLA–DR7 and –DW53 with rheumatic fever in Brazil. These apparently differing results concerning HLA antigens and susceptibility to rheumatic fever prompt speculation that the reported associations might involve genes close to, but not identical with, an unknown gene for that susceptibility. Alternatively, and more likely, susceptibility to acute rheumatic fever is polygenic, and the D8/17 antigen might be associated with only one of the genes (i.e. those of the MHC complex encoding for DR antigens) conferring susceptibility. While the explanation remains to be determined, it is none the less true that the presence of the D8/17 antigen appears to identify a population at special risk for contracting acute rheumatic fever.

Aetiological considerations

While a large body of evidence, both immunological and epidemiological, has implicated the group A streptococcus in the induction of the disease process, the exact pathological mechanisms involved still remain obscure. At least three main theories have been proposed.

The first is concerned with the question of whether persistence of the organism is important. Despite several controversial reports, no investigators have been able consistently to demonstrate live organisms in cardiac tissues or valves in rheumatic fever.

The second theory revolves around the question of whether the deposition of toxic products is required. Although an attractive hypothesis, little or no experimental evidence has been obtained in its support. For example, Halbert et al. (1961) suggested that streptolysin O (an extracellular product of group A streptococci) is cardiotoxic and might be carried to the site by circulating complexes containing streptolysin O and antibody. However, in spite of an intensive search for these products (J.B. Zabriskie, unpublished data), no such complexes have been identified *in situ*.

Renewed interest in these extracellular toxins has recently emerged with the observation by Schlievert et al. (1987) that certain streptococcal pyrogenic toxins (A and C) may act as superantigens. These antigens may stimulate large numbers of T cells through their unique interaction between MHC class II and T-cell receptors of specific V_β types. This interaction does not involve the usual concept of antigen presentation in the context of the MHC complex. Once activated, these cells induce the production of tumour necrosis factor, interferon-γ, and a number of interleukin moieties, thereby contributing to the initiation of pathological damage. Further-more, it has been suggested (Paliard et al. 1991) that in certain disease states such as rheumatoid arthritis, autoreactive cells of specific V_β lineage may 'home' to the target organ. Although an attractive hypothesis, no data on the role of these superantigens in rheumatic fever have as yet emerged.

Perhaps the best evidence to date favours the concept that, in the genetically susceptible individual, there is an abnormal host immune response (both humoral and cellular) to those streptococcal antigens cross-reactive with mammalian tissues. The evidence supporting this concept may be divided into three broad categories as follows.

1. Employing a wide variety of methods, numerous investigators have documented the presence of heart-reactive antibodies in serum from rheumatic fever. The incidence of these antibodies has varied from a low of 33 per cent to a high or 85 per cent in various series. While these antibodies are seen in other individuals (notably those with uncomplicated streptococcal infections and patients with post-streptococcal glomerulonephritis), the titres are always lower than in rheumatic fever and decrease with time during the convalescent period (Zabriskie 1985).
2. Serum in rheumatic fever also contains higher titres of antibodies to both myosin and tropomyosin than serum from patients with uncomplicated streptococcal infections. These myosin affinity-purified antibodies also cross-react with M-protein moieties, suggesting this molecule could be the antigenic stimulus for the production of myosin antibodies in these sera (Cunningham et al. 1988).
3. Finally, as indicated above, autoimmune antibodies are a prominent finding in another major clinical manifestation of acute rheumatic fever, chorea, and these antibodies are directed against the cells of the caudate nucleus. The titre of this antibody corresponds with clinical disease activity (Husby et al. 1976).

While not necessarily autoimmune in nature, the presence of elevated amounts of immune complexes has been well documented both in serum and joints in acute rheumatic fever. These amounts, which may be as high as those seen in classical post-streptococcal glomerulonephritis, may be responsible for immune-complex vasculitis seen in acute rheumatic fever and may provide the initial impetus for vascular damage, followed by the secondary penetration of autoreactive antibodies. Support for the concept is found in the close clinical similarity of arthritis in rheumatic fever to experimentally induced serum sickness in animals or the arthritis secondary to drug hypersensitivity. Deposition of host immunoglobulin and complement is also seen in the cardiac tissues of patients with acute rheumatic fever, suggesting autoimmune deposition of immunoglobulins in or near the Aschoff lesions.

At a cellular level, there is now ample evidence for the presence of both lymphocytes and macrophages at the site of pathological damage in the heart in patients with acute rheumatic fever (Kemeny et al. 1989). The cells are predominantly CD4+ helper lymphocytes during acute stages of the disease (4 : 1). The ratio of CD4+/CD8+ lymphocytes (2 : 1) more closely approximates the normal ratio in valvular specimens in chronic rheumatics. A majority of these cells express Ia antigens. A potentially important finding has been the observation that macrophage-like fibroblasts present in the diseased valves express Ia antigens (Amoils et al. 1986) and might be the antigen-presenting cells for the CD4+ lymphocytes.

There was greater reactivity to streptococcal antigens in preparations of mononuclear cells from peripheral blood of patients with acute rheumatic fever than in these cells isolated from patients with nephritis (Read et al. 1986). This abnormal reactivity peaked at 6 months after the attack but could persist for as long as 2 years after the initial episode. Once again the reactivity was specific only for those strains associated with acute rheumatic fever, suggesting an abnormal humoral and cellular response to streptococcal antigens unique to rheumatic fever-associated streptococci.

Support for the potential pathological importance of these T cells is further strengthened by the observation that lymphocytes obtained from experimental animals sensitized to cell membranes but not cell walls are specifically cytotoxic for syngeneic embryonic cardiac myofibrils *in vitro*. In humans, normal mononuclear cells primed *in vitro* by M-protein molecules from a rheumatic fever-associated strain were also cytotoxic for myofibrils but specificity solely for cardiac cells was lacking (Dale and Beachey 1987). Similar studies have not yet been done with lymphocytes from patients with active acute rheumatic fever.

Clinical features of acute rheumatic fever

The clinical presentation of acute rheumatic fever is rather variable, and the lack of a single pathognomonic feature has resulted in the development of the revised Jones criteria, as illustrated in Table 2 (Jones Criteria Update 1992), which are used to establish a diagnosis.

It should be noted that these criteria were established only as guidelines for the diagnosis and were never intended to be 'etched in stone'. Thus, depending on the age, geographical location, and ethnic population, emphasis on one or the other criterion for the diagnosis of acute rheumatic fever may be more or less important. Manifestations of rheumatic fever that are not clearly expressed pose a dilemma because of the importance of clearly identifying a first rheumatic attack in order to establish the need for prophylaxis (see below). Some of the isolated manifestations, particularly polyarthritis, may be difficult or impossible to distinguish from other diseases, especially at their onset. The diagnosis can be made, however, when 'pure' chorea is the sole manifestation, because of the rarity with which this syndrome is due to any other cause.

Arthritis

In the classic, untreated case the arthritis of rheumatic fever affects several joints in quick succession, each for a short time. The legs are usually affected first and later the arms. The terms 'migrating' or 'migratory' are often used to describe the polyarthritis of rheumatic fever, but these designations are not meant to signify that the inflammation necessarily disappears in one joint when it appears in another. Rather, the various localizations usually overlap in time, and the onset, as opposed to the full course of the arthritis, 'migrates' from joint to joint.

Joint involvement is more common, and also more severe, in teenagers and young adults than in children. It occurs early in the rheumatic illness, and is usually the earliest symptomatic manifestation of the disease, although asymptomatic carditis may precede it. Rheumatic polyarthritis may be excruciatingly painful, but is almost always transient. The pain is usually more prominent than the objective signs of inflammation.

When the disease was allowed to express itself fully, unchecked by anti-inflammatory treatment, over half of patients studied show a true polyarthritis, with inflammation in any of from 6 to 16 joints. Classically, each joint is maximally inflamed for only a few days, or a week at the most: the inflammation decreases, perhaps lingering for another week or so, and then disappears completely. Radiographs taken at this point may show a slight effusion but most probably will be unremarkable.

Table 2 Revised Jones criteria for diagnosis of acute rheumatic fever[a]

Major manifestations	Minor manifestations
Carditis	Fever
Polyarthritis	Arthralgia
Chorea	Previous rheumatic fever or rheumatic heart disease
Erythema marginatum	
Subcutaneous nodules	
Laboratory findings	
1. Elevated acute-phase reactants:	
(a) C-reactive protein	
(b) Erythrocyte sedimentation rate	
2. Prolonged P–R interval rate	
Supporting evidence of proceeding streptococcal infection	
1. Increased ASO or other streptococcal antibodies	
2. Positive throat culture of group A haemolytic streptococci	
3. Recent scarlet fever	

[a] Jones Criteria Update (1992). ASO, antistreptolysin O.

In routine practice, however, many patients with arthritis and/or arthralgias are treated empirically with salicylates or other non-steroidal anti-inflammatory drugs. Accordingly, arthritis subsides quickly in the joint(s) already affected and does not 'migrate' to new joints. Thus, therapy may deprive the diagnostician of a useful sign. In a large series of patients with rheumatic fever and associated arthritis, most of whom had been treated, involvement of only a single large joint was common (25 per cent). One or both knees were affected in 76 per cent, and one or both ankles in 50 per cent. Elbows, wrists, hips, or small joints of the feet were involved in 12–15 per cent of patients, and shoulder or small joints of the head were affected in 7–8 per cent. Joints rarely affected were the lumbosacral (2 per cent), cervical (1 per cent), sternoclavicular (0.5 per cent), and temporomandibular (0.5 per cent). Involvement of the small joints of the hands or feet alone occurred in only 1 per cent of these patients.

Analysis of the synovial fluid in well-documented cases of rheumatic fever with arthritis generally reveals a sterile inflammatory fluid. There may be a decrease of the complement components C1q, C3, and C4, indicating their consumption by immune complexes in the joint fluid.

Post-streptococcal reactive arthritis

A number of investigators (e.g. Fink 1991) have raised the question of whether post-streptococcal migratory arthritis, in the absence of carditis both in adults and children, is really acute rheumatic fever, for the following reasons.

1. The latent period between the antecedent streptococcal infection and the onset of acute rheumatic fever is shorter (1–2 weeks) than the 3–4 weeks usually seen in classical acute rheumatic fever.
2. The response of the arthritis to aspirin and other non-steroidal medications is poor in comparison to the dramatic response seen in classical acute rheumatic fever.
3. Evidence of carditis is not usually seen in these patients and the arthritis is rather severe.
4. Extra-articular manifestations such as tenosynovitis and renal abnormalities are often seen in these patients.

While these cases (admittedly rare) do exist, migratory arthritis without evidence of other major Jones criteria, if supported by two minor manifestations (see Table 3), must still be considered acute rheumatic fever, especially in children. Variations in the response to aspirin in these children often are not recorded with serum salicylate concentrations, and an unusual clinical course is not sufficient to exclude the diagnosis of acute rheumatic fever; appropriate prophylactic measures should be therefore taken (reviewed by Gibofsky and Zabriskie 1994). Support for this concept may be found in the work of Crea and Mortimer (1959), in which 50 per cent of the children with signs of migratory arthritis alone went on to develop significant valvular damage after a long follow-up.

Table 3 Physical signs and symptoms of acute rheumatic fever, Rockefeller University Hospital, 1950–1970

	RHD (*n* = 40) (%)	No RHD (*n* = 47) (%)	Total (*n* = 87) (%)	Bland and Jones (1951) (%)
Carditis	100	83.0	90.1	65.3
Arthritis	67.5	68.1	67.8	41.0
Epistaxis	0.0	10.6	5.7	27.4
Chorea	5.0	2.1	3.4	51.8
Pericarditis	2.5	4.3	3.4	13.0
Nodules	7.5	0.0	3.4	8.8
Erythema marginatum	0.0	4.3	2.3	7.1

Rheumatic fever also occurs in adults. Although migratory arthritis is a common presenting symptom, a recent outbreak in San Diego Naval Training Camp (Wallace et al. 1989) revealed a 30 per cent incidence of valvular damage in these patients.

The importance of clearly defining this reactive arthritis as a variant of rheumatic fever has obvious implications for secondary prophylactic treatment. As suggested by some investigators, post-streptococcal reactive arthritis is a benign condition without need for prophylaxis. Yet as these patients by and large do fulfil the Jones criteria (one major, two minor), they should be considered as having rheumatic fever and treated as such.

Carditis

Cardiac valvular and muscle damage can manifest in a variety of signs or symptoms, including organic heart murmurs, cardiomegaly, congestive heart failure, or pericarditis. Mild to moderate chest discomfort, pleuritic chest pain, or a pericardial friction rub are indications of pericarditis. On clinical examination, the patient can have new or changing organic murmurs, most commonly mitral regurgitant murmurs, and occasionally aortic regurgitant murmurs and/or systolic ejection murmurs, caused by acute valvular inflammation and deformity. Rarely, a Carey Coombs mid-diastolic murmur caused by rapid flow over the mitral valve is heard. If the valvular damage is severe enough, together with concurrent cardiac dysfunction, congestive heart failure can ensue, which is the most life-threatening clinical syndrome of acute rheumatic fever. Congestive heart failure needs to be treated intensively and quickly with a combination of anti-inflammatory drugs, diuretics and, occasionally, steroids to acutely decrease the cardiac inflammation. Electrocardiographic abnormalities include all degrees of heart block, including atrioventricular dissociation, but first-degree heart block is not associated with a poor prognosis. Second- or third-degree heart block can occasionally be symptomatic. If heart block is associated with congestive heart failure, a temporary pacemaker can be placed if indicated. The most common manifestation of carditis is cardiomegaly, as seen on radiographs.

In the population of patients recently reviewed from our institution, The Rockefeller University Hospital, who were diagnosed with acute rheumatic fever between 1950 and 1970, with an average of 20 years of follow-up, 90 per cent had evidence of carditis at diagnosis (Table 3). In a classic review of 1000 patients (Bland and Jones 1951), only 65 per cent were diagnosed with carditis. The addition of Doppler sonography to the clinical evaluation of patients during the recent Utah outbreak increased the proportion diagnosed with carditis from 72 to 91 per cent (Minisch et al. 1997; Veasy 2001). These more recent studies indicate that, with more sensitive measurements of cardiac dysfunction and applying strict criteria to the echocardiac findings, almost all patients with acute rheumatic fever have signs of acute carditis. They also point out that the cardiac manifestations and congestive failure are more related to inflammation of the leaflets and valvular tissues than to the myocarditis. Repair of the valvular damage in most cases allows the return of normal cardiac function.

Rheumatic heart disease

Rheumatic heart disease is the most severe outcome of acute rheumatic fever. Usually occurring 10–20 years after the original attack, it is the major cause of acquired valvular disease in the world. The mitral valve is mainly involved and the aortic valve less often. Mitral stenosis is a classic finding in rheumatic heart disease and can manifest as a combination of mitral insufficiency and stenosis, secondary to severe calcification of the mitral valve. When symptoms of left atrial enlargement are present, mitral valve replacement may become necessary.

In various studies, the incidence of rheumatic heart disease in patients with a history of acute rheumatic fever has varied. In the classic study of Bland and Jones (1951), after 20 years, one-third of patients had no murmur, another one-third had died, and the remaining one-third was alive with rheumatic heart disease. A majority of the patients who died had rheumatic heart disease. While the dogma is that patients with rheumatic heart disease invariably have had more than one attack of acute rheumatic fever, recent analysis of our patients at the Rockefeller University Hospital disproves this. The population studied was 87 patients who had had only one documented attack of acute rheumatic fever, without any evidence (clinical or laboratory) of a recurrence during a 20-year follow-up under close supervision. Over 80 per cent had carditis at admission and approximately 50 per cent now have organic murmurs (Table 3). Thus, valvular damage manifesting as organic murmurs later in life is still likely to occur in 50 per cent of the patients if they presented with evidence of carditis at initial diagnosis. All of the patients in our population who ended up with rheumatic heart disease had carditis at diagnosis.

Chorea

Sydenham's chorea, chorea minor, or 'St Vitus dance' is a neurological disorder consisting of abrupt, purposeless, non-rhythmic involuntary movements, muscular weakness, and emotional disturbances. They disappear during sleep, but may occur at rest and may interfere with voluntary activity. Initially, it may be possible to suppress these movements, which may affect all voluntary muscles, with the hands and face usually the most obvious. Grimaces and inappropriate smiles are common. Handwriting usually becomes clumsy and provides a convenient way of following the patient's course. Speech is often slurred. The movements are commonly more marked on one side and are occasionally completely unilateral (hemichorea).

The muscular weakness is best revealed by asking the patient to squeeze the examiner's hands: the pressure of the patient's grip increases and decreases continuously and capriciously, a phenomenon known as relapsing grip, or milking sign.

The emotional changes manifest themselves in outbursts of inappropriate behaviour, including crying and restlessness. In rare cases, the psychological manifestations may be severe and may result in transient psychosis.

The neurological examination fails to reveal sensory losses or involvement of the pyramidal tract. Diffuse hypotonia may be present.

Chorea may follow streptococcal infections after a latent period, which is longer, on the average, than the latent period of other rheumatic manifestations. Some patients with chorea have no other symptoms, but other patients develop chorea weeks or months after arthritis. In both cases, examination of the heart may reveal murmurs.

Skin lesions

Sub-cutaneous nodules

The sub-cutaneous nodules of rheumatic fever are firm and painless. The overlying skin is not inflamed and can usually be moved over the nodules. The diameter of these round lesions varies from a few millimetres to 1 or even 2 cm. They are located over bony surface or prominences, or near tendons; their number varies from a single nodule to a few dozen and averages three or four; when numerous, they are usually symmetrical. These nodules are present for one or more weeks, rarely for more than a month. They are smaller and more short-lived than the nodules of rheumatoid arthritis. Although in both diseases the elbows are most frequently involved, the rheumatic nodules are more common on the olecranon, and the rheumatoid nodules are usually found 3 or 4 cm distal to it. Rheumatic sub-cutaneous nodules generally appear only after the first few weeks of illness, usually only in patients with carditis.

Erythema marginatum

Erythema marginatum is an evanescent, non-pruritic skin rash, pink or faintly red, usually affecting the trunk, sometimes the proximal parts or the limbs, but not the face. The lesion extends centrifugally while the skin in the centre returns gradually to normal; hence, the name 'erythema marginatum'. The outer edge of the lesion is sharp, whereas the inner edge is diffuse. Because the margin of the lesion is usually continuous, making a ring, it is also known as 'erythema annulare'.

The individual lesions may appear and disappear in a matter of hours, usually to return. A hot bath or shower may make them more evident or may even reveal them for the first time.

Erythema marginatum usually occurs in the early phase of the disease. It often persists or recurs, even when all other manifestations of disease have disappeared. Occasionally, the lesions appear for the first time or, more probably, are noticed for the first time, late in the course of the illness or even during convalescence. This disorder usually occurs only in patients with carditis.

The minor manifestations of rheumatic fever

Temperature is increased in almost all rheumatic attacks and ranges from 38.4 to 40°C. Usually fever decreases in about a week without antipyretic treatment, and may become low grade for another week or two. Fever rarely lasts for more than 3–4 weeks.

Abdominal pain

The abdominal pain of rheumatic fever resembles that of other conditions associated with acute microvascular mesenteric inflammation and is non-specific. It usually occurs at or near the onset of the rheumatic attack, so that other manifestations may not yet be present to clarify the diagnosis. In many cases, it may mimic acute appendicitis.

Epistaxis

In the past, epistaxis occurred most prominently and severely in patients with severe and protracted rheumatic carditis. Early clinical studies reported a frequency as high as 48 per cent, but it probably occurs even less frequently now (see Table 3). Although epistaxis has been correlated in the past with the severity of rheumatic inflammation, it is difficult to assess retrospectively the possible thrombasthenic effect of large doses of salicylates administered for prolonged periods in protracted attacks.

Rheumatic pneumonia

Rheumatic pneumonia may appear during the course of severe rheumatic carditis. This inflammatory process is difficult or impossible to distinguish from pulmonary oedema or the alveolitis associated with respiratory distress syndrome due to a variety of pathophysiological states.

Laboratory findings

The diagnosis of rheumatic fever cannot readily be established by laboratory tests. Nevertheless, tests may be helpful in two ways: first in demonstrating that an antecedent streptococcal infection has occurred and second in documenting the presence or persistence of an inflammatory process. Serial chest radiographs may be helpful in following the course of carditis and the electrocardiogram may reflect the inflammatory process on the conduction system.

Throat cultures are usually negative by the time rheumatic fever appears but an attempt should be made to isolate the organism. It is our practice to take three throat cultures during the first 24 h, before giving antibiotics. Streptococcal antibodies are more useful because: (i) they reach a peak titre at about the time of onset of rheumatic fever; (ii) they indicate true infection rather than transient carriage; and (iii) by performing several tests for different antibodies, any significant recent streptococcal infection can be detected. To demonstrate a rising titre, it is useful to take a serum specimen when the patient is first seen and another one 2 weeks later for comparison.

The specific antibody tests most frequently used to diagnosis streptococcal infections are those directed against extracellular products. They include antistreptolysin O, anti-DNAse B, antihyaluronidase, anti-NADase (anti-DPNase), and antistreptokinase. Antistreptolysin O has been the most widely used test and is generally available in hospitals in the United States.

Titres of antistreptolysin O vary with age, season, and geographical region. They reach peak levels in the young, school-age population. Titres of 200–300 Todd units/ml are common, therefore, in healthy children of elementary-school age. After a streptococcal pharyngitis, the antibody response peaks at about 4–5 weeks, which is usually during the second or third week of rheumatic fever (depending on how early it is detected). Thereafter, antibody titres fall off rapidly in the next several months, and, after 6 months, they decline more slowly. Since only 80 per cent of documented rheumatics exhibit a rise in the titre of antistreptolysin O, it is recommended that other antistreptococcal antibody tests be performed in the absence of a positive titre. These include anti-DNAse B, hyaluronidase, or streptozyme, which is a combination of various streptococcal antigens.

Streptococcal antibodies, when increased, support but do not prove the diagnosis of acute rheumatic fever, nor are they a measure of rheumatic activity. Even in the absence of intercurrent streptococcal infection, titres decline during the rheumatic attack despite the persistence or severity of rheumatic activity.

Acute-phase reactants

Acute-phase reactants are elevated during acute rheumatic fever, just as they are during other inflammatory conditions. Both the C-reactive protein and erythrocyte sedimentation rate are almost invariably abnormal during the active rheumatic process, if it is not suppressed by antirheumatic drugs. Pure chorea and persistent erythema marginatum are exceptions. Particularly when treatment has been discontinued or is being tapered off, the C-reactive protein or erythrocyte sedimentation rate are useful in monitoring 'rebounds' of rheumatic inflammation, which indicate that the rheumatic process is still active. If either remains normal a few weeks after discontinuing antirheumatic therapy, the attack may be considered ended unless chorea appears. Even then, usually, there will be no exacerbation of the systemic inflammation and chorea will be present as an isolated manifestation.

Anaemia

A mild normochromic normocytic anaemia of chronic infection or inflammation may be seen during acute rheumatic fever. Suppressing the inflammation usually improves the anaemia, thus iron therapy is usually not indicated.

Clinical course and treatment of acute rheumatic fever

The mainstay of treatment for acute rheumatic fever has always been anti-inflammatory agents, most commonly aspirin. Dramatic improvement in symptoms is usually seen after the start of therapy. Usually 80–100 mg/kg/day in children and 4–8 g/day in adults is required for an effect to be seen. Aspirin concentrations can be measured and 20–30 mg/dl is the therapeutic range. The duration of anti-inflammatory therapy can vary but the treatment should be maintained until all symptoms are absent and laboratory values are normal. If severe carditis is also present, as indicated by significant cardiomegaly, congestive heart failure or third-degree heart block, steroid therapy can be instituted. The usual dosage is 2 mg/kg/day of oral prednisone during the first 1–2 weeks. Depending on clinical and laboratory improvement, the dosage is then tapered over the next 2 weeks and during the last week aspirin may be added in the dosage recommended above sufficient to achieve 20–30 mg/dl.

Whether or not signs of pharyngitis are present at the time of diagnosis, antibiotic therapy with penicillin should be started and maintained for at least 10 days, in doses recommended for the eradication of a streptococcal pharyngitis. In addition, all family contacts should be cultured and treated for streptococcal infection, if positive. If compliance is an issue, depot penicillins, such as benzathine penicillin G 600 000 units in children, 1.2 million units in adults, should be given. Recurrences of acute rheumatic fever are most common within 2 years of the original attack but can occur at any time. The risk of recurrence decreases with age. Recurrence rates have been decreasing, from 20 to 2–4 per cent in recent outbreaks. This might be due to better surveillance and treatment.

Prophylaxis

Antibiotic prophylaxis with penicillin should be started immediately after the resolution of the acute episode. The optimal regimen consists of oral penicillin VK 250 000 units twice a day, or depot intramuscular injection of 1.2 million units penicillin G every 4 weeks. Recent data suggest, however, that injections every 3 weeks are more effective than every 4 weeks in preventing recurrences of acute rheumatic fever (Lue et al. 1986). If the patient is allergic to penicillin, erythromycin 250 mg/day can be substituted.

The end-point of prophylaxis is unclear; most believe it should continue at least until the patient is a young adult, which is usually 10 years from an acute attack with no recurrence. In our opinion, individuals with documented evidence of rheumatic heart disease should be on continuous prophylaxis indefinitely since our experience has been that rheumatic fever can recur even in the fifth or sixth decades. Another potential problem for recurrences is the presence in the household of young children who could transmit new group A streptococcal infections to rheumatic-susceptible individuals.

Obviously, the alternative to long-term prophylaxis in an individual with rheumatic fever will be the introduction of streptococcal vaccines designed not only to prevent recurrent infections in rheumatic-susceptible individuals but also to prevent streptococcal disease in general. While it is not within the scope of this chapter to discuss the prospects for these vaccines (see review by Fischetti 1989), at least a few words are appropriate. Immunization of mice with either C-repeat peptides of M protein or 'cloned' M protein in a vaccinia virus vector protected them against intranasal infection with homologous or heterologous strains of group A streptococci. Whether or not these antigens and/or vectors are protective in man is being investigated. One of the major problems will be to avoid using those parts of the molecule that are cross-reactive with mammalian tissues.

Conclusion

In spite of its disappearance in many areas, rheumatic fever continues to be a serious problem in those geographical areas where two-thirds of the world's population lives. Even in developed countries with full access to medical care, and better nutrition and housing, the recent resurgence of rheumatic fever emphasizes the need for continued vigilance by physicians and other health officials in both diagnosing and treating the disease. The importance of early diagnosis and therapy cannot be overemphasized. Although the joint manifestations are transient and self-limiting, the cardiac sequelae are chronic and life-threatening. Whether the resurgence represents a change in the virulence of the organism or failure to recognize the importance and need for adequate treatment of an antecedent streptococcal infection is an area of intense debate and will therefore require careful and controlled epidemiological surveillance.

Nevertheless, rheumatic fever remains one of the few autoimmune disorders known to occur as a result of infection with a specific organism. The confirmed observation of an increased frequency of a B-cell alloantigen in several populations of rheumatics suggests that it might be possible to identify rheumatic fever-susceptible individuals at birth. If so, then from a public health standpoint: (i) these individuals would be prime candidates for immunization with any streptococcal vaccine that might be developed in the future, (ii) careful monitoring of streptococcal disease in the susceptible population could lead to early and effective antibiotic strategies, resulting in disease prevention, and (iii) in individuals previously infected, who later present with subtle or non-specific manifestations of the disease, the presence or absence of the marker could be of value in arriving at a diagnosis.

The continued study of rheumatic fever as a prime example of microbial–host interactions also has important implications for the study of autoimmune diseases in general and rheumatic diseases in particular. Further insights into this intriguing host–parasite relation may shed additional light on those diseases where infection is assumed to have occurred but has not as yet been identified.

References

Amoils, B. et al. (1986). Aberrant expression of HLA-DR antigen on valvular fibroblasts from patients with acute rheumatic carditis. *Clinical and Experimental Immunology* **66**, 84–94.

Ayoub, E.A., Barrett, D.J., Maclaren, N.K., and Krischer, J.P. (1986). Association of class II human histocompatibility leucocyte antigens with rheumatic fever. *Journal of Clinical Investigation* **77**, 2019–26.

Bessen, D., Jones, K.F., and Fischetti, V.A. (1989). Evidence for the distinct classes of streptococcal M protein and their relationship to rheumatic fever. *Journal of Experimental Medicine* **169**, 269–83.

Bland, E.F. and Jones, T.D. (1951). Rheumatic fever and rheumatic heart disease: a twenty year report on 1000 patients followed since childhood. *Circulation* **4**, 836–43.

Crea, M.A. and Mortimer, E.A. (1959). The nature of scarlatinal arthritis. *Pediatrics* **23**, 879–84.

Cunningham, M.W. et al. (1988). Human monoclonal antibodies reactive with antigens of the group A streptococcus and human heart. *Journal of Immunology* **141**, 2760–6.

Dale, J.B. and Beachey, E.H. (1985). Multiple cross reactive epitopes of streptococcal M proteins. *Journal of Experimental Medicine* **161**, 113–22.

Dale, J.B. and Beachey, E.H. (1987). Human cytotoxic T lymphocytes evoked by group A streptococcal M proteins. *Journal of Experimental Medicine* **166**, 1825–35.

Faarber, P. et al. (1984). Cross reactivity of anti DNA antibodies with proteoglycans. *Clinical and Experimental Immunology* **55**, 402–12.

Fillit, H.M., McCarty, M., and Blake, M. (1986). Induction of antibodies to hyaluronic acid by immunization of rabbits with encapsulated streptococci. *Journal of Experimental Medicine* **164**, 762–76.

Fink, C.W. (1991). The role of streptococcus in post streptococcal reactive arthritis and childhood polyarteritis nodosa. *Journal of Rheumatology* **18**, 14–20.

Fischetti, V.A. (1989). Streptococcal M protein: molecular design and biological behavior. *Clinical and Microbiology Reviews* **2**, 285–314.

Froude, J., Gibofsky, A., Buskirk, D.R., Khanna, A., and Zabriskie, J.B. (1989). Cross reactivity between streptococcus and human tissue: a model of molecular mimicry and autoimmunity. *Current Topics in Microbiology and Immunology* **145**, 5–26.

Gibofsky, A. and Zabriskie, J.B. (1994). Rheumatic fever: new insights into an old disease. *Bulletin on the Rheumatic Diseases: Arthritis Foundation* **42**, 5–7.

Goldstein, I. and Caravano, R. (1967). Determination of anti group A streptococcal polysaccharide antibodies in human sera by an hemagglutination technique. *Proceedings of the Society of Experimental Biology and Medicine* **124**, 1209–12.

Goldstein, I., Rebeyrotte, P., Parlebas, J., and Halpern, B. (1968). Isolation from heart valves of glycopeptides which share immunological properties with *Streptococcus haemolyticus* group A polysaccharides. *Nature* **219**, 866–8.

Gordis, L. (1985). The virtual disappearance of rheumatic fever in the United States: lessons in the rise and fall of disease. *Circulation* **72**, 1155–62.

Guilherme, L., Weidenbach, W., Kiss, M.H., Snitcowsky, R., and Kalil, J. (1991). Association of human leucocyte class II antigens with rheumatic fever or rheumatic heart disease in a Brazilian population. *Circulation* **83**, 1995–8.

Halbert, S.P., Bircher, R., and Dahle, E. (1961). The analysis of streptococcal infections. V. Cardiotoxicity of streptolysin O for rabbits *in vivo*. *Journal of Experimental Medicine* **113**, 759–84.

Heymer, B., Schleifer, K.H., Read, S.E., Zabriskie, J.B., and Krause, R.M. (1976). Detection of antibodies to bacterial cell wall peptidoglycan in human sera. *Journal of Immunology* **117**, 23–6.

Husby, G., van de Rijn, I., Zabriskie, J.B., Abdin, Z.H., and Williams, R.C., Jr. (1976). Antibodies reacting with cytoplasm of subthalmic and caudate nuclei neurons in chorea and acute rheumatic fever. *Journal of Experimental Medicine* **144**, 1094–110.

Jones Criteria Update (1992). Guidelines for diagnosis of rheumatic fever. *Journal of the American Medical Association* **268**, 2069–70.

Kaplan, E.L., Johnson, D.R., and Cleary, P.P. (1989). Group A streptococcal serotypes isolated from patients and sibling contacts during the resurgence of rheumatic fever in the United States in the mid 1980s. *Journal of Infectious Diseases* **159**, 101–3.

Kemeny, E., Grieve, T., Marcus, R., Sareli, P., and Zabriskie, J.B. (1989). Identification of mononuclear cells and T cell subsets in rheumatic valvulitis. *Clinical Immunology and Immunopathology* **52**, 225–37.

Khanna, A.K., Buskirk, D.R., Williams, R.C., Jr., Gibofsky, A., Crow, M.K., and Menon, A. (1989). Presence of a non-HLA B cell antigen in rheumatic fever patients and their families as defined by a monoclonal antibody. *Journal of Clinical Investigation* **83**, 1710–16.

Kingston, D. and Glynn, L.E. (1971). A cross-reaction between *Streptococcus pyogenes* and human fibroblasts, endothelial cells and astrocytes. *Immunology* **21**, 1003–16.

Lue, H.C., Mil-Wham, W., Hsieh, K.H., Lin, G.J., Hsieh, R.P., and Chou, F.F. (1986). Rheumatic fever recurrences: controlled study of 3 week versus 4 week benzathine penicillin prevention programs. *Journal of Pediatrics* **108**, 299–304.

Maharaj, B., Hammond, M.G., Appadoo, B., Leary, W.P., and Pudifin, D.J. (1987). HLA-A, B, DR and DQ antigens in black patients with severe chronic rheumatic heart disease. *Circulation* **765**, 259–61.

Markowitz, M. (1987). Rheumatic fever: recent outbreaks of an old disease. *Connecticut Medicine* **51**, 229–33.

Minich, L.L., Tani, L.Y., Pagotta, L.T., Shaddy, R.E., and Veasy, L.G. (1997). Doppler echocardiography distinguishes between physiologic and pathologic 'silent' mitral regurgitation in patients with rheumatic fever. *Clinical Cardiology* **20**, 924–6.

Paliard, X. et al. (1991). Evidence for the effects of superantigen in rheumatoid arthritis. *Science* **253**, 325–9.

Patarroyo, M.E. et al. (1979). Association of a B cell alloantigen with susceptibility to rheumatic fever. *Nature* **278**, 173–4.

Pope, R.M. (1989). Rheumatic fever in the 1980s. *Bulletin on the Rheumatic Diseases, Arthritis Foundation* **38**, 1–8.

Potter, E.V., Svartman, M., Mohammed, I., Cox, R., Poon-King, T., and Earle, D.P. (1978). Tropical acute rheumatic fever and associated streptococcal infections compared with concurrent acute glomerulonephritis. *Journal of Pediatrics* **92**, 325–33.

Read, S.E. et al. (1986). Serial studies on the cellular immune response to streptococcal antigens in acute and convalescent rheumatic fever patients in Trinidad. *Journal of Clinical Immunology* **6**, 433–41.

Salvadori, L.G., Blake, M.S., McCarty, M., Tai, J.Y., and Zabriskie, J.B. (1995). Group A streptococcus-liposome ELISA antibody titers to group A polysaccharide and opsonophagocytic capabilities of the antibodies. *Journal of Infectious Diseases* **171**, 593–600.

Sargent, S.J., Beachey, E.H., Corbett, C.E., and Dale, J.B. (1987). Sequence of protective epitopes of streptococcal M proteins shared with cardiac sarcolemmal membranes. *Journal of Immunology* **139**, 1285–90.

Schlievert, P.M., Johnson, L.P., Tomai, M.A., and Handley, J.P. (1987). Characterization and genetics of group A streptococcal pyrogenic exotoxins.

In *Streptococcal Genetics* (ed. J. Ferretti and R. Curtisis), pp. 136–42. Washington DC: ASM.

Stollerman, G.H., ed. *Rheumatic Fever and Streptococcal Infection* New York: Grune and Stratton, 1975, p. 70.

Veasy L.G. (2001). Time to take soundings in acute rheumatic fever. *Lancet* **357**, 1994–5.

Veasy, L.G. et al. (1987). Resurgence of acute rheumatic fever in the intermountain area of the United States. *New England Journal of Medicine* **316**, 421–7.

Wallace, M.R., Garst, P.D., Papadimos, T.J., and Oldfield, E.C. (1989). The return of acute rheumatic fever in young adults. *Journal of the American Medical Association* **262**, 2557–61.

Whitnack, E. and Bisno, A.L. (1980). Rheumatic fever and other immunologically mediated cardiac diseases. In *Clinical Immunology* Vol. II (ed. C. Parker), pp. 894–929. Philadelphia PA: Saunders.

Zabriskie, J.B. (1985). Rheumatic fever: the interplay between host genetics and microbe. *Circulation* **71**, 1077–86.

6.3 Rheumatoid arthritis

6.3.1 Immunopathogenesis of rheumatoid arthritis

Ravinder N. Maini and Marc Feldmann

Historical review

The delineation of rheumatoid arthritis as a disease entity in the contemporary medical literature began to emerge in the eighteenth century. Initially, clinical observations sought to distinguish the disorder from other prevalent joint diseases, such as gout and rheumatic fever, and emphasized distinctive features, for example, its chronicity, joint deformities, female sex distribution, and disability. Thus, Sydenham (1676), Landry-Beauvais (1800), Brodie, and others were in all probability describing rheumatoid arthritis in their writings, but it was Alfred Baring Garrod (1859) who first used the term 'rheumatoid' arthritis (Garrod 1859; and for reviews see Short 1974; Fraser 1982).

The definition of rheumatoid arthritis and its separation from other forms of chronic polyarthritis did not end with Garrod, and has continued to evolve since. A proportion of patients who might previously have been diagnosed as having rheumatoid arthritis would now be readily reclassified as having polyarthritis seen in the context of ankylosing spondylitis, Reiter's syndrome, psoriatic arthritis, or inflammatory bowel disease. The uniform lack of rheumatoid factor (seronegativity), spinal involvement, and HLA-B27 positivity has linked these disorders into the so-called seronegative spondyloarthropathies. It is of special historical interest to note that until the late 1950s, despite striking differences in clinical features, ankylosing spondylitis was termed rheumatoid spondylitis by North American physicians in the belief that it was part of the disease spectrum of rheumatoid arthritis. This view was essentially based on the striking histopathological similarity to rheumatoid arthritis of the synovitis and erosive arthropathy of diarthrodial joints in ankylosing spondylitis. However, the inflammatory lesion at the point of tendon and ligamentous attachments to bone (enthesopathy) and the association with HLA-B27 proved to be sufficiently distinctive to constitute a basis for differentiation from rheumatoid arthritis.

The possibility that rheumatoid arthritis may result from an infection has had its proponents since the early part of the century. In the early days of modern medicine, rheumatoid arthritis, like other diseases of unknown causes, was thought to result from foci of infection (Hunter 1901; Wilcox 1935). The belief that rheumatoid arthritis may result from infection with *Mycobacterium tuberculosis* is alleged to have motivated Forrestier in France (Forrestier 1935) to use gold salts, which have some antimicrobial activity, in its therapy. An alternative concept of the aetiology of rheumatoid arthritis arose from microscopical observations of 'fibrinoid' change in rheumatoid joints and nodules. Fibrinoid change in connective tissue in systemic lupus and systemic sclerosis had prompted Klemperer et al. (1942) to consider that these diseases might result from diffuse primary degeneration of collagen. This led to the inclusion of rheumatoid arthritis in the group of 'collagen diseases'; however, the development of this new theory was hampered by the observation that the hydroxyproline and collagen content of subcutaneous nodules in rheumatoid arthritis was normal (Ziff et al. 1953).

The discovery by Waaler over half a century ago (Waaler 1940) of IgM rheumatoid factor in the blood of patients with rheumatoid arthritis was the first immunological marker of rheumatic disease to be recognized and served to distinguish it from other forms of inflammatory arthritis. However, a proportion of patients with the clinical features of rheumatoid arthritis who are persistently seronegative for rheumatoid factor, and do not satisfy the diagnostic criteria of spondyloarthropathy, still remain in the category 'seronegative rheumatoid arthritis'. It is possible that this serologically defined sub-group may eventually prove to have a different aetiological basis.

The relatively recent historical description of rheumatoid arthritis has prompted the speculation that it is a disease of modern times. A great deal of interest has therefore focused on seeking evidence of the occurrence of rheumatoid arthritis in medieval and ancient times. Examination of ancient medical writings and medieval paintings has yielded evidence which has satisfied some researchers that rheumatoid arthritis was indeed prevalent in these periods (Short 1974; Dequeker 1987; Dieppe 1988). However, subjectivity of judgement is an obvious problem in assessing such evidence and there appears to be a dearth of convincing descriptions, given that in contemporary life rheumatoid arthritis is such a common and ubiquitous cause of disability and pain. Another approach in establishing the antiquity of rheumatoid arthritis has been an attempt to gauge its prevalence by using palaeontographic methods. Fossil remains of archaic Indian skeletons found in Alabama and Kentucky in the United States, dated as several thousand years old, have been described as exhibiting changes consistent with an erosive arthritis compatible with rheumatoid arthritis (Rothschild and Woods 1990). However, the basis of ascribing the changes to rheumatoid arthritis has been challenged and the lack of rheumatoid pathology in a study of 800 skeletons excavated in the West Country in England has been used as an argument highlighting the lack of this disorder in ancient times (Rogers and Dieppe 1990).

The implication of the claim that rheumatoid arthritis is a relatively modern disease is the possibility that it might have become widespread as a result of an environmental trigger factor which in itself was new. A report from South Africa purporting to demonstrate an increased prevalence of rheumatoid arthritis in Xhosa tribesmen living in urban surroundings compared with their cousins in rural areas (Solomon et al. 1975) has been interpreted as a recapitulation in a contemporary setting of a global scenario unfolding over the past two centuries. The insight that the epidemiology of acquired immunodeficiency syndrome (AIDS) has provided into how new diseases of man become established, has provided an arena for renewed interest in the possibility that the environmental factor responsible could be an infectious agent.

Aetiology

Rheumatoid arthritis is a disease of unknown cause, but current thinking favours the notion that interplay among genetic factors, sex hormones, and possibly an infectious agent or another immune activating agent initiates an autoimmune disease mechanism that culminates in a disease with inflammatory and destructive features.

Genetic factors

Genetic factors were implicated by population studies that showed a slight increase in the frequency of rheumatoid arthritis in first-degree relatives of patients with rheumatoid arthritis, especially if seropositive for rheumatoid factor (Lawrence 1970). Concordance rates of disease in identical twins in hospital-based studies were estimated to be of the order of 30 per cent, compared with 5 per cent in non-identical twins (Lawrence 1970), although the figures are lower in community-based studies (Silman et al. 1989), again supporting the concept of a genetic contribution, but arguing against the proposition that rheumatoid arthritis results from a dominant single-gene disorder. The rates of prevalence in the general population, families, and twins have in fact led to the conclusion that rheumatoid arthritis is a polygenic disease, and that non-inherited factors are also of great importance.

Attempts at identifying the genes involved in predisposition to rheumatoid arthritis took a step forward when tissue typing for HLA class II antigen of Caucasian patients showed that 60–70 per cent of patients with rheumatoid arthritis were HLA–DR4 positive by cellular or serological techniques compared with 20–25 per cent of control populations (Statsny 1976, 1978; Panayi et al. 1979). The patients with more severe rheumatoid arthritis, especially those with systemic complications such as vasculitis and Felty's syndrome, were even more likely to have HLA–DR4 than patients with less aggressive disease confined to joints (Ollier et al. 1984; Westedt et al. 1986).

The increased frequency of HLA–DR4 has also been reported in American black subjects, Japanese, Asian North Indians, and Latin Americans. In Israeli Jews and an Indian immigrant community in the United Kingdom an increased frequency of HLA–DR1 has been found. The increase of HLA–DR4 or –DRl cannot, however, be found in all races and ethnic groups, and a notable exception was a study of Greek patients in whom no HLA associations could be discovered, irrespective of disease severity or serological status (reviewed by Goldstein and Arnett 1987).

Typing by mixed leucocyte culture has defined several HLA–DR4 subtypes. It is of considerable interest that while the subtypes HLA–Dw4 and –Dw14 are associated with rheumatoid arthritis in several studies, Dw15 is only associated with rheumatoid arthritis in the Japanese, while Dw10 and Dw13 are not associated with rheumatoid arthritis in any ethnic group. Another study has shown that in *DR4* homozygotes, *Dw4/Dw14* individuals were at greater risk of developing rheumatoid arthritis than *Dw4/Dw4* (Wordsworth et al. 1992). The significance of this is discussed below.

At the phenotypic level, the importance of HLA class II molecules lies in their participation in a trimolecular reaction involving the HLA antigen-binding cleft formed by the α and β chains of an antigen-presenting cell binding to a processed linear peptide antigen of at least nine amino acids, and the HLA–antigen complex in turn binding to the variable portion of the T-cell receptor. Several research techniques have been used in an attempt to define the similarity of HLA class II molecules common to all patients with rheumatoid arthritis, including patients who are not necessarily HLA–DR4 positive. These include, for example, genotyping of DNA and nucleotide sequencing, using the polymerase chain reaction and enzymatic digestion for restriction fragment length polymorphisms. At the level of expressed surface proteins, HLA epitopes have been sought by using monoclonal antibodies and alloreactive T-cell clones (see Goldstein and Arnett 1987). These studies have lent support to the concept that susceptibility to rheumatoid arthritis is related to a 'shared epitope' on the HLA molecules (Gregersen et al. 1987; Hammer et al. 1995).

Nucleotide sequencing of *HLA DR*β_1 exons coding amino acid residues 70–74 has revealed that HLA–DR4 subtypes Dw4, Dw14, and Dw15 share similarities with each other (with a conservative substitution of glutamine with lysine at position 71 in Dw4) and with HLA–DRl (Table 1)

Table 1 HLA–DR associations with rheumatoid arthritis defined by *DR*β_1 sequence position 70–74

DR type	Sequence[a]					Association
	70	71	72	73	74	
DR4–w4	Q	K	R	A	A	Positive
–w14	Q	R	R	A	A	Positive
–w15	Q	R	R	A	A	Positive
DR1	Q	R	R	A	A	Positive
DR4–w10	D	E	R	A	A	Negative
–w13	Q	R	R	A	E	Negative

[a] O, glutamine; K, lysine; R, arginine; A, alanine; D, aspartic acid; E, glutamic acid.

(Winchester and Gregersen 1988). The sequence predicts susceptibility to rheumatoid arthritis and, for example, is associated with rheumatoid arthritis in 83 per cent of Caucasians in Britain (Wordsworth et al. 1989). In contrast, negative associations are observed in individuals who are DR4w10, in whom the charged basic amino acids glutamine and arginine in positions 70 and 71 are replaced by the acidic amino acids aspartic and glutamic acid. In Dw13 individuals, in whom a negative association is also observed, arginine is substituted for glutamic acid in position 74. Molecular modelling studies suggest that amino acid residues 70–74 are located in the α-helix forming the wall of the peptide-binding groove, and thus likely to be involved in antigen binding and subsequent interaction with T-cell receptors (Fig. 1). Acidic substitutions could profoundly alter protein structures and thereby alter affinity for peptide antigens. The predictions that protein structures on the HLA molecule are important in susceptibility to rheumatoid arthritis are supported by serotyping with alloantisera and monoclonal antibodies as well as reactivity with homozygous T cells and T-cell clones (Goronzy et al. 1986; Winchester and Gregersen 1988). However, whether the susceptibility to rheumatoid arthritis is due to permissive binding of specific peptides such as those on autoantigens or on environmental antigens, whether superantigens may initiate disease by binding specifically to the HLA molecules (Herman et al. 1991), or whether selection or tolerance of the T-cell repertoire are also involved, remains to be elucidated (Goronzy and Weyand 1995).

The evidence that *Dw4/Dw14* heterozygotes are more likely to develop rheumatoid arthritis than are *Dw4* homozygotes (Wordsworth et al. 1992), and the evidence that individuals expressing DR4 (and not DR1) are more likely to have severe disease, challenges the concept that sequences 70–74 are the only HLA–D regions that influence disease expression. This is despite the sequence identity of DR1 and DR4w4 in these positions, and a conservative substitution in Dw14 (Table 1). It has been hypothesized that the severity of disease and extra-articular complications are related to homozygosity and the density of disease-associated MHC molecules which critically influence the selection of the T-cell repertoire and tolerance to antigens (Weyand et al. 1992; Goronzy and Weyand 1993). In contrast to the focus in HLA–DR, David and his colleagues have produced data on transgenic mice which suggests that HLA–DQβ1 polymorphism determines the severity of collagen induced arthritis, and based on these data, have suggested that the importance of HLA–DQ alleles need to be further examined (Bradley et al. 1997). A further refinement suggests that the DRβ1 coded peptides modulate pathogenic responses dependent on antigen presentation by HLA–DR molecules (Zanelli et al. 1995).

Although HLA genes are of obvious importance in rheumatoid arthritis, it has been calculated from studies of HLA in multicase families that they may only account for 37 per cent of the genetic factors involved (Deighton et al. 1989). However, a recent reanalysis has suggested that up to 60 per cent of susceptibility could be determined genetically (Macgregor and Silman 1994). Other susceptibility genes have been sought, and associations with T-cell receptors in gene polymorphisms and deletions of immunoglobulin genes have been observed (Olee et al. 1991). However, TCR gene expression

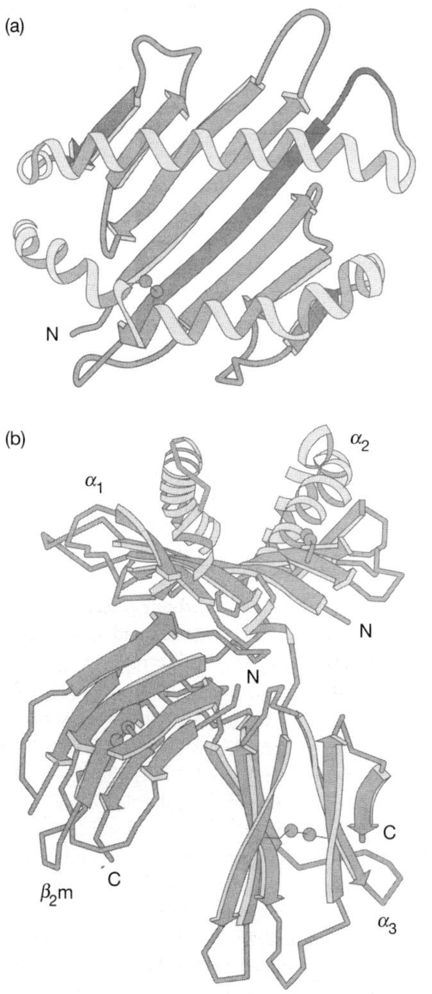

Fig. 1 Structure of HLA. (a) View of peptide-binding groove as seen by T-cell receptor. (b) From side.

widely studied, results enormously diverse. Attempts to use TCR peptides for therapy have not yet been successful (Moreland et al. 1998).

Environmental factors

Population and twin studies strongly suggest that non-inherited, presumably environmental, factors such as smoking and infections may play a part in the aetiology of rheumatoid arthritis, although rearrangement of the $\alpha\beta$ genes on T-cell receptors may also contribute to the non-inherited component. As discussed above, although prevalence rates of rheumatoid arthritis from world-wide studies are similar, a population survey designed to seek effects of the environment showed that urbanized tribal South African black subjects suffered from rheumatoid arthritis more than their rural cousins. However, the classical clue of case clustering suggesting an infectious background has not been found for rheumatoid arthritis in any study, unlike Lyme disease. Attempts at demonstrating microbial organisms directly from joints have had a chequered history, since in all instances claims of positive findings—for example, of mycoplasma, diphtheroids, and viruses—have either been attributed to laboratory contamination or have been refuted on grounds of a lack of reproducibility.

Other studies have sought to implicate microbes in the aetiology of rheumatoid arthritis by seeking evidence of immune hyper-reactivity to microbial antigens. Increased antibody titres to Epstein–Barr virus (EBV) antigens and an induced rheumatoid arthritis nuclear antigen have suggested that this ubiquitous virus, known to infect the majority of people by the late teens, may be of aetiological importance (Venables et al. 1981; Venables 1988). Its persistence in B lymphocytes of patients with rheumatoid arthritis in greater than normal amounts because of impaired cellular immunity could lead to the hyper-reactivity of B cells, and autoantibody production typical of the disease. Sequence similarity of an EBV capsid antigen to the HLA–DR β_1 susceptibility sequence QKRAA (Table 1) (Roudier et al. 1988) has suggested a possible explanation for the increased persistence of EBV in rheumatoid arthritis, while immunological cross-reactivity of EBV nuclear antigens to the autoantigens collagen, actin, and cytokeratin and to an antigen in the synovial membrane have suggested mechanisms for the induction of autoimmunity and for localization of immune cells to joints (Baboonian et al. 1991). However, these data fail to explain why only a small proportion of individuals infected with EBV might develop rheumatoid arthritis, and conversely, that there are well-documented patients with rheumatoid arthritis who have not been infected with EBV (Venables et al. 1981).

At least three bacteria have attracted attention in recent years as candidate agents in the aetiology of rheumatoid arthritis. The first, *M. tuberculosis*, gained current interest following the studies of Cohen et al. (1985) on an animal model of rheumatoid arthritis (see Adjuvant arthritis in Animal models below). In these studies, mycobacterial protein showed immunological cross-reactivity and sequence similarity to a cartilage link protein, a finding which suggested a possible reason for the localization of the immune response to joints (van Eden et al. 1985). The link with human rheumatoid arthritis was suggested by the demonstration of reactivity of synovial T cells to mycobacterial antigens in rheumatoid arthritis (Holoshitz et al. 1986). The mycobacterial 65-kDa protein was subsequently shown to belong to the family of heat-shock proteins (hsp65) which are expressed in a variety of bacteria and also in the inflamed synovium of rheumatoid arthritis (van Eden et al. 1988). Whether human hsp is a major target of T-cell autoreactivity in rheumatoid arthritis, however, is unproven, as there are significant differences in sequence and epitopes expressed by bacterial and human hsp (Gaston et al. 1989). Arguing against a role is the fact that identical responses to hsp65 are found in other inflammatory sites, for example, pleural effusion (Res et al. 1990). Attempts to suppress rheumatoid arthritis by vaccination with T cells derived from joints, in a protocol similar to that successfully used in adjuvant arthritis, could have provided support for the importance of mycobacterial immunity, but attempts have not been successful (Van Laar et al. 1991).

In a further study seeking a mechanism dependent on molecular mimicry, antigens homologous to the amino acid sequence QKRAA (see Table 1) present in the hsp DNAj of *Escherichia coli* were reported to elicit T-cell responses only in patients with rheumatoid arthritis (Albani et al. 1995). It was suggested by these workers that activated T cells may cross-react with autologous DNA heat-shock proteins that are expressed in the joints.

The third bacterium proposed as a candidate aetiological agent is *Proteus mirabilis*. Increased levels of IgG antibody to the organism have been detected in patients with rheumatoid arthritis but not ankylosing spondylitis or control subjects (Ebringer et al. 1989). It has been claimed that persistence of the organism in the urinary tracts, especially of women, may provide the nidus of infection that triggers a deleterious immune response culminating in rheumatoid arthritis.

The similarity of retrovirus-induced caprine arthritis to rheumatoid arthritis has attracted interest in the possibility that retroviruses may be of aetiological importance (Trabandt et al. 1992). Retroviral GAG proteins have been demonstrated immunohistochemically in the synovium of patients with rheumatoid arthritis (Ziegler et al. 1989), and a transgenic mouse carrying the human T-cell leukaemia virus type I (HTLV-1) that developed chronic arthritis with synovial inflammation and joint erosion similar to rheumatoid arthritis has been described (see section on 'Animal models'). The arthropathy associated with HTLV-1 in Japan appears to be distinct from rheumatoid arthritis (reviewed in Brand et al. 1999).

Parvovirus B19 has also been proposed by several groups over the years to be possibly involved (e.g. Takahashi et al. 1989), but the consensus is that while parvovirus causes forms of arthritis, which in it chronic form may resemble clinical features of rheumatoid arthritis, it is not a cause of rheumatoid arthritis (Moore 2000).

Other aetiological factors

Apart from the possible role that infectious agents may play, increased prevalence in females and a notable onset of rheumatoid arthritis in the premenopausal or post-partum period, and the protective effect of the contraceptive pill, presumably because of its progesterone content, have suggested that sex hormones may accelerate or retard its onset (Lahita 1990). Other aetiological factors that have been considered include diet (Buchanan et al. 1991) and stress (Adler 1985), but their role in initiating disease is debatable, and may be more significant in altering disease expression and outcome.

Autoimmunity

Autoantibodies

The discovery of the autoantibody, IgM rheumatoid factor, in the blood of patients with rheumatoid arthritis was the principal reason for its inclusion in the group of autoimmune diseases. Although high-titre IgM rheumatoid factor is relatively specific for a diagnosis of rheumatoid arthritis in the context of chronic polyarthritis, its occurrence in many connective tissue diseases with or without arthritis (e.g. primary Sjögren's syndrome and SLE) and in chronic infections has raised doubts about the role it might play in the pathogenesis of rheumatoid arthritis. However, rheumatoid factor-secreting plasma cells of IgG, IgA, and IgM class can be demonstrated in the rheumatoid synovium (reviewed by Maini et al. 1987), thus implicating them at the site of disease. Indeed, cells of the B-lymphocyte lineage constitute 10–15 per cent of the population of mononuclear cells in rheumatoid arthritis, produce autoantibodies, are a source of immune complexes that fix complement, and can act as efficient antigen-presenting cells. It seems likely that they contribute to perpetuation of the disease (Andrew et al. 1991). Rheumatoid factors may be involved in the induction of cytokine production (Chantry et al. 1989). The cell-membrane receptor Fcγ RIIIa has been implicated as important for triggering of TNF in macrophages by IgG-RF complexes (Abrahams et al. 2000).

IgG in patients with rheumatoid arthritis shows markedly reduced glycosylation, with a galactose 'pocket' in the Fc region (Parekh et al. 1985), in association with low levels of B-cell galactosyl transferase (Axford et al. 1987). It has been suggested that this glycosylation defect could result in conformational changes in the Fc region, rheumatoid factors more readily aggregating such molecules. Passive transfer of an acute synovitis in T-cell-primed mice has been shown to be enhanced using IgG containing autoantibodies to type II collagen when the antibodies are present as the agalactosyl glycoform. (Raddemacher et al. 1994), demonstrating that agalactosyl IgG glycoforms are directly associated with pathogenicity in murine collagen-induced arthritis. However, the role of such glycosylation defects in the aetiology or pathogenesis of rheumatoid arthritis has yet to be established, and it is not disease specific being also found in Crohn's disease (Dube et al. 1990), so it is likely to be secondary to inflammation or cytokine production.

Autoantibodies that occur in rheumatoid arthritis but are not specific for the disease include natural autoantibodies, antinuclear antibodies, anticollagen antibodies, antiphospholipid antibodies, and antineutrophil cytoplasmic antibodies.

Antinuclear antibodies detected by indirect immunofluorescence occur in up to 40 per cent of sera from patients with rheumatoid arthritis. Antibodies to histones, which also react as rheumatoid factors as a result of an epitope shared with IgG-Fc, have also been described in rheumatoid sera (Hannestad and Stollar 1978). Precipitating antibodies to soluble cellular antigen have been described in rheumatoid vasculitis (Venables et al. 1979). An antibody (detected by Western blotting) to a ribonucleoprotein termed RA33, present in soluble nuclear extracts, has been found in 36 per cent of rheumatoid sera, including early in disease, but also occurs in sera from mixed connective tissue disease and systemic lupus. Partial sequencing of RA33 shows it to be identical to the A2 protein of the heterogeneous nuclear ribonucleoprotein (hnRNP) complex (Steiner et al. 1992; Hassfeld et al. 1995).

Antiphospholipid antibodies of IgM class (Morris and Mackworth-Young 1996) and antineutrophil cytoplasmic antibodies (Mulder et al. 1993) have been detected in up to one-third of rheumatoid sera.

Another set of antibodies in rheumatoid arthritis are directed against antigens present in cartilage only, such as collagen types II, IX, and XI, and chondrocyte-specific antigens. The published data on the frequency of these antibodies are variable in different series, possibly as a result of the differing derivation of collagen (both homologous and heterologous collagens are used and are not identical), lack of purity of antigens, interference from serum factors, and the wide variety of techniques for detection. In one study, antibodies to collagen II occurred in 29 per cent of patients with rheumatoid arthritis, while antibodies to types IX and XI were present in 40 per cent (Charriere et al. 1988). However, antibodies to collagens II and XI were also equally frequent in osteoporosis and Paget's disease, whereas anticollagen IX was relatively restricted to rheumatoid arthritis. Antibodies to collagen I and II are produced locally in rheumatoid joints (Tarkowski et al. 1989). Antibodies to chondrocyte membrane antigens occur in rheumatoid arthritis but have been poorly characterized so far (Mollenhauer et al. 1988). A recent set of studies suggests that a glycoprotein (gp39), synthesized by chondrocytes, but also present in inflammatory cells, is a specific T-cell autoantigen in rheumatoid arthritis (Rijnders et al. 1996; Cope et al. 1999; Patil et al. 2001).

Autoantibodies that appear to be specific for rheumatoid arthritis have also been described. For example, antibodies to the antigen Sa, a 50-kDa protein present in human placenta, spleen, and rheumatoid joints, and occurring in about 40 per cent of rheumatoid sera, but also found in early disease have been described (Menard et al. 2000). Also disease specific are antibodies to a p68 antigen identified as BiP, a chaperone protein localized in the endoplasmic reticulum (Bläß et al. 2001; Corrigall et al. 2001). T-cell immunity to BiP appears to prevent the induction of experimental murine arthritis (Corrigall et al. 2001).

Two IgG-class autoantibodies detected by immunofluorescent microscopy described over 30 years ago appeared to show high specificity (>90 per cent) for rheumatoid arthritis. The first, referred to as antiperinuclear factor (APF), was demonstrated as an antibody binding to spherical keratohyaline granules present in buccal mucosal epithelial cells (Nienhuis and Mandema 1964). The second antibody activity in rheumatoid serum, termed antikeratin antibody (AKA) was found to bind to the keratinized stratified epithelium of rat oesophagus (Young et al. 1979). In subsequent studies evidence has accumulated suggesting that APF and AKA recognize epitopes expressed by filaggrin β, a protein present in cytoskeletal structures of epithelial cells (Berthelot et al. 1994; Sebbag et al. 1995). Immunoblot and enzyme linked immunosorbent assays (ELISA) using filaggrin purified from human skin and recombinant filaggrin have been developed and a sensitivity of 50–60 and 99 per cent specificity for rheumatoid arthritis has been claimed (Vincent et al. 1998).

The autoantigenicity of filaggrin appears to require the deimination of arginine residues into citrulline by the enzyme peptidylarginine deiminase during differentiation of epithelial cells. A mixture of citrullinated peptides or a single citrullinated cyclical peptide (anticitrullinated peptide antibodies) in ELISA appear to be equally sensitive and specific for rheumatoid arthritis, supporting the hypothesis that the autoimmune reaction is critically dependent on the presence of citrulline-containing proteins rather than filaggrin per se (Schellekens et al. 1998, 2000). It has been proposed that the target antigens in rheumatoid joints are in fact deiminated forms of fibrin (Masson-Bessiere et al. 2001), thus implicating the autoantibodies in the immunopathology of disease.

Induction

In the context of autoimmune diseases in general, as in rheumatoid arthritis, environmental agents are seen as triggers rather than as being directly involved in the disease process. However, how environmental agents induce autoimmunity is not understood. Various hypotheses have been proposed of which the concept of 'antigenic mimicry' is the most popular.

'Antigenic mimicry' implies that an immune response to an extrinsic antigen (usually microbial), closely resembling an autoantigen, induces an immune response that cross-reacts with the autoantigen. If the response is to be long lasting, then the autoantigen must perpetuate it as the extrinsic antigen is eliminated. Despite the popularity of this concept, there are as yet no definite examples in human autoimmunity. Mimicry can occur in autoimmunity, it is the mechanism by which heterogeneous or chemically treated autoantigens can induce experimental autoimmune diseases, for example, thyroiditis by using thyroglobulin, or collagen arthritis (see below).

Another concept, proposed by Bottazzo, Feldmann, and colleagues (reviewed in Feldmann 1987, 1989), was that a local immune response, to any environmental agents, may release enough cytokines into the environment to upregulate local antigen-presenting capacity, so allowing autoantigens, otherwise 'hidden' from the immune system because of lack of HLA class II expression, to be presented to immunocompetent T cells that have escaped elimination or induction of tolerance. This was first proposed for endocrine autoimmune diseases, with the suggestion that the endocrine epithelium becomes the critical source of (atypical) antigen-presenting capacity and of autoantigen. Substantial evidence has since accumulated that this scheme may apply in both experimental models and human disease. Transgenic mice, producing interferon-γ in their islets of Langerhans under the control of the insulin promoter, develop an immune, T-cell-dependent diabetes, with autoreactive T cells lysing islets and rejecting transplanted islets (Sarvetnick et al. 1990). In human Graves' thyroiditis, the antigen-presenting capacity of thyrocytes has been documented, as well as the presence of activated autoantigen-reactive T cells, and of local cytokines needed to maintain both antigen-presenting function and T-cell activation (reviewed in Feldmann et al. 1991). In rheumatoid arthritis, abundant antigen-presenting function resides in macrophages, dendritic cells, B cells, endothelium, and possibly activated T cells, although which of these is most deeply involved in antigen presentation in rheumatoid arthritis is not known. The presence of CD5+ B lymphocytes and their descendants may contribute significantly to local antigen-presenting function by binding to autoantibody containing immune complexes in their immunoglobulin receptor (Andrew et al. 1991).

What are the important autoantigens in rheumatoid arthritis? In a local autoimmune disease the autoimmune response is localized by the restricted distribution of critical autoantigens. This can be shown in Graves' disease where antigens synthesized by thyroid epithelial cells—thyroglobulin, thyroid peroxidase, and thyroid-stimulating hormone receptor—are targets of both T- and B-cell recognition (Dayan et al. 1991). In rheumatoid arthritis, cartilage autoantigens such as collagen type II, type IX, and type XI recognized by T and B cells would fulfil this role. These antigens as well as other cartilage- or chondrocyte-specific antigens could be of importance in the initial localization to synovial joints. A report of benefit following daily intake of a preparation of purified chicken type II collagen, has excited interest in the possibility of induction of 'bystander' T-cell tolerance by regulating T cells to joints from the gut lymphoid system (Trentham et al. 1993). Subsequent reports of other clinical trials have also not yielded significant results (Gimsa et al. 1997). T cells recognizing hsp65 or the antigen implicated in the autologous mixed lymphocyte reaction, which have been described in rheumatoid arthritis, could not have this role because the antigens are ubiquitous in cell types in most tissues, but may be of importance in maintaining the disease process, and in the extra-articular manifestations.

It is not clear whether rheumatoid arthritis should be considered as a single disease, with all cases having the same aetiology, or whether it should be viewed as a syndrome, with a range of aetiological factors initiating the same pathogenetic mechanism, and so producing a similar constellation of features.

Pathology

Introduction

The most pronounced and invariant pathology is in the synovial joints. There is a typical distribution, the small joints of the hands and feet, knees, and hips being most often implicated, symmetrically. In the different joints there are minor differences in pathology, but there is an overall pattern. There are also extra-articular manifestations, such as nodules and systemic disease.

Involvement of synovial joints

While attempts have been made to study the early events in rheumatoid arthritis, this is difficult, and so the pathology that is well known is from established cases. The involvement of synovial joints in rheumatoid arthritis is both of the synovial fluid and membrane (Zvaifler et al. 1994). Synovial fluid volumes are increased, and the cellularity increased; the predominant cell is the polymorph, which is only rarely seen in the lining layer of the synovial membrane. The other major cells in the synovial fluid and membrane are T cells and macrophages, with dendritic cells and cells of the B-lymphocyte lineage in small numbers. Typical numbers in acute cases are about 10^6/ml of polymorphs, and $1–3 \times 10^5$/ml of mononuclear cells. The exact relationship of the cells in the fluid to those in the membrane is not clear. Those in the fluid originate from the membrane, but how they reach the fluid is not clear. Whether they can re-enter the membrane or directly damage cartilage is also not known.

The involvement of synovial membrane is summarized in Fig. 2. There are several key features:

1. The lining layer, normally two cells thick, is much thickened with increased numbers of both type A (macrophage-like) cells and type B (fibroblast-like) cells, both expressing activation markers.

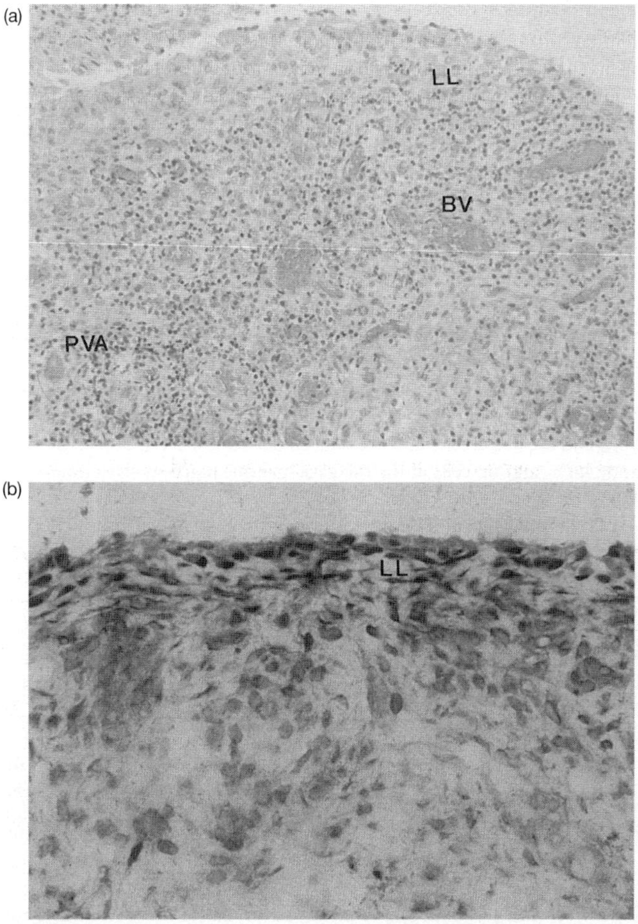

Fig. 2 Synovial membrane from a rheumatoid joint. (a) Haematoxylin–eosin staining of paraffin-embedded tissue (original magnification $\times$100) showing lining layer (LL) hypercellularity, prominent blood vessels (BV), and perivascular aggregates (PVA) of lymphocytes. The perivascular T lymphocytes are predominantly CD4+, CD45RO+, and CD29+ and a proportion bear activation markers HLA–DR and IL-2 receptors. CD8+ T cells are distributed in interaggregate areas, as are plasma cells. (b) Tumour necrosis factor-α (TNF-α), IL-1α, β, and IL-6 are located in LL and in deeper layers: this cryostat section stained with F(ab$'$)$_2$ anti-TNF-α and developed with an immunoperoxidase method shows intracytoplasmic TNF-α.

2. The deeper layers are of increased cellularity, with perivascular accumulations and follicles. These are rich in T cells particularly CD4+ cells. CD8+ T cells are more frequently found in between perivascular accumulations, as are the abundant plasma cells and infrequent B cells. Macrophages are found in the follicles and in between. There are few polymorphs and dendritic cells in the membrane, the majority of which accumulate in fluid.
3. The rheumatoid synovium is particularly vascular. There are markedly increased numbers of vessels, and in some instances high-endothelial venules develop, as in lymph nodes. There are new vessels formed by angiogenesis which can be distinguished by cell surface markers, such as $\alpha V\beta 3$.
4. Many of the cells, of all types, in the rheumatoid joint are activated. Thus HLA class II expression is found on nearly all the cell types, at an increased level, compared with that in normal or osteoarthritic joints. T cells are about 50 per cent class II positive, providing strong evidence of their activation status. B cells are positive, but typically plasma cells are not, as these lose the capacity to express class II. Macrophages express class II, as is often the case when activated, and class II-expressing fibroblasts and endothelial cells can also be seen.

Of interest is the HLA–DQ expression in rheumatoid arthritis, which is significantly greater than in other types of joint inflammation, for example, Reiter's syndrome (Barkley et al. 1989a). The meaning of this difference is not clearly understood, as the relative roles of the commonest class II antigen, HLA–DR, compared with the less common DQ and DP molecules are not known. Certain evidence allies HLA–DQ-restricted T cells to the suppressive immunoregulatory lineage (Sasazuki et al. 1986). However, some workers have presented evidence that DQ might be of pathogenic relevance (Bradley et al. 1997).

Other markers of activation abound. On the macrophage lineage, expression of CD11b (CR3) is increased, as is the related CD11c (p150/95). CD11a (lymphocyte function associated antigen-1) is increased on macrophages and many cell types. On T cells, expression of very late antigen (VLA) is increased, as is class II on a major proportion. In contrast interleukin (IL)-2 receptor is much less apparent. Endothelial cell expression of the adhesion molecules (AMs) ICAM-1 (intercellular), VLA-1, and ELAM-1 (endothelium–leucocyte) is increased. Tumour necrosis factor (TNF) receptors, also markers of activation, are upregulated in rheumatoid joints and are detectable on more than 80 per cent of T cells, on cells of the lining layer, and on cells at the cartilage–pannus junction (Deleuran et al. 1992; Brennan et al. 1995).

A common feature of activated cells is their increased production of cytokines and expression of cytokine receptors. This is the case in rheumatoid synovium, and the details will be discussed under pathogenesis.

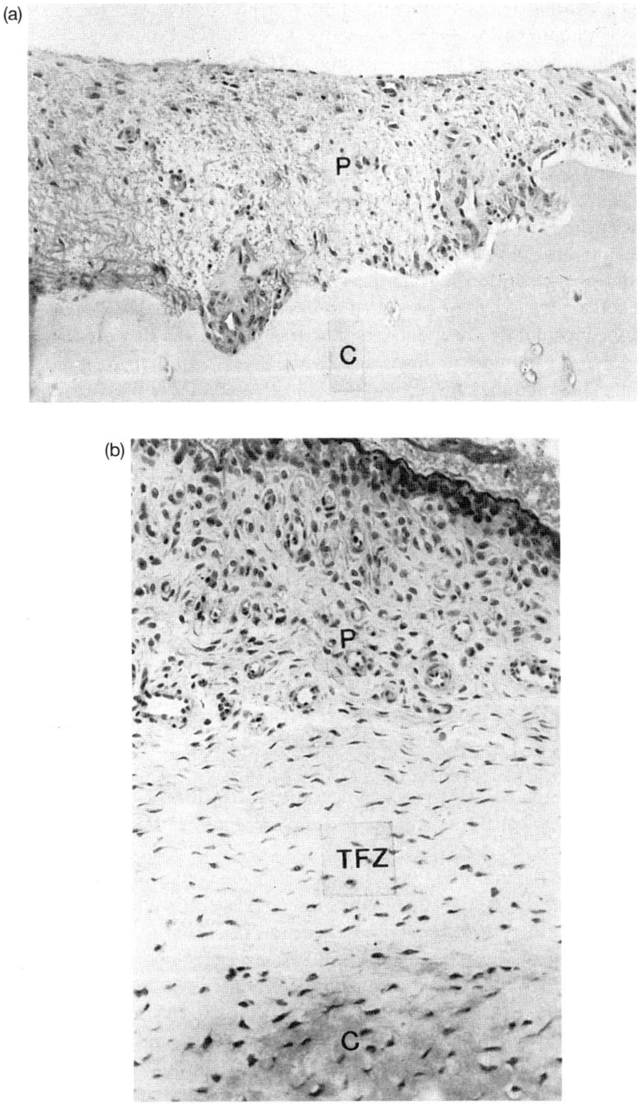

Fig. 3 Two types of cartilage–pannus junction seen in rheumatoid joints. (a) A distinct, well-defined margin can be seen between pannus (P) and cartilage (C). (b) A transitional fibroblastic zone (TFZ) separates a cellular, vascular pannus (P) from the underlying cartilage (C). Safranin O stain; original magnification ×46. (Reproduced with permission from Allard et al. 1987, figure 1.)

Pannus

The junction between synovial tissue, cartilage, and the bare area of bone within the capsule of the joint is the site of early erosive damage in rheumatoid arthritis. This site becomes filled and overlaid by vascular tissue termed pannus. The lining layer of pannus is in continuity with the lining layer of hypercellular synovium and has been regarded as being derived from it. The cellular pannus forms a distinct junction with underlying cartilage (see Fig. 3), which shows many characteristics of degradation, including loss of matrix and water content, and chondrocyte depletion. The conventional view is that pannus has an invasive degradative effect on underlying cartilage, mediated by the secretions of enzymes such as metalloproteinases. This is associated with further loss of cartilage as a result of enzymatic destruction of matrix by chondrocytes themselves mediated by aggrecanases (Torterella 1999), coupled with a lack of synthesis of newly formed matrix. Pannus also appears to erode adjacent bone by a similar process involving degradation of bone matrix, but in addition involving active bone resorption by osteoclasts.

A second morphologically distinct type of pannus may also be observed, especially in the marginal cartilage area of weight-bearing joints. This consists of vascular pannus overlying cartilage with an indistinct, intervening, multilayered zone of fibroblast-like cells (Fig. 3). In contrast, the underlying cartilage of this pannus does not show degradative changes with loss of matrix. This type of pannus could represent a fibrotic healing phase, but has alternatively been termed a 'transitional' fibroblastic zone because the cytoplasm of these cells contains cartilage components such as keratan sulfate, chondroitin sulfate, and collagen type II (Allard et al. 1991). These cells may be derived from chondrocytes as a result of metaplastic change. However, the possibility has been raised that cells with the same phenotype resident in the subperiosteum, contiguous to synovium in normal joints, may give rise to the transitional fibroblastic zone in rheumatoid arthritis (Allard et al. 1990). The finding of proinflammatory cytokines capable of inducing the degradation of cartilage (such as IL-l and TNF) in pannus cells contiguous with cartilage in the invasive type of erosion contrasts with absence of these cytokines in the transitional fibroblastic zone (Chu et al. 1991a,b). Instead, the latter type of pannus shows the presence of only transforming growth factor-β (TGF-β), as this factor stimulates collagen and matrix production its presence is compatible with the proposal that the tissue is in an anabolic state of healing or differentiation.

Extra-articular manifestations

Local

These are more common in long-standing and severe cases. Rheumatoid nodules are the most common, and are found in areas susceptible to trauma, such as elbows. They consist of a palisade of macrophages surrounding fibrous tissue.

Systemic

There are disagreements about the extent and frequency of systemic manifestations, and whether rheumatoid arthritis is always manifest systemically. Elevated concentrations of acute-phase proteins such as C-reactive protein, serum amyloid A, or complement components are found in most cases, and these suggest that their production in liver is increased. IL-6 can activate the liver to produce many acute-phase proteins, and it is currently assumed that the increased production of IL-6 (and IL-1) in rheumatoid arthritis (reviewed in Feldmann et al. 1996) is responsible.
In more severe cases there may be:

1. vasculitis;
2. fibrosis of the lungs, which may progress to significant fibrotic impairment of lung function;
3. granuloma formation as characterized by nodule formation;
4. serositis as characterized by pericarditis and pleurisy, commonly asymptomatic;
5. Felty's syndrome: enlargement of the spleen with lymphadenopathy, fever, leg ulcers, and susceptibility to bacterial infections.

There is evidence that severity and extra-articular manifestations may be associated with a double dose of the shared epitope, especially in DR4/DR14 (Wordsworth et al. 1992).

Pathogenesis

Introduction

Describing the pathogenesis of a chronic disease, such as rheumatoid arthritis, for which there are no very accurate animal models, is difficult. It is possible to describe, on the basis of human studies, the events occurring when the disease is well established. Accurate description of early events is not possible, only informed speculation can be made. As the pathology—the morphological description of what has happened—has been discussed, consideration of the pathogenesis will be itemized in relation to how these changes may have evolved.

Cell recruitment

The vast majority of the increased number of cells in the rheumatoid joint are of lymphohaemopoietic origin, as shown by immunostaining techniques, and their presence in the rheumatoid joint implies that there are mechanisms for increasing cell input, and also for increasing retention. This increase in cellularity is accompanied by angiogenesis in the synovial membrane, thus increasing delivery of cells and molecules to areas of inflammation (Folkman 1995). Neovascularization involves angiogenic cytokines such as vascular endothelial growth factor (VEGF), an endothelial-specific mitogen which promotes the growth of new blood vessels (Colville-Nash and Scott 1992) and also renders the vasculature hyperpermeable *in vivo* (Ferrara et al. 1991). Much work has focused on the endothelium in rheumatoid arthritis, as blood-borne cells would first have to adhere and migrate through endothelium. Augmented expression of adhesion molecules capable of binding lymphocytes, polymorphs, and monocytes has been noted: ICAM-1, E-selectin, and vascular cell adhesion molecule (VCAM-1) are all increased at various pathological sites. Isolated rheumatoid synovial endothelial cells constitutively express ICAM-1 and E-selectin and this expression is upregulated by IL-1 and TNF (Abbot et al. 1992). Immunohistochemical techniques have shown that VCAM-1, ICAM-1, and E-selectin are highly expressed by rheumatoid synovial vascular endothelial cells and cells in the lining layer (Koch et al. 1992; Morales-Ducret et al. 1992).

Local differentiation of T cells in rheumatoid arthritis synovial membrane has been suggested by the predominance of T cells with the phenotype of memory cells (CD45RO+, CD29), however, increased expression of VLA-4 on CD45RO+ T cells could indicate selective migration of memory T cells into the inflamed synovial membrane. In fact CD45RO+ T cells have been shown to have a better adherence to endothelial cells than CD45RO− T cells (Pitzalis et al. 1987). In addition, synovial T cells in rheumatoid arthritis have a significantly greater capacity to migrate trans-endothelially compared with those from normal or rheumatoid arthritis peripheral blood (Cush et al. 1992).

Equally important in cell recruitment is the action of chemotactic factors, which promote the migration of cells into a site. Some of these mediators have been identified within rheumatoid joints including representatives of the two families of chemokines, the C-X-C(α) chemokines such as IL-8 (Brennan et al. 1990a), and the C-C(β) chemokines such as RANTES (regulated upon activation, T-cell expressed, and secreted) (Rathanaswami et al. 1993), MCP-1 (monocyte chemoattractant protein 1) (Koch et al. 1992; Akahoshi et al. 1993), MIP-1α (macrophage inflammatory protein-α) (Koch et al. 1994), and MIP-1β (Villiger et al. 1992). As the majority of the cells in the rheumatoid arthritis synovium are macrophages and T lymphocytes, β-chemokines are likely to be important but neutrophil chemoattractants such as IL-8, GROα (melanoma growth-stimulating activity), and ENA-78 (epithelial neutrophil activating peptide) are likely to play a role in neutrophil accumulation within the joint fluid. Split complement components C3a and C5a present in rheumatoid arthritis joints (Jose et al. 1990; Abbink et al. 1992) are also chemotactic for neutrophils.

SDF-1, which is produced by synovial fibroblasts, is believed to be of importance in T-cell retention and lack of apoptosis (Buckley et al. 2000).

There is a new, nomenclature for chemokines, which is more systematic. In this terminology:

GROα = CXCL1, ENA-78 = CXCL5, IL-8 = CXCL8, MCP = CCL2, MIP-1α = CCL3, MIP-1β = CCL4, RANTES = CCL5

T-cell activation in rheumatoid arthritis

The T lymphocyte is one of the most common cells in active rheumatoid arthritis, with an abundance ranging from 20 to 50 per cent of the cells extracted from synovial membrane. CD4+ cells are more abundant than CD8+ in the membrane, but not necessarily in the synovial fluid. The CD4+ cells tend to concentrate in perivascular nodules, whereas the CD8+ are more diffusely scattered. CD4+ cells have been sub-divided into subsets, depending on their CD45 expression. In normal blood, about one-half is CD45RA+, indicating a 'virgin state'. Essentially all the cells in the rheumatoid joint lack CD45RA and express CD45RO/CD29, indicating a 'primed' or 'memory' state (Pitzalis et al. 1987). This is not surprising, as there is evidence for an ongoing immune response, as judged by the expression of T-cell activation markers, such as HLA class II (on 50 per cent), and IL-2 receptors on fewer cells (2–12 per cent) (Brennan et al. 1988a; Londei et al. 1989).

T lymphocytes may also be classified according to their T-cell receptor for antigen. In normal blood the great majority (more than 95 per cent) express a heterodimer of α and β chains, whereas a minority use γ and δ chains. Of interest was the observation (Brennan et al. 1988b) that there was selective enrichment of $\gamma\delta$ T cells in active rheumatoid joints. and that some of the $\gamma\delta$ T cells recognize mycobacterial antigens (Holoshitz et al. 1989). However, elevated $\gamma\delta$ cell numbers have not been confirmed in all studies. In patients who have augmented $\gamma\delta$ T cells in their blood there is a trend towards increased amounts of CD5+ B cells (Brennan et al. 1989c).

An important question is whether T cells have a critical role in rheumatoid arthritis. Firestein and Zvaifler (1990), based on low or absent levels of T-cell cytokines in the rheumatoid synovial environment, have proposed that T cells may not be important in the chronic established phase of disease. Indeed, in controlled clinical trials of rheumatoid arthritis with anti-T-cell (e.g. anti-CD4, anti-CD5) monoclonal antibodies, no beneficial effects were observed (Olsen et al. 1994; Van der Lubbe et al. 1995). However, our opinion is that in a prolonged, chronic, asynchronous disease with profound immunoregulation, the quantity of cytokines detected need not reflect their importance. Various lines of evidence support this possibility. First is the abundance of T cells in rheumatoid joints. Virtually none are present in normal joints. Second is their partially activated status and proximity to antigen-presenting cells (see above). Third is the fact that the proportions of different types of T cells present in rheumatoid joints are not the same as in blood (as discussed above), indicating that it is not a reflection of passive trafficking in an inflammatory response. Fourth is the observation that antigen-specific T cells are present, are activated, and persist in rheumatoid joints. For example, we found that collagen type II-specific T cells were present, and expressing IL-2 receptors, in three operative specimens in a patient with rheumatoid arthritis, over a period of more than 4 years (Fig. 4) (Londei et al. 1989). Finally, T-helper 1(Th1) cells appear to predominate in the joint and interferon-γ and IL-2 are expressed, albeit at low levels, but with unexpectedly high IL-10 production (Buchan et al. 1988b; Simon et al. 1994; Cohen et al. 1995). It is of interest that recent studies have identified regulating T cells as those making large amounts of IL-10.

A restricted pattern of V_β chains of the T-cell receptor was observed in rheumatoid joints by one group of workers, suggesting the possibility that activation of lymphocytes was mediated by superantigens (Paliard et al. 1991). However, other laboratories have not confirmed this observation. Thus, whereas Paliard et al. (1991) reported low $V_\beta14$ in blood of patients with rheumatoid arthritis compared with the level found in joints, Howell et al. (1991) reported that multiple V_β gene families were transcribed in patients, although sequence similarities were found, in keeping with the hypothesis that superantigen may play a role in rheumatoid arthritis. Clearly much more work is needed in this area if it is to be understood, but noting that all known autoimmune diseases and models are T-cell dependent, it is very likely that rheumatoid arthritis is T-cell dependent even in its later stages.

T-macrophage contact maybe of major importance in the cell interactions involved in perpetuating the cytokine imbalance in the rheumatoid synovium. Dayer and colleagues reported that activated T cells can activate macrophages to induce the production of IL-1, TNF-α as well as matrix metalloproteases (Isler et al. 1993; Lacal et al. 1994). This work has been reproduced by others, and it was found that depending on the mode of T-cell activation, the cytokines generated differed. Thus, McInnes et al. (1996) found that with T cells activated with IL-15, there was production of TNF-α. Sebbag et al. (1997) and Parry et al. (1997) found that while both antigen-activated T cells and those activated by a cocktail of cytokines (IL-6, TNF, and IL-2) induced TNF-α, only the former type of T cells induced the inhibitory cytokine IL-10. These results suggest that T cells may be of importance in the maintenance of rheumatoid arthritis cytokine synthesis, and especially that cytokine-activated T cells (IL-15 or IL-6/TNF/IL-2 cocktail) maybe responsible for the relative lack of inhibitory cytokines such as IL-10. To evaluate whether rheumatoid arthritis T cells resemble the ones activated by antigen or by cytokines, attempts were made to differentiate how these cells activate macrophages. It was found that *in vitro* cytokine activated T cells, like *in vivo* derived rheumatoid synovial T cells, drive TNF-α production in an NF$\kappa\beta$ dependent and P13 kinase independent fashion, in contrast to antigen activated T cells. These findings indicate that the cytokine activated subset of T cells may be of importance in disease maintenance. The well-established association with HLA–DR genes and the shared epitope suggest that antigen-activated T cells may also be involved, probably at disease initiation or in the shaping of the T-cell repertoire. An endogenous serum regulator of the interaction between T-cells and macrophages, which blocks IL-1 and TNF production has been described (Hyka et al. 2001) and has been identified as apolipoprotein A-1,

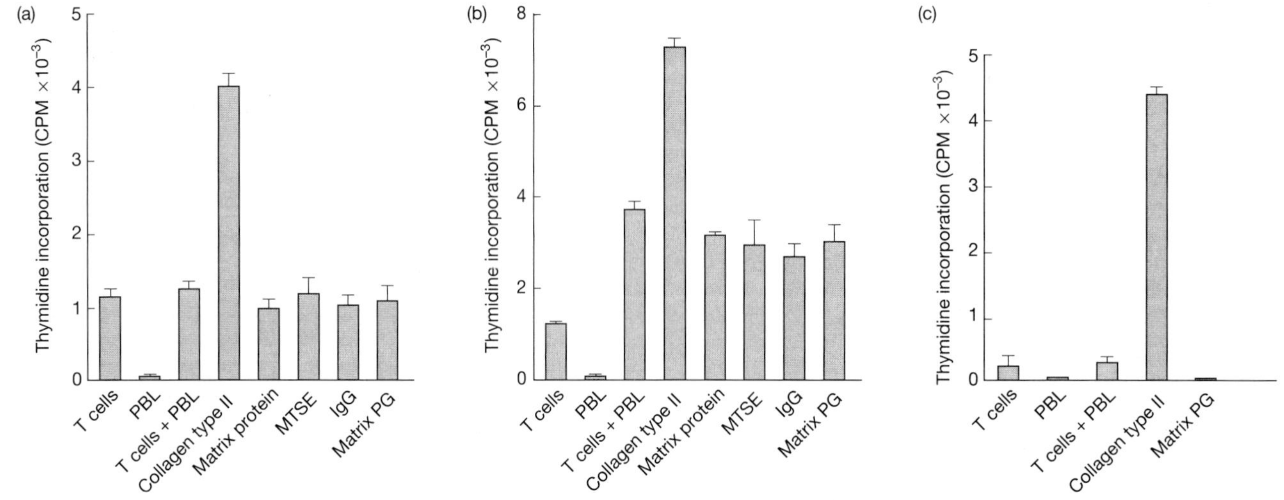

Fig. 4 Proliferative response of collagen type II-specific clones. (a) Clone 4 from the first synovial membrane. (b) Clone 55 with autologous mixed lymphocyte reactivity, from the first synovial membrane. (c) Clone B8 from the second synovial preparation. Results are the arithmetic means ± SEM of a representative experiment from each clone. In other experiments, collagen type I was also used, but there was no response from any of the clones. Cloned T cells (10^4), 2×10^4 irradiated, autologous, peripheral blood, mononuclear cells were cultured with or without the antigen indicated. Antigens were used at 100 μg/ml, except MTSE which was at 1 μg/ml. These were the optimal concentrations. PBL, peripheral blood lymphocytes; PG, proteoglycan; MTSE, mycobacterial tuberculosis soluble extract. (Reproduced with permission from Londei et al. 1989.)

a structural component of low-density lipoprotein. The importance of interactions of T cells with macrophages and fibroblasts has been emphasized and have recently been published (Dayer and Burger 1999).

Whilst the function of T cells in rheumatoid arthritis is unresolved, much can be learned from investigations that define the role of T cells in induction and perpetuation of experimental models of arthritis. Collagen-induced arthritis is a CD4+ T-cell dependent disease as demonstrated by T-cell depletion (Ranges et al. 1985). However, unlike adjuvant arthritis, it is not readily transferred with T cells or T-cell clones. In the case of collagen-induced arthritis, transfer from histoincompatible DBA/1 mice to mice with subacute combined immunodeficiency has demonstrated that T and B cells act in synergy in the full expression of disease (Williams et al. 1992b; Taylor et al. 1995).

B-cell lineage

Plasma cells are abundant in rheumatoid arthritis. Some, but not all are involved in the production of rheumatoid factors. Rheumatoid factor immune complexes have been shown to induce the production of cytokines such as IL-1 and TNF (Fig. 5) (Chantry et al. 1989), this may operate via FcRIIIa (Abrahams et al. 2000).

The specificity of the antibodies produced in rheumatoid joints has been investigated by the cell fusion technique using the human B-cell fusion partner, SPAZ4. Large numbers of hybridomas producing IgM and IgG were detected (Maini 1989). While a few of these were 'polyreactive', and some produced rheumatoid factors, the majority did not bind to a battery of autoantigens tested. However, it has been claimed that the majority of rheumatoid joints contain B cells producing antibody to collagen type II and IgG Fc (Tarkowski et al. 1989).

In examining the B-cell repertoire activated in rheumatoid joints, attempts are being made to ascertain whether there is any evidence of a restricted use of certain genes selected from among the multiple heavy-chain *V* genes available in the genome. In one such study, analysed by Northern blotting, an over-representation of V_H4 was noted (Brown et al. 1992). Such over-representation may result from dominance of a B-cell subset in diseased tissues or from selection pressures created by specific antigens or superantigens. Alternatively, regulatory elements in flanking regions active in rheumatoid arthritis may favour recombination of particular individual gene elements and so skew the B-cell repertoire activated (Brown et al. 1995). As primed B cells recognizing antigen present antigen to T cells more efficiently than do macrophages (Lanzavecchia et al. 1985) and are probably important in the development and maintenance of the immune network in neonatal and adult life (reviewed by Plater-Zyberk et al. 1992), a greater understanding of the role of B cells should illuminate the pathogenesis of rheumatoid arthritis.

A new model of spontaneous arthritis has been developed by Benoist, Mathis, and their colleagues (Kouskoff et al. 1996). This model was generated by serendipitously crossing the autoimmunity susceptible non-obese diabetic (NOD) mouse with a C57BL/6 mouse transgenic for a T-cell receptor recognizing bovine ribonuclease presented by I-A^{K}. However, in the NOD MHC context a peptide of a ubiquitously derived protein glucose-6-phosphate isomerase (GPI) is recognized, and antibodies to GPI develop (Matsumoto et al. 1999). This animal model has many of the features of human rheumatoid arthritis, with a chronic inflammation of may synovial joints, leading to joint destruction. Antibodies to GPI are pathogenic, as their transfer into normal mice leads to the onset of arthritis as soon as 24 h. An interesting question is how the antibody to an ubiquitous antigen only causes inflammation in joints. The pathology resembles rheumatoid arthritis, but is not clear to what extent this disease resembles human rheumatoid arthritis. For example, serum transfer from rheumatoid patients has not been reported to be successful in humans. A recent preliminary study with few controls has suggested that antibodies to GPI may also be present in patients with rheumatoid arthritis (Schaller et al. 2001). The depletion of B cells by a combination of a specific therapeutic antibody, cyclophosphamide, and corticosteroids in a preliminary non-randomized and uncontrolled clinical trial has fuelled speculation that B cells may be of pathogenic importance (Edwards and Cambridge 2001).

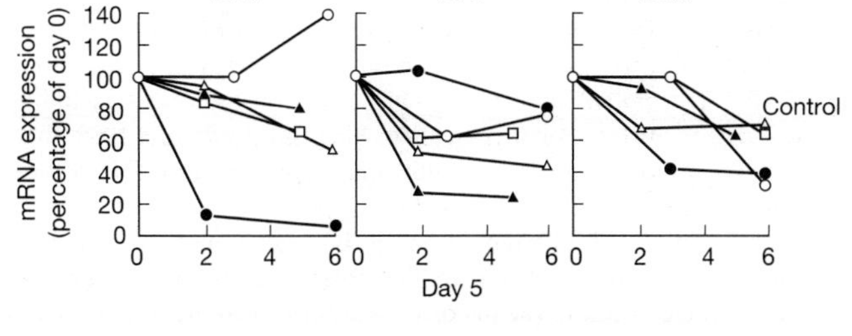

Fig. 5 Fresh isolated synovial membrane and synovial fluid cells obtained from five patients were placed in culture at 1 × 10^6/ml in the presence or absence of mediators (IFN-γ and IL-2). Cells were harvested at the times indicated for the determination of cytoplasmic RNA. The results are expressed as percentages of the basal level. (●), Patient 1; (△), Patient 2; (▲), Patient 3; (□), Patient 4; (○), Patient 5. (Reproduced with permission from Kissonerghis et al. 1989.)

Antigen-presenting cells

There are abundant cells with antigen-presenting capacity in human rheumatoid joints. Which of these are of major importance in different stages of disease is a controversial question. Macrophages and monocytes represent some 30–50 per cent of the cell pool, and there is evidence for their activation, for example, increased expression of HLA–DQ, and diminished CD14. Dendritic cells are present in increased numbers. Regrettably, due to lack of specific markers for human dendritic cells, their numbers are not easy to quantify. However, cell separation studies by several groups have all demonstrated increased numbers of dendritic cells in rheumatoid synovial fluid, comprising up to 5–7 per cent of the mononuclear cells, whereas synovial tissue contained fewer dendritic cells (March 1987; Tsai et al. 1989). Dendritic cells from rheumatoid synovial fluid were potent antigen-presenting cells, but not more so than normal activated dendritic cells. The importance of dendritic cells in rheumatoid arthritis was recently reviewed (Thomas and Lipsky 1996; Thomas 1998). CD5+ B cells have Fc receptors and many produce rheumatoid factors. These may permit CD5 B cells to take up immune complexes and present the relevant antigens. The possible importance of CD5+ B cells in antigen presentation in rheumatoid arthritis has been discussed (Maini 1989). Chondrocytes can be activated to express HLA class II and may be critical in the early events of rheumatoid arthritis. ICAM-l expression in chondrocytes, which facilitates antigen-presenting cell function, has been reported (Davies et al. 1992).

Cell interaction

The importance of cell interactions in the rheumatoid joint can be inferred from the immunohistological studies, which show close appositions of T cells and antigen-presenting cells in nodules and in other sites throughout the synovial membrane. However, there are very few T cells in the pannus, suggesting that different interactions may prevail in this specialized site.

Dissociated cells from rheumatoid joints, placed in tissue culture, in the absence of any extrinsic stimulus, rapidly reform into aggregates. This suggests that interactions are of critical importance in the disease process. Experimentally, one can demonstrate that these cell interactions are of importance *in vitro*. We have noted that rheumatoid synovial cells, placed in culture and in the absence of extrinsic stimulation, retain many features of active rheumatoid arthritis. Thus expression of HLA class II persists *in vitro*, at both the protein and mRNA levels, provided that the whole mixture of joint cells is cultured (Fig. 5). If only the adherent cells (chiefly fibroblasts) are cultured, class II expression apparently does not persist in culture (Teyton et al. 1987). Below, the persistence of cytokine production in cell cultures from rheumatoid joint not extrinsically stimulated is discussed.

The role of T cells in the persistence of class II expression has been studied by depleting T cells using a combination of lysis with antibody and complement, and antibody-coated magnetic beads. Even with an incomplete depletion of cells, a marked reduction in class II expression was noted after 6 days in culture (Brennan et al. 2001; Hawrylowicz et al. unpublished observations). This emphasizes the importance of cell interactions, but does not clarify which T cells are of critical importance, nor which are the critical antigen-presenting cells.

Cytokine expression

As rheumatoid arthritis is mostly manifest in synovial joints, which are the sites of inflammation and destruction, cytokine production in the joints has been investigated by several groups. However, cytokines can also be detected in blood cells by immunostaining, for example, IL-1α (Barkley et al. 1989b). Whether other cytokines can also be detected in the blood cells remains to be established. Elevated serum concentrations of cytokines have been reported, for example, IL-l β (Eastgate et al. 1988), but their reproducibility and significance remain to be established in view of the presence of serum cytokine inhibitors. The first evidence of cytokine expression in rheumatoid arthritis was the detection of IL-1 bioactivity in synovial fluid (Fontana et al. 1982). Other cytokines are also present, for example, TNF-α (reviewed by Feldmann et al. 1996).

Rheumatoid joints contain a wide variety of activated cell types, and so it would be expected that many cytokines would be produced locally in the joint. When we began studies on the expression of cytokines in rheumatoid joints in 1985, slot blotting and cDNA hybridization were used to obtain maximum data on cytokine expression from a small number of cells. With these techniques 2×10^6 cells were used, and could provide data on about six, or sometimes up to 10 cytokines. By densitometry, relative quantification was possible. Further advantages of this technique are its specificity for individual cytokines, ease of performance (same technique for all cytokines), and its resistance to artefacts caused by rheumatoid factors (a problem in binding assays), and to 'toxic' components of synovial fluid in bioassays (Buchan et al. 1988a,b). A disadvantage is that the amounts of cytokine mRNA being measured do not always correlate with the amounts of cytokine protein produced. This is especially a problem with cytokines known to be regulated post-transcriptionally, for example, TNF-α. If this type of work was to be begun again, obviously the polymerase chain reaction (PCR) would be used, for its much greater sensitivity (Brenner et al. 1989). However, the use of PCR is not without problems; for example, quantification is very difficult and contamination frequent. Using PCR to explore cytokine expression in rheumatoid arthritis has yielded the same results as slot blotting, that is, predominance of IL-1α and abundance of TNF-α, IL-6, etc. (Brennan et al. 1989a). In situ hybridization has yielded analogous results (Firestein et al. 1990), and also provides information about localization, but quantification is difficult.

It is not surprising that virtually all the cytokines sought have been detected, because of the wide variety of activated cells. Table 2 summarizes the cytokine expression in the rheumatoid joint. There are some interesting generalizations that can be made. For example, cytokines that are predominantly macrophage products are abundant, at both the mRNA and protein level, for example, IL-1, IL-6, TNF, and IL-8. In contrast, cytokines produced by T cells are detectable at the mRNA level, but barely detectable at the protein level, for example, interferon-γ, lymphotoxin, and IL-2. The reasons for this discrepancy are not yet known, but TGF-β which inhibits cytokine production post-transcriptionally or IL-10 may be responsible. Local consumption of cytokines by cells with high-affinity receptors may also contribute, as, for example, there are free and cell-bound IL-2 receptors in rheumatoid joint cells (Symons et al. 1988).

Cytokines are essential for many processes in rheumatoid arthritis, such as cell growth and expression of HLA class II (reviewed in Feldmann et al. 1996). However, it is not clear which cytokines are of major importance in different processes. A critical step in the generation of an immune or inflammatory reaction is activation of macrophages and induction of HLA class II expression. Interferon-γ is potentially the most effective cytokine at inducing such expression in the absence of other factors (Portillo et al. 1989). However, negligible amounts of interferon-γ (or other T-cell lymphokines) are produced by rheumatoid synovial cells (Firestein and Zvaifler 1987; Brennan et al. 1989a) suggesting that other factors alone or in combination with this interferon-γ are involved. One possible candidate is the haemopoietic growth factor, granulocyte–macrophage colony-stimulating factor (GM-CSF), which induces HLA–DR expression on human monocytes (Chantry et al. 1990) and which could be an important macrophage activator and induce HLA class II expression in the rheumatoid joint (Alvaro-Garcia et al. 1989). However, the most significant inhibition of that expression which we observed in the rheumatoid synovial cultures was with anti-TNF antibody (unpublished observation), and was greater than that with antibodies to interferon-γ or GM-CSF. This is unlikely to be a direct effect, as TNF by itself does not induce the expression of HLA class II (e.g. Pujol-Borell et al. 1987). This suggests that many different cytokines may work together to induce this expression (Sadeghi et al. 1992a,b) or that other, as yet undefined, molecules may be involved. Alternatively (or in addition) cell–cell interactions through cell adhesion molecules may be necessary to maintain this. Of interest is the observation that TNF-α is a potent inducer of many adhesion molecules including ICAM-1 and VCAM-1 (Pober et al. 1986; Rice and Bevilacqua 1989). The expression of adhesion molecules is downregulated after anti-TNF-α therapy (Paleolog et al. 1996; Tak et al. 1996).

Table 2 Summary of cytokines produced by rheumatoid synovial cells

Cytokine[a]	mRNA	Protein
IL-1α	+	+
IL-1β	+	+
TNF-α	+	+
LT	+	−
IL-2	+	−
IL-3	−	−
IL-4	?	−
IFN-γ	+	−
GM-CSF	+	+
IL-8	+	+
G-CSF	+	?
M-CSF	−	?
TGF-β	+	+
EGF	+	+
PDGF-A	+	+
PDGF-B	+	+

[a] EGF, epidermal growth factor; G-CSF, granulocyte colony-stimulating factor; GM-CSF, granulocyte-macrophage CSF; IL, interleukin; LT, lymphotoxin; M-CSF, macrophage CSF; PDGF, platelet-derived growth factor; TGF, transforming growth factor; TFN, tumour necrosis factor. After Brennan et al. (1991).

The activation and differentiation of B cells is also mediated by cytokines, of which IL-4 and IL-6 are the most important. IL-4 is a potent B-cell growth factor but in the majority of published studies is detected in negligible amounts in rheumatoid synovial cells or in synovial fluid. In contrast, high levels of IL-6 have been detected both in rheumatoid synovial fluid and in cells from rheumatoid synovial membrane (Hirano et al. 1988; Field et al. 1991). The presence of high levels of IL-6 in rheumatoid joints may explain the large numbers of plasma cells and few B cells in the synovium and the production of autoantibodies including rheumatoid factors.

Lymphotoxin and TNF-α can also act as a B-cell growth factor (Kehrl et al. 1987). The presence of immune complexes containing rheumatoid factor may further contribute to the pathogenesis of rheumatoid arthritis by inducing the production of IL-1 as shown by Chantry et al. (1989) (Fig. 6). The 'cytokine synthesis inhibitor', IL-10, which inhibits T-cell production of interferon-γ, is also a potent B-cell stimulator (Moore et al. 1990).

T-cell growth is controlled by cytokines. For many years, after the discovery of 'T-cell growth factor' and the purification, cloning, and expression of IL-2, it was thought that all T-cell growth was mediated by IL-2. Subsequent work has shown that the position is much more complex. IL-4, initially, described as a B-cell stimulating factor, is also a potent growth factor for many T cells, and IL-7, described as a pre-B growth factor, is also highly active (e.g. Londei et al. 1990). T-cell activation is found in rheumatoid arthritis, with many cells expressing HLA class II (20–50 per cent), and a few (2–12 per cent) expressing IL-2 receptors. IL-15 is a more recently described T-cell growth factor, produced by antigen-presenting cells, whose receptors are present on resting cells. It is present in rheumatoid arthritis synovium and SF, and activates synovial T cells (McInnes et al. 1996, 1998). However, the mechanism of T-cell growth is unclear, as while IL-2 mRNA is found (Buchan et al. 1988b), the protein is not readily detectable. This could be due to absorption by cell-bound receptors, IL-2 inhibitors such as the soluble IL-2 receptor (Symons et al. 1991), or post-transcriptional regulation. IL-4 is also not readily detectable, for possibly the same reasons. IL-7 in rheumatoid joints, is a candidate for T-cell growth regulation in rheumatoid arthritis. A synergy between all these cytokines could permit T-cell growth in the presence of low protein levels of each of these mediators. This possibility requires investigation using cells from rheumatoid joints in culture.

Fibrosis is an important component and complication of rheumatoid arthritis. It participates in deformation of joints, but pulmonary fibrosis can be a damaging systemic complication. Which cytokine drives the fibrosis in the rheumatoid joint (or other tissues) is not currently known.

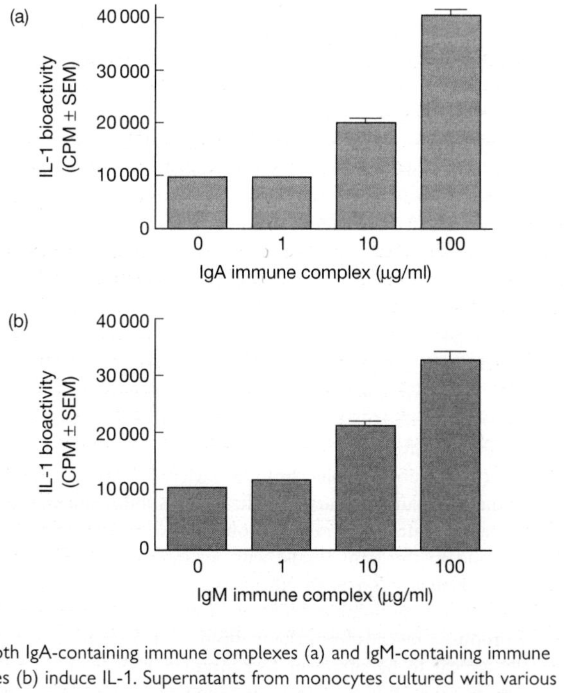

Fig. 6 Both IgA-containing immune complexes (a) and IgM-containing immune complexes (b) induce IL-1. Supernatants from monocytes cultured with various concentrations of immune complex for 24 h were assayed for IL-1 bioactivity using the thymocyte comitogenic assay. Data is shown as [^{3}H]-thymidine incorporation (mean ± SEM of triplicate cultures). Proliferation due to phytohaemagglutinin antigen alone was 3486 ± 450 c.p.m. For both immune complexes significant ($p < 0.01$) interleukin could be detected at concentrations as low as 10 μg/ml. (Reproduced with permission from Chantry et al. 1989.)

There are abundant candidates present in the rheumatoid joint, for example, IL-1α and -β, TNF-α, which may act indirectly via induction by platelet-derived growth factor (Raines et al. 1989), and TGF-α and -β. The extensive fibroblast growth family may also be important.

Cytokine regulation

Initial studies of the expression of IL-1 in rheumatoid joints revealed that all samples contained IL-1 mRNA. After the experimental activation of normal cells *in vitro*, expression of IL-1 mRNA (and the expression of other cytokines) is brief (24–48 h), so the fact that all samples from rheumatoid arthritis were positive suggested that cytokine production in the rheumatoid joint may be relatively stable and persistent. In a chronic disease only persistent features can be relevant to the maintenance of the disease process, so the consistence and persistence of cytokine production suggested that it was of importance in the pathogenesis (Buchan et al. 1988a).

Cytokine persistence was directly tested *in vitro* by culturing dissociated cells from rheumatoid joints in the absence of extrinsic stimulation. The initial results showed that both IL-1α and IL-1β mRNA persisted for up to the 5-day culture period (Fig. 7) (Buchan et al. 1988a). This indicates that the signals necessary to regulate cytokine production are present in the culture, and so can be analysed experimentally.

Neutralizing antibodies were chosen as the tool to investigate the signals involved in regulating the production of IL-1. The strongest non-microbial signals for the regulation of this production were the cytokines TNF-α and TNF-β (lymphotoxin), so neutralizing antibodies to these two cytokines were used. The results were clear cut; anti-TNF-α but not anti-TNF-β or control rabbit Ig inhibited IL-1 production after the first day of culture [Fig. 8(a)] (Brennan et al. 1989b). Assays at the mRNA level show more rapid kinetics, but the lack of an early effect on the amount of IL-1 protein indicates that already ongoing synthesis of IL-1 was not affected, but that subsequent activation was blocked. As a control, the same antibodies were used on cultures of cells from osteoarthritic joints. Despite the presence of immunoreactive TNF-α there was no effect of anti-TNF-α on the low levels of IL-1 in osteoarthritis [Fig. 8(b)]. This is now known to be caused by the TNF in osteoarthritis not being biologically active, neutralized by the abundant soluble TNF-receptors, which is the endogenous inhibitor (Cope 1992; Dayer 1993).

The finding that TNF-α was the single dominant signal regulating the production of IL-1 was surprising. It had been anticipated that multiple signals may be of importance, including immune complexes and perhaps other non-cytokine signals. However, samples from the first seven patients behaved in this way, regardless of their therapy. This led us to investigate

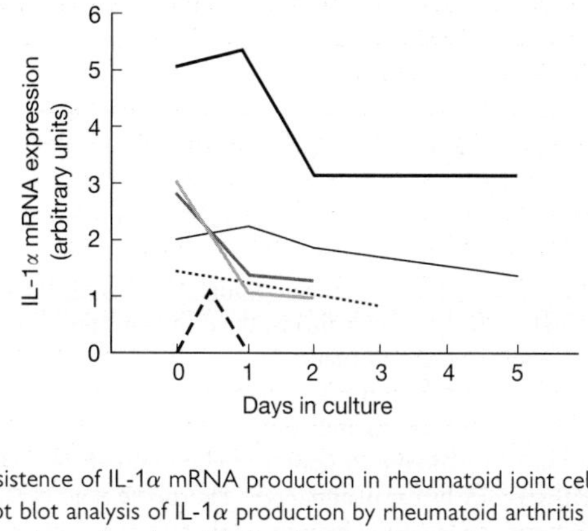

Fig. 7 Persistence of IL-1α mRNA production in rheumatoid joint cells in culture. Slot blot analysis of IL-1α production by rheumatoid arthritis synovial fluid mononuclear cells cultured in the absence of extrinsic antigen. SF and SM mononuclear cells were cultured for 0–5 days, the RNA extracted, blotted on to nitrocellulose, and probed with IL-1α. Integral values were calculated. Different symbols represent different patients. ----- is IL-1α mRNA from mitogen-activated peripheral blood mononuclear cells. (Reproduced with modification from Buchan et al. 1988a.)

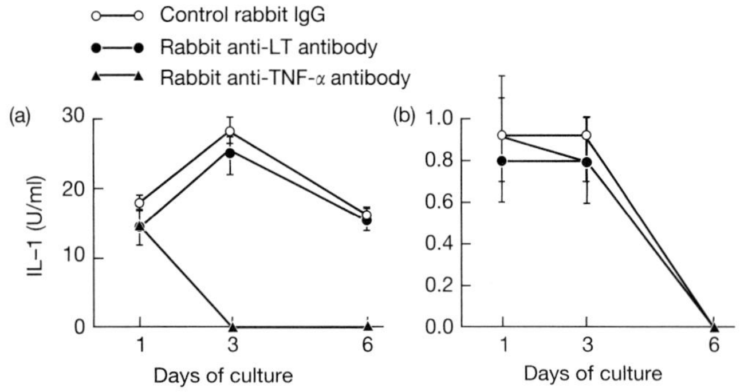

Fig. 8 (a) Effect of anti-TNF-α on rheumatoid arthritis joint cell culture. (b) Lack of effect of anti-TNF-α on osteoarthritis joint cell cultures. (Reproduced with modification from Brennan et al. 1989a.)

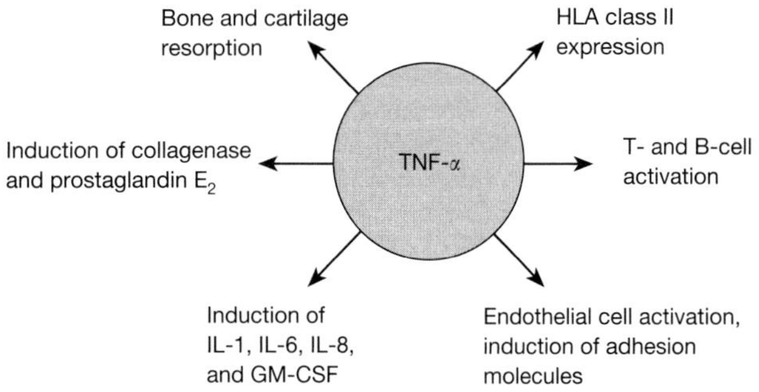

Fig. 9 Effects mediated by TNF-α in rheumatoid arthritis.

what other effects of anti-TNF-α on the disease process may be. It has been postulated that GM-CSF is an important cytokine in rheumatoid arthritis, as it is an inducer of class II on monocytes, and induces cytokine production and macrophage activation (Alvaro-Garcia et al. 1989). It was therefore of interest to determine which cytokine regulates the production of GM-CSF in cell cultures from rheumatoid joints. Anti-TNF-α markedly inhibited the production of GM-CSF, but more slowly than inhibition of IL-1, being virtually complete only by day 5 (Alvaro-Garcia et al. 1991; Haworth et al. 1991). We have also found that anti-TNF partially inhibits class II expression and also the aggregation normally found in these cultures. A summary of the effects of TNF in rheumatoid joints is shown in Fig. 9.

The above results obtained in rheumatoid arthritis documenting the effects of TNF-α on other pro-inflammatory cytokines are analogous to those now described in the response of mice to systemic Gram-negative bacteria. Production of TNF-α, IL-1, and IL-6 was monitored; peaks of TNF-α preceded those of IL-1 then IL-6. Anti-TNF-α abrogated the production of IL-1 and IL-6 in this animal model (Fong et al. 1989). Thus, it seems likely that in rheumatoid arthritis, the dominant position of TNF-α recapitulates the physiological situation.

Following the demonstration that anti-TNF can inhibit the production *in vitro* of IL-1 and other proinflammatory cytokines (IL-6, GM-CSF, IL-8) (Feldmann et al. 1996) and the successful amelioration of collagen-induced arthritis in DBA/1 mice by use of anti-TNF (Thorbecke et al. 1992; Williams et al. 1992a), we formulated the hypothesis that TNF-α is at the apex of a cytokine cascade. This gave the rationale to blockade TNF in 20 patients with active rheumatoid arthritis, in an open phase I/II trial lasting 8 weeks (Elliott et al. 1993).

The monoclonal antibody used was a chimeric (mouse Fv, human IgG1) neutralizing antibody produced by Centocor, Inc (now known as infliximab). The benefits of anti-TNF treatment were evident in all patients within a few days and lasted 8–26 weeks (median 12 weeks). Improvements in clinical parameters included reduction in pain and morning stiffness, falls in swollen and tender joint counts, increased erythrocyte sedimentation rate, and reduced C-reactive protein and serum amyloid A. Following this initial success a randomized, double-blind, placebo-controlled, multicentre trial of anti-TNF in 73 patients was undertaken, the results of which confirmed the open study (Elliott et al. 1994) and supported the hypothesis that TNF is of major importance in the pathogenesis of rheumatoid arthritis (Figs 10 and 11). The long-term control of signs and symptoms in approximately 60 per cent of patients not responding to conventional therapies by infliximab and etanercept (a p75-TNF receptor linked to human Fcγ1 fusion protein) has been demonstrated in Phase III trials (reviewed by Maini and Taylor 2000; Feldmann and Maini 2001; Taylor et al. 2001). Of special interest is the radiographic data demonstrating prevention of bone erosions over a 1 year period by etanercept in early disease, and arrest of cartilage narrowing and bone erosions in long-standing refractory disease by a combination of infliximab and methotrexate (Bathon et al. 2000; Lipsky et al. 2000). Anti-TNF therapy (infliximab and etanercept) has been approved for the treatment of severe rheumatoid arthritis in the United States and Europe in 1998 and 2000, respectively.

The mechanism of the anti-inflammatory action of anti-TNF-α antibody is under examination in current studies. A rapid decrease of serum IL-6 following anti-TNF demonstrates the effect of anti-TNF antibody on downregulation of other cytokines (Maini et al. 1995). A second, and possibly more important, effect of TNF blockade is in reducing the cellularity of the synovium (Maini et al. 1995). This is accompanied by an increase in peripheral blood lymphocyte count and a decrease in expression of adhesion molecules in synovial biopsies taken before and after therapy (Tak et al. 1996). There is an associated decrease in circulating levels of E-selectin and ICAM-1 (Paleolog et al. 1996) and of chemokines IL-8 and MCP-1 (Taylor et al. 2000). Direct evidence of a reduction in polymorphonuclear cell retention in inflamed joints has been obtained by imaging 111-indium labelled cells (Taylor et al. 2000). The arrest and possible healing of structural changes in 39–54 per cent of patients treated with infliximab and methotrexate for 1 year (Lipsky et al. 2000) have suggested that TNF-α is involved in both cartilage and bone damage. Viewed together, these data suggest that anti-TNF therapy reduces cell traffic into joints by reducing leucocyte–endothelium interactions, thereby reducing the mass of inflammatory tissue and its clinicopathological consequences. This topic is discussed in more detail in a recent review (Feldmann and Maini 2001).

Cytokine antagonists

In 1989, TNF-binding protein, capable of inhibiting the action of TNF, was discovered in the blood and urine of febrile patients (Seckinger et al. 1989; Engelmann et al. 1990; Feldmann and Maini 2001). This was subsequently found to be derived from the extracellular domain of the two TNF receptors, probably by proteolytic cleavage. On account of the proposed role of TNF-α in the pathogenesis of rheumatoid arthritis, the role of TNF inhibitor was explored, with the expectation that low levels of soluble TNF receptors may be involved.

Analysis of serum samples from a variety of arthritic patients has revealed that in rheumatoid arthritis the TNF inhibitor system is enhanced, and there are elevated levels of both soluble TNF receptors (p55 and p75) in serum and in the joint fluids, with an intermediate rise in levels in seronegative arthritis and osteoarthritis (Cope et al. 1992). However, these upregulated levels of soluble TNF receptors do not neutralize fully the TNF-α produced by cells from rheumatoid joints in culture, whereas they generally appear to be sufficient to neutralize TNF-α produced by cells from osteoarthritic joints in culture (Brennan et al. 1995). Thus, in arthritis there appears to be an attempt at homeostasis, which, however, is inadequate (Cope and Maini 1995). Other soluble cytokine receptors that in the fluid phase would act as cytokine antagonists have been described, for example, soluble IL-1 (Symons et al. 1991), -2 (p55), -4, -6, and -7 receptors and soluble interferon-γ receptor, which may act as regulators of the

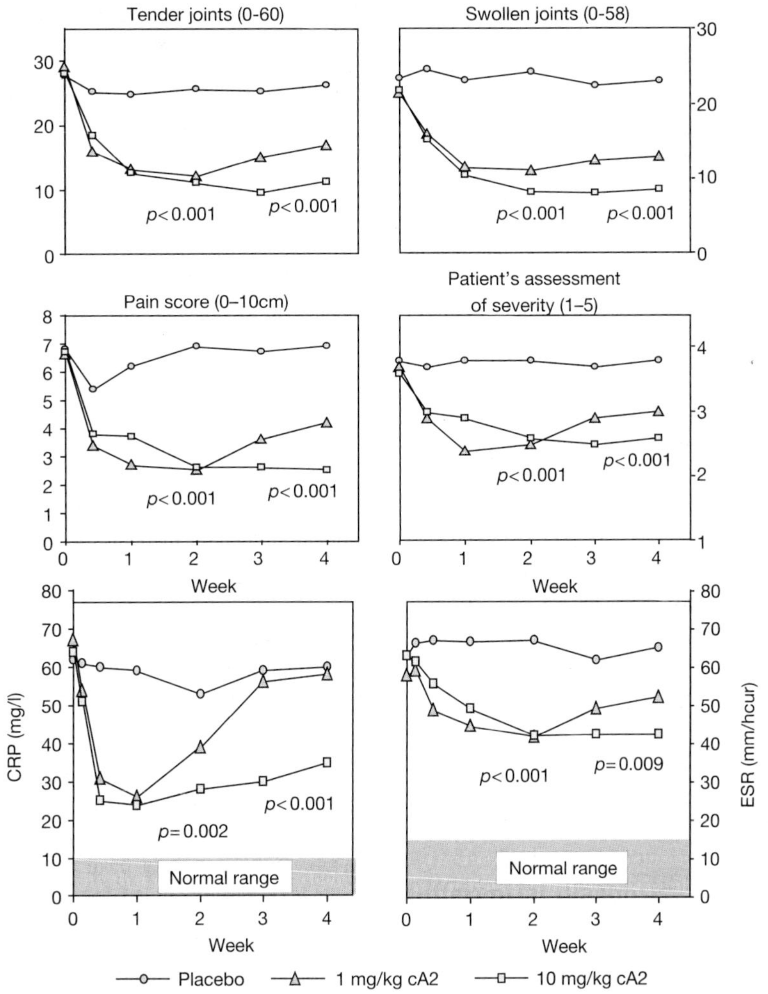

Fig. 10 Changes in clinical assessments in 73 patients treated with placebo (o), 1 mg/kg (Δ), or 10 mg/kg (□) anti-TNF monoclonal antibody in a randomized, double-blind trial (p values represent significance versus placebo: $+ \, p < 0.05$; § $p < 0.01$; $* \, p < 0.001$). [Reprinted with permission from Elsevier Science (*Lancet*, 1994, **344**, 1105–10).]

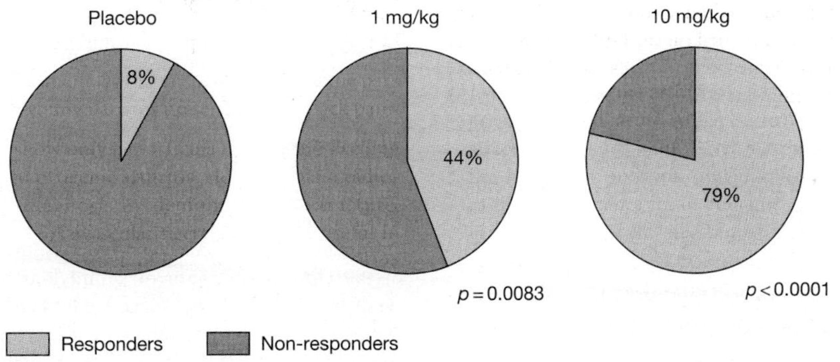

Fig. 11 Overall clinical responses to placebo, 1 mg/kg, or 10 mg/kg anti-TNF monoclonal antibody in 73 patients, 4 weeks after treatment, in a randomized, double-blind trial (p values represent significance versus placebo). (Reproduced by kind permission from articles by Elliott et al. 1994 and Maini et al. 1995.)

cytokine network. An IL-18 binding protein is particularly abundant (Novick et al. 2001).

There is so far only one cytokine inhibitor described which acts as a receptor antagonist, that is, the IL-1 receptor antagonist, which is produced in rheumatoid joints (Arend 1991). This is a member of the IL-1 family, with 30 per cent homology to IL-1β. The physiological role of this molecule is unclear, as quantities greatly in excess of those of IL-1 are necessary to exert inhibitory effects, far larger than are physiologically present *in vivo*. Its role may be simply to localize the effects of IL-1 in the environment in which the cytokine is produced. Whatever the exact physiological roles of IL-1 receptor antagonist and soluble TNF receptor, these natural agents with the capacity to interfere with cytokine action have therapeutic activity in rheumatoid arthritis (Arend and Dayer 1995; Elliott and Maini 1996; Taylor et al. 2001).

Immune suppression in rheumatoid arthritis

Despite the evidence for an ongoing autoimmune response at both the T- and B-cell level, there is also considerable evidence that the systemic immune response is suppressed in patients with rheumatoid arthritis. This has been demonstrated as a reduced response to tuberculin (purified protein derivative) testing (Emery 1984; Kingsley et al. 1987), in IL-2 production, or in T-cell proliferative or cytokine production. Serial studies have shown that the degree of immune suppression is more severe as the patients are clinically more ill. The mechanisms of this suppression are not understood, but could lead eventually to new forms of therapy aimed at reinforcing the endogenous mechanisms of immune suppression.

A number of molecules found in the joints in rheumatoid arthritis may be important contributors to this process. These include prostaglandins and TGF-β. Other potential candidates not yet known to be present include oncostatin M, IL-10, and IL-4. Prostaglandins are produced in the inflammation of rheumatoid arthritis. However, most non-steroidal anti-inflammatory drugs interfere with the production of prostaglandins, and this does not overcome the endogenous suppression, which accordingly is mostly caused by other agents. TGF-β is found in large amounts in supernatants of synovial cell cultures (10–20 ng/ml) of which 1–2 ng/ml is bioactive (Brennan et al. 1990b). There is thus sufficient TGF-β to influence immune functions of T and B cells, and cytokine production. However, appropriate neutralizing experiments on synovial cell cultures remain to be done. Oncostatin M is growth inhibitory for a variety of cell types, is produced by activated T cells and macrophages, and so may be expected to be present. IL-10, a product of T and B cells, can interfere with antigen-presenting capacity and with the production of interferon-γ. IL-10 has been demonstrated in rheumatoid joints and *in vitro* studies reveal that it is apparently exerting a suppressive effect on endogenous production of TNF-α and IL-1 (Katsikis et al. 1993). The beneficial effect of administration of recombinant IL-10 in established collagen-induced arthritis supports its possible therapeutic potential (Walmsley et al. 1996).

Animal models (see Chapter 3.4)

Research in unravelling the factors that initiate rheumatoid arthritis, understanding the perpetuation of disease, and devising new strategies for therapy or prevention has to some extent depended on concepts developed and validated in animal models. Recent clinical studies have raised questions that have increased, rather than diminished, the complementary value of the use of animal models. However, there is as yet no ideal animal model of rheumatoid arthritis that exhibits all key features, namely:

1. predictable and spontaneous development of an erosive, chronic, symmetrical arthritis punctuated by flares;
2. female preponderance;
3. association with the MHC homologue of HLA–DR4 or –DR1;
4. high frequency of circulating IgM rheumatoid factor;
5. synovitis with a cellular response, profile of local production of cytokines, proteases, and inflammatory mediators identical to that observed in rheumatoid arthritis;
6. cartilage and bone degeneration with pannus formation;
7. response to disease-modifying antirheumatoid drugs akin to that observed in rheumatoid arthritis.

Despite reservations, the ensuing section gives examples of existing and new models of rheumatoid arthritis, which have contributed to our understanding of this disease.

Collagen-induced arthritis

The distribution of collagen II is essentially restricted to cartilage and the vitreous humour of the eye. Intradermal injection of native collagen II in Freund's adjuvant (but not of collagen types I and III or denatured type II) induces a polyarthritis in rats (Trentham et al. 1977), mice (Courtenay et al. 1980), and monkeys (Cathcart et al. 1986). Heterologous or autologous type II collagens are effective but the former leads to a destructive yet self-limiting disorder, whereas the latter is characterized by a chronic remitting and exacerbating course of disease (Holmdahl et al. 1986; Boissier et al. 1987). Malfait et al. (2001) have demonstrated that the response of this chronic model to drugs more closely resembles that of human rheumatoid arthritis. T- and B-cell responses to multiple epitopes on collagen II occur, and disease of a milder variety than in the immunized animals has been transferred into syngeneic animals by serum and/or T cells. Rheumatoid factor is detectable and villous synovitis with increased cellularity of the lining layer, infiltration of deeper layers with mononuclear cells (predominantly CD4+ T cells), and pannus formation echo the changes observed in rheumatoid arthritis. The best-documented susceptible mouse, the DBA/l, bears the *H-2q* haplotype; H-2^r mice are also susceptible, but H-2^d mice are resistant to collagen arthritis. Although a polygenic disease, it is of considerable interest that the HLA class II molecules mapping to I-A (the mouse homologue of human HLA DQ) appear to be the element controlling susceptibility and immune responses to type II collagen in DBA/1 (Holmdahl et al. 1989). The importance of non-MHC genes, for example, genes regulating complement synthesis and the expression of IgG subclass isotypes, has been deduced from other studies.

The collagen arthritis has significant similarities to rheumatoid arthritis and its importance lies in the ability of an immune response to a constituent of cartilage to induce disease. As B- and T-cell-specific responses to collagen II occur in a proportion of patients with rheumatoid arthritis, especially, and sometimes exclusively, when lymphocytes from the synovial membrane are studied, the model provides evidence that collagen immunity might perpetuate rheumatoid disease. The model has provided useful data on the arthritogenic epitopes on type II collagen and therapeutic manipulations have provided evidence that antibodies directed against CD4+ T cells (Ranges et al. 1985), B cells (Helfgott et al. 1984), and TNF-α (Williams et al. 1992a) are effective in ameliorating established disease.

Adjuvant arthritis

A single intradermal injection of Freund's complete adjuvant (containing *M. tuberculosis*) in the footpad or tail of rats induces a severe arthropathy involving the wrists, ankles, paws, and caudal part of the spine and tail (Pearson 1956). The arthropathy in its developed stage consists of synovitis with villous formation, pannus eroding cartilage and bone, marked periostitis with new bone formation, and inflammation and fibrosis of periarticular tissues. After peaking, the inflammatory arthritis declines and is followed by fibrous and bony ankylosis of joints. Extra-articular features can be prominent and include balanitis, conjunctivitis, and cutaneous lesions resembling psoriasis. Although the disease in diarthrodial joints has some similarity to rheumatoid arthritis, the other features are reminiscent of the clinical spectrum of spondyloarthropathies, especially Reiter's syndrome. This is further suggested by a consistent lack of IgM rheumatoid factor. Susceptibility is strain dependent; for example, Lewis rats are most susceptible, and Fisher rats are less so. Susceptibility is believed to involve multiple genes with no convincing role for the MHC genes.

The major interest in the model springs from the demonstration that the disease is mediated by T cells that recognize mycobacterial peptides (Cohen et al. 1985). Furthermore, there is evidence for molecular mimicry between a mycobacterial antigen and cartilage antigens (van Eden et al. 1985), and this is believed to be the key factor in localization of the disease to joints. The relevant antigen has been defined and is a mycobacterial nonapeptide present in a 65-kDa mycobacterial protein that belongs to the family of hsp65 (van Eden et al. 1988). The nonapeptide stimulates T-cell clones of the CD4 phenotype, termed A2b and A2c, derived from a parent line, A2, obtained from a rat with adjuvant arthritis. Following *in vivo* inoculation into irradiated syngeneic Lewis rats, A2b causes a severe arthritis, whereas A2c protects from disease induction and causes a rapid remission (Cohen et al. 1985). When hsp65 or the nonapeptide are given before Freund's adjuvant, the rats are protected from the disease.

The possibility that T cells equivalent to the suppressive clones isolated from adjuvant arthritis are present in the inflammatory exudate of rheumatoid arthritis has prompted optimism that T-cell vaccination may prove to be a promising therapy. Activated T cells, treated with hydrostatic pressure, or T-cell receptors cross-linked with glutaraldehyde are used as surrogate suppressor–inducers in vaccination protocols. However, preliminary trials have not shown any benefit in rheumatoid arthritis (Van Laar et al. 1991).

Streptococcal cell-wall arthritis

A single injection intraperitoneally of an aqueous suspension of group A streptococcal cell-wall fragments into rats induces a polyarthritis (Cromartie et al. 1977). The arthritis involves wrists, ankles, and other joints, spares the axial skeleton, and is biphasic with an early phase reaching its maximum at 3 days, followed by the onset of a chronic arthritis 2–4 weeks later. Lewis (LEW/N) female rats are the most susceptible to this form of arthritis and exhibit many pathological features of rheumatoid arthritis—a villous synovial thickening with surface fibrin, thickening of the synovial lining layer, polymorph exudation into joint fluid, mononuclear cell infiltrates with a predominance of CD4+ T cells, angiogenesis, and fibroblast proliferation with pannus formation and associated erosion of underlying cartilage and bone. Low titres of IgM rheumatoid factor are detectable. The active proinflammatory constituent of streptococcal cell-wall is its peptidoglycan component, which has extensive pathophysiological effects involving many cell types; the smallest active subunit of peptidoglycan is muramyl dipeptide, which is itself an activator of macrophages and endothelial cells. Persistence of streptococcal cell-wall owing to its protective carbohydrate side chains, is believed to contribute to the initiation and perpetuation of disease.

The importance of T cells in the pathogenesis of the disease has been demonstrated by transfer of arthritis to nude, T-cell deficient, inbred Lewis rats. Like rheumatoid arthritis, the T-cell abnormalities include depressed responses to mitogen and defective production of IL-2. As hsp65 protects against arthritis induced by streptococcal cell-wall (van den Broek et al. 1989), it has been suggested that this protein may be the host protein target for the T-cell response. However, the molecular basis of this has not been resolved. Although HLA class II molecules are rapidly induced in endothelial cells in inflamed tissues, the role of MHC antigen-associated susceptibility is ambiguous because a related strain of rats (the Fisher strain) with the same histocompatibility locus is relatively resistant to arthritis.

Of considerable interest are the observations on the hypothalamoadrenal axis in the arthritis induced by streptococcal cell-wall. In susceptible female Lewis rats there is an abnormally low gene expression at the mRNA level of the corticotrophin-releasing hormone and encephalin, with a deficient response of adrenal corticotrophic hormone and adrenal corticosteroid (Sternberg et al. 1989a,b). In contrast, Fisher rats, resistant to arthritis, show relatively rapid and efficient responses from the hypothalamoadrenal axis. That these neuroendocrine responses are important in the pathogenesis of disease is suggested by the observation that giving corticosteroid in small doses simultaneously administered with streptococcal cell-wall improves the course of the induced arthritis and, conversely, blockade of the glucocorticoid receptor with RU 486 accelerates disease in resistant Fisher rats (Sternberg et al. 1989a).

Other models of arthritis

The transient inflammatory arthritis of serum sickness in rabbits induced by antigen and mediated by antigen–antibody complexes (Dixon et al. 1958) had antedated the description of chronic arthritis in the rabbit knee induced by intra-articular injection of protein antigens such as fibrin, heterologous gammaglobulin, and ovalbumin into previously sensitized animals that had received antigen in Freund's adjuvant (Dumonde and Glynn 1962). One aspect of interest in the latter model was the demonstration that the arthritis was dependent on antigen–antibody complexes sequestered in cartilaginous tissues (Jasin 1975) which could act as a depot of persistent immunogen and gave rise to a cellular immune response. The induction of arthritis by a similar protocol in neonatally thymectomized or bursectomized chickens demonstrated that arthritis was inducible by both thymus-dependent T and bursa-dependent B cells; however, the fully developed lesion required an intact thymus and bursa (Oates et al. 1972).

Infective agents as a cause of arthritis have attracted much interest; and mycoplasmas (Decker and Barden 1975) and erysipelotherix (Drew 1972) are both well-described causes of chronic arthritis in swine. In the former model, a chronic arthritis persisted long after viable organisms could be cultured from joints, blood, or lymph nodes and non-viable antigen persisted for longer periods, and it was suggested that this might have been responsible for the destructive arthritis. In a model of swine arthritis resembling rheumatoid arthritis studied in Sweden, introduction of fish meal in the diet was causative of arthritis and evidence was obtained that this was associated with population of the gut by *Clostridium perfringens* (Mansson et al. 1971). Immune responses to the clostridium were demonstrable, but the organism could not be isolated from the joints and as such represented a form of reactive arthritis.

Caprine arthritis, mainly involving large joints, has generated interest in the arthritogenic potential of the causative lentivirus, which is a lentiform retrovirus, as is the human immunodeficiency virus (Crawford et al. 1980). In this disease, possibly acquired by ingestion of milk by goat kids, the virus is harboured by mononuclear phagocytes. Encephalitis also occurs and this feature makes it distinct from rheumatoid arthritis. Chronic destructive joint lesions are described, and these resemble rheumatoid arthritis, as does the mononuclear cell infiltrate in the synovium. However, the lentivirus cannot be isolated from joints. In contrast to rheumatoid arthritis, mononuclear cells rather than polymorphs are dominant in joint fluids and, also unlike rheumatoid arthritis, high levels of interferon activity are demonstrable. Studies of the tropism for joints and the pathogenesis of the inflammatory reaction provide insight into the pathways that might prove important in devising investigations of the possibility that retroviruses may cause rheumatoid arthritis.

The MRL/lpr mouse is generally regarded as a model of systemic lupus and develops a multisystem disease characterized by glomerulonephritis, vasculitis, and antibodies to double-stranded DNA and Sm antigen, associated with marked lymphoproliferation involving a T cell with an $\alpha\beta$ heterodimer receptor, but lacking CD4 and CD8 antigens (Andrews et al. 1978). This mouse strain, however, also develops an arthritis of the hind limbs with invasion of cartilage by pannus, high levels of rheumatoid factor, and anticollagen type II antibodies; therefore in some respects it shows features of rheumatoid arthritis. Production of rheumatoid factor appears to be under the control of the lymphoproliferation gene. The early destruction of articular tissue is at the marginal junction of the synovium with cartilage and bone, in association with proliferation of fibroblastic cells, and antedates an inflammatory response (O'Sullivan et al. 1985). This spontaneous model of arthritis appears to be of importance in delineating the relationship between autoimmunity and non-immune cellular responses in the synovium and pannus invasion of cartilage and bone, as well as understanding the genetic regulation of rheumatoid factor.

Transgenic mice offer the possibility of assessing *in vivo* the effect of introduced genes on the development of disease. Two models have recently been published which may shed insight into the mechanism of arthritis. The simplest to evaluate is the introduction of a modified human TNF-α gene, under its own promoter, into fertilized ova. The modification of the gene was replacement of the TNF-α 3′ untranslated region, which has been shown to confer mRNA instability, with the 3′ untranslated region of β-globin, which has a very stable mRNA. With this deregulated TNF-α production, it was found that the mice developed a progressive arthritis by

4 weeks of age. The arthritis was preventable by the injection of antihuman TNF-α monoclonal antibody from birth onwards. The arthritis is characterized by sub-chondral erosions and frequent fibrosis, but further analysis is necessary to establish how closely this disease resembles rheumatoid arthritis (Keffer et al. 1991). This model, however, confirms the hypothesis that TNF-α is intimately involved in the arthritic process.

Transgenic mice carrying the human T-cell leukaemia virus-1 genome also develop a chronic erosive arthritis (Iwakura et al. 1991). In this model, approximately one-third of the mice highly expressing the transgene developed arthritis with synovial inflammation and cartilage erosion, closely resembling a pannus. Low levels of rheumatoid factor were occasionally detected. It was of interest that the mRNA of the *Tax* gene, a trans-acting transcriptional activator, was highly expressed in the joints. Thus, it is likely that the arthritis is the result of increased cytokine expression in the joints. Supporting this is the preliminary observation, cited in Iwakura et al. (1991), that IL-1α mRNA is expressed in the joints of these mice, as it is in rheumatoid arthritis.

Conclusions

Our understanding of the pathogenesis of rheumatoid arthritis in molecular terms has progressed rapidly in the past few years. This has provided a number of molecular targets, and therapeutic trials based on these targets have been initiated. The first of these was CD4, and monoclonal anti-CD4 has been used by a number of groups, with beneficial though transient results in a proportion of patients.

Attempts are being made to devise peptide-based therapies which will selectively block the critical HLA peptide-presenting genomes. Neutralization of cytokines such as TNF-α and IL-1 with antibodies or soluble receptors has been successfully applied in clinical trials and has set the stage for an era of promising new therapeutic interventions.

These (and more) therapeutic trials will have an important benefit in helping to evaluate ideas concerning the pathogenesis of rheumatoid arthritis, and even if (as is likely) they are not totally successful, they will contribute to refining our concepts of the pathogenesis of the disease and to more effective therapies.

References

Abbink, J.J. et al. (1992). Relative contribution of contact and complement activation to inflammatory reactions in arthritic joints. *Annals of the Rheumatic Diseases* **51**, 1123–8.

Abbot, S.E. et al. (1992). Isolation and culture of synovial microvascular endothelial cells: characterization and assessment of adhesion molecule expression. *Arthritis and Rheumatism* **35**, 401–6.

Abrahams, V.M. et al. (2000). Induction of tumor necrosis factor alpha production by adhered human monocytes: a key role for Fc gamma receptor type IIIa in rheumatoid arthritis. *Arthritis and Rheumatism* **43**, 608–16.

Adler, R. (1985). Psychoneuroimmunologic contributions to the study of rheumatic diseases. In *Immunology of Rheumatic Diseases* (ed. S. Gupta and N. Talal), pp. 669–96. New York: Plenum Medical Book Company.

Akahoshi, T. et al. (1993). Expression of monocyte chemotactic and activating factor in rheumatoid arthritis. *Arthritis and Rheumatism* **36**, 762–71.

Albani, S. et al. (1995). Positive selection in autoimmunity: abnormal immune responses to a bacterial DNAJ antigenic determinant in patients with early rheumatoid arthritis. *Nature New Medicine* **1**, 448–52.

Allard, S.A., Muirden, K.D., Camplejohn, K.L., and Maini, R.N. (1987). Chondrocyte-derived cells and matrix at the rheumatoid cartilage-pannus junction identified with monoclonal antibodies. *Rheumatology International* **7**, 153–9.

Allard, S.A., Bayliss, M.T., and Maini, R.N. (1990). The synovial–cartilage junction of the normal human knee: implications for joint destruction and repair. *Arthritis and Rheumatism* **33**, 1170–9.

Allard, S.A., Bayliss, M.T., and Maini, R.N. (1991). Correlation of histopathological features of pannus with patterns of damage in different joints in rheumatoid arthritis. *Annals of the Rheumatic Diseases* **50**, 278–83.

Alvaro-Garcia, J.M., Zvaifler, N.J., and Firestein, G.S. (1989). Cytokines in chronic inflammatory arthritis. IV. Granulocyte/macrophage colony stimulating factor-mediated induction of class II MHC antigen on human monocytes: a possible role in rheumatoid arthritis. *Journal of Experimental Medicine* **170**, 865–75.

Alvaro-Garcia, J.M. et al. (1991). Cytokines in chronic inflammatory arthritis. VI. Analysis of the synovial cells involved in granulocyte-macrophage colony stimulating factor production and gene expression in rheumatoid arthritis and its regulation by IL-1 and TNFα. *Journal of Rheumatology* **146**, 3365–71.

Andrew, E.M. et al. (1991). The potential role of B lymphocytes in the pathogenesis of rheumatoid arthritis. *British Journal of Rheumatology* **30** (Suppl. 1), 47–52.

Andrews, B.S. et al. (1978). Spontaneous murine lupus-like syndrome. *Journal of Experimental Medicine* **148**, 1198–215.

Arend, W.F. (1991). Interleukin-l receptor antagonist—a new member of the IL-1 family. *Journal of Clinical Investigation* **88**, 1445–51.

Arend, W.D. and Dayer, J.-M. (1995). Inhibition of the production and effects of interleukin-1 and tumor necrosis factor in rheumatoid arthritis. *Arthritis and Rheumatism* **38**, 151–60.

Arner, E.C. et al. (1999). Aggrecanase. A target for the design of inhibitors of cartilage degradation. *Annals of the New York Academy of Science* **878**, 92–107.

Axford, J.S. et al. (1987). Reduced B-cell galactosyltransferase activity in rheumatoid arthritis. *Lancet* **ii**, 1486–8.

Baboonian, C. et al. (1991). Cross-reaction of antibodies to a glycine–alanine repeat sequence of Epstein–Barr virus nuclear antigen-1 with collagen, cytokeratin, and actin. *Annals of the Rheumatic Diseases* **50**, 772–5.

Barkley, D. et al. (1989a). Increased expression of HLA–DQ antigens by interstitial cells and endothelium in the synovial membrane of rheumatoid arthritis patients compared with reactive arthritis patients. *Arthritis and Rheumatism* **32**, 955–63.

Barkley, D., Feldmann, M., and Maini, R.N. (1989b). The detection by immunofluorescence of distinct cell populations producing interleukin-1α and interleukin-1β in activated human peripheral blood. *Journal of Immunological Methods* **120**, 277–83.

Bathon, J.M. et al. (2000). A comparison of etanercept and methotrexate in patients with early rheumatoid arthritis. *New England Journal of Medicine* **343**, 1586–93.

Berthelot, J.-M. et al. (1994). APF (antiperinuclear factor). In *Manual of Biological Markers of Disease* (ed. R.N. Maini and W.J. Van Venrooij), B1.2, pp. 1–9. Dordrecht: Kluwer.

Boissier, M.C. et al. (1987). Experimental autoimmune arthritis in mice. I. Homologous type II collagen is responsible for self-perpetuating chronic polyarthritis. *Annals of the Rheumatic Diseases* **46**, 691–700.

Bläß, S. et al. (2001). The stress protein BiP is overexpressed and is a major B and T cell target in rheumatoid arthritis. *Arthritis and Rheumatism* **44**, 761–71.

Bradley, D.S. et al. (1997). HLA–DQB1 polymorphism determines incidence, onset, and severity of collagen-induced arthritis in transgenic mice. Implications in human rheumatoid arthritis. *Journal of Clinical Investigation* **100**, 2227–34.

Brand, A. et al. (1999). Human retrovirus-5 in rheumatic disease. *Journal of Autoimmunity* **13**, 149–54.

Brennan, F.M. et al. (1988a). Heterogeneity of T cell receptor idiotypes in rheumatoid arthritis. *Clinical and Experimental Immunology* **73**, 417–23.

Brennan, F.M. et al. (1988b). T cells expressing $\gamma\delta$ chain receptors in rheumatoid arthritis. *Journal of Autoimmunity* **1**, 319–26.

Brennan, F.M. et al. (1989a). Cytokine production in culture by cells isolated from the synovial membrane. *Journal of Autoimmunity* **2** (Suppl.), 177–86.

Brennan, F.M. et al. (1989b). Inhibitory effect of TNFα antibodies on synovial cell interleukin-1 production in rheumatoid arthritis. *Lancet* **ii**, 244–7.

Brennan, F.M. et al. (1989c). Co-ordinate expansion of 'fetal type' lymphocytes (TCR $\gamma\delta$ + T and CD5 + β) in rheumatoid arthritis and primary Sjögren's syndrome. *Clinical and Experimental Immunology* **77**, 175–8.

Brennan, F.M. et al. (1990a). Detection of interleukin 8 biological activity in synovial fluids from patients with rheumatoid arthritis and production of IL-8 mRNA by isolated synovial cells. *European Journal of Immunology* **20**, 2141.

Brennan, F.M. et al. (1990b). Detection of transforming growth factor β in rheumatoid arthritis synovial tissue: lack of effect on spontaneous cytokine production in joint cell cultures. *Clinical and Experimental Immunology* **81**, 278–85.

Brennan, F.M. et al. (1995). TNF inhibitors are produced spontaneously by rheumatoid and osteoarthritis synovial joint cell cultures: evidence of feedback control of TNF action. *Scandinavian Journal of Immunology* **42**, 158–65.

Brennan, F.M. et al. (2001). Evidence that rheumatoid arthritis synovial T cells are similar to cytokine activated T cells: involvement of P13 kinase and NF-κB pathways in TNFα production in rheumatoid arthritis. *Arthritis and Rheumatism* **46**, 31–41.

Brenner, C.A. et al. (1989). Message amplification phenotyping (MAPPing): a technique to simultaneously measure multiple mRNAs from small number of cells. *BioTechniques* **7**, 1096–2003.

Brown, C.M.S. et al. (1992). Immunoglobulin heavy chain variable region gene utilization by B cell hybridomas derived from rheumatoid synovial tissue. *Clinical and Experimental Immunology* **89**, 230–8.

Brown, C.M.S. et al. (1995). Sequence analysis of immunoglobulin heavy-chain variable region genes from the synovium of a rheumatoid arthritis patient shows little evidence of mutation but diverse CDR3. *Immunology* **84**, 367–74.

Buchan, G. et al. (1988a). Interleukin-1 and tumour necrosis factor mRNA expression in rheumatoid arthritis: prolonged production of IL-1α. *Clinical and Experimental Immunology* **73**, 449–55.

Buchan, G. et al. (1988b). Detection of activated T cell products in the rheumatoid joint using cDNA probes to interleukin 2, IL-2 receptor and interferon γ. *Clinical and Experimental Immunology* **71**, 295–301.

Buchanan, H.M. et al. (1991). Is diet important in rheumatoid arthritis? *British Journal of Rheumatology* **30**, 125–34.

Buckley, C.D. et al. (2000). Persistent induction of the chemokine receptor CXCR4 by TGF-beta 1 on synovial T cells contributes to their accumulation within the rheumatoid synovium. *Journal of Immunology* **165**, 3423–39.

Cathcart, E.S. et al. (1986). Experimental arthritis in a non-human primate. 1. Induction by bovine type II collagen. *Laboratory Investigation* **54**, 26–31.

Chantry, D. et al. (1989). Mechanism of immune complex mediated damage: induction of interleukin 1 by immune complexes and synergy with interferon γ and tumour necrosis factor α. *European Journal of Immunology* **19**, 189–92.

Chantry, D. et al. (1990). Granulocyte–macrophage colony stimulating factor induces both HLA–DR expression and cytokine production by human monocytes. *Cytokine* **2**, 60–7.

Charriere, G. et al. (1988). Antibodies to type I, II, IX, XI collagen in the serum of patients with rheumatic diseases. *Arthritis and Rheumatism* **3I**, 325–32.

Chu, C.Q. et al. (1991a). Localization of tumor necrosis factor α in synovial tissues and at the cartilage–pannus junction in patients with rheumatoid arthritis. *Arthritis and Rheumatism* **34**, 1125–32.

Chu, C.Q. et al. (1991b). Transforming growth factor β_1 in rheumatoid synovial membrane and cartilage/pannus junction. *Clinical and Experimental Immunology* **86**, 380–6.

Cohen, I.R. et al. (1985). T lymphocyte clones illuminate pathogenesis and effect therapy of experimental arthritis. *Arthritis and Rheumatism* **28**, 841–5.

Cohen, S.B.A. et al. (1995). High level of interleukin-10 production by the activated T cell population within the rheumatoid synovial membrane. *Arthritis and Rheumatism* **38**, 946–52.

Colville-Nash, P.R. and Scott, D.L. (1992). Angiogenesis and rheumatoid arthritis: pathogenic and therapeutic implications. *Annals of the Rheumatic Diseases* **51**, 919–25.

Cope, A.P. and Maini, R.N. (1995). Soluble tumor necrosis factor receptors in arthritis. *Journal of Rheumatology* **22**, 382–4.

Cope, A. et al. (1992). Increased levels of soluble tumor necrosis factor receptors in the sera and synovial fluids of patients with rheumatic diseases. *Arthritis and Rheumatism* **35**, 1160–9.

Cope, A. et al. (1999). T cell responses to a human cartilage autoantigen in the context of rheumatoid arthritis-associated and non-associated HLA-DR4 alleles. *Arthritis and Rheumatism* **42**, 1497–507.

Corrigall, V.M. et al. (2001). The human endoplasmic reticulum molecular chaperone BiP is an autoantigen for rheumatoid arthritis and prevents the induction of experimental arthritis. *Journal of Immunology* **166**, 1492–8.

Courtenay, J.S. et al. (1980). Immunisation against heterologous type II collagen induces arthritis in mice. *Nature* **283**, 666–8.

Crawford, T.B. et al. (1980). Chronic arthritis in goats caused by a retrovirus. *Science* **207**, 997–9.

Cromartie, W.J. et al. (1977). Arthritis in rats after systemic injection of streptococcal cells or cell walls. *Journal of Experimental Medicine* **146**, 1585–602.

Cush, J.J. et al. (1992). The intrinsic migratory capacity of memory T cells contributes to their accumulation in rheumatoid synovium. *Arthritis and Rheumatism* **35**, 1434–44.

Davies, M.E., Sharma, H., and Pigott, R. (1992). ICAM-1 expression on chondrocytes in rheumatoid arthritis: induction by synovial cytokines. *Mediators of Inflammation* **1**, 71–4.

Dayan, C.M. et al. (1991). Autoantigen recognition by thyroid-infiltrating T cells in Graves' disease. *Proceedings of the National Academy of Sciences USA* **88**, 7415–19.

Dayer, J.M. and Burger, D. (1999). Cytokines and direct cell contact in synovitis: relevance to therapeutic intervention. *Arthritis Research* **1**, 17–20.

Decker, J.L. and Barden, J.A. (1975). *Mycoplasma hyortinis* of swine: a model for rheumatoid arthritis? *Rheumatology* **6**, 338–45.

Deighton, C.M. et al. (1989). The contribution of HLA to rheumatoid arthritis. *Clinical Genetics* **36**, 178–82.

Deleuran, B.W. et al. (1992). Localization of tumor necrosis factor receptors in the synovial tissue and cartilage–pannus junction in patients with rheumatoid arthritis: implications for local actions of tumor necrosis factor α. *Arthritis and Rheumatism* **35**, 1170–8.

Dequeker, J. (1987). Rheumatic diseases in visual arts. (General review.) In *Art History and Antiquity of Rheumatic Diseases* (ed. T. Appelboom), p. 84. Brussels: Elsevier.

Dieppe, P.A. (1988). Did Galen describe rheumatoid arthritis? *Annals of the Rheumatic Diseases* **47**, 84–5.

Dixon, F.J. et al. (1958). Pathogenesis of serum sickness. *Archives of Pathology* **65**, 18–22.

Drew, R.A. (1972). Erysipelothrix arthritis in pigs as a model of rheumatoid arthritis. *Proceedings of the Royal Society of Medicine* **65**, 42–6.

Dube, R. et al. (1990). Agalactosyl IgG in inflammatory bowel disease: correlation with C-reactive protein. *Gut* **31**, 431–4.

Dumonde, D.C. and Glynn, L.E. (1962). The production of arthritis in rabbits by an immunological reaction to fibrin. *British Journal of Experimental Pathology* **43**, 373–83.

Eastgate, J.A. et al. (1988). Correlation of plasma interleukin-1 levels with disease activity in rheumatoid arthritis. *Lancet* **ii**, 706–9.

Ebringer, A., Khalafpour, S., and Wilson, C. (1989). Rheumatoid arthritis and *Proteus*: a possible aetiological association. *Rheumatism International* **9**, 223–8.

van Eden, W., Holoshitz, J., Nevo, Z., Frenkel, A., Klajman, A., and Cohen, I.R. (1985). Arthritis induced by a T lymphocyte clone that responds to mycobacterium tuberculosis and to cartilage proteoglycans. *Proceedings of the National Academy of Sciences USA* **82**, 5117–20.

van Eden, W. et al. (1988). Cloning of the mycobacterial epitope recognized by T lymphocytes in adjuvant arthritis. *Nature* **331**, 171–3.

Edwards, J.C.W. and Cambridge, G. (2001). Sustained improvement in rheumatoid arthritis following a protocol designed to deplete B lymphocytes. *Rheumatology* **40**, 205–11.

Elliott, M.J. and Maini, R.N. (1996). What are the prospects for therapy based on cytokines and anticytokines in rheumatoid arthritis? In *Cytokines in Autoimmunity* (ed. F.M. Brennan and M. Feldmann), pp. 239–56. Austin TX: R.G. Landes.

Elliott, M.J. et al. (1993). Treatment of rheumatoid arthritis with chimeric monoclonal antibodies to tumor necrosis factor α. *Arthritis and Rheumatism* **36**, 1681–90.

Elliott, M.J. et al. (1994). Randomised double-blind comparison of chimeric monoclonal antibody to tumour necrosis factor α (cA2) versus placebo in rheumatoid arthritis. *Lancet* **344**, 1105–10.

Engelmann, H., Novick, D., and Wallach, D. (1990). Two tumour necrosis factor-binding proteins purified from human urine. *Journal of Biological Chemistry* **265** (3), 1531–6.

Feldmann, M. (1987). Regulation of HLA class II expression and its role in autoimmune disease. *Autoimmunity and Autoimmune Disease* Vol. 129. Ciba Foundation Symposium, pp. 88–108. Chichester: Wiley.

Feldmann, M. (1989). Molecular mechanisms involved in human autoimmune diseases: relevance of chronic antigen presentation, class II expression and cytokine production. *Immunology* (Suppl. 2), 66–71.

Feldmann, M. and Maini, R.N. (2001). Anti TNFα therapy of rheumatoid arthritis: What have we learned? *Annual Review of Immunology* **19**, 163–96.

Feldmann, M. et al. (1991). Cytokine assays: role in evaluation of the pathogenesis of autoimmunity. *Immunological Reviews* **119**, 105–23.

Feldmann, M., Brennan, F.M., and Maini, R.N. (1996). Role of cytokines in rheumatoid arthritis. *Annual Review of Immunology* **14**, 397–440.

Ferrara, N. et al. (1991). The vascular endothelial growth factor family of polypeptides. *Journal of Cell Biochemistry* **47**, 211–18.

Field, M. et al. (1991). Interleukin-6 in the synovial membrane in rheumatoid arthritis. *Rheumatism International* **11**, 45–50.

Firestein, G.S. and Zvaifler, N.J. (1987). Peripheral blood and synovial fluid monocyte activation in inflammatory arthritis. II. Low levels of synovial fluid and synovial tissue interferon suggest that γ-interferon is not the primary macrophage activating factor. *Arthritis and Rheumatism* **30**, 864–71.

Firestein, G.S. and Zvaifler, N.J. (1990). How important are T cells in chronic rheumatoid synovitis? *Arthritis and Rheumatism* **33**, 768–73.

Firestein, G.S., Alvaro-Garcia, J.M., and Maki, R. (1990). Quantitative analysis of cytokine gene expression in rheumatoid arthritis. *Journal of Immunology* **144**, 3347–53.

Folkman, J. (1995). Angiogenesis in cancer, vascular, rheumatoid and other disease. *Nature Medicine* **1**, 27–30.

Fong, Y. et al. (1989). Antibodies to cachectin/tumour necrosis factor reduce interleukin 1β and interleukin 6 appearance during lethal bacteremia. *Journal of Experimental Medicine* **170**, 1627–33.

Fontana, A. et al. (1982). Interleukin 1 activity in the synovial fluid of patients with rheumatoid arthritis. *Rheumatology International* **2**, 49–53.

Forrestier, J. (1935). Rheumatoid arthritis and its treatment by gold salts. *Journal of Laboratory and Clinical Medicine* **20**, 827–40.

Fraser, K.J. (1982). Anglo-French contributions to the recognition of rheumatoid arthritis. *Annals of the Rheumatic Diseases* **41**, 335–43.

Garrod, A.B. *Nature and Treatment of Gout and Rheumatic Gout.* London: Walton and Maberly, 1859.

Gaston, J.S. et al. (1989). *In vitro* response to a 65 kDa mycobacterial protein by synovial T cells from inflammatory arthritis patients. *Journal of Immunology* **143**, 2494–500.

Gimsa, U. et al. (1997). Type II collagen serology: a guide to clinical responsiveness to oral tolerance? *Rheumatology International* **16**, 237–40.

Goldstein, R. and Arnett, F.C. (1987). The genetics of rheumatic disease in man. *Rheumatic Disease Clinics of North America* **13** (3), 487–510.

Goronzy, J. and Weyand, P.M. (1993). Interplay of T lymphocytes and HLA–DR molecules in rheumatoid arthritis. *Current Opinion in Rheumatology* **5**, 169–77.

Goronzy, J. and Weyand, P.M. (1995). T and B cell dependent pathways in rheumatoid arthritis. *Current Opinion in Rheumatology* **7**, 214.

Goronzy, J., Weyand, P.M., and Fathman, C.G. (1986). Shared T cell recognition sites on human histocompatibility leukocyte antigen class II molecules of patients with seropositive rheumatoid arthritis. *Journal of Clinical Investigation* **77**, 1042–9.

Gregersen, P.K., Silver, J., and Winchester, R.J. (1987). The shared epitope hypothesis. An approach to understanding the molecular genetics of susceptibility to rheumatoid arthritis. *Arthritis and Rheumatism* **30**, 1205–13.

Hammer, J. et al. (1995). Peptide binding specificity of HLA–DR4 molecules: correlation with rheumatoid arthritis association. *Journal of Experimental Medicine* **181**, 1847–55.

Hannestad, K. and Stollar, B.D. (1978). Certain rheumatoid factors react with nucleosomes. *Nature* **275**, 671–3.

Hassfeld, W. et al. (1995). Autoimmune response to the spliceosome: an immunologic link between rheumatoid arthritis, mixed connective tissue disease and systemic lupus erythematosus. *Arthritis and Rheumatism* **38**, 777–85.

Haworth, C., Brennan, F.M., Chantry, D., Turner, M., Maini, R.N., and Feldmann, M. (1991). Expression of granulocyte-macrophage colony-stimulating factor in rheumatoid arthritis: regulation by tumour necrosis factor α. *European Journal of Immunology* **21**, 2575–9.

Helfgott, S.M., Bazin, H., Dessein, A., and Trentham, D.E. (1984). Suppressive effects of anti-μ serum on the development of collagen arthritis in rats. *Clinical Immunology and Immunopathology* **31**, 403–11.

Herman, A., Kappler, J.W., Marrack, P., and Pullen, A.M. (1991). Superantigens: mechanism of T-cell stimulation and role in immune responses. *Annual Review of Immunology* **9**, 745–72.

Hirano, T. et al. (1988). Excessive production of interleukin 6/B cell stimulatory factor-2 in rheumatoid arthritis. *European Journal of Immunology* **18**, 1797–801.

Holmdahl, R., Jansson, L., Larsson, E., Rubin, K., and Klareskog, L. (1986). Homologous type II collagen induces chronic and progressive arthritis in mice. *Arthritis and Rheumatism* **29**, 106–13.

Holmdahl, R., Karlsson, M., Andersson, M.E., Rask, L., and Andersson, L. (1989). Localisation of a critical restriction site on the 1-A beta chain which determines susceptibility to collagen-induced arthritis. *Proceedings of the National Academy of Sciences USA* **86**, 9475–9.

Holoshitz, J. et al. (1986). T lymphocytes of rheumatoid arthritis patients show increased reactivity to a fraction of mycobacteria cross-reactive with cartilage. *Lancet* **11**, 305–9.

Holoshitz, J., Koning, F., Coligan, J.E., De Bruyn, J., and Strober, S. (1989). Isolation of CD4–CD8- mycobacteria-reactive T lymphocyte clones from rheumatoid arthritis synovial fluid. *Nature* **339**, 226–9.

Howell, M.D. et al. (1991). Limited T-cell receptor β chain heterogeneity among interleukin-2 receptor-positive T cells suggests a role for superantigen in rheumatoid arthritis. *Proceedings of the National Academy of Sciences USA* **88**, 10921–5.

Hunter, W. *Oral Sepsis as a Cause of Septic Conditions.* London: Cassell, 1901.

Hyka, N. et al. (2001). Apolipoprotein A-I inhibits the production of interleukin-1 beta and tumor necrosis factor-alpha by blocking contact-mediated activation of monocytes by T lymphocytes. *Blood* **97**, 2381–91.

Isler, P. et al. (1993). Cell surface glycoproteins expressed on activated human T cells induce production of interleukin-1 beta by monocytic cells: a possible role of CD69. *European Cytokine Network* **4**, 15–23.

Iwakura, Y. et al. (1991). Induction of inflammatory arthropathy resembling rheumatoid arthritis in mice transgenic for HTLV. *Science* **253**, 1026–8.

Jasin, H.E. (1975). Mechanism of trapping of immune complexes into joint collagenous tissues. *Clinical and Experimental Immunology* **22**, 473–85.

Jose, P.J., Moss, I.K., Maini, R.N., and Williams, T.J. (1990). Measurement of the chemotactic complement fragment C5a in rheumatoid synovial fluids by radioimmunoassay: role of C5a in the acute inflammatory phase. *Annals of the Rheumatic Diseases* **49**, 747–52.

Katsikis, P., Chu, C.Q., Brennan, F.M., Maini, R.N., and Feldmann, M. (1993). Immunoregulatory role of interleukin-10 (IL-10) in rheumatoid arthritis. *Journal of Experimental Medicine* **179**, 1517–27.

Keffer, J. et al. (1991). Transgenic mice expressing human tumour necrosis factor: a predictive gene model of arthritis. *EMBO Journal* **10**, 4025–31.

Kehrl, J.H., Alvarez-Mon, M., Delsing, G.A., and Fauci, A.S. (1987). Lymphotoxin is an important T cell derived growth factor for human B cells. *Science* **238**, 1144–7.

Kingsley, G.M., Pitzalis, C., and Panayi, G.S. (1987). Abnormal lymphocyte reactivity to self—major histocompatibility antigens in rheumatoid arthritis. *Journal of Rheumatology* **14**, 667–73.

Kissonerghis, A.M., Maini, R.N., and Feldmann, M. (1989). High rate of HLA class II mRNA synthesis in rheumatoid arthritis joints and its persistence in culture: down-regulation by recombinant interleukin 2. *Scandinavian Journal of Immunology* **29**, 73–82.

Klemperer, P., Pollack, A.D., and Baehr, G. (1942). Diffuse collagen disease: acute disseminated lupus erythematosus and diffuse systemic sclerosis. *Journal of the American Medical Association* **119**, 331–2.

Koch, A.E. et al. (1992). Enhanced production of monocyte chemoattractant protein-1 in rheumatoid arthritis. *Journal of Clinical Investigation* **90**, 772–9.

Koch, A.E. et al. (1994). Macrophage inflammatory protein-1α. *Journal of Clinical Investigation* **93**, 921–8.

Kouskoff, V. et al. (1996). Organ-specific disease provoked by systemic autoimmunity. *Cell* **87**, 811.

Lacraz, S. et al. (1994). Direct contact between T lymphocytes and monocytes is a major pathway for induction of metalloproteinase expression. *Journal of Biological Chemistry* **269**, 22027–33.

Lahita, R.G. (1990). Sex hormones and the immune system. Part 1: Human data. *Baillière's Clinical Rheumatology* **4**, 1–12.

Lanzavecchia, A. et al. (1985). Antigen-specific interaction between T and B cells. *Nature* **314**, 537–9.

Lawrence, J.S. (1970). Rheumatoid arthritis: nature or nurture? *Annals of the Rheumatic Diseases* **29**, 357–69.

Lipsky, P.E. et al. (2000). Infliximab and methotrexate in the treatment of rheumatoid arthritis. *New England Journal of Medicine* **343**, 1594–602.

Londei, M. et al. (1989). Persistence of collagen type II specific T cell clones in the synovial membrane of a patient with rheumatoid arthritis. *Proceedings of the National Academy of Sciences USA* **86**, 636–40.

Londei, M. et al. (1990). Interleukin 7 is a growth factor for mature human T cells. *European Journal of Immunology* **20**, 425–8.

Macgregor, A.J. and Silman, A. (1994). An analysis of the relative contribution of genetic and environmental factors to rheumatoid arthritis susceptibility. *Arthritis and Rheumatism* **37** (Suppl.), S169.

Maini, R.N. (1989). Exploring immune pathways in rheumatoid arthritis. *British Journal of Rheumatology* **28**, 466–79.

Maini, R.N., Plater-Zyberk, C., and Andrew, E.M. (1987). Autoimmunity in rheumatoid arthritis: an approach via a study of B lymphocytes. *Rheumatic Diseases Clinics of North America* **13**, 319–38.

Maini, R.N. et al. (1995). Monoclonal anti-TNFα antibody as a probe of pathogenesis and therapy of rheumatoid disease. *Immunology Reviews* **144**, 195–223.

Maini, R.N. and Taylor, P.C. (2000). Anti-cytokine therapy for rheumatoid arthritis. *Annual Review of Medicine* **51**, 207–29.

Malfait, A.-M. et al. (2001). Chronic relapsing homologous collagen-induced arthritis in DBA/1 mice as a model for testing disease-modifying and remission-inducing therapies. *Arthritis and Rheumatism* **44**, 1215–24.

Mansson, I., Norberg, R., Olhagen, B., and Bjorklund, N.E. (1971). Arthritis in pigs induced by dietary factors: microbiological, clinical, and histologic studies. *Clinical and Experimental Immunology* **9**, 677–93.

March, L.M. (1987). Dendritic cells in the pathogenesis of rheumatoid arthritis. *Rheumatism International* **7**, 93–100.

Masson-Bessiere, C. et al. (2001). The major synovial targets of the rheumatoid arthritis-specific antifilaggrin autoantibodies are deiminated forms of the alpha- and beta-chains of fibrin. *Journal of Immunology* **166**, 4177–84.

Matsumoto, I. et al. (1999). Arthritis provoked by linked T and B cell recognition of a glycolytic enzyme. *Science* **286**, 1732–5.

McInnes, I.B. et al. (1996). Interleukin-15 mediates T cell-dependent regulation of tumor necrosis factor-alpha production in rheumatoid arthritis. *Nature Medicine* **3**, 189–95.

McInnes, I.B. et al. (1998). Interleukin 15: a proinflammatory role in rheumatoid arthritis synovitis. *Immunology Today* **19**, 75–9.

Menard. H.A. et al. (2000). Insights into rheumatoid arthritis derived from the Sa immune system. *Arthritis Research* **2**, 429–32.

Mollenhauer, J., von der Mark, K., Burmester, G., Gluckert, K., Lütjen-Drecoll, E., and Brune, K. (1988). Serum antibodies against chondrocyte cell surface proteins in osteoarthritis and rheumatoid arthritis. *Journal of Rheumatology* **15**, 1811–17.

Moreland, L.W. et al. (1998). T cell receptor peptide vaccination in rheumatoid arthritis: a placebo-controlled trial using a combination of Vbeta3, Vbeta 14 and Vbeta17 peptides. *Arthritis and Rheumatism* **41**, 1906–10.

Morris, V. and Mackworth-Young, C. (1996). Antiphospholipid antibodies: clinical aspects. In *Autoantibody Manual. Manual of Biological Markers of Disease*, C2.5 (ed. W.J. van Venrooij and R.N. Maini), pp. 1–14. Dordrecht: Kluwer Academic Publishers.

Moore, T.L. (2000). Parvovirus-associated arthritis. *Current Opinion in Rheumatology* **12**, 289–94.

Moore, K.W., Vieiva, P., Fiorentino, D.F., Trounstine, M.L., Khan, T.A., and Mosmann, T.R. (1990). Homology of cytokine synthesis inhibitory factor (IL-10) to the Epstein–Barr virus gene BCRF 1. *Science* **248**, 1230–4.

Morales-Ducret, J., Wayner, E., Elices, M.J., Alvaro-Garcia, J.M., Zvaifler, N.J., and Firestein, G.S. (1992). Alpha 4/beta 1 integrin (VLA-4) ligands in arthritis: I. Vascular cell adhesion molecule 1 expression in synovium and on fibroblast-like synoviocytes. *Journal of Immunology* **149**, 1424–31.

Mulder, A.H., Horst, G., van-Leeuwen, M.A., Limburg, P.C., and Kalleberg, C.G. (1993). Antineutrophil cytoplasmic antibodies in rheumatoid arthritis. Characterization and clinical correlations. *Arthritis and Rheumatism* **36**, 1054–60.

Nienhuis, R.L.F. and Mandema, E. (1964). A new serum factor in patients with rheumatoid arthritis: the perinuclear factor. *Annals of the Rheumatic Diseases* **23**, 302–5.

Novick, D. et al. (2001). A novel IL-18BP ELISA shows elevated serum IL-18BP in sepsis and extensive decrease of free IL-18. *Cytokine* **14**, 334–42.

Oates, C.M., Maini, R.N., Payne, L.N., and Dumonde, D.C. (1972). Possible role of lymphokines in the development of ectopic lymphoid foci in the chicken. *Advances in Experimental Medicine and Biology* **29**, 611–18.

Olee, T. et al. (1991). Molecular basis of an autoantibody-associated restriction fragment length polymorphism that confers susceptibility to autoimmune diseases. *Journal of Clinical Investigation* **88**, 193–203.

Ollier, W. et al. (1984). HLA antigen associations with extra-articular rheumatoid arthritis. *Tissue Antigens* **24**, 279–91.

Olsen, N.J. et al. (1994). Multicenter trial of an anti-CD5 immuno-conjugate in rheumatoid arthritis (RA). *Arthritis and Rheumatism* **37**, S295.

O'Sullivan, F.X., Fassbender, H.G., Gay, S., and Koopman, W.J. (1985). Etiopathogenesis of the rheumatoid arthritis-like disease in MRL/ lpr mice. 1. The histomorphologic basis of joint destruction. *Arthritis and Rheumatism* **28**, 529–36.

Paleolog, E.M., Hunt, M., Elliott, M.J., Woody, J.N., Feldmann, M., and Maini, R.N. (1996). Monoclonal anti-tumour necrosis factor α antibody deactivates vascular endothelium in rheumatoid arthritis. *Arthritis and Rheumatism* **39**, 1082–91.

Paliard, X. et al. (1991). Evidence for the effects of a superantigen in rheumatoid arthritis. *Science* **253**, 325–9.

Panayi, G.S., Woolley, P.H., and Batchelor, J.H. (1979). HLA–DRW4 and rheumatoid arthritis. *Lancet* **i**, 730–4.

Parekh, R.B. et al. (1985). Association of rheumatoid arthritis and primary osteoarthritis with changes in the glycosylation pattern of total serum IgG. *Nature* **316**, 452–7.

Patil, N.S. et al. (2001). Autoantigenic HCgp39 epitopes are presented by the HLA–DM-dependent presentation pathway in human B cells. *Journal of Immunology* **166**, 33–41.

Pearson, C.M. (1956). Development of arthritis, periarthritis, and periostitis in rats given adjuvants. *Proceedings of the Society of Experimental Biology and Medicine* **91**, 95–101.

Pitzalis, C., Kingsley, G., Murphy, J., and Panayi, G. (1987). Abnormal distribution of the helper-inducer and suppressor-inducer T lymphocyte subsets in the rheumatoid joint. *Clinical Immunology and Immunopathology* **45**, 252–8.

Plater-Zyberk, C., Maini, R.N., Brennan, F.M., and Feldmann, M. (1992). CD5+ B and double-negative T cells in rheumatoid arthritis. In *Rheumatoid Arthritis* (ed. J. Smolen, J. Kalden, and R.N. Maini), pp. 122–36. Berlin: Springer.

Pober, J.S. et al. (1986). Overlapping patterns of activation of human endothelial cells by interleukin 1, tumour necrosis factor, and immune interferon. *Journal of Immunology* **137**, 1893–6.

Portillo, G., Turner, M., Chantry, D., and Feldmann, M. (1989). Effect of cytokines on HLA–DR and IL-1 production by a monocytic tumour, THP-1. *Immunology* **66**, 170–5.

Pujol-Borrell, R. et al. (1987). HLA class II induction in human islet cells by interferon-γ plus tumour necrosis factor of lymphotoxin. *Nature* **326**, 304–6.

Raddemacher, T.W., Williams, P., and Dwek, R.A. (1994). Agalactosyl glycoforms of IgG autoantibodies are pathogenic. *Proceedings of the National Academy of Sciences USA* **91**, 6123–7.

Raines, E.W., Dower, S.K., and Ross, R. (1989). Interleukin 1 mitogenic activity for fibroblasts and smooth muscle cells is due to PDGK AA. *Science* **243**, 393–7.

Ranges, G.E., Stiram, S., and Cooper, S.M. (1985). Prevention of type II collagen-induced arthritis by *in vivo* treatment with anti-L_3T_4. *Journal of Experimental Medicine* **162**, 1105–10.

Rathanaswami, P., Hachicha, M., Sadick, M., Schall, T.J., and McColl, S.R. (1993). Expression of the cytokine RANTES in human rheumatoid synovial fibroblasts. Differential regulation of RANTES and interleukin-8 genes by inflammatory cytokines. *Journal of Biological Chemistry* **268**, 5834–9.

Res, P.C., Telgt, D., van Laar, J.M., Pool, M.O., Breedveld, F.C., and De Vries, R.R. (1990). High antigen reactivity in mononuclear cells from sites of chronic inflammation. *Lancet* **336**, 1406–8.

Rice, G.E. and Bevilacqua, M.P. (1989). An inducible endothelial cell surface glycoprotein mediates melanoma adhesion. *Science* **326**, 1303–6.

Rijnders, A., Boots, A., Verheijden, G., de Keijser, F., and Veijs, E. Identification of a key autoantigen in rheumatoid arthritis. Sixteenth European Workshop for Rheumatology Research, Stockholm, 1996.

Rogers, J. and Dieppe, P.A. (1990). Skeletal paleopathology and the rheumatic diseases. Where are we now? *Annals of the Rheumatic Diseases* **49**, 885–6.

Rothschild, B.M. and Woods, R.J. (1990). Symmetrical erosive peripheral polyarthritis in arctic Indians: the origin of rheumatoid in the New World. *Seminars in Arthritis and Rheumatism* **19**, 278–84.

Roudier, J., Rhodes, G., Petersen, J., Vaughan, J., and Carson, D.A. (1988). The Epstein–Barr virus glycoprotein gp110, a molecular link between HLA–DR4, HLA–DR1, and rheumatoid arthritis. *Scandinavian Journal of Immunology* **27**, 367–71.

Sadeghi, R., Hawrylowicz, C.M., Chernajovsky, Y., and Feldmann, M. (1992a). Synergism of glucocorticoids with granulocyte macrophage colony stimulating factor (GM-CSF) but not interferon g (interferon–γ) or interleukin-4 (IL-4) on induction of HLA class II expression on human monocytes. *Cytokine* **4**, 287–97.

Sadeghi, R., Feldmann, M., and Hawrylowicz, C.M. (1992b). Upregulation of HLA class II, but not intercellular adhesion molecule 1 (ICAM-1) by granulocyte-macrophage colony stimulating factor (GM-CSF) or interleukin-3 (IL-3) in synergy with dexamethasone. *European Cytokine Network* **3**, 373–80.

Sarvetnick, N. et al. (1990). Loss of pancreatic islet tolerance induced by B cell expression of interferon-γ. *Nature* **346**, 844–7.

Sasazuki, T. et al. (1986). HLA-linked immune suppression maps within HLA–DQ subregion. In *Regulation of Immune Gene Expression* (ed. M. Feldmann and A. McMichael), pp. 197–206. New Jersey: Humana Press.

Schaller, M., Burton, D.R., and Kitzel, H.J. (2001). Autoantibodies to GPI in rheumatoid arthritis : linkage between an animal model and human disease. *Nature Immunology* **2**, 746–53.

Schellekens, G.A. et al. (1998). Citrulline is an essential constituent of antigenic determinants recognized by rheumatoid arthritis-specific autoantibodies. *Journal of Clinical Investigation* **101**, 273–81.

Schellekens, G.A. et al. (2000). The diagnostic properties of rheumatoid arthritis antibodies in recognizing a cyclic citrullinated peptide. *Arthritis and Rheumatism* **43**, 155–63.

Sebbag, M. et al. (1995). The anti-perinuclear factor and the so-called anti-keratin antibodies are the same rheumatoid arthritis-specific autoantibodies. *Journal of Clinical Investigation* **95**, 2672–9.

Seckinger, P., Isaaz, S., and Dayer, J.M. (1989). Purification and biologic characterisation of a specific tumour necrosis factor inhibitor. *Journal of Biological Chemistry* **264**, 11966–73.

Short, C.L. (1974). The antiquity of rheumatoid arthritis. *Arthritis and Rheumatism* **17**, 193–205.

Silman, A.J., Ollier, W., Hayton, R.M., Holligan, S., and Smith, K. (1989). Twin concordance rates for rheumatoid arthritis: preliminary results from a nationwide study. *British Journal of Rheumatology* **28** (Suppl. 2), 95.

Simon, A.K., Seipelt, E., and Sieper, J. (1994). Divergent T-cell cytokine patterns in inflammatory arthritis. *Proceedings of the National Academy of Sciences USA* **91**, 8562–6.

Solomon, L., Robin, G., and Valkenburg, H.A. (1975). Rheumatoid arthritis in an urban South African negro population. *Annals of the Rheumatic Diseases* **34**, 128–35.

Statsny, P. (1976). Mixed lymphocyte cultures in rheumatoid arthritis. *Journal of Clinical Investigation* **57**, 1148–57.

Statsny, P. (1978). Association of the B cell alloantigen DRW4 with rheumatoid arthritis. *New England Journal of Medicine* **97**, 664–761.

Steiner, G. et al. (1992). Purification and partial sequencing of the nuclear autoantigen RA33 shows that it is indistinguishable from the A2 protein of the heterogenous nuclear ribonuclearprotein complex. *Journal of Clinical Investigation* **90**, 1061–6.

Sternberg, E.M. et al. (1989a). Inflammatory mediator-induced hypothalamic–pituitary–adrenal axis activation is defective in streptococcal cell wall arthritis-susceptible Lewis rats. *Proceedings of the National Academy of Sciences USA* **86**, 2374–8.

Sternberg, E.M. et al. (1989b). A central nervous system defect in biosynthesis of corticotropin-releasing hormone is associated with susceptibility to streptococcal cell-wall induced arthritis in Lewis rats. *Proceedings of the National Academy of Sciences USA* **86**, 4771–5.

Symons, J.A., Wood, N.C., Di Giovine, F.S., and Duff, G.W. (1988). Soluble IL-2 receptor in rheumatoid arthritis. *Journal of Immunology* **141**, 2612–18.

Symons, J.A., Eastgate, J.A., and Duff, G.W. (1991). Purification and characterization of a novel soluble receptor for interleukin 1. *Journal of Experimental Medicine* **174**, 1251–4.

Tak, P.P. et al. (1996). Reduction in cellularity and expression of adhesion molecules in rheumatoid synovial tissue after anti-TNFα monoclonal antibody treatment. *Arthritis and Rheumatism* **39**, 1077–81.

Takahashi, Y. et al. (1989). Human parvovirus B19 as a causative agent for rheumatoid arthritis. *Proceedings of the National Academy of Sciences USA* **95**, 8227–32.

Tarkowski, A. et al. (1989). Secretion of antibodies to types I and II collagen by synovial tissue cells in patients with rheumatoid arthritis. *Arthritis and Rheumatism* **32**, 1087–96.

Taylor, P.C., Maini, R.N., and Plater-Zyberk, C. (1995). The role of the B cells in the adoptive transfer of collagen-induced arthritis from DBA/1 (H-2^q) to SCID (H-2^d) mice. *European Journal of Immunology* **25**, 763–9.

Taylor, P.C. et al. (2000). Reduction of chemokine levels and leukocyte traffic to joints by tumor necrosis factor α blockade in patients with rheumatoid arthritis. *Arthritis and Rheumatism* **43**, 38–47.

Taylor, P.C., Williams, R.O., and Maini, R.N. (2001). Immunotherapy for rheumatoid arthritis. *Current Opinion in Immunology* **13**, 611–16.

Teyton, L. et al. (1987). HLA DR, DQ and DP antigen expression in rheumatoid synovial cells: a biochemical and quantitative study. *Journal of Immunology* **138**, 1730–8.

Thomas, R. and Lipsky, P. (1996). Presentation of self-peptides by dendritic cells: implications for the pathogenesis of rheumatoid arthritis. *Immunology Today* **39**, 183.

Thorbeck, G.J. et al. (1992). Involvement of endogenous tumour necrosis factor alpha and transforming growth factor beta during induction of collagen type II arthritis in mice. *Proceedings of the National Academy of Sciences USA* **89**, 7375–9.

Trabandt, A., Gay, R.E., and Gay, S. (1992). Oncogene activation in rheumatoid synovium. *Acta Pathologica, Microbiologica et Immunologica Scandinavica* **100**, 861–75.

Trentham, D.E., Townes, A.S., and Kang, A.H. (1977). Autoimmunity to type II collagen: an experimental model of arthritis. *Journal of Experimental Medicine* **146**, 857–68.

Trentham, D.E. et al. (1993). Effects of administration of oral type II collagen on rheumatoid arthritis. *Science* **261**, 1727–30.

Tsai, V., Bergroth, V., and Zvaifler, N.J. (1989). Dendritic cells in health and disease. In *T cell Activation in Health and Disease* (ed. M. Feldmann, R.N. Maini, and J.N. Woody), pp. 33–44. New York: Academic Press.

Van den Broek, M.F., Hogervast, E.J., van Bruggen, M.C., van Eden, W., van der Zee, R., and van den Berg, W.B. (1989). Protection against streptococcal cell-wall-induced arthritis by pretreatment with the 65 kD mycobacterial heat shock protein. *Journal of Experimental Medicine* **170**, 449–66.

Van der Lubbe, P.A., Djikmans, B.A.C., Markusse, H.M., Nassander, U., and Breedveld, F.C. (1995). A randomized, double-blind, placebo-controlled study of CD4 monoclonal antibody therapy in early rheumatoid arthritis. *Arthritis and Rheumatism* **38**, 1097–106.

Van Laar, J.M., Miltenburg, A.M., Verdonk, M.J., Daha, M.R., de Vries, R.R., and Breedveld, F.C. (1991). T cell vaccination in rheumatoid arthritis. *British Journal of Rheumatology* **30** (Suppl. 2), 28–9.

Venables, P.J.W. (1988). Epstein–Barr virus infection and autoimmunity in rheumatoid arthritis. *Annals of the Rheumatic Diseases* **47**, 265–9.

Venables, P.J.W., Erhardt, C.C., Mumford, P., and Maini, R.N. (1979). The occurrence of antibodies to extractable nuclear antigens (ENA) in extra-articular disease in rheumatoid arthritis (RA). *Annals of the Rheumatic Diseases* **39**, 146–53.

Venables, P.J.W., Roffe, L.M., Erhardt, C.C., Maini, R.N., Edwards, J.M.B., and Porter, A.D. (1981). Titers of antibodies to RANA in rheumatoid arthritis and normal sera. *Arthritis and Rheumatism* **24**, 1459–69.

Villiger, P.M., Terkeltaub, R., and Lotz, M. (1992). Production of monocyte chemoattractant protein 1 by inflamed synovial tissue and cultured synoviocytes. *Journal of Immunology* **149**, 722–7.

Vincent, C. et al. (1998). Immunoblotting detection of autoantibodies to human epidermis filaggrin: a new diagnostic test for rheumatoid arthritis. *Journal of Rheumatology* **25**, 838–46.

Waaler, E. (1940). On the occurrence of a factor in human serum activating the specific agglutination of sheep blood corpuscles. *Acta Pathologica et Microbiologica Scandinavica* **17**, 172–6.

Walmsley, M. et al. (1996). IL-10 inhibits progression of established collagen-induced arthritis. *Arthritis and Rheumatism* **39**, 495–503.

Westedt, M.L., Breedveld, F.C., Schreuder, G.M.T., d'Amato, J., Cats, A., and de Vries, R.R.P. (1986). Immunogenetic heterogeneity of rheumatoid arthritis. *Annals of the Rheumatic Diseases* **45**, 534–8.

Weyand, C.M., Xie, C., and Goronzy, J.J. (1992). Homozygosity for the HLA–DRB1 allele selects for extra-articular manifestations in rheumatoid arthritis. *Journal of Clinical Investigation* **89**, 2033–9.

Wilcox, W.H. *Reports on Chronic Rheumatic Disease* Vol. 1, No. 72. London: Lewis, 1935.

Williams, R.O., Feldmann, M., and Maini, R.N. (1992a). Anti-tumor necrosis factor ameliorates joint disease in murine collagen-induced arthritis. *Proceedings of the National Academy of Sciences USA* **89**, 9784–8.

Williams, R.O., Plater-Zyberk, C., Williams, D.G., and Maini, R.N. (1992b). Successful transfer of collagen-induced arthritis to severe combined immunodeficiency (SCID) mice. *Clinical and Experimental Immunology* **88**, 455–60.

Winchester, R.J. and Gregersen, P.K. (1988). The molecular basis of susceptibility to rheumatoid arthritis: the conformational equivalence hypothesis. *Springer Seminars in Immunopathology* **10**, 119–39.

Wordsworth, B.P., Lanchbury, J.S.S., Sakkas, L.I., Welsh, K.I., Panayi, G.S., and Bell, J.I. (1989). HLA–DR4 subtype frequencies in rheumatoid arthritis indicate that DRbl is the major susceptibility locus within the HLA class II region. *Proceedings of the National Academy of Sciences USA* **86**, 10049–53.

Wordsworth, B.P. et al. (1992). HLA heterozygosity contributes to susceptibility to rheumatoid arthritis. *American Journal of Human Genetics* **51**, 585–91.

Young, B.J.J., Mallya, R.K., Leslie, R.D.G., Clark, C.J.M., and Hamlin, T.J. (1979). Anti-keratin antibodies in rheumatoid arthritis. *British Medical Journal* **ii**, 97–9.

Zanelli, E., Gonzalez-Gay, M.A., and David, C.S. (1995). Could HLA–DRβ1 be the protective locus in rheumatoid arthritis? *Immunology Today* **16**, 274–8.

Ziegler, B., Gay, R.E., Huang, G., Fassbender, H.G., and Gay, S. (1989). Immunohistochemical localisation of HTLV-1 pk and p24-related antigens in synovial joints of patients with rheumatoid arthritis. *American Journal of Pathology* **135**, 1–5.

Ziff, M., Kantor, T., Bien, E., and Smith, A. (1953). Studies on the composition of fibrinoid material of subcutaneous nodule of rheumatoid arthritis. *Journal of Clinical Investigation* **32**, 1253–9.

Zvaifler, N.J., Boyle, D., and Firestein, G.S. (1994). Early synovitis, synoviocytes and mononuclear cells. *Seminars in Arthritis and Rheumatism* **23** (6, Suppl. 2) 11–16.

6.3.2 Rheumatoid arthritis—the clinical picture

Marjonne C.W. Creemers and Leo B.A. van de Putte

Introduction

Rheumatoid arthritis (RA) is a chronic systemic inflammatory disease. The main characteristic is a persistent synovitis of diarthrodial joints, often symmetrical in distribution, resulting in pain, stiffness, and loss of function. In many cases, ongoing synovitis results in joint destruction and deformities. RA has a wide clinical spectrum, which varies from mild joint symptoms to severe inflammation and damage to joints. In addition, being a systemic rather than a localized disease, a wide variety of extra-articular features may develop, for example, rheumatoid nodules, vasculitis, lymphadenopathy, serositis, and amyloidosis. Serological studies often show the presence of rheumatoid factor, an autoantibody directed against the Fc-fragment of autologous IgG. The aetiology is unknown, but risk factors for onset and severity have been identified. In the past 15 years or so, new insights into the course of the disease have been developed and more effective therapeutic agents for its treatment have become available. As a result, patients are currently treated earlier with a beneficial influence on disease progression at least as shown in short-term studies (van der Heide et al. 1996; Stenger et al. 1998). It seems likely that these developments may have lead to a change in the clinical picture, including extra-articular features, such as amyloidosis (Hazenberg and van Rijswijk 2000a). Since there is no exact definition of RA, criteria to classify the disease have been delineated. These are dominated by signs and symptoms of locomotor disease.

Classification and diagnosis

Criteria are needed for both epidemiological studies and clinical trials. For these purposes, the classification criteria of the American Rheumatism Association (ARA) were developed (Ropes et al. 1956), which in 1987 were replaced by the criteria of the American College of Rheumatology (ACR) (Arnett et al. 1988) (Table 1). Against the 'gold standard' of physician diagnosis, this 1987 ACR criteria set has a sensitivity in the range of 77–95 per cent and a specificity in the range of 85–98 per cent (Bernelot Moens et al. 1992). RA is diagnosed if at least four out of seven criteria are present. It should be noticed that, in contrast to the original ARA criteria scheme, the ACR criteria do not contain exclusion criteria. The ACR criteria were developed by observing a number of 'typical' patients considered to suffer from RA by experienced rheumatologists. The mean disease duration was 7.7 years. Evidence suggests that the 1987 ACR criteria have important limitations when used for case recognition in prospective studies which require a set of criteria sensitive to the presence of early disease (McGregor and Silman 1998). They may best be used in clinical trials aimed at patients with well-established disease.

Since data are emerging that (very) early treatment may considerably improve the disease, early diagnosis becomes mandatory (Symmons and Harrison 2000). There are, however, no accepted criteria for early RA, although recent data from early arthritis clinics may be helpful in this respect. In one study, investigators looked for a number of items including disease duration, morning stiffness, arthritis of three or more joints, bilateral tenderness of feet, presence of IgM rheumatoid factor, antibodies against cyclic citrullinated peptide (antiCCP), and erosive disease at the first visit. The likelihood of the development of RA was shown to increase with the number of items present at baseline (Visser et al. 2000).

Epidemiology

Since RA lacks a pathognomonic test, the diagnosis of RA rests on a composite of clinical and laboratory observations. In epidemiological studies

Table 1 The revised criteria of 1987 (ARA/ACR)

Criteria	Comment
1. Morning stiffness	Duration >1 h lasting >6 weeks
2. Arthritis of at least three areas[a]	Soft tissue swelling or exudation lasting >6 weeks
3. Arthritis of hand joints	Wrist, metacarpophalangeal joints or proximal interphalangeal joints lasting >6 weeks
4. Symmetrical arthritis	At least one area, lasting >6 weeks
5. Rheumatoid nodules	As observed by a physician
6. Serum rheumatoid factor	As assessed by a method positive in less than 5% of control subjects
7. Radiographic changes	As seen on anteroposterior films of wrists and hands

[a] Possible areas: proximal interphalangeal joints, metacarpophalangeal joints, wrist, elbow, knee, ankle, metatarsophalangeal joints. At least four criteria must be fulfilled. No exclusions.

criteria sets must be relied upon. Such studies in patients with RA can be divided into those dealing with descriptive epidemiology (incidence, prevalence, and survival) and others dealing with risk factors associated with the disease (Gabriel 2001).

Descriptive epidemiology of RA

The prevalence of RA is approximately 0.5–1 per cent in diverse populations worldwide. However, an unusually high prevalence of the disease has been reported in certain North American Indian tribes, while the disease is rare in rural Africans and rural and urban Chinese (Silman and Hochberg 1993). RA affects women more often than men. The annual incidence is approximately 0.2–0.4 per 1000 in females and 0.1–0.2 per 1000 in males. This female excess is possibly greatest in the younger age groups. Furthermore, the incidence of the disease increases with age (Silman and Hochberg 1993) although both the Norfolk Arthritis register (Symmons et al. 1994) and the Rochester Epidemiology Program (Gabriel et al. 1999a–b) report a decrease in incidence of RA in women over 80 years of age. Biases in reporting, however, cannot be excluded in these data. Table 2 gives an overview of studies on the incidence of RA. A declining incidence from 1960 onwards has been observed in women in the Rochester Epidemiology Program (Linos et al. 1980; Gabriel et al. 1999a) and in both women and men among Pima Indians (Jacobsson et al. 1994). However, in Finland, while the incidence of rheumatoid factor positive RA remained constant, only the incidence of rheumatoid factor negative RA declined (Kaipiainen-Seppanen et al. 1996).

Patients with RA have a significantly increased risk of death compared with age- and sex-matched controls without RA from the same community. The determinants of this excess mortality remain unclear; however, reports suggest increased risk from gastrointestinal, respiratory, cardiovascular, infectious, and haematologic diseases among RA patients compared with controls (Myllykangas-Luosujärvi 1995; Gabriel 2001). An overview of the results of RA mortality studies, shows that the standardized mortality ratios in these studies varied from 1.28 to 2.98. Two recent studies do not show increased mortality (Lindquist and Eberhardt 1999; Kroot et al. 2000), possibly reflecting earlier and more effective treatment.

Risk factors with RA

Risk factors contributing to the development or severity of the disease course of RA include genetics, infectious agents, oestrogens, smoking, coffee consumption, and formal education.

Genetics

The familial nature of RA has long been recognized, suggesting that either genetic or environmental risk factors are important in the aetiology of the disease. Clear evidence to support a genetic influence comes from twin studies indicating an excess risk of disease concordance among co-twins of monozygotic (MZ) when compared with dizygotic (DZ) affected twins. This excess risk implies a genetic influence, since it is assumed that both types of twins share a similar environment. A large Finnish study showed a concordance for RA in MZ twins of 12 per cent compared with 4 per cent in DZ pares (Aho et al. 1986). Compared with the background disease prevalence of approximately 1 per cent in non-relatives, these twin studies indicate that genetic factors substantially contribute to the disease. A recent study examined familial aggregation of RA in the Netherlands and analysed the effect of proband characteristics on the concordance rate for RA (Barrera et al. 1999). European-wide cross-sectional hospital-based surveys were used to identify familial RA, that is, affected sib-pair families. The estimated prevalence for familial RA was 9.8 per cent and familial aggregation of RA was estimated to occur preferentially in large siblings. Probands with familial RA were more often rheumatoid factor positive and had a longer follow-up period. Male gender and history of joint replacements were associated with higher concordance for RA.

Genetic studies have focused primarily on the role of the major histocompatibility complex (MHC) locus in RA, namely HLA–DR4 and HLA–DR1, later on being refined to as alleles coding for a 'shared epitope' (SE) on the HLA–DRB1 molecule (see Chapter 6.3.1). It seems that variation in the population prevalence of SE-encoding alleles partly explains the heterogeneity in the geographical distribution of RA. There remains some dispute whether genetic factors determine an individual's susceptibility to RA per se or the severity of the disease once it develops. Several studies of RA patients show that HLA alleles are more strongly associated with features of severe disease, such as rheumatoid factor positivity, erosions, and nodules (Ollier and McGregor 1995). Although the overall genetic influence on disease features is far from clear.

Reproductive and hormonal factors

Several observations pointed to the importance of endocrine factors. There is a clear-cut preponderance of women compared to men in developing RA before but also after the menopause. Pregnancy itself seems to be associated with a reduced risk of newly developing RA (Hazes 1991), whereas the risk is increased in the 12 months after delivery (Silman et al. 1992). The latter may be related to breast feeding, as supported by a case–control study of women developing RA the first 12 months after pregnancy; exposure to breast feeding after the first pregnancy increased the risk of RA five-fold (Brennan and Silman 1994).

A number of studies have indicated that oral contraceptives offer a protective effect against the development of RA, although other studies did not find such an effect. The same holds true for post-menopausal oestrogen use and RA. Most of the evidence points to a protective role of oestrogen in aetiology of RA, but additional research is needed (Gabriel 2001).

Other risk factors

There is no conclusive evidence of an association of RA with a number of putative triggers, including Epstein–Barr virus, parvovirus, proteus, cytomegalo virus (CMV), retroviruses, mycoplasma, and mycobacteria. Studies on lifestyle factors in RA provide conflicting information and are often difficult to interpret. Several studies have indicated that smoking may

Table 2 Incidence of rheumatoid arthritis (Gabriel et al. 2001)

Author	County/region	Years of study	Age range (years)	Sample size	Annual incidence rate per 100 000 population
Uhlig et al. (1998)	Oslo, Norway	1988–1993	20–79	550	25.7 O 36.7 F 13.8 M
Symmons et al. (1994)	Manchester, United Kingdom	1990–1991	15–85+	104	35.9 F 14.3 M
Kaipiainen-Seppanen et al. (1996)	Finland	Four 1-year periods: 1975, 1980, 1985, and 1990	16–85+	1321	1975: 29.0 1980: 35.5 1985: 35.0 1990: 29.5
Gabriel et al. (1999a)	Olmsted County, Minnesota	1955–1985	35–85+	425	75.3 O (95% CI: 68.0–82.5) 98.1 F (95% CI: 87.1–109.1) 49.7 M (95% CI: 40.5–58.9)
Jacobsson et al. (1994)	Pima Indians, Arizona	1965–1990	25–65+	78	1966–1973: 8.9 O[a], 11.5 F[a], 5.9 M[a] 1974–1982: 6.2 O[a], 7.5 F[a], 4.6 M[a] 1983–1990: 3.8 O[a], 4.9 F[a], 2.7 M[a]
Drosos et al. (1997)	Northwest Greece (Ioannina)	1987–1995	16–75+	428	24.0 O 36.0 F 12.0 M
Dugowson et al. (1991)	Seattle, Washington	1987–1990	18–64 (women only)	81	23.9 F

[a] Cases per 1000 person years at risk.

Note: F = female; M = male; O = overall.

be an independent risk factor in the development of RA (Silman et al. 1996). A recent study from Finland showed data supporting that coffee consumption is related to both rheumatoid factor positivity and development of RA (Heliövaara et al. 2000).

Several studies have indicated an association between adverse socioeconomic status and worse disease outcome in RA. Low levels of formal education have also been associated with increased mortality as well as poor clinical status in patients with RA. However, other studies did not confirm these observations. Most of the evidence points to a low level of formal education as a risk factor for RA. So far, the mechanisms involved remain unknown (Gabriel 2001).

Disease course

The natural course of RA is not fully known, because patients are always treated with NSAIDs and often with DMARDs. In controlled studies, the effects of DMARDs was studied and remissions were observed in 10 per cent of patients, chronic progressive disease in 40–70 per cent and a course showing remissions and exacerbations in 20–40 per cent (Ten Wolde et al. 1996).

The onset of the disease may be either abrupt/acute or gradual/insidious or anywhere between these extremes (Fleming et al. 1976). A gradual onset is present in 50 per cent of the cases and usually starts with systemic features, such as fatigue, generalized weakness, loss of weight, and subfebrility, followed by synovitis and evolving to chronic disease. An abrupt onset of the disease is less common (10–25 per cent) and functional outcome in these patients is contradictory, that is, in one study these cases showed a better functional outcome (Fleming et al. 1976), while in another study there appeared to be no difference after an 11-year follow-up. The latter was confirmed in a Finnish study of 235 RA patients in which radiographically evident damage was equal in groups with different onset of disease types (Luukkainen et al. 1983). In a minority of patients there is a 'malignant' onset and a relentless disease course cannot be controlled by any antirheumatic drug regimen. In some 10 per cent of the patients the onset of RA has been preceded by a positive rheumatoid factor test (Aho et al. 1991) or by palindromic rheumatism for several years. In addition, mild or transient RA occurs, having a favourable course, and is probably underreported (Masi et al. 1983).

Involvement of individual joints

Rheumatic diseases often show characteristic, be it not diagnostic, patterns of joint involvement. This is the wrists, fingers, knees, and feet are the most commonly affected joints (Fig. 1). Severe disease is frequently associated with involvement of large joints, such as the shoulders, elbows, and knees.

Hand and wrist

The hand joints affected by RA have many characteristic features, which when present in combination may be almost pathognomonic. Boggy and tender swelling of proximal interphalangeal and metocarpophalangeal joints, wrists, and caput ulnae are common early signs (Fig. 2). Tenosynovitis of extensor, and more often flexor tendon sheets, with or without nodules are other features. Interosseal muscle atrophy is often seen early. Pain is prominent and may contribute to muscle atrophy. Limitation of motion, in particular dorsal flexion of wrist and finger flexion is common. Compression of the median nerve in the carpal tunnel as a result of flexor tenosynovitis, may be the presenting symptom of RA and is frequent in the early phase of the disease. Atrophy of the thenar muscle may be seen after long-standing compression of the median nerve. Pain elicited by tangential squeezing of MCP joints is an important diagnostic clue for RA. Distal interphalangeal (DIP) joint involvement occurs, but is rare and should be distinguished from coincidental osteoarthritis.

Occasionally, massive diffuse swelling of both hands may be seen, commonly associated with an acute onset. Pitting oedema, especially of the dorsal hand is characteristic and is not uncommon in seronegative elderly persons. This remitting seronegative symmetrical synovitis with pitting oedema (RS3PE) syndrome, may have a relatively benign prognosis (McCarthy et al. 1985). If a somewhat similar picture is associated with signs of sympathetic overactivity and shoulder stiffness, reflex dystrophy should be considered as a differential diagnosis.

As the disease progresses, signs of irreversible tissue damage appear: ulnar deviation of the fingers (Fig. 3) beginning with the index and fifth finger,

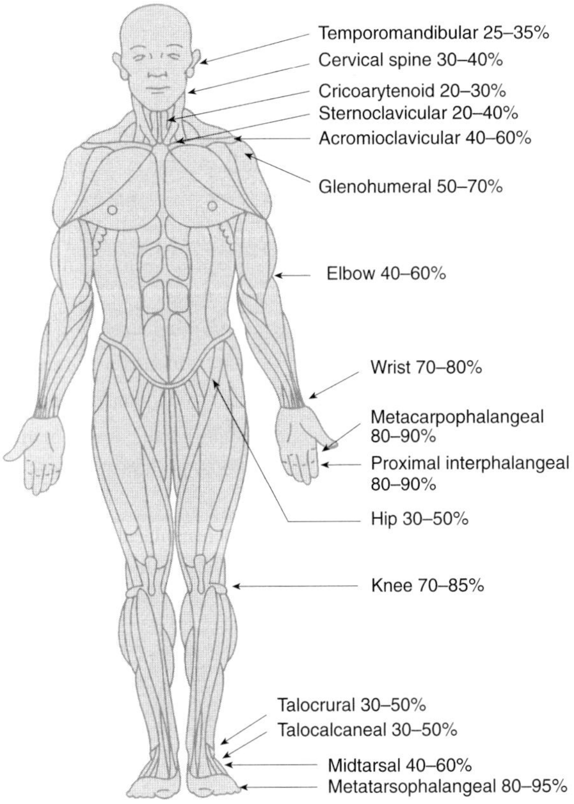

Fig. 1 Joint involvement in long-standing RA (Maddison 1998).

volar subluxation of metocarpophalangeal joints, loosening of the distal radioulnar joint with dorsal protusion of the ulnar head, as well as swan-neck and buttonhole (boutonnière) deformities of the fingers occur in various combinations. Destruction of cartilage and bone as well as weakening and rupture of tendons and joint linings are all contributing factors in the pathogenesis of hand deformities. Inability to make a fist, pinch thin objects, and loss of grip strength are important functional consequences of severe hand involvement in rheumatoid arthritis. Decrease in grip strength in RA patients is caused by a number of factors including active synovitis, reflex inhibition of muscular contraction secondary to pain, altered joint position, flexor tenosynovitis, muscular weakness, and occasionally oedema.

Since the function of the thumb is so important for hand function, damage to the thumb may have a marked influence on daily activities. Three types of deformities may affect the thumb: the flail interphalangeal (IP) joint, the boutonnière (buttonhole) thumb (S-shaped thumb), and the infrequently occurring 'duckbill' thumb.

The hand in RA may reveal other extra-articular features. Raynaud's phenomenon may be seen in a minority of patients, and palmar erythema in more. The presence of digital and nail-fold infarcts indicate rheumatoid vasculitis (RV) and is seen in more severe forms of RA usually associated with the presence of rheumatoid factor.

Elbow

Involvement of the elbow is present in half or more of the patients seen by specialists and may become a major problem in 10–20 per cent. Loss of extension usually develops early, sometimes without the patients noticing anything abnormal. Active synovitis is readily palpated at the site of the groove normally present between the olecranon and the lateral epicondyle. Bulging tenderness and flexion contracture are typical findings. These abnormalities may disappear after intra-articular injection of glucocorticoids. Epicondylitis and olecranon bursitis may also be present. Passive pronation and supination are painful in elbow synovitis. Destructive changes can be diagnosed by feeling crepitation when the radial head moves during this procedure. Severe loss of flexion, usually late in the disease, may have a major impact on self-care activities. The olecranon bursa and proximal extensor surface of the ulnae are sites of predilection for rheumatoid nodules. In patients with large effusions of the elbow joint, peri-articular cysts may rupture into the forearm. Compression of the ulnar

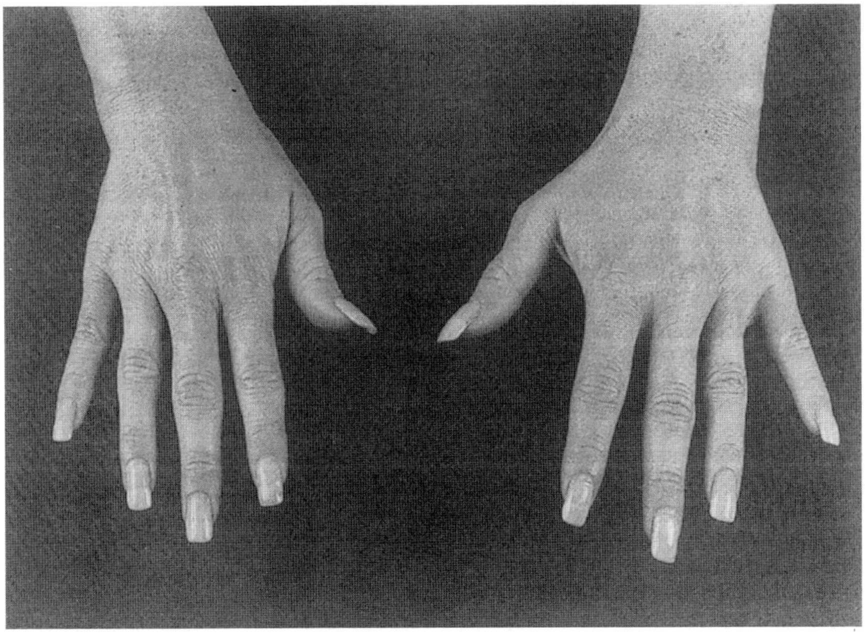

Fig. 2 Arthritis in early RA (Firestein et al. 2000).

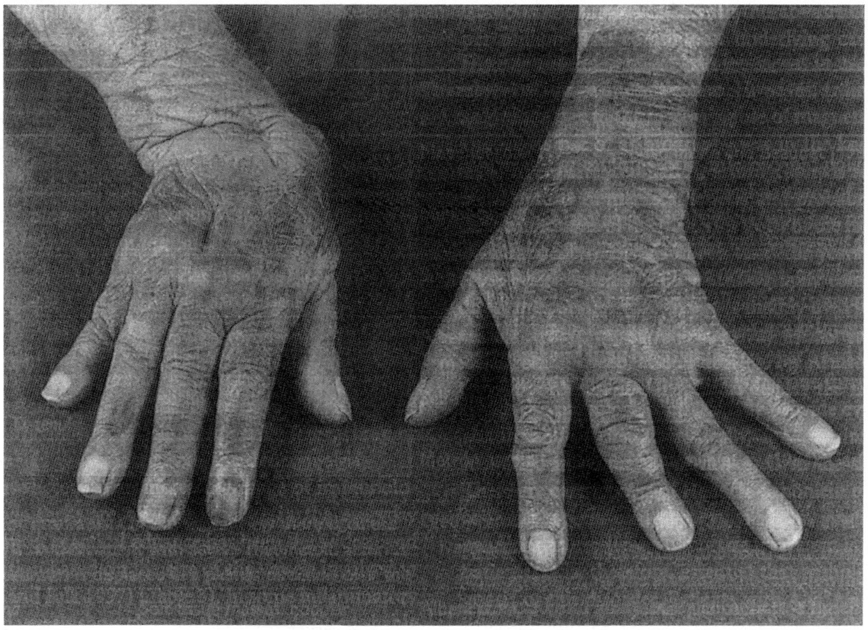

Fig. 3 Hand deformities of RA (Firestein et al. 2000).

nerve posteromedially to the elbow may result in paraesthesias in the fourth and fifth fingers.

Shoulder

The shoulder joints are involved in a majority of patients with established RA, especially with increasing disease duration. Synovitis of the glenohumeral joint causes tenderness on cranial palpation from below the axilla. It also results in pain with active and passive motion.

Acromioclavicular synovitis is not uncommon, giving local tenderness and a painful arch above 100° of abduction. Occasionally, synovitis is present in the sternoclavicular joint. Rotator cuff tendinitis with various degrees of supraspinatus injury is most common and causes considerable shoulder dysfunction, painful arch from 50 to 100° of abduction, and night pain. It may be difficult to distinguish inflammatory from degenerative abnormalities. Subarcromial bursitis is also common, and may present with a palpable swelling. It is suggested that ultrasound is useful for differentiation between chronic synovitis and bursitis/tendinitis in patients with chronic shoulder complaints. Another advantage of ultrasound is that it may also discriminate between tendinitis and tendon rupture which obviously has an impact on therapeutic intervention. For daily activities, it is often possible for patients to compensate mildly decreased shoulder function in the presence of relatively good functional capacity of elbow, wrists, and hands.

Foot and ankle

Initial foot and ankle involvement occurs in 17 per cent of the cases. During the course of the disease, virtually all patients develop forefoot involvement. Most frequently, the earliest erosions are seen in the metatarsophalangeal joints (Eberhardt et al. 1990). Pain in the forefoot elicited by walking is a well-recognized presenting manifestation of RA (Luukkainen et al. 1983), and often causes difficulties in ambulation. In the hindfoot, the talonavicular joint consisting of the talus, calcaneus, talonavicular, and calcaneocuboid joint, is the most commonly involved. Arthritis of the subtalar and calcaneacuboid joint may also be present. Synovitis of the ankle joint, formed by the distal ends of the tibia and fibula and the proximal aspect of the body of the talus, may manifest itself by swelling over the anterior side of the joint, which has to be differentiated from superficial linear swelling of the tendon sheets. Talocalcaneal synovitis is diagnosed by causing pain on passive pronation or supination. Synovitis of the mid-tarsal joint gives rise to pain on rotating the foot while keeping the heel fixed. Foot deformities develop with time, for example, lateral deviation of toes, hammertoes, cock-up toes (Plate 99), and valgus deformity of the ankle. Bursitis, corn-formation, and tendinitis are also common. Nodules on the Achilles tendon are not uncommon and may be troublesome.

Knee

The knee joint is the largest joint in humans. Although not often inflamed at onset of RA, gonarthritis at some stage occurs in approximately 80 per cent or more of all cases. Synovitis is usually easy to identify by tenderness and swelling. Other signs are the presence of synovial fluid effusion, which may be demonstrated by the patella click or the bulge sign. Gonarthritis often leads to quadriceps athrophy and flexion contracture of the joint, both of which should initiate prompt and vigilant therapy. The knee joint communicates with bursae in the fossa poplitea which may become distended and merge into a large Baker's cyst. This may grow and dissect its way down into the calf muscle or rarely into the thigh, and sometimes rupture, causing diffuse swelling and pain and may be mistaken for deep-vein thrombosis. A haemorrhagic 'crescent' sign in the skin about the ankle below the malleoli is characteristic of synovial rupture and is not a feature of thrombophlebitis (Kraag et al. 1976). In exsudate containing knee joints, intra-articular pressure may increase as much as 1100 mmHg (Geborek et al. 1989). This will contribute to decreased muscular function, impede circulation through the synovial membrane, and lead to local lactic acidosis and may be a pathogenic factor in the rupture of Baker's cysts. The natural course of long-standing knee involvement is often valgus instability, flexion contracture, and inability to walk. Increased intra-articular pressure may also contribute to bone erosion (Monsees et al. 1985).

Hip

Hip joint involvement is less common and was formerly considered to be a late manifestation. However, once it starts, the arthritis often leads to severe disability with pain on weight bearing and limitation of motion, in particular abduction and rotation. In a prospective study of recent onset RA, hip involvement was found in about 20 per cent of the patients. Fifteen of 113 patients underwent total hip replacement after a median disease duration of 4 years (Eberhardt et al. 1995). Thus, joint failure is more common in the hip than in the knee in the early phase of RA.

Involvement of the hip must be distinguished from peri-articular bursitis or subtrochanteric bursitis, which is characterized by local tenderness, painful motion, and responsiveness to local infiltration with glucocorticoids (Raman and Haslock 1982).

Cervical spine

Cervical involvement in RA patients is common and may ultimately lead to serious complications, particularly at the C1–C2 level, the most important being cervical cord compression. Some form of damage of the cervical spine may occur in up to 30 per cent of RA patients, predominantly in patients with severe erosive disease (Paimela et al. 1997). The most important cause of cervical involvement in RA is chronic inflammation of synovial joints of the cervical spine leading to damage of peri-articular structures and subluxation (see under 'Complications').

The cricoarytenoid joint

Synovitis of the cricoarytenoid joint is a well-recognized manifestation in RA, occurring in two-thirds of patients in a contemporary hospital-based study (Geterud 1991). Symptoms include sensation of a foreign body, hoarseness and weak voice, as well as stridor, particularly at night. This may become severe and eventually cause suffocation. The condition can be detected by palpating local tenderness and finding the vocal cords tender, red, and swollen as well as immovable on laryngoscopic examination. Laryngeal obstruction can be assessed by computed tomography (CT). The condition is amenable to surgical correction (Geterud 1991).

Patient at risk for involvement of the cricoarytenoid joint, should have a laryngoscopic evaluation before surgery under general anaesthesia.

The temporomandibular joint

This joint is affected in approximately one-fourth of patients, usually symmetrically, and causing no major disability. In fact, patients with unequivocal, palpable synovial swelling, or tenderness often do not report pain on chewing unless specifically asked for. In severe destructive cases of RA, however, attrition of joint cartilage and bone causes malalignment of the teeth with malocclusion (Chalmers and Blair 1973).

Extra-articular features

RA is characterized by chronic synovial inflammation and pannus formation involving small and large joints. However, numerous extra-articular manifestations occur, particularly in male patients who are ANA and RF positive (Cimmino et al. 2000). Some features occur early in the disease, like general fatigue, low grade fever, and weight loss and can predominate the clinical picture, thus causing diagnostic problems. Weight loss has been related to high levels of TNF in both the initial presentation of RA and during flares of the disease (Roubenoff et al. 1992). Extra-articular manifestations can be detected in almost any organ system, causing considerable disease-related morbidity and interference with quality of life. In a study of 587 outpatients of a rheumatology clinic, 40.9 per cent of the patients suffered from extra-articular features, sicca syndrome, and nodules being most common (Cimmino et al. 2000).

In addition, patients tend to develop more than one extra-articular feature; pulmonary involvement, vasculitis and nodules frequently coexist (Scott 1981). A compilation of symptoms and associated extra-articular features is presented in Table 3.

Extra-articular manifestations of RA in a hospital-based population were predicted by the presence of ANA and the presence of nodules before the diagnosis of RA or the development of nodules in the first 2 years of the disease (Turesson et al. 2000).

Table 3 Symptoms and associated extra-articular RA features

Skin	Nodules Ulceration	Nodulosis, methotrexate therapy vasculitis, Felty's syndrome
Cardio-respiratory	Dyspnoea, dry cough	Interstitial lung, BOOP[a] methotrexate constrictive pericarditis, myocarditis
	Hoarse/painful throat	Cricoarytenoid arthritis
Neurological	Paraesthesias	Entrapment, mononeuritis, cervical myelopathy (AAS)[b]
	Muscle weakness	Disuse atrophy, neuropathy, steroid use
Eye	Dry eye Blurred vision Red eye	Sjögren's syndrome Keratitis/corneal melt, drug therapy Scleritis, episcleritis
General	Fever	Infections, including joint flare of arthritis, interstitial lung disease, BOOP
	Lymphadenopathy	Flare of arthritis, joint sepsis, lymphoma, methotrexate
Urinalysis	Haematuria/proteinuria	Amyloidosis, glomerulonephritis, drug

[a] BOOP = bronchiolitis obliterans-organizing pneumonia.

[b] AAS = atlantoaxial subluxation.

Nodules

Rheumatoid nodules occur in about 25 per cent of patients with RA (Ziff 1990), and reflect high levels of disease activity and severity. Typically, they are present at pressure areas throughout the skin, like extensor areas of the forearm (Plate 99), finger joints, ischial and sacral prominences, occipital scalp, and Achilles tendon. Rheumatoid nodules are firm and frequently adherent to the underline periosteum. Rarely, they are the first presenting symptom of the disease and occasionally are present in internal organs, for example, lungs, gallbladder, and heart. A rheumatoid nodule is composed of three histological zones: (i) an inner central necrotic zone, (ii) a surrounding zone of palisading cells (predominantly macrophages), and (iii) an outer zone with perivascular infiltration of chronic inflammatory cells (Ziff 1990). The lesion is thought to be the result of small vessel vasculitis with fibrinoid necrosis. Local collagenase and proteinase production may explain the central necrosis (Palmer et al. 1987). Nodules may regress during effective treatment with DMARDs as disease activity reduces. However, methotrexate has been reported to induce or aggravate nodulosis, especially over finger tendons, despite reduction of disease activity (Jeurissen et al. 1989; Combe et al. 1993).

Haematological features

Several types of anaemia can occur in RA, as well as lymphopaenia, eosinophilia, and thrombopaenia (see 'Laboratory investigations').

Lymphadenopathy is frequently seen in active RA and sometimes is the presenting symptom of the disease. It may mimic Hodgkin's disease and give rise to diagnostic problems. Lymph nodes are generally present in the axillary, inguinal, and epitrochlear areas, usually being mobile and nontender. They will decrease parallel with decrease of disease activity. Biopsy shows follicular reactive hyperplasia.

Felty's syndrome

Felty's syndrome is defined as RA in combination with splenomegaly and leucopaenia. It is seen in less than 1 per cent of hospital RA patients and occurs in the same frequency in males and females (Goldberg and Pinals 1980; Breedveld et al. 1987a). The syndrome characteristically occurs in patients with long-standing, seropositive, nodular, and destructive RA. Leg ulcers, hyperpigmentation, serositis, and peripheral neuropathy is frequently seen in patients with Felty's syndrome. Remarkably often active joint disease is absent. Hepatomegaly and lymphadenopathy are common. The diagnosis is established when white cell counts of less than $2 \times 10^9/mm^3$ are found on three consecutive occasions. Thrombocytopaenia and to a lesser extend anaemia may also be present. Asymptomatic Felty's syndrome may be present and thus undiagnosed for several years. Increased susceptibility to infection has been reported and repeated upper and lower respiratory tract infections account for the slightly increased mortality in this syndrome (Voskuyl et al. 1995). In addition to this, there is an increased risk for lymphoproliferative malignancies in these patients (Gridley et al. 1994).

The management of Felty's syndrome is still under investigation. In a review (Rashba et al. 1996) methotrexate, haematopoietic growth factors, and splenectomy appeared to be the most efficacious in increasing granulocyte count and improving clinical outcome. Treatment with DMARDs might improve cytopaenia and reduce the susceptibility to infection (Dillon et al. 1986). Splenectomy is still controversial: it might improve hematologic abnormalities although granulocytopaenia can re-occur and/or persist. It is indicated in case of serious infections due to neutropaenia.

Vasculitis

A large number of extra-articular features have been reported in RV (Table 4) (Bacon and Carruthers 1995). The most frequently observed features are chronic deep skin ulcers and nailfold lesions (Fig. 4). The latter occur in about 5 per cent of patients and are not associated with a worse prognosis.

RV should be suspected in advanced disease associated with fever, weight loss, and fatigue. RV can be present without active joint disease. Frequently, other extra-articular features are present like episcleritis, pleural, and pericardial effusions (Voskuyl et al. 1996), a raised ESR, a low serum albumin, and sometimes liver enzymes disturbances. The annual incidence of RV was estimated to be 12.5 per million population (Watts et al. 1994). Capillaries, small venules, veins, arterioles, medium-sized arteries are most frequently involved (Bacon and Carruthers 1995), but large vessels can also be affected (Gravallese et al. 1989).

Obliterative endarteritis, small vessel (or leucocytoclastic) vasculitis, and medium-sized vessel (or polyarteritis nodosa type) vasculitis are seen histologically. To establish the diagnosis a full thickness skin and muscle biopsy must be performed. Serological tests are of limited value for the diagnosis of RV. In the past several autoantibodies have been suggested to be present, more frequently in patients with RV compared to patients without (see table on autoantibodies). However, none of them is pathognomonic. Some reports are contradictory. Antinuclear antibodies are present in a large proportion of RV patients (Scott et al.1981; Quismorio et al. 1983; Coremans et al. 1992).

If large vessels are affected, skin ulceration develops, often on lower extremities, or where skin is exposed to pressure, for example, IP joints of the toes, over bunions, ankles, elbows and, in bedridden patients, the buttocks. These ulcerations may be very painful, come in crops, and tend to grow and become chronic. Superinfection frequently occurs being particularly a great risk for patients with joints prostheses (see 'Bacterial arthritis'). In severe cases, ulcerations may form over subcutaneous nodules.

Cutaneous vasculitis or leucocytoclastic vasculitis, seen as palpable purpura (Plate 100), heals as a rule and responds to conventional DMARD therapy (Heurkens et al. 1991). Large vessel vasculitis requires prompt treatment with corticosteroids and cytotoxic drugs. In addition to drug treatment, pressure ulcers should be treated by eliminating pressure, frequent bathing in soda or betadine water, and careful local bandage therapy. It is difficult to determine whether pressure is the only cause of such ulcers, and vasculitis should be regarded in case of any irregularly shaped purpuric lesions and nonhealing ulcers.

RV develops relatively frequent in males and its estimated lifetime risk is 9:1 compared to 38:1 for females (Watts et al. 1994). Mortality in RV patients is slightly increased (Voskuyl et al. 1996). Risk factors associated with increased mortality reported are cutaneous vasculitis (including skin ulcers, rash, and gangrene), neuropathy affecting three or four extremities and depressed level of serum C4 complement (Puechal et al. 1995).

Table 4 Rheumatoid vasculitis

	Clinical features
Nervous system	Seizures Aseptic meningitis Stroke Mononeuritis multiplex Polyneuropathy (sensory/motor)
Eye	Episcleritis Sjögren's syndrome
Skin	Nailfold lesions Digital infarcts Urticaria Gangrene Ulcers Nodules Purpura
Heart	Aortitis Pericarditis Valve lesions Coronary arteritis
Lungs	Pleuritis Fibrosing alveolitis Nodules
Kidney	Glomerulonephritis Haematuria Proteinuria
Gastrointestinal tract	Bowel infarcts Bowel ulcers (Ischaemic) colitis
Systemic	Weight loss Fever Hepatomegaly Splenomegaly

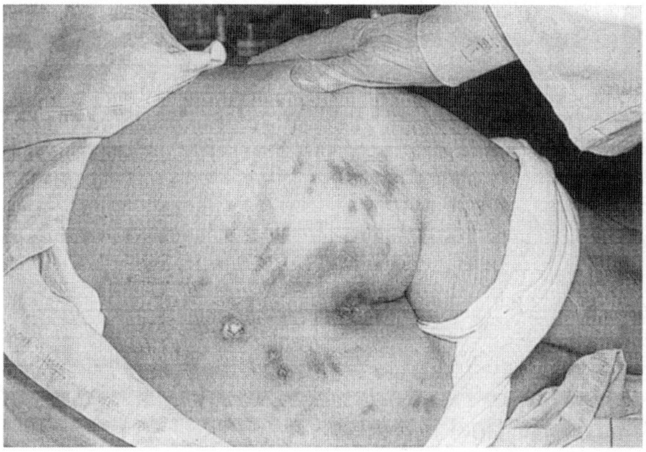

Fig. 4 Deep skin ulcers.

Secondary Sjögren's syndrome

Sjögren's syndrome in RA has been reported with a prevalence varying from 11 to 62 per cent. It occurs predominantly in patients with longstanding RA, especially in seropositive, erosive disease (Moutsopoulos et al. 1979; Andonopoulos et al. 1987). Clinical features of the syndrome may become manifest at any time of the disease; and its treatment is essentially the same as for patients with primary Sjögren's syndrome (see Chapter 6.9). An increased incidence of lymphoreticular malignancies has been reported in patients with Sjögren's syndrome in RA, non-Hodgkin lymphoma being responsible for this increase (Kauppi et al. 1997).

In general, fewer extra-glandular features are seen in secondary Sjögren's syndrome compared to primary Sjögren's syndrome; although pulmonary involvement, especially pulmonary fibrosis, alveolitis, and lymphocytic pneumonitis has been observed more frequently in secondary Sjögren's syndrome in RA patients (Andonopoulos et al. 1987). In a majority of RA patients with secondary Sjögren's syndrome, antinuclear antibodies are present, occasionally SS-A autoantibodies and seldom SS-B autoantibodies (Andonopoulos et al. 1987).

Pulmonary involvement

Pulmonary involvement in RA includes pleurisy, pleural effusion, nodules, interstitial lung disease, and obstructive airway disease. Post-mortem studies in RA patients of longer duration have identified pulmonary involvement, mainly pleural, in as much as 75 per cent of the patients (Shannon and Gale 1992). Pleural effusions are the most common manifestation, mostly occurring in male patients with nodular RA during active disease. Usually, pleural effusions are small and symptomatic, sometimes it is the beginning of clinically significant extra-articular disease. Pulmonary nodules (Kelley 1993) are histologically identical to those found in the skin, occurring more often in men, and mostly in the upper lobes and right middle lobe. Caplan's syndrome, that is, pulmonary nodulosis and pneumoconiosis, is characterized by multiple nodules, greater than 1 cm. It is seen in men extensively exposed to coal dust, silica, and asbestos (Kelley 1993). Diffuse interstitial pulmonary fibrosis tends to occur more often in seropositive male patients with long-standing nodular disease. Its clinical picture and course is identical to idiopathic pulmonary fibrosis. Bronchiolitis obliterans with organizing pneumonia (BOOP) is a specific type of interstitial pneumonia. It has been associated with RA, responds well to therapy with glucocorticoids, and has a generally good prognosis (Anaya et al. 1995). Finally, low-dose weekly methotrexate may rarely lead to life-threatening pneumonitis (Barrera et al. 1994).

Cardiac involvement

Cardiac involvement in RA includes pericarditis, myocardial disease, coronary artery vasculitis, valve lesions, amyloidosis, and conduction abnormalities, as well as accelerated atherosclerosis. Pericardial disease is most common and histologically looks similar to pleural involvement. Usually, it is an asymptomatic feature (Carrao et al. 1995; Guedes et al. 2001). Symptomatic disease can be treated with NSAIDs, and mostly becomes asymptomatic during effective treatment of active joint disease. Evolution into constrictive pericarditis is rare and ultimately may necessitate pericardectomy. Myocardial disease may be associated with nodulosis or amyloidosis and may manifest itself as congestive heart failure. Nodules can also lead to conduction disturbances as well as to valve lesions, mimicking endocarditis (Carrao et al. 1995). Mitral valve regurgitation was found in 80 per cent of RA patients as compared to 37 per cent of matched-controls in a study using transesophageal sonography (Guedes et al. 2001). Coronary arteritis may occur as part of systemic vasculitis in RA.

Gastrointestinal involvement

The gastrointestinal (GI) tract is relatively spared in RA; manifestations seen are usually due to vasculitis, amyloidosis, and as a result of drug toxicity. Drug-related events include peptic ulcer disease and liver function abnormalities. Elevation of liver enzymes (especially serum glutamic oxaloacetic transaminase and alkaline phosphatase) can be seen during active RA (Fernandes et al. 1979). In up to 65 per cent of patients with Felty's syndrome liver involvement may be present. The histology varies from portal fibrosis to nodular regenerative hyperplasia (Thorne et al. 1982).

Other GI complaints can be a result of secondary Sjögren's syndrome, for example, xerostomia, dysphagia, nausea, and chronic epigastric pain.

Renal involvement

Renal involvement of clinical significance is unusual in RA. However, in a study of 110 RA patients with suspicion for renal disease undergoing renal biopsy, 40 per cent of the patients showed histologically mesangial glomerulonephritis, especially those patients with haematuria. Amyloidosis was found in 33 patients, most of them having nephrotic syndrome (Helin et al. 1995). In about 25 per cent of RA patients, microalbuminuria is present and reflects disease activity (Pedersen et al. 1995). Other renal manifestations may be related to RV. In addition, various forms of renal disease can be induced by antirheumatic drugs, especially gold, cyclosporine, D-penicillamine, and NSAIDs.

Ocular involvement

Ocular involvement is frequently present in RA patients and includes keratoconjunctivitis sicca (KCS), episcleritis, scleritis, uveitis, episcleral nodulosis, corneal melt, and peripheral ulcerative keratitis (PUK). The most common eye disease is KCS, which has been reported in about 35 per cent of patients (Andonopoulos et al. 1989; Matsuo et al. 1997). Symptoms and treatment are described in 'Secondary Sjögren's syndrome'. Severity of symptoms does not necessarily correlate with the disease activity of RA (Matsuo et al. 1997).

Scleritis and episcleritis both present as a red eye and prompt evaluation is necessary in order to prevent vision loss due to scleritis. Both are strongly associated with systemic manifestations and nodular disease (Jayson and Jones 1971). Scleritis is a form of RV and is very painful, gives blurred vision, and may last for months to years (Tessler 1985). Untreated, scleritis may progress into scleromalacia. Episcleritis (Fig. 5) is typically a mild and usually self-limiting disease, not affecting vision. Other conditions affecting the eye in RA are uveitis, episcleral nodulosis, corneal melt, and PUK. Although rare, they may require local or systemic corticosteroids and immune suppression. Diplopia is a rare symptom in RA, which can be

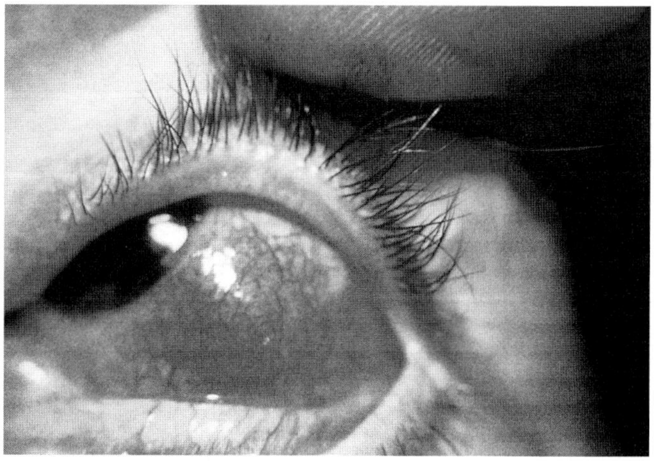

Fig. 5 Episcleritis in RA.

attributed to inflammation and thickening of the superior oblique tendons (Cooper 1990). In addition, drugs used in the treatment of RA can affect the eye as well: glucocorticosteroids may cause cataract, and glaucoma, gold may deposit in conjunctiva and cornea; and chloroquine derivatives can induce kerato- and retinopathy.

Muscular involvement

Muscular weakness in RA patients can be caused by muscular atrophy secondary to joint inflammation, by an inflammatory myopathy, by motor neuropathies (see 'Complications') and can be iatrogenic. Isometric, isokinetic, and aerobic capacity are markedly reduced in RA patients (Ekdahl and Broman 1992).

Inflammatory myopathies occur rarely, mostly affecting type II or fast-twitch muscle fibres (Halla et al. 1984), the histology usually showing non-specific changes and sometimes coexistent vasculitis. Slight to moderate elevation of muscle enzymes or even normal enzyme levels have been observed. Intramuscular rheumatoid nodules can be seen.

The iatrogenic causes of muscular atrophy and/or weakness are corticosteroids, D-penicillamine, and hydroxychloroquine.

Bone

Generalized and peri-articular osteoporosis secondary to RA occur frequently and are associated with an increased fracture risk (Cooper et al. 1995). Bone loss has recently been attributed to osteoclast activation as a result of the inflammatory process, especially in early RA (Cough et al. 1994, 1998). In addition to this, immobility and corticosteroid use are also important contributing factors (Cooper et al. 1995). Methotrexate osteopathy is an uncommon finding causing bone pain, osteoporosis, and fractures, typically located in the distal tibia (Preston et al. 1993; Zonneveld et al. 1996).

Generalized secondary osteoporosis and fractures will be dealt in 'Complications' below.

Complications

RA can be associated with serious complications contributing to severe illness and increased mortality. These complications may relate to the disease itself (including extra-articular manifestations) or its treatment.

Infections

Infections occur more frequently in RA patients (Nived et al. 1985), being related either to the disease itself, the presence of Felty's syndrome (Voskuyl et al. 1996) or iatrogenic, that is, drugs, surgery, the presence of joint prosthesis, etc. Septic arthritis occurs more frequently in RA patients (28–38 per 100 000 per year) than in the general population (five per 100 000 per year), and especially in RA patients with joint prostheses (40–68 per 100 000 per year) (Kaandorp 1997; Goldenberg 1998). *Staphylococcus aureus* is the most frequent infecting organism varying from 44 to 80 per cent of cases of RA patients (Kaandorp 1997; Goldenberg 1998). Streptococci groups B, C, and G occur frequently in immune-compromised hosts (Goldenberg 1998). The presence of RA itself is a risk factor for the development of septic arthritis; additional risk factors are age over 80 years, diabetes mellitus, hip and/or knee prosthesis, joint surgery and skin infection (Kaandorp et al. 1995) (see Chapter 6.2.1).

Infections in general occur more frequently in RA patients (Nived et al. 1985). Treatment with systemic glucocorticoids increases the risk of infection, dependent on the dose and duration of treatment (Dale and Petersdorf 1973). Concomitant treatment with immunosuppressive drugs may contribute to this increased frequency. Methotrexate is associated with an increased occurrence of infections in RA patients compared to treatment with other DMARDs (Singh et al. 1994; van der Veen et al. 1994), especially in patients with severe RA (Boerbooms et al. 1995). Regular intra-articular injections increase the risk of infection in patients with RA (Gray et al. 1981), although the absolute risk is low (Kaandorp et al. 1995).

Neurological complications

RV (see Table 4), entrapment neuropathy, and atlantoaxial joint subluxation are the three main groups of neurological complications in RA. Mononeuritis multiplex is usually bilateral and most common in the legs. The sudden onset of motor neuropathy signals the presence of aggressive RV and poor prognosis (Geirson et al. 1987). Other manifestations of RV involve the central nervous system and may become manifest as a stroke, seizure, haemorrhage, encephalopathy, and aseptic meningitis. Amyloidosis and nodules are found in the dura mater and the choroids plexus of the brain (Markenson et al. 1979; Matsuki et al. 1994). Extradural nodules may result in nerve root compression and myelopathy.

Entrapment neuropathy is the most frequent neurological complication in RA, carpal tunnel syndrome being the most common. Phalen's sign and Tinel's sign are not very specific and sensitive and EMG nerve conduction tests are more specific in order to verify the diagnosis, especially in atypical presentations. Carpal tunnel syndrome may be caused by (teno) synovitis, nodules, secondary osteoarthritis, and amyloidosis. Signs of sensory median nerve compression are nocturnal paraesthesia of the first to third fingers and medial side of the fourth finger, although pain radiating to the lower arm can also be the presenting symptom. There are two sites where nerve entrapment may occur, that is, in the carpal tunnel and under the pronator teres muscle. Other entrapment neuropathies are of the ulnar nerve, radial nerve, the anterior and posterior tibial nerves at the fibular head, and in the tarsal tunnel. The latter causing burning feet and intrinsic foot weakness (Goodgold et al. 1965).

Cervical spine subluxation

Chronic non-specific inflammation in RA leads to destructive lesions in the cervical spine (Marks and Sharp 1981). Synovitis is present in the odontoid-atlas joint, uncovertebral joint, and the interlaminar joints (facet joints), ultimately leading to cervical spine instability and eventually serious, sometimes life-threatening complications. Radiographically, subluxation of the atlantoaxial joint (AAS) or C1–C2 subluxation is present in about 30 per cent of RA patients with severe RA (Paimela et al. 1997). The degree of erosive changes in the peripheral joints and the acute phase response in time correlates closely with the degree of AAS (Fujiwara et al. 1998). AAS may produce progressive cervical myelopathy. Symptoms include paraesthesia, numbness, and muscular weakness. In severe cases this can result in spastic paralysis, paraplegia, tetraplegia, sensory loss and also loss of bladder control, faecal incontinence, and syncope. Physical examination may reveal upper motor-neuron weakness, hyperreflexia, and a positive Babinski sign; the last often in connection with cough or vomiting. Occipital headache may occur in the absence of any visible spinal abnormality, but the reverse can also be seen: severe lesions without any complaints. Alarm symptoms include sensory disturbances, muscle weakness, loss of sphincter control, and spontaneous muscle cramps and Lhermitte's sign.

There are several types of subluxation. The *anterior subluxation* of the atlas is the most common in RA. This results from synovitis of the synovial articulation between the transverse ligament of the atlas and the posterior aspect of the odontoid. The transverse ligament prevents a forward slip of C1 on C2, and damage by chronic synovitis may induce laxity of the ligament, and/or erosions of the dens. Normally, the space between the odontoid process and the arch of the atlas measures 3 mm or less; in RA patients it may exceed 10 mm (Fig. 6). *Vertical subluxation* may result from synovitis of the apophyseal joint in the occipitoatlantal area. Destruction of the lateral atlantoaxial joints or of bone around the foramen magnum may cause vertical subluxation. In this form of subluxation, the odontoid may move up through the foramen magnum leading to damage of the upper

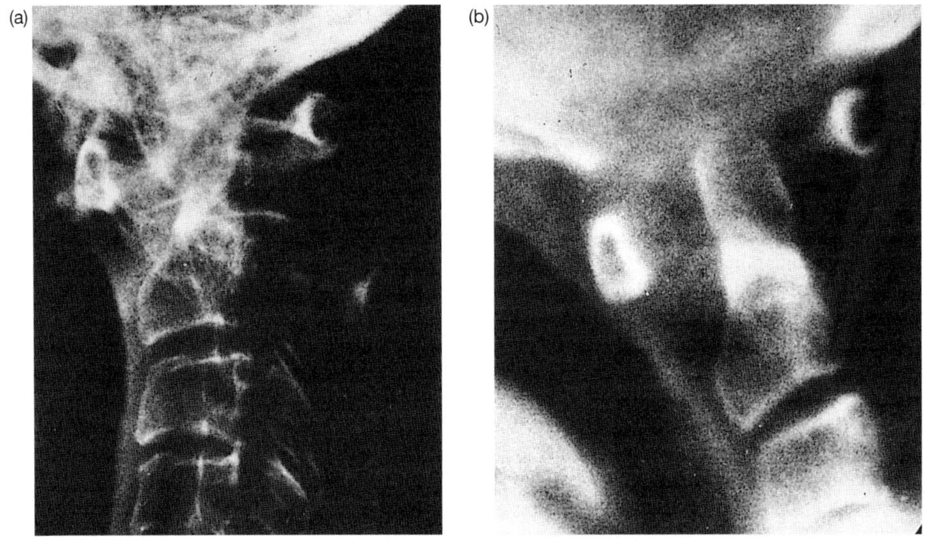

Fig. 6 C1–C2 subluxation. (a) A lateral film of the cervical spine in flexion in a 68-year-old woman with a long history of rheumatoid arthritis shows a marked increase in the distance between the anterior arch of the atlas and odontoid process, measuring 10.2 mm; normally, it should not exceed 3 mm. (b) Trispiral tomogram demonstrates atlantoaxial subluxation in detail.

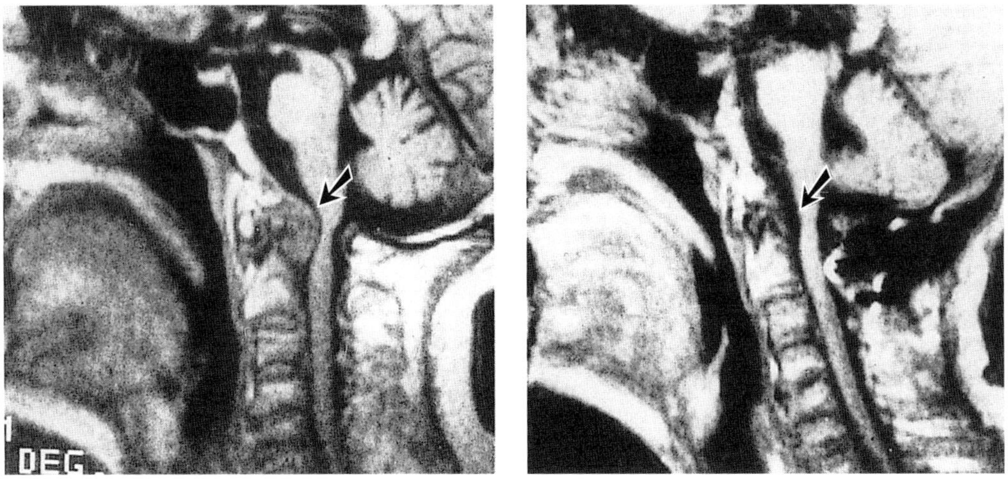

Fig. 7 Preoperative MRI (left) and 4 months postoperative MRI (right) after successful surgical fusion. Arrows indicate periodontoid pannus.

cervical cord and medulla. Basilar invagination, which may be fatal, can occur by penetration of the odontoid process in the foramen magnum, putting pressure on the brainstem.

Screening for cervical pathology usually includes radiographs in flexion/extension, and also an open mouth anteroposterior to detect on occasional fracture or the odontoid process or significant atlantoaxial. MRI is valuable for the assessment of spinal cord damage (Breedveld et al. 1987b) (Fig. 7), especially with the neck in flexion and extension (Jacobsen and Riise 2000). Damage of the cervical spine needs not to be confined to the C1–C2 level. It may occur also at lower levels, namely C2–C5.

Treatment consists of stabilizing the cervical spine by either neck collar or surgical fixation, the latter being absolutely necessary in case of pyramidal signs and/or severe neck pain (Crockard 1995).

In patients with RA, who require surgery under general anaesthesia, the presence of cervical subluxation presents a risk. Therefore, flexion/extension cervical radiographs should be taken pre-operatively in suspected patients.

Tendon and ligament damage

'Spontaneous' rupture may be caused by the destructive process in RA involving ligaments and tendons, or by attrition over roughened bone created by erosion or osteophytes. The most common sites of clinically significant involvement are hands, wrists, shoulders, neck, knees, and feet. Rheumatoid nodules can be present causing pain and stenosing tenosynovitis. Joint deformity is often complicating the clinical examination and the patient may not notice tendon rupture in a hand deformed by RA if great loss of function already exists. However, sudden loss of active flexion or extension in the finger is usually the result of an attrition rupture (Ertel et al. 1988). In the hand tendon rupture may affect flexor and extensor tendons, more frequently in the extensor tendons. Extensor tendon rupture can also occur at the wrist. The goal of treatment should be prevention of further ruptures, restoration of hand function, and reconstructive surgery at an early stage.

Weakening of ligaments causes joint instability and in the hand subluxation of metacarpophalangeal joints, allowing ulnar drift and volar subluxation. Loosening or destruction of the distal radioulnar ligament gives instability volar luxation of the radius and carpus, and prominence of the ulnar head (piano-key sign). Relaxation of the central slip in PIP joints can result in two different types of finger deformities: boutonnière deformity and swan-neck deformity. The rotator cuff of the shoulder can rupture as well as the supraspinate tendon. Rupture of the supraspinate muscle results in shrugging of the shoulder when attempting abduction movement. At the knee, damage to the lateral end cruciate ligaments combined with loss of cartilage causes instability and pain, detectable by means of the 'anterior drawer sign'.

Amyloidosis

Secondary amyloidosis, also called systemic AA amyloidosis, is caused by systemic deposition of the acute phase reactant serum amyloid A (SAA) protein in a fibrillar structure. It is associated with chronic inflammation and the most common cause is RA (Hazenberg and van Rijswijk 2000a). In longstanding RA, depending on the severity of the disease 5–20 per cent of RA patients develop AA amyloidosis (Husby 1985; Kobayashi et al. 1996). In the past, it was believed that deposition of serum amyloid A was irreversible; however, in some patients clinical improvement has been reported after effective treatment of the chronic inflammatory process. In scintigraphic studies with radiolabelled serum amyloid P component regression was demonstrated in some patients (Hawkins 1994). Almost any organ can be affected by amyloid deposits and the clinical picture depends on the severity of involvement of these organs.

In patients with symptomatic AA amyloidosis, restrictive heart failure and renal involvement causing proteinuria are the complications having the main clinical consequences. In such cases prognosis is poor. Recently, it has been reported that AA amyloidosis shows a decreasing incidence in RA (Hazenberg and van Rijswijk 2000a), also reflected in a decreasing number of RA patients in dialysis treatment of end-stage renal disease due to AA amyloidosis (Kaipiainen-Seppanen et al. 2000) (see Chapter 6.12.1 on Amyloidosis). This may be explained either by a true decline in AA amyloidosis due to a more effective treatment of chronic inflammation, that is, more aggressive treatment in an earlier phase of the disease, earlier joint replacement therapy leading to removal of substantial amounts of inflamed tissue, and a decrease in the burden of comorbidity such as tuberculosis, recurrent urinary, and pulmonary infections (Hazenberg and van Rijswijk 2000b). In the pre-clinical phase, deposition of AA amyloidosis can be demonstrated using abdominal subcutaneous fat aspiration (Hazenberg et al. 1999). Treatment of AA amyloidosis is mainly focused on reducing chronic inflammation and supportive therapy in order to delay target organ failure, that is, restrictive heart failure and renal failure (Gillmore et al. 1997). In the past, colchicine has been used in inflammatory bowel disease and chlorambucil in juvenile idiopathic arthritis to treat amyloidosis.

Osteoporosis

Generalized and peri-articular osteoporosis are common in chronic RA. Contributing factors include immobility, corticosteroid therapy, postmenopausal status, low body weight, sun deprivation, poor diet, and persistent osteoclast activation in correlation with disease activity (Lane et al. 1992; Gough et al. 1994, 1998; Cooper et al. 1995). Patients with early RA who have high levels of acute phase reactants and high disease activity were more at risk for generalized bone loss (Gough et al. 1998). Peri-articular bone loss occurs in inflamed joints in RA. Rheumatoid synovial tissue produces inflammatory cytokines, amongst others IL-6, TNF, IL-1, and enzymes like metalloproteinase. These cytokines may induce maturation and activation of osteoclasts leading to bone resorption (Thomson et al. 1987). Metalloproteinase causes direct resorption of bone (Grillet et al. 1997). These inflammatory mediators also account for the development of systemic osteoporosis. Stress fractures can occur and may be misdiagnosed as pain related to RA itself. Abnormal biomechanics and muscle weakness are additional risk factors.

The relative risk for vertebral deformities is increased in RA: in a cross-sectional study 12.1 per cent of RA patients had vertebral fractures compared with 6.2 per cent of the age- and gender-matched controls (odds ratio 2 : 1, 95 per cent confidence interval 1.2–3.7) (Spector et al. 1993).

Glucocorticoids can induce bone loss in RA. Glucocorticoids, administered to improve joint discomfort (and prevent erosions), accelerate bone loss. However, in patients with RA glucocorticoids may also control inflammation for short periods (<6 months) and induce reversible bone loss (Laan et al. 1993a,b).

In addition, the lower end of the fibula may be fractured causing pain around the ankle joint, and femoral neck fractures can be seen, only after minor trauma and misdiagnosed as hip arthritis. Several guidelines for prevention and treatment of secondary osteoporosis in RA as well as for corticosteroid induced osteoporosis have been published (Eastell 1995; ACR 1996; Bijlsma 1997). In general, they recommend prophylactic therapy with bisphosphonates, or calcium and vitamin D (see Chapter 6.16.1 on Osteoporosis). An uncommon disorder is methotrexate induced osteopathy, causing bone pain, osteoporosis, and fracture typically in the distal tibia (Preston et al. 1993; Zonneveld et al. 1996). This already occurs in adults using low-dose methotrexate.

Comorbidity and mortality

Comorbidity

A high frequency of coexisting disease has been reported in RA in three studies (Berkanovic and Hurwicz 1990; Gabriel et al. 1999b; Kroot et al. 2001). The advanced mean age of the patients at disease onset as well as the chronic nature of RA are contributing factors. Coexisting disease is being defined as comorbidity if it is not apparently related to RA. Cardiovascular disease in the form of (chronic) congestive heart failure, myocardial infarction and hypertension is that most frequently found. This form of comorbidity might also be related to an increased mortality (Wållberg-Jonsson et al. 1999) and may be associated with considerable disability. Important comorbidities in RA are summarized in Table 5. It should be noted that patients with arthritis tend to have more comorbidity than non-arthritic

Table 5 Distributions of comorbidities and demographics of patients

	Berkanovic (1990)	Gabriel et al. (1999a–c)	Kroot (2001)[a]
No. of patients	288	450	106
Mean age (SD)	NA	64.7	53.7
% Male	NA	23	40
% Patients with comorbidity	54	49	27
	(%)	(%)	(%)
Cardiovascular disease including hypertension	33	31	27
Lung disease	7	12	18
Renal disease	1	6	6
Cancer	2	11	6
Gastrointestinal disease	12	11	6
Diabetes	6	7	6
Neurological disease	2	13	1
Peripheral vascular disease	2	12	4

[a] Only study in early RA disease.

Note: Cardiovascular disease occurs most often next to lung disease. There is a slight difference between the first two studies and the third one, probably due to the fact that the latter study included only early RA patients. NA = not available.

patients; male sex, age, and comorbidity present at diagnosis of RA being significant predictors of increased comorbidity (Gabriel et al. 1999b).

Mortality

The death rate usually is expressed as the standard mortality ratio (number of deaths attributed to a disease in a given time period divided by deaths of the total population). In mortality records, the rheumatic disorder is often not recorded in the death certificate. Therefore, usually studies of cohorts of RA patients provide the most valuable information (Vandenbroucke et al. 1984; Pincus et al. 1994). Up to now, four inception cohorts of recent onset RA have been published, which report data upon mortality rates (Corbett et al. 1993; Lindquist and Eberhardt 1999; Kroot et al. 2000). The first two studies provide data of patients included before 1975 and show an increased mortality rate. The other two studies report data from patients included since 1985 and did not find an increased mortality rate for a follow-up period of up to 13 and 10 years, respectively (Lindquist and Eberhardt 1999; Kroot et al. 2000). The difference might be explained by the dramatic change in treatment forms and strategies since the late 1980s. A large number of other studies have reported increased mortality in RA, which could mainly be attributed to infections, especially respiratory infections, renal disease, GI disease, lymphoproliferative disorders, and RA as a disease itself (Suzuki et al. 1994; Anderson 1996). In another study of 1666 RA patients who had died, 47 deaths were attributed to antirheumatic medication: 30 of them due to side-effects of NSAIDs, 11 due to glucocorticoid use. Six other cases could be attributed to DMARDs: fatal bone marrow suppression (two patients on MTX and two on sulfasalazine), one lymphoma (azathioprine), and one hydroxychloroquine intoxication (Myllykangas-Luosojärvi et al. 1995). Predictors of increased mortality were low educational level and poor functional status (Suzuki et al. 1994). Severe long-standing RA was associated with an increased number of deaths due to cardiovascular disease (Wållberg-Jonsson et al. 1999). Male sex and age as reviewed in 25 studies, did not show a clear association with mortality in RA (Anderson 1996). No increased mortality figures due to cancer have been found so far, except for the risk of lymphoma, which is related to the duration and severity of the disease (Bäcklund et al. 1998).

Laboratory abnormalities

RA is a chronic systemic immuno-inflammatory disease, which results in abnormalities of connective tissue metabolism. Characteristic immuno-inflammatory abnormalities distinguish the disease from other arthritides. Laboratory tests in a disease like RA should be essentially clinically useful, that is, specific and sensitive and be helpful for making a diagnosis and prognosis, monitoring the course of the disease, and be helpful in therapeutic monitoring (Table 6).

Rheumatoid factor

In the 1940s, high levels of antibodies, later called rheumatoid factor (RF), were detected in patients with chronic polyarthritis that is nowadays classified as RA. RF remains up till now the most important laboratory aid in the establishment of the diagnosis of RA and is the only serologic indicator included in the ARA/ACR criteria. RF is found in 75–80 per cent of RA patients. RF is an autoantibody specific for antigenic epitopes of the Fc-portion of IgG antibody. RFs are usually of the IgM isotype; however, in RA IgG, IgA, and IgE RFs can be detected. The classical Waaler-Rose test uses sheep erythrocytes coated with rabbit IgG. A more sensitive test is the latex-fixation test in which particles, coated with aggregated human IgG, visibly agglutinate by IgM-RF. The highest serum dilution causing agglutination is the titre. A titre greater than1 : 80 is considered positive. RF can also be measured by radioimmunoassay, indirect immunofluorescence, enzyme-linked immunoabsorbent assay (ELISA) (Smiley et al. 1968), and laser nephelometry.

Table 6 Laboratory assessments and their value for diagnosis, disease activity, prognosis, and radiological progression

	Diagnosis	Disease activity	Prognosis	Radiological progression
Hb (↓)	—	×	—	—
ESR (↑)	—	×	—	×
CRP (↑)	—	×	×(AUC)	×(AUC)
Serum amyloid A (↑)	—	×	—	—
Plasmaviscosity, ferritine (↑)	—	×	—	—
RF	×	—	×	×
APF	×	—	—	—
Anti-CCP Ab	×	—	—	—
AKA	×	—	—	—

Note: See text for abbreviations. ENA and antihistone are present in RA with RV especially predicting severity of extra-articular disease.

In a study of 8287 outpatients, RF tested by latex fixation yielded a sensitivity of 78 per cent and a specificity of 97.9 per cent (Wolfe et al. 1991).

High titre of RF is usually associated with severe disease as well as with extra-articular features and nodulosis. Presence of RF has been found to predict radiographic progression (Aman et al. 2000; Uhlig et al. 2000).

Other autoantibodies in RA

Antikeratinized epithelium antibody (AKA), antiperinuclear factor (APF), and anticyclic citrulline containing peptide antibodies (anti-CCP) may be useful diagnostic markers in RA and be also positive in RF negative RA patients. They are present early in the disease and may indicate a more severe disease. AKA binds to a 40-kDa neutral/acidic isoform of basic filaggrin in human epidermis (Simon et al. 1993), with a high specificity for RA (95–100 per cent) but a low sensitivity (60 per cent). APF labels specifically the perinuclear factor, a component of the so called keratohyaline granules, surrounding the nuclei of differentiating human buccal mucosal cells (Vincent et al. 1999). It is suggested that AKA and APF are overlapping specifities. APF is highly specific and sensitive in RA, 86 and 96 per cent, respectively (Janssens et al. 1988; Sebbag et al. 1995).

In addition, recent studies have revealed that APF antibodies (and AKA) specifically bind to substrates containing the modified amino acid citrulline (Schellekens et al. 1998) (see Chapters 5.4 and 6.3.1). This anti-CCP-antibody can be measured using a peptide-based ELISA and appears to be highly specific for RA (96–98 per cent) (Schellekens et al. 2000). The combination of the anti-CCP and the IgM-RF ELISAs resulted in a significantly higher positive predictive value of 91 per cent and showed a positive predictive value of 91 per cent for erosive disease in early RA (Schellekens et al. 2000). It is suggested that RF negative patients, positive for APF, have a poor prognosis (Westgeest et al. 1987; Schellekens et al. 2000). Numerous other autoantibodies can be found in RA. The reader is referred to Chapter 6.3.1.

Acute phase reactants

The acute phase response can be assessed by measuring the erythrocyte sedimentation rate (ESR), C-reactive protein (CRP), serum amyloid A (SAA), and plasma viscosity (van Leeuwen and van Rijswijk 1994). ESR and CRP are most frequently used for disease activity measurement. Both measures correlate with the disease activity, especially joint swelling, but not with pain. ESR is the cheapest test, but can easily be influenced by anaemia and hyperglobulinaemia frequently present. CRP is more sensitive. Persistent elevated acute phase response is associated with an increased rate of radiographic progression and also predicts radiographic progression (van Leeuwen et al. 1993; Plant et al. 2000). In fact, the time-integrated CRP correlates significantly with the rate of radiographic progression in both early and longstanding RA (van Leeuwen and van Rijswijk 1994).

Haematological abnormalities

Anaemia is a frequently occurring extra-articular manifestation of RA, being mostly of the normochromic and normocytic type. Anaemia is multifactorial, reflected in dimorphic appearance and wide red cell distribution or width (RDW). Anaemia of chronic disease (ACD) and iron deficiency anaemia (IDA) are the most important types of anaemia in RA patients. The latter can occur as a consequence of G1 occult blood loss due to NSAIDs. In addition, inefficient erythropoiesis, reduced reponse of bone marrow to erythropoietin (EPO), shortened red cell lifespan, and peripheral destruction of erythrocytes by inflamed synovium have been described (Vreugdenhil et al. 1990). Evaluation of body iron stores can distinguish between ACD and IDA. Ferritin levels are higher in ACD. Frequently, anaemia is of a mixed type, and differentation between the two types may not always be easy. ACD is not usually responsive to iron therapy whilst IDA is. Mean corpuscular volume is low in IDA and normal in ACD. The 'gold standard' to differentiate between both is bone marrow examination. ACD can be regarded as the result of current and past (chronic) inflammation and is associated with a higher disease activity. In a cohort of 225 early RA patients, 64 per cent of them had an anaemia of which 23 per cent was due to IDA and 77 per cent due to ACD (Peeters et al. 1996). Anaemia can also be drug-induced. Anti-folate drugs, such as methotrexate and sulfasalazine may induce a megaloblastic anaemia. Gold therapy can result in aplastic anaemia. Rarely autoimmune haemolytic anaemia is seen in RA.

Extra-articular disease and high titres of RF are sometimes associated with eosinophilia. This also can be induced by drug use, especially gold. Lymphopaenia was seen in 15 per cent of cases of one study; it was related to severity of the disease, but was not influenced by therapy (Symmons 1989).

Platelets are frequently increased as a result of the acute phase response; however, no increased incidence of thromboembolic manifestations does occur. Less commonly, platelets may be depleted, related either to adverse events of drugs or Felty's syndrome.

Tissue specific markers for disease activity

During the last decade an increasing number of tissue-specific markers for organ involvement/damage have been identified and assays for clinical use have become available. Many of these markers are still under investigation and currently have no established role in diagnosis, monitoring, or prognostication of the disease (Wollheim and Saxne 1992; Poole 1994; Young-Min et al. 2001).

Synovial fluid and tissue

Synovial fluid (SF) contains a specific amount of extravasated plasma supplemented with high molecular weight molecules, especially hyaluronan (Simkin 1995). SF analysis can play an important role in the differential diagnosis of inflammatory versus non-inflammatory arthropathies, infections, and crystal-induced arthropathies. Many different cells, almost every type of cytokine and joint matrix molecules are present in inflammatory SF. Synovial tissue (ST) in early arthritis has been studied for reasons of diagnosis, prognosis, and treatment monitoring. It is suggested that immunohistochemical analysis of ST specimens from early arthritis patients can be used to differentiate RA from non-RA patients. The number of plasma cells, B cells, and macrophages are characteristically increased in RA patients (Kraan 1999). Its practical value however, has to be established yet.

Imaging

In RA osteoarticular involvement concerns mostly the appendicular skeleton and the cervical spine. Imaging is important for diagnosis, as well as for establishment of disease progression and outcome and evaluation of extra-articular involvement. In fact, radiological scores of hands and feet are the most frequently used outcome measures to establish the disease modifying efficacy of treatment (see 'Assessment'). Imaging modalities used in RA are conventional radiography, sonography, magnetic resonance imaging (MRI), CT, bone scintigraphy, and arthrography.

X-rays

Conventional radiography is sufficient for accurate evaluation of diagnosis, severity, and outcome in RA. High-resolution images are needed to detect erosions (Chapter 5.6.1). Under- and overexposed films result in loss of detection of erosive disease. Features, seen on X-ray are periarticular swelling, erosions, osteoporosis, cysts, subluxations, periosteal reactions, and joint space narrowing (loss of cartilage), ankylosis, reactive sclerosis, and osteophytes. Distribution of damage in RA is in order of frequency: hands, feet, knees, hip, cervical spine, shoulders, and elbows (Resnick 1976, Brower 1998). Each joint can be viewed in different ways and dependent on the view erosions can be seen easy or missed. Of increasing importance is the early detection of erosions, which appear mostly first in the feet and later in the hands (van der Heijde et al. 1992; Plant et al. 1994). Early erosions indicate aggressive disease and predict outcome (Plant et al. 1994). In the hands and feet juxta-articular osteoporosis due to hyperaemia is first seen, followed by erosions, joint space narrowing, and subluxation. First metatarsophalangeal (MTP) joints (Fig. 8) and then metacarpophalangeal joints (MCP) show erosive disease. The proximal interphalangeal joints (PIP) follow (Fig. 9) (van der Heijde et al. 1992; Plant et al. 1994). Remarkably, healing of erosive changes has been described, seen as recortication and subsequent filling in with bone, and osteoarthritis with sclerosis and osteophyte formation (Rau and Herborn 1996).

In the wrists erosions progress to large subchondral erosions (Monsees et al. 1985) and in late stage loss of joint space of all carpal bones is seen, and eventually bony ankylosis. Larger joints in RA can also be affected,

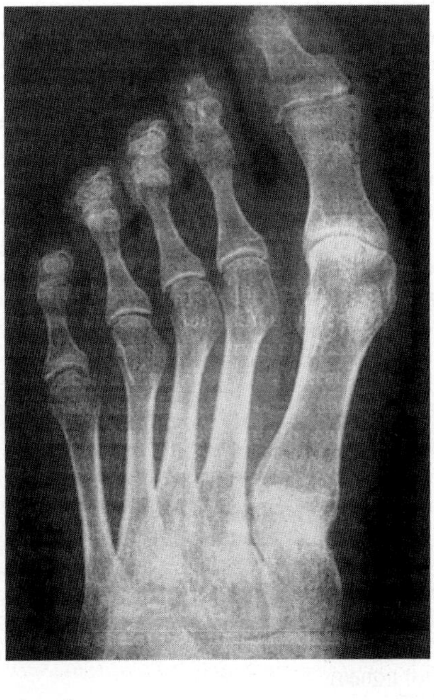

Fig. 8 Metatarsal erosion.

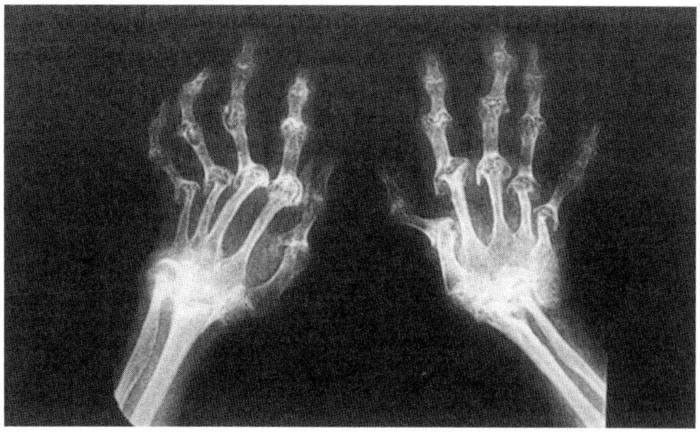

Fig. 9 Hands, advanced radiographic damage.

usually bilaterally and symmetrically. All three compartments of the knee—medial, lateral, and patellofemoral—show uniform loss of cartilage and marginal erosion. The hips migrate in a superomedial direction in the acetabulum due to uniform concentric loss of cartilage, leading to acetabular protrusion (Resnick 1975). In the shoulder, erosive lesions can occur at the superior lateral aspect of the humoral head adjacent to the greater tuberosity, as well as cysts. In addition, cartilage loss leads to medial migration of the humeral head and upward migration due to rotator cuff tears.

Other joints including elbow, ankle, sternoclavicular, and temporomandibular joints can be involved (Resnick 1976; Brower 1988), initially seen as periarticular osteoporosis, followed by erosions and cartilage loss. The sacroiliac joints can be involved as well, usually in a late stage of the disease. Involvement can be seen radiographically as ankylosis and erosions.

Radiographs of the cervical spine are important to evaluate vertical or horizontal C1–C2 subluxation, especially the flexed lateral view (see C1–C2 instability under 'Complications'). Discovertebral destruction and apophysial involvement have been observed (Martel 1977).

Ultrasound

In the last decade ultrasound examination of joints and periarticular tissues has become increasingly important (Schmidt 2001). Its role in evaluation of severity and progression of the disease still has to be established. In early disease, erosions are detected in 6.5-fold more patients (Wakefield et al. 2000). With this technique erosions are seen as a cortical defects with an irregular floor in longitudinal and transversal planes (Wakefield et al. 2000). Especially in those joints affected early, MCP2 and MTP5, ultrasound examination appeared to be superior to radiography (Grassi et al. 2001). The technique is very useful in establishing an accurate diagnosis of tendonitis, tendon ruptures, popliteal cysts, joint effusions, and rotator cuff tears (Ghozlan and Vacher 2000).

Magnetic resonance imaging

MRI allows visualization of bone and soft tissues. Erosive changes are frequently detected in early disease even before they appear in conventional radiographs, like with sonography (Klarlund et al. 2000). Bone marrow oedema, may precede the development of erosions (McQueen 2000). However, MRI is not always easily available all over the world, is costly and, in addition, time consuming (Ghozlan and Vacher 2000). In cervical spine involvement, MRI is the modality of choice to visualize soft tissues and the cervical medulla, especially with the neck in a flexed and extended position (Jacobsen and Riise 2000).

Other techniques

Bone scintigraphy reveals areas with increased blood flow to bone as foci of increased radiopharmaceutical uptake as 'hot spots' and in this way detects arthritis (Brussatis 1990).

Arthrography nowadays plays a minor role in evaluation of RA patients and is largely replaced by ultrasound examination. Popliteal cysts and rotator cuff tears have been demonstrated with this technique. In ruptured cysts with extravasated material into soft tissue, arthrography might be preferable to sonography (Good 1964).

Imaging of extra-articular involvement

Pulmonary involvement, vasculitis, and nodulosis are extra-articular features in which imaging techniques can be helpful for diagnosis and establishing severity and progression.

Plain chest X-rays are first choice for screening for pulmonary involvement such as pleural effusion, nodulosis, interstitial fibrosis, and pneumonitis.

High-resolution computed tomography (HR-CT) in addition to conventional CT can be used to detect interstitial lung disease (Kalden-Nemeth and Manger 2000).

Vasculitis of the central nerve system can be visualized either by MRI or single-photon emission computer tomography (SPECT) of the brain (see Section 6.10).

Interventional radiology

Imaging techniques can be helpful for diagnostic and therapeutic intervention. Especially sonography is easy to perform and cheap compared to CT and MRI. Ultrasonic guided puncture of joint or bursa effusion has been used to obtain fluid for analysis and for injection of steriods and for anaesthetics in the shoulder, hip, and subacromial and psoas bursae (Ghozlan and Vacher 2000).

Assessment

RA is a disease with a highly variable presentation between patients and during the course of the disease, within individual patients. Symptoms and signs can be attributed to joint inflammation, locomotor damage, extra-articular involvement, and complications, next to systemic features such as subfebrile temperatures, weight loss, and fatigue. Joint complaints include swelling, pain, and stiffness. Evaluation of different aspects of the disease, therefore, is complicated and this has lead to an incredible large number of variables used (van Riel and van de Putte 1994). Accurate judgement of the disease process with regard to activity, severity, extent, and outcome is of major importance in both daily clinical practice and (randomized) clinical trials (van Riel and van Gestel 1999). Standardization of assessments is necessary to make results interchangeable and prevent non-uniformity. During the last decade, attempts have been made for consensus about a minimal set of variables measuring disease activity (van Riel 1992; Felson et al. 1993). These attempts have resulted in a core set of variables and development of criteria for response (Felson 1995; van Gestel et al. 1996) and remission (Prevoo et al. 1993). Variables used for assessment include different aspects of the disease and in general can be divided in two catagories (Fries 1983):

1. *Process variables:* measuring what actually happens along the way or the disease state at a given time point reflecting the actual disease activity;
2. *Outcome variables:* reflecting the end result of the processes.

It has been reported that levels of acute phase reactants, for instance, predict radiographic damage (van Leeuwen et al. 1993) if they are evaluated in a time-integrated manner. In clinical trials, efficacy is also evaluated in a time-integrated manner (Pham et al. 1999). One of the major difficulties of variables is that they often reflect a mixture of process and outcome of the disease.

In general, early in the disease, variables largely reflect process and in the later stages, increasingly, outcome (Guillemin et al. 1992). In addition, none of the variables is disease specific and abnormalities can be caused amongst others by comorbidity (see Table 5).

Disease activity measures

The 'core set' is a set of standardized measures covering the variable presentation of the disease (Table 7), and thus assessing disease activity. The core set includes several components and does not give a single value for disease activity. Another approach for assessing disease activity is by using indices of disease activity, which combine different variables into one value. The different variables of the core set will be described below.

Joint scores

Several joint scores using swelling and tenderness have been developed. They differ in grading for tenderness, the number of joints scored, weighting of joint surface areas, and measured combinations of abnormalities.

Articular indices reported can either be physician or patient assessed. The existing of different articular indices makes comparibility difficult. Physicians' and patients' assessed disease activity indices/variables correlate about 0.6–0.8 (Stucki et al. 1995; Prevoo et al. 1996a,b). This indicates that measurements are not identical and thus cannot replace each other. The 28-joint score, not graded and weighted, is valid, reproducible (a small intra- and interobserver variability), and consumes little time (Fuchs et al. 1989; Prevoo et al. 1993; Fuchs and Pincus 1994; Smolen et al. 1995).

Acute phase reactants

ESR and CRP are the most frequently used variables. They correlate with disease activity (van Leeuwen et al. 1993; van der Heijde et al. 1993a) and can predict in a time-integrated manner radiographic progression (van Leeuwen et al. 1993).

Pain

Pain can be measured using scales or questionnaires. Scales can be ordinal or continuous. The Likert scale, grading pain in a number of categories, is ordinal (Felson et al. 1993), whilst a visual analogue scale (VAS) is continuous. They are associated but not equivalent. The sensitivity to change is larger in a continuous scale, but a VAS needs more instruction and is less reliable in illiterate patients.

Table 7 Assessment variables

Clinical measurements	Process	Outcome	Core set
Joint scores			
Swollen	+	–	+
Tender	+	±	+
Pain scores (visual analogue?)	+	±	+
Stiffness	+	–	–
Fatigue	+	±	–
Global score of disease activity			
Physician	+	–	+
Patient	+	–	+
Grip strength	+	+	–
Acute phase response (ESR, CRP)	+	–	+
Radiographic damage	–	+	+
Functional disability	+[a]	+[a]	+
Extra-articular symptoms	+	–	–

[a] Dependent on the phase of the disease

Note: Reference: van Riel (1992), Guillemin et al. (1992), Felson (1993), van Riel and van de Putte (1994), Tugwell (1994).

Global disease activity

Global disease activity can be measured in the same way using a VAS or a Likert scale. Both physician and patient are assessed and considered valid instruments (Felson 1995).

Functional disability

Functional disability can be assessed by judgement of the physician, a standardized observation, or self-reported assessments. Judgement by a physician shows large interobserver variation and standardized observation is time-consuming. Self-reported assessments are most popular and a lot of questionnaires are available. All are efficient and sensitive, although there are slight differences (Liang et al. 1985).

Arthritis impact measurement scales

The Stanford Health Assessment Questionnaire (HAQ) (Fries et al. 1980) and the Arthritis Impact Measurement Scales (AIMS) (Meenan et al. 1980) are the two most frequently used questionnaires, which are sensitive to change (Ward 1993). The modified HAQ has been reported to predict increased morbidity and mortality (Wolfe 1988). Functional disability at start of the disease predicts functional status at 1 year of disease duration (Jansen et al. 2000).

Radiographic assessment

Radiographic damage is considered the 'gold standard' for assessment of outcome and used in clinical trials as primary outcome or end point. Methods developed for assessment of radiographic damage, in general, judge joint space narrowing and erosions. Other features that can be judged are osteoporosis, malalignment, subluxation, ankylosis, cysts, dislocation, and soft tissue swelling, but these variables are inconsistent and depend on the technique used.

In general, radiographs of hands and feet are used since these include the joints affected earliest and may be a good measure of general joint damage (Kuper et al. 1997). The two most commonly used radiographic scores are the Sharp score (Sharp et al. 1971) and the Larsen score (Larsen et al. 1977), both being validated and sensitive to change. A number of modifications of these methods have been published (van der Heijde et al. 1992; Larsen 1995), which adds scoring of feet (van der Heijde et al. 1992), reduction of the number of scored joints, and quantification of the degree of erosions and/or joint space narrowing (Rau et al. 1998) and weighting of joint (Genant 1983).

One of the major problems of both Larsen and Sharp methods as well as of the modifications is the 'ceiling effect', that is, when the maximum score in a joint is reached, further damage cannot be quantified (Kuper et al. 1999). In addition there is still discussion going on regarding the manner of scoring in time, that is, random order, sequential, or paired-order (van der Heijde et al. 1999).

Newer imaging techniques still have to prove their value in scoring joint damage both in daily practice and clinical trials.

Indices

Indices of disease activity are being developed to combine disease activity measures into a single expression of disease activity. Combined measures have the advantage of unambiguous interpretation of disease activity, comparibility, and increased power. Their disadvantage is not being able to show the individual components easily and calculations may be complex. Indices can measure actual disease activity or change in disease activity (van Riel and van de Putte 1994).

The Disease Activity Score (DAS) 28 (van der Heijde et al. 1993b; Prevoo et al. 1995) measures current disease activity. It comprises 28-joint counts for tenderness and swelling, the ESR, and a VAS for general health. The DAS has been validated in several studies (Fuchs 1993; Prevoo et al. 1995, 1996a,b).

Clinical trials versus daily clinical practice

Clinical trials are designed to evaluate efficacy of treatment in groups of selected patients. Disease activity measures should be valid, reproducible, and well tolerated by the patient.

Two sets of improvement criteria have been developed:

1. criteria based upon the core set of disease activity variables (preliminary ACR improvement criteria) (Felson 1995). Response is defined as a 20 per cent response from base-line in a number of core set variables;
2. criteria based upon an index of disease activity (EULAR response criteria) (van Gestel et al. 1996), which includes changes in disease activity as well as current disease state.

The absence or a very low level of disease activity—remission—is the ultimate goal of therapy and has been defined in remission criteria (Prevoo et al. 1996a,b). The ARA remission criteria are dichotomous, based upon judgement of rheumatologists, and the other approach defines remission as a continuous variable using the DAS (van Gestel et al. 1996).

Recently, improvement in patients in clinical trials has been proposed by the numeric ACR criteria (ACRn). Based upon this ACRn, area under the curve (ACR AUC) have been developed and utilized in clinical studies (Schiff et al. 1999; Bathon et al. 2000). A dominating disadvantage of the ACR AUC is the highly important value of baseline, and in addition the lack of validation of this ACRn (van Riel and van Gestel 2001).

The monitoring of disease course in daily clinical practice is quite different from that in clinical trials. Often a global way of assessment is performed, based upon the patients' history and a global joint assessment. Laboratory values are not available at the time of actual judgement of disease activity. The DAS28 could be a good instrument for monitoring actual disease activity. In addition, as measures of outcome, the HAQ and regular taken radiographs, scored according to methods as described above, should be done in order to assess process as well as outcome of the disease in daily clinical practice.

Table 8 Factors influencing the management of rheumatoid arthritis (Hazes and Cats; Klippel, Dieppe Textbook)

Patient	Disease	Drugs	Care providers
Age	Serum factors	Azathioprine	Rheumatologist
Sex	Radiologic lesions	Gold	Nurse
Medical history	Extra-articular manifestations	Cyclophosphamide	Occupational therapist
		Methotrexate	
Family	Disease progression	Leflunomide	Social worker
Education		Sulfasalazine	Physical therapist
Occupation		Antimalarials	Orthopaedic
Social network		Cyclosporine	surgeon
			Podiatrist

Therapeutic principles

Details about pharmacotherapy of RA as well as other therapeutic modalities are described in Chapter 6.3.3. However, it is appropriate that the therapeutic *principles* and the way they are related to clinical features of RA, are stated too.

Clinical features and their assessment have an increasing impact on the management of the disease, specifically the following aspects:

- Management has to take into account the stage of the disease, since for example, treatment of early-stage disease usually is dominated by pharmacotherapy, whereas end-stage disease, in addition, requires a number of other therapeutic modalities.
- Factors related to both patient and disease may considerably influence management of RA. In Table 8 a number of these factors are compiled.
- Clinical assessment (see 'Assessment') has now become an integral part of drug treatment monitoring, especially in the more powerful, fast acting forms of treatment that have become available.

RA being essentially a chronic *inflammatory* condition, pharmacotherapy is the cornerstone of treatment. However, for a considerable number of patients pharmacotherapy alone is sub-optimal. For this reason, other treatment modalities remain important, and are often offered to the patient in the form of a multidisciplinary approach.

Pharmacotherapeutic principles

Management of RA has changed substantially in the past 15 years as a result of new insights into the course of the disease and proliferation of the number of therapeutic agents for its treatment. Treatment goals have changed from mere symptom modification to, in addition, control of the disease process. Drugs used in the treatment of RA have been traditionally divided in so-called first- and second-line drugs. First-line drugs include NSAIDs, which have a rapid suppressive effect on signs of inflammation, including pain and stiffness. They do not however, influence progression of radiographic joint damage. In contrast, second-line drugs, also called DMARDs, influence the disease process more fundamentally by decreasing disease activity, slowing down the progression of joint damage, and preserving functional capacity. Another class of drugs, glucocorticosteroids, usually considered a separate category, are still indispensable in the treatment of at least some patients with RA. Finally, the recent development of the 'biologicals' has revolutionized the treatment. TNFα blocking agents especially are increasingly being used either as monotherapy or in combination with other DMARDs.

Increasing armamentarium of antirheumatic drugs

For a potentially life-long disease, it is important to have a great armamentarium of drugs, especially since there is a great variation among individual patients in clinical response and toxic side-effects.

The category of NSAIDs has recently been extended by specific inhibitors of cyclooxygenase (COX) 2 that have shown in short-term studies to have advances over the conventional NSAIDs (see Chapter 4.5). Conventional NSAIDs block both COX1 and COX2, thereby affecting COX1 mediated housekeeping functions of the COX system, like gastric mucosal protection and renal blood flow. So far, in short-term studies COX2 specific inhibitors have shown to lead to fewer gastric ulcers (Bombardier et al. 2000; Silverstein et al. 2000). However, results of long-term studies have to be awaited before the full spectrum of beneficial and toxic effects have become apparent. Of considerable importance is the increase in number of DMARDs in the last 10–15 years. Table 9 gives an overview of currently available DMARDs for RA. Conventionally used DMARDs like parenteral gold and D-penicillamine, were rather toxic, and probably most important, very slow acting, that is, the time from starting the therapy to the onset of clinical efficacy often lasted 3–6 months. Drugs like methotrexate and sulfasalazine, which have been rediscovered in the 1970s and 1980s, and lately leflunomide (Smolen et al. 1999), all have a faster mode of action, often showing clinical efficacy after 3–6 weeks. This allows for more effective titration towards efficacy. Virtually all those drugs have been shown to be able to suppress disease activity as well as slowing down progression of radiographic joint damage. Although toxicity remains a major problem, long-term studies show that individual drugs are mostly stopped because of inefficacy (Sokka and Hannonen 1999). An interesting question is whether one of the DMARDs is better than the other. In comparing 'composite efficacy' on the one hand and drop-outs from toxicity on the other hand, Felson et al. (1992) found that methotrexate and sulfasalazine performed somewhat better than the other DMARDs in a meta-analysis of available studies.

Table 9 Second-line agents for RA (from Wijnands and van Riel 1995)

Azathioprine
Cyclophosphamide
Hydroxycholoroquine
Methotrexate
Oral gold (auranofin)
Parenteral gold (aurothioglucose or sodium aurothiomalate)
D-Penicillamine
Sulfasalazine
Cyclosporine
Leflunomide

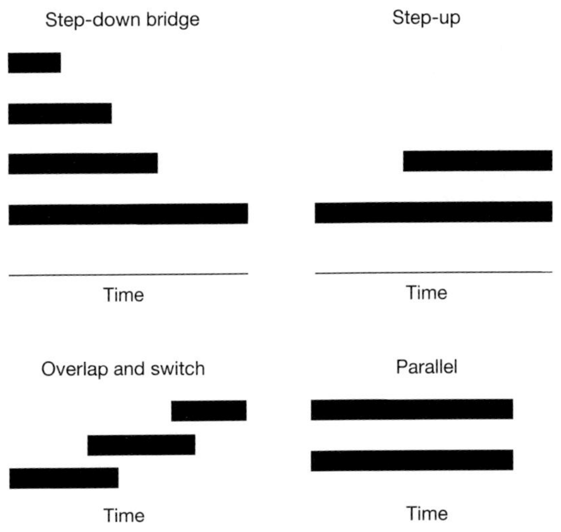

Fig. 10 Designs for combination therapy.

Early treatment

Probably the greatest advance in recent DMARD treatment of RA has been the early use of these drugs, be it as monotherapy or in combinations (van de Putte et al. 1998). Several observations have lead to change in therapeutical attitude. Radiographic studies have indicated that (irreversible) damage to joints starts relatively early in the disease (van der Heijde et al. 1992); on the other hand, many short- and intermediate-term studies now have indicated that DMARD therapy can at least decrease progression of joint damage. In addition, it has been shown that RA not only leads to morbidity but may also affect survival. One of the determinants was severity of the disease as indicated by the extend and severity of polyarthritis. Although not yet proven, it may result from these observations that adequate suppression of polyarthritis will benefit survival. Finally, a recent meta-analysis study by Anderson et al. (2000) concludes that less treatment is required in the early phase to suppress the disease, than when treatment is started later on in the process.

Radiographic follow-up studies have indicated that initial benefit of early treatment in terms of slowing down joint damage, are still present, several years later (van der Heijde, 1989).

Combination therapies

Recently, some combinations have been shown to be better than monotherapy. Combination therapy may be applied according to different designs. These designs are summarized in Fig. 10. One of the first successful combination therapy studies was designed according to the so-called step-up design (Tugwell et al. 1995). This form of therapy probably is most frequently used in current daily practice. Another design is the step-down variant, in which two or more DMARDs are started and subsequently tapered down. A classical example is the study by Boers et al. (1997). Other designs include the parallel design and the bridging design. Although the step-down and parallel design may be useful in severe disease, so far in clinical practice the step-up and bridging variants are most frequently used. Interestingly several studies have shown that combination of DMARDs does not lead to more toxicity (Boers et al. 1997; Haagsma et al. 1997).

Target-oriented therapies

Modern biotechnology has allowed for the development of target-oriented therapies, directed towards targets of interest. In principle, therapies have been aimed at either eliminating proinflammatory cells or molecules, or adding anti-inflammatory agents. Interestingly, although T cells were thought to play an important role in the pathogenesis, so far anti-T-cell therapies have not been consistently successful (van der Lubbe et al. 1995). The most impressive clinical data have come from studies aimed at blocking TNFα, a cytokine at the top of the cytokine cascade (Maini et al. 1999; Moreland et al. 1999; Bathon et al. 2000; Lipsky et al. 2000). TNF blocking therapies show already clinical effects within days of administration. These agents have to be given at regular intervals, and therefore suppress inflammation rather than cure the disease. Problems experienced so far with these agents include amongst others increased susceptability to infections, development of antibodies against the agents, which may be overcome by concurrent use of immunosuppressants like methotrexate (Maini et al. 1998) and, seldomly, development of autoimmune syndromes. Long-term studies are eagerly awaited. Therefore, and because these agents are very expensive, they are currently reserved for people who have failed at least one DMARD, including methotrexate (Smolen et al. 2000).

Corticosteroids

These can be used in different ways. Low-dose oral corticosteroids are frequently used when DMARD therapy is insufficiently effective. The well-known side-effects of corticosteroids over time have tempered the initial enthusiasm. Interest in systemic corticosteroids was renewed when treatment with lower doses was proposed as so-called bridge therapy, which aims to relieve symptoms of RA during the period between initiation of DMARDs and onset of clinical efficacy or to combat intercurrent disease flares. Finally, corticosteroids are used frequently locally. Systemic corticosteroids may have a modest effect on radiographic progression (Kirwan et al. 1995).

Side-effects prevention

Since currently available drugs and treatment strategies seem to be more effective than in the past, interest in side-effect prevention has grown (Wijnands and van Riel 1995). One recent placebo-controlled study of folate or folinic acid co-medication in patients treated with methotrexate, indicated that especially liver toxicity was significantly less in the group with co-medication, allowing for over 20 per cent more patients continuing their treatment on effective doses (van Ede et al. 2001). Since osteoporosis has always been a limiting factor in prolonged steroid therapy, the observation that it can be influenced by concomitant bisphosphonate therapy is of clinical importance (Wallach et al. 2000). Another contribution to side-effect prevention is the development of COX2 specific drugs, which will hopefully decrease the incidence of long-term complications. Of course of major importance in preventing side-effects is experience with antirheumatic drugs and knowledge of risk factors for side-effect development. In this respect, fast-acting drugs are easier to handle, allowing for titration towards efficacy and (temporarily) reduction of the dose in case of side-effects.

Table 10 Members of the multidisciplinary team (from Wijnands and van Riel, 1995)

Rheumatologist
Nurse
Occupational therapist
Physical therapist
Social worker
Psychologist/psychiatrist
Neurologist
Orthopaedic surgeon
General physician
Podiatrist

The multidisciplinary approach

With respect to treatment, the ideal situation in a disease like RA is to suppress the inflammatory process completely by pharmacotherapeutic means, there being no need for other treatment modalities. However, despite improvements in drug treatment in the recent decades, the disease still has significant physical, psychological, and socio-economic consequences for the patient. The wide spectrum of available treatment modalities, including current pharmacotherapy, physical therapy (Hazes et al. 1996), and occupational therapy, the ever increasing number of surgical interventions, the increased awareness of patients, and the reduced opportunities for hospitalization indicate a continued need for the multidisciplinary approach. Although traditionally done in an in-patient setting, this form of treatment is also effective in an out-patient setting (Vliet Vlieland et al. 1997).

In most cases, the rheumatologist is the coordinating person of the team. Members of such a team are compiled in Table 10. The relative accents of multidisciplinary treatment will depend on individual needs of the patients. Surgical treatment modalities include synovectomy, arthrodesis, joint replacement, and resection arthroplasty. Early synovectomy is nowadays less popular. An extensive overview of available forms of orthopaedic surgical treatments is found in Chapters 7.1 and 7.2.

Management of end-stage disease

Since treatment possibilities for active inflammatory RA definitely have improved, and destructive lesions are known to be largely irreversible, it is important to make a distinction between end-stage disease (dominated by joint destruction) and early and established active inflammatory disease. Table 11 compiles the relative role of different therapeutic modalities in the management of RA related to the stage of the disease. It appears from this table that extensive drug therapy in end-stage disease may be somewhat less important, whereas reconstructive surgical interventions and joint replacements are definitely more important. However, detection of active inflammation in this stage of the disease may be hampered by difficulties in clinical assessment and data have suggested that for many patients pharmacotherapy has to be continued (Ten Wolde et al. 1996). Important principles in end-stage RA are:

- Assessment should make a distinction between destructive lesions and active synovitis.
- When present, treat the inflammatory process as optimal as possible.
- Primary goals should include preservation and maximization of function and prevention of disability. Physical, rehabilitative, and occupational therapy as well as orthopaedic surgery are important tools in this respect.
- In case these treatments still leave considerable disability, remaining handicaps should be overcome by adapting the environment.

Table 11 Role of therapeutic regimens in the management of RA related to the stage of disease

Therapeutic regimen	Early and established disease	End-stage disease
Conservative therapy		
Patient education	+ + +	+
Rest		
Systemic/therapeutic	+	+
Local/protective	+ +	+ +
Physical therapy		
Maintenance range of motion	+ +	+
Prevention of disuse atrophy of muscle, support of condition	+	+ +
Occupational therapy		
Joint protection	+ +	+
Adaptation	+	+ +
Drug therapy		
NSAIDs	+ +	+ +
Second-line drugs	+ +	+
Corticosteroids (systemic)	+	±
Intra-articular therapy	+ +	+
Surgical intervention		
Therapeutic (synovectomy)	+	–
Reconstructive	+	+ +
Joint replacement	–	+ + +

References

ACR (1996). Task force on osteoporosis guidelines. Recommendations for the prevention and treatment of glucocorticoid-induced osteoporosis. *Arthritis and Rheumatism* 39, 1791–801.

Aho, K. et al. (1986). Occurrence of rheumatoid arthritis in a nationwide series of twins. *Journal of Rheumatology* 13, 899–902.

Aho, K. et al. (1991). Rheumatoid factors antedating clinical rheumatoid arthritis. *Journal of Rheumatology* 18, 1282–4.

Aman, S. et al. (2000). Prediction of disease progression in early rheumatoid arthritis by ICP, IRF and CRP. A comparative 3 year follow up study. *Rheumatology* 39, 1009–13.

Anaya, J.M. et al. (1995). Pulmonary involvement in rheumatoid arthritis. *Seminars in Arthritis and Rheumatism* 24, 242–54.

Anderson, S.T. (1996). Mortality in rheumatoid arthritis: do age and gender make a difference? *Seminars in Arthritis and Rheumatism* 25, 291–6.

Anderson, J.J. et al. (2000). Factors predicting response to treatment in rheumatoid arthritis: the importance of disease duration. *Arthritis and Rheumatism* 43, 22–9.

Andonopoulos, A.P. et al. (1987). Secondary Sjögren's syndrome in rheumatoid arthritis. *Journal of Rheumatology* 14, 1098–103.

Andonopoulos, A.P. et al. (1989). Sjögren's syndrome in rheumatoid arthritis and progressive systemic sclerosis. A comparative study. *Clinical and Experimental Rheumatology* 7, 203–5.

Arnett, F. et al. (1988). The American Rheumatism Association 1987 revised criteria for the classification of rheumatoid arthritis. *Arthritis and Rheumatism* 31, 315–24.

Bäcklund, E. et al. (1998). Disease activity and risk of lymphoma in patients with rheumatoid arthritis: tested case–control study. *British Journal of Rheumatology* 317, 180–1.

Bacon, P.A. and Carruthers, D.M. (1995). Vasculitis associated with connective tissue disorders. *Rheumatic Diseases Clinics of North America* 21, 1077–96.

Barrera, P. et al. (1994). Methotrexate-related pulmonary complications in rheumatoid arthritis. *Annals of the Rheumatic Diseases* 53, 434–9.

Barrera, P. et al. (1999). Familial aggregation of rheumatoid arthritis in the Netherlands. A cross-sectional hospital-based survey. European Consortium on Rheumatoid Arthritis Families (ECRAF). *Rheumatology (Oxford)* 38, 415–22.

Bathon, J.M. et al. (2000). Comparison of etanercept and methotrexate in patients with early rheumatoid arthritis. *New England Journal of Medicine* **343**, 1586–93.

Berkanovic, E. and Hurwicz, M.-L. (1990). Rheumatoid arthritis and comorbidity. *Journal of Rheumatology* **17**, 888–92.

Bernelot Moens, H.J., van de Laar, M.A., and van der Korst, J.K. (1992). Comparison of the sensitivity and specificity of the 158 and 1987 criteria for rheumatoid arthritis. *Journal of Rheumatology* **19** (2), 198–203.

Bijlsma, J.W.J. (1997). Prevention of glucocorticoid-induced osteoporosis. *Annals of the Rheumatic Diseases* **56**, 507–9.

Boerbooms, A.M. et al. (1995). Infections during low-dose methotrexate treatment in rheumatoid arthritis. *Seminars in Arthritis and Rheumatism* **24**, 411–21.

Boers, M. et al. (1997). Randomised comparison of combined step-down prednisolone, methotrexate and sulphasalazine alone in early rheumatoid arthritis. *Lancet* **350**, 309–18.

Bombardier, C. et al. (2000). Comparison of upper gastrointestinal toxicity of rofecoxib and naproxen in patients with rheumatoid arthritis. *New England Journal of Medicine* **343**, 1520–8.

Breedveld, F.C. et al. (1987a). Factors influencing the incidence of infections in Felty's syndrome. *Archives of Internal Medicine* **147**, 915–20.

Breedveld, F. et al. (1987b). Magnetic resonance imaging in the evaluation of patients with rheumatoid arthritis and subluxation of the cervical spine. *Arthritis and Rheumatism* **26**, 624–9.

Brennan, P. and Silman, A.J. (1994). Breast-feeding and the onset of rheumatoid arthritis. *Arthritis and Rheumatism* **37**, 808–13.

Brower, A.C. (1988). Rheumatoid arthritis. In *Arthritis in Black and White* (ed. A.C. Brower), pp. 137–65. Philadelphia PA: W.B. Saunders.

Brussatis, F. (1990). Degenerative Skeletterkrankungen. Nuklearmedizinische Diagnostik. In *Nuklearmedizin in der Orthopädie* (ed. F. Brussatis and K. Hahn), pp. 134–48. Berlin: Springer.

Carrao, S. et al. (1995). Cardiac involvement in rheumatoid arthritis: evidence of silent heart disease. *European Heart Journal* **16**, 253–6.

Chalmers, I.M. and Blair, G.S. (1973). Rheumatoid arthritis of the temporomandibular joint. *Quarterly Journal of Medicine* **42**, 369–86.

Cimmino, M.A. et al. (2000). Extra-articular manifestations in 587 patients with rheumatoid arthritis. *Rheumatology International* **19** (6), 213–17.

Combe, B. et al. (1993). Accelerated nodulosis and systemic manifestations during methotrexate therapy for rheumatoid arthritis. *European Journal of Medicine* **2**, 153–6.

Cooper, C. et al. (1990). Brown's syndrome: an unusual ocular complication in rheumatoid arthritis. *Annals of the Rheumatic Diseases* **49**, 188–9.

Cooper, C., Coupland, M., and Mitchell, M. (1995). Rheumatoid arthritis, corticosteroid therapy and hip fracture. *Annals of the Rheumatic Diseases* **54**, 49–52.

Corbett, M. et al. (1993). Factors predicting death, survival and functional outcome in a prospective study of early RA after 15 years. *British Journal of Rheumatology* **32**, 717–23.

Coremans, I.E.M. et al. (1992). Anti-lactoferrin antibodies in patients with rheumatoid arthritis associated with vasculitis. *Arthritis and Rheumatism* **35**, 1466–75.

Cough, A.K.S. et al. (1994). Generalised bone loss in patients with early rheumatoid arthritis. *Lancet* **344**, 23–7.

Cough, A.K.S. et al. (1998). Osteoclastic activation is the principal mechanism leading to secondary osteoporosis in rheumatoid arthritis. *Journal of Rheumatology* **25**, 1282–9.

Crockard, H.A. (1995). Surgical management of rheumatoid problems. *Spine* **20**, 2584–90.

Dale, D.C. and Petersdorf, R.G. (1973). Corticosteroids and infectious diseases. *Medical Clinics of North America* **57**, 1277–87.

Dillon, A.M. et al. (1986). Parenteral gold therapy in the Felty syndrome: experience with 20 patients. *Medicine* **65**, 112.

Drosos, A.A. et al. (1997). Epidemiology of adult rheumatoid arthritis in northwest Greece, 1987–1995. *Journal of Rheumatology* **24**, 2129–33.

Dugowson, C.E. et al. (1991). Rheumatoid arthritis in women. Incidence rates in Group Health Cooperative, Seattle, Washington, 1987–1989. *Arthritis and Rheumatism* **34**, 1502–7.

Eastell, R. (1995). On behalf of a UK consensus group meeting on osteoporosis. Management of corticosteroid-induced osteoporosis. *Journal of Internal Medicine* **237**, 439–47.

Eberhardt, K.B. et al. (1990). Early rheumatoid arthritis—onset, course and prognosis over 2 years. *Rheumatology International* **10**, 135–42.

Eberhardt, K.H. et al. (1995). Hip involvement in early rheumatoid arthritis. *Annals of the Rheumatic Diseases* **54**, 45–8.

Ekdahl, C. and Broman, G. (1992). Muscle strength, endurance and aerobic capacity in rheumatoid arthritis: a comparative study with healthy subjects. *Annals of the Rheumatic Diseases* **51**, 35–40.

Ertel, A.N. et al. (1988). Flexor tendon ruptures in patients with rheumatoid arthritis. *Journal of Hand Surgery* **13**, 860–6.

Felson, D.T. (1995). American College of Rheumatology preliminary definition of improvement in rheumatoid arthritis. *Arthritis and Rheumatism* **38**, 727–35.

Felson, D.T., Anderson, J.J., and Meenan, R.F. (1992). Use of short-term efficacy/toxicity tradeoffs to select second-line drugs in rheumatoid arthritis. A meta-analysis of published clinical trials. *Arthritis and Rheumatism* **35**, 1117–25.

Felson, D.T. et al. (1993). The American College of Rheumatology preliminary core set of disease activity measures for rheumatoid arthritis clinical trials. *Arthritis and Rheumatism* **36**, 729–40.

Fernandes, L. et al. (1979). Studies on the frequency and pathogenesis of liver involvement in rheumatoid arthritis. *Annals of the Rheumatic Diseases* **38**, 501–6.

Firestein, G.S. et al., ed. *Rheumatoid Arthritis*. Oxford: Oxford University Press, 2000.

Fleming, A., Crown, J.M., and Corbett, M. (1976). Early rheumatoid disease, I. onset, II. patterns of joint involvement. *Annals of the Rheumatic Diseases* **35**, 357–63.

Fries, J.F. et al. (1980). Measurement of patient outcome in arthritis. *Arthritis and Rheumatism* **23**, 137–45.

Fries, J.F. (1983). Towards an understanding of patients outcome measurement. *Arthritis and Rheumatism* **26**, 697–704.

Fuchs, H.A. (1993). The use of the disease activity score in the analysis of clinical trials in rheumatoid arthritis. *Journal of Rheumatology* **20**, 1863–6.

Fuchs, H.A. and Pincus, T. (1994). Reduced joint counts in controlled clinical trials in rheumatoid arthritis. *Arthritis and Rheumatism* **37**, 470–5.

Fuchs, H.A. et al. (1989). Simplified 28-joint count quantitative articular index in rheumatoid arthritis. *Arthritis and Rheumatism* **32**, 531–7.

Fujiwara, K. et al. (1998). Cervical lesions related to the systemic progression in rheumatoid arthritis. *Spine* **23**, 2052–6.

Gabriel, S. (2001). The epidemiology of rheumatoid arthritis. *Rheumatic Disease Clinics of North America* **27**, 269–81.

Gabriel, S.E., Crowson, C.S., and O'Fallon, W.M. (1999b). Comorbidity in arthritis. *Journal of Rheumatology* **26**, 2475–9.

Gabriel, S.E., Crowson, C.S., and O'Fallon, W.M. (1999a). The epidemiology of rheumatoid arthritis in Rochester, MN, 1955–1985. *Arthritis and Rheumatism* **42**, 415–20.

Geborek, P., Moritz, U., and Wollheim, F.A. (1989). Joint capsular stiffness in knee arthritis. Relationship to intra-articular volume, hydrostatic pressures, and extensor muscle function. *Journal of Rheumatology* **16**, 1351–8.

Geirson, A.J., Sturfelt, G., and Truedsson, L. (1987). Clinical and serological features of severe vasculitis in rheumatoid arthritis—prognostic implications. *Annals of the Rheumatic Diseases* **46**, 727–33.

Genant, H.K. (1983). Methods of assessing radiographic change in rheumatoid arthritis. *American Journal of Medicine* **75** (6A), 35–47.

Geterud, Å. Rheumatoid arthritis in the larynx. A clinical and methodological study. PhD thesis, University of Gothenburg, Sweden, 1991.

Ghozlan, R. and Vacher, H. (2000). Where is imaging going in rheumatology? *Baillière's Clinical Rheumatology* **14**, 617–33.

Gillmore, J.D., Hawkins, P.N., and Pepys, M.B. (1997). Amyloidosis: a review of recent diagnostic and therapeutic developments. *British Journal of Rheumatology* **99**, 245–56.

Goldberg, J. and Pinals, R.S. (1980). Felty's syndrome. *Seminars in Arthritis and Rheumatism* **10**, 52–65.

Goldenberg, D.L. (1998). Septic arthritis. *Lancet* **351**, 197–202.

Good, A.E. (1964). Rheumatoid arthritis, Bakers' cyst and thrombophlebitis. *Arthritis and Rheumatism* **7**, 56–64.

Goodgold, J., Kopell, H.P., and Speilholz, N.I. (1965). The tarsal tunnel syndrome. *New England Journal of Medicine* **273**, 472–745.

Gough, A.K.S. et al. (1994). Generalized bone loss in patients with early rheumatoid arthritis. *Lancet* **344**, 23–7.

Gough, A.K.S. et al. (1998). Osteoclastic activation is the principle mechanism leading to secondary osteoporosis in rheumatoid arthritis. *Journal of Rheumatology* **25**, 1282–9.

Grassi, W. et al. (2001). Ultrasonography in the evaluation of bone erosions. *Annals of the Rheumatic Diseases* **60**, 98–103.

Gravallese, E.M. et al. (1989). Rheumatoid aortitis: a rarely recognized but clinically significant entity. *Medicine (Baltimore)* **68**, 95–106.

Gray, R.G., Tenenbaum, J., and Gottlieb, N.L. (1981). Local corticosteroid injection treatment in rheumatic disorders. *Arthritis and Rheumatism* **10**, 231–54.

Gridley, G. et al. (1994). Incidence of cancer among men with the Felty syndrome. *Annals of Internal Medicine* **120**, 35–9.

Grillet, B. et al. (1997). Gelatinase B in chronic synovitis: immunolocalization with a monoclonal antibody. *British Journal of Rheumatology* **36**, 744–7.

Guedes, C. et al. (2001). Cardiac manifestations of rheumatoid arthritis: a case–control transesophageal echocardiography study in 30 patients. *Arthritis Care and Research* **45**, 129–35.

Guillemin, F., Briançon, S., and Pourel, J. (1992). Functional disability in rheumatoid arthritis: two different models in early and established disease. *Journal of Rheumatology* **19**, 366–9.

Haagsma, C.J. et al. (1997). Combination of sulfasalazine and methotrexate versus the single components in early rheumatoid arthritis: a randomized, controlled, double-blind, 52 week clinical trial. *British Journal of Rheumatology* **36**, 1082–8.

Halla, J.T. et al. (1984). Rheumatoid myositis. *Arthritis and Rheumatism* **27**, 737–43.

Hawkins, P.N. (1994). Studies with radiolabelled serum amyloid P component provide evidence for turnover and regression of amyloid deposits *in vivo*. *Clinical Science* **87**, 289–95.

Hazenberg, B.P.C. et al. (1999). A quantitive method for detecting deposits of amyloid A protein in aspirated fat tissue of patients with arthritis. *Annals of the Rheumatic Diseases* **58**, 96–102.

Hazenberg, B.P.C. and van Rijswijk, M.H. (2000a). Aspects cliniques de l'amylose AA. In *Les amyloses* (ed. G. Grateau, M.D. Benon, and M. Delpech), pp. 377–427. Paris: Flammarian.

Hazenberg, B.P.C. and van Rijswijk, M.H. (2000b). Where has secondary amyloid gone? *Annals of the Rheumatic Diseases* **59**, 577–9.

Hazes, J.M.W. (1991). Pregnancy and its effect on the risk of developing rheumatoid arthritis. *Annals of the Rheumatic Diseases* **50**, 71–2.

Hazes, J.M.W. and Ende van den, C.H.M. (1996). How vigorously should we exercise our rheumatoid arthritis patients? *Annals of the Rheumatic Diseases* **55**, 861–2.

Helin, H.J. et al. (1995). Renal biopsy findings and clinicopathological correlations in rheumatoid arthritis. *Arthritis and Rheumatism* **38**, 242–7.

Heliövaara, M. et al. (2000). Coffee consumption, rheumatoid factor and the risk of rheumatoid arthritis. *Annals of the Rheumatic Diseases* **8**, 631–5.

Heurkens, A.H.M., Westedt, M.L., and Breedveld, F.C. (1991). Prednisone plus azathioprine treatment in patients with rheumatoid arthritis complicated by vasculitis. *Archives of Internal Medicine* **151**, 224–54.

Husby, G. (1985). Amyloidosis and rheumatoid arthritis. *Clinical and Experimental Rheumatology* **3**, 173–80.

Jacobsen, E.A. and Riise, T. (2000). MRI of cervical spine with flexion and extension used in patients with rheumatoid arthritis. *Scandinavian Journal of Rheumatology* **29**, 249–54.

Jacobsson, L.T.H. et al. (1994). Decreasing incidence and prevalence of rheumatoid arthritis in Pima Indians over a twenty-five-year period. *Arthritis and Rheumatism* **37**, 1158–65.

Jansen, L.M.A. et al. (2000). Predictors of functional status in patients with early rheumatoid arthritis. *Annals of the Rheumatic Diseases* **59**, 223–6.

Janssens, X. et al. (1988). The diagnostic significance of the antiperinuclear factor for rheumatoid arthritis. *Journal of Rheumatology* **15**, 1346–50.

Jayson, M.I.V. and Jones, D.E.P. (1971). Scleritis and rheumatoid arthritis. *Annals of the Rheumatic Diseases* **30**, 343–7.

Jeurissen, M.E.C., Boerbooms, A.M.T., and van de Putte, L.B.A. (1989). Eruption of nodulosis and vasculitis during methotrexate therapy for RA. *Clinical Rheumatology,* **8**, 418–19.

Kaandorp, C.J.E. et al. (1995). Risk factors for septic arthritis in patients with joints disease: a prospective study. *Arthritis and Rheumatism* **38**, 1819–25.

Kaandorp, C.J.E. et al. (1997). Incidence and sources of native and prosthetic joint infection: a community based prospective survey. *Annals of the Rheumatic Diseases* **56**, 470–5.

Kaipiainen-Seppanen, O. et al. (1996). Incidence of rheumatoid arthritis in Finland during 1980–1990. *Annals of the Rheumatic Diseases* **55**, 608–11.

Kaipiainen-Seppanen, O. et al. (2000). Intensive treatment of rheumatoid arthritis reduces need for dialysis due to secondary amyloidosis. *Scandinavian Journal of Rheumatology* **29**, 232–5.

Kalden-Nemeth, D. and Manger, B. (2000). Imaging. In *Rheumatoid Arthritis Frontiers in Pathogenesis and Treatment* (ed. G.S. Firestein, G.S. Panayi, and F.A. Wollheim), pp. 257–74. Oxford: Oxford University Press.

Kauppi, M., Pukkala, E., and Isomäki, H. (1997). Elevated incidence of hematologic malignancies in patients with Sjögren's syndrome compared with patients with rheumatoid arthritis (Finland). *Cancer Causes and Control* **8**, 201–4.

Kelley, C.A. (1993). Rheumatoid arthritis: classical lung disease. *Baillière's Clinical Rheumatology* **7**, 1–16.

Kirwan, J.R. and the Arthritis and Rheumatism Council Low-Dose Glucocorticoid Study Group (1995). The effect of glucocorticoids on joint destruction in rheumatoid arthritis. *New England Journal of Medicine* **333**, 142–6.

Klarlund, M. et al. (2000). Magnetic resonance imaging, radiography, and scintigraphy of finger joints: one year follow up of patients with early arthritis. *Annals of the Rheumatic Diseases* **59**, 521–8.

Kobayashi, H. et al. (1996). Secondary amyloidosis in patients with rheumatoid arthritis: diagnostic and prognostic value of gastroduodenal biopsy. *British Journal of Rheumatology* **35**, 44–9.

Kraag, G. et al. (1976). The hemorrhage crescent sign of acute synovial rupture. *Annals of Internal Medicine* **85**, 477–8.

Kraan, M.C. et al. (1999). Immunohistological analysis of synovial tissue for differential diagnosis in early arthritis. *Rheumatology (Oxford)* **38**, 1074–80.

Kroot, E.J.A. et al. (2000). No increased mortality in patients with rheumatoid arthritis, up to 10 years of follow up from disease onset. *Annals of the Rheumatic Diseases* **59**, 954–8.

Kroot, E.J.A. et al. (2001). Chronic comorbidity in patients with early rheumatoid arthritis; a descriptive study. *Journal of Rheumatology* **28**, 1511–17.

Kuper, H.H. et al. (1997). Radiographic damage in large joints in early rheumatoid arthritis: relationship with radiographic damage in hands and feet, disease activity, and physical disability. *British Journal of Rheumatology* **36**, 855–60.

Kuper, H.H. et al. (1999). Influence of a ceiling effect on the assessment of radiographic progression in rheumatoid arthritis during the first 6 years of disease. *Journal of Rheumatology* **26**, 268–76.

Laan, R.F.J.M. et al. (1993a). Bone mineral density in patients with recent onset rheumatoid arthritis: influence of disease activity and functional capacity. *Annals of the Rheumatic Diseases* **52**, 21–6.

Laan, R.F.J.M. et al. (1993b). Low dose prednisone induces rapid reversible axial bone loss in patients with rheumatoid arthritis. *Annals of Internal Medicine* **119**, 963–8.

Lane, N.E. and Goldring, S.R. (1998). Bone loss in rheumatoid arthritis: what role does inflammation play? *Journal of Rheumatology* **25**, 1251–3.

Larsen, A., Dale, K., and Eek, M. (1977). Radiographic evaluation of rheumatoid arthritis and related conditions by reference films. *Acta Radiologica Diagnosis* **18**, 481–91.

Larsen, A. (1995). How to apply Larsen score in evaluating radiographs of rheumatoid arthritis. *Arthritis and Rheumatism* **22**, 1974–5.

Liang, M.H. et al. (1985). Comparative measurement efficiency and sensibility of five health status instruments for arthritis research. *Arthritis and Rheumatism* **28**, 542–7.

Lindqvist, E. and Eberhardt, K. (1999). Mortality in rheumatoid arthritis patients with disease onset in the 1980s. *Annals of the Rheumatic Diseases* **58**, 11–14.

Linos, A. et al. (1980). The epidemiology of rheumatoid arthritis in Rochester, Minnesota: a study of incidence, prevalence, and mortality. *American Journal of Epidemiology* **111** (1), 87–98.

Lipsky, P.E. et al. (2000). Infliximab and methotrexate treatment of rheumatoid arthritis. *New England Journal of Medicine* **343**, 1594–602.

Luukkainen, R., Isomäki, H., and Kajander, A. (1983). Prognostic value of the type of onset of rheumatoid arthritis. *Annals of the Rheumatic Diseases* **42**, 274–5.

Maddison, P.J. et al., ed. *Oxford Textbook of Rheumatology* 2nd edn. Oxford: Oxford University Press, 1998.

Maini, R. et al. (1998). Therapeutic efficacy of multiple intravenous infusions of anti-tumor necrosis alpha monoclonal antibody combined with low-dose weekly methotrexate in rheumatoid arthritis. *Arthritis and Rheumatism* **41**, 1552–63.

Maini, R. et al. (1999). Infliximab (chimeric anti-tumor necrosis factor alpha monoclonal antibody) versus placebo in rheumatoid arthritis patients receiving concomitant methotrexate: a randomised phase III trial. ATTRACT Study Group. *Lancet* **354**, 1932–9.

Markenson, J.A. et al. (1979). Rheumatoid meningitis: a localized immune process. *Annals of Internal Medicine* **90**, 786–9.

Marks, J.S. and Sharp, J. (1981). Rheumatoid cervical myelopathy. *Quarterly Journal of Medicine* **50**, 307–19.

Martel, W. (1977). Pathogenesis of cervical discovertebral destruction in rheumatoid arthritis. *Arthritis and Rheumatism* **20**, 1217–25.

Masi, A.T., Feigenbaum, S.L., and Kaplan, S.B. (1983). Articular patterns in the early course of rheumatoid arthritis. *American Journal of Medicine* **75** (Suppl. 6A), 16–26.

Matsuki, Y. et al. (1994). Amyloidosis secondary to rheumatoid arthritis associated with plexiform change in bilateral temporal lobes. *Internal Medicine* **33**, 764–7.

Matsuo, T. et al. (1997). Incidence of ocular complications in rheumatoid arthritis and the relation to keratoconjunctivitis sicca to its systemic activity. *Scandinavian Journal of Rheumatology* **26**, 113–16.

McCarty, D.J. et al. (1985). Remitting seronegative symmetrical synovitis with pitting edema. (RS3PE) syndrome. *Journal of the American Medical Association* **2545**, 2763–7.

McGregor, A.J. and Silman, A.J. (1998). Rheumatoid arthritis. Classification and epidemiology. In *Rheumatology* 2nd edn. (ed. J.H. Klippel and P.A. Dieppe), pp. 521–6. London: Mosby.

McQueen, F.M. (2000). Magnetic resonance imaging in early inflammatory arthritis: what is its role? *Rheumatology* **39**, 700–6.

Meenan, R.F., German, P.M., and Mason, J.M. (1980). Measuring health status in arthritis: the arthritis impact measurement scales. *Arthritis and Rheumatism* **23**, 146–52.

Monsees, B. et al. (1985). Pressure erosions of bone in rheumatoid arthritis: a subject review. *Radiology* **155**, 53–9.

Moreland, L.W. et al. (1999). Etanercept therapy in rheumatoid arthritis. A randomized, controlled trial. *Annals of Internal Medicine* **130**, 478–86.

Moutsopoulos, H.M. et al. (1979). Differences in the clinical manifestation of sicca syndrome in the presence and absence of rheumatoid arthritis. *American Journal of Medicine* **66**, 733–6.

Myllykangas-Luosujärvi, R.A., Aho, K., and Isomäki, H.A. (1995). Mortality in rheumatoid arthritis. *Seminars in Arthritis and Rheumatism* **25**, 193–202.

Nived, O., Sturfelt, G., and Wollheim, F. (1985). Systemic lupus erythematosus and infection. A controlled and prospective study including an epidemiological group. *Quarterly Journal of Medicine* **55**, 271–87.

Ollier, W.E. and MacGregor, A. (1995). Genetic epidemiology of rheumatoid arthritis. *British Medical Bulletin* **51**, 267–85.

Paimela, L. et al. (1997). Progression of cervical spine changes in patients with early RA. *Journal of Rheumatology* **24**, 1280–4.

Palmer, D.G. et al. (1987). Macrophage migration and maturation within rheumatoid nodules. *Arthritis and Rheumatism* **30**, 729–36.

Pedersen, L.M. et al. (1995). Microalbuminuria in patients with rheumatoid arthritis. *Annals of the Rheumatic Diseases* **54**, 189–92.

Peeters, H.R.M. et al. (1996). Course and characteristics of anemia in patients with rheumatoid arthritis of recent onset. *Annals of the Rheumatic Diseases* **55**, 162–8.

Pham, B. et al. (1999). Validity of area-under-the-curve analysis to summarize effect in rheumatoid arthritis clinical trials. *Journal of Rheumatology* **26**, 712–16.

Pincus, T. et al. (1994). Prediction of long-term mortality in patients with rheumatoid arthritis according to simple questionnaire and joint count measures. *Annals of Internal Medicine* **120**, 26–34.

Plant, M.J. et al. (1994). Measurement and prediction of radiologic progression in early rheumatoid arthritis. *Journal of Rheumatology* **21**, 1808–13.

Plant, M.J. et al. (2000). Relationship between time-integrated C-reactive protein levels and radiologic progression in patients with rheumatoid arthritis. *Arthritis and Rheumatism* **43**, 1473–7.

Poole, R. (1994). Immunochemical markers of joint inflammation, skeletal damage and repair: where are we now? *Annals of the Rheumatic Diseases* **53**, 3–5.

Preston, S.J. et al. (1993). Methotrexate osteopathy in rheumatic disease. *Annals of the Rheumatic Diseases* **52**, 582–5.

Prevoo, M.L.L. et al. (1993). Validity and reliability of joint indices. A longitudinal study of patients with recent onset rheumatoid arthritis. *British Journal of Rheumatology* **32**, 584–94.

Prevoo, M.L.L. et al. (1995). Modified disease activity scores that include twenty eight joint counts. *Arthritis and Rheumatism* **38**, 44–8.

Prevoo, M.L.L. et al. (1996a). Remission in a prospective study of patients with rheumatoid arthritis. American Rheumatism Association preliminary remission criteria in relation to the disease activity score. *British Journal of Rheumatology* **35**, 1101–5.

Prevoo, M.L.L. et al. (1996b). Validity and reproducibility of self-administered joint counts. A large prospective longitudinal follow-up study in patients with rheumatoid arthritis. *Journal of Rheumatology* **23**, 841–5.

Puechal, X. et al. (1995). Peripheral neuropathy with necrotizing vasculitis in rheumatoid arthritis. *Arthritis and Rheumatism* **38**, 1618–29.

Quismorio, F.P. et al. (1983). IgG rheumatoid factors and anti-nuclear antibodies in rheumatoid vasculitis. *Clinical and Experimental Immunology* **53**, 333–40.

Raman, D. and Haslock, I. (1982). Trochanteritic bursitis—a frequent cause of 'hip' pain in rheumatoid arthritis. *Annals of the Rheumatic Diseases* **41**, 602–3.

Rashba, E.J., Rowe, J.M., and Packman, C.H. (1996). Treatment of the neutropenia of Felty syndrome. *Blood Review* **10**, 177–84.

Rau, R. and Herborn, G. (1996). Healing phenomena of erosive changes in rheumatoid arthritis patients undergoing disease-modifying antirheumatic drug treatment. *Arthritis and Rheumatism* **39**, 162–8.

Rau, R. et al. (1998). A new method for scoring radiographic changes in RA. *Journal of Rheumatology* **25**, 2094–106.

Resnick, D. (1975). Patterns of migration of the femoral head in osteoarthritis of the hip: roentgenographic–pathologic correlation and comparison with rheumatoid arthritis. *Am J Roentgenol Radium Ther Nucl Med* **124** (1), 62–74.

Resnick, D. (1976). Rheumatoid arthritis. In *Bone and Joint Imaging* 2nd edn. (ed. D. Resnick), pp. 195–209. Philadelphia PA: W.B. Saunders.

Ropes, M.W. et al. (1956). Proposed diagnostic criteria for rheumatoid arthritis. *Bulletin of Rheumatic Diseases* **7**, 121–4.

Roubenoff, R. et al. (1992). Rheumatoid cachexia, depletion of lean body mass in rheumatoid arthritis. Possible association with tumor necrosis factor. *Journal of Rheumatology* **19**, 1505–10.

Schellekens, G.A. et al. (1998). Citrulline is an essential constituent of antigenic determinants recognized by rheumatoid arthritis-specific auto-antibodies. *Journal of Clinical Investigation* **101**, 273–81.

Schellekens, G.A. et al. (2000). The diagnostic properties of rheumatoid arthritis antibodies recognizing a cyclic citrullinated peptide. *Arthritis and Rheumatism* **43**, 155–63.

Schiff, M. et al. (1999). Comparison of ACR response, numeric ACR and ACR ANC as measures of clinical improvement in rheumatoid arthritis clinical trials. *Arthritis and Rheumatism* **42** (Suppl.), 881.

Schmidt, W.A. (2001). Value of sonography in diagnosis of rheumatoid arthritis. *Lancet* **357**, 1056–7.

Scott, D.G.I., Bacon, P.A., and Tribe, C.R. (1981). Systemic rheumatoid vasculitis: a clinical and laboratory study of 50 cases. *Medicine (Baltimore)* **60**, 288–97.

Sebbag, M. et al. (1995). The antiperinuclear factor and the so-called antikeratin antibodies are the same rheumatoid arthritis—specific autoantibodies. *Journal of Clinical Investigation* **95**, 2672–9.

Shannon, T.M. and Gale, E. (1992). Non-cardiac manifestations of rheumatoid arthritis in the thorax. *Journal of Thorax Imaging* **7**, 19–29.

Sharp, J.T. et al. (1971). Method of scoring the progression of radiologic changes in rheumatoid arthritis. Correlation of radiologic, clinical and laboratory abnormalities. *Arthritis and Rheumatism* **14**, 706–20.

Silman, A.J., Kay, A., and Brennan, P. (1992). Timing of pregnancy in relation to the onset of rheumatoid arthritis. *Arthritis and Rheumatism* **35**, 152–5.

Silman, A.J. and Hochberg, M.C. *Epidemiology of the Rheumatic Diseases.* Oxford: Oxford University Press, 1993.

Silman, A.J., Newman, J., and MacGregor, A.J. (1996). Cigarette smoking increases the risk of rheumatoid arthritis: results from a nationwide study of disease discordant twins. *Arthritis and Rheumatism* **39**, 732–5.

Silverstein, F.E. et al. (2000). Gastrointestinal toxicity with celecoxib versus nonsteroidal anti-inflammatory drugs for osteoarthritis and rheumatoid arthritis. The CLASS study, a randomized controlled trial. *Journal of the American Medical Association* **284**, 1247–55.

Simkin, P.A. (1995). Synovial perfusion and synovial fluid solutes. *Annals of the Rheumatic Diseases* **54**, 424–8.

Simon, M. et al. (1993). The cytokeratin filament-aggregating protein filaggrin is the target of the so-called 'antikeratin antibodies', autoantibodies specific for rheumatoid arthritis. *Journal for Clinical Investigation* **92**, 1387–93.

Singh, G. et al. (1994). Toxicity profile of disease modifying antirheumatic drugs and rheumatoid arthritis. *Journal of Rheumatology* **18**, 188–94.

Smiley, J.D., Sachs, C., and Ziff, M. (1968). *In vitro* synthesis of immunoglobulin by rheumatoid synovial membrane. *Journal for Clinical Investigation* **47**, 624–32.

Smolen, J.S. et al. (1995). Validity and reliability of the 28-joint count for the assessment of rheumatoid arthritis activities. *Arthritis and Rheumatism* **38**, 38–43.

Smolen, J.S. et al. (1999). Efficacy and safety of leflunomide compared with placebo sulfasalazine in active rheumatoid arthritis: a double-blind, randomised, multicentre trial. *Lancet* **353**, 259–66.

Smolen, J. et al. (2000). Consensus statement on the initiation and continuation of tumor necrosis factor blocking therapies in rheumatoid arthritis. *Annals of the Rheumatic Diseases* **59**, 504–5.

Sokka, T. and Hannonen, P. (1999). Utility of disease modifying antirheumatic drugs in 'sawtooth' strategy. A prospective study of early rheumatoid arthritis patients up to 15 years. *Annals of the Rheumatic Diseases* **58**, 618–22.

Spector, T.D. et al. (1993). Risk of vertebral fracture in women with rheumatoid arthritis. *British Journal of Rheumatology* **306**, 58.

Stenger, A.A.M.E. et al. (1998). Early effective suppression of inflammation in rheumatoid arthritis reduces radiographic progression. *British Journal of Rheumatology* **37**, 1157–63.

Stucki, G. et al. (1995). Comparison of the validity and reliability of self-reported articular indices. *British Journal of Rheumatology* **34**, 760–6.

Suzuki, A. et al. (1994). Cause of death in 81 autopsied patients with rheumatoid arthritis. *Journal of Rheumatology* **21**, 33–6.

Symmons, D.P.M. (1989). Lymphopenia in rheumatoid arthritis. *Journal of the Royal Society of Medicine* **82**, 462–3.

Symmons, D. and Harrison, B. (2000). Early inflammatory polyarthritis: results from the Norfolk Arthritis Register with a review of the literature. I. Risk factors for the development of inflammatory polyarthritis and rheumatoid arthritis. *Rheumotology* **38**, 835.

Symmons, D.P.M. et al. (1994). The incidence of rheumatoid arthritis in the United Kingdom: Results from the Norfolk Arthritis Register. *British Journal of Rheumatology* **33**, 735–9.

Ten Wolde, S. et al. (1996). Randomised placebo-controlled study of stopping second-line drugs in rheumatoid arthritis. *Lancet* **347**, 347–52.

Tessler, H.H. (1985). The eye in rheumatic disease. *Bulletin of the Rheumatic Diseases* **35**, 1–8.

Thomson, B.M., Mundy, G.R., and Chambers, T.J. (1987). Tumour necrosis factor alpha and beta induce osteoblastic cells to stimulate osteoclastic bone resorption. *Journal of Immunology* **138**, 775–9.

Thorne, C. et al. (1982). Liver disease in Felty's syndrome. *American Journal of Medicine* **73**, 35–40.

Tugwell, P. et al. (1995). Combination therapy with cyclosporine and methotrexate in severe rheumatoid arthritis. *New England Journal of Medicine* **333**, 137–41.

Turesson, C. et al. (2000). Predictors of extra-articular manifestations in rheumatoid arthritis. *Scandinavian Journal of Rheumatology* **29**, 358–64.

Uhlig, T. et al. (1998). The incidence and severity of rheumatoid arthritis, results from a county register in Oslo, Norway. *Journal of Rheumatology* **25**, 1078–84.

Uhlig, T. et al. (2000). The course of rheumatoid arthritis and predictors of psychological, physical and radiographic outcome after 5 years of follow up. *Rheumatology* **39**, 732–41.

van de Putte, L.B.A. et al. (1998). Early treatment of rheumatoid arthritis: rationale, evidence and implications. *Annals of the Rheumatic Diseases* **57**, 511–12.

van der Heide, A. et al. (1996). The effectiveness of early treatment with 'second-line' antirheumatics: a randomized, controlled trial. *Annals of Internal Medicine* **8**, 699–707.

van der Heijde, D.M.F.M. et al. (1989). Effects of hydroxychloroquine and sulphasalazine on progression of joint damage in rheumatoid arthritis. *Lancet* **13**, 1036–8.

van der Heijde, D.M.F.M. et al. (1992). Biannual radiographic assessment of hands and feet in a three-year prospective follow-up of patients with early rheumatoid arthritis. *Arthritis and Rheumatism* **35**, 26–34.

van der Heijde, D.M.F.M. et al. (1993a). Validity of single variables and indices in measure disease activity in rheumatoid arthritis. *Journal of Rheumatology* **20**, 535–7.

van der Heijde, D.M.F.M. et al. (1993b). Development of a disease activity score based on judgement in clinical practice by rheumatologists. *Journal of Rheumatology* **20**, 579–81.

van der Heijde, D.M.F.M. et al. (1999). Reading radiographs in chronological order, in pairs or as single films has important implications for the discriminative power of rheumatoid arthritis clinical trials. *Rheumatology (Oxford)* **38**, 1213–20.

van der Lubbe, P.A. et al. (1995). A randomized, double-blind, placebo-controlled study of DC4 monoclonal antibody therapy in early rheumatoid arthritis. *Arthritis and Rheumatism* **38**, 1097–106.

van der Veen, M.J. et al. (1994). Infection rate and use of antibiotics in patients with rheumatoid arthritis treated with methotrexate. *Annals of the Rheumatic Diseases* **53**, 224–8.

van Ede, A.E. et al. (2001). Effect of folic or folinic acid supplementation on the toxicity and efficacy of methotrexate in rheumatoid arthritis. *Arthritis and Rheumatism* **44**, 151–2.

van Gestel, A.M. et al. (1996). Development and validation of the European League Against Rheumatism response criteria for rheumatoid arthritis. *Arthritis and Rheumatism* **39**, 34–40.

van Leeuwen, M.A. et al. (1993). The acute-phase responses in relation to radiographic progression in early rheumatoid arthritis: a prospective study during the first 3 years of the disease. *British Journal of Rheumatology* **32**, 9–13.

van Leeuwen, M.A. and van Rijswijk, M.H. (1994). Acute phase proteins in the monitoring of inflammatory disorders. *Baillière's Clinical Rheumatology* **8**, 531–52.

van Riel, P.L.C.M. (1992). Provisional guidelines for measuring disease activity in clinical trials in rheumatoid arthritis. *British Journal of Rheumatology* **31**, 793–6.

van Riel, P.L.C.M. and van de Putte, L.B.A. (1994). Clinical assessment and clinical trials in rheumatoid arthritis. *Current Opinion in Rheumatology* **6**, 132–9.

van Riel, P.L.C.M. and van Gestel, A.M. (1999). Are measures of outcome helpful indicators? In *Challenges in Rheumatoid Arthritis* (ed. H.A. Bird and M.L. Snaith), pp. 93–105. Oxford: Blackwell Science.

van Riel, P.L.M.C. and van Gestel, A.M. (2001). Area under the curve for the American College of Rheumatology improvement criteria: a valid addition to existing criteria in rheumatoid arthritis? (Letter). *Arthritis and Rheumatism* **7**, 1719–22.

Vandenbroucke, J.P., Hazevoet, H.M., and Cats, A. (1984). Survival and cause of death in rheumatoid arthritis: a 25 year prospective follow-up. *Journal of Rheumatology* **11**, 158–61.

Vincent, C. et al. (1999). Anti-perinuclear factor compared with the so called antikeratin antibodies to human epidermis filaggrin, in the diagnosis of arthritides. *Annals of the Rheumatic Diseases* **58**, 42–8.

Visser, H. et al. (2000). How to diagnose rheumatoid arthritis early? A prediction model for persistent (erosive) disease. *Arthritis and Rheumatism* **43**, 154.

Vliet Vlieland, T.P.M., Breedveld, F.C., and Hazes, J.M.W. (1997). The two-year follow-up of a randomized comparison of in-patient multidisciplinary team care and routine out-patient care for active rheumatoid arthritis. *British Journal of Rheumatology* **36**, 82–5.

Voskuyl, A.E. et al. (1995). The mortality of rheumatoid vasculitis compared to rheumatoid arthritis. *Arthritis and Rheumatism* **39**, 266–71.

Voskuyl, A.E. et al. (1996). Factors associated with the development of vasculitis in rheumatoid arthritis: results of a case–control study. *Annals of the Rheumatic Diseases* **55**, 190–2.

Vreugdenhil, G. et al. (1990). Anaemia in rheumatoid arthritis: the role of iron, vitamin B12, and folic acid deficiency, and erythropoietin responsiveness. *Annals of the Rheumatic Diseases* **49**, 93–8.

Wakefield, R.J. et al. (2000). The value of sonography in the detection of bone erosions in patients with rheumatoid arthritis. *Arthritis and Rheumatism* **43**, 2762–70.

Wallach, S. et al. (2000). Effects of risedronate treatment on bone density and vertebral fracture in patients on corticosteroid therapy. *Calcification Tissue International* **67**, 277–85.

Wållberg-Jonsson, S. et al. (1999). Extent of inflammation predicts cardiovascular disease and overall mortality in seropositive rheumatoid arthritis. A retrospective cohort study from disease onset. *Journal of Rheumatology* **26**, 2562–71.

Ward, M.W. (1993). Clinical measures in rheumatoid arthritis: which are most useful in assessing patients? *Journal of Rheumatology* **21**, 17–21.

Watts, R.A. et al. (1994). The incidence of rheumatoid vasculitis in the Norwich Health Authority. *British Journal of Rheumatology* **33**, 832–3.

Westgeest, A.A.A. et al. (1987). Antiperinuclear factor: indicator of more severe disease in seronegative rheumatoid arthritis. *Journal of Rheumatology* **14**, 893–7.

Wijnands, M.J.H. and van Riel, P.L.C.M. (1995). Management of adverse effects of disease modifying antirheumatic drugs. *Drug Safety* **13**, 219–27.

Wiles, N.J. et al. (2001). Reduced disability at five years with early treatment of inflammatory polyarthritis. *Arthritis and Rheumatism* **44**, 1033–42.

Wolfe, F., Cathey, M.A., and Roberts, F.K. (1991). The latex test revisited. *Arthritis and Rheumatism* **34**, 951–60.

Wollheim, F.A. and Saxne, T. (1992). Markers of cartilge destruction. In *Rheumatoid Arthritis—Recent Research Advances* (ed. J. Smolen). Berlin: Springer-Verlag.

Young-Min, S.A., Cawston, T.E., and Griffiths, I.D. (2001). Markers of joint destruction: principles, problems, and potential. *Annals of the Rheumatic Diseases* **60**, 545–8.

Ziff, M. (1990). The rheumatoid nodule. *Arthritis and Rheumatism* **33**, 761–7.

Zonneveld, I.M. et al. (1996). Methotrexate osteopathy in long-term, low-dose methotrexate treatment for psoriasis and rheumatoid arthritis. *Archives of Rheumatology* **132**, 184–7.

6.3.3 Rheumatoid arthritis—management

Sarah J. Bingham, Mark A. Quinn, and Paul Emery

The importance of accurate (and early) diagnosis

Recent evidence (see below) supports the concept that the optimal outcome of therapy in rheumatoid arthritis (RA) is likely to be achieved with early, accurate diagnosis and appropriate intervention. However, the very early diagnosis of RA can be difficult. RA may be indistinguishable from other conditions such as post-viral arthropathies, early spondyloarthropathy, and other self-limiting arthritides that may satisfy the 1987 American College of Rheumatology (ACR) classification criteria for RA (Arnett et al. 1988). The important questions to answer in early polyarthritis are: (i) Is it inflammatory? (ii) Is it persistent? (iii) Is it structurally damaging? The last is relevant only if there is persistent inflammation, but is important in confirming the need for intervention. If present, the physician will have greater confidence in instituting potentially toxic therapies.

Is it inflammatory?

Distinguishing early inflammatory arthritis from non-inflammatory disease in the very early stages may be difficult. Acute phase markers may be normal in upto 50 per cent and radiographs in upto 80 per cent of early RA patients. Serology can be unhelpful or even confusing. Often the only factors that differentiate inflammatory disease are clinical and are given in Table 1. Frequently a number of factors are used to determine if it is inflammatory, important is a classical history, but also examination findings and supportive serology.

Is it persistent?

Having established that inflammatory arthritis is present, the next issue is to differentiate self-limiting from persistent disease. Of the parameters that have been examined, which include rheumatoid factor, C-reactive protein (CRP), HLA–DRB1 status, and ACR classification criteria for RA, symptom duration greater than 12 weeks (Green et al. 1999) or 14 weeks (Tunn and Bacon 1993) appears to be the best single predictor of persistence. In disease of short duration the level of CRP, ACR criteria, etc. have poor predictive value (Green et al. 1999). After 12 weeks, conventional predictors of persistence are more reliable and are detailed in Table 2. Genetics or more specifically the presence of the shared-epitope has little value in predicting disease persistence in the total population of patients with early polyarthritis (Harrison et al. 1998), but may be of use in patients seronegative for rheumatoid factor (Green et al. 1999). New imaging methods such as ultrasound (US) and magnetic resonance imaging (MRI) may also allow even earlier diagnosis, by sensitively diagnosing synovitis, allowing earlier diagnosis of persistence (see later).

Is it damaging?

Plain radiographs of the hands and feet are the standard method of assessing damage. The first sites most commonly affected are the fifth metatarsal

Table 1 Early symptoms and signs of RA

Joint swelling
Symmetrical symptoms
MCP and MTP involvement
Significant early morning stiffness
Good response to NSAIDs

Table 2 Factors which determine persistence in early inflammatory polyarthritis

Symptoms >12 weeks
RF positivity
Wrist/MCP/PIP involvement or large joints
Female sex
ACR RA criteria, only if >12 weeks of symptoms

head and ulnar styloid process. Published data suggest upto 40 per cent (Hannonen et al. 1993) of patients have irreversible erosive damage on plain radiographs at presentation at standard clinics (after less than 6 months of symptoms) and even with the early arthritis clinic (EAC) approach, 25 per cent of early RA patients are erosive at outset (van der Horst-Bruinsma et al. 1998). However, new imaging techniques demonstrate bone changes occur even earlier than was first thought. Bone oedema, the MRI precursor to erosions, can be seen in patients after less than 4 weeks of symptoms (McGonagle et al. 1999a) and ultrasound has shown to detect 6.5 times as many erosions in 7.5 times more patients than plain radiography in the metacarpophalangeal (MCP) joints in early RA (Wakefield et al. 2000). Damage is therefore more widespread in early disease than conventional radiography detects. The new imaging modalities are likely to have a role in the future for earlier detection of damage.

The consequences of damage can be measured indirectly as functional impairment, quality of life and also, more recently work disability or job loss. In terms of function almost all patients will exhibit impairment prior to introduction of therapy. The extent of disability at presentation is proportional to inflammatory activity (Devlin et al. 1997) but also functional reserve, and therefore age. In early disease disability appears reversible; however, if therapy is delayed more than 2 years, functional impairment is likely to be permanent (Munro et al. 1998). A major reason for this is that disability in late disease is determined by joint damage rather than inflammatory activity and therefore is less amenable to therapy.

What evidence is there to support early treatment?

Synovitis is widespread

Both US and MRI (Conaghan et al. 1998a) have demonstrated that synovitis is more widespread at presentation than is detected by conventional clinical examination in early RA. In early oligoarthritis, US has also shown sub-clinical synovitis to be widespread, with upto 50 per cent actually having polyarticular disease and the presence of sub-clinical disease correlated with persistence and poor outcome (Wakefield et al. 1998). In support of these findings both arthroscopy (Kraan et al. 1998) and blind biopsy (Fitzgerald et al. 1991) have demonstrated evidence of synovial inflammation in clinically normal knees of RA patients.

Spontaneous remission is rare

The number of patients whose disease remits without therapy is unknown. Longitudinal studies in RA suggest the sustained remission rate is between 5 and 7 per cent (Harrison et al. 1996a; Eberhardt and Fex 1998), which can be increased to approximately 35 per cent with more aggressive therapeutic approaches (Boers et al. 1997; Quinn et al. 2001a). There are further difficulties in assessing remission, as the definition is variable and often subjective, actually representing low disease activity as opposed to true absence of disease or cure. The most widely used definition is that of ACR remission (Pinals et al. 1981). This utilizes a number of parameters subjective and objective but includes measures that are not necessarily disease specific. Widespread synovitis in patients satisfying ACR remission criteria using both MRI and US has been demonstrated (Brown et al. 2001). True spontaneous remission (representing absence of disease) virtually never occurs in correctly diagnosed RA patients. The only time for remission appears to be very early on and baseline parameters have so far have been unable to predict which patients will remit (Harrison et al. 1996a).

Inflammation = damage

Measures of the acute phase response, particularly CRP, correlate with progression of radiographic damage, loss of function, and bone mineral density (Gough et al. 1994a; Fex et al. 1997; van Leeuwen et al. 1997). Suppression of CRP results in at least stabilization of the respective parameters (Dawes et al. 1986; Stenger et al. 1998), consistent with the paradigm: inflammation × time = damage.

From longitudinal MRI studies in early RA, synovitis precedes MRI bone oedema and subsequent erosion development, furthermore erosions occur only in joints with synovitis (McGonagle et al. 1999a). This accords with other published work where radiographic progression correlates with the presence of clinically detected synovitis (Boers et al. 2000). More importantly, it has been demonstrated that if synovitis is adequately suppressed, MRI shows reduced bone oedema and absence of new bony lesions (Conaghan et al. 1999). It therefore appears that the adequate suppression of synovitis prevents progression of bone damage.

In summary, at presentation damage may have already occurred, synovitis may be more widespread than is clinically apparent, spontaneous remission is rare and risk of job loss is high. Therefore, there appears little benefit from withholding therapy or adopting a 'wait and see' approach once the diagnosis of persistent synovitis has been correctly made. But what evidence is there to suggest that intervention at this stage is effective and alters outcome?

Patients treated early do well

Patients, who present early to rheumatologists, do better than those presenting late. In an analysis of 1435 patients from 11 different studies, disease duration was of foremost importance in predicting response to disease modifying antirheumatic drug (DMARD) therapy (Anderson et al. 2000). Patients presenting with less than 1 year disease duration showed a response in 53 per cent, whereas later groups 1–2, 2–5, 5–10, and over 10 years showed diminished response with time. In a study of 448 RA patients, those who present with less than 5 years disease, maintained a lower mortality ratio over 21.5 years of follow up compared to late presenters (Symmons et al. 1998). Other studies looking at any DMARD use versus non-steroidal anti-inflammatory drug (NSAID) or no therapy, strongly favour DMARD use with respect to long-term disability index (Fries et al. 1996) and also deformed/damaged joint and radiographic score (Abu-Shakra et al. 1998).

DMARD treatment is not necessarily more toxic

In practical terms, 90 per cent of patients diagnosed with RA are treated with DMARDs within 3 years of diagnosis (Emery and Salmon 1995); therefore the majority of patients are eventually subjected to potential DMARD toxicity and early introduction is unlikely to result in over exposure. NSAIDs have been compared to DMARDs by calculating a toxicity index derived from symptoms, abnormal laboratory measures, and hospitalizations related to treatment (Fries et al. 1991, 1993). The comparisons show that some commonly used NSAIDs have toxicity indices considerably greater than intramuscular (IM) gold and hydroxychloroquine (HCQ) and comparable to methotrexate (MTX) and azathioprine (AZA). In context, DMARD toxicity is no worse than that of long-term NSAID use. From this evidence delaying use of DMARDs on toxicity grounds is unfounded.

How to make a diagnosis/classification

Disease diagnosis and classification in the early stages, as already briefly discussed, can be difficult. The principle reason for this is that the classical features of RA such as radiographic erosions, rheumatoid nodules, and clinical findings, for example, wrist/MCP subluxation, ulnar deviation, and wasting of the interossei occur late and are absent at the time of presentation in the majority of patients. Thus, the very fact that both nodules and radiographic changes are included in the ACR classification criteria of RA reduces the sensitivity of the criteria in early disease (Harrison et al. 1998; Green et al. 1999). However, once disease is established the criteria have greater discriminant validity. It must be remembered that these criteria were not devised for, nor intended for use in, early RA. Therefore, in early disease, evidence of persistent inflammation, the pattern of joint involvement, with or without supportive laboratory data should be sufficient for the

Table 3 Persistent inflammatory symmetrical arthritis (PISA) scoring system[a]

Prognostic factor	Score
RF positive	1
HLA–DR1 or DR4	1
CRP >20 mg/l	1
Female sex	1
HAQ raw score >4 and ≤11	1
HAQ raw score >11	2
Score	Total = out of 6

[a] PISA is a prerequisite for this scoring system.
A score of ≥3 indicates poor prognosis.

institution of therapy. Such a pragmatic approach, will identify patients at risk of permanent damage and has led to an alternative classification which targets patients with persistent inflammatory symmetrical arthritis (PISA, Table 3) (Emery 1997). The essential prerequisite is persistent inflammation (and not the clinical diagnosis of RA) although the majority of such patients ultimately have RA and prognosis can be predicted using the PISA score.

New imaging modalities such as MRI and US are increasingly available. Such tools, as already described, have greater sensitivity for detecting both synovitis and erosions compared to clinical diagnosis or conventional radiography and may have an impact on diagnosis and management (Karim et al. 2001). These modalities should allow earlier classification of IA and possibly true targeted earlier intervention. An anatomical explanation for 'good prognosis RA' has already been reported using MRI assessment of metacarpophalangeal joints (McGonagle et al. 1999b). Findings of intrasynovial disease and bone oedema distinguished poor prognosis from good prognosis patients who had predominantly capsular and extra-articular pathology.

Future classifications of arthritis may also include synovial appearances at arthroscopy, and features seen on histopathology and immunohistochemistry. Differences have been reported in macroscopic synovial vascularity in early rheumatoid and psoriatic arthritis (Reece et al. 1999) and also RA and spondyloarthropathy (Baeten et al. 2000). Differential expression of the pro-angiogenic factors VEGF (Fearon et al. 1999) and serum matrix metalloproteinases (MMP-9) (Fraser et al. 2001) in these arthropathies may explain the resulting differences in macroscopic appearance and may therefore have future use for classification purposes.

Prognostic factors

Disease presentation

The type of presentation may be prognostic in RA. Patients with an acute presentation and high CRP tend to have a good prognosis (van der Heijde et al. 1992; Green et al. 1999). One explanation is a misclassification of patients with self-limiting symmetrical small joint arthritides, for example, post-viral arthropathy, etc. as RA or a true sub-group of RA patients. Such patients differ from the classical insidious disease onset characteristic of the majority of RA patients and may have a different pathogenesis (McGonagle et al. 1999b).

Rheumatoid factor

Rheumatoid factor (RF) has been the most consistent predictor of poor prognosis across both inflammatory polyarthritis and RA cohort studies with outcome measured by functional deterioration/radiographic damage. However, it is not specific for RA being found in other connective tissue diseases, transiently during some infections and in upto 15 per cent of the population aged more than 65 (Maddison 1993). It is present in 75 per cent of patients with RA.

In a large early polyarthritis cohort of 486 patients, RF seropositivity predicted both radiological erosions and poor functional outcome and seronegativity best predicted remission at 3 years (Harrison et al. 2001). Similarly studies have found RF negativity to be the best predictors of self-limiting disease in early undifferentiated arthritis in cohorts of 65 and 532 patients, respectively (Tunn and Bacon 1993; Wolfe et al. 1993). In established RA, findings are equally consistent with RF positivity predicting both short-term radiological progression in the first year (van der Heide et al. 1995a) and long-term damage after 6 years (Möttönnen et al. 1998). In early RA, RF seropositivity has been shown to have a relative risk for the development of erosions at 1 year of 13.49 (sensitivity 95 per cent, specificity 39 per cent) (Gough et al. 1994b). In a retrospective study to investigate the effect of age (under 60 versus over 60) on outcome after 5 years of disease RF positive patients (of both age groups) had suffered significantly more disease activity and radiographic damage than those seronegative for RF (van Schardenburg et al. 1993). The mortality of the seropositive patients (but not seronegative) was higher than in the general population with the relative risk of dying six times greater in seropositive patients. RF is also a significant predictor of short- and long-term functional disability as assessed by the Health Assessment Questionnaire (HAQ) (van der Heide et al. 1995b).

These studies indicate that RF seropositivity at the onset of RA is associated with a more progressive disease course resulting in increased disability and radiological progression. In addition, it is possible to increase the predictive value of the RF by combining it with other factors such as the shared-epitope, a measure of acute phase response, the haemoglobin level, and the number of platelets. Once disease is established, the differences between seronegative and positive patients seem to diminish (Panayi et al. 1987).

Since the introduction of isotype specific assays for RF a number of studies have been published concerning the clinical value of isotype analysis. All isotypes of RF have been shown to be associated with a more progressive disease course. However, IgA RF appears to be more specifically associated with the development of erosions in early disease and a persistent disease course, although with a reduced sensitivity (van Zeben et al. 1992).

In summary, the presence of RF in a patient with symmetrical small joint disease indicates persistent disease and poor prognosis. The major value of RF has been in the predicting severity and its association with a high frequency of systemic and extra-articular manifestations.

C-reactive protein

The CRP is generally accepted as the most accurate measure of the acute phase response and hence of tissue inflammation. In the normal individual the basal concentration is extremely low or undetectable. In response to inflammation the concentration can rapidly increase upto 1000-fold. The CRP is not affected by the confounding factors that influence the ESR and plasma viscosity. However, as a prognostic marker CRP has limitations; it is non-specific and can only be interpreted in the light of clinical information, the elevated CRP must be attributable to the symptoms and signs and not coincidental, furthermore there is a significant interpatient variation to a given stimulus. Also a patient's CRP concentration can increase many times from basal level and still lie within the normal range whilst being markedly abnormal for that individual. Of concern also is that upto 50 per cent of patients may have a normal CRP at time of diagnosis (Emery 1997). Whereas a single CRP measurement is somewhat unhelpful, there is substantial evidence that a persistently elevated acute phase response is associated with an increased rate of radiological progression, poor functional outcome, and the development of generalized osteoporosis (Scott et al. 1987; Gough et al. 1994a; van Leeuwen et al. 1997). In addition, a fall in CRP in response to second line therapy represents the first objective sign of clinical improvement (Sheeran et al. 1990). It has been argued that using time-integrated values of CRP measurements (i.e. area under the curve) is the most accurate method for quantifying the fluctuating activity of the acute phase response and a significant correlation with radiological damage has been shown (Plant et al. 2000).

The shared-epitope

Many studies have looked at the prognostic utility of the shared-epitope or HLA–DRB1*04 alleles. Several longitudinal studies suggest a correlation between possession of the shared-epitope and both radiographic progression (Gough et al. 1994b) and persistence (Harrison and Symmons 2000). However, the literature can be conflicting (Harrison et al. 1999; Rau et al. 2000). Such variability between studies can be explained by the selection of patients and new therapeutic approaches. Patients with early, untreated disease will differ from those with chronic disabling disease. For example, patients seen late in disease have already been selected for poor prognosis and subsequently the prevalence of the shared-epitope will be high, upto 80 per cent. Many of these patients will also have poor prognostic clinical features and the comparator group without the shared-epitope will be small and therefore have little power to show a difference. Paradoxically it has also been shown that possession of the shared-epitope a predictor of a favourable response to triple therapy (O'Dell et al. 1998). The latter suggests new approaches to treatment may influence the natural progression of RA. Subsequently, as therapies become more effective the prognostic utility of the shared-epitope may diminish. Recent studies have consistently shown that the shared-epitope has particular prognostic utility in seronegative patients for both disease severity (Rau et al. 2000; Mattey et al. 2001) and persistence (Harrison et al. 1999).

Functional impairment and radiography

Several studies have demonstrated baseline functional impairment, measured using the HAQ, to be the best predictor of future disability (Harrison et al. 1996b; Eberhardt and Fex 1998). Similar studies show radiographic erosions at presentation predict further radiographic damage (van der Heijde et al. 1992). However, in essence such functional and radiographic data are somewhat self-fulfilling, as severe disease at baseline is predicting subsequent severe disease. Of perhaps more utility and far greater prognostic potential are the newer imaging methods of US and MRI, which have greater sensitivity in detecting both synovitis and boney changes at an early stage. These modalities have far greater prognostic potential.

Age/sex/smoking

Age at disease onset would appear to influence functional outcome but not radiographic outcome (van Schardenburg et al. 1993). This is likely to result from reduced functional reserves in the elderly population. In a study of late onset (>65 years) versus early onset disease (<65 years), however, no differences in disease course were found, with RF, DR4, and elevated acute phase predicting damage irrespective of age (Pease et al. 1999).

In determining the impact of sex on outcome, several studies have reported worse prognosis for females in terms of function (Eberhardt and Fex 1998), radiographic damage (Feigenbaum et al. 1979), and higher remission rates in males.

Several papers have identified an increase risk of developing RA in smokers (Heliövaara et al. 1993; Uhlig et al. 1999). Published associations with smoking include poor prognosis and a higher incidence of extra-articular manifestations such as vasculitis, interstitial lung disease, nodules, sicca symptoms, and neuropathy, but other studies examining smoking in RA have failed to show significant prognostic results in terms of function and damage (Harrison et al. 2001).

Anti-CCP/MMPs

Recently, data have supported the use of serological tests for RA in diagnosis and prognosis. Anti-cyclic citrullinated peptide (anti-CCP) antibodies are a collective term for antibodies that recognize filagrin. Not only have they shown high specificity (Schellekens et al. 2000) but also prognostic utility in terms of damage and functional disability (Kroot et al. 2000). However, what these antibodies add in real terms over and above measurement of RF is still to be confirmed. MMP-3 may also be useful in predicting damage in early RA (Posthummus et al. 1999).

Assessing and monitoring disease activity

Two validated composite measures which utilize both subjective and objective assessments are available and have been advocated for use in monitoring patients in the outpatient clinic. The first are the ACR improvement criteria based on the ACR core set of disease activity variables (Felson et al. 1995). These criteria are dependent on improvement from baseline variables. ACR 20, ACR 50, and ACR 70 response represent a 20, 50, and 70 per cent improvement from baseline, respectively. The improvement score is based on percentage improvement of the swollen and tender joint counts in addition to three out of five of the remaining variables (Table 4). In this example, the reduction in tender joint count is the limiting variable. Such data are of greatest utility when therapeutic efficacy is being assessed in clinical trials, the purpose for which they were originally designed. In clinical practice simply demonstrating an improvement from outset, may still leave the patient with an unacceptable level of inflammation. Also, while useful in established disease where disease is often widespread, the clinical utility of these criteria are diminished when applied to early patients where disease is in evolution (Quinn et al. 2001b).

Perhaps of greater clinical utility is the Disease Activity Score (DAS) (van der Heijde et al. 1990). This provides a composite measure of disease activity based on joint counts, ESR, and patient global assessment of general health rather than measuring response. This is not dependent on baseline parameters to show a difference and therefore provides a more absolute measure of disease severity, which can be followed over time. The DAS28 based on joint counts of 28 joints is easier to use in the clinic and does not utilize Ritchie Index like the original DAS (Prevoo et al. 1995). However, in early disease it may not be as sensitive as the DAS based on the 68 count. The DAS has proven prognostic utility with respect to both function and radiographic progression (van der Heijde et al. 1992).

Whether such composite measures are superior to their individual components remains a subject for debate. Predictors of prognosis such as CRP, joint counts, and imaging may all have prognostic utility individually, at present it is unclear how frequently and successfully these could be used as single monitoring measures. Such parameters may be sufficient individually for monitoring purposes.

Joint counts are utilized globally in clinical RA trials. Unfortunately, clinical examination is considerably less sensitive than US or MRI in detecting synovitis. Further problems exist in late disease when distinguishing between synovitis and bony swelling and noting the considerable subjectivity of measures of tenderness and swelling. Radiographs are commonly

Table 4 An example of an ACR improvement calculation

Parameter	Baseline score	Follow-up score	Per cent improvement
Swollen joint count	10	2	80
Tender joint count	5	3	40
HAQ (raw score)	16	10	38
Patients' pain VAS	76	24	68
Patients' disease activity VAS	90	28	69
Physicians disease activity VAS	65	10	85
CRP (mg/l)	32	6	81
ACR improvement score			40

used for monitoring, usually annually in the early years of disease until damage progression is reduced. A significant problem is the lag time between inflammatory joint disease and the appearance of radiographic erosions. Another problem highlighted by the findings from US and MRI is that in using a two-dimensional modality to assess a three-dimensional defect accuracy and sensitivity are lost. While perhaps of limited use in assessing an individual patient, for the purposes of clinical trials they provide an objective outcome measure of cumulative damage. A number of scoring systems and subsequent modifications, based on joint space narrowing and erosions, have been produced with the Larsen and Sharp methods being the most commonly used (Sharp et al. 1971; Larsen et al. 1977). Using these scoring systems, therapeutic arms can be compared in a blinded fashion by independent assessors removing any patient or investigator bias.

There is obvious potential of both US and MRI for monitoring disease activity in RA. Both modalities offer improved sensitivity and accuracy of joint assessment for synovitis and damage. MRI, however, is likely to be limited due to cost and availability. US, however, offers a relatively cheap, easy to learn, non-invasive, three-dimensional imaging modality which can be performed in the outpatient setting. Multiple joints can be assessed at any one time and both synovitis and erosions quantified. It is unlikely that US will be used for all patients, but may be most useful in cases where there clinical uncertainty such as a discrepancy between symptoms and signs.

Surrogate markers—health status questionnaires

These measures assess the impact of disease on an individual. In an ideal disease model for RA, disease activity would reflect functional impairment and functional impairment would reflect quality of life. Unfortunately due to the nature of RA this statement is only partially true. A number of self-administered questionnaires are available to assess function in RA. The most widely used is the Stanford HAQ (Fries et al. 1980). Using this tool two patterns of functional impairment emerge in RA. In early RA, prior to the development of irreversible bone damage, disability correlates with inflammatory activity. However, in established disease, when joint damage has occurred, function is largely determined by extent of damage (Guilleman et al. 1992). Deterioration of functional status is an indicator of therapeutic failure and is likely to result in both disability and even job loss. Patients exhibiting progressive functional loss should be targeted with aggressive treatment regimes.

Principles of management

For many years drugs used in patients with RA produced such a high withdrawal rate due to both toxicity and lack of efficacy that there was some doubt whether they had any impact on disease progression. With better study design and more efficient use of drugs it is now clear that DMARDs do alter the disease course as evidenced by retardation of bony erosions and improvement in function (Stenger et al. 1998). Until recently, standard treatment for RA consisted of sequential monotherapy with different DMARDs which replace each other as the individual drugs became toxic or ineffective. However, add-on studies in which a second (and in some cases a third) drug was added to patients who were partial responders to a single agent have shown additional efficacy without unacceptable toxicity over monotherapy (Bingham and Emery 2001) (see below). There is now sufficient data to indicate that patients with aggressive disease resistant to monotherapy may benefit from the initiation of combination therapy. It is imperative to identify patients with inadequate response and unacceptable disease activity in order to target more aggressive therapy to these patients. The period of time spent with active synovitis must be reduced to a minimum to prevent progression of joint damage and hence disability (see above).

A major change occurred with the licensing of biological anticytokine therapies. These drugs are not yet universally available due to cost constraints. In addition, the long-term safety of such drugs still requires confirmation. Therefore, these drugs are currently used most commonly in patients with aggressive disease that is not responsive to conventional therapy. A working definition of failed conventional therapy has been proposed (Bingham and Emery 2000) where documented lack of response to monotherapy, combination therapy with methotrexate, sulfasalazine, and hydroxychloroquine, a trial of parenteral methotrexate and leflunomide (LEF) is required before consideration of biological therapy, although these guidelines will be continuously updated.

Non-steroidal anti-inflammatory drugs

NSAIDs are widely used for relief of pain and stiffness in RA. These are usually the first drugs commenced following disease onset and often prior to assessment by a rheumatologist. NSAIDs are normally prescribed concomitantly with simple analgesics and disease modifying agents throughout the course of disease. A wide range of NSAIDs is available and new compounds are continuously being developed that claim to have improved safety and efficacy profiles (see Chapter 4.5.1).

NSAIDs can have a dramatic effect on hand joint inflammation and function early in disease. Therapy with NSAIDs during the early phase of disease may mask the symptoms and signs if inflammatory arthritis that can lead to a misdiagnosis or delay in accurate assessment (Marzo-Ortega et al. 2000). Therefore assessment off NSAIDs is valuable in equivocal cases. There are also beneficial effects which might include a possible direct affect on the synovium (Quinn et al. 2000).

Conventional disease modifying antirheumatic drugs (Table 5)

Sulfasalazine

Sulfasalazine (SSA) is used in many centres as the first-line DMARD. Efficacy has been shown in several placebo-controlled trials (Box and Pullar 1997). SSA reduces the rate of bone erosions in early (van der Heijde et al. 1989) and established disease (Pullar et al. 1987). Two large meta-analyses of studies comparing SSA with other DMARDs have suggested that SSA was as effective as injectable gold, penicillamine, and methotrexate (MTX) in reducing ESR and tender joint count and increasing grip strength. It was significantly better than antimalarials, oral gold, and azathioprine (Felson et al. 1991).

SSA is generally well tolerated. Serious side-effects are most common in the first 12 weeks of therapy and include leucopaenia and hepatotoxicity; these necessitate cessation of therapy. Gastrointestinal upset is common but can usually be improved by dose reduction. Increased antinuclear antibody titre can occur in some patients, but overt clinical lupus is unusual. If a significant rise in titre occurs SSA should be discontinued.

Methotrexate

MTX is used commonly (increasingly first-line) both alone and in combination with other DMARDs (commonly SSA and/or hydroxychloroquine, HCQ). It is normally given with folic acid to reduce the incidence of toxicity. It is well tolerated and therapy is continued significantly longer than other DMARDs (Kremer and Lee 1988). Several studies and a meta-analysis (Tugwell et al. 1989) have confirmed the efficacy of MTX monotherapy compared to placebo and MTX has superior efficacy compared to azathioprine and oral gold in double-blind positively controlled studies (Weinblatt et al. 1990; Jeurissen et al. 1991). MTX has been shown to reduce the progression of erosions when used first line (Rich et al. 1999). MTX is normally given orally once a week, but can also be given parenteraly if there is concern regarding bioavailibity or in order to prevent gastric toxicity (Hamilton and Kremer 1997). The dose of MTX must be reduced in renal impairment and its use is contraindicated in the presence of significant renal disease. Concomitant NSAIDs reduce renal clearance of MTX.

Table 5 Conventional disease modifying agents

Drug[a]	Mechanisms of action	Effect	Metabolism	Major side-effects
AZA	Interferes with adenine and guanine ribonucleotides via suppression of inosinic acid synthesis	Decreased T-cell number (CD8) and function, reduced B-cell function, decreased IL-2	Cleaved to 6-mercaptopurine (6-MP) which is metabolized to thioinosinic and thioguanylic acid through the action of hypoxanthine phosphoridosyltransferase. Two distinct populations of AZA metabolizers: fast and slow, leading to a four-fold variation in the rate of clearance. The enzyme which metabolizes 6-MP (thiopurine methyltransferase) exhibits genetic polymorphism with a small subset of the population producing low levels leading to increased toxicity (usually bone marrow suppression)	Hypersensitivity reactions, marrow suppression, hair loss, increased infection risk, nausea
Chlorambucil	Metabolized to phenylacetic acid mustard, which cross-links DNA	Decreased lymphocyte replication	Chlorambucil and its metabolites are renally excreted	Marrow suppression (usually granulocytopaenia or isolated thrombocytopaenia) and infertility. Increased risk of cutaneous and haematological malignancy
CTX	DNA cross-linking	Decreased lymphocyte replication	Renal excretion of CTX and its metabolites	Gastrointestinal upset, malignancy, infertility, bone marrow toxicity, and haemorrhagic cystitis
CYA	Complexes with cytoplasmic cyclophilin which then binds calcineurin, an intracellular phosphatase	Decreased IL-2 and hence cellular immune amplification. Decreased B-cell response to T-cell dependent antigens. Decreased IFN-γ and NK function	Metabolized in the liver by cytochrome P-450 mixed-function oxidase to at least 15 metabolites, some of which have immuno-suppressive properties. Elimination is via the biliary system	Increased serum creatinine and urea, renal impairment, hypertrichosis, tremor, hypertension, hepatic impairment, GI upset
Gold	Inhibits transcription factor AP-1 binding. Formation of aurocyanide in polymorphonuclear cell phagocytosis	Effects on polymorphonuclear cell, monocyte and macrophage phagocytosis. Decreased HLA class II expression on monocytes. Inhibition of synovial cell proliferation. Reduced IL-1 induced lymphocyte proliferation	Mainly excreted unchanged in the urine	Hypersensitivity reaction, proteinuria, blood disorders
HCQ	Alkalinizing lysosomes and interfering with protease function and release. Inhibition of IL-1 release and RNA and DNA synthesis	Effects on lysosome function and antigen processing in lymphocytes, macrophages, fibroblasts, and polymorphs. Decreased IL-1	Metabolized in the liver and then renally excreted	GI upset, headache, rash, retinopathy
Lef	Active metabolite inhibits hydroorotate dehydrogenase inhibiting cell cycle of activated cells	Decreased lymphocyte immune functions. Inhibition of antigen processing	The active metabolite is further metabolized and then renally excreted	Hypertension, leucopaenia, hepatic impairment, GI upset, headache, hair loss, rash
MTX	Inhibits 5-aminoimidazole-carboxamide-ribonucleotide-transformase increasing adenosine levels. Inhibits dihydrofolate reductase leading to lack of purine nucleotides	Reduced leukocyte trafficking, inhibition of T-cell and macrophage function. Decreased IL-1 and IL-2 production	MTX and its metabolites mainly eliminated via the kidney	Marrow suppression, hepatic impairment, pneumonitis, GI upset, stomatitis, headache, fatigue, malaise
D-Pen	Exchange reactions in or on cell surface receptor sulfydryl groups. Inhibits binding of transcription factor AP-1	Modulates activities of T-cells, NK cells, monocytes, and macrophages	Cleared largely through oxidation to form disulfides with plasma albumin, L-cystine, homocysteine and itself. Patients with impaired sulfoxidation status have increased risk of toxicity	Nausea, rash, marrow suppression, proteinuria, haematuria, haemolytic anaemia, lupus-like syndrome, myasthenia gravis-like syndrome
SSA	Scavenge proinflammatory reactive oxygen species. Lowers prostenoid levels (e.g. leukotriene B_4)	Reduced numbers of activated lymphocytes	Sulfapyridine and 5-aminosalicylic acid liberated from sulfasalazine in the colon. Sulfapyridine is metabolized by N^4-acetylation, ring hydroxylation and subsequent gluconuration	Rash, GI upset, marrow suppression, hepatotoxicity, orange urine/tears, reversible decreased spermatogenesis, rarely renal failure, increased ANA titre

[a] AZA, azathioprine; CTX, cyclophosphamide; CYA, cyclosporin A; HCQ, hydroxychloroquine; Lef, leflunomide; MTX, methotrexate; DPA, D-penicillamine; SSA, sulfasalazine.

Antimalarials (hydroxychloroquine and chloroquine)

HCQ has low efficacy when used as monotherapy, but is sometimes used as first line therapy in mild disease. Recently, its use in severe disease has increased following studies showing additional efficacy of combination therapy (with SSA and MTX) in patients with refractory disease (see below). The use of chloroquine has declined due to its higher toxicity profile. The majority of adverse events are transient and not serious.

Leflunomide

LEF, is currently licensed only as monotherapy, although studies are underway with combination therapy with SSA or MTX (see below). In clinical studies, LEF has shown efficacy comparable with SSA and MTX in terms of reduced disease activity and radiological progression that may persist for beyond 2 years (Smolen et al. 1999; Strand et al. 1999; Emery et al. 2000).

The incidence of toxicity appears to be most common during the first 2–4 weeks of therapy and may be related to the loading dose.

Gold therapy

Injectable gold (sodium aureothiomalate) and oral gold (auranofin) are no longer first line therapies and tend to be used in patients who have failed treatment with MTX and SSA. Aureothiomalate has superior efficacy to auranofin and equal efficacy to SSA although its use tends to be limited by therapeutic escape and a high incidence of toxicity (Sambrook et al. 1982). Toxicity is more common with injectable gold than the oral preparation.

Renal toxicity is the most common side effect; therapy should be avoided in renal impairment and is contra-indicated in severe renal disease. Minor proteinuria ($<$300 mg/l) occurs in 10 per cent of patients and usually responds to suspension of gold therapy, but treatment should be discontinued if the proteinuria persists or rises above 300 mg/l. Rarely nephrotic syndrome develops which always resolves, but may take months or years. Occasionally, membranous glomerulonephritis occurs with more severe proteinuria and haematuria.

Cyclosporin A

Cyclosporin monotherapy has been shown to be efficacious in the treatment of RA (Tugwell 1992) and to reduce radiographic progression (Førre 1994). Double-blind controlled trials show cyclosporin A (CYA) to be as effective as DPA, chloroquine, or azathioprine (Furst 1995). In an open study of patients with RA of less than 3 years duration, CYA was better than chloroquine (van den Borne et al. 1996) and comparable to parenteral gold in retarding joint progression (Zeidler et al. 1998).

CYA can commonly reduce glomerular filtration rate (GFR) and should be avoided in patients with pre-existing renal disease. Doses of CYA greater than 5 mg/kg/day or a marked ($>$50 per cent) increase in serum creatinine have been associated with increased renal damage on biopsy (Kowal et al. 1990). Hypertension can commonly occur, but potassium-sparing antihypertensives should be avoided as CYA can induce hyperkalaemia. In addition, calcium-channel blockers may increase CYA concentrations.

Azathioprine

AZA is occasionally used in patients with severe refractory disease not responsive to other conventional medications. AZA has a complicated metabolism (Table 5). In addition to the principal toxicities of AZA (marrow suppression and gastrointestinal upset), hypersensitivity reactions can occur, which in severe case manifests as multiple organ failure (Brown et al. 1997).

Cyclophosphamide

Cyclophosphamide (CTX) pulse therapy (usually intravenous) is used for the management of rheumatoid vasculitis. CTX is sometimes used in patients with severe refractory joint disease although there is little evidence to support this. Two small studies have shown that CTX can retard bone destruction (Clements 1991).

The urological toxicity of CTX is due to its metabolite acrolein, which is excreted in the urine. The risk of haemorrhagic cystitis can be reduced by co-administration of mesna with each pulse and assuring adequate patient hydration, neither of which is possible with continuous oral administration.

D-Penicillamine

The use of D-penicillamine (DPA) in the treatment of RA is declining, as more efficacious therapies are now available. Mild proteinuria is common (30 per cent) and may resolve despite continued treatment. Heavy proteinuria and nephrotic syndrome due to membranous glomerulonephritis (GN) may occur and can persist for months or years after cessation of drug. DPA can induce Goodpasture's syndrome or systemic lupus erythematosus (SLE), both of which can cause rapidly progressive (crescentic) GN indicated by the presence of haematuria.

Chlorambucil

Chlorambucil is occasionally used in patients with refractory joint disease, vasculitis, and secondary amyloid. Chlorambucil has been shown to be efficacious in one double-blind randomized placebo-controlled trial and several open studies (Cannon et al. 1985; Tsokos 1987).

Antibiotics

Although evidence supporting the role of an infectious agent in RA is currently lacking, antibiotics have been used in treatment. The observed efficacy may be due to mechanisms of action in addition to antimicrobial effects. The tetracyclines have several effects including decreased phagocytosis by PMNs and monocytes, inhibition of lymphocyte proliferation and inhibition of interferon-gamma (IFN-γ) production. In addition, tetracyclines inhibit matrix metalloproteinases. The most promising results regarding efficacy were seen with minocycline, however, its use has recently declined following reports of drug-induced lupus (Elkayam et al. 1999).

Combination therapy with conventional DMARDs

Following studies showing increased efficacy of additional therapy, combination therapy is increasingly being used in patients with disease that does not respond adequately to monotherapy (Bingham and Emery 2001).

Combinations including MTX, MTX with SSA +/− HCQ

In a study of patients with an insufficient response to SSA alone, the addition of MTX in combination was found to be superior to switching to MTX monotherapy (Haagsma et al. 1994). Triple therapy with MTX, SSA, and HCQ has been shown to be significantly superior to MTX alone (O'Dell et al. 1996a). Patients on MTX alone who withdrew from this study due to inefficacy subsequently improved when commenced on MTX, SSA, and HCQ (O'Dell et al. 1996b). Therefore, adding SSA and HCQ to therapy for patients failing MTX alone appears to be beneficial. Recently, the same group has published results of a 2-year study comparing MTX/SSA/HCQ with MTX/HCQ or MTX/SSA (O'Dell et al. 2002). Triple therapy was well tolerated and superior in efficacy to therapy with MTX/HCQ or MTX/SSA. In a further study, the effects of therapy with MTX or SSA or HCQ, or MTX/SSA or MTX/HCQ, or all three drugs have been compared (Calguneri et al. 1999). All groups improved, but responses were greater and much more significant in the patients who were given combination therapies and triple therapy was the most efficacious overall.

Combination therapy has also been shown to be efficacious in early disease. Therapy with SSA, MTX, and prednisolone was found to be more efficacious than SSA alone (Boers et al. 1997). Dougados et al. (1999) found a significant reduction in disease activity score (DAS) occurred in DMARD native patients given SSA and MTX compared to SSA and MTX alone.

Combination therapy with MTX/SSA/HCQ/prednisolone in early disease appears to be more likely to induce disease remission at 1 and 2 years compared to SSA with or without prednisolone (Möttönen et al. 1999). In another study, the combination of MTX and SSA offered no advantage over MTX or SSA alone (Haagsma et al. 1997).

MTX and CYA

The combination of MTX and CYA has been shown to be efficacious in the treatment of RA in a randomized double-blind, placebo-controlled study and a subsequent open label extension phase (Tugwell et al. 1995; Stein et al. 1997). In the treatment of early RA, aggressive therapy with CYA, MTX, and intra-articular steroids have been shown to be more effective than monotherapy with SSA (Proudman et al. 2000).

MTX and LEF

In two studies (one open and one randomized placebo-controlled) combination therapy with LEF and MTX has been shown to be more efficacious than MTX alone (Weinblatt et al. 1999a; Kremer et al. 2000a). Both studies found an increased incidence of toxicity in the combination therapy groups and recently, the increased risk of liver toxicity with MTX/LEF combination therapy has be highlighted in patients without adequate blood test monitoring.

Other combinations with MTX

Combination therapy with MTX and intramuscular gold has been found to be advantageous in an open study (Rau et al. 1998), but the combination of MTX and AZA offers increased toxicity without increased efficacy (Wilkens and Stablein 1996).

Other combination therapy

Combination therapy with IM gold and CYA induced improvements in clinical markers of disease activity were seen and disease flared in most patients at 6 months when CYA was withdrawn suggesting therapeutic benefit (Benson et al. 1994). A non-significant advantage of combination therapy with HCQ and IM gold has been shown, but half the combination group withdrew due to adverse events (mainly rash) (Scott et al. 1989). A study of combination therapy with SSA and LEF is currently underway (RELIEF study).

Corticosteroids

In most patients, steroids rapidly reduce the level of inflammation, but are associated with significant toxicity when a high cumulative dose is given. Short-term steroids can be useful when waiting for DMARDs to start working and anecdotal evidence suggests that a new disease modifying agent is more likely to be successful if the inflammatory load is already reduced. In the COBRA study, combination therapy with prednisolone, SSA, and MTX was significantly superior to SSA alone, but this effect was lost on the withdrawal of prednisolone at 28 weeks (Boers et al. 1997), suggesting steroids played a significant role in response. The use of oral prednisolone (7.5 mg) in early disease has been shown to reduce the rate of erosion (Kirwan et al. 1995). Two studies in early disease have shown that a more targeted application of steroids with intra-articular injections is superior to DMARDs alone in the short-term (Conaghan et al. 1998b; Proudman et al. 2000). Steroids induce many serious side-effects, the incidence of which is dependent on the total cumulative dose. Toxic effects include osteoporosis, diabetes, hypertension, centropedal weight gain, arteriosclerosis, and cataracts. Steroids should be used at the lowest possible dose and wherever possible should be used in conjunction with a steroid-sparing DMARD. Calcium, vitamin D, hormone replacement therapy, and biphosponates have all been used to prevent steroid-induced bone loss. Such protective agents should be commenced at the same time as continuous oral steroids as the maximal speed of bone mineral density loss occurs during the first 6 months of therapy.

Biological therapy

Recently, a new generation of biological disease modifying agents has been developed. These drugs consist of either humanized monoclonal antibodies or receptor antagonists and are targeted against specific cytokines or cell surface molecules. So far agents have been developed specific for the cytokines tumour necrosis factor alpha (TNF-α) and interleukin (IL-1), T-cell surface molecules CD52w (CAMPATH), CD4, and CTLA4 and B-cell surface molecule CD20.

Anti-cytokine therapies (Table 6)

TNF-α blockade

TNF-α is a pivotal cytokine in the pathogenesis of RA (see Chapter 6.3.1). Two agents that inhibit the actions of this cytokine have been licensed in the United Kingdom (infliximab and etanercept) and a third is likely to be licensed in the near future (adalimumab). Further agents are currently under going phase three trials.

Infliximab

Infliximab (Remicade®) is given by intermittent intravenous infusion with concomitant MTX therapy which reduces the induction of human antichimeric A2 (HACA) antibodies and maintains efficacy (Maini et al. 1998). The ATTRACT study showed infliximab and MTX to be highly efficacious in patients with an inadequate response to MTX (Maini et al. 1999). The licensed dose is 3 mg/kg given at 0, 2, 6 weeks and then 8-weekly. In the ATTRACT study, infliximab markedly reduced the rate of joint damage in all the treatment groups (Lipskey et al. 2000).

Adverse events include headache, nausea, upper respiratory tract infection, abdominal pain, and pharyngitis (Lipskey et al. 2000). Antidouble stranded DNA (dsDNA) antibodies developed in 16 per cent of patients after treatment with infliximab in the ATTRACT trial (Maini et al. 1999). One patient had to withdraw from the study after developing a drug- induced lupus syndrome, but a further analysis of 156 patients receiving infliximab revealed that although IgM dsDNA antibodies may develop, the occurrence

Table 6 Biological therapies directed against pathogenic cytokines

Target	Name	Construct	Administration	Status
TNF-α	Infliximab (Remicade®)	Chimeric monoclonal antibody	Intravenous infusion concomitant MTX	Licensed for RA and Crohn's disease
	Etanercept (Enbrel®)	TNFR : Fc fusion protein	Subcutaneous injections, +/−MTX	Licensed for RA
	Adalimumab	Human monoclonal antibody	Subcutaneous injections	Phase III trials
IL-1	Anakinra	Recombinant receptor antagonist	Subcutaneous injections	Licensed for RA

of a drug-induced lupus syndrome is rare (Charles et al. 2000). Analysis of 2-year data form the ATTRACT study suggests infliximab with MTX is safe (Lipskey et al. 2000). However, post-licensing surveillance in the United States has revealed a small number of patients developing *Mycobacterium tuberculosis* infections with unusual presentations (Gershon et al. 2000).

Etanercept

Etanercept (Enbrel®) is given by subcutaneous injection (25 mg twice a week) and has been shown to be efficacious as monotherapy in the treatment of RA (Moreland et al. 1999). A subsequent study has shown superior efficacy of combination therapy with etanercept and MTX over MTX alone in patients with a partial response to MTX (Weinblatt et al. 1999b). Etanercept has been shown to be superior to MTX in terms of efficacy and retardation of radiographic progression in patients with early RA (<1 year) (Bathon et al. 2000). Etanercept effectively reduces the rate of joint damage (Moreland et al. 2001).

In clinical studies, etanercept was well tolerated; adverse events included mild injection site reactions and mild upper respiratory tract symptoms (cough, rhinitis, sinusitis, and pharyngitis). A small number of patients developed anti-dsDNA antibodies, but no patients developed any symptoms of systemic lupus. Long-term data suggest etanercept is safe and effective either alone or in combination with MTX (Kremer et al. 2000b; Moreland et al. 2001).

Adalimumab

This is a fully humanized anti-TNF-α antibody that is currently undergoing phase III trials. It is given by subcutaneous injection. Early data suggest comparable safety and efficacy to infliximab and etanercept (Keystone et al. 2001; Schattenkirchner et al. 2001).

Interleukin-1 receptor antagonist (IL-1ra)

Evidence is emerging that IL-1 is also a pivotal cytokine driving inflammation in RA (see Chapter 4.1). IL-1ra is a naturally occurring receptor antagonist that inhibits the effects of IL-1 by irreversibly binding to the IL-1 receptor (IL-1RI). Recombinant IL-1ra (Anakinra) has been shown to be clinically effective and reduce the rate of joint erosion (Bresnihan 2001; Watt and Cobby 2001) and has just been licensed in the United Kingdom. Combination therapy with IL-1ra and MTX is effective in patients with active RA (Cohen et al. 2002).

Practical use of TNF-α antagonists

Choice of patient

The high cost and possible long-term toxicity of these therapies necessitate targeting to appropriate patients. Consensus guidelines for selection of patients for TNF-α antagonists are set out in Table 7. In the first instance eligible patients are logically those with disease resistant to therapy with conventional drugs. In addition, patients must have active disease capable of response as demonstrated by a modified DAS28 of greater than 5.1.

Choice of agent

Currently there is no data comparing the clinical efficacy and safety of infliximab and etanercept. Therefore, the choice of anti-TNF therapy depends on:

1. patient preference regarding self-injection versus hospital-based infusion;
2. previous toxicity with methotrexate; infliximab should be given with methotrexate;
3. capacity of day unit facilities for infliximab infusions.

Monitoring

The major side-effects of these treatments are increased risk of infection, injection site/infusion reactions and potential increased long-term risk of malignancy. Long-term surveillance of patients who receive biological therapies is imperative to detect any side-effects such as lymphoid malignancy

Table 7 British Society of Rheumatology Consensus Guidelines for selection of patients for TNF-α antagonists (British Society for Rheumatology, 2001)

Eligibility:

1. Active RA—DAS28 >5.1 (Prevoo et al. 1995)
2. Failure of standard therapy—failed therapy with 2 or more standard DMARDs (including MTX)
   Failure defined as:
   (a) treatment for at least 6 months, with at least 2 months at standard target dose (unless limited by toxicity)
   (b) treatment for <6 months, where treatment was withdrawn because of drug intolerance or toxicity, but normally after at least 2 months at therapeutic doses

Exclusion criteria:

1. Pregnant or breast feeding women
2. Active infection
3. Patients at high risk of infection including
   (a) leg ulcers
   (b) previous TB unless the patient has completed full course of anti-TB therapy in the modern therapeutic era. Patients without adequate modern therapy of radiological evidence of previous TB without a clinical episode may be counselled regarding the risks of recurrence and anti-TB prophylaxis should be considered
   (c) septic arthritis of a native joint within the last 12 months
   (d) sepsis of a prosthetic joint within the last 12 months or indefinitely if the joint remains in situ
   (e) persistent or recurrent chest infections
   (f) indwelling urinary catheter
4. Previous malignancy or pre-malignancy excluding:
   (a) basal cell carcinoma
   (b) malignancies diagnosed and treated more then 10 years previously (where the probability of cure is very high)

or chronic infections including tuberculosis. All patients exposed to TNF-α antagonists in the United Kingdom are entered onto a national database coordinated by the British Society of Rheumatology.

Combination therapy with anticytokine therapies

Animal studies have suggested TNF-α and IL-1 act synergistically and combination therapy with anti-IL-1 and anti-TNF-α was found to be more potent than anti-TNF-α alone in animal studies. Therefore, a double-hit approach inhibiting TNF-α and IL-1β in humans is likely to be beneficial.

Anti-B-cell therapies

Rituximab

Rituximab is a depleting humanized monoclonal antibody directed against CD20 on B cells. It has been shown to be effective in a small study of patients with severe refractory RA (Edwards and Cambridge 2001). A single intravenous infusion given with a pulse of cyclophosphamide and methylprednisolone was effective for upto 27 months without serious toxicity. A placebo-controlled double-blind randomized study is currently underway.

Other therapies

Autologous stem cell transplantation

In recent years, autologous stem cell transplantation (SCT) has been investigated as a possible therapy for a wide range of autoimmune diseases including RA (Bingham et al. 2000b). Interest in this technique arose following animal studies and case reports of patients entering remission from their autoimmune disease following transplantation for a coincidental haematological disease. Recent improvements in mortality and morbidity associated with SCT have allowed this procedure to be used for therapy of the autoimmune disease itself. However, this procedure is considered appropriate only for those patients for whom there is no reasonable therapeutic alternative.

Prosorba

The Prosorba column consists of *Staphylococcus* protein A bound to inert silica matrix and it binds IgG and IgG–antigen complexes. Several studies have indicated the removal of circulating immune complexes in this way may be beneficial in patients with severe RA refractory to conventional DMARDs (Gendreau et al. 2001).

Non-pharmacological therapy

Multidisciplinary team

RA is a complex disease resulting in multiple problems for the patient both physically and psychologically and therefore a multidisciplinary team of allied health experts should ideally be available. Several studies have assessed the benefit of a specialised programme for rehabilitation of patients with inflammatory arthritis (Spiegel et al. 1986; Solomon et al. 1997; Vliet Vlieland and Hazes 1997). Most of the studies were inconclusive, partly due to poor study design (Clarke 1999). Inpatient programmes however, did show some advantage. In general, evidence to support many non-pharmacological therapies is currently lacking. This does not mean, however, that such treatments are ineffective. Further research is required to provide an evidence base for this type of management.

The nurse practitioner

The rheumatology nurse practitioner plays a central role in patient management, often co-ordinating treatment by other medical staff and therapists. The increasing use of combination DMARD therapy and biologics requires adequate patient counselling, education, and monitoring for their safe administration. The nurse practitioner often provides vital psychological support for patients at all stages of their disease.

The physiotherapist

Physiotherapy improves patients' mobility, independence, and self-esteem in addition to providing specific medical benefits such as improving post-operative outcome following joint replacement. Several studies have shown that the majority of RA sufferers will show an improvement in function and a lessening of pain if they exercise (Lyngberg et al. 1988) and a prolonged course of hand exercises induced significant improvements compared to a control group (Brighton et al. 1993). Hydrotherapy, when compared to seated immersion, land exercises, and relaxation, gave the best results in terms of physical and psychological parameters, which persisted for at least 3 months (Hall et al. 1996). Prolonged hydrotherapy over 4 years maintain grip strength better than in controls and patients also had a better general functional outcome (Stenstrom et al. 1991).

The occupational therapist

Independent living is facilitated by the use of aids and adaptations both in the home and in the work place. Although, many such interventions seem appropriate and use common sense, there is little supportive evidence. In addition, occupational therapists can give advice regarding joint protection. One recent study showed significant improvements in pain, disease status and functional ability in a group receiving joint protection advice compared to those receiving standard RA education (Hammond and Freeman 2001).

The podiatrist

Patients with RA can develop multiple and complex foot disorders and assessment by a podiatrist is essential in many patients. Intervention, including correction of deformity and/or abnormal pressure distribution, can improve patient pain and mobility. The prevention and early treatment of foot ulceration is extremely important especially in the era of biological therapies.

Non-surgical intra-articular interventions

Arthroscopy and joint lavage

Joint lavage followed by intra-articular steroid has been shown to be of benefit for joints resistant to blind injection of steroid (Sharma et al. 1996). In addition, visual exploration of the joint and synovial biopsy can aid diagnosis and patient management (Reece et al. 1999).

Chemical and radiosynovectomy

Although these treatments are popular in Europe they are used infrequently in the United Kingdom and there is little published evidence in support of their use. In 1998, a small study showed improvement in nine of ten patients with RA treated with radiosynovectomy (Alsono-Ruiz et al. 1998).

Surgery

The most frequently performed surgical operation is total hip arthroplasty, which is performed for pain relief and to increase range of movement and mobility with highly significant improvement in quality of life. Other joints that are routinely replaced are the knee and shoulder and more recently the elbow, metacarpal–phalangeal and interphalangeal joints. Wrist fusion is also occasionally performed for pain relief. Surgical synovectomy of the wrist and other joints such as the knee may be performed in the presence of persistent synovitis. Other operations include tendon repair, correction of digital deformity, and cervical spine fusion. Close collaboration between the rheumatologist and orthopaedic and neurosurgical units is required to provide optimal surgical management of patients with RA in terms of optimal time of referral and available procedures.

References

Abu-Shakra, M. et al. (1998). Clinical and radiographic outcomes of rheumatoid arthritis patients not treated with disease modifying drugs. *Arthritis and Rheumatism* **41**, 1190–5.

Alsono-Ruiz, A. et al. (1998). Efficacy of radiosynovectomy of the knee in rheumatoid arthritis: evaluation with magnetic resonance imaging. *Clinical Rheumatology* **17**, 277–81.

Anderson, J.J. et al. (2000). Factors predicting response to treatment in rheumatoid arthritis. The importance of disease duration. *Arthritis and Rheumatism* **43**, 22–9.

Arnett, F.C. et al. (1988). The American Rheumatism Association 1987 revised criteria for the classification of rheumatoid arthritis. *Arthritis and Rheumatism* **3**, 315–24.

Baeten, D. et al. (2000). Comparative study of the synovial histology in rheumatoid arthritis, spondyloarthropathy, osteoarthritis: influence of disease duration and activity. *Annals of the Rheumatic Diseases* **59**, 945–53.

Bathon, J. et al. (2000). A comparison of etanercept and methotrexate in patients with early rheumatoid arthritis. *New England Journal of Medicine* **343**, 1586–93.

Benson, W., Tugwell, P., and Robert, R.M. (1994). Combination treatment of cyclosporin with methotrexate and gold in rheumatoid arthritis (2 pilot studies). *Journal of Rheumatology* **21**, 2034–8.

Bingham, S. and Emery, P. (2000) Resistant rheumatoid arthritis clinics—a necessary development? *Rheumatology* **39**, 2–5.

Bingham, S. and Emery, P. (2001). Combination therapy in rheumatoid arthritis. *Springer Seminars in Immunopathology* **23** (1–2), 165–83.

Bingham, S.J., Snowden, J.A., and Emery, P. (2000). Autologous blood stem cell transplantation as therapy for autoimmune diseases. *Annals of Medicine* **32**, 615–21.

Boers, M. et al. (1997). Randomised comparison of combined step-down prednisolone, methotrexate and sulphasalazine with sulphasalazine alone in early rheumatoid arthritis. *Lancet* **350**, 309–18.

Boers, M., Kostense, P.J., and COBRA Trial Group (2000). In early rheumatoid arthritis presence of inflammation in individual hand joints predicts (progression of) damage in that joint. *Arthritis and Rheumatism* **43** (Suppl.), S115.

van den Borne, B.E. et al. (1996). Low dose cyclosporin in early rheumatoid arthritis: effective and safe after two years of therapy when compared to chloroquine. *Scandinavian Journal of Rheumatology* **25**, 307–16.

Box, S.A. and Pullar, T. (1997). Sulphasalazine in the treatment of rheumatoid arthritis. *British Journal of Rheumatology* **36**, 382–6.

Bresnihan, B. (2001). The safety and efficacy of interleukin-1 receptor antagonist in the treatment of RA. *Seminars in Arthritis and Rheumatism* **30** (5 Suppl. 2), 17–20.

Brighton, S.W., Lubbe, J.E., and van der Merwe, C.A. (1993). The effect of a long-term exercise programme on the rheumatoid hand. *British Journal of Rheumatology* **32**, 392–5.

British Society for Rheumatology. *Guidelines for Prescribing TNF-α Blockers in Adults with RA*. London: British Society for Rheumatology, 2001.

Brown, A.K. et al. (2001). Ultrasonography detects synovitis in the majority of RA patients satisfying ACR remission criteria. *Rheumatology* **40** (Suppl.), 70.

Brown, G. et al. (1997). Azathioprine-induced multisystem organ failure and cardiogenic shock. *Pharmacotherapy* **17**, 815–18.

Calguneri, M. et al. (1999). Combination therapy versus monotherapy for the treatment of patients with rheumatoid arthritis. *Clinical and Experimental Rheumatology* **17**, 699–704.

Cannon, G.W. et al. (1985). Chlorambucil therapy in rheumatoid arthritis: clinical experience in 28 patients and literature review. *Seminars in Arthritis and Rheumatism* **15**, 106–18.

Charles, P.J. et al. (2000). Assessment of antibodies to double stranded DNA induced rheumatoid arthritis patients following treatment with infliximab, a monoclonal antibody to tumour necrosis factor α. *Arthritis and Rheumatism* **43**, 2383–90.

Clarke, A.K. (1999). Effectiveness of rehabilitation in arthritis. *Clinical Rehabilitation* **13** (Suppl. 1), 51–62.

Clements, P.J. (1991). Alkylating agents. In *Second Line Agents in the Treatment of Rheumatic Diseases* (ed. J. Dixon and D.E. Furst). New York: Marcel Dekker.

Cohen, S. et al. (2002). Treatment of rheumatoid arthritis with anakinra, a recombinant human interleukin-1 receptor antagonist, in combination with methotrexate: results of a twenty-four week, multicenter, randomised, double-blind, placebo controlled trial. *Arthritis and Rheumatism* **46**, 574–8.

Conaghan, P.G. et al. (1998a). MCPJ assessment in early RA: a comparison between X-ray, MRI, high-resolution ultrasound and clinical examination. *Arthritis and Rheumatism* **41** (Suppl.), S246.

Conaghan, P.G. et al. (1998b). Intra-articular corticosteroids prevent progression of erosions in methotrexate treated early arthritis. *Arthritis and Rheumatism* **41** (Suppl.), S238.

Conaghan, P.G. et al. (1999). Reversal of bony damage in early rheumatoid arthritis patients treated with IA corticosteroids and methotrexate: an MRI and ultrasonographic study. *Annals of the Rheumatic Diseases* **58** (Suppl.), 75.

Dawes, P.T. et al. (1986). Rheumatoid arthritis: treatment which controls the C-reactive protein and erythrocyte sedimentation rate reduces radiological progression. *British Journal of Rheumatology* **25**, 44–9.

Devlin, J. et al. (1997). The acute phase and function in early RA. CRP levels correlate with functional outcome. *Journal of Rheumatology* **24**, 9–13.

Dougados, M. et al. (1999). Combination therapy in early rheumatoid arthritis: a randomised controlled double-blind 52-week trail of sulphasalazine and methotrexate compared with the single components. *Annals of the Rheumatic Diseases* **58**, 220–5.

Eberhardt, K. and Fex, E. (1998). Clinical course and remission rate in patients with early rheumatoid arthritis: relationship to outcome after 5 years. *British Journal of Rheumatology* **37**, 1324–9.

Edwards, J.C. and Cambridge, G. (2001). Sustained improvement in rheumatoid arthritis following a protocol designed to deplete B-lymphocytes. *Rheumatology* **40**, 205–11.

Elkayam, O., Yaron, M., and Caspi, D. (1999). Minocycline induced autoimmune syndromes: an overview. *Seminars in Arthritis and Rheumatism* **28**, 392–7.

Emery, P. (1997). Prognosis in inflammatory arthritis: the value of HLA genotyping and oncological analogy. The Dunlop Dotteridge Lecture. *Journal of Rheumatology* **24**, 1436–42.

Emery, P. and Salmon, M. (1995). Early rheumatoid arthritis: time to aim for remission? *Annals of the Rheumatic Diseases* **54**, 944–7.

Emery, P. et al. (2000). A comparison of the efficacy and safety of leflunomide and methotrexate for the treatment of rheumatoid arthritis. *Rheumatology* **39**, 655–65.

Fearon, U. et al. (1999). Synovial cytokine and growth factor regulation of MMPs/TIMPs: implications for erosions and angiogenesis in early rheumatoid and psoriatic arthritis patients. *Annals of the New York Academy of Sciences* **878**, 619–21.

Feigenbaum, S.L. et al. (1979). Prognosis in rheumatoid arthritis—a longitudinal study of newly diagnosed younger adult patients. *American Journal of Medicine* **66**, 377–84.

Felson, D.T. et al. (1995). American College of Rheumatology preliminary definition of improvement in rheumatoid arthritis. *Arthritis and Rheumatism* **38**, 727–35.

Felson, D.T., Anderson, J.J., and Meenan, R.F. (1991). The comparative efficacy and toxicity of second-line drugs in RA. Results of two meta-analyses. *Arthritis and Rheumatism* **34**, 1342–3.

Fex, E., Eberhardt, K., and Saxne, T. (1997). Tissue derived macromolecules and markers of inflammation in serum in early rheumatoid arthritis: relationship to development of joint destruction in hands and feet. *British Journal of Rheumatology* **36**, 1161–5.

Fitzgerald, O. et al. (1991). Morphometric analysis of blood vessels in synovial membranes obtained from clinically affected and unaffected knee joints of patients with rheumatoid arthritis. *Annals of the Rheumatic Diseases* **50**, 792–6.

Førre, Ø. (1994). The Norwegian Arthritis Study Group. Radiologic evidence of disease modification in rheumatoid arthritis patients treated with cyclosporine. Results of a 48-week multicenter study comparing low-dose cyclosporine with placebo. *Arthritis and Rheumatism* **37**, 506–12.

Fraser, A. et al. (2001). Matrix metalloproteinase-9, apoptosis and vascular morphology in early arthritis. *Arthritis and Rheumatism* **44** (9), 2024–8.

Fries, J.F. et al. (1980). Measurement of patient outcome in arthritis. *Arthritis and Rheumatism* **23**, 137–45.

Fries, J.F., Williams, C.A., and Bloch, D.A. (1991). The relative toxicity of non-steroidal anti-inflammatory drugs. *Arthritis and Rheumatism* **34**, 1353–60.

Fries, J.F. et al. (1993). The relative toxicity of disease-modifying antirheumatic drugs. *Arthritis and Rheumatism* **36**, 297–306.

Fries, J. et al. (1996). Reduction in long-term disability in patients with rheumatoid arthritis by disease-modifying antirheumatic drug-based treatment strategies. *Arthritis and Rheumatism* **39**, 616–22.

Furst, D.E. (1995). Cyclosporin, leflunomide and nitrogen mustard. Innovative treatment approaches for rheumatoid arthritis. *Clinical Rheumatology* **9**, 711–29.

Gendreau, R.M. et al. (2001). A randomised double-blind sham controlled trial of the Prosorba column for the treatment of refractory RA. *Therapeutic Apheresis* **5**, 79–83.

Gershon, S. et al. (2000). Postlicense reports of infection during use of etanercept and infliximab. *American College of Rheumatology Annual Scientific Meeting.* Late Breaking Abstract.

Gough, A.K.S. et al. (1994a). Generalised bone loss in patients with early rheumatoid arthritis. *Lancet* **344**, 23–7.

Gough, A. et al. (1994b). Genetic typing of patients with inflammatory arthritis at presentation can be used to predict outcome. *Arthritis and Rheumatism* **37**, 1166–70.

Green, M.J. et al. (1999). Persistence of mild early inflammatory arthritis: the importance of disease duration, rheumatoid factor and the shared epitope. *Arthritis and Rheumatism* **42**, 2184–8.

Guilleman, F., Briancon, S., and Pourel, J. (1992). Functional disability in rheumatoid arthritis: two different models in early and late disease. *Journal of Rheumatology* **19**, 366–9.

Haagsma, C.J. et al. (1994). Combination of methotrexate and sulphasalazine versus methotrexate alone: a randomised open clinical trial in rheumatoid arthritis patients resistant to sulphasalazine therapy. *British Journal of Rheumatology* **33**, 1049–55.

Haagsma, C.J. et al. (1997). Combination of sulphasalazine and methotrexate versus the single components in early rheumatoid arthritis: a randomised controlled double-blind 52 week clinical trial. *British Journal of Rheumatology* **36**, 1082–8.

Hall, J. et al. (1996). A randomised and controlled study of hydrotherapy in rheumatoid arthritis. *Arthritis Care Research* **9**, 206–15.

Hamilton, R.A. and Kremer, J.M. (1997). Why intramuscular methotrexate may be more efficacious than oral dosing in patients with rheumatoid arthritis. *British Journal of Rheumatology* **36**, 86–90.

Hammond, A. and Freeman, K. (2001). One-year outcomes of a randomised controlled trial of an educational-behavioural joint protection programme for people with rheumatoid arthritis. *Rheumatology* **40**, 1044–51.

Hannonen, P. et al. (1993). Sulfasalazine in early rheumatoid arthritis. a 48 week double-blind, prospective, placebo-controlled study. *Arthritis and Rheumatism* **36**, 1501–9.

Harrison, B. and Symmons, D. (2000). Early inflammatory polyarthritis: results from the Norfolk Arthritis Register with a review of the literature. II. Outcome at 3 years. *Rheumatology* **39**, 939–49.

Harrison, B.J. et al. (1996a). Natural remission in inflammatory polyarthritis: issues of definition and prediction. *British Journal of Rheumatology* **35**, 1096–100.

Harrison, B.J. et al. (1996b). Inflammatory polyarthritis in the community is not a benign disease: predicting functional disability one year after presentation. *Journal of Rheumatology* **23**, 1326–31.

Harrison, B.J. et al. (1998). The performance of the 1987 ARA classification criteria for rheumatoid arthritis in a population based cohort of patients with early inflammatory arthritis. *Journal of Rheumatology* **25**, 2324–30.

Harrison, B.J. et al. (1999). The influence of HLA–DRB1 alleles and rheumatoid factor on disease outcome in an inception cohort of patients with early inflammatory arthritis. *Arthritis and Rheumatism* **42**, 2174–83.

Harrison, B.J. et al. (2001). The association of cigarette smoking with disease outcome in patients with early inflammatory polyarthritis. *Arthritis and Rheumatism* **44**, 323–30.

van der Heide, A. et al. (1995a). Prediction of progression of radiological damage in newly diagnosed rheumatoid arthritis. *Arthritis and Rheumatism* **38**, 1466–75.

van der Heide, A. et al. (1995b). Is it possible to predict the first year extent of pain and disability for patients with rheumatoid arthritis? *Journal of Rheumatology* **22**, 1466–70.

van der Heijde, D.M.F.M. et al. (1989). Effects of hydroxychloroquine and sulphasalazine on progression of joint damage in rheumatoid arthritis. *Lancet* **1**, 1036–8.

van der Heijde, D.M.F.M. et al. (1990). Judging disease activity in clinical practice in rheumatoid arthritis: first step in development of a disease activity score. *Annals of the Rheumatic Diseases* **49**, 916–20.

van der Heijde, D.M.F.M. et al. (1992). Prognostic factors for radiographic damage and physical disability in early rheumatoid arthritis. A prospective follow up study of 147 patients. *British Journal of Rheumatology* **31**, 519–25.

van der Horst-Bruinsma, I. et al. (1998). Diagnosis and course of early-onset arthritis: results of a special early arthritis clinic compared to routine patient care. *British Journal of Rheumatology* **37**, 1084–8.

Heliövaara, M. et al. (1993). Smoking and the risk of rheumatoid arthritis. *Journal of Rheumatology* **20**, 1830–85.

Jeurissen, M.E. et al. (1991). Methotrexate versus azathioprine in the treatment of rheumatoid arthritis: a 48-week randomised, double blind trial. *Arthritis and Rheumatism* **34**, 961–72.

Karim, Z. et al. (2001). The impact of ultrasonography on diagnosis and management of patients with musculoskeletal conditions. *Arthritis and Rheumatism* **44**, 2932–3.

Keystone, E. et al. (2001). The fully human anti-TNF monoclonal antibody, adalimumab (D2E7), dose ranging study: the 24-week clinical results in patients with active RA on methotrexate therapy (the Amada trial). *Annals of the Rheumatic Diseases* **60**, 67.

Kirwan, J.R. et al. (1995). The effects of glucocorticoids on joint destruction in rheumatoid arthritis. *New England Journal of Medicine* **333**, 142–6.

Kowal, A., Carstens, J.H., Jr., and Schnitzer, T.J. (1990). Cyclosporin in rheumatoid arthritis. In *Immunomodulators in the Rheumatic Diseases* (ed. D.E. Furst and M.E. Weinblatt), pp. 61–98. New York: Marcel Dekker.

Kraan, M.C. et al. (1998). Asymptomatic synovitis precedes clinically manifest arthritis. *Arthritis and Rheumatism* **41**, 1481–8.

Kremer, J.M. and Lee, J.K. (1988). A long-term prospective study of the use of methotrexate in rheumatoid arthritis: update after a mean of 53 months. *Arthritis and Rheumatism* **31**, 577–84.

Kremer, J.M. et al. (2000a). The combination of leflunomide (LEF) and methotrexate (MTX) in patients with active rheumatoid arthritis (RA) who are failing on MTX treatment alone: a double blind placebo (PLC) controlled study. *Arthritis and Rheumatism* **43** (Suppl.), S224.

Kremer, J.M. et al. (2000b). Etanercept (Enbrel) in addition to methotrexate in rheumatoid arthritis (RA): long-term observations. *Arthritis and Rheumatism* **43** (Suppl.), S270.

Kroot, E.J. et al. (2000). The prognostic value of anti-cyclic citrullinated antibody in patients with recent onset rheumatoid arthritis. *Arthritis and Rheumatism* **43**, 1831–5.

Larsen, A., Dale, K., and Eek, M. (1977). Radiographic evaluation of rheumatoid arthritis and related conditions by standard reference films. *Acta Radiologica* **18**, 481–91.

van Leeuwen, M.A. et al. (1997). Individual relationship between progression of radiological damage and the acute phase response in early rheumatoid arthritis. Towards development of a decision support system. *Journal of Rheumatology* **24**, 20–7.

Lipskey, P. et al. (2000). Infliximab and methotrexate in the treatment of rheumatoid arthritis. *New England Journal of Medicine* **343**, 1594–602.

Lyngberg, K., Danneskiold-Samsoe, B., and Halskov, O. (1988). The effect of physical training on patients with rheumatoid arthritis: changes in disease activity, muscle strength and aerobic capacity. A clinically controlled minimized cross-over study. *Clinical and Experimental Rheumatology* **6**, 253–60.

Maddison, P.J. (1993). Autoantibody profile: rheumatoid factor. In *The Oxford Textbook of Rheumatology* (ed. P.J. Maddison, D.A. Isenberg, P. Woo, and D.N. Glass), pp. 394–5. Oxford: Oxford University Press.

Maini, R.N. et al. (1998). Therapeutic efficacy of multiple intravenous infusions of anti-tumour necrosis factor α monoclonal antibody combined with low-dose weekly methotrexate in rheumatoid arthritis. *Arthritis and Rheumatism* **41**, 1552–63.

Maini, R. et al. (1999). Infliximab (chimeric anti-tumour necrosis factor α antibody) versus placebo in rheumatoid arthritis patients receiving concomitant methotrexate: a randomised phase III trial. *Lancet* **354**, 1932–9.

Marzo-Ortega, H. et al. (2000). Non-steroidal anti-inflammatory drugs alter the presentation of early inflammatory arthritis. *Rheumatology* **39** (Suppl. 1), 42.

Mattey, D.L. et al. (2001). Independent association of rheumatoid factor and the HLA–DRB1 shared epitope with radiographic outcome in rheumatoid arthritis. *Arthritis and Rheumatism* **44**, 1529–33.

McGonagle, D. et al. (1999a). The relationship between synovitis and bone changes in early untreated rheumatoid arthritis. *Arthritis and Rheumatism* **42**, 1706–11.

McGonagle, D. et al. (1999b). An anatomical explanation for good prognosis rheumatoid arthritis. *Lancet* **353**, 123–4.

Moreland, L.W. et al. (1999). Etanercept therapy in rheumatoid arthritis. A randomized, controlled trial. *Annals of Internal Medicine* **130**, 478–86.

Moreland, L.W. et al. (2001). Long-term safety and efficacy of etanercept in patients with rheumatoid arthritis. *Journal of Rheumatology* **28**, 1238–44.

Möttönnen, T. et al. (1998). Only high disease activity and positive rheumatoid factor indicate poor prognosis in patients with rheumatoid arthritis treated with 'saw-tooth' strategy. *Annals of the Rheumatic Diseases* **57**, 533–9.

Mottonen, T. et al. (1999). Comparison of combination therapy with single drug therapy in early rheumatoid arthritis: a randomised trial. *Lancet* **353**, 1568–73.

Munro, R. et al. (1998). Improved functional outcome in patients with early rheumatoid arthritis treated with intramuscular gold: results of a five year prospective study. *Annals of the Rheumatic Disease* **57**, 88–93.

O'Dell, J.R. et al. (1996a). Treatment of rheumatoid arthritis with methotrexate, sulfasalazine and hydroxychloroquine, or a combination of these medications. *New England Journal of Medicine* **334**, 1287–91.

O'Dell, J.R. et al. (1996b). Efficacy of triple DMARD therapy in patients with RA with suboptimal response to methotrexate. *Journal of Rheumatology* **23** (Suppl. 44), 72–4.

O'Dell, J.R. et al. (1998). HLA–DRB1 typing in rheumatoid arthritis: predicting response to specific treatments. *Annals of the Rheumatic Diseases* **57**, 209–13.

O'Dell, J., Leff, R., Paulsen, G., Haire, C., Mallek, J., Eckhoff, P., Fernandez, A., Blakely, K., Wees, S., Stoner, J., Hadley, S., Felt, J., Palmer, W., Waytz, P., Churchill, M., Klassen, L., and Moore, G. (2002). Treatment of rheumatoid arthritis with methotrexate and hydroxychloroquine, methotrexate and sulphasalazine, or a combination of the three medications. Results of a two-year randomised, double-blind, placebo-controlled trial. *Arthritis and Rheumatism* **46**, 1164–70.

Panayi, G.S. et al. (1987). Seronegative and seropositive rheumatoid arthritis: similar diseases. *British Journal of Rheumatology* **26**, 172–80.

Pease, C. et al. (1999). Does the age of onset of rheumatoid arthritis influence phenotype? A prospective study of outcome and prognostic factors. *Rheumatology* **38**, 228–34.

Pinals, R.S. et al. (1981). Preliminary criteria for clinical remission in rheumatoid arthritis. *Arthritis and Rheumatism* **24**, 1138–42.

Plant, M.J. et al. (2000). Relationship between time integrated C-reactive protein levels and radiographic progression in patients with rheumatoid arthritis. *Arthritis and Rheumatism* **43**, 1473–7.

Posthummus, M.D. et al. (1999). Serum levels of matrix metalloproteinase-3 in relation to the development of radiological damage in patients with early rheumatoid arthritis. *Rheumatology* **38**, 1081–7.

Prevoo, M.L.L. et al. (1995). Modified disease activity scores that include twenty-eight joint counts: development and validation in a prospective longitudinal study of patients with rheumatoid arthritis. *Arthritis and Rheumatism*, **38**, 44–8.

Proudman, S.M. et al. (2000). Treatment of poor prognosis early rheumatoid arthritis. A randomised study of treatment with methotrexate, cyclosporin A and intraarticular corticosteroids compared with sulfasalazine alone. *Arthritis and Rheumatism* **43**, 1809–19.

Pullar, T., Hunter, J.A., and Capell, H.A. (1987). Effect of sulphasalazine on the radiological progression of rheumatoid arthritis. *Annals of the Rheumatic Diseases* **46**, 398–402.

Quinn, M. et al. (2000). NSAIDs reduce synovial volume in early RA: a double blind randomised MRI study. *Arthritis and Rheumatism* **43** (Suppl.), S226.

Quinn, M.A. et al. (2001a). Early rheumatoid arthritis: 12 month results from a large secondary care multi-centre study using step-up combination therapy. *Rheumatology* **40** (Suppl.), 37.

Quinn, M.A. et al. (2001b). Using improvement criteria, may lead to overtreatment in early RA. *Rheumatology* **40** (Suppl.), 81.

Rau, R. et al. (1998). Long-term combination therapy of refractory and destructive rheumatoid arthritis with methotrexate (MTX) and intramuscular gold or other disease modifying antirheumatic drugs compared to MTX monotherapy. *Journal of Rheumatology* **25**, 1485–92.

Rau, R. et al. (2000). The effect of HLA–DRB1 genes, rheumatoid factor and treatment on radiographic disease progression in rheumatoid arthritis over 6 years. *Journal of Rheumatology* **27**, 2566–75.

Reece, R.J. et al. (1999). Distinct vascular patterns of early synovitis in psoriatic, reactive and rheumatoid arthritis. *Arthritis and Rheumatism* **42**, 1481–4.

Rich, E., Moreland, L.W., and Alarcon, G.S. (1999). Paucity of radiographic progression in rheumatoid arthritis treated with methotrexate as the first disease modifying anti-rheumatic drug. *Journal of Rheumatology* **26**, 259–61.

Sambrook, P.N. et al. (1982). Terminations of treatment with gold sodium thiomalate in rheumatoid arthritis. *Journal of Rheumatology* **9**, 932–51.

van Schaardenburg, D. et al. (1993). Outcome of rheumatoid arthritis in relation to age and rheumatoid factor at diagnosis. *Journal of Rheumatology* **20**, 45–52.

Schattenkirchner, M. et al. (2001). Long-term use of the fully human anti-TNF antibody adalimumab (D2E7) in DMARD-refractory rheumatoid arthritis. *Annals of the Rheumatic Diseases* **60**, 66.

Schellekens, G.A. et al. (2000). The diagnostic properties of rheumatoid arthritis antibodies recognising a cyclic citrullinated peptide. *Arthritis and Rheumatism* **43**, 155–63.

Scott, D.L. et al. (1987). Long term outcome of treating rheumatoid arthritis: results after 20 years. *Lancet* **8542**, 1108–11.

Scott, D.L. et al. (1989). Combination therapy with gold and hydroxychloroquine in rheumatoid arthritis: a prospective, randomized, placebo-controlled study. *British Journal of Rheumatology* **28**, 128–33.

Sharma, A. et al. (1996). Arthroscopic lavage treatment in rheumatoid arthritis of the knee. *Journal of Rheumatology* **23**, 1872–4.

Sharp, J.T. et al. (1971). Methods of scoring the progression of radiologic changes in rheumatoid arthritis: correlation of radiologic, clinical and laboratory abnormalities. *Arthritis and Rheumatism* **14**, 706–20.

Sheeran, T.P. et al. (1990). The effect of bed rest and intra-articular steroid on the acute phase response in active rheumatoid arthritis. *British Journal of Rheumatology* **29**, 2–11.

Smolen, J.S. et al. (1999). Efficacy and safely of leflunomide compared with placebo and sulphasalazine in active rheumatoid arthritis: a double blind, randomised, multi-centre trial. *Lancet* **353**, 259–66.

Solomon, D.H. et al. (1997). Costs, outcomes and patient satisfaction by provider types for patients with rheumatic and musculo-skeletal conditions: a critical review of the literature and proposed methodologic standards. *Annals of Internal Medicine* **127**, 52–60.

Spiegel, J.S. et al. (1986). Rehabilitation for rheumatoid arthritis patients: a controlled trial. *Arthritis and Rheumatism* **29**, 628–37.

Stein, C.M. et al. (1997). Combination treatment of severe rheumatoid arthritis with cyclosporine and methotrexate for forty-eight weeks: an open-label extension study. The Methotrexate–Cyclosporine Combination Study Group. *Arthritis and Rheumatism* **40**, 1843–51.

Stenger, A.A.M.E. et al. (1998). Early effective suppression of inflammation in rheumatoid arthritis reduces radiographic progression. *British Journal of Rheumatology* **37**, 1157–63.

Stenstrom, C.H. et al. (1991). Intensive dynamic training in water for rheumatoid arthritis functional class II—a long-term study of effects. *Scandinavian Journal of Rheumatology* **20**, 358–65.

Strand, V. et al. (1999). Treatment of active rheumatoid arthritis with leflunomide compared to placebo and methotrexate. *Archives of Internal Medicine* **159**, 2542–50.

Symmons, D. et al. (1998). Long term mortality outcome in patients with rheumatoid arthritis: early presenters continue to do well. *Journal of Rheumatology* **25**, 1072–7.

Tsokos, G.C. (1987). Immunomodulatory treatments in patients with rheumatic diseases: mechanism of action. *Seminars in Arthritis and Rheumatism* **17**, 24–38.

Tugwell, P. (1992). Cyclosporine in rheumatoid arthritis: documented safety and efficacy. *Seminars in Arthritis and Rheumatism*, **21** (Suppl. 3), 30–8.

Tugwell, P. et al. (1989). Methotrexate in RA. *Annals of Internal Medicine* **110**, 581–3.

Tugwell, P. et al. (1995). Combination therapy with cyclosporine and methotrexate in severe rheumatoid arthritis. *New England Journal of Medicine*, **333**, 137–41.

Tunn, E.J. and Bacon, P.A. (1993). Differentiating persistent from self-limiting symmetrical synovitis in an early arthritis clinic. *British Journal of Rheumatology* **32**, 97–103.

Uhlig, T., Hagen, K.B., and Kvien, T.K. (1999). Current tobacco smoking and the risk of rheumatoid arthritis. *Journal of Rheumatology* **42**, 910–17.

Vliet Vlieland, T.P. and Hazes, J.M. (1997). Efficacy of multidisciplinary team care programs in rheumatoid arthritis. *Seminars in Arthritis and Rheumatism* **27**, 110–22.

Wakefield, R.J. et al. (1998). High resolution ultrasound defined subclinical synovitis—a predictor of outcome in early oligoarthritis? *Arthritis and Rheumatism* **41** (Suppl.), S246.

Wakefield, R.J. et al. (2000). The value of sonography in the detection of bone erosion in patients with rheumatoid arthritis: a comparative study with conventional radiography. *Arthritis and Rheumatism* **43**, 2762–70.

Watt, I. and Cobby, M. (2001). Treatment of rheumatoid arthritis patients with interleukin-1 receptor antagonist: radiologic assessment. *Seminars in Arthritis and Rheumatism* **30** (5 Suppl. 2), 21–5.

Weinblatt, M.E. et al. (1990). Low-dose methotrexate compared with auranofin in adult rheumatoid arthritis. *Arthritis and Rheumatism* **33**, 330–8.

Weinblatt, M.E. et al. (1999a). Pharmacokinetics, safety and efficacy of the combination of methotrexate and leflunomide in patients with active rheumatoid arthritis. *Arthritis and Rheumatism* **42**, 1322–7.

Weinblatt, M.E. et al. (1999b). A trial of etanercept, a recombinant tumor necrosis factor receptor: Fc fusion protein, in patients with rheumatoid arthritis receiving methotrexate. *New England Journal of Medicine* **340**, 253–9.

Wilkens, R.F. and Stablein, D. (1996). Combination treatment of rheumatoid arthritis using azothioprine and methotrexate: a 48-week controlled clinical trial. *Journal of Rheumatology* **23** (Suppl. 44), 64–8.

Wolfe, F. et al. (1993). The prognosis of rheumatoid arthritis and undifferentiated polyarthritis syndrome in the clinic: a study of 1141 patients. *Journal of Rheumatology* **20**, 2005–9.

van Zeben, D. et al. (1992). Clinical significance of rheumatoid factors in early rheumatoid arthritis: results of a follow up study. *Annals of the Rheumatic Diseases* **51**, 1029–35.

Zeidler, H.K. et al. (1998). Progression of joint damage in early active severe rheumatoid arthritis during 18 months of treatment: comparison of low-dose cyclosporin and parenteral gold. *British Journal of Rheumatology* **37**, 874–82.

6.3.4 Polyarticular rheumatoid factor positive (seropositive) juvenile idiopathic arthritis*

Alberto Martini

Polyarticular rheumatoid factor positive (seropositive) juvenile idiopathic arthritis (JIA) is identical on clinical, genetic, and laboratory grounds, to adult seropositive rheumatoid arthritis and is considered its equivalent in childhood. However, at variance with adults, where seropositive disease represents the most frequent form of chronic arthritis, seropositive polyarticular JIA is responsible for only a tiny proportion of childhood chronic arthritis.

* The figures in this chapter were supplied by Dr B. Ansell.

Epidemiology

Out of the 1831 children with chronic arthritis recorded in the British Pediatric Rheumatology Group National Diagnostic Register, 55 (3 per cent) had seropositive polyarticular JIA (Symmons et al. 1996). Of the 2071 children recorded in a US Pediatric Rheumatology Disease Registry, only 20 (less than 1 per cent) had seropositive polyarticular JIA (Bowyer et al. 1996).

As in adults, seropositive polyarticular JIA is much more frequent in females than in males with a female/male ratio of 12.8 in the British registry and of 5.7 in the above-mentioned US registry. Seropositive polyarticular disease occurs very rarely in the first years of life and usually has its onset in late childhood or in adolescence. The mean age at onset in the British registry was 9.0 years (range 1.5–15.9) and in the US registry 8.9 ± 4.5 years.

In other parts of the world (such as South Africa, India, and Thailand) as well as among African American and Canadian aboriginal populations, polyarticular seropositive JIA appears to be considerably more frequent, accounting for up to 15–20 per cent of patients with JIA (Andersson-Gäre 1999). The reasons for this increased frequency of seropositive polyarticular JIA in these countries remains speculative and could include: (i) a selection bias towards more severe cases, since these data come from clinical series rather than from epidemiological studies; (ii) differences in genetic predisposition, as suggested by Oen et al. (1998) for Canadian First Nations (Aboriginal) population; (iii) differences in environmental factors such as polyclonal activation of the immune system caused by frequent infections.

Genetics

Since seropositive polyarticular JIA is a quite rare disorder only relatively small series of patients have been studied. However, the results are consistent with what found in adult seropositive arthritis. In a study of 52 Caucasian patients (Clemens et al. 1983), all showing erosive disease by 5 years from onset, 62 per cent were DR4 positive in contrast to 29 per cent of patients with seronegative arthritis and 27 per cent of normal British adult population. About one-fourth of patients had a family history of seropositive rheumatoid arthritis. The same result was obtained in a smaller Scandinavian study in which 53 per cent of the patients were DR4-positive (Forre et al. 1983). Nepom et al. (1984) and subsequently Vehe et al. (1990) confirmed the presence of an association with DR4 and found an increase in the number of patients homozygous for DR4, particularly for the combination Dw4 (DRB1*0401) and Dw14 (DRB1*0404); they suggested that homozygosity for HLA–DR4 positive susceptibility alleles may be related to the earlier onset of the disease in children.

Clinical manifestations

Few studies have been specifically devoted to seropositive polyarticular JIA. The largest group of patients with seropositive JIA has been reported by Ansell (1983). This study included 138 patients, of whom approximately two-thirds had been followed for at least 10 years.

The usual presentation is that of a symmetric polyarthritis involving the small joints of the hands and feet and often developing insidiously. Ansell and Wood (1976) noted that a combination of soft tissue swelling of the wrists and carpi with involvement of metacarpophalangeal and proximal interphalangeal and metatarsophalangeal joints is closely associated with the persistent presence of rheumatoid factor. The large joints, usually knees and ankles, can also be involved early but usually in association with small joint involvement. Hip involvement may occur in the early phase of the disease.

Tendon involvement is frequent. Flexor tenosynovitis of the hand may give rise, much more often than in other forms of JIA, to tendon nodules, and cause finger triggering. Rupture of the extensor tendons, a very rare feature in other forms of JIA, may occur. Rheumatoid nodules, which are much less common in other JIA subsets, occurs in the classic sites (extensor surface of the forearm and elbow) in about one-third of patients during the first year of disease (Ansell 1983).

Oligoarticular onset asymmetric JIA associated with the presence of elevated and persistent titres of rheumatoid factor has been occasionally reported (Sailer et al. 1997). Early erosive disease, early hip involvement, and tendon rupture have all been observed in these patients. Whether this very small and unusual subset of patients belong to polyarticular seropositive JIA or represents a separate entity is unclear.

Tiredness, moderate loss of weight, and general malaise are not uncommon. Low-grade fever and lymphadenopathy are rare. Erythrocyte sedimentation rate and C-reactive protein are elevated and correlate with disease activity. Moderate normochromic and normocytic anaemia may be present. Rheumatoid factor is positive by definition. Although antinuclear antibodies (ANAs) may be positive, their presence is not associated with an increased risk of chronic anterior uveitis, a complication that is characteristic of other ANA positive forms of JIA but not of seropositive polyarticular disease.

In conclusion, seropositive polyarticular JIA is clinical identical to seropositive adult disease and these patients meet the criteria for diagnosis of adult RA. In particular, they have prominent morning stiffness, symmetrical arthritis involving three or more joint areas, frequent involvement of the wrist, metacarpophalangeal and proximal interphalangeal joints, rheumatoid nodules and, as outlined below, erosive radiological changes.

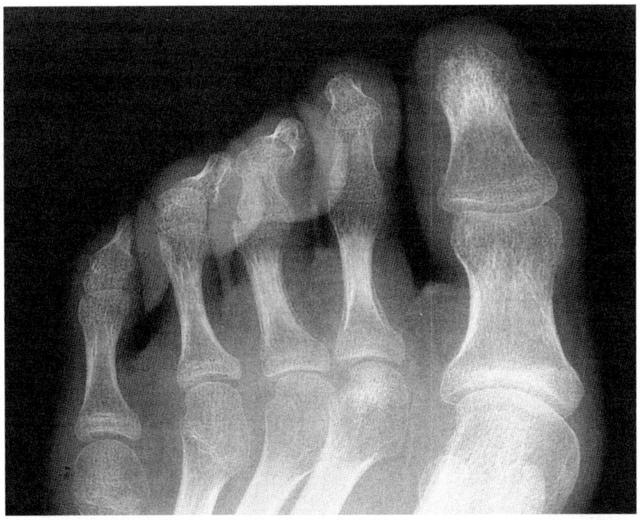

Fig. 1 Periostitis along the proximal phalanx of the second and third toe; note also the severity of the osteoporosis.

Course

The course is characterized, as in adults, by progressive and diffuse joint involvement with severe generalized stiffness; virtually any joint can be involved. Radiological changes tend to occur early, in particular, in the hands and feet. Periostitis along the shafts of the metacarpals and metatarsals and at the bases of the proximal phalanges may be seen radiologically usually between 3 and 6 months (Ansell and Kent 1977) (Fig. 1). On X-ray, protrusio, sometime severe, may occur within months from the first hip symptoms (Ansell 1983) (Fig. 2). By 5 years, the general picture is often that of a severe deforming arthritis. Williams and Ansell (1985) studied retrospectively a total of 81 patients followed for an average of 11 years. Only in some patients, where the disease was controlled, healing of erosions could occur (Fig. 3). However, 5 years from onset all but three patients were affected by erosive disease. The wrist and metacarpophalangeal joints were the common early sites affected by erosions and also the sites of the most severe change (Fig. 4). In the feet the pattern of joint involvement was similar to that found in the hand although the changes were often less severe. Erosion of the hip or knee was present in 30 out of 70 patients and replacement had been performed in eight hips of five patients. After 10 years of disease, the distribution of joint damage was similar. Fusion of carpal bones had occurred in half of the patients studied. Out of 41 patients in the 10 years follow-up, seven had received a total of 12 hip replacements and three patients had received total knee replacements, one being bilateral. Approximately 50 per cent of patients had some degree of atlanto-axial subluxation (Fig. 5). Overall, the joint damage showed a distribution of changes similar to adult seropositive disease with the additional feature of more common distal interphalangeal joint erosion and fusion of the carpal bones.

Severe extra-articular manifestations are rare but can be responsible for severe morbidity during the course of the disease. Severe aortic regurgitation requiring aortic valve replacement has been reported (Leak et al. 1981; Delgado et al. 1988). Although uncommon this complication requires regular cardiac appraisal in the routine assessment of patients. Most patients had long-standing, severe, erosive disease; however, aortic incompetence was seen to occur as early as 2 years from onset. In some patients, echocardiography showed a dilated aortic root that was presumed to be on the basis of aortitis. Rheumatoid nodules in the valve cusps have been demonstrated. Aortic valve regurgitation may remain stable for several years but sudden deterioration in cardiac function can occur at any time (Fig. 6) and coronary artery occlusion, presumably secondary to aortitis, may develop with further compromise of cardiac function.

Pulmonary manifestations are very uncommon. Two cases have been reported in which lymphocytic interstitial pneumonitis preceded the onset of polyarticular seropositive JIA (Lovell et al. 1984; Uziel et al. 1998). Interestingly, both cases were characterized by an unusually precocious

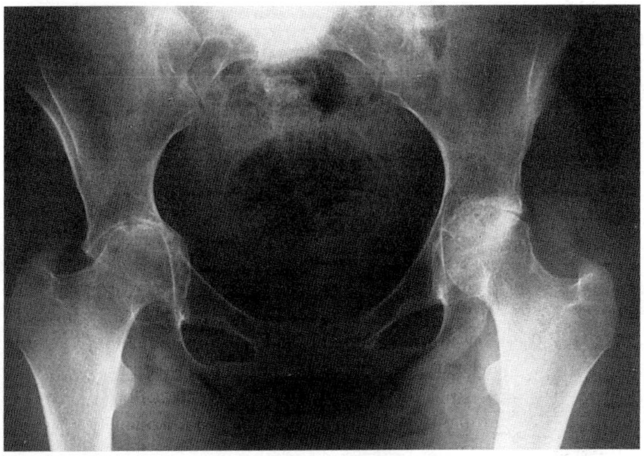

Fig. 2 Both hips were painful and limited in this 14-year-old girl with seropositive disease of 2-years duration. The right shows protrusio with marked narrowing of joint space and erosions; on the left the disease is less advanced.

disease onset, at 5 and at 3.5 years of age, respectively. Pulmonary fibrosis is also of very rare occurrence (Atreya et al. 1980) (Fig. 7). One case of bronchiolitis obliterans in a child receiving chrysotherapy has been reported (Pegg et al. 1994). Felty's syndrome (Rosenberg et al. 1984; Toomey and Hepburn 1985) as well as vasculitis (Ansell 1977) are also exceedingly rare in children with seropositive polyarticular JIA. Although rare, JIA associated Sjögren's syndrome has been reported (Stillman and Barry 1977; Anaya et al. 1995).

Two of the patients followed for at least 10 years by Ansell died from renal failure due to amylodosis (Ansell 1983).

Diagnosis

According to ILAR criteria (Petty et al. 1998) the diagnosis of rheumatoid factor positive polyarticular JIA require the presence, in a child, of arthritis affecting five or more joints during the first 6 months of disease, associated with positive rheumatoid factor test (as routinely defined in a laboratory using the WHO standard) at least on two occasions, 3 months apart, during the first 6 months of observation. Exclusion criteria include the absence of rheumatoid factor and the presence of systemic features. Using standard tests, IgM rheumatoid factor can be detectable within a few weeks from

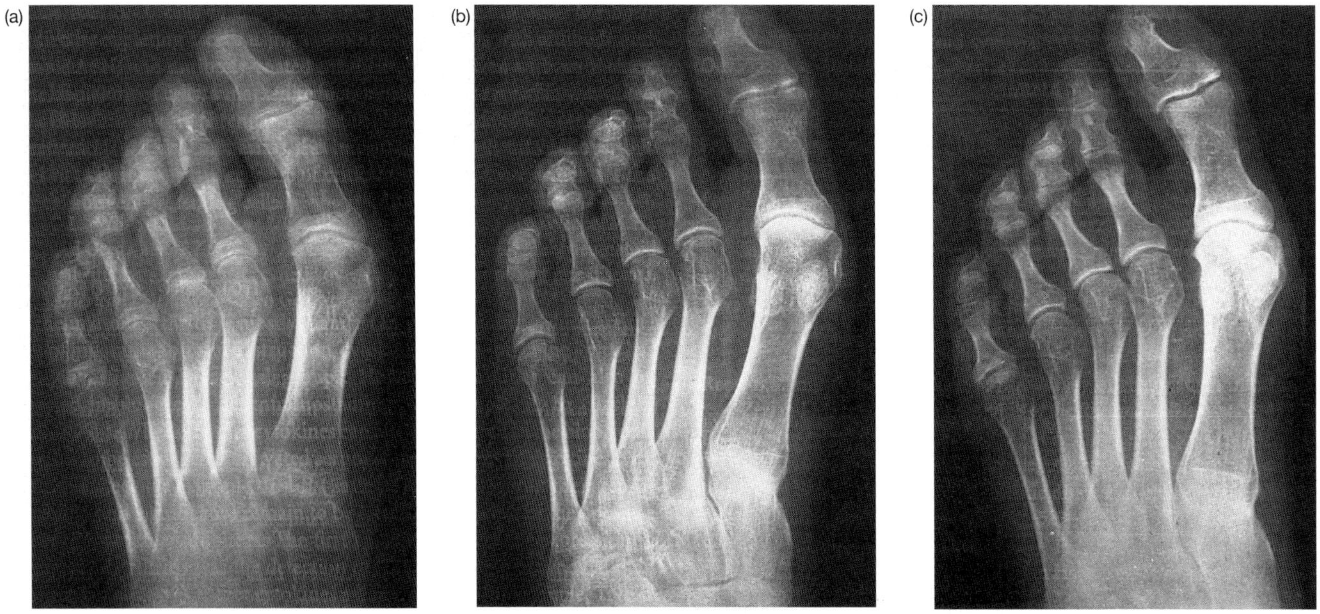

Fig. 3 (a) Radiograph of feet at presentation with disease duration of 3.5 months; note the erosions in the fifth metatarsals and periostitis along the fourth, third, and second proximal phalanges as well as irregularity in the shape of the first metatarsal head. Therapy was commenced at this time and continued. (b) Eighteen months from the first picture there has been healing of the erosions in the fifth metatarsophalangeal joint and improvement in overall porosity with no new erosive changes. (c) This improvement has been maintained during the further 3-year treatment period.

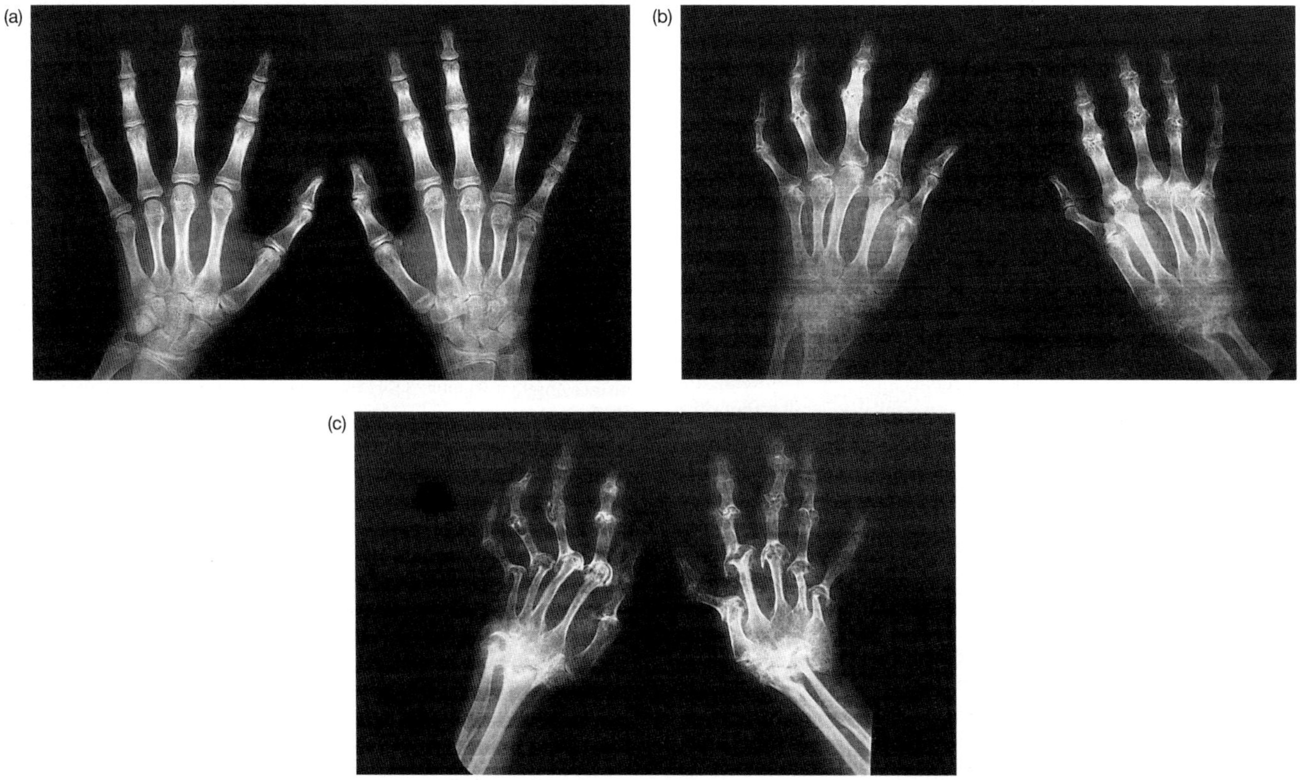

Fig. 4 (a) At presentation, this girl (aged 13.5 years) had crowding of the carpus and changes between the distal row of the carpus; the bases of the metacarpi and particularly the head of the second metacarpals on both sides are thinning. (b) 5 years from onset there has been gross destructive arthritis affecting the carpus which is fusing all metacarpophalangeal joints, and proximal and distal interphalangeal joints. (c) Twenty years from onset destruction has occurred, particularly in the metacarpophalangeal joints and at the wrists.

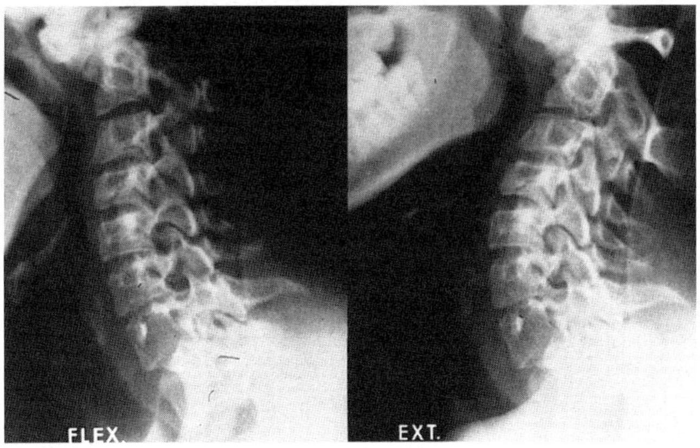

Fig. 5 Atlanto-axial subluxation causing compression on the cord but with selectively little change elsewhere in the cervical spine.

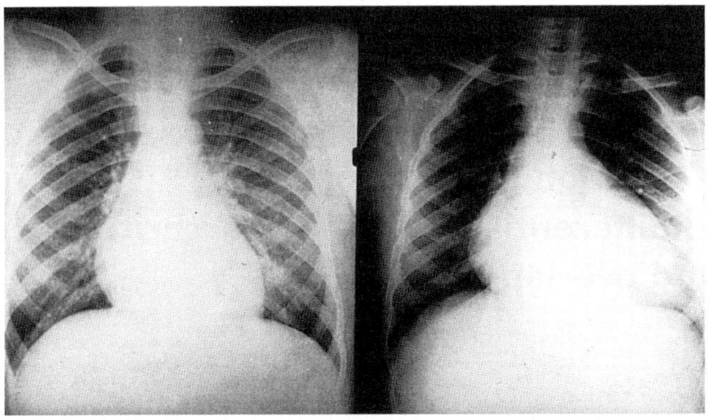

Fig. 6 Rapidly increasing cardiac silhouette over 4 months in a girl who had been noted to have a diastolic murmur 7 months before.

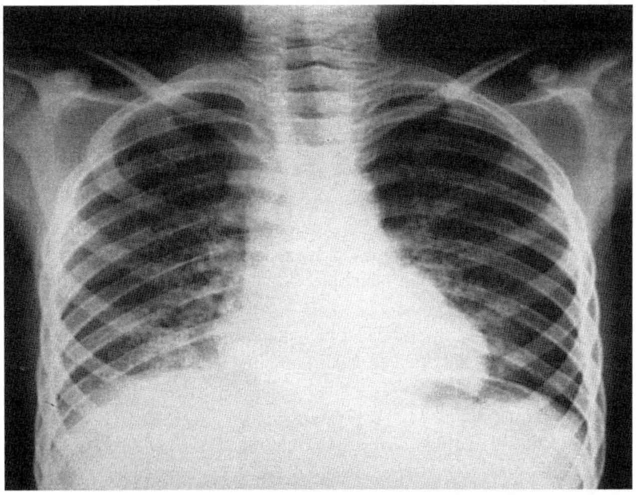

Fig. 7 This 15-year-old patient presented with increasing dyspnoea. Although seropositive, relatively mild juvenile rheumatoid arthritis of some 5-years duration was present affecting the hands and feet only. The duration of the chest symptoms could not be adequately assessed, but he had finger clubbing at presentation.

disease onset and in the majority by 3 months titres tend to rise as the disease become established; it is exceptional for the rheumatoid factor to become positive after more than 1 year of illness (Ansell 1987).

Rheumatoid factor may be transiently positive in several infectious diseases that may cause arthritis including viral infections and sub-acute bacterial endocarditis; on the other hand, rheumatoid factor may be persistently positive in chronic inflammatory conditions such as sarcoidosis or in connective tissue diseases such as systemic lupus erythematosus or overlap syndromes that may cause arthritis. All such conditions have to be excluded before assuming that a child has seropositive polyarticular JIA.

Treatment

Unlike seronegative JIA, no specific controlled trial has been performed in seropositive polyarticular JIA to evaluate drug efficacy. However, since the disease is considered the childhood equivalent of seropositive adult rheumatoid arthritis, the results obtained in studies performed in adults can also be considered valid for childhood disease. Therefore, principles of management are essentially the same as in adults.

Non-steroidal anti-inflammatory drugs of common use in children are described in the previous section on seronegative polyarthritis. Low-dose methotrexate, which is the first-choice remission-inducing agent, appears to be well tolerated in children with JIA (Ravelli and Martini 2000). As in adults, antitumour necrosis factor agents are effective and well tolerated (Lovell et al. 2000). As in other childhood diseases, corticosteroids, where indicated, should be used at the lowest effective dosage, possibly on an alternate day regimen and, if daily treatment is needed, administered once daily in the morning. These measures reduce the risk of suppression of the hypothalamic pituitary adrenal axis and the risk of toxicity including the negative effect on statural growth.

Of course, as in other forms of arthritis, physiotherapy is of great importance in maintaining position and function of the joints. Since the disease often follows a destructive course, collaboration with orthopaedic services is particularly important in disease management. About half of the orthopaedic surgical procedures performed in patients with JIA in a referral centre concerned patients with polyarticular seropositive disease (Ansell 1983).

Two specific paediatric instruments that are very useful to assess functional ability (Childhood Health Assessment Questionnaire or CHAQ) and quality of life (Child Health Questionnaire or CHQ) during treatment have been translated in many languages and cross-culturally adapted and validated (Martini and Ruperto 2001).

Since the disease often occurs in adolescents, particular attention should be paid to the handling of problems that are peculiar to this delicate age. Development of independence, of self-confidence and self-esteem can be profoundly affected by the physical limitation and the alteration of the body image produced by the disease especially in relation with peer relationships, school achievements, and vocational expectations. In this respect, management of the disease needs careful, sympathetic handling, as well as the cooperation of the family and the involvement of school teachers.

Summary

Polyarticular rheumatoid factor positive (seropositive) juvenile idiopathic arthritis (JIA) on clinical, genetic and laboratory grounds, is identical to adult seropositive rheumatoid arthritis and is considered its equivalent in childhood. However, at variance with adults, seropositive polyarticular JIA is responsible for only a small (≤3%) proportion of childhood chronic arthritis.

As in adults, the disease often follows a rapidly destructive course and requires prompt treatment. Extra-articular manifestations are rare but can be responsible for additional severe morbidity. The therapeutic approach does not differ from that in adults and often includes the early indication of methotrexate and antitumour necrosis factor agents. As in other childhood diseases, drug (such as corticosteroids) usage has to take into account toxicity specifically related to paediatric age. Since the disease often occurs in adolescents, special attention should be paid to psychological implications.

References

Anaya, J.-M., Ogawa, N., and Talal, N. (1995). Sjögren's syndrome in childhood. *Journal of Rheumatology* **22**, 1152–8.

Andersson-Gäre, B. (1999). Juvenile arthritis. Who gets it, where and when? A review of current data on incidence and prevalence. *Clinical and Experimental Rheumatology* **17**, 367–74.

Ansell, B.M. (1977). Juvenile chronic polyarthritis. *Arthritis and Rheumatism* **20** (Suppl.), 176–8.

Ansell, B.M. (1983). Juvenile chronic arthritis with persistently positive tests for rheumatoid factor (sero-positive juvenile rheumatoid arthritis). *Annales de Pédiatrie* **30**, 545–50.

Ansell, B.M. (1987). Juvenile chronic arthritis. *Scandinavian Journal of Rheumatology* **66** (Suppl.), 47–50.

Ansell, B.M. and Kent, P.A. (1977). Radiological changes in juvenile chronic polyarthritis. *Skeletal Radiology* **1**, 129–44.

Ansell, B.M. and Wood, P.H.N. (1976). Prognosis in juvenile chronic polyarthritis. *Clinic in Rheumatic Diseases* **2**, 397–412.

Athreya, B.H., Doughty, R.A., Bookspan, M., Schumacher, H.R., Sewell, E.M., and Chatten, J. (1980). Pulmonary manifestations of juvenile rheumatoid arthritis. *Clinics in Chest Medicine* **1**, 361–74.

Bowyer, S., Roettcher, P., and the members of the Paediatric Rheumatology Database Research Group (1996). Pediatric rheumatology clinic populations in the United States: results of a 3 year survey. *Journal of Rheumatology* **23**, 1968–74.

Clemens, L.E., Albert, E., and Ansell, B.M. (1983). HLA studies in IgM rheumatoid factor positive childhood arthritis. *Annals of the Rheumatic Diseases* **42**, 431–4.

Delgado, E.A., Petty, R.E., Malleson, P.N., Patterson, M.W.H., D'Orsogna, L., and LeBlanc, J. (1988). Aortic valve insufficiency and coronary artery narrowing in a child with polyarticular juvenile rheumatoid arthritis. *Journal of Rheumatology* **15**, 144–7.

Forre, O., Dobloug, J.H., Hoyeraal, H.M., and Thorsby, E. (1983). HLA antigens in juvenile arthritis: genetic basis for different subtypes. *Arthritis and Rheumatism* **26**, 35–8.

Leak, A.M., Millar-Craig, M.W., and Ansell, B.M. (1981). Aortic regurgitation in seropositive juvenile arthritis. *Annals of the Rheumatic Diseases* **40**, 229–34.

Lovell, D., Lindsley, C., and Langston, C. (1984). Lymphoid interstitial pneumonia in juvenile rheumatoid arthritis. *Journal of Pediatrics* **105**, 947–50.

Lovell, J.D. et al. (2000) Etanercept in children with polyarticular juvenile rheumatoid arthritis. *New England Journal of Medicine* **342**, 763–9.

Martini, A. and Ruperto, N., ed. (2001). Quality of life in juvenile idiopathic arthritis patients compared to healthy children. *Clinical and Experimental Rheumatology* **19** (Suppl. 23), S1–172.

Nepom, B.S., Nepom, G.T., Mickelson, E., Schaller, J.G., Antonelli, P., and Hansen, J.A. (1984). Specific HLA–DR4-associated histocompatibility molecules characterize patients with seropositive juvenile rheumatoid arthritis. *Journal of Clinical Investigation* **74**, 287–91.

Oen, K. et al. (1998). Juvenile rheumatoid arthritis in a Canadian First Nations (Aboriginal) population: onset subtypes and HLA associations. *Journal of Rheumatology* **25**, 783–90.

Pegg, S.J., Lang, B., Mikhail, E.L., and Hughes, D.M. (1994). Fatal bronchiolitis obliterans in a patient with juvenile rheumatoid arthritis receiving chrysotherapy. *Journal of Rheumatology* **21**, 549–51.

Petty, R.E. et al. (1998). Revision of the proposed classification criteria for juvenile idiopathic arthritis: Durban, 1997. *Journal of Rheumatology* **25**, 1991–4.

Ravelli, A. and Martini, A. (2000). Methotrexate in juvenile idiopathic arthritis: answers and questions. *Journal of Rheumatology* **27**, 1830–3.

Rosemberg, A.M., Mitchell, D.M., and Card, R.T. (1984). Felty's syndrome in a child. *Journal of Rheumatology* **1984**, 835–7.

Sailer, M., Cabral, D., Petty, R.E., and Malleson, P.N. (1997). Rheumatoid factor positive, oligoarticular onset juvenile rheumatoid arthritis. *Journal of Rheumatology* **24**, 586–8.

Stillman, J.S. and Barry, P.E. (1977). Juvenile rheumatoid arthritis. *Arthritis and Rheumatism* **20** (Suppl.), 171–5.

Symmons, D.P.M., Jones, M., Osborne, J., Sills, J., Southwood, T.R., and Woo, P. (1996). Pediatric rheumatology in the United Kingdom: data from the British Pediatric Rheumatology Group National Diagnostic Register. *Journal of Rheumatology* **23**, 1975–80.

Toomey, K. and Hepburn, B. (1985). Felty syndrome in juvenile arthritis. *Journal of Pediatrics* **106**, 254–5.

Uziel, Y., Hen, B., Cordoba, M., and Wolach, B. (1998). Lymphocytic interstitial pneumonitis preceding polyarticular juvenile rheumatoid arthritis. *Clinical and Experimental Rheumatology* **16**, 617–19.

Vehe, R.K., Begovich, A.B., and Nepom, B.S. (1990). HLA susceptibility genes in rheumatoid factor positive juvenile rheumatoid arthritis. *Journal of Rheumatology Supplement* **26** (Suppl.), 11–15.

Williams, R.A. and Ansell, B.M. (1985). Radiological findings in seropositive juvenile chronic arthritis (juvenile rheumatoid arthritis) with particular reference to progression. *Annals of the Rheumatic Diseases* **44**, 685–93.

6.4 Spondyloarthropathies

6.4.1 Spondyloarthropathy, undifferentiated spondyloarthritis, and overlap

Eric Veys and Herman Mielants

Introduction

Spondyloarthropathy is a group of chronic autoimmune disorders (Schumacher and Bardin 1998) including ankylosing spondylitis (van der Linden and van der Heijde 1998), reactive arthritis (Keat 1999), psoriatic arthritis (Espinoza et al. 1992), arthritis associated with inflammatory bowel disease (De Keyser et al. 1998), acute anterior uveitis (Rosenbaum 1992), and undifferentiated spondyloarthropathies (Zeidler et al. 1992). A childhood form juvenile spondyloarthropathy also exists (Veys et al. 1995). The spondyloarthropathies share common clinical, radiological, and genetic features that are clearly distinct from other inflammatory rheumatic diseases.

History and terminology

Wright and Moll introduced the concept initially using the term *seronegative polyarthritis* (Wright and Moll 1976), which was eventually changed to *spondyloarthropathy*. The term relates not only to the spine and the peripheral joints but also refers to other structures, which are involved in the disease process (the enthesis, the eye, the gut) (François et al. 1995; Braun and Sieper 1996). The adjective seronegative is useless, since the absence of the rheumatoid factor is the primary characteristic of patients included in the concept and the term is confusing with its most common use in relation to HIV infection.

Characteristics of the spondyloarthropathies

These common characteristics, which are essential in the recognition of the spondyloarthropathy concept, are listed in Table 1.

Absence of the rheumatoid factor and rheumatoid nodules

The co-existence of spondyloarthropathy and rheumatoid arthritis in the same patient may occur (Luthra et al. 1976). Histologically proven rheumatoid nodules are not, however, found in spondyloarthropathies and remain characteristic for rheumatoid arthritis.

Peripheral arthritis

The peripheral arthritis in the spondyloarthropathies is generally pauciarticular, asymmetrical, and involves preferentially the small and large weight-bearing joints of the lower limbs. The number of involved joints is clinically less important than the asymmetry, keeping in mind that the fewer involved joints, the better the chance of observing an asymmetrical pattern; the larger the number of involved joints, the smaller the chance of finding an asymmetrical pattern. In general, the arthritis is non-erosive and self-resolving, in some patients the arthritis becomes chronic and erosive (Fig. 1) (Mielants et al. 1990a).

In contrast to rheumatoid arthritis, distal interphalangeal joint involvement in spondyloarthropathies is common. Dactylitis is a specific peripheral manifestation of the spondyloarthropathies and comprises tenosynovitis of the flexor tendon, often accompanied by arthritis of the proximal interphalangeal and distal interphalangeal joint of the same digit or toe (sausage finger or toe) (Fig. 2). Peripheral arthritis is the key feature of undifferentiated spondyloarthropathies, reactive arthritis, and juvenile spondyloarthropathies. In ankylosing spondylitis peripheral joint involvement varies according to authors but a prevalence of up to 40 per cent is reported (Gran et al. 1997). The hips and the shoulders are the most frequently involved peripheral joints in ankylosing spondylitis. Peripheral arthritis other than hip and shoulders in spondyloarthropathies, is a distinct entity from the axial involvement not related to the presence of HLA-B27. The pattern of the peripheral arthritis is clearly asymmetrical even in patients in whom the peripheral involvement is polyarticular, as in a majority of the cases with long-standing psoriatic arthritris.

Table 1 Characteristics of the spondyloarthropathy concept

1. Absence of the rheumatoid factor and rheumatoid nodules
2. Peripheral arthritis
3. Spinal inflammation: inflammatory back pain, sacroiliitis with or without spondylitis
4. Peripheral enthesitis
5. Clinical overlap between different entities of the group
6. Familial aggregation
7. Association with HLA-B27

Spinal inflammation: inflammatory back pain and sacroiliitis with or without spondylitis

Inflammatory back pain is often the earliest sign of inflammatory spinal involvement in spondyloarthropathies. Inflammatory back pain is defined by insidious onset before the age of 45 years, improvement by exercise, association with morning stiffness and duration of at least 3 months (Calin et al. 1977). Inflammatory back pain is present in more than 90 per cent of patients with ankylosing spondylitis, in 50–80 per cent of patients with undifferentiated spondyloarthropathies (Zeidler et al. 1992), in 11 per cent of the patients with inflammatory bowel diseases (Protzer et al. 1996), and in 70 per cent of patients with reactive arthritis (Fox et al. 1979).

Sacroiliitis is the cornerstone for the classification of ankylosing spondylitis; without sacroiliitis the definite diagnosis of ankylosing spondylitis cannot be made. Few patients with typical spinal lesions of ankylosing spondylitis without sacroiliitis have been described (Khan et al. 1985). Sacroiliitis affects up to 40 per cent of the patients with reactive arthritis (Leirisalo-Repo et al. 1994), 20 per cent of the psoriatic arthritis patients (Torre Alonso et al. 1991), 20 per cent of the patients with inflammatory bowel disease (de Vlam et al. 2000), and 50–70 per cent of the patients with undifferentiated spondyloarthropathy (Mau et al. 1988). Sacroilitis in ankylosing spondylitis is no different from the sacroiliac involvement in other forms of spondyloarthropathies, except for the more frequent unilateral involvement in the latter diseases.

The spondylitis is characterized radiologically by the presence of squaring, erosions, syndesmophytes, zygapophyseal joint involvement, discitis and ankylosis. Usually the spondylitis develops at a later stage of the disease than the sacroiliitis. The spondylitis in ankylosing spondylitis cannot be distinguished from the spondylitis in the other forms of spondyloarthropathy, except for the asymmetrical appearance of the syndesmophytes in the latter diseases. Radiological signs of spondylitis are seen in 62 per cent of the ankylosing spondylitis patients with a higher frequency in male compared to female patients (Gran et al. 1997). Differences are seen between HLA-B27 positive and HLA-B27 negative ankylosing spondylitis patients (Mielants et al. 1993). Spondylitis evolves to bamboo spine in about 20 per cent of the ankylosing spondylitis patients but less frequently in females than in males (Gran et al. 1997). Spondylitis affects up to 26 per cent of the patients with reactive arthritis (Leirisalo-Repo 1998), 20 per cent of the patients with psoriatic arthritis (Scarpa et al. 1988), and 20 per cent with inflammatory bowel disease (de Vlam et al. 2000).

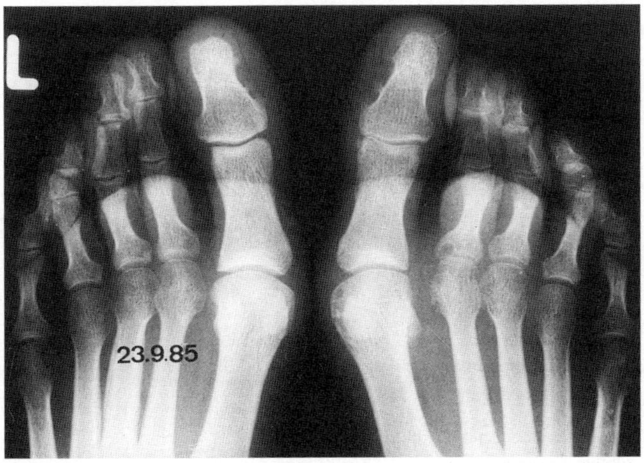

Fig. 1 Erosive lesions of MTP joints I and II right (pauciarticular and asymmetric) in a patient with spondyloarthropathy.

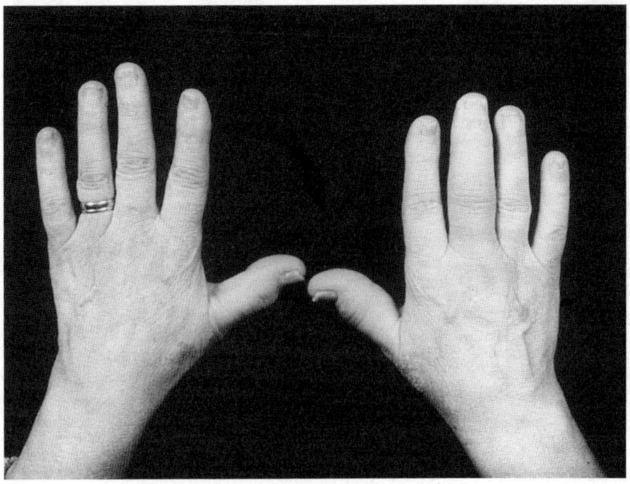

Fig. 2 Sausage finger: third finger right.

Peripheral enthesitis

Inflammation at the enthesis, the attachment of a tendon, joint capsule, ligament, or fascia to bone, is a specific pathological characteristic of the spondyloarthropathies (Ball 1971). Inflammation at the enthesis causes a focal osteitis with local destruction, followed by the formation of granulation tissue, which is replaced by bone in the final phase (Ball 1971). Repeated episodes of inflammation, destruction, and osseous repair result in bone apposition, the enthesophyte. In the spine the enthesitis is localized at the intervertebral disc, the zygapophyseal joints. The most frequently involved peripheral entheses are the insertion of the fascia plantaris at the calcaneum, the insertion of the Achilles' tendon at the posterior surface of the calcaneum and the insertion of the ligamentum patellae at the tuberositas tibiae (Fig. 3). Peripheral enthesitis can cause pain but may be also asymptomatic. Peripheral enthesitis occurs in 20 per cent of the patients with spondyloarthropathy and is seen in all forms of spondyloarthropathy. Isolated enthesitis in association with HLA-B27 is reported as the presenting symptom in some cases (Olivieri et al. 1989). In ankylosing spondylitis, the prevalence varies from one study to the other from 25 to 54 per cent (Gerster et al. 1977; Resnick et al. 1977) and may antedate peripheral arthritis and spinal symptoms in juvenile onset forms (Burgos-Vargas et al. 1997). Peripheral enthesitis is found in up to 40 per cent of the patients with reactive arthritis (Kvien et al. 1994), in 20–50 per cent of the patients with pauciarticular juvenile arthritis (Gerster and Piccinin 1985; Mielants et al. 1993), in 6 per cent of the patients with inflammatory bowel disease (Scarpa et al. 1992; de Vlam et al. 2000), and in 20 per cent of patients with psoriatic arthritis (Oriente et al. 1994).

Overlap between the different clinical entities of the spondyloarthropathy concept

There is a definite clinical overlap between the different diseases which are included in the spondyloarthropathy concept (Moll et al. 1974). The diseases share not only many clinical and radiological locomotor manifestations, such as inflammatory back pain, peripheral arthritis, enthesitis, sacroiliitis, and spondylitis, but also extra-articular manifestations in the eye, at the mucosal level, and in the skin. Acute anterior uveitis which is linked to HLA-B27 is the most common extra-articular manifestation of spondyloarthropathy and occurs in 20–40 per cent of the patients during the course of the disease (Banares et al. 1998).

Mucosal involvement in patients with spondyloarthropathy is seen in the gastrointestinal and urogenital tracts. Mucocutaneous changes in the mouth are seen in 10 per cent of patients with chlamydia-induced reactive arthritis (Amor et al. 1983). Inflammatory gut lesions are found in 65 per cent of the patients with undifferentiated spondyloarthropathy, in 90 per cent of the patients with intestinal triggered reactive arthritis, and in 60 per cent of the patients with ankylosing spondylitis, with a higher prevalence in patients with peripheral involvement (Mielants et al. 1989). Gut inflammation is also observed in psoriatic arthritis (Schatteman et al. 1995), in late onset pauciarticular juvenile chronic arthritis (Mielants et al. 1993), and in acute anterior uveitis (Mielants et al. 1990b).

Other mucosal localization (urethritis, balanitis, cervicitis) occurs, especially in urogenital reactive arthritis but is rare in other subgroups. Prostatitis is quite common in urogenital reactive arthritis and in ankylosing spondylitis (Wollenhaupt et al. 1995). Balanitis, cervicitis, and urethritis are often asymptomatic. Similar lesions can also be observed in the oral mucosa. Skin involvement, such as erythema nodosum, keratoderma blennorrhagica, pyoderma gangrenosum, and psoriatic-like lesions occur with variable frequencies (Wollenhaupt et al. 1995).

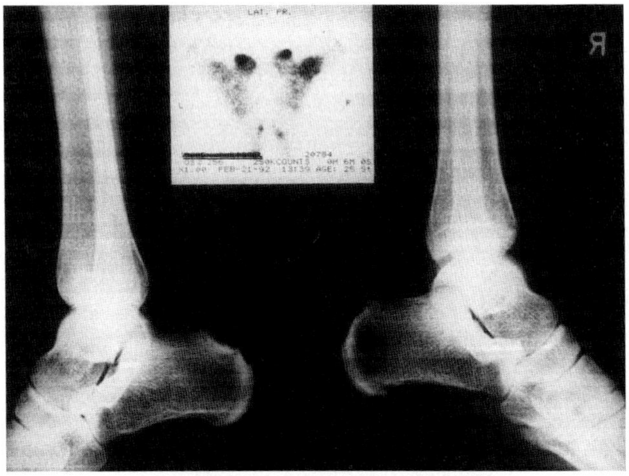

Fig. 3 Bilateral enthesitis of the Achilles' tendon insertion; on the left side important erosion. In the middle of the figure: technetium-scan of both feet; high uptake at the insertion of the Achilles' tendon.

Familial aggregation

Evidence for familial aggregation in each of the disorders may be derived from multiple pedigree studies (Wright 1978; Hochberg et al. 1978). Sixteen per cent of the patients with spondyloarthropathy have a first or second degree relative with inflammatory axial pain or peripheral arthritis (Hochberg et al. 1978). An increased prevalence of ankylosing spondylitis and subclinical sacroiliitis is reported in relatives of patients with inflammatory bowel disease, reactive arthritis, and juvenile chronic arthritis (Calin and Fries 1975; Mielants et al. 1986).

Association with HLA-B27

The discovery of an association between HLA-B27 and ankylosing spondylitis and related disorders broadened the interest and understanding of these diseases (Brewerton et al. 1973; Schlosstein et al. 1973). The strong association of the spondyloarthropathies with HLA-B27 reinforces the familial aggregation and the clinical overlap amongst the different entities of the concept. The prevalence of ankylosing spondylitis and spondyloarthropathies in a population correlates directly with the prevalence of HLA-B27 and there may be differences amongst HLA-B27 and disease association according to the different ethnic groups. The association of HLA-B27 seems especially linked to the presence of spondylitis and sacroiliitis rather than to the presence of peripheral arthritis.

The frequency of HLA-B27 in the various diseases of the spondyloarthropathy concept is given in Table 2.

Table 2 Frequency of HLA-B27 in the different spondyloarthropathies

Disease	HLA-B27 positivity (%)
Ankylosing spondylitis	>90
Reactive arthritis	70–90
Psoriatic arthritis	
With peripheral arthritis	a to 25
With sacroiliitis or spondylitis	70
Inflammatory bowel diseases	
With peripheral arthritis	a
With spondylitis or sacroiliitis	50–70
Undifferentiated spondyloarthropathy	80
Idiopathic anterior uveitis	70
Late onset pauciarticular chronic juvenile arthritis	
Without sacroiliitis	25
With sacroiliitis	40–60

a Denotes equal to normal population.

Classification criteria

Classification criteria for several disorders belonging to the spondyloarthropathy already exist; for ankylosing spondylitis: the Rome criteria (Kellgren 1962), the New York criteria (Bennett and Burch 1968), the van der Linden criteria (van der Linden et al. 1984); for psoriatic arthritis (Vasey and Espinoza 1984). There is a consensus that these criteria are too restricted, as there is a need to emphasize the existence of a much wider disease spectrum. This radiographically detected sacroiliitis in the absence of symptoms would not be included in the existing classifications. Some patients who clearly are part of the spondyloarthropathy concept, such as those who, for example, present an asymmetric sacroiliitis together with a dactylitis or an anterior uveitis, would also be excluded from these classifications. For this reason the European Spondyloarthropathy Study Group (ESSG) has proposed a set of criteria for the entire spondyloarthropathy group of patients (Dougados et al. 1991). Patients with clearly defined disease entities such as reactive arthritis or ankylosing spondylitis on the one hand and those with undifferentiated spondyloarthropathy on the other would be selected by these criteria. Patients with inflammatory spinal pain or asymmetrical synovitis predominantly of the lower limb, together with at least one of the following: positive family history, psoriasis, inflammatory bowel disease, enthesopathy, alternate buttock pain, or sacroiliitis correspond to the ESSG criteria and should be classified as spondyloarthropathy (Table 3).

Parallel to the ESSG criteria, Amor et al. (1991) have developed a point-scale with comparable sensitivity and specificity (Table 4). By their simplicity, the ESSG criteria are more useful in general medicine.

Table 3 European Spondyloarthropathy Study Group (ESSG) criteria

Inflammatory spinal pain or
Synovitis (asymmetrical[a] or predominantly in the lower limbs[a])
and
One or more of the following
Positive family history
Psoriasis
Inflammatory bowel disease
Enthesopathy
Alternate buttock pain
Sacroiliitis

[a] Without sacroiliitis, sensitivity = 77%, specificity = 89%; with sacroiliitis, sensitivity = 86%, specificity = 87%.

Table 4 Criteria for diagnosing spondyloarthropathies (Amor 1991)

	Points
A. Clinical symptoms or past history of	
1. Lumbar or dorsal pain during the night or morning stiffness of the lumbar or dorsal spine	1
2. Asymmetrical oligoarthritis	2
3. Buttock pain—if affecting alternatively the right or the left buttock	1 or 2
4. Sausage-like toe or digit	2
5. Heel pain or other well-defined enthesopathic pain	2
6. Iritis	2
7. Non-gonococcal urethritis or cervicitis accompanying or within 1 month before onset of arthritis	1
8. Acute diarrhoea accompanying, or within 1 month before, the onset of arthritis	1
9. Presence or history of psoriasis and/or balanitis and/or inflammatory bowel disease (ulcerative colitis, Crohn's disease)	2
B. Radiological findings	
10. Sacroiliitis (grade ≥ 2 if bilateral, grade ≥ 3 if unilateral	3
C. Genetic background	
11. Presence of HLA-B27 and/or familial history of ankylosing spondylitis, Reiter's syndrome, uveitis, psoriasis, or chronic enterocolopathies	2
D. Response to treatment	
12. Clear-cut improvement of rheumatic complaints with non-steroidal anti-inflammatory drugs (dramatic improvement or relapse of the pain in NSAIDs discontinued)	2

A patient will be considered as suffering from a spondyloarthropathy if the sum of the 12 criteria is at least 6.

Diseases belonging to the spondyloarthropathy concept

The diseases included in the spondyloarthropathy concept are listed in Table 5. They all will be described in subsequent paragraphs and chapters (see Chapters 6.4.2, 6.4.3, 6.4.5, and 1.3.12).

Previously the late onset pauciarticular juvenile chronic arthritis was considered as a disease belonging to the concept like the others, but it seems preferable to consider that this group is as heterogeneous as in the adult, in which we must recognize different subgroups as juvenile ankylosing spondylitis, juvenile psoriatic arthritis, juvenile inflammatory bowel disease, juvenile acute anterior uveitis, and juvenile undifferentiated spondyloarthropathies.

At present Whipple's disease is no longer included in the concept since the incidence of sacroiliitis and spondylitis as well as the relationship with HLA-B27 is controversial (Feurle et al. 1979; Dobbins 1987). Moreover, the pattern of peripheral joint is mostly polyarticular and symmetrical in contrast with the pauciarticular asymmetric involvement in the spondyloarthropathies (Helliwell and Wright 1987).

There is some debate as to whether or not Behçet's syndrome is a spondyloarthropathy. Lack of familial association with other diseases included in the concept, the association with HLA-B51 rather than with HLA-B27, the lack of low back pain and the intermittent reports about the incidence of sacroiliitis resulted in the exclusion of Behçet's disease from the spondyloarthropathy concept (Hamuryudan et al. 1997). Nonetheless, the simultaneous presence of spondyloarthropathy and Behçet's disease may occur in the same patient. The same question can be asked about the classification of the arthritis occurring in coeliac disease. The peripheral involvement is polyarticular and symmetric, without predominance of the lower limbs, the arthritis disappears when the patient is kept on a gluten-free diet and does not relapse if adherence to the diet. Axial involvement is rare (Lubrano et al. 1996) and the relation with HLA-B27 is inconstant (Bourne et al. 1985). Consequently, the arthritis in coeliac disease should probably be excluded from the spondyloarthropathy concept.

SAPHO (synovitis, acne pustulosis, hyperostosis, and osteomyelitis) syndrome groups joint and bone involvement associated with dermatological disorders, such as palmoplantar pustulosis and pustular psoriasis (Chamot et al. 1987). The association with sacroiliitis, bowel disease, and

Table 5 Diseases included in the spondyloarthropathy concept

Ankylosing spondylitis
Reactive arthritis (enterogenic and urogenital)
Psoriatic arthritis
Inflammatory bowel disease
Acute anterior uveitis
Synovitis acne pustulosis hyperostosis osteomyelitis (SAPHO) syndrome
Undifferentiated spondyloarthropathies
Juvenile spondyloarthropathies

psoriasis links SAPHO with the concept of spondyloarthropathy (Kahn and Khan 1994).

A number of patients correspond to the characteristics of the spondyloarthropathies but cannot be classified in one of the diseases listed in Table 5. They are included in the concept and are labelled as undifferentiated spondyloarthropathy (Mielants et al. 1989; Khan and van der Linden 1990). Careful investigation for associated conditions like psoriasis (by careful clinical observation in the hair region and umbilical region and of the nails) and inflammatory bowel disease (by performing ileocolonoscopy with biopsy) and the discovery of other unexpected disease associations will reduce the number of patients with undifferentiated spondyloarthropathy and will enable their classification into one of the well-defined subgroups. Clinical research and further improvement of the knowledge of the pathogenesis of the spondyloarthropathies in the future may end with the disappearance of the subgroup of the undifferentiated spondyloarthropathies.

Description of the diseases included in the spondyloarthropathy concept

Ankylosing spondylitis (see Chapter 6.4.3)

Psoriatic arthritis (see Chapter 6.4.4)

Reactive arthritis (see Chapter 6.4.5)

Inflammatory bowel disease

Inflammatory joint disease is generally considered an enteropathic arthritis if the gastrointestinal tract is directly involved in the pathogenesis. A wide spectrum of other rheumatic diseases may be accompanied by intestinal complication, but cannot be classified as enteropathic arthritides.

The most common enteropathic arthritides belong to the concept of spondyloarthropathies; Whipple's disease and coeliac disease can cause joint involvement but are not considered spondyloarthropathies. Idiopathic inflammatory bowel disease, Crohn's disease, and ulcerative colitis are the specific diseases linked to the concept.

Epidemiology

The prevalence of ulcerative colitis ranges from 50 to 100 individuals per 100 000 in the general population. The disease seems to be more frequent in Whites than in non-Whites, and more frequent in the Jewish population. The prevalence of Crohn's disease has increased during the last few decades to about 75 per 100 000. Ongoing epidemiological studies suggest that the true prevalence may have been underestimated by 27–35 per cent (Mayberry et al. 1989). These studies also suggest the existence of patients with subclinical inflammatory bowel disease.

Peripheral arthritis, enthesitis, sacroiliitis, and axial involvement are the most frequent extra-intestinal manifestations occurring in about 40 per cent of the patients (de Vlam et al. 2000) but skin, eye, and other organs can be involved.

Intestinal symptoms

The most frequent abdominal manifestations of ulcerative colitis are diarrhoea and blood loss. In distal locations, there can be passage of blood with each bowel movement. With more extensive colon involvement, the blood will be mixed with a soft, liquid, and sometimes mucopurulent stool. Diarrhoea is practically always present.

Crohn's disease is characterized by the classic triad of diarrhoea, abdominal pain, and weight loss. Disease onset may be insidious and progression subclinical. Diarrhoea consists mainly of frequent watery bowel movements and typically follows meals. The stool volume depends on the anatomic location of the disease. Intestinal bleeding is uncommon. Abdominal pain is present in the majority of patients and described as cramping, predominantly in the right lower quadrant of the abdomen. Pain is usually not reported as severe.

Weight loss is a common feature and is in the range of 10–20 per cent of body weight. General debility is a common complaint together with low grade fever.

In the later stages of Crohn's disease perianal involvement appears, with fistulae and abscesses. The finding of a tender abdominal mass may be a sign of an intra-abdominal abscess or fistulae.

In ulcerative colitis abdominal pain, rectal cramps and fever are less frequent than in Crohn's disease, and considerable weight loss is distinctly uncommon.

Peripheral arthritis

The frequency of peripheral arthritis in inflammatory bowel disease ranges from 17 to 20 per cent with a higher prevalence in Crohn's disease (Gravallese et al. 1988).

In studies from gastrointestinal units arthritis was described in 10 per cent of inflammatory bowel disease patients (Orchard et al. 1998; de Vlam et al. 2000) but this prevalence is underestimated since in a rheumatological clinic articular involvement was described in 65 per cent of patients with ulcerative colitis (Scarpa et al. 1992).

The sex ratio in inflammatory bowel disease is equal, and peak age is between 25 and 44 years. In both diseases, the arthritis is pauciarticular, generally asymmetric, and frequently transient and migratory. Large and small joints, predominantly of the lower limbs, are involved. The arthritis usually is non-destructive, and many attacks subside within 6 weeks. Recurrences are common. Dactylitis may occur. Enthesopathies, especially inflammation of the Achilles tendon or of the insertion of the plantar fascia, are known manifestations and also may involve the knee or other sites. Clubbing and, rarely, periostitis may occur in Crohn's disease. The peripheral arthritis becomes chronic in some cases, and destructive lesions of small joints and hips may occur.

In most cases of Crohn's disease, intestinal symptoms antedate or coincide with the joint manifestations, but the articular symptoms may precede the intestinal symptoms by years.

In the Oxford study (Orchard et al. 1998) enteropathic peripheral arthropathy without axial involvement was subdivided into pauciarticular and symmetrical polyarticular involvement.

Relationship between arthritis and gut inflammation

In most cases gut symptoms antedate or coincide with the joint manifestations; in a recent study 13 per cent of the patients had articular symptoms 10–36 months before inflammatory bowel disease diagnosis (Orchard et al. 1998). In a prospective study 8 out of 129 (6 per cent) spondyloarthropathy patients without clinical manifestations of inflammatory bowel disease at onset developed Crohn's disease during a follow-up period of up to 9 years (Mielants et al. 1995). Colonic involvement increases the susceptibility to peripheral arthritis.

A temporal relationship between attacks of arthritis and flares of bowel diseases is more frequent in ulcerative colitis than in Crohn's disease; this was only found in patients with the typical pauciarticular involvement and not in those with polyarticular arthritis (Orchard et al. 1998), suggesting that this last form is less disease related.

Axial involvement

There is no significant difference between the axial involvement in Crohn's disease and ulcerative colitis. The true prevalence of sacroiliitis is difficult to estimate since the onset is frequently insidious. Prevalence rates of 10–15 per cent for sacroiliitis and of 7–12 per cent for spondylitis have been described, although the real figures are probably higher. Ten per cent of patients with inflammatory bowel disease attending a gastroenterology unit fulfilled the criteria for ankylosing spondylitis and an additional 18 per cent of patients had asymptomatic sacroiliitis detected by conventional X-ray (de Vlam et al. 2000). The male to female ratio is 3 : 1, which is comparable to uncomplicated ankylosing spondylitis, which the clinical picture closely resembles.

The onset of axial involvement does not parallel that of bowel disease and frequently precedes it. Its course is also totally independent of the course of the gut disease; neither colectomy in ulcerative colitis nor surgery in Crohn's disease alter the course of any associated sacroiliitis or spondylitis.

Extra-intestinal and extra-articular features

Skin lesions, specifically erythema nodosum and pyoderma gangrenosum, are frequently associated and occur in 10–21 per cent of patients. Erythema nodosum (Plate 101) parallels the activity of the bowel disease and tends to occur in patients with active peripheral arthritis of the pauciarticular form; it is probably a manifestation of Crohn's disease. Pyoderma gangrenosum (Plate 102) is less common and more severe. It is not related to bowel and joint diseases and is probably an associated disorder (Schorr-Lesnick et al. 1988). Clubbing is also reported in Crohn's disease.

Eye involvement is the most frequent extra-articular feature of inflammatory bowel disease, occurring in between 10 and 20 per cent of the patients. The most typical presentation is the acute anterior uveitis seen in other spondyloarthropathies, acute in onset, unilateral, transient but with recurrences. In these forms, choroid and retina are spared and the visual prognosis is good (Rosenbaum et al. 1992). It is more associated with the axial form of spondyloarthropathy and with HLA-B27.

A chronic form, bilateral, posterior, with insidious onset and chronic duration is, however, also described (Lyons and Rosenbaum 1997); in these cases cataract, glaucoma, cystoid macular oedema, and posterior synechiae can occur. Episcleritis, scleritis, and granulomatous uveitis have also been described.

Secondary amyloidosis with involvement of major organs is described in Crohn's disease, is uncommon but usually lethal.

Laboratory and radiographic findings

Raised inflammatory serum parameters (especially C-reactive protein), marked thrombocytosis, and a hypochromic anaemia due to chronic inflammation are common findings. The synovial fluid analysis is non-specific and consistent with inflammatory arthritis, with a cell count varying from 1500 to 50 000/mm^3 (1.5–50 $\times$ 10^9/l). Cultures are negative.

As a rule, radiographs of the peripheral joints show no erosive lesions. However, erosive lesions of MCP and MTP joints have been described, and these only differ from the arthritis seen in rheumatoid arthritis by their pauciarticular and asymmetric distribution. Adjacent bone proliferation is frequently present. The radiographic appearance of the enthesopathies is similar to that found in other spondyloarthropathies.

The axial involvement of inflammatory bowel disease is indistinguishable from that of uncomplicated ankylosing spondylitis, although the frequency of asymmetric sacroiliitis is higher and the ankylosis of zygoapophyseal joints is more seldom (Helliwel et al. 1998) (Fig. 4).

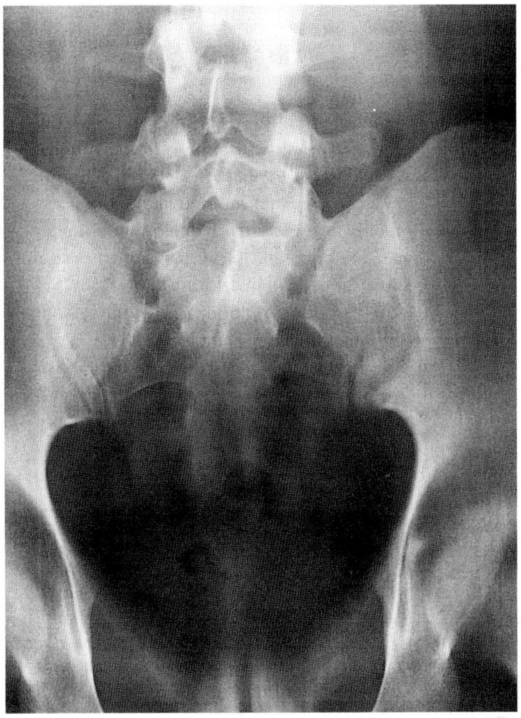

Fig. 4 Asymmetric sacroiliitis; only widening, blurring and erosions at the left sacroiliac joint.

Genetics

There is substantial evidence favouring a genetic cause for inflammatory bowel disease. Familial aggregation of Crohn's disease and ulcerative colitis has been frequently described (Kirsner 1973). Both diseases are believed to be genetically linked, since both occur within the same families.

Recently a susceptibility locus for Crohn's disease has been mapped to chromosome 16. A mutation of NOD2, a gene that encodes a protein which activates nuclear factor NF-κB and is related to response to bacterial liposaccharides, was associated with Crohn's disease (Hugot et al. 2001; Ogura et al. 2001).

The pauciarticular form of inflammatory bowel disease was associated with HLA–DRB1*0103, B35, and B27 while the polyarticular form was associated with HLA-B44 (Orchard et al. 2000). No accepted association of the peripheral arthritis with HLA-antigens has been identified and presence of the shared epitope for rheumatoid arthritis (QRRAA) was only found in inflammatory bowel disease patients with peripheral synovitis and not in those without (de Vlam et al. 2000).

Sacroiliitis and spondylitis in inflammatory bowel disease are associated with HLA-B27 but to a lesser degree than in uncomplicated ankylosing spondylitis (33 versus 71 per cent). Interestingly, ankylosing spondylitis patients lacking the HLA-B27 antigen are at a higher risk of developing inflammatory bowel disease than are HLA-B27 positive ankylosing spondylitis patients.

Uveitis (see Chapter 1.3.12)

Undifferentiated spondyloarthropathy

Definition and terminology

The nosology of undifferentiated spondyloarthropathies has been introduced to describe patients presenting clinical, biological, radiological, and genetic features of spondyloarthropathy, who cannot be classified in the well-defined clinical disease categories such as ankylosing spondylitis, psoriatic arthritis, reactive arthritis, and enteropathic arthritis. Patients can present with a wide spectrum of disease manifestations of varying degrees of severity. Typical presentations are a patient with mono- or pauciarthritis, or a patient developing an inflammatory enthesitis in the feet or a dactylitis, more seldom a form of chronic or relapsing inflammatory low back pain, or combinations of these manifestations. Any of articular and extra-articular characteristic manifestations of spondyloarthropathy described above may develop without the patient necessarily fulfilling diagnostic criteria for a distinct subgroup.

Prevalence

Undifferentiated spondyloarthropathy is a frequent disease. In a population study undifferentiated spondyloarthropathy was estimated at 0.67 per cent of the white population (Braun et al. 1998).

On 217 consecutive spondyloarthropathy patients undergoing ileocolonoscopy, excluding psoriatic arthritis and inflammatory bowel disease, the diagnosis of undifferentiated spondyloarthropathy was made slightly less than diagnosis of ankylosing spondylitis (40 versus 42 per cent) (Mielants et al. 1995a,b,c). The male/female ratio is about 2/1 to 3/2 with an onset which varies between 12 and 70 years. There is an important familial predisposition: in first degree relatives of patients with ankylosing spondylitis, 38 per cent had inflammatory low back pain (Calin et al. 1983) whereas 9 per cent of HLA-B27 positive relatives of ankylosing spondylitis patients had chronic inflammatory low back pain without radiological changes (Khan et al. 1985).

A family history of spondyloarthropathy was present in 14 per cent of patients with undifferentiated spondyloarthropathy (Collantes et al. 2000).

Clinical features and diagnosis

The diagnosis of undifferentiated spondyloarthropathy can be made if patients present chronic inflammatory low back pain (Calin et al. 1977) without the presence of bilateral radiological sacroiliitis stage II or other radiological abnormalities in the spine, or if they present with a relapsing or chronic inflammatory mono- or pauciarthritis, or a dactylitis, or an inflammatory tendinitis (Achilles tendon or fascia plantaris) and fulfil the ESSG or Amor criteria. The good response of these locomotor symptoms to NSAID is an important diagnostic feature and will be present in 49 per cent of the patients (Collantes et al. 2000).

The presence of HLA-B27 suggests the diagnosis of undifferentiated spondyloarthropathy, but its absence does not exclude it. The prevalence of HLA-B27 in undifferentiated spondyloarthropathy is estimated to be 80 per cent (Zeidler et al. 1992). Patients should be rheumatoid factor negative and most will have raised inflammatory serum parameters during disease manifestations.

Radiologically sacroiliitis can be present, but should be asymmetrical or may not exceed stage I (pseudo-widening and blurring of sacroiliac joints). Spinal lesions without sacroiliitis are seldom observed, although zygoapophyseal joint involvement at a certain level and squaring can be present and be the first manifestation of spinal involvement (de Vlam et al. 1999).

The peripheral arthritis is mostly non-erosive and self-resolving, in some patients the arthritis becomes chronic and erosive (Mielants et al. 1990).

Differential diagnosis has to be made with other inflammatory joint diseases and with the other forms of spondyloarthropathy. Differential diagnosis with an early form of rheumatoid arthritis (in a mono- or pauciarticular form) can be difficult, especially when no specific serum factors are detectable: needle arthroscopy can reveal macroscopical and histological differences and presence of specific markers such as expression of integrins ($\alpha V\beta 3$ was decreased in the synovial lining and $\alpha V\beta 5$ was increased in the sublining in rheumatoid arthritis compared to spondyloarthropathy) and of citrullinated peptides, which were only found in rheumatoid arthritis synovium, could be useful in differential diagnosis (Baeten et al. 2000).

Other related diseases should be excluded by careful clinical and radiological examination. The presence of psoriatic lesions in the scalp or nails should be investigated. A familial history of psoriasis or inflammatory bowel disease should be recorded, symptoms of urogenital or intestinal inflammation should be sought, and a search for specific infectious agents (such as *Chlamydia*, *Yersinia*) in stools or urine or for specific antibodies in serum performed.

Ileocolonoscopic studies revealed the prevalence of gut inflammation on histology in 70 per cent of patients with undifferentiated spondyloarthropathy, most of them describing no clinical intestinal symptoms (Mielants et al. 1989). A small but significant number of undifferentiated spondyloarthropathy patients with chronic inflammatory gut lesions developed clinical overt inflammatory bowel disease on follow-up 2–9 years after ileocolonoscopy (Mielants et al. 1995a,b,c) suggesting that a number of patients with undifferentiated spondyloarthropathy have subclinical Crohn's disease.

Course and prognosis

Undifferentiated spondyloarthropathy can occur at an early stage of spondyloarthropathy, an abortive form of spondyloarthropathy not developing the classical picture, an overlap of spondyloarthropathy or a specific subcategory of spondyloarthropathy (Zeidler et al. 1992). Different authors have studied the evolution of undifferentiated spondyloarthropathy and confirm the hypothesis of those four possibilities. In a review study 2–9 years later 31 out of 51 patients went into clinical remission and can be considered as abortive forms, 9 developed ankylosing spondylitis, 3 inflammatory bowel disease and can be considered as an early stage or an overlap syndrome, and 8 remained as an undifferentiated spondyloarthropathy and can be considered a specific subcategory (Mielants et al. 1995a,b,c).

The remission rate was comparable in other studies: 34 per cent (Schattenkircher and Kruger 1987) and 41 per cent (Nissila et al. 1983) underlying the relative good prognosis of this disease entity.

Persistent oligoarthritis without developing an other form of spondyloarthropathy was observed in up to 26 per cent of patients (Mau et al. 1987). Evolution to ankylosing spondylitis was observed in 25–59 per cent.

Risk factors for a patient with undifferentiated spondyloarthropathy to develop ankylosing spondylitis are the presence of inflammatory axial pain, persistence of high inflammatory serum parameters, presence of HLA-B27, and the presence of chronic gut inflammation on ileocolonoscopy (Mielants et al. 1995a,b). Risk factors for the development of inflammatory bowel disease are identical, except for the presence of HLA-B27 (Mielants et al. 1995a,b,c). Only undifferentiated spondyloarthropathy patients with chronic inflammatory gut lesions developed ankylosing spondylitis or inflammatory bowel disease.

SAPHO (synovitis, acne, pustulosis, hyperostosis, and osteitis) (see Chapter 6.4.5)

Juvenile spondyloarthropathy (see Chapter 6.4.2)

Etiopathogenic considerations

These considerations must deal with the linkage with HLA-B27 and the role of bacterial pathogens (Lopez de Castro 1998; Allen et al. 1999; Yu 1999). A major pathophysiological clue is provided by reactive arthritis, the subgroup of the spondyloarthropathies which is known to be triggered by infections of the gut or the urogenital tract with bacterial strains such as *Yersinia enterocolitica*, *Salmonella typhimurium* and *enteridis*, *Shigella flexneri*, *Campylobacter jejuni*, and *Chlamidia trachomatis* (Burmester et al. 1995). The importance of intestinal pathogens has further been illustrated by the HLA-B27 transgenic rat model, in which arthritis and colitis do not develop in germ-free conditions (Taurog et al. 1994, 1999).

In human there is compelling evidence that gut inflammation and increased gut permeability play a role not only in reactive arthritis but also in other types of spondyloarthropathies (Mielants et al. 1988, 1995a,b), while both bacterial antigens and T cells reactive with those antigens have been demonstrated in the joint (Hermann et al. 1989, 1993; Granfors et al. 1990). Correlating the bacterial hypothesis with the MHC class I linkage, it has been proposed that HLA-B27 is involved in the activation of cytotoxic T lymphocytes by presenting either specific bacterial peptides or arthritogenic self-peptides crossreacting with bacterial antigens. Alternatively, HLA-B27 itself could share peptide sequence homologies with bacterial antigens that could trigger cytotoxic T lymphocytes (molecular mimicry) (Lopez-Larrea et al. 1998). However, HLA-B27 has also effects which are independent from its antigen presenting function: it impairs bacterial elimination, leading to defective host defense with persistence of bacterial antigens (Laitio et al. 1997), and it alters intracellular signalling and the secretion of pro-inflammatory cytokines (Ikawa et al. 1998). Finally, HLA-B27 appears to be particularly sensitive to misfolding during the intracellular assembly process (Mear et al. 1999; Colbert 2000), thereby triggering inflammation through two different pathways. First, misfolding can induce the activation of NF-κB and the secretion of pro-inflammatory cytokines (Baeuerle and Henkel 1994), or lower the threshold of NF-κB activation by other stimuli such as lipopolysaccharides (Pentinen et al. 1999). Second, misfolding can lead to the formation of HLA-B27 heavy chain homodimers and, consequently, potentially immunogenic structures that could be recognized by T helper cells (Khare et al. 1996; Allen et al. 1999).

In summary, interactions at multiple levels between bacterial infections and genetic factors appear to activate both the innate and the acquired immunity in spondyloarthropathy. Emerging insights in these interactions, in the role of defective host defense and in the etiopathogenic relationship between joint and gut will allow better understanding of the disease and provide new opportunities for experimental therapeutic interventions in spondyloarthropathy (De Keyser et al. 2000).

Treatment

Nearly all patients with spondyloarthropathy take non-steroidal anti-inflammatory drugs (NSAID) for control of pain and stiffness. However, their use is sometimes limited by major side-effects and drug interactions. The only disease-modifying agent that has been demonstrated to be useful for SpA is sulfasalazine: the drug has a proven beneficial effect on gastrointestinal symptoms in inflammatory bowel disease (Dick et al. 1964; Van Hees et al. 1981); although it also has been found to have a favourable effect on articular symptoms in SpA patients, this effect appears to be modest for peripheral arthritis and enthesitis, and imperceptible for spondylitis (Dougados et al. 1995; Clegg et al. 1999). In patients with PsA methotrexate has become the most widely used therapy (Cuellar and Espinoza 1997). Although cyclosporin has a proven effect on skin disease in psoriasis (Ellis et al. 1991), the only data in patients with PsA come from a 1-year prospective trial which compared cyclosporin to methotrexate, and showed that both treatments were effective (Spadaro et al. 1995); however, no double-blind, placebo-controlled trials were performed with this agent in PsA.

Tumour necrosis factor α in the treatment of spondyloarthropathies

Recently, the use of biological therapies that block tumour necrosis factor α (TNFα) has opened a new avenue for the treatment of patients with SpA. Infliximab (Remicade™, Centocor, Malvern, PA, USA) is a chimeric anti-TNFα monoclonal IgG1 antibody, neutralizing the soluble cytokine as well as blocking the membrane bound cytokine (Knight et al. 1993). Infliximab has been approved by the health authorities in the United States (FDA) and Europe (EMEA) for use as a treatment for therapy-resistant moderate to severe CD and CD with fistulas, and for therapy-resistant rheumatoid arthritis (RA). In both diseases the effect of TNFα blockade with infliximab has been well documented (Targan et al. 1997; Kavanaugh et al. 1998; Maini et al. 1999; Present et al. 1999).

However, studies with infliximab in inflammatory bowel disease have not evaluated the effect on associated rheumatological manifestations such as spondylitis, synovitis, or enthesitis in patients with concomitant SpA. From a clinical point of view, we observed a fast and significant improvement of articular as well as axial inflammation in four patients with SpA associated with CD treated with infliximab (Van den Bosch et al. 2000). The observations in these patients suggested that refractory joint manifestations in CD might be a potential indication for infliximab treatment, and warranted further investigation of the therapeutic potential of TNFα blockade in patients with other subtypes of SpA. Moreover, observations in poly-articular psoriatic arthritis (Antoni et al. 1999; Mease et al. 2000) suggested a beneficial role of TNFα blockade on articular symptoms and skin disease. With respect to the expression of TNFα in the joints of patients with SpA, few data exist: however, in sacroiliac joint biopsy specimens from patients with ankylosing spondylitis, abundant TNFα message was identified by in situ hybridization (Braun et al. 1995).

In consequence, a pilot study was set up to evaluate the efficacy of TNFα blockade with infliximab in patients with different subtypes of active SpA (Van den Bosch et al. 2000): this was an open-label study in 21 patients who received a loading dose regimen of three infusions of infliximab (5 mg/kg) at week 0, 2, and 6. All the measured variables improved significantly, with most parameters reaching statistical significance already at day 3. During this pilot trial, the beneficial effect was maintained up to day 84 (6 weeks after the third infusion). In this study, no significant adverse events were observed. Minor side-effects, such as nausea, dizziness, headache, and fatigue were reported, but none of these caused interruption or discontinuation of the treatment. After the initial loading dose all patients were entered in a maintenance regimen protocol consisting of an infusion of 5 mg/kg infliximab every 14 weeks. The significant improvement of all disease manifestations was maintained over a 1 year follow-up period (Kruithof et al. 2002). The beneficial effects of TNFα blockade were confirmed in an open German study in AS (Brandt et al. 2000), and in a double-blind study in SpA (Van den Bosch et al. 2002).

A major concern with TNFα blockade is the occurrence of infections or malignancies. In the 1-year follow-up study, 12 infectious episodes were noted: eight patients had an episode of self-limiting upper respiratory tract infection, whereas in four patients the infections (one otitis media, one vaginal candidiasis, one tooth abscess, and one pyelonephritis) required antibiotic or antimycotic treatment. None of these infections were life-threatening, nor did they require hospitalization. No malignancies were reported. During the 1-year follow-up 12 patients (57 per cent) developed antinuclear antibodies (ANA); in four of these patients (19 per cent) antibodies to double stranded DNA (anti-dsDNA) were detected by the Crithidia luciliae assay. However, no lupus-like symptoms were observed. This is consistent with the data in rheumatoid arthritis where the incidence of ANA and anti-dsDNA after treatment with infliximab is, respectively, 53 and 14 per cent (Charles et al. 2000).

In eight patients with treatment-resistant SpA that were treated with infliximab at week 0, 2, and 6, synovial biopsies were obtained at week 0, 2, and 12 (Baeten et al. 2001). Histological analysis indicated that the synovial lining layer thickness tended to decrease, with a significant reduction of CD55+ synoviocytes at week 12. In the sublining layer, vascularity was reduced at week 12, with a decreased endothelial expression of vascular cell adhesion molecule 1 (VCAM-1) and E-selectin. The number of neutrophils and CD68+ macrophages in the sublining layer was decreased at weeks 2 and 12, whereas the CD20+ lymphocytes (B cells) and plasma cells were clearly increased. Although these preliminary data need to be confirmed in a larger cohort, they suggest distinct immunomodulatory mechanisms of TNFα blockade in SpA, and confirm the clinical improvement in the peripheral arthritis, seen in these patients.

References

Allen, R.L. et al. (1999). HLA-B27 can form a novel beta 2-microglobulin-free heavy chain homodimer structure. *Journal of Immunology* **162**, 5045–8.

Allen, R.L., Bowness, P., and McMichael, A. (1999). The role of HLA-B27 in spondylarthritis. *Immunogenetics* **50**, 220–7.

Amor, B., Bouchet, H., and Delrieu, F. (1983). National survey on reactive arthritis by the French Society of Rheumatology. *Revue du Rhumatisme et des maladies ostéoarticulaires* **50**, 733–43.

Amor, B. et al. (1991). Evaluation des critères de spondylarthropathies d'Amor et Liesseg: une étude transversale de 2228 patients. *Annales de Médecine Interne* **142**, 85–9.

Antoni, C. et al. (1999). Succesful treatment of severe psoriatic arthritis with infliximab. *Arthritis and Rheumatism* **42** (Suppl. 9), A1801.

Baeten, D. et al. (2000). A comparative study of the synovial histology in rheumatoid arthritis, spondylarthropathy and osteoarthritis: influence of disease duration and activity. *Annals of the Rheumatic Diseases* **59**, 945–53.

Baeten, D. et al. (2001). Immunomodulatory effects of anti-tumor necrosis factor α therapy on synovium in spondylarthropathy: histologic findings in eight patients from an open-label pilot study. *Arthritis and Rheumatism* **44**, 186–95.

Baeuerle, P.A. and Henkel, T. (1994). Function and activation of NF-kappa B in the immune system. *Annual Review of Immunology* **12**, 141–9.

Ball, J. (1971). Enthesopathy of rheumatoid and ankylosing spondylitis. *Annals of the Rheumatic Diseases* **30**, 213–23.

Banares, A. et al. (1998). Eye involvement in the spondylarthropathies. *Rheumatic Diseases Clinics of North America* **24**, 771–84.

Bennett, P.H. and Burch, T.A. (1968). The epidemiological diagnosis of ankylosing spondylitis. In *Population Studies of the Rheumatic Diseases* (ed. P.H. Bennett and P.H.N. Wood), pp. 305–13. New York: Exerpta Medica Foundation.

Bourne, J.T. et al. (1985). Arthritis and coeliac disease. *Annals of the Rheumatic Diseases* **44**, 592–8.

Brandt, J. et al. (2000). Successful treatment of active ankylosing spondylitis with the anti-tumor necrosis factor monoclonal antibody infliximab. *Arthritis and Rheumatism* **43**, 1346–52.

Braun, J. and Sieper, J. (1996). The sacroiliac joint in the spondylarthropathies. *Current Opinion in Rheumatology* **8**, 275–87.

Braun, J. et al. (1995). Use of immunohistologic and in situ hybridization techniques in the examination of sacroiliac joint biopsy specimens from patients with ankylosing spondylitis. *Arthritis and Rheumatism* **38**, 499–505.

Braun, J. et al. (1998). Prevalence of spondylarthropathies in HLA-B27 positive and negative blood donors. *Arthritis and Rheumatism* **41**, 58–67.

Brewerton, D.A. et al. (1973). Ankylosing spondylitis and HLA-B27. *Lancet* **1**, 904–7.

Burgos-Vargas, R., Pacheco-Tena, C., and Vazques-Mellado, J. (1997). Juvenile-onset spondylarthropathies. *Rheumatic Diseases Clinics of North America* **23**, 569–98.

Burmester, G.R. et al. (1995). Immunology of reactive arthritides. *Annual Review of Immunology* **13**, 229–35.

Cabral, D.A., Malleson, P.N., and Petty, R.E. (1995). Spondylarthropathies of childhood. *Pediatric Clinics of North America* **42**, 1051–70.

Calin, A. and Fries, J.F. (1975). Striking prevalence of ankylosing spondylitis in 'healthy' W27 positive males and females. *New England Journal of Medicine* **293**, 835–9.

Calin, A. et al. (1977). Clinical history as a screening test for ankylosing spondylitis. *Journal of the American Medical Association* **237**, 2613–14.

Calin, A. et al. (1983). Genetic differences between B27 positive patients with ankylosing spondylitis and B27 positive healthy controls. *Arthritis and Rheumatism* **26**, 1460–4.

Chamot, A.M. et al. (1987). Le syndrome acné pustulose hyperostose ostéite (SAPHO). Résultat d'une enquête nationale. *Revue du Rhumatisme* **54**, 187–96.

Charles, P.J. et al. (2000). Assessment of antibodies to double-stranded DNA induced in rheumatoid arthritis patients following treatment with infliximab, a monoclonal antibody to tumor necrosis factor α. *Arthritis and Rheumatism* **43**, 2383–90.

Clegg, D.O., Reda, D.J., and Abdellatif, M. (1999). Comparison of sulfasalazine and placebo for the treatment of axial and peripheral articular manifestations of the seronegative spondylarthropathie: a Department of Veterans Affairs cooperative study. *Arthritis and Rheumatism* **42**, 2325–9.

Colbert, R.A. (2000). HLA-B27 misfolding: a solution to the spondylarthropathy conundrum? *Molecular Medicine Today* **6**, 224–30.

Collantes, E. et al. (2000). Can some cases of 'possible' spondylarthropathy be classified as 'definite' or 'undifferentiated' spondylarthropathy? Value of criteria for spondylarthropathies. *Joint, Bone, Spine* **67**, 516–20.

Cuellar, M.L. et al. (1997). Methotrexate use in psoriasis and psoriatic arthritis. *Rheumatic Diseases Clinics of North America* **23**, 797–809.

De Keyser, F. et al. (1998). Bowel inflammation and the spondylarthropathies. *Rheumatic Diseases Clinics of North America* **24**, 785–813.

De Keyser, F. et al. (2000). Opportunities for immune modulation in the spondylarthropathies with special reference to gut inflammation. *Inflammation Research* **49**, 47–54.

De Vlam, K., Mielants, H., and Veys, E.M. (1999). Involvement of the zygapophyseal joint in ankylosing spondylitis: relation to the bridging syndesmophyte. *Journal of Rheumatology* **26**, 1738–45.

De Vlam, K. et al. (2000). Spondylarthropathy is underestimated in inflammatory bowel disease: prevalence and HLA association. *Journal of Rheumatology* **27**, 2860–5.

Dick, A.P. et al. (1964). Controlled trial of sulfasalazine in the treatment of ulcerative colitis. *Gut* **5**, 437–42.

Dobbins, W.O. (1987). HLA antigens in Whipple's disease. *Arthritis and Rheumatism* **30**, 102–5.

Dougados, M. et al. (1991). The European Spondylarthropathy Study Group preliminary criteria for the classification of spondylarthropathies. *Arthritis and Rheumatism* **34**, 1218–26.

Dougados, M. et al. (1995). Sulfasalazine in the treatment of spondylarthropathy: a randomized, multicenter, double-blind, placebo-controlled study. *Arthritis and Rheumatism* **38**, 618–27.

Ellis, C.N. et al. (1991). Cyclosporine for plaque-type psoriasis: results of a multidose, double-blind trial. *New England Journal of Medicine* **324**, 277–84.

Espinoza, L.R., Cuellar, M.L., and Sileira, L.H. (1992). Psoriatic arthritis. *Current Opinion in Rheumatology* **4**, 470–8.

Feurle, G.E. et al. (1979). HLA-B27 and defects in T-cell system in Whipple's disease. *European Journal of Clinical Investigations* **9**, 385–9.

Fox, R. et al. (1979). The chronicity of symptoms and disability in Reiter's syndrome: an analysis of 131 consecutive patients. *Annals of Internal Medicine* **91**, 190–3.

François, R.J., Eulderink, F., and Bywaters, E.G.L. (1995). Commented glossary for rheumatic spinal diseases, based on pathology. *Annals of the Rheumatic Disesases* **54**, 615–25.

Gerster, J.C. and Piccinin, P. (1985). Enthesiopathy of the heels in juvenile onset seronegative B-27 positive spondylarthropathies. *Journal of Rheumatology* **12**, 310–14.

Gerster, J.C. et al. (1977). The painful heel: comparative study in rheumatoid arthritis, ankylosing spondylitis, Reiter's syndrome and generalized osteoarthrosis. *Annals of the Rheumatic Diseases* **36**, 343–8.

Gran, J.T. and Skomsvoll, J.F. (1997). The outcome of ankylosing spondylitis: a study of 100 patients. *British Journal of Rheumatology* **36**, 766–71.

Granfors, K. et al. (1990). Salmonella lipopolysaccharide in synovial cells of patients with reactive arthritis. *Lancet* **35**, 685–8.

Gravallese, E.M. and Kantrowitz, F.G. (1988). Arthritic manifestations of inflammatory bowel disease. *American Journal of Gastroenterology* **83**, 703–9.

Hamuryudan, V., Özdogan, H., and Yazici, H. (1997). Other forms of vasculitis and pseudovasculitis. *Baillière's Clinical Rheumatology* **11**, 345–55.

Helliwell, P.S. and Wright, V. (1987). Seronegative spondarthritides. *Baillière's Clinical Rheumatology* **1**, 491–523.

Helliwell, P.S., Hickling, P., and Wright, V. (1998). Do the radiological changes of classic ankylosing spondylitis differ from the changes found in spondylitis associated with inflammatory bowel disease, psoriasis and reactive arthritis? *Annals of the Rheumatic Diseases* **57**, 135–40.

Hermann, E. et al. (1989). Response of synovial fluid T cell clones to *Yersinia enterocolitica* antigens in patients with reactive arthritis. *Clinical and Experimental Rheumatology* **75**, 365–70.

Hermann, E. et al. (1993). HLA-B27-restricted CD8 T cells derived from synovial fluids of patients with reactive arthritis and ankylosing spondylitis. *Lancet* **342**, 645–50.

Hochberg, M.C., Bias, W.B., and Arnett, F.C. (1978). Family studies in HLA-B27 associated arthritis. *Medicine* **57**, 463–75.

Hugot, J.P. et al. (2001). Association of NOD2 leucine-rich repeat variants with susceptibility to Crohn's disease. *Nature* **411**, 599–603.

Ikawa, T. et al. (1998). Expression of arthritis-causing HLA-B27 on Hela cells promotes induction of c-fos in response to *in vitro* invasion by *Salmonella typhimurium*. *Journal of Clinical Investigations* **101**, 263–72.

Kahn, M.F. and Khan, M.A. (1994). The SAPHO syndrome. *Baillière's Clinical Rheumatology* **8**, 333–62.

Kavanaugh, A.F. et al. (1998). Anti-tumor necrosis factor-α monoclonal antibody therapy for rheumatoid arthritis. *Rheumatic Diseases Clinics of North America* **24**, 593–614.

Keat, A. (1999). Reactive arthritis. *Advances in Experimental Medicine and Biology* **455**, 201–6.

Kellgren, J.H. (1962). Diagnostic criteria for population studies. *Bulletin on the Rheumatic Diseases* **3**, 291–2.

Khan, M.A. et al. (1985). Spondylitic disease without radiologic evidence of sacroiliitis in relatives of HLA-B27 positive ankylosing spondylitis patients. *Arthritis and Rheumatism* **28**, 40–3.

Khan M.A. and van der Linden, S.M. (1990). A wider spectrum of spondylarthropathies. *Seminars in Arthritis and Rheumatism* **20**, 107–13.

Khare, S.D. et al. (1996). HLA-B27 heavy chains contribute to spontaneous inflammatory disease in B27/human beta2-microglobulin (beta2m) double transgenic mice with disrupted mouse beta2m. *Journal of Clinical Investigations* **98**, 2746–55.

Kirsner, J.B. (1973). Genetic aspects of inflammatory bowel disease. *Clinical Gastroenterology* **2**, 557–62.

Knight, D.M. et al. (1993). Construction and initial characterization of a mouse-human chimeric anti-TNF antibody. *Molecular Immunology* **30**, 1443–53.

Kruithof, E. et al. (2002). Repeated infusions of infliximab, a chimeric anti-TNFα monoclonal antibody, in patients with active spondylarthropathy: one-year follow-up. *Annals of the Rheumatic Diseases* **61**, 207–12.

Kvien, T.K. et al. (1994). Reactive arthritis: incidence, triggering agents and clinical presentations. *Journal of Rheumatology* **21**, 115–22.

Laitio, P. et al. (1997). HLA-B27 modulates intracellular survival of *Salmonella enteridis* in human monocytic cells. *European Journal of Immunology* **27**, 1331–8.

Leirisalo-Repo, M. (1998). Prognosis, course of disease and treatment of the spondylarthropathies. *Rheumatic Diseases Clinics of North America* **24**, 537–51.

Leirisalo-Repo, M. et al. (1994). High frequency of silent inflammatory bowel disease in spondylarthropathy. *Arthritis and Rheumatism* **37**, 23–31.

van der Linden, S.M., Valkenburg, H.A., and Cats, A. (1984). Evaluation of diagnostic criteria for ankylosing spondylitis. A proposal for modification of the New York criteria. *Arthritis and Rheumatism* **27**, 361–8.

van der Linden, S. and van der Heijde, D. (1998). Ankylosing spondylitis. Clinical features. *Rheumatic Diseases Clinics of North America* **24**, 663–76.

Lopez de Castro, J.A. (1998). The pathogenic role of HLA-B27 in chronic arthritis. *Current Opinion in Immunology* **10**, 59–66.

Lopez-Larrea, C., Gonzalez, S., and Martinez-Borra, J. (1998). The role of HLA-B27 polymorphism and molecular mimicry in spondylarthropathy. *Molecular Medicine Today* **4**, 540–9.

Lubrano, E. et al. (1996). The arthritis of coeliac disease: prevalence and pattern in 200 adult patients. *British Journal of Rheumatology* **35**, 1314–18.

Luthra, H.S., Ferguson, R.H., and Conn, D.L. (1976). Coexistence of ankylosing spondylitis and rheumatoid arthritis. *Arthritis and Rheumatism* **19**, 111–14.

Lyons, J.L. and Rosenbaum, J.T. (1997). Uveitis associated with inflammatory bowel disease compared with uveitis associated with spondylarthropathy. *Archives of Ophthalmology* **115**, 61–4.

Maini, R.N. et al. (1999). Infliximab (chimeric anti-tumour necrosis factor α monoclonal antibody) versus placebo in rheumatoid arthritis patients receiving concomitant methotrexate: a randomised phase III trial. *Lancet* **354**, 1932–9.

Mau, W. et al. (1987). Outcome of a possible ankylosing spondylitis in a 10 years follow-up study. *Clinical Rheumatology* **6** (Suppl. 2), 60–6.

Mau, W. et al. (1988). Clinical features and prognosis of patients with possible ankylosing spondylitis. Results of a 10 years follow up. *Journal of Rheumatology* **15**, 1109–14.

Mayberry, J.F. et al. (1989). Epidemiological study of asymptomatic inflammatory bowel disease: the identification of cases during a screening programme for colorectal cancer. *Gut* **30**, 481–3.

Mear, J.P. et al. (1999). Misfolding of HLA-B27 as a result of its B pocket suggests a novel mechanism for its role in susceptibility to spondylarthropathies. *Journal of Immunology* **163**, 6655–70.

Mease, P.J. et al. (2000). Etanercept in the treatment of psoriatic arthritis and psoriasis: a randomised trial. *Lancet* **356**, 385–90.

Mielants, H. et al. (1986). Familial aggregation in seronegative spondylarthritis of enterogenic origin. A family study. *Journal of Rheumatology* **13**, 126–8.

Mielants, H. et al. (1988). Ileonoscopic findings in seronegative spondylarthropathies. *British Journal of Rheumatology* **27**, S95–105.

Mielants, H. et al. (1989). Subclinical involvement of the gut in undifferentiated spondylarthropathies. *Clinical and Experimental Rheumatology* **7**, 499–504.

Mielants, H. et al. (1990a). Destructive lesions of small joints in seronegative spondylarthropathies: relation to gut inflammation. *Clinical and Experimental Rheumatology* **8**, 23–7.

Mielants, H. et al. (1990b). HLA-B27 positive idiopathic acute anterior uveitis: a unique manifestation of subclinical gut inflammation. *Journal of Rheumatology* **17**, 841–2.

Mielants, H. et al. (1993a). A prospective study of patients with spondylarthropathy with special reference to HLA-B27 and to gut histology. *Journal of Rheumatology* **20**, 1353–8.

Mielants, H. et al. (1993b). Gut inflammation in children with late onset pauciarticular juvenile arthritis and evolution to adult spondylarthropathy—a prospective study. *Journal of Rheumatology* **20**, 1567–72.

Mielants, H. et al. (1995a). The evolution of the spondylarthropathies in relation to gut histology. I. Clinical aspects. *Journal of Rheumatology* **22**, 2266–72.

Mielants, H. et al. (1995b). The evolution of the spondylarthropathies in relation to gut histology. II. Histological aspects. *Journal of Rheumatology* **22**, 2273–8.

Mielants, H. et al. (1995c). The evolution of the spondylarthropathies in relation to gut histology. III. Relation between gut and joint. *Journal of Rheumatology* **22**, 2279–84.

Moll, J.M.H. et al. (1974). Association between ankylosing spondylitis, psoriatic arthritis, Reiter's disease, the intestinal arthropathies of Behçet's syndrome. *Medicine* **53**, 343–64.

Nissila, M. et al. (1983). Prognosis of inflammatory joint disease. *Scandinavian Journal of Rheumatology* **12**, 33–6.

Ogura, Y. et al. (2001). A frameshift mutation in NOD2 associated with susceptibility to Crohn's disease. *Nature* **411**, 603–6.

Olivieri, I. et al. (1989). Isolated HLA-B27 associated peripheral enthesitis. *Journal of Rheumatology* **16**, 1519–21.

Orchard, T.R., Wordsworth, B., and Jewell, D.P. (1998). Peripheral arthropathies in inflammatory bowel disease: their articular distribution and natural history. *Gut* **42**, 387–91.

Orchard, T.R. et al. (2000). Clinical phenotype is related to HLA genotype in the peripheral arthropathies of inflammatory bowel disease. *Gastroenterology* **118**, 274–8.

Oriente, P., Biondi-Oriente, C., and Scarpa, R. (1994). Psoriatic arthritis: clinical manifestations. *Baillière's Clinical Rheumatology* **25**, 1352–7.

Pentinen, M.A. et al. (1999). MHC Class I molecules modulate LPS-induced NF-kB activation in U937 human monocytic cells. *Arthritis and Rheumatism* **42**, S385.

Present, D.H. et al. (1999). Infliximab for the treatment of fistulas in patients with Crohn's disease. *New England Journal of Medicine* **340**, 1398–405.

Protzer, U. et al. (1996). Enteropathic spondylarthropathy in chronic inflammatory bowel disease: prevalence, pattern of manifestation and HLA association. *Medizinische Klinik* **91**, 330–5.

Resnick, D. et al. (1977). Calcaneal abnormalities in articular disorders: rheumatoid arthritis, ankylosing spondylitis, psoriatic arthritis and Reiter's syndrome. *Radiology* **125**, 355–66.

Rosenbaum, J.T. (1992). Acute anterior uveitis and spondylarthropathies. *Rheumatic Diseases Clinics of North America* **18**, 143–51.

Scarpa, R. et al. (1988). The clinical spectrum of psoriatic spondylitis. *British Journal of Rheumatology* **27**, 123–7.

Scarpa, R. et al. (1992). The arthritis of ulcerative colitis: clinical and genetic aspects. *Journal of Rheumatology* **19**, 373–7.

Schatteman, L. et al. (1995). Gut inflammation in psoriatic arthritis: a prospective ileocolonoscopic study. *Journal of Rheumatology* **22**, 680–3.

Schattenkircher, M. and Kruger, K. (1987). Natural course and prognosis of HLA-B27 positive oligoarthritis. *Clinical Rheumatology* **6** (Suppl. 2), 83–6.

Schlosstein, L.P. et al. (1973). High association of an HLA antigen, W27, with ankylosing spondylitis. *New England Journal of Medicine* **288**, 704–6.

Schorr-Lesnick, B. and Brandt, L.J. (1988). Selected rheumatologic and dermatologic manifestations of inflammatory bowel disease. *American Journal of Gastroenterology* **83**, 216–23.

Schumacher, H.R. and Bardin, T. (1998). The spondylarthropathies: classification and diagnosis. Do we need terminologies? *Baillière's Clinical Rheumatology* **12**, 551–65.

Spadaro, A. et al. (1995). Comparison of cyclosporin A and methotrexate in the treatment of psoriatic arthritis: a one-year prospective study. *Clinical and Experimental Rheumatology* **13**, 589–93.

Targan, S.R. et al. (1997). A short-term study of chimeric monoclonal antibody cA2 to tumor necrosis factor alpha for Crohn's disease. Crohn's Disease cA2 Study Group. *New England Journal of Medicine* **337**, 1029–35.

Taurog, J.D. et al. (1994). The germfree state prevents development of gut and joint inflammatory disease in HLA-B27 transgenic rats. *Experimental Medicine* **180**, 2359–64.

Taurog, J.D. et al. (1999). Inflammatory disease in HLA-B27 transgenic rats. *Immunological Reviews* **169**, 209–23.

Torre Alonso, J.C. et al. (1991). Psoriatic arthritis (PA): a clinical, immunological and radiological study of 180 patients. *British Journal of Rheumatology* **30**, 245–50.

Van den Bosch, F. et al. (2000a). Crohn's disease associated with spondylarthropathy: effect of TNF-α blockade with infliximab on the articular symptoms. *Lancet* **356**, 1821–2.

Van den Bosch, F. et al. (2000b). Effects of a loading dose regimen of 3 infusions of chimeric antibody to tumour necrosis factor α (infliximab) in spondylarthropathy: an open pilot study. *Annals of the Rheumatic Diseases* **59**, 428–33.

Van den Bosch, F. et al. (2002). Randomized double-blind comparison of chimeric monoclonal antibody to tumor necrosis factor α (infliximab) versus placebo in active spondylarthropathy. *Arthritis and Rheumatism* **46**, 755–65.

Van Hees, P.A.M. et al. (1981). Effect of sulfasalazine in patients with active Crohn's disease: a controlled double-blind study. *Gut* **22**, 404–9.

Vasey, F.B. and Espinoza, L.R. (1984). Psoriatic arthritis. In *Spondylarthropathies* (ed. A. Calin), pp. 151–84. Orlando FL: Grune and Stratton.

Veys, E.M. et al. (1993). Juvenile spondylarthropathies in 1992. *Journal of Rheumatology* **20** (Suppl. 37), 19–25.

Wollenhaupt, J. et al. (1995). Manifestations of Chlamydia induced arthritis in patients with silent versus symptomatic urogenital chlamydial infection. *Clinical and Experimental Rheumatology* **13**, 453–8.

Wright, V. (1978). Seronegative polyarthritis. *Arthritis and Rheumatism* **21**, 618–33.

Wright, V. (1980). Relationship between ankylosing spondylitis and other spondylarthritides. In *Ankylosing Spondylitis* (ed. J.M.H. Moll). Edinburgh: Churchill Livingstone.

Wright, V. and Moll, J.M.H. (1976). Psoriatic arthritis. In *Seronegative Polyarthritis* (ed. V. Wright and J.M.H. Moll), pp. 169–23. Amsterdam: North Holland Publishing Co.

Yu, D.T. (1999). Pathogenesis of reactive arthritis. *Internal Medicine* **38**, 97–101.

Zeidler, H., Mau, W., and Khan, M.A. (1992). Undifferentiated spondylarthropathies. *Rheumatic Disease Clinics of North America* **18**, 187–202.

6.4.2 Spondyloarthritis in childhood

Wietse Kuis and Taunton R. Southwood

Clinical features and classification

Classification of the spondyloarthropathies in the context of the juvenile idiopathic arthritides (JIA) of childhood is challenging. The spondyloarthropathies, as a group, are dynamic diseases that may continue to evolve during childhood before reaching full clinical expression during the adult years. It is frequently difficult to distinguish early or undifferentiated spondyloarthropathy from other forms of juvenile arthritis. For example, a child with arthritis in a peripheral joint may not be suspected of having a spondyloarthropathy until classical signs of axial involvement develop during adulthood.

The term spondyloarthropathy (derived from the Greek *sphondylos*: vertebra) may be misleading to use in a paediatric context, for three reasons. First, only a small minority develop classical sacroiliac or lumbosacral vertebral arthritis during the juvenile years. Second, spondyloarthropathy classically does not cover one of the commoner sites of spinal involvement in childhood, that of the cervical spine (which is often seen in other forms of JIA including oligoarthritis, polyarthritis, or systemic arthritis). Finally, psoriatic arthritis, which is grouped with the spondyloarthropathies in adults, in children appears to have less in common with spondyloarthropathy than with other forms of childhood arthritis (Southwood et al. 1989). The most recent proposed classification of the spondyloarthropathy group of diseases in childhood specifically excludes psoriatic arthritis (Petty et al. 1998).

This poses a diagnostic challenge: to identify characteristic clinical features that predate the onset of back and sacroiliac symptoms, and therefore allow the prediction of outcome with some accuracy. The spondyloarthropathy spectrum is clinically manifest by a number of features including peripheral arthritis, enthesitis, extra-articular disease (inflammatory bowel disease, acute anterior uveitis, skin involvement) and the presence of HLA-B27 (Petty 1990). Recognition of this constellation of features may predict the onset of axial inflammation in later years.

This chapter will cover the classifications that have been proposed for the juvenile spondyloarthropathy spectrum, followed by an outline of the recognizable patterns of clinical features associated with specific subgroups of this disease; ankylosing spondylitis, inflammatory bowel disease, Reiter's syndrome, and psoriatic arthritis.

Classifications of the spondyloarthropathy spectrum in childhood

Only three classifications of spondyloarthropathy have been formulated specifically for the paediatric age spectrum, enthesitis-related arthritis (ERA) (Table 1), seronegative enthesopathy and arthropathy (SEA) syndrome (Table 2), and atypical spondyloarthropathies in children (Hussein et al. 1989: Table 3). All three recognized the major factors that characterize

Table 1 Enthesitis-related arthritis (Petty et al. 1998)

Definitions
1. Arthritis and enthesitis or
2. Arthritis or enthesitis with at least two of the following:
   (a) Sacroiliac joint tenderness and/or inflammatory lumbosacral pain
   (b) Presence of HLA-B27
   (c) Onset of arthritis in a male after age 6[a] years
   (d) Ankylosing spondylitis, enthesitis related arthritis, sacroiliitis with inflammatory bowel disease, Reiter's syndrome, or acute anterior uveitis in a first-degree relative

Exclusions
1. Psoriasis in the patient or a first-degree relative
2. Presence of IgM rheumatoid factor on at least two occasions more than 3 months apart
3. Presence of systemic arthritis

[a] Modified after Murray et al. (1999).

Table 2 Seronegative arthritis and enthesitis syndrome (Rosenberg and Petty 1982)

Onset of musculoskeletal symptoms before age 17 years
Absence of rheumatoid factors and antinuclear antibodies
Presence of enthesitis
Presence of arthralgia or arthritis

Table 3 Atypical spondyloarthropathies in childhood (Hussein et al. 1989)

Major criteria
1. A family history of spondyloarthropathy or oligoarthritis
2. Enthesopathy
3. Arthritis of digital joints including big toes
4. Sacroiliitis
5. Presence of HLA-B27 gene
6. Recurrent arthralgia or arthritis

Minor criteria
1. Age of onset after 10 years of age
2. Male sex
3. Only lower extremities affected
4. Acute iritis or conjunctivitis
5. Arthritis of hips
6. Onset following idiopathic enteritis

childhood forms of the disease, the presence of enthesitis and the absence of spondylitis. Particular emphasis was placed on enthesitis, which is defined as inflammation at one or more *entheses*, the sites of attachment of tendon, ligament, fascia, or joint capsule, into bone (Table 1).

The classification criteria for ERA form part of the ILAR proposal for development of classification criteria for JIA (Petty et al. 1998). The umbrella term JIA is defined as definite arthritis of unknown aetiology that begins before the sixteenth birthday and persists for at least 6 weeks. Seven categories of JIA have been defined, including oligoarthritis (persistent and extended), polyarthritis rheumatoid factor negative, polyarthritis rheumatoid factor positive, systemic arthritis, ERA, psoriatic arthritis, and undifferentiated arthritis. The principle of the classification is that all categories of JIA are mutually exclusive, and this is reflected in the list of exclusions for each category. For ERA, the 'inclusion' criteria of enthesitis, sacroiliac joint tenderness, low back pain, HLA-B27, and a family history of ankylosing spondylitis and related diseases are also 'exclusion' criteria for all the other categories of JIA. In the same way, the presence of psoriasis or other psoriatic inclusion criteria are exclusion criteria for ERA.

There have been several published reviews of the ILAR classification criteria, including the ERA criteria. Merino et al. (2001) examined ERA against the European Spondyloarthropathy Study Group (ESSG) preliminary criteria for juvenile spondyloarthropathy. They reported that the proposed ILAR criteria allocated only 84.8 per cent of the patients classified by traditional criteria, with the main conundra being a family history of psoriasis ($n = 12$) and polyarticular onset of disease in patients with ERA ($n = 5$).

Table 4 Amor criteria for classification of spondyloarthropathies

Criterion	Points
Clinical	
Lumbar or thoracic night pain or stiffness	1
Asymmetric oligoarthritis	2
Buttock pain alternating in site or triggered by pelvic movement	1
Sausage digit	2
Enthesopathy	2
Iritis	2
Non-specific urethritis or cervicitis within 1 month before onset	1
Diarrhoea within 1 month before onset	1
Psoriasis, balanitis, or chronic enterocolitis	2
Radiologic	
Sacroiliitis (≥stage 2 if bilateral; ≥stage 3 if unilateral)	3
Genetic	
Presence of HLA-B27, family history of pelvospondylitis, Reiter's syndrome, psoriasis, uveitis, or chronic enterocolitis	2
Therapeutic	
Amelioration of pain within 48 h of treatment with NSAID	1
A definite diagnosis of spondyloarthropathy is confirmed if 6 or more points are present	

Table 5 Classification criteria of the ESSG (Dougados et al. 1991)

Inflammatory spinal pain
or
Synovitis (asymmetric or predominantly in lower limbs)
plus
One of the following:
Positive family history
Psoriasis
Inflammatory bowel disease
Urethritis, cervicitis, or diarrhoea within 1 month before arthritis
Buttock pain alternating between right and left gluteal areas
Enthesopathy
Sacroiliitis

Similar findings were reported from Canada, although only one patient with spondyloarthropathy could not be classified as ERA using ILAR criteria (Ramsey et al. 2000), and from France, where there appeared to be a significant number of exclusions from ERA and psoriatic arthritis, in comparison with the other groups (Hofer et al. 2001).

The diagnostic criteria for atypical spondyloarthropathies were studied in 26 children (Table 3). Cases were classified according to criteria that were shown to be sensitive in differentiating atypical spondyloarthropathies from other forms of arthritis in children. When four of the six major criteria were present, 96.1 per cent of the patients were correctly classified as having atypical spondyloarthropathy, with a sensitivity of 84.6 per cent and a specificity of 100 per cent. The same diagnostic accuracy was achieved when three major and three minor criteria were present (Hussein et al. 1989).

Two classifications of spondyloarthropathy in adults have also been applied to children; the Amor criteria (Amor et al. 1990) for classification of spondyloarthropathies (Table 4) and the classification criteria of the ESSG (Table 5). Both recognize the presence of psoriasis as a criterion, which may render them less useful for the paediatric age group.

Epidemiology of the spondyloarthropathy spectrum in childhood

Andersson Gare et al. (1987) reported that 5 per cent of Swedish children with chronic arthritis were classified as having spondyloarthropathy, but a large survey of 1742 patients from North America suggested that spondyloarthropathy spectrum diseases were more frequent, accounting for 13 per cent of referred rheumatic conditions in childhood, with an incidence rate of 2.0 per 100 000 children at risk, compared with 4.0 per 100 000 for other forms of chronic arthritis (Denardo et al. 1994). A survey of paediatric rheumatology centres in Austria by Huemer et al. (2001) found a similar mean annual incidence of juvenile spondyloarthropathy; 2.9 per 100 000 children, compared to 4.28 and 0.48 per 100 000 children for other forms of JIA and paediatric systemic lupus erythematosus, respectively.

An estimated 5–8 per cent of children with arthritis attending paediatric rheumatology clinics have ankylosing spondylitis (Ladd et al. 1971). The prevalence of juvenile ankylosing spondylitis can also be extrapolated from the numbers of adult patients who report that onset occurred before they were 16 years old. Lawrence et al. (1989) reported an estimated prevalence of ankylosing spondylitis in populations from the United States ranging from 129 per 100 000 (Carter et al. 1979) to 222 per 100 000 (Mikkelsen et al. 1967). Generally 10–19 per cent of cases begin before the sixteenth year (Hart and Maclagan 1955). The prevalence depends on the ethnic origins of the population studied. For example, Burgos-Vargas et al. (1989) described a Mexican-Mestizo population in which ankylosing spondylitis was diagnosed from 1980 to 1987 in which 54 per cent had onset of symptoms before 16 years of age. The sum of these data suggests that the prevalence of juvenile ankylosing spondylitis is approximately 12–18 per 100 000. These figures are higher than those reported for juvenile spondyloarthropathies in general, suggesting that they may be an overestimate (Olivieri et al. 1992).

Enthesitis-related arthritis

ERA is a new term, and few studies have reported on the clinical features and outcome of patients with this disease. For the purposes of this chapter, the term ERA is presumed to encompass patients previously diagnosed as having the SEA syndrome, undifferentiated and atypical spondyloarthropathy, and HLA-B27 positive arthritis.

Several descriptive studies of children who eventually developed an identifiable spondyloarthropathy highlighted a number of linking clinical features (Schaller 1977, 1983, 1985; Jacobs et al. 1982). A family history of spondyloarthropathy (defined as inflammatory low back disease) was described in up to 60 per cent of patients. There was a strong male predominance in patients with reported male/female ratios of up to 10 : 1, although this has been disputed in a large retrospective survey of 379 adults with ankylosing spondylitis who developed musculoskeletal symptoms during childhood, which reported a ratio of 2.6 : 1 (Gomez et al. 1997). Antecedent insults included febrile illnesses and musculoskeletal trauma. The arthritis was typically of late onset as only 40 per cent of children were symptomatic by their ninth year. The earliest recorded onset was 12 months of age. The arthritis involved few joints and was asymmetrical, predominantly affecting the large weight bearing joints of the lower limbs. Extra-articular manifestations occurred in over 40 per cent of patients, including urethritis, symptomatic iritis, conjunctivitis, and keratoderma blennorrhagicum. Enthesopathy was prominent in 75 per cent of patients.

Clinical features

Rosenburg and Petty (1982) described 39 children (35 boys and 4 girls) with a SEA syndrome. The mean age of onset of the first musculoskeletal symptom was 9.8 years (range 1–16 years). This group included 13 patients who fulfilled diagnostic criteria for juvenile ankylosing spondylitis, inflammatory bowel disease, reactive arthritis, or Reiter's syndrome. The remaining 26 did not have one of these identifiable diseases, but did have the combination of enthesitis and arthritis or arthralgia. Principle sites of enthesitis included the calcaneal insertions of the plantar fascia and Achilles tendons, the metatarsal heads and base of the fifth metatarsal, the ischial tuberosities, iliac crests, and patella tendon insertions. Low back pain and stiffness were present in only nine patients, but many had abnormal flattening of the lumbar curve on forward flexion. HLA typing of 32 children demonstrated that 23 (72 per cent), including the eight patients with juvenile ankylosing spondylitis and one with Reiter's syndrome, were HLA-B27 positive.

Ankylosing tarsitis has been identified in up to 80 per cent of patients with SEA syndrome and 87 per cent of those with juvenile ankylosing spondylitis (Levi et al. 1990; Burgos-Vargas 1991). These patients develop inflammation of synovial sheaths and bursae, tendons, entheses, and joints of the feet, leading to radiographic or MRI evidence of ankylosis. Additionally, non-traumatic atlantoaxial subluxation has been reported in two HLA-B27 positive children with SEA syndrome (Foster et al. 1995).

The systemic manifestations of ERA and the undifferentiated spondyloarthropathies have not been as extensively studied as those of ankylosing spondylitis, even in childhood. The association of cardiac abnormalities with ankylosing spondylitis is undisputed (see next section), but in ERA and other forms of HLA-B27 associated arthritis it is less clear. Huppertz et al. (2000) investigated 40 patients (including one with ankylosing spondylitis) using electrocardiogram, echocardiography with pulsed and colour-flow Doppler at rest and at the termination of bicycle exercise and compared their results to a control group negative for HLA-B27.

Four patients with HLA-B27 associated arthritis had aortic regurgitation (0 controls). After the exercise component, late diastolic flow velocity was significantly increased in HLA-B27 positive patients, even those with relatively mild articular disease. Case reports have also highlighted cardiac involvement. Rapidly progressive aortic insufficiency with aneurysmal dilatation of ascending aorta was described in a 15-year-old boy with juvenile spondyloarthropathy (Kim et al. 1997). A 13-year-old boy who developed both aortic and mitral incompetence responsive to anti-inflammatory medication has been reported (Lee et al. 2001).

Other systemic complications associated with juvenile spondyloarthropathy include eye inflammation, pulmonary fibrosis, and bowel inflammation without overt colitis. Acute iritis is one of the classification criteria for ERA. Additionally, episcleritis has been associated with juvenile spondyloarthropathy in a case series of 12 children (Read et al. 1999). In 18 children with spondyloarthropathy and normal chest radiographs, Camiciottoli et al. (1999) found that one-third had evidence of functional impairment on pulmonary function testing (reduced forced vital capacity in four and reduced DLCO in two). There was no correlation with disease activity or progression over a 2-year follow-up period. Mielants et al. (1996) demonstrated that 80 per cent of children with late onset oligoarthritis had histological evidence of gut inflammation, which, on repeat ileocolonoscopy, had resolved entirely with remission of the arthritis.

HLA-B27 has been associated with a number of different musculoskeletal diseases in children and it is unclear if all of these form part of the spondyloarthropathy spectrum. For example, there have been reports of children with isolated dactylitis (Siegel and Baum 1988), isolated peripheral enthesitis (Olivieri et al. 1990; Olivieri and Pasero, 1992), and isolated hip flexion contractures (Bowyer 1995). The interpretation of a positive HLA-B27 result must take into account the occurrence of the gene in at least 8 per cent of the non-arthritic childhood population.

Outcome

There have been several long-term follow-up studies of patients with SEA syndrome. Cabral et al. (1992) reported 11 years (mean, range 2.5–23.5 years) follow-up data on 36 of the original 39 patients described by Rosenberg and Petty (1982). Assessment of outcome in the patients who did not have ankylosing spondylitis, inflammatory bowel disease, reactive arthritis, or Reiter's syndrome in the original study revealed that the disease had progressed to definite or probable ankylosing spondylitis in half (12 patients). The presence of arthralgia was less specific than arthritis for predicting a spondylitic outcome.

Burgos-Vargas and Clark (1989) reported 20 Mexican patients with SEA syndrome, and compared their outcome after at least 5 years follow-up with 25 patients with JIA (polyarthritis) and 28 patients with definite ankylosing spondylitis of juvenile onset. Radiographic evidence of sacroiliitis type was found in four patients with SEA syndrome before the third year of follow-up. From the third to the fifth year of follow-up, back complaints and radiographically confirmed sacroiliitis fulfilling the diagnostic criteria for ankylosing spondylitis developed in an increasing proportion of the patients (47.1–75 per cent) and ultimately affected 92.3 per cent. Other than the absence of back problems at the initial presentation, no significant differences in outcome were seen between the group with SEA syndrome and the group with juvenile ankylosing spondylitis. Olivieri et al. (1992) reported that only one of 11 Caucasian HLA-B27 positive children (9.1 per cent) with SEA syndrome developed bilateral sacroiliitis after 5 years of disease. Ethnic and environmental factors were thought to have contributed to the discrepancy between these findings and those of the Mexican population reported by Burgos-Vargas and Clark (1989).

Systematic studies of the radiographic or MR images of the sacroiliac joints in HLA-B27 positive children with chronic arthritis have been rarely performed. Bollow et al. (1998) evaluated 130 children with arthritis and detected acute or chronic sacroiliitis in 35 (27 per cent) using dynamic MRI of the sacroiliac joints. Three spondyloarthropathy groups were considered; undifferentiated juvenile spondyloarthropathy (n = 41, 88 per cent HLA-B27 positive) of which 41 per cent had sacroiliitis changes, differentiated juvenile spondyloarthropathy (16 with reactive arthritis, 9 with ankylosing spondylitis and 3 with psoriatic arthritis, 97 per cent HLA-B27 positive), of which 52 per cent had MRI abnormalities, and late onset oligoarthritis (n = 30, 93 per cent HLA-B27 positive), of which 10 per cent had MRI changes. None of the disease or normal controls had MRI abnormalities. Plain radiographs of the sacroiliac joints appeared to be less sensitive than MRI in this study.

Minden et al. (2000) reviewed 171 children with spondyloarthropathy (n = 28) or other forms of arthritis (n = 143). Patients with ERA (older onset oligoarthritis and HLA-B27 positive) had a lower probability of remission (17 per cent at 5 years follow-up) compared with HLA-B27 negative patients. Oligoarthritis and systemic arthritis carried the best chance of 5-year remission (54 and 38 per cent, respectively) and polyarthritis the worst outlook (15 per cent). In a study of 19 patients with juvenile spondyloarthropathy, predictors of joint erosions were long duration of elevated erythrocyte sedimentation rate, long disease duration before first admission, and long disease duration before treatment with a slow-acting antirheumatic drug (Flato et al. 1998).

A number of investigators have reported the outcome of children with arthritis who are HLA–B27 positive. Jacobs et al. (1982) described 58 patients who were followed for a mean of 5 years. Arthritis at the initiation of the illness was often transient and recurrent, oligoarticular, and asymmetric in distribution, and occurred primarily in the knees and ankles. Hip signs were noted in only seven of the patients at onset, but the hips were ultimately affected in 36 per cent. Radiographs of the sacroiliac joints were obtained for 43 of the patients, 10 of whom showed signs of sacroiliitis after a mean symptomatic period of 5 years (range 1–12 years). Other radiographic findings included periostitis, severe osteopaenia, calcaneal erosions, or spurs. Rapid destruction of a single joint occurred in three patients.

Prieur (1987) reported a study of 65 children with HLA-B27 associated arthritis. There were 45 boys and 20 girls, with a mean age of onset of symptoms of 10 years (range 2.5–16 years). Just over a quarter of the patients (27 per cent) had arthritis in an upper limb during the first 6 months of disease. Enthesitis was present in 10 patients and dactylitis in one-third. After 5 years' follow-up, 32 per cent had fulfilled criteria for ankylosing spondylitis (seven patients), Reiter's syndrome (two patients), psoriatic arthritis (nine patients), and Crohn's arthritis (three patients).

Thirty-six HLA-B27 positive children with arthritis who had been followed for a mean of 8.9 years were described by Sheerin et al. (1988). Five patients had an initial diagnosis of juvenile ankylosing spondylitis (14 per cent), and 24 (67 per cent) initially had peripheral arthritis without axial involvement. The most frequently involved joint was the knee (15 patients) followed by the ankle (eight patients), and the foot (five patients). During the follow-up period, 22 patients had symptoms consistent with enthesitis, although it was demonstrable in only 16 patients (44 per cent). Eight patients (22 per cent) had extra-articular manifestations: acute iritis (four patients), inflammatory bowel disease (one), psoriasis (two) and localized scleroderma (one). One of the patients with psoriasis had recurrent episodes of urethritis suggestive of incomplete Reiter's syndrome. Of the 28 patients in whom radiographs of sacroiliac joints were taken, 13 had normal results. A clinical course consistent with juvenile ankylosing spondylitis ultimately developed in 27 of the 36 patients. The presence of HLA-B27 itself has been proposed as a poor prognostic factor in juvenile arthritis. In 91 patients who had arthroplasty for juvenile arthritis, 39 were HLA-B27 positive. They underwent arthroplasty an average of 2.9 years earlier than the HLA-B27 negative patients (Savolainen et al. 1998).

The dearth of quality of life studies in juvenile spondyloarthropathies is likely to improve with the development and validation of the juvenile arthritis quality of life questionnaire for children with arthritis, particularly the juvenile spondyloarthropathy group (Duffy et al. 1997). General fitness rates are reduced in older children with spondyloarthropathies even in remission (Hebestreit et al. 1998). A worrying report from Au et al. (2001) has suggested that HLA-B27 is associated an increased risk of acute leukaemia in carriers, but the long-term follow-up data on children with juvenile spondylitis is insufficient to contribute to this data.

Juvenile ankylosing spondylitis

The diagnosis of juvenile ankylosing spondylitis depends on criteria formulated for use in adults (Table 6, Bennett and Burch 1967). Althougth these have not been validated for the paediatric population, there is a small proportion of children with arthritis who fulfil the criteria. In a survey of 44 patients fulfilling New York ankylosing spondylitis criteria, with symptom onset during childhood, only 14 (32 per cent) rapidly progressed to full-blown ankylosing spondylitis within 3 years of presentation. The main predictor of this outcome was polyarthritis at onset (Burgos-Vargas et al. 1996).

Clinical features

Juvenile ankylosing spondylitis commonly presents as an arthritis affecting the large joints of the lower limbs, particularly the knees, ankles, and tarsal joints, often associated with enthesopathy (Bywaters 1976; Ansell 1980; Burgos-Vargas and Vazquez-Mellado 1995).

Although it is rare for the hips to be the sole site involved at presentation, there is a small group of children in whom recurrent, transient hip symptoms eventually develop into ankylosing spondylitis. The early course of the disease is frequently episodic, and other features of an undifferentiated spondyloarthropathy may be present. Inflammation of the entheses may be prominent early in the disease course. The most common sites include Achilles tendon insertions, peripatella insertions including the quadriceps and patella tendons, and the insertions of the plantar fascia into calcaneum and metatarsal heads. Subtalar and mid-tarsal arthritis is not uncommon. Tarsometatarsal arthritis is sometimes associated with hindfoot involvement and results in a supination deformity. Indeed, spontaneous fusion and complete obliteration of the tarsometatarsal joints may occur (Levi et al. 1990; Burgos-Vargas 1991) (Fig. 1.) Pernicious hip involvement leading eventually to total hip arthroplasty is one of the most common peripheral articular complications of juvenile ankylosing spondylitis (Calin and Elswood 1988). In a study of 147 patients with ankylosing spondylitis, 22 juvenile ankylosing spondylitis patients had a higher frequency of ankle ($p = 0.012$) and knee ($p = 0.001$) involvement, heel enthesitis ($p = 0.001$), and total hip replacement ($p = 0.038$) (Sampaio-Barros et al. 2001).

The joints of the arms are much less commonly affected, but occasionally the shoulders are involved. In contrast to adults with ankylosing spondylitis, most affected children do not report pain in the axial skeleton initially. Only 12–24 per cent have pain, stiffness, or limitation of motion of the lumbosacral spine or sacroiliac joint within the first year of disease

Table 6 New York criteria for the diagnosis of ankylosing spondylitis (AS)

Clinical criteria
1. Limitation of lumbar spine motion in all three planes
2. Pain or history of pain at the dorsolumbar junction or lumbar spine
3. Limitation of chest expansion to 2.5 cm or less at the level of the fourth intercostal space
Definite AS
1. Grade 3–4 bilateral sacroiliac arthritis on radiograph with at least 1 clinical criterion, or
2. Grade 3–4 unilateral or grade 2 bilateral sacroiliac arthritis on radiograph with criterion 1 or criteria 2 and 3
Probable AS
1. Grade 3–4 bilateral sacroiliac arthritis on radiograph without clinical criteria

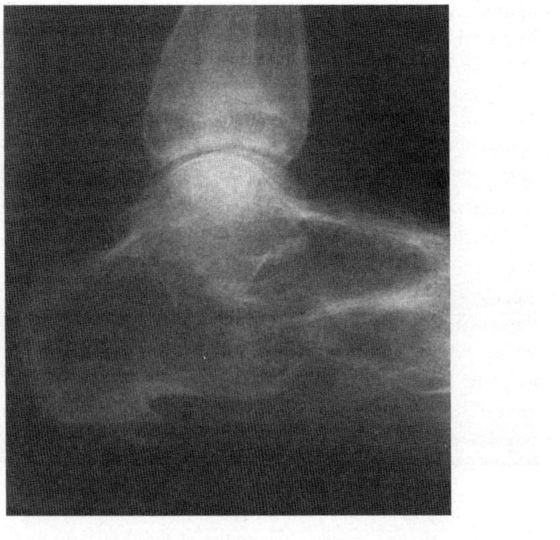

Fig. 1 Radiograph of ankle and hindfoot of the patient also illustrated in Fig. 2. The subtalar and talonavicular articulations are ankylosed. A calcaneal spur is present from long-standing plantar fasciitis.

(Burgos-Vargas and Petty 1992). This may be due in part to the rather poorly localized symptoms of inflammation in these areas, which may cause pain in the buttock, groin, thigh, or back. Evidence of sacroiliac involvement can be elicited by pressure over the sacroiliac joints of by compression of the joints using manoeuvres such as Patrick's test or Gaenselen's sign (Hoppenfield 1976). Serial follow-up with Schober's measurements and measurement of chest expansion can reveal progressive restriction of the range of motion of the axial skeleton. Most patients develop axial involvement 5–10 years after the onset of symptoms. Definite involvement of the spine and sacroiliitis in patients with juvenile ankylosing spondylitis occurred after a mean of 7.3 ± 2 years in a series of 35 patients (Burgos-Vargas and Vazquez-Mellado 1995). Serial plain radiographs of the sacroiliac joints may be helpful in monitoring the course of the disease (Fig. 2). It is important to note that interpretation of plain radiographs of the sacroiliac joints is fraught with difficulty in the child and adolescent. The first reliable sign is sclerosis of the lateral border of the sacroiliac joint, but without experience this would be difficult to differentiate from normality (Azouz and Duffy 1995). Several authors have suggested that magnetic resonance imaging improves the detection rate of sacroiliitis (Azouz and Duffy 1995; Bollow et al. 1998; Pepmueller and Moore 2000).

Several studies have compared juvenile with adult ankylosing spondylitis (Garcia-Morteo et al. 1983; Marks et al. 1987; Burgos-Vargas et al. 1989). Significant differences noted were peripheral arthritis at onset, precocious hip destruction, and the insidious late development of axial involvement, all observed in the juvenile form. Pulmonary disease, IgA nephropathy, and cauda equina syndrome have not been reported in children.

The systemic complications of juvenile ankylosing spondylitis include acute iritis (Ladd et al. 1971; Ansell 1980; Hafner 1987), aortic valve insufficiency (Stewart et al. 1978; Reid et al. 1979; Stamato et al. 1995), C1–C2 subluxation (Reid and Hill 1978), and amyloidosis (Ansell 1980). The frequency of aortic valve insufficiency ranges from 8 to 30 per cent, the latter detected by imaging with colour Doppler ultrasound (Gerster et al. 1987; Stamato et al. 1995). Jimenez-Balderas et al. (2001) compared juvenile (n = 20) and adult (n = 31) ankylosing spondylitis using two-dimensional echocardiography. Cardiomyopathy, demonstrated by left ventricular ejection fraction, was found in 25 per cent of juvenile cases, compared with 32.2 per cent adult cases, in association with an increased mitral valve gradient. There was a lower frequency of aortic problems in the juvenile cases. Others have confirmed mitral regurgitation in 5 per cent of juvenile ankylosing spondylitis patients (Stamato et al. 1995).

Outcome

The long-term outcome of juvenile ankylosing spondylitis is variable. Garcia-Morteo et al. (1983) found no juvenile-onset patients who retained full functional capacity after a mean disease duration of 15 years. Twelve patients (50 per cent) were in class II, seven in class III, and five in class IV, using the Steinbroker classification. In contrast, the functional outcome of patients with the disease appears to be reasonably good, with a large proportion in employment (73 per cent) or continuing education (Marks et al. 1987). Most patients (95 per cent) require long-term anti-inflammatory therapy and have persistent peripheral arthritis. Calin and Eastwood (1988) followed 135 patients with juvenile ankylosing spondylitis and reported that 74 per cent remained in full time employment, a higher proportion than a comparable number of patients with adult-onset disease (54 per cent).

(a)

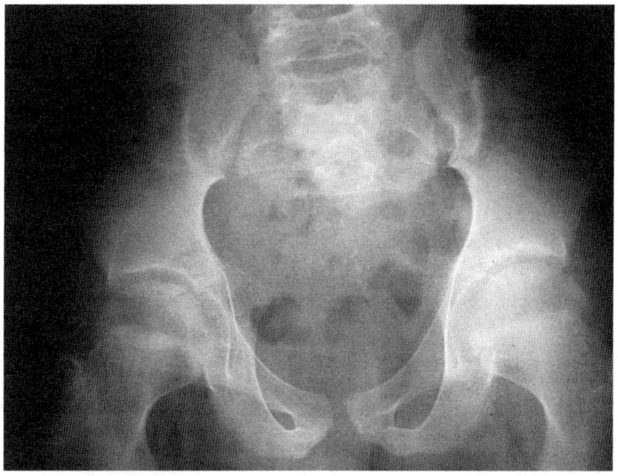

(b)

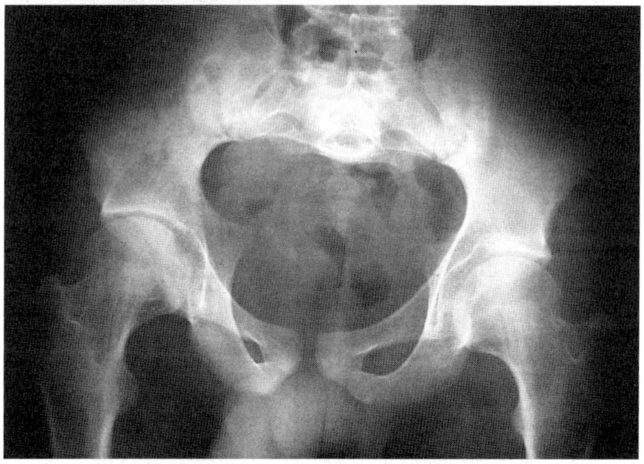

Fig. 2 (a) Radiograph of pelvis in a 14-year-old boy demonstrating normal sacroiliac joints. He was initially diagnosed as oligoarthritic. (b) Radiograph of the same patient after 4 years of disease activity. Note the sclerosis and erosion of the sacroiliac joints. The patient did not specifically complain of back pain but had limited lumbar flexion on Schober's testing.

Inflammatory bowel disease associated arthritis

Peripheral arthritis and spondylitis are among the most common extra-articular manifestations of chronic inflammatory bowel disease. Although inflammatory bowel disease is divided into two major clinicopathological types, Crohn's disease and ulcerative colitis, the common articular complications of each sub-type are the same. In most series of adult patients, the prevalence of joint involvement is 2–22 per cent for both Crohn's colitis and ulcerative colitis (Gavallese and Kantrowitz 1988). Two reviews of arthritis associated with inflammatory bowel disease in children revealed similar prevalence: 9–21 per cent of patients with ulcerative colitis and 10–16 per cent of patients with Crohn's disease (Lindsley and Schaller 1974; Passo et al. 1986). A study of 40 children with either oligoarthritis, inflammatory bowel disease related arthritis or spondyloarthropathy by Picco et al. (2000) found evidence of abnormal intestinal permeability in all groups, although significantly higher in the latter two groups. There was a positive correlation between intestinal permeability and gastrointestinal symptoms.

Clinical features

The peripheral arthritis involves few joints, usually the large weight-bearing joints of the lower limbs, but occasionally involving joints of the upper limbs. The duration of attacks ranges from 2 days to 12 weeks, and averages about 1 month. These attacks occasionally precede the onset of bowel symptoms but usually coincide with or occur after the onset of bowel inflammation. After the initial attack, episodes of peripheral arthritis frequently occur during exacerbations or active periods of bowel disease. Passo et al. (1986) noted eight patients with Crohn's disease who had episodes of arthritis at times when they were free of bowel symptoms. These patients had anaemia and hypoalbuminaemia, however, suggesting that sub-clinical bowel inflammation may have been present. Importantly, most flares of bowel disease were not accompanied by arthritic manifestations. There was no correlation between the severity of the bowel inflammation and the occurrence of arthritis. Treatment of the bowel inflammation was usually associated with resolution of the peripheral arthritis.

Lindsley and Schaller (1974) described five children with inflammatory bowel disease, all of whom had classical signs of ankylosing spondylitis (low back pain and loss of motion and radiographic evidence of arthritis in the sacroiliac joints and lumbar spine). The symptoms were persistent and progressive, resulting in permanent impairment. Destructive hip disease was seen in four of these patients and all five had peripheral arthritis, including hip inflammation at some time during follow-up. Joint symptoms preceded bowel symptoms in two of the patients by 3 months and 8 years; one had concurrent onset of bowel and joint symptoms. The activity of the spondylitis and peripheral arthritis appeared to progress independently of the bowel symptoms. Treatment of the bowel inflammation was not effective in the treatment of the spondylitis, observations that have been supported by case reports (Unsal et al. 1997). These patients are more likely to carry the HLA-B27 antigen, but there are few reproducible data on HLA typing in children with spondylitis and inflammatory bowel disease. In adult patients, the prevalence of HLA-B27 positivity is 53–75 per cent, considerably lower than the 90–95 per cent prevalence seen in idiopathic ankylosing spondylitis (Gavallese and Kantrowitz 1988).

Reiter's syndrome

Prevalence

There are no estimates of the prevalence of Reiter's syndrome in the child population. Although fewer than 100 childhood cases have been described, reactive arthritis often goes unreported and probably many more cases have been encountered. There are several reviews of the literature and summaries of the data (Lockie and Hunder 1971; Iverson et al. 1975; Singsen et al. 1977; Rosenberg and Petty 1979; Cuttica et al. 1992). There is undoubtedly a considerable overlap between Reiter's syndrome and reactive arthritis.

Clinical manifestations

The clinical syndrome in children is similar to that described in adult patients. The individual features of arthritis, urethritis, conjunctivitis, keratoderma blennorrhagicum, circinate balanitis, and oral mucosal ulcers may occur sequentially over a period of several weeks. Singsen et al. (1977) reported seven boys in a 2-year period who developed the triad of urethritis, arthritis, and conjunctivitis over a range of 4–24 days (mean 11 days). The evolution of signs and symptoms occurs asynchronously in many children. Whereas adult Reiter's syndrome often follows venereal infection, most cases of childhood Reiter's syndrome are preceded by enteric infection with species of *Salmonella, Shigella, Yersinia,* or *Campylobacter.* There are also individual reports of *Clostridium difficile* and parasitic infestation provoking Reiter's syndrome. A 14-year-old female was reported with Reiter's syndrome following a urinary tract infection with *Escherichia coli* (Thomas and Roberton 1994). In 1992, Cuttica et al. (1992) reported the largest series of children with Reiter's syndrome and confirmed that diarrhoea antedated the onset of arthritis in 18 per 26 (69 per cent) patients; no patient reported venereal disease. The majority of patients (69 per cent) had oligoarticular involvement of lower extremities. Spine involvement was seen in six patients (23 per cent). The full triad of arthritis, conjunctivitis, and urethritis was seen in 9 per 16 (35 per cent). Reiter's syndrome in most children is a short-lived condition characterized by complete resolution of the signs and symptoms; however, a protracted course and recurrent disease have been described (Iverson et al. 1975; Singsen et al. 1977; Southwood and Gaston 1993). In Cuttica's series, mean duration of follow-up was 28.5 months (range 2–13.5 years); 15 per 26 (58 per cent) were in complete remission when last seen, seven (27 per cent) had a sustained course, three (11.5 per cent) had a fluctuating course, and only one child had a relapsing course. Functional outcome was grade I to II in 96 per cent. Radiographic erosions were noted in 4 per 26 (15 per cent) peripheral joints and sacroiliitis in 5 per 26 (21 per cent) (Cuttica et al. 1992). The long-term outcome of Reiter's syndrome in children is not well documented, although a proportion of cases undoubtedly progress to ankylosing spondylitis.

Juvenile psoriatic arthritis

Juvenile psoriatic arthritis has been traditionally grouped with the spondyloarthropathies, but there is emerging evidence that the clinical and laboratory features of this disease have greater similarity to oligoarthritis with an asymmetrical polyarticular course. Important dissimilarities to the spondyloarthropathies are the lack of association with HLA-B27 and the relatively rare outcome of ankylosing spondylitis. The classification criteria proposed as part of the ILAR task force on classification in juvenile arthritis (Petty et al. 1998) modified the Vancouver criteria by removing the minor criterion of atypical psoriatic rash (Table 7).

Foeldvari and Bidde (2000) found that the presence of a family history of psoriatic arthritis was the most frequent reason for being unable to classify patients in one of the sub-categories of the ILAR proposal.

Prevalence

Most estimates of the prevalence of psoriasis in the general population range from 1 to 2 per cent (Baker 1966). In children, its estimated prevalence is approximately 0.3 per cent (Farber and Carsen 1966). The onset of psoriasis is frequently between 5 and 15 years of age with one-third of all cases starting by the age of 15 years. Based on a population study by Hellegren (1969), Lawrence et al. (1989) calculated that approximately 4.5 per cent of those with psoriasis have psoriatic arthritis. They further suggested that the prevalence of psoriatic arthritis in the United States is 0.67 per cent; accordingly, about 160 000 persons in the United States have psoriatic arthritis. Cassidy and Petty (1995) estimated the prevalence of juvenile psoriatic arthritis at between 10 and 15 cases per 1 000 000 based on population studies reported by Espinoza (1985), making it approximately one-tenth as common as juvenile idiopathic arthritis (Lambert et al. 1976; Calabro 1977; Sills 1980; Shore and Ansell 1982; Hamilton et al. 1990; Truckenbrodt and Hafner 1990).

Overall, juvenile psoriatic arthritis accounts for 2–8 per cent of chronic arthritic conditions in childhood (Lambert et al. 1976; Ansell 1977; Sills 1980). However, on using more liberal criteria for the diagnosis, Kuster and Quoss (1983) reported that it might account for as much as 40 per cent of juvenile chronic arthritis. Biondi Oriente et al. (1994) studied the frequency of juvenile psoriatic arthritis from a dermatological perspective. They reviewed 425 patients with psoriasis whose skin disease began before 31 years of age (according to the Lambert and Ansell criteria, the onset of

Table 7 Proposed ILAR classification criteria for juvenile idiopathic arthritis: juvenile psoriatic arthritis

Inclusion criteria
1. Arthritis and psoriasis or
2. Arthritis and at least two of the following
(a) Dactylitis
(b) Nail pitting or onycholysis
(c) Psoriasis in a first degree relative
Exclusion criteria
1. Arthritis in an HLA-B27 positive male with arthritis onset after 6 years of age
2. Ankylosing spondylitis, enthesitis related arthritis, sacroiliitis with inflammatory bowel disease, Reiter's syndrome, acute anterior uveitis in a first degree relative
3. Presence of IgM rheumatoid factor on at least two occasions more than 3 months apart
4. Presence of systemic arthritis

psoriasis in juvenile arthritis patients could occur up to 15 years after the onset of arthritis). Five patients with onset of arthritis before 16 years were identified; a prevalence of 1 per cent. However, considering only the 85 patients who developed psoriasis during the paediatric age span, the prevalence of psoriatic arthritis was 6 per cent. All had a family history of psoriasis and arthritis preceded psoriasis in two cases. The interval between the onset of cutaneous and articular involvement never exceeded 8 years (Biondi Oriente et al. 1994).

Clinical characteristics

Juvenile psoriatic arthropathy is a heterogeneous group of arthritic conditions that poses classification problems. The majority of affected children resemble cases of juvenile chronic arthritis and a smaller fraction juvenile spondyloarthropathy. Additionally, there are probably children who have coincidental psoriasis and juvenile chronic arthritis (Petty 1994). Juvenile psoriatic arthritis has been defined by Lambert et al. (1976) as 'an inflammatory arthritis commencing prior to the age of 16 years associated with psoriasis either preceding the onset of arthritis or occurring within the subsequent 15 years and usually with an absence of rheumatoid factor in the serum'. The psoriasis (nail and cutaneous manifestations) may lag behind the onset of arthritis by several months to years. Patients with conventionally defined psoriatic arthritis constituted 6 per cent of the juvenile arthritis population; indeed, according to the revised criteria, psoriatic arthritis constitutes approximately 19 per cent of the chronic arthritides of childhood. Shore and Ansell (1982) also described children without skin lesions but with probably juvenile psoriatic arthritis. Their 12 patients had asymmetrical arthritis of both upper and lower limbs, and a positive family history of psoriasis; eight of the 12 had significant nail pitting. They suggested that such patients should be regarded as having 'probably juvenile psoriatic arthritis'. In the 5 years of follow-up, half of these patients developed overt psoriasis.

Juvenile psoriatic arthritis differs from the other spondyloarthropathies in that females are affected more often than males (1.5 : 1), but with marked variability among series (range 2 : 8 to 1 : 1.3, female/male) (Lambert et al. 1976; Shore and Ansell 1982; Southwood et al. 1989; Hamilton et al. 1990; Truckenbrodt and Hafner 1990). Simultaneous onset of arthritis and psoriasis is relatively uncommon. Most studies listed above show that the onset of arthritis is oligoarticular but an asymmetrical polyarthritis evolves over the ensuing years. Sacroiliitis occurs in a significant number of cases (11–47 per cent) but is not inevitable (Southwood et al. 1989; Hamilton et al. 1990). The knee is the most commonly affected joint; dactylitis, tendonitis, and involvement of the distal interphalangeal joints are also extremely common. Dactylitis, distal interphalangeal inflammation, and the associated classical psoriatic nail changes are sometimes obvious (Plates 103 and 104). The course of the disease tends to be more severe than that of oligoarthritis; it is less severe, however, than the polyarticular course of juvenile chronic arthritis, especially in patients positive for rheumatoid factor. Overall, Steinbroker functional class I or II outcomes are common (Lambert et al. 1976; Calabro 1977). Fewer than 10–15 per cent of patients evolve into functional classes III or IV (Shore and Ansell 1982).

Chronic iridocyclitis similar to that seen in juvenile arthritis developed in 8–17 per cent of reported patients with psoriatic arthritis (Sills 1980; Shore and Ansell 1982; Southwood et al. 1989; Truckenbrodt and Hafner 1990). Most patients with chronic iridocyclitis have also been positive for antinuclear antibody, which draws a closer association with juvenile chronic arthritis than the typical spondyloarthropathies that manifest acute iritis.

No strong HLA association with juvenile psoriatic arthritis has been demonstrated. Hamilton et al. (1990) showed increased frequency of HLA-A2 and -B17, a possible increase in HLA–DR7 and no increase in HLA-B27. Southwood et al. (1989) found increased HLA–DR8 and decreased frequencies of HLA–DR4; HLA-B27 was found in eight patients (23 per cent) five of whom had clinical features of spondyloarthropathy (back pain, limited range of motion in the back and sacroiliitis). Ansell et al. (1993) confirmed the heterogeneity of 70 patients: HLA-B27 was increased in frequency, particularly in boys with older onset. HLA-A2, HLA–DR5, and HLA–DRw8 were found to be increased in early-onset cases. Other class I HLA genes associated with juvenile onset psoriasis (Cw6 and B57) have not been associated with arthritic complications, but Hohler et al. (1996) found that the TAP gene ('transporter associated with antigen processing') TAP1*0101, but no TAP2 gene polymorphism, was associated with the psoriasis in 60 patients with juvenile psoriatic arthritis.

Outcome

Roberton et al. (1996) reviewed the disease course of 63 children (44 girls, median age at onset 4.5 years; 19 boys, median age at onset 10.1 years). Antinuclear antibody was present in 50 per cent. Thirty-eight children were followed for more than 5 years, 18 for more than 10 years, and 7 for more than 15 years. Forty-four children had active arthritis; 32 per cent were in functional class I, 38 per cent in class II, 22 per cent in class III, and 8 per cent in class, IV. Of the 46 patients with oligoarticular onset, 21 remained oligoarticular and 25 became polyarticular. Arthritis in the small joints of the hands and feet increased in frequency, with arthritis eventually occurring in proximal interphalangeal joints in 63 per cent, metacarpophalangeal or metatarsophalangeal joints in 55 per cent, and distal interphalangeal joints in 27 per cent. Dactylitis occurred in 35 per cent, most commonly in second toes and index fingers. Nine patients (14 per cent) developed chronic anterior uveitis. Eleven of 24 patients (46 per cent) who initially had probable juvenile psoriatic arthritis evolved to definite juvenile psoriatic arthritis after a median of 2.1 years. Five developed psoriasis and the remainder developed additional minor criteria.

References

Amor, B., Dougados, M., and Mijiyawa, M. (1990). Criteria of the classification of spondylarthropathies. *Revue du rhumatisme et des maladies Osteo-articulaires* **57** (2), 85–9.

Andersson Gare, B., Fasth, A., Andersson, J., Berglund, G., Ekstrom, H., Eriksson, M., Hammaren, L., Holmquist, L., Ronge, E., and Thilen, A. (1987). Incidence and prevalence of juvenile chronic arthritis: a population survey. *Annals of the Rheumatic Diseases* **46**, 277–81.

Ansell, B.M. (1977). Juvenile chronic polyarthritis. *Arthritis and Rheumatism* **20** (Suppl.), 176–8.

Ansell, B.M. (1980). Juvenile spondylitis and related disorders. In *Ankylosing Spondylitis* (ed. J.M. Moll), pp. 120–36. London: Churchill Livingstone.

Ansell, B., Beeson, M., Hall, P., Bedford, P., and Woo, P. (1993). HLA and juvenile psoriatic arthritis. *British Journal of Rheumatology* **32**, 836–7.

Au, W.Y., Hawkins, B.R., Cheng, N., Lie, A.K., Liang, R., and Kwong, Y.L. (2001). Risk of haematological malignancies in HLA–B27 carriers. *British Journal of Haematology* **115**, 320–2.

Azouz, E.M. and Duffy, C.M. (1995). Juvenile spondyloarthropathies: clinical manifestations and medical imaging. *Skeletal Radiology* **24** (6), 399–408.

Baker, H. (1966). Epidemiological aspects of psoriasis and arthritis. *British Journal of Dermatology* **78**, 249–61.

Bennett, P.H. and Burch, T.A. (1967). New York symposium on population studies in the rheumatic diseases: new diagnostic criteria. *Bulletin of Rheumatic Diseases* **17**, 453–8.

Biondi Oriente, C., Scarpa, R., and Oriente, P. (1994). Prevalence and clinical features of juvenile psoriatic arthritis in 425 psoriatic patients. *Acta Dermatologie Venereologie (Stockholm)* **186** (Suppl.), 109–10.

Bollow, M., Biedermann, T., Kannenberg, J., Paris, S., Schauer-Petrowski, C., Minden, K., Schontube, M., Hamm, B., Sieper, J., and Braun, J. (1998). Use of dynamic magnetic resonance imaging to detect sacroiliitis in HLA-B27 positive and negative children with juvenile arthritides. *Journal of Rheumatology* **25**, 556–64.

Bowyer, S. (1995). Hip contracture as the presenting sign in children with HLA-B27 arthritis. *Journal of Rheumatology* **22**, 165–7.

Burgos-Vargas, R. (1991). Ankylosing tarsitis: clinical features of a unique form of tarsal disease in the juvenile onset spondyloarthropathies. *Arthritis and Rheumatism* (Suppl.), S196.

Burgos-Vargas, R. and Clark, P. (1989). Axial involvement in the seronegative enthesopathy and arthropathy syndrome and its progression to ankylosing spondylitis. *Journal of Rheumatology* **16**, 192–7.

Burgos-Vargas, R. and Petty, R.E. (1992). Juvenile ankylosing spondylitis. *Rheumatic Diseases Clinics of North America* **18**, 123–42.

Burgos-Vargas, R. and Vazquez-Mellado, J. (1995). The early clinical recognition of juvenile-onset ankylosing spondylitis and its differentiation from juvenile arthritis. *Arthritis and Rheumatism* **36**, 186–91.

Burgos-Vargas, R., Naranjo, A., Castillo, J., and Katona, G. (1989). Ankylosing spondylitis in the Mexican Mestizo patterns of disease according to age at onset. *Journal of Rheumatology* **16**, 186–91.

Burgos-Vargas, R., Vazquez-Mellado, J., Cassis, N., Duarte, C., Casarin, J., Cifuentes, M., and Lino, L. (1996). Genuine ankylosing spondylitis in children: a case-control study of patients with early definite disease according to adult onset criteria. *Journal of Rheumatology* **23**, 2140–7.

Bywaters, E.G.L. (1976). Ankylosing spondylitis in childhood. *Clinical Rheumatic Diseases* **21**, 387–95.

Cabral, D.A., Oen, K., and Petty, R.E. (1992). SEA syndrome revisited: a longterm follow up of children with a syndrome of seronegative enthesopathy and arthropathy. *Journal of Rheumatology* **19**, 1282–5.

Calabro, J.J. (1977). Psoriatic arthritis in children. *Arthritis and Rheumatism* **20**, (Suppl.), 415–17.

Calin, A. and Elswood, J. (1988). The natural history of juvenile-onset ankylosing spondylitis: a 24 year retrospective case control study. *British Journal of Rheumatology* **27**, 91–3.

Camiciottoli, G., Trapani, S., Ermini, M., Falcini, F., and Pistolesi, M. (1999). Pulmonary function in children affected by juvenile spondyloarthropathy. *Journal of Rheumatology* **26**, 1382–6.

Carter, E.T., McKenna, C.H., and Brian, D.D. (1979). Epidemiology of ankylosing spondylitis in Rochester, Minnesota 1935–1973. *Arthritis and Rheumatism* **22**, 365–70.

Cassidy, J.T. and Petty, R. (1995). Spondyloarthropathy. In *The Textbook of Pediatric Rheumatology* 3rd edn. (ed. J.T. Cassidy and R.E. Petty), pp. 224–59. Philadelphia PA: Saunders.

Cuttica, R.J., Scheines, E.J., Garay, S.M., Romanelli, M.D., and Cocco, J.A.M. (1992). Juvenile onset Reiter's syndrome. A retrospective study of 26 patients. *Clinical and Experimental Rheumatology* **10**, 285–8.

Denardo, B.A., Tucker, L.B., Miller, L.C., Szer, I.S., and Schaller, J.G. (1994). Demography of a regional pediatric rheumatology patient population. Affiliated Children's Arthritis Centers of New England. *Journal of Rheumatology* **21**, 1553–61.

Dougados, M. et al. (1991). The European Spondylarthropathy Study Group preliminary criteria for the classification of spondylarthropathy. *Arthritis and Rheumatism* **34** (10), 1218–27.

Duffy, C.M., Arsenault, L., Duffy, K.N., Paquin, J.D., and Strawczynski, H. (1997). The Juvenile Arthritis Quality of Life Questionnaire—development of a new responsive index for juvenile rheumatoid arthritis and juvenile spondyloarthritides. *Journal of Rheumatology* **24**, 738–46.

Espinoza, L.R. (1985). Psoriatic arthritis: further epidemiologic and genetic considerations. In *Psoriatic Arthritis* (ed. L.H. Gerber and L.R. Espinoza), pp. 9–32. Orlando FA: Grune and Stratton.

Farber, E.M. and Carsen, R.A. (1966). Psoriasis in childhood. *California Medicine* **105**, 415–20.

Flato, B., Aasland, A., Vinje, O., and Forre, O. (1998). Outcome and predictive factors in juvenile rheumatoid arthritis and juvenile spondyloarthropathy. *Journal of Rheumatology* **25**, 366–75.

Foeldvari, I. and Bidde, M. (2000). Validation of the proposed ILAR classification criteria for juvenile idiopathic arthritis. International League of Associations for Rheumatology. *Journal of Rheumatology* **27**, 1069–72.

Foster, H.E., Cairns, R.A., Burnell, R.H., Malleson, P.N., Roberton, D.M., Tredwell, S.J., Petty, R.E., and Cabral, D.A. (1995). Atlantoaxial subluxation in children with seronegative enthesopathy and arthropathy syndrome: 2 case reports and a review of the literature. *Journal of Rheumatology* **22**, 548–51.

Garcia-Morteo, O., Maldonado-Cocco, A., Suarez-Almazor, M.E., and Garay, E. (1983). Ankylosing spondylitis of juvenile onset: comparison with adult onset disease. *Scandinavian Journal of Rheumatology* **12**, 246–8.

Gavallese, E.M. and Kantrowitz, F.G. (1988). Arthritis manifestations of inflammatory bowel disease. *American Journal of Gastroenterology* **84**, 703–9.

Gerster, J.C., Payot, M., and Piccinin, P. (1987). Clinical and echocardiographic assessment in juvenile-onset. *British Journal of Rheumatology* **26**, 155–6.

Gomez, K.S., Raza, K., Jones, S.D., Kennedy, L.G., and Calin, A. (1997). Juvenile onset ankylosing spondylitis—more girls than we thought? *Journal of Rheumatology* **24**, 735–7.

Hafner, R. (1987). Die juvenile spondarthritis. Retrospektive untersuchung on 91 patienten. *Monatsschrift Kinderheilkund* **135**, 41–6.

Hamilton, M.L., Gladman, D.D., Shore, A., Laxer, R.M., and Silverman, E.D. (1990). Juvenile psoriatic arthritis and HLA antigens. *Annals of the Rheumatic Diseases* **49**, 694–7.

Hart, F.D. and Maclagan, N.F. (1955). Ankylosing spondylitis. A review of 184 cases. *Annals of the Rheumatic Diseases* **14**, 77.

Hebestreit, H., Muller-Scholden, J., and Huppertz, H.I. (1998). Aerobic fitness and physical activity in patients with HLA-B27 positive juvenile spondyloarthropathy that is inactive or in remission. *Journal of Rheumatology* **25**, 1626–33.

Hellegren, L. (1969). Association between arthritis and psoriasis in total populations. *Acta Rheumatologica* **15**, 316–26.

Hofer, M.F., Mouy, R., and Prieur, A.M. (2001). Juvenile idiopathic arthritides evaluated prospectively in a single center according to the Durban criteria. *Journal of Rheumatology* **28**, 1083–90.

Hohler, T., Weinmann, A., Schneider, P.M., Rittner, C., Schopf, R.E., Knop, J., Hasenclever, P., Meyer zum Buschenfelde, K.H., and Marker-Hermann, E. (1996). TAP-polymorphisms in juvenile onset psoriasis and psoriatic arthritis. 1. *Human Immunology* **51**, 49–54.

Hoppenfield, S. (1976). Physical examination of the lumbar spine and extremities. In *Physical Examination of the Spine and Extremities* (ed. S. Hoppenfield), pp. 261–2. New York: Appleton-Century-Croft.

Huemer, C., Huemer, M., Dorner, T., Falger, J., Schacherl, H., Bernecker, M., Artacker, G., and Pilz, I. (2001). Incidence of pediatric rheumatic diseases in a regional population in Austria. *Journal of Rheumatology* **28**, 2116–19.

Huppertz, H., Voigt, I., Muller-Scholden, J., and Sandhage, K. (2000). Cardiac manifestations in patients with HLA-B27-associated juvenile arthritis. *Pediatric Cardiology* **21**, 141–7.

Hussein, A., Abdul-Khaliq, H., and von de Hardt, H. (1989). Atypical spondyloarthropathies in children: proposed diagnostic criteria. *European Journal of Pediatrics* **148**, 513–17.

Iverson, J.M.I., Nanda, B.S., Hancock, J.A.H., Pownall, P.J., and Wright, V. (1975). Reiter's disease in three boys. *Annals of the Rheumatic Diseases* **34**, 364–8.

Jacobs, J.C., Berdon, W.E., and Johnson, A.D. (1982). HLA–B27-associated spondylarthritis and enthesopathy in childhood: clinical, pathologic and radiographic observations in 58 patients. *Pediatrics* **100**, 521–8.

Jimenez-Balderas, F.J., Garcia-Rubi, D., Perez-Hinojosa, S., Arellano, J., Yanez, P., Sanchez, M.L., Camargo-Coronel, A., and Zonana-Nacach, A. (2001). Two-dimensional echo Doppler findings in juvenile and adult onset ankylosing spondylitis with long-term disease. *Angiology* **52**, 543–8.

Kim, T.H., Jung, S.S., Sohn, S.J., Park, M.H., and Kim, S.Y. (1997). Aneurysmal dilatation of ascending aorta and aortic insufficiency in juvenile spondyloarthropathy. *Scandinavian Journal of Rheumatology* **26**, 218–21.

Kuster, R.M. and Quoss, I. (1983). Juvenile psoriatic arthritis and spondylitis with or without psoriasis: probable and definite courses. *Zeitschrift für Rheumatologie* **42**, 310 (abstract).

Ladd, J.R., Cassidy, J.T., and Martel, W. (1971). Juvenile ankylosing spondylitis. *Arthritis and Rheumatism* **14**, 579–90.

Lambert, J.R., Ansell, B.M., Stephenson, E., and Wright, V. (1976). Psoriatic arthritis in childhood. *Clinical Rheumatic Disease* **2**, 339–52.

Lawrence, R.C., Hochberg, M.C., Kelsey, J.L., McDuffie, F.C., Medsger, T.A., Jr., Felts, W.R., and Shulman, L.E. (1989). Estimates of the prevalence of selected arthritic and musculoskeletal diseases in the United States. *Journal of Rheumatology* **16**, 427–41.

Lee, S.J., Im, H.Y., and Schueller, W.C. (2001). HLA–B27 positive juvenile arthritis with cardiac involvement preceding sacroiliac joint changes. *Heart* **86**, E19.

Levi, S., Ansell, B.M., and Klenerman, L. (1990). Tarsometatarsal involvement in juvenile. *Foot and Ankle Journal* **11**, 90–2.

Lindsley, C.B. and Schaller, J.G. (1974). Arthritis associated with inflammatory bowel disease in children. *Journal of Pediatrics* **84**, 16–20.

Lockie, G.N. and Hunder, G.G. (1971). Reiter's syndrome in children: a case report and review. *Arthritis and Rheumatism* **14**, 767–72.

Marks, S.H., Barnett, M., and Calin, A. (1987). A case–control study of juvenile and adult onset ankylosing spondylitis. *Journal of Rheumatology* **9**, 739–41.

Merino, R., De Inocencio, J., and Garcia-Consuegra, J. (2001). Evaluation of ILAR classification criteria for juvenile idiopathic arthritis in Spanish children. *Journal of Rheumatology* **28**, 2731–6.

Mielants, H., Veys, E.M., Covelier, C., and De Vos, M. (1996). Course of gut inflammation in spondylarthropathies and therapeutic consequences. *Bailliere's Clinical Rheumatology* **10** (1), 147–64.

Mikkelsen, W.M., Dodge, H.J., Duff, I.F., and Kato, H. (1967). Estimates of the prevalence of rheumatic diseases in the population of Tecumseh, Michigan, 1959–60. *Journal of Chronic Disease* **20**, 351–69.

Minden, K., Kiessling, U., Listing, J., Niewerth, M., Doring, E., Meincke, J., Schontube, M., and Zink, A. (2000). Prognosis of patients with juvenile chronic arthritis and juvenile spondyloarthropathy. *Journal of Rheumatology* **27**, 2256–63.

Murray, K.J., Moroldo, M.B., Donnelly, P., Prahalad, S., Passo, M.H., Giannini, E.H., and Glass, D.N. (1999). Age-specific effects of juvenile rheumatoid arthritis-associated HLA alleles. *Arthritis and Rheumatism* **42**, 1843–53.

Olivieri, I. and Pasero, G. (1992). Longstanding isolated juvenile onset HLA-B27 associated peripheral enthesitis. *Journal of Rheumatology* **19**, 164–5.

Olivieri, I., Barbieri, P., Gemignani, G., and Pasero, G. (1990). Isolated juvenile onset HLA-B27 associated peripheral enthesitis. *Journal of Rheumatology* **17**, 567–8.

Olivieri, I., Foto, M., Ruju, G.P., Gemignani, G., Giustarini, S., and Pasero, G. (1992). Low frequency of axial involvement in Caucasian pediatric patients with seronegative enthesopathy and arthropathy syndrome after 5 years of disease. *Journal of Rheumatology* **19**, 469–75.

Passo, M.H., Fitzgerald, J.F., and Brandt, K.D. (1986). Arthritis associated with inflammatory bowel disease in children: relationship of joint disease to activity and severity of bowel lesion. *Digestive Diseases and Sciences* **31**, 492–7.

Pepmueller, P.H. and Moore, T.L. (2000). Juvenile spondyloarthropathies. *Current Opinion in Rheumatology* **12** (4), 269–73.

Petty, R.E. (1990). HLA-B27 and rheumatic diseases of childhood. *Journal of Rheumatology* **17**, 7–10.

Petty, R.E. (1994). Juvenile psoriatic arthritis, or juvenile arthritis with psoriasis? *Clinical Experimental Rheumatology* **12** (Suppl. 10), S55–8.

Petty, R.E., Southwood, T.R., Baum, J., Bhettay, E., Glass, D.N., Manners, P., Maldonado-Cocco, J., Suarez-Almazor, M., Orozco-Alcala, J., and Prieur, A.M. (1998). Revision of the proposed classification criteria for juvenile idiopathic arthritis: Durban 1997. *Journal of Rheumatology* **25** (10), 1991–4.

Picco, P., Gattorno, M., Marchese, N., Vignola, S., Sormani, M.P., Barabino, A., and Buoncompagni, A. (2000). Increased gut permeability in juvenile chronic arthritides. A multivariate analysis of the diagnostic parameters. *Clinical Experimental Rheumatology* **18**, 773–8.

Prieur, A.M. (1987). HLA B27 associated chronic arthritis in children: review of 65 cases. *Scandinavian Journal of Rheumatology* **66** (Suppl.) 51–6.

Ramsey, S.E., Bolaria, R.K., Cabral, D.A., Malleson, P.N., and Petty, R.E. (2000). Comparison of criteria for the classification of childhood arthritis. *Journal of Rheumatology* **27**, 1283–6.

Read, R.W., Weiss, A.H., and Sherry, D.D. (1999). Episcleritis in childhood. *Ophthalmology* **106**, 2377–9.

Reid, G.D. and Hill, R.H. (1978). Atlanta-axial subluxation in juvenile ankylosing spondylitis. *Journal of Pediatrics* **93**, 531–2.

Reid, G.D., Patterson, M.W.H., Patterson, A.C., and Cooperberg, P.L. (1979). Aortic insufficiency in association with juvenile ankylosing spondylitis. *Journal of Pediatrics* **95**, 78–80.

Roberton, D.M., Cabral, D.A., Malleson, P.N., and Petty, R.E. (1996). Juvenile psoriatic arthritis: followup and evaluation of diagnostic criteria. *Journal of Rheumatology* **23**, 166–70.

Rosenberg, A.M. and Petty, R.E. (1979). Reiter's disease in children. *American Journal of Diseases of Children* **133**, 394–8.

Rosenberg, A.M. and Petty, R.E. (1982). A syndrome of seronegative enthesopathy and arthropathy in children. *Arthritis and Rheumatism* **25**, 1041–7.

Sampaio-Barros, P.D., Bertolo, M.B., Kraemer, M.H., Neto, J.F., and Samara, A.M. (2001). Primary ankylosing spondylitis: patterns of disease in a Brazilian population of 147 patients. *Journal of Rheumatology* **28**, 560–5.

Savolainen, H.A., Lehtimaki, M., Kautiainen, H., Aho, K., and Anttila, P. (1998). HLA-B27: a prognostic factor in juvenile chronic arthritis. *Clinical Rheumatology* **17** (2), 121–4.

Schaller, J.G. (1977). Ankylosing spondylitis of childhood onset. *Arthritis and Rheumatism* **20**, 398–401.

Schaller, J.G. (1983). Pauciarticular arthritis of childhood (pauciarticular juvenile arthritis). *Annales de Pediatrie* **30**, 557–63.

Schaller, J.G. (1985). The spondyloarthropathies (variant diseases). In *Practice of Pediatrics* Vol. 8 (ed. V.E. Kelly), pp. 1–10. Philadelphia PA: Harper and Row.

Sheerin, K.A., Giannini, E.H., Brewer, E.J., Jr., and Barron, K.S. (1988). HLA-B27 associated arthropathy in childhood: longterm clinical and diagnostic outcome. *Arthritis and Rheumatism* **31**, 1165–70.

Shore, A. and Ansell, B.M. (1982). Juvenile psoriatic arthritis—an analysis of 60 cases. *Journal of Pediatrics* **4**, 529–35.

Siegel, D.M. and Baum, J. (1988). HLA-B27 associated dactylitis in children. *Journal of Rheumatology* **15**, 976–7.

Sills, E.M. (1980). Psoriatic arthritis in childhood. *Johns Hopkins Medical Journal* **146**, 49–53.

Singsen, B.H., Bernstein, B.H., Koster-King, K.G., Glovsky, M.M., and Hanson, V. (1977). Reiter's syndrome in childhood. *Arthritis and Rheumatism* **20** (Suppl.) 402–7.

Southwood, T.R. and Gaston, J.S.H. (1993). The evolution of immune responses to Yersinia in a case of HLA B27 associated juvenile arthritis. *British Journal of Rheumatology* **32**, 845–8.

Southwood, T.R., Petty, R.E., Malleson, P.N., Delgado, E.A., Hunt, D.W., Wood, B., and Schroeder, M.L. (1989). Psoriatic arthritis in children. *Arthritis and Rheumatism* **32**, 1007–13.

Stamato et al. (1995). Prevalence of cardiac manifestations of juvenile ankylosing spondylitis. *American Journal of Cardiology* **75**, 744–6.

Stewart, S.R., Robbins, D.L., and Castles, J.J. (1978). Acute fulminant aortic and mitral insufficiency in ankylosing spondylitis. *New England Journal of Medicine* **299**, 1448–9.

Thomas, D.G. and Roberton, D.M. (1994). Reiter's syndrome in an adolescent girl. *Acta Paediatrica* **83**, 339–40.

Truckenbrodt, H. and Hafner, R. (1990). Die psoriasisarthritis intramuscular kinkesalter. *Zeitschrift für Rheumatologie* **49**, 88–94.

Unsal, E., Eroglu, Y., Buyukgebiz, B., Kupelioglu, A., and Cevik, N.T. (1997). A case of juvenile ankylosing spondylitis and Crohn's disease. *Turkish Journal of Pediatrics* **39**, 277–80.

6.4.3 Ankylosing spondylitis

Andrei Calin

Introduction

Ankylosing spondylitis continues to excite attention. It is so much more than an inflammatory spinal disorder. Thanks to its dramatic relationship with HLA-B27 and tantalizing link to putative infective triggers, the condition is studied around the world by clinicians, microbiologists, immunogeneticists, and others.

Historical review

As summarized elsewhere (Calin 1988), the condition has a long, intriguing history.

Diagnostic criteria

Criteria for the classification and diagnosis of different rheumatic diseases have been developed to help different clinicians in different locations use the same diagnostic labels for similar groups of patients. Originally, criteria were formulated in Rome in 1961 and later revised in New York in 1966 (Bennett and Burch 1968) (Table 1). The most frequent means of satisfying these is a radiographic demonstration of grade 3 or 4 bilateral sacroiliitis (Fig. 1), together with a history of back pain. Most would consider a patient as having ankylosing spondylitis if symptomatic and with sacroiliitis. However, we do recognize ankylosing spondylitis *sine* sacroiliitis on the one hand or atypical forms of disease on the other.

The disease is considered primary if no other rheumatological disorder is present, or secondary if the sacroiliitis is related to psoriatic arthropathy, inflammatory bowel disease, or Reiter's syndrome. Many patients are wrongly diagnosed as mechanical back pain or other inappropriate labels. A single anteroposterior film of the pelvis is sufficient to define the radiological entity. More sophisticated investigations such as the use of magnetic resonance imaging are always expensive and may be inappropriate and unhelpful (Braun et al. 1994).

Table 1 Criteria for ankylosing spondylitis

Rome criteria	
Clinical criteria	
1.	Low back pain >3 months, relieved by rest
2.	Thoracic pain and stiffness
3.	History of iritis
4.	Limited motion of lumbar spine
5.	Limited chest expansion
Radiological criteria	
1.	Bilateral sacroiliitis
Ankylosing spondylitis is diagnosed if bilateral sacroiliitis plus one clinical criterion, or four out of five clinical criteria, are present	
New York criteria	
Clinical criteria	
1.	Limited movement of lumbar spine in three planes
2.	Pain in lumbar spine or at dorsolumbar junction
3.	Chest expansion <2.5 cm
Radiological criteria	
1.	Bilateral sacroiliitis, grade 3–4
2.	Unilateral sacroiliitis, grade 3–4, or bilateral sacroiliitis, grade 2

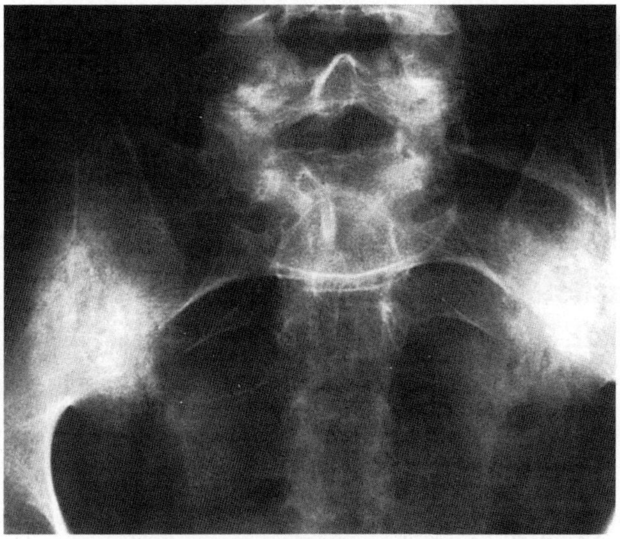

Fig. 1 Pelvic radiograph (anteroposterior view) revealing grade IV sacroiliitis. Note marked juxta-articular sclerosis and destruction of joint with fusion.

We defined the qualitative nature of pain in patients with inflammatory spinal disease, that is, ankylosing spondylitis: (Calin and Fries 1977) (i) patients are typically below 40 years of age at onset; (ii) the onset is insidious; (iii) duration has been at least 3 months at first attendance; (iv) there is an association with morning stiffness; and (v) improvement occurs with exercise. For those with three or more of these features a pelvic radiograph should elucidate whether there is evidence of sacroiliitis. HLA-B27 typing has led to immense strides in the understanding of the spondyloarthropathy group but should not be considered a diagnostic test or necessary for the diagnosis of ankylosing spondylitis. A patient with symptomatic sacroiliitis lacking HLA-B27 still has ankylosing spondylitis and, moreover, the test is frequently negative in secondary forms of ankylosing spondylitis, where only some 50 per cent of those with enteropathic spondylitis or psoriatic spondylitis carry the antigen. Moreover, the link with B27 is less impressive in some non-white ethnic groups. Occasionally, sacroiliitis is seen as a chance finding in the absence of pain. Presumably the precipitating trigger has been pulled, but symptoms have never reached a threshold noticed by patient or physician. A review of Bayesian theory reminds us that HLA-B27 typing can only be helpful when we are 50 per cent certain of the diagnosis!

The clinician perhaps should simply treat with a non-steroidal anti-inflammatory drug if a diagnosis of ankylosing spondylitis appears possible, rather than relying on further testing with more sophisticated imaging. (Calin 1980, 1982).

In epidemiological and familial studies, patients are sometimes found with unilateral sacroiliitis, dactylitis, syndesmophytes, and other stigmata of 'undifferentiated spondyloarthropathy'.

Until the specific environmental trigger(s), gene(s), and biological mechanism(s) leading to disease pathogenesis are fully elucidated, the obsessional use of criteria for classification may be inappropriate.

Epidemiology

The search for an explanation for this increased heritability took a dramatic step forward in 1973 with two reports of the association between ankylosing spondylitis and HLA-B27. Indeed, the link between HLA-B27 and ankylosing spondylitis could elucidate several observations:

1. The family clustering: HLA-B27 is inherited as an autosomal codominant characteristic, 50 per cent of first-degree relatives of probands with HLA-B27 possessing the antigen.
2. Uveitis is a common accompaniment of ankylosing spondylitis: HLA-B27 is found in some 40 per cent of individuals with acute unilateral self-limiting uveitis, even in the absence of underlying rheumatological disease.
3. Many patients with Reiter's disease develop sacroiliitis: overall, some 80 per cent of patients with reactive arthropathy are HLA-B27 positive, those developing sacroiliitis and ascending spinal disease being more closely linked to HLA-B27. Whether the sacroiliitis in such patients should be considered a complication of Reiter's syndrome or a further manifestation of the HLA-B27 status remains unclear.
4. Juvenile arthropathy, psoriatic arthropathy, and inflammatory bowel disease can all be associated with sacroiliitis and ankylosing spondylitis and it is known that HLA-B27 is increased in these groups who have a spondyloarthropathy picture.

In terms of the link between HLA-B27 and the spondyloarthropathies:

1. Some 5–10 per cent of HLA-B27 positive individuals develop ankylosing spondylitis after an unknown environmental event and 20 per cent of subjects with HLA-B27 develop reactive arthropathy after contact with an arthritogenic agent (chlamydia, salmonella, etc.).
2. Up to 5 per cent of Caucasian patients with ankylosing spondylitis are not HLA-B27 positive.

3. Only 50 per cent of those with psoriatic or enteropathic spondylitis are B27 positive.
4. The association between ankylosing spondylitis and HLA-B27 in non-Caucasians (around 50 per cent) is much less than that seen in Caucasians.
5. Relatives of probands with both sacroiliitis and HLA-B27, even when B27 positive, frequently remain disease free.
6. The Pima and Haida Indians, both with a high frequency of HLA-B27, develop ankylosing spondylitis frequently but Reiter's syndrome rarely. By contrast, the Navaho Indians and Alaskan Inupiat Eskimos develop Reiter's syndrome more frequently than ankylosing spondylitis. Similarly, ankylosing spondylitis and Reiter's syndrome tend to 'breed true' within Caucasian families (Calin et al. 1984).
7. HLA-B27 relatives of HLA-B27-positive patients are 20 times more likely to develop ankylosing spondylitis than are HLA-B27-positive relatives of healthy HLA-B27 subjects, but the specific risk depends on sex of index case (i.e. paternal or maternal and sex of offspring) (Calin 1999a). The distribution of HLA-B27 among different healthy and disease groups is summarized elsewhere (Calin 1989; Calin and Elswood 1989a; De Castro 1994; Inman and Schfield 1994; Braun and Sieper 1996; Khan 1996; Lopez-Larrea et al. 1996; Scofield 1996; Toivanen and Toivanen 1996).
8. Some 23 subtypes of HLA-B27 are now recognized.

Table 2 Major differences between ankylosing spondylitis in men and in women

	Males	Females
Family history	+	++
Association with psoriasis	++	+
Association with inflammatory bowel disease	++	+++
HLA-B27	>90%	>90%
Disease activity	++	+++
Function (severity)	++	+++
Peripheral joint disease:		
Initial	+	++
Subsequent	+	+++
Spinal ankylosis[a]	++	+
Cervical spine symptoms	+	++
Osteitis pubis	+	+++

[a] Skipping thoracic and lumbar spine in females.

Prevalence (see van der Linden and van der Heijde 1996)

With the increased awareness and interest in the disease, many patients who previously were thought to have other disorders are now recognized as having ankylosing spondylitis. The true prevalence of ankylosing spondylitis and spondyloarthritis appears to be in the region of 0.25–1 per cent with a peak of 2 per cent in northern Norway. The figures contrast sharply with older data reporting a ratio of ankylosing spondylitis to rheumatoid disease of about 1 : 15. The true figure now approaches 1 : 1.

Studies of blood donor populations suggest that up to 20 per cent of HLA-B27-positive individuals develop symptomatic ankylosing spondylitis, many of whom did not carry a diagnosis (Calin 1975; Braun 1999).

The prevalence and nature of spondyloarthropathy varies in different ethnic groups. For example, Boyer et al. (1994) identified 104 cases of spondyloarthropathy in an Eskimo population, a prevalence of 2.5 per cent in adults aged 20 years and over. They found undifferentiated spondyloarthropathy and reactive arthropathy to be more common than ankylosing spondylitis per se. Strikingly, there was an equal sex distribution. Elsewhere, Alexeeva et al. (1994) studied the prevalence of spondyloarthritis amongst the native population of Chukotaa in Russia. Among these circumpolar subjects, they found the prevalence of spondyloarthropathy to be 2.5 per cent, with 1 per cent having ankylosing spondylitis. HLA-B27 occurred in 34 per cent of the population.

Delay in diagnosis

Until recently delays of between 5 and 10 years were recorded between the onset of symptoms and the diagnosis at last being made.

Sex distribution

In our large series in Britain (some 6200 cases, based in Bath), the sex ratio is in the region of 2.5 to 1 in favour of men, a figure confirmed by other studies. Distinguishing features between men and women with disease are discussed below (and see Table 2) (Will et al. 1990a; Kennedy et al. 1993).

Racial distribution

Ankylosing spondylitis roughly follows the distribution of HLA-B27. For example, in the American Indian where HLA-B27 prevalences have been reported ranging from 18 to 50 per cent, ankylosing spondylitis is particularly frequent, whereas the condition is less common in the Black American, where HLA-B27 has a prevalence of 3–4 per cent, and correspondingly rarer in Black Africans, where HLA-B27 occurs in under 1 per cent. In Sub-Saharan Africa, the situation is dramatically changing. Although ankylosing spondylitis itself remains unusual, the other spondyloarthritides have become progressively more prevalent with the advent of HIV. The story has been recently reviewed by McGill and Njobvu (2001). Of note, among the Fula population of Gambia HLA-B27 has a relatively high prevalence of 6–68 per cent of whom are B*2705 positive while the remainder carry B*2703. The apparent low prevalence of ankylosing spondylitis amongst this population suggests either the rarity of an environmental trigger (an unlikely explanation), or the presence of additional genetic or environmental protective factors. Meanwhile, there appears to be an ever-increasing prevalence of psoriatic and reactive type arthritides associated with HIV.

Age distribution (see Kennedy and Calin 1994)

Sacroiliac and spinal disease usually develop in the late teenage years or in the early twenties in primary ankylosing spondylitis, whereas in those with secondary forms of disease, older ages at onset are seen. Interestingly, in the developing world, ankylosing spondylitis occurs more frequently at a younger age, teenagers with onset of disease being frequently found. Our studies (Will et al. 1990b, 1992) have suggested that within France and Britain the age at onset of ankylosing spondylitis is increasing. The fact that different studies using different epidemiological techniques have produced these findings is of particular interest.

Pathological features (see Francois et al. 2001)

The unique pathology of ankylosing spondylitis and the spondyloarthritides was clearly defined by Ball (1971) and developed further by Bywaters (1984). In contrast to the situation in rheumatoid disease, the primary pathological site is the enthesis (insertion of ligaments and capsules into bone) rather than the synovium. In addition, the enthesopathic change is characterized by fibrosis and ossification rather than joint destruction and instability. In the spine, enthesopathic changes at the site of insertion of the outer fibres of the anulus fibrosus result in squaring of vertebral bodies (Fig. 2), vertebral end-plate destruction, and syndesmophyte formation

(Fig. 3). The enthesis is a metabolically active site, perhaps explaining why early changes in ankylosing spondylitis occur during growth in the teenage years. We still do not understand why the enthesis preferentially becomes affected, or why the sacroiliac joints are almost universally involved in the disease. Osteoporosis is an early phenomenon and may explain much of the poor posture and disability (see below).

Apart from enthesitis, synovitis, subchondral bone marrow changes and cartilage proliferation are seen and within the subentheseal bone marrow and synovium CD8 positive T cells may play a central role. Imaging of early changes is achieved best by ultrasonography or magnetic resonance imaging (MRI).

It is said that when plain radiographs are normal early in the disease process, MRI can detect cartilage abnormalities, subchondral bone marrow oedema and inflammation in and around the sacroiliac joints. However, adequate control films are not yet available.

In summary, ossification occurs in the region of the discs, the epiphyseal, and sacroiliac joints, and extraspinal sites, initiated by lesions at the site of ligamentous insertion. Synovitis itself does occur in peripheral joints and a proliferative synovitis can mimic that seen in rheumatoid disease.

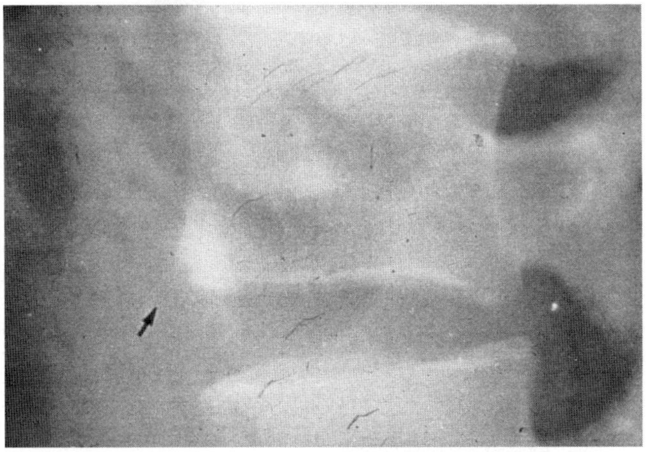

Fig. 2 Squaring of lumbar vertebral body in ankylosing spondylitis. Note sclerosis of bone at site of enthesopathic change at insertion of anterior fibres of the annulus fibrosis.

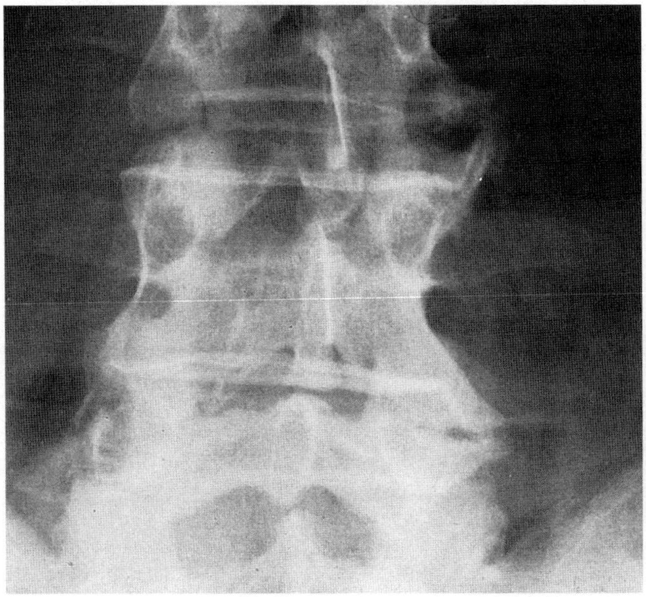

Fig. 3 Note syndesmorphytes between vertebral bodies. These are vertically directed new bone lesions associated with normal joint space.

Clinical features

Ankylosing spondylitis will only be diagnosed when there is a high index of suspicion in a patient presenting with back pain of an inflammatory nature. In any such individual the differential diagnosis relates to mechanical dysfunction. The two conditions are contrasted in Table 3.

We have demonstrated a striking loss of bone mineral content in early disease (Will et al. 1990c). Juxta-articular and generalized osteoporosis are well recognized in rheumatoid disease but the relative role of hormonal factors, immobility, drug therapy, and the disease process is unclear. Although it has long been recognized that patients with severe ankylosing spondylitis may develop a dorsal kyphosis with some anterior wedging of the vertebrae, early osteoporosis has not until now been recognized. Whether the pattern of bone loss relates to tumour necrosis factor or other mediators remains unclear. HLA-B27-positive brothers of HLA-B27-positive patients have normal bone density. To what extent this early osteoporosis in patients who have normal spine mobility should be considered an early pathological marker, with changes at the enthesis being secondary in nature, is unknown.

Spinal symptoms

Late spinal complications

Few patients progress relentlessly to the classical late 'bamboo spine' (Figs 4 and 5). The fused spine may fracture (Fig. 6) following trivial or even unrecognized injury and microfractures and clinical fractures are relatively common in severe ankylosing spondylitis. The spinal deformity may make it difficult to see a fracture site, particularly in the low neck (C6–7), and special views (via axilla) may be required. The fracture may be clinically

Table 3 Differential findings in mechanical and inflammatory back pain

	Mechanical	Inflammatory
Past history	±	++
Family history	−	+
Onset	Acute	Insidious
Age (years)	15–90	<40
Sleep disturbance	±	++
Morning stiffness	+	+++
Involvement of other systems	−	+
Effect of exercise	Worse	Better
Effect of rest	Better	Worse
Radiation of pain	Anatomic (S1, L5)	Diffuse (thoracic, buttock)
Sensory symptoms	+	−
Motor symptoms	+	−
Scoliosis	+	−
Range of movement decreased	Asymmetrically	Symmetrically
Local tenderness	Local	Diffuse
Muscle spasm	Local	Diffuse
Straight-leg raising	Decreased	Normal
Sciatic nerve stretch	Positive	Absent
Hip involvement	−	+
Neurodeficit	+	−
Other systems	−	+

silent or a dramatic event which can be fatal. A sudden exacerbation of back pain, spontaneously or following mild trauma, may relate to a fracture or a localized defect of the vertebral end plate (destruction of the disc–bone border). Spondylodiscitis is the term given to this lesion and may require rest and analgesia, with pain decreasing over 2 or 3 weeks. This contrasts with the usual exercise programme required for patients. The nature of spondylodiscitis and its prevalence has recently been defined in a cross-sectional study of over 100 patients, some 12 per cent of whom had radiological evidence of discitis, though often asymptomatic in nature (Kabasakal et al. 1994). A further complication of discitis is that of a pseudoarthrosis where adventitious movement creates pain and debility. Surgical fusion may be needed.

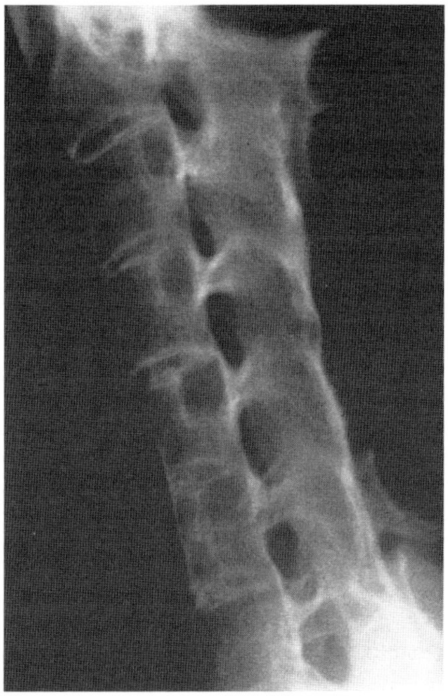

Fig. 4 Cervical spine in severe ankylosing spondylitis. Note fusion of facetal joints and anterior fusion of bodies with squaring of vertebrae.

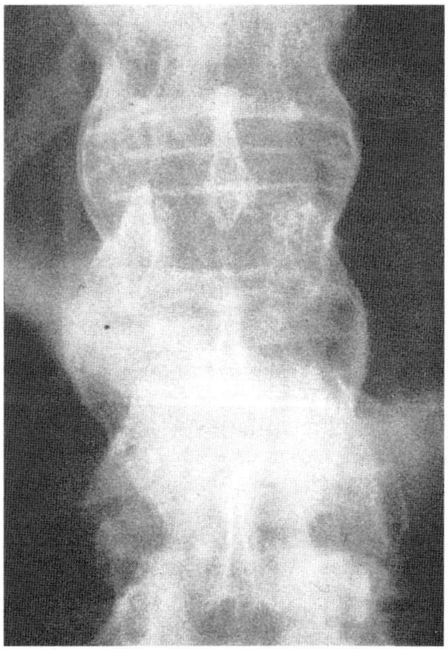

Fig. 5 Fused lumbar spine vertebrae with syndesmorphytes linking vertebrae.

Extraspinal joint disease

Some 20–40 per cent of patients have peripheral joint disease at some stage during their illness. This may be asymmetric and often affects the lower limbs predominantly. Hip (Fig. 7) ankylosis and shoulder disease may provide major disability, with temporomandibular joint dysfunction occurring in upto 10 per cent of patients. HLA–DR4 may be associated with peripheral joint disease.

We have recently shown that there is a striking inverse correlation between the age at onset of disease and hip involvement; the vast majority of individuals requiring a total hip replacement having onset of disease during the teenage years. Hip involvement in those with onset in the twenties

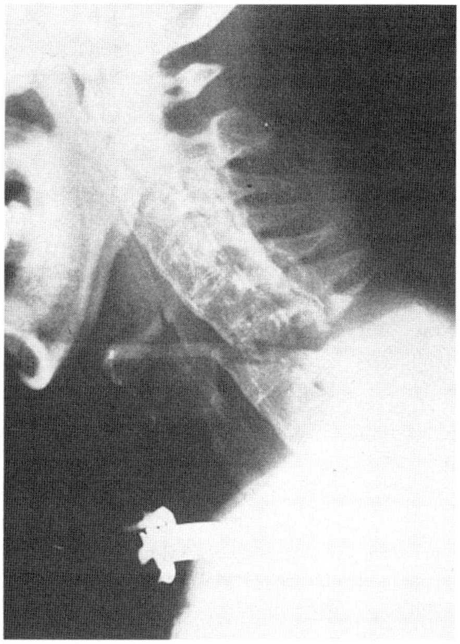

Fig. 6 Fracture of fused cervical spine in ankylosing spondylitis following minimal trauma—note defect in C6.

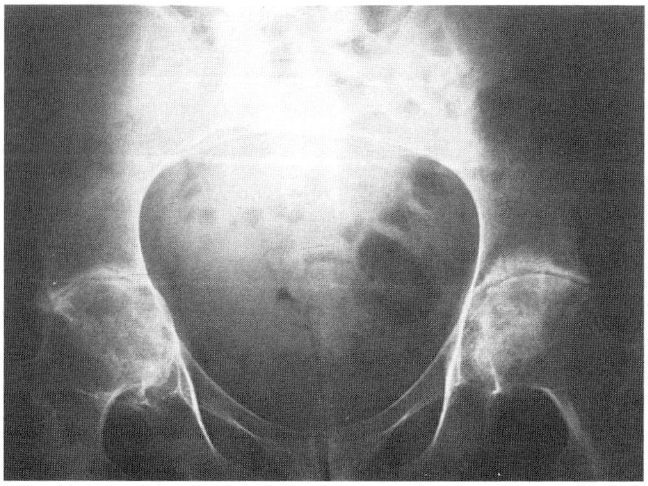

Fig. 7 Bilateral hip arthropathy in a female with ankylosing spondylitis. Note joint space reduction and erosive change in heads of femora.

or later is vanishingly rare. For those requiring hip replacement, bilateral surgery is frequent. The long-term outcome for those with total hip replacements is excellent, the majority doing well 20 years after surgery. Even those in whom the primary replacement fails do well following revision arthroplasty (Sweeney et al. 2001).

Enthesopathic lesions

In view of the pathological disorder, it is not surprising that patients have insertional tendinitis at any site typified by involvement of the Achilles tendon, intercostal muscle insertions, plantar fasciitis, and dactylitis.

Apart from low back pain some patients have a 'pluritic' type of chest pain that may cause sleep disturbance and anxiety. This pain is worse on inspiration and relates to an insertional tendinitis of the small costosternal and costovertebral muscles.

Extra-articular disease

Until recently, ankylosing spondylitis was predominantly considered to be a spinal disease with little constitutional systemic involvement. It is now recognized that the disorder may affect all body systems and indeed may not be immunologically silent.

General symptoms

Constitutional features include fatigue, weight loss, low-grade fever, hypochromic or normochromic anaemia, and increased inflammatory mediators. For many patients, fatigue is the major component. We have shown (Calin et al. 1993a) that in a comparison of pain, stiffness, and fatigue, the three major features of ankylosing spondylitis, the last of these has been a major component for a large minority. Exercise and anti-inflammatory drugs are good for both the pain and stiffness but, to date, fatigue remains a frustrating symptom to treat, although amitriptyline therapy may help (Koh et al. 1997). Certain features such as an arthropathy and uveitis can occur at any time in the course of the disease; other problems are predominantly associated with severe chronic involvement. Examples of the latter include aortic regurgitation, cord compression, upper lobe pulmonary fibrosis, and amyloid deposition.

Eye disease

Iritis (Plate 105) occurs in up to 40 per cent of patients with ankylosing spondylitis. Although the visual episodes are often self-limiting, local steroid drops or systemic therapy may be required. Uveitis is a marker for greater radiological involvement (Edmunds and Calin 1991; Pavy et al. 2001). We failed to define any obvious environmental trigger even in those with recurrent disease.

Pulmonary involvement

Chronic infiltrative and fibrotic changes in the upper lobe of the lungs may occur. This upper lobe pulmonary fibrosis is well recognized. Cough, sputum, and dyspnoea may develop. Radiographs reveal usually bilateral upper lobe pulmonary fibrosis, sometimes with cyst formation and parenchial destruction. The lesions can be invaded by aspergillus with changes mimicking tuberculosis. Dense fibrosis can occur. Treatment is of no avail and death may follow massive haemoptysis.

A rigid chest wall may result from fusion of the thoracic joints but pulmonary ventilation is usually well maintained by the diaphragm. Court-Brown and Doll (1965) noted deaths from respiratory causes to be some three times higher than in a control population.

Cardiovascular disease

Cardiovascular involvement is well recognized. The stated prevalence of this complication varies from 3.5 per cent of cases within 15 years to 10 per cent with upto 30 years duration. Although heart disease occurs more frequently in those with more severe spondylitis, cardiac conduction defects and other abnormalities may occur in those with minimal disease.

Aortic incompetence, cardiomegaly, and persistent defects in cardiac conduction are the most common findings with complete atrioventricular block occasionally occurring. Pericarditis has been described and cardiac involvement can range from being clinically silent to dominating the picture.

Upto 20 per cent of patients with ankylosing spondylitis may have anatomic evidence of involvement of the aortic valve but few of these have clinically detectable valvular dysfunction. Scar tissue and intimal fibrous proliferation may affect the aortic valve cusps and aorta. Scar tissue may extend below the base of the aortic valve producing a subaortic fibrous ridge.

Amyloidosis

Amyloid is an occasional complication of ankylosing spondylitis. In one study, 3 of 35 patients were found to have amyloid on routine rectal biopsy. Although relatively common, the event is rarely of clinical significance.

Renal disease

There appears to be no impairment of renal glomerular function in ankylosing spondylitis, in spite of the recognized pathological changes. In a study of 38 consecutive patients with severe ankylosing spondylitis, investigation of glomerular function failed to show any marked abnormality (Calin 1975). Nevertheless, immunoglobulin A (IgA) nephropathy is well recognized; of relatively little clinical significance.

Neurological syndromes

Involvement of the cauda equina may occur in the later stages of the disease. The syndrome presents with insidious onset of leg and buttock pain with sensory and motor impairment in association with bowel and bladder dysfunction. Lumbar diverticulae are found on MRI scanning. Unfortunately, treatment appears to be of little avail, but in a single case report, the value of a peritoneal shunt (in one of our patients) was suggested.

Bowel disease (see Wollheim 2001)

There is an intimate relationship between the bowel and ankylosing spondylitis. Low-grade bowel inflammation has been described (on ileocolonoscopy) in the absence of symptoms. The relevance of these findings remains unclear, although we know that the HLA–B27-positive transgenic rat develops a picture typical of spondyloarthropathy with a major degree of bowel involvement. Rats raised in a germ-free milieu develop neither bowel nor joint disease.

Physical examination

Spinal mobility is symmetrically decreased but may be normal in the earlier stages of disease. A variety of measurements have been described, although the modified Schober is the most useful. The distraction of a line drawn from the midpoint between the posterior iliac spines to an arbitrary site 10 cm above this point is measured and the distraction noted on forward flexion. In a normal individual, this 10-cm line increases by some 50–100 per cent whereas a patient with active disease may only have a distraction of some 20 per cent or less. Lateral spinal flexion may be measured by noticing the distraction on contralateral flexion of a line drawn in the midaxillary plane. Chest expansion can be reduced, although this may only occur late in the disease. Moreover, in the female—for obvious reasons—chest expansion is difficult to measure. Intermalleolar straddle on abducting the legs is a useful measurement of non-specific pelvic inflammation, and neck mobility can be measured. A formal evaluation (the Bath Ankylosing Spondylitis Metrology Index, BASMI; Jenkinson et al. 1994) has been validated.

There may be muscle spasm with loss of the normal lumbar lordosis, while some individuals may present with pain but no physical abnormality. Peripheral joints may be normal or grossly involved—particularly in women, who tend to have more peripheral joint disease than men.

Radiological evaluation

The five grades of sacroiliitis introduced by the New York Criteria range from 0 to 4. These are summarized in Table 4. Grade 0 refers to normal joints with clear sacroiliac margins and uniform joint space. There is no juxta-articular sclerosis. Grade 1 signifies suspicious change but no definite abnormality, while grades 2 and 3 relate to an increasing degree of sacroiliitis, as defined by blurring of the joint margin, juxta-articular sclerosis, decreased joint width, and erosive change. Grade 4 describes complete fusion or ankylosis of the joints with or without residual sclerosis.

A single anteroposterior view radiograph of the pelvis is sufficient. Sacroiliitis does not occur as an age-related phenomenon although degenerative change of the sacroiliac joints may occur. Osteitis condensans ilii, a sclerotic condition of unknown cause producing dense bone in one or both iliacs but not the sacrum, may confuse the unwary. However, typically this iliac change allows the joint margin to be defined more clearly and therefore there should be no confusion between the two conditions. It is not unknown for an individual patient to have both sacroiliitis and osteitis condensans ilii.

Patients with bilateral, grade 4 sacroiliitis but no extrapelvic disease are frequently seen. Why some patients do not have progressive disease above the pelvic rim remains unclear, although genetics is likely to have a prominent role (Brophy 2001; Brophy et al. 2001).

In view of the enthesopathic nature of the disease, it is not surprising that radiological changes occur elsewhere. Thus, vertebral squaring may occur, vertebral end-plate collapse may be seen, and varying degrees of ossification develop. The radiological changes may be contrasted with those seen in diffuse idiopathic hyperostosis (Table 5). Likewise syndesmophytes must be differentiated from osteophytes; the latter associated with disc-space narrowing. In essence, syndesmophytes move in a vertical direction whereas osteophytes are typically horizontal. McEwen et al. (1971) have defined the radiological differences between primary ankylosing spondylitis and the secondary spondyloarthropathies, as summarized in Table 6. The Bath Ankylosing Spondylitis Radiology Index allows for a simple and rapid assessment of entire spine and hips (Pande et al. 1995; Mackay et al. 1998; Calin et al. 1999b; Doran et al. 2000; Mackay et al. 2000).

Radionuclide scanning may be more sensitive than radiography but the change is non-specific and is likely to confuse rather than help. Likewise computed tomography and MRI is expensive, usually unnecessary and not obviously specific for spondyloarthritis. The radiographic features of enthesitis include soft tissue swelling, peri-insertional osteopaenia, bone cortex irregularity, adjacent periostitis, entheseal soft tissue calcification and neoostosis. Ultrasonography may reveal swelling of entheses and peritendinous soft tissues and distention of adjacent bursae. MRI reveals inflammation of bone adjacent to insertion and other soft tissue changes. Dynamic, Gadolinium-enhanced MRI and short TAU inversion recovery and other fat-suppression techniques show inflammatory responses associated with enthesopathy. Flexor tenosynovitis may be seen in association with dactylitis.

Ankylosing spondylitis and diffuse idiopathic skeletal hyperostosis are compared in Table 6. Osteoporosis is now well recognized as is the consequence (i.e. compression fractures).

Table 4 Sacroiliac changes in ankylosing spondylitis[a]

Grade	
0 Normal	Grade depends on degree
1 Suspicious	of blurring of joint margins,
2 Minimal sacroiliitis	juxta-articular scoliosis,
3 Moderate sacroiliitis	erosive change, and
4 Ankylosis	narrowing

[a] According to New York criteria.

Table 5 Differentiating features of diffuse idiopathic skeletal hyperostosis (DISH) and ankylosing spondylitis. Of note osteoporosis is an early and dramatic finding in ankylosing spondylitis (Will et al. 1989)

	DISH	Ankylosing spondylitis
Usual age of onset (years)	>50	<40
Thoracolumbar kyphosis	±	++
Limitation of spinal mobility	±	++
Pain	±	++
Limitation of chest expansion	±	++
Radiography		
Hyperostosis	+	+
SI joint erosion	−	++
SI joint (synovial) obliteration	±	++
SI joint (ligamentous) obliteration	+	++
Apophyseal joint obliteration	−	++
ALL ossification	++	±
PLL ossification	+	?
Syndesmophytes	−	++
Enthesopathies (whiskering) with erosions	−	++
Enthesopathies (whiskering) without erosions	++	+
HLA-B27 (White patients) (%)	8	95
HLA-B27 (Black patients) (%)	2	50

Note: SI, sacroiliac; ALL, anterior longitudinal ligament; PLL, posterior longitudinal ligament.

Laboratory abnormalities

Apart from the presence of HLA-B27 in over 95 per cent of white patients, the majority have no evidence of change in laboratory tests. In fact, there is little correlation between erythrocyte sedimentation rate and other so-called

Table 6 Radiographic changes in primary and secondary forms of ankylosing spondylitis

	Primary ankylosing spondylitis—and ankylosing spondylitis associated with inflammatory bowel disease	Ankylosing spondylitis associated with Reiter's syndrome and psoriatic arthropathy
Sacroiliac changes	Symmetrical	Asymmetrical
Osteitis pubis	++	+
Facetal joint involvement	+++	+
Squaring of vertebrae	++	+
Syndesmophytes	+++	+
Ossification	++	+
Spread	Ascending	Random

mediators of inflammatory disease and disease activity as defined by clinical symptoms and findings. Serum alkaline phosphatase may be elevated and we and others have described elevated serum creatinine phosphokinase levels. Circulating immune complexes may be found and one study suggested that psoriasis-associated retrovirus-like particles may be present. Likewise antibodies to proteoglycan occur and antibodies to heat shock protein are described. Interleukin-6 (IL-6) and acute phase reactants have recently been compared (Tutuncu et al. 1994). IL-6 is more frequently raised in disease, compared to the situation with erythrocyte sedimentation rate, plasma viscosity, or C-reactive protein (approximately 80 per cent compared with 50 per cent). HLA-B27 itself is now known to have at least 23 sub-types (HLA-B*2701–2723), B*2706 and 09 may have a protective role or at least are less frequently associated with disease (Feltkamp et al. 2001).

Intriguingly, HLA-B27 does provide the host with some good news. Specifically, subjects with this antigen are less likely to progress to frank AIDS following HIV infection—an example whereby B27 has, perhaps in the past, provided benefit in society. Indeed, it has always been thought that there must be some protective value of such an antigen explaining its persistence in society—in spite of the association with a chronic disease (Goulder et al. 1997).

Ankylosing spondylitis in women

The disease is frequently missed in women unless a high degree of suspicion exists. The major differences between the disease in men and women are summarized in Table 2. Women tend to have more peripheral joint involvement and the spinal disease progresses less rapidly. However, dramatic spinal involvement in women as in men is sometimes seen. Historically, the delay in diagnosis is greater in women than men. Interestingly, the sex distribution of primary ankylosing spondylitis favouring men in the ratio of 2.5 to 1 is even greater in psoriatic spondylitis (4 to 1), but for those with enteropathic disease the ratio is equal. Age is also a factor (Kennedy et al. 1993; Kennedy and Calin 1994).

Aetiology (see Khan 1996; Sieper et al. 2000; Reveille et al. 2001; Rudwaleit et al. 2001)

The cause of ankylosing spondylitis remains unknown. For the last decade interest has focused on a specific klebsiella serotype and the putative relationship between this organism and HLA-B27-positive lymphocytes of patients. However, it appears more likely that many different organisms can precipitate disease in susceptible individuals. The relationship between HLA-B27, other genes, and the environment is under intense scrutiny. There are several recognized facts that must be taken into consideration:

1. Approximately 5–10 per cent of HLA-B27-positive individuals develop ankylosing spondylitis—a similar percentage to those who develop reactive arthropathy following infection with an arthritogenic organism.
2. Relatives of healthy HLA-B27-positive subjects only rarely develop disease while those of HLA-B27- positive patients are more likely to do so.
3. Both ankylosing spondylitis and Reiter's syndrome breed true within families.
4. The prevalence of ankylosing spondylitis follows the distribution of HLA-B27—where the latter is rare the association is less close.
5. Some 5 per cent of individuals with ankylosing spondylitis are HLA-B27 negative.
6. Certain ethnic groups such as the Haida and Pima are likely to develop ankylosing spondylitis while others such as the Navaho and Inupiat Eskimo develop Reiter's syndrome. In other communities, atypical forms of disease typically occur, known as undifferentiated spondyloarthritis.
7. HLA-B27 is heterogeneic with some 25 alleles or subtypes recognized, encoding 23 different protein products (B*2701 to B*2723). To date few differences have been found between HLA-B27-positive patients and HLA-B27-positive controls. HLA*2706 and 09 may protect against disease in the Orient and in Sardinia, respectively (Lopez-Larrea et al. 1996).
8. Serum IgA and secretory IgA are raised in spondylitics.
9. Iliocolonoscopic biopsy evaluation of the distal small bowel reveals some clinical inflammation in both HLA–B27-positive and -negative individuals, regardless of bowel symptoms.
10. Diet may modify arthritis in animals and perhaps in humans.
11. Silent carriage of certain microorganisms can precipitate disease in reactive arthritis.
12. There is influence from genetic loci on additional chromosomes in terms of susceptibility and severity (see below).
13. There is apparent sharing of homologous amino-acid sequence by HLA-B27 (host antigen residue 72–77) and *Klebsiella pneumoniae* (residues 188–193). Moreover, there is cross-reactivity between plasmid and HLA-B27 and between HLA-B27 and heat shock protein.
14. The link between psoriasis, inflammatory bowel disease, and ankylosing spondylitis is intriguing. Those with skin or bowel involvement often have both conditions.
15. Sulfasalazine, which is efficacious in the management of inflammatory bowel disease, has some effect in modifying the disease process in ankylosing spondylitis, at least in those with peripheral joint disease.
16. That ankylosing spondylitis is not immunologically silent is now recognized. Immunoglobulin allotypes are similar to those of controls.
17. Animal models are of major value. The adjuvant rat and the HLA-B27-positive transgenic rat and mice models will certainly further elucidate the situation. The latter suggests that HLA-B27 itself is of paramount importance.
18. Calin et al. (1993b) compared familial ankylosing spondylitis with sporadic diseases and determined that familial disease tended to be milder than the sporadic version, suggesting that the latter had fewer susceptibility but more severity genes in contrast to the former, a story taken further by Brophy et al. (2001) and Hamersma et al. (2001).
19. Sibling and twin studies reveal that a substantial proportion of susceptibility to spondyloarthropathy arises from genes outside the HLA region on chromosome 6. The role of these other genetic loci remains unclear, but we accept that a Th2 cytokine pattern (low TNFα, low interferon-γ, and high IL-10) dominates in the joints and presumably cytokine production is under genetic control influenced by recognized polymorphisms. An aberrant immune response to bacteria or autoantigens may trigger arthropathy. Moreover, T cells with specificity for bacteria-derived proteins or peptides can be demonstrated in synovial fluid and peripheral blood. In terms of cytokine secretion, there are preliminary data suggesting that in reactive arthropathy those with a low TNFα production have a chronic course, while subjects with high T-cell secretion of TNFα are more likely to have a self-limited pattern of disease. Conceivably, those with an impaired Th1 cytokine response with little TNFα production and increased production of IL-10 may have an inadequate immune response to eliminate the intracellular bacteria.

The TNF gene itself is located on the short arm of chromosome 6 within the HLA Class 3 region. Within this locus there are several polymorphic areas including five microsatellites and several promotor polymorphisms. Conflicting data regarding genetic results can perhaps be explained by variations in linkage disequilibrium in different communities. Almost certainly, in the future a clearly defined picture will emerge regarding interactions of multiple cytokines and cytokine receptor polymorphisms while potential candidate genes will become apparent.

20. Substantial evidence favours a direct role for HLA-B27 but the underlying molecular basis remains poorly defined. Moreover, B27 contributes less than 50 per cent of the total genetic risk for disease and other potential genes include proteosome genes, transporter associated with antigen processing (TAP) genes, TNFα genes and major histocompatibility complex (MHC) class 1 chain-related gene A (MICA) as well as non-MHC genes on other chromosomes (e.g. IL-1 RA, IL-6, IL-10, and CYP2D6). Genome wide screens have identified other chromosomal areas of interest including 1P, 2Q, 6P, 9Q, 10Q, 16Q, and 19Q. The concordance rate of ankylosing spondylitis for HLA-B27 positive monozygotic twin pairs is considerably higher (63 per cent) than among HLA-B27 dizygotic twin pairs (24 per cent) indicating that B27 alone is not capable of explaining the genetic epidemiology of the disease.

HLA class 2 genes are also implicated in the pathogenesis of spondyloarthritis. HLA–DR1 increases the risk for disease, while DR8 may be associated with uveitis. The poor metabolizer genotype of cytochrome P450 2D6 (CYP2D6) gene located on the long arm of chromosome 22 (22Q) is associated with disease.

We have shown (Calin et al. 1999a) that the influence of female sex (i.e. maternal influence) is greater than that of male sex in determining increased susceptibility to ankylosing spondylitis in children. Moreover, the striking maternal effect is greatest for women with younger age at onset—a phenomenon not seen in men. Further, the sex ratio of affected children depends on the sex of the affected parent.

Elsewhere, we have shown that there is no linkage of the X chromosome with susceptibility to ankylosing spondylitis, but it is noted that the androgen receptor gene is located on chromosome X and relates to androgen receptor transactivation function.

Prognosis

The outcome for an individual patient is difficult to define. Some patients have disease limited to the pelvis while others have progressive intractable inflammation of spine and elsewhere. HLA-B27 homogeneity is not associated with more severe disease. In an attempt to define entry variables leading to poor outcome we have shown that some 15 per cent of patients younger than 15 years of age at onset require one or more total hip replacements within 18 years compared with only 1 per cent of those in their late twenties. Clearly the developing hip is at particular risk. For those who require a total hip replacement, hip survival is excellent, with 70–80 per cent functioning well at 15–20 years (Sweeney et al. 2001).

Sib pairs concordant for disease (Calin and Elswood 1989a) have a similar disease process from the radiological standpoint but for the fact that the age at onset appears to be determined by environmental rather than genetic factors (i.e. the sib pairs share the same calendar date at onset rather than a similar age at onset). The younger sib is more likely to develop hip involvement as discussed above. By contrast, offspring concordant for disease with their parent develop a disorder that relates only little to the prior generation. Lehtinen (1993) has studied the nature of mortality and causes of death in 398 patients with ankylosing spondylitis. There are no major surprises. Patients died from cardiovascular causes, amyloidosis, and sometimes the effect of treatment. Elsewhere, data suggest a higher death rate from violent causes (Calin 1998).

In an attempt to define predictive factors in spondyloarthropathy, Amor et al. (1994) suggested that early hip involvement, an erythrocyte sedimentation rate over 30, poor initial response to non-steroidal anti-inflammatory drug treatment, a decreased Schober, the presence of dactylitis or oligo-articular disease, and age at onset below 16 years were all associated with a worse prognosis. We would agree but also add lower social–educational background. In addition, sporadic disease (Calin et al. 1993b) would appear to have a worse prognosis than the familial disorder.

The story is further complicated because we have to develop an understanding not only of the natural history of ankylosing spondylitis but also of the effect of treatment. As discussed (Calin 1994), the situation in ankylosing spondylitis is infinitely more difficult than that for rheumatoid disease or systemic lupus erythematosus. In the study of outcome, in spondylitis, we do not have the advantage of valuable laboratory tests. We therefore need to rely much more on what the patient tells us. Happily, we know from data provided by Hidding et al. (1994) that there is an excellent correlation between the self-report of symptoms and observed status in patients with ankylosing spondylitis, in contrast to the situation in those with fibromyalgia and, to a lesser extent, rheumatoid arthritis.

Defining disease status in ankylosing spondylitis

We have developed and validated self-administered instruments that define disease status in ankylosing spondylitis (Garrett et al. 1994) and functional ability (Calin et al. 1994). The Bath Ankylosing Spondylitis Disease Activity Index and the Bath Ankylosing Spondylitis Functional Index, together, define with clarity and simplicity the clinical status of patients with this condition. These two self-administered instruments, in addition to an objective measurement (the Bath Ankylosing Spondylitis Metrology Index) will allow many more studies in terms of natural history and response to management. The Metrology Index (Jenkinson et al. 1994) consists of five simple measurements of cervical rotation, tragus to wall distance, lateral spinal flexion, modified Schober, and intermalleolar distance. Finally, we have produced the Bath Ankylosing Spondylitis Global Status, which allows the definition of the different components of clinical well-being, or otherwise, to be defined and compared (Pande et al. 1995), and the Bath Radiology Index (BASRI). In recent years we have further focused on the nature of hip disease in the condition and now can address both BASRI(s) and BASRI(h) in terms of pure spinal disease or with the addition of hip involvement, respectively (Mackay et al. 1998, 2000; Calin et al. 1999b).

Management: general considerations

The majority of patients with ankylosing spondylitis have good prognosis for a successful life pattern, despite chronic discomfort over many years. The disease progresses to severe and total ankylosis in relatively few patients. A summary of treatment is given in Box 1.

The patients should stop smoking. Swimming is the best routine sport to pursue. For those few individuals with relentless disease, admission to an active rehabilitation unit is advisable. Hydrotherapy and aggressive remedial exercises provide benefit over the short-term and our ongoing studies are addressing the long-term outcome in a controlled study.

Postural exercise

The patient must realize that the aim of therapy is to maintain normal posture and physical activity. A hard bed and one pillow should be used. Extension exercises should remind the patient that the natural tendency of the disease is towards flexion and loss of height. A hot shower provides decreased stiffness and allows the exercise regimen to be followed. During the day, adequate attention must be given to the position of work, the style of chairs, and the chance for mobility.

One major difficulty for the patient with ankylosing spondylitis is that of fatigue. Our study suggests that low-dose amitriptyline at night may ameliorate this phenomenon (Koh et al. 1996), and indeed improve function and decrease disease activity.

Therapy (see Braun et al. 2001)

Phenylbutazone was for a long time the drug of choice but this agent has fallen into disrepute, although we still favour its use in those with severe disease who do not respond to indomethacin or other agents. Indomethacin is usually considered the drug of choice and we use the slow-release

Box 1 Treatment of ankylosing spondylitis

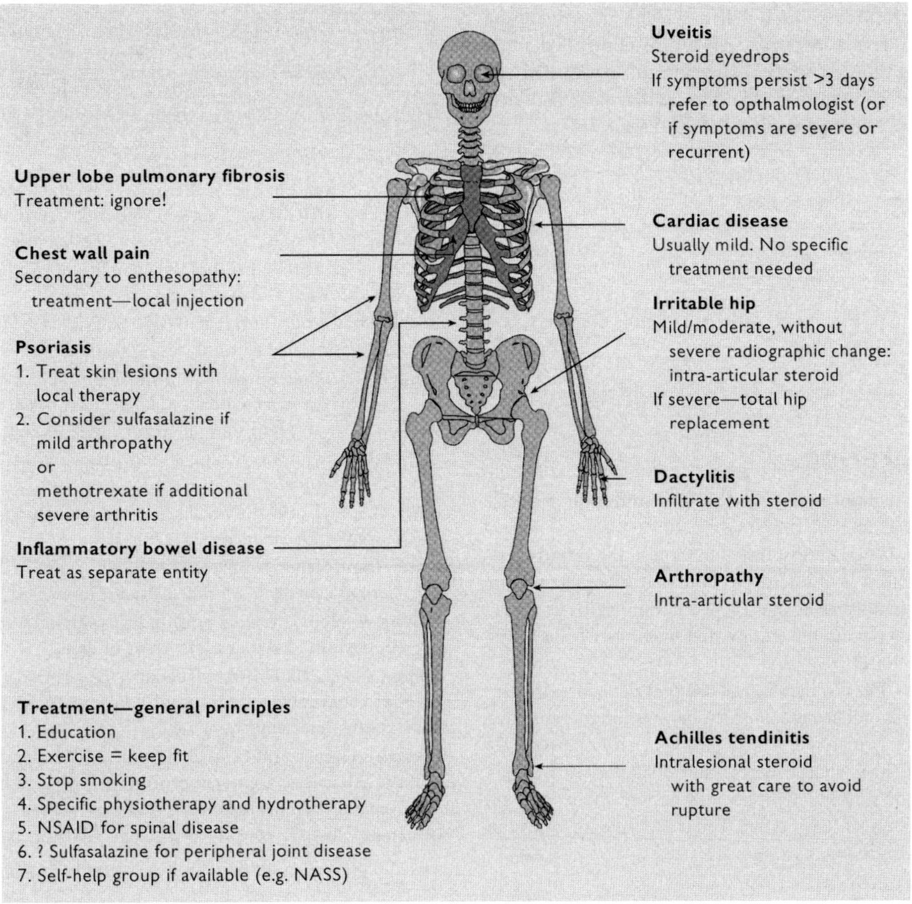
Uveitis
Steroid eyedrops
If symptoms persist >3 days refer to opthalmologist (or if symptoms are severe or recurrent)
Upper lobe pulmonary fibrosis
Treatment: ignore!
Cardiac disease
Usually mild. No specific treatment needed
Chest wall pain
Secondary to enthesopathy: treatment—local injection
Irritable hip
Mild/moderate, without severe radiographic change: intra-articular steroid
If severe—total hip replacement
Psoriasis
1. Treat skin lesions with local therapy
2. Consider sulfasalazine if mild arthropathy or methotrexate if additional severe arthritis
Dactylitis
Infiltrate with steroid
Inflammatory bowel disease
Treat as separate entity
Arthropathy
Intra-articular steroid
Treatment—general principles
1. Education
2. Exercise = keep fit
3. Stop smoking
4. Specific physiotherapy and hydrotherapy
5. NSAID for spinal disease
6. ? Sulfasalazine for peripheral joint disease
7. Self-help group if available (e.g. NASS)
Achilles tendinitis
Intralesional steroid with great care to avoid rupture

preparation of 75 mg given once at night or twice daily. Patients are advised to titrate the dosage downwards, some requiring one tablet every other night or simply one tablet once or twice weekly. Indeed, it is likely that although indomethacin has been available for some 30 years, there is no newer non-steroidal anti-inflammatory drug with greater efficacy.

Sulfasalazine has been shown in a meta-analysis to be efficacious when compared with placebo. The improvement is perhaps not dramatic and needs to be weighed against the relative cost and the inevitable need for blood testing. In a European-wide study of sulfasalazine in patients with ankylosing spondylitis, reactive arthropathy, and psoriatic spondyloarthropathy, we have shown that sulfasalazine has a small role to play, particularly in those with peripheral stigmata (Dougados et al. 1995). We have focused on patients' perception of drug risks and preparedness to take this risk (O'Brien et al. 1990a,b). Outcome studies relating to a controlled evaluation of inpatient compared with outpatient management, and studies of improved outcome with enhanced outpatient treatment (video support, exercises, etc.) are becoming available (Sweeney et al. 2000). At last, we do have access to newer drug therapies. For those individuals who cannot tolerate Indomethacin or Phenylbutazone in terms of gastrointestinal toxicity, it is almost certain that the Cox-2 specific inhibitors (Rofecoxib and Celecoxib) together with the next generation newer Coxibs will provide the patient with a comparably efficacious but safe agent. However, at last, we have evidence that the newer biologics will have an important role to play in this condition. Specifically, anti-TNF both in the form of Infliximab and Etanercept clearly control disease better than was hitherto possible. Around the world, several major multicentre multinational studies are now underway attempting to define the best regimen for the anti-TNF agents. Of note, TNFα has been detected in the inflamed gut and sacroiliac joints of patients with chronic inflammatory bowel disease and spondyloarthropathy. Not surprisingly, anti-TNF has been studied in inflammatory bowel disease as well as spondyloarthritis, and at least for certain forms of Crohn's disease, Infliximab appears to have a major effect. Both Etanercept and Infliximab are being used in psoriatic arthropathy and no doubt psoriatic spondyloarthropathy. Inevitably, cost continues to be a major concern but hopefully, over the next years, this will reduce and for the first time patients will be able to enjoy drugs that really do modify the disease process. However, even if the process is dampened down, we still do not have a drug that turns off the disease process and the search for the real magic bullet will continue.

The use of bisphosphonates is also intriguing. In the United Kingdom, we are about to start a multicentre study evaluating Alendronate 70 mg once per week versus placebo in ankylosing spondylitis in the hope that not only will the bone status be enhanced, but also the inflammatory disease reduced in activity. For example, we do have evidence that pulsed intravenous Pamidronate therapy can reduce BASDAI, BASFI, and BAS-G by around 45 per cent, together with a decline in ESR and CRP (Maksymowych et al. 2001). Further formal studies will elucidate the role of such agents in this condition.

Surgical treatment is indicated, particularly for hip replacements, but also vertebral wedge osteotomies may be done in order to correct deformity. In terms of total hip replacement, we have revealed outstandingly good outcome for both primary hip replacements and even revision hip replacements over 10, 15, and 20 years. Nevertheless, tragically, we still meet patients for whom a total hip replacement is mandatory, whereas the orthopaedic surgeon has encouraged a delay in treatment suggesting that the patient is 'too young'. No age is too young for a total hip replacement, given that there can be a major improvement in quality of life for 20- or 30-year-olds without waiting for a magical later date (Sweeney et al. 2001).

Radiotherapy

Radiotherapy may be of limited value but it has fallen into disrepute because of the risk of leukaemia. A retrospective case–controlled study comparing those who had received radiotherapy and those who had not (Calin and Elswood 1989c) showed that radiotherapy may have had little more than minimal effect in altering the course of the disease.

Genetic counselling

Family members of patients with ankylosing spondylitis and other HLA-B27-related arthropathies are advised against routine typing. However, it is important for the family and physician to have knowledge regarding the disease in order that this can be recognized early on in family members, and appropriate management introduced.

Further considerations

The socio-economic consequences of ankylosing spondylitis are well recognized (e.g. Boonen et al. 2001).

The inter-relationship between uveitis, inflammation of the skin, bowel, and joints is self-evident and it is of interest to note that sulfasalazine, for example, has a role to play in decreasing the risk of anterior uveitis in ankylosing spondylitis as well as having the minor role in terms of the joints (Benitez Del Castillo et al. 2001).

Both CD4 positive and CD8 positive T cells are prevalent in sacroiliac joint and entheseal structures, but bacteria or microorganism remnants have not been recognized in biopsy material. A Th2 profile or an impaired Th1 status appears to be dominant in spondyloarthritis, unlike that of rheumatoid disease. Moreover, gut mucosal lymphocytes appear to be actively involved in the disease process. It may be that TNFα blockade reverses the relative anergic state of Th1 cells.

The National Ankylosing Spondylitis Society

In Britain, there is a flourishing patient association known as the National Ankylosing Spondylitis Society (NASS) and this has now been followed in many other countries around the world. All patients should be directed to their national association where membership provides excellent educational material, newsletters, and advice about everyday and professional activities. For information regarding NASS or the international body contact The Director, Mr Fergus Rogers, National Ankylosing Spondylitis Society, PO Box 179, Mayfield, East Sussex, TN20 6ZL. Tel.: 01435-873527, fax: 01435-873027, E-mail: nasslon@aol.com.

Summary

Ankylosing spondylitis is a common disease. There are still many aspects of the disorder that remain poorly understood, both in terms of aetiology and natural history. For example, an epidemiological study suggested that even in the absence of specific and recognized complications, the death rate in patients with ankylosing spondylitis is greater than in matched controls (Radford et al. 1977). Nevertheless the physician and patient can usually remain optimistic about the long-term outlook. The vast majority of patients are following a satisfying professional, personal, and family life. Further, with the advent of the new biologics and the possibility of value from bisphosphonates, improved function and quality of life is beginning to be a serious possibility.

References

Alexeeva, L., Krylov, M., Vturin, V., Mylov, N., Erdesz, S., and Benevolenskaya, L. (1994). Prevalence of spondylarthropathies and HLA-B27 in the native population of Chukotka, Russia. *Journal of Rheumatology* **21**, 2298–300.

Amor, B., Silva Santos, R., Nahal, R., Listrat, V., and Dougados, M. (1994). Predictive factors for the longterm outcome of spondylarthropathies. *Journal of Rheumatology* **21**, 1883–7.

Armas, J., Stevenson, F.K., Spellerberg, M.B., and Calin, A. (1990). Release of cell surface MHC class II antigen into synovial fluid: correlation with disease type and severity. *British Journal of Rheumatology* **29** (Suppl. 1), 23.

Ball, J. (1971). Enthesopathy of rheumatoid and ankylosing spondylitis. *Annals of the Rheumatic Diseases* **30**, 213.

Benitez Del Castillo, J.M. et al. (2001). Sulfasalazine in the prevention of anterior uvetis associated with ankylosing spondylitis. *Eye* **14**, 340–3.

Bennett, P.H. and Burch, T.A. *Population Studies of the Rheumatic Diseases* Excerpta Medica Foundation, Amsterdam, 1968, pp. 456–7.

Boonen A. et al. (2001) Employment, work disability, and work days lost in patients with ankylosing spondylitis—a cross sectional study of Dutch patients. *Annals of the Rheumatic Diseases* **60**, 353–8.

Boyer, G.S. et al. (1994). Prevalence of spondylarthropathies in Alaskan Eskimos. *Journal of Rheumatology* **21**, 2292–7.

Braun, J. and Sieper, J. (1996). The sacroiliac joint in the spondyloarthropathies. *Current Opinion in Rheumatology* **8**, 275–87.

Brophy, S. (2001). Factors affecting susceptibility and severity in ankylosing spondylitis. PhD thesis, University of Bath.

Brophy, S. et al. (2001). Towards defining the genetic determinants of disease severity in ankylosing spondylitis. *British Journal of Rheumatology* **40** (Suppl. 1), 17 (abstract supplement).

Burney, R.O. et al. (1994). Analysis of the MCH Class II encoded components of the HLA Class I antigen processing pathways in ankylosing spondylitis. *Annals of the Rheumatic Diseases* **53**, 58–60.

Bywaters, E.G.L. (1984). Pathology of the spondylarthropathies. In *Spondylarthropathies* (ed. A. Calin), pp. 43–68. Orlando FL: Grune and Stratton.

Calin, A. (1975). Renal glomerular function in ankylosing spondylitis. *Scandinavian Journal of Rheumatology* **4**, 241–3.

Calin, A. (1980). HLA-B27—to type or not to type. *Annals of Internal Medicine* **92**, 208–11 (editorial).

Calin, A. (1982). HLA–B27 in 1982. Reappraisal of a clinical test. *Annals of Internal Medicine* **96**, 114–15.

Calin, A. (1988). The history of the seronegative spondylarthropathies. In *The Antiquity of the Erosive Arthropathies.* ARC Conference Proceedings No. 5.

Calin, A. (1989). Ankylosing spondylitis. In *Textbook of Rheumatology* 3rd edn. (ed. W.N. Kelley, E.D. Hards, S. Ruddy, and C.G. Sledge), pp. 1021–37. Philadelphia PA: W.B. Saunders.

Calin, A. (1994). Can we define the outcome of ankylosing spondylitis and the effect of physiotherapy management? *Journal of Rheumatology* **21**, 184–5, (editorial).

Calin, A. (1998). Survival, alcohol and deaths in ankylosing spondylitis. *British Journal of Rheumatology* **37** (6), 600–1 (editorial).

Calin, A. and Elswood, J. (1989a). Relative role of genetic and environmental factors in disease expression: sib-pair analysis in ankylosing spondylitis. *Arthritis and Rheumatism* **32**, 77–81.

Calin, A. and Elswood, J. (1989b). The outcome of 138 total hip replacements and 12 revisions in ankylosing spondylitis: high success rate after a mean follow-up of 7.5 years. *Journal of Rheumatology* **16**, 955–8.

Calin, A. and Elswood, J. (1989c). Retrospective case–control analysis of 376 irradiated patients with ankylosing spondylitis. *Journal of Rheumatology* **16**, 1443–5.

Calin, A. and Fries, J.F. (1977). The clinical history as a screening test in ankylosing spondylitis. *Journal of the American Medical Association* **237**, 2613–14.

Calin, A., Marder, A., Marks, S., and Burns, T. (1984). Familial aggregation of Reiter's syndrome and ankylosing spondylitis: a comparative study. *Journal of Rheumatology* **11**, 672–7.

Calin, A., Elswood, J., Rigg, S., and Skevington, S.M. (1988). Ankylosing spondylitis—an analytical review of 1500 patients: the changing pattern of disease. *Journal of Rheumatology* **15**, 1234–8.

Calin, A., Edmunds, L., and Kennedy, L.G. (1993a). Fatigue in ankylosing spondylitis—why is it ignored? *Journal of Rheumatology* **20**, 991–5.

Calin, A., Kennedy, L.G., Edmunds, L., and Will, R. (1993b). Familial versus sporadic ankylosing spondylitis: two differing diseases. *Arthritis and Rheumatism* **36**, 676–81.

Calin, A. et al. (1994). A new approach to defining functional ability in ankylosing spondylitis: the development of the Bath Ankylosing Spondylitis Functional Index. *Journal of Rheumatology* **21**, 2281–5.

Calin, A. et al. (1999a). Impact of sex on inheritance of ankylosing spondylitis: a cohort study. *Lancet* **354**, 1687–90.

Calin, A. et al. (1999b). A new dimension to outcome: application of the Bath Ankylosing Spondylitis Radiology Index. *Journal of Rheumatology* **26**, 988–92.

Court-Brown, W.M. and Doll, R. (1965). Mortality from cancer and other causes after radiotherapy for ankylosing spondylitis. *British Journal of Medicine* **2**, 1327.

Dawkins, R.C. et al. (1981). Prevalence of ankylosing spondylitis and radiological abnormalities of the sacroiliac joints in HLA-B27 positive individuals. *Journal of Rheumatology* **8**, 1025.

Doran, M. et al. (2000). Predictors of radiological progression in ankylosing spondylitis. *Arthritis and Rheumatism* **43** (9), Abs. No. 1202, S267 (Abstract Supplement Annual Scientific Meeting, ACR).

Dougados, M. et al. (1995). Sulphasalazine in the treatment of spondylarthropathy: a randomized, multicentre, double-blind, placebo-controlled study. *Arthritis and Rheumatism* **38**, 618–27.

Edmunds, L. and Calin, A. (1991). New light on uveitis in ankylosing spondylitis. *Journal of Rheumatology* **18**, 50–2.

Feltkamp, T.E.W. et al. (2001). Spondyloarthropathies in eastern Asia. *Current Opinion in Rheumatology* **13**, 285–90.

Garrett, S., Jenkinson, T., Kennedy, L.G., Whitelock, H., Gaisford, P., and Calin, A. (1994). A new approach to defining disease status in ankylosing spondylitis: The Bath Ankylosing Spondylitis Disease Activity Index. *Journal of Rheumatology* **21**, 2286–91.

Goulder, P.J.R., Phillips, R.E., Colbert, R.A., McAdam, S., Ogg G., Nowak, M.A. et al. (l997). Late escape from an immunodominant cytotoxic T-lymphocyte response associated with progression to AIDS. *Nature Medicine* **3** (2), 212–17.

Hamersma, J. et al. (2001). Is disease severity in ankylosing spondylitis genetically determined? *Arthritis and Rheumatism* **44**, 1396–400.

Hidding, A. et al. (1994). Comparison between self-report measures and clinical observations of functional disability in ankylosing spondylitis, rheumatoid arthritis and fibromyalgia. *Journal of Rheumatology* **21**, 818–23.

Inman, R.D. and Schfield, R.H. (1994). Etiopathogenesis of ankylosing spondylitis and reactive arthritis. *Current Opinion in Rheumatology* **6**, 360–70.

Jenkinson, T.R., Mallorie, P.A., Whitelock, H.C., Kennedy, L.G., Garrett, S.L., and Calin, A. (1994). Defining spinal mobility in ankylosing spondylitis (AS). The Bath AS Metrology Index. *Journal of Rheumatology* **21**, 1694–8.

Kabasakal, Y., Garrett, S.L., and Calin, A. (1994). The epidemiology of spondylodiscitis in ankylosing spondylitis—a controlled study. *British Journal of Rheumatology* **33** (51), 122.

Kabasakal, Y., Garrett, S.L., and Calin, A. (1995). Outcome of total hip replacement (THR) in ankylosing spondylitis (AS): a thirteen year follow-up study. *British Journal of Rheumatology* **34** (51), 114.

Kabasakal, Y., Garrett, S.L., and Calin, A. (1996). The epidemiology of spondylodiscitis in ankylosing spondylitis—a controlled study. *British Journal of Rheumatology* **35**, 660–3.

Kennedy, L.G. and Calin, A. (1994). Sex ratios and age at onset in probands and secondary cases in the spondylarthropathies. *Journal of Rheumatology* **20**, 1900–4.

Kennedy, L.G., Will, R., and Calin, A. (1993). Sex ratio in the spondylarthopathies and its relationship to phenotypic expression, mode of inheritance and age at onset. *Journal of Rheumatology* **20**, 1062–3.

Khan, M.A., ed. *Spine. Ankylosing Spondylitis and Related Spondylarthropathies* 4, No. 3. Philadelphia PA: Hanley and Belfus, 1990.

Khan, M.A. (1996). Spondylarthropathies. Editoral overview. *Current Opinion in Rheumatology* **8**, 267–8.

Koh, W.H., Pande, I., Jones, S., Samuels, A., and Calin, A. (1996). A placebo-controlled study of low dose amitriptyline in ankylosing spondylitis. *British Journal of Rheumatology* **35** (Suppl. 1), 288 (abstract).

Koh, W.H., Pande, I., Samuels, A., Jones, S.D., and Calin, A. (1997). Low dose amitriptyline in ankylosing spondylitis: a short-term, double-blind, placebo-controlled study. *Journal of Rheumatology* **24** (11), 2158–61.

Lehtinen, K. (1993). Mortality and causes of death in 398 patients admitted to hospital with ankylosing spondylitis. *Annals of the Rheumatic Diseases* **52**, 174–7.

Lopez-Larrea, C., Gonzalez-Roces, S., and Alvarez, V. (1996). HLA-B27 structure, function, and disease association. *Current Opinion in Rheumatology* **8**, 296–308.

Mackay, K. et al. (1998). The Bath Ankylosing Spondylitis Radiology Index (BASRI): a new validated approach to disease assessment. *Arthritis and Rheumatism* **41** (12), 2263–70.

Mackay, K. et al. (2000). The development and validation of a radiographic grading system for the hip in ankylosing spondylitis: the Bath Ankylosing Spondylitis Hip Index (BASRI-h). *Journal of Rheumatology* **27** (12), 2866–72.

McEwen, C. et al. (1971). Ankylosing spondylitis and spondylitis accompanying ulcerative colitis, regional enteritis, psoriasis, and Reiter's disease. *Arthritis and Rheumatism* **14**, 291.

Maksymowych, W.P. et al. (2001). Clinical and radiological amelioration of refractory peripheral spondyloarthritis by pulse intravenous pamidronate therapy. *Journal of Rheumatology* **28**, 144–55.

McGill, P.E. and Njobvu, P.D. (2001). Rheumatology in Sub-Saharan Africa. *Clinical Rheumatology* **20**, 163–7.

O'Brien, B.J., Elswood, J., and Calin, A. (1990a). Perception of prescription drug risks: a survey of patients with ankylosing spondylitis. *Journal of Rheumatology* **17**, 503–57.

O'Brien, B., Elswood, J., and Calin, A. (1990b). Willingness to accept risk in the treatment of rheumatic disease. *Journal of Epidemiology and Community Health* **44**, 249–52.

Pande, I., Mackay, K., Chatfield, K., and Calin, A. (1995). The Bath Ankylosing Spondylitis Radiology Index (BASRI): a new validated approach to disease assessment. *British Journal of Rheumatology* **34** (Suppl. 2), 37 (abstract).

Pavy, S., Brophy, S., Hickey, S. and Calin, A. (2001). Iritis: is it a predictor of long term outcome in ankylosing spondylitis? Abstract ACR, San Francisco CA.

Radford, E.P., Doll, R., and Smith, P.G. (1977). Mortality among patients with ankylosing spondylitis not given X-ray therapy. *New England Journal of Medicine* **297**, 572.

Scofield, R.H. (1996). Etiopathogenesis and biochemical and immunologic evaluation of spondyloarthropathies. *Current Opinion in Rheumatology* **8**, 309–15.

Sweeney, S., Gupta, R., Taylor G., and Calin A. (2001). Total hip arthroplasty in ankylosing spondylitis: outcome in 340 patients. *Journal of Rheumatology* **28**, 1862–6.

Sweeney, S., Taylor G., and Calin A. (2002). The effect of home-based exercise intervention package on outcome in ankylosing spondylitis: a randomized controlled trial. *Journal of Rheumatology* **29**, 763–6.

Toivanen, A. and Toivanen, P. (1996). Reactive arthritis. *Current Opinion in Rheumatology* **8**, 334–40.

Tutuncu, Z.N., Bilgic, A., Kennedy, L.G., and Calin, A. (1994). Interleukin-6. Acute phase reactants in clinical status and ankylosing spondylitis. *Annals of the Rheumatic Diseases* **53**, 425–6.

van der Linden, S. and van der Heijde, M.F.M. (1996). Current and epidemiologic aspects of ankylosing spondylitis and spondyloarthropathies. *Current Opinion in Rheumatology* **8**, 269–74.

Will, R., Palmer, R., Bhalla, A.K., Ring, F., and Calin, A. (1989). Marked osteoporosis is present in early ankylosing spondylitis and may be a primary pathological event. *Lancet* **ii**, 1483–4.

Will, R. et al. (1990a). Is there sexual inequality in ankylosing spondylitis? The study of 498 women and 1201 men. *Journal of Rheumatology* **17**, 1649–52.

Will, R., Amor, B., and Calin, A. (1990b). The changing epidemiology of rheumatic diseases: should ankylosing spondylitis now be included? *British Journal of Rheumatology* **29**, 299–300.

Will, R., Palmer, R., Bhalla, A.K., Ring, F., and Calin, A. (1990c). Marked osteoporosis is present in early ankylosing spondylitis and progresses in late disease. *Proceedings 2nd Bath Conference on Osteoporosis and Bone Mineral Measurement*, 25–27 June.

Will, R., Calin, A., and Kirwan, J. (1992). Increasing age at presentation for patients with ankylosing spondylitis. *Annals of the Rheumatic Diseases* **52**, 340–42.

6.4.4 Psoriatic arthritis

Dafna D. Gladman

Introduction

Psoriatic arthritis is an inflammatory arthritis, associated with psoriasis (Wright and Moll 1976). Its original definition as seronegative for rheumatoid factor, has been replaced by 'usually seronegative' since as many as 15 per cent of the general population, particularly over age 60, may have a positive rheumatoid factor, and rheumatoid factor may be present in more than 10 per cent of patients with psoriasis who do not have arthritis (Gladman et al. 1986). The majority of patients with psoriatic arthritis run a benign course. However, in about one-fifth of the patients, a chronic, progressive, deforming arthritis may develop, resulting in significant joint destruction and limitation of daily activities.

Epidemiology

Psoriasis is a chronic skin condition which affects 1–3 per cent of the population (Greaves and Weinstein 1995). The association between psoriasis and arthritis might be fortuitous. Since psoriasis is a common condition, and arthritis, particularly osteoarthritis, is quite prevalent, it is conceivable that psoriasis and some unrelated form of arthritis may occur in the same patient. Indeed, some patients with psoriasis do present with a coincidental rheumatoid arthritis, or osteoarthritis. Cats (1990) has argued that psoriasis is just a measure of disease expression in certain patients with peripheral arthritis and spondyloarthropathy. However, epidemiologic evidence described below supports the notion that psoriatic arthritis is a distinct form of arthritis associated with psoriasis.

Although the first description of arthritis associated with psoriasis was provided by Aliberti (Eccles and Wright 1985; O'Neill and Silman 1994), psoriatic arthritis was considered to be a variant of rheumatoid arthritis until the middle of the twentieth century. Epidemiological studies have confirmed the association between psoriasis and arthritis. These studies have shown an increased frequency of arthritis among patients with psoriasis and an increased prevalence of psoriasis among patients with arthritis. Thus, 6–42 per cent of patients with psoriasis may have psoriatic arthritis (Table 1), while the prevalence of arthritis in the general population is about 3 per cent. Likewise, the prevalence of psoriasis among patients with seronegative arthritis is reported to be 20 per cent, while arthritis occurs in only 2–3 per cent of the general population (Eccles and Wright 1985; O'Neill and Silman 1994).

Estimates of the prevalence of psoriatic arthritis range from 0.04 per cent in the Faroe Islands (Lomholt 1963) to 1.2 per cent in a Swedish study (Hellgren 1969). Lawrence et al. (1989) estimated the prevalence of psoriatic arthritis in the United States to be 0.67 per cent. A recent report from Olmstead County (Mayo Clinic) suggests a frequency of 0.1 per cent (Shbeeb et al. 2000). This variation may be due to the fact that there are no validated diagnostic or classification criteria for psoriatic arthritis (Gladman 1995).

Table 1 The prevalence of psoriatic arthritis among patients with psoriasis

Author (year)	Centre	Number of patients studied	% with arthritis
Leczinsky (1948)	Sweden	534	7
Vilanova (1951)	Barcelona	214	25
Little et al. (1975)	Toronto	100	32
Leonard et al. (1978)	Rochester	77	39
Green et al. (1981)	Cape Town	61	42
Scarpa et al. (1984)	Naples	180	34
Stern (1985)	Boston	1285	20
Zanelli and Wilde (1992)	Winston-Salem	459	17
Falk and Vandbakk (1993)	Kautokeino	35	17
Barišic-Druško et al. (1994)	Osijek region	553	10
Salvarani et al. (1995)	Reggio-Emilia	205	36

The discovery of the rheumatoid factor and its association with rheumatoid arthritis helped separate psoriatic arthritis as a distinct entity, since patients with arthritis and psoriasis tended to be seronegative. Radiologic features in psoriatic arthritis were found to be different from those of rheumatoid arthritis (Avila et al. 1960). A female preponderance was found in rheumatoid arthritis, whereas the gender ratio among patients with psoriatic arthritis was almost equal (Wright and Moll 1976; Eccles and Wright 1985; O'Neill and Silman 1994). Unlike patients with rheumatoid arthritis, patients with psoriatic arthritis may present with a spondyloarthropathy. Psoriatic arthritis is therefore classified with the seronegative spondyloarthropathies.

The frequency of psoriatic arthritis has been reported in 6–42 per cent of patients with psoriasis (Leczinsky 1948; Little et al. 1975; Leonard et al. 1978; Green et al. 1981; Scarpa et al. 1984; Stern 1985; Zanelli and Wilde 1992; Falk and Vandbakk 1993; Barišic-Druško et al. 1994; Salvarani et al. 1995; Baek et al. 2000). Since psoriasis may affect 1–3 per cent of the population, and as many of 30 per cent of psoriatic patients may develop psoriatic arthritis, almost 1 per cent of the population may suffer from psoriatic arthritis, which is the expected prevalence of rheumatoid arthritis, and close to the estimated prevalence of 0.67 per cent reported for psoriatic arthritis in the United States (Lawrence et al. 1989).

Little et al. (1975) and Leonard et al. (1978) suggested that psoriatic arthritis was more common in patients with severe psoriasis. However, psoriatic arthritis may precede the diagnosis of psoriasis in about 15 per cent of the patients (Wright and Moll 1976; Kammer et al. 1979; Gladman et al. 1987; Jones et al. 1994) (Table 2), and the highest prevalence of psoriatic arthritis was recorded among patients attending an outpatient dermatology clinic in Cape Town (Green et al. 1981). Patients with active psoriatic arthritis included in a multicentre drug trial had mild psoriasis and severity of skin and joint disease did not correlate strongly among these 225 patients (Cohen et al. 1999). A cross-sectional study of 70 patients with psoriatic arthritis suggested a correlation between the extent of skin and joint severity only among patients with simultaneous onset of skin and joint manifestations (Elkayam et al. 2000).

Clinical features

Psoriatic arthritis affects women and men almost equally, usually in their third or fourth decade (Wright 1956; Kammer et al. 1979; Green et al. 1981; Scarpa et al. 1984; Gladman et al. 1987). Nail lesions proved to be the only clinical feature that may identify patients with psoriasis destined to develop arthritis (Gladman et al. 1986). These lesions occur in close to 90 per cent of

Table 2 Clinical features of psoriatic arthritis in large reported series

Feature	Roberts et al. (1976)	Kammer et al. (1979)	Scarpa et al. (1984)	Gladman et al. (1987)	Helliwell et al. (1991)	Torre-Alonso et al. (1991)	Veale et al. (1994)	Jones et al. (1994b)	Trabace (1994)
No. of patients	168	100	62	220	50	180	100	100	58
M/F	67/101	47/53	29/33	104/116	32/18	99/81	59/41	43/57	35/33
Age of onset	36–45	33–45	40–60	37	39	39	34	37.6	42
Asymmetric oligoarthritis (%)	53	54[a]	16	11[b]	14	37	43	26[c]	50
Symmetric polyarthritis (%)	54[a]	25[a]	39	19[d]	78	35	33	63	40
Distal (%)	17	[e]	7.5	12	0	0	16	1	[e]
Back (%)	5	21	21	2[f]	6	7	4	6	[e]
Mutilans (%)	5	[e]	2.3	16	2	4	2	4	[e]
Sacroiliitis (%)	[e]	[e]	16	27	36	20	15	6	43
Joints before skin (%)	16	30	[e]	17	[e]	15	[e]	18	[e]

[a] Includes patients with only distal joints involved.

[b] 14 including symmetric oligoarthritis.

[c] Four were symmetric.

[d] Forty including asymmetric polyarthritis.

[e] Unspecified.

[f] Thirty-three including peripheral joint + back involvement.

patients with psoriatic arthritis (Little et al. 1975; Wright and Moll 1976; Kammer et al. 1979; Green et al. 1981; Gladman et al. 1987) and in 46 per cent of patients with psoriasis uncomplicated by arthritis (Gladman et al. 1986).

Psoriatic arthritis is inflammatory in nature. It may affect any peripheral joint, as well as the axial skeleton and the sacroiliac joints. Patients usually present with pain, associated with stiffness, which is more marked in the morning, and improves with activity. Morning stiffness of more than 30-min duration is documented in more than half the patients (Gladman et al. 1987). Evidence of inflammation may be detected clinically by the presence of stress pain or joint line tenderness, as well as effusions (Gladman et al. 1990a), although these signs may not be as easily detectable as they are in rheumatoid arthritis, since patients with psoriatic arthritis are less tender than patients with rheumatoid arthritis (Buskila et al. 1992). The inflamed joints in patients with psoriatic arthritis may have a purplish-red discoloration, a feature which is not often seen in rheumatoid arthritis. The effusions in psoriatic arthritis joints tend to be tense, and are often difficult to detect. There is no predilection to particular joints, with the exception of the distal interphalangeal joints. Features which appear to differentiate psoriatic arthritis from rheumatoid arthritis clinically are shown in Table 3.

The spondyloarthropathy may present with an inflammatory type of back pain, associated with stiffness and improves with activity. Clinical evidence of sacroiliitis may be obtained by specific tests, including the Gaenslen's manoeuvre, the FABER (flexion, abduction, external rotation of the hip) test and direct pressure over the sacroiliac joints (Gladman et al. 1987; Hanly et al. 1988). Some patients have restricted range of back movements documented by a reduction of flexion-extension as well as lateral flexion and rotation (Gladman et al. 1987; Hanly et al. 1988). Unlike ankylosing spondylitis, many of the patients with psoriatic spondyloarthropathy are asymptomatic, and demonstrate full range of back movement (Gladman et al. 1987, 1992b, 1993; Hanly et al. 1988).

Table 3 Comparison between psoriatic arthritis and rheumatoid arthritis

	Psoriatic arthritis	Rheumatoid arthritis
Female preponderance	Uncommon	Common
DIP involvement	Common	Uncommon
Symmetry	Less common	Common
Erythema over affected joint	Common	Uncommon
Back involvement	Common	Uncommon
Enthesopathy	Common	Uncommon
Skin lesions	Common	Uncommon
Nail lesions	Common	Uncommon
Rheumatoid factor	Uncommon	Common
Osteopaenia	Uncommon	Common
Osteolysis	Common	Uncommon
Ankylosis	Common	Uncommon

Clinical spectrum of psoriatic arthritis

In their seminal work Wright and Moll (1976) presented five clinical patterns of psoriatic arthritis: distal arthritis, involving the distal interphalangeal (DIP) joints (Fig. 1); an asymmetric oligoarthritis involving small- or medium-sized joints in an asymmetric distribution (Fig. 2); a symmetric polyarthritis, indistinguishable from rheumatoid arthritis; arthritis mutilans, which is a deforming, destructive, and disabling form of arthritis (Figs 3 and 4); and a spondyloarthropathy (Figs 5 and 6). Similar descriptions have been reported by others (Kammer et al. 1979; Scarpa et al. 1984; Gladman et al. 1987; Helliwell et al. 1991; Torre-Alonso et al. 1991; Jones et al. 1994; Veale et al. 1994b). The frequency of the various patterns has varied in the literature (Table 2). Although initially the most common pattern was thought to be asymmetric oligoarthritis (Wright and Moll 1976), polyarthritis has emerged as the most frequent clinical subset of psoriatic arthritis. In comparison with rheumatoid arthritis, psoriatic arthritis tends to be characterized as an asymmetric form of arthritis. Helliwell et al. (1991) suggested a method for defining symmetrical involvement in patients with psoriatic arthritis, such that for each level of joints if the ratio of the number of matched pairs to the total number of joints was more than 0.5, then the distribution was considered

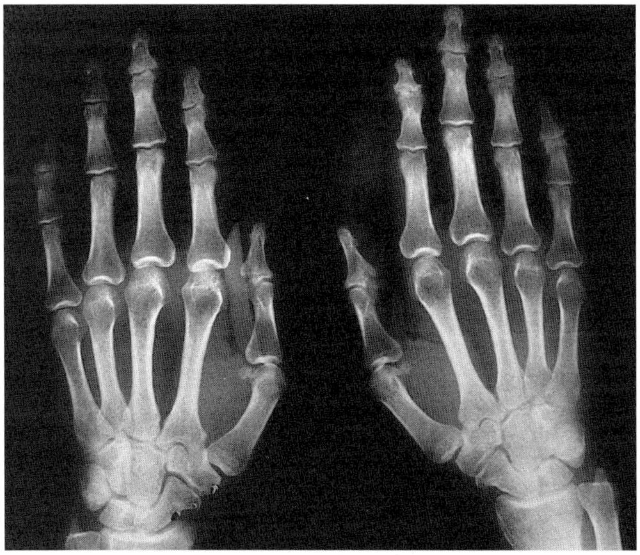

Fig. 1 Distal arthritis, involving the DIP joints, with erosions and joint space narrowing.

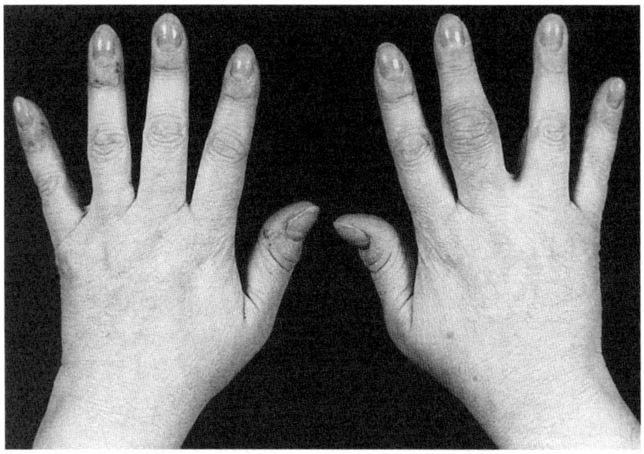

Fig. 2 An asymmetric oligoarthritis involving the third PIP joint on the right. Note the psoriatic lesions in the periungual areas of the left fourth and fifth fingers.

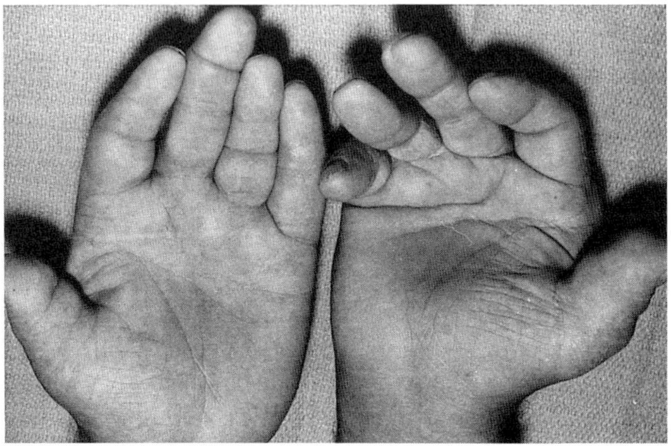

Fig. 3 Arthritis mutilans, which is a deforming, destructive and disabling form of arthritis, showing the inability to fully use the hands.

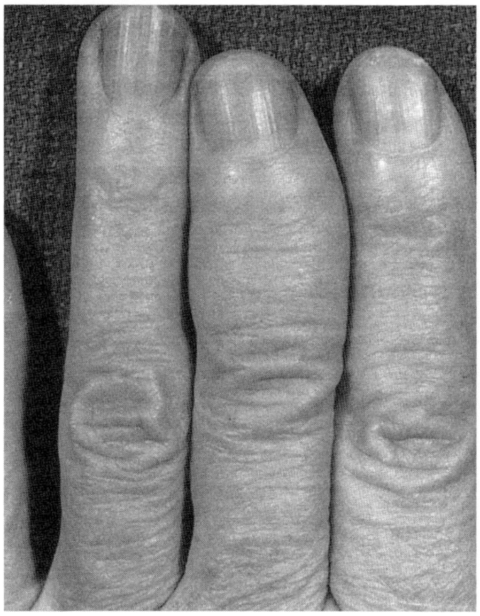

Fig. 4 Telescoping of the third DIP joint, seen in patients with psoriatic arthritis, which may be part of arthritis mutilans.

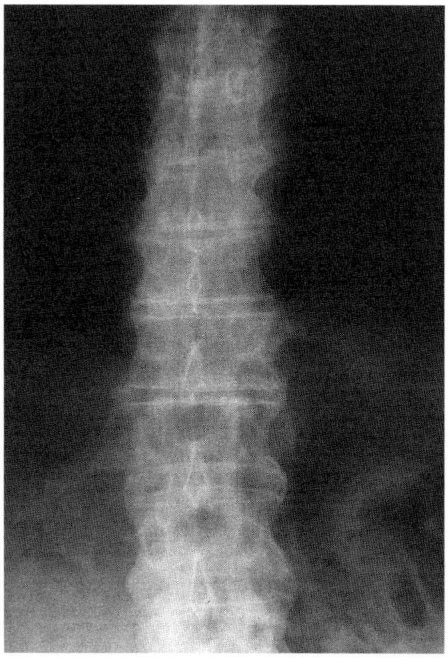

Fig. 5 Thoraco-lumbar spine in a patient with psoriatic spondyloarthropathy demonstrating syndesmophytes.

symmetrical. Jones et al. (1994) showed that using this method more patients were found to have a symmetrical arthritis, and Helliwell et al. (2000) found no difference in symmetry between patients with rheumatoid arthritis and psoriatic arthritis. They confirmed that symmetry was a function of the total number of joints involved. Although the distal pattern has been described as typical for psoriatic arthritis, its frequency has varied widely, and some investigators have not been able to identify patients with isolated distal joint involvement. It has also been recognized that the patterns may change with time in individual patients (Gladman 1992). A patient may present initially

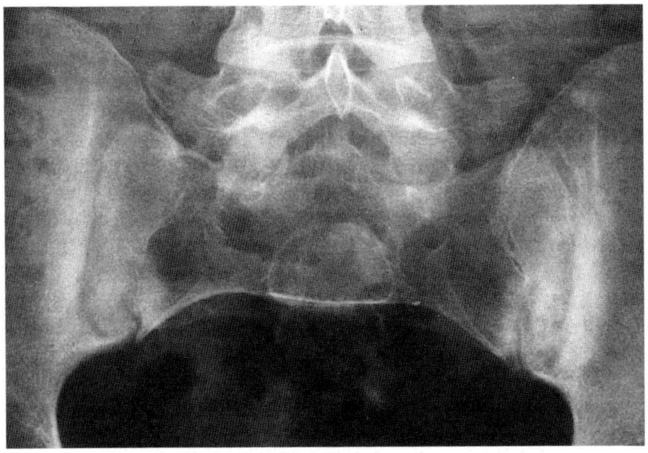

Fig. 6 Bilateral sacroiliitis in a patient with psoriatic spondyloarthropathy.

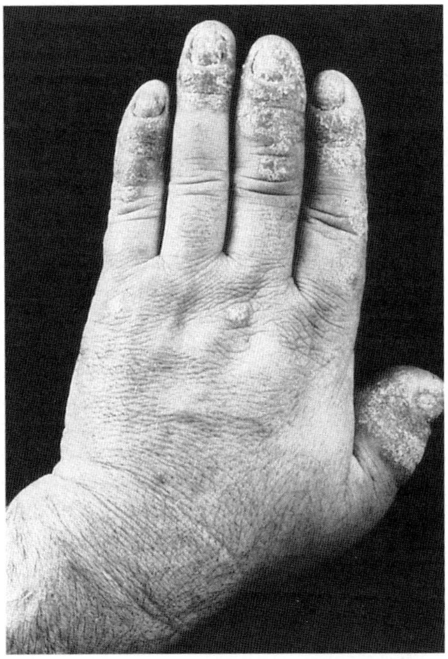

Fig. 7 Dactylitis, which presents as swelling of a whole digit, with inflammation involving DIP, PIP, and occasionally the MCP joints, involving the thumb and third finger. Note the psoriatic skin and nail lesions.

with an oligoarthritis which later becomes polyarticular, or develop an initial polyarthritis, which persists in only a few joints. Indeed, Jones et al. (1994) documented these changes in pattern over time in over 60 per cent of their patients with psoriatic arthritis. A Spanish study suggested that only two clinical associations could be defined, namely axial arthritis and peripheral arthritis, in a cross-sectional study of psoriatic arthritis (Marsal et al. 1999). Unless radiographs are performed on all patients, joints that had been previously involved may not be identified, and the spondyloarthropathy may be missed (Little et al. 1975; Gladman et al. 1987; Hanly et al. 1988; Battistone et al. 1999).

A typical feature of psoriatic arthritis is the development of dactylitis, which presents as a swelling of a whole digit, with inflammation involving distal and proximal interphalangeal, and occasionally the metacarpophalangeal joints (Fig. 7). Dactylitis occurs in over one-third of the patients (Gladman et al. 1987), and appears to result from extensive inflammation and effusion in the joints of a particular digit, with an associated tenosynovitis. Ultrasonography demonstrated the presence of both synovitis and tenosynovitis in digits affected by dactylitis (Kane et al. 1999).

Tenosynovitis is also a feature of psoriatic arthritis. As in the other spondyloarthropathies, such as Reiter's syndrome and ankylosing spondylitis, Achilles tendinitis, heel pain, and plantar fasciitis are common among patients with psoriatic arthritis. Enthesitis, or inflammation at sites of tendon insertion, is frequent, particularly at the Achilles tendon, the insertion of the plantar fascia, and ligamentous insertions around the pelvic bones. These are commonly diagnosed radiologically as spurs (Fig. 8). Recent studies support a role for ultrasonography in identifying involvement of the tendons and entheses in patients with psoriatic arthritis (Lehtinen et al. 1994; Galluzzo et al. 2000). Isolated enthesitis and dactylitis may constitute a specific subset of psoriatic arthritis, even in the absence of peripheral joint involvement (Salvarani et al. 1997). McConagle et al. (1999) proposed that psoriatic arthritis be considered an enthesopathic disease.

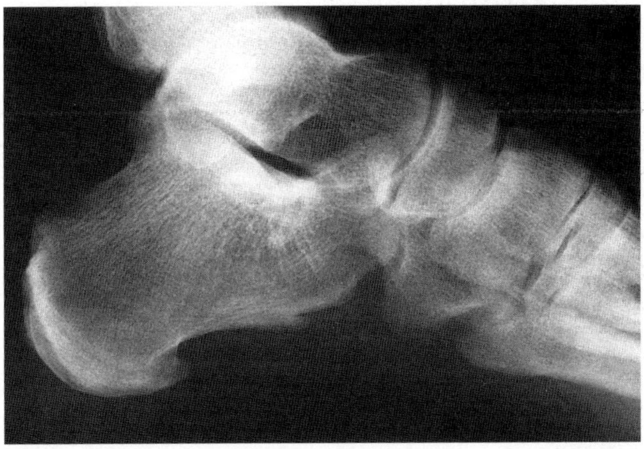

Fig. 8 Spur formation at the insertion of the plantar fascia, representing enthesitis.

The spondyloarthropathy of psoriatic arthritis

The frequency of spinal involvement in psoriatic arthritis has varied from 2 per cent, as isolated back disease, to as high as 78 per cent, when associated with peripheral arthritis (Wright and Moll 1976; Lambert and Wright 1977; Kammer et al. 1979; Scarpa et al. 1984; Gladman et al. 1986, 1987; Hanly et al. 1988; Moll 1994; Battistone et al. 1999; Baek et al. 2000). Lambert and Wright (1977) found that 40 per cent of 130 patients with psoriatic arthritis had back involvement, based on back pain and reduced spinal mobility. Gladman et al. (1987) documented spinal involvement, based on both clinical and radiological evidence, in 35 per cent of their patients at their first visit to the psoriatic arthritis clinic. This number increased to 51 per cent at follow-up (Gladman et al. 1992b). In both studies, patients with spinal involvement tended to be male and older than patients without back involvement. Among patients participating in a multicentre trial who underwent sacroiliac radiography, 78 per cent were found to have at least grade 2 sacroiliitis (Battistone et al. 1999). Among Korean patients with psoriatic arthritis, spondyloarthropathy was detected in 50 per cent, and it may even be higher if the patients with psoriasis who had radiographic changes of sacroiliitis were included among the psoriatic arthritis group (Baek et al. 2000).

The spondyloarthropathy of patients with psoriatic arthritis is less severe than that seen in ankylosing spondylitis (Hanly et al. 1988; Scarpa et al. 1988; Scarpa 2000). This is evidenced by the lower frequency of symptomatic neck and back disease, as well as less limitation of movement and grade 4 sacroiliitis in patients with psoriatic arthritis compared to those with ankylosing spondylitis (Gladman et al. 1993). Moreover, among patients with psoriatic spondyloarthropathy, there are gender-related differences in disease expression, with more advanced spondyloarthropathy noted among men (Gladman et al. 1992b).

The cervical spine in psoriatic arthritis received special attention in two recent studies. Salvarani et al. (1992a) studied 57 patients with psoriatic arthritis, of whom 70 per cent had radiological evidence of cervical spine disease. They identified a high prevalence (23 per cent) of atlanto-axial subluxation. Jenkinson et al. (1994) detected cervical spine disease in 57 per cent of their patients with psoriatic arthritis, of whom only three had atlanto-axial subluxation. The majority of their patients had spondylitic type changes with apophysial joint narrowing or fusion and syndesmophytes. In both these studies, neck involvement was related to prolonged disease duration. Jeannou et al. (1999) found the frequency of neck pain much higher among 30 patients with psoriatic arthritis (73 per cent) than in 30 controls of the same age but who had 'common low back pain' (26 per cent). Moreover, among the psoriatic arthritis patients the neck pain was inflammatory in nature in 63.6 per cent compared with only 12.5 per cent of the controls. However, on radiographs none of their subjects had syndesmophytes while three patients had atlanto-axial subluxation.

Extra-articular features

Skin psoriasis

Skin psoriasis consists of an erythematous scaly area that varies from a localized plaque on the elbows and knees to an incapacitating, generalized skin involvement with significant effect on the cardiovascular and heat regulating mechanism (Goodfield 1994). The skin lesions are classified as: typical psoriasis vulgaris, with major involvement of the extensor surfaces; inverse psoriasis, affecting the flexural areas; pustular psoriasis, which may be localized to the palms and soles, or may be of the more generalized serious form called Von Zambush, and which may pose a threat to life; and the erythrodermic generalized group. The majority of patients with psoriatic arthritis demonstrate the classic psoriasis vulgaris pattern (Wright et al. 1979; Gladman et al. 1986, 1987). All areas of the skin may be affected, including the mucosa and the nails. Nail lesions include pitting, ridging, and onycholysis (Wright and Moll 1976). Two or all of these features in the same patient are in favour of a psoriatic origin for the nail dystrophy (Eastmond and Wright 1979). As already mentioned, nail lesions are particularly common among patients with psoriatic arthritis (Gladman et al. 1986). Nail lesions were associated with DIP joint disease in one study (Cohen et al. 1999).

Other extra-articular features

The extradermal extra-articular features of psoriatic arthritis are similar to the features described in other seronegative spondyloarthropathies and include iritis, which may occur in 7 per cent of the patients (Gladman et al. 1987). Uveitis associated with psoriatic arthritis was more insidious in onset, posterior, persistent, and more likely to be bilateral than when associated with other spondyloarthropathy (Paiva et al. 2000). Mouth ulcers, urethritis, colitis, and aortic valve disease may also complicate psoriatic arthritis (Wright and Moll 1976). A case of a patient with psoriatic arthritis with pyoderma gangrenosum was described (Smith and White 1994), and we have seen a case in our psoriatic arthritis clinic. The development of lymphoedema of the upper limb in patients with psoriatic arthritis has also been described (Mulherin et al. 1993). Cantini et al. (2001) identified distal extremity swelling with pitting oedema in 39/183 (21 per cent) psoriatic arthritis patients and in 18/366 (4.9 per cent) rheumatology clinic controls which excluded spondyloarthropathy ($p < 0.0001$). They concluded that upper or lower distal extremity swelling with pitting oedema due to tenosynovitis, usually unilateral, is a common feature in psoriatic arthritis patients and may represent the first, isolated manifestation of the disease.

Laboratory investigations in psoriatic arthritis

There are no specific laboratory tests diagnostic for psoriatic arthritis. Anaemia occurred in 14 per cent of the patients presenting to the psoriatic arthritis clinic (Gladman et al. 1987), and at a higher level at follow-up (Gladman et al. 1990b), and was thought to represent the untoward effect of these drugs. Elevated white-cell counts and other acute phase reactants, may also be present (Gladman et al. 1987). Elevated sedimentation rates may be seen in more than 40 per cent of patients with psoriatic arthritis, and likely reflect both joint and skin inflammation (Gladman et al. 1986, 1987). Hyperuricaemia occurred at least once in 20.7 per cent of a cohort of 265 patients with psoriatic arthritis followed prospectively over a 6-year period (Bruce et al. 2000). Although it has been thought to result from the high turnover of skin cells there was no correlation between skin severity and uric acid levels. Since both psoriasis and gout may occur in young males, one must rule out the possibility that the arthritis is crystal induced, before making the diagnosis of psoriatic arthritis in a patient with psoriasis. On the other hand, the presence of an acute monoarthritis, even in the first metatarsophalangeal joint in the presence of psoriasis does not mean the patient has gout. In both these situations, a careful search for negatively birefringent, uric acid crystal should be carried out on the fluid obtained by joint aspiration.

Patients with psoriatic arthritis are usually seronegative for rheumatoid factor. However, in each series of patients with psoriatic arthritis there are about 10–15 per cent of the patients who have a positive rheumatoid factor, albeit in a low titre. In addition, patients with psoriasis uncomplicated by arthritis demonstrate the same frequency of positive rheumatoid factor, despite the fact that they are younger on average than the patients with psoriatic arthritis (Gladman et al. 1986). Antinuclear factor has also been demonstrated in the sera of patients with uncomplicated psoriasis and patients with psoriatic arthritis, in the same frequency (Gladman et al. 1986). Whether this antinuclear antibody reflects the presence of antibodies to stratum corneum antigens is unclear (Gladman 1985).

Radiologic features of psoriatic arthritis

Radiologic abnormalities may be seen in both peripheral joints and the axial skeleton in patients with psoriatic arthritis (Resnick and Niwayama 1981). The features commonly associated with psoriatic arthritis and which help differentiate it from rheumatoid arthritis include: absence of juxta-articular osteoporosis; the predilection for distal interphalangeal joints; 'whittling' (lysis) of terminal phalanges (Fig. 9); lack of symmetry; gross destruction of isolated joint; 'pencil-in-cup' appearance (Fig. 10); ankylosis (Fig. 10); fluffy periostitis (Fig. 11); both classical and atypical spondylitis (Wright and Moll 1971; Resnick and Niwayama 1981; Figs 5–7). However, a direct comparison of radiographs of patients with rheumatoid arthritis and patients with psoriatic arthritis matched for age and disease duration, the differences were not obvious (Rahman et al. 2001).

Diagnosis of psoriatic arthritis

There are no available diagnostic criteria for psoriatic arthritis (Gladman 1995). The European Spondyloarthropathy Study Group preliminary criteria for the classification of the spondyloarthropathies were only 65 per cent sensitive for psoriatic arthritis (Salvarani et al. 1995). A new classification based on a comparison of clinical and laboratory features of 100 patients with psoriatic arthritis, 80 patients with ankylosing spondylitis, and 80 patients with rheumatoid arthritis identified nine criteria which were 95 per cent sensitive and 98 per cent specific for psoriatic arthritis in the study population (Fournie et al. 1998). These criteria include the presence of psoriasis either in the patient or a relative, distal joint arthritis, inflammatory spinal involvement, asymmetric oligoarthritis, enthesitis, the presence of one

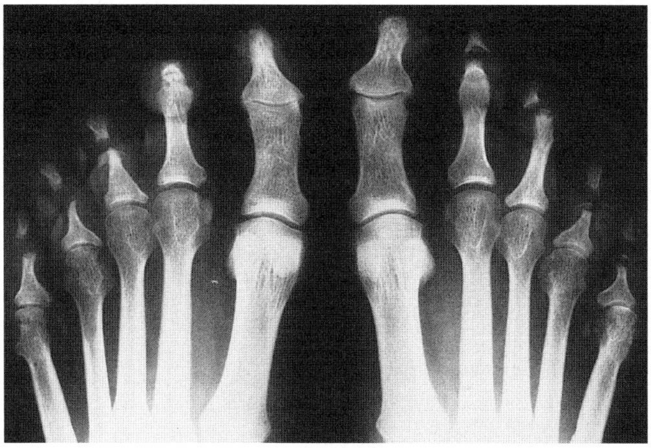

Fig. 9 'Whittling' (lysis) of terminal phalanges of the first and second toes bilaterally.

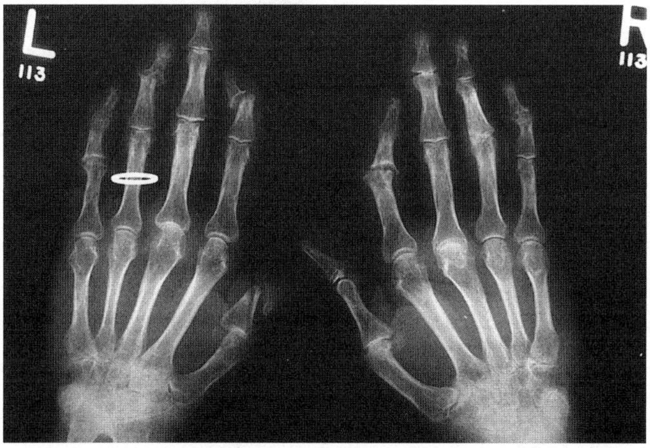

Fig. 10 'Pencil-in-cup' appearance seen in its early phase in the second right PIP, the fifth right DIP, and the left fifth DIP. Fully developed changes are seen in the left index DIP and the left thumb IP joints. In addition, ankylosis is seen in the right DIP joint.

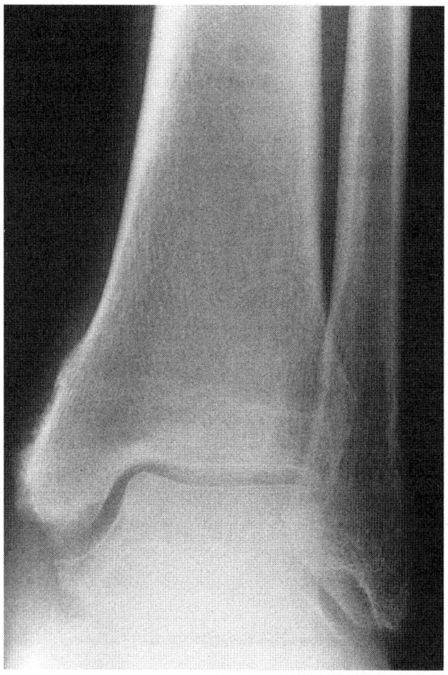

Fig. 11 Fluffy periostitis in the distal end of the tibia.

of five radiological digit criteria, the presence of a relevant HLA antigen, and a negative rheumatoid factor. The proposed criteria would be difficult to achieve at the bedside as they require both laboratory and radiological evidence. Moreover, the criteria still require confirmation in an additional, larger patient cohort.

Nonetheless, the diagnosis of psoriatic arthritis is generally based on the definition of the disease: an inflammatory arthritis in the presence of psoriatic skin lesions, usually seronegative for rheumatoid factor. In a patient with psoriasis, the development of an inflammatory arthritis makes the diagnosis easier. The clinical and radiologic features described above help identify the patient with psoriatic arthritis who had not previously demonstrated skin lesions. Thus, a patient who presents with an asymmetric oligoarthritis, or an inflammatory polyarthritis which includes distal interphalangeal joints, or peripheral arthritis with a spondyloarthropathy, should be investigated for the presence of psoriasis, and psoriatic arthritis should clearly be considered in the differential diagnosis. The presence of dactylitis is certainly helpful, as is the presence of enthesitis. The skin lesions may be minimal, and indeed 'hidden'. One must therefore search for these lesions, particularly in the umbilical area, the anal cleft, the groin, the scalp, and the ears. Nail lesions are not always recognized by the patient, and should be looked for carefully. The common occurrence of distal joint involvement means that psoriatic arthritis needs to be differentiated from osteoarthritis. The distal interphalangeal lesions in patients with psoriatic arthritis are inflammatory in nature, and tend to be swollen, such that for the most part they can be differentiated clinically as softer than the hard bony enlargement of Heberden's nodes. The presence of more proximal joint involvement, particularly the wrist and metacarpophalangeal joints, also helps distinguish psoriatic arthritis from osteoarthritis. However, osteoarthritis is a common condition, particularly with advancing age, and a patient may have Heberden's nodes complicating pre-existing psoriatic arthritis. Reiter's disease occasionally presents a diagnostic difficulty. The skin lesions in pustular psoriasis may be indistinguishable both clinically and pathologically from those of Reiter's syndrome, and the clinical features of the arthritis and the spondyloarthropathy are similar. Psoriatic arthritis tends to be polyarticular, which may help. Iritis and mucous membrane lesions may be more common in Reiter's disease.

Pathogenesis of psoriatic arthritis

Although the exact pathogenesis of psoriatic arthritis remain to be elucidated, factors thought to be important include environmental genetic and immunologic (Gladman 1992; Abu-Shakra and Gladman 1994).

Genetic factors

A family history of the skin or joint disease in first-degree family members is obtained in more than 40 per cent of patients with psoriatic arthritis (Gladman et al. 1986, 1987). Moll and Wright (1973) identified the prevalence of psoriatic arthritis among first-degree relatives of 88 probands with the disease at 5.5 per cent compared to the calculated prevalence in the UK population of 0.1 per cent. Population based studies and twin studies support the genetic contribution in psoriasis (Espinoza 1985; Eastmond 1994). Segregation studies in psoriasis conclude that a polygenic or a multifactorial pattern is the most likely mode of inheritance (Bhalerao and Bowcock 1998).

Population studies in psoriasis revealed an increased frequency of HLA antigens B13, B17, B37, Cw6, and DR7 (Espinoza 1985; Gladman et al. 1986; Eastmond 1994). In psoriatic arthritis, increased frequencies of HLA-B13, B17, B27, B38, B39, DR4, and DR7 have been reported (Espinoza 1985;

Gladman et al. 1986; Sakkas et al. 1990). Gladman et al. (1986) compared 158 patients with psoriatic arthritis to 101 patients with uncomplicated psoriasis. They found that the HLA-B7 or -B27 antigen were more common among patients with psoriatic arthritis, whereas B17, Cw6, and DR7 were more common among patients with uncomplicated psoriasis. HLA-B27 has clearly been associated with back disease in psoriatic arthritis, thus lending further credence to its grouping with the HLA-B27-associated spondyloarthropathy. HLA–DR4 appears to be associated with the peripheral articular pattern of psoriatic arthritis (Gladman et al. 1986). No specific T-cell receptor genes unique to the disease were identified (Sakkas et al. 1990), but immunoglobulin heavy chain gene (IgH) on chromosome 14q32 may confer susceptibility to arthritis in patients with psoriasis (Sakkas et al. 1991).

Several genetic loci have been identified in family investigations in psoriasis, including loci on chromosome 17q (Tomfohrdre et al. 1994; Nair et al. 1997), 4q (Matthews et al. 1996), 6p (Burden et al. 1996; Trembath et al. 1997; Leder et al. 1998; Samuelsson et al. 1999; Veal et al. 2001), and 1p (Veal et al. 2001). The strongest association by far is with loci on chromosome 6p. An analysis of all families for whom complete data was available in the literature suggests that HLA-B locus is in linkage disequilibrium with the PSORS1 gene (Leder et al. 1998). However, the exact location and nature of PSOR1 on 6p is unclear. Similar studies are currently underway for psoriatic arthritis.

Environmental factors

Infection

Support for the role of bacterial antigens in the pathogenesis of psoriasis and psoriatic arthritis comes from indirect observations of enhanced humoral and cellular immunity to Gram-positive bacteria typically found in the psoriatic plaques (Vasey 1985). However, psoriatic plaques often get secondarily infected, thus the cause–effect relationship of bacteria and psoriasis is complicated. Moreover, investigators have demonstrated that there is no specific role for streptococcal responsive synovial T lymphocytes psoriatic arthritis (Grilington et al. 1993; Thomssen et al. 2000). However, Prinz (2001) recently pointed out the possibility that an infectious agent may have triggered the psoriatic process, and the immunological response seen in patients with both psoriasis and psoriatic arthritis may be the result of molecular mimicry between streptococcal antigens and epidermal autoantigens.

The exacerbation of psoriasis and psoriatic arthritis seen in the context of acquired immunodeficiency virus infection is intriguing (Vasey et al. 1989). The possibility that psoriatic arthritis might be virus induced has been proposed (Luxembourg et al. 1987). Hepatitis C virus has been detected more commonly among patients with psoriatic arthritis, but its role in the pathogenesis of the disease cannot be confirmed (Taglione et al. 1999).

Trauma

In almost all accounts of psoriatic arthritis, there are reports of patients whose arthritis developed after trauma. However, the majority of the reports are anecdotal case reports (Punzi et al. 1998). A case series was reported by Scarpa et al. (1992) who found that trauma of some type preceded the diagnosis of psoriatic arthritis in 9 per cent of the cases, whereas in rheumatoid arthritis it was found in only 1 per cent of the patients, suggesting a role for trauma in some patients with psoriatic arthritis. Whether this represents an internal Koebner phenomenon (the appearance of psoriasis at sites of cutaneous injury due to trauma) is unclear. However, substance P, a neuropeptide, and vasoactive intestinal peptide are over expressed in psoriatic skin lesions and in psoriatic synovium (Veale et al. 1993a).

Immunological mechanisms

The clinical and pathological features of both psoriasis and psoriatic arthritis support the role of immunological factors in the pathogenesis of these conditions. The inflammatory nature of the disease, the cellular infiltrates seen both in skin and joint lesions, and the deposition of immunoglobulins in the epidermis as well as the synovial membrane, all support an immune mechanism (Panayi 1994).

Psoriasis is characterized histologically by keratinocyte proliferation, vascular changes and the presence of T lymphocytes in affected skin (Gottlieb 1988). T lymphocytes, particularly CD8+ cells, are thought to play a prime role in its pathogenesis. Activated T cells have been noted in the affected tissues (both skin and joints) in psoriatic arthritis by most investigators (Gladman 1993; Veale et al. 1993b, 1994a; Panayi 1994). In an animal model, a severe combined immunodeficient (SCID) mouse with grafted unaffected human skin, injection of activated T cells from affected individuals causes psoriasis to develop in the grafted and surrounding skin (Wrone-Smith and Nickoloff 1996). A predominance of CD8+ T lymphocytes with clonal expansion was documented in the synovial fluid from patients with psoriatic arthritis (Costello et al. 1999). Examination of T-cell antigen receptor beta chain variable (TCRβV) gene repertoires in skin and synovium reveal common expansions in both sites, suggesting that a common antigen may act as a trigger for disease in both tissues (Tassiulas et al. 1999). Psoriatic arthritis synovial explants produced more IL-1β, IL-2, IL-10, IFN-γ, and TNF-α than those of rheumatoid arthritis or osteoarthritis. Levels of IL-1β, IFN-γ, IL-10 were higher in synovial tissue than dermal plaques from patients with psoriatic arthritis (Ritchlin et al. 1998). Thus, cytokines secreted from activated T cells and other mononuclear proinflammatory cells induce proliferation and activation of synovial and epidermal fibroblasts, leading to the fibrosis reported in patients with long-standing psoriatic arthritis. This is also consistent with the prominent ankylosis seen both clinically and radiologically in patients with psoriatic arthritis. The effect of anticytokine therapy further supports the role of cytokines in this disease. Anti-TNF agents have been shown to work in both psoriasis (Chaudhari et al. 2001) and psoriatic arthritis (Mease et al. 2000).

The role of metabolites of arachidonic acid, such as prostaglandins and particularly leukotrienes, in the pathogenesis of both psoriasis and psoriatic arthritis has been proposed. Increased levels of leukotriene B4 in the psoriatic skin lesions have been noted, and injections of this compound has caused intraepidermal microabscesses. Greaves and Camp (1988) proposed an integrated approach to inflammation of human skin, considering both the lipoxygenase system, platelet activating factor and cytokines. However, studies in both psoriasis (Soyland et al. 1993) and psoriatic arthritis (Veale et al. 1994c) failed to demonstrate clinical improvement in either skin or joint manifestations in patients treated with fish oil.

Treatment of psoriatic arthritis

The treatment modalities employed in psoriatic arthritis are in part based on the pathogenetic mechanisms discussed above. These are based on control of inflammation, and an attempt to modify the immunological mechanisms thought to be operating in this disease (Gladman and Brockbank 2000).

The treatment of psoriasis

The treatment of psoriatic arthritis includes treatment for the skin condition as well as treatment for the joint disease. The skin lesions are treated by topical medications, aimed at controlling the inflammation and skin proliferation, including tar, anthralin, and corticosteroids. In refractory cases, systemic medications such as methotrexate PUVA (psoralen and ultraviolet A light), retinoic acid derivatives, and more recently cyclosporin are used (Greaves and Weinstein 1995).

The treatment of psoriatic arthritis

Non-steroidal anti-inflammatory therapy

The initial treatment for psoriatic arthritis consists of non-steroidal anti-inflammatory drugs (NSAIDs), including enteric-coated acetylsalicylic acid (ECASA), ibuprofen, naproxen, indomethacin, tolmetin, piroxicam, diclofenac sodium, and other NSAIDs (Gladman and Brockbank 2000).

In patients with significant peripheral arthritis, medications such as ECASA, ibuprofen, naproxen, or diclofenac sodium might be preferred. However, for the spondyloarthropathy, indomethacin or tolmetin would be more appropriate. The latter two drugs would also be appropriate if morning stiffness is prolonged, and may be used in conjunction with other NSAIDs. Several of the NSAIDs have been incriminated in exacerbating the psoriasis, perhaps through the prostaglandin mechanism. It may therefore be necessary to change medications if an exacerbation of psoriasis occurs. The newer cyclooxygenase-2 (COX-2) selective inhibitors recently released for the treatment of rheumatoid arthritis and osteoarthritis, including celecoxib, rofeocoxib, and mobicoxib have not been adequately tested in psoriatic arthritis, and do not appear to be any more effective that the previously available NSAIDs. It remains to be determined whether they have an adverse effect on the skin lesions.

Disease modifying drugs for psoriatic arthritis

If the arthritis persists despite the use of non-steroidal anti-inflammatory medications, disease-modifying antirheumatic drugs are added.

Gold

Gold has been studied in a controlled fashion in psoriatic arthritis, using either intramuscular (Dowart et al. 1978) or oral (Carrett and Calin 1989) preparations. Intramuscular preparation has been proven superior to the oral gold in patients with psoriatic arthritis (Palit et al. 1990). However, although gold may control the inflammatory process in patients with psoriatic arthritis, it has not prevented progression of erosive disease over a 2-year period (Mader et al. 1995).

Penicillamine

Penicillamine has also been used successfully in psoriatic arthritis (Roux et al. 1979). Both gold and penicillamine are quite slow acting, however, requiring at least 6 months for a therapeutic effect. Therefore, other medications, whose onset of action is faster have been tried.

Antimalarials

Although physicians have been reluctant to use antimalarials because of anecdotal reports of flares of psoriasis, and despite the lack of controlled trials, both chloroquine phosphate and hydroxychloroquine have been used (Kammer et al. 1979). Indeed, chloroquine has been shown to reduce disease activity in patients with psoriatic arthritis over a period of 6 months, and the frequency of psoriatic flares was no greater than that observed in the control group (Gladman et al. 1992a).

Methotrexate

Methotrexate, which has been found to be effective in controlling the skin psoriasis, has been used in psoriatic arthritis since 1964, when Black et al. (1964), performed a double-blind study of 21 patients using parenteral methotrexate. There have been two controlled trials using low-dose weekly methotrexate in psoriatic arthritis. Willkens et al. (1984) demonstrated improvement in grip strength, morning stiffness, and joint count in patients with psoriatic arthritis, and physician global assessment was improved in the methotrexate group at 3 months, but only physician global assessment was significantly higher in the methotrexate group compared with the placebo. Zacharias and Zacharias (1987) found significant improvement in pain and functional scores as well as a decrease in the erythrocyte sedimentation rate during treatment with low-dose weekly methotrexate for psoriatic arthritis. Espinoza et al. (1992), in a retrospective uncontrolled study of 40 patients with psoriatic arthritis treated with a mean of dose of 11.2 mg/week of methotrexate during a mean period of 34 months, found that 37 per cent of the patients had an excellent response (no evidence of active synovitis) while 58 per cent had a good response (no more than four active joints and a decrease of at least 50 per cent in the number of those previously involved). Only two patients had discontinued the drug because of toxicity; one leucopaenia and the other stomatitis. Eleven patients developed liver test abnormalities; however, cirrhosis related to methotrexate was not noted. Abu-Shakra et al. (1995) found that while methotrexate reduced the actively inflamed joint count in patients with psoriatic arthritis, it did not prevent disease progression in these patients over a period of 2 years of treatment. Nonetheless, methotrexate is used regularly for the treatment of psoriatic arthritis, particularly in the face of severe psoriasis. Methotrexate has an advantage over gold and penicillamine since it is effective within a few weeks. In addition, because it is given as an intermittent dose, once a week, patients prefer to take it over medications that are required daily, and often in repeated doses. Concerns about severe liver disease resulting from methotrexate therapy which resulted from reports in the late 1960s and early 1970s seem to have been alleviated since more judicious use of intermittent dose has become commonplace. The use of either folic acid or folinic acid has also reduced some of the side-effects of methotrexate.

Sulfasalazine

Sulfasalazine has been shown in several double-blind placebo-controlled trials to be effective in psoriatic arthritis (Farr et al. 1990; Fraser et al. 1993; Combe et al. 1996; Clegg et al. 1998). However, the effect has been modest (Jones et al. 2000). A recent study in an outpatient clinic reported that 44 per cent of the patients who started on sulfasalazine were unable to tolerate it, and that there was no long-term advantage in terms of erosive disease (Rahman et al. 1998).

Azathioprine

Azathioprine has also been used in psoriatic arthritis (Levy et al. 1972; Lee et al. 2001), but since its effect on the psoriasis is not well recognized, it has not been as useful as it is in rheumatoid arthritis. The use of azathioprine in patients with psoriatic arthritis who had not responded or were unable to tolerate methotrexate was recently described (Lee et al. 2001) with encouraging results. However, compared to other medications used azathioprine was not found to have an advantage in preventing damage in patients with psoriatic arthritis.

Retinoids

Retinoids have only been studied in uncontrolled fashion, since it is difficult to blind both patients and observers to their side-effects (Klinkhoff et al. 1989). While these drugs may be effective against both skin and joint manifestations, their toxicity appears high.

Cyclosporin A

Cyclosporin A has been studied as a therapeutic option for both psoriasis and psoriatic arthritis (Gupta et al. 1989; Salvarani et al. 1992b). In a comparative study with methotrexate, there was significant improvement in the skin and joints of both groups, with no significant difference between them. However, there was a higher withdrawal rate in those patients on cyclosporin (Spadarao et al. 1995). Although it has been suggested that it is effective and safe, NSAIDs cannot be used concomitantly. Moreover, its adverse effects, particularly on the kidney, preclude its wide spread use.

Steroids

Oral steroids are usually avoided in psoriatic arthritis, since upon dose reduction they can cause significant flares of the skin psoriasis (Griffith 1997). However, intra-articular steroids may be used at any time, especially when there is a joint which is particularly inflamed. We tend to avoid injecting joints which are surrounded by psoriatic plaques because of fear of causing infections.

Anti-TNF agents in psoriatic arthritis

The development of anti-TNF agents for the treatment of rheumatoid arthritis which was based on a proposed role for TNF in the pathogenesis of the inflammatory process opened up new avenues for the treatment of both skin and joint manifestations of psoriatic arthritis. Etanercept is a recombinant human protein, consisting of two TNF receptor p75 fused with the FC domain of human IgG1. Consequently it binds TNF and inactivates it. A double-blind controlled trial of 60 patients with psoriatic arthritis, half of whom were also on methotrexate demonstrated a remarkable improvement in the psoriatic arthritis response criteria (87 per cent compared to 27 per cent in the placebo group) which was much better than in the study of sulfasalazine in psoriatic arthritis for which the criteria were developed (Clegg et al. 1998; Mease et al. 2000). A follow-up open-label study further demonstrated the efficacy of etanercept in patients who were randomized to placebo in the original trial. In this group 65 per cent responded to etanercept. A larger multicentre randomized controlled trial of etanercept in psoriatic arthritis is currently being completed. Etanercept is given subcutaneously at a dose of 25 mg twice a week. Patients can self-inject. It is relatively safe, with injection site reactions being the commonest side-effects. However, there is a concern about susceptibility to infection. Infliximab is a human/mouse chimeric anti-TNF-α antibody that blocks TNF from reaching its receptor. It has also been proven effective in rheumatoid arthritis. Infliximab is also given parenterally, however, it is given by infusion which is more difficult for the patients since they require to attend a medical centre at 6–8-week interval for at least 2 h. Infliximab was recently demonstrated to be effective in the treatment of severe psoriasis (Chaudhari et al. 2001). There are few case series of its use in psoriatic arthritis. It was given to 10 patients in Germany with good response (Antoni et al. 2002). We have had an opportunity to treat 15 patients with severe psoriatic arthritis with infliximab. Seven of the 15 demonstrated greater than 70 per cent reduction in the number of actively inflamed joints. The majority demonstrated excellent response of their skin. However, five patients had to discontinue the drug because of adverse effects, which included infection, rectal bleeding, and allergic reactions. Infliximab has been associated with allergic reactions that are thought to result from antibody formation to the foreign protein. Recently, there has been concern about reactivation of pulmonary tuberculosis by anti-TNF agents. It is possible that newer anti-TNF agents such as a completely human anti-TNF antibody and TNF receptor to p55 as well as p75 will be available for the treatment of psoriatic arthritis.

There are other biologic agents currently under study for psoriasis, including an anti-CD11 antibody, CTLA4-Ig. They have yet to be investigated for psoriatic arthritis.

Dietary modification

Based on the proposed pathogenesis of both psoriasis and psoriatic arthritis, there may be a role for fish oil preparations or specific immunomodulators in the treatment of both psoriasis and psoriatic arthritis. However, a placebo controlled trial of Efamol marine demonstrated no efficacy in psoriatic arthritis (Veale et al. 1994c). The use of oral vitamin D_3 for the treatment of psoriatic arthritis has also been proposed (Huckins et al. 1990).

Other medications

Psoralen and ultraviolet A light has been used in psoriatic arthritis with some success (Perlman et al. 1979). Later, the use of extracorporeal photochemotherapy has been proposed (de Misa et al. 1994). Buskila et al. (1991) described a woman with psoriatic arthritis, who experienced a remarkable improvement of her arthritis while she was taking bromocriptine for primary infertility due to hyperprolactinaemia. Others have also reported similar results. Peptide T has also been advocated for the treatment of psoriatic arthritis, but information is currently available only from case reports (Abu-Shakra and Gladman 1994).

Physiotherapy and occupational therapeutic modalities should be used both for symptomatic relief and to avoid development of deformities. Patients may require splints, and need to be instructed as to energy conservation and joint protection. In patients with spondyloarthropathy, specific back exercises may be necessary.

Surgery

Surgery is reserved for patients whose joints have become deformed and damaged. Of 444 patients with psoriatic arthritis followed prospectively 31 (7 per cent) had musculoskeletal surgery at an average of 13 years after the onset of joint disease. A high number of actively inflamed joints and advanced radiological damage at first assessment were highly predictive of subsequent surgery (Zangger et al. 1998). Seventy-one procedures were performed in 43 patients at one centre during a 10 year period (Zangger et al. 2000). Among patients with polyarticular disease, a variety of procedures were performed including complex hand and foot surgery, hip replacements, and fusion of individual joints, whereas patients with oligoarticular disease tended to have hip and knee replacements. Four procedures led to complications: (i) an infection in a hip arthroplasty, which required removal of the prosthesis; (ii) a malunion of an ankle arthrodesis, which required correction; (iii) a lack of fixation in a PIP joint, which was corrected within 12 days, and (iv) a death from an undiagnosed hepatic hemangioma. An approach to the treatment of tempomandibular joint disease in psoriatic arthritis has been described (Peterson and Shepherd 1992). Hicken et al. (1994) reported their experience of 27 forefoot and toe arthroplasty or arthrodesis procedures in 17 patients with psoriatic arthritis collected over a 15-year period. The operations were considered successful in 89 per cent of the cases but they did not use standardized methods for assessing functional outcome. Complications occurred in a patient who had a local infection associated with a local flare of psoriasis and required corrective surgery, another patient who required an additional procedure, and a third patient who had delayed union.

The course and prognosis of psoriatic arthritis

The course of psoriatic arthritis is variable. There are patients who have few episodes and who recover completely (Gladman et al. 2001), but in many the disease is persistent. Roberts et al. (1976) concluded in their follow-up study that 'apart from the deforming group the arthritis was not notably progressive'. However, there was time lost from work in at least 60 per cent of all patients, and radiologic progression was recorded in about 15 per cent. Stern (1985) noted that more than 50 per cent of the patients with psoriatic arthritis had some limitation on their daily activities, and they were twice as likely to be unemployed as patients with other joint disease. Hanly et al. (1988) and Gladman et al. (1990b), suggested that the disease is progressive, based on the increased number of deformed and damaged joints observed in their patients, who were followed according to a standard protocol in the University of Toronto Psoriatic Arthritis Clinic, where clinical measures of inflammatory activity as well as damage have been validated (Gladman et al. 1990a). Coulton et al. (1989) reported on the outcome of 40 patients hospitalized for psoriatic arthritis who were followed for a mean of 8 years. At the end of that period, none of the patients died. However, 35 per cent of their patients were in Steinbrocker's classes III and IV, supporting the notion that a proportion of patients with psoriatic arthritis become disabled. Clear evidence of progression of deformities was demonstrable when patients were compared at presentation and at follow-up based on duration of follow-up at the psoriatic arthritis clinic (Gladman 1994). Gladman et al. (1995) studied 305 patients who entered the psoriatic arthritis clinic with less than 10 deformed joints, and identified clinical indicators for progression through four stages: no deformities, 1–4 deformities, 5–9 deformities, and 10 or more deformities. Patients who had five or more effused joints at presentation to the clinic were more likely to progress, as were patients treated with disease-modifying drugs, while patients who had a low erythrocyte sedimentation rate were less likely to develop more deformities during follow-up. There was no correlation with disease duration. Moreover, Gladman and Farewell (1995) demonstrated that the HLA antigens B27 in the presence of HLA–DR7, HLA-B39, and HLA–DQw3, in the absence of HLA–DR7 were more important than the clinical features in predicting such progression. The same investigators further demonstrated that the number of actively inflamed joint at each visit is an important predictor of subsequent clinical damage in patients with psoriatic arthritis (Gladman and Farewell 1999).

Psoriatic arthritis may no longer be considered a mild form of arthritis. Patients with psoriatic arthritis have an increased mortality risk compared to the general population (Wong et al. 1997). While the causes of death are similar to those of the population at large, previously active and severe disease are predictors for early mortality among patients with psoriatic arthritis (Gladman et al. 1998).

Nonetheless, the arthritis-specific Health Assessment Questionnaire (HAQ) and the generic Medical Outcome Survey Short Form 36 (SF-36) in patients with psoriatic arthritis does not give the same high scores seen in rheumatoid arthritis (Jones et al. 1994; Blackmore et al. 1995; Husted et al. 2001). This may very well be due to the fact that the questionnaires correlate highly with pain, which is less likely to be an issue for patients with psoriatic arthritis than for patients with rheumatoid arthritis (Buskila et al. 1992). However, the quality of life in patients with psoriatic arthritis was found to be lower than in patients with uncomplicated psoriasis (Lundberg et al. 2000).

Approach to the management of psoriatic arthritis

The overall approach to a patient with psoriatic arthritis includes confirming the diagnosis, assessing the extent of disease activity in terms of both joint and skin disease, and assessing the degree of damage that has occurred. This involves a careful history, physical examination, laboratory assessment, and radiological evaluation. The goal of treatment is control of inflammation which will hopefully lead to control of symptoms, and prevention of deformities and damage, so that the patient may continue to lead active and productive life.

Once the diagnosis has been made and the patient assessed, the management approach begins with patient education. It is explained to the patient that he/she suffers from an inflammatory arthritis, that treatment is aimed at controlling inflammation and therefore medications need to be taken regularly. The role of daily stresses on exacerbations of both skin and joint disease is reviewed. The need to treat both skin and joint manifestations of the disease is also discussed. These topics often need to be repeated during follow-up.

The actual therapeutic approach is then tailored to the individual patient (Box 1). A patient who has mild disease, with minimal skin lesions and mild arthritis without deformities, is treated with topical ointments for the skin, and NSAIDs for the joints. The trendency is to use enteric-coated acetylsalicylicacid, ibuprofen, naproxen, or diclofenac for polyarticular disease, and for those patients who complain of pain. In patients with oligoarticular disease, and those with spondyloarthropathies, indomethacin or tolmetin are used. While there is no scientific proof to support this approach, it seems to be empirically correct. However, since patients vary both in their response to and tolerance of different NSAIDs, this sequence is often changed. For individuals who clearly express aversion to taking pills, those NSAIDs that can be given once daily are chosen. The selective COX-2 inhibitors may provide gastroprotection, but are not superior to the other NSAIDs in their anti-inflammatory activity.

Intra-articular corticosteroid injections are used for individual joints. It is found that in psoriatic arthritis, the inflammation is intense and deformity can ensue rapidly. Patients are educated to call immediately when a red hot joint appears, and to present themselves for joint injections. Although some people feel that intra-articular steroids are not as effective in seronegative disease as they are in rheumatoid arthritis, this is not always the case. It has been possible to control severe inflammation and prevent damage in joints which were injected early (as judged by what happened to other joints in the same individual). This applies to both large and small joints in this disease. Joint injections as an adjunct to systemic therapy is used, as well, at any point in the disease, provided the joint is not completely destroyed.

In a patient with active and severe arthritis second-line medications are used early. Antimalarials, sulfasalazine, methotrexate, gold, and azathioprine have been used, for this type of patient. If the patient demonstrates a spondyloarthropathy, sulfasalazine is given first preference, since it seems to control spinal disease as well as peripheral disease, whereas the other medications have not been shown to be as effective for spinal involvement. More recently, the ability of the anti-TNF agents to control psoriatic arthritis has been tested, and these drugs have been made more easily available and accessible. These drugs could be used as early as possible in patients presenting with highly inflammatory disease.

In a patient who has severe psoriasis, even if the arthritis is not that severe, methotrexate is first used, since it has been shown to be effective for both components of the disease. If the methotrexate is not tolerated, then either sulfasalazine (unless there is sulfa allergy) or azathioprine is used. If the methotrexate is tolerated, but not completely effective, either an antimalarial or sulfasalazine is added. In patients with severe psoriasis and mild arthritis PUVA which works well for the skin is used, and has worked well for the joints.

The use of cyclosporin A and retinoids is reserved for patients with severe psoriasis and arthritis who either refuse to take methotrexate, or are unable to tolerate it. These drugs are more toxic than the others and need to be used with caution.

Box 1 Therapeutic approach to the management of psoriatic arthritis

Type of presentation	NSAIDs	Second line	Intra-articular
Mild skin; mild joint	Yes	No	p.r.n.
Mild skin; moderate joint	Yes	Sulfasalazine, methotrexate, antimalarials, gold, azathioprine	p.r.n.
Severe skin; mild joint	Yes	Methotrexate, sulfasalazine, cyclosporin A, PUVA, retinoids	p.r.n.
Severe skin; severe joint	Yes	Methotrexate, sulfasalazine, azathioprine, PUVA, cyclosporin A, retinoids	p.r.n.

References

Abu-Shakra, M. and Gladman, D.D. (1994). Aetiopathogenesis of psoriatic arthritis. *Rheumatology Reviews* **3**, 1–7.

Abu-Shakra, M., Gladman, D.D., Thorne, J.C., Long, J., Gough, J., and Farewell, V.T. (1995). Longterm methotrexate therapy in psoriatic arthritis: clinical and radiologic outcome. *Journal of Rheumatology* **22**, 241–5.

Antoni, C., Dechant, C., Hanns-Martin Lorenz, P.D., Wendler, J., Ogilvie, A., Lueftl, M., Kalden-Nemeth, D., Kalden, J.R., and Manger, B. (2002). Open-label study of Infliximab treatment for psoriatic arthritis: clinical and magnetic resonance imaging measurements of reduction of inflammation. *Arthritis and Rheumatism* **47**, 506–12.

Avila, R. et al. (1960). Psoriatic arthritis. A roentgenologic study. *Radiology* **75**, 691–702.

Baek, H.J. et al. (2000). Spondylitis is the most common pattern of psoriatic arthritis in Korea. *Rheumatology International* **19**, 89–94.

Battistone, M.J., Manaster, B.J., Reda, D.J., and Clegg, D.O. (1999). The prevalence of sacroiliitis in psoriatic arthritis: new perspectives from a large, multicenter cohort. A Department of Veterans Affairs Cooperative Study. *Skeletal Radiology* **28**, 196–201.

Bhalerao, J. and Bowcock, A.M. (1998). The genetics of psoriasis: a complex disorder of the skin and immune system. *Human Molecular Genetics* **7** (10), 1537–45.

Barišic-Druško, V. et al. (1994). Frequency of psoriatic arthritis in general population and among psoriatics in department of dermatology. *Acta Dermato Venerologica (Stockholm)* **74** (Suppl. 186), 107–8.

Black, R.L., O'Brien, W.M., Van Scott, E.J., Auerbach, R., Eisen, A.Z., and Bunim, J.J. (1964). Methotrexate therapy in psoriatic arthritis. Double blind study on 21 patients. *Journal of the American Medical Association* **189**, 743–7.

Blackmore, M., Gladman, D.D., Husted, J., Long, J., and Farewell, V.T. (1995). Measuring health status in psoriatic arthritis. *Journal of Rheumatology* **22**, 886–92.

Bruce, I.N., Schentag, C., and Gladman, D.D. (2000). Hyperuricemia in psoriatic arthritis (PsA) does not reflect the extent of skin involvement. *Journal of Clinical Rheumatology* **6**, 6–9.

Burden, A.D. et al. (1996). Linkage to chromosome 6p and exclusion of chromosome 17q in familial psoriasis in Scotland. *British Journal of Dermatology* **135**, 815–51.

Buskila, D. et al. (1991). Improvement of psoriatic arthritis in a patient treated with bromocriptine for hyperprolactinemia. *Journal of Rheumatology* **18**, 611–12.

Buskila, D. et al. (1992). Patients with rheumatoid arthritis are more tender than those with psoriatic arthritis. *Journal of Rheumatology* **19**, 1115–19.

Cantini, F. et al. (2001). Distal extremity swelling with pitting edema in psoriatic arthritis: a case–control study. *Clinical and Experimental Rheumatology* **19**, 291–6.

Carrett, S. and Calin, A. (1989). Evaluation of auranofin in psoriatic arthritis: a double blind placebo controlled trial. *Arthritis and Rheumatism* **32**, 158–65.

Cats, A. (1990). Psoriasis and Arthritis. *Cutis* **46**, 323–9.

Chaudhari, U., Romano, P., Mulcahy, L.D., Dooley, L.T., Baker, D.G., and Gottlieb, A.B. (2001). Efficacy and safety of infliximab monotherapy for plaque-type psoriasis: a randomised trial. *Lancet* **357**, 1842–7.

Clegg, D.O. et al. (1998). Comparison of sulfasalazine and placebo in the treatment of psoriatic arthritis. A Department of Veterans Affairs Cooperative Study. *Arthritis and Rheumatism* **39**, 2013–20.

Cohen, M.R., Reda, D.J., and Clegg, D.O. (1999). Baseline relationships between psoriasis and psoriatic arthritis: analysis of 221 patients with active psoriatic arthritis. Department of Veterans Affairs Cooperative Study Group on Seronegative Spondyloarthropathies. *Journal of Rheumatology* **26**, 1752–6.

Combe, B., Goupille, P., Kuntz, J.L., Tebib, J., Liote, F., and Bregeon, C. (1996). Sulphasalazine in psoriatic arthritis: a randomized, multicentre, placebo-controlled study. *British Journal of Rheumatology* **35**, 664–8.

Costello, P., Bresnihan, B, O'Farrell, C., and Fitzgerald, O. (1999). Predominance of CD8+ T lymphocytes in psoriatic arthritis. *Journal of Rheumatology* **26**, 1117–24.

Coulton, B.L., Thomson, K., Symmons, D.P.M., and Popert, A.J. (1989). Outcome in patients hospitalised for psoriatic arthritis. *Clinical Rheumatology* **2**, 261–5.

Dowart, B.B., Gall, E.P., Schumacher, H.R., and Krauser, R.E. (1978). Chrysotherapy in psoriatic arthritis: efficacy and toxicity compared to rheumatoid arthritis. *Arthritis and Rheumatism* **21**, 513–15.

Eastmond, C.J. (1994). Genetics and HLA antigens. *Baillière's Clinical Rheumatology* **8**, 263–76.

Eastmond, C.J. and Wright, V. (1979). The nail dystrophy of psoriatic arthritis. *Annals of the Rheumatic Diseases* **38**, 226–8.

Eccles, J.T. and Wright, V. (1985). The history and epidemiologic definition of psoriatic arthritis as a distinct entity. In *Psoriatic Arthritis* (ed. L.H. Gerber and L.R. Espinoza), pp. 1–8. Orlando FL: Grune & Stratton.

Elkayam, O., Ophir, J., Yaron, M., and Caspi, D. (2000). Psoriatic arthritis: interrelationships between skin and joint manifestations related to onset, course and distribution. *Clinical Rheumatology* **19**, 301–5.

Ellis, C.N. et al. (1991). Cyclosporin for-plaque-type psoriasis. Results of a multidose, double-blind trial. *New England Journal of Medicine* **324**, 277–84.

Espinoza, L.R. (1985). Psoriatic arthritis: further epidemiologic and genetic considerations. In *Psoriatic Arthritis* (ed. L.H. Gerber and L.R. Espinoza), pp. 9–32. Orlando FL: Grune & Stratton.

Espinoza, L.R. et al. (1992). Psoriatic arthritis: clinical response and side effects of methotrexate therapy. *Journal of Rheumatology* **19**, 872–7.

Falk, E.S. and Vandbakk, Ø. (1993). Prevalence of psoriasis in a Norwegian Lapp population. *Acta Dermato Venerologica (Stockholm)* **73**, 6–9.

Farr, M., Kitas, G.D., Waterhouse, L., Jubb, R., Felix-Davies, D., and Bacon, P.A. (1990). Sulphasalazine in psoriatic arthritis: a double-blind placebo-controlled study. *British Journal of Rheumatology* **29**, 46–9.

Fournie, B. et al. (1998). Proposed classification criteria of psoriatic arthritis. A preliminary study in 260 patients. *Revue du Rhumatisme (English Edition)* **66**, 446–56.

Fraser, S.M. et al. (1993). Sulphasalazine in the management of psoriatic arthritis. *British Journal of Rheumatology* **32**, 923–5.

Galluzzo, E. et al. (2000). Sonographic analysis of the ankle in patients with psoriatic arthritis. *Scandinavian Journal of Rheumatology* **29**, 52–5.

Gladman, D.D. (1985). Immunologic factors in the pathogenesis of *psoriatic arthritis*. In Psoriatic Arthritis (ed. L.H. Gerber and L.R. Espinoza), pp. 33–44. Orlando FL: Grune & Stratton.

Gladman, D.D. (1992). Psoriatic arthritis: recent advances in pathogenesis and treatment. *Rheumatology Disease Clinics of North America* **18**, 247–56.

Gladman, D.D. (1993). Toward unravelling the mystery of psoriatic arthritis. *Arthritis and Rheumatism* **36**, 881–4.

Gladman, D.D. (1994). Natural history of psoriatic arthritis. *Baillière's Clinical Rheumatology* **8**, 379–94.

Gladman, D.D. (1995). Classification criteria for psoriatic arthritis. *Baillière's Clinical Rheumatology* **9**, 319–29.

Gladman, D.D. and Brockbank, J. (2000). Psoriatic arthritis. *Expert Opinion on Investigational Drugs* **9**, 1511–22.

Gladman, D.D. and Farewell, V.T. (1995). The role of HLA antigens as indicators of disease progression in psoriatic arthritis (PSA): multivariate relative risk model. *Arthritis and Rheumatism* **38**, 845–50.

Gladman, D.D. and Farewell, V.T. (1999). Progression in psoriatic arthritis: role of time varying clinical indicators. *Journal of Rheumatology* **26**, 2409–13.

Gladman, D.D., Anhorn, K.A.B., Schachter, R.K., and Mervart, H. (1986). HLA antigens in psoriatic arthritis. *Journal of Rheumatology* **13**, 586–92.

Gladman, D.D., Shuckett, R., Russell, M.L., Thorne, J.C., and Schachter, R.K. (1987). Psoriatic arthritis (PSA)—an analysis of 220 patients. *Quarterly Journal of Medicine* **62**, 127–41.

Gladman, D.D., Farewell, V., Buskila, D., Goodman, R., Hamilton, L., Langevitz, P., and Thorne, J.C. (1990a). Reliability of measurements of active and damaged joints in psoriatic arthritis. *Journal of Rheumatology* **17**, 62–4.

Gladman, D.D., Stafford-Brady, F., Chang, C.H., Lewandowski, K., and Russell, M.L. (1990b). Clinical and radiological progression in psoriatic arthritis. *Journal of Rheumatology* **17**, 809–12.

Gladman, D.D., Blake, R., Brubacher, B., and Farewell, V.T. (1992a). Chloroquine therapy in psoriatic arthritis. *Journal of Rheumatology* **19**, 1724–6.

Gladman, D.D., Brubacher, B., Buskila, D., Langevitz, P., and Farewell, V.T. (1992b). Psoriatic spondyloarthropathy in men and women: a clinical, radiographic, and HLA study. *Clinical Investigational Medicine* **15**, 371–5.

Gladman, D.D., Brubacher, B., Buskila, D., Langevitz, P., and Farewell, V.T. (1993). Differences in the expression of spondyloarthropathy: a comparison between ankylosing spondylitis and psoriatic arthritis. Genetic and gender effects. *Clinical Investigational Medicine* **16**, 1–7.

Gladman, D.D., Farewell, V.T., and Nadeau, C. (1995). Clinical indicators of progression in psoriatic arthritis (PSA): multivariate relative risk model. *Journal of Rheumatology* **22**, 675–9.

Gladman, D.D., Farewell, V.T., Husted, J., and Wong, K. (1998). Mortality studies in psoriatic arthritis. Results from a single centre. II. Prognostic indicators for mortality. *Arthritis and Rheumatism* **41**, 1103–10.

Gladman, D.D., Ng Tung Hing, E., Schentag, C.T., and Cook, R. (2001). Remission in psoriatic arthritis. *Journal of Rheumatology* **28**, 1045–8.

Goodfield, M. (1994). Skin lesions in psoriasis. *Baillière's Clinical Rheumatology* **8**, 295–316.

Gottlieb, A.B. (1988). Immunologic mechanisms in psoriasis. *Journal of American Academy of Dermatology* **18**, 1276–380.

Greaves, M.W. and Camp, R.D.R. (1988). Prostaglandins, leukotrienes, phospholipase, platelet activating factor, and cytokines: an integrated approach to inflammation of human skin. *Archives of Dermatology* **280** (Suppl.), S33–41.

Greaves, M.W. and Weinstein, G.D. (1995). Treatment of psoriasis. *New England Journal of Medicine* **322**, 581–8.

Green, L., Meyers, O.L., Gordon, W., and Briggs, B. (1981). Arthritis in psoriasis. *Annals of the Rheumatic Diseases* **40**, 366–9.

Griffith, C.E.M. (1997). Therapy for psoriatic arthritis: sometimes a conflict for psoriasis. *British Journal of Rheumatology* **36**, 409–12.

Grilington, F.M., Skinner, M.A., Birchall, N.M., and Tan, P.L.I. (1993). $\gamma\delta+$ T cells from patients with psoriatic and rheumatoid arthritis respond to streptococcal antigen. *Journal of Rheumatology* **20**, 983–7.

Gupta, A.K., Matteson, E.I., Ellis, C.N., Ho, V.C., Tellner, D.C., Voorhees, J.J., and McCune, W.J. (1989). Cyclosporin in the treatment of psoriatic arthritis. *Archives of Dermatology* **125**, 507–10.

Hanly, J.G., Russell, M.L., and Gladman, D.D. (1988). Psoriatic spondyloarthropathy: a long term prospective study. *Annals of the Rheumatic Diseases* **47**, 386–93.

Hellgren, L. (1969). Association between rheumatoid arthritis and psoriasis in total populations. *Acta Rheumatologica Scandinavica* **15**, 316–26.

Helliwell, P., Marchesoni, A., Peters, M., Barker, M., and Wright, V. (1991). A re-evaluation of the osteoarticular manifestations of psoriasis. *British Journal of Rheumatology* **30**, 339–45.

Helliwell, P.S. et al. (2000). Joint symmetry in early and late rheumatoid and psoriatic arthritis: comparison with a mathematical model. *Arthritis and Rheumatism* **43**, 865–71.

Hicken, G.J., Kitaoka, H.B., and Valente, R.M. (1994). Foot and ankle surgery in patients with psoriasis. *Clinical Orthopedics and Related Research* **300**, 204–6.

Huckins, D., Felson, D.T., and Holick, M. (1990). Treatment of psoriatic arthritis with oral 1,25-dihydroxyvitamin D3: a pilot study. *Arthritis and Rheumatism* **33**, 1723–7.

Husted, J.A., Gladman, D.D., Farewell, V.T., and Cook, R.J. (2001). Health-related quality of life of patients with psoriatic arthritis: a comparison with patients with rheumatoid arthritis. *Arthritis and Rheumatism* **45**, 151–18.

Jeannou, J., Goupille, P., Avimadje, M.A., Zerkak, D., Valat, J.P., and Fouquet, B. (1999). Cervical spine involvement in psoriatic arthritis. *Revue du Rhumatisme (English Edition)* **66**, 695–700.

Jenkinson, T. et al. (1994). The cervical spine in psoriatic arthritis: a clinical and radiological study. *British Journal of Rheumatology* **33**, 255–9.

Jones, S.M., Armas, J.B, Cohen, M.G., Lovell, C.R., Evison, G., and McHugh, N.J. (1994). Psoriatic arthritis: outcome of disease subsets and relationship of joint disease to nail and skin disease. *British Journal of Rheumatology* **33**, 834–9.

Jones, G., Crotty, M., and Brooks, P. (2000). Interventions for psoriatic arthritis (Cochrane review). *Cochrane Database System Reviews* **3**, CD000212.

Kammer, G.M., Soter, N.A., Gibson, D.J., and Schur, P.H. (1979). Psoriatic arthritis. A clinical, immunologic and HLA study of 100 patients. *Seminars in Arthritis and Rheumatism* **9**, 75–97.

Kane, D., Greaney, T., Bresnihan, B., Gibney, R., and FitzGerald, O. (1999). Ultrasonography in the diagnosis and management of psoriatic dactylitis. *Journal of Rheumatology* **26**, 1746–51.

Klinkhoff, A.V., Gertner, E., Chalmers, A. Gladman, D.D., Stewart, W.D., Schachter, G.D., and Schachter, R.K. (1989). Pilot study of etretinate in psoriatic arthritis. *Journal of Rheumatology* **16**, 789–91.

Lambert, J.B. and Wright, V. (1977). Psoriatic spondylitis: a clinical and radiological description of the spine in psoriatic arthritis. *Quarterly Journal of Medicine* **46**, 411–25.

Lawrence, R.C. et al. (1989). Estimates of the prevalence of selected arthritis and musculoskeletal diseases in the United States. *Journal of Rheumatology* **16**, 427–41.

Leczinsky, C.G. (1948). The incidence of arthropathy in a ten-year series of psoriasis cases. *Acta Dermato Venerologica* **28**, 483–7.

Leder, R.O., Mansbridge, J.N., Hallmayer, J., and Hodge, S.E. (1998). Familial psoriasis and HLA-B: unambiguous support for linkage in 97 published families. *Human Heredity* **48**, 198–211.

Lee, J.C.T., Gladman, D.D., Schentag, C.T., and Cook, R.J. (2001). The long-term use of azathioprine in patients with psoriatic arthritis. *Journal of Clinical Rheumatology* **7**, 160–5.

Lehtinen, A., Traavisainen, M., and Leirisalo-Repo, M. (1994). Sonographic analysis of enthesopathy in the lower extremities of patients with spondyloarthropathy. *Clinical and Experimental Rheumatology* **12**, 143–8.

Leonard, D.G., O'Duffy, J.D., and Rogers, R.S. (1978). Prospective analysis of psoriatic arthritis in patients hospitalized for psoriasis. *Mayo Clinic Proceedings* **53**, 511–18.

Levy, J.J. et al. (1972). A double-blind controlled evaluation of azathioprine treatment in rheumatoid arthritis and psoriatic arthritis. *Arthritis and Rheumatism* **15**, 116–17.

Little, H., Harvie, J.N., and Lester, R.S. (1975). Psoriatic arthritis in severe psoriasis. *Canadian Medical Association Journal* **112**, 317–19.

Lomholt, G. Psoriasis: prevalence, spontaneous course and genetics. A census study on the prevalence of skin diseases in the Faroe Islands. Copenhagen: GEC CAD, 1963.

Lundberg, L., Johannesson, M., Silverdahl, M., Hermansson, C., Lindberg, M. (2000). Health-related quality of life in patients with psoriasis and atopic dermatitis measured with SF-36, DLQI and a subjective measure of disease activity. *Acta Dermato Venerologica* **80**, 430–4.

Luxembourg, A., Cailla, H., Roux, H., and Roudier, J. (1987). Do viruses play an etiologic role in ankylosing spondylitis and psoriatic arthritis? *Clinical Immunology and Immunopathology* **45**, 292–5.

Mader, R. et al. (1995). Injectable gold for the treatment of psoriatic arthritis—long term follow-up. *Clinical Investigational Medicine* **18**, 139–43.

Marks, J.M. (1980). Psoriasis: utilizing the treatment options. *Drugs* **19**, 429–36.

Marsal, S., Armadans-Gil, L., Martinez, M., Gallardo, D., Ribera, A., and Lience, E. (1999). Clinical, radiographic and HLA associations as markers for different patterns of psoriatic arthritis. *Rheumatology (Oxford)* **38**, 332–7.

Matthews, D. et al. (1996). Evidence that a locus for familial psoriasis maps to chromosome 4q. *Nature Genetics* **13**, 231.

McGonagle, D. et al. (1999). Psoriatic arthritis. *Arthritis and Rheumatism* **42**, 1080–6.

Mease, P.J., Goffe, B.S., Metz, J., VanderStoep, A., Finck, B., and Burge, D.J. (2000). Etanercept in the treatment of psoriatic arthritis and psoriasis: a randomised trial. *Lancet* **356**, 385–90.

de Misa, R.F. et al. (1994). Psoriatic arthritis: one year of treatment with extracorporeal photochemotherapy. *Journal of the American Academy of Dermatology* **30**, 1037–8.

Moll, J.M. (1994). The place of psoriatic arthritis in the spondarthritides. *Baillière's Clinical Rheumatology* **8**, 395–417.

Moll, J.M. and Wright, V. (1973). Familial occurrence of PsA. *Annals of Rheumatic Diseases* **32**, 181–201.

Mulherin, D.M., FitzGerald, O., and Bresnihan, B. (1993). Lymphedema of the upper limb in patients with psoriatic arthritis. *Seminars in Arthritis and Rheumatism* **22**, 350–6.

Nair, R.P. et al. (1997). Evidence for two psoriasis susceptibility loci (HLA and 17q) and two novel candidate regions (16q and 20p) by genome-wide scan. *Human Molecular Genetics* **6**, 1349–56.

O'Neill, T. and Silman, A.J. (1994). Historical background and epidemiology. *Baillière's Clinical Rheumatology* **8**, 245–61.

Paiva, E.S., Macaluso, D.C., Edwards, A., and Rosenbaum, J.T. (2000). Characterisation of uveitis in patients with psoriatic arthritis. *Annals of Rheumatic Diseases* **59**, 67–70.

Palit, J. et al. (1990). A multicentre double-blind comparison of auranofin, intramuscular gold thiomalate and placebo in patients with psoriatic arthritis. *British Journal of Rheumatology* **29**, 280–3.

Panayi, G. (1994). Immunology of psoriasis and psoriatic arthritis. *Baillière's Clinical Rheumatology* **8**, 419–27.

Perlman, S.G. et al. (1979). Photochemotherapy and psoriatic arthritis. A prospective study. *Annals of Internal Medicine* **91**, 717–22.

Peterson, A.W. and Shepherd, J.P. (1992). Facia lata interpositional arthroplasty in the treatment of tempomandibular joint ankylosis caused by psoriatic arthritis. *International Journal of Oral Maxillofactory Surgery* **21**, 137–9.

Prinz, J.C. (2001). Psoriasis vulgaris—a sterile antibacterial skin reaction mediated by cross-reactive T cells? An immunological view of the pathophysiology of psoriasis. *Clinical and Experimental Dermatology* **26**, 326–32.

Punzi, I. et al. (1998). Clinical, laboratory and immunogenetic aspects of post-traumatic psoriatic arthritis: a study of 25 patients. *Clinical and Experimental Rheumatology* **16**, 277–81.

Rahman, P., Gladman, D.D., Zhou, Y., and Cook, R.J. (1998). The use of sulfasalazine in psoriatic arthritis: a clinic experience. *Journal of Rheumatology* **25**, 1957–61.

Rahman, P., Nguyen, E., Cheung, C., Schentag, C.T., and Gladman, D.D. (2001). Comparison of radiological severity in psoriatic arthritis and rheumatoid arthritis. *Journal of Rheumatology* **28**, 1041–4.

Resnick, D. and Niwayama, G., ed. Psoriatic arthritis. In *Diagnosis of Bone and Joint Disorders*, pp. 1103–29. Philadelphia PA: W.B. Saunders Co, 1981.

Ritchlin, C. et al. (1998). Patterns of cytokine production in psoriatic synovium. *Journal of Rheumatology* **25**, 1544–52.

Roberts, M.E.T., Wright, V., Hill, A.G.S., and Mehra, A.C. (1976). Psoriatic arthritis: A follow-up study. *Annals of the Rheumatic Diseases* **35**, 206–19.

Roux, H., Schiano, A., Maestracci, D., and Serratrice, G. (1979). Notre experience du traitement du rheumatisme psoriasique par la D-penicillamine. *Revue du Rheumatisme* **46**, 631–3.

Sakkas, L.I., Loqueman, N., Bird, H., Vaughan, R.W., Welsh, K.I., and Panayi, G.S. (1990). HLA class II and T cell receptor gene polymorphisms in psoriatic arthritis and psoriasis. *Journal of Rheumatology* **17**, 1487–90.

Sakkas, L.I. et al. (1991). Immunoglobulin heavy chain gene polymorphism in Italian patients with psoriasis and psoriatic arthritis. *British Journal of Rheumatology* **30**, 449–50.

Salvarani, C. et al. (1992a). The cervical spine in patients with psoriatic arthritis: a clinical, radiological and immunogenetic study. *Annals of the Rheumatic Diseases* **51**, 73–7.

Salvarani, C. et al. (1992b). Low dose cyclosporin A: relation between soluble interleukin-2 receptors and response to therapy. *Journal of Rheumatology* **19**, 74–9.

Salvarani, C. et al. (1995). Prevalence of psoriatic arthritis in Italian patients with psoriasis. *Journal of Rheumatology* **22**, 1499–503.

Salvarani, C. et al. (1997). Isolated peripheral enthesitis and/or dactylitis: a subset of psoriatic arthritis. *Journal of Rheumatology* **24**, 1106–10.

Samuelsson, L. et al. (1999). A genome-wide search for genes predisposing to familial psoriasis by using a stratification approach. *Human Genetics* **105**, 523–9.

Scarpa, R. (2000). Discovertebral erosions and destruction in psoriatic arthritis. *Journal of Rheumatology* **27**, 975–8.

Scarpa, R., Oriente, P., Pulino, A., Torella, M., Vignone, L., Riccio, A., and Biondi-Oriente, C. (1984). Psoriatic arthritis in psoriatic patients. *British Journal of Rheumatology* **23**, 246–50.

Scarpa, R., Oriente, P., Pucino, A., Vignone, L., Cosentini, E., Minerva, A., and Biondi-Oriente, C. (1988). The clinical spectrum of psoriatic spondylitis. *British Journal of Rheumatology* **27**, 123–37.

Scarpa, R. et al. (1992). Interplay between environmental factors, articular involvement, and HLA-B27 in patients with psoriatic arthritis. *Annals of the Rheumatic Diseases* **51**, 78–9.

Shbeeb, M., Uramoto, K.M., Gibson, L.E., O'Fallon, W.M., and Gabriel, S.E. (2000). The epidemiology of psoriatic arthritis in Olmsted County, Minnesota, USA, 1982–1991. *Journal of Rheumatology* **27**, 1247–50.

Soyland, E. et al. (1993). Effect of dietary supplementation with very-long-chain n-3 fatty acids in patients with psoriasis. *New England Journal of Medicine* **328**, 1812–16.

Smith, D.L. and White, C.R., Jr. (1994). Pyoderma gangrenosum in association with psoriatic arthritis. *Arthritis and Rheumatism* **37**, 1258–60.

Spadarao, A. et al. (1995). Comparison of cyclosporin A and methotrexate in the treatment of psoriatic arthritis: a one-year prospective study. *Clinical and Experimental Rheumatology* **13**, 589–93.

Stern, R.S. (1985). The epidemiology of joint complaints in patients with psoriasis. *Journal of Rheumatology* **12**, 315–20.

Taglione, E. et al. (1999). Hepatitis C virus infection: prevalence in psoriasis and psoriatic arthritis. *Journal of Rheumatology* **26**, 370–2.

Tassiulas, I. et al. (1999). Clonal characteristics of T cell infiltrates in skin and synovium of patients with psoriatic arthritis. *Human Immunology* **60**, 479–91.

Thomssen, H., Hoffmann, B., Schank, M., Elewaut, D., Meyer zum Buschenfelde, K.H., and Marker-Hermann, E. (2000). There is no disease-specific role for streptococci-responsive synovial T lymphocytes in the pathogenesis of psoriatic arthritis. *Medical Microbiology and Immunology (Berlin)* **188**, 203–7.

Tomfohrdre, J. et al. (1994). Gene for familial psoriasis susceptibility mapped to the distal end of human chromosome 17q. *Science* **264**, 1141–5.

Torre-Alonso, J.C. et al. (1991). Psoriatic arthritis (PA): a clinical, immunological and radiological study of 180 patients. *British Journal of Rheumatology* **30**, 245–50.

Trabace, S., Cappellacci, S., Ciccarone, P., Liaskos, S., Polito, R., and Zorzin, L. (1994). Psoriatic arthritis: a clinical, radiological and genetic study of 58 Italian patients. *Acta Dermato Venerelogica* **186** (Suppl.), 69–70.

Trembath, R.C. et al. (1997). Identification of a major susceptibility locus on chromosome 6p an evidence for further disease loci revealed by two stage genome-wide search in psoriasis. *Human Molecular Genetics* **6**, 813–20.

Vasey, F.B. (1985). Etiology and pathogenesis of psoriatic arthritis. In *Psoriatic Arthritis* (ed. L.H. Gerber and L.R. Espinoza), pp. 45–57. Orlando FL: Grune & Stratton.

Vasey, F.B., Seleznick, M.J., Fenske, N.A., and Espinoza, L.R. (1989). New signposts on the road to understanding psoriatic arthritis. *Journal of Rheumatology* **16**, 1405–7.

Veal, C.D. et al. (2001). Identification of a novel psoriasis susceptibility locus at 1p and evidence of epistasis between PSORI1 and candidate loci. *Journal of Medical Genetics* **38**, 7–13.

Veale, D., Barrell, M., and Fitzgerald, O. (1993a). Mechanisms of joint sparing in a patient with unilateral psoriatic arthritis and a long-standing hemiplegia. *British Journal of Rheumatology* **32**, 413–16.

Veale, D., Yanni, G., Rogers, S., Barnes L, Bresnihan, B., and Fitzgerald, O. (1993b). Reduced synovial membrane macrophage numbers, ELAM-1 expression, and lining layer hyperplasia in psoriatic arthritis as compared with rheumatoid arthritis. *Arthritis and Rheumatism* **36**, 893–900.

Veale, D.J., Barnes, L., Rogers, S., and FitzGerald, O. (1994a). Immunohistochemical markers for arthritis in psoriasis. *Annals of the Rheumatic Diseases* **53**, 450–4.

Veale, D., Rogers, S., and Fitzgerald, O. (1994b). Classification of clinical subsets in psoriatic arthritis. *British Journal of Rheumatology* **33**, 133–8.

Veale, D.J. et al. (1994c). A double-blind placebo controlled trial of efamol marine on skin and joint symptoms of psoriatic arthritis. *British Journal of Rheumatology* **33**, 954–8.

Vilanova, X. and Pinol, J. (1951). Psoriasis arthropathica. *Rheumatism* **7**, 197–208.

Willkens, R.F. et al. (1984). Randomized, double-blind, placebo controlled trial of low-dose pulse methotrexate in psoriatic arthritis. *Arthritis and Rheumatism* **27**, 376–81.

Wong, K., Gladman, D.D., Husted, J., Long, J., and Farewell, V.T. (1997). Mortality studies in psoriatic arthritis. Results from a single centre. I. Risk and causes of death. *Arthritis and Rheumatism* **40**, 1868–72.

Wright, V. (1956). Psoriasis and Arthritis. *Annals of the Rheumatic Diseases* **15**, 348–53.

Wright, V. and Moll, J.M.H. (1971). Psoriatic arthritis. *Bulletin of Rheumatic Diseases* **21**, 627–32.

Wright, V. and Moll, J.M.H., ed. Psoriatic arthritis. In *Seronegative Polyarthritis* pp. 169–223. Amsterdam: North Holland Publishing Co., 1976.

Wright, V., Roberts, M.C., and Hill, A.G.S. (1979). Dermatological manifestations in psoriatic arthritis: a follow-up study. *Acta Dermato Venerologica* **59**, 235–40.

Wrone-Smith, T. and Nickoloff, B.J. (1996). Dermal injection of immunocytes induces psoriasis. *Journal of Clinical Investigation* **98**, 1878–87.

Zacharias, H. and Zacharias, E. (1987). Methotrexate treatment of psoriatic arthritis. *Acta Dermato Venerologica* **67**, 270–3.

Zanelli, M.D. and Wilde, J.S. (1992). Joint complaints in psoriasis patients. *International Journal of Dermatology* **31**, 488–91.

Zangger, P., Gladman, D.D., and Bogoch, E.R. (1998). Musculoskeletal surgery in psoriatic arthritis. *Journal of Rheumatology* **25**, 725–9.

Zangger, P., Esufali, Z.H., Gladman, D.D., and Bogoch, E.R. (2000). Type and outcome of reconstructive surgery for different patterns of PsA. *Journal of Rheumatology* **27**, 967–74.

6.4.5 Reactive arthritis and enteropathic arthropathy

J.S. Hill Gaston

Definitions

The term 'reactive arthritis' is often used rather loosely to cover any form of arthritis which can be linked to preceding infection. This produces a large group of diseases with little in common as far as their clinical features or pathogenesis are concerned, for example, post-viral arthritis, post-streptococcal reactive arthritis, and Lyme disease. It is preferable to reserve the term 'reactive arthritis' for a clearly identified clinical syndrome which falls naturally within the spondyloarthropathies on clinical, immunogenetic, and pathogenetic grounds. This syndrome is usually triggered by a relatively small number of organisms and forms an important part of the differential diagnosis of acute oligo- and mono-arthritis (Table 1). Other forms of arthritis seen in relation to infection are best termed 'post-infectious'. In the past, reactive arthritis and post-infectious arthritis were proposed as terms to distinguish arthritis in which the organism could not be identified in the joint (reactive) from those in which it could (post-infectious) (Toivanen and Toivanen 1999), but this is no longer valid in view of recent investigations showing that organisms can indeed be demonstrated in reactive arthritis joints (see below).

There are several examples of disorders linking the gastrointestinal tract and arthritis, reactive arthritis following gastroenteritis being an obvious example, along with the arthritis associated with Crohn's disease or ulcerative colitis. Both of these are classified within the spondyloarthropathies, but other forms of arthritis are sometimes included in the 'enteropathic' grouping such as Whipple's disease, arthritis associated with coeliac disease, and other syndromes. This chapter will be divided into two sections, the first dealing with reactive arthritis, and the second with other forms of enteropathic arthritis.

Reactive arthritis

Historical perspective

An association between urethritis and arthritis has been known for nearly 500 years. Many authors attribute the first description of reactive arthritis to van Forest in the 1500s and a description in Spanish literature by Lopez de Hinojosos in Mexico City in 1578 has been recognized (Aceves-Avila et al. 1998). By the beginning of the nineteenth century the syndrome was clearly recognized, but inevitably in a pre-bacteriological era 'venereal arthritis' encompassed both post-gonococcal arthritis and true reactive arthritis. Nevertheless, some of the case descriptions, particularly those which mention prominent eye involvement, very likely represent reactive arthritis. Brodie described six cases in 1818 and a recent survey of early case records in London hospitals shows the condition was commonly recognized from 1820 onwards, accounting for a significant proportion of hospital admissions (Storey and Scott 1998).

A link between gastrointestinal infection and reactive arthritis was noted in the early years of the twentieth century and outbreaks of dysentery in the trenches of World War I led to classical descriptions by Fiessinger and Leroy in 1916, and also by Hans Reiter. Although the term 'Leroy–Fiessinger–Reiter syndrome' is sometimes encountered, it is the name of Reiter which has come to be associated with reactive arthritis and the terms have often been used interchangeably. There are several cogent reasons for bringing this practice to an end and abandoning the term 'Reiter's syndrome'. First, Reiter was clearly not the first to describe reactive arthritis; disease associated with dysentery was first reported by Vossius in 1904. Second, Reiter did not shed any useful light on its pathogenesis, erroneously attributing it to spirochetal infection. Third and more practically, the triad of arthritis, conjunctivitis, and urethritis/cervicitis has often been taken to imply that Reiter's syndrome is the form of reactive arthritis secondary to genitourinary infection, missing the point that the urethritis in his original description was also 'reactive' following bacillary dysentery. There are no prognostic implications associated with the classical triad and therefore no clinical value in singling out Reiter's syndrome as a sub-section of reactive arthritis. Lastly, several authors have felt the eponym inappropriate in view of some dubious aspects of Reiter's later medical career (Wallace and Weisman 2000).

Table 1 Infections that trigger arthritis

Reactive arthritis	Post-infectious arthritis
Common triggering infections	**Post-viral arthritis**
Salmonella	Parvovirus
Campylobacter	Rubella
Yersinia	Mumps
Shigella flexneri	HIV
Chlamydia trachomatis	Hepatitis B and C
Occasional triggering infections	Arboviruses
Chlamydia pneumoniae	Other case reports (e.g. Herperviruses)
Clostridium difficile	**Bacterial infection**
M. bovis BCG (intravesical)	Streptococcal
Mycoplasma spp. (e.g. *U. urealyticum*)	Rheumatic fever
Rare triggering infections	Post-streptococcal arthritis
Many case reports of infection, particularly of the intestine, including:	Neisseria
Giardia	Gonoccal arthritis
Crptosporidium	Meningococcal arthritis
Shigella sonnei	Lyme disease (*Borrelia* spp.)
Chlamydia psittaci	Brucella
Hafnia alvei	Whipple's disease (*Tropheryma whippelii*)
Vibrio parahaemolyticus etc.	

Case definition

Classification criteria for reactive arthritis present difficulties. Since reactive arthritis is one of the spondyloarthropathies, criteria such as those devised by Amor et al. (1990) or the European Spondyloarthropathy Study Group (Dougados et al. 1991) can be applied. Many cases of reactive arthritis, however, do not have sufficient features to satisfy the Amor criteria and, whilst most cases would meet the ESSG criteria, these are very wide ranging and do not allow reactive arthritis to be distinguished from undifferentiated spondyloarthropathy. Criteria proposed in the past have often emphasized urethritis or cervicitis, in an attempt to delineate Reiter's syndrome (Willkens et al. 1981). Unfortunately all current criteria fail to deal adequately with cases with no preceding symptomatic gastrointestinal or genitourinary infection. In these cases, a link to preceding infection depends on adequate laboratory investigation (see below). Whilst diagnostic and classification criteria continue to be debated (Hulsemann and Zeidler 1999; Pachecotena et al. 1999), a suggested working definition is presented in Table 2. This groups patients with: (i) classical clinical features (oligoarthritis, predominantly of the lower limbs with extra-articular signs, including enthesitis) and proven infection with one of the organisms known to trigger reactive arthritis, *irrespective* of preceding symptoms; (ii) patients in whom preceding infection is proven, even though the arthritis has no diagnostic features; and (iii) patients with classical clinical features in whom a bacteriological diagnosis cannot be proven. This avoids separating patients with identical clinical manifestations on the basis of the skills of the microbiological laboratory, or failing to include patients with new inflammatory disease of joints or entheses after proven, but asymptomatic, infection with reactive arthritis-associated organisms. The latter are often seen in follow-up of cohorts of patients infected in food poisoning outbreaks. Indeed in a recent series, the proportion of patients in whom a triggering infection could be identified after appropriate investigations was very similar in patients with a preceding symptomatic infection and those with no such history (Fendler et al. 2001). Practically, it is worth considering the diagnosis of reactive

Table 2 Working definition of reactive arthritis

Classical clinical features: asymmetric oligoarthritis, lower limbs predominate enthesitis extra-articular signs and proven infection by *Salmonella, Camplyobacter, Yersinia,* Shigella, or *Chlamydia trachomatis* (whether symptomatic or not)
Classical clinical features and proven infection by other organisms (e.g. *Clostridium difficile, Mycobacterium bovis* BCG)
Any acute inflammatory arthritis (including monoarthritis) and proven infection by ReA-associated bacteria
Classical clinical features and preceding diarrhoea or urethritis/cervicitis, infection not proven

arthritis in any patient presenting for the first time with acute oligo- or monoarticular synovitis in whom no other diagnosis (sepsis, crystal arthropathies, etc.) is evident. This allows an adequate history, physical examination, and diagnostic tests to be performed, so that a definite diagnosis of reactive arthritis can be made.

Epidemiology

Given the difficulties in case definition, accurate epidemiological studies on incidence and prevalence present problems. There are two possible approaches. In the first, the proportion of patients with reactive arthritis can be measured in clinics designed to examine all cases of early synovitis. One such study in Oslo measured an incidence of 9.6 per 100 000, equally divided between cases due to *Chlamydia trachomatis* and enteric infection (Kvien et al. 1994). Previous estimates of chlamydia-induced arthritis of 5 per 100 000 have also been recorded (Kvien et al. 1995). The difficulty with this approach is that it cannot take account of mild cases not referred to early synovitis clinics, or cases where arthritis is short lived. The alternative approach has been to take advantage of food poisoning outbreaks where an entire population infected with an organism at a particular time is followed up prospectively. Patients are sent questionnaires on the occurrence of subsequent arthritic symptoms, and those reporting symptoms examined by a rheumatologoist. Although the incidence of reactive arthritis in food poisoning outbreaks varies substantially, several series report an incidence of 5–25 per cent (Tertti et al. 1984; Inman et al. 1988; Mattila et al. 1998; Ekman et al. 2000; McColl et al. 2000), with an additional percentage of patients developing arthritic symptoms but not meeting criteria for reactive arthritis. These figures are interesting in relation to a recent comprehensive UK study on the community incidence of enteric infections in a population of 460 000 (Wheeler et al. 1999). This showed a combined incidence of campylobacter, salmonella, and yersinia infection confirmed by stool culture of 17.7 per 1000. Interestingly, particularly for yersinia, the number of cases identified in the community survey was substantially higher than those from the same population who presented to their family physician. This means that many of the cases of yersinia infection were too mild to require medical attention. Combining these results would give an estimate of reactive arthritis in the community of 100–200 per 100 000, and this would not include cases induced by chlamydia. Although a large proportion of these cases might have relatively trivial self-limiting disease, the figures suggest that the incidence calculated on the basis of patients seen at early synovitis clinics is a serious underestimate.

The incidence of reactive arthritis may be declining, and for chlamydia-associated arthritis this has been attributed to increased use of barrier contraceptives because of fears of HIV infection (Iliopoulos et al. 1995). However, the overall incidence of chlamydia infection has not declined substantially in western countries—the incidence in the United Kingdom nearly doubled through the 1990s to 50 000 cases per year. This suggests that other factors may be affecting the incidence of chlamydia-induced arthritis. Infections with salmonella and campylobacter have also increased substantially in recent years without a notable increase in the incidence of reactive arthritis, again pointing to additional factors affecting the incidence of arthritis. These could include prior exposure to related organisms, for example, infection with *Chlamydia pneumoniae,* which has declined with improved socio-economic conditions. Previously, many patients infected with *C. trachomatis* would previously have experienced *C. pneumoniae* infection in childhood and might be primed to make an arthritogenic immune response to chlamydia antigens.

Pathogenesis

Since reactive arthritis is a member of the spondyloarthropathy group, pathogenesis of these conditions can be considered together, and is discussed elsewhere (see Chapters 6.4.1, 6.4.2, and 6.4.3). However, its clear association with infection by known bacteria, and its usual acute presentation, means that reactive arthritis lends itself to investigation, and much work has been done in the last 20 years. From this, three factors have emerged as critical to pathogenesis: the infecting organism, the immune response elicited by infection, particularly that mounted by T lymphocytes, and genetic influences, principally HLA B27. Interestingly, all of these are important in rodent HLA B27 transgenic models of spondyloarthropathy (Khare et al. 1995; Taurog et al. 1999); arthritis requires infection (gut flora rather than specific pathogens), T lymphocytes (especially CD4+ T cells), and an appropriate genetic background apart from transgenic B27 since disease incidence varies in different rodent strains.

The list of bacteria which *commonly* cause reactive arthritis is quite short (Table 1). Another set of organisms has been implicated in reactive arthritis on multiple occasions, but their contribution to reactive arthritis incidence is relatively small. Lastly, there are many single case reports implicating particular infections. In these cases, there is always uncertainty about whether the organism provoked true reactive arthritis or simply a post-infectious arthritis, but where extra-articular features are present (as distinct from only B27), the reports are convincing. It is noticeable that even very similar organisms such as *Shigella flexnerii* and *Shigella sonnei* are associated with very different rates of reactive arthritis (common in the former and very rare in the latter). These observations indicate that specific properties of the bacterium play an important role in disease induction.

Contrary to previous expectations, there is now substantial evidence that bacteria or their antigens reach affected joints. Bacterial antigens were first demonstrated in phagocytic cells within the joint using immunofluorescence and immunoblotting techniques (Granfors et al. 1989, 1990; MerilahtiPalo et al. 1991). This has been shown for salmonella, yersinia, and shigella, and since phagocytic cells and peripheral blood were also shown to contain antigen (Granfors et al. 1998), it seems likely that there is traffic from the site of infection to the affected joint. Most studies to demonstrate nucleic acids of enteric bacteria in reactive arthritis joints have been negative (Nikkari et al. 1992, 1999; Ekman et al. 1999), but recently, using the more sensitive technique of RT PCR, ribosomal RNA from *Yersinia pseudotuberculosis* was unequivocally demonstrated in a reactive arthritis joint (Gaston et al. 1999). The demonstration of bacterial RNA is particularly important since unlike DNA this has a relatively short half life and its presence implies that live, transcriptionally active organisms can reach the joint. Evidence that intact *C. trachomatis* reaches the joint is much stronger, with detection by both PCR and RT PCR (Taylor-Robinson et al. 1992; Schumacher et al. 1997) and the demonstration of organisms (albeit with atypical morphology) by electron microscopy or immunofluorescence (Schumacher et al. 1988). Interestingly, in all these studies evidence for organisms or their antigens in the joint has been obtained long after the initial infection, strongly suggesting that these organisms can persist at low levels, perhaps in sites such as gut associated lymphoid tissue. This persistence may relate to their ability to survive intracellularly. Such persistence has been demonstrated, even after 'curative' antibiotics, but dormant intracellular organisms which divide infrequently may be relatively insensitive to conventional antibiotics.

Affected joints in reactive arthritis have a substantial infiltrating T-cell population, including both CD4+ and CD8+ T cells (BeacockSharp et al. 1998). Some of these T cells may have trafficked from the gut or genitourinary tract because the synovium shares 'addressins' (molecules which determine which T cells are recruited) with the mucosal associated lymphoid tissue (Salmi et al. 1995). Prominent responses to arthritis triggering bacteria have been demonstrated in both populations, most work having been done on the experimentally more tractable CD4+ T cells (Gaston et al. 1989; Sieper et al. 1993). Organism-specific clones have been obtained and their specificities identified (Gaston et al. 1990; Viner et al. 1991; Mertz et al. 1994); in several studies bacterial hsp60 has emerged as a major target antigen (Gaston et al. 1989; Hermann et al. 1991), although this is a common feature of cell-mediated responses to intracellular bacteria. Whether any of these T-cell responses causes arthritis is unclear. The attractive idea that bacteria-specific CD8 T cells restricted by HLA B27 would make an autoreactive response to a joint-specific antigen has not yet received experimental support, although yersinia-reactive, B27-restricted T-cell clones have been isolated from reactive arthritis joints (Hermann et al. 1993). Analysis of T-cell receptor expression has shown expansions of multiple clones in both CD4+ and CD8+ subsets of blood and joint (Allen et al. 1997), with CD8+ expansions commonest in the joint. It may be that both subsets are involved in disease. Interestingly, in the reactive arthritis which frequently occurs in HIV-infected individuals in Sub-Saharan Africa, the arthritis is associated with modest diminution in CD4+ T-cell counts rather than profound levels of CD4 T-cell depletion (Njobvu et al. 1998), suggesting that CD4 T cells are required for arthritis—an observation in agreement with B27 transgenic models (Khalil et al. 1997). The cytokines produced by synovial bacteria-specific T cells are generally proinflammatory (interferon-γ, IL-17) (Schlaak et al. 1992; Kotake et al. 1999). IL-4 producing T cells have been demonstrated in some studies, leading to the suggestion that this is an inappropriate T cell response which would inhibit clearance of the organism from the joint (Simon et al. 1994). However, in view of the dominance of interferon-γ producing T cells this seems unlikely.

HLA B27 is associated with the occurrence of reactive arthritis (Aho et al. 1973; Brewerton et al. 1973), but more strikingly with severe disease (Ekmal et al. 2000). Patients with prolonged course, recurrent attacks or evolution to chronic arthropathy are very likely to be B27+ (Leirisalo-Repo et al. 1997). However, B27 is not necessary for reactive arthritis to develop and ascertaining B27 status is not useful diagnostically, although it may help predict prognosis. How B27 acts remains frustratingly unclear. As noted, the idea that disease depends on B27-restricted autoreactive T cells has neither been proven nor refuted. Various experiments have pointed to an influence of HLA B27 on intracellular infection (Granfors 1998; Ikawa et al. 1998). Conversely, others have highlighted unusual properties of HLA B27 which might interact with intracellular infection; these include relatively slow transit from the endoplasmic reticulum to the surface (Mear et al. 1999), a tendency for expression of B27 molecules which do not contain bound peptide and could therefore receive exogenous peptides from microorganisms (Benjamin et al. 1991), and the expression of either free HLA B27 heavy chains or homodimers of heavy chains linked by disulfide bonding through the cysteine at position 67 (Allen et al. 1999).

Clinical features

Preceding illness

A history of urethritis (dysuria or discharge) or diarrhoea must be specifically sought for several reasons. The interval between these symptoms and the development of arthritis means that patients may not connect these apparently unrelated events. Secondly, preceding infection may be virtually asymptomatic. Chlamydia infection in women is notoriously silent, and in men these symptoms or a sexual history are often not volunteered spontaneously. Of gastrointestinal infections, salmonella is likely to produce symptoms in those who go on to reactive arthritis (Mattila et al. 1998), whereas in yersinia-related arthritis many patients have sub-clinical or mild gastrointestinal symptoms (Leirisalo et al. 1982).

Arthritis

Reactive arthritis is usually an asymmetric oligoarthritis, generally involving less than six joints, with a tendency to affect the lower limbs preferentially. However, any joint can be affected and a proportion of patients have monoarthritis. Some patients may have arthralgias at sites in addition to those affected by synovitis. Affected joints generally become rapidly hot and swollen and large effusions can develop in the knee. The evolution of joint involvement is such as to make septic arthritis or crystal-induced arthritis likely differential diagnoses. There is a real possibility of patients being treated for a culture-negative septic arthritis if a full history is not obtained from the patient or careful examination made for features of reactive arthritis, particularly extra-articular signs. The arthritis also has features seen in other forms of spondyloarthropathy; thus dactylitis, resembling that seen in psoriatic arthritis occurs in reactive arthritis. Many patients experience low back or buttock pain often due to acute sacroiliitis. The arthritis is generally most severe in the first few weeks following its onset, followed by substantial improvement over the next few weeks. However, mild but significant symptoms often persist 6–12 months before full resolution. Patients need reassurance during this phase that complete resolution is still probable. In addition, not all patients experience a 'monophasic' disease and both exacerbations and involvement of new joints can occur, even in those in whom the disease eventually settles completely.

Extra-articular disease

One of the characteristic features of spondyloarthropathies is the presence of enthesitis (inflammation of ligamentous and tendinous insertions) and it has even been argued that synovitis in spondyloarthropathies is secondary to enthesitis (McGonagle et al. 1998). Whether or not this is so, the presence of enthesitis is often helpful in making a diagnosis of reactive arthritis, with the Tendo Achilles insertion and plantar fascia the commonest sites of involvement. Enthesitis may be mild, particularly in relation to active synovitis at other sites, and so the patient may not report symptoms, particularly if not weight-bearing. Other ligamentous insertions involving the pelvis and chest wall may be symptomatic, and some low back symptoms may represent enthesitis.

Conjunctivitis is a classical feature of reactive arthritis but is usually painless and often transitory. It may not be evident when the patient presents with arthritis and a history should be sought from the patient (or relatives who may have noticed red eyes). Persistent eye inflammation and painful eyes raises the question of acute anterior uveitis but this is much less common in reactive arthritis. It requires full ophthalmological assessment.

Skin and mucous membranes can be involved. Keratoderma blennorhagica is histologically identical to psoriasis, and is most commonly seen on the soles of the feet, although it can also involve the hands and trunk. Its site, and the fact that it is painless, means that again it needs to be sought directly since patients may not have noticed it. Balanitis is also asymptomatic and may not be readily apparent, particularly in uncircumcised males. The occurrence of balanitis, like urethritis, does not imply a genitourinary aetiology for the reactive arthritis. Ulcerative lesions in the mouth and soft palate are also seen but, again, are usually asymptomatic. Lastly, erythema nodosum has been noted in reactive arthritis associated with yersinia (Plates 106–108).

In general, extra-articular disease is associated with severity of arthritis, a less favourable prognosis, and HLA B27 positivity. The most severe extra-articular manifestations are aortitis and cardiac conduction disorders but fortunately these are rare. Table 3 shows the frequency of joint and extra-articular involvement in a number of series of reactive arthritis patients.

Differential diagnoses

Differential diagnoses are listed in Table 4. In patients who present with an acute arthritis, the principal differential diagnoses are septic arthritis and crystal arthropathies. Other forms of post-infectious arthritis enter the differential, particularly post-gonococcal or post-meningococcal arthritis, along with arthritis due to streptococci and Lyme disease. Whilst streptococcal infection rarely gives rise to rheumatic fever, except under conditions

Table 3 Frequency (%) of extra-articular signs in reactive arthritis[a]

Lesion	Enteric infection	Sexually acquired infection
Keratoderma and psoriaform lesions	1–2	10–30
Circinate balanitis	5–25; higher in Shigella	40–70
Conjunctivitis	6–20; higher in Shigella	25–40
Oral ulcers	2–5	10–30
Erythema nodosum	7 (mainly Yersinia)	0
Reactive urethritis	10–30	N/A

[a] Data from Angulo and Espinoza (1998) combined with other published series.

Table 4 Differential diagnosis of reactive arthritis

Septic arthritis
Post-infectious arthritis Lyme disease Post-streptococcal or Neisseria infection Viral arthritis
Crystal arthropathies
Other spondyloarthopathies SAPHO
Behçet's disease
Sarcoidosis
Trauma, sports injury

of social deprivation, an inflammatory oligoarthritis strongly resembling reactive arthritis is seen (Deighton 1993) but classical extra-articular features are not present. In sub-acute disease, it is sometimes difficult to distinguish reactive arthritis from other forms of spondyloarthropathy, particularly if there is no history of preceding infection and no laboratory evidence to implicate specific infections. The term 'undifferentiated spondyloarthropathy' is rightly applied to these cases, with the possibility that psoriasis or inflammatory bowel disease will declare themselves as time goes on.

One condition with some similarities to the spondyloarthropathies, including reactive arthritis, is the SAPHO syndrome, a term introduced by Chamot and colleagues in 1987, for patients with arthritis/osteitis together with various skin conditions. The condition was previously often termed chronic recurrent multifocal osteomyelitis; the eponym comprises: Synovitis, Acne (particularly major forms such as Acne conglobata, Acne fulminans or even hidradenitis suppurativa), Palmoplantar pustulosis (50–60 per cent have this or another form of psoriasis), Hyperostosis, and Osteitis. Thus features in common with reactive arthritis include sterile synovitis, pustulosis, enthesopathy (e.g. anterior chest pain) and involvement of the sacroiliac joint (33 per cent of patients). A minority of SAPHO patients also have inflammatory bowel disease, mainly Crohn's disease. The relationship of SAPHO to other spondyloarthropathies has been debated but no striking association with HLA-B27 has been demonstrated. The involvement of bacteria, particularly *P. acnes* has been postulated, and is an attractive possibility in view of the skin pathology. Like reactive arthritis the joint and bone lesions are generally sterile, though there are reports of the isolation of *P. acnes* or its demonstration by PCR, so there may be similar pathogenic mechanisms at work in both diseases even if they have different underlying genetic susceptibility factors (Kahn 1994; Hayem 1999).

Laboratory investigations

Investigations are directed towards excluding the major differential diagnoses, and thereafter trying to establish the organism responsible for triggering the disease.

General investigations

In acute reactive arthritis severe enough to present to hospital, there is usually a major acute phase response (ESR $>$ 100, CRP 100–200 mg/l) and neutrophilia. Other biochemical investigations are not generally helpful, although serum urate should be checked. Classical autoantibodies such as rheumatoid factor and antinuclear antibodies are absent, and although positive anti-neutrophil cytoplasmic antibodies have been described (Schultz et al. 2000), they are not diagnostically useful. The antibodies are not directed against proteinase-3 or myeloperoxidase, unlike those seen in Wegener's granulomatosis and microscopic polyangiitis.

Microbiology

Tests to exclude septic arthritis or other forms of post-infectious arthritis

Microscopy, Gram stain and culture of synovial fluid is the single most important investigation to diagnose septic arthritis, together with blood cultures and culture of any other possible site of infection, including throat swab for streptococci. Application of PCR techniques may establish the triggering agent in reactive arthritis (see below), but may also be helpful in the diagnosis of mycobacterial infection, borreliosis and Whipple's disease. Antibody responses to streptococcal antigens, including both anti-streptolysin and anti-DNaseB should be sought, along with antibodies to *Borrelia* in patients who have been in endemic areas. Viral antibodies may also be checked.

Identification of reactive arthritis associated organisms

An excellent account of microbiological tests useful in the diagnosis of reactive arthritis is available (Wollenhaupt et al. 1998). By definition, reactive arthritis and associated bacteria are not cultured from affected joints, but the organisms may be identified by culture of stool in enteric arthritis and of swabs from the genitourinary tract or urine in chlamydia infection. Nucleic acid amplification techniques are now favoured for diagnosing chlamydia infection and avoid invasive swabs whilst maintaining high sensitivity. Their use should allow a higher proportion of patients with chlamydia-induced reactive arthritis to be positively diagnosed. There is much interest in using PCR to identify organisms in infected joints, and chlamydia has been found in synovium or synovial fluid of a high proportion of patients with chlamydia-induced arthritis. Nevertheless, identification of chlamydia in an inflamed joint does not establish a diagnosis of chlamydia-triggered reactive arthritis, since chlamydiae have been demonstrated by PCR in patients with other forms of inflammatory arthritis, including rheumatoid disease (Schumacher et al. 1988, 1999). This result is not surprising since, in populations in whom chlamydia infection is frequent, chlamydiae may well traffic to affected joints in the same way that they do in reactive arthritis. Attempts to demonstrate enteric organisms in affected joints by PCR have generally been negative, although a recent study established that this could occur for yersinia-triggered disease (Gaston et al. 1999). The possibility of reactive arthritis triggered by *C. pneumoniae* is now under investigation (Hannu et al. 1999) and PCR studies may help to clarify its role. Again the question of non-specific trafficking of an organism to an inflamed joint arises, particularly since this organism is known to disseminate, having been isolated from many arterial sites, particularly those affected by atherosclerosis (Saikku 2000).

Serological techniques can also be used to establish preceding infection. Current chlamydia serology is unsatisfactory since there are difficulties in distinguishing antibodies to *C. trachomatis* and *C. pneumoniae*, and the incidence of antibodies to the latter can be very high in the general population. Specialized techniques measuring antibody bound to purified organisms, and comparing the titre of antibodies to *C. trachomatis* and *C. pneumoniae* can establish specificity, but are not used routinely. New techniques using recombinant chlamydial antigens may in the near future allow more specific and sensitive serological testing for chlamydial infection.

There are also problems with the serology of enteric infections, mainly because the general population commonly encounters organisms such as salmonella and campylobacter in foods such as chicken and eggs and may develop antibodies (Maki et al. 1992). In acute disease, measurement of specific IgM (the Widal test) can be useful but has low sensitivity. Since high titres of IgG antibodies to organisms such as salmonella or campylobacter are not uncommon in the general population, it is preferable to demonstrate a rising titre of IgG antibodies or high levels of persistent IgA antibodies to the organism of interest. IgA has a shorter half-life than IgG, so persistence of high titres of specific IgA antibodies are often taken to indicate persistent infection (Granfors and Toivanen 1986), and therefore more useful in making a diagnosis of reactive arthritis than IgG antibodies which merely confirm previous encounter with the organism. In the near future, antibodies to recombinant antigens may allow more accurate serological diagnosis, particularly if arthritis is associated with hyper-responsiveness to particular protiens, as seen in chronic Lyme disease in which OspA is targetted (Kalish et al. 1993).

Reactive arthritis triggering organisms also elicit prominent T-cell mediated responses and the possibility of these being useful diagnostically has been considered (Fendler et al. 1998). The responses are most easily detectable in synovial fluid, but because they only demonstrate T-cell memory for the organism, they cannot provide more than supporting evidence that a particular episode of arthritis is due to an organism recognized by synovial fluid T cells. They may have some negative diagnostic value—it would be very unusual for a patient to have chlamydia-triggered reactive arthritis without a T-cell response to chlamydia being detectable in the joint. However, as noted in discussion of PCR tests, patients with rheumatoid arthritis can become infected with reactive arthritis associated organisms and will then have organism-specific T cells detectable in their affected joints.

In summary, for routine investigation of reactive arthritis stool should be cultured, chlamydia sought by PCR of urine, and antibodies to yersinia and camplyobacter measured. Other tests require further study for their validation.

Tissue typing

HLA B27 testing has no diagnostic value since reactive arthritis often occurs in B27-negative patients. However, it is still worth performing to help establish prognosis since this is less favourable in B27+ patients. These may warrant earlier treatment with disease modifying drugs (see below) or closer follow-up to detect chronic spondyloarthropathy.

Radiology

Radiological examination of acutely affected joints is not helpful in the diagnosis of reactive arthritis, but may aid in establishing differential diagnoses, for example, by showing chondrocalcinosis. Chest X-ray may reveal hilar adenopathy in sarcoidosis, or occasionally in yersinia infection which can cause a sarcoid-like illness. Although sacro-iliac joint involvement is common acutely in reactive arthritis, radiographic abnormality is not, and scintigraphy is useful to show activity at this site if there is doubt about the clinical diagnosis. This may also show inflammation at other entheses as may magnetic resonance imaging. Indeed, the latter has been used to document the predominance of involvement of entheses in the spondyloarthropathies (McGonagle et al. 1998). Ultrasonography is also useful to demonstrate enthesitis and to distinguish oedema of tendon and ligament insertions from bursitis (Lehtinen et al. 1994). In patients in whom disease persists, radiological changes can develop, with erosion of affected joints including the sacro-iliac joints, and the formation of new bone, which can be seen as either periostitis in the hands and feet or spur formation at entheses such as the plantar ligament insertion. Erosions may also be present at these same sites. In chronic reactive arthritis, paravertebral ossification may be seen in the lumbar spine; unlike ankylosing spondylitis this is often asymmetric. Atlanto-axial subluxation has also been described in chronic reactive arthritis.

Treatment

Symptomatic treatment

Patients require conventional measures to treat acutely inflamed joints, including non-steroidal drugs, joint aspiration with injection of depot steroid preparations (when septic arthritis has been excluded), together with analgesia and physiotherapy to maintain range of motion and regain the muscle power and bulk which is lost during acute inflammation. In severe disease, systemic corticosteroids may be used but injection of affected joints is preferable. Extra-articular disease does not call for specific treatment with the exception of uveitis which requires topical steroids. Of the triggering infections only chlamydia infection requires specific treatment in its own right, with conventional short term antibiotic regimes using tetracyclines or azithromycin.

Specific treatment

Current opinion on the pathogenesis of reactive arthritis would suggest two specific treatment strategies. If disease is maintained by persistent infection and trafficking of triggering organisms to affected joints and entheses, long-term antibiotics should hasten resolution of the disease. On the other hand, if disease is mainly maintained by an aberrant immune response triggered by infection but later directed against components of the joint, immunosuppressive treatment would be indicated. Unfortunately, evidence from therapeutic trials does not yet allow us to distinguish definitively between these hypotheses.

There have been several trials of prolonged doses of antibiotics in reactive arthritis. The first trial using lymecycline did not show efficacy overall, but a sub-group of patients with chlamydia-induced arthritis had a decreased duration (Lauhio et al. 1991). Patients with chronic yersinia infection, diagnosed by showing organisms in intestinal mucosa or gut lymphoid tissue, and with wider symptomatology than reactive arthritis, responded to ciprofloxacin in an uncontrolled trial. These findings prompted controlled trials but those in enteric reactive arthritis have shown no therapeutic advantage of three months treatment with ciprofloxacin (Sieper et al. 1999; Wakefield et al. 1999; YliKerttula et al. 2000). This does not necessarily imply that disease is not maintained by persistent infection since organisms may be relatively resistant to ciprofloxacin when not actively dividing. When tetracycline was used to treat episodes of non-gonococcal urethritis very promptly, there was a decrease in the number of episodes of reactive arthritis, but in this instance treatment begins prior to the onset of arthritis (Bardin et al. 1992). Animal models support the idea that arthritis might be prevented by early administration of antibiotics, although the window of opportunity may be small (Zhang et al. 1996). Currently, there is no evidence to suggest that patients presenting with reactive arthritis benefit from prolonged antibiotics but trials with different agents and design continue.

Disease modifying agents used in rheumatoid disease have also been tested in reactive arthritis, although such patients have often been included in larger groups with other forms of spondyloarthropathy (Dougados et al. 1995). One difficulty in these trials is that the rate of spontaneous remission in reactive arthritis is high and therefore large numbers of patients would need to be tested to have adequate power to show a therapeutic effect. If extrapolation from other forms of spondyloarthropathy is justified, both sulfasalazine and methotrexate should be useful, but the effect of sulfasalazine is relatively modest (Egsmose et al. 1997). Intravenous pamidronate may be useful in peripheral arthritis of spondyloarthropathy (Maksymowych et al. 2001). Therapies directed against TNFα, having proved useful in other forms of spondyloarthropathy (Brandt et al. 2000; Mease et al. 2000; VandenBosch et al. 2000), have recently been tested in a few patients with severe prolonged reactive arthritis and been effective, but further follow-up is awaited. It is reasonable to withhold disease modifying drugs for the first three months and reserve their use for those whose disease is not settling (particularly if they are B27+) or who have involvement of new joints.

Prognosis

Many of the patients with reactive arthritis are young, otherwise healthy, and used to an active life-style. To these individuals reactive arthritis, even when self-limiting, is a major life event, particularly since cases seen in hospital practice commonly take months to resolve. Patients therefore need considerable reassurance that there is an 80 per cent chance of complete resolution of their symptoms within the first year, with a further 10 per cent settling in the following year. Prognosis is less favourable in those who have disease severe enough to require hospitalization and who are B27+. Progression to chronic disease in 16 per cent was recorded in one series, with recurrent attacks of reactive disease in a further 22 per cent (Leirisalo-Repo et al. 1997; Leirisalo-Repo 1998). The tendency to trivialize the disease because its prognosis is generally so much better than that of rheumatoid arthritis needs to be resisted. Although many reactive arthritis patients may have future episodes of gastroenteritis or urethritis without recurrence of arthritis, it is advisable for patients to minimize their risk of recurrent infection, particularly younger patients who may need advice on foreign travel and barrier contraception.

Enteropathic arthropathy

Whilst reactive arthritis due to enteric infection falls within the definition of enteropathic arthritis, this section will discuss forms of arthritis other than reactive arthritis which are associated with gut inflammation. These include others within the spondyloarthropathy group, along with the arthritis associated with coeliac disease, and Whipple's disease (Utsinger et al. 1996).

Spondyloarthropathies associated with gut inflammation

Crohn's disease and ulcerative colitis

The association between inflammatory bowel disease (IBD) and arthropathy has long been recognized (Wright and Watkinson 1965; Haslock and Wright 1973). Although estimates of the incidence of arthritis vary, several large series from different geographical areas suggest approximately 10 per cent of IBD patients have peripheral arthritis, with a somewhat higher incidence in Crohn's disease as compared to ulcerative colitis. An additional proportion of patients (~5 per cent) have axial disease indistinguishable from ankylosing spondylitis, whilst asymptomatic sacroiliitis is even commoner (15–20 per cent). Arthritis in IBD is associated with other extra-gastrointestinal features, and is present in 30–60 per cent of patients with uveitis or skin lesions such as erythema nodosum and pyoderma gangrenosum. Arthritis is also commonly accompanied by enthesopathy, as seen in other spondyloarthropathies.

The idea of linkage between spondyloarthopathies and IBD is given greater credence by ileocolonoscopy studies which have shown that approximately 60 per cent of patients with ankylosing spondylitis or undifferentiated spondyloarthopathy have sub-clinical inflammatory lesions in the gut (Leirisalo-Repo et al. 1994; Mielants et al. 1996); a proportion of these patients progress to overt clinical inflammatory bowel disease. The situation has been further clarified by a recent sub-classification of the peripheral arthritis of IBD into patients with less than five involved joints (Type I) and those with five or more involved joints (Type II) (Orchard et al. 1998). Type I patients mainly have assymetric involvement of predominantly lower limb joints (often a monoarthritis, particularly at onset), whereas Type II patients have symmetric polyarticular small joint involvement in a rheumatoid-like distribution. Further analysis suggests that only Type I patients can be regarded as falling within the spondyloarthopathy group. Like reactive arthritis, 80 per cent have self-limiting disease and active arthritis is associated with relapse of inflammatory bowel disease in 80 per cent. In contrast, 80 per cent of Type II patients have persistent disease and a much less marked association between active arthritis and IBD relapse. These clinical observations are underpinned by the associations with the relatively rare MHC class II allele, HLA–DRB*0103 seen in both Type I arthritis (relative risk 12) and reactive arthritis due to enteric infection (Orchard et al. 2000). The same allele has also been found to be increased in IBD patients with ankylosing spondylitis, and with IBD and uveitis. An association with B27 was also described, but weaker for Type I disease than for reactive arthritis. In contrast Type II disease showed no association with either B27 or DRB*0103, but instead a weak association with HLA-B44.

The pathogenesis of the peripheral arthritis in IBD likely has many features in common with reactive arthritis; whereas specific pathogens are required to provoke the gastrointestinal inflammation which produces reactive arthritis in the presence of susceptibility genes (HLA B27 and others), the same genes predispose to arthritis in response to the gastrointestinal inflammation of IBD, itself likely to be an aberrant response to normal gut bacteria or possibly LPS (Hugot et al. 2001; Ogura et al. 2001). As in reactive arthritis, further genetic influences, again including B27, may lead to chronicity with established sacro-iliitis and axial disease, rather than self-limiting arthritis, but unlike classical ankylosing spondylitis, HLA B27 is only found in 50 per cent of the IBD patients with spondylitis, suggesting that other genetic factors can substitute for B27. In a different genetic background, other patterns of arthritis are seen, including rheumatoid-like Type II arthritis, but also rarer diseases such as the SAPHO syndrome (Hayem et al. 1999).

Treatment is directed at the underlying IBD, and for Type I peripheral arthritis effective control of IBD allows resolution of arthritis. This is not the case for Type II arthritis and spondylitis, and these require treatment in their own right. NSAIDs and methotrexate, which are generally appropriate in the management of inflammatory arthritis, can both exacerbate IBD (although methotrexate is also sometimes used to treat IBD). In contrast, sulfasalazine, and more recently, anti-TNFα drugs, are useful for both IBD and its associated arthritis.

Pouchitis

Patients treated by proctocolectomy for ulcerative colitis commonly have a pouch fashioned by ileo-anal anastomosis to avoid ileostomy. The pouch develops inflammation in 20–40 per cent of patients, possibly due to bacterial overgrowth, and this 'pouchitis' responds to antibiotics, particularly metronidazole. A proportion of patients with pouchitis also develop an arthritis which has features of spondyloarthopathy including lower limb involvement, enthesitis and sacroiliitis (Balbir-Gurman et al. 2001). Other extra-articular features such as iritis and erythema nodosum have been described. The development of pouchitis and associated arthritis is much commoner in patients operated on for ulcerative colitis than in those requiring colectomy for familial polyposis, perhaps indicating a genetic predisposition to make inflammatory responses to gut flora. Some authors have described a close relationship between the severity of pouchitis and arthritis (similar to Type I arthritis in inflammatory bowel disease) with recovery following pouch removal in some cases. Clinically significant arthritis associated with pouchitis is relatively uncommon, but a larger proportion (30 per cent) of patients complain of arthralgia involving hands and knees; in these cases a relationship with pouch inflammation is not evident (Thomas et al. 1999).

Coeliac disease

Inflammatory arthritis complicating coeliac disease has been recognized for two decades (Bourne et al. 1992), but is relatively rare. The disease is generally an oligo- or monoarthritis, with preferential involvement of lower limb joints. Lumbar spine and sacro-iliac joint involvment have also been described, but there is no clear association with HLA B27. The best evidence that the arthritis is causally related to coeliac disease and not an incidental finding is the observation that both respond to a gluten-free diet. Joint symptoms can precede gastrointestinal symptoms; indeed coeliac disease can be silent in one-third of cases with arthritis, so that investigation of unexplained seronegative arthritis by measuring anti-endomysial antibodies is appropriate, followed by endoscopy and biopsy in antibody-positive patients. This approach is justified since untreated coeliac disease carries an increased risk of lymphoma. Note that measuring antibodies to gliadin is much less satisfactory since such antibodies are sometimes present in patients with polyclonal increases in immunoglobulins, such as those with RA (Ferreira et al. 1992). There is controversy on whether coeliac disease occurs with increased frequency in juvenile idiopathic arthritis (JIA); investigation has estimated that 1–3 per cent JIA patients have underlying coeliac disease.

Whipple's disease

Understanding of this disease has been advanced enormously by the discovery of the causative organism, using the molecular approach of amplifying bacterial ribosomal RNA genes which have sequences which are conserved in all bacteria (Relman et al. 1992). This allows the use of 'universal' primers which amplify all bacteria. Sequencing the product allows particular bacteria to be identified since rRNA genes also possess species-specific sequences. In the case of the Whipple's bacillus, a previously undescribed sequence was identified by PCR, and consistently found in jejunal biopsies from Whipple's disease patients. The organism has been named *Tropheryma whippelii* and is related to actinomycetes. It is not uncommon in the environment, and can be found in normal individuals' saliva or duodenal secretions (but not normal jejunal biopsies), but does not usually establish infection, suggesting that Whipple's patients have some impairment of their immune response. Whilst bacteria have long been implicated in Whipple's disease, identification of a specific organism has allowed more accurate diagnosis and indicates that there are patients, including some with arthropathy, who do not have the histological changes in the gut previously required for diagnosis. PCR has shown the presence of the organism in the joints (O'Duffy et al. 1999), and also in the eye in patients with uveitis (Michel et al. 1997).

Whipple's disease is a systemic disorder, and the commonest triad of symptoms is weight loss, diarrhoea, and arthritis. Spondyloarthropathy features are absent, although a high frequency of HLA B27 has been observed in some series. The arthritis can precede other features by several years, and PCR diagnosis may allow cases to be identified and treated before they develop systemic symptoms. The diagnosis should be considered in patients with persistent seronegative oligoarthritis. The infection can also involve CNS, heart valves and lungs; treatment is with long courses of trimethoprim/sulphamethoxazole, and its efficacy can be monitored by determining which patients remain PCR positive. These have persistent infection and may fail to improve clinically or relapse.

References

Aceves-Avila, F.J. et al. (1998). Descriptions of Reiter's disease in Mexican medical texts since 1578. *Journal of Rheumatology* **25**, 2033–4.

Aho, K. et al. (1973). HLA-antigen 27 and reactive arthritis. *Lancet* **ii**, 157–9.

Allen, R.L. et al. (1997). Multiple T cell expansions are found in the blood and synovial fluid of patients with reactive arthritis. *Journal of Rheumatology* **24**, 1750–7.

Allen, R.L. et al. (1999). Cutting edge: HLA-B27 can form a novel beta(2)-microglobulin-free heavy chain homodimer structure. *Journal of Immunology* **162**, 5045–8.

Amor, B., Dougados, M., and Mijiyawa, M. (1990). Criteres de classification des spondylarthropathies. *Revue du Rhumatisme et des Maladies Osteoarticulaires* **57**, 85–9.

Angulo, J. and Espinoza, L. (1998). The spectrum of skin, mucosa and other extra-articular manifestations. *Baillière's Clinical Rheumatology* **12**, 649–64.

Balbir-Gurman, A., Schapira, D., and Nahir, M. (2001). Arthritis related to ileal pouchitis following total proctocolectomy for ulcerative colitis. *Seminars in Arthritis and Rheumatism* **30**, 242–8.

Bardin, T. et al. (1992). Antibiotic treatment of venereal disease and Reiter's syndrome in a Greenland population. *Arthritis and Rheumatism* **35**, 190–4.

BeacockSharp, H., Young, J.L., and Gaston, J.S.H. (1998). Analysis of T cell subsets present in the peripheral blood and synovial fluid of reactive arthritis patients. *Annals of the Rheumatic Diseases* **57**, 100–6.

Benjamin, R., Madrigal, J., and Parham, P. (1991). Peptide binding to empty HLA B27 molecules of viable human cells. *Nature* **351**, 74–7.

Bourne, J. et al. (1992). Arthritis and coeliac disease. *Annals of the Rheumatic Diseases* **44**, 592–8.

Brandt, J. et al. (2000). Successful treatment of active ankylosing spondylitis with the anti-tumor necrosis factor alpha monoclonal antibody infliximab. *Arthritis and Rheumatism* **43**, 1346–52.

Brewerton, D.A. et al. (1973). Reiter's disease and HLA-27. *Lancet* **2**, 996–8.

Chamot, A.M., Benhamou, C.L., Kahn, M.F., Beraneck, L., Kaplan, G., and Prost, A. (1987). Acne-pustulosis-hyperostosis-osteitis syndrome. Results of a national survey—85 cases. *Revue du Rhumatisme et des Maladies Osteoarticulaires* **54**, 187–96.

Deighton, C. (1993). Beta-haemolytic streptococci and reactive arthritis in adults. *Annals of the Rheumatic Diseases* **52**, 475–82.

Dougados, M. et al. (1991). The European Spondylarthropathy Study Group preliminary criteria for the classification of spondylarthropathy (see comments). *Arthritis and Rheumatism* **34**, 1218–27.

Dougados, M. et al. (1995). Sulfasalazine in the treatment of spondylarthropathy: a randomized, multicenter, double-blind, placebo-controlled study. *Arthritis and Rheumatism* **38**, 618–27.

Egsmose, C. et al. (1997). Limited effect of sulphasalazine treatment in reactive arthritis. A randomised double blind placebo controlled trial. *Annals of the Rheumatic Diseases* **56**, 32–6.

Ekman, P., Kirveskari, J., and Granfors, K. (2000). Modification of disease outcome in Salmonella-infected patients by HLA-B27. *Arthritis and Rheumatism* **43**, 1527–34.

Ekman, P. et al. (1999). Detection of *Salmonella infantis* in synovial fluid cells of a patient with reactive arthritis. *Journal of the Rheumatology* **26**, 2485–8.

Fendler, C. et al. (1998). Bacteria-specific lymphocyte proliferation in peripheral blood in reactive arthritis and related diseases. *British Journal of Rheumatology* **37**, 520–4.

Fendler, C. et al. (2001). Frequency of triggering bacteria in patients with reactive arthritis and undifferentiated oligoarthritis and the relative importance of the tests used for diagnosis. *Annals of the Rheumatic Disease* **60**, 337–43.

Ferreira, M. et al. (1992). Endomysial antibody: is it the best screening test for coeliac disease? *Gut* **33**, 1633–7.

Gaston, J. et al. (1989). *In vitro* responses to a 65 kD mycobacterial protein by synovial T cells from inflammatory arthritis patients. *Journal of Immunology* **143**, 2594–600.

Gaston, J.S.H. et al. (1989). Synovial T lymphocyte recognition of organisms that trigger reactive arthritis. *Clinical and Experimental Immunology* **76**, 348–53.

Gaston, J.S.H. et al. (1990). Recognition of a mycobacteria specific epitope in the 65 kD heat shock protein by synovial fluid derived T cell clones. *Journal of Experimental Medicine* **171**, 831–41.

Gaston, J.S.H., Cox, C., and Granfors, K. (1999). Clinical and experimental evidence for persistent Yersinia infection in reactive arthritis. *Arthritis and Rheumatism* **42**, 2239–42.

Granfors, K. (1998). Host-microbe interaction in reactive arthritis: Does HLA-B27 have a direct effect? *Journal of Rheumatology* **25**, 1659–61.

Granfors, K. and Toivanen, A. (1986). IgA-anti-yersinia antibodies in yersinia-triggered reactive arthritis. *Annals of the Rheumatic Diseases* **45**, 561–5.

Granfors, K. et al. (1989). Yersinia antigens in synovial fluid cells from patients with reactive arthritis. *New England Journal of Medicine* **320**, 216–21.

Granfors, K. et al. (1990). Salmonella lipopolysaccharide in synovial cells from patients with reactive arthritis. *Lancet* **335**, 685–8.

Granfors, K. et al. (1998). Persistence of Yersinia antigens in peripheral blood cells from patients with Yersinia enterocolitica O:3 infection with or without reactive arthritis. *Arthritis and Rheumatism* **41**, 855–62.

Hannu, T., Puolakkainen, M., and Leirisalo-Repo, M. (1999). *Chlamydia pneumoniae* as a triggering infection in reactive arthritis. *Rheumatology (Oxford)* **38**, 411–14.

Haslock, I. and Wright, V. (1973). The musculoskeletal complications of Crohn's disease. *Medicine* **52**, 217–25.

Hayem, G. et al. (1999). SAPHO syndrome: a long-term follow-up study of 120 cases. *Seminars in Arthritis and Rheumatism* **29**, 159–71.

Hermann, E. et al. (1991). Synovial fluid derived Yersinia reactive T cells responding to human 65 kDa heat shock protein and heat stressed antigen presenting cells. *European Journal of Immunology* **21**, 2139–43.

Hermann, E. et al. (1993). HLA-B27-restricted CD8 T-cells derived from synovial fluids of patients with reactive arthritis and ankylosing spondylitis. *Lancet* **342**, 646–50.

Hugot, J.P. et al. (2001). Association of NOD2 leucine-rich repeat variants with susceptibility to Crohn's disease. *Nature* **411**, 599–603.

Hulsemann, J.L. and Zeidler, H. (1999). Diagnostic evaluation of classification criteria for rheumatoid arthritis and reactive arthritis in an early synovitis outpatient clinic. *Annals of the Rheumatic Disease* **58**, 278–80.

Ikawa, T. et al. (1998). Expression of arthritis-causing HLA-B27 on HeLa cells promotes induction of c-fos in response to *in vitro* invasion by *Salmonella typhimurium*. *Journal of Clinical Investigation* **101**, 263–72.

Iliopoulos, A. et al. (1995). Change in the epidemiology of Reiter's syndrome (reactive arthritis) in the post-AIDS era? An analysis of cases appearing in the Greek army. *Journal of Rheumatology* **22**, 252–4.

Inman, R.D. et al. (1988). Postdysenteric reactive arthritis: a clinical and immunologic study following an outbreak of Salmonellosis. *Arthritis and Rheumatism* **31**, 1377–83.

Kahn, M.F. and Khan, M.A. (1994). The SAPHO syndrome. *Baillière's Clinical Rheumatology* **8**, 333–62.

Kalish, R., Leong, J., and Steere, A. (1993). Association of treatment-resistant chronic Lyme arthritis with HLA–DR4 and antibody reactivity to OspA and OspB of Borrelia burgdorferi. *Infection and Immunity* **61**, 2774–9.

Khalil, A. et al. (1997). HLA-B27 transgenic mice lacking CD4 gene have decreased incidence of spontaneous inflammatory disease. *Arthritis and Rheumatism* **40**, S330.

Khare, S.D., Luthra, H.S., and David, C.S. (1995). Spontaneous inflammatory arthritis in HLA-B27 transgenic mice lacking beta(2)-microglobulin: a model of human spondyloarthropathies. *Journal of Experimental Medicine* **182**, 1153–8.

Kotake, S. et al. (1999). Gamma interferon and interleukin-10 gene expression in synovial tissues from patients with early stages of Chlamydia-associated arthritis and undifferentiated oligoarthritis and from healthy volunteers. *Infection and Immunity* **67**, 2682–6.

Kvein, T. et al. (1995). The natural history of reactive arthritis. *Rheumatology in Europe* **24**, 15–19.

Kvien, T.K. et al. (1994). Reactive arthritis—incidence, triggering agents and clinical presentation. *Journal of Rheumatology* **21**, 115–22.

Lauhio, A. et al. (1991). Double-blind, placebo-controlled study of three-month treatment with lymecycline in reactive arthritis with special reference to chlamydia arthritis. *Arthritis and Rheumatism* **34**, 6–14.

Lehtinen, A., Taavitsainen, M., and Leirisalo-Repo, M. (1994). Sonographic analysis of enthesopathy in the lower extremities of patients with spondylarthropathy. *Clinical and Experimental Rheumatology* **12**, 143–8.

Leirisalo, M. et al. (1982). Followup study on patients with Reiter's disease and reactive arthritis, with special reference to HLA-B27. *Arthritis and Rheumatism* **25**, 249–59.

Leirisalo-Repo, M. et al. (1994). High frequency of silent inflammatory bowel disease in spondylarthropathy. *Arthritis and Rheumatism* **37**, 23–31.

Leirisalo-Repo, M. (1998). Prognosis, course of disease, and treatment of the spondyloarthropathies. *Rheumatic Diseases Clinics of North America* **24**, 737–51, viii.

Leirisalo-Repo, M. et al. (1997). Long term prognosis of reactive salmonella arthritis. *Annals of the Rheumatic Disease* **56**, 516–20.

Maki, I.O. et al. (1992). Salmonella antibodies in healthy populations in Finland and the UK. How many Salmonella-triggered reactive arthritides are there? *British Journal of Rheumatology* **32**, 262–3.

Maksymowych, W.P. et al. (2001). Clinical and radiological amelioration of refractory peripheral spondyloarthritis by pulse intravenous pamidronate therapy. *Journal of Rheumatology* **28**, 144–55.

Mattila, L. et al. (1998). Reactive arthritis following an outbreak of *Salmonella bovismorbificans* infection. *Journal of Infection* **36**, 289–95.

McColl, G.J. et al. (2000). HLA-B27 expression and reactive arthritis susceptibility in two patient cohorts infected with *Salmonella typhimurium. Australian and New Zealand Journal of Medicine* **30**, 28–32.

McGonagle, D., Gibbon, W., and Emery, P. (1998). Classification of inflammatory arthritis by enthesitis. *Lancet* **352**, 1137–40.

McGonagle, D. et al. (1998). Characteristic magnetic resonance imaging entheseal changes of knee synovitis in spondylarthropathy. *Arthritis and Rheumatism* **41**, 694–700.

Mear, J.P. et al. (1999). Misfolding of HLA-B27 as a result of its B pocket suggests a novel mechanism for its role in susceptibility to spondyloarthropathies. *Journal of Immunology* **163**, 6665–70.

Mease, P.J. et al. (2000). Etanercept in the treatment of psoriatic arthritis and psoriasis: a randomised trial. *Lancet* **356**, 385–90.

Merilahti-Palo, R. et al. (1991). Bacterial antigens in synovial biopsy specimens in yersinia-triggered reactive arthritis. *Annals of the Rheumatic Diseases* **50**, 87–90.

Mertz, A. et al. (1994). The evolutionarily conserved ribosomal protein L23 and the cationic urease beta-subunit of *Yersinia enterocolitica* O : 3 belong to the immunodominant antigens in Yersinia-triggered reactive arthritis: implications for autoimmunity. *Molecular Medicine* **1**, 44–55.

Michel, M. et al. (1997). Whipple's disease presenting as corticosteroid-resistant uveitis: Report of six cases. *Arthritis and Rheumatism* **40**, S145.

Mielants, H. et al. (1996). Course of gut inflammation in spondylarthropathies and therapeutic consequences. *Baillière's Clinical Rheumatology* **10**, 147–64.

Nikkari, S. et al. (1992). Yersinia triggered reactive arthritis. Use of polymerase chain reaction and immunocytochemical staining in the detection of bacterial components from synovial specimens. *Arthritis and Rheumatism* **35**, 682–7.

Nikkari, S. et al. (1999). Salmonella-triggered reactive arthritis: use of polymerase chain reaction, immunocytochemical staining, and gas chromatography-mass spectrometry in the detection of bacterial components from synovial fluid. *Arthritis and Rheumatism* **42**, 84–9.

Njobvu, P. et al. (1998). Spondyloarthropathy and human immunodeficiency virus infection in Zambia. *Journal of Rheumatology* **25**, 1553–9.

O'Duffy, J.D. et al. (1999). Whipple's arthritis—direct detection of *Tropheryma whippelii* in synovial fluid and tissue. *Arthritis and Rheumatism* **42**, 812–17.

Ogura, Y. et al. (2001). A frameshift mutation in NOD2 associated with susceptibility to Crohn's disease. *Nature* **411**, 603–6.

Orchard, T., Wordsworth, B., and Jewell, D. (1998). Peripheral arthropathies in inflammatory bowel disease: their articular distribution and natural history. *Gut* **42**, 387–91.

Orchard, T.R. et al. (2000). Clinical phenotype is related to HLA genotype in the peripheral arthropathies of inflammatory bowel disease. *Gastroenterology* **118**, 274–8.

Pachecotena, C. et al. (1999). A proposal for the classification of patients for clinical and experimental studies on reactive arthritis. *Journal of Rheumatology* **26**, 1338–46.

Relman, D.A. et al. (1992). Identification of the uncultured bacillus of Whipple's disease. *New England Journal of Medicine* **327**, 293–301.

Saikku, P. (2000). Epidemiologic association of Chlamydia pneumoniae and atherosclerosis: the initial serologic observation and more. *Journal of Infectious Diseases* **181**, S411–13.

Salmi, M. et al. (1995). Dual binding capacity of mucosal immunoblasts to mucosal and synovial endothelium in humans: Dissection of the molecular mechanisms. *Journal of Experimental Medicine* **181**, 137–49.

Schlaak, J. et al. (1992). Predominance of Th1 type T cells in synovial fluid of patients with Yersinia induced reactive arthritis. *European Journal of Immunology* **22**, 2771–6.

Schultz, H. et al. (2000). BPI-ANCA is found in reactive arthritis caused by Yersinia and Salmonella infection and recognise exclusively the C-terminal part of the BPI molecule. *Scandinavian Journal of the Rheumatology* **29**, 226–31.

Schumacher, H. et al. (1997). Surveying for evidence of synovial *Chlamydia trachomatis* by polymerase chain reaction (PCR). A study of 411 synovial biopsies and synovial fluids. *Arthritis and Rheumatism* **40**, S270.

Schumacher, H.R. et al. (1988). Light and electron microscope studies on the synovial membrane in Reiter's syndrome. *Arthritis and Rheumatism* **31**, 937–46.

Schumacher, H.R. et al. (1999). Chlamydia trachomatis nucleic acids can be found in the synovium of some asymptomatic subjects. *Arthritis and Rheumatism* **42**, 1281–4.

Sieper, J. et al. (1993). T-cells are responsible for the enhanced synovial cellular immune response to triggering antigen in reactive arthritis. *Clinical and Experimental Immunology* **91**, 96–102.

Sieper, J. et al. (1999). No benefit of long-term ciprofloxacin treatment in patients with reactive arthritis and undifferentiated oligoarthritis—a three-month, multicenter, double-blind, randomized, placebo-controlled study. *Arthritis and Rheumatism* **42**, 1386–96.

Simon, A.K., Seipelt, E., and Sieper, J. (1994). Divergent T-cell cytokine patterns in inflammatory arthritis. *Proceedings of the National Academy of Sciences (USA)* **91**, 8562–6.

Storey, G.O. and Scott, D.L. (1998). Arthritis associated with venereal disease in nineteenth century London. *Clinical Rheumatology* **17**, 500–4.

Taurog, J.D. et al. (1999). Inflammatory disease in HLA-B27 transgenic rats. *Immunology Reviews* **169**, 209–23.

Taylor-Robinson, D. et al. (1992). Detection of *Chlamydia trachomatis* DNA in joints of reactive arthritis patients by polymerase chain reaction. *Lancet* **340**, 81–2.

Tertti, R. et al. (1984). An outbreak of Yersinia pseudotuberculosis infection. *Journal of Infectious Disease* **149**, 245–50.

Thomas, P.D. et al. (1999). Extraintestinal manifestations of ulcerative colitis following restorative proctocolectomy. *European Journal of Gastroenterology and Hepatology* **11**, 1001–5.

Toivanen, P. and Toivanen, A. (1999). Two forms of reactive arthritis? *Annals of the Rheumatic Disease* **58**, 737–41.

Utsinger, P., Weiner, S., and Utsinger, J. (1996). Human models: Whipple's disease, coeliac disease and jejunoileal bypass. *Baillière's Clinical Rheumatology* **10**, 77–103.

VandenBosch, F. et al. (2000). Crohn's disease associated with spondyloarthropathy: effect of TNF-alpha blockade with infliximab on articular symptoms. *Lancet* **356**, 1821–2.

Viner, N. et al. (1991). Isolation of Yersinia specific T cell clones from the synovial membrane and synovial fluid of a patient with reactive arthritis. *Arthritis and Rheumatism* **34**, 1151–7.

Wakefield, D. et al. (1999). Ciprofloxacin treatment does not influence course or relapse rate of reactive arthritis and anterior uveitis. *Arthritis and Rheumatism* **42**, 1894–7.

Wallace, D. and Weisman, M. (2000). Should a war criminal be rewarded with eponymous distinction? The double life of Hans Reiter. *Journal of Clinical Rheumatology* **6**, 49–54.

Wheeler, J.G. et al. (1999). Study of infectious intestinal disease in England: rates in the community, presenting to general practice, and reported to national surveillance. The Infectious Intestinal Disease Study Executive. *British Medical Journal* **318**, 1046–50.

Willkens, R. et al. (1981). Reiter's syndrome: evaluation of preliminary criteria for definitive disease. *Arthritis and Rheumatism* **24**, 844–9.

Wollenhaupt, J., Schnarr, S., and Kuijpers, J.G. (1998). Bacterial antigens in reactive arthritis and spondarthritis. Rational use of laboratory testing in diagnosis and follow-up. *Baillière's Clinical Rheumatology* **12**, 627–47.

Wright, V. and Watkinson, G. (1965). The arthritis of ulcerative colitis. *British Medical Journal* **2**, 670–5.

YliKerttula, T. et al. (2000). Effect of a three month course of ciprofloxacin on the outcome of reactive arthritis. *Annals of the Rheumatic Diseases* **59**, 565–70.

Zhang, Y. et al. (1996). Antibiotic prophylaxis and treatment of reactive arthritis: lessons from an animal model. *Arthritis and Rheumatism* **39**, 1238–43.

6.5 Arthropathies primarily occurring in childhood

6.5.1 Juvenile idiopathic arthritis

David D. Sherry, Elizabeth D. Mellins, Christy I. Sandborg, and Vivian E. Saper

Pauciarticular-onset juvenile idiopathic arthritis (JIA) is the most commonly encountered subset of the chronic childhood arthritides, accounting for 40–50 per cent of children with chronic arthritis. By definition, its onset occurs before the age of 16 years, active synovitis of at least one joint is present continuously for a minimum of 6 weeks by American Rheumatism Association criteria (Brewer et al. 1977) or for 3 months by European League Against Rheumatism criteria (Wood 1978), and a total of four or fewer joints are involved during the first 6 months of disease. Some of the characteristics which make this disease entity quite distinct from other forms of juvenile or adult arthritis include its striking predilection for pre-school-age girls, the tendency for involvement of large joints excluding the hip and shoulder, the frequent occurrence of chronic anterior uveitis, the presence of antinuclear antibodies, and unique immunogenetic associations.

Epidemiology

Pauciarticular-onset JIA is a rheumatic disease distinctly of childhood, and the vast majority of patients are female toddlers. Overall, the disease affects an estimated 20–30 per 100 000 children (Gare et al. 1987). The female to male ratio is 4:1 (Petty 1979), and may be as high as 7.5:1 among children with iridocyclitis and chronic arthritis (Spalter 1975). The age at onset peaks sharply between 1 and 3 years, but ranges from as young as a few months of age to the teenage years (see Fig. 1 and Cassidy and Petty 2001). Only a limited number of cases in adults have been reported (Chaouat et al. 1990; Kenesi-Laurent et al. 1991), and the absence of HLA–DR5 and of eye involvement in patients in the latter series raises the possibility that

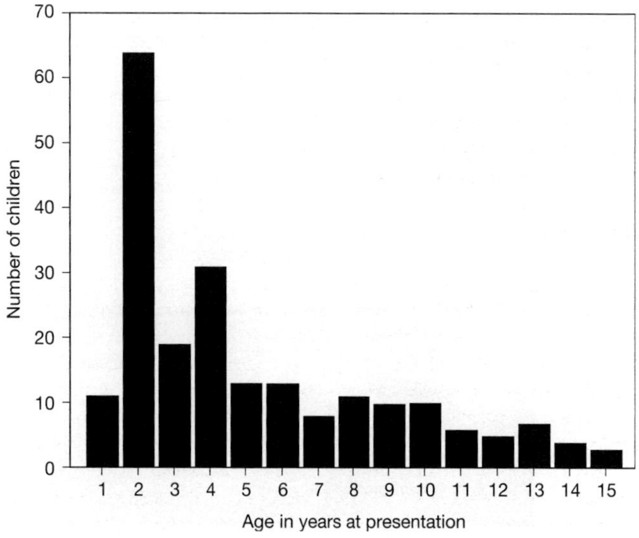

Fig. 1 Age at onset in 215 consecutive children with pauciarticular-onset juvenile chronic arthritis (Sharma and Sherry 1999).

pauciarticular arthritis in adults represents a distinct disease entity. Pauciarticular-onset JIA is a more common subtype of JIA in Caucasian, as compared to non-Caucasian patients (Oen and Cheang 1996).

Clinical features

JIA is always a diagnosis of exclusion, as there are no pathognomonic signs, symptoms, or laboratory investigations. Nevertheless, the classic clinical picture is quite recognizable: an otherwise healthy female toddler who has arthritis in only a few joints, such as one knee and one ankle [see Fig. 2(a)]. Clinical features are usually mild compared with other forms of JIA, reactive arthritis, or joint infections (Morrissy 1990; Sherry 1990; Cassidy and Petty 2001). Non-articular inflammation is rare, except for chronic asymptomatic uveitis (see below). In one study, 26 per cent of patients presented without pain (Sherry et al. 1990). Most children will complain of morning stiffness, gelling, or pain with use, but typically are not incapacitated and limit their activities only modestly. Constitutional signs and symptoms are not a part of pauciarticular-onset JIA and, if present, virtually exclude this diagnosis.

The knee is the most frequently involved joint followed by the ankle (Table 1) (Schaller and Wedgwood 1972; Ansell 1976). Children may have arthritis involving only one or two small joints of the hand, although this is not the usual pattern. It is not rare for patients with pauciarticular-onset arthritis to develop disease of the temporomandibular joint (Strabrun 1991) or cervical spine; the latter can produce torticollis. Shoulder involvement is exceedingly rare; arthritis of the hip is so rare that the diagnosis is suspect and should be made only after extensive evaluation for other causes. Occasionally, a child will have five or six joints affected over the first 6 months, but never evolve into the typical polyarticular pattern. Although meeting criteria for polyarticular-onset JIA, these children have a disease more like the pauciarticular-onset disease in terms of their risk for chronic uveitis and long-term prognosis.

Laboratory features

No particular laboratory abnormalities are diagnostic of pauciarticular-onset JIA. Acute-phase reactants are usually normal to slightly elevated but

Table 1 Pattern of joint involvement at presentation in 215 consecutive children with pauciarticular-onset arthritis (Sharma and Sherry 1999)

	(%)
Single joint	58
Two joints	24
Three joints	13
Four joints	5
Knee	56
Ankle	20
Small hand joint	10
Small foot joint	6
Wrist	4
Elbow	2.8
Hip	1.4
Temporomandibular	0.3

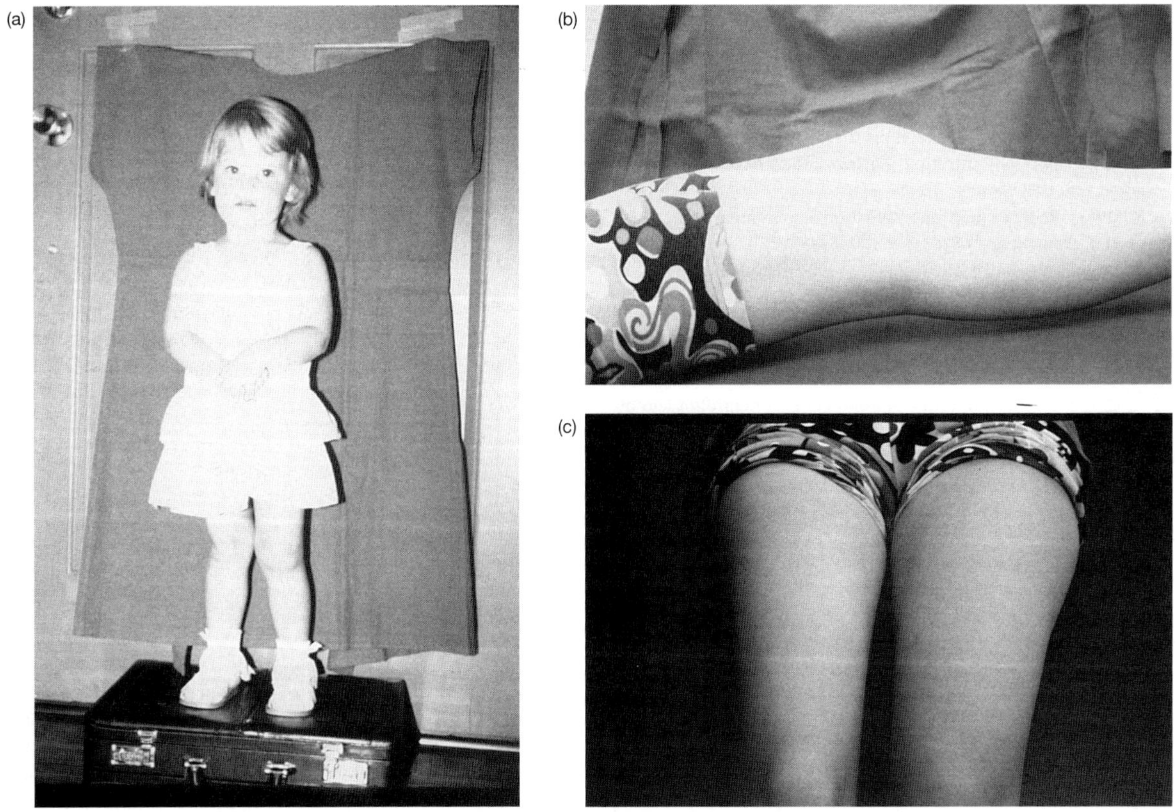

Fig. 2 Clinical features of pauciarticular-onset juvenile idiopathic arthritis. (a) Archetypical patient with pauciarticular-onset JIA. Note generally healthy young girl with involvement of a single knee. (b) Unilateral flexion contracture as seen frequently. To evaluate for subtle flexion contraction, especially in children with hypermobility, lift both heels equally high and observe for unequal knee height. (c) Thigh atrophy in unilateral disease. This may be a permanent sequela.

occasionally the erythrocyte sedimentation rate will be markedly elevated. This should prompt an extensive search for infection or occult inflammation, such as inflammatory bowel disease or leukaemia. Reactive or viral arthritis may also produce high erythrocyte sedimentation rates. A highly elevated erythrocyte sedimentation rate has been associated with a more severe course (Guillaume et al. 2000).

Antinuclear antibodies (ANA) are present in 40–75 per cent of children with pauciarticular-onset JIA, depending on the analytical technique employed and are in a homogeneous, or, less commonly, a speckled pattern. Antibodies to histones are relatively common; one report identified them in 42 per cent of patients with uveitis-negative, pauciarticular-onset disease (Malleson et al. 1992). ANA titres are usually low, less than or equal to three dilutions beyond the threshold of normal. Higher titres, especially in the older patient, should be investigated for specific autoantigens. Most studies find no connection between the titre of ANA and disease activity. There is no evidence that ANA precede the development of pauciarticular-onset JIA; in fact, most healthy children with an isolated positive ANA will not develop any rheumatic disease when followed over several years (Cabral et al. 1992).

Rheumatoid factor is distinctly rare, occurring in less than 5 per cent of these children and portends a polyarticular, prolonged course with a high risk of erosive arthritis. Non-classical rheumatoid factors (IgG and IgA) have been reported, but the significance of these is unknown.

Synovial fluid or a synovial biopsy are usually obtained only as an aid to excluding other diagnoses. Synovial fluid most often contains less than 25 000 white blood cells/mm^3, mostly polymorphonuclear cells. The glucose concentration in synovial fluid is within 10 per cent of the serum glucose concentration; protein concentration is elevated.

A synovial biopsy has features similar to those of adult rheumatoid arthritis, with hyperplasia and hypertrophy of the synovial lining, and vascular endothelial hyperplasia with lymphocytic and plasma cell infiltration. Progression of these inflammatory changes to pannus formation and cartilaginous and eventually bony erosion, although uncommon in pauciarticular-onset arthritis, can occur and is indistinguishable pathologically from other forms of juvenile or adult rheumatoid arthritis (Cassidy and Petty 2001).

Radiographs taken early in the disease process reveal joint effusion or soft tissue swelling. Over time, juxta-articular osteoporosis occurs, followed in more severe cases by joint space narrowing and ultimately erosions. However, many bones are cartilaginous in young children (such as the carpals) or have cartilaginous epiphyses. As these ossify, the articular surface may appear quite irregular or multiple ossification centres may occur, giving the appearance of an erosion. Magnetic resonance imaging can be helpful in both early cases and late cases for determining the extent of synovitis and joint damage (Lamer and Sebag 2000).

Course

In most children with pauciarticular-onset arthritis, the disease remains pauciarticular. Although synovitis may develop in new joints over time, the total number of affected joints remains below five. A relatively short course of active arthritis, usually 2–5 years, is typical. Some of these children will have a subsequent episode of chronic arthritis, sometimes many years after the original episode. Each episode seems to mimic the first in terms of joints affected and duration of disease.

An important minority will eventually develop arthritis in many joints, with earlier studies showing about 20 per cent of all children with disease of pauciarticular onset will later be classified as functional stage III or IV (Stoeber 1981; Cush and Fink 1987; Wallace and Levinson 1991). There is a growing impression among paediatric rheumatologists that a larger number of children with pauciarticular-onset JIA have long-term, active synovitis than was formerly appreciated (Cush and Fink 1987), and this number may not be reflected in the functional classification data. One study showed that patients with two to four arthritic joints at onset, had upper extremity arthritis, or an elevated erythrocyte sedimentation rate were more likely to develop a polyarticular course (Guillaume et al. 2000). It is generally only those converting to a polyarticular course who develop marked joint destruction, similar to those with polyarticular-onset JIA. A patient whose disease remains pauciarticular for 5 years is unlikely to progress to polyarticular involvement.

Complications

Articular complications

Children with pauciarticular-onset JIA are at risk of developing juxta-articular muscle atrophy, bony enlargement of the joint, or leg length inequality [Fig. 2(b) and (c)]. When knee synovitis starts before the age of 3 years, quadriceps muscle atrophy may continue years after disease is past (Vostrejs and Hollister 1988). Bony overgrowth around the affected joint is primarily of cosmetic concern. In those children with unilateral knee involvement, bony overgrowth may lead to a significant leg length discrepancy. When disease begins before 3 years of age, a longer leg develops on the affected side (Vostrejs and Hollister 1988), whereas when disease onset is after the age of 9 years, premature epiphyseal closure can occur, resulting in a shorter leg on the involved side (Simon et al. 1981). Mechanically, a longer leg on the involved side may be a problem, since the child will flex the arthritic knee to keep the pelvis level, thus exacerbating a flexion contracture. Rarely, a severe flexion contracture may progress to subluxation. Synovial cysts, especially in the popliteal space, are not uncommon (Szer et al. 1992) and acute onset of intense limb pain and swelling suggests a ruptured cyst.

Ocular complications

In addition to musculoskeletal complications, a chronic, insidious, and potentially blinding uveitis can occur in children with pauciarticular-onset JIA. Described first in a case report in 1910 (Ohm 1910), the association of chronic uveitis and juvenile arthritis is now firmly established and available data suggest it is observed worldwide (Rosenberg 1987). The ocular inflammation characteristically affects the anterior uveal tract (the iris and ciliary body); involvement of the posterior uveal tract (the choroid) is infrequent (Key and Kimure 1975).

Prevalence studies of uveitis in paediatric patients with pauciarticular arthritis in the United States and Britain suggest that approximately 20 per cent develop chronic uveitis (Sherry et al. 1991). Uveitis is also seen in a small fraction of patients with polyarticular onset (5 per cent) and more rarely in those with systemic-onset disease (Key and Kimure 1975; Chylack 1977). The risk of uveitis is associated with the pauciarticular mode of onset of arthritis and not with the later extent of articular disease. In two independent studies, polyarticular disease developed in about 45 per cent of pauciarticular-onset patients with uveitis (Kanski and Shun-shin 1984; Wolf et al. 1987). Children with uveitis thus appear to contribute disproportionately to the group with pauciarticular-onset whose disease becomes polyarticular.

In addition to pauciarticular onset of arthritis, other risk factors for the uveitis associated with JIA have been identified (Table 2). The highest risk group for developing uveitis is ANA-positive females whose pauciarticular-onset disease began before the age of 2 years (Chylack et al. 1979). It is not known why ANA are a serological marker of those at risk. Interestingly, these antibodies are not found in patients with chronic anterior uveitis without juvenile chronic arthritis, although this disease has otherwise similar characteristics, including a female preponderance (Rosenberg and Romanchuk 1990). In children with uveitis associated with chronic arthritis, the titre of the ANA is usually intermediate (less than 1:640) and does not correlate with the severity of ocular disease (Kanski 1977). No differences in reactivity to defined nuclear antigens are found in the ANA of children with and without uveitis (Malleson et al. 1989).

The uveitis is commonly asymptomatic, even in the face of substantial damage to the eye. In reported series, pain and redness of the eye occur in up to 25 per cent of patients; visual disturbance, photophobia, and headache

Table 2 Risk factors associated with uveitis in juvenile idiopathic arthritis

Female gender	
Female–male ratio	4.7–7.5 : 1[a]
Young onset age of arthritis	
Mean onset age (years)	4.0
Oligoarthritis	
Percentage with pauciarticular-onset arthritis	86.6
Percentage with polyarticular-onset arthritis	12.6
Percentage with systemic-onset arthritis	0.8
Antinuclear antibody positivity	
Percentage positive	80–90[b]

[a] Reviewed in Cassidy and Petty (2001).

[b] The percentage of uveitis patients with detectable antinuclear antibodies has risen to 90+ per cent since 1975 when sensitive assays became available (Wolf et al. 1987).

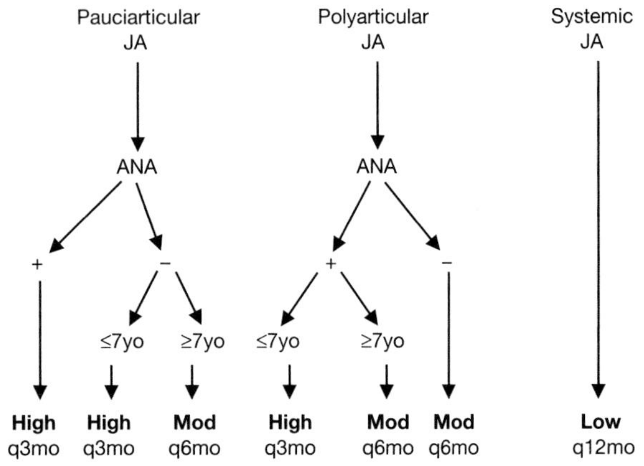

Fig. 3 Uveitis surveillance: recommended frequency of slit-lamp examinations. (American Academy of Pediatrics Section on Rheumatology and Section of Ophthalmology 1993.)

are less frequent (Cassidy and Petty 2001). Detection of disease generally requires slit-lamp ophthalmological examination, which is an essential component of routine surveillance and is recommended at frequent intervals for at least the first 4 years (Fig. 3). Biomicroscopic signs of active disease include the presence of inflammatory cells and protein flare in the anterior chamber of the eye and fresh keratitic precipitates. On the initial rheumatological evaluation, one should look carefully for evidence of earlier uveitis, such as pupillary irregularities and punctate corneal deposits (Plate 109). If present, immediate ophthalmic evaluation is appropriate.

In most children, uveitis and arthritis develop at different times. Uveitis is documented before onset of arthritis in 10 per cent of affected children (Rosenberg 1987), but asymptomatic (and undetected) uveitis may precede arthritis more often. Among routinely screened children with chronic arthritis, uveitis is usually detected within 7 years (median, 2 years) of the onset of arthritis (Kanski and Shun-shin 1984). However, uveitis has developed up to 34 years after joint symptoms (Cassidy et al. 1977).

The uveitis associated with pauciarticular JA is chronic, rarely lasting less than 2 years and often more than 15 years (Smiley 1976). In a study of 20 patients, the course was remitting and relapsing in 60 per cent, persistent in 20 per cent, and limited to a single episode in 20 per cent. Both eyes are involved in roughly two-thirds of patients (Rosenberg 1987), but both are not necessarily coincidentally inflamed. Moreover, children with uveitis of one eye rarely develop involvement of the second eye after more than 1 year of unilateral disease (Kanski 1990). Eye and joint disease evolve independently, and the overall severity of each is likely to differ (Leak and Ansell 1987). In many cases, uveitis persists years after the arthritis has become inactive (Key and Kimure 1975).

A variety of ocular complications can occur in the uveitis associated with JIA (Plate 109). Posterior synechiae, which are fibrous bands adhering the iris to the lens, give the pupil a star-burst or irregular appearance. Band keratopathy, a layer of calcium deposits in Bowman's membrane of the cornea, is another characteristic sequela. The pathogenesis of this condition is unknown and active iritis may persist for years without the development of keratopathy. Glaucoma is a common complication that may result from prolonged intraocular inflammation and/or from steroid treatment (Foster et al. 2000). Other complications include cataracts, and rarely, phthisis bulbi. Approximately 40 per cent of affected eyes progress to 20/200 visual acuity or below, and approximately 10 per cent of affected eyes will become blind (Rosenberg 1987).

Differential diagnosis

Conditions that may simulate pauciarticular-onset JIA can be classified into four major categories: monoarticular conditions, short-lived inflammatory conditions, spondyloarthropathies, and complaints of pain without joint inflammation. A list of these conditions, along with some of their distinguishing features, is given in Table 3.

Monoarticular conditions

Monoarticular conditions are the most difficult to sort out and include several requiring immediate intervention. However, it is not uncommon for careful examination of a child with monoarticular complaints to reveal involvement of other joints. When a single joint is involved, pauciarticular-onset JIA is a frequent cause, but the conditions described in Table 3 should also be considered.

Short-lived inflammatory conditions

These conditions cause inflammation in one or several joints which can simulate pauciarticular-onset JIA, and include inflammatory reactions to a number of viral and bacterial infections. However, the inflammation is relatively fleeting, usually lasting 1–4 weeks, but occasionally up to 8 weeks. When initially evaluating a child, one need not withhold anti-inflammatory treatment in order to establish a diagnosis. Only rarely would JIA respond so well as to go into complete remission in such a short time. Lyme arthritis can mimic pauciarticular-onset JIA and the long interval between infection and onset of arthritis can obscure the diagnosis. Patients with a possible exposure history should be tested for Lyme antibodies which are almost universally positive in Lyme arthritis (Tugwell 1996).

Spondyloarthropathies

These conditions are discussed at length in Chapter 6.4.2, and are contrasted with pauciarticular-onset JIA in Table 3. Briefly, unlike pauciarticular-onset disease, they occur predominantly in adolescents, boys are much more commonly affected, the arthritis is usually limited to the lower extremity and involves both large and small joints, enthesitis is common, and HLA-B27 is highly associated (Rosenberg and Petty 1982; Burgos-Vargas et al. 1997). Heel pain is often noted in spondyloarthropathies but is uncommon in pauciarticular-onset arthritis. Furthermore, the iritis that occurs with the spondyloarthropathies, in contrast to that of pauciarticular-onset disease, is typically acute and painful, leading to scleral injection and photophobia.

Pain complaints without joint inflammation

Many children present with musculoskeletal pain that does not emanate from the joint. Younger children in particular may not localize their pain accurately. These conditions can be persistent and underlying arthritis may

Table 3 Differential diagnosis of pauciarticular-onset juvenile chronic arthritis

Condition	Distinguishing features
Monoarticular	
Septic arthritis	Child is ill, high ESR, very painful, joint can be erythematous
	Haemophilus influenza predominates in children under 5 years of age, *Staphylococcus aureus* in those over 5 years
Tuberculosis	Pulmonary disease present
	Lower extremity predominates including hip
	Rapid joint destruction, may be insidious in onset
Trauma	History of direct blow or forced hyperextension
without intra-articular bleeding	Swelling in 12–24 h, short-lived
with intra-articular bleeding	Swelling in 2 h, very painful, may have adjacent fracture
Pigmented villonodular synovitis	Repeated bleeding into joint causes synovial fluid to be haemorrhagic
Foreign-body synovitis	History of injury; organic material present in synovium
Isolated hip inflammation or pain	Older children usually affected
	Most of these conditions have typical radiographic features
Patellofemoral joint disease	Adolescent females more commonly affected
	Tenderness of undersurface of the patella
Palindromic rheumatism	Episodic and migratory
Thalassaemia	Episodic and migratory; anaemic
Short-lived inflammatory conditions (usually last 3–6 weeks, occasionally up to 8 weeks)	
Lyme disease	Exposure in an endemic area, rash, fever, other signs of Lyme disease (neurological, cardiac), positive Lyme serology
Viral arthritis	May be associated with rash or immunization
	Rubella, varicella, parvovirus infection have been implicated
Reactive arthritis (including Reiter's)	History of preceding infection (upper respiratory, gastrointestinal, streptococcal, rarely venereal)
	Conjunctivitis, urethritis (dysuria or sterile pyuria)
	Usually older males (over 8 years old)
	May have rash, fever, or enthesitis
Post-streptococcal; acute	Preceding streptococcal infection
rheumatic fever	Migratory arthritis
	May have other signs of rheumatic fever including carditis, erythema migrans, nodules, chorea
Cystic fibrosis	Chronic pulmonary infection, usually with *Pseudomonas* spp.; rash
Spondyloarthropathies (Usually affect older children (over 8 years old); boys more than girls; may have acute iritis, most have enthesitis, frequently HLA-B27 positive, ESR often higher than expected clinically)	
Ankylosing spondylitis	Sacroiliac joint involvement; back pain; back limitation; decreased chest excursion
Psoriatic arthritis	Rash; pitting or other nail changes
Arthritis of inflammatory bowel disease	Bloody diarrhoea, high ESR
Pain complaints without joint inflammation (notable for lack of true arthritis)	
Hypermobility	Nocturnal pain in the popliteal space; can occur after specific activities; four of five criteria present:
	(1) thumb adducts to touch forearm
	(2) fingers hyperextend to parallel forearm
	(3 and 4) elbows or knees hyperextend beyond 10°
	(5) when standing, can bend over and touch palms to floor
Reflex neurovascular dystrophy	Usually pre- to adolescent females with signs of autonomic dysfunction
	More pain and disability than expected or than affect would indicate; incongruent, cheerful affect
	May have abnormal bone scan
Psychogenic musculoskeletal pains	Similar to reflex neurovascular dystrophy but without signs of autonomic dysfunction
	Hyperaesthesia common
Bone pain	Tenderness to palpation of the tibia, ulna, or other assessable bones
	Malignancy can cause some arthritis
	May be episodic
Avulsion fractures	Point-specific pain, such as at tibial tuberosity (Osgood–Schlatter), inferior pole of patella (Sinding–Larson–Johansson); or Achilles tendon insertion (Sever)
Aseptic necrosis	Point-specific pain with radiographic changes, at tarsal navicular (Köhler), carpal lunate (Kienböck), or second or third metatarsal head (Frieberg)
Osteoid osteoma	Site-specific pain, relieved by aspirin
	Abnormal radiograph and bone scan
	50% in tibia
Enthesitis without arthritis	Usually older children (over 8 years old)
	Boys more than girls
	May have acute iritis
	Often HLA-B27 positive

be suspected, but true arthritis is never seen. The most common examples are listed in Table 3.

Treatment

As pauciarticular-onset JIA often affects the joints and eyes of very young children, a team approach which provides expertise in paediatric rheumatology, ophthalmology, physical therapy, and sometimes psychosocial issues is optimal. The overall guiding principles in treating these children is to keep the joint(s) as normal as possible while the disease is active so that once it becomes quiescent, the child is left with minimal complications and to treat ocular inflammation early and thoroughly.

Control of intra-articular inflammation is paramount (Emery 1993) as this can minimize, but not necessarily eliminate, articular complications. Initially either the joint is injected or non-steroidal anti-inflammatory drugs (NSAIDs) are given (see Table 4; Ansell 1983; Silver 1988; Duffy et al. 1989; Hollingworth 1993). COX-2 inhibitors are increasingly being used in inflammatory arthritis, and may likely become an important therapy once approved for children (Golden and Abramson 1999). Once the diagnosis is established, intra-articular corticosteroid injection is very helpful since it may quickly resolve the inflammation (Eich et al. 1994; Huppertz et al. 1995). Triamcinolone hexacetonide is the agent of choice since its effectiveness persists longer than other preparations, generally 1 year or more in this subtype (Breit et al. 2000). During this time, if there is no evidence of synovitis, administering NSAIDs is unnecessary. Treating children initially and repeatedly (average of 3.25 injections over 42 months) was associated with the lack of leg length discrepancy and less thigh atrophy compared to treating with just NSAIDs (Sherry et al. 1999). Specific indications for intra-articular injections include synovial cysts, one or two joints with arthritis, marked pain or dysfunction due to a very limited number of arthritic joints, or when NSAIDs are incompletely effective, not tolerated or contra-indicated. Synovial cysts usually resolve after steroid injection of the adjacent joint (Allen et al. 1986) as these cysts communicate with the joint.

Some joints may not respond to an initial injection but respond well to a second attempt. If needed, joint injection can be repeated. The maximum number of injections per year and total has not been studied and some authors recommend no more than three injections per year per joint. In these recalcitrant cases, we will continue to inject as needed but add in more aggressive treatment (see below). Intra-articular steroids may lead to localized cutaneous atrophy, hypopigmentation, or intra-articular calcifications, but these are rarely of clinical significance. Infection due to the injection is estimated to occur once per 50 000 to 100 000 injections.

While a few studies have demonstrated the effectiveness of particular NSAIDs, such as aspirin, tolmetin, and naproxen (Levinson et al. 1977; Moran et al. 1979; Kvien et al. 1984), there are no consistent findings as to relative efficacy and tolerance. Therefore, the choice of non-steroidal drug is largely empirical, often dictated by the availability of liquid preparations for small children or by individual response. Less frequent dosing enhances compliance, and COX-2 inhibitors may avoid gastrointestinal side-effects with similar efficacy to traditional NSAIDs (Golden and Abramson 1999).

Most NSAIDs are tolerated well by children, with little clinical evidence of gastritis. Chemical hepatitis is their most common untoward effect, with aspirin the leading cause (Bernstein et al. 1977). Aspirin is used less frequently than before possibly due to the higher incidence of adverse effects (Cron et al. 1999). We recommend close monitoring when liver function tests such as aspartate aminotransferase reach a level greater than three times normal, and we generally will stop the medication when the level rises to four times normal.

Pseudoporphyria, a skin disorder characterized by skin fragility, vesiculation, and scarring, has recently been reported as a side-effect of NSAIDs, particularly naproxen, among patients with juvenile chronic arthritis (Levy et al. 1990; Lang and Finlayson 1994). Both excessive sun exposure and fair complexion seem to increase risk for this complication. Scarring can also occur in the absence of blistering (Wallace et al. 1994).

The association of aspirin with Reye's syndrome, though controversial, is of concern, and it is prudent to interrupt aspirin therapy when influenza or varicella infection is suspected. It is not necessary or practical, however, to stop the drug during every viral syndrome in young children. It has been

Table 4 Non-steroidal anti-inflammatory drug use in children with juvenile idiopathic arthritis

NSAID	Total daily dose	Maximum daily dose	No. of doses/day	Liquid[a]	Approved[b]
Salicylic acids					
Aspirin	80–100 mg/kg/day	5200 mg	4 or 3		✓
Choline magnesium trilisate	50 mg/kg/day	4500 mg	2	✓	✓
Acetic acids					
Indomethacin	1.5–3 mg/kg/day	200 mg	4 or 3[c]	✓	
Sulindac	300–400 mg/day (adult)	400 mg	2		
Tolmetin	30–50 mg/kg/day	1800 mg	4 or 3		✓
Diclofenac	2.5 mg/kg/day	225 mg	2		
Propionic acids					
Naproxen	10–20 mg/kg/day	100 mg	2	✓	✓
Fenoprofen	40 mg/kg/day	3200 mg	4 or 3		
Ibuprofen	40 mg/kg/day	3200 mg	4 or 3	✓	✓
Fenamic acids					
Meclofenamate	3–7.5 mg/kg/day	400 mg	4 or 3		
Oxicams					
Piroxicam	0.25–0.4 mg/kg/day	20 mg (adult)	1		
Cox II specific agents					
NSAID					
Celexicob	Not determined	400 mg	2	×	×
Rofecoxib	Not determined	50 mg	1	✓	×

[a] Available as liquid preparations.

[b] Approved for use in children by the United States Federal Drug Administration.

[c] Twice daily for slow-release form.

recommended that children treated with aspirin receive an annual influenza immunization (Committee on Infectious Diseases 2000) and we extend this recommendation to include patients on chronic NSAID therapy. Idiosyncratic reactions to all of the NSAIDs can occur. Neurological complications such as depression or personality changes are uncommon, and can be difficult to detect in very young children. Close attention to parental concerns is warranted. While children often take NSAIDs for years without side effects, potentially severe complications can occur, such as blood dyscrasias or renal papillary necrosis. Therefore we recommend careful monitoring during their use, including a complete blood count with platelet count, aspartate aminotransferase, alanine aminotransferase, blood urea nitrogen, creatinine, and urinalysis at least twice a year while on a stable dose.

For children who develop prolonged arthritis, extension to polyarticular disease or destructive joint changes, more aggressive therapy is indicated. As in children with polyarticular or systemic-onset JIA, early recognition and aggressive treatment of destructive disease is critical for optimal outcome. While pauciarticular-onset JIA most often carries a favourable prognosis, it is important to monitor patients closely to identify those who will progress to more severe disease. For example, radiographs of affected joints should be obtained yearly in patients with persistent arthritis. Unlike typical adult rheumatoid arthritis, radiographic signs of destructive joint disease may not become evident in JIA until many years into the disease course.

For those patients requiring further disease-modifying drugs, there are several options (Rosenberg 1989; Gabriel and Levinson 1990; Giannini et al. 1993), although few studies have been done in pauciarticular-onset JIA. Methotrexate has been used in some pauciarticular-onset patients with good results (Truckenbrodt and Häfner 1986; Wallace et al. 1989; Giannini et al. 1992); its safety and efficacy make it an increasingly attractive option. We currently will often use methotrexate if NSAIDs and multiple injections have failed. Sulfasalazine is a good choice in patients with mild to moderate persistent disease (Gedalia et al. 1993). There is some controversy as to the effectiveness of hydroxychloroquine, and one study found no difference between it and placebo (Van Kerckhove et al. 1988). Similarly, good data on the use of gold and penicillamine are scant. Methotrexate is usually given at a dose between 0.3 and 0.6 mg/kg per week as a single oral or subcutaneous dose. An occasional patient is given as much as 1 mg/kg per week. We monitor blood counts, liver enzymes, and renal function monthly. The role of liver biopsy in ascertaining toxicity is controversial and presently we do not recommend it (Walker et al. 1993). Folic and/or folinic acid may be helpful in limiting side effects, without interfering with efficacy, although appropriate timing of folinic acid doses is important (Ravelli et al. 1999). Inflammatory cytokine inhibitors such as the TNF inhibitors, etanercept or infliximab, have been shown to be very effective in adult rheumatoid arthritis (Maini et al. 1998) and polyarticular-course JIA that is unresponsive to methotrexate (Lovell et al. 2000). Because pauciarticular-onset JIA generally is more responsive to treatment than other forms of juvenile arthritis, this class of drugs is indicated infrequently. Additionally new medications such as the pyrimidine inhibitor leflunomide are currently being tested in children with chronic arthritis.

In those patients whose arthritis completely resolves, the question of when to stop medication arises. The length of treatment depends on the severity and duration of the arthritis; in general, the more difficult it is to achieve remission, the longer the treatment will continue after remission. However, there is a paucity of data to support this recommendation. We generally will continue either sulphasalazine or methotrexate for at least 1–2 years after remission has been documented. We define remission as the complete clinical absence of active synovitis or iritis, in addition to the lack of the variably present conventional signs and symptoms of morning stiffness, increased erythrocyte sedimentation rate, or joint pain.

Aggressive use of physical therapy by a therapist specifically experienced in the treatment of this disease is recommended to keep range and strength as normal as possible. Children may unconsciously substitute the use of unaffected muscle groups during play and exercise, thus normal play activities are not an acceptable alternative to directed physical therapy. Since age-appropriate exercise programmes require experience and creativity, it is important to utilize the services of a therapist knowledgeable in paediatrics.

Orthotic devices can be very useful in appropriate patients. We have mostly used these in children with markedly pronated ankles due to subtalar arthritis. A few children have tenacious flexion contractures that require serial night splinting or even serial casting to correct. Serial casting is usually carried out three times a week for up to a month. Casting under anaesthesia is done infrequently but can be of great help in difficult situations. Where there is length inequality, shoe lifts on the short side improve gait, encourage full knee extension on the longer side, and help maintain quadriceps and vastus medialis strength.

Surgical intervention is rarely necessary. Synovectomy for chronic arthritis is controversial and long-term benefit is limited. In one well-designed study, synovectomy did not prevent progressive joint destruction in adult rheumatoid arthritis (Arthritis Foundation Committee on Evaluation of Synovectomy 1988). Although the complications of arthroscopic synovectomy are much lower than with the open procedure, the effort required in rehabilitation makes this procedure inappropriate for younger children. Chemical and irradiation synovectomies in children have not been adequately studied. The rare child with subluxation of the knee may require surgical correction; long-term outcome is uncertain regardless of surgery. Leg length inequality can, rarely, persist into adolescence and is amenable to growth-stopping procedures on the long leg (Simon et al. 1981).

Eye involvement may prove to be more of a therapeutic challenge than joint disease. Corticosteroid eye drops and mydriatics to prevent synechiae are the typical initial regimen and are generally thought to be effective in preserving vision in eyes with minimal inflammation (Wolf et al. 1987). Nonetheless, in one study, 42 per cent of children had not responded to topical steroids after 6 months, despite early detection and treatment of disease (Chylack 1977). Unresponsive disease is usually treated with subtenon injections of steroid or with oral prednisone; however, these increase the risk of cataract formation and glaucoma. Although adjunctive use of NSAIDs may permit a reduction in steroid dose (Olson et al. 1988), subcutaneous methotrexate at 1 mg/kg/week can produce an excellent response (Weiss et al 1998). Experience with immunosuppressive therapy such as azathioprine or chlorambucil is limited (reviewed in Kanski 1990); cyclosporin A has been used in severe, refractory uveitis. A recent report on the use of etanercept (a TNF-blockade) in treatment resistant uveitis suggests that further study of this modality is warranted (Reiff et al. 2001). Band keratopathy may require chelation with EDTA or corneal scraping. Treatment of glaucoma is initially topical, but systemic therapy with carbonic anhydrase therapy or surgery may be required (Foster et al 2000). Surgical intervention may also be necessary for cataracts. In the past, surgical treatment has been only marginally successful in these children, but results with microsurgical techniques and laser therapy are improving (Flynn et al. 1988; Kanski 1990).

The psychosocial aspects of pauciarticular-onset JIA bear some mention, especially as they may affect the ability to deliver therapy. The vast majority of patients are young and resilient and do quite well psychologically. They are not particularly limited and are able to carry out developmental tasks without difficulty. However, control issues may become a source of persistent strife between child and parent. This is especially true of the young child who may dislike taking medicine or exercising and the adolescent who is beginning to individuate from the family. The degree of other stresses in the family, particularly parental dysfunction, may contribute more to the state of psychological health of children with JIA than the disease itself (Daltroy et al. 1992). Appropriate attention to psychosocial issues can potentially have a dramatic impact on the well being of the child.

The child with pauciarticular-onset JIA is best cared for by an interdisciplinary team consisting of members who are experienced with the complications of this disease and intimately familiar with each other's roles (Brewer et al. 1989). This will enhance both family education and team communication. This team should include physicians (a paediatric rheumatologist, ophthalmologist, and orthopaedist), nurses, physical and occupational therapists, a social worker, and, as needed, other health professionals such as a nutritionist. It is with such a team that a uniform, consistent plan of therapy can be initiated and appropriately altered if complications arise.

Prognosis

Over 80 per cent of children with pauciarticular-onset chronic arthritis suffer little or no musculoskeletal disability at 15-year follow-up (Ansell and Wood 1976; Stoeber 1981; Dequecker and Mardjuadi 1982). Remission rates have varied from 36 per cent after 8 years in one study to 65 per cent after 26 years in another (Guillaume et al. 2000; Zak and Pedersen 2000). In this latter study, 78 per cent of those children who remained pauciarticular went into remission since those with a polyarticular course fared poorer. The majority of the children whose disease becomes polyarticular do so within the first 5 years of onset. It has been hoped that certain HLA genes might be associated with the subset of children who progress to a polyarticular course and thus predict those at high risk, but at this time there is no consensus that particular genes are helpful in predicting disease course in an individual child (see below).

The outcome of uveitis associated with pauciarticular-onset JIA varies from remission without residua to significant visual loss. A critical determinant affecting outcome is the extent of disease at initial examination. Eyes which are normal or have mild uveitis at first evaluation do significantly better than those with posterior synechiae. In addition, early onset of uveitis in relationship to arthritis correlates with poor outcome. Ocular prognosis is of greatest concern if uveitis is documented before the onset of arthritis, as progression to symptomatic disease implies significant injury to the eye. These results strongly suggest that early intervention beneficially influences outcome (Wolf et al. 1987). However, a small minority of patients relentlessly progress, even with appropriate screening and management (Nguyen and Foster 1998). There may also be a subgroup of patients with a more benign form of the disease (Smiley 1976). Kanski (1977) reported that 8 out of 26 eyes with continuing active uveitis for more than 10 years remained free of complications or visual loss. Unfortunately, no particular features distinguish these subsets of children at disease onset. The overall prognosis for vision among patients with the uveitis associated with juvenile arthritis has apparently improved in recent years (Sherry et al. 1991; Cassidy and Petty 2001). This observed decrease in disease severity is probably due to more comprehensive detection of uveitis, including benign disease, and to more timely treatment.

Aetiology

The aetiology of pauciarticular-onset JIA is unknown. However, the available evidence supports two main ideas: that the disease occurs in genetically susceptible individuals and that dysregulation of the immune response is important in pathogenesis. Genetic susceptibility appears to require inheritance of susceptible alleles at several genetic loci, including, but not restricted to, certain genes of the HLA complex. This topic is discussed in detail in the next section on immunogenetics. A number of immune alterations have been reported in children with pauciarticular arthritis and these are discussed below. However, for the most part, we do not know if these findings represent primary immune abnormalities that contribute to pathogenesis or secondary phenomena resulting from the disease process. Ultimately, any satisfactory model of pathogenesis of pauci-JIA must account for the two most striking features of the disease: the preponderance of young female patients and the frequent association of uveitis. The former suggests a possible contribution of an X-linked gene; the latter may reflect tropism of an infectious agent or involvement of an autoantigen common to the eye and the joint. However, experimental evidence to support these hypotheses is lacking at the present time.

The finding that certain genes of the HLA complex confer risk for pauciarticular JIA implies a role for T cells in disease development, and indeed, clonally expanded $CD4^+$ T cells accumulate in affected joints of pauciarticular-JIA patients. The predominant synovial T-cell clones generally differ from predominant clones in peripheral blood, are found at multiple sites of inflammation within single patients, and persist over time (reviewed in Thompson et al. 1998). These findings may reflect an antigen or superantigen driven expansion of T cells at the site of disease or a highly selective recruitment of peripheral blood T cells that survive in the joint. In pauciarticular JIA, many synovial $CD4^+$ cells express the chemokine receptor CCR5, which is expressed by cells in association with Th1 polarization (Wedderburn et al. 2000). In all JIA subtypes, synovial $CD4^+$ T cells early in disease are also enriched for $CCR4^+$ cells, which are associated with the Th2 phenotype and IL-4 production (Thompson et al. 2001); this finding may be unique to JIA, since this early phenomenon has not yet been observed in RA. In combined data for pauciarticular-JIA and spondyloarthropathy patients, increased synovial tissue levels of the Th2 cytokine, IL-4, have been observed in JIA that remains pauciarticular and perhaps relates to the more benign outcome in this JIA subtype (Murray et al. 1998).

In addition to T cells, other arms of the immune system also appear involved in autoimmune responses in pauciarticular JA. Examples of B cell autoimmunity include the presence of ANA and antibodies to a putative oncogene (the DEK nuclear protein), elevated levels of circulating immune complexes, and altered *in vitro* immunoglobulin synthesis (Miller 1990). Interestingly, IgA deficiency and pauciarticular-onset disease have been associated (Barkley et al. 1979). Aberrant activation of the alternate complement pathway is suggested by the finding of an increased C3d/C3 ratio in pauci-JA patients. A correlation between C3d/C3 ratios and the titre of IgG antibodies to lipid A was also observed in pauciarticular-onset disease, implicating these antibodies in disease pathology (Olds and Miller 1990). Altered expression of fas, a cell surface receptor that initiates programmed cell death, has been noted in mononuclear cells of pauci-JIA patients (Haas et al. 1999). Myeloid-related proteins 8 and 14, secreted by neutrophils and monocytes after interaction with activated endothelial cells, are found in the synovial fluid and serum of pauci-JA patients in correlation with active disease (Frosch et al. 2000). Despite this wide variety of apparent immune deviations, other indices of immune function, such as lymphocyte subpopulation ratios and responses to T-cell mitogens, are usually normal in these patients.

The possibility that JIA represents a chronic infection or is initiated by an environmental trigger has prompted the search for candidate microorganisms. No single pathogen has been consistently identified with the development of this disease (Phillips 1988). Rubella virus has been isolated from lymphoreticular cells of seven out of 19 children with chronic rheumatic disease, including two of six with pauciarticular-onset disease (Chantler et al. 1985). Persistence of rubella virus in these patients may reflect an aetiological role for the virus or a state of immunodeficiency in the patients. In two small series, antibody to peptidoglycan, a constituent of bacterial cell walls, was elevated in 25–50 per cent of pauciarticular patients with chronic uveitis (Burgos-Vargas et al. 1986; Moore et al. 1989). This finding may be relevant to disease aetiology because humoral immunity to streptococcal cell wall preparations has been implicated in the pathogenesis of chronic synovitis in animal models (Greenblat et al. 1980). Alternatively, these antibodies may reflect a state of altered immune reactivity in children with JIA. Of related interest, antibody responses to immunization with bacteriophage were observed in a study of children with each type of JIA (Ilowite et al. 1987). Another possible role for an infectious agent is in disease initiation through 'molecular mimicry'; this hypothesis has gained some support, based on the observation that HLA alleles that confer susceptibility to pauci-JIA share stretches of amino acid sequence with proteins from Ebstein–Barr virus (Albani 1994).

The aetiology of the associated uveitis is likewise unknown, but it also appears to be an immune mediated disorder, occurring in genetically susceptible individuals. Animal models of acute uveitis implicate TNFα in disease pathogenesis (Reiff et al. 2001). Human histopathological studies show non-granulomatous, inflammatory infiltration, including plasma cells and lymphocytes. Ocular fluids from affected eyes contain elevated immunoglobulin levels (Rahi et al. 1977; Sabetes et al. 1979) and ANA (Rahi et al. 1977). The antigenic stimulus that initiates or maintains this process has not been identified. Inflammation of both the joint and eye occur in several diseases (e.g. Kawasaki's disease, seronegative spondyloarthropathies, inflammatory bowel disease). The possibility that collagen acts as an autoantigen at both sites has been investigated in patients with JIA, but studies have failed to demonstrate a heightened immune response to collagen in children with uveitis (Rosenberg 1987). In one study, 29 per cent of patients with pauciarticular-onset juvenile chronic arthritis and uveitis were found to have serum antibodies to a low-molecular-weight fraction of bovine iris proteins. However, the presence of these antibodies did not correlate with severity of uveal inflammation (Hunt et al. 1993). Paradoxically, 30 per cent of children with this chronic arthritis and uveitis manifest a humoral response to a retinal antigen, S (Petty et al. 1987). Immunization with this protein induces an acute uveitis in animal models, but its role in chronic uveitis is unclear, as there is at present no animal model of chronic uveitis.

Immunogenetics

Several lines of evidence indicate that genetic factors are involved in disease susceptibility (summarized in Maksymowych and Glass 1988; Cassidy and Petty 2001). Multiple cases of pauciarticular-onset JIA within one family are unusual, but some have been reported. In addition, concordance for disease is increased in twins; in many cases, clinical disease manifestations between twins are similar (Clemens et al. 1985). Lastly, a large number of studies indicate that certain genes within the *HLA* complex contribute to disease susceptibility (the *HLA* association studies discussed below are reviewed in Nepom 1991; Nepom and Glass 1992; De Inocencio et al. 1993; Fernandez-Vina et al. 1994). These reported *HLA* associations are quite complex, in contrast to those of many other rheumatic diseases where a single allele or family of alleles confers disease risk. In pauciarticular-onset juvenile chronic arthritis, not only are a number of different alleles associated with disease, but products of different loci are involved and the risks from each are additive. It appears that one gene is insufficient for disease expression and that gene–gene interactions influence whether disease develops. In addition, the HLA genes associated with pauci-JA have a well-defined 'window-of-effect' during which time they contribute risk; 80 per cent of the risk is complete by the sixth year of life (Murray et al. 1999).

Initial studies described *HLA* class I associations with pauciarticular disease, with *HLA A2*, the most consistently identified allele. The consensus of more recent studies using precise DNA-based HLA typing techniques is that alleles of the class II loci are most strongly associated. However, it appears that the *HLA A2*0201* allele remains significantly associated with disease even after class II associations are taken into account (Fernandez-Vina et al. 1994).

Among *HLA* class II genes, several alleles of the *DRB1* locus are the most reproducibly associated with disease. *DR8* (primarily the *DRB1*0801* allele in many studies) shows the strongest correlation, with relative risks of approximately 4–12. In a number of different North American and Northern and Southern European populations, *DR8* accounts for approximately 25–50 per cent of patients. The *DR8* association is intriguing, since this allele is infrequent (3–10 per cent) in control Caucasian populations, and has not been primarily associated with other autoimmune conditions. *DR5* is also consistently associated with pauciarticular-onset juvenile chronic arthritis, with a relative risk of about 2–7 in most studies. Several *DR5* alleles are present among patients, but *DRB1*1104* alleles are most significantly increased (Melin-Aldana et al. 1992; Haas et al. 1994). *DR6* has been variably reported to be increased in some populations; the *DRB1*1301* allele appears primarily responsible for this association.

Interestingly, juvenile pauciarticular-onset arthritis was one of the first diseases shown to be associated with an allele of the *DPB1* locus. *DPB1*0201* contributes to disease susceptibility, and this effect is independent of the *DRB1* contribution. Possessing *DPB1*0201* may not by itself provide enough susceptibility to lead to disease expression; instead, it adds to the risk conferred by the *DRB1* susceptibility alleles.

The initial HLA studies were done using population-based, case-controlled methods, which reveal disease associations. More recently, linkage of *HLA–DR5, 6,* and *8* alleles and *HLA-A2* to pauci-JIA has been confirmed in family studies using the transmission disequilibrium test (Glass and Giannini 1999). The linkage of *HLA-DR8* has been further corroborated by a study of affected sibling pairs (Prahalad et al. 2000). In contrast, *DR4*, which is the *HLA* type most highly associated with both adult and juvenile rheumatoid factor-positive rheumatoid arthritis, and *DR7* are almost never seen in pauciarticular-onset juvenile chronic arthritis; these alleles are thus thought to provide protection for this disease.

In addition to HLA genes, a number of non-HLA genes whose products have immunological functions are reported to be associated with JA, although these associations are not as robust or consistent as HLA associations (reviewed in Glass and Giannini 1999). A susceptibility factor has been mapped to the TNFA/TNFB gene region in HLA–DRB1*11 individuals with early onset pauciarticular disease. Studies of polymorphism of T-cell receptor genes reveal an increased frequency of the Vβ-6.1B allele in pauciarticular patients who possess the DQA1*0101 allele. Both findings imply that particular HLA alleles interact with other susceptibility alleles in certain disease subsets. Associations have also been observed with regulatory regions of cytokine genes, including IL-1A and IL-10. Polymorphisms within promoter regions can result in differential regulation of gene transcription, with the consequence that certain individuals will produce more cytokine than others. A 'high expressor' promotor allele of *NRAMP1*, a macrophage activation gene, has been found to be associated with pauciarticular JIA in Latvian children (Sanjeevi et al. 2000). An interesting possibility is that some of the JIA-associated alleles of non-HLA genes may predispose broadly to autoimmunity. Indeed, summarizing data from genome-wide searches in several autoimmune diseases, greater than 10 chromosomal loci/genes common to multiple diseases have been identified (Glass and Giannini 1999).

Many investigators have hoped that disease-associated alleles will allow prediction of clinical manifestations of pauciarticular-onset juvenile chronic arthritis, such as which patients are at increased risk for uveitis or progression to polyarticular disease. While an association of iritis, ANA, and *DR5* has been observed by some groups, other studies have not consistently borne this out. *DR8* has also been variably associated with the occurrence of uveitis. Similarly, attempts to link *HLA* alleles to severity of joint disease have been confusing. *DR8, DR5*, and a *DR6* haplotype have all been reported to be increased among patients with mild or persistently pauciarticular arthritis. Some reports correlate genes on the *DQA1*0101/DRB1*0101* haplotype with severe arthritis. Another associates an interleukin 1α allele with chronic iridocyclitis (McDowell et al. 1995). Pauciarticular-onset JA with polyarticular course is associated with a 'low producer' IL-10 promotor allele, whereas persistent pauciarticular JIA is not (Crawley et al. 1999). Although at present none of these associations is strong enough for use in predicting specific manifestations in an individual patient, it is hoped that further elucidation of immunogenetic associations with specific aspects of this disorder will ultimately lead to improved understanding of disease pathogenesis as well as clinical utility in the management of patients.

Summary

The typical child with pauciarticular-onset JIA is a female toddler with chronic arthritis in a couple of large joints. Up to 70 per cent have antinuclear antibodies present, and 20 per cent will develop chronic asymptomatic uveitis. Education, physical therapy, intra-articular steroids, and non-steroidal agents are usually required, but complications or severe disease may necessitate further therapy. Ocular disease requires prompt, intensive therapy and thus requires vigilant surveillance with periodic ophthalmologic examinations. Many children have joint disease that is active for only a few years and 80 per cent suffer no major functional disability at 15 years after onset. The remaining 20 per cent can have widespread destructive arthritis.

References

Albani, S. (1994). Infection and molecular mimicry in autoimmune diseases of childhood. *Clinical and Experimental Rheumatology* **12** (Suppl. 10), S35–41.

Allen, R.C., Gross, K.R., Laxer, R.M., Malleson, P.N., Beauchamp, R.D., and Petty, R.E. (1986). Intraarticular triamcinolone hexacetonide in the management of chronic arthritis in children. *Arthritis and Rheumatism* **29**, 997–1001.

American Academy of Pediatrics Section on Rheumatology and Section of Ophthalmology (1993). Guidelines for ophthalmologic examinations in children with juvenile rheumatoid arthritis. *Pediatrics* **92**, 295–6.

Ansell, B.M. (1976). Joint manifestations in children with juvenile chronic polyarthritis. *Arthritis and Rheumatism* **20**, 204–6.

Ansell, B.M. (1983). The medical management of chronic arthritis in childhood. *Annals of the Academy of Medicine (Singapore)* **12**, 168–73.

Ansell, B.M. and Wood, P.H.N. (1976). Prognosis in juvenile chronic polyarthritis. *Clinics in the Rheumatic Diseases* **2**, 397–412.

Arthritis Foundation Committee on Evaluation of Synovectomy (1988). Multicenter evaluation of synovectomy in the treatment of rheumatoid arthritis. Report of the results at the end of five years. *Journal of Rheumatology* **15**, 764.

Barkley, D.O., Hohermuth, H.J., Howard, A., Webster, D.B., and Ansell, B.M. (1979). IgA deficiency in juvenile chronic polyarthritis. *Journal of Rheumatology* **6**, 219–24.

Bernstein, B.H., Singsen, B.H., King, K.K., and Hanson, V. (1977). Aspirin-induced hepatotoxicity and its effect on juvenile rheumatoid arthritis. *American Journal of Diseases of Children* **131**, 659–63.

Breit, W., Frosch, M., Meyer, U., Heinecke, A., and Ganser, G. (2000). A subgroup-specific evaluation of efficacy of intraarticular triamcinolone hexacetonide in juvenile chronic arthritis. *Journal of Rheumatology* **27**, 2696–702.

Brewer, E.J., Jr. et al. (1977). Current proposed revision of JRA criteria. *Arthritis and Rheumatism* **20**, 195–9.

Brewer, E.J., Jr., McPherson, M., Magrab, P.R., and Hutchins, V.L. (1989). Family-centered, community-based, coordinated care for children with special health care needs. *Pediatrics* **83**, 1055–60.

Burgos-Vargas, R., Howard, A., and Ansell, B.M. (1986). Antibodies to peptidoglycan in juvenile onset ankylosing spondylitis and pauciarticular onset juvenile arthritis associated with chronic iridocyclitis. *Journal of Rheumatology* **13**, 760–2.

Burgos-Vargas, R., Pacheco-Tena, C., and Vazquez-Mellado, J. (1997) Juvenile-onset spondyloarthropathies. *Rheumatic Diseases Clinics of North America* **23**, 569–98.

Cabral, D.A., Petty, R.E., Fung, M., and Malleson, P.N. (1992). Persistent antinuclear antibodies in children without identifiable inflammatory rheumatic or autoimmune disease. *Pediatrics* **98**, 441–4.

Cassidy, J.T. and Petty, R.E. *Textbook of Pediatric Rheumatology* 4th edn. Philadelphia PA: W.B. Saunders, 2001.

Cassidy, J.T., Sullivan, D.B., and Petty, R.E. (1977). Clinical patterns of chronic iridocyclitis in children with JRA. *Arthritis and Rheumatism* **20**, 224–7.

Chantler, J.K., Tingle, A.J., and Petty, R.E. (1985). Persistent rubella virus infection associated with chronic arthritis in children. *New England Journal of Medicine* **313**, 1117–23.

Chaouat, D., Chaouat, Y., and Aron-Rosa, D. (1990). Pauciarticular juvenile chronic arthritis with ocular involvement and antinuclear antibody presenting in an adult woman. *British Journal of Rheumatology* **29**, 236–7.

Chylack, L.T., Jr. (1977). The ocular manifestations of juvenile rheumatoid arthritis. *Arthritis and Rheumatism* **20**, 217–23.

Chylack, L.T., Dueker, D.K., and Philaja, D.J. (1979). Ocular manifestations of juvenile rheumatoid arthritis: pathology, fluorescein iris angiography and patient care patterns. In *Juvenile Rheumatoid Arthritis* (ed. J.J. Miller), pp. 149–63. Littleton: Publishing Sciences Group.

Clemens, L.E., Albert, E., and Ansell, B.M. (1985). Sibling pairs affected by chronic arthritis of childhood: evidence for a genetic predisposition. *Journal of Rheumatology* **12**, 108.

Committee on Infectious Diseases. *2000 Red Book: Report of the Committee on Infectious Diseases* (ed. L. K. Pickering) 25th edn., p. 356. Elk Grove Village IL: American Academy of Pediatrics, 2000.

Crawley, E., Kay, R., Sillibourne, J., Patel, P., Hutchinson, I., and Woo, P. (1999). Polymorphic haplotypes of the interleukin-10 5' flanking region determine variable interleukin-10 transcription and reassociated with particular phenotypes of juvenile rheumatoid arthritis. *Arthritis and Rheumatism* **42**, 1101–8.

Cron, R.Q., Sharma, S., and Sherry, D.D. (1999). Current treatment by United States and Canadian pediatric rheumatologists. *Journal of Rheumatology* **26**, 2036–8.

Cush, J.J. and Fink, C.W. (1987). Clinical outcome of pauciarticular onset juvenile arthritis. *Arthritis and Rheumatism* **30**, S34.

Daltroy, L.H. et al. (1992). Psychosocial adjustment in juvenile arthritis. *Journal of Pediatic Psychology* **17**, 277–89.

De Inocencio, J., Giannini, E.H., and Glass, D.N. (1993). Can genetic markers contribute to the classification of juvenile rheumatoid arthritis? *Journal of Rheumatology* **20** (Suppl. 40), 12–18.

Dequecker, J. and Mardjuadi, A. (1982). Prognostic factors in juvenile chronic arthritis. *Journal of Rheumatology* **9**, 909–15.

Duffy, C.M., Laxer, R.M., and Silverman, E.D. (1989). Drug therapy for juvenile arthritis. *Comprehensive Therapy* **15**, 48–59.

Eich, G.F., Halle, F., Hodler, J., Seger, R., and Willi, U.V (1994). Juvenile chronic arthritis: imaging of the knees and hips before and after intraarticular steroid injection. *Pediartic Radiology* **24**, 558–63.

Emery, H.M. (1993). Treatment of juvenile rheumatoid arthritis. *Current Opinion in Rheumatology* **5**, 629–733.

Fernandez-Vina, M., Fink, C.W., and Stastny, P. (1994). HLA associations in juvenile arthritis. *Clinical and Experimental Rheumatology* **12**, 205–14.

Flynn, H.W., Davis, J.L., and Culbertson, W.W. (1988). Pars plena lensectomy and vitrectomy for complicated cataracts in juvenile rheumatoid arthritis. *Ophthalmology* **95**, 1114–19.

Foster, C.S., Havrlikova, K., Baltatzis, S., Christen, W.G., and Merayo-Lloves, J. (2000). Secondary glaucoma in patients with juvenile rheumatoid arthritis-associated iridocyclitis. *Acta Ophthalmologica Scandinavia* **78**, 576–9.

Frosch, M., Strey, A., Vogl, T., Wulffraat, N.M., Kuis, W., Sunderkotter, C., Harms, E., Sorg, C., and Roth, J. (2000). Myeloid-related proteins 8 and 14 are specifically secreted during interaction of phagocytes and activated endothelium and are useful markers for monitoring disease activity in pauciarticular-onset juvenile rheumatoid arthritis. *Arthritis and Rheumatism* **43**, 628–37.

Gabriel, C.A. and Levinson, J.E. (1990). Advanced drug therapy in juvenile rheumatoid arthritis. *Arthritis and Rheumatism* **33**, 587–90.

Gare, B.A. et al. (1987). Incidence and prevalence of juvenile chronic arthritis: a population survey. *Annals of the Rheumatic Diseases* **46**, 277–81.

Gedalia, A., Barash, J., Press, J., and Buskila, D. (1993). Sulphasalazine in the treatment of pauciarticular-onset juvenile chronic arthritis. *Clinical Rheumatology* **12**, 511–14.

Giannini, E.H. et al. (1992). Methotrexate in resistant juvenile rheumatoid arthritis. *New England Journal of Medicine* **326**, 1043–9.

Giannini, E.H. et al. (1993). Comparative efficacy and safety of advanced drug therapy in children with juvenile rheumatoid arthritis. *Seminars in Arthritis and Rheumatism* **23**, 34–46.

Glass, D.N., Giannini, E.H. (1999). Juvenile rheumatoid arthritis as a complex genetic trait. *Arthritis and Rheumatism* **42**, 2261–8.

Golden, B.D. and Abramson, S.B. (1999) Selective cyclooxygenase-2 inhibitors. *Rheumatic Diseases Clinics of North America* **25**, 359–78.

Greenblat, J.J., Hunter, N., and Schwab, J.H. (1980). Antibody response to streptococcal cell wall antigens associated with experimental arthritis in rats. *Clinical and Experimental Immunology* **42**, 450–7.

Guillaume, S., Prieur, A-M., Coste, J., and Job-Deslandre, C. (2000). Long-term outcome and prognosis in oligoarticular-onset juvenile idiopathic arthritis. *Arthritis and Rheumatism* **43**, 1858–65.

Haas, J.P., Truckenbrodt, H., Paul, C., Hoza, J., Scholz, S., and Albert, E.D. (1994). Subtypes of HLA–DRB1*03, *08, *011, *12, *13 and *14 in early onset pauciarticular juvenile chronic arthritis (EOPA) with and without iridocyclitis. *Clinical and Experimental Rheumatology* **12** (Suppl. 10), S7–14.

Haas, J.P., Frank, C., Haefner, R., Herrmann, M., Spath, H., and Ruder, H. (1999). Inverted ratio of m-fas/s-fas expression in early onset pauciarticular juvenile chronic arthritis. *European Journal of Immunogenetics* **26**, 325–9.

Hollingworth, P. (1993). The use of non-steroidal anti-inflammatory drugs in paediatric rheumatic diseases. *British Journal of Rheumatology* **32**, 73–7.

Hunt, D.W., Petty, R.E., and Millar, F. (1993). Iris protein antibodies in serum of patients with juvenile rheumatoid arthritis and uveitis. *International Archives of Allergy and Immunology* **100**, 314–18.

Huppertz, H-I., Tschammler, A., Horwitz, A.E., and Schwab, K.O. (1995). Intraarticular corticosteroids for chronic arthritis in children: efficacy and effects on cartilage and growth. *Journal of Pediatrics* **127**, 317–21.

Ilowite, N.T., Wedgewood, R.J., Rose, L.M., Clark, E.A., Lindgren, C.G., and Owen, M.J. (1987). Impaired *in vivo* and *in vitro* antibody responses to bacteriophage OX174 in juvenile rheumatoid arthritis. *Journal of Rheumatology* **14**, 957.

Kanski, J.J. (1977). Anterior uveitis in juvenile rheumatoid arthritis. *Archives of Ophthalmology* **95**, 1794–7.

Kanski, J.J. (1990). Uveitis in juvenile chronic arthritis. *Clinical and Experimental Rheumatology* **8**, 499–503.

Kanski, J.J. and Shun-shin, G.A. (1984). Systemic uveitis syndromes in childhood: analysis of 340 cases. *Ophthalmology* **91**, 1247–51.

Kenesi-Laurent, M.A., Kaplan, G., and Kahn, M.F. (1991). Oligoarthrites de l'adulte avec facteurs anti-nuclearies. Originalite du syndrome, rapports avec l'oligoarthrite juvenile. *Revue du Rhumatisme et des Maladies Osteo-articulaires* **58**, 1–6.

Key, S.N. and Kimure, S.J. (1975). Iridocyclitis associated with juvenile rheumatoid arthritis. *American Journal of Ophthalmology* **80**, 425–9.

Kvien, T.K., Høyeraal, H.M., and Sandstad, B. (1984). Naproxen and acetylsalicylic acid in the treatment of pauciarticular and polyarticular juvenile rheumatoid arthritis. *Scandinavian Journal of Immunology* **13**, 342–50.

Lamer, S., and Sebag, G.H. (2000). MRI and ultrasound in children with juvenile chronic arthritis. *European Journal of Radiology* **33**, 85–93.

Lang, B.A. and Finlayson, L.A. (1994). Napoxen-induced pseudoporphyria in patients with juvenile rheumatoid arthritis. *Journal of Pediatrics* **124**, 639–42.

Leak, A.M. and Ansell, B.M. (1987). The relationship between ocular and articular disease activity in juvenile rheumatoid arthritis complicated by chronic anterior uveitis. *Arthritis and Rheumatism* **30**, 1196–7.

Levinson, J.E. et al. (1977). Comparison of tolmetin sodium and aspirin in the treatment of juvenile rheumatoid arthritis. *Journal of Pediatrics* **91**, 799–804.

Levy, M.L., Barron, K.S., Eitchenfield, A., and Honig, P.J. (1990). Naproxen-induced pseudoporphyria in juvenile chronic arthritis. *Journal of Pediatrics* **117**, 660–4.

Lovell, D.J. et al. (2000). Etanercept in children with polyarticular juvenile rheumatoid arthritis. Pediatric Rheumatology Collaborative Study Group. *New England Journal of Medicine* **342**, 763–9.

Maini, R.N. et al. (1998). Therapeutic efficacy of multiple intravenous infusions of anti-tumor necrosis factor alpha monoclonal antibody combined with low-dose weekly methotrexate in rheumatoid arthritis. *Arthritis and Rheumatism* **41**, 1552–63.

Maksymowych, W.P. and Glass, D.N. (1988). Population genetics and molecular biology of the childhood chronic arthropathies. *Baillière's Clinical Rheumatology* **2**, 649–71.

Maksymowych, W.P. et al. (1992). Polymorphism in a T-cell receptor viable gene is associated with susceptibility to a juvenile rheumatoid arthritis subset. *Immunogenetics* **35**, 257–62.

Malleson, P., Petty, R.E., Fung, M., and Candido, E.P.M. (1989). Reactivity of antinuclear antibodies with histones and other antigens in juvenile rheumatoid arthritis. *Arthritis and Rheumatism* **32**, 919–23.

Malleson, P.N., Fung, M.Y., Petty, R.E., Mackinnon, M.J., and Schroeder, M.-L. (1992). Autoantibodies in chronic arthritis of childhood: relations with each other and with histocompatibility antigens. *Annals of the Rheumatic Diseases* **51**, 1301–6.

McDowell, T.L., Symons, J.A., Ploski, R., Førre, Ø., and Duff, G.W. (1995). A genetic association between juvenile rheumatoid arthritis and a novel interleukin-1α polymorphism. *Arthritis and Rheumatism* **38**, 221–8.

Melin-Aldana, H. et al. (1992). Human leukocyte antigen-DRB1*1104 in the chronic iridocyclitis of pauciarticular juvenile rheumatoid arthritis. *Journal of Pediatrics* **121**, 56–60.

Miller, J.J. (1990). Immunologic abnormalities of juvenile arthritis. *Clinical Orthopaedics and Related Research* **259**, 23–30.

Moore, T.L., El-Najdawi, E., and Dorner, R.W. (1989). Antibody to streptococcal cell wall peptidoglycan-polysaccharide polymers in sera of patients with juvenile rheumatoid arthritis but absent in isolated immune complexes. *Journal of Rheumatology* **16**, 1069–73.

Moran, H. et al. (1979). Naproxen in juvenile chronic polyarthritis. *Annals of the Rheumatic Diseases* **38**, 152.

Morrissy, R.T., ed. *Lovell and Winter's Pediatric Orthopaedics* 3rd edn. Philadelphia PA: Lippincott, 1990.

Murray, K.J., Grom, A.A., Thompson, S.D., Lieuwen, D., Passo, M.H., and Glass, D.N. (1998). Contrasting cytokine profiles in the synovium of different forms of juvenile rheumatoid arthritis and juvenile spondyloarthropathy: prominence of interleukin 4 in restricted disease. *Journal of Rheumatology* **25**,1388–98.

Murray, K.J., Moroldo, M.B., Donnelly, P., Prahalad, S., Passo, M.H., Giannini, E.H., and Glass, D.N. (1999). Age-specific effects of juvenile rheumatoid arthritis-associated HLA alleles. *Arthritis and Rheumatism* **42**, 1843–53.

Nepom, B. (1991). The immunogenetics of juvenile rheumatoid arthritis. *Rheumatic Diseases Clinics of North America* **17**, 825–42.

Nepom, B.S. and Glass, D.N. (1992). Juvenile rheumatoid arthritis and HLA: Report of the Park City III Workshop. *Journal of Rheumatology* **19**, 70–4.

Nepom, B.S., Malhotra, U., Schwarz, D.A., Nettles, J.W., Schaller, J.G., and Concannon, P. (1991). HLA and T cell receptor polymorphisms in pauciarticular juvenile rheumatoid arthritis. *Arthritis and Rheumatism* **34**, 1260–7.

Nguyen, Q.D., and Foster, C.S. (1998). Saving the vision of children with juvenile rheumatoid arthritis-associated uveitis. *Journal of the American Medical Association* **280**, 1133–4.

Oen, K.G. and Cheang, M. (1996) Epidemiology of chronic arthritis in childhood. *Seminars in Arthritis and Rheumatism* **26**, 575–91.

Ohm, J. (1910). Bandformige Hornhauttrubung bei einem neunjahrigen Madchen und ihre Behandlung mit subkonjunktivalen Jodkaliumeinspritzungen. *Klinische Monatsblatter für Augenheilkunde* **48**, 243.

Olds, L.C. and Miller, J.J. (1990). C3 activation products correlate with antibodies to lipid A in pauciarticular juvenile arthritis. *Arthritis and Rheumatism* **33**, 520.

Olson, N.Y., Lindsley, C.B., and Godfrey, W.A. (1988). Nonsteroidal anti-inflammatory drug therapy in chronic childhood iridocyclitis. *American Journal of Diseases of Children* **142**, 1289–92.

Petty, R.E. (1979). Epidemiology of juvenile rheumatoid arthritis. In *Juvenile Rheumatoid Arthritis* (ed. J.J. Miller), pp. 11–31. Littleton: Publishing Sciences Group.

Petty, R.E., Hunt, D.W.C., Rollins, D.F., Schroeder, M.L., and Puterman, M.L. (1987). Immunity to soluble retinal antigen in patients with uveitis accompanying juvenile rheumatoid arthritis. *Arthritis and Rheumatism* **30**, 287–93.

Phillips, P.E. (1988). Evidence implicating infectious agents in rheumatoid arthritis and juvenile rheumatoid arthritis. *Clinical and Experimental Rheumatology* **6**, 87–94.

Prahalad, S., Ryan, M.H., Shear, E.S., Thompson, S.D., Giannini, E.H., and Glass, D.N. (2000). Juvenile rheumatoid arthritis: linkage to HLA demonstrated by allele sharing in affected sibpairs. *Arthritis and Rheumatism* **43**, 2335–8.

Rahi, A.S.H., Kanski, J.J., and Fielder, A. (1977). Immunoglobulins and antinuclear antibodies in aqueous humor from patients with juvenile rheumatoid arthritis (Still's disease). *Transactions of the Ophthalmological Society of the United Kingdom* **97**, 217–22.

Ravelli, A., Migliavacca, D., Viola, S., Ruperto, N., Pistorio, A., and Martini, A. (1999). Efficacy of folinic acid in reducing methotrexate toxicity in juvenile idiopathic arthritis. *Clinical and Experimental Rheumatology* **17**, 625–7.

Reiff, A., Takei, S., Sadeghi, S., Stout, A., Shaham, B., Bernstein, B., Gallagher, K., and Stout, T. (2001). Etanercept therapy in children with treatment-resistant uveitis. *Arthritis and Rheumatism* **44**, 1411–15.

Rosenberg, A.M. (1987). Uveitis associated with juvenile rheumatoid arthritis. *Seminars in Arthritis and Rheumatism* **16**, 158–73.

Rosenberg, A.M. (1989). Advanced drug therapy for juvenile rheumatoid arthritis. *Pediatrics* **114**, 171–8.

Rosenberg, A.M. and Petty, R.E. (1982). A syndrome of seronegative enthesopathy and arthropathy in children. *Arthritis and Rheumatism* **25**, 1041–7.

Rosenberg, A.M. and Romanchuk, K.G. (1990). Antinuclear antibodies in arthritis and nonarthritic children with uveitis. *Journal of Rheumatology* **17**, 60–1.

Sabetes, R., Smith, T., and Apple, D. (1979). Ocular histopathology in juvenile rheumatoid arthritis. *Annals of Ophthalmology* **11**, 733–7.

Sanjeevi, C.B., Miller, E.N., Dabadghao, P., Rumba, I., Shtauvere, A., Denisova, A., Clayton, D., and Blackwell, J.M. (2000). Polymorphism at NRAMP1 and D2S1471 loci associated with juvenile rheumatoid arthritis. *Arthritis and Rheumatism* **43**, 1397–404.

Schaller, J. and Wedgwood, R.J. (1972). Juvenile rheumatoid arthritis: a review. *Pediatrics* **50**, 940–53.

Sharma, S. and Sherry, D.D. (1999). Joint distribution at presentation in children with pauciarticular arthritis. *Journal of Pediatrics* **134**, 642–3.

Sherry, D.D. (1990). Limb pain in childhood. *Pediatrics in Review* **12**, 39–46.

Sherry, D.D., Bohnsack, J., Salmonson, K., Wallace, C.A., and Mellins, E. (1990). Painless juvenile rheumatoid arthritis. *Journal of Pediatrics* **116**, 921–3.

Sherry, D.D., Mellins, E.D., and Wedgwood, R.J. (1991). Decreasing severity of chronic uveitis in children with pauciarticular arthritis. *American Journal of Diseases of Children* **145**, 1026–8.

Sherry, D.D., Stein, L.D., Reed, A.M., Schanberg, L.E., and Kredich, D.W. (1999). Prevention of leg length discrepancy in young children with pauciarticular juvenile rheumatoid arthritis by treatment with intraarticular steroids. *Arthritis and Rheumatism* **42**, 2330–4.

Silver, R.M. (1988). Nonsteroidal anti-inflammatory drugs in the management of juvenile arthritis. *Journal of Clinical Pharmacology* **28**, 566–70.

Simon, S., Whiffen, J., and Shapiro, F. (1981). Leg-length discrepancies in monoarticular and pauciarticular juvenile rheumatoid arthritis. *Journal of Bone and Joint Surgery* **63A**, 209–15.

Smiley, W.K. (1976). The eye in juvenile chronic polyarthritis. *Clinical Rheumatology* **2**, 413.

Spalter, H.F. (1975). The visual prognosis in juvenile rheumatoid arthritis. *Transactions of the American Ophthalmological Society* **73**, 554.

Stoeber, E. (1981). Prognosis in juvenile chronic arthritis. *European Journal of Pediatrics* **135**, 225–8.

Strabrun, A.E. (1991). Impaired mandibular growth and micrognathic development in children with juvenile rheumatoid arthritis. A longitudinal study of lateral cephalographs. *European Journal of Orthodontics* **13**, 423–34.

Szer, I.S., Klein-Gitelman, M., DeNardo, B.A., and McCauley, R.G.K. (1992). Ultrasonography in the study of prevalence and clinical evolution of popliteal cysts in children with knee effusions. *Journal of Rheumatology* **19**, 458–62.

Thompson, S.D., Luyrink, L.K., Graham, T.B., Tsoras, M., Ryan, M., Passo, M.H., and Glass, D.N. (2001). Chemokine receptor CCR4 on CD4(+) T cells in juvenile rheumatoid arthritis synovial fluid defines a subset of cells with increased IL-4: IFN-gamma mRNA Ratios. *Journal of Immunology* **66**, 6899–906.

Thompson, S.D., Murray, K.J., Grom, A.A., Passo, M.H., Choi, E., and Glass, D.N. (1998). Comparative sequence analysis of the human T cell receptor beta chain in juvenile rheumatoid arthritis and juvenile spondylarthropathies: evidence for antigenic selection of T cells in the synovium. *Arthritis and Rheumatism* **41**, 482–97.

Truckenbrodt, H. and Häfner, R. (1986). Methotrexate therapy in juvenile rheumatoid arthritis: a retrospective study. *Arthritis and Rheumatism* **29**, 800–7.

Tugwell, P., Dennis, D.T., Weinstein, A., Wells, G., Shea, B., Nichol, G., Hayward, R., Lightfoot, R., Baker, P., and Steere, A.C. (1996). Laboratory evaluation in the diagnosis of Lyme disease. *Annals of Internal Medicine* **127**, 1109–23.

Van Kerckhove, C., Giannini, E.H., and Lovell, D.J. (1988). Temporal patterns of response to D-penicillamine, hydroxychloroquine, and placebo in juvenile rheumatoid arthritis patients. *Arthritis and Rheumatism* **31**, 1252–8.

Vostrejs, M. and Hollister, J.R. (1988). Muscle atrophy and leg length discrepancies in pauciarticular juvenile rheumatoid arthritis. *American Journal of Diseases of Children* **142**, 343–5.

Walker, A.M. et al. (1993). Determinants of serious liver disease among patients receiving low-dose methotrexate for rheumatoid arthritis. *Arthritis and Rheumatism* **36**, 329–35.

Wallace, C.A. and Levinson, J.E. (1991). Juvenile rheumatoid arthritis: outcome and treatment for the 1990s. In *Rheumatic Diseases Clinics of North America* (ed. B.H. Athreya), pp. 891–906. Philadelphia PA: W.B. Saunders.

Wallace, C.A., Bleyer, W.A., Sherry, D.D., Salmonson, K.L., and Wedgwood, R.J. (1989). Toxicity and serum levels of methotrexate in children with juvenile rheumatoid arthritis. *Arthritis and Rheumatism* **32**, 677–81.

Wallace, C.A., Farrow, D., and Sherry, D.D. (1994). Increased risk of facial scars in children taking non-steroidal antiinflammatory drugs. *Journal of Pediatrics* **125**, 819–22.

Wedderburn, L.R., Patel, A., Robinson, N., Versani, H., and Woo, P. (2000). Selective recruitment of polarized T cells expressing CCR5 and CXCR3 to the inflamed joints of children with juvenile idiopathic arthritis. *Arthritis and Rheumatism* **43**, 765–74.

Weiss, A.H., Wallace, C.A., and Sherry, D.D. (1998). Methotrexate for resistant chronic uveitis in children with juvenile rheumatoid arthritis. *Journal of Pediatrics* **133**, 266–8.

Wolf, M.D., Lichter, P.R., and Ragsdale, C.G. (1987). Prognostic factors in the uveitis of juvenile rheumatoid arthritis. *Ophthalmology* **94**, 1242–8.

Wood, P.H.N. (1978). Special meeting on: nomenclature and classification of arthritis in children. In *The Care of Rheumatic Children* (ed. E. Munther), p. 47. Basel: EULAR.

Zak, M. and Pedersen, F.K. (2000). Juvenile chronic arthritis into adulthood: a long-term follow-up study. *Rheumatology* **39**, 198–204.

6.5.2 Systemic-onset juvenile chronic arthritis

Ronald M. Laxer and Rayfel Schneider

Introduction

In 1897, Still highlighted the unique features of systemic arthritis and differentiated it from both rheumatoid arthritis in adults and other forms of juvenile idiopathic arthritis (JIA) (Still 1897). Much remains to be learned about the aetiology, pathogenesis, and treatment of this severe, and potentially fatal, form of JIA.

Although arthritis is required to confirm the diagnosis of systemic arthritis, true joint inflammation may not be present at the onset of the disease. In fact, patients with otherwise classic features of systemic arthritis have developed arthritis as late as 9 years after the onset (Calabro et al. 1976). In addition to chronic arthritis, the American College of Rheumatology classification criteria require 2 weeks of intermittent fever spikes to at least 103°F (Brewer et al. 1977). The ILAR criteria also include chronic arthritis and fever for 2 weeks (documented to be quotidian for at least 3 days) in addition to at least one of the following: evanescent, erythematous rash, generalized lymphadenopathy, hepato-megaly or splenomegaly and serositis (Petty et al. 1998).

Epidemiology

The prevalence of JIA approximates to 50 cases per 100 000 and systemic arthritis accounts for about 10–20 per cent of these patients, with a reported range of 5–43 per cent (Hanson et al. 1977; Andersson Gare and Fasth 1992; Peterson et al. 1996). Even within a given region, the prevalence of systemic arthritis may change over time.

In contrast to the two to three-fold female predominance for all JIA, there is an almost equal sex incidence in systemic arthritis. Females may be more commonly affected when the disease begins after age 10 years (Ansell and Wood 1976). Systemic arthritis may occur at any age from the neonatal period to adolescence. The mean age at onset is 4–6 years (Schaller 1977).

The non-articular features of systemic arthritis make a viral aetiology an attractive hypothesis, but there is little direct evidence to support this. Seasonal variation in disease onset, with a higher incidence in the late spring, summer, and autumn, has been reported (Lindsley 1987), but is not corroborated by others, except for a similar variation in a specific geographic region in a Canadian study (Feldman et al. 1996). Interestingly, disease severity was found to correlate with a seasonal onset in a small Israeli study (Uziel et al. 1999).

HLA associations

HLA studies have demonstrated genetic heterogeneity in patients with systemic arthritis. Inconsistent and weak associations have been reported for a variety of class I antigens. Stronger associations have been reported for class II antigens, including DR5 (relative risk 4–7), DR8 (relative risk 4–5), and DR4 (relative risk 2–5) (De Inocencio et al. 1993). Unlike rheumatoid factor positive arthritis, there has not been a striking association with DR4 homozygosity and there are conflicting reports regarding the prognostic significance of DR4 in systemic arthritis. The DR4 association with systemic arthritis does not appear to hold true for all systemic disease populations (Nepom and Glass 1992). Associations with Dw7 (Stasny and Fink 1979) and DPBI polymorphism (Paul et al. 1995) have also been reported.

Clinical features

Extra-articular manifestations

The hallmark of systemic arthritis is the systemic toxicity and extra-articular features that occur during 'attacks' or flares of disease.

Fever

Fever is absolutely essential to make a diagnosis. A typical fever pattern occurs in the majority of cases, and is described as a quotidian, or occasionally double quotidian, fever pattern (Fig. 1). During typical flares, the temperature will spike rapidly in the late afternoon or early evening, to at least 39°C, only to return fairly quickly to normal, or often below normal, even without antipyretic treatment. Occasionally, the classic fever pattern is only established when anti-inflammatory treatment is begun. Characteristically, the patient will appear toxic during the spike of fever, may have chills and rigors, and will complain of severe arthralgias and myalgias. Frequently, rash is present only during the fever spikes. When the fever subsides, the patient is usually much more comfortable and appears less toxic. The fever must be present for at least 2 weeks to satisfy classification criteria and may persist for months even with treatment. Rarely, fever may follow the development of arthritis.

Rash

The rash of systemic arthritis is a salmon-pink colour and is most prominent over the trunk and proximal upper and lower limbs, although it can be generalized. Individual lesions are 3–5 mm in diameter and often demonstrate central clearing [Plate 110(a)]. The rash may coalesce into large lesions. The rash is usually macular but can be urticarial and pruritus occurs in 10 per cent of patients. While the rash typically comes and goes with the spikes of fever (evanescent), it may be persistent and even occur without fever or other systemic manifestations. The rash may also demonstrate the Koebner phenomenon, the exaggeration of rash in areas of minor trauma or scratching [Plate 110(b)]. Histologically, the lesion typically shows a sparse, perivascular infiltrate with a predominance of polymorphonuclear leucocytes (Isdale and Bywaters 1956).

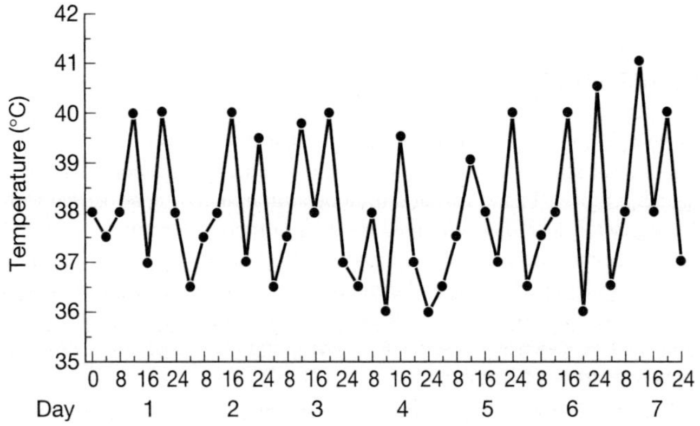

Fig. 1 Temperature chart of a patient demonstrating daily (quotidian), or double-daily, fever spikes with rapid return to below the baseline of 37°C.

Reticuloendothelial involvement

Reticuloendothelial hyperplasia with hepatomegaly, splenomegaly, and generalized lymphadenopathy is a common feature of systemic arthritis. Mild elevations of serum transaminases occur frequently and are usually not clinically significant. Liver histology in systemic arthritis is characterized by non-specific periportal inflammatory cell infiltration and Kupfer cell hyperplasia. Hypertransaminasaemia may reflect disease activity or the effect of treatment with potentially hepatotoxic medications, including salicylates, non-steroidal anti-inflammatory drugs (NSAIDs), or methotrexate.

Patients with systemic arthritis may rarely develop hepatomegaly with acute, severe hepatic dysfunction and even fulminant hepatic failure (Hadchouel et al. 1985). This potentially life-threatening syndrome has been associated with macrophage activation syndrome.

Serositis

Involvement of serosal surfaces is one of the hallmarks of systemic arthritis. Pericardial involvement is most common and pleuritis is more common than peritonitis. Pericarditis is frequently asymptomatic and is best detected by two-dimensional (2D) echocardiography. In one series, nine out of 57 patients had symptomatic pericardial involvement, which was isolated in five cases, but associated with myocarditis in the remaining four (Goldenberg et al. 1992). Cardiac involvement usually occurs within the first year, but it can occur later. Occasionally, patients present only with pericarditis and fever before diagnosis. Therefore, pericardiocentesis may be performed, both for relief of symptoms and diagnosis. Manifestations include tachycardia (out of keeping with the fever), anterior chest pain, and a pericardial friction rub. More severe involvement may lead to dyspnoea, tachypnoea, and even congestive heart failure. Rarely, cardiac tamponade and constrictive pericarditis may result (Goldenberg et al. 1990). The electrocardiogram may be normal, but may show ST wave elevation, or non-specific ST segment changes. The chest radiograph may show enlargement of the cardiothoracic silhouette.

Pleuritis is much less common than pericarditis. Occasionally, large pleural effusions associated, almost invariably, with pericarditis, may dominate the clinical picture. Sterile peritonitis may cause severe abdominal pain.

Arthritis

Most patients have arthritis at disease onset, or have arthralgias or myalgias with the fever spikes and duration from the onset of fever to the development of arthritis may range from just a few weeks to several years. Patients with only arthralgias, or no joint symptoms, pose substantial diagnostic challenges. Most patients develop arthritis within 3 months of disease onset. Chronic, persistent arthritis evolves in half to two-thirds of patients (Schaller and Wedgwood 1972; Calabro et al. 1976). In more than 75 per cent of patients, the wrists, knees, and ankles are involved and the cervical spine, hips, and temporomandibular joints are characteristically involved. Torticollis, secondary to cervical spine involvement, may be a presenting feature (Uziel et al. 1998). Hip involvement occurs in about 50 per cent of patients, is almost always bilateral and usually associated with polyarthritis. The hip and wrist joints are the most frequent sites of progressive and advanced destructive changes (Figs 2a, b and 3), which may occur as early as the first year after onset (Svantesson et al. 1983). Almost one-third of patients who have hip involvement require total hip

(a)

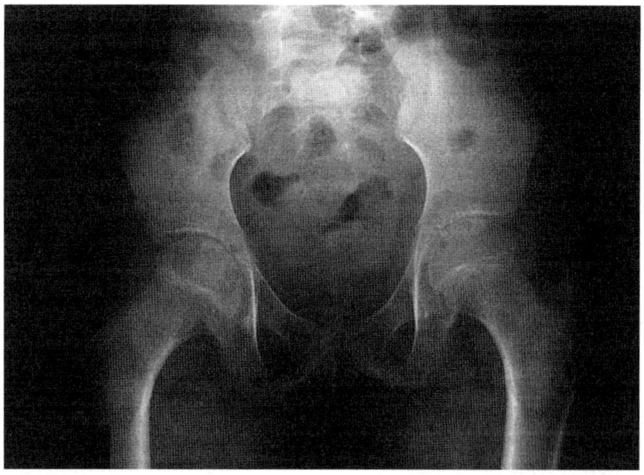

(b)

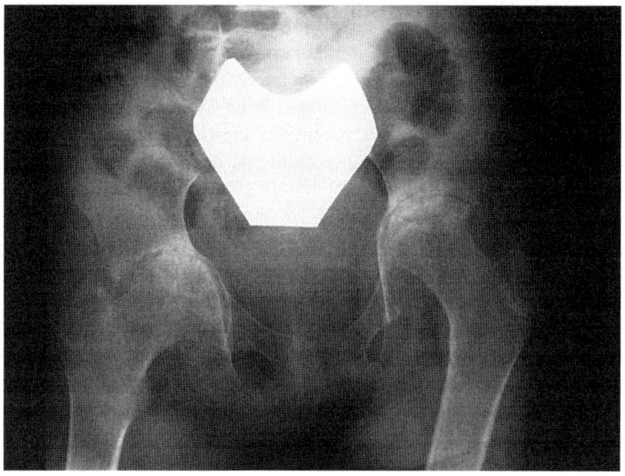

Fig. 2 Girl with systemic arthritis since 7 years. Hip radiographs show: (a) at 33 months after disease onset, osteopaenia, joint space narrowing, and erosions; (b) at 4.5 years after disease onset, increased loss of joint space, protrusio acetabulae, subchondral irregularity and erosions, and sclerosis of both sides of the joints. There is also flattening of the left femoral head.

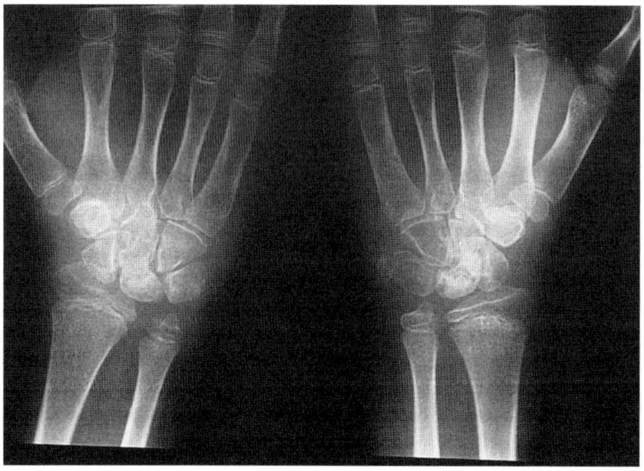

Fig. 3 Same patient as in Fig. 2. Wrist radiographs show advanced changes 2 years after disease onset with moderate narrowing of the carpus, sclerosis, carpal irregularity and erosions, and deformity of the distal radial epiphysis.

arthroplasty (Hayem et al. 1994). The hands are more commonly affected than the feet. Cricoarytenoid arthritis may cause laryngeal stridor. Tenosynovitis of the carpus and tarsus is common.

Less common features

Many organ systems can be involved. Pleuritis is the most frequent pulmonary manifestation, but parenchymal disease occurs occasionally (Athreya et al. 1980). Reduced muscle strength may play a part in the respiratory abnormalities (Knook et al. 1999).

Myocarditis, although rare, can be a serious event with considerable mortality. It has been reported to occur in up to 12 per cent of a series of patients with systemic arthritis from Brazil and symptoms include tachycardia, dyspnoea, and congestive heart failure (Goldenberg et al. 1992). Typically, this occurs during systemic flares of disease and usually with pericarditis. Myocarditis should be suspected in patients who have tachycardia out of keeping with fever or anaemia, cardiomegaly, and congestive heart failure. Diagnosis can be made by electrocardiography, showing increased PR interval and low voltages and echocardiography, showing reduced ventricular function. Digitalis has been used with good effect (Goldenberg et al. 1992), but should be used with caution as it may precipitate arrhythmias. Cardiac murmurs are common, resulting from anaemia and fever, but valvular disease itself is only rarely seen.

Macrophage activation syndrome (also see Chapter 6.12.7)

Macrophage activation syndrome (MAS) is an uncommon, but dramatic, complication of systemic arthritis, characterized by fever, hematocytopaenias, hepatic dysfunction, disseminated intravascular coagulopathy, and encephalopathy. It may run a fulminant course and is associated with considerable morbidity and mortality. It has been reported under a variety of names including 'consumptive coagulopathy' (Silverman et al. 1983), a syndrome of 'acute hemorrhagic, hepatic and neurological manifestations' (Hadchouel et al. 1985) and likely includes reports of viralinduced hemophagocytic syndromes in children with systemic arthritis. In fact, the clinical and laboratory features are very similar to those seen in hemophagocytic lymphohistiocytosis (HLH) secondary to viral infections.

Macrophage activation syndrome in systemic arthritis can be precipitated by changes in medications, including gold, sulfasalazine, hydroxychloroquine, and methotrexate (Ravelli et al. 2001) and has occurred following autologous stem cell transplantation (Wulffraat and Kuis 2001). Changes in NSAIDs have occasionally been implicated. The occurrence of MAS is unpredictable and may occur at disease onset in association with active disease or during periods of remission. Typical clinical features include the rapid onset of sustained high fever, different from the quotidian fever of active disease, hepatosplenomegaly, lymphadenopathy, bruising and mucosal bleeding, drowsiness, and even coma. Respiratory distress with pulmonary involvement and haematuria and proteinuria with renal failure may ensue. Early recognition of MAS is critical to reducing mortality. In contrast to a flare, MAS may be heralded by the rapid evolution of severe pancytopaenia and a decreasing ESR. Transaminases, which may be mildly elevated with active disease, can rise sharply. Fibrinogen, often elevated in active disease, may be low or normal, in association with elevations of D-dimers and prolongation of the prothrombin time (PT) and partial thromboplastin time (PTT), associated with clotting factor deficiencies. Marked elevations of serum ferritin and elevated triglycerides are also seen. Macrophage and T cell-derived cytokines are elevated, especially interferon-γ and tumour necrosis factor (TNF)-α, as well as soluble TNF receptors 1 and 2 (de Benedetti et al. 1997b). Diagnosis is best confirmed by evidence of histiocytic consumption of red cells and platelets in the bone marrow or lymph nodes.

Prompt treatment with high-dose corticosteroids should be instituted and intravenous pulse corticosteroids are recommended. Cyclosporine has been reported to be rapidly effective when corticosteroids have failed

(Mouy et al. 1996). Etanercept has been reported to be effective (Prahalad et al. 2001). Severe multisystem involvement may be associated with poor prognosis and warrants further immunosuppressive therapy. Etoposide is used for other types of HLH and has been successful in treating MAS (Fishman et al. 1995).

Other clinical features

Central nervous system manifestations are dominated by irritability and lethargy during fever spikes. Occasional cases of central nervous system vasculitis have been documented, as have cases of aseptic neutrophilic meningitis during systemic flares of disease (Blockmans et al. 2000). Autopsy series have shown perivascular infiltrates of chronic inflammatory cells in the brain. Fatal cerebral oedema, secondary to inappropriate ADH secretion, has been reported and patients presenting with fever, lethargy, and vomiting are at increased risk of this syndrome (Schneider et al. 2000). Fatal encephalopathy may accompany MAS.

Renal involvement may occur as a complication of treatment, or may indicate the onset of amyloidosis. Mild abnormalities, including proteinuria and mild haematuria may be seen, but significant renal disease is rarely a component of systemic arthritis and its presence should raise suspicion about an alternative diagnosis. Renal disease in children with systemic arthritis may follow treatment with intravenous immunoglobulin (Uziel et al. 1996). Significant proteinuria is an indication to exclude amyloidosis with appropriate tissue biopsies.

Ocular involvement is distinctly unusual relative to other forms of JIA, but asymptomatic uveitis does occasionally occur. It is recommended that patients with systemic arthritis be screened annually for the development of uveitis (Anonymous 1993). Tenosynovitis of the superior oblique muscle (Brown's syndrome) has been reported (Wang et al. 1984).

Amyloidosis (also see Chapter 6.12.1)

Amyloidosis occurs most frequently in the systemic sub-type of JIA and is associated with significant morbidity and mortality. Although rarely reported in North America, approximately 9–10 per cent of patients with systemic arthritis in European series have developed this complication (Ansell and Wood 1976; Svantesson et al. 1983). The reason for this discrepancy in incidence is unclear. No HLA allele has been associated with amyloidosis, but a restriction fragment length polymorphism, related to the amyloid-P component gene, has been associated with the development of amyloidosis in patients (Woo et al. 1987). Serum amyloid-A protein is usually elevated in amyloidosis, but is not predictive of its development. However, persistent elevation of the C-reactive protein level may predict the development of amyloidosis (Gwyther et al. 1982). Fortunately, the incidence of amyloidosis seems to be diminishing in patients with JIA. This is thought to be due to earlier recognition and diagnosis of the disease and earlier and more aggressive pharmacologic management (Savolainen and Isomaki 1993).

David et al. (1993), reported that 57 per cent of patients with amyloidosis had systemic-onset disease. The interval between the onset of disease and the diagnosis of amyloidosis varied widely from 1.5 to 25 years. Ninety per cent of patients had active synovitis at the time of diagnosis. Age at disease onset and duration of disease activity were not related to the development of amyloidosis (Schnitzer and Ansell 1977). The diagnosis should be suspected in patients with persistent proteinuria. The clinical features are generally accompanied by laboratory evidence of acute-phase reaction with anaemia, thrombocytosis, elevation of the erythrocyte sedimentation rate and C-reactive protein, hypergammaglobulinaemia, and hypoalbuminaemia. Confirmation of amyloidosis is most reliably achieved by renal, rectal, or even subcutaneous fat biopsy. Scintigraphy, using a radio-iodinated serum amyloid-P component, has been shown to be a useful, non-invasive technique for detecting amyloid deposits in both suspected and occult sites and may be useful in monitoring the response to therapy (Hawkins et al. 1993).

Treatment is aimed at controlling the underlying inflammatory process since no therapy has been effective in removing amyloid deposits. Treatment with chlorambucil significantly improves the survival rate (David et al. 1993; Savolainen 1999), but its potential toxicities include malignancy and infertility. There is no conclusive role for other immunosuppressive agents.

Growth and nutrition

Children with systemic arthritis frequently have abnormalities of growth (Fig. 4). The systemic features of the disease are associated with hypercatabolism, anorexia with poor energy and nutrient intake. In addition, daily intake of corticosteroids equal to, or greater than, 5 mg/m^2 results in growth delay (Allen 1996). While alternate-day steroid therapy suppresses growth to a lesser degree than daily treatment, this is often difficult to achieve in severely ill patients. Bernstein et al. (1977) have documented that patients with systemic arthritis treated with corticosteroids, had lower growth velocities than a similar group of systemic lupus erythematosus patients treated with steroids, suggesting that the disease itself has a growth suppressing effect.

Levels of growth hormone in children with systemic arthritis have been reported as both normal and reduced (Allen et al. 1991). Low levels of insulin-like growth factors, which mediate the effects of growth hormone, as well as insulin growth factor binding protein-3, have been reported (Tsatsoulis et al. 1999).

Reduced levels of IGF-1 may correlate with disease activity and may explain the growth delay associated with active disease. The NSE/hIL-6 murine model produces high levels of interleukin (IL)-6, an important inflammatory mediator in patients with systemic arthritis (de Benedetti et al. 1997a). These mice

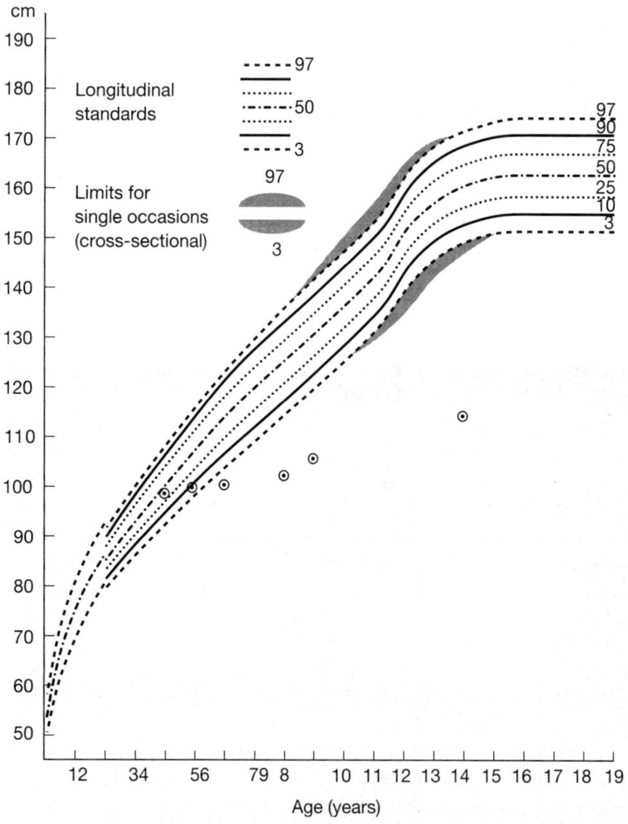

Fig. 4 Growth curve of a 15-year-old girl with severe systemic-onset juvenile arthritis, requiring long-term, high-dose prednisone treatment, showing severe growth delay.

have significant growth delay, with reduced levels of IGF-1 that correlate with IL-6 levels.

Studies of growth hormone treatment in children with juvenile arthritis have shown increased height velocities in the majority of patients (Touati et al. 1998; Al-Mutair et al. 2000). It is unclear whether the ultimate height reached will be altered with growth hormone treatment. Most importantly, suppression of disease activity with medications other than corticosteroids and adequate nutrition must be achieved. Currently, treatment with growth hormone should be reserved for patients in prospective studies and whose growth is significantly below the third percentile.

Laboratory features

The common laboratory abnormalities of systemic-onset juvenile chronic arthritis reflect an activation of the acute-phase response.

Characteristic haematological abnormalities include anaemia, thrombocytosis, and leucocytosis. The anaemia is a reflection of chronic disease and typically results in a hypochromic microcytic smear. Haemoglobin levels are frequently below 100 g/l and may occasionally drop quickly to levels as low as 50 g/l. Serum ferritin is usually increased and, since it is an acute-phase reactant, is not helpful in detecting iron deficiency. Elevated serum transferrin receptor concentration, which is not influenced by chronic inflammation, may be a more reliable marker of iron deficiency anaemia (Kivivuori et al. 2000). Bone marrow examination usually shows a reactive marrow, with an increased number of plasma cells with stainable iron. Examination of the mechanisms underlying anaemia in systemic arthritis suggests an abnormal response to cellular mediators of haematopoiesis. There appears to be normal growth of erythroid colonies and erythropoietin is appropriately regulated. However, there is a defect in iron supply for erythropoiesis (Cazzola et al. 1996), which is most likely mediated by IL-6.

Leucocytosis with a left shift and thrombocytosis are also hallmarks of systemic arthritis, and normal counts should raise suspicion about the diagnosis. White blood cell counts as high as 70×10^9/l may be seen. Similarly, thrombocytosis is characteristic of active disease and platelet counts may exceed 1000×10^9/l. Rarely, both leucopaenia and/or thrombocytopaenia can occur, either as isolated events (Lin and Jaing 1999), with pancytopaenia, or as part of a disseminated intravascular coagulation-like syndrome.

The erythrocyte sedimentation rate is raised, often to greater than 100 mm/h (Westergren). Polyclonal hypergammaglobulinaemia is often observed, although not necessarily at onset; however, both transient and persistent IgA deficiency has been reported (Pelkonen et al. 1983). Other indicators of acute-phase reaction include elevated C-reactive protein (Gwyther et al. 1982) and significant hypoalbuminaemia. Serum complement levels are often raised. Dyslipoproteinaemia has been observed (Ilowite et al. 1989).

There may be evidence of a sub-clinical coagulopathy. Activated factor VIIa, D-dimer, and thrombin–antithrombin III complex levels may be elevated and D-dimer levels correlate with systemic disease activity (Bloom et al. 1998). Elevated soluble TNF receptor levels have been correlated with prolongation of the PTT and a decrease in prothombin activity (de Benedetti et al. 1997b). However, in contrast to MAS, fibrinogen and platelet counts are typically elevated in active disease. Von Willebrand factor elevations may reflect endothelial cell activation (Inamo et al. 1995).

Synovial fluid analysis may not differ from that of other JIA sub-types, but leucocyte counts as high as 100×10^9/l with polymorphonuclear predominance may be seen in the absence of infection, especially with active systemic disease.

Virtually all children with systemic arthritis are seronegative for antinuclear antibody and rheumatoid factor. Antineutrophil cytoplasmic antibodies occur occasionally (Mulder et al. 1997).

Abnormalities of immunoregulation, cell number and function and cytokines have been reported. Levels of IL-1 are raised and, in one study, correlated with disease activity (Martini et al. 1986). Mangge et al. (1995) reported that levels of IL-1b were uniquely raised in systemic arthritis, compared with other sub-types, while others have demonstrated that IL-1b levels are lower that those seen in polyarticular JIA (de Benedetti et al. 1995; Rooney et al. 1995). IL-1 receptor antagonist levels are markedly elevated and correlate with systemic features, severity of arthritis and C-reactive protein concentration (de Benedetti et al. 1995).

Levels of sIL-2R are elevated and appear to be higher in systemic arthritis than other types of JIA and correlate with disease activity (Silverman et al. 1991; Lipnick et al. 1993). Studies of circulating TNF-α levels have yielded conflicting results, but some have shown elevated TNF-α levels which correlate with disease activity (Mangge et al. 1995). Soluble TNF receptor p55 and p75 levels have been elevated more consistently and are also associated with disease activity. A TNF-α single nucleotide polymorphism has been associated with systemic arthritis in a cohort of Japanese children (Date et al. 1999).

There is now compelling evidence that dysregulation of IL-6 plays a prominent role in the cytokine network imbalance and may be associated with many of the systemic symptoms, the arthritis and the laboratory features. IL-6 has been invoked as a critical cytokine in producing fever, thrombocytosis, elevated C-reactive protein levels, serum amyloid A, generalized osteopaenia (by the stimulation of osteoclasts), microcytic anaemia, and growth failure (de Benedetti and Martini, 1998). Circulating and synovial fluid levels are markedly elevated and significantly higher than in other JIA sub-types. Studies of the unique quotidian fever pattern of systemic arthritis show that IL-6 concentrations rise and fall with the temperature spikes and defervences (Rooney et al. 1995; Prieur et al. 1996). There are no similar temporal elevations of TNF-α, or IL-1, with fever. In addition, IL-6 induces IL-1 receptor antagonist expression and IL-1 receptor antagonist levels peak about 1 h after the IL-6 peak and also correlate with fever. Soluble IL-6 receptor levels are also significantly increased in systemic arthritis and correlate with fever in limited longitudinal studies (Keul et al. 1998). Recently, Pignatti et al. (2001) have reported that IL-10, which typically inhibits IL-6 production by monocytes, demonstrates reduced inhibition of IL-6 in children with systemic arthritis.

The hypothesis that IL-6 overproduction is genetically determined is supported by the finding of a single nucleotide polymorphism in the promoter region of the IL-6 gene and the demonstration that two genotypes predispose to higher and lower IL-6 production, respectively. There is a significant association of this polymorphism with systemic arthritis and the low responder genotype is less common in this disease, especially in children whose disease onset is under 6 years of age (Fishman et al. 1998).

Levels of soluble E-selectin and soluble ICAM-1 are elevated in active disease (de Benedetti et al. 2000). Serum levels of monocyte chemoattractant protein-1 and IL-8 are also significantly increased and have been associated with systemic symptoms (de Benedetti et al. 1999). Macrophage inhibitory factor (MIF) is increased in serum and synovial fluid in systemic arthritis, compared to other sub-types and a single nucleotide polymorphism for MIF is associated with systemic arthritis (Donn et al. 2001).

Radiological features

The frequency of radiological abnormalities described by Lang et al. (1995) are shown in Table 1. Similar findings were reported by Cassidy and Martel (1977), with a significantly greater frequency of early periosteal new bone formation (50 per cent) and epiphyseal and vertebral compression fractures (attributed to the use of corticosteroids). Cervical spondylitis with narrowing, irregularity and fusion of the apophyseal joints is also common. Ankylosis most commonly affects the C2–C3 level, but may include the entire cervical spine (Fig. 5). Cervical spine ankylosis has been reported to be more frequent in systemic arthritis than in other sub-types (Espada et al. 1988). Other typical sites of ankylosis are the wrist and tarsus. It is noteworthy that metaphyseal rarefaction, a typical radiological finding of acute leukaemia, has been described in systemic arthritis (Martel et al. 1962).

A striking finding in the study by Lang et al. (1995), was the early appearance of destructive changes. Subtle changes of subchondral irregularity and sclerosis seemed to portend the development of erosions. These early destructive changes may be followed by progressive polyarticular disease.

Table 1 Frequency of radiological abnormalities in 42 patients with systemic juvenile chronic arthritis

Radiological feature	Percentage
Soft tissue swelling/osteopaenia	81
Joint space narrowing	50
Growth abnormalities	48
Erosions	43
Subluxation	21
Ankylosis	19
Joint destruction	14
Protrusio acetabulae	10
Periosteal new bone formation	10

Modified from Lang et al. (1995).

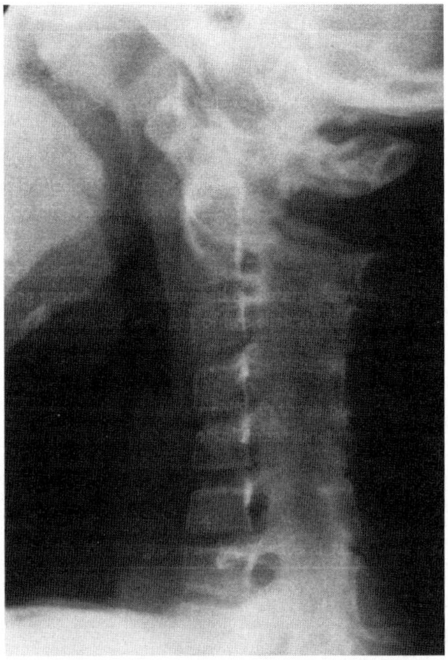

Fig. 5 Boy with systemic arthritis since 3.5 years. Cervical spine radiograph taken 5 years after disease onset shows ankylosis of the apophyseal joints (C2–C5).

Table 2 Important differential diagnoses of systemic onset juvenile rheumatoid arthritis (JRA)

Clinical conditions	Differentiating clues
Infections	
Septic arthritis	Cultures, joint fluid aspiration, for gonococcal septic arthritis a history of sexual activity, tenosynovitis, and a pustular rash
Infective endocarditis	Valvular heart disease, mucocutaneous lesions, nephritis, positive blood cultures
Viral	History of infectious contact, absence of leucocytosis, lymphocytosis with atypical lymphocytes, viral serology, culture or PCR
Post-infectious syndromes	
Acute rheumatic fever	Preceding pharyngeal infection, migratory arthritis, red and very painful joints, valvular heart lesions, streptococcal serology
Reactive arthritis	Preceding infection (pharyngeal, gastrointestinal, genital urinary), mucosal lesions, enthesitis, cultures, and serology
Connective tissue disease	
Systemic lupus erythematosus	Malar rash, photosensitivity, mucosal lesions, nephritis, cerebritis, leucopaenia, lymphopaenia, thrombocytopaenia, and low complement
Dermatomyositis	Characteristic rash, persistent proximal muscle weakness, elevated muscle enzymes, abnormal EMG, MRI of muscles, calcinosis
Vasculitis	
Systemic vasculitis	Subcutaneous nodules, mucosal lesions, palpable purpura, nephritis, sinusitis, pulmonary nodules, infiltrates or haemorrhage, positive ANCA
Kawasaki disease	Conjunctivitis, extremity changes, prominent cervical adenopathy without diffuse adenopathy, coronary artery lesions
Malignancy	Pain out of keeping with clinical findings, night pain, low white blood cell count and platelet count, elevated LDH, metaphyseal rarefaction, bone marrow aspirate and biopsy, lymph node biopsy
Inflammatory bowel disease	Weight loss, growth delay, diarrhoea, abdominal pain, mucosal lesions, family history
Sarcoidosis	Increased calcium, ACE, erythema nodosum, hilar lymphadenopathy
CINCA	Very early onset, abnormal epiphyses, chronic meningitis and ocular findings, severe growth delay
Periodic fever syndromes	Characteristic fever patterns, family history, gene studies

Unusual radiological findings include large humeral cysts, soft tissue calcification unrelated to intra-articular corticosteroid injections and shoulder synovial cysts (Lang et al. 1995).

Differential diagnosis

Many of the classic signs and symptoms are often lacking and the clinician must be astute enough to recognize clues that lead to this diagnosis. One of the most important clues is the variation in the clinical signs and symptoms that can occur over a 24-h period. Children may appear very well throughout most of the day, only to look toxic with rash, arthralgia and myalgia at the time of a fever spike.

In order to make a diagnosis of JIA, a number of exclusions must be made. Malignancies may be especially difficult to diagnose in children who have received even a very short course of corticosteroids for a presumptive diagnosis of JIA. The diagnostic workup must be focused to exclude the entities considered in the American Rheumatism Association classification criteria (Brewer et al. 1977). It is vital to ensure that the child's temperature is recorded and plotted every 4 h to document the intermittent fever pattern. The recommended diagnostic investigations are summarized in Table 2.

Disease course and prognosis

Patients with systemic arthritis may follow a monocyclic course, with complete remission within 2–3 years of disease onset, a polycyclic course characterized by exacerbations of systemic disease activity, or a course of persistent polyarthritis (Calabro et al. 1976; Lomater et al. 2000). The mean duration of active disease is 5–6 years, but some patients have persistent disease activity well into their adult years. Long-term follow up studies suggest that 40–50 per cent of patients followed for at least 10 years still have active disease (Wallace and Levinson 1991). Fifty per cent of patients will have recurrent episodes of fever of variable duration (Schaller 1977) and one-third of patients may have fever for more than 1 year after disease onset (Svantesson et al. 1983). North American series report that few patients will have active, systemic features for more than 5 years (Calabro et al. 1976; Baum et al. 1980). However, two large European studies (Prieur et al. 1984; Hafner and Truckenbrodt 1986) reported that 25–30 per cent had persistent systemic symptoms 10–15 years after disease onset. Occasionally, patients may have recurrences of active disease following prolonged remissions.

Progressive, destructive arthritis occurs in at least one-third of patients (Schaller 1977; Mozziconacci et al. 1983; Cabane et al. 1990), with 25–50 per cent of patients in functional class III or IV after long-term follow-up (Ansell and Wood 1976; Hafner and Truckenbrodt 1986; Lomater et al. 2000). This sub-group of patients would seem to have the worst outcome of all patients with JIA. One report of 14 patients with systemic arthritis, who were followed for more than 10 years, is more optimistic (David et al. 1994). These patients had relatively good functional and psychological outcomes, with none in modified Steinbrocker classes III or IV, but total hip replacement surgery was required in 57 per cent.

Predicting the disease course and outcome is difficult. Several long-term studies have suggested the following to be possible predictors of poor outcome: disease onset under 5–8 years of age; female sex; persistent disease activity for 1–5 years, which may be associated with amyloidosis; cardiac disease; thrombocytosis; accelerated radiological changes; raised IgA levels (Mozziconacci et al. 1983; Svantesson et al. 1983; Hull 1988). The cumulative duration of active periods of disease is predictive of the severity of disability (Lomater et al. 2000). It is important to identify those patients who might benefit from early aggressive treatment before destructive joint changes have ensued. We identified persistence of systemic symptoms and a platelet count of more than 600×10^9/l at 6 months after disease onset as poor prognostic indicators. Three-quarters of our patients with both of these predictors developed joint destruction (Schneider et al. 1992). A subsequent study of 104 children with systemic arthritis showed persistent systemic symptoms and platelet counts greater than 600×10^9/l at 6 months predicted poor functional outcome, as evaluated by the CHAQ (Spiegel et al. 2000). Generalized lymphadenopathy, age less than 8 years at onset and polyarticular arthritis with hip involvement at 6 months, predicted poor articular outcome (Modesto et al. 2001).

Mortality

There are more deaths amongst patients with systemic arthritis than any other sub-type of JIA with a reported mortality of 8–14 per cent in several large earlier European studies (Ansell and Wood 1976; Prieur et al. 1984; Hafner and Truckenbrodt 1986). Amyloidosis has been associated with almost half the deaths in European patients with JIA and with only 13 per cent of deaths amongst North American patients. This may account for the higher mortality in European series. The declining incidence of amyloidosis has contributed to a reduction in the mortality rate to 2–5 per cent (Kobayashi et al. 1993; Lomater et al. 2000). Infection is the most common cause of death in North American patients and is often associated with corticosteroid therapy. MAS has emerged as a significant cause of death and could include the deaths previously attributed to liver failure. Most deaths occur within the first 10 years of disease onset.

Management (Box 1)

The lack of randomized placebo-controlled trials in patients with systemic arthritis makes it difficult to evaluate the efficacy of any therapy. Because of increased medication-related toxicity in these patients, all therapeutic

Box 1 Guidelines to the pharmacological management of patients with systemic-onset juvenile arthritis

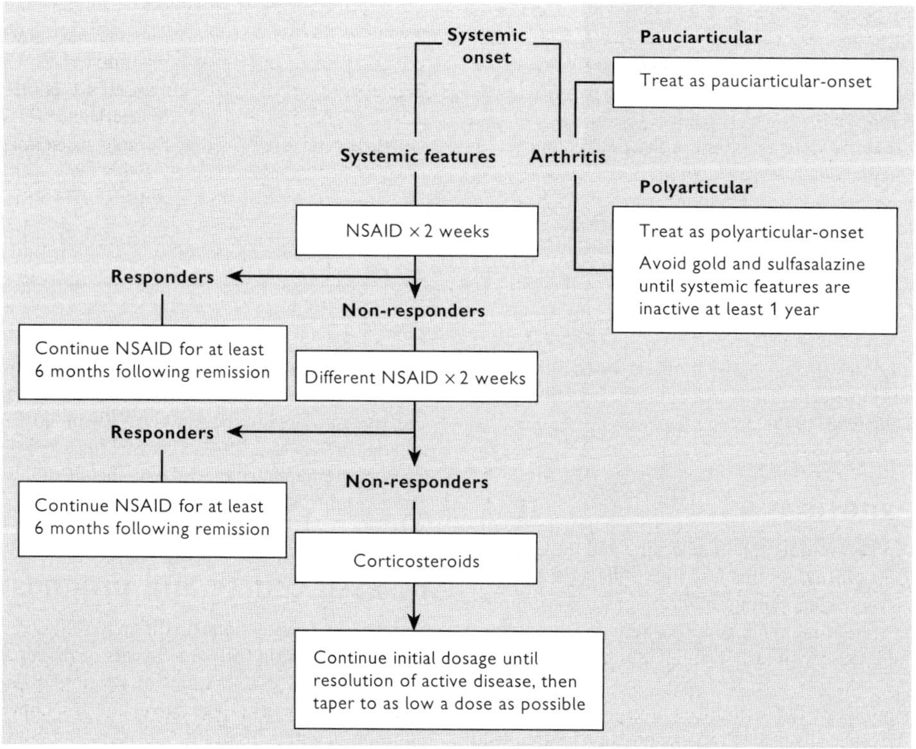

interventions must be carefully monitored. The approach to the management of systemic arthritis must be a co-ordinated one, involving all members of the health care team. In addition to the articular and extra-articular features of the disease, growth and psychosocial development must be carefully monitored. The effects of disease activity and corticosteroid treatment on bone density are substantial and can lead to significant morbidity. The significant financial burdens placed upon families with a chronically ill child must not be overlooked.

Extra-articular features

Initial attempts to control fever should be with NSAIDs. Many paediatric rheumatologists in North America have moved away from salicylates, because of their increased hepatotoxicity relative to other NSAIDs and the potential for Reye's syndrome. Success in controlling fevers has been achieved with both ibuprofen and indomethacin. Because NSAIDs are protein bound, it is essential that the serum albumin be measured and the dose reduced if hypoalbuminaemia is present. Failing to do so will result in excessive free drug, which can result in toxicity. A minimum of a 1-week trial of a NSAID should be given before it is deemed to have failed. If the patient is not too ill, a second NSAID trial should be attempted.

At least 50 per cent of patients will have an inadequate response to NSAIDs. When NSAIDs fail to control systemic toxicity, corticosteroid treatment is indicated. If used in high enough doses, steroids will virtually always be effective. However, as they have significant side effects and do not limit the duration of active disease or alter the long-term prognosis, they must be used judiciously. At times, patients, parents, and physicians may have to be willing to settle for some fever provided that the peaks are not too high and not associated with severe systemic toxicity or profound anaemia. Patients requiring steroids require at least 1 mg/kg/day and often in divided doses. Occasionally, symptoms may be so severe that the daily dose may be better administered in three or four doses over a 24-h period for a short period of time. High-dose alternate-day prednisone has been reported to be effective (Kimura et al. 2000a). High-dose, intravenous pulse methylprednisolone may also be used with severe flares, but provide short-term benefit only. A protocol of intravenous methylprednisolone mini-pulses has been reported to be effective on early clinical and laboratory parameters of inflammation, lasting as long as 6 months. This protocol resulted in a significantly lower cumulative dose of corticosteroid over a 6-month period than in a similar group of patients started on 1 mg/kg/day (Picco et al. 1996).

While the presence of lymphadenopathy, hepatosplenomegaly and rash usually correlate with more active systemic symptoms and are an indication of active disease, these alone do not justify an increase in treatment. Anaemia is common in patients with systemic arthritis and is usually a result of chronic disease. Maintenance doses of iron supplementation may raise the haemoglobin concentration slightly, but are rarely of great benefit. Rarely, during acute systemic flares, the haemoglobin concentration may fall rapidly to as low as 40–50 g/l, necessitating blood transfusion in addition to corticosteroid therapy, particularly in the face of cardiac compromise.

Several agents have been attempted to manage the systemic features and reduce steroid toxicity. Methotrexate, which has proven efficacy for polyarticular JIA, is much less consistently effective in controlling systemic features (Speckmaier et al. 1989; Halle and Prieur 1991). An early open-label study, with high-dose intravenous immunoglobulin (IVIG), reported an impressive improvement in both articular and extra-articular disease and in laboratory abnormalities, as well as in a reduction in the dose of steroids over a 6-month time period (Silverman et al. 1990). A second open-label study did not seem to show any long-term benefit of IVIG, although there was an improvement in the laboratory markers of active disease (Prieur et al. 1990). The Pediatric Rheumatology Collaborative Study Group trial did not show a statistically significant improvement in patients treated with IVIG, compared to placebo, although there was a trend towards overall improvement in the IVIG-treated group (Silverman et al. 1994). However, many patients entered the trial so early in the disease course that spontaneous remissions may have occurred. Finally, Uziel et al. (1996) reported that IVIG might be effective in some patients. IVIG should probably be reserved for patients whose systemic symptoms are not controlled by steroids, or who have significant steroid toxicity prior to the use of other potentially more toxic agents. Very preliminary data on the use of the TNF antagonist etanercept suggest that it may help systemic features in some patients, but many patients fail to respond (Higgins et al. 2000; Kimura et al. 2000b; Schmeling et al. 2001). One case report on the use of infliximab showed short-term benefit on fever control (Elliott et al. 1997).

Serositis, as with the fever of systemic arthritis, will often respond to NSAIDs. Indomethacin seems to be especially effective for the treatment of pericarditis. Corticosteroids in low to moderate doses (0.5–1 mg/kg/day) are usually sufficient to control serositis if NSAIDs are not effective. We have found intravenous pulse methylprednisolone, 30 mg/kg/day (maximum 1 g) daily for 3 days, to be rapidly effective and without toxicity, although of only short-term benefit. If there is significant compromise of cardiac function, pericardiocentesis may be required. Some authors recommend a pleural or pericardial drain for several days. Ventricular tachycardia, complicating pericardiocentesis, has resulted in a few deaths (Goldenberg et al. 1990). Myocarditis may be of such severity that congestive heart failure ensues. Treatment with high-dose oral or intravenous pulse corticosteroids, together with other supportive measures, is indicated.

Articular disease

Some children with systemic arthritis have arthritis that is only problematic during flares of systemic disease. These children generally have a good outcome and respond well to management of the systemic components of the illness. However, the subset of children with persistent polyarticular disease, even in the absence of systemic manifestations, has progressive erosive disease difficult to treat with the standard first and second line agents. Unfortunately, no adequately controlled studies have been conducted in this group of children and our current approach is based largely on anecdotal experience.

Management of the chronic systemic arthritis follows the same principles of management of arthritis in other forms of JIA. Intra-articular corticosteroid injections have a definite role in sytemic arthritis, but are generally less effective than in other JIA sub-types, with a shorter duration of response (Breit et al. 2000). The benefit of intra-articular corticosteroids in the presence of uncontrolled systemic disease is particularly short-lived. Increased drug-related toxicity is perhaps unique to patients with systemic arthritis. This may be seen with salicylates, NSAIDs, and disease-modifying antirheumatic drugs, including gold (Silverman et al. 1983; Hadchouel et al. 1985) and sulfasalazine (Cassidy 1990; Hertzberger-Ten Cate and Cats 1991). In fact, many authors consider that both gold and sulfasalazine are contraindicated in patients with systemic arthritis, particularly if the disease is systemically active. Currently, methotrexate is the drug of choice for most patients with JIA, including systemic arthritis, needing second-line agents (Giannini et al. 1992). However, it is unclear how effective methotrexate is for systemic arthritis and there is little evidence that it has any effect on systemic symptoms. In fact, systemic patients may be less responsive to methotrexate than patients with other types of JIA (Speckmaier et al. 1989; Halle and Prieur 1991). Early treatment (within 2 years of onset), before the development of radiographical lesions at the time of starting methotrexate, may improve the response (Ravelli et al. 1994). Increasing doses of methotrexate to 0.46–1.2 mg/kg/week did not result in significant improvement over standard doses in two open series (Wallace and Sherry 1992; Reiff et al. 1995). While a retrospective case series suggested that weekly methotrexate at a dose of 0.7 mg/kg/week led to an improvement in systemic symptoms over a period of 3–15 months (Al-Sewairy et al. 1998), these findings were not duplicated in a placebo-controlled trial (Woo et al. 2000). Furthermore, early institution of methotrexate, which is thought to result in improved outcomes in JIA, did not alter the progressive course of systemic patients with prognostic indicators of a poor functional outcome (Spiegel et al. 2000).

The methotrexate toxicity profile in patients with systemic arthritis is similar to that of patients with other forms of JIA. However, the general susceptibility of the liver in patients with systemic disease, as well as the frequent use of many other medications in these patients, suggests that extra careful attention should be paid to looking for signs of toxicity. One case of accelerated nodulosis (Falcini et al. 1997), two cases of macrophage activation syndrome (Ravelli et al. 1996, 2001), and one of Hodgkin's disease (Padeh et al. 1997), following methotrexate use in systemic arthritis, have been reported.

Early studies of cyclosporin in systemic arthritis (Bjerkhoel and Forre 1988; Ostensen et al. 1988) showed only minimal effect on synovitis and systemic symptoms persisted in several patients. The toxicity of cyclosporin seemed to outweigh the benefits. However, a more recent study using somewhat lower doses did document efficacy at recommended doses of 5 mg/kg/day in two divided doses (Pistoia et al. 1993). Improvement in terms of reduction of arthritis, fever and prednisone dose was noted as early as 1 month after starting treatment. Fourteen patients with systemic arthritis who received cyclosporine, with or without methotrexate, were reported (Reiff et al. 1997). The authors concluded that cyclosporin resulted in fever reduction, improved morning stiffness and was steroid sparing. Patients who received cyclosporin, together with methotrexate, seemed to have better results. However, there was a high incidence of infections and reduced renal function. Thus, the authors suggested starting at a relatively low-dose (2.5–3 mg/kg/day) and to reduce the dose for any rise in serum creatinine beyond 30 per cent. Lomater et al. (2000) have also commented that 21 of 26 patients treated with cyclosporin had side-effects. It is unclear whether cyclosporin is truly remitting, if patients will be able to discontinue cyclosporin and what the long-term efficacy and toxicity are.

Chlorambucil has been used in those patients who also develop amyloidosis, with significantly improved survival (David et al. 1993), but systemic features may not be well controlled (Manners and Ansell 1986). In addition, the risk of leukaemia seems to be particularly increased with this alkylating agent. Azathioprine may be somewhat effective (Kvien et al. 1986).

Combination therapy with monthly intravenous methylprednisolone and cyclophosphamide and weekly methotrexate has been reported in two separate open-label studies (Shaikov et al. 1992; Wallace and Sherry 1997). While the preliminary data showed that patients improved, no long-term results are available. Given the concern about toxicity with cyclophosphamide treatment, the long-term follow-up of these patients should be reported before this approach can be recommended in the standard management.

The TNF antagonist etanercept was shown to prevent flares in patients with polyarticular JIA, who either had an inadequate response to, or were intolerant of methotrexate when compared to placebo (Lovell et al. 2000). While some patients with systemic polyarticular juvenile arthritis do respond to Etanercept, the response does not appear to be as beneficial as with other subtypes (Higgins et al. 2000; Kimura et al. 2000b).

Thalidomide, another agent with anti-TNF properties, has been reported in a small group of children with systemic arthritis who had failed methotrexate, cyclosporin, and etanercept. At a mean follow-up of 5.2 months on a dose of 3 mg/kg/day, there was a significant improvement in the joint count and laboratory abnormalities. No adverse events were reported (Lehman et al. 2002).

There remain a number of patients who do not seem to have an appropriate response to any of the agents discussed above and who also suffer intolerable medication-related toxicity, particularly from corticosteroid treatment. It is for these patients that treatment with stem cell transplantation has been suggested. In some patients, the responses have been dramatic (Wulffraat et al. 1999), with resolution of disease activity, reduction in corticosteroid treatment and resumption of growth. Nevertheless, there has also been significant mortality (14 per cent) associated with this treatment (Wulffraat and Kuis 2001). Patient selection and induction regime are just two factors that must be better understood before this treatment can be recommended as anything more than experimental.

Adult-onset Still's disease

In 1971, Bywaters described an entity in adults that appeared virtually identical in clinical and laboratory manifestations to systemic arthritis and coined the term adult-onset Still's disease (AoSD) (Bywaters 1971). AoSD has been described at all ages and has a worldwide distribution. Females outnumber males slightly. The majority of cases occur before the age of 40, but cases have been reported up to age 70. Several sets of criteria have been proposed for the classification or diagnosis of AoSD. Those of Yamaguchi et al. (1992) were found to have the highest degree of sensitivity (Masson et al. 1996). Risk factors for AoSD were studied in a case control series of 60 patients. Stressful life events in the year preceding the onset of AoSD were the only identified risk factors (Sampalis et al. 1996). Many infectious agents have been associated with AoSD, but none has been proven to be consistently positive.

The fever pattern is identical to that of systemic arthritis (Fig. 1). Approximately 90 per cent of patients have a rash that is evanescent and may demonstrate a Koebner phenomenon. The rash may be pruritic. Occasionally fixed eruptions may occur. Urticarial rashes can also occur. One important feature not well appreciated in systemic arthritis is a complaint of a severe sore throat during flares of disease (Nguyen and Weisman 1997). While arthritis is not necessarily present at the onset, arthralgias are present in virtually all patients with fever spikes. Initial series described the arthritis as being quite mild, but chronic arthritis with disability may be a sequel in up to 40 per cent of cases (Elkon et al. 1982; Cush et al. 1987; Cabane et al. 1990; Pouchot et al. 1991; Lin et al. 2000). As in the childhood form, hepatosplenomegaly and lymphadenopathy are common. Weight loss is frequently observed (Ohta et al. 1987; Mok et al. 1998). Pericarditis is the most common cardiac manifestation and tamponade may rarely occur. Pulmonary abnormalities are occasionally observed (Cheema and Quismorio 1999). Abdominal pain may relate to hepatitis, adenitis, and sterile peritonitis. Abnormal liver function tests have been reported in up to 76 per cent of patients (Pouchot et al. 1991). Neurological involvement, including neutrophilic meningitis, may occur during systemic flares (Blockmans et al. 2000), or as a result of infection, or complications of therapy (Wouters and van de Putte 1986). The differential diagnosis should be approached in the same way as that for systemic arthritis and include thorough searches for infection and malignancy, including lymphoma and carcinoma.

The disease may follow several courses (Cush et al. 1987; Pouchot et al. 1991). In one series, patients with either a monocyclic or polycyclic systemic course had articular manifestations that manifested primarily during systemic exacerbations and had a good functional outcome. On the other hand, patients with a chronic articular course do not fare as well. Those patients with a polyarticular onset, axial arthritis, need for steroids within 2 years of onset, a history suggestive of childhood attacks and the presence of a rash seems to be at a greater overall risk for progressive joint damage and an unfavourable outcome (Cush et al. 1987; Pouchot et al. 1991). Involvement of the carpus with ankylosis (Medsger and Christy 1975) is particularly common, as is tarsal ankylosis, and involvement of the cervical spine and hips, with rapid progression of destructive disease.

The laboratory abnormalities, like those of systemic arthritis, are nonspecific and include leucocytosis with neutrophilia, normochromic, normocytic anaemia, and thrombocytosis. Eosinophilia appears to be common in Japanese cases (Ohta et al. 1987). Hypoalbuminaemia, hypergammaglobulinaemia, and increased serum complement levels are commonly observed. Raised serum levels of hepatic transaminases, while common, are usually transient and reflect active disease. Hyperferritinaemia is thought to be an especially important marker of active disease (Fautrel et al. 2001). The proinflammatory cytokine, IL-18, was reported to be markedly elevated in a group of 16 patients with AoSD and correlated with both active disease and serum ferritin level (Kawashima et al. 2001). This cytokine may drive the over-production of IL-6, interferon-γ and TNF-α, which are also elevated in patients with AoSD (Hoshino et al. 1998; Stambe and Wicks 1998). Levels of macrophage-colony stimulating factor were also found to be elevated in a group of patients with AoSD (Matsui et al. 1999). No consistent HLA associations have been identified (Wouters et al. 1986; Pouchot et al. 1991), nor was HLA-DR typing able to discriminate patients who developed chronic arthritis from those who remained systemic (Fujii et al. 1998).

The treatment of AoSD should follow along the same lines as those of systemic arthritis. Initial attempts at fever control should be made with either high-dose salicylates (100 mg/kg/day), or other NSAIDs, particularly indomethacin. The majority of patients will ultimately require moderate to high-dose glucocorticoid therapy at some time during their course. In one series with a median follow-up of 10 years, 50 per cent of patients still required treatment with second-line agents (gold, hydroxychloroquine, or methotrexate) and one-third of these continued to require low-dose prednisone (Sampalis et al. 1995). There is a suggestion that dexamethasone may be effective in controlling systemic features not controlled with high-dose prednisolone (Koizumi et al. 2000). Similarly, IVIG may be tried to avoid the need for corticosteroids, or to potentially reduce the dose (Mahmud and Hughes 1999). Several second-line agents may be effective in patients who are not controlled on NSAIDs and low-dose corticosteroids. Low-dose weekly methotrexate leads to improvement in articular and systemic features in most patients, but hepatotoxicity and infectious complications remain significant concerns (Kraus and Alarcon-Segovia 1991; Aydintug et al. 1992; Fujii et al. 1997; Fautrel et al. 1999). The response may depend on the patients' immunogenetic phenotype (Fujii et al. 1997). Cyclosporine has also been reported to be effective at doses below 5 mg/kg/day (Marchesoni et al. 1997).

The role of etanercept in AoSD treatment was reported in a prospective study of 12 patients, three of whom had childhood onset disease. Ten of 12 completed a 6-month trial of 25 mg etanercept biweekly. Seven of 12 met the ACR 20 criteria, four met the ACR 50 criteria and two met the ACR 70 criteria. Of three patients with systemic features, only one improved and the arthritis did not improve in any of these patients. The etanercept treatment was well tolerated (Husni et al. 2002).

The use of the TNF antagonist infliximab has been reported in three patients with AoSD (Cavagna et al. 2001), but the role of TNF antagonists in AoSD is not clear at the current time. One patient has been reported who achieved a partial remission lasting 1 year following autologous stem-cell transplantation, but relapse with synovitis appeared 15 months post-transplant (Lanza et al. 2000).

Death may result in a very small number of patients from a wide variety of causes, including liver involvement and systemic amyloidosis (Ohta et al. 1987; Reginato et al. 1987). In comparison to same-sex siblings, patients with AoSD had significantly higher levels of pain, psychological disability, and physical disability. Despite these problems, educational achievement, occupational prestige, social functioning, social support, annual family income, and days lost from work did not differ between patients and same-sex siblings (Sampalis et al. 1995).

References

Allen, D.B. (1996). Growth suppression by glucocorticoid therapy. *Endocrinology and Metabolism Clinics of North America* **25**, 699–717.

Allen, R.C., Jimenez, M., and Cowell, C.T. (1991). Insulin-like growth factor and growth hormone secretion in juvenile chronic arthritis. *Annals of the Rheumatic Diseases* **50**, 602–6.

Al-Mutair, A., Bahabri, S., Al-Mayouf, S., and Al-Ashwal, A. (2000). Efficacy of recombinant human growth hormone in children with juvenile rheumatoid arthritis and growth failure. *Journal of Pediatric Endocrinology & Metabolism* **13**, 899–905.

Al-Sewairy, W., Al-Mazyed, A., Al-Dalaan, A., Al-Balaa, S., and Bahabri, S. (1998). Methotrexate therapy in systemic-onset juvenile rheumatoid arthritis in Saudi Arabia: a retrospective analysis. *Clinical Rheumatology* **17**, 52–7.

Andersson Gare, B. and Fasth, A. (1992). Epidemiology of juvenile chronic arthritis in Southwestern Sweden: a 5 year, prospective population study. *Pediatrics* **90**, 950–8.

Anonymous (1993). American Academy of Pediatrics Section on Rheumatology and Section on Ophthalmology: guidelines for ophthalmologic examinations in children with juvenile rheumatoid arthritis. *Pediatrics* **92**, 295–6.

Ansell, B.M. and Wood, P.H.N. (1976). Prognosis in juvenile chronic polyarthritis. *Clinics in Rheumatic Diseases* **2**, 397–412.

Athreya, B.H., Doughty, R.R., Bookspan, M., Schumacher, H.R., Sewell, E.M., and Chatten, J. (1980). Pulmonary manifestations of juvenile rheumatoid arthritis. A report of eight cases and review. *Clinics in Chest Medicine* **1**, 361–74.

Aydintug, A.O., D'Cruz, D., Cervera, R., Khamashta, M.A., and Hughes, G.R. (1992). Low dose methotrexate treatment in adult Still's disease. *Journal of Rheumatology* **19**, 431–5.

Baum, J., Alerkseer, L.S., Brewer, E.J., Jr., Dolgopolova, A.V., Mudholkar, G.S., and Patel, K. (1980). Juvenile rheumatoid arthritis. A comparison of patients from the USSR and USA. *Arthritis and Rheumatism* **23**, 977–84.

Bernstein, B.H., Stobie, D., Singsen, B.H., Koster-King, K., Kornreich, H.K. and Hanson, V. (1977). Growth retardation in juvenile rheumatoid arthritis (JRA). *Arthritis and Rheumatism* **20**, 212–16.

Bjerkhoel, F. and Forre, O. (1988). Cyclosporin treatment of a patient with severe systemic juvenile rheumatoid arthritis. *Scandinavian Journal of Rheumatology* **17**, 483–6.

Blockmans, D.E., Knockaert, D.C., and Bobbaers, H.J. (2000). Still's disease can cause neutrophilic meningitis. *Neurology* **54**, 1203–5.

Bloom, B.J., Tucker, L.B., Miller, L.C., and Schaller, J.G. (1998). Fibrin D-dimer as a marker of disease activity in systemic onset juvenile rheumatoid arthritis. *Journal of Rheumatology* **25**, 1620–5.

Breit, W., Frosch, M., Meyer, U., Heinecke, A., and Ganser, G. (2000). A subgroup-specific evaluation of the efficacy of intra-articular triamcinolone hexacetonide in juvenile chronic arthritis. *Journal of Rheumatology* **27**, 2696–702.

Brewer, E.J., Jr. et al. (1977). Current proposed revision of JRA Criteria. JRA Criteria Subcommittee of the Diagnostic and Therapeutic Criteria Committee of the American Rheumatism Section of The Arthritis Foundation. *Arthritis and Rheumatism* **20**, 195–9.

Bywaters, E.G. (1971). Still's disease in the adult. *Annals of the Rheumatic Diseases* **30**, 121–33.

Cabane, J. et al. (1990). Comparison of long term evolution of adult onset and juvenile onset Still's disease, both followed up for more than 10 years. *Annals of the Rheumatic Diseases* **49**, 283–5.

Calabro, J.J., Holgerson, W.B., Sonpal, G.M., and Khoury, M.I. (1976). Juvenile rheumatoid arthritis: a general review and report of 100 patients observed for 15 years. *Seminars in Arthritis and Rheumatism* **5**, 257–98.

Cassidy, J.T. (1990). Management of JCA: slow-acting anti-rheumatic drugs. In *Pediatric Rheumatology Update* (ed. P. Woo, P.H. White, and B.M. Ansell), pp. 66–80. New York: Oxford University Press.

Cassidy, J.T. and Martel, W. (1977). Juvenile rheumatoid arthritis: clinicoradiologic correlations. *Arthritis and Rheumatism* **20**, 207–11.

Cavagna, L., Caporali, R., Epis, O., Bobbio-Pallavicini, F., and Montecucco, C. (2001). Infliximab in the treatment of adult Still's disease refractory to conventional therapy. *Clinical and Experimental Rheumatology* **19**, 329–32.

Cazzola, M. et al. (1996). Defective iron supply for erythropoiesis and adequate endogenous erythropoietin production in the anemia associated with systemic-onset chronic arthritis. *Blood* **87**, 4824–30.

Cheema, G.S. and Quismorio, F.P., Jr. (1999). Pulmonary involvement in adult-onset Still's disease. *Current Opinions in Pulmonary Medicine* **5**, 305–9.

Cush, J.J., Medsger, T.A., Jr., Christy, W.C., Herber, D.C., and Copperstein, L.A. (1987). Adult-onset Still's disease. Clinical course and outcome. *Arthritis and Rheumatism* **30**, 186–94.

Date, Y. et al. (1999). Identification of a genetic risk factor for systemic juvenile rheumatoid arthritis in the 5′-flanking region of the TNF-α gene and HLA genes. *Arthritis and Rheumatism* **42**, 2577–82.

David, J., Vouyiouka, O., Ansell, B.M., Hall, A., and Woo, P. (1993). Amyloidosis in juvenile chronic arthritis: a morbidity and mortality study. *Clinical and Experimental Rheumatology* **11**, 85–90.

David, J. et al. (1994). The functional and psychological outcomes of juvenile chronic arthritis in young adulthood. *British Journal of Rheumatology* **33**, 876–81.

de Benedetti, F. and Martini, A. (1998). Editorial: Is systemic juvenile rheumatoid arthritis an interleukin 6 mediated disease? *Journal of Rheumatology* **25**, 203–7.

de Benedetti, F., Pignatti, P., Massa. M., Sartirana, P., Ravelli, A., and Martini, A. (1995). Circulating levels of interleukin 1 beta and of interleukin 1 receptor antagonist in systemic juvenile chronic arthritis. *Clinical and Experimental Rheumatology* **13**, 779–84.

de Benedetti, F. et al. (1997a). Interleukin 6 causes growth impairment in transgenic mice through a decrease in insulin-like growth factor-I: a model for stunted growth in children with chronic inflammation. *Journal of Clinical Investigation* **99**, 643–50.

de Benedetti, F. et al. (1997b). Soluble tumour necrosis factor receptor levels reflect coagulation abnormalities in systemic juvenile chronic arthritis. *British Journal of Rheumatology* **36**, 581–8.

de Benedetti, F. et al. (1999). Interleukin 8 and monocyte chemoattractant protein-1 in patients with juvenile rheumatoid arthritis. Relation to onset types, disease activity, and synovial fluid leukocytes. *Journal of Rheumatology* **26**, 425–31.

de Benedetti, F. et al. (2000). Circulating levels of soluble E-selectin, P-selectin and intercellular adhesion molecule-1 in patients with juvenile idiopathic arthritis. *Journal of Rheumatology* **27**, 2246–50.

De Inocencio, J., Giannini, E.H., and Glass, D.N. (1993). Can genetic markers contribute to the classification of juvenile rheumatoid arthritis? *Journal of Rheumatology* **40**, 12–18.

Donn, R.P., Shelley, E., Ollier, W.E., and Thomson, W. (2001). A novel 5′-flaking region polymorphism of macrophage migration inhibitory factor is associated with systemic-onset juvenile idiopathic arthritis. *Arthritis and Rheumatism* **44**, 1782–5.

Elkon, K.B. et al. (1982). Adult-onset Still's disease. Twenty-year followup and further studies of patients with active disease. *Arthritis and Rheumatism* **25**, 647–54.

Elliott, M.J., Woo, P., Charles, P., Long-Fox, A., Woody, J.N., and Maini, R.N. (1997). Suppression of fever and the acute-phase response in a patient with juvenile chronic arthritis treated with monoclonal antibody to tumour necrosis factor-alpha (cA2). *British Journal of Rheumatology* **36**, 589–93.

Espada, G., Babini, J.C., Maldonado-Cocco, J.A., and Garcia-Morteo, O. (1988). Radiologic review: the cervical spine in juvenile rheumatoid arthritis. *Seminars in Arthritis and Rheumatism* **17**, 185–95.

Falcini, F. et al. (1997). Methotrexate-associated appearance and rapid progression of rheumatoid nodules in systemic-onset juvenile rheumatoid arthritis. *Arthritis and Rheumatism* **40**, 175–8.

Fautrel, B. et al. (1999). Corticosteroid sparing effect of low dose methotrexate treatment in adult Still's disease. *Journal of Rheumatology* **26**, 373–8.

Fautrel, B. et al. (2001). Diagnostic value of ferritin and glycosylated ferritin in adult onset Still's disease. *Journal of Rheumatology* **28**, 322–9.

Feldman, B.M. et al. (1996). Seasonal onset of systemic-onset juvenile rheumatoid arthritis. *Journal of Pediatrics* **129**, 513–18.

Fishman, D., Rooney, M., and Woo, P. (1995). Successful management of reactive haemophagocytic syndrome in systemic-onset juvenile chronic arthritis. *British Journal of Rheumatology* **34**, 888.

Fishman, D. et al. (1998). The effect of novel polymorphisms in the interleukin-6 (IL-6) gene on IL-6 transcription and plasma IL-6 levels, and an association with systemic-onset juvenile chronic arthritis. *Journal of Clinical Investigation* **102**, 1369–76.

Fujii, T. et al. (1997). Methotrexate treatment in patients with adult onset Still's disease—retrospective study of 13 Japanese cases. *Annals of Rheumatic Diseases* **56**, 144–8.

Fujii, T., Suwa, A., Mimori, T., and Akizuki, M. (1998). Chronic arthritis and carpo: metacarpal ratio in Japanese patients with adult Still's disease. *Journal of Rheumatology* **25**, 2402–7.

Giannini, E.H. et al. (1992). Methotrexate in resistant juvenile rheumatoid arthritis. Results of the U.S.A.–U.S.S.R. double-blind, placebo-controlled trial. The Pediatric Rheumatology Collaborative Study Group and The Cooperative Children's Study Group. *New England Journal of Medicine* **326**, 1043–9.

Goldenberg, J. et al. (1990). Cardiac tamponade in juvenile chronic arthritis: report of two cases and review of publications. *Annals of the Rheumatic Diseases* **49**, 549–53.

Goldenberg, J. et al. (1992). Symptomatic cardiac involvement in juvenile rheumatoid arthritis. *International Journal of Cardiology* **34**, 57–62.

Gwyther, M., Schwarz, H., Howard, A., and Ansell, B.M. (1982). C-reactive protein in juvenile chronic arthritis: an indicator of disease activity and possibly amyloidosis. *Annals of the Rheumatic Diseases* **41**, 259–62.

Hadchouel, M., Prieur, A.M., and Griscelli, C. (1985). Acute hemorrhagic, hepatic and neurologic manifestations in juvenile rheumatoid arthritis: possible relationship to drugs or infection. *Journal of Pediatrics* **106**, 561–6.

Hafner, R. and Truckenbrodt, H. (1986). Course and prognosis of systemic juvenile chronic arthritis—retrospective study of 187 patients. *Klinische Padiatrie* **198**, 401–7.

Halle, F. and Prieur, A.M. (1991). Evaluation of methotrexate in the treatment of juvenile chronic arthritis according to the subtype. *Clinical and Experimental Rheumatology* **9**, 297–302.

Hanson, V., Kornreich, H., Bernstein, B., King, K.K., and Singsen, B. (1977). Prognosis of juvenile rheumatoid arthritis. *Arthritis and Rheumatism* **20**, 279–84.

Hawkins, P.N. et al. (1993). Serum amyloid P component scintigraphy and turnover studies for diagnosis and quantitative monitoring of AA amyloidosis in juvenile rheumatoid arthritis. *Arthritis and Rheumatism* **36**, 842–51.

Hayem, F., Calede, C., Hayem, G., and Kahn, M.F. (1994). Involvement of the hip in systemic-onset forms of juvenile chronic arthritis. Retrospective study of 28 cases. *Revue du Rhumatisme (Ed. Francaise)* **61**, 583–9.

Hertzberger-Ten Cate, R. and Cats, A. (1991). Toxicity of sulfasalazine in systemic juvenile chronic arthritis. *Clinical and Experimental Rheumatology* **9**, 85–8.

Higgins, G.C., Jones, K., and Rennebohm, R.M. (2000). Variable response of systemic juvenile rheumatoid arthritis to Etanercept. *Arthritis and Rheumatism* **43**, S257.

Hoshino, T. et al. (1998). Elevated serum interleukin 6, interferon-γ, and tumor necrosis factor-α levels in patients with adult Still's disease. *Journal of Rheumatology* **25**, 396–8.

Hull, R.G. (1988). Outcome in juvenile arthritis. *British Journal of Rheumatology* **27**, 66–71.

Husni, M.E. et al. (2002). Etanercept in the treatment of adult patients with Still's disease. *Arthritis and Rheumatism* **46**, 1171–6.

Iiowite, N.T., Samuel, P., Beseler, L., and Jacobson, M.S. (1989). Dyslipoproteinemia in juvenile rheumatoid arthritis. *Journal of Pediatrics* **114**, 823–6.

Inamo, Y., Pemberton, S., Tuddenham, E.G., and Woo, P. (1995). Increase of activated factor VIIA and haemostatic molecular markers in juvenile chronic arthritis. *British Journal of Rheumatology* **34**, 466–9.

Isdale, I.C. and Bywaters, E.G.L. (1956). The rash of rheumatoid arthritis and Still's disease. *Quarterly Journal of Medicine* **99**, 377–87.

Kawashima, M. et al. (2001). Levels of interleukin-18 and its binding inhibitors in the blood circulation of patients with adult-onset Still's disease. *Arthritis and Rheumatism* **44**, 550–60.

Keul, R., Heinrich, P.C., Muller-Newen, G., Muller, K., and Woo, P. (1998). A possible role for soluble IL-6 receptor in the pathogenesis of systemic onset juvenile chronic arthritis. *Cytokine* **10**, 729–34.

Kimura, Y., Fieldston, E., Devries-Vandervlugt, B., Li, S., and Imundo, L. (2000a). High dose, alternate day corticosteroids for systemic onset juvenile rheumatoid arthritis. *Journal of Rheumatology* **27**, 2018–24.

Kimura Y, Li, S., Ebner-Lyon, L., and Imundo, L. (2000b). Treatment of systemic JIA with Etanercept: results of a survey. *Arthritis and Rheumatology* **43**, S257.

Kivivuori, S.M., Pelkonen, P., Ylijoki, H., Verronen, P., and Siimes, M.A. (2000). Elevated serum transferrin receptor concentration in children with juvenile chronic arthritis as evidence of iron deficiency. *Rheumatology* **39**, 193–7.

Knook, L.M., de Kleer, I.M., van der Ent, C.K., van der Net, J.J., Prakken, B.J., and Kuis, W. (1999). Lung function abnormalities and respiratory muscle weakness in children with juvenile chronic arthritis. *European Respiratory Journal* **14**, 529–33.

Kobayashi, T., Tanaka, S., Maeda, M., Okubo, H., Matsuyama, T., and Watanabe, N. (1993). A study of prognosis in 52 cases with juvenile rheumatoid arthritis. *Acta Paediatrica Japonica* **35**, 439–46.

Koizumi, R., Tsukada, Y., Ideura, H., Ueki, K., Maezawa, A., and Nojima, Y. (2000). Treatment of adult Still's disease with dexamethasone, an alternative to prednisolone. *Scandinavian Journal of Rheumatology* **29**, 396–8.

Kraus, A. and Alarcon-Segovia, D. (1991). Fever in adult onset Still's disease. Response to methotrexate. *Journal of Rheumatology* **18**, 918–20.

Kvien, T.K., Hoyeraal, H.M., and Sandstad, B. (1986). Azathioprine versus placebo in patients with juvenile rheumatoid arthritis: a single center double blind comparative study. *Journal of Rheumatology* **13**, 118–23.

Lang, B.A., Schneider, R., Reilly, B.J., Silverman, E.D., and Laxer, R.M. (1995). Radiologic features of systemic onset juvenile rheumatoid arthritis. *Journal of Rheumatology* **22**, 168–73.

Lanza, F. et al. (2000). Prolonged remission state of refractory adult onset Still's disease following CD34-selected autologous peripheral blood stem cell transplantation. *Bone Marrow Transplantation* **25**, 1307–10.

Lehman, T.J, Striegel, K.H., and Onel, K.B. (2002). Thalidomide therapy for recalcitrant systemic onset juvenile rheumatoid arthritis. *Journal of Pediatrics* **140**, 125–7.

Lin, S.J. and Jaing, T.H. (1999). Thrombocytopenia in systemic-onset juvenile chronic arthritis: report of two cases with unusual bone marrow features. *Clinical Rheumatology* **18**, 241–3.

Lin, S.J., Chao, H.C., and Yan, D.C. (2000). Different articular outcomes of Still's disease in Chinese children and adults. *Clinical Rheumatology* **19**, 127–30.

Lindsley, C.B. (1987). Seasonal variation in systemic onset juvenile rheumatoid arthritis. *Arthritis and Rheumatism* **30**, 838–9.

Lipnick, R.N., Sfinkakis, P.P., Klipple, G.L., and Tsokos, G.S. (1993). Elevated soluble CD8 antigen and soluble interleukin-2 receptors in the sera of patients with juvenile rheumatoid arthritis. *Clinical Immunology and Immunopathology* **68**, 64–7.

Lomater, C., Gerloni, V., Gattinara, M., Mazzotti, J., Cimaz, R., and Fantani, F. (2000). Systemic onset juvenile idiopathic arthritis: a retrospective study of 80 consecutive patients followed for 10 years. *Journal of Rheumatology* **27**, 491–6.

Lovell, D.J. et al. (2000). Etanercept in children with polyarticular juvenile rheumatoid arthritis. Pediatric Rheumatology Collaborative Study Group. *New England Journal of Medicine* **16**, 763–9.

Mahmud, T. and Hughes, G.R. (1999). Intravenous immunoglobulin in the treatment of refractory adult Still's disease. *Journal of Rheumatology* **26**, 2067–8.

Mangge, H. et al. (1995). Serum cytokines in juvenile rheumatoid arthritis. Correlation with conventional inflammation parameters and clinical subtypes. *Arthritis and Rheumatism* **38**, 211–20.

Manners, P.J. and Ansell, B.M. (1986). Slow-acting antirheumatic drug use in systemic onset juvenile chronic arthritis. *Pediatrics* **77**, 99–103.

Marchesoni, A., Ceravolo, G.P., Battafarano, N., Rosetti, A., Tosi, S., and Fantini, F. (1997). Cyclosporin A in the treatment of adult onset Still's disease. *Journal of Rheumatology* **24**, 1582–7.

Martel, W., Holt, J.F., and Cassidy, J.T. (1962). Roentgenologic manifestations of juvenile rheumatoid arthritis. *American Journal of Roentgenology* **88**, 400–23.

Martini, A. et al. (1986). Enhanced interleukin 1 and depressed interleukin 2 production in juvenile arthritis. *Journal of Rheumatology* **13**, 598–603.

Masson, C. et al. (1996). Comparative study of 6 types of criteria in adult Still's disease. *Journal of Rheumatology* **23**, 495–7.

Matsui, K. et al. (1999). High serum level of macrophage-colony stimulating factor (M-CSF) in adult-onset Still's disease. *Rheumatology* **38**, 477–8.

Medsger, T.A., Jr. and Christy, W.C. (1975). Selective carpo-metacarpal arthritis with early ankylosis in adult onset Still's disease. *Arthritis and Rheumatism* **18**, 526–7.

Modesto, C. et al. (2001). Systemic onset juvenile chronic arthritis, polyarticular pattern and hip involvement as markers for a bad prognosis. *Clinical and Experimental Rheumatology* **19**, 211–17.

Mok, C.C., Lau, C.S., and Wong, R.W. (1998). Clinical characteristics, treatment, and outcome of adult onset Still's disease in southern Chinese. *Journal of Rheumatology* **25**, 2345–51.

Mouy, R., Stephan, J.L., Pillet, P., Haddad, E., Hubert, P., and Prieur, A.M. (1996). Efficacy of cyclosporine A in the treatment of macrophage activation syndrome in juvenile arthritis: report of five cases. *Journal of Pediatrics* **129**, 750–4.

Mozziconacci, P., Prieur, A.M., Hayem, F., and Oury, C. (1983). Articular prognosis of the systemic form of chronic juvenile arthritis (100 cases). *Annales de Pediatrie* **30**, 553–6.

Mulder, L. et al. (1997). Antineutrophil cytoplasmic antibodies in juvenile chronic arthritis. *Journal of Rheumatology* **24**, 568–75.

Nepom, B.S. and Glass, D.N. (1992). Juvenile rheumatoid arthritis and HLA: report of the Park City III workshop. *Journal of Rheumatology* **33** (Suppl.), 70–4.

Nguyen, K.H. and Weisman, M.H. (1997). Severe sore throat as a presenting symptom of adult onset Still's disease: a case series and review of the literature. *Journal of Rheumatology* **24**, 592–7.

Ohta, A., Yamaguchi, M., Kaneoka, H., Nagayoshi, T., and Hiida, M. (1987). Adult Still's disease: review of 228 cases from the literature. *Journal of Rheumatology* **14**, 1139–46.

Ostensen, M., Hoyeraal, H.M., and Kass, E. (1988). Tolerance of cyclosporine A in children with refractory juvenile rheumatoid arthritis. *Journal of Rheumatology* **15**, 1536–8.

Padeh, S., Sharon, N., Schiby, G., Rechavi, G., and Passwell, J.H. (1997). Hodgkin's lymphoma in systemic onset juvenile rheumatoid arthritis after treatment with low dose methotrexate. *Journal of Rheumatology* **24**, 2035–7.

Paul, C. et al. (1995). Immunogenetics of juvenile chronic arthritis. I. HLA interaction between A2, Dr5/8-DR/DQ, and DPB1*0201 is a general feature of all subsets of early onset pauciarticular juvenile chronic arthritis II. DPB1 polymorphism plays a role in systemic juvenile chronic arthritis. *Tissue Antigens* **45**, 280–3.

Pelkonen, P., Savilahti, E., and Makela, A.L. (1983). Persistent and transient IgA deficiency in juvenile rheumatoid arthritis. *Scandinavian Journal of Rheumatology* **12**, 273–9.

Peterson, L.S., Mason, T., Nelson, A.M., O'Fallon, W.M., and Gabriel, S.E. (1996). Juvenile rheumatoid arthritis in Rochester, Minnesota 1960–1993. Is the epidemiology changing? *Arthritis and Rheumatism* **39**, 1385–90.

Petty, R.E. et al. (1998). Revision of the proposed classification criteria for juvenile idiopathic arthritis: Durban, 1997. *Journal of Rheumatology* **25**, 1991–4.

Picco, P., Gattorno, M., Buoncompagni, A., Pistoia, V., and Borrone, C. (1996). 6-Methylprednisolone 'mini-pulse': a new modality of glucocorticoid treatment in systemic onset juvenile chronic arthritis. *Scandinavian Journal of Rheumatology* **25**, 24–7.

Pignatti, P., Vivarelli M., Meazza, C., Rizzolo, M.G., Martini, A., and de Benedetti, F. (2001). Abnormal regulation of interleukin 6 in systemic juvenile idiopathic arthritis. *Journal of Rheumatology* **28**, 1670–6.

Pistoia, V. et al. (1993). Cyclosporin A in the treatment of juvenile chronic arthritis and childhood polymyositis–dermatomyositis. Results of a preliminary study. *Clinical and Experimental Rheumatology* **11**, 203–8.

Pouchot, J. et al. (1991). Adult Still's disease: manifestations, disease course, and outcome in 62 patients. *Medicine* **70**, 118–36.

Prahalad, S., Bove, K.E., Dickens, D., Lovell, D.J., and Grom, A.A. (2001). Etanercept in the treatment of macrophage activation syndrome. *Journal of Rheumatology* **28**, 2120–4.

Prieur, A.M., Bremard-Oury, C., Griscelli, C., and Mozziconacci, P. (1984). Prognosis of the systemic forms of juvenile chronic arthritis. Apropos of 100 cases. *Archives Francaise de Pediatrie* **41**, 91–7.

Prieur, A.M., Adleff, A., Debre, M., Boulate, P., and Griscelli, C. (1990). High dose immunoglobulin therapy in severe juvenile chronic arthritis: long-term follow-up in 16 patients. *Clinical and Experimental Rheumatology* **8**, 603–8.

Prieur, A.M., Roux-Lombard, P., and Dayer, J.M. (1996). Dynamics of fever and the cytokine network in systemic juvenile arthritis. *Revue du Rhumatisme English Edition* **63**, 163–70.

Ravelli, A. Ramenghi, B., de Fuccia, G., Ruperto, N., Zontal, L., and Martini, A. (1994). Factors associated with response to methotrexate in systemic-onset juvenile chronic arthritis. *Acta Paediatrica* **83**, 428–32.

Ravelli, A., de Benedetti, F., Viola, S., and Martini, A. (1996). Macrophage activation syndrome in systemic juvenile rheumatoid arthritis successfully treated with cyclosporine. *Journal of Pediatrics* **128**, 275–8.

Ravelli, A., Caria, M.C., Buratti, S., Malattia, C., Temporini, F., and Martini, A. (2001). Methotrexate as a possible trigger of macrophage activation syndrome in systemic juvenile idiopathic arthritis. *Journal of Rheumatology* **28**, 865–7.

Reginato, A.J., Schumacher, H.R., Jr., Baker, D.G., O'Connor, C.R., and Ferreiros, J. (1987). Adult onset Still's disease: experience in 23 patients and literature review with emphasis on organ failure. *Seminars in Arthritis and Rheumatism* **17**, 39–57.

Reiff, A., Shaham, B., Wood, B.P., Bernstein, B.H., Stanley, P., and Szer, I.S. (1995). High dose methotrexate in the treatment of refractory juvenile rheumatoid arthritis. *Clinical and Experimental Rheumatology* **13**, 113–18.

Reiff, A. et al. (1997). Preliminary evidence for Cyclosporin A as an alternative in the treatment of recalcitrant juvenile rheumatoid arthritis and juvenile dermatomyositis. *Journal of Rheumatology* **24**, 2436–43.

Rooney, M., David, J., Symons, J., di Giocine, F., Carsani, J., and Woo, P. (1995). Inflammatory cytokine responses in juvenile chronic arthritis. *British Journal of Rheumatology* **34**, 454–60.

Sampalis, J.S. et al. (1995). A controlled study of the long-term prognosis of adult Still's disease. *American Journal of Medicine* **98**, 384–8.

Sampalis, J.S. et al. (1996). Risk factors for adult Still's disease. *Journal of Rheumatology* **23**, 2049–54.

Savolainen, H.A. (1999). Chlorambucil in severe juvenile chronic arthritis: long-term followup with special reference to amyloidosis. *Journal of Rheumatology* **26**, 898–903.

Savolainen, H.A. and Isomaki, H.A. (1993). Decrease in the number of deaths from secondary amyloidosis in patients with juvenile rheumatoid arthritis. *Journal of Rheumatology* **20**, 1201–3.

Schaller, J. (1972). Arthritis as a presenting manifestation of malignancy in children. *Journal of Pediatrics* **81**, 793–7.

Schaller, J.G. (1977). Juvenile rheumatoid arthritis: Series 1. *Arthritis and Rheumatism* **20**, 165–70.

Schaller, J. and Wedgwood, R.J. (1972). Juvenile rheumatoid arthritis: a review. *Pediatrics* **50**, 940–53.

Schmeling, H., Mathony, K., John, V., Keysser, G., Burdach, S., and Horneff, G. (2001). A combination of etanercept and methotrexate for the treatment of refractory juvenile idiopathic arthritis: a pilot study. *Annals of the Rheumatic Diseases* **60**, 410–12.

Schneider, R. et al. (1992). Prognostic indicators of joint destruction in systemic-onset juvenile rheumatoid arthritis. *Journal of Pediatrics* **120**, 200–5.

Schneider, R., Silverman, E.D., Feldman, B., Spiegel, L., and Laxer, R.M. (2000). Acute fatal neurologic events in severe systemic-onset juvenile rheumatoid arthritis (SoJRA). *Arthritis and Rheumatism* **43**, S119.

Schnitzer, T.J. and Ansell, B.M. (1977). Amyloidosis in juvenile chronic polyarthritis. *Arthritis and Rheumatism* **20**, 245–52.

Shaikov, A.V., Maximov, A.A., Speransky, A.I., Lovell, D.J., Giannini, E.H., and Solovyev, S.K. (1992). Repetitive use of pulse therapy with methylprednisolone and cyclophosphamide in addition to oral methotrexate in children with systemic juvenile rheumatoid arthritis—preliminary results of a longterm study. *Journal of Rheumatology* **19**, 612–16.

Silverman, E.D., Miller, J.J., III, Bernstein, B., and Shafai, T. (1983). Consumption coagulopathy associated with systemic juvenile rheumatoid arthritis. *Journal of Pediatrics* **103**, 872–6.

Silverman, E.D. et al. (1990). Intravenous gamma globulin therapy in systemic juvenile rheumatoid arthritis. *Arthritis and Rheumatism* **33**, 1015–22.

Silverman, E.D., Laxer, R.M., Nelson, D.L., and Rubin, L.A. (1991). Soluble interleukin-2-receptor in juvenile rheumatoid arthritis. *Journal of Rheumatology* **18**, 1398–402.

Silverman, E.D. et al. (1994). Intravenous immunoglobulin in the treatment of systemic juvenile rheumatoid arthritis: a randomized placebo controlled trial. *Journal of Rheumatology* **21**, 2353–8.

Speckmaier, M. et al. (1989). Low-dose methotrexate in systemic onset juvenile chronic arthritis. *Clinical and Experimental Rheumatology* **7**, 647–50.

Spiegel, L. et al. (2000). Early predictors of poor functional outcome in systemic-onset juvenile rheumatoid arthritis: a multicenter cohort study. *Arthritis and Rheumatism* **43**, 2402–9.

Stambe, C. and Wicks, I.P. (1998). TNFα and response of treatment-resistant adult-onset Still's disease to thalidomide. *The Lancet* **352**, 544–5.

Stasny, P. and Fink, C.W. (1979). Different HLA-D associations in adult and juvenile rheumatoid arthritis. *Journal of Clinical Investigation* **63**, 124–30.

Still, G.F. (1897). On a form of chronic joint disease in children. *Medical-chirurgical Transactions* **80**, 47–59.

Svantesson, H., Akesson, A., Eberhardt, K., and Elborgh, R. (1983). Prognosis in juvenile rheumatoid arthritis with systemic onset. A follow-up study. *Scandinavian Journal of Rheumatology* **12**, 139–44.

Touati, G., Prieur, A.M., Riuz, J.C., Noel, M., and Czernichow, P. (1998). Beneficial effect of one-year growth hormone administration to children with juvenile chronic arthritis on chronic steroid therapy. I. Effects on growth velocity and body composition. *Journal of Clinical Endocrinology and Metabolism* **83**, 403–9.

Tsatsoulis, A., Siamopoulou, A., Petsoukis, C., Challa, A., Bairaktari, E., and Seferiadis, K. (1999). Study of growth hormone secretion and action in growth-retarded children with juvenile chronic arthritis (JCA). *Growth Hormone and IGF Research* **9**, 143–9.

Uziel, Y., Laxer, R.M., Schneider, R., and Silverman, E.D. (1996). Intravenous immunoglobulin therapy in systemic onset juvenile rheumatoid arthritis: a followup study. *Journal of Rheumatology* **23**, 910–18.

Uziel, Y., Rathaus, V., Pomeranz, A., Solan, H., and Wolach, B. (1998). Torticollis as the sole initial presenting sign of systemic onset juvenile rheumatoid arthritis. *Journal of Rheumatology* **25**, 166–8.

Uziel, Y. et al. (1999). Seasonal variation in systemic onset juvenile rheumatoid arthritis in Israel. *Journal of Rheumatology* **26**, 1187–9.

Wallace, C.A. and Levinson, J.E. (1991). Juvenile rheumatoid arthritis: outcome and treatment for the 1990s. *Rheumatic Diseases Clinics of North America* **17**, 891–905.

Wallace, C.A. and Sherry, D.D. (1992). Preliminary report of higher dose methotrexate treatments in juvenile rheumatoid arthritis. *Journal of Rheumatology* **19**, 1604–7.

Wallace, C.A. and Sherry, D.D. (1997). Trial of intravenous pulse cyclophosphamide and methylprednisolone in the treatment of severe systemic-onset juvenile rheumatoid arthritis. *Arthritis and Rheumatism* **40**, 1852–5.

Wang, F.M., Wertenbaker, C., Behrens, M.M., and Jacobs, J.C. (1984). Acquired Brown's syndrome in children with juvenile rheumatoid arthritis. *Ophthalmology* **91**, 23–6.

Woo, P., O'Brien, J., Robson, M., and Ansell, B.M. (1987). A genetic marker for systemic amyloidosis in juvenile arthritis. *Lancet* **2**, 767–9.

Woo, P. et al. (2000). Randomized, placebo-controlled, crossover trial of low-dose oral methotrexate in children with extended oligoarticular or systemic arthritis. *Arthritis and Rheumatism* **43**, 1849–57.

Wouters, J.M. and van de Putte, L.B. (1986). Adult-onset Still's disease; clinical and laboratory features, treatment and progress of 45 cases. *Quarterly Journal of Medicine* **61**, 1055–65.

Wouters, J.M., Reekers, P., and van de Putte, L.B. (1986). Adult-onset Still's disease. Disease course and HLA associations. *Arthritis and Rheumatism* **29**, 415–18.

Wulffraat, N.M. and Kuis, W. (2001). Treatment of refractory juvenile idiopathic arthritis. *Journal of Rheumatology* **28**, 929–31.

Wulffraat, N., van Royen, A., Bierings, M., Vossen, J., and Kuis, W. (1999). Autologous haemopoietic stem-cell transplantation in four patients with refractory juvenile chronic arthritis. *Lancet* **353**, 550–3.

Yamaguchi, M. et al. (1992). Preliminary criteria for classification of adult Still's disease. *Journal of Rheumatology* **19**, 424–30.

6.5.3 Rheumatoid factor-negative polyarthritis in children ('seronegative polyarthritis')

Anne-Marie F. Prieur

The classification of childhood arthritis has recently been a matter of debate. During the last three decades, the most accepted diagnostic criteria were either those of the European League Against Rheumatism (EULAR) (Wood 1978) (referred to as juvenile chronic arthritis) or those of the American College of Rheumatology (ACR), previously the American Rheumatism Association (ARA) (Brewer et al. 1977) (referred to as juvenile rheumatoid arthritis). In the EULAR criteria, polyarthritis with positive rheumatoid factor (RF) was excluded, while in the ACR proposal, patients with positive RF were included in the group of polyarticular onset. In an effort of unifying the language and for designing more homogeneous groups of patients, the International League of Associations of Rheumatologists (ILAR) Taskforce on the Classification of Childhood Arthritis considered new classification proposals. The term 'juvenile idiopathic arthritis' (JIA) was adopted to overcome any semantic discussions and to indicate that childhood arthritides are of unknown origin. Six different categories were recognized: systemic arthritis, oligoarthritis, RF-negative polyarthritis, RF-positive polyarthritis, enthesitis related arthritis (ERA), and psoriatic arthritis. A seventh category was proposed for children fitting with more than one category, and those fitting in no category (Petty et al. 1998). In this classification, RF-negative polyarthritis was recognized as an autonomous group. In a prospective study evaluating over 3 months 194 children with JIA, 15 per cent fitted with the criteria for RF-negative polyarthritis (Hofer et al. 2001). By definition, polyarthritis occurs before the age of 16 years with the involvement of a minimum of five joints. The proposed diagnostic criteria do not take into account the type of course, which is extremely important for the prognosis and outcome. Oligoarticular onset with a polyarticular course will not be considered in this chapter.

The RF-positive group represents the early onset of adult rheumatoid arthritis and all data available in adults are also true in children (see Chapter 6.3.4). It is uncommon and occurs in less than 10 per cent of children. Polyarticular onset that is RF-negative is the most common and is extremely heterogeneous. Some sub-groups are easy to identify, but others need further evaluation to establish convenient and precise criteria for classification. It is the author's personal view that four sub-groups can be identified in the RF-negative group (Table 1). The following discussion is based on the author's experience of more than 20 years in a paediatric rheumatology clinic with an annual referral of more than 1200 patients, one-third of them being first-time referrals.

Frequent manifestations of RF-negative polyarthritis

Extra-articular manifestations

Extra-articular manifestations may be present. Fever can be observed in one-third of patients. It is generally low grade or a high fever often of short duration. In the Durban criteria, long-lasting swinging fever as described in systemic arthritis is an exclusion criteria as well as the presence of rheumatoid factor. In very young children, a transient rash lasting 1 or 2 days can occur in the early stages. There is generally no lymphadenopathy, hepatosplenomegaly, or visceral involvement.

Joint manifestations

Joint manifestations dominate the clinical presentation. Generally, the mode of onset is rapidly progressive. The child is referred to the specialist often after several weeks of worsening joint stiffness and/or swelling.

A joint is a complex organ (Chapter 3.5) made up of synovial membrane, articular cartilage, fibrous capsule, ligaments, tendons with their site of attachment on bone (the enthesis), bursas, and tendon sheaths. In children, the joints also have growth cartilage. All these structures may be inflamed during the rheumatic process and chronic inflammation results in joint alterations and deformities. Chronic swelling and limited motion results in local demineralization. Muscular wasting is a consequence of the limitation of motion and it reduces joint motility. Chronic hyperaemia may induce local accelerated growth and growth cartilage fusion. Cartilage and bone erosions are late manifestations. There is potential for cartilage generation in children, which may delay severe functional impairment.

Upper limb involvement

Deformities in the hands and wrists are the consequence of an imbalance between the modified cartilage surfaces, local accelerated growth of bones, and modification of the forces between tendons and ligaments. Reduced carpal length, joint space reduction, and erosions can lead to carpal fusion. A carpal dislocation due to bone lysis is rare but can be observed in severe cases. Radial or ulnar growth reduction induces radial or ulnar deviation.

Table 1 A proposed classification of sub-groups of RF-negative polyarthritis

	I	II	III	IV
M/F ratio	1/7	1/1	1/1	3/1
Approximate frequency (%)	40	25	20	15
Age at onset (years)	2–3	>8	>6	8–9
Clinical characteristics	Diffuse synovitis (small and large joints)	Boggy synovitis and tenosynovitis; mild pain	Mild or no synovitis; marked stiffness	Lower limb predominence
Biological inflammation	Marked	Marked	Mild, if any	Marked
Specific features	Positive ANA; negative RF; risk of CAU	None	None	Incomplete ERA
Genetic markers	HLA–DR8; HLA–DR11	?	?	HLA-B27
Prognosis	Poor	Late reduction of joint motion	Progressive stiffness	Risk of ERA, and/or JAS
Therapeutic indications	MTX, Etanercept	DMARDs	Physiotherapy	Sulfasalazine

(a)

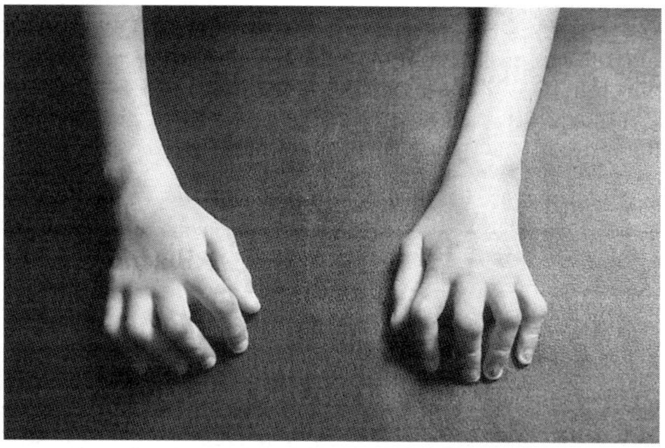

(b)

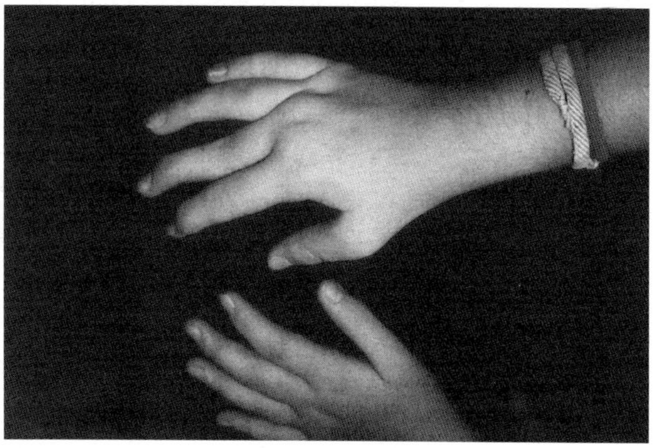

Fig. 1 (a) Boutonnière deformity and (b) swan-neck deformity of fingers.

Small joint and associated tendon involvement results in boutonnière or swan-neck deformities of the fingers (Fig. 1).

Flexion contracture is the first manifestation of elbow involvement. It may be mild and of little functional significance. Limitation of supination is very common. The shoulders are frequently involved in severe cases, leading to limitation of movement, particularly abduction and external rotation of the glenohumeral joint. In severe cases, growth disturbances and humeral head modifications are observed.

Lower limb involvement

Lower limb involvement may have significant functional consequences. Individual deformities can affect the performance of other lower limb joints. The foot is a complex joint with many articular surfaces in several planes. Foot deformities may also be increased by hip and knee involvement. Tenosynovitis and bursitis are nearly as common as ankle synovitis (Fig. 2). Subtalar joint involvement most often results in valgus deformity or, less commonly, in a varus deformity. As in the carpal area, bony fusion of the tarsus may occur. Mid-tarsal involvement affects the equilibrium of the foot. Metatarsal joint involvement leads to valgus toe deformities.

Flexion contracture of the knee is common, being particularly rapid and severe in the very young child. In the absence of correction, it may rapidly induce a posterior subluxation of the tibia due to capsular retraction [Fig. 3(a)]. The overgrowth of the epiphysis induces an accelerated growth of the limb and consequently flexion contracture of the knee [Fig. 3(b)]. In severe cases, the patella may fuse to the anterior femoral surface.

Hip involvement is characterized by flexion contracture and limitation of motion, particularly of abduction and rotation. This is secondary to the muscle spasm, mainly of the adductors, induced by local synovitis. Chronic inflammation induces anatomic modifications of the bone, with femoral head overgrowth, principally in the external part, and decreased development of the neck, which appears shorter and wider [Fig. 4(a)]. Later, aseptic necrosis of the femoral head may occur. Acetabular modifications with erosions or protrusions are possible [Fig. 4(b)]. Joint abnormalities at one site in the lower limb may have a reciprocal effect in aggravating deformities at other sites. For example, hip contracture induces a compensatory lumbar lordosis, knee overgrowth increases flexion contractures, and valgus of the knee increases talus deformity.

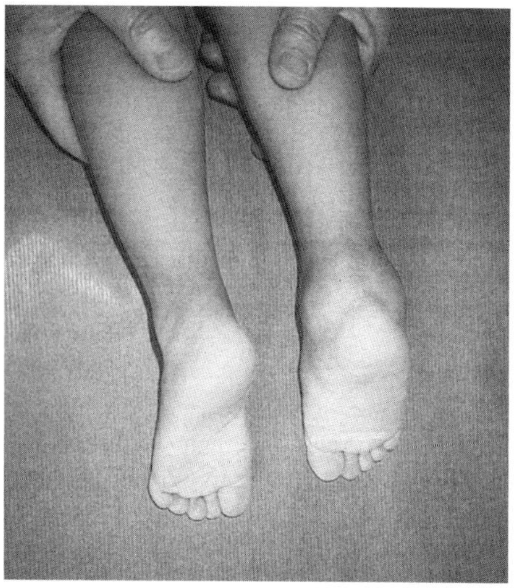

Fig. 2 Retromalleolar tenosynovitis, predominantly on the right side.

Spine

Spine involvement is generally clinically expressed at the cervical level. Torticolis and limitation of motion are common. Radiological changes develop progressively with apophyseal joint fusion most often of the C2–C3 vertebrae, but also of the other cervical spaces. Intervertebral instability below (Fig. 5) and above the fused cervical segment may occur. Subluxation of the atlas on the axis can be observed. A surgical arthrodesis is indicated in case of spinal cord compression. Anaesthetists should be aware of possible difficulties during intubation. Although rarely mentioned, synovitis of the thoracic and lumbar apophyseal joints is possible. A high frequency of spinal scoliosis is described in these children.

Temporomandibular joint

Temporomandibular joint involvement is common. It is often discovered at routine examination. It reduces the normal growth of the mandible and results in micrognathia (Fig. 6). Dental malocclusion is common and may warrant surgical correction when growth is completed.

Laboratory abnormalities

Laboratory features are non-specific in RF-negative polyarthritis. Acute-phase reactants and erythrocyte sedimentation rate can be elevated or normal. The leucocytosis is normal or increased, as is the platelet count. Low blood-cell counts are unusual and suggest an alternative diagnosis. Positive antinuclear antibodies (ANAs) may be present in a sub-group of patients (see below). The presence of ANAs was not included in the Durban criteria proposals, but it was considered to be discussed in future studies for disease characterization (Petty et al. 1998).

Specific features of sub-groups of RF-negative polyarthritis

Polyarthritis positive for ANAs

Although less frequent than the oligoarticular type with positive ANAs, this group of patients represents about 40 per cent of the polyarticular onset in

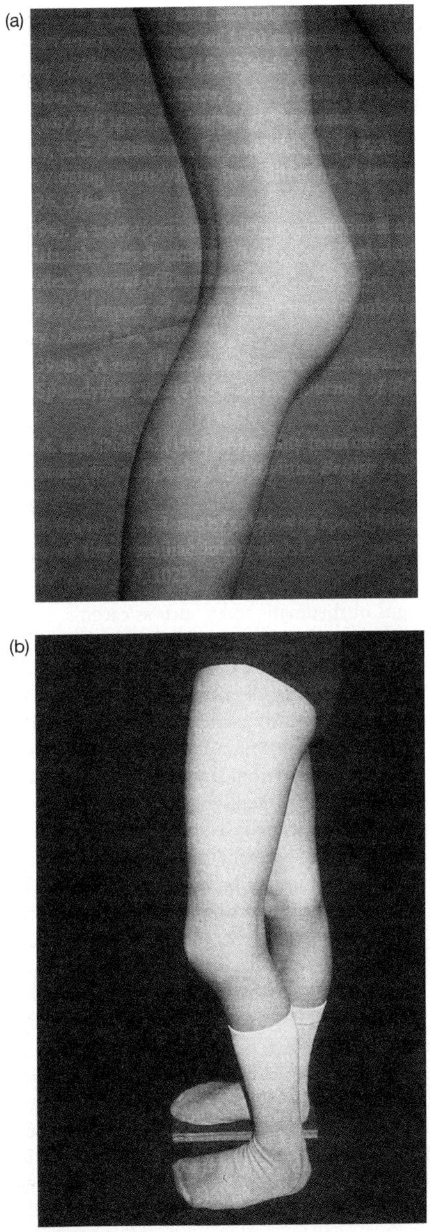

Fig. 3 (a) Posterior tibial subluxation. (b) Increased growth of the left lower limb due to chronic inflammation of the knee.

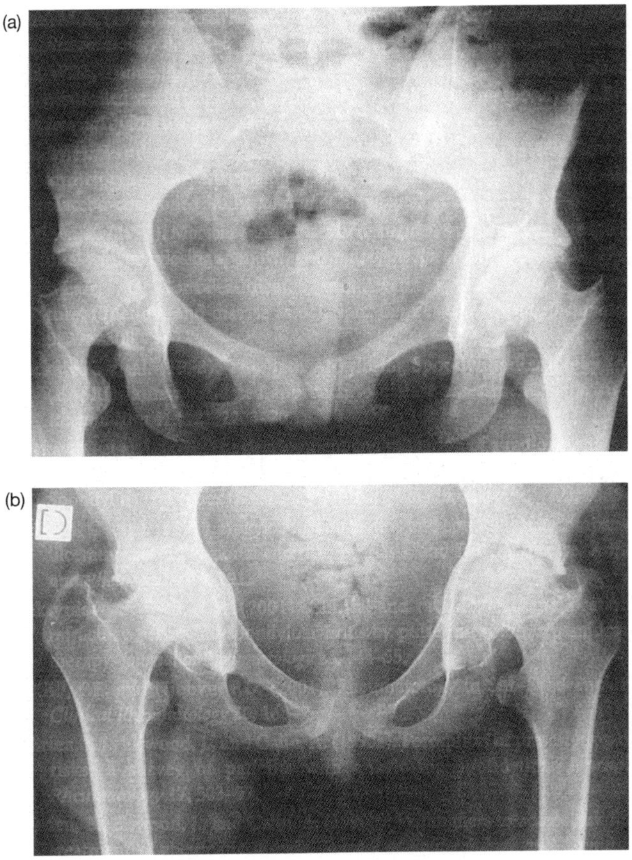

Fig. 4 (a) Chronic involvement of the hip with shortened femoral neck, irregular head, and joint space narrowing; (b) with acetabular protrusion.

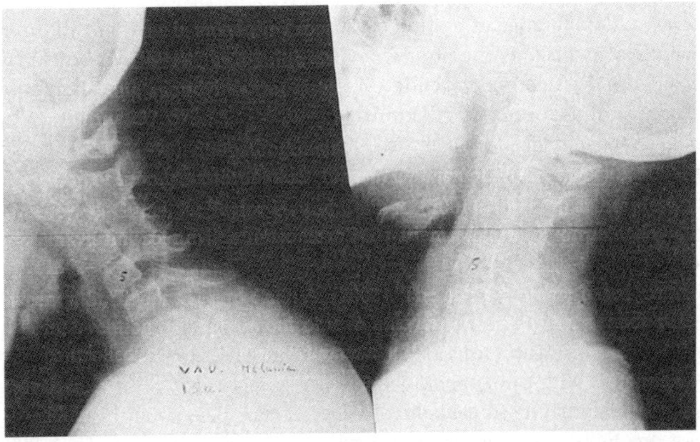

Fig. 5 Cervical spine fusion with underlying hypermobility.

our clinic. In a series of 136 children with arthritis positive for ANAs, 21 were polyarticular at onset. As in the oligoarticular-onset group with ANAs, there is a female preponderance, although the proportion of boys is higher than in the oligoarticular type. The disease is observed in very young children, two-thirds of the children reviewed in our series (Peralta and Prieur 1990) are less than 3 years old at onset. There is a risk of eye involvement as in the oligoarticular type (21 compared with 42 per cent). To my knowledge, no prognostic study of this particular group of polyarticular onset has been reported. In our experience, very young children with symmetrical involvement of both large and small joints within the first 3 months have a poorer outcome than those with symmetrical polyarticular involvement predominantly of large joints but not necessarily at the same time.

The presence of ANAs in the serum characterizes this sub-group of patients. The most frequently used substrate for diagnosis is the HEp-2 cell. The titres of ANAs are usually low and there are no obvious correlations between the titre of the autoantibody and the severity of the disease. The specificity of these ANAs is antihistone (Malleson et al. 1989; Pauls et al. 1989), but there are discrepancies in the frequencies of histone subtypes recognized by the autoantibodies. Anti-H1 and anti-H3 are the most commonly described (Pauls et al. 1989). The autoreactivity to histone fragments is demonstrated to several fragments within H3 and H4 (Tuaillon et al. 1990). The sera from 138 children with juvenile chronic arthritis were tested with 34 histone peptides covering the full length of the four core histones, and two peptides from H1. No correlation was found either with disease sub-type or activity, or with the presence of chronic anterior uveitis (Stemmer et al. 1995). A significant association between the presence of ANAs and the presence of high mobility protein 1 (HMG-1) was found in females with ANAs (Rosenberg and Cordeiro 2000).

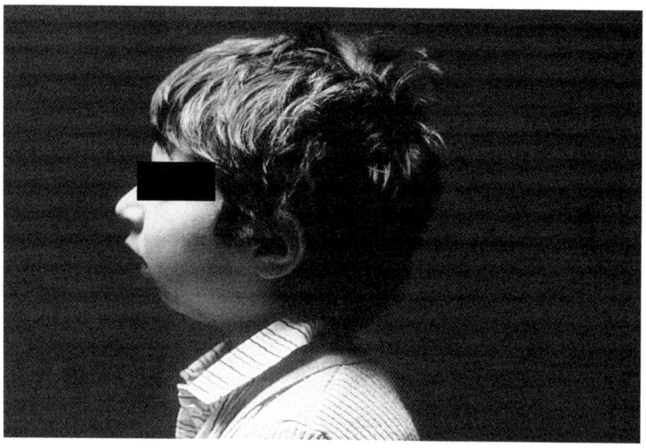

Fig. 6 Microretrognathia.

Polyarthritis with boggy synovitis

Some children may present with very thick pannus involving joints in a symmetrical manner. Tenosynovitis is common. Pain remains mild and functional impairment is late. Laboratory tests show often a high erythrocyte sedimentation rate (>40 mm/h), marked leucocytosis, and increased levels of acute-phase reactants. There are no autoantibodies. Boys and girls are equally affected.

'Dry' polyarthritis

This group of patients is roughly the counterpart of the previous group. The diagnosis is often delayed as there is no joint swelling but very progressive stiffness. These joint manifestations lead to gait abnormalities including limping. It is not unusual for these children to be referred to a paediatric neurologist, or even to a psychiatrist! However, osteoarticular examination reveals a limited range of motion because of articular stiffness but without obvious synovitis or with minor synovitis. Joint stiffness seems to be due to capsular and tendon contraction. Muscle wasting occurs. The laboratory profile is normal or mildly inflammatory. There are no autoantibodies.

Polyarthritis with spondyloarthropathy features (see Chapter 6.5.1)

Some older patients, particularly boys, can present with polyarthritis (more than four joints), most often in the lower limbs. According to the Durban criteria, patients with polyarthritis meeting the criteria for ERA are excluded from this sub-group (see Chapter 6.5.1). But patients with RF-negative polyarthritis with only one of the following: sacro-iliac joint tenderness and/or inflammatory spinal pain, presence of HLA-B27, family history in at least one first- or second-degree relative of medically confirmed HLA-B27 associated disease, anterior uveitis that is usually associated with pain, redness, or photophobia, onset of arthritis in a boy after the age of 8 years of age must be classified as RF-negative polyarthritis. Exclusion criteria as proposed in the Durban criteria were not enough sensitive since among 194 patients that we evaluated prospectively, eight met the diagnositic criteria for both ERA and RF-negative polyarthritis (Hofer et al. 2001). Joint pain is often marked. Non-steroidal anti-inflammatory drugs (NSAIDs) induce rapid pain relief (Amor et al. 1990). There are no autoantibodies in this group of patients, except for the occasional presence of antinuclear antibodies. In rare cases, there may be inflammatory bowel disease or reactive arthritis (Reiter's syndrome) with eye and mucosal manifestations. These features were not considered as exclusion in the Durban criteria for RF-negative polyarthritis. Psoriatic arthritis is considered as a separate group of disease in the Durban criteria. However, patients with RF-negative polyarthritis who have first degree relative with psoriasis must be studied for confirming or not if they may belong to the group of psoriatic arthritis.

Differential diagnosis

Other juvenile idiopathic arthritis

Exclusions for RF-negative polyarthritis were defined in the ILAR classification (Petty et al. 1998): systemic arthritis, presence of RF, presence of enthesitis, or at least two of sacro-iliac joint tenderness, inflammatory spinal pain, presence of HLA-B27, family history in at least one first- or second-degree relative of medically confirmed HLA-B27 associated disease, anterior uveitis that is usually associated with pain, redness, or photophobia, onset of arthritis in a boy after the age of 8 years of age, presence of psoriasis.

Polyarthritis related to an infectious agent

Viruses may induce a joint reaction, particularly in very young children. It may be preceded by an upper respiratory tract infection, with or without fever. Synovial fluid analysis shows a majority of lymphocytes. Joint involvement generally lasts less than 2 weeks. Parvovirus B19, hepatitis, and rubella are among the most common causes of arthritis. Rubella vaccination may be followed by a polyarthritis which can last several weeks. Streptococcal infection or acute rheumatic fever may cause a migratory arthritis (see Chapter 6.2.12). Other signs of rheumatic fever, such as carditis, chorea, and eruption, may be present. Treatment consists of anti-inflammatory drugs, aspirin, and/or corticosteroids, and penicillin for at least 5 years. Although this condition now occurs very rarely, we should be aware of its possible resurgence. Lyme borreliosis (see Chapter 6.2.4) can be considered when the child has had a tick bite in an endemic area. Typical clinical symptoms are a flu-like illness with erythema chronicum migrans. Some weeks later other symptoms can occur, including neurological, cardiac, ocular, and articular manifestations. Joint involvement is less frequent in Europe than in North America. The diagnosis and treatment is described in Chapter 6.2.4.

Acute infections of the joint or bone are usually easily diagnosed (see Chapter 6.2.2). However, a polyarthritis-like disease can occur in immunodeficiencies (see Chapter 6.2.11). The most frequent immunodeficiency in which this is observed is the X-linked humoral deficiency or Bruton's disease, which occurs in young boys with a history of upper respiratory tract, pulmonary, or gut infection. The diagnosis is made by the absence of serum immunoglobulins. A multifocal, bacterial joint infection should be ruled out first and treated. However, non-bacterial joint swelling is possible, probably resulting from chronic virus infection. Immunoglobulin infusion generally improves chronic joint involvement. Other immunodeficiencies such as acquired humoral deficiencies, or Wiskott–Aldrich and ataxia telangiectasia, can also be complicated by non-bacterial arthritis. In the latter, joint manifestations are rarely the initial symptom.

Connective tissue disorders

Autoimmune rheumatic disorders such as systemic lupus erythematosus must also be considered. Polyarthritis is nearly always present in systemic lupus erythematosus and is one of the eleven diagnostic criteria of the ACR (see Chapter 6.6.1). The presence of skin manifestations, serositis, and renal involvement should prompt laboratory investigations to confirm the diagnosis. Cytopaenia, anti-DNA antibodies, and decreased complement are the usual findings. Polyarthritis is also prominent in overlap syndromes and mixed connective tissue disease (see Chapter 6.11). Polymyositis or dermatomyositis are usually easily diagnosed, but a joint component is possible.

Systemic vasculitic syndromes

Systemic vasculitic syndromes (see Chapter 6.10.9) are not exceptional. Kawasaki disease is generally observed in very young children, but the joint symptoms are of secondary importance to the extra-articular manifestations. Polyarteritis nodosa may cause a very severe and painful polyarthritis associated with myalgia. As well as the painful joints, skin involvement includes nodules, with typical changes of medium-sized arteries on biopsy. Cutaneous and articular features without visceral involvement are possible.

The differential diagnosis of RF-negative polyarthritis from other forms of systemic vasculitis such as Wegener's granulomatosis, lymphomatoid granulomatosis, Henoch–Schönlein purpura, and hypocomplementaemic vasculitis is generally easy. Arthritis can occur in relapsing polychondritis. The diagnosis is generally obvious with inflammation of auricular cartilage and nasal chondritis with a saddle-nose deformity.

Behçet's syndrome (see Chapter 6.10.8) can occur in children. These patients may have polyarthritis. The diagnosis is made on the basis of possible familial clustering and ethnic origin, when genital and oral ulcerations are present. Inheritance is autosomal recessive. These children can also develop ocular, intestinal, and neurological manifestations (Koné-Paut et al. 1999). Familial Mediterranean fever (see Chapter 6.12.2) occurs in Sephardic Jews, Armenians, Greeks, Turks, and Arabs. Inheritance is also autosomal recessive and the gene has been mapped on the short arm of chromosome 16. Clinical manifestations include fever, skin rash, serositis, abdominal pain, and possibly arthritis. Colchicine is an effective therapy in preventing attacks and the occurrence of renal amyloidosis.

Sarcoid arthritis produces a distinctive syndrome in children under the age of 4 years, sometimes in the first year of life. The triad of skin rash, uveitis, and huge proliferation of boggy synovium with tenosynovitis is highly suggestive of sarcoid arthritis. Skin or synovial biopsy shows the typical sarcoid granulomata. Joint involvement is relatively painless. CARD15 mutations were recently identified in some familial cases suggesting that the entity referred as Blau syndrome (Blau 1985) is different from familial sarcoidosis. The later seems to be characterized by more frequent visceral involvement (Miceli-Richard et al. 2001). Systemic corticosteroids are often necessary to control uveitis and arthritis. Polyarthritis can be observed in the adult type of sarcoidosis in older children.

Haematological disorders

In early childhood, joint involvement in sickle-cell disease may result in hand–foot syndrome. Swelling of the hands and feet is extremely painful. Later, migratory arthritis can be observed. Bone pain can be due to either bone infarction or to osteomyelitis. The diagnosis is based on ethnic origin and haemoglobin electrophoresis. Constitutional bleeding disorders such as haemophilias can be manifested by joint haemorrhage. Generally, the deficiency of clotting factor is identified. Modern therapeutic management aims to prevent haemarthrosis and joint destruction.

Acute leukaemia may induce bone pain and joint swelling due to infiltrates of leukaemic cells. The diagnosis must be confirmed rapidly by examination of a bone marrow smear and specific therapy started without delay. Neuroblastoma with bone metastasis must also be considered in a young child with osteoarticular pain.

Other causes of polyarticular manifestations

Patients with chronic, recurrent, multifocal osteomyelitis can present with bone pain. There is no joint swelling and careful examination localizes the pain to the metaphyseal area. Radiography confirms the diagnosis by the presence of osteolytic lesions in the metaphysis. The lesion is sterile and antibiotics have no effect. The course may be long and relapsing (Beretta-Picoli et al. 2000).

Patients with hip pain are sometimes referred as having possible polyarthritis. In an adolescent, the possibility of lamellar coxitis should be ruled out. It is generally unilateral and the laboratory screen is normal, while radiography shows narrowing of the hip space. The cause is unknown and the prognosis is unpredictable. Similarly, Legg–Calvé–Perthes' disease induces osteonecrosis of the femoral head in young boys around the age of 7 years. It is generally unilateral, rarely bilateral. Radiographs are normal at onset, but scintigraphy or MRI may show necrosis at this stage. Orthopaedic management is required. In younger children, transient synovitis of the hip is frequent. It occurs around 6 years of age and may be preceded by upper respiratory tract infection. An increased erythrocyte sedimentation rate is frequent. Bed rest with traction and NSAIDs are necessary. Recovery occurs within a few days. Occasionally hip dysplasia is evident. Some patients develop recurrent episodes of transient synovitis of the hip.

Diabetic arthropathy is observed in uncontrolled diabetes. Exceptionally, it may be the first manifestation of diabetes. Diabetic cheiroarthropathy with progressive flexion contractures of the fingers, as a result of increased deposition of collagen in the tissues, is well recognized. Idiopathic juvenile osteoporosis is a painful disease. There are no joint manifestations. Usually, there are no abnormalities of phosphocalcium metabolism. Recovery occurs in adolescence, sometimes with sequellae resulting from spontaneous fractures or vertebral collapse.

Immunogenetics

Most of the immunogenetic studies in polyarticular-onset juvenile arthritis separate the group of 'seropositive' and 'seronegative' forms. RF-positive polyarticular arthritis in children and adults are both associated with HLA–DRB1*04 (Ploski et al. 1993). Several authors have observed an association between RF-negative polyarticular arthritis in children and HLA–DR8, mainly involving the HLA–DRB1*0801 sub-type (Morling et al. 1985; Hall et al. 1989; Fernandez-Vina et al. 1990; Barron et al. 1992; Ploski et al. 1993). Ethnic differences may be observed in some populations, such as the studies on Italian (Fantini et al. 1987) and Czech children (Cerna et al. 1994) in which no correlation with HLA–DR8 could be found.

HLA–DR8, in fact, is associated with several forms of juvenile arthritis including early-onset oligoarticular forms (Malagon et al. 1991) and juvenile spondyloarthropathies (Ploski et al. 1995). In contrast, HLA–DPB1*0201 is associated with the oligoarticular, but not with the polyarticular forms. The frequency of HLA–DPB1*0301 is increased significantly in patients with polyarticular arthritis and juvenile spondyloarthropathies. This association between HLA–DRB1*0801 and HLA–DPB1*0301 in polyarticular-onset disease has been confirmed by several authors. This combination, rarely observed in the normal population or in the oligoarticular types of disease, suggests an interaction between these two alleles, conferring an increased susceptibility to the polyarticular expression of the disease.

However, there are discrepancies between the studies, probably due to various factors including ethnic background, the absence of clinical homogeneity of the patients, the definition of each clinical sub-group, and the number of patients studied. It is evident that uniformly agreed criteria for the improved sub-grouping of patients is still required. Using statistical techniques such as latent class analysis of appropriate clinical and laboratory variables provides a new tool for identifying HLA haplotypes associated to homogeneous categories of JIA (Thomas et al. 2000).

Management

The principles of management are those of any childhood chronic disease of the joints, namely to offer pain relief, maintain satisfactory joint function, minimize drug toxicity, and allow the child to grow and be educated as normally as possible. It is sometimes difficult to meet all these requirements and complete trust between the family and the paediatric team must be established.

Another difficulty is the need to document accurately the efficacy of the drugs. It cannot be concluded from many publications because of the number of patients, and of the different methodology. A working network is now available for trials in paediatric rheumatology allowing to progress more rapidly with a sufficient number of patients through the Paediatric Rheumatology International Trial Organization (PRINTO) (Giannini et al. 1997).

Non-steroidal anti-inflammatory drugs

The use of NSAIDs remains the basis of treatment. In children, only a certain number of drugs have been studied and their licence for use varies in different countries. Acetylsalicylic acid and other NSAIDs such as diclofenac, ibuprofen, and naproxen are available for use in most countries. Recommended doses are indicated in Table 2. In general, all NSAIDs have similar efficacy but tolerance may vary. Aspirin induces the most frequent

Table 2 Non-steroidal anti-inflammatory drugs

Name	Dose per kg body weight per day (maximum daily dose)
Acetyl salicylic acid	50–100 mg (4 g)
Naproxen	15–20 mg (1.5 g)
Ibuprofen	40–60 mg (2.4 g)
Ketoprofen	3–5 mg (300 mg)
Fenoprofen	40–50 mg (3.2 g)
Flurbiprofen	4–5 mg (300 mg)
Diclofenac	2–3 mg (200 mg)
Sulindac	4–6 mg (400 mg)
Piroxicam	0.3 mg
Indomethacin	1–3 mg (200 mg)
Tolmetin	20–30 mg (1.8 g)

Table 3 Slow-acting antirheumatic drugs in children

Name	Dose	Side-effects
Aurothiomalate (Myocrisin®)	Weekly: 0.5 mg, then 1 mg/kg body weight for 3–6 months	Rash Cytopaenia
Aurothiosulfate (Allochrysin®) (intramuscular)	Monthly: 1 g/kg body weight	Bone marrow aplasia
D-Penicillamine (oral)	5, for 1 month, then 10 mg/kg body weight per day (if necessary 15 mg/kg per day)	Rash Cytopaenia Proteinuria Pneumopathy Autoimmunity: myasthenia, lupus
Hydroxychloroquine (oral)	5–7 mg/kg body weight per day (max. 200 mg)	Retinopathy Cutaneaous symptoms Neuropathies Cytopaenia
Methotrexate	10 mg/m^2/week	Increased transaminases Cytopaenia Nausea, aphtae Pulmonary manifestations
Etanercept (subcutaneous route)	0.4 mg/kg twice a week (max. 25 mg)	Local skin irritation increases the risk of infection, contraindicated in neurological diseases

side-effects, as shown in a comprehensive study (Barron et al. 1982). The few available pharmacokinetic studies in older children have shown only minor differences to adults. The half-life in synovial fluid is longer than in plasma (Hallé et al. 1991). NSAIDs are usually rapidly effective. The most frequent side-effects are gastrointestinal (mainly abdominal pain), cutaneous (urticaria, rash, and hypersensitivity), and haematological (anaemia). Rare cases of renal damage and disorders of the central nervous system (headache and dizziness) have been reported. Allergic reactions can also occur. Macrophage activation syndrome is exceptional in polyarticular disease, but it must be borne in mind, particularly when aspirin is used (Prieur and Stephan 1994).

Disease modifying drugs

Disease modifying drugs can be indicated in the polyarticular forms of JIA. These treatments all take several weeks to work and carry a risk of side-effects that are now well documented in adults. Their use in children must take account of age and the clinical presentation. An improvement is usually observed during the first 6 months, and there is no point in continuing treatment if no result is obtained after this period. Table 3 summarizes the main preparations, their doses, and side-effects.

In fact, published results on disease modifying drugs are only mediocre. A meta-analysis of 6-month efficacy on disease activity confirmed the lack of spectacular improvement (Giannini et al. 1991). In addition, most of these studies did not distinguish between the different categories of juvenile arthritis. There is no evidence that combinations of disease modifying drugs are effective in children, although this has not been studied in children in a systematic fashion.

Methotrexate is one of the most widely used immunomodulatory agents. The use of methotrexate in children with rheumatic diseases was proposed when its efficacy and acceptable tolerability were established in adults. The recommended dose, based on a double-blind, placebo-controlled trial, is 10 mg/m^2 per week (Giannini et al. 1992), but certain authors propose higher doses for particularly resistant forms (Wallace et al. 1991).

The tolerability of methotrexate in children is acceptable (Graham et al. 1992). In combination with NSAIDs, the level of methotrexate in the blood can increase (Dupuis et al. 1990). A few cases of severe liver damage have been reported (Keim et al. 1990). Side-effects, which are generally mild, must be monitored every 1 or 2 months. Many patients (almost 30 per cent) show increased transaminase levels. Values usually return to normal when the dose is reduced or treatment is suspended. After a few months of treatment, nausea is fairly frequent immediately after methotrexate intake, and these patients may benefit from a switch to the intramuscular route. Oral aphthae, cytopaenia, and pulmonary manifestations are observed rarely.

Methotrexate seems to have clear efficacy in some cases, especially in pauciarticular juvenile chronic arthritis with the presence of ANAs (Hallé and Prieur 1991). A European, multicentre, double-blind trial confirms this observation (Woo et al. 2000).

Steroids

Steroids are a very powerful tool but often have unacceptable side-effects in children. They can be given systemically or locally.

Systemic steroids generally are not indicated in the polyarticular form of juvenile chronic arthritis (Prieur 1993). In severe crippling cases, they can be used to improve the functional status. The side-effects of systemic steroids are the main problem in paediatric use. Rapid weight gain can only be avoided by a strict diet, which must be not only sodium-free but also restricted in slow-resorption carbohydrates. The most troublesome cutaneous side-effects are permanent striae, but these are rare if weight gain is controlled by dieting. Arterial hypertension and diabetes can develop. Osteoporosis can lead to very painful vertebral collapse which necessitates immobilization in a corset. Aseptic joint necrosis, especially of the hips, is far from rare and complicates underlying diseases that can also involve the joints. The onset of steroid-induced cataracts must be monitored closely. Finally, above all in children, daily steroid therapy arrests growth. This is overcome by alternate-day dosing when possible.

Intra-articular steroid injections have modified totally the prognosis of joint manifestations. They can be used in polyarticular forms when stiffness and flexion contractures cannot be controlled by general therapy. Among the many available products, only triamcinolone hexacetonide gives satisfactory results. It is fairly potent and must therefore be used with care to avoid local complications (mainly cutaneous atrophy at the injection site). This procedure is straightforward for large joints such as the knee, but general anaesthesia may be necessary for small and/or tight joints, especially in the very young child. An experienced practitioner must treat the joints of small children. In general, the volume injected must be adapted to the volume of the joint, and the product must not be injected 'under pressure'. The joint must be rested with a splint for 3 days. Needless to say, the potency of this preparation contraindicates its use for injecting tendon sheaths, where only water-soluble steroids can be used.

Uveitis, a frequent complication of polyarticular forms of juvenile chronic arthritis with ANAs, is treated with steroid-based eye drops and mydriatic agents.

Cytotoxic drugs

Cytotoxic treatments may be of value in severe forms. However, their efficacy is often difficult to determine objectively because of the small number of sound, prospective, multicentre trials. Ideally, as in oncology, multicentre protocols should be established to accelerate the assessment of the efficacy and tolerability of experimental treatments.

Azathioprine at a dose of 2–2.5 mg/kg body weight per day, is used by certain specialists. It is generally well tolerated. However, the possible long-term risk of cancer must be borne in mind, and this agent should probably only be used in severe cases (Silman et al. 1988). In juvenile arthritis, azathioprine appears to be slightly more effective than placebo (Kvien et al. 1985).

Alkylating agents can be considered in exceptional cases when classical treatments fail to control disease progression. However, chlorambucil (0.2 mg/kg) has a very high mutagenic risk (Prieur et al. 1979). It is thus only recommended for life-threatening complications such as secondary amyloidosis, which hardly ever complicates polyarticular juvenile chronic arthritis. Similarly, the indication for cyclophosphamide in the polyarticular forms is only for exceptional cases.

Cyclosporine A is effective in adult rheumatoid arthritis at doses below 5 mg/kg body weight per day. Studies involving patients with juvenile chronic arthritis have failed to show marked improvement, but further trials are required. The paediatric side-effects of cyclosporine A are identical to those observed in adults.

Intervention on the cytokine network

The possibility of intervention on the cytokine network, the imbalance of which being responsible at least in part of the chronic inflammation represents a very promising issue. The most intersting results are at the present time obtained by using TNFα inhibitors. Infliximab (Remicade®) is mainly used in adult RA with very good results. The recombinant p75 sTNF: Fc fusion protein (etanercept) was used in 69 children with polyarticular

Box 1 RF negative polyarthritis—therapeutic scheme

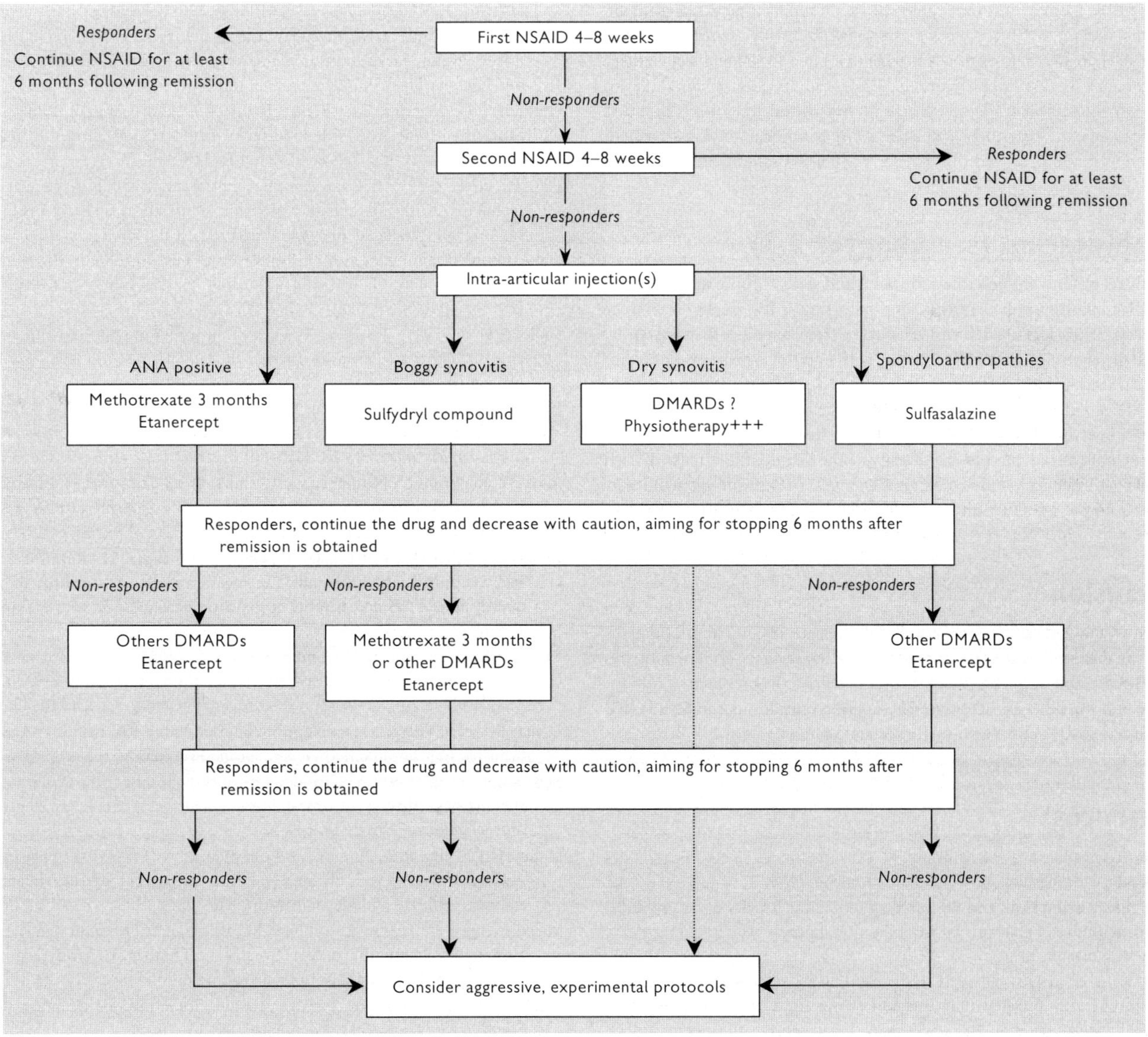

course of JIA. Subcutaneous injections of 0.4 mg/kg etanercept was administered for three months. Seventy-four per cent responded significantly. The responders were then enrolled in a double-blind study versus placebo. Under placebo, a flare after a median time of 28 days occured in 21 among 26 patients, while in the treated group, a flare occured in 7 of 25 patients after a median time of 116 days. The main adverse effects were injection-site reactions and infections in the open-label part of the study. In the double-blind study, there was no difference in the frequencies of adverse events between patients receiving etanercept and those receiving placebo (Lovell et al. 2000). In an extended trial, the response was maintained in children who continued etanercept, and the patients who relapsed under placebo were responding again to the drug. More publications on etanercept efficacy are now available in children. The tolerance is generally good. Skin reactions are possible (Skytta et al. 2000). One case of diabetes mellitus was observed in a systemic-onset JIA (Bloom 2000).

Surgery (see Chapter 7.1)

Surgery plays an increasing role in the management of chronic rheumatic diseases when the medical means are insufficient. The orthopaedic surgeon must participate in the therapeutic discussion. The technical approaches are numerous. Arthroscopy is now efficient for small joints, with adapted equipment. It allows intra-articular examination, biopsies, and synovectomy. Surgery in the form of soft tissue release, osteotomies, surgical realignment, and arthrodesis may be necessary to treat fixed joint deformities. Surgical treatment of growth deformities is mandatory when functional impairment and secondary mechanical problems in adjacent joints develop. Finally, joint arthroplasty must be considered when joint destruction and joint failure lead to major handicap. Anaesthetists must be aware of cervical spine involvement and temporomandibular arthritis, which may make intubation difficult.

Rehabilitation (see Chapter 2.3)

Physical treatments are necessary for any child with chronic arthritis. The techniques involve applied heat (water, paraffin, or hot packs) to induce muscle relaxation. Flexion deformities must be stretched out either actively by the child or passively by the child, parent, or therapist. Correct positioning of the joint must be obtained at rest with appropriate splinting. Prone positions should be recommended for reading or watching television. Each joint requires a specific technique of rehabilitation to prevent deformities. The treatment must be adapted to the severity of the disease, the impact of each joint on total function, and radiological changes. In cases of surgical intervention, both pre-operative and post-operative rehabilitation are necessary.

Conclusion

RF-negative polyarthritis is now a well-defined category in childhood arthritides. Further studies are necessary for evaluating several different subtypes already predictable according to age at onset, gender, the presence of autoantibodies and the HLA associations. Therapeutic indications can be adapted to the different RF-negative polyarthritis sub-groups as shown in Box 1.

References

Amor, B., Dougados, M., and Mijiyawa, M. (1990). Critères de classification des spondylarthropathies. *Revue du Rhumatisme* **57**, 85–9.

Barron, K.S., Person, D.A., and Brewer, E.J. (1982). The toxicity of non steroidal antiinflammatory drugs in juvenile rheumatoid arthritis. *Journal of Rheumatology* **9**, 149–55.

Barron, K. et al. (1992). DNA analysis of HLA–DR, DQ, and DP alleles in children with polyarticular juvenile rheumatoid arthritis. *Journal of Rheumatology* **19**, 1611–16.

Beretta-Piccoli, B.C., Sauvain, M.J., Gal, I., Schibler, A., Saurenmann, T., Kressebuch, H., and Bianchetti, M.G. (2000). Synovitis, acne, pustulosis, hyperostosis, osteitis (SAPHO) syndrome in childhood: a report of ten cases and review of the literature. *European Journal of Pediatrics* **159**, 594–601.

Blau, E.B. (1985). Familial granulomatous arthritis, iritis and rash. *Journal of Pediatrics* **107**, 689–93.

Bloom, B.J. (2000). Development of diabetes mellitus during etanercept therapy in a child with systemic-onset juvenile rheumatoid arthritis. *Arthritis and Rheumatism* **43**, 2606–8.

Brewer, E.J., Jr. et al. (1977). Current proposed revision of JRA criteria. *Arthritis and Rheumatism* **20**, 195–9.

Cerna, M. et al. (1994). Class II alleles in juvenile arthritis in Czech children. *Journal of Rheumatology* **21**, 159–64.

Dupuis, L.C. et al. (1990). Methotrexate–non steroidal antiinflammatory drug interaction in children with arthritis. *Journal of Rheumatology* **17**, 1469–73.

Fantini, F. et al. (1987). HLA phenotypes in Italian children affected with juvenile chronic arthritis. *Clinical and Experimental Rheumatology* **5**, 17.

Fernandez-Vina, M.A., Finck, C.W., and Stastny, P. (1990). HLA antigens in juvenile arthritis. Pauciarticular and polyarticular juvenile arthritis are immunogenetically distinct. *Arthritis and Rheumatism* **33**, 1787–94.

Giannini, E.H. et al. (1991). Meta-analysis of antirheumatic drug trials in juvenile rheumatoid arthritis. *Arthritis and Rheumatism* **34**, S152.

Giannini, E.H. et al. (1992). Methotrexate in resistant juvenile rheumatoid arthritis. *New England Journal of Medicine* **326**, 1043–9.

Giannini, E.H., Ruperto, N., Ravelli, A., Lovell, D.J., Felson, D.T., and Martini, A. (1997). Preliminary definition of improvement in juvenile arthritis. *Arthritis and Rheumatism* **40**, 1202–9.

Graham, L.D., Myones, B.L., Rivas-Chalon, R.F., and Pachman, L.M. (1992). Morbidity associated with long-term methotrexate therapy in juvenile rheumatoid arthritis. *Journal of Pediatrics* **120**, 468–73.

Hall, P.J. et al. (1989). HLA and complement C4 antigens in polyarticular onset seronegative juvenile chronic arthritis: association of early onset with HLA–DRw8. *Journal of Rheumatology* **16**, 55–9.

Hallé, F. and Prieur, A.M. (1991). Evaluation of methotrexate in the treatment of juvenile chronic arthritis according to the subtype. *Clinical and Experimental Rheumatology* **9**, 297–302.

Hallé, F. et al. (1991). Pharmacokinetics of pirprofen in children with juvenile chronic arthritis. *European Journal of Drug Metabolism and Pharmacokinetics* **16**, 29–34.

Hofer, M., Mouy, R., and Prieur, A.M. (2001). Juvenile idiopathic arthritides evaluated prospectively in a single center according to the Durban criteria. *Journal of Rheumatology* **28**, 1083–90.

Keim, D., Ragadale, C., Heidelberger, K., and Sullivan, D. (1990). Hepatic fibrosis in the use of methotrexate for juvenile arthritis. *Journal of Rheumatology* **17**, 846–8.

Koné-Paut, I., Geisler, I., Wechsler, B., Ozen, S., Ozdogan, H., Rozenbaum, M., and Touitou, I. (1999). Familial aggregation in Behçet's disease: high frequency in siblings and parents of pediatric probands. *Journal of Pediatrics* **135**, 89–93.

Kvien, T.K., Hoyeraal, H.M., and Sandstad, B. (1985). Azathioprine versus placebo in patients with juvenile rheumatoid arthritis: a single center double-blind comparative study. *Journal of Rheumatology* **13**, 118–23.

Lovell, D.J. et al. (2000). Etanercept in children with polyarticular rheumatoid arthritis. *New England Journal of Medicine* **342**, 763–9.

Malagon, C. et al. (1991). The iridocyclitis of early onset pauciarticular juvenile rheumatoid arthritis: outcome in immunogenetically characterized patients. *Journal of Rheumatology* **19**, 160–3.

Malleson, P., Petty, R.E., Fun, M., and Candido, P.M. (1989). Reactivity of antinuclear antibodies with histones and other antigens in juvenile rheumatoid arthritis. *Arthritis and Rheumatism* **32**, 919–23.

Miceli-Richard, C., Lesage, S., Rybojad, M., Prieur, A.M., Manouvrier-Hanu, S., Hafner, R., Chamaillard, M., Zouali, H., Thomas, G., and Hugot, J.P. (2001). CARD15 mutations in Blau syndrome. *Nature Genetics* **29**, 19–20.

Morling, N. et al. (1985). HLA antigen frequencies in juvenile chronic arthritis. *Scandinavian Journal of Rheumatology* **14**, 209–16.

Pauls, J.D., Silverman, E., Laxer, R.M., and Fritzler, M.J. (1989). Antibodies to histones H1 and H5 in sera of patients with juvenile rheumatoid arthritis. *Arthritis and Rheumatism* **32**, 877–83.

Peralta, J.L. and Prieur, A.-M. (1990). Arthrite chronique juvénile avec présence d'anticorps antinucléaires sériques. *Archives de Pediatrie* **47**, 497–502.

Petty, R. et al. (1998). Revision of the proposed classification criteria for juvenile idiopathic arthritis: Durban, 1997. *Journal of Rheumatology* **25**, 1991–5.

Ploski, R. et al. (1993). HLA class II alleles and heterogeneity of juvenile rheumatoid arthritis: DRB1*0101 may define a novel subset of the disease. *Arthritis and Rheumatism* **36**, 465–72.

Ploski, R., Flato, B., Vinje, O., Maksymowych, W., Forre, O., and Thorsby, E. (1995). Association to HLA–DRB1*08, HLA–DPB1*0301 and homozygosity fo an HLA-linked proteasome gene in juvenile ankylosing spondylitis. *Human Immunology* **44**, 88–96.

Prieur, A.-M. and Stephan, J.-L. (1994). Macrophage activation syndrome in pediatric rheumatic diseases. *Revue du Rhumatisme (English Edition)* **6**, 385–8.

Prieur, A.-M., Balafrej, M., Griscelli, C., and Mozziconacci, P. (1979). Résultats et risques à long terme des traitements immunosuppresseurs dans l'arthrite chronique juvénile. *Revue du Rhumatisme* **46**, 85–90.

Rosenberg, A.M. and Cordeiro, D.M. (2000). Relationship between sex and antibodies to high mobility group proteins 1 and 2 in juvenile idiopathic arthritis. *Journal of Rheumatology* **27**, 2489–93.

Skytta, E., Pohjankoski, H., and Savoilanen, A. (2000). Etanercept and urticaria in patients with juvenile idiopathic arthritis. *Clinical and Experimental Rheumatology* **18**, 533–4.

Silman, A.J. et al. (1988). Lymphoproliferative cancer and other malignancy in patients with azathioprine. A 20 year follow-up study. *Annals of the Rheumatic Diseases* **47**, 988–92.

Stemmer, C., Tuaillon, N., Prieur, A.-M., and Muller, S. (1995). Mapping of B-cell epitopes by antibodies to histones in subsets of juvenile chronic arthritis. *Clinical and Experimental Immunopathology* **76**, 82–9.

Thomas, E., Barrett, J.H., Donn, R.P., Thomson, W., and Southwood, T.R. (2000). Subtyping of juvenile idiopathic arthritis using latent class analysis. British Paediatric Rheumatology Group. *Arthritis and Rheumatism* **43**, 1496–503.

Tuaillon, N. et al. (1990). Antibodies from patients with rheumatoid arthritis and juvenile chronic arthritis analysed with core histone synthetic peptides. *International Archives of Allergy and Immunology* **91**, 297–305.

Wallace, C., Sherry, D., and Salmonson, K. (1991). Treatment of juvenile rheumatoid arthritis with higher dose methotrexate. *Arthritis and Rheumatism* **34**, S152.

Woo, P., Southwood, T.R., Prieur, A.M., Dore, C.J., Grainger, J., David, J., Ryder, C., Hasson, N., Hall, A., and Lemelle, I. (2000). Randomized, placebo-controlled, crossover trial of low-dose oral methotrexate in children with extended oligoarticular or systemic arthritis. *Arthritis and Rheumatism* **43**, 1849–57.

Wood, P.H.N. (1978). Special meeting on nomenclature and classification of arthritis in children. In *The Care of Rheumatic Children* (ed. E. Munthe), p. 47. Basel: European League Against Rheumatism.

6.6 Systemic lupus erythematosus

6.6.1 Systemic lupus erythematosus in adults—clinical features and aetiopathogenesis

Michael R. Ehrenstein and David A. Isenberg

Introduction

Systemic lupus erythematosus (SLE) has taken the mantle of syphilis as the great mimic of other conditions. It is probably better to think of it as a group of related disorders rather than a single disease entity. By analogy, it might also be compared to the Hydra monster of ancient Greek mythology (Fig. 1). This beast, one of the offsprings of Echidne and Typhon was notoriously unpleasant and possessed numerous heads. It was said that cutting off one head led to the growth of two or three others. By analogy, lupus presents in many unpleasant guises and the successful treatment of, say, joint pain in lupus may be followed by the emergence of skin rash or pleuropericardial involvement. There is another analogy with lupus as no one could agree precisely how many heads the Hydra had or about their appearance—similarly there remains disagreement as to how disease activity in lupus should best be assessed.

Definition and classification of lupus

SLE is perhaps best defined as a clinical syndrome, with a complex multifactorial aetiology characterized by inflammation and the involvement of most of the body's organs or systems. It is characterized by remissions and exacerbations and although the musculoskeletal system and skin are invariably affected, it frequently gives rise to manifestations in the kidney, heart, lungs, and central nervous system. The diversity among its clinical features is matched by an apparent serological diversity.

The American College of Rheumatology (ACR) has published three sets of criteria in 1971, 1982, and 1997. Strictly speaking the criteria are for the classification of the disease rather than use as a diagnostic tool, although in practice there is blurring of this distinction. The 1997 criteria are set out in Table 1.

The variable clinical and serological expression of lupus make it easy to obtain a distorted view of the disease. Patients present to a variety of

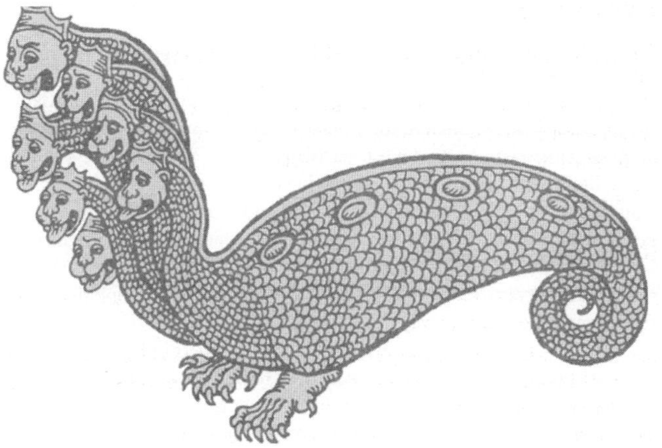

Fig. 1 The Hydra—a useful analogy of lupus (see text).

Table 1 Revised criteria of the American College of Rheumatology for the classification of SLE[a]

1. Malar rash
2. Discoid rash
3. Photosensitivity
4. Oral ulcers
5. Arthritis
6. Serositis:
   (a) pleuritis or
   (b) pericarditis
7. Renal disorder:
   (a) proteinuria >0.5 g/24 h or 3+, persistently, or
   (b) cellular casts
8. Neurological disorder:
   (a) seizures or
   (b) psychosis (having excluded other causes, e.g. drugs)
9. Haematologic disorder:
   (a) Haemolytic anaemia or
   (b) Leucopaenia or $<4.0 \times 10^9$/l on two or more occasions
   (c) Lymphopaenia or $<1.5 \times 10^9$/l on two or more occasions
   (d) Thrombocytopaenia $<100 \times 10^9$/l
10. Immunological disorders:
    (a) Raised antinative DNA antibody binding or
    (b) AntiSm antibody or
    (c) Positive finding of antiphospholipid antibodies based on
        (1) an abnormal serum level of IgG/IgM anticardiolipin antibodies;
        (2) a positive test result for lupus anticoagulant using a standard method, or
    (d) A false positive serologic test for syphilis known to be positive for at least 6 months and confirmed by *Treponema pallidum* immobilization or fluorescent treponemal antibody absorption test
11. Antinuclear antibody in raised titre

[a] '... A person shall be said to have SLE if four or more of the 11 criteria are present, serially or simultaneously, during any interval of observation.' Tan et al. (1982).

specialists each of whom will see a different spectrum of its clinical features. Thus, bias among the reporting physicians must be borne in mind when assessing reports about lupus. A broad overview of the cumulative percentage incidence of SLE features in five large series is shown in Table 2. The incidence of some clinical features varies between ethnic groups. For example, a study of 137 Chinese SLE patients in Hong Kong reported a relatively low incidence of arthritis (71 per cent) compared with other groups but a high incidence of renal involvement (70 per cent) (Lee et al. 1993).

Epidemiology and natural history

Lupus is a worldwide disease. Although it has been estimated that approximately 1 in 250 black women in the United States and the West Indies, about 1 in 1000 Chinese, and 1 in 4300 Caucasians in New Zealand have systemic lupus, there are some curiously conflicting data. In particular, it seems that lupus is rare in most parts of Africa (Nived and Sturfelt 1997). Two studies from urban centres in the United Kingdom have highlighted the significant variation in the prevalence of lupus among different ethnic groups sharing much the same environment. The study from Nottingham (Hopkinson et al. 1993), while noting a prevalence of 45.4/100 000 per year among women (3.7/100 000 per year in men), implied that the numbers of lupus patients of Afro-Caribbean and Asian origin were over-represented, but did not quote any figures. In contrast, the study from Birmingham (Johnson et al. 1995) reported prevalence rates of 36.2, 90.6, and 206 per 100 000 among women of Caucasian, Asian, and Afro-Caribbean origin, respectively.

The important genetic contribution to the aetiology of lupus is emphasized by the study of twin concordance reported by Deapen et al. (1992). Of 107 twin pairs studied concordance among monozygotic pairs was found to be 24 per cent compared to 2 per cent among dizygotic pairs. While the figure for monozygotic twins is lower than previously reported, it is still 12 times that for the dizygotic pairs and may in fact be an underestimate, as not all of the twins were personally examined by the authors and long-term follow-up of the pairs was restricted.

It is widely agreed that lupus is approximately 10–20 times more common in women than men. There is also little dispute that the overwhelming majority of lupus patients will develop their disease between the ages of 15 and 40.

Although, in the early part of the century, lupus was considered a serious and frequently fatal disease, perceptions of it have changed considerably. The now widely available tests for measuring antinuclear antibodies have eased identification of milder cases. The introduction of corticosteroids and immunosuppressive drugs, dialysis, and renal transplantation has improved the chances of survival in the more serious cases. However, as will be discussed, lupus continues to cause considerable morbidity and 10–20 per cent of patients succumb from either the disease, a side-effect of its treatment, or both within 15 years of follow-up.

Clinical features

Non-specific features

Lupus, in common with many other chronic diseases, is accompanied by a variety of non-specific or general features. Of these, lethargy is frequently the most disabling and the least likely to attract the sympathy of the physician! It is, however, invariably present in active lupus but may also be due to anaemia, hypothyroidism, or fibromyalgia. The last of these has been reported in 20–30 per cent of lupus patients in North America (e.g. Wang et al. 1998) but is much less common (<10 per cent) in the United Kingdom (Taylor et al. 2000). Careful examination frequently reveals the presence of lymphadenopathy, especially in the axillae, which persists long after patients have gone into remission. On occasion, it may be so prominent in the neck or under the arms that a biopsy has to be taken to exclude any more sinister pathology. Patients with active lupus may experience weight loss and, on occasion, nausea. Most of these general features will improve when treatment is commenced.

Musculoskeletal involvement

Arthralgia occurs in about 90 per cent of patients with SLE. The joint pain is polyarticular and frequently symmetrical, episodic, and flitting in nature. It is accompanied in about half the patients by early morning stiffness. Very often, the patient's symptoms outweigh the objective signs and major synovial effusions are rare. Severe clinically overt arthritis with joint deformity is probably confined to around 10 per cent of these patients (Spronk et al. 1992). Furthermore, unlike patients with rheumatoid arthritis, the deformities (Fig. 2) are usually related to an intense tenosynovitis and less frequently to synovial hypertrophy, with or without bone erosion. These deformities in the hands are known as Jaccoud's arthropathy which is generally a reversible subluxation. Magnetic resonance imaging scanning (MRI) is useful in distinguishing Jaccoud's arthropathy from frank arthritis (Ostendorf et al. 2003).

Because of the relatively mild joint involvement it is uncommon for 'lupus joints' to be examined histologically but a 'lupus synovium' has been described with a characteristic minor cellular inflammation, occasional haemotoxylin bodies, and non-specific vasculitis and perivasculitis. Synovial fluid examination usually reveals a low white count (<3000 cells/mm^3), in which mononuclear cells predominate. The fluid is occasionally positive for rheumatoid factor or antinuclear antibodies. Immune complex deposition has been described in synovial tissues and is thought to be responsible for the observed inflammatory lesions. Approximately 2–3 per cent of patients classified as having lupus also meet the ACR's criteria for rheumatoid arthritis with erosive disease.

An occasional complication of joint involvement in lupus is spontaneous tendon rupture, which is generally confined to the patella or Achilles

Table 2 Cumulative percentage incidence of systemic lupus features—a comparison of several large studies

Feature	Dubois and Tuffanelli (1964) (520 cases)	Estes and Christian (1971) (150 cases)	Thumboo et al. (1998) (381 Chinese cases)	Tan et al. (1982) (177 cases)	Moss et al. (2002) (300 cases)
Female sex	89	91	93	NA[a]	92
Caucasian	58	52	0	NA	67
Afro-Caribbean	23	47	0	NA	15
Malar rash	72	81	63	57	74
Discoid rash			7	18	
Photosensitivity	33	NA	32	43	48
Alopecia	21	37	NA	56	17
Oral ulcers	9	7	19	27	28
Arthritis/arthralgia	92	95	62	86	96
Pleurisy	45	45	21	52	51
Pericarditis	31			18	
Renal	40	53	56	51	31
Neuropsychiatric	26[b]	59	14	20	25
Haemolytic anaemia	NA	14	NA	18	2[c]
Sjögren's syndrome	<2	NA	NA	NA	12
Antinuclear antibody	NA	87	93	99	94
LE cells	76	78	NA	73	NA
Anti-dsDNA antibody	NA	NA	86	67	60
Wassermann reaction	NA	24	NA	15	NA
Rheumatoid factor	57	21	NA	NA	20
Leucopaenia	43	66	80	46	42
Lymphopaenia	NA	NA		NA	77
Thrombocytopaenia	7	19		21	18

[a] NA, not available.

[b] Central nervous system involvement only.

[c] 2% with haemoglobin <8 g/dl but 5% with haemoglobin <10 g/dl.

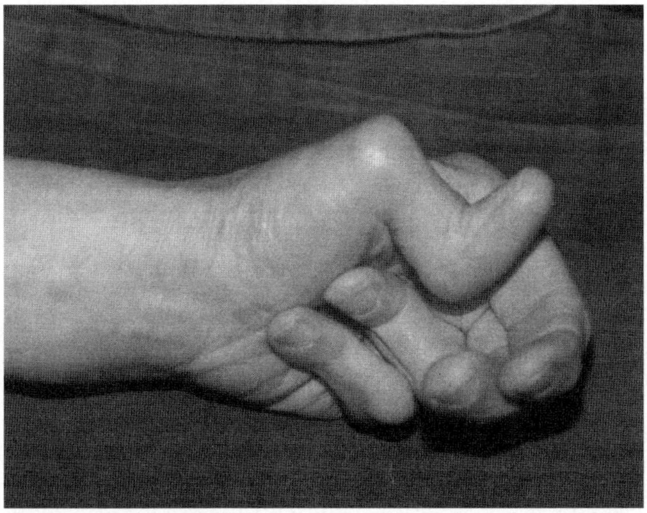

Fig. 2 Severe hand deformity in a lupus patient due to chronic tenosynovitis, not an erosive arthritis.

tendons (Furie and Chartash 1988). Its aetiology is not well understood, but in some cases at least it seems to be related to inflammatory changes in and around the tendon as a result of the underlying disease process. It is also possible that corticosteroid therapy is in part responsible.

Other, less common, musculoskeletal features include subcutaneous nodules (present in around 5 per cent of SLE patients and indistinguishable from those found in patients with rheumatoid arthritis), calcinosis (less common in lupus than in scleroderma or dermatomyositis), chondritis, and avascular necrosis. The last of these features occurs in 4–9 per cent of lupus patients, most cases being associated with prior corticosteroid therapy but not, as was once suspected, with the presence of antiphospholipid antibodies (Mok et al. 2000). In many instances, the avascular necrosis occurs at multiple sites.

Myalgia, muscle weakness, and tenderness have been reported in upto 60 per cent of lupus patients, although a true myositis is confined to about 5 per cent of these patients (Isenberg and Snaith 1981). Treatment with corticosteroids and chloroquine may cause a myopathy, but in the main the myalgia experienced by lupus patients seems to be a complication of adjacent joint involvement.

Histologically a vacuolar myopathy has been described in lupus. This is identified by the presence of plump, swollen sarcolemmal nuclei with other prominent vacuolated nuclei, centrally located within the muscle fibre. Immunoglobulin deposition is often seen in the muscles of patients with lupus (Isenberg 1983) but this is irrespective of whether they have clinically overt muscle disease and seems to relate better to muscle fibre damage as a secondary event, rather than to a primary inflammatory myopathy.

Dermatological involvement

Although lupus takes its name from the classic butterfly rash found over the bridge of the nose and malar bones [see Plate 111(a)], this is actually found in only about one-third of patients with systemic lupus. There are, however,

Table 3 Cutaneous manifestations in SLE

Common (20–50% approximately)	Butterfly rash Photosensitivity Non-specific maculopapular lesions Chronic discoid lesion Non-scarring alopecia Purpura/petechiae
Less common (5–20% approximately)	Mucous membrane lesions Urticaria Diffuse hyperpigmentation Leg ulcer Subcutaneous nodules
Occasional (<5%)	Periorbital oedema Jaundice Severe scarring alopecia Pruritis Bullae Panniculitis Psoriaform lesions

numerous other forms of dermatological involvement (Pistiner et al. 1992, and see Table 3). These include maculopapular rashes and discoid lesions [Plate 111(b)], splinter haemorrhages, dilated capillaries at the nail base, bullous lesions, angioneurotic oedema, and buccal and nasal ulceration [Plate 111(c)]. Vasculitis affecting the fingers and toes is common and frequently causes pain and tenderness [Plate 111(d)]. Many lupus rashes are photosensitive and thus not surprisingly, photosensitivity is commonest in white females. It is important to advise patients with SLE to avoid sun exposure and use sunscreen even when driving with an arm exposed through an open window.

Alopecia is a common feature of lupus. Although the lack of precision in interpreting and reporting it led to this feature being deleted from the 1982 revised ARA criteria for lupus, it remains an important component of SLE. It is usually diffuse but non-scarring, and more often a cause of limited upset. In contrast severe, scarring alopecia is uncommon but can be quite devastating for those who develop it.

Among the less common but important dermatological features of lupus are diffuse hyperpigmentation, usually most prominent on the light exposed and extensor surfaces of the body, and lupus panniculitis. The latter is a form of lipoatrophy which usually takes the form of a relapsing nodular, non-suppurative lesion. The nodules resemble those seen in Weber–Christian disease. The skin overlying the nodules may ulcerate and scars invariably remain after healing takes place.

A variant of SLE known as subacute cutaneous lupus erythematosus has been described. Early reports suggested that there were two types, annular and papulosquamous, and that the condition was associated with anti-Ro antibodies and HLA–DR3. Other evidence (Callen and Klein 1988) suggests that this group of patients is less distinctive but generally easily controlled.

Immunoglobulin (IG) deposition at the dermal/epidermal junction has been recognised for some 40 years. These immunoglobulins are usually of the IgG or IgM isotype. Intriguingly, these depositions may be identified in areas of skin that are not light exposed (such as the buttocks) and which have no rash. This forms the basis of the so-called lupus band test (see Plate 112). Complement components may also be found at the dermal/epidermal junction.

Cardiovascular and pulmonary involvement

Involvement of the heart in lupus has been recognized for approximately a century. The names of Libman and Sachs are regarded as synonymous with cardiac involvement, following their classic descriptions of non-bacterial verrucous endocarditis. Many studies have confirmed the effects of lupus on the heart. These may be subdivided into pericardial, myocardial, or endocardial/valvular involvement.

Pericardial disease

Pericardial disease is the most common component of heart involvement in lupus. A pericardial rub is, however, also more common than significant accumulations of pericardial fluid. Mandell (1987) reviewed 22 studies of pericardial involvement in lupus and concluded that whereas 29 per cent of the patients had clinical evidence of the disease, echocardiography revealed abnormalities in 37 per cent and necropsy studies showed that 66 per cent of lupus patients had pericardial involvement. Abnormalities of the electrocardiogram, notably of the T waves are detectable in up to 75 per cent of patients. Echocardiographic findings more commonly show pericardial thickening than large effusion. The results of pericardial fluid analyses may mimic those seen in bacterial pericarditis, and on occasions this latter diagnosis is difficult to distinguish. Studies of pericardial fluid have shown the presence of an antinuclear antibody, LE cells, and even hypocomplementaemia.

When large pericardial effusions have been discovered there may be further underlying complicating factors such as uraemia and viral or bacterial infection. Constrictive pericarditis can develop within a few weeks of the first appearance of a pericardial effusion. There is some evidence that corticosteroid therapy may contribute to the development of constriction.

Histological abnormalities vary from occasional foci of fibrinoid degeneration and inflammatory infiltrates, to far more extensive lesions. Immune complex components have also been found throughout the pericardial tissue, even in areas where histologically the pericardium looks normal. There is no diagnostic pathological finding for lupus pericarditis with the possible exception of hematoxylin bodies.

Myocardial disease

True myocardial involvement is less frequent than pericardial disease. The results of investigations and necropsy studies suggest that involvement is more common than is suspected clinically. Clinical myocarditis, usually defined by combinations of unexplained tachycardia, congestive heart failure, arrythmias, prolongation of the PR interval on electrocardiogram, or cardiomegaly without pericardial effusion or valvular disease, occurs in up to 15 per cent of lupus patients. Echocardiographic studies have suggested that myocardial function can reversibly deteriorate in parallel with flares of generalized lupus activity.

Histological studies of myocardium have indicated that a mild non-specific perivascular infiltration with lymphocytes and neutrophils is relatively common. Intimal proliferation of the smaller intramyocardial arteries is also commonly reported, together with hyalinized vessels that may reflect either previous arteritis or primary thrombosis. The latter is of particular interest in view of the recognized links with antiphospholipid antibodies. The propensity for corticosteroid therapy to increase the risk factors such as hypertension, hypercholesterolaemia, and obesity for coronary artery disease has been emphasized recently (reviewed in Urowitz and Gladman 2000). In contrast, hydroxychloroquine was associated with a lowered serum cholesterol.

Valves

Conduction defects and rhythm disturbances are recognized as occasional features of lupus, but have rarely been found in more than 10 per cent of patients.

Systolic murmurs have been recorded in upto a third of lupus patients, but in the majority of cases this probably represents the hypodynamic circulation secondary to the chronic anaemia often found in these individuals. In contrast, diastolic murmurs are rather rare.

The classic endocarditis described by Libman and Sachs (1924), although identified in up to 50 per cent of autopsied cases, rarely causes clinically significant lesions. Histologically small (1–4 cm) vegetations (verrucae) comprising proliferating and degenerating valve tissue with fibrin and thrombi are seen. A prospective echocardiographic study of 132 consecutive lupus patients reported a prevalence of valvular lesions of 22.7 per cent (Khamashta et al. 1990). These lesions were most commonly found adjacent to the edges of the mitral and aortic valves and have been shown to contain immunoglobulin and complement components, notably within the walls of the small junctional vessels in the active portions of the verrucous endocardial lesions. These deposits might therefore represent immune complexes deposited via the circulation. In the above report, the valve vegetations were associated with the presence of antiphospholipid antibodies. Leung et al. (1990) also found a correlation between antiphospholipid antibodies and both valvular abnormalities and isolated left ventricular dysfunction in a study using M-mode, two dimensional, and Doppler echocardiography.

In Mandell's review (1987) of the reports of haemodynamically significant valvular disease in lupus, aortic incompetence and mitral regurgitation were the most frequently found among the paucity of published case reports.

Bacterial endocarditis has been reported on a number of occasions in lupus patients. It has not been determined whether the most likely cause is a consequence of the underlying immunopathology of the disease or the predisposition to infection. However, reports of bacterial endocarditis in lupus patients do antedate corticosteroid therapy, suggesting that in some patients at least it is the primary immunopathology which predisposes to secondary bacterial infection. As most of the lesions of Libman–Sachs endocarditis are too small to be accurately assessed by echocardiography, any vegetations which can be identified in a lupus patient who is febrile should certainly raise the possibility of bacterial endocarditis.

Accelerated atherosclerosis

Linked to some of the clinical features described above it is now recognized that patients with lupus have an increased risk of developing accelerated atherosclerosis. Furthermore this is an increasingly important cause of morbidity and mortality. For example, Manzi et al. (1999) using B-mode ultrasound reported that 40 per cent of their lupus patients had evidence of focal carotid artery plaque.

The precise aetiopathogenesis of accelerated atherosclerosis in lupus is uncertain, but likely to be multifactorial. Elevated lipid levels (especially early in the course of the disease), corticosteroid therapy (which tend to increase lipid levels whereas antimalarials do the opposite), the chronic inflammation that characterizes lupus, raised plasma homocysteine levels, and elevated antiphospholipid antibodies (and other pro-coagulant effects) are all likely contributors. Reduced paraoxonase activity (an enzyme that regulates oxidation of low density lipoprotein) may also be involved (Delgado Alves et al. 2002).

Pulmonary disease

The nature and features of pulmonary disease are indicated in Table 4. The commonest feature is pain due to pleurisy, which affects approximately half of lupus patients at some time. This pain may be uni- or bilateral and is usually present at the costophrenic angles anteriorly or posteriorly. Pleural effusions, usually small, also uni- or bilateral, straw-coloured, with a protein level generally more than 3 g/dl, high mononuclear cell count but normal glucose level, are found in one-fourth of the patients. Low levels of pleural fluid complement are quite common compared to effusions in other conditions such as heart failure and cancer but a positive antinuclear antibody is very infrequently recorded.

Table 4 Major pulmonary manifestations in lupus

1. Pleuritic pain/pleuritis is present in 40–60%
2. Pleural effusions are found in 20–30%. These are usually small volume, straw coloured, white cell count 3–5000/mm^3 mostly mononuclear cells and lymphocytes, glucose levels approximate to those in the blood (unlike RA in which the levels are lower), ANA may be detected, protein content varies from 2.75 to 6.4 g%
3. CXR and lung function tests (and autopsy findings!) invariably indicate a greater degree of pulmonary involvement than is evident clinically
4. Interstitial fibrosis, pulmonary vasculitis, and interstitial pneumonitis are found in upto one-fifth of the patients
5. Pulmonary hypertension is unusual and has been linked to the presence of antiphospholipid antibodies

Parenchymal involvement attributable to lupus were reported in 18 per cent of patients (Haupt et al. 1981). These patients had interstitial fibrosis, pulmonary vasculitis, and interstitial pneumonitis. However, many pulmonary lesions such as alveolar haemorrhage, alveolar wall necrosis, and oedema, previously attributed to direct lupus involvement, are probably secondary to factors such as concurrent infection, congestive heart failure, renal failure, and oxygen toxicity. A true lupus pneumonitis is recognized but is rare (<2 per cent).

Almost as uncommon is clinically symptomatic diffuse interstitial lung disease. Its manifestations resemble those found in patients with scleroderma and rheumatoid arthritis who may also develop this complication. Thus, the slow onset of a chronic non-productive cough with shortness of breath is usually present. Occasionally, a more acute presentation occurs after an episode of acute lupus pneumonitis.

There is great interest in antiphospholipid antibodies and thrombotic events in SLE. It is accepted that around 10 per cent of patients develop thrombophlebitis and/or a pulmonary embolus. Antiphospholipid antibodies should be sought in patients with these presenting symptoms and also the small number who present with pulmonary hypertension. However, in the largest study to date from a single centre the 18 patients with lupus who had pulmonary hypertension (out of 419 studied) showed no association with anticardiolipin antibodies (Li and Tam 1999). This study did show, contrary to earlier much more pessimistic reports, that the prognosis was variable and a few of their patients improved markedly.

Well recognized, but also uncommon, are patients with the so-called 'shrinking lung syndrome' (Hoffbrand and Beck 1965). It is evident that diaphragmatic dysfunction makes a significant contribution to this syndrome.

Abnormal pulmonary function tests (described in detail in Chapter 1.3.5), notably diminished total lung capacity and flow rates, often show more serious involvement than expected. Haemoptysis is unusual, although commoner than major pulmonary haemorrhage, which, while rare, may be life-threatening.

In the relatively few cases studied, immune complex deposition has been correlated with histological evidence of inflammatory lesions in the pleural and pericardial membrane.

Renal involvement

In many older published series renal disease has been most common cause of death in lupus patients. However, the clinical symptoms suggesting renal involvement, notably ankle swelling, shortness of breath related to secondary heart failure, and 'frothy' urine, rarely become evident until substantial damage has been done. Thus, careful monitoring of the blood pressure for hypertension, the urine for protein, protein/creatinine ratio, red cells or casts, and the plasma for raised creatinine and urea levels is most important. The World Health Organization (WHO) have sub-divided renal lupus into six major categories according to biopsy-derived information (Table 5 and Plate 113). In brief, the major manifestations are defined as minimal or mesangial change; mild or focal proliferative; severe or diffuse proliferative, and membranous. The glomerulus appears to bear the brunt of the attack in lupus. The range of glomerular changes include swelling, proliferation of mesangial, endothelial, and parietal epithelial cells, with infiltration by monocytes and polymorphonuclear leucocytes. In addition immune complexes, foci of necrosis, and haemotoxylin bodies can be identified in the glomeruli of lupus patients. While the WHO score has been widely adopted, it has drawbacks. It does not, for example, consider tubulo-interstitial disease and makes no allowances for varying degrees of severity within individual categories. Neither does it recognize the recently described overlap of lupus nephritis and the multiple small thrombi associated with antiphospholipid antibodies (see Plate 113). In addition the type of lupus nephritis may change over time.

The role of renal biopsy in the management of lupus nephritis

There is a difference of opinion as to precisely when renal biopsy should be undertaken in lupus patients, and about its value. The ability of lupus nephritis to transform from one variety to another and for the same biopsy to have more than one histological appearance, is partly responsible for the conflict. In addition, few studies of the relationships between renal histology and clinical outcome have actually directly addressed the question as to what information the renal histology adds to the clinical data. Goulet et al. (1993) used regression tree techniques to show that combinations of serum creatinine, 24 h urine protein levels, nephrotic syndrome, and duration of prior renal disease provide accurate prognostic information about lupus nephritis without recourse to biopsy.

The biopsy itself is not without its problems, including quite heavy haematuria on occasion. In our experience over a 22-year period, this complication has occurred twice (approximately 2 per cent of all our lupus patient renal biopsies) resulting in a nephrectomy on one occasion. It is obviously most important to assess the clotting capability of the lupus patient before undertaking the biopsy. Fries et al. (1978) found that renal biopsy contains important prognostic information but that it was less than that of even the simplest clinical classification. Whiting-O'Keefe et al. (1982) applied a stepwise regression analysis to data collected over a 12-month period after renal biopsy in 130 lupus patients to see if biopsy added any useful information to the clinical data. They found the histological classification did not add significantly to the predictive power of the 'before biopsy' model, but that certain features, notably the percentage of glomeruli which had undergone sclerosis in the presence of sub-endothelial deposits on electron microscopy did increase the ability to predict the effect of 12 months of treatment of lupus nephritis. These authors felt that renal biopsy did not add important prognostic information over and above the clinical history examination and laboratory tests. A more recent study (Blanco et al. 1994) emphasized that chronicity markers notably hyalinosis, tubular atrophy, and glomerular sclerosis on light microscopy and sub-epithelial, mesangial, and intramembranous deposits on electron microscopy are the best indicators of a poor prognosis. More worryingly, Schwartz et al. (1993) cast doubt upon the ability of pathologists to reproduce activity and chronicity scores accurately.

Table 5 WHO classification of SLE glomerulonephritis

I	Normal glomeruli (a) Nil (by all techniques) (b) Normal by light microscopy, but deposits by electron or immunofluorescence microscopy
II	Pure mesangial alterations (mesangiopathy) (a) Mesangial widening and/or mild hypercellularity (+) (b) Moderate hypercellularity (++)
III	Focal segmental glomerulonephritis (associated with mild or moderate mesangial *alterations)* (a) 'Active' necrotizing lesions (b) 'Active' and sclerosing lesions (c) Sclerosing lesions
IV	Diffuse glomerulonephritis (severe mesangial, endocapillary, or mesangiocapillary proliferation, and/or extensive sub-endothelial deposits) (a) Without segmental lesions (b) With 'active' necrotizing lesions (c) With 'active' and sclerosing lesions (d) With sclerosing lesions
V	Diffuse membranous glomerulonephritis (a) Pure membranous glomerulonephritis (b) Associated with lesions of Category II (a or b) (c) Associated with lesions of Category III (a–c) (d) Associated with lesions of Category III (a–d)
VI	Advanced sclerosing glomerulonephritis

In contrast, Stamenkovic et al. (1986) described treatment based on renal histology of 56 lupus patients. The mean follow-up period from first biopsy was 8.2 years, by which time 5.3 per cent were dialysis dependent, but nearly 95 per cent had resumed normal renal function. They found that the biopsy provided valuable information about the state of the kidney, independent of the clinical stage of the disease, and have argued that biopsy alone can improve predictions about 'renal survival' in lupus. McLaughlin et al. (1994) in a long-term follow-up study of 123 SLE patients who had a renal biopsy between 1970 and 1984 showed that the biopsy was helpful in assessing prognosis in patients with normal serum creatinine. In those with an elevated serum creatinine, the biopsy did not contribute additional information about the risk of dying.

Various attempts to introduce activity and chronicity indices have been made but their utility remains controversial. However, we support the views of Melvin Schwartz that 'the development of a rational treatment program for a patient with lupus nephritis is contingent upon . . . information provided by the renal biopsy with respect to . . . its severity, and the presence of chronicity and evidence of past damage' (Schwartz 1999).

Thus, it can be recommended that patients with lupus who have haematuria and/or proteinuria and those with diminished glomerular filtration rate should be seriously considered for renal biopsy. However, as the above review of the controversy about the significance (and reproducibility in reporting) of renal biopsies indicates, the information they provide about prognosis should not be overestimated. The opinion of a pathologist with experience in assessing these biopsies is strongly advised.

Nervous system involvement

Features of neurological disease range from the common, relatively harmless migraine headaches, to major psychotic episodes and grand mal seizures, recognized in some lupus patients.

Manifestations of lupus affecting the nervous system can be sub-divided into central, or cerebral effects, peripheral lesions and psychological aspects. A significant development in this area has been the establishment of a neuropsychiatric nomenclature by an ad hoc committee of the American College of Rheumatology (1999). This has defined 12 central and 7 peripheral nervous system features and is already being widely utilized (Table 6).

Central/cerebral involvement

Upto 30 per cent of lupus patients suffer from migraine, although this may be manifested by teichopsia alone. Of much greater concern are the grand

Table 6 Neuropsychiatric syndromes observed in SLE

Central nervous system
Aseptic meningitis
Cerebrovascular disease
Demyelinating syndrome
Headache (including migraine and benign intracranial hypertension)
Movement disorder (chorea)
Myelopathy
Seizure disorders
Acute confusional state
Anxiety disorder
Cognitive dysfunction
Mood disorder
Psychosis
Peripheral nervous system
Acute inflammatory demyelinating polyradiculoneuropathy (Guillain–Barré syndrome)
Autonomic disorder
Mononeuropathy, single/multiplex
Myasthenia gravis
Neuropathy, cranial
Plexopathy
Polyneuropathy

mal seizures which may be an initial manifestation of lupus in perhaps 5 per cent of cases, but are present in around 20 per cent of patients eventually. It may be difficult to be certain whether the seizures represent true cerebral disease, or a manifestation of more general problems. They may, for example, be secondary to uraemia and other biochemical disturbances associated with renal involvement. Similarly, hemiplegia (and transverse myelitis) may be consequent upon primary neurological disease or could be secondary to hypertension, or associated with the more recently recognized antiphospholipid antibodies. Cerebellar disease and aseptic meningitis were uncommon. A variety of organic brain syndromes with impaired temporal–spatial orientation, poor memory, and intellectual deficit are all well recognized and remain difficult management problems.

There has been a resurgence of interest in a small group of lupus patients, who suffer from the movement disorders chorea or ballismus. On occasion, chorea due to lupus may be difficult to differentiate from that due to rheumatic fever. However, in the more recently described patients links with the presence of antiphospholipid antibodies have been stressed. This problem is discussed in more detail later in the chapter.

Ocular lesions in lupus are well recognized. These include conjunctivitis, episcleritis, and cytoid bodies (white patches seen on retinal examination). In addition, retinal haemorrhage, and occasional papilloedema (usually found in association with malignant hypertension) and macular degeneration have all been described. The potential retinal toxicity of antimalarial drugs is discussed later in the chapter.

Peripheral neuropathy

Upto 10 per cent of patients with lupus develop a peripheral neuropathy in the course of their disease. These are usually sensory, occasionally sensorimotor. Cranial nerve involvement is less common, usually associated with active systemic disease and manifested by visual defects, tinnitus, vertigo, nystagmus, ptosis, and facial palsies. Feinglass et al. (1976) reported that the most commonly affected cranial nerves in their study were VII, III, VI, V, and IX in order of decreasing frequency. Optic neuritis was also uncommon, although it may, on rare occasions, be a presenting feature.

Psychological aspects

It has been claimed that up to 70 per cent of lupus patients suffer a variety of psychiatric abnormalities. However, this label includes depression and anxiety, and most studies have failed to separate the non-specific psychological stresses associated with a debilitating and sometimes painful disease like lupus, from those specifically caused by the disease itself. Whatever the precise cause, a report of seven suicides in patients with lupus serves to emphazise that depression must be taken very seriously in SLE (Matsukawa et al. 1994).

A lack of significant correlation between indices of general disease activity and psychiatric morbidity has been acknowledged by several authors. However, as with other aspects of lupus, more detailed testing, in this case using psychometric tests and nuclear MRI, has been claimed to identify subtle degrees of impairment which may not be immediately evident clinically. Thus, using a variety of standardized neuropsychological tests, Hanley et al. (1993) identified cognitive impairment in 21 per cent of their SLE patients compared to 4 per cent of their rheumatoid and healthy controls.

Emotional lability, personality change, impairment of judgement, and difficulty in performing simple tests of cognitive function such as recall of serial numbers, all suggest organic involvement in lupus. The major psychoses, notably paranoia, schizophrenia, and hypomania, are also well documented. During the 1950s and 1960s after the introduction of corticosteroids, a concern was expressed that in large doses, these drugs, given to patients for therapeutic purposes, might actually be responsible for some of the psychiatric manifestations. Later studies have tended to discount this possibility. For example, Feinglass et al. (1976) considered that only two of 140 patients had a steroid induced psychosis.

Investigations of neurological disease

It seems generally agreed that examination of the cerebrospinal fluid in neuropsychiatric disease is not very useful, apart from ruling out concomitant infection. Lupus patients may show moderately raised cell counts, some increase in protein and IgG levels, and occasionally low CSF glucose. Its potential use, however, is limited by the need for serial determinations. A range of autoantibodies including antiSm, antineuronal, antilymphocytotoxic and, most recently, antiribosomal-P has been linked to nervous system involvement. Invariably hopes raised in the initial reports have been dashed by later studies. For example, in 1987 in a retrospective study, antiribosomal-P protein antibodies were reported to be strongly correlated with lupus psychosis (Bonfa et al. 1987). Since then there have been over a dozen other studies [most reviewed by Fox and Isenberg (1997)] with conflicting findings and on balance there seems little value in a single measurement of anti-P antibodies to identify patients with lupus psychosis or in undertaking serial estimations to predict impending CNS relapse. In contrast, there is increasing support for the notion that antiphospholipid antibodies are linked, possibly pathogenetically so (e.g. Karassa et al. 2000). However, when brain infarction is suspected as a cause for a sudden cerebral event, it is clearly worthwhile testing for antiphospholipid antibodies. Sustained high levels of anticardiolipin antibodies (but not raised anti-dsDNA or low C3 levels) were found to correlate well with various neuropsychiatric tests in patients with lupus (Menon et al. 1999).

Electroencephalographic (EEG) studies have been shown by some to be helpful during flares of cerebral disease. The most commonly observed abnormality was diffuse slow wave activity but focal changes have been found in some 30 per cent of the patients studied. EEG changes tend to be associated with seizure activity or focal neurological signs, although on occasion these findings have been reported in patients with purely psychiatric symptoms. More recent, studies have looked at visual, auditory, and somato-sensory evoked potentials. These tests have still to acquire widespread acceptance.

Computed tomography (CT) has been used to analyse lupus patients for approximately 15 years. Unfortunately, the results have been conflicting. Thus diffuse cerebral abnormalities have been found in some patients with active disease, but not in others. CT is, however, very helpful in distinguishing between cerebral infarction and cerebral haemorrhage. It has also been claimed that many patients with neuropsychiatric manifestations of lupus have increased cerebral atrophy as evidenced by enlarged sulci either with or without ventricular enlargement. In fact, corticosteroids may promote this atrophy.

MRI provides a preferred means of investigating cerebral lupus. It is exceptionally sensitive for large lobar infarcts, cranial haemorrhage, and transverse myelitis and is useful for excluding associated conditions such as brain abscess and mycotic aneurisms. Figure 3 shows a patient who presented with severe depression, yet who had multiple small infarcts visible on MRI despite normal EEG and CT scans. High-intensity spots are the most common MRI brain abnormality report in SLE, present in at least one-third of lupus patients (Ishikawa et al. 1994). However, these spots are neither specific for neuropsychiatric lupus nor do they show good correlation with CNS disease.

A range of other imaging modalities including magnetic resonance spectroscopy (MRS), proton MRS, and ^{31}P-MRS are now being used to analyse CNS abnormalities in patients with lupus. More recently single photon emission tomography (SPECT) scanning has been used (Oku et al. 2003). Definitive results are awaited. No method of CNS imaging appears to distinguish reliably between small ischaemic lesions and vasculitis.

Haematopoietic involvement

Virtually all patients with lupus have some haematological abnormalities (Keeling and Isenberg 1993). For example, a normochromic, normocytic anaemia, the 'anaemia of chronic disease', is present in upto 70 per cent of lupus patients. Levels of ferritin in these patients are usually normal. In some individuals other factors contribute to anaemia, including end stage renal disease and non-steroidal anti-inflammatory drugs (NSAIDs). Coombs' positive haemolytic anaemia occurs in approximately 10 per cent of all lupus patients. Much less frequently, a microangiopathic haemolytic anaemia with disseminated intravascular coagulation has been described. It should be noted that a positive Coombs' test is not always associated with haemolysis. An association between pure red cell aplasia and SLE has also now been established.

Leucopaenia ($<4 \times 10^9$/l) and lymphopaenia ($<1.5 \times 10^9$/l) are the most frequent abnormalities of the white blood cell count in lupus patients. Estimates for the former have ranged from approximately 45 to 65 per cent and for the latter up to 80 per cent. Both T and B lymphocytes are reduced while null cells are increased. Lymphocytotoxic antibodies have been found in over one-third of lupus patients. In contrast, leukocytosis is rare in lupus in the absence of infection or major corticosteroid therapy.

There are at least three types of clinical presentation of thrombocytopaenia associated with lupus. Of these, chronic thrombocytopaenia ($<100 \times 10^9$/l) has been detected in approximately 20 per cent of most series. This is rarely associated with bleeding episodes in lupus patients, unlike those rarer cases of acute thrombocytopaenia, where the fall in the platelet count may be both dramatic and life threatening. Finally, some lupus patients may present with what initially appears to be an idiopathic thrombocytopaenia, usually treated successfully with corticosteroids, which only several years later is followed by other manifestations of the disease.

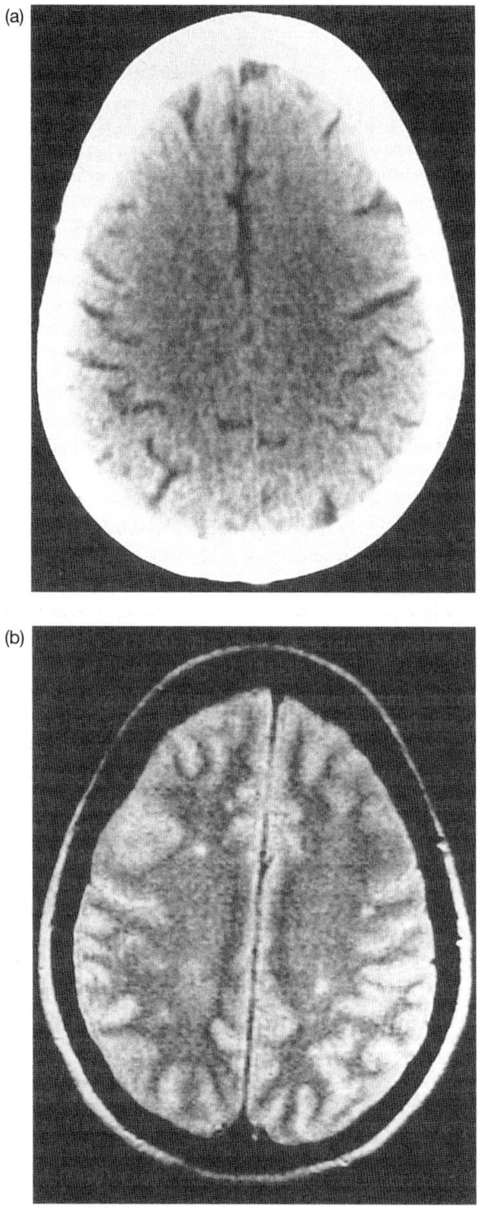

Fig. 3 Equivalent brain sections seen on CT scanning (a) and MRI scanning (b) in a patient with neuropsychiatric disease. Although some widening of the sulci is seen in (a), several discrete ischaemic areas are present in (b) which are not demonstrated on CT scanning.

Gastrointestinal disease

Gastrointestinal diseases include mouth ulcers, dysphagia, anorexia, nausea, vomiting, haemorrhage, and abdominal pain (Sultan et al. 1999). Most published series indicate that approximately 20–25 per cent of lupus patients have recurrent crops of mouth ulcers which are characterized histopathologically by hyperkeratosis, keratotic plugging, and inflammatory perivascular infiltrate and intraepithelial micro-abscesses. In contrast, dysphagia is generally reported in less than 10 per cent of lupus patients. Assessing the true incidence of peptic ulcer disease in patients with lupus is complicated by the fact that virtually all patients with the disease require treatment with NSAIDs and corticosteroids. Gastrointestinal vasculitis, if present, is usually accompanied by evidence of active disease in other organs. However, its true incidence is likely to be less than 2 per cent of patients. The differential diagnosis of abdominal pain ranges from mesenteric and hepatic artery thrombosis (perhaps linked to the presence of antiphospholipid antibodies) to abdominal problems such as appendicitis and rare complications such as pancreatic abscesses. The drugs used to treat patients with lupus often complicate determining the cause of abdominal pain.

Hepatomegaly, which can be detected in upto one-fourth of patients with lupus, is usually a minor degree of enlargement only and rarely accompanied by major abnormalities in liver function tests. Splenomegaly is found in approximately 10 per cent of the patients, though again the spleen is rarely greatly enlarged.

Other manifestations of lupus

Vascular lesions, notably Raynaud's phenomenon, cutaneous vasculitis, and ulcers and gangrene of the fingers (Fig. 4) and toes are all well recognized in lupus patients. Approximately one-third of patients have Raynaud's

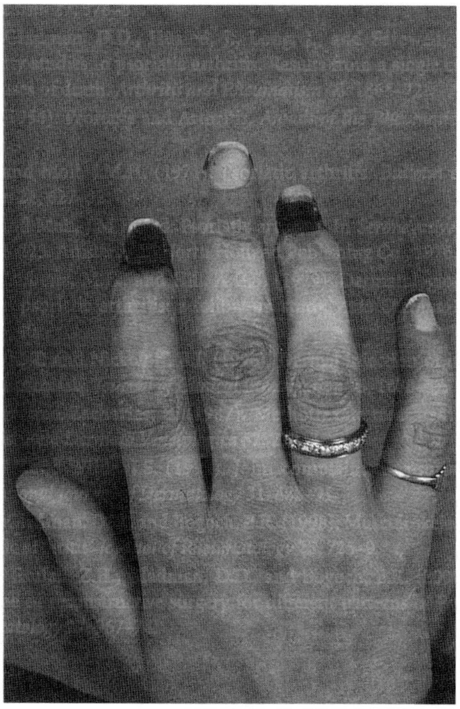

Fig. 4 Gangrene affecting two terminal digits in a young female patient with lupus.

phenomenon, which may antedate the onset of the disease by several years. It is generally relatively easy to control with vasodilating drugs, but on rare occasions it may be associated with gangrene of the extremities . Unlike the older population, which suffers gangrene due to atherosclerosis, the potential for recovery in the lupus patient is better as the patients are much younger. Active vasculitis in lupus may manifest as necrotic ulcers, small cutaneous infarction, or lupus profundus. Leg ulcers have been recorded in up to 5 per cent of lupus patients, most commonly around or just above the malleoli.

Apart from the autoantibodies detected in lupus (described later in this chapter) a number of other common blood tests are frequently abnormal in lupus patients. For example, hypoalbuminaemia has been described in upto 50 per cent of lupus patients, and hypergammaglobulinaemia in upto 60 per cent. IgG and IgM levels, in particular, have been reported to be elevated in lupus patients; IgA and IgE levels much less frequently so.

The erythrocyte sedimentation rate is increased in the vast majority of these patients, over 90 per cent in some series. Occasionally, however, normal levels are found even in the presence of active disease. In contrast, C-reactive protein (CRP) levels are generally, although not always, normal in lupus patients except for those with a concurrent infection, serositis, or severe arthritis.

Lupus and the risk of infection

As indicated in the section on the relationship between lupus and malignancy, the combined effect of the disease itself and its treatment is to encourage infection. It is often impossible to apportion responsibility for such infections to one or the other, but there are major consequences for outcome. In addition, a variety of (generally) non-fatal infectious diseases, such as herpes zoster (Kahl 1994), salmonella (Abramson et al. 1985), and candida (Sieving et al. 1975), are quite common.

Diseases complicating lupus

Sjögren's syndrome is present in upto 20 per cent of patients. The dryness of the eyes and mouth differs little from those cases of primary disease although antibodies to Ro and La are present less frequently. Sjögren's syndrome is reviewed fully in Chapter 6.9. Autoimmune thyroid disease (generally hypo- rather than hyperthyroid) has been identified in 5–10 per cent of lupus patients. However, antibodies to thyroglobulin and thyroid microsomes have been found in upto one-third of the patients. The treatment of under or overactive autoimmune thyroid disease in patients who also have lupus is similar to those without it. Likewise myositis also detectable in up to 5 per cent of lupus patients is treated no differently from patients with the idiopathic disease. A smaller percentage of lupus patients (perhaps no more than 1 per cent) has myasthenia gravis. This may antedate or postdate the onset of the lupus itself.

Much has been written as to whether systemic lupus and rheumatoid arthritis can coexist. It is certainly very rare to have lupus glomerulonephritis occurring in patients with seropositive erosive rheumatoid arthritis. However, it is generally accepted that 1 or 2 per cent of patients do have an erosive arthropathy, suggesting that an overlap between these two conditions may exist in some individuals.

Lupus in special situations

Pregnancy and lupus

Even in healthy individuals pregnancy results in drastic immunological changes. These have been the subject of much interest in the past few years. Oestrogens, for example, are thought to decrease T-suppressor cell function, while androgens have the opposite effect. Oestrogens also tend to increase immune complex clearance thus decreasing their renal deposition. The CD5+ B lymphocytes are also thought to be under oestrogen control. Progesterone is thought to have immunosuppressive properties and its production increases throughout pregnancy. Prolactin, another hormone associated with pregnancy, is a known modulator of lymphocyte responses to antigen in rodents, and human B and T cells are known to have receptors for it. It is thus evident that the effects of pregnancy on the immune system in general are complex and therefore not surprising that lupus patients with their significantly disordered immune system may suffer deleterious effects during pregnancy.

There are many conflicting data about the effect of pregnancy on the lupus patient. Despite earlier reports suggesting that sterility might be common among lupus patients, more recent studies have noted that sterility and fertility were little changed by lupus. An exception to this are those patients in renal failure who do have reduced fertility. Similarly, whereas some reports of an increase in maternal mortality in lupus patients during pregnancy were described in the 1950s and 1960s, the current view is that the majority of pregnancies do not adversely affect the lupus mother. Thus in a case control study of 46 patients with 79 pregnancies lupus flares occurred no more frequently than in non-pregnant controls (Urowitz et al. 1993). The frequency of non-renal complications during pregnancy is relatively low but is a little higher in the period immediately after parturition. Flares of disease, especially renal involvement, may require the introduction of or increase in corticosteroids, and on occasion the baby may have to be induced as early as 30 weeks of gestation.

In contrast to the relatively encouraging outcome for the lupus mother, foetal outcome is much less certain. A combination of spontaneous abortion and still birth causes a foetal mortality of around 20 per cent. Upto 25 per cent of babies born to mothers with lupus may have to be delivered prematurely, for a combination of reasons relating to foetal distress as well as maternal ill health.

In the past decade, the link between recurrent spontaneous abortion and the presence of antiphospholipid antibodies has been established. This is discussed in detail elsewhere in the chapter. The precise mechanism of these foetal deaths remains uncertain.

Lupus mothers who have antibodies to Ro and/or La also appear to be prone to develop the so-called neonatal lupus syndrome. Approximately one in 20 women who have either of these antibodies will have a child with this syndrome, which is notable for its congenital conduction defects or skin rashes. This subject is discussed in detail in Chapter 6.6.3.

Lupus in males

Although lupus in males, especially Caucasian males, is uncommon, many different groups have attempted to identify characteristics of male lupus patients that distinguish them from women with the disease. No clearly identifiable criteria have been identified. As discussed by Isenberg and Malick (1994), virtually every claim of a distinctive feature in one series is rebutted in others. In the United States, however, it has been reported that the prognosis is worse for male lupus patients. Among males with lupus there appears to be no evidence of androgen deficiency, although in one large series 50 per cent had elevated plasma oestrogen levels (Muller et al. 1983) although corticosteroid administration might have been expected to decrease these values.

Individuals with Klinefelter's syndrome, who have an unusual XXY karyotype, are said to be more susceptible to SLE. Abnormalities in oestradiol metabolism in these patients may be linked to the persistent oestrogenic stimulation which might explain the predisposition.

Several families in which SLE predominates in males have been described (Lahita et al. 1983) where sons may have inherited the disease from their fathers analogous to disease in the BXSB mouse, an experimental model of lupus, which is described later in this chapter.

Lupus in the elderly

It is clearly a matter of opinion at which point lupus in the middle aged becomes lupus in the elderly! Most reports have taken 50 or 55 years as a cut-off, although there has been very little attempt to relate chronological age to the menopause, a fact which may well be important in the aetiology of the disease in these patients.

There are conflicting reports about the patterns of presentation, organ involvement, serological findings, and prognosis in this group. It appears that the clinical onset of lupus in the elderly is more insidious, milder, has a lower incidence of severe renal and neurological complications, a lower frequency of antibodies to double-stranded DNA and hypocomplementaemia, but an increased frequency of serositis, interstitial lung disease, and antibodies to Ro and La (e.g. Ho et al. 1998). The last of these features suggests that the overlap between lupus and Sjögren's syndrome is frequent in an elderly population.

Among less frequent modes of presentation in the elderly, a polymyalgia rheumatica-like picture has been described, and neuropsychiatric manifestations which might easily be confused with other types of organic disease are important in this group. The time between onset of disease and presentation, and between presentation and diagnosis, are increased compared to younger lupus patients, although this should change with increasing awareness that lupus can occur for the first time well into old age—the oldest case reported so far was diagnosed aged 87.

The antiphospholipid antibodies syndrome and lupus

Associations between anticardiolipin antibodies and the lupus anticoagulant with SLE have attracted considerable interest in the past 15 years.

Anticardiolipin antibodies are part of an overlapping spectrum of antiphospholipid antibodies of which the lupus anticoagulant is part. Detailed analysis of anticardiolipin antibodies has distinguished two major varieties. In patients with infectious diseases the antibodies recognize epitopes on cardiolipin itself. However, in many lupus patients the antibodies are probably binding to a complex or neo-epitope formed by phospholipid and a plasma cofactor β_2-glycoprotein 1 (Galli et al. 1990). Thus, β_2-glycoprotein 1 dependency was noted for anticardiolipin (40 per cent), antiphosphatidyl serine (20 per cent), and antiphosphatidylinositol (18 per cent) antibodies but not for syphilis or normal sera (Matsuda et al. 1994).

The following clinical features are widely believed to be associated with lupus patients who have these antiphospholipid antibodies:

- venous and arterial thrombosis;
- thrombocytopaenia;
- cerebral disease (including cerebrovascular accident, transient ischaemic attacks, chorea, amaurosis fugax);
- recurrent foetal loss;
- pulmonary hypertension; and
- livedo reticularis.

A meta-analysis undertaken by Love and Santoro (1990) suggests caution in the interpretation of the published results. In their analysis of 29 published series, they estimated an average frequency of 34 per cent for the lupus anticoagulant and 44 per cent for anticardiolipin antibodies in studies representing over 1000 lupus patients. However, anticardiolipin antibodies are also prevalent in patients with a wide variety of diseases other than idiopathic lupus, including drug-induced lupus, rheumatoid arthritis, and acute infection. In lupus patients, a statistically significant association has been shown between the presence of either antibody and a history of thrombosis, neurological disorders, and thrombocytopaenia (see also Chapter 6.6.4 on 'The antiphospholipid antibody syndrome'). In a large prospective cohort study of 389 primiparous women assessed at study entry and delivery, 24 per cent were antiphospholipid antibody positive, 15.8 per cent of whom had foetal loss compared with 6.5 per cent of antibody negative patients (Lynch et al. 1994). Elevated IgG antiphospholipid antibody levels were statistically associated with recurrent foetal loss but not with low birth weight, neonatal distress, and maternal complications.

A small cohort of lupus patients with anticardiolipin antibodies has been shown to develop impaired renal function due to multiple small thrombi (Leaker et al. 1991). These patients have minimal proteinuria and only gradually increasing renal damage. This type of pathology may coincide with the more typical glomerulonephritis.

A number of contentious issues about antiphospholipid antibodies remain. For example, the precise links with other autoantibodies have been the subject of debate. It is widely accepted that anticardiolipin antibodies are associated with the biologically false-positive Venereal Disease Research Laboratory test. However, early studies undertaken with monoclonal antibodies which suggested significant overlap between those binding cardiolipin and DNA were not supported by studies in lupus patients. Although low affinity (generally IgM) antibodies to DNA may bind cardiolipin, higher affinity (generally IgG) antibodies to DNA do not. This would imply separate sub-populations of anti-DNA and antiphospholipid antibodies. This is probably an oversimplification, as a single amino acid substitution can convert an antiphospholipid antibody into an anti-DNA antibody, supporting the view that these antibodies are very closely related (Diamond and Scharff 1984).

Table 7 Summary of malignancies reported in large series of patients with SLE

Cohort origin	Number of patients followed-up	Number of malignancies	SIR[a]	Comments	Reference
Chicago	616	30	2.0 (1.4, 2.9)	State cancer registry Lung cancer increased overall, breast cancer in Caucasians	Ramsey-Goldman et al. (1998)
Denmark	1588	102	1.3 (1.1, 2.9)	Used a national cancer registry. Overall cancer risk increased including non-Hodgkin's lymphoma	Mellemkjaer et al. (1997)
Finland	206	15	2.6 (1.5, 4.4)	Used a national cancer registry. Overall cancer risk increased	Pettersson et al. (1992)
London	276	16	1.16 (0.5, +2.1)	Regional cancer registry. No overall cancer risk but an increased risk of Hodgkin's lymphoma	Sultan et al. (2000)
Pittsburgh	412	20	1.4 (0.9, 2.2)	No overall cancer risk	Sweeney et al. (1995)
Toronto	724	24	1.1 (0.7, 1.6)	No overall cancer risk	Abu-Shakra et al. (1996)

[a] SIR, standardized incidence rate.

Neither the lupus anticoagulant nor anticardiolipin antibodies appear to correlate with age, duration of disease, or a variety of well-known lupus clinical features, including polyarthritis, vasculitis, or serositis.

Lupus and malignancy

Given that the immune system is so disordered in patients with lupus and that many patients are treated with major immunosuppressive drugs there has been much recent interest in whether there is an increased risk of malignancy in SLE. Table 7 reviews several published series. There is an overall lack of agreement as to whether malignancy is increased and, if it is, which cancers are to be found more commonly. However, to date there is little support for the notion that immunosuppressive drugs lead to a high risk of malignancy in patients with lupus. Because the overall risk is low, the question of a link to malignancy can only be answered by large multicentre studies. These are currently being carried out by the Systemic Lupus Erythematosus International Collaborating Clinics group.

Assessing patients with lupus

Activity assessment

The assessment of disease activity in lupus is clearly central to patient management, but for many years there was no consensus on its measurement. However, in the past 12 years, more determined attempts to compare and contrast some of the different activity indices have been undertaken. Thus, the SLAM (Systemic Lupus Activity Measures), SLEDAI (Systemic Lupus Erythematosus Disease Activity Index), and ECLAM (European Community Lupus Activity Measure) are three global score systems that have been shown to correlate well with each other (Vitali et al. 1992). They also correlate well with the British Isles Lupus Assessment Group (BILAG) system, which was established to provide more detailed information about disease activity in each of eight organs or systems (Hay et al. 1993). The BILAG index is based upon the principle of the 'physician's intention to treat'. There has been an encouraging international effort to compare the SLAM, SLEDAI, and BILAG systems in combined studies of both 'paper' and real patients. These systems have repeatedly been shown to correlate with one another and to be reliable in evaluating disease activity in SLE. They have also been shown to be sensitive to change in disease activity over time (Gladman et al. 1994). Information about these three indices and a comparison between them, based on an assessment of real, as opposed to 'paper' patients by seven different physicians is shown in Table 8.

Table 8 Correlations (*r* values) between the three SLE activity indices[a]

	VAS	SLEDAI	SLAM
SLEDAI	0.261	0.732	
SLAM	0.209	0.732	
BILAG	0.162	0.763	0.797

[a] VAS, visual analogue scale completed by the observer. Figures are based on real patient assessments by seven different physicians.

BILAG—British Isles Lupus Assessment Group. This activity index is based on the physician's 'intention of treat' the patient. Lupus activity is divided into eight areas: general features, locomotor system, nervous system, renal involvement, dermatological involvement, pleuropericardial disease, vasculitis, and haematological involvement. Within each system the patients are designated A (action) implying that major immunosuppressive therapy needs to be initiated or increased; B (beware) the patient is known to have active disease but the therapy does not require alteration; C (contentment) remission in symptoms in that organ/system; D (discount) there is no current involvement in this organ/system, or E there is no (evidence) of activity in the organ/system now or previously. See Hay et al. (1993) for further details.

SLAM (systemic lupus activity measures) devised by Dr Liang (Boston) and SLEDAI (systemic lupus erythematosus diseased activity index) described by Drs Urowitz, Gladman, and Bombadier are two good global score indices [see Liang et al. (1988) for further discussion].

Damage assessment

Equally constructive have been attempts by 'lupologists' to agree an index that distinguishes damage (due to lupus or its treatment) from disease activity. The distinction in not simply an academic one. For example, a patient with shortness of breath may have active but reversible vasculitis which could improve with major immunosuppressive therapy. Alternatively, the symptom may be due to fibrosis causing irreversible damage for which there would be no requirement for such treatment. Thus, a SLICC (systemic lupus international collaborating clinics) damage index has been developed (see Table 9) and is currently being assessed by many groups in North America and Europe.

The damage index records the number of items of permanent change that have affected an individual patient since the onset of the disease. Damage is distinguished in 12 organs or systems, and for a feature to be regarded as due to damage it must have persisted for at least 6 months. In a 10-year retrospective study of 80 patients with SLE, it was shown that renal damage at 1 year was predictive of end stage renal failure and that pulmonary damage at 1 year was predictive of death by the end of the study. This study also demonstrated that Afro-Caribbean patients had significantly higher mean renal damage in the course of 10 years compared to the Caucasian patients (Stoll and Isenberg 1996). Amongst a range of later studies, an analysis of 263 patients also followed up for 10 years, the damage at 1 year was highly predictive ($p = 0.002$) of mortality by the end of the study, principally due to renal and cardiovascular disease (Rahman et al. 2001). In a comparison of 86 SLE patients with disease onset after the age of 54 and 155 matched for gender and ethnic origin with disease onset before the age of 40, the SLICC/ACR Damage Index scores were higher in the late-onset group at both 1 and 5 years and a difference in the pattern of organ damage was noted. While damage to the skin, kidneys, and CNS ocurred with similar frequency, late onset disease was characterised by significantly more cardiovascular, ocular, and musculoskeletal damage, and malignancy (Maddison et al. 2001).

Health status assessment

An important principle, now widely recognized, is that patients' perceptions of their lupus are frequently different from those of their clinicians. Although no lupus specific measure has been designated to date, two measures to assess health status in patients with SLE have been used in a wide variety of studies. These measures were developed from questionnaires initially devised by the Rand Corporation. From over 200 items initially selected for study, the medical outcome survey Short Form-20 (SF-20) (literally 20 questions) and subsequently the Short Form-36 have been developed. The SF-36 is almost as quick and easy to complete as the SF-20 and being broader in its range of questions has generally found wider acceptance. It records concerns about physical function, role limitations, physical problems, emotional problems, social function, mental health, general health perception, vitality, and pain. It is now widely used for a range of lupus patient studies [reviewed in Isenberg and Ramsey-Goldman (1999)]. The three elements described above, that is, assessment of activity, damage and status, form the core of assessments now being undertaken in a series of new therapeutic trials described later in this chapter. The development of a drug responder index, which the SLICC group and others are working towards, clearly requires the recognition of these three elements, together with an accurate assessment of side-effects and cost.

Immunopathology of lupus

In this section, we review the immunopathology of the disease both in strains of lupus-prone mice and in humans by describing the specificity of autoantibodies, dysregulation, and abnormalities at the cellular level, and the genetic background that predisposes to the autoimmune response.

Table 9 SLICC damage index[a]

Item	Score	
Ocular (either eye, by clinical assessment)		
Any cataract ever	1	
Retinal change OR optic atrophy	1	
Neuropsychiatric		
Cognitive impairment (e.g. memory deficit, difficulty with calculation, poor concentration, difficulty in spoken or written language, impaired performance level)	1	
OR major psychosis	1	
Seizures requiring therapy for 6 months	1	
Cerebral vascular accident ever (score 2 if > once), or resection not for malignancy	1	2
Cranial or peripheral neuropathy (excluding optic)	1	
Transverse myelitis	1	
Renal		
Estimated or measured glomerular filtration rate <50%	1	
Proteinuria 24 h, ≥ 3.5 g	1	
OR		
End stage renal disease (regardless of dialysis or transplantation)		3
Pulmonary		
Pulmonary hypertension (right ventricular prominence, or loud P2)	1	
Pulmonary fibrosis (physical and radiograph)	1	
Shrinking lung (radiograph)	1	
Pleural fibrosis (radiograph)	1	
Pulmonary infarction (radiograph) OR resection not for malignancy	1	
Cardiovascular		
Angina OR coronary artery bypass	1	
Myocardial infarction ever (score 2 if > once)	1	2
Cardiomyopathy (ventricular dysfunction)	1	
Valvular disease (diastolic murmur, or a systolic murmur > 3/6)	1	
Pericarditis for 6 months OR percardiectomy	1	
Peripheral vascular		
Claudication for 6 months	1	
Minor tissue loss (pulp space)	1	
Significant tissue loss ever (loss of digit or limb, including resection not for malignancy) score 2 if > one site	1	2
Venous thrombosis with swelling, ulceration, OR venous stasis	1	
Gastrointestinal		
Infarction or resection of bowel below duodenum, spleen, liver, or gallbladder ever, for whatever cause (score 2 if > one site)	1	2
Mesenteric insufficiency	1	
Chronic peritonitis	1	
Musculoskeletal		
Muscle atrophy or weakness	1	
Deforming or erosive arthritis (including reducible deformities, excluding avascular necrosis)	1	
Osteoporosis with fracture or vertebral collapse (excluding avascular necrosis)	1	
Avascular necrosis (score 2 if > once)	1	2
Osteomyelitis	1	
Ruptured tendon	1	
Skin		
Scarring chronic alopecia	1	
Extensive scarring or panniculum other than scalp and pulp space	1	
Skin ulceration (excluding thrombosis) for more than 6 months	1	
Premature gonadal failure	1	
Diabetes (regardless of treatment)	1	
Malignancy (exclude dysplasia) (score 2 if > one site)	1	2

[a] Damage (non-reversible change, not related to active inflammation) occurring since onset of lupus, ascertained by clinical assessment and present for at least 6 months unless otherwise stated. Repeat episodes mean at least 6 months apart to score 2. The same lesion cannot be scored twice. [The development of this index is described in Gladman et al. (1996).]

Experimental models of lupus

Several strains of mice spontaneously develop clinical and serological symptoms that resemble lupus. Recently, the number of these mouse models of lupus has significantly increased as a variety of single gene knockouts (and gene overexpression) has resulted in lupus-like disease (Table 10). The most striking aspect of these observations is the range of unrelated molecules whose dysregulation results in lupus-like disease. This observation reinforces the point that lupus can arise through different immunological pathways which include effects on B and T lymphocyte function and clearance of apoptotic cells and their products. The 'older' models of lupus, are summarized in Table 11. Two of the traditional strains, the MRL/lpr mouse and the moth-eaten mouse, have a single gene defect, the absence of fas and protein tyrosine phosphatase SHP-1, respectively, which significantly accelerates disease in a specific susceptible genetic background. A significant effort is currently underway to identify the susceptibility genes that contribute to disease in the NZB/W mice, often considered to be the mouse strain that most closely resembles human lupus. In NZB mice, susceptibility loci on chromosomes 1, 4, 7, and 13 have been repeatedly identified in different mapping studies as contributing to nephritis and, although the most important NZW contribution to disease in NZB/W mice comes from the MHC locus, background non-MHC genes clearly play a role. Amongst the lupus prone mice 31 susceptibility loci have been identified distributed among 21 non-overlapping genomic intervals, clearly illustrating the complexity of the genetic basis for susceptibility to systemic autoimmunity (Wakeland et al. 1999). In the NZB/NZW-related NZM2410 lupus-prone strain, three recessive loci, Sle1, Sle2, and Sle3 on chromosomes 1, 4, and 7, respectively, are sufficient to produce 'full blown' lupus nephritis on a C57Bl6 non-autoimmune background. An area of chromosome 1 appears to be important, containing several susceptibility genes (Morel et al. 2001).

Awareness of the contrasts between human and mouse lupus is important, but information gleaned from these mouse models has the potential to guide investigations in human lupus as well as inform on immunopathological processes. In the last edition of this book it was said: 'comparison of inbred mouse strains with outbred humans may not be relevant genetically' but as mentioned in the genetics section below corresponding (syntenic) loci have now been identified in humans and mice suggesting that the same genes may predispose to human and mouse lupus.

F1 hybrids between an autoimmune strain (NZB) and a non-autoimmune strain (SWR) have an accelerated autoimmune disease with a high incidence of nephritis. All females are dead by 1 year of age. These mice have IgG2b anti-dsDNA antibodies which are cationic and deposit in the glomerular basement membrane. The pathogenic antibodies are derived from the normal SWR parent and carry a nephritogenic idiotypic marker which is not found in the circulation of either parent. The normal parents have deleted 50 per cent of their T-cell receptor Vβ chains and are I-E negative (equivalent to HLA–DR in humans) thus they have peripheral T cells with I-E reactive T-cell receptors. The autoimmune parent and the F1 offspring are I-E positive. Autoimmunity arises from the expression of 'forbidden' T-cell receptors by double negative T-helper cells and suggests an abnormality in thymic selection/deletion.

The Yaa (Y-chromosome-linked autoimmune acceleration) gene accelerates disease in MRL+/+ mice. These mice have increased levels of gp70–anti-gp70 immune complexes but no increase in the levels of circulating antibodies to DNA. Disease expression may be controlled by at least four genes, three of which have been mapped to chromosomes 7 and 17. Hyperproliferation of B (but not T) lymphocytes is found in Yaa mice.

Autoantibodies in SLE

The serological hallmark of SLE is the presence of circulating autoantibodies directed against a wide variety of nuclear, cytoplasmic, and plasma membrane antigens which are outlined in Table 12. Autoantibodies with new specificities are continuosly identified, for example, anti-ASE-1, a 55-kDa nucleolar autoantigen, associated with serositis (Edworthy et al. 2000). Among the first 300 patients with lupus under our care 99 per cent had a positive ANA with a titre 1 : 40 (unpublished observations). The most

Table 10 More recent mouse models of lupus from gene targeting experiments

KO mouse	Background mouse	Antibodies	Glomerular nephritis	Other features	Putative function
Autoimmunity through lack of clearance of apoptotic cells					
Serum amyloid P	129 × C57BL/6	ANA DNA Chromatin Histone	Immune complex GN		Binds apoptotic cells and nuclear debris, targeting chromatin for catabolism in the liver
DNase-1	C57BL/6	ANA ssDNA dsDNA Histone Nucleosome	Immune complex GN IgG and C3 deposits		Removal of DNA from autoantigenic nucleoprotein complexes
C1q	129/ × C57BL/6	ANA ENA-Sm	Proliferative GN C3 and apoptopic body deposits		Promotes clearance of dying cells
Mer	C57BL/6	Anti-DNA		Blind	Mer a macrophage receptor tyrosine kinase required for phagocytosis and clearance of apoptotic cells
Serum IgM	129 × C57BL/6	dsDNA Cardiolipin Myeloperoxidase	Immune complex GN C3 and IgG deposits		Alteration in antigen clearance
Negative regulators of B-cell activation					
FcγRIIB	129 × C57BL/6	ANA DNA Chromatin	Glomerular sclerosis IgG deposits	Systemic vasculitis, anaemia	Inhibitory receptor gating of BCR Induces B cell apoptosis
CD22	129 × C57BL/6	Serum IgM, IgG dsDNA	Immune complex GN		Negative regulator BCR
	129 × BALB/c	Cardiolipin Myeloperoxidase			
Lyn	E14 × C57BL/6	10-fold increase in serum IgM NP-IgM ab ANA	FSGS Crescentic GN Deposits IgG	Pancytopaenia, haemolytic anaemia, vasculitis	Negative signal transduction molecule in the BCR pathway Triggering elimination of autoreactive B cells
Dysregulated B- and T-cell proliferation					
Eμ-bcl-2–22 transgene	C57BL/6 × SJL	ANA Histone dsDNA Sm RNP Serum IgM and IgG	Immune complex GN IgM, IgG, C3 deposits	Lymphadenopathy, splenomegaly	Expansion B-cell population Accumulation autoreactive B-cell precursors
BAFF(Blys/ THANK/zTNF 4/TALL-1) transgene	C57BL/6J × DBA	Serum IgM and IgG Rh factor Cryoglobulin ssDNA dsDNA ANA	Immune complex GN C3 and IgG deposits	Lymphadenopathy, splenomegaly, enlarged Peyers patches	Proliferation of activated autoreactive B cells Supression of protective effect of dendritic cells against autoreactive T cells
Point mutation inhibitory wedge CD45	129 × C57BL/6	dsDNA Increased serum IgG2a and IgA	Diffuse membrano proliferative GN	Splenomegaly Lymphadenopathy including gut	Inappropriate lymphocyte activation Polyclonal T- and B-cell activation
P21	C57BL/6 × 129/5V	dsDNA ANA Histone ssDNA	Immune complex GN IgG deposits	Lymphadenopathy	Sustained CD4+ and CD8+ T-cell proliferation Exposure to antinuclear antigens from excess apoptotic bodies
PD-1	C57BL/6	IgG3	Proliferative GN Deposits of IgG3, C3, PAS +ve material	Arthritis	Negative regulation of antigen stimulated T-cell response Decreases clonal expansion Accelerates cell death following antigen stimulation
PD-1	BALB/c			Pancarditis thrombosis	
Cbl-b	C57BL/6	dsDNA	Interstitial nephritis	Leucocyte infiltration of vital organs	Negative molecular adaptor on lymphocyte activation pathway

Continued

Table 10 Continued

KO mouse	Background mouse	Antibodies	Glomerular nephritis	Other features	Putative function
Enzymes affecting TCR recruitment					
Mgat5	129		GN		Enhanced TCR recruitment Sustained T-cell activation
M11	C57BL/6	ANA	Immune complex GN		Enhanced TCR recruitment Sustained T-cell activation
Lack of apoptosis of activated B and T cells					
Pten +/−	129 × C57BL/6	ANA dsDNA ssDNA Histone Increased serum IgG	Immune complex GN, segmental sclerosis	Lymphomas, splenomegaly, lymphadenopathy	Negatively regulates Akt survival signals and thus promotes Fas-mediated cell death

Table 11 Lupus-prone mouse strains

Strain	Symptoms	Autoantibodies	Defects
(NZB × NZW)F1	F >> M renal defects hypergamma-globulinaemia	dsDNA ssDNA	TNF deficiency nephritis delayed by administration of TNFα
NZB	Autoimmune haemolytic anaemia	RBC	
MRL+/+	F >> M, late onset renal disease lymphadenopathy	Sm, histones, DNA, RF	
MRL-lpr/lpr	Early onset similar to +/+	Sm, histones DNA, RF	lpr gene accelerates, neonatal thymectomy delays disease onset
BXSB	Males only haemolytic anaemia glomerulonephritis lymphadenopathy	DNA, thymocytes, RBC	Y chromosome factor Early thymic atrophy
Moth-eaten	M + F glomerulonephritis hair loss, infection	DNA, thymocytes, RBC	Immunosuppression
(SWR × NZB)F1	F >> M, early onset lethal glomerulo-nephritis	IgG_{2b} anti-DNA	Pathogenic antibodies

Note: M, male; F, female; RBC, red blood cells; TNF, tumour necrosis factor.

widely studied autoantibody in lupus binds to dsDNA, a subset of which are pathogenic.

Antibodies to dsDNA are usually of the IgG isotype. Studies of kidney biopsies from patients with glomerulonephritis show deposition of IgG and complement components indicating a localised immune response and subsequent inflammation. Eluates from affected kidneys show that the IgG has specificity for dsDNA though other lupus associated antibody specificities are also present such as Ro and Clq. These nephritogenic antibodies are cationic in charge, clonally restricted and high affinity but even armed with this information it is not possible to predict which antibodies are pathogenic. Only a proportion of both mouse and human monoclonal anti-DNA antibodies can cause nephritis when transferred into non-autoimmune mice (Ehrenstein 1999; Madaio 1999). Different monoclonal autoantibodies, when administered to mice, resulted in various patterns of immunoglobulin deposition and histological profiles.

However, some high-affinity IgG anti-dsDNA antibodies did not cause nephritis. The clear implication from these experiments is that the different clinical and histological presentations of lupus nephritis may in part be due to differences in the specificity of the autoantibodies produced.

It is unclear what are the defining characteristics that govern the nephritogenicity of a particular antibody; it does not appear simply to reflect the affinity for DNA. Indeed, rarely, lupus nephritis can occur in patients without any evidence of circulating anti-DNA antibodies and, conversely, persistent high serum titres of IgG anti-dsDNA antibodies can occur without clinical evidence of renal injury. In one study, the pathogenicity of a monoclonal anti-DNA antibody was lost after site-directed mutagenesis of its antigen binding region despite retaining DNA binding activity (Katz et al. 1994). One explanation for the imperfect association between binding to DNA and pathogenicity is that the nephritogenic antinuclear antibodies are cross-reacting with glomerular antigens. One candidate glomerular antigen is the acidic alpha-actinin, binding to this molecule has shown some correlation to pathogenicity as opposed to non-pathogenic, anti-DNA antibodies (Mostoslavsky et al. 2001). An alternative mechanism whereby antibodies can cause nephritis is through the deposition of immune complexes, that is, antibody plus nuclear antigens. To what extent direct binding to glomerular antigens or immune complexes contribute to nephritis in lupus is still unclear. In a series of studies (reviewed by Kalsi et al. 1999) using seven human hybridomas derived monoclonal anti-DNA antibodies

Table 12 Autoantibodies in SLE

Antibody	Antigen/epitope	Prevalence (%)	Clinical and other associations
Intracellular			
DNA	dsDNA (ssDNA) (Z DNA)	40–90	IgG, cationic, present in renal eluates. Pathogenic cross-reactions: LAMP/ glomerular heparin sulfate
Histone	H1, 2A, 2B, 3, 4	30–80	Drug induced lupus + α-ssDNA
Sm	A, B/B′	Overall ~35 Afro-Caribbean 50–70 Caucasian 10–20	SLE specific Afro-Caribbean 80% Sm+ also DR2+
U1RNP	D, N, 68 kDa ribonucleoprotein	20–35	Mild disease
Ro/SS-A	60, 52 kDa protein bound to cytoplasmic RNA (hY1–hY5)	25–40	Renal involvement, DR4 DR2 DQw1(= DQw6) DQw2, DQw3—protective?
La/SS-B	47 kDa protein bound to variety of RNA [Pol III transcripts, viral (EBV, CMV, adeno) U1RNA (Pol II) hY RNA]	10–15	DR3 (2° SS) κ chain allotype (Km1)
Heatshock proteins	hsp70 hsp90	40 50	IgM > IgG Surface expression of hsp90 on monocytes and CD4+ T cells and B lymphocytes + ↑ cytoplasmic expression in lymphocytes and monocytes
Cellmembrane			
Cardiolipin	Phospholipids DNA	20–40	Recurrent abortion Thrombosis
Neuronal antigen	Expressed on neuronal cell line grown *in vitro*	70–90 (+CNS) ~10 (–CNS)	In serum and CNS some cross-react with lymphocyte cell surface
Lymphocyte	T cells >> B cells HLA components CD4+ CD8+	~74 (IgM) ~47 (IgG)	Cytotoxic (80%) some cross-react with cell surface antigens of CNS
Red cell	Non-Rh related	<10	Haemolytic anaemia
Platelet		<10	ITP
Extracellular			
RF	Fc region of IgG	~25	Usually IgM, cross-react with histones, Ro/SS-A
C1q	Complement component	~56	Rising titres precede renal involvement (prolif GN)

Note: LAMP, lymphocyte-associated membrane protein; RNP, ribonucleoprotein; MHC, major histocompatibility complex; HSP, heat shock protein; CSF, cerebrospinal fluid; CNS, central nervous system; RF, rheumatoid factor; 2° SS, secondary Sjögren's syndrome; ITP, idiopathicthrombocytopaenic purpura; prolif GN, proliferative glomerulonephritis.

(six were high affinity anti-dsDNA) two were shown in SCID mice to bind exclusively to glomeruli resulting in significant proteinuria. Electron microscopic studies showed that one of these antibodies (RH14) induced glomerular basement membrane thickening and fusion of the foot processes, two of the early features of lupus nephritis.

One intriguing claim that has arisen (or perhaps been revisited) from studies of monoclonal anti-DNA antibodies is that some of these immunoglobulins can penetrate living cells and react directly with the nucleus (Madaio and Yanase 1998). It has been proposed that this subset of antibodies bind to myosin 1 on the cell surface, become internalized, cause glomerular hypercellularity, and subsequently proteinuria. Indeed, a peptide derived from one of these antibodies has been shown to be able to act as a vector for the intranuclear delivery of macromolecules. These autoantibodies are not specific for glomerular cells, but have the ability to penetrate a wide variety of cells. It has been speculated that after these antibodies have been internalized, they modulate the process of apoptosis through an interaction with DNase I. This modulation of apoptosis could have a major impact on inflamed tissues and perhaps explain the glomerular hypercellularity observed when these antibodies are administered to normal mice. A human monoclonal IgG antibody (B3) with specificity for dsDNA, which is also an *in vivo* cell penetrator was derived from a patient with active lupus.

A number of other autoantibodies are worth noting with respect to lupus. Antibodies to Sm, which are essential for the splicing of pre-mRNAs in eukaryotes, are specific to lupus though found much less frequently than anti-dsDNA antibodies. These antibodies to Sm as well as antibodies to U1RNP but not directed to dsDNA, Ro/La or cardiolipin are more frequently associated with Afro-Caribbeans than Caucasians (Isenberg et al. 1997). Antibodies to U1RNP are usually associated with mild disease, a lower incidence of renal involvement, and the MHC haplotype, DR4.

Antibodies to Ro and La are more frequently associated with Sjögren's syndrome secondary to a diagnosis of lupus. These antibodies are also found in mothers with children who have congenital heart block and cutaneous disease. Recent evidence has demonstrated that apoptotic human foetal cardiac myocytes express Ro and La on their surface and promote the secretion of TNFα by macrophages (Miranda-Carus et al. 2000).

Claims have been made suggesting an association of autoantibodies to ribosomal P protein in SLE patients with cerebral involvement and psychosis but these findings remain controversial.

Autoantibodies to C1q may be elevated in SLE and are indicative of proliferative glomerulonephritis. Recent evidence suggests that the measurement of antiC1q, anti-DNA and anticardiolipin antibodies are highly specific for glomerulonephritis in lupus patients (Siegert et al. 1999; Loizou et al. 2000).

Abnormalities and dysregulation at the cellular level

SLE is characterized by multiple functional defects among cells of the immune system—T and B lymphocytes, natural killer cells, and accessory cells (antigen presenting cells) (Table 13). Numbers of circulating lymphocytes may be altered profoundly. Hyperactive B cells are increased in number,

Table 13 Cellular abnormalities and cytokine dysregulation

Monocyte/ macrophages	**↓ TNFα production—genetic defect**
Lymphocytes	
B cells	↑ nos. activated B cells → hypergammaglobulinaemia → IgG autoantibodies reactive with self antigens (cell membrane, cytoplasmic proteins, nuclear antigens, extracellular proteins) and non-self (polyclonal)
	↑ IL-2R, ↓ CR1 expression, ↑ surface expression of hsp90 but not hsp70 compared to normal cells
T cells	↓ CD4+CD45R+ (subset Th, suppressor/inducer)
	↑↑ CD4-8-TCRαβ+Th (escape thymic deletion since double negative?)
In vivo	Activated T cells are Class II + (DP, DR)
	Defective suppression
	Impaired cytotoxicity
	Activated peripheral T cells (only 15% → anti-DNA help), cloned → Tγδ cells reactive with hsp 60
In vitro	and → help to anti-DNA+ B cells (not class II restricted) (blocked by Ab to hsp65 but not hsp70)
Cytokines	
IL-1	↓ Does not activate T cells? Insufficient production by accessory cells or defective T-cell IL-1 receptor. Not corrected by addition of IL-1 *in vitro*
IL-2	Normal or ↓ IL-2 production by CD4+ and CD8+ T cells. Impairment not reversed by addition of IL-2. IFN-γ +IL-2 restores T-cell proliferation *in vitro*? Functional activity versus level of IL-2. Low affinity IL-2 receptors expressed on CD4+ T cells. Administration of rIL-2 exacerbates disease
IL-4	↑ IL-4 (Ag primed T cells → IL-4 → all B cells)
IL-6	No response to inflammation/acute phase reactants
IL-10	↑ in patients. Administration accelerates disease in NZB/W mice
IL-12	↑ in patients (one report shows ↓ levels), drives IFN-gamma-dependent autoimmune kidney disease in MRL-Fas(lpr) mice
IL-16	↑ in patients, correlates with disease activity
IL-17	↑ in patients
IL-18	↑ in patients, lymphocytes hyperresponsive to IL-18
B cell (BlyS) stimulator	Increased levels in lupus serum. Inhibition leads to improved survival in murine models of lupus
TGFβ	Increased tissue expression in renal nephritis. Antibodies against IL-10 delay disease onset and ↑ TNFα
TNFα	MHC linked production: protective therefore levels are critical
IFNγ	Normal levels produced. NK cells refractory. Absence in lpr mice leads to abolition of disease

Note: IL-2R, IL-2 receptor; hsp, heat shock protein; Th, T-helper cell; MHC, major histocompatibility complex; NK, natural killer cells.

expressing elevated levels of CD86, with coexistent T lymphocytopaenia. Numbers of both lymphocyte populations are extremely variable and fluctuate between normal and abnormal levels with respect to disease activity and duration.

The increase in activated B cells contributes to the hypergammaglobulinaemia associated with reactivity to self-antigens outlined in Table 12. On circulating, B-cell receptors for the cytokine, IL-2, are increased while CR1 (the receptor for C3b) expression is decreased. Evidence from animal models of lupus demonstrate that B cells play a role both as the source of high affinity pathogenic antibodies and as antigen presentation cells. Lupus-prone mice made deficient in B cells do not develop autoimmune disease and have a normal lifespan. Altering the expression of molecules that control B cell activation. One particular population of B lymphocytes that has attracted recent interest are the CD1 positive, marginal zone B cells which are expanded at an early stage in NZB/W mice (Zeng et al. 2000). These B cells appear to interact with antiCD1 T cells which in turn are able to influence disease in NZB/NZW mice. The CD1 family of MHC class I-like proteins present lipid antigens to T cells. Double-negative (DN) T cells, which are increased in lupus patients, provide help for CD1c+ B cells for IgG production and are restricted by CD1c (Sieling et al. 2000). IgG helper activity for CD1c+ B cells was weaker or undetectable among the DN T cells from healthy donors. DN T-cell help for IgG production was mediated through CD1c, IL-4, and CD40.

Among the two major T cell populations, CD4+ (helper/inducer) and CD8+ (suppressor/cytotoxic) there is a marked reduction of a subset of T cells bearing the CD4+ and CD45R+ phenotype. This population of cells helps to induce suppression by providing a signal to the CD8+ population. The reduction in this subset may explain the failure of T cells to suppress the hyperactive B cells. Anti-T-cell autoantibodies may be responsible for the depletion of this particular subset. CD45 autoantibodies mediate neutralization of activated T cells from lupus patients through anergy or apoptosis (Mamoune et al. 2000). A study has reported that the titre of anti-T-cell antibodies is directly proportional to the ratio of CD4/CD8 killing and that flares of disease are associated with an increase in CD4/CD8 killing and disease remission is accompanied by a corresponding decrease in the ratio. Parallel changes in anti-T-cell titres reflect the disease activity (Yamada et al. 1993).

T lymphocytes from lupus patients demonstrate increased downstream signalling following activation, and yet have reduced T-cell receptor zeta chain, a critical signalling molecule. This may be partly explained by the increased expression of FcεRIγ chain in a large proportion of SLE T cells (Enyedy et al. 2001). Another defect that has been well described in T cells is the deficient synthesis of IL-2 when T cells are stimulated by mitogens, this defect also extending to NK cells. This defect may be explained by the finding that freshly isolated SLE T cells demonstrate a TCR-mediated defect in the activation of NF-κB (Wong et al. 1999).

The appearance of class II molecules, usually HLA–DR, on T cells is taken as a marker of activation. Peripheral T cells with increased expression of HLA–DP at the cell surface and as m-RNA transcripts have been found in lupus patients. The frequency of HLA–DP expression exceeded that of HLA–DR and correlated well with disease activity. The ratio of HLA–DP+ T cells is inversely proportional to the extent of IL-2 production during *in vitro* response to mitogen (Hishikawa et al. 1990; Kanai et al. 1993).

Antigen-specific T cells have now been cloned from patients with SLE. Nucleosome specific T cells have attracted much interest, and peptide autoepitopes in core histones of nucleosomes are recurrently recognized by the autoimmune T cells derived from lupus patients (Lu et al. 1999). HLA–DR restricted T cells have also been cloned from a lupus patient and shown to induce IgG anti-DNA antibodies *in vitro* from high density (activated) B cells from DR-matched patients with lupus, and IgM antiDNA antibodies from B cells from DR-matched normal individuals (Murakami et al. 1992).

A number of studies have shown that SLE patients exhibit deficient antigen presenting cell (APC) function for allogeneic T cells, deficient APC function for the presentation of exogenous antigen, and reduced stimulation of autologous T cell proliferation in the autologous mixed lymphocyte reaction (MLR). The frequencies of dendritic cells (DC) in peripheral blood are consistently reduced in SLE patients compared with healthy controls (Scheinecker et al. 2001). This reduction results mainly from diminished proportions of CD11c+ DC. These observations may explain the reduction in CD4+ T cells since mature CD4+ T cells need peripheral class II MHC expression, such as is found on DCsm, for survival.

Cytokines

Cytokines in lupus can be classified according to whether they are pro- or anti-inflammatory. An inflammatory reaction such as occurs in lupus can thus be understood in terms of an imbalance of these opposing cytokines, or their inhibitory receptors. It is likely that this balance of cytokines not only determines disease severity but also the particular organ involvement. For example, one report suggests that interleukin-6 (IL-6) is increased in the cerebrospinal fluid (CSF) of patients with central nervous system (CNS) involvement in SLE but not in patients with SLE who lack neurological symptoms. Similarly, TGFβ has been implicated in preventing renal disease and decreased levels have been found in renal tissue. The characterization of different subsets of T-helper cells is directly related to their cytokine profiles and several autoimmune diseases may now be classified according to the predominance of a particular T-helper cell subset (Dean et al. 2000).

Table 14 summarizes the major differences between Th1 and Th2 cells in terms of cytokine profiles and function and outlines the cytokines found in serum or produced spontaneously after stimulation of peripheral blood mononuclear cells. Th1 cells support cell mediated immunity while Th2 cells provide B cell help and also suppress cell mediated immunity. The balance between cytokines from Th1 and those from Th2 cells is thus critical in determining the outcome of the immune response and any imbalance could have profound pathological effects.

At a most simplistic level SLE could be expected to be a disease where Th2 cells predominate resulting in too much help for B cells and overproduction of antibodies. In support of this concept, increased levels of IL-10 have been found in lupus patients and this cytokine suppresses Th1 cells and thus impairs cell mediated immunity, a characteristic feature of SLE. In mice continuous administration of anti-IL-10 delays the onset of disease.

Tumour necrosis factor (TNFα) is produced by T (Th1) and B lymphocytes, natural killer cells, and mononuclear phagocytic cells. Another cytokine (TNFβ), originally called lymphotoxin, is produced by activated lymphocytes. The genes for both TNFα and -β are closely linked and located within the major histocompatibility complex (MHC). *In vitro* TNFα production by mitogen activated peripheral blood lymphocytes varies according to the HLA Class II haplotype of the donor. Elevated production is found in DR3 and DR4 subjects whereas low production is found in DR2 and DQw1 positive donors. The DR2, DQw1 genotype in lupus patients is associated with lupus nephritis. DR3+ lupus patients are not predisposed to lupus nephritis and have elevated levels of TNFα production. The DR4 haplotype is associated with high TNFα inducibility and negatively correlated with lupus nephritis (Jacob et al. 1990a).

Table 14 T-cell subsets and cytokines

		Th1	Th2
Subsets of CD41 T cells			
Function		Cell mediated immunity	B cell help
Cytokines		IFNγ	IL-4
		IL-10 (humans only)	IL-10
		IL-12	
		TNFα	
Cytokine	**Serum level**[a]	**Spontaneous**	**Stimulation *in vitro***
Cytokine profiles in patients with active SLE			
IFN-γ	↑	Low	↓
TNF-α	↑ (or normal)	↓ (DR2 DQw1; ↑ nephritis) ↑ (DR3,4; ↓ nephritis)	↓
IL-1	n.d.[b]	↑ PBM production	↓ monocyte production
IL-2	↑	Low	↓
IL-4	n.d.	Low	Low
IL-6	↑	↑	—
IL-10	↑ (or normal)	↑ (or normal)	Normal
IL-12	?	Normal	↓

[a] Serum levels of cytokines are difficult to interpret since these may be affected by soluble cytokine receptors which are shed from cells. Among the known shed receptors are those for IL-1, IL-2, IL-6, TNFα, and IFNγ. Soluble TNFαR and IL-2R levels are increased in SLE and correlate with disease activity and lupus nephritis.

[b] n.d. = not detected.

High levels of TNFα are more frequently associated with RA and as such therapeutic benefit has been reported using monoclonal antibodies to TNFα. In one study 14 per cent of rheumatoid arthritis patients treated with anti-TNF therapy developed IgM antidsDNA antibodies. Only 1 of the 156 patients who were treated with anti-TNF developed a self-limiting clinical lupus syndrome associated with IgG antiDNA antibodies (Charles et al. 2000).

Both macrophage and natural killer (NK) cell mediated cytotoxicity are frequently impaired in lupus patients. Interferon-γ (IFN-γ) induced enhancement of both types of cytotoxicity is also impaired despite normal levels of IFN-γ production by lupus Th1 cells. SLE NK cells fail to release soluble factors necessary for killing. Recombinant interferon-γ (rIFN-γ) has been used to induce remission in patients with RA but exacerbated disease in both lupus patients (Machold and Smolen 1990) and lupus-prone strains of mice (Jacob et al. 1990b).

Accessory cells in lupus seem to produce insufficient amounts of IL-1 to provide the necessary activation signal for T cells. This effect cannot be overcome *in vitro* by the addition of exogenous IL-1 suggesting that a defect may exist at the level of the IL-1 receptor on T cells. Alternatively, the defect could exist at a distal point in some biochemical pathway.

Both CD4+ and CD8+ T cells have been described to produce either normal or decreased amounts of IL-2 in response to exogenous antigens, mitogens, allo- and autoantigens. Reduced IL-2 generation would have a profound effect on T-cell responses. This impairment is not reversed by the addition of exogenous IL-2. However, *in vitro* treatment of SLE accessory cells with IFN-γ plus the addition of IL-2 has been shown to restore T-cell proliferation and the expression of T suppressor activity. The variability of experimental data in this context raises the question of whether IL-2 functional activity varies between patients rather than merely reflecting levels of IL-2.

Studies *in vitro* on the response to IL-2 of the CD4+T-cell subset (helper/inducer) indicate that there is altered expression of IL-2 receptors. The CD8+ T-cell subset (suppressor/cytotoxic) has IL-2 receptors but fails to respond as there is no IL-2 signal from CD4+ T cells. This is a secondary defect. The primary disorder relates to the CD4+ subset which expresses IL-2 receptors of low affinity. Functional IL-2 receptors are of high affinity. Variable synthesis of both types of receptors may be governed by altered intracellular synthesis and/or transport.

Apoptosis

Apoptosis appears to have a dual role in lupus pathogenesis. First, this process is an important mechanism for deletion of autoreactive lymphocytes and secondly, apoptosis results in the availability of autoantigens which can be presented to the immune system. It is the latter that has generated most interest in recent years. Normally apoptotic cells are rapidly cleared by macrophages but recent evidence had demonstrated that these is a profound defect in this clearance pathway in lupus patients. When macrophages from a sub-group of SLE patients were differentiated *in vitro*, they displayed markedly impaired phagocytosis of apoptotic cells, leading to the accumulation of secondary necrotic cells (Herrmann et al. 1998). Evidence from a number of animal models has suggested that the clearance of apoptotic cells lies at the the heart of the pathogenesis of lupus (Walport 2000). Thus, a lupus type phenotype occurs in mice lacking C1q, which, together with other complement proteins, helps to clear immune complexes and apoptotic cells2. Deletion of the gene encoding serum amyloid P component (Sap), which binds chromatin and may mask it from the immune system, results in antinuclear autoimmunity and glomerulonephritis. A similar phenotype is observed in mice lacking secreted IgM, implicated in clearing effete cells. Mice that lack DNAase1 develop lupus autoimmunity, the ability of DNAase to digest DNA prevents an immune response. The importance of removing apoptotic cells is explained by the appearance of a variety of nuclear autoantigens which are sequestered in blebs on the surface of apoptotic cells, and may become accessible for dendritic cells (DCs) (Andrade et al. 2000). Remarkably, DCs but not macrophages efficiently cross-present antigen derived from apoptotic cells to autologous cytotoxic T cells (Albert et al. 1998). In individuals with a defective clearance, sun exposure may result in accumulation of non-ingested apoptotic cells and nuclear autoantigens in the skin, which is a highly immune-competent tissue. This fact presumably explains the disease and flare inducing capabilities of exposure to ultraviolet light.

Evidence from murine models of lupus have suggested that lupus can arise from failure to delete autoreactive lymphocytes. The *Fas* protein has been intimately linked with apoptosis and is normally expressed on the cell surface (CD95). MRL-*lpr/lpr* mice have an endogenous retroviral DNA sequence integrated into the *Fas* gene which results in incorrect membrane expression of the *Fas* protein and loss of apoptosis. This abnormality would result in failure of self-reactive T cells to undergo apoptosis in the thymus and may account for the accumulation of double negative T cells (CD4−CD8) which infiltrate many tissues in these mice. Although defects in the apoptotic gene *Fas* lead to autoimmunity in mice, conflicting evidence has been found in lupus patients which might arise from differences in the study populations. A recent study demonstrated increased levels of *in vitro* apoptosis in SLE in a patient population with inactive disease and without use of immunosuppressive medication, factors which might have influenced results from previous studies (Bijl et al. 2001).

Bcl-2 is a proto-oncogene located at the inner membrane of mitochondria, the ER and the nuclear membrane and exerts a regulatory function during development and maintenance of adult tissue by preventing apoptosis in specific cell types. It is involved in T-cell development and thymic selection and is found in long-lived B lymphocytes within the follicular mantle zone. Over-expression of *bcl-2* in mice leads to increased B-cell longevity and an increased response to foreign antigens, and, in some genetic backgrounds autoimmunity. It is peripheral rather than central tolerance that is defective in these mice. Elevated Bcl-2 levels have been found in lymphocytes derived from a proportion of lupus patients and that a number of cytokines (IL-2, IL-4, IL-7, and IL-15) can increase this expression, and prevent cellular apoptosis, preferentially in lupus patients (Graninger et al. 2000). However, more compelling are the data from Herrmann et al. (1998) who have shown that although there is little wrong with apoptosis per se in patients with lupus, there is a major defect in the removal of apoptotic cells. This could lead to the undue persistence of potential autoantigens. Injection of apoptotic B cells into lupus prone mice leads to an exacerbation of their lupus (Trebeden-Negre et al. 2003).

Cell adhesion molecules

Interest in the adhesive mechanisms which facilitate cell–cell and cell–matrix interactions has expanded considerably over the past few years. Adhesion is mediated by several molecules which vary in affinity and structure on the surface of the cells which express them. Adhesion molecules belong to one of three main families; (i) selectins, (ii) integrins, or (iii) the Ig superfamily. As leucocytes roll in the direction of blood flow random contact is made with the endothelium. Transient adhesion of leucocytes to the endothelium occurs through low affinity binding to E-selectins. The cells become activated and then bind with higher affinity to vascular integrins. Once cells are firmly attached transendothelial migration occurs and under the influence of extravascular chemoattractants sub-endothelial migration into the extracellular matrix occurs.

Upregulation of the surface expression of three distinct adhesion molecules, E-selectin, VCAM-1, and ICAM-1, has been shown in biopsies from non-lesional, non-sun exposed skin from 16 patients with SLE. Levels of adhesion molecules were directly correlated with disease activity and in serial biopsy specimens decreased with clinical improvement (Belmont et al. 1994). Another study showed that the levels of CD14, ICAM-1, and E-selectin were elevated in active lupus and that the levels of these adhesion molecules in lupus were similar to patients with sepsis (Egerer et al. 2000). These findings suggest that excessive complement activation in association with edendothelial cells induces leucocyte–endothelial cell adhesion and leuco-occlusive vasculopathy. Furthermore, UV irradiation of keratinocytes *in vitro* induces release of epidermal and dermal cytokines and increases ICAM-1 expression which *in vivo* may lead to vascular activation culminating in the photosensitive lupus syndromes (Norris 1993). Autoantibodies to endothelium are present in lupus patients and have been correlated with disease severity. Human monoclonal antibodies with endothelial specificity bind to and then activate endothelium (Yazici et al. 2001).

Soluble forms of adhesion molecules are elevated in the circulation of patients with SLE compared to healthy controls. Elevated levels of soluble ICAM-1 (sICAM-1) have been reported to show significant association with skin involvement and disease activity (Sfikakis et al. 1994). Lupus patients also have elevated levels of a soluble form of VCAM-1 (Wellicome et al. 1993). The importance of these observations may become apparent from studies in murine lupus which have demonstrated upregulation of ICAM-1 in nephritic MRL-*lpr/lpr* and NZB/W kidneys, particularly in the brush borders of proximal tubules, glomerular mesangium and endothelium of larger vessels (Wuthrich et al. 1990). Mrl/mpj-fas(lpr) lupus mouse strain made deficient in ICAM-1 have reduced tissue inflammation and prolonged survival (Bullard et al. 1997). Similarly VCAM-1 is also upregulated in MRL-*lpr/lpr* kidneys, not only in the endothelium but also in cortical tubules and glomeruli. Kidney tissue sections from nephritic MRL-*pr/lpr* mice also display increased adhesiveness for T cell and macrophage cell lines which can be blocked by monoclonal antibodies to ICAM-1 and VCAM-1 (Wuthrich 1992). The expression of ICAM-1 and VCAM-1 are induced by TNFα and IL-1 in MRL/lpr mice (McHale et al. 1999).

Genetic components

The idea that genetic factors may play a role in susceptibility to SLE stems from the high rate of concordance for disease in monozygotic twins, increased frequency of SLE and immunological abnormalities in relatives of SLE patients, and the prevalence of SLE among certain ethnic groups. The genes which may influence or predispose to SLE include those which determine sex, colour, complement haplotype, tissue type (HLA), antibody variable regions, and T-cell receptors (TCR) (Table 15). The recent development of densely mapped genetic markers spanning the entire genome has drastically changed the study of genetic predisposition. Chromosomal regions containing possible susceptibility loci can be identified by linkage analysis based on the genetic location, without prior knowledge of the function of the genes. Both mouse and human loci have been identified and in some cases the same regions have been associated with SLE.

Six genome scans have been published to date for SLE, their results varying substantially presumably because of heterogeneity of sample populations and differing methods of analysis. These studies have identified several chromosomal regions indicating possible linkages with SLE. In some cases chromosomal regions containing genes already known to be associated were identified, for example, FcγRIIA on 1q23 and in other cases the same region has been identified in humans and mice, for example, Sle1, Lbw7, and Nba2 on chromosome 1 map to a region syntenic to human chromosome 1q21–1q23 (Tsao 2000). It is interesting to note that none of the chromosome 1 regions were identified in the Icelandic patients. Other regions have been identified as a cluster of autoimmune loci, for example, 19q which has linkage to MS and IDDM and contains candidate genes such as CD22, a negative regulator of B-cell activation, and TGFβ which plays numerous roles in controlling immune reactions.

Sex and ethnic background

At the most basic genetic level SLE affects females more than males and shows an ethnic bias in that Afro-Caribbeans are more affected than

Table 15 Genetic components associated with SLE

	Genetic factors		
Complement	C1, C4 deficiencies (>75% prevalence, severe disease)		
	C2 deficiency (~35% prevalence, severity similar to non-C deficient lupus patients)		
	C4 50–80% of patients partially deficient		
	CR1 deficiencies (acquired rather than genetic)		
MHC associations	HLA-A1, B8, DR3—English/Irish patients		
	DR3 and DQw2—antiRo/La antibodies		
	DQw1—antiRo antibodies		
	DQw6, 7, 8—lupus anticoagulant		
	DR2—Afro-Caribbean patients with antiSm		
	DR2, DQw1 (DQw6), DQ2—susceptibility to nephritis		
	DR4, DQw3—protective?		
	DRw8—early onset SLE (<20 years)		
	Decreased expression of Class II on APC		
	Susceptibility may depend upon a single amino acid substitution (Histidine→ tyrosine at position 30 in sequence of DQw1.19b β gene from single SLE patient compared to healthy control)		
T-cell receptor			
Man	Little data on human TCR family usage		
	AntiRo response related to TCR β gene product in SLE		
	Genomic DNA restriction fragment length polymorphism in humans no deletions, insertions in TCR α, β, γ chain genes		
Mouse	Cβ deletion in TCR of NZW and NZB × NZW F1 mice		
	(a) normal TCR—MW 90 kDa		
	(b) 'light' TCR—MW 70–85 kDa		
	latter increases as animals age and as disease and lymphadenopathy develop		
Antibody V genes			
Germ-line encoded	Human monoclonal antiDNA/Sm germline encoded but use same V gene families as Ab to non-self. Thus may not need somatic mutation. Genetic predisposition to develop antiSm Ab in SLE patients and first-degree healthy relatives		
Somatic mutation	↑ Somatic mutation (e.g. low concordance between homozygous twins) Autoantibody response generally IgG. Somatic mutation increases with immunoglobulin class switch		
Idiotypic analysis	Preferential use of V gene family with or without autoantibody activity (proband versus family members). Specific deposition of anti-DNA pathogenic/nephritogenic idiotypes in kidney:		
		16/16	*IdGN*
	% SLE	42	75
	% disease controls	0	6
Ethnic origin	Blacks >> Whites. Most probably linked to MHC		
Sex and endocrine factors?	Females >> Males. Oestrogen enhances the immune response. Testosterone is immunosuppressive		

Orientals, in turn more affected than Caucasians. These basic differences are reflected in other ways. Sex hormones are known to influence disease in both mice and humans with autoimmune disease. Androgens are immunosuppressive and oestrogens are immunoenhancing. This explains the susceptibility of women to autoimmune diseases compared to men. For example, androgens reduce while oestrogens enhance the spontaneous antibody production in mixed strains of mice (NZB × CBA and NZB × C3H). In MRL-*pr/lpr* r mice testosterone treatment reduces lupus-like symptoms without affecting lymphoproliferation. In humans where pregnancy occurs during active disease, exacerbations often occur as oestrogen levels rise.

Complement

SLE is associated with deficiencies of the early classical pathway of complement components C1, C4, and C2. The strength of the association is inversely correlated with the position of these complement components in the classical activation pathway. Thus, deficiency in C1q leads to a lupus like disease in 95 per cent of cases, C4 57 per cent , and C2 10 per cent. C3 deficiency leads to a somewhat different clinical picture of recurrent pyogenic infections, membranoproliferative glomerulonephritis, and rashes. The mechanism that links these deficiencies in the early components of complement are not entirely clear. Perhaps the most favoured explanation is that these factors promote the clearance of apoptotic cells as discussed above (Walport 2000). Two alleles are inherited for each complement thus component deficiencies may be partial or complete (homozygous). Congenital deficiencies of C2 and C4 are frequently in linkage disequilibrium with HLA–DR3 and –DR2, HLA haplotype associated with SLE.

Mannose-binding protein (MBP) is an acute phase protein that activates both the classical and alternative complement pathways. A defective allele, incapable of activating complement, has been associated with SLE in several ethnic populations. (e.g. Sullivan et al. 1996). Complement receptors, CR1

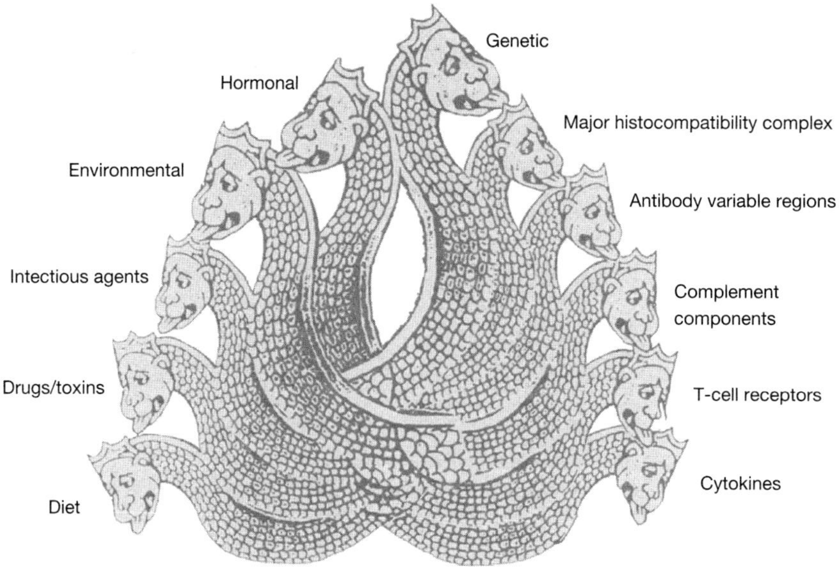

Fig. 5 The Hydra—an analogy of the multiple factors involved in lupus.

and CR2, have been studied in SLE. The CR1 ligands are C3b and C4b bound to immune complexes. The receptor is present on peripheral B lymphocytes, erythrocytes, monocytes, and tissue macrophages and binds, internalises, processes, and transports immune complexes which have activated complement. Low expression of CR1 on erythrocytes and peripheral blood leucocytes was described in SLE patients and their healthy family members (Walport and Lachmann 1988). This was originally interpreted as an inherited defect which could predispose to SLE. More recently, this defect is thought to be acquired as normal erythrocytes infused into SLE patients also showed a decrease in CR1 receptors. Levels of CR1 deficiency in SLE patients correlate with disease activity. Controversy still abounds in this area as to the precise nature of this defect and is confounded further by the possibility of a functional defect of CR1 receptors on polymorphonuclear neutrophils.

Complement receptor 2, CR2 (CD21), has recently been described on peripheral T cells in healthy individuals. The ligands for CR2 are C3d, and EBV. The receptor is present on mature, circulating and lymph nodecells, follicular dendritic cells, and on 10–40 per cent of peripheral blood CD4+ or CD8+ T cells. In patients with active or inactive SLE, B cell CR2 expression is significantly diminished. This may be a consequence of the activated state of SLE B cells reflecting the loss of CR2 as cells differentiate into Ig-secreting cells and then plasma cells or the levels may be modulated by high levels of circulating immune complexes or cytokines. Expression of CR2 on T cells from patients with inactive SLE is similar to that found in healthy individuals but is increased in some patients with active lupus (90 per cent of CD4+ and CD8+ peripheral T cells expressing increased levels of CR2). In this context CR2 is important in signalling and its increased expression on T cells may play a role in cell adhesion or cytotoxicity (Levy et al. 1992). CR2-linked inhibitors can be targeted to the lupus kidney to prevent complement activation (Song et al. 2003).

Major histocompatibility complex

The associations between the MHC and SLE must take into account the ethnic origin of the patient. A recent report highlights this aspect by demonstrating that only in Caucasian patients of English/Irish descent is SLE associated with an MHC extended haplotype (HLA-B8; SCO1; DR3) (Schur et al. 1990). In American Blacks, DRw52b is positively associated with renal disease and negatively associated with antinuclear RNP antibodies. DR3 (DRw17) and DQw2 are highly associated with the ability to produce antiRo/antiLa antibodies. These antibodies are associated with sub-acute cutaneous lupus, lymphopaenia, neonatal lupus, and complete congenital heart block. DR4 is associated with the ability to make antiRNP and with a reduced risk for lupus nephritis. In contrast to the protection conferred by DR4, DR2 confers susceptibility to nephritis. Associations with DQw1 and with DQβ1.AZH and DQβ2 are more recent findings. Early onset SLE (~20 years) is associated with DRw8 and the frequency of neuropsychiatric involvement correlates negatively with a DQβ fragment (Reveille et al. 1989). Compared to the normal ethnic population, Afro-Caribbean patients with antibodies to Sm have an increased frequency of DR2 and a reduced frequency of DR3, regardless of anti-DNA antibody status (Olsen et al. 1993).

DQw7 correlates significantly with lupus anticoagulant although there are patients who have lupus anticoagulant but lack the DQw7 haplotype. However, these patients all have DQw8. Amino acids in position 71–77 of the third hypervariable region of DQB1 chains were identical in DQw7, DQw6, and DQw8 individuals leading to the proposal that this region might constitute the 'epitope' for mediation of this autoimmune response (Arnett et al. 1991). For a more complete description of the known associations between MHC class II genes and autoantibody subsets, the reader is referred to an excellent review by Arnett and Reveille (1992).

Summary

In the introduction to this chapter, an analogy was drawn between SLE and the Hydra monster of Greek legend. In Fig. 5, this analogy is reiterated to confirm the multiple factors involved in the aetiology and pathogenesis of lupus. It is evident that this remarkable disease presents a wide spectrum of clinical features and is characterized by multiple autoantibodies, although clearly not due to random polyclonal B-cell activation. While lupus for some patients causes a relatively mild set of problems, for many others it has significant morbidity and for a small subset, an increased risk premature death.

References

Abramson, S., Kramer, S.B., Radin, A., and Holzman, R. (1985). Salmonella bacteremia in systemic lupus erythematosus. Eight year experience at a municipal hospital. *Arthritis and Rheumatism* **28**, 75–9.

Abu-Shakra, M., Gladman, D.D., and Urowitz, M. (1996). Malignancy in systemic lupus erythematosus. *Arthritis and Rheumatism* **39**, 1250–6.

Albert, M.L. et al. (1998). Dendritic cells acquire antigen from apoptotic cells and induce class I-restricted CTLs. *Nature* **392**, 86–9.

Andrade, F., Casciola-Rosen, L., and Rosen, A. (2000). Apoptosis in systemic lupus erythematosus. Clinical implications. *Rheumatic Diseases Clinics of North America* **26** (2), 215–27.

Arnett, F., Olsen, M., Anderson, K., and Reveille, J.D. (1991). Molecular analysis of major histocompatibility complex alleles associated with the lupus antioagulant. *Journal of Clinical Investigation* **87**, 1490–5.

Arnett, F.C. and Reveille, J.D. (1992). Genetics of systemic lupus erythematosus. *Rheumatic Diseases Clinics of North America* **18**, 865–92 (review).

Belmont, H.M., Buyon, J., Giorno, R., and Abramson, S. (1994). Up-regulation of endothelial cell adhesion molecules characterizes disease activity in systemic lupus erythematosus. The Schwartzman phenomenon revisited. *Arthritis and Rheumatism* **37**, 376–83.

Bijl, M., Horst, G., Limburg, P.C., and Kallenberg, C.G. (2001). Anti-CD3-induced and anti-Fas induced apoptosis in systemic lupus erythematosus (SLE). *Clinical and Experimental Immunology* **123** (1), 127–32.

Blanco, F.J., De La Mata, J., Lopez-Fernandez, J.I., and Gomez-Reino, J.J. (1994). Light, immunofluorescence and electron microscopy renal biopsy findings as predictors of mortality in 85 Spanish patients with systemic lupus erythematosus. *British Journal of Rheumatology* **33**, 260–6.

Bonfa, E. et al. (1987). Association between lupus psychosis and anti-ribosomal P protein antibodies. *New England Journal of Medicine* **317**, 265–71.

Bullard, D.C., King, P.D., Hicks, M.J., Dupont, B., Beaudet, A.L., and Elkon, K.B. (1997). Intercellular adhesion molecule-1 deficiency protects mrl/mpj-fas(lpr) mice from early lethality. *Journal of Immunology* **159**, 2058.

Callen, J.P. and Klein, J. (1988). Subacute cutaneous lupus erythematosus. *Arthritis and Rheumatism* **31**, 1007–13.

Charles, P.J., Smeenk, R.J., De Jong, J., Feldmann, M., and Maini, R.N. (2000). Assessment of antibodies to double-stranded DNA induced in rheumatoid arthritis patients following treatment with infliximab, a monoclonal antibody to tumor necrosis factor alpha: findings in open-label and randomised placebo-controlled trials. *Arthritis and Rheumatism* **43**, 2383–90.

Dean, G.S., Tyrrell-Price, J., Crawley, E., Isenberg, D.A. (2000). Cytokines and systemic lupus erythematosus. *Annals of the Rheumatic Diseases* **59**, 243–51.

Deapen, D. et al. (1992). A revised estimate of twin concordance in systemic lupus erythematosus. *Arthritis and Rheumatism* **35**, 311–18.

Delgado Alves, J., Ames, P.R.J., Donohue, S., Stanger, L., Noorooz-Zadeh, J., Ravirajan, C.I., and Isenberg, D.A. (2002). Antibodies to high density lipoprotein and B2 glycoprotein 1 are inversely correlated with paraoxonase activity in systemic lupus erythematosus and primary anti-phospholipid syndrome. *Arthritis and Rheumatism* **46**, 2686–94.

Diamond, B. and Scharff, M. (1984). Somatic mutation of the T15 heavy chain gives rise to an antibody with autoantibody specificity. *Proceedings of the National Academy of Sciences USA* **81**, 841–4.

Dubois, E.L. and Tuffanelli, D.L. (1964). Clinical manifestations of systemic lupus erythematosus. Computer analysis of 250 cases. *Journal of the American Medical Association* **190**, 104–11.

Edworthy, S., Fritzler, M., Whitehead, C., Martin, L., and Rattner, J.B. (2000). ASE-1: an autoantigen in systemic lupus erythematosus. *Lupus* **9**, 681–7.

Egerer, K., Feist, E., Rohr, U., Pruss, A., Burmester, G.R., and Dorner, T. (2000). Increased serum soluble CD14, ICAM-1 and E-selectin correlate with disease activity and prognosis in systemic lupus erythematosus. *Lupus* **9**, 614–21.

Ehrenstein, M.R. (1999). Antinuclear antibodies and lupus: causes and consequences. *Rheumatology* **38**, 691–3.

Enyedy, E.J., Nambiar, M.P., Liossis, S.N., Dennis, G., Kammer, G.M., and Tsokos, G.C. (2001). Fc epsilon receptor type I gamma chain replaces the deficient T cell receptor zeta chain in T cells of patients with systemic lupus erythematosus. *Arthritis and Rheumatism* **44**, 1114–21.

Estes, D. and Christian, C.L. (1971). The natural history of systemic lupus erythematosus by prospective analysis. *Medicine* **50**, 85–95.

Feinglass, E.J., Arnett, F.C., Dorsch, D.A., Zizic, T.M., and Stevens, M.B. (1976). Neuropsychiatric manifestations of systemic lupus erythematosus: diagnosis, clinical spectrum and relationship to other features of the disease. *Medicine* **55**, 323–37.

Fox, R.A. and Isenberg, D.A. (1997). The clinical relevance of antibodies to ribosomal P—where are we now? *Japanese Journal of Rheumatology* **7**, 235–46.

Fries, J., Porta, J., and Liang, M.H. (1978). Marginal benefit of renal biopsy in systemic lupus erythematosus. *Archives of Internal Medicine* **138**, 1386–9.

Furie, R.A. and Chartash, E.K. (1988). Tendon rupture in systemic lupus erythematosus. *Seminars in Arthritis and Rheumatism* **18**, 127–33.

Galli, M., Comfurius, P., Manssen, C., Hemker, H.C., De Baets, M.H., Van Breda-Vriesman, P.J.G., Barbui, T., Zwaal, R.F.A., and Beuers, E.M. (1990). Anticardiolipin antibodies (ACA) directed not to cardiolipin but to a plasma protein cofactor. *Lancet* **335**, 1544–7.

Gladman, D.D. et al. (1994). Sensitivity to change of 3 systemic lupus erythematosus disease activity indices: international validation. *Journal of Rheumatology* **21**, 1468–71.

Gladman, D., Ginzler, E., Goldsmith, C., Fortin, P., Liang, M.H., Urowitz, M., Bacon, P., Bombardieri, S., Hanley, J., Hay, E., Isenberg, D.A., Jones, J., Kalunian, K., Maddison, P., Nived, O., Petri, M., Richter, S., Sanchez-Guerrero, J., Snaith, M.L., Sturfelt, G., Symmons, D., and Zoma, A. (1996). The development and initial validation of the Systemic Lupus International Collaborating Clinics/American College of Rheumatology damage index for systemic lupus erythematosus. *Arthritis and Rheumatism* **39**, 363–9.

Goulet, J.R., Mackenzie, T., Lewinton, C., Hayslett, J.P., Campi, A., and Esdaile, J.M. (1993). The long term prognosis of lupus nephritis: the impact of disease activity. *Journal of Rheumatology* **20**, 59–65.

Graninger, W.B., Steiner, C.W., Graninger, M.T., Aringer, M., Smolen, J.S. (2000). Cytokine regulation of apoptosis and Bcl-2 expression in lymphocytes of patients with systemic lupus erythematosus. *Cell Death and Differentiation* **7**, 966–72.

Guldner, H.H., Netter, H.J., Szostecki, C., Jaeger, E., and Will, H. (1990). Human anti-p68 autoantibodies recognise a common epitope of nuclear ribonucleoprotein and influenza B virus. *Journal of Experimental Medicine* **171**, 819–29.

Hanley, J.G. et al. (1993). Cognitive impairment and autoantibodies in systemic lupus erythematosus. *British Journal of Rheumatology* **32**, 291–6.

Haupt, P.M., Moore, W.G., and Hutchins, G.M. (1981). The lung in systemic lupus erythematosus. Analysis of the pathologic changes in 120 patients. *American Journal of Medicine* **71**, 791–7.

Hay, E.M. et al. (1993). The BILAG index: a reliable and valid instrument for measuring clinical disease activity in systemic lupus erythematosus. *Quarterly Journal of Medicine* **86**, 447–58.

Herrmann, M., Voll, R.E., Zoller, O.M., Hagenhofer, M., Ponner, B.B., and Kalden, J.R. (1998). Impaired phagocytosis of apoptotic cell material by monocyte-derived macrophages from patients with systemic lupus erythematosus. *Arthritis and Rheumatism* **41** (7), 1241–50.

Hishikawa, T., Tokano, Y., and Sekigawa, I. (1990). T cells and deficient interleukin 2 production in patients with systemic lupus erythematosus. *Clinical Immunology and Immunopathology* **55**, 285– 96.

Ho, C.T.K., Mok, C.C., Lau, C.S., and Wong, R.W.S. (1998). Late onset systemic lupus erythematosus in southern Chinese. *Annals of the Rheumatic Diseases* **57**, 437–40.

Hoffbrand, B.I. and Beck, E.R. (1965) 'Unexplained' dyspnoea and shrinking lungs in systemic lupus erythematosus. *British Medical Journal* **1**, 1273–7.

Hopkinson, N.D., Doherty, M., and Powell, R.J. (1993). The prevalence and incidence of systemic lupus erythematosus in Nottingham, UK, 1989–1990. *British Journal of Rheumatology* **32**, 110–15.

Isenberg, D.A. (1983). Immunoglobulin deposition in skeletal muscle in primary muscle disease. *Quarterly Journal of Medicine* **52**, 297–310.

Isenberg, D.A. and Malick, J. (1994). Male lupus—the Loch Ness revisited. *British Journal of Rheumatology* **33**, 307–8.

Isenberg, D. and Ramsey-Goldman, T. (1999). Assessing patient swith lupus: towards drug responder Index. *Rheumatology* **38**, 1045–9.

Isenberg, D.A. and Snaith, M.L. (1981). Muscle disease in SLE: a study of its nature, frequency and cause. *Journal of Rheumatology* **8**, 917–24.

Isenberg, D.A., Garton, M., Reichlin, M.W., and Reichlin, M. (1997). Long term follow up of autoantibody profiles in black female lupus patients and clinical comparisons with Caucasian and Asian patients. *British Journal of Rheumatology* **36**, 229–33.

Ishikawa, O., Ohnishi, K., Miyachi, Y., and Ishizaka, H. (1994). Cerebral lesions in systemic lupus erythematosus detected by magnetic resonance imaging. Relationship to anti-cardiolipin antibody. *Journal of Rheumatology* **21**, 87–90.

Jacob, C.O., Fronek, Z., Lewis, G.D., Koo, M., Hansen, J.A., and McDevitt, H.O. (1990a). Heritable major histocompatibility complex class II-associated differences in relevance to genetic predisposition to systemic lupus erythematosus. *Proceedings of the National Academy of Sciences USA* **87**, 1233–7.

Jacob, C.O., van der Meide, P.H., and McDevitt, H.O. (1990b). *In vivo* treatment of (NZB × NZW) F1 lupus-like nephritis with monoclonal antibody to γ interferon. *Journal of Experimental Medicine* **166**, 798–803.

Johnson, A.E., Gordon, C., Palmer, R.G., and Bacon, P.A. (1995). The prevalence and incidence of systemic lupus erythematosus (SLE) in Birmingham, UK, related to ethnicity and country of birth. *Arthritis and Rheumatism* **38**, 551–8.

Kahl, L.E. (1994). Herpes zoster infections in systemic lupus erythematosus: risk factors and outcome. *Journal of Rheumatology* **21**, 84–6.

Kalsi, J.K., Ravirajan, C.T., Rahman, A., and Isenberg, D.A. (1999). Structure–function analysis and the molecular origins of anti-DNA antibodies in SLE. Expert review. In *Molecular Medicine*, 1–28. Cambridge: Cambridge University Press.

Kanai, Y., Tokano, Y., Tsuda, H., Hashimoto, H., Okumura, K., and Hirose, S. (1993). HLA-DP positive T cells in patients with polymyositis/dermatomyositis. *Journal of Rheumatology* **20**, 77–9.

Karassa, F.B., Ionannidis, J.P.A., Toulomi, G., Boki, K.A., and Moutsopoulos, H.M. (2000). Risk factors for central nervous system involvement in systemic lupus erythematosus. *Quarterly Journal of Medicine* **93**, 169–74.

Katz, J.B., Limpanasithikul, W., and Diamond, B. (1994). Mutational analysis of an autoantibody: differential binding and pathogenicity. *Journal of Experimental Medicine* **180**, 925–32.

Keeling, D.M. and Isenberg, D.A. (1993). Haematological manifestations of systemic lupus erythematosus. *Blood Reviews* **7**, 199–207.

Khamashta, M.A., Cerbera, R., Asherson, R.A., Font, J., Gil, A., Cottar, D.J., Vasques, J.J., Paré, C., Ingelmo, M., Oliver, J., and Hughes, G.R.V. (1990). Association of antibodies against phospholipids with heart valve disease in systemic lupus erythematosus. *Lancet* **335**, 1541–4.

Lahita, R.G., Chiorazzi, N., Gibofsky, A., Winchester, R.J., and Kunkel, H.G. (1983). Familial systemic lupus erythematosus in males. *Arthritis and Rheumatism* **26**, 39–44.

Leaker, M., McGregor, A., Griffiths, M., Snaith, M., Neild, G., and Isenberg, D.A. (1991). Insidious loss of renal function in patients with anti-cardiolipin antibodies and absence of overt nephritis. *Annals of the Rheumatic Diseases* **30**, 422–5.

Lee, S.S., Li, C.S., and Li, P.C.K. (1993). Clinical profile of Chinese patients with systemic lupus erythematosus. *Lupus* **2**, 105–9.

Leung, W.H., Wong, K.L., Lau, C.P., Wong, C.K., and Liu, H.W. (1990). Association between antiphospholipid antibodies and cardiac abnormalities in patients with systemic lupus erythematosus. *American Journal of Medicine* **89**, 411–19.

Levy, E., Ambrus, J., Kahl, L., Molina, H., Tung, K., and Holers, V.M. (1992). T lymphocyte expression of complement receptor 2 (CR2/CD21): a role in adhesive cell–cell interactions and dysregulation in a patient with systemic lupus erythematosus (SLE). *Clinical and Experimental Immunology* **90**, 235–44.

Li, E.K. and Tam, L. (1999). Pulmonary hypertension in systemic lupus erythematosus: clinical association and survival in 18 patients. *Journal of Rheumatology* **26**, 1923–9.

Liang, M.H., Sacher, S.A., Robert, W.N., and Esdaile, J.M. (1988). Measurement of systemic lupus erythematosus activity in clinical research. *Arthritis and Rheumatism* **31**, 817–25.

Libman, E. and Sachs, B. (1924). A hitherto undescribed form of valvular and mural endocarditis. *Archives of Internal Medicine (Chicago)* **33**, 701–9.

Loizou, S., Samarkos, M., Norsworthy, P.J., Cazabon, J.K., Walport, M.J., and Davies, K.A. (2000). Significance of anticardiolipin and anti-beta(2)-glycoprotein I antibodies in lupus nephritis. *Rheumatology (Oxford)* **39** (9), 962–8.

Love, P.E. and Santoro, S.A. (1990). Anti-phospholipid antibodies: anticardiolipin and the lupus anticoagulant in systemic lupus erythematosus (SLE) and in non-SLE disorders. *Annals of Internal Medicine* **112**, G82–98.

Lu, L., Kaliyaperumal, A., Boumpas, D.T., and Datta, S.K. (1999). Major peptide autoepitopes for nucleosome-specific T cells of human lupus. *Journal of Clinical Investigation* **104**, 345–55.

Lynch, A., Malar, R., Murphy, J., Davila, G., Santos, M., Rutledge, J., and Emlen, W. (1994). Anti-phospholipid antibodies in predicting adverse pregnancy outcome—a prospective study. *Annals of Internal Medicine* **15**, 470–5.

Machold, K.P. and Smolen, J.S. (1990). Interferon-γ induced exacerbation of systemic lupus erythematosus. *Journal of Rheumatology* **17**, 831–2.

Madaio, M.P. (1999). The role of autoantibodies in the pathogenesis of lupus nephritis. *Seminars in Nephrology* **19**, 48–56.

Madaio, M.P. and Yanase, K. (1998). Cellular penetration and nuclear localization of anti DNA antibodies: mechanisms, consequences, implications and applications. *Journal of Autoimmunity* **11** (5), 535–8.

Maddison, P., Farewell, V., Isenberg, D.A., Aranow, C., Bae, S.C., Barr, S., Buyon, J., Fortin, P., Ginzler, E., Gladman, D., Hanley, J., Manzi, S., Nived, O., Petri, M., Ramsey-Goldman, R., and Sturfelt, G. (2001). The rate and pattern of organ damage in late-onset systemic lupus erythematosus. *Journal of Rheumatology* **29**, 913–17.

Mamoune, A., Kerdreux, S., Durand, V., Saraux, A., Goff, P.L., Youinou, P., and Corre, R.L. (2000). CD45 autoantibodies mediate neutralization of activated T cells from lupus patients through anergy or apoptosis. *Lupus* **9** (8), 622–31.

Mamula, M.J., Fatenejad, S., and Craft, J. (1994). B cells process and present lupus autoantigens that initiate autoimmune T cell responses. *Journal of Immunology* **152**, 1453–61.

Mandell, B. (1987). Cardiovascular involvement in systemic lupus erythematosus. *Seminars in Arthritis and Rheumatism* **17**, 120–41.

Manzi, S. et al. (1999). Prevalence and risk factors of carotid plaque in women with systemic lupus erythematosus. *Arthritis and Rheumatism* **42**, 51–60.

Matsuda, J., Saitoh, N., Gohchi, I., Gotoh, M., and Tsukamoto, M. (1994). Detection of β2-glycoprotein 1-dependent antiphospholipid antibodies and anti-β2-glycoprotein 1 antibody in patients with systemic lupus erythematosus and in patients with syphilis. *International Archives of Allergy and Immunology* **103**, 239–44.

Matsukawa, Y., Sawada, S., Hayama, T., Usui, H., and Horie, T. (1994). Suicide in patients with systemic lupus erythematosus: a clinical analysis of seven suicidal patients. *Lupus* **3**, 31–5.

McHale, J.F., Harari, O.A., Marshall, D., and Haskard, D.O. (1999). TNF-alpha and IL-1 sequentially induce endothelial ICAM-1 and VCAM-1 expression in MRL/lpr lupus-prone mice. *Journal of Immunology* **163**, 3993–4000.

McLaughlin, J.R., Bombardier, C., Farewell, V.T., Gladman, D.A., and Urowitz, M.B. (1994). Kidney biopsy in systemic lupus erythematosus. III. Survival analysis, controlling for clinical and laboratory variables. *Arthritis and Rheumatism* **4**, 559–67.

Mellemkjaer, L., Andersen, V., Linet, M.J., Gridley, G., Hoover, R., and Olsen, J.H. (1997). Non-Hodgkin's lymphoma and other cancers among a cohort of patients with SLE. *Arthritis and Rheumatism* **40**, 761–8.

Menon, S., Jameson-Shortall, E., Newman, S.P., Hall-Craggs, M.R., Chinn, R., and Isenberg, D.A. (1999). A longitudinal study of anticardiolipin antibody levels and cognitive functioning in systemic lupus erythematosus. *Arthritis and Rheumatism* **42**, 735–41.

Miranda-Carus, M.E., Askanase, A.D., Clancy, R.M., Di Donato, F., Chou, T.M., Libera, M.R., Chan, E.K., and Buyon, J.P. (2000). Anti-SSA/Ro and anti-SSB/La autoantibodies bind the surface of apoptotic fetal cardiocytes and promote secretion of TNF-alpha by macrophages. *Journal of Immunology* **165** (9), 5345–51.

Mok, M.Y., Farewell, V.T., and Isenberg, D.A. (2000). Risk factors for avascular necrosis of bone in patients with systemic lupus erythematosus: is there a role for anti-phospholipid antibodies? *Annals of the Rheumatic Diseases* **59**, 462–7.

Morel, L., Blenman, K.R., Croker, B.P., and Wakeland, E.K. (2001). The major murine systemic lupus erythematosus susceptibility locus, Sle1, is a cluster of functionally related genes. *Proceedings of the National Academy Sciences USA* **98** (4), 1787–92.

Moss, K., Ioannou, Y., Sultan, S.M., Haq, I., and Isenberg, D.A. (2002). Outcome of a cohort of 300 patients with systemic lupus erythematosus attending a dedicated clinic for over two decades. *Annals of the Rheumatic Diseases* **61**, 409–13.

Mostoslavsky, G., Fischel, R., Yachimovich, N., Yarkoni, Y., Rosenmann, E., Monestier, M., Baniyash, M., and Eilat, D. (2001). Lupus anti-DNA autoantibodies cross-react with a glomerular structural protein: a case for tissue injury by molecular mimicry. *European Journal of Immunology* **4**, 1221–7.

Muller, M.H., Urowitz, M.B., Gladman, D.D., and Killinger, D.W. (1983). Systemic lupus erythematosus in males. *Medicine (Baltimore)* **62**, 327–34.

Murakami, M., Kumagai, S., Sugita, M., Iwai, K., and Imura, H. (1992). *In vitro* induction of IgG anti-DNA antibody from high density B cells of systemic lupus erythematosus patients by an HLA–DR-restricted T cell clone. *Clinical and Experimental Immunology* **90**, 245–50.

Nakamura, M., Tsunematsu, T., and Tanigawa, Y. (1998). TCR-alpha chain-like molecule is involved in the mechanism of antigen-non-specific suppression of a ubiquitin-like protein. *Immunology* **94**, 142–8.

Nived, O. and Sturfelt, G. (1997). Does the black population in Africa get SLE? If not why not. In *Controversies in Rheumatology* (ed. D.A. Isenberg and L.B. Tucker), pp. 65–74. London: Martin Dunitz Ltd.

Norris, D.A. (1993). Pathomechanisms of photosensitive lupus erythematosus. *Journal of Investigative Dermatology* **100**, 58S–68S (review).

Oku, K., Atsumi, T., Furukawa, S., Horita, T., Sakai, Y., Jodo, S., Amasaki, Y., Ichikawa, K., Amengual, O., and Koike, T. (2003). Cerebral imaging by magnetic resonance imaging and single photon emission computed tomography in systemic lupus erythematosus with central nervous system involvement. *Rheumatology* **42**, 773–7.

Olsen, M.L., Arnett, F.C., and Reveille, J.D. (1993). Contrasting molecule patterns of MHC class II alleles associated with the anti-Sm and anti-RNP precipitin autoantibodies in systemic lupus erythematosus. *Arthritis and Rheumatism* **36**, 94–104.

Ostendorf, B., Scherer, A., Specker, C., Modder, V., and Schneider, M. (2003). Jaccoud's arthropathy in systemic lupus erythematosus. *Arthritis and Rheumatism* **48**, 157–65.

Pettersson, T., Pukkala, I., Teppo, L., and Friman, C. (1992). Increased risk of cancer in patients with systemic lupus erythematosus. *Annals of the Rheumatic Diseases* **31**, 427–39.

Pistiner, M., Wallace, D.J. Nessim, S., Metzger, A.L., and Klinenberg, J.R. (1992). Lupus erythematosus in the 1980s: a survey of 570 patients. *Seminars in Arthritis and Rheumatism* **21**, 358–63.

Rahman, P., Gladman, D.S., Urowitz, M.B., Hallett, D., and Tam, L.S. (2001). Early damage as measured by the SLICC/ACR damage index is a predictor of mortality in systemic lupus erythematosus. *Lupus* **10**, 93–6.

Ramsey-Goldman, R., Mattai, S.A., and Schilling, E. (1998). Increased malignancy in patients with systemic lupus erythematosus. *Journal of Investigative Medicine* **46**, 217–22.

Reveille, J.D., Schrohenloher, R.E., Acton, R.T., and Barger, B.O. (1989). DNA analysis of HLA-DR and DQ genes in American blacks with systemic lupus erythematosus. *Arthritis and Rheumatism* **32**, 1243–51.

Scheinecker, C., Zwolfer, B., Koller, M., Manner, G., and Smolen, J.S. (2001). Alterations of dendritic cells in systemic lupus erythematosus: phenotypic and functional deficiencies. *Arthritis and Rheumatism* **44** (4), 856–65.

Schur, P.H., Marcus-Bagley, D., Awdeh, Z., Yunis, E.J., and Alper, C.A. (1990). The effect of ethnicity on major histocompatibility complex complement allotypes and extended haplotypes in patients with systemic lupus erythematosus. *Arthritis and Rheumatism* **33**, 985–92.

Schwartz, M. (1999). The pathological classification of lupus nephritis In *Lupus Nephritis* (ed. E.J. Lewis, M. Schwartz, and S.M. Korbet), pp. 126–58. Oxford: Oxford University Press.

Schwartz, M.M., Lan, S., Bernstein, J., Hill, G.S., Holley, K., and Lewis, E.J. (1993). Irreproducability of the activity and chronicity indices limits their utility in the management of lupus nephritis. *American Journal of Kidney Disease* **21**, 374–7.

Sfikakis, P.P., Charalambopoulos, D., Vayiopoulos, G., Oglesby, R., Sfikakis, P., and Tsokos, G.C. (1994). Increased levels of intercellular adhesion moleculel in the serum of patients with systemic lupus erythematosus. *Clinical and Experimental Rheumatology* **12**, 5–9.

Siegert, C.E., Kazatchkine, M.D., Sjoholm, A., Wurzner, R., Loos, M., and Daha, M.R. (1999). Autoantibodies against C1q: view on clinical relevance and pathogenic role. *Clinical and Experimental Immunology* **116** (1), 4–8.

Sieling, P.A., Porcelli, S.A., Duong, B.T., Spada, F., Bloom, B.R., Diamond, B., and Hahn, B.H. (2000). Human double-negative T cells in systemic lupus erythematosus provide help for IgG and are restricted by CD1c. *Journal of Immunology* **165**, 5338–44.

Sieving, R.R., Kauffman, C.A., and Watanakunakorn, C. (1975). Deep fungal infection in systemic lupus erythematosus—three cases reported, literature reviewed. *Journal of Rheumatology* **2**, 61–72.

Song, H., He, C., Knaak, C., Guthridge, J.M., Holers, V.M., and Tomlinson, S. (2003). Complement receptor 2-mediated targeting of complement inhibitors to sites of complement activation. *Journal of Clinical Investigation* **111**, 1875–85.

Spronk, P.E., ter Borg, E.J., and Kallenberg, C.G.M. (1992). Patients with systemic lupus erythematosus and Jaccoud's arthropathy: a clinical subset with an increased C reactive protein response. *Annals of the Rheumatic Diseases* **51**, 358–61.

Stamenkovic, I., Favre, H., Doneth, A., Assimacopoulos, A., and Chatelanet, F. (1986). Renal biopsy in systemic lupus erythematosus irrespective of clinical findings. Long term follow up. *Clinical Nephrology* **26**, 109–15.

Stoll, T. and Isenberg, A. (1966). SLICC/ACR damage index is valid and renal and pulmonary organ scores are predictors of severe outcome in patients with systemic lupus erythematosus. *British Journal of Rheumatology* **35**, 248–51.

Sullivan, K.E., Wooten, C., Goldman, D., and Petri, M. (1996). Mannose-binding protein genetic polymorphisms in black patients with systemic lupus erythematus. *Arthritis and Rheumatism* **39**, 2046–51.

Sultan, S.M., Ioannou, Y., and Isenberg, D.A. (1999). A review of gastrointestinal manifestations of systemic lupus erythematosus. *Rheumatology* **38**, 917–32.

Sultan, S.M., Ioannou, Y., and Isenberg, D.A. (2000). Is there an association of malignancy with SLE? An analysis of 276 patients under long-term review. *Rheumatology* **39**, 1147–52.

Sweeney, D.M., Manzi, S., and Janosky, J. (1995). Risk of malignancy in women with SLE. *Journal of Rheumatology* **22**, 1478–82.

Tan, E.M., Cohen, A.S., Fries, J.F., Masi, A.T., McShane, D.J., Rothfield, N.F., Schaller, J.G., Talal, N., and Winchester, R.J. (1982). The 1982 revised criteria for the classification of systemic lupus erythematosus. *Arthritis and Rheumatism* **25**, 1271–7.

Taylor, J. et al (2000). Lupus patients with fatigue—is there a link with fibromyalgia syndrome? *Rheumatology* **39**, 620–3.

Theofilopoulos, A.N., Singer, P.A., Kofler, R., Kono, D.H., Duchosal, M.A., and Balderas, R.S. (1989). B and T cell antigen receptor repertoires in lupus/arthritis murine models. *Springer Seminars in Immunopathology* **11**, 335–68.

Thumboo, J., Fong, K.Y., Chng, H.H., Koh, E.T., Chia, H.P., Leong, K.H., Koh, W.H., Howe, H.S., Leong, K.P., Wong, M.H., Chew, S.M., Chai. P., Goh, L.H., Goon, T.J., Lau, T.L., Lim, W.S., Pek, W.Y., Tong, K.L., Yang, W.L., Feng, P.H., and Boey, M.L. (1998). The effects of ethnicity on disease pattern in 472 Orientals with systemic lupus erythematosus. *Journal of Rheumatology* **25**, 1299–304.

Trebeden-Negre, H., Weill, B., Fournier, C., and Batteux, F. (2003). B cell apoptosis accelerates the onset of murine lupus. *European Journal of Immunology* **33**, 1603–12.

Tsao, B.P. (2000). Lupus susceptibility genes on human chromosome 1. *International Review of Immunology* **19** (4–5), 319–34.

Urowitz, M.B. and Gladman, D.A. (2000). Accelerated atheroma in lupus—background. *Lupus* **9**, 161–5.

Urowitz, M.B., Gladman, D.D., Farewell, V.T., Stewart, J., and McDonald, J. (1993). Lupus and pregnancy studies. *Arthritis and Rheumatism* **36**, 1392–7.

Vitali, C. et al. (1992). Disease activity in SLE: report of the consensus study group of the European Workshop for Rheumatology Research III: development of a computerised clinical chart and its application to the comparison of different indices of disease activity. *Clinical and Experimental Rheumatology* **10**, 549–54.

Wakeland, E.K., Wandstrat, A.E., Liu, K., and Morel, L. (1999). Genetic dissection of systemic lupus erythematosus. *Current Opinion in Immunology* **11**, 701–7.

Walport, M.J. (2000). Lupus, DNase and defective disposal of cellular debris. *Nature Genetics* **25** (2), 135–6.

Walport, M.J. and Lachmann, P.J. (1988). Erythrocyte complement receptor type I, immune complexes and the rheumatic diseases. *Arthritis and Rheumatism* **31**, 153–8.

Wang, B., Gladman, D.D., and Urowitz, M.B. (1998). Fatigue in lupus is not correlated with disease activity. *Journal of Rheumatology* **25**, 892–5.

Wellicome, S.M., Kapahi, P., Mason, J.C., Lebranchu, Y., Yarwood, H., and Haskard, D.O. (1993). Detection of a circulating form of vascular cell adhesion molecule-1: raised levels in rheumatoid arthritis and systemic lupus erythematosus. *Clinical and Experimental Immunology* **92**, 412–18.

Whiting-O'Keefe, Q., Henke, J.E., Sheard, M.A., Hopper, J., Jr., Biava, C.G., and Epstein, W.V. (1982). The information content from renal biopsy in systemic lupus erythematosus. Stepwise linear regression analysis. *Annals of Internal Medicine* **96**, 718–27.

Wong, H.K., Kammer, G.M., Dennis, G., and Tsokos, G.C. (1999). Abnormal NF-kappa B activity in T lymphocytes from patients with systemic lupus erythematosus is associated with decreased p65-RelA protein expression. *Journal of Immunology* **163**, 1682–9.

Wuthrich, R.P. (1992). Vascular cell adhesion molecule (VCAM-1) expression in murine lupus nephritis. *Kidney International* **42**, 903–14.

Wuthrich, R.P., Jevnikar, A.M., Takei, F., Glimcher, L.H., and Kelley, V.E. (1990). Intercellular adhesion molecule-1 (ICAM-1) expression is upregulated in autoimmune murine lupus nephritis. *American Journal of Pathology* **136**, 441–50.

Yamada, A., Minota, S., Nojima, Y., and Yazaki, Y. (1993). Changes in subset specificity of anti-T cell autoantibodies in systemic lupus erythematosus. *Autoimmunity* **14**, 269–73.

Yazici, Z.A., Raschi, E., Patel, A., Testoni, C., Borghi, M.O., Graham, A.M., Meroni, P.L., and Lindsey, N. (2001). Human monoclonal antiendothelial cell IgG-derived from a systemic lupus erythematosus patient binds activates human endothelium *in vitro*. *International Immunology* **13**, 349–57.

Zeng, D., Lee, M.K., Tung, J., Brendolan, A., and Strober, S. (2000). Cutting edge: a role for CD1 in the pathogenesis of lupus in NZB/NZW mice. *Journal of Immunology* **164** (10), 5000–4.

6.6.2 SLE—management in adults

David A. Isenberg and Anisur Rahman

The challenge of managing SLE

There are many possible manifestations of systemic lupus erythematosus (SLE) which often fluctuate markedly over time. The most severe manifestations are not necessarily the most symptomatic. It is necessary to control the patient's symptoms and to suppress the underlying disease adequately. The correct regimen of drugs to achieve both these goals, and to balance the need to treat aggressively on occasions mindful of the possible long term side effects of the agents used is essential.

The exact cause of the disease is not known. It is clear that SLE arises from abnormalities of the immune system, and that autoantibodies probably play an important role in causing its clinical features. Therapy targeted at those abnormalities remains problematic. Thus, treatment of SLE continues to rely upon the use of broad spectrum immunosuppressive agents with all their inherent difficulties.

Patients tend to be young and often female. Since the disease is suppressed but not cured by treatment, such patients may be faced with the prospect of taking potent drugs for years. The social and psychological effects of both the chronic disease and the necessity for continuing treatment must be recognized and addressed by physicians and patients. Potential effects of the drugs upon fertility or pregnancy are particularly important.

Non-pharmacological management

General measures which may be useful for patients with SLE include the avoidance of excessive sunlight. This is particularly important in fair-skinned people since solar radiation may not only cause photosensitive rash, but also a more general flare of symptoms. Rest as appropriate, a low-fat diet with added fish oil, and avoidance of oestrogen-containing contraceptive pills are also advised. Vaccinations apart from 'live' vaccines in patients on greater than 10 mg prednisolone and/or immunosuppressives are safe but the use of hormone replacement in patients past the menopause is still controversial.

Pharmacological management

Patients with SLE are treated with four main groups of drugs, often in combination. These are:

- non-steroidal anti-inflammatory drugs (NSAIDs),
- antimalarials,
- corticosteroids,
- cytotoxic drugs.

Recommendations about precisely when to commence therapy, the initial dose of a given drug, the likely response of a given symptom, and the duration of treatment vary widely. In Table 1, the broad indications for use of these four types of drugs are shown. In Table 2, suggestions are provided as to the initial doses and duration of treatment with the antimalarials, corticosteroids, and cytotoxic drugs. These are intended purely as guidelines and there will be patients who require larger doses for longer periods of time. Both Tables 1 and 2 make the point that different regimens of drugs are suitable for different manifestations of the disease.

Treatment with NSAIDs and antimalarials

In general, the patient with mildly active lupus can be managed with combinations of NSAIDs and antimalarials. Lupus patients are at no lesser risk of gastrointestinal and renal complications of the NSAIDs than other patients, and thus careful monitoring is required.

Hydroxychloroquine (Plaquenil) is the antimalarial drug of choice. It is commonly used in cases where the main symptoms are fatigue, rash, and arthralgia, without evidence of major organ involvement. The efficacy of hydroxychloroquine in such cases was supported by a small randomized controlled trial (Canadian Hydroxychloroquine Study Group 1991). Patients with SLE who discontinued hydroxychloroquine were more likely to suffer flares of rash, arthralgia, and fatigue than those who continued taking the drug. Retinal toxicity sufficient to cause reduced visual acuity occurs in about 1 in 1800 cases. Although a recent review found no conclusive evidence that regular retinal monitoring by an ophthalmologist is necessary when taking hydroxychloroquine (Silman and Shipley 1997), many units choose to carry out such monitoring every 6–9 months.

Whereas many patients with cutaneous SLE respond well to hydroxychloroquine, a minority may require treatment with a combination of hydroxychloroquine and quinacrine or with more potent agents such as dapsone or thalidomide.

Treatment with corticosteroids

Corticosteroids in the main are required when NSAIDs and antimalarials are insufficient to relieve the patient's symptoms. Thus, these drugs (usually in moderate doses up to 30 mg/day) may be used in severe arthritis, pleuritis, or pericarditis. Corticosteroids are used at higher dosages where SLE causes more severe effects, which may in some cases be life threatening. Examples are autoimmune haemolytic anaemia and thrombocytopaenia, nephritis, and a wide range of neuropsychiatric problems.

Corticosteroids are usually prescribed and taken by mouth but may also be given intramuscular or intravenously. Intravenous pulse therapy has been widely used in the past 20 years. If given over a 15–20 min period there is a danger of reactive arthropathy, and in our experience intravenous pulses are best given slowly over a 3–4 h period. We use pulse therapy: for example, 1 g on 3 successive days for patients with severe disease not responding to oral corticosteroids. Although some claims have been made

Table 1 Drug therapy in systemic lupus

	NSAID	Antimalarial	Corticosteroids	Cytotoxic agents
Malaise	+	+	+	−
Fever	+	−	+	−
Serositis	+	−	+	−
Arthralgia	+	+	+	−
Arthritis	+	+	+	+
Myalgia	+	+	+	−
Myositis	−	−	+	+
Malar/discoid rash	−	+	+	−
Pneumonitis	−	−	+	+
Carditis	−	−	+	+
Vasculitis	−	−	+	+
CNS disease	−	−	?[a]	?
Renal	−	−	+	+
Haemolytic anaemia	−	−	+	+
Thrombocytopaenia	−	−	+	+
Raynaud's	−	−	?	?
Alopecia	−	−	?	?

[a] Widely prescribed but doubts remain that steroids are beneficial in many cases.

Note: + = usually beneficial; − = not beneficial; ? = dubious/controversial.

Table 2 Recommendations for drug usage in lupus

Symptom	Drugs to try	Dose and duration
Arthralgia	Non-steroidal anti-inflammatory drugs	No special recommendations
Myalgia Lethargy Arthralgia	Hydroxychloroquine	Start 400 mg/day for 3–4 months then reduce to 200 mg/day for 3–4 months, then to 200 mg five times week for 3–4 months; repeat courses may be necessary and retinal checks every 6–9 months are generally recommended
Arthritis Pleuritis Pericarditis	Prednisolone	20–40 mg per day initially for 2–4 weeks, reducing in 5–10 mg increments per week, if patient is responding; treatment is likely to be required for several months
Autoimmune haemolytic anaemia/thrombocytopaenia	Prednisolone often accompanied by azathioprine	60–80 mg prednisolone for 1–2 weeks reducing in 10 mg increments in response to the blood test results; aim for 2.5–3 mg/kg azathioprine; treatment will last for several months
Renal	Prednisolone plus azathioprine or cyclophosphamide	Depending upon the severity of the renal lesion, anything from 30–80 mg/day is required; cyclophosphamide can be given by intravenous boluses (750 mg–1 g) monthly for 6 months, then every 3 months for 2 years; some groups prefer prednisolone and azathioprine at 2–3 mg/kg in the first instance; treatment is likely to be required for several years
Central nervous system	Prednisolone plus an appropriate drug, e.g. an antidepressant, anticonvulsant, etc.	Controversial—but 20–100 mg prednisolone have been prescribed (sometimes accompanied by azathioprine or intravenous cyclophosphamide pulses); treatment is likely to be required for months

about its advantages the evidence that anything more than a temporary benefit is obtained is controversial.

Evidence that alternate day oral steroid regimes reduce the number or the severity of side effects compared to daily use is lacking. The major side effects, however, if corticosteroids are prescribed, are increased risk of infection, osteoporosis, diabetes, hypertension, Cushingoid facies, abdominal striae, and insomnia. They are thus no panacea. It is important to take these side effects into account in planning a course of high dose corticosteroids. For example, a patient with diabetes will need closer monitoring of his or her blood glucose level and may have to take a higher dose of antidiabetic medication. The risk of osteoporosis must be considered in all patients who are going to take 7.5 mg prednisolone/day or more for a period of several months. Patients are advised to take calcium and vitamin D supplements to reduce the risk of corticosteroid-induced osteoporosis. Some will be offered bisphosphonates, such as alendronate or residronate, which have a greater protective effect on bone but also have more side effects. The introduction of DEXA scanning offers a simple and effective way of monitoring bone loss, and should be repeated every 18–24 months in those on regular oral steroids.

Cytotoxic drugs

Various controlled trials of cytotoxic drugs in lupus have been reported. The group from the National Institutes of Health at Bethesda has argued strongly that intravenous boluses of cyclophosphamide, monthly for 6 months and subsequently every 3 months for 2 years are the treatment of choice in patients with severe renal involvement (Boumpas et al. 1991, 1992, 1993). The problems of side-effects with this drug (profound nausea, alopecia, infertility especially in patients over 30, neoplasia, bladder toxicity, and bone marrow suppression) have made others more wary about its routine use. In common with many European groups, we prefer to use steroids and maintenance azathioprine in the first instance for patients with mild/moderately active renal disease. Occasionally, however, we have seen patients being treated with steroids and azathioprine for other manifestations who develop severe renal disease and require cyclophosphamide urgently. Whatever immunosuppressive regime is chosen a key element in managing renal lupus is controlling the blood pressure. Very often, in severe cases, a combination of antihypertensives (e.g. a diuretic, an angiotensin converting enzyme inhibitor, and a beta blocker) is required for adequate control.

For those patients in whom renal failure develops in spite of immunosuppressive therapy dialysis and/or renal transplantation are required. Unfortunately, as Stone et al. (1997) have reviewed, lupus patients who receive renal transplants do not fare as well as those patients whose end stage renal disease has other causes. However, it is rare for a lupus patient with a transplanted kidney to develop lupus nephritis in the new organ.

Azathioprine may also be used as a steroid-sparing agent in cases where it proves difficult to reduce the dose of oral prednisolone without causing a flare of symptoms. A patient, for example, who normally develops severe pleuritic pain at doses of prednisolone below 10 mg daily, may remain free of symptoms on 5 mg prednisolone and 100 mg azathioprine daily.

There have been surprisingly few studies of methotrexate in the treatment of SLE. Most of these studies have been retrospective and of relatively few patients. There are some data to suggest that methotrexate may be useful for mildly active disease and as a 'steroid sparer' (Carneiro and Sato 1999) and to treat antimalarial resistant lupus arthritis (Rahman et al. 1998).

Mycophenolate mofetil is a relatively new immunosuppressive drug, which is sometimes used in cases of severe SLE that have proved resistant to other cytotoxic agents. A combination of prednisolone and mycophenolate mofetil has been compared with prednisolone and oral cyclophosphamide in the treatment of renal SLE (Chan et al. 2000). Both regimes were equally effective but mycophenolate had fewer major side-effects. Use of this agent is likely to increase in the future, especially as it lacks some of the more troublesome side-effects of cyclophosphamide.

A flow diagram of the way we use drugs to treat the various aspects of lupus is shown in Boxes 1 and 2.

The main side-effects of drugs used commonly in SLE are shown in Table 3, together with the measures that can be taken to prevent them.

Other 'standard' treatments

Plasma exchange

In the late 1970s and early 1980s there was a great vogue for using plasma exchange (Wei et al. 1983). The concept was that the removal of circulating, presumptively pathogenic, immune complexes offered a therapeutic advantage. In practice, it became evident that in some patients a 'rebound'

Box 1 Flow diagram of the management of non-renal systemic lupus that forms the basis of our practice

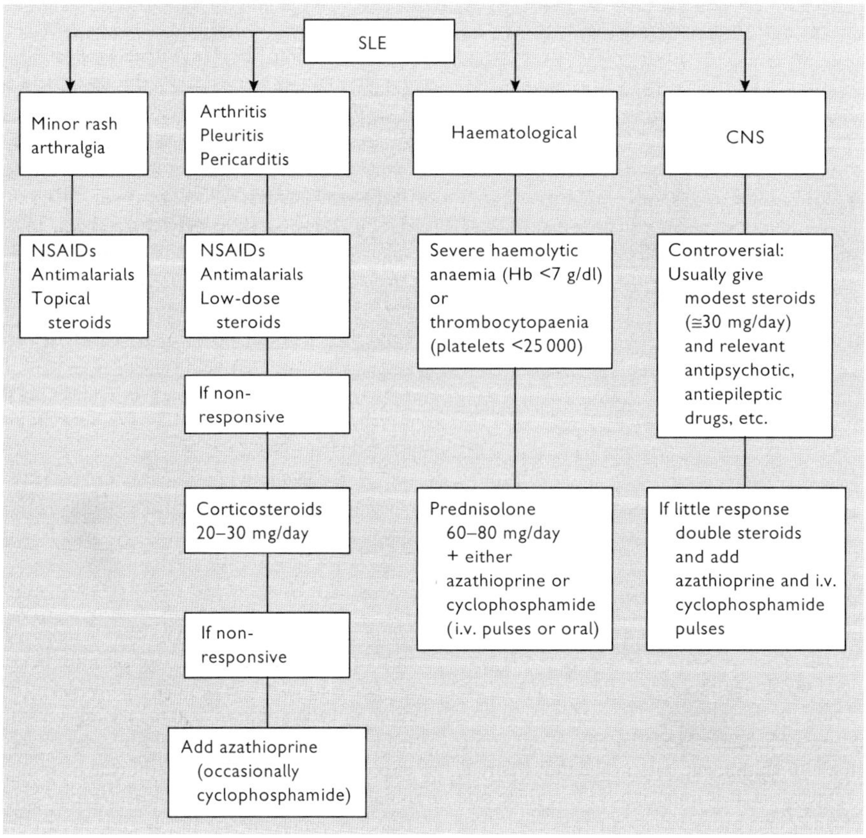

Box 2 Flow diagram of the management of renal SLE based on our own practice

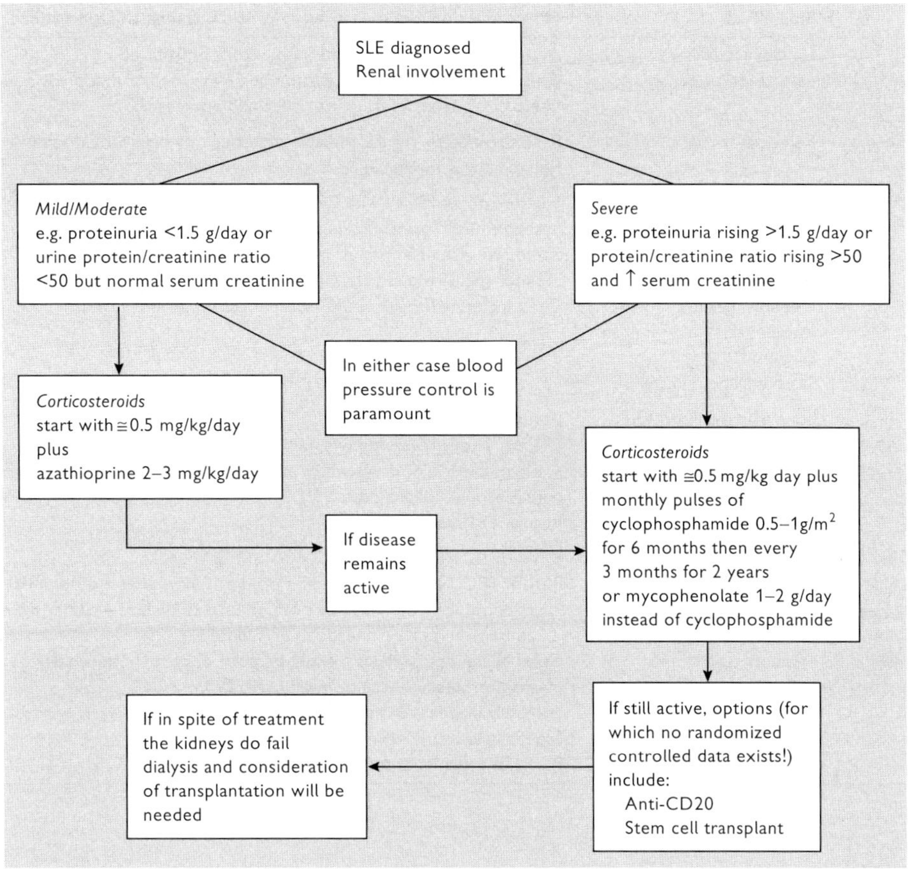

phenomenon occurred in which patients' symptoms and signs dramatically improved but returned within a few days or weeks. This form of treatment requires good venous access, much patience on the part of both physician and patient, and is extremely expensive. As reviewed elsewhere (McClure and Isenberg 1997) controlled studies failed to provide convincing evidence of real benefit. Even combining plasma exchange with subsequent pulse cyclophosphamide did not provide additional clinical benefit compared to pulse cyclophosphamide alone (Schroeder et al. 1997).

Lymphoid irradiation

Fractionated total lymphoid irradiation has been shown to improve survival in some murine models of lupus. This treatment has not found widespread acceptance in patients. Another form of radiation using ultraviolet A1, has been shown to reduce disease activity in patients in a provisional study (McGrath 1994).

Diet therapy

Many lupus patients are anxious to know if some form of dietary modification might be of help. Supplementation of the diet by fish oils has been shown to be beneficial. In a double-blind cross-over study in which all the lupus patients were put on to low-fat diets, those who were concurrently taking 10 g of fish oil per day were shown to have done significantly better over a 6 month period (Walton et al. 1991).

Intravenous high-dose gammaglobulins

Intravenous high-dose gammaglobulins (IvIg) may be effective in the treatment of immune thrombocytopaenic purpura, immune neutropaenia, and myasthenia gravis. This treatment has also been used with moderate success in lupus patients with low platelet counts. It has recently been claimed that monthly IvIg may be a useful alternative to intravenous cyclophosphamide in the treatment of lupus nephritis (Boletis et al. 1999). A randomized control trial is needed to confirm this claim. When this approach does not work for patients with thrombocytopaenia, splenectomy is beneficial in four or five out of six cases, provided the problem has not been left to become long term and chronic (Hakim et al. 1998).

Cyclosporin/neoral therapy

Following the failure of original attempts to use cyclosporin (because the dose was too high and caused nephrotoxicity) (Isenberg et al. 1981), there was something of a moratorium on its use in patients with SLE. Recently, several investigators (e.g. Caccavo et al. 1997) have shown that a dose of 2.5–5 mg/kg does provide reasonable disease control and enables steroid reduction over long term follow-up. However, hypertrichosis develops in the majority of patients and it is best avoided in the presence of significant renal disease.

Sex hormone therapy

Given the marked predilection of lupus for females, it is not surprising that attempts have been made to treat the condition by manipulating the level of sex hormones.

However, the clinical use of sex hormones in lupus and other autoimmune diseases has neither been extensive nor particularly successful. One drug, Danazol, an androgen with reduced virilizing capacity has been used by several groups; as is so often the case with new drugs, the initial optimism has given way to the view that it adds little to the treatment of lupus. Another androgen, dehydroepiandrosterone (DHEA) was shown in a single study to reduce the requirement for steroids in patients with SLE.

Table 3 Major side-effects of drugs commonly used in SLE

Drug	Side effect	Notes and possible measures to protect against this side-effect
NSAIDs	Gastrointestinal irritation/bleeding	Avoid using NSAID in patients with history of GI bleed Co-prescribe H2 blocker or proton pump inhibitor or misoprostol Use COX-2 selective drug (e.g. rofecoxib or celecoxib)
Hydroxychloroquine	Retinopathy	Rare side-effect—regular retinal monitoring may help early diagnosis Retinopathy is reversible by stopping the drug
Corticosteroids	Osteoporosis	Measure bone density with DEXA scan. Prescription of calcium/vitamin D supplements for most patients on long term steroids Some may also need oral or i.v. bisphosphonates
	Hypertension	Monitor regularly and treat with standard antihypertensives
	Diabetes mellitus	Checking urine for glucose is usually sufficient for monitoring
	Weight gain	
	Hirsutism	
	Susceptibility to infection	
Azathioprine	Bone marrow toxicity	Regular FBC measurements Effect is usually reversible when drug is stopped Avoid co-prescibing drugs which potentiate the effect of azathioprine (e.g. allopurinol and captopril)
	Liver dysfunction	Regular LFT measurements Effect is usually reversible when the drug is stopped
Cyclophosphamide	Bone marrow toxicity	Regular FBC. Nadir in white count occurs 10 days after a dose of i.v. cyclophosphamide. This value can be used to deduce whether the next dose can be given safely or needs to be reduced
	Haemorrhagic cystitis	Good hydration (i.v. fluids if giving i.v. pulse of cyclophosphamide) Mesna is protective—can be given orally or i.v.
	Increased risk of malignancy	Especially bladder carcinoma and lymphoma
	Infertility and amenorrhoea	Especially in women over the age of 30
	Nausea	Powerful antiemetics such as granisetron may be necessary

Newer forms of therapy

A variety of biological agents are being investigated as potential therapies for patients with SLE. These reagents have been developed to interfere with a range of immunological reactions including T cell activation, T cell–B cell collaboration, anti-dsDNA antibody production, deposition of anti-dsDNA antibody complexes, complement activation and deposition, and cytokine activation and modulation. Recently stem cell transplantation has been attempted (Traynor et al. 2000) and anti-CD20 therapy is being used in some centres (Leandro et al. 2002). For a more comprehensive review of these and other possible approaches including bromocryptine and leflunomide, the reader is referred to Remer et al. (2001).

LJP 394

LJP 394 is a drug that has been developed specifically to inactivate B cells which produce anti-dsDNA antibodies. The drug consists of four oligonucleotides, each 20 bases in length, which are attached to an inert scaffold. When these nucleotides bind surface Ig anti-dsDNA molecules on B cells, they can cross link those molecules. This leads to anergy or deletion of the B cells rather than activation, because the drug molecule does not carry any T-cell epitopes and cannot recruit T-cell help. More recently, it was demonstrated that treatment with LJP 394 delayed time to renal flare and reduced number of renal flares, but only in those patients who possessed high affinity antibodies to the drug (Alarcon Segonia et al. 2003).

LJP 394 has been shown to reduce serum anti-dsDNA antibodies and lengthen life in mouse models of SLE (Coutts et al. 1996). In a recent clinical trial, only weekly intravenous doses of 10 or 50 mg consistently reduced anti-dsDNA levels in patients with SLE and the effect on disease activity was no better than placebo. In a larger trial, there was no evidence that the drug reduced the rate of renal flares of SLE (Furie et al. 2001). More recently, it was demonstrated that treatment with LJP 394 delayed time to renal flare and reduced number of renal flares, but only in those patients who possessed high affinity antibodies to the drug (Alarcon Segovia et al. 2003).

Anti-cytokine agents

Evidence from animal studies and cytokine measurements in patients suggests that a number of cytokines may be involved in the pathogenesis of SLE. This raises the possibility that drugs which either promote or antagonize the effects of these cytokines might be useful in treating the disease. IL-10 levels are consistently elevated in the blood of patients with SLE, and monoclonal anti-IL-10 antibodies have recently been used to treat six patients with SLE for 21 days each (Llorente et al. 2000). These patients reported improvements of the skin and joints, which persisted for up to 6 months in the majority of cases. Anticytokine drugs, however, are expensive and their utility in more severe forms of SLE, such as glomerulonephritis, has not been demonstrated. Anti-TNFα drugs used in rheumatoid arthritis may be associated with the production of anti-dsDNA antibodies and, rarely, the development of a lupus-like syndrome (Ioannou and Isenberg 2000).

Anti-CD40 ligand antibody

The interaction between CD40, which is present on antigen presenting cells, and CD40 ligand (L) expressed on T cells provides an important costimulus to the activation of T cells. This interaction also has significant effects on B cells for example augmenting B-cell responses to cytokines and causing antibody isotype switching. Monoclonal antibodies to CD40L have been used to treat patients with lupus and in at least one case found to be safe and well tolerated (Davis 2001). However, fears about this approach causing major vascular events (e.g. infarcts and strokes) have yet to be allayed (Boumpas et al. 2003).

Leflunomide

Leflunomide is known to inhibit the pyrimidine synthesis pathway, thus blocking RNA and DNA synthesis in T- and B cells and inhibiting proliferation of these cells. The first studies of this drug in the treatment of SLE have appeared (e.g. Remer et al. 2001). It appears to be safe and reasonably efficacious in short-term studies. However, randomized controlled long-term studies are needed.

Management in special situations

Pregnancy

Since most patients with SLE are women during the child bearing years it is not surprising that the question of managing pregnancy is a significant issue for many. It is important to recognize that around 25 per cent of lupus patient pregnancies do not go to full term (i.e. well in excess of the figure of approximately 10 per cent of pregnancies in healthy women). Those patients with antiphospholipid antibodies are especially likely to suffer recurrent miscarriages. Those with anti-Ro or anti-La antibodies have a small (1 : 20) chance of having a child with the neonatal lupus syndrome. Those patients with renal disease have to be watched very closely during pregnancy and on occasion it may be hard to distinguish a renal flare from pre-eclamptic toxaemia. We strongly recommend co-managing SLE patients with an interested obstetrician. The overall guide to management is shown in Box 3.

Coincident antiphospholipid antibody syndrome (APS)

Perhaps 10 per cent of patients with SLE also have APS and even more (around 25 per cent) have antiphospholipid antibodies. The 'balance of disease' may go in either direction and on occasion we have seen a patient deemed to have primary APS develop SLE over time. Mainly, however, in our experience SLE is diagnosed first.

Managing the APS component of those with both conditions is little different from patients who have primary APS. Problems may arise in particular when an overlap patient of this type presents with hypertension and mild proteinuria. Invariably a renal biopsy will be needed to ascertain to what extent the kidneys have been affected by multiple small thrombi and/or 'lupus' glomerulonephritis. In some patients, therapy with both immunosuppressives and long-term anticoagulants is needed.

Box 3 Flow diagram of the management of SLE in pregnancy

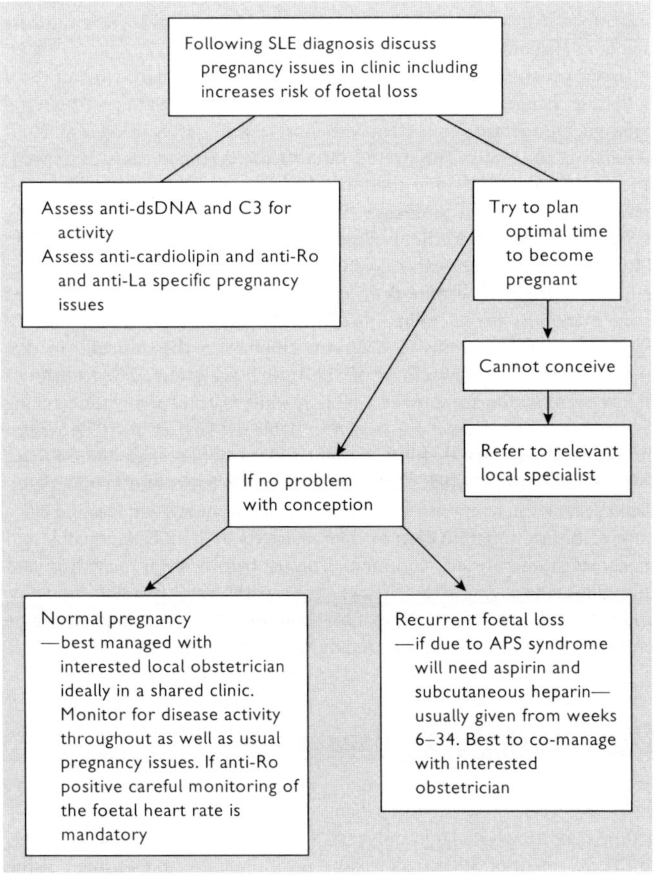
Following SLE diagnosis discuss pregnancy issues in clinic including increases risk of foetal loss
Assess anti-dsDNA and C3 for activity
Assess anti-cardiolipin and anti-Ro and anti-La specific pregnancy issues
Try to plan optimal time to become pregnant
Cannot conceive
Refer to relevant local specialist
If no problem with conception
Normal pregnancy —best managed with interested local obstetrician ideally in a shared clinic. Monitor for disease activity throughout as well as usual pregnancy issues. If anti-Ro positive careful monitoring of the foetal heart rate is mandatory
Recurrent foetal loss —if due to APS syndrome will need aspirin and subcutaneous heparin— usually given from weeks 6–34. Best to co-manage with interested obstetrician

Other situations

With the recognized increase in atherosclerosis observed in patients with lupus (see Chapter 6.6.1) it has become more important to monitor lipid levels over time. Advice on other modifiable risk factors such as exercise and cessation of smoking may be beneficial. Plaquenil has been shown to lower these levels and lower the risk of thrombotic events (Petrie et al. 1996) but if insufficient a statin is likely to be required.

Prognosis and survival

Studies on duration of disease and overall survival rates have frequently been confounded by the numbers of patients lost to follow-up and inadequate attention paid to the ethnic group, age of onset, and socio-economic status of individual patients. With these possible confounding factors in mind, and the division of lupus patients into those with overt nephritis and those without, it is reasonable to state that the five year survival in lupus is presently 90 per cent or greater, but at 15 years only 60 per cent of those with nephritis will still be alive compared to around 85 per cent of those without nephritis. In the United States, it has been claimed that black lupus patients, males, those from poorer socio-economic groups and possibly children, have poorer survival, especially if nephritis is present. It has also been suggested that there exists a bimodal mortality curve. Patients who die within 5 years usually have very active disease, with a requirement for substantial doses of steroids and other immunosuppressives. Those patients dying much later tend to do so from cardiovascular disease and possibly infection. Overall, most lupus patients die from active generalized disease, malignancy, sepsis, nephritis, and cardiovascular disease. Evidence that lupus patients may be more predisposed to malignancy has been discussed in a previous chapter.

Summary

Over the last 50 years, the prognosis of SLE has improved considerably. The introduction of corticosteroids and later of cytotoxic drugs were the major contributors to this improvement. Nevertheless, the treatment and general management of lupus continues to present a challenge. While lupus may for some patients represent a relatively mild set of problems, many others require large doses of immunosuppressive drugs, which carry long-term concerns about side-effects. New drugs, with actions more closely targeted to the pathogenesis of SLE are being introduced. The role of cardiovascular disease as a cause of death in patients with SLE is increasingly recognized and will present further challenges in the future.

References

Alarcon Segovia, D. et al. (2003). LJP394 for the prevention of renal flare in patients with systemic lupus erythematosus. *Arthritis and Rheumatism* **48**, 442–54.

Boletis, J.N. et al. (1999). Intravenous immunoglobulin compared with cyclophosphamide for proliferative lupus nephritis. *Lancet* **354**, 569–70.

Boumpas, D.T. et al. (1991). Pulse cyclophosphamide for severe neuropsychiatric lupus. *Quarterly Journal of Medicine* **81**, 975–84.

Boumpas, D.T. et al. (1992). Controlled trial of methylprednisolone versus two regimens of pulse cyclophosphamide in severe lupus nephritis. *Lancet* **340**, 741–5.

Boumpas, D.T. et al. (1993). Risk for sustained amenorrhoea in patients with systemic lupus erythematosus receiving intermittent pulse cyclophosphamide therapy. *Annals of Internal Medicine* **119**, 366–9.

Boumpas, D.T. et al. (2003). A short course of BG9588 (anti-CD40 ligand antibody) improves serologic activity and decreases hematuria in patients with proliferative lupus glomerulonephritis. *Arthritis ad Rheumatism* **48**, 719–27.

Caccavo, D. et al. (1997). Long term treatment of systemic lupus erythematosus with cyclosporin A. *Arthritis and Rheumatism* **40**, 27–35.

Canadian Hydroxychloroquine Study Group (1991). A randomized study of the effect of withdrawing hydroxychloroquine sulphate in systemic lupus erythematosus. *New England Journal of Medicine* **324**, 150–4.

Carneiro, J.R.M. and Sato, E.M. (1999). Double blind randomized, placebo controlled clinical trial of methotrexate in systemic lupus erythematosus. *Journal of Rheumatology* **26**, 1275–9.

Chan, T.M. et al. (2000). Efficacy of mycophenolate mofetil in patients with diffuse proliferative lupus nephritis. *New England Journal of Medicine* **343**, 1156–62.

Coutts, S.M. et al. (1996). Pharmacological intervention in antibody mediated disease. *Lupus* **5**, 158–9.

Davis, J.C., Jr. (2001). Phase 1 clinical trial of a monoclonal antibody against CD40-Ligand (IDEC-131) in patients with systemic lupus erythematosus. *Journal of Rheumatology* **28**, 95–101.

Furie, R.A. et al. (2001). Treatment of systemic lupus erythematosus with LJP 394. *Journal of Rheumatology* **28**, 257–65.

Hakim, A., Machin, S.J., and Isenberg, D.A. (1998). Autoimmune thrombocytopenia in primary antiphospholipid syndrome and systemic lupus erythematosus: the response to splenectomy. *Seminars in Arthritis and Rheumatism* **28**, 20–5.

Ioannou, Y. and Isenberg, D.A. (2000). Current evidence for the induction of autoimmune rheumatic manifestations by cytokine therapy. *Arthritis and Rheumatism* **43**, 1431–42.

Isenberg, D.A. et al. (1981). Cyclosporin A for the treatment of systemic lupus erythematosus. *International Journal of Immunopharmacology* **3**, 163–9.

Leandro, M.J. et al. (2002). An open study of B lymphocyte depletion in systemic lupus erythematosus. *Arthritis and Rheumatism* **46**, 2673–7.

Llorente, L. et al. (2000). Clinical and biologic effects of anti-interleukin-10 monoclonal antibody administration in systemic lupus erythematosus. *Arthritis and Rheumatism* **43**, 1790–800.

McClure, C.E. and Isenberg, D.A. (1997). Does plasma exchange have any part to play in the management of SLE? In *Controversies in Rheumatology* (ed. D.A. Isenberg and L.B. Tucker), pp. 75–86. London: Martin Dunitz.

McGrath, H., Jr. (1994). Ultra-violet-A1 irradiation decreases clinical disease activity and autoantibodies in patients with systemic lupus erythematosus. *Clinical and Experimental Rheumatology* **12**, 129–35.

Petrie, M. (1996). Hydroxychloroquine use in the Baltimore Lupus Cohort: effects on lipids, glucose and thrombosis. *Lupus* **5** (Suppl. 1), 516–22.

Rahman, P. et al. (1998). Efficacy and tolerability of methotrexate in antimalarial resistant lupus arthritis. *Journal of Rheumatology* **25**, 243–6.

Remer, C.F., Weisman, M.H., and Wallace, D.J. (2001). Benefits of leflunomide in systemic lupus erythematosus: a pilot observational study. *Lupus* **10**, 480–3.

Silman, A. and Shipley, M. (1997). Ophthalmologic monitoring for hydroxychloroquine toxicity: a scientific review of the available data. *British Journal of Rheumatology* **36**, 599–601.

Stone, J.H., Amend, and W.J.C., and Criswell, L.A. (1997). Outcome of renal transplantation in systemic lupus erythematosus. *Seminars in Arthritis and Rheumatism* **27**, 17–26.

Traynor, A.E. et al. (2000). Treatment of severe systemic lupus erythematosus with high dose chemotherapy and haemopoietic stem-cell transplantation: a phase 1 study. *Lancet* **356**, 701–7.

Walton, A.J.E. et al. (1991). Dietary fish oil reduces the severity of symptoms in patients with SLE. *Annals of the Rheumatic Diseases* **33**, 463–6.

Wei, N., Klippel, J.H., and Husto, D.P. (1983). Randomised trial of plasma exchange in mild SLE. *Lancet* **i**, 17–22.

6.6.3 Paediatric systemic lupus erythematosus

Earl D. Silverman and Diane Hebert

Systemic lupus erythematosus (SLE) in children and adolescents has many features in common with adult-onset SLE. This chapter, rather than fully reviewing all the possible presentations and manifestations of SLE will highlight the differences between paediatric SLE and adult-onset lupus. This chapter will not cover topics such as immunopathogenesis, cytokines, and animal models which are outlined in Chapter 6.6.1, nor will it cover antiphospholipid antibodies in depth. Rather, it should serve as a complementary chapter and will place its emphasis on unique features and provide an overview of general features of paediatric SLE. We suggest reading both chapters on SLE. A separate section of this chapter will cover neonatal lupus erythematosus.

Incidence

The epidemiological data on paediatric SLE is limited. The best data suggests an incidence of six cases per 100 000 white females of less than 15 years of age as compared with an overall incidence of 25 cases per 100 000 white females of all ages. The incidence rate rapidly rose to 18.9 cases per 100 000 white females aged between 15 and 25 years. Therefore, the incidence of SLE beginning prior to age 19 is likely between 6 and 18.9 cases per 100 000 in white females, and higher in black (20–30 per 100 000) and Puerto Rican females (16–36.7 per 100 000) (Siegel and Lee 1973). Most series of SLE patients with a large number of paediatric cases state that 20 per cent of all cases of SLE have onset prior to age 18 (Kaufman et al. 1986; Reeves and Lahita 1987). It is likely that the incidence of SLE beginning prior to age 18 is 10–20 cases per 100 000 children and adolescents, with an overall prevalence of 10–20 cases per 10 000 people less than 18 years old. These rates are higher in Hispanic, black, and oriental people.

In our patients, we found a male : female ratio of paediatric SLE of 1 : 4.4 with little change in the ratio for pre-pubertal as compared to post-pubertal children. Our data are consistent with most larger reviews (King et al. 1977; Lehman et al. 1989). The overall ratio of male : female cases of approximately 1 : 4.5 suggests that there is a higher percentage of male cases in paediatric SLE than in adult cases of SLE.

In most case series, the average age at diagnosis varied from 11 to 14 years (median 12.2 years). The youngest reported case of SLE was in a 9-month-old girl. The time from onset of symptoms to diagnosis varied from 8 months to 3.3 years (median 1.2 years). This median time of 1.2 years from symptoms to diagnosis emphasizes the difficulty in diagnosis or the lack of awareness of SLE in this age group. The features of SLE at presentation are shown in Table 1; while features at any time during the course of the disease are shown in Table 2 (King et al. 1977; Caeiro et al. 1981; Yancey et al. 1981; Schaller 1982; Glidden et al. 1983; Emery 1986; Kaufman et al. 1986; Lehman et al. 1989; Lacks and White 1990). General systemic symptoms such as fever, malaise, and weight loss and evidence of diffuse inflammation as demonstrated by lymphadenopathy and hepatosplenomegaly are common. This is true both at diagnosis and throughout the course of the disease. Nephropathy, fever, lymphadenopathy, and the requirement for the use of corticosteroids have been reported to be more common in children than in adults (Tucker et al. 1995).

Musculoskeletal disease

Arthritis and arthralgia are among the most common symptoms occurring in 70–90 per cent of cases. Most patients with arthritis have a symmetric polyarthritis affecting both large and small joints. The arthritis usually responds to the treatment of other major organ involvement or to treatment of the

Table 1 Clinical features: at diagnosis

	Other series (%)	Our series (%)
Fever	60–90	55
Arthritis	60–88	78
Any skin rash	60–78	79
Malar rash	22–60	36
Renal	20–80	61
Cardiovascular	5–30	14
Pulmonary	18–40	18
Central nervous system	5–30	25
Gastrointestinal	14–30	19
Hepatosplenomegaly	16–42	30
Lymphadenopathy	13–45	34

Table 2 Clinical features: at anytime during the course

	Other series (%)	Our series (%)
Fever	80–100	86
Arthritis	60–90	80
Any skin rash	60–90	86
Malar rash	30–80	38
Renal	48–100	69
Cardiovascular	25–60	17
Pulmonary	18–81	18
Central nervous system	26–44	34
Gastrointestinal[a]	24–40	24
Hepatosplenomegaly	19–43	30
Lymphadenopathy[a]	13–45	34

[a] Not included in follow-up data in many paediatric series.

general systemic symptoms. Severely painful joints are common and usually the pain is out of proportion to the physical findings. In most cases, there is no radiographic evidence of joint destruction or of deformity. However, in 1–2 per cent of cases of lupus arthritis there is a deforming erosive arthritis as seen in seropositive juvenile chronic arthritis. A more common cause of joint deformities is secondary to ligamentous laxity and periarticular fibrosis, the so-called Jaccoud's arthritis. This can result in deformity of the hand with multiple joint subluxations but with good preservation of function. Radiographs show only osteoporosis without evidence of erosions or joint space loss. Jaccoud's arthritis is more of a periarticular rather than an articular disease and is usually restricted to the hands. Tenosynovitis is common. Of particular interest have been the reports of patients with definite juvenile chronic arthritis that develop SLE years later. Initial reports had shown a transformation from polyarticular rather than systemic juvenile chronic arthritis to SLE (Saulsbury et al. 1982); however, we and others, have seen transformation from systemic juvenile-onset chronic arthritis to SLE (Citera et al. 1993).

Myalgia, as part of the generalized disease process, occurs in approximately 50–60 per cent of paediatric cases, while true myositis with proximal muscle weakness or tenderness occurs in less than 10 per cent of cases. Primary muscle involvement must be differentiated from muscle weakness secondary to steroid treatment. In contrast to clinically detectable muscle involvement, a pathology study in adults, demonstrated evidence of immune deposits in one-third of all patients.

The other steroid-induced musculoskeletal side-effects include avascular necrosis, osteoporosis with fracture or vertebral body collapse, and growth failure if prolonged high-dose steroids are required. Growth failure may be alleviated partially by alternate-day dose regimens but even using these it still remains a problem.

Avascular necrosis occurs in approximately 10–15 per cent of paediatric cases and appears to be more common in children than adults. In our experience, avascular necrosis occurs more commonly in SLE than other paediatric autoimmune diseases where prolonged high-dose steroids are used. Usually avascular necrosis is related to the dose and duration of therapy and the use of early prolonged high dose steroids but there have been case reports of it developing prior to or without steroid usage. Although it was initially proposed that there was an increased risk of avascular necrosis in patients with antiphospholipid antibodies, this association does not appear to be true after adjustment for steroid dosage (Mok et al. 2000). Magnetic resonance imaging is a very sensitive way to determine avascular necrosis. However, it may be too sensitive and some stage I lesions may regress.

The last musculoskeletal side-effect of steroid therapy is osteoporosis and fractures secondary to steroid-induced osteoporosis. This appears to occur less commonly in children than adults and may reflect relative differences in bone mineral content between the groups. The incidence of vertebral collapse is probably related not only to steroid dose and duration but also to the amount of weight gain and physical activity. There are few studies on bone mineral density in paediatric SLE. In one small study, there was an inverse correlation with bone mineral density and cumulative steroid dose but not disease activity or disease duration. These results are similar to most studies in adults which suggest that steroid dose and/or duration of steroid therapy are the most significant factors related to decreased bone mineral density. The role of therapy for glucocorticoid-induced osteoporosis is more controversial in children than in adults. Bisphosphanates, a mainstay of therapy for post-menopausal osteoporosis and steroid-induced osteoporosis in adults, are usually stated to be contraindicated in women of child-bearing potential. This encompasses the majority of paediatric patients. Suggested preventive therapies should include a diet high in calcium and supplemented if required and adequate doses of vitamin D. However, following an osteoporosis-induced fracture, the use of bisphosphonates and calcitonin should be considered.

Treatment of musculoskeletal involvement

The arthritis of SLE frequently occurs with disease flares elsewhere and usually responds to the treatment for the more serious complication. However, if isolated, the use of a non-steroidal anti-inflammatory drug with an antimalarial drug (usually hydroxychloroquine at a dose of 5 mg/kg) has a high success rate. The only word of caution is that SLE patients seem to be more susceptible to hepatotoxicity induced by non-steroidal anti-inflammatory drugs, particularly aspirin. The major side-effects of hydroxychloroquine are retinal macular deposition of the drug, which, if progressive, can lead to blindness; and gastrointestinal distress. Therefore, ophthalmologic examination every 6 months are required. Although myocardial, muscle, and neurotoxicities are rare, the incidence of these side-effects is increased in patients with renal insufficiency as the drug is at least partial excreted in the urine. Antimalarials should be used with caution in patients with decreased renal function. Prednisone at low to moderate dose may be required. For suggested therapy of arthritis (see Box 1).

Mucocutaneous involvement

Cutaneous involvement has been reported in 50–80 per cent of patients at the time of diagnosis and in up to 85 per cent of patients during the course of the disease. A malar rash, in the classic 'butterfly distribution', is the most common rash. The rash may be mild, requiring no treatment, but can be severe and cosmetically unacceptable requiring treatment with steroids, either topically or systemic, and/or antimalarial drugs. The appearance of a malar rash often heralds a disease flare and while usually non-scarring it

Box 1 Arthritis therapy flow chart

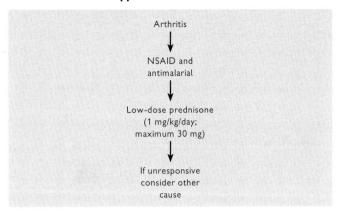

Arthritis
↓
NSAID and antimalarial
↓
Low-dose prednisone (1 mg/kg/day; maximum 30 mg)
↓
If unresponsive consider other cause

Box 2 Therapy flow chart for dermatological involvement

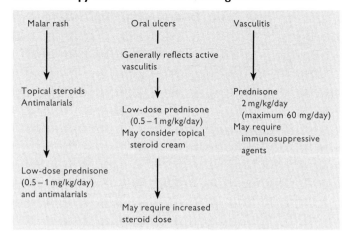

Malar rash
↓
Topical steroids
Antimalarials
↓
Low-dose prednisone (0.5 – 1 mg/kg/day) and antimalarials

Oral ulcers
↓
Generally reflects active vasculitis
↓
Low-dose prednisone (0.5 – 1 mg/kg/day)
May consider topical steroid cream
↓
May require increased steroid dose

Vasculitis
↓
Prednisone
2 mg/kg/day
(maximum 60 mg/day)
May require immunosuppressive agents

can be present as a crusted or scaling lesion. A photosensitive rash only occurs in approximately one-third of paediatric patients. The photosensitive rash can occur not only on the face but also in any sun-exposed area, especially the arms and legs (Plate 114). This photosensitive rash may be maculopapular or papulosquamous and may be associated with anti-Ro and anti-La antibodies. The other anti-Ro/La antibody-associated rash is annular erythema which is commonly photosensitive and occurs on the face or neck (Deng et al. 1984) (Plate 115). True discoid lupus lesions are seen rarely in patients under the age of 18 years. In patients with a photosensitive rash, sun exposure may not only exacerbate the skin disease but may cause a systemic flare. Therefore, we recommend avoidance of sunbathing along with the use of sun-blocking agents, with high sun protecting factor (SPF) blocking both ultraviolet A and B wavelengths, and protective clothing including long-sleeved shirts and hats.

A true vasculitic skin rash has been reported in 10–20 per cent of patients. It occurs commonly in fingers or toes and can result in splinter haemorrhages and digital infarcts. Chilblains are common cutaneous lesions seen in children particularly in countries with cold, damp weather. It can be difficult to differentiate chilblains from vasculitic lesions and both can occur in patients with SLE.

A vasculitic process causes oral or nasal ulcers and they are probably a reflection of alterations seen in other vascular beds. Even when isolated, they may signify active disease. Painless ulcers are more common on the hard palate but may occur on the soft palate. A petechial rash on the hard palate may precede true ulceration while a chronic sore throat may represent mildly active vasculitis. Similarly, hyperaemia of the nasal mucosa usually precedes ulceration or perforation (Plate 116). These lesions occur in 10–20 per cent of patients. For suggested therapy of mucocutaneous disease see Box 2. In addition to therapies listed in the table, open label studies have shown that thalidomide may be effective in refractory cutaneous lesions. Advise regarding teratogenic effects of this drug must be given.

Although rare, bullous lesions, including lesions consistent with pemphigus, may be the prominent dermatologic manifestation. Patients with C1q deficiency and other complement component deficiencies can present with prominent cutaneous features. Recurrent infection may also be an important symptom in these patients and may be a clue to the diagnosis of an accompanying complement deficiency.

Alopecia, is common and occurs in 30–50 per cent of paediatric patients. Diffuse hair loss during washing or brushing is more common than patchy hair loss. In some patients there is a delay in the hair loss, which may follow a disease flare or increase after the introduction of steroids. Rarely is the hair loss significant enough to cause a cosmetic problem. Scarring is unusual.

Raynaud's phenomenon appears to be less common in paediatric than adult lupus, occurring in only 10–20 per cent of patients. In some patients local therapy including avoidance of cold, use of insulated mittens rather than gloves, and hand/feet warmers will suffice. However, many patients will have more severe disease requiring the use of calcium-channel blocking agents or other vasodilating medication. Paediatric patients appear to tolerate calcium-channel blocking agents better than adults do. Raynaud's phenomenon may precede overt clinical SLE by months and may initially involve only a few digits and later involve all fingers and toes.

Central nervous system

Involvement of the central nervous system (CNS) occurs in 20–70 per cent of paediatric patients. CNS involvement can occur in isolation or it may be associated with disease flares in other organs. Although patients may have CNS disease at presentation of their SLE, up to 25 per cent of patients will not demonstrate their initial CNS involvement until more than 1 year after presentation (Steinlin et al. 1995). The most frequent disease correlations are between central nervous disease and vasculitis and thrombocytopaenia. Table 3 lists the different manifestations of nervous system involvement seen.

Neuropsychiatric SLE

Psychosis, with or without overt hallucinations or organic brain syndrome, occurs in 30–50 per cent of patients with CNS disease. Patients with neuropsychiatric SLE (NP-SLE) generally exhibit poor concentration/attention or other features of organic brain syndrome. The hallucinations may be auditory, visual, or tactile and these patients frequently suffer from some degree of paranoia (Steinlin et al. 1995). Suicidal ideation is common. However, many patients present with mild affective or mood disorders. The difficulty is determining whether the abnormalities detected are a direct result of the disease, secondary to steroid treatment, or 'reactive' to the disease or changes in body image. Although affective disorders occur less frequently than cognitive impairment (see below), it must be recognized that patients can present with a major affective disorder with very few other signs of lupus.

It can be very difficult to differentiate NP-SLE-induced cognitive impairment and concentration difficulties from other causes of poor school performance. Defects in cognitive function may reflect active disease or residual defects from previous central nervous involvement. There has been an association of cognitive function abnormalities and antiphospholipid antibodies (Carbotte et al. 1986). To date there has been few studies in paediatric SLE. The studies suggest that cognitive function defects are common (Papero et al. 1990).

Seizures occur in approximately 10–40 per cent of paediatric cases and may be the presenting sign. Generalized seizures are more common than focal seizures. Seizures are generally easily treated with anticonvulsant medication and usually do not require high-dose steroids for control and status epilepticus is very rarely seen. Seizures may not be primary but rather

Table 3 Neuropsychiatric lupus

Psychiatric
Psychosis
Depression
Central nervous system
Organic brain syndrome
Cognitive function deficits
Seizures
Cranial nerve palsy
Optic atrophy
Papilloedema
Parkinson-like syndrome
Coma
Headache—unremitting or migrainous
Transverse myelitis
Aseptic meningitis
Cerebrovascular accident—infarction
Pseudotumour cerebri
Movement disorders
Chorea
Hemmiballismus
Cerebellar ataxia
Tremor
Hemiparesis
Peripheral nervous system
Peripheral neuropathy
Guillain–Barré syndrome
Paraparesis
Myasthenia-like syndrome
Infection
Bacterial
Viral
Fungal
Opportunistic

secondary to metabolic disturbances caused by uraemia, hypertension, cerebral infarction, or central nervous infection. Structural abnormalities should be ruled-out in all patients with new onset or increasing frequency of seizures.

Movement disorders including chorea, cerebellar ataxia, hemiballismus, tremor, and Parkinsonian-like movements, occur in 5–10 per cent of cases. Interestingly chorea appears to be over-represented in the paediatric age group. In one review of 52 cases of SLE-associated chorea, 34 had chorea that developed before the age of 18 years, with the chorea preceding other manifestations of SLE by more than 1 year in 20 per cent of all cases (Bruyn and Padberg 1984). The association of chorea and antiphospholipid antibodies is well established. The decline in the incidence of rheumatic fever means that the diagnosis of SLE or antiphospholipid antibody syndrome should be considered in all patients presenting with chorea.

Neuropathies

Both cranial and peripheral neuropathies occur, with cranial nerve involvement being the more common. Cranial nerve involvement usually affects cranial nerves II, III, IV, and VI and less frequently facial palsy (VII), trigeminal neuropathy (V) or nystagmus and vertigo (VIII) occur. When peripheral neuropathies occur, a sensory or mixed sensorimotor involvement is more common than an isolated motor neuropathy. However, mononeuritis or mononeuritis multiplex can occur and isolated cases of Guillain–Barré-like syndrome have been seen. One study suggested that there is a high incidence of neurophysiological evidence without clinical evidence of a neuropathy in an unselected population of paediatric patients with SLE (Loh et al. 2000).

Paresis is less common in children than adults and hemiparesis is rarely seen. Transverse myelitis may present with acute paraplegia or quadriplegia and may be the presenting sign of SLE. In many patients with transverse myelitis, multiple investigations including evidence of complement activation are negative.

Headache

Headache requires a separate category as this is a common symptom occurring in up to 75 per cent of patients. The most common type of headache is an intermittent tension headache and may be related to musculoskeletal disease or general constitutional symptoms (Sfikakis et al. 1998). The significance of headache in the absence of other neurological symptoms is controversial. The differentiation of the type of headache is important. The severe, unremitting lupus headache is the most serious and may reflect active disease or may represent cerebral vein thrombosis (see below). A migrainous headache secondary to SLE must be differentiated from non-lupus associated vascular (Isenberg et al. 1982). Conversely, a migraine headache may reflect active central nervous SLE (Miguel et al. 1994). A headache may be the presentation of pseudotumour cerebri with or without leucoencephalopathy, which has been described as the presenting diagnosis in paediatric SLE. SLE should be considered in children who present with idiopathic intracranial hypertension.

Most worrying is the association of severe headache with cerebral vein thrombosis. Although cerebral vein thrombosis has been felt to be rare, we have frequently seen this complication in patients with severe headache. The headache associated with cerebral vein thrombosis may occur without any other neurological manifestation (Uziel 1995). We recommend neuroimaging studies for patients with persistent or severe headaches.

Autonomic nervous system

Many studies in adults with SLE had demonstrated mild to severe, asymptomatic autonomic nerve dysfunction with incidences up to 50 per cent and it has been suggested that autoantibodies directed against autonomic nervous system tissue may be important (Maule et al. 1997). Neither the clinical significance of these abnormalities nor the prevalence of these abnormalities in paediatric patients is known.

Investigation

Abnormalities of cerebrospinal fluid (CSF) cell count, protein, and complement levels have been described. However, the findings are inconsistent. It has been suggested that measurements of the integrity of the blood–brain barrier and of immunoglobulin synthesis in the CSF may correlate with neuropsychiatric SLE, but the demonstration of these abnormalities is not specific for SLE. It has been suggested that measurement CSF levels of soluble interleukin-2 receptor, tumour necrosis factor-alpha, or interleukin-1-beta levels may differentiate stroke associated with SLE from other causes of stroke (Gilad et al. 1997). Others have suggested that CSF interleukin-6 and prolactin levels could differentiate patients with NP-SLE from patients without CNS involvement (Jara et al. 1998). However, there is great overlap of the individual values obtained from patients with and without CNS involvement and none of these studies have been in a paediatric population. In contrast, the simplest test, examination and culture of cerebrospinal fluid, remains important when the possibility of infection or haemorrhage exists. An elevated CSF protein and/or white blood cell count, in the absence of infection, is suggestive of cerebritis. However, most patients with NP-SLE have normal CSF cell counts, protein, and glucose and the most common abnormality is only an increased opening pressure.

One prospective adult study suggested that a combination of the measurement of antineuronal antibodies with a large battery of sophisticated neurophysiological cognitive function tests correlated well with fluctuations of disease (Long et al. 1989). Our limited experience has suggested that this combination of testing may be of benefit in diagnosis and disease monitoring. However, cognitive function testing requires more time and expertise than is routinely available. Furthermore, longitudinal studies of cognitive function may be required to determine whether a defect is old, permanent, or temporary.

Serial measurement of more routine autoantibodies and routine blood tests may not correlate with NP-SLE (Miguel et al. 1994). Patients may have normal serology and complement levels despite active CNS-SLE. One paediatric study demonstrated that the majority of patients had normal serum complement levels at initial presentation of CNS disease (Quintero-Del-Rio and Van 2000). The presence of the antiribosomal P antibodies may distinguish depression secondary to SLE from other causes including reactive, steroid-induced or other non-SLE causes of depression. We found that antiribosomal P antibodies were specific for psychosis secondary to SLE but they had a low sensitivity in SLE patients with psychosis and a low specificity for psychosis in our SLE population (Press et al. 1996).

Electroencephalogram are frequently normal and when abnormal the changes are usually non-specific and generally unhelpful (Steinlin et al. 1995). The exception may be the demonstration of focal abnormalities in patients with seizures.

Radiological investigation may be helpful in demonstrating specific structural lesions such as infarction, embolus, and subdural or intracranial haemorrhage. However, neither computed tomography (CT) nor magnetic resonance imaging (MRI) has been shown to be consistently helpful in measuring overall CNS disease activity. The most common abnormalities are cerebral atrophy and non-specific changes. The use of MRI to determine the presence of diffuse disease activity in the CNS remains controversial (Jarek et al. 1994). MR spectroscopy, currently a research tool, may reflect metabolic disturbances in patients with CNS disease but further studies are required. Interestingly, similar to nuclear medicine single-photon-emission computed tomography (SPECT) brain scans (see below), MR spectroscopy frequently is in the face of abnormal CNS examination.

Persistent or severe headache should be investigated for the presence of intracranial thrombosis and in particular cerebral vein thrombosis. The best investigation is by a combination of CT and MRI scans (Uziel 1995). The diagnosis of cerebral vein thrombosis may be confirmed by the absence of flow on a MR venogram.

SPECT scanning, a measurement of brain functional activity and indirectly of cerebral blood flow, has been advocated to be of benefit in assessing CNS-SLE in both adults and children (Holman 1991). However the ability of this test to differentiate active CNS-SLE from active disease without overt CNS manifestations is controversial. Many patients without overt CNS disease may have an abnormal SPECT scan (Russo et al. 1998). Whether the perfusion abnormalities in patients without overt CNS disease reflects subclinical CNS dysfunction or the generalized disease process, remains to be determined. In addition, SPECT scans frequently remain abnormal despite clinical CNS remission. The classic pattern seen in patients with CNS-SLE, or other rheumatic illnesses, is one of diffuse patchy rather than focal abnormalities.

Treatment of central nervous system disease

The therapy of CNS disease varies with the manifestation. Currently, the treatment of isolated cognitive disorders is controversial, although these defects may be steroid-responsive. Obviously when infection is present the therapy is dictated by the microbiological identification of the organism. It must be remembered that these patients are susceptible to encapsulated organisms, Gram-negative organisms, and opportunistic infections.

Active psychosis and/or organic brain syndrome are potentially life-threatening complications and should be treated aggressively with high-dose corticosteroids. These patients frequently require immunosuppressive therapy with azathioprine or cyclophosphamide. Psychotropic drugs may also be needed for the control of the psychosis. We do not recommend the isolated use of psychotropic medication without the use of steroids. For suggested therapy of severe CNS disease see Box 3.

Box 3 Flow chart for therapy of central nervous system disease

CNS

↓ Severe disease including psychosis and organic brain syndrome

Controversial but our recommendation is:
Prednisone 2 mg/kg in divided doses
when appropriate:
Neuroleptic drugs
Anticonvulsants

↓

May double prednisone or
pulse i.v. methylprednisolone
Frequently requires
azathioprine for successful
steroid taper
May require pulse
cyclophosphamide

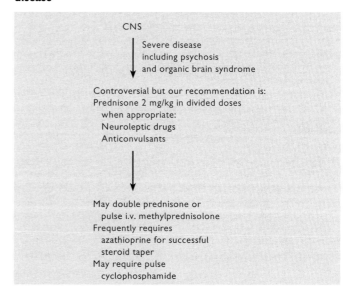

Treatment of seizures should be directed at finding their cause. Anticonvulsant medication may be required to control the seizures, but in many cases it is needed only for a short-term if the underlying cause of the seizure can be corrected.

As previously described, headaches can occur for a variety of reasons in these patients. The treatment is therefore dictated by the cause. Persistent headache resistant to analgesia may reflect active SLE or may be secondary to an intracranial thrombosis (in particular cerebral vein thrombosis). The management of 'lupus' headache secondary to active SLE requires better control of the SLE, which may include the use of steroids. We suggest that cerebral vein thrombosis requires long-term anticoagulation (Uziel 1995).

Renal disease

In a literature review of 540 children followed at centres other than our own, 72 per cent developed nephritis during the course of their disease, similar to our overall incidence of 61 per cent in 138 children with SLE.

The prognosis is related to the World Health Organization (WHO) morphological classification of the lesion (Table 4). It has been our practice to biopsy any child with clinical or laboratory evidence of renal involvement as the WHO classification influences our patient management; an approach that is supported by the experience of others. In the report by Platt et al. (1982), only 59 per cent of the children with diffuse proliferative lupus nephritis (DPLN) were alive without endstage renal failure 10 years after diagnosis compared with an 85 per cent 10-year survival rate for all 70 children with SLE. Other paediatric series have demonstrated 44–91 per cent five year survival. Our long-term outcome of lupus nephritis, at a median follow-up of 11 years, demonstrated a 94 per cent survival rate and a 91 per cent survival rate for patients with DPLN. Most of the patients in our series received azathioprine early in the treatment of DPLN (vide infra). Similarly, Nossent et al. (2000) reported that adult patients with DPLN treated with azathioprine had a similar long-term to the outcome previously reported for patients treated with intravenous pulse cyclophosphamide.

The most commonly seen form of SLE nephritis is DPLN which occurs in approximately 40–45 per cent of children (Table 5). Patients may undergo histological transformation to DPLN from focal proliferative (FPLN) and mesangial lupus nephritis months to years after initial diagnosis.

Table 4 WHO classification of lupus nephritis[a]

I	Normal A Nil (by all techniques) B Normal by light microscopy, but deposits present by electron microscopy
II	Pure mesangiopathy A Mesangial widening and/or mild hypercellularity (+) B Moderate hypercellularity (++)
III	Focal segmental glomerulonephritis (associated with mild or moderate mesangial alterations) A Active necrotizing lesions B Active and sclerosing lesions C Sclerosing lesions
IV	Diffuse glomerulonephritis (severe mesangial, endocapillary, or mesangiocapillary proliferation and/or extensive subendothelial deposits. Mesangial deposits are present invariably and subepithelial deposits often, and can be numerous) A Without segmental lesions B With active necrotizing lesions C With active and sclerotic lesions D With sclerosing lesions
V	Diffuse membranous glomerulonephritis A Pure membranous glomerulonephritis B Associated with lesions of Category II (A or B)
VI	Advanced sclerosing glomerulonephritis

[a] From Churg, J., Bernstein, J., and Glassock, R.J. (1995). Lupus nephritis, In *Renal Diseases. Classification and Atlas of Glomerular Diseases* (ed. J. Churg, J. Bernstein, and R.J. Glassock), p. 151. New York: Igaku-Shoin.

Table 5 Histological patterns of SLE nephritis at HSC

	General (%)[a] (n = 368)	Seven paediatric series (%)[b] (n = 424)	HSC 1979–1995 (%) (n = 79)
Mesangial	27	24	19
Focal proliferative	18	24	20
Diffuse proliferative	39	44	39
Membranous	16	8	22

[a] Data obtained from Pollak and Pirani (1993).

[b] Data obtained from King et al. (1977), Abeles et al. (1980), Platt et al. (1982), Glidden et al. (1983), Cameron (1994), Yang et al. (1994), Cassidy et al. (1997).

Table 6 Clinical manifestations at the time of biopsy of children with DPLN[a]

	Mean ± 1SD	Median	Range	Percentage
Age (years)	13 ± 4	14	4–17	
Female				67
Microhaematuria				100
Proteinuria (mg/kg/day)	46 ± 36	35	3–129	
⩾50				50
25–49				10
⩽24				40
Serum albumin (g/l)	30 ± 7	30	16–47	
⩾35				30
26–34				50
⩽25				20
GFR[b] ml/min/1.73 m^2	95 ± 33	102	17–151	
⩾100				52
60–99				33
⩽59				14
Hypertension				33
C3[c] (g/l)	0.47 ± 0.15	0.49	0.09–0.70	

[a] Diffuse proliferative lupus nephritis diagnosed at our institution since 1979; clinical data available on 29/33 children.

[b] GFR, glomerular filtration rate determined by ^{99}Tc-DPTA or Schwartz equation.

[c] C3, third component of complement; normal value is 0.8–1.8 g/l in our laboratory.

The profile of 29 children at the time of biopsy-confirmed DPLN illustrates this point (Table 6).

Severe proteinuria, even in the nephrotic range, does not always predict the presence of DPLN. Three children in our series had nephrotic syndrome with minimal glomerular histological changes consistent with the diagnosis of mesangial lupus nephritis. Electron microscopy revealed fusion of the foot processes of the glomerular epithelial cells. Similarly membranous lupus nephritis may present with nephrotic range proteinuria. Membranous nephritis occurs in approximately 20–25 per cent of patients with nephritis (Sorof et al. 1998). A diagnosis of SLE should be considered in any child with membranous nephropathy, a form of nephropathy that is rare in children.

Focal necrotizing lesions, even in patients with FPLN, is a bad prognostic sign. These lesions were present in 50 per cent of our patients with biopsy-proven FPLN, all of whom required treatment with a cytotoxic drug before their disease could be controlled adequately. In a long-term follow-up study of childhood lupus nephritis of all classes, renal insufficiency was reported in 53 per cent of patients who had focal necrotizing glomerular lesions on the initial biopsy (McCurdy et al. 1992).

Another important consideration is the presence of chronic damage. It has been reported that patients with any evidence of chronic damage at initial biopsy have a higher chance of developing end stage renal disease (ESRD) than who do not (Austin et al. 1984). Patients with the combination of cellular crescents and interstitial have the poorest long-term outcome. In our series, most patients who have developed ESRD all had advanced chronic disease on the renal biopsy at the initial presentation.

Acute interstitial inflammation, frequently neglected, is commonly observed in patients with DPLN (75 per cent in our series) where it may or may not be associated with tubulointerstitial immune deposits. Significant interstitial inflammation may be seen without DPLN (Fig. 1). A positive correlation between the number of interstitial mononuclear cells and both renal function and the degree of chronic renal damage and a poor outcome has been shown (Alexopoulos et al. 1990). Cases of hyporeninemic hypoaldosteronism have been reported in children with SLE nephritis as a result of distal tubular dysfunction (Hataya et al. 1999).

A variety of renal vascular lesions may be observed in SLE patients, including those associated with vascular immune complex deposits, non-inflammatory necrotizing vasculopathy, thrombotic microangiopathy, and true renal vasculitis (Appel et al. 1994). Studies of renal vascular lesions in childhood SLE have not been published. In adults the presence of vascular lesions suggests a worse prognosis compared to patients without vascular lesions.

Regular evaluation of the urine is important in all SLE patients. Many patients with renal involvement develop urinary abnormalities within 3 years of diagnosis, but a longer lag period can occur (Tucker et al. 1995).

Hypertension is common and an elevated blood pressure prior to steroid therapy suggests that the patient has DPLN or renovascular disease. Hypertension may be associated with a poorer renal outcome and may itself

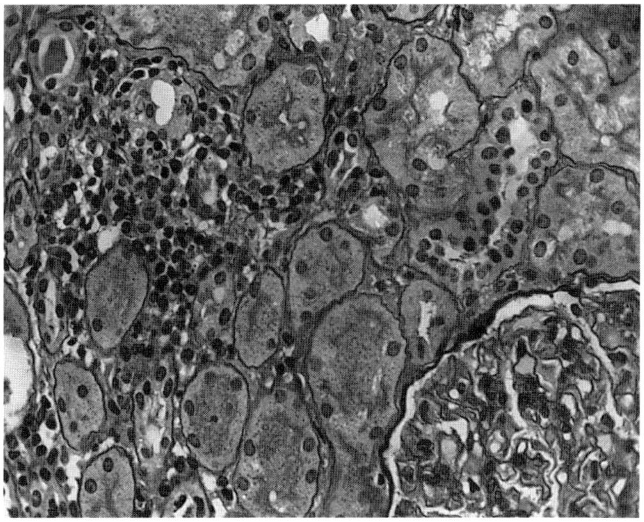

Fig. 1 Light photomicrograph of the renal biopsy of a 14-year-old girl with lupus nephritis illustrating the presence of interstitial inflammation. In this patient, immunofluorescence and electron microscopy demonstrated the presence of immune deposits along tubular basement membranes. Interstitial inflammation is a common finding in lupus nephritis and often occurs in the absence of extraglomerular immune complex deposition.

play a role in the development renal insufficiency. Aggressive antihypertensive therapy is warranted in all patients.

Rarely patients can present with haematuria due to a bleeding diathesis and Factor II deficiency should be considered in patients with gross haematuria (Eberhard et al. 1994).

Urological manifestations of SLE are not widely recognized but may be seen. Urinary frequency may occur as a result of chronic autoimmune interstitial cystitis and an obstructive uropathy has been described. However, it is always important to rule out an infectious cause, particularly in immunosuppressed patients.

Treatment of nephritis

The therapy of SLE nephritis should be directed by histologic lesion.

The majority of patients with mesangial lupus nephritis require a relatively short course of treatment with low-dose steroids. The long-term outcome of these patients is excellent and the side-effects of steroid therapy must be weighed against the excellent prognosis (if the lesion does not transform).

It had been suggested that patients with FPLN may be successfully managed with steroids alone; however, more recent data, and our personal experience, suggests that most, if not all, patients require cytotoxic agents. The requirement for the addition of cytotoxic therapy is particularly important when focal segmental necrotizing lesions are present (Najafi et al. 2001). The outcome likely depends on the percentage of glomeruli involved and the degree and severity of the necrotizing lesion. Controversy still remains in the therapy of patients with DPLN. The evaluation of treatment protocols for DPLN is impeded by the need to follow adequate number of patients for long periods of time. We have developed treatment guidelines:

1. Initial treatment always includes high-dose steroids (prednisone 2 mg/kg/day; maximum 60 mg/day), divided three times daily for 4 weeks, consolidated to once daily for a further 2 weeks and then tapered slowly over several months. Patients remain on low-dose alternate day prednisone, with immunosuppressive agent, for years in an attempt to minimize the risk of subsequent relapses.
2. Azathioprine (2–3 mg/kg/day) is initiated within the first month of diagnosis. Although many studies in adults (some studies in paediatrics) demonstrate the efficacy of cyclophosphamide in DPLN (Yan et al. 1995; Lehman and Onel 2000), our data, the data of others and meta-analyses of the therapy of DPLN all suggest that the majority of patients do well without the use of cyclophosphamide (Felson and Anderson 1984; Bansal and Beto 1997; Niaudet 2000; Nossent and Koldingsnes 2000). Since the long-term toxicities of cyclophosphamide (especially malignancy and infertility) are correlated with the lifetime accumulated dose, we are reluctant to use this drug initially in children. The age at the initiation of cyclophosphamide therapy and the cumulative dose of therapy are major determinants of long-term complications of cyclophosphamide therapy. A 'compromise' alternative may be initial 'induction' with 6 months of pulse therapy with cyclophosphamide, followed by maintenance therapy with azathioprine or mycophenolate mofetil (MMF).
3. We currently reserve intravenous pulse cyclophosphamide for azathioprine failures or patients who present in renal failure. When used alone, we have seen a sustained remission in only a minority of patients treated with cyclophosphamide at our institution, however, others have reported a better response (Yan et al. 1995; Lehman and Onel 2000). We have seen a good response to 6 months of intravenous cyclophosphamide followed by long-term azathioprine in patients who have presented in renal failure. We suggest that cyclophosphamide should be reserved for patients who have failed a trial of azathioprine, who are non-compliant with azathioprine, or who present with renal failure.
4. The chronicity index should be taken into consideration when making decisions about the use of cytotoxic drugs. If advanced chronic disease is present indicating that endstage renal disease is inevitable and severe extrarenal manifestations of SLE are not present, then cytotoxic drugs may not be justified. The survival of SLE patients on dialysis and following renal transplantation is very good (Nossent et al. 1991). The risk of recurrent lupus nephritis in renal allografts is very low.
5. Intravenous methylprednisolone, at a dose of 30 mg/kg (maximum 1000 mg) daily for 3 consecutive days, monthly for 6 months may be used as adjunctive therapy. Short-term results are good but a sustained long-term benefit has not been demonstrated.
6. Plasmapheresis may be considered in patients presenting with acute fulminating renal disease but long-term therapy is not justified.
7. Methotrexate therapy may be useful in selected patients with long-term disease that is difficult to control (Abud-Mendoza et al. 1993). Methotrexate should be restricted to patients with good renal function to avoid serious drug toxicity.
8. MMF has been shown to have good short-term results in patients with DPLN (Chan et al. 2000). Similar to azathioprine, MMF may be used long-term following an initial 6-month course of pulse cyclophosphamide. MMF should be considered in patients who are intolerant of azathioprine. Further investigations should be undertaken to study MMF in paediatric DPLN.

Close follow-up of patients with renal involvement, with urinalysis and quantification of urinary protein excretion rates is essential. Persistent proteinuria 1 year after the initiation of treatment suggests a poor long-term prognosis although clearing of proteinuria as be reported up to 2 years after onset. Measurement of serum complement profile, particularly levels for the third component of complement (C3) and anti-DNA antibody levels may be useful markers of renal disease activity. Although we do not consider serological abnormalities alone (i.e. hypocomplementaemia, increasing anti-DNA antibody levels) an indication to re-treat a patient, clinically active disease frequently ensues and these patients need to be followed closely (Fig. 2).

Preservation of renal function is the obvious goal. Unfortunately, obtaining an accurate measurement of the glomerular filtration rate is not easy. Taking inulin clearance as the 'gold standard', Meyers and his colleagues (Shemesh et al. 1985) have demonstrated that creatinine clearance determinations

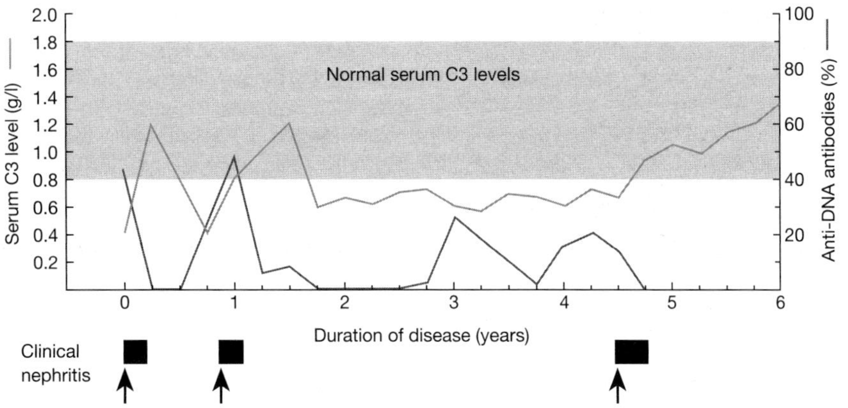

Fig. 2 Schematic summary of the clinical course of a girl with congenital C4 deficiency who developed SLE at 4 years of age associated with diffuse proliferative lupus nephritis. The value of monitoring serum C3 levels (solid line) is highlighted by her clinical course. Initial prednisone therapy (arrow) failed to maintain the C3 level in the normal range. She developed a clinical relapse of nephritis 10 months after the initial presentation, which was treated with prednisone and azathioprine (arrow). One year later the C3 level fell below the normal range. However, she remained clinically well for 3.5 years before a second renal flare occurred (arrow).

Table 7 Creatinine clearance is an unreliable measure of glomerular filtration rate in lupus nephritis[a]

Inulin clearance (ml/min per 1.73 m^2)	*n*	Creatinine/inulin clearance
>80	13	1.20 ± 0.08
40–80	10	1.57 ± 0.11
<40	21	2.21 ± 0.16

[a] As illustrated by the study of Shemesh et al. (1985) the creatinine clearance does not provide an accurate measure of the true glomerular filtration rate (assessed by inulin clearance rates) in patients with lupus nephritis. The more severe the reduction in renal function, the greater is this discrepancy.

overestimate the glomerular filtration rate during the acute phase of lupus nephritis, probably as a result of tubular secretion of creatinine (Table 7). Isotopic tests (e.g. ^{99}Tc-DTPA) appear to provide a more accurate measure of glomerular filtration rate in these patients.

The optimal treatment of patients with lupus membranous nephropathy is unknown. We agree with Appel et al. (1987) that the long-term outcome of these patients is less favourable than was suggested originally. A subset of these patients will develop chronic renal failure and should be treated with high-dose steroids. Less clear is the indication for alkylating agents. Sloan et al. (1996) reported that long-term prognosis in patients with SLE membranous nephritis was determined by the degree of associated glomerular inflammation seen on biopsy. The only patient at our institution with membranous SLE who developed endstage renal disease had diffuse endocapillary proliferation. Cyclosporine, with appropriate monitoring, has been successfully used in patients with membranous nephritis (Hallegua et al. 2000). Our short-term experience has been similar with good control of initial nephrotic range proteinuria and preservation of renal function. Angiotensin converting enzyme inhibitors may also be used to reduce proteinuria. These drugs have been shown to be safe in children and their use to preserve renal function requires further examination.

For an overview of suggested therapy for renal disease see Box 4.

Haematological involvement

Anaemia, thrombocytopaenia, and leucopaenia are very common laboratory abnormalities seen in 50–75 per cent of patients. The most common anaemia is normochromic normocytic, which when persistent usually becomes a microcytic and hypochromic anaemia. The serum ferritin may be normal or elevated, as ferritin production is increased as part of the acute-phase response.

The Coombs' test is positive in approximately 30–40 per cent of patients but less than 10 per cent of patients have overt haemolysis. Haemolysis is seen generally only in the presence of immunoglobulin in addition to complement on the surface of erythrocytes. The likely explanation for the lack of haemolysis when only complement is present is that red blood cells bind immune complexes through their C3b receptor (Wilson et al. 1989). In addition, complement activation products, C4d and C3b, may non-specifically coat red blood cells and therefore, can be detected in a Coombs' test. For an overview of suggested therapy for anaemia see Box 5.

Thrombocytopaenia is present in 15–45 per cent and in our experience, it may be the initial presentation in up to 15 per cent of paediatric cases. The thrombocytopaenia is usually secondary to peripheral destruction rather than bone marrow suppression. The development of SLE may take 20 years or more. Most patients with idiopathic thrombocytopaenic purpura and autoimmune haemolytic anaemia, so-called Evans syndrome, will probably develop SLE.

Despite the high incidence of thrombocytopaenia in paediatric SLE, bleeding is unusual and usually occurs only when the platelet count is less than 10 000. Most patients with thrombocytopaenia will respond to steroid or intravenous immunoglobulin therapy. Cyclophosphamide may be required for resistant cases (Lipnick et al. 1990). Splenectomy is very controversial, as some reports have suggested not only a lack of effect but also an unacceptably high increase in infections in patients postsplenectomy. These findings are not universal and splenectomy may have a role in resistant, persistent life-threatening thrombocytopaenia. For an overview of suggested therapy for thrombocytopaenia see Box 5.

Thrombotic thrombocytopaenia purpura (TTP) is an uncommon diagnosis in children. These children present with a microangiopathic haemolytic anaemia and evidence of neurologic disease and renal disease. Classic TTP with all three components, as opposed to haemolytic–uraemic syndrome (HUS), is rarely seen in children and most patients have haematologic involvement plus either neurologic or renal disease. We have recently reviewed our cases of TTP and the literature and found that, unlike what is seen adults, TTP in childhood is commonly associated with SLE (Brunner et al. 1999). HUS has also been associated with SLE.

In addition to thrombocytopaenia, acquired abnormalities of platelet function have been described. These include serum inhibitors that decrease aggregation and block uptake and storage of adenosine diphosphate and serotonin. Collagen-induced aggregation may be absent and adenosine

Box 4 Therapy flow chart for renal disease

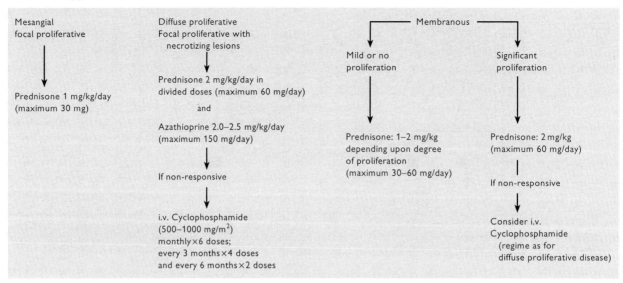

Mesangial focal proliferative
↓
Prednisone 1 mg/kg/day (maximum 30 mg)

Diffuse proliferative
Focal proliferative with necrotizing lesions
↓
Prednisone 2 mg/kg/day in divided doses (maximum 60 mg/day)
and
Azathioprine 2.0–2.5 mg/kg/day (maximum 150 mg/day)
↓
If non-responsive
↓
i.v. Cyclophosphamide ($500–1000\ mg/m^2$)
monthly × 6 doses;
every 3 months × 4 doses
and every 6 months × 2 doses

Membranous
→ Mild or no proliferation
↓
Prednisone: 1–2 mg/kg depending upon degree of proliferation (maximum 30–60 mg/day)

→ Significant proliferation
↓
Prednisone: 2 mg/kg (maximum 60 mg/day)
↓
If non-responsive
↓
Consider i.v. Cyclophosphamide (regime as for diffuse proliferative disease)

Box 5 Flow chart for treatment of haematological disease

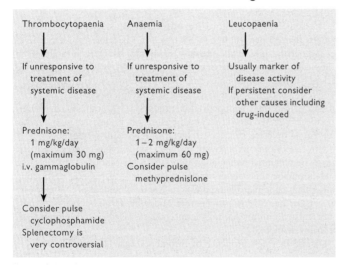

Thrombocytopaenia
↓
If unresponsive to treatment of systemic disease
↓
Prednisone: 1 mg/kg/day (maximum 30 mg)
i.v. gammaglobulin
↓
Consider pulse cyclophosphamide
Splenectomy is very controversial

Anaemia
↓
If unresponsive to treatment of systemic disease
↓
Prednisone: 1–2 mg/kg/day (maximum 60 mg)
Consider pulse methyprednislone

Leucopaenia
↓
Usually marker of disease activity
If persistent consider other causes including drug-induced

diphosphate and adrenaline-induced aggregation impaired (Decker et al. 1979). These defects generally present as purpura while overt bleeding is rare.

Leucopaenia is seen in 20–40 per cent of cases of paediatric SLE. Both lymphopaenia and granulocytopaenia can be seen. In many patients lymphopaenia is a sensitive marker of general disease activity and will rarely if ever require specific therapy. A lymphopaenia may also be secondary to therapy with azathioprine or cyclophosphamide. Granulocytopaenia is usually secondary to a central depression of granulopoiesis or splenic sequestration and more rarely antigranulocyte antibodies. Drugs including prednisone, azathioprine, and cyclophosphamide decrease granulocyte function and/or numbers. All of these problems probably contribute to the increased susceptibility to infection seen in SLE patients.

An interesting association is the development of SLE in adolescents with sickle-cell anaemia or sickle cell/beta thalassaemia; the SLE usually develops prior to the age of 18 (Katsanis et al. 1987). Interestingly, improvement of both the SLE and sickle cell anaemia has been described following therapy with hydroxyurea.

Following thrombocytopaenia, the presence of the lupus anticoagulant is the most common coagulation defect. This abnormality presents with an elevated partial thromboplastin time and occurs in 20–30 per cent of paediatric cases. Patients with the lupus anticoagulant do not bleed but rather have an increased incidence of deep vein thrombosis, thromboemboli, and less commonly arterial thrombosis. More details are given in Chapters 6.6.1 and 6.6.4. When a venous or arterial thrombosis occurs, then patients should be treated with anticoagulation with heparin followed by warfarin. We suggest that the international normalized ratio (INR) should be maintained long-term at around 2.0–3.0. The full spectrum of diseases associated with antiphospholipid antibodies and the lupus anticoagulant, the so-called antiphospholipid antibody syndrome (APS), is fully discussed in Chapters 6.6.1 and 6.6.4. The clinical syndromes are similar in adults and children except that chorea as the sole manifestation of these autoantibodies is more common in children than in adults. These patients with chorea are at risk for later thrombosis or other manifestations of the antiphospholipid antibody syndrome. Most studies, including our own study, have demonstrated that patients with the lupus anticoagulant with or without high titre anticardiolipin antibodies are at high risk for thrombosis and/or thrombocytopaenia (Berube et al. 1998). A particularly worrisome complication of antiphospholipid antibodies is the development of the catastrophic antiphospholipid antibody syndrome. These patients usually present with multiple microangiopathic thrombotic changes in multiple organs. There is usually a rapid progression to death and adult respiratory distress syndrome is common. Unlike what occurs in patients with APS, patients with catastrophic APS rarely have large vessel thrombosis. A high index of suspicion is required to entertain this diagnosis.

Specific inhibitors of other factors of the coagulation cascade have been described. The most common of these is prothrombin deficiency which is associated usually with the lupus anticoagulant. These patients, unlike those with the anticoagulant only, present with bleeding and a prolonged prothrombin and partial thromboplastin time. Prothrombin deficiency appears to be more common in paediatric SLE and a review of our patients demonstrated this abnormality in approximately 4 per cent of our SLE patients (Eberhard et al. 1994). As expected these patients presented with bleeding rather than clotting. We have found that the prothrombin deficiency will rapidly respond to steroid therapy. More rarely a steroid-responsive acquired von Willebrand's defect has been described.

Splenomegaly is quite common occurring in 20–30 per cent of paediatric cases. In our series of patients, splenomegaly was seen commonly in patients less than 10 years of age and may be the result of the generalized inflammatory state. Functional asplenia has been described and this abnormality of splenic function may increase the incidence of sepsis.

Cardiac involvement

Symptomatic pericarditis is the most common cardiac manifestation occurring in approximately 5–25 per cent of patients and is commonly associated with pleuritis (De Inocencio and Lovell 1994). Echocardiographic studies in children suggest that echocardiographic abnormalities can be seen in between 32 and 68 per cent of patients. In most patients, the echocardiogram demonstrated asymptomatic pericarditis (Guevara et al. 2001). Most cases of pericarditis will rapidly respond to either non-steroidal anti-inflammatory drugs alone, or low to moderate dose of corticosteroids. We suggest the initial use of indomethacin at a dose of 3 mg/kg/day divided into three doses. Indomethacin appears to work well in patients with SLE and is well tolerated in the paediatric patient.

The diagnosis of myocarditis or endocarditis is uncommon, with clinically detectable or significant myocarditis in less than 10 per cent of patients (Badui et al. 1985). When present, myocarditis frequently occurs in the presence of pericarditis but can be rarely seen without evidence of other cardiac involvement. Occasionally, patients with myocarditis may present with first degree atrioventricular block or arrhythmia. Libman–Sacks endocarditis has been detected in up to 50 per cent of all hearts at autopsy, while echocardiographic evidence of small vegetations may occur in 2–5 per cent of cases. The vegetations commonly occur at valvular rings and commissures. However, clinically significant lesions causing aortic or mitral stenosis or regurgitation are very rare.

Atherosclerotic heart disease and myocardial infarction are becoming increasing common with greater steroid usage and longevity of patients (Rubin et al. 1985). Patients in the paediatric age group, without other risk factors except SLE and its therapy, have been described with acute myocardial infarction. We have found that 16 per cent of asymptomatic paediatric patients had evidence of abnormal myocardial perfusion. These abnormalities tended to be reversible and were associated with active SLE (Gazarian et al. 1998). Hyperlipidaemia can either be the result of a primary hyperlipidaemia of SLE or secondary to treatment with steroids, which alters lipid profiles including cholesterol, triglycerides, and both high- and low-density lipoprotein levels (Ilowite et al. 1988). Although myocardial infarction during childhood or adolescence is rare, the incidence of myocardial infarction in young adults (under 25 years of age) with initial onset of SLE in the paediatric age is increasing.

Pulmonary involvement

Pulmonary involvement is common in paediatric SLE occurring in 25–75 per cent of cases depending on whether symptomatic or asymptomatic involvement is described. The manifestations range from severe life-threatening pulmonary haemorrhage or infection to asymptomatic abnormalities of pulmonary function tests (see Table 8 for a complete list of pulmonary complications). Decreased carbon monoxide diffusing capacity is the most common abnormality in both paediatric and adults patients; in one paediatric series it was seen in 100 per cent of unselected patients although more recent studies suggested that only 50 per cent of patients have any abnormal diffusing capacity (Al-Abbad et al. 2001). The next most common abnormality in pulmonary function testing is a restrictive pattern in 35–60 per cent of cases, while an obstructive defect is uncommon as is asymptomatic pleural involvement. The functional defects are probably secondary to chronic fibrotic changes that in turn are secondary to mild subclinical lupus pneumonitis, as suggested by the diffusing capacity abnormalities and restrictive rather than obstructive defects. These abnormalities rarely require specific therapy and although they are usually asymptomatic the changes generally persist. With the advent of high-resolution CT the percent of patients with asymptomatic pulmonary involvement may be as high as 75 per cent with evidence of chest X-ray abnormalities in less than 50 per cent of patients with CT scan abnormalities. The most common abnormal finding on CT scan was interstitial lung disease.

Table 8 Pulmonary involvement in childhood SLE

Pleuritis
Diaphragm involvement including shrinking lungs
Pneumonitis (acute or chronic)
Vasculitis
Pulmonary haemorrhage
Pulmonary emboli
Isolated pulmonary function test abnormalities
Drug-induced changes
Pulmonary hypertension

In contrast to what is seen in asymptomatic patients, pleural and/or pericardial involvement are commonly seen in patients complaining of respiratory symptoms. In the most recent review of paediatric patients, chest X-ray revealed that the majority of patients with respiratory symptoms had either pleural effusions or pericardial effusions with cardiomegaly. Less commonly alveolar infiltrates, interstitial infiltrates and/or lung abscesses were seen. However, isolated pleuritis, presenting as chest pain, can occur during a systemic flare and may be unilateral. When the pleuritis is mild, treatment can consist of anti-inflammatory doses of non-steroidals, but usually prednisone, at a low to moderate dose, is required. Similar to patients with pericarditis, antimalarials may be of benefit.

Dyspnoea, a common symptom, can be secondary to acute or chronic pneumonitis, pulmonary infection, pulmonary haemorrhage, or shrinking lung syndrome. The dramatic presentation of acute pneumonitis with fever, cough, dyspnoea, hypoxia, and chest pain occurs in only 3–10 per cent of patients. Pulmonary haemorrhage has a high mortality but occurrs in less than 5 per cent of patients (Nadorra and Landing 1987). Pulmonary haemorrhage may be the initial presenting sign in children with SLE and SLE should be considered in all patients with evidence of a pulmonary haemorrhage. Pulmonary haemorrhage or acute pneumonitis must be differentiated from congestive heart failure, pulmonary infection, and non-cardiogenic pulmonary oedema secondary to medication side-effects, uraemia, pancreatitis, or sepsis. The clinical differentiation of acute SLE pneumonitis from pulmonary haemorrhage may be aided by a fall in haemoglobin, the presence of haemoptysis, and an increased carbon monoxide diffusing capacity on pulmonary function tests seen in pulmonary haemorrhage.

In the acutely ill patient, the possibility of pulmonary infection must be considered. There is an increased incidence of infection even prior to steroid or immunosuppressive treatment. In addition to the more common bacterial and viral causes of pneumonia, these patients are at risk for opportunistic infection. When patients present with acute respiratory failure and fever, we recommend treatment with broad-spectrum antibiotics and high-dose steroids including pulse therapy. The use of bronchial washings obtained via bronchoscopy should be considered early, especially if intubation is required and identification of the organism using the polymerase chain reaction should be attempted. If the above-mentioned opportunistic infections are suspected clinically, then antifungal, antiprotozoan, antilegionella, antipneumocystis, and even antinocardia therapy should be considered. If the patient does not improve quickly then a diagnostic open lung biopsy is necessary.

In contrast to acute pneumonitis, chronic or interstitial pneumonitis has an insidious onset. Clinically significant disease is uncommon and usually follows long-standing SLE. When severe, most patients have clinically evident pulmonary involvement and present with cough and chest pain leading to dyspnoea and a decreased diffusing capacity. In adults, high-resolution CT scanning revealed that honey-combing and/or a ground glass appearance of the lung was common in patients with persistent respiratory symptoms without evidence of these changes on routine CT scan in many of these patients. An autopsy study of 26 paediatric patients with SLE showed

Box 6 Flow chart for therapy of cardiovascular and pulmonary disease

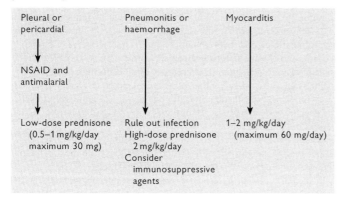

Pleural or pericardial	Pneumonitis or haemorrhage	Myocarditis
↓	↓	↓
NSAID and antimalarial		
↓		
Low-dose prednisone (0.5–1 mg/kg/day maximum 30 mg)	Rule out infection High-dose prednisone 2 mg/kg/day Consider immunosuppressive agents	1–2 mg/kg/day (maximum 60 mg/day)

a mild chronic interstitial pneumonitis in all patients, with additional pulmonary lesions in 18 patients (Nadorra and Landing 1987). Most of the chronic lesions were asymptomatic prior to death.

A more unusual cause of dyspnoea is the shrinking lung syndrome. This disorder is diagnosed by chest radiography that demonstrates an elevated diaphragm in the clinical setting of dyspnoea, which might be mild. A paediatric review demonstrated radiographic evidence of an elevated diaphragm in 12 per cent of patients (Delgado et al. 1990).

Difficult to treat, pulmonary hypertension fortunately is rare and is seen usually only with long-standing disease. These patients present with classic signs and symptoms of primary pulmonary hypertension but it may evolve from one of five processes: (i) primary or idiopathic pulmonary hypertension of SLE; (ii) secondary to pulmonary artery thrombosis or recurrent emboli; (iii) secondary to chronic left ventricular failure; (iv) secondary to chronic hypoxic from diffuse interstitial lung disease; and (v) obstruction of peripheral pulmonary vasculature secondary to vasculitis. An overview of suggested therapy for cardiovascular and pulmonary disease is given in Box 6.

Gastrointestinal disease

Gastrointestinal involvement occurs in 20–40 per cent of patients. The most common complaint is abdominal pain that can result from peritoneal inflammation (serositis), vasculitis, pancreatitis, malabsorption, pseudo-obstruction, paralytic ileus, and/or direct bowel wall involvement (enteritis). The presentation of serositis may vary from mild crampy or colicky pain to severe pain with a rigid abdomen. It can be difficult to differentiate peritoneal inflammation as a manifestation of the underlying SLE from infective peritonitis.

Lupus-associated enteropathy may be divisible into two types; an acute ischaemic enteritis and a protein-losing enteropathy, each presenting distinct radiographic features. Bowel wall inflammation presenting as crampy, abdominal pain, and diarrhoea can be caused by a primary enteritis or be secondary to a mesenteric vasculitis or thrombosis. The latter two are generally more acute and may be accompanied by bloody diarrhoea and nausea or vomiting. These disorders must be differentiated because vasculitis with thrombosis may require urgent surgery owing to the risk of bowel ischaemia, while most cases of non-thrombotic enteritis will respond to steroids. Involvement of other organ systems may aid in the diagnosis as there is an association of severe enteritis with central nervous system disease and lupus cystitis (Orth et al. 1983; Eberhard et al. 1991a). A protein-losing enteropathy may present with abdominal pain, diarrhoea, oedema, and hypoalbuminaemia. We and others have seen patients with asymptomatic pneumatosis cystoides intestinalis. Abdominal X-rays show the characteristic multiple round translucencies along the wall of the ascending and transverse colon. We treated our patient with intravenous antibiotics and bowel rest while other patients have been treated successfully with oral antibiotics. As our patient and the patients described in the literature were asymptomatic and the X-rays were done for other reasons, it is not clear whether pneumatosis cystoides intestinalis is a more common gastrointestinal manifestation than has been reported.

An autopsy study of 26 young patients reported that prior to death 65 per cent of patients had abdominal pain and 46 per cent gastrointestinal bleeding. Dysphagia and symptoms of reflux were unusual. A gastrointestinal 'vasculopathy' was commonly found with ischaemic lesions, and a non-specific infiltrate was found in 96 per cent. In 20 per cent of the cases, autopsy findings of ischaemic bowel were clinically asymptomatic (Nadorra et al. 1987).

Pancreatitis, although it must always be considered, is a uncommon with an overall incidence of less than 5 per cent. In order to determine the incidence of pancreatic dysfunction in SLE, we prospectively evaluated pancreatic function and performed pancreatic ultrasonography in 36 patients. We did not find any significant pancreatic pathology over the 2-year study period and could not find any association of pancreatic function abnormalities with steroid or azathioprine use (Eberhard et al. 1992).

Liver disease

Hepatomegaly occurs in 40–50 per cent of paediatric patients, while abnormalities of liver function tests (LFTs) may occur in up to 25 per cent. However, the elevation of liver enzymes is usually mild to moderate and they tend to resolve when the disease becomes inactive. Liver membrane autoantibodies (LMA) may seen in the majority of patients with active SLE and abnormal LFTs. When abnormal LFTs persist other causes should be sought.

When there is marked elevation of LFTs another cause must be sought as the clinical features of autoimmune hepatitis, so-called 'lupoid hepatitis', may mimic SLE (Miller 1977). Both these diseases preferentially occur in adolescent females. Many patients with autoimmune hepatitis have clinical features of SLE including a malar rash, arthritis, and serological features including anti-DNA antibodies, and hypergammaglobulinaemia. It is likely that LFT abnormalities, in the presence of anti-DNA or other specific autoantibodies seen in SLE, with clinical features of SLE, such as arthritis and malar rash, is SLE with the liver as the major target. These patients rarely have nephritis or CNS disease. When jaundice is a prominent feature in a known SLE patient then a second disease such as obstruction, haemolysis, or viral hepatitis is probably the cause.

Liver involvement may be part of the generalized vasculitis and may explain the increased salicylate sensitivity seen in 10–20 per cent of SLE patients. However, salicylate toxicity rarely results in significant, permanent pathological changes. A similar percentage of patients with systemic juvenile arthritis, another disease with systemic vasculitis, develop salicylate sensitivity. An increased incidence of hepatotoxicity to other drugs including azathioprine, and even cyclophosphamide, has been reported. Rarely systemic vasculitis has resulted in hepatic rupture secondary to liver infarction. These patients present with an acute abdomen and usually have evidence of active vasculitis and Raynaud's phenomenon elsewhere.

Endocrine involvement

Thyroid involvement is the most common endocrine organ involved in SLE. In a prospective study we found that antithyroid antibodies were present in 45 per cent of paediatric patients and clinical hypothyroidism was present in 15 per cent (Eberhard et al. 1991b). Hyperthyroidism, although less common than hypothyroidism, occurs with an increased incidence in SLE patients than the general paediatric population. Steroid-induced diabetes mellitus occurs in up to 10 per cent of patients but a lower percentage require insulin treatment. There does not appear to be an increased incidence of diabetes mellitus in the absence of steroid therapy. Delayed puberty and menstrual abnormalities are seen commonly. However, these abnormalities are probably secondary to chronic illness and active disease, rather than as a direct result of the disease process. Rarely, hypoparathyroidism has been reported in association with SLE. This diagnosis should be considered in the presence of unexplained hypocalcaemia.

Infection and immunization

Patients with SLE are particularly susceptible to infection with streptococcus pneumonia in contrast to the general healthy paediatric population where pneumococcal infections of the soft tissues and blood are uncommon. It has been postulated that abnormal neutrophil function and hypocomplementaemia may be the predisposing factors leading to invasive pneumococcal disease. Although the mechanisms are not well elucidated, patients with SLE produce low, non-protective concentrations of anti-pneumococcal antibodies.

As outlined in the sections on individual organ involvement, patients with SLE are susceptible to infection with opportunistic organisms. Invasive fungal should be considered in patients with persistent meningitis even at diagnosis.

Viruses may have a role in the development of SLE or viral infections may be mistake for SLE. The clinical picture of SLE can overlap that of Epstein–Barr virus (EBV) infection and patients with EBV can have renal involvement (Dror et al. 1998). Many viral infections present with cervical adenopthay. Kikuchi disease, necrotizing lymphadenitis, can be mistaken for SLE and it can present with cervical lymphadenopathy, fatigue, and fever. Infection with human parvovirus B19 (HPV-B19) is common in the paediatric age group. Infection with HPV-B19 may mimic the clinical picture of SLE and these patients may have serology suggestive of SLE (Moore et al. 1999). It has also been suggested that HPV-B19 infection may trigger true SLE. As can be seen, the differentiation of EBV and HPV-19 from SLE can be difficult and the role of these viruses in inciting SLE still remains to be determined.

Important questions, particularly in younger children, are whether immunizations are safe and effective in children with SLE and which immunizations should be given. There are no specific studies in children to address this question and therefore the data must be extrapolated from studies in adults. The majority of patients with SLE appear to respond well to immunization with tetanus toxoid and *Haemophilus influenzae* type B vaccines but not as well to pneumococcal vaccination. There is no evidence that the overall lupus disease activity is affected by immunization (Battafarano et al. 1998). It is suggested that when patients are on high-dose steroids or significant immunosuppression then immunization with live viral vaccines should be deferred.

Autoantibodies

The hallmark of SLE is the production of autoantibodies. There is a long list of antibodies directed against histone, non-histone, RNA-binding, cytoplasmic, and nuclear proteins. Many articles have reviewed the structure and function of the autoantigens and their role in autoimmune disease. A good review of autoantibodies is found in Chapter 6.6.4 and therefore, in this section we will focus on the limited literature regarding specific autoantibodies and disease manifestation in paediatric SLE.

The most common autoantibody is antinuclear which is seen in up to 100 per cent of patients. Anti-DNA antibodies are present in 60–90 per cent of cases. A paediatric study demonstrated that a lower percentage of paediatric SLE patients had IgG and higher percentage of IgM anti-DNA antibodies than adults (Shergy et al. 1989). Similarly there was an increased percentage of paediatric patients with IgM anti-Sm, anticardiolipin and anti-70-kDa ribonucleoprotein antibodies when compared with adult SLE patients. In enzyme-linked immunosorbent assays (ELISA), the overall incidence of anti-Sm antibodies is 50–60 per cent, anticardiolipin antibodies 50 per cent of patients, and anti-70 kDa ribonucleoprotein antibodies 70–90 per cent of patients.

Rheumatoid factor has been seen in 12–29 per cent of patients by conventional methods. Anticardiolipin antibodies may be present in up to 50 per cent of patients and the lupus anticoagulant is present in approximately 20 per cent of cases. No studies have examined the incidence of anti-Ro and/or anti-La antibodies in paediatric patients, but similar to adults, the presence of anti-Ro and anti-La antibodies defines a population which is at risk of a photosensitive rash and subacute cutaneous lupus.

As previously stated in the haematology section, the presence of anticardiolipin antibodies, the lupus anticoagulant, and antiphospholipid antibodies is associated with an increased risk of thrombosis. These autoantibodies are common in paediatric patients and these patients are at increased risk for thrombosis (Shergy et al. 1988; Ravelli et al. 1994). In our experience, thrombosis may occur in 30–50 per cent of patients with detectable antiphospholipid antibodies. Furthermore, these patients are at risk for the development of other manifestations of the antiphospholipid antibody syndrome including chorea, avascular necrosis, epilepsy, migraine headache, and livedo reticularis (Ravelli et al. 1994).

Antiribosomal P antibodies have been addressed in more detail in the section on central nervous system disease. These antibodies appear to be present in approximately 15 per cent of all patients with SLE and there is an increased incidence of antiribosomal P antibodies in patients with psychosis. In patients with psychosis titres of antiribosomal P antibodies may vary with disease activity in the central nervous system. These autoantibodies may be either IgM or IgG.

Neonatal lupus erythematosus

Neonatal lupus erythematosus (NLE) or the so-called neonatal lupus erythematosus syndrome (NLS) is a disease of the foetus/newborn defined by the demonstration of maternal autoantibodies and characteristic clinical features. NLE is assumed to be the result of foetal and/or neonatal damage caused by the transplacental passage of maternal IgG autoantibodies. The major clinical manifestations are cardiac and dermatological, with complete congenital heart block (CCHB) being the most significant lesion (Watson et al. 1984; Lee et al. 1986). More rarely haemolytic anaemia, thrombocytopaenia, neutropaenia, urinary abnormalities, neurologic involvement, and liver dysfunction are seen (Watson et al. 1984; McCune et al. 1987). Most early reports suggested that children with NLE are born to mothers with anti-Ro antibodies. However, in larger studies, we and others have demonstrated that the presence of anti-La antibodies in association with anti-Ro antibodies was a more specific disease maker, especially in patients CCHB. The presence of maternal anti-La antibodies was associated with a greater relative risk for the development of congenital heart block in the offspring than the presence of maternal anti-Ro antibodies alone (Buyon and Winchester 1990; Silverman et al. 1991). In addition, antibodies directed against 52-kDa Ro were more specific than antibodies directed against the 60-kDa form in determining the risk of development of NLE, although other studies have suggested the importance of antinative 60-kDa Ro antibodies (Buyon et al. 1993; Reichlin et al. 1994).

The clinical spectrum

Cardiac lesions

The characteristic cardiac lesion of NLE is isolated CCHB although there have been case reports of CCHB in association with endomyocardial fibroelastosis, valvular insufficiency, and patent ductus arteriosus. It is estimated that CCHB occurs in 1 in 14 000 live births. Ho et al. (1986) described the histopathology of eight hearts with complete congenital heart block, seven of which were associated with maternal anti-Ro antibodies.

The histopathology of the cardiac lesion suggests either early interference with normal organogenesis, or intrauterine inflammatory lesions resulting in subsequent scarring (Carter et al. 1974). The inflammatory lesion hypothesis is supported by the pathological demonstration of fibrosis at the chordae tendinae and the ventricular (Weber and Myers 1994).

Congenital heart block was described originally as a relatively benign condition. However, studies of large series of patients with this condition are not as optimistic. Of our more than 100 patients with CCHB, almost all have required pacemaker therapy. The pacemaker may not be necessary neonatally but rather in later life. We have had neonatal and later deaths as a result of pacemaker failure. A follow-up report of 14 children with congenital heart block showed that three of the children (21 per cent) died neonatally of congestive heart failure secondary to the block and a further five required pacemakers (McCune et al. 1987). Therefore, although congenital heart block has been described as being benign, most series have demonstrated both intrauterine and neonatal deaths with the potential for further deaths to occur secondary to pacemaker failure. The most serious consequence of CCHB is the development of hydrops foetalis and intrauterine death. An intrauterine heart rate of less than 55 beats/minute has been associated with poor outcome.

Skin lesions

The skin lesions of NLE are very similar to those of subacute cutaneous lupus erythematosus in which at least 80 per cent of patients have anti-Ro antibodies. Both Ro and La antigens have been documented in human skin (Lee et al. 1985), and exposure to ultraviolet light increases the expression of Ro on the surface of keratinocytes (LeFeber et al. 1984). This feature may explain the photosensitive nature of the skin rash in both NLE and subacute cutaneous lupus erythematosus (Plate 117). However, the skin rash may be present at birth or in non-sun exposed areas such as palms and soles. There is a predilection for the rash to develop around the eyes which cannot be explained by sun exposure alone. The rash of NLE is usually transient and usually heals well without evidence of residual scarring. However, in approximately 10 per cent of cases telangiectasia will develop in the area of the temples (Neiman et al. 2000). These telangiectasiae in the temple region may develop without previous evidence of a rash in this area.

Although cutaneous NLE is almost universally associated with anti-Ro and/or anti-La antibodies, there have been reports of the condition with anti-U1 ribonucleoprotein antibodies, instead of anti-Ro or anti-La antibodies. In our prospective study, we demonstrated maternal anti-Ro antibodies in 100 per cent of cutaneous NLE patients, while anti-La antibodies were present in 75 per cent of sera. The pathology of cutaneous NLE demonstrates the typical histology of subacute cutaneous lupus with epidermal basal cell damage and immunoglobulin deposition at the dermoepidermal junction.

Liver disease

Enlargement of the liver, spleen, or both occurs in approximately 30 per cent of cases of NLE. The enlargement of these organs may be secondary to congestive heart failure, but there may also be primary hepatic enlargement. In most reported cases, the liver disease is associated with other clinical manifestations of NLE. These patients presented with liver enlargement, elevated levels of hepatic enzymes, and evidence of cholestasis (Laxer et al. 1990). The histological changes seen on biopsy include giant cell transformation, ductal obstruction, and extramedullary haematopoiesis. The liver changes generally are not severe and recovery from the liver disease usually occurs despite the presence of residual fibrosis on repeat biopsy. However, we and others have seen cases of severe intrahepatic cholestasis secondary to NLE (Rosh et al. 1993). Hepatic involvement with elevated liver function tests may be the only manifestation of NLE in up to 20 per cent of cases.

Other disease manifestations

Haematological problems occasionally occur including thrombocytopaenia, neutropaenia, and mild haemolytic anaemia. Although usually seen in conjunction with other manifestations of NLE, haematologic involvement may occur in isolation. The thrombocytopaenia rarely causes bleeding and is not usually associated with antiplatelet antibodies. The haematologic abnormalities tend to resolve without specific treatment within 3–4 months. However, it has been reported that high-dose steroids or intravenous immunoglobulins have been required in the rare life-threatening bleeds associated with thrombocytopaenia and NLE.

Urinary abnormalities include transient pyuria or urethritis, but to date there have been no cases of nephritis. We and others have seen children with chondrodysplasia punctae associated with other features of NLE. A diverse group of CNS manifestations have been described which include myelopathy, a vasculopathy, and hydrocephalus.

Treatment

Cutaneous NLE rarely requires treatment as usually it is self-limited and usually heals without scarring. In the unusual case with more severe or scarring lesions, topical steroids may be required. Rarely laser therapy is required to treat severe telangiectasia. The liver disease of NLE will usually spontaneously resolve by the age of six months and does not require steroid treatment. However, if the cholestasis is severe, these infants may require a formula high in medium-chain triglycerides.

The treatment or prevention of congenital heart block is much more complex than the treatment of cutaneous NLE. Previously, it had been suggested that all mothers at risk for delivering a child with congenital heart block should be treated with plasmapheresis and dexamethasone throughout the pregnancy. However, this form of treatment will subject both the mother and the foetus to significant risks during the pregnancy, and up to 90 per cent of mothers will deliver a normal child without congenital heart block, despite having previously delivered a child with this. Therefore, the current recommendation is to monitor the foetus using foetal echocardiography to assess the developing heart, prior to the initiation of potentially toxic treatment.

Once intrauterine CCHB is detected, it is our current practice to treat all cases of uncomplicated autoantibody-associated intrauterine CCHB with maternal administration of a fluorinated corticosteroid (dexamethasone is our drug of choice). If there is no response with an increase in heart rate or reversal of the CCHB after 10 weeks of therapy, then we discontinue the dexamethasone. Most foetuses will tolerate a ventricular rate of 60 beats per minute or more. When congenital heart block and foetal hydrops is discovered during gestation, treatment of the mother with dexamethasone with or without plasmapheresis may reverse the foetal congestive heart failure but not the heart block. However, the efficacy of this therapy in altering the natural history of congenital heart block is controversial and unproven. Maternal therapy with digoxin, furosemide, and/or sympathomimetics may be used to reverse the hydrops foetalis. If this therapy fails then early delivery is required. The use of direct foetal therapy via the umbilical cord is still experimental. Prospective collaborative studies are required to determine the population at risk for CCHB and how to prevent it.

Children diagnosed with or suspected of having CCHB should be delivered in a high-risk neonatal centre which can provide cardiac pacing. If the foetal bradycardia is recognized as congenital heart block rather than foetal distress, then unnecessary early, emergency delivery may be prevented.

References

Abeles, M., Urman, J.D., Weinstein, A., Lowenstein, M., and Rothfield, N.F. (1980). Systemic lupus erythematosus in the younger patient: survival studies. *Journal of Rheumatology* **7**, 515–22.

Abud-Mendoza, C., Sturbaum, A.K., Vazquez-Compean, R., and Gonzalez-Amaro, R. (1993). Methotrexate therapy in childhood systemic lupus erythematosus. *Journal of Rheumatology* **20**, 731–3.

Al-Abbad, A.J. et al. (2001). Echocardiography and pulmonary function testing in childhood onset systemic lupus erythematosus. *Lupus* **10**, 32–7.

Alexopoulos, E., Seron, D., Hartley, R.B., and Cameron, J.S. (1990). Lupus nephritis: correlation of interstitial cells with glomerular function. *Kidney International* **37**, 100–9.

Appel, G.B., Cohen, D.J., Pirani, C.L., Meltzer, J.I., and Estes, D. (1987). Long-term follow-up of patients with lupus nephritis. A study based on the classification of the World Health Organization. *American Journal of Medicine* **83**, 877–85.

Appel, G.B., Pirani, C.L., and D'Agati, V. (1994). Renal vascular complications of systemic lupus erythematosus. *Journal of the American Society of Nephrology* **4**, 1499–515.

Austin, H.A., III, Muenz, L.R., Joyce, K.M., Antonovych, T.T., and Balow, J.E. (1984). Diffuse proliferative lupus nephritis: identification of specific pathologic features affecting renal outcome. *Kidney International* **25**, 689–95.

Badui, E. et al. (1985). Cardiovascular manifestations in systemic lupus erythematosus. prospective study of 100 patients. *Angiology—Journal of Vascular Diseases* **36**, 431–41.

Bansal, V.K. and Beto, J.A. (1997). Treatment of lupus nephritis: a meta-analysis of clinical trials. *American Journal of Kidney Diseases* **29**, 193–9.

Battafarano, D.F. et al. (1998). Antigen-specific antibody responses in lupus patients following immunization. *Arthritis and Rheumatism* **41**, 1828–34.

Berube, C. et al. (1998). The relationship of antiphospholipid antibodies to thromboembolic events in pediatric patients with systemic lupus erythematosus: a cross-sectional study. *Pediatric Research* **44**, 351–6.

Brunner, H.I. et al. (1999). Close relationship between systemic lupus erythematosus and thrombotic thrombocytopenic purpura in childhood. *Arthritis and Rheumatism* **42**, 2346–55.

Bruyn, G.W. and Padberg, G. (1984). Chorea and systemic lupus erythematosus. *European Neurology* **23**, 435–48.

Buyon, J.P. and Winchester, R. (1990). Congenital complete heart block. *Arthritis and Rheumatism* **33**, 609–14.

Buyon, J.P. et al. (1993). Identification of mothers at risk for congenital heart block and other neonatal lupus syndromes in their children. *Arthritis and Rheumatism* **36**, 1263–73.

Caeiro, E., Michielson, F.M.C., Bernstein, R., Hughes, G.R., and Ansell, B.M. (1981). Systemic lupus erythematosus in childhood. *Annals of the Rheumatic Diseases* **40**, 325–31.

Cameron, J.S. (1994). Lupus nephritis in childhood and adolescence. *Pediatric Nephrology* **8**, 230–49.

Carbotte, R.M., Denburg, S.D., and Denburg, J.A. (1986). Prevalence of cognitive impairment in systemic lupus erythematosus. *Journal of Nervous and Mental Disease* **174**, 357–64.

Carter, J.B., Blieden, L.C., and Edwards, J.E. (1974). Congenital heart block. *Archives of Pathology* **97**, 51–7.

Chan, T.M. et al. (2000). Efficacy of mycophenolate mofetil in patients with diffuse proliferative lupus nephritis. Hong Kong–Guangzhou Nephrology Study Group. *New England Journal of Medicine* **343**, 1156–62.

Citera, G., Espada, G., and Maldonado Cocco, J.A. (1993). Sequential development of 2 connective tissue diseases in juvenile patients. *Journal of Rheumatology* **20**, 2149–52.

Decker, J.L., Steinberg, A.D., Reinertsen, J.L., Plotz, P.H., Balow, J.E., and Klippel, J.H. (1979). Systemic lupus erythematosus: evolving concepts. *Annals of Internal Medicine* **91**, 587–604.

De Inocencio, J. and Lovell, D.J. (1994). Cardiac function in systemic lupus erythematosus. *Journal of Rheumatology* **21**, 2147–56.

Delgado, E.A., Malleson, P.N., Pirie, G.E., and Petty, R.E. (1990). The pulmonary manifestations of childhood onset systemic lupus erythematosus. *Seminars in Arthritis and Rheumatism* **19**, 285–93.

Deng, J.-S., Sontheimer, R.D., and Gilliam, J.N. (1984). Relationships between antinuclear antibodies and anti-Ro/SSA antibodies in subacute cutaneous lupus erythematosus. *Journal of the American Academy of Dermatology* **11**, 494–9.

Dror, Y. et al. (1998). Systemic lupus erythematosus associated with acute Epstein–Barr virus infection. *American Journal of Kidney Diseases* **32**, 825–8.

Eberhard, A., Shore, A., Silverman, E., and Laxer, R. (1991a). Bowel perforation and interstitial cystitis in childhood systemic lupus erythematosus: a case report. *Journal of Rheumatology* **18**, 746–7.

Eberhard, A., Laxer, R., Eddy, A., and Silverman, E. (1991b). Presence of thyroid abnormalities in children with systemic lupus erythematosus. *Journal of Pediatrics* **119**, 277–9.

Eberhard, A., Couper, R., Durie, P., and Silverman, E. (1992). Exocrine pancreatic function in children with systemic lupus erythematosus. *Journal of Rheumatology* **19**, 964–7.

Eberhard, A., Sparling, C., Sudbury, S., Ford, P., Laxer, R., and Silverman, E. (1994). Hypoprothrombinemia in childhood systemic lupus erythematosus. *Seminars in Arthritis and Rheumatism* **24**, 12–18.

Emery, H. (1986). Clinical aspects of systemic lupus erythematosus in childhood. *Pediatric Clinics of North America* **33**, 1177–90.

Felson, D.T. and Anderson, J. (1984). Evidence for the superiority of immunosuppressive drugs and prednisone over prednisone alone in lupus nephritis. Results of a pooled analysis. *New England Journal of Medicine* **311**, 1528–33.

Gazarian, M. et al. (1998). Assessment of myocardial perfusion and function in childhood systemic lupus erythematosus. *Journal of Pediatrics* **132**, 109–16.

Gilad, R. et al. (1997). Cerebrospinal fluid soluble interleukin-2 receptor in cerebral lupus. *British Journal of Rheumatology* **36**, 190–3.

Glidden, R.S., Mantzouranis, E.C., and Borel, Y. (1983). Systemic lupus erythematosus in childhood: clinical manifestations and improved survival in fifty-five patients. *Clinical Immunology and Immunopathology* **29**, 196–210.

Guevara, J.P. et al. (2001). Point prevalence of cardiac abnormalities in children with systemic lupus erythematosus. *Journal of Rheumatology* **28**, 854–9.

Hallegua, D. et al. (2000). Cyclosporine for lupus membranous nephritis: experience with ten patients and review of the literature. *Lupus* **9**, 241–51.

Hataya, H. et al. (1999). Distal tubular dysfunction in lupus nephritis of childhood and adolescence. *Pediatric Nephrology* **13**, 846–9.

Ho, Y.S., Esscher, E., Anderson, R.H., and Michaelsson, M. (1986). Anatomy of congenital complete heart block and relation to maternal anti-Ro antibodies. *American Journal of Cardiology* **58**, 291–4.

Holman, B.L. (1993). Functional imaging in systemic lupus erythematosus: an accurate indicator of central nervous system involvement? *Arthritis and Rheumatism* **36**, 1193–5.

Ilowite, N.T., Samuel, P., Ginzler, E., and Jacobson, M.S. (1988). Dyslipoproteinemia in pediatric systemic lupus erythematosus. *Arthritis and Rheumatism* **31**, 859–63.

Isenberg, D.A., Meyrick-Thomas, D., Snaith, M.L., McKeran, R.O., and Royston, J.P. (1982). A study of migraine in systemic lupus erythematosus. *Annals of the Rheumatic Diseases* **41**, 30–2.

Jara, L.J. et al. (1998). Prolactin and interleukin-6 in neuropsychiatric lupus erythematosus. *Clinical Rheumatology* **17**, 110–14.

Jarek, M.J., West, S., Baker, M.R., and Rak, K.M. (1994). Magnetic resonance imaging in systemic lupus erythematosus patients without a history of neuropsychiatric lupus erythematosus. *Arthritis and Rheumatism* **37**, 1609–13.

Katsanis, E., Hsu, E., Luke, K.-H., and McKee, J.A. (1987). Systemic lupus erythematosus and sickle hemoglobinopathies: a report of two cases and review of the literature. *American Journal of Hematology* **25**, 211–14.

Kaufman, D.B., Laxer, R.M., Silverman, E.D., and Stein, L. (1986). Systemic lupus erythematosus in childhood and adolescence—the problem, epidemiology, incidence, susceptibility, genetics, and prognosis. *Current Problems in Pediatrics* **16**, 555–624.

King, K.K., Kornreich, H.K., Bernstein, B.H., Singsen, B.H., and Hanson, V. (1977). The clinical spectrum of systemic lupus erythematosus in childhood. *Arthritis and Rheumatism* **20** (Suppl.), 287–94.

Lacks, S. and White, P. (1990). Morbidity associated with childhood systemic lupus erythematosus. *Journal of Rheumatology* **17**, 941–5.

Laxer, R.M. et al. (1990). Liver disease in neonatal lupus. *Journal of Pediatrics* **116**, 238–42.

Lee, L.A., Harmon, C.E., Huff, J.C., Norris, D.A., and Weston, W.L. (1985). The demonstration of SS-A/Ro antigen in human fetal tissues and in neonatal and adult skin. *Journal of Investigative Dermatology* **85**, 143–6.

Lee, L.A., Norris, D.A., and Weston, W.L. (1986). Neonatal lupus and the pathogenesis of cutaneous lupus. *Pediatric Dermatology* **3**, 491–7.

LeFeber, W.P. et al. (1984). Ultraviolet light induces binding of antibodies to selected nuclear antigens on cultured keratinocytes. *Journal of Clinical Investigation* **74**, 1545–51.

Lehman, T.J.A. et al. (1989). Intermittent intravenous cyclophosphamide therapy for lupus nephritis. *Journal of Pediatrics* **144**, 1055–60.

Lehman, T.J. and Onel, K. (2000). Intermittent intravenous cyclophosphamide arrests progression of the renal chronicity index in childhood systemic lupus erythematosus. *Journal of Pediatrics* **136**, 243–7.

Lipnick, R.N., Tsokos, G.C., Bray, G.L., and White, P.H. (1990). Autoimmune thrombocytopenia in pediatric systemic lupus erythematosus: alternative therapeutic modalities. *Clinical and Experimental Rheumatology* **8**, 315–19.

Loh, W.F. et al. (2000). Neurological manifestations of children with systemic lupus erythematosus. *Medical Journal of Malaysia* **55**, 459–63.

Long, A.A., Denburg, S.D., Carbotte, R.M., Singal, D.P., and Denburg, J.A. (1989). Serum lymphocytotoxic antibodies and neurocognitive function in systemic lupus erythematosus. *Annals of the Rheumatic Diseases* **49**, 249–53.

Maule, S. et al. (1997). Autonomic nervous dysfunction in systemic lupus erythematosus (SLE) and rheumatoid arthritis (RA): possible pathogenic role of autoantibodies to autonomic nervous structures. *Clinical and Experimental Immunology* **110**, 423–7.

McCune, A.B., Weston, W.L., and Lee, L.A. (1987). Maternal and fetal outcome in neonatal lupus erythematosus. *Annals of Internal Medicine* **106**, 518–23.

McCurdy, D.K. et al. (1992). Lupus nephritis: prognostic factors in children. *Pediatrics* **89**, 240–6.

Miguel, E.C. et al. (1994). Psychiatric manifestations of systemic lupus erythematosus: clinical features, symptoms, and signs of central nervous system activity in 43 patients. *Medicine* **73**, 224–32.

Miller, J.J.I. (1977). Drug-induced lupus-like syndrome in children. *Arthritis and Rheumatism* **20** (Suppl.), 308–11.

Mok, M.Y. et al. (2000). Risk factors for avascular necrosis of bone in patients with systemic lupus erythematosus: is there a role for antiphospholipid antibodies? *Annals of the Rheumatic Diseases* **59**, 462–7.

Moore, T.L. et al. (1999). Parvovirus infection mimicking systemic lupus erythematosus in a pediatric population. *Seminars in Arthritis and Rheumatism* **28**, 314–18.

Nadorra, R.L. and Landing, B.H. (1987). Pulmonary lesions in childhood onset systemic lupus erythematosus: analysis of 26 cases, and summary of literature. *Pediatric Pathology* **7**, 1–18.

Nadorra, R.L., Nakazato, Y., and Landing, B.H. (1987). Pathologic features of gastrointestinal tract lesions in childhood-onset systemic lupus erythematosus: study of 26 patients, with review of the literature. *Pediatric Pathology* **7**, 245–59.

Najafi, C.C. et al. (2001). Significance of histologic patterns of glomerular injury upon long-term prognosis in severe lupus glomerulonephritis. *Kidney International* **59**, 2156–63.

Neiman, A.R. et al. (2000). Cutaneous manifestations of neonatal lupus without heart block: characteristics of mothers and children enrolled in a national registry. *Journal of Pediatrics* **137**, 674–80.

Niaudet, P. (2000). Treatment of lupus nephritis in children. *Pediatric Nephrology* **14**, 158–66.

Nossent, H.C., Swaak, T.J.G., and Berden, J.H.M. (1991). Systemic lupus erythematosus after renal transplantation: patient and graft survival and disease activity. *Annals of Internal Medicine* **114**, 183–8.

Nossent, H.C. and Koldingsnes, W. (2000). Long-term efficacy of azathioprine treatment for proliferative lupus nephritis. *Rheumatology (Oxford)* **39**, 969–74.

Orth, R.W., Weisman, M.H., Cohen, A.H., Talner, L.B., Nachtsheim, D., and Zvaifler, N.J. (1983). Lupus cystitis: primary bladder manifestations of systemic lupus erythematosus. *Annals of Internal Medicine* **98**, 323–6.

Papero, P.H., Bluestein, H.G., White, P., and Lipnick, R.N. (1990). Neuropsychologic deficits and antineuronal antibodies in pediatric systemic lupus erythematosus. *Clinical and Experimental Rheumatology* **8**, 417–24.

Platt, J.L., Burke, B.A., Fish, A.J., Kim, Y., and Michael, A.F. (1982). Systemic lupus erythematosus in the first two decades of life. *American Journal of Kidney Diseases* **11**, 212–22.

Pollak, V.E. and Pirani, C.L. (1993). *Dubois' Lupus Erythematosus* 4th edn. (ed. D.J. Wallace and B.H. Hahn), pp. 525–41. Philadelphia: Lea and Ferbiger.

Press, J. et al. (1996). Antiribosomal P antibodies in pediatric patients with systemic lupus erythematosus and psychosis. *Arthritis and Rheumatism* **39**, 671–6.

Quintero-Del-Rio, A.I. and Van, M. (2000). Neurologic symptoms in children with systemic lupus erythematosus. *Journal of Child Neurology* **15**, 803–7.

Ravelli, A., Martini, A., and Burgio, G.R. (1994). Antiphospholipid antibodies in paediatrics. *European Journal of Pediatrics* **153**, 472–9.

Reeves, W.H. and Lahita, R.G. (1987). Clinical presentation of systemic lupus erythematosus in the adult. In *Systemic Lupus Erythematosus* (ed. R.G. Lahita), pp. 355–75. New York: John Wiley.

Reichlin, M. et al. (1994). Concentration of autoantibodies to native 60-kd Ro/SS-A and denatured 52-kd Ro/Ss-A in eluates from the heart of a child who died with congenital complete heart block. *Arthritis and Rheumatism* **37**, 1698–703.

Rosh, J.R., Silverman, E.D., Groisman, G., Dolgin, S., and LeLeiko, N.S. (1993). Intrahepatic cholestasis in neonatal lupus erythematosus. *Journal of Pediatric Gastroenterology and Nutrition* **17**, 310–12.

Rubin, L.A., Urowitz, M.B., and Gladman, D.D. (1985). Mortality in systemic lupus erythematosus: the bimodal pattern revisited. *Quarterly Journal of Medicine* **55**, 87–98.

Russo, R. et al. (1998). Single photon emission computed tomography scanning in childhood systemic lupus erythematosus. *Journal of Rheumatology* **25**, 576–82.

Saulsbury, F.T., Kesler, R.W., Kennaugh, J.M., Barber, J.C., and Chevalier, R.L. (1982). Overlap syndrome of juvenile rheumatoid arthritis and systemic lupus erythematosus. *Journal of Rheumatology* **9**, 610–12.

Schaller, J. (1982). Lupus in childhood. *Clinics in the Rheumatic Diseases* **8**, 219–28.

Shemesh, O., Golbetz, H., Kriss, J.P., and Myers, B.D. (1985). Limitations of creatinine as a filtration marker in glomerulopathic patients. *Kidney International* **28**, 830–8.

Shergy, W.J., Kredich, D.W., and Pisetsky, D.S. (1988). The relationship of anticardiolipin antibodies to disease manifestations in pediatric systemic lupus erythematosus. *Journal of Rheumatology* **15**, 1389–94.

Shergy, W.J., Kredich, D.W., and Pisetsky, D.S. (1989). Patterns of autoantibody expression in pediatric and adult systemic lupus erythematosus. *Journal of Rheumatology* **16**, 1329–34.

Siegel, M. and Lee, S.L. (1973). The epidemiology of systemic lupus erythematosus. *Seminars in Arthritis and Rheumatism* **3**, 1–54.

Sfikakis, P.P. et al. (1998). Headache in systemic lupus erythematosus: a controlled study. *British Journal of Rheumatology* **37**, 300–3.

Silverman, E.D., Mamula, M., Hardin, J.A., and Laxer, R.M. (1991). Importance of the immune response to the Ro/La particle in the development of congenital heart block and neonatal lupus erythematosus. *Journal of Rheumatology* **18**, 120–4.

Sloan, R.P., Schwartz, M.M., Korbet, S.M., Borok, R.Z., and the Lupus Nephritis Collaborative Study Group (1996). Long-term outcome in systemic lupus erythematosus membranous glomerulonephritis. *Journal of the American Society of Nephrology* **7**, 299–305.

Sorof, J.M. et al. (1998). Increasing incidence of childhood class V lupus nephritis. *Journal of Rheumatology* **25**, 1413–18.

Steinlin, M.I. et al. (1995). Neurologic manifestations of pediatric systemic lupus erythematosus. *Pediatric Neurology* **13**, 191–7.

Tucker, L.B., Menon, S., Schaller, J.G., and Isenberg, D.A. (1995). Adult- and childhood-onset systemic lupus erythematosus: a comparison of onset, clinical features, serology and outcome. *British Journal of Rheumatology* **34**, 866–72.

Uziel, Y., Laxer, R.M., Blaser, S., Andrew, M., Scneider, R., and Silverman, E.D. (1995). Cerebral vein thrombosis in childhood systemic lupus erythematosus. *Journal of Pediatrics* **126**, 722–7.

Watson, R.M., Lane, A.T., Barnett, N.K., Bias, W.B., Arnett, F.C., and Provost, T.T. (1984). Neonatal lupus erythematosus. A clinical, serological and immunologenic study with review of the literature. *Medicine Baltimore* **63**, 362–78.

Weber, H.S. and Myers, J.L. (1994). Maternal collagen vascular disease associated with fetal heart block and degenerative changes of the atrioventricular valves. *Pediatric Cardiology* **15**, 204–6.

Wilson, W.A., Armatis, P.E., and Perez, M.C. (1989). C4 concentrations and C4 deficiency alleles in systemic lupus erythematosus. *Annals of the Rheumatic Diseases* **48**, 600–4.

Yan, D.C. et al. (1995). Intravenous cyclophosphamide pulse therapy on children with severe active lupus nephritis. *Chung Hua Min Kuo Hsiao Erh Ko I Hsueh Hui Tsa Chih* **36**, 203–9.

Yancey, C.L., Doughty, R.A., and Athreya, B.H. (1981). Central nervous system involvement in childhood systemic lupus erythematosus. *Arthritis and Rheumatism* **24**, 1389–95.

6.6.4 The antiphospholipid antibody syndrome

Munther A. Khamashta and Graham R.V. Hughes

Introduction

In 1983, few rheumatologists would have predicted the interest that the introduction of the anticardiolipin test would generate (Harris et al. 1983). New autoantibodies turn up frequently in patients with systemic lupus erythematosus and there may have seemed little reason why anticardiolipin antibodies should have merited any more than passing interest. However, their association with an unusual combination of clinical complications that included venous and arterial thrombosis, pregnancy loss, and thrombocytopaenia attracted the attention of investigators from a variety of disciplines (Hughes 1983).

During the last two decades, considerable progress has been made in understanding antiphospholipid antibodies and the disorder with which they are associated, but many questions remain unanswered, particularly those of pathogenesis and optimal treatment (Khamashta 2000a). A chronology of the major developments in the unfolding of the antiphospholipid syndrome story is listed in Table 1.

Detection of antiphospholipid antibodies

Antiphospholipid antibodies are detected by a variety of laboratory tests, the most useful for identifying patients with the antiphospholipid syndrome being the lupus anticoagulant and the anticardiolipin antibody tests. These antibodies are distinct and separable immunoglobulins present alone or in combination in the plasma of people with the antiphospholipid syndrome. The autoantibodies sometimes bind phospholipids utilized in the Venereal Disease Research Laboratories (VDRL) test; hence, some patients may have a false-positive test for syphilis. However, the VDRL test is not positive frequently enough to make it valuable in diagnosing the antiphospholipid syndrome.

The lupus anticoagulant is a functional assay measuring the ability of antiphospholipid antibodies to prolong clotting via their inhibition of the conversion of prothrombin to thrombin or the activation of factor X (both reactions are catalyzed by phospholipids). Tests for the lupus anticoagulant have been difficult to standardize, and no single test appears to be adequate. The test begins with an attempt to demonstrate an abnormal coagulation screening test, such as a prolonged activated partial thromboplastin time, dilute Russell viper venom time, or kaolin clotting time. If any of these is positive, the test is repeated, using a sample in which the patient's plasma has been mixed with normal plasma. If the patient's disorder is a clotting deficiency, the test should become normal. If, on the other hand, lupus anticoagulant or some other clotting inhibitor is present, the clotting time will remain prolonged. The presence of lupus anticoagulant is confirmed by the return to normal of the clotting test after addition of freeze–thawed platelets or excess phospholipids, either of which bind the antibodies. The lupus anticoagulant test must be performed on platelet-poor plasma.

The most sensitive test for antiphospholipid antibodies is the anticardiolipin antibody test, introduced in 1983 and extensively improved since that time (Tincani et al. 2000). This test uses enzyme-linked immunosorbent assay to determine antibody binding to solid plates coated either with cardiolipin or other phospholipids. Serum or plasma samples may be used for the anticardiolipin assay. The availability of reference sera which are isotype specific (IgG and IgM) has greatly improved interlaboratory testing and quantification of anticardiolipin antibodies. IgA anticardiolipin reference sera are also now available. Many laboratories currently measure all three isotypes and sensitive kits are commercially available. Flow cytometry has also been used to test for anticardiolipin antibodies. This system allows the simultaneous measurement of antiphospholipid antibody isotypes with different phospholipid specificity.

In general, lupus anticoagulant antibodies are more specific for the antiphospholipid syndrome, whereas anticardiolipin antibodies are more sensitive. The specificity of anticardiolipin antibodies for antiphospholipid syndrome increases with the titre and is higher for the IgG than for the IgM isotype. However, some patients may have only a positive IgM test, and a few are only IgA positive.

In most laboratories, there is substantial concordance between lupus anticoagulant activity and anticardiolipin antibodies, with approximately 70 per cent of patients with definite antiphospholipid syndrome having both lupus anticoagulant and anticardiolipin antibodies. However, these antibodies may not be identical, either because they detect different epitopes altogether, or because they have different affinities to various epitopes in different test systems. Thus, multiple antiphospholipid antibody tests (most commonly lupus anticoagulant and IgG and IgM anticardiolipin antibodies) should be used in seeking the diagnosis of antiphospholipid syndrome.

The observation that many anticardiolipin antibodies are directed at an epitope on β_2-glycoprotein I led to the development of anti-β_2-glycoprotein I antibody immunoassays (Matsuura et al. 1994). Although their presence is not currently included in the criteria for the antiphospholipid syndrome (Wilson et al. 1999), anti-β_2-glycoprotein I antibodies are strongly associated with thrombosis and other features of the antiphospholipid syndrome. Indeed, in some patients with clinical features of antiphospholipid syndrome, anti-β_2-glycoprotein I antibodies are the sole antibodies detected (Cabral et al. 1996).

The clinical utility of antiphospholipid antibody assays for autoantibodies to phospholipids other than cardiolipin and to phospholipid-binding proteins other than β_2-glycoprotein I remains unclear (Bertolaccini et al. 1998a,b).

Table 1 Antiphospholipid antibodies and the antiphospholipid syndrome—history

1906	Wasserman reaction (reagin)
1941	Reagin binds cardiolipin
1952	False-positive test for syphillis
1952	Lupus anticoagulant
1960s	Lupus anticoagulant: association with thrombosis
1970s	Lupus anticoagulant is due to immunoglobulin
1975	Lupus anticoagulant: association with recurrent miscarriages
1983	Anticardiolipin antibodies
1983–1985	Detailed clinical description of the antiphospholipid syndrome
1985	Antiphospholipid syndrome—separate entity from lupus
1989	Lupus anticoagulant and anticardiolipin: separate antibody sub-groups
1990	Phospholipid-binding proteins (β_2-glycoprotein I)
1990s	Animal models for antiphospholipid syndrome
1999	Classification criteria for the antiphospholipid syndrome

Clinical features

The antiphospholipid syndrome is a non-inflammatory autoimmune disease. The most critical pathologic process is thrombosis, which results in most of the clinical features suffered by these patients. Any organ can be affected in this disorder; thus, the range of clinical features is extremely wide (Table 2). However, this syndrome is best defined as the occurrence of recurrent vascular thrombosis and/or pregnancy losses associated with persistently elevated levels of antiphospholipid antibodies.

Table 2 Clinical features of the antiphospholipid syndrome

Major features
Venous thrombosis: deep venous thrombosis, Budd–Chiari syndrome, and pulmonary thromboembolism
Arterial thrombosis: strokes, transient ischaemic attacks, multi-infarct dementia, and myocardial infarction
Pregnancy complications: recurrent pregnancy loss, intrauterine growth restriction, pre-eclampsia, and abruption
Associated clinical features
Thrombocytopaenia
Leg ulcers, livedo reticularis, thrombophlebitis, and Sneddon's syndrome
Heart valve lesions
Transverse myelitis, chorea, and epilepsy
Haemolytic anaemia, Coombs' positivity, and Evans' syndrome
Pulmonary hypertension
Cognitive impairment
Chronic headache
Others (less common)
Splinter haemorrhages
Labile hypertension and accelerated atherosclerosis
Ischaemic necrosis of bone
Bone marrow necrosis
Addison's disease
Guillain–Barré syndrome and pseudo-multiple sclerosis
Aumaurosis fugax
Sensorineural hearing loss
Renal artery and vein thrombosis and microangiopathy
Retinal artery and vein thrombosis
Digital gangrene

Thrombosis

Arterial and venous thrombosis can be present in the antiphospholipid syndrome, distinguishing this from other prothrombotic states such as protein C, protein S, or antithrombin III deficiency, where only venous thrombosis occurs. Vessels of all sizes may be affected, and the vascular pathological appearance has consistently been of bland occlusion without inflammatory infiltrate (Lie 1994). Thus, it is unlikely that thrombotic occlusion of blood vessels in patients with the antiphospholipid syndrome is caused by vasculitis, which may be seen in other patients with autoimmune rheumatic disorders. The distinction is important not only for discovering the pathogenesis of the vascular lesions, but also for the choice of treatment.

In the venous circulation, thrombosis of the deep veins of the lower extremities has been reported most frequently (occasionally after the use of oral contraceptive pills containing oestrogen). It is often recurrent and may be accompanied by pulmonary embolism. It has been estimated that up to 19 per cent of patients with deep vein thrombosis and/or pulmonary thromboembolism are suffering from antiphospholipid coagulopathy and may demonstrate a positive lupus anticoagulant test, antibodies to cardiolipin, or both. Some patients with antiphospholipid antibodies also have pulmonary hypertension, perhaps caused by recurrent pulmonary emboli or intravascular thromboses. Other reported venous sites of thrombosis include the axillary, ocular, renal, hepatic and sagittal veins, and the inferior vena cava. The antiphospholipid syndrome is now considered one of the most frequent causes of the Budd–Chiari syndrome (Plate 118) (Espinosa et al. 2001). Antiphospholipid antibodies have been implicated in the development of adrenal vein thrombosis leading to Addison's disease. Venous events usually occur at single sites and these can recur at the same or different sites, months or years apart.

Unlike other known clotting disorders, arterial thromboses are a major feature of the antiphospholipid syndrome. Occlusion of the intracranial arteries has been reported most frequently, with the majority of patients presenting with stroke and transient ischaemic attacks. However, cerebral infarction may be silent. Magnetic resonance imaging scans show changes that vary from single lesions to multiple widely-scattered infarcts. In some patients, untreated recurrent cerebral thrombosis has led to multi-infarct dementia and psychiatric and cognitive impairment have been prominent in the presentation of some patients with the antiphospholipid syndrome (Menon et al. 1999). Antiphospholipid antibodies are now internationally recognized as an important aetiological factor and may be present in 7 per cent of all patients who have suffered a stroke. They should be sought especially in young patients with strokes, where they may account for up to 18 per cent. Since emboli from heart valve vegetations may be responsible for cerebral infarction, it is advisable to perform echocardiograms on patients with antiphospholipid syndrome who present with transient ischaemic attacks or stroke. Other arterial thromboses have involved the retina, coronary, mesenteric, and peripheral arteries. The clinical presentation depends on the anatomic site occluded. Malignant hypertension with renal insufficiency secondary to thrombosis of the renal glomeruli and renal thrombotic microangiopathy (without classical lupus nephritis) has also been associated with the presence of antiphospholipid antibodies (Amigo et al. 1992). As with venous thrombosis, arterial events occur at single sites usually and can recur months or years later.

Pregnancy complications

Recurrent spontaneous pregnancy losses are one of the most consistent complications of the antiphospholipid syndrome. Losses can occur at any stage of pregnancy, although miscarriages associated with antiphospholipid antibody are strikingly frequent during the second and third trimester (about 50 per cent of cases). This differs from the pattern of pregnancy loss in the normal population, which usually occurs during the first trimester and is most often due to non-immunological factors, that is, morphological or chromosomal abnormalities. The rate of miscarriage in patients positive for antiphospholipid antibody is still uncertain, although the epidemiology is being studied and, increasingly, testing for this antibody is becoming a routine investigation in women with recurrent miscarriages. Fewer than 2 per cent of apparently normal pregnant women have either anticardiolipin antibody or lupus anticoagulant in any titre and less than 0.2 per cent have high titre antibody. Hence, screening normal pregnant women has little value. Previous pregnancy history is of importance in determining the significance of a positive laboratory test for antiphospholipid antibodies. It has been estimated that if a patient with lupus has a positive lupus anticoagulant, or at least moderate levels of IgG anticardiolipin antibodies, the risk of spontaneous miscarriage during the first pregnancy is 30 per cent and if she has a history of at least two spontaneous miscarriages, the risk is 70 per cent during the following pregnancy. The risk of foetal loss is directly related to the antibody titre, particularly the IgG anticardiolipin, although many women with recurrent miscarriages have IgM anticardiolipin antibodies only. It is impossible to predict which women are likely to develop complications in pregnancy, and some women with persistently elevated antiphospholipid antibody titres and a history of thromboses have no foetal complications at all. Previous obstetric outcome remains the most important predictor of future risk (Branch et al. 1992; Lima et al. 1996; Shehata et al. 2001).

In pregnancies that do not end in miscarriage or foetal loss, there is a high incidence of intrauterine growth restriction, placental abruption, and premature delivery. The most recent classification criteria for antiphospholipid syndrome have been amended to highlight the fact that not only foetal loss but premature birth before 34 weeks as a result of pre-eclampsia, placental abruption, or intrauterine growth restriction, and positive lupus anticoagulant or anticardiolipin antibody may allow the patient to be labelled as having antiphospholipid syndrome (Wilson et al. 1999).

It is important to note that units that manage patients with severe manifestations of antiphospholipid syndrome such as thrombosis and previous stillbirth (Branch et al. 1992; Lima et al. 1996), have a higher incidence of complications in pregnancy than those that recruit women predominantly from recurrent miscarriage clinics (Kutteh 1996; Rai et al. 1997). In our unit we run a multidisciplinary team service, where most antiphospholipid syndrome cases have either been identified by rheumatology (association with systemic lupus erythematosus) or haematology (previous thrombosis) colleagues. Many patients are referred for specialist management after previous poor obstetric outcome. Our live birth rate is 70–80 per cent, and in a previous study from our unit, the incidence of pre-eclampsia was 18 per cent, the percentage of babies born with birth weights less than the tenth centile for gestational age was 31 per cent, and the percentage of infants delivered prematurely (<37 weeks) with a mean gestation of approximately 34 weeks was about 43 per cent. Approximately 70 per cent of these women were delivered by caesarean section, and 7 per cent of babies died in the neonatal period as a result of problems related to prematurity (Lima et al. 1996).

Other manifestations

Thrombocytopaenia is common in patients with antiphospholipid antibodies, though rarely severe enough to cause haemorrhage. The platelet count often remains stable for many years; then, for reasons that are often obscure, the count drops, sometimes catastrophically. Occasionally, patients with the antiphospholipid syndrome may present only with severe thrombocytopaenia and later develop pregnancy loss or thrombosis. This form of presentation was observed in a very small number of our patients with the syndrome (Cuadrado and Hughes 2001). Some patients with antiphospholipid antibodies and thrombocytopaenia also develop haemolytic anaemia with positive direct Coombs' test. This is widely known as Evans' syndrome.

Epilepsy and chorea are less frequent manifestations of the antiphospholipid syndrome and have, intriguingly, been seen to improve in some patients treated with anticoagulants. Transverse myelopathy, though rare, is strongly associated with the presence of antiphospholipid antibodies (Alarcon-Segovia et al. 1989). Occasionally, in some patients with bizarre, transient/recurrent neurologial signs (resembling multiple sclerosis), antiphospholipid antibodies have been detected in the absence of other immunological abnormalities. Its recognition is important as anticoagulation therapy may be effective in these patients (Cuadrado et al. 2000). Migraine is a common finding in patients with the antiphospholipid syndrome, and often pre-dates the diagnosis by many years. However, several prospective studies have not demonstrated a significant statistical association between migraine headaches and the presence of antiphospholipid antibodies (Cuadrado and Hughes 2001).

Heart valve disease, particularly mitral valve involvement, is strikingly associated with antiphospholipid antibodies (Khamashta et al. 1990). In some cases, this is due to a combination of valvular thrombosis and degeneration. In our prospective echocardiographic studies, the valves were involved in more than one-third of the patients with lupus or primary antiphospholipid syndrome. Most patients with heart valve disease associated with antiphospholipid antibodies are asymptomatic, though heart insufficiency requiring surgical valve replacement has been reported. Emboli from sterile valvular vegetations can cause multiple cerebral lesions. Large intracardiac thrombosis associated with antiphospholipid antibodies can mimic atrial myxoma.

One of the most striking physical signs in patients positive for antiphospholipid antibody is livedo reticularis (Plate 119), sometimes widespread, sometimes subtle, for example, confined to a small area on the back of the wrist. Many cases of Sneddon's syndrome, defined as the clinical triad of stroke, livedo reticularis, and hypertension, may represent undiagnosed antiphospholipid syndrome. More dramatic skin manifestations associated with vascular thrombosis include widespread skin ulceration, notably in the lower extremities. Clinically, some patients with antiphospholipid antibodies may develop nail splinter haemorrhages and clubbing, posing major diagnostic difficulties, in those with heart valve disease, in differentiating from bacterial endocarditis.

Avascular necrosis of bone is an uncommon complication in lupus patients and clearly associated with high steroid dosage. We have noted an increased risk of avascular necrosis in individuals positive for antiphospholipid antibody, possibly as a result of small arterial occlusions, notably of the head of the femur.

Many patients with the antiphospholipid syndrome seem to develop widespread arteriopathy. The systemic narrowing of major arteries is similar in many respects to the widespread endarterial disease seen in some patients after heart–lung transplantation. Thus, antiphospholipid antibodies might be associated with accelerated vascular disease, including atherosclerosis (George et al. 2001).

Epidemiology

The epidemiology of antiphospholipid antibodies is still being investigated worldwide. Efforts are being made in clinics throughout the world to assess the importance of this factor in recurrent abortion, stroke, myocardial infarction, epilepsy, and so on. Prospective studies have shown an association between antiphospholipid antibodies and the first episode of venous thrombosis (Ginsburg et al. 1992), the first myocardial infarction (Vaarala et al. 1995), and the first ischaemic stroke (Brey et al. 2001). A critical issue, therefore, is the identification of patients with antiphospholipid antibodies who are at increased risk for a thrombotic event.

Many patients have laboratory evidence of antiphospholipid antibodies without clinical consequence. Antiphospholipid antibodies, using standardized techniques, are detected in less than 1 per cent of apparently normal individuals and in up to 3 per cent of the elderly population without clinical manifestations of the antiphospholipid syndrome. Among patients with systemic lupus erythematosus, the prevalence of antiphospholipid antibodies is much higher, ranging from 30 to 40 per cent (Cervera et al. 1999). For otherwise healthy control subjects, there are insufficient data to determine what percentage of those with antiphospholipid antibodies will eventually have a thrombotic event or a complication of pregnancy consistent with the antiphospholipid syndrome. In contrast, the antiphospholipid syndrome may develop in 50–70 per cent of patients with both systemic lupus erythematosus and antiphospholipid antibodies after 10–20 years of follow-up (Shah et al. 1998; Petri 2000).

The specificities of antiphospholipid antibodies probably differ in various disorders. Large retrospective studies of patients with thrombotic complications suggest that those with high concentrations of IgG anticardiolipin antibodies appear to be at greatest risk for thrombosis, whereas the risk of clotting appears to be much lower in patients with infection-related or drug-induced antiphospholipid antibodies.

Genetic analyses and modelling studies strongly support a genetic basis for disease in families with the antiphospholipid syndrome and suggest an autonomic dominant model of inheritance (Goel et al. 1999). HLA studies have suggested associations with DR7, DR4, DRw53, DQw7, and C4 null alleles.

Definition and classification criteria

An international consensus statement on classification criteria for definite antiphospholipid syndrome was published after a workshop in Sapporo, Japan, 1998 (Wilson et al. 1999). These criteria have recently been validated (Lockshin et al. 2000). A patient with the antiphospholipid syndrome must meet at least one of two clinical criteria (vascular thrombosis or complications of pregnancy) and at least one of two laboratory criteria (anticardiolipin antibody or lupus anticoagulant) (Table 3). The purpose of the

Table 3 Criteria for the classification of definite antiphospholipid syndrome

Clinical criteria

1. *Vascular thrombosis*
   One or more clinical episodes of arterial, venous, or small vessel thrombosis in any tissue or organ, confirmed by imaging or histopathology in the absence of significant evidence of inflammation in the vessel wall
2. *Pregnancy morbidity*
   (a) one or more unexplained deaths of a morphologically normal foetus at or beyond the tenth week of gestation, or
   (b) one or more premature births of a morphologically normal neonate at or before the thirty-fourth week of gestation, due to severe pre-eclampsia, eclampsia or placental insufficiency, or
   (c) three or more unexplained consecutive spontaneous abortions before the tenth week of gestation (maternal anatomic or hormonal abnormalities and chromosomal causes excluded)

Laboratory criteria

1. *Anticardiolipin antibodies*
   IgG and/or IgM anticardiolipin antibody, in medium or high titre, on two or more occasions, at least 6 weeks apart, measured by a standardized enzyme-linked immunosorbent assay for β_2-glycoprotein I-dependent anticardiolipin antibodies
2. *Lupus anticoagulant*
   Lupus anticoagulant present in plasma, on two or more occasions at least 6 weeks apart, detected according to the guidelines of the International Society on Thrombosis and Haemostasis

Note: Definite antiphospholipid syndrome may be diagnosed if at least one of the clinical criteria and at least one of the laboratory criteria are met. Modified from Wilson et al. (1999).

classification criteria was to facilitate studies of treatment and causation, and focused on defining a category of 'definite' antiphospholipid syndrome. 'Probable' or 'possible' categories were excluded due to lack of supportive prospective studies or experimental evidence. Other features of antiphospholipid syndrome such as thrombocytopaenia, haemolytic anaemia, transient cerebral ischaemia, transverse myelopathy or myelitis, livedo reticularis, cardiac valve disease, multiple sclerosis-like syndrome, chorea, and migraine were felt by the workshop to not have as strong an association and were excluded as classification criteria. This should not deter the clinicians from making the diagnosis or administering therapy if other causes of such features have been excluded.

Many of the patients reported to have the syndrome have lupus and can be regarded as having secondary antiphospholipid syndrome. Some patients do not have any underlying systemic disease. These patients may be regarded as having primary antiphospholipid syndrome. For research and classification purposes, the term primary is useful, although there appear to be few differences in complications related to antiphospholipid antibody or in antibody specificity in the presence or absence of systemic lupus erythematosus (Cervera et al. 2002). Although some patients with primary antiphospholipid syndrome progress to systemic lupus, most do not show such progression.

A minority of patients with the antiphospholipid syndrome present with an acute and devastating syndrome characterized by multiple simultaneous vascular occlusions throughout the body, often resulting in death. This syndrome, termed 'catastrophic antiphospholipid syndrome', is defined by the clinical involvement of at least three different organ systems over a period of days or weeks with histopathological evidence of multiple occlusions of large or small vessels (Asherson et al. 2001). Although the same clinical manifestations seen with primary and secondary antiphospholipid syndrome occur as part of catastrophic antiphospholipid syndrome, there are important differences in prevalence and in the calibre of the vessels predominantly affected. Ischaemia of the kidneys, bowels, lungs, heart and/or brain are most frequent, but rarely adrenal, testicular, splenic, pancreatic, or skin involvement have been described. Occlusion of small vessels (thrombotic microangiopathy) is characteristic resulting in symptoms related to dysfunction of the affected organs. Depending on the organs involved, patients may present with hypertension and renal impairment, acute respiratory distress syndrome, alveolar haemorrhage and capillaritis, confusion and disorientation, or abdominal pain and distension secondary to bowel infarction. Precipitating factors of catastrophic antiphospholipid syndrome include infections, surgical procedures, withdrawal of anticoagulant therapy, and the use of drugs such as oral contraceptives.

Differential diagnosis

Careful family and personal history and physical examination of patients with unexplained thromboses are of the utmost importance as thrombotic events and, notably, venous thromboses often have explanations other than the antiphospholipid syndrome (Hunt and Ames 2000).

The most striking feature of the antiphospholipid syndrome is the frequent observation of life-threatening thrombosis in the setting of thrombocytopaenia. A number of other conditions can result in thrombocytopaenia and thrombosis, including heparin-induced thrombocytopaenia and thrombotic thrombocytopaenic purpura.

Heparin-induced thrombocytopaenia develops in 1–5 per cent of patients receiving standard heparin and somewhat less frequently in those who receive preparations of low molecular weight. This is due to the presence of an antibody which binds to platelet factor 4 and heparin. Approximately 10–20 per cent of patients with substantial heparin-induced thrombocytopaenia have venous or arterial thrombosis, including pulmonary, cardiac, and cerebral thrombosis. Thrombocytopaenia typically develops approximately a week after exposure in persons not previously treated with heparin and sooner in those with previous exposure.

Thrombotic thrombocytopaenic purpura is associated with neurological syndromes, but it is chiefly a microvascular disorder and confusion, seizures, or changes in the level of consciousness are more frequent than isolated, cerebral, large vessel thrombosis. Microangiopathic haemolysis with evidence of schistocytes in peripheral blood is usually a prominent finding. Elevation in the serum level of lactate dehydrogenase is found in nearly all cases and is a sensitive marker of the severity of the disorder.

Antiphospholipid syndrome has been identified as a cause of first, second, and third trimester pregnancy losses as well as intrauterine growth restriction and pre-eclampsia. One of the major advances in the field of thrombophilia in the last few years have been the recognition that other thrombophilic states, such as Factor V Leiden mutation and prothrombin 20210A mutation, also predispose to second and third trimester losses, as well as intrauterine growth restriction and pre-eclampsia (Kupfermic et al. 1999). It is important when considering the late pregnancy morbidity associated with antiphospholipid antibodies to check that the history concurs with that of placental insufficiency. We have a number of women referred to our clinic with the diagnosis of antiphospholipid syndrome on the basis of pregnancy loss where antiphospholipid antibodies were an incidental finding. These women have proved to have pregnancy loss due to other causes such as premature labour secondary to an incompetent cervix (Stone et al. 2002). Thus, history-taking and obtaining the post-mortem findings in previous pregnancy losses are very important.

Pathogenesis

There is now good evidence, mainly from animal models, that antiphospholipid antibodies can be pathogenic rather than a simple serological marker for antiphospholipid syndrome. Passive transfer and active immunization of BALB/c mice with human or mouse anticardiolipin monoclonal antibodies induced features of the antiphospholipid syndrome (Pierangeli et al. 2000; Sherer and Shoenfeld 2000). Also, atherosclerosis in a susceptible mouse model (the LDL-receptor knockout mouse) was accelerated by immunization with human anticardiolipin antibodies from an antiphospholipid syndrome patient, providing additional evidence for a causal pathogenic effect (George et al. 2001). However, a direct causal relationship between antiphospholipid antibodies and thrombotic manifestations or pregnancy losses in humans has not yet been proven.

Mechanisms of thrombosis

Antiphospholipid antibodies alone apparently are unable to induce thrombotic manifestations per se. In this regard, a two-hit hypothesis has been suggested: antiphospholipid antibodies (first hit) increases the risk of thrombotic events that occur in the presence of another thrombophilic condition (second hit) (Meroni and Riboldi 2001).

Precisely how antiphospholipid antibodies relate to thrombosis is unknown. Several mechanisms have been proposed to explain the prothrombotic nature of the antiphospholipid syndrome. The range of possible mechanisms include effects of antiphospholipid antibodies on platelet membranes, on endothelial cells, and on clotting components such as antithrombin III, protein C, and protein S (Table 4) (Rand 2002).

Great interest has centred on the role of phospholipid-binding proteins as a clue to the mechanism of thrombosis in antiphospholipid syndrome. The better characterized β_2-glycoprotein I. It is now accepted that antiphospholipid antibodies can react with endothelial cells, mainly through the binding to β_2-glycoprotein I expressed on cell membranes. Exogenous β_2-glycoprotein I can bind to endothelial cells at the putative phospholipid binding site located in the fifth domain of the molecule. Binding of antiphospholipid antibodies induces activation of endothelial cells and thus a procoagulant state, as assessed by upregulation of the expression of adhesion molecules, the secretion of cytokines and the metabolism of prostacyclins (Meroni et al. 2000). Anti-β_2-glycoprotein I-mediated endothelial cell activation may also play a role in the accelerated atherosclerosis associated with antiphospholipid syndrome. Recent findings showing that statins, the cholesterol lowering drugs, are able to inhibit such activation *in vitro* open new therapeutic modalities (Meroni et al. 2001).

The oxidation of phospholipids may be necessary for antiphospholipid antibody recognition. Autoantibodies to oxidized LDL occur in association with anticardiolipin antibodies and some anticardiolipin antibodies cross-react with oxidized LDL. Moreover, anticardiolipin antibodies bind to oxidized but not reduced cardiolipin, suggesting that anticardiolipin antibodies recognize oxidized phospholipids, phospholipid-binding proteins, or both (George et al. 2001). Elevated levels of antioxidized LDL antibodies have been proposed to be markers for arterial thrombosis in the antiphospholipid syndrome.

Another theory proposes that antiphospholipid antibodies upregulate the expression of endothelin-I. Atsumi et al. (1998) reported that plasma levels of endothelin-1 peptide, the most potent endothelium-derived contracting factor, significantly correlated with the history of arterial thrombosis in patients with antiphospholipid syndrome.

Mechanisms by which antiphospholipid antibodies interfere with the regulatory functions of prothrombin, protein C, annexin V, and tissue factor have also been proposed (Rand 2002). Interestingly, plasma levels of tissue factor and tissue factor pathway inhibitor, were found significantly elevated in patients with antiphospholipid syndrome, suggesting an *in vivo* upregulation of tissue factor pathway (Dobado-Berrios et al. 2001).

An alternative route by which antiphospholipid antibodies might promote thrombosis is by platelet activation leading to enhanced platelet adhesion. The increase in thromboxane A_2 urinary metabolites was reported as indirect evidence in favour of pathogenic interaction between antiphospholipid antibodies and platelets. However, the ability of antiphospholipid antibodies to activate platelets directly is still debated.

It remains unclear which cellular phospholipids and phospholipid-binding proteins are targeted by antiphospholipid antibodies *in vivo*. The absence of anionic phospholipids on the cell surface and the apparent lack of reactivity of antiphospholipid antibodies with intact cells suggest that perturbation of the cell membrane may be required for antiphospholipid antibodies to bind to cells. Indeed, some antiphospholipid antibodies react with activated platelets and apoptotic cells, which have undergone a loss of the normal asymmetric distribution of membrane phospholipids and expose anionic phospholipids on their cell surface. Binding of antiphospholipid antibodies to apoptotic cells is dependent on β_2-glycoprotein I, as is induction of antiphospholipid antibodies by apoptotic cells (Levine et al. 2002).

It was recently shown by Gharavi et al. (2002) that a synthetic peptide which shares structural similarity with the putative phospholipid binding region of the β_2-glycoprotein I molecule, and shares high homology to cytomegalovirus, is able to induce antiphospholipid antibodies in mice. Some of the antibodies exhibited binding to cultured endothelial cells *in vitro* or had lupus anticoagulant activity, and some were pathogenic *in vivo*, resulting in a significant increase in the number of leucocytes adhering to endothelial cells and enhanced thrombus formation.

Table 4 Proposed mechanisms of thrombosis mediated by antiphospholipid antibody

Decrease of prostacyclin production and/or release by endothelial cells
Inhibition of factor XII/prekallikrein-mediated fibrinolytic activity
Decrease of protein C activation
Decrease of free protein S levels
Interference with thrombomodulin function on endothelial cells
Decrease of antithrombin III activation
Increase of platelet activation and aggregation
Interference with the function of plasma β_2-glycoprotein I
Increase of tissue factor expression on monocytes and on endothelial cells
Inhibition of tissue factor pathway inhibitor
Decrease of function of annexin V
Direct injury to endothelium
Complement activation
Induction of apoptosis on vascular cells
Vascular activation and release of von Willebrand factor multimer
Increase of endothelin-1
Increase of plasminogen activator inhibitor-1
Cross-reactivity to oxidized LDL

Mechanisms of pregnancy loss

The mechanism of pregnancy loss associated with antiphospholipid antibody remains uncertain. Progressive thrombosis of the microvasculature of the placenta and subsequent infarction resulting in placental insufficiency, foetal growth restriction and, ultimately, foetal loss, is a plausible explanation. One of the most intriguing hypothesis as to how this might occur relates to antiphospholipid displacement of annexin V proteins from trophoblast surfaces (Rand et al. 1997). Not all placentas examined, however, have shown areas of thrombosis or infarction and other mechanisms may be operative in these patients. Recently, *in vitro* studies showed that antiphospholipid antibodies may impair trophoblastic invasion and hormone production, thereby promoting not only early miscarriages but also foetal loss and uteroplacental insufficiency (Di Simone et al. 2000). These findings provide strong evidence for a defective placentation mediated directly by antiphospholipid antibodies that is not necessarily associated with thrombotic phenomena (Stone et al. 2001). Another, recent, work points to the complement system as having a major role in antiphospholipid syndrome-related pregnancy loss, showing that C3 activation is required for foetal loss in a murine model (Holers et al. 2002).

Treatment

One of the reasons for the widespread interest in the antiphospholipid syndrome has been its effect on approaches to therapy. Before its recognition, most features of systemic lupus erythematosus were attributed to inflammatory phenomena, requiring anti-inflammatory measures such as corticosteroids. Now it is recognized that features as diverse as fits, miscarriage, endocardial disease, and hypertension may all be the result of a thrombotic process. This concept has spread beyond the confines of systemic lupus, and pinpointing antiphospholipid-associated thrombosis and taking appropriate anticoagulation measures have become important considerations in specialties as diverse as neurology and obstetrics. Table 5 shows our preferred treatment for the different clinical features associated with antiphospholipid antibodies.

Primary thromboprophylaxis

The controversy over whether or not prophylactic treatment is indicated for patients with antiphospholipid antibodies who have no history of thrombosis remains unresolved. Although low-dose aspirin (75–100 mg daily) has been considered to be a logical first option, the Physician Health Study showed that low-dose aspirin (325 mg daily) use in men with anticardiolipin antibodies did not protect against deep venous thrombosis or pulmonary embolism (Ginsburg et al. 1992). In contrast, aspirin may provide protection against thrombosis in patients with systemic lupus erythematosus (Wahl et al. 2000) and in women with the antiphospholipid syndrome and previous pregnancy loss (Erkan et al. 2001).

Hydroxychloroquine may be protective against the development of thrombosis in antiphospholipid antibody-positive patients with systemic lupus erythematosus (Petri 2000). The antiplatelet effects of hydroxychloroquine/chloroquine are well known and these drugs were widely used for prophylaxis of deep vein thrombosis and pulmonary thromboembolism after hip surgery during the 1970s and 1980s. However, the need for a regular review by an ophthalmologist for the early detection of retinal toxicity is a limiting factor for the long-term use of antimalarials in the primary thromboprophylaxis of antiphospholipid antibody-positive individuals.

Low intensity oral anticoagulation (international normalized ratio, INR~1.5) might be an option for the primary prevention of thrombosis in antiphospholipid antibody-positive individuals. This regime has been shown to be effective in the thromboprophylaxis of other prothrombotic states, which include central venous catheterization, stage IV breast cancer, and men at risk for ischaemic heart disease. A prospective, randomized clinical trial comparing aspirin alone with aspirin plus low-intensity warfarin (INR~1.5) in patients with antiphospholipid antibodies who have never had thrombosis is currently underway in the United Kingdom (Khamashta 2000b). Until these results are available, we suggest that individuals with a persistently positive anticardiolipin antibody (moderate/high titres) and/or unequivocally positive lupus anticoagulant tests, take low-dose aspirin (75–100 mg daily) indefinitely. Prophylaxis with heparin administered subcutaneously should certainly be given to cover high-risk situations, such as surgery and long-haul flights.

The most important prophylactic therapy may be the avoidance or reduction of other risk factors for thrombosis such as smoking, obesity, high blood pressure, hypercholesterolaemia, and oestrogen-containing oral contraceptive pills. Oestrogen replacement therapy also increases the risk of arterial and venous thromboembolism and, therefore, should be avoided.

Prevention of recurrent thrombosis

There is now good evidence that antiphospholipid syndrome patients with thrombosis will be subject to recurrences, and these can be prevented by long-term anticoagulation (Khamashta et al. 1995; Krnic-Barrie et al. 1997; Brunner et al. 2002). Many patients with the antiphospholipid syndrome in whom anticoagulation has been stopped, have had major recurrent thrombosis. It is not clear, however, whether prolonged anticoagulation is necessary in antiphospholipid syndrome patients whose first thrombotic episode developed in association with surgery, oral contraceptive pill, pregnancy, or other circumstantial thrombotic risk factors.

Most patients requiring long-term anticoagulant therapy respond well to warfarin targeted to an INR of 2.0–3.0. However, the optimal intensity of anticoagulation therapy is uncertain for patients with antiphospholipid-associated thrombosis. There are reports based on retrospective analyses of observational studies, that patients with antiphospholipid syndrome and thrombosis are inadequately protected from recurrent thrombotic episodes if treated at a targeted INR of 2.0–3.0 (Rosove and Brewer 1992; Khamashta et al. 1995). In the largest retrospective study of 147 antiphospholipid antibody-associated thromboses followed up for 10 years, a recurrent thrombosis occurred in 69 per cent of patients. High intensity warfarin (INR~3.0) was the most effective therapeutic option in the secondary prevention of venous and arterial thromboses in these patients (Khamashta et al. 1995). Some dispute this and prefer to advocate an INR of 2.0–3.0 for those with venous thrombosis (Schulman et al. 1998), reserving intensive anticoagulation (INR 3.0–4.0) for those with recurrent venous thrombosis or arterial thrombosis.

The description of the antiphospholipid syndrome in 1983 provided a new insight into vascular aspects of neurological disease. Here, for the first time, was a common pro-thrombotic disorder, which resulted in arterial as well as venous thrombosis. The cerebral circulation appears to be particularly targeted, with strokes and transient ischaemic attacks, movement disorders, epilepsy, myelopathy, and migraine being major manifestations. Anectdotally, the initiation of adequate anticoagulant therapy coincides with rapid, often dramatic, amelioration of symptoms. It is not uncommon for patients with antiphospholipid syndrome to 'know' precisely when their INR has fallen—the headaches, dysarthria, memory disturbance, and

Table 5 Preferred treatment for the different clinical manifestations associated with antiphospholipid antibodies

Clinical situation	Suggested treatment
1. Asymptomatic individuals	Observation ± low-dose aspirin
2. Thrombotic events	
Deep vein thrombosis ± pulmonary embolism	Long-term warfarin (INR 2.5–3.0)
Large vessel arterial occlusion (i.e. stroke)	Long-term warfarin (INR~3.0)
Recurrent thrombosis	Long-term warfarin (INR~3.0) ± low-dose aspirin
Catastrophic antiphospholipid syndrome	Oral anticoagulants (INR~3.0) + plasmapheresis ± corticosteroids or immunosuppressives
3. Pregnancy	
No previous history of thrombosis/miscarriage	Observation ± low-dose aspirin
Previous thrombosis	Low-molecular-weight heparin + low-dose aspirin
Recurrent early miscarriage	Low-dose aspirin
Late foetal loss/severe pre-eclampsia/intrauterine growth restriction	Low-molecular-weight heparin + low-dose aspirin

neurological features predictably returning when the INR drops, for example, below 3.0.

Concerns exist over the validity of the INR in the control of oral anticoagulant dosing if lupus anticoagulant is present. The inhibitor occasionally increases the prothrombin time and, in turn, the INR, which may thus not reflect the true degree of anticoagulation. This phenomenon seems to be more likely when certain recombinant thromboplastin reagents are used and can usually be circumvented by careful selection of the thromboplastin to be used for the prothrombin-time test (Lawrie et al. 1997).

A significant number of patients require high doses of warfarin (upto 25 mg/day) to maintain the INR in therapeutic range (3.0–4.0). In our experience, most of these patients were receiving other drugs and, notably, azathioprine at the same time as warfarin therapy. An important drug interaction has been pointed out between azathioprine and warfarin. When azathioprine is reduced or discontinued, anticoagulation may increase with the potential for bleeding if the INR is not carefully monitored in these patients.

High-intensity oral anticoagulation therapy carries an inevitable risk of serious haemorrhage. In antiphospholipid syndrome, serious bleeding complications may occur, but their risk is not higher than that observed in other thrombotic conditions warranting oral anticoagulation (Ruiz-Irastorza et al. 2002).

The role of steroids and immunosuppressive drugs in treatment of patients with antiphospholipid antibodies and thrombosis is uncertain. Such drugs have severe side-effects when given for prolonged periods and antiphospholipid antibodies are not always suppressed by these agents. Furthermore, in our series of patients with the antiphospholipid syndrome, corticosteroids and immunosuppressive therapy, prescribed in some patients to control lupus activity, did not prevent further thrombotic events (Khamashta et al. 1995). The use of these drugs is probably justified only in patients with repeated episodes of thrombosis despite adequate anticoagulant therapy, that is, catastrophic antiphospholipid syndrome. In this rare but life-threatening condition, plasmapheresis has also been used with varying success (Asherson et al. 2001).

The use of intra-arterial fibrinolysis has been described to be of benefit in patients with acute myocardial infarction associated with antiphospholipid antibodies. Prostacyclin analogues (iloprost) were also successfully used in patients with severe ischaemic necrotic toes associated with antiphospholipid syndrome. Elective pulmonary thromboendarterectomy can be very effective and lifesaving in selected patients with chronic large-vessel thromboembolic pulmonary hypertension (Khamashta 2000a).

Prevention of pregnancy loss

The management of pregnancy in women known to have antiphospholipid syndrome is the subject of much debate and, as yet, there have been very few randomized controlled trials. Anticoagulation in one form or another is the preferred treatment rather than steroids (once widely recommended). The current choices lie between aspirin, heparin, or both (Shehata et al. 2001). Recently, two prospective trials showed that heparin plus low-dose aspirin is more effective than aspirin alone for achieving live births among women with antiphospholipid antibodies and first trimester recurrent pregnancy loss (Kutteh 1996; Rai et al. 1997). A third prospective trial of antiphospholipid antibody-positive women with repeated pregnancy loss, but no history of thrombosis or systemic lupus erythematosus, found similar live birth rates (~80 per cent), using either low-dose aspirin or placebo (Pattison et al. 2000), suggesting that treatment may be unnecessary in some women. The optimal treatment for women with one or more late pregnancy losses (second/third trimester) but no history of thromboembolism, is controversial, but some studies have suggested that heparin therapy in addition to low-dose aspirin may contribute to improved foetal outcome in these women (Levine et al. 2002).

Intravenous immunoglobulin has also been used during pregnancy, usually in conjunction with heparin and low-dose aspirin, especially in women with particularly poor past obstetric histories or recurrent pregnancy loss during heparin treatment. However, a randomized, controlled, pilot study of intravenous immunoglobulin treatment during pregnancy in unselected antiphospholipid syndrome cases found no benefit to this expensive therapy compared to heparin and low-dose aspirin (Branch et al. 2000). It is currently unclear whether intravenous immunoglobulin may play a role in 'refractory' cases. Therefore, it would seem prudent to limit its use to salvage therapy in women who develop obstetric complications despite aspirin and heparin.

Women with antiphospholipid syndrome and previous thromboembolism are usually treated with long-term warfarin. These women are at extremely high risk in pregnancy and the puerperium and should, therefore, be given antenatal thromboprophylaxis with subcutaneous heparin. The change from warfarin to heparin should be achieved prior to 6 weeks gestation to avoid warfarin embryopathy. For the benefit of the foetus, warfarin should ideally be converted to subcutaneous heparin prior to conception. Some women prefer to continue with warfarin until the first missed period, and then convert at this time. Heparin does not cross the placenta and is not known to cause any adverse foetal effects. However, long-term use of heparin in pregnancy has been associated with osteoporosis in the mother. Many centres are now using low molecular weight heparin, since it has increased bioavailability, has a longer half-life and can, therefore, conveniently be given once daily. It seems to have no greater deleterious effect on bone density than occurs physiologically during pregnancy (Sanson et al. 1999). Heparin should be continued intrapartum and post-partum until women are re-warfarinized. Both warfarin and subcutaneous heparin are compatible with breast-feeding.

Most authorities agree that one of the main reasons for the improving outcome of antiphospholipid syndrome pregnancies is closer obstetric surveillance. Viable antiphospholipid pregnancies have a high incidence of obstetric and foetal complications, including intrauterine growth restriction, prematurity, and pre-eclampsia, hence, close monitoring including uterine artery Doppler scans, and timely delivery may improve foetal outcome in these women.

Some clinicians are convinced that antiphospholipid antibodies are associated with infertility. Additionally, some clinicians recommend that infertile women who have antiphospholipid antibodies and are undergoing *in vitro* fertilization should be treated with heparin to improve the rate of pregnancy. However, this recommendation has not been adequately substantiated by evidence (Branch and Hatasaka 1998).

Management of other manifestations of antiphospholipid syndrome

Mild thrombocytopaenia with platelet counts between 100 000 and 150 000/mm^3 are common in patients with antiphospholipid antibody and usually does not require intervention. In a minority of cases it can be severe. In these cases, corticosteroid therapy should always be the treatment of choice. Several drugs have been used successfully to treat steroid-resistant thrombocytopaenia in antiphospholipid syndrome patients, including aspirin, intravenous gammaglobulin infusion, danazol, chloroquine, and dapsone. Splenectomy has been safely and successfully performed in some patients (Hakim et al. 1998; Galindo et al. 1999).

Chronic headache is a common feature in antiphospholipid syndrome and usually responds to conventional treatment. In some of our patients with antiphospholipid syndrome, headache improved remarkably with low-dose aspirin and, in the very resistant cases, warfarin may be an alternative therapy (Cuadrado and Hughes 2001).

Transverse myelitis and multiple sclerosis-like illnesses have been described in antiphospholipid syndrome. Anecdotally, most clinicians dealing with antiphospholipid syndrome or lupus with antiphospholipid syndrome have seen patients initially labelled as 'probable multiple sclerosis'. Certainly the ischaemic changes produced by the antiphospholipid syndrome in white matter may be indistinguishable on MRI from those of multiple sclerosis. Therefore, in some of these patients with multiple sclerosis-like illness, the importance of a treatable differential diagnosis—antiphospholipid syndrome—cannot be understated.

There is a high prevalence of heart valve lesions in patients with antiphospholipid antibodies. In some cases, valvular damage may result in significant haemodynamic compromise requiring surgery. Both biological and mechanical valves have been implanted with favourable results. Regardless of the valve type used, all patients with antiphospholipid syndrome and valve prosthesis require full anticoagulation.

It is important to distinguish the thrombotic microangiopathy that some patients with antiphospholipid syndrome can suffer, from inflammatory forms of renal involvement. The physician can face this problem mainly in patients with systemic lupus erythematosus and management with oral anticoagulation or steroids will depend on the histological findings. The outcome of kidney transplantation in patients with systemic lupus erythematosus and end-stage renal failure appears to be similar to that of patients with renal failure from other causes. However, the presence of antiphospholipid antibodies seems to be associated with a poorer prognosis. Post-transplant thromboembolic phenomena, recurrence of thrombotic microangiopathy in the graft despite anticoagulation, and thrombosis of the graft's renal vein, have all been reported (McIntyre and Wagenknecht 2001).

Prognosis

The long-term prognosis in patients with antiphospholipid syndrome is primarily influenced by the risk of recurrent thrombosis (Amigo 2001). Although there are a number of studies of prognostic factors in systemic lupus erythematosus, only a few have addressed the possible role of antiphospholipid antibodies. Lupus patients with antiphospholipid syndrome are reported to have higher mortality rates, independently of other variables (Cervera et al. 1999; Williams et al. 2002). Shah et al. (1998) reported on the 10-year follow-up of 52 patients with positive anticardiolipin antibodies seen in 1986. These included 31 patients with antiphospholipid syndrome, of whom 10 had primary antiphospholipid syndrome, and 21 had systemic lupus erythematosus with anticardiolipin antibodies but without clinical features of the syndrome. Despite antithrombotic treatment, 29 per cent of the antiphospholipid syndrome patients had further thrombotic events. In addition, half of the patients with the antibody but without the syndrome subsequently developed antiphospholipid syndrome. The mortality at 10 years was 10 per cent and four of the five deaths were directly related to thrombosis. Erkan et al. (2000) found that the prognosis of patients with primary antiphospholipid syndrome is poor. One-third of patients had organ damage and one-fifth were unable to perform everyday activities.

Antiphospholipid syndrome in childhood

There have been relatively few reports of clinical associations of antiphospholipid antibodies in children and the spectrum of clinical findings remains at present unknown. Antiphospholipid antibodies in childhood-onset systemic lupus erythematosus have been described in several small clinical reports, occurring in one-third of the patients. The clinical manifestations are similar to those encountered in adults, particularly recurrent deep-vein thrombosis, strokes, and chorea. Devastating thrombotic complications of the antiphospholipid syndrome in children have been reported including digital ischaemia and myocardial infarction. The risk of maternal transmission of antiphospholipid antibodies to infants during pregnancy is unknown, though there have been several case reports of thrombotic events in neonates of mothers with the antiphospholipid syndrome (Avcin et al. 2002).

There is general agreement that long-term anticoagulation is needed in children who experienced an antiphospholipid-related thrombosis to prevent recurrences, but there is no consensus about the duration and intensity of this therapy. Given that the risk of recurrence might be lower in antiphospholipid-positive children compared with adults, and considering the higher risk of haemorrhage during play and sports, it was suggested that intermediate-intensity anticoagulation therapy targeted at an INR of 2.0–2.5 be performed in paediatric patients who have experienced an antiphospholipid-related thrombosis (Tucker 2000).

References

Alarcon-Segovia, D. et al. (1989). Antiphospholipid antibodies and the antiphospholipid syndrome in systemic lupus erythematosus: a prospective analysis of 500 consecutive patients. *Medicine (Baltimore)* **68**, 353–65.

Amigo, M.C. et al. (1992). Renal involvement in primary antiphospholipid syndrome. *Journal of Rheumatology* **19**, 1181–5.

Amigo, M.C. (2001). Prognosis in antiphospholipid syndrome. *Rheumatic Disease Clinics of North America* **27**, 661–9.

Asherson, R.A. et al. (2001). Catastrophic antiphospholipid syndrome. Clues to the pathogenesis from a series of 80 patients. *Medicine (Baltimore)* **80**, 355–77.

Atsumi, T. et al. (1998). Arterial disease and thrombosis in the antiphospholipid syndrome. A pathogenic role for endothelin 1. *Arthritis and Rheumatism* **41**, 800–7.

Avcin, T., Cimaz, R., and Meroni, P.L. (2002). Recent advances in antiphospholipid antibodies and antiphospholipid syndromes in pediatric populations. *Lupus* **11**, 4–10.

Bertolaccini, M.L. et al. (1998a). Multiple antiphospholipid tests do not increase the diagnostic yield in antiphospholipid syndrome. *British Journal of Rheumatology* **37**, 1229–32.

Bertolaccini, M.L. et al. (1998b). Autoantibodies to human prothrombin and clinical manifestations in 207 patients with systemic lupus erythematosus. *Journal of Rheumatology* **25**, 1104–8.

Branch, D.W. and Hatasaka, H. (1998). Antiphospholipid antibodies and infertility: fact or fallacy. *Lupus* **7** (Suppl. 2), S90–4.

Branch, D.W. et al. (1992). Outcome of treated pregnancies in women with antiphospholipid syndrome: an update of the Utah experience. *Obstetrics and Gynecology* **80**, 614–20.

Branch, D.W. et al. (2000). A multicenter, placebo-controlled pilot study of inravenous immune globulin treatment of antiphospholipid syndrome during pregnancy. *American Journal of Obstetrics and Gynecology* **182**, 122–7.

Brey, R.L. et al. (2001). β_2-glycoprotein I-dependent anticardiolipin antibodies and the risk of ischemic stroke and myocardial infarction: the Honolulu Heart Program. *Stroke* **32**, 1701–6.

Brunner, H.I. et al. (2002). Long-term anticoagulation is preferable for patients with antiphospholipid antibody syndrome. Result of a decision analysis. *Journal of Rheumatology* **29**, 490–501.

Cabral, A.R. et al. (1996). The antiphospholipid/cofactor syndromes: a primary variant with antibodies to β_2-glycoprotein I but no antibodies detectable in standard antiphospholipid assays. *American Journal of Medicine* **101**, 472–81.

Cervera, R. et al. (1999). Morbidity and mortality in systemic lupus erythematosus during a 5 year period: a multi-centre prospective study of 1000 patients. *Medicine (Baltimore)* **78**, 167–75.

Cervera, R. et al. (2002). Antiphospholipid syndrome: clinical and immunologic manifestations and patterns of disease expression in a cohort of 1000 patients. *Arthritis and Rheumatism* **46**, 1019–27.

Cuadrado, M.J. and Hughes, G.R.V. (2001). Hughes (antiphospholipid) syndrome: clinical features. *Rheumatic Disease Clinics of North America* **27**, 507–24.

Cuadrado, M.J. et al. (2000). Can neurologic manifestations of Hughes (antiphospholipid) syndrome be distinguished from multiple sclerosis? *Medicine (Baltimore)* **79**, 57–68.

Di Simone, N. et al. (2000). Antiphospholipid antibodies affect trophoblast gonadotropin secretion and invasiveness by binding directly and through adhered β_2-glycoprotein I. *Arthritis and Rheumatism* **43**, 140–50.

Dobado-Berrios, P.M. et al. (2001). The role of tissue factor in the antiphospholipid syndrome. *Arthritis and Rheumatism* **44**, 2467–76.

Erkan, D. et al. (2000). Primary antiphospholipid syndrome: functional outcome after 10 years. *Journal of Rheumatology* **27**, 2817–21.

Erkan, D. et al. (2001). High thrombosis rate after fetal loss in antiphospholipid syndrome: effective prophylaxis with aspirin. *Arthritis and Rheumatism* **44**, 1466–7.

Espinosa, G. et al. (2001). Budd–Chiari syndrome secondary to antiphospholipid syndrome. Clinical and immunologic characteristics of 43 patients. *Medicine (Baltimore)* **80**, 345–54.

Galindo, M., Khamashta, M.A., and Hughes, G.R.V. (1999). Splenectomy for refractory thrombocytopenia in the antiphospholipid syndrome. *Rheumatology* **38**, 848–53.

George, J., Haratz, D., and Shoenfeld, Y. (2001). Accelerated atheroma, antiphospholipid antibodies, and the antiphospholipid syndrome. *Rheumatic Disease Clinics of North America* **27**, 603–10.

Gharavi, A.E. et al. (2002). Antiphospholipid antibodies induced in mice by immunization with a cytomegalovirus-derived peptide cause thrombosis and activation of endothelial cells *in vivo*. *Arthritis and Rheumatism* **46**, 545–52.

Ginsburg, K.S. et al. (1992). Anticardiolipin antibodies and the risk for ischemic stroke and venous thrombosis. *Annals of Internal Medicine* **117**, 997–1002.

Goel, N. et al. (1999). Familial antiphospholipid antibody syndrome. *Arthritis and Rheumatism* **42**, 318–27.

Hakim, A.J., Machin, S.J., and Isenberg, D.A. (1998). Autoimmune thrombocytopenia in primary antiphospholipid syndrome and systemic lupus erythematosus: the response to splenectomy. *Seminars in Arthritis and Rheumatism* **28**, 20–5.

Harris, E.N. et al. (1983). Anticardiolipin antibodies: detection by radioimmunoassay and association with thrombosis in systemic lupus erythematosus. *Lancet* **ii**, 1211–14.

Holers, V.M. et al. (2002). Complement C3 activation is required for antiphospholipid antibody-induced fetal loss. *Journal of Experimental Medicine* **195**, 211–20.

Hughes, G.R.V. (1983). Thrombosis, abortion, cerebral disease and lupus anticoagulant. *British Medical Journal* **287**, 1088–9.

Hunt, B.J. and Ames, P.R.J. (2000). Antiphospholipid syndrome: differential diagnosis. In *Hughes Syndrome—Antiphospholipid Syndrome* (ed. M.A. Khamashta), pp. 449–56. London: Springer.

Khamashta, M.A., ed. *Hughes Syndrome—Antiphospholipid Syndrome.* London: Springer, 2000a.

Khamashta, M.A. (2000b). Primary prevention of thrombosis in subjects with positive antiphospholipid antibodies. *Journal of Autoimmunity* **15**, 249–53.

Khamashta, M.A. et al. (1990). Association of antiphospholipid antibodies with heart valve disease in systemic lupus erythematosus. *Lancet* **335**, 1541–4.

Khamashta, M.A. et al. (1995). The management of thrombosis in the antiphospholipid-antibody syndrome. *New England Journal of Medicine* **332**, 993–7.

Krnic-Barrie, S. et al. (1997). A retrospective review of 61 patients with antiphospholipid syndrome. *Archives of Internal Medicine* **157**, 2101–8.

Kupferminc, M.J. et al. (1999). Increased frequency of genetic thrombophilia in women with complications of pregnancy. *New England Journal of Medicine* **340**, 9–13.

Kutteh, W.H. (1996). Antiphospholipid antibody-associated recurrent pregnancy loss: treatment with heparin and low-dose aspirin is superior to low-dose aspirin alone. *American Journal of Obstetrics and Gynecology* **174**, 1584–9.

Lawrie, A.S. et al. (1997). Monitoring of oral anticoagulant therapy in lupus anticoagulant positive patients with the antiphospholipid syndrome. *British Journal of Haematology* **98**, 887–92.

Levine, J.S., Branch, D.W., and Rauch, J. (2002). The antiphospholipid syndrome. *New England Journal of Medicine* **346**, 752–63.

Lie, J.T. (1994). Vasculitis in the antiphospholipid syndrome: culprit or consort? *Journal of Rheumatology* **21**, 397–9.

Lima, F. et al. (1996). A study of sixty pregnancies in patients with the antiphospholipid syndrome. *Clinical and Experimental Rheumatology* **14**, 131–6.

Lockshin, M.D., Sammaritano, L.R., and Schwartzman, S. (2000). Validation of the Sapporo criteria for antiphospholipid syndrome. *Arthritis and Rheumatism* **43**, 440–3.

Matsuura, E. et al. (1994). Anticardiolipin antibodies recognize β_2-glycoprotein I structure altered by interacting with an oxygen modified solid phase surface. *Journal of Experimental Medicine* **179**, 457–62.

McIntyre, J.A. and Wagenknecht, D.R. (2001). Antiphospholipid antibodies. Risk assessment for solid organ, bone marrow, and tissue transplantation. *Rheumatic Disease Clinics of North America* **27**, 611–31.

Menon, S. et al. (1999). A longitudinal study of anticardiolipin antibody levels and cognitive functioning in systemic lupus erythematosus. *Arthritis and Rheumatism* **42**, 735–41.

Meroni, P.L. and Riboldi, P. (2001). Pathogenic mechanisms mediating antiphospholipid syndrome. *Current Opinion in Rheumatology* **13**, 377–82.

Meroni, P.L. et al. (2000). Endothelial activation by aPL: a potential pathogenetic mechanism for the clinical manifestations of the syndrome. *Journal of Autoimmunity* **15**, 237–40.

Meroni, P.L. et al. (2001). Statins prevent endothelial cell activation induced by antiphospholipid (anti-β_2-glycoprotein I) antibodies—effect on the proadhesive and proinflammatory phenotype. *Arthritis and Rheumatism* **44**, 2870–8.

Pattison, N.S. et al. (2000). Does aspirin have a role in improving pregnancy outcome for women with the antiphospholipid syndrome? A randomized controlled trial. *American Journal of Obstetrics and Gynecology* **183**, 1008–12.

Petri, M. (2000). Epidemiology of the antiphospholipid antibody syndrome. *Journal of Autoimmunity* **15**, 145–51.

Pierangeli, S.S., Gharavi, A.E., and Harris, E.N. (2000). Experimental thrombosis and antiphospholipid antibodies: new insights. *Journal of Autoimmunity* **15**, 241–7.

Rai, R. et al. (1997). Randomized controlled trial of aspirin and aspirin plus heparin in pregnant women with recurrent miscarriage associated with phospholipid antibodies. *British Medical Journal* **314**, 253–7.

Rand, J.H. et al. (1997). Pregnancy loss in the antiphospholipid-antibody syndrome—a possible thrombogenic mechanism. *New England Journal of Medicine* **337**, 154–60.

Rand, J.H. (2002). Molecular pathogenesis of the antiphospholipid syndrome. *Circulation Research* **90**, 29–37.

Rosove, M.H. and Brewer, P.M.C. (1992). Antiphospholipid thrombosis: clinical course after the first thrombotic event in 70 patients. *Annals of Internal Medicine* **117**, 303–8.

Ruiz-Irastorza, G. et al. (2002). Bleeding and recurrent thrombosis in antiphospholipid syndrome: analysis of a series of 66 patients treated with high-intensity oral anticoagulation. *Archives of Internal Medicine* **162**, 1164–9.

Sanson, B.J. et al. (1999). Safety of low-molecular weight heparin in pregnancy: a systematic review. *Thrombosis and Haemostasis* **81**, 668–72.

Schulman, S. et al. (1998). Anticardiolipin antibodies predict early recurrence of thromboembolism and death among patients with venous thromboembolism following anticoagulant therapy. *The American Journal of Medicine* **104**, 332–8.

Shah, N.M. et al. (1998). Outcome of patients with anticardiolipin antibodies: a 10 year follow-up of 52 patients. *Lupus* **7**, 3–6.

Shehata, H.A., Nelson-Piercy, C., and Khamashta, M.A. (2001). Management of pregnancy in antiphospholipid syndrome. *Rheumatic Disease Clinics of North America* **27**, 643–59.

Sherer, Y. and Shoenfeld, Y. (2000). Antiphospholipid syndrome: insight from animal models. *Current Opinion in Hematology* **7**, 321–4.

Stone, S., Khamashta, M.A., and Poston, L. (2001). Placentation, antiphospholipid syndrome and pregnancy outcome. *Lupus* **10**, 67–74.

Stone, S. et al. (2002). Antiphospholipid antibodies do not a syndrome make. *Lupus* **11**, 130–3.

Tincani, A. et al. (2000). Overview on anticardiolipin ELISA standardization. *Journal of Autoimmunity* **15**, 195–7.

Tucker, L.G. (2000). Antiphospholipid antibodies and antiphospholipid syndrome in children. In *Hughes Syndrome—Antiphospholipid Syndrome* (ed. M.A. Khamashta), pp. 155–66. London: Springer.

Vaarala, O. et al. (1995). Anti-cardiolipin antibodies and risk of myocardial infarction in a prospective cohort of middle-aged men. *Circulation* **91**, 23–7.

Wahl, D.G., et al. (2000). Prophylactic antithrombotic therapy for patients with systemic lupus erythematosus with or without antiphospholipid antibodies. *Archives of Internal Medicine* **160**, 2042–8.

Williams, F.M.K. et al. (2002). Critical illness in systemic lupus erythematosus and the antiphospholipid syndrome. *Annals of the Rheumatic Diseases* **61**, 414–21.

Wilson, W.A., et al. (1999). International consensus statement on preliminary classification criteria for definite antiphospholipid syndrome: report of an international workshop. *Arthritis and Rheumatism* **42**, 1309–11.

6.7 Scleroderma and related disorders in adults and children

Carol M. Black and Christopher P. Denton

'Scleroderma', a word meaning hard skin, is a part of many syndromes including localized, limited, and generalized scleroderma (Table 1). Most of these disorders can occur at any stage of life, although the pattern of scleroderma occurring in childhood is different from that in the adult (see below). Scleroderma or systemic sclerosis has been confused with other diseases that have cutaneous features resembling it, for example, scleromyxoedema, scleroedema, and primary amyloidosis (Table 2).

The milestones in the history of scleroderma (see Table 3) bear testimony to the gradual realization of the heterogeneity of the disorder. For a more detailed discussion of the fascinating history of this disease the reader is referred to the excellent historical review by Rodnan, the 'father' of modern-day clinical scleroderma (Rodnan and Benedek 1962).

The group of syndromes called localized scleroderma includes morphoea (limited and guttate), linear scleroderma with the *en coup de sabre* variety, and generalized morphoea. These syndromes predominate in childhood and are almost never associated with systemic involvement but may demonstrate abnormal autoimmune serology and inflammatory histological changes in skin.

Raynaud's phenomenon is classified as either primary or secondary (the terms Raynaud's disease and Raynaud's syndrome should be abandoned and replaced by these more accurate, simple descriptive terms) and can be a forerunner of the autoimmune rheumatic diseases such as generalized scleroderma (see below).

When generalized scleroderma is called systemic sclerosis the term is preferable to progressive systemic sclerosis because not all cases are progressive. It is characterized pathologically by the overproduction of several elements of the connective tissue, notably collagen, widespread vascular damage with the development of microvascular obliteration, and tissue infiltration of mononuclear inflammatory cells often in a perivascular distribution (Prescott et al. 1992). It embraces a clinical spectrum ranging from widespread skin thickening (diffuse scleroderma) to skin thickening either limited to the face and distal extremities (limited scleroderma) or absent (systemic sclerosis *sine* scleroderma).

There is no single diagnostic test for systemic sclerosis and, for the purposes of separating it from other autoimmune rheumatic diseases and identifying cases to permit comparison of reported series, preliminary criteria were developed and published in 1980 (Subcommittee for Scleroderma Criteria of the American Rheumatism Association Diagnostic and Therapeutic Criteria Committee 1980; Pope and Bellamy 1993). These criteria, which remain preliminary, had a high sensitivity and specificity for diffuse cutaneous systemic sclerosis, but they are less sensitive for the limited cutaneous subset. In addition they do not take account of the hallmark autoantibodies now recognized in the disease.

Classification of systemic sclerosis is difficult (Masi 1988), and a number of different systems have been proposed (LeRoy et al. 1988). Currently, the most widely used classification defines two subsets, based on the extent of skin involvement together with a number of reliable clinical laboratory and natural history associations. The two-subset model divides the disease into limited cutaneous systemic sclerosis and diffuse cutaneous systemic sclerosis (Table 4) (LeRoy et al. 1988). The term limited cutaneous systemic sclerosis is preferable to CREST [Calcinosis, Raynaud's, (O)Esophageal dysphagia, Sclerodactyly, Telangiectasia syndrome], because cutaneous manifestations often extend beyond sclerodactyly and calcinosis may be present only late or radiologically. Diffuse cutaneous systemic sclerosis, is much more rapid in onset, with organ failure often present within 5 years of the first symptoms. It is appreciated that some patients do not have significant or extensive skin involvement at the early stages of their disease. The concept of limited systemic sclerosis has been proposed, including patients with negligible skin involvement but with hallmark antibodies and nailfold capillary abnormalities and often some evidence of visceral involvement such as oesophageal reflux (LeRoy and Medsger 2001).

The subset distinction is important as the natural history and frequency of complications differ as outlined in Table 5. Within each subset, there is great variability in the pace of the disease: for example, some patients with diffuse cutaneous systemic sclerosis develop extensive internal-organ complications within 2–4 years; others have widespread skin disease but only grumbling internal organ involvement. Similarly, whilst most patients with limited cutaneous systemic sclerosis have some internal organ involvement

Table 1 Spectrum of scleroderma and scleroderma-like syndromes

Localized	
Morphoea	
Localized	One or more skin lesion, often on truncal areas
Generalized	Widespread skin lesions, can be reminiscent of diffuse cutaneous systemic sclerosis, but Raynaud's unusual, no visceral manifestations and skin changes are less likely to be acral
Linear scleroderma	The most common form occurring in childhood. Skin changes follow a dermatomal distribution, especially on the limbs and lead to important secondary growth defects
en coup de sabre	Midline or parasaggittal variant of linear scleroderma which manifests in childhood and is associated often with defects in underlying fascial and skeletal structures
Systemic	
Limited cutaneous systemic sclerosis	Skin sclerosis distal to the wrists (or ankles), over the face and neck Often long-standing Raynaud's phenomenon
Diffuse cutaneous systemic sclerosis	Truncal and acral skin involvement. Presence of tendon friction rubs. Onset of skin changes (puffy or hidebound) within 1 year of onset of Raynaud's phenomenon
Overlap syndromes	Features of systemic sclerosis together with those of at least one other autoimmune rheumatic disease, e.g. SLE, RA, or polymyositis
Systemic sclerosis *sine scleroderma*	Vascular or fibrotic visceral features without skin sclerosis ($<$1% cases)
Raynaud's phenomenon	
Autoimmune Raynaud's phenomenon	Raynaud's phenomenon associated with antinuclear antibodies usually also abnormal nailfold capillaroscopy. Approximately 10% of cases develop features of a definite autoimmune rheumatic disease
Primary Raynaud's phenomenon	Vasospastic symptoms with normal nailfold capillaroscopy and negative autoimmune serology and no other underlying medical/mechanical cause

Table 2 Differential diagnosis for scleroderma

Skin sclerosis
Infiltrative disorders
Amyloidosis
Scleromyxoedema
Scleroedema of Buschke
Lichen sclerosis and atrophicus
Metabolic disorders
Myxoedema
Porphyria cutanea tarda
Congenital porphyrias
Acromegaly
Phenylketonuria
Inflammatory
Overlap connective tissue diseases
Eosinophilic fasciitis
Chronic graft versus host disease
Sarcoidosis
Acral vasospasm
Raynaud's phenomenon
Primary Raynaud's phenomenon
Other autoimmune rheumatic disorders
SLE
Rheumatoid disease
Dermato/polymyositis
Other vascular disease
Haematological
Cryoglobulinaemia
Cold agglutinin disease
Hyperviscosity syndrome
Systemic vasculitis
Buerger's disease (thromboangiitis obliterans)
Macrovascular disease

Table 3 History of scleroderma

c. 400 BC	Hippocrates	Described an Athenian with indurated unpinchable skin Insufficient detail to ascertain whether this was scleroderma
1753	Curzio	Description of young woman of Naples with 'excessive hardness of the skin'—possibly scleroderma, but probably scleroedema of Buschke
1847	Gintrac	First use of the name 'sclérodermie'
1847	Forget	First description of joint involvement in scleroderma
1854	Addison	First description of linear scleroderma
1862	Raynaud	Description of 'local asphyxia and symmetrical gangrene of the extremities'
1878	Weber	Coexistence of scleroderma and calcinosis noted
1892	Osler	Tendency for scleroderma patients to die of pulmonary or renal disease noted
1893	Hutchinson	Association of scleroderma and Raynaud's phenomenon noted
1903	Ehrmann	Association of scleroderma and dysphagia noted
1910	Thibierge and Weissenbach	'Rediscovery' of the coexistence of scleroderma and calcinosis
1924	Matsui	First clear description of visceral involvement, with sclerosis of lungs, gastrointestinal tract and kidneys
1943	Weiss	Clear description of myocardial involvement in scleroderma
1945	Goetz	Coined the term 'progressive systemic sclerosis'
1964	Winterbauer	Described the CREST subset (calcinosis, Raynaud's, oesophagitis, sclerodactyly, and telangiectasia)

with gastro-oesophageal reflux, a minority of patients develop pulmonary vascular disease or severe mid-gut involvement. Although major visceral complications generally occur later in lcSSc than diffuse disease, they may occur as early as 5–7 years after diagnosis. Subsetting accurately represents a well-established clinical approach to risk-stratification in systemic sclerosis.

Epidemiological considerations

Scleroderma is an uncommon disorder and virtually all of the descriptive epidemiology is derived from retrospective or prospective reviews of patients attending hospitals or institutions serving a defined denominator population: there is only one true population-based study (Maricq et al. 1989). A summary of salient epidemiological data is given in Table 6. Although there are apparently different disease frequencies between populations some of these may be accounted for by methodological factors. Interestingly, although the prevalence in the United Kingdom was previously estimated in a large west midlands population as several fold lower than in Maricq's study other reports observe a higher frequency, in line with that in North America and Australia. Currently, the best estimate for UK prevalence overall is approximately 120 per million of the population. Its relative rarity suggests that the genetic and/or environmental exposures necessary for disease susceptibility occur infrequently in the population. Scleroderma has a female excess (4F : 1M overall, and in the child-bearing years 15F : 1M). A number of geographical clusters have been reported. Clustering has been described close to international airports in the United Kingdom (Silman 1995), with a variety of autoimmune rheumatic diseases in the Republic of Georgia (Freni-Titulaer et al. 1989), and a clearer cluster of systemic sclerosis in a region of Italy close to Rome (Valesini et al. 1993). In North America, a high prevalence has been observed in one population of Choctaw native Americans in Oklahoma. There is growing evidence for a genetic basis for this high prevalence and on-going studies are defining this in detail (Tan et al. 2000). Finally, again in contrast to other autoimmune rheumatic diseases, a growing number of environmental agents have been implicated in systemic sclerosis (see Table 7).

Aetiology and pathogenesis

Systemic sclerosis is almost certainly multifactorial involving genetic and environmental factors (Briggs et al. 1990). Systemic sclerosis occurs mostly in females and gender may be the strongest genetic marker. There are several lines of evidence indicating familial or genetic predisposition to systemic sclerosis. Although rare, there are familial clusters of systemic sclerosis and related diseases, particularly Raynaud's phenomenon. Autoantibodies associated with systemic sclerosis are found in high frequency in blood relatives of patients with systemic sclerosis, although the incidence of antinuclear antibodies in spouses suggests an environmental component. Thirty-six per cent of relatives with antinuclear antibodies had clinical features of autoimmune rheumatic disease not observed in spouses (Briggs et al. 1993). The presence of autoantibodies in the blood of patients' spouses in the UK study was not confirmed in an Australian study. Many centres worldwide have observed abnormal frequencies of the major histocompatibility complex (MHC) antigens associated with systemic sclerosis. The association is complex (see Table 8) and the strongest link is between HLA–DR52a and patients with systemic sclerosis who have lung fibrosis (relative risk 16.7).

As one of the primary roles of MHC class II molecules is the presentation of processed antigen to the T-cell receptor on helper T lymphocytes

Table 4 Clinical features of the major systemic sclerosis subsets

Diffuse cutaneous SSc (dcSSc)
Inflammatory features more prominent at onset. Raynaud's often develop later. Skin sclerosis proximal to wrists/elbows and truncal. Prominent pruritis and constitutional symptoms. Tendon friction rubs associated with progressive disease. Significant visceral disease more frequent than in lcSSc. Renal, pulmonary fibrosis (secondary PHT), cardiac, gut. Disease activity appears to remain fairly constant over many years, with prominent vasospastic symptoms. Approximately one-third of SSc cases

Limited cutaneous SSc (lcSSc)
Long standing Raynaud's, skin changes hands, face, neck. Compared with dcSSc renal disease less frequent, isolated pulmonary hypertension, severe gut disease and interstitial lung fibrosis (if antitopoisomerase-1 present). Florid telangiectasis and calcinosis (especially ACA positive). Disease activity appears to be maximal in first 3 years from onset then often plateaus and skin involvement may stabilize or improve. The majority (≈60%) of cases are classified to this subset

Systemic sclerosis sine scleroderma
A small proportion (<2%) of SSc cases manifest vascular (Raynaud's phenomenon) and visceral manifestations including gastrointestinal disease, scleroderma renal crisis or pulmonary fibrosis. Typical disease associated autoantibodies are generally present

Pre-scleroderma/limited systemic sclerosis
Inclusion of patients with Raynaud's phenomenon, abnormal nailfold capillaroscopy and a hallmark autoantibody (e.g. anticentomere, antitopoisomerase-1, or anti-RNA polymerase I/III) within as a subset of systemic sclerosis is controversial. These cases may represent a subset of 'autoimmune Raynaud's' and a proportion probably remain stable. This makes the term limited systemic sclerosis more appropriate than 'pre-scleroderma'. Frequency of this group of patients very difficult to ascertain

resulting in an antigen-specific immune response, autoantibody subsets in scleroderma might be expected to show correlations with class II MHC polymorphism and indeed they do, although again, they appear to be complex. Anticentromere antibody was initially reported to be associated with HLA–DR5 (–DR11), –DR4 (–D13 sub-types), –DR1, and –DR8. These findings appear to reflect linkage disequilibrium of *HLA–DR5* (*–DR11*) and many *HLA–DR4* (*–D13* sub-types) with *HLA–DQ7*, and *–DR1* with *–DQ5*. These HLA–DR specificities share no unique amino acid sequences, which raised the possibility that another linked gene might be more highly correlated with this antibody response. More recently, in a study by Reveille et al. (1992b), oligotyping showed that the anticentromere antibody response was most closely associated with *HLA–DQB1* alleles in linkage disequilibrium with *HLA–DR1*, *–DR4*, *–DR5* (*DR11*), and *–DR8*. These *HLA–DQB1* alleles had in common a polar tyrosine or a glycine at position 26 of the outermost domain of the HLA–DQB molecule, as opposed to a hydrophobic leucine residue. In a British study (Briggs et al. 1993) implication of the *HLA–DQB1* locus was inferred, as virtually all of the anticentromere antibody-positive patients had either HLA–DR1 or –DR4. However, McHugh et al. (1994) have indicated that, although at least one *HLA–DQB1* allele not coding at position 26 of the first domain appears necessary, it may not be sufficient for the generation of anticentromere antibody. Reveille and colleagues have also extended the known associations of antitopoisomerase antibodies with HLA–DR5, –DR2, and –DR52a to include four *HLA–DQB1* alleles (Reveille et al. 1992a). Japanese workers have found a similar allele association (Kuwana et al. 1993). Localization of 'susceptible epitopes', however, has been less definitive. Suggestions include an American population in which a tyrosine at position 30 or the TRAELDT sequence spanning positions 71–77 of the *HLA–DQB1* outermost domain is seen (Reveille et al. 1992a,b), and a Japanese population with systemic sclerosis in which a tyrosine at position 26 of the *HLA–DQB1* outermost domain is present (Kuwana et al. 1993). In a British study, an HLA–DPB1 association was suggested, with the presence of an acidic amino-acid residue at position 69 in the third hypervariable region of the outermost domain. Autoantibodies to the anti-Pm/Scl antigen (see below) are nearly 100 per cent correlated with the presence of the *HLA DR3-DQw2* haplotype (Reveille et al. 1992a,b). Studies examining class II MHC associations with antitopoisomerase-1 antibodies in a number of populations suggest association with HLA–DRB1 and HLA–DQB1 alleles. Interestingly, T-cell

Table 5 Characteristic findings in the early and late stages of systemic sclerosis subsets

Diffuse cutaneous	*Early (<3 years from onset)*	*Late (>3 years from onset)*
Constitutional	Malaise, fatigue, weight loss	Minimal; weight often regained
Vascular	Raynaud's often relatively mild	Raynaud's more severe, increased telangiectasia
Cutaneous	Rapid progression involving arms, trunk and face. Pruritis	Stable or regression. Trophic and ischaemic ulcers. Pruritis decreases
Gastrointestinal	Dysphagia, heartburn	More
Cardiorespiratory	Maximum risk for myocarditis, pericardial effusion, interstitial pulmonary fibrosis	Reduced risk of new involvement but progression of existing established visceral fibrosis
Renal	Maximum risk period for scleroderma renal crisis	Reduced risk of crisis but chronic renal impairment may be progressive
Limited cutaneous	*Early (<3 years from onset)*	*Late (>3 years from onset)*
Constitutional	None	Only secondary to visceral complications
Vascular	Raynaud's typically severe and long-standing	Raynaud's persists, often causing digital ulceration or telangiectasia gangrene
Cutaneous	Mild sclerosis with little progression prominent	Slow progression of skin involvement. Calcinosis ulceration from ischaemia and underlying calcinosis
Gastrointestinal	Dysphagia, heartburn	More pronounced symptoms, midgut and anorectal complications are prevalent
Cardiorespiratory	Involvement unusual	Isolated pulmonary hypertension occurs most often at this stage. Patients may develop interstitial lung fibrosis, especially if antitopoisomerase-1 autoantibody positive
Renal	No involvement	Rarely involved

Table 6 Epidemiological facts in systemic sclerosis

Mortality	USA 1969–1977	1.5 males and 3.5 females per million population
	UK 1974–1985	1.0 males and 4.0 females per million population
Incidence (new cases detected/population at risk/time period)	Rates variable	2–10 per million population per year
	Pittsburgh study 1963–1982	19.1 per million per year
	UK 1980–1985	3.7 per million population per year
Prevalence (number of cases living at particular time or during time interval)	Estimates	
	1985 (USA)	253 per million (community)
	1986 (USA)	290 per million (point prevalence)
	1986 (UK)	31 per million (hospital/community)
	1988 (Australia)	126 per million (hospital study)
	2000 (UK)	120 per million (hospital/community)
Survival		
Cumulative survival using life-table methods	Overall	60–70% at 5 years
		40–50% at 10 years
	By subset	
	Limited cutaneous	80% at 10 years
		50% at 12 years
	Diffuse cutaneous	30% at 6 years
		15% at 12 years

Table 7 Environmental agents implicated in the development of scleroderma

Agent	Occupational exposure
Silica	Stone masons
Organic chemicals	
Aliphatic hydrocarbons	
Chlorinated	
Vinyl chloride	Plastic manufacture
Trichloroethylene	Dry cleaning
Perchloroethylene	
Non-chlorinated	
Naphtha-*n*-hexane	
Aromatic hydrocarbons	
Benzene	
Toluene	
Xylene	
Mixtures (diesel fuel, white spirit)	
Epoxy resins	
Foam insulin (urea-formaldehyde)	
Metaphenylene diamine (biogenic amine)	
Toxic oil (aniline-treated rapeseed oil)	
Drugs	
L-5-hydroxytryptophan	
Pentazocine	
Carbidopa	
Appetite suppressants	
Diethylpropion hydrochloride	
Mazindol	
Fenfluramine	
Bleomycin	
Cocaine	
Amide-type local anaesthetics	

activation assays using recombinant topoisomerase-1 peptides have confirmed these associations, demonstrating that only patients with certain class II haplotypes can generate a T-cell proliferative response to disease-associated epitopes (Kuwana et al. 1999). Recently, in a mixed UK population, association with topoisomerase-1 has been linked to HLA–DPB1*1301 (Gilchrist et al. 2001).

Table 8 Genetic associations in systemic sclerosis

	Autoantibody association[a]	Clinical association
HLA Class II		
HLA–DRB1*11	ATA	dcSSc, lung fibrosis
HLA–DPB1*1301	ATA	dcSSc, lung fibrosis
HLA–DQB1*0201	ARA	dcSSc, renal involvement
HLA–DQB1*0505	ACA	lcSSc
HLA–DQB1*0101	ACA	lcSSc
Cytokines		
CXCR-2		Increased frequency of two non-coding region polymorphisms in SSc
TGFβ3		Microsatellite markers at this locus associate with dcSSc
TGFβ2		Microsatellite markers at this locus associate with SSc
Extracellular matrix components		
TIMP1		Microsatellite markers at this locus associate with SSc
Fibronectin		Linkage of single nucleotide polymorphism haplotypes with lung fibrosis in SSc
Fibrillin-1		Linkage of fibrillin single nucleotide polymorphism haplotypes with SSc in Native American and Japanese patients with SSc

[a] ATA, antitopoisomerase-1; ACA, anticentromere antibody.

Important racial and ethnic differences in the frequencies of these autoantibodies have been described, with Western Europeans and North American Whites having a significantly higher frequency of anticentromere autoantibodies and a lower frequency of antitopoisomerase-1 than American Blacks, Choctaw native Americans, Thai, and Italians (Kallenberg 1994). Particular forms of the disease may not be so strongly influenced by gender. For example, certain chemically induced systemic sclerosis-like disorders tend to be associated with males, partly due to an occupational bias. The range of known agents that can induce a systemic sclerosis-like disease is large and growing (Table 7), although it must be noted that in formal epidemiological studies, no excess was found. It is almost certain that sporadic cases can follow certain occupational exposures, but that both the absolute and attributable risks are low. There are some MHC associations with the environmentally induced cases, for example toxic oil syndrome is characterized by a raised incidence of HLA–DR4, while vinyl chloride disease is primarily associated with HLA–DR5, HLA–DR3 being a marker of severity. There is (see Table 8) inconsistency in the frequencies for genetic markers of susceptibility between patients from different study centres. This may reflect at least in part different agents present at these various geographical locations. Another environmentally induced, systemic sclerosis-like condition is the eosinophilic–myalgic syndrome associated with the oral ingestion of the essential amino acid L-tryptophan (discussed elsewhere). Although there has been much speculation about a possible association of silicone-containing cosmetic prostheses and the development of connective tissue disease several well-conducted studies and reviews have failed to show any statistically significant association between these and systemic sclerosis. Hochberg (1994) has carefully reviewed the epidemiological aspects of the literature and has reasonably concluded that none of the available studies has demonstrated a statistical association between augmentation mammoplasty with silicone gel-filled prostheses and scleroderma or other autoimmune rheumatic disorders.

Autoimmune considerations

An increasing number of immune abnormalities are being reported in systemic sclerosis and the designation of systemic sclerosis as an autoimmune disease now has widespread support. Some of the clinical features of scleroderma bear similarities to other autoimmune disorders such as systemic lupus erythematosus, dermatomyositis, and rheumatoid arthritis, and there are also patients who have overlap syndromes or who have sequential development of more than one autoimmune rheumatic disease. Cases of familial systemic sclerosis and familial associations of systemic sclerosis with other autoimmune diseases such as rheumatoid arthritis and systemic lupus erythematosus occur and have already been mentioned.

There is considerable evidence that abnormalities in both humoral and cell-mediated immunity occur in systemic sclerosis, although the precise importance of these immunological events in the pathogenesis remains uncertain (Table 9). The lack of a generalized immune dysfunction in systemic sclerosis suggests that the derangement of immune-cell dysfunction may be specific to certain antigens or cell types (Lupoli et al. 1990).

The association of systemic sclerosis with particular major HLA antigens and the close association of certain HLA alleles with scleroderma-specific antibodies (see Table 8) is indirect evidence for T-cell involvement in systemic sclerosis. There is considerable evidence for T-cell activation in systemic sclerosis, including an increased ratio of circulating CD4+ : CD8+ cells (Degiannis et al. 1990; White 1994), reflecting an increased number of CD4+ and/or a reduced number of CD8+ lymphocytes. A particular role for $\gamma\delta$ T-cells has been suggested (White 1994) and others have reported increased numbers of lymphokine-activated killer and natural killer cells (Kantor et al. 1992) in blood samples from patients with systemic sclerosis. Furthermore, several studies have found increased soluble interleukin-2 receptor in scleroderma, sometimes appearing to correlate with disease activity (Kahaleh 1991). Support for the possibility that activated T-cells are important in pathogenesis is provided by the presence of infiltrates of CD3+, CD4+, CD450+, interleukin 2-producing, HLA–DR-positive+, leucocyte function-associated antigen-1-positive+, a/β T cells in lesional tissues (Prescott et al. 1992). Also, chronic graft-versus-host disease in humans shows several histological and clinical similarities with systemic sclerosis, and is known to be a T-cell-mediated process. Humoral abnormalities in systemic sclerosis are most clearly reflected by the presence of autoantibodies with well-defined target epitopes; mapping of the precise binding sites for some of these is currently being undertaken in several centres (Bona and Rothfield 1994). Although circulating immune complexes have been reported in systemic sclerosis, most studies have not found functional complement abnormalities, probably because most systemic sclerosis-associated autoantibodies do not activate the complement cascade (White 1994).

About 97 per cent of systemic sclerosis patients have detectable antinuclear antibodies when HEp-2 lines are used as the detection tissue (Table 10). Characteristic staining patterns for antinuclear antibodies within the nuclear and subnuclear structures are relatively specific and can be confirmed by more sophisticated tests. A diffusely grainy pattern of staining is associated with the presence of antibodies to topoisomerase-1 (Scl-70), the major DNA uncoiling enzyme. An anticentromere staining pattern occurs in up to 80 per cent of patients with the limited form of systemic sclerosis. Antigens recognized by positive sera have been identified as CENP-A, CENP-B, and CENP-C, with molecular weights of 19, 80, and 140 kDa, respectively (Earnshaw et al. 1986). A correlation has been shown (Jabs et al. 1993) between anticentromere antibodies and aneuploidy in patients with systemic sclerosis, and it is possible that anticentromere antibodies could disrupt centromere function and allow chromosomes to segregate inappropriately during mitosis, leading to a high rate of chromosomal breakage and sister chromatid exchange, although to date no correlation has been found between the presence of anticentromere antibody and chromosomal changes. Anti-RNA polymerase (RNAP) antibodies occur mainly in patients with diffuse disease, and antibodies against RNAPI, -II, and -III have been described (Bona and Rothfield 1994). The RNAPs are multiprotein complexes and are components of the transcription complex (Reeves et al. 1994). Each RNAP is composed of collections of smaller proteins shared by other RNAPs and two large distinct proteins. RNAPI synthesizes ribosomal RNA precursors in the nucleoli, whereas RNAPs II and III are found in the nuclei. RNAPII synthesizes most of the small nuclear RNAs found in ribonucleoprotein particles that mediate pre-mRNA splicing and synthesize precursors of mRNA, and RNAPIII synthesizes small RNAs including single-strand ribosomal RNA and transfer RNA. Other autoantibodies have also been detected in systemic sclerosis as well as localized scleroderma, such as those reacting against the microfibrillar protein fibrillin-1 and antibodies against a number of different cytokines. These reactivities appear more likely to be related to abnormal protein expression or processing for these antigens and may provide insight into the biochemical processes which are perturbed in scleroderma spectrum disorders although it seems unlikely that they are directly involved in disease pathogenesis.

It would appear that certain of these antibodies are closely related to particular HLA alleles, for example, it has recently been shown that class II MHC haplotype is an important factor determining *in vitro* responsiveness to topoisomerase antigen, both in patients with systemic sclerosis and in healthy control individuals (Kuwana et al. 1995). It is important to consider

Table 9 Summary of evidence for immune system involvement in systemic sclerosis

Immunogenetic associations (see Table 8)
Autoantibody associations (see Table 10)
Increased circulating levels of soluble CD4, soluble IL2 receptor and lymphocyte-derived cytokines (IL2, IL4, IL6, IL8) in some patients
Cellular and humoral immune responses to extracellular matrix components including laminin, collagen type I, and fibrillin-1
Perivascular T cell infiltrates in active dcSSc skin biopsies
Restricted T cell receptor gene expression in lymphocytes from bronchoalveolar lavage samples in SSc associated fibrosing alveolitis
Increased tissue expression of lymphocyte binding cell surface adhesion molecules and enhanced lymphocyte-fibroblast interactions in SSc
Clinical and pathological similarities with chronic graft-versus-host disease

Table 10 Autoantibodies in scleroderma

Antigen	Molecular identity	Immunofluorescence pattern	Frequency	Clinical association
Topoisomerase-1 (Scl 70)	100 kDa protein degrades to 70 kDa	Nuclear (diffuse fine speckles)	35% dcSSc 10–15% lcSSc	Associated with diffuse skin involvement, renal disease in dcSSc and especially with lung fibrosis in both subsets of SSc
Kinetochore centromere	17, 80, and 140 kDa proteins at inner and outer kinetochore plates	Centromere	60% lcSSc; upto 25% primary biliary cirrhosis	Almost restricted to lcSSc subset. These patients are at risk of isolated pulmonary hypertension, severe gut disease but relatively protected from lung fibrosis
RNA polymerases I and III	Complex of proteins 13–210 kDa. Antibodies may coexist	Nucleolar (punctate)	20% dcSSc	Associated with diffuse skin involvement and especially with renal involvement in both subsets
Fibrillarin	34 kDa protein forming a component of U3RNP	Nucleolar (clumpy) staining coilin bodies	5%	Occurs in both major subsets. Associated with poor outcome in dcSSc with cardiac disease, pulmonary hypertension, renal involvement and myositis
PM-Scl	Complex of 11 proteins 20–110 kDa	Nucleolar (homogeneous)	3%	High frequency of myositis. In childhood may associate with milder disease but renal involvement increased in adult SSc
To or Th	40 kDa protein associated with 7.2 and 8.2 kDa RNAs	Nucleolar (homogeneous)	$<$2%	Occurs in SSc and localized scleroderma. Clinical associations not defined
U1 RNP	70 kDa protein associated with small nuclear RNP complex	Speckled antinuclear	8% SSc 3% dcSSc 14% lcSSc	Higher frequency in Black patients with SSc. Associated with joint involvement and lung fibrosis in SSc
Mitochondrial M2	70 kDa protein dihydrolipoamide acyltransferase	Cytoplasmic (rod like)	15–20% lcSSc	Associated with development of primary biliary cirrhosis (positive in 95% of PBC)

that there may be racial differences in HLA associations for the various autoantibodies (see Table 8).

The antinuclear antibody profile is not as clear-cut in juveniles as in the adult form, although some trends are emerging. Serum antinuclear antibodies have been reported in 25–55 per cent of juveniles with localized scleroderma, the association being most marked in the linear group and in patients with extensive cutaneous lesions. Antibodies to single-stranded DNA also appear to be correlated with the extent of localized disease, whereas antibodies to double-stranded DNA are rarely found. It is interesting that in the generalized form of childhood scleroderma no anticentromere antibodies have been reported, even in those children with disease identical to that found in the adult.

A pathogenetic role for autoantibodies in systemic sclerosis has long been sought. Defined epitopes seem to be targets for the autoantibodies and there has been recent work showing homology between target autoantigens in systemic sclerosis and retroviral proteins, suggesting molecular mimicry, which may have significance in disease pathogenesis. There are reports that some of these antibodies are also able to enter intracellular compartments (Ma et al. 1991) and thereby to mediate intracellular events, such as the reported ability of anticentromeric antibodies to disrupt the centromere. It has been suggested that some of the autoantibodies in serum from systemic sclerosis may mediate antibody-dependent cytotoxicity, and potential effector cells have been found in the skin of some patients (White 1994).

Macrophages, mast cells, eosinophils, and basophils are found in increased numbers and in an activated state in tissues of patients with systemic sclerosis. These cells are capable of producing soluble mediators and can thereby modify endothelial and fibroblast function; for example, mast cells produce histamine and tryptase, which stimulate proliferation and matrix synthesis by fibroblasts.

The initiating stimulus in idiopathic scleroderma is unknown, although the identification of chemical precipitants for environmentally induced systemic sclerosis as discussed above (e.g. vinyl chloride and epoxy resin) may provide some clues to the processes involved, particularly in view of the similar immunogenetic associations for both idiopathic and chemically induced disease (Black et al. 1983). The most obvious major targets for the immune response in systemic sclerosis are endothelial cells and the fibroblasts. Stimulation of collagen synthesis could involve an increasing number of cytokines known to modulate the properties of fibroblasts. It is possible that cascades of such cytokines or autocrine/paracrine loops stimulate or maintain the disease process. It is now appreciated that the repertoire of mediators and cytokines produced by immune cells, fibroblasts, and endothelial cells is large. It is possible that the aberrant properties of connective tissue cells (e.g. excess synthesis of collagen, fibronectin, and glycosaminoglycans) and the endothelial-cell damage and vasculopathy, are consequences of the immunological events in systemic sclerosis.

Pathogenesis

The pathogenesis of systemic sclerosis is still uncertain, it is likely that the development of both the fibrous and the vascular lesion is complicated and a number of key events (Fig. 1).

Fibrosis is a hallmark of a number of diseases that includes scleroderma, pulmonary fibrosis, atherosclerosis, liver cirrhosis, and keloids. Excess deposition of collagen and extracellular matrix protein in the skin and internal organs of patients with systemic sclerosis was first demonstrated histopathologically many years ago, and this was confirmed by physical and biochemical means. Subsequently, techniques for culturing fibroblasts have

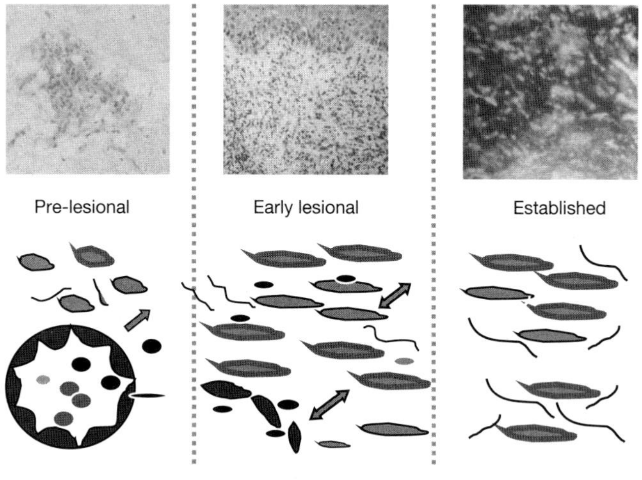

Fig. 1 Hypothesis for pathogenesis of the scleroderma lesion. Complex interactions between cells of the immune system, vasculature, and connective tissue matrix lead to the development of an activated fibrogenic fibroblast phenotype. Three separate phases in development of the established fibrotic lesion can be identified. Activated fibroblasts have bold outlines. Perivascular emigration of inflammatory mononuclear cells activates fibroblasts and leads to excessive extracellular matrix deposition. Later, a persistent fibrotic population of cells persist independent of ongoing inflammation.

provided valuable insight into the mechanisms involved in the synthesis of extracellular matrix components.

The observation that skin fibroblasts from scleroderma, or at least a subset of them, synthesize increased quantities of fibronectin, proteoglycan core proteins, and particularly collagen types I and III and to a lesser degree IV and VI was inferred from *ex vivo* studies of skin biopsies but the intriguing finding that this phenotype of matrix overproduction persists in tissue culture and could be passed on at cell division has provided a paradigm for the mechanisms underlying the development of fibrosis secondary to vascular and immunological perturbation (LeRoy 1974). Overproduction of type I collagen is a reflection of increased transcriptional activation of the two pro(I)collagen genes and of increased transcript stability. Transcriptional regulation of collagen genes has itself been a major area of biological study and a number of important *cis*-acting regulatory regions and factors interacting with these regions have been identified. More recent studies have implicated several ubiquitous transcription factors in collagen gene activation in systemic sclerosis fibroblasts including the heterotrimeric factor CBF, the GC-sequence binding protein Sp1 (Ihn and Tamki 2000) and most recently Smad proteins and their co-activators (Jimenez and Saitta 1999). It seems likely that upstream regulators of these factors are disturbed in systemic sclerosis and that this leads to greater levels or more active phosphorylated forms of the transcription factors. Another possibility is that genetic differences in these factors or their regulation contribute to severity or susceptibility to scleroderma, as part of the polygenic background to this disease.

Profibrotic cytokines are likely to be involved in the initiation of fibrosis in scleroderma and constitutive alterations in the production of some growth factors or responsiveness to their actions has been observed in scleroderma fibroblasts. One of the most potent of these is connective tissue growth factor and there is a body of evidence now suggesting that this could be an important autocrine factor in the maintenance of the scleroderma fibroblast phenotype. Modern molecular genetic methods are now being applied to understanding scleroderma as for other diseases. This includes approaches such as high-density genetic marker maps being used in pedigree and association studies to identify disease-associated loci and especially the application of methods for parallel assessment of and protein gene expression. Different studies have identified various genes, including established candidates already suggested by linkage studies and novel factors such as protease nexin-1 (Strehlow et al. 1999) and CTGF (Shi-Wen 2000). Some loci implicated by these studies are listed in Table 8.

Vascular lesions

The most prevalent clinical manifestation of vascular abnormality is Raynaud's phenomenon, which is present in over 95 per cent of systemic sclerosis patients. In addition, nailfold capillaroscopy is generally altered in systemic sclerosis at the time of diagnosis. Indeed, the combination of Raynaud's phenomenon and characteristic nailfold capillary dilatation or drop-out offers one of the earliest opportunities to diagnose patients as they develop systemic sclerosis and it has been proposed that these patients, especially when they also carry a hallmark autoantibody reactivity such as anticentromere or antitopoisomerase-1 reactivity comprise a specific pre-scleroderma clincial subset of the disease (Ihata et al. 2000). It has also prompted re-classification of some of these cases as limited systemic sclerosis (LeRoy and Medsger 2001).

The pathological features of vascular damage, immune cell activation, and fibrosis are believed to be closely linked in scleroderma (Denton et al. 1996). In both localized and generalized disease many histological features are often shared but the remainder of this discussion will focus on systemic sclerosis. Detailed studies suggest that in both the skin and internal organs one of the earliest features is endothelial cell injury, initially at the ultrastructural level (Freemont et al. 1992), and that this is temporally and spatially associated with activation of perivascular fibroblasts and subsequent deposition of increased amounts of structurally normal extracellular matrix components. Inflammation is associated with early lesions leading to tissue oedema and leucocytic infiltration. Mononuclear cells predominate with monocytes/macrophages amongst the earliest cells within lesional tissue (Kraling et al. 1995) followed later by lymphocytes, mainly carrying phenotypic markers of activated T-lymphocytes and including a significant proportion of Ro+ 'memory' cells.

Many factors may be important in the vascular damage but it is the endothelial cell that is thought to have a pivotal role. The endothelium is now known to produce numerous molecules and to regulate many aspects of vascular stability including control of vascular tone, permeability, thrombotic potential, and leucocyte trafficking (Pearson 1990; Kahaleh and Mattuci-Cerinic 1995). The precise role of vascular pathology in the pathogenesis of systemic sclerosis remains uncertain. There is considerable evidence that endothelial cell activation and damage are early events in lesional and prelesional tissues but their importance in initiating or sustaining abnormalities in other cell types remains uncertain.

Data suggest that angiogenesis might be altered in scleroderma. The classical telangiectatic lesions of limited cutaneous disease which are also common especially at later stages of diffuse cutaneous systemic sclerosis are consistent with local disruption of angiogenesis. The established fibrotic skin of scleroderma is relatively avascular and it is an attractive hypothesis that perhaps angiogenesis in scleroderma may be inadequate and perturbed. Elevated circulating levels of inhibitors of angiogenesis have been reported although tissue expression of angiogenic factors have not been shown to be consistently altered.

Oxidant stress in scleroderma pathogenesis

There is considerable evidence that oxidant stress may play a role in pathogenesis of systemic sclerosis. It is potentially involved in the fragmentation of autoantigens to expose cryptic epitopes and facilitate the development of antibodies. This has been shown for RNA polymerases and topoisomerase-1 and may be catalyzed by heavy metal ions (Casciola-Rosen et al. 1997). There is some data to support an additional association between heavy metal exposure and the development of autoantibodies. The combination of an appropriate HLA haplotype and exposure to appropriate immunogenic epitopes offers a unifying hypothesis to link different hallmark events in scleroderma. Since tissue hypoxia may occur secondary to Raynaud's phenomenon and the vasculopathy of scleroderma, perhaps in concert with the relative tissue hypoxia of the established lesional tissue it is possible that oxidant stress may promote disease development. Moreover, there is additional evidence that oxidative modification of proteins may also facilitate the development of scleroderma (Arnett et al. 2000). Antioxidant strategies for therapy offer an exciting possibility for treatment and are being pursued.

Microchimerism in scleroderma pathogenesis

The observation that foetal cells and even naked foetal DNA may persist in the maternal circulation after pregnancy has fuelled the hypothesis that some of these foetal cells may become reactivated and that scleroderma could represent a graft-versus-host disease. Indeed it has even been suggested that maternal cells passed to the foetus may persist, allowing an alloreactive process to be implicated in male patients with scleroderma. Although the concept is attractive there is only weak evidence to support it and recent data suggest that differences between scleroderma and control levels of foreign DNA are at most quantitative rather than absolute.

Experimental models for scleroderma

There are several established animal models for scleroderma, each demonstrating some features of the disease. The early vascular events of scleroderma, including endothelial cell apoptosis are demonstrated in the UCD2000 tight skin chicken model. Fibrosis in this condition remains localized although scleroderma-associated hallmark autoantibodies have been reported at later stages. The two tight-skin mouse models for scleroderma, types 1 and 2, designated Tskl and Tsk2 are both genetically determined. Tskl is a spontaneous mutant strain demonstrating fibrosis in the skin and some internal organs (though not the lungs) from around 10 days old. It has been mapped to a partial reduplication at the fibrillin-1 gene locus on chromosome 2. This leads to secretion of a larger-than-normal fibrillin-1 protein although the mechanism by which this leads to generalized connective tissue fibrosis is unclear. Recent association of human systemic sclerosis with microsatellite marker haplotypes near the fibrillin-1 locus, and detection of anti-fibrillin autoantibodies in scleroderma-spectrum disorders have revived interest in the Tskl model (Tan et al. 2001). In contrast, the precise genetic basis for Tsk2 has not yet been confirmed, although it has been mapped to a 25 kb region of chromosome 1. There are reports that an inflammatory cell infiltrate may precede the development of skin fibrosis and the induced nature of this strain by an environmental mutagen (ethylnitrosourea) similar to some agents associated with development of human disease and in these respects it is possible that Tsk2 is a more complete, though less well characterized animal model. Chronic murine GVHD occurs after bone marrow engraftment in susceptible strains across certain H-2 differences. This model is clearly immunologically determined and has prominent mononuclear cell infiltrates in the skin and viscera. It has been shown to be treatable using agents which neutralize TGFβ isoforms (McCormick et al. 1999). Two other models have recently been described, first induction of skin sclerosis by bleomycin (Yamamoto et al. 1999), again only in certain mouse strains that are resistant to lung disease, and a hybrid mouse strain in which the IFNgamma receptor knock-out line is backcrossed with a pro-inflammatory line. Other genetically modified mice are now been characterized, which may further illuminate pathogenic processes *in vivo* and allow the role of key pathways and gene products in the development of scleroderma to be assessed.

The clinical picture

Scleroderma, as discussed earlier, is not one condition but a spectrum of heterogeneous conditions occurring at any age and including localized and systemic forms. Within each subtype the rate of progression and extent of damage varies. It is increasingly realized that, whilst localized and systemic forms of scleroderma are most often discrete there are some overlap syndromes between localized scleroderma and systemic sclerosis, and that localized scleroderma may occasionally coexist with related pathologies such as eosinophilic fasciitis. In addition, there are sclerotic conditions induced by a variety of occupational, environmental, and metabolic stimuli.

Childhood-onset scleroderma is rare in comparison to the adult disease and to juvenile chronic arthritis. Fewer than 3 per cent of all cases of scleroderma are childhood-onset, and such children comprised fewer than 3 per cent of all patients seen in a paediatric rheumatology clinic. Ascertainment of childhood scleroderma may be biased by referral patterns and subspecialty orientation. In a paediatric rheumatology centre, systemic sclerosis is seen much less frequently than localized scleroderma, approximately 1 case to every 15 of localized disease. In a busy dermatology clinic, morphoea is more commonly seen and scleroderma *en coup de sabre* may be misdiagnosed as alopecia areata: consequentially, the real prevalence of these conditions is unknown. Like its adult counterpart, childhood-onset scleroderma occurs in all races, with a female predominance. There appears to be no significant familial incidence. HLA studies with sufficient numbers of children in each group are only now being undertaken, and preliminary information presented would suggest that the HLA associations in the childhood disease are quite different from those found in adult scleroderma.

Localized scleroderma

This is separated from systemic sclerosis not only by the absence of vasospasm, structural vascular damage, and involvement of internal organs, but also by the distribution of the dermal lesions, which may, depending on the subtype, follow a dermatomal pattern. The varied clinical features have led to the separation of three main varieties of localize scleroderma, morphoea, linear, and *en coup de sabre.*

Morphoea

This may be circumscribed or generalized. In circumscribed morphoea (Plate 120) there may be just one or two lesions with no generalized spread. The changes often begin with small, violaceous, or erythematous skin lesions, which enlarge and progress to firm 'hidebound' skin with variable degrees of hypo- or hyperpigmentation. These lesions eventually settle into a waxy, white appearance with subsequent atrophy. Pruritis is often a problem with the early lesion. Lesions vary in diameter between 1 and 10 cm. The condition generally resolves within 3–5 years, although sometimes a patch may persist for over 25 years. In generalized morphoea, there are many patches covering a large surface area. The acral parts are usually spared, but the trunk and legs are often involved. Generalized morphoea can be disfiguring and may continue to extend, resulting in contractures, disability, and troublesome ulceration that may occasionally become malignant. In guttate morphoea there are multiple small, hypopigmented, and pigmented papules 2–10 mm in diameter, with minimal sclerosis, and the lesions closely resemble those of lichen sclerosus et atrophicus. These lesions usually localize to the neck, shoulders, and anterior chest wall.

Linear scleroderma

The sclerotic areas occur in a linear, band-like pattern, often in a dermatomal distribution (Plate 121). They often cross joint lines, and are associated with atrophy of the soft tissue, muscle, periosteum, bone, and occasionally synovium; they can lead to extensive growth defects in a limb or a part thereof, which can be extremely disfiguring. Fixed valgus or various deformities also occur, and scoliotic changes in the spine can develop as a result of inequalities in limb length. If the toes or fingers are involved, 'hammer toes' or 'claw hand' may develop. All of these changes are much more noticeable in a growing child and most cases of linear systemic sclerosis tend to occur in childhood, as do most cases of *en coup de sabre*, a specialized form of linear disease. Lesions generally predominate on one side of the body although some degree of contralateral involvement is often present at later stages, suggesting that there may be a systemic process operating.

En coup de sabre

Linear scleroderma occurring on the face or scalp may assume a depressed, ivory appearance. The lesion was considered originally reminiscent of the scar from a sabre wound so it was termed *coup de sabre*. The linear lesion is often associated with hemiatrophy of the face on the same side. It may also be associated with vascular abnormalities of the brain and also with morphoea lesions elsewhere. There is clinical overlap between this form of linear scleroderma and specific localized growth defects such as idiopathic hemifacial atrophy (Parry–Romberg syndrome). In the latter the overlying skin may be texturally normal or there may be skin changes resembling those of scleroderma. It is not uncommon for patients to present with morphoea and then later develop linear lesions. This evolution should be anticipated extremely carefully, as the linear lesions tend to have much greater morbidity than the circumscribed patches of morphoea. The linear lesions may be quietly progressive for a long period, and lengthy follow-up is important.

In addition, in children there has been described a small group with morphoea and/or linear lesions who also have a synovitis, which can be demonstrated by infrared thermography. These patients have a raised erythrocyte sedimentation rate, rheumatoid factor, and circulating autoantibodies. Such cases are unusual, but they have an accelerated course with rapid development of contractures. At the time of presentation, there may only be a small area of localized or linear scleroderma, distant from the joint symptoms. The erythrocyte sedimentation rate and rheumatoid factor are usually normal, but autoantibodies are often present. There is both a clinical and a biochemical association, the nature of which is unclear, between localized scleroderma and eosinophilic fasciitis, in which large sclerotic patches may also occur.

Evaluation of all forms of scleroderma is difficult. In the localized forms, charting of the involved areas is often cumbersome and imprecise. However, the size of the lesion can be recorded, leg length, limb circumferences, and posture can be monitored, and muscle function and neurological status assessed. Charting of new lesions is also essential. In addition, thermography can be used to assess the activity of localized disease (Birdi et al. 1992) and high-frequency ultrasound or MRI have also been used to determine the depth of localized scleroderma lesions.

Raynaud's phenomenon and its relationship with systemic sclerosis

The overall prevalence of Raynaud's phenomenon has been variably assessed as between 3 and 10 per cent of adults worldwide, although it may affect as many as 20 per cent of young women. The prevalence varies somewhat depending on climate, skin colour, ethnic background, and occupational exposure to vibrating machines (Belch 1990).

The clinical syndrome was first described by Maurice Raynaud in 1862 as episodic digital ischaemia provoked by cold and emotion. It is classically manifest by episodic pallor of the digits followed by cyanosis, suffusion, and/or pain and tingling. This blanching reflects digital arterial vasospasm, the cyanosis the deoxygenation of static venous blood, and the redness reactive hyperaemia following the return of blood flow. Continuous blanching, blueness, or pain is not Raynaud's phenomenon and to have implications for autoimmune rheumatic disease the phenomenon must be biphasic and episodic. Important clues to secondary Raynaud's on clinical evaluation are: the development of Raynaud's either in very young children or after the age of 45 years; severe symptoms occurring all year round; digital ulcerations, which rarely, if ever occur in primary Raynaud's; asymmetry of symptoms; and the reoccurrence of chilblains in an adult. Two simple, inexpensive, non-invasive procedures have high predictive power for detecting patients in the Raynaud's group who will have systemic sclerosis in the future; serum autoantibody determination and nailfold capillary microscopy. The antinuclear antibodies were discussed earlier in the chapter and the presence of disease-specific autoantibodies plus abnormal nailfold capillaries is a powerful predictive tool (Spencer-Green 1998).

Autoantibodies

A prospective study of primary Raynaud's and undifferentiated autoimmune rheumatic disease, using the immunoblot method, found that the presence of antinuclear antibodies at the time of entry into the study was associated with the evolution of an autoimmune rheumatic disease, usually scleroderma. Furthermore, in those who initially presented with Raynaud's disease alone, anticentromere antibody had a predictive value for the development of limited cutaneous systemic sclerosis (sensitivity 60 per cent, specificity 98 per cent) and Scl-70 for diffuse cutaneous systemic sclerosis (sensitivity 38 per cent, specificity 100 per cent). Antinucleolar antibodies now being characterized biochemically are present in many patients with scleroderma and further definition may improve their diagnostic specificity. Thus, it seems that the presence of antinuclear antibodies, particularly anticentromere antibody and Scl-70, in a patient with apparent Raynaud's disease may mark the probability of later progression to one of the subsets of systemic sclerosis.

Nailfold capillaroscopy

The most distal parts of the skin and its appendages receive their nutrient blood supply from capillary loops that arise from and return to a vascular plexus deeper in the skin. These capillary loops can be seen in the skinfold of the fingernail, where the capillary is visible over its long axis (Fig. 2). Direct observation of the nailfold capillary bed dates back almost 70 years

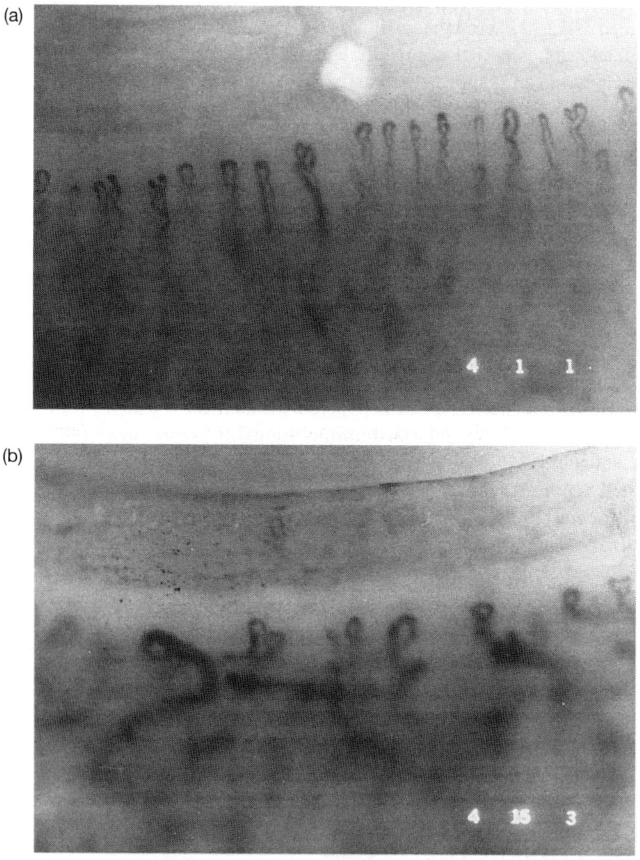

Fig. 2 (a) Photographs of normal nailfold capillaries showing normal spacing, orientation, and indentations. (b) Photograph of nailfold capillaries of a patient with scleroderma showing avascular areas and capillaries that are dilated and irregular in shape and distribution with disturbed orientation. Original magnification ×65. (By courtesy of Dr Frances Lefford, Department of Anatomy and Developmental Biology, University College, London.)

and was introduced by German investigators. Recent refinements have permitted permanent photographic recording of a row of horizontal capillary loops at the nailfold, just proximal to the cuticle (Carpentier and Maricq 1990). The characteristic patterns seen in patients destined to develop autoimmune rheumatic disease are enlargement of capillary loops, loss of capillaries, either diffusely or adjacent to enlarged capillaries. Small areas of haemorrhage around disordered capillaries are also seen in some cases.

Comment

A metaanalysis of studies examining the extent to which abnormal nailfold capillaroscopy and positive antinuclear antibody reactivity associate with evolution form isolated Raynaud's phenomenon into a connective tissue disease suggest an overall 10 year rate of around 10 per cent. Tests for autoantibodies and nailfold capillaroscopy together detect more than 90 per cent of patients destined to have generalized systemic sclerosis. Of the 3–10 per cent of the population with Raynaud's phenomenon, upto 15 per cent are positive for one or both procedures. Conversely, these tests are even stronger as negative predictors of progression, and so a patient with isolated Raynaud's phenomenon and entirely normal nailfold capillaroscopy and no antinuclear antibodies almost never progresses to develop a significant connective tissue disease (Spencer-Green 1998).

There is little evidence that symptomatic treatment of Raynaud's phenomenon in any way influences the evolution of scleroderma. However, once the mechanisms of fibrosis and vascular damage are better understood, the predictive power of these two tests, possibly coupled with other serological or genetic markers, ought to allow for a more preventive approach. It is important to appreciate that some patients with little skin involvement demonstrate typical capillaroscopic and serological features of systemic sclerosis and may also have other features such as oesophageal reflux. These patients have previously been designated as 'autoimmune Raynaud's' but it has been suggested that the term limited systemic sclerosis might be more appropriate. Prospective studies to determine the natural history and frequency with which more significant visceral complications develop are needed.

Cutaneous involvement (Plates 122 and 123)

The changes in the skin usually proceed through three phases: early, established, late. The early stage can be difficult to diagnose and a high level of suspicion is needed in the oedematous phase when the only feature may be puffiness of the hands and feet, most marked in the mornings. Oedema may be dependent and can lead to symptoms of neural compression including carpal tunnel syndrome. The face may feel slightly taut at this stage and Raynaud's may be present. On examination there is a non-pitting oedema with intact epidermal and dermal appendages. The subsequent, often sudden, development of firm, taut, hidebound skin proximal to the metacarpophalangeal joints, adherent to deeper structures such as tendons and joints, causing limitation of their movement and subsequent contractures, permits a definitive diagnosis in over 90 per cent of patients. The skin may be coarse, pigmented, and dry at this stage. The epidermis thins, hair growth ceases, sweating is impaired, and skin creases disappear.

Changes limited to the fingers alone (sclerodactyly) do not carry the same implication. The classical changes, once fully developed, can remain static for many years. Careful mapping of the degree and extent of skin involvement is the single best clinical technique for detecting the patient at risk for life-threatening involvement of internal organs. A number of scoring systems to quantify skin sclerosis have been developed. The most widely applied is a modification of that proposed by Rodnan, consisting of a 0–3 grading at 17 skin sites (maximum score 51). The original Rodnan skin score assessed 22 sites grade 0–3. In this grading, normal skin scores 0, mild (or equivocal) thickening scores 1, established (or definite) thickening without fixation to deeper tissues scores 2, and severe thickening with fixation to deep tissues (hide-bound) areas are scored 3. The sites assessed in the modified skin score are summarized in Table 11).

Table 11 Standardized assessment of skin involvement in systemic sclerosis using a modified Rodnan skin score

Site	**Maximum score**	
Face	3	
Neck	3	
Anterior chest	3	
Abdomen	3	
Back–upper	3	
Back–lower	3	
Sub-total	18	
	Right	**Left**
Upper arm	3	3
Forearm	3	3
Hand	3	3
Fingers	3	3
Thigh	3	3
Leg	3	3
Foot	3	3
	21	21
Maximum	60	

Scoring of each skin region determined by skin thickness and tethering:

0 = normal
1 = possible thickening
2 = definite thickening but mobile
3 = skin more thickened and fixed to deeper tissues 'hide-bound'

Scoring system assessing 17 sites (omitting neck and back) with maximum of 54 is also widely used to avoid these sites which are often hard to accurately score

The interobserver variability in the use of the modified Rodnan skin score in studies from both the United Kingdom and United States is similar (Clements et al. 1990). An overall within-patient variability in scoring (derived from multiple examinations) is about five skin-thickness units. Although recent controlled trials of D-penicillamine and recombinant human relaxin have both failed to demonstrate significant therapeutic benefit these well studies and prospectively collected patient cohorts have provided a clearer insight into the natural history of skin involvement in systemic sclerosis, emphasizing that after 2 or 3 years there is often plateauing of skin score or improvement even without effective treatment. Also the use as a surrogate for outcome is supported by secondary analyses confirming that skin score at presentation reflects disease outcome at later time-points.

Taut hypo- or hyperpigmented skin proximal to the elbows, knees, or clavicles determines diffuse cutaneous systemic sclerosis and such patients require more frequent multisystem evaluation. Patients with diffuse cutaneous systemic sclerosis have a preponderance of visceral involvement in the first 5 years of symptoms. Skin biopsy is usually no more sensitive than the experienced touch in diagnosing the full-blown disease, but may provide useful suggestive information in the early oedematous phase. In the early phase there are collections of mononuclear cells in the dermis, particularly around blood vessels. The soluble products of these monocytes and lymphocytes may have pathogenetic significance in the disease process. In the classic phase, fibrosis replaces the cellular infiltrate and may extend deep into the connective tissue to surround tendons, nerves, muscle bundles, and joint capsules. In the final stage, the fibrosis may be less evident, with epidermal thinning and loss of appendages the major findings.

Systemic features of disease

General manifestations

The patient with systemic sclerosis must cope with a complex set of symptoms that range from features common to chronic diseases through to complaints attributable to specific visceral involvement; fatigue and lethargy are common throughout the illness, although usually more pronounced in its early phases. Weight loss is almost universal in the diffuse cutaneous form and is less common in the limited variety. Fever is uncommon and if present, other causes such as infection or underlying malignancy should be excluded. Reactive depression is a frequent accompaniment to this often relentless and disfiguring disorder. Patients often feel isolated and support groups provide an invaluable service.

Gastrointestinal tract

The gastrointestinal tract is probably the most commonly involved internal organ system in systemic sclerosis. Over 90 per cent of patients with limited cutaneous and diffuse cutaneous systemic sclerosis have oesophageal hypomotility and serious gastrointestinal disease has been estimated to occur in 50 per cent of patients with limited cutaneous systemic sclerosis. It is probable that when systemic sclerosis affects an area of the gastrointestinal tract it does so in a sequential manner with progressive dysfunction (Cohen et al. 1980; Greydanus and Camilleri 1989). This concept is important when designing therapeutic regimens. The earliest lesion is neural dysfunction. The basis for this lesion is uncertain, although in the oesophagus there is both physiological and anatomical evidence that it is due to arteriolar changes in the vasa nervorum (D'Angelo et al. 1969; Russell et al. 1982; Greydanus and Camilleri 1989). An alternative explanation would be compression of nerve fibres by fibrous tissue (Dessein et al. 1992). The final lesion, as with all other organs in systemic sclerosis, is muscle fibrosis superimposed on neural dysfunction and atrophy. At this stage, restoration of function is not possible.

The earliest clinical symptoms may be quite subtle. Patients can often recall a specific event when there was difficulty in swallowing a pill or bolus of hard food. They may also experience retrosternal discomfort or even overt pain, which can be nocturnal. Measurement of lower oesophageal pressure is frequently unacceptable to the patient and therefore in clinical practice, the oesophageal transit time (quantitative oesophageal scintigraphy) is usually the preferred screening test. It is non-invasive, cost-effective, and is highly acceptable to patients. In those who have an abnormal scan and those who have frank dysphagia or heartburn, barium studies and/or direct oesophagoscopy may be required to identify structural divisions such as hiatus hernia and oesophageal strictures. Barrett's metaplasia and oesophageal stricture are relatively rare, but the former must be regularly assessed endoscopically. Therapies available for oesophageal disease are numerous and their place in management is summarized in Table 12.

Small-bowel disease with hypomotility is a major problem in scleroderma and can lead to weight loss, cachexia, malabsorption, and death. The classical symptoms are of a change in bowel pattern, with loose, frequent, floating, foul-smelling stools, and abdominal distension, but a patient may also present with weight loss (otherwise unexplained) or a nutritional anaemia. Once the disease is established, bacterial overgrowth with its associated malabsorption is a recurring problem, often punctuated by abrupt episodes of distension and adynamic ileus (pseudo-obstruction). Management of such patients is difficult and includes the rotational use of antibiotics, attempts to stimulate the bowel directly with prokinetics including erythromycin or domperidone, and on occasion total parenteral nutrition. Atony and hypomotility of the rectum and sigmoid colon is frequent and occurs early. It is often missed clinically because patients are reluctant to discuss their symptoms. Constipation is usually manageable with the use of dietary manipulation

Table 12 Gastrointestinal tract pathology in systemic sclerosis

Site	Disorder	Symptom	Investigation	Treatment
Mouth	Tight skin	Cosmetic	None	Facial exercises
	Dental caries	Toothache	Dental radiograph	Dental treatment
	Sicca syndrome	Dry mouth	Salivary gland biopsy	Artificial saliva
Oesophagus	Dysmobility/oesophageal spasm	Dysphagia	Barium swallow Oesophageal scintigraphy	Proton-pump inhibitors Minimize NSAID and calcium channel blocker use
	Reflux oesophagitis	Heartburn	Manometry	Elevate head of bed
	Stricture	Dysphagia	Endoscopy	Avoid late meals
Stomach	Gastric paresis	Anorexia	Scintigram	Proton-pump inhibitors
	NSAID-related ulcer	Nausea	Endoscopy	Metoclopramide, domperidone
		Early satiety	Barium meal	
Small bowel	Hypomotility	Weight loss	Barium follow through	Rotational antibiotics
	Stasis	Post-prandial bloating	^{14}C glycocholate or hydrogen breath test	Erythromycin
	Bacterial overgrowth	Malabsorption; steatorrhoea	Jejunal aspiration	Domperidone, metoclopramide; octreotide (low dose)
	NSAID enteropathy		Faecal microscopy	Oral nutritional supplements; enteral or parenteral nutritional support
	Pseudo-obstruction	Abdominal pain; distension	Plain abdominal radiograph	Conservative management: 'drip and suck'
	Pneumatosis intestinalis	Diarrhoea with blood; benign pneumoperitoneum	Plain abdominal radiograph	
Large bowel	Hypomotility	Alternating constipation and diarrhoea	Barium enema	Dietary manipulation; stool expanders for constipation; loperamide for diarrhoea
	Colonic pseudodiverticula	Rare perforation	Barium enema	Resection as a last resort
	Pseudo-obstruction	Abdominal pain; distension	Plain abdominal radiograph	Conservative management: 'drip and suck'
Anus	Sphincter involvement	Faecal incontinence	Rectal manometry	Protective measures; sacral nerve stimulation

and stool volume expanders. Codeine can cause constipation and should be avoided.

Surgery to the large bowel or any other part of the gastrointestinal tract must be viewed with great caution. Careful manometry and radiographic localization of affected segments of stomach, small intestine, and colon may allow judicious surgical resection or venting procedures, but these are not without risk and are not always successful.

Pancreatic exocrine function is frequently reduced, but rarely to an extent that is clinically important. Primary biliary cirrhosis may occur and it is associated with the subgroup of limited cutaneous systemic sclerosis. As the gastrointestinal manifestations of systemic sclerosis are frequent, and debilitating if not life-threatening, the goal in this area must be early detection, support, and control, thus permitting as active a life as possible.

Cardiac disease

It is likely that cardiac involvement from scleroderma, although important and potentially life-threatening, is underdiagnosed. This partly reflects uncertainty about its frequency and also the intrinsic difficulties of detection of some specific manifestations such as paroxysmal arrhythmia or cardiac fibrosis. Although it has been recognized for many years that cardiac involvement was an important complication the precise prevalence has not been determined. Early studies used a simple weighted scoring system for gross ECG or abnormalities and demonstrated an association between the presence of these abnormalities and mortality. More recently abnormal long axis function has been suggested to be an indicator of myocardial fibrosis. Comprehensive assessment using multiple modalities and examining patients who did not have cardiac symptoms suggested that almost 50 per cent of patients attending hospital clinics with established systemic sclerosis may have abnormalities in at least one cardiac investigation.

Pericarditis is well recognized as a complication of systemic sclerosis. It is particularly seen in the context of severe diffuse cutaneous systemic sclerosis and is probably most frequently encountered in patients with established or imminent scleroderma renal crisis. Echocardiographic studies often reveal small haemodynamically insignificant effusions in scleroderma patients. Therapeutic pericardiocentesis is only occasionally required.

Fibrotic changes in the myocardium in scleroderma have been demonstrated in biopsy specimens and at necropsy. However, the precise prevalence of this complication is unclear (Follansbee et al. 1986). Non-invasive imaging techniques such as MRI or spiral CT scanning may allow this to be determined more precisely. Indirect clues of cardiac involvement may be deduced from ECG or echocardiographic studies.

Inflammatory disease of the cardiac muscle is almost certainly underdiagnosed in patients with systemic sclerosis. It is likely that an inflammatory phase occurs in the majority of cases in which fibrosis ultimately develops, drawing analogy with the better understood sequence of pathogenic events in skin or lung fibrosis in this disease. This inflammatory process should probably be viewed as distinct from more significant myocarditis occurring in some cases with severe progressive dcSSc.

Electrophysiological cardiac abnormalities are well recognized in scleroderma. Fixed or persistent conduction defects may be easily detected but intermittent problems especially arrhythmias are much more difficult to diagnose. This means that this potentially important group of complications are likely to be under-reported. Most survival studies for scleroderma demonstrate an increase in mortality above that explicable by the frequency of life-threatening renal, pulmonary or small intestinal disease, and occult cardiac pathology is likely to be an important contributor to this increased mortality. A mechanism contributing to cardiac rate and rhythm disturbances is a cardiac autonomic neuropathy and there is some evidence to support this based upon analysis of circadian heart rate variability. These may arise from either of the preceding pathological processed. Conduction defect are the most frequently observed disturbances. Typical features include QTc prolongation on 12 lead ECG. Later conduction tissue fibrosis may lead to varying degrees of heart block including first- or second-degree block or complete heart block necessitating pacemaker implantation. Bundle branch blocks may reflect abnormalities in the conducting tissues or be complications of ventricular strain. Thus, RBBB may be seen in association with PHT and LBBB may occur in when there is left ventricular strain from hypertension or cardiac muscle disease. Paroxysmal dysrhythmias are much more difficult to detect than conduction abnormalities and it is likely that serious arrhythmias from occult cardiac disease are an important cause of sudden unexplained death in patients with systemic sclerosis.

The treatment of the cardiac manifestations of systemic sclerosis is primarily supportive, empirical, and of moderate value (see Table 13). Caution is necessary when treating patients with large pericardial effusions in diffuse scleroderma to avoid intravascular volume depletion, because of their predisposition to develop renal failure. Patients with systemic sclerosis and coexisting coronary arterial disease are often not good candidates for bypass surgery because of the distal vascular and interstitial disease that will reduce flow despite the presence of a satisfactory graft.

Peripheral vascular disease

There have been several reports that macrovascular disease may be increased in patients with systemic sclerosis. This is largely based upon case reports and small series. Large cross-sectional case–control studies or longitudinal prospective cohort studies will be necessary to confirm the association. At present, even if this occurs it is possible that it may only be found in certain populations or ethnic groups. However, it is plausible given the number of common aetiopathogenic mechanisms between the processes of atherosclerosis and systemic sclerosis including endothelial cell perturbation, activation and damage, and subsequent fibroproliferation. One possibility is that common aetiological agents predispose to both conditions.

Large vessel disease has important implications for organ-based complications of systemic sclerosis such as renal disease, peripheral ischaemia, and bowel involvement. Some non-invasive studies have suggested large vessel flow abnormalities in cerebral and renal circulation in systemic sclerosis, and by analogy with the results of studies investigating cardiac and pulmonary blood flow variations attributable to vasomotor instability in these vascular beds it is certainly plausible that episodic vasospasm is not restricted to the extremities in this disease.

Both symptomatic and asymtomatic macrovascular disease are have been reported to be increased in systemic sclerosis compared with a population control group (Youseff et al. 1993; Ho et al. 2000). A recent study from Australia has attempted to define more precisely the pattern of macrovascular disease in systemic sclerosis and interestingly a particular predilection for the ulnar artery was observed. Clearly, this particular pattern of involvement is likely to be directly relevant to the development of severe digital ischaemia. It may also suggest that factors related to the vasospastic or skin sclerosis components of the disease might be involved in the development of coexisting macrovascular disesae. Other post-mortem studies have reported that cerebrovascular disease, especially with vascular calcification, may be disproportionately severe in patients with limited cutaneous systemic sclerosis compared with macrovascular disease at other sites.

Pulmonary involvement

Pulmonary involvement is now the major cause of death in scleroderma. A study (Altmann et al. 1990) on patients with diffuse skin disease, pulmonary involvement but no cardiac or renal disease found a median survival of 78 months with 60 per cent dead at 5 years. Early diagnosis enabling the institution of effective therapy to halt disease progression is therefore a critical aim in the management of the patient with systemic sclerosis. The two major clinical manifestations of lung involvement are fibrosing alveolitis and pulmonary vascular disease. Other potential complications include aspiration pneumonia, pleural disease, spontaneous pneumothorax, drug-induced pneumonitis, associated pneumoconiosis, and neoplasm. Pulmonary fibrosis occurs in more than three-quarters of the patients with systemic sclerosis and pulmonary vascular disease in approximately 50 per cent. Autopsy studies have always yielded higher percentages than clinical studies.

Table 13 Cardiopulmonary manifestations of systemic sclerosis

	Pathology	Frequency	Clinical features	Investigation	Treatment
Lung disease					
Pulmonary fibrosis	Alveolitis with predilection for lung bases. Inflammatory infiltrate precedes development of established fibrosis. At biopsy most patients show an NSIP histological pattern	Overall around 25% of SSc. Strongly associated with anti-topoisomerase-1 autoantibody and with HLAD3/DR52a in both dcSSc and lcSSc. Overall more frequent in diffuse subset	Dry cough, exertional dyspnoea, bibasal crepitation. Finger clubbing uncommon	CXR often normal (high kV more sensitive). Restrictive pattern of PFT (low FVC and DLCO). HRCT and BAL most useful investigations. DTPA clearance accelerated. Thoracoscopic lung biopsy valuable in atypical cases	Most often treated with immunosuppression (cyclophosphamide, azathioprine) and corticosteroids. Data from retrospective studies encouraging, definitive controlled trials underway in Europe and USA
Pleural disease	Effusions and pleurisy uncommon except in overlap syndromes or renal crisis	Rare	Chest pain, dyspnoea	CXR	NSAIDs or low-dose prednisolone
Pneumothorax	Rupture of cyst into pleural cavity	Rare	Chest pain, dyspnoea	CXR	Intercostal drainage. Expansion may be poor, especially if lung fibrosis. Pleuradesis
Bronchiectasis	Suppurative inflammation of airways	Rare	Chronic productive cough	CT scan	Antibiotics, postural drainage
Lung carcinoma	Overall probably increased risk, especially scar type (alveolar cell)	Rare	Variable	Conventional resolution CT scan/bronchoscopy; biopsy	Dismal prognosis. Late diagnosis often due to associated lung pathology
Pulmonary hypertension	Isolated (no fibrosis) or secondary to lung fibrosis	10–15% overall	Exertional breathlessness, chest pain, loud pulmonary P2, syncope, right heart failure	ECG, PFT (low DLCO preserved FVC in isolated PHT), Doppler-echocardiography to estimate peak PAP. Right heart catheter definitive	Outcome for severe disease (NYHA III/IV) improved by parenteral/inhaled prostanoids or oral bosentan. Anticoagulation and vasodilators may be helpful
Cardiac disease					
Arrhythmias	Re-entry mechanism or inflammation	Uncertain	Palpitation, syncope	ECG—especially 24 h with symptom diary; stress test	Treat only if haemodynamically significant
Conduction defects	Local fibrosis	10% on ECG	Syncope	ECG	May require pacemaker
Pericardial disease	Inflammation or effusion	10% clinically; 30% at autopsy	Chest pain, dyspnoea	ECG, echocardiogram	NSAID, corticosteroids, drainage, fenestration
Myocardial involvement	Myocarditis Myocardial fibrosis	Rare 30–50% dcSSc	Congestive cardiac failure, arrhythmias	ECG, echocardiogram, MUGA, gated cardiac MRI	Management of heart failure. Immunosuppression/ corticosteroids if myocarditis

Pulmonary fibrosis

Interstitial lung disease often develops insidiously but established fibrosis is irreversible and early diagnosis is therefore vital and in the future genetic markers may help to identify this group at presentation. Pulmonary manifestations of systemic sclerosis are listed in Table 13.

The most common symptoms of respiratory involvement are breathlessness, especially on exertion, and a dry cough. Chest pain is infrequent and haemoptysis rare, and if either is present then the presence of additional pathology should be sought. On physical examination the most frequent finding is of bilateral basal crepitations. The classical radiographic features consist of reticulonodular shadowing, usually symmetrical and most marked at the lung bases. However, the chest radiograph is an insensitive indicator of fibrosing alveolitis, and should be used only as an initial screen or to exclude infection or aspiration secondary to oesophageal abnormalities. There are many mildly symptomatic patients with normal chest radiographs despite interstitial lung disease, and lung function tests are more discriminatory. The single-breath diffusion test (*DLco*) is abnormal in over 70 per cent of patients with diffuse cutaneous systemic sclerosis (including asymptomatic patients with no complaints and an unremarkable chest radiograph). A reduction in *DLco* is the earliest proven abnormality in patients with systemic sclerosis who develop interstitial lung disease; lung function tests that show normal volumes but reduced transfer of gases in the face of normal imaging are suggestive of pure pulmonary vascular disease. Measurement of the alveolar–arterial oxygen difference during exercise also appears to be a sensitive indicator of lung disease in systemic sclerosis.

The application of thin (3 mm)-section, high-resolution CT scanning of the lungs has been of immense value for definition and assessment of diffuse lung diseases and has revealed the character and distribution of fine structural abnormalities not visible on chest radiographs (Harrison et al. 1989) (Fig. 3). Using this technique, the earliest detectable abnormality is usually a narrow, often ill-defined, subpleural crescent of increased density in the posterior segments of the lower lobes. When more extensive, the shadowing often takes on a more characteristic reticulonodular appearance yet frequently retaining

(a)
(b)
(c)
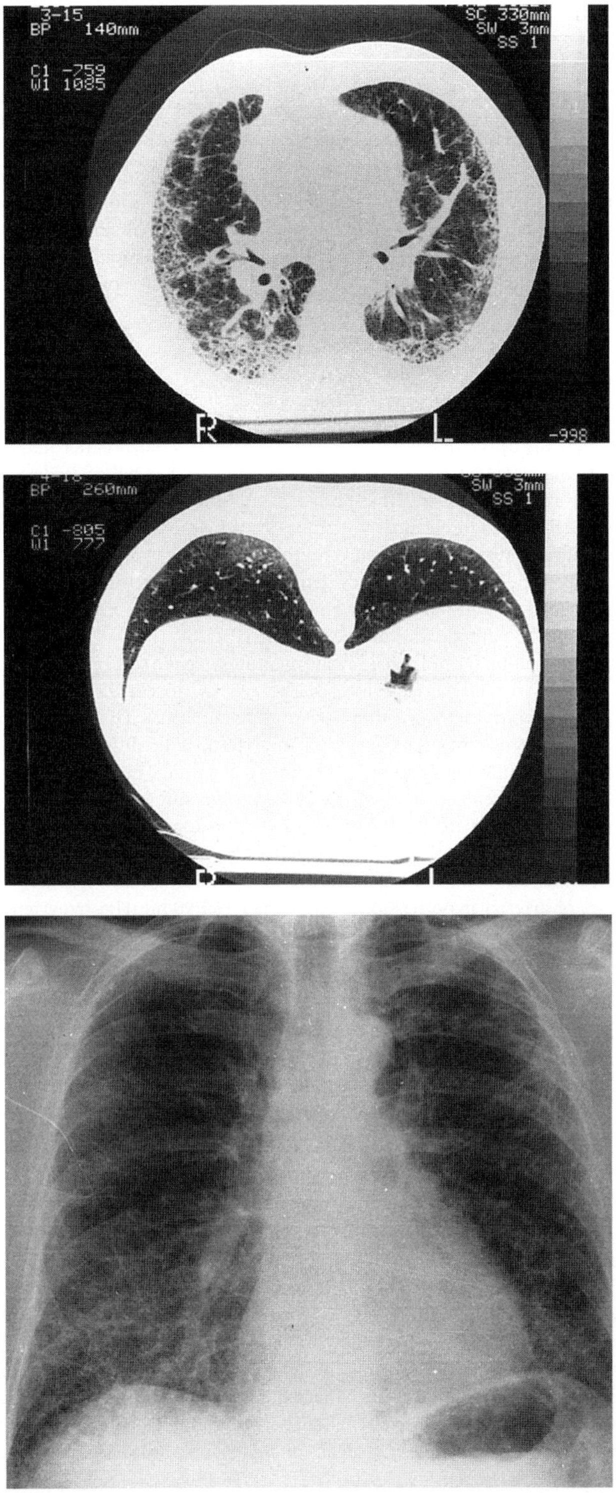

Fig. 3 Thin-section CT scan images illustrating: (a) ground-glass appearance of early pulmonary involvement posteriorly, associated with a normal chest radiograph; (b) extensive honeycomb shadowing and cystic air spaces involving both lower lobes, with corresponding chest radiographic appearances of advanced interstitial lung disease (bibasilar reticulonodular shadowing) (c). (With grateful acknowledgement to Drs A. Wells, R. du Bois, and B. Strickland, Departments of Respiratory Medicine and Radiology, Royal Brompton Hospital, London.)

a subpleural distribution. It also becomes associated with fine, honeycomb air spaces and ultimately larger, cystic air spaces—an appearance that mirrors the macroscopic appearance. In a semiquantitative comparison of the predictive value of these CT appearances to mirror the biopsy evidence of an inflammatory alveolitis, a 'ground glass' pattern of opacification on CT was associated with a predominantly cellular biopsy whereas a reticular pattern of abnormality was found in patients whose subsequent lung biopsy confirmed a particularly fibrotic disease process (Muller and Miller 1990; Wells et al. 1992). CT scans also confirm the presence of pleural disease or mediastinal lymphadenopathy, which is commonly present. It is important to perform prone as well as supine scans, particularly in more subtle cases, to exclude the contribution of gravity to the radiographic appearances from vascular and interstitial pooling in the dependent areas. In addition to identifying early disease, high-resolution CT scanning can identify a pattern of disease that predicts a better response to therapy and a better prognosis (Wells et al. 1993a,b). Furthermore, the extent of disease present, as defined by CT within the lavaged lobe, correlates with the predominant type of inflammatory cell obtained by bronchoalveolar lavage of that same lobe: lymphocytes are present in excess before CT identifies disease; eosinophils appear as the lung becomes abnormal; neutrophils are found in most abundance when at least 50 per cent of the lavaged lobe is involved in the disease process (Wells et al. 1994).

In predicting the histological pattern CT, although useful, has not replaced lung biopsy as the 'gold standard' investigation (Plate 124). As yet, patients who appear to have early changes on CT should still be considered for a thoracoscopic biopsy for staging of the disease. Drawing analogy from studies of idiopathic pulmonary fibrosis (IPF), lung biopsies can be classified as non-specific interstitial pneumonia (NSIP) or usual interstitial pneumonia (UIP) (Katzenstein and Myers 1998). In systemic sclerosis, the predominant histological pattern is NSIP whereas in IPF the majority show UIP. Outside the context of systemic sclerosis there is a better long-term outcome for NSIP and this may have important implications for systemic sclerosis-associated lung disease.

The use of DTPA clearance in the management of systemic sclerosis has been the subject of extensive study and has been shown to be of value. It identifies early disease and also identifies a group of patients whose disease will run a more stable, non-progressive course, that is, those with normal clearance (Wells et al. 1993a,b). The speed of clearance of the isotope is dependent upon the integrity of the epithelial barrier and therefore anything that disrupts this, either inflammation or fibrosis, will increase the rate of clearance. DTPA clearance is highly sensitive: cigarette smoking will produce increased clearance rates and the test is, therefore, only of value in non-smokers or those who have given up smoking for at least 1 month before the assessment. In systemic sclerosis, clearance of DTPA may be abnormal even when chest radiography and pulmonary function tests are normal (Harrison et al. 1989). In established disease, clearance is enhanced in comparison with normal individuals. Furthermore, changes in clearance can predict subsequent changes in pulmonary function tests (Wells et al. 1993a,b).

The definition and assessment of lung fibrosis in systemic sclerosis has now reached the stage that the extent, pattern and activity of lung disease can be reliably assessed (Veeraraghavan et al. 2001). Unfortunately, whilst this provides a number of validated tools to assess outcome treatments remain uproven. Corticosteroids and cyclophosphamide are the most widely used treatments and the studies that have been performed, and whilst several suggest benefit no trial has been prospective, placebo controlled, and of sufficient rigor to confirm efficacy. Fortunately, both in North America and the United Kingdom there are now studies to assess oral or parenteral cyclophosphamide and the results of these studies are eagerly awaited.

Pulmonary hypertension

Pulmonary vascular disease complicates up to 15 per cent of cases of systemic sclerosis and occurs in several contexts. The most important of these is its occurrence as isolated pulmonary hypertension (PHT), occurring in up to 10 per cent of patients with limited cutaneous systemic sclerosis and a smaller proportion of those with diffuse cutaneous systemic sclerosis. There are serological associations for both types, ACA being more common in patients with limited cutaneous systemic sclerosis and antifibrillarin (anti-U3RNP) being associated with this complication in diffuse systemic sclerosis. The pathology of isolated PHT in systemic sclerosis is very similar to that of idiopathic or familial PHT and the latter has been used as a treatment paradigm for systemic sclerosis-associated disease. Patients with associated pulmonary fibrosis may develop secondary PHT, as in other forms of interstitial lung disease, and this may require consideration in managing these cases as it is important to determine the contribution of the two pathologies. Other situations in which PHT occurs include associated cardiac disease with diastolic dysfunction.

Current treatment and investigation of PHT occurring in the context of systemic sclerosis requires first that the diagnosis is made. The first indication may be from symptoms, which typically include exertional breathlessness and less often chest pain or syncope. In general, patients with systemic sclerosis will undergo regular monitoring of pulmonary function, Doppler-echocardiography and ECG examination. In the majority of cases, the clinical suspicion of pulmonary vascular disease will arise due to abnormal tests as outlined above. Definitive diagnosis requires exclusion of related pathologies such as thromboembolic disease (by ventilation: perfusion lung scan, spiral CT scan or pulmonary angiography, and establishment that the mean PA pressure is above 25 mmHg at rest or 30 mmHg upon exercise. Although there is a reasonably good correlation between estimated peak PA pressure using Doppler-echocardiography and measurements at right heart catheterization at low and high values, this is not always true between 30 and 50 mmHg and caution must be used. For this reason, and the additional information which it yields, right heart catheterization has become mandatory for optimal management of these cases. It allows pulmonary venous hypertension to be identified using the PCWP and the pulmonary vascular resistance, cardiac output (cardiac index), and pulmonary artery pressures to be measured.

All patients with PHT should receive oral anticoagulation and if appropriate, diuretic therapy (usually spironolactone) and digoxin. If there is evidence of sustained hypoxia (arterial saturation consistently below 90 per cent on air) long-term low-dose oxygen can be helpful by reducing hypoxia induced pulmonary vasoconstriction. Typically, 2 l/min using nasal cannulae is given. Pulmonary vascular disease has become much more important to detect now that there are licensed treatments for use both in the PHT and in connective tissue disease associated PHT. The first agent shown to be effective was parenteral prostacyclin in the form of Flolan in two controlled clinical trials. This is given as a long-term treatment using an ambulatory pump and permanent indwelling central venous line. More recently, other routes of administration have also been shown to improve symptoms including subcutaneous infusion and inhaled routes. More exciting still were results of the BREATHE-1 study which suggest that bosentan a relatively well tolerated orally active agent is also an effective treatment for PHT. Bosentan is a broad-spectrum endothelin (ET) receptor antagonist and elevated serum and tissue levels of ET have been clearly demonstrated in systemic sclerosis, providing a rationale to this treatment. The complex nature of the diagnosis of PHT and determining its basis together with the need to diagnose early, when surrogate markers such as DLCO on pulmonary function testing or evidence of right-sided abnormalities on echocardiography may be equivocal justifies having a low threshold for right heart catheterization. This allows the diagnosis to be confirmed using pressure measurements at rest and during exercise and also allows cardiac index and pulmonary vascular resistance to be directly measured. These variables often change before significantly elevated pressures can be detected non-invasively for instance by Doppler-echocardiography. Nevertheless this test is valuable for use in non-selected patients and particularly in those with clinical features suggesting PHT. If on testing pulmonary function there is an isolated marked decrease in diffusing capacity for carbon monoxide (<50 per cent of predicted normal) in the absence of significant restrictive ventilatory abnormalities then pulmonary hypertension is to be strongly suspected. Non-invasive investigative tools such as gated cardiac MRI and exercise echocardiography hold promise for the future but are not yet widely available. Pathologically, pulmonary arteries of all sizes show marked intimal and medial hyperplasia; of great interest is the finding by Follansbee et al. (1990) that although the clinical syndrome seems confined to the group with limited cutaneous systemic sclerosis, intimal thickening and narrowing, albeit to a lesser degree, occurred in patients with diffuse cutaneous systemic sclerosis. In addition to the obstructive vascular lesions, the pulmonary vasculature appears to be abnormally reactive, with significant pulmonary vasoconstriction occurring on exposure to cold, again analogous to a peripheral Raynaud's phenomenon. That systemic sclerosis can be an overwhelmingly vascular disease is perhaps nowhere more convincingly demonstrated than in the subset of patients with severe PHT. It has an extraordinarily poor prognosis; death is usually due to rapidly progressive respiratory insufficiency accompanied by severe right-ventricular hypertrophy and failure.

Renal disease

This remains one of the most important complications of scleroderma and is amenable to treatment, although the prognosis is much better if appropriate management is instituted early. As with PHT, renal scleroderma is mainly a vascular disease. Both post- and ante-mortem studies suggest that epithelial and endothelial renal lesions occur before there is clinical evidence of renal disease in systemic sclerosis (Kovalchik et al. 1978), and certainly precede any histological evidence of fibrosis. This supports the view that epithelial, and particularly endothelial, damage are important early events in the pathogenesis of scleroderma (Prescott et al. 1992). The best characterized pattern of renal involvement in systemic sclerosis is an acute or subacute renal hypertensive crisis. This generally occurs in patients with diffuse systemic sclerosis within 5 years of disease onset. The overall incidence of scleroderma renal crisis is uncertain, with differences in the reported frequency even in series from the same unit. This variation probably reflects differences in incidence in the various subsets of systemic sclerosis. In high-risk patients, the incidence may be as great as 20 per cent but overall is probably less than 10 per cent (Steen 1984). Traub (1984) proposed the following criteria to diagnose scleroderma renal crisis: abrupt onset of arterial hypertension greater than 160/90 mmHg; hypertensive retinopathy of at least grade III severity; and rapid deterioration of renal function and elevated plasma renin activity. Other typical features include the presence of a microangiopathic haemolytic blood film and hypertensive encephalopathy, often complicated by generalized convulsions. It is generally considered important to perform a renal biopsy, once hypertension has been adequately controlled, especially if renal replacement therapy is being contemplated. This allows histological confirmation of the diagnosis and the exclusion of other causes for renal failure of abrupt onset, such as glomerulonephritis or the haemolytic–uraemic syndrome. Histologically, systemic sclerosis renal crisis typically shows fibrinoid necrosis, mucoid, or fibromucoid proliferative intimal lesions (when extensive, termed onion skinning) in renal arteries, particularly the arcuate and interlobular vessels; glomerular thrombi occur and ultimately glomerulosclerosis (Plate 125). The extent of the glomerular lesion can be useful in predicting the eventual degree of functional recovery. Patients usually present with the clinical features of severe hypertension, including headaches, visual disturbances, hypertensive encephalopathy (especially seizures), and pulmonary oedema. Occasionally a similar pattern of renal dysfunction occurs without hypertension (normotensive renal crisis), suggesting that the pathological features are not simply the end-organ consequences of raised arterial pressure (Helfrich et al. 1989).

Management of renal systemic sclerosis requires a high index of suspicion to enable early diagnosis and treatment of the renal crisis. Creatinine clearance or isotope glomerular filtration rate should be checked twice yearly in diffuse cutaneous systemic sclerosis for the first 5 years and annually thereafter. In limited cutaneous systemic sclerosis, there is much less risk and a less frequent measurement of the glomerular filtration rate is sufficient. Blood pressure should be well controlled (often antihypertensive treatments also help Raynaud's symptoms) and in diffuse cutaneous systemic sclerosis the use of angiotensin-converting enzyme inhibitors is particularly appropriate since there is some anecdotal evidence that they protect from hypertensive crisis (Steen et al. 1990). High-dose corticosteroids have now been formally demonstrated in a case–control study to increase the risk of renal crisis in diffuse cutaneous systemic sclerosis and doses above 20 mg prednisolone equivalent daily should be avoided (Steen et al. 1994).

Once diagnosed, an acute renal crisis in systemic sclerosis must be treated as a medical emergency. The patient should be admitted immediately and reasonable control of the blood pressure is a priority. Extreme caution must be taken, however, to avoid a precipitous or excessive drop in arterial pressure and also to prevent relative or actual hypovolaemia associated with vasodilatation of constricted vascular beds, both of which can further diminish renal perfusion and compound the renal lesion of systemic sclerosis with acute tubular necrosis. For this reason, powerful parenteral antihypertensives (e.g. intravenous nitroprusside or labetolol) should be avoided; an internal jugular or subclavian venous cannula should be inserted to monitor central venous filling pressure, and an indwelling arterial cannula for pressure monitoring should be considered. Hypertension should be treated with angiotensin-converting enzyme inhibitors (captopril or enalapril up to maximum dose) and calcium-channel blockers (starting with long-acting nifedipine initially), aiming to reduce both diastolic and systolic pressure by 20 mmHg in the first 48 h and ultimately maintaining diastolic pressure at 80–90 mmHg. Intravenous prostacyclin, which is believed to help the microvascular lesion without precipitating hypotension, is often administered from diagnosis. Fish-oil capsules are sometimes prescribed in view of their unproven but theoretically beneficial properties (McCarthy and Kenny 1992). Renal function should be closely monitored by twice-weekly creatinine clearance and daily serum creatinine estimations. Regular full blood counts, clotting screening, and estimations of fibrin degradation product are important to monitor the degree of microangiopathic haemolytic anaemia, which often reflects the activity of the disease process. Short-term haemodialysis should be given if necessary and peritoneal dialysis often works well if long-term renal replacement therapy is needed. Interestingly, it has been observed that after a renal crisis, skin sclerosis and other features of systemic sclerosis improve (Denton et al. 1994), particularly if a patient is undergoing maintenance dialysis. The reason for this is unknown; it may result from the removal or inactivation of circulating mediators or simply reflect the natural history of the disease. It should be remembered that there is also often considerable recovery in renal function after an acute crisis, sometimes allowing dialysis to be discontinued, and improvement can continue for up to 2 years. Therefore any decisions regarding renal transplantation should not be made before this time.

Musculoskeletal system

Muscle

Skeletal muscle is often involved in scleroderma (Russell 1988). In many instances, the weakness and atrophy results from disuse secondary to joint contractures or chronic disease. However, about 20 per cent have a chronic myopathy is characterized by mild weakness and atrophy of muscles, minimal elevation of creatine phosphokinase, few or no changes on electromyography, and subtle histological features showing focal replacement of myofibrils with collagen and perimysial and epimysial fibrosis without inflammatory change. This form of myopathy is often unresponsive to anti-inflammatory mediation. A minority of patients exhibit an inflammatory myositis, indistinguishable from polymyositis; caution must be observed if this occurs in the context of early diffuse disease, when treatment with high-dose steroids might precipitate renal failure, and an alternative treatment should be considered. An atypical inflammatory myositis that requires special histochemical stains to demonstrate the differences in fibre size and composition has been reported in association with myocarditis in a few cases of systemic sclerosis. This form of myopathy, which can last for many years, is often unresponsive to non-steroidal or glucocorticoid anti-inflammatory medications.

Joints

A symmetrical polyarthritis, usually seronegative, anodular, and nonerosive, is the presenting feature in a small number of patients destined ultimately to develop systemic sclerosis. By 2 years, frequently much earlier, the synovitis has subsided and classic cutaneous systemic sclerosis is present, often developing abruptly over 1–3 months.

The fibrosis characteristic of the classical disease affects the tendons (causing tendon friction rubs), the ligaments, and joint capsules, restricting movement; fibrosis is also found in the synovium. The synovium in systemic sclerosis is often covered by an excessive amount of fibrin; the reason for this is unknown. Joint destruction is unusual. Management of soft tissue and joint problems is closely linked to skin care and to overall skeletal mobility. True bone changes in the form of distal tufts are usually a late change occurring in the second and third decade of the disease, and are thought to be due to a lack of a vascular supply adequate enough to preserve viable bone. This can occur in patients with long-standing Raynaud's phenomenon without connective tissue disease. Other sites of bone reabsorption, for example, the mandible and ribs, have been recorded late in the disease.

Other organ involvement

Other organs involved in systemic sclerosis are listed in Table 14.

Systemic sclerosis and pregnancy

The greater incidence of scleroderma in women has focused interest on the potential interrelations between scleroderma, hormones, and pregnancy. It is of interest that women with Raynaud's phenomenon have an increased likelihood of low birthweight babies and fertility problems both before and after the onset of disease. It is unknown whether these findings are a reflection of the vasospasm affecting pregnancy or whether they reflect a common aetiological link.

The question of pregnancy in systemic sclerosis can be approached from two angles: the effect of scleroderma on pregnancy and its outcome, and the effect of pregnancy on the development and course of systemic sclerosis (Black 1990).

Case–controlled studies have provided conflicting evidence on the outcome of pregnancy. British and Italian studies have shown an increase in the spontaneous abortion rate in women destined to develop systemic sclerosis. The British workers also found a higher rate of infertility, habitual abortion, and a higher probability that the pregnancy would end in stillbirth or neonatal death. An American study, however, showed only an increase in intrauterine growth retardation and prematurity, but not in miscarriage or foetal death.

The outcome of the pregnancy for the mother is also a subject of discussion. The American workers found no increase in maternal morbidity or mortality. However, the 23 case reports since 1932 (which may well select more interesting and thus severe cases) gave nine deaths, eight in patients with diffuse cutaneous systemic sclerosis, and at least five due to renal failure. Disease progressed in 12 of these patients, regressed in two, regressed during pregnancy but progressed afterwards in two, and developed during the pregnancy in one. In reports of larger series, totalling 103 pregnancies (mainly in women with limited disease), the disease developed during pregnancy in nine, progressed in 32, remitted in 11, and was stable in 35. There were 24 spontaneous abortions, five perinatal deaths, six cases of toxaemia, and two maternal deaths. These reports reinforce the worse prognosis in diffuse disease. Of some encouragement are three more recent case reports. One describes a successful pregnancy in a patient with renal involvement, controlled with angiotensin-converting enzyme inhibitors throughout. The second patient, who had a renal crisis 6 years before treated with angiotensin-converting enzyme inhibitors for 5 years, managed without therapy to reach 38 weeks' gestation before becoming hypertensive and needing caesarean section for delivery of a healthy baby. The third case described a patient with limited cutaneous systemic sclerosis, livedoid vasculitis with foot ulceration, and a positive ribonucleoprotein autoantibody, and three previous spontaneous abortions, one neonatal

Table 14 Other organ involvement in scleroderma

Organ	Effect	Pathological process	Frequency
Thyroid	Spectrum of autoimmune diseases—especially hypothyroidism. May precede or follow onset of SSc	>30% have antithyroid antibodies	20–40%
Liver	Primary biliary cirrhosis	Antimitochondrial antibodies in up to 20% of patients with SSc. ACA 95% of PBC	3% of lcSSc
Nervous system	Cranial neuropathy	Microvasculopathy of vasa nervorum	Trigeminal or glossopharyngeal neuralgia commonest neurological change. Painless sensory trigeminal neuropathy also occurs
	Median nerve compression	Very frequent in dcSSc due to tendinitis in carpal tunnel	Often the first diagnosis in early dcSSc. Generally improves later in disease but surgical decompression frequently performed prior to diagnosis of SSc
	Peripheral neuropathy		
	Autonomic neuropathy		
Sexual dysfunction	Erectile dysfunction (male); dyspareunia (female)	Complex mechanism including structural vascular changes, autonomic dysfunction and psychosexual factors	Under recognized and of major morbidity

death (28 weeks' gestation), and a 4-year period of secondary infertility. She was delivered of a healthy baby at 33 weeks, taking nifedipine before and throughout pregnancy for the foot ulceration.

The most feared complication in pregnancy is renal disease, which usually presents with hypertension especially in the third trimester, and is thus difficult to distinguish from toxaemia. Renal scleroderma should be considered in all but the most typical cases of pre-eclamptic toxaemia. In contrast to ordinary pre-eclamptic toxaemia, patients with systemic sclerosis can be vulnerable in the post-partum period, and must be watched very carefully.

Advice to patients with systemic sclerosis at pregnancy is difficult, since studies are limited and retrospective. Patients with diffuse skin involvement, especially with lung, renal, or cardiac involvement, tend to have a worse prognosis, and should be offered therapeutic abortion. The patient with limited disease should be told of the possible development of complications, and the variable and unpredictable outcome, and may then request abortion. Very close monitoring of any patient with systemic sclerosis is then necessary throughout pregnancy.

Management of systemic sclerosis

There have been major advances in treating many of the organ-specific complications of systemic sclerosis. Thus, critical ischaemia and severe Raynaud's phenomenon are improved by parenteral prostacyclin analogues; the management and outcome of scleroderma renal crisis has been transformed by use of ACEI agents and the morbidity from oesophagitis has been drastically cut by use of proton pump inhibitors. Added to this are the exciting developments in treating pulmonary hypertension and several encouraging retrospective studies suggesting that immunosuppression using cyclophosphamide may be effective in slowing the progression of systemic sclerosis-associated fibrosing alveolitis. Added to these developments is a much clearer understanding of the heterogeneity and natural history of the major subsets of systemic sclerosis and an appreciation that risk stratification, the use of serological markers and proactive regular screening of patients for early signs of complications. Together, these factors make systemic sclerosis a much more manageable disease than ever.

These positive developments must be tempered by the assertion that so far no agent has been proven to be an effective disease modifying therapy. There have now been many pilot studies and several well-controlled Phase II and III studies of promising candidate treatments. These include treatments directed towards the immunological activation which is believed to drive early systemic sclerosis and targeting the fibrotic process that is the predominant pathology of established systemic sclerosis.

The choice and evaluation of any treatment regimen are not easy because the disease is complex and the pathogenesis poorly understood; the disorder is heterogeneous and its extent, severity, and rate of progression are highly variable—therapy must therefore be closely tailored to the individual patient systems involved; there is a tendency towards spontaneous stabilization and/or regression after a few years, particularly within the more benign and numerically larger subset of limited cutaneous systemic sclerosis; and there is a paucity of both clinical and laboratory features for ascertaining improvement (or deterioration) in the disease, especially with respect to visceral change.

Efforts over the last several years in trying to develop effective disease modifying treatments for systemic sclerosis have ensured that there is now a robust infrastructure for conducting prospective clinical trials in systemic sclerosis and much more insight that previously into the nature of the end-points that are likely to yield interpretable data during a clinical trial and appreciation of the likely requirements of licensing bodies in demonstrating that agents are beneficial in systemic sclerosis.

Ultimately, it is hoped that a better understanding of the pathogenesis of systemic sclerosis, especially in its aggressive diffuse form, will identify key factors, pathways, or processes that can be targeted therapeutically. It is possible that targets will be stage or subset specific. There are already examples of pilot studies of anticytokine therapies using neutralizing antibodies or soluble receptors. Ultimately, small molecules that inhibit key pathways are likely to be the most successful form of treatment but these are presently a long-way off.

Immunomodulatory therapy

The rationale for immunosuppressive treatment for systemic sclerosis is based upon several premises. This is reviewed in the discussion of pathogenesis earlier in the chapter. It is generally considered that immunosuppressive strategies are most likely to be effective in the early stages of systemic sclerosis at the time that inflammatory features are prominent. A large number of agents have been tries but none has been shown in clinical trials to be definitely effective. The various agents evaluated are listed in Table 15, together with a summary of the extent of formal evaluation. It is noteworthy that the extend of immunosuppression ranges form specific and relatively mild such as the induction of oral tolerance to type I collagen at one extreme to non-specific and very profound at the other end of the spectrum such as immunoablation with autologous peripheral stem cell rescue. Several immunosuppressive treatments are currently being evaluated in clinical trials. It is disappointing that a large study of methotrexate therapy in systemic sclerosis showed some trends of improvement in skin score and global measures of systemic sclerosis severity but was statistically underpowered.

It must be remembered that segregation of potential therapies may be artificial and it is likely that immunosuppressive or antimetabolic agents also affect non-immune cell components of the disease process such as fibroblasts or vascular cells and agents whose primary mode of action is believed to be antifibrotic also modulate immune cell function. Good examples of this are the interferons and D-penicillamine. It is nevertheless helpful when considering agents to classify them to aid study design so that sage and subset of systemic sclerosis can be appropriately considered.

Long-term high-dose steroids have no place in the management of systemic sclerosis; indeed they are potentially toxic (Steen et al. 1994) and may precipitate 'hypertensive renal crisis'. Steroid usage has been restricted to patients with myositis, symptomatic serositis, the early oedematous phase of the skin disease, and refractory arthritis and tenosynovitis. The lowest possible but therapeutically effective dose should be sought.

Antifibrotic agents

Although many current strategies used to treat systemic sclerosis are immunomodulatory, it is clear from earlier discussions of pathogenesis that the most effective agents for establishes disease are likely to have antifibrotic activity. Unfortunately, no agent has yet been shown to be effective. Some are still in use although they have not been shown to be effective in controlled trials and should perhaps be abandoned. Some potential novel agents and those previously used are listed in Table 16.

In the absence of proven disease-modifying therapies and because of the severe and disabling nature of the worst forms of scleroderma a number of novel approaches are currently being considered. These include strategies to modulate immunological activation in early systemic sclerosis, ranging from immunoablation with reconstitution using autologous peripheral stem cells at one extreme, to induction of oral tolerance using native bovine type I collagen, at the other.

It is likely that successful management of scleroderma will require not only suppression of immune events but also antifibrotic treatments, especially in later stage disease. Hence, a number of novel antifibrotic therapies are also currently under evaluation include the plant alkaloid halofuginone, recombinant human relaxin, and the antibiotic minocycline. Oxidant stress is implicated in the pathogenesis of scleroderma and so a number of antioxidant agents have been considered as potential therapies. In theory such an approach might influence the vascular, fibrotic, and immunological aspects of the disease.

Finally, advances in understanding the pathogenic processes which underlie the development and progression of systemic sclerosis raises the possibility of identifying key molecular mediators which are central to the disease and which might provide specific targets for therapeutic modulation.

Another drug that has been tried in a very small study is minocycline. This agent has a number of properties in addition to being an antibiotic.

Table 15 Immunomodulatory strategies for disease-modifying treatment of systemic sclerosis

Agent	Clinical trial data	Reference
Cyclosporin A	Open study, 10 patients. Improvement in skin score	Clements et al. (1994)
Methotrexate	Placebo-controlled trial 30 patients. Significant improvement in skin score. Larger North American study inconclusive	van den Hoogen et al. (1996); Pope et al. (2001)
Cyclophosphamide	Open study, 5 patients. Symptomatic improvement	Tyndall et al. (2001)
Immunoablation/stem cell transplantation	On going studies USA and Europe	Tyndall (2001)
Extracorporeal photopheresis	Recent open study 6/16 case showed improvement	Krasagakis et al. (1998)
Antithymocyte globulin (ATG)	Open study, 13 patients with mycophenolate mofetil. Skin score improved	Tarkowski and Lindgren (1994); Stratton et al. (2000)
Thalidomide	Pilot studies underway	None yet
Rapamycin	Anecdotal benefit	None yet
Oral tolerization to type I collagen	Favourable pilot data. Trial on going in USA	Postlethwaite et al. (2000)

Table 16 Antifibrotic strategies for disease-modifying treatment of systemic sclerosis

Agent	Clinical trial data	Reference
D-penicillamine	High versus low dose study in USA 134 patients, no apparent benefit	Clements et al. (1999)
Interferon-α	Placebo controlled trial (35 patients). Better outcome in placebo group	Black et al. (1999)
Relaxin	Placebo controlled dose-escalation study (30 patients stable scleroderma) encouraging improved global assessment score. Large phase III study negative. Considered ineffective	Seibold et al. (2000)
Interferon-γ	Open study (44 patients) showed minor improvements in skin sclerosis	Grassegger et al. (1998)
Anticytokine therapy	Pilot studies of anti-TGFβ1 antibodies are now underway	None yet
Halofuginone	Plant alkaloid with *in vitro* and *in vivo* potential to downregulate collagen (I) gene expression. Little human data available	None yet
Prolylhydroxylase inhibition	Pilot studies underway using topical formulations for skin fibrosis. Systemic administration likely to be toxic	None yet

These include an ability to inhibit metalloproteinases—although this would not be helpful in a systemic fibrotic disease. The pilot study of minocycline was widely reported in the lay-press and to determine usefulness a larger formal evaluation is essential. A controlled clinical trial is currently underway to evaluate this treatment and the results are eagerly awaited.

Difficulties in conducting clinical trials in scleroderma are well recognized. These include clinical heterogeneity, absence of any treatment of proven efficacy to use as an active-control arm and a reluctance of patients with a life-threatening disorder to participate in placebo-controlled studies. To try and improve trials guidelines for evaluating disease-modifying treatments in systemic sclerosis have been published by the American College of Rheumatology. Although the current climate of evidence-based medicine has encouraged critical appraisal of current treatment approaches for systemic sclerosis, one drawback is that agents may be inadequately evaluated. It is possible that effective therapies risk of being discarded due to under powered studies giving false-negative results. To avoid this trials will almost certainly have to be multicentre and perhaps even multinational. Currently consortia of clinicians around the world are vigorously improving the infrastucture for multicentre clinical trials, under the auspices of the Scleroderma Clinical Trials Consortium (SCTC) in the United States and the European Scleroderma Club. Up-to-date information regarding on going studies is available at the SCTC web-site, http://www.sctc-online.org.

Vascular therapies in systemic sclerosis

The third major process underlying systemic sclerosis is a vasculopathy, as discussed above. Clinically this is most clearly observed in the Raynaud's phenomenon present in over 97 per cent of cases. Treatments for Raynaud's phenomenon can also be regarded as potential modifiers of the disease process, although only agents with potential for modulating endothelial cell properties or inducing microvascular remodelling are likely to have a significant effect on the underlying disease. However, vasospasm is an aspect of the disease that can be relieved, though the response is variable. This idiosyncratic response may reflect the stage of the disease. If structural damage is present and severe, the patient will respond rather poorly to vasodilators alone. In uncomplicated cases, simple measures may suffice. As the attacks become more frequent, prolonged oral drug therapy, possibly on an intermittent basis, may be needed. Intravenous therapy and limited surgery are restricted to the most severe cases (Table 17).

Because of the widespread vascular damage there has been a search to find drugs to protect injured endothelial cells and to prevent platelet aggregation and subsequent release of platelet-derived mediators. This search has been disappointing to date. Ketanserin, a serotonin antagonist, although useful in Raynaud's phenomenon, does not improve structural vascular disease. Dipyridamole and aspirin, although reducing the circulating plasma concentrations of β-thromboglobulin or circulating platelet aggregates, were not clinically effective in a randomized double-blind trial. Captopril, the angiotensin-converting enzyme inhibitor that has been so successful in the treatment of renal crisis, has been considered for the primary and possibly prophylactic treatment of vascular disease.

Our own approach to the management for some of the important subgroups of patients within the scleroderma spectrum of disorders is summarized below and in Box 1. The management of localized scleroderma in adults and children is summarized in Table 18.

Our approach to management of Raynaud's and scleroderma

Raynaud's phenomenon without other features of autoimmune rheumatic disease

At presentation

Detailed history and examination to look for evidence of asymptomatic autoimmune rheumatic disease. Thoracic-inlet radiographic imaging to exclude simple structural lesion (e.g. cervical rib). Baseline nailfold capillaroscopy and autoantibody profile (antinuclear antibodies, extractable nuclear antigen, anticentromere antibody) are important to determine whether the patient has primary Raynaud's phenomenon or is likely to develop features of an autoimmune rheumatic disease in the future. Infrared thermography with a standard cold challenge can be used to confirm diagnosis in equivocal cases and assess severity of vasospasm.

Follow-up

If capillaroscopy and autoantibodies are normal/negative, then simple approaches with advice on non-pharmacological relief (hand-warmers, thermal gloves), supplemented as necessary by vasodilator drugs. If the Raynaud's is of short duration (i.e. $<$2 years) the patient is followed annually until the fourth year after onset of symptoms. If capillaroscopy or autoantibody studies are positive, then give the same advice and treatment but follow-up at 6 months, and then yearly for 5 years, with repeat capillaroscopy and autoimmune profile. Discharge from regular follow-up at 5 years if no other disease features have developed, and Raynaud's has not required parenteral vasodilator drugs.

Diffuse cutaneous systemic sclerosis

At presentation

History and physical examination generally establish the diagnosis. Assess the extent of visceral disease by baseline hand and chest radiography, lung function tests, oesophageal motility study (scintigraphy or barium swallow), creatinine kinase, creatinine clearance and urinary protein excretion, Doppler echocardiography (with estimation of pulmonary arterial systolic pressure), and electrocardiogram. High-resolution CT lung scan, DTPA clearance, and bronchoscopy with studies of bronchoalveolar lavage fluid are usually performed in highly specialized units. Right-heart catheter studies and open lung biopsies are occasionally necessary to supplement the information obtained from other less invasive investigations. Once diagnosis is confirmed, tissue typing and autoantibody profiles may be useful to identify groups with poor prognosis. Raynaud's symptoms, if prominent, can respond well to intravenous

Table 17 Treatment options for Raynaud's phenomenon

Treatment	Examples	Comments
Simple measures		
Non-drug	Hand warmers. Protective clothing	Universally helpful; also useful to minimize cold exposure and ambient temperature changes in work environment
Pharmacological	Evening primrose oil	Evening primrose oil has been shown effective in controlled clinical trials
	Fish oil capsules	Theoretical benefit due to increased synthesis of vasodilator prostanoids
	Antioxidant vitamins	Potentially reduces oxidant stress which may contribute to Raynaud's symptoms and pathology
Oral vasodilators		
Calcium channel blockers	Nifedipine; nicardapine; diltiazem; amlodipine	Variable and differential response to different agents. Slow titration of dose reduced the severity of side-effects. Try each drug for at least 3 weeks if possible
5-HT antagonists	Ketanserin	5HT receptor antagonist. Limited availability
	Fluoxetine	Readily available. Fewer vasodilatory side-effects that calcium channel blockers. Depletes platelet 5HT levels. ACEI blocks formation of angiotensin II. Need to observe renal function. Cough may be troublesome
Angiotensin antagonists	Quinapril; captopril; enalapril; losartan	Well tolerated, potential remodelling potential by blocking fibrogenic effects of angiotensin II
Topical vasodilators	GTN patches	Shown effective in short-term use but systemic effects often cause headaches
Parenteral vasodilators	Iloprost; Flolan; prostaglandin E1	Effective at healing ulcers and reducing severity and frequency of Raynaud's attacks. Expensive and limited long-term duration of benefit
Antibiotics	Flucloxacillin; erythromycin	Important adjunct to vasodilator therapy for secondary infection of digital ulcers. Prolonged treatment necessitated by poor tissue perfusion
Surgical procedures		
Lumbar sympathectomy	Chemical or operative	Fore severe lower limb Raynaud's
Radical microarteriolysis	Division of adventitia of digital arteries. Sometimes termed digital sympathectomy	Useful treatment for individual critically ischaemic digits
Debridement, amputation	Surgical or autoamputation	Surgery should be as conservative as possible to allow maximum possibility of spontaneous healing

Box 1 Algorithm summarizing therapy for the multisystem manifestations of systemic sclerosis

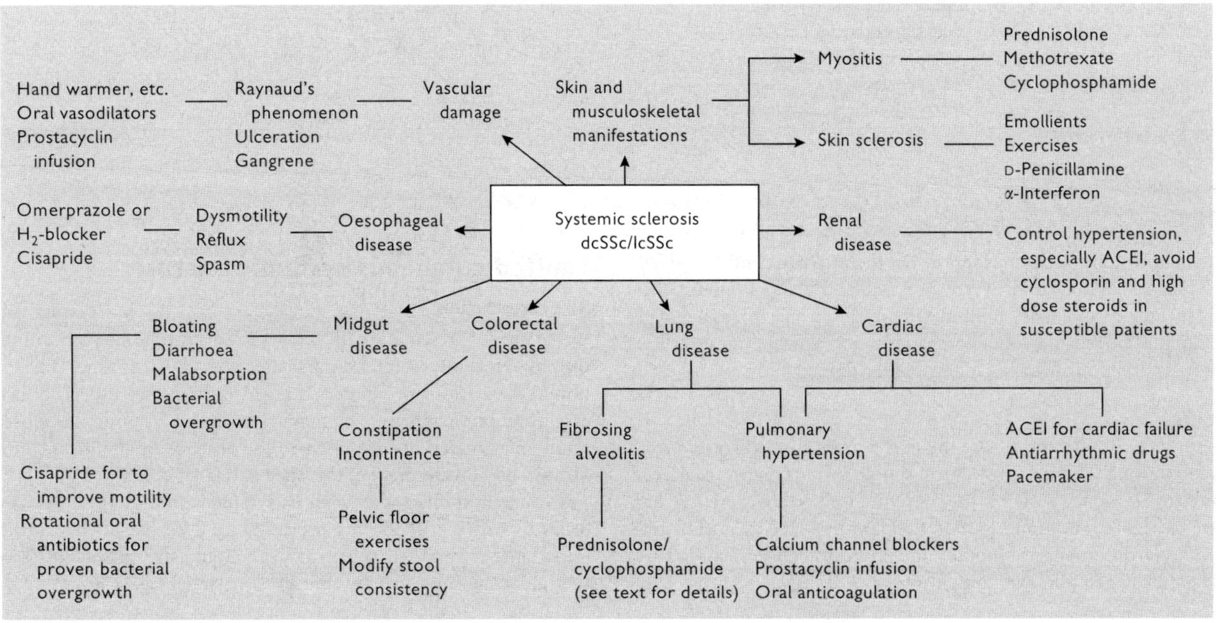

Table 18 Management of localized scleroderma in adults and children

Pattern of disease	Clinical features	Treatment	Prognosis
Localized morphoea	One or a few circumscribed sclerotic plaques with hypo- or hyperpigmentation and an inflamed violaceous border	Often unnecessary Serial measurement to assess progress	Good prognosis; lesions less active within 3 years but pigmentary changes often persist
Generalized morphoea	Widespread pruritic lesions, often symmetrical and following the distribution of superficial veins	Suppress inflammatory component using corticosteroids: in children oral doses up to 15 mg/day have been used. Intravenous infusions often effective Methotrexate or other immunosuppressive maintenance therapy often used, although benefit not proven in controlled trials. Vitamin D containing creams may be useful Topical corticosteroids rarely helpful. PUVA has been used	Internal organ pathology very rare; Raynaud's sometimes associated and antinuclear antibody present in 5% of cases. This does not necessarily imply systemic pathology Generally improves within 5 years of onset, although textural and pigmentary changes may persist
Linear scleroderma	Sclerotic areas occurring in a linear distribution often on limbs and asymmetrical; in childhood can lead to growth defect. MRI imaging confirms the depth of lesions and associated musculoskeletal defects. Serial measurements of limb length and girth essential to monitor progression	Suppress inflammatory component using corticosteroids: in children oral doses up to 15 mg/day have been used. Intravenous infusions often effective Methotrexate or other immunosuppressive maintenance therapy often used, although benefit not proven in controlled trials. Vitamin D containing creams may be useful Physiotherapy and appropriate regular exercise important to minimize growth defect in childhood-onset disease Surgical correction of limb defects may be considered when disease is inactive	Long-term effects of childhood onset form are minimized by effective suppression of the inflammatory process and by good physiotherapy Ultimately, the disease tends to resolve, but it can remain active for many years
En coup de sabre	Linear scleroderma affecting the face or scalp, often involving the underlying subcutaneous tissues, muscles, periostium and bone. Cerebral abnormalties also reported including intracranial calcification. May coexist with hemifacial atrophy (Parry–Romberg syndrome)	Therapeutic options as for linear scleroderma; systemic treatment only for active inflammatory lesions	Scarring, growth defects and alopecia persist but the inflammatory component usually resolves

prostacyclin infusions. Immunosuppressive therapy (e.g. antithymocyte globulin) may be considered for severe cases within 3 years of onset. Other strategies include maintenance immunosuppression using mycophenolate mofetil, monthly intravenous cyclophosphamide, or oral methotrexate. There are no proven antifibrotic therapies for established disease.

Follow-up

This is especially important during the first 5 years from disease onset. Vigilant monitoring for renal involvement should include regular checks of blood pressure, 6-monthly 24-h urine collection for protein excretion and creatinine clearance. Six-monthly lung function tests and electrocardiograms, with yearly oesophageal motility and echocardiographic studies are generally performed in our own unit.

Limited cutaneous systemic sclerosis

At presentation

By the time of presentation the history is usually of some years duration and the physical signs, even if minimal, are generally diagnostic. Diligent attention to the assessment of internal organs is necessary, especially as the disease duration lengthens. The main risks in this scleroderma subset are of pulmonary hypertension, often in the absence of significant interstitial fibrosis, and involvement of the small and large bowel.

Treatment in this group is largely symptomatic and as yet no satisfactory drugs to halt the underlying processes are available. It may, however, be important to treat these patients at an asymptomatic stage in the hope of preventing or slowing down the chronic vascular damage. Current treatment in this group is directed mainly towards the vascular features (Raynaud's phenomenon and pulmonary vascular disease, when present) and gastrointestinal complications. Reflux oesophagitis is almost universal but fortunately responds well to proton-pump inhibitors such as omeprazole, which we prefer to use rather than H_2-blockers, although the latter also often give good symptomatic relief. Oesophageal spasm may respond to cisapride. In contrast, although midgut disease and anorectal complications are less frequent, they are far more difficult to manage.

Follow-up

Annual follow-up is generally undertaken, with assessment of visceral disease, including renal function by creatinine clearance. These patients often require long-term vasodilator therapy, usually intensified during the winter months. Later in the disease (especially after 10 years of established limited cutaneous systemic sclerosis), PHT more likely. Patients carrying antitopoisomerase-1 (Scl-70) antibody are particularly susceptible to lung fibrosis and their lung function should be carefully monitored.

Education and support forms a particularly important component of the management of patients with systemic sclerosis, who should be made aware of the various support groups and the importance of non-pharmacological aspects of care including appropriate exercises, skin care, and the importance of being in a stable, warm ambient temperature.

Conclusion

Currently therefore, although there is no curative treatment for scleroderma, a careful consideration of the subset and stage of disease of the individual patient can maximize the use of the drugs currently available. It is hoped, more importantly, that the level and degree of activity of research into the cause and pathogenesis of the condition may eventually result in early rational effective treatment.

Acknowledgement

The authors are grateful to Dr Aine Burns, Consultant Nephrologist at the Royal Free Hospital, London, for her help with the section on renal disease in scleroderma.

References

Altmann, R.D., Medsger, T.A., Jr., Bloch, D.A., and Michel, B.A. (1990). Predictors of survival in systemic sclerosis (scleroderma). *Arthritis and Rheumatism* **34**, 403–13.

Arnett, F.C., Fritzler, M.J., Ahn, C., and Holian, A. (2000). Urinary mercury levels in patients with autoantibodies to U3-RNP (fibrillarin). *Journal of Rheumatology* **27** (2), 405–10.

Belch, J.J.F. (1990). Raynaud's phenomenon. *Current Opinions in Rheumatology* **2**, 937–41.

Birdi, N. et al. (1992). Childhood linear scleroderma: a possible role of thermography for evaluation. *Journal of Rheumatology* **19**, 968–72.

Black, C.M. (1990). Systemic sclerosis and pregnancy. *Baillière's Clinical Rheumatology* **4**, 105–24.

Black, C.M. et al. (1983). Genetic susceptibility to scleroderma-like syndrome induced by vinyl chloride. *Lancet* **i**, 53–5.

Black, C.M., Silman, A.J., Herrick, A.I., Denton, C.P., Wilson, H., Newman, J., Pompon, L., and Shi-Wen, X. (1999). Interferon-alpha does not improve outcome at one year in patients with diffuse cutaneous scleroderma: results of a randomized, double-blind, placebo-controlled trial. *Arthritis and Rheumatism* **42** (2), 299–305.

Blann, A.D., Illingworth, K., and Jayson, M.I.V. (1993). Mechanisms of endothelial cell damage in systemic sclerosis and Raynaud's phenomenon. *Journal of Rheumatology* **20**, 1325–30.

Bocchieri, M.H. and Jimenez, S.A. (1990). Animal models of fibrosis. *Rheumatic Disease Clinics of North America* **16**, 153–67.

Bona, C. and Rothfield, N. (1994). Autoantibodies in scleroderma and tightskin mice. *Current Opinions in Immunology* **6**, 931–7.

Briggs, D., Black, C.M., and Welsh, K.I. (1990). Genetic factors in scleroderma. *Rheumatic Disease Clinics of North America* **16**, 31–51.

Briggs, D., Stephens, C., Vaughan, R., Welsh, K.I., and Black, C.M. (1993). A molecular and serologic analysis of the major histocompatibility complex and complement component C4 in systemic sclerosis. *Arthritis and Rheumatism* **36**, 943–54.

Carpentier, P.H. and Maricq, H.R. (1990). Microvasculature in systemic sclerosis. *Rheumatic Disease Clinics of North America* **16**, 75–91.

Casciola-Rosen, L., Wigley, F., and Rosen, A. (1997). Scleroderma autoantigens are uniquely fragmented by metal-catalyzed oxidation reactions: implications for pathogenesis. *Journal of Experimental Medicine* **185** (1), 71–9.

Clements. P.J., Lachenbruch, P.A., Ng, S.C., Simmons, M., Sterz, M., and Furst, D.E. (1990). Skinscore: a semi-quantitative measure of cutaneous involvement that improves prediction of prognosis in systemic sclerosis. *Arthritis and Rheumatism* **33**, 1256–63.

Clements, P.J. et al. (1994). Cyclosporine in systemic sclerosis. Results of a forty-eight week open safety study in ten patients. *Arthritis and Rheumatism* **36**, 75–83.

Clements, P.J., Furst, D.E., Wong, W.K., Mayes, M., White, B., Wigley, F., Weisman, M.H., Barr, W., Moreland, L.W., Medsger, T.A., Jr., Steen, V., Martin, R.W., Collier, D., Weinstein, A., Lally, E., Varga, J., Weiner, S., Andrews, B., Abeles, M., and Seibold, J.R. (1999). High-dose versus low-dose D-penicillamine in early diffuse systemic sclerosis: analysis of a two-year, double-blind, randomized, controlled clinical trial. *Arthritis and Rheumatism* **42** (6), 1194–203.

Cohen, S., Laufer, I., Snape, W.J., Shiau, Y.-F., Levine, G.M., and Jimenez, S.A. (1980). The gastrointestinal manifestations of scleroderma: pathogenesis and management. *Gastroenterology* **79**, 155–66.

D'Angelo, W.A., Fries, J.F., Masi, A.T., and Shulman, L.E. (1969). Pathologic observations in systemic sclerosis (scleroderma). *American Journal of Medicine* **46**, 428–40.

Degiannis, D., Seibold, J., Czarnecki, M., Raskova. J., and Raska, K. (1990). Soluble and cellular markers of immune activation in patients with systemic sclerosis. *Clinical Immunology and Immunopathology* **56**, 259–70.

Denton, C.P., Abdullah, A., Sweny, P., and Black, C.M. (1994). Acute renal failure occurring in scleroderma treated with cyclosporin A—a report of three cases. *British Journal of Rheumatology* **33**, 90–2.

Denton, C.P., Xu, S., Welsh, K.I., Pearson, J.D., and Black, C.M. (1996). Scleroderma fibroblast phenotype is modulated by endothelial cell co-culture. *Journal of Rheumatology* **23** (4), 633–8.

Dessein, P.H., Joffe, B.I., Metz, R.M., Millar, D.L., Lawson, M., and Stanwix, A.E. (1992). Autonomic dysfunction in systemic sclerosis: sympathetic overactivity and instability. *American Journal of Medicine* **93**, 143–50.

Earnshaw, W.C., Bordwell, B., Marino, C., and Rothfield, N. (1986). Three human chromosomal autoantigens are recognised by sera from patients with anticentromere antibodies. *Journal of Clinical Investigation* **77**, 426–30.

Follansbee, W.P. (1986). The cardiovascular manifestations of systemic sclerosis (scleroderma). *Current Problems in Cardiology* **11**, 242–98.

Follansbee, W.P. et al. (1990). Myocardial fibrosis in systemic sclerosis (scleroderma): a case controlled clinicopathologic study. *Journal of Rheumatology* **17**, 656–62.

Freemont, A.J., Hoyland, J., Fielding, P., Hodson, N., and Jayson, M.I. (1992). Studies of the microvascular endothelium in uninvolved skin of patients with systemic sclerosis: direct evidence for a generalized microangiopathy. *British Journal of Dermatology* **126** (6), 561–8.

Freni-Titulaer, L.J.W. et al. (1989). Connective tissue disease in south eastern Georgia: a case–control study. *American Journal of Epidemiology* **129**, 404–9.

Gilchrist, F.C., Bunn, C., Foley, P.J., Lympany, P.A., Black, C.M., Welsh, K.I., and du Bois, R.M. (2001). Class II HLA associations with autoantibodies in scleroderma: a highly significant role for HLA-DP. *Genes and Immunity* **2** (2), 76–81.

Grassegger, A., Schuler, G., Hessenberger, G., Walder-Hantich, B., Jabkowski, J., MacHeiner, W., Salmhofer, W., Zahel, B., Pinter, G., Herold, M., Klein, G., and Fritsch, P.O. (1998). Interferon-gamma in the treatment of systemic sclerosis: a randomized controlled multicentre trial. *British Journal of Dermatology* **139** (4), 639–48.

Greydanus, M.P. and Camilleri, M. (1989). Abnormal post-cibal gastric and small bowel motility due to neuropathy or myopathy in systemic sclerosis. *Gastroenterology* **96**, 110–15.

Harrison, N.K. et al. (1989). Pulmonary involvement in systemic sclerosis: the detection of early changes by thin section CT scan, bronchoalveolar lavage and 99mTc-DTPA clearance. *Respiratory Medicine* **83**, 403–14.

Helfrich, D.J., Banner, B., Steen, V.D., and Medsger, T.A., Jr. (1989). Renal failure in normotensive patients with systemic sclerosis. *Arthritis and Rheumatism* **32**, 1128–34.

Ho, M., Veale, D., Eastmond, C., Nuki, G., and Belch, J. (2000). Macrovascular disease and systemic sclerosis. *Annals of the Rheumatic Diseases* **59** (1), 39–43.

Hochberg, M.C. (1994). Silicone breast implants and rheumatic disease. *British Journal of Rheumatology* **33**, 601–2.

Ihata, A., Shirai, A., Okubo, T., Ohno, S., Hagiwara, E., and Ishigatsubo, Y. (2000). Severity of seropositive isolated Raynaud's phenomenon is associated with serological profile. *Journal of Rheumatology* **27** (7), 1686–92.

Ihn, H. and Tamki, K. (2000). Increased phosphorylation of transcription factor Sp1 in scleroderma fibroblasts: association with increased expression of the type I collagen gene. *Arthritis and Rheumatism* **43** (10), 2240–7.

Jabs, E.W., Tuck-Muller, I.C.M., Anhalt, G.J., Earnshaw, W.C., Wise, R.W., and Wigley, F. (1993). Cytogenetic survey in systemic sclerosis and association with autoantibodies to RNA polymerases I and III. *Journal of Clinical Investigation* **91**, 1399–404.

Jimenez, S.A. and Saitta, B. (1999). Alterations in the regulation of expression of the alpha 1(I) collagen gene (COL1A1) in systemic sclerosis (scleroderma). *Springer Seminars in Immunopathology* **21** (4), 397–414 (Review).

Kahaleh, M.B. (1991). Soluble immunologic products in scleroderma sera. *Clinical Immunology and Immunopathology* **58**, 139–44.

Kahaleh, M.B. and Mattuci-Cerinic, M. (1995). Raynaud's phenomenon and scleroderma: dysregulated neuroendothelial control of vascular tone. *Arthritis and Rheumatism* **38**, 1–4.

Kallenberg, C.G. (1994). Antitopoisomerase and anticentromere antibodies in the sclerodermatous complex. *Clinical Reviews in Allergy* **12**, 221–35.

Kantor, T.V., Whiteside, T.L., Friberg, D., Buckingham, R.B., and Medsger, T.A., Jr. (1992). Lymphokine activated killer cells and natural killer cell activities in patients with systemic sclerosis. *Arthritis and Rheumatism* **35**, 694–9.

Katzenstein, A.L. and Myers, J.L. (1998). Idiopathic pulmonary fibrosis: clinical relevance of pathologic classification. *American Journal of Respiratory and Critical Care Medicine* **157** (4 Pt 1), 1301–15.

Kovalchik, M.T., Guggenheim, S.J., Robertson, J.S., and Steigerwald, J.C. (1978). The kidney in progressive systemic sclerosis: a prospective study. *Annals of Internal Medicine* **89**, 881–7.

Kraling, B.M., Maul, G.G., and Jimenez, S.A. (1995). Mononuclear cellular infiltrates in clinically involved skin from patients with systemic sclerosis of recent onset predominantly consist of monocytes/macrophages. *Pathobiology* **63** (1), 48–56.

Krasagakis, K., Dippel, E., Ramaker, J., Owsianowski, M., and Orfanos, C.E. (1998). Management of severe scleroderma with long-term extracorporeal photopheresis. *Dermatology* **196** (3), 309–15.

Kuwana, M., Kaburaki, J., Okano, Y., Inoko, H., and Tsuji, K. (1993). The HLA–DR and DQ genes control the autoimmune response to DNA topoisomerase 1 in systemic sclerosis (scleroderma). *Journal of Clinical Investigation* **92**, 1296–301.

Kuwana, M., Medsger, T.A., and Wright, T.M. (1995). T cell proliferative response induced by DNA topoisomerase 1 in patients with systemic sclerosis and healthy donors. *Journal of Clinical Investigation* **96**, 586–96.

Kuwana, M., Inoko, H., Kameda, H., Nojima, T., Sato, S., Nakamura, K., Ogasawara, T., Hirakata, M., Ohosone, Y., Kaburaki, J., Okano, Y., and Mimori, T. (1999). Association of human leukocyte antigen class II genes with autoantibody profiles, but not with disease susceptibility in Japanese patients with systemic sclerosis. *Internal Medicine* **38** (4), 336–44.

Langevitz, P., Buskila, D., Gladman, D.D., Darlington, G.A., Farewell, V.T., and Lee, P. (1992). HLA alleles in systemic sclerosis: associations with pulmonary hypertension and outcome. *British Journal of Rheumatology* **31**, 609–13.

Le Hir, M., Martin, M., and Haas, C. (1999). A syndrome resembling human systemic sclerosis (scleroderma) in MRL/lpr mice lacking interferon-gamma (IFN-gamma) receptor (MRL/lprgammaR-/-). *Clinical and Experimental Immunology* **115** (2), 281–7.

LeRoy, E.C. (1974). Increased collagen synthesis by scleroderma skin fibroblasts *in vitro*. A possible defect in regulation or activation of scleroderma fibroblasts. *Journal of Clinical Investigation* **54**, 880–9.

LeRoy, E.C. and Medsger, T.A., Jr. (2001). Criteria for the classification of early systemic sclerosis. *Journal of Rheumatology* **28** (7), 1573–6 (Review).

LeRoy, E.C. et al. (1988). Scleroderma (systemic sclerosis): classification, subsets, and pathogenesis. *Journal of Rheumatology* **15**, 202–5.

Lupoli, S., Amlot, P., and Black, C.M. (1990). Normal immune responses in systemic sclerosis. *Journal of Rheumatology* **17**, 323–37.

Ma, J., Chapman, G.V., Chen, S.L., Melick, G., Penny, R., and Briet, S.N. (1991). Antibody penetration of viable human cells: I. Increased penetration of human lymphocytes by anti-RNP IgG. *Clinical and Experimental Immunology* **84**, 83–91.

Maricq, H.R. et al. (1989). Prevalence of scleroderma spectrum disorders in the general population of South Carolina. *Arthritis and Rheumatism* **32**, 998–1006.

Masi, A.T. (1988). Classification of systemic sclerosis (scleroderma): relationship of cutaneous subgroups in early disease to outcome and serologic reactivity. *Journal of Rheumatology* **15**, 894–8.

McCarthy, G.M. and Kenny, D. (1992). Dietary fish oil in rheumatic diseases. *Seminars in Arthritis and Rheumatism* **21**, 318–75.

McCormick, L.L., Zhang, Y., Tootell, E., and Gilliam, A.C. (1999). Anti-TGF-beta treatment prevents skin and lung fibrosis in murine sclerodermatous graft-versus-host disease: a model for human scleroderma. *The Journal of Immunology* **163** (10), 5693–9.

McHugh, N.J. et al. (1994). Anti-centromere antibodies (ACA) in systemic sclerosis patients and their relatives: a serological and HLA study. *Clinical and Experimental Immunology* **96**, 267–74.

Muller, N.L. and Miller, R.R. (1990). Computed tomography of chronic diffuse infiltrative lung disease. *American Review of Respiratory Disease* **142**, 1206–15; 1440–8.

Pearson, J.D. (1990). The endothelium: its role in systemic sclerosis. *Annals of the Rheumatic Diseases* **50**, 866–71.

Pope, J.E. and Bellamy, N. (1993). Outcome measurements in scleroderma clinical trials. *Seminars in Arthritis and Rheumatism* **23**, 22–33.

Pope, J.E., Bellamy, N., Seibold, J.R., Baron, M., Ellman, M., Carette, S., Smith, C.D., Chalmers, I.M., Hong, P., O'Hanlon, D., Kaminska, E., Markland, J., Sibley, J., Catoggio, L., and Furst, D.E. (2001). A randomized, controlled trial of methotrexate versus placebo in early diffuse scleroderma. *Arthritis and Rheumatism* **44** (6), 1351–8.

Postlethwaite, A.E., McKown, K.M., Carbone, L.D., Bustillo, J., Seyer, J.M., and Kang, A.H. (2000). Induction of immune tolerance to human type I collagen in patients with systemic sclerosis by oral administration of bovine type I collagen. *Arthritis and Rheumatism* **43** (5), 1054–61.

Prescott, R.J., Freemont, A.J., Jones, C.J., Hoyland, J., and Fielding, P. (1992). Sequential dermal microvascular and perivascular changes in the development of scleroderma. *Journal of Pathology* **166**, 255–63.

Reveille, J.D. et al. (1992a). Association of amino acid sequences in the HLA–DQB1 first domain with the anti-topoisomerase I autoantibody response in scleroderma (progressive systemic sclerosis). *Journal of Clinical Investigation* **90** (3), 973–80.

Reveille, J.D., Owerbach, D., Goldstein, R., Moreda, R., Isern, R.A., and Arnett, F.C. (1992b). Association of polar amino acids at position 26 of the HLA–DQB1 first domain with the anticentromere autoantibody response in systemic sclerosis (scleroderma). *Journal of Clinical Investigation* **89**, 1208–13.

Rodnan, G.P. and Benedek, T.G. (1962). An historical account of the study of progressive systemic sclerosis (diffuse scleroderma). *Annals of Internal Medicine* **57**, 305–19.

Rook, A.H. et al. (1992). Treatment of systemic sclerosis with extracorporeal photochemotherapy. Results of a multicenter trial. *Archives of Dermatology* **128** (3), 337–46.

Russell, M.L. (1988). Muscle and nerve in systemic sclerosis (scleroderma). In *Systemic Sclerosis: Scleroderma* (ed. C.M. Black and M.I.V. Jayson), pp. 241–7. Chichester: Wiley.

Russell, M.L., Friesen, D., Henderson, R.D., and Hanna, W.M. (1982). Ultrastructure of the oesophagus in scleroderma. *Arthritis and Rheumatism* **25**, 1117–23.

Saitta, B., Gaidarova, S., Cicchillitti, L., and Jimenez, S.A. (2000). CCAAT binding transcription factor binds and regulates human COL1A1 promoter activity in human dermal fibroblasts: demonstration of increased binding in systemic sclerosis fibroblasts. *Arthritis and Rheumatism* **43** (10), 2219–29.

Seibold, J.R., Korn, J.H., Simms, R., Clements, P.J., Moreland, L.W., Mayes, M.D., Furst, D.E., Rothfield, N., Steen, V., Weisman, M., Collier, D., Wigley, F.M., Merkel, P.A., Csuka, M.E., Hsu, V., Rocco, S., Erikson, M., Hannigan, J., Harkonen, W.S., and Sanders, M.E. (2000). Recombinant human relaxin in the treatment of scleroderma. A randomized, double-blind, placebo-controlled trial. *Annals of Internal Medicine* **132** (11), 871–9.

Shi-Wen, X., Pennington, D., Holmes, A., Leask, A., Bradham, D., Beauchamp, J.R., Fonseca, C., du Bois, R.M., Martin, G.R., Black, C.M., and Abraham, D.J. (2000). Autocrine overexpression of CTGF maintains fibrosis: RDA analysis of fibrosis genes in systemic sclerosis. *Experimental Cell Research* **259** (1), 213–24.

Silman, A.J. (1995). Scleroderma. *Ballière's Clinical Rheumatology* **9**, 471–8.

Spencer-Green, G. (1998). Outcomes in primary Raynaud phenomenon: a meta-analysis of the frequency, rates, and predictors of transition to secondary diseases. *Archives of Internal Medicine* **158** (6), 595–600.

Steen, V.D., Powell, D.L., and Medsger, T.A., Jr. (1988). Clinical correlations and prognosis based on serum autoantibodies in patients with systemic sclerosis. *Arthritis and Rheumatism* **31**, 196–203.

Steen, V.D., Constantino, J.P., Shapiro, A.P., and Medsger, T.A., Jr. (1990). Outcome of renal crisis in systemic sclerosis: relation to the availability of converting enzyme inhibitors (ACE). *Annals of Internal Medicine* **113**, 352–7.

Steen, V.D., Conte, C., and Medsger, T.A., Jr. (1994). Case-control study of corticosteroid use prior to scleroderma renal crisis. (Abstract). *Arthritis and Rheumatism* **37** (Suppl.), S360.

Stratton, R.J., Wilson, H., and Black, C.M. (2001). Pilot study of anti-thymocyte globulin plus mycophenolate mofetil in recent-onset diffuse scleroderma. *Rheumatology (Oxford)* **40** (1), 84–8.

Strehlow, D., Jelaska, A., Strehlow, K., and Korn, J.H. (1999). A potential role for protease nexin 1 overexpression in the pathogenesis of scleroderma. *Journal of Clinical Investigation* **103** (8), 1179–90.

Subcommittee for Scleroderma Criteria of the American Rheumatism Association Diagnostic and Therapeutic Criteria Committee (1980). Preliminary criteria for the classification of systemic sclerosis (scleroderma). *Arthritis and Rheumatism* **23**, 581–90.

Tan, F.K. and Arnett, F.C. (2000). Genetic factors in the etiology of systemic sclerosis and Raynaud phenomenon. *Current Opinion in Rheumatology* **12** (6), 511–19.

Tan, F.K., Wang, N., Kuwana, M., Chakraborty, R., Bona, C.A., Milewicz, D.M., and Arnett, F.C. (2001). Association of fibrillin 1 single-nucleotide polymorphism haplotypes with systemic sclerosis in Choctaw and Japanese populations. *Arthritis and Rheumatism* **44** (4), 893–901.

Tarkowski, A. and Lindgren, I. (1994). Beneficial effects of anti-thymocyte globulin in severe cases of progressive systemic sclerosis. *Transplantation Proceedings* **26**, 3197–9.

Traub, Y.M. et al. (1984). Hypertension and renal failure (scleroderma renal crisis) in progressive systemic sclerosis. Report of a 25 year experience with 68 cases. *Medicine* **62**, 335–52.

Tyndall, A., Passweg, J., and Gratwohl, A. (2001). Haemopoietic stem cell transplantation in the treatment of severe autoimmune diseases 2000. *Annals of the Rheumatic Diseases* **60** (7), 702–7.

Valesini, G., Litta, A., Bonavita, M.S., Luan, F.L., Purpura, M., Mariani, M., and Balsano, F. (1993). Geographical clustering of scleroderma in a rural area in the province of Rome. *Clinical and Experimental Rheumatology* **11** (1), 41–7.

van den Hoogen, F.H., Boerbooms, A.M., Swaak, A.J., Rasker, J.J., van Lier, H.J., and van de Putte, L.B. (1996). Comparison of methotrexate with placebo in the treatment of systemic sclerosis: a 24 week randomized double-blind trial, followed by a 24 week observational trial. *British Journal of Rheumatology* **35** (4), 364–72.

Varai, G., Earle, L., Jimenez, S.A., Steiner, R.M., and Varga, J. (1998). A pilot study of intermittent intravenous cyclophosphamide for the treatment of systemic sclerosis associated lung disease. *Journal of Rheumatology* **25** (7), 1325–9.

Veeraraghavan, S., Nicholson, A.G., and Wells, A.U. (2001). Lung fibrosis: new classifications and therapy. *Current Opinions in Rheumatology* **13** (6), 500–4.

Wells, A.U., Hansell, D.M., Corrin, B., Harrison, N.K., Goldstraw, P., Black, C.M., and du Bois, R.M. (1992). High resolution computed tomography as a predictor of lung histology in systemic sclerosis. *Thorax* **47**, 738–42.

Wells, A.U., Hansell, D.M., Harrison, N.K., Lawrence, R., Black, C.M., and du Bois, R.M. (1993a). Clearance of inhaled 99m-Tc DTPA predicts the clinical course of fibrosing alveolitis. *European Respiratory Journal* **6**, 797–802.

Wells, A.U., Hansell, D.M., Rubens, M.B., Cullinan, P., Black, C.M., and du Bois, R.M. (1993b). The predictive value of appearances on thin section computed tomography in fibrosing alveolitis. *American Review of Respiratory Disease* **148**, 1076–82.

Wells, A.U. et al. (1994). Fibrosing alveolitis associated with progressive systemic sclerosis: the relationship between bronchoalveolar lavage cellularity and computed tomographic appearances. *American Journal of Respiratory and Critical Care Medicine* **150**, 462–8.

White, B. (1994). Immunologic aspects of scleroderma. *Current Opinion in Rheumatology* **6**, 612–15.

Yamamoto, T., Takagawa, S., Katayama, I., Yamazaki, K., Hamazaki, Y., Shinkai, H., and Nishioka, K. (1999). Animal model of sclerotic skin. I: local injections of bleomycin induce sclerotic skin mimicking scleroderma. *Journal of Investigative Dermatology* **112** (4), 456–62.

Youssef, P., Englert, H., and Bertouch, J. (1993). Large vessel occlusive disease associated with CREST syndrome and scleroderma. *Annals of the Rheumatic Diseases* **52**, 564–9.

6.8 Polymyositis and dermatomyositis

6.8.1 Polymyositis and dermatomyositis in adults

Ira N. Targoff

Introduction

Polymyositis (PM) and dermatomyositis (DM) are forms of 'idiopathic inflammatory myopathy', along with inclusion body myositis (IBM), and several rare forms. Inflammatory myopathy may also be induced by drugs or infections. By clinical definition, DM is distinguished from PM by the presence of a characteristic rash. Weakness affecting skeletal muscle is the major clinical manifestation of most patients, although the skin rash or other extra-muscular features may predominate in some.

Wagner first described a case as PM in 1863, while Unverricht first used the term DM in 1887. Early studies often included cases that would not fit our present concept. The wide acceptance of the diagnostic criteria of Bohan and Peter (Bohan et al. 1977) has served to standardize subsequent studies and promote recognition.

Epidemiology

Incidence and prevalence

Estimates of the annual incidence of PM/DM have ranged from 1 to 9 cases/million/year, with a recent estimate of 7.4 from Australia (Patrick et al. 1999). The prevalence is approximately 2–10 cases per 100 000.

The incidence appears to increase over time, reflecting either better detection and recognition, or a true increase.

PM is more frequent than DM in most studies of adults (Bohan et al. 1977; Arnett et al. 1996; Hill et al. 2001). The ratio, 1.5–2 : 1, varies with the population, referral patterns, and criteria for DM, and some studies find DM to be more common (Love et al. 1991). Overlap syndromes with other autoimmune rheumatic diseases (ARD) occur in 15–20 per cent.

Risk factors

PM and DM are four-fold more common in African-American patients than in Caucasian patients. The female:male ratio is 2 : 1 overall, but lower in myositis with malignancy, and higher during the childbearing years (5 : 1) and in patients with overlap syndromes (Bohan et al. 1977). PM and DM may begin at almost any age, but the peak in adults is usually from 40 to 60 years, with 29 per cent aged 65 or over (Marie et al. 1999). The mean age of onset in a Scandinavian study was 55–57 years (Hill et al. 2001).

Cases of adult PM and DM among family members are rare, but have been observed (Rider et al. 1998). A family history of myopathy should lead one to reassess the diagnosis. Other autoimmune disease in relatives of PM and DM patients is not unusual (Ginn et al. 1998).

Temporal and geographic factors

Most studies have not found variation in the incidence of adult-onset PM/DM with time of year, but certain autoantibody-defined sub-groups show seasonal differences in the onset of myositis: anti-Jo-1-associated myositis begins more often in the spring, and anti-SRP-myositis more often in the autumn (Targoff 2000).

PM and DM occur in all parts of the world. Areas with greater than expected incidence suggesting possible environmental factors have been observed (Patrick et al. 1999). DM may increase relative to PM in lower latitudes (Brouwer et al. 2001), and certain myositis autoantibodies may differ in prevalence in different regions or populations.

Clinical picture

Classification

Several classification systems have been proposed to define sub-groups of patients with idiopathic inflammatory myopathies that are more clinically homogeneous, and able to predict course and responsiveness. Disagreement remains, however, due to our lack of knowledge of aetiology.

Many studies have used the clinical classification of Bohan and Peter (Table 1), or modifications. Although useful, it does not separate PM and DM when they occur in association with a malignancy, an ARD, or in children. Also, it does not recognize IBM (see 'Inclusion body myositis'), or other distinctive forms of myositis (Table 1). Other classifications emphasize histological patterns, which can reflect differing pathogenetic mechanisms in PM, DM, and IBM (Dalakas 1991). Thus, patients may have DM by muscle histology, without overt skin lesions. Certain specific autoantibodies can also define subgroups of patients that differ in clinical features, response to therapy, prognosis, and HLA from the overall myositis population (Love et al. 1991).

Table 1 Classification of idiopathic inflammatory myopathies[a]

I	Primary idiopathic polymyositis
II	Primary idiopathic dermatomyositis
III	Polymyositis or dermatomyositis with malignancy
IV	Juvenile dermatomyositis (or polymyositis)
V	Overlap syndrome of polymyositis or dermatomyositis with another connective tissue disease
VI	Inclusion body myositis[b]
VII	Rare forms of idiopathic myositis
	(a) Granulomatous myositis
	(b) Eosinophilic myositis
	(c) Focal myositis
	(d) Orbital myositis

[a] Classes I–V correspond to Bohan and Peter's original classification (Bohan et al. 1977).

[b] Patients with inclusion body myositis in association with malignancy or other connective tissue diseases should be considered to be Class VI.

Clinical features

Myositis

Weakness

Muscle weakness is the main clinical feature of both PM and DM, occurring in almost all patients. It usually develops insidiously over weeks to months, generally more slowly in PM than in DM. More indolent cases may be seen, progressing over years, although some of these PM cases may be unrecognized IBM (Amato et al. 1996). More rapid onset also occurs occasionally.

The weakness is typically symmetrical, affecting the large proximal muscles around the shoulders, hips, thighs, trunk, and neck. The lower extremities are often involved first, but in most patients both upper and lower extremity involvement occurs. Patients often have impairment in performance of daily activities such as standing from a chair, getting out of a car, climbing stairs, reaching or working overhead, or combing hair. The gait may be affected. Sitting from a supine position, or raising the head off the pillow may become difficult. Weakness of distal muscles is uncommon, but may occur late in the course (~10 per cent) (Love et al. 1991). Patients may note impairment of chewing or dysphagia. Involvement of the face is unusual, and involvement of extraocular muscles is rare, and suggests other diagnoses. Within regions of weakness, there is usually diffuse involvement, unlike some myopathies in which weakness and atrophy may be selective for specific muscles.

Other muscle manifestations

Myalgia and muscle tenderness occur in approximately 50 per cent. They are usually not prominent, but may be more severe when myositis develops acutely. Atrophy may occur with chronic disease (9 per cent) (Love et al. 1991), more in PM than in DM. Contractures may occur with disease of long duration.

Examination

Muscle strength should be assessed as part of initial evaluation and later monitoring of progress (Miller et al. 2001). Simple activities, such as walking, squatting, standing from a chair without using the arms, sitting up or raising the head from a supine position, should be observed and multiple repetitions timed. Deltoids, biceps, iliopsoas, quadriceps, and other proximal muscles should be manually tested, and graded by systems such as the Medical Research Council scale. In order to overcome insensitivity and subjectivity, and standardize and quantify such testing, there is continuing interest in assessing muscle strength by mechanical means (Stoll et al. 1995). Muscle strength testing depends on effort, and may be complicated by fatigue or pain of arthritis or myalgia.

Cutaneous manifestations

Rash

The DM rash most commonly precedes the weakness by weeks to months, or occurs simultaneous with it. Ninety per cent of adult DM patients may have the rash at presentation, while only half have weakness (Bohan et al. 1977). The activity of the rash may parallel that of the weakness or may be independent, and may persist after the myositis resolves.

Gottron's lesions

Erythematous or violaceous, sometimes scaly, papules or plaques (Gottron's papules) or macular patches (Gottron's sign) over the metacarpophalangeal, proximal, and less often distal interphalangeal joints (Plate 126) (Drake et al. 1996), and/or over the extensor surfaces of the knees, wrists, elbows, or medial malleoli occur in 70–80 per cent of DM patients, and are the most DM-specific feature. Telangiectasia and atrophy can occur. Erythema may extend from the joints along the course of the extensor tendons (linear extensor erythema) (Franks, Jr. 1988) (Plate 127).

Erythematous and/or poikilodermatous rash

A macular erythematous or violaceous eruption may involve the upper chest, neck, shoulders, extremities, hands, scalp, and face. Atrophy and scale may occur, and poikiloderma may develop, varied hyper- and hypopigmentation with atrophy and fine telangiectasias. Typical of DM are the 'V'-sign [involvement at the anterior base ('V') of the neck] (36 per cent), and the 'shawl'-sign (back of neck, upper torso, and shoulders) (22 per cent) (Love et al. 1991). Scalp involvement is frequent, sometimes resembling psoriasis or seborrhoeic dermatitis. Rash on the malar areas, forehead, and chin may lead to confusion with lupus, although the nasolabial folds may be involved. The distribution still suggests photosensitivity, and exacerbation or development of new lesions can occur after sun exposure or therapeutic UV light (Sontheimer 1996).

Heliotrope

The heliotrope sign, found in about 30–60 per cent of DM, is a purplish, lilac-coloured (like the heliotrope flower) suffusion around the eyes, particularly the upper eyelids and surrounding area (Plate 128), often associated with periorbital edema. It is characteristic of DM, but a similar appearance may occasionally be seen in allergy, trichinosis, lupus, or other conditions (Drake et al. 1996).

Other cutaneous features (non-defining)

Periungual telangiectasia and haemorrhages are common. Nailfold capillaries may show marked changes similar to those in scleroderma, including thrombosis and haemorrhage, giant capillary loops, and capillary loss, that may parallel disease activity (Plate 129). The cuticles may be thickened, roughened, and irregular (Plate 130).

Hyperkeratosis and scaling with fissuring and hyperpigmentation may appear as dirty horizontal lines along the lateral and palmar aspects of the fingers ('mechanic's hands') (Plate 131), a lesion that is strongly associated with antisynthetase autoantibodies (Love et al. 1991).

Although more common in children, calcinosis can occur in adults. It can be extensive, and usually occurs late. The cutaneous ulcers that are associated with severe vasculopathy in children may also rarely be seen in adults.

Linear, erythematous lesions labeled 'centripetal flagellate erythema' have been associated with DM (Nousari et al. 1999). Papular or plaque-like mucinosis may occur. Rarely, vesico-bullous lesions or hyperkeratotic lesions that resemble pityriasis rubra pilaris (Lupton et al. 2000) can be seen, with a suggested association with malignancy. Other rare manifestations include panniculitis, which can show membranocystic changes, and erythroderma.

Amyopathic dermatomyositis

There is increasing recognition of patients with typical cutaneous DM who do not develop myositis. Some of the patients have subclinical myositis, and some later develop overt myositis, but some have no sign of myositis for years (Sontheimer 1999). 'Amyopathic DM' (or 'DM sine myositis') is applied to those with rash but no clinical myositis for at least 2 years without treatment. Such patients require different criteria for diagnosis (Drake et al. 1996). The risk of malignancy and systemic complications appears similar to classical DM.

Manifestations in other systems

Systemic signs

Fatigue and malaise are common and must be distinguished from muscle weakness. Weight loss may occur. Fevers are seen in about 40 per cent overall, more commonly with antisynthetases (87 versus 23 per cent without antibody) (Love et al. 1991).

Pulmonary disease

Pulmonary involvement resulting from muscle weakness, treatment, or the underlying disease, occurs in 40–50 per cent of patients (Targoff 1990; Marie et al. 1999).

Respiratory muscle weakness

Significant respiratory muscle weakness develops in 4–7 per cent of patients, but a measurable decrease in respiratory muscle strength may be more common (Targoff 1990). Both inspiratory and expiratory muscles may be affected, including the diaphragm, with reduced vital capacity and elevated residual volume. Respiratory failure requiring assisted ventilation may result, and may develop rapidly, but usually responds to treatment. Most such patients have had involvement of the pharyngeal and tongue muscles with dysphagia and impaired speech. Patients at risk should be monitored closely, often using serial measures of expiratory pressure or peak flow.

Pharyngeal and tongue involvement increase the risk of aspiration, as does impaired cough and difficulty turning or sitting up in bed. Most patients with aspiration have had dysphagia. Pneumonia related to respiratory muscle weakness or oesophageal involvement is more common in elderly patients (21.7 per cent) (Marie et al. 1999).

Pulmonary complications of treatment

Opportunistic lung infections such as pneumocystis carinii pneumonia may result from treatment of myositis with high doses of corticosteroids and immunosuppressive agents (Kadoya et al. 1996), particularly if lymphocyte counts are low. Methotrexate hypersensitivity pneumonitis occurs in myositis, presenting acutely with fever, cough, dyspnoea, and interstitial infiltrates. Pulmonary reactions may also rarely occur with azathioprine. These conditions can be difficult to distinguish from disease-related pneumonitis.

Interstitial lung disease

Interstitial lung disease (ILD) is found in 10–40 per cent of PM and DM overall, and may be more frequent in Japanese patients (Hirakata and Nagai 2000). There is a higher frequency in patients with antisynthetases and certain overlap syndromes (Targoff 1990; Love et al. 1991; Marguerie et al. 1992) than in other myositis patients. Some have a fulminant course, resembling acute respiratory distress syndrome, with fever and rapidly progressive dyspnoea that may be fatal within weeks (Clawson and Oddis 1995). Others have a more chronic course, and a third group has asymptomatic involvement. Chest X-ray shows a reticulonodular pattern, often more prominent in the bases, and pulmonary function tests show a restrictive defect with decreased diffusing capacity and hypoxaemia with exercise, early signs that can be used to assess progress.

The severity is unrelated to that of the myositis, even occurring in amyopathic DM. It may precede or follow myositis (Douglas et al. 2001). Limitations from ILD may mask muscle weakness, but elevated creatine kinase (CK), myositis autoantibodies, or the DM rash may reveal the underlying disease.

Lung histology shows interstitial mononuclear cell infiltrates (Fig. 1) with a variable amount of fibrosis. The patterns observed may vary, and include bronchiolitis obliterans organizing pneumonia, which appears to have the best prognosis, usual interstitial pneumonitis, which may be more frequent in PM than DM, non-specific interstitial pneumonitis, and diffuse alveolar damage, which usually has the worst prognosis (Hirakata and Nagai 2000). Douglas et al. (2001) found non-specific interstitial pneumonia to be the predominant pattern; 18 had it, of the 22 biopsied (out of 70 with myositis and ILD). Pulmonary hypertension may occur in association with interstitial fibrosis. Pulmonary vasculitis may also occur.

There have been numerous case reports of spontaneous pneumomediastinum in DM. It is usually associated with ILD, of uncertain mechanism, although an association with cutaneous ulcers suggests a relation to DM vasculopathy (Kono et al. 2000).

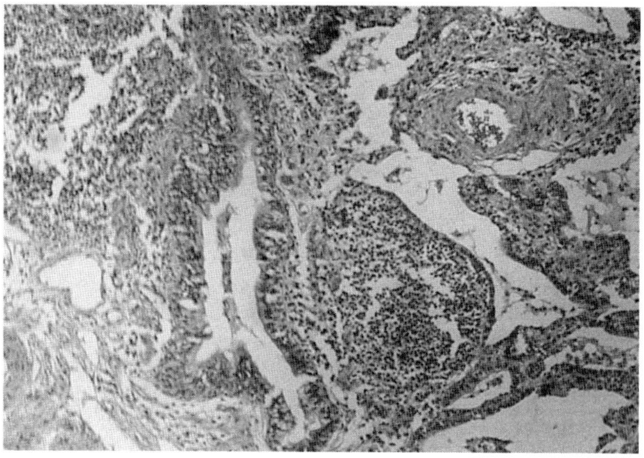

Fig. 1 Lung pathology from a patient with anti-Jo-1 positive polymyositis, showing severe mononuclear cell infiltration and thickening of the interstitium.

Cardiac disease

Signs of cardiac involvement in PM and DM may be found in more than 70 per cent. It is commonly asymptomatic, but can contribute to mortality. The activity of the cardiac disease may be independent of the myositis. The major manifestations include conduction disturbances, arrhythmias, and myocarditis.

Although electrocardiographic abnormalities are frequent, most are minor non-specific ST–T wave changes (Lie 1995). Only occasionally does advanced heart block occur, requiring a pacemaker. Fibrosis of the conducting system correlates with conduction disturbance in some cases, and inflammation has been seen. The most common arrhythmias seen are extrasystoles and tachyarrhythmias, usually mild. Palpitations occur in 26 per cent, more in PM (57 per cent) than in DM (19 per cent) (Love et al. 1991).

Although myocarditis similar to that in skeletal muscle can be seen in up to 30 per cent of patients at autopsy, and small vessel disease may occur, clinical congestive heart failure is uncommon. Diastolic dysfunction was found in 42 per cent of PM and DM (Gonzalez-Lopez et al. 1996).

Pericardial effusions can be seen in 5–25 per cent of PM/DM by echocardiogram, but are usually asymptomatic. Significant pericarditis without SLE overlap is rare.

Gastrointestinal disease

Dysphagia may occur in up to 30 per cent, particularly with more severe disease (Spiera and Kagen 1998). It was more common in older patients (34.8 versus 16.1 per cent) (Marie et al. 1999). It increases the risk of aspiration and has been associated with a poor prognosis. Dysphagia can result from weakness of swallowing muscles (pharyngeal muscles or striated muscles of the upper oesophagus), correlating with disease activity and responding to treatment. Regurgitation of liquids into the nose can occur with attempted swallowing. Nasal speech or hoarseness may be associated. Histology is similar to that of other striated muscle. It may occasionally be the presenting complaint.

Abnormal upper and lower oesophageal motility abnormalities may occur, as in scleroderma, that do not respond to treatment. Decreased lower oesophageal sphincter pressure may lead to dysphagia, heartburn, reflux, and stricture. Gastric emptying may also be delayed.

Cricopharyngeal muscle dysfunction from inflammation or fibrosis may lead to a distinctive dysphagia marked by a sensation of food sticking in the back of the throat, or coughing with swallowing, and may require surgical myotomy (Oddis 2000b).

Intestinal vasculitis with perforation, as well as pneumatosis cystoides intestinalis, well recognized in juvenile DM, are rare in adults, but they can occur.

Malignancy

Association

Recent population studies have confirmed the association of DM with an increased risk of malignancy (Buchbinder 2001; Hill et al. 2001), ranging from 6 to 43 per cent. Some studies have also found an increased risk in PM. Malignancy may be antecedent, concurrent, or subsequent to myositis onset.

In a recent pooled analysis of data from Sweden, Denmark, and Finland, 32 per cent of 618 DM and 15 per cent of 914 PM patients had cancer (Hill et al. 2001); 18.6 per cent had cancer after DM diagnosis (standardized incidence ratio or SIR 3.0, 95 per cent confidence interval 2.5–3.6), and 10.4 per cent after PM diagnosis (SIR 1.3, CI 1.0–1.6). The risk of cancer was greatest in the first year (SIR 13.5 DM, 2.6 PM), but was still significantly elevated for DM after 5 years. The risk for cancer in the year prior to DM diagnosis was also greatly increased (SIR 9.8). The risk in DM was greatest after age 45, but there was some risk for DM under 45. An Australian study showed similar results, with an SIR for DM of 6.2, and for PM of 2.0 (Buchbinder et al. 2001).

The activity of the myositis may appear linked to that of the malignancy ('paraneoplastic', about 1/5 of DM-cancers), either because the myositis resolves with treatment of the cancer, remains resistant until the cancer is resected, or flares with cancer recurrence. This supports the validity of an association, but more often the cancer and myositis have an independent course. The mechanism for the association of DM and malignancy, even in paraneoplastic cases, is unknown.

Tumours

A wide variety of tumours have been reported in myositis. Tumours that are frequent in the general population (lung, breast, etc.) are frequent in DM. However, ovarian cancer is over-represented. Hill et al. (2001) found that in DM, the increase in risk for ovarian cancer was greatest of any type (SIR 10.5), with only lung cancers more frequent. In the elderly, however, 50 per cent with DM and malignancy had a colon tumour (Marie et al. 1999). In Taiwan, nasopharyngeal carcinomas were the most common type seen (Chen et al. 2001), a tumour that is common in the population. Hill et al. (2001) also found that DM patients have a significant increase in lung, pancreatic, stomach, colorectal, and breast cancers, and non-Hodgkin's lymphomas. In PM, only lung, bladder, and lymphoma were significantly increased.

Evaluation

The extent of testing that should be performed to uncover an occult malignancy in recent-onset DM is controversial. All agree with the importance of a thorough initial evaluation including history, physical examination, stool occult blood testing, screening mammography and gynaecologic examination, and routine laboratory tests and chest X-ray. Any abnormalities should be pursued, and the evaluation should be repeated yearly, at least for 2–3 years. In addition, most would give special attention to excluding ovarian cancer in women. Ovarian cancer can be difficult to detect in DM, and transvaginal ultrasound and serum CA-125 levels have been recommended (Whitmore et al. 1997).

There is disagreement as to the extent of further searching recommended in the absence of abnormalities. Those at higher risk may warrant further investigation, including those with resistant disease, or weight loss. The highest risk is in DM patients over age 45 with no overlap signs or myositis autoantibodies. Cutaneous ulcerations may also indicate risk.

Other features, overlap syndromes, and associated conditions

Raynaud's phenomenon may occur in PM or DM without overlap, more commonly in antisynthetase patients. Such patients may also develop a subluxing polyarthritis with associated calcinosis (Oddis et al. 1990). Monoarthritis, however, should raise suspicion of infection in immunosuppressed myositis patients.

Patients with myositis may have overlap syndromes with other ARDs, particularly lupus (~ 50 per cent), scleroderma (20 per cent), or Sjögren's syndrome (Love et al. 1991) (Plate 134). Patients with certain autoantibodies such as anti-PM-Scl, anti-U1RNP, or anti-Ku, are more likely to have overlap syndromes involving myositis. Patients with lupus and PM or DM can have myositis that is similar to, and as severe as, patients without overlap (Garton and Isenberg 1997).

Renal disease is very rare in PM or DM without overlap, but focal mesangial proliferative glomerulonephritis has been seen. Renal injury more often occurs from myoglobinuria.

A variety of other autoimmune conditions have been reported in association with PM and DM. Of note are apparent associations with primary biliary cirrhosis, myasthenia gravis (including cases with thymoma), Graves' or Hashimoto's disease, inflammatory bowel disease, celiac disease, Behçet's disease, thrombotic thrombocytopaenic purpura, and others.

Myositis indistinguishable from PM may occur as part of graft-versus-host disease (Parker et al. 1996). It can be confused with other causes for weakness after transplant, and may respond to corticosteroids.

Pregnancy and PM/DM

Active PM/DM appears to confer increased risk to both mother and foetus, with potential for exacerbation or onset during or after pregnancy (Kanoh et al. 1999). In established PM/DM, controlled at the time of pregnancy, most patients do not have flares, and many pregnancies are successful. Patients should optimally be in remission before becoming pregnant. If treatment is needed during pregnancy, prednisone is often used. Intensive evaluation for malignancy in pregnant patients without other indications would be inadvisable. No effect on fertility is apparent.

Laboratory investigations

Muscle factors

Enzymes

Creatine kinase

Serum levels of enzymes released from damaged muscle can be helpful for diagnosis and disease monitoring (Rider and Miller 1995). CK is the most widely used due to its sensitivity, relative specificity for muscle, ready availability, and correlation with disease activity. Elevated CK levels are seen in most adults (80–90 per cent) when first seen, and in up to 95 per cent at some time during their course (Bohan et al. 1977). The mean increase of CK is about 10-fold, with the potential to rise over 100-fold. CK elevations may precede clinical exacerbations by about 6 weeks. A fall in CK usually indicates improvement, and can precede recovery of strength by 3–4 weeks. There is a general correlation of CK level and disease activity for most individuals over time.

CK may be normal in some adults despite active myositis (Rider and Miller 1995), more often in DM than PM. Lesser elevations may be seen in chronic disease, especially with severe atrophy, but elevations may still occur. Patients with myositis–lupus overlap had comparable CK levels to those of isolated myositis (Garton and Isenberg 1997). Enzymatic measurement of CK could be falsely reduced if an inhibitor is present. Steroids may lower the CK level even if they do not suppress disease activity. Levels that are within the normal range in patients with active disease may still be higher than the baseline for that individual. It has been suggested that a normal CK in patients with active disease or with interstitial lung disease may be a poor prognostic sign, but many see no relation (Rider and Miller 1995).

CK may be elevated in a wide variety of conditions leading to muscle necrosis (Table 2), but not usually in simple atrophy as in disuse, denervation, steroid myopathy, or hyperthyroidism. Unaccustomed strenuous exercise may raise the CK level in normal people, as can physical injury to muscle, including intramuscular injections or electromyography (EMG).

Table 2 Causes of elevated CK levels

1. Strenuous prolonged exercise
2. Muscle trauma
   (a) Injury
   (b) Needlestick
   (c) EMG
   (d) Surgery
3. Diseases affecting muscle
   (a) Myositis
      (i) Infectious
      (ii) Idiopathic
   (b) Metabolic
   (c) Dystrophy
   (d) Myocardial infarction[a]
   (e) Rhabdomyolysis
   (f) Amyotrophic lateral sclerosis (effect on muscle indirect)
4. Drugs
   (a) Toxic myopathy
   (b) Induction of myositis (D-penicillamine)
   (c) Direct elevation of CK (inhibition of excretion) barbiturates, morphine, diazepam
5. Endocrine and metabolic abnormalities
   (a) Hypothyroidism
   (b) Hypokalaemia
   (c) Hyperosmolar state or ketoacidosis
   (d) Diabetic nephrotic syndrome
   (e) Renal failure
6. Others
   (a) CNS disease[b]
      (i) Cerebral ischaemia
      (ii) Head injury
      (iii) Psychosis
      (iv) Delirium tremens
   (b) Tumours (gastrointestinal, bronchial, others[b])
   (c) Pneumococcal sepsis
7. Normal
   (a) Ethnic group
   (b) Increased muscle mass
   (c) Technical artefact

[a] Elevated proportion of CK-MB.

[b] Predominantly or elevated proportion of CK-BB.

Drugs can raise the CK level through a variety of mechanisms, including toxic effects, induction of myositis or myopathy, or decreasing excretion of CK. Various myopathies, as well as carrier states, may increase CK, including dystrophies, metabolic myopathies, and others. Gastrointestinal or lung tumours can raise CK-BB. The normal range for CK is higher for men than for women, and higher for African-Americans than for Caucasians (Kagen 2000).

Serum CK-MB isoenzyme can be elevated in 50 per cent of myositis patients without evident cardiac involvement (Erlacher et al. 2001), and severe cardiac involvement may occur despite normal CK-MB. Regenerating or chronically stressed skeletal muscle fibres are the likely source of the CK-MB. Macro CK type 1, a complex of antibody with CK, can occur in myositis.

Other enzymes

Several other enzymes released during muscle damage may be helpful for disease monitoring. Most patients will have an elevation of at least one serum enzyme at some time during their course. Aldolase is usually elevated in PM and DM, in some cases when CK is not, but is not as specific for muscle and does not correlate as well with disease activity. Lactic dehydrogenase (LDH) is also elevated (predominantly LDH-5, although LDH-1 may increase), as are AST and ALT, and correlate with muscle inflammation, but are usually less sensitive than CK, particularly in adult PM.

Carbonic anhydrase III, an isoenzyme found exclusively in skeletal and not cardiac muscle, rises in myositis.

Myoglobin

Myoglobin is unique to skeletal and cardiac muscle, and is detectable in the serum of most patients with active myositis (Kagen 2000). It rises with exacerbation and falls with remission, and can predict exacerbation in some cases. It has the advantages of tissue specificity, rapid clearance, and sensitive, non-enzymatic detection. There may be diurnal variation.

Other muscle factors

Cardiac troponin-I is not expressed in normal, regenerating, or myositis skeletal muscle. Serum cardiac troponin-T can be elevated in myositis without evident cardiac involvement, but not usually the serum cardiac troponin-I (Erlacher et al. 2001).

Creatine excretion rises with muscle disease due to defects in muscle uptake and retention. The creatine/(creatinine + creatine) ratio in a 24 h urine sample (normal <6 per cent) is elevated in most myositis patients, and can vary with disease activity. Its clinical utility is limited; elevations may persist in inactive disease due to atrophy, and measurement is difficult to obtain.

Measures of muscle mass correlate with strength, but not necessarily inflammation; they can be used to provide a longer-term view. 3-Methyl histidine excretion, reflecting skeletal muscle protein turnover, and total body potassium, measuring total body mass, have been used in studies but are not in current clinical use. Dual X-ray absorptiometry may be used in the future.

Autoantibodies

Indirect immunofluorescence is positive in 50–80 per cent of patients with PM or DM (Love et al. 1991), more in overlap and less in malignancy. Nuclear speckled patterns are most common, nucleolar may be seen. Cytoplasmic patterns suggest an antisynthetase or anti-SRP (Plate 132). A high ANA titre favours PM or DM over other myopathies, and a myositis-specific autoantibody strongly supports it (see 'Autoantibodies' under 'Aetiology and pathogenesis'). Antisynthetases may alert the physician to an increased risk for ILD, or suggest underlying PM or DM in patients who present with extramuscular features.

A general correlation of anti-Jo-1 titre with disease activity has been observed, and in some cases a rise in anti-Jo-1 predicted exacerbation. Occasional disappearance of anti-Jo-1 correlates with disease remission. The usefulness of titres as an index of disease activity is not established, but they may provide support if serial measurements are available.

Other tests

The erythrocyte sedimentation rate is elevated in about half of active cases, but is poorly correlated with disease activity or response to treatment. Similarly, the CRP may be normal or slightly high despite active disease. Rheumatoid factor is positive in approximately 10–20 per cent of patients, most commonly in the overlap group. Circulating immune complexes and cryoglobulins have been reported in some patients, but their significance is unclear. Elevated gamma globulins may be seen; hypogammaglobulinaemia should raise the suspicion of echovirus or other infection. Patients with PM with monoclonal gammopathies have been described, including some in which sarcolemmal deposition of paraprotein was found. Complement is usually normal, although myositis has occurred in C2 deficiency.

Serum markers intended to reflect the activity of ILD have been described, and have been elevated in the serum of myositis patients with lung disease, such as KL-6 (Hirakata and Nagai 2000) or cytokeratin 19, and may have future utility.

Table 3 The diagnosis of polymyositis and dermatomyositis

Criteria for the diagnosis of polymyositis and dermatomyositis[a]

1. Compatible weakness
   Symmetrical proximal muscle weakness, developing over weeks to months
2. Elevated serum muscle enzymes
   CK, aldolase
3. Electromyographic findings typical of PM or DM
   Most common:
   Myopathic potentials: low amplitude, short duration, polyphasic potentials
   Most characteristic:
   Triad of
   (a) myopathic potentials;
   (b) fibrillations, positive sharp waves, increased insertional activity;
   (c) complex repetitive discharges
4. Muscle biopsy findings typical of PM or DM
   Necrosis, phagocytosis, regeneration, inflammation
5. Dermatologic features of DM
   (a) Gottron's papules or sign, involving finger joints, knees, elbows, and/or medial malleoli;
   (b) heliotrope sign;
   (c) erythematous and/or poikilodermatous rash

Other useful diagnostic findings

1. Autoantibodies:
   (a) myositis-specific autoantibodies: low sensitivity, high specificity (Table 8);
   (b) positive ANA: sensitivity 60%
2. Imaging:
   (a) MRI: increased signal on T_2 images;
   (b) MRS: elevated Pi/PCr ratio
3. Other dermatologic findings: nailfold capillary changes, calcinosis, mechanic's hands

[a] From Targoff et al. (1997).

Diagnosis

The criteria of Bohan and Peter (Bohan et al. 1977) (Table 3), often with modifications such as that of Dalakas (Dalakas 1991), have been widely used for diagnosis and clinical studies. Muscle enzymes, EMG, and muscle biopsy remain essential in evaluation of patients and establishing the diagnosis of PM and DM. Autoantibody testing and magnetic resonance imaging (MRI) can also greatly aid in diagnosis. Recent attempts have been made to devise new criteria that take advantage of newer tests and other features (Tanimoto et al. 1995; Targoff et al. 1997). Even when the criteria are satisfied, other causes of muscle disease must be excluded.

Electromyography

EMG and nerve conduction studies can provide evidence that a process is myopathic and consistent with myositis, and can help to exclude neuropathies and certain myopathies. EMG may reveal muscle involvement in patients presenting with rash or extramuscular features. Ninety per cent of patients with active myositis have an abnormal EMG (Bohan et al. 1977). Testing of multiple muscles is important, since involvement may be limited. This can demonstrate the distribution of involvement, which can sometimes help to direct biopsies to the contralateral side. Paraspinal muscle involvement is common, and may be the only abnormal area.

Motor unit action potentials are typically myopathic (low amplitude, short duration). Polyphasic potentials, complex potentials with increased turns, are increased. Over time, long-duration, high amplitude polyphasic potentials may be seen, attributed to reinnervation of regenerating fibres. Patients with myositis have early recruitment and full interference patterns (more fibres required to achieve a given force), in contrast to the decreased recruitment and interference seen in neuropathies.

Spontaneous activity at rest is seen in 3/4 of patients, associated with active inflammation; it is less common with chronic disease, and may subside with treatment. Increased insertional activity is very common, as are fibrillations and positive sharp waves, attributed to damage to intramuscular nerves or motor end plates, or to segmental muscle fibre necrosis. Complex repetitive discharges may also be seen in 1/3 – 1/2 of patients. They start and stop abruptly, and usually have constant amplitude. Single-fibre EMG in myositis shows increased jitter and blocking, although less prominent than in myasthenia gravis.

Imaging

MRI

Numerous studies have demonstrated the value of MRI in PM/DM for diagnosis and assessment of disease activity. MRI can sensitively identify areas of muscle inflammation, atrophy, or fatty replacement (Park and Olsen 2000). It is non-invasive and can be repeated sequentially. Use is often limited by cost or availability, but in certain situations it can provide critical information that may not be available by other methods, affecting treatment decisions (Park et al. 1994).

T_2-weighted images can best show areas of active muscle inflammation, where increased water content is seen as increased intensity, not visible with T_1-weighted images. Increased fat is seen on both images. Fat suppression is used to improve image contrast. Gadolinium is not helpful. The thighs are most often studied.

By MRI, involvement is often focal, with differences in intensity between and within muscles, and can thus be more sensitive than biopsy for detecting clinical activity (Park et al. 1994). Atrophy is correlated with disease duration. Fatty infiltration is more common in PM than DM, and in chronic disease. PM may show more tendency to extend to posterior as well as anterior thigh muscles (Park and Olsen 2000).

MR signal intensity may vary with disease activity, thus helping assess therapeutic response; abnormalities can return to normal within months on treatment (Park et al. 1994). MRI may show increased intensity in active disease, even when enzymes and other tests are normal, although false negatives may occur.

Magnetic resonance spectroscopy

P-31 magnetic resonance spectroscopy (MRS) can be used to assess energy utilization and reserve by measuring phosphate metabolites in muscle. The inorganic phosphate to phosphocreatine (Pi/PCr) ratio rises in myopathies indicating a decrease in energy reserve, and is correlated with disease activity (Park et al. 1994). PCr and ATP are decreased at rest, decrease further with exercise, and show delayed recovery to baseline. The decline of ATP with exercise may contribute to fatigue, and impaired energy utilization may contribute to weakness.

While not specific, MRS may help monitor disease activity and response to therapy. It can be abnormal in some patients with normal CK (Park et al. 1994), but can continue abnormal in some patients whose inflammation has resolved, reflecting persistent muscle abnormalities. MRS can be more useful for assessing disease status. Even patients with amyopathic DM and normal MRI may show reduced oxidative capacity by MRS with exercise (Park et al. 1995).

Other methods

Ultrasound of muscle is abnormal in about 80 per cent of patients, most often due to fat and atrophy (Park and Olsen 2000). It is less expensive and more readily available than MRI, but is less sensitive and specific. It may help direct the biopsy.

Technetium-99m and thallium uptake may be increased in muscles affected by active PM. Although non-specific, this also might be useful for directing a biopsy. Gallium-67 scanning has been used in the diagnosis of macrophagic myofasciitis (Cherin et al. 2000), and Lyme disease and other infections. Scanning with indium-labelled antimyosin can reveal areas of muscle necrosis in myositis (Lofberg et al. 1998) and correlates with disease activity.

Biopsy

Indications

In most cases, when PM or DM is suspected, muscle biopsy should be performed. It can provide the most convincing evidence supporting the diagnosis, and can definitively exclude certain relevant conditions. However, in patients with proximal weakness, elevated enzymes, and a typical EMG, a biopsy may not be necessary if a DM rash, myositis-specific autoantibodies, or connective tissue disease overlap syndrome with specific antibodies (anti-U_1RNP, anti-PM-Scl) is present (Targoff et al. 1997).

Methods

Open muscle biopsy gives the best picture of the muscle architecture. The large specimen may decrease sampling error, allow proper orientation, and provide enough muscle for all studies. Complications from the procedure are unusual (bleeding, infection, nerve damage, etc.), but it leaves a significant scar. Needle biopsy causes substantially less morbidity, is often more easily arranged, and is adequate for diagnosis of myositis in most cases. Multiple specimens may be taken through the same incision site for enzyme histochemistry and electron microscopy, and to reduce sampling error. However, processing of samples is more difficult, more artefact is encountered, and open biopsy is required for certain functional enzyme studies.

The best information is obtained from muscle with active disease but not end-stage fibrosis or atrophy. Muscles with trauma from EMG or intramuscular injection should not be used for biopsy. The quadriceps or deltoid are most often used due to accessibility. EMG, MRI, ultrasound, and Tc scans have been used to direct the biopsy to areas of disease activity, but MRI gives the best resolution.

Electron microscopy should be performed when IBM or mitochondrial myopathies are considerations. Enzyme histochemistry may be helpful to exclude metabolic myopathies. Coordination with the pathologist can optimize processing and evaluation of specimens.

Muscle pathology

Inflammation is a hallmark of myositis. The infiltrates are predominantly lymphocytes, but include macrophages, plasma cells, and sometimes eosinophils, basophils, and neutrophils. The amount of inflammation is variable, and up to 25 per cent may show no inflammation, usually attributed to a focal process.

In PM, inflammatory infiltrates more often predominate in the endomysial area around the muscle fibres, usually without perifascicular atrophy (Plate 133). Necrosis of individual muscle fibres may be observed. The fibres appear swollen with homogeneous contents, losing the normal striations of the contractile proteins. There is invasion of mononuclear cells, phagocytosis, and regeneration (Fig. 2), the latter marked by sarcoplasmic basophilia, large vesicular, internalized nuclei, and prominent nucleoli. In later stages, there is atrophy, fibrosis, and fatty replacement. Steroid treatment may enhance type II fibre atrophy.

In typical DM, infiltration predominates in the perimysial area (around the fascicles) and around small blood vessels, sometimes extending into the endomysial area. Microvascular changes are often seen, with perifascicular atrophy (decreased fibre size at the periphery of the fascicle), a characteristic feature of DM (Fig. 3) (Dalakas 1991). This may result from capillary loss, which is greater in the perifascicular region, or to a direct effect of perifascicular inflammation. It is most common in juvenile DM (90 per cent), but occurs in adult DM (50 per cent). Circumscribed areas of myofibrillar loss are also typical, attributed to ischaemic damage. Some patients without a DM rash clinically can have this histologic picture. Perifascicular atrophy and inflammation have also been noted in patients with PM and anti-Jo-1 autoantibodies, without capillary loss (Mozaffar and Pestronk 2000).

Electron microscopy shows endothelial cell injury, with swelling, hyperplasia, vacuolization, degeneration, and regeneration. There is endothelial cell necrosis and capillary thrombosis, and loss of capillaries resulting in

(a)

(b)

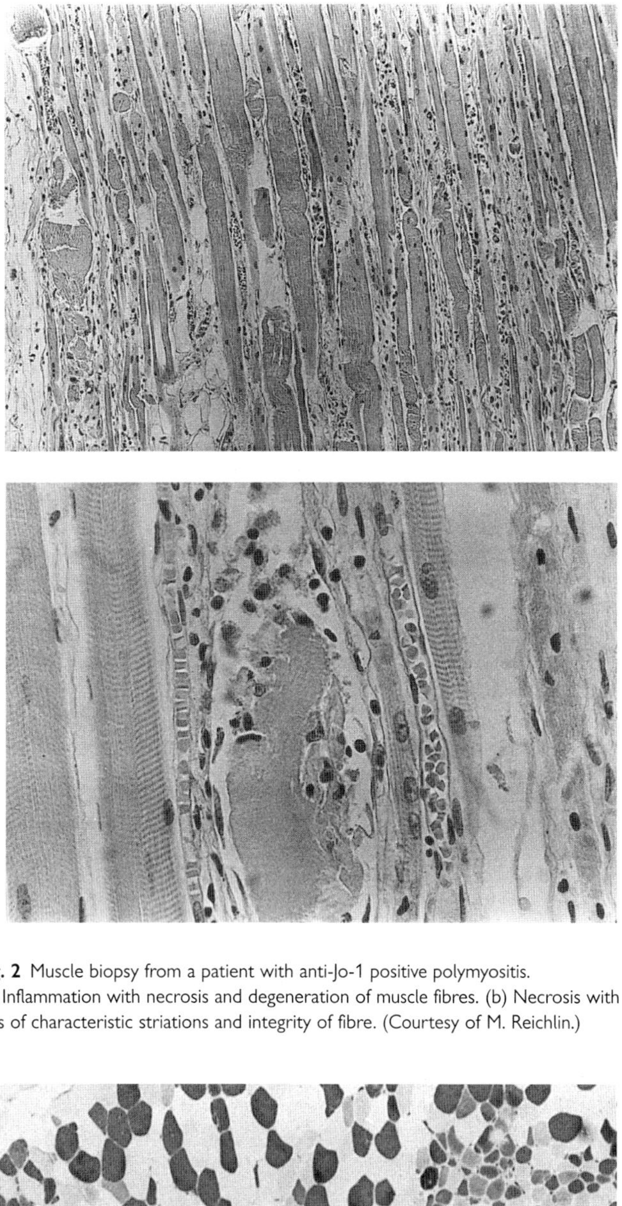

Fig. 2 Muscle biopsy from a patient with anti-Jo-1 positive polymyositis. (a) Inflammation with necrosis and degeneration of muscle fibres. (b) Necrosis with loss of characteristic striations and integrity of fibre. (Courtesy of M. Reichlin.)

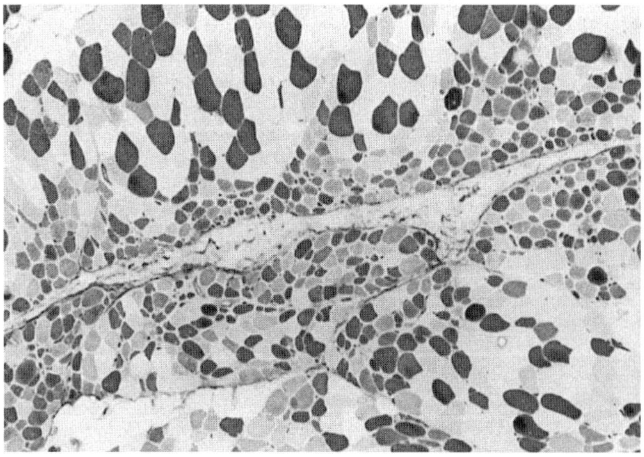

Fig. 3 Muscle biopsy (ATPase stain) from a patient with dermatomyositis. The pattern of perifascicular atrophy is evident.

decreased capillary density (Emslie-Smith and Engel 1990). The endothelial cells contain characteristic tubuloreticular inclusions ('undulating tubules'). These may be seen in other tissues and can be induced by interferon-α; they may occur in other diseases, although usually not PM.

Skin pathology

A skin biopsy should be taken from lesional skin. Vacuolar degeneration of the basal cell layer is seen. There is often a mild mononuclear cell infiltrate in the upper dermis and dermal–epidermal junction. There may be basement membrane thickening. Oedema and increased mucin can be seen in the dermis. With poikiloderma, there is telangiectasia and epidermal atrophy. In Gottron's papules, typical DM changes may be seen, with less atrophy, but more epidermal change such as acanthosis.

These findings may resemble SLE, but the dermal–epidermal infiltrate is milder in DM, and there is more dermal mucin. Immunoglobulin deposition is much less prominent in DM; the lupus band test is usually negative (Magro and Crowson 1997).

Differential diagnosis

The rash makes diagnosis of DM easier than PM. In PM or less typical DM, other conditions that can cause muscle weakness, myalgias, or elevated CK levels must be excluded and the role of medications should be considered. Patients with risk factors should be tested for retroviral infection.

In patients with weakness without systemic features, other myopathies or neuropathies should be considered. In patients with weakness and signs of acute illness or connective tissue disease, such as fever, arthritis, etc., the major conditions to be distinguished may be infectious or rheumatic. Conditions to be excluded are listed in Table 4.

HIV

Patients with HIV infection may develop myositis indistinguishable from PM, sometimes before other HIV manifestations. Weakness, myalgia, and elevated CK are seen, but rarely a rash. EMG shows myopathy, and biopsy shows inflammation with lymphocytic infiltration and necrosis (Dalakas 1993). HIV-PM may be part of the diffuse infiltrative lymphocytosis syndrome.

The pathogenesis of HIV-myositis has similarities to idiopathic PM. CD8+ cytotoxic T cells and macrophages predominate, with very few CD4+ cells. There is endomysial infiltration, surrounded and invaded fibres, and expression of MHC-1 on most muscle fibres, consistent with cell mediated attack (Dalakas 1993). Numerous studies failed to find HIV inside intact muscle fibres, but it was found in cells infiltrating muscle. HIV-myositis must be distinguished from the myopathy of zidovudine. Zidovudine inhibits mitochondrial DNA synthesis, resulting in muscle mitochondrial toxicity, with ragged red fibres.

HIV has also been associated with a wasting syndrome that may occasionally represent an unrecognized myopathy. Patients with AIDS are also at risk for myositis from other infections, such as tuberculosis or microsporidia, and for pyomyositis.

Human T-cell lymphotropic virus type I

Human T-cell lymphotropic virus type I (HTLV-1) has also been associated with myositis, clinically similar to PM, with or without HTLV-1-associated myelopathy. It may be a major cause of PM in endemic areas such as Jamaica, but is infrequent in PM patients in non-endemic areas. As with HIV, studies of infiltrating lymphocytes and MHC-1 expression suggest T-cell mediated cytotoxicity. Infiltrating cells were positive for virus, but HTLV-1 did not infect muscle cells *in vitro* (Sherman et al. 1995).

Bacterial pyomyositis

Pyomyositis has been well known in tropical areas for many years, most commonly affecting young males, with one or more spontaneous muscle abscesses, usually from *Staphylococcus aureus*. Pyomyositis in non-tropical areas is increasingly reported, often non-Staphylococcal, affecting older patients, diabetics, or the chronically ill (Gomez-Reino et al. 1994). Pyomyositis also occurs in AIDS, most often due to Staphylococci in men with very low CD4 counts. Diagnosis can be made with ultrasound, CT, or MRI.

Table 4 Differential diagnosis of PM/DM

I Other forms of inflammatory myopathy (myositis)
  A Infectious myositis:
    1. Viruses:
      (a) Retroviruses:
        (i) HIV: PM-like myositis, other infections
        (ii) HTLV-1
      (b) Picornaviruses (enteroviruses):
        (i) Echovirus (In Ig deficiency)
        (ii) Coxsackie virus
      (c) Other viruses:
        (i) Influenza
        (ii) Hepatitis B or C
        (iii) Others (EBV, CMV, adenovirus, etc.)
    2. Bacteria:
      (a) Pyomyositis
      (b) Lyme myositis
      (c) Other (TB, mycoplasma, leprosy, strep, etc.)
    3. Protozoa: toxoplasmosis, American trypanosomiasis
    4. Parasites: trichinosis, cysticercosis
    5. Fungi: candida
  B Idiopathic:
    1. Inclusion body myositis
    2. Autoimmune rheumatic diseases
      (a) Scleroderma
      (b) SLE
      (c) Sjögren's syndrome
      (d) RA
      (e) Vasculitis (PAN, Wegener's, RA)
      (f) Polymyalgia rheumatica
    3. Other idiopathic myositis
      (a) Granulomatous myositis (giant cell, sarcoid, etc.)
      (b) Eosinophilic myositis
      (c) Eosinophilia–myalgia and toxic oil syndromes
      (d) Focal myositis
      (e) Orbital myositis

II Other myopathies
  A Dystrophies
    1. Limb-girdle
    2. Fascio-scapulo-humeral
  B Congenital myopathies
    1. Congenital myopathies (nemaline rod, central core, etc.)
    2. Mitochondrial myopathies
  C Metabolic
    1. Myophosphorylase deficiency (McArdles's)
    2. Phosphofructokinase deficiency
    3. Myoadenylate deaminase deficiency
    4. Acid maltase deficiency
    5. Lipid storage diseases
      (a) Carnitine deficiency
      (b) Carnitine palmitoyl transferase deficiency
    6. Carcinomatous myopathy
    7. Acute rhabdomyolysis

III Other neurological disorders
  A Motor neuron diseases
  B Myasthenia gravis or Eaton-Lambert
  C Guillain–Barre syndrome
IV Endocrine/metabolic disorders
  A Thyroid
    1. Hypothyroidism
    2. Hyperthyroidism
  B Hypercortisolism
    1. Endogenous
    2. Steroid myopathy
  C Parathyroid
    1. Hypoparathyroidism
    2. Hyperparathyroidism
  D Metabolic
    1. Hypocalcaemia
    2. Hypokalaemia
  E Diabetes and neurological complications
  F Malnutrition

V Drugs (see Table 5)

Other neurological conditions

Diseases with exclusively diffuse motor involvement, such as amyotrophic lateral sclerosis or myasthenia gravis, can resemble PM. Fasciculations and prominent atrophy may be clues in the former, and extraocular or eyelid muscle involvement in the latter.

A family history of myopathy is against PM/DM. A few hereditary myopathies may present in adults (Table 4). Selective muscle involvement, lack of response to therapy, and myotonia are clues, and biopsy should help. Mitochondrial myopathy may sometimes present in adults with pure limb myopathy, suggested by 'ragged red fibres' on biopsy, due to subsarcolemmal accumulation of abnormal mitochondria. Genetic defects in glycogen or glucose metabolism usually present with episodic fatigue, cramping, or pain related to exercise. Some, however, such as deficiencies of myophosphorylase (McArdle's disease), phosphofructokinase, myoadenylate deaminase, or acid maltase, may have an atypical presentation with late onset progressive weakness. Biopsy may show increased glycogen deposition; if suspected, enzyme histochemistry should be performed. The forearm ischaemic exercise test is often used to screen for such disorders; several cause impaired rise in lactate but not ammonia, while myoadenylate deaminase causes impaired rise in ammonia but not lactate.

An entity recently described in France, macrophagic myofasciitis, can also cause a picture resembling PM (Cherin et al. 2000). Myalgia was more common than weakness, and CK and EMG were not consistently abnormal. Infiltration by sheets of large macrophages was seen. Fibre damage was not prominent, with no necrosis. Treatment with steroids and antibiotics helped.

Granulomatous myositis is rare, and commonly associated with sarcoidosis (Prayson 1999). Eosinophilic myositis can also cause a picture resembling PM, and can occur as part of the hypereosinophilic syndrome. These conditions can be distinguished by biopsy. Inclusion body myositis is discussed below. Other idiopathic inflammatory myopathies, such as focal myositis or orbital myositis, are unlikely to be confused with PM.

Drug-induced myopathies

Numerous drugs can induce myopathy (Table 5). Most have a toxic effect but the picture of weakness, myalgia, and elevated CK, often with EMG changes of myopathy, can look like myositis (Zuckner 1994). D-penicillamine may induce autoimmune myositis (see below).

Colchicine may cause a non-inflammatory, vacuolar neuromyopathy (Kuncl et al. 1987), most often occurring with maintenance therapy at usual doses with renal insufficiency. A rise in CK is a sensitive indicator. *Chloroquine*, and less often *hydroxychloroquine*, can cause vacuolar myopathy with characteristic myeloid and curvilinear bodies (Estes et al. 1987). Cardiomyopathy and neuropathy with loss of reflexes may be seen. Case reports of vacuolar myopathy with other drugs have appeared.

Muscle toxicity is a common side-effect with *cholesterol-lowering agents*. It is most common with HMG-CoA-reductase inhibitors such as *lovastatin*, but can also occur with fibrates or nicotinic acid. It can be more severe with combination therapy or with cyclosporine as after heart transplant. Renal insufficiency may predispose to fibrate myopathy.

Alcohol abuse may lead to either an acute necrotizing myopathy with prominent pain and high CKs, or a chronic myopathy with proximal-muscle weakness, atrophy, and milder CK elevation (Charness et al. 1989). Several drugs of abuse, including cocaine, may lead to myopathy, CK elevation, or rhabdomyolysis. Abuse of ipecac in bulimia can induce a proximal, PM-like myopathy, and as with other drug abuse, may be hidden.

In the eosinophilia–myalgia syndrome associated with L-tryptophan ingestion, proximal myopathy was seen in two-thirds of patients. Aldolase was sometimes elevated, but not CK. Mononuclear and eosinophilic interstitial infiltrate (perimyositis) was seen, but fibre necrosis was rare.

Several case reports have described a picture resembling DM with hydroxyurea therapy, and treatment with interferon-α can cause myositis (Dietrich et al. 2000).

Table 5 Drugs causing myopathy

I	Implicated in autoimmune myopathy 1. D-Penicillamine 0.2–1.4% of RA patients taking drug; well documented 2. Cimetidine Case report of inflammatory myopathy 3. L-Tryptophan Eosinophilia–myalgia syndrome 4. Zidovudine Mitochondrial changes and myositis; role in myositis unclear
II	Myopathy with weakness, myalgia, elevated CK 1. Colchicine Neuromyopathy, elevated CK; when normal doses used with renal insufficiency 2. Chloroquine/hydroxychloroquine Vacuolar myopathy, curvilinear bodies 3. Lipid-lowering agents (a) Lovastatin and other statins Frequency may be higher with lovastatin; increases when used in combination with cyclosporine (30%), and some increase with clofibrate, gemfibrozil (5%), or niacin (b) Clofibrate (c) Gemfibrozil (d) Niacin 4. Cyclosporine 5. Alcohol 6. Ipecac, emetine 7. Vincristine 8. Aminocaproic acid 9. Carbimizole, propyl-thiouracil 10. NSAIDs Rare; aspirin, phenylbutazone
III	Rhabdomyolysis picture 1. Alcohol 2. Drugs of abuse Trauma, muscle crush, and direct drug effect (a) Cocaine (b) Amphetamines (c) Heroin (d) Phencyclidine (e) Barbiturates 3. Lovastatin 4. Anaesthetics Malignant hyperthermia 5. Psychotropics Neuroleptic-malignant syndrome
IV	Muscle effects, normal CK 1. Diuretics, etc. Drug-induced hypokalaemia 2. Corticosteroids CK usually normal
V	Interferon-α

Endocrine and steroid myopathies

Hypothyroidism is a common cause for elevated CK level with or without weakness, and can resemble PM. Thyroid function should be tested in all patients when myositis is considered. Hypokalaemia from any cause can lead to myopathy with CK elevation; severe hypokalaemic myopathy has been associated with chronic licorice ingestion (Table 5).

Corticosteroid excess may lead to proximal muscle weakness, associated with accentuated type II fibre atrophy. Its onset is usually insidious, with lower extremity predominance. It is more likely with higher doses for extended periods, with multiple daily doses or longer acting fluorinated preparations. It usually improves if the dose is lowered. An acute form can occur associated with high-dose intravenous therapy and neuromuscular blocking agents in patients on respirators (Zuckner 1994). Steroid myopathy can be confused with recurrent myositis. Elevated CK, increased spontaneous activity on EMG, and inflammation by MRI or biopsy should all be absent in pure steroid myopathy. It may develop while the myositis is still active, indicating the likely need for a steroid-sparing drug. Often, if the situation is not life-threatening, dosage reduction is tried.

Aetiology and pathogenesis

Aetiology

Abundant evidence supports an autoimmune pathogenesis for PM and DM, but the reason it develops is unknown. It is generally felt that an inciting factor acts in a genetically susceptible host. Different inciting agents, such as D-penicillamine, HIV infection, various malignancies, and connective tissue diseases, can lead to similar-appearing autoimmune inflammatory myopathies.

Potential aetiologic factors

Infection

A variety of infections can induce a syndrome resembling PM in humans or animals, suggesting that unrecognized infections may lead to some cases of idiopathic PM. Viruses could induce autoimmune myositis through persistent infection, molecular mimicry, presentation or alteration of muscle antigens, production of immune complexes, immune dysregulation, or other mechanisms.

A variety of viruses such as influenza can cause myositis, but efforts to culture viruses from muscle in typical PM and DM have been unsuccessful. Picornaviruses, small RNA viruses that include enteroviruses [Coxsackie (CV), echo] and animal viruses such as encephalomyocarditis (EMC), have been suspected as possible aetiologic factors in myositis and myocarditis, in part due to their muscle tropism, evident in animal models and human infection. For example, enteroviral infection, particularly echovirus, can cause a dermatomyositis-like syndrome, usually with meningoencephalitis, in patients with agammaglobulinaemia. Some studies have found antibodies to CV to be more frequent in myositis, but attempts to demonstrate the virus in muscle have been conflicting. Some in situ hybridization studies suggested virus, but the reactive material was not further confirmed as viral, and subsequent studies found no enterovirus. Most studies using PCR have been negative for enterovirus and other viruses (Leff et al. 1992). Thus, a role for ongoing picornavirus infection seems unlikely for most cases, but a potential role exists for isolated cases, or as an initiating agent.

Persistent skin infection with parvovirus B19 has been found in adult patients with DM (Crowson et al. 2000), as well as in muscle of a DM patient, and a pathogenetic role has been suggested. Patients with myositis and hepatitis C have been reported, but a pathogenetic role is uncertain.

The similarity of HIV and HTLV-1 myositis to idiopathic myositis suggests that PM and DM may be induced by unidentified retroviruses, but no evidence of retrovirus was found by PCR (Leff et al. 1992).

Toxoplasma gondii infection can cause a myositis resembling PM (Ytterberg 1994). Antibodies to *Toxoplasma* were more frequent in PM patients than controls, including IgM antibodies suggesting recent infection. The significance of such tests is unclear, and a role for *Toxoplasma* in the PM of those patients has not been established. No *Toxoplasma* DNA was found by PCR in three PM patients with elevated titres. Active *Toxoplasma* infection is not found in the muscle in most typical PM by culture or biopsy. It remains possible that some cases of apparently idiopathic PM result from unrecognized *Toxoplasma* or related infection.

Non-infectious

Environmental factors D-Penicillamine can induce a PM-like inflammatory myopathy. The mechanism is unknown, and there is no clear relation to dose or duration. It usually responds when the drug is stopped, but steroids are often needed and deaths have occurred. A case with anti-Jo-1 has even been reported. This emphasizes that ingested environmental agents could induce idiopathic PM. However, it is more frequent among Japanese and Asian Indian patients than Caucasian patients, and HLA–DR associations differed (DR2 versus DR4). Thus, genetic background may affect susceptibility to the aetiologic agent.

Environmental toxins are of potential significance in inducing autoimmune myositis (Love and Miller 1993). Possible examples include the natural fish toxin ciguatera, or silica exposure. Although cases of DM have occurred after bovine collagen dermal implants, a causal role has not been shown, and there was no increase in expected frequency of DM. Cases of PM or DM have occurred in patients with silicone breast implants or after immunization, but the aetiologic role of these factors is unknown.

Genetic factors Associations with MHC genes indicate the importance of genetic susceptibility in PM and DM (Shamim et al. 2000). HLA–DR3 has been associated with PM in several studies, such as that of Love et al. (1991) (DR3 = 45 per cent in PM/DM versus 23 per cent in controls). DRB1*0301, DQA1*0501, and DQB1*0201 were increased in Caucasians with PM more than DM (Arnett et al. 1996). In African-Americans and Mexican-Americans, DQA1*0501 and *0401 were still increased in myositis. The MHC association with DQA1*0501 and *0401 was stronger in patients with antisynthetases. Anti-PM-Scl is most common among Caucasians, and is rare in Japanese patients. It is strongly associated with DR3, including all of 22 patients in one study (Marguerie et al. 1992). Anti-Mi-2 has a strong association with DR7 (75 versus 16 per cent without MSA), and anti-SRP with DR5 (57 versus 20 per cent) (Love et al. 1991).

Rider et al. (1999) recently confirmed the strong association of DRB1*0301, DQA1*0501, and related DRB1's in Whites. This was not seen in Koreans, for whom DRB1*14 and Gm21 were protective. It was emphasized that despite similar clinical and autoantibody profiles for Whites and Koreans, there were no shared immunogenetic markers.

The high frequency of autoimmune diseases in relatives of PM and DM patients suggests an unrecognized genetic factor predisposing to autoimmunity (Ginn et al. 1998). Potential predisposing genes have been found for juvenile DM at or near the TNF-α, IL-1ra, and IL-1-α genes, and their role in adult DM is uncertain (Shamim et al. 2000). Genetic factors are also suggested by differences in myositis in different countries and ethnic groups noted in recent studies of French Canadian (Uthman et al. 1996) and Polish (Hausmanowa-Petrusewicz et al. 1997) populations.

Pathogenetic mechanisms

Cellular immunity

Lymphocytes in inflammatory infiltrates in muscle have been characterized using monoclonal antibodies to cell surface markers (Hohlfield et al. 1997). Such studies reveal that a cellular immune attack on muscle fibres is a prominent pathogenetic process in PM but not in DM (Messner 2000).

In PM, CD8+ T-cells are more abundant in the endomysial areas. In moving from the perivascular to the endomysial area, the proportion of CD8+ suppressor/cytotoxic T-cells increases, and that of CD4+ T- and B-cells decreases (Arahata and Engel 1984). Many non-necrotic muscle fibres are surrounded and invaded by mononuclear cells. A majority of surrounding and most of the invading cells are CD8+ T-lymphocytes (Engel and Arahata 1984), a high proportion being activated cytotoxic cells. Many cells show CD45RO indicating memory T-cells. Immunoelectron microscopy confirms the direct involvement of CD8+ T-cells and macrophages in fibre injury, by becoming apposed against the fibre, sending 'spike-like processes' into the fibre, then displacing and replacing the fibre (Hohlfeld et al. 1997; Messner 2000). Necrotic fibres become infiltrated predominantly by macrophages. Many endomysial (not perimysial) cells may show perforin and granzyme A, granule proteins of cytotoxic T-cells that may participate in fibre damage. The perforin is distributed toward the fibre, suggesting attack on an antigen (Hohlfeld et al. 1997).

Studies of the T-cell receptors (TCR) of the infiltrating lymphocytes also suggest an antigen-directed T-cell attack in PM, with TCR rearrangements and marked restriction in V-gene usage, although some differences in V-genes used were seen. The findings suggest local clonal expansion, evidently in response to a muscle antigen, presumably on the muscle surface, that remains unidentified (Hohlfeld et al. 1997).

Several studies have looked for apoptosis of muscle cells as a pathogenetic mechanism in myositis, but most studies do not find this. Apoptosis was expected in view of the inflammatory processes observed, with release of granzyme, expression of Fas and Fas ligand, and other conditions. Apoptosis inhibitory proteins have been identified in myositis muscle (FLIP, IAP-like protein) which may explain this (Nagaraju 2001).

While expression of MHC-1 antigens on muscle fibres is normally low or absent, in PM muscle many fibres strongly express MHC-1. This could promote T-cell mediated attack, and, consistent with this, is present on all surrounded and invaded fibres. However, it is also seen in areas distant from cellular infiltrates, and is seen in DM where such fibres are rare. It could also be a primary factor leading to autoimmunity against muscle, as evidenced by a recent transgenic mouse model in which expression of MHC-1 in muscle leads to myositis (Nagaraju et al. 2000). Studies of expression of MHC Class II molecules on muscle fibres in myositis are conflicting (Hohlfeld et al. 1997; Nagaraju 2001), but they can be induced *in vitro*, and could further promote muscle antigen presentation.

Overexpression of ICAM-1 can be induced on fibres under attack in myositis, which may be induced by cytokines. The complementary marker LFA-1 is expressed on infiltrating T-cells. This may contribute to the immune response against muscle. ICAM-1 can also be expressed on endothelial cells, fibroblasts, and infiltrating cells. VCAM-1 and LFA-3 can also be expressed on endothelial cells. ICAM-1 and VCAM-1 can be expressed on skin endothelial cells. Serum levels of ICAM-1 and VCAM-1 are reported to be elevated and correlate with disease activity.

Cytokines could be important in the development, enhancement, or perpetuation of the autoimmune response, or in tissue injury and cytotoxicity (Nagaraju 2001). Interferon-γ (IFN-γ) can enhance MHC-1 and ICAM-1 expression and induce MHC-2 expression on cultured muscle fibres *in vitro*. IFN-γ can inhibit proliferation and differentiation, an effect enhanced by TNF-α (Kalovidouris et al. 1993). IFN has been seen in myositis muscle in some studies, and PM has occurred after IFN therapy.

Studies of myositis muscle have consistently shown expression of TGF-β, but its role is uncertain. IL-1-α and -β are also frequently found (Lundberg and Nyberg 1998). Expression was prominent in endothelial cells, suggesting that these cells are important in pathogenesis of PM as well as DM. Other cytokines are found less frequently or consistently (Lundberg and Nyberg 1998; Nagaraju 2001). The β-CC chemokine MIP-1-α was found frequently in myositis muscle, and less often MIP-1-β and RANTES (Adams et al. 1997); these may enhance the inflammation.

Serum levels of IL-1-α and IL-2 receptor are elevated in active disease, possibly reflecting activated lymphocytes. IL-1-ra was also elevated in some patients (Gabay et al. 1994). A potential role for IL-1-α and TNF in juvenile DM has been suggested by enhanced disease in patients with genetic polymorphisms that may lead to increased expression.

Strength can return with treatment sooner than would be expected if regeneration were required. Inflammation may not correlate with weakness, which may persist in inactive disease. The weakness may relate to muscle cell dysfunction. Cytokines such as IL-1, and expression of MHC-1, may persist, and contribute to muscle dysfunction (Nyberg et al. 2000).

Humoral immunity

Microvascular injury

T-cell attack on muscle fibres does not appear to be a significant process in DM. DM biopsies show a higher proportion of B-cells and a lower proportion of CD8+ T-cells. There is intense B-cell and CD4+ T-cell infiltrate in the perivascular area, suggesting a local humoral response (Arahata and Engel 1984). There is little endomysial infiltrate, and non-necrotic surrounded and invaded fibres are rare.

Vasculopathy involving the small vessels and capillaries, with loss of capillaries leading to ischaemic damage and perifascicular atrophy, is an important mechanism of muscle injury in DM (Emslie-Smith and Engel 1990). It is generally not found in typical PM. Approximately 10 per cent with evidence of this process do not have a DM rash, but many still consider these patients to have DM.

Microvascular damage in muscle appears to be mediated by complement. Membrane attack complex (MAC) of complement is deposited in muscle microvasculature in DM but not PM or IBM, indicating local activation of complement (Emslie-Smith and Engel 1990). It is greater in areas where ischaemic damage is recent (fibres with 'punched-out' central myofibrillar loss) than in those with perifascicular atrophy (a later change), and is less evident in longstanding disease.

Muscle biopsies from DM patients that show little or no structural change by routine examination often still show vascular abnormalities, including endothelial cell injury, microtubular inclusions, decreased capillary density, and MAC deposition (Emslie-Smith and Engel 1990). Biopsies showing overt DM have even lower capillary density and more advanced vascular changes, including capillary necrosis. This early involvement suggests that the microvasculature is the primary target in DM.

The factors leading to complement activation are not known. Deposition of immunoglobulin in muscle blood vessels, not seen in normals, has been found in DM in some studies, but is not specific.

The C5b-9 MAC deposition is also found in vessels of the skin lesions of most DM patients (Magro and Crowson 1997), although this was also seen in 21 per cent of lupus. It also occurred at the dermal epidermal junction and at the keratinocyte to a variable degree.

Autoantibodies

Autoantibodies to nuclear and cytoplasmic antigens are found in up to 89 per cent of patients (Targoff 2000) (Plate 132). The specificities of these antibodies have been studied in detail, and are heterogeneous (Table 6). About half of patients have autoantibodies of recognized specificity, some of which are found primarily in myositis, referred to as 'myositis-specific autoantibodies' (MSAs). Others have an association with myositis, but may be found in other conditions ('myositis-associated autoantibodies', MAAs). Most MSAs are associated with a characteristic clinical picture, and an individual most often has only a single MSA, so that MSAs can define clinical subgroups (Love et al. 1991; Targoff 2000).

MSAs (a) *Antisynthetases:* About 25 per cent of PM and DM patients have antibodies to an aminoacyl-tRNA synthetase, an enzyme that attaches one specific amino acid to its cognate tRNAs. Six antisynthetases have been found in myositis sera (Table 6), but usually an individual patient has antibodies to only one, with antihistidyl-tRNA synthetase (anti-Jo-1) by far the most common, found in approximately 20 per cent.

A group of clinical features have been associated with anti-Jo-1 and other antisynthetases in several studies (Table 7) (Marguerie et al. 1990; Love et al. 1991). The most striking feature is ILD, found in 50–90 per cent with anti-Jo-1. Two-third of patients with anti-Jo-1 have inflammatory polyarthritis (Oddis et al. 1990), usually mild and responsive to treatment, but 1/3 may have finger deformity, usually non-erosive, occasionally with calcinosis. Raynaud's phenomenon (62 per cent), fever (87 per cent), and mechanic's hands (71 per cent) are other important features (Love et al. 1991). Sclerodactyly (72 per cent) and sicca (59 per cent) may also occur. Response to therapy may be less complete, with more relapses. 1/3–1/2 have the DM rash, less with anti-Jo-1 than others. The set of clinical features associated with antisynthetases has been referred to as the 'antisynthetase syndrome' (Targoff 2000). It may resemble overlap syndromes, but the myositis is usually more prominent, significant ILD is more frequent, and SLE features are unusual.

ILD can dominate the clinical picture. Occasionally, ILD (or rarely arthritis) occurs without overt myositis. This is more common with anti-PL-12, and possibly anti-OJ and anti-KS, than with anti-Jo-1, and possibly more

Table 6 Autoantibodies in PM/DM

Antibody	Antigen	% of all PM/DM	Myositis sub-group[a]
Myositis-specific antibodies		30–40	
Anticytoplasmic			
Antisynthetase	Aminoacyl-tRNA synthetases	20–30	
Anti-Jo-1	Histidyl-tRNA synthetase	18–20	Antisynthetase syndrome[b]
Anti-PL-7	Threonyl-tRNA synthetase	<3	Antisynthetase syndrome
Anti-PL-12	Alanyl-tRNA synthetase/tRNA^{ala}	<3	Antisynthetase syndrome
Anti-OJ	Isoleucyl-tRNA synthetase	<2	Antisynthetase syndrome
Anti-EJ	Glycyl-tRNA synthetase	<2	Antisynthetase syndrome
Anti-SRP	Signal recognition particle	≤5	PM
Antinuclear			
Anti-Mi-2	Nucleosome remodelling complex	8	DM[d]
Anti-56 kD	56 kD nuclear protein	80	All
Anti-hPMS1	DNA mismatch repair	ND	ND
Anti-MJ	Nuclear protein	ND	Juvenile DM
Myositis-associated antibodies			
Antitranslation			
Anti-KJ	Unidentified translation factor	<1	PM, Raynaud's, ILD
Anti-Fer	Elongation factor 1 α	<1	ND[c]
Myositis overlap antibodies			
Anti-PM-Scl	Nucleolar/nucleolar protein complex	8	PM/DM—scleroderma overlap
Anti-U1RNP	U1 small nuclear ribonucleoprotein	12	PM/DM—overlap syndromes
Anti-U2RNP	U2 small nuclear ribonucleoprotein	<2	PM—scleroderma overlap
Anti-U5RNP	U5 small nuclear ribonucleoprotein	<2	PM
Anti-Ku	DNA binding protein dimer	<2	PM–scleroderma or SLE
Anti-Ro60	RNA-protein particle	10	SLE; Sjögren's overlap
Anti-Ro52	RNA-protein particle	20	SLE; Sjögren's
Anti-La/SSB	RNA-protein	5–7	SLE; Sjögren's overlap

[a] Most characteristic sub-group is shown, but most may occur in others.

[b] Antisynthetase syndrome: see Table 7.

[c] ND, not determined.

[d] Higher frequency (14%) and occurence in PM when recombinant ELISA used (Brouwer et al. 2001).

Table 7 Features of antisynthetase syndrome

	Love et al. (1991) (*n* = 47)	Marguerie et al. (1991) (*n* = 29)
Myositis	100%	83%
Arthritis/arthralgia	94%	90%
Interstitial lung disease	89%	79%
Raynaud's phenomenon	62%	93%
Fever	87%	NR
Flares during taper	60%	NR
Mechanic's hands	71%	NR
Sclerodactyly	NR	72%
Sicca	NR	59%
Myalgia	84%	NR
Calcinosis	NR	24%
DM rash	54%	38%
Anti-Ro/SSA	25%	24%
HLA–DR3	73%	NR
Mortality	21%	17%
F:M ratio	2.7	1.4
% Anti-PL-12	2	21

NR, not recorded.

common in Japanese than American patients. Anti-Jo-1 has been highly specific for patients with one or more manifestations of this syndrome.

Muscle histology in anti-Jo-1 patients was found to differ in pattern from typical PM and DM. The primary finding was perimysial connective tissue fragmentation and inflammation, with perifasciular atrophy, but without capillary loss (Mozaffar and Pestronk 2000). Endomysial inflammation was not prominent.

(b) *Anti-SRP:* Antibodies to other cytoplasmic antigens are found in a small proportion of PM/DM patients (Table 6), the most important of which is antibody to the signal recognition particle (anti-SRP), a ribonucleoprotein involved in protein translocation into the endoplasmic reticulum. Anti-SRP is found almost exclusively in PM (Targoff 2000), with no increase in ILD, arthritis, or Raynaud's phenomenon. Some patients with anti-SRP have an acute, fulminant course, resistant to treatment (Love et al. 1991). Cardiac involvement can occur. One study found individual patients who had both anti-Jo-1 and anti-SRP, but this is unusual (Brouwer et al. 2001).

Rarely, myositis patients with other anticytoplasmic autoantibodies have been found, such as anti-KJ, associated with a clinical picture similar to that of antisynthetases.

(c) *Anti-Mi-2:* Antinuclear autoantibodies are more common than anticytoplasmic, but most are less studied. Anti-Mi-2, which reacts with a nuclear antigen that is part of a protein complex ('nucleosome remodelling deacetylase') involved in chromosomally mediated regulation of transcription (Targoff 2000), is strongly associated with DM. In most studies, 95 per cent with anti-Mi-2 have DM, although use of sensitive recombinant ELISAs may decrease its specificity (Brouwer et al. 2001). No increase in ILD or Raynaud's is seen.

Myositis associated autoantibodies Several autoantibodies are seen in patients with myositis overlap syndromes. Although not myositis-specific, these antibodies can be very helpful in evaluating patients with suspected myositis, and some may have similar significance for the disease.

(a) *Anti-PM-Scl:* Anti-PM-Scl reacts with a protein complex of 11 polypeptides in the nucleolus and nucleus labeled the 'exosome', involved in RNA processing. Patients with anti-PM-Scl most commonly have an overlap syndrome with features of myositis and scleroderma that some have called 'scleromyositis', although some patients have only one of the diseases. The DM rash and calcinosis may occur (Marguerie et al. 1992). Cutaneous scleroderma is usually limited when present. The myositis is often mild and tends to be responsive to treatment. In Japan, anti-PM-Scl is rare, but anti-Ku is commonly found in PM-SSc overlap. In the United States, anti-Ku is more common in SLE and scleroderma.

(b) *Anti-snRNPs:* Among myositis patients, anti-U1RNP is found in 5–15 per cent, often with overlap features such as Raynaud's, arthritis or dactylitis. Among anti-U1RNP patients, myositis is often seen as part of overlap syndromes or SLE. Anti-Sm may occur, usually with SLE overlap. Anti-Sm-negative patients with antibodies specific for individual Sm snRNPs other than U1 (anti-U2RNP, anti-U4/6RNP, anti-U5RNP), often have overlap syndromes involving myositis.

(c) *Anti-Ro/SSA:* Although anti-Ro60 occurs in a small proportion of myositis patients, a recent surprising finding was the high frequency of myositis patients with anti-Ro52 (25 per cent), often in the absence of anti-Ro60 (Brouwer et al. 2001). They are much more frequent in patients with antisynthetases.

Other myositis autoantibodies A high proportion of myositis patient sera, up to 87 per cent, were found to react with a 56 kDa protein of nuclear ribonucleoprotein particles (Targoff 2000). Although common in all sub-groups, it was seen more in DM than PM. The antigen has not been characterized further. The titre varied with disease activity. This promises to be a useful antibody when tests are more widely available. Other new antibodies associated with DM (anti-MJ, anti-155kd) have been described in preliminary reports. Also recently described was a new antibody to PMS-1, a protein involved in DNA repair (Casciola-Rosen et al. 1999). This antibody was found in a small proportion of myositis patients but appears to be specific.

Antiendothelial cell antibodies can occur, and are of interest in view of the endothelial injury in DM, but they are not disease specific and the antigens are not well characterized. Other autoantibodies have been described in myositis but are either rare or non-specific (Targoff 2000).

Significance The reason for production of these antibodies is unknown, and may relate to aetiologic factors (Targoff 1994). HLA and other genetic factors seem to be important. Production appears to be driven and perpetuated by the recognized antigens, but they may not initiate the responses. One hypothesis has been molecular mimicry with myositis-inducing viruses. This suggests that the specificity of the responses derives from a unique initiating event, not secondary to muscle damage. Recent findings have suggested other possibilities. In a transgenic mouse model, the forced expression of MHC-1 led to myositis that became self-perpetuating (Nagaraju et al. 2000). In some mice, anti-Jo-1 was produced, suggesting that the autoantibody can arise from particular muscle inflammatory processes, or the MHC-1 itself, without a specific stimulus. The reason these particular antigens are targeted remains unknown. It was noted that most autoantigens, including most myositis antigens, are particularly likely to be cleaved during apoptosis by granzyme B, when compared to proteins that have not been found to be autoantigens (Casciola-Rosen et al. 1999). The reason for myositis specificity, when the antigens are in all tissues, and the reason different antisynthetases are associated with a similar clinical syndrome, remain unknown.

It is not known if the antibodies play a direct role in pathogenesis (Targoff 1994). The fact that some of the transgenic mice had myositis without autoantibodies suggests that they are epiphenomena, not required for pathogenesis. MSAs can occur in PM, for which there is little evidence of humoral muscle injury. However, the recent finding of distinctive histology associated with anti-Jo-1 suggests that the antibody may contribute to muscle pathology, or may mark a unique syndrome with fundamental differences in pathogenetic mechanisms (Mozaffar and Pestronk 2000).

Animal models

Experimental autoimmune myositis

Certain strains of guinea pig, rat, or mouse develop myositis, with minimal weakness or rash, as a result of immunizations with homologous or heterologous muscle homogenates in adjuvant. Inflammation and necrosis occur, but no vascular changes or perifascicular atrophy. Muscle damage is mediated by cellular immune mechanisms. The histology resembles human PM, but with more macrophages in the inflammatory infiltrate. Myositis and 'C protein' may be antigens (Kohyama and Matsumoto 1999). SJL/J mice are uniquely susceptible to EAM, and with ageing, develop a similar and more severe myositis spontaneously, possibly holding clues into aetiologic factors.

Viral models

Neonatal Swiss mice infected with CV-B1 Tuscon strain develop an acute illness followed by a chronic inflammatory myositis resembling PM (Messner 2000). Myositis progresses beyond the period in which virus can be cultured (6 months versus 2 weeks), but viral nucleic acid persists longer than culturable virus. Production of the myositis depends on the strain of virus and of mouse used, and requires cell-mediated immunity. A myotropic strain of encephalomyocarditis virus causes myositis and myocarditis in adult mice (Messner 2000), also dependent on strain of virus and genetics of mouse. Viral persistence may be important. Theiler's murine encephalomyelitis virus has also been studied as a mouse model of myositis. Thus, picornaviruses can produce immune-mediated myositis, supporting their potential as aetiologic agents in some cases of idiopathic myositis. A condition resembling DM occurs spontaneously in collies and Shetland sheep dogs, who develop muscle weakness and an erythematous, scaly rash over the periorbital areas, face, and distal extremities. Muscle histology shows inflammation, necrosis, and regeneration. The model has significant differences from human myositis.

Transgenic mouse

As noted, expression of MHC-1 on mouse muscle resulted in inflammatory myositis with similarities to PM (Nagaraju et al. 2000). H-2Kb expression was designed to be prevented by administration of doxycycline. Clinical weakness developed 2 months after it was stopped, and became more severe over the next 2–4 months. There were no rashes. Muscle enzymes rose and inflammation, degeneration, and regeneration were seen. ICAM-1 and MIP-1α were secondarily expressed, and may have helped perpetuate the myositis after readministration of doxycycline.

Management

Treatment should be started promptly, since significant delay has been associated with poorer outcome. Treatment is most urgent in patients with rapid onset of severe weakness, dysphagia, respiratory insufficiency, myocardial involvement, or systemic signs. Most cases can be managed outside the hospital, but admission may be required for patients with respiratory insufficiency or severe dysphagia, those requiring intravenous medications, or clarification of diagnosis.

A general approach to treatment is outlined in Table 8. Guidelines for initial treatment, dosage reduction, and choice of agents should be adapted

Table 8 A strategy for treatment

We generally use the following strategy for treatment of the myositis in patients with newly diagnosed, active, idiopathic PM or DM:

(1) *Initial treatment:* Prednisone, 1 mg/kg/day (≥ 60 mg/day), in divided doses. With severe or rapidly progressive weakness, or concerning features (significant dysphagia, respiratory muscle weakness), start with high-dose pulse methyl-prednisolone (1 g/day for 3 days). In very severe cases, consider IVGG

(2) *Continuing treatment:* Prednisone dose is consolidated to a single daily morning dose after the acute period (initial response is seen, patient is stabilized). Continue for at least 1 month, and the CK returns to normal

- (a) If inadequate response of CK and strength by 4–8 weeks: begin second-line agent
  - —Begin with MTX, if no contraindication, at 10 mg/week, and gradually increase until response, or 20 mg/week oral or 30 mg/week S.C. or i.v.
  - —If contraindication, or failure of MTX, go to other second line agent, depending on individual patient factors (severity, age, associated illness, etc.):
    - Less severe (able to wait months for response, no antisynthetases, no anti-SRP):
      - Switch to AZA
    - More severe, options are:
      - Add AZA
      - or switch to cyclosporine (especially if also failed AZA)
      - or add monthly IVGG (especially if problems tolerating other meds; rapid response required; or fails two second-line agents)
    - Refractory:
      - Combination MTX and AZA
      - Tacrolimus
      - Cyclophosphamide and/or chlorambucil
      - Consider mycophenolate
      - Consider fludarabine
- (b) If CK responds but strength not recovering as expected: further evaluation needed. MRI may help. Addition of MTX or other second-line agent, along with steroid taper, is considered
- (c) If CK and strength improve, begin taper of prednisone
  - —Consolidate to single dose if not already done
  - —Decrease dose such that maintenance level (5–10 mg/day) achieved by 6 months if no exacerbation (≈25% per month)
  - —If steroid side-effects occur, convert to alternate-day or add steroid sparing agent
  - —Continue maintenance dose prednisone at >5 mg/day for at least 1 year, then taper gradually by approximately 1 mg per 3 months until stopped

(3) *Other considerations*

- (a) Rehabilitation: begin with passive range of motion. Cautiously add resistive exercises when CK normalizes and slowly advance
- (b) ILD: if progressive and requiring treatment, and high-dose prednisone tried first. If no response, cyclophosphamide is considered, either as i.v. pulse (0.5–1.0 g/m^2/month) or daily oral, with latter used for more severe cases or failures of i.v. Consider cyclosporine or tacrolimus for cyclophosphamide failure or contraindication
- (c) Myositis in SLE or SSc: in patients with anti-PM-Scl or anti-U1RNP who have mild myositis requiring treatment but no other indication, lower initial dose prednisone (≈30 mg/day) is considered
- (d) Cutaneous DM without myositis: watch for myositis, especially in first 2 years, with prompt treatment as above if seen. Topical steroids and sunscreens initially. Hydroxychloroquine 200–400 mg/day for non-responders who require additional treatment. If no myositis, moderate-dose steroids or MTX are used only when indicated for the cutaneous lesions themselves
- (e) Urgent situation such as respiratory failure: IVGG and/or high-dose pulse methylprednisolone used at any point (plus supportive care)

to the situation of the patient. Many patients are given a trial of corticosteroids alone, but initial therapy with a combination of steroids and immunosuppressives also has some support (Oddis 2000a).

Corticosteroids

While not demonstrated by prospective randomized controlled trials, the effectiveness of steroids in improving muscle strength is generally accepted, and readily apparent from observation of treated patients.

Initial treatment

Treatment is usually begun at high doses (prednisone 1 mg/kg/day, usually 60–80 mg/day, or equivalent), often in divided doses, considered to increase effectiveness. Adequate initial treatment has been associated with better responses. The daily amount is usually consolidated to a single morning dose after the acute period or before beginning dosage taper.

The frequent side-effects of high-dose steroids have prompted alternative regimens. It was recently suggested that a lower dose (0.5 mg/kg/day or less), usually in combination with an immunosuppressive agent, could be equally effective (Nzeusseu et al. 1999). Such an approach could be considered for patients with mild disease, or risk factors for side-effects. Other approaches have included use of high-dose intravenous 'pulse' methylprednisolone, in regimens such as 1 g/day for 3 days, with lower maintenance doses (Oddis 2000a). Pulse methylprednisolone is also used for more rapid response in severely ill patients, or for exacerbations during steroid taper. Although some have used alternate-day steroids in milder cases from the outset to reduce side-effects, it is less reliable.

Response

Monitor patients closely during treatment for degree of improvement, new complications, or side-effects. Muscle strength assessed by manual muscle testing and observation of activities, and CK levels are helpful (Kagen 2000). The response to steroids tends to be slower than that in SLE or RA. A high initial dose is usually continued for 1–2 months, until a response is seen, with substantial improvement in CK and strength (Oddis 2000b). It may take longer to achieve the full effect and recover to normal strength. The CK usually normalizes weeks to months earlier than the strength, generally indicating adequate suppression of disease activity. CK levels in the high normal range may indicate disease activity and may decrease with treatment.

If there is no improvement or persistent weakness, the disease may be resistant, but other possibilities include: (i) incorrect diagnosis: the basis for the diagnosis should be reviewed, and further evaluation considered, such as repeat biopsy looking for IBM or metabolic myopathy; (ii) malignancy: myositis with malignancy may be responsive, but failure to respond or weight loss on steroids should suggest a more extensive search; (iii) steroid myopathy: when CK falls but weakness persists, consider steroid myopathy; (iv) permanent loss of strength, despite complete suppression of disease activity, more likely if there was prolonged delay before treatment, atrophy, or prominent fibrosis. Persistent elevation of the CK usually means that the disease has not been controlled. Occasional patients have resolution or stabilization of weakness while CK remains elevated, and MRI may help assess whether inflammation remains.

Dosage reduction

The dose is tapered slowly to a maintenance level over about 6 months, which can be achieved by 25 per cent reduction per month (Table 8) to a maintenance level (such as prednisone 5–10 mg/day or 10–20 mg every other day), sometimes continued for a year, or tapered slowly over 1–2 years. Some recommend routine conversion to an alternate-day regimen after the initial high-dose regimen.

Exacerbations of disease are common. If CK elevation occurs after initial response, causes other than disease flare should be considered, particularly when no other signs are present. Exacerbation without CK elevation may occur, even if the CK was elevated originally, but steroid myopathy should be considered. Other tests, such as MRI, EMG, or repeat needle biopsy, can help assess disease activity in these cases. Exacerbation is usually treated with an increase in steroid dosage and/or addition of an immunosuppressive agent.

The side-effects of corticosteroids in PM/DM are similar to those in other situations. Steroid myopathy poses a special problem, as noted. Steroid-induced hypokalaemia may also lead to further weakness and should be avoided. The usually prolonged course increases risks of osteoporosis and preventive measures should be instituted. Aseptic necrosis is a risk. Gastric protection is commonly used. Diabetes, hypertension, cataracts, and opportunistic infections may be seen.

Immunosuppressives

Indications for immunosuppressive agents include: (i) failure to respond to high-dose steroids; (ii) persistent disease activity after prolonged therapy despite initial improvement; (iii) inability to taper the steroids without recurrence; or (iv) severe steroid side-effects. Immunosuppressives would be considered earlier in those with more severe disease or poor prognostic signs. Recent trends are toward earlier introduction of immunosuppressive agents to reduce the risk of steroid side-effects and improve response, with some recommending combination steroids and immunosuppressive agent as initial treatment (Oddis 2000b).

Methotrexate (MTX) and azathioprine (AZA) are the immunosuppressives used most in myositis. Retrospective analysis (Joffe et al. 1993) suggests a higher response rate and more rapid onset of effect with MTX. However, AZA may have less toxicity. MTX should be used with caution in antisynthetase patients due to the frequent lung involvement, but has been used with success (Joffe et al. 1993).

Methotrexate

MTX is typically begun at 7.5–10 mg/week, and can be increased if needed to 20–25 mg/week orally, or higher parenterally. Doses up to 50 mg/week were used in older studies. Intramuscular injections should generally be avoided when monitoring CK levels. Approximately 70 per cent of myositis patients respond, usually between 3 weeks and several months. MTX should be avoided in renal insufficiency, hepatic damage, or alcoholism. The monitoring guidelines for RA can be difficult to follow due to elevation of enzymes due to muscle injury. One study of 10 DM patients (Zieglschmid-Adams et al. 1995) found hepatic fibrosis in two, on usual doses; diabetes was a risk factor. Other side-effects include stomatitis, infections, teratogenicity, bone marrow suppression, and gastrointestinal bleeding, among others. Folic acid supplements are helpful, and folinic acid might be considered for the higher doses.

Azathioprine

Response rates with an adequate course of AZA are similar to those with methotrexate, about 75 per cent. Patients beginning therapy with AZA plus prednisone had better long-term outcome with less disability and less prednisone requirement than those receiving prednisone alone (Bunch 1981). It is used orally at 1.5–3.0 mg/kg/day, with doses of 100–150 mg/day being most common. An adequate trial requires 3–6 months. Steroids may be gradually reduced as response occurs. Cytopaenias or bone marrow suppression may occur, and complete blood counts including platelets must be monitored. The risk of inducing malignancy appears low in myositis. Other side-effects are similar to those in other situations.

Alkylating agents

Cyclophosphamide is generally reserved for those who have failed to respond to other agents, or have manifestations such as severe interstitial lung disease (Oddis 2000b). There is higher risk of malignancy, bone marrow suppression, infertility, and haemorrhagic cystitis. Monthly i.v. pulse cyclophosphamide was found to have poor efficacy and high toxicity in a group of long-standing, refractory patients (Cronin et al. 1989), but others have had more success. It has been used also in brief courses of 0.5 g i.v. pulses at 1–2 week intervals. Chlorambucil has been used with success in DM patients resistant to other treatment, but carries similar long-term malignancy risk.

Cyclosporine

Several case reports or small series have described beneficial effects of cyclosporine, including in severe, resistant disease (Oddis 2000a). Cyclosporine at 3–3.5 mg/kg/day was recently compared to MTX 7.5–15 mg/week as a second agent in patients being treated with steroids. Response favored MTX but not significantly, but the effects of these agents are hard to separate from those of the steroids (Vencovsky et al. 2000). Cyclosporine, usually 5 mg/kg/day, also appeared to be effective as initial therapy in DM, with responses in a mean of 8.6 weeks. Nephrotoxicity is the greatest concern; dosage reduction for creatinine rise more than 30 per cent over baseline is recommended. Tacrolimus (FK506) was effective in refractory patients (Oddis 2000a).

Combination therapy

A recent crossover study compared the combination of MTX and AZA to high-dose intravenous MTX with leucovorin rescue in refractory patients (Villalba et al. 1998). There were patients who responded with both regimens, but the combination appeared to be more effective, whether given as the first stage or after the trial of IV-MTX. Combination MTX/cyclosporine has had success but has not been studied systematically in adults.

Intravenous gammaglobulin

High-dose intravenous gamma globulin (IVGG) has been shown to be efficacious in DM in a double-blind, crossover, placebo-controlled trial (Dalakas 1998). Nine of 12 had major improvement with IVGG versus 0 of 11 with placebo. None worsened with IVGG, versus 5 of 11 with placebo. The rash improved in most. There are a number of reports and series describing success in PM as well.

A major advantage of IVGG is its low risk. Testing for IgA deficiency to avoid anaphylaxis, for high viscosity due to its significant rise with IVGG, and for renal impairment, have been recommended. Although transmission of hepatitis C has occurred, current risk is felt to be low.

The monthly dose that has been studied is 2 g/kg/day, given over 2–5 days. The effectiveness of an individual treatment appears to be of limited duration (usually 4–6 weeks). Prolonged monthly courses may have continuing effect. Whether prolonged courses can have long-term benefit after cessation is not yet clear, although exacerbations and tachyphylaxis may occur. Tapering and maintenance regimens are empiric; reduction to 0.8 g/kg/month was effective in one PM patient, a dose that could be administered in 1 day. The major impediment to more widespread use is the very high cost.

In DM, by repeat biopsies, capillary density increased, MAC deposition was prevented, and expression of ICAM-1 on endothelial cells and MHC-1 on muscle fibres was normalized. Thus, IVGG acts on early pathogenetic mechanisms, not simply on symptoms. IVGG blocked deposition of activated C3 fragments *in vitro* (Basta and Dalakas 1994), suggesting that it works in DM by binding fragments, protecting muscle capillaries from complement-mediated injury. Other mechanisms are likely to be operative in PM. If persistent infection is a factor, this could be a target for IVGG, but effects on the immune system are more likely.

Experimental

Case reports and collected series have described improvement with plasmapheresis, but most patients have received other treatments, so the independent contribution of plasmapheresis was unclear. In a controlled, double-blind trial, no improvement was seen in strength or functional outcome with plasmapheresis or leukapheresis (12 treatments in 1 month) (Miller et al. 1992). Prednisone was used, but not immunosuppressives. CPK fell from direct removal, without correlation with improvement. Sub-groups of patients might still benefit from these procedures, or they may enhance the benefit of other treatments.

There are no published studies at this time regarding the use in myositis of the newer agents developed for RA. Preliminary anecdotal reports suggest benefit from anti-TNF agents in some patients; caution would be advised in lupus overlap. There is no information available regarding anakinra, although cytokine studies noted above suggest a rationale.

Autologous stem cell transplant was successful in an anti-Jo-1 patient.

A pilot study of the adenine analogue fludarabine in myositis (Adams et al. 1999) showed significant response in 4/16 refractory patients, and a suggestion of benefit in another four.

Total body irradiation (150 rads over 5 weeks) has been successful in some cases, resulting in prolonged responses in some cases resistant to other treatments (Oddis 2000b). However, some have not responded, and at least one patient died. Late malignancy is a concern. Irradiation is a treatment of last resort.

Treatment of extramuscle manifestations

Dermatomyositis rash

The DM rash may respond to treatment of the myositis with steroids or immunosuppressives. If DM lesions persist, hydroxychloroquine 200–400 mg/day may be helpful. It would not be expected to help the myositis. If unsuccessful, quinacrine 100 mg qd might be considered, or isotretinoin (0.5–1.0 mg/kg/day) (Oddis 2000b), with caution to avoid it in pregnancy. Mycophenolate mofetil was reportedly effective in four patients with severe refractory skin manifestations. IVIG is effective, including in reduced dose (0.1 g/kg/day × 5 days). The rash may be photosensitive, and sunscreens are recommended. Topical steroids are commonly used, but are often unsuccessful. For cutaneous ulcerations, IVGG has been effective.

Treatment of amyopathic DM is controversial. Sunscreens, topical therapy, and hydroxychloroquine are usually tried. Other agents such as MTX are usually added only if justified for the cutaneous manifestations. Improvement of skin lesions with MTX (average maximal 20 mg/week orally) was noted in two of three amyopathic DM, and all seven DM (Zieglschmid-Adams et al. 1995). If not treated, patients must be followed closely, especially in the first 2 years, to avoid delay in treatment if myositis appears.

Calcinosis

Calcinosis is more of a problem in juvenile DM but may occur in adults. Several treatments may be tried, such as diltiazem, probenecid, alendronate, or low dose warfarin, but none is of consistent or proven benefit. Surgical excision can be helpful if necessary, and an inflammatory component may respond to colchicine. Treatment of the disease helps prevent calcinosis, but it does not affect established calcinosis.

Interstitial lung disease

Treatment for ILD should be considered for clinically significant active and progressive disease. ILD is sometimes amenable to treatment, but can be unresponsive and contribute to mortality. Treatment is more effective when the biopsy shows active inflammation, or possibly bronchiolitis obliterans organizing pneumonia. Prednisone is usually used initially, but cytotoxic agents are often needed. Cyclophosphamide has been successful in case reports (Oddis 2000b), both orally and by i.v. pulse. Cyclosporine and tacrolimus have been effective (Oddis 2000a).

Gastrointestinal

Dysphagia resulting from pharyngeal weakness usually responds to treatment of the myositis. In resistant or very severe cases, IVGG may be effective. Supportive treatment may be necessary with tube or parenteral alimentation (Oddis 2000b). In persistent dysphagia, cricopharyngeal muscle dysfunction should be considered, and cricopharyngeal myotomy may be needed. Distal oesophageal and lower dysmotility will generally not respond to immunosuppression, but measures similar to those used in oesophageal reflux and scleroderma can be helpful.

Rehabilitation

Passive range of motion exercises should be started early to help prevent joint contractures. When acute inflammation subsides, active exercise, cautiously introduced and slowly advanced, may help recover lost strength from disease, immobility, and steroid-related atrophy. Several recent studies have shown that active, resistive exercise can benefit stable patients without exacerbating muscle injury (Alexanderson et al. 2000), and can be considered even if some disease activity remains. It may help to start with isometric exercises. The patient may also require assistance with activities of daily living and assistive devices while severely disabled, and possibly vocational rehabilitation if permanent disability develops.

Prognosis

Mortality

Current survival rates are higher than those prior to corticosteroids, and improvement continues due to many factors, including better general medical care and use of medications. Better recognition of myositis may lead to inclusion of milder cases or exclusion of other diseases.

Five-year survival between 1970 and 1981 was 80.4 per cent in the United States (Hochberg et al. 1986), and may now be up to 90 per cent (Oddis 2000b), but was 71 per cent in a recent Spanish study. The most common causes of mortality are malignancy, infection, and cardiac and lung manifestations. Factors which increase mortality include older age of onset, cardiac involvement, or ILD. Dysphagia has been associated with increased mortality in some studies. Anti-SRP and antisynthetase autoantibodies were associated with decreased survival, the latter possibly related to ILD (Love et al. 1991). Disease severity has not correlated with poor prognosis. Mortality is increased in the elderly (47.8 versus 7.3 per cent), due to pneumonia related to respiratory and oesophageal weakness, and malignancy (Marie et al. 1999).

Recovery of strength

Prognosis for recovery of full strength is worse if treatment is delayed (Joffe et al. 1993), or if the course is chronic and progressive. Patients whose treatment begins more than 6–12 months after onset may not recover full strength even with complete suppression of disease activity. Older patients may respond less well and may require longer treatment. In general, those with adult DM do better than those with pure PM, and those with overlap syndromes do best (Joffe et al. 1993). Steroid side-effects of compression fracture and avascular necrosis add significantly to disability (Clarke et al. 1995). Antisynthetase patients usually respond initially, but both antisynthetase and anti-SRP patients have a higher frequency of incomplete response and flare with taper.

Inclusion body myositis

IBM is a distinct clinicopathological entity, comprising 15–28 per cent of idiopathic myositis, although it may be overrepresented in referral centers due to treatment resistance. It usually begins after 50, and is the most common muscle disease beginning in this group (Felice and North 2001). It is two- to three-fold more common in males. It can be difficult to distinguish from PM, and is often misdiagnosed at first; this, plus insidious onset, lead to a time to diagnosis of 3–6 years.

Clinical picture

The onset is insidious and progression is slow. Distal weakness is common, seen eventually in 50–95 per cent (Love et al. 1991). It more often involves lower extremities before upper, with leg weakness the most common first symptom (71 per cent) (Felice and North 2001). There is prominence of involvement of the anterior thighs, seen in almost all patients; the forearm flexors, involved in most; and the anterior foreleg. Grip strength is affected early, and patients may eventually be unable to close the hand. Asymmetry occurs more often (61 per cent) than in PM and DM. Falling is a common problem (96 versus 1–17 per cent in PM/DM), possibly related to the severe quadriceps weakness. The knee reflex is reduced or absent within 5 years in most patients. Atrophy is common, especially affecting the thigh and forearm. There have been suggestions of an associated neuropathy, but recent studies have not supported this. Half may have dysphagia at presentation, and cricopharyngeal dysfunction is common.

Laboratory

The CK is usually elevated but typically less than 10-fold normal. The EMG picture usually shows myopathy similar to that of PM, with myopathic potentials and fibrillations, but some show a higher than expected frequency of neuropathic (polyphasic, high-amplitude) potentials, and a portion may have abnormal nerve conduction, consistent with a neuropathic component. MRI typically shows focal, predominantly anterior thigh involvement as observed clinically.

Pathology

The distinctive features of IBM on light microscopy are vacuoles rimmed by basophilic material, and small, refractile, eosinophilic cytoplasmic, and nuclear inclusions. Cytoplasmic inclusions, usually near vacuoles, are composed of distinctive filaments of 15–21 nm. Smaller inclusions are found in the nucleus.

IBM usually shows typical features of inflammatory myopathy, with endomysial inflammatory infiltrates, necrosis and regeneration. In some patients (≈10 per cent), inflammation is very sparse or not evident, despite the presence of inclusions and vacuoles. The inflammatory features are more prominent in the early stages, and the vacuoles are more abundant later, possibly accounting for some initial misdiagnosis. Grouped atrophic fibres and hypertrophied fibres are seen, reminiscent of neuropathy and usually not seen in PM/DM.

The vacuoles and inclusions are seen also in a hereditary myopathy that may take an autosomal dominant or recessive form, which may have different patterns of muscle involvement. 'Hereditary inclusion body myopathy' (hIBM) usually does not show inflammation, in contrast to 'sporadic inclusion body myositis' (sIBM). Rimmed vacuoles can be seen in a variety of other inherited myopathies (Griggs et al. 1995).

Diagnosis

The characteristic histologic features must be demonstrated, and confirmed by electron microscopy or amyloid stain, to establish the diagnosis of 'definite' IBM. If seen, along with the typical inflammatory picture, the diagnosis is established without requirement for clinical criteria. However, these features are not always evident, even in retrospect. Diagnostic criteria have therefore been proposed that allow a diagnosis of 'possible IBM' if these clinical features are observed: slow progression, older onset, typical distribution (including forearm flexor and quadriceps weakness), modest CK elevation (<12 fold), and a consistent inflammatory myopathy by EMG and biopsy. Resistance of PM to treatment should lead to consideration of IBM. Of note is that patients with resistant PM as a group share some key features with IBM, such as lower CK elevations and distal weakness (Amato et al. 1996). IBM can also be mistaken for other conditions, such as motor neuron disease or fascioscapulohumeral dystrophy (Felice and North 2001).

Aetiology and pathogenesis

As with PM/DM, viruses have been suspected, although cultures are usually negative. The inclusions of IBM resemble viral structures such as nucleocapsid proteins of paramyxovirus, but despite early supportive studies, the presence of mumps virus proteins was excluded by PCR and other techniques (Leff et al. 1992).

Both sIBM and hIBM show twisted tubulofilaments that are paired helical filaments similar to those seen in Alzheimer's disease. β amyloid deposits are also seen. Numerous other proteins that have been associated with Alzheimer's disease have also been found, including phosphorylated tau, ubiquitin, ApoE, and others (Askanas and Engel 2001; Oldfors and Fyhr 2001). These findings suggest non-autoimmune mechanisms in IBM, an attractive hypothesis in view of the limited response to immunosuppression. Vacuolation suggestive of IBM can be produced in transgenic mice with expression of mutant β amyloid precursor protein.

Cases of IBM with malignancy have been reported (Oddis 2000b), and an increased frequency of malignancy has been noted, with an SIR of 2.4 (Buchbinder et al. 2001). A small percentage of patients have an association with connective tissue diseases. Otherwise, features such as arthritis or Raynaud's are not usually found. Antinuclear antibodies are found in about 20 per cent, less than PM but more than normal. One study found MSAs or MAAs in several IBM patients (Brouwer et al. 2001), but other studies did not (Love et al. 1991).

The strongest evidence of autoimmunity is the finding of non-necrotic fibres surrounded and invaded by lymphocytes. As in PM, analysis of infiltrating lymphocytes suggests T cell-mediated immune attack on muscle fibres. Such fibres are more abundant than vacuolated fibres, at least at first. However, the possibility that this response is secondary has not been excluded. TCRs showed frequent Vβ3 and Vβ6, which was polyclonal in one of three patients suggesting possible superantigen stimulation, but other evidence suggested an antigen-driven response as seen in PM (Hohlfeld et al. 1997). Muscle fibres in IBM usually show expression of MHC-1 antigen, consistent with the cytotoxic T-cell response, but it is not seen in non-inflammatory biopsies.

HLA–DR3 was significantly associated with sIBM (92 per cent); the susceptibility gene may be between HLA–DR and C4 (Oldfors and Fyhr 2001). Other genes have been studied but no other associations found. The gene for an autosomal recessive form of hIBM that spares the quadriceps has been identified in the chromosome 9p12–13 region (Eisenberg et al. 2001).

Mitochondrial abnormalities are more common in sIBM than normal elderly (Santorelli et al. 1996), with multiple mitochondrial deletions in 73 per cent of patients, but also in 47 per cent of diseased controls. However, this may not be a primary pathology.

Treatment

Patients with IBM do not respond to treatment as well as those with PM. They are less likely to show any response, and those that do will usually not return to normal. Response is more likely when autoimmune features are seen, inflammation is more prominent by biopsy, CK is higher, or when extensive atrophy has not yet occurred (Leff et al. 1993). Retrospective analyses suggest that treatment may slow or stop deterioration, and a small proportion of patients may improve (Cherin 1999). A trial of therapy is generally worthwhile, with recognition of limitations. Some patients benefit from prednisone, but more aggressive therapy appears to do better. As with PM, MTX, and AZA are most often used, or combinations (Cherin 1999). Improvement in CK does not necessarily predict a clinical response. IVGG has been studied both alone and with corticosteroids, and does not provide clinically significant benefit, although individual patients may respond noticeably, and more for dysphagia (Dalakas 1998).

Prognosis

Over time, weakness will progress in most patients, with gradually increasing disability, but progression is very slow. Patients often need assistance with usual activities within 10 years, and may be wheelchair bound within 15, although more prolonged courses may be seen.

References

Adams, E.M. et al. (1997). The predominance of beta (CC) chemokine transcripts in idiopathic inflammatory muscle diseases. *Proceedings of the Association of American Physicians* **109**, 275–85.

Adams, E.M. et al. (1999). A pilot study: use of fludarabine for refractory dermatomyositis and polymyositis, and examination of endpoint measures. *Journal of Rheumatology* **26**, 352–60.

Alexanderson, H. et al. (2000). The safety of a resistive home exercise program in patients with recent onset active polymyositis or dermatomyositis. *Scandinavian Journal of Rheumatology* **29**, 295–301.

Amato, A.A. et al. (1996). Inclusion body myositis: clinical and pathological boundaries. *Annals of Neurology* **40**, 581–6.

Arahata, K. and Engel, A.G. (1984). Monoclonal antibody analysis of mononuclear cells in myopathies. I. Quantitation of subsets according to diagnosis and sites of accumulation and demonstration and counts of muscle fibres invaded by T cells. *Annals of Neurology* **16**, 193–208.

Arnett, F.C. et al. (1996). Interrelationship of major histocompatibility complex class II alleles and autoantibodies in four ethnic groups with various forms of myositis. *Arthritis and Rheumatism* **39**, 1507–18.

Askanas, V. and Engel, W.K. (2001). Inclusion-body myositis: newest concepts of pathogenesis and relation to aging and Alzheimer disease. *Journal of Neuropathology and Experimental Neurology* **60**, 1–14.

Basta, M. and Dalakas, M.C. (1994). High-dose intravenous immunoglobulin exerts its beneficial effect in patients with dermatomyositis by blocking endomysial deposition of activated complement fragments. *Journal of Clinical Investigation* **94**, 1729–35.

Bohan, A. et al. (1977). A computer-assisted analysis of 153 patients with polymyositis and dermatomyositis. *Medicine (Baltimore)* **56**, 255–86.

Brouwer, R. et al. (2001). Autoantibody profiles in the sera of European patients with myositis. *Annals of the Rheumatic Diseases* **60**, 116–23.

Buchbinder, R. et al. (2001). Incidence of malignant disease in biopsy proven inflammatory myopathy. A population-based cohort study. *Annals of Internal Medicine* **134**, 1087–95.

Bunch, T.W. (1981). Prednisone and azathioprine for polymyositis: long-term followup. *Arthritis and Rheumatism* **24**, 45–8.

Casciola-Rosen, L. et al. (1999). Cleavage by granzyme B is strongly predictive of autoantigen status: implications for initiation of autoimmunity. *Journal of Experimental Medicine* **190**, 815–26.

Charness, M.E., Simon, R.P., and Greenberg, D.A. (1989). Ethanol and the nervous system. *New England Journal of Medicine* **321**, 442–54.

Chen, Y.J., Wu, C.Y., and Shen, J.L. (2001). Predicting factors of malignancy in dermatomyositis and polymyositis: a case–control study. *British Journal of Dermatology* **144**, 825–31.

Cherin, P. (1999). Treatment of inclusion body myositis. *Current Opinion in Rheumatology* **11**, 456–61.

Cherin, P. et al. (2000). Gallium-67 scintigraphy in macrophagic myofasciitis. *Arthritis and Rheumatism* **43**, 1520–6.

Clarke, A.E. et al. (1995). A longitudinal study of functional disability in a national cohort of patients with polymyositis/dermatomyositis. *Arthritis and Rheumatism* **38**, 1218–24.

Clawson, K. and Oddis, C.V. (1995). Adult respiratory distress syndrome in polymyositis patients with the anti-Jo-1 antibody. *Arthritis and Rheumatism* **38**, 1519–23.

Cronin, M.E. et al. (1989). The failure of intravenous cyclophosphamide therapy in refractory idiopathic inflammatory myopathy. *Journal of Rheumatology* **16**, 1225–8.

Crowson, A.N., Magro, C.M., and Dawood, M.R. (2000). A causal role for parvovirus B19 infection in adult dermatomyositis and other autoimmune syndromes. *Journal of Cutaneous Pathology* **27**, 505–15.

Dalakas, M.C. (1991). Polymyositis, dermatomyositis, and inclusion-body myositis. *New England Journal of Medicine* **325**, 1487–98.

Dalakas, M.C. (1993). Retroviruses and inflammatory myopathies in humans and primates. *Bailliere's Clinical Neurology* **2**, 659–91.

Dalakas, M.C. (1998). Controlled studies with high-dose intravenous immunoglobulin in the treatment of dermatomyositis, inclusion body myositis, and polymyositis. *Neurology* **51**, S37–S45.

Dietrich, L.L., Bridges, A.J., and Albertini, M.R. (2000). Dermatomyositis after interferon alpha treatment. *Medical Oncology* **17**, 64–9.

Douglas, W.W. et al. (2001). Polymyositis–dermatomyositis associated interstitial lung disease. *American Journal of Respiratory and Critical Care Medicine* **164**, 1182–5.

Drake, L.A. et al. (1996). Guidelines of care for dermatomyositis. American Academy of Dermatology. *Journal of the American Academy of Dermatology* **34**, 824–9.

Eisenberg, I. et al. (2001). The UDP-N-acetylglucosamine 2 epimerase *N*-acetylmannosamine kinase gene is mutated in recessive hereditary inclusion body myositis. *Nature Genetics* **29**, 83–7.

Emslie-Smith, A.M. and Engel, A.G. (1990). Microvascular changes in early and advanced dermatomyositis: a quantitative study. *Annals of Neurology* **27**, 343–56.

Engel, A.G. and Arahata, K. (1984). Monoclonal antibody analysis of mononuclear cells in myopathies. II: Phenotypes of autoinvasive cells in polymyositis and inclusion body myositis. *Annals of Neurology* **16**, 209–15.

Erlacher, P. et al. (2001). Cardiac troponin and beta-type myosin heavy chain concentrations in patients with polymyositis or dermatomyositis. *Clinica Chimica Acta* **306**, 27–33.

Estes, M.L. et al. (1987). Chloroquine neuromyotoxicity: clinical and pathologic perspective. *American Journal of Medicine* **82**, 447–55.

Felice, K.J. and North, W.A. (2001). Inclusion body myositis in Connecticut: observations in 35 patients during an 8-year period. *Medicine (Baltimore)* **80**, 320–7.

Franks, A.G., Jr. (1988). Important cutaneous markers of dermatomyositis. *Journal of Musculoskeletal Medicine* **5**, 39–63.

Gabay, C. et al. (1994). Elevated serum levels of interleukin-1 receptor antagonist in polymyositis/dermatomyositis. A biologic marker of disease activity with a possible role in the lack of acute-phase protein response. *Arthritis and Rheumatism* **37**, 1744–51.

Garton, M.J. and Isenberg, D.A. (1997). Clinical features of lupus myositis versus idiopathic myositis: a review of 30 cases. *British Journal of Rheumatology* **36**, 1067–74.

Ginn, L.R. et al. (1998). Familial autoimmunity in pedigrees of idiopathic inflammatory myopathy patients suggests common genetic risk factors for many autoimmune diseases. *Arthritis and Rheumatism* **41**, 400–5.

Gomez-Reino, J.J. et al. (1994). Nontropical pyomyositis in adults. *Seminars in Arthritis and Rheumatism* **23**, 396–405.

Gonzalez-Lopez, L. et al. (1996). Cardiac manifestations in dermato-polymyositis. *Clinical and Experimental Rheumatology* **14**, 373–9.

Griggs, R.C. et al. (1995). Inclusion body myositis and myopathies. *Annals of Neurology* **38**, 705–13.

Hausmanowa-Petrusewicz, I. et al. (1997). Clinical, serologic, and immunogenetic features in Polish patients with idiopathic inflammatory myopathies. *Arthritis and Rheumatism* **40**, 1257–66.

Hill, C.L. et al. (2001). Frequency of specific cancer types in dermatomyositis and polymyositis: a population-based study. *Lancet* **357**, 96–100.

Hirakata, M. and Nagai, S. (2000). Interstitial lung disease in polymyositis and dermatomyositis. *Current Opinion in Rheumatology* **12**, 501–8.

Hochberg, M.C., Feldman, D., and Stevens, M.B. (1986). Adult onset polymyositis/dermatomyositis: an analysis of clinical and laboratory features and survival in 76 patients with a review of the literature. *Seminars in Arthritis and Rheumatism* **15**, 168–78.

Hohlfeld, R. et al. (1997). Cellular immune mechanisms in inflammatory myopathies. *Current Opinion in Rheumatology* **9**, 520–6.

Joffe, M.M. et al. (1993). Drug therapy of the idiopathic inflammatory myopathies: Predictors of response to prednisone, azathioprine, and methotrexate and a comparison of their efficacy. *American Journal of Medicine* **94**, 379–87.

Kadoya, A. et al. (1996). Risk factors for *Pneumocystis carinii* pneumonia in patients with polymyositis/dermatomyositis or systemic lupus erythematosus. *Journal of Rheumatology* **23**, 1186–8.

Kagen, L.J. (2000). History, physical examination, and laboratory tests in the evaluation of myopathy. In *Diseases of Skeletal Muscle* (ed. R.L. Wortmann), pp. 255–66. Philadelphia PA: Lippincott Williams & Wilkins.

Kalovidouris, A.E., Plotkin, Z., and Graesser, D. (1993). Interferon-gamma inhibits proliferation, differentiation, and creatine kinase activity of cultured human muscle cells. II. A possible role in myositis. *Journal of Rheumatology* **20**, 1718–23.

Kanoh, H. et al. (1999). A case of dermatomyositis that developed after delivery: the involvement of pregnancy in the induction of dermatomyositis. *British Journal of Dermatology* **141**, 897–900.

Kohyama, K. and Matsumoto, Y. (1999). C-protein in the skeletal muscle induces severe autoimmune polymyositis in Lewis rats. *Journal of Neuroimmunology* **98**, 130–5.

Kono, H. et al. (2000). Pneumomediastinum in dermatomyositis: association with cutaneous vasculopathy. *Annals of the Rheumatic Diseases* **59**, 372–6.

Kuncl, R.W. et al. (1987). Colchicine myopathy and neuropathy. *New England Journal of Medicine* **316**, 1562–8.

Leff, R.L. et al. (1992). Viruses in idiopathic inflammatory myopathies: absence of candidate viral genomes in muscle. *Lancet* **339**, 1192–5.

Leff, R.L. et al. (1993). The treatment of inclusion body myositis: a retrospective review and a randomized, prospective trial of immunosuppressive therapy. *Medicine (Baltimore)* **7233**, 225–35.

Lie, J.T. (1995). Cardiac manifestations in polymyositis/dermatomyositis: how to get to the heart of the matter. *Journal of Rheumatology* **22**, 809–11.

Lofberg, M. et al. (1998). Antimyosin scintigraphy compared with magnetic resonance imaging in inflammatory myopathies. *Archives of Neurology* **55**, 987–93.

Love, L.A. and Miller, F.W. (1993). Noninfectious environmental agents associated with myopathies. *Current Opinion in Rheumatology* **5**, 712–18.

Love, L.A. et al. (1991). A new approach to the classification of idiopathic inflammatory myopathy: myositis-specific autoantibodies define useful homogeneous patient groups. *Medicine (Baltimore)* **70**, 360–74.

Lundberg, I.E. and Nyberg, P. (1998). New developments in the role of cytokines and chemokines in inflammatory myopathies. *Current Opinion in Rheumatology* **10**, 521–9.

Lupton, J.R. et al. (2000). An unusual presentation of dermatomyositis: the type Wong variant revisited. *Journal of the American Academy of Dermatology* **43**, 908–12.

Magro, C.M. and Crowson, A.N. (1997). The immunofluorescent profile of dermatomyositis: a comparative study with lupus erythematosus. *Journal of Cutaneous Pathology* **24**, 543–52.

Marguerie, C. et al. (1990). Polymyositis, pulmonary fibrosis and autoantibodies to aminoacyl-tRNA synthetase enzymes. *Quarterly Journal of Medicine* **77**, 1019–38.

Marguerie, C. et al. (1992). The clinical and immunogenetic features of patients with autoantibodies to the nucleolar antigen PM-Scl. *Medicine (Baltimore)* **71**, 327–36.

Marie, I. et al. (1999). Influence of age on characteristics of polymyositis and dermatomyositis in adults. *Medicine (Baltimore)* **78**, 139–47.

Messner, R.P. (2000). Pathogenesis of idiopathic inflammatory myopathies. In *Diseases of Skeletal Muscle* (ed. R.L. Wortmann), pp. 111–27. Philadelphia PA: Lippincott Williams & Wilkins.

Miller, F.W. et al. (1992). Controlled trial of plasma exchange and leukapheresis in polymyositis and dermatomyositis. *New England Journal of Medicine* **326**, 1380–4.

Miller, F.W. et al. (2001). Proposed preliminary core set measures for disease outcome assessment in adult and juvenile idiopathic inflammatory myopathies. *Rheumatology* **40**, 1262–73.

Mozaffar, T. and Pestronk, A. (2000). Myopathy with anti-Jo-1 antibodies: pathology in perimysium and neighbouring muscle fibres. *Journal of Neurology, Neurosurgery and Psychiatry* **68**, 472–8.

Nagaraju, K. (2001). Update on immunopathogenesis in inflammatory myopathies. *Current Opinion in Rheumatology* **13**, 461–8.

Nagaraju, K. et al. (2000). Conditional up-regulation of MHC class I in skeletal muscle leads to self-sustaining autoimmune myositis and myositis-specific autoantibodies. *Proceedings of the National Academy of Sciences USA* **97**, 9209–14.

Nousari, H.C. et al. (1999). 'Centripetal flagellate erythema': a cutaneous manifestation associated with dermatomyositis. *Journal of Rheumatology* **26**, 692–5.

Nyberg, P. et al. (2000). Increased expression of interleukin 1 alpha and MHC class I in muscle tissue of patients with chronic, inactive polymyositis and dermatomyositis. *Journal of Rheumatology* **27**, 940–8.

Nzeusseu, A. et al. (1999). Functional outcome of myositis patients: can a low-dose glucocorticoid regimen achieve good functional results? *Clinical and Experimental Rheumatology* **17**, 441–6.

Oddis, C.V. (2000a). Current approach to the treatment of polymyositis and dermatomyositis. *Current Opinion in Rheumatology* **12**, 492–7.

Oddis, C.V. (2000b). Idiopathic inflammatory myopathies. In *Diseases of Skeletal Muscle* (ed. R.L. Wortmann), pp. 45–85. Philadelphia PA: Lippincott Williams & Wilkins.

Oddis, C.V., Medsger, T.A., Jr., and Cooperstein, L.A. (1990). A subluxing arthropathy associated with the anti-Jo-1 antibody in polymyositis/dermatomyositis. *Arthritis and Rheumatism* **33**, 1640–5.

Oldfors, A. and Fyhr, I.M. (2001). Inclusion body myositis: genetic factors, aberrant protein expression, and autoimmunity. *Current Opinion in Rheumatology* **13**, 469–75.

Park, J.H. and Olsen, N.J. (2000). Skeletal muscle imaging for the evaluation of myopathies. In *Diseases of Skeletal Muscle* (ed. R. L. Wortmann), pp. 293–312. Philadelphia PA: Lippincott Williams & Wilkins.

Park, J.H. et al. (1994). Magnetic resonance imaging and P-31 magnetic resonance spectroscopy provide unique quantitative data useful in the longitudinal management of patients with dermatomyositis. *Arthritis and Rheumatism* **37**, 736–46.

Park, J.H. et al. (1995). Use of magnetic resonance imaging and P-31 magnetic resonance spectroscopy to detect and quantify muscle dysfunction in the amyopathic and myopathic variants of dermatomyositis. *Arthritis and Rheumatism* **38**, 68–77.

Parker, P. et al. (1996). Polymyositis as a manifestation of chronic graft-versus-host disease. *Medicine (Baltimore)* **75**, 279–85.

Patrick, M. et al. (1999). Incidence of inflammatory myopathies in Victoria, Australia, and evidence of spatial clustering. *Journal of Rheumatology* **26**, 1094–100.

Prayson, R.A. (1999). Granulomatous myositis. Clinicopathologic study of 12 cases. *American Journal of Clinical Pathology* **112**, 63–8.

Rider, L.G. and Miller, F.W. (1995). Laboratory evaluation of the inflammatory myopathies. *Clinical and Diagnostic Laboratory Immunology* **2**, 1–9.

Rider, L.G. et al. (1998). Clinical, serologic, and immunogenetic features of familial idiopathic inflammatory myopathy. *Arthritis and Rheumatism* **41**, 710–19.

Rider, L.G. et al. (1999). Genetic risk and protective factors for idiopathic inflammatory myopathy in Koreans and American whites: a tale of two loci. *Arthritis and Rheumatism* **42**, 1285–90.

Santorelli, F.M. et al. (1996). Multiple mitochondrial DNA deletions in sporadic inclusion body myositis: a study of 56 patients. *Annals of Neurology* **39**, 789–95.

Shamim, E.A., Rider, L.G., and Miller, F.W. (2000). Update on the genetics of the idiopathic inflammatory myopathies. *Current Opinion in Rheumatology* **12**, 482–91.

Sherman, M.P. et al. (1995). Identification of human T cell leukemia/lymphoma virus type I antibodies, DNA, and protein in patients with polymyositis. *Arthritis and Rheumatism* **38**, 690–8 (see comments).

Sontheimer, R.D. (1996). Photoimmunology of lupus erythematosus and dermatomyositis: a speculative review. *Photochemistry and Photobiology* **63**, 583–94.

Sontheimer, R.D. (1999). Cutaneous features of classic dermatomyositis and amyopathic dermatomyositis. *Current Opinion in Rheumatology* **11**, 475–82.

Spiera, R. and Kagen, L. (1998). Extramuscular manifestations in idiopathic inflammatory myopathies. *Current Opinion in Rheumatology* **10**, 556–61.

Stoll, T. et al. (1995). Muscle strength assessment in polymyositis and dermatomyositis evaluation of the reliability and clinical use of a new, quantitative, easily applicable method. *Journal of Rheumatology* **22**, 473–7.

Tanimoto, K. et al. (1995). Classification criteria for polymyositis and dermatomyositis. *Journal of Rheumatology* **22**, 668–74.

Targoff, I.N. (1990). Inflammatory muscle disease. In *The Lung in Rheumatic Diseases* (ed. G.W. Cannon and G.A. Zimmerman), pp. 303–28. New York: Marcel Dekker.

Targoff, I.N. (1994). Immune manifestations of inflammatory muscle disease. *Rheumatic Disease Clinics of North America* **20**, 857–80.

Targoff, I.N. (2000). Autoantibodies and muscle disease. In *Diseases of Skeletal Muscle* (ed. R.L. Wortmann), pp. 267–91. Philadelphia PA: Lippincott Williams & Wilkins.

Targoff, I.N. et al. (1997). Classification criteria for the idiopathic inflammatory myopathies. *Current Opinion in Rheumatology* **9**, 527–35.

Uthman, I., Vazquez-Abad, D., and Senecal, J.L. (1996). Distinctive features of idiopathic inflammatory myopathies in French Canadians. *Seminars in Arthritis and Rheumatism* **26**, 447–58.

Vencovsky, J. et al. (2000). Cyclosporine A versus methotrexate in the treatment of polymyositis and dermatomyositis. *Scandinavian Journal of Rheumatology* **29**, 95–102.

Villalba, L. et al. (1998). Treatment of refractory myositis: a randomized crossover study of two new cytotoxic regimens. *Arthritis and Rheumatism* **41**, 392–9.

Whitmore, S.E. et al. (1997). Serum CA-125 screening for ovarian cancer in patients with dermatomyositis. *Gynecologic Oncology* **65**, 241–4.

Ytterberg, S.R. (1994). The relationship of infectious agents to inflammatory myositis. *Rheumatic Disease Clinics of North America* **20**, 995–1016.

Zieglschmid-Adams, M.E. et al. (1995). Treatment of dermatomyositis with methotrexate. *Journal of the American Academy of Dermatology* **32**, 754–7.

Zuckner, J. (1994). Drug-related myopathies. *Rheumatic Disease Clinics of North America* **20**, 1017–32.

6.8.2 Polymyositis and dermatomyositis in children

Lauren M. Pachman

Introduction

Muscle damage in association with an inflammatory infiltrate is recognized in an increasing range of diseases, including those with genetic causes of muscle dysfunction. In North America and Europe, the most common of the inflammatory myopathies in children are associated with acute viral infections, while chronic myositis is often seen as juvenile dermatomyositis (JDM) or polymyositis (JPM). Inflammatory myopathy is also found in other autoimmune diseases, with or without other rheumatic findings, and in parasitic or bacterial infection.

Recent evidence suggests that genetic and infectious factors may play a part in disease susceptibility and disease outcome. The primary clinical feature of both JDM and JPM is chronic and progressive weakness of proximal muscles. In JDM, the vasculopathy and distinctive skin manifestations are associated commonly with muscle involvement; in JPM the skin is spared. Fulfillment of the criteria of Bohan and Peter (1975) establishes the diagnosis of either type of myopathy (Table 1). Newer proposed criteria include MRI evidence of muscle damage. Myositis is often a part of other autoimmune rheumatic diseases and, therefore, it is essential to exclude such conditions as systemic lupus erythematosus, mixed connective tissue disease, juvenile chronic arthritis (especially of systemic onset), the spondyloarthropathies, and Sjögren's syndrome.

Epidemiology

Demographic data

A bimodal age distribution of populations of combined polymyositis (CPM)/dermatomyositis (DM) is seen in the spectrum of inflammatory myopathy, with a childhood peak (at 5–9 years of age, and an adult peak (at 45–64 years of age) (Medsger et al. 1970). In the United Kingdom and Ireland, five times as many girls were diagnosed as boys, with an incidence of 1.9 per million children under the age of 16 years (Symmons et al. 1995) and JDM is the most common of the autoimmune rheumatic diseases. In the United States, Caucasian children with JDM account for 71 per cent of the reported patients followed by 12 per cent in Hispanic children and 9 per cent in children of African-American origin, and twice as many girls as boys are affected (Mendez et al. 2003), although the gender ratio is reversed in the Middle East. JDM occurs at least 20–30 times more often than JPM. In

Table 1 Criteria for diagnosis of JDM and JPM in childhood[a]

1. Symmetric, often progressive, proximal muscle weakness
2. Characteristic electromyographic (EMG) triad seen in myositis
   Short duration, small, low amplitude polyphasic potentials
   Fibrillation potentials, seen even at rest
   Bizarre high-frequency repetitive discharges
3. Elevations of serum levels of muscle-associated enzymes
   Creatine kinase (CK)
   Aldolase
   Lactate dehydrogenase (LD)
   Transaminases (ALT/SGPT and AST/SGOT)
4. Evidence of chronic inflammation in muscle biopsy
   Necrosis of Type I and Type II muscle fibres
   Degeneration and regeneration of myofibres with variation in myofibre size
   Interstitial or perivascular mononuclear cells
5. Characteristic rashes of dermatomyositis
   Scaly erythematous eruptions over the metacarpal-phalangeal or interphalangeal joints (Gottron's papules)
   Periorbital purplish discoloration (Heliotrope rash)
   Erythematous scaly rashes over the face, neck (V-sign), upper back and arms (shawl-sign), and extensor tendons (linear extensor erythema) and other extensor surfaces

Definite disease = all criteria 1–4, except for dermatomyositis in which any 3 of the first 4 criteria plus the rash are adequate;
Probable disease = any 3 of the first 4 criteria, except for dermatomyositis in which any 2 of the first 4 criteria plus the rash are adequate;
Possible disease = any 2 of the first 4 criteria, except for dermatomyositis in which any 1 of the first 4 criteria plus the rash is adequate.

[a] Bohan and Peter (1975).

marked contrast to earlier reports of one-third mortality and one-third morbidity (Bitnum et al. 1964), both of these adverse outcomes have decreased since the advent of steroid therapy, while malignancy or interstitial lung disease remain rare in children (Hiketa et al. 1992). Only sporadic cases of children with both an inflammatory myopathy and malignancy have been cited (Sherry et al. 1993). A 2.9 per cent mortality rate was documented in Japan, during a 10-year period (1973–1983) (Hidano et al. 1986).

JDM disease onset in children appears to vary by year, and perhaps by season. A comparison of disease onset of JDM and PM in Memphis, Tennessee, revealed a seasonal onset (February–April) in 55 per cent of the children (Medsger et al. 1970), which was supported by a later study documenting a January–June time frame for JDM disease onset (Christensen et al. 1986). In the United Kingdom and Ireland (Symmons et al. 1995), and in Canada, (Rosenberg 1994) clustering was observed as well, suggesting an environmental influence. A National Institutes of Health JDM Research Registry of over 323 children with newly diagnosed JDM in the United States (1994–1999) did not identify a particular season when the first symptom (rash and/or weakness) was recognized, but the incidence of JDM appeared to vary by year (Mendez et al. 2003).

Infectious agents and juvenile dermatomyositis

There are several lines of evidence that suggest that JDM may be associated with an antecedent illness, although the specific nature of the agent(s) may vary and have yet to be identified. Reports of antecedent illness in the 3 months prior to the first definite symptom of JDM were greater ($p = 0.03$) than that recalled on interview in an age–region matched national United States case–control study (Pachman et al. 1997). The NIAMS JDM Research Registry data showed that the antecedent symptoms were primarily upper respiratory in nature, requiring antibiotic usage in over 50 per cent (Pachman et al. 1999). Evidence from gene expression profiles from muscle of untreated children with JDM compared with paediatric muscle biopsies proven to be normal, or from children with Duchenne muscular dystrophy, documented a marked increase in IFNα/β inducible immune response genes (some as high as 90-fold), only in the JDM muscle, which was comparable to a viral resistance model (Tezak et al. 2002).

Several agents have been associated with the onset (and on occasion, flare) of JDM. The most prominent are the RNA picornaviruses, group A β-haemolytic streptococci, and *Toxoplasma gondii.* There is inconsistent evidence of increased antibody to CVB in sera taken from children within 3 months of diagnosis of JDM living in the same region, but with disease onset at differing times (Christensen et al. 1986; Pachman et al. 1995). Enteroviral RNA was identified in the muscle of English patients with polymyositis/dermatomyositis (Bowles et al. 1987), but viral RNA was not found in myositis cases from the United States, either in Jo-1 positive adults (Leff et al. 1992), or untreated children with active JDM (Pachman et al. 1995). Other infectious agents have been implicated in JDM, including toxoplasmosis and hepatitis B, but there is no confirmed evidence of these infections in JDM (Christensen et al. 1986; Pachman et al. 1997). Theiler's murine encephalomyelitis virus (TMEV) was identified in an adult with PM, but not in JDM (Rosenberg et al. 1989). In addition, the pathogenesis of JDM may include molecular mimicry, for a protein such as streptococcal type 5M protein stimulates lymphocytes from children with recurrent JDM, and streptococcal infection can induce JDM disease flares (Massa et al. 2002). Taken together, the above data suggest that the probable antigen induced aetiology of JDM may be multifactorial.

Clinical presentation

Cutaneous findings

In JDM, the rash may predate (25 per cent) or follow (25 per cent) the onset of symmetrical weakness in proximal muscles. The rash has a violaceous or heliotrope hue, and is almost always seen on the eyelid, where small infarctions may develop (Plate 135) as well as the malar region, crossing the bridge of the nose. Oedema may be generalized or localized to the periorbital region, and resolves with appropriate therapy. Eyelid telangiectasia, which may persist, is found in 50–90 per cent of affected children. Sunlight may exacerbate the skin manifestations alone or may activate symptoms of myositis. Erythema may involve the upper anterior thorax (shawl area), the extensor surfaces of the arms and legs, medial malleoli of the ankles, as well as the buttocks, in the absence of raised serum concentrations of muscle-derived enzymes (see below). The skin over the knuckles is often either hypertrophic or pale red, evolving into colourless bands of atrophic skin (Gottron's sign). The hypertrophic areas (alligator skin) can also appear on the extensor aspect of the elbows or knees, or the medial aspect of the eyelid. The peripheral lipoatrophy may not be tender despite a lymphohistiocytic infiltrate, while acanthosis nigricans, associated with insulin-resistant diabetes, may occasionally be found in the skin folds. Diffuse vasculopathy (nailbed telangiectasia, infarction of oral epithelium and skin folds, or digital ulceration) is associated with more severe disease. Calcinosis is seen in 23 per cent of cases at diagnosis (Pachman et al. 1998), and appears to be associated with disease severity and duration (Pachman et al. 1985).

Musculoskeletal symptoms

Proximal muscle weakness as evidenced by difficulty in climbing stairs, getting up from a chair, combing hair, or using the hands to push off the body in an attempt to stand (Gower's sign). Weakness of the neck flexors is a particularly sensitive indicator, and muscle pain on compression is present in 60 per cent of children at diagnosis. Fatigue is common, and is also seen in the dystrophies (most commonly those of Duchenne and Becker) as well. The most frequent symptoms of JDM at diagnosis are listed in Table 2. The child is more comfortable when the limbs are flexed, promoting the development of contractures. The use of MRI-directed biopsies minimizes error in sampling uninvolved areas in this focal disease (Hernandez et al. 1993), and detects occult subcutaneous changes. The MRI may normalize several months after the muscle enzymes return to the normal ranges, and P-32

Table 2 Juvenile dermatomyositis symptoms at diagnosis

Rash	79 (100)
Weakness	79 (100)
Muscle pain	58 (73)
Fever	51 (65)
Dysphagia	35 (44)
Hoarseness	34 (43)
Abdominal pain	29 (37)
Arthritis	28 (35)
Calcifications	18 (23)
Melena	10 (13)

Source: Pachman et al. (1998b).

spin MRI can reflect mitochondrial damage in the muscle (Park et al. 2001). Decreased bone density (associated with a depressed serum osteocalcin) is frequent in untreated JDM and places the child at risk of bony fracture (Reed et al. 1990), which is further augmented by steroid administration.

Gastrointestinal involvement

Impairment of the flow of secretions associated with decreased oesophageal motility is a very poor prognostic sign. Radiographic contrast studies show retained barium in a widened atonic, pyriform sinus and/or airway penetration. Oesophageal reflux may result in aspiration pneumonia and appropriate precautions should be taken to prevent this (e.g. using thickened foods, raising the bed head, and bronchial drainage). Smooth muscle dysfunction can also result in decreased lower-gastrointestinal dysmotility, making constipation an annoying symptom. Involvement of the masseter may result in difficulty in chewing; chronic masseter/bussal fat pad atrophy is often apparent once long standing disease has become quiescent. Vasculopathy affects any part of the gastrointestinal tract; in severe disease there is weight loss and mucosal ulceration with life-threatening perforation. In the young child, soft palate involvement is often revealed by nasal, high-pitched speech (e.g. by saying 'E') and usually resolves.

Cardiorespiratory abnormalities

The ECG demonstrates asymptomatic conduction diagnosis in over half the children with definite JDM, which usually resolves. Decreased ventilatory capacity, with abnormal diffusion of carbon dioxide was found in 78 per cent of children with JDM (sero negative for tRNA synthetase antibody who tested 20 years later) who had no respiratory complaints (Pachman and Cooke 1980). The decrease in ventilatory capacity can be associated with diminished speech volume and several of our children have developed vocal cord nodules. Myositis-specific antibodies (MSA) (Love et al. 1991) are rare in children, and, while not cost effective (Feldman et al. 1996), can help to guide therapy. For example, antibodies such tRNA synthetases or signal recognition protein (SRP) are highly associated with an unremitting disease course. The few children with Jo-1 (Rider and Miller 1997) are similar to adults and are characterized by dyspnoea on exertion, a pulmonary perfusion deficit with evidence of pulmonary fibrosis and disease flares with the reduction of therapy. The most common MSA in children is Mi-2 (an anti-helicase antibody), which may be associated with pulmonary disease in later life.

Genitourinary involvement

Massive breakdown of muscle elements as well as primary compromise of the renal parenchyma itself, can occur in children and requires prompt hydration and monitoring of renal function. If unchecked, renal failure can occur. Necrosis of the ureter has been reported, involving the middle one-third (iliac) segment, which is more vulnerable to vascular compromise as a consequence of inflammation. This vulnerability occurs because of the relatively sparse blood supply to this region compared with the upper (lumbar) or lower (pelvic) segments (Borrelli et al. 1988).

Eye signs

The most common findings are dilated vessels at the margin of the upper eyelid, which may persist for years. In active disease, transient retinal exudates and 'cotton wool' spots may occur after the occlusion of small vessels, leading to intraretinal oedema with injury to retinal nerve fibres, optic atrophy, and sustained visual loss. Isolated orbital myositis, a rare form of focal myositis, can also be seen in children. Children treated with steroids should be monitored for both glaucoma and for the development of sublenticular cataracts, which may resolve as the steroids are tapered. If there is a family history of red–green colour blindness, the use of hydroxychloroquine should be avoided.

Other disease manifestations

Vasculopathy involving the central nervous system may be associated with depression and/or wide mood swings, which may be exacerbated by steroid therapy (see below). It is not usual for a child with JDM to present with Raynaud's phenomenon; these symptoms are found more frequently in overlap syndromes and are associated with antibodies to ribonucleoprotein or Pm/Scl.

Differential diagnosis of juvenile dermatomyositis

General

The differential diagnosis of this inflammatory myopathy includes many of the major neuromuscular disorders of infancy and childhood as well as metabolic and infectious diseases, which can be symptomatic at any age. Table 3 presents most of the potential candidates for consideration.

Skin

Many of the other autoimmune diseases exhibit some of the cutaneous signs of JDM. As in systemic lupus, exposure to sun can exacerbate both the malar rash as well as the systemic complaints in children with dermatomyositis. Gottron's sign can be mimicked by psoriatic lesions, accompanied by healing foci of hypopigmentation found in areas usually unaffected in JDM, such as the pretibial region. These rashes may clear with sun exposure, rather than becoming more prominent. We have observed that psoriasis can emerge, once the JDM symptoms have resolved. Telangiectasia, a prominent feature of scleroderma, also occurs in overlap syndromes. Capillary end loop destruction, which results in avascularity, can be monitored using nailfold capillary microscopy and helps differentiate JDM from some of the other vasculopathies (Pachman et al. 2000a).

Muscle complaints

Weakness of symmetrical proximal muscles is the predominant symptom, but pain on muscle compression in not uncommon. Other conditions associated with muscle cramps and contractures include hypothyroidism, uraemia, and electrolyte imbalance such as hypokalemia. Pain that awakens the child at night should be investigated for another cause such as malignancy, osteoid osteoma, or osteomyelitis. Weakness can be associated with hormonal derangements, either endogenous or iatrogenic, such as in adrenal, thyroid, pituitary, or parathyroid dysfunction, or after long-term high-dose steroid administration. Metabolic muscle diseases include defects of glycolysis (e.g. phosphofructokinase deficiency) and are associated with contractures, exercise intolerance, myoglobinuria, and a positive ischaemic lactate test. There may be a defect in lipid metabolism such as a carnitine deficiency state, which may be exacerbated by non-steroidal anti-inflammatory

Table 3 Classification of the major neuromuscular disorders of infancy and childhood

1.	Drug- and toxin-induced myopathies
	Corticosteroids
	Lipid lowering drugs
	Colcichine
	Chloroquine
	L-Tryptophan (eosinophilia myalgia syndrome)
	Ethanol
	D-Penicillamine
	Ipecac
	Zidovudine (AZT)
2.	Endocrine diseases
	Hypothyroidism
	Acromegaly
	Hyperthyroidism
	Diabetes mellitus
3.	Neurologic disorders
	Amyotrophic lateral sclerosis
	Multiple sclerosis
	Motor neuron disease
	Myasthenia gravis
	Guillain-Barré syndrome
4.	Other connective tissue diseases
	Polymyalgia rheumatica
	Systemic sclerosis
	Rheumatoid arthritis
	Tendinitis and overuse syndromes
5.	Metabolic abnormalities
	Hypokalaemia
	Hypercalcaemia
6.	Inherited metabolic defects
	Acid maltase deficiency
	Phosphorylase deficiency (McArdle disease)
	Lipid metabolic defects (carnitine or carnitine palmityltransferase deficiency)
	Phosphofructokinase deficiency
7.	Dystrophies
	Duchenne/Becker
	Limb-girdle
	Dysferlin
	Fascioscapulohumeral
	Myotonic
8.	Infectious myopathies
	Bacterial (pyomyositis)
	Parasitic
	Viral, including HIV and HTLV-I and -II
9.	Mitochondrial myopathies

Source: Pachman (2003).

drugs; or a myalgia syndrome, which can be detected by a positive ischaemic ammonia test. Inclusion-body myositis, which often runs a steroid-resistant course, has also been described in both the familial and sporadic forms in children.

Acute infectious viral myositis in children, most frequently attributed to influenza A or B, is differentiated clinically from chronic myositis by its localization to the muscles of the calf, severe pain, and rapid resolution in 1–4 weeks (Mejlszenkier et al. 1973). Adults with HIV or HTLV-1 may also have muscle complaints, as do the children with these illnesses.

Other autoimmune rheumatic disorders may also be accompanied by inflammatory muscle disease. For example, children with systemic-onset juvenile arthritis, spiking fevers, and an evanescent rash may complain on muscle compression and have an MRI positive for muscle involvement. Children with antibody to RNP or PM/Sc are less likely to have complete resolution of their symptoms, requiring long-term therapy.

Electromyogram

Evidence of an inflammatory myopathy on electromyography is not specific to JDM and is similar in other autoimmune rheumatic disorders which have a myopathic component. Selection of a focal site of active involvement is facilitated by MRI. Once the location of the electrodes has been chosen (not the site of a future biopsy), insertional irritability, followed by spontaneous electrical activity at rest is often observed, but may be also seen in the muscular dystrophies and in early acute myositis. Abnormal early full recruitment of muscle fibres with moderate effort occurs in about 45 per cent of patients with JDM, and bizarre, high-frequency discharges occur in 15–20 per cent of patients tested. Reduced motor unit activity is seen in Duchenne muscular dystrophy as well as in JDM.

Pathophysiology of juvenile dermatomyositis

Vascular findings

The vasculopathy of this disease may occur in the absence of a prominent inflammatory component, and is very characteristic of children with JDM (Banker and Victor 1966). In JDM, damage to capillaries, venules, and small arteries causes loss of the capillary network resulting in structural change in the nailfold capillary bed as well as in muscle, with a subsequent decrease in the capillary/fibre ratio.

Muscle pathology

The muscle pathology in JDM also reflects vascular compromise and capillary dropout (Silver and Maricq 1989), with perifascicular atrophy of both type I and type II fibres (Plate 136). Muscle biopsies from JDM children have altered mitochondria as a consequence of cytotoxic damage and/or ischaemia, suggesting a cytotoxic mechanism (Engel and Arahata 1986). We have identified an increased number of CD56+ cells in untreated muscle biopsies taken from JDM patients with symptoms for less than 3 months duration (Pachman et al. 1998a, 2000c) in association with activation of the TRAIL pathway of apoptosis. The range of mechanism(s) of target damage are not yet clearly defined for untreated children of varying genetic backgrounds at different stages of disease duration and activity.

Pathological calcification in soft tissues

The aetiology of the pathological calcification must be clinically differentiated from other conditions in which calcinosis occurs, such as in heterotopic calcinosis or following trauma. The genetic background of the child may predispose the development of calcification, for JDM children with an A polymorphism at the -308 promoter region of the TNFα gene locus not only synthesize more TNFα, but have an increased frequency of pathological calcifications (Pachman et al. 2000b). Sepsis is not uncommon in this event and is a major contributor to morbidity and mortality. Calcinosis is accompanied by increased urinary excretion of γ-carboxyglutamic acid (GLA), found in the vitamin K-dependent coagulation pathway (Lian et al. 1982). Calcifications are not associated with antinuclear antibody, immune complexes, or class II HLA antigens (Pachman et al. 1985). Their composition includes hydroxyapatite, macrophages, IL-6, and TNFα (Mukamel et al. 2001), in addition to components also found in calcified heart valves (Pachman et al. 2001).

Immunological, genetic, and haematological data

Immunological data

Children with active untreated JDM are lymphopaenic (O'Gorman et al. 1995), and have an increased percentage of B cells (defined by anti-CD19 monoclonal antibody) (Eisenstein et al. 1997). The increased percentage of B cells is often correlated with an elevated disease activity score (Bode et al. 2002), and frequently remain elevated despite normalization of serum levels of muscle enzymes (Pachman 1995). The CD4:CD8 cell ratio is increased (decrease in circulating CD8+ cells) and non-CD19 positive cells (T cells) that are ICAM-1 positive are depleted from the circulation (O'Gorman et al. 2000). Clonal expansion of T cells in the muscle of children with new-onset untreated JDM is also observed (Pachman et al. 1998a).

Humoral immunity may be abnormal in a minority of patients: in early disease, IgM (Pachman and Cooke 1980) or IgG (O'Gorman et al. 1995) may be elevated or IgA deficiency may be present (Pachman and Cooke 1980). Tests for a spectrum of antibodies with tissue or organ specificity were negative when comparing sera from patients with newly diagnosed JDM with age-/sex-matched controls. Only the antinuclear antibodies (ANA) and antibody to the polymyositis antigen-1 (PM-1) were more frequent in patients than controls (Pachman et al. 1985). The ANA has a speckled and cytoskeletal pattern in 60–70 per cent of children (often in modest titres), often with a specificity for a 56 kDa protein (Cambridge et al. 1994), and is found in association with the DQA1*0501 allele (Lutz et al. 2001).

Complement activation has been implicated in several studies that included children with JDM (Kissel et al. 1991). Immune complexes may be present, with complement activation (despite normal levels of total complement, C3 and C4) accompanied by increased plasma levels of fibrinopeptide A and von Willebrand factor antigen (Scott and Arroyave 1987). Neopterin levels (T-cell dependent macrophage product) are increased in about 60 per cent of active JDM (DeBenedetti et al. 1993).

Genetic studies

Maternal factors appear to play an important role in susceptibility to JDM. Two independent groups reported the increased frequency of maternal chimerism in males who developed JDM (Arlett et al. 2000; Reed et al. 2000). Records of JDM affecting more than one family member are sporadic, but the disease has been reported in monozygotic twins, who developed muscle-related abnormalities 2 weeks after an upper respiratory tract infection (Harati et al. 1986). There is a stronger association of the HLA antigen, DQA1*0501 in all racial groups (Reed et al. 1991; Reed and Stirling 1995), than with HLA B8 (Friedman et al. 1983a) or DR3 (Friedman et al. 1983b). The DQA1*0501 allele is in close proximity to the TNFα-308 region, and polymorphism in this area is associated with prolonged disease duration, pathological calcifications (Pachman et al. 2000b), and increased production of TNFα by both isolated peripheral blood mononuclear cells, as well as muscle fibres in biopsies from untreated children with JDM (Fedczyna et al. 2001), which may contribute to the vasculopathy of the disease.

Haematological data

In children with JDM, the usual indicators of an acute-phase reaction are often within normal range, although children with acute severe disease or infected sites of calcinosis may have elevated values. The lymphopaenia is commonly accompanied by a normal platelet count and a mild microcytic anaemia may be present. The von Willebrand factor antigen, released from damaged endothelial cells, is correlated with disease activity in some but not all children. These clues to disease activity—the MRI, neopterin, von Willebrand factor antigen, and peripheral lymphocyte phenotype—are of substantial aid in characterizing the ongoing inflammatory process.

Course and therapy

Course

The outcome of JDM has improved greatly since the 1960s when one-third of the children died, one-third were crippled, and the remainder recovered (Bitnum et al. 1964). Several types of disease course have been described—monocyclic, recurrent, and continuous (Spencer et al. 1984). The magnitude of the initial creatine kinase appears to be a direct correlate of disease severity (van Rossum et al. 1994). The frequency of calcinosis in some series (which was associated with loss of mobility) has decreased from over 60 per cent of cases to undetectable (Callen et al. 1994), while late disease recurrence after years of apparent inactivity may dispose to calcification. Despite evidence of persistent rash and weakness (Huber et al. 2000), as well as arthritis (Tse et al. 2001), the children achieve good socio-economic status as adults (Chalmers et al. 1982). Polymorphism at the TNFα-308 allele is associated with a prolonged JDM disease course (requiring immunotherapy for 36 months or more) (Pachman 2000b). Partial lipodystrophy in JDM has been reported by many observers, and a recent investigation suggests that 25 per cent of patients with JDM already have this condition (Huemer et al. 2001).

Therapy

There is continuing controversy over the type, duration, and route of medication to be instituted. Recommendations are imperfect and there is a lack of long-term outcome data. Medical practices have changed in the recent past, and it is not known how this change will affect the children's course in the future—both the consequences of the autoimmune disease and its therapy. A summary of one approach to the treatment of JDM is given in Box 1.

High-dose intravenous intermittent (pulse) methylprednisolone (IVMP) has been used for the treatment of JDM over the past 2 decades (Miller 1980). JDM children receiving IVPM therapy compared with 2 mg/kg of

Box 1 An approach to the evaluation and treatment of juvenile dermatomyositis

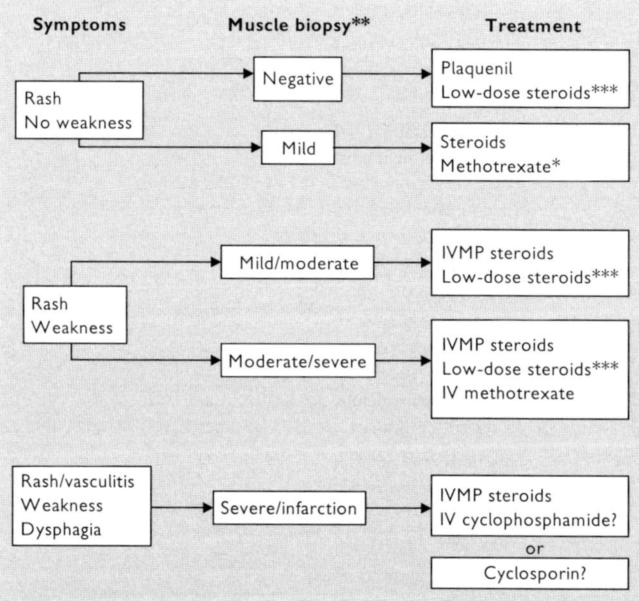

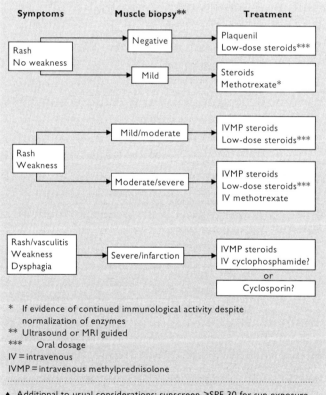

* If evidence of continued immunological activity despite normalization of enzymes
** Ultrasound or MRI guided
*** Oral dosage
IV = intravenous
IVMP = intravenous methylprednisolone

- Additional to usual considerations: sunscreen >SPF 30 for sun exposure, Ca^{2+} in diet
- If positive for Jo-1, myositis-associated antibody, perform pulmonary function tests with DLCO
- If osteocalcin is low, consider bone mineral density, exogenous 1,25 vitamin D
- If immunosuppression leads to low IgG, may require replacement of IV IgG (0.4 g/kg every 4 weeks)
- Other considerations: evaluation of renal and cardiac function

oral prednisone/day had a shorter disease course with respect to persistence of rash (1.5 versus 3.9 years), weakness (1.5 versus 2.7 years), and did not have calcinosis or growth retardation, although the frequency of cataracts was the same in both groups (Callen et al. 1994). A subset of this group with a monocyclic disease course was subjected to a cost analysis: the intravenously treated group had two disease-free years, but their bill was about US$10 000 higher than those given oral therapy (Klein-Gitelman et al. 2000). Cost differences associated with long-term outcomes are not known. We and others (Al Mayouf et al. 2000) have found that the addition of methotrexate early in the therapy has shortened the duration of immunosuppression required.

In our centre, the child with active JDM is thoroughly evaluated on admission. If there is evidence of dysphagia or difficulty in handling secretions, then IV methotrexate at a starting dose of 15 mg/M^2, is administered immediately following the IVMP (30 mg/kg/day, 1 g maximum, in 100 ml D5W, given over at least 30 min with monitoring of vital signs every 15 min for 30 min after the infusion is completed). Low-dose oral steroids, at 0.5 mg/day are given in the morning on the days that the IVMP is not infused. The protocol for each child is individual and IVMP is administered on a frequent basis until all the laboratory tests normalize. The use of IVMP is not without some side-effects. In an analysis of the drug usage over a 5-year period in which 213 children with various types of serious rheumatic disease were given over 2622 doses, 46 children (22 per cent) experienced an adverse reaction. Behavioural changes (21 children) ranged from euphoria to emotional lability. There was one case of anaphylaxis (Klein-Gitelman and Pachman 1998).

When there is severe skin involvement, hydroxychloroquine (7 mg/kg/day) is given if there is no family history of red–green colour blindness. Topical agents to lessen dryness help the occasional pruritis as do topical steroids, which should be used sparingly. For breaks in the integument, a 'skin substitute' (e.g. 'second skin', duoderm) should be considered. Sepsis secondary to infected calcinosis must be treated aggressively.

Children with severe disease, or those who do not respond to steroids, have been treated with methotrexate for the past 2 decades. Use of this drug (IV, weekly) in doses that start at 15 mg/M^2/week has reduced the morbidity of the disease (Miller L.C. et al. 1992). Complaints of nausea may be circumvented by dividing the dose given within a 24-h period or by using antiemetic agents. The function of the liver and bone marrow must be monitored. If the child's condition deteriorates, cyclosporine A is started, and the trough levels monitored, as well as potential toxic damage. For an acute non-responsive vasculitic state, intravenous cyclophosphamide therapy, starting at 500 mg/m^2 every 3 weeks (following adequate hydration), with mesna for bladder protection, is instituted and the methotrexate is discontinued. As with immunosuppression regimes, levels of IgG must be checked on a periodic basis to ensure that they are adequate; if not, replacement therapy (0.4 g/kg every 3–4 weeks) may be needed to prevent recurrent infections. On rare occasions, we have used ECMO, and have rescued a child with severe disease.

When considering therapies other than steroids, high-dose (not replacement) intravenous gammaglobulin may initially ameliorate the inflammatory process, especially the rash (Roifman et al. 1987) if given early in the disease course. Plasmapheresis alone does not appear to be effective in adults (Miller et al. 1992) and no data is available for children. Formal evaluation of the efficacy of cyclosporin has been proposed (Heckmatt et al. 1989) but has been hampered by coexisting therapies (Pistoia et al. 1993). FK506 has been useful in the therapy of adults with Jo-1 myopathy (Oddis 2000), but no published data are available for children. Preliminary data concerning the use of entanercept in five children with chronic JDM symptoms (<36 months) was not encouraging, but the subjects were not selected on the basis of their TNFα-308A allele (Miller et al. 2000).

There are no successful therapies for long-standing calcinosis in children with inactive disease, although there is one report of alondronate inducing their resolution (Mukamel et al. 2001), it has not been confirmed. Pathological calcifications may diminish with control of the inflammation. Osteoporosis, a consequence of disease activity as well as corticosteroid therapy, can be slowed or reversed in children using a calcium-sufficient diet, and the addition of thrice-weekly (Monday, Wednesday, Friday) 1,25-vitamin D, in conjunction with disease control. This may aid in calcium absorption from the gastrointestinal tract in the face of steroid therapy (which inhibits calcium absorption).

Combined drug treatment (to suppress inflammation) and physiotherapy (gentle, passive stretching) are required in the early phase of the disease, and more intensive, graded physiotherapy is effective later in the disease, once the inflammation has abated. Prevention of sunburn, both by avoidance and barriers (clothing, UVA/UVB PABA-free sunblocks over SPF 30) helps keep the disease in remission.

In summary, juvenile dermatomyositis, characterized by a genetically restricted and immunologic mediated vasculopathy, elicited in response to a probable antigenic agent, is under intense investigation. These are exciting times, for as more knowledge of the specific pathophysiology of the disease(s) is accrued, more effective therapeutic interventions will be devised.

Acknowledgements

This work was supported in part by grants, P60-AR-30692, R01-AR-4-3978, and NO1-AR-4-2219, from the National Institute of Arthritis, Musculoskeletal and Skin disorders, and from the Arthritis Foundation, as well as children with JDM and their families.

References

Al Mayouf, S., Al Mazyed, A., and Bahabri, S. (2000). Efficacy of early treatment of severe juvenile dermatomyositis with intravenous methylprednisolone and methotrexate. *Clinical Rheumatology* **19**, 138–41.

Artlett, C.M. et al. (2000). Chimeric cells of maternal origin in juvenile idiopathic inflammatory myopathies. Childhood myositis heterogeneity collaborative group. *Lancet* **356**, 2155–6.

Banker, B.Q. and Victor, M. (1966). Dermatomyositis (systemic angiopathy) of childhood. *Medicine* **45**, 261–89.

Bitnum, C., Dawschnor, C.W., and Travis, L.B. (1964). Dermatomyositis. *Journal of Pediatrics* **64**, 101–31.

Bode, R.K. et al. (2003). Disease activity score for children with Juvenile Dermatomyositis (JDM): reliability and validity evidence. *Arthritis Care Research* **49**, 7–15.

Bohan, A. and Peter, J.B. (1975). Polymyositis and dermatomyositis (parts 1 and 2). *New England Journal of Medicine* **292**, 344–7, 403–7.

Borrelli, M.P. et al. (1988). Ureteral necrosis in dermatomyositis. *Journal of Urology* **139**, 1275–7.

Bowles, N.E. et al. (1987). Dermatomyositis, polymyositis, and coxsackie-B-virus infection. *Lancet* **ii**, 1004–7.

Callen, A.M. et al. (1994). Intermittent high-dose intravenous methylprednisolone (IV pulse) therapy prevents calcinosis and shortens disease course in juvenile dermatomyositis (JDMS). *Arthritis and Rheumatism* **37**, R10.

Cambridge, G. et al. (1994). Juvenile dermatomyositis: serial studies of circulating autoantibodies to a 56 kD nuclear protein. *Clinical and Experimental Rheumatology* **12**, 451–7.

Chalmers, A., Sayson, R., and Walters, K. (1982). Juvenile dermatomyositis: medical, social and economic status in adulthood. *Canadian Medical Association Journal* **126**, 31–3.

Christensen, M.L. et al. (1986). Prevalence of coxsackie B virus antibodies in patients with juvenile dermatomyositis. *Arthritis and Rheumatism* **29**, 1365–70.

DeBenedetti, F. et al. (1993). Correlations of serum neopterin concentrations with disease activity in juvenile dermatomyositis. *Archives of the Diseases of Children* **69**, 232–5.

Eisenstein, D.M., O'Gorman, M.R., and Pachman, L.M. (1997). Correlations between change in disease activity and changes in peripheral blood lymphocyte subsets in patients with juvenile dermatomyositis. *Journal of Rheumatology* **24**, 1830–2.

Engel, A.G. and Arahata, K. (1986). Mononuclear cells in myopathies: quantitation of functionally distinct subsets, recognition of antigen-specific cell-mediated cytotoxicity in some diseases, and implications for the pathogenesis of the different inflammatory myopathies. *Human Pathology* **17**, 704–21.

Fedczyna, T.O., Lutz, J., and Pachman, L.M. (2001). Expression of TNFα by muscle fibers in biopsies from children with untreated juvenile dermatomyositis: association with the TNFα-308A allele. *Clinical Immunology* **100**, 236–9.

Feldman, B.M. et al. (1996). Clinical significance of specific autoantibodies in juvenile dermatomyositis. *Journal of Rheumatology* **23**, 1794–7.

Friedman, J.M. et al. (1983a). Immunogenetic studies of juvenile dermatomyositis: HLA antigens in patients and their families. *Tissue Antigens* **21**, 45–9.

Friedman, J.M. et al. (1983b). Immunogenetic studies of juvenile dermatomyositis: HLA–DR antigen frequencies. *Arthritis and Rheumatism* **26**, 214–16.

Harati, Y., Niakan, E., and Bergman, E.W. (1986). Childhood dermatomyositis in monozygotic twins. *Neurology* **36**, 721–3.

Heckmatt, J.Z. et al. (1987). Cyclosporin in juvenile dermatomyositis. *Lancet* 1063–6.

Hernandez, R.J., Sullivan, D.B., and Chenevert, T.L. (1993). MR imaging in children with dermatomyositis: musculoskeletal findings and correlation with clinical and laboratory findings. *American Journal of Roentgenology* **161**, 359–66.

Hidano, A., Keneka, K., and Arai, Y. (1986). Survey of the prognosis for dermatomyositis with special reference to its associated malignancy and pulmonary fibrosis. *Journal of Dermatology* **13**, 233–41.

Hiketa, T. et al. (1992). Juvenile dermatomyositis: a statistical study of 114 patients with dermatomyositis. *Journal of Dermatology* **19**, 470–6.

Huber, A.M. et al. (2000). Medium- and long-term functional outcomes in a multicenter cohort of children with juvenile dermatomyositis. *Arthritis and Rheumatism* **43**, 541–9.

Huemer, C. et al. (2001). Lipodystrophy in patients with juvenile dermatomyositis—evaluation of clinical and metabolic abnormalities. *Journal of Rheumatology* **28**, 610–15.

Kissel, J.T. et al. (1991). The relationship of complement-mediated microvasculopathy to the histologic features and clinical duration of disease in dermatomyositis. *Archives of Neurology* **48**, 26–30.

Klein-Gitelman, M.S. and Pachman, L.M. (1998). Intravenous pulse corticosteroids (CS): adverse reactions are more variable than expected in children. *Journal of Rheumatology* **25**, 1995–2002.

Klein-Gitelman, M.S., Waters, T., and Pachman, L.M. (2000). The economic impact of intermittent high-dose intravenous versus oral corticosterol treatment of juvenile dermatomyositis. *Arthritis Care and Research* **13**, 360–8.

Leff, R.L. et al. (1992). Viruses in idiopathic inflammatory myopathies: absence of candidate viral genomes in muscle. *Lancet* **339**, 1192–5.

Lian, J.B. et al. (1982). Gamma-carboxyglutamate excretion and calcinosis in juvenile dermatomyositis. *Arthritis and Rheumatism* **25**, 1094–100.

Love, L.A. et al. (1991). A new approach to the classification of idiopathic inflammatory myopathy: myositis-specific autoantibodies define useful homogeneous patient groups. *Medicine (Baltimore)* **70**, 360–74.

Lutz, J.L. et al. (2001). The association of the DQA1*0501 allele and antibody to a 56kD nuclear protein in sera from patients with juvenile dermatomyositis (JDM). *Arthritis and Rheumatism* **44**, S293.

Massa, M. et al. (2002). Self-epitopes shared between human skeletal myosin and Streptococcus pyogenes M5 protein are targets of immune responses in active juvenile dermatomyositis. *Arthritis and Rheumatism* **46**, 3015–25.

Medsger, T.A., Jr., Dawson, W.N., Jr., and Masi, A.T. (1970). The epidemiology of polymyositis. *American Journal of Medicine* **48**, 715–23.

Mejlszenkier, J.D., Safran, A.E., and Healy, J.J. (1973). The myositis of influenza. *Archives of Neurology* **29**, 441–3.

Mendez, E.P. et al. (2003). U.S. incidence of JDM 1995–98: results from the NIAMS Registry. *Arthritis Care Research* **49**, 300–5.

Miller, J.J., III (1980). Prolonged use of large intravenous steroid pulses in the rheumatic diseases of children. *Pediatrics* **65**, 989–94.

Miller, F.W. et al. (1992). Controlled trial of plasma exchange and leukapheresis in polymyositis and dermatomyositis. *New England Journal of Medicine* **326**, 1380–4.

Miller, L.C. et al. (1992). Methotrexate treatment of recalcitrant childhood dermatomyositis. *Arthritis and Rheumatism* **35**, 1143–9.

Miller, M.L. et al. (2000). Experience with etanercept in chronic juvenile dermatomyositis (JDM). *Arthritis and Rheumatism* **43**, 1883.

Mukamel, M., Horev, G., and Mimouni, M. (2001). New insight into calcinosis of juvenile dermatomyositis: a study of composition and treatment. *Journal of Pediatrics* **138**, 763–6.

Oddis, C.V. (2000). Current approach to the treatment of polymyositis and dermatomyositis. *Current Opinion in Rheumatology* **6**, 492–7.

O'Gorman, M.R.G. et al. (1995). Flow cytometric analysis of the lymphocyte subsets in peripheral blood of children with untreated active juvenile dermatomyositis. *Clinical, Diagnostic and Laboratory Immunology* **2**, 205–8.

O'Gorman, M.R.G. et al. (2000). Decreased CD54(ICAM-1) positive non-CD19+ lymphocytes in the peripheral blood of untreated children with active symptoms of juvenile dermatomyositis. *Clinical, Diagnostic and Laboratory Immunology* **7**, 693–7.

Pachman, L.M. (2003). Juvenile dermatomyositis and other inflammatory myopathies in children. In *Neuromuscular Disorders of Infancy and Childhood: A Clinician's Approach* (ed., H.R. Jones, Jr., D.C. De Vivo, B.T. Darras, and M.A. Woburn), pp. 901–37. Philadelphia PA: Butterworth-Heinemann.

Pachman, L.M. and Cooke, N. (1980). Juvenile dermatomyositis: a clinical and immunologic study. *Journal of Pediatrics* **96**, 226–34.

Pachman, L.M. et al. (1985). Immunogenetic studies of juvenile dermatomyositis. III. Study of antibody to organ-specific and nuclear antigens. *Arthritis and Rheumatism* **28**, 151–7.

Pachman, L.M. et al. (1995). Lack of detection of enteroviral RNA or bacterial DNA in MRI directed muscle biopsies from twenty children with active untreated juvenile dermatomyositis. *Arthritis and Rheumatism* **38**, 1513–18.

Pachman, L.M. et al. (1997). New-onset juvenile dermatomyositis: comparisons with a healthy cohort and children with juvenile rheumatoid arthritis. *Arthritis and Rheumatism* **40**, 1526–33.

Pachman, L.M. et al. (1998a). Evidence of a TCR Vβ 8 motif and increased CD56+ NK cells in muscle biopsies (MBx) from DQA1*0501 positive untreated children with juvenile dermatomyositis (JDM) very early in their disease course. *Pediatric Research* **43**, 338A.

Pachman, L.M. et al. (1998b). Juvenile dermatomyositis at diagnosis: clinical characteristics of 79 children. *Journal of Rheumatology* **25**, 1198–204.

Pachman, L.M. et al. (1999). Parent report of antecedent illness and environmental factors before onset of juvenile dermatomyositis (JDM): NIAMS JDM research registry data. *Arthritis and Rheumatism* **42**, 395.

Pachman, L.M. et al. (2000a). The rash of juvenile dermatomyositis (JDM) is associated with derangement of capillaries. *Arthritis and Rheumatism* **43**, 1884, S380.

Pachman, L.M. et al. (2000b). TNFalpha-308A allele in juvenile dermatomyositis: association with increased production of tumor necrosis factor alpha, disease duration, and pathologic calcifications. *Arthritis and Rheumatism* **43**, 2368–77.

Pachman, L.M. et al. (2000c). Increased CD8+and CD56+ lymphocytes in untreated juvenile dermatomyositis (JDM) muscle biopsies (MBx) are associated with a short compared with a long disease duration. *Arthritis and Rheumatism* **43**, 772.

Pachman, L.M. et al. (2001). Expression of bone matrix proteins (osteopontin, bone sialoprotein, osteonectin, and bone acidic-glycoprotein) in muscle biopsies from children with untreated juvenile dermatomyositis. *Arthritis and Rheumatism* **44**, 1267.

Park, J.H. et al. (2001). Muscle abnormalities in juvenile dermatomyositis patients: P-31 magnetic resonance spectroscopy studies. *Arthritis and Rheumatism* **43**, 2359–67.

Pistoia, V. et al. (1993). CyclosporinA in the treatment of juvenile chronic arthritis and childhood polymyositis–dermatomyositis. Results of a preliminary study. *Clinical and Experimental Rheumatology* **11**, 203–8.

Reed, A.M. and Stirling, J.D. (1995). Association of the HLA–DQa1*0501 allele in multiple racial groups with juvenile dermatomyositis. *Human Immunology* **44**, 131–5.

Reed, A.M. et al. (1990). Abnormalities in serum osteocalcin values in children with chronic rheumatic diseases. *Journal of Pediatrics* **116**, 574–80.

Reed, A.M., Pachman, L.M., and Ober, C. (1991). Molecular genetic studies of major histocompatibility complex genes in children with juvenile dermatomyositis: increased risk associated with HLA–DQA1*0501. *Human Immunology* **32**, 235–40.

Reed, A.M. et al. (2000). Chimerism in children with juvenile dermatomyositis. *Lancet* **356**, 2156–7.

Rider, L.G. and Miller, F.W. (1997). Classification and treatment of the juvenile idiopathic inflammatory myopathies. *Rheumatic Diseases Clinics of North America* **23**, 619–55.

Roifman, C.M. et al. (1987). Reversal of chronic polymyositis following intravenous immune serum globulin therapy. *Journal of the American Medical Association* **258**, 513–15.

Rosenberg, A.M. (1994). Geographical clustering of childhood dermatomyositis in Saskatchewan. *Arthritis and Rheumatism* **37**, S402.

Rosenberg, N.L. et al. (1989). Evidence for a novel picornavirus in human dermatomyositis. *Annals of Neurology* **26**, 204–9.

Scott, J.P. and Arroyave, C. (1987). Activation of complement and coagulation in juvenile dermatomyositis. *Arthritis and Rheumatism* **30**, 572–6.

Sherry, D.D., Haas, J.E., and Milstein, J.M. (1993). Childhood polymyositis as a paraneoplastic phenomenon. *Pediatric Neurology* **9**, 155–6.

Silver, R.M. and Maricq, H.R. (1989). Childhood dermatomyositis: serial microvascular studies. *Pediatrics* **83**, 278–83.

Spencer, C.H. et al. (1984). Course of treated juvenile dermatomyositis. *Journal of Pediatrics* **105**, 399–408.

Symmons, D.P., Sills, J.A., and Davis, S.M. (1995). The incidence of juvenile dermatomyositis: results from a nation-wide study. *British Journal of Rheumatology* **34**, 732–6.

Tezak, T. et al. (2002). Expression profiling in DQA1*0501 children with juvenile dermatomyositis: A novel model of pathogenesis. *Journal of Immunology* **168**, 4154–63.

Tse, S. et al. (2001). The arthritis of inflammatory childhood myositis syndromes. *Journal of Rheumatology* **28**, 192–7.

Van Rossum, M.A.J. et al. (1994). Juvenile dermato/polymositis: a retrospective analysis of 33 cases with special focus on initial CPK levels. *Clinical and Experimental Rheumatology* **12**, 339–42.

6.9 Sjögren's syndrome

Athanasios G. Tzioufas, Pierre Youinou, and Haralampos M. Moutsopoulos

Introduction

Sjögren's syndrome is a chronic autoimmune disease of unknown aetiology, characterized by lymphocyte infiltration of exocrine glands resulting in xerostomia and keratoconjunctivitis sicca. This syndrome is particularly interesting among the autoimmune diseases for two reasons. First, it has a broad clinical range extending from autoimmune exocrinopathy to extraglandular (systemic) disease affecting the lungs, kidneys, blood vessels, and muscles; it may occur alone (primary Sjögren's syndrome) or in association with other autoimmune diseases (secondary Sjögren's syndrome) (Table 1). Second, it is a disorder in which a benign autoimmune process can terminate in a lymphoid malignancy. Thus, Sjögren's syndrome is a 'crossroads disease' that offers potential insight into the mechanisms whereby immunological dysregulation may predispose to malignant transformation of B cells that are already involved in an autoimmune process.

Table 1 Association of Sjögren's syndrome with other autoimmune diseases

Rheumatoid arthritis
Systemic lupus erythematosus
Systemic sclerosis
Mixed connective tissue disease
Primary biliary cirrhosis
Myositis
Vasculitis
Thyroiditis
Chronic active hepatitis
Mixed cryoglobulinaemia

Historical review (Moutsopoulos et al. 1980)

The clinical features of the disorder were first described by Hadden in 1888. Four years later, Mikulicz described the case of a German farmer who suffered from bilateral enlargement of the parotid glands. A biopsy of the parotid showed an intense, focal, lymphocytic infiltrate that is known today as the hallmark of the disease. In the 1920s, Gougerot described the disease in France and in 1933, Sjögren, a Swedish ophthalmologist, wrote the classic monograph on the disease in which he emphasized that the eye manifestations are local findings of a systemic disorder. In 1953, Morgan and Castleman showed that the histopathological findings in Sjögren's syndrome and Mikulicz disease are identical. In the 1960s, the diverse clinical range of the syndrome was recognized and the study of its autoantibodies was initiated. The genetic predisposition to the disease was substantiated with the study of HLA in the 1970s. In the 1980s, with progress in molecular biology, the specificity of autoantibodies to the cellular components Ro(SSA) and La(SSB), and the composition of the focal lymphocytic infiltration of the exocrine glands, were dissected. The last few years, several studies have pointed the central role of the epithelial cell in the pathogenesis of the disease, and suggested that the aetiologic name of the syndrome should be 'autoimmune epithelitis' (Moutsopoulos 1994).

Epidemiology

The syndrome primarily affects women (nine women to every one man), mainly in the fourth and fifth decades of life. However, it can occur in people of all ages, including children and elderly persons. In an epidemiologic study, performed in a closed rural population in Greece and included 837 females (age range from 18 to 90 years), the prevalence of definite and probable primary Sjögren's syndrome was 0.6 and 3 per cent, respectively (Dafni et al. 1997). In a cross-sectional population-based survey performed on 1000 adults, aged 18–75 years, in the United Kingdom it was found that Sjögren's syndrome affects approximately 3–4 per cent of adults and it appears to be associated with a clinically significant impairment of patients health (Thomas et al. 1998). In another epidemiological study of 705 Swedish adults, the calculated prevalence for the disease was 2.7 per cent (Jacobsson et al. 1989).

Aetiology and pathogenesis

Over the past two decades, research in immunopathology, autoantibodies, immunogenetics, and viruses has further refined the concepts of the pathophysiology and pathogenesis of Sjögren's syndrome. One may speculate that the disease develops in three steps: first, autoimmunity may be triggered by a given environmental factor that acts on a particular genetic background; second, the autoimmune reactivity becomes chronic through abnormal immune regulatory mechanisms; and third, the lesion occurs as a consequence of the continuing inflammatory process.

The triggering of autoimmunity

Environment

Autoimmune reactions against host tissue following viral infection have been reported in both man and experimental animals. Viruses are therefore suspected as being major contributing factors in certain autoimmune disorders.

Hepatitis C virus (HCV) infection may produce a chronic lymphocytic sialadenitis, which mimics that observed in Sjögren's syndrome. HCV RNA has been detected in salivary glands of patients with chronic HCV infection by in situ hybridization (Arrieta et al. 2001), while chronic lymphocytic sialadenitis was developed spontaneously in two independent lines of transgenic animals carrying the HCV envelope genes (Koike et al. 1997). Approximately 50 per cent of patients infected with HCV have been reported, in one study, to present with histological changes compatible with Sjögren's syndrome in their minor salivary glands (Haddad et al. 1992). In some cases, the clinical picture of primary Sjögren's syndrome and chronic HCV infection is indistinguishable (Ramos-Casals et al. 2001). On the other hand, patients with Sjögren's syndrome do not usually have antibodies to HCV in their sera (Vitali et al. 1992b).

Human immunodeficiency virus-I (HIV-I) and the human T-lymphotrophic virus type 1 (HTLV-1) can infect the epithelial cells in salivary glands and produce chronic sialadenitis (Papadopoulos and Moutsopoulos 1992). Transgenic mice bearing the *tax* gene of the HTLV-1 develop an autoimmune exocrinopathy resembling that of Sjögren's syndrome: an initial increase and proliferation of the acinar epithelial cells is followed by a gradual infiltration of lymphocytes and plasma cells, leading to destruction of the acini (Green et al. 1989). Other studies have failed to demonstrate an aetiological relation between Sjögren's syndrome and human retrovirus 5 (HRV 5) (Rigby et al. 1997).

The c-*myc* proto-oncogene is involved in the pathogenesis of B-cell malignancies and especially Burkitt's lymphoma caused by EBV. Skopouli et al. (1992), using in situ hybridization with specific c-*myc* probes, have demonstrated the expression of c-*myc* mRNA in minor salivary glands of patients with Sjögren's syndrome. The minor labial salivary glands of normal individuals and of patients with rheumatoid arthritis and sarcoidosis did not show this picture. Immunostaining of the hybridized tissue with monoclonal antibodies and correlation with the clinicoserological and histological findings showed that the proto-oncogene is expressed on the acinar epithelial cells and its appearance is correlated strongly with the duration of disease as well as with the intensity of the T-cell infiltration. The epithelial cells of the exocrine glands in Sjögren's syndrome have an increased rate of apoptosis (Polihronis et al. 1998). Programmed cell death (apoptosis) can occur after several extrinsic or intrinsic triggering factors, among them viral infections. Apoptosis of the epithelial cell is mediated through the Fas–Fas ligand interaction and the perforin/granzyme B pathway. The periepithelial lymphocytic infiltrates in the immunopathological lesion possess cytotoxic properties against the epithelial cells, a finding similar to that observed in the response against virus infected host cells. Thus, CD8+ T lymphocytes were located around the acinar epithelial cells. The majority of these CD8+ T lymphocytes possess a unique integrin, alpha E beta 7 (CD103). The acinar epithelial cells adherent with alpha E beta 7 (CD103)+ CD8+ T lymphocytes were apoptotic (Fujihara et al. 1999). Furthermore, the existence of a CD4+ cytotoxic cell population which expressed perforin mRNA has been demonstrated in the lymphocytic infiltration of minor salivary glands of patients with Sjögren's syndrome (Xanthou et al. 1999). Experiments in different cell lines have shown that apoptotic cells can release intracellular autoantigens, which in turn can prime an autoimmune response (Casiola-Rosen et al. 1994).

All the above data suggest viral involvement in Sjögren's syndrome. Transient or persistent infection of the epithelial cells by a putative virus may be the initiating event; accumulation of T and B cells, which eventually prime a local autoimmune response using autoantigens provided by the epithelial apoptotic cells may be the second step; and monoclonal expansion of B cells under selective antigenic or T-cell-induced pressures the final step.

Genetic background (immunogenetics)

It is well known that members of the family of patients with Sjögren's syndrome have a higher prevalence of the syndrome and a higher incidence of serological autoimmune abnormalities than age- and sex-matched controls (Mann 1987).

Numerous investigators have shown associations between primary Sjögren's syndrome and factors encoded by the major histocompatibility complex; HLA–DR3 has been reported in 50–80 per cent of patients with Sjögren's syndrome (Mann 1987). The ethnic origin of the patients, studied so far, influences the association with the HLA–DR phenotype. Using a DNA sequence-specific, oligonucleotide probe typing of Israeli Jewish and Greek non-Jewish patients with Sjögren's syndrome (Tambur et al. 1993), it was found that the majority of patients in both groups presented either *DRBI**1101* or *DRBI*1104* alleles that were linked in a linkage disequilibrium with *DRBI*0301* and *DQA1*0501*. Molecular analysis of *DQB1* and *DQA1* alleles found in American Caucasian and American Black patients with Sjögren's syndrome revealed high frequencies of *DQB1*0201* and *DQA1*0501* (Reveille et al. 1991). Therefore, the majority of patients with Sjögren's syndrome, independent of their racial and ethnic background, carry a common allele, the *DQA1*0501* allele. Furthermore, it has been shown that a glutamine residue at position 34 of the outermost domain of the *DQA1* and/or leucine at position 26 of the outermost domain of the *DQB1* chain have a 'gene dosage' role in the anti-Ro/SSA and anti-La/SSB antibody response. The *DQA1*0501* gene is one of the genes that possess glutamine at position 34 and is found in the majority of patients with anti-Ro/SSA and anti-La/SSB. Taken together, it appears that the DQA1*0501 molecule is probably an important determining factor for the predisposition of certain individuals to primary Sjögren's syndrome.

Development and continuation of the autoimmune process

The two major autoimmune phenomena observed in Sjögren's syndrome are the B-lymphocyte hyper-reactivity and the focal lymphoplasmacytic infiltrates in the exocrine glands. Numerous studies have sought to describe and delineate (a) the nature of these phenomena, and (b) the mechanisms involved in their perpetuation.

Humoral studies

Polyclonal hyper-reactivity

The most common serological finding in Sjögren's syndrome is hypergammaglobulinaemia. The increased amount of immunoglobulins in these patients often contains a number of autoantibodies directed against non-organ-specific antigens such as other immunoglobulins (rheumatoid factor), antinuclear antibodies (which usually give a speckled pattern on immunofluorescence), cellular antigens [Ro(SSA), La(SSB), RANA], and organ-specific antigens such as salivary ductal cells, thyroid gland cells, and gastric mucosa. Recently, new sets of autoantibodies directed against the cytoskeletal protein α-fordrin (Witte et al. 2000), the proteasomes (Feist et al. 1999), and the muscarinic receptors M3 (Bacman et al. 1996), have been described in primary Sjögren's syndrome. The most common autoantibodies to cellular antigens in patients with Sjögren's syndrome are directed against two ribonucleoprotein antigens known as Ro or SSA and La or SSB. These autoantibodies are not specific for the syndrome and may be found in other autoimmune diseases, especially systemic lupus erythematosus (see Chapter 6.6.1). Anti-Ro and anti-La are detected by immunodiffusion in approximately 45 and 20 per cent, respectively, of patients with Sjögren's syndrome but in upto 95 and 85 per cent, respectively, by more sensitive techniques such as enzyme-linked immunosorbent assay. Characterization of these ribonucleoproteins has led to the observation that the fine specificity of antibodies to the polymorphic forms of Ro differs in Sjögren's syndrome and systemic lupus (reviewed in Chapter 5.4). Sera with anti-Ro or anti-La reactivity contain antibodies against many different linear and conformational antigenic determinants of these autoantigens (Moutsopoulos et al. 2000).

The presence of anti-Ro(SSA)/La(SSB) autoantibodies is associated with certain clinical manifestations of primary Sjögren's syndrome: they are correlated with earlier onset and longer duration of disease, recurrent enlargement of the parotids, and with splenomegaly/lymphadenopathy and vasculitis. In addition, the incidence of these antibodies correlates with the intensity of the infiltration of minor salivary glands (Manoussakis et al. 1986).

Oligomonoclonal hyper-reactivity

Patients with primary Sjögren's syndrome and extraglandular manifestations have usually monoclonal immunoglobulins or light chains in their serum and urine (Moutsopoulos et al. 1983, 1985). Furthermore, a significant proportion of patients have mixed monoclonal cryoglobulins (type II), containing an IgM-κ monoclonal rheumatoid factor (Tzioufas et al. 1986) (Fig. 1).

The above data suggest that patients with Sjögren's syndrome express circulating monoclonal immunoglobulins very early in the disease, together with the polyclonal B-cell activation. Monoclonality is observed more often in those patients with systemic, extraglandular disease. Serial follow-up studies have shown that the presence of mixed monoclonal (type II) cryoglobulinaemia correlates with lymphoma in patients with primary Sjögren's syndrome (Tzioufas et al. 1996).

The presence of circulating monoclonal immunoglobulins is associated with a monoclonal B-cell expansion in the salivary glands. This has been demonstrated by a peroxidase–antiperoxidase bridge technique for the detection of intracytoplasmic immunoglobulins in the salivary lymphocytic infiltrates. Seven of 12 patients with Sjögren's syndrome with

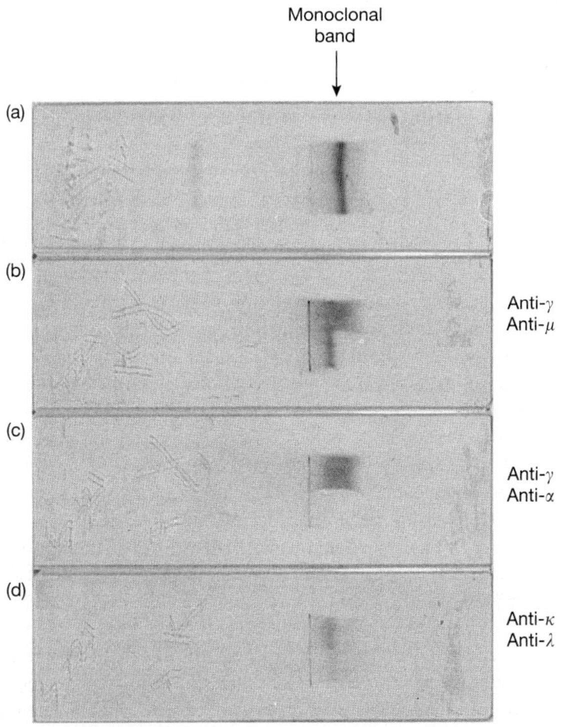

Fig. 1 (a) High-resolution agarose gel electrophoresis of the cryoglobulins of a Sjögren's syndrome patient reveals a monoclonal band. (b–d) Immunofixation, using anti-human κ, λ light, and α, γ, μ heavy chains, identified the monoclonal bands as an IgM-κ monoclonal immunoglobulin.

cryoprecipitable IgM-κ monoclonal immunoglobulins had a predominance of κ-positive plasma cells in the minor salivary glands, while patients without cryoglobulins or with polyclonal cryoglobulins had almost equal numbers of κ- and λ-positive cells (Moutsopoulos et al. 1990). Immunogenotypic studies, have shown that in the lymphoepithelial lesion there are rearrangements of oligo- or monoclonal immunoglobulin genes. Cloning and sequencing of the variable part [V(H)-D-J(H)] of the immunoglobulin heavy chain genes expressed in B cells derived from labial salivary glands and lymph nodes from Sjögren's syndrome patients revealed that a clonal B-cell expansion takes place in both the salivary glands and lymph nodes of patients with Sjögren's syndrome who do not have histological evidence of developing lymphoma (Gellrich et al. 1999).

P53 is a transcription factor, inducing cell cycle arrest in the G1 phase or apoptosis after DNA damage. Inactivation of the P53 gene, caused by mutations or deletions can lead to its tumour suppressor activity and is considered as the most common molecular event in human malignancies. Sequence analysis of the p53 gene on DNA samples obtained from labial salivary glands biopsy samples of seven patients with Sjögren's syndrome and from four patients with Sjögren's syndrome and in situ non-Hodgkin's lymphoma (NHL) revealed that the p53 gene from patients with Sjögren's syndrome and in situ NHL had two novel mutations in exon 5. These mutations were single-base substitutions and most probably are functional, since exon 5 is included in the coding region of the p53 gene (Tapinos et al. 1999). The novel mutations of the p53 gene implicate dysregulation of this tumour suppressor gene as a possible mechanism for lymphoma development in Sjögren's syndrome.

Taken all together, it seems that the lymphomagenesis in Sjögren's syndrome is a multistep process where the chronic ongoing antigenic stimulation leads to an oligoclonal B-cell expansion, which takes place in the immunopathologic lesion of the disease. In a following step, a partial or complete inhibition of the antineoplastic regulatory mechanisms (e.g. p53 mutations), could transform the oligoclonal B-cell process into a malignant lymphoma.

Lymphocyte studies

Peripheral blood lymphocytes

The absolute number of the total lymphocytes as well as T and B cells in peripheral blood does not differ substantially from that observed in normal individuals. Although decreased numbers of CD4+ and CD8+ T cells have been reported, this finding has not been substantiated by other investigators (Fauci and Moutsopoulos 1981). In a recent study it was shown that the number of CD4+ T lymphocytes was decreased, while their expression of Fas and HLA–DR was significantly increased in patients with primary Sjögren's syndrome compared with healthy controls. An increased rate of spontaneous, anti-CD3-, or anti-Fas-induced apoptosis was observed in the T cells of Sjögren's syndrome patients, and this was correlated with the decreased CD4+ T cell number (Zeher et al. 1999).

Peripheral blood B lymphocytes from patients with Sjögren's syndrome and normal controls, unlike lymphocytes from patients with systemic lupus, did not spontaneously secrete increased amounts of immunoglobulins. Thus, the activated B cells in patients with systemic lupus are distributed widely but in patients with Sjögren's syndrome they are probably localized to, and infiltrate, organs such as the exocrine glands.

Tissue lymphocytes

The majority of the infiltrating lymphocytes are T cells, while B lymphocytes constitute 20–25 per cent of the round cells. Monocytes, macrophages, as well as natural killer cells, make up less that 5 per cent. Studies of T-lymphocyte sub-populations have shown that 60–70 per cent of the T lymphocytes bear the CD4 phenotype and exhibit the memory/inducer marker (CD45 Ro). Almost all infiltrating T cells express the α T-cell receptor (TCR) (Skopouli et al. 1991). Analysis of the receptor repertoire of the infiltrating T lymphocytes from minor salivary-gland biopsies of patients with Sjögren's syndrome by a quantitative polymerase chain reaction revealed that the repertoire of the *TCR V* gene was not restricted, although $V_{\beta 2}$ and $V_{\beta 13}$ were predominantly expressed in the inflammatory infiltrates (Sumida et al. 1992). T cells in the lesion are activated as it is attested by the membrane expression of HLA class II molecules, interleukin-2 receptor (IL-2r), lymphocyte function associated antigen a_1 (LFA-1), and interleukin (IL-2) production (Skopouli et al. 1991; Fox et al. 1994; Boumba et al. 1995).

B lymphocytes infiltrating the labial salivary glands are activated, since they are able to produce increased amount of immunoglobulins with autoantibody activity (Tengner et al. 1998). In addition, evaluation with an immunoperoxidase technique of the isotypes of intracytoplasmic immunoglobulins of the plasma cells infiltrating the salivary glands of patients with Sjögren's syndrome showed that the IgG and IgM isotype predominates, in contrast to the plasma cells of the normal salivary glands, where the IgA isotype is dominant (Lane et al. 1983). This observation prompted some investigators to support the notion that quantitation of cells containing IgA and IgG intracytoplasmic immunoglobulins may serve as diagnostic criterion with high specificity and sensitivity for Sjögren's syndrome (Bodeuitsch et al. 1992).

Immunopathology

As clearly shown in the previous sections, both the B and the T lymphocytes that contribute to the tissue lesion of primary Sjögren's syndrome are activated. This is of particular interest since the classic antigen-presenting cells, monocytes/macrophages, are poorly represented in this lesion. These findings suggest that possibly another cell may play the part of the antigen presenter in the immunopathological lesion of Sjögren's syndrome. Several recent studies suggest that the glandular or acinar epithelial cells perform this function; these are summarized in the following list.

1. Histopathological studies in newly diagnosed cases of Sjögren's syndrome reveal that the focal lymphocytic infiltrates start around the ducts.
2. Staining of the labial salivary glands with anti-class-II HLA monoclonal antibodies showed that the ductal and acinar epithelial cells inappropriately express these molecules (Skopouli et al. 1991). Interferon-γ (IFN-γ) and tumour necrosis factor-α (TNF-α) have been shown to upregulate the expression of both histocompatibility antigen classes on the surface of epithelial and other cells. These cytokines are produced locally by the activated T cell. Therefore, it is not known whether the HLA–DR expression and possible antigen presentation by epithelial cells predates, or is a consequence of, the lymphocytic infiltration.
3. Studies on the expression of proto-oncogene mRNA in the minor salivary glands of patients with Sjögren's syndrome revealed that c-*myc*, in contrast to c-*fos* and c-*jun*, is selectively expressed by the epithelial glandular cells (Skopouli et al. 1992). Since the expression of the c-*myc* is so restricted, this phenomenon cannot be attributed to microenvironmental factors. The expression of HLA class II antigen and c-*myc* by epithelial cells may indicate a specific way of activating these cells.
4. The salivary gland epithelial cells express B7 molecules (Manoussakis et al. 1999). These molecules are expressed on classic antigen presenting cells and play a critical role in the regulation of immune responses by providing activation or inhibitory signals to T cells, through the ligation with CD28 or CTLA4 receptors, respectively. In a recent study, it was shown that B7 molecules expressed in the epithelial cells of primary Sjögren's syndrome patients are functional inducing co-stimulation signal in CD4+ T cells (Kapsogeorgou et al. 2001a).
5. Acinar epithelial cells coexpress accessory adhesion molecules and autoantigens, which in conjunction with the expression of class II antigen may potentially prime an autoimmune response. In fact, translocation and membrane localization of the nuclear antigen La/SSB has been observed in conjunctival epithelial cells of patients with Sjögren's syndrome (Yannopoulos et al. 1992). In addition, the infiltrating lymphocytes express a diverse array of cell adhesion molecules (lymphocyte function-associated antigen 1 and 3, CD2), while the intercellular adhesion molecule-1 (ICAM-1) is detected on acinar epithelial cells adjacent to sites of intense inflammation. ICAM-1 is also expressed spontaneously in epithelial cell lines derived from minor salivary glands of patients with Sjögren's syndrome (Kapsogeorgou et al. 2001b).
6. In recent years, cytokine production in the immunopathological lesion of Sjögren's syndrome has been studied extensively by in situ hybridization and reverse-transcriptase, quantitative, polymerase chain reaction (Fox et al. 1994; Boumba et al. 1995). Both techniques demonstrated the presence of proinflammatory cytokines IL-1 and IL-6 in the labial salivary glands of patients with Sjögren's syndrome. In addition, using in situ hybridization and immunohistochemistry it was shown that lymphoid chemokines are produced by the epithelial cells in the chronic inflammatory lesion of Sjögren's syndrome patients (Xanthou et al. 2001). Lymphoid chemokines are a newly defined set of chemokines which orchestrate leucocyte microenvironmental homing and contribute to the formation of lymphoid structures. The expression pattern of both proinflammatory cytokines and lymphoid chemokines in minor salivary glands, points further to the role of epithelial cells in the pathogenesis of Sjögren's syndrome and reinforces the concept that this cell is an active counterpart in the inflammatory response rather than a target of the immune-mediated injury.

Pathology

The common finding in all affected organs in patients with Sjögren's syndrome is a potentially progressive lymphocytic infiltration. These infiltrates cause functional disability of the affected organs, producing the various clinical manifestations.

The salivary glands are the best-studied organs, because (i) they are affected in almost all patients, and (ii) they are readily accessible. Microscopic examination of the enlarged major salivary glands reveals a benign lymphoepithelial lesion, characterized by lymphocytic replacement of the salivary epithelium and the presence of epimyoepithelial islands, which are composed of keratin-containing epithelial cells. Sometimes, the salivary gland biopsy does not show benign lymphoepithelial lesions, but instead contains various degrees of focal lymphocytic infiltration [defined as focal aggregates of 50 or more lymphocytes and histiocytes (Daniels et al. 1987)].

The need for a practical and easy way to assess the salivary component of Sjögren's syndrome led to the introduction of labial gland biopsy. The histopathological characteristics of the biopsy of the minor salivary glands include (i) focal aggregates of at least 50 lymphocytes/plasma cells and macrophages, adjacent to and replacing the normal acini, and (ii) the consistent presence of these foci in all or most of the glands in the specimen (Plate 137). Larger foci often show the formation of germinal centres but epimyoepithelial islands are very uncommon. These lesions are, in fact, typical findings for a chronic lymphocytic sialadenitis. However, a biopsy of minor salivary glands can be very specific for Sjögren's syndrome if it is obtained through normal-appearing mucosa, includes 5–10 glands, separated from the surrounding connective tissue, and shows focal lymphocytic infiltrates in all or most of the glands in the specimen, with a focus score above a chosen diagnostic threshold. Therefore, several methods of scoring the number of foci have been applied (reviewed in Daniels et al. 1987). Chisholm and Mason used a semiquantitative method to assess inflammation in salivary gland biopsies from 40 patients with several autoimmune diseases; only in patients with Sjögren's syndrome was there more than one focus of lymphocytes per 4 mm^2 of gland. Using a modification of this method, Greenspan et al. enumerated scores from 1 to 12 foci/4 mm^2 and found a significant positive correlation between a higher score and larger foci in biopsies of minor salivary glands of patients with Sjögren's syndrome. In another study by Tarpley et al. grading of 86 biopsies from primary and secondary Sjögren's syndrome showed, by qualitative criteria, larger lymphocytic foci in the primary syndrome. Minor salivary gland biopsy of a patient with Sjögren's syndrome, showing moderate and large focal lymphocytic infiltrates around the acini and ducts.

Although there is no perfect diagnostic criterion for the salivary component of Sjögren's syndrome, the finding of the characteristic focal sialadenitis in biopsies of minor salivary glands is the best single criterion in terms of its disease specificity, convenience, availability, and low risk.

Animal models

Spontaneously induced disease with features resembling those of human Sjögren's syndrome has been recognized in autoimmune strains of mice that develop a lupus-like syndrome. These include the NZB, NZB/NZW, and MRL/1pr, MRL/n (lacking the *lpr* gene) strains. All experimental animals have various degrees of lymphoplasmacytic infiltration in the lacrimal and salivary glands, with the milder form in the NZB mice and the more severe form in the MRL/n mice. Antibodies to Ro(SSA) and/or La(SSB) autoantigens were not detected in their sera.

The non-obese diabetic (NOD) mouse is not only the prototypic model for human insulin-dependent diabetes, but it may also be utilized (Humphreys-Beher et al. 1994) as an animal model for the study of Sjögren's syndrome. It has indeed been determined that such mice develop sialadenitis with morphologically similar exocrinopathy as in human Sjögren's syndrome. The salivary and lacrimal glands are characterized by foci of inflammatory cells, where $\alpha\beta$T cells predominate largely over $\gamma\delta$T cells. Importantly, these infiltrating T cells comprise a vast majority of CD4+ T cells. It is surprising that, unlike what has been described in the human disease, inflammation is far worse in lacrimal glands of males, whereas immune reaction is much greater in salivary tissues of females (Toda et al. 1999).

A variety of autoantibodies have been reported in the NOD mouse model, along with a 1.4-fold increase in serum IgG level, compared to the Balb/c controls (Humphreys-Beher et al. 1993). Seventy per cent of the affected mice produce antibodies to cytoplasmic and/or nuclear components of HEp-2 cells. Unexpectedly, the anti-nuclear antibody pattern is limited to the anti-Ro/SSA reactivity, with the 52-kDa protein as the main target (Skarstein et al. 1995). Other autoantibodies have been described, most notably those directed towards the 120-kDa chain of α fodrin (Yanagi et al. 1998) and towards various hither to unidentified salivary gland proteins.

Although T cells, particularly the IL-2 and IFN-γ-producing cells (i.e. the Th1 cells), seem to be endowed with the key role in the pathophysiology of NOD mouse Sjögren's syndrome, apoptosis of epithelial cells appear to be one of the triggering events, as described in human disease. A potential apoptotic process dependent on Fas/Fas L has been reported to occur in NOD-scid secretory epithelial cells, even in the absence of lymphocytic infiltration. In this respect, worth noting is that salivary gland epithelial cells in NOD and NOD-scid mice overexpress the pro-apoptotic molecules *Bax* and caspase 3; the former could possibly be responsible for activation of the latter (Masago et al. 2001). In conclusion, the NOD mouse models for Sjögren's syndrome do not reproduce exactly the human pathophysiology. They are, nonetheless, important to gain further insight into the understanding of the disease.

Clinical picture

Sjögren's syndrome can occur alone (primary) or in association with other autoimmune diseases (secondary). The initial manifestation of primary Sjögren's syndrome can be non-specific and a median time of 6 years elapse from the initial symptoms to the full-blown development of the syndrome (Skopouli et al. 2000). The clinical picture of the disease occurs as a consequence of the two major autoimmune phenomena which characterize the syndrome; the periepithelial invasion by autoreactive T cells in glandular and extraglandular tissues are usually observed early and have a chronic and benign course (Fig. 2). On the other hand, extraepithelial manifestations attributed to immune-complex deposition such as skin vasculitis, glomerulonephritis, and peripheral neuropathy are appeared later and associated with increased morbidity.

Glandular manifestations

Oral component

Symptoms and signs

The principal oral symptom of Sjögren's syndrome is dryness (xerostomia). Patients describe this as difficulty in swallowing dry food, inability to speak continuously, changes in sense sensation, a burning sensation, an increase in dental caries (Fig. 3), and problems in wearing complete dentures. Examination shows a dry, erythematous, sticky oral mucosa, and often dental caries, while saliva from the major glands is either not expressible or is cloudy. Atrophy of the filiform papillae of the tongue is apparent (Fig. 4) and in some cases overgrowth of *Candida* is observed.

Enlargement of the parotids or other major salivary glands occurs in 50 per cent of patients with the primary syndrome, but is uncommon in those with Sjögren's syndrome and rheumatoid arthritis (see below). In many patients, the salivary gland swelling is episodic, but some have chronic persistent enlargement. The swelling of the parotids may begin unilaterally but often becomes bilateral. In Table 2, conditions other than Sjögren's syndrome causing parotid enlargement are depicted.

Diagnosis

A variety of medical conditions other than Sjögren's syndrome can cause xerostomia (Table 3). To evaluate the oral component of the syndrome, various tests are used with different specificity and sensitivity for the disease.

Sialometry

Salivary flow rates can be measured clinically for whole saliva or for separate secretions from the parotid or submandibular and sublingual glands, with or without stimulation. Patients with clinically overt Sjögren's syndrome have reduced flow. However, flow rates depend on many factors such as age,

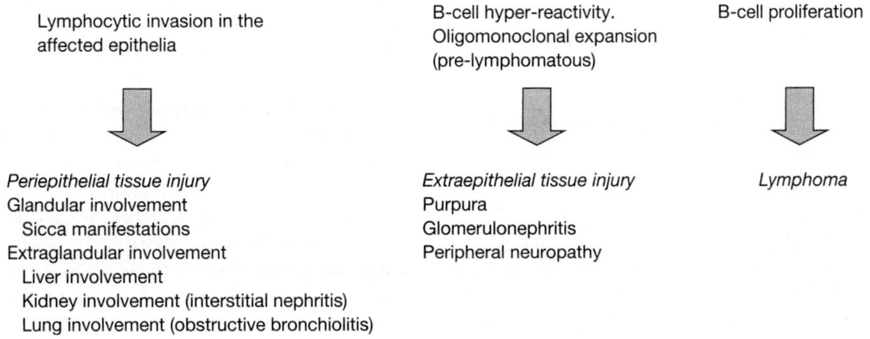

Fig. 2 The spectrum of primary Sjögren's syndrome.

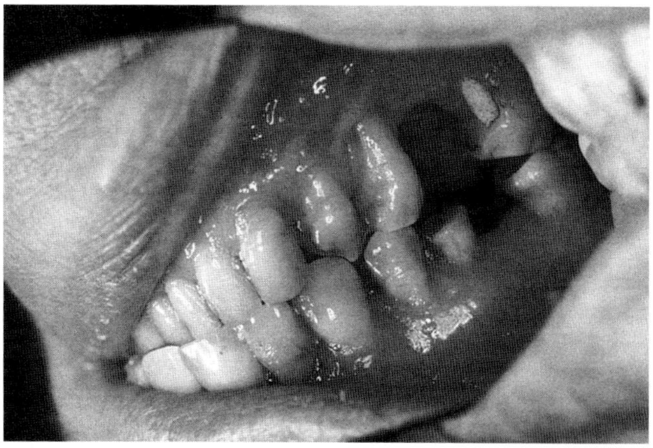

Fig. 3 Dental caries in Sjögren's syndrome; note also the remarkable periodontitis in both lower and upper teeth.

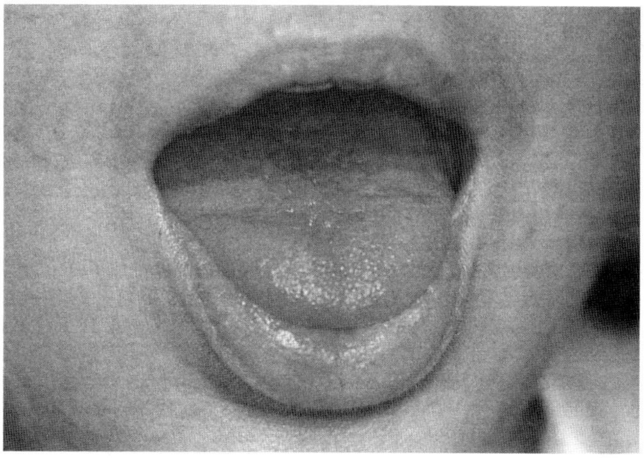

Fig. 4 Dry tongue of a patient with Sjögren's syndrome. Note the remarkable atrophy of filiform papillae.

Table 2 Differential diagnosis of parotid gland enlargement

Unilateral
Salivary gland neoplasm
Bacterial infection
Chronic sialadenitis
Bilateral
Viral infection (mumps, influenza, Epstein–Barr, coxsackie A, cytomegalovirus, HIV)
Sjögren's syndrome
Sarcoidosis
Miscellaneous (diabetes mellitus, hyperlipoproteinaemia, hepatic cirrhosis, chronic pancreatitis, acromegaly, gonadal hypofunction)
Recurrent parotitis of childhood

sex, medication, and time of day. Therefore, setting a cut-off point between the normal and abnormal is difficult because of the wide range of flow rates among normal individuals (Skopouli et al. 1989).

Sialography

This is a radiocontrast method of assessing anatomical changes in the salivary ductal system. It has been widely used in patients with Sjögren's syndrome, in whom various degrees of sialectasis have been found. Sialography using oil-based contrast material causes pain and swelling of the parotid glands. Vitali et al. (1988) described sialography with water-soluble media in 84 patients with primary and secondary Sjögren's syndrome and compared it with the findings of minor salivary gland biopsy, as well as with the patients' clinical and the serological picture. They reported that sialography was as sensitive and specific as the biopsy.

Table 3 Causes of xerostomia

Drugs
Psychotherapeutic
Parasympatholytic
Antihypertensive
Viral infections
Dehydration
Diabetes mellitus
Trauma
Psychogenic
Irradiation
Congenital (absent or malformed glands)

Scintigraphy

Isotope scanning provides a functional evaluation of all the salivary glands by observing the rate and density of uptake of the [$^{99}Tc^{m}$] pertechnetate and the time taken for it to appear in the mouth during a 60-min period after intravenous injection. In patients with Sjögren's syndrome the uptake of the label by the glands and the secretion of labelled saliva is delayed or absent. In a study of 320 patients with oral dryness who had primary or secondary Sjögren's syndrome, graft-versus-host disease, and other autoimmune diseases, scanning had high sensitivity but no well-established disease specificity (Parrago et al. 1987).

Sialochemistry

Chemical and immunological factors in saliva of patients with Sjögren's syndrome have been examined extensively in the past. So far, the results are conflicting and controversial (Baum and Fox 1987), offering very limited diagnostic value.

Ocular component

Ocular involvement is a major glandular manifestation of Sjögren's syndrome. Diminished tear secretion leads to the destruction of the corneal and bulbar conjunctival epithelium termed keratoconjunctivitis sicca. The patients usually complain of a burning, foreign-body sensation, a sandy or scratchy sensation under the lids, itchiness, redness, and photosensitivity. Clinical signs include dilation of the bulbar conjunctival vessels, pericorneal injection, irregularity of the corneal image, and sometimes enlargement of the lacrimal glands. All tests for the evaluation of this condition are very sensitive but not specific for Sjögren's syndrome, as keratoconjunctivitis sicca may occur in a number of other conditions.

The Schirmer's test is used for the evaluation of tear secretion. The test is made with strips of filter paper 30 mm in length. The strip is slipped beneath the inferior lid, with the remainder of the paper hanging out. After 5 min the length of paper wetted is measured. Wetting of less than 5 mm is a strong indication of diminished secretion. The presence of decreased tear secretion is not diagnostic of keratoconjunctivitis sicca. In contrast, it can easily be diagnosed using rose bengal staining. Rose bengal is an aniline compound that stains the devitalized or damaged epithelium of both the cornea and conjunctiva. Slit-lamp examination after rose bengal staining shows a punctate pattern of filamentary keratitis (Plate 138).

The break-up time of tears is another useful measure. A drop of fluorescein is instilled in the eye and the time between the last blink and appearance of dark, non-fluorescent areas in the tear film is measured. An overly rapid break-up of the tear film indicates an abnormality of either the mucin or the lipid layer (Kincaid 1987).

Systemic (extraglandular) manifestations

Extraglandular (systemic) manifestations are seen in more than one-third of patients with primary Sjögren's syndrome (Moutsopoulos et al. 1980; Skopouli et al. 2000) (Table 4). Patients with primary Sjögren's syndrome complain most often of being easily fatigued, of low-grade fever, and of myalgias and arthralgias.

The extraglandular features are divided into those produced from the lymphocytic invasion in epithelial tissues of non-exocrine organs, such as kidneys (interstitial nephritis), liver, and lungs and the extraepithelial manifestations, which include glomerulonephritis, peripheral neuropathy, and palpable purpura. It is now recognized that these two entities have a different natural history, prognosis, outcome, and therapy.

Arthritis

Seventy per cent of patients with primary Sjögren's syndrome complain of arthralgias, while one-fourth of patients develop arthritis (Skopouli et al. 2000). In contrast to rheumatoid arthritis, radiographs of the hand usually do not reveal pathological changes (Tsampoulas et al. 1990).

Raynaud's phenomenon

This occurs in 35 per cent of patients with primary Sjögren's and usually precedes sicca manifestations by many years. Patients with the primary syndrome and Raynaud's phenomenon present with swollen hands, but, in contrast to those with scleroderma, they do not experience digital ulcers and telangiectasias are not seen. In addition, these patients present non-specific nailfold capillary abnormalities in higher frequency than patients without Raynaud's phenomenon (Tektonidou et al. 1999). Radiographs of the hands of these patients may show small tissue calcifications (Skopouli et al. 1990). Non-erosive arthritis has also been shown to be significantly more frequent in patients with Raynaud's phenomenon than in those without (Youinou et al. 1990).

Table 4 Incidence of extraglandular manifestations in primary Sjögren's syndrome (Skopouli et al. 2000)

Clinical feature	% of patients
Easy fatigue	95
Fever	44
Arthralgias	75
Arthritis	23
Raynaud's phenomenon	48
Lymphadenopathy	32
Splenomegaly	7
Purpura	
Non-palpable	3
Palpable	8
Pulmonary involvement	29
Nephritis	
Interstitial	9
Glomerulonephritis	2
Primary biliary cirrhosis	4
Peripheral neuropathy	2
Central nervous system	0
Lymphoma	4

Skin involvement

Cutaneous lesions are seen frequently in patients with primary Sjögren's syndrome. Patients with dry skin complain of dermal stinging and itching. Nasal dryness with crusting, vaginal dryness syndrome with dyspareunia, and cheilitis have also been described. Flat purpura is usually seen in patients with hypergammaglobulinaemia, while palpable purpura is a manifestation of skin vasculitis and is observed in 7 per cent of patients (Skopouli et al. 2000). Other cutaneous manifestations include skin hyper- or hypopigmentation, patchy alopecia, and pernio-like lesions. Some Japanese patients with Sjögren's syndrome may present with annular erythema affecting mainly the face and the trunk; it extends centrifugally and fades without leaving pigmentation (Teramoto et al. 1989).

Pulmonary involvement

Manifestations from the trachea to the pleura have been described in patients with Sjögren's syndrome. These are frequent but rarely important clinically. They can present with a range of symptoms from dry cough secondary to dryness of the tracheobronchial mucosa (xerotrachea) to dyspnoea from interstitial disease or even airway obstruction (Constantopoulos and Moutsopoulos 1987).

Evaluation of 61 consecutive, non-smoking patients with primary Sjögren's syndrome by pulmonary function tests and arterial blood gases revealed that the major finding was a small airways obstruction, which was frequently associated with mild hypoxaemia. Chest radiography showed mild, interstitial-like changes in 45 per cent of patients. Lung high-resolution computed tomography in patients with abnormal chest radiography revealed either thickened bronchial walls at the segmental level or a mild interstitial pattern distributed around the bronchi. Transbronchial and/or endobronchial biopsy specimens in 10 of the 11 sufficient tissue samples disclosed peribronchial and/or peribronchiolar mononuclear inflammation, while in only two patients interstitial inflammation coexisted (Papiris et al. 1999). Interstitial lung disease is rather uncommon.

Lymphoma should always be suspected when lung nodules or hilar and/or mediastinal lymphadenopathy are found on chest radiographs.

Pleural effusions are usually found in Sjögren's syndrome associated with other rheumatic disorders and not in the primary syndrome.

Gastrointestinal and hepatobiliary features

Patients with Sjögren's syndrome often complain of dysphagia, owing to dryness of the pharynx and oesophagus, or to abnormal oesophageal motility. Nausea and epigastric pain are also common complaints. Biopsies of gastric mucosa show chronic atrophic gastritis and lymphocytic infiltrates, similar to those described in minor salivary glands. In addition, patients with Sjögren's syndrome have hypopepsinogenaemia, an elevated serum gastrin, low serum vitamin B_{12}, and antibodies to parietal cells. Acute or chronic pancreatitis has been reported rarely. In contrast, sub-clinical pancreatic involvement is a rather common finding, as illustrated by the fact that hyperamylasaemia is found in one-fourth of patients with the syndrome (Trevino et al. 1987).

The prevalence and nature of liver involvement was studied in 300 patients with Sjögren's syndrome (Skopouli et al. 1994). Seven per cent had antimitochondrial antibodies and 5 per cent had elevated liver enzymes. Patients with antimitochondrial antibodies had elevated liver enzymes and no evidence of hepatitis B and C viral infection. Eleven out of 17 patients with antimitochondrial antibodies underwent liver biopsy. The histopathological picture disclosed in seven specimens was a mild intrahepatic bile duct inflammation, an 'autoimmune cholangiitis' affecting small and medium-sized bile ducts, without, however, evidence of 'piecemeal' necrosis (Fig. 5). These histological features are similar with those observed in stage I of primary biliary cirrhosis.

There is also a high incidence of Sjögren's syndrome in patients with primary biliary cirrhosis: sicca manifestations have been described in approximately half of a group of patients with primary biliary cirrhosis; among these, 10 per cent had severe clinical features of dryness (Tsianos et al. 1990).

Renal involvement

Overt kidney disease is found in approximately 5 per cent of patients with Sjögren's syndrome (Goules et al. 2000). The patients may present either interstitial nephritis or glomerulonephritis. Interstitial nephritis is usually an early feature of the syndrome, while glomerulonephritis is a late sequelae. Approximately 35 per cent of patients have an abnormal urine acidification test suggesting a sub-clinical involvement of renal tubules. The renal biopsy reveals interstitial lymphocytic infiltration. When interstitial nephritis is clinically apparent the patients present with hyposthenuria and hypokalaemic, hyperchloraemic distal tubular acidosis. Distal tubular acidosis can be silent or can present with recurrent renal colic and/or hypokalaemic muscular weakness. Untreated renal tubular acidosis leads to renal stones, nephrocalcinosis, and compromised renal function (Fig. 6). Less commonly, these patients have proximal tubular acidosis with Fanconi syndrome. Glomerulonephritis in Sjögren's syndrome has been described in few patients the histological type may be membranous, membranoproliferative or messangioproliferative. Glomerulonephritis is associated with cryoglobulinaemia and hypocomplementaemia (Kassan and Talal 1987).

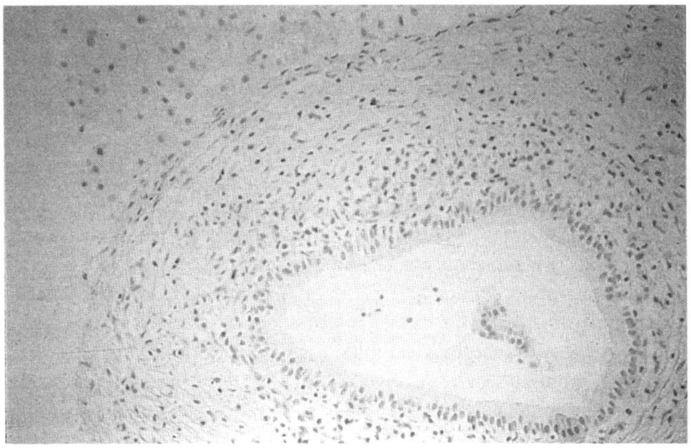

Fig. 5 Periportal inflammation in liver biopsy of a patient with Sjögren's syndrome.

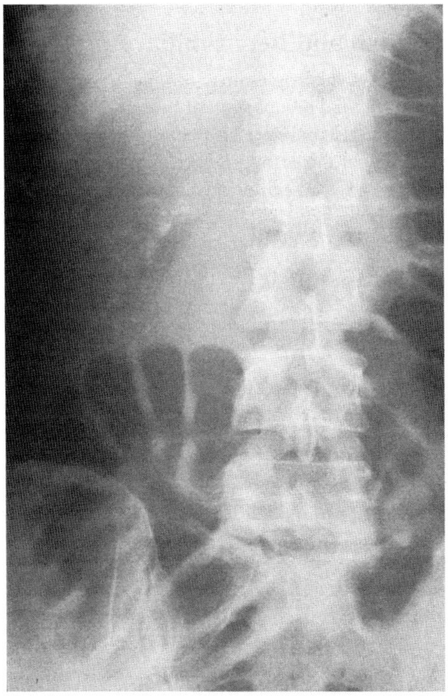

Fig. 6 Abdominal radiograph of a patient with Sjögren's syndrome reveals nephrocalcinosis of the right kidney.

Vasculitis

Vascular involvement is found in approximately 5 per cent of patients with Sjögren's syndrome. It affects small and medium-sized vessels. The most common manifestations are purpura, recurrent urticaria, skin ulcerations, and mononeuritis multiplex. However, cases of systemic vasculitis with visceral involvement affecting kidney, lung, gastrointestinal tract, spleen, breast, and the reproductive tract have been described (Alexander 1987a; Tsokos et al. 1987). There are two histopathological types of vasculitis, according to the type of the infiltrating cell—the mononuclear and the neutrophil type. The latter is associated with hypergammaglobulinaemia, high titres of rheumatoid factor, antibodies to Ro(SSA) cellular antigen, and hypocomplementaemia (Alexander 1987a). In another classification of vascular involvement (Tsokos et al. 1987), the small-vessel vasculitis was of the hypersensitivity type, that is leucocytoclastic and lymphocytic, while the medium-vessel vasculitis was acute necrotizing and simulated polyarteritis nodosa but without the formation of aneurysms. Endarteritis obliterans was seen in patients with a long-standing history of vasculitis.

Neuromuscular involvement

Neurological manifestations of Sjögren's syndrome include peripheral sensory or sensorimotor neuropathy as a consequence of vascular involvement. Cranial neuropathy, usually affecting single nerves such as the trigeminal or the optic, has been well documented. Involvement of the central nervous system in the syndrome is a matter of considerable controversy. Over the last decade some investigators have described a high proportion of such involvement, which before had been unrecognized internationally. They found that this disease was multifocal, recurrent, and progressive. The clinical signs included hemiparesis, hemisensory deficits, seizures, movement disorders, and transverse myelopathy. Some patients presented with diffuse brain injury expressed as encephalopathy, aseptic meningitis, and dementia (Alexander 1987b). On the other hand, others have failed to demonstrate severe central involvement in 55 patients with primary and 50 with secondary Sjögren's syndrome (Binder et al. 1988). Eighteen of these patients had mild neurological abnormalities confined to the secondary syndrome; all were characteristics of the underlying rheumatic disorders. A study of 63 consecutive patients with primary Sjögren's syndrome revealed that 17 had a mild sensory or sensorimotor neuropathy while one patient with past history of hypertension had had a mild episode (Andonopoulos et al. 1990a), suggesting that peripheral neuropathy is a rather common finding in Sjögren's syndrome whereas central nervous disease must be rare.

Many patients with the primary syndrome complain of myalgia, but muscle enzymes are usually normal of slightly elevated. Polymyositis with extensive necrosis of muscle fibres and invasion of macrophages into the affected muscle, as well as inclusion body myositis, have been described in Sjögren's syndrome (Leroy et al. 1990).

Other manifestations

Autoimmune thyroid disease has been described in some patients with primary Sjögren's syndrome. In a study by Karsh et al. (1980), half of the patients with Sjögren's syndrome presented with antithyroid antibodies and signs of altered thyroid function as evaluated by a basal thyroid-hormone stimulation test. In a recent study, it was shown that thyroid disease can be seen in more than one-third of patients with primary Sjögren's syndrome, but no significant differences were observed when the prevalence of thyroid disease was compared with that in a control group of similar age and gender (Ramos-Casals et al. 2000).

Sjögren's syndrome may also associated with interstitial cystitis (Van de Merwe et al. 1993), which is a non-bacterial disease of the bladder producing constant or intermittent, long-lasting symptoms, such frequent micturition, nocturia, and suprapubic or perineal pain. Bladder biopsy discloses intense inflammation in the mucosa and submucosa with lymphoid cells and mast cells. Lymphoid cell infiltrates contain CD4+ T cells as well as B-cell nodules with germinal centres. Detrusor fibrosis can be seen in the later stages of the disease.

Mild normochromic and normocytic anaemia is a common finding; leucopaenia and thrombocytopaenia are relatively rare features. An elevated erythrocyte sedimentation rate is found in approximately 70 per cent of patients (Moutsopoulos et al. 1980). In contrast, raised levels of C-reactive protein are not detected in patients with primary Sjögren's syndrome but are found in those with Sjögren's syndrome and rheumatoid arthritis (Table 5).

Lymphoproliferative disease

Patients with Sjögren's syndrome have a 44 times higher relative risk of developing lymphoma, compared with age-, sex-, and race-matched normal controls (Kassan et al. 1978).

The prevalence of NHL in Sjögren's syndrome is 4.3 per cent. The median time between Sjögren's syndrome diagnosis and lymphoma development is 7.5 years. The predictive factors for lymphoma development in Sjögren's syndrome include persistent parotid gland enlargement, lymphadenopathy, splenomegaly, palpable purpura, glomerulonephritis, mixed monoclonal cryoglobulinaemia (type II cryoglobulinaemia), and low levels of the C4 complement component (Tzioufas et al. 1996; Skopouli et al. 2000). These patients should be closely followed by their physicians for lymphoma development.

In a large European multicentre study (Voulgarelis et al. 1999), the clinical picture and the outcome of patients with Sjögren's syndrome and lymphoma were studied. The lymphomas in Sjögren's syndrome patients are NHLs, originating from the B cell. The majority of lymphomas are marginal zone B-cell lymphomas, a term which includes the mucosa-associated lymphoid tissue (MALT) and monocytoid B-cell lymphomas. Other types of NHL include the follicle center and large B-cell lymphomas. Lymphomas in Sjögren's syndrome arise frequently in epithelial extranodular sites, mainly in the salivary glands. Other sites such as the stomach, lung, nasopharynx, and liver, can also be involved. Lymph node involvement is common and usually associated with extranodular involvement. In 85 per cent of patients, lymphoma appears in the peripheral lymph nodes. The presenting symptoms are attributed to persistent major salivary gland enlargement, mostly the parotid glands. Patients with Sjögren's syndrome and lymphoma do not usually present B symptoms (i.e. fever, fatigue, and night sweats), while their performance status is good. Approximately 60 per cent of lymphomas in Sjögren's syndrome are localized and the majority are of low grade histologic type. These lymphomas may remain local for many years and regress spontaneously without treatment. Transition from a low-grade to a high-grade lymphoma can be seen. Most high-grade lymphomas in salivary glands are diffuse large B-cell lymphomas. Cases of lymphoblastic and Burkitt's type lymphomas have been also described.

Table 5 Laboratory findings in Greek patients with primary Sjögren's syndrome (Skopouli et al. 2000)

	% of patients
Anaemia	16
Haemolytic anaemia	3
Leucopaenia	12
Hypergammaglobulinaemia	47
Rheumatoid factor	61
Antinuclear antibodies	89
aRo/SSA	56
aLa/SSB	30
aU1RNP	2
adsDNA	4
Cryoglobulinaemia	14
Low C_3 levels (<50 mg/dl)	2
Low C_4 levels (<20 mg/dl)	17

Secondary Sjögren's syndrome

The association of Sjögren's syndrome with rheumatoid arthritis was first described by Henrik Sjögren in 1933. During the following years, it became evident that sicca manifestations can also be found in other autoimmune rheumatic diseases, such as systemic lupus erythematosus and progressive systemic sclerosis. In addition, manifestations of Sjögren's syndrome have been described in polymyositis, polyarteritis nodosa, and primary biliary cirrhosis (see Table 1) (Moutsopoulos et al. 1980).

The incidence of clinically overt Sjögren's syndrome in patients with rheumatoid arthritis is around 5 per cent. Using a special questionnaire, however, 20 per cent of patients with rheumatoid arthritis registered complaints of dry eyes and/or xerostomia (Andonopoulos et al. 1987). The diagnosis of rheumatoid arthritis usually preceded that of Sjögren's syndrome by many years. Patients with the arthritis and the syndrome usually present with keratoconjunctivitis sicca, while enlargement of the parotids or other major salivary glands is less common than in primary Sjögren's syndrome.

Patients with primary Sjögren's syndrome and those with systemic lupus may have similar disease manifestations such as arthralgias, rash, peripheral neuropathy, and glomerulonephritis. These observations prompted Heaton in 1959 to conclude that Sjögren's syndrome was a benign form of systemic lupus. The diagnosis is usually obtained histologically; approximately 20 per cent of patients with systemic lupus have lymphocytic infiltrates in biopsies from their minor salivary glands (Andonopoulos et al. 1990b).

Dry eyes and mouth are found in approximately 20 per cent of unselected patients with scleroderma. Subjective xerostomia could be due to fibrosis of the exocrine glands. In fact, in biopsies from minor salivary glands of 44 unselected patients with scleroderma, 38 per cent had fibrosis while only 22 per cent had lymphocytic infiltration compatible with Sjögren's syndrome (Andonopoulos et al. 1989).

Diagnosis and differential diagnosis

Since the initial definition and the proposed criteria of Sjögren's syndrome by Bloch et al. (1965), several sets of criteria have been used by different groups for the diagnosis of Sjögren's syndrome. As a result, patients with Sjögren's syndrome had often been missed at diagnosis, or classified incorrectly due both to the great variability at disease presentation and to the lack of well-defined and commonly accepted diagnostic criteria.

A prospective concerted action involving 26 centres in 12 European countries led to a study with the goal of obtaining validated criteria for the diagnosis of Sjögren's syndrome. The study resulted in: (i) the validation of a simple six-item questionnaire for determination of dry eyes and mouth, useful in the initial screening for Sjögren's syndrome, and (ii) the definition of a new set of criteria for Sjögren's syndrome. The sensitivity and specificity of both questionnaire and diagnostic criteria were determined, exhibiting good discrimination between patients and controls. Hence, using this set of criteria, a general agreement can be reached on the diagnosis of Sjögren's syndrome (Table 6) (Vitali et al. 1993).

Differential diagnosis must be, of course, from other diseases responsible for dry eyes, xerostomia, and parotid enlargement. Sarcoidosis is one disease that can mimic the clinical picture of Sjögren's syndrome (Drosos et al. 1989). However, the biopsy of minor salivary glands reveals non-caseating granulomas in sarcoidosis, while there is a lack of autoantibodies to Ro(SSA) or La(SSB). Other medical conditions that can mimic the syndrome are lipoproteinaemias (types II, IV, and V), chronic graft-versus-host disease, amyloidosis. Viral infections with HIV, HTLV-I, and HCV

Table 6 International classification criteria for Sjögren's syndrome

I	Ocular symptoms: a positive response to at least one of the following questions: (a) Have you daily, persistent, troublesome dry eyes for more than three months? (b) Do you have a recurrent sensation of sand or gravel in the eyes? (c) Do you use tear substitutes more than three times a day?
II	Oral symptoms: a positive response to at least one of the following questions: (a) Have you had a daily feeling of dry mouth for more than three months? (b) Have you had recurrently or persistently swollen salivary glands as an adult? (c) Do you frequently drink liquids to aid in swallowing dry food?
III	Ocular signs: objective evidence of ocular involvement defined as a positive result for at least one of the following two tests. (a) Schirmer's test performed without anaesthesia ($\leq$5 mm in 5 min) (b) Rose bengal score or other ocular dye score ($\geq$4 according to van Bijsterveld's scoring system)
IV	Histopathology in minor salivary glands, obtained through normal-appearing mucosa, focal lymphocytic sialodenitis, evaluated by an expert histopathologist, with a focus score $\geq$1, defined as a number of lymphocytic foci that are adjacent to normal-appearing mucous acini and contain more than 50 lymphocytes per 4 mm^2 of glandular tissue.
V	Salivary gland involvement: objective evidence of salivary gland involvement defined by a positive result for at least one of the following diagnostic tests: (a) Unstimulated whole salivary flow ($\leq$1:5 ml in 15 min) (b) Parotid sialography showing the presence of diffuse sialectasias (punctate, cavitary, or destructive pattern), without evidence of obstruction in the major ducts (c) Salivary scintigraphy showing delayed uptake, reduced concentration, and/or delayed excretion of tracer
VI	Autoantibodies: presence of the following autoantibodies: (a) Antibodies to SSA/Ro or SSB/La antigens, or both

may produce chronic sialadenitis and a clinical picture similar with that of primary Sjögren's syndrome. Patients with HIV infection present with sicca manifestations, parotid gland enlargement, pulmonary involvement and lymphadenopathy. These patients had an increased prevalence of HLA–DR5 alloantigen (Itescu et al. 1990). The two diseases can be easily distinguished since patients with HIV infection are usually young males, have no autoantibodies to Ro(SS-A) and La(SS-B) and the lymphocytic infiltrates of the salivary glands consist of CD8+ T cells. HCV may produce a chronic lymphocytic sialadenitis which mimics Sjögren's syndrome (Haddad et al. 1992). These patients have a higher mean age, a lower prevalence of parotid gland enlargement and a higher prevalence of liver involvement, compared to patients with primary Sjögren's syndrome (Ramos-Casals et al. 2000). On the other hand, Sjögren's syndrome patients did not possess increased frequency of antibodies to HCV in their sera (Vitali et al. 1992).

Prognostic factors and outcome

The prognostic factors of outcome and survival in Sjögren's syndrome have recently been determined. Skopouli et al. (2000), studied the evolution of the clinical picture and laboratory profile, the incidence and predictors for systemic disease, as well as the impact of the clinical features on overall survival, in a prospective cohort study of 261 Greek patients with primary Sjögren's syndrome followed for a 10-year period. The results were compared with the general Greek population, adjusting for age and sex. The glandular manifestations of the syndrome were typically present at the time of diagnosis and the serological profile of the patients, did not change substantially during the follow-up. Arthritis, Raynaud's phenomenon, and the periepithelial extraglandular manifestations such as interstitial nephritis, obstructive bronchiolitis and liver involvement usually appeared early during the process of the disease and have a favourable outcome. The extraepithelial features of the disease, including palpable purpura, glomerulonephritis, as well as decreased C4 complement levels and mixed monoclonal cryoglobulinaemia were identified as adverse prognostic factors. The overall mortality of patients with primary Sjögren's syndrome compared with the general population was increased only in patients with adverse predictors. In another survival study performed by Martens et al. (1999) in residents of Olmsted County, Minnesota, United States, between 1976 and 1992, 50 cases with primary Sjögren's syndrome and 24 with secondary Sjögren's syndrome were identified. An average of 7.2 years of follow-up was available for patients with primary Sjögren's syndrome and 9.9 years for patients with secondary Sjögren's syndrome. Increased mortality was found in patients with secondary, but not primary Sjögren's syndrome.

Therapy (Box 1)

Sjögren's syndrome is a chronic, multisystem disease. Therefore, patients with Sjögren's syndrome should be followed regularly for significant functional deterioration, signs of complications and significant changes in the course of the disease. The patient should be informed that regular outpatient visits, and close collaboration with the outpatient clinics for rheumatology, ophthalmology, and oral medicine, give the most satisfactory results.

Treatment of sicca manifestations is aimed at symptomatic relief and limiting the damaging local effects of chronic xerostomia and keratoconjunctivitis sicca either by substitution or stimulation of the missing secretions (Moutsopoulos and Vlachoyiannopoulos 1993).

Keratoconjunctivitis sicca is treated with fluid replacement supplied as often as necessary. To replace deficient tears, there are several readily available ophthalmic preparations (Tearisol; Liquifilm; 0.5 per cent methylcellulose; Hypo Tears). In severe cases, it may be necessary for patients to use these as often as every 30 min. If corneal ulceration is present, eye-patches and boric acid ointment are recommended. Certain drugs that may cause further deterioration of lacrimal and salivary function, such as diuretics, antihypertensive drugs and antidepressants, should be avoided. The low levels of humidity in air-conditioned environments, as well as windy or dry climates, must be avoided. Soft contact lenses may help to protect the cornea, especially in the presence of filaments. However, the lenses themselves require wetting and the patients must be followed very carefully due to the increased risk of infection. Local stimulators for tear secretion using a cyclic adenosine monophosphate (AMP) derivative, 3-isobutyl-1-methyl-xanthine can be administered as eye drops (Gilbard et al. 1991). In severely dry eyes punctual cauterization should be used. Lateral tarsorraphy is indicated to decrease the ocular surface in a case of severe dryness. When corneal perforation occurs, corneal transplantation is recommended.

Treatment of xerostomia is difficult. Stimulation of salivary flow by sugar-free, highly flavoured lozenges has been found to be rather helpful. Most patients carry water and use sugarless lemon drops or chewing-gum. These must be sugar free, because of the risk of rampant dental caries. Adequate oral hygiene after meals is essential for the prevention of dental disease. Topical oral treatment with fluoride enhances dental mineralization and retards damage to tooth surfaces. In rapidly progressive dental disease, fluoride can be directly applied to the teeth from plastic trays that are used at night. Propionic acid gels may be used to treat vaginal dryness. Bromhexine given orally at high doses (48 mg/day) has been suggested to improve sicca manifestations. However, frequent ingestion of fluids, particularly with meals, is often the best solution.

Pilocarpine hydrochloride (5 mg, four times daily) can also improve sicca manifestations, via its muscarinic, cholinergic activity (Fox 1992). Flushing and sweating are possible side-effects.

Patients with Sjögren's syndrome often complain of parotid gland swelling. If the gland becomes tender with permanent enlargement, infection should be ruled out and treatment with tetracycline orally should be

Box 1 Treatment of Sjögren's syndrome

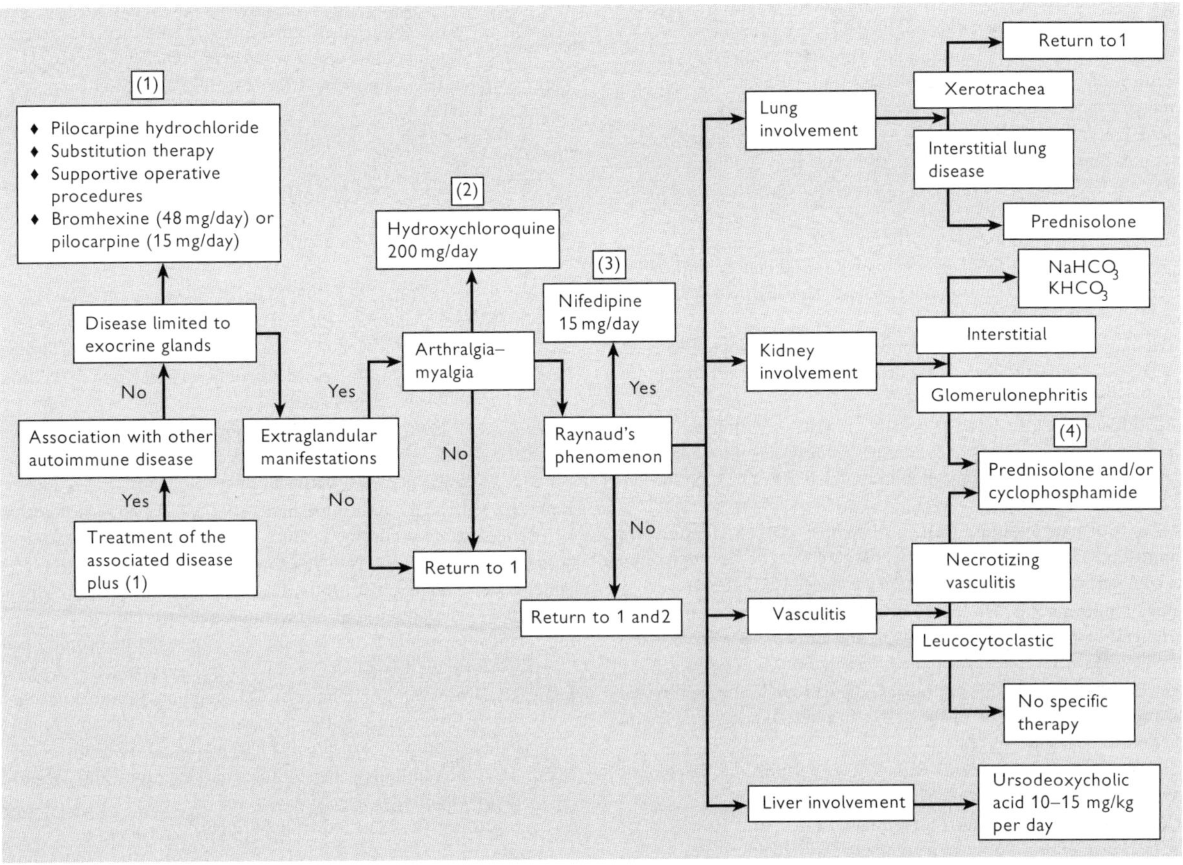

recommended (500 mg, four times daily). Local moist heat, a short course of small doses of steroids and non-steroidal anti-inflammatory drugs are usually helpful in resolving this problem. If the gland remains tender, lymphoma should be ruled out by biopsy.

Preliminary studies showed that hydroxychloroquine, which is efficacious and safe in other autoimmune diseases, may be useful in treating Sjögren's patients. A dose of 200 mg/day partially corrects hypergammaglobulinaemia and decreases the titre of IgG antibodies to La/SSB antigen. Furthermore, hydroxychloroquine decreased the erythrocyte sedimentation rate and increased the haemoglobin (Fox et al. 1988).

Corticosteroids (prednisolone 0.5–1 mg/kg per day) or other immunosuppressive agents (i.e. cyclophosphamide) are indicated for the treatment of life-threatening extraglandular manifestations, particularly when renal or severe pulmonary involvement and systemic vasculitis are present.

Treatment of Sjögren's syndrome-associated lymphoma depends on the staging and histologic type. The low grade marginal zone lymphomas are usually localized and can be treated with local therapy such as surgical removal. The overall survival of patients with low grade lymphomas is 6.3 years and does not differ among treated and untreated patients. Therefore, it is recommended that in these patients a wait and watch policy should be followed. In patients with high-grade lymphoma, a combined chemotherapy using cyclophosphamide, doxorubicin, vincristine, and prednisone (CHOP) should be undertaken.

References

Alexander, E.L. (1987a). Inflammatory vascular disease in Sjögren's syndrome. In *Sjögren's Syndrome: Clinical and Immunological Aspects* (ed. N. Talal, H.M. Moutsopoulos, and S.S. Kassan), pp. 102–24. Berlin: Springer.

Alexander, E.L. (1987b). Neuromuscular complications of primary Sjögren's syndrome. In *Sjögren's Syndrome: Clinical and Immunological Aspects* (ed. N. Talal, H.M. Moutsopoulos, and S.S. Kassan), pp. 61–82. Berlin: Springer.

Andonopoulos, A.P., Drosos, A.A., Skopouli, F.N., Acritidis, N.C., and Moutsopoulos, H.M. (1987). Secondary Sjögren's syndrome in rheumatoid arthritis. *Journal of Rheumatology* **1**, 1098–103.

Andonopoulos, A.P., Drosos, A.A., Skopouli, F.N., and Moutsopoulos, H.M. (1989). Sjögren's syndrome in rheumatoid arthritis and progressive systemic sclerosis: a comparative study. *Clinical and Experimental Rheumatology* **7**, 203–5.

Andonopoulos, A.P., Lagos, G., Drosos, A.A., and Moutsopoulos, H.M. (1990a). The spectrum of neurological involvement in Sjögren's syndrome. *British Journal of Rheumatology* **29**, 21–3.

Andonopoulos, A.P., Skopouli, F.N., Dimou, G.S., Drosos, A.A., and Moutsopoulos, H.M. (1990b). Sjögren's syndrome in systemic lupus erythematosus. *Journal of Rheumatology* **17**, 201–4.

Arrieta, J.J. et al. (2001). In situ detection of hepatitis C virus RNA in salivary glands. *American Journal of Pathology* **158**, 259–64.

Bacman, S., Sterin-Borda, L., Camusso, J.J., Arana, R., Hubscher, O., and Borda, E. (1996). Circulating antibodies against rat parotid gland M3 muscarinic receptors in primary Sjögren's syndrome. *Clinical and Experimental Immunology* **104**, 454–9.

Baum, B.J. and Fox, P.C. (1987). Chemistry of saliva. In *Sjögren's Syndrome: Clinical and Immunological Aspects* (ed. N. Talal, H.M. Moutsopoulos, and S.S. Kassan), pp. 25–34. Berlin: Springer.

Binder, A., Snaith, M.L., and Isenberg, D. (1988). Sjögren's syndrome: a study of its neurological complications. *British Journal of Rheumatology* **27**, 275–80.

Bloch, K.J., Buchanan, W.W., Wohl, M.J., and Bunim, J.J. (1965). Sjögren's syndrome: a clinical, pathological and serological study of sixty-two cases. *Medicine (Baltimore)* **44**, 187–231.

Bodeuitsch, C. et al. (1992). Quantitative immunohistologic criteria are superior to the lymphocytic focus score criterion for the diagnosis of Sjögren's syndrome. *Arthritis and Rheumatism* **35**, 1075–87.

Boumba, D., Skopouli, F.N., and Moutsopoulos, H.M. (1995). Cytokine mRNA expression in the labial salivary gland tissues from patients with primary Sjögren's syndrome. *British Journal of Rheumatology* **34**, 326–33.

Casciola-Rosen, L.A., Anhalt, G., and Rosen, A. (1994). Autoantigens targeted in systemic lupus erythematosus are clustered in two populations of surface structures on apoptotic keratinocytes. *Journal of Experimental Medicine* **179**, 1317–30.

Constantopoulos, S.H. and Moutsopoulos, H.M. (1987). The respiratory system in Sjögren's syndrome. In *Sjögren's Syndrome: Clinical and Immunological Aspects* (ed. N. Talal, H.M. Moutsopoulos, and S.S. Kassan), pp. 83–9. Berlin: Springer.

Dafni, U., Tzioufas, A.G., Staikos, P., Skopouli F.N., and Moutsopoulos, H.M. (1997). The prevalence of Sjögren's syndrome in a close rural community. *Annals of the Rheumatic Diseases* **56**, 521–5.

Daniels, T.E., Aufdemorte, T.B., and Greenspan, J.S. (1987). Histopathology of Sjögren's syndrome. In *Sjögren's Syndrome: Clinical and Immunological Aspects* (ed. N. Talal, H.M. Moutsopoulos, and S.S. Kassan), pp. 266–86. Berlin: Springer.

Drosos, A.A., Constantopoulos, S.H., Phsychos, D., Stefanou, D., Papadimitriou, C.S., and Moutsopoulos, H.M. (1989). The forgotten cause of sicca complex; sarcoidosis. *Journal of Rheumatology* **16**, 1548–51.

Fauci, A.S. and Moutsopoulos, H.M. (1981). Polyclonally triggered B-cells in the peripheral blood of normal individuals and in patients with SLE and primary Sjögren's syndrome. *Arthritis and Rheumatism* **24**, 577–84.

Feist, E. et al. (1999). Autoantibodies in primary Sjögren's syndrome are directed against proteasomal subunits of the alpha and beta type. *Arthritis and Rheumatism* **42**, 697–702.

Fox, R.I. (1992). Treatment of patients with Sjögren's syndrome. *Rheumatic Disease Clinics of North America* **18**, 699–709.

Fox, R.I., Chan, E., Bentol, L., Fong, S., Freidlaender, M., and Howell, F.W. (1988). Treatment of primary Sjögren's syndrome with hydroxychloroquine. *American Journal of Medicine* **85** (Suppl. 4A), 62–7.

Fox, R.I. et al. (1994). Cytokine mRNA expression in salivary biopsies of Sjögren's syndrome. *Journal of Immunology* **152**, 5532–9.

Fujihara, T., Fujita, H., and Tsubota, K. (1999). Preferential localization of CD8+ alpha E beta 7+ T cells around acinar epithelial cells with apoptosis in patients with Sjögren's syndrome. *Journal of Immunology* **163**, 2226–35.

Gellrich, S. et al. (1999). Analysis of V(H)-D-J(H) gene transcripts in B cells infiltrating the salivary glands and lymph node tissues of patients with Sjögren's syndrome. *Arthritis and Rheumatism* **42**, 240–7.

Gilbard, J.P., Rossi, S.R., Heyda, K.G., and Dartt, D.A. (1991). Stimulation of tear secretion and treatment of dry eye disease with 3-isobutyl-1-methylxanthine. *Archives in Ophthalmology* **109**, 672–5.

Green, J.E., Hinricks, S.H., Vogel, J., and Jay, G. (1989). Exocrinopathy resembling Sjögren's syndrome in HTLV-1 *tax* transgenic mice. *Nature* **341**, 72–4.

Goules, A., Masouridi, S., Tzioufas, A.G., Ioannidis, J.P., Skopouli, F.N., and Moutsopoulos, H.M. (2000). Clinically significant and biopsy-documented renal involvement in primary Sjögren syndrome. *Medicine (Baltimore)* **79**, 241–9.

Haddad, J. et al. (1992). Lymphocytic sialadenitis of Sjögren's syndrome associated with chronic hepatitis C virus liver disease. *Lancet* **339**, 321–3.

Humphreys-Beher, M.G., Brinkley, L., Purushotham, K.R., Wang, P.L., Nakagawa, Y., Dusek, D., Kerr, M., Chegini, N., and Chan, E.K. (1993). Characterization of antinuclear antibodies present in the serum from non-obese diabetic mice. *Clinical Immunology and Immunopathology* **68**, 350–6.

Humphreys-Beher, M.G., Hu, Y., Nakagawa, Y., Wang, P.L., and Purushotham, K.R. (1994). Utilization of the non-obese mouse as an animal model for the study of secondary Sjögren's syndrome. *Advances in Experimental and Medical Biology* **350**, 631–6.

Itescu, S. et al. (1990). A diffuse infiltrative CD8 lymphocytosis syndrome in human immunodeficiency virus (HIV) infection: a host immune response associated with HLA-DR5. *Annals of Internal Medicine* **112**, 3–10.

Jacobsson, L. et al. (1989). Dry eyes or mouth—an epidemiological study in Swedish adults with special reference to primary Sjögren's syndrome. *Journal of Autoimmunity* **2**, 521–7.

Kapsogeorgou, E.K., Moutsopoulos, H.M., and Manoussakis, M.N. (2001a). Functional expression of a costimulatory B7.2 (CD86) protein on human salivary gland epithelial cells that interacts with the CD28 receptor, but has reduced binding to CTLA4. *Journal of Immunology* **166**, 3107–13.

Kapsogeorgou, E.K., Dimitriou, I.D., Abu-Helu, R.F., Moutsopoulos, H.M., and Manoussakis, M.N. (2001b). Activation of epithelial and myoepithelial cells in the salivary glands of patients with Sjögren's syndrome: high expression of intercellular adhesion molecule-1 (ICAM-1) in biopsy specimens and cultured cells. *Clinical and Experimental Immunology* **124**, 126–33.

Karsh, J., Pavlidis, N., Neintraub, B.D., and Moutsopoulos, H.M. (1980). Thyroid disease in Sjögren's syndrome. *Arthritis and Rheumatism* **23**, 1326–9.

Kassan, S.S. and Talal, N. (1987). Renal disease with Sjögren's syndrome. In *Sjögren's Syndrome: Clinical and Immunological Aspects* (ed. N. Talal, H.M. Moutsopoulos, and S.S. Kassan), pp. 96–102. Berlin: Springer.

Kassan, S.S. et al. (1978). Increased risk of lymphoma in sicca syndrome. *Annals of Internal Medicine* **89**, 888–92.

Kincaid, M.C. (1987). The eye in Sjögren's syndrome. In *Sjögren's Syndrome: Clinical and Immunological Aspects* (ed. N. Talal, H.M. Moutsopoulos, and S.S. Kassan), pp. 25–34, Berlin: Springer.

Koike, K., Moriya, K., and Ishibashi, K. (1997). Sialadenitis histologically resembling Sjögren syndrome in mice transgenic for hepatitis C virus envelope genes. *Proceedings of National Academy of Sciences (USA)* **94**, 233–6.

Lane, H.C., Callahay, T.R., Jaffe, E.S., Fauci, A.S., and Moutsopoulos, H.M. (1983). The presence of intracytoplasmic infiltrates of the minor salivary glands of patients with primary Sjögren's syndrome. *Clinical and Experimental Rheumatology* **1**, 237–9.

Leroy, J.P., Drosos, A.A., Yannopoulos, D.I., Youinou, P., and Moutsopoulos, H.M. (1990). Intravenous pulse cyclophosphamide therapy in myositis and Sjögren's syndrome. *Arthritis and Rheumatism* **33**, 1579–81.

Mann, D. (1987). Immunogenetics of Sjögren's syndrome. In *Sjögren's Syndrome: Clinical and Immunological Aspects* (ed. N. Talal, H.M. Moutsopoulos, and S.S. Kassan), pp. 235–43. Berlin: Springer.

Manoussakis, M.N., Tzioufas, A.G., Pange, P.J.E., and Moutsopoulos, H.M. (1986). Serological profiles in subgroups of patients with Sjögren's syndrome. *Scandinavian Journal of Rheumatology* **61** (Suppl.), 89–92.

Manoussakis, M.N. et al. (1999). Expression of B7 costimulatory molecules by salivary gland epithelial cells in patients with Sjögren's syndrome. *Arthritis and Rheumatism* **42**, 229–39.

Martens, P.B., Pillemer, S.R., Jacobsson, L.T., O'Fallon, W.M., and Matteson, E.L. (1999). Survivorship in a population based cohort of patients with Sjögren's syndrome, 1976–1992. *Journal of Rheumatology* **26**, 1296–300.

Masago, R., Aiba-Masago, S., Talal, N., Zuluaga, F.J., Al-Hashimi, I., Moody, M., Lau, C.A., Peck, A.B., Brayer, J., Humphreys-Beher, M.G., and Dang, H. (2001). Elevated proapoptotic Bax and caspase 3 activation in the NOD-scid model of Sjögren's syndrome. *Arthritis and Rheumatism* **44**, 693–702.

Moutsopoulos, H.M. (1994). Sjögren's syndrome autoimmune epithelitis. *Clinical Immunology and Immunopathology* **72**, 162–5.

Moutsopoulos, H.M. and Vlachoyiannopoulos, P.G. (1993). What would I do if I had Sjögren's syndrome. *Rheumatology Review* **2**, 17–23.

Moutsopoulos, H.M. et al. (1980). Sjögren's syndrome (sicca syndrome): current issues. *Annals of Internal Medicine* **92**, 212–26.

Moutsopoulos, H.M., Steinberg, A.D., Fauci, A.S., Lane, H.C., and Papadopoulos, N.M. (1983). High incidence of free monoclonal λ light chains in the sera of patients with Sjögren's syndrome. *Journal of Immunology* **130**, 2263–5.

Moutsopoulos, H.M., Costello, R., Drosos, A.A., Mavridis, A.K., and Papadopoulos, N.M. (1985). Demonstration and identification of monoclonal proteins in the urine of patients with Sjögren's syndrome. *Annals of the Rheumatic Diseases* **44**, 109–12.

Moutsopoulos, H.M., Tzioufas, A.G., Bai, M.K., Papadopoulos, N.M., and Papadimitriou, C.S. (1990). Serum IgMκ monoclonicity in patients with Sjögren's syndrome is associated with an increased proportion of κ-positive plasma-cells infiltrating the labial minor salivary glands. *Annals of the Rheumatic Diseases* **49**, 929–31.

Moutsopoulos, N.M., Routsias, J.G., Vlachoyiannopoulos, P.G., Tzioufas, A.G., and Moutsopoulos, H.M. (2000). B-cell epitopes of intracellular autoantigens: Myth and reality. *Molecular Medicine* **6**, 141–51.

Papadopoulos, G.K. and Moutsopoulos, H.M. (1992). Slow viruses and the immune system in the pathogenesis of local tissue damage in Sjögren's syndrome. *Annals of the Rheumatic Diseases* **51**, 136–8.

Parrago, G., Rain, G.D., Brochierion, C., and Rocher, F. (1987). Scintigraphy of the salivary glands in Sjögren's syndrome. *Journal of Clinical Pathology* **40**, 1463–7.

Papiris, S.A., Maniati, M., Constantopoulos, S.H., Roussos, C., Moutsopoulos, H.M., and Skopouli, F.N. (1999). Lung involvement in primary Sjögren's syndrome is mainly related to the small airway disease. *Annals of the Rheumatic Diseases* **58**, 61–4.

Polihronis, M., Tapinos, N.I., Theocharis, S.E., Economou, A., Kittas, C., and Moutsopoulos, H.M. (1998). Modes of epithelial cell death and repair in Sjögren's syndrome (SS). *Clinical and Experimental Immunology* **114**, 485–90.

Ramos-Casals, M. et al. (2000). Thyroid disease in primary Sjögren syndrome. Study in a series of 160 patients. *Medicine (Baltimore)* **79**, 103–8.

Ramos-Casals, M. et al. (2001). Hepatitis C virus infection mimicking primary Sjögren syndrome. A clinical and immunologic description of 35 cases. *Medicine (Baltimore)* **80**, 1–8.

Reveille, J.D., Macleod, M.J., Whittington, K., and Arnett, F.C. (1991). Specific amino acid residues in the second hypervariable region of HLA–DQA1 and DQB1 chain genes promote the Ro(SSA)/La(SSB) autoantibody responses. *Journal of Immunology* **146**, 3871–5.

Rigby, S.P., Griffiths, D.J., Weiss, R.A., and Venables, P.J. (1997). Human retrovirus-5 proviral DNA is rarely detected in salivary gland biopsy tissues from patients with Sjögren's syndrome. *Arthritis and Rheumatism* **40**, 2016–21.

Skarstein, K., Wahren, M., Zaura, E., Hattori, M., and Jonsson, R. (1995). Characterization of T cell receptor repertoire and anti-Ro/SSA autoantibodies in relation to sialadenitis of NOD mice. *Autoimmunity* **22**, 9–16.

Skopouli, F.N., Siouna-Fatourou, H.I., Ziciadis, C., and Moutsopoulos, H.M. (1989). Evaluation of unstimulated whole saliva flow rate and stimulated parotid flow as confirmatory tests for xerostomia. *Clinical and Experimental Rheumatology* **7**, 127–9.

Skopouli, F.N. et al. (1990). Raynaud's phenomenon in primary Sjögren's syndrome. *Journal of Rheumatology* **17**, 618–20.

Skopouli, F.N., Fox, P.C., Galanopoulou, V., Atkinson, J.C., Jaffe, E.C., and Moutsopoulos, H.M. (1991). T-cell subpopulation in the labial minor salivary gland histopathologic lesion of Sjögren's syndrome. *Journal of Rheumatology* **18**, 210–14.

Skopouli, F.N., Kousvelari, E., Mertz, P., Jaffe, E.S., Fox, P.C., and Moutsopoulos, H.M. (1992). c-*myc* mRNA expression in minor salivary glands of patients with Sjögren's syndrome. *Journal of Rheumatology* **19**, 693–9.

Skopouli, F.N., Barbatis, C., and Moutsopoulos, H.M. (1994). Liver involvement in primary Sjögren's syndrome. *British Journal of Rheumatology* **33**, 745–8.

Skopouli, F.N., Dafni, U., Ioannidis, J.P., and Moutsopoulos, H.M. (2000). Clinical evolution, and morbidity and mortality of primary Sjögren's syndrome. *Seminars in Arthritis and Rheumatism* **29**, 296–304.

Sumida, T. et al. (1992). T-cell receptor repertoire of infiltrating T-cells in lips of Sjögren's syndrome patients. *Journal of Clinical Investigation* **89**, 681–5.

Tambur, A.R. et al. (1993). Molecular analysis of HLA class II genes in primary Sjögren's syndrome: a study of Israeli and Greek non-Jewish patients. *Human Immunology* **36**, 235–42.

Tapinos, N.I., Polihronis, M., and Moutsopoulos, H.M. (1999). Lymphoma development in Sjögren's syndrome: novel p53 mutations. *Arthritis and Rheumatism* **42**, 1466–72.

Tengner, P., Halse, A.K., Haga, H.J., Jonsson, R., and Wahren-Herlenius, M. (1998). Detection of anti-Ro/SSA and anti-La/SSB autoantibody-producing cells in salivary glands from patients with Sjögren's syndrome. *Arthritis and Rheumatism* **41**, 2238–48.

Tektonidou, M., Kaskani, E., Skopouli, F.N., and Moutsopoulos, H.M. (1999). Microvascular abnormalities in Sjögren's syndrome: nailfold capillaroscopy. *Rheumatology (Oxford)* **38**, 826–30.

Teramoto, N. et al. (1989). Annular erythema: a possible association with primary Sjögren's syndrome. *Journal of the American Academy of Dermatology* **20**, 596–601.

Thomas, E., Hay, E.M., Hajeer, A., and Silman, A.J. (1998). Sjögren's syndrome. A community-based study of prevalence and impact. *British Journal of Rheumatology* **37**, 1069–76.

Toda, I., Sullivan, B.D., Rocha, E.M., da Silveira, L.A., Wickam, L.A., and Sullivan, D.A. (1999). Impact of gender on exocrine gland inflammation in mouse models of Sjögren's syndrome. *Experimental Eye Research* **69**, 355–66.

Trevino, H., Tsianos, E.B., and Schenkers, S. (1987). Gastrointestinal and hepatobiliary features in Sjögren's syndrome. In *Sjögren's Syndrome: Clinical and Immunological Aspects* (ed. N. Talal, H.M. Moutsopoulos, and S.S. Kassan), pp. 89–95. Berlin: Springer.

Tsampoulas, C.G. et al. (1990). Hand radiographic changes in patients with primary and secondary Sjögren's syndrome. *Scandinavian Journal of Rheumatology* **15**, 333–9.

Tsianos, E.B. et al. (1990). Sjögren's syndrome in patients with primary biliary cirrhosis. *Hepatology* **11**, 730–4.

Tsokos, M., Lazarou, S.A., and Moutsopoulos, H.M. (1987). Vasculitis in primary Sjögren's syndrome: histologic classification and clinical presentation. *American Journal of Clinical Pathology* **88**, 26–31.

Tzioufas, A.G., Manoussakis, M.N., Costello, R., Silis, M., Papadopoulos, N.M., and Moutsopoulos, H.M. (1986). Cryoglobulinemia in autoimmune rheumatic diseases: evidence of circulating monoclonal cryoglobulins in patients with primary Sjögren's syndrome. *Arthritis and Rheumatism* **29**, 1098–104.

Tzioufas, A.G., Boumba, D.S., Skopouli, F.N., and Moutsopoulos, H.M. (1996). Mixed monoclonal cryoglobulinemia and monoclonal rheumatoid factor cross-reactive idiotypes as predicting factors for lymphoma development in primary Sjögren's syndrome. *Arthritis and Rheumatism* **39**, 767–72.

Van de Merwe, J.P., Kamerling, R., Arendsen, H.S., Mulder, A.H., and Hooijkaas, H. (1993). Sjögren's syndrome in patients with interstitial cystitis. *Journal of Rheumatology* **20**, 962–6.

Vitali, C. et al. (1988). Parotid sialography and minor salivary gland biopsy in the diagnosis of Sjögren's syndrome: a comparative study of 84 patients. *Journal of Rheumatology* **15**, 262–7.

Vitali, C. et al. (1992). Anti hepatitis C virus antibodies in primary Sjögren's syndrome: false positive results are related to hyper-γ-globulinemia. *Clinical and Experimental Rheumatology* **10**, 103–4.

Vitali, C. et al. (1993). Preliminary criteria for the classification of Sjögren's syndrome. Results of a prospective concerted action supported by the European Community. *Arthritis and Rheumatism* **36**, 340–8.

Voulgarelis, M., Dafni, U.G., Isenberg, D.A., and Moutsopoulos, H.M. (1999). Malignant lymphoma in primary Sjögren's syndrome: a multicenter, retrospective, clinical study by the European Concerted Action on Sjögren's syndrome. *Arthritis and Rheumatism* **42**, 1765–72.

Witte, T. et al. (2000). IgA and IgG autoantibodies against alpha-fodrin as markers for Sjögren's syndrome. Systemic lupus erythematosus. *Journal of Rheumatology* **27**, 2617–20.

Xanthou, G., Tapinos, N.I., Polihronis, M., Nezis, I.P., Margaritis, L.H., and Moutsopoulos, H.M. (1999). CD4 cytotoxic and dendritic cells in the immunopathologic lesion of Sjögren's syndrome. *Clinical and Experimental Immunology* **118**, 154–63.

Xanthou, G., Polihronis, M., Tzioufas, A.G., Paikos, S., Sideras, P, and Moutsopoulos, H.M. (2001). 'Lymphoid' chemokine messenger RNA expression by epithelial cells in the chronic inflammatory lesion of the salivary glands of Sjögren's syndrome patients: possible participation in lymphoid structure formation. *Arthritis and Rheumatism* **44**, 408–18.

Yanagi, K., Ishimaru, N., Haneji, N., Saegusa, K., Saito, I., and Hayashi, Y. (1998). Anti-120-kDa alpha-fodrin immune response with Th1-cytokine profile in the NOD mouse model of Sjögren's syndrome. *European Journal of Immunology* **28**, 3336–45.

Yannopoulos, D.I. et al. (1992). Conjunctival epithelial cells from patients with Sjögren's syndrome inappropriately express major histocompatibility complex molecules, La/SSB antigen and heat shock proteins. *Journal of Clinical Immunology* **12**, 259–65.

Youinou, P., Pennec, Y.L., Katsikis, P., Jouquan, J., Faugment, P., and LeGoll, P. (1990). Raynaud's phenomenon in primary Sjögren's syndrome. *British Journal of Rheumatology* **29**, 205–7.

Zeher, M., Szodoray, P., Gyimesi, E., and Szondy, Z. (1999). Correlation of increased susceptibility to apoptosis of CD4+ T cells with lymphocyte activation and activity of disease in patients with primary Sjögren's syndrome. *Arthritis and Rheumatism* **42**, 1673–81.

6.10 Vasculitis

6.10.1 Classification and epidemiology of vasculitis

David G.I. Scott and Richard A. Watts

Introduction

The vasculitides are a heterogeneous group of relatively uncommon diseases which can arise de novo [e.g. Wegener's granulomatosis (WG)] or as a secondary feature of an established clinical disease such as rheumatoid arthritis (RA).

The word vasculitis means inflammation of blood vessels, that is, the blood vessel is the primary site of inflammation. The pathological consequence of such inflammation is often destruction of the vessel wall, seen on histology as fibrinoid necrosis (Plate 139), hence the term 'necrotizing vasculitis'.

Vasculitis can occasionally be localized and clinically insignificant but more commonly is generalized and potentially life-threatening, especially when small muscular arteries are involved. Muscular arteries may develop focal or segmental lesions. The former (affecting part of the vessel wall) may lead to aneurysm formation and possibly rupture; segmental lesions (affecting the whole circumference) are more common and lead to stenosis or occlusion with distal infarction. Small-vessel vasculitis, by contrast, most commonly affects the skin and rarely causes dysfunction of internal organs. Widespread small-vessel vasculitis may cause problems, especially in the kidney, when sufficient numbers of adjacent vessels are affected with significant release of inflammatory mediators or where overall perfusion is threatened.

The aetiology of vasculitis is unknown but is clearly multifactorial; among the influences on disease expression are ethnicity, genes (HLA and others), gender, and environment (UV light, infections, toxins, drugs, allergy, smoking, etc.). In this chapter, we will review the available evidence and attempt to identify important epidemiological factors involved in the major vasculitic syndromes using current classification criteria. This has been structured around a classification system based on the size of vessels predominantly involved (Table 1) which has evolved from a number of other classifications which will also be reviewed.

Classification of vasculitis

Classification of vasculitis is confusing because of the considerable overlap between the different vasculitic syndromes and because the cause of the vasculitis is usually unknown.

Historical

Kussmaul and Maier (1866) are credited with the first description of 'periarteritis nodosa' when they described a 'new disease' characterized by numerous nodules along the course of small muscular arteries. Earlier descriptions suggest that formal recording of the disease is at least 200 years old [reviewed by Matteson (2000)].

Zeek (1952) reviewed the literature relating to vasculitis and periarteritis nodosa and used the generic term 'necrotizing angiitis' to indicate the specific damage to the blood vessel wall rather than the presence of anti-inflammatory cells alone; she classified these into five distinct entities: (i) hypersensitivity angiitis, (ii) allergic granulomatous angiitis, (iii) rheumatic arteritis, (iv) periarteritis nodosa, and (v) temporal arteritis. Most modern classifications are based on Zeek's work, which essentially combined histological changes and clinical features. Notable omissions from Zeek's classification were WG and Takayasu's arteritis; these were not fully described in the English literature until after 1953, and also the early description of microscopic polyangiitis (MPA) by Davson et al. (1948), which was not generally recognized until the 1990s.

Current classification

The American College of Rheumatology (ACR) in 1990, addressing the previous problem of lack of uniformity, proposed criteria for the classification of seven different vasculitides with sensitivities varying from 71.0 to 95.3 per cent and specificities of 78.7–99.7 per cent (Fries et al. 1990). The most sensitive and specific criteria were found in Churg–Strauss syndrome (CSS), giant cell arteritis, and Takayasu's arteritis; hypersensitivity (leucocytoclastic) vasculitis was the least well-defined condition. The ACR criteria are not perfect; they were established by comparing patients with different types of vasculitis, but not with patients prior to the diagnosis of vasculitis, or with other systemic diseases or even with other connective tissue diseases. The reliability of these criteria when used in patients in whom vasculitis is only suspected is poor (Rao et al. 1998).

In 1994, consensus definitions for the commoner forms of vasculitis were proposed at the Chapel Hill Consensus Conference (CHCC) (Table 2). These provided important and useful definitions of disease but were not

Table 1 Classification of systemic vasculitis

Dominant vessels involved	Primary	Secondary
Large arteries	Giant cell arteritis Takayasu's arteritis Isolated CNS angiitis	Aortitis associated with RA Infection (e.g. syphilis)
Medium arteries	Classical PAN Kawasaki's disease	Infection (e.g. hepatitis B) Hairy cell leukaemia
Small vessels and medium arteries	Wegener's granulomatosis[a] Churg–Strauss syndrome[a] Microscopic polyangiitis[a]	Vasculitis secondary to RA, SLE, SS Sjögren's syndrome Drugs, malignancy Infection (e.g. HIV)
Small vessels (leucocytoclastic)	Henoch–Schönlein purpura Essential mixed cryoglobulinaemia Cutaneous leucocytoclastic angiitis	Drugs[b] Infection (e.g. hepatitis B, C)

[a] Diseases most commonly associated with ANCA (antimyeloperoxidase and antiproteinase 3 antibodies), a significant risk of renal involvement, and which are most responsive to immunosuppression with cyclophosphamide.

[b] Sulfonamides, penicillins, thiazide diuretics, and many others.

Note: CNS, central nervous system; HIV, human immunodeficiency virus; PAN, polyarteritis nodosa; RA, rheumatoid arthritis; SLE, systemic lupus erythematosus; SS, Sjögren's syndrome. Reproduced from Watts and Scott (2002).

Table 2 Names and definitions of vasculitides adopted by the Chapel Hill Consensus Conference on the nomenclature of systemic vasculitis[a]

Large-vessel vasculitis	
Giant cell (temporal) arteritis	Granulomatous arteritis of the aorta and its major branches, with a predilection for the extracranial branches of the carotid artery. *Often involves the temporal artery. Usually occurs in patients older than 50 and often is associated with polymyalgia rheumatica*
Takayasu's arteritis	Granulomatous inflammation of the aorta and its major branches. *Usually occurs in patients younger than 50*
Medium-sized vessel vasculitis	
Polyarteritis nodosa[b] (classic polyarteritis nodosa)	Necrotizing inflammation of medium-sized or small arteries without glomerulonephritis or vasculitis in arterioles, capillaries, or venules
Kawasaki's disease	Arteritis involving large, medium-sized, small arteries, and associated with mucocutaneous lymph node syndrome. *Coronary arteries are often involved. Aorta and veins may be involved. Usually occurs in children*
Small-vessel vasculitis	
Wegener's granulomatosis[c]	Granulomatous inflammation involving the respiratory tract, and necrotizing vasculitis affecting small to medium-sized vessels (e.g. capillaries, venules, arterioles, and arteries). *Necrotizing glomerulonephritis is common*
Churg–Strauss syndrome[c]	Eosinophil-rich and granulomatous inflammation involving the respiratory tract, necrotizing vasculitis affecting small to medium-sized vessels, and associated with asthma and eosinophilia
Microscopic polyangiitis[b] (microscopic polyarteritis)[c]	Necrotizing vasculitis, with few or no immune depositis, affecting small vessels (i.e. capillaries, venules, or arterioles). *Necrotizing arteritis involving small- and medium-sized arteries may be present. Necrotizing glomerulonephritis is very common. Pulmonary capillaritis often occurs*
Henoch–Schönlein purpura	Vasculitis, with IgA-dominant immune deposits, affecting small vessels (i.e. capillaries, venules, or arterioles). *Typically involves skin, gut, and glomeruli, and is associated with arthralgia or arthritis*
Essential cryoglobulinaemic vasculitis	Vasculitis, with cryoglobulin immune deposits, affecting small vessels (i.e. capillaries, venules, or arterioles), and associated with cryoglobulins in serum. *Skin and glomeruli are often involved*
Cutaneous leucocytoclastic angiitis	Isolated cutaneous leucocytoclastic angiitis without systemic vasculitis or glomerulonephritis

[a] Large vessel refers to the aorta and the largest branches directed towards the major body regions (e.g. to the extremities and the head and neck); medium-sized vessel refers to the main visceral arteries (e.g. renal, hepatic, coronary, and mesenteric arteries); small vessel refers to venules, capillaries, arterioles, and the intraparenchymal distal arterial radicals that connect with arterioles. Some small- and large-vessel vasculitides may involve medium-sized arteries, but large and medium-sized vessel vasculitides do not involve vessels smaller than arteries. Essential components are represented by normal type; italicized type represents usual, but not essential, components.

[b] Preferred term.

[c] Strongly associated with antineutrophil cytoplasmic antibodies.

Source: Reproduced from Jeanette et al. (1994) with permission.

considered appropriate for diagnosis or classification of patients as no specific criteria were produced (Jeanette et al. 1994). This attempt was the first to define MPA (not included in the ACR study) and hence this definition has been used in some epidemiological studies. We have shown, for example, that the currently available criteria/definitions often identify different patients (Watts et al. 1996). The implication of these developments is that any study must identify the criteria/definitions on which the diagnosis has been based.

The ACR classification criteria and the CHCC definitions did not specifically include ANCA. Antibodies to neutrophil cytoplasmic antigens, particularly those against proteinase 3 (PR3), are now well recognized to be strongly associated with WG and those against myeloperoxidase (MPO) with MPA, CSS, and idiopathic necrotizing glomerulonephritis. The CHCC definitions group all the small vasculitides together which have been separated in the classification system outlined in Table 1. We strongly believe that the diseases WG, CSS, and MPA should be separated in classification systems from the other small vasculitides because they (i) often involve small- and sometimes medium-sized arteries, (ii) are the diseases most commonly associated with ANCA, (iii) are associated with the highest risk of glomerulonephritis, and (iv) respond best to immunosuppression with cyclophosphamide. The aetiology of these diseases is probably unrelated to immune complex formation, in contrast to pure small vessel vasculitis such as Henoch–Schönlein purpura (HSP) and essential mixed cryoglobulinaemia. This classification also reflects broad therapeutic strategies (Table 3), with the medium- and small-vessel groups responding best to immunosuppression with cyclophosphamide in addition to corticosteroids, the large-vessel group requiring moderate to high-dose corticosteroids, usually alone, and the small-vessel group only sometimes requiring corticosteroids at a low dose.

Epidemiology

The lack of any clear understanding of the aetiology of the systemic vasculitides and the problems with classification systems outlined above have hampered accurate epidemiological studies. Most studies are hospital based from tertiary/university referral centres with ill-defined denominator populations. There may in addition be referral bias: patients seen in tertiary hospitals may not be representative of those seen either at district hospitals or in the community, especially in terms of disease severity of age spectrum. Prospective population based estimates of incidence and prevalence are few.

The epidemiology of the primary systemic vasculitides (WG, CSS, MPA, and polyarteritis) has been most widely studied in the Norwich Health Authority with data collected prospectively from 1988. Incidence rates adjusted for age and sex to the 1992 population show an overall annual incidence of primary systemic vasculitis of 19.8 per million [95 per cent confidence intervals (CI) 15.8–24.6]. The point prevalence on 31 December 1997 was 144.5 per million (95 per cent CI 110.4–185.3). Primary systemic vasculitis was more common in males (23.3 per million) than females (16.4 per million). The age and sex specific incidence showed a clear increase with age with an overall peak in the 65–74 year age group (60.1 per million) (Watts et al. 2000). Using the same classification criteria on three populations—Norwich, United Kingdom; Tromso, North Norway; and Lugo, North-west Spain—confirmed the older age at onset (compared with previous studies) and showed a similar overall incidence and pattern of vasculitis in terms of age- and sex-distribution. MPA was more common and WG less common in southern Europe while CSS appeared to be more common in Norwich. The importance of such comparative data from well-defined populations may provide further insights into the role of environmental or genetic factors in the pathogenesis of vasculitis which will be

Table 3 Relationship between vessel size and response to treatment

Dominant vessels involved	Corticosteroids alone	Cyclophosphamide + corticosteroids	Others
Large arteries	+++	−	+
Medium arteries	+	++	++[a]
Small vessels and medium arteries	+	+++	−
Small vessels	+	−	++

[a] Includes plasmapheresis, antiviral therapy for hepatitis B-associated vasculitis, and intravenous immunoglobulin for Kawasaki's disease.

Source: Reproduced from Watts and Scott (2002).

explored further within the context of each individual disease as seen below (Watts et al. 2001).

Large-vessel vasculitis

Giant cell arteritis and polymyalgia rheumatica (see Chapters 6.10.5 and 6.10.6)

Giant cell arteritis (GCA) and polymyalgia rheumatica (PMR) are two closely related disorders, which in some patients coexist. GCA is a vasculitic disease in which the characteristic feature is the presence of giant cells in a biopsy of the temporal artery. Although the ACR criteria for GCA (Hunder et al. 1990) do not require histological evidence of arteritis, many studies only report biopsy positive cases. Clearly, the biopsy rate and intensity of histological search for evidence of vasculitis will influence the reported incidence. Furthermore, many of the studies have been hospital based and retrospective. Prospective studies from Scandinavia have reported annual incidence figures for biopsy proven GCA of 15–35 per 100 000 individuals aged over 50 years and a similar rate has been reported from Olmsted County (Minnesota, United States of America) (Table 4). In the United Kingdom the incidence of GCA in the over 65-year-olds may be as high as four per 1000 in general practice (Kyle et al. 1985). There is an increasing incidence with age, peaking in persons aged 80 years or greater; very few cases occur in those aged less than 50 years. Most series report a greater incidence in women with a female to male ratio of around 2 : 1.

Time trends

Several studies have suggested an increase in the incidence of GCA and PMR with time. In Olmsted County, there has been a steady increase in the annual incidence of GCA between 1950 and 1991, with an increase from 7.3/100 000 to 19.1/100 000 inhabitants aged greater than 50 years. The predicted rate of increase was 2.6 per cent every 5 years.

Geographical factors

The majority of studies have come from Scandinavia or from populations with the same ethnic background (Olmsted County includes a significant population of Scandinavian ancestry). Studies from southern Europe (Italy and Spain) and France have consistently reported lower incidence rates than those from Scandinavia. Jews from Jerusalem also seem to have a very low incidence. Multiple regression analysis correcting for the effect of increasing incidence with time suggests that there is a significant trend to increasing incidence with more northerly latitude (Fig. 1). In the United States, there is only one study from a population other than Olmsted County, this is from Tennessee and reports a lower incidence in the southern Caucasian population. This trend is similar to that seen in multiple sclerosis and RA.

Ethnic differences

PMR and GCA are uncommon in non-Caucasians although there is little substantive epidemiological data. The Tennessee study reported a low incidence in African-Americans (Smith et al. 1983).

Cardiovascular risk factors

Cardiovascular risk factors for GCA/PMR were reported in a prospective case–control study in France. Smoking was associated with a six-fold increase and previous atheromatous disease with 4.5-fold increase in women with GCA (Duhaut et al. 1998). This was an independent effect. Only smoking was a risk factor for PRM in women. For men no significant cardiovascular risk factors for GCA or PMR were identified.

Environmental factors

The Olmsted County study identified peaks in incidence occurring every 7 years, a finding that would be consistent with an infectious aetiology. In Denmark, peak incidences were correlated with the occurrence of epidemics of *Mycoplasma pneumoniae* infection (Elling et al. 1996). Using a matched case–control method Russo et al. (1995) showed a correlation between infection and onset of GCA but could not identify a specific infection.

Cimmino and colleagues reported an increased prevalence of antibodies to respiratory syncytial virus and adenovirus in Italian patients (Cimmino 1997), and more recently a French group performed a large case–control study suggesting that reinfection with human parainfluenza virus (HPIV) (a virus known to induce human multinucleated giant cells) is associated with the onset of GCA (Duhaut et al. 1999). No association was seen with other viruses that induce multinucleated giant cells, such as measles virus, herpes simplex virus, Epstein–Barr virus, and respiratory syncytial virus, nor was there an association with temporal artery biopsy negative patients and PMR.

Parvovirus B19 infection occurs in epidemic cycles similar to those seen for GCA. Gabriel and colleagues have recently demonstrated, by PCR, the presence of parvovirus B19 DNA in temporal artery biopsy specimens from GCA patients (Gabriel et al. 1999). The aetiological significance of this is at present unclear.

In summary, no unifying hypothesis has emerged. Cimmino has proposed that infrared and UVA solar radiation damages the internal elastic lamina of superficial arteries, this facilitates the localization of an unknown aetiological antigen (possibly viral protein). Antigenic peptides are then presented in the context of class II MHC molecules, macrophages and CD4+ T lymphocytes are stimulated, which results in GCA or PMR depending on the pattern of cytokine profiles. This process is accentuated in elderly females with specific HLA–DRB1 alleles (Cimmino 1997).

Takayasu's arteritis

Takayasu's arteritis (described world-wide) is usually considered to be more common in Asia. In most series, there appears to be an excess of patients of Asian descent. The peak age of disease onset is in the third decade and the disease is more common in women.

The ACR classification criteria for the diagnosis of Takayasu's arteritis are given in Table 5 (Arend et al. 1990). Takayasu's arteritis is clearly distinguished from giant cell arteritis by age. A high erythrocyte sedimentation rate, carotid artery tenderness, and/or hypertension lack specificity and sensitivity to differentiate patients with Takayasu's arteritis from other forms of arteritis.

Table 7 Annual incidence of polyarteritis nodosa

Diagnosis	Year	Place	Incidence (million)	Reference
PAN	1972–1980	Bristol/Bath, UK	4.6	Scott et al. (1982)
PAN[a]	1988–1998	Lugo, Spain	6.2	Watts et al. (2001)
PAN[a]	1988–1998	Norwich, UK	9.7	Watts et al. (2001)
PAN[a]	1988–1998	Tromso, Norway	4.4	Watts et al. (2001)
PAN[a]	1992–1996	Kristiansand, Norway	6.6	Haugeberg et al. (1998)
PAN	1951–1967	Olmsted County, MN, USA	7.0	Kurland et al. (1969)
PAN	1957–1971	Michigan, USA	2.0	Sack et al. (1975)
PAN	1976–1979	Olmsted County, MN, USA	9.0	Kurland et al. (1984)
PAN[b]	1993–1996	Kuwait	16.0	El-Reshaid et al. (1997)
PAN[b]	1988–1997	Lugo, Spain	0.9	Watts et al. (2001)
PAN[b]	1988–1998	Norwich, UK	0.0	Watts et al. (2001)
PAN[b]	1988–1998	Tromso, Norway	0.5	Watts et al. (2001)
PAN[c]	1974–1985	Alaska	77.0	McMahon et al. (1989)
PAN[b]	1998	Germany	1.0	Reinhold-Keller et al. (2002)

[a] ACR (1990) criteria.

[b] Chapel Hill Consensus definition.

[c] Hepatitis B positive.

Table 8 Annual incidence of microscopic polyangiitis

Diagnosis	Year	Place	Incidence (per million)	Reference
MPA[a,b]	1971–1993	Lund, Sweden	2.5	Westman et al. (1998)
MPA	1980–1986	Leicester, UK	0.5	Andrews et al. (1990)
MPA	1987–1989	Leicester, UK	3.0	Andrews et al. (1990)
MPA[a]	1984–1989	Heidelberg, Germany	1.5	Andrassy et al. (1991)
MPA[b]	1988–1998	Lugo, Spain	11.6	Watts et al. (2001)
MPA[b]	1988–1998	Norwich, UK	8.4	Watts et al. (2001)
MPA[b]	1988–1998	Tromso, Norway	2.7	Watts et al. (2001)
MPA[a,b]	1993–1996	Kuwait	24.0	El-Reshaid et al. (1997)
MPA[a]	1998	Germany	2.5	Reinhold-Keller et al. (2002)

[a] Renal involvement only.

[b] Chapel Hill Consensus definition.

study undertaken in Norfolk showed that silica was particularly associated with MPA/pANCA. Propylthiouracil and hydralazine are drugs known to be associated with vasculitis and propylthiouracil particularly associated with ANCA. Our case–control study also showed an association between farming exposure and vasculitis with odds ratios as high as nine (Lane et al. 2003).

Wegener's granulomatosis (see also Chapter 6.10.2)

Wegener first described a disease characterized by necrotizing granulomata of the upper and lower respiratory tract, focal glomerulonephritis, and necrotizing systemic vasculitis [reviewed by Matteson (2000)]. Respiratory tract disease may precede systemic and renal vasculitis by many months or years. De Remee classified WG on the basis of organs involved (E–L–K)—E, ear, nose, throat; L, lung; K, kidney involvement (DeRemee et al. 1976). This classification has proved useful in staging patients with the disease, but pre-supposes a progression from E–L–K, which does not always occur.

The ACR (1990) classification criteria for the diagnosis of WG are shown in traditional format in Chapter 6.10.2.

The CHCC definition restricts the term WG to patients with necrotizing granulomatous inflammation (Table 2). Neither the CHCC nor the ACR classification scheme address the issue of limited disease.

The annual incidence of WG since 1986 in Europe is in the range of 2–11/million [reviewed in Watts and Scott (2002)], but there are no comparable figures from elsewhere in the world. The prevalence of WG in the United States was estimated to be 26.0 per million in 1986–1990 (Cotch et al. 1996). The incidence of WG may be increasing. A study from Leicester, United Kingdom, reported an increase in the annual incidence of WG from 0.7 per million (1980–1986) to 2.8 per million (1987–1989). This was partially attributed to an increase in diagnostic awareness following the introduction of assays for ANCA in 1987. A recent Norwegian study reported an increase from 5 per million to 12 per million over the last 15 years. We did not observe any significant change during the 10 year period in our Norwich study (reviewed in Watts and Scott 2002).

The pathogenesis of WG is unknown. Duna et al. (1998) studied self-reported exposure to heat, fumes, and particulates. There was a higher incidence of exposure in WG patients compared with normal control subjects, but no difference between WG patients and patients with other types of lung disease. Our case–control study showed an association between silica exposure (particularly agricultural silica) and WG, solvents, and also farm exposure as documented with MPA. The strongest association in terms of ANCA was for cANCA (PR3) with sheep and chickens, and for pANCA/MPO with cows (Lane et al. 2003).

WG has been linked to parvovirus B19 and *Staphylococcus aureus* infection. Nasal carriage of *S. aureus* has been associated with increased risk of relapse in WG (Stegeman et al. 1996).

Clusters of WG occurring in families have been described [reviewed in Nowack et al. (1999)]. In most clusters no more than two people have been affected, usually one parent and a child or two siblings. Distant family members are rarely reported. The occurrence of clusters in first degree relatives and not in more distant family members suggests that environmental triggers play an important role in the aetiology as parents and children or siblings share their environment as well as genetic background.

Churg–Strauss syndrome

Churg and Strauss (1951) described the post-mortem features of 13 patients who died following an illness characterized by asthma, eosinophilia, fever, systemic upset, and granulomatous necrotizing vasculitis. Lanham in 1984, provided a clinical definition of CSS as a triad of asthma, eosinophilia ($>1 \times 10^9$/l), and systemic vasculitis involving two or more extra pulmonary organs (Lanham et al. 1984). In their experience extravascular granulomata were not essential for the diagnosis of CSS. They also noted a triphasic pattern of illness with allergic rhinitis, evolving into asthma, followed by peripheral blood eosinophilia and eosinophilic tissue infiltrates, and finally a systemic vasculitis phase. The granulomata may be localized and associated with a variety of systemic manifestations. Furthermore, the necrotizing vasculitis may be indistinguishable from that found in classical PAN and/or MPA.

The ACR criteria for the diagnosis of CSS are given in Table 9 (Masi et al. 1990). These criteria do not include some common clinical features of CSS such as rash or cardiac involvement, as they gave poor discrimination. The combination of asthma and eosinophilia are both sensitive and highly specific for the diagnosis of CSS.

The CHCC definition of CSS (Chapter 6.10.2) includes the presence of asthma and eosinophilia (Jeanette et al. 1994). The presence of conspicious eosinophils in inflammatory infiltrates is not alone a discriminating feature as they can occur in other types of vasculitis including WG and MPA.

The UK annual incidence of CSS as defined by the ACR criteria was 2.8 per million, in Lugo (Spain), 1.1 per million during 1988–1997, and in Tromso (Norway) 0.5 per million (Watts et al. 2001).

Environmental factors

The majority of cases of CSS are idiopathic; inhaled antigens, vaccination, and desensitization have been reported as triggering factors (Guillevin et al. 1999). Drugs including sulfonamides, penicillin, anticonvulsants, and thiazides have also been associated with the syndrome. Recently Wechsler et al. (1998) reported eight patients with glucocorticosteroid-dependent asthma receiving the sulfidopeptide-leukotriene antagonist zafirlukast, who developed CSS associated with corticosteroid withdrawal. Two patients probably had pre-existing CSS with asthma, neuropathy, and infiltrates. In the other patients, zafirlukast improved asthma control sufficiently to permit reduction in glucocorticoid dose. CSS became apparent within days or months of the dose reduction. Although allergic vasculitis due to zafirlukast is possible, it is more likely that reduction of steroid dose unmasked underlying CSS.

Kawasaki's disease

Kawasaki's disease (mucocutaneous lymph node syndrome) (KD) is an acute vasculitis, which predominately affects infants and young children. The condition was first recognized in Japan in 1967 (Kawasaki 1967). Coronary vasculitis is a major cause of morbidity and mortality. There is no laboratory test for the diagnosis of KD and the diagnosis is therefore based on standard clinical criteria, as defined by the American Heart Association (1990). KD occurs in both epidemic and endemic forms worldwide. The occurrence of epidemic KD has lead to speculation that the condition is caused by an infectious agent.

Geographical factors

In Japan, nationwide epidemiological surveys carried out between 1970 and 1992 found a total of 116 848 cases. The annual incidence of KD in 1991–1992 in Japan was 900 per million in children aged less than 5 years (Yanagawa et al. 1995), because KD is rare in children aged over 5 years.

A recent study by Gardner-Medwin et al. (2002) found an annual incidence in the United Kingdom of 55 per million in children aged less than 5 years.

Ethnic factors

The incidence of KD has always been considered to be higher in Japanese and other Asiatic populations. In the Washington State study, the annual incidence (appears to be increasing with time) was greatest in Asian Americans aged less than 5 years (333 per million) compared with Black Americans (234 per million) and Caucasians (127 per million) (Davis et al. 1995). This difference was also documented in the UK series with Asian children (of Indian, Pakistani, or Bangladeshi origin) showing an incidence of 146 per million compared with Blacks (59 per million) and White Caucasians (46 per million) (Gardner-Medwin et al. 2002). This UK study is important as the Asian Americans were all of oriental origin, whereas none of the UK Asians were.

Table 9 ACR 1990 criteria for the classification of Churg–Strauss syndrome (traditional format)

Criterion	Definition
1. Asthma	History of wheezing or diffuse high-pitched rales on expiration
2. Eosinophilia	Eosinophilia >0% on white blood cell differential count
3. History of allergy[a]	History of seasonal allergy (e.g. allergic rhinitis) or other documented allergies, including food, contactants, and others, except for drug allergy
4. Mononeuropathy or polyneuropathy	Development of mononeuropathy, multiple mononeuropathies, or polyneuropathy (i.e. glove/stocking distribution) attributable to a systemic vasculitis
5. Pulmonary infiltrates, non-fixed	Migratory or transitory pulmonary infiltrates on radiographs (not including fixed infiltrates), attributable to a systemic vasculitis
6. Paranasal sinus abnormality	History of acute or chronic paranasal sinus pain or tenderness or radiographic opacification of the paranasal sinuses
7. Extravascular eosinophils	Biopsy including artery, arteriole, or venule, showing accumulations of eosinophils in extravascular areas

[a] History of allergy, other than asthma or drug related, is included only in the tree classification set and not in the traditional format criteria set, which requires four or more of the other six items listed here. The presence of any four or more criteria yields a sensitivity of 85.0% and a specificity or 99.7%.

Small-vessel vasculitis

Henoch–Schönlein purpura and hypersensitivity vasculitis

William Heberden of London first described what became known as 'Henoch–Schönlein purpura' in his Commentarii de Marlbaun published in 1801. Schönlein later described a childhood illness characterized by acute purpura and arthritis. Henoch (1874) described the additional features of colicky abdominal pain and nephritis (reviewed by Matteson 2000). Vasculitis due to allergic or hypersensitivity mechanisms has been considered a distinct entity since the 1940s (Zeek 1952). The ACR (1990) considered HSP and hypersensitivity vasculitis (HSV) (leucocytoclastic vasculitis) to be separate conditions. The criteria for HSV were not sensitive (71.0 per cent) or specific (78.5 per cent) (Fries et al. 1990). There is considerable overlap between the ACR and CHCC criteria. The CHCC definition for HSP makes a much better distinction between HSP and cutaneous leucocytoclastic angiitis (their preferred term for cutaneous vasculitis; they did not consider hypersensitivity vasculitis), because they included the presence of IgA deposits in the definition (Jeanette et al. 1994).

The annual incidence of HSP in children is 204 per million for all children under 17 years, or 221 per million in children under 14 years. The estimated annual incidence is highest between the ages of 4 and 6 years with a mean age of onset of 6.4 years and a median of 4.8 years. Black children have a significantly lower annual incidence of HSP than White or Asian populations with a sex ratio of male to female of 1.2 : 1 (Gardner-Medwin et al. 2002). The incidence of HSP in adults is significantly lower.

Secondary vasculitis

Vasculitis occurring in the presence of autoimmune rheumatic disease or infection is usually considered to be secondary (Table 1). This most typically occurs in patients with RA, SLE, or Sjögren's syndrome and in our experience is more common than primary vasculitis. Rheumatoid vasculitis has established criteria and there are some data on its frequency (see Chapter 6.10.4).

Systemic rheumatoid vasculitis

Vasculitis as a complication of RA was first described in 1898, in a patient with histological evidence of vascular inflammation of the vas nervorum. The early clinical descriptions in the 1940s and 1950s were of the classical features of peripheral gangrene and mononeuritis multiplex. Since then a wider spectrum of disease has been recognized to include carditis, scleritis, nodules, and systemic disease (Scott et al. 1981). All sizes of vessel may be involved, from aorta to capillaries. Small-vessel vasculitis can occur in isolation as small nail edge or nail fold lesions, which are considered to be benign but may herald or coexist with major arterial disease. Systemic rheumatoid vasculitis usually occurs in patients with long-standing rheumatoid factor-positive erosive RA. Males with RA are at greater risk than females.

Scott and Bacon (1984) proposed criteria for the definition of systemic rheumatoid vasculitis. An obligatory criterion was the presence of established RA as defined by the ACR. This should prevent confusion with other forms of either primary or secondary vasculitis as such patients are unlikely to meet the ACR criteria for the diagnosis of RA. However, these criteria have not been validated formally.

Time trends

Systemic rheumatoid vasculitis first became widely recognized and reported during the 1960s, a period when glucosteroids were widely used for the management of RA. It has been suggested that RA is becoming less severe and that therefore the frequency of RA should also be declining. During 1988–1997 in Norfolk we calculated the annual incidence to be 12.5 per million (Watts et al. 1999), suggesting an increase over the previous UK study from Bath/Bristol in the 1970s, which reported 6 per million [reviewed by Watts and Scott (2002)].

Methotrexate has been linked with development of cutaneous vasculitis and nodules in a small proportion of patients, but a case–control study suggested that the frequency (5.4 per cent) was the same in methotrexate-treated patients and those not receiving methotrexate (Kaye et al. 1996).

Conclusions

The systemic vasculitides are a group of important inflammatory conditions resulting in inflammation and necrosis of blood vessel walls. They are associated with significant morbidity as well as mortality, particularly MPA. They are commoner than previously believed with an annual incidence of primary systemic vasculitis of 20/million per year. The most common forms are systemic rheumatoid vasculitis and WG.

The primary vasculitides are also seen in a much older population than was previously reported.

Classification criteria and disease definitions are now well established, which has led to conformity between different centres, allowing geographical comparisons. The numbers of studies are still relatively small and further understanding of these diseases, particularly in the Indian subcontinent and the Far East, may be important in areas where other infections are common, particularly TB.

Studies of epidemiology have suggested some important avenues for research in terms of environmental factors, particularly the role of silica and potential infections associated with farming.

Data, however, is still essentially descriptive at this stage but further epidemiological studies will hopefully shed further light on aetiopathogenesis.

References

American Heart Association Committee on Rheumatic Fever, Endocarditis and Kawasaki Disease (1990). Diagnostic guidelines for Kawasaki disease. *American Journal of Diseases of Childhood* **144**, 1218–19.

Andrassy, K. et al. (1991). Rapidly progressive glomerulonephritis: analysis of prevalence and clinical course. *Nephron* **59**, 206–12.

Andrews, M. et al. (1990). Systemic vasculitis in the 1980s – is there an increasing incidence of Wegener's granulomatosis and microscopic polyarteritis. *Journal of Royal Colloidal Physics* **24**, 284–8.

Arend, W.P. et al. (1990). The American College of Rheumatology 1990 criteria for the classification of Takayasu's arteritis. *Arthritis and Rheumatism* **33**, 1129–34.

Churg, J. and Strauss, L. (1951). Allergic granulomatosis, allergic angiitis, and periarteritis nodosa. *American Journal of Pathology* **27**, 277–301.

Cimmino, M.A. (1997). Genetic and environmental factors in polymyalgia rheumatica. *Annals of the Rheumatic Disease* **56**, 576–7.

Cotch, M.F. et al. (1996). The epidemiology of Wegener's granulomatosis: estimates of the five year period prevalence, annual mortality and geographic disease distribution from population based data sources. *Arthritis and Rheumatism* **39**, 87–92.

Davis, R.L. et al. (1995). Kawasaki syndrome in Washington State. Race specific incidence rates and residential proximity to wataer. *Archives of Pediatric and Adolescent Medicine* **149**, 66–9.

Davson, J., Ball, J., and Platt, R. (1948). The kidney in periarteritis nodosa. *Quarterly Journal of Medicine* **17**, 175–202.

DeRemee, R.A. et al. (1976). Wegener's granulomatosis: anatomic correlates—a proposed classification. *Mayo Clinic Proceedings* **51**, 777–81.

Duhaut, P. et al. (1998). Giant cell arteritis and cardiovascular risk factors. A multi-centre, prospective case–control study. *Arthritis and Rheumatism* **41**, 1960–5.

Duhaut, P. et al. (1999). Giant cell arteritis, polymyalgia rheumatica, and viral hypothesis: a multicenter, prospective case–control study. *Journal of Rheumatology* **26**, 361–9.

Duna, G.F. et al. (1998). Wegener's granulomatosis: role of environmental exposures. *Clinical and Experimental Rheumatology* **16**, 669–74.

Elling, P., Olsson, A.T., and Elling, H. (1996). Synchronous variations of the incidence of temporal arteritis and polymyalgia rheumatica in different regions of Denmark, association with epidemics of *Myoplasma pneumoniae* infection. *Journal of Rheumatology* **23**, 112–19.

El-Reshaid, K. et al. (1997). The spectrum of renal disease associated with microscopic polyangiitis and classical polyarteritis nodosa in Kuwait. *Nephrology Dialysis Transplantation* **12**, 1874–82.

Fries, J.F. et al. (1990). The American College of Rheumatology 1990 criteria for the classification of vasculitis: summary. *Arthritis and Rheumatism* **33**, 1135–6.

Gabriel, S.E. et al. (1999). The role of parvovirus B19 in the pathogenesis of giant cell arteritis. *Arthritis and Rheumatism* **42**, 1255–8.

Gardner-Medwin, J.M. Dolezalova, P., Cummins, C., and Southwood, T.R. (2002). Incidence of Henoch–Schönlein purpura, Kamasaki disease, and rare vasculitides in children of different ethnic origins. *Lancet* **360** (9341), 1197–202.

González-Gay, M.A. and Garcia-Porrua, C. (1999). Systemic vasculitis in adults in North Western Spain 1988–97. Clinical and epidemiological aspects. *Medicine* **78**, 292–308.

Guillevin, L. et al. (1999). Churg–Strauss syndrome: clinical study and long-term follow up of 96 pateints. *Medicine* **78**, 26–37.

Haugeberg, G. et al. (1998). Primary vasculitis in a Norwegian community hospital: retrospective study. *Clinical Heumatology* **17**, 364–8.

Hunder, G.G. et al. (1990). The American College of Rheumatology 1990 criteria for the classification of giant cell arteritis. *Arthritis and Rheumatism* **33**, 1122–8.

Jeanette, J.C. et al. (1994). Nomenclature of systemic vasculitides. Proposal of an international consensus conference. *Arthritis and Rheumatism* **37**, 187–92.

Kawasaki, T. (1967). Acute febrile mucocutaneous syndrome with lymphoid involvement with specific desquamation of the fingers and toes in children: clinical observations in 50 cases. *Japanese Journal of Allergology* **16**, 178–222.

Kaye, O. et al. (1996). The frequency of cutaneous vasculitis is not increased in patients with rheumatoid arthritis treated with Methotrexate. *Journal of Rheumatology* **23**, 253–7.

Kurland, J.T. et al. (1984). The epidemiology of systemic arteritis. In *The Epidemiology of Rheumatic Diseases* (ed. R.C. Lawrence and L.E. Shulman), pp. 196–205. New York: Gower Publishing.

Kussmaul, A. and Maier, R. (1866). Über eine bisher nicht beschreibene eigenthümliche Arterienerkrankung (Periarteris nodosa), die mit Morbus Brightü und rapid fortschreitender allgemeiner Muskellähmung einhergeht. *Deutsche Archive Klinical Medizine* **1**, 484–514.

Kyle, V. et al. (1985). Polymyalgia rheumatica/giant cell arteritis in a Cambridge general practice. *British Medical Journal Clinical Research Edition* **291**, 385–7.

Lane, S.E., Watts, R.A., Bentham, G, Innes, N.J., and Scott, D.G. (2003). Are environmental factors important in primary systemic vasculitis? A case control study. *Arthritis and Rheumatism* **48**, 814–23.

Lanham, J.G. et al. (1984). Systemic vasculitis in asthma and eosinophilia: a clinical approach to the Churg–Strauss syndrome. *Medicine (Baltimore)* **63**, 65–81.

Lightfoot, R.W. et al. (1990). The American College of Rheumatology 1990 criteria for the classification of polyarteritis nodosa. *Arthritis and Rheumatism* **33**, 1088–93.

Masi, A.T. et al (1990). The American College of Rheumatology 1990 criteria for the classification of Churg–Strauss syndrome (allergic granulomatosis and angiitis). *Arthritis and Rheumatism* **33**, 1094–100.

Matteson, E.L. (2000). Notes on the history of eponymic idiopathic vasculitis: the diseases of Henoch and Schönlein, Wegener, Churg and Strauss, Horton, Kawasaki, Takayasu, Behçet and Kawasaki. *Arthritis Care and Research* **13**, 237–45.

McMahon, B.J. et al. (1989). Hepatitis B—associated polyarteritis nodosa in Alaskan eskimos: clinical and epidemiological features and long-term follow up. *Hepatology* **9**, 97–101.

Nowack, R. et al. (1999). Familial occurrence of systemic vasculitis and rapidly progressive glomerulonephritis. *American Journal of Kidney Disease* **34**, 364–73.

Rao, J.K., Allen, N.B., and Pincus, T. (1998). Limitations of the 1990 American College of Rheumatology Classification Criteria in the diagnosis of vasculitis. *Annals of Internal Medicine* **129**, 345–52.

Reinhold-Keller, E. et al. (2000). No difference in the incidences of vasculitides between north and south Germany: first results of the German vasculitis register. *Rheumatology* **41**, 540–9.

Russo, M.G. et al. (1995). Correlation between infection and the onset of the giant cell arteritis (temporal) arteritis syndrome. *Arthritis and Rheumatism* **38**, 374–80.

Sack, M., Cassidy, J.T., and Bole, G.G. (1975). Prognostic factors in polyarteritis. *Journal of Rheumatology* **2**, 411–20.

Scott, D.G.I. et al. (1982) Systemic vasculitis in a district general hospital 1972–80: clinical and laboratory features, classification and prognosis of 80 cases. *Quarterly Journal of Medicine* **203**, 292–11.

Scott, D.G.I. and Bacon, P.A. (1984). Intravenous cyclophosphamide plus methyl-prednisolone treatment in systemic rheumatoid vasculitis. *American Journal of Medicine* **76**, 377–84.

Scott, D.G.I., Bacon, P.A., and Tribe, C.R. (1981). Systemic rheumatoid vasculitis: a clinical and laboratory study of 50 cases. *Medicine (Baltimore)* **60**, 288–97.

Smith, C.A., Fidler, W.J., and Pinals, R.S. (1983). The epidemiology of giant cell arteritis. Report of a ten year study in Shelby County, Tennessee. *Arthritis and Rheumatism* **26**, 1214–19.

Stegeman, C.A. et al. (1996). Trimethoprim–sulphamethoxazole (co-trimoxazole) for the prevention of relapses in Wegener's granulomatosis. *New England Journal of Medicine* **335**, 16–20.

Tidman, M. et al. (1998). Patients hospitalised because of small vessel vasculitides with renal involvement in the period 1975–95: organ involvement, anti-neutrophil cytoplasmic antibodies patterns, seasonal attack rates and fluctuation of annual frequencies. *Journal of Internal Medicine* **244**, 133–41.

Watts, R.A. and Scott, D.G.I. (2002). Epidemiology of vasculitis. In *Vasculitis* (ed. G.V. Ball and S.L. Bridges, Jr.), pp. 211–26. Oxford: Oxford University Press.

Watts, R.A. et al. (1996). Effect of classification on the incidence of polyarteritis nodosa and microscopic polyangiitis. *Arthritis and Rheumatism* **39**, 1208–12.

Watts, R.A. et al. (1999). Epidemiology of systemic rheumatoid vasculitis (SRV)—a ten year study. *Arthritis and Rheumatism* **42**, S173 (abstract).

Watts, R.A. et al. (2000). Epidemiology of systemic vasculitis—a ten year study in the United Kingdom. *Arthritis and Rheumatism* **43**, 414–19.

Watts, R.A. et al. (2001). Annual incidence of primary systemic vasculitis in three regions of Europe. *Annals of the Rheumatic Diseases* **60**, 1156–7 (letter).

Wechsler, M.E. et al. (1998). Pulmonary infiltrates, eosinophilia, and cardiomyopathy following corticosteroid withdrawal in patients with asthma receiving Zafirlukast. *Journal of the American Medical Association* **279**, 455–7.

Westman, K. et al. (1998). Relapse rate renal survival and cancer morbidity in patients with Wegener's granulomatosis or microscopic polyangiitis and enal involvement. *Journal of the American Society of Nephrology* **9**, 842–52.

Yanagawa, H. et al. (1995). Epidemiologic pictures of Kawasaki disease in Japan from the nationwide incidence survey in 1991 and 1992. *Paediatrics* **95**, 475–9.

Zeek, P.M. (1952). Periarteritis nodosa: a critical review. *American Journal of Clinical Pathology* **22**, 777–90.

6.10.2 Clinical features of primary ANCA-associated vasculitis

Wolfgang L. Gross and Eva Reinhold-Keller

ANCA-associated vasculitis

Vasculitis is a clinicopathological process characterized by inflammation and necrosis of blood vessels. The clinical spectrum ranges from primary disease (primary systemic vasculitis, PSV) to a secondary component of some other primary systemic disease, such as systemic lupus erythematosus (SLE). The clinical and pathological features are variable and depend on the site and type of blood vessels affected. One approach to classifying non-infectious vasculitides is to categorize them in part according to the predominant type of vessels affected. Small vessel vasculitis thus affects vessels smaller than arteries, such as arterioles, venules, and capillaries. Vessels of skin, respiratory tract, kidneys, gut, peripheral nerves, and skeletal muscle are often involved, but the frequency varies among the various entities of PSV [for review, see Gross et al. (2000b)].

Classifications based on the size of the affected vessels ignore the fact that many vasculitis syndromes do not respect vessel size boundaries. So aetiological factors (e.g. cryoglobulinaemic vasculitis due to hepatitis C virus) and markers of immunopathogenetic mechanisms [e.g. IC deposition in situ, or autoantibodies to neutrophil components (ANCA) in blood] can provide further aid in differentiating the various PSV.

Small vessel vasculitis associated with antineutrophil cytoplasmic antibodies (ANCA) will be described in subsequent chapters.

Wegener's granulomatosis

Historical background

Wegener's granulomatosis (WG) was recognized as a distinct clinicopathological entity 60 years ago. Of unknown aetiology, WG is a granulomatous disorder associated with systemic necrotizing vasculitis. Classic WG involves predominantly the triad of upper airways (E), the lung (L), and the kidneys (K) according to the ELK-classification (DeRemee et al. 1976). However, *formes frustes* of WG confined to E or to both E and L as a purely granulomatous process without clinical evidence of systemic vasculitis are also known and have been designated 'limited disease', 'initial phase', or 'localized WG' (Carrington and Liebow 1966; Nölle et al. 1989).

'Classic WG' syndrome is a generalized disease process that usually begins with an *initial phase* of variable duration with symptoms limited mostly to the upper and/or lower respiratory tracts [for review, see Wegener (1990)]. Since these limited forms of WG are being detected with increasing frequency, due partly to greater physician awareness and partly to more sophisticated diagnostic procedures, it is now evident that they follow a rather subacute or protracted chronic course of unpredictable duration before transforming into the *generalized phase:* the latter is characterized by systemic necrotizing vasculitis, usually with renal and pulmonary involvement. If untreated, it can turn into the fulminant form (e.g. renal–pulmonary syndrome), which carries a devastating prognosis. Rheumatic complaints, and eye or peripheral nerve involvement are frequently an ominous herald of the onset of the vasculitic phase, which is usually also associated with constitutional (B-) symptoms such as malaise, weight loss, fever, and night sweats. In this phase, non-specific markers of inflammation, for example, erythrocyte sedimentation rate (ESR) and C-reactive protein (CRP), are usually elevated and cANCA (proteinase3 ANCA = PR3-ANCA), which has a 90 per cent specificity for WG, is detectable in 95 per cent of sera (Nölle et al. 1989; Gross and Csernok 1995).

Because of the potentially life-threatening course of the ANCA-associated vasculitides, such as generalized WG, microscopic polyangiitis (MPA), or Churg–Strauss syndrome (CSS), 'standard' treatment (NIH) standard therapy/Fauci's scheme consisting of daily 'low-dose' cyclophosphamide (CYC, 2–4 mg/day) plus glucocorticoids (GC) is generally considered to be of most benefit to the majority of patients. This view has been challenged in recent years by data indicating (i) the variability of clinical course and aggressiveness in the same disease entity, (ii) continued morbidity despite CYC plus GC therapy, (iii) a high incidence of relapse among patients thought to be 'cured', and (iv) the alarming range of treatment-related morbidity and mortality induced by the 'standard protocol' (Anderson et al. 1992; Hoffman et al. 1992; Reinhold-Keller et al. 2000).

Improved diagnostic procedures, including computed tomography (CT) imaging of the lung and magnetic resonance imaging (MRI) of the head (Greenan et al. 1992; Muhle et al. 1997; Reuter et al. 1998), immunodiagnostic methods such as ANCA assays, and detection of cytokine/cytokine-receptor molecules such as the sIL-2R, have enhanced diagnostic precision by clarifying the anatomic distribution of involvement and the clinical activity of the disease (Nölle et al. 1989; Schmitt et al. 1993). Consequently, it is now possible to design stage-adapted and disease activity-related therapeutic protocols.

Terms and definitions

Usually, generalized ('full-blown', classic) WG (Fig. 1) is described as a distinct clinicopathological entity characterized by lesions induced by necrotizing granulomatous inflammation in the upper (ENT-region) and the lower respiratory tracts (including the lung), and by vasculitis involving various additional organs (Wegener 1939). According to the original criteria of Godman and Churg (1954), WG characteristically involves the *triad* of airway, lung, and kidney.

The 'ELK-classification' (DeRemee et al. 1976) has proved to be useful in clinical practice. Patients are classified according to the extent of the organ system involvement observed during disease course. The 'extended' ELK-classification is now the basis for the 'disease extension index (DEI)' used in clinical studies and in the daily practice (de Groot et al. 2001a).

The American College of Rheumatology 1990 criteria for the classification of WG (ACR criteria) were developed by comparing 85 WG patients with 722 control patients with other forms of vasculitis. For the traditional format classification, four criteria were selected (Fig. 1) (Leavitt et al. 1990).

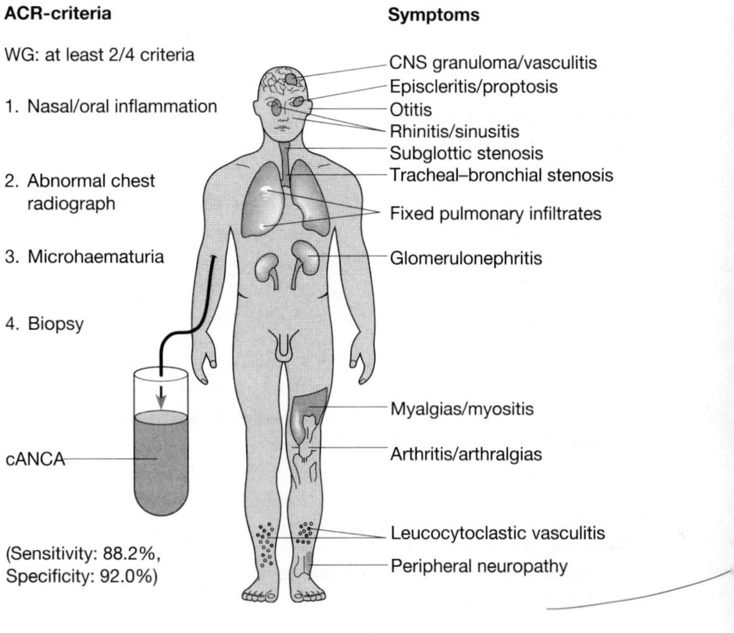

Fig. 1 Schematic representation of the characteristic clinical symptoms of WG and the ACR 1990 classification criteria.

The Chapel Hill Consensus Conference on the Nomenclature of Systemic Vasculitis (CHC definitions) (Jennette et al. 1994) defined WG as follows: granulomatous inflammation involving the respiratory tract, and necrotizing vasculitis affecting small- to medium-sized vessels (e.g. capillaries, venules, arterioles, and arteries). Necrotizing glomerulonephritis (GN) is common. The disease is often associated with ANCA.

Course of disease

Although, until the last decade, WG was generally regarded as an invariably serious and fatal disease, perceptions of it have changed (Hoffman et al. 1992). Improved diagnostic procedures, including high-resolution CT imaging of the lung and MRI of the head, as well as immunodiagnostic methods, such as ANCA assays, have enhanced diagnostic precision by clarifying clinical manifestations in the E or L region, and the anatomic distribution of involvement *(disease extension)* and clinical *disease activity* (Luqmani et al. 1994; de Groot et al. 2001a). Thus, in addition to full-blown forms of WG with possible fatal outcome, indolent and/or less aggressive and life-threatening variants have been found to be more frequent than once thought. In addition, the introduction of immunosuppressive drugs, dialysis, and renal transplantation have led to a dramatic improvement in survival rates in serious cases.

In their updated analysis of 158 patients with WG, Hoffman et al. (1992) emphasized the variability of the disease course prior to diagnosis. In many cases, WG followed a confusing and indolent course (upto 16 years), particularly in patients without renal manifestation before a definite diagnosis was established. The median and mean periods from onset of symptoms to diagnosis of WG were 4.7 and 15 months, respectively. Diagnosis of WG was made within 3 months after onset of symptoms in only 42 per cent of patients. This is surprising because earlier studies had reported a median survival of only 5 months (Walton 1958). In Great Britain, 265 WG patients were observed between 1975 and 1985 (Anderson et al. 1992). The mean intervals from onset of symptoms to presentation and from presentation to diagnosis were both approximately 7 months. Correct diagnosis was often missed for many years (range: <1–188 months). The mean survival of 4.2 years, which was shorter if renal disease was present, in patients receiving no drug treatment in the first 3 months after establishment of diagnosis (10 per cent) indicates that these variants must have been very mild. Furthermore, it is striking that the median survival of 72 patients treated with GC alone during the first 3 months exceeded 12 years. Unfortunately, the authors did not indicate the number of patients in the different treatment groups, nor their disease activity and extent. They also provided no information on the treatment beyond the first 3 months. A large study on 155 WG patients from a single centre observed over a median of 7 years described a median survival of more than 21 years. Kidney or lung involvement at diagnosis was predictive of a three- to five-fold higher mortality (Reinhold-Keller et al. 2000). An overview of the clinical outcome and characteristics is given in Table 1.

Clinical features

Although generalized WG is a systemic disease with multiple organ system involvement (Fig. 1), it is essentially a respiratory–renal syndrome. These two organ systems are largely responsible for the clinical course and outcome of the disease.

Along with the *triad* of necrotizing granulomas of the upper (E) and lower respiratory tracts (L), plus GN (i.e. renal vasculitis; K), *generalized WG* may also involve joints (A), skin (S), peripheral nerves (P), skeletal muscle (A), heart (H), brain (C), and eyes (EY), mostly as vasculitis of the small vessels.

Retrospective analyses have shown that in half of patients WG characteristically begins in the upper respiratory tract *(initial phase/localized WG)* as the sole sign of disease preceding symptoms of generalized disease. These and pulmonary features may evolve over several months and even years and can be followed by the overt presentation of systemic vasculitis (generalized phase WG), including glomerular disease. Because of the sometimes long evolution, the diagnosis 'WG' may not be made until some time after respiratory presentation. In contrast, WG sometimes starts without obvious granulomatous lesions as a purely small vessel vasculitis. It is important to realize that there are overlapping features shared by WG and MPA, combined with the subsequent development over time of inflammatory lesions (e.g. GN followed by skin vasculitis followed by pulmonary vasculitis—and lastly, followed by obvious granulomatous lesions in the respiratory tract).

Table 1 Clinical characteristics and outcome in Wegener's granulomatosis [modified from Reinhold-Keller et al. (2000)]

	Hoffman et al. (1992)	Anderson et al. (1992)	Matteson et al. (1996)	Reinhold-Keller (2000)
No. of patients, *n*	158	265	77	155
Male/female (%)	50/50	55/45	64/36	49/51
Age at diagnosis (years)	41 (mean)	50 (mean)	45 (mean)	48
cANCA[a] positive (%)	88	n.i.	n.i.	84
Mortality (%)	20	56	36	14
Median survival (years)	n.i.	8.5	n.i.	21.7
Death due to WG and/or its therapy (%)	13	n.i.	n.i.	12
Death due to infections (%)	3	12	10	3
Involved organ systems at onset or diagnosis/over the whole course (%)[b]				
ENT	73/92	75/n.i.	n.i.	93/99
Kidney	18/77	60/n.i.	n.i./73	54/70
Lung	45/85	63/n.i.	n.i./53	55/66
Eye	15/52	14/n.i.	n.i.	40/61
Heart	n.i./8	n.i.	n.i./14	13/25
Skin	13/46	25/n.i.	n.i.	21/33
PNS	n.i./15	n.i.	n.i./c	21/40
CNS	n.i./8	n.i.	n.i./c	6/11
Rheum. complaints	32/67	20/n.i.	n.i.	61/77
'Initial phase' (localized WG) at diagnosis (%)	n.i.	22	n.i.	15

[a] Classic antineutrophil cytoplasmic antibodies.

[b] In the study of Hoffman et al. (1992) information only on the onset of disease, in that of Anderson et al. at presentation.

c Involvement of both peripheral and central nervous system 31%.

In any case, a strict *diagnosis of WG depends* on (i) characteristic clinical symptoms, (ii) the demonstration of characteristic granulomas and vasculitis in biopsy material, and/or (iii) the detection of characteristic ANCA, that is, cANCA (PR3-ANCA) or less frequently (<10 per cent) pANCA (MPO-ANCA), in the serum. It is noteworthy that *each* of these 'characteristics' can be observed in similar disorders, and that diagnosis should not rely on any one of these variables alone (Lamprecht et al. 2000).

Initial phase WG or localized WG ['initial stage'; E, L, EL according to the ELK classification 'purely' granulomatous WG: for review, see Gross et al. (2000a)]. In most instances the ENT-region is affected first. Characteristically there are no clinical signs of systemic vasculitis. Initial phase WG patients account for 10 per cent of the vasculitis patients in a rheumatological unit.

The earliest *nasal manifestations* (E) usually include nasal obstruction (mucosal swelling), serosanguineous discharge, and epistaxis. Examination reveals granulation (Plate 140) and there may be thick crusts, which upon removal reveal friable mucosa or even septal perforation. In many patients, the clinical diagnosis can be confirmed by the characteristic histology obtained from nasal biopsy (Devaney et al. 1990; Del Bueno and Flint 1991). In addition to the symptoms described, facial pain, nosebleeds, nasal chondritis, saddling of the nose (Plate 141), and *paranasal sinus involvement* (chronic sinusitis) typically occur.

In the *oral cavity and oropharynx* (E), gingival involvement can lead to ulcerative stomatitis, frank ulcerations (Plate 142), or hyperplastic gingivitis. Laryngeal symptoms such as hoarseness and/or increasing stridor are frequently due to reddish, friable, circumferential narrowing just below the cords and extending for 3–5 cm.

Otological manifestations (E) of WG include involvement of the external ear (chondritis, sometimes with secondary ear lobe atrophy) or middle ear (serous otitis media; suppurative otitis media, mastoiditis). Sometimes, peripheral facial nerve palsy occurs.

Eye symptoms (EY) in WG—excluding those arising from small vessel vasculitis (!) which are seen only in generalized WG (e.g. 'red eye')—derive from the granulomatous lesions (obstruction of the nasolacrimal duct) and masses developing retro-orbitally (protrusio bulbi; optical nerve compression: Plate 143 and Fig. 2). Less frequently, orbital involvement may result from the spread of a purulent sinusitis due, for example, to secondary bacterial infection (Duncker et al. 1993).

The *tracheo-bronchial tree* (L) may also be involved in this locoregionally restricted and not yet generalized process of granulomatous inflammation: subglottic pseudotumor and/or stenosis leading to stridor and dyspnoea (Plate 144); bronchial stenosis, which may cause atelectasis and/or obstructive pneumonia. Single or multiple nodules with or without cavitation (Fig. 3) are found incidentally in the lung of hitherto asymptomatic persons (Hoffman et al. 1992).

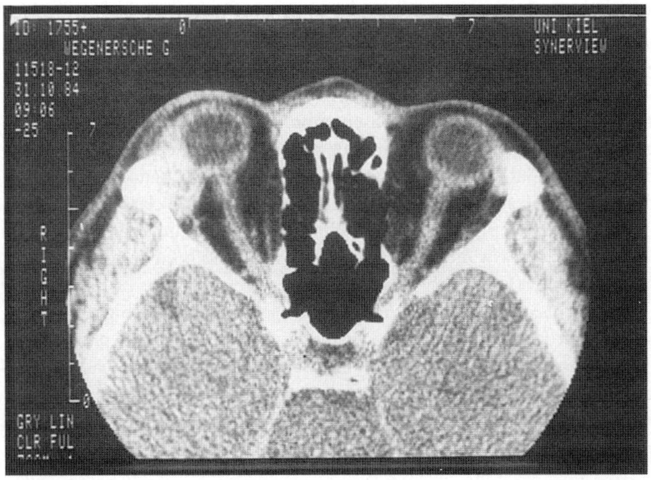

Fig. 2 Protrusio bulbi induced by retro-orbital granulomatous masses (CT scan).

Because of the regionally restricted symptomatology (mostly confined to the ENT-region: E or less frequently lower respiratory tract), the *initial stage* is often puzzling to the diagnostician. It frequently takes years until WG is suspected and a histological diagnosis of WG is finally made. Fever can occur, perhaps caused by the underlying inflammatory disease, although it appears to be more commonly associated with secondary bacterial infection mostly caused by *Staphylococcus aureus* of the involved paranasal sinus.

Generalized WG ('systemic' WG; E, L, K stage according to the ELK-classification): the transition from the initial stage to the *active generalized phase* with its frequent fulminant course is heralded by the *indirect symptoms* of systemic vasculitis: weight loss, fever, night sweats (constitutional symptoms; similar to 'B-symptomatology' in Hodgkin's disease). Clinically, this combination of fatigue, malaise, and anorexia, together with uncharacteristic rheumatic complaints (A; polymyalgia, arthralgia: see below) and the striking laboratory abnormalities typical of this phase (ESR and CRP maximally elevated, leucocytosis, thrombocytosis), warrants close scrutiny to ensure early recognition of the imminent complications which, if untreated, lead to the life-threatening situations described below. *Direct signs* of the small vessel vasculitis characteristically found in generalized WG are 'red eye' (EY; due to episcleritis, scleritis), palpable purpura of the lower extremities (S; due to leucocytoclastic vasculitis of the skin), peripheral neuropathy (P; due to the vasculitis of the vasa nervorum) and, most dangerous of all, renal involvement, which ranges from mild focal and segmental GN with minimal haematuria and little diminution of the glomerular filtration rate to fulminant diffuse necrotizing and crescentic GN (K; rapidly progressive GN: RPGN) with haematuria, pyuria, and red cell casts leading within several days or a few weeks to oligo-anuria and dialysis. In addition—or separately—pulmonary symptoms (L) can arise which may ultimately lead to pulmonary haemorrhage and severe respiratory insufficiency. In fulminant WG, all of the symptoms described here can occur together (e.g. as a pulmonary–renal syndrome) or separately (alveolar haemorrhage syndrome without GN; RPGN without alveolar haemorrhage, etc.). In these situations only rapid diagnosis and immediate immunosuppressive treatment can restrain this life-threatening condition and prevent end-stage renal failure or death.

Most WG patients, however, follow a clinical course lying between these extremes (initial phase versus fulminant generalized disease).

Otological manifestations in generalized WG—in addition to those described for initial phase WG—characteristically include hearing loss due to sensorineural deafness usually induced by the small vessel vasculitis of the cochlear vessels and/or the vasa nervorum of the acoustic nerve. Vestibular impairment as manifested by vertigo can additionally occur. Similarly, peripheral facial nerve palsy can be induced by the otitis media (including mastoiditis) and the vasculitis.

Eye manifestations (EY) in the generalized stage of WG are episcleritis—'red eye'—(Plate 145), optic nerve vasculitis, and retinal artery occlusion, all due to the now prominent vasculitic process in addition to the granulomatous lesions described above.

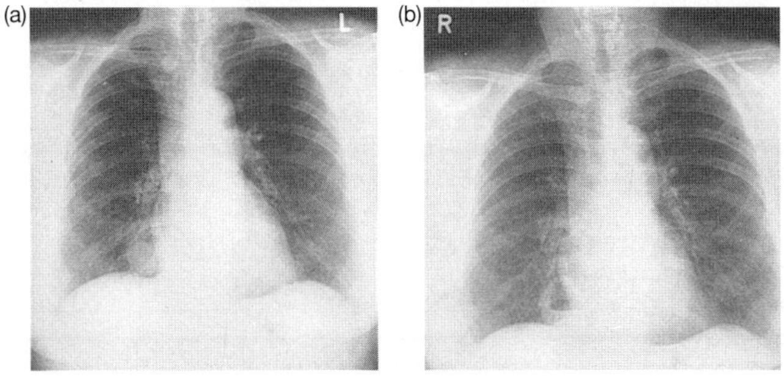

Fig. 3 Nodules in the lung usually consist of rounded lesions (a) with well-defined margins and (b) they tend to cavitate.

The *bronchial tree and lung* (L) are usually involved in the systemic phase of WG. In addition to the stenotic processes and nodules—this kind of pulmonary involvement itself is more typical of the initial phase of WG and rather asymptomatic—localized or diffuse infiltrates should alert to the possibility of an alveolar haemorrhage resulting from the predominantly alveolar capillaritis. The three most consistent features for clinical recognition of alveolar haemorrhage are haemoptysis, infiltrates on the chest roentgenogram, and anaemia. X-ray typically shows an alveolar or mixed alveolar–interstitial pattern. A distribution like that in pulmonary oedema is most common, but focal and sometimes migratory infiltrates are also observed (Fig. 4). However, the clinical and roentgenographic manifestations of immune alveolar haemorrhage are similar regardless of their aetiology. Such patients usually also have an RPGN (Plate 146) and thus typically present a pulmonary–renal vasculitic syndrome. Immunohistochemistry on lung biopsies or kidney specimens reveal only a few or no immunodeposits, thus excluding IC-mediated and antibasement membrane antibody-mediated pulmonary and pulmonary–renal vasculitic syndromes. Most patients with such 'pauci-immune' pulmonary–renal vasculitic syndromes have either cANCA (PR3-ANCA) or less frequently pANCA induced by myeloperoxidase (MPO) antibodies (MPO-ANCA).

Abnormalities of pulmonary function include obstruction to airflow, reduced lung volumes, and diffusing capacity abnormalities.

Kidney involvement (K) in generalized WG shows considerable variation. At one extreme lies RPGN, which is a major indicator of poor prognosis (see above). The most common manifestation of renal disease, however, is asymptomatic (micro-)haematuria with a nephritic urinary sediment and little if any renal function impairment; this erythrocyturea is due to focal segmental GN (Plate 146). Immunohistologically, the glomeruli typically have no deposits of immunoglobulin; likewise, there is little ultrastructural evidence for IC deposits. This has led to the term 'pauci-immune necrotizing and crescentic glomerulonephritis'. It is noteworthy that very similar lesions due to 'microscopic' vessel inflammation are seen in other 'ANCA-associated vasculitides' (e.g. MPA) (Wegener 1990; Jennette and Falk 1994). Impaired renal function predicts poor outcome (Reinhold-Keller et al. 2000).

Neurological involvement occurs in upto 50 per cent of cases. The CNS (C) is affected in only about 10 per cent of patients, much more often—affecting almost half of patients—the peripheral nervous system (P), mostly in the lower extremities. In a recently published study (de Groot et al. 2001b), 56 out of 128 patients were found to have a polyneuropathy (PNP), 31 a distal symmetric PNP, 25 a mononeuritis multiplex. Involvement of the peripheral nervous system in most patients occurred within the first 2 years of disease. In some cases the PNP was the only initial symptom of WG preceding other organ manifestations.

Clinical manifestations in the heart (H) are not common in generalized WG. However, asymptomatic pericardial effusions frequently occur and frank peri-(pan) carditis, severe granulomatous giant-cell myocarditis, and cardiomyopathy have been described.

Rheumatic complaints (A), ranging from mild myalgias and/or arthralgias to frank arthritis and/or myositis, represent the second most frequent symptom complex (after ENT-region symptoms) in generalized WG. These rheumatic manifestations were described in two-thirds of patients in a large series of WG cases! Twenty-eight per cent had non-erosive and non-deforming polyarthritis. Sacroilitis was found in three of 50 and relapsing polychondritis in two of 50 WG patients. Rheumatoid factor was present in half of the patients with generalized WG tested. In our own series of 186 patients with WG (148 biopsy-proven), we found episodes with arthralgia, myalgia, or arthritis in two-thirds of cases as the presenting symptom and in three-fourths of all cases over time. Thus, rheumatic complaints have been found to belong to the main symptom complex (Fig. 6). They are more frequent than symptoms of the eye, skin, or nervous system. The most common complaint is myalgia (45 per cent), followed by frank arthritis (21 per cent), mainly in the larger joints. Approximately 90 per cent of WG patients suffering from rheumatic symptoms have a generalized form of the disease and the rheumatic symptoms usually occur together with the constitutional symptoms typically associated with active vasculitis.

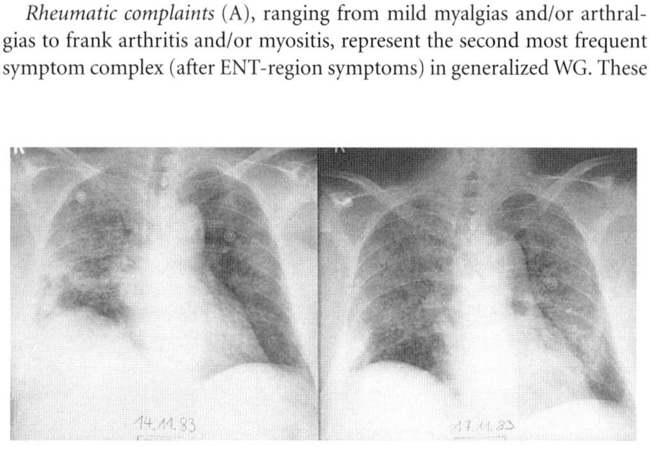

Fig. 4 Roentgenographic manifestation of alveolar haemorrhage in WG.

Skin involvement (S) in systemic WG usually occurs as palpable purpura due to leucocytoclastic vasculitis (Plate 147). Less frequent are necrotic papules due to necrotizing vasculitis. Livedo reticularis and pyoderma gangrenosum are occasionally seen, sometimes as the presenting feature [Frances et al. 1994; for review, see Csernok and Gross (2000)].

An overview of the organ systems involved in four large WG cohorts is provided in Table 1.

In addition to this broad spectrum of symptoms, a wide variety of other manifestations, including involvement of the breast, ovaries, prostate, urethral duct, etc., have been described, mostly in the form of case reports.

Subsets of WG and 'WG-like diseases'

Besides patients with *formes frustes*, for example, localized WG as described above, there are patients with biopsy proven *active generalized WG* fulfilling the CHC definition and ACR criteria for WG who remain consistently ANCA negative in serum or plasma over their whole course of disease ranging from 5 to more than 9 years. Their clinical hallmark is a severe central nervous system (CNS) manifestation, for example, meningeal involvement with favourable response to immunosuppressive therapy (Reinhold-Keller et al. 2001). A further 'new' subset seems to be the co-existence of two different granulomatous diseases in one patient (Lamprecht et al. 2000). Some patients have Crohn's disease (as substantiated by typical Crohn's epithelioid cell granuloma) *plus* necrotizing palisading granulomas restricted to the ENT tract typical of WG. In addition, we have seen a young woman with generalized WG for many years who developed a Löfgren syndrome while her WG was in complete remission. Furthermore, fewer than 10 per cent of WG patients are MPO-ANCA positive whereas the great majority are PR3-ANCA positive. These MPO-ANCA-positive WG patients suffer less frequently from renal and other extra-renal involvement than patients with 'classic' PR3-ANCA-positive WG (Schönermarck et al. 2001). Some patients with characteristic symptoms and typical histological features of WG and who fulfilled both the ACR criteria and the CHC definitions (Moins-Teisserenc et al. 1999) were, however, also constantly ANCA-negative (in many different assays and reference labs) over the years of observation and did not respond to conventional immunosuppressive treatment (Moins-Teisserenc et al. 1999). It has been shown that this 'WG-like syndrome' is the consequence of a TAP I/II defect which leads to low surface expression of HLA class I molecules. Despite a clinical phenotype resembling WG, the immunopathogenesis of this disease is clearly different from WG. Thus, it has been designated 'WG-like syndrome' (Lamprecht et al. 2000).

In conclusion, there is a *clinicopathologic entity* with a highly specific seromarker (ANCA) and a broad range of disease expression plus, apparently, previously unknown *other diseases* which mimic (at least in part histologically) WG.

Laboratory investigations

Up to the mid-1980s, no disease-specific laboratory marker for WG existed. Disease activity was evaluated according to the clinical picture and general *indices of inflammation* (ESR, CRP), leucocytosis (usually with no or only moderate eosinophilia: <10 per cent!), thrombocytosis, and normochromic normocytic anaemia. In the *initial phase of WG*, all of these parameters are only slightly elevated, but they become maximally elevated in the fulminant *generalized stage of WG* (Gross and Csernok 1995).

In contrast to the family of *other autoimmune rheumatic diseases* (e.g. SLE), generalized WG is associated with no or only mild hypergammaglobulinemia, no or only low-titre antinuclear-antibody (ANA), no complement consumption (indeed slight elevations may occur as acute phase proteins), but with a rheumatoid factor positive in upto 50 per cent of patients. In addition, cryoglobulins are characteristically absent. *Indices for organ lesions*, for example, kidney involvement, have to be monitored by appropriate tests, for example, urine analysis (haematuria, proteinuria, serum creatinine, etc.).

ANCA represent a class of antibodies directed against various neutrophil granule constituents and against monocytic antigens [for review, see Gross and Csernok (1995)]. Since their first description two main immunofluorescent staining patterns of ANCA have been found: the classic cytoplasmic pattern [Plate 148(a)] with accentuated fluorescence intensity in the area within the nuclear lobes (cANCA) and the perinuclear pattern [pANCA, Plate 148(b)]. In vasculitis, cANCA is a seromarker for WG and pANCA is a marker for MPA; the cytoplasmic pattern associated with WG is characteristically induced by PR3-ANCA, and the perinuclear pattern seen in MPA is typically induced by MPO-ANCA. However, the associations are not absolute and PR3-ANCA are sometimes seen in MPA and MPO-ANCA in WG (Schönermarck et al. 2001).

The sensitivity of ANCA for WG has been reported to range from 28 to 92 per cent (Rao et al. 1995). This broad variation reflects the different criteria that were applied to establish the diagnosis of WG. Several series have shown a high specificity of cANCA for WG, ranging from 80 to 100 per cent. The use of more sensitive PR3-ANCA-specific methods of detection has confirmed that the cANCA phenomenon in WG is always associated with PR3-ANCA (Hagen et al. 1998; Specks 2000). Despite these findings, a positive cANCA/PR3-ANCA test result, which may be useful in suggesting the possibility of WG, should not be used instead of biopsy to make the diagnosis. How closely the ANCA titre follows the disease activity is controversely discussed and whether a rise of the ANCA titre necessarily predicts a relapse of WG. Given the possibility that the disease may not worsen and the toxicity of treatment may be considerable, treatment should not be changed based on a rising ANCA titre alone. However, such a finding should prompt a careful examination for any objective evidence of active disease and frequent patient monitoring.

In addition, cytokines, cytokine-receptor molecules, and adhesion molecules have been shown to be associated with clinical disease activity when measured in serum and/or plasma [for review, see Csernok and Gross (2000)]. Soluble IL-2 receptor (sIL-2R) serum levels were found to be higher in patients with generalized rather than initial phase WG and may indicate a higher risk of relapse in these patients if still elevated in remission.

Investigation of the diagnostic value of the markers of endothelial perturbation and damage, such as von Willebrand's factor and thrombomodulin, has demonstrated that plasma levels of these parameters reflected the course of clinical activity more closely than cANCA (Boehme et al. 1996).

Monitoring disease activity and disease extension

Because generalized WG is a multisystem disease with a high rate of relapse (Hoffman et al. 1992; Gordon et al. 1993; Reinhold-Keller et al. 2000), it is especially important that the clinical aspects of disease activity and disease extension be monitored on a regular and controlled basis by an *interdisciplinary team* of physicians, ENT surgeons, ophthalmologists, neurologists, and radiologists (Table 2; Reinhold-Keller et al. 2000) combined with a programme of standardized patient education. An important aspect of the patient education is training in early detection of relapse, which if detected should result in a physician visit as soon as possible.

The value of ESR and CRP levels albeit non-specific indices of *disease activity* is generally accepted. In the initial phase of disease, both tests may be normal, although secondary and opportunistic infections can lead to elevated levels of both. cANCA titres seem to correlate with disease activity in many patients (Nölle et al. 1989). Consequently, changes in cANCA titre remain one of the most important markers of disease activity, and the only one that is specific for WG. In contrast to ESR and CRP levels, the cANCA-titre does not rise during a secondary infection. Highly elevated sIL-2R levels are found in patients with increased disease activity and may be an

Table 2 Regular interdisciplinary staging to assess the extent and activity of WG [from Reinhold-Keller et al. (2000)]

Organ system	Manifestations	Score	Standardized examination
E	Upper respiratory tract (including subglottic/oral)	2	ENT-specialist, MRI of the head (sinoscopy, biopsy)
L	Lung	2	X-ray, high resolution CT of the chest (bronchoscopy, incl. bronchoalveolar lavage, biopsy)
K	Kidney	2	Urinary analysis, serum creatinine, ultrasound (biopsy)
EY	Inflammatory eye involvement (no granulomatous changes)	2	Ophthalmologist, MRI of the head (fluorescence angiography)
H	Heart	2	ECG, X-ray, echocardiography (thallium scintigraphy, coronary angiography, myocardial biopsy)
S	Skin	2	Dermatologist's opinion (biopsy)
GI	Gastrointestinal tract	2	Ultrasound (endoscopy, incl. biopsy, angiography)
P	Peripheral nervous system	2	Neurologist, EMG, ENG (MRI of muscles, biopsy)
C	Central nervous system	2	Neurologist, MRI of the head (cerebrospinal fluid, angiography, ultrasound of extra- and intracranial vessels)
A	Rheumatic complaints	2	X-ray, joint ultrasound, scintigraphy (joint puncture, EMG, muscle-MRI, biopsy)
B	Constitutional symptoms	1	Fever >38%, weight loss >10% of body weight, fatigue, night sweats

Note: MRI, magnetic resonance imaging scan; CT, computerized tomography scan; EMG, electromyography; ENG, electroneurography; ( ), procedures that are optional, if standard procedures yield findings that need further specification.

indicator of imminent relapse in patients in complete clinical remission [for review, see Csernok and Gross (2000)].

The value of MRI of the *head* in determining *disease extension* is now widely recognized (Greenan et al. 1992; Muhle et al. 1997). MRI can not only demonstrate extension of the granulomatous lesions within the upper respiratory tract not detectable by nasal endoscopy or conventional X-ray, but can also reveal intracerebral granuloma (Fig. 5) and/or grey and white matter infarcts following vasculitis.

In patients with obvious *lung* involvement or in patients under immunosuppression with suspected opportunistic infection, bronchoalveolar lavage (BAL) analysis can help in obtaining a histological diagnosis from transbronchial biopsy specimens and in demonstrating WG-specific disease activity when neutrophils are markedly increased. BAL can also reveal *Pneumocystis carinii* or cytomegalovirus or other infections (Jarrousse et al. 1993; Schnabel et al. 1999). High-resolution CT findings may be a useful adjunct to clinical scoring of disease activity in WG and suspected lung involvement (Reuter et al. 1998).

For patients in whom cytotoxic agents have been previously employed, continued surveillance combined with standardized patient education must include evaluation of signs and symptoms that suggest toxicities (haemorrhagic cystitis, bladder cancer, myelodysplasia, lymphoma, etc.). Because of the possibility of 'silent' relapse, especially in the kidneys and lungs, urine analysis (sediment!), and chest X-ray should be performed at frequent intervals if there are even minor clinical symptoms.

Pathology and pathogenesis

WG is a clinicopathological entity closely associated with cANCA, particularly those induced by the PR3 antibodies, whose diagnosis requires specific clinical and pathological criteria and/or the presence of (PR3)-ANCA in the serum.

Until recently, autopsy pathology provided most of the tissue for the morphological investigations that led to the model of the *classic pathological triad* of granulomatous inflammation, necrosis, and vasculitis (Godman and Churg 1954). As a matter of fact, however, only biopsy from open lung biopsies exhibits this triad. More commonly, only one or two elements of the triad are seen in extra-airway biopsies. Therefore, a pathological study was performed on 126 head and neck biopsies from 70 patients with WG to work out criteria for the diagnosis of WG based on head and neck biopsies (Devaney et al. 1990). The following criteria were proposed:

1. If all three major pathological criteria are met, it may be considered diagnostic if there is clinical involvement of E, L, K, or either L or K.
2. If two major pathological criteria are met, it may be considered diagnostic if there is typical clinical involvement of the lung as well as kidney (ELK); however, if only one of these sites is involved (E, L, or K), the diagnosis may be considered as probable and further biopsies should be performed.
3. If only one of the major pathological criteria is met, histology may be considered as suggestive of WG if the patient has typical clinical evidence of WG (E, L, K). It is suspicious for WG if the patient has only one additional site of disease (E and L or E and K).

The diagnostic value and limitations of orbital biopsy in WG have recently been delineated.

WG begins with granulomatous changes, as Fienberg's group (1981) was able to establish after decades of research [for review, see Wegener (1990)]. More recently, open lung biopsies were studied to determine the histogenesis of pulmonary lesions and to identify early lesions (Mark et al. 1988). The earliest microscopic lesion is a small focus of necrosis of collagen. This is followed by accumulation of histiocytes and their aggregation around the necrosis to form palisading granuloma. Progression continues from micronecrosis, usually with neutrophils forming 'microabscesses', to widespread macronecrosis and later to fibrosis. Collagen in many structures of the lung was observed to become necrotic. This included walls of blood vessels and conducting airways, alveolar walls, and pleura. The primary process, therefore, is not restricted to blood vessels, although WG is often described as a primary vasculitis. The study outlines the major criteria for histologic diagnosis of WG based on lung biopsies. The major discriminating features are palisading granulomas or palisading histiocytes in vascular walls and in extravascular tissue, microabscesses, or fibrinoid necrosis in vascular walls, leucocytoclastic capillaritis, diffuse granulomatous tissue, and granulomatous bronchiolitis. Granulomatous inflammation must be present in any case.

Palisading granuloma should be distinguished from a compact, circumscribed, rounded granuloma of tuberculoid or sarcoidal type. Palisading granuloma is virtually pathognomonic of WG. By contrast, the observation of a granuloma of the tuberculoid or sarcoidal type is strong evidence against WG. Like chronic granulomatous inflammation in response to a known cause (e.g. tuberculosis), palisading histiocytes and diffuse granulomatous tissue may constitute signs of good host response in WG. Fibrinoid necrosis of collagen within scars suggests active disease in the face of repair and prior to host response.

From the morphological point of view, the second major feature of WG, *vasculitis*, is even more polymorphic. Vasculitis generally originates in granulomas of the respiratory tract. In many cases the anatomical picture is dominated by a necrotizing vasculitis similar to the microscopic form of polyarteritis. Vessels of many types can be affected in WG, resulting in various clinical expressions. Less frequently, the histological picture resembles that seen in classic polyarteritis nodosa (PAN), giant-cell (Horton's type) arteritis, and other vasculitic disorders.

Characteristically, *acute vasculitis* exhibits segmental necrotizing lesions in the walls of arteries, arterioles, capillaries, and venules. Commonly involved vessels include arteries and arterioles in skeletal and cardiac muscle as well as in liver and kidneys, post-capillary venules and arterioles in the skin, and capillaries in the pulmonary alveoli and renal glomeruli.

The third feature of the classic triad, involvement of the kidneys, is also characterized by a variety of clinical and anatomical pictures [for review, see Jennette and Falk (1994)]. As in other affected organs, the kidneys exhibit scattered granulomas in addition to variably disseminated vasculitic

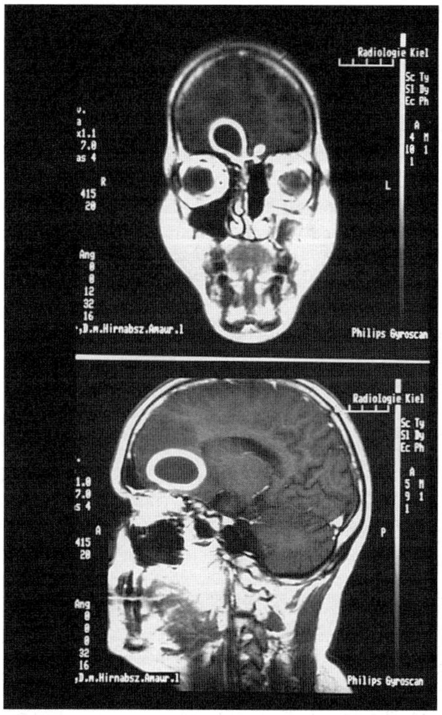

Fig. 5 Intracerebral spread of contiguous granulomatous lesion (frontal lobe) from the sinuses.

processes and often marked interstitial inflammatory infiltration. Glomerular involvement is frequent and is characterized histologically by segmental fibrinoid necrosis and crescent formation. No ultrastructural evidence of IC localization can be found (*pauci-immune necrotizing and crescentic GN*). Glomerular basement membranes and Bowman's capsule are often disrupted in areas of necrosis. Injury to the glomerular capillary wall is an important initiating event in the formation of glomerular crescents. Thus, the extent of renal capillaritis determines the number of crescents that ultimately lead to RPGN.

Immunopathology

Although the primary immunopathogenic events that cause WG remain unclear, advances in molecular and cellular immunology have defined many of the effector mechanisms that play a role in disease and provide possible areas for therapeutic interventions in the future.

In WG, the circumstantial evidence supports an autoimmune inflammatory process, characterized by an early lesion involving neutrophils and endothelial cells as both targets and active participants and ANCA, which may enhance immunoinflammatory events that contribute to disease [for review, see Csernok et al. (1999a)].

Autoantibodies against proteinase3 are highly specific for WG and since their titre follows clinical disease activity in many cases, it is believed that PR3-ANCA are of immunopathogenic relevance. It has been shown that the autoantibody interferes with the biological functions of PR3 (e.g. by inhibition of elastinolytic activity) as well as with enzyme inhibitors (e.g. alpha-1-antitrypsin) of PR3. ANCA also activate neutrophils when PR3 is accessible on the cell membrane by engaging the Fcγ receptors to produce reactive oxygen species and to degranulate. As a unifying construct, it was proposed that priming doses of proinflammatory cytokines, such as those produced during infection, induce surface expression of ANCA target antigens. Binding of ANCA to these antigens leads to neutrophil degranulation and endothelial cell injury with subsequent vascular damage. Through these mechanisms a variety of pathways may be brought into play, all leading to vascular injury. The effects of ANCA that lead to enhancement of neutrophils and endothelial cell activation and injury are summarized in Fig. 6 (ANCA–cytokine-sequence theory).

There are a few animal models for ANCA-related vasculitis that resemble WG or MPA [for review, see Heeringa et al. (1998)]. A model of proliferative GN resembling the renal involvement characteristic of MPA has been developed. Immunization of Brown Norway rats with MPO and subsequent localized perfusion with neutrophil lysosomal extract and H_2O_2, have provided substantial insights into the cellular and molecular mechanisms leading to the development of vasculitis and GN. It is important to mention that induction of MPO-ANCA alone did not cause disease manifestations. Additional factors (infections?) inducing priming/activation of neutrophils, monocytes and endothelial cells with subsequent release of products (enzymes, oxygen species, etc.) are required. MPO-ANCA production occurs spontaneously in an inbred strain of mice (SCG/kj) that spontaneously develops GN and necrotizing vasculitis. Recently, Harper et al. (1998) demonstrated that 22 per cent of female MRL-lpr mice develop MPO-ANCA. Anti-MPO monoclonal antibodies derived from these mice are polyreactive and react with double-stranded DNA. They bind to a conformational epitope on human MPO which is also expressed by activated human neutrophils. These mice develop a clinical syndrome of vasculitis and GN that is distinct from IC disease. The results suggest that a subset of MRL-lpr mice develops ANCA-related vasculitis rather than SLE and may be used as a model for human MPA.

In another model, purified human PR3-ANCA injected into Balb/c mice caused production of mouse antibodies against human PR3-ANCA (Ab1), followed during the next month by production of anti-Ab1 antibodies (Ab2) that recognized human PR3. At the time of anti-Ab2 production the mice developed renal and pulmonary vasculitis similar to that in WG, suggesting a link between the two events. However, it is not clear from these experiments whether the antibodies (Ab2) also recognize murine PR3. Jenne et al. (1997) recently identified and characterized murine PR3. Despite the strong similarities between human and murine PR3, PR3-ANCA from WG patients did not recognize the natively folded murine PR3, indicating that the endogenous murine homologue does not present any of the epitopes required for the study of human ANCA-induced vasculitis in mice. Consequently, it is unlikely that disease observed in mice after immunization with PR3-ANCA is caused by pathogenic antibodies against mouse PR3.

So far *no* satisfactory animal model for ANCA-associated vasculitis has been developed. None of the experimental models completely mimics the

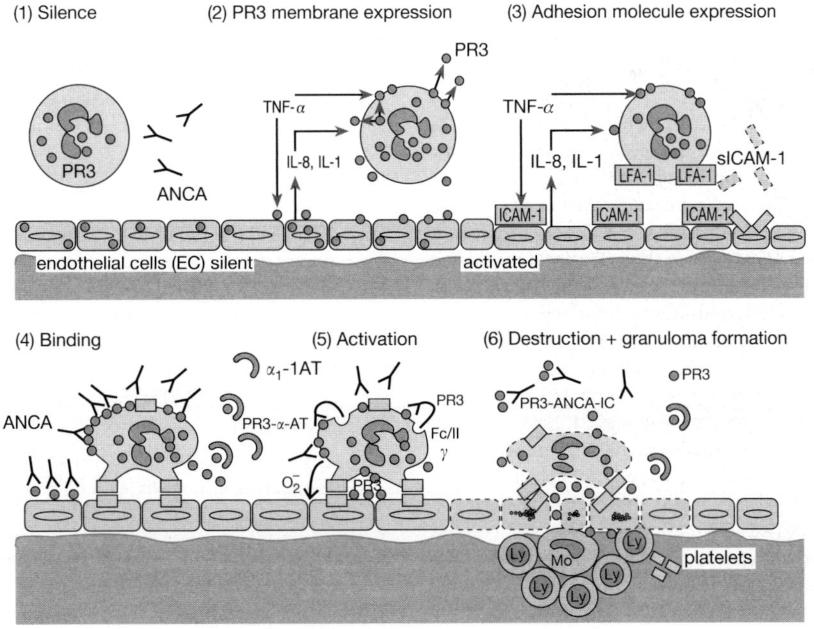

Fig. 6 Pathophysiological model of ANCA-mediated vasculitis: *(ANCA–cytokine sequence theory).*

human ANCA-associated diseases. Furthermore, all of the *in vivo* animal models suggest, but do not definitively prove, that ANCA are pathogenic.

Granuloma formation

WG begins with granulomatous changes. The primary granulomas form and develop in connective tissue, but without vascular involvement (Fienberg 1981). In his last paper on this topic, Friedrich Wegener wrote in 1990: the vasculitis that accompanies the granulomatous disease is a secondary feature that represents a later stage. Thus, insights into the leading immunopathogenic mechanisms in WG should come from studies concentrating on cells from the *pathergic granuloma* or its surroundings (e.g. BAL). Highly elevated soluble CD30 (sCD30) levels have been detected in the plasma of WG patients (Wang et al. 1997). This finding in association with the variable numbers of eosinophils in the granuloma, the moderate blood eosinophilia, and the slight elevation of IgE and the autoimmune phenomena (cANCA) led to the working hypothesis that WG is a Th2-associated condition. On the other hand, studies on T cells from peripheral blood have clearly shown that these cells exhibit increased secretion of IFN-γ but not of IL-4, IL-5, and IL-10, thus demonstrating that at least the periphery shows a Th1 response (Ludviksson et al. 1998).

The Th1 pattern is the main cytokine profile exhibited by T-cell clones isolated from nasal biopsy specimens displaying granulomatous inflammation and—to a lesser extent—by T-cell clones and T-cell lines generated from BAL cells (Csernok et al. 1999b). These findings fit well in the concept that T cells play a triggering role in the pathogenesis of WG and demonstrate the existence of a clear-cut *Th1 polarization of the immune response* in the granulomatous inflammation. Analysis of the phenotype of inflammatory cells by immunochemistry in nasal biopsies from patients with localized/initial and generalized WG have demonstrated the presence of CD26, an operational Th1 marker, which is a dipeptidylpeptidase predominantly expressed by CD4+ T cells (Müller et al. 2000).

As mentioned above, WG typically begins with a granulomatous inflammation in the respiratory tract without vasculitis and if untreated leads ultimately to 'full-blown' WG mainly as a consequence of the subsequent vasculitic disease. Considered in this manner, WG is a granulomatous diseases that evolves into a Th2-dominated vasculitic disease. Its remains to be determined by which mechanism the putative Th1/Th2 switch occurs during the disease process. In the light of ongoing advances in the development of immunotherapy modalities, it is imperative that these studies are performed in future.

Outcome

Since the introduction of the so-called standard therapy consisting of daily CYC (2–4 mg/kg/day) plus GC, the prognosis of patients with WG has greatly improved. In the largest study, consisting of 158 WG patients from the National Institutes of Health (NIH), 80 per cent of patients survived for a mean of 8 years under this therapy (Hoffman et al. 1992). The latter report on this cohort, however, revealed a high rate of therapy-related morbidity and mortality with a high relapse rate. In two further multicentre studies of WG, mortality rates over comparable periods was two- to three-fold higher (36 and 56 per cent; see Table 1) [for review, see Reinhold-Keller et al. (2000)]. In a recently published study on 155 WG patients from a single centre over a median of 7 years, the mortality rate was only 13 per cent, and the estimated median survival time after diagnosis was 21.7 years (95 per cent CI 15.60–27.86; Table 2; Reinhold-Keller et al. 2000). Significant predictors at diagnosis for a higher mortality were age greater than 50 years (relative risk, RR: 5.45), kidney involvement with impaired renal function (RR: 5.4), and lung involvement (RR: 3.75). Similar to the NIH cohort, more than 90 per cent of all patients of this cohort were treated with daily CYC, but in contrast to the NIH cohort it was combined with mesna to reduce the urotoxicity. Under the latter regime the risk of CYC-induced cystitis can be reduced by 2/3 compared to CYC therapy without mesna (Reinhold-Keller et al. 2000). In both cohorts, more than 80 per cent of all deaths were related to WG and/or its therapy. In addition, the relapse rates in both cohorts were high and amounted to 50 per cent in the NIH cohort and 64 per cent in the German cohort. Patients who were followed for more than 5 years 71 per cent of these patients even suffered from one or more relapses (Reinhold-Keller et al. 2000).

Since WG has changed from a disease with a mostly fatal outcome to a treatable although chronic and often relapsing disease like other chronic diseases, its socio-economic impact and long-term effect on quality of life are becoming increasingly important. Little data exists on this topic. Hoffman et al. (1998) reported on 60 WG patients, in 80 per cent of whom the disease had compromised their normal activity of daily living. Thirty-one per cent of formerly employed patients became permanently disabled. The results are similar in a other study on 60 younger WG patients (Reinhold-Keller et al. 2002): 27 per cent became permanently unemployed because of WG. Only the gender was predictive of unemployment: women had a nearly three-fold higher risk of losing their job than men, independent of severity or duration of disease.

Microscopic polyangiitis

Historical background

In 1923 Friedrich Wohlwill described two patients with systemic vasculitis in which histological examination showed nongranulomatous small vessel vasculitis and associated crescentic GN as an only microscopic recognizable form of 'periarteriitis'. Wainwright and Davson described six cases in 1950 characterized by a high frequency of necrotizing and crescentic GN. In three of these cases necrotizing granulomas were seen. Around the same time Zeek et al. (1948) distinguished hypersensitivity angiitis from classic PAN pain. An indolent course before admission and diagnosis is observed in many cases. General symptoms and rheumatic complaints are noted months before recognition of full-blown disease with life-threatening conditions (Savage et al. 1985). All of the patients had clinical evidence of hypersensitivity to sulfonamides and/or foreign proteins, and all had necrotizing GN without crescent formation. In 1954 Godman and Churg clarified the relationship between PAN and some types of small vessel vasculitis. They postulated that the 'microscopic form of periarteritis' is distinct from 'periarteritis nodosa' and closely related to WG. In contrast to periarteritis nodosa, which is a disease of arteries, microscopic polyarteritis involves many different types of vessels (Godman and Churg 1954). Savage et al. (1985) diagnosed microscopic polyarteritis in 34 patients on the basis of the defined criteria (Table 3). All had non-granulomatous small vessel vasculitis and associated focal segmental necrotizing GN, usually with crescent

Table 3 Clinical findings in microscopic polyangiitis in 34 patients (Savage et al. 1985)

	Patients (%)
Glomerulonephritis	100
'Vasculitic general symptoms'	76
Rheumatic complaints	65
Vasculitic skin efflorescence	44
Episcleritis	24
Lung involvement (pulmonary complications) (haemoptysis, infiltrations, etc.)	32
Gastrointestinal problems	32
ENT-symptoms (mucocutaneous ulcers, sinusitis, epistaxis, hypacusis)	21
Neurological deficits	18
Cardiovascular complications	3

formation. In the renal biopsies immunodeposits were observed in only a minority of the cases. In 1990 the ACR issued criteria for the classification of seven major vasculitis disorders. The term 'microscopic polyarteritis' was not used, so the ACR gave no guidelines for this particular disease.

Jennette et al. (1994) published the names and definitions for vasculitis disorders proposed at an international consensus conference at Chapel Hill. They distinguished MPA entirely on the basis of histologic and immunological criteria, and proposed the term 'microscopic polyangiitis' to connote a small vessel vasculitis with few or no ICs (pauci-immune), even if medium-sized arteries are involved. They grouped WG, MPA, and CSS in the category of ANCA-associated small vessel vasculitis, although few patients with typical clinical and pathological features of these diseases remain ANCA negative. Thus, more than half a century after Wohlwill's first description, the diagnosis of MPA is still confusing because of the lack of uniform criteria and the inclusion of MPA cases with groups of PAN or WG cases.

Terms and definitions

MPA is a necrotizing systemic vasculitis with few or no immunodeposits in situ that mainly affects small vessels (i.e. capillaries, venules, and arterioles). Necrotizing crescentic GN and haemorrhagic pulmonary capillaritis are frequent manifestations and are the most important causes of morbidity and mortality [for review, see Jennette et al. (2001)].

Clinical features

MPA's clinical manifestations are very similar to that of generalized WG with regard to the organs involved by the vasculitic process; it however does not include granuloma. The clinical features of MPA are extremely variable and non-specifiable (see Table 3). Common signs and symptoms include GN, lung capillaritis with pulmonary haemorrhage often in combination, purpura, peripheral neuropathy, myalgias, arthralgias, and abdominal pain. An indolent course before admission and diagnosis is observed in many cases. General symptoms and rheumatic complaints are noted months before recognition of full-blown disease with life-threatening conditions (Savage et al. 1985).

Kidney

Most patients have renal involvement (80 per cent) with impairment at admission; renal function deteriorates rapidly thereafter, finally leading to RPGN. Renal biopsy typically shows GN with crescent formation. Immunochemistry can differentiate this form from IC or antibasement membrane, antibody-induced GN due to the absence of immune deposits (pauci-immune GN) [for review, see Balow and Fauci (1993); Van der Woude and Ferrario (1999)].

Lung

Alveolar haemorrhage is an important factor for morbidity and mortality. Haemoptysis starts within 1 month of admission in most patients, but sometimes has been present for much longer. The radiological feature of pulmonary haemorrhage is alveolar shadowing in the absence of pulmonary oedema or infection. An elevated carbon monoxide transfer coefficient is also indicative of alveolar haemorrhage, which is clinically diagnosed by BAL [for review, see Schnabel et al. (1999)].

Some patients may present with an interstitial process mimicking idiopathic pulmonary fibrosis. Matsumoto et al. (1993) also found diffuse alveolar damage and interstitial fibrosis and considered them to be complications of the vasculitis. An 'idiopathic' pulmonary fibrosis can be the first sign of MPA and precede the MPA as systemic vasculitis (Fig. 7; Becker-Merok et al. 1999; Mansi et al. 2001).

In fulminant MPA, RPGN and alveolar haemorrhage occur together as a pulmonary–renal syndrome. The pulmonary–renal syndrome is clinically indistinguishable from that of Goodpasture's syndrome, of WG, and of other vasculitides or collagen-vascular diseases affecting the lung and the kidney.

A retrospective study of 29 patients with MPA and alveolar haemorrhage recruited between 1995 and 1998 was recently published by Lauque et al. (2000). In 27/29 patients, a pauci-immune necrotizing GN was also observed. The most frequent clinical pulmonary features were dyspnoea (90 per cent), cough (90 per cent), and haemoptysis (90 per cent). The dyspnoea was severe in 69 per cent of patients and required immediate mechanical ventilation in three patients. Opacities with an alveolar filling pattern were seen in 28/29 patients, bilateral in 26 patients. Nine patients (31 per cent) died after a median follow-up of 6 months, five patients exclusively due to vasculitis. The 5-year survival was 68 per cent.

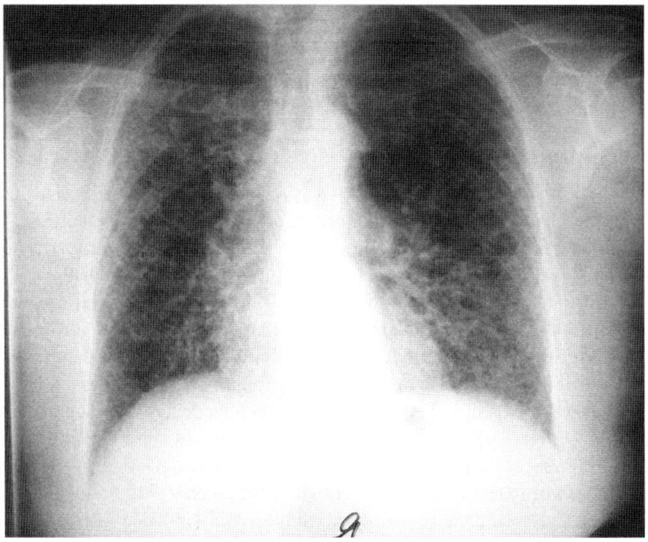

Fig. 7 Female patient with MPA with an involvement of lung, kidney, peripheral nervous system, and rheumatic complaints diagnosed at the age of 62 years. Pulmonary fibrosis at the time of diagnosis showing an increase of granulocytes in the bronchoalveolar lavage.

Other clinical features

Musculoskeletal symptoms similar to those in WG occur in 50–72 per cent of patients. All other vasculitic symptoms described for generalized WG can also occur. Ear, nose, and throat lesions are common, but do not lead to histological granulomatous masses or lesions. However, patients with WG have more widespread extrarenal organ involvement than MPO-ANCA-positive patients. Patients with MPA are about 10 years older than patients with WG at the time of diagnosis (Franssen et al. 2000).

Laboratory investigations

The general laboratory findings with increase of acute phase reactants are very similar to those of in WG. In MPA, however, cANCA or PR3-ANCA are seen in a very low percentage of patients. pANCA with specificity for MPO are most commonly found (50–80 per cent). MPO-ANCA are also present in about 80 per cent of patients with active idiopathic (pauci-immune) necrotizing crescentic GN. MPO-ANCA have also been described in low frequencies and usually with low titres in other autoimmune diseases, such as SLE, drug-induced GN, sarcoidosis, and in infections. A recently published meta-analysis of the diagnostic performance of MPO-ANCA (Choi et al. 2001) revealed for combined indirect immunofluorescence and MPO-ELISA a specificity for systemic vasculitis of 99.4 per cent, but a low sensitivity of 31.5 per cent. MPO-ANCA appear to follow the clinical course of MPA less closely than PR3-ANCA follow that of WG.

Treatment

Treatment has not yet been definitively established and different strategies have been proposed. Most investigators treat MPA similar to generalized

WG. Considering the high frequency of renal involvement most patients have to be treated intensively with high-dose corticosteroids and CYC. In patients with RPGN which has led to renal failure (creatinine >500 mmol/l) plasma exchange may be useful (for details see Chapter 4.5.2).

Pathology

The basic *acute vascular lesion* of MPA is segmental vascular necrosis with infiltration by neutrophils and monocytes, often accompanied by leucocytoclasia and fibrinoid necrosis, causing varying degrees of haemorrhage. Dermal venulitis is associated with purpura, alveolar capillaritis with pulmonary haemorrhage, GN with haematuria, etc. The earliest arterial lesions have segmental fibrinoid necrosis with varying degrees of neutrophilic leucocyte infiltration and the acute capillaritis usually has increased numbers of neutrophils in alveolar or glomerular capillaries. Immunohistological or electron-microscopical examination only of lung or kidney tissue distinguishes between MPA and Goodpasture's syndrome because the latter has linear staining of the capillary basement membrane for IgG whereas the former does not (pauci-immune vasculitis). In the *chronic phase*, non-specific features of alveolar damage with scattered haemosiderin-laden macrophages are seen and interstitial fibrosis can occur.

In the kidney, the process primarily affects the glomeruli. Early capillary thrombosis results in segmental necrosis of glomerular tufts, capillary rupture, and bleeding into Bowman's space which, in turn, triggers the accumulation and proliferation of monocytes and epithelial cells with the formation of crescents. The amount of immunoglobulin deposited is small, giving rise to the term pauci-immune GN. Ultrastructural studies have shown that the earliest changes affect the vascular endothelium with swelling, necrosis, and adherence, suggesting that the endothelium itself is a target for initial injury. In the lung the typical finding is haemorrhagic pulmonary capillaritis *without* granuloma formation. Involvement of medium and large vessel occurs in about half of patients with MPA.

Immunopathology

The *aetiology* of MPA is not known. Various drugs have been described as a trigger (see 'Wegener's granulomatosis'). Recent advances have been made in the understanding of relevant mechanisms of inflammation, particularly the role of the endothelium and interactions with inflammatory mediators and immune effector cells. As in WG, experimental *in vitro* evidence suggests an autoimmune inflammatory process characterized by an early lesion involving neutrophils and endothelial cells as both targets and effective participants. Priming of neutrophils and endothelium cells by proinflammatory cytokines allows anti-MPO autoantibodies (MPO-ANCA) to activate neutrophils in the same way PR3-ANCAs do in Wegener's vasculitis. These activated neutrophils probably damage the endothelium [for review, see Harper and Savage (2000)].

Outcome

The 5-year survival rate is between 60 and 80 per cent (Guillevin et al. 1999). An increase in mortality was observed in patients with proteinuria (>1 g/day), pulmonary haemorrhage, and renal insufficiency. The relapse rate in MPA seems to be lower than in WG patients. A long-term study of 107 patients with MPA and necrotizing crescentic GN found that relapse occurred in 29 per cent within 18 months of the end of immunosuppressive therapy. A further study including 67 MPA patients and 56 WG patients revealed relapse rates of 40 and 47 per cent, respectively (Westman et al. 1998).

Renal

Renal survival post-transplantation in patients with MPA (or WG) is the same as for other causes of end-stage renal disease. Relapses occur less often than in dialysed or non-dialysed patients. However, there is still a substantial relapse rate in the ANCA-associated small vessel vasculitis population after transplantation (Schmitt et al. 1993; Allen et al. 1998; Nachman et al. 1999).

Churg–Strauss syndrome

Historical background

Churg–Strauss syndrome was originally described in 1949 as *allergic granulomatosis*. Prior to that an association between asthma, peripheral blood eosinophilia, and 'periarteritis nodosa' had been noted in 1939 by Rackemann and Greene. Similarly, other authors noted proceeding severe asthma in the course of PAN in upto 18 per cent of patients until in 1951 Jacob Churg and Lotte Strauss reported 13 cases of severe asthma with a uniform clinical picture, including fever, hypereosinophilia, and evidence of vascular disturbances in other organ systems (Churg and Strauss 1951). Pathological examination revealed tissue infiltration by eosinophils, necrotizing vasculitis, and extravascular granulomas. These findings suggested that the clinico-pathological complex described as 'allergic granulomatosis, allergic angiitis and aeriarteritis' was distinct from classic PAN and given the eponymous name '*Churg–Strauss syndrome*'.

Terms and definitions

In their 1951 paper defining the new syndrome, Churg and Strauss noted the constellation of asthma, fever, hyper-eosinophilia, systemic vasculitis, interstitial eosinophilic infiltrates, and extravascular granulomas occurring in multiple sites including the heart, lungs, liver, spleen, skin, peripheral nerves, gastrointestinal tract, and kidneys.

Criteria for *classification of the vasculitis syndrome* were recently developed by comparing 20 patients who had this diagnosis with 787 patients with other forms of vasculitis. Six features were selected for the *ACR criteria*: asthma, eosinophilia (>10 per cent) in the blood, mononeuropathy (including multiplex) or polyneuropathy, non-fixed pulmonary infiltrates (chest X-ray), paranasal sinus abnormality, and biopsy specimens containing a blood vessel with extravascular eosinophils (Masi et al. 1990), see Table 4.

In the *definition of vasculitides* adopted by the 1992 Chapel Hill Consensus Conference on the nomenclature of systemic vasculitis CSS is characterized by the presence of asthma and eosinophilia and belongs to the group of *small vessel vasculitis* which is strongly associated with ANCA.

Table 4 ACR 1990 criteria for the classification of Churg–Strauss syndrome

Criteria	Definition
1. Asthma	History of wheezing or diffuse high-pitched rales on expiration
2. Eosinophilia	Eosinophilia >10% on white blood cell differential count
History of allergy[a]	History of seasonal allergy (e.g. allergic rhinitis) or other documented allergies, including food, contactants, and others, *except* for drug allergy
3. Mononeuropathy or polyneuropathy	Development of mononeuropathy, multiple mononeuropathies, or polyneuropathy (i.e. glove/stocking distribution) attributable to a systemic vasculitis
4. Pulmonary infiltrates, non-fixed	Migratory or transitory pulmonary infiltrates on radiographs (not including fixed infiltrates)
5. Paranasal sinus abnormality	History of acute or chronic paranasal sinus pain or tenderness or radiographic opacification of the paranasal sinuses
6. Extravascular eosinophils	Biopsy including artery, arteriole, or venule, showing accumulations of eosinophils in extravascular areas

[a] History of allergy, other than asthma or drug-related, is included only in the tree classification criteria set and not in the traditional format criteria set, which requires four or more of the other six items listed here.

Source: From Masi et al. (1990), with permission.

By definition there is an 'eosinophil-rich and granulomatous inflammation involving the respiratory tract, and necrotizing vasculitis affecting small- to medium-sized vessels, and associated with asthma and eosinophilia'.

A broader and more inclusive definition was proposed by Lanham et al. (1984). The authors' proposal is based on three criteria: asthma, a peak peripheral blood eosinophil count in excess of 1.5×10^9/l, and systemic vasculitis involving two or more extrapulmonary organs.

The existence of *limited forms* of CSS, analogous to the *formes frustes* of WG, has also been postulated (Lie 1993; Churg et al. 1995).

Clinical features

Although CSS was first distinguished from PAN and then from WG (Henochowicz et al. 1986; Schmitt et al. 2001), the main organ systems affected apart from the respiratory tract and the lung include the heart, the nervous system, the skin, the gut, and kidneys (Table 5; Lhote et al. 1998). Compared with WG and/or MPA, CSS has more frequent cardiac and neurologic involvement and less frequent severe renal disease. Coronary arteritis and myocarditis are the principal causes of morbidity and mortality and account for approximately 50 per cent of deaths. However, there are eosinophilic variants of WG [for review, see Gross (2002)]. In these patients, in addition to pathergic necrosis, granulomatous inflammation, and vasculitis, intense stromal eosinophilia can be observed in the absence of peripheral blood eosinophilia or clinical asthma.

Three phases of the disease have been identified (Lanham et al. 1984). A prodromal phase, which may persist for years, consists of allergic diseases (e.g. allergic rhinitis and nasal polyposis), which is frequently followed by asthma. The second phase of the disease is characterized by the onset of peripheral blood and tissue eosinophilia, frequently causing a picture resembling Löffler's syndrome, chronic eosinophilic pneumonia, or eosinophilic gastroenteritis. The eosinophilic infiltrative disease may remit over years before the third phase of full-blown disease, consisting of a life-threatening systemic vasculitis, is reached. However, clinical experience has demonstrated that these three phases do not necessarily have to follow one another in that order.

The ACR criteria for the classification of CSS are given in Table 4. Because these criteria were developed to enable discrimination of the various primary vasculitides, they used those symptoms most typical of the underlying entity while ignoring some common clinical features of CSS such as rash or cardiac involvement. The ACR criteria should thus not be used as diagnostic criteria.

Allergic rhinitis

About two-thirds of all cases studied had allergic upper respiratory tract disease. The principal symptoms are rhinorrhoea, sneezing, nasal obstruction, and recurrent sinusitis with radiological evidence of pansinusitis in upto 80 per cent of cases. Many patients require upper respiratory tract surgery, principally nasal polypectomy.

Asthma

Asthma is the central feature of CSS and precedes the systemic manifestations in nearly all cases. Compared to common asthma, it begins relatively late in life, at a mean age of 35 years. Asthmatic attacks usually increase until the onset of vasculitis. Asthma may abate during the vasculitic illness.

Pulmonary infiltrates

Pulmonary infiltrates frequently occur in the vasculitic phase, as well as in the prodromal illness. They are generally transient and patchy without segmental or lobar distribution and have no predilection for any region of the lung. These infiltrates are found in upto 77 per cent of patients (Fig. 8). In contrast to WG or MPA, CSS rarely involves alveolar haemorrhage. Massive bilateral nodular infiltrates can arise in CSS and may become confluent but, in contrast to WG, rarely cavitate. Pleural effusions occur in 27 per cent of cases and typically contain large numbers of eosinophils (Choi et al. 2000).

Cardiac involvement

Whereas renal and lung involvement appear to be negative prognostic factors in WG or MPA, in CSS most deaths occur from cardiac involvement. Manifestations include cardiac arrest, myocardial infarction, valvular heart disease, congestive heart failure, pericardial effusion, and acute or chronic constrictive pericarditis. Indeed, 60 per cent of the post-mortem examinations in the initial study by Churg and Strauss revealed cardiac lesions and in the study by Lanham et al. (1984) cardiac disease accounted for 48 per cent of deaths. Cardiac involvement is common and occurs in upto 84.6 per cent of patients. Morphologically in a series of 39 autopsy reports manifestations of granulomatous vasculitis of the coronary arteries or granulomatous myocarditis were found in 62 per cent of cases. Eosinophilic

Table 5 Clinical features of Churg–Strauss syndrome based on 372 patients from the literature, expressed as percentage of the studies population [from Lhote et al. (1998), with permission]

	Chumbley et al. (1977)	Literature review	Lanham et al. (1984)	Guillevin et al. (1996)	Gaskin et al. (1991)	Haas et al. (1991)	Abu-Shakra et al. (1994)[a]	Guillevin et al. (1999)
Patients (*n*)	30	138	16	43	21	16	12	96
Male/female	2.3	1.09	3	1.3	2	3	1	0.88
Mean age (years)	47	38	38	43.2	46.5	42.5	48	48.2
range	(15–69)			(7–66)	(23–69)	(17–74)	(28–70)	(17–74)
Asthma	100	100	100	100	100	100	100	100
General symptoms			72		100	100	70	
Pulmonary infiltrates	26.6	74	72	77	43	62	58	38
Allergic rhinitis	70	9	70	21		10	83	47
Mononeuritis multiplex	63.3	64	66	67	70	75	92	78
Gastrointestinal disease	16.6	62	59	37	58	56	8	33
Cardiovascular disease		52	47	49	15	56	42	30
Arthritis, arthralgia	20	46	51	28	43	31	42	41
Myalgias			68			43	33	54
Cutaneous diseases	66.6				50	68	67	51
Purpura		46	48	28		25		31
Nodules	26.6	33	30	21		25		19
Renal disease		42	49	16	80	31	8	16
Pleural effusion		29	29	2.3		25		

[a] Neurology patients.

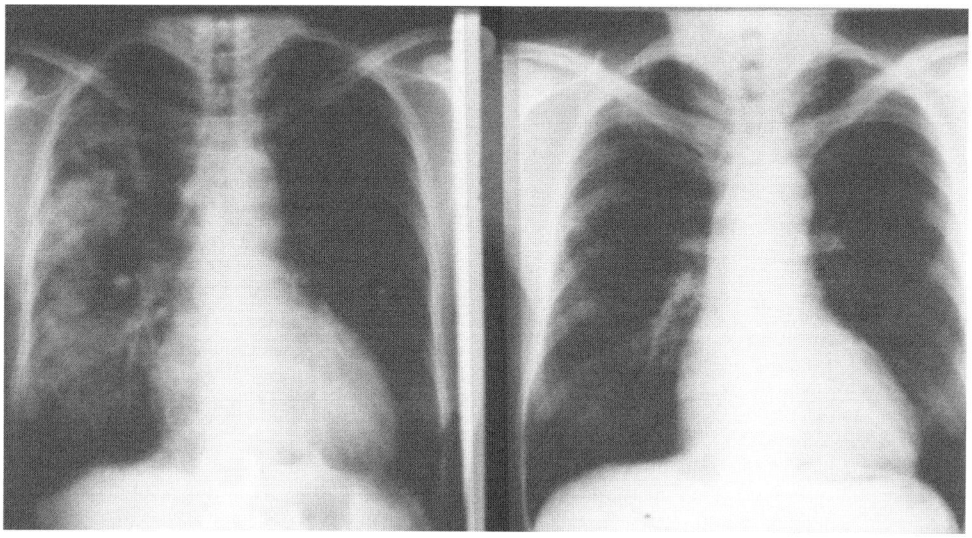

Fig. 8 Female patient with CSS with an involvement of the lung, upper respiratory tract, and heart diagnosed at the age of 39 years. Pulmonary infiltrates at the time of diagnosis (left) with an eosinophilia of 30% in the bronchoalveolar lavage (right), after immunosuppressive therapy.

endomyocarditis can be seen when additional immunofluorescence investigations are done to find eosinophil major basic protein (MBP) in the foci of necrosis within the granulomas (Ramakrishna et al. 2000). Diffusely hypokinetic ventricular walls with decreased ejection fraction (<35 per cent) have been associated with cardiac thrombus formation. The potential for stroke in CSS due to cardioembolic phenomena has been noted (Sehgal et al. 1995), as has the recurrence of CSS in a transplanted heart.

Neuropathy

Peripheral neuropathy, both mononeuritis multiplex and polyneuropathy, is found in up to 75 per cent of CSS patients and in a clinical setting with vasculitis, neuropathy is highly suggestive of the diagnosis (for review, see Gross 2002). In a French series of 16 patients with CSS, 12 had peripheral neuropathies as the most prominent organ symptom. Of 47 patients seen at the Mayo Clinic, 29 (62 per cent) had neurological involvement. Peripheral neuropathy was detected in 25 patients, 17 had multiple mononeuropathy, seven had distal symmetric polyneuropathy, and one had an asymmetric polyneuropathy (Sehgal et al. 1995).

While peripheral nerve disease is often an early manifestation of CSS, CNS involvement is most common late in the course of fulminant disease. Thus, the majority of cases in an autopsy series (Churg and Strauss 1951) had major CNS manifestations. Cerebral haemorrhage or infarction is the second most common cause of death with cerebral vasculitis or hypertension. Of the Mayo Clinic series cited above, three patients had cerebral infarctions. Asthma preceded the onset of neurologic involvement in all cases (mean duration 6.7 years).

Cutaneous disease

Rash is one of the most common features of the vasculitic phase, occurring in 70 per cent of cases. Purpura is seen in nearly half of cases and subcutaneous nodules in 30 per cent. The scalp and the extensor side of the arms are typical sites for nodules. The nodular lesions termed 'CSS granuloma' are highly specific when they have an eosinophilic core.

Renal involvement

Many patients (16–49 per cent) have renal involvement but only a minority has severe disease. due Perhaps to a selection bias, the Hammersmith group from a nephrological unit reported a series of 90 CSS patients in whom renal involvement was more common (84 per cent) and often severe. Three patients had nephrotic syndrome, four had serum creatinine greater than 500 μmol/l, and two required dialysis. Focal segmental GN was the predominant lesion on biopsy (85 per cent), often with necrotizing features and crescent formation. Treatment with high-dose prednisolone was not always sufficient to stop the progression to more severe vasculitis.

Gastrointestinal disease

Eosinophilic gastroenteritis may precede or coincide with the vasculitic phase of CSS. Digestive tract symptoms, including abdominal pain, diarrhoea and gastrointestinal bleeding, can occur in upto two-thirds of patients. Mesenteric intestinal ischaemia and small bowel necrosis with perforation of small intestine can resemble the gastrointestinal features of PAN. So abdominal pain may reflect severe disease due to bowel perforation with peritonitis following mesenteric vasculitis. Severe gastrointestinal tract involvement is a criterion for poor prognosis in CSS.

Musculoskeletal involvement

Arthritis or arthralgia occur in about half of cases usually in the vasculitic phase. Any joint may be affected and the arthralgias are often migratory. There is no destructive or erosive arthritis, myalgias and clinically obvious myositis are only occasional features of CSS.

Other organ involvement

Comparing to WG or MPA an eye involvement is rarely observed (<10 per cent) (Schmitt et al. 2001).

Diagnosis

Diagnosis depends on the combination of characteristic clinical and histological features and, in most cases, characteristic peripheral hypereosinophilia.

The *differential diagnosis* of CSS includes—if vasculitis is present—primarily PAN and WG (Schmitt et al. 2001). Many similarities also exist between CSS and hypereosinophilic syndrome. However, it is usually easy to distinguished CSS from this syndrome based on the latter's characteristic clinical features, including endomyocardial fibrosis, the absence of asthma and vasculitis, resistance to corticosteroids, morphological absence of granuloma and different immunological features (unusual T-cell phenotypes: CD3− CD4+ CD8− T cells and so called double-negative CD3+ CD4− CD8− T cells; high interleukin (IL)-5 production by these abnormal clones of T cells [for review, see Gross (2002)].

Laboratory investigations

Typical laboratory findings in CSS include a normochromic normocytic anaemia, leucocytosis with prominent eosinophilia (>10 per cent), and an acute phase response. Eosinophilia is constant and often more than 10^9/l. Elevated serum IgE is observed in 75 per cent of patients. Low levels of circulating IgE ICs, rheumatoid factor, and ANA have also been described. Complement and/or cryoglobulin levels are usually unremarkable.

The clinical value of ANCA in CSS is questionable. Due to the relative rarity of CSS many reports are based on a small number of patients. Summarizing the available data, Eustace et al. (1999) showed that of 82 CSS patients tested for ANCA, 52 per cent (!) were negative, 23 were pANCA positive, and 12 were cANCA positive in the indirect immunofluorescence test. In most of the pANCA-positive patients, the antibody was directed against MPO (MPO-ANCA). In a recent review, the prevalence of ANCA in CSS was reported to be about 25 per cent for cANCA and 50 per cent for pANCA, the remaining 25 per cent having no ANCA [for review, see Saviage et al. (1999)].

Monitoring disease activity and disease manifestation

Disease activity has to be evaluated according to the clinical picture and laboratory parameters. During the vasculitic phase, the heart is a major target of the disease and the major cause of death in CSS. Any sign of cardiac involvement is an indication for immediate therapy. The earliest manifestation is usually seen in the electrocardiogram or echocardiogram, cardiac failure and/or cardiomyopathy can be demonstrated.

A life-threatening situation is created by alveolar haemorrhage syndrome, which can be detected by chest X-ray and documented by BAL. Although this is—in comparison with WG or MPA—a rare complication of CSS, it is an indication for aggressive therapy. Asthma usually responds well to small doses of GC.

Severe peripheral neuropathy is rather frequent and has to be evaluated by a neurologist, usually by measuring the nerve-conduction-time. Nerve biopsy is unnecessary in most cases. Digestive tract symptoms usually need to be investigated by endoscopy and sometimes by coeliac-angiography. As described for cardiac disease, severe gastrointestinal tract involvement is a criterion for poor prognosis in CSS.

Detection of renal involvement is equally important. Active sediment should be sought first, followed by analysis of renal function.

ESR and CRP are generally accepted indices of disease activity. In addition, the eosinophil count in peripheral blood is of significant importance. Most cases have moderate (<1500–5000 cells/mm^3) or severe eosinophilia (>5000 cells). Various serum markers of lymphocyte activation (e.g. sIL-2R), cytokine production (i.e. IL-10), endothelial cell damage (e.g. soluble thrombomodulin), eosinophil activation markers (e.g. eosinophil cationic protein, ECP) and ANCA, were found to be associated with active disease [for review, see Gross (2002)].

Pathology and pathogenesis

The pathological triad of CSS is infiltration by eosinophils, formation of granulomas, and necrotizing vasculitis. Vasculitis affects both arteries and veins, and is characterized by fibrinoid necrosis, inflammation with many eosinophils, and the tendency to form granulomas in and around the vascular wall. The first phase of early disease is characterized by marked perivascular oedema with sparse infiltration of tissue by eosinophilic leucocytes, and oedema of the vascular wall, most evident in deep intima close to the media. The early fibrinoid vasculitis resembles that seen in PAN. It appears that in CSS the 'fibrinoid' vasculitis attracts eosinophils and later macrophages or monocytes, while in PAN and WG the early cell is predominantly the neutrophilic leucocyte. The small vessel vasculitis is usually of the leucocytoclastic type, with neutrophilic or eosinophilic exudates.

The tissue eosinophilia, which is usually quite intense, may be construed as the counterpart of blood eosinophilia. However, tissue infiltration without significant blood eosinophilia is occasionally seen in other vasculitides such as PAN and WG. The characteristic feature of CSS is a progression of inflammation to a special type of granuloma ('allergic'). This begins as a necrosis in a densely packed focus of eosinophils, with scattering of this specific granules and nuclear debris. The underlying parenchyma also undergoes necrosis, with disintegration of the collagenous stroma. Multinucleated giant cells may be found nearby as well as an accumulation of 'epitheliod' cells. Macrophages and giant cells around the necrotic centre form a palisading formation. The granuloma is surrounded by inflammatory cells, mainly eosinophils.

Whereas IC deposition was earlier favoured as the mechanism of vasculitis injury in CSS (IC vasculitis), recent studies have found no evidence of immune protein deposits, for example, in the vascular walls of epineuronal vessels [for review, see Peen et al. (2000); Gross 2002] demonstrated the presence of MBP in muscle fibres undergoing necrosis in a small bowel biopsy.

Immunopathology

Aetiologically, hyper-responsiveness to an antigenic stimulus seems to underlie the syndrome. In asthmatics, cysteinyl leukotriene receptor type I-antagonists are reported to trigger the disease. Many of these case reports noted that CSS was diagnosed following reduction in the dose of systemic GC, suggesting that the reduced GC dose was the factor that precipitated the 'unmasking' of the vasculitis process. An alternative hypothesis is that CSS represents a hypersensitivity reaction to this class of medication (zafirlukast, montelukast, pranlukast).

Type I hypersensitivity reactions occur in CSS. Typical examples of allergic reactions are rhinitis and bronchial asthma, which are characteristically found in this disease. In full-blown disease, the characteristic pathological findings are blood and tissue *eosinophilia*, extravascular granulomas, and necrotizing vasculitis.

Observation of CSS in cases of parasitic disease (e.g. ascaris, trichinosis, etc.) suggests that immunological stimulation of IgE and eosinophils is involved in its pathogenesis. Many patients present with severe peripheral blood eosinophilia (>5000 cells/mm^3) and marked tissue eosinophil infiltration. Immunofluorescence examination of involved tissues for the presence of eosinophil granule MBP, a molecule of known toxic and costimulatory activities, indicates that MBP deposition occurs in CSS (Peen et al. 2000). Eosinophil activation with release of granule proteins can be detected in the serum and in biopsy specimens, for example, from small bowel. Direct nerve injury can be caused in part by MBP, a highly phlogistic cationic protein enriched with arginine, and eosinophil-derived neurotoxin and/or ECP, which are neurotoxic. One key advance was the recognition that eosinophilia is orchestrated by the Th2 sub-class of CD4+ T cells. Th2 cells produce IL-4, -5, -9, and -13 and are the immunopathological hallmark of allergic disease. More recently it was demonstrated that the cytokine production pattern of T-cell lines from CSS is that of Th2 cells [for review, see Gross (2002)]. In addition, impairment of CD95 ligand-mediated killing of lymphocytes and eosinophils in CSS was recognized to result from variations in CD95 receptor isoform expression. Drugs that block Th2-cell activity (e.g. interferon α) have been successfully used in the treatment of CSS [for review, see Gross (2002)].

On the other hand, evidence for a direct role of immediate type of hypersensitivity in the pathogenesis of vasculitis is rather circumstantial and other mechanisms, including deposition of IgE-containing circulating IC, have to be considered. Elevated serum levels of IgE-laden circulating IC and deposition of various Ig classes and C3 in renal biopsies have been observed.

CSS has been associated with immunotherapy for allergic disease, for example, with administration of allergen extracts. Many drugs can cause pulmonary eosinophilia. However, despite the frequency of drug-related pulmonary eosinophilia, drugs have only really been implicated in the development of CSS. Wechsler et al. (1998) described eight patients with asthma in whom clinical signs and symptoms suggestive of CSS developed when oral corticosteroids were tapered after treatment with zafirlukast, cysteinyl leukotriene receptor type I antagonist. All eight patients had pulmonary infiltrates, characterized as patchy, diffuse alveolar infiltrates in the one case that was described in detail. The peripheral blood eosinophil count ranged from 19 to 72 per cent (2800–16 000 qmm). All of the patients had evidence of cardiac involvement and six had sinusitis. Fever and myalgia were common. Only two patients had evidence of neuropathy. All of the patients had tissue eosinophilia on biopsy. Similar cases have been described in patients in whom orally administered corticosteroids were being taken during or after treatment with montelukast or pranlukast, further cysteinyl leukotriene receptor antagonists. Whether the development of CSS after administration of the leukotriene receptor antagonists is an idiosyncratic reaction to the drugs or the results from corticosteroid withdrawal in patients with pre-existing CSS is unknown.

Outcome

Based on a prospective study of 342 patients with CSS and PAN, a French group searched for *prognostic factors*. Among all parameters evaluated, the following five had significant prognostic value and were responsible for higher mortality and thus formed the basis for the five factor score: proteinuria greater than 1 g/day, renal insufficiency (creatinaemia >140 μmol/l), cardiomyopathy, gastrointestinal tract involvement, and central nervous system involvement. When the FFS was 0, mortality at 5 years was 12 per cent; when FFS equalled 1, mortality was 26 per cent; when the FFS was less than or equal to 2, mortality was 46 per cent (Guillevin et al. 1996). However, these data have to be regarded with some caution since PAN and CSS differ in their morbidity and mortality (Abu-Shakra et al. 1994).

References

Abu-Shakra, M., Smythe, H., Lewtas, J., Badley, E., Weber, D., and Keystone, E. (1994). Outcome of polyarteritis nodosa and Churg–Strauss syndrome. An analysis of twenty-five patients. *Arthritis and Rheumatum* **37**, 1798–803.

Allen, A., Pusey, C., and Gaskin, G. (1998). Outcome of renal replacement therapy in antineutrophil cytoplasmic antibody-associated systemic vasculitis. *Journal of the American Society of Nephrology* **9**, 1258–63.

Anderson, G., Crane, M., Douglas, A.C., Gibbs, A.R., Coles, E.T., Geddes, D.M., Peel, E.T., and Wood, J.B. (1992). Wegener's granuloma. A series of 265 British cases seen between 1975 and 1985. A report by a sub-committee of the British Thoracic Society Research Committee. *Quarterly Journal of Medicine* **302**, 427–38.

Balow, J.E. and Fauci, A.S. (1993). Vasculitis diseases of the kidney: polyarteritis nodosa, Wegener's granulomatosis, allergic angiitis and granulomatosis, and other disorders. In *Disease of the Kidney* Vol. 2, 5th edn. (ed. R.W. Schrier and C.W. Gottschalk), pp. 2335–60.

Becker-Merok, A., Nossent, J.C., and Ritland, N. (1999). Fibrosing alveolitis predating microscopic polyangiitis. *Scandinavian Journal of Rheumatology* **28**, 254–6.

Boehme, M.W., Schmitt, W.H., Youinou, P., Stremmel, W.R., and Gross, W.L. (1996). Clinical relevance of elevated serum thrombomodulin and soluble E-selectin in patients with Wegener's granulomatosis and other systemic vasculitides. *American Journal of Medicine* **101**, 387–94.

Carrington, C.B. and Liebow, A.A. (1966). Limited forms of angiitis and granulomatosis of Wegener's type. *American Journal of Medicine* **41**, 497–527.

Choi, Y.H., Im, J.G., Han, B.K., Kim, J.H., Lee, K.Y., and Myoung, N.H. (2000). Thoracic manifestation of Churg-Strauss syndrome: radiologic and clinical findings. *Chest* **117**, 117–24.

Choi, H.K., Liu, S., Merkel, P.A., Colditz, G.A., and Niles, J.L. (2001). Diagnostic performance of antineutrophil cytoplasmic antibody tests for idiopathic vasculitides: metaanalysis with a focus on antimyeloperoxidase antibodies. *Journal of Rheumatology* **28**, 1584–90.

Churg, J. and Strauss, L. (1951). Allergic granulomatosis, allergic angiitis and periarteritis nodosa. *American Journal of Pathology* **27**, 277–301.

Churg, A., Brallas, M., Cronin, S.R., and Churg, J. (1995). Formes frustes of Churg–Strauss syndrome. *Chest* **108**, 320–3.

Csernok, E., Müller, A., and Gross, W.L. (1999a). Immunopathology of ANCA-associated vasculitis. *Internal Medicine* **38** (10), 759–65.

Csernok, E., Trabandt, A., Müller, A., Wang, G.C., Moosig, F., Paulsen, J., Schnabel, A. and Gross, W.L. (1999b). Cytokine profiles in Wegener's granulomatosis: predominance of type 1 (Th1) in the granulomatous inflammation. *Arthritis and Rheumatism* **42**, 742–50.

Csernok, E. and Gross, W.L. (2000). Primary vasculitides and vasculitis confined to skin: clinical features and new pathogenic aspects. *Archives of Dermatological Research* **292** (9), 427–36.

de Groot, K., Gross, W.L., Herlyn, K., and Reinhold-Keller, E. (2001a). Development and validation of a disease extent index for Wegener's granulomatosis. *Clinical Nephrology* **55**, 31–8.

de Groot, K., Schmidt, D.K., Arlt, A.C., Gross, W.L., and Reinhold-Keller, E. (2001b). Standardized neurologic evaluations of 128 patients with Wegener granulomatosis. *Archives of Neurology* **58**(8), 1215–21.

DeRemee, R.A., McDonald, T.J., Harrison, E.G.J.R., and Coles, D.T. (1976). Wegener's granulomatosis. Anantomic correlates, a proposed classification. *Mayo Clinic Proceedings* **51**, 777–81.

Del Buono, E.A. and Flint, A. (1991). Diagnostic usefulness of nasal biopsy in Wegener's granulomatosis. *Human Pathology* **22**, 107–10.

Devaney, K.O., Travis, W.D., Hoffman, G., Leavitt, R., Lebovics, R., and Fauci, A.S. (1990). Interpretation of head and neck biopsies in Wegener's granulomatosis. *American Journal of Surgical Pathology* **14** (6), 555–64.

Duncker, G., Nölle, B., Asmus, R., Koltze, H., and Rochels, R. (1993). Orbital involvement in Wegener's granulomatosis. In *ANCA-Associated Vasculitides* (ed. W.L. Gross), pp. 315–18. New York: Plenum Press.

Eustace, J.A., Nadasdy, T., and Choi, M. (1999). Disease of the month. The Churg–Strauss syndrome. *Journal of the American Society of Nephrology* **10** (9), 2048–55.

Fienberg, R. (1981). The protracted superficial phenomenon in pathergic (Wegener's) granulomatosis. *Human Pathology* **12**, 458–67.

Frances, C., Huong Du, L.T., Piette, J.C., Saada, V., Boisnic, S., Wechsler, B., Bletry, O., and Godeau, P. (1994). Wegener's granulomatosis: dermatological manifestations in 75 cases with clinicopathologic correlation. *Archives of Dermatology* **130**, 861.

Franssen, C.F.M., Stegemann, C.A., Kallenberg, C.G.M., Gans, R.O.B., De Jong, P.E., Hoorntje, S.J., and Cohen Tervaert, J.W. (2000). Antiproteinase 3- and antimyeloperoxidas-associated vasculitis. *Kidney International* **57**, 2195–206.

Godman, G.C. and Churg, J. (1954). Wegeners granulomatosis. Pathology and review of the literature. *Archives of Pathology and Laboratory Medicine* **58**, 533–53.

Gordon, M., Luqmani, R.A., Adu, D., Greaves, I., Richards, N., Michael, J., Emery, P., Howie, A.J., and Bacon, P.A. (1993). Relapses in patients with a systemic vasculitis. *Quarterly Journal of Medicine* **86**, 779–89.

Greenan, T.J., Grossman, R.I., and Goldberg, H.I. (1992). Cerebral vasculitis: MR imaging and angiographic correlation. *Radiology* **182**, 65–72.

Gross, W.L. and Csernok, E. (1995). Antineutrophil cytoplasmic autoantibodies (ANCA). Immunodiagnostic and pathophysiological aspects. *Current Opinion in Rheumatology* **7** (1), 11.

Gross, W.L., Schnabel, A., and Trabandt, A. (2000a). New perspectives in pulmonary angiitis. From pulmonary angiitis and granulomatosis to ANCA associated vasculitis. *Sarcoidosis Vasculitis and Diffuse Lung Disease* **17** (1), 33–52.

Gross, W.L., Trabandt, A., and Reinhold-Keller, E. (2000b). Diagnosis and evaluation of vasculitis. *Rheumatology (Oxford)* **39** (3), 245–52.

Gross, W.L. (2002). Churg–Strauss syndrome: update on recent developments. *Current Opinion in Rheumatology* **14** (1), 11–14.

Guillevin, L., Lhote, F., Gayraud, M., Cohen, P., Jarrousse, B., Lortholary, O., Thibult, N., and Casassus, P. (1996). Prognostic factors in polyarteritis nodosa and Churg–Strauss syndrome. A prospective study in 342 patients. *Medicine (Baltimore)* **75**, 17–28.

Guillevin, L., Durand-Gasselin, B., Cevallos, R., Gayraud, M., Lhote, F., Callard, P., Amouroux, J., Casassus, P., and Jarrousse, B. (1999). Microscopic polyangiitis: clinical and laboratory findings in eighty-five patients. *Arthritis and Rheumatisom* **42** (3), 421–30.

Hagen, E.C., Daha, M.R., Hermans, J., Andrassy, K., Csernok, E., Gaskin, G., Lesavre, P., Lüdemann, J., Rasmussen, N., Sinico, R.A., Wiik, A., and van der Woude, F.J. (1998). Diagnostic value of standardized assays for anti-neutrophil cytoplasmic antibodies in idiopathic systemic vasculitis. EC/BCR project for ANCA assay standardization. *Kidney International* **53**, 743–53.

Harper, J.M., Thiru, S., Lockwood, C.M., and Cooke, A. (1998). Myeloperoxidase autoantibodies distinguish vasculitis mediated by anti-neutrophil cytoplasm antibodies from immune complex disease in MRL/Mp- lpr/lpr mice: a spontaneous model for human microscopic angiitis. *European Journal of Immunology* **28**, 2217–26.

Harper, L. and Savage, C.O. (2000). Pathogenesis of ANCA-associated systemic vasculitis. *Journal of Pathology* **190**, 349–59.

Henochowicz, S., Eggensperger, D., Pierce, L., and Barth, W. (1986). Necrotizing systemic vasculitis with features of both Wegener's granulomatosis and Churg–Strauss vasculitis. *Arthritis and Rheumatisom* **29**, 565–9.

Heeringa, P., Brouwer, E., Cohen Tervaert, J.W., Weening, J.J., and Kallenberg, C.G. (1998). Animal models of anti-neutrophil cytoplasmic antibody associated vasculitis. *Kidney International* **53**, 253–63.

Hoffman, G.S., Kerr, G.S., Leavitt, R.Y., Hallahan, C.W., Lebovics, R.S., Travis, W.D., Rottem, M., and Fauci, A.S. (1992). Wegener granulomatosis: an analysis of 158 patients. *Annals of Internal Medicine* **116**, 488–98.

Hoffman, G.S., Drucker, Y., Cotch, M.F., Locker, G.A., Easley, K., and Kwoh, K. (1998). Wegener's granulomatosis: patient-reported effects of disease on health, function, and income. *Arthritis and Rheumatisom* **41**, 2257–62.

Jarrousse, B., Guillevin, L., Bindi, P., Hachulla, E., Leclerc, P., Nilson, B., Rèmy, P., Rossert, J., and Jacquot, C. (1993). Increased risk of *Pneumocystis carinii* pneumonia in patients with Wegener's granulomatosis. *Clinical and Experimental Rheumatology* **11**, 615–21.

Jenne, D.E., Frohlich, L., Hummel, A.M., and Specks, U. (1997). Cloning and functional expression of the murine homologue of proteinase 3: implications for the design of murine models of vasculitis. *FEBS Letters* **408**, 187–90.

Jennette, J.C. and Falk, R.J. (1994). The pathology of vasculitis involving the kidney. *American Journal of Kidney Diseases* **24**, 130–41.

Jennette, J.C., Falk, R.J., Andrassy, K., Bacon, P.A., Churg, J., Gross, W.L., Hagen, E.C., Hoffman, G.S., Hunder, G.G., Kallenberg, C.G.M., McCluskey, R.T., Sinico, R.A., Rees, A.J., Van Es, L.A., Waldherr, R., and Wiik, A. (1994). Nomenclature of systemic vasculitides. Proposal of an International Consensus Conference. *Arthritis and Rheumatisom* **37**, 187–92.

Jennette, J.C., Thomas, D.B., and Falk, R.J. (2001). Microscopic polyangiitis (microscopic polyarteritis). *Seminars in Diagnostic Pathology* **18** (1), 3–13.

Lamprecht, P., Trabandt, A., and Gross, W.L. (2000). Clinical and immunological aspects of Wegener's granulomatosis (WG) and other syndromes resembling WG. *The Israel Medical Association Journal* **2**, 621–6.

Lanham, J., Elkon, K., Pusey, C., and Hughes, G. (1984). Systemic vasculitis with asthma and eosinophilia: a clinical approach to the Churg–Strauss syndrome. *Medicine* **63**, 65–81.

Lauque, D., Cadranel, J., Lazor, R., Pourrat, J., Ronco, P., Guillevin, L., and Cordier, J.F. (2000). Microscopic polyangiitis with alveolar haemorrhage. A study of 29 cases and review of the literature. Groupe d'Etudes et de Recherche sur les Maladies 'Orphelines' Pulmonaires (GERM'O'P). *Medicine (Baltimore)* **79** (4), 222–33.

Leavitt, R.Y., Fauci, A.S., Bloch, D.A., Michel, B.A., Hunder, G.G., Arend, W.P., Calabrese, L.H., Fries, J.F., Lie, J.T., Lightfoot, R.W., Masi, A.T., McShane, D.J., Mills, J.A., Stevens, M.B., Wallace, S.L., and Zvaifler, N.J. (1990). The American College of Rheumatology 1990 criteria for the classification of Wegener's granulomatosis. *Arthritis and Rheumatism* **33**, 1101–7.

Lhote, F., Cohen, P., and Guillevin, L. (1998). Polyarteritis nodosa, microscopic polyangiitis and Churg–Strauss syndrome. *Lupus* **7**, 238–58.

Lie, J.T. (1993). Limited forms of Churg–Strauss syndrome. *Pathology of Annulare* **28**, 199–220.

Ludviksson, B.R., Sneller, M.C., Chua, K.S., Talar-Williams, C., Langford, C.A., Ehrhardt, R.O., Fauci, A.S., and Strober, W. (1998). Active Wegener's granulomatosis is associated with HLA–DR+ CD4+ T cells exhibiting an unbalanced Th1-type T cell cytokine pattern: reversal with IL-10. *Journal of Immunology* **160**, 3602–9.

Luqmani, R.A., Bacon, P.A., Moots, R.J., Janssen, B.A., Pall, A., Emery, P., Savage, C., and Adu, D. (1994). Birmingham vasculitis activitiy score (BVAS) in systemic necrotizing vasculitis. *Quarterly Journal of Medicine* **87**, 671–8.

Mansi, I.A., Opran, A., Sondhi, D., Ayinla, R., and Rosner, F. (2001). Microscopic polyangiitis presenting as idiopathic pulmonary fibrosis: is antineutrophilic cytoplasmic antibody testing indicated? *American Journal of Medical Science* **321**(3), 201–2.

Mark, E.J., Matsubara, O., Tan-Liu, N.S., and Fienberg, R. (1988). The pulmonary biopsy in the early diagnosis of Wegener's (pathergic) granulomatosis: a study based on 35 open lung biopsies. *Human Pathology* **19**, 1065–71.

Masi, A.T. et al. (1990). The American college of rheumatology 1990 criteria for the classification of Churg–Strauss syndrome (allergic granulomatosis and angiitis). *Arthritis and Rheumatisom* **33**, 1094–100.

Matsumoto, T., Homma, S., Okada, M., Kuwabara, N., Hoshi, T., Uekusa, T., and Saiki, S. (1993). The lung in polyarteritis nodosa: a pathologic study of 10 cases. *Human Pathology* **24** (7), 717–24.

Moins-Teisserenc, H.T., Gadola, S.D., Cella, M., Dunbar, P.R., Exley, A., Blake, N., Baykal, C., Lambert, J., Bigliardi, P., Willemsen, M., Jones, M., Buechner, S., Colonna, M., Gross, W.L., Cerundolo, V., and Baycal, C. (1999). Association of a syndrome resembling Wegener's granulomatosis with low surface expression of HLA class-I molecules. *Lancet* **6**, 354(9190), 1598–603.

Müller, A., Trabandt, A., Gloeckner-Hofmann, K., Seitzer, U., Csernok, E., Schonermarck, U., Feller, A.C., and Gross, W.L. (2000). Localized Wegener's granulomatosis: predominance of CD26 and IFN-gamma expression. *Journal of Pathology* **192**, 113–20.

Muhle, C., Reinhold-Keller, E., Richter, C., Duncker, G., Beigel, A., Brinkmann, G., Gross, W.L., and Heller, M. (1997). MRI of the nasal cavity, the paranasal sinuses and orbits in Wegener's granulomatosis. *European Radiology* **7** (4), 566–70.

Nachman, P.H., Segelmark, M., Westman, K., Hogan, S.L., Satterly, K.K., Jennette, J.C., and Falk, R. (1999). Recurrent ANCA-associated small vessel vasculitis after transplantation: a pooled analysis. *Kidney International* **56** (4), 1544–50.

Nölle, B., Specks, U., Lüdemann, J., Rohrbach, M.S., DeRemee, R.A., and Gross, W.L. (1989). Anticytoplasmic autoantibodies: their immunodiagnostic value in Wegener's granulomatosis. *Annals of Internal Medicine* **111**, 28–40.

Peen, E., Hahn, P., Lauwers, G., Williams, R.C., Jr., Gleich, G., and Kephart, G.M. (2000). Churg–Strauss syndrome: localization of eosinophil major basic protein in damaged tissues. *Arthritis and Rheumatisom* **43** (8), 1897–900.

Ramakrishna, G., Connolly, H.M., Tazelaar, H.D., Mullany, C.J., and Midthun, D.E. (2000). Churg–Strauss syndrome complicated by eosinophilic endomyocarditis. *Mayo Clinic Proceedings* **75**, 631–5.

Rao, J.K., Weinberger, M., Oddone, E.Z., Allen, N.B., Landsman, P., and Feussner, J.R. (1995). The role of antineutrophil cytoplasmic antibody (c-ANCA) testing in the diagnosis of Wegener granulomatosis. A literature review and meta-analysis. *Annals of Internal Medicine* **123**, 925–32.

Reinhold-Keller, E., Beuge, N., Latza, U., de Groot, K., Rudert, H., Nölle, B., Heller, M., and Gross, W.L. (2000). An interdisciplinary approach to the care of patients with Wegener's granulomatosis: long-term outcome in 155 patients. *Arthritis and Rheumatisom* **43** (5), 1021–32.

Reinhold-Keller, E., de Groot, K., Arlt, A., Holl-Ullrich, K., Feller, A., and Gross, W.L. (2001). Severe CNS manifestations as the clinical hallmark in three patients with generalized Wegener's granulomatosis consistently negative for antineutrophil cytoplasmic antibodies (ANCA). *Clinical and Experimental Rheumatology* **19**, 541–9.

Reinhold-Keller, E., Herlyn, K., Wagner-Bastmeyer, R., Gutfleisch, J., Peter, H., Raspe, H., and Gross, W.L. (2002). Effect of Wegener's granulomatosis (WG) on work disability, need of medical care, and qualitiy of life in patients younger than 40 years at diagnosis of WG. *Arthritis Care and Research* **47**, 320–5.

Reuter, M., Schnabel, A., Wesner, F., Tetzlaff, K., Risheng, Y., Gross, W.L., and Heller, M. (1998). Pulmonary Wegener's granulomatosis: correlation between high-resolution CT findings and clinical scoring of disease activity. *Chest* **114** (2), 500–6.

Savage, C.O., Winearls, C.G., Evans, D.J., Rees, A.J., and Lockwood, C.M. (1985). Microscopic polyarteritis: presentation, pathology and prognosis. *Quarterly Journal of Medicine* **56**, 467–83.

Savige, J., Gillis, D., Benson, E., Davies, D., Esnault, V., Falk, R.J., Hagen, E.C., Jayne, D., Jennette, J.C., Paspaliaris, B., Pollock, W., Pusey, C., Savage, C.O., Silvestrini, R., van der Woude, F., Wieslander, J., and Wiik, A. (1999). International consensus statement on testing and reporting of antineutrophil cytoplasmic antibodies (ANCA). *American Journal of Clinical Pathology* **111** (4), 507–13.

Schmitt, W.H., Haubitz, M., Mistry, N., Brunkhorst, R., Erbsloh-Möller, B., and Gross, W.L. (1993). Renal transplantation in Wegener's granulomatosis. *Lancet* **342** (8875), 860.

Schmitt, W.H., Linder, R., Reinhold-Keller, E., and Gross, W.L. (2001). Improved differentiation between Churg–Strauss syndrome and Wegener's granulomatosis by an artificial neural network. *Arthritis and Rheumatisom* **44** (8), 1887–96.

Schnabel, A., Reuter, M., Gloeckner, K., Müller-Quernheim, J., and Gross, W.L. (1999). Bronchoalveolar lavage cell profiles in Wegener's granulomatosis. *Respiratory Medicine* **93** (7), 498–506.

Schönermarck, U., Lamprecht, P., Csernok, E., and Gross, W.L. (2001). Prevalence and spectrum of rheumatic diseases associated with proteinase 3-antineutrophil cytoplasmic antibodies (ANCA) and myeloperoxidase-ANCA. *Rheumatology* **40**, 178–84.

Sehgal, M., Swanson, J.W., DeRemee, R.A., and Colby, T.V. (1995). Neurologic manifestations of Churg–Strauss syndrome. *Mayo Clinic Proceedings* **70**, 337–41.

Specks, U. (2000). What you should know about PR3-ANCA. Conformational requirements of proteinase 3 (PR3) for enzymatic activity and recognition by PR3-ANCA. *Arthritis Research* **2** (4), 263–7.

Van der Woude, F.J. and Ferrario, F. (1999). Renal involvement in ANCA-associated systemic vasculitis. *Journal of Nephrology* **12** (2), 105–28.

Wainwright, J. and Davson, J. (1950). The renal appearance in the microscopic form of periarteritis nodosa. *Journal of Pathology* **62**, 189–96.

Walton, E.W. (1958). Giant-cell granuloma of the respiratory tract (Wegener's granulomatosis). *British Medical Journal* **2**, 265–9.

Wang, G., Hansen, H., Tatsis, E., Csernok, E., Lemke, H., and Gross, W.L. (1997). High plasma levels of the soluble form of CD30 activation molecule reflect disease activity in patients with Wegener's granulomatosis. *American Journal of Medicine* **102**, 517–23.

Wechsler, M.E., Garpestad, E., Flier, S.R., Kocher, O., Weiland, D.A., Polito, A.J., Klinek, M.M., Bigby, T.D., Wong, G.A., Helmers, R.A., and Drazen, J.M. (1998). Pulmonary infiltrates, eosinophilia, and cardiomyopathy following corticosteroid withdrawal in patients with asthma receiving zafirlukast. *Journal of the American Medical Association* **279**, 455–7.

Wegener, F. (1939). Über eine eigenartige rhinogene Granulomatose mit besonderer Beteiligung des Arteriensystems und der Nieren. *Beiträge zur Pathologie* **102**, 36–68 (in German).

Wegener, F. (1990). Wegener's granulomatosis. Thoughts and observations of a pathologist. *European Archives of Otorhinolaryngology* **247**, 133–42.

Westman, K.W., Bygren, P.G., Olsson, H., Ranstam, J., and Wieslander, J. (1998). Relapse rate, renal survival, and cancer morbidity in patients with Wegener's granulomatosis or microscopic polyangiitis with renal involvement. *Journal of the American Society of Nephrology* **9** (5), 842–52.

Wohlwill, F. (1923). Über die nur mikroskopisch erkennbare Form der Periarteriitis nodosa. *Virchows Archives* **246**, 377–411.

Zeek, P.M., Smith, C.C., and Weeter, J.C. (1948). Studies on periarteritis nodosa III. The differentiation between vascular lesions of periarteritis nodosa and hypersensitivity. *American Journal of Pathology* **24**, 889–917.

6.10.3 Treatment of primary ANCA-associated vasculitis

David Jayne and Niels Rasmussen

Introduction

The primary ANCA-associated vasculitides are potentially fatal if untreated. Immunosuppressive therapy, introduced in the 1960s, saves lives, salvages organ function, and has changed the outcome of vasculitis to that of a chronic disorder with accumulating incapacity. Current treatments are toxic and contribute to morbidity and mortality. Therapy in a particular patient therefore requires a balanced assessment of the dangers posed by the disease and the potential treatments. Such assessments have been limited by differences in disease classification, a paucity of long-term outcome studies, and limited understanding of prognostic factors. Over the last decade, consensus over disease classification and results of controlled, clinical trials have harmonized approaches to therapy. These now provide a basis to assess longer-term outcomes, and evaluate the quality of care and the potential of newer drugs as they become available.

Historical aspects

Prior to the introduction of steroids, the 1-year mortality of vasculitis with vital organ involvement was over 75 per cent. In a retrospective review of 55 cases of Wegener's granulomatosis, Walton (1958) reported a 1-year mortality of 82 per cent, largely due to renal failure. A Medical Research Council trial from 1960 found reduced mortality of polyarteritis with cortisone at 1 year, but after 3 years, steroid associated mortality had eroded any benefit over no intervention (MRC 1960). Leib found a reduction in 5-year mortality to 50 per cent with steroids in polyarteritis nodosa and a further reduction with the use of immunosuppressives to 12 per cent. Although cytotoxic drugs had been used in various forms since the mid-1950s, the reports by Fauci et al. (1983) from the National Institutes of Health confirmed the position of cyclophosphamide in induction regimens for systemic vasculitis with a remission rate of 93 per cent in 85 patients with Wegener's granulomatosis. Retrospective studies from single centres have reported varying survival rates with immunosuppressive therapy from 75 per cent at 12 months to 87 per cent at 8 years with heterogeneity in disease presentations and therapeutic protocols accounting for the difference (Hoffman et al. 1992).

Approaches to treatment

The vasculitides associated with ANCA—Wegener's granulomatosis, microscopic polyangiitis, and renal-limited vasculitis—have strong similarities in their presentation, pathology, and response to treatment. This has led to their being grouped together in recent therapeutic trials (Rasmussen et al. 1995). Within this diagnostic grouping clinical presentations have been subdivided according to disease severity (Table 1) (Rasmussen et al. 1995). These classifications are empirical and await confirmation through the identification of prognostic markers or common aetiological factors. Treatment phases include remission induction by high-dose therapy to arrest active vasculitis and remission maintenance with lower-dose therapy to prevent relapse.

Induction of remission

Localized disease

Treatments for localized vasculitis (Table 1) have included corticosteroids alone and immunomodulators such as dapsone, hydroxychloroquine, and oxpentyfylline. The demonstration of the efficacy of sulfamethoxazole/trimethoprim in reducing remission in Wegener's granulomatosis has suggested its use as sole therapy in this sub-group (Stegeman et al. 1996).

Early systemic disease

This sub-grouping mainly includes 'limited Wegener's granulomatosis', patients with organ involvement confined to the respiratory tract (Table 1). Historical protocols have used the combination of cyclophosphamide and steroids but recent experience with methotrexate has found remission rates of 60–70 per cent (Table 2) (Sneller et al. 1995; de Groot et al. 1998). Relapse rates on continued methotrexate have varied between studies from 12 to 35 per cent; and are influenced by previous cyclophosphamide treatment and concomitant steroid dosing. Progression of mild renal vasculitis (i.e. haematuria without declining renal function) was prevented in one study; other

Table 1 Sub-grouping of patients at presentation according to disease severity (Rasmussen et al. 1995)

Clinical sub-group	Constitutional symptoms	Typical ANCA status	Threatened vital organ function	Serum creatinine (μmol/l)
Localized	No	Positive or negative	No	<120
Early systemic	Yes	Positive or negative	No	<120
Generalized	Yes	Positive	Yes	<500
Severe renal	Yes	Positive	Yes	>500
Refractory	Yes	Positive or negative	Yes	Any

Table 2 Therapeutic trials of methotrexate for Wegener's granulomatosis

Study	Number	Follow-up (months)	Remission rate	Relapse rate
Sneller et al. (1995)	41	?	71%	34%
de Groot et al. (1996)	33	18	Cyclophosphamide induction	12%
de Groot et al. (1998)	17	25	59% Partial 35% full	20%
Stone (1999)	19		89% Partial 79% full	50%
Langford (2000)	42	76	20/21 with renal involvement	10% Renal progression
Rheinhold-Keller (2002)	72	25	Cyclophosphamide induction	36% 16 Renal

studies have found this feature to predict a poor therapeutic response or have noted a high frequency of new renal vasculitis occurring during methotrexate remission maintenance therapy. Intravenous administration of methotrexate may be more efficient than oral administration.

Thus methotrexate (Table 3a) may be an alternative to cyclophosphamide for this sub-group but a proportion will develop progressive disease and require conversion to cyclophosphamide. Moreover, a majority will relapse within 6 months after withdrawal of the consensus treatment (Table 3a), suggesting an extension of remission therapy.

Generalized/renal disease

The empirical introduction of daily oral cyclophosphamide became popular during the 1970s but was only recently subjected to randomized trial (Guillevin et al. 1991). Retrospective data from the North Carolina glomerulonephritis study group compared patients with microscopic polyangiitis treated with cyclophosphamide to those treated with steroids alone and found improved renal survival and a lower relapse rate in those receiving cyclophosphamide (Falk et al. 1990). A consensus statement in 1995 selected the combination of daily oral cyclophosphamide for 1 year and a tapering dose of prednisolone as the 'standard' treatment for this sub-group (Table 3b) (Rasmussen et al. 1995). With this regimen a remission rate of 93 per cent at the expense of a severe adverse effect rate of 26 per cent was obtained (Jayne 2003). The potential superiority of pulsed cyclophosphamide has been assessed in four trials and summarized in a pooled analysis (de Groot et al. 2001). This found good remission rates with pulsed cyclophosphamide but relapse rates were higher than for daily oral administration with a 50 per cent lower cumulative cyclophosphamide exposure

Table 3 Consensus standard and alternative treatment regimens for (Rasmussen et al. 1995; Jayne and Rasmussen 1997)

(a) Treatment regimen for 'early systemic' vasculitis

Induction phase			
0–3 months	Prednisolone 1 mg/kg/day (tapering)	'Standard regimen' cyclophosphamide 2 mg/kg/day	'Alternative regimen' methotrexate 15–25 mg/week
Early remission phase			
3–12 months	0.2 tapering to 0[a]	'Standard regimen' cyclophosphamide 1.5 tapering to 0	'Alternative regimen' methotrexate 25 tapering to 0[a]
Later remission phase			
12–18 months	0[a]		0[a]

(b) Treatment regimen for 'generalized' vasculitis

Induction phase			
0–3 months	Prednisolone 1 mg/kg/day (tapering)	Cyclophosphamide 2 mg/kg/day	
Early remission phase			
3–12 months	0.2	'Standard regimen' cyclophosphamide 1.5	'Alternative regimen' azathioprine 2
Later remission phase			
12–18 months	0.075 (tapering)	Azathioprine 1.5	

(c) Long-term remission therapy for renal vasculitis

	'Standard regimen'		'Alternative regimen'	
18–24 months	Prednisolone 5 mg/day tapering to 0	Azathioprine 1 mg/kg/day tapering to 0	Prednisolone 5 mg/day	Azathioprine 1 mg/kg/day
25–40 months	0	0	Prednisolone 5 mg/day	Azathioprine 1 mg/kg/day
40–48 months	0	0	Prednisolone 5 mg/day tapering to 0	Azathioprine 1 mg/kg/day tapering to 0

(d) Regimen for 'pulsed' cyclophosphamide in systemic vasculitis

Time (weeks)	Pulse no.	Route	Dosage (mg/kg)
0	1	Intravenous (i.v)	15
2	2	i.v.	15
4	3	i.v.	15
7	4	i.v. or oral	15
10	5	i.v. or oral	15
13	6	i.v. or oral	15
16	7	i.v. or oral	15
19	8	i.v. or oral	15
22	9	i.v. or oral	15
25	10	i.v. or oral	15

(e) Pulsed cyclophosphamide dose (mg/kg/pulse) reductions for renal function and age

Age (years)	Creatinine (μmol/l)	
	150–300	300–500
<60	15	12.5
>60 and <70	12.5	10
>70	10	7.5

[a] See text.

and less frequent severe toxicity. The choice between pulsed and daily oral cyclophosphamide remains controversial and will be influenced by concurrent steroid doses, patient age, disease severity, and the proposed duration of cyclophosphamide as well as local experience.

Severe renal disease

Many patients with systemic vasculitis present in renal failure and require dialysis. Early intervention to reverse renal inflammation is likely to minimize damage. This theory is supported by the observation that the recovery level of serum creatinine, reflecting surviving nephrons, is related to long-term renal survival (Hogan et al. 1996). More intensive therapy with high- dose intravenous steroids or plasma exchange has been used to 'rescue' renal function. Studies using plasma exchange have pointed to increasing the chances of regaining dialysis independence (Table 4) (Pusey et al. 1991). A consensus statement has suggested that either pulsed methylprednisolone (3 g over 3 days) or plasma exchange (seven, 4-l exchanges within 14 days) are reasonable additions to the protocols for generalized vasculitis (Rasmussen et al. 1995). A rationale for plasma exchange in vasculitis was based on its success in antiglomerular basement membrane disease and a presumed immune complex aetiology even though immune deposits in most primary systemic vasculitides are typically scanty or absent (Lockwood et al. 1977). The discovery of ANCA and its potential pathogenetic role has provided a new rationale for their physical removal in these disorders. A small randomized study of Wegener's granulomatosis of varying severity reported improved outcomes beyond the kidney with plasma exchange (Szpirt et al. 1996). Other mechanisms for the effect of plasma exchange include the removal of cytokines and coagulation factors and alternative indications have included diffuse pulmonary haemorrhage and refractory vasculitis (Jayne 1998).

Remission maintenance

Over 50 per cent of patients will have a relapse of vasculitis and this possibility has a major influence on their long-term care. Relapse is more common in Wegener's granulomatosis than microscopic polyangiitis and with PR3-ANCA as opposed to MPO-ANCA (Boomsma et al. 2000). In view of the toxicity of long-term cyclophosphamide, early substitution after 3–6 months, with either methotrexate or azathioprine is attractive (de Groot et al. 1996). The role of azathioprine for this indication in generalized vasculitis has been confirmed by a randomized comparison with continued cyclophosphamide (Jayne 2003). Relapse rates of 16 per cent were similar between both limbs upto the 18-month duration of the trial (Table 3b). The optimal duration of maintenance therapy is undetermined and the dangers of cumulative drug toxicity need to be balanced against the potential consequences of relapse. Prolonged therapy for 2–4 years has been proposed in cases with moderate renal impairment where renal relapse may lead to end-stage renal failure (Table 3c). The development of relapse despite these therapies, or drug intolerance which occurs in almost 10 per cent, has prompted the current evaluation of alternative immunosuppressives, including leflunomide, mycophenolate mofetil, and cyclosporin (Nowack et al. 1999).

Table 4 Renal survival in prospective trials including patients presenting with renal failure due to renal vasculitis. Treatment with or without plasma exchange

	No.	Plasma exchange	No plasma exchange
Glockner (1988)	12	5/8	3/4
Pusey et al. (1991)	19	10/11	3/8
Cole (1992)	11	3/4	2/7
Levy (1994)	20	9/11	5/9
Guillevin (1995)	8	4/6	1/2
Haubitz (1998)	22	6/12	2/10
Total	92	37/52 (67%)[a]	16/40 (40%)

[a] $p = 0.01$.

Relapse

The severity of relapse has been classified as major or minor according to whether vital organ function is threatened. Recent studies have treated minor relapse with an increase in prednisolone to 0.5 mg/kg/day and continued azathioprine or methotrexate. Major relapse has been treated by a return to cyclophosphamide and high dose steroids as for induction regimens. In a trial of generalized vasculitis, 10 of the 21 relapses were classified as major (Jayne 2003).

Infection and relapse

Due to the association of infection and death, systemic antibiotic treatment plays an important role in the management of these diseases. A majority of deaths in the initial phase of disease is due to infectious complications (Neild 1990). The causative organisms include bacteria, fungi, and viruses. An aggressive approach to microbiological diagnosis and relevant antibiotic treatment in the initial phase is therefore mandatory. Vasculitis may occur as a consequence of infection, such as endocarditis, and intercurrent infection can provoke relapse of primary vasculitis. Infection is predisposed by immunosuppressive treatment and by structural damage to epithelial surfaces caused by previous vasculitis, where it may mimic relapse. Colonization of the upper respiratory tract by *Staphylococcus aureus* in Wegener's granulomatosis increases the risk of disease relapse, and this observation has drawn attention to the possibility of an infectious aetiology for this vasculitis (Stegeman et al. 1994). Long-term antibiotic therapy with sulfamethoxazole/trimethoprim in Wegener's granulomatosis reduces the risk of respiratory tract relapse in a placebo-controlled study when added to conventional immunosuppression (Stegeman et al. 1996). Sulfamethoxazole/trimethoprim was less effective in controlling disease activity in Wegener's granulomatosis when used in place of immunosuppression at various stages of disease in a prospective study of 72 patients (Reinhold-Keller et al. 1990). An alternative approach to the control of bacterial nasal carriage has used the cyclical application of the topical antibiotic mupirocin.

ANCA and relapse

An association between ANCA titre and relapse exists but the strength of this association and the role changes in ANCA should play in dictating treatment remain controversial (Boomsma et al. 2000). An early study in Wegener's granulomatosis randomized patients in remission to treatment intensification or no change in therapy on the basis of a rise in ANCA titre (Cohen Tervaert et al. 1990). Subsequent relapse was frequent in the latter group and was not seen in the group treated on the basis of the ANCA titre; the cumulative exposure to immunosuppression was lower in the treatment intensification group. Other studies have consistently reported a high frequency of ANCA positivity at the time of relapse, and an increased relapse risk in those with persistent ANCA positivity during remission or in those whose ANCA becomes positive during remission. While further interventional studies based on ANCA specificity and persistence are anticipated, a common response to the increased risk of relapse is to reduce the period between clinic reviews in order to diagnose relapse as early as possible. With newer ANCA assays the positive predictive value of a rise in ANCA for subsequent relapse is approximately 75 per cent. Both the erythrocyte sedimentation rate (ESR) and C-reactive protein (CRP) are of value in sequential monitoring but lack prognostic value for vasculitis relapse.

Persistent/grumbling disease

Several strategies have been used in this setting without comparison in randomized trials. They can be grouped as further immunosuppression, lymphocyte depletion, and immunomodulation. Pulsed cyclophosphamide does not appear to offer an advantage over daily administration for this subset, indeed patients failing pulsed treatment have been salvaged by changing to daily oral dosing. Mycophenolate mofetil has been successful in vasculitis resistant to cyclophosphamide. Lymphocyte depletion using antithymocyte globulin or monoclonal anti-CD 52 (CAMPATH-1H), has led to remission in small open studies, some of these remissions have been long lasting (Lockwood et al. 1993; Hagen et al. 1995). While the role of this approach awaits larger studies these results have indicated the importance of the T-cell to the pathogenesis of vasculitis and they are the first drugs since cyclophosphamide to induce sustained remission of aggressive disease. Pooled, intravenous immunoglobulin (IVIg) is of proven benefit in the childhood vasculitis, Kawasaki disease. It has several modes of action of potential importance in vasculitis: it contains antibodies which inhibit ANCA, has regulatory effects at both B- and T-cell levels and interacts with inflammatory factors such as complement and cytokines. A placebo-controlled trial of relapsing or persistent ANCA-associated vasculitis found improved disease control in IVIg treated patients (Jayne et al. 2000). This effect was only observed upto 3 months suggesting that repeated dosing, possibly at 3-month intervals, would be necessary for a sustained effect.

Newer approaches to treatment

Several immunosuppressive agents have been reported to be beneficial in anecdotal case reports including etoposide in Wegener's and interferon-α for Churg–Strauss angiitis. Immunomodulatory agents, such as, thalidomide, oxpentyffiline, and colchicine have also been used. The pyrimidine antagonist, leflunomide, the TNF antagonists, infliximab and etanercept, and the antiproliferative drugs, deoxyspergualin and anisperimus are the focus of ongoing studies in vasculitis (Stone et al. 2001). Anti-TNF therapy offers the opportunity for a rapid onset and may be an alternative to high-dose steroids in the acute situation.

Developments of plasma exchange including semi-specific immunoabsorption with L-tryptophan or protein-A columns remove ANCA without depletion of non-immunoglobulin plasma proteins and appear of comparable efficacy to plasma exchange. The production of recombinant ANCA autoantigens will permit the development of ANCA specific extra-corporeal immunoabsorption, which has the theoretical advantage of removing pathogenetic factors without depletion of regulatory antibodies or unrelated immunoglobulins (Griffin et al. 1997). Immunoablation using high-dose cytotoxic medication followed by stem cell rescue has led to prolonged remission in refractory vasculitis. Bone marrow allografting has also corrected vasculitis in a genetically prone mouse. The further development of this technology in vasculitis depends on the safety of the procedure and identification of suitable patients before organ damage has taken place.

Adverse effects

The toxicity of treatment contributes to the chronic morbidity and mortality of vasculitis. The National Institutes of Health experience with Wegener's granulomatosis reported a contribution of treatment toxicity to permanent damage in over 50 per cent of their patients (Hoffman et al. 1992). A recent trial of generalized vasculitis reported an adverse-effect frequency of 1.3 episodes per patient with 26 per cent having severe or life-threatening adverse effects within the first 18 months.

Infections

Infectious adverse effects are the most common cause of death or severe morbidity and their frequency is associated with leucopaenia, age, and concomitant steroid dosage. *Pneumocystis carinii* pneumonia rates of upto 20 per cent have been found which have prompted advice for routine prophylaxis with low dose sulfamethoxazole/trimethoprim in centres where this infection is common (Guillevin et al. 1997). Adverse effects, in particular leucopaenia, are reduced with methotrexate as compared to cyclophosphamide.

Organ toxicity and cancer

Urothelial toxicity of cyclophosphamide metabolites is known to cause cystitis and bladder cancer. In a historical cohort, 73/145 developed non-glomerular haematuria and seven (5 per cent) bladder cancer (Talar-Williams et al. 1996). These patients were collected over a time period when prolonged daily oral cyclophosphamide was standard therapy. The frequency of haematuria was related to the duration or total dose of cyclophosphamide with a 50 per cent rate after 40 months or 120 g. None of the 72 patients without haematuria developed bladder cancer. Of particular concern is the rise in bladder cancer risk with longer follow-up, which was estimated in this study to be 5 per cent at 10 years and 16 per cent at 15 years. Haemorrhagic cystitis is rare in pulse cyclophosphamide-treated patients, being reported in only one case from the reviewed studies (de Groot et al. 2001). A Swedish study found an 11-fold increase in bladder cancer rates in patients receiving oral cyclophosphamide for more than 1 year, and an increase in dermatological malignancy related to azathioprine and steroid exposure Rare cases of pneumonitis, hepatotoxicity, and myelosuppression are seen with methotrexate, but have been reversible.

Gonadal failure

Gonadal failure is associated with the total cyclophosphamide dose and is manifested by amenorrhoea, premature menopause, or higher FSH levels in treated males. Sperm bank deposits have been recommended before cyclophosphamide treatment. Data from the use of cyclophosphamide in 39 women with lupus nephritis has shown that the risk of infertility is related to age and duration of treatment with an incidence of 12 per cent in those under 25 years and 60 per cent in those over 30. LH-RH antagonists protect rats from cyclophosphamide-induced infertility and are under investigation human studies.

Bone demineralization

Steroid-induced bone disease is common due to the high cumulative exposure and the age of the patient population. Consensus documents have recommended monitoring bone density, bisphosphonates are becoming routinely used in older patients. Cyclical etidronate protects against steroid-induced bone loss in giant cell arteritis, newer alternatives such as risendronate or alendronate may be more effective. It is suspected, but unproven that cardiovascular disease is more prevalent in small vessel vasculitides: there are abnormalities of vascular function in large arteries even during disease remission. Such large-vessel disease is likely to be further exacerbated by steroids, due to effects on blood pressure, glucose and lipid metabolism.

References

Boomsma, M.M. et al. (2000). Prediction of relapses in Wegener's granulomatosis by measurement of antineutrophil cytoplasmic antibody levels: a prospective study. *Arthritis and Rheumatism* **43**, 2025–33.

Cohen Tervaert, J.W. et al. (1990). Prevention of relapses in Wegener's granulomatosis by treatment based on antineutrophil cytoplasmic antibody titre. *Lancet* **336**, 709–11.

Cole, E. et al. (1992). A prospective randomized trial of plasma exchange as additive therapy in idiopathic crescentic glomerulonephritis. The Canadian Apheresis Study Group. *American Journal of Kidney Diseases* **20**, 261–9.

de Groot, K. et al. (1996). Therapy for the maintenance of remission in sixty-five patients with generalized Wegener's granulomatosis. Methotrexate versus trimethoprim/sulfamethoxazole. *Arthritis and Rheumatism* **39**, 2052–61.

de Groot, K., Muhler, M., Reinhold-Keller, E., Paulsen, J., and Gross, W.L. (1998). Induction of remission in Wegener's granulomatosis with low dose methotrexate. *Journal of Rheumatology* **25**, 492–5.

de Groot, K., Adu, D., and Savage, C. (2001). The value of pulse cyclophosphamide in ANCA-associated vasculitis: meta-analysis and critical review. *Nephrology Dialysis Transplantation* **16**, 2018–27.

Falk, R.J., Hogan, S., Carey, T.S., and Jennette, J.C. (1990). Clinical course of anti-neutrophil cytoplasmic autoantibody-associated glomerulonephritis and systemic vasculitis. The Glomerular Disease Collaborative Network. *Annals of Internal Medicine* **113**, 656–63.

Fauci, A.S., Haynes, B.F., Katz, P., and Wolff, S.M. (1983). Wegener's granulomatosis: prospective clinical and therapeutic experience with 85 patients for 21 years. *Annals of Internal Medicine* **98**, 76–85.

Glockner, W.M. et al. (1988). Plasma exchange and immunosuppression in rapidly progressive glomerulonephritis: a controlled, multi-center study. *Clinical Nephrology* **29**, 1–8.

Griffin, S.C.P., Elliott, J., Brownlee, A., Short, A., Barclay, A., Moguilevsky, N., Bollen, A., and Lockwood, C.M. (1997). Recombinant human autoantigens as an extracorporeal immunoadsorbent in therapeutic apheresis. *Japanese Journal of Apheresis* **16**, 17–22.

Guillevin, L. et al. (1991). Long-term followup after treatment of polyarteritis nodosa and Churg–Strauss angiitis with comparison of steroids, plasma exchange and cyclophosphamide to steroids and plasma exchange. A prospective randomized trial of 71 patients. The Cooperative Study Group for Polyarteritis Nodosa. *Journal of Rheumatology* **18**, 567–74.

Guillevin, L. et al. (1995). Corticosteroids plus pulse cyclophosphamide and plasma exchanges versus corticosteroids plus pulse cyclophosphamide alone in the treatment of polyarteritis nodosa and Churg–Strauss syndrome patients with factors predicting poor prognosis. A prospective, randomized trial in sixty-two patients. *Arthritis and Rheumatism* **38**, 1638–45.

Guillevin, L. et al. (1997). A prospective, multicenter, randomized trial comparing steroids and pulse cyclophosphamide versus steroids and oral cyclophosphamide in the treatment of generalized Wegener's granulomatosis. *Arthritis and Rheumatism* **40**, 2187–98.

Hagen, E.C. et al. (1995). Compassionate treatment of Wegener's granulomatosis with rabbit anti-thymocyte globulin. *Clinical Nephrology* **43**, 351–9.

Haubitz, M. et al. (1998). Intravenous pulse administration of cyclophosphamide versus daily oral treatment in patients with antineutrophil cytoplasmic antibody-associated vasculitis and renal involvement: a prospective, randomized study. *Arthritis and Rheumatism* **41**, 1835–44.

Hoffman, G.S. et al. (1992). Wegener granulomatosis: an analysis of 158 patients. *Annals of Internal Medicine* **116**, 488–98.

Hogan, S.L., Nachman, P.H., Wilkman, A.S., Jennette, J.C., and Falk, R.J. (1996). Prognostic markers in patients with antineutrophil cytoplasmic autoantibody-associated microscopic polyangiitis and glomerulonephritis. *Journal of the American Society of Nephrology* **7**, 23–32.

Jayne, D. (1998). Pulmonary–renal syndrome. *Seminars in Respiratory and Critical Care Medicine* **19**, 69–77.

Jayne, D.R. and Rasmussen, N. (1997). Treatment of antineutrophil cytoplasm autoantibody-associated systemic vasculitis: initiatives of the European Community Systemic Vasculitis Clinical Trials Study Group. *Mayo Clinic Proceedings* **72**, 737–47.

Jayne, D.R. et al. (2000). Intravenous immunoglobulin for ANCA-associated systemic vasculitis with persistent disease activity. *Quarterly Journal of Medicine* **93**, 433–9.

Jayne, D., Rasmussen, N., Andrassy, K., Bacon, P., Cohen Tervaert, J.W., Dadoniene, J., Ekstrand, A., Gaskin, G., Gregorini, G., de Groot, K., Gross, W., Hagen, E.C., Mirapeix, E., Pettersson, E., Siegert, C., Sinico, A., Tesar, V., Westman, K., and Pusey, C. (2003). A randomized trial of maintenance therapy for vasculitis associated with antineutrophil cytoplasmic autoantibodies. *New England Journal of Medicine* **394**, 36–44.

Langford, C.A., Talar-Williams, C., and Sneller, M.C. (2000).Use of methotrexate and glucocorticoids in the treatment of Wegener's granulomatosis. Long-term renal outcome in patients with glomerulonephritis. *Arthritis and Rheumatism* **43**, 1836–40.

Lockwood, C.M., Thiru, S., Isaacs, J.D., Hale, G., and Waldmann, H. (1993). Long-term remission of intractable systemic vasculitis with monoclonal antibody therapy. *Lancet* **341**, 1620–2.

Lockwood, C.M. et al. (1977). Plasma-exchange and immunosuppression in the treatment of fulminating immune-complex crescentic nephritis. *Lancet* **1**, 63–7.

Neild, G. (1990). Infectious complications in the management of systemic vasculitis and rapidly progressive glomerulonephritis. *APMIS* **18** (Suppl. 19), 56–60.

Nowack, R., Gobel, U., Klooker, P., Hergesell, O., Andrassy, K., and van der Woude, F.J. (1999). Mycophenolate mofetil for maintenance therapy of Wegener's granulomatosis and microscopic polyangiitis: a pilot study in 11 patients with renal involvement. *Journal of the American Society of Nephrology* **10**, 1965–71.

Pusey, C.D., Rees, A.J., Evans, D.J., Peters, D.K., and Lockwood, C.M. (1991). Plasma exchange in focal necrotizing glomerulonephritis without anti-GBM antibodies. *Kidney International* **40**, 757–63.

Rasmussen, N.J.D., Abramowicz, D., Andrassy, K., Bacon, P.A., Cohen Tervaert, J.W., Dadonienė, J., Feighery, C., van Es, L.A., Ferrario, F.G.G., Gregorini, G., de Groot, K., Gross, W.L., Grönhagen-Riska, C., Guillevin, L., He, C., Heigl, Z.J.H., Kallenberg, C.G.M., Landais, P., Lesavre, P., Lockwood, C.M., and Luqmani, R. (1995). European therapeutic trials in ANCA-associated systemic vasculitis: disease scoring, consensus regimens and proposed clinical trials. *Clinical and Experimental Immunology* **101** (Suppl. 1), 29–34.

Reinhold-Keller, E., De Groot, K., Rudert, H., Nolle, B., Heller, M., and Gross, W.L. (1996). Response to trimethoprim/sulfamethoxazole in Wegener's granulomatosis depends on the phase of disease. *Quarterly Journal of Medicine* **89**, 15–23.

Reinhold-Keller, E. et al. (2002). High rate of renal relapse in 71 patients with Wegener's granulomatosis under maintenance of remission with low-dose methotrexate. *Arthritis and Rheumatism* **47**, 326–32.

Report to the Medical Research Council by the Collagen Diseases and Hypersensitivity Panel (1960). Treatment of polyarteritis nodosa with cortisone: results after three years. *British Medical Journal* **1399**, 1400.

Sneller, M.C., Hoffman, G.S., Talar-Williams, C., Kerr, G.S., Hallahan, C.W., and Fauci, A.S. (1995). An analysis of forty-two Wegener's granulomatosis patients treated with methotrexate and prednisone. *Arthritis and Rheumatism* **38**, 608–13.

Stegeman, C.A., Cohen Tervaert, J.W., de Jong, P.E., and Kallenberg, C.G. (1996). Trimethoprim–sulfamethoxazole (co-trimoxazole) for the prevention of relapses of Wegener's granulomatosis. Dutch Co-Trimoxazole Wegener Study Group. *New England Journal of Medicine* **335**, 16–20.

Stegeman, C.A., Tervaert, J.W., Sluiter, W.J., Manson, W.L., de Jong, P.E., and Kallenberg, C.G. (1994). Association of chronic nasal carriage of Staphylococcus aureus and higher relapse rates in Wegener granulomatosis. *Annals of Internal Medicine* **120**, 12–17.

Stone, J.H., Tun, W., and Hellman, D.B. (1999). Treatment of non-life threatening Wegener's granulomatosis with methotrexate and daily prednisone as the initial therapy of choice. *Journal of Rheumatology* **26**, 1134–9.

Stone, J.H., Uhlfelder, M.L., Hellmann, D.B., Crook, S., Bedocs, N.M., and Hoffman, G.S. (2001). Etanercept combined with conventional treatment in Wegener's granulomatosis: a six-month open-label trial to evaluate safety. *Arthritis and Rheumatism* **44**, 1149–54.

Szpirt, W.M., Rasmussen, N., and Petersen, J. (1996). Plasma exchange and cyclosporin A in Wegener's granulomatosis: a controlled study. *International Journal of Artificial Organs* **10**, 501.

Talar-Williams, C. et al. (1996). Cyclophosphamide-induced cystitis and bladder cancer in patients with Wegener granulomatosis. *Annals of Internal Medicine* **124**, 477–84.

Walton, E. (1958). Giant cell granuloma of the respiratory tract (Wegener's granulomatosis). *British Medical Journal* **2**, 265–70.

6.10.4 Secondary vasculitis and vasculitis mimics

Richard A. Watts and David G.I. Scott

Introduction

Vasculitis may be either a primary event [e.g. Wegener's granulomatosis (WG)] or secondary to established rheumatic disease, malignancy, or to other exogenous stimuli such as drugs and infection. There are also a number of conditions that can mimic vasculitis.

Infection and vasculitis

The idea that infection could trigger vasculitis was first suggested over 100 years ago. A wide variety of organisms have been implicated (Table 1). Possible mechanisms for infection related vasculitis include: (i) direct microbial toxicity either by endothelial invasion (e.g. rickettsia, bartonella, or cytomegalovirus) or the effect of microbial toxins on endothelium; (ii) immune mediated by either humoral (immune complex, e.g. hepatitis C and cryoglobulinaemia) or cellular responses (Somer and Finegold 1995). Infection may also be a consequence of intensive immunosuppression for primary vasculitis.

Bacterial infections

Direct endothelial invasion by pyogenic organisms (e.g. staphylococcus and streptococcus) is a well-recognized cause of vasculitis. The spectrum of bacteria associated with vasculitis has changed over the past two decades with more unusual infections being reported, for example, *Mycobacterium fortuitum*, enterobacteriaceae, and Salmonella. There is a predisposing condition in around 60 per cent of cases of which the most common is diabetes mellitus (Oskoui et al. 1993). Infection often occurs at a site of previous damage by atherosclerosis or surgery.

The vascular response to direct infection depends on the organism and site of infection. In large arteries, infection leads to an erosive arteritis with mycotic aneurysm formation. Aortitis is an uncommon manifestation of *Streptococcus pneumoniae* infection (Fig. 1). Salmonella aortitis is well recognized and usually presents with fever together with abdominal and back pain. The most frequent site involved is the abdominal aorta followed by the thoracic aorta. Predisposing conditions include hypertension, diabetes mellitus, and myelodysplastic syndrome (Soravia-Dunand et al. 1999). Treatment is with intravenous antibiotics combined with surgery.

Table 1 Infection and vasculitis

Vessel involved	Infection	
Large arteries	Bacterial	*Staphylococcus, Salmonella, Mycobacteria, Streptococcus*
	Spirochaetal	*Treponema pallidum*
	Fungal	*Coccidiomycosis*
Medium arteries	Bacterial	Group A *Streptococcus, Mycobacteria*
	Viral	HBV, HCV, HIV, parvovirus B19
Small vessels and medium arteries	Bacterial	*Streptococcus*
	Viral	HBV, HCV, HIV, CMV
Small vessel (leucocytoclastic)	Bacterial	*Staphylococcus, Salmonella, Mycobacteria, Streptococcus, Yersinia, Neisseria*
	Viral	HIV, CMV, herpes zoster, parvovirus B19, HBV, HCV
	Rickettsiae	

Source: Adapted from Somer and Finegold (1995) (with permission).

Direct bacterial infection of small arteries and arterioles infection causes a necrotizing vasculitis or thrombosis. *Neisseria gonorrhoeae, N. meningitides,* and *Streptobacillus moniliformis,* for example, may directly infect vascular endothelium causing maculopapular or purpuric skin lesions. Biopsies of early lesions show a small vessel vasculitis with mononuclear cells, neutrophils, leucocytoclasis, and necrosis. The organisms can be cultured from an aspirate of the lesions.

Mycobacterial infections

Vessels of any size can be involved in tuberculous infection, with veins more often affected than arteries (Somer and Finegold 1995). The typical clinical lesion is erythema nodosum. Tuberculous vasculitis of large and small vessels is a granulomatous panarteritis or thrombophlebitis. Acid-fast bacilli may be found in or adjacent to the vessel wall.

The vascular lesions of *M. leprae* infection are focal in distribution and involve arteries and veins with equal frequency. The most common site is small vessels, for example, erythema nodosum leprosum or the vasa vasorum of large vessels. The clinical consequences of vasculitis are rarely significant.

Viral infections

Viral infection may followed by several different outcomes: (i) viral clearance, (ii) latency with periodic reactivation, for example, herpes zoster, or (iii) persistent viral replication with stable or progressive course, for example, hepatitis B and C.

Hepatitis B virus (HBV) infection has been firmly associated with polyarteritis nodosa (PAN) for 30 years. In areas endemic for hepatitis B infection upto 95 per cent of cases are associated with HBV infection (McMahon et al. 1989). In France, falling HBV infection rates have been correlated with a decrease in HBV-associated PAN (Guillevin 1999). Only 2/13 patients with PAN in Spain (seen 1988–1997) were positive for HBV (González-Gay and Garcia-Porrua 1999). In our population (Norwich, United Kingdom), HBV infection is rare and we have not seen a case of HBV-associated PAN since 1988. The clinical characteristics of HBV-associated PAN are similar to those observed in non-HBV-associated classic PAN apart from more frequent gastrointestinal involvement, extraglomerular renovascular disease with malignant hypertension, and orchitis in HBV-associated PAN. HBV-associated PAN should be identified, because therapy is antiviral therapy in addition to

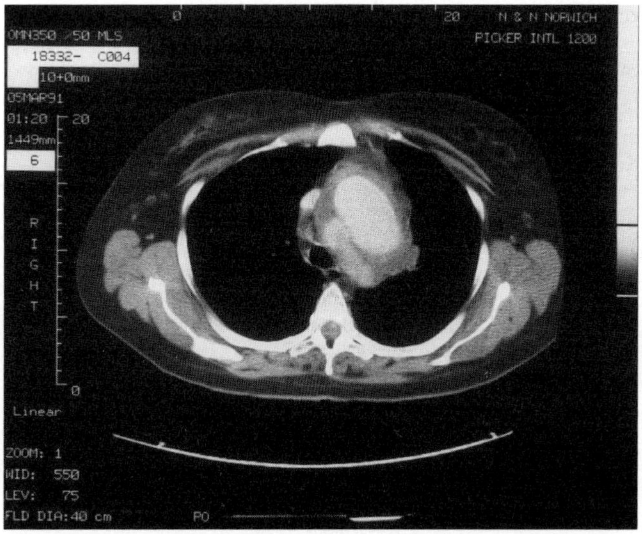

Fig. 1 Thoracic CT scan showing an aneurysm of the descending aorta. *Pneumococcus pneumoniae* was cultured from the resected vessel [from Chakravarty et al. (1992), with permission].

conventional immunosuppressive therapy, possibly in combination with plasma exchange (Guillevin 1999).

Hepatitis C virus (HCV) was first identified in 1989. There is a strong association between HCV infection and essential mixed cryoglobulinaemia, with 80–90 per cent of such patients positive for anti-HCV antibodies. Circulating HCV RNA has been identified in the peripheral blood of patients with cryoglobulinaemia. HCV has been identified within cutaneous vasculitic lesions and has been selectively concentrated together with specific antibody in cryoprecipitates.

The most common clinical features of both HCV associated and non-HCV associated cryoglobulinaemic vasculitis are given in Table 2. The majority of patients have hypocomplementaemia (90 per cent) and circulating rheumatoid factor (70 per cent). They are ANCA negative. Hypocomplementaemia is a useful distinguishing feature from ANCA-associated systemic vasculitis. HCV infection has also been associated with a PAN-type vasculitis with involvement of medium-sized arteries and a necrotizing vasculitis (Cacoub 2001).

Antiviral therapy with interferon-alpha is effective in patients with HCV associated cryoglobulinaemia (Lamprecht et al. 1999). Sustained elimination of HCV RNA is required for long-term suppression of vasculitis, and maintenance antiviral therapy is therefore required. Severe or life threatening disease should be treated with steroids, cyclophosphamide with or without plasma exchange (Lamprecht et al. 1999).

Human immunodeficiency virus (HIV) infection has been associated with a wide variety of autoimmune and inflammatory vascular conditions. Vasculitis may either be directly related to HIV infection or be a consequence of secondary opportunistic infection particularly with cytomegalovirus or tuberculosis (Chetty 2001). A number of patterns of vasculitis have been described including PAN-like, hypersensitivity vasculitis, large-vessel disease (Chetty 2001). Vasculitis usually occurs in late HIV infection and treatment is difficult; combinations of antiviral therapy and apheresis have been proposed.

Parvovirus B19, cytomegalovirus, and herpes zoster are the major other viruses that have been implicated in the pathogenesis of vasculitis (Somer and Finegold 1995). They have been associated with most types of vasculitis usually in isolated case reports or small series. Parvovirus has been associated with PAN and HSP. Herpes zoster has been associated with granulomatous cerebral vasculitis. Epidemiological studies of parvovirus B19 in PAN and WG have not supported a causal association (Nikkari et al. 1994).

Table 2 Clinical symptoms in HCV and non-HCV-associated cryoglobulinaemic vasculitis

Common symptoms in CV (>70%)	Purpura (less often: urticaria, livedo, exanthem, acral necrosis, leg ulcers) Arthralgias, arthritis Weakness
Frequent symptoms in CV (40–70%)	Polyneuropathy (subacute, distal, symmetrical or asymmetrical, motor and/or sensory polyneuropathy, acute mononeuritis multiplex; note electrophysiological variables may be altered in upto 80% of patients) Sub-clinical lymphocytic alveolitis (usually T-lymphocytic alveolitis)
Less common symptoms in CV (<40%)	Meltzer's triad (purpura, arthralgia, weakness) Renal involvement (nephrotic syndrome or nephritic urinary sediment due to mesangial proliferative GN, membranoproliferative GN, membranous GN, endocapillary GN, rapidly progressive GN) Secondary Sjögren's syndrome Secondary Raynaud's phenomenon CNS involvement (cerebrovascular accident, cerebral vasculitis, diffuse encephalopathy, cranial neuropathy, hearing loss) Gastrointestinal involvement (abdominal pain, haemtochezia, diarrhoea, haemetemesis, and intestinal infarction) Cardiac involvement (coronary arteritis, myocarditis) Pulmonary–renal syndrome Retinal involvement Temporal arteritis Polyarteritis nodosa Myalgia/myositis

Note: CV, cryoglobulinaemic vasculitis; GN, glomerulonephritis.

Source: Adapted from Lamprecht et al. (1999) (with permission).

Spirochaetal infection

Treponema pallidum is well recognized as a cause of aortitis, with aneurysm formation and development of aortic incompetence. The primary histological changes are in the vasa vasorum with endarteritis and perivascular infiltration with lymphocytes and plasma cells. Infection occurs early in disease and organisms lie dormant in the aortic wall. Spirochaetes can, however, only rarely be detected in tissue. Symptomatic aortic disease occurs as a feature of tertiary syphilis. Diagnosis is based on the radiographic appearances and serological tests. *Borrelia burgdorferi* infection (Lyme disease) may cause a mild vasculitis as part of disseminated infection but major vasculitis is rare.

Rickettsial infection

Vascular lesions are a prominent feature of some rickettsial infections, particularly Rocky Mountain spotted fever, epidemic typhus, and scrub typhus. In humans the organism are usually found in vascular endothelium and in some cases vascular smooth muscle. The pathology of the vascular lesion in *Rickettsia rickettsii* (Rocky Mountain spotted fever) follows a characteristic pattern. In the early stages, endothelial cell swelling is seen in association with intracellular rickettsiae. Later vasculitis with increased vascular permeability, haemorrhage, and occasionally thrombosis occurs with immunoglobulin and complement deposition.

Fungal infections

Fungal infections may cause vasculitis by direct spread into the vessel wall with formation of a mycotic aneurysm. This usually occurs in patients who are already severely immunocompromised from other diseases. Fungi such as *Coccidiodes immitis* may also cause a local CNS vasculitis, presenting acutely with stroke-like lesions, these patients have a high mortality and require aggressive antifungal therapy (Williams et al. 1992).

Vasculitis and malignancy

Vasculitis has been associated with haematological and more rarely solid malignancies (Plate 149). The recognition of this association is important, as vasculitis may be the first sign of malignancy. Vasculitis associated with lymphoproliferative disorders may be confined to the skin or more rarely be systemic. In a series of 172 adults with cutaneous vasculitis, only four (2.3 per cent) were associated with malignancy. All four malignancies were haematological (Blanco et al. 1998). Experience suggests that malignancy is slightly more common, seven malignancies (including three solid tumours) were observed in a prospective cohort of 84 patients seen between 1990 and 1994 (Watts et al. 1998). Possible mechanisms include immune complex formation, tumour antigens acting as a sensitizing antigen, malignant cell products stimulating vascular inflammation, and direct invasion.

Hamidou and colleagues analysed the frequency of ANCA and vasculitis in a prospective cohort study of 60 patients with myelodysplastic syndromes and 140 patients with lymphoid malignancies (Hamidou et al. 2000). The overall frequency of ANCA was similar to that found in the general French population. Sixty patients had myelodysplasia, of which, six had ANCA-negative systemic vasculitis, one ANCA-positive systemic vasculitis, one giant cell arteritis, and one relapsing polychondritis. Of the 140 patients with lymphoid malignancies, two patients had ANCA-negative systemic vasculitis, two had leucocytoclastic vasculitis in association with tuberculous infection, and one giant cell arteritis. There was no association with HBV or HCV infection.

Hairy cell leukaemia is a rare lymphoproliferative disease characterized by the presence of mononuclear cells with hair-like cytoplasmic projections in peripheral blood, bone marrow, spleen, and liver. Hairy cell leukaemia has been strongly associated with systemic necrotizing vasculitis, especially PAN and cutaneous leucocytoclastic vasculitis (Hasler et al. 1995). Direct infiltration of vessel walls by hairy cells has been seen in some cases. In the majority of cases, the leukaemia is diagnosed first and the interval between the two diagnoses may be several years. The vasculitis is not usually the cause of death, which is due to complications of leukaemia and its therapy.

Malignancies have also been associated with other specific types of vasculitis including adult onset Henoch–Schönlein purpura (HSP) (Pertuiset et al. 2000). Compared with HSP patients without malignancy those with malignancy were more likely to be older, male, have more joint involvement, and fewer preceding infections.

Tatsis and colleagues compared the frequency of malignancies in 477 WG patients with 479 rheumatoid arthritis (RA) patients (Tatsis et al. 1999). Cancer was found in 23 WG patients compared with 18 RA patients. Seven patients with renal cell carcinoma were found in the WG group and only one in the RA group. Simultaneous occurrence of cancer was found in 14 WG patients (5/7 renal carcinoma patients) and only one in the RA group. Proteinase 3 could not be identified in samples of malignant tissue from the WG patients. The frequency of other cancers was not different from the control population. Malignancy might sometimes therefore be the trigger for development of WG. Malignancy may be a complication of therapy especially bladder cancer following cyclophosphamide therapy and lymphoma after azathioprine or other immunosuppressive therapy.

Vasculitis may also mimic malignancy. A large mass of inflammatory tissue associated with constitutional symptoms may be misdiagnosed as a malignancy. The differentiation between lymphoma and WG of the upper airways can be particularly difficult.

Drugs and vasculitis

Drug-induced vasculitis is probably one of the commoner causes of vasculitis. A very wide range of drugs together with vaccines and desensitization procedures has been reported as causing a vasculitic reaction; however, many of these are isolated case reports and it is not possible to conclusively prove a causal relationship. Recently, more definite associations have been described in particular with propylthiouracil, hydrallazine, and leucotriene antagonists. A number of recreational drugs have been reported to cause vasculitis, including heroin, cocaine, and metamphetamine. They have been particularly associated with cerebral vasculitis. The majority of patients develop an isolated small-vessel vasculitis; medium vessel involvement occurs uncommonly. Large vessel involvement is rare. The frequency of drug-induced hypersensitivity vasculitis is unknown, but may account for 10–20 per cent of cutaneous vasculitis.

A number of different terms have been used to describe drug-induced vasculitis, including hypersensitivity vasculitis, allergic vasculitis, serum sickness, leucocytoclastic vasculitis, and cutaneous vasculitis. The pathogenesis is generally thought to be immune mediated, but there are specific pathogenic mechanisms, immune complex formation, hypocomplementaemia, and cell-mediated mechanisms with T-cell activation.

The clinical and pathological presentation of drug-induced vasculitis is indistinguishable from other types of small-vessel vasculitis. The most common skin lesion is purpura which may be palpable, this occurs in 50 per cent of cases, with urticarial lesions occurring in 10 per cent. The rash is symmetrical and often affects the extremities. The lesions are the same age and disappear within several weeks of drug withdrawal. They may scar or leave haemosiderosis. Involvement of extracutaneous organs is in most series uncommon, but has been reported in up to 50–60 per cent of cases (Mullich et al. 1977). This is probably an overestimate, reflecting the specialist referral of more severe cases. The most common histological appearance is a leucocytoclastic vasculitis. Other laboratory findings are non-specific with leucocytosis, hypocomplementaemia, and raised acute phase response. An eosinophilia is suggestive of a drug aetiology but is also a typical feature of the Churg–Strauss syndrome (CSS). ANCA may be present and sometimes reflects systemic involvement.

Vasculitis associated with ANCA has been attributed to a number of drugs including hydralazine, and propylthiouracil and is especially associated with anti-MPO specificity (Choi et al. 2000). Choi and colleagues reviewed their 30 patients with the highest titre MPO-ANCA and found that 10 patients had been exposed to hydralazine and three to propylthiouracil. In addition two patients each had been exposed allopurinol and penicillamine. The clinical and histological features were typical of ANCA associated vasculitis. The target antigens were elastase and lactoferrin.

The leukotriene inhibitors (zafirlukast, montelukast, and pranlukast) are recently introduced therapies for asthma. Wechsler et al. (2000) described 12 patients with steroid dependent asthma who developed CSS following withdrawal of steroids permitted by zafirlukast or montelukast. All the patients fulfilled the criteria for CSS. Whether this represents unmasking of previously unrecognized CSS or an allergic reaction triggering CSS is uncertain, but the former is more likely. The incidence rate is similar with both zafirlukast and montelukast (60/million patient years), and also to that observed in an asthmatic population not treated with the leukotriene inhibitors. Furthermore, a similar phenomenon has been described in patients receiving high-dose inhaled steroids and salmeterol. Cases have not been observed in steroid (either oral or inhaled) naive patients.

The therapy of drug-induced hypersensitivity is unclear. The majority of cases respond simply to withdrawal of the inducing drug. Reported cases tend to reflect the severe end of the spectrum and reported therapies include corticosteroids, plasmapheresis, and cyclophosphamide.

Serum sickness

Serum sickness is an immune complex mediated phenomenon occurring after repeated administration of heterologous proteins, characterized by arthritis, vasculitis, and nephritis. Hyperimmune heterologous sera are no longer in therapeutic use; antilymphocyte or antithymocyte globulins are still used in the treatment of autoimmune disease or allograft rejection. Monoclonal antibodies (mAb) of murine or rat origin have recently been developed for treatment of autoimmune disease. Use of rodent mAbs invariably results in an antiglobulin response with detectable levels of human antirodent antibodies (Isaacs 2001). Development of an antiglobulin response has not prevented repeated courses of therapy; however, they may become less effective and potentially result in anaphylactic reaction. The concomitant use of methotrexate prolongs the duration of action of chimeric anti-TNF-alpha antibody (Infliximab) when used to treat RA (Maini et al. 1998). The use of humanized antibodies should reduce the antiglobulin response, although it is still possible for an anti-idiotypic or antiallotypic response to develop. Serum sickness may also occur after administration of intravenous or intracardiac streptokinase or anisolyated plasminogen streptokinase activator complex.

Vaccination

Vaccine-induced vasculitis has been rarely described after some antiviral vaccines. Vasculitis occurring after recombinant HBV vaccination has been reported in 13 cases (Le Hello et al. 1999). Initial clinical features developed within 6–7 weeks of vaccination. Involved organs were most typically skin, joints, retina, and muscle; renal involvement was not seen. Vaccine induced vasculitis, in particular CSS, has been noted following tetanus, influenza, HBA, rubella, and small pox vaccination (Guillevin et al. 1999).

Desensitization

Desensitization or hyposensitization therapy is a specific treatment for IgE related allergies including allergic rhinitis, asthma, and bee stings.

Increasing doses of allergen are injected subcutaneously. CSS may rarely occur within a few weeks or months of desensitization to candida, polymicrobial antigens, and acarian (Guillevin et al. 1999).

Vasculitis mimics

The presenting features of the systemic vasculitides are protean and diagnosis is based on a combination of clinical, laboratory, and histopathological features. Clinical features alone are not always diagnostic and a variety of other diseases can mimic systemic vasculitis (Table 3). These mimics usually present with multiorgan illness or evidence of vascular damage, or a combination of both. Biopsy of involved organs is, therefore, important to identify non-inflammatory vascular changes such as embolism or thrombosis. Angiographic features including aneurysms, though typical of PAN, can occur in other conditions such as myxoma and bacterial endocarditis.

Cholesterol crystal embolism

Cholesterol crystal embolism has been recognized for more than a century; however, it remains underdiagnosed. Risk factors for cholesterol embolism are male sex, age more than 60 years, Caucasian, hypertension, tobacco use, and diabetes mellitus (Scolari et al. 2000). Cholesterol embolism may occur spontaneously or after trauma to the aortic wall during vascular surgery or angiographic procedures. Other aetiological factors include anticoagulation therapy with either heparin or warfarin and thrombolysis. The clinical consequences of cholesterol crystal embolism are variable. Embolization may be completely asymptomatic and the diagnosis made at renal biopsy, or cause an ischaemic digit or a multisystem disease that mimics systemic vasculitis. The distribution of end organ damage depends on the location of the original atherosclerotic plaques.

Clinically significant renal involvement occurs in around 50 per cent of patients (Scolari et al. 2000), the onset of renal disease after the triggering event may be immediate but can be more insidious with a delay of weeks or months. There may be acute renal impairment following massive embolization, alternatively there may be a gradual deterioration in renal function due to crystal embolic showers, or an ischaemic nephropathy.

Cutaneous manifestations are typically ischaemic digits, particularly the toes from abdominal atheroma emboli and livedo reticularis affecting the legs. The ischaemic toe usually presents as sudden onset of a small, cool, cyanotic and painful area of the foot (usually the toe). The lesions are tender to touch and may progress to ulceration, digital infarction, and gangrene. The peripheral pulses are usually well preserved despite the digital cyanosis. Other common features include abdominal pain, central nervous system involvement, fever, and weight loss.

Laboratory investigations are often non-specific including uraemia, thrombocytopaenia, eosinophilia, elevated ESR, hypocomplementaemia, and disseminated intravascular coagulation. ANCA is not usually detected in the serum (Scolari et al. 2000). Diagnosis is based on the clinical features with a typical history, supported by histological demonstration of the typical cholesterol clefts or cholesterol emboli in vessels.

Treatment is aimed at halting the progression of tissue ischaemia and prevention of further embolization. Anticoagulation should be avoided as this may exacerbate embolization. Antiplatelet therapy is unsuccessful.

Table 3 Vasculitis masquerades

Systemic multisystem disease
Infection
Subacute bacterial endocarditis
Neisseria
Rickettsiae
Malignancy
Metastatic carcinoma
Paraneoplastic
Other
Sweet syndrome
Occlusive vasculopathy
Embolic
Cholesterol crystals
Atrial myxoma
Infection
Thrombotic
Antiphospholipid syndrome
Procoagulant states
Calciphylaxis
Others
Ergot
Radiation
Degos
Severe Raynaud's
Acute digital loss
Angiographic
Aneurysmal
Fibromuscular dysplasia
Neurofibromatosis
Occlusion
Coarctation

Calciphylaxis

Calciphylaxis is rare, but potentially fatal. It occurs in patients with chronic renal failure with secondary hyperparathyroidism. Disturbance of calcium and phosphate metabolism results in painful necrosis of skin, subcutaneous tissue, and acral gangrene. Appearance of the lesions is distinctive but the pathogenesis remains uncertain. Correction of hyperphosphataemia or occasionally hypercalcaemia is vital, and parathyroidectomy may be of benefit (Mathur et al. 2001).

Embolism

Cardiac myxoma

Cardiac myxoma are rare benign tumours most commonly found in the left atrium (90 per cent of cases). Constitutional symptoms and systemic embolization may lead to an erroneous diagnosis of vasculitis (Boussen et al. 1991).

Systemic manifestations seen in 90 per cent of cases include: fever, weight loss, Raynaud's phenomenon, clubbing, elevated acute phase proteins, and hypergammaglobulinaemia. Systemic embolization occurs in 40 per cent; emboli may be large enough to occlude the aortic bifurcation, smaller emboli may remain viable and invade the vessel wall resulting in aneurysm formation that mimics PAN. The diagnosis is made by echocardiography, which should be performed on all cases of suspected systemic vasculitis. Treatment is by surgical resection of the primary tumour and any emboli.

Infective endocarditis

Infective endocarditis is associated with both a true vasculitis and embolic phenomenon. True vasculitic lesions are caused either by an immune complex vasculitis, the infectious agent or mycotic aneurysm formation by septic emboli where there is direct invasion of the vessel wall. Petechiae, strokes, splenic infarcts, and glomerulonephritis are the most extra-cardiac common features. There is an immunological response with elevation of acute phase proteins, hypergammaglobulinaemia, and autoantibody formation. The diagnosis is made by blood culture and echocardiography.

Fibromuscular dysplasia

Fibromuscular dysplasia is a vascular disease that affects small to medium arteries. It is a non-inflammatory, non-atherosclerotic condition that occurs in younger people and women. Renal artery involvement occurs in 60–75 per cent, cervicocranial arteries in 25–30 per cent, visceral arteries in 9 per cent, and peripheral arteries in 5 per cent of cases (Begelman and Olins 2000). Classification is dependent on the dominant arterial wall layer involved: intimal, medial, and adventitial. The aetiology is unknown, but there is a strong genetic component. Clinical manifestations reflect the arterial tree involved with renovascular hypertension, renal infarction, dissection, transient ischaemic attacks, and stroke. The diagnosis is made on the typical angiographic appearances with the classic 'string of beads appearance'. Fibromuscular dysplasia in particular diffuse intimal disease can occasionally be difficult to distinguish from vasculitis. There should not, however, be evidence of an acute phase response. Symptomatic stenotic lesions are treated by percutaneous transluminal angioplasty or bypass grafting, together with antiplatelet drugs.

Chronic ergotism

Epidemic ergotism occurs after ingestion of grain contaminated with ergot (*Claviceps purpurea*) (Christopoulos et al. 2001). Since mediaeval times epidemics have been described in which painful gangrene of the peripheries occurred with loss of extremities. Critical mesenteric ischaemia can occur. Chronic ergotism can occur following long-term use of ergotamine tartrate to treat migraine. Peripheral, carotid, coronary, and visceral ischaemia may develop. The angiographic appearances may simulate vasculitis with irregular, long or short segmental stenosis. The diagnosis is dependent on a history of ergot consumption. The lesions may not be fully reversible on withdrawal of ergot.

Köhlmeier–Degos disease

Köhlmeier–Degos disease (malignant atrophic papulosis) is a rare and lethal condition, which involves skin, gut, and the nervous system. The typical skin lesions are circular, porcelain white with a depressed centre 4–8 mm in diameter with a slightly elevated erythematosus margin. The arterial lesion is luminal stenosis or occlusion due to intimal proliferation and consequent thrombosis (Magrinat et al. 1989). Presentation is with acute abdominal pain (in association with the skin lesion), leading to bowel infarction. The multisystem nature of Köhlmeier–Degos disease mimics a vasculitis. The diagnosis is made on biopsy.

Cryofibrinogenaemia

Cryofibrinogenaemia occurs when a cryoprecipitate occurs in plasma, which has been anticoagulated with oxalate, citrate, or edetic acid. The cryoprecipitate is a complex, which includes a number of plasma proteins including fibrin, fibrinogen, and fibrin split products. The cryofibrinogen is consumed in the clotting process and therefore unlike a cryoglobulin does not precipitate in cooled serum. Cryofibrinogenaemia may be asymptomatic but can present with purpura, skin necrosis, ulcers, gangrene, arthralgias, glomerulonephritis, or a leucocytoclastic vasculitis (Blain et al. 2000), and thus mimic a systemic vasculitis. Cryofibrinogenaemia may be primary or secondary to malignancy, infection, or a connective tissue disease. Treatment is by cold avoidance and treatment of the underlying condition, combined with immunosuppression, plasmapheresis, and/or fibrinolytic drugs.

Radiation vasculopathy

Radiation has been known to cause vascular injury since the early 1900s. Acute vascular injury occurs within hours of large doses of radiation and presents with hypotension, shock, and death. Chronic radiation vasculopathy present with: (i) internal injury and mural thrombosis occurring within 5 years; (ii) progressive sclerosis of arterioles and arteries occurring within 10 years and which can lead to luminal occlusion; and (iii) accelerated atherosclerosis with a latency of 20 years. The endothelial cell is the most radiation sensitive part of the vascular system.

Clinically, the manifestations depend on the organs included in the field of radiation, and the dose and type of radiation used. Features include arterial stenosis and occlusion, rupture, and aneurysms formation. The angiographic appearance is similar to those seen on atherosclerosis. Radiation vasculopathy can be distinguished from systemic vasculitis by the history of irradiation and the lack of an acute phase response.

Inflammatory rheumatic disease

Rheumatoid vasculitis

RA complicated by vasculitis was first described over 100 years ago, in a patient with involvement of the vasa nervorum. The classical association with peripheral gangrene and mononeuritis multiplex was clearly established in the 1940s and 1950s (Bywaters 1957). However, a broader spectrum of disease is now recognized including pericarditis, scleritis, nodules, and systemic disease.

The annual incidence of systemic rheumatoid vasculitis (SRV) was estimated in Norfolk during 1988–1997 to be 12.5 per million with a greater incidence in males than females. Over this 10-year period there has been a trend towards a reduction in incidence. Whether this reflects a change in the severity of rheumatoid disease or changing disease management with lower use of corticosteroids and more frequent use of methotrexate is speculative.

There are no validated diagnostic criteria for the definition of SRV. Scott and Bacon (1984) proposed criteria for the definition of SRV: the presence of peripheral gangrene or ulceration, neuropathy, positive biopsy, or extra-articular disease in a patient with RA.

The major clinical features of SRV are given in Table 4. Development of rheumatoid vasculitis is associated with male gender, extra-articular features, and a severe disease course as assessed by joint damage and the requirement for disease modifying therapy. The strongest association is with the presence of rheumatoid factor.

Three main patterns of rheumatoid vasculitis can be identified:

1. isolated nailfold vasculitis due to digital endarteritis with intimal proliferation;
2. venulitis and small-vessel arteritis characterized by rash, skin eruptions, or purpura;
3. necrotizing arteritis of small- and medium-sized arteries with involvement of internal organs and peripheral nerves.

Cutaneous lesions are common including transient typical isolated small nail fold or nail edge lesions. These reflect mainly small vessel involvement, and may easily be missed. The reported frequency reflects the intensity of the search and they have been reported in 34 per cent of men and 18 per cent of women with classical RA attending hospital (Golding et al. 1964). In our experience, patients presenting with isolated nailfold vasculitis have a low risk of progressing from localized to systemic disease (Watts et al. 1995).

Leg ulcers occur commonly in RA patients and are usually multifactorial. Vasculitic ulcers are typically painful, deep punched out lesions of acute onset and occur in association with other evidence of vasculitis. They occur in sites not typically associated with venous stasis ulceration, such as the sacrum or foot. Biopsies are rarely obtained because of fears about poor wound healing. Chronic superficial ulcers should not be considered a feature of SRV without other evidence of SRV (either histological or clinical).

Neurological involvement is common with development of acute mononeuritis multiplex or peripheral neuropathy often in association with nailfold lesions. A distal symmetric sensory or sensori-motor pattern is more common than mononeuritis multiplex. Peripheral neuropathy is attributable to development of necrotizing vasculitis of the vasa nervorum.

SRV is associated with significant mortality and morbidity, and this has led to the early use of immunosuppressive regimens. Corticosteroids alone are usually ineffective and rapid changes in dose have been implicated in the pathogenesis and induction of SRV and may predispose patients to vascular occlusion. Azathioprine in combination with prednisolone may be effective in the treatment of SRV (Heurkins et al. 1991) but no controlled data exist. A comparison of azathioprine and prednisolone in the treatment of isolated

Table 4 Clinical features at presentation of patients with systemic rheumatoid vasculitis

	Norwich (%)	Bath[a] (%)
n	47	50
Rheumatoid factor	42 (89)	47 (94)
Erosions	32 (68)	NA
Nodules	16/28 (57)	43/50 (86)
Systemic	23 (49)[b]	41 (82)
Weight loss	16	41
Malaise	13	NA
Cutaneous	42 (89)	44 (88)
Infarct	33	26
Ulcer	21	12
Purpura	7	28
Gangrene	16	7
Neurological	18 (38)	21 (42)
PN	16	14
MNM	6	7
Stroke	2	2
Pulmonary	13 (28)	17 (34)
Fibrosis	8	9
Pleurisy/effusion	6	8
Infiltrates	0	NA
Renal	12 (25)	12 (24)
Protein/haematuria	8	6
Raised creatinine	1	2
Ophthalmic	12 (25)	8 (16)
Scleritis	11	7
CVS	9 (19)	17 (34)
Pericarditis	5	7
Aortic incomp	2	2
MI	2	3
Gastrointestinal	2 (4)	5 (10)

[a] From Scott et al. (1981).

[b] $p < 0.001$ (Norwich versus Bath).

Note: PN, peripheral neuropathy; MNM, mononeuritis multiplex; MI, myocardial infarction; NA, data not available. [From O'Gradaigh et al. (2000) with permission.]

nailfold vasculitis showed no significant advantage over conventional therapy (Heurkins et al. 1991). Cyclophosphamide combined with corticosteroids has become the standard treatment for SRV. Isolated nailfold vasculitis does not require specific therapy as the risk of progression to systemic disease is low; however, the patient should be kept under close observation.

Spondyloarthopathies

Aortitis may complicate the seronegative spondyloarthropathies in particular ankylosing spondylitis and Reiter's syndrome. The aortic ring and ascending aorta are the typical sites of involvement but distal aortitis has been described. Aortic incompetence occurs in up to 5 per cent of cases of ankylosing spondylitis, 2.5 per cent of cases of Reiter's syndrome, and probably less frequently in the other seronegative spondyloarthropathies (Townend et al. 1991).

Echocardiography shows thickening of the aortic leaflets, subaortic echodense bumps, and aortic root densities. Histologically, there is thickening of the aortic valve cusps and aorta, together with lymphocytic infiltration in the aortic wall and fibrosis of the aortic root. These changes can be difficult to distinguish from lesions occurring in syphilitic aortitis (Townend 1991).

Treatment of the inflammatory process with immunosuppressive agents has been suggested but no controlled data exists as their benefit in this situation in particular whether the need for aortic valve replacement can be delayed or prevented.

Systemic lupus erythematosus

Vascular involvement in systemic lupus erythematosus (SLE) can vary from a mild focal deposition of fibrinoid in the vessel wall, leading to proliferation and luminal narrowing without endothelial damage to more destructive lesions with damage to both the elastic and muscular elements of the wall and eventual necrosis. Thrombosis is uncommon in this setting. In the antiphospholipid syndrome (APS) the primary lesion is thrombotic without evidence of vessel wall abnormality.

Vasculitic skin lesions occur with a cumulative prevalence of 40 per cent (Morrow et al. 1999). These are usually found at the fingertips or toes, or on the extensor surface of the forearm. When they occur around the malleoli, they may lead to tender, deep leg ulcers, which may be slow to heal. Vasculitis causing neurological, renal, or cardiac involvement is rare.

Sjögren's syndrome

Vasculitis with purpura or urticaria is an uncommon feature of Sjögren's syndrome occurring in up to 17 per cent of patients (Morrow et al. 1999). The purpuric rash has a predilection for the legs. Histologically, there is a neutrophilic infiltrate, with low complement, elevated gamma globulins, and raised titres of anti-Ro and rheumatoid factor. Patients with hypergammaglobulinaemia may have recurrent episodes of cutaneous vasculitis.

Antiphospholipid antibody syndrome

APS may present catastrophically with recurrent arterial and venous thrombosis, peripheral gangrene, and organ infarction. This may mimic systemic vasculitis but the pathology is thrombotic (Lie 1994). The diagnosis may be made by the presence of anticardiolipin antibodies in the typical clinical setting. Treatment is with anticoagulation rather that immunosuppression.

References

Begelman, S.M. and Olins, J.W. (2000). Fibromuscular dysplasia. *Current Opinion in Rheumatology* **12**, 41–7.

Blain, H. et al. (2000). Cryofibrinogenaemia: a study of 49 patients. *Clinical Experimental Immunology* **120**, 253–60.

Blanco, R. et al. (1998). Cutaneous vasculitis in children and adults. Associated diseases and etiologic factors in 303 patients. *Medicine (Baltimore)* **77**, 403–18.

Boussen, K. et al. (1991). Embolisation of cardiac myxoma masquerading as polyarteritis nodosa. *Journal of Rheumatology* **18**, 283–5.

Bywaters, E.G.L. (1957). Peripheral vascular obstruction in rheumatoid arthritis and its relationships to other vascular lesions. *Annals of the Rheumatic Diseases* **16**, 84–103.

Cacoub, P. (2001). Systemic vasculitis in patients with hepatitis C. *Journal of Rheumatology* **28**, 109–18.

Chakravarty, K. and Scott, D. (1992). Mycotic aneurysm of the aortic arch masquerading as systemic lupus erythematosus. *Annals of the Rheumatic Diseases* **51**, 1079–81.

Chetty, R. (2001). Vascultides associated with HIV infection. *Journal of Clinical Pathology* **54**, 275–8.

Choi, H.K. et al. (2000). Drug associated anti-neutrophil cytoplasmic antibody positive vasculitis. *Arthritis and Rheumatism* **43**, 405–13.

Christopoulos, S., Szilagyi, A., and Kahn, S.R. (2001). Saint Anthony's fire. *Lancet* **358**, 1694.

Golding, J., Hamilton, M., and Gill, R. (1964). Arteritis of rheumatoid arthritis. *British Journal of Dermatology* **77**, 207–10.

Gonzalez-Gay, M.A. and Garcia-Porrua, C. (1999). Systemic vasculitis in adults in northwestern Spain, 1988–1997. Clinical and epidemiologic aspects. *Medicine (Baltimore)* **78**, 292–308.

Guillevin, L. (1999). Virus associated vasculitis. *Rheumatology* **38**, 588–90.

Guillevin, L. et al. (1999). Churg Strauss Syndrome. Clinical study and long term follow up of 96 patients. *Medicine (Baltimore)* **78**, 26–37.

Hamidou, M.A. et al. (2000). Prevalence of rheumatic manifestations and anti-neutrophil cytoplasmic antibodies in haematological malignancies. A prospective study. *Rheumatology (Oxford)* **39**, 417–20.

Hasler, P., Kistler, H., and Gerber, H. (1995). Vasculitides in hairy cell leukaemia. *Seminars in Arthritis and Rheumatism* **25**, 134–42.

Heurkins, A., Westedt, M., and Breedfeld, F. (1991). Prednisolone plus azathioprine treatment in patients with rheumatoid arthritis complicated by vasculitis. *Archives of Internal Medicine* **15**, 2249–54.

Isaacs, J.D. (2001). From bench to bedside: discovering rules for antibody design, and improving serotherapy with monoclonal antibodies. *Rheumatology (Oxford)* **40**, 724–38.

Lamprecht, P., Gause, A., and Gross, W. (1999). Cryoglobulinaemic vasculitis. *Arthritis and Rheumatism* **42**, 2507–16.

Le Hello, C. et al. (1999). Suspected hepatitis B vaccination related vasculitis. *Journal of Rheumatology* **26**, 191–4.

Lie, J. (1994). Vasculitis in the antiphospholipid syndrome: culprit or consort? *Journal of Rheumatology* **21**, 397–9.

Magrinat, G., Kerwin, K.S., and Gabriel, D.A. (1989). The clinical manifestations of Degos syndrome. *Archives of Pathology Laboratory Medicine* **113**, 354–62.

Maini, R. et al. (1998). Therapeutic efficacy of multiple intravenous infusions of anti-tumor necrosis factor alpha monoclonal antibody combined with low-dose weekly methotrexate in rheumatoid arthritis. *Arthritis and Rheumatism* **41**, 1552–63.

Mathur, R.V., Shortland, J.R., and El Nahas, A.M. (2001). Calciphylaxis. *Postgraduate Medical Journal* **77**, 557–61.

McMahon, B.J. et al. (1989). Hepatitis B-associated polyarteritis nodosa in Alaskan Eskimos: clinical and epidemiological features and long-term follow up. *Hepatology* **9**, 97–101.

Morrow, J. et al. *Autoimmune Rheumatic Disease.* Oxford: Oxford University Press, 1999.

Mullich, F.G. et al. (1977). Drug related vasculitis. *Human Pathology* **10**, 313–25.

Nikkari, S. et al. (1994). Wegener's granulomatosis and parvovirus B19 infection. *Arthritis and Rheumatism* **37**, 1707–8.

O'Gradaigh, D., Watts, R.A., and Scott, D.G.I. (2000). Extra-articular features of rheumatoid arthritis. In *Rheumatoid Arthritis: New Frontiers in Pathogenesis and Treatment* (ed. G.S. Firestein, G.S. Panayi, and F.A. Wollheim), pp. 227–42. Oxford: Oxford University Press.

Oskoui, R. et al. (1993). Salmonella aortitis. *Archives of Internal Medicine* **153**, 517–25.

Pertuiset, E. et al. (2000). Adult Henoch–Schönlein purpura associated with malignancy. *Seminars in Arthritis and Rheumatism* **29**, 360–7.

Scolari, F. et al. (2000). Cholesterol crystal embolism: a recognizable cause of renal disease. *American Journal of Kidney Disease* **36**, 1089–99.

Scott, D. and Bacon, P. (1984). Intravenous cyclophosphamide plus methyl prednisolone in the treatment of systemic rheumatoid vasculitis. *American Journal of Medicine* **76**, 377–84.

Scott, D.G.I., Bacon, P.A., and Tribe, C.R. (1981). Systemic rheumatoid vasculitis: a clinical and laboratory study of 50 cases. *Medicine* **60**, 288–97.

Somer, T. and Finegold, S. (1995). Vasculitides associated with infections, immunization and antimicrobial drugs. *Clinical Infectious Diseases* **20**, 1010–36.

Soravia-Dunand, V., Loo, V., and Salit, I. (1999). Aortitis due to Salmonella: report of 10 cases and comprehensive review of the literature. *Clinical Infectious Diseases* **29**, 862–8.

Tatsis, E. et al. (1999). Wegener's granulomatosis associated with renal cell carcinoma. *Arthritis and Rheumatism* **42**, 751–6.

Townend, J. et al. (1991). Acute aortitis and aortic incompetence due to systemic rheumatological disorders. *International Journal of Cardiology* **33**, 253–8.

Watts, R., Carruthers, D., and Scott, D. (1995). Isolated nailfold vasculitis in rheumatoid arthritis. *Annals of the Rheumatic Diseases* **54**, 927–9.

Watts, R. et al. (1998). Cutaneous vasculitis in a defined population—clinical and epidemiological associations. *Journal of Rheumatology* **25**, 920–4.

Wechsler, M. et al. (2000). Churg–Strauss syndrome in patients receiving montelukast as treatment for asthma. *Chest* **117**, 708–13.

Williams, P.L. et al. (1992). Vasculitic and encephalitic complications associated with *Coccidioides immitis* infection of the central nervous system. *Clinical Infectious Diseases* **14**, 673–82.

6.10.5 Large vessel vasculitis/giant cell arteritis

Elisabeth Nordborg and Claes Nordborg

Introduction

The clinical and pathological features of systemic vasculitic disorders depend on the site of the lesions and the type of blood vessels involved. Diseases in which vasculitis is a primary process are called primary systemic vasculitides. The spectrum of systemic vasculitides has been organized according to the predominant size of the vessels affected; large vessels are defined as the aorta and its main branches such as the subclavian, carotid, renal, mesenteric, and femoral arteries (Jennette et al. 1994). The two most important forms of large vessel vasculitis are giant cell (temporal) arteritis (GCA) and Takayasu's arteritis (TA). Sharing a number of clinical and pathologic features, these entities are related, but are distinct disorders. Although, the understanding of the pathogenetic mechanisms leading to vascular inflammation in GCA, has increased during the last few years, much less is known about the pathogenesis of TA. Histologically, both disorders, display a granulomatous inflammation with infiltration of lymphocytes and macrophages, and with the formation of giant cells, characteristically distributed in patchy and scattered lesions. Systemic symptoms (fever, malaise, and weight loss) are common in both diseases, but clear differences exist between the two disorders. TA, typically, affects young women from Asian countries, whereas GCA is restricted to elderly people, mainly of Caucasian origin. GCA is the most common primary systemic vasculitis in the Western world, with an annual incidence in individuals aged over 50 years of about 200 per million.

In contrast to GCA, the inflammation in TA frequently targets intracranial arteries as well as renal and pulmonary arteries. The vascular symptoms in GCA are mainly due to the inflammation of branches of the external carotid artery, in particular its superficial temporal division, although necropsy studies have shown aortic involvement in the majority of cases (Östberg 1972). Aortic involvement often leads to aneurysm formation in GCA, whereas aortic stenoses are more common in TA (Evans et al. 1994a,b). Corticosteroids are the first choice of drug treatment in both TA and GCA. However, in steroid-responsive patients in TA remission is often achieved and maintained on an alternate-day regimen, whereas every day therapy with prednisolone is recommended in GCA.

Large vessel vasculitis may occur as a secondary feature in other disorders, predominantly bacterial, fungal, mycobacterial, or spirochetal infections, the aorta being the primary target.

Furthermore, secondary vessel vasculitides are frequent in patients with autoimmune disease such as rheumatoid arthritis, systemic lupus, seronegative spondyloarthopathies, and juvenile idiopathic arthritis. The vasculitic process in these disorders particularly affects medium-sized and small vessels; large vessel involvement is rare. Hence, the secondary vasculitis associated with other rheumatic diseases is not traditionally refferred to the group of large vessel vasculitides.

Giant cell arteritis

GCA in a historical perspective

GCA may be a very old disorder. Around 1000 AD, the Mesopotamian physician Ali Ibn Isa noticed a relationship between the inflamed temporal artery, headache, and visual symptoms, and even recommended its removal for treatment (Wood 1936). Some European paintings from the fifteenth and sixteenth centuries are considered to show examples of temporal arteritis [*Jan van Eyck* 'The Holy Virgin with Canon Van der Paele' (1436), *Piero di Cosimo* 'Lorenzo Giambetti' (1502) (Plate 150)]. In modern times GCA was first clinically observed in 1890, by Sir Jonathan Hutchinson, a British surgeon, who described an 80-year-old man with 'painful, red streaks on his head, which prevented him from wearing his hat'. The red streaks were the temporal arteries and Hutchinson named the disease 'arteritis of the aged' (Hutchinson 1890). In 1932 Horton made the first histological description of this granulomatous arteritis and defined the clinical profile; the disease was named Horton's arteritis (Horton et al. 1932). Gilmour called attention to the characteristic histological hallmarks of this disorder including the presence of multinucleated giant cells (Gilmore 1941). Since then the names temporal arteritis and GCA have been used synonymously.

The modern history of GCA runs along two paths, that of temporal arteritis and that of polymyalgia rheumatica. In the 1950s and 1960s, muscle pain of the girdles was recognized as a frequent symptom in biopsy-positive GCA, which prompted Hamrin (1972), to propose the name polymyalgia arteritica. At present, most Scandinavian clinicians consider polymyalgia rheumatica to be a manifestation of a generalized arteritis and usually include it as a special form of GCA. However, almost 50 years later there is still a debate as to the relationship between the two. In this volume, polymyalgia rheumatica and temporal (giant cell) arteritis are dealt with in separate chapters.

Classification of GCA

The aetiology of GCA is unknown and a specific diagnostic test for this form of arteritis is lacking. Therefore, its diagnosis depends on the presence of a combination of clinical and pathological findings. In 1990, the American College of Rheumatology (ACR) formed classification criteria (Hunder et al. 1990), comparing data from 593 patients with symptoms and clinical findings of other known vasculitides, with those from 214 patients with a clear diagnosis of GCA. The ACR criteria set is most efficient for the distinction of GCA from other vasculitides but are not purely diagnostic. They allow, for the first time, comparison of patients in a uniform manner. Thus, the criteria are widely used in clinical research.

In a case of suspected vasculitis, the finding of three of the following five criteria were associated with a GCA diagnosis of 94 per cent sensitivity and 91 per cent specificity:

- age greater than or equal to 50 years at the time of disease onset;
- localized headache of new onset;
- tenderness or decreased pulse of the temporal artery;
- ESR greater than 50 mm/h (Westergren);
- biopsy, which includes an inflamed artery with a predominance of mononuclear cells or a granulomatous process with multinucleated giant cells.

Disease occurrence

Incidence and geographic variation

GCA is not an uncommon form of vasculitis. However, the incidence varies greatly between different geographic regions. The highest incidence rates have been reported from Scandinavia and Minnesota, United States, with a population of mainly north European descent (Nordborg 2000). Swedish epidemiological studies have recorded the average annual incidence rate of biopsy-positive GCA to be between 16.8 and 22.2 per 100 000 inhabitants over 50 years of age (1973–1995) (Petursdottir et al. 1999). Recently, even higher incidence rates were found in Iceland, and the highest figures worldwide, 32.8 per 100 000 inhabitants aged 50 years and older, were documented in Norway, using the ACR criteria (Haugeberg et al. 2000a,b). Interestingly, a geographical gradient of GCA frequency has been observed, implying a statistically verified increase in frequency by latitude north (Watts et al. 2001). These results are in accordance with earlier epidemiological reports from various parts of Europe. GCA is rarely seen in blacks and it is distinctly infrequent in Asian countries.

Time trends

An increase in annual incidence rates with time, has been reported from several centres (Machado et al. 1988; Petursdottir et al. 1999). Changes in classification criterias, shift from retrospective to prospective study design, or an increased access to temporal arteries could not explain these results. A longer life-expectancy of the general population or an increased degree of medical attention may have contributed. The report by Östberg on GCA in an autopsy material indicates that GCA may be considerably more common than is clinically apparent (Östberg 1971).

Disease risk factors

Age

Essentially, GCA is not diagnosed in people younger than 50 years. The likelihood of getting the disorder increases continuously with age. GCA is about 20 times more common among people in their ninth decade compared with people aged between 50 and 60 years (Bengtsson and Malmvall 1981). GCA is thus a disease of elderly people, which suggests that factors related to the ageing of the arterial wall and the immune system might be involved in its pathogenesis (Nordborg et al. 2000). Exactly how the ageing of the immune system affects immune reactivity in GCA patients has not been investigated.

A decline in immunocompetence with age, has been attributed to a deteriorating thymic function, resulting in an increased risk of infections and a reduced antitumour immunity. Elderly people also have a higher incidence of clonal disorders and they more frequently produce autoantibodies.

Gender

There is a clear female predominance in GCA with a two- to four-fold overweight in women compared with men. Since GCA is a disorder among elderly females the question might be raised of whether sex hormones are involved in its pathogenesis. Interestingly, a recent epidemiological study revealed that the number of pregnancies was lower among GCA patients than among controls, suggesting that the hyperoestrogenic state during pregnancy might protect the artery wall (Duhaut et al. 1999). Oestrogen displays a wide variety of mechanisms which, theoretically, may be related to GCA. It is thus known to preserve a normal vessel wall by stimulating as well as inhibiting the growth of vascular smooth-muscle cells. Moreover, there is evidence that oestrogen influences the immune system (Cutolo et al. 1995).

Genetic factors

GCA almost exclusively affects Caucasians. Subjects of Northern European descent, and in particular people of Nordic heritage, seem to be most susceptible to develop GCA, irrespective of their place of residence; similar incidence rates are reported from Scandinavia and Minnesota, United States, two regions of similar ethnic composition. Studies of HLA antigens have shown a significant association with class II antigens DR4; HLA–DRB1*0401 was found to be the most frequent allele in patients with GCA. One study disclosed a disease-related HLA-amino acid sequence mapped to the antigen-binding area of the HLA molecule, which differed from the sequences associated with rheumatoid arthritis, which are located in the third hypervariable region (Weyand et al. 1994). As yet, these data have not been confirmed by others.

GCA and arterial degeneration

Morphologically, there is no reason to believe that atherosclerosis is a risk factor or initiator of GCA. Atherosclerosis is seldom seen in temporal arteries.

Instead, in the general population, a morphologically distinct type of arterial degeneration is encountered, indicating media atrophy and minute calcifications of the internal elastic membrane (IEM) (Nordborg et al. 2000). The age and sex distribution of these calcifications is similar to that of GCA, that is, they are more common in women and they increase with age. Using light- and electron microscopy, the inflammatory process of GCA appears to start with the formation of foreign-body giant cells, which attack the IEM calcifications. The presence of this degenerative lesion in the general population might thus explain the age and sex distribution of this disorder. It remains, however, to be elucidated why only a minority of the population react against their IEM calcifications.

Environmental risk factors

Non-randomness in geographic and ethnic distribution of GCA is suggestive of genetic risk determinants, but it could also indicate a contribution by environmental factors. *Clustering* of disease incidence, as well as *rhythmic* annual and seasonal *fluctuations*, may indicate the involvement of epidemic infections or other exogenous aetiological factors (Petursdottir et al. 1999). Serological studies regarding influenza A and B, mumps, adeno-, rota-, and enterovirus, Q-fever, *Mycoplasma pneumoniae* and *Chlamydia* revealed no difference in seroprevalence between GCA cases and controls, although most investigations were performed on small series of patients. The seroprevalence was also similar in cases and controls regarding viruses known to induce giant cells in humans such as the herpes virus group, Epstein–Barr virus, measles, respiratory syncytial virus, and parainfluenza types 1, 2, and 3. An association between *Chlamydia pneumoniae* (TWAR) and atherosclerosis has been suggested (Kou et al. 1995). Its role in GCA was recently addressed. One study detected *C. pneumoniae* in the inflamed temporal artery specimens, but in none of the controls, using immunohistochemical staining and PCR techniques (Wagner et al. 2000). In contrast Haugeberg et al. (2000a) did not detect this organism in a large sample of biopsy-proven GCA. Furthermore, the epidemiology of *C. pneumoniae* does not support the hypothesis that it plays a role in the pathogenesis of GCA; the seroprevalence was low in Scandinavian countries and its sex distribution showed a clear predilection for men. Consequently, *C. pneumoniae* does not relate statistically to the high prevalence of GCA in Scandinavian women. To date, there is no convincing evidence that GCA is a truly infectious vasculitis, although possibly environmental factors such as infections might trigger the immune system in a susceptible host, as suggested by Russo et al. (1995), who found a correlation between *different* infections and the onset of GCA in a clinical retrospective study.

Pathology

GCA is an inflammatory vasculopathy of medium-sized and large arteries, with a distinct tropism for arteries with well-developed elastic membranes, essentially sparing the microvessels. At highest risk are the upper extremity branches of the aorta and the cranial arteries.

Histologically, GCA is characterized by chronic inflammation including varying amounts of lymphocytes, histiocytes, and multinucleated giant cells. Despite its name, pathological specimens contain giant cells in, at most, two-thirds of the cases and this finding is not a prerequisite for the diagnosis. The inflammation does not affect the involved arteries in a uniform fashion, and the 'skip phenomenon' is the rule rather than the exception. Thus, in a single vessel, severely inflamed segments alternate with normal ones, sometimes at intervals of a fraction of a millimetre. The disease causes luminal narrowing of the affected vessels resulting in end-organ ischaemia and, in the aorta, weakening of the wall with aneurysm formation and a risk of rupture (Evans et al. 1994a,b).

Pathogenesis

GCA as an antigen-driven disease. The adventitia—port of entry of inflammatory cells?

The IEM has repeatedly been addressed as the most plausible target for the inflammatory reaction in GCA. Degradation of elastic fibres in the arterial wall in GCA was observed long ago. The striking concentration of the inflammatory reaction around the IEM has given rise to the theory of a reaction towards elastin as the aetiopathogenetic mechanism. However, no antielastin antibodies have been found in serum from GCA patients. During the past years, new information has been presented concerning the pathogenesis of GCA. Morphologically, the inflammatory process of GCA appears to start with a focal foreign-body giant cell reaction directed at calcified elastin in both temporal arteries and the aorta (Petursdottir et al. 1996; Nordborg and Nordborg 1998; Nordborg et al. 2000). Others have concluded that the antigen is located in the adventitia, since activated T cells, HLA–DR, and IL-2 receptor were mainly found there, together with a clonal proliferation of a minority of the CD4+ T cells (Weyand 1996). Histological and immunocytochemical studies have shown that macrophages, CD4+ T lymphocytes, and multinucleated giant cells comprise the dominant cell types in GCA. CD8+ T cells are less numerous and B lymphocytes are infrequent. Granulocytes are generally not involved in the arterial lesion. The expression of HLA–DR and IL-2 receptors by the CD4+ T cells indicates that they are in an activated state, due to recent activation by antigen recognition (Cid et al. 1989). The yet unknown antigen (or antigens) initiates the proliferation and migration of the CD4+ T cells into the adventitia, of which a minority expands clonally (Wagner et al. 1996). Due to the preferential location in the *adventitia* of CD4+ T cell and since these cells express IL-2 receptors and accumulate around microvessels, the adventitia was proposed to control the entry of the invading cells, via the vasa vasorum. Some of the CD4+ T cells produce interferon-γ, hereby attracting monocytes/macrophages to the arterial wall. A few of the macrophages fuse at the intima–media junction to form multinucleated giant cells. Moreover, macrophages produce metalloproteinases and inducible nitric oxide synthase, contributing to the destruction of the IEM and further damage of the vessel wall. The function of the multinucleated giant cells has been further elucidated. Apart from its phagocytosing properties, it also displays a secretory role by producing growth factors, such as vascular endothelial growth factors (VEGF), which stimulate growth of new capillaries both in the adventitia and at the intima–media junction. One other growth factor produced by giant cells and invading monocytes/macrophages in particular, is the platelet derived growth factors (PDGF), which is abundantly expressed in the inflamed tissue, contributing to growth, migration, and matrix production by myofibroblasts and to their proliferation resulting in an increase in intima thickness.

Clinical features

Comprehensive in-depth prospective clinical investigations have been reported from several centres during the last decades, contributing greatly to what we consider as classical knowledge today (Bengtsson and Malmvall 1981; Hunder 1997). Beside systemic signs of inflammation, the clinical features are most variable depending on which vessels are affected by the inflammatory process.

At presentation, the symptoms might be misinterpreted as an infectious disorder since over 90 per cent of the patients are febrile. The temperature curve does not follow a characteristic pattern. Chills and fever spikes of 39°C have been reported, although some develop subfebrility. Other common symptoms are weight loss, fatigue, and anorexia. The referring physician may have made a tentative diagnosis of virosis, pneumonia, malignancy, or fever of unknown origin. In larger series, about 20 per cent of the patients report an acute onset of the disease, often specifying a certain day when the symptoms started. However, in the majority of cases the onset is more insidious, progressing during some weeks or even months.

Systemic symptoms alone are more uncommon. Muscular discomfort from shoulders, neck, and/or hips is reported in about half the patients with GCA. Cranial symptoms usually manifest in various ways, headache being the most common sign. The headache in GCA is sometimes superficial or mild, resembling tension headache, but at times it is very severe, with burning sensations and paroxysms of lanciating pain; even the slightest pressure when resting the head on a pillow or combing the hair will give rise to intense pain. Scalp tenderness is a very specific diagnostic symptom encountered in only 2–3 per cent of patients without GCA. Most often the cranial symptoms are specific, localized to one or both temporal regions or in the forehead or occiput. Difficulties in opening and closing the mouth or complaint of pain on mastication or swallowing might give rise to a suspicion of a disease of the temporomandibular joint (Plate 151). At examination some patients show tenderness along the carotid vessels. Moreover, the temporal artery may appear swollen, sometimes nodular and tender with diminished pulsations. Exceptionally, the occipital arteries are swollen and painful. Not only tender, swollen arteries, but also clinically normal vessels may show histological inflammation. Since GCA is a generalized disease, mainly affecting medium-sized and large arteries, it may cause ischaemic lesions in various organs. GCA may thus be life-threatening by affecting vessels such as the coronaries, or the cerebral arteries. It may also cause aortic rupture. Fatal GCA cases might be less often detected today due to decreasing frequencies of autopsies and the fact that microscopic examination of the arteries is not routinely performed.

Hamrin contributed to our knowledge concerning the engagement of the aorta and its large branches by his meticulous clinical examinations reporting murmurs over large arteries and by describing the aortic arch syndrome, defined as a difference in blood pressure between the arms exceeding 25 mmHg (Hamrin 1972). Evans calculated that the risk for GCA patients to get thoracic aortic aneurysms was 17.3 times (95 per cent confidence interval 7.9–33) the risk in the general population (Evans et al. 1994a,b). The corresponding risk for abdominal aortic aneurysms was 2.4 (95 per cent CI 0.8–5.5). In Göteborg, Sweden aortic aneurysms were found in 6 per 90 patients (Andersson et al. 1986). Cerebral infarction has been reported in less than 10 per cent of consecutive patients with biopsy-proven GCA. Manifestations of occlusive changes in large arteries such as extremity claudication or Raynaud's phenomenon are present in 10–15 per cent. Peripheral neuropathies or mononeuropathies may affect upper or lower extremities.

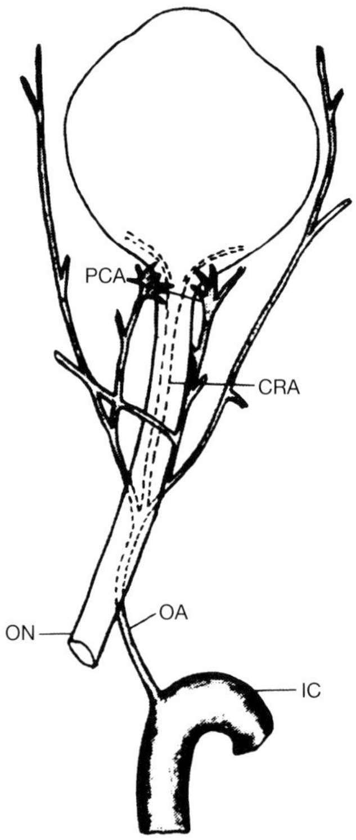

Fig. 1 Artery supply of the eye. IC, internal carotid artery; OA, ophthalmic artery; CRA, central retinal artery; PCA, posterior ciliary artery; ON, optic nerve.

Visual impairment in GCA

Permanent visual loss is one of the most dreaded manifestations of GCA, often occurring early or even as the very first clinical sign of the disease. Blindness might be partial or complete. Other visual symptoms include transient or permanent diplopia or ptosis. Loss of vision in GCA is caused by inflammatory lesions in the arteries supplying the eye, thereby compromising the blood flow to the optic nerve head (anterior ischaemic optic neuropathy, AION) or the retina (retinal stroke). The ophthalmic artery arises from the internal carotid artery and its branches supply the eye (Fig. 1). Two or three short posterior ciliary arteries are the only sources of blood to the optic nerve head. Involvement of one of these vessels results in sectorial defects. The central retinal artery supplies the retina. The eye muscles receive blood from the branches of the opthalmic artery which anastomose abundantly with vessel branches from the external carotid artery which possibly explains the transient nature of diplopia due to eye muscle paralysis.

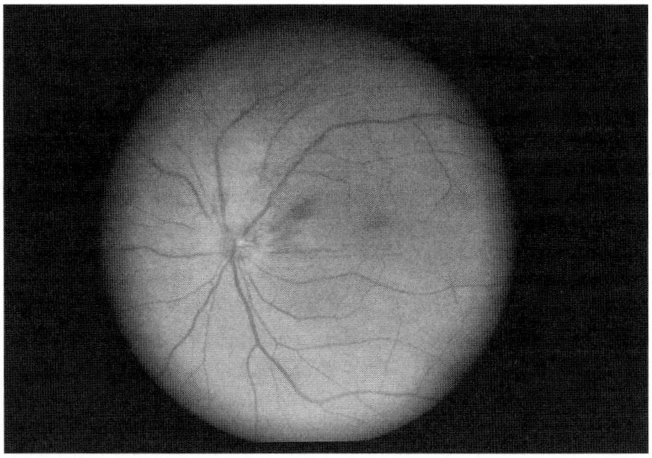

Fig. 2 AION in a 76-year-old male patient with biopsy-proven temporal arteritis. Note the prominent oedema of the optic disc. Its inferior sectors are swollen and pale, and surrounded by haemorrhages.

Fundoscopic findings in GCA

Early fundoscopic examination is most valuable. In the acute phase of AION, the optic disc is pale and swollen whereas the retina appears almost normal (Fig. 2). Within 4–6 weeks, the optic disc becomes atrophic, with a chalky appearance. If the arteritic process strikes the central retinal artery, the retina will appear greyish swollen due to ischaemic damage of the ganglion cells and a contrasting red zone, 'cherry red spot', can be seen in the macula. In patients without eye involvement, the ophthalmologic examination is generally normal.

Visual outcome in GCA

In early reports, the incidence of visual loss in GCA was about 30–60 per cent, whereas in more recent studies the outcome is more favourable with an estimation of blindness in 7–15 per cent. Most amaurotic cases experience the visual loss *before* the institution of corticosteroid therapy and the visual impairment is usually non-progressive. Hence, visual loss that has not occurred within 1 week after start of treatment, is exceptional (Hayreh 1991). The transient visual loss, *amaurosis fugax*, indicates a medical emergency, prompting immediate corticosteroid treatment, to avoid permanent blindness. Unfortunately, bilateral involvement of the eyes does still occur, with affection of the second eye within a week after the first one, unless therapy is instituted. AION causes 80–90 per cent of the visual deficit in GCA patients. Once established, visual impairment usually becomes permanent, although, a certain improvement after the start of corticosteroid therapy has been reported. The probability to develop further visual loss after treatment was started was only 1 per cent over a 5-year follow-up (Hunder 1997).

Laboratory investigations

There are no specific laboratory tests for the detection of GCA. Moderate normochromic anaemia accompanied with a slight leucocytosis and thrombocytosis is frequently seen. Eosinophilia is not observed. The erythrocyte sedimentation rate (ESR) is generally markedly elevated and parallells other acute-phase proteins, such as C-reactive protein (CRP), fibrinogen, and haptoglobin. An ESR greater than 50 mm/h was required as one of three criteria to make the diagnosis, according to the 1990 ACR set of criteria. In about 10 per cent of the patients, the ESR is below 50 or even normal, also in patients displaying arteritis on their temporal artery biopsy. Therefore, an ESR of more than 30 mm/h is usually regarded as significant in most centres. The ESR correlates with the disease activity in GCA, although CRP, usually falls more rapidly, and is often normalized within a week after treatment has been started (Hunder 1997). Levels of circulating IL-6 were shown to normalize within a few hours on corticosteroid treatment. However, so far, the clinical use of IL-6 has not been evaluated, and the ESR is still regarded the best laboratory test to follow disease activity and as a guide for treatment.

Rheumatoid factors, antinuclear antibodies, or other specific antibodies are not found in sera of GCA patients. Liver function tests are mildly abnormal, with an increase in alkaline phosphatase as the most common abnormality; liver biopsy rarely shows portal or intralobular inflammation with focal liver cell necrosis or small epitheloid cell granulomas. Renal functional tests are characteristically normal and so are muscle enzymes. Muscle biopsies show normal histology.

The plasma levels of von Willebrand factor (vWF) are increased in patients with GCA. Unlike the acute phase protein levels, vWF does not decrease with corticosteroid therapy (Cid et al. 1996). Elevated levels of circulating vWF have been suggested to be a marker of endothelial dysfunction in vasculitis. Persistent high levels of vWF might reflect sub-clinical disease with continued endothelial activation due to the stimulation by cytokines released from circulating monocytes. However, the serum level of vWF was neither a helpful guide in clinical management nor useful in the prediction of relapse or the risk of vascular complications (Nordborg et al. 1991). Furthermore, multiple conditions affect the vWF concentration, especially in elderly patients; vWF is, for example, associated with atherosclerosis and its risk factors. The consequence of continued high concentrations of vWF in GCA during therapy is not yet known. Provided that more sensitive assays become available, one or more parameters might be helpful in the future to differentiate between clinically silent cases with a remaining corticosteroid requiring inflammatory activity and those with true remission.

Diagnosis

The ACR criteria of 1990, have not been considered truly diagnostic. The histological confirmation of a positive temporal artery biopsy is still the most well-established means to make the diagnosis. GCA is an important differential diagnosis in patients over 50 years, presenting with systemic illness, in particular if additional symptoms, suggestive of underlying arteritis are apparent. Such symptoms should be asked for also when patients present with polymyalgia rheumatica. Furthermore, palpation of the vessels of head, neck, and arms and the auscultation for arterial bruits are mandatory, besides blood pressure measurement in both arms.

Since the symptoms are often non-specific in GCA, a large number of other conditions must be considered such as chronic arthritides, connective tissue diseases, endocrinopathies, malignancies, and infections. A temporal artery biopsy should always be carried out on subjects presenting symptoms suggestive of GCA. Selecting nodular, swollen, or tender segments of the temporal artery increases the chance of getting histological proof. The high rate of negative biopsies can be attributed to the focal, patchy nature of the inflammatory lesions. Lesions may be as short as some 100 μm. It is, therefore, important to remove 3–5 cm long segments of the artery and to examine it carefully at short intervals. Current data show that the inflammatory infiltrate remains in the vessel wall for at least 2 weeks after the start of corticosteroid treatment and sometimes much longer (Evans et al. 1994a,b). An angiographic examination of the aortic arch and its branches should be performed in patients with symptoms of large artery involvement. The typical pattern in GCA includes stenoses or occlusions with a smooth, tapered appearance, alternating with areas of normal or increased vessel calibre. Angiography has traditionally been the diagnostic modality used, but there is an increasing reliance upon non-invasive procedures such as computed tomography (CT), magnetic resonance imaging (MRI), and ultrasonography. Ultrasonography was shown to detect signs of vasculitis with high sensitivity and specificity. Still, the use of modern high-resolution scanners is essential. Compared with angiography, CT and MRI scanning are considered to be better diagnostic methods when it comes to the detection of aneurysmal disease. Furthermore, standard CT imaging with contrast enhancement, certain MRI sequences, as well as ultrasound permit the identification of oedema and other inflammatory markers in the vessel wall, which is important for the evaluation of disease activity.

Treatment

Once the diagnosis of GCA has been established, treatment with glucocorticosteroids should be instituted. The purpose of the treatment is two-fold. On the one hand it aims at preventing vascular catastrophes, and on the other, at relieving painful symptoms (Box 1). A characteristic feature of GCA is the prompt improvement of symptoms within the first week upon the initiation of corticosteroid therapy. In fact, in the absence of a rapid response the correctness of the diagnosis should be questioned. Opinions vary when it comes to the initial dosage. Most centres agree that 40–60 mg of prednisolone, given as a single morning dose, is an appropriate starting dose, provided there are no occular symptoms. In patients with occular symptoms or severe vascular complications, 0.5 g methylprednisolone should be administered intravenously, twice daily or more often during the first days. Generally, a reduction of 5 mg each week during the first months is recommended, although, relapses require more extended treatment. When the dosage is 15 mg/day, a further reduction by 2.5 mg every 2–4 weeks is recommended, with close monitoring of clinical and laboratory status. Most patients reach a maintenance dosage of 2.5–7.5 mg/day of prednisolone within the first year. Once the disease is stable, a reduction of the maintenance dosage by a further 1 mg/month is sometimes possible. Other treatment schedules of corticosteroids such as intramuscular methylprednisolone or alternate day administration have not been successful in GCA; furthermore, such treatment did not minimize the development of steroid-induced osteoporosis. Despite, the confirmed preventive effect on fatal vascular complications, long-term corticosteroid therapy is associated with well-known co-morbidities, such as diabetes mellitus, vertebral crush fractures, hip fractures, cataract, and peptic ulcer. Therefore, corticosteroid-sparing therapy has been requested in GCA. Various approaches, including combined therapy with cytotoxic agents (azathioprine, methotrexate, cyclosporin) have been suggested. To date, the majority of available studies in this field are inconclusive. Methotrexate is the drug that holds the best promise. Controlled studies will reveal whether new drugs such as leflunomide, mycophenolate, and biological TNF α blocking agents may be successful in the treatment of GCA.

Bone-sparing agents including calcium and vitamin D should be given generously to patients with GCA and in combination with other bone sparing agents, guided by the results of bone density of hip and/or lumbar spine by DEXA (dual X-ray absorptiometry).

In conclusion, corticosteroids remain the cornerstone in the treatment of GCA. There is at present little evidence that corticosteroids can be replaced by other compounds, emphasizing the unique role of steroid-mediated immunosuppression in this form of vasculitis.

Disease course and outcome

Fatal complications, such as rupture of aortic aneurysms, cerebral and myocardial infarction, stresses the importance of detecting GCA at an early stage. The preventive effect of corticosteroid treatment is indicated by a significantly reduced risk of severe occular catastrophes, as well as the favourable long-term outcome in follow-up studies. The overall mortality rate is not increased compared with the general population (Hunder 1997).

Box 1 Flow diagram of the management of giant cell arteritis that forms the basis of our practice

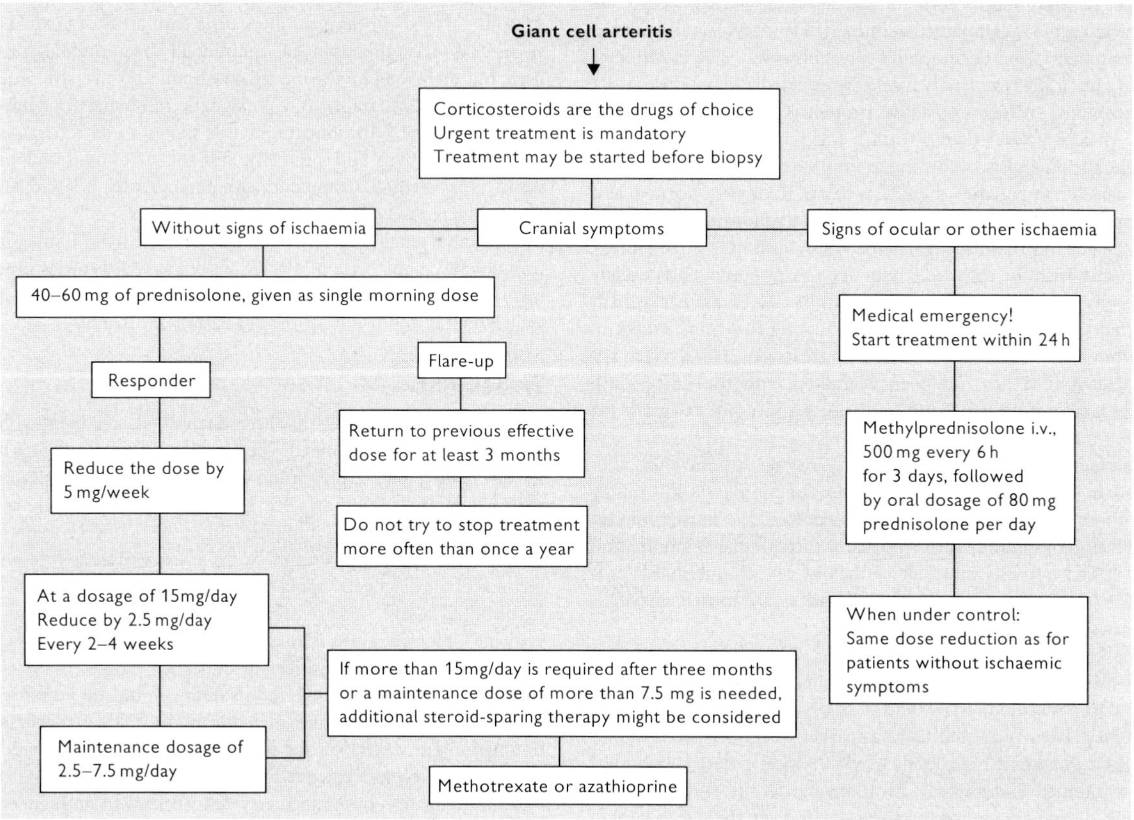

Traditionally, GCA has been considered to be fairly benign, running a self-limiting course. Although corticosteroid therapy can eventually be discontinued in most patients, the disease course is, however, unpredictable. The median duration of treatment is about 5 years, whereas a shorter disease course of 2 years was reported from the United States (Andersson et al. 1986; Hunder 1997).

Although corticosteroid treatment suppresses the symptoms of GCA, there is no absolute proof that the treatment actually influences the duration of the disease. Thus, GCA, shows a remarkable tendency to relapse and lesions showing active arteritis have been found in patients considered to be in clinical remission for months or even years. Evans and colleagues recently demonstrated that patients considered to be in clinical remission run an increased risk of developing aortic aneurysms late in the disease course (Evans et al. 1994a,b). Thus, pathogenetic processes may progress long after clinical remission. The reason why some patients develop a self-limiting response to a supposed antigen while others have an active response for years, or sometimes indefinitely, is not known.

Takayasu's disease

In 1908, Takayasu reported peculiar arteriovenous anastomoses around the optic papillae in a 21-year old woman (Takayasu 1908). It was later realized that this was the ocular manifestation of a type of large vessel vasculitis, which is frequent in Japan. TA (pulseless disease, aortic arch arteritis, or nonspecific aorto-arteritis) is a chronic granulomatous panarteritis with a predilection for the aorta and its major branches. The inflammation of the blood vessels generally causes stenosis or occlusion, although aortic aneurysms may also develop (Kerr 1994).

Epidemiology

The disease typically affects young women (10–30 years in 70–90 per cent), although children and individuals over 40 years of age have been reported. There is a female:male ratio of about 4 : 1 (Kerr 1994). The incidence and prevalence are not known in detail. Large series have been reported from Japan, India, China, Thailand, and Korea (Hata et al. 1996; Hoffman 1996). It is infrequent in Caucasian populations, with an incidence of 2.6 per million inhabitants a year in North America (Kerr 1994), even rarer in other European countries. However infrequent it may be outside Asia and South America, a diagnosis of TA cannot be excluded on the basis of age, race, or gender.

Aetiology and pathogenesis

The aetiology and pathogenesis of TA are unknown. It has been linked to a variety of infectious agents including spirochetes, bacteria, mycobacteria, and viruses. There is, however, no convincing evidence that any of them play an aetiopathogenetic role. Occasionally, an association with other autoimmune diseases such as juvenile rheumatoid arthritis, adult Still's disease, systemic lupus erythematosus, erythema nodosum, inflammatory bowel disease, and spodylarthropathies have been reported. Whether these links reflect true aetiopathogenetic association or chance occurrence is unclear.

TA targets large arteries with well-developed elastic membranes. In contrast to GCA, the inflammation frequently involves intracranial arteries (Kerr 1994). The cellular infiltrates tend to be localized in the adventitia and the outer part of the media with a marked inflammation of the vasa vasorum. Cytotoxic T lymphocytes, recognizing heat-shock proteins, have been proposed to be responsible for tissue destruction. The scarce availability of samples from involved tissues has largely restricted the application of modern immunohistochemical and molecular techniques in the investigation of this disorder.

Genetic factors in TA

The strong predilection for young women, a high incidence in Asian and South American countries, as well as familial clustering, suggest that host genetic factors govern the susceptibility to TA. There is no clear association with class II HLA antigens but class I antigens are prevalent with a positive association to HLA-B5 in India and to one of its variants, B52, in patients from Japan and Korea (Kerr 1994). However, there is no such association in North American or Mexican patients.

The variation of disease expression in different ethnic settings might indicate a heterogenous group of vascular disorders. Detailed genetic studies might help to identify whether Eastern and Western TA are similar or distinct disease entities.

Clinical description

The clinical presentation is related to a combination of various non-specific systemic symptoms and the particular vessels involved. Constitutional symptoms such as malaise, fever, and night sweats are regularly recorded. Traditionally, TA has been characterized as a disease of progressive clinical stages with an initial systemic phase, followed by an active vascular inflammatory phase, subsequently ending up with a fibrous pulseless 'burned-out' stage. Although progressive stages might occur in some patients, increasing evidence have shown that such a scheme is of limited value and does not accurately reflect the status of the blood vessel inflammation. Furthermore, in the large series from the National Institutes of Health, only a minority of patient reported 'stages' of the disease (Kerr 1994). The most prevalent vascular symptoms in this large cohort were upper extremity claudication, hypertension, pain over the carotid arteries (caritodynia), dizziness, and visual abnormalities. More than 50 per cent expressed musculoskeletal manifestations such as myalgias and chest wall pain. Although synovites are characteristically mild, joint pain may be severe. Other vessel-related features include abdominal pain, ischaemic cardiac, or renal disease and pulmonary hypertention. In contrast to patients with GCA, intracranial arteries are major targets in TA. Cutaneous lesions resembling erythema nodosum are occasionally seen, whereas ischaemic retinopathy, originally reported by Takayasu, is rare. Vascular symptoms depend both on the anatomical location of the involved artery and on the nature of the lesion, be it stenotic or occlusive. Symptoms such as dizziness, syncope, visual changes, vertigo, and arm claudication are more common in patients from Japan and the United States, whereas, hypertention is more characteristic in Indian patients due to a higher frequency of abdominal aortic and renal artery stenosis (Kerr 1994; Hata et al. 1996). This ethnic and geographical variation in TA-disease expression may indicate aetiopathogenetic heterogeneity.

Diagnosis of TA

TA should be considered when a young patient presents with ischaemic symptoms related to large vessels and/or hypertension, in particular if systemic symptoms are also present. The diagnosis of TA is commonly delayed (Kerr 1994). At the time of admission, approximately 20 per cent of patients are clinically asymptomatic. A careful physical examination is mandatory in patients with TA. Bruits over the aorta and its major branches is found in about one-third of the patients, as is hypertension, related to the involvement of renal arteries or stenosis of the thoracic or upper abdominal aorta. Reduced or absent pulses of large arteries as well as a blood pressure discrepancy of more than 20 mmHg between the arms or legs are commonly seen. Laboratory tests show non-specific changes related to chronic inflammation such as anaemia, elevated sedimentation rate, hypoalbuminaemia, and hypergammaglobulinaemia. The ESR is not helpful in assessing the disease. One-third of the patients with clinically active disease presented with normal ESR, whereas in 56 per cent the ESR remained elevated despite clinical remission (Kerr 1994). Invasive angiography remains the best method to assess the extent and severety of the lesions and it is essential for the planning of interventional treatment such as bypass grafting and percutaneous angioplasty. Whereas angiography displays luminal changes, it does not distinguish between stenosis caused by active inflammation and fibrous scarring. Moreover, invasive methods carry a risk of complications. Technical improvement of non-invasive methods, such as CT and MRI, will permit serial evaluation of the inflammatory progression of the vessel wall and permit its comparison with clinical parameters, thus assessing if vascular changes are related to active clinical disease or not.

According to the 1990 classification criteria proposed by the ACR (Arend et al. 1990), at least three of the following six criteria are required to achieve a diagnosic sensitivity of 90.5 per cent and a specificity of 97.8 per cent; age less than 40 years, claudication of the extremities, decreased brachial artery pulse, blood pressure difference greater than 10 mmHg between the right and left arm, bruits over subclavian arteries or aorta or arteriographic abnormality. The existing diagnostic criteria of TA are not perfect, since they are not always fulfilled in patients with lesions restricted to the aorta, the renal arteries, or the pulmonary arteries. Moreover, previous criteria regarded age less than 40 years as obligatory.

Since the clinical expression varies between ethnic groups, the classification schemes adopted in the United States may not be valid in other parts of the world. The major challenge for the future in the management of TA includes better diagnostic criteria as well as improved monitoring of disease activity.

Treatment and course of disease

Treatment guidelines, have been suggested from Japan and the United States (Kerr 1994; Hoffman 1996). Corticosteroids (prednisolone) is the recommended first choice treatment of TA. While most patients with GCA respond satisfactorily to corticosteroid therapy, treatment failure is not uncommon in TA. Systemic symptoms respond well, but those related to occlusion or stenosis due to active vasculitis, such as claudication and extremity pain, have been reported to respond less well in about 20 per cent of the patients (Kerr 1994). A remitting and relapsing course is characteristic. Incomplete initial response and relapse during tapering of corticosteroids calls for additional treatment. Methotrexate may control constitutional symptoms and stabilize vascular lesions by symptomatic and angiographic criteria. Most TA patients suffer substantial morbidity during the progress of the disease including cardiac symptoms with aortic insufficiency, coronary artery disease, or congestive heart failure. The long-term outcome varies between different studies. Disease-related mortality is usually caused by congestive heart failure, cerebrovascular events, myocardial infarction, aortic aneurysm rupture, or renal failure. Statistically significant predictors of poor outcome include a progressive disease course, as well as the presence of major complications such as Takayasu's retinopathy, secondary hypertention, aortic valve insufficiency, and aneurysms (Ishikawa and Maetoni 1994).

Surgical treatment is required in up to 50 per cent of the cases (Kerr 1994) due to renal artery stenosis, extremity ischaemia, stenosis of cerebral vessels, aortic regurgitation, and coronary artery stenosis. Outcome figures were improved if the surgical intervention was performed during an inactive stage of the disease.

Cogan's syndrome

Cogan's syndrome is a rare disease of young people, with a median age at onset of 24 years (Vollertsen et al. 1986). In typical cases, the initial manifestations are ocular (interstitial keratitis) and audiovestibular, generally appearing within a couple of months. Systemic vasculitis is rare, but aortitis with aneurysm formation or aortic insufficiency, which develops in about 10 per cent, is the most serious manifestation, accounting for the majority of deaths. Audiovestibular symptoms such as partial or total hearing loss, vertigo, and ataxia, characteristically appear abruptly. With time the vestibular symptoms usually improve, whereas hearing rarely returns to normal.

Since no definite serologic or histologic markers exist, the diagnosis of Cogan's syndrome is entirely clinical. Non-specific constitutional features are common, including anaemia, leucocytosis, fever, malaise, and weight loss.

The acute audiovestibular symptoms usually respond to high doses of corticosteroids, although the addition of a cytotoxic agent, such as methotrexate or cyclosporine is sometimes required. The interstitial keratitis usually responds to topical corticosteroids. The course and outcome of the disease are variable, with periods of flares and remissions during many years. Unfortunately, nearly half of the patients become totally deaf (Vollertsen et al. 1986). Aortic valve replacement and surgical repair of aortic aneurysms may be required.

Other vasculitides affecting large vessels

The key to a correct diagnosis of the many different forms of vasculitis is a high index of suspicion. Aortic lesions and involvement of large vessels that may mimic GCA, TA, or Cogan's syndrome may occur in other vasculitides, most of them very rare such as relapsing polychondritis, spondyloarthropathies, Behçet's disease, polyarteritis nodosa, and Buerger's disease. Other causes of large vessel involvement are the infection-related arteritides, among which syphilis was reported to be the most common cause during the nineteenth century. Studying 20 591 autopsies in Malmö, Sweden, during 1957–1971 Östberg found that of 443 aortic aneurysms, 85 per cent were caused by atherosclerosis, 8 per cent by syphilis, and 7 per cent by GCA (Östberg 1972). Other microorganisms may exceptionally cause large vessel arteritis, including bacteria (Staphylococcus, Streptococcus, Pneumococcus, Klebsiella, Pseudomonas, Salmonella, Haemophilus, and *Mycobacterium tuberculosis*) and fungi (Candida, Aspergillos, Coccidioides, and Histoplasma).

References

Andersson, R., Malmvall, B.E., and Bengtsson, B.Å. (1986). Long-term survival in giant cell arteritis including temporal arteritis and polymyalgia rheumatica. A follow-up study of 90 patients treated with corticosteroids. *Acta Medica Scandinavica* **220**, 361–4.

Arend, W.P. et al. (1990). The American College of Rheumatology 1990 criteria for the classification of Takayasu arteritis. *Arthritis and Rheumatism* **33**, 1129–34.

Bengtsson, B.Å. and Malmvall, B.E. (1981). The epidemiology of giant cell arteritis including temporal arteritis and polymyalgia rheumatica. Incidences of different clinical presentations and eye complications. *Arthritis and Rheumatism* **24**, 899–904.

Cid, M.C. et al. (1989). Immunohistochemical analysis of lymphoid and macrophage cell subsets and their immunologic activation markers in temporal arteritis. *Arthritis and Rheumatism* **32**, 884–930.

Cid, M.C. et al. (1996). Von Willebrand Factor in the outcome of temporal arteritis. *Annals of the Rheumatic Diseases* **55**, 927–30.

Cutolo, M., Sulli, A., Seriolo, B., Accardo, S., and Masi, A.T. (1995). Estrogens, the immune response and autoimmunity. *Clinical and Experimental Rheumatology* **13**, 217–26.

Duhaut, P. et al. (1999). Giant cell arteritis and polymyalgia rheumatica: are pregnancies a protective factor? A prospective multicentre case–control study. *Rheumatology* **38**, 118–23.

Evans, J.M., Batts, K.P., and Hunder, G.G. (1994a). Persistent giant cell arteritis despite corticosteroid treatment. *Mayo Clinic Proceedings* **69**, 1060–1.

Evans, J.M., Bowles, C., Björnsson, J., Mullany, C.G., and Hunder, G.G. (1994b). Thoracic aortic aneurysm and rupture in giant cell arteritis. *Arthritis and Rheumatism* **37**, 1539–47.

Gilmore, J.R. (1941). Giant cell arteritis. *Journal of Pathology and Bacteriology* **53**, 263–77.

Hamrin, B. (1972). Polymyalgia arteritica. *Acta Medica Scandinavica* **192** (Suppl.), 533.

Hata, A., Noda, M., Moriwaki, R., and Numano, F. (1996). Angiographic findings of Takayasu's arteritis: new classification. *International Journal of Cardiology* **54** (Suppl.), 155–63.

Haugeberg, G., Bie, R.B., and Nordbo, S.A. (2000a). Chlamydia pneumoniae was not detected in temporal artery biopsies from patients with temporal arteritis. *Scandinavian Journal of Rheumatology* **29**, 127–8.

Haugeberg, G., Paulsen, P.Q., and Bie, R.B. (2000b). Temporal arteritis in Vest Agder County in Southern Norway: incidence and clinical findings. *Journal of Rheumatology* **27**, 2624–7.

Hayreh, S.S. (1991). Ophthalmic features of giant cell arteritis. *Clinical Rheumatology* **5**, 431–69.

Hoffman, G.S. (1996). Takayasu's arteritis: lessons from the American National Institutes of Health experience. *International Journal of Cardiology* **54** (Suppl.), 83–6.

Horton, B.T., Magath, T.B., and Brown, G.F. (1932). An undescribed form of arteritis of the temporal vessels. *Mayo Clinic Proceedings* **7**, 700–1.

Hunder, G.G. (1997). Giant cell arteritis and polymyalgia rheumatica. *Medical Clinics of North America* **81**, 195–219.

Hunder, G.G. et al. (1990). The American College of Rheumatology 1990 criteria for the classification of giant cell (temporal) arteritis. *Arthritis and Rheumatism* **33**, 1122–8.

Hutchinson, J. (1890). Diseases of the arteries. On a peculiar form of thrombotic arteritis of the aged which is sometimes productive of gangrene. *Archives of Surgery* **1**, 323–9.

Ishikawa, K. and Maetoni, S. (1994). Long-term outcome for 120 Japanese patients with Takayasu's disease: clinical and statistical analyses of related prognostic factors. *Circulation* **90**, 1855.

Jennette, J.C. et al. (1994). Nomenclature of systemic vasculitides. Proposal of an international consensus conference. *Arthritis and Rheumatism* **37**, 187–92.

Kerr, G.S. (1994). Takayasu's arteritis. *Current Opinion in Rheumatology* **6**, 32–8.

Kou, C.C. et al. (1995). *Chlamydia pneumoniae* (TWAR) review. *Clinical Microbiology Review* **8**, 451–61.

Machado, E.B.V. et al. (1988). Trends in incidence and clinical presentation of temporal arteritis in Olmsted county, Minnesota, 1950–85. *Arthritis and Rheumatism* **31**, 745–9.

Nordborg, C., Nordborg, E., and Petursdottir, V. (2000). Giant cell arteritis. Epidemiology, etiology and pathogenesis. Review article. *Acta Pathologica, Microbiologica et Immunologica Scandinavica (APMIS)* **108**, 713–24.

Nordborg, E. (2000). Epidemiology of biopsy-positive giant cell arteritis: an overview. *Clinical and Experimental Rheumatology* **18** (Suppl. 20), 15–17.

Nordborg, E. and Nordborg, C. (1998). The inflammatory reaction in giant cell arteritis. An immunohistochemical study. *Clinical and Experimental Rheumatology* **16**, 165–8.

Nordborg, E., Andersson, R., Tengborn, L., Eden, S., and Bengtsson, B.Å. (1991). Von Willebrand Factor and plasminogen activator inhibition in giant cell arteritis. *Annals of the Rheumatic Diseases* **50**, 316–20.

Östberg, G. (1971). Temporal arteritis in a large necropsy series. *Annals of the Rheumatic Diseases* **30**, 224.

Östberg, G. (1972). Morphological changes in large arteries in polymyalgia arteritica. *Acta Medica Scandinavia* **533**, 135–64.

Petursdottir, V., Nordborg, E., and Nordborg, C. (1996). Atrophy of the aortic media in giant cell arteritis. *Acta Pathologica, Microbiologica et Immunologica Scandinavica (APMIS)* **104**, 191–8.

Petursdottir, V., Johansson, H., Nordborg, E., and Nordborg, C. (1999).The epidemiology of biopsy-positive giant cell arteritis: special reference to cyclic fluctuations. *Rheumatology* **38**, 1208–12.

Russo, M.G., Waxman, J., Abdoh, A.A., and Serebro, L.H. (1995). Correlation between infection and the onset of the giant cell (temporal) arteritis syndrome. A trigger mechanism? *Arthritis and Rheumatism* **38**, 374–80.

Takayasu (1908). Case with unusual changes of the central vessels of the retina. *Acta Societatis Ophthalmologica Japonica* **21**, 554.

Vollertsen, R.S., Mc Donald, T.J., Younge, B.R., Banks, P.M., Stanson, A.W., and Ilstrup, D.M. (1986). Cogan's syndrome: 18 cases and a review of the literature. *Mayo Clinic Proceedings* **61**, 344–61.

Wagner, A.D, Björnsson, J., Bartley, G.B., Goronzy, J.J., and Weyand, C.M. (1996). Interferon-γ-producing T cells in giant cell vasculitis represent a minority of tissue-infiltrating cells and are located distant from the site of pathology. *American Journal of Pathology* **148**, 1925–33.

Wagner, A.D. et al. (2000). Detection of *Chlamydia pneumoniae* in giant cell vasculitis and correlation with the topographic arrangement of tissue-infiltrating dendritic cells. *Arthritis and Rheumatism* **43**, 1543–51.

Watts, R.A., Gonzalez-Gay, M., Lane, S.E., Garcia-Porrua, C., Bentham, G., and Scott, D.G. (2001). Geoepidemiology of systemic vasculitis. *Annals of the Rheumatic Diseases* **60**, 170–2.

Weyand, C.M. (1996). Correlation of the topographical arrangement and the functional pattern of tissue-infiltrating macrophages in giant cell arteritis. *Journal of Clinical Investigation* **98**, 1642–9.

Weyand, C.M, Hunder, N.N., Hicok, K.C., Hunder, G.G., and Goronzy, J.J. (1994). HLA–DRB1 alleles in polymyalgia rheumatica, giant cell arteritis and rheumatoid arthritis. *Arthritis and Rheumatism* **37**, 514–20.

Wood, C.A. *A memorandum Book of a Tenth Century Oculist, a Translation of Tadkivat of Ali Ibn Isa.* Chicago IL: Northwestern University Press, 1936.

6.10.6 Polymyalgia rheumatica

B. Dasgupta and Shubhada Kalke

Introduction

Polymyalgia rheumatica (PMR) and giant cell arteritis (GCA) are inflammatory rheumatic diseases predominantly seen in the elderly. Their importance derives from:

(i) the high prevalence (many surveys list PMR as the commonest rheumatic indication for long-term steroid intake) (Walsh et al. 1996),

(ii) the difficulties in disentangling PMR from other causes of the polymyalgic syndrome,

(iii) the neuro-ophthalmic complications of GCA, and

(iv) the need for careful disease assessment to maintain an acceptable balance between benefits and risks of long-term steroid therapy.

History

PMR and GCA have probably been present in Europe for several centuries. In the tenth century, Ali Ibn Isa, an Arab physician from Baghdad described temporal artery inflammation associated with headaches and visual disturbances. Jan van Eyck's portrait of Canon Van der Paele in 1436 and the portrait of Francesco Gambetti by Piero di Cosimo in 1505 are impressive representations of temporal arteritis (Dequeker 1987). There are indications in the literature that Canon Van der Paele had symptoms suggestive of PMR.

Bruce described PMR as senile rheumatic gout (Bruce 1988). Bagratuni described the articular manifestations in 1953 but the term PMR was coined by Barber (Barber 1957; Bagratuni 1963). It was felt that the disease was a mild form of rheumatoid arthritis (RA), which did not progress to erosive inflammation.

Hutchinson reported an elderly man with painful temporal arteries, and Horton described the pathology of temporal arteritis (Hutchinson 1890; Horton et al. 1932). The link between the two conditions has been recognized for the last 40 years (Poulley and Hughes 1960). Hamrin used the term polymyalgia arteritica for both diseases (Hamrin et al. 1964).

Definitions

PMR is characterized by pain and stiffness, usually of sudden onset, affecting the limb girdle areas (shoulder, hip), neck, and torso. Some definitions stipulate minimum disease duration and others include a rapid response to low dose steroids. There is also a need to exclude other conditions, for example, RA, chronic infection, inflammatory muscle disease, and neoplasia. GCA (also known as temporal arteritis) affects the cranial branches of arteries arising from the aortic arch, most typically the superficial temporal artery. Both conditions are characterized by an acute phase response. The diagnostic criteria for PMR are summarized in Table 1 (see classification criteria for GCA in Chapter 6.10.5).

Epidemiology

GCA is the commonest of the vasculitides and PMR is even commoner. Age and female sex are risk factors for PMR and GCA. There is an increasing incidence with successive decades and the female preponderance increases in the older age groups. The age adjusted incidence rates for these linked conditions is 2.5–3 times higher in females than in males. Both conditions are common in Caucasians especially of Northern European stock and in populations of Anglo-Saxon origin. They are rare among Asians and Blacks. There appears to be a positive correlation between incidence and the latitude of the geographic area. This reflects in the high incidence figures from Northern Europe such as the Scandinavian countries and from northern parts of the United States. There are wide variations in incidence rates. The annual incidence rate of PMR varies in different studies from 12.7 to 68.3 and that of GCA from 9.3 to 27 per 100 000 persons aged 50 and older (Table 2). An increased incidence has been noted with age with both PMR and GCA. There is a suggestion of a cyclical pattern with GCA but not with PMR. Siblings with GCA are at increased risk of getting the disease. According to studies in Minnesota and Gothenburg, the incidence of GCA in females is increasing (Nordborg 1995). There is also suggestion that the overall incidence of PMR and GCA has increased in recent years. This may be related to greater awareness of the disease but real epidemiological changes cannot be excluded (Cimmino and Zaccaria 2000).

Environmental agent

Both PMR and GCA may be linked to environmental agents. Their acute onset, association with infections and vaccinations, occurrence in conjugal pairs, and presence of antibodies to intermediate filaments may suggest such an association. There are reports of links with adenovirus, respiratory syncytial virus, *Mycoplasma pneumoniae*, parvovirus B19, *Chlamydia pneumoniae*, and human parainfluenza virus (HPIV) (Cimmino et al. 1993; Gabriel et al. 1999). A prospective case controlled study by Duhaut et al. found a serological association with HPIV type I-IgM titres in French patients with both PMR and GCA, especially in the biopsy positive subset of GCA patients at onset of disease. In this study there was no difference between cases and controls for IgM and IgG serology for measles, respiratory syncytial, and herpes simplex viruses 1 and 2 (Duhaut et al. 1999a,b).

Chlamydia pneumoniae was found by PCR and immunohistochemistry of temporal artery specimens in GCA (Wagner et al. 2000) although this has not been confirmed by other studies. Serological studies for hepatitis B virus, herpes simplex virus, varicella-zoster, Epstein–Barr virus, influenza A and B, parainfluenza type 3, mumps, measles, rotavirus, enterovirus, rubella, leptospira, and Q fever have showed no positive association (Duhaut et al. 2000).

Other environmental risk factors may play a role in development of the disease. There is some evidence that smoking and history of arterial disease are independently associated with PMR/GCA. Null parity and prolonged sun exposure (actinic hypothesis) in genetically predisposed people with skin sensitivity have been described as risk factors. It is suggested that ageing of the immune and neuroendocrine systems may lead to breakdown of tolerance, increased susceptibility to infections and triggering or

Table 1 Diagnostic criteria for PMR

Criteria	Chaung et al. (Mayo clinic) 1982	Healey (Masson clinic) 1984	Bird et al. 1979	Jones and Hazleman 1981
1. Age ≥50 years	+	+	≥65 years	+
2. Bilateral aching of neck, shoulders, pelvic girdle	+ Any two	+ Any two	+ Shoulder pain and/or stiffness	+ Shoulder and pelvic girdle pain without weakness
3. Morning stiffness >1 h	+	+	+	+
4. Duration of symptoms	≥1 month	≥1 month	2 weeks	≥2 months unless treated
5. ESR > 40 mm/h	+	+	+	ESR > 30/ CRP > 6 mg/L
6. Depression and/loss of weight	–	–	+	–
7. Exclusion of other diagnosis	+	+	–	+
8. Rapid response to prednisolone (≤20 mg/day)	–	+	–	+
9. Others	–	–	Bilateral upper arm tenderness	–
Diagnosis	All criteria need to be fulfilled	All criteria need to be fulfilled	Any 3 or 1 plus positive temporal artery biopsy	All criteria need to be fulfilled

Table 2 Epidemiology of PMR and GCA

Country and study	Annual incidence per 100 000 aged 50 or older	
	PMR	GCA
Olmsted County, Minnesota 1972–1992 (Machado et al. 1988)	52.2, prevalence 600	17.8, prevalence 200
Reggio-Emelia, Italy, 1980–1988 (Salvarani et al. 1991)	12.7	6.9
Denmark, 1982–1994 (Elling et al. 1996)	41.3	20.4
South-Norway, 1987–1994 (Gran and Myklebust 1997)	112.6	29
UK, >65 years (Kyle et al. 1985)	400	
Northwestern Spain, 1987–1996 (Gonzalez-Gay et al. 1999)	18.7 (13.5)	

perpetuation of inflammation as a result of relative cortisol deficiency in the elderly (Stevens and Hughes 1995).

Immunogenetics

Familial aggregation and racial differences suggest a role of heredity in susceptibility to PMR and GCA. Early studies showed links between both PMR and GCA and HLA–DR4. DR4 negative patients with PMR/GCA have increased frequency of DR3, DR8, and DR13. There is no difference between HLA–DR4 positive and DR4 negative patients in their clinical presentations.

Weyand et al. have identified a conserved amino acid sequence within the second hypervariable region of the DRB1 in GCA that maps to the antigen binding cleft of HLA–DR (Weyand et al. 1999). Dababneh et al. in 1998 reported the association of HLA–DRB1*0401 with GCA regardless of PMR status (Dababneh et al. 1998). The association of HLA–DRB1*0101 and *0102 though present, was less strong. Patients with isolated PMR showed significant association with DRB1*13 and *14. A weak association between presence of the RA DRB1 shared epitope and GCA (but not with isolated PMR) was seen in this study. The same group in another study has reported association of GCA with higher frequency of relapses with HLA–DR4*0401 (Gonzalez-Gay et al. 1999). A study from Northern Italy does not confirm these findings (Salvarani et al. 1999).

Other genetic polymorphisms have also been studied as factors in susceptibility to PMR/GCA. Such associations have been described with polymorphisms of the tumour necrosis factor gene, interleukin-I gene cluster, and intercellular adhesion molecule-1 (ICAM-1) (Boiardi et al. 2000; Makki et al. 2000; Mattey et al. 2000). Serum soluble (ICAM-1) has been found to be elevated in PMR. Elevated levels of the chemokine RANTES have been reported in PMR, which normalizes with steroid treatment (Pulsatelli et al. 1998).

Immunopathogenesis

The immunogenetic associations suggest a role for cell-mediated immunity in the pathogenesis of these conditions. The levels of CD8 positive T lymphocytes in the peripheral blood (percentage and absolute numbers) may be reduced in PMR (Dasgupta et al. 1989). It is unclear how this relates to disease pathogenesis since the level of CD8 T cells may not be a good indicator of disease activity in PMR and is unable to predict the safe withdrawal of steroids (Corrigal et al. 1997).

Antibodies to intermediate filaments may be found in PMR and GCA. This may suggest an environmental hypothesis since these antibodies are found in viral infections (Dasgupta et al. 1989). Antibodies to cardiolipin and beta 2 GPI have been described in small numbers in both PMR and GCA. Larger longitudinal studies are required to prove whether these may relate to vascular complications. Monoclonal gammopathies have been reported in PMR though changes in the disease activity do not correlate with levels of paraproteinaemia (Stevens and Hughes 1995).

Cytokines may be involved in the pathogenesis. Interleukin-6 (IL-6) and interleukin-1 receptor antagonist levels are significantly increased in untreated PMR and remain elevated compared with controls during therapy (Dasgupta and Panayi 1990; Uddhammar et al. 1998). High levels of interleukin-10 have been reported with mild forms of PMR (Straub et al. 1999). Gamma interferon is reported to correlate with ischaemic symptoms and interleukin-2 with polymyalgic symptoms in cytokine analysis of temporal artery biopsies in GCA.

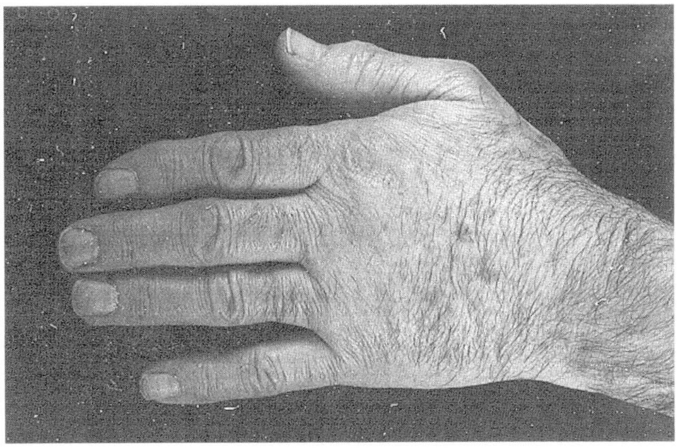

Fig. 1 Hand oedema in the RS3PE syndrome.

Pathology

The pathology in GCA suggests an ongoing local immune response and is described in detail in Chapter 6.10.5. Arteries that originate from the arch of aorta are most commonly affected but any artery or vein can be affected. Superficial temporal, ophthalmic, posterior ciliary, and vertebral arteries are most commonly involved (Plate 152).

Histological changes of inflammation in temporal artery biopsies have been noted in 6–50 per cent PMR patients without overt arteritic symptoms. There are reports of lymphocytic synovitis in the knees, shoulders, and sternoclavicular joints in PMR (Hunder 1997). The majority of the infiltrate consists of macrophages and T cells but no B cells. The T cells are CD45RO positive (Meliconi et al. 1996). There is intense HLA class II staining in lining layer, macrophages, and lymphocytes, but not in the blood vessels. It is suggested that the distribution of soft tissue and bone changes in PMR and remitting seronegative symmetrical synovitis with peripheral oedema are reminiscent of spondyloarthropathy, and that these could be relate to capsular or entheseal pathology (McGonagle et al. 2000). Muscle biopsies in PMR are normal or show non-specific type II muscle fibre atrophy.

Table 3 Neurological manifestations of temporal arteritis

Common
Headache
Amaurosis fugax
Ischaemic optic neuropathy
Less common
Transient ischaemic attacks
Cerebral infarctions
Acute confusional states
Multi-infarct dementia
Ischaemic cervical myelopathy
Ischaemic mononeuropathy

Clinical features

Polymyalgia rheumatica

Arthralgias and myalgias usually develop abruptly and involve proximal parts of extremities. Shoulder girdle pain and morning stiffness are the predominant features at onset in the majority (70–95 per cent). Neck, hip, axial musculature, and tendinous attachments are involved less commonly and only occasionally seen at the onset. The symptoms may be unilateral initially but become subsequently bilateral. Patients may experience significant disability with activities of daily living because of pain and stiffness. Muscle strength is usually unimpaired. In later stages, muscle atrophy or contracture of the shoulder capsule may develop leading to limitation of active and passive movement.

Systemic features like fever, malaise, anorexia, fatigue, and weight loss may occur in up to a third of patients. Although the symptoms are predominantly proximal, peripheral involvement may also occur. This often takes the form of transient synovitis of knees, wrists, and sternoclavicular joints, the remitting, symmetrical seronegative synovitis (RS3PE) syndrome, distal extremity swelling with or without pitting oedema (Fig. 1), carpal tunnel syndrome, and tenosynovitis (Salvarani et al. 1996).

Giant cell arteritis

Headache is the main symptom in more than two-thirds of the patients. It is characteristically a sudden onset, severe, predominantly temporal headache but occasionally may be occipital or even non-localized. The temporal artery may be thickened, tender, red or even non-pulsatile. Scalp tenderness, localized or diffuse, may be present. Tender scalp nodules may develop and there are reports of scalp necrosis. Intermittent claudication of the muscles of mastication, muscles of the tongue and extremities is sometimes seen. A low-grade fever may be seen and patients may present as pyrexia of unknown origin.

Visual symptoms are important early manifestations and include transient and permanent visual loss, diplopia, and ptosis. Early fundoscopy may show slight pallor and oedema of optic disc, scattered cotton-wool exudates, and small haemorrhages due to ischaemic neuritis. Optic atrophy may develop later. Permanent visual loss may be seen in 0–20 per cent of the cases. Risk of permanent visual loss is reported in patients with transient visual loss, jaw claudication, or both. Other neurological manifestations may occur (Table 3).

Large arteries may be involved in 10–15 per cent of the cases, presenting with upper extremity claudication, absent pulses in the neck and arms, Raynaud's and bruits over the carotid, subclavian axillary, and brachial arteries. Thoracic artery aneurysm and dissection of the aorta may rarely complicate GCA. Angina pectoris, congestive heart failure, and myocardial infarction secondary to coronary arteritis have been reported (Hunder 1997).

Relationship between PMR and GCA

PMR is reported in 40–60 per cent patients with GCA and as part of the initial symptom complex in 20–40 per cent. In patients presenting with polymyalgia, the reports of GCA have been between 0 and 80 per cent. This extreme variability depends on whether the diagnosis of GCA is based on clinical grounds or arterial histology and may be biased by clinical practice. For example, the high Scandinavian figures of GCA may be due to biopsing all patients diagnosed as PMR even in the absence of cephalic symptoms. Ten to fifteen per cent of patients with PMR without symptoms of arteritis have been documented to have abnormal temporal artery biopsy. PMR may occur before, simultaneously, or after GCA.

Investigations

Laboratory

Acute phase reactants like ESR and CRP are commonly elevated. So far there is little evidence that there is any difference between the two in measuring disease activity. The initial response of CRP to the corticosteroid treatment has been reported as a prognostic factor in PMR.

Often there is normocytic normochromic anemia, high platelet count, mildly elevated alkaline phosphatase, and mild abnormalities of transaminases, decreased serum albumin, and increased $\alpha 2$ globulins. Renal function is normal and autoantibodies are negative. Patients with PMR and GCA have increased levels of von Willebrand factor even during steroid therapy.

Approximately 7 per cent of patients with PMR may have no evidence of an acute phase response. Some studies suggest that this figure may be as high as 22 per cent. This syndrome of PMR with normal ESR is considered more benign with less systemic features (Proven et al. 1999).

Imaging

Ultrasonography (US) in PMR and MRI may show glenohumoral effusion and subacromial bursitis in significant number of patients. Coari et al. studied 90 shoulders with RA, 32 with PMR, 122 with periarticular disorders, and 108 controls. They described significant glenohumeral effusion in PMR, involvement of both articular and periarticular structures in RA, and only the tendons in periarticular disorders (Coari et al. 1999). Lange studied 32 patients more than 60 years of age and found shoulder joint inflammation in 61 per cent with PMR and 63.2 per cent of patients with elderly onset RA (Lange et al. 2000). Recent Italian studies report as high as 100 per cent subacromial bursitis in PMR but this needs further confirmation. There are also reports of hip synovitis and trochanteric bursitis in PMR.

MRI of hands and feet done in seven patients showed tenosynovitis in five and joint synovitis in three. MRI has also confirmed shoulder and hip synovitis and subacromial bursitis in these patients (Cantini et al. 1999). A case of MR angiography showing stenotic bilateral temporal arteries has been reported (Mitomo et al. 1998). Arthroscopy of the shoulder has shown synovitis in upto 89 per cent of patients (Brooks and MoGee 1997).

Colour duplex ultrasonography has been described in 30 patients with temporal arteritis. Seventy three per cent showed a dark halo around the lumen of temporal arteries which disappeared after a mean of 16 days, 80 per cent showed stenoses or occlusion, 93 per cent showed halo, stenoses or occlusion (Plate 153) (Schmidt et al. 1997).

Temporal 67-gallium uptake was significantly higher when studied in 24 patients with temporal arteritis (19 biopsy positive and 5 biopsy negative) and was found to have 94 per cent specificity and 90 per cent positive predictive value for the diagnosis. The uptake normalized after steroid treatment for 6 months when patients were in remission (Genereau et al. 1999).

Angiography is useful for documenting large vessel involvement in the form of stenotic areas, occlusions, and collaterals in some patients (Stanson et al. 1976). A preliminary report used PET scan as a non-invasive technique to evaluate large vessel vasculitis (Blockmans et al. 1999).

Temporal artery biopsy however remains the gold standard for the diagnosis of temporal arteritis though US, gallium scans, and MR angiography are non-invasive investigations and may have promising results. Biopsy positive cases appear to have more severe disease than biopsy negative cases at the time of diagnosis and during follow-up (Duhaut et al. 1999a,b).

Differential diagnosis

There are many features of these related conditions that predispose the unwary clinician to diagnostic error. The main symptoms of PMR (pain and stiffness in girdle areas and neck) and GCA (headaches) can occur as a presentation of many other conditions. An acute phase response, again a feature of PMR and GCA, can occur in many other settings such as neoplasia, RA, and infection.

Both conditions, even PMR without GCA, are regarded as urgent indications for the start of steroid therapy. Many clinicians use a response to steroids as the main defining feature. This encourages diagnostic error since steroids are potent anti-inflammatory agents that can mask symptoms from a host of conditions ranging from osteoarthritis, rotator cuff problems, RA, cancer, infection, migraine, and intracranial tumour—especially if used in traditional high doses. An audit of rheumatologist's diagnosis in patients referred with suspected PMR to the rheumatology clinic showed that of 53 referrals 18 had PMR, 5 GCA, 6 RA (all seronegative and non-erosive), 7 OA (AC joint, glenohumeral, cervical spine, hip, and generalized), periarticular shoulder lesions (3), malignancy (2), hypothyroidism (1), fibromyalgia (4), transient myalgia (3), and infections (3) (Kalke and Dasgupta 2000).

PMR is usually diagnosed and treated in primary care and is listed as the commonest diagnosis for long-term steroids in the community. In view of the serious toxicity of long-term steroid administration it is important to exclude mimicking conditions before steroids are started. In many of these conditions long term low dose steroids are not indicated and may adversely affect outcome. For example, GCA needs high-dose steroids, RA needs methotrexate, infections need antibiotics, cancers need appropriate quick workup and referral, and the non-inflammatory conditions such as OA and periarticular lesions need management with advice, physiotherapy, and local therapy such as injections. Steroids can mask and delay diagnosis in all these conditions and we do not feel that immediate prescription of steroids in all patients with suspected PMR (without GCA) is a desirable practice. A thorough clinical evaluation is more important and this may need to be complemented by appropriate relevant investigations.

We outline an approach to a patient presenting proximal pain and stiffness (the polymyalgic syndrome) (Fig. 2) and clues to a non-PMR diagnosis (Table 4). Various mimics have been reported in the medical literature. In the main these are malignancies (especially myeloma), the seronegative arthritides, and other connective tissue diseases (Gonzalez-Gay et al. 2000). There are case reports on myelodysplastic syndome, spinal cord haemangioma, C5 radiculopathy, infections such as Lyme disease, bacterial endocarditis, and quinidine induced rheumatic syndromes.

Treatment

Corticosteroids are the treatment of choice for PMR and GCA. Oral steroids are the common practice but intravenous methylprednisolone can be used for neuro-ophthalmic manifestations of GCA. Most cases of PMR can be effectively controlled with an initial daily dose of 10–15 mg depending on disease severity. The dose is generally reduced thereafter by 1 mg a month depending on clinical and laboratory responses. In GCA, the treatment is initiated at variable doses of 40–80 mg daily. It can be reduced to 40 mg by the end of 1 month, by 5 mg every 1–2 weeks thereafter till the dose of 20 mg is reached. Further reduction could be by 2.5 mg every 2–4 weeks while monitoring clinical symptoms and ESR or CRP. There is uncontroversial evidence that the cumulative steroid dosage is directly related to incidence of steroid side effects. This makes the case for using minimum effective steroid doses in both PMR and GCA (Kyle and Hazleman 1989).

PMR can also be treated effectively with intramuscular depot methylprednisolone acetate using a regimen of 120 mg every 3 weeks for first 12 weeks and thereafter by monthly injections reduced by 20 mg every 12 weeks. This has the advantage of much lower cumulative dose compared with oral prednisolone and translates into lower steroid related toxicity. We found lower fracture rates (3.3 per cent in injection group versus 26.7 per cent in oral group) and less weight gain though bruising was higher. Some patients with severe symptoms may still require oral steroids (Dasgupta et al. 1998).

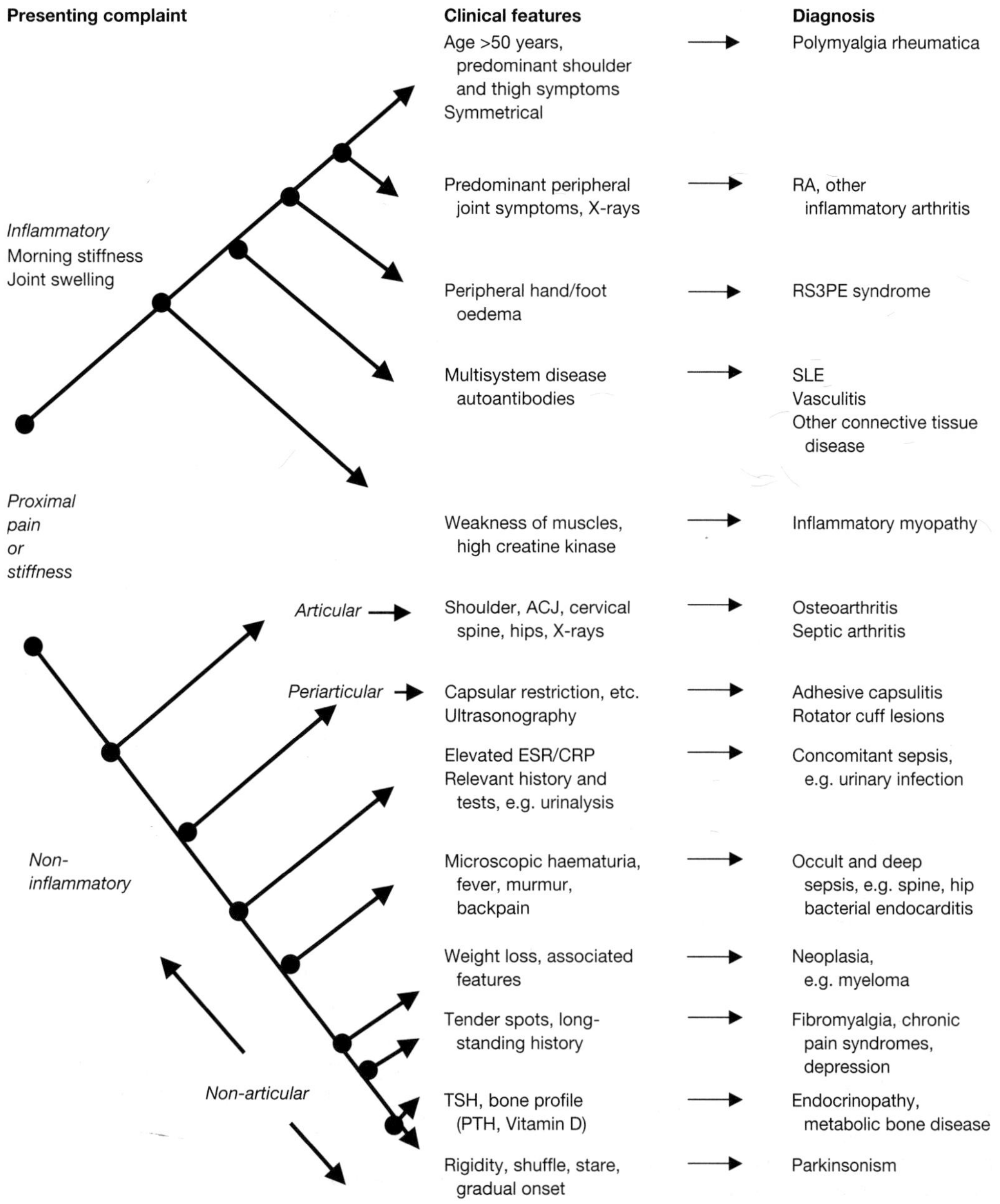

Fig. 2 Approach to the evaluation of proximal pain and stiffness.

Table 4 Clues to a non-PMR diagnosis

Age of onset <50 years
Chronic onset
Absence of upper limb involvement
Absence of inflammatory stiffness
Normal ESR and CRP
Incomplete response to 15 mg/day of prednisolone

Deflazacort has not been found to be more efficacious or associated with reduced toxicity in PMR. In PMR the anti-inflammatory equipotency between deflazacort and prednisolone is approximately 1.4. There are isolated reports of success of azathioprine and methotrexate in PMR and GCA as steroid sparing agents in resistant cases, but not with cyclosporine. Trials using methotrexate yielded mixed results but this may be due to low dosage, small sample size, and higher dropouts and patient selection.

There is also no consensus on appropriate outcome measures to be used for trials in PMR and GCA. Patient based outcome measures have not been used although in pilot study we have shown the validity of HAQ and its ability to measure change in disease activity in PMR (Kalke et al. 2000). Further outcome studies are in progress evaluating the following measures in PMR: morning stiffness, pain scale, modified HAQ, short form-36, physician's and patients' global assessment, and the acute phase response.

There is evidence that inflammation as well as treatment with steroids may have deleterious effect on the bone mass and prophylaxis is advised especially with high-risk groups (Dolan et al. 1997). It is very important to recognize high-risk osteoporotic complications at a very early stage of steroid therapy. It is our regular practice to co-prescribe calcium and vitamin D with low-dose steroids. We use bisphosphonates with long-term large dosage (>15 mg/day prednisolone), history of previous fractures, other risk factors for osteoporosis or deteriorating bone density.

We recommend bone densitometry at start of treatment and then every year while the patient remains on high steroid doses (prednisolone >7.5 mg daily). The frequency of follow-up scans depends on future fracture risk, that is, other risk factors (e.g. previous fragility fractures), initial bone density, co-morbidities, and steroid dosage.

Outcome

PMR has a self-limiting course of about 1–2 years, though a smaller proportion of patients may run a chronic course and require longer duration of treatment. Narvaez et al. (1999) estimated that 50 per cent patients with PMR require prednisolone therapy for 2 years, 30 per cent longer than 3 years, and 18 per cent longer than 4 years, whereas 50 per cent of patients with both PMR and GCA require treatment for more than 4 years. Increasing age at diagnosis, female sex, higher baseline ESR, and lower daily corticosteroid dose are reported to be risk factors associated with prolonged therapy and lower rate of clinical remission. The coexistence of temporal arteritis and occurrence of at least one relapse are also associated with prolonged therapy. The rate of relapse ranges from 25 to 60 per cent. Patients are reported to relapse frequently during first year and when the dosage of prednisolone was reduced from 7.5 to 5 mg. Kyle et al. (1985) have suggested that patients should be seen more frequently in first 6 months as relapses are common during this period of steroid reduction (54 per cent).

Corticosteroid related side-effects develop in about one-third patients and in two-thirds if weight gain is included. The deleterious effect on bone density has already been discussed. Gastrointestinal bleeding and infection are responsible for fatal events. The adverse effects are related to higher initial dose (>30 mg/day) and cumulative dose. Higher morbidity and mortality is reported in GCA but not in PMR.

Gabriel et al. (1997) have described the adverse outcomes of steroid and NSAID therapy in 232 patients with PMR followed for an average of 8 years. Sixty-five per cent of patients treated with steroids alone had at least one adverse event compared to 80 per cent of patients treated with steroids and NSAIDs. The three variables that independently increased risk of adverse events were age, cumulative steroid dose (>1800 mg prednisolone), and female sex. Risks of diabetes mellitus, vertebral, femoral neck, and hip fractures are reported to be 2–5 times greater in patients with PMR on steroids compared to age and sex matched normal controls. Secondary amyloidosis and dissecting aortic aneurysm have been reported in PMR. There are cases reported in association with bronchiolitis obliterans, organizing pneumonia, posterior scleritis, and pulmonary fibrosis.

Summary

PMR and GCA are related diseases seen in the elderly. A diligent evaluation is required before starting steroids. Treatment should be with minimum effective corticosteroid doses with appropriate measures for osteoporosis. Patients should be carefully followed to assess disease activity, to monitor steroid toxicity, and to look for other diagnoses that may manifest later in the course of the disease.

References

Bagratuni, L. (1953). A rheumatic syndrome occuring in the elderly. *Annals of the Rheumatic Diseases* **12**, 98–104.

Barber, H.S. (1957). Myalgic syndrome with constitutional effects: polymyalgia rheumatica. *Annals of the Rheumatic Diseases* **16**, 230–7.

Bird, H.A., Esselinckx, W., Dison, A.S.J., Mowat, A.G., and Wood, P.H.N. (1979). An evaluation of polymyalgia rheumatica. *Annals of the Rheumatic Diseases* **38**, 434–9.

Blockmans, D. et al. (1999). New arguments for a vasculitic nature of polymyalgia rheumatica using positron emission tomography. *Rheumatology (Oxford)* **38**, 444–7.

Boiardi, L., Salvarani, C., Timms, J.M., Macchioni, P.L., and di Giovine, F.S. (2000). Interleukin 1 Cluster and tumour necrosis factor-alpha gene polymorphisms in polymyalgia rheuamatica. *Clinical and Experimental Rheumatology* **8**, 675–81.

Brooks, R.C. and McGee, S.R. (1997). Diagnostic dilemmas in polymyalgia rheumatica. *Archives of Internal Medicine* **157**, 162–8.

Bruce, W. (1988). Senile rheumatic gout. *British Medical Journal* **2**, 811–13.

Cantini, F. et al. (1999). Remitting seronegative symmetrical synovitis with pitting oedema (RS3PE) syndrome: a prospective follow up and magnetic resonance imaging study. *Annals of the Rheumatic Diseases* **58**, 230–6.

Chaung, T.Y., Hunder, G.G, Ilstrup, D.M., and Kirkland, L.T. (1982). Polymyalgia rheumatica: a 10 year epidemiologic and clinical study. *Annals of Internal Medicine* **97**, 672–80.

Cimmino, M.A. and Zaccaria, A. (2000). Epidemiology of polymyalgia rheumatica. *Clinical and Experimental Rheumatology* **18**, S9–11.

Cimmino, M.A., Grazi, G., Balistreri, M., and Accardo, S. (1993). Increased prevalence of antibodies to adenovirus and respiratory syncyitial virus in polymyalgia rheumaica. *Clinical and Experimental Rheumatology* **11**, 309–13.

Coari, G., Paoletti, F., and Iagnocco, A. (1999). Shoulder involvement in rheumatic diseases. Sonographic findings. *Journal of Rheumatology* **26**, 668–73.

Corrigall, V.M., Dolan, A.L., Dasgupta, B., and Panayi, G.S. (1997). The sequential analysis of T lymphocyte subsets and interleukin-6 in polymyalgia rheumatica patients as predictors of disease remission and steroid withdrawal. *British Journal of Rheumatology* **36**, 976–80.

Dababneh, A., Gonzalez-Gay, M.A., Garcia-Porrua, C., Hajeer, A., Thomson, W., and Ollier, W. (1998). Giant cell arteritis and polymyalgia rheumatica can be differentiated by distinct patterns of HLA class II association. *Journal of Rheumatology* **25**, 2140–5.

Dasgupta, B. and Panayi, G.S. (1990). Interleukin-6 in serum of patients with polymyalgia rheumatica and giant cell arteritis. *British Journal of Rheumatology* **29**, 456–8.

Dasgupta, B., Duke, O., Timms, A.M., Pitzalis, C., and Panayi, G.S. (1989). Selective depletion and activation of CD8+ lymphocytes from peripheral blood of patients with polymyalgia rheumatica and giant cell arteritis. *Annals of the Rheumatic Diseases* **48**, 307–11.

Dasgupta, B., Dolan, A.L., Panayi, G.S., and Fernandes, L. (1998). An initially double-blind controlled 96 week trial of depot methylprednisolone against oral prednisolone in the treatment of polymyalgia rheumatica. *British Journal of Rheumatology* **37**, 189–95.

Dequeker, J. (1987). Rheumatic diseases in visual art. General review. In *Art, History and Antiquity of Rheumatic Diseases* (ed. T. Appelboom), pp. 31–7. Brussels: Elsevier.

Dolan, A. et al. (1997). Effects of inflammation and treatment on bone turnover and bone mass in polymyalgia rheumatica. *Arthritis and Rheumatism* **40**, 2022–9.

Duhaut, P. et al. (1999a). Giant cell arteritis, polymyalgia rheumatica, and viral hypotheses: a multicenter, prospective case–control study. *Journal of Rheumatology* **26**, 361–9.

Duhaut, P. et al. (1999b). Biopsy proven and biopsy negative temporal arteritis: differences in clinical spectrum at the onset of the disease. *Annals of the Rheumatic Diseases* **58**, 335–41.

Duhaut, P., Bosshard, S., and Dumontet, C. (2000). Giant cell arteritis and polymyalgia rheumatica: role of viral infections. *Clinical and Experimental Rheumatology* **18**, S22–3.

Elling, P., Olsson, A.T., and Elling, H. (1996). Synchronous variations of the incidence of temporal arteritis and polymyalgia rheumatica in different regions of Denmark; association with epidemics of *Mycoplasma pneumoniae* infection. *Journal of Rheumatology* **23**, 112–19.

Gabriel, S.E., Sunku, J., Salvarani, C., O'Fallon, M., and Hunder, G. (1997). Adverse outcomes of antiinflammatory therapy among patients with polymyalgia rheumatica. *Arthritis and Rheumatism* **40**, 1873–8.

Gabriel, S.E., Espy, M., Erdman, D.D., Bjornsson, J., Smith, T.F., and Hunder, G. (1999). The role of parvovirus B19 in the pathogenesis of giant cell arteritis: a preliminary evaluation. *Arthritis and Rheumatism* **42**, 1255–8.

Genereau, T. et al. (1999). Temporal 67gallium uptake is increased in temporal arteritis. *Rheumatology (Oxford)* **38**, 709–13.

Gonzalez-Gay, M.A., Garcia-Porrua, C., Vazquez-Caruncho, M., Dababneh, A., Hajeer, A., and Ollier, W.E. (1999). The spectrum of polymyalgia rheumatica in northwestern Spain: incidence and analysis of variables associated with relapse in a 10 year study. *Journal of Rheumatology* **26**, 1326–32.

Gonzalez-Gay, M.A., Garcia-Porrua, C., Salvarani, C., Olivieri, I., and Hunder, G.G. (2000). The spectrum of conditions mimicking polymyalgia rheumatica in Northwestern Spain. *Journal of Rheumatology* **27**, 2179–84.

Gran, J. and Myklebust, G. (1997). The incidence of polymyalgia rheumatica and temporal arteritis in the county of Aust Agder, south Norway: a prospective study. 1987–94. *Journal of Rheumatology* **24**, 1739–43.

Hamrin, B., Jonsson, N., and Landberg, T. (1964). Arteritis in polymyalgia rheumatica. *Lancet* **1**, 397–401.

Healey, L.A. (1984). Long term follow up of polymyalgia rheumatica: evidence for synovitis. *Seminars in Arthritis and Rheumatism* **13**, 322–8.

Horton, B.T., Magath, T.B., and Brown, G.E. (1932). A undescribed form of arteritis of temporal vessels. *Proceedings of the Staff Meetings of the Mayo Clinic* **7**, 700–1.

Hunder, G.G. (1997). Giant cell arteritis and polymyalgia rheumatica. *Medical Clinics of North America* **81**, 195–219.

Hutchinson, J. (1889–1890). Diseases of the arteries No1. On a peculiar form of thrombotic arteritis of the aged which is sometimes productive of gangrene. *Archives of Surgery (London)* **1**, 323–9.

Jones, J.G. and Hazleman, B.L. (1981). Prognosis and management of polymyalgia rheumatica. *Annals of the Rheumatic Diseases* **40**, 1–5.

Kalke, S. and Dasgupta, B. (2000). The accuracy of diagnosis in polymyalgia rheumatica (PMR): results from a PMR referral Clinic. *Arthritis and Rheumatism* **43**, S365.

Kalke, S., Mukerjee, D., and Dasgupta, B. (2000). A study of Health Assessment Questionnaire (HAQ) to evaluate functional status in polymyalgia rheumatica. *Rheumatology (Oxford)* **39**, 883–5.

Kyle, V. and Hazleman B.L. (1989). Treatment of polymyalgia rheumatica and giant cell arteritis. II. Relation between steroid dose and steroid associated side effects. *Annals of the Rheumatic Diseases* **48**, 662–6.

Kyle, V., Silverman, B., Silman, A., King, H., Oswald, N., and Reiss, B. (1985). Polymyalgia rheumatica/giant cell arteritis in a Cambridge general practice. *British Medical Journal (Clinical Research Edition)* **10**, 385–7.

Lange, U., Piegsa, M., Teichmann, J., and Neeck, G. (2000). Ultrasonography of the glenohumeral joints—a helpful instrument in differentiation in elderly onset rheumatoid arthritis and polymyalgia rheumatica. *Rheumatology International* **19**, 185–9.

Machado, E.B.V., Michet, C.J., and Ballard, D.J. (1988). Trends in incidence and clinical presentation of temporal arteritis in Olmsted County, Minnesota, 1950–85. *Arthritis and Rheumatism* **31**, 745–9.

Makki, R.F., al Sharif, F., González-Gay, M.A., García-Porrúa, C., Ollier, W.E., and Hajeer, A.H. (2000). RANTES gene polymorphism in polymyalgia rheumatica, giant cell arteritis and rheumatoid arthritis. *Clinical and Experimental Rheumatology* **18**, 391–3.

Mattey, D.L., Hajeer, A.H., Dababneh, A., Thompson, W., Gonzalez-Gay, M.A., Gracia Porrua, C., and Oliver, W.E. (2000). Association of giant cell arteritis and polymyalgia rheumatica with different tumour necrosis factor microsatellite polymorphisms. *Arthritis and Rheumatism* **43**, 1749–55.

McGonagle, D., Pease, C., Marzo-Ortega, H., O'Connor, P., and Emery, P. (2000). The case for classification of polymyalgia rheumatica and remitting seronegative symmetrical synovitis with pitting edema as primarily capsular/entheseal based pathologies. *Journal of Rheumatology* **27**, 837–40 (editorial).

Meliconi, R. et al. (1996). Leucocyte infiltration in synovial tissue from the shoulder of patients with polymyalgia rheumatica. Quantitative analysis and influence of corticosteroid treatment. *Arthritis and Rheumatism* **39**, 1199–207.

Mitomo, T., Funyu, T., Takahashi, Y., Murakami, K., Koyama, K. Kamio (1998). Giant cell arteritis and magnetic resonance angiography. *Arthritis and Rheumatism* **41**, 1702.

Narvaez, J., Nolla-Sole, J.M., Clavaguera, M.T., Valverde-Garcia, J., and Roig-Escofet, D. (1999). Long term therapy in polymyalgia rheumatica: effect of coexistent temporal arteritis. *Journal of Rheumatology* **26**, 1945–52.

Nordborg, E., Nordborg, C., Malmavall, B., Andersson, R., and Bengtsson, B. (1995). Giant cell arteritis. *Rheumatic Disease Clinics of North America* **21**, 1013–26.

Poulley, J. and Hughes, J.P. (1960). Giant cell arteritis or arteritis of the aged. *British Medical Journal* **2**,1562–7.

Proven, A., Gabriel, S.E., O'Fallon, W.M. and Hunder, G.G. (1999). Polymyalgia rheumatica with low erythrocyte sedimentation rate at diagnosis. *Journal of Rheumatology* **26**, 1333–7.

Pulsatelli, L., Meliconi, R., Boiardi, L., Macchioni, P., Salvarani, C., and Facchini, A. (1998). Elevated serum concentrations of the chemokine RANTES in patients with polymyalgia rheumatica. *Clinical and Experimental Rheumatology* **16**, 263–8.

Salvarani, C. et al. (1991). Epidemiology and immunologic aspects of polymyalgia rheumatica and giant cell arteritis in Northern Italy. *Arthritis and Rheumatism* **34**, 351–6.

Salvarani, C., Gabriel, S., and Hunder, G.G. (1996). Distal extremity swelling with pitting oedema in polymyalgia rheumatica. Report on nineteen cases. *Arthritis and Rheumatism* **39**, 73–80.

Salvarani, C. et al. (1999). HLA–DRB1, DQA1, and DQB1 alleles associated with giant cell arteritis in northern Italy. *Journal of Rheumatology* **26**, 2395–9.

Schmidt, W.A., Kraft, H.E., Vorpahl, K., Volker, L., and Gromnica-Ihle, E.J. (1997). Color duplex ultrasonography in the diagnosis of temporal arteritis. *New England Journal of Medicine* **337**, 1336–42.

Stanson, A.W., Klein, R.G., and Hunder, G.G. (1976). Extracranial angiographic findings in giant cell (temporal) arteritis. *American Journal of Roentgenology* **127**, 957–63.

Stevens, R.J. and Hughes, R.A. (1995). The aetiopathogenesis of giant cell arteritis. *British Journal of Rheumatology* **34**, 960–5.

Straub, R.H. et al. (1999). Favorable role of interleukin 10 in patients with polymyalgia rheumatica. *Journal of Rheumatology* **26**, 1318–25.

Uddhammar, A., Sundqvist, K.G., Ellis, B., and Rantapaa-Dahlqvist, S. (1998). Cytokines and adhesion molecules in patients with polymyalgia rheumatica. *British Journal of Rheumatology* **37**, 766–9.

Wagner, A.D., Gerard, H.C., Fresemann, T., Schmidt, W.A., Gromnica-Ihle, E., Hudson, A.P., and Zeidler, H. (2000). Detection of Chlamydia pneumoniae in giant cell vasculitis and correlation with the topographic arrangement of tissue-infiltrating dendritic cells. *Arthritis and Rheumatism* **43**, 1543–51.

Walsh, L.J., Wong, C.A., Pringle, M., and Tattersfield, A.E. (1996). Use of corticosteroids in the community and the prevention of secondary osteoporosis: a cross sectional study. *British Medical Journal* **313**, 344–6.

Weyand, C.M. and Goronzy, J.J. (1999). Arterial wall injury in giant cell arteritis. *Arthritis and Rheumatism* **42**, 844–53.

6.10.7 Other vasculitides including small-vessel vasculitis

Miguel A. Gonzalez-Gay and Carlos Garcia-Porrua

Introduction

The term small-vessel vasculitis encompasses a wide spectrum of clinical syndromes characterized by predominant cutaneous involvement and a different grade of systemic manifestations. All these conditions share the presence of vascular inflammation and blood vessel damage with inflammation of small blood vessels including arterioles capillaries and postcapillary venules. However, a frequent overlap in the size of vessels involved is observed. Thus, the distinction between small blood vessel vasculitides mainly restricted to arterioles, capillaries, and postcapillary venules and those that also involve medium-size arteries is often difficult (Lie et al. 1990; Stone and Nousari 2001).

Controversy also exists on the definition and classification of small-vessel vasculitis. Some authors only include within this group of conditions those vasculitides characterized by leucocytoclastic changes (Lie 1994). Their histology shows infiltration of neutrophils within and around blood vessel walls, leucocytoclasia (degranulation and fragmentation of neutrophils leading to the production of nuclear 'dust'), fibrinoid necrosis of the damaged vessel walls, and necrosis, swelling, and proliferation of the endothelial cells (Plate 154). However, although the term 'leucocytoclastic' is used to describe the majority of vasculitides involving the skin, the presence of leucocytoclasia is merely an expression of a significant neutrophilic infiltrate, which may also be found in non-vasculitic conditions involving the skin such as, for example, in cutaneous infections or in Sweet syndrome. Other authors, however, accept a wider term for small-vessel vasculitis, without the requirement of evidence of leucocytoclastic vasculitis, if an inflammatory infiltration within the vessel walls is observed along with at least one of the features described before (Gibson and Su 1995). In these cases, small vessel vasculitis is considered to be present regardless of the type of predominant inflammatory infiltration. Thus, besides the typical neutrophilic pattern of inflammatory cells, other patterns such as those due to a predominance of eosinophils, mononuclear cell, or a mixed pattern of vascular inflammatory infiltration may be observed. In these cases, small- vessel vasculitides may be classified in two different categories according to the presence or absence of leucocytoclastic changes (Table 1).

In addition, although some authors (Lie 1994) considered within the group of leucocytoclastic vasculitis only those vasculitides involving predominantly small blood vessels, the Chapel Hill Conference Consensus (CHCC) Proposal included within the term of small-vessel vasculitis other vasculitides such as Wegener's granulomatosis, microscopic polyangiitis, or Churg–Strauss syndrome where necrotizing vasculitis involving small- and medium-sized arteries is also present (Jennette et al. 1994).

In this chapter only the group of vasculitides involving exclusively small blood vessels will be discussed.

Table 1 Classification of small-vessel vasculitis

Leucocytoclastic vasculitis
Primary
Hypersensitivity vasculitis (cutaneous leucocytoclastic angiitis)
Henoch–Schönlein purpura
Urticarial (hypocomplementemic) vasculitis
Cryoglobulinaemic vasculitis[a]
Erythema elevatum diutinum and granuloma faciale
Hypergammaglobulinaemic purpura of Waldeström
'ANCA-associated' vasculitides[a]
Microscopic polyangiitis
Wegener granulomatosis
Churg–Strauss syndrome
Secondary
Malignancy (paraneoplastic vasculitides)
Infection
Drugs
Collagen vascular diseases
Most frequently:
Systemic lupus erythematosus[a]
Sjögren's syndrome[a]
Rheumatoid arthritis[a]
Behçet's disease[b]
Other conditions (uncommon)
Inflammatory bowel disease
Bowel bypass syndrome
Primary biliary cirrhosis
Cystic fibrosis
Sarcoidosis
Patients with HIV or AIDS
Others (non-leucocytoclastic vasculitis)
Primary
Nodular vasculitis
Livedo vasculitis
Pityriasis lichenoides
Secondary
Related to drugs

Note: ANCA, antineutrophil cytoplasmic antibodies.

[a] Conditions in which a frequent overlap of small- and medium-sized blood vessel involvement is observed.

[b] Besides small blood vessels, medium- and large-sized blood vessels may be involved.

Leucocytoclastic vasculitis

Pathogenesis

These conditions are known to be related to circulating immune complexes (Lie et al. 1990). Antibodies are formed and then bound to antigens. Soluble immune complexes not removed by the mononuclear-phagocyte system may become lodged between the endothelial cells of the vessel walls. The vascular damage is due to the deposition of those immune complexes in vessel walls with activation of the complement cascade. Release of vasoactive amines increases vascular permeability. The immune complexes promote platelet aggregation and are capable of activating complement leading to the release of chemotactic factors, in particular C5a, which in turn recruit polymorphonuclear leucocytes at the site of deposition. The release of lysosomal enzymes due to the ingestion of immune complexes by the polymorphonuclear leucocytes results in vessel damage. Membrane-attack complexes are also required for the endothelial damage. In this regard, raised serum concentration of C5b-9 complex has been found significantly elevated in many patients with leucocytoclastic vasculitis. As a consequence, increased permeability, oedema, and haemorrhage occur. Finally, mononuclear cells clean the tissues.

In most leucocytoclastic vasculitides, immune complexes are constituted by IgG or IgM. However, Henoch–Schönlein purpura (HSP) is a vasculitis due to IgA-mediated inflammation of small vessels. In HSP IgA-dominant immune deposits in the wall of the small vessels and in the renal glomeruli is observed. HSP is associated with abnormalities involving only IgA1 but not IgA2 sub-class of IgA. Abnormalities involving the glycosylation of the hinge region of IgA1 may be responsible of the clinical and histopathologic features of HSP.

Clinical features: general considerations

Cutaneous involvement is the typical finding in patients with leucocytoclastic vasculitis. In Western countries, after giant cell arteritis, they constitute the second most common group of primary vasculitides (Gonzalez-Gay and Garcia-Porrua 2001). The pattern of skin involvement is initially a maculopapular rash that may be followed by other skin lesion, in particular by palpable purpura. This term, palpable purpura, has frequently been considered synonymous of small sized cutaneous leucocytoclastic vasculitis [Plate 155(a)]. It is due to extravasation of erythrocytes through damaged blood vessel walls into the tissues. These lesions do not blanch with pressure on the skin. A post-inflammatory hyperpigmentation is generally seen in the phase of resolution of the disease. Other skin lesions such as non-palpable macules and patches, urticaria, bullous lesions, vesicules, splinter haemorrhages, ulcerations, or non-specific changes may also be observed in these vasculitides. Combination of these different lesions is common [Plate 155(b)]. Nevertheless, a purpuric component is generally present. The increased hydrostatic pressure predisposes certain areas of involvement. This fact explains that skin lesions are more common on the legs and buttocks.

Main clinical syndromes

Hypersensitivity vasculitis and cutaneous leucocytoclastic angiitis

The concept of inflammatory vascular disease secondary to allergic of hypersensitivity mechanisms as distinct nosologic entity was proposed by

Zeek et al. (1948). The term hypersensitivity vasculitis (HV) was then used in several classifications of vasculitides. It is characterized by a prominent involvement of the skin, generally as a maculopapular rash or palpable purpura, frequently precipitated by the use of drugs, and the existence of infiltration of the small blood vessels with polymorphonuclear leucocytes and leucocytoclasia. Lesions tend to be about the same age, occurring around the same time. Deep ulceration is uncommon as, like HSP, this vasculitis involves the small blood vessels of the superficial papillary dermis. Complement levels are normal but in 50 per cent of the cases with vasculitis limited to skin direct immunofluorescence shows granular deposition of C3, IgG, and especially IgM in and around superficial dermal blood vessels. Some difficulties have arisen in defining HV as a distinct syndrome, as sometimes no precipitating event can be found and similar clinical and pathologic pictures may be observed as manifestation of several processes such as infections, malignancies, other systemic vasculitides, and in most of the connective tissue diseases. Moreover, the 1990 American College of Rheumatology (ACR) classification criteria for HV have proved to have relatively low sensitivity and specificity (Calabrese et al. 1990). Thus, the CHCC definitions did not use the term HV and considered the categories of microscopic polyangiitis and cutaneous leucocytoclastic angiitis (CLA) that may comprise most patients included within the category of HV (Jennette et al. 1994). The term CLA defines an isolated cutaneous leucocytoclastic vasculitis limited to skin. Due to this, the diagnosis of CLA is one of the exclusion as, although occasionally associated synovitis is present, other features of systemic vasculitides must be absent (Stone and Nousari 2001).

Hypersensitivity vasculitis is more common in adults. In northwest Spain HV was more common in men (Gonzalez-Gay and Garcia-Porrua 2001). In Norwich (UK), in contrast, both HV and CLA were more common in women (Watts et al. 1998). The annual incidence of biopsy-proven HV in adults from Spain was 29.7/million. The incidence of CLA in adults from Norwich was 15.4/million. In unselected series a wide spectrum of drugs, in particular antibiotic and non-steroidal anti-inflammatory drugs, have been considered to be precipitating events. In these cases, HV is generally limited to skin with few and usually mild systemic complications and excellent outcome. Most patients have a single episode, which resolves spontaneously (Garcia-Porrua et al. 2001b). In these cases removal of the precipitating drug and bed rest may obviate the need to treat the cutaneous manifestations. Joint symptoms usually respond to non-steroidal anti-inflammatory drugs. Colchicine and dapsone have also been used. Non-responders have been treated with a short course of corticosteroids or azathioprine. However, no clear evidence exists about the benefit of more aggressive therapies.

Henoch–Schönlein purpura ('anaphylactoid purpura')

The term most commonly used is named after Schönlein (1837), who described the association between arthralgia and purpuric cutaneous lesions in a child and Henoch (1874), who described a syndrome of purpura, severe abdominal colic, and melena, and a few years later referred to nephritis as a complication of this syndrome. The diagnosis is confirmed by the demonstration of IgA deposition in and around blood vessels walls on direct immunofluorescence studies.

It is the most common vasculitis in children and an infrequent condition in adults. The annual incidence in children ranges between 130 and 180 cases per million. In adults, in contrast, the annual incidence generally ranges between 8 and 14 cases per million (Gonzalez-Gay and Garcia-Porrua 2001). The disease is observed predominantly in children between the ages of 2 and 10. Boys slightly outnumber girls. Peaks in autumn, fall, and winter have been described. In at least 50 per cent of cases in the paediatric age an upper respiratory tract infection may precede the onset of the disease. Thus, beta-haemolytic streptococcus group A is the organism most frequently isolated. A rash of erythematous papules or more rarely a pruriginous itchy an urticarial rash that is followed by palpable purpura is the most common initial manifestation. The rash occurs in all the cases but it is not always the presenting sign. It is more commonly petechial or purpuric with contiguous erythematous plaques, often associated with macular, papular or vesicular elements. The distribution of the purpura is roughly symmetrical, where it typically appears on the lower extremities and then it reaches the thighs and buttocks [Plate 155(c)]. In young children, facial involvement and subcutaneous oedema of the hands, feet, scalp, and ears may be observed in up to 45 per cent of the cases as an early manifestation of the disease. Skin necrosis, especially in adults may develop in areas of severe haemorrhage that suffer significant pressure.

Gastrointestinal complications have been described in up to 75 per cent of the series. Abdominal pain, frequently colicky, is caused by peritoneal or visceral purpura leading to submucosal and mucosal extravasation of blood and oedema fluid, which may further lead to ulceration of the bowel mucosa and eventual bleeding into the lumen (Plate 156). Stools may show occult blood. Melena and haematemesis have been reported in up to 50 and 15 per cent of the patients, respectively. Other gastrointestinal complications are shown in Table 2. As with gastrointestinal complications, joint manifestations may also precede the development of palpable purpura by several days in up to 25 per cent of the cases (Gonzalez-Gay and Garcia-Porrua 2002). Transient arthralgias or arthritis, often associated with oedema, mainly in the large joints of the lower extremities, are observed in more than 50 per cent of cases (Calviño et al. 2001).

Macroscopic or microscopic haematuria, either isolated or in association with proteinuria, is observed in 30–80 per cent of the cases (Kaku et al. 1998). It generally occurs within the first 3 months after the onset of the disease (Calviño et al. 2001). However, it may be observed later, generally in the setting of relapses of the palpable purpura. Microscopic haematuria may persist for months or even years. The initial haematuria may be associated with hypertension and elevation of serum creatinine as in cases of nephritic syndrome. However, the most severe clinical presentation is that of mixed nephritic and nephrotic syndromes with haematuria, hypertension, and renal insufficiency associated with severe proteinuria and hypoalbuminaemia.

In Table 2, other less common clinical manifestations of HSP are described.

Table 2 Clinical features of Henoch–Schönlein purpura

Common clinical manifestations
Symmetrical purpura (mainly on the lower extremities)
Gastrointestinal complications
Abdominal pain (colicky)
Melena and haematemesis
Joint manifestations
Arthralgias or arthritis (mainly in the lower extremities)
Renal manifestations
Macroscopic or microscopic haematuria
Proteinuria (almost invariably associated with haematuria)
Other less common complications
Gastrointestinal
Acute intussusception
Haemorrhage and shock
Malabsorption
Exudative enteropathy and haemorrhagic ascites
Renal complications
Nephrotic syndrome
Mixed nephritic and nephrotic syndromes
Renal insufficiency (more frequent in adults)
Extrarenal genitourinary manifestations
Scrotal swelling, orchitis, testicular torsion
Bladder haemorrhage
Neurologic complications
Headache, encepalopathy, seizures, or subdural haematomas
Intracranial haemorrhage, intraparenchimal bleeding
Vasculitis involving the cerebral parenchyma
Peripheral neuropathy
Pulmonary complications
Pulmonary haemorrhage

The natural history of HSP is a self-limiting disease in most cases. Long-term morbidity and mortality of HSP are almost invariably related to renal involvement. In unselected children from northwest Spain, the outcome was generally good and nephrotic syndrome was the best predictor for renal sequelae (Calviño et al. 2001). In unselected adults from the same area the presence of haematuria at disease onset, and the persistence of renal manifestations during the course of the disease were significant indicators of the possible development of long-term renal sequelae (Garcia-Porrua et al. 2001a). Renal biopsies may include minimal changes or glomerulonephritis, which is often indistinguishable from IgA nephropathy [Plate 157(a)]. The prognosis is poor if patients with HSP, generally adults, present with rapidly progressive glomerulonephritis [Plate 157(b)].

Treatment of HSP is largely supportive. Besides bed rest, non-steroidal anti-inflammatory drugs can improve joint pain. High-dose corticosteroids have been used in patients with severe gastrointestinal manifestations (Gonzalez-Gay and Garcia-Porrua 2002). However, the use of corticosteroids in the prevention of nephritis is controversial (Saulsbury 1993; Kaku et al. 1998). Patients with severe nephritis have been treated with various therapeutic modalities including corticosteroids (oral or pulse therapy) alone or in combination with immunosuppressive agents, plasmapheresis, high-dose intravenous immunoglobulin therapy, and danazol (Szer 1996; Gonzalez-Gay and Garcia-Porrua 2002). However, in most cases the absence of randomized placebo-controlled studies makes it difficult to draw definitive conclusions about the therapeutic modalities for HSP nephritis. For a minority of patients who progress to end-stage renal insufficiency, renal transplantation may be considered.

Urticarial vasculitis

In contrast to the typical palpable purpura observed in most small-vessel leucocytoclastic vasculitides, urticarial skin lesions characterize urticarial vasculitis (UV). Lesions may be several centimetres in diameter, non-pruritic, frequently associated with a painful or burning sensation. They are located centripetally, more commonly in trunk and proximal extremities. Unlike common urticaria, the skin lesions of UV persist for more than 48 h and resolve with purpura and hyperpigmentation (Mehregan et al. 1992). A neutrophilic vasculitis of the vessels in the superficial papillary dermis and perivascular oedema is generally observed. Positive IgG immunofluorescence around blood vessel at the basement membrane zone is frequently observed in cases with hypocomplementia (Stone and Nousari 2001). The incidence and the aetiology are unknown. It is more common in women (by 2 : 1) in the fifth decade of life (Gibson and Su 1995). Based on the measurement of complement two categories have been described: hypocomplementic, associated with decreased C3 and C4 serum levels and CH50, described by McDuffie et al. (1973) and normocomplementemic. Hypocomplementemia is observed in 35–64 per cent of the patients with UV (Mehregan et al. 1992). Systemic manifestations such as arthralgia or arthritis, abdominal pain, angio-oedema, obstructive pulmonary disease, renal involvement, or ocular symptoms are more common in patients with hypocomplementemia (McDuffie et al. 1973; Mehregan et al. 1992). It has been associated with collagen vascular diseases, complement deficiencies, viral infections, serum sickness, reactions to drugs, haematologic neoplasia, more rarely with solid tumours, and with sun exposure or cold. Of note, UV has been reported in patients with systemic lupus erythematosus and sometimes it may be an early form of this disease. In general, patients with UV have a chronic but benign course. The average course is 3 years (Gibson and Su 1995). Results of treatment of UV have been inconsistent. Antihistamines, non-steroidal anti-inflammatory drugs, in particular indomethacin, antimalarials, dapsone, colchicine, plasmapheresis, gold, and cytostatics have proved to be useful in small series (Mehregan et al. 1992). Corticosteroids, initially at high dose, have provided relief in a high proportion of patients.

Cryoglobulinaemic vasculitis

Cryoglobulins are cold-precipitating immunoglobulins. Three sub-types can be distinguished based on the presence of rheumatoid factor activity and monoclonality: type I in which the cryoglobulin fraction is a single monoclonal immunoglobulin; type II which has mixed cryoglobulins with monoclonal component (usually IgM rheumatoid-like factor) combined with polyclonal component (generally IgG); and type III constituted by mixed polyclonal cryoglobulins (with one or more components) (Lamprecht et al. 1999). Type I generally accompanies lymphoproliferative and myeloproliferative disorders and is more likely to be associated with hyperviscosity than with vasculitis. Type II and Type III are associated with immune-complex vasculitides that predominantly affect small vessels (Jennette et al. 1994). However, medium-sized or sometimes large vessels may also be involved. Types II and III may also be associated with lymphoproliferative or autoimmune diseases and with viral (mainly hepatitis C virus) and bacterial infections. Cryoglobulinaemic vasculitides are the consequence of cryoglobulinaemia. In this regard, although at present mixed cryoglobulinaemia may be found in more than 50 per cent of patients with hepatitis C virus infection, the frequency of vasculitis in these patients is much lower (Agnello 1998).

The definition of 'essential' mixed cryoglobulinaemic vasculitis has been recently reconsidered. Cases where clinical signs of infections, autoimmune, or lymphoproliferative diseases are absent will meet this category. The disease is more common in women. In patients with cryoglobulinaemic vasculitis recurrent palpable purpura, generally involving the lower extremities, arthralgias, or arthritis and weakness are almost invariably present (Gorevic et al. 1980). Peripheral neuropathy and sub-clinical lymphocytic alveolitis are observed in 40–70 per cent of the cases. Renal complications, manifested as nephritic or nephrotic syndrome, secondary Sjögren's syndrome, Raynaud's phenomenon, central nervous system, gastrointestinal, cardiac and retinal involvement have been described in less than 40 per cent of the cases (Lamprecht et al. 1999). Low serum C4 levels are generally observed. Serum levels of C3 fluctuate with the course of the disease. High titres of rheumatoid factor are found in most patients.

Cryoglobulinaemic vasculitis associated with infectious endocarditis or other bacterial infections requires specific antibiotic therapy. In those secondary to connective tissue or lympho-myeloproliferative diseases treatment of the underlying condition is required. There is no consensus on how to treat essential cryoglobulinaemic vasculitis. Interferon-alpha was shown to be effective in some patients with 'essential' hepatitis C virus negative cryoglobulinaemic vasculitis (Casato et al. 1998). In these cases, cyclophosphamide, azathioprine, and methotrexate have also been used. Additional plasmapheresis or cryofiltration have been considered in rapidly deteriorating courses, generally for neurologic symptoms or in rapidly progressive glomerulonephritis. Interferon-alpha has specifically been recommended in hepatitis C virus-associated cryoglobulinaemic vasculitis, when a clinical remission was obtained or in chronic phases of the disease (Lamprecht et al. 1999).

Other primary leucocytoclastic vasculitides

Erythema elevatum diutinum is an uncommon disease, more frequent in women, characterized by non-purpuric prominent and persistent oedematous erythematous papules and plaques on the extensor surface of the extremities (backs of hands, elbows, or knees) that heal over months or years with fibrosis (Gibson and Su 1995). Treatment with dapsone has yielded good results.

As the former condition, granuloma faciale is also a rare and localized chronic leucocytoclastic vasculitis, which presents with single or multiple pink to brown smooth papules and plaques on the face. Lesions persist for years. A zone of normal collagen below the epidermis and the presence of eosinophils may be useful in differentiating this condition from erythema elevatum diutinum. Intralesional steroids may be useful.

Hypergammaglobulinaemic purpura of Waldeström is another leucocytoclastic vasculitis characterized by long-standing purpura, hyperglobulinaemia, and increased erythrocyte sedimentation rate.

Secondary leucocytoclastic vasculitis

Small-sized cutaneous vasculitis may be associated with malignancy. Vasculitis may antedate the discovery of the neoplasia, coincide, appear after the malignancy has already been diagnosed or give a clue to a recurrence. Lymphoproliferative disorders, leukaemia, or even solid tumours must be suspected in those patients with unexplained chronic relapsing course of skin purpura, in particular if anaemia is present (Gonzalez-Gay and Garcia-Porrua 1999).

An association between infection and systemic vasculitis has also been described. Gram-positive cocci (Staphylococcus and Streptococcus) and *Neisseria meningitidis* and *N. gonorrhoea* are the most common bacteria associated with vasculitis (Somer and Finegold 1995). In some patients, a vasculitis, in particular a small-sized cutaneous vasculitis, may be the presenting sign of a concealed life-threatening bacterial infection. In this case, leucocytosis with either low-grade or high fever are generally present (Gonzalez-Gay and Garcia-Porrua 1999).

Small-vessel cutaneous vasculitis may occur in the context of connective tissue diseases, especially in the disease flare and it may be related to a worse prognosis (Bacon and Carruthers 1995).

Non-leucocytoclastic vasculitis

Nodular vasculitis

It is characterized by recurrent subcutaneous nodules, generally presenting as bluish-red plaques, which occur in women from 30 to 60 years of age. It involves the arteries and veins of the panniculus with perivascular lymphocytic infiltration and granulomatous changes. The aetiology is unknown. The legs are predominantly affected, in particular in the posterolateral regions. Lesions may ulcerate, evolve slowly and generally heal with little atrophy or scarring within 2–6 weeks. However, they may erupt at irregular intervals for months or years (Gibson and Su 1995). Bed rest, non-steroidal anti-inflammatory drugs, and low doses of prednisone have been used. Treatment with potassium iodide has proved to be useful.

Livedo vasculitis

It is a thrombogenic vasculopathy characterized by a flat network of intersected blue–red lines (Lotti et al. 1998). Ischaemic damage is due to vascular occlusion and the histology shows hyalinized thickening of the small blood vessels of the middle and deep dermis, with endothelial proliferation and intraluminal thrombosis. It occurs more commonly on the legs, arms, and lower trunk. Lesions are asymptomatic and evolve to stellate ivory white scars with surrounding erythema, telangiectasia, and hyperpigmentation. Ulceration is uncommon. It must be differentiated from the necrotizing livedo reticularis seen in larger vessel vasculitides, hyperviscosity states, and cholesterol emboli. The course is chronic with frequent recurrences. Bed rest and some medications such as low-dose anticoagulation with heparin or coumadin, low-dose aspirin, and pentoxifylline have been used.

Pityriasis lichenoides

There is an acute form, usually a self-limiting disorder, characterized by crops of oedematous pink papules that show an early central necrosis and heal with scarring. Lymphocytic perivascular infiltration and endothelial swelling, generally without fibrinoid necrosis is observed. Chronic forms, with crops of lesions that last for months or years, have also been described. Ultraviolet B irradiation has yielded good results (Rogers 1992).

Secondary to drugs

Besides leucocytoclastic vasculitis, drugs may be the cause of a vasculitis where the infiltrate is composed mainly of lymphocytes. Lymphocytic

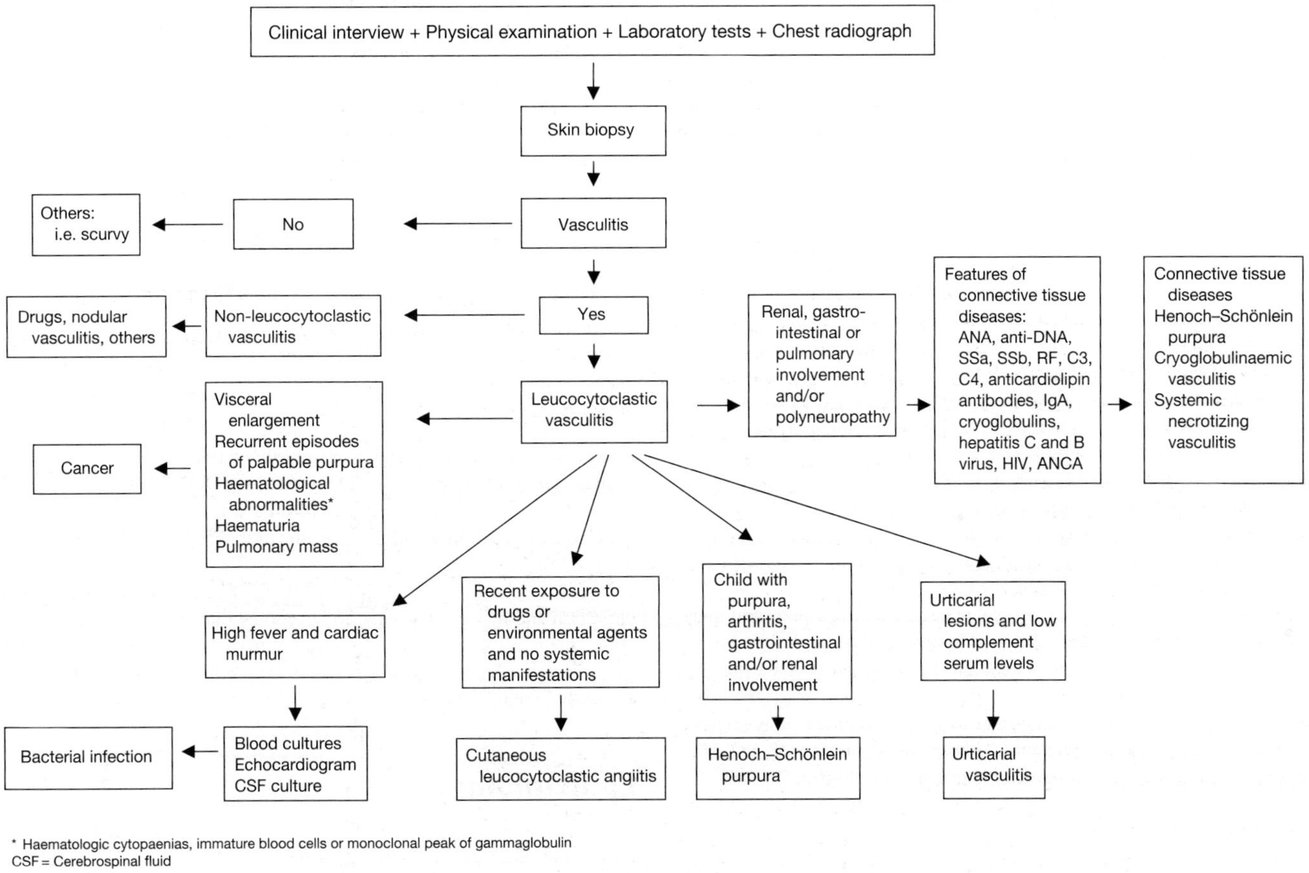

Fig. 1 Diagnostic approach of small-vessel vasculitis.

vasculitis is probably a reactive process and drug reaction was considered to be the cause in 17 per cent of the cases described by Massa and Su (1984). It may present as maculopapules, petechiae, infarctions, erythema or urticaria. Non-leucocytoclastic vasculitides with predominant eosinophil infiltration in the vessel walls may also be related to drugs.

Diagnostic approach (algorithm work-up)

As the presence of purpura does not always indicate the diagnosis of small-sized blood vessel vasculitis, skin biopsy specimens for routine microscopy and direct immunofluorescence are required in patients presenting with cutaneous lesions. Clinical decisions, however, should not be delayed until the result is available. A careful clinical history should search for data regarding ingestion of drugs, presence of pre-existing symptoms suggestive of chronic or acute disorders, autoimmune diseases, and history of recent or a chronic infection. Physical examination, routine laboratory tests, and chest radiograph should be performed in all the cases. Moreover, in the presence of specific symptoms or signs of an underlying systemic disorder additional examinations and laboratory tests should be performed (Fig. 1).

References

Agnello, V. (1998). Mixed cryoglobulinemia after hepatitis C virus: more and less ambiguity. *Annals of the Rheumatic Diseases* **57**, 701–2.

Bacon, P.A. and Carruthers, D.M. (1995). Vasculitis associated with connective tissue disorders. *Rheumatic Diseases Clinics of North America* **21**, 1077–96.

Calabrese, L.H. et al. (1990). The American College of Rheumatology 1990 criteria for the classification of hypersensitivity vasculitis. *Arthritis and Rheumatism* **33**, 1108–13.

Calviño, M.C., Llorca, J., Garcia-Porrua, C., Fernandez-Iglesias, J.L., Rodriguez-Ledo, P., and Gonzalez-Gay, M.A. (2001). Henoch–Schönlein purpura in children from Northwest Spain: a 20-year epidemiologic and clinical study. *Medicine (Baltimore)* **80**, 279–90.

Casato, M., Lagana, B., Pucillo, L.P., and Quinti, I. (1998). Interferon for hepatitis C virus negative type II mixed cryoglobulinemia. *New England Journal of Medicine* **338**, 1386–7.

Garcia-Porrua, C., Gonzalez-Louzao, C., Llorca, J., and Gonzalez-Gay, M.A. (2001a). Predictive factors for renal sequelae in adults with Henoch–Schönlein purpura. *Journal of Rheumatology* **28**,1019–24.

Garcia-Porrua, C., Llorca J., Gonzalez-Louzao, C., and Gonzalez-Gay, M.A. (2001b). Hypersensitivity vasculitis in adults: a benign disease usually limited to skin. *Clinical and Experimental Rheumatology* **19**, 85–8.

Gibson, L.E. and Su, W.F. (1995). Cutaneous vasculitis. *Rheumatic Diseases Clinics of North America* **21**, 1097–113.

Gonzalez-Gay, M.A. and Garcia-Porrua, C. (1999). Systemic vasculitis in adults in Northwestern Spain, 1988–1997: clinical and epidemiologic aspects. *Medicine (Baltimore)* **78**, 292–308.

Gonzalez-Gay, M.A. and Garcia-Porrua, C. (2001). The epidemiology of the vasculitides. *Rheumatic Diseases Clinics of North America* **27**, 729–49.

Gonzalez-Gay, M.A. and Garcia-Porrua, C. (2002). Henoch–Schönlein purpura. In *Vasculitis* Chapter 35 (ed. G.V. Ball and S.L. Bridges, Jr.), pp. 476–94. Oxford: Oxford University Press.

Gorevic, P.D. et al. (1980). Mixed cryoglobulinemia: clinical aspects and long-term follow up of 40 patients. *American Journal of Medicine* **69**, 287–308.

Henoch, E.H.H. (1874). Über eine eigentümliche Form von Purpura. *Berliner Klinische Wochenschrift* **ii**, 641–3.

Jennette, J.C. et al. (1994). Nomenclature of systemic vasculitides: proposal of an international consensus conference. *Arthritis and Rheumatism* **37**, 187–92.

Kaku, Y., Nohara, K., and Honda, S. (1998). Renal involvement in Henoch–Schönlein purpura: a multivariate analysis of prognostic factors. *Kidney International* **53**, 1755–9.

Lamprecht, A., Gause, A., and Gross, W.L. (1999). Cryoglobulinemic vasculitis. *Arthritis and Rheumatism* **42**, 2507–16.

Lie, J.T. (1994). Nomenclature and classification of vasculitis: plus ça change, plus c'est la meme chose. *Arthritis and Rheumatism* **37**, 181–6.

Lie, J.T. and Members and Consultants of the American College of Rheumatology Subcommittee on classification of vasculitis (1990). Illustrated histopathologic classification criteria for selected vasculitis syndromes. *Arthritis and Rheumatism* **33**, 1074–87.

Lotti, T., Ghersetich, I., Comacchi, C., and Jorizzo, J.L. (1998). Cutaneous small-vessel vasculitis. *Journal of the American Academy of Dermatology* **39**, 667–87.

Massa, M.C. and Su, W.P.D. (1984). Lymphocytic vasculitis: is it a specific clinicopathologic entity? *Journal of Cutaneous Pathology* **11**, 132–9.

McDuffie, F.C. et al. (1973). Hypocomplementemia with cutaneous vasculitis and arthritis: possible immunocomplex syndrome. *Mayo Clinic Proceedings* **48**, 340–8.

Mehregan, D.R., Hall, M.J., and Gibson, L.E. (1992). Urticarial vasculitis: a histopathologic and clinical review of 72 cases. *Journal of the American Academy of Dermatology* **26**, 441–8.

Rogers, M. (1992). Pityriasis lichenoides and lymphomatoid papulosis. *Seminars in Dermatology* **11**, 73–9.

Saulsbury, F.T. (1993). Corticosteroid therapy does not prevent nephritis in Henoch–Schönlein purpura. *Pediatric Nephrology* **7**, 69–71.

Schönlein, J.L. *Allgemeine und specielle Pathologie und Therapie* Vol., 3rd edn. Wurzburg Herisau, 1837.

Somer, T. and Finegold, S.M. (1995). Vasculitides associated with infections, immunizations and antimicrobial drugs. *Clinical Infectious Diseases* **20**, 1010–36.

Stone, J.H. and Nousari, H.C. (2001). 'Essential' cutaneous vasculitis: what every rheumatologist should know about vasculitis of the skin. *Current Opinion in Rheumatology* **13**, 23–34.

Szer, I.S. (1996). Henoch–Schönlein purpura: when and how to treat. *Journal of Rheumatology* **23**, 1661–5.

Watts, R.A., Jolliffe, V.A., Grattan, C.E.H., Elliot, J., Lockwood, M., and Scott, D.G.I. (1998). Cutaneous vasculitis in a defined population—clinical and epidemiological associations. *Journal of Rheumatology* **25**, 920–4.

Zeek, P.M., Smith, C.C., and Weeter, J.C. (1948). Studies on periarteritis nodosa. III. The differentiation between the vascular lesions of periarteritis nodosa and hypersensitivity. *American Journal of Pathology* **24**, 889–917.

6.10.8 Behçet's syndrome

Hasan Yazici, Sebahattin Yurdakul, and İzzet Fresko

Introduction

Behçet's syndrome is a systemic vasculitis of unknown aetiology with a peculiar geographic distribution. Most cases are clustered around the countries of the Mediterranean basin, the Middle East, and the Far East. Its most dreaded complication, eye disease, is one of the leading causes of blindness in these areas.

In 1937, Behçet described in detail three patients with oral and genital ulceration and hypopyon uveitis, and proposed that this was a distinct entity. Subsequently, it was realized that many other clinical manifestations were part of this syndrome (Sakane et al. 1999). Table 1 gives the more important of these manifestations.

Epidemiology

The usual onset of the syndrome is in the third or fourth decade. The onset is rare in children and after the age of 45.

The male/female ratio is approximately equal but the syndrome has a more severe course in men. Based on case registries, the prevalence is about 1 : 300 000 in Northern Europe and 1 : 10 000 in Japan. The prevalence may

Table 1 Clinical findings in Behçet's syndrome

Lesion	Prevalence (%)
Aphthous ulcerations	97–100
Genital lesions	80–90
Skin lesions	80
Eye lesions	50
Arthritis	40–50
Thrombophlebitis	25
Neurological involvement	1–15
Gastrointestinal involvement	0–25

be higher in Mediterranean countries. In Turkey, based on two spot surveys among the adult population, the prevalence rates were 8 and 37 : 10 000 (Yurdakul et al. 1988). On the other hand, again from Turkey, no cases were detected among a nation-wide survey of 47 000 children (Ozen et al. 1998). This places the prevalence among children to less than 1 : 15 000, with 95 per cent confidence (Yazici et al. 2001a) even in the face of a recent awareness of childhood cases (Kone-Paut et al. 1998).

Clinical features

Skin and mucosal involvement

Oral aphthae

Behçet's syndrome only rarely occurs without oral ulceration, frequently also the first manifestation of the syndrome. The majority of oral ulcers in Behçet's syndrome are indistinguishable from those seen in recurrent oral ulceration, but tend to be multiple and occur more frequently. Large (major) ulcers are less frequent and herpetiform ulcers are rare. Major ulcers, however, can be very troublesome because they heal with scarring, which can even occlude the oropharynx. The minor ulcers do not as a rule leave scars. The histology reveals non-specific ulceration with necrotic material.

Genital ulceration

In the male, 90 per cent of the genital ulcers occur on the scrotum and almost always leave scars. Urethritis is not observed. In the female, the labia (major and minor) are commonly affected. Histologically, they are indistinguishable from oral aphthae.

Skin lesions

The skin lesions of Behçet's syndrome can be divided into three main types: (a) Nodular lesions resembling erythema nodosum. These are similar to idiopathic erythema nodosum and those due to other conditions (e.g. sarcoidosis). It has recently been shown that more elements of vasculitis are observed on histological sections of these lesions when compared to idiopathic erythema nodosum or to erythema nodosum due to other causes (Demirkesen et al. 2001). Sometimes superficial thrombophlebitis can be clinically indistinguishable from erythema nodosum. (b) Papulopustular lesions also called acneiform lesions or simply acne. Most papulopustular lesions are histologically very similar to ordinary acne. However, they differ from the latter in their propensity to occur also in the extremities in addition to the face and the trunk. (c) Others that represent various forms of vasculitis such as leucocytoclastic vasculitis, necrotizing arteritis of the small and medium arteries, superficial thrombophlebitis (quite difficult clinically to differentiate from the erythema nodosum lesions), unclassifiable papules and pustules, and Sweet syndrome (Jorizzo et al. 1995).

The pathergy reaction (Plate 158), a curious hyperreactivity of the skin to a needle prick, is peculiar to this syndrome. The only other condition in which it is known to be positive with any consistency is pyoderma gangrenosum. After a skin puncture with a needle, a papule or a pustule forms in 24–48 h.

Pathergy is seldom found among patients in Northern Europe or the United States. In patients from Japan and Turkey it is positive in around 60–70 per cent when tested repeatedly.

The mechanism of the pathergy reaction is still obscure. Surgical cleaning of the skin considerably dampens this reaction, which suggests that more than disrupting the integrity of the epidermis and dermis is operational. Immunophenotypic analysis of skin biopsy specimens of positive pathergy reactions suggest that the reaction consists of a delayed hypersensitivity reaction independent of a specific antigen (Gül 2001).

The pathergy phenomenon in Behçet's syndrome is not confined to the skin; various tissues are known to be hyperreactive to surgical trauma, and it is not uncommon to have attacks of uveitis after eye surgery and synovitis after an arthrocentesis. However, it has been shown that wound healing after biopsy induced trauma is normal in patients with Behçet's syndrome.

The propensity for inflammation in Behçet's syndrome can also be observed in the response these patients have to intradermal injections of monosodium urate crystals (Çakir et al. 1991).

Eye involvement (Plate 159)

This is one of the most serious manifestations. Its overall prevalence is about 50 per cent. Males and those with younger age of onset have an increased prevalence. Females are less severely affected. Disease is bilateral in 90 per cent of the patients with ocular involvement. The onset of eye disease is usually within 2–3 years of the development of the syndrome.

Eye disease in Behçet's syndrome consists of a chronic relapsing posterior and anterior uveitis. Isolated anterior uveitis is found in only 10 per cent of those with ocular involvement.

Hypopyon uveitis (Plate 159) is very typical of Behçet's syndrome, although occasionally it can be observed in Reiter's syndrome. It is an accumulation of white cells and debris in the anterior chamber that precipitates to form a layer due to gravity. Hypopyon is seen in 20 per cent of patients with eye disease and as a rule is almost always associated with severe retinal disease.

The basic retinal lesion is a vasculitis, which can lead to exudates, haemorrhages, venous thrombosis, papillooedema, and macular disease that frequently results in a hole. The pars plana is also involved. During an acute flare there is a marked influx of fibrin, inflammatory cells, and cellular debris into the vitreous. After each flare there is usually some residual structural damage in the form of retinal changes, vitreal opacities, posterior synechiae, and cataracts. Secondary glaucoma frequently develops. The extent of these structural changes determines the course of eye disease in Behçet's syndrome.

Musculoskeletal system

Involvement of the joints is seen in about one-half of the patients in the form of arthritis or arthralgia. There is usually a mono or oligoarticular involvement but symmetrical disease of the wrist or elbow, which can be confused with rheumatoid arthritis, may occasionally occur. Usually lasting a few weeks, it seldom leads to chronic synovitis and deformity. Erythema of the overlying skin is not seen. Erosions are uncommon. The synovial fluid is inflammatory (see below) and the histological changes are non-specific (Yurdakul et al. 1983).

Knees are the most commonly affected joints, followed in frequency by ankles, wrists, and elbows. Back pain is quite rare in Behçet's syndrome and an increased prevalence of sacroiliac joint involvement has not been found in controlled studies. A recent study has shown that patients with Behçet's syndrome who had arthritis also had more acne lesions compared to controls suggesting a link with the reactive arthritides (Diri et al. 2001).

Local or generalized myositis is occasionally found in Behçet's syndrome. The muscle enzymes are not raised in the local forms and the histological features are indistinguishable from those of polymyositis.

Another musculoskeletal manifestation associated with Behçet's syndrome is aseptic necrosis of the bone. This is possibly related to vasculitis and not necessarily to steroid use.

Neurological involvement

There is much variation in the reported prevalence rates of neurological involvement. Most patients have parenchymal involvement with pyramidal signs, hemiparesis, behavioural changes, sphincter disturbances, and less frequently brainstem signs and pyramidocerebellar syndrome. The remaining have non-parenchymal disease with increased intracranial pressure due to dural sinus thrombosis. Dementia can develop in an occasional patient. In the majority of the cases, headaches can be related to the basic pathology only if there are other associated signs and symptoms in the central nervous system. As is true with eye involvement, the most severe forms of central nervous involvement are seen in the male. Parenchymal involvement has a more severe course (Akman-Demir et al. 1999).

The findings in cerebrospinal fluid are usually non-specific. An inflammatory cerebrospinal fluid indicates a severe prognosis.

The most common site of involvement is the brainstem. Hemispheric, meningeal, and spinal cord lesions are also seen. The lesions are best demonstrated by magnetic resonance imaging. In contrast to the other vasculitides, peripheral nerve disease is quite unusual (Siva et al. 2001).

Cardiovascular and pulmonary involvement

Cardiac involvement

Endocarditis, myocarditis, and pericarditis can all occur but are rare. Right-sided intracardiac thrombi along with endomyocardial fibrosis have also been reported and cases with coronary vasculitis and ventricular aneurysms have been documented.

Venous lesions

Involvement of the veins is one of the main manifestations of Behçet's syndrome. In fact, Behçet's syndrome, together with systemic lupus and Buerger's disease, is one of the few vasculitides that can involve the venous side of the circulatory system along with the arterial side. Furthermore, in contrast to the other two, it can involve the vena cavae.

Thrombophlebitis occurs in 25 per cent of all patients. More frequent in the calf, it is also seen in veins of the upper extremity. A frequent outcome of thrombosis in the lower extremities is a chronic stasis dermatitis associated with recurring skin ulcers. Thrombosis of the iliac veins and both vena cavae is less frequent and seen almost only in male patients. Occlusion of the suprahepatic veins can cause a Budd–Chiari syndrome. This carries high mortality.

Pulmonary embolism is rare in Behçet's syndrome even though thrombophlebitis is seen in one-fourth of the patients. The thrombi in this syndrome involve long segments and seem to be adherent to the vessel wall.

Arterial lesions (Fig. 1)

Aneurysms of the abdominal aorta, carotid, femoral, and the popliteal can be seen (Koç et al. 1992). The rupture of these aneurysms is frequently fatal. The basic pathology is thought to be a vasculitis of the vasa vasorum. There is a high recurrence rate after reconstructive surgery of the aneurysms of the peripheral vessels.

The basic pulmonary pathology in Behçet's syndrome is also related to vasculitis. Pulmonary vascular changes in the form of arterial aneurysms, arterial and venous thromboses, and pulmonary infarcts are found (Efthimiou et al. 1986; Hamuryudan et al. 1994). The classic radiographic finding is the non-cavitating mass lesion.

Pulmonary arterial aneurysms in Behçet's syndrome carry a grave prognosis with the terminating event usually being the rupture of an aneurysm into a bronchus.

Gastrointestinal involvement

While gastrointestinal involvement is seen in about one-third of patients from Japan it is quite rare among patients in Turkey (Bayraktar et al. 2000). The basic pathology is that of mucosal ulceration. This is most commonly seen in the ileum, followed by the caecum and other parts of the colon.

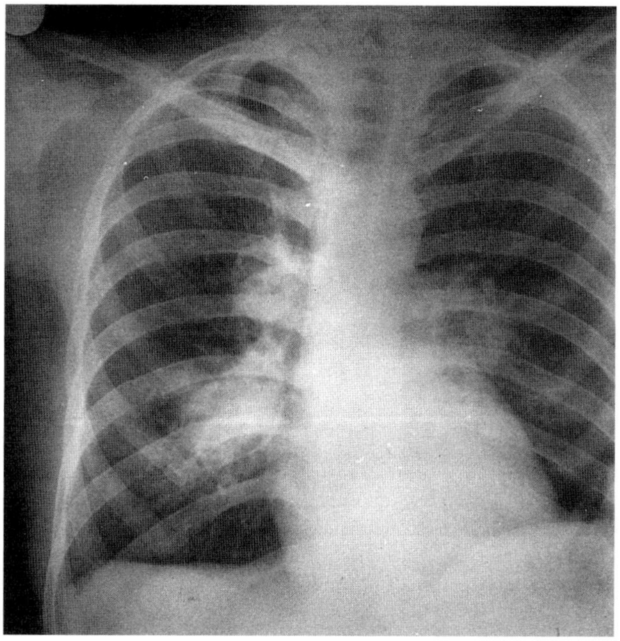

Fig. 1 Pulmonary artery aneurysms.

Histologically, the ulcers are indistinguishable from those found in ulcerative colitis. The usual symptoms are abdominal pain and melena. A mass is often palpable in the abdomen. The ileocaecal ulcers have the worst prognosis, with a distinct tendency to perforate.

Hepatic problems are not common in Behçet's syndrome except when an associated Budd–Chiari syndrome is present.

Other clinical features

Renal involvement is seen much less frequently than one would expect in a systemic vasculitis. There are occasional reports of glomerulonephritis. Epididymitis and voiding dysfunction are well-recognized symptoms (Cetinel et al. 1998).

Amyloidosis of the AA type is seen sporadically, usually presents with nephrotic syndrome and carries a grave prognosis (Melikoglu et al. 2001).

Diagnosis

The full-blown syndrome is easy to identify; the so-called incomplete forms sometimes cause problems. The main conditions that should be considered in the differential diagnosis are shown in Table 2 (Barnes and Yazici 1999).

Using the presence of recurrent oral ulceration as mandatory, together with proper exclusions, International Study Group criteria (International Study Group for Behçet's Disease 1990) require involvement of two other organ systems for a diagnosis, or more correctly classification, of Behçet's syndrome. In this scheme a positive pathergy test can replace involvement of an organ system.

Laboratory investigations

There are no laboratory findings specific for Behçet's syndrome. A moderate anaemia of chronic disease and leucocytosis are seen in 15 per cent of the patients. The erythrocyte sedimentation rate is only mildly elevated, as is the C-reactive protein. Neither correlates well with disease activity.

The synovial fluid is usually inflammatory. The cell count is between 5000 and 50 000 mm^3 with neutrophils predominating. Despite this high cell count the mucin clot is usually good.

Table 2 Highlights of the clinical manifestations of Behçet's syndrome and differential diagnosis (Barnes and Yazici 1999)

Manifestation	Comment	Differential diagnosis
Mouth ulcers	Similar in appearance to common aphthous ulcers, more frequent and frequently multiple	Reiter's syndrome—painless ulceration
Genital ulcers	Most commonly scrotal or vulval, painful, recurrent, and usually with scarring. Urethral discharge and penile lesions very rare	Reiter's syndrome
Skin	Acneiform lesions as common acne in appearance and histology but also at uncommon sites such as the extremities. Erythema nodosum like lesions leaving pigmentation. Not psoriasis	Seronegative arthropathies; inflammatory bowel disease; sarcoidosis
Eyes	Panuveitis and retinal vasculitis, usually bilateral occuring within about 2 years of the onset of the disease. Conjunctivitis and sicca syndrome most unusual	Seronegative arthropathies
Joints	Monoarthritis in 50%, otherwise oligoarticular or polyarticular, involving relatively few joints; may be symmetrical; knees most frequently; intermittent resolving in 2–4 weeks or chronic and continuous; not involving sacroiliac joints or spine; deformity and erosions rare. Inflammatory synovial fluid with good mucin clot	Inflammatory arthropathies
Peripheral arterial and venous disease	Sub-clinical peripheral large vein disease uncommon, usually involves large segments with skip areas without embolization; arteritis with occlusion and/or pseudoaneurysms; microaneurysms of the polyarteritic type very uncommon	Other vasculitides
Neurological involvement	Peripheral neuropathy with isolated cerebellar involvement very unusual, headaches with dural sinus thrombosis; vascular central nervous system lesions including transverse myelitis-type manifestation. Multiple sclerosis with aphthous ulcers a problem but no plaques on magnetic resonance imaging	Multiple sclerosis
Pulmonary involvement	Haemoptysis associated with pulmonary artery aneurysm; pulmonary artery occlusion; pleural involvement uncommon; interstitial involvement very rare	Pulmonary embolism; any cause of haemoptysis
Gastrointestinal involvement	Severe abdominal pain; ulcerative lesions at any level but mainly in the ileocaecal region; mild gastrointestinal symptoms should not be associated with Behçet's syndrome	Inflammatory bowel disease
Cardiac disease	Pericarditis, valve lesions, and coronary artery involvement uncommon; rarely intracardiac thrombi	Valve lesions in seronegative arthropathies

Serum immunoglobulins are sometimes elevated, while autoantibodies are absent. Complement levels may be high. Despite the pauci-immune nature of the basic disease process, antineutrophilic antibodies are not a feature of Behçet's syndrome.

Genetics and pathogenesis

Behçet's syndrome is an inflammatory vasculitis. Immunologically mediated mechanisms seem to be important in the pathogenesis (Yazici et al. 2001b), but the precise mechanisms that initiate and sustain the increased inflammatory state that characterizes the syndrome remain unknown.

Most cases are sporadic and do not show a Mendelian inheritance pattern. Familial cases exist and a sibling recurrence risk ratio (λ_s) of 11.4–52.5 has been recently reported (Gül 2001).

HLA-B51 has been associated with Behçet's syndrome especially in areas where the syndrome shows the highest prevalence such as the Mediterranean Basin and the Far East but the strength of this association decreases in patients from the United Kingdom and the United States. Genes in linkage disequilibrium with HLA-B51 such as MHC class I chain related gene A (MICA) have also been linked to the syndrome but recent analyses in different ethnic groups have shown that HLA-B51 itself still confers the highest susceptibility.

The direct role of HLA-B51 in the pathogenesis of Behçet's syndrome is not known. Cross-reaction with self-peptides (Retinal S) and HLA-B51 has been implicated as a potential mechanism (Direskeneli 2001) and it is not yet known if additional gene(s) are involved.

An infectious aetiology has been implicated in the pathogenesis since the original description of Behçet's syndrome. Herpes simplex virus Type I (Sakane et al. 1999) and streptococci (*S. oralis*) have been held reponsible but a direct link between these organisms and Behçet's syndrome has not been shown. The cellular and humoral immune response to mycobacterial heat shock proteins (HSP65) and to their human homologues—coupled with the production of uveitis in Lewis rats with some of these proteins—have been proposed as a unifying mechanism that bridges the role of different microorganisms (Stanford et al. 1994; Direskeneli 2001).

Behçet's syndrome does not have the features of a classical autoimmune disorder such as female predominance, hypergammaglobulinaemia, and a coexistent Sjögren's syndrome but various abnormalities of the immune system are noted. Neutrophil hyperreactivity in the form of increased superoxide production, endothelial adhesion, chemotaxis, and phagocytosis have been reported and an animal model has linked increased superoxide production to the presence of HLA-B51 (Takeno et al. 1995). However, recent reports have shown that neutrophil hyperreactivity in Behçet's syndrome is debatable. An increased cellular immune response with a Th1 cytokine predominance (Frassanito et al. 1999) and an increased proportion of $\delta\gamma+$ T lymphocytes (Freysdottir et al. 1999) that are thought to play important roles in mucosal defense have been reported. However, the evidence for a specific antigen or superantigen in eliciting this response has been inconclusive.

A non-specific hyperreactivity as exemplified by the pathergy phenomenon constitutes an important feature of Behçet's syndrome. The spontaneous or induced overproduction of proinflammatory cytokines from mononuclear cells in Behçet's syndrome may also constitute an aspect of this non-specific hyperreactivity (Mege et al. 1993).

No consistent coagulation abnormality has been found in Behçet's syndrome. Increased Factor V Leiden and prothrombin gene G20210A mutations have been observed mainly in patients with venous thrombosis but their exact roles in the pathogenesis have been inconclusive. Antiendothelial cell antibodies, antiphospholipid antibodies, and various endothelial cell activation markers have also been reported (Leiba et al. 2001).

Management

There are several important features of Behçet's syndrome that have to be taken into consideration when planning the management: (a) the usual course of the syndrome in any organ system is that of exacerbations and remissions with the overall activity generally abating with the passage of time; thus, the principal aim is to prevent irreversible structural damage, which is the outcome of the early stormy course; (b) being young and male are separate and additive negative prognostic factors; (c) eye disease usually has its onset, if at all, either initially or within the first few years; (d) the syndrome can be fatal, especially in the young male; and (e) there are many patients with Behçet's syndrome who do not need any treatment but reassurance.

Immunosuppressive drugs are the main line of treatment for eye involvement. Although corticosteroids have been used for a long time, there is no formal evidence that they are effective. Their short-term use over a few months, however, may shorten the duration of an attack.

Azathioprine at 2.5 mg/kg/day is useful in maintaining visual acuity and perhaps more importantly in preventing the emergence of new eye disease. Its early use in the disease course leads to a better long-term outcome (Hamuryudan et al. 1998a) and it is important that treatment is begun well before structural changes appear in the eye. Cyclosporin A is an effective and rapidly acting drug in the uveitis of Behçet's syndrome. Problems with cyclosporin A are the potential nephrotoxicity, especially at doses greater than 5 mg/kg/day, and the very frequent relapses after cessation of therapy. The high cost is another problem. Eye disease in remission for 2 years or more usually needs no further treatment. Young males, in general, need to be treated more vigorously. Once initiated, the usual course for cytotoxic or cyclosporin A therapy is a minimum of 2 years, after which attempts at discontinuation are made. There is the concern that this medication not only tends to accelerate the development of central nervous system (CNS) symptoms but also can cause CNS symptoms that can be confused with those in Behçet's syndrome. Thus, its use is not recommended in patients with CNS disease. In some patients, after a course for 6–8 months of combined azathioprine and cyclosporin A, treatment is continued with azathioprine only. In more resistant cases azathioprine is used in combination with cyclosporin A (both at conventional doses) for extended periods of time. Our uncontrolled experience with this mode of therapy in severe eye disease is quite favourable.

Data are accumulating which suggest that interferon alpha is effective remedy for various manifestations of Behçet's syndrome including eye disease (Kotter et al. 1998).

Structural damage to the eye can be managed surgically (i.e. vitrectomy) at specialized centres. However, results are not uniformly satisfactory. There is always the problem of new attacks of inflammation in surgically handled tissue in Behçet's syndrome. Also, the already established disease in the retina cannot be helped by surgery. Local mydriatics should be used in the acute stage to prevent synechiae.

The oral and genital ulcers are usually well controlled by immunosuppressives and steroids. However, these should be reserved for more severe cases. Often, a local steroid preparation that adheres to fresh ulceration (such as triamcinolone acetonide oral paste) is all that is required.

A recent 2-year controlled trial has shown that colchicine is more effective than placebo in the treatment of mucocutaneous and joint symptoms and that this effect is especially prominent among the females (Yurdakul et al. 2001). Most notably colchicine did not have any effect on the genital ulcerations among the male.

Thalidomide at a dose of 100 mg daily can induce dramatic relief from oral and genital ulcers (Hamuryudan et al. 1998b). Relapses are a rule after stopping treatment. Teratogenesis and polyneuropathy are the drawbacks of chronic thalidomide use.

Cyclophosphamide, either 2–2.5 mg/kg/day orally or 500–1500 mg weekly or monthly intravenous boluses, is required to treat those patients with severe cutaneous, arterial, or pulmonary vasculitis, or those with arterial aneurysms or vena caval involvement. There is no formal experience with any therapy for central nervous disease; however, steroids and immunosuppressives are again used.

Gastrointestinal involvement is initially managed by sulfasalazine at a dosage of 2–6 g/day. Sometimes surgery is required, with resection of large segments of bowel. Usually, a good portion of uninvolved area should also be removed to prevent recurrences. Surgery is also mandatory for aneurysms of peripheral vessels (Tüzün et al. 1997).

There is debate whether to use heparin or oral anticoagulants for the thrombophlebitis of Behçet's syndrome. Pulmonary embolism is seldom observed, as explained above. In this setting, antiplatelet drugs (i.e. aspirin) are probably sufficient. We also use azathioprine in thrombophlebitis of Behçet's syndrome as an agent to suppress the disease activity in general.

Combination of these drugs with steroids or the combination of azathioprine and cyclosporin A can be tried in cases resistant to a single agent.

Preliminary experience suggests that the new anti-TNF agents, etanercept, and infliximab, have the potential to be useful in the treatment of Behçet's syndrome.

In the absence of any hard data it is customary to stop treatment in a patient in remission after 2–4 years.

Prognosis

The disease intensity usually abates with the passage of time. On the other hand, Behçet's syndrome is a significant cause of increased mortality, especially due to bleeding pulmonary artery aneurysms, among the young and male patients (Yazici et al. 1996).

Other causes of mortality in Behçet's syndrome are ruptured peripheral aneurysms, severe central nervous system disease, Budd–Chiari syndrome, and finally intestinal ulceration and perforation especially prominent among the Japanese.

References

Akman-Demir, G. et al. (1999). Clinical patterns of neurological involvement in Behçet's disease: evaluation of 200 patients. *Brain* **122**, 2171–82.

Barnes, C.G. and Yazici, H. (1999). Behçet's syndrome. *Rheumatology (Oxford)* **38**, 1171–6.

Bayraktar, Y., Ozaslan, E., and Van Thiel, D.H. (2000). Gastrointestinal manifestations of Behçet's disease. *Journal of Clinical Gastroenterology* **30**, 144–54.

Çakir, N. et al. (1991). Response to intradermal injection of monosodium urate crystals in Behçet's syndrome. *Annals of the Rheumatic Diseases* **50**, 634–6.

Cetinel, B. et al. (1998). Urologic screening for men with Behçet's syndrome. *Urology* **52**, 863–5.

Demirkesen, C. et al. (2001). Clinicopathological evaluation of nodular lesions of Behçet's disease. *American Journal of Clinical Pathology* **116**, 341–6.

Direskeneli, H. (2001). Behçet's disease: infectious aetiology, new autoantigens and HLA-B51. *Annals of the Rheumatic Diseases* **60**, 996–1002.

Diri, E. et al. (2001). Papulopustular skin lesions are seen more frequently in patients with Behçet's syndrome who have arthritis: a controlled and masked study. *Annals of the Rheumatic Diseases* **60**, 1074–6.

Efthimiou, J. et al. (1986). Pulmonary disease in Behçet's syndrome. *Quarterly Journal of Medicine* **58**, 259–80.

Frassanito, M.A. et al. (1999). Th1 polarization of the immune response in Behçet's disease: a putative pathogenetic role of interleukin-12. *Arthritis and Rheumatism* **42**, 1967–74.

Freysdottir, J., Lau, S., and Fortune, F. (1999). Gammadelta T cells in Behçet's disease (BD) and recurrent aphthous stomatitis (RAS). *Clinical and Experimental Immunology* **118**, 451–7.

Gül, A. (2001). Behçet's disease: an update on the pathogenesis. *Clinical and Experimental Rheumatology* **19** (Suppl. 24), S6–12.

Hamuryudan, V. et al. (1994). Pulmonary arterial aneurysms in Behçet's syndrome: a report of 24 cases. *Rheumatology (Oxford)* **33**, 48–51.

Hamuryudan, V. et al. (1998a). Azathioprine in Behçet's syndrome: effects on long-term prognosis. *Arthritis and Rheumatism* **40**, 769–74.

Hamuryudan, V. et al. (1998b). Thalidomide in the treatment of the mucocutaneous lesions of the Behçet syndrome. A randomized, double-blind, placebo-controlled trial. *Annals of Internal Medicine* **128**, 443–50.

International Study Group for Behçet's Disease (1990). Criteria for diagnosis of Behçet's disease. *Lancet* **335**, 1078–80.

Jorizzo, J.L. et al. (1995). Mucocutaneous criteria for the diagnosis of Behçet's disease: an analysis of clinicopathologic data from multiple international centers. *Journal of the American Academy of Dermatology* **32**, 968–76.

Koç, Y. et al. (1992). Vascular involvement in Behçet's disease. *Journal of Rheumatology* **19**, 402–10.

Kone-Paut, I. et al. (1998). Clinical features of Behçet's disease in children: an international collaborative study of 86 cases. *Journal of Pediatrics* **132**, 721–5.

Kotter, I. et al. (1998). Treatment of ocular symptoms of Behçet's disease with interferon alpha 2a: a pilot study. *British Journal of Ophthalmology* **82**, 488–94.

Ozen, S. et al. (1998). Prevalence of juvenile chronic arthritis and familial Mediterranean fever in Turkey: a field study. *Journal of Rheumatology* **25**, 2445–9.

Leiba, M. et al. (2001). Behçet's disease and thrombophilia. *Annals of the Rheumatic Diseases* **60**, 1081–5.

Mege, J.L. et al. (1993). Overproduction of monocyte derived tumor necrosis factor alpha, interleukin (IL) 6, IL-8 and increased neutrophil superoxide generation in Behçet's disease. A comparative study with familial Mediterranean fever and healthy subjects. *Journal of Rheumatology* **20**, 1544–9.

Melikoglu, M. et al. (2001). A reappraisal of amyloidosis in Behçet's syndrome. *Rheumatology (Oxford)* **40**, 212–15.

Sakane, T. et al. (1999). Behçet's disease. *New England Journal of Medicine* **341**, 1284–91.

Siva, A. et al. (2001). Behçet's disease: diagnostic and prognostic aspects of neurological involvement. *Journal of Neurology* **248**, 95–103.

Stanford, M.R. et al. (1994). Heat shock protein peptides reactive in patients with Behçet's disease are uveitogenic in Lewis rats. *Clinical and Experimental Immunology* **97**, 226–31.

Takeno, M. et al. (1995). Excessive function of peripheral blood neutrophils from patients with Behçet's disease and from HLA-B51 transgenic mice. *Arthritis and Rheumatism* **38**, 426–43.

Tüzün, H. et al. (1997). Management of aneurysms in Behçet's syndrome: an analysis of 24 patients. *Surgery* **121**, 150–6.

Yazici, H. et al. (1996). The ten-year mortality in Behçet's syndrome. *Rheumatology (Oxford)* **35**, 139–41.

Yazici, H. et al. (2001a). The 'zero patient' design to compare the prevalences of rare diseases. *Rheumatology (Oxford)* **40**, 121–2.

Yazici, H., Yurdakul, S., and Hamuryudan, V. (2001b). Behçet disease. *Current Opinion in Rheumatology* **13**, 18–22.

Yurdakul, S. et al. (1983). The arthritis of Behçet's disease: a prospective study. *Annals of the Rheumatic Diseases* **42**, 505–15.

Yurdakul, S. et al. (1988). The prevalence of Behçet's syndrome in a rural area in northern Turkey. *Journal of Rheumatology* **15**, 820–2.

Yurdakul, S. et al. (2001). A double blind trial of colchicine in Behçet's syndrome. *Arthritis and Rheumatism* **44**, 2686–92.

6.10.9 Vasculitis in children

Seza Ozen

Vasculitis is an inflammatory, destructive process affecting vessels. The common vasculitides of childhood, such as Henoch–Schönlein purpura (HSP) and Kawasaki disease (KD) are considerably more benign and self-limited compared to those in adults. A consistent and comprehensive classification of the vasculitides that takes into account both clinical and histopathological aspects is still not available (Cassidy and Petty 1995). Among the current classifications, the nomenclature for systemic vasculitis introduced by the Chapel Hill Consensus Conference (CHCC) (Jennette et al. 1994) has, in spite of some problems, gained widespread acceptance (Table 1). These criteria have been suggested for use in classification not for diagnosis. Other classifications include those of the American College of Rheumatology Subcommittee on Classification of Vasculitis (Hunder et al. 1990). This chapter will discuss childhood vasculitides in the context of the CHCC classification. Polyarteritis nodosa (PAN) will be discussed under one heading.

Table 1 Classification of vasculitides in childhood [modified from Jennette et al. (2001), reprinted by permission of Wiley-Liss, Inc., a subsidiary of John Wiley and Sons, Inc.]

Primary vasculitides
Predominantly large-vessel
Takayasu disease (giant cell arteritis)
Predominantly medium-sized vessel
Kawasaki disease
PAN: Classic PAN, systemic PAN, cutaneous PAN
Predominantly small vessel involvement
PAN: microscopic PAN and systemic PAN
Wegener's granulomatosis
Henoch–Schönlein purpura
Churg–Strauss syndrome
Cutaneous leucocytoclastic vasculitis
Secondary vasculitides

Primary vasculitides

Predominantly large vessel

Takayasu disease

Takayasu's arteritis is a segmental inflammatory arteritis leading to stenosis and aneurysms of large muscular arteries, mainly the aorta and its major branches (Hall et al. 1985). Females are affected more than males. Many reports have drawn attention to the association of Takayasu's arteritis with tuberculosis.

A patient is classified as Takayasu's arteritis if three of the following six are present: (i) age less than 40 years, (ii) claudication of extremities, (iii) decreased brachial artery pulse, (iv) blood pressure difference greater than 10 mmHg, (v) bruit over subclavian arteries or aorta, and (vi) arteriogram abnormality (Arend et al. 1990).

Clinical and laboratory features

The presenting symptoms of the patients are fever, night sweats, anorexia, weight loss, and musculoskeletal symptoms. Symptoms related to hypertension and pulse deficits often emerge (Hall et al. 1985). The type of vascular involvement seems to differ according to the geographic area: obstructive lesions seem to be more common in the United States, western Europe, and Japan, whereas aneurysms appear to be more common in south east Asia and Africa (Cassidy and Petty 1995).

Acute phase reactants are elevated. Although plain radiographs may be helpful, diagnosis requires the demonstration of the arteritis and typical findings by magnetic resonance or conventional angiography.

Treatment

Corticosteroids are used in acute disease (Hoffman et al. 1994). As with other vasculitides cyclophosphamide is an effective alternative. Recent adult and childhood reports have emphasized the use of methotrexate as a steroid sparing agent (Hoffman et al. 1994). A positive tuberculin test would justify antituberculous therapy. Subsequent reconstructive surgery and transluminal angioplasty may be employed for the vascular complications.

Predominantly medium-sized vessel

Kawasaki disease

KD has been increasingly recognized since it was first described by Tomisaku Kawasaki in 1967 (Kawasaki 1967). It is a disease of childhood, about 80 per cent of the cases occurring in children younger than 5 years of age with the highest included in the first 3 years of life. In a nationwide survey in Japan, the incidence was as high as 102–108 per 100 000 (Yanagawa et al. 1998). The incidence in diverse areas outside Japan has been reported as 6–10 per 100 000 children younger than 5 years of age (Barron et al. 1999). In epidemic years the figures increase three- to six-fold. KD is 1.5 times more common in boys.

The epidemiological and clinical features of the disease strongly suggest an infectious aetiology. Outbreaks are expected to occur when a new group of susceptible children are added to the population (Barron et al. 1999). The role of infectious agents and superantigens in the development and triggering of KD has been suggested (Petty and Cassidy 2001).

The CHCC criteria has categorized the disease as medium-vessel vasculitis, however, the coronary arteriolar branches are small sized.

Clinical features and diagnosis

Diagnosis of KD relies on a set of diagnostic criteria (Dillon 1998). These criteria are:

- Fever persisting for at least 5 days;
- Changes in peripheral extremities being reddening of palms and soles, oedema in the initial stage and membranous desquamation of the skin of hands and feet in the convalescent phase (Plate 160);
- Polymorphous exanthema;
- Bilateral conjunctival injection;
- Changes of lips and oral cavity: reddening of lips, diffuse injection of oral, and pharyngeal mucosa;
- Cervical lymphadenopathy: acute, non-purulent.

Either five of the six criteria or four criteria plus coronary angiogram by 2D-echocardiography are required for the diagnosis (Japan Kawasaki Disease Research Committee 1984). Cardiac disease may range from coronary aneurysms and thrombosis to myocarditis, pericarditis, and cardiac tamponade.

Children with KD are very irritable. Arthralgia and/or arthritis are common. Features suggesting an upper respiratory tract infection such as cough, coryza, otitis media, may occur as well as diarrhoea, vomiting, ileus, jaundice, dysuria, pneumonitis, uveitis, convulsions, and meningitis (Petty and Cassidy 2001).

However, there are problems with the current criteria. In all reported series, at least 10 per cent of the KD patients do not fulfil the five criteria and constitute the atypical cases. These patients present a problem to the clinician. Another problem with these criteria is in the low specificity; that is, a number of patients with other diseases may fulfil the criteria. Most important of these are adenoviral infections. KD should also be differentiated from streptococcal scarlet fever, Stevens Johnson syndrome, and toxic shock syndrome.

Laboratory investigations

Acute phase reactants, leucocyte and thrombocyte counts are characteristically elevated early in the course of the disease. Occasionally, the platelet count may be low during the early phase; however, it almost always rises markedly by the second week (Cassidy and Petty 1995). Pyuria with negative culture may be present. Although antineutrophil cytoplasmic antibody (ANCA) and antiendothelial cell antibody may be detected in KD, their diagnostic value is not clear. Echocardiograms should be performed to detect any cardiac complications in all cases at diagnosis and follow-up.

Treatment and prognosis

Pharmacological treatment of KD consists of aspirin 80–100 mg/kg, reduced when the platelet count returns to normal.

Since it has been shown that intravenous immunoglobulin (IVIG) treatment reduces the incidence of coronary aneurysms, it has become the mainstay of treatment. IVIG is given as a single dose (2 g/kg) or 400 mg/kg/day for 4 days, within the first 10–12 days (Barron et al. 1999). In a retrospective analysis, 77 per cent fully responded to a single IVIG treatment; 10 out of 15 patients responded to subsequent re-treatment (Wallace et al. 2000). In the remaining patients the disease progression was blocked after methylprednisolone and/or cyclophosphamide. Although the use of steroids remains controversial, it should be considered in children unresponsive to IVIG (Petty and Cassidy 2001). A management plan for KD is given below (Petty and Cassidy 2001).

- Make diagnosis admit to hospital
-

Evaluation	*Treatment*
Cardiac status	Aspirin
CNS status	If platelets <400 000: 80 mg/kg/day in four doses
Fluid and electrolyte status	If platelets >400 000: 3–5 mg/kg/day
Urinalysis	IVIG: 2 g/kg
Ophthalmologic status	Keep in hospital until afebrile or for complications
Monitor cardiac status	Repeat IVIG once. If no clinical response give IV methylprednisolone (2-week intervals until stable, then 1-month intervals until normal)
Monitor ESR and platelet count	Maintain low dose aspirin until ESR and platelets are normal if no coronary abnormalities, for 2 years if there have been abnormalities but are no longer present, and indefinitely if coronary artery disease persists

- Repeat echo at 6–8 weeks

KD is essentially a self-limited disease, morbidity and mortality are defined by the cardiac involvement. The occurrence of cardiac aneurysms decreased from 20–25 per cent to less than 2 per cent with treatment. Patients who develop cardiac complications need long-term follow-up into adult life, since vascular dysfunction may persist with regressed aneurysms (Iemura et al. 2000).

Polyarteritis nodosa of childhood

PAN is characterized by necrotizing vasculitis of small- and/or medium-sized arteries. Cassidy and Petty (2001) have defined PAN as a clinical syndrome that is characterized by the presence of fibrinoid necrosis of small to medium-sized arteries. The CHCC has defined PAN in two entities as classic and microscopic forms, which will be discussed below (Jennette et al. 1994). However, there are a considerable number of children with necrotizing vasculitis who do not necessarily fit in within these two entities defined for adults, but fulfil the classification criteria suggested by the ACR and Ozen et al. (Lightfoot et al. 1990; Ozen et al. 2001) or who have overlapping features of the aforementioned forms.

PAN should be suspected in any child with fever of unknown origin, dermal findings, myalgia, unexplained pulmonary, cardiovascular, nervous system, or renal disease. Classification criteria for the disease have attempted to cover this multisystem involvement (Lightfoot et al. 1990; Ozen et al. 1992). However, the sensitivity and specificity of both sets of criteria may need to be improved. Both lack the presence of ANCA, which has emerged as an important marker for the disease.

The association with streptococcal infection is a remarkable feature that has been commented on in various paediatric patients (David et al. 1993; Bont et al. 1998), this association is less common in adults (Dillon 1998).

General features of systemic PAN in childhood

The average ages of patients were 9.3 and 7.5 years in two series both including infants (Dillon 1990; Ozen et al. 1992). Children almost always have constitutional symptoms such as malaise, fever, and/or weight loss. Severe myalgia and arthralgia were present in 56–81 per cent, whereas renal involvement was present in 65–80 per cent (Fink 1977; Ozen et al. 1992). A number of patients do not have typical presentations of microscopic or classic PAN, but have inflammation in varying-sized arteries of skin, musculoskeletal, and other organ systems (Plate 161) (Watts et al. 1996; Bakkaloglu et al. 2001).

In a recent evaluation of paediatric patients six had crescentic necrotizing glomerulo-nephritis with/without pulmonary involvement confirming microscopic PAN. Ten had typical changes in renal angiograms without small-vessel involvement (Bakkaloglu et al. 2001). Nine had features hard to classify within the categories of CHCC.

Classical PAN Classical PAN is defined as the necrotizing inflammation of predominantly medium-sized arteries, frequently leading to aneurysm formation (Fig. 1). The main clinical feature is organ infarction occurring mostly in kidneys and gut. Hypertension due to renal artery aneurysms is a frequent manifestation in childhood patients. On the other hand these patients may also have skin disease where small vessels are also involved, creating difficulties in categorization according to the CHCC definition.

Hepatitis B has been implicated in this disease. Guillevin et al. (1996) have shown that patients with abnormal angiograms had significantly more hypertension, more orchitis, more HBs antigenaemia and negative ANCA.

Microscopic polyarteritis or polyangiitis The predominant feature is rapidly progressive renal involvement. Pulmonary vascular disease may accompany in some causing a 'pulmonary–renal disease'.

The renal disease manifests as nephritic and/or nephrotic features or renal insufficiency (Besbas et al. 2000). The hallmark of the disease is the necrotizing glomerulonephritis on renal biopsy.

Laboratory findings

Patients with PAN, frequently have leucocytosis, thrombocytosis, and almost always elevated ESR and C-reactive protein. A urinalysis must be obtained in all cases to be tested for haematuria, proteinuria, and casts.

Diagnostic work-up of these patients would also include ANCA (Wong et al. 1992). In microscopic PAN, the ANCA predominantly shows a perinuclear pattern of antibody staining using the indirect immunofluorescence technique (Wong et al. 1992). An ELISA test will frequently show that the autoantibody is directed against myeloperoxidase. On the other hand ANCA is not always present in other forms of childhood PAN and if ANCA directed against myeloperoxidase is present, it is of lower titres. Thus a negative ANCA would not exclude the diagnosis.

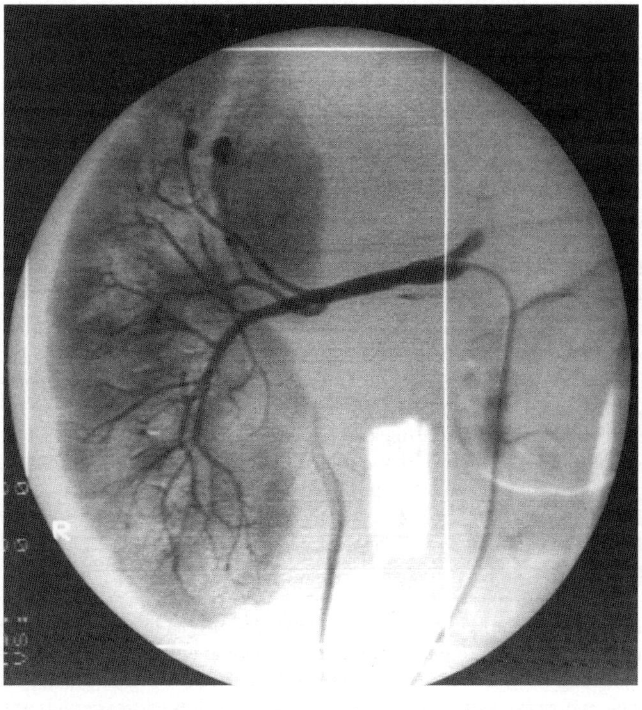

Fig. 1 Classical PAN, renal angiogram demonstrating aneurysms.

A biopsy of the involved organ system showing necrotizing arteritis, or a conventional or magnetic resonance angiogram is indicated for definite diagnosis.

Treatment of systemic PAN in childhood

Corticosteroids remain the basis of treatment. In severe organ involvement intravenous pulses of methylprednisolone are indicated. Systemic disease and renal involvement necessitates cyclophosphamide for induction of remission (Besbas et al. 2000). In a child, the cumulative dose of immunosuppressives remains a major concern of the paediatricians. When data from large studies were compiled, a cumulative dose of up to 200–250 mg/kg was considered safe for most children in terms of gonadal toxicity (Latta et al. 2001). This would be roughly equal to 3.5 months of oral cyclophosphamide at a dose of 2 mg/kg/day. Thus, after 3 months cyclophosphamide is switched to azathioprine if remission is achieved. Switching to azathioprine has proved successful in adult studies as well (Jayne 2001). Uncontrolled studies have suggested that plasma exchange and intravenous prostacyclin may be beneficial (Dillon 1998).

In classic PAN that is associated with HBs antiviral treatment is required.

Mortality has been reported to be as high as 20 per cent in some childhood series, although better with current therapies (Fink 1977; Dillon 1990). However, in some childhood series, the outcome has been substantially better; a good prognosis is especially prominent in those associated with a streptococcal infection who do not present typical patterns defined in adult patients in the CHCC. In these patients the beneficial role of penicillin deserves controlled studies. This effect is especially striking in cutaneous PAN.

Cutaneous PAN

A topic overlooked by most adult criteria is cutaneous PAN. Cutaneous PAN is characterized by crops of painful skin nodules and livedo reticularis and sometimes non-specific musculoskeletal findings such as myalgia, arthralgia (Dillon 1998). There is often a history of preceding streptococcal infection (David et al. 1993; Bont et al. 1998). Constitutional symptoms are absent and the acute phase reactants are often normal. The concern with cutaneous PAN is that it may evolve into systemic PAN. Any constitutional symptom or organ involvement should alert the physician for the development of systemic PAN.

Skin biopsy reveals necrotizing vasculitis. Non-steroidal anti-inflammatory drugs and short courses of low-dose oral corticosteroids have been used. Relapses are frequent.

Predominantly small-vessel involvement

Wegener's granulomatosis

Wegener's granulomatosis is characterized by glomerulonephritis accompanied by granulomatous lesions of the respiratory tract. It is rare in childhood.

Clinical and laboratory findings and features and diagnosis

Patients frequently present with malaise, fever, sinusitis, epistaxis, and haematuria. Diagnosis according to the ACR criteria requires two out of the four following criteria: (i) nasal–oral inflammation, (ii) abnormal chest X-ray, (iii) microhaematuria, and (iv) granulomatous inflammation on biopsy (Leavitt et al. 1990).

Pulmonary involvement may be in the form of nodules, fixed infiltrates or cavities (Leavitt et al. 1990). The skin disease may be in the form of palpable purpura, papules, vesicles, ulcers, and nodules (Rottem et al. 1993). Most features in children are similar to those of adults; however, some features such as subglottic stenosis and nasal deformity are more common in children (Rottem et al. 1993). Multifocal infiltrates with or without small peripheral nodules were the commonest thoracic CT manifestations (McHugh et al. 1991). Differential diagnosis includes PAN, Churg–Strauss syndrome, relapsing polychondritis, and the recently defined TAP deficiency syndrome.

In patients with kidney involvement the findings range from proteinuria and/or haematuria to impairment of renal function. In Wegener's granulomatosis ANCA displays a cytoplasmic-staining pattern by immunofluorescence and is against serine proteinase 3.

Treatment

Treatment is similar to that for patients with microscopic PAN. In a prospective study the NIH has suggested treatment with oral cyclophosphamide, where the dose was tapered when remission was sustained. Prednisone was started concurrently (Rottem et al. 1993). Although there are no controlled studies in children, trimethoprim–sulfamethaxazole prophylaxis is suggested.

Prognosis has been dramatically improved with immunosuppressive therapy. However, a significant proportion of patients are still subject to permanent morbidity and mortality from both the disease and treatment (Rottem et al. 1993). The course is complicated with relapses. Stegmayer et al. (2000) have reported that 80 per cent of their young patients relapsed within a period of 4–120 months.

Henoch–Schönlein purpura

HSP is a leucocytoclastic vasculitis involving the small vessels only. HSP is the most common form of vasculitis of childhood in many geographical areas and mainly under the age of 25. It is often preceded by an upper respiratory tract infection and a wide variety of pathogens including streptococci have been implicated in the aetiology (Bagga and Dillon 2001).

Clinical features and diagnosis

Diagnosis depends on the characteristic features of the disease: the typical non-thrombocytopaenic palpable purpura (present in almost all), abdominal pain reflecting the gastrointestinal involvement (in 63–100 per cent of the patients), arthralgia and/or arthritis (in 47–84 per cent of the patients), and renal involvement (in 37–51 per cent of the patients) (Saulsbury 1993; Bagga and Dillon 2001). Crops of palpable purpura are most manifest on pressure bearing areas and extensor surfaces (Plate 162). Cutaneous oedema of the scalp and extremities is also quite typical. Early morbidity and mortality is associated with gastrointestinal involvement whereas late morbidity is associated with renal involvement (White et al. 1999).

Laboratory findings

There is no specific laboratory test and the diagnosis is clinical. There may be a moderate leucocytosis and acute phase reactants are usually mildly elevated. Serum IgA is increased in almost half of the patients and some may have circulating immune complexes (White et al. 1999).

Renal involvement often manifests as haematuria and/or proteinuria. In 5–10 per cent of the patients, the involvement is severe necessitating immunosuppression (Szer 1996). The characteristic finding on renal biopsy is IgA deposition mainly in the glomerular mesangium.

Treatment

The optimal management of gastrointestinal and renal involvement has not yet been determined (Szer 1996). Joint complaints respond well to nonsteroidal anti-inflammatory agents. Cutaneous manifestations are often self-limited however they may have a relapsing pattern. The family should be cautioned against severe gastrointestinal involvement, such as fresh bleeding that may be a sign of intussusception. For severe gastrointestinal involvement uncontrolled studies favour a short course of oral corticosteroids.

Urinary symptoms such as haematuria and mild proteinuria would not require immunosuppressive treatment but should be followed closely. Clinical features of rapidly progressive glomerulonephritis and/or nephrotic range proteinuria necessitate a biopsy: more than 50 per cent crescentic glomerulonephritis leads to renal failure in 50 per cent of patients with HSP (White et al. 1999). Thus, in these patients we use an intensive approach with corticosteroids and oral cyclophosphamide for 3 months (Oner et al. 1995). Management is summarized as follows:

- Admit for severe GIS or renal disease
- *Evaluate* / *Treat*

Evaluate	*Treat*
GIS examination	Oral prednisone 1 mg/kg/day for GIS
Check stool for blood	Bleeding or severe pain
Urinalysis, proteinuria	NSAID for arthritis
Monitor renal function test	If renal crescents on biopsy oral
Renal biopsy for nephrotic proteinuria and/or impaired renal function	Prednisone (tapered after a month) + cyclophosphamide (3 months)
CNS and pulmonary status	Pulse steroid and cyclophosphamide for CNS and pulmonary disease (rare)

Follow-up (depends on persistence and recurrence of findings)

There are no studies proving the use of steroids for mild renal disease (White et al. 1999). The protective role of steroids is also debatable (Mollica et al. 1992; Saulsbury 1993). We still need more data to decide on the role of therapy in this potentially 'self-limited' disease.

Churg-Strauss syndrome (allergic granulomatosis)

Churg–Strauss syndrome is a small-vessel vasculitis defined by: allergic rhinitis, asthma, peripheral eosinophilia, peripheral neuropathy, pulmonary infiltrations, chronic sinusitis, and biopsy proven eosinophilic vasculitis. It is very rare in childhood. All childhood-onset patients had peripheral eosinophilia and almost all had asthma (Louthrenoo et al. 1998). Cardiac, renal, and nervous involvement may also occur. Corticosteroids are the main therapy. Immunosuppressives were added in most reported cases. Mortality is very high.

Cutaneous leucocytoclastic vasculitis

This is small-vessel vasculitis confined to the skin. Histologically the lesion is a leucocytoclastic angiitis (Jennette and Falk 1997). The definition requires the exclusion of any systemic feature.

Drugs and other causes should be considered in the aetiology. Drug-induced vasculitis develops within 7–21 days after treatment begins (Jennette and Falk 1997). Treatment is often symptomatic however, steroids may be indicated although they have not been proven to alter the course of the disease.

Miscellaneous

Behçet's disease

Behçet's disease is a vasculitis affecting arteries and venules with special tendency to thrombosis. The course of the disease is characterized by exacerbations and remissions with a poorer prognosis in males (Yazici et al. 1998). There is clinical and laboratory data suggesting an association with streptococci (Ozen 1999). About 1–2 per cent of the Behçet's disease patients are children. Definite Behçet's disease is diagnosed in a patient with recurrent oral ulceration plus two of the following: recurrent genital ulceration, eye lesions, skin lesions, and positive pathergy test (International Study Group, 1990). A striking feature in children is the high frequency of family history, present in 15–20 per cent of the patients (Kone-Paut et al. 1998; Uziel et al. 1998).

Vascular complications may occur in the form of arterial aneurysms, or thrombosis in the veins or arteries. Pulmonary arterial involvement is the most severe complication of the disease. There are no controlled studies evaluating treatment in Behçet's disease in children. We thus depend on adult experience (Yazici et al. 1998). For the vasculitis corticosteroids and cyclophosphamide are indicated.

Secondary vasculitides

Since vasculitis is defined as inflammation of the blood vessels, practically any process accompanied by this feature may be termed as secondary vasculitis. Infectious agents may act as triggering factors through various mechanisms such as molecular mimicry, or through direct damage, or by immune-mediated damage to the vessel by immune complex deposition, or by a bystander damage to the blood vessel (Ozen 1999). Among viral causes, hepatitis-B and HIV associated vasculitis are probably the best described in children (Athreya 1995).

The other causes of secondary vasculitides include vasculitis secondary to malignancy, cryoglobulinaemia, or to other rheumatic diseases such as systemic lupus erythematosus, dermatomyositis.

Recently it has been recognized that patients with familial Mediterranean fever (FMF) may also have features of vasculitis and an increased incidence of PAN (Ozdogan et al. 1997; Ozen 1999; Ozen et al. 2001). FMF is an autoinflammatory disease characterized by attacks of fever and serositis. When compared to other PAN patients, those associated with FMF, tended to be younger at onset, had a better prognosis, and some had overlapping features. The clinical features of PAN in FMF patients are thus suggested to be different and may be a feature of FMF per se (Ozen et al. 2001).

Conclusion

Nature has been kind to children; although childhood vasculitides such as HSP and KD are more common than the adult vasculitides, it is remarkable that they are more benign and self-limited diseases as compared to those in adults. One of the reasons for the substantial frequency of vasculitides in childhood maybe because that childhood is the time when we first encounter the common micro-organisms, and that these microbial agents are crucial in the aetiopathogenesis of vasculitis. Indeed, the role of infectious agents in the aetiopathogenesis of these diseases is evident.

Early diagnosis and effective treatment options have improved the prognosis in vasculitides. However, the physician should be aware of the additional issues of the growing child when managing the disease.

References

Arend, W.P. et al. (1990). The ACR 1990 criteria for the classification of Takayasu arteritis. *Arthritis and Rheumatism* **33**, 1129–35.

Athreya, B.H. (1995). Vasculitis in children. *Pediatric Clinics of North America* **42**, 1239–61.

Bagga, A. and Dillon, M.J. (2001). Leukocytoclastic vasculitis. In *Textbook of Pediatric Rheumatology* (ed. J.T. Cassidy and R.E. Petty), p. 569. Philadelphia PA: W.B. Saunders & Co.

Bakkaloglu, A. et al. (2001). The significance of ANCA in microscopic polyangiitis and classic polyarteritis nodosa. *Archives of Disease in Childhood* **85**, 427–30.

Barron, K.S. et al. (1999). Report of the NIH workshop on Kawasaki disease. *Journal of Rheumatology* **26**, 170–90.

Besbas, N. et al. (2000). Renal involvement in PAN: evaluation of 25 Turkish children. *Pediatric Nephrology* **14**, 325–7.

Bont, K. et al. (1998). The clinical spectrum of post-streptococcal syndrome with arthritis in children. *Clinical and Experimental Rheumatology* **16**, 750–2.

Cassidy, J.T. and Petty, R.E. (1995). Vasculitis. In *Textbook of Pediatric Rheumatology* (ed. J.T. Cassidy and R.E. Petty), pp. 365–422. Philadelphia PA: W.B. Saunders & Co.

David, J., Ansell, B.M., and Woo, P. (1993). Polyarteritis nodosa associated with streptococcus. *Archives of Disease in Childhood* **69**, 685–8.

Dillon, M.J. (1990). Vaculitis syndromes. In *Pediatric Rheumatology Update* (ed. P. Woo, P.H. White, and B.M. Ansell), pp. 227–42. New York: Oxford University Press.

Dillon, M. (1998). Primary vasculitis in children. In *Oxford Textbook of Rheumatology* 2nd edn. (ed. P.J. Maddison, D.A. Isenberg, P. Woo, and D.N. Glass), pp. 1402–12. Oxford: Oxford University Press.

Fink, C.W. (1977). Polyarteritis and other diseases with necrotizing vasculitis in childhood. *Arthritis and Rheumatism* **20**, 378–84.

Guillevin, L. et al. (1996). ANCA, abnormal angiograms and pathological findings in polyarteritis nodosa and Churg–Strauss syndrome. *British Journal of Rheumatology* **35**, 958–64.

Hall, S. et al. (1985). Takayasu arteritis. A study of 32 North American patients. *Medicine* **64**, 89–99.

Hoffman, G.S. et al. (1994). Treatment of glucocorticoid resistant or relapsing Takayasu arteritis with methotrexate. *Arthritis and Rheumatism* **37**, 578–82.

Hunder, G.G. et al. (1990). The American College of Rheumatology 1990 criteria for the classification of vasculitis: introduction. *Arthritis and Rheumatism* **33**, 1065–7.

Iemura, M. et al. (2000). Long term consequences of regressed coronary aneurysms after Kawasaki disease: vascular wall morphology and function. *Heart* **83**, 307–11.

Japan Kawasaki Disease Research Committee. *Diagnostic Guidelines of Kawaski Disease* (4th revised edn.). Tokyo: Japan Red Cross Medical Centre, 1984.

Jayne, D. (2001). Update on the European vasculitis study group trials. *Current Opinion in Rheumatology* **13**, 48–55.

Jennette, J.C. and Falk, R.J. (1997). Small vessel vasculitis. *New England Journal of Medicine* **337**, 1513–22.

Jennette, J.C. et al. (1994). Nomenclature of systemic vasculitides. Proposal of an international consensus conference. *Arthritis and Rheumatism* **37**, 187–92.

Kawasaki, T. (1967). Acute febrile mucocutaneous syndrome with lymphoid involvement with specific desquamation of fingers and toes in children. *Japanese Journal of Allergy* **16**, 178–222.

Kone-Paut, I. et al. (1998). Epidemiological features of Behçet's syndrome in children: an international collaborative survey of 86 cases. *Journal of Pediatrics* **132**, 721–5.

Latta, K., von Schnakenburg, C., and Ehrich, J.H.H. (2001). A meta-analysis of cytotoxic treatment for frequently relapsing nephrotic syndrome in children. *Pediatric Nephrology* **16**, 271–82.

Leavitt, R.Y. et al. (1990). The ACR 1990 criteria for the classification of Wegener's granulomatosis. *Arthritis and Rheumatism* **33**, 1101.

Lightfoot, R.W., Jr. et al. (1990). The ACR 1990 criteria for the classification of polyarteritis nodosa. *Arthritis and Rheumatism* **33**, 1088.

Louthrenoo, W. et al. (1998). Childhood Churg–Strauss syndrome. *Journal of Rheumatology* **26**, 1387–93.

Mollica, F. et al. (1992). Effectiveness of early prednisone treatment in preventing the development of nephropathy in anaphylactoid purpura. *European Journal of Pediatrics* **151**, 140–4.

Oner, A., Tinaztepe, K., and Erdogan, O. (1995). The effect of triple therapy on rapidly progressive type of Henoch–Schönlein nephritis. *Pediatric Nephrology* **9**, 6–10.

Ozdogan, et al. (1997). Vasculitis in familial Mediterranean fever. *Journal of Rheumatology* **24**, 323–7.

Ozen, S. (1999). Vasculopathy, Behçet's disease and familial Mediterranean fever. *Current Opinion in Rheumatology* **11** (5), 393–8.

Ozen, S. et al. (1992). Diagnostic criteria for polyarteritis nodosa in childhood. *Journal of Pediatrics* **2**, 206–9.

Ozen, S. et al. (2001). Polyarteritis nodosa associated with familial mediterranean fever: is it an association? *Seminars in Arthritis and Rheumatism* **30**, 281–7.

Petty, R.E. and Cassidy, J.T. (2001). Kawasaki disease. In *Textbook of Pediatric Rheumatology* (ed. J.T. Cassidy, and R.E. Petty), p. 580. Philadelphia PA: W.B. Saunders & Co.

Rottem, M. et al. (1993). Wegener granulomatosis in children and adolescents: clinical presentation and outcome. *Journal of Pediatrics* **122**, 26.

Saulsbury, F.T. (1993). Corticosteroid therapy does not prevent nephritis in HSP. *Pediatric Nephrology* **7**, 69–71.

Stegmayer, B.G. et al. (2000). WG in children and young adults. A case study of 10 patients. *Pediatric Nephrology* **14**, 208–13.

Szer, I.S. (1996). Henoch–Schönlein purpura: when and how to treat. *Journal of Rheumatology* **23**, 1661–5.

Uziel, Y. et al. (1998). Juvenile Behçet's syndrome in Israel. *Clinical Experimental Rheumatology* **16**, 502–5.

Wallace, C.A. et al. (2000). Initial intravenous gammaglobulin treatment failure in Kawasaki disease. *Pediatrics* **105**, E78.

Watts, R.A. et al. (1996). Effect of classification on the incidence of polyarteritis nodosa and microscopic polyangiitis. *Arthritis and Rheumatism* **39**, 1208–12.

White, R.H.R., Yoshikawa, N., and Feehally, J. (1999). IgA nephropathy and Henoch–Schönlein nephritis. In *Pediatric Nephrology* (ed. T.M. Barratt, E.D. Avner, and W.E. Harmon), pp. 691–706. Baltimore MD: Lippincott Williams and Wilkins.

Wong, S.-N., Shah, V., and Dillon, M.J. (1992). ANCA in childhood systemic vasculitis. *Journal of the American Society of Nephrology* **3**, 668.

Yanagawa, H. et al. (1998). Results of the nationwide epidemiologic survey of Kawasaki disease in 1995 and 1996 in Japan. *Pediatrics* **102**, E65.

Yazici, H., Yurdakul, S., and Hamuryudan, V. (1998). Behçet's syndrome. In *Oxford Textbook of Rheumatology* 2nd edn. (ed. P.J. Maddison, D.A. Isenberg, P. Woo, and D.N. Glass), pp. 1394–402. Oxford: Oxford University Press.

6.11 Overlap syndromes in adults and children

Enrique Roberto Soriano and Neil John McHugh

Introduction

Autoimmune rheumatic diseases (connective tissue diseases) are an overlapping group of disorders of unknown aetiology. Their classification depends on identifying clusters of clinical and laboratory features. At least three problems arise when attempting to classify individual patients into one of the defined autoimmune rheumatic diseases early on in their disease or when they present with clinical overlaps: (i) most of the clinical or laboratory features are not exclusive to one disease; (ii) many of the symptoms and signs that define the autoimmune rheumatic diseases do not occur concurrently, but rather occur sequentially; (iii) as many as 25 per cent of patients with autoimmune rheumatic disease present with an overlap syndrome with typical features of more than one disorder.

The terms undifferentiated connective tissue disease, overlap syndrome, and even mixed connective tissue disease (MCTD), have been used for patients who are not comfortably placed within any one of the defined autoimmune rheumatic diseases. These terms are not interchangeable, but unfortunately are often applied loosely. This chapter will describe some of the more common overlap conditions, and what is known concerning environmental triggers. Mixed connective tissue disease is discussed at some length reflecting the large proportion of studies in this area, although there is debate as to whether this disease is a distinct entity or a disease in evolution. Mention will be made of attempts to define more homogeneous subsets of connective tissue disease by knowledge of immunogenetic and serological profiles.

Undifferentiated autoimmune rheumatic disease

Criteria for the diagnosis of undifferentiated connective tissue disease are not yet established. The term is best applied to those patients with features strongly suggestive of an autoimmune rheumatic disease but who do not fulfil criteria for any one disorder. The features usually include Raynaud's phenomenon, polyarthritis, rash, and myalgia (Alarcon 2000). Undifferentiated connective tissue disease may develop into a well-defined autoimmune rheumatic disease, may persist unchanged over time, or the symptoms may even disappear. Raynaud's phenomenon is probably the most frequent clinical feature of undifferentiated autoimmune rheumatic disease. In Alarcon's (2000) study most of the patients who entered the cohort with isolated Raynaud's phenomenon remained undifferentiated, with only 13 per cent evolving into defined CTDs.

Overlap syndrome

The term overlap syndrome has been used when two or more autoimmune rheumatic diseases, or some of their unique manifestations, occur in the same individual simultaneously. Features that are characteristic of certain defined autoimmune rheumatic diseases are given in Table 1. The overlap may consist of full expression of the features of two or more conditions, or more commonly may be limited to one or more manifestations of each disease. In the latter case, the diagnosis of undifferentiated connective tissue disease may equally apply.

Serological subsets

A characteristic feature of autoimmune rheumatic diseases is the presence of autoantibodies. As autoantibodies are associated with particular clinical features, knowledge of the autoantibody profile may help in diagnosis and prognosis. The best-known example is the association of anti-U1RNP antibodies with MCTD, which will be further discussed. Other examples include the association of anti-Ro (SS-A) and anti-La (SS-B) antibodies with Sjögren's syndrome, antiphospholipid antibodies with the antiphospholipid syndrome, and antibodies to tRNA synthetases with the antisynthetase syndrome (Fig. 1). Also, in most cases there are strong associations between autoantibody-defined subsets of disease and HLA genes that may explain, at least, in part, the genetic basis for disease susceptibility (Table 2).

Table 1 Features usually restricted to one autoimmune rheumatic disease, and less common in others

Systemic lupus erythematosus	Systemic sclerosis	Poly/dermatomyositis	Rheumatoid arthritis
Malar rash	Scleroderma	Myositis	Erosive arthritis
Photosensitivity	Oesophageal hypomobility	Heliotrope rash	Subcutaneous nodules
Glomerulonephritis	Telangiectasia	Gottron's papules	Rheumatoid factor
Central nervous system disease	Antitopoisomerase 1 antibodies	Antisynthetase antibodies	
Anti-Sm antibodies		Anti-Mi-2 antibodies	
Anti-double-stranded DNA			

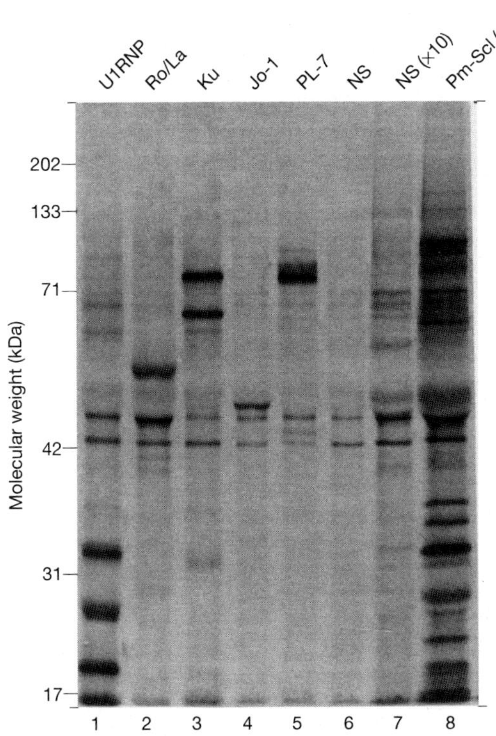

Fig. 1 Proteins immunoprecipitated using sera containing autoantibodies that are associated with overlap syndromes; anti-U1RNP with MCTD, anti-Ro/La antibodies with SLE/Sjögren's syndrome, anti-Ku with SLE or scleroderma, anti-Jo-1 (histidyl-tRNA synthetase) and anti-PL-7 (threonyl-tRNA synthetase) with the antisynthetase syndrome, and anti-Pm-Scl with polymyositis/scleroderma/arthritis. NS, normal serum.

Table 2 Recognized clusters of clinical overlaps, autoantibodies, and HLA class II alleles

Overlap syndrome	Autoantibody specificity	HLA class II allele
Mixed connective tissue disease	U1RNP	HLA–DR4 (DRB1 *0401) HLA–DQ3 (DQB1 *0301) (Kuwana et al. 1995)
Polymyositis, intersititial lung disease, Raynaud's, arthritis	Jo-1 (histidyl-tRNA synthetase) and less often other tRNA synthetases	HLA–DR3, DRw52 (Goldstein et al. 1990)
Systemic sclerosis, polymyositis	PM-Scl Ku U2RNP	HLA–DR3 (Marguerie et al. 1992)

Mixed connective tissue disease

Definition

Mixed connective tissue disease was first described by Sharp and coworkers (Sharp et al. 1971, 1972) as an 'apparently distinct rheumatic disease syndrome' in which the clinical characteristics included a combination of features similar to those of systemic lupus erythematosus (SLE), scleroderma, and polymyositis. The spectrum has been broadened by some to include features of rheumatoid arthritis (Sullivan et al. 1984). Mixed connective tissue disease was considered unique, as it was associated with autoantibodies to a ribonuclease-sensitive component of extractable nuclear antigen, now known as U1RNP.

There remains debate as to whether MCTD is a distinct disease, a disease in evolution, or a subset of another autoimmune rheumatic disease such as SLE (McHugh et al. 1990; Citera et al. 1995; Smolen and Steiner 1998; Isenberg and Black 1999). Diagnosis that is dependent on a single serological finding may suffer from ascertainment bias. Many patients with the clinical features 'characteristic' of MCTD do not have anti-U1RNP antibodies (Lazaro et al. 1989), and conversely anti-U1RNP antibodies may appear in other conditions (McHugh et al. 1990). Also many features, such as the abscence of cerebral, pulmonary, and renal involvement, and good response to a very small dose of corticosteroids, thought to make patients with MCTD clinically distinct have not held true over time (Nimelstein et al. 1980). In spite of these long-standing concerns the term MCTD is considered by some to be a syndrome that has a core of manifestations associated with a serological marker. Three revised and distinct sets of diagnostic criteria have been proposed (Table 3).

Epidemiology

Mixed connective tissue disease is a disease of the second to fourth decades of life with a mean age of onset of 35 years in adults (Sharp et al. 1972), and 10 years in children (Singsen et al. 1977). Women are affected more often than men at all ages, and represent around 80 per cent of patients. The incidence of MCTD in adults remains unknown. In a nationwide, prospective, hospital-based study for 4 years in Finland in children aged 0–15 years, the annual incidence rate for MCTD was 0.10/100 000 compared with 0.37 for SLE, 0.30 for polymyositis/dermatomyositis, and 0.05 for scleroderma (Pelkonen et al. 1994).

Clinical features (Table 4)

General symptoms

The typical patient is a 20- to 30-year-old female presenting with Raynaud's phenomenon, arthralgias/arthritis, swollen hands and/or puffy fingers, in association with a high titre, speckled pattern, antinuclear antibody (ANA) (Plate 163). Other presenting symptoms may include fatigue, fever, serositis, mild myositis, aseptic meningitis, or unexplained lymphadenopathy.

Vascular involvement

Raynaud's phenomenon is present in 75–100 per cent of adults and children (Table 4), and is often the first symptom to appear. Ischaemic necrosis and ulcerations of the fingertips are rare but may occur. Nailfold capillaroscopy shows capillary dilatation and capillary loss (avascular areas) in 50–90 per cent of patients and may be associated with pulmonary disease (Sullivan et al. 1984). Dystrophic, branched 'bushy' capillaries may be especially characteristic. Raynaud's in children develops early in the course of the disease and frequently persists over years, being the main symptom of the disease during the long term in 24 per cent of patients (Hartmut 1997).

Skin

Swelling of the hands, particularly of the fingers leading to a sausage appearance (Fig. 2), occurs more frequently in adults than in children. The skin of the hands may be taut and thick and histologically resembles scleroderma. Scleroderma extending more proximally is not usually a feature of MCTD. Sclerodermatous skin changes have been reported in 52–86 per cent of children, mostly in the form of sclerodactyly without fingertip ulcerations or pitting scars (Hartmut 1997). Other less frequent cutaneous manifestations are alopecia, depigmentation, telangiectasia, erythema nodosum, and chronic discoid lesions.

Joints

Polyarthralgia is an early symptom and occurs in most patients. A symmetrical polyarthritis most often involving hands and wrists may mimic rheumatoid arthritis but is less deforming and erosive. Nonetheless, the

Table 3 Diagnostic criteria for MCTD

Sharp (1987)	Kasukawa et al. (1987)	Alarcon-Segovia and Cardiel (1989)
Major criteria 1. Myositis, severe 2. Pulmonary involvement (a) CO diffusing capacity < % or (b) Pulmonary hypertension (c) Proliferative vascular lesions on biopsy 3. Raynaud's phenomenon or oesophageal hypomotility 4. Swollen hands 5. Highest observed anti-ENA > 1:10 000 and anti-U1RNP positive and anti-Sm negative	I Common symptoms 1. Raynaud's phenomenon 2. Swollen fingers or hands II Anti-nRNP antibodies III Mixed findings A. SLE-like findings 1. Polyarthritis 2. Lymphadenopathy 3. Facial erythema 4. Pericarditis or pleuritis 5. Leucocytopaenia (<4000 mm^{-3}) or thrombocytopaenia (<100 000 mm^{-3}) B. PSS-like findings 1. Sclerodactyly 2. Pulmonary fibrosis, restrictive change of lung (% VC < 80%) or reduced diffusion capacity (DLCO < 70%) 3. Hypomobility or dilatation of oesophagus C. PM-like findings 1. Muscle weakness 2. Increased serum level of myogenic enzymes (CPK) 3. Myogenic pattern in EMG	1. Serological Positive anti-nRNP at a haemagglutination titre of 1:1600 or higher 2. Clinical Oedema of hands Synovitis Myositis (laboratory or biopsy proven) Raynaud's phenomenon (2 or 3 colour phase) Acrosclerosis (with or without proximal scleroderma)
Definite = four majors	Requirements for MCTD 1. Positive in either one or two common symptoms 2. Positive anti-nRNP antibodies 3. Positive in one or more findings in two or three disease categories of A, B, and C	1. Serological 2. At least three clinical findings 3. Association of oedema of the hands, Raynaud's phenomenon, and acrosclerosis requires at least one of the other two criteria

Note: PN, polymyositis; PSS, progressive systemic sclerosis; SLE, systemic lupus erythematosus.

Table 4 Frequent clinical features in adults and children with MCTD

Feature	Adults (%)					Children (%)	
	Bennett and O'Connell (1980) (*n* = 20)	Sullivan et al. (1984) (*n* = 34)	Prakash et al. (1985) (*n* = 81)	Kitridou et al. (1986) (*n* = 30)	Burdt et al. (1999) (*n* = 47)	Singsen et al. (1977) (*n* = 14)	Hartmut (1997) (*n* = 33)
Raynaud's	75	91	79	83	96	78	94
Arthritis	100	85	62	97	96	93	97
Swollen hands	75	85[a]	—	60	66	14	85[b]
Sclerodactyly	20	85[a]	54	60	49	78	52
Myositis	35	79	48[c]	53	51	50	70
Oesophageal dysmotility	47	74	49[d]	60	66	??	6
Lymphadenopathy	50	50	26	17	—	50	—
Pleuritis	—	35	6	23	43[e]	14	21[f]
Renal[g]	20	26	—	40	11	50	21
Cardiac	35	26	—	—	43[e]	64	6
Neurological	55	6	—	20	17	21	0

[a] Swollen hands and sclerodactyly were considered together.

[b] Puffy fingers.

[c] Defined as muscle weakness, 44/55 patients had abnormal electromyograms.

[d] Only 39/81 patients were studied.

[e] Pleuritis/pericarditis were considered together.

[f] Lung involvement.

[g] Clinical and/or histological evidence of renal involvement.

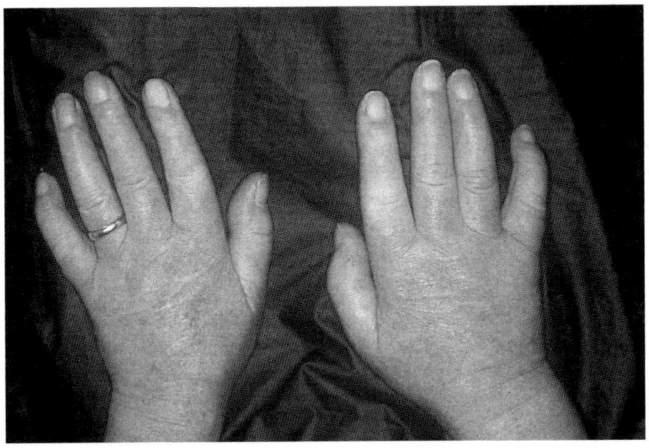

Fig. 2 Typical 'sausage-shaped' swollen fingers of a patient with MCTD.

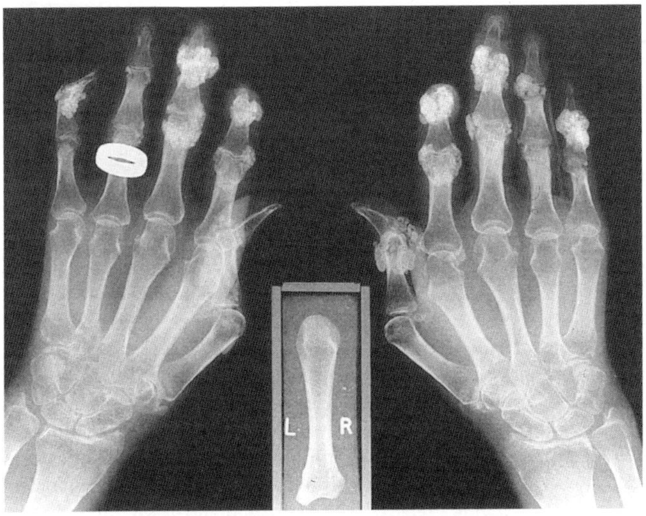

Fig. 3 Prominent periarticular calcification in a patient with MCTD.

development of Jaccoud's deformities of the hands and feet (Reilly et al. 1990), swan neck changes, and flexion contractures are not rare. Erosions are found in about 60 per cent of adult patients (Bennett and O'Connell 1980; Catoggio et al. 1983), and in upto 57 per cent of children (Hartmut 1997), and are usually small, punched-out, and asymetrically distributed. Prominent periarticular calcification is not uncommon (Fig. 3). Avascular necrosis of bone may occur in children (Tiddens et al. 1993) and adults (O'Connell and Bennett 1977). Minute, multiple peritendinous nodules may be found adjacent to the flexor tendons of the forearms and the extensor tendons of the hands (Babini et al. 1985). About 9–57 per cent of children have functional joint limitations that may be long-standing (Hartmut 1997).

Muscle

Myalgias are common and about two-thirds of patients develop an inflammatory myopathy that is identical clinically and histologically to polymyositis (Sharp et al. 1972; Bennett and O'Connell 1980). Very often myositis may occur acutely in a patient who has other mild features and prompts the diagnosis of MCTD. In children, myositis is usually an early manifestation of disease and generally causes no serious problems for the patients in the long term. Muscles of the upper limb are involved more frequently in children than those of the lower limb (Hartmut 1997).

Gastrointestinal tract

Gastrointestinal involvement is similar to that in systemic sclerosis, with heartburn and dysphagia the most common symptoms. Oesophageal manometry is abnormal in upto 85 per cent of patients (Marshall et al. 1990). Extensive gastrointestinal tract involvement with malabsorption, colonic and small bowel perforations due to vasculitis, acute pancreatitis (Marshall et al. 1990), duodenal haemorrhage, pneumatosis intestinalis and pneumoperitoneum (Bennett and O'Connell 1980), haemobilia due to vasculitis of the gallbladder, protein-losing enteropathy, and secretory diarrhoea have all been reported. Hepatomegaly and splenomegaly are found in about 25 per cent of patients but major liver involvement is uncommon. The spectrum of gastrointestinal involvement is similar in children, although gastrointestinal involvement in children and adolescents seems to be more frequent than clinical symptoms indicate (Weber et al. 2000).

Keratoconjunctivitis sicca

Sicca symptoms are not uncommon in adults and children. Sialectasia was found in 82 per cent of 39 adults with MCTD studied by parotid sialography (Ohtsuka et al. 1992), although 50 per cent of these patients also fulfilled criteria for Sjögren's syndrome. Recurrent parotid gland swelling has been reported in 24–67 per cent of children, although accompained by sicca symptomatology in only a minority of them (Hartmut 1997).

Neurological involvement

Trigeminal sensory neuropathy may occur in upto 10 per cent of patients and may be an early manifestation of the disease (Sullivan et al. 1984). Involvement of the central nervous system is rare in adults although an aseptic meningitis-like syndrome has been reported (Bennett and O'Connell 1980). Other occasional findings are headaches, seizures, peripheral neuropathy, spinal cord involvement, transverse myelitis, hypertrophic cranial pachymeningitis, and demyelination. Three of the 14 children reported by Singsen et al. (1977) had cerebral involvement. Chronic headache and depression has also been frequently found in children (Hartmut 1997).

Heart

Major cardiovascular abnormalities are uncommon. Pericarditis may occur in upto 20 per cent of patients and pericardial tamponade has been reported (Bennett and O'Connell 1980). Electrocardiogram abnormalities are more common (Alpert et al. 1983; Oetgen et al. 1983), and cardiac conduction defects have been described. Echocardiographic changes including pericardial effusions, mitral valve prolapse, and right ventricle enlargement have been found in 38–60 per cent of patients (Alpert et al. 1983; Oetgen et al. 1983). Heart involvement seems to play a secondary role in children with mixed connective tissue disease. Pericarditis, myocarditis, and aortic stenosis have been reported occasionally (Hartmut 1997). Intimal hyperplasia of coronary arteries and inflammatory cell infiltrates of the myocardium may be found in both adults and children (Singsen et al. 1977; Alpert et al. 1983).

Lungs

Pleuropulmonary involvement is common and may be clinically inapparent. The most common clinical findings are dyspnoea, pleuritic pain, and bibasilar rales (Table 5). Children may present with reduced exercise tolerance. Chest radiograph abnormalities include basal interstitial fibrosis, pleural effusion, pneumonic infiltrates, and pleural thickening (Sullivan et al. 1984), and high-resolution computed tomography have shown the presence of ground-glass attenuation, non-septal linear opacities, and perhipheral and lower lobe predominance as the more frequent abnormalities (Kozuka et al. 2001). Abnormalities of pulmonary function test are very common and may include a restrictive pattern, small airway involvement, and respiratory muscle weakness. They are also quite prevalent in children, even in those clinically asymptomatic (Hartmut 1997). Interstitial lung disease usually responds to corticosteroids but rapidly progressive cases have been reported.

Pulmonary hypertension is frequent in MCTD, may be difficult to detect and is a major cause of death (Table 6) (Burdt et al. 1999). The presence of

Table 5 Pulmonary involvement in adults with MCTD

Feature	Sullivan et al. (1984) (n = 34) (%)	Prakash et al. (1985) (n = 81) (%)
Asymptomatic	33	75
Dyspnoea	58	16
Pleuritic pain	40	7
Bibasilar rales	42	—
Cough	24	5
Abnormal chest radiograph	30	21
Restrictive pulmonary function tests	41	69
Decreased diffusing capacity	72	69

Table 6 Reported causes of death in MCTD

Presumed cause of death	Death			
	Adults (n = 42)	%	Children (n = 17)	%
Pulmonary hypertension	20	48	2	12
Septicaemia	3	7	7	41
Sudden death	3	7	—	—
Cardiac (myocardial infarction/myocarditis)	2	5	2	12
Pulmonary embolus	1	2	—	—
Pulmonary vasculitis	1	2	—	—
Scleroderma-like renal crisis	1	2	1	6
Glomerulonephritis	—	—	1	6
Cerebral	—	—	3	18
Gastrointestinal bleeding	—	—	1	6
Others, possibly unrelated	9	21	—	—
Unknown	2	5	—	—
Total number of death/total number of patients	42/257	16	17/224	8

Note: Data taken from Bennett and O'Connell (1980); Nimelstein et al. (1980); Grant et al. (1981); Sullivan et al. (1984); Prakash et al. (1985); Kitridou et al. (1986); Hartmut (1997) and Burdt et al. (1999).

scleroderma-type capillary changes on nailfold capillary microscopy may be predictive of the development of pulmonary hypertension (Sullivan et al. 1984). Histological findings show proliferative vascular abnormalities resembling those found in the CREST syndrome. Pulmonary hypertension seems less frequent in children, although it is a major cause of death in this population (Table 6).

Kidney

In their initial report Sharp et al. (1972) stressed the paucity of renal involvement but later reports have found a prevalence of upto 50 per cent in adults and children (Table 4, and Bennett and Spargo 1977). Nephrotic syndrome associated with membranous nephropathy is the most common presentation and may respond to high-dose corticosteroid therapy (Kitridou et al. 1986). The characteristic renal lesion is an immune-deposit nephritis. Renal crisis is a rare manifestation but should be suspected in a patient with accelerated hypertension as the treatment with angiotensin-converting enzyme inhibitor may be effective. Renal involvement has been observed in upto 47 per cent of children, mainly in those with a lupus-like course (Hartmut 1997). These children had more frequently anti-ds DNA antibodies, antibodies against the D polypeptide of the Sm antigen, HLA–DR2, and low titre of anti-U1RNP antibodies (Hartmut 1997). Glomerular and vascular deposition of amyloid material have been reported (Piirainen et al. 1989).

Laboratory findings

The most common laboratory features in adults and children are listed in Table 7. A moderate anaemia of chronic inflammation is usually present. Frank haemolytic anaemia and severe thrombocytopaenia may occur but are rare complications. Thrombocytopaenia may be associated with anticardiolipin antibodies, which have been found in 15 per cent of patients. The clinical features associated with the antiphospholipid syndrome seemed to be more rare than in SLE, perhaps because most anticardiolipin antibodies were beta-2-glycoprotein I independent (Hoffman and Greidinger 2000). Hypergammaglobulinaemia is more frequent than in SLE. Hypocomplementaemia and cryoglobulins are present in about one-third of patients but neither seem specifically associated with renal or other organ involvement. An elevated creatine phosphokinase may be associated with aseptic meningitis and trigeminal neuropathy in addition to myositis (Bennett and O'Connell 1980).

Autoantibodies

The presence of autoantibodies to the ribonuclease-sensitive component of extractable nuclear antigen (ENA) by a haemagglutination test is a characteristic serological feature of MCTD. The autoantibodies are now termed anti-U1RNP antibodies. The presence of these autoantibodies is suggested by a high titre, coarse speckled, nuclear pattern on an indirect immunofluorescence screen for ANAs (Plate 163). Immunodiffusion tests are now more commonly used than haemagglutination to confirm the presence of anti-U1RNP antibodies. The ribonuclease-resistant component of ENA is recognized by anti-Sm antibodies, which frequently coexist with anti-U1RNP antibodies. The absence of anti-Sm antibodies and anti-DNA antibodies in sera positive for anti-U1RNP is also felt to be an important discriminatory finding (Table 3) as anti-Sm and anti-DNA antibodies are more specific for SLE.

Anti-U1RNP and anti-Sm antibodies recognize polypeptides on small ribonucleoproteins that participate in the formation of spliceosomes and process RNA. Anti-U1RNP antibodies selectively immunoprecipitate the U1RNA by recognition of 70 kDa, A and C polypeptides, which are unique to the U1RNP particle, whereas anti-Sm antibodies immunoprecipitate the abundant uridine-rich small RNAs U1, U2, U5, and U4/U6 by recognition of core polypeptides found on all these RNAs. Precise characterization of the autoantibody specificity may be obtained by the technique of Western blotting (Fig. 4). Some studies have suggested that the clinical picture of MCTD is associated with an immune response to U1RNP that is quantitatively and qualitatively distinctive from that seen in other CTD (Maddison 2000).

Pathogenesis

It is likely that environmental factors trigger MCTD in genetically susceptible individuals. Various environmental agents have been reported including drugs such as procainamide, toxins such as polyvinyl chloride (Kahn et al. 1989), and silicone implants (Kumagai et al. 1984). Familial cases are rare but autoimmune conditions including MCTD may cluster in families, suggesting the inheritance of a common autoimmune diathesis.

An inbalance in cytokine synthesis could be an important factor resulting in excessive autoantibody production. An increase in both type 1 and type 2 cytokines including an increase in interleukin 10, interferon gamma, and tumour necrosis factor alpha these has been reported (Jury et al. 2001).

Table 7 Laboratory features in adults and children with MCTD

Feature	Adults (%)			Children (%)	
	Bennett and O'Connell (1980) (*n* = 20)	Sullivan et al. (1984) (*n* = 34)	Prakash et al. (1985) (*n* = 81)	Singsen et al. (1977) (*n* = 14)	Tiddens et al. (1993) (*n* = 14)
Anaemia	75	24	—	Most	64
Leucopaenia	75	21	—	64	43
High ESR	100	—	—	100	—
Hypergammaglobulinaemia	75	53	73	60	—
High creatine kinase	43	—	—	—	50
Positive direct Coombs'	60	—	—	—	—
Positive rheumatoid factor	25	59	49	64	57
Low complement	—	32	5	—	—
Positive LE cell	—	18	—	—	—
Thrombocytopaenia	—	—	—	50	21
Positive ANA	100[a]	100	93	100	100
Anti-U1RNP	100[a]	100	100	100	100
Anti-dsDNA	0	23	4	0	21

[a] By definition patients had positive ANA, RNPase-sensitive ENA haemagglutination test, negative anti-Sm, and negative anti-ds DNA.

Note: ANA, antinuclear antibodies; ESR, erythrocyte sedimentation rate; LE, lupus erythematosus.

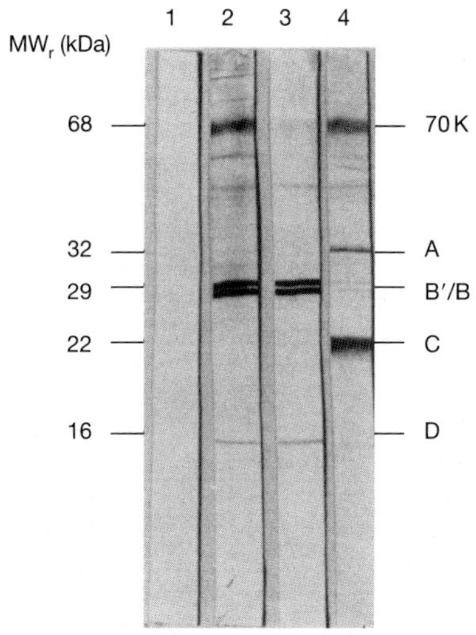

Fig. 4 Immunoblot showing the U1RNP and Sm antigenic peptides. Lane 1, normal serum; lane 2, anti-U1RNP and anti-Sm serum; lane 3, anti-Sm serum; lane 4, anti-U1 RNP and anti-Sm serum.

Recently, there have been reports that patients with distinct clinical rheumatic disease manifestations recognize apoptotically and oxidatively modified forms of the U1-70 kDa autoantigen. Strong recognition of apoptotically modified U1-70 kDa was associated with lupus skin disease, whereas oxidative cleavage was associated with Raynaud's phenomenom. This finding suggests that immune recognition of modified forms of self-antigens may be relevant to the pathogenesis of some rheumatic diseases (Hoffman and Greidinger 2000).

Histopathology

Proliferative vascular changes may be widespread and involve organs not clinically affected. The vascular changes are similar to systemic sclerosis but accompanied by less fibrosis. There is a predilection for intimal thickening of large arteries including coronary, pulmonary, renal, and aortic arteries (Singsen et al. 1980; Alpert et al. 1983; Sullivan et al. 1984). Skin biopsies show dermal thickening with hypertrophy of collagen bundles, thickening of blood vessel walls, and a perivascular mononuclear cell infiltration.

Longitudinal studies in mixed connective tissue disease

Long-term follow-up studies have shown that after many years of disease, features of only one autoimmune rheumatic disease (mainly scleroderma or SLE) predominate over the 'overlap' features present earlier in the course of the disease, which has cast doubt on MCTD being a separate entity. However, many of the patients that fulfil carefully selected criteria for MCTD at the time of diagnosis will still fulfil them at long-term follow-up. Most of the patients originally described by Sharp et al. (1972) developed either systemic sclerosis or SLE of variable severity on long-term follow-up, although five of 25 patients were virtually asymptomatic (Nimelstein et al. 1980). More recently a study of a cohort of 47 patients followed for a mean of 15 years showed a favourable otucome in 62 per cent of patients, while only 38 per cent had continued active disease or died, with death associated with pulmonary hypertension (Brudt et al. 1999). In this cohort MCTD rarely evolved into SLE or systemic sclerosis. In a series of 14 children with MCTD followed for nearly 10 years, features of SLE and polymyositis became less prominent, but scleroderma-like symptoms and joint abnormalities persisted (Tiddens et al. 1993). A revision of 191 paediatric patients retrieved from the literature showed remissions in around 5 per cent, a favourable outcome (absence of organ involvement, minor residual symptoms or signs) in around 70 per cent and an unfavourable outcome (clinically evident organ involvement, disability due to joint malfunction, severe Raynaud's phenomenon, severe vasculitis, severe adverse drug reactions, or death) in the remaining 25–30 per cent of children (Hartmut 1997).

Scleroderma-like skin abnormalities in adults and children are less responsive to treatment than initially thought and in most cases will persist, or may develop in patients who are initially diagnosed as having seronegative rheumatoid arthritis (Bennett and O'Connell 1980). Therefore, the clinical features of MCTD do appear to evolve with time; skin and pulmonary lesions persist in adults whereas skin and joint involvement are prominent in children. The differentiation of MCTD into SLE or systemic sclerosis may be determined by the immunogenetic background (Gendi et al. 1995).

Studies in patients with anti-U1RNP antibodies

About 50 per cent of patients with anti-U1RNP antibodies do not have MCTD, even with extended follow-up (Table 8). High titres of anti-U1RNP antibodies are associated more strongly with the development of MCTD (Lundberg and Hedfors 1991). Virtually all patients with MCTD will fulfil criteria for another autoimmune rheumatic disease at some stage in their illness. In our experience, patients with anti-U1RNP antibodies who fulfil criteria for MCTD without fulfilling criteria for SLE or systemic sclerosis are extremely rare (McHugh et al. 1990). Nonetheless, studies that exclude MCTD once another autoimmune rheumatic disease is diagnosed (Calderon et al. 1984; Van Den Hoogen et al. 1994) may be misleading, as such patients may still be said to have the former disease. In the context of SLE, the presence of anti-U1RNP antibodies is associated with Raynaud's phenomenon, swollen fingers, myositis, pulmonary involvement, and less renal disease (Reichlin and Mattioli 1972; McHugh et al. 1990; Maddison 2000). In patients with an overlap syndrome, the presence of anti-U1RNP antibodies may be associated with Raynaud's phenomenon and pulmonary hypertension (Lazaro et al. 1989).

Prognosis

The prognosis may not be as favourable as originally reported (Table 6). The major cause of mortality appears to be pulmonary hypertension in adults, and infection in children (Table 6). Pulmonary hypertension is not always progressive, however (Burdt et al. 1999). One-third of the 34 patients followed by Sullivan et al. (1984) had very severe disease requiring repeated courses or sustained high doses of corticosteroids and four patients died. A more favourable course is suggested in Burdt et al.'s (1999) study. In children the presence of reactivity to the Sm D polypeptide is associated with a poorer prognosis.

Management

Management of MCTD depends on manifestations of the disease. A suggested approach to management is outlined in Fig. 5. Raynaud's phenomenon is managed as in scleroderma, with emphasis on the patient keeping warm, avoiding trauma to the fingers, and discouragement of cigarette smoking. Vasodilators such as calcium channel blockers, angiotensin-converting enzymes, pentoxifylline, and ketanserin are effective in some patients. Intravenous prostacyclin may be used for acute ischaemic digital lesions.

Oesophageal involvement may respond to corticosteroids, although such treatment is rarely justified. More often, antacids, H_2-antagonists, and omeprazole are required. Fatigue, fever, lymphadenopathy, arthralgia, and myalgia may respond to non-steroidal anti-inflammatory drugs in conventional doses. The addition of antimalarial agents early in the course of the disease is becoming a more widespread practice. Low-dose corticosteroids (less than 20 mg of prednisolone per day) may be needed if general symptoms do not respond to other measures. The development of an erosive polyarthritis may warrant the introduction of methotrexate or azathioprine. Myositis in MCTD may respond to lower doses of corticosteroids than polymyositis/dermatomyositis (Nimelstein et al. 1980; Catoggio and Soriano 2000).

The management of renal disease remains controversial, although knowledge of histology may help in the decision. High-dose corticosteroids were effective for nephrotic syndrome and proteinuria in about two-thirds of patients described by Kitridou et al. (1986). However, cytotoxic drugs are probably indicated for those patients with more proliferative lesions, or those patients who require large corticosteroid doses for long periods of time.

Antiphospholipid antibodies should be sought in patients with pulmonary hypertension, and anticoagulation therapy considered when these antibodies are present. Corticosteroids and cytotoxic drugs should be considered at an early phase because of the poor prognosis associated with pulmonary hypertension in MCTD and its usually rapid progression. There are reports of patients responding to chlorambucil, cyclophosphamide, and cyclophosphamide and cyclosporin A, and even plasmapheresis and autologous peripheral blood stem cell transplantation (Myllykangas-Luosujarvi et al. 2000). Recurrent episodes of pulmonary vasoconstriction may contribute to the development of pulmonary hypertension in patients with diffuse systemic sclerosis, the CREST syndrome, and MCTD. Patients should follow the same management plan as primary pulmonary hypertension. Anticoagulation should be added if the patients have antiphospholipid antibodies. If there is no contraindication for anticoagulation, warfarin

Table 8 Outcome in patients with anti-U1RNP antibodies

	Method of detection	*n*	Follow-up (years)	Disease duration (years)	Definitive diagnosis						
					MCTD	SLE	UCTD	PSS	RA	PM	Others
Sharp et al. (1976)	Haemagglutination	100	NS	NS	74	12	6	8	—	—	—
Maddison et al. (1978)	Immunodiffusion	43	1–12	NS	5	30	4	1	1	—	2
Rasmussen et al. (1987)	Haemagglutination	97	Mean 9	NS	42	22	11	7	9	6	—
Lemmer et al. (1982)	Immunodiffusion haemagglutination	44	NS	1–16	11	10	20	1	—	2	—
Lundberg et al. (1992)	CIE	32	Mean 5.4	Mean 10.1	17	5	5	—	1	—	4
Catoggio et al. (1983)	Immunodiffusion	37	Median 4	Median 9	17	11	3	2	4	—	—
Van Den Hoggen et al. (1994)	CIE immunoblot	46	Mean 15	Mean 17	24	11	—	7	4	—	—
Total (%)		399			190 (47)	101 (25)	49 (12)	26 (6.5)	19 (5)	8 (2)	6 (1.5)

Note: MCTD, mixed connective tissue disease; SLE, systemic lupus erythematosus; UCTD, undifferentiated connective tissue disease; PSS, progressive systemic sclerosis; RA, rheumatoid arthritis, PM, polymyositis; CIE, counterimmunoelectrophoresis; NS, not stated.

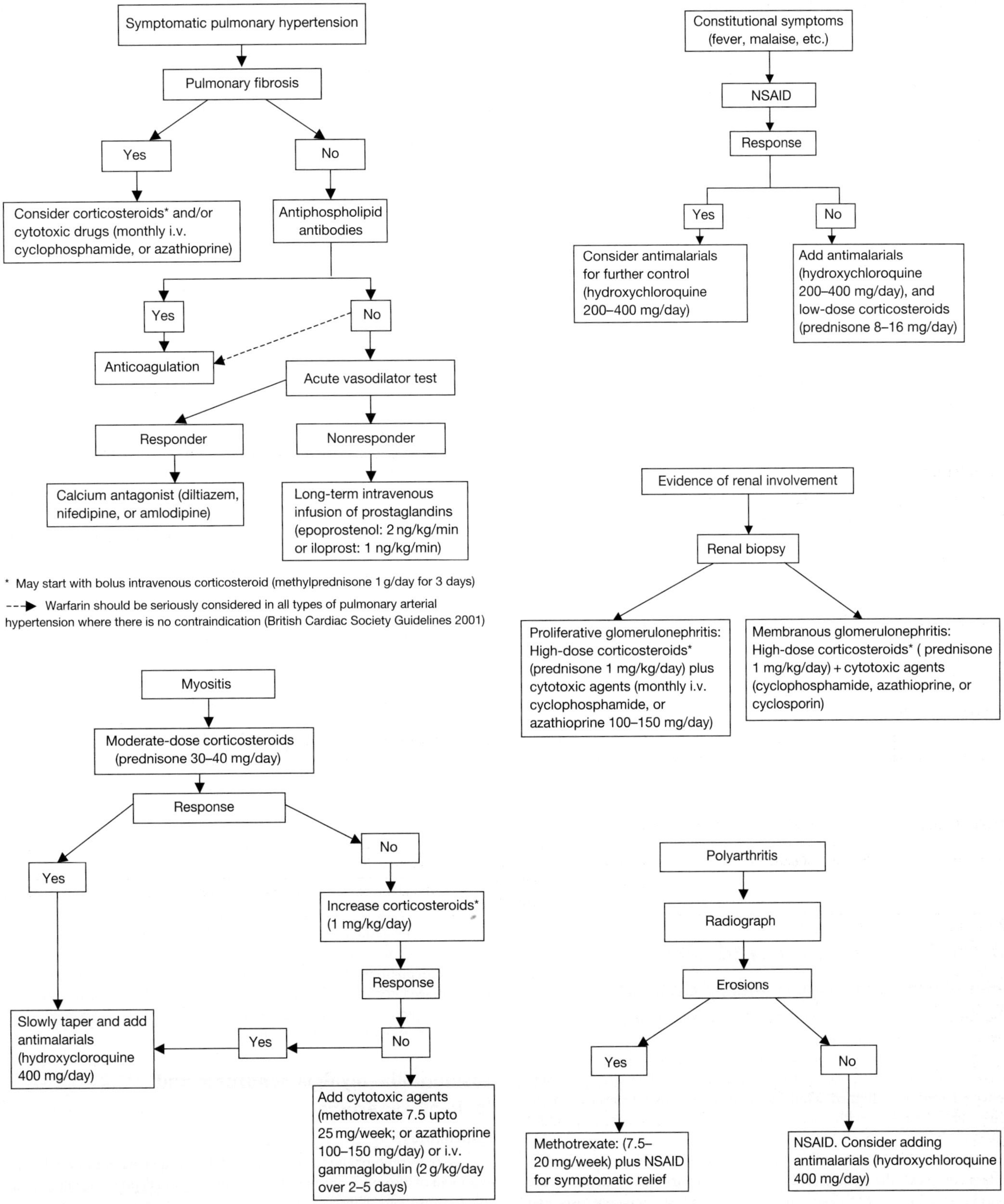

Fig. 5 Management of overlap syndrome.

should be seriously considered even in patients without these antibodies (British Cardiac Society Guidelines 2001). Calcium antagonists should only be used in those patients with a positive acute vasodilator response. Patients with pulmonary fibrosis may benefit from immunosuppressive therapy. Treatment of pulmonary hypertension with continuous infusion of prostacyclin had shown significant reductions in mean pulmonary artery pressure and increases in cardiac output in patients with secondary pulmonary hypertension (Hoffman and Gredinger 2000; British Cardiac Society Guidelines 2001).

Polymyositis overlap syndromes

Anti-tRNA synthetases syndrome

Autoantibodies are found in the majority of patients with polymyositis and dermatomyositis. The most frequent autoantibody is anti-Jo-1, which is directed against histidyl-tRNA synthetase, one of the 20 different enzymes that attaches the tRNA with its specific amino acid (Mathews and Bernstein 1983; Jury et al. 2001). Anti-Jo-1 is found in 15–20 per cent of all myositis patients, and very rarely in dermatomyositis (Jury et al. 2001).

A characteristic group of clinical features is associated with this group of autoantibodies. The 'antisynthetase syndrome' is characterized by myositis, interstitial lung disease, arthritis, and Raynaud's phenomenon (Targoff 1992). A particular cutaneous feature is the presence of hyperkeratosis and fissuring along the lateral aspects of the fingers, the so-called 'mechanic's (or machinist's) fingers' (Plate 164).

This syndrome is discussed in detail elsewhere in this book.

Rhupus

The existence of patients with a clinical picture resembling both rheumatoid arthritis and SLE has long been recognized.

The appearance of nodules or an erosive arthropathy in patients with SLE (Cohen and Webb 1987) suggests a genuine overlap between the two conditions. The term 'rhupus' has been used to describe such patients (Panush et al. 1988). 'Rhupus' does not seem to occur more frequently than expected than the chance concurrence of SLE and rheumatoid arthritis (Panush et al. 1988). Some of the patients described in these earlier studies had overlap features and if serological techniques had been available for detecting anti-U1RNP antibodies, they may have fulfilled criteria for MCTD. Immunogenetic factors may determine which clinical features become most prominent (Brand et al. 1992).

Scleroderma overlap syndromes

Scleroderma and primary biliary cirrhosis

The association between systemic sclerosis and primary biliary cirrhosis is well recognized (Murray-Lyon et al. 1970; Reynolds et al. 1971). Scleroderma occurs in 4–17 per cent of patients with primary biliary cirrhosis. Scleroderma in primary biliary cirrhosis is usually the CREST syndrome, now better referred to as limited cutaneous systemic sclerosis. Conversely, upto 5 per cent of patients with scleroderma have clinical evidence of primary biliary cirrhosis (Jury et al. 2001).

Antimitochondrial antibodies (directed against the pyruvate dehydrogenase complex), the serological hallmark of primary biliary cirrhosis, are found in 15–25 per cent of sera from patients with systemic sclerosis, and anticentromere antibodies, the serological hallmark of the CREST syndrome, are found in upto 30 per cent of sera from patients with primary biliary cirrhosis (Reynolds et al. 1971; Jury et al. 2001). The serological overlap between primary biliary cirrhosis and systemic sclerosis is more prevalent than the clinical overlap, although subclinical hepatic involvement may not be evident without liver biopsy. The serological overlap is not because of cross-reactivity between mitochondrial and centromere-associated antigens, which are independent antigenic targets (Whyte et al. 1994).

Patients with primary biliary cirrhosis also have a high prevalence of Sjögren's syndrome or keratoconjunctivitis sicca.

Scleroderma–polymyositis overlap

In the series of patients with polymyositis reported by Bohan et al. (1977), 21 per cent of 153 patients had another autoimmune rheumatic disorder and were classified as type V polymyositis. The most frequently associated autoimmune rheumatic disease was scleroderma (36 per cent). The diagnosis of MCTD was not considered, especially as detailed serological investigation was not available. However, anti-U1RNP antibodies were present in 25–33 per cent of a later series of similar patients (Hochberg et al. 1986).

Other autoantibody specificities may also be associated with the scleroderma–polymyositis overlaps. Anti-Ku antibodies are associated with the polymyositis–scleroderma overlap syndrome in Japan, but are less frequent in the United States; conversely anti-Pm-Scl antibodies are more frequent in polymyositis–scleroderma overlap in the United States but not in Japan (Targoff 1992). This might be explained by the fact that anti-Pm-Scl antibodies are closely associated with HLA–DR3 seen in 30 per cent of the healthy White population, but in less than 1 per cent of the healthy Japanese population (Ioannou et al. 1999). In general, anti-Pm-Scl antibodies are found in 8 per cent of myositis patients and 3 per cent of scleroderma patients (Targoff 1992). Among 22 patients with anti-Pm-Scl antibodies, polymyositis/dermatomyositis alone was present in 55 per cent, scleroderma without polymyositis/dermatomyositis in 5 per cent, and myositis–scleroderma overlap in 41 per cent (Reichlin et al. 1984).

The prognosis of patients with type V polymyositis is no different from that in polymyositis alone, in that the response to steroid therapy and the long-term outcome is generally favourable (Ioannou et al. 1999).

Eosinophilia–myalgia syndrome, toxic oil syndrome, eosinophilic fasciitis

The eosinophilia–myalgia syndrome (EMS) was first defined in 1989 (Centers for Disease Control 1989) as a new epidemic in association with the ingestion of L-tryptophan preparations (Kilbourne et al. 1996), traced to a single Japanese manufacturer (Kilbourne et al. 1996). However, this has been recently questioned by epidemilogists who have identified a number of methodological problems in the early reports associating EMS with L-tryptophan, and many questions remain regarding this syndrome (Clauw and Pincus 1996; Horwitz and Daniels 1996; Shapiro 1996). The clinical picture and the pathological features strongly resemble those of the Spanish toxic oil syndrome (TOS). Toxic oil syndrome was another epidemic that occurred in Spain in 1981 and was associated with the ingestion of adulterated rapeseed cooking oil. The presence of eosinophilia and fasciitis link these two epidemics with eosinophilic fasciitis. However, no toxin has been associated with eosinophilic fasciitis.

Eosinophilia–myalgia syndrome and toxic oil syndrome

Epidemiology

The use of L-tryptophan was widespread in the United States in 1989 for the treatment of insomnia, pre-menstrual syndrome, and depression, being available to consumers without a prescription. The surveillance case definition of EMS was as follows: eosinophil count greater than 1000 mm^{-3}, incapacitating myalgia, and exclusion of other infectious or neoplastic illnesses that could account for the other two findings (Hertzman 1996). Investigators have questioned whether these criteria are specific enough for surveillance studies, and most agree that they are inadequate for diagnostic purposes in an individual patient (Clauw and Pincus 1996; Hertzman 1996; Shapiro 1996).

National surveillance data from the United States in 1990 showed that 84 per cent of affected patients were female, 97 per cent were non-Hispanic white, and 87 were aged 35 years or older (Swygert et al. 1990). The female preponderance is more likely due to ingestion patterns rather than gender susceptibility. Two risk factors for developing EMS were older age and the quantity of tryptophan consumed. However, there may have been over reliance on a history of L-tryptophan ingestion in making the diagnosis of EMS. The incidence of EMS in the general population is low, even among L-tryptophan users (Hertzman 1996).

Toxic oil syndrome occurred in Spain in 1981 affecting more than 20 000 individuals with about 500 deaths. Epidemiological investigations implicated the use of aniline-denatured rapeseed oil that was sold and reprocessed illegally (Kilbourne et al. 1988).

Clinical features and histology

The more common clinical and laboratory manifestations of EMS and TOS are summarized in Table 9. By definition all patients had severe myalgia with an elevated peripheral eosinophil count. Myalgia was generally diffuse, although could be localized, and accompanied by severe episodic muscle cramps. The acute phase is followed by a chronic phase, characterized by varying degrees of dermal and subcutaneous sclerosis, persistent myalgia and muscle cramps, neuropathy and neurocognitive symptoms (Silver 1996). By contrast, patients with TOS presented as an atypical pneumonia, with non-productive cough, pleuritic chest pain, headache, fever, and bilateral pulmonary infiltrates. Gastrointestinal findings and striking eosinophilia became prominent within the first month.

The most prominent histological feature in both conditions was a perimysial and epimysial inflammatory infiltrate consisting of mononuclear cells, histiocytes, and eosinophils, epineural perivascular inflammation, and fibrosis with axonal degeneration (Silver 1996). Later in the course of the disease, muscle fibre atrophy consistent with denervation was observed in both conditions.

Pulmonary involvement was a major feature in both conditions. Toxic oil syndrome was characterized by an acute onset of cough and dyspnoea. Radiographic and pathological changes in TOS were consistent with a non-inflammatory non-cardiogenic pulmonary oedema, and 250 deaths occurred from this complication (Hertzman and Abaitua Borda 1993). Acute respiratory involvement in EMS occurred less frequently and was characterized by an interstitial pneumonitis that resolved spontaneously or was highly responsive to corticosteroids (Hertzman and Abaitua Borda 1993).

Pulmonary hypertension developed in the intermediate stage of both conditions (1–12 months) in 8 per cent of patients with TOS and in 5 per cent of patients with EMS, indicating a vasculitic pulmonary process occurring during the actue phase of disease (Silver 1996). Progressive or chronic pulmonary disease has not been seen in most patients with EMS (Silver 1996).

The most frequent cutaneous manifestations in the acute phase of EMS and TOS were diffuse erythematous macules over the trunk and extremities that are sometimes pruritic or urticarial. Histologically, the subcutaneous and dermal changes could not be distinguished from eosinophilic fasciitis; however, the pancutaneous nature of the eosinophilia–myalgia syndrome lesion and the perineural involvement distinguish it from the otherwise similar histopathologic characteristics seen in eosinophilic fasciitis (Silver 1996).

The central nervous system has been involved much less frequently than the peripheral nervous system during the acute phase of EMS (Silver 1996). The existence of chronic central nervous system involvement is controversial.

The laboratory findings are shown in Table 9. The most characteristic finding was the presence of eosinophilia in peripheral blood, usually within the first week. Antinuclear antibodies were found in 40 per cent of patients with EMS and in a minority of patients with TOS. Normal creatine kinase levels were seen in almost all patients, although isolated elevation of serum aldolase was reported in 58 per cent of patients with EMS (Silver 1996).

Table 9 Prevalence of selected clinical and laboratory findings in EMS and TOS

Feature	EMS (Swygert et al. 1990), $n = 1075$ (%)	TOS (Kilbourne et al. 1983), $n = 121$ (%)
Myalgia	100[b]	55.5
Arthralgia	73	8.4
Rash	60	64.7
Peripheral oedema	59	64.7
Cough	59[a]	68.1
Dyspnoea	59[a]	42
Fever	36	68.1
Scleroderma-like skin	32	—
Alopecia	28	5
Neuropathy	28	39.5
Hepatomegaly	5	37
Leucocytosis	85	71.1
Eosinophilia (>500 mm^{-3})	100[b]	77.7
Elevated ESR	33	38.8
Elevated aldolase	46	55.4
Elevated creatine kinase	10	—
Abnormal chest radiograph	21	87.6
Abnormal liver function test	43	41.3

[a] Cough and dyspnoea taken together (Swygert et al. 1990).

[b] By definition all patients had incapacitating myalgia and eosinophil count of more than 1.0×10^9 cells (Swygert et al. 1990).

Aetiology and pathogenesis

Eosinophilia–myalgia syndrome

The epidemic nature of EMS, and its association with batches of L-tryptophan originating from a single manufacturer, suggested a contaminant. A single absorbance peak labelled 'peak E', or peak 97, and later identified as 1,1′-ethylidene bis(tryptophan) (EBT), was found consistently in L-tryptophan lots associated with EMS. A second contaminant (peak UV-5) has been identified as 3-(phenylamino)alanine (PAA) and related to L-tryptophan associated with cases of EMS (Clauw 1996). Of interest, PAA is chemically similar to 3-phenylamino-1,2-propanediol, an aniline derivative implicated in the development of TOS.

Both cellular and humoral autoimmune mechanisms have been implicated in the pathogenesis of EMS. A hypothetical model is that the initial trigger (tryptophan contaminant or metabolite) activates inflammatory cells, which are induced to secrete cytokines (IL-5, GM-CSF, transforming growth factor-β) that cause activation of eosinophils and fibroblasts. Activated eosinophils may release cytokines and toxic granule proteins (including major basic protein), which may contribute to tissue injury. Activated fibroblasts produce increased amounts of collagen and other extracellular matrix components resulting in the characteristic fibrosis (Silver 1996).

Toxic oil syndrome

Fatty acid anilides have been proposed as the aetiological agents in TOS. Fatty acid anilides may alter arachidonic acid metabolism or impair fibrinolytic activity in endothelial cells leading to the early intimal lesions seen in these patients.

Prognosis

The disease-related mortality rate for the first year was 2.7 per cent for EMS and 1.5–3.6 per cent for TOS (Kaufman 1993; Swygert et al. 1993). Toxic oil syndrome was more severe than EMS in its acute stages (Kaufman 1993). Progressive polyneuropathy and myopathy accounted for 67 per cent of deaths in patients with EMS. Older age and involvement of more than one organ system, in particular neuromuscular, pulmonary, and cardiovascular sequelae, suggested a poor prognosis (Swygert et al. 1993).

Long-term morbidity was frequent in both syndromes. The clinical status of patients with the EMS 2–4 years after its description was studied (Pincus 1996): persistent symptoms such as fatigue (76 per cent), myalgia (69 per cent), poor memory (69 per cent), poor sleep (67 per cent), muscle cramping, and numbness (66 per cent) were reported in most patients (Pincus 1996). Almost no patient experienced new signs of acute inflammation more than 1 year after the onset of disease

In an 8-year follow-up study of 332 patients with TOS, only 9 per cent achieved full remission (Alonso-Ruiz et al. 1993). The severity of the chronic manifestations was variable, but was mild in most of the cases (Alonso-Ruiz et al. 1993). Muscle cramps and chronic musculoskeletal pain were the most common symptoms.

Management

A variety of medical regimens, mainly non-steroidal anti-inflammatory agents and corticosteroids, have been used to treat patients with EMS and TOS. Although acute symptoms such as oedema, acute pulmonary disease, and eosinophilia responded to corticosteroid treatment, such treatment was not associated with long-term improvement in symptoms. Corticosteroids may have been life saving in cases of acute respiratory failure due to non-cardiogenic pulmonary oedema in TOS.

Eosinophilia–myalgia syndrome in children

Eosinophilia–myalgia syndrome occasionally has been identified among children, including a neonate with persistent eosinophilia whose mother ingested tryptophan during pregnancy (Hatch et al. 1991). More recently a case of EMS was reported in a child with phenylketonuria who developed the syndrome after ingesting a specialized infant formula containing contaminated tryptophan (Springer et al. 1992).

Eosinophilic fasciitis

Eosinophilic fasciitis is a relatively uncommon idiopathic disease, first described by Shulman (1974), and characterized by fasciitis and peripheral blood eosinophilia. It shares similar clinical and histological features with EMS and TOS, but significant internal organ involvement is uncommon. Also, there are differences that distinguish eosinophilic fasciitis from systemic sclerosis: the absence of Raynaud's phenomenon, normal nailfold capillaries, sparing of the dermis, infrequent visceral involvement, absence of the serological features characteristic of systemic sclerosis, and the development of haematological complications, such as aplastic anaemia and thrombocytopaenia, seldom reported in typical systemic sclerosis (Maddison 1991). The age of onset is 30–40 years (mean: 47; range: 11–72), and in half of the patients a history of recent strenuous exertion can be recalled (Lakhampal et al. 1988).

Cutaneous manifestations are the most common presenting feature and usually evolve through three stages: pitting oedema, *peau d'orange*, and induration. These stages are often present simultaneously in different areas of the body (Maddison 1991). The arms and legs are affected most commonly and simultaneous involvement of hands and feet is not uncommon. Localized morphoea may occur in other areas, especially in children (Miller 1992). Synovitis is not uncommon and may be the presenting feature. Low-grade myositis may be present, although serum creatine kinase levels are usually normal.

Eosinophilic fasciitis has been associated with malignancy and may present as a paraneoplastic syndrome (Naschitz et al. 1994), which remits with successful cancer surgery. Haematological malignancies are overrepresented, and aplastic anaemia in particular has a high associated mortality (Hoffman et al. 1982). Eosinophilic fasciitis associated with malignancy has a female predominance and usually fails to respond to corticosteroids (Naschitz et al. 1994).

Peripheral eosinophilia, sometimes impressive, is the most striking laboratory feature. Eosinophilia may be transient and the diagnosis should not be dismissed because of its absence. Diagnosis is confirmed by a cutaneous biopsy to include tissue extending from the epidermis to skeletal muscle and the deep fascia. Characteristic histological findings are a widespread inflammatory infiltrate involving the deep fascia and septae of the subdermal fat as well as the dermal layer and a normal epidermis.

The cause of eosinophilic fasciitis is unknown. Of interest is the association with strenuous exertion, especially in men. After the description of EMS associated with L-tryptophan, some retrospective studies have found an association of eosinophilic fasciitis with the consumption of L-tryptophan (Martin et al. 1991), while others have not (Varga et al. 1991). More than half of patients with eosinophilic fasciitis respond to corticosteroids, although complete remission is achieved in only 15 per cent. There may be spontaneous remissions. Other agents such as cimetidine, hydroxychloroquine, colchicine, D-penicillamine, and cyclosporin A have been used with variable results. In children, two-thirds of patients developed cutaneous fibrosis (Farrington et al. 1993).

References

Alarcon, G.S. (2000). Unclassified or undifferentiated connective tissue disease. *Baillière's Clinical Rheumatology* **14**, 125–37.

Alarcon-Segovia, D. and Cardiel, M.H. (1989). Comparison between 3 diagnostic criteria for mixed connective tissue disease. Study of 593 patients. *Journal of Rheumatology* **16**, 328–34.

Alonso-Ruiz, A., Calabozo, M., Perez-Ruiz, F., and Mancebo, L. (1993). Toxic oil syndrome: a long-term follow-up of a cohort of 332 patients. *Medicine (Baltimore)* **72**, 285–95.

Alpert, M.A. et al. (1983). Cardiovascular manifestations of mixed connective tissue disease in adults. *Circulation* **68**, 1182–93.

Babini, S.M., Maldonado-Cocco, J.A., Barcelo, H.A., and Garcia-Morteo, O. (1985). Peritendinous nodules in overlap syndrome. *Journal of Rheumatology* **12**, 160–4.

Bennett, R.M. and Spargo, B.H. (1977). Immune complex nephropathy in mixed connective tissue disease. *American Journal of Medicine* **63**, 534–41.

Bennett, R.M. and O'Connell, D.J. (1980). Mixed connective tissue disease: a clinicopathologic study of 20 cases. *Seminars in Arthritis and Rheumatism* **10**, 25–50.

Bohan, A., Peter, J.B., Bowman, R.L., and Pearson, C.M. (1977). A computer-assisted analysis of 153 patients with polymyositis and dermatomyositis. *Medicine (Baltimore)* **56**, 255–86.

Brand, C.A., Rowley, M.L, Tate, B.D., Muirden, K.D., and Whittingham, S.F. (1992). Coexistent rheumatoid arthritis and systemic lupus erythematosus. Clinical, serological and phenotypic features. *Annals of the Rheumatic Diseases* **51**, 173–6.

British Cardiac Society Guidelines and Medical Practice Committee, and approved by the British Thoracic Society and the British Society of Rheumatology (2001). Recommendations on the management of pulmonary hypertension in clinical practice. *Heart* (Suppl. 1), 1–13.

Burdt, M.A., Hoffman, R.W., Deutscher, S.L., Wang, G.S., Johnson, J.C., and Sharp, G.C. (1999). Long-term outcome in mixed connective tissue disease. Longitudinal clinical and serologic findings. *Arthritis and Rheumatism* **42**, 899–909.

Calderon, L., Rodriguez-Valverde, V., Sanchez-Andrade, S., Riestra, J.L., and Gomez-Reyno, J. (1984). Clinical profiles of patients with antibodies to nuclear ribonucleoprotein. *Clinical Rheumatology* **8**, 483–92.

Catoggio, L.J. and Soriano, E.R. (2000). Inflammatory muscle disease: therapeutic aspects. *Baillière's Clinical Rheumatology* **14**, 55–71.

Catoggio, L.J., Evison, G., Harkness, J.A.L., and Maddison, P.J. (1983). The arthropathy of systemic sclerosis (scleroderma); comparison with mixed connective tissue disease. *Clinical and Experimental Rheumatology* **1**, 101–12.

Centers for Disease Control (1989). Eosinophilia–myalgia syndrome New Mexico. *Morbidity and Mortality Weekly Report* **38**, 765–7.

Citera, G., Lazaro, M.A., and Maldonado Cocco, J.A. (1995). Mixed connective tissue disease: fact or fiction? *Lupus* **4**, 255–7.

Clauw, D.J. (1996). Animal models of the eosinophilia–myalgia syndrome. *Journal of Rheumatology* **23**, 93–8.

Clauw, D.J. and Pincus, T. (1996). The eosinophilia–myalgia syndrome: what we know, what we think we know, and what we need to know. *Journal of Rheumatology* **23**, 2–6.

Cohen, M.G. and Webb, J. (1987). Concurrence of rheumatoid arthritis and systemic lupus erythematosus: report of 11 cases. *Annals of the Rheumatic Diseases* **46**, 853–8.

Farrington, M.L., Haas, J.E., Nazar-Stewart, V., and Mellins, E.D. (1993). Eosinophilic fasciitis in children frequently progress to scleroderma-like cutaneous fibrosis. *Journal of Rheumatology* **20**, 128–32.

Gendi, N.S.T., Welsh, K.I., Van Venrooij, W.J., Vancheeswaran, R., Gilroy, J., and Black, C. (1995). HLA type as a predictor of mixed connective tissue disease differentiation. Ten-year clinical and immunogenetic followup of 46 patients. *Arthritis and Rheumatism* **38**, 259–66.

Goldstein, R. et al. (1990). HLA-D region genes associated with autoantibody responses to histidyl-transfer RNA synthetase (Jo-1) and other translation-related factors in myositis. *Arthritis and Rheumatism* **33**, 1240–8.

Grant, K.D., Adams, L.E., and Hess, E.V. (1981). Mixed connective tissue disease—a subset with sequential clinical and laboratory features. *Journal of Rheumatology* **8**, 587–98.

Hartmut, M. (1997). Course of mixed connective tissue disease in children. *Annals of Medicine* **29**, 359–64.

Hatch, D.L., Garona, J.E., Goldman, L.R., and Walker, K.O. (1991). Persistent eosinophilia in an infant with probable intrauterine exposure to L-tryptophan-containing supplements. *Pediatrics* **88**, 810–13.

Hertzman, P.A. (1996). Criteria for the definition of the eosinophilia–myalgia syndrome. *Journal of Rheumatology* **23**, 7–12.

Hertzman, P.A. and Abaitua Borda, I. (1993). The toxic oil syndrome and the eosinophilia–myalgia syndrome: pursuing clinical parallels. *Journal of Rheumatology* **20**, 1707–10.

Hochberg, M.C., Feldman, D., and Stevens, M.B. (1986). Adult onset polymyositis/dermatomyositis: an analysis of clinical and laboratory features and survival in 76 patients with a review of the literature. *Seminars in Arthritis and Rheumatism* **15**, 168–78.

Hoffman, R.W. and Greidinger, E.L. (2000). Mixed connective tissue disease. *Current Opinion in Rheumatology* **12**, 386–90.

Hoffman, R., Young, N., Ershler, W.B., Mazur, E., and Gewirtz, A. (1982). Diffuse fasciitis and aplastic anemia: a report of four cases revealing an unusual association between rheumatologic and hematologic disorders. *Medicine* **61**, 373–81.

Horwitz, R.I. and Daniels, S.R. (1996). Bias or biology: evaluating the epidemiologic studies of L-tryptophan and the eosinophilia–myalgia syndrome. *Journal of Rheumatology* **23**, 60–72.

Ioannou, Y., Sultan, S., and Isenberg, D.A. (1999). Myositis overlap syndromes. *Current Opinions in Rheumatology* **11**, 468–74.

Isenberg, D. and Black, C. (1999). Naming names! Comment on the article by Smolen and Steiner. *Arthritis and Rheumatism* **42**, 191–12.

Jury, E.C., D'Cruz, D., and Morrow, W.J.W. (2001). Autoantibodies and overlap syndromes in autoimmune rheumatic disease. *Journal of Clinical Pathology* **54**, 340–7.

Kahn, M.F., Bourgeois, P., Aeschlimann, A., and de Truchis, P. (1989). Mixed connective tissue disease after exposure to polyvinyl chloride. *Journal of Rheumatology* **16**, 533–5.

Kasukawa, R. et al. (1987). Preliminary diagnostic criteria for classification of mixed connective tissue diseases. In *Mixed Connective Tissue Diseases and Anti-nuclear Antibodies* (ed. R. Kasukawa and G.C. Sharp), pp. 41–7. Amsterdam: Excerpta Medica.

Kaufman, L.D. (1993). Eosinophilia–myalgia syndrome: morbidity and mortality. *Journal of Rheumatology* **20**, 1644–6.

Kilbourne, E.M. et al. (1983). Clinical epidemiology of toxic-oil syndrome. *New England Journal of Medicine* **309**, 1408–14.

Kilbourne, E.M. et al. (1988). Chemical correlates of pathogenicity of oils related to the toxic oil syndrome epidemic in Spain. *American Journal of Epidemiology* **127**, 1210–27.

Kilbourne, E.M., Philen, M.R., Kamb, M.L., and Falk, H. (1996). Tryptophan produced by Showa Denko and epidemic eosinophilia–myalgia syndrome. *Journal of Rheumatology* **23**, 81–8.

Kitridou, R.C., Akmal, M., Turkel, S.B., Ehresmann, G.R., Quismorio, F.P., Jr., and Massry, S.G. (1986). Renal involvement in mixed connective tissue disease: a longitudinal clinicopathologic study. *Seminars in Arthritis and Rheumatism* **16**, 135–45.

Kozuka, T. et al. (2001). Pulmonary involvement in mixed connective tissue disease: high-resolution CT findings in 41 patients. *Journal of Thoracic Imaging* **16**, 94–8.

Kumagai, Y., Shiokawa, Y., Medsger, T.A., and Rodnan, G.P. (1984). Clinical spectrum of connective tissue disease after cosmetic surgery. *Arthritis and Rheumatism* **27**, 1–12.

Kuwana, M., Okano, Y., Kaburaki, J., Tsuji, K., and Inoko, H. (1995). Major histocompatibility complex class II gene associations with anti-U1 small nuclear ribonucleoprotein antibody. *Arthritis and Rheumatism* **38**, 396–405.

Lakhampal, S., Ginsburg, W.W., Michet, J.J., Doyle, J.A., and Breanndan Morre, S. (1988). Eosinophilic fasciitis: clinical spectrum and therapeutic response in 52 cases. *Seminars in Arthritis and Rheumatism* **17**, 221–31.

Lazaro, M.A. et al. (1989). Clinical and serologic characteristics of patients with overlap syndrome: is mixed connective tissue disease a distinct clinical entity? *Medicine (Baltimore)* **68**, 58–65.

Lemmer, J.P., Curry, N.H., Mallory, J.H., and Waller, M.V. (1982). Clinical characteristics and course in patients with high titer anti-RNP antibodies. *Journal of Rheumatology* **9**, 536–42.

Lundberg, I. and Hedfors, E. (1991). Clinical course of patients with anti-RNP antibodies. A prospective study of 32 patients. *Journal of Rheumatology* **18**, 1511–19.

Lundberg, I., Nennesmo, I., and Hedfors, E. (1992). A clinical, serological, and histopathological study of myositis patients with and without anti-RNP antibodies. *Seminars in Arthritis and Rheumatism* **22**, 127–38.

Maddison, P.J. (1991). Mixed connective tissue disease, overlap syndromes, and eosinophilic fasciitis. *Annals of the Rheumatic Diseases* **50**, 887–93.

Maddison, P.J. (2000). Mixed connective tissue disease: overlap syndromes. *Baillière's Best Practice and Research in Clinical Rheumatology* **14**, 111–24.

Marguerie, C. et al. (1992). The clinical and immunogenetic features of patients with autoantibodies to the nucleolar antigen PM-Scl. *Medicine (Baltimore)* **71**, 327–36.

Marshall, J.B. et al. (1990). Gastrointestinal manifestations of mixed connective tissue disease. *Gastroenterology* **98**, 1232–8.

Martin, R.W., Duffy, J., and Lie, J.T. (1991). Eosinophilic fascitis associated with use of L-tryptophan: a case control study and comparison of clinical and histopathologic features. *Mayo Clinic Proceedings* **66**, 892–8.

Mathews, M.B. and Bernstein, R.M. (1983). Myositis autoantibody inhibits histidyl-tRNA synthetase: a model for autoimmunity. *Nature* **304**, 177–9.

McHugh, N., James, I., and Maddison, P. (1990). Clinical significance of antibodies to a 68 kDa U1RNP polypeptide in connective tissue disease. *Journal of Rheumatology* **17**, 1320–8.

Miller, J.J., III. (1992). The fasciitis–morphea complex in children. *American Journal of Diseases in Children* **146**, 733–6.

Murray-Lyon, I.M., Thompson, R.P.H., Ansell, I.D., and Williams, R. (1970). Scleroderma and primary biliary cirrhosis. *British Medical Journal* **iii**, 258–9.

Myllykangas-Luosujarvi, R., Jantunen, E., Kaipiainen-Seppanen, O., Mahlamaki, E., and Nousiainen, T. (2000). Autologous peripheral blood stem cell transplantation in a patient with severe mixed connective tissue disease. *Scandinavian Journal of Rheumatology* **29**, 326–7.

Naschitz, J.E. et al. (1994). Cancer associated fasciitis panniculitis. *Cancer* **73**, 231–5.

Nimelstein, S.H., Brody, S., Mcshane, D., and Holman, H.R. (1980). Mixed connective tissue disease: a subsequent evaluation of the original 25 patients. *Medicine (Baltimore)* **59**, 239–48.

O'Connell, D.J. and Bennett, R.M. (1977). Mixed connective tissue disease—clinical and radiological aspects of 20 cases. *British Journal of Radiology* **50**, 620–5.

Oetgen, W.J., Mutter, M.L., Lawless, O.J., and Davia, J.E. (1983). Cardiac abnormalities in mixed connective tissue disease. *Chest* **83**, 185–8.

Ohtsuka, E., Nonaka, S., Shingu, M., Yasuda, M., and Nobunaga, M. (1992). Sjögren syndrome and mixed connective tissue disease. *Clinical and Experimental Rheumatology* **10**, 339–44.

Panush, R.S., Edwards, L., Longley, S., and Webster, E. (1988). 'Rhupus' syndrome. *Archives of Internal Medicine* **148**, 1633–6.

Pelkonen, P.M. et al. (1994). Incidence of systemic connective tissue diseases in children: a nationwide prospective study in Finland. *Journal of Rheumatology* **21**, 2143–6.

Pincus, T. (1996). Eosinophilia–myalgia syndrome: patient status 2–4 years after onset. *Journal of Rheumatology* **23**, 19–25.

Piirainen, H.I., Helve, A.T., Tornroth, T., and Pettersson, T.E. (1989). Amyloidosis in mixed connective tissue disease. *Scandinavian Journal of Rheumatology* **18**, 165–8.

Rasmussen, E.K., Ullman, S., Horer-Madsen, M., Sorensen, S.F., and Halberg, P. (1987). Clinical implications of ribonucleoprotein antibody. *Archives of Dermatology* **123**, 601–5.

Reichlin, M. and Mattioli, M. (1972). Correlation of a precipitin reaction to an RNA protein antigen and a low prevalence of nephritis in patients with systemic lupus erythematosus. *New England Journal of Medicine* **286**, 908–11.

Reichlin, M. et al. (1984). Antibodies to a nuclear/nucleolar antigen in patients with polymyositis-overlap syndrome. *Journal of Clinical Immunology* **4**, 40–4.

Reilly, P.A., Evison, G., McHugh N.J., and Maddison, P.J. (1990). Arthropathy of hands and feet in systemic lupus erythematosus. *Journal of Rheumatology* **17**, 777–84.

Reynolds, T.B., Denison, E.K., Frankl, H.D., Lieberman, F.L., and Peters, R.L. (1971). Primary biliary cirrhosis with scleroderma, Raynaud's phenomena, and telangiectasis. *American Journal of Medicine* **67**, 302–12.

Shapiro, S. (1996). Epidemiologic studies of the association of L-tryptophan with the eosinophilia–myalgia syndrome: a critique. *Journal of Rheumatology* **23**, 44–59.

Sharp, G.C. (1987). Diagnostic criteria for classification of MCTD. In *Mixed Connective Tissue Diseases and Anti-nuclear Antibodies* (ed. R. Kasukawa and G.C. Sharp), pp. 23–32. Amsterdam: Excerpta Medica.

Sharp, G.C. et al. (1971). Association of autoantibodies to different nuclear antigens with clinical patterns of rheumatic disease and responsiveness to therapy. *Journal of Clinical Investigation* **50**, 350–9.

Sharp, G.C., Irvin, W.S., Tan, E.M., Gould, R.G., and Holman, H.R. (1972). Mixed connective tissue disease—an apparently distinct rheumatic disease syndrome associated with a specific antibody to an extractable nuclear antigen (ENA). *American Journal of Medicine* **52**, 148–59.

Sharp, G.C. et al. (1976). Association of antibodies to ribonucleoprotein and Sm antigens with mixed connective-tissue disease, systemic lupus erythematosus and other rheumatic diseases. *New England Journal of Medicine* **295**, 1149–54.

Shulman, L.E. (1974). Diffuse fasciitis with hypergammaglobulinaemia and eosiniphilia in a new syndrome. *Journal of Rheumatology* **1** (Suppl.), 46.

Silver, R.M. (1996). Pathophysiology of the eosinophilia–myalgia syndrome. *Journal of Rheumatology* **23**, 26–36.

Singsen, B.H., Bernstein, B.H., Kornreich, H.K., Koster King, K., Hanson, V., and Tan, E.M. (1977). Mixed connective tissue disease in childhood. A clinical and serologic survey. *Journal of Pediatrics* **90**, 893–900.

Singsen, B.H., Swanson, V.L., Bernstein, B.H., Heuser, E.T., Hanson, V., and Landing, B.H. (1980). A histologic evaluation of mixed connective tissue disease in childhood. *American Journal of Medicine* **68**, 710–17.

Smolen, J.S. and Steiner, G. (1998). Mixed connective tissue disease: to be or not to be? *Arthritis and Rheumatism* **41**, 768–77.

Springer, M.A., Bock, H.G., Philen, R.M., Hill, R.H., Jr., and Crawford, L.V. (1992). Eosinophilia–myalgia syndrome in a child with phenylketonuria. *Pediatrics* **90**, 630–3.

Sullivan, W.D. et al. (1984). A prospective evaluation emphasizing pulmonary involvement in patients with mixed connective tissue disease. *Medicine (Baltimore)* **63**, 92–107.

Swygert, L.A., Maes, E.F., Sewell, L.E., Miller, L., Falk, H., and Kilbourne, E.M. (1990). Eosinophilia–myalgia syndrome. Results of national surveillance. *Journal of the American Medical Association* **264**, 1698–703.

Swygert, L.A., Back, E.E., Auerbach, S.B., Sewell, L.E., and Falk, H. (1993). Eosinophilia–myalgia syndrome: mortality data from the US national surveillance system. *Journal of Rheumatology* **20**, 1711–17.

Targoff, I.N. (1992). Autoantibodies in polymyositis. *Rheumatic Disease Clinics of North America* **18**, 455–82.

Tiddens, H.A.W.M. et al. (1993). Juvenile-onset mixed connective tissue disease: longitudinal follow-up. *Journal of Pediatrics* **122**, 191–7.

Van Den Hoogen, F.H.J. et al. (1994). Long-term follow-up of 46 patients with anti-(U1)snRNP antibodies. *British Journal of Rheumatology* **33**, 1117–20.

Varga, J., Griffin, R., Newman, J.H., and Jimenez, S.A. (1991). Eosinophilic fasciitis is clinically distinguishable from the eosinophilia–myalgia syndrome and is not associated with L-tryptophan use. *Journal of Rheumatology* **18**, 259–63.

Weber, P., Ganser, G., Frosch, M., Roth, J., Hulskamp, G., and Zimmer, K.P. (2000). Twenty-four hour intraesophageal pH monitoring in children and adolescents with scleroderma and mixed connective tissue disease. *Journal of Rheumatology* **27**, 2692–5.

Whyte, J., Hough, D., Maddison, P.J., and McHugh, N.J. (1994). The association of primary biliary cirrhosis and systemic sclerosis is not accounted for by cross reactivity between mitochondiral and centromere antigens. *Journal of Autoimmunity* **7**, 413–24.

6.12 Miscellaneous inflammatory conditions

6.12.1 Amyloidosis

P.N. Hawkins

Introduction

Amyloidosis is a disorder of protein folding in which normally soluble proteins are deposited as abnormal, insoluble fibrils that disrupt tissue structure and cause disease (Dobson et al. 2001). Some 20 different unrelated proteins can form amyloid *in vivo*, and amyloidosis is classified clinically according to the fibril protein type (Table 1). In systemic amyloidosis deposits may occur in all tissues except the brain, and are present in blood vessels throughout the body. Systemic amyloidosis is potentially fatal although its prognosis has been improved by haemodialysis, kidney, liver, and heart transplantation, and by increasingly effective treatment of the various conditions that underlie amyloid deposition. There are also various local forms of amyloidosis in which deposits are confined to specific foci or to a particular organ or tissue. These may be clinically silent or trivial, or they may be associated with serious disease, such as heart failure in senile cardiac amyloidosis, or haemorrhage in local respiratory or urogenital tract amyloid. In addition there are important diseases associated with local amyloid deposition in which the pathogenetic role of the amyloid is still unclear, for example, Alzheimer's disease, the prion disorders, and type 2 diabetes mellitus. Although these conditions will not be discussed here, it should be recognized that therapeutic strategies aimed at inhibiting amyloid fibrillogenesis and/or promoting regression of amyloid deposits in systemic amyloidosis may also be applicable to localized amyloidosis and vice versa.

In addition to the fibrils, amyloid deposits always contain the plasma protein serum amyloid P component (SAP), because it undergoes specific

Table 1 Classification of amyloidosis

Type	Fibril precursor protein	Clinical syndrome
AA	Serum amyloid A protein	Reactive systemic amyloidosis associated with acquired or hereditary chronic inflammatory diseases. Formerly known as secondary amyloidosis
AL	Monoclonal immunoglobulin light chains	Systemic amyloidosis associated with myeloma, monoclonal gammopathy, occult B cell dyscrasia. Formerly known as primary amyloidosis
ATTR	Normal plasma transthyretin	Senile systemic amyloidosis with prominent cardiac involvement
ATTR	Genetically variant transthyretin, e.g. Met30Val and about 80 other point mutations	Familial amyloid polyneuropathy, usually with systemic amyloidosis. Sometimes prominent amyloid cardiomyopathy or nephropathy
Aβ_2-M	β_2-Microglobulin	Periarticular and, occasionally, systemic amyloidosis associated with renal failure and long-term dialysis
Aβ	β-Protein precursor (and rare genetic variants)	Cerebrovascular and intracerebral plaque amyloid in Alzheimer's disease. Occasional familial cases
AApoAI	Apolipoprotein AI (genetic variants, including Gly26Arg, Trp50Arg, Leu60Arg, Leu90Pro, Arg173Pro, Leu174Ser, Leu178His and several deletion mutations)	Autosomal dominant systemic amyloidosis. Predominantly non-neuropathic with prominent visceral involvement
AFib	Fibrinogen α chain (genetic variants, including Glu526Val, Arg554Leu, and frame shift mutations at codons 522 and 524)	Autosomal dominant systemic amyloidosis. Non-neuropathic with prominent visceral involvement
ALys	Lysozyme (genetic variants, including Asp67His, Ile56Thr, and Trp64Arg)	Autosomal dominant systemic amyloidosis. Non-neuropathic with prominent visceral involvement
ACys	Cystatin C (genetic variant Leu68Gln)	Hereditary cerebral haemorrhage with cerebral and systemic amyloidosis
AGel	Gelsolin (genetic variants Asp187Asn, Asp187Tyr)	Autosomal dominant systemic amyloidosis. Predominant cranial nerve involvement with lattice corneal dystrophy
AIAPP	Islet amyloid polypeptide	Amyloid in islets of Langerhans in type II diabetes mellitus and insulinoma

Note: Amyloid composed of peptide hormones, prion protein, and unknown proteins, not included.

calcium-dependent binding to amyloid fibrils (Pepys et al. 1997). SAP contributes to amyloidogenesis (Botto et al. 1997), and radiolabelled SAP is a specific, quantitative, and highly informative tracer for scintigraphic imaging of systemic amyloid deposits (Hawkins et al. 1990a). The treatment of amyloidosis comprises measures to support impaired organ function, including dialysis and transplantation, along with vigorous efforts to control underlying conditions responsible for production of fibril precursors (Gillmore et al. 1997). Serial SAP scintigraphy has demonstrated that reduction of the supply of amyloid fibril precursor proteins leads to regression of amyloid deposits and clinical benefit in many cases.

Pathogenesis

Amyloid fibril formation involves substantial refolding of the native structures of the various fibril precursor proteins to generate structures that are rich in β-sheet, and which autoaggregate in a highly ordered manner to form the fibrils (Booth et al. 1997; Sunde et al. 1997). Amyloid deposition occurs *in vivo* under several conditions. First, when a normal protein is present for sufficient time at an abnormally high concentration, such as serum amyloid A protein (SAA) or β_2-microglobulin (β_2-M). Secondly, with an ordinary concentration of a normal, but inherently amyloidogenic, protein over a very prolonged period, as in the case of transthyretin in senile systemic amyloidosis. Thirdly, when there is an acquired or inherited variant protein with abnormal amyloidogenic structure, such as some monoclonal immunoglobulin light chains or variants of transthyretin, lysozyme, apolipoprotein AI, fibrinogen A α-chain, etc.

Amyloid fibrils

Regardless of their very diverse protein subunits, amyloid fibrils of different types are remarkably similar. Straight, rigid, non-branching, of indeterminate length and 10–15 nm in diameter. They are insoluble in physiological solutions, relatively resistant to proteolysis, and bind Congo red dye producing pathognomonic green birefringence when viewed in polarized light. Electron microscopy reveals that each fibril consists of two or more protofilaments, the precise number varying with the fibril type. The X-ray diffraction patterns of the different *ex vivo* amyloid fibrils, and of synthetic fibrils formed *in vitro*, that have been studied demonstrate the presence of a common core structure within the filaments, in which the subunit proteins are arranged in a stack of twisted antiparallel β-pleated sheets lying with their long axes perpendicular to the fibril long axis. Recent observations show that many different proteins, including molecules totally unrelated to amyloidosis *in vivo*, can be refolded after denaturation *in vitro* to form typical, stable, Congophilic cross β fibrils. Although it is not clear why only the 20 or so known amyloidogenic proteins adopt the amyloid fold and persist as fibrils *in vivo*, a major unifying theme that is currently emerging is that in all cases studied the precursors are relatively destabilized. Even under physiological or other conditions they may encounter *in vivo*, they populate partly unfolded states, involving loss of tertiary or higher order structure that readily aggregate with retention of β-sheet secondary structure into protofilaments and fibrils. Once the process has started, seeding may also play an important facilitating role, so that amyloid deposition may progress exponentially as expansion of the amyloid template 'captures' further precursor molecules.

Glycosaminoglycans

Amyloidotic organs contain more glycosaminoglycans than normal tissues, some of which is a tightly bound, integral part of the amyloid fibrils. These fibril-associated glycosaminoglycans are heparan sulfate and dermatan sulfate in all forms of amyloid which have been investigated. Fibrils isolated by water extraction and separated from other tissue components contain 1–2 per cent by weight of glycosaminoglycan, none of which is covalently associated with the fibril protein. Interestingly, in systemic amyloid A protein (AA) and immunoglobulin light chain (AL) amyloidosis, the only forms in which this has been studied so far, there is marked restriction of the heterogeneity of the glycosaminoglycan chains, suggesting that particular subclasses of heparan and dermatan sulfates are involved. Immunohistochemical studies demonstrate the presence of proteoglycan core proteins in all amyloid deposits, and that these are closely related to fibrils at the ultrastructural level. However, in isolated fibril preparations much of the glycosaminoglycan material is free carbohydrate chains and it is not yet clear whether this represents aberrant glycosaminoglycan metabolism related to amyloidosis or is just an artefact.

The significance of glycosaminoglycans in amyloid remains unclear, but their universal presence, intimate relationship with the fibrils, and restricted heterogeneity all suggest that they may be important. Glycosaminoglycans are known to participate in the organization of some normal structural proteins into fibrils and they may have comparable fibrillogenic effects on certain amyloid fibril precursor proteins.

Serum amyloid P component

All amyloid deposits in all species contain the non-fibrillar glycoprotein amyloid P component (AP). AP is identical to and derived from the normal circulating plasma protein, SAP, a member of the pentraxin protein family which includes C-reactive protein (CRP). Human SAP is secreted only by hepatocytes and is a trace constituent of plasma present at a steady concentration of around 20–30 mg/l. Within the amyloid deposits it is by far the most abundant protein apart from the fibrils themselves.

SAP consists of five identical non-covalently associated subunits, each with a molecular mass of 25 462 Da, which are non-covalently associated in a pentameric disc-like ring. SAP is a calcium-dependent ligand binding protein, the best defined specificity of which is for the 4,6-cyclic pyruvate acetal of β-D-galactose, but it also binds avidly and specifically to DNA, chromatin, glycosaminoglycans, particularly heparan and dermatan sulfates, and all known types of amyloid fibrils. This latter interaction is responsible for the unique, specific, accumulation of SAP in amyloid deposits. In addition to being a plasma protein, SAP is also a normal constituent of certain extracellular matrix structures. It is covalently associated with collagen and/or other matrix components in the *lamina rara interna* of the human glomerular basement membrane and is present on the microfibrillar mantle of elastin fibres throughout the body.

The SAP molecule is highly resistant to proteolysis and, although not itself a proteinase inhibitor, its binding to amyloid fibrils *in vitro* protects them against proteolysis. Once bound to amyloid fibrils *in vivo*, SAP persists for very prolonged periods and is not catabolized at all, in contrast to its rapid clearance from the plasma, half life 24 h, and prompt catabolism in the liver. These observations suggest that SAP may contribute to persistence of amyloid deposits *in vivo* and indeed SAP knockout mice show retarded and reduced induction of experimental AA amyloidosis, confirming that SAP is significantly involved in pathogenesis of amyloidosis.

Other proteins in amyloid

A number of plasma proteins, other than the fibril proteins themselves and SAP, have been detected immunohistochemically in some amyloid deposits. These include α_1-antichymotrypsin, some complement components, apolipoprotein E, and various extracellular matrix or basement membrane proteins. None of these match the universality, quantitative or selective importance of SAP, and their role, if any, in pathogenesis of amyloid deposition or its effects is not known.

Mechanisms by which amyloid cause disease

The mechanisms by which amyloid deposits damage tissues and compromise organ function are poorly understood. Massive deposits, which may amount to kilograms, are structurally disruptive and incompatible with normal function, as are strategically located small deposits, for example, in the glomeruli or nerves. However, the relationship between quantity of amyloid and organ dysfunction differs greatly between individuals, and there is a strong impression that the rate of new amyloid deposition is at least as important a determinant of progressive organ failure as the amyloid load itself. *In vitro* studies have suggested that isolated amyloid fibrils, and in particular newly formed fibrils, are toxic and may induce death of cultured cells both by necrosis and apoptosis.

Major unanswered questions concern the tissue distribution and time of appearance of amyloid deposits as well as their variable clinical consequences. Although many features among the various forms of amyloidosis overlap, the clinical phenotype associated with a particular fibril type can also be enormously variable, even between families with identical amyloidogenic mutations, and even within single kindreds. There are clearly major genetic and environmental influences on *in vivo* amyloidogenesis, other than simply the presence of an amyloidogenic variant protein, but there are few clues to the nature of these factors.

Acquired systemic amyloidosis

Acquired systemic amyloidosis is the cause of death in more than 1 in 1500 patients in the United Kingdom, and is probably much underdiagnosed among the elderly population, which is at greatest risk of its development. Systemic AL amyloidosis is the most serious and commonly diagnosed form, and presently outnumbers referrals of AA amyloidosis to the UK National Amyloidosis Centre by a factor of about 7:1. Although less serious, dialysis related β_2-M amyloidosis affects about one million patients receiving long-term renal replacement therapy world-wide, and causes much suffering. Senile systemic amyloidosis, which predominantly involves the heart, occurs in about one-quarter of individuals over the age of 80 years, a sector of the population that is ever rising.

Reactive systemic amyloidosis, AA amyloidosis

AA amyloidosis is a complication of chronic infections and inflammatory diseases, and indeed any condition that stimulates overproduction of the acute phase protein, SAA. The amyloid fibrils are composed of AA protein, an *N*-terminal fragment of SAA, and AA amyloidosis occurs in about 1–5 per cent of patients with rheumatoid arthritis, juvenile idiopathic arthritis, and Crohn's disease. Most patients present with nephropathy, and although liver and gastrointestinal involvement may occur at a late stage, the heart and nerves are very rarely affected.

AA fibril protein

The AA protein is a single non-glycosylated polypeptide chain usually of mass 8000 Da and containing 76 residues corresponding to the *N*-terminal portion of the 104 residue SAA protein. Smaller and larger AA fragments, even whole molecules, have also been reported in AA fibrils. SAA is an apolipoprotein of high density lipoprotein particles and is the polymorphic product of a set of genes located on the short arm of chromosome 11. SAA is highly conserved in evolution and is a major acute phase reactant. Most of the SAA in plasma is produced by hepatocytes in which the synthesis is under transcriptional regulation by cytokines, especially interleukin (IL)-1, IL-6, and tumour necrosis factor. After secretion SAA rapidly associates with high density lipoproteins from which it displaces apolipoprotein AI. The circulating concentration can rise from normal levels of upto 3 mg/l to over 1500 mg/l within 24–48 h of an acute stimulus, and with ongoing chronic inflammation can remain persistently high.

Amyloid AA protein is derived from circulating SAA by proteolytic cleavage, which can be produced by macrophages and by a variety of proteinases. However, it is not known whether in the process of AA fibrillogenesis, cleavage of SAA occurs before and/or after aggregation of monomers. Persistent overproduction of SAA causing sustained high circulating levels is a necessary condition for deposition of AA amyloid but it is not known why only some individuals in this state get amyloid. In mice, only one of the three major isoforms of murine SAA, is the precursor of AA in amyloid fibrils.

more extensive deposits in the heart, affecting ventricles and atria and situated in the interstitium and vessel walls, cause significant impairment of cardiac function and may be fatal. The TTR involved is probably usually of the normal wild-type but cases with TTR variants have been described, which may be hereditary clinical cardiac amyloidosis associated with wild-type TTR is extremely rare before 65 years of age.

Hereditary systemic amyloidosis

Hereditary systemic amyloidosis is caused by deposition of genetically variant proteins as amyloid fibrils, and is associated with mutations in the genes for TTR, cystatin C, gelsolin, apolipoprotein AI, apolipoprotein AII, lysozyme, and fibrinogen A α-chain. These diseases are all inherited in an autosomal dominant pattern with variable penetrance, and present clinically at various times from the teens to old age, though usually in adult life. By far the commonest hereditary amyloidosis is caused by TTR variants and usually presents as familial amyloid polyneuropathy with peripheral and autonomic neuropathy. Cystatin C amyloidosis presents as cerebral amyloid angiopathy with recurrent cerebral haemorrhage and clinically silent systemic deposits, and has been reported only in Icelandic families. Gelsolin amyloidosis presents with cranial neuropathy but is also extremely rare. Apolipoprotein AI, lysozyme and fibrinogen α-chain amyloidosis present as non-neuropathic systemic amyloidosis that can affect any or all the major viscera, with renal involvement usually being prominent. These latter conditions are readily misdiagnosed as acquired AL amyloidosis, and are less rare than previously thought.

Familial amyloidotic polyneuropathy

Familial amyloidotic polyneuropathy (FAP) is caused by point mutations in the gene for the plasma protein TTR and is an autosomal dominant syndrome with peak onset between the third and sixth decades (Benson and Uemichi 1996). The disease is characterized by progressive and disabling peripheral and autonomic neuropathy and varying degrees of visceral amyloid involvement. Severe cardiac amyloidosis is common. Deposits within the vitreous of the eye are well recognized but renal, thyroid, spleen, and adrenals deposits are usually asymptomatic. There are well-recognized foci in Portugal, Japan, and Sweden, and FAP has been reported in most ethnic groups throughout the world. There is considerable phenotypic variation in the age of onset, rate of progression, involvement of different systems and disease penetrance generally, although within families the pattern is often quite consistent. More than 80 variant forms of TTR are associated with FAP, the most frequent of which is the substitution of methionine for valine at residue 30.

Familial amyloid polyneuropathy with predominant cranial neuropathy

Originally described in Finland but now reported in other ethnic groups, this is a very rare autosomal dominant form of hereditary amyloidosis that presents in adult life with cranial neuropathy, lattice corneal dystrophy, and a mild distal peripheral neuropathy. There may be skin, renal, and cardiac manifestations but these are usually covert and life expectancy approaches normal. The mutant gene responsible encodes a variant form of gelsolin, which is an actin-modulating protein. The functional role of circulating gelsolin is unknown but may be related to clearance of actin filaments released by apoptotic cells. There is no specific treatment for this disorder, which is progressively disfiguring and very distressing its late stages.

Hereditary non-neuropathic systemic amyloidosis

Ostertag (1932) first described the syndrome of hereditary systemic amyloidosis in a German family. He reported two families with autosomal dominantly inherited renal amyloidosis without neuropathy. This disorder is now known to be caused by mutations in the genes for lysozyme, apolipoprotein AI, and fibrinogen A α-chain (Benson et al. 1993). A single family with this phenotype has also been reported with a stop-codon mutation in the gene for apolipoprotein A11 that results in a 21-residue extension at the *C*-terminus of the protein.

Lysozyme amyloidosis

Hereditary non-neuropathic systemic amyloidosis has been described in association with three lysozyme variants (Booth et al. 1997), the substitution of hisidine for aspartic acid at position 67, threonine for isoleucine at position 56, and arginine for tryptophan at position 64. Most patients present in middle age with proteinuria, very slowly progressive renal impairment and sometimes hepatosplenomegaly with or without purpuric rashes. Virtually all patients have substantial gastrointestinal amyloid deposits, and although these are often asymptomatic, they are important since gastrointestinal haemorrhage or perforation is a frequent cause of death.

Apolipoprotein AI amyloidosis

Apolipoprotein AI is a major constituent of high density lipoprotein. Eleven amyloidogenic variants are known, eight of which are single amino acid substitutions, two are deletions, and one a deletion/insertion. Depending on the mutation patients can present with massive abdominal visceral amyloid involvement, predominant cardiomyopathy, or an FAP-like syndrome. Several of the variants in the *C*-terminal region are also associated with hoarseness due to laryngeal amyloid deposits. The majority of patients eventually develop renal failure but despite extensive hepatic amyloid deposition liver function usually remains well preserved. Normal wild-type apolipoprotein AI amyloid is itself weakly amyloidogenic, and is the precursor of small amyloid deposits that occur quite frequently in aortic atherosclerotic plaques.

Fibrinogen A α-chain amyloidosis

Fibrinogen A α-chain was first isolated from amyloid fibrils in 1993. Four amyloidogenic mutations have been described in eight unrelated kindreds. These include two frame shifting deletion mutations, and a leucine for arginine substitution at codon 554. However, much the commonest mutation results in the substitution of valine for glutamic acid at position 526 (Uemichi et al. 1994). We have lately shown that this mutation is unexpectedly frequent in the northern European population, and that, overall, it has quite low penetrance. Indeed, most patients with this form of hereditary amyloidosis do not give a family history of similar disease. Five per cent of patients referred to the UK National amyloidosis Centre with a diagnosis of acquired AL amyloidosis have been shown on further investigation to have hereditary fibrinogen A α-chain valine 526 amyloidosis. Most patients present in middle age with proteinuria or hypertension and over the following 4–10 years progress to end-stage renal failure. Amyloid deposition is seen in the kidneys, spleen, and sometimes the liver but is usually asymptomatic in the latter two sites. The majority of patients have an excellent outcome on dialysis and the limited experience with renal transplantation is extremely encouraging.

Diagnosis of amyloidosis

The diagnosis of amyloidosis usually requires histological confirmation (Hawkins 1994). The pathognomonic tinctorial property of amyloidotic tissue is apple green/red birefringence when stained with Congo red dye and viewed under intense cross-polarized light. Immunohistochemical staining of amyloid containing tissue sections is the most accessible method for characterizing the amyloid fibril protein type (Plate 165). However, histology cannot provide information about the overall whole body load or distribution of amyloid deposits, nor does it permit monitoring of the natural history of amyloidosis or its response to treatment. In order to overcome these problems we developed radiolabelled human SAP as a specific, non-invasive, quantitative *in vivo* tracer for amyloid deposits, and have used it as a routine tool in our clinical practice for 10 years (Hawkins et al. 1988, 1990a). We have performed over 3000 studies, and scintigraphy and metabolic turnover studies with labelled SAP have contributed greatly to knowledge of amyloidosis and, especially its diagnosis, monitoring and response to treatment.

Histochemical diagnosis of amyloid

Biopsy

The diagnosis of amyloid is usually made following a biopsy of the kidneys, liver, heart, bowel, peripheral nerve, lymph node, skin, thyroid, or bone marrow. When amyloidosis is suspected clinically, biopsy of subcutaneous fat or rectum is the less invasive. Amyloid is present in these sites in 50–80 per cent of cases of systemic AA or AL. Alternatively, a clinically affected tissue may be biopsied directly, which has a higher yield but a greater risk of haemorrhage and other complications.

Congo red and other histochemical stains

Many cotton dyes, fluorochromes, and metachromatic stains have been used, but Congo red staining, and its resultant green birefringence when viewed with high intensity polarized light, is the pathognomonic histochemical test for amyloidosis. The stain is unstable and must be freshly prepared every 2 months or less. Thick sections of 5–10 μm and inclusion in every staining run of a positive control tissue containing modest amounts of amyloid are critical.

Immunohistochemistry

Although many amyloid fibril proteins can be identified immunohistochemically, the demonstration of amyloidogenic proteins in tissues does not, on its own, establish the presence or type of amyloid. Congo red staining and green birefringence are always required and immunostaining may then enable the amyloid fibril protein to be classified. Antibodies to SAA are commercially available and virtually always stain AA deposits, as is the case with antibodies to β_2-M in haemodialysis-associated amyloid. In AL amyloid the deposits are stainable with antibodies to κ or λ immunoglobulin light chains in only about half of all cases, probably because the light-chain fragment in the fibrils is chiefly the *N*-terminal variable domain, which is unique for each monoclonal protein. Immunohistochemical staining of TTR, and other hereditary amyloid fibril proteins may require pre-treatment of sections with formic acid, alkaline guanidine, or deglycosylation, and, even then, may not give definitive results in some cases.

Electron microscopy

Amyloid fibrils cannot always be convincingly identified ultrastructurally, and a diagnosis of amyloidosis made through electron microscopy alone should be regarded with caution since other fibrillar deposition diseases occur.

Problems of histological diagnosis

The tissue sample must be adequate (e.g. the inclusion of submucosal vessels in a rectal biopsy specimen), and failure to find amyloid does not exclude the diagnosis. The unavoidable sampling problem means that biopsy cannot reveal the extent or distribution of amyloid. Experience with Congo red staining is required if clinically important false-negative and false-positive results are to be avoided. Immunohistochemical staining requires positive and negative controls, including demonstration of specificity of staining by absorption of positive antisera with isolated pure antigens.

Non-histological investigations

Two-dimensional echocardiography showing small, concentrically hypertrophied ventricles, generally impaired contraction, dilated atria, homogeneously echogenic valves, and 'sparkling' echodensity of ventricular walls is virtually diagnostic of cardiac amyloidosis (Fig. 1). However, clinically significant restrictive diastolic impairment may be difficult to detect even by comprehensive Doppler and other functional studies. Imaging after injection of isotope-labelled calcium-seeking tracers has poor sensitivity and specificity and is of no routine clinical value.

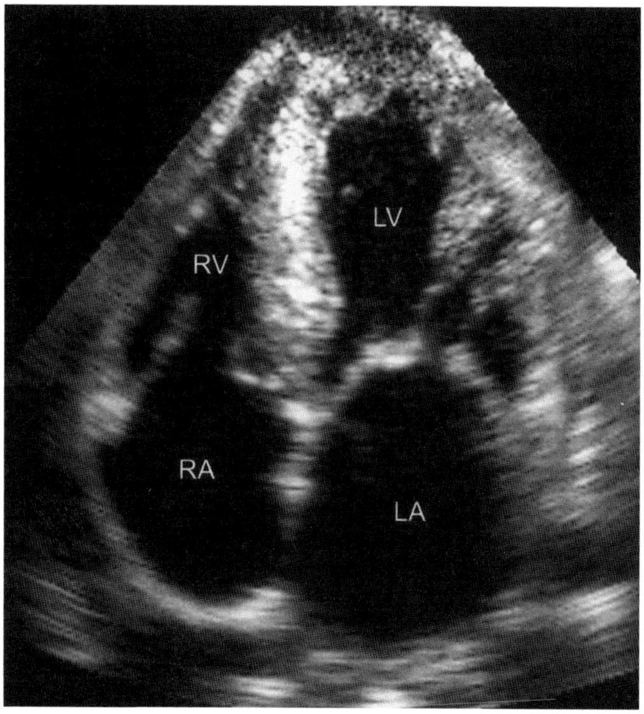

Fig. 1 Echocardiographic four chamber view in a patient with cardiac AL amyloidosis showing concentric thickening of the ventricular walls, dilated atria and thickened valves. Doppler flow studies demonstrated restrictive physiology, but systolic function was relatively well preserved.

In cases of known or suspected hereditary amyloidosis the gene defect must be characterized. If amyloidotic tissue is available the fibril protein may be known and the corresponding gene can then be studied, but if no tissue containing amyloid is available, screening of the genes for known amyloidogenic proteins must be undertaken.

Biochemical and immunochemical screening tests for the presence in the plasma of amyloidogenic variant protein products of mutant genes also exist, but molecular genetic analysis of DNA is the most direct approach. However, it remains essential to corroborate DNA findings by confirming one way or another that the respective protein is indeed the main constituent of the amyloid.

Radiolabelled serum amyloid P component scintigraphy and natural history of amyloid

The universal presence in amyloid deposits of AP, derived from circulating SAP, is the basis for use of radioisotope-labelled SAP as a diagnostic tracer in amyloidosis (Hawkins et al. 1988, 1990a). No localization or retention of labelled SAP occurs in healthy subjects or in patients with diseases other than amyloidosis. Radio-iodinated SAP has a short half life (24 h) in the plasma and is rapidly catabolized with complete excretion of the iodinated breakdown products in the urine. However, in patients with systemic or localized extracerebral amyloidosis, the tracer rapidly and specifically localizes to the deposits, in proportion to the quantity of amyloid present, and persists there without breakdown or modification (Fig. 2). For clinical purposes, highly purified SAP is isolated from the plasma of single accredited donors and is oxidatively iodinated with the pure gamma emitter ^{123}Iodine. The dose of radioactivity administered (<4 mSv) is well within accepted safety limits. In addition to the images, the uptake of tracer into various organs can be precisely and repeatedly quantified (Hawkins et al. 1990b, 1993a).

Important observations regarding amyloid, which have been made for the first time *in vivo*, include the following: the different distribution of amyloid

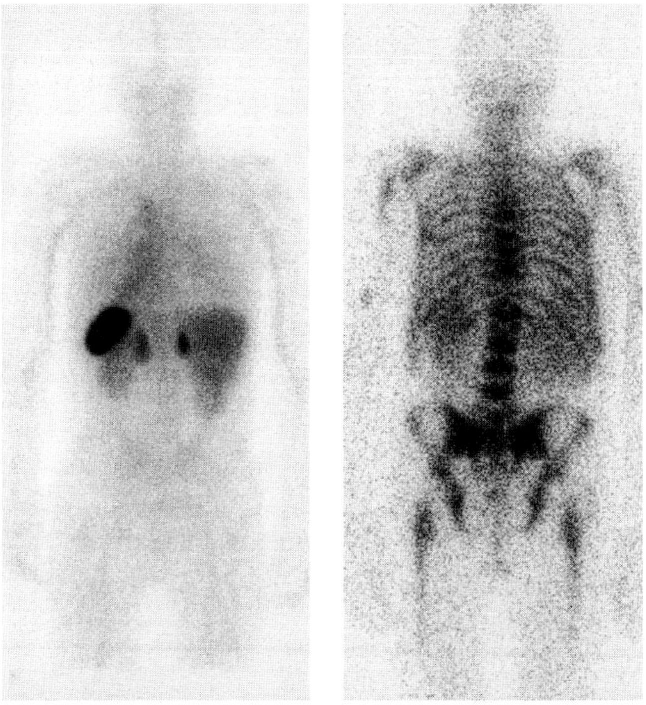

Fig. 2 Posterior whole body ^{123}I-serum amyloid P component scintigraphy demonstrating systemic amyloid deposits in the spleen, adrenal glands, and kidneys of a patient with AA amyloidosis (left), and throughout the bones of a patient with AL amyloidosis (right). Major uptake of I^{123}-SAP into bones only occurs in amyloidosis of AL type.

in different forms of the disease; amyloid in anatomic sites not available for biopsy (adrenals, spleen); major systemic deposits in forms of amyloid previously thought to be organ-limited; a poor correlation between the quantity of amyloid present in a given organ and the level of organ dysfunction; a non-homogeneous distribution of amyloid within individual organs; and evidence for rapid progression and regression of amyloid deposits with different rates in different organs. The impression that amyloid deposition is irreversible and inexorably progressive is misleading, and largely reflects the persistent nature of the acquired or hereditary conditions that underlie it. Many case reports have described improvement in organ function, suggesting regression of amyloid, when underlying conditions have been controlled, and serial SAP scintigraphy has systematically shown regression of amyloid under these circumstances. This has been observed when supply of amyloid fibril precursor proteins has been reduced in AA amyloidosis by vigorous control of rheumatic inflammation (Hawkins et al. 1993b), in AL amyloidosis with clonal suppression by cytotoxic drugs (Gillmore et al. 1999b), in haemodialysis associated amyloidosis after renal transplantation (Tan et al. 1996), and in hereditary TTR (Rydh et al. 1998) and fibrinogen A α-chain amyloidosis following liver transplantation (Gillmore et al. 2000). It is now clear that amyloid deposits exist generally in a state of dynamic turnover, with encouraging implications for patient management.

Labelled SAP studies thus make a valuable contribution to the diagnosis and management of patients with systemic amyloidosis, and are now performed routinely at the National Health Service National Amyloidosis Centre at the Royal Free Hospital, London.

Management of systemic amyloidosis

Although no treatments yet exist that specifically promote the mobilization of amyloid, there have been substantial recent advances in management of systemic amyloidosis, in particular active measures to support failing organ function whilst attempts are made to reduce the supply of the amyloid fibril precursor protein. Control of the primary disease process, or removal of the source of the amyloidogenic precursor, frequently results in regression of existing deposits and recovery or preservation of organ function (Table 3). This strongly supports aggressive intervention, and relatively toxic drug regimes or other radical approaches are justified by the poor prognosis. However, clinical improvement in amyloidosis is often delayed long after the underlying disorder has remitted, reflecting very gradual regression of the deposits and slow recovery of organ function. Continuing production of the amyloid precursor protein should be monitored as closely as possible long-term, to determine the requirement for and intensity of treatment for the underlying primary condition. In AA amyloidosis this involves frequent estimation of the plasma SAA level, and in AL amyloidosis requires monitoring of monoclonal plasma cell proliferation and immunoglobulin light chain production.

AA amyloidosis

The treatment of AA amyloidosis ranges from potent anti-inflammatory and immunosuppressive drugs in patients with rheumatoid arthritis, to life-long prophylactic colchicine in familial Mediterranean fever, and surgery in conditions such as refractory osteomyelitis and Castleman's disease tumours. The outcome in AA amyloidosis is chiefly determined by the extent to which the underlying acute phase response can be suppressed in the long-term, by whatever means may be appropriate for the respective inflammatory disease.

In a long-term study performed in our centre (Gillmore et al. 2001), amyloidotic organ function and survival were studied prospectively for 12–117 months in 80 patients with systemic AA amyloidosis in whom serum SAA concentration was measured monthly, and the visceral amyloid deposits were evaluated annually by SAP scintigraphy. The causative underlying inflammatory diseases were treated as vigorously as possible. Amyloid deposits regressed in 25 out of 42 patients whose median SAA values were sustained within the reference range (<10 mg/l), and amyloidotic organ function stabilized or improved in 39 of these cases (Fig. 3). Outcome varied substantially between patients whose median SAA concentration exceeded 10 mg/l, but amyloid load increased and organ function deteriorated in most patients whose SAA remained above 50 mg/l. The survival at 10 years estimated by Kaplan–Meier analysis was 90 per cent in patients whose median SAA was under 10 mg/L, and 40 per cent among those whose median SAA exceeded this value ($p < 0.0009$).

Cytotoxic alkylating drugs are frequently used to treat patients with AA amyloidosis secondary to rheumatic disease (Berglund et al. 1993; Gillmore et al. 2001). Many patients have been treated with oral chlorambucil but cyclophosphamide, azathioprine, and other disease modifying therapies have also been used with some success. Chlorambucil has been prescribed for over 30 years to children with juvenile rheumatoid arthritis complicated by AA amyloidosis, and has dramatically improved the prognosis (Schnitzer and Ansell 1977). More than 90 per cent of patients managed in this way are alive 10 years after the diagnosis of amyloidosis, and renal function can be preserved in a substantial proportion of cases (David 1991). More than half of adult patients with AA amyloidosis complicating inflammatory arthritis also respond extremely well to chlorambucil treatment. The protocol for treatment with oral chlorambucil used in our centre comprises a starting dose of 2 mg daily, increased by 2 mg increments every 6–8 weeks, upto a dose of 6–8 mg daily, until plasma SAA concentration has fallen substantially or borderline total leucopaenia occurs. A response may take upto 6 months, and slow progressive reduction in dose is advised after one year in patients who have responded. Chlorambucil is not licensed for this indication in the United Kingdom, causes permanent infertility in males, and premature menopause in women. It is potentially teratogenic and carcinogenic, although these risk are relatively small even following long-term treatment.

Many patients with AA amyloidosis now have a prolonged life expectancy, and although the amyloid deposits frequently regress following successful

Table 3 Principles of treatment in systemic amyloidosis

Disease	Objective of treatment	Example of treatment
AA amyloidosis	Suppress acute phase response, thereby reducing SAA production	Immunosuppression in rheumatoid arthritis, colchicine in familial Mediterranean fever
AL amyloidosis	Suppress production of monoclonal light chains	Chemotherapy for myeloma and monoclonal gammopathy
Hereditary amyloidosis	Reduce/eliminate production of genetically variant amyloidogenic protein	Orthotopic liver transplantation for variant transthyretin associated FAP, and selected cases of fibrinogen A α-chain amyloidosis

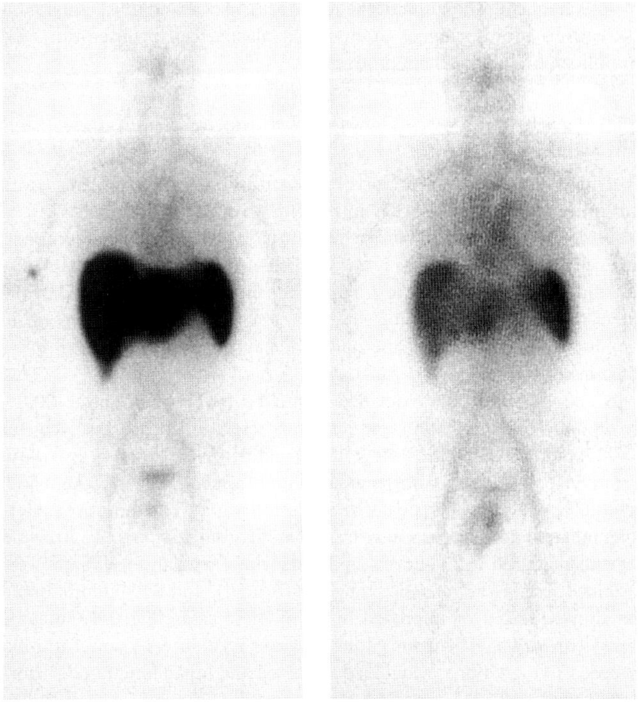

Fig. 3 Serial anterior ^{123}I-serum amyloid P component scintigraphy demonstrating regression of hepatic and splenic AA amyloid deposits in a patient with rheumatoid arthritis, which remitted completely following treatment with oral chlorambucil. The scan on the left was obtained at presentation and the follow-up scan on the right was performed 2 years later.

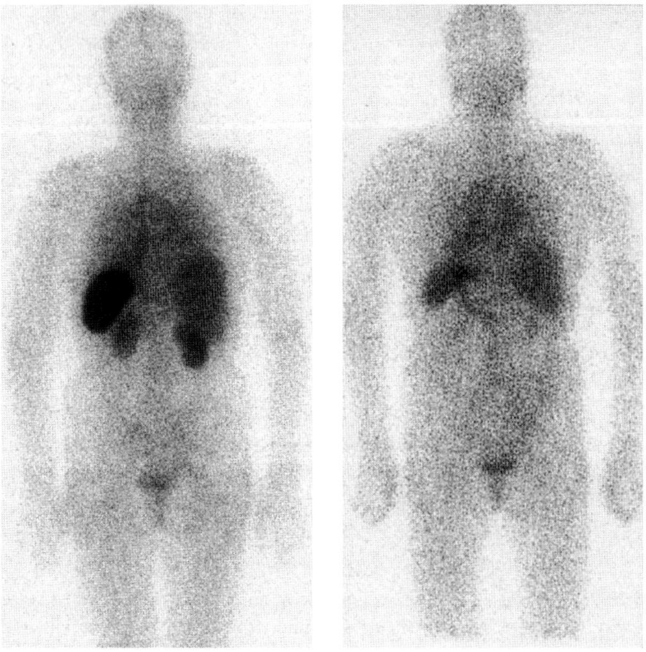

Fig. 4 Serial posterior ^{123}I-serum amyloid P component scintigraphy demonstrating regression of splenic and renal AL amyloid deposits in a patient whose low grade monoclonal gammopathy was suppressed by high dose melphalan and stem cell rescue. The scan on the left was obtained at presentation in 1998 and the follow-up scan on the right was performed 3 years later.

treatment, follow-up SAP scintigraphy has shown that substantial deposits remain present in some such patients for decades, long after the function of amyloidotic organs has recovered. It is important to recognize that such patients remain at increased risk of acute renal failure under intercurrent stresses including dehydration, surgery, or pregnancy. They also may re-accumulate damaging quantities of amyloid extremely rapidly should they develop a further acute phase response, probably because their amyloid deposits serve as template for ongoing amyloid deposition as soon as a supply of SAA is available in the plasma.

AL amyloidosis

Treatment of AL amyloidosis is based on that for myeloma, although the plasma cell dyscrasias in AL are often very subtle. The aim of treatment is to suppress the underlying clonal B-cell dyscrasia and, therefore, production of the AL amyloid fibril precursor protein. There are, however, many challenges. Many patients have very advanced multi-system disease at diagnosis which limits therapeutic options and may be accompanied by a prognosis that is too short for treatment to produce benefit. Amyloid regression does occur (Fig. 4), but clinical or functional improvement may be delayed for months or even years after suppression of the monoclonal light chain production. Unfortunately, regression of cardiac amyloid seems to be particularly slow, and evaluating a response of the underlying disease to treatment is often hampered by the very subtle nature of monoclonal gammopathies in AL amyloidosis.

However, many patients with AL amyloidosis do benefit from chemotherapy. Prolonged low intensity cytotoxic regimes such as oral melphalan and prednisolone are effective in about 20 per cent of patients (Kyle et al. 1997). Dose intensive infusional chemotherapy regimes such as vincristine, doxorubicin (Adriamycin) and dexamethasone ('VAD'), and autologous peripheral blood stem-cell transplantation are presently being evaluated with very promising early results (Comenzo et al. 1998). Rigorous selection of patients for stem cell transplantation is essential as treatment related mortality is high in individuals with multiple amyloidotic organ involvement. Patients with autonomic neuropathy, severe cardiac amyloidosis, a large whole body amyloid load at SAP scintigraphy or a history of gastrointestinal bleeding, and over 55 years are also at increased risk.

β_2-Microglobulin amyloidosis

The disabling arthralgia of β_2-M amyloidosis may respond partially to non-steroidal anti-inflammatory drugs or corticosteroids, but the only really effective treatment for this condition is renal transplantation (Drüeke 1998). Serum levels of β_2-M fall rapidly following transplantation and this is usually accompanied by a very rapid and substantial improvement in symptoms. Although prospective SAP scintigraphy has shown that β_2-M amyloid deposits can gradually regress, the resolution of symptoms within days or weeks of renal transplantation implicates other factors. These may include the anti-inflammatory properties of immunosuppression after transplantation, and some effect of discontinuation of the dialysis procedure itself. In contrast to the symptoms, radiological bone cysts heal very slowly indeed, and unsurprisingly amyloid can be demonstrated histologically many years after renal transplantation. Within a few years of renal transplantation, arthralgic symptoms may reappear very rapidly if the graft is lost, providing further evidence that dialysis is required for the clinical expression of disease associated with β_2-M amyloid deposits. Possible explanations of this phenomenon are that newly deposited β_2-M amyloid is more damaging than old, or that the cytokine modulating effects of dialysis are involved. Certainly, β_2-M amyloid deposits are unusual in that they are often associated with a degree of inflammation and macrophage infiltration.

The risks of developing symptomatic β_2-M amyloidosis may be increased in patients dialyzed using less 'biocompatible' cuprophane membranes, and the use of more permeable membrane systems that remove β_2-M more efficiently may be relatively protective (Miyata et al. 1998).

Drug treatment of established disease includes non-steroidal anti-inflammatory analgesics, systemic, and intra-articular corticosteroid therapy, but none of these is especially effective and long-term steroid therapy is particularly undesirable in this population of patients. Surgery may be required to relieve carpal tunnel compression, stabilize the cervical spine or to treat bone fractures.

Hereditary amyloidosis

Hepatic transplantation is effective in familial amyloid polyneuropathy associated with TTR gene mutations since the variant amyloidogenic protein is produced mainly in the liver (Holmgren et al. 1993). Successful liver transplantation has now been reported in hundreds of patients with this condition and although the peripheral neuropathy usually only stabilizes, autonomic function can improve substantially and the associated visceral amyloid deposits have been shown to regress in most cases. Important questions remain about the timing of the procedure but, so far, early intervention seems advisable. Disappointingly in a few cases, there is evidence that wild-type TTR, an inherently but weakly amyloidogenic protein, may continue to be deposited after liver transplantation, on the existing 'template' of amyloid (Stangou et al. 1998). This may occur to a clinically important extent in the heart and in the vitreous, but seems to be mutation-specific and usually does not happen in the bulk of FAP patients who have the TTR Met30 variant.

Fibrinogen is also synthesized only in the liver and hepatic transplantation therefore has a potential role in the management of hereditary fibrinogen A α-chain amyloidosis. Successful, and most likely curative, liver transplants have been performed in a small number of these patients who have had unusually severe and early onset disease. However, renal support including renal transplantation offers most patients with hereditary fibrinogen A α-chain amyloidosis an excellent quality of life and a relatively normal life expectancy.

The most common forms of hereditary apolipoprotein AI amyloidosis present with slowly progressive renal disease, which is probably managed optimally by renal transplantation. Although this does not alter the supply of the amyloidogenic precursor protein, which is produced in the liver and small intestine, renal and other solid organ grafts are rarely damaged by 'recurrent' amyloid deposition in the medium to long-term.

Hereditary lysozyme amyloidosis usually runs an exceptionally slow course, and patients with renal failure merit strong consideration for renal transplantation (Gillmore et al. 1999a).

Supportive measures

Supportive therapy remains critical in systemic amyloidosis, with the potential for delaying target organ failure, maintaining quality of life and prolonging survival whilst the underlying process can be treated. Rigorous control of hypertension is vital in renal amyloidosis. Surgical resection of amyloidotic tissue is occasionally beneficial but, in general, a conservative approach to surgery, anaesthesia and other invasive procedures is advisable. Should any such procedure be undertaken, meticulous attention to blood pressure and fluid balance is essential. Amyloidotic tissues may heal poorly and are liable to bleed. Diuretics and vasoactive drugs should be used cautiously in cardiac amyloidosis because they can reduce cardiac output substantially. Dysrhythmias may respond to conventional pharmacological therapy or to pacing. Replacement of vital organ function, notably dialysis, may be necessary and cardiac, renal, and liver transplant procedures have a role in selected cases.

New approaches

Improved understanding of the protein folding mechanisms underlying amyloid fibrillogenesis, and recognition that relative instability of the precursor molecules is a key factor in amyloidogenesis, have identified novel therapeutic possibilities. These include investigation of small molecules, peptides, and glycosaminoglycan analogues that bind to and stabilize fibril precursors, or interfere with refolding and/or aggregation into the cross-β core structure common to amyloid fibrils. Some of these agents have already been shown to be effective in experimental murine AA amyloidosis. Our own efforts to develop specific therapy are focused on the avid binding of SAP to amyloid fibrils which significantly contributes to pathogenesis of amyloidosis (Botto et al. 1997). The removal of SAP from amyloid deposits may facilitate their clearance, and we have identified a pharmacological compound that inhibits the SAP–fibril interaction, and which is presently being evaluated in clinical trials at the Royal Free Hospital.

References

Benson, M.D. and Uemichi, T. (1996). Transthyretin amyloidosis. *Amyloid: The International Journal of Experimental and Clinical Investigation* **3**, 44–56.

Benson, M.D. et al. (1993). Hereditary renal amyloidosis associated with a mutant fibrinogen α-chain. *Nature Genetics* **3**, 252–5.

Berglund, K., Thysell, H., and Keller, C. (1993). Results, principles and pitfalls in the management of renal AA-amyloidosis; a 10–21 year follow-up of 16 patients with rheumatic disease treated with alkylating cytostatics. *Journal of Rheumatology* **20**, 2051–7.

Booth, D.R. et al. (1997). Instability, unfolding and aggregation of human lysozyme variants underlying amyloid fibrillogenesis. *Nature* **385**, 787–93.

Botto, M. et al. (1997). Amyloid deposition is delayed in mice with targeted deletion of the serum amyloid P component gene. *Nature Medicine* **3**, 855–9.

Comenzo, R.L. et al. (1998). Dose-intensive melphalan with blood stem-cell support for the treatment of AL (amyloid light-chain) amyloidosis: survival and responses in 25 patients. *Blood* **91**, 3662–70.

David, J. (1991). Amyloidosis in juvenile chronic arthritis. *Clinical and Experimental Rheumatology* **9**, 73–8.

Dobson, C.M., Ellis, R.J., and Fersht, A.R., ed. (2001). Protein misfolding and disease. In *Philosophical Transactions of the Royal Society of London B.* Vol. 356, pp. 127–227. London: The Royal Society.

Drüeke, T.B. (1998). Dialysis-related amyloidosis. *Nephrology, Dialysis, Transplantation* **13**, 58–64.

Gillmore, J.D., Hawkins, P.N., and Pepys, M.B. (1997). Amyloidosis: a review of recent diagnostic and therapeutic developments. *British Journal of Haematology* **99**, 245–56.

Gillmore, J.D. et al. (1999a). Hereditary renal amyloidosis associated with variant lysozyme in a large English family. *Nephrology, Dialysis, Transplantation* **14**, 2639–44.

Gillmore, J.D. et al. (1999b). Serum amyloid P component scintigraphy in AL amyloidosis. In *Amyloid and Amyloidosis 1998* (ed. R.A. Kyle and M.A. Gertz), pp. 148–50. Pearl River NY: Parthenon Publishing.

Gillmore, J.D. et al. (2000). Curative hepatorenal transplantation in systemic amyloidosis caused by the Glu526Val fibrinogen α-chain variant in an English family. *Quarterly Journal of Medicine* **93**, 269–75.

Gillmore, J.D. et al. (2001). Amyloid load and clinical outcome in AA amyloidosis in relation to circulating concentration of serum amyloid A protein. *Lancet* **358**, 24–9.

Hawkins, P.N. et al. (1988). Diagnostic radionuclide imaging of amyloid: biological targeting by circulating human serum amyloid P component. *Lancet* **i**, 1413–18.

Hawkins, P.N., Lavender, J.P., and Pepys, M.B. (1990a). Evaluation of systemic amyloidosis by scintigraphy with ^{123}I-labeled serum amyloid P component. *New England Journal of Medicine* **323**, 508–13.

Hawkins, P.N., Wootton, R., and Pepys, M.B. (1990b). Metabolic studies of radioiodinated serum amyloid P component in normal subjects and patients with systemic amyloidosis. *Journal of Clinical Investigation* **86**, 1862–9.

Hawkins, P.N. et al. (1993a). Scintigraphic quantification and serial monitoring of human visceral amyloid deposits provide evidence for turnover and regression. *Quarterly Journal of Medicine* **86**, 365–74.

Hawkins, P.N. et al. (1993b). Serum amyloid P component scintigraphy and turnover studies for diagnosis and quantitative monitoring of AA amyloidosis in juvenile rheumatoid arthritis. *Arthritis and Rheumatism* **36**, 842–51.

Holmgren, G. et al. (1993). Clinical improvement and amyloid regression after liver transplantation in hereditary transthyretin amyloidosis. *Lancet* **341**, 1113–16.

Kyle, R.A. and Greipp, P.R. (1983). Amyloidosis (AL): clinical and laboratory features in 229 cases. *Mayo Clinic Proceedings* **58**, 665–83.

Kyle, R.A. and Gertz, M.A. (1995). Primary systemic amyloidosis: clinical and laboratory features in 474 cases. *Seminars in Hematology* **32**, 45–59.

Kyle, R.A. et al. (1997). A trial of three regimens for primary amyloidosis: colchicine alone, melphalan and prednisone, and melphalan, prednisone, and colchicine. *New England Journal of Medicine* **336**, 1202–7.

Miyata, T. et al. (1998). Beta-2 microglobulin in renal disease. *Journal of the American Society of Nephrology* **9**, 1723–35.

Ostertag, B. (1932). Demonstration einer eigenartigen familiaren 'Paramyloidose'. *Zentralblatt fur allgemeine Pathologie und Pathologische Anatomie* **56**, 253–4.

Pepys, M.B. et al. (1997). Amyloid P component. A critical review. *Amyloid: The International Journal of Experimental and Clinical Investigation* **4**, 274–95.

Rydh, A. et al. (1998). Serum amyloid P component scintigraphy in familial amyloid polyneuropathy: regression of visceral amyloid following liver transplantation. *European Journal of Nuclear Medicine* **25**, 709–13.

Schnitzer, T.J. and Ansell, B.M. (1977). Amyloidosis in juvenile chronic polyarthritis. *Arthritis and Rheumatism* **20**, 245–52.

Solomon, A., Weiss, D.T., and Pepys, M.B. (1992). Induction in mice of human light chain-associated amyloidosis. *American Journal of Pathology* **140**, 629–37.

Stangou, A.J. et al. (1998). Progressive cardiac amyloidosis following liver transplantation for familial amyloid polyneuropathy: implications for amyloid fibrillogenesis. *Transplantation* **66**, 229–33.

Sunde, M. et al. (1997). Common core structure of amyloid fibrils by synchrotron X-ray diffraction. *Journal of Molecular Biology* **273**, 729–39.

Tan, S.Y. et al. (1996). Long term effect of renal transplantation on dialysis-related amyloid deposits and symptomatology. *Kidney International* **50**, 282–9.

Uemichi, T., Liepnieks, J.J., and Benson, M.D. (1994). Hereditary renal amyloidosis with a novel variant fibrinogen. *Journal of Clinical Investigation* **93**, 731–6.

Wetzel, R. (1997). Domain stability in immunoglobulin light chain deposition disorders. *Advances in Protein Chemistry* **50**, 183–242.

6.12.2 Familial Mediterranean fever

Avi Livneh, Mordechai Pras, and Pnina Langevitz

History

A genetic disease with a gene frequency as high as that of familial Mediterranean fever (FMF) in Sephardi Jews must have existed for hundreds or thousands of years. Nevertheless, in the first half of the twentieth century only a few isolated characteristic cases could be traced in medical publications (Janeway and Mosenthal 1908; Alt and Barker 1930). The reason why a disease with such dramatic manifestations has only recently been recognized may be connected to the exposure of the affected population to advanced medical facilities and research, partly due to migrations.

Siegal (1945) was the first to describe the abdominal attacks as a separate disease entity. Later, many typical cases were included in the heterogeneous case collection, termed 'periodic disease' by Reimann (1949). French physicians described many typical cases of FMF in Jewish patients deriving from North Africa (Mamou and Cattan 1952; Benhamou et al. 1954). They were the first to perceive the familial nature and the fatal renal lesion of the disease.

Tel Hashomer Hospital served in the early 1950s as a referral centre for the new immigrants to Israel. Cases that appeared on the wards with recurrent, short-lived episodes of fever, accompanied by peritoneal, pleural, or arthritic inflammation, caught the attention of the group led by Prof. Harry Heller, who defined the clinical features of the disease and its diagnostic criteria, established its genetic nature, mode of transmission, and ethnic distribution, emphasized the role of amyloidosis, and coined the name 'familial Mediterranean fever' (Heller et al. 1958, 1961; Sohar et al. 1961, 1967).

Diagnosis

At present, a specific diagnostic laboratory test for FMF is still missing and the diagnosis is based on clinical manifestations, taking into account the specific features of the attacks, ethnicity, inheritance, development of nephropathic AA amyloidosis, and response to colchicine. Attempts at formulating these factors into more rigid rules resulted in several sets of diagnostic criteria (Livneh et al. 1997; Pras 1998). Table 1 demonstrates the most commonly applied one.

Table 1 Criteria for diagnosis of familial Mediterranean fever[a] (Livneh et al. 1997)

Major criteria
I Typical[b] attacks presenting by at least one of the following:
1. Peritonitis (generalized)
2. Pleuritis (unilateral) or pericarditis
3. Monoarthritis (hip, knee, ankle)
4. Fever alone
II Incomplete[c] abdominal attacks
Minor criteria
1. Incomplete chest attacks
2. Incomplete joint attack
3. Exertional leg pain
4. Favourable response to colchicine

[a] Diagnosis requires ≥1 major or ≥2 minor.

[b] Typical attacks are recurrent (at least three times in the same site), febrile (>38°C rectal), and short (12 h to 3 days).

[c] Incomplete attacks are recurrent but differ from typical attacks by one or two features of the following: (i) temperatures lower than 38°C; (ii) shorter or longer than typical attacks (no less than 6 h or more than a week); (iii) peritoneal irritation is not detected during the abdominal attacks; (iv) the abdominal attack is limited to one area; (v) the arthritis involves joints other than those specified.

Table 2 Episodic febrile illnesses simulating familial Mediterranean fever

1. Hyper IgD syndrome (HIDS)
2. Familial Hibernian fever (FHF)/TNF receptor-associated periodic syndromes (TRAPS)
3. Muckle Well's syndrome/familial cold-induced urticaria
4. Behçet's disease
5. Pelvic inflammatory disease (PID)
6. Inflammatory bowel disease (IBD)
7. Juvenile chronic arthritis (JCA)
8. Syndrome of periodic fever, aphthous stomatitis, pharyngitis, and adenitis (PFAPA)
9. Cyclic neutropaenia
10. Relapsing fever
11. Lymphoma
12. Factitious fever

In most instances, the diagnosis is straightforward. In some patients, however, fulfilment of diagnostic criteria may require measurement of rectal temperature, examination by physician during the acute attacks to document the presence of peritonitis, pleuritis, or arthritis, and employment of a therapeutic trial with colchicine (Livneh and Langevitz 2000). In atypical history, exclusion of another episodic febrile disease, such as those appearing in Table 2, may be required.

The genetics of familial Mediterranean fever

The disease may become manifest as early as during the first year of life, although in most cases onset is later. In two-thirds of our patients, the first manifestations appeared during the first decade of life; by the end of the second decade 90 per cent are affected. Only rarely is the onset delayed beyond the age of 40 (Tamir et al. 1999). Among our 6000 patients there are only about 200 Ashkenazi Jews and the disease is rare in other Jewish ethnic groups (Yemenite and Iranian). Table 3 shows the prevalence of FMF, calculated by the number of patients and the size of the total population in each ethnic sub-group (Yuval et al. 1995).

The peculiar ethnic restriction and the familial aggregation in FMF suggest a genetic aetiology. Analysis of 229 of our families led us to conclude that the disease is due to a single, recessive autosomal gene (Sohar et al. 1967). A twin study showed 100 per cent concordance, suggesting a minimal role for environmental factors in disease expression (Shohat et al. 1992).

In 1992, the FMF gene (MEFV) was located to the short arm of chromosome 16 (Pras et al. 1992), and 5 years later, the FMF gene was cloned by two independent groups of researchers (The French FMF Consortium 1997; The International FMF Consortium 1997). The gene is 10 kb long and consists of 10 exons. The protein product was called pyrin/marenostrin. It is predicted to be 781 amino acid long, but its function is yet unknown. At present, 30 disease associated mutations have been identified, mostly in exon 10. Only upto 50 per cent of our patients are homozygous or compound heterozygous to the studied mutations. The remaining patients carry either one mutation or none of the mutations, precluding the use of mutations detection as a diagnostic test. Many unaffected individuals were found to carry two mutations (phenotype III) suggesting a low penetrance of some mutation or a pre-clinical state (Kogan et al. 2001). Altogether these findings suggest an important role for additional genetic factors in the expression of the disease. Phenotype–genotype correlations revealed an association between the missense mutations, changing methionine in position 694 either to valine or to isoleucine and a more severe disease that may be complicated with amyloidosis (Livneh et al. 1999; Shinar et al. 2000). Modifier genes contributing to disease outlook started to emerge (Cazeneuve et al. 2000; Touitou et al. 2001). One surprising finding is the extremely high carrier state frequency among Jewish and Arab sub-populations in Israel, reaching 1 : 3 in Iraqi Jews, 1 : 4 in North African Jews, 1 : 7 in Ashkenazi Jews, and 1 : 10 in Arabs (Shinawi et al. 2000; Stoffman et al. 2000; Kogan et al. 2001). These findings suggest a biological benefit to carriers of MEFV mutations.

Table 3 Prevalence of familial Mediterranean fever

Ethnic Jewish origin	Total population	Number of FMF patients	Prevalence of FMF
Algeria, Morocco, Tunis	613 500	866	1:700
Libya	76 900	310	1:250
Turkey	91 100	87	1:1000
Iraq	266 300	261	1:1000
Ashkenazi	867 500	22+	1:40 000

The clinical picture

Attacks

The febrile, painful attacks that are the hallmark of the disease are characterized by marked elevation of body temperature, acute inflammation of the peritoneum, synovia or pleura, a duration of 12–48 h and complete health between attacks (Sohar et al. 1967). Repeated attacks at irregular intervals and in an unpredictable sequence are typical of the disease. During the illness, a patient will probably encounter several forms of attacks, but the recurrence of one type over many years is not uncommon.

The most frequent manifestation is the abdominal attack, experienced by 90 per cent of patients; in 68 per cent of these it is the presenting sign (Sohar et al. 1967). They are marked by the sudden onset of fever (often with chills) and pain spreading over the entire abdomen from variable points of origin. As the attack gains in intensity, guarding, rebound tenderness, board-like rigidity, distension, and absence of peristalsis appear. Multiple, small fluid levels in the small bowel on radiography combine to suggest an acute abdominal catastrophe. After 6–12 h the signs and symptoms recede, and within 24–48 h the attack is usually over, leaving the patient as well as before.

Organization of the exudate may result in fibrous adhesions, which in rare cases may give rise to mechanical ileus and ascites, and cause sterility in some affected women.

The pleural attack has been experienced by 45 per cent of our patients, and in 5 per cent it was the presenting sign (Sohar et al. 1967). It assumes the picture of an acute febrile pleuritis, resembling the peritoneal attacks in its abrupt onset, rapid resolution, and unpredictable recurrence. Breathing is painful and breath sounds are diminished on the affected side. There may be radiological evidence of a small exudate in the costophrenic angle, which is difficult to aspirate and which resolves within 48 h. No sequelae of clinical significance have been noted.

Pericarditis is a rare feature of FMF. We observed clinical attacks of pericarditis in 27 out of 4000 of our patients (Kees et al. 1997). On M-mode echocardiography, pericardial involvement was reported to be more common than in the general population (Dabestani et al. 1982). Only rarely may permanent sequelae or protracted attacks evolve (Livneh et al. 1996).

The articular attack is the second most common form of attack. It was experienced by 75 per cent of the patients in our series, and was the presenting symptom in 16 per cent. Arthritic attacks may recur for years as the only feature of the disease, before other forms appear (Sohar et al. 1967). As a rule, large joints are involved, particularly those of the lower extremities. Arthritic attacks of FMF may present in two forms: acute, or chronic and protracted. In the acute form the onset is abrupt, fever ranges from 38 to 40°C, and the affected single joint is tender, swollen, and held immobile because of the severe pain. Redness and local heat are frequently less marked than would be expected in such an acute process. The signs and symptoms usually peak in 1–2 days and then gradually subside, usually within 1–7 days, leaving no residue. The attacks can sometimes be precipitated by minor trauma or effort, such as prolonged walking. Synovial effusion is often demonstrable. The synovial fluid is sterile and varies in its appearance from cloudy to purulent, depending upon the acuteness and severity of the synovitis.

About 5 per cent of patients experience protracted attacks, which persist for more than a month. Usually the hip or knee are involved (Sohar et al. 1967; Sneh et al. 1977), but episodes in other joints, such as the ankle and rarely, the temporomandibular or the sternoclavicular, may also assume a protracted course. The involved joint remains markedly swollen and painful, presenting a picture of chronic monoarthritis or in rare cases, chronic oligoarthritis. The affected knee joint, in extreme cases, resembles a fluid bag from which upto 200 ml can be drained (Fig. 1). After several weeks or months, sometimes even after a year or more, the pain and swelling subside spontaneously. During such protracted attacks in a joint, short attacks involving other joints, the abdomen, or chest may occur (Sohar et al. 1967).

In some protracted cases, especially in the hips, damage to the joints with permanent deformity occurred. In 27 of our patients, there was residual incapacity in the affected joint (21 in the hips). Seven hips showed radiologically typical aseptic necrosis of the femoral head, and in 14, sclerosis and narrowing of the joint space was observed. Most of these hips eventually required total joint replacement (Sneh et al. 1977) (Fig. 2). A cementless hip prostheses is recommended in such patients because a relatively high percentage of aseptic loosening of the cemented hip prosthesis was noted (Salai et al. 1993). Among 160 patients with protracted arthritis we found a small group of 11 in whom the HLA-B27 was negative, who nevertheless fulfilled the criteria for seronegative spondyloarthropathy (Langevitz et al. 1997).

Pain in the lower extremities, induced by efforts such as walking or standing, is very common in FMF. It may be located in the soles, heels, ankles, shins, calf muscles, or a combination of these. The pain subsides after a night's rest, or NSAID, and usually it is not associated with swelling or signs of inflammation.

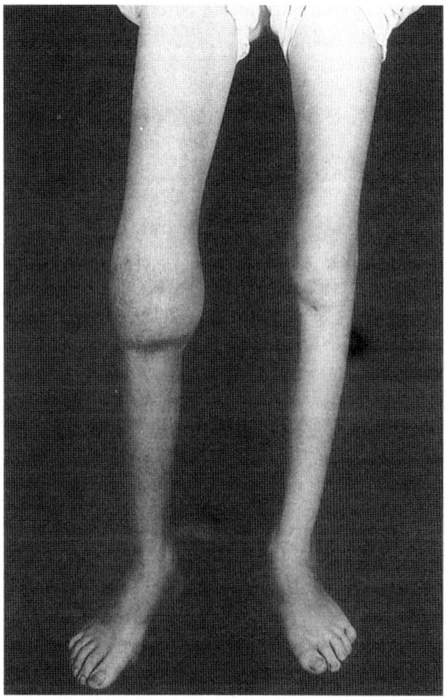

Fig. 1 Protracted arthritis of right knee, which lasted 11 months.

Short febrile attacks of muscle pain in one or several muscle groups may also occur, though uncommonly. Generalized muscle pain occurs in FMF as part of fibromyalgia, accompanying the course of the disease in 30 per cent of the patients (Langevitz et al. 1994b) and as part of non-specific constitutional symptoms of the febrile attack in any site affected by the disease (Livneh et al. 1996).

In 14 of about 3000 of our patients, a syndrome of protracted febrile myalgia developed, characterized by severe, debilitating myalgia accompanied by fever, abdominal pain, a high erythrocyte sedimentation rate, leucocytosis, and hyperglobulinaemia. In a few patients a mild, short-lasting, vasculitic, non-thrombocytopaenic purpura with a deposition of IgA in small vessel walls was noted. The attacks lasted 6–8 weeks, but they subsided promptly after a high dose of prednisone (Langevitz et al. 1994a). Colchicine induced myopathy in rare cases, especially in transplanted patients treated with cyclosporin (Yussim et al. 1994), may be erroneously confused with an attack of protracted febrile myalgia.

Erysipelas-like erythema is one of the most characteristic manifestations of FMF. It was reported in 11 per cent of affected children, usually combined with arthritis. Rather sharply bordered red patches, hot, tender, and swollen, and 10–35 cm^2 in area, appear on the skin of the lower extremities. They are usually located between the knee and ankle, or on the dorsum of the foot or ankle region, and are also accompanied by abrupt elevation of body temperature and last about 24–48 h (Sohar et al. 1967). Histological examination reveals oedema of the superficial dermis, sparse perivascular infiltrates of lymphocytes, neutrophils and nuclear dust and deposits of C3, and occasionally IgM and fibrinogen in the wall of small vessels (Barzilai et al. 2000).

Scrotal attacks (acute, unilateral, painful swelling and redness of the 'testis' due to inflammation of the tunica vaginalis) have been recognized as a form of attack in children or young adults. It subsides spontaneously after 12–24 h, without anatomical residue (Eshel et al. 1988).

Elevation of body temperature, sometimes to 40°C for a few hours, occurs frequently, especially in children, as the only expression of an attack (Sohar et al. 1967). This phenomenon is often falsely attributed to viral infection, pharyngitis, or tonsillitis. PFAPA (Table 2) is an important consideration in the differential diagnosis of such an attack (Padeh et al. 1999).

Mild splenomegaly of 1–4 cm, unrelated to amyloidosis, was found in many patients. In some patients the liver was also palpable. None showed clinical or laboratory malfunction of these organs.

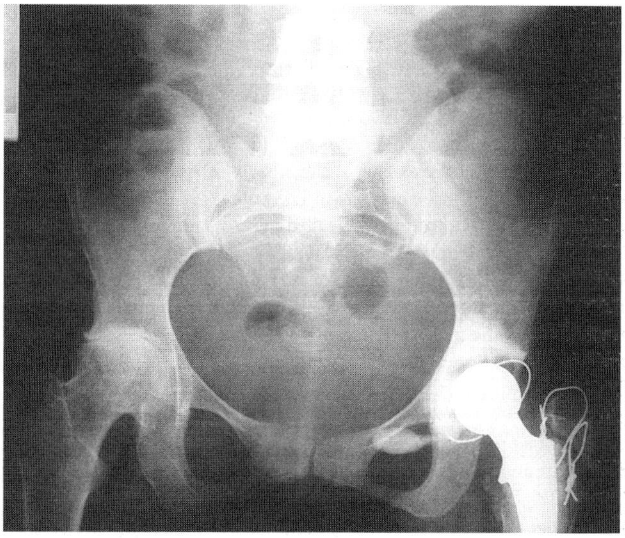

Fig. 2 Results of protracted arthritis of both hips in a 17-year-old girl. State following hip arthroplasty of left hip. Narrowing of the joint space, sclerosis, and aseptic necrosis of the lateral aspect can be seen in the right hip.

Allied conditions

Henoch–Schönlein purpura occurred in over 40 of our patients, mostly children and young adults. In most of them, the disease was characterized by a prolonged and severe course and was treated with steroids.

Polyarteritis nodosa has been reported in 15 cases of FMF (Glikson et al. 1989). Common peculiar manifestations of PAN in FMF include young age at onset, precipitation by streptococcal infection, presentation with muscle pain and association with perinephric haematoma. Fifteen cases in approximately 10 000 patients with FMF are 300 times higher than the expected frequency.

Behçet's disease was discerned in 40 out of 4000 of our patients (Schwartz et al. 2000), 16 with complete agreement with the international set of criteria for diagnosis of Behçet's disease. Patients with this combination were clinically and demographically comparable with patients suffering from each of the conditions alone.

A relatively high incidence of fibromyalgia (30 per cent) was found in patients with FMF, especially in those who suffers from back and leg/foot pain (Langevitz et al. 1994b).

Various types of glomerulonephritis were reported in few patients with FMF, including post-streptococcal glomerulonephritis, diffuse mesangial proliferative glomerulonephritis with IgA and IgM deposits, and also rapidly progressive glomerulonephritis (Said et al. 1992).

In seven of 4000 FMF patients Crohn's disease was also noted. The clinical picture of these patients was characterized by severe FMF with extra-abdominal manifestations. Most had a third disease entity, usually FMF-associated spondyloarthropathy (Fidder et al. 2000). Interestingly, in most patients, the onset of Crohn's disease was significantly late (40 versus 25 years in Crohn's disease without FMF).

Amyloidosis

A genetically determined, AA-type amyloidosis, clinically manifested as nephropathy (Sohar et al. 1967; Levine et al. 1972) is the fatal manifestation in patients with FMF. Its clinical presentation occurs at an early age; 90 per cent of the patients who died from amyloidosis were under 40 and six were under 10 (Sohar et al. 1967). Subsequent evaluation showed ethnic differences in the prevalence of amyloidosis, reaching 60 per cent of untreated individuals in North African Jews, Armenians, and Turks (the highest prevalence among all diseases predisposing reactive amyloidosis), yet much lower in other Jewish ethnic groups and in Armenians living in the United States (Schwabe and Peters 1974; Pras et al. 1982; Livneh et al. 1996). The amyloidosis of FMF is not directly related to the frequency or intensity of the recurrent inflammatory attacks. In some patients it occurs before the appearance of the febrile attacks (phenotype II) and in a few it is the only manifestation of the disease (Blum et al. 1962).

Clinically, the amyloid nephropathy passes through several stages—proteinuric, nephrotic, azotaemic, and uraemic. There is a preclinical stage but it can only be diagnosed by repeated rectal and renal biopsies or is inadvertently found in an occasional Congo red-stained appendectomy specimen. In less than 10 per cent of patients, uraemia may precede proteinuria or coincide with it, probably reflecting an atypical amyloid deposition. Persistent proteinuria in an otherwise healthy patient with FMF has proved to be a certain indication of renal amyloidosis. Kidney tissue is the best source of pathological evidence for amyloid involvement. Histological confirmation may also be obtained from extrarenal tissues through rectal, bone marrow, gingival, and mouth labial biopsies (Livneh et al. 1996).

Clinical evidence of extrarenal amyloidosis was scant, when patients died from renal failure before the chronic dialysis advent, manifested mainly by clinical and laboratory evidence of intestinal malabsorbtion. Following prolongation of life by chronic dialysis and renal transplantation, amyloid deposition in other organs has become more pronounced. In recent years we have observed extrarenal amyloid deposition that interfered with the normal function of certain organs (Table 4). The deposition of amyloid in the small bowel is a particularly grave consequence that caused the death of six patients.

Table 4 Extrarenal amyloidosis in familial Mediterranean fever

Amyloid cardiomyopathy
Giant hepatomegaly
Amyloid goitre
Addison's disease
Fatal malabsorption

Peculiar to amyloid nephropathy, hypertension complicates only 35 per cent of the affected patients, mostly late in the course of the disease (Livneh et al. 1996). A tendency to renal vein thrombosis in the nephrotic stage of the disease presenting with aggravating proteinuria, loin pain, and rapidly progressive renal failure was reported (Reuben et al. 1997). Finally, pregnancy may have a deleterious effect on amyloid nephropathy in patients with more advanced renal failure at conception (Livneh et al. 1993).

Laboratory tests

Laboratory findings are meagre and non-specific. The white blood cell count is increased during the attacks. The erythrocyte sedimentation rate is accelerated, and acute-phase proteins such as α_2-globulin reactive protein, serum amyloid A, and fibrinogen are increased, especially during attacks, but occasionally also in between (Sohar et al. 1967). Special attention is given to serum amyloid A because its *N*-terminal is AA protein, which is part of the AA amyloid fibril. During attacks, very high concentrations of serum amyloid A are observed, which decrease gradually in the days following an attack. However, even during remissions the serum amyloid A is often two or three times normal. This is specifically true in patients with amyloidosis (Knecht et al. 1985).

Increased levels of immunoglobulins is inconsistently observed in FMF patients, with IgA being the most commonly elevated one. IgD is elevated in 10 per cent of the patients, precluding differentiation of hyper IgD syndrome from FMF based on high levels of IgD alone. Cytokines found to be associated with the acute inflammatory response in FMF include tumour necrosis factor, interleukin-1, interleukin-6, interleukin-8, interferon γ, and others (Gang et al. 1999). Mild anaemia with a low serum iron is common. Low levels of haemoglobin (7–10 g per cent) were found in some patients. Haematuria, mostly only microscopic, has been observed in several patients during and between attacks. The synovial fluid is very turbid in FMF arthritis. Most cells are neutrophils and their count may reach 100 000 per microlitre. Turbidity and neutrophil predominance also characterize the peritoneal fluid during the acute abdominal attack (Sohar et al. 1967).

Imaging is not diagnostic, and findings in FMF attacks are similar to findings in acute peritonitis, pleuritis, and arthritis of any other cause. The damage detected in radiograms of a chronic joint of FMF is indistinguishable from that of aseptic necrosis (Sohar et al. 1975). In CT, amyloidotic kidney is denser than endstage kidney in other nephropathics and has coarse parenchymal calcification (Apter et al. 2001).

Treatment (Table 5)

Until 1973, therapeutic measures were restricted to alleviating pain. Daily prophylactic treatment with colchicine was suggested by Goldfinger (1972) and confirmed by double-blind studies (Zemer et al. 1974). The dose required to prevent attacks is not body weight-dependent. Treatment is started with 1 mg colchicine/day. This dose is increased if necessary to 1.5–2 mg, until remission from attacks is achieved. If doses of 2 mg/day do not produce remission, further elevation of the dose usually does not help. Omission of a daily dose may be followed promptly by an attack.

Table 5 Approach to the management of familial Mediterranean fever

Clinical characteristics	Colchicine	Additional therapies
To control febrile attacks and prevention of amyloidosis	Continuous 1–2 mg daily	
Amyloid nephropathy		
Normal blood creatinine	2 mg daily	
Abnormal creatinine	1 mg daily	
Acute arthritis	Increase the usual dose by 0.5 mg	NSAIDs for 1–2 weeks
Protracted arthritis	1.5–2 mg	NSAIDs for months, intra-articular corticosteroids
Seronegative spondyloarthropathy	1.5–2 mg	NSAIDs, DMARDs
Protracted febrile myalgia	1.5–2 mg	Corticosteroids 1 mg/kg per day

Note: DMARD, disease-modifying antirheumatic drug; NSAID, non-steroidal anti-inflammatory drug.

Sixty-five per cent of patients enjoy a complete remission of attacks, if they adhere to their daily dose of colchicine. Partial remission, defined as a significant decrease in the frequency and severity of the attacks, is experienced by an additional 30 per cent. In 5 per cent of treated patients, the attack rate remains unchanged. They are maintained on 2 mg/day to prevent amyloidosis.

Our experience showed that continuous prophylactic treatment with colchicine in patients inhibits the development of nephropathic amyloidosis (Zemer et al. 1986). None of the patients who started treatment without proteinuria has developed amyloidosis during the follow-up period of 21 years, while a control group of non-compliant patients showed the same rate of amyloidosis as would be expected in the natural history of the disease. In patients with established nephropathic amyloidosis, colchicine may reverse proteinuria, even in the nephrotic range if administered before uraemia has developed and in an appropriate dose (>1.5 mg/day; Livneh et al. 1994). This favourable effect of colchicine is not associated with a significant reduction in the amyloid load.

Side-effects of colchicine are generally mild. Diarrhoea and abdominal pain are the most common, and usually prove transient and easily controllable. Long-term experience with children reveals that in none of the treated patients has colchicine caused any deviation from normal in physical examination, routine laboratory tests, linear growth, or sexual development (Zemer et al. 1991). There is no data that shows that colchicine in the doses used affects fertility in patients with FMF. By preventing febrile attacks, colchicine treatment may improve spermatogenesis known to be deranged by high body temperature. Fertility may be impaired in women with FMF, probably due to the induction of early miscarriages or to pelvic adhesions that develop after frequent abdominal attacks (Ismachovich et al. 1973). Colchicine, by preventing the abdominal attacks, may lessen the rate of early miscarriages and the development of pelvic adhesions. Four pregnancies producing infants with Down syndrome were reported in colchicine-treated patients (Rabinovitch et al. 1992; and our unpublished data). Although this is not higher than expected, routine amniocentesis to exclude chromosomal aberrations in colchicine-treated patients is recommended.

Kidney transplantation is the treatment of choice in the endstage disease of FMF. A daily dose of 1.5–2.0 mg colchicine appears to protect the renal graft from amyloidosis (Livneh et al. 1992). Cyclosporin, given to most renal transplanted patients, is avoided or prescribed in a lower dose in FMF-amyloidosis, because it almost invariably precipitates colchicine intoxication (Yussim et al. 1994).

References

Alt, H.L. and Barker, H. (1930). Fever of unknown origin. *Journal of the American Medical Association* **94**, 1457–61.

Apter, S. et al. (2001). Abdominal CT findings in nephropathic amyloidosis of familial Mediterranean fever. *Amyloid* **8**, 58–64.

Barzilai, A. et al. (2000). Erysipelas-like erythema of familial Mediterranean fever: clinicopathologic correlation. *Journal of the American Academy of Dermatology* **42**, 791–5.

Benhamou, E., Albou, A., and Griguer, P. (1954). Remarques cliniques biologiques et therapeutiques sur la maladie periodique (a propos de 24 cas personels). *Bulletin et Memoires de la Societe Medical des Hopitaux de Paris* **70**, 254–8.

Blum, A. et al. (1962). Amyloidosis as the sole manifestation of familial Mediterranean fever (FMF). *Annals of Internal Medicine* **57**, 795–9.

Cazeneuve, C. et al. (2000). Identification of MEFV-independent modifying genetic factors for familial Mediterranean fever. *American Journal of Human Genetics* **67**, 1136–41.

Dabestani, A. et al. (1982). Pericardial disease in familial Mediterranean fever. *Chest* **81**, 592–5.

Eshel, G., Zemer, D., and Bar-Yochai, A. (1988). Acute orchitis in familial Mediterranean fever. *Annals of Internal Medicine* **109**, 164–5.

Fidder, H.H. et al. (2000). Crohn's disease in patients with familial Mediterranean fever. *Clinical and Experimental Rheumatology* **18**, 300.

Gang, N. et al. (1999). Activation of the cytokine network in familial Mediterranean fever. *Journal of Rheumatology* **26**, 890–7.

Glikson, M. et al. (1989). Polyarteritis nodosa and familial Mediterranean fever. A report of two cases and review of the literature. *Journal of Rheumatology* **16**, 536–9.

Goldfinger, S.E. (1972). Colchicine for familial Mediterranean fever. *New England Journal of Medicine* **287**, 1302.

Heller, H., Sohar, E., and Sherf, L. (1958). Familial Mediterranean fever. *Archives of Internal Medicine* **102**, 50–71.

Heller, H., Sohar, E., and Gafni, J. (1961). Amyloidosis in familial Mediterranean fever. *Archives of Internal Medicine* **107**, 539–50.

Ismachovich, B. et al. (1973). The causes of sterility in females with familial Mediterranean fever. *Sterility and Fertility* **24**, 844–7.

Janeway, T.C. and Mosenthal, H.D. (1908). An unusual paroxysmal syndrome probably allied to recurrent vomiting with a study of the nitrogen metabolism. *Transactions of the Association of American Physicians* **23**, 504–18.

Kees, S. et al. (1997). Attacks of pericarditis as a manifestation of familial Mediterranean fever (FMF). *Quarterly Journal of Medicine* **90**, 643–7.

Knecht, A., De Beer, F.C., and Pras, M. (1985). Serum amyloid A protein in familial Mediterranean fever. *Annals of Internal Medicine* **102**, 71–2.

Kogan, A. et al. (2001). Common MEFV mutations among Jewish ethnic groups in Israel: high frequency of carrier and phenotype III states and absence of a perceptible biological advantage of the carrier state. *American Journal of Medical Genetics* **102**, 272–6.

Langevitz, P. et al. (1994a). Protracted febrile myalgia in patients with familial Mediterranean fever. *Journal of Rheumatology* **21**, 1708–9.

Langevitz, P. et al. (1994b). Fibromyalgia in familial Mediterranean fever. *Journal of Rheumatology* **21**, 1335–7.

Langevitz, P. et al. (1997). Seronegative spondyloarthropathy in familial Mediterranean fever. *Seminars in Arthritis and Rheumatism* **27**, 67–72.

Levine, M. et al. (1972). The amino acid sequence of a major non-immunoglobulin component of some amyloid fibrils. *Journal of Clinical Investigation* **51**, 2773–6.

Livneh, A. and Langevitz, P. (2000). Diagnostic and treatment concerns in familial Mediterranean fever. *Baillière's Clinical Rheumatology* **14**, 477–98.

Livneh, A. et al. (1992). Colchicine prevents kidney transplant amyloidosis in familial Mediterranean fever. *Nephron* **60**, 418–22.

Livneh, A. et al. (1993). Effect of pregnancy on renal function in amyloidosis of familial Mediterranean fever. *Journal of Rheumatology* **20**, 1519–23.

Livneh, A. et al. (1994). Colchicine treatment of AA amyloidosis of familial Mediterranean fever. An analysis of factors affecting outcome. *Arthritis and Rheumatism* **37**, 11804–11.

Livneh, A. et al. (1996). The changing face of familial Mediterranean fever. *Seminars in Arthritis and Rheumatism* **26**, 612–27.

Livneh, A. et al. (1997). Criteria for the diagnosis of familial Mediterranean fever. *Arthritis and Rheumatism* **40**, 1884–90.

Livneh, A. et al. (1999). MEFV mutation analysis in patients suffering from amyloidosis of familial Mediterranean fever. *Amyloid* **6**, 1–7.

Mamou, H. and Cattan, R. (1952). La maladie periodique (sur 14 cas personnels dont 8 compliques de nephropathies). *La Semaine des Hopitaux de Paris* **28**, 1062–70.

Padeh, S. et al. (1999). Periodic fever, aphthous stomatitis, pharyngitis, and adenopathy syndrome: clinical characteristics and outcome. *Journal of Pediatrics* **135**, 98–101.

Pras, M. (1998). Familial Mediterranean fever: from the clinical syndrome to the cloning of the pyrin gene. *Scandinavian Journal of Rheumatology* **24**, 92–7.

Pras, M. et al. (1982). Variable incidence of amyloidosis in familial Mediterranean fever among different ethnic groups. *Johns Hopkins Medical Journal* **150**, 22–6.

Pras, E. et al. (1992). Mapping of a gene causing familial Mediterranean fever to the short arm of chromosome 16. *New England Journal of Medicine* **326**, 1509–13.

Rabinovitch, O. et al. (1992). Colchicine treatment in conception and pregnancy: two hundred thirty-one pregnancies in patients with familial Mediterranean fever. *American Journal of Reproductive Immunology* **28**, 245–6.

Reimann, H.A. (1949). Periodic disease. Periodic fever, periodic abdominalgia, cyclic neutropenia, intermittent arthralgia, angioneurotic edema, anaphylactoid purpura and periodic paralysis. *Journal of the American Medical Association* **141**, 175–82.

Reuben, A., Hirsch, M., and Berlyne, G.M. (1977). Renal vein thrombosis as a major cause of renal failure in familial Mediterranean fever. *Quarterly Journal of Medicine* **46**, 243–58.

Said, R. et al. (1992). Spectrum of renal involvement in familial Mediterranean fever. *Kidney International* **41**, 414–19.

Salai, M. et al. (1993). Total hip replacement in familial Mediterranean fever. *Bulletin of the Hospital for Joint Diseases* **53**, 25–8.

Schwabe, A.D. and Peters, R.S. (1974). Familial Mediterranean fever in Armenians, analysis of 100 cases. *Medicine* **53**, 453–62.

Schwartz, T. et al. (2000). Behçet's disease in familial Mediterranean fever: characterisation of the association between the two diseases. *Seminars in Arthritis and Rheumatism* **29**, 286–95.

Shinar, Y. et al. (2000). Genotype–phenotype assessment of common genotypes among patients with familial Mediterranean fever. *Journal of Rheumatology* **24**, 1703–7.

Shinawi, M. et al. (2000). Familial Mediterranean fever: high gene frequency and heterogeneous disease among an Israeli Arab population. *Journal of Rheumatology* **27**, 1492–5.

Shohat, M. et al. (1992). Twin studies in familial Mediterranean fever. *American Journal of Medical Genetics* **44**, 179–82.

Siegal, S. (1945). Benign paroxysmal peritonitis. *Annals of Internal Medicine* **22**, 1–21.

Sneh, E. et al. (1977). Protracted arthritis in familial Mediterranean fever. *Rheumatology and Rehabilitation* **16**, 102–6.

Sohar, E. et al. (1961). Genetics of familial Mediterranean fever. *Archives of Internal Medicine* **107**, 529–38.

Sohar, E. et al. (1967). Familial Mediterranean fever. A survey of 470 cases and review of literature. *American Journal of Medicine* **43**, 227–53.

Sohar, E., Pras, M., and Gafni, J. (1975). Familial Mediterranean fever and its articular manifestations. *Clinics in Rheumatic Diseases* **1**, 195–209.

Stoffman, N. et al. (2000). Higher than expected carrier rates for familial Mediterranean fever in various Jewish ethnic groups. *European Journal of Human Genetics* **8**, 307–10.

Tamir, N. et al. (1999). Late onset familial Mediterranean fever (FMF): a subset with distinct clinical, demographic, and molecular genetic characteristics. *American Journal of Medical Genetics* **87**, 30–5.

The French FMF Consortium (1997). A candidate gene for familial Mediterranean fever. *Nature Genetics* **17**, 25–31.

The International FMF Consortium (1997). Ancient missense mutations in new members of the RoRet gene family are likely to cause familial Mediterranean fever. *Cell* **90**, 797–807.

Touitou, I. et al. (2001). The MICA region determines the first modifier locus in familial Mediterranean fever. *Arthritis and Rheumatism* **44**, 163–9.

Yussim, A. et al. (1994). Gastrointestinal, hepatorenal and neuromuscular toxicity caused by cyclosporine–colchicine interaction in renal transplantation. *Transplantation Proceedings* **26**, 2825–6.

Yuval, Y. et al. (1995). Dominant inheritance in two families with familial Mediterranean fever. *American Journal of Medical Genetics* **57**, 455–7.

Zemer, D. et al. (1974). A controlled trial of colchicine in preventing attacks of familial Mediterranean fever. *New England Journal of Medicine* **291**, 932–4.

Zemer, D. et al. (1986). Colchicine in the prevention and treatment of the amyloidosis of familial Mediterranean fever. *New England Journal of Medicine* **314**, 1001–5.

Zemer, D. et al. (1991). Long-term colchicine treatment in children with familial Mediterranean fever. *Arthritis and Rheumatism* **34**, 973–7.

6.12.3 Periodic fevers

Michael F. McDermott

Introduction

Recurrent fevers associated with abdominal discomfort, joint pains, and muscle aches have afflicted mankind throughout recorded history. Medical advances in the nineteenth and twentieth centuries helped to identify microbial pathogens (e.g. spirochaete infections and mosquito-borne malarial and dengue fevers) as the underlying cause of many of these diseases, particularly in tropical regions. However, there also exists a group of rare inherited disorders (both autosomal dominant and recessive) that cluster within families and are characterized by intermittent self-limiting inflammatory episodes with fever, synovial/serosal inflammation, skin rashes, and conjunctivitis. This group of disorders has been called the 'periodic fevers', even though the intervals between attacks may vary considerably. No infectious or autoimmune cause has yet been found, and all these diseases tend to follow Mendelian patterns of inheritance. The most common autosomal recessive condition is familial Mediterranean fever (FMF, MIM249100—MIM refers to the Mendelian Inheritance in Man classification number), with hyperimmunoglobulinaemia D (HIDS, MIM260920) being much less common. Among the autosomal dominant recurrent fever syndromes, there is familial Hibernian fever (FHF, MIM142680), which has been renamed TRAPS (for tumour necrosis factor receptor-associated periodic syndrome), and two related conditions: familial cold urticaria (FCU, MIM120100) and Muckle–Wells syndrome (MWS, MIM191900). All these conditions were originally thought to have a restricted ethnic distribution, with FMF being particularly prevalent in the Middle East while the other conditions were reported mostly among Western European populations and their descendants. However, autosomal dominant periodic fevers have now been reported in most ethnic groups, including Middle-Eastern, Asian, Native American, and African populations.

The clinical features of this group of disorders have exercised the minds of physicians since the beginning of the nineteenth century. In 1806, Heberden described 'pains which are regularly intermittent, the fits of which return periodically as those of ague', and in 1895 Osler reported a condition associated with pains in the abdomen, chest, and limbs (Osler 1895). Other case reports of what were almost certainly periodic fevers date from the early twentieth century, for example, a Jewish child who most probably suffered from FMF (Janeway and Mosenthal 1908). In 1945, a report by Siegal of recurrent fevers in five patients was probably the first accurate clinical description of FMF (Siegal 1945). The blanket term 'periodic fevers' was introduced to cover all pyrexial illnesses in this disease category (Reimann 1948) and the FMF coinage was introduced in 1958 (Heller et al. 1958).

In 1957, a periodic fever was reported in five successive generations of a single family (Bouroncle and Doan 1957), and Mendelian dominant inheritance was proposed in these individuals, as the illness was transmitted vertically from one of the parents to approximately half the children. The term 'familial Hibernian fever' (FHF, MIM249100) was introduced in 1982 to describe an autosomal dominant periodic illness in an Irish–Scottish family, 'Hibernia' being the ancient Roman name for Ireland (Williamson et al. 1982). MWS is a rare disorder in which progressive sensorineural deafness, skin rashes, and amyloidosis are combined in a dominantly inherited syndrome (Muckle and Wells 1962). FCU is characterized by maculopapular exanthem, painful swollen joints, chills, and fever after exposure to cold (Kile and Rusk 1940). As skin biopsy reports generally do not demonstrate urticaria in FCU, it has been proposed that the condition be renamed 'familial cold autoinflammatory syndrome' (FCAS) (Hoffman et al. 2001a).

A further step in the overall classification of periodic fevers was taken in 1984 when 'hyperimmunoglobulinaemia D and periodic fever syndrome' (HIDS) (van der Meer et al. 1984) was described. This is a rare autosomal recessive condition, initially reported in six Dutch patients who suffered from recurrent fevers and abdominal pain since childhood, with headaches and lymphadenopathy. The condition has also been described in other European populations, including French and Italian, and in one Japanese patient (Prieur and Griscelli 1984; Drenth et al. 1994; Scolozzi 1995).

Significant conceptual breakthroughs in our understanding of the molecular basis of inflammatory mechanisms in general have occurred since 1997, with successive identification of the genetic anomalies in all the known periodic fever syndromes. The FMF susceptibility gene, *MEFV* (*ME*diterranean *FeV*er), encodes a previously unknown protein (variously termed pyrin or marenostrin) (The French FMF Consortium 1997; The International FMF Consortium 1997). Following upon this landmark discovery, mutations in the tumour necrosis factor receptor 1 gene (*TNFRSF1A* for tumor necrosis factor receptor superfamily 1A) were reported in FHF (McDermott et al. 1999). Given that these mutations were found in a range of ethnic groups in addition to Irish, the term FHF was replaced by the acronym TRAPS, so that all cases with documented *TNFRSF1A* mutations, regardless of ethnic background, could be included in this classification.

An intermediary enzyme in cholesterol metabolism and isoprenoid biosynthesis, mevalonate kinase (MK), is mutated in HIDS patients (Drenth et al. 1999; Houten et al. 1999), but the mechanisms whereby this leads to recurrent fevers and lymphadenopathy remain a major challenge. A protein with homology to pyrin/marenostrin, called cryopyrin, is mutated in both FCU/FCAS and MWS (Hoffman et al. 2001b).

This series of discoveries has served to emphasize the distinct pathophysiological and genetic differences among these disorders, despite marked similarities in their inflammatory phenotypes. The basis of the episodic nature of the attacks of fever remains unclear, but may reflect intermittent exposure to infection, physical exertion, environmental agents, or indeed psychological stress. Hormonal factors are also undoubtedly involved in the aetiology of TRAPS, given that the disease often flares up in the premenstrual and post-partum periods, with remission during pregnancy.

Genetically complex disorders such as Behçet's disease (BD), juvenile-onset systemic rheumatoid arthritis (RA), and systemic lupus erythematosus (SLE), may also present with recurrent fevers. BD is a polygenic disease associated with particular HLA genotypes, and there is evidence that *MEFV* mutations may act as additional susceptibility factors in BD susceptibility (Touitou et al. 2000). Conversely, the presence of BD may increase the likelihood of a single *MEFV* mutation causing FMF (Livneh et al. 2001).

A new disease classification entitled 'autoinflammatory syndromes' has been proposed for the large group of disorders characterized by spontaneous attacks of systemic inflammation in the apparent absence of a self-directed immune process due to autoantigenic exposure (Galon et al. 2000). Conditions found in this disease category include granulomatous disorders such as Crohn's disease (MIM266600) and Blau syndrome (MIM186580), as well as periodic fevers.

Epidemiology

FMF primarily affects Jews (Sephardic more frequently than Ashkenazi), Anatolian Turks, Armenians, and Arabs (Table 1) (Chapter 6.12.2). Relatively few epidemiological studies have been done on TRAPS and HIDS, but tertiary referrals to specialized units suggest that TRAPS is the more prevalent of the two. It has also become apparent that the TRAPS phenotype encompasses patients of diverse ethnic backgrounds, including Dutch–Indonesian (Simon et al. 2001), Israeli Arab (Aganna et al. 2002), Argentinian Arab, and Puerto Rican. However, a disproportionate percentage of TRAPS referrals continue to be of Irish–Scottish descent (Aksentijevich et al. 2001).

The exact prevalence of FCU/FCAS is unknown, but over 10 families have been reported in Europe and North America. MWS is also found mostly in descendants of northern European populations, but a syndrome combining features of both FCU/FCAS and MWS has been reported in an Indian family (McDermott et al. 2000).

Clinical features and differential diagnosis

A diagnosis of periodic fever requires a high index of suspicion, and is based on clinical criteria of acute, remitting attacks, and family history (Table 1). These diseases have several features in common, including an acute-phase response during attacks, as indicated by raised C reactive protein, alpha-1 antitrypsin, SAA protein, and haptoglobin, with polymorphonuclear leucocytosis. White blood cell counts may exceed 30 000/mm^3, with neutrophils predominating, and in severe attacks there may be a significant infiltration of neutrophils into sites of inflammation. There is continuous fever (usually sudden in onset in the case of FMF and HIDS), with temperatures higher than 39°C. This pattern of fever is different from that encountered in Still's disease, where it is intermittent. Sterile peritonitis, which may resemble acute abdomen, is a very common presentation in both FMF and TRAPS, but is not a feature of HIDS (Table 1). A neutrophilic exudate is revealed at laparotomy on these patients, but the appendix is normal. However, abdominal pain may also be severe in HIDS, and is often accompanied by diarrhoea and vomiting. As the tunica vaginalis is an extension of the peritoneal sac, inguinal hernias and acute scrotal pain may also be observed in some males with TRAPS (McDermott et al. 1997), as well as in a small percentage of FMF patients (Table 1).

The specific clinical features that help to distinguish between different types of periodic fever are of particular importance. These include longer duration of attacks, and periorbital oedema specific to TRAPS; cutaneous involvement is usually confined to the legs and feet in FHF, but all over the body, except for the face, in TRAPS (Toro et al. 2000). The most frequently reported symptoms in TRAPS include fever lasting a week or more, abdominal or chest pain, red, swollen eyes, and a migratory erythematous skin rash with muscle tenderness underneath. Lymphadenopathy, particularly of the cervical nodes, is a major physical sign during an attack of HIDS, but is unusual in FMF, and uncommon in TRAPS.

Table 1 A differential diagnostic approach to patients with recurrent episodes of fever and a positive family history

	FMF	TRAPS	HIDS	MWS	FCU/FCAS	CINCA/NOMID
Mode of inheritance	Autosomal recessive	Autosomal dominant	Autosomal recessive	Autosomal dominant	Autosomal dominant	Autosomal dominant
Age of onset	90% by 20 years 50–65% by 10 years	Usually in childhood	96% by 10 years	85% by 20 years 60–75% by 10 years	95% by 6 months	Neonatal period
Ethnic background	Jews, Arabs, Armenians, Turks, Italians, Greeks	Most ethnic backgrounds	Mostly Northern European, mainly Dutch and French	Northern European	Only reported in Northern European and French–Canadians	Most ethnic backgrounds
Fever	Abrupt onset and defervescence	During attacks	Abrupt onset, gradual decrease	During severe attacks	With most attacks	Variable
Abdominal involvement	Peritonitis in 85%, constipation more common than diarrhoea	Pain, diarrhoea or constipation, vomiting	Severe pain, vomiting, diarrhoea	Infrequent abdominal pain	No	No
Joint involvement	Monoarticular non-erosive, asymmetric 5% protracted arthritis	Arthralgia common	Oligo-articular symmetric, no protracted arthritis	Arthralgia, non-destructive, occasional arthritis	Primarily arthralgia, occasional arthritis	Arthropathy, epiphyseal bone formation
Skin involvement	Erysipeloid rash of lower leg	Migratory erythematous rash, with myalgia	Polymorphic maculo-papular	Urticarial maculo-papular exanthem	Maculo-papular. resembles urticaria	Persistent skin rash, urticaria-like
Scrotal pain, inguinal hernia	Rare episodes in childhood	Common in some families	None reported	None reported	None reported	None reported
Myalgia	20% have myalgia in attacks	Painful myalgia beneath rash and near affected joints	Rarely	Occasionally	Occasionally	Occasionally
Lymphadenopathy	Uncommon	May occur	Common cervical, axillary, inguinal	May be significant	None reported	None reported
Pleurisy	In 1/3 of cases	May occur	None reported	No	No	No
Vasculitis	Henoch–Schönlein purpura, polyarteritis nodosa	Perivascular infiltrations	Leucocytoclastic vasculitis	No	No	No
Amyloidosis	Frequent in absence of colchicine in patients homozygous for M694V mutation	Up to 15%. Most, but not all, are cysteine mutations	Low risk	Up to 35%	Infrequent, but has been reported	Rare

Continued

Table 1 Continued

	FMF	TRAPS	HIDS	MWS	FCU/FCAS	CINCA/NOMID
Splenomegaly	10–50% of patients; 100% if patient has amyloidosis	May occur	With attacks in children	No	No	No
Neurological involvement	Rare, apart from headache	Rare	Yes, with severe cases of mevalonic aciduria	Sensori-neural deafness	No	Chronic meningitis, mental retardation
Duration of attacks	1–3 days	Days to weeks	3–7 days	Usually 2–3 days	1–2 days, may be longer	Variable
Distinguishing features (not always present)	Ethnic background	Periorbital oedema, migratory rash, and myalgia	Lymphadenopathy (cervical)	Deafness, amyloidosis	Attacks after exposure to cold, conjunctivitis	Distinctive facies with frontal bossing and protruding eyes
Chromosome	16p13	12p13	12q24	1q44	1q44	1q44
Serum IgD level	Elevated in 10–20%	Elevated in approximately 10%	May exceed 100 IU/ml (14 mg/dl), not always present	Normal	Normal	Normal
Gene involved	*MEFV*	*TNFRSF1A*	Mevalonate kinase (*MVK*)	*CIAS1/NALP3/PYPAF1*	*CIAS1/NALP3/PYPAF1*	*CIAS1/NALP3/PYPAF1*
Laboratory findings	Cloudy sterile exudates	Low level of sTNFRSF1A (however not consistent and may mislead clinician)	During attacks mevalonate increased in urine	Neutrophilia	Neutrophilia	Neutrophilia
Treatment	Oral colchicine to prevent attacks and amyloidosis	Etanercept, oral or intravenous steroids	No prophylaxis; may respond to steroids	Promising preliminary data with Anakinra	Promising preliminary data with Anakinra	Trial of Anakinra initiated
Prognosis	Excellent with prophylaxis colchicine to prevent amyloidosis	Awaiting outcome of Etanercept trial on prevention of disease progression	No effect on longevity	Awaiting outcome of Anakinra trial	Awaiting outcome of Anakinra trial	Awaiting outcome of Anakinra trial

FCU/FCAS has been classified as one of the physical urticarias, but it is clinically different from the more common acquired cold urticaria (ACU) (Hoffman et al. 2001a). Furthermore, skin biopsies taken during attacks in FCU/FCAS patients show an intense polymorphonuclear leucocyte infiltrate without mast cells, whereas mast cells are present in biopsies from ACU patients. Disease onset usually occurs during the first 6 months of life in FCU/FCAS patients, and conjunctivitis is relatively common. In periodic fevers, in general, the arthralgia is usually asymmetric. Arthritis, when present, is often monoarticular and non-erosive, affecting the larger joints in FMF; however, it is often polyarticular in HIDS.

Systemic diseases resembling periodic fevers must also be considered in the differential diagnosis. The absence of joint deformity and spontaneous resolution of arthralgia make a diagnosis of juvenile idiopathic arthritis (JIA) less likely. Neurological involvement in children with FMF is relatively uncommon, but magnetic resonance imaging studies have revealed abnormal brain scans in TRAPS patients with severe neurological involvement. Systemic amyloidosis of the AA type is a serious complication of FMF (in the absence of colchicine therapy), TRAPS, and MWS, but is very rarely found in HIDS.

In addition to DNA-based diagnostic tests, which may only be done in specialized centres, a number of laboratory tests are generally available. These include the presence of moderate levels of mevalonate in the urine and elevated polyclonal serum IgD (greater than 100 U/ml) in most, but not all, cases of HIDS, and, for TRAPS patients, low serum levels of TNFRSF1A (sTNFRSF1A) between attacks of fever.

Genetics and pathophysiology

FMF

Mutations of the *MEFV* gene, encoding pyrin/marenostrin, which appears to be predominantly expressed in neutrophils, cause FMF (Chapter 6.12.2). At least 29 mutations have been identified at this time, and while most of these are located in exon 10, some are also dispersed within exons 1, 2, 3, 5, and 9 (Bernot et al. 1998; Aksentijevich et al. 1999).

TRAPS

Unlike FMF, the susceptibility gene for FHF turned out to be a well-characterized molecule (*TNFRSF1A*, or *TNFR1* as it was formerly known). Six different missense mutations of the TNFRSF1A extracellular domains were described in the initial series, five of which involved cysteine residues. Over 20 *TNFRSF1A* mutations have been identified, and cysteine mutations are no longer in the majority (Dodé et al. 2000; Jadoul et al. 2001; Simon et al. 2001; Nevala et al. 2002). The range of mutations include a splice-junction mutation (c.193-14 G $\rightarrow$ A) between exons 2 and 3 (Aksentijevich et al. 2001), a less penetrant R92P mutation (Aganna et al. 2001), and two substitutions (P46L and R92Q), present in approximately 1 per cent of chromosomes in healthy subjects. The increased frequency of P46L and R92Q among TRAPS patients, as well as functional studies, suggest that these are low-penetrance mutations rather than benign polymorphisms. The R92Q variant is also more frequently found in patients with early arthritis (Aksentijevich et al. 2001), and all *TNFRSF1A* mutations described so far, have been confined to the extracellular domains.

In general, low levels of soluble TNFRSF1A (sTNFRSF1A) are found in the serum of affected individuals between febrile attacks and reduced cleavage of the mutant TNFRSF1A from the cell surface has been demonstrated in some, though not all, TRAPS patients. The disease phenotype relates to altered function of this key receptor in TNF homeostasis but the condition is unlikely to be solely caused by sTNFRSF1A concentrations at 50 per cent of normal, as such levels might be expected to deal with most physiological insults. Other possible pathogenic mechanisms include dysfunction of intracellular TNF signalling, and altered transcription factor activation.

HIDS

Both HIDS and its related more severe disease, mevalonic aciduria (MA), are caused by a deficiency of the MK enzyme, resulting from mutations in the MK gene (*MVK*). In MA, which is characterized by mental retardation and dysmorphism in addition to the clinical features of HIDS, enzymatic activity is virtually absent, leading to considerably higher urinary mevalonate excretion than in HIDS. Modestly increased levels of mevalonate are found in the urine during attacks of HIDS (Frenkel et al. 2000), but not in the intervening periods. There is slight residual MK activity in HIDS patients, which may be just sufficient to avoid development of the more severe disease phenotype (Houten et al. 2001).

In HIDS, the mutations are located to different exons all along the *MVK* gene, unlike MA, where mutations are mainly clustered to a couple of exons. Most HIDS patients are compound heterozygotes for two mutations, and the majority share a common mutation (*V377I*) (Houten et al. 2001). The second most common mutation is *I268T*, and it has been proposed that diagnostic screening in HIDS should be directed at these two more common mutations (Cuisset et al. 2001). However, a small number of HIDS patients do not possess *V377I*, and there is often difficulty in demonstrating genotype–phenotype relationships, as at least three mutations (*I268T*, *H20P*, and *V377I*) are involved in both HIDS and MA, and there may be clinical overlap between these two diseases (Cuisset et al. 2001; Houten et al. 2001).

MWS and FCU/FCAS syndrome

MWS syndrome was linked initially to chromosome 1q44 (Jung et al. 1996) and this genetic interval was also independently implicated in three further studies of both FCU/FCAS and MWS families (Cuisset et al. 1999; Hoffman et al. 2000; McDermott et al. 2000). Mutations in a single gene (variously termed *CIAS1* for cold-induced autoinflammatory syndrome 1 encoding crypoyrin, *PYPAF1* for a pyrin containing Apaf-1 like protein, and *NALP3*) are involved in both these conditions (Hoffman et al. 2001b). However, a clinical distinction continues to be made between these MWS and FCU/FCAS, based on a considerably higher incidence of amyloidosis and hearing loss in MWS (Table 1).

Defective cellular apoptosis and Nuclear Factor kappa B (NFκB) activation—a unifying theme in the pathogenesis of periodic fevers

Apoptosis is a process of cellular suicide, also called programmed cell death, that occurs during development, ageing, and different pathological processes. A key apoptotic pathway is initiated by ligation of various membrane bound 'death receptors', with subsequent activation of a family of intracellular proteases, termed caspases. These enzymes bring about elimination of unwanted cellular debris, which is a normal means of maintaining homeostasis of cells and tissues. The TNF cytokine regulates apoptosis mainly through TNFRSF1A ligation, with intracellular signalling through a death domain called the TNFR-associated death domain (TRADD). Alternatively, TNF may also activate a cell-survival response by activation of the NFκB with transcription of NFκB dependent genes, for example, cytokines like interleukin 1. This coordinated activation of numerous genes in response to pathogens and pro-inflammatory cytokines is central to the development of acute and chronic inflammatory states. The elements controlling this delicate 'ying yang' balance between TNF-dependent cellular survival and annihilation are very poorly understood.

The *N*-terminal pyrin domain, which is integral to both pyrin/marenostrin and crypoyrin/NALP3 proteins, is another member of the death domain-fold superfamily (Fairbrother et al. 2001), and has been shown to interact with an apoptosis-associated speck-like recruitment domain (ASC), also involved in caspase recruitment and regulation of NFkB transcription factor (Manji et al. 2002). Therefore, mutations involving TNFRSF1A, pyrin/marenostrin, or CIASl/NALP3 molecules might all be postulated to result in defective apoptosis and transcriptional regulation, albeit through different intracellular signalling pathways. Such defects may be central to the over-exuberant inflammatory response seen in some periodic fevers. The mechanisms underlying the HIDS phenotype appear to be distinct from these processes and are currently unknown.

Other causes of recurrent febrile illnesses

Infectious disease may also cause recurrent fevers, as in brucellosis, malaria, and leishmaniasis. Recurrent infections with a 21-day periodicity are a consistent feature of cyclic haematopoiesis; the attacks are due to a temporary reduction in circulating neutrophil levels (Horwitz et al. 1999). There are also some systemic inflammatory disorders without obvious infectious, autoimmune, or hereditary cause, which could be regarded as non-hereditary autoinflammatory diseases. The Periodic Fever Aphtous stomatitis, Pharyngitis and Adenitis (PFAPA) syndrome is a childhood disorder characterized by monthly episodes of fever, lasting about 4 days, and usually accompanied by chills, cervical lymphadenopathy, pharyngitis, and aphtous stomatitis (Padeh et al. 1999). The diagnosis is based solely on clinical findings and no specific test is available. The chronic infantile neurologic cutaneous and articular (CINCA) syndrome is characterized by perinatal onset, and occasionally a family history (Prieur 2001) (Chapter 6.12.8).

Therapy

Prior to the availability of DNA-based tests, many people with periodic fevers remained undiagnosed, and were exposed to unnecessary investigations and operative interventions. Patients suffering from these diseases are benefiting from recent developments including carrier testing and improved therapy; furthermore, genetic counselling for parents is being considered (Ben-Chetrit and Sagi 2001). However, FMF screening usually tests for known mutations, and detection rates often do not exceed 80 per cent, even in specialized centres. Screening for the presence of TRAPS is usually concentrated on exons 2–5 of the *TNFRSF1A* gene.

The current treatment of choice for FMF is daily colchicine (Zemer 1986), a neutrophil-suppressive agent that has been used for FMF since 1972 (Goldfinger 1972). The efficacy of this drug has been demonstrated in double-blind trials (Dinarello et al. 1974; Zemer et al. 1986); in young children it is best to start with a low dose (0.3 mg/day) and gradually increase the levels, as needed, to control symptoms. In adults and older children the effective dose of colchicine is 1–2 mg/day, regardless of body weight; it is generally a safe drug despite some reported side-effects.

Newly developed TNF-inhibitors such as etanercept (Enbrel), which is a recombinant p75 TNFR : Fc fusion protein (formerly TNFR2 protein) have been used for the treatment of TRAPS (Galon et al. 2000). Etanercept is given subcutaneously at a dosage of 25 mg twice weekly in adults, and 0.4 mg/kg in children. The more common side-effects include injection site reactions and bacterial infections. Of more serious concern is the possibility of demyelination during anti-TNF therapy (Mohan et al. 2001) and a small number of active cases of tuberculosis have been reported in patients treated with a humanized anti-TNF antibody called infliximab (Remicaide) (Keane et al. 2001). A study is being carried out on the efficacy and safety profile of etanercept in the long-term treatment of TRAPS.

Anakinra (Kineret), which is a selective antagonist of the IL-1 cytokine by causing inhibition of IL-1 binding to type I receptor (IL-1RI), is an effective therapy for MWS and FCU (Hawkins et al. 2003), but its effectiveness in CINCA remains to be ascertained.

There has been more difficulty in finding an effective therapy for HIDS. A clinical trial of statins, which reduce the concentration of mevalonate by inhibiting the hydroxymethyl-glutaryl-CoA reductase enzyme, has recently been initiated and steroids may also be useful in severe cases (de Dios Garcia-Diaz and Alvarez-Blanco 2001). There is no effective therapy for MWS and FCU/FCAS at this time.

The 'periodic fevers' constitute a dynamic and expanding area of research, and further advances may be anticipated, particularly in the area of therapy. These may include small molecules taken orally to modulate specific protein–protein interactions, as well as, possibly, gene therapy, once some challenging technical hurdles have been overcome.

References

Aganna, E. et al. (2001). Tumor necrosis factor receptor associated periodic syndrome (TRAPS) in a Dutch family. Evidence for a *TNFRSF1A* mutation with reduced penetrance. *European Journal of Human Genetics* **9**, 63–6.

Aganna, E. et al. (2002). An Israeli Arab patient with a de novo *TNFRSF1A* mutation causing tumor necrosis factor receptor associated periodic syndrome (TRAPS). *Arthritis and Rheumatism* **46**, 245–9.

Aganna, E. et al. (2003). Heterogeneity amongst patients with tumor necrosis factor receptor associated periodic syndrome (TRAPS) phenotypes. *Arthritis and Rheumatism* **48**, 2632–44.

Aksentijevich, I. et al. (1999). Mutation and haplotype studies of familial Mediterranean fever reveal new ancestral relationships and evidence for a high carrier frequency with reduced penetrance in the Ashkenazi Jewish population. *The American Journal of Human Genetics* **64**, 949–62.

Aksentijevich, I. et al. (2001). The TNF receptor-associated periodic syndrome (TRAPS): new mutations in *TNFRSF1A*, ancestral origins, genotype–phenotype studies, and evidence for further genetic heterogeneity of periodic fevers. *The American Journal of Human Genetics* **69**, 301–14.

Ben-Chetrit, E. and Sagi, M. (2001). Genetic counselling in familial Mediterranean fever: has the time come? *Rheumatology* **40**, 606–9.

Bernot, A. et al. (1998). Non-founder mutations in the MEFV gene establish this gene as the cause of familial Mediterranean fever (FMF). *Human Molecular Genetics* **8**, 1317–25.

Bouroncle, B.A. and Doan, C.A. (1957). 'Periodic fever': occurrence in five generations. *American Journal of Medicine* **23**, 502–6.

Cuisset, L. et al. (1999). Genetic linkage of the Muckle–Wells syndrome to chromosome 1q44. *American Journal of Human Genetics* **65**, 1054–9.

Cuisset, L. et al. (2001). Molecular analysis of MVK mutations and enzymatic activity in hyper-IgD and periodic fever syndrome. *European Journal of Human Genetics* **9**, 260–6.

de Dios Garcia-Diaz, J. and Alvarez-Blanco, M.J. (2001). Glucocorticoids but not NSAID abort attacks in hyper-IgD and periodic fever syndrome. *Journal of Rheumatology* **28**, 925–6.

Dinarello, C.A. et al. (1974). Colchicine therapy for familial Mediterranean fever. A double-blind trial. *New England Journal of Medicine* **291**, 934–7.

Dodé, C. et al. (2000). A novel missense mutation (C30S) in the gene encoding tumor necrosis factor receptor 1 linked to autosomal-dominant recurrent fever with localized myositis in a French family. *Arthritis and Rheumatism* **43**, 1535–42.

Drenth, J.P., Haagsma, C.J., and van der Meer, J.W. (1994). Hyperimmunoglobulinemia D and periodic fever syndrome. The clinical spectrum in a series of 50 patients. International Hyper-IgD Study Group. *Medicine (Baltimore)* **73**, 133–44.

Drenth, J.P.H. et al. (1999). Mutations in the gene encoding mevalonate kinase cause hyper-IgD and periodic fever syndrome. *Nature Genetics* **22**, 178–81.

Fairbrother, W.J. et al. (2001). The PYRIN domain: a member of the death domain-fold superfamily. *Protein Science* **10**, 1911–18.

Frenkel, J. et al. (2000). Clinical and molecular variability in childhood periodic fever with hyperimmunoglobulinaemia D. *Rheumatology (Oxford)* **40**, 579–84.

Galon, J. et al. (2000). TNFRSFIA mutations and autoinflammatory sydromes. *Current Opinion in Immunology* **12**, 479–86.

Goldfinger, S.E. (1972). Colchicine for familial Mediterranean fever. *New England Journal of Medicine* **287**, 1302.

Heller, H., Sohar, E., and Sherf, L. (1958). Familial Mediterranean fever. *Archives of Internal Medicine* **102**, 50–71.

Hoffman, H.M. et al. (2000). Identification of a locus on chromosome 1q44 for Familial Cold Urticaria. *American Journal of Human Genetics* **66**, 1693–8.

Hoffman, H.M., Wanderer, A.A., and Broide, D.H. (2001a). Familial cold autoinflammatory syndrome: phenotype and genotype of an autosomal dominant periodic fever. *Journal of Allergy and Clinical Immunology* **108**, 615–20.

Hoffman, H.M. et al. (2001b). Mutation of a new gene encoding a putative pyrinlike protein causes familial cold autoinflammatory syndrome and Muckle–Wells syndrome. *Nature Genetics* **29**, 301–5.

Horwitz, M. et al. (1999). Mutations in ELA2, encoding neutrophil elastase, define a 21-day biological clock in cyclic haematopoiesis. *Nature Genetics* **23**, 433–6.

Houten, S.M. et al. (1999). Mutations in MVK, encoding mevalonate kinase, cause hyperimmunoglobulinemia D and periodic fever syndrome. *Nature Genetics* **22**, 175–7.

Houten, S.M. et al. (2001). Organization of the mevalonate kinase (MVK) gene and identification of novel mutations causing mevalonic aciduria and hyperimmunoglobulinaemia D and periodic fever syndrome. *European Journal of Human Genetics* **9**, 253–9.

Jadoul, M. et al. (2001). Autosomal-dominant periodic fever with AA amyloidosis: novel mutation in tumor necrosis factor receptor 1 gene. *Kidney International* **59**, 1677–82.

Janeway, T.C. and Mosenthal, H.O. (1908). An unusual paroxysmal syndrome, probably allied to recurrent vomiting, with a study of the nitrogen metabolism. *Transactions of the Association of American Physicians* **23**, 504–18.

Jung, M. et al. (1996). A locus for familial cold urticaria maps to distal chromosome 1q: familial cold urticaria and Muckle–Wells syndrome are probably allelic. *The American Journal of Human Genetics* **59**, 1281 (abstract).

Keane, J. et al. (2001). Tuberculosis associated with infliximab, a tumor necrosis factor alpha-neutralizing agent. *New England Journal of Medicine* **345**, 1098–104.

Kile, R.L. and Rusk, H.A. (1940). A case of cold urticaria with unusual family history. *Journal of the American Medical Association* **114**, 1067–8.

Livneh, A. et al. (2001). A single mutated MEFV allele in Israeli patients suffering from familial Mediterranean fever and Behçet's disease (FMF–BD). *European Journal of Human Genetics* **9**, 191–6.

Manji, G.A. et al. (2002). PYPAF1: A PYRIN-containing Apaf1-like protein that assembles with and regulates activation of NF-kB. *Journal of Biological Chemistry* **277** (13), 11570–5.

McDermott, E.M., Smillie, D.M., and Powell, R.J. (1997). Clinical spectrum of familial Hibernian fever: a 14-year follow-up study of the index case and extended family. *Mayo Clinic Proceedings* **72**, 806–17.

McDermott, M.F. et al. (1999). Germline mutations in the extracellular domains of the 55 kDa TNF receptor (TNF-R1) define a family of dominantly inherited autoinflammatory syndromes. *Cell* **97**, 133–44.

McDermott, M.F. et al. (2000). An autosomal dominant periodic fever associated with AA amyloidosis in a north Indian family maps to distal chromosome 1q. *Arthritis and Rheumatism* **43**, 2034–40.

Mohan, N. et al. (2001). Demyelination occurring during anti-tumor necrosis factor alpha therapy for inflammatory arthritides. *Arthritis and Rheumatism* **44**, 2862–9.

Muckle, T.J. and Wells, M. (1962). Urticaria, deafness and amyloidosis: a new heredo-familial syndrome. *Quarterly Journal of Medicine* **31**, 235–48.

Nevala, H. et al. (2002). A novel mutation in the third extracellular domain of the TNF receptor 1 (*TNFRSF1A*) in a Finnish family with autosomal dominant recurrent fever. *Arthritis and Rheumatism* **46** (4), 1061–6.

Osler, W. (1895). On the visceral complications of erythema exudativum multiforme. *American Journal of Medical Sciences* **110**, 629–46.

Padeh, S. et al. (1999). Periodic fever, aphthous stomatitis, pharyngitis, and adenopathy syndrome: clinical characteristics and outcome. *Journal of Pediatrics* **135**, 98–101.

Prieur, A.M. (2001). A recently recognised chronic inflammatory disease of early onset characterised by the triad of rash, central nervous system involvement and arthropathy. *Clinical and Experimental Rheumatology* **19**, 103–6.

Prieur, A.M. and Griscelli, C. (1984). (Nosologic aspects of systemic forms of very-early-onset juvenile arthritis. Apropos of 17 cases). *La Semaine des Hopitaux* **60**, 163–7.

Reimann, H.A. (1948). Periodic disease. Probable syndrome including periodic fever, benign paroxysmal peritonitis, cyclic neutropenia, and intermittent arthralgia. *Journal of the American Medical Association* **136**, 239–44.

Sarrauste de Menthiere, C. et al. (2003). INFEVERS: the Registry for FMF and hereditary inflammatory disorders mutations. *Nucleic Acids Research* **31**, 282–5.

Scolozzi, R. (1995). Hyper-IgD syndrome (HIDS). *Recenti Progressi in Medicina* **86**, 243–7.

Siegal, S. (1945). Benign paroxysmal peritonitis. *Annals of Internal Medicine* **22**, 1–21.

Simon, A. et al. (2001). Familial periodic fever and amyloidosis due to a new mutation in the TNFRSF1A gene. *American Journal of Medicine* **110**, 313–16.

The French FHF Consortium (1997). A candidate gene for familial Mediterranean fever. *Nature Genetics* **17**, 25–31.

The International FMF Consortium (1997). Ancient missense mutations in a new member of the *RoRet* gene family are likely to cause familial Mediterranean fever. *Cell* **90**, 797–807.

Toro, J.R. et al. (2000). Tumor necrosis factor receptor-associated periodic syndrome: a novel syndrome with cutaneous manifestations. *Archives of Dermatology* **136**, 1487–94.

Touitou, I. et al. (2000). MEFV mutations in Behçet's disease. *Human Mutation* **16**, 271–2.

van der Meer, J.W.M. et al. (1984). Hyperimmunoglobulinemia D and periodic fever. A new syndrome. *Lancet* **I**, 1087–90.

Williamson, L.M. et al. (1982). Familial hibernian fever. *The Quarterly Journal of Medicine* **204**, 469–80.

Zemer, D. et al. (1986). A controlled trial of colchicine in preventing attacks of familial Mediterranean fever. *New England Journal of Medicine* **291**, 932–4.

6.12.4 Panniculitis

Jeffrey P. Callen

Panniculitis refers to inflammation within the subcutaneous fat (Patterson 1987). Panniculitis is probably a dynamic process that progresses through inflammation with neutrophils to lymphocytes to histiocytes and ends with fibrosis (Ter Poorten and Thiers 2002). The panniculitis can become granulomatous when in the histiocytic phase. The exact nature of the infiltrate perhaps depends upon when the biopsy is taken in relation to the age of the lesion being sampled. The panniculitides have been divided into four categories based on histopathological criteria: (i) septal panniculitis, (ii) lobular panniculitis, (iii) mixed with septal and lobular components, and (iv) panniculitis with vasculitis. Table 1 presents one of the currently accepted classifications for the panniculitides. Frequently, the panniculitides are associated with systemic disease. Often, the separation of one syndrome from another is possible only after a period of observation (Black 1988).

Erythema nodosum

The prototypic septal panniculitis is erythema nodosum (Soderstrom 1982). A relatively common process, erythema nodosum is usually acute and self-limited. Erythema nodosum occurs most commonly in young adult women between the ages of 20 and 30, but any age or sex can be affected, including children (Kakourou et al. 2001). The typical clinical presentation is the sudden onset of one or more tender, erythematous nodules on the anterior tibial surface (Plate 166). The eruption is often preceded by a prodrome of fever, malaise, and/or arthralgias. The nodules are deep and are better palpated than visualized. As the lesions age they may soften and develop an ecchymotic appearance. Over a 4–6 week period, the lesions eventually heal without scar formation. Ulceration of the primary process is extremely rare.

Although erythema nodosum is usually an acute process, many patients with chronic or recurrent disease have been described primarily in middle-aged (mean 45–50 years) women. Terms such as chronic erythema nodosum, erythema nodosum migrans, or subacute nodular migratory

Table 1 Classification of the panniculitides

Septal panniculitis—erythema nodosum, Villanova's disease—subacute nodular migratory panniculitis
Lobular panniculitis
Webber–Christian disease—relapsing febrile nodular non-suppurative panniculitis (controversy about the existence of this entity)
Rothman–Makai syndrome—lipogranulomatosis subcutanea
Subcutaneous fat necrosis of the new born
Post-steroid panniculitis
Enzymatic panniculitis
Pancreatic
α_1-Antitrypsin deficiency
Calcifying panniculitis (calciphylaxis) associated with haemodialysis
Physical or factitial panniculitis
Cytophagic histiocytic panniculitis and subcutaneous T-cell lymphoma
Lipodystrophy syndromes
Connective panniculitis—scleroderma or inflammatory myopathy associated
Lipodermatosclerosis—sclerosing panniculitis
Mixed panniculitis—lupus erythematosus panniculitis (lupus profundus)
Panniculitis with vasculitis
Small-vessel vasculitis
Medium-sized vessel vasculitis
Nodular vasculitis (erythema induratum)
Polyarteritis nodosa

Table 2 Some aetiological causes of or associations with erythema nodosum

Infections
Streptococcal pharyngitis
Tuberculosis
Valley fever (coccidioidomycosis)
Blastomycosis
Histoplasmosis
Psittacosis
Yersinia colitis
Salmonella gastroenteritis
Cat scratch fever
Leprosy
Drugs
Antibiotics—penicillins, sulfonamides
Birth control pills
Systemic processes or diseases
Pregnancy
Sarcoidosis
Inflammatory bowel disease
Collagen–vascular disorders—dermatomyositis, lupus erythematosus, scleroderma
Malignancy (rare)
Sweet's syndrome
Idiopathic

panniculitis (Vilanova's disease) have been used to characterize these patients (Prestes et al. 1990). The disease is often present for several years, and is most common on the legs. As with acute erythema nodosum, accompanying symptoms may be present, but are usually a result of the associated condition.

Causative or associated conditions are present in about 60 per cent of patients with acute, or recurrent erythema nodosum, but may be much less in patients with chronic erythema nodosum. The associated conditions can be broken into three broad categories: infectious diseases, therapeutic agents, or systemic diseases (usually inflammatory). Garcia-Porrua et al. (2000) and Psychos et al. (2000) reported that sarcoidosis accounted for 20 and 28 per cent of the cases, an infection for 34 and 18 per cent of the patients, respectively, usually in the upper respiratory tract, and often β-haemolytic streptococcal infection (Garty and Poznanski 2000); an unknown cause occurred in roughly 35 per cent of the patients. A few patients in each study were noted to have Sweet's syndrome, Behçet's disease, pregnancy, drugs, or inflammatory bowel disease as associated processes/causes. Some of the known associations are listed in Table 2.

The infectious agents associated with erythema nodosum primarily tend to affect the respiratory or gastrointestinal tracts and are most often bacterial or fungal in origin. The most common drugs linked with the disease are antibiotics and oral contraceptives. Pregnancy, particularly in its second trimester, is a known association; and erythema nodosum will recur with subsequent pregnancies or with oral contraceptive use. A specific variant of sarcoidosis is associated with erythema nodosum, known as Löfgren's syndrome. This is an acute, often self-resolving variant in which erythema nodosum occurs in association with bilateral hilar lymphadenopathy, arthritis, and anterior uveitis (Mana et al. 1999). Crohn's disease (granulomatous colitis and regional enteritis) and ulcerative colitis have been associated with erythema nodosum. Patients with these inflammatory bowel diseases develop erythema nodosum that parallels the activity of the bowel disease. Panniculitis can occur with the collagen–vascular diseases (Winkelmann 1983), but it may not be best to classify the process as erythema nodosum (see below).

Weber–Christian disease

The existence of Weber–Christian disease has often been questioned. Traditionally, this process is characterized by multiple recurrent subcutaneous nodules (Plate 167), with accompanying fever (Panush et al. 1985). Histopathologically, the disease is characterized by a lobular panniculitis with an early neutrophilic infiltrate, fat degeneration, foamy histiocytes, and giant-cell formation. Eventually, fibrosis occurs, and this, in addition to the destruction of fat, results in the clinical finding of an atrophic scar. Other clinical features that commonly occur are arthralgias and myalgias. Some patients also have recurrent abdominal pain. In addition to the skin lesions, any area of the body containing fat can be affected by Weber–Christian disease. Several cases of mesenteric panniculitis have been reported, as has involvement of the heart, lungs, liver, and/or kidneys (Lemley et al. 1991). The disease is chronic, but can result in death in 10–15 per cent of cases. Some of the patients with Weber–Christian disease have had multiple surgical procedures because of an acute inflammatory lesion in the presence of fever.

The laboratory abnormalities associated with Weber–Christian disease include an elevated sedimentation rate, anaemia, leucopaenia or leucocytosis, depression of complement components, and evidence of circulating immune complexes. There have been several reports of α_1-antitrypsin deficiency in patients with Weber–Christian disease (Breit et al. 1983). In addition, patients who have lupus erythematosus, pancreatic disease, or factitial panniculitis (Diesk and Pannush 1981) have been misdiagnosed as this form of panniculitis. White and Winkelmann (1998) retrospectively studied 30 cases diagnosed as Weber–Christian panniculitis and found that 26 could be classified as another form of panniculitis including erythema nodosum (12), post-phlebitic syndrome (6), factitial panniculitis (5), and one case each of cytophagic panniculitis, lymphoma, or leukaemia. This report suggests that when followed and studied closely most of the patients with Weber–Christian disease have another panniculitic syndrome.

Panniculitis associated with α_1-antitrypsin deficiency

Several groups of patients with a lobular or septal panniculitis have been found to have a deficiency of α_1-antitrypsin (Smith et al. 1987). In a study of

96 patients with panniculitis, Smith et al. (1989) found 15 patients with α_1-antitrypsin deficiency. Clinical differences include more frequent ulceration and drainage, and the presence of preceding trauma. Histopathological differences include greater amounts of fat necrosis and destruction of elastic tissue and a splaying of neutrophils between collagen bundles. The recognition of these patients is important because debridement of the lesion should be avoided; these patients should be evaluated for pulmonary and/or liver disease and should be counselled to avoid smoking; therapy with α_1-proteinase inhibitor concentrate may be helpful.

Pancreatic panniculitis

Some patients with pancreatic diseases develop subcutaneous fat necrosis (lobular panniculitis) (Plate 168), with accompanying polyarthritis and osseous intramedullary fat necrosis (Wilson et al. 1983). A variety of changes have been implicated in the development of this process including pancreatitis, pancreatic carcinoma (acinar cell), pancreatitis secondary to cholelithiasis, post-traumatic lesions, pancreatic ischaemia, pancreatic pseudocyst (Zimmerman-Gorska et al. 1986), and a pancreatic difusum (a congenital pancreatic abnormality) (Huber and Asaad 1986). It is not clear whether the elevated lipase in the circulation is primarily involved in the pathogenesis of the fat necrosis, or whether its presence follows the fat necrosis (Simkin et al. 1983). Histopathologically there is extensive fat necrosis with a basophilic alteration of lipocytes. Ghost cells with absent nuclei are also common. Treatment centres on non-specific measures for control of the panniculitis (see below) and reduction of the pancreatic inflammation or removal of a pancreatic tumour.

Calcifying panniculitis of renal failure

Patients with renal failure often have abnormal calcium–phosphorus metabolism. Rarely, these patients develop acute, erythematous, tender indurated nodules as a manifestation of calciphylaxis (Ivker et al. 1995). The panniculitic lesions can progress to necrosis and ulceration (Plate 169). Laboratory evaluation reveals a normal calcium level and hyperphosphataemia with elevated calcium–phosphorus product. This condition must be differentiated from metastatic calcification. The prognosis is poor, and treatment is aimed at a correction of the calcium–phosphorus imbalance. Parathyroidectomy may at times be helpful.

Post-steroid panniculitis

Panniculitis following withdrawal of corticosteroid therapy is a rare entity that seems to be limited to children (Roenigk et al. 1964). Patients reported have been treated with corticosteroids for a wide array of problems including leukaemia, nephrotic syndrome, rheumatic carditis, and encephalopathy. Interestingly, the panniculitis may clear upon re-administration of the corticosteroids. The pathogenesis of this rare complication is not understood.

Lipoatrophic panniculitis

Several conditions have been described in children that often result in lipoatrophy following the inflammatory reaction. There exists a spectrum that perhaps includes Rothman–Makai syndrome (lipogranulomatosis subcutanea), lipoatrophic panniculitis, lipophagic panniculitis of childhood (Winkelmann et al. 1989; Melchiorre et al. 2000), and localized lipoatrophy (atrophic connective tissue disease panniculitis) (Peters and Winkelmann 1980). These children tend to have multiple erythematous lesions, most commonly on the extremities, which resolve with subcutaneous atrophy (Plate 170) (Roth et al. 1989). The patients often are febrile. They may have associated 'autoimmune' phenomena such as juvenile chronic arthritis, Hashimoto's thyroiditis, or diabetes mellitus (Billings et al. 1987). There is no known effective therapy, but some patients have responded to oral corticosteroids, oral antimalarials, or oral dapsone.

Histiocytic cytophagic panniculitis

Histiocytic cytophagic panniculitis was described by Crotty and Winkelmann (1981) as a chronic histiocytic disease of the subcutaneous fat, with accompanying inflammatory panniculitis, fever, serositis, and 'reticuloendotheliomegaly'. This is an extremely rare entity, having been reported in a small number of patients. The process may be a primary skin disorder of unknown cause, but has also been linked to neoplastic processes such as lymphoma and malignant histiocytosis (Barron et al. 1985). Histopathologically, the fat contains both T cells and histiocytes (Perniciaro et al. 1994). Haemorrhagic complications, perhaps due to thrombocytopaenia, have occurred in half of the patients (Crotty and Winkelmann 1981). Alegre and Winkelmann (1989) have suggested that aggressive therapy with cytotoxic agents be used early in this process. Recently Craig et al. (1998) has suggested that there are two, perhaps distinct, patterns of disease, one that is benign (termed cytophagic histiocytic panniculitis) and one that is malignant (termed subcutaneous T-cell lymphoma). In both instances the haemophagocytic syndrome may occur, but in cytophagic histiocytic panniculitis there is often a response to prednisone and/or cyclosporin. Some of these patients perhaps have EB virus within their lesions. The diagnosis of subcutaneous T-cell lymphoma is at times very difficult to confirm (Weenig et al. 2001).

Factitial panniculitis

Factitial panniculitis from external trauma or from the injection of foreign substances is not uncommon, and should be considered in any patient with panniculitis and unusual clinical or histopathological features (Plate 171). In traumatic lesions an organizing haematoma is often demonstrated histopathologically; whereas with the injection of foreign material, refractile bodies, or a 'Swiss cheese' effect are encountered. Occasionally, spectroscopic and/or chromatographic techniques are necessary to identify the causative injected material.

Lupus erythematosus panniculitis (lupus profundus)

This is a rare manifestation of chronic cutaneous lupus erythematosus occurring in less than 3 per cent of cases of systemic lupus erythematosus, and less than 1 per cent of cases with cutaneous lupus erythematosus (Izumi 1985). The lesions are tender, red–blue, subcutaneous nodules (Plate 172) that may eventually ulcerate or atrophy. Calcification may occur in late lesions (Plate 173). The lesions tend to occur on the face, upper arms, thighs, and/or buttocks (Martens et al. 1999). The lesions may underlie a typical lesion of discoid lupus erythematosus. Trauma may initiate or worsen these lesions. Facial lesions are common, and in a recent report, lupus panniculitis accounted for peri-parotid swelling and was confused clinically with a possible neoplastic process (White et al. 1993). Histopathological changes include a panniculitis that is both lobular and septal. The overlying epidermis and dermis often demonstrate changes of lupus erythematosus, in which case the diagnosis of lupus erythematosus panniculitis can be histopathologically confirmed. Although one-half of the patients have four or more of the criteria for systemic lupus erythematosus, the activity of the panniculitic lesion does not seem to follow the course of the systemic disease.

Sclerosing panniculitis

Jorizzo et al. (1991) coined the term sclerosing panniculitis to describe a group of patients with well-circumscribed, indurated, inflammatory plaques of the lower extremity (Plate 174). These lesions most frequently occur in women and are often accompanied by signs of venous insufficiency. There may be a history of prior thrombophlebitis (Alegre et al. 1988). Histopathologically, this disorder is characterized by fat necrosis, sclerosis, and a lobular panniculitis. Fat microcysts with foci of membranous fat necrosis are also commonly observed in the later stages of the disease. Sclerosing panniculitis is probably a manifestation of venous insufficiency and thus therapy should include support stockings, elevation, and rest. Measures for the prevention of phlebitis are also warranted. Low-dose aspirin or other non-steroidal anti-inflammatory drugs may be helpful. Intralesional injection of triamcinolone acetonide may also be helpful.

Panniculitis with vasculitis

Nodular vasculitis, polyarteritis nodosa (both cutaneous and systemic varieties), and small-vessel vasculitis may involve subcutaneous vessels and result in inflammatory or ischaemic changes in the subcutaneous fat. Erythema induratum is a form of nodular vasculitis thought to be due to tuberculosis.

Evaluation

The evaluation of the patient with panniculitis should include a careful history, physical examination, and a deep incisional biopsy. Findings from this examination will usually allow appropriate classification. Patients with erythema nodosum should be screened for the possibility of infection of the upper respiratory tract, and a throat swab for a rapid streptococcal screen, a skin test with PPD (purified protein derivative), and a chest radiograph should be obtained. Inflammatory bowel disease or infectious enteritis are usually symptomatic and thus it is rarely necessary to perform endoscopic or radiographic procedures in these patients. In patients in whom Weber–Christian disease or pancreatic panniculitis are being considered, tests for enzymatic abnormalities such as amylase, lipase, or α_1-antitrypsin deficiency should be ordered. In all patients the possibility of a coexistent collagen vascular disease should be considered.

Treatment

The treatment of erythema nodosum and other panniculitides first involves assessment of a causative disease and its treatment. In the absence of a treatable disorder, therapy is symptomatic (Callen 1985). Acute erythema nodosum is often self-limited, thus non-toxic therapies are advised. Bed rest and leg elevation are very helpful in controlling symptomatology. In patients who need to continue to be ambulatory, support stockings or tights may be helpful (Lehman 1980). Aspirin or other non-steroidal anti-inflammatory agents may be helpful. My experience with aspirin has not produced results prior to toxicity and therefore my choice is to use oral indomethacin at a dosage of 25–75 mg/day (Barr and Robinson 1981).

In patients with chronic erythema nodosum or frequent recurrences, oral potassium iodide at a dosage of 300–900 mg/day has been useful in open clinical trials. My experience with 15 patients with erythema nodosum treated with oral potassium iodide has yielded control of the disease in 10 patients (unpublished observation). Furthermore, in some of the responding patients, when the drug is stopped or the dosage is lowered, the disease has relapsed, only to respond again with reinstitution of therapy. Other therapies that may be considered include oral corticosteroids, colchicine (Lupton et al. 1988), or an immunosuppressive agent. Systemic corticosteroids, which are almost always effective, are often complicated by iatrogenic Cushing's syndrome. Colchicine has not been effective in any of the patients who were treated. Azathioprine and cyclosporin have been used successfully in some patients. One adjunctive therapy that can be helpful is intralesionally injected triamcinolone acetonide (3–5 mg/ml).

There is no specific therapy for Weber–Christian disease. Reports have centred on the use of anti-inflammatory agents including aspirin, non-steroidal anti-inflammatory drugs, oral corticosteroids, antimalarials, and immunosuppressives including cyclophosphamide and cyclosporin (Usuki et al. 1988). In addition, colchicine, dapsone, and potassium iodide may be effective in individual cases. Non-steroidal therapies such as potassium iodide, colchicine, or dapsone could be used to begin with. When these agents fail, the use of either azathioprine or methotrexate can be considered. If the patient is found to have α_1-antitrypsin deficiency then either doxycycline or replacement therapy has been reported to be effective.

Patients with cytophagic histiocytic panniculitis should be aggressively treated with corticosteroids and/or immunosuppressive agents. Despite this treatment, many patients develop either the haematophagocytic syndrome or subcutaneous T-cell lymphoma, and multiple deaths have been reported in this seemingly benign inflammatory process.

Patients with lupus erythematosus panniculitis may respond to antimalarials or to intralesional injections of triamcinolone. Corticosteroids and/or immunosuppressives are rarely necessary for lupus erythematosus panniculitis.

Conclusion

Panniculitides form a wide array of syndromes that perhaps can be separated on the basis of clinical features, associated disorders, and/or histopathological features. Unfortunately, several of the syndromes have overlapping features, the pathogenesis is not understood for most, and therapeutic options are similar for all. The differential diagnosis often depends on an adequate specimen for histopathological investigation. Thus, a deep, fusiform, incisional biopsy or a wedge biopsy, often including fascia, should be performed. Furthermore, a biopsy of the youngest lesion should be taken. Sections should be serially cut to identify the pattern of the panniculitis: lobular, septal, vasculitis, or mixed. The patient should be tested for underlying processes including ingestants, infections, malignancy, and autoimmune disorders. Treatment, in the absence of an underlying disease, is aimed at control of the inflammatory reaction with agents such as non-steroidal anti-inflammatory drugs, corticosteroids, dapsone, potassium iodide, antimalarials, colchicine, or immunosuppressive agents.

References

Alegre, V.A. and Winkelmann, R.K. (1989). Histiocytic cytophagic panniculitis. *Journal of the American Academy of Dermatology* **20**, 177–85.

Alegre, V.A., Winkelmann, R.K., and Aliaga, A. (1988). Lipomembranous changes in chronic panniculitis. *Journal of the American Academy of Dermatology* **131**, 241–5.

Barr, W.G. and Robinson, J.A. (1981). Chronic erythema nodosum treated with indomethacin. *Annals of Internal Medicine* **95**, 695.

Barron, D.R., Davis, P.R., Pomeranz, J.R., Hines, J.D., and Park, C.H. (1985). Cytophagic histiocytic panniculitis. *Cancer* **29**, 2538–42.

Billings, J.K., Milgramm, S.S., Gupta, A.K., Headington, J.T., and Rasmussen, J.E. (1987). Lipoatrophic panniculitis: a possible autoimmune inflammatory disease of fat. *Archives of Dermatology* **123**, 1662–6.

Black, M.M. (1988). Panniculitis: problems with diagnosis. *Australasian Journal of Dermatology* **29**, 79–84.

Breit, S.N., Clark, P., Robinson, J.P., Luckhurst, E., Daekins, R.L., and Penny, R. (1983). Familial occurrence of α_1-antitrypsin deficiency and Weber–Christian disease. *Archives of Dermatology* **119**, 198–202.

Callen, J.P. (1985). Erythema nodosum. In *Current Therapy in Dermatology* (ed. T.T. Provost and E.R. Farmer), pp. 159–60. St Louis MO: Mosby.

Craig, A.J., Cualing, H., Thomas, G., Lamerson, C., and Smith, R. (1998). Cytophagic histiocytic panniculitis—a syndrome associated with benign and malignant panniculitis: case comparison and review of the literature. *Journal of the American Academy of Dermatology* **39**, 721–36.

Crotty, C. and Winkelmann, R.K. (1981). Cytophagic histiocytic panniculitis with fever, cytopenia, liver failure, and terminal hemorrhagic diathesis. *Journal of the American Academy of Dermatology* 4, 181–94.

Diesk, A. and Pannush, R.S. (1981). Factitial Weber–Christian disease: a case report. *Journal of Rheumatology* 8, 129–32.

Garcia-Porrua, C., Gonzalez-Gay, M.A., Vazquez-Caruncho, M., Lopez-Lazaro, L., Lueiro, M., Fernandez, M.L., Alvarez-Ferreira, J., and Pujol, R.M. (2000). Erythema nodosum: etiologic and predictive factors in a defined population. *Arthritis and Rheumatism* 43, 584–92.

Garty, B.Z. and Poznanski, O. (2000). Erythema nodosum in Israeli children. *Israeli Medical Association Journal* 2, 145–6.

Huber, R.M. and Asaad, D.M. (1986). Panniculitis associated with a pancreas difusum. *Journal of the American Academy of Dermatology* 14, 331–4.

Ivker, R.A., Woosley, J., and Briggaman, R.A. (1995). Calciphylaxis in three patients with end-stage renal disease. *Archives of Dermatology* 131, 63–8.

Izumi, A.K. (1985). Lupus erythematosus panniculitis. *Clinics in Dermatology* 3, 69–78.

Jorizzo, J.L., White, W.L., Zanolli, M.D., Greer, K.E., Solomon, A.R., and Jetton, R.L. (1991). Sclerosing panniculitis: a clinicopathologic assessment. *Archives of Dermatology* 127, 544–8.

Kakourou, T., Drosatou, P., Psychou, F., Aroni, K., and Nicolaidou, P. (2001). Erythema nodosum in children: a prospective study. *Journal of the American Academy of Dermatology* 44, 17–21.

Lehman, D.W. (1980). Control of chronic erythema nodosum with naproxen. *Cutis* 26, 66–7.

Lemley, D.E. et al. (1991). Cardiac manifestations of Weber–Christian disease: report and review of the literature. *Journal of Rheumatology* 18, 756–60.

Lupton, G.P., Slagel, G.A., and Distelmeier, M.R. (1988). Treatment of nodular vasculitis with colchicine. *Journal of the Association of Military Dermatology* 14, 24–6.

Mana, J., Gomez-Vaquero, C., Montero, A., Salazar, A., Marcoval, J., Valverde, J., Manresa, F., and Pujol R. (1999). Lofgren's syndrome revisited: a study of 186 patients. *American Journal of Medicine* 107, 240–5.

Martens, P.B., Moder, K.G., and Ahmed, I. (1999). Lupus panniculitis: clinical perspectives from a case series. *Journal of Rheumatology* 26, 68–72.

Melchiorre, L.P., Jr., Rose, C.D., Hyde, P.M., Yussen, P.S., and Connard, K.A. (2000). Lipophagic granulomatous panniculitis with lipoatrophy mimicking arthritis with pitting edema. *Journal of Rheumatology* 27, 504–6.

Panush, R.S., Vonker, R.A., Diesk, A., Langley, S., and Caldwell, J.R. (1985). Weber–Christian disease. *Medicine* 64, 181–90.

Patterson, J.W. (1987). Panniculitis: new findings in the third compartment. *Archives of Dermatology* 123, 1615–18.

Perniciaro, C., Winkelmann, R.K., and Ehrhardt, D.R. (1994). Fatal systemic cytophagic histiocytic panniculitis: a histopathological and immunohistochemical study of multiple organ sites. *Journal of the American Academy of Dermatology* 31, 901–5.

Peters, M.S. and Winkelmann, R.K. (1980). Localized lipoatrophy (atrophic connective tissue disease panniculitis). *Archives of Dermatology* 116, 1363–8.

Prestes, C.A., Winkelmann, R.K., and Su, W.P.D. (1990). Septal granulomatous panniculitis: comparison of the pathology of erythema nodosum migrans (migratory panniculitis) and chronic erythema nodosum. *Journal of the American Academy of Dermatology* 22, 477–83.

Psychos, D.N., Voulgari, P.V., Skopouli, F.N., Drosos, A.A., and Moutsopoulos, H.M. (2000). Erythema nodosum: the underlying conditions. *Clinical Rheumatology* 19, 212–16.

Roenigk, H.H., Haserick, J.R., and Arundell, F.D. (1964). Post steroid panniculitis. Report of a case and review of the literature. *Archives of Dermatology* 90, 387–91.

Roth, D.E., Schickler, K., and Callen, J.P. (1989). Annular atrophic connective tissue panniculitis of the ankles. *Journal of the American Academy of Dermatology* 21, 1152–6.

Simkin, P.A., Brunzell, J.D., Wisner, D., Fiechter, J.R., Cardin, J.S., and Wilkins, R.F. (1983). Free fatty acids in the pancreatic arthritis syndrome. *Arthritis and Rheumatism* 26, 127–32.

Smith, K.C., Pittelkow, M.R., and Su, W.P.D. (1987). Panniculitis associated with severe α-1-antitrypsin deficiency. *Archives of Dermatology* 123, 1655–61.

Smith, K.C., Su, W.P.D., Pittelkow, M.R., and Winkelmann, R.K. (1989). Clinical and pathologic correlations with 96 patients with panniculitis, including 15 patients with deficient levels of α_1-antitrypsin. *Journal of the American Academy of Dermatology* 21, 1192–6.

Soderstrom, R.M. (1982). Erythema nodosum: an update. *Current Concepts in Skin Diseases.* Spring, 3–7.

Ter Poorten, M.C. and Thiers, B.H. (2002). Panniculitis. *Dermatologic Clinics of North America* 20, 421–33.

Usuki, K., Kitamura, K., Urabe, A., and Takakin, F. (1988). Successful treatment of Weber–Christian disease by cyclosporin A. *American Journal of Medicine* 85, 276–8.

Weenig, R.H., Ng, C.S., and Perniciaro, C. (2001). Subcutaneous panniculitis-like T-cell lymphoma. An elusive case presenting as lipomembranous panniculitis and a review of 72 cases in the literature. *American Journal of Dermatopathology* 23, 206–15.

White, J.W. and Winkelmann, R.K. (1998). Weber–Christian panniculitis: a review of 30 cases with this diagnosis. *Journal of the American Academy of Dermatology* 39, 56–62.

White, W.L., Sherertz, E.F., Berg, D., and Clark, R.E. (1993). Periparotid lupus erythematosus panniculitis. *Archives of Pathology and Laboratory Medicine* 117, 535–9.

Wilson, H.A., Askar, A.D., Neiderhizer, D.H., Johnson, M., Andrew, B.S., and Hoskins, L.C. (1983). Panniculitis with atrophy and subcutaneous fat necrosis. *Arthritis and Rheumatism* 26, 121–6.

Winkelmann, R.K. (1983). Panniculitis in connective tissue diseases. *Archives of Dermatology* 119, 336–44.

Winkelmann, R.K., McEvoy, M.T., and Peters, M.S. (1989). Lipophagic panniculitis of childhood. *Journal of the American Academy of Dermatology* 21, 971–8.

Zimmerman-Gorska, I., Urbaniak, M., and Karwowski, A. (1986). Coexistence of arthritis, subcutaneous fat necrosis, and pseudocyst of pancreas. *Rheumatology International* 6, 45–58.

6.12.5 Neutrophilic dermatoses

Jeffrey P. Callen

The neutrophilic dermatoses are a group of non-infectious disorders characterized by the presence of an angiocentric, vessel-based, primary neutrophilic inflammatory cell infiltrate (Table 1) (Jorizzo 1988). These disorders can be further divided into those which lead to destruction of vessel walls (vasculitis) and those that do not destroy the vessels. The disorders to be discussed in this chapter will be those in which the vessel wall is not destroyed. For a full discussion of Behçet's disease see Chapter 6.10.8, for vasculitides see Chapters 6.10.1–6.10.9, and for familial Mediterranean fever see Chapter 6.12.2. The remaining disorders are linked by the presence of similar associated processes, massive cutaneous neutrophilic infiltrates, occasionally overlapping clinical features, and similar approaches to therapy.

Sweet's syndrome (acute febrile neutrophilic dermatosis)

In 1964, R.D. Sweet described a group of patients with one or more attacks of painful, erythematous plaques, accompanied by fever, arthralgias, and leucocytosis (Sweet 1964). The histopathological correlate was a massive neutrophilic infiltration of the dermis in the absence of vessel wall destruction or demonstrable infection. Sweet termed the process acute febrile neutrophilic dermatosis, but it has become known as Sweet's syndrome (Cohen and Kurzrock 2000).

Table 1 Non-infectious neutrophilic dermatoses

I *Non-angiocentric*
Psoriasis
Reiter's syndrome
Subcorneal pustular dermatosis
Acne fulminans
Blastomycosis-like pyoderma (pyoderma vegetans)
II *Angiocentric*
(A) Vessel wall destruction
1. Leucocytoclastic vasculitis
2. Polyarteritis nodosa
(B) No vessel wall destruction
1. Acute febrile neutrophilic dermatosis (Sweet's syndrome)
(a) Typical
(b) Atypical (cancer-associated) variant
2. Pyoderma gangrenosum
(a) Typical
(b) Atypical (cancer-associated) variant
3. 'Pustular vasculitis'
(a) Behçet's disease
(b) Bowel-associated dermatosis–arthritis syndrome
4. Rheumatoid neutrophilic dermatosis
5. Pyostomatitis vegetans
6. Pustular eruption of ulcerative colitis
7. Familial Mediterranean fever
8. Neutrophilic eccrine hidradenitis

Source: Derived from Jorizzo (1988).

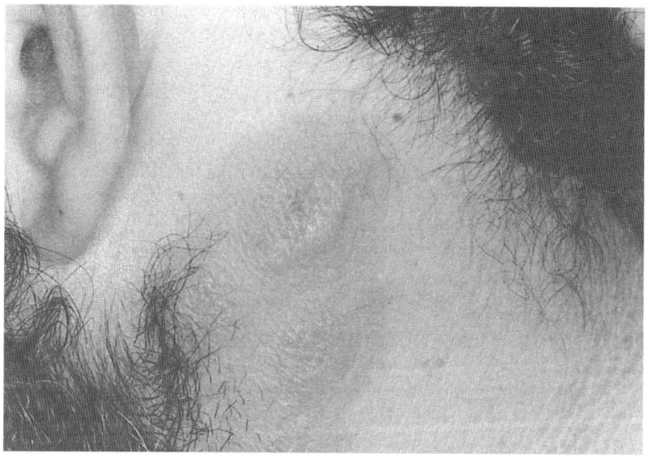

Fig. 1 Sweet's syndrome. This patient developed erythematous plaques with a central mammillated 'microvesicular' surface.

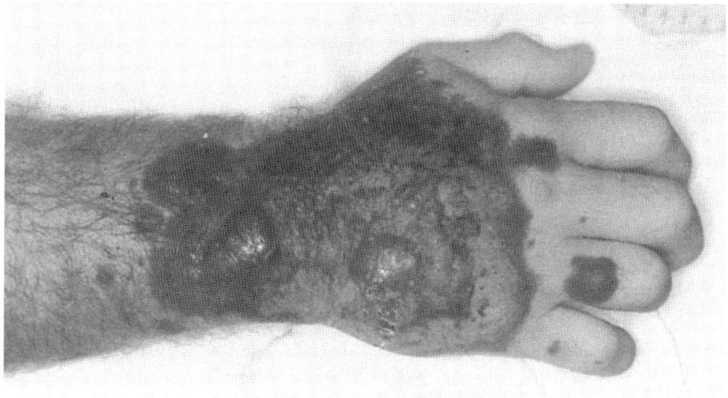

Fig. 2 Sweet's syndrome in a patient with acute myelogenous leukaemia. The purpura is due to bleeding into the lesions associated with thrombocytopaenia.

This syndrome is more frequent in women (3.7 : 1) between the ages of 30 and 70 years (mean age 52.6 years). Children with Sweet's syndrome have also been reported (Boatman et al. 1994). The disease may be preceded by symptoms suggestive of an upper respiratory tract infection. The characteristic lesion is a well-defined, erythematous plaque with a mammillated surface, which may give the clinical impression of microvesiculation (Fig. 1). The lesions usually heal without scar formation. Pustules may stud the surface or may be a major feature of the process. An uncommon clinical variant is a tender, erythematous nodule, which clinically resembles erythema nodosum (Cohen et al. 1992). Genital lesions have been reported, but are rare (Banet et al. 1994). The lesions occur in crops, and may be initiated by a variety of traumatic injuries (pathergy) such as a needle stick, wound debridement, or burn. Fever and malaise occurs in most patients, and myalgias and/or arthralgias in about half. Headache, nausea, vomiting, diarrhoea, and/or conjunctivitis may also occur in some patients. Untreated lesions resolve over 6–8 weeks; however, many patients continue to produce new lesions chronically or recurrently.

The laboratory findings include a leukocytosis, ranging from 10 000 to 20 000/mm^3, composed of mature neutrophils. The remainder of the blood count is normal, except in patients with leukaemia-associated Sweet's syndrome. The erythrocyte sedimentation rate is frequently elevated. Biopsy reveals a dense dermal infiltrate composed of mature polymorphonuclear leucocytes, often more pronounced in perivascular areas. The classic description suggests that the vessel walls are spared, however, Malone et al. (2002) demonstrated that vascular inflammation is frequent and correlates with the age of the lesion. Immunofluorescence microscopy has been negative in a small number of cases reported.

Sweet's syndrome has been reported in association with a variety of diseases that can be subdivided into four groups: (i) classic or idiopathic, (ii) parainflammatory, either infectious diseases or disorders of the immune system, (iii) paraneoplastic, and (iv) pregnancy associated (Cohen and Kurzrock 2000). While idiopathic cases are the most frequent, paraneoplastic Sweet's syndrome is the most frequently identified association and myelogenous leukaemia or preleukaemic states such as a myelodysplastic syndrome account for most of the paraneoplastic conditions. Sweet's syndrome is not clinically or histopathologically different among the four groups; however, in the presence of leukaemia or myelodsyplasia, the patients tend to be anaemic or thrombocytopaenic and may have haemorrhagic lesions (Fig. 2). Parainflammatory Sweet's syndrome has also been reported primarily in conjunction with inflammatory bowel disease, but rheumatoid arthritis, Behçet's disease, sarcoidosis, thyroiditis, and erythema nodosum have also been reported (Cohen and Kurzrock 2000). The strongest links for infections are those of the upper respiratory tract, but HIV, hepatitis, mycobacteria, cytomegalovirus, and salmonella have all been reported. There are several drugs that have been reported to be associated with Sweet's syndrome, including granulocyte-colony stimulating factor, minocycline, nitrofurantoin, trimethoprim-sulfamethoxazole, carbamazepine, hydralazine, and all-*trans*-retinoic acid.

Recent reports have focused on extracutaneous disease that may occur in patients with Sweet's syndrome as well as other neutrophilic dermatoses (Vignon-Pennamen 2000). Neutrophilic infiltration of the lungs, myocardium, muscles (Marie et al. 2001), central nervous system (Hisanaga et al. 1999), eyes (Newman and Frank 1993), and bone has been reported in multiple patients. Pulmonary infiltrates that might even cavitate have been reported (Brown et al. 2000). The eye disease that seems to be frequently reported is known as peripheral ulcerative keratitis (Wilson et al. 1999). The bony lesion that occurs is known as multifocal sterile osteomyelitis.

The pathogenesis of Sweet's syndrome is not known. Tests for circulating immune complexes, tissue-bound immunoglobulins, or complement have generally been negative. Kemmett and Hunter (1990) reported perinuclear antineutrophil cytoplasmic antibodies (p-ANCA) in six patients with Sweet's syndrome, but believed this to be an epiphenomenon. Von den Driesch (1994) was unable to demonstrate p- or c-ANCA in any of his 10 patients who were tested. Studies of neutrophil function have not shown a consistent abnormality. Furthermore, abnormalities of T cells and proinflammatory cytokines such as γ-interferon or interleukin-8 have not been reproducibly reported.

The diagnosis of Sweet's syndrome is one of exclusion. Infections, neoplasia, vasculitis, and factitial disease must be excluded. The lesion at times is difficult to differentiate from erythema nodosum, erythema elevatum diutinum, and small-vessel vasculitis. In addition, in my opinion there is overlap with several other neutrophilic dermatoses such as pustular eruption of ulcerative colitis, bowel bypass syndrome, and rheumatoid neutrophilic dermatosis. Lastly, patients with Behçet's disease or inflammatory bowel disease may have Sweet-like lesions and there may be confusion regarding nomenclature and classification of such patients.

Sweet's syndrome is usually an acute, steroid-responsive, self-limited disease. In general, a 2-week tapering course of oral prednisone (40–60 mg/day) is effective. One or more exacerbations requiring brief reinstitution of corticosteroids are common. From Sweet's initial report and the many later ones, it appears that the process can follow a chronic course, and the use of steroid-sparing agents should be considered. In reports of individual or small groups of patients, dapsone, potassium iodide, indomethacin, doxycycline, clofazimine, colchicine, metronidazole, isotretinoin, methotrexate, chlorambucil, cyclosporin (von den Driesch et al. 1994), and pulse dosage of methylprednisolone have been successfully used (Callen 2002).

Pyoderma gangrenosum

Pyoderma gangrenosum (PG) is an uncommon, ulcerative, cutaneous condition with distinctive clinical characteristics (Callen 1998). Frequently there is an associated systemic disease. The diagnosis is made by exclusion of other processes that may cause cutaneous ulcers. Like patients with Sweet's syndrome, patients with pyoderma gangrenosum are often pathergic, with lesions sometimes developing after minor trauma.

There are two variants that account for most of the cases of PG—the typical (classical) form and the atypical, more superficial form (Bennett et al. 2000). These two differ in their clinical manifestations, their associations with systemic diseases and their responsiveness to corticosteroids.

The ulcerations of typical (classical) PG are frequently clinically characteristic. The border is well defined with a deep erythematous to violaceous colour (Fig. 3). The lesion extends peripherally and often the border overhangs the ulceration (undermined) as the inflammatory process spreads within the dermis. The lesions may be single, or may occur in crops, often beginning as a discrete pustule with a surrounding inflammatory erythema. The lesions may occur on any surface, but are most common on the legs. Pain is a prominent feature and is sometimes so severe that narcotics are required for symptomatic relief. As the lesion heals, scar formation occurs and the resulting scar is often described as cribriform. These patients frequently have an association with inflammatory bowel disease or a polyarthritis.

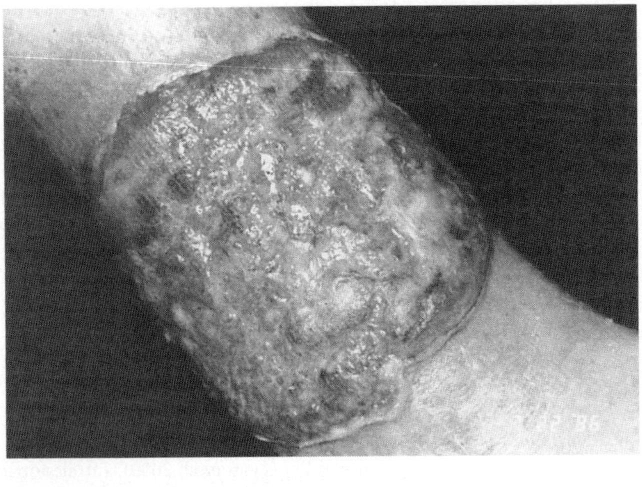

Fig. 3 Pyoderma gangrenosum. Typical large ulceration with an undermined violaceous border.

Several variants other than the classical and atypical forms have been described. The pustular eruption of ulcerative colitis was first reported by O'Loughlin and Perry (1978). In this process the patient is acutely ill with fever and develops multiple sterile pustules (Fenske et al. 1983; Callen and Woo 1985). The lesions may regress without scarring, or some may progress into a typical lesion of PG. Biopsy of the early lesion reveals sheets of mature polymorphonuclear leucocytes.

Peristomal PG is a recently recognized variant that occurs primarily in patients with inflammatory bowel disease, but may also occur in patients who have had abdominal surgery for cancer with the creation of an ileostomy, colostomy, or urostomy (Hughes et al. 2000). The ulceration (Plate 175) may occur as an early or late phenomenon. Perhaps irritation from the ileostomy or colostomy appliance is involved in the induction of this process (pathergy). These ulcerations must be differentiated from infections, dermatitis, or extension of the underlying bowel disease (Crohn's only). Patients with this variant may be discovered to have active inflammation of the bowels and thus even those with a history of ulcerative colitis whose entire large colon has been resected or those patients that develop the process following cancer surgery should be studied for the possibility that Crohn's disease is present. These patients may respond to excision of actively inflamed bowel (Sheldon et al. 2000), to antibiotics such as dapsone or metronidazole, to topical agents such as superpotent corticosteroids or tacrolimus (Lyon et al. 2000), to infliximab as used for Crohn's disease (Hughes et al. 2000), or may require more aggressive therapies.

Vulvar PG is another variant (McCalmont et al. 1991). Except for its location, the ulceration is otherwise typical of PG. This variant should be differentiated from Behçet's disease.

Another variant is pyostomatitis vegetans. This process is one in which chronic, pustular, eventually vegetative erosions develop on the mucous membranes, most notably in the oral cavity (Van Hale et al. 1985). Most of these patients have had inflammatory bowel disease, and some have had ulcerative skin lesions similar to PG (Storwick et al. 1994).

A condition known as malignant pyoderma is distinguished from PG by three features: (i) lesions predominantly on the head and neck (atypical for PG), (ii) lack of associated systemic diseases, and (iii) the absence of undermined borders and surrounding erythema (Perry et al. 1968). The distinctiveness of this variant has been questioned (Wernikoff et al. 1987).

Lastly, there is a variant known as atypical or bullous PG. In this, the ulceration is more superficial, there is often a bullous, blue-grey margin (Plate 176), and the upper extremities and face are more commonly affected (Perry and Winkelmann 1962). In rare instances patients may have typical PG on the legs and atypical PG on the arms/hands. An entity termed pustular vasculitis of the dorsal hands (later termed neutrophilic dermatosis of the dorsal hands) is in my view a variant of atypical PG (Galaria et al. 2000). Atypical PG has been reported primarily with haematological disease, primarily myelodysplastic conditions (Bennett et al. 2000), or acute myelogenous leukaemia. At times the separation of atypical PG from leukaemia-associated Sweet's syndrome is difficult.

The histopathological features of PG are not specific, but are useful in ruling out other causes of cutaneous ulceration. There is controversy over what is the initial histopathological change, with some classifying the process as a neutrophilic dermatosis (Jorizzo 1988), and others believing that the initial changes involve lymphocytic infiltrate, endothelial cell swelling, and fibrinoid necrosis of the vessel wall (a lymphocytic vasculitis) (Su et al. 1986). Regardless, the lesion does not involve a leucocytoclastic vasculitis, nor is granuloma formation compatible with a diagnosis of PG.

The aetiology and pathogenesis of PG are not understood, but a variety of abnormalities of the immune system have been described. Although

Table 2 Diseases associated with pyoderma gangrenosum

Common associations
Inflammatory bowel disease
Chronic ulcerative colitis
Regional enteritis, granulomatous colitis (Crohn's disease)
Arthritis
Seronegative with inflammatory bowel disease
Seronegative without inflammatory bowel disease
Rheumatoid arthritis
Spondylitis
Osteoarthritis
Psoriatic arthritis
Haematological diseases
Myelocytic leukaemias
Hairy cell leukaemia
Myelofibrosis, myeloid metaplasia
Monoclonal gammopathy (IgA)
Rarely reported associations
Chronic active hepatitis
Myeloma
Polycythaemia rubra vera
Paroxysmal nocturnal haemoglobinuria
Takayasu's arteritis
Primary biliary cirrhosis
Systemic lupus erythematosus
Wegener's granulomatosis
Hidradenitis suppurativa
Acne conglobata
Solid tumours
Thyroid disease
Pulmonary disease
Sarcoidosis
Diabetes mellitus
Deficiency of the seventh component of complement (C7)

associated conditions are common (Table 2), perhaps a quarter to a half of the patients has 'idiopathic' disease. The most common associated conditions are inflammatory bowel disease, arthritis, paraproteinaemia, and haematological malignancy and their frequency varies with the clinical variant of PG that is present.

Initial reports of PG emphasized the association with ulcerative colitis (Perry 1959). Eventually, it has become recognized that regional enteritis and Crohn's disease (granulomatous colitis) are found with PG as often as ulcerative colitis (Powell et al. 1985; Prystowsky et al. 1989). In the most recent accounts, inflammatory bowel disease has constituted about 15–20 per cent of the associated phenomena. In addition, early reports stressed the relationship of PG to the activity of the bowel disease, and even suggested that some patients' PG lesions may benefit from surgical resection of the inflamed bowel (ulcerative colitis only) (Cox et al. 1986). Callen et al. (1989) have reported PG in association with inactive terminal ileitis, and Talansky et al. (1983) also have reported lack of effect of bowel resection in some patients with PG and ulcerative colitis.

Arthritis is a frequent finding with PG. In some of the later reports, arthritis has been the most frequent associated condition (Powell et al. 1985; Prystowsky et al. 1989). Five of the nine patients with arthritis reported by Prystowsky et al. (1989) had inflammatory bowel disease associated arthritis. In general, the arthritis associated with PG is a symmetrical polyarthritis, which may be seronegative or seropositive. Spondylitis, although it may occur in conjunction with inflammatory bowel disease associated with PG, has not been reported independently with PG.

A variety of malignancies have been reported with PG, most commonly myelogenous leukaemia or preleukaemia. This association may be more common with the atypical variants of PG. Although a variety of solid tumours have been reported, their presence is probably coincidental.

Table 3 Diagnostic evaluation of the patient with pyoderma gangrenosum

Careful history and thorough physical examination
Skin biopsy with tissue taken for cultures (bacterial, fungal, and/or viral)
Studies of the gastrointestinal tract
Studies for possible abnormal serum proteins, antiphospholipid antibodies
Complete blood count, examination of the peripheral smear, and possible bone marrow examination

Paraproteinaemia, in general a benign variety, has been reported with PG. With newer techniques of protein separation, it appears that 15 per cent of patients with PG may have a benign monoclonal gammopathy, most often of IgA variety (Murray 1983; Prystowsky et al. 1989). The development of myeloma inpatients with PG has been reported (Jackson and Callen 1997), but is very rare.

The diagnostic evaluation (Table 3) of the patient presumed to have PG has two objectives: (i) to rule out other causes of cutaneous ulceration, and (ii) to determine whether there is a treatable, systemic, associated disorder. There is not a specific laboratory or histopathological test that is diagnostic. Moreover, some of the associated disease processes may be clinically silent.

The differential diagnoses of ulcerative cutaneous lesions include: (i) infectious diseases, (ii) halogenodermas, (iii) vasculitis, (iv) insect bites, (v) venous or arterial insufficiency (including occlusive disease associated with antiphospolipid antibodies), and (vi) factitial ulcerations. Cultures should be taken from both exudates and tissues.

To test for the presence of an associated disorder, another series of examinations should be made. A thorough historical evaluation and examination of the gastrointestinal tract should be undertaken in conjunction with a gastroenterologist. Radiographic procedures may include an upper gastrointestinal series and a barium enema. Flexible sigmoidoscopy or colonoscopy, or both, may also be done, with appropriate biopsies being taken. A complete blood count, careful evaluation of the peripheral smear, and possibly a bone marrow aspirate or biopsy will help rule out the presence of an associated haematological malignant process. Serum protein electrophoresis, serum immunodiffusion studies, and possibly, serum and urine immunoelectrophoresis will help to eliminate a diagnosis of an associated monoclonal gammopathy or myeloma. Multiple reports of PG-like leg ulcers in patients with antiphospholipid antibodies have appeared and tests such as VDRL, anticardiolipin antibody, and partial thromboplastin time are now standard in the evaluation of a patient with PG.

There is not a uniformly effective treatment for PG. Although systemic treatment may affect the underlying disease process in some patients with chronic ulcerative colitis (Mir-Madjlessi et al. 1985), it sometimes becomes necessary to consider colectomy. Some patients' skin lesions will respond to bowel resection or therapies aimed at control of the bowel disease (e.g. infliximab for Crohn's disease), but there are patients with presumed ulcerative colitis in whom total colectomy, including removal of the rectosigmoid colon, does not lead to a remission (Talansky et al. 1983). It is possible that in retrospect the more appropriate diagnosis for the inflammatory bowel disease was Crohn's colitis rather than ulcerative colitis.

In mild cases of PG, local measures, such as dressings, elevation, rest, topical agents, or intralesional injections may be sufficient to control the disease process. Compresses, wet to dry dressings, or the newer bio-occlusive semi-permeable dressings may be useful. Cleansing or therapies with antibacterial agents such as hydrogen peroxide or benzoyl peroxide have been reported to be beneficial in an occasional patient. Hyperbaric oxygen has also been reported, in a small number of cases, to be effective. Superpotent topical corticosteroids or topical tacrolimus might be beneficial, particularly in those patients with peristomal PG (Lyon et al. 2000). Intralesional injections of corticosteroids may be beneficial in some patients. Other topical approaches include the use of sodium cromoglycate, nitrogen mustard, and 5-aminosalicyclic acid (Callen 1998).

In patients who do not respond to topical or local therapies, or in whom a severe, rapid course warrants the use of a systemic agent, sulfonamides, sulfones, or corticosteroids have been the most commonly used agents. Perry (1959) reported that oral sulfasalazine is effective in patients both with and without inflammatory bowel disease. Dapsone in doses of up to 400 mg/day has often been used as a monotherapy, or as an adjunctive steroid-sparing agent. Usually the drug is administered in lower doses (100–150 mg/day), and the usual precautions and pretherapy evaluation are necessary. The mechanism of action of the sulfonamides and sulfones in this process is not understood, but effects on the polymorphonuclear leucocyte may be a factor. Another antileprosy agent, clofazimine, has also been reported to be successful in some patients with PG. Finally, several other antibiotics have been used successfully in individual cases; these include minocycline and rifampicin.

Systemic corticosteroids have been used extensively in patients with PG and its variants are generally believed to be very effective. Usually, large doses (40–120 mg/day) are necessary in order to induce a remission of the disease. These doses, used over the long term, will frequently result in steroid-related side-effects. In the studies by Holt et al. (1980), six of their 12 patients treated with corticosteroids developed serious steroid complications, and four of these six died as a result of the therapy. To avoid the complications of long-term steroid use, Johnson and Lazarus (1982), and subsequently others, have used pulse therapy with 1 g of methylprednisolone given intravenously each day for a period of 5 days. Maintenance of the remission was accomplished with oral corticosteroids every other day. Prystowsky et al. (1989) have reported the experience of Lazarus with a further eight patients. They found that remissions occurred in five of the patients, and that they were usually able to remove oral corticosteroid therapy and often lower the dose of other therapies. Pulse therapy is not without side effects, which include sudden death. In the hands of Prystowsky et al., and my experience with three patients, this therapy has primarily resulted in transient hyperglycaemia; however, it should only be used with great caution and proper monitoring.

Immunosuppressive agents have been suggested for use in patients who fail to respond to other therapies, particularly systemic corticosteroids, or who develop steroid-related side effects. Individual reports using oral azathioprine, cyclophosphamide, chlorambucil, cyclosporin tacrolimus, or methotrexate have suggested that, at least in some patients, these agents may be successful (Matis et al. 1992; Burruss et al. 1996; Callen 1998). Intravenous pulses of cyclophosphamide or immunoglobulin have also been successful in individual patients. The mode of action of the immunosuppressive agents is not understood.

With the introduction of biologic therapies for inflammatory bowel disease and rheumatoid arthritis there are now reports of the effectiveness of the antitumour necrosis factor a monoclonal antibody (infliximab) for patients with PG (Tan et al. 2001). Thalidomide may also be useful for individual patients (Federman and Federman 2000). Lastly, although generally it is recommended that surgery be avoided, some patients have successfully been grafted with bioengineered skin when pretreated with an immunosuppressive agent (de Imus et al. 2001).

Rheumatoid neutrophilic dermatitis

Ackerman (1978) described a neutrophilic dermatosis in patients with rheumatoid arthritis. Most patients have seropositive rheumatoid arthritis, but recent reports by Gay-Corsier et al. (2000) and Brown et al. (2001) suggest that the process may occur in seronegative patients. This is apparently a rare manifestation of rheumatoid arthritis, and has only been reported in a small number of patients (Scherbenske et al. 1989; Sanchez and Cruz 1990; Lowe et al. 1992). The patients are described as having symmetric, erythematous nodules and plaques on the extensor surfaces of the joints. There is an apparent predilection for the dorsa of the hands and arms. It is not clear whether this condition is clinically or histopathologically distinct, specifically, whether it can be differentiated from Sweet's syndrome or the atypical variant of PG. An effective therapy includes corticosteroids, dapsone, and colchicine.

Bowel-associated dermatosis–arthritis syndrome

Patients who had undergone bowel bypass surgery for morbid obesity have occasionally developed scattered pustular lesions and arthritis. This became known as the bowel bypass syndrome, and was felt to be an immune-complex disease caused by bacterial overgrowth in the blind loop. Treatment with antibiotics was often effective in clearing the cutaneous lesions and improving the joint symptoms. Later, Jorizzo et al. (1983) coined the term 'bowel-bypass syndrome without bowel bypass' or 'bowel-associated dermatosis–arthritis syndrome'. They reported on four patients with this syndrome of whom two had blind loops due to Billroth II procedures, one had ulcerative colitis, and one had Crohn's disease. Dicken (1984) reported two similar patients who had had Roux-en Y procedures with resultant blind loops. These patients present with a widespread eruption, characterized by pustules on an erythematous or necrotic base. The lesions may be few in number, or may be extensive. Ulceration is rare. The appearance of the lesions is often accompanied by fever, arthralgias or a true inflammatory arthropathy, and myalgias. The arthritis accompanying this process is generally symmetrical, non-deforming, and most frequently involves the small joints such as the wrists, ankles, metacarpophalangeal, proximal interphalangeal, and metatarsophalangeal joints. Histopathologically, the disease resembles Sweet's syndrome. In fact, only after the report by Jorizzo et al. (1983) did we recognize that a patient reported by our group (Bechtel and Callen 1981) probably would have been more correctly diagnosed as having the bowel-associated dermatosis–arthritis syndrome (Plate 177) rather than Sweet's syndrome, because of his prior Billroth II procedure. This disease is presumed to be due to immune complexes (Jorizzo et al. 1984) and while anti-inflammatory therapy is at times helpful, antibiotics frequently control the process, or bowel surgery (to remove 'blind' loops) will reverse it.

Neutrophilic eccrine hidradenitis

Neutrophilic eccrine hidradenitis is a recently described entity that is characterized by erythematous papules, plaques, or nodules most often on acral skin (Bachmeyer and Aractingi 2000). However, the clinical presentation may be varied and includes periorbital inflammation, pustular presentations and disseminated disease. The histopathologic examination of the lesion reveals neutrophilic infiltration that surrounds necrotic eccrine glands. The process is primarily linked to acute myelogenous leukaemia and usually occurs during chemotherapy with cytarabine or an anthracyclin; however, there are instances in which the presence of neutrophilic eccrine hidradenitis heralds the onset of the leukaemia. The process is self-limiting.

References

Ackerman, A. *Histologic Diagnosis of Inflammatory Skin Diseases: A Method by Pattern Analysis.* Philadelphia PA: Lea & Febiger, 1978, pp. 449–50.

Bachmeyer, C. and Arbactingi, S. (2000). Neutrophilic eccrine hidradentitis. *Clinics in Dermatology* **18**, 319–30.

Banet, D.E., McClave, S.A., and Callen, J.P. (1994). Oral metronidazole, an effective treatment for Sweet's syndrome in a patient with associated inflammatory bowel disease. *Journal of Rheumatology* **21** (9), 1766–8.

Bechtel, M.A. and Callen, J.P. (1981). Acute febrile neutrophilic dermatosis (Sweet's syndrome). *Archives of Dermatology* **117**, 664–6.

Bennett, M.L., Jackson, J.M., Jorizzo, J.L., Fleischer, A.B., White, W.L., and Callen, J.P. (2000). Pyoderma gangrenosum. A comparison of typical and atypical forms with an emphasis on time to remission. Case review of 86 patients from 2 institutions. *Medicine (Baltimore)* **79**, 37–46.

Boatman, B.W., Taylor, R.C., Klein, L.E., and Cohen, B.A. (1994). Sweet's syndrome in children. *Southern Medical Journal* **87**, 193–6.

Brown, T.S., Marshall, G.S., and Callen, J.P. (2000). Cavitating pulmonary infiltrate in an adolescent with pyoderma gangrenosum: a rarely recognized extracutaneous manifestation of a neutrophilic dermatosis. *Journal of the American Academy of Dermatology* **43**, 108–12.

Brown, T.S., Fearneyhough, P., Burruss, J.B., and Callen, J.P. (2001). Seronegative rheumatoid neutrophilic dermatosis. *Journal of the American Academy of Dermatology* **45**, 596–600.

Burruss, J.B., Farmer, E., and Callen, J.P. (1996). Chlorambucil is an effective corticosteroid-sparing agent for recalcitrant pyoderma gangrenosum. *Journal of the American Academy of Dermatology* **35**, 720–4.

Callen, J.P. (1998). Pyoderma gangrenosum. *Lancet* **351**, 581–5.

Callen, J.P. (2002). Neutrophilic dermatoses. *Dermatologic Clinics of North America* **20**, 409–19.

Callen, J.P. and Woo, T.Y. (1985). Vesiculopustular eruption in a patient with ulcerative colitis. *Archives of Dermatology* **121**, 339–44.

Callen, J.P., Case, J.D., and Sager, D. (1989). Chlorambucil—an effective corticosteroid-sparing therapy for pyoderma gangrenosum. *Journal of the American Academy of Dermatology* **21** (3 pt 1), 515–19.

Cohen, P.R. and Kurzrock, R. (2000). Sweet's syndrome: a neutrophilic dermatosis classically associated with acute onset and fever. *Clinics in Dermatology* **18**, 265–82.

Cohen, P.R., Holder, W.R., and Rapini, R.P. (1992). Concurrent Sweet's syndrome and erythema nodosum: a report, world literature review and mechanism of pathogenesis. *Journal of Rheumatology* **19**, 814–20.

Cox, N.H., Peebles-Brown, A., and Mackie, R.M. (1986). Pyoderma gangrenosum occurring 10 years after protocolectomy for ulcerative colitis. *British Journal of Hospital Medicine* **36**, 363–5.

de Imus, G., Golomb, C., Wilkel, C., Tsoukas, M., Nowak, M., and Falanga, V. (2001). Accelerated healing of pyoderma gangrenosum treated with bioengineered skin and concomitant immunosuppression. *Journal of the American Academy of Dermatology* **44**, 61–6.

Dicken, C.H. (1984). Bowel-associated dermatosis–arthritis syndrome: bowel bypass syndrome without bowel bypass. *Mayo Clinic Proceedings* **59**, 43–6.

Federman, G.L. and Federman, D.G. (2000). Recalcitrant pyoderma gangrenosum treated with thalidomide. *Mayo Clinic Proceedings* **75**, 842–4.

Fenske, N.A. et al. (1983). Vesiculopustular eruption of ulcerative colitis. *Archives of Dermatology* **119**, 664–9.

Galaria, N.A., Junkins-Hopkins, J.M., Kligman, D., and James, W.D. (2000). Neutrophilic dermatosis of the dorsal hands: pustular vasculitis revisited. *Journal of the American Academy of Dermatology* **43**, 870–4.

Gay-Corsier, F., Dayer, J.M., Charaz, P., and Hauser, C. (2000). Rheumatoid neutrophilic dermatitis/Sweet's syndrome in a patient with seronegative rheumatoid arthritis. *Dermatology* **201**, 185–7.

Hisanaga, K., Hosokawa, M., Sato, N., Mochizuki, H., Itoyama, Y., and Iwasaki, Y. (1999). Neuro-Sweet disease. Benign recurrent encephalitis with neutrophilic dermatosis. *Archives of Neurology* **56**, 1010–13.

Holt, P.J.A. et al. (1980). Pyoderma gangrenosum. *Medicine* **59**, 114–33.

Hughes, A.P., Jackson, M.J., and Callen, J.P. (2000). Clinical features and treatment of peristomal pyoderma gangrenosum. *Journal of the American Medical Association* **284**, 1546–8.

Jackson, J.M. and Callen, J.P. (1997). Pyoderma gangrenosum associated with IgA myeloma. *Journal of Cutaneous Medicine and Surgery* **2**, 100–3.

Johnson, R.B. and Lazarus, G.S. (1982). Pulse therapy. *Archives of Dermatology* **118**, 76–84.

Jorizzo, J.L. (1988). Neutrophilic dermatoses: Sweet's syndrome and pyoderma gangrenosum. In *Inflammation: Basic Principles and Clinical Correlates* (ed. J.I.Gallin, I.M. Goldstein, and R. Synderman), pp. 785–802. New York: Raven Press.

Jorizzo, J.L. et al. (1983). Bowel bypass syndrome without bowel bypass: bowel-associated dermatosis–arthritis syndrome. *Archives of Internal Medicine* **143**, 457–61.

Jorizzo, J.L. et al. (1984). Bowel-associated dermatosis–arthritis syndrome: immune complex-mediated vessel damage and increased neutrophil migration. *Archives of Internal Medicine* **144**, 738–40.

Kemmett, D. and Hunter, J.A.A. (1990). Sweet's syndrome: a clinicopathologic review of twenty-nine cases. *Journal of the American Academy of Dermatology* **23**, 503–7.

Lowe, L., Kornfeld, B., Clayman, J., and Golitz, L.E. (1992). Rheumatoid neutrophilic dermatosis. *Journal of Cutaneous Pathology* **19**, 48–53.

Lyon, C.C., Smith, A.J., Beck, M.H., Wong, G.A.E., and Griffiths, C.E.M. (2000). Parastomal pyoderma gangrenosum: clinical features and management. *Journal of the American Academy of Dermatology* **42**, 992–1002.

Malone, J.C., Slone, S.P., Willis-Frank, L.A., Fearneyhough, P.K., Lear, S.C., Goldsmith, L.J., Hood, A.F., and Callen, J.P. (2002). Vascular inflammation (vasculitis) in Sweet's syndrome—a clinicopathologic study of 28 biopsies from 21 patients. *Archives of Dermatology* **138**, 345–9.

Marie, I., Levesque, H., Joly, P., Reumont, G., Courvile, P., Baudrimont, M., Baubion, D., Cailleux, N., and Courtois, H. (2001). Neutrophilic myositis as an extracutaneous manifestation of neutrophilic dermatosis. *Journal of the American Academy of Dermatology* **44**, 137–9.

Matis, W.L., Ellis, C.N., Griffiths, C.E.M., and Lazarus, G.S. (1992). Treatment of pyoderma gangrenosum with cyclosporine. *Archives of Dermatology* **128**, 1060–4.

McCalmont, C.S., Leshin, B., White, W.L., Greiss, F.C., Jr., and Jorizzo, J.L. (1991). Vulvar pyoderma gangrenosum. *International Journal of Gynecology and Obstetrics* **35**, 175–8.

Mir-Madjlessi, S.H., Taylor, J.S., and Farmer, R.G. (1985). Clinical course and evolution of erythema nodosum and pyoderma gangrenosum in chronic ulcerative colitis: a study of 42 patients. *American Journal of Gastroenterology* **80**, 615–20.

Murray, J.C. (1983). Pyoderma gangrenosum and IgA gammopathy. *Cutis* **32**, 503–7.

Newman, W.P. and Frank, H.J. (1993). Pyoderma gangrenosum of the orbit. *Eye* **7**, 89–94.

O'Loughlin, S. and Perry, H.O. (1978). A diffuse pustular eruption associated with ulcerative colitis. *Archives of Dermatology* **114**, 1061–4.

Perry, H.O. (1959). Pyoderma gangrenosum. *Southern Medical Journal* **62**, 899–908.

Perry, H.O. and Winkelmann, R.K. (1962). Bullous pyoderma gangrenosum and leukemia. *Archives of Dermatology* **106**, 901–5.

Perry, H.O. et al. (1968). Malignant pyoderma. *Archives of Dermatology* **98**, 561–74.

Powell, F.C. et al. (1985). Pyoderma gangrenosum: a review of 86 patients. *Quarterly Journal of Medicine* **55**, 173–86.

Prystowsky, J.H., Kahn, S.N., and Lazarus, G.S. (1989). Present status of pyoderma gangrenosum. *Archives of Dermatology* **125**, 57–64.

Sanchez, J.L. and Cruz, A.(1990). Rheumatoid neutrophilic dermatosis. *Journal of the American Academy of Dermatology* **22**, 922–5.

Scherbenske, J.M., Benson, P.M., and Lupton, G.P. (1989). Rheumatoid neutrophilic dermatosis. *Archives of Dermatology* **125**, 1105–8.

Sheldon, D.G., Sawchuck, L.L., Kozarek, R.A., and Thirlby, R.C. (2000). Twenty cases of peristomal pyoderma gangrenosum. Diagnostic implications and management. *Archives of Surgery* **135**, 564–9.

Storwick, G.S., Prihoda, M.B., Fulton, R.J., and Wood, W.S. (1994). Pyodermatitis–pyostomatitis vegetans: a specific marker for inflammatory bowel disease. *Journal of the American Academy of Dermatology* **31**, 336–41.

Su, W.P.D. et al. (1986). Histopathologic and immunopathologic study of pyoderma gangrenosum. *Journal of Cutaneous Pathology* **13**, 323–30.

Sweet, R.D. (1964). An acute febrile neutrophilic dermatosis. *British Journal of Dermatology* **76**, 349–56.

Talansky, A.L. et al. (1983). Does intestinal resection heal the pyoderma gangrenosum of inflammmatory bowel disease? *Journal of Clinical Gastroenterology* **108**, 580–1.

Tan, M.-H., Gordon, M., Lebwohl, O., George, J., and Lebwohl, M.G. (2001). Improvement of pyoderma gangrenosum and psoriasis associated with Crohn disease with anti-tumor necrosis factor α monoclonal antibody. *Archives of Dermatology* **137**, 930–3.

Van Hale, H.M. et al. (1985). Pyostomatitis vegetans: a reactive mucosal marker for inflammatory disease of the gut. *Archives of Dermatology* **121**, 94–8.

von den Driesch, P. (1994). Sweet's syndrome (acute febrile neutrophilic dermatosis). *Journal of the American Academy of Dermatology* **31**, 535–56.

von den Driesch, P. et al. (1994). Sweet's syndrome: therapy with cyclosporin A. *Clinical and Experimental Dermatology* **19**, 274–7.

Vignon-Pennamen, M.D. (2000). The extracutaneous manifestations in the neutrophilic dermatoses. *Clinics in Dermatology* **18**, 339–48.

Wernikoff, S. et al. (1987). Malignant pyoderma or pyoderma gangrenosum of the head and neck? *Archives of Dermatology* **123**, 371–5.

Wilson, D.M., John, G.R., and Callen, J.P. (1999). Peripheral ulcerative keratitis—an extracutaneous neutrophilic disorder: report of a patient with rheumatoid arthritis, pustular vasculitis, pyoderma gangrenosum, and Sweet's syndrome with an excellent response to cyclosporine therapy. *Journal of the American Academy of Dermatology* **40**, 331–4.

6.12.6 Sarcoidosis

Barry Bresnihan

Sarcoidosis is a multisystem disease most commonly affecting young adults, characterized by the presence of multiple non-caseating granulomas in involved tissues. Symptoms depend on the severity of disease and may resemble other diseases like lymphoma and tuberculosis.

Aetiology

Acute sarcoidosis occurs more frequently during spring months, suggesting environmental agents more common in spring may be involved (Poukkula et al. 1986). Localized outbreaks of sarcoidosis suggest an infectious agent (Jawad et al. 1989; Veale and FitzGerald 1990) and occupation may be relevant (Parks et al. 1979; Edmondstone 1988).

Genetic factors may be important, as there is an increased incidence of sarcoidosis within families. The British Thoracic and Tuberculosis Association (1973) reported 121 cases of sarcoidosis among 59 families. An association between the angiotensin converting enzyme (ACE) DD-genotype and sarcoidosis susceptibility is reported in Afro-Americans, but not Caucasians (Maliarik et al. 1998). An association exists between HLA B8 DR3 in Whites of European ancestry and acute sarcoidosis with arthritis (Hedfors and Lindstrom 1983; Kremer 1986). This genetic profile is associated with many autoimmune diseases (Rybicki et al. 1997). HLA–DR 17(3) is associated with acute sarcoidosis and good prognosis (Berlin et al. 1997). The ACE DD-genotype was associated with poor prognosis in Finnish patients with sarcoidosis (Pietinalho et al. 1999). Prevalence, clinical manifestations, and outcome vary widely in different areas (Milman and Selroos 1990; Newman et al. 1997; Rybicki et al. 1997).

Pathology

The characteristic histological feature of sarcoidosis is a well-defined granuloma, the central area of which is occupied by lymphocytes, predominantly CD4+ mononuclear phagocytes and their progeny (Fig. 1). Caseation is absent, but a small area of fibrinoid necrosis may be present. The outer zone of the granuloma is formed by CD4+ and CD8+ lymphocytes, fibroblasts, mast cells, and other immunoregulatory cells. Sarcoid granulomas are divided into early, intermediate and late, and size varies between 150 and 300 μm.

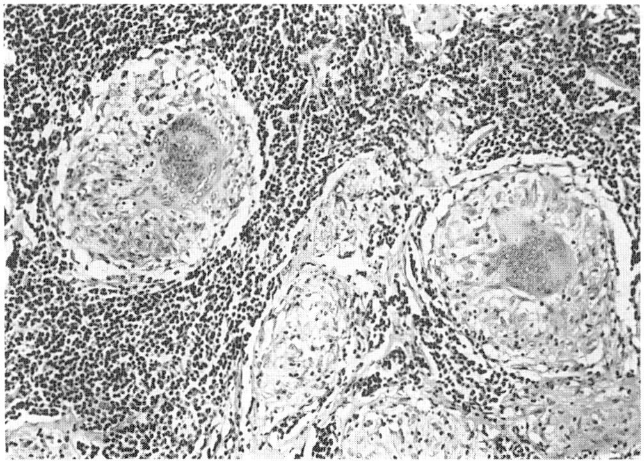

Fig. 1 Sarcoid granuloma. Two well formed non-caseating granulomas are demonstrated in lymph node tissue. Central multinucleated giant cells are present, surrounded by epithelioid cells and some lymphocytes.

Evidence suggests sarcoidosis is the consequence of an antigen-driven, cell-mediated immune response (Agostini et al. 2000; Barnard and Newman 2001). For example, lung type II alveolar epithelial cells, resident alveolar macrophages, and pulmonary dendritic cells function as antigen presenting cells, these cells produce proinflammatory cytokines. IL-12 induces differentiation of CD4+ T lymphocytes into Th1 cells, promoting the release of IFN-γ and IL-2, characteristic of antigen-activated T-cells in a delayed-type hypersensitivity immune response. IL-15 acts synergistically with IL-2 and TNFα, stimulating T lymphocyte proliferation. Dendritic cells are rich sources of IL-12 and may play an important role in the generation of Th1 cells. Pulmonary dendritic cells encounter and process antigen within lung, migrate to the regional lymph nodes, and present the antigen to naive T lymphocytes. Upon activation, T lymphocytes undergo clonal expansion and differentiation into effector and memory T lymphocytes. In sarcoidosis, most T lymphocytes appear to have been previously stimulated, and have migrated back to the affected organ. Studies of the T-cell receptor (TCR) repertoire suggest sarcoidosis is initiated by an antigen-specific immune response (Silver et al. 1996; Trentin et al. 1997).

The release of inflammatory cytokines recruits peripheral blood monocytes to affected organs, where they differentiate into exudate macrophages with an enhanced antigen-presenting capacity releasing TNFα and IL-1β, which promote granuloma formation. TNFα upregulates endothelial cell adhesion molecule expression, stimulates T lymphocyte release of IFN-γ, and enhances T lymphocyte proliferation. IL-1 may participate in granuloma formation by stimulating macrophage production of IL-8 and granulocyte macrophage-colony stimulating factor (GM-CSF) that promotes monocyte differentiation and proliferation. The result is an amplification loop involving antigen recognition, proinflammatory cytokine release, cell activation, and granuloma formation.

Epidemiology

Sarcoidosis is recognized more often in developed than in underdeveloped countries, in Western more than in Far Eastern countries, and in Northern Europe more than in Southern Europe. Moreover, the prevalence within a given region may vary. In the United States, the incidence of sarcoidosis was estimated to be 10.9 per 100 000 population for Caucasians, and 35.5 per 100 000 for Afro-Americans (Rybicki et al. 1997). In Nordic countries an incidence of 15–20 per 100 000 population was reported (Milman and Selroos 1990).

General clinical features

Approximately 50 per cent of patients with sarcoidosis present with pulmonary symptoms (Sharma 1984). A further approximately 20 per cent, present with an abnormal routine chest X-ray, but minimal symptoms. Approximately 25 per cent present with non-specific constitutional symptoms and less than 10 per cent present with features confined to extra-pulmonary systems.

Acute (subacute) sarcoidosis

Acute sarcoidosis may present as an explosive onset illness usually characterized by fever, erythema nodosum, and hilar lymphadenopathy. The association between the last two is often referred to as Lofgren's syndrome (Lofgren 1953) and has a high rate of spontaneous remission and a good prognosis. Chest radiographic appearances return to normal within 1 year of presentation for more than 60 per cent of patients with acute sarcoidosis and rarely recurs.

Chronic sarcoidosis

Chronic sarcoidosis has a subtle onset with an insidious and highly variable clinical course and fibrosis of organs commonly occurs. Chest radiographic appearances include extensive parenchymal infiltration and pulmonary function tests confirm a restrictive lung defect. Fibrosis is induced by cells that participate in the inflammatory response, but it is not known why sarcoidosis becomes chronic in some patients and not others. Clinical manifestations in chronic sarcoidosis include:

- lung—parenchymal disease;
- skin—lupus pernio, skin plaques, or nodules;
- eye—uveitus, conjunctivitis, keratoconjunctivitis sicca;
- lymphatic system—peripheral lymphadenopathy, spenomegaly;
- bone marrow infiltration;
- liver—hepatic granulomata, portal hypertension, hepatic failure;
- kidney—nephrocalcinosis, renal calculi, granulomatous infiltration, glomeral disease, renal arteritis;
- heart—cardiomyopathy, conduction abnormalities;
- nervous system—cranial and peripheral neuropathy, papilloedema, intracerebal lesion, meningitis, seizures, spinal cord involvement, psychiatric disorders;
- endocrine—pituitary, hypothalamus, thyroid, parathyroid, adrenal;
- reproductive organs—ovaries, testes;
- gastrointestinal tract and pancreas;
- salivary and lacrimal glands;
- nose, tonsils, larynx.

Diagnosis

There are no definitive diagnostic tests specific for sarcoidosis. Diagnosis is dependent on clinical appearance, histological demonstration of non-caseating granulomas, and exclusion of other causes. Trans-bronchial lung biopsy is highly sensitive and selective and has become the most widely employed diagnostic technique (Pettersson 2000). Open lung biopsy and medistinal lymph node biopsy are also highly sensitive and selective options, but are more invasive. Other sources for histological diagnosis include scalene nodes, liver, spleen, skin, synovium, muscle, conjunctiva, and the lacrimal and minor salivary glands.

Sarcoidosis was proven histologically in 63 per cent of patients clinically diagnosed with Lofgren's syndrome (Maña et al. 1999). None of the patients without a histologically proven diagnosis developed an alternative disease during follow-up. In a typical case of Lofgren's syndrome, routine biopsy to confirm sarcoidosis is not required, but patients should be followed until resolution of hilar adenopathy. In cases where clinical or radiological appearances are not typical, histological confirmation is strongly recommended to exclude lymphoma, other malignancy, and tuberculosis.

ACE catalyses the conversion of angiotensin I to vasoactive angiotensin II and inactivates bradykinin. It is produced by epitheliod cells in sarcoid granulomas and alveolar macrophages. Elevated levels of serum ACE have been reported in sarcoidosis and other granulomatous and non-granulomatous diseases (Studdy and James 1983; Ainslie and Benatar 1985; Costabel and Yeschler 1997). However, initial serum ACE levels do not predict outcome, but serum ACE levels can be used to monitor the disease and treatment.

Computerized tomography (CT) scans of the thorax are indicated if sarcoidosis is suspected and clinical or chest radiograph findings are atypical or inconclusive. CT scans may show factors undetectable on plain radiography.

Bronchoalveolar lavage (BAL) provides samples of alveolar secretions useful in differential diagnosis, clinical evaluation, and assessing treatment. BAL fluid samples typically demonstrate elevated lymphocyte counts with marked increases in the CD4/CD8 T lymphocyte ratio (Barnard and Newman 2001), usually accompanied by an increase in macrophage numbers.

Gallium-67 citrate scanning of lungs is a sensitive method for detecting granuloma formation in sarcoidosis (Nosal et al. 1979; Beaumont et al. 1982) and reflects disease activity and response to therapy (Line et al. 1981; Klech et al. 1982; Lawrence et al. 1983; Baughmann et al. 1984). Lung uptake of gallium-67 is greatest in acute disease with high serum ACE levels, but does not correlate with pulmonary function measurements, nor clinical course and outcome. It is uncertain why gallium-67 accumulates at sites of granulomatous inflammation. Skin anergy, characterized by a negative tuberculin test, is a typical but not diagnostic feature of sarcoidosis. The Kveim–Siltzbach test is not in general use as the material is not widely available.

Musculoskeletal manifestations

Joint disease

Distinctive patterns of arthropathy are associated with sarcoidosis (Newman et al. 1997; Maña et al. 1999). In acute sarcoidosis, transient flitting arthralgias may precede the emergence of fever, erythema nodosum (Fig. 2), and hilar adenopathy (Fig. 3). Approximately 65 per cent of patients with acute sarcoidosis demonstrate articular features. Signs of inflammation are present, with marked erythema and tenderness of joints, causing pain and limited motion. Arthritis is usually symmetric and migratory, persisting for periods between 3–4 days and 3–4 months. It can be difficult to distinguish erythema nodosum from articular and periarticular inflammation. Ultrasonography has demonstrated that ankle swelling more often represents periarticular swelling and oedema than synovial inflammation (Kellner et al. 1992). Joint effusions are not always detectable, but when present are usually only mildly inflammatory with less than 1000 leucocytes/mm^3, predominantly lymphocytes, and large mononuclear cells. Occasionally, an inflammatory effusion is aspirated with leucocyte counts of more than 40 000/mm^3, predominantly neutrophils. Needle biopsy specimens of synovial membrane in acute sarcoid arthropathy demonstrate mild non-specific synovitis (Kremer 1986) consistent with the clinical impression that much of the inflammation is periarticular.

Chronic arthritis is rare but most frequent in Afro-American populations (Pettersson 2000) and a history of erythema nodosum is usual. Chronic monoarticular arthritis usually involves large joints unless secondary to osseous disease (Schriber and Firooznia 1975). Chronic polyarthritis is more

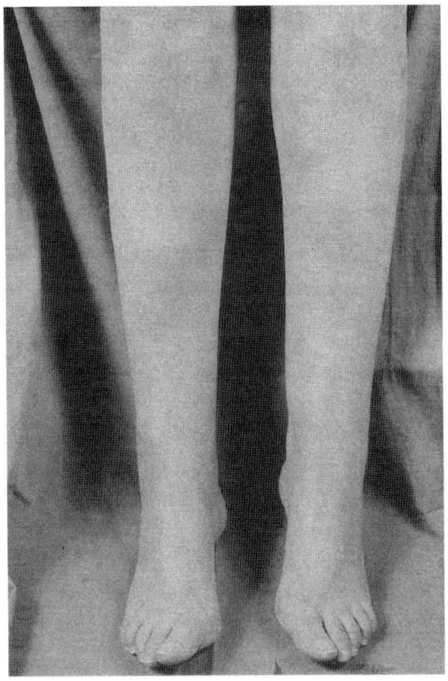

Fig. 2 Erythema nodosum is characteristic of acute sarcoidosis. Tender red swellings appear on the thighs and upper limbs. Resolving erythema nodosum resembles painful bruises. Erythema nodosum usually resolves fully within 3–6 weeks.

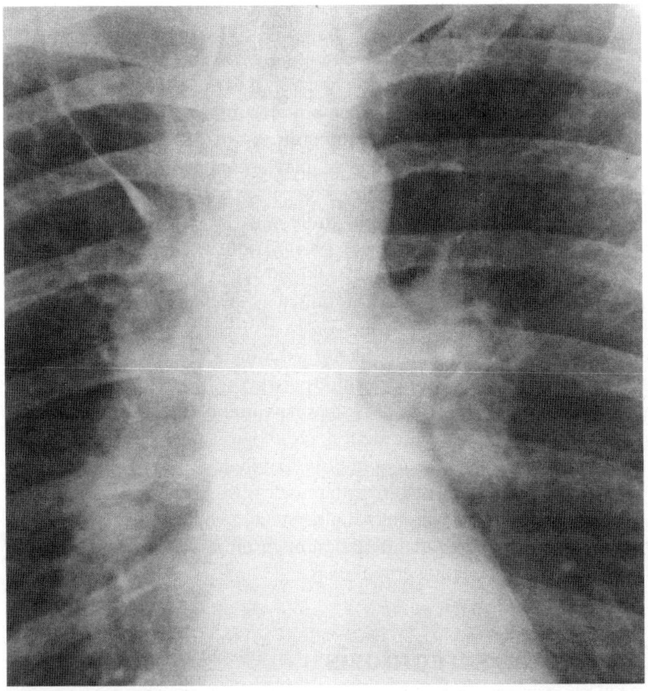

Fig. 3 Bilateral hilar lymphadenopathy due to sarcoidosis may be discovered on routine chest radiography in asymptomatic individuals. It also frequently presents in acute sarcoidosis with fever, erythema nodosum, and arthritis.

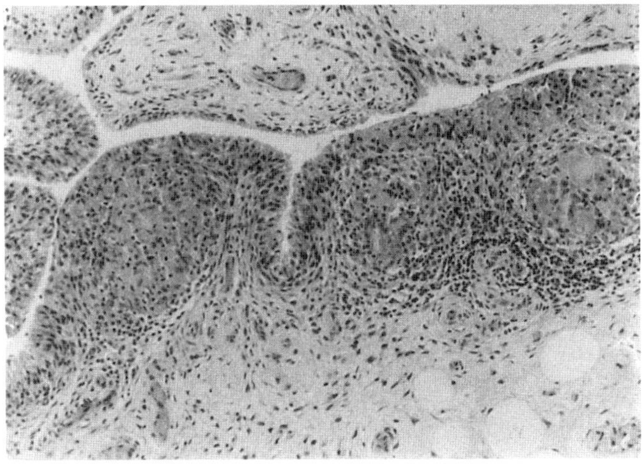

Fig. 4 Chronic synovitis in sarcoidosis, demonstrating synovial lining layer thickening, mononuclear cell infiltration, and non-caseating granuloma formation.

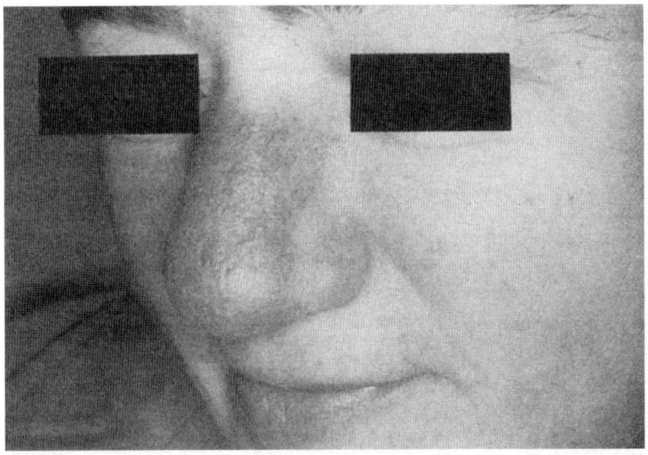

Fig. 5 Lupus pernio, presenting as a bluish-red or violaceous swelling of the nose extended onto the cheek, is characteristic of chronic sarcoidosis and is frequently associated with bone lesions.

frequently observed in women than men. Chronic sarcoid arthritis is characterized by synovial thickening and effusions. Histological examination of synovial membrane may reveal typical non-caseating granulomata (Fig. 4); however, some patients with chronic arthritis have non-specific histological features in synovial membrane (Palmer and Schumacher 1984).

Bone disease

Bone involvement occurs in approximately 5 per cent of patients with sarcoidosis (Neville et al. 1977). Bone cysts containing characteristic granulomata are most frequently observed in hands and feet (Sokoloff and Bunim 1959; Gumpel et al. 1967; James et al. 1976), but are occasionally observed in long bones, pelvis, vertebrae, and the skull (Perlman et al. 1978; Franco-Saenz et al. 1979). Bone lesions are most frequent in persistent disease and particularly so in lupus pernio (Fig. 5). Sarcoidosis limited to osseous disease of fingers and toes has been described (Schriber and Firooznia 1975). Bone lesions can be asymptomatic and may be absent even when obvious bony swelling is present. Bone scanning techniques may be more sensitive than routine radiography at detecting early osseous sarcoidosis (Reginato et al. 1976).

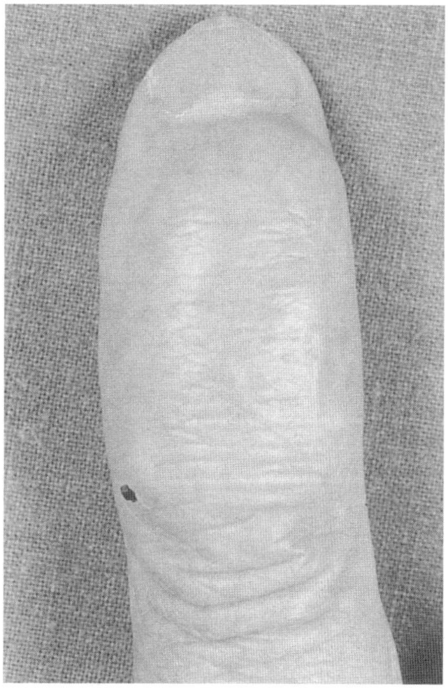

Fig. 6 Sacroid dactylitis caused by granuloma formation in phalanges and surrounding soft tissue.

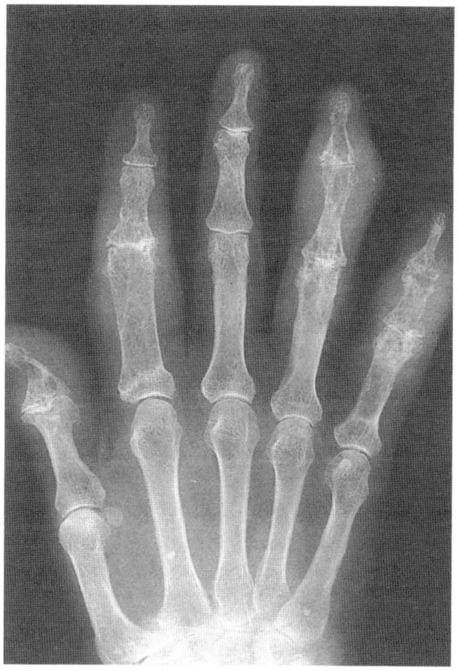

Fig. 8 Bone sarcoidosis involving four digits sparing the middle finger. Soft tissue swelling, bone cysts, and joint space narrowing are prominent. There is expansion of the second proximal phalanx.

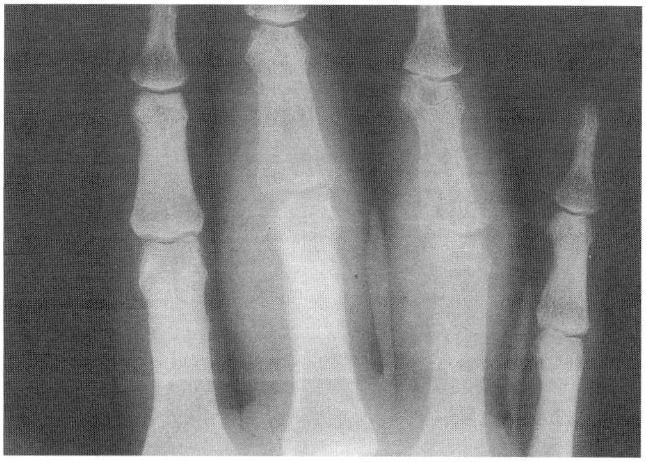

Fig. 7 Bone sarcoidosis of middle and distal phalanges. Several lytic lesions and cortical defects are present.

The most characteristic presentation of osseous sarcoidosis is swollen sausage-like digits with cyst formation in the phalanges (Fig. 6). Radiological examination demonstrates lytic lesions of various sizes, ranging from minute cortical defects to intra-osseous cysts causing diffusely expanded phalanges or cysts in phalangeal or metatarsal heads (Figs 7 and 8). Rarer radiographic changes include thickening of cortical bone with fine reticular lace-like changes of the trabecular pattern and acrosclerosis of distal phalanges or, rarely, gross bony destruction. Osseous sarcoidosis may cause secondary articular changes in the joints of the hands and feet.

Vertebral sarcoidosis may present with back pain or neurological impairment from cord compression. Radiologic examination of the spine demonstrates lytic or sclerotic changes in one or more vertebrae at any level. Pathological fracture is a complication of long bone involvement and skull involvement may appear as multiple lytic defects associated with overlying soft tissue swellings containing granulomata.

Muscle disease

In the early acute stages of sarcoidosis, asymptomatic granulomatous muscle involvement is common, especially in the presence of erythema nodosum, with a prevalence rate ranging between 50 and 80 per cent (Pettersson 2000). Random muscle biopsy is a useful diagnostic procedure for patients presenting with erythema nodosum, but generous sampling and examination of multiple tissue sections.

Symptomatic muscular sarcoidosis may accompany acute sarcoidosis, characterized by fever, severe muscle pain, and tenderness involving proximal upper and lower limb girdle muscles (Wallace et al. 1958; Hinterbuchner and Hinterbuchner 1964; Gardiner-Thorp 1972; Douglas et al. 1973; Lynch and Bansal 1973; Stjernbery et al. 1981). Histological appearances in acute symptomatic muscular sarcoidosis are identical to those in asymptomatic patients and consist of characteristic granulomatous lesions located between apparently normal muscle fibres. The electromyographic features are those of idiopathic polymyositis. A number of patients with isolated sarcoid muscle disease may have granulomata without clinical manifestations and systematic clinical, radiological, and histological evaluation usually reveals evidence of multisystem disease.

A chronic insidious myopathy with muscle wasting and weakness may be associated with chronic persistent multisystem sarcoidosis. Palpable muscle nodules are another rare manifestation of chronic sarcoidosis. Biopsy will demonstrate non-caseating granulomas.

Childhood sarcoidosis

Juvenile sarcoidosis is rare and there are two distinct forms (Hetherington 1982). Older children present with similar features to adults, but children under 4 present a distinct form of the disease, characterized by rash, uveitis, and arthritis/tenosynovitis (Rasmussen 1981; Hetherington 1982; Rosenberg et al. 1983; Clarke 1987). Arthritis usually affects knees

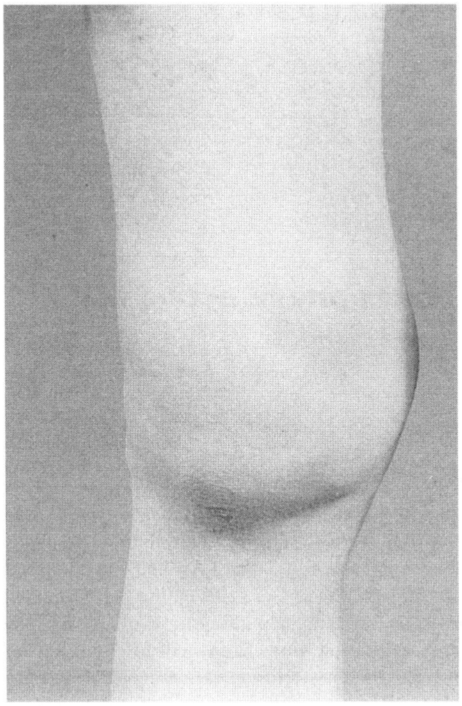

Fig. 9 Chronic sarcoid arthritis with prominent synovial thickening of the knee joint in a 5-year-old boy who also had uveitis.

and ankles and is characterized by boggy synovial or tendon sheath thickening and effusion, causing minimal pain and limitation (Fig. 9). Sarcoid arthritis in children usually follows an indolent clinical course with minimal or no constitutional symptoms, although severe late complications have been described (Fink and Cimaz 1997).

Treatment

Acute sarcoidosis with erythema nodosum and hilar lymphadenopathy is a self-limiting illness, the arthralgias and arthritis are transient, and symptoms are usually relieved by rest and NSAIDs. Occasionally, a short course of corticosteroid therapy may be justified for very acute symptoms. Exacerbations of chronic arthritis are associated with active multisystem disease. Therapeutic decisions depend on severity of non-articular features and most patients will require corticosteroids for control of systemic disease. There are anecdotal reports that disease-modifying drugs, including hydroxychloroquine, methotrexate, azathioprine, cyclosporine, cyclophosphamide, and thalidomide, may be effective (Pettersson 2000). In osseous sarcoidosis and asymptomatic muscle disease, therapy is not indicated for asymptomatic patients. Corticosteroids are prescribed for symptomatic osseous sarcoidosis and healing of lytic and destructive lesions has been documented. Corticosteroids are also recommended for symptomatic patients with muscle disease, though uncertainties remain regarding efficacy, particularly in chronic sarcoid myopathy. Evidence-based treatment protocols for chronic musculoskeletal manifestations of sarcoidosis have not yet been proposed.

References

Agostini, C., Adami, F., and Semenzato, G. (2000). New pathogenetic insights into the sarcoid granuloma. *Current Opinion in Rheumatology* **12**, 71–6.

Ainslie, G.M. and Benatar, S.R. (1985). Serum angiotensin converting enzyme in sarcoidosis: sensitivity and specificity in diagnosis: correlations with disease activity, duration, extra-thoracic involvement, radiographic type and therapy. *Quarterly Journal of Medicine* **55**, 253–70.

Barnard, J. and Newman, L.S. (2001). Sarcoidosis: immunology, rheumatic involvement, and therapeutics. *Current Opinion in Rheumatology* **13**, 84–91.

Baughmann, R.P., Frenandez, M., Bosken, C.H., Mantil, J., and Hurtubise, P. (1984). Comparison of gallium-67 scanning, cronchoalveolar lavage and serum angiotensin-converting enzyme levels in pulmonary sarcoidosis: predicting response to therapy. *American Review of Respiratory Diseases* **129**, 676–81.

Beaumont, D., Herry, S.Y., Sapene, M., Bourguet, P., Larzul, J.J., and DeLabarthe, B. (1982). Gallium 67 in the evaluation of sarcoidosis: correlation with serum angiotensin converting enzyme and bronchoalveolar lavage. *Thorax* **37**, 11–18.

Berlin, M., Fogdell-Hahn, A., Olerup, O., Eklund, A., and Grunewald, J. (1997). HLA–DR predicts the prognosis in Scandinavian patients with pulmonary sarcoidosis. *American Review of Respiratory and Critical Care Medicine* **156**, 1601–5.

British Thoracic and Tuberculosis Association (1973). Familial association in sarcoidosis. *Tubercle* **54**, 87–98.

Clarke, S.K. (1987). Sarcoidosis in children. *Pediatric Dermatology* **4**, 291–9.

Costabel, U. and Yeschler, H. (1997). Biochemical changes in sarcoidosis. *Clinics in Chest Medicine* **18**, 827–42.

Douglas, A.C., MacLeod, J.G., and Matthews, J.D. (1973). Symptomatic sarcoidosis of skeletal muscle. *Journal of Neurology, Neurosurgery and Psychiatry* **36**, 1034–40.

Edmonstone, W.M. (1988). Sarcoidosis in nurses: is there an association? *Thorax* **43**, 342–3.

Fink, C.W. and Cimaz, R. (1997). Early onset sarcoidosis: not a benign disease. *Journal of Rheumatology* **24**, 174–7.

Franco-Saenz, R., Ludwig, G.D., and Henderson, L.W. (1979). Sarcoidosis of the skull. *Annals of Internal Medicine* **72**, 929–31.

Gardiner-Thorp, C. (1972). Muscle weakness due to sarcoid myopathy: six case reports and an evaluation of steroid therapy. *Neurology* **22**, 917–27.

Gumpel, J.M., Johns, C.J., and Shulman, L.E. (1967). The joint disease of sarcoidosis. *Annals of the Rheumatic Diseases* **26**, 194–205.

Hedfors, E. and Lindstrom, F. (1983). HLA-B8/DR3 in sarcoidosis. Correlation to acute onset disease with arthritis. *Tissue Antigens* **22**, 200–3.

Hetherington, S. (1982). Sarcoidosis in young children. *American Journal of Diseases in Children* **136**, 13–15.

Hinterbuchner, C.N. and Hinterbuchner, L.P. (1964). Myopathic syndrome in muscular sarcoidosis. *Brain* **87**, 355–66.

James, D.G., Neville, E., and Carstairs, L.S. (1976). Bone and joint sarcoidosis. *Seminars in Arthritis and Rheumatism* **6**, 53–81.

Jawad, A.S.M., Hamour, A.A., Wenley, W.G., and Scott, D.G. (1989). An outbreak of acute sarcoidosis with arthropathy in Norfolk. *British Journal of Rheumatology* **28**, 178 (letter).

Kellner, H., Spathling, S., and Herzer, P. (1992). Ultrasound findings in Lofgren's syndrome: is ankle swelling caused by arthritis, tenosynovitis or periarthritis? *Journal of Rheumatology* **19**, 38–41.

Klech, H., Kohn, H., Dummer, F., and Mostbeck, A. (1982). Assessment of activity in sarcoidosis; sensitivity and specificity of 67 gallium scintigraphy, serum ace levels, chest roentgenography and blood lymphocytes populations. *Chest* **6**, 732–8.

Kremer, J.M. (1986). Histologic findings in siblings with acute sarcoid arthritis; assocation with the HLA B8, DR3 phenotype. *The Journal of Rheumatology* **13**, 593–7.

Lawrence, E.C., Teague, R.B., Gottlieb, M.S., Jhingran, S.G., and Lieberman, J. (1983). Serial changes in markers of disease activity with corticosteroid treatment in sarcoidosis. *American Journal of Medicine* **74**, 746–7.

Line, B.R., Hunninghake, G.W., Keogh, B.A., Jones, A.E., Johnston, G.S., and Crystal, R.G. (1981). Gallium-67 scanning to stage the alveolitis of sarcoidosis; correlation with clinical studies, pulmonary function studies and bronchoalveolar lavage. *American Review of Respiratory Diseases* **123**, 440–6.

Lofgren, S. (1953). Primary pulmonary sarcoidosis. I. Early signs and symptoms. *Acta Medica Scandinavica* **145**, 424–31.

Lynch, P.G. and Bansal, D.V. (1973). Granulomatous polymyositis. *Journal of the Neurological Sciences* **18**, 1–9.

Maliarik, M.J., Rybicki, B.A., Malvitz, E., Sheffer, R.G., Major, M., Popovich, J., Jr., and Iannuzzi, M.C. (1998). Angiotensin-converting enzyme gene polymorphism and risk of sarcoidosis. *American Journal of Respiratory and Critical Care in Medicine* **158**, 1566–70.

Maña, J., Gomez-Vaquero, C., Montero, A., Salazar, A., Marcoval, J., Valverde, J., Manresa, F., and Pujol, R. (1999). Lofgren's syndrome revisited: a study of 186 patients. *American Journal of Medicine* **107**, 240–5.

Milman, N. and Selroos, O. (1990). Pulmonary sarcoidosis in the Nordic countries 1950–1982: epidemiology and clinical picture. *Sarcoidosis* **7**, 50–7.

Neville, E., Carstairs, L.S., and James, D.G. (1977). Sarcoidosis of bone. *Quarterly Journal of Medicine* **46**, 215–27.

Newman, L., Rose, C., and Maier, L. (1997). Sarcoidosis. *New England Journal of Medicine* **336**,1224–34.

Nosal, A., Schleissner, L.A., Mishkin, F.S., and Lieberman, J. (1979). Angiotensin-converting enzyme and gallium scan in non-invasive evaluation in sarcoidosis. *Annals of Internal Medicine* **90**, 328–31.

Palmer, D.G. and Schumacher, H.R. (1984). Synovitis with non-specific histologic changes in synovium in chronic sarcoidosis. *Annals of the Rheumatic Diseases* **43**, 778–82.

Parks, D.R., Bryan, V.M., Oi, V.M., Oi, V.T., and Hervenberg, L.A. (1979). Antigen specific identification and cloning of hybridomas with a fluorescence activated cell sorter (FACS). *Proceedings of the National Academy of Sciences of the USA* **76**, 1962–6.

Perlman, S.F., Damergis, J., Witorsch, P., Cooney, F.D., Cunther, S.F., and Barth, W.F. (1978). Vertebral sarcoidosis with paravertebral ossification. A case report. *Arthritis and Rheumatism* **21**, 271–6.

Pettersson, T. (2000). Sarcoid and erythema nodosum arthropathies. *Baillierés Clinical Rheumatology* **14**, 461–76.

Pietinalho, A., Furuya, K., Yamaguchi, E., Kawakami, Y., and Selroos, O. (1999). The angiotensin-converting enzyme DD gene is associated with poor prognosis in Finnish sarcoidosis patients. *European Respiratory Journal* **13**, 723–6.

Poukkula, A., Huhti, E., Lilja, A., and Saloheimo, M. (1986). Incidence and clinical picture of sarcoidosis in a circumscribed geographical area. *British Journal of Diseases of Chest* **80**, 138–47.

Rasmussen, J.E. (1981). Sarcoidosis in young children. *Journal of the American Academy of Dermatology* **5**, 566–70.

Reginato, A.J., Schiappaccasse, V., Guzman, L., and Claure, H. (1976). 99m Technetium-pyrophosphate scintiphotography in bone sarcoidosis. *The Journal of Rheumatology* **3**, 426–35.

Rosenberg, A.M., Yee, E.H., and MacKenzie, J.W. (1983). Arthritis in childhood sarcoidosis. *The Journal of Rheumatology* **10**, 987–90.

Rybicki, B.A., Maliarik, M.J., Major, M., Popovich, J., Jr., and Iannuzzi, M.C. (1997). Genetics of sarcoidosis. *Clinics in Chest Medicine* **18**, 707–17.

Schriber, R.A. and Firooznia, H. (1975). Extensive phalangeal cystic lesions. Sarcoidosis limited to the hands and feet? *Arthritis and Rheumatism* **18**, 123–8.

Sharma, O.P. (1984). Clinical features. In *Sarcoidosis—Clinical Management*, pp. 22–4. London: Butterworths.

Silver, R.F., Crystal, R.G., and Moller, D.R. (1996). Limited heterogeneity of biased T-cell receptor Vβ gene usage in lung but not blood T cells in active pulmonary sarcoidosis. *Immunology* **88**, 516–23.

Sokoloff, L. and Bunim, J.J. (1959). Clinical and pathological studies of joint involvement in sarcoidosis. *New England Journal of Medicine* **260**, 841–7.

Stjernbery, N., Cajander, S., Truedsson, H., and Uddenfeldt, P. (1981). Muscle involvement in sarcoidosis. *Acta Medica Scandanavia* **209**, 213–16.

Studdy, P.R. and James, D.G. (1983). The sensitivity and specificity of serum angiotensin-converting enzyme in sarcoidosis and other diseases. In *Ninth International Conference on Sarcoidosis and other Granulomatous Disorders* (ed. J. Chretien, J. Marsac, and J.C. Saltiel), pp. 679–81. Paris: Pergamon Press.

Trentin, L., Zambello, R., Facco, M., Tassinara, C., Sancetta, R., Siviero, M., Cerutti, A., Cipriani, A., Marcer, G., Majori, M., Pesci, A., Agostini, C., and Semenzato, G. (1997). Selection of T lymphocytes bearing limited T-cell receptor Vβ regions in the lung of patients with hypersensitivity pneumonitis and sarcoidosis. *American Journal of Respiratory and Critical Care in Medicine* **155**, 587–96.

Veale, D. and FitzGerald, O. (1990). Acute sarcoid arthropathy—an infective cause? *British Journal of Rheumatology* **29**, 158–9.

Wallace, S.L., Lattes, R., Malia, J.P., and Ragan, C. (1958). Muscle involvement in Boeck's sarcoid. *Annals of Internal Medicine* **48**, 497–511.

6.12.7 Macrophage activation syndrome

Alexei Grom

Introduction

In rheumatology, the term '*macrophage activation syndrome*' refers to a set of clinical symptoms caused by the excessive activation and proliferation of well-differentiated macrophages. It was first described as a complication of systemic onset juvenile rheumatoid arthritis (soJRA) (Hadchouel et al. 1985; Stephan et al. 1993). The pathognomonic features of this syndrome are found in bone marrow aspiration: numerous, well-differentiated macrophages (or histiocytes) actively phagocytosing haematopoietic elements. Such cells may be found in various organs and may account for many of the systemic features of this syndrome. Since in many cases, macrophage activation syndrome (MAS) is triggered by infections or modifications in the drug therapy, the term '*reactive haemophagocytic lymphohistiocytosis*' has also been used to classify this condition.

In turn, *haemophagocytic lymphohistiocytosis* (HLH) is a more general term, which applies to a spectrum of disease processes characterized by accumulations of histologically benign well-differentiated mononuclear cells with a macrophage phenotype (Favara et al. 1997). Since such mononuclear phagocytes represent a subset of histiocytes that are distinct from Langerhans cells, this entity should be distinguished from Langerhans cell histiocytosis as well as other dendritic cell disorders. HLH can be further divided into at least two major groups of conditions which are often difficult to distinguish from each other: primary, or *familial haemophagocytic lymphohistiocytosis* (FHLH), and secondary. The group of secondary haemophagocytic disorders includes *infection associated HLH* (IAHLH) and *malignancy associated HLH*. Although there are many clinical similarities between MAS of soJRA, IAHLH, and FHLH, the exact relationships between these conditions are not understood. This chapter is focused on MAS presenting as a complication of a systemic rheumatic disease.

Although MAS can occur in almost any paediatric or adult rheumatologic disorder, it is by far most common in soJRA. Thus, Hadchouel et al. (1985) described seven JRA patients who acutely presented with a haemorrhagic syndrome associated with mental status changes, hepatosplenomegaly, increased serum levels of liver enzymes, and a sharp fall in blood cell counts and erythrocyte sedimentation rate (ESR). Six of these patients had the systemic form of JRA. Since in most of these patients bone marrow aspiration revealed the presence of numerous non-neoplastic histiocytes with prominent haematophagocytic activity, the authors suggested that this severe complication might be induced by excessive activation of macrophages. The term 'macrophage activation syndrome' was eventually introduced by Stephan et al. in 1993 in a follow-up article originating from the same centre. Over the following years, few more reports from various countries described a number of patients with very similar symptoms (Davies et al. 1994; Fishman et al. 1995; Mouy et al. 1996; Ravelli et al. 1996; Quesnel et al. 1997; Prahalad et al. 2001; Sawhney et al. 2001). As in the original report, most of those patients had a systemic form of JRA. A life-threatening nature of this syndrome was stressed in all the reports.

More recently, MAS has been also observed in a small number of patients with polyarticular JRA (Hadchouel et al. 1985; Sawhney et al. 2001), systemic lupus erythematosus, rheumatoid arthritis, sarcoidosis (Reiner and Spivak 1988), dermatomyositis, and CINCA syndrome (Sawhney et al. 2001). The reason for increased incidence of MAS in soJRA is unclear.

Epidemiology

The exact incidence of MAS is not known. One retrospective review of all cases of MAS from a single tertiary level paediatric rheumatology unit, identified nine patients diagnosed between 1980 and 2000 (Sawhney et al. 2001). Seven of these patients had soJRA, one had enthesitis related arthritis, and one had CINCA syndrome. During the same period of time, the unit cared for 103 patients with soJRA, 37 with enthesitis related arthritis, and three with CINCA syndrome. Based on these observations, about 7 per cent of soJRA patients followed by the unit developed MAS. These numbers, however, may underestimate the true incidence of MAS since many patients with milder forms of this syndrome remain undiagnosed.

Based on our own experience and review of the literature, MAS occurs with equal frequency in boys and girls. There appears to be no racial predilection, and it may occur almost at any age. The youngest MAS patient reported to date was 12 months old (Silverman et al. 1983). Although most patient develop this syndrome sometime during the course of their primary rheumatic disease, MAS occurring at the initial presentation of a rheumatic illness have been described as well. The vast majority of patients have an active primary rheumatic disease prior to developing MAS. One report, however, described a patient whose polyarticular JRA was not active at the time of MAS presentation (Davies et al. 1994).

Triggers

In the early reports, the triggering of macrophage activation was linked to either recent modifications in the drug therapy or viral infections (Hadchouel et al. 1985; Stephan et al. 1993). For instance, in the series reported by Hadchouel et al. three of seven JRA patients with MAS, had an acute episode after the second injection of gold salts. Gold preparations were implicated in the development of MAS in other reports as well (Jacobs et al. 1984). Salicylates as possible triggers, were also mentioned in few reports, although their role is less clear (Silverman et al. 1983; Stephan et al. 1993).

Among the infectious triggers, viral illnesses, particularly EBV and other members of Herpes family, appear to be most commonly reported. It is now evident, however, that development of MAS can be precipitated by virtually any infectious agent: bacterial, fungal, and even parasitic (Reiner and Spivak 1988). In many patients, triggering events are not identified.

Clinical features

The clinical findings in MAS are dramatic. Typically, patients with a chronic condition become acutely ill with persistent fever, mental status changes, lymphadenopathy, hepatosplenomegaly, liver dysfunction, easy bruising, and mucosal bleeding. These clinical symptoms are associated with precipitous fall in all three blood cell lines (leucocytes, erythrocytes, and platelets) and ESR. Many patients develop a fulminant disease course with the need for intensive care support including ventilation.

Coagulation abnormalities

Haemorrhagic syndrome resembling disseminated intravascular coagulation (DIC) is the most striking abnormality in MAS. Haemorrhagic skin rashes from mild petechiae to extensive echimotic lesions, epistaxis, bleeding from gums, haematoemesis secondary to upper gastrointestinal bleeding, and rectal bleeding, are most commonly described clinical symptoms caused by coagulation abnormalities observed in MAS (Hadchouel et al. 1985; Stephan et al. 1993). Further laboratory evaluation reveals prolonged prothrombin and partial thromboplastin times, marked hypofibrinogenaemia, and moderated deficiency of vitamin K-dependent clotting factors. A decrease in Factor V levels is usually mild. Fibrin degradation products may be present as well.

Neurological manifestations

Neurologic involvement has been described in several reports. Mental status changes, seizures, and coma are the most common manifestations of CNS disease (Hadchouel et al. 1985; Stephan et al. 1993). EEG is often abnormal with periodic slow waves. Cerebrospinal fluid pleocytosis with mildly elevated protein has been noted in some studies (Hadchouel et al. 1985). CT evaluation of encephalopathy was performed in some series (Stephan et al. 1993), and was suggestive of brain infarcts in one patient (Reiner and Spivak 1988).

Liver involvement

Liver involvement is another cardinal feature of the syndrome. Significant hepatomegaly is consistently present. Some patients develop mild jaundice. Liver function tests reveal high serum transaminases activity and mildly elevated levels of serum bilirubin. Serum ammonia levels are typically normal or mildly elevated. Moderate hypoalbuminaemia has been consistently reported as well (Silverman et al. 1983).

Other clinical manifestations

Significant deterioration in renal function has been noted in several series (Stephan et al. 1993; Sawhney et al. 2001), and was associated with particularly high mortality in one report (Sawhney et al. 2001). Pulmonary infiltrates have been mentioned in several reports (Davies et al. 1994; Mouy et al. 1996), but to what extent they can be attributed to MAS is not clear.

Laboratory findings

Profound decrease in at least two of the three blood cells lines (i.e. leucocytes, erythrocytes, and platelets) is the most common feature of MAS (Hadchouel et al. 1985). The fall in platelet count is usually most dramatic. Since bone marrow aspiration typically reveals significant hypercellularity and normal megakaryocytes, such cytopaenias do not seem to be secondary to inadequate production of cells. Increased destruction of the cells by phagocytosis and consumption at the inflammatory sites are more likely explanations.

Precipitous fall in ESR is another characteristic laboratory feature, which probably reflects the degree of hypofibrinogenaemia.

Hypertriglyceridaemia is often seen in MAS patients, and is likely to be induced by high levels of TNF-α observed in this syndrome. One of the metabolic effects of TNF-α is stimulation of hepatic lipogenesis and inhibition of synthesis of lipoprotein lipase, an enzyme needed to release fatty acids from circulating lipoproteins so that they can be used by the tissues. The same pathogenic mechanism appears to be responsible for the development of fatty changes in the liver.

Low levels of fibrinogen and vitamin K-dependent clotting factors, probably reflective of the degree of liver dysfunction, are consistently reported.

Tissue histology

The most common histopathologic finding in patients with this syndrome is a proliferation of cytologically benign yet actively phagocytic histiocytes (Plate 178). Although the demonstration of haemophagocytic histiocytes in the bone marrow or lymph nodes is virtually diagnostic, negative reports may occur due to sampling difficulties or timing of the procedure (Sawhney et al. 2001). The histiocytosis generally involves the bone marrow, the sinusoids and the medullary cords of the lymph nodes, the red pulp of the spleen, and the sinusoids, and portal tracts of the liver (Reiner and Spivak 1988). The lymph nodes reportedly show diffuse architectural disorganization and lymphoid depletion. The histiocytes may also be found in various organs

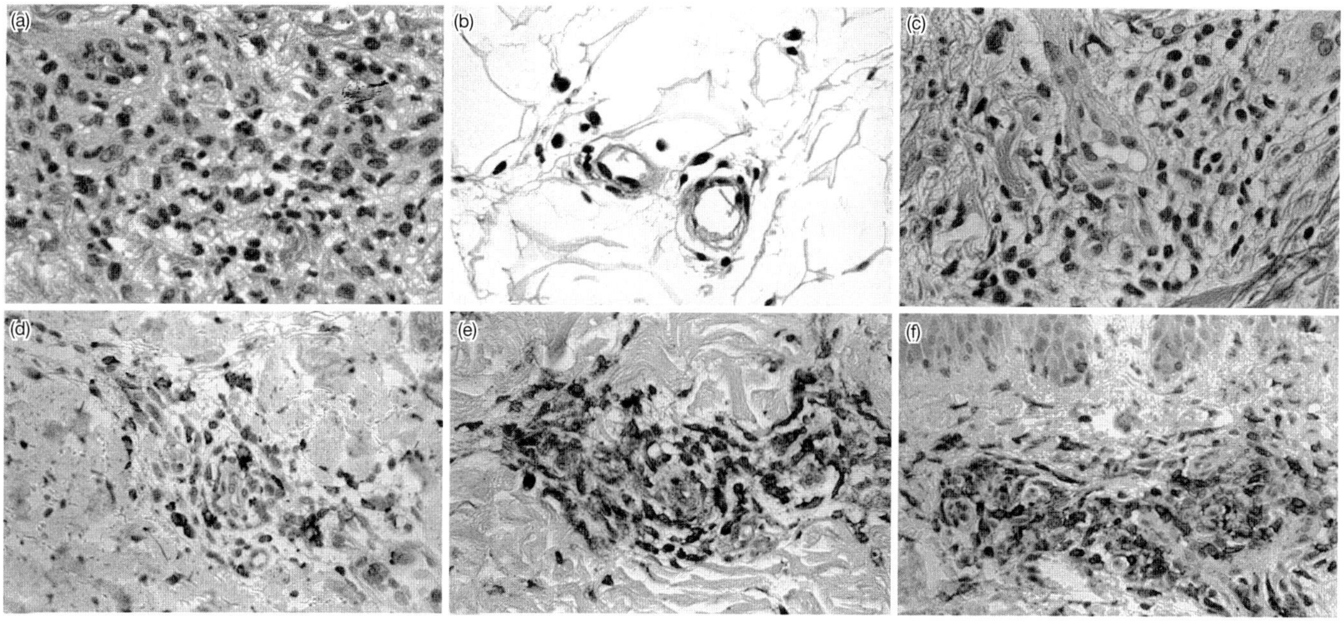

Fig. 1 Skin biopsy specimen from a MAS patient. (a–c) Show leucocytoclastic vasculitis in superficial dermis (H&E stain); (d–f) show immunostaining for macrophages (CD68+), T-lymphocytes, and factor XIIIa positive cells respectively.

and may account for many of the systemic features of this syndrome. Thus, post-mortem evaluation of one of the patients with MAS revealed extensive infiltration by non-malignant histiocytes of the heart, adrenal glands, liver, pancreas, and meninges (Reiner and Spivak 1988). In addition to sinusoidal and periportal histiocytic infiltration, histological evaluation of the liver often reveals severe diffuse fatty changes and marked Kupffer cell hyperplasia (Hadchouel et al. 1985).

The most common cutaneous manifestations of MAS are panniculitis and purpura (Smith et al. 1992; Prahalad et al. 2001). Most biopsy specimens show oedema and haemorrhage with a lymphohistiocytic infiltrate and prominent histiocytic cells occasionally showing erythrophagocytosis (Fig. 1).

Schuval et al. (1993) have recently described two patients with *histiocytic cytophagic panniculitis* associated with systemic manifestations such as fever and hepatosplenomegaly. At some point during the course of their disease, both patients acutely developed pancytopaenias that responded to cyclosporin A. Although these patients did not have apparent coagulation abnormalities, activation of macrophages did play a role in the pathogenesis of their diseases, suggesting that there may be a significant overlap between the pathogenic mechanisms involved in MAS and histiocytic cytophagic panniculitis (Schuval et al. 1993).

Pathogenesis

Immunological mechanisms

While the aetiology of MAS is unknown, it appears that there is an underlying abnormality in immunoregulation that contributes to the lack of control of an exaggerated immune response.

Clinically, MAS has similarities with other conditions, such as familial and virus-associated haemophagocytic lymphohistiocytosis. The most consistent immunologic abnormality described in those patients has been global impairment of cytotoxic function. Thus, Egeler et al. (1996) showed that most patients with FHLH had normal quantitative serum immunoglobulin levels. Phenotypic analysis of lymphocyte subsets showed that the majority of patients had surprisingly normal absolute lymphocyte counts and normal distribution of mature T-cell subsets. CD4/CD8 ratios were normal in most patients. In contrast, the NK function was markedly decreased or absent in the majority of patients. Cytotoxic activity of CD8+ cells was also defective (Egeler et al. 1996).

One sub-type of FHLH, accounting for approximately 30 per cent of cases in the United States, has been recently associated with mutations in the perforin gene leading to decreased expression of this protein (Stepp et al. 1999). It is of great interest that defective perforin function has been described in some patients with soJRA as well (Wulffraat et al. 2000), suggesting that there may be a common pathogenic mechanisms in both FHLH and MAS of soJRA. There is increasing evidence that perforin, a cytotoxic protein that lymphocytes secrete to kill virus-infected cells, may also control lymphocyte and/or macrophage proliferation (Stepp et al. 1999; Badovinac et al. 2000). Therefore, in both conditions perforin deficiency may lead to persistent lymphocyte activation associated with production of large quantities of IFN-γ and GM-CSF, two important macrophage activators. Subsequently, the sustained macrophage activation results in tissue infiltration and in the production of high levels of TNF-α, IL-1, and IL-6, which play a major role in the various clinical symptoms and tissue damage. A report on successful treatment of JRA associated MAS by cyclosporin A with transient exacerbation of MAS by conventional-dose G-CSF, does support this hypothesis (Quesnel et al. 1997).

Another possible pathogenic mechanism in MAS is impaired ability of regulatory T cells and NKT cells to downregulate activation of macrophages. The increased occurrence of MAS in soJRA patients after autologous stem cell transplantation that involves profound T-cell depletion (Wulffraat et al. 2000), is certainly consistent with this scenario.

In a recent study of cytotoxic function in familial and EBV-associated HLH, two major patterns of immunologic abnormalities were delineated: (i) normal or decreased numbers of NK cells, very low NK activity with low (or absent) levels of perforin expression in all cytotoxic cell lines, and (ii) very low numbers of NK cells, low NK activity, but mildly increased levels of perforin expression in CD8+ and CD56+ cytotoxic cells. The first pattern was most characteristic of FHLH, while the second was more often observed in virus-associated HLH. It was noted, however, that there was a significant overlap between the two patterns (Kogawa et al. 2002). This study was eventually expanded to include seven soJRA patients with MAS (Grom et al. 2003).

It showed that even in this small group of patients, there was significant heterogeneity in terms of the underlying immunologic abnormalities. Four of these patients had decreased NK activity and mildly increased levels of perforin expression in CD8+ and CD56+ cytotoxic cells, a pattern somewhat similar to that in virus-associated reactive lymphohistiocytosis. Two of the soJRA/MAS patients, however, had decreased NK activity associated with very low levels of perforin expression in all cytotoxic cell populations, a pattern indistinguishable from that in FHLH carriers. This last observation raises a question whether there may be a genetic predisposition for MAS, at least in some soJRA patients. It has been also reported, however, that in several soJRA patients with a history of MAS, perforin expression and NK activity returned to normal levels after autologous stem cell transplantation, suggesting that the described immunologic abnormalities may be also induced by the underlying disease, that is, systemic JRA (Wulffraat et al. 2000).

Regardless of the underlying immunopathogenic mechanisms, very low NK function is consistently observed in all MAS patients. What also becomes clear from these studies is that whatever the primary immunologic aberrations are, they all lead to a common final pathway involving abnormal interactions of NK and/or T cells with macrophages. It appears that this common pathway is associated with either persistent lymphocyte activation associated with production of large quantities of cytokines capable of stimulating or impaired ability of regulatory T cells and NK cells to downregulate macrophages.

Coagulopathy

In the early reports, the coagulation abnormalities observed in this syndrome have been interpreted by several authors as 'consumption coagulopathy' triggered by the vasculitic component of the disease (Silverman et al. 1983). Others have proposed that severe liver dysfunction induced by macrophages infiltrating the liver parenchyma is central to its pathogenesis (Stephan et al. 1993). Indeed, liver disease may result in a complex coagulopathy caused by decreased synthesis of clotting factors, such as fibrinogen. The liver also produces inhibitors of coagulation such antithrombin III, protein C and S, and is the clearance site for activated coagulation factors and fibrinolytic enzymes. Thus, patients with severe liver dysfunction are 'hypercoagulable' and predisposed to developing DIC and may develop systemic pathological fibrinolysis. For these reasons, coagulation defects in advanced liver disease are often difficult to distinguish from those in DIC.

An MAS patients reported by Prahalad et al. however, developed severe acute haemorrhagic diathesis in the absence of significant liver dysfunction. The vasculitic component in the skin lesions was not prominent (Prahalad et al. 2001). The most striking feature was the intense perivascular infiltration of the dermis with activated macrophages and T cells, a pattern consistent with the observations described by Smith et al. (1992). There is ample evidence that activated macrophages themselves may have significant procoagulant activity. Thus, in an inflammatory response, they can be induced to produce fibrin stabilizing factor XIIIa and haemostatic tissue factor. Tissue factor expressed on monocytes and on TNF-α-stimulated vascular endothelial cells, has been shown to be central to the pathogenesis of DIC accompanying septicaemia. Massive accumulation of activated macrophages in the skin lesions in the patient described by Prahalad et al. (2001) suggests that similar mechanisms may be relevant to the development of coagulation abnormalities in MAS as well.

A possible role for TNF-α in the development of coagulopathy in MAS has been suggested in many reports. Indeed, increased serum levels of TNF-α, a major macrophage-derived pro-inflammatory cytokine, have been demonstrated in several cases of MAS (Stephan et al. 1993; Ravelli et al. 1996). Furthermore, excessive amounts of TNF-α have been implicated in the pathogenesis of disseminated intravascular coagulation in both clinical and experimental situations. The importance of TNF-α in the development of coagulation abnormalities in soJRA was also stressed by de Benedetti et al. (1997) in a study that demonstrated strong correlation between the serum levels of soluble TNF receptors and prolongation of PTT and decrease in prothrombin activity.

Differential diagnosis

MAS is a serious complication of systemic JRA associated with considerable morbidity and death. Deterioration is often rapid and a fatal outcome is frequent. Therefore, the early recognition of this syndrome and immediate therapeutic intervention to produce a rapid clinical response are critical.

MAS can be clinically differentiated from a typical JRA exacerbation by several features that are apparent early in the course of this syndrome (Grom and Passo 1996). Patients with an exacerbation of systemic JRA usually have a spiking daily (quotidian) or double-daily (double quotidian) fever, evanescent rash, generalized lymphadenopathy, and hepatosplenomegaly. Symptoms of polyserositis and arthritis may also be present. A marked polymorphonuclear leucocytosis and thrombocytosis and increased ESR with hyperfibrinogenaemia are common features that reflect the activity of inflammation. Mild elevation of liver enzyme activity is also common. In contrast, persistent unremitting fever (which is different from the quotidian fever of systemic JRA), mental status changes, and moderately elevated liver enzyme activity (occasionally seen with hyperbilirubinaemia), accompanied by a sharp fall in ESR in association with hypofibrinogenaemia, relative leucopaenia, thrombocytopaenia, prolonged prothrombin time, and easy bleeding, should rise suspicion of MAS. The diagnosis is confirmed by demonstration of haemophagocytic histiocytes in bone marrow and lymph nodes.

Several features of MAS, that is, a combination of encephalopathy and hepatic dysfunction, might be reminiscent of Reye syndrome. The diagnosis of Reye syndrome, however, is based on a combination of viral prodrome, unexplained vomiting, behavioural changes, and unusual chemical profile consisting of rapid coordinated increase in serum aminotransferase levels, blood ammonia, and prothrombin time, with minimal alteration in serum bilirubin. Haemorrhagic syndrome having features of DIC has never been described in Reye syndrome. Conversely, hyperammonaemia, an important feature of Reye syndrome, is usually very mild in MAS patients (Hadchouel et al. 1985).

Thrombotic thrombocytopaenic purpura is another important consideration; however, microangiopathic anaemia is a key feature in the former, and not recognized in MAS. It is also important to differentiate MAS from malignancy associated haemophagocytic lymphohistiocytosis and malignant histiocytic disorders. It is generally held that the histopathologic features which distinguish malignant histiocytes from the syndrome of haemophagocytic lymphohistiocytosis are the cytological immaturity of the histiocytes, less haemophagocytosis, less bone marrow involvement, greater effacement of nodal architecture, and absence of lymphoid depletion (Reiner and Spivak 1988). Some other important differential diagnoses include sepsis and side-effects of medications.

Management

In MAS, the clinical picture quickly evolves into a fulminant process associated with high mortality. In our clinic, to achieve rapid reversal of coagulation abnormalities, we often start with IV methylprednisolone pulse therapy (30 mg/kg daily for 3 consecutive days) followed by 2–3 mg/kg/day in four divided doses. After normalization of haematological abnormalities and resolution of coagulopathy, steroids are tapered slowly to avoid relapses of macrophage activation. Not uncommonly, however, macrophage activation syndrome appears to be corticosteroid resistant with deaths being reported even among patients treated with massive doses of steroids.

Parental administration of cyclosporin A in patients with corticosteroid resistant MAS, was recently proposed by Stephan et al. (1996). From the primary effect of cyclosporin A, largely but not entirely confined to T cells, a wide variety of other effects are mediated (see Table 1), leading to profound and therapeutically useful immunosuppression (Schreiber and Crabtree 1992). In the MAS patients reported by Stephan et al. (1993), Ravelli et al. (1996), and Mouy et al. (1996) parental administration of cyclosporin A (2–8 mg/kg/day) not only provided rapid control of symptoms but also allowed to avoid excessive use of corticosteroids.

Table 1 Immunosuppressive effects of cyclosporin A

T cells	
↓ Transcription of 'early activation' genes	
Macrophages	
↓ IL-6, IL-1, and TNF-α production	
↓ Tissue factor expression	
↓ NO and PGE2 production	
Dendritic cells	
↓ Expression of co-stimulatory molecules	

There have been anecdotal reports on the use of some other medications in corticosteroid-resistant cases. For instance, etoposide, a podophyllotoxin derivative that inhibits mitotic activity by inhibiting DNA type II topoisomerase, was successfully used to treat MAS in one report (Fishman et al. 1995) but induced severe bone marrow suppression in another (Stephan et al. 1993).

A suggested role for TNF-α in the development of coagulation abnormalities, provided a rationale for the use of TNF-α inhibitors in one corticosteroid resistant case of MAS (Prahalad et al. 2001). The administration of etanercept in conjunction with corticosteroids resulted in a fast resolution of coagulopathy. This medication should not be used, however, when an infectious agent is suspected as a possible trigger of MAS.

Course

Without treatment MAS is often fatal, particularly when associated with coagulation abnormalities. Early administration of high-dose corticosteroids and cyclosporin A dramatically improves the outcome of this condition. In five patients reported by Mouy et al. (1996) the administration of cyclosporin A resulted in a rapid resolution of symptoms: in each case, fever resolved within 24 h and haematologic disturbances within a few days. Full normalization of biochemical parameters, however, may take up to several weeks.

Some soJRA patients may have several reoccurrences of MAS. Whether the underlying immunologic abnormalities that predispose such patients to develop recurrent MAS are genetic or induced by the primary rheumatic disease, still remains to be determined.

References

Badovinac, V.P. et al. (2000). Regulation of antigen-specific CD8(+) T cell homeostasis by perforin and interferon-gamma. *Science* **290**, 1354–8.

de Benedetti, F. et al. (1997). Soluble tumour necrosis factor receptor levels reflect coagulation abnormalities in systemic juvenile chronic arthritis. *British Journal of Rheumatology* **36**, 581–8.

Davies, S.V. et al. (1994). Epstein–Barr virus-associated haemophagocytic syndrome in a patient with juvenile chronic arthritis. *British Journal of Rheumatology* **33**, 495–7.

Egeler, R.M. et al. (1996). Characteristic immune abnormalities in hemophagocytic lymphohistiocytosis. *Journal of Pediatric Hematology and Oncology* **18**, 340–5.

Favara, B.E. et al. (1997). Contemporary classification of histiocytic disorders. The WHO Committee on Histiocytic/Reticulum Cell Proliferations. Reclassification Working Group of the Histiocyte Society. *Medical and Pediatric Oncology* **29**, 157–66.

Fishman, D., Rooney, M., and Woo, P. (1995). Successful management of reactive haemophagocytic syndrome in systemic-onset juvenile chronic arthritis. *British Journal of Rheumatology* **34**, 888.

Grom, A.A. and Passo, M. (1996). Macrophage activation syndrome in systemic juvenile rheumatoid arthritis. *Journal of Pediatrics* **129**, 630–2.

Grom, A.A. et al. (2003). Natural killer cell dysfunction in patients with systemic-onset juvenile rheumatoid arthritis and macrophage activation syndrome. *Journal of Pediatrics* **142**, 292–6.

Hadchouel, M., Prieur, A.M., and Griscelli, C. (1985). Acute hemorrhagic, hepatic, and neurologic manifestations in juvenile rheumatoid arthritis: possible relationship to drugs or infection. *Journal of Pediatrics* **106**, 561–6.

Jacobs, J.C. et al. (1984). Consumption coagulopathy after gold therapy for JRA. *Journal of Pediatrics* **105**, 674–5.

Kogawa, K. et al. (2002). Perforin expression in cytotoxic lymphocytes from patients with hemophagocytic lymphohistiocytosis and their family members. *Blood* **99**, 61–6.

Mouy, R. et al. (1996). Efficacy of cyclosporine A in the treatment of macrophage activation syndrome in juvenile arthritis: report of five cases. *Journal of Pediatrics* **129**, 750–4.

Prahalad, S. et al. (2001). Etanercept in the treatment of macrophage activation syndrome. *Journal of Rheumatology* **28**, 2120–4.

Quesnel, B. et al. (1997). Successful treatment of juvenile rheumatoid arthritis associated haemophagocytic syndrome by cyclosporin A with transient exacerbation by conventional-dose G-CSF. *British Journal of Haematology* **97**, 508–10.

Ravelli, A. et al. (1996). Macrophage activation syndrome in systemic juvenile rheumatoid arthritis successfully treated with cyclosporine. *Journal of Pediatrics* **128**, 275–8.

Reiner, A.P. and Spivak, J.L. (1988). Hematophagic histiocytosis. A report of 23 new patients and a review of the literature. *Medicine* **67**, 369–88.

Sawhney, S., Woo, P., and Murray, K.J. (2001). Macrophage activation syndrome: a potentially fatal complication of rheumatic disorders. *Archives of Disease in Childhood* **85**, 421–6.

Schreiber, S.L. and Crabtree, G.R. (1992). The mechanism of action of cyclosporin A and FK506. *Immunology Today* **13**, 136–42.

Schuval, S.J. et al. (1993). Panniculitis and fever in children. *Journal of Pediatrics* **122**, 372–8.

Silverman, E.D. et al. (1983). Consumption coagulopathy associated with systemic juvenile rheumatoid arthritis. *Journal of Pediatrics* **103**, 872–6.

Smith, K.J. et al. (1992). Cutaneous histopathologic, immunohistochemical, and clinical manifestations in patients with hemophagocytic syndrome. *Archives of Dermatology* **128**, 193–200.

Stephan, J.L. et al. (1993). Macrophage activation syndrome and rheumatic disease in childhood: a report of four new cases. *Clinical and Experimental Rheumatology* **11**, 451–6.

Stepp, S.E. et al. (1999). Perforin gene defects in familial hemophagocytic lymphohistiocytosis. *Science* **286**, 1957–9.

Wulffraat, N.M. et al. (2000). Autologous hemopoietic stem-cell transplantation for children with refractory autoimmune disease. *Current Rheumatology Reports* **2**, 316–23.

6.12.8 The chronic, infantile, neurological, cutaneous, and articular syndrome

Anne-Marie F. Prieur

With increasing knowledge in paediatric rheumatology, new inflammatory entities have been more accurately defined. Syndromes thought to belong to the systemic-onset type of juvenile chronic arthritis, now appear to differ from it by their particular clinical sites and courses. Syndromes resembling systemic-onset juvenile arthritis occurring during the first year of life were stressed several years ago by Prieur and Griscelli (1983). The children in question all had high fever, skin rash, and polyarthritis, but careful analysis of the symptoms allowed then to distinguish various entities. Among these, a group of patients displayed a chronic syndrome that also involved the central nervous system, including the eye and other sensory organs. The autonomy of this syndrome, which in Europe is designated as chronic, infantile, neurological, cutaneous, and articular syndrome (CINCA), is now accepted, although its cause remains a mystery. CINCA is now more often recognized all around the world.

Clinical presentation

Background

In definitive descriptions of CINCA, the first symptoms occur in early infancy and are often present at birth. The course of the disease is chronic, with intermittent flare-ups associated with fever, and enlargement of lymph nodes and spleen. There have been individual case reports of a disease with these characteristics (Campbell and Clifton 1950; Lorber 1973; Ansell et al. 1975, Lampert et al. 1975; Fajardo et al. 1982), mostly preceding our suggestion that this could be a specific syndrome (Prieur and Griscelli 1981), and others have since confirmed its autonomy (Hassink and Goldsmith 1983; Yarom et al. 1985; Kaufman and Lovell 1986; Inamo et al. 1994; De Cunto et al. 1997; Miura et al. 1997; Milewska-Bobula et al. 1998). A comprehensive description of the disease is given in Prieur et al. (1987). The syndrome is now more easily identified and more fully documented (Torbiak et al. 1989).

The CINCA syndrome is often sporadic, but some families where more than one member is affected are known (see also Campbell and Clifton 1950; Ansell et al. 1975).

Perinatal events

The frequency of perinatal events is an important feature of this syndrome. These have been identified in half of the neonates in whom details of perinatal period are known. After generally uneventful pregnancies (except for minor viral infections in a few cases), half of the babies are premature. The average birth weight is 2600 g (range 1700–4700 g) after a 38-week pregnancy (range 33–42 weeks). Five instances of anomaly in the umbilical cord have been found (umphaloceles or umphalitis). In one case, a histological study of the placenta showed thickened vessel walls with thrombosis and microcalcifications, and infiltration of the umbilical cord by polymorphonuclear cells. There was no evidence of infection in any of the infants.

Signs and symptoms

The association of skin rash, joint involvement, and central nervous manifestations is most often present.

Rash

The rash is present at birth in three-fourths of the children or occurs within the first 6 months after birth in the others. In a few patients, it has been noticed later or information on this period of life is lacking. The clinical expression is similar in all patients, although variable in intensity. It resembles the rash of Still's disease but is more intense, often having the appearance of a non-pruritic urticaria (Fig. 1). The rash is exacerbated during flare-ups of other symptoms of the disease. Skin biopsy shows a normal epidermis, mild inflammation in the dermis, and perivascular aggregation of polymorphonuclear cells with some eosinophils. No immunoglobulin or complement deposits have been found by immunofluorescence.

Central nervous and sensory anomalies

These are important manifestations of this syndrome. They are usually discovered at the onset of symptoms that could be related to a chronic meningeal irritation, such as headaches, vomiting, seizures, or transitory episodes of hemiplegia. A chronic meningitis is identified in most patients investigated; these patients had a mild leucocytosis with polymorphs

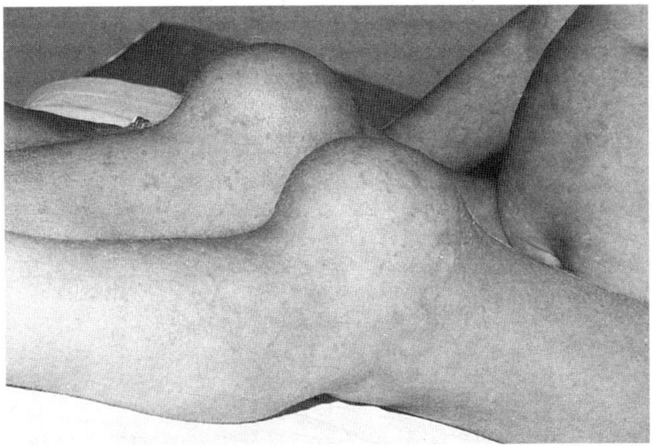

Fig. 1 The skin rash and patella overgrowth with knee deformity. [Reproduced from Prieur et al. (1987), with permission.]

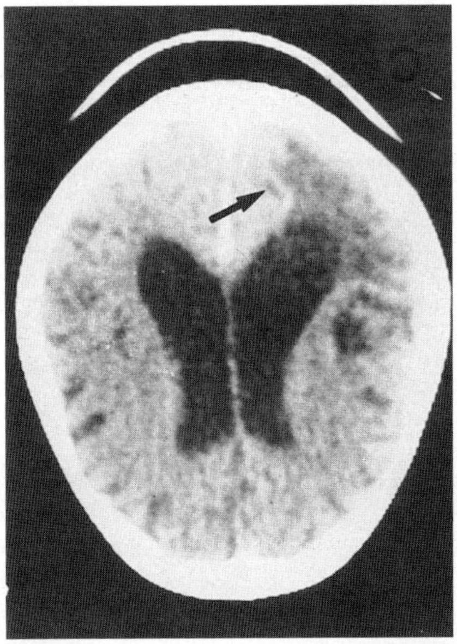

Fig. 2 CT scan: enlargement of ventricles with an area of cerebral change of probable vascular origin. [Reproduced from Prieur et al. (1987), with permission.]

(and sometimes eosinophils), and/or increased protein concentrations in the cerebrospinal fluid (CSF). In few patients, CSF was found normal (Hunttenlocher et al. 1995). Extensive attempts to demonstrate chronic infection, including electron microscopy of cells in the CSF, have been negative. Clinical follow-up of the central nervous involvement often shows an increase in the meningeal irritation, with headaches and sometimes seizures. When tested, a cerebral hyperpressure is present. Cerebral imaging often reveals a mild ventricular dilatation (Fig. 2). A low IQ has been noticed in several patients.

The skull has an increased cranial volume and there is delay in the closure of the anterior fontanelle. In some patients, there are calcifications of the faulx and dura (Fig. 3).

Sensory anomalies are progressive. Varying degrees of perceptive deafness are present in older children, often requiring the use of a hearing aid. Eye involvement can be severe: optic atrophy, papillitis, conjunctivitis, keratitis, uveitis, and chorioretinitis have been observed and can lead to a progressive

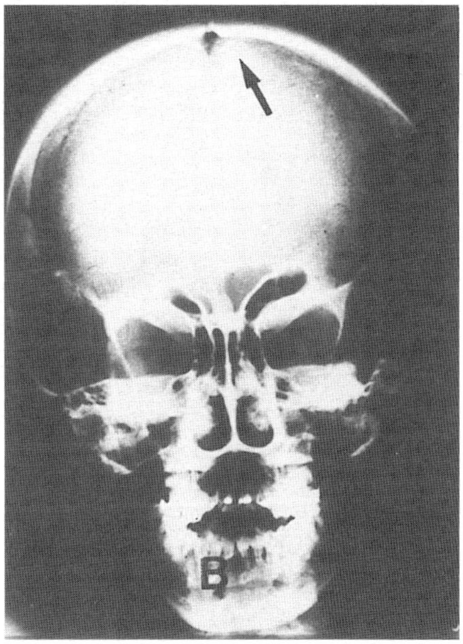

Fig. 3 Calcifications on the faulx and dura in a 12-year-old patient. [Reproduced from Prieur et al. (1987), with permission.]

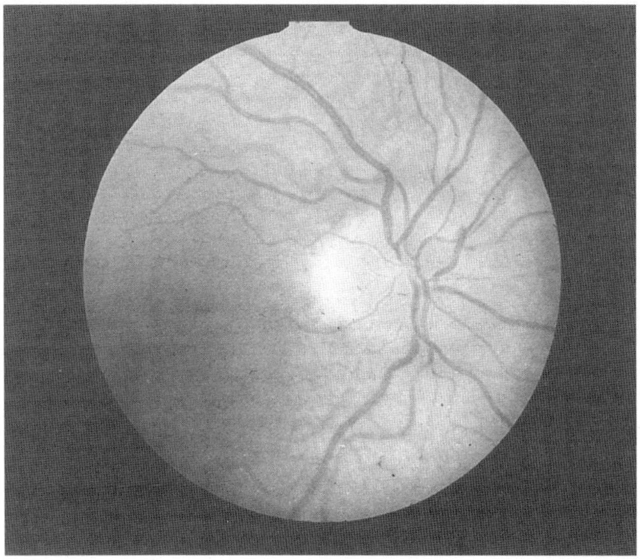

Fig. 4 Papillitis.

visual defect (Fig. 4). A stout evaluation of 31 patients underlined the frequency of optic disc changes and that ocular features in CINCA are definitely different from those of chronic uveitis observed in juvenile arthritis (Dollfus et al. 2000). Hoarseness is frequent.

Joint involvement

The severity of joint involvement varies among patients. The knees are most frequently affected (see Fig. 1), then elbows, wrists, ankles, and small joints of the hand. In some patients, the joint symptoms are mild, and manifest as transitory inflammation during flare-ups. In this group, the first articular manifestations are generally observed after the age of 2 years. In other patients, the arthropathy may present as early as 10 days of age (Hassink and Goldsmith 1983). The main finding is an overgrowth of the epiphyseal plate of the bone, resulting in hard bony enlargement. The synovial fluid exudate may show a non-specific inflammatory reaction. Progressive contractures and limitation of motion due to patellar and/or epiphyseal overgrowth occur (see Fig. 1).

The radiographic anomalies of affected joints are progressively more characteristic with increasing age in half of the patients. The first finding is swelling of periarticular soft tissues, sometimes with early periosteal reaction of the diaphysis (Kaufman and Lovell 1986). The most characteristic modifications are in the metaphysis and epiphysis of long bones, giving an irregular ossification with abnormal trabeculae. These anomalies may involve growth cartilage plates (Fig. 5); one biopsy showed an irregular metachromasia and completely disorganized columns of cartilaginous cells. Surprisingly, no inflammatory cells were found in the abnormal cartilage. In the other half of the patients, there is no radiographic anomalies.

Morphological changes

These patients have morphological changes in common. A progressive growth retardation with height below the third percentile is very frequent, but no defect in growth hormone has been found. The heads of these patients have a similar appearance, with enlargement (often with frontal bossing) and blond hair making these unrelated children look like siblings. The adults also resemble each other. A saddle-back nose is frequent. Our adult patients looks surprisingly like one of the patients in the first published descriptions in 1950 (Campbell and Clifton 1950). There is also clubbing of the fingers and toes. Hands and feet appear short and thick. In some patients, the palms and soles have a wrinkled appearance.

Follow-up

Long-term follow-up reveals a slow worsening of most symptoms despite various therapeutic trials. Non-steroidal anti-inflammatory drugs induce pain relief. Steroids are partially effective for fever and pain, but not for skin lesions or joint disease. Immunosuppressive drugs have no dramatic effect; disease-modifying drugs are ineffective. Physiotherapy improves the functional status in patients with severe arthropathy. We observed secondary amyloidosis in two patients: a young boy who died with renal failure, and an adult, father of one of our patients. These children may reach adulthood, although eight deaths have been reported in children with this syndrome. The causes of death in five of the children were: secondary amyloidosis (Prieur et al. 1987); sepsis (Fajardo et al. 1982); leukaemia, possibly related to chlorambucil therapy (Prieur and Griscelli 1981); and subacute necrotizing leucoencephalopathy after head injury (Lampert 1986). An adult died of gangrene of the foot (Warin 1977).

Pathogenesis

The pathophysiology of this syndrome is now better understood with reports of gene defects (Aksentijenich et al. 2002; Feldmann et al. 2002). There are indications of a non-specific inflammation: hypochromic anaemia, leucocytosis with a predominance of polymorphonuclear neutrophils and eosinophils, high platelet counts, and an increase in erythrocyte sedimentation rate and other acute-phase reactants. A polyclonal stimulation of immunoglobulin synthesis has been found in all patients. Surprisingly, no circulating immune complexes have been detected; no autoantibodies or immunodeficiency have been found. The microscopic architecture of the lymph nodes is preserved except for features of chronic inflammation, with an infiltration of the subcortical T-cell region by polymorphonuclear cells and often eosinophils. Extensive investigations for an infectious agent have been unsuccessful. Evidence of a retroviral infection was sought in leucocytes and cells from CSF in a recently diagnosed patient, but the outcome was negative.

This disorder is an unremitting inflammatory process that begins at birth. Most of the organs or tissues involved, except cartilage, show chronic inflammation. Cartilage may be the target organ in this syndrome, with the clustering of growth retardation, anomalies of ossification of skull and epiphyses, saddle-back nose, hoarseness suggesting laryngeal localization, and progressive deafness. Indeed, some indications of such a mechanism

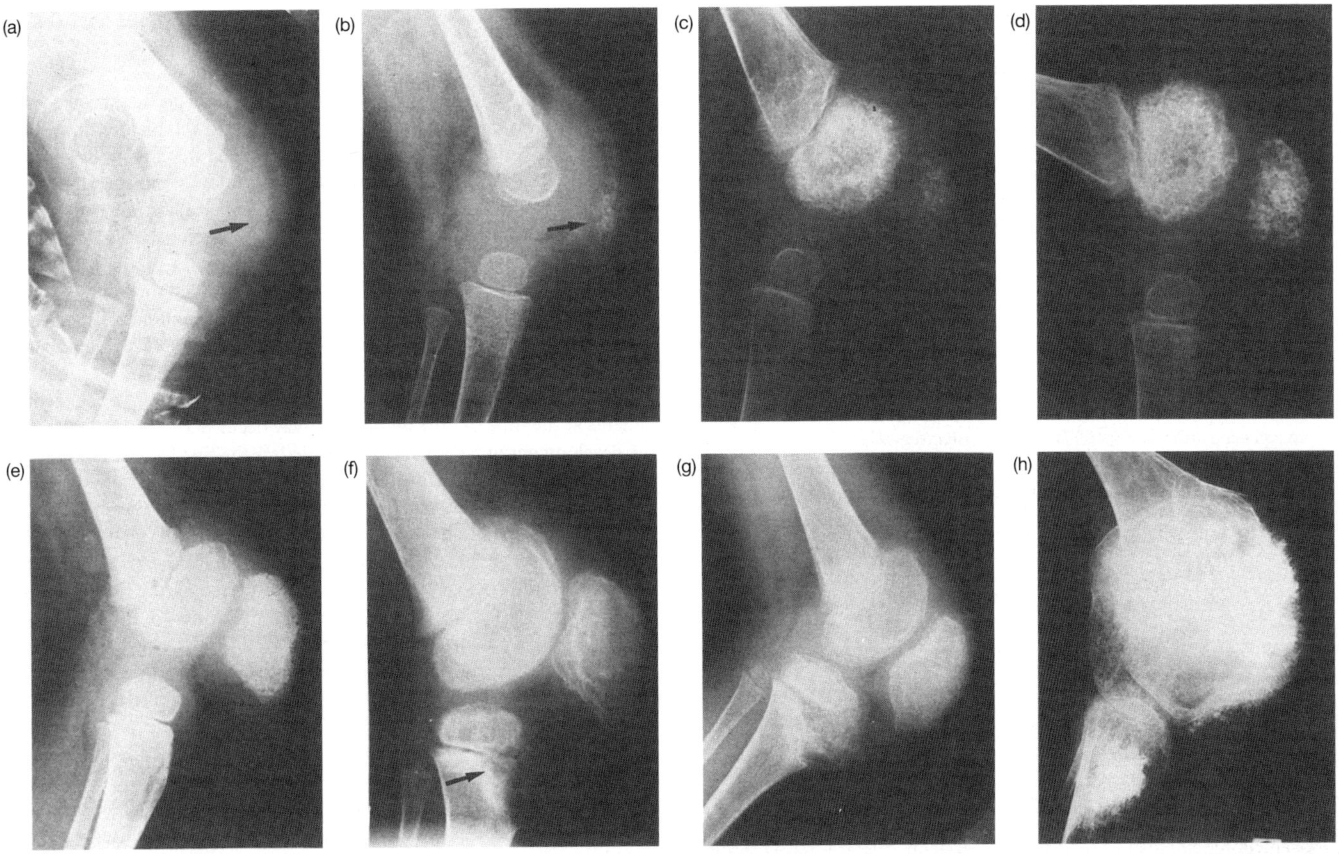

Fig. 5 Follow-up of radiographic anomalies in the knee at various ages: (a) 1 year; (b) 1 year and 6 months; (c) 2 years and 6 months; (d) 3 years and 9 months; (e) 5 years; (f) 6 years (arrow: late modification of tibial growth cartilage); (g) 8 years; (h) 33 years (another patient). [Reproduced from Prieur et al. (1987), with permission.]

were suggested by the presence of a toxic effect of the serum from these patients on normal human cartilage cells in culture (Prieur et al. 1988). However, the origin of this disease remains unknown, even though one may speculate on an initiating event that takes place before birth. It represents an original and new disorder that must be distinguished from previously described rheumatic diseases of childhood.

References

Aksentijenich, I. et al. (2002). De novo CIAS1 mutations, cytokine activation, and evidence for genetic heterogeneity in patients with neonatal-onset multisystem inflammatory disease (NOMID). A new member of the expanding family of pyrin-associated autoinflammatory diseases. *Arthritis and Rheumatism* **46**, 3340–8.

Ansell, B.M., Bywaters, E.G.L., and Elderkin, F.M. (1975). Familial arthropathy with rash, uveitis and mental retardation. *Proceedings of the Royal Society of Medicine* **68**, 584–5.

Campbell, A.M.G. and Clifton, F. (1950). Adult toxoplasmosis in one family. *Brain* **73**, 281–90.

De Cunto, C.L., Liberatore, D.I., San Roman, J.L., Goldberg, J.C., Morandi, A.A., and Feldman, G. (1997). Infantile-onset multisystem inflammatory disease: a differential diagnosis of systemic juvenile rheumatoid arthritis. *Journal of Pediatrics* **130**, 551–6.

Dollfus, H., Hafner, R., Hofmann, H.M., Russo, R.A., Denda, L., Gonzales, L.D., DeCunto, C., Premoli, J., Melo-Gomez, J., Jorge, J.P., Vesely, R., Stubna, M., Dufier, J.L., and Prieur, A.M. (2000). Chronic infantile neurological cutaneous and articular/neonatal onset multisystem inflammatory disease syndrome: ocular manifestations in a recently recognized chronic inflammatory disease of childhood. *Archives of Ophthalmology* **118**, 1386–92.

Fajardo, J.E., Geller, T.J., Koenig, H.M., and Kleine, M.L. (1982). Chronic meningitis, polyarthritis, lymphadenitis and pulmonary hemosiderosis. *Journal of Pediatrics* **101**, 738–40.

Feldmann, J. et al. (2002). Chronic infantile neurological cutaneous and articular syndrome is caused by mutations in CIAS1, a gene highly expressed in polymorphonuclear cells and chondrocytes. *American Journal of Human Genetics* **71**, 198–203.

Hassink, S.G. and Goldsmith, T.J. (1983). Noeonatal onset multisystem inflammatory disease. *Arthritis and Rheumatism* **26**, 668–73.

Huttenlocher, A., Frieden, I.J., and Emery, H. (1995). Neonatal onset multisystem inflammatory disease. *Journal of Rheumatology* **22**, 1171–3.

Inamo, Y., Kin, H., Fujita, Y., Ochiai, T., and Okuni, M. (1994). Chronic, infantile, neurological, cutaneous and articular syndrome in Japan; two case reports. *Clinical and Experimental Rheumatology* **12**, 447–9.

Kaufman, R.A. and Lovell, D.J. (1986). Infantile-onset multisystem inflammatory disease: radiologic findings. *Radiology* **160**, 741–6.

Lampert, F. et al. (1975). Infantile chronic relapsing inflammation of the brain, skin and joints. *Lancet* **i**, 1250–2 (letter).

Lorber, J. (1973). Syndrome for diagnosis: dwarfing; persistently open fontanelle; recurrent meningitis; recurrent subdural effusions with temporary alternate-sided hemiplegia; high tone deafness; visual defect with pseudopapilloedema; slowing intellectual development; recurrent acute polyarthritis; erythema marginatum, splenomegaly and iron resistant hypochromic anemia. *Proceedings of the Royal Society of Medicine* **66**, 1070–1.

Milewska-Bobula, B., Lipka, B., Rowecka-Trzebicka, K., Rostropowicz-Denisiewicz, K., Romicka, A., and Witwicki, J.M. (1998). Chronic, infantile, neurologic, cutaneous and articular syndrome (CINCA) in an infant. *Archives de Pédiatrie* **5**, 1094–7.

Miura, M., Okabe, T., Tsubata, S., Takizawa, N., and Sawaguchi, T. (1997). Chronic infantile neurological cutaneous articular syndrome in a patient from Japan. *European Journal of Pediatrics* **156**, 624–6.

Prieur, A.M. and Griscelli, C. (1981). Arthropathy with rash, chronic meningitis, eye lesions and mental retardation. *Journal of Pediatrics* **99**, 79–83.

Prieur, A.M. and Griscelli, C. (1983). Aspect nosologique des formes systémiques de l'arthrite juvénile à début très précoce: a propos de dix-sept observations. *Annales de Pediatrie (Paris)* **30**, 565–9.

Prieur, A.M. et al. (1987). A chronic, infantile, neurological, cutaneous and articular (CINCA) syndrome: a specific entity analysed in 30 patients. *Scandinavian Journal of Rheumatology* **66**, 57–68.

Prieur, A.M., Cournot-Witmer, G., Plachot, J.J., Griscelli, C., and Corvol, M.T. (1988). *In vitro* study of growth cartilage in children with the infantile onset neurologic, cutaneous and articular syndrome. Inhibitory effect of patient's sera on cultured normal human chondrocyte metabolism. *Arthritis and Rheumatism* **31**, 578.

Torbiak, R.P., Dent, P.B., and Colkshott, W.P. (1989). NOMID—a neonatal syndrome of multisystem inflammation. *Skeletal Radiology* **18**, 359–64.

Warin, R.P. (1977). Familial vasculitis (life-long morbiliform urticaria, neurological changes and arthritis). *British Journal of Dermatology* **97**, 30–1.

Yarom, A., Rennebohm, R.M., and Levinson, J.E. (1985). Infantile multisystem inflammatory disease: a specific syndrome? *Journal of Pediatrics* **106**, 390–6.

6.12.9 Multicentric reticulohistiocytosis

Peter J. Maddison

Multicentric reticulohistiocytosis is a rare systemic disease that is recognized clinically by the combination of typical papular and nodular skin lesions and a severe and destructive polyarthritis, although virtually any organ system of the body can be involved. The term 'multicentric reticulohistiocytosis' was introduced by Goltz and Layman (1954) to distinguish the disorder from solitary cutaneous nodules, termed reticulohistiocytomas, which have identical histological appearances but are not associated with systemic disease. There are a number of synonyms, which include lipoid dermatoarthritis, reticulohistiocytosis, giant-cell reticulohistiocytosis, and normocholesterolaemic xanthomatosis. At one time it was thought to be a lipid-storage disease but no consistent abnormality of serum or intracellular lipids has been identified. It is thought generally that the histiocytes and giant cells that characterize the lesions contain a non-specific accumulation of glycoprotein and lipids, and that this disease is a histiocytic granulomatous reaction to an unknown stimulus (Campbell and Edwards 1991). However, in one case, type VI collagen inclusions usually found in lymphohistiocytic neoplasms were demonstrated, supporting the concept of a proliferative rather than an inflammatory background for this condition (Fortier-Beaulieu et al. 1993).

Clinical features

Multicentric reticulohistiocytosis is primarily a disorder of adults, about three times more common in women (Barrow and Holubar 1969), with a mean age at onset in the fifth decade. About 85 per cent of reported cases are Caucasians, but it can also occur in other ethnic groups. Typical cases have been reported in adolescence (Raphael et al. 1989), but in most instances the childhood form differs from that in adults as having a marked tendency to involve the eye (glaucoma, uveitis, and cataracts), and a lack of giant cells in tissue sections, the last feature being considered an essential feature of multicentric reticulohistiocytosis (Zayid and Farraj 1973).

Skin nodules and a destructive polyarthritis are the most common features (Barrow and Holubar 1969). Arthritis is frequently the presenting feature. It has a similar distribution to rheumatoid arthritis, including the temporomandibular joints and atlantoaxial involvement (Gold et al. 1975), but also affects the distal interphalangeal joints. Commonly involved sites are the hands (75 per cent), knees (70 per cent), shoulders (65 per cent), wrists (65 per cent), hips (60 per cent), ankles (60 per cent), elbows (60 per cent), feet (60 per cent), and spine (50 per cent). Often it has a persistent course with progressive joint destruction, sometimes leading to the picture of arthritis mutilans with 'opera glass' deformities of the hand developing in approximately 40 per cent. Radiographs of the joints show symmetrical erosions resembling rheumatoid arthritis. However, osteoporosis is not marked and there is often prominent involvement of the distal interphalangeal joints, and the spread of erosions from the periphery of the joint produces apparent widening of the joint space (Fig. 1). Analysis of joint fluid shows low to moderate cell counts, mostly with a preponderance of mononuclear cells but sometimes of neutrophils. Synovial biopsy shows the presence of lipid-laden giant cells and histiocytes, as found in the involved skin.

Mucocutaneous involvement is apparent in approximately 90 per cent of patients at the time of presentation but may occur in the months following the development of arthritis. Occasionally it is the first feature. Skin lesions consist of numerous, usually non-pruritic, skin-coloured, yellowish or red-brown nodules, ranging from a few millimetres to several centimetres in diameter. Occasionally, however, pruritus is a feature, and can be severe and precede the overt lesions. The nodules mostly involve the hands in a periungual distribution, together with nodules scattered on the fingers and on the face, where lesions develop on the ears, at the corners of the mouth, and the side of the nose adjacent to the alae (Plate 179). Extensive involvement of the face produces a leonine facies. Lesions can also occur on the forehead, chest, back, and over the olecranon process and knees. Xanthelesma develops in approximately 25 per cent. The oral mucous membranes are involved in approximately half, with, for example, numerous flesh-coloured papules on the buccal mucosa, sides of the tongue, surface of the palate, and gingiva. Occasionally the pharynx and larynx are affected (Katz and Anderson 1988). To date there have been no reports of vaginal or perianal involvement.

Although multicentric reticulohistiocytosis usually affects the skin and joints, a large variety of systemic features can occur, reflecting the potential involvement of most tissues and organs of the body. There are also reported associations with various types of malignancy and with co-existent autoimmune disease. Constitutional manifestations occur in about one-third of patients, and include fever and weight loss: Cases have been reported with pericarditis, pulmonary involvement, and myositis. There have also been case reports of lymph node enlargement, splenomegaly, marrow infiltration resulting in pancytopaenia, salivary gland involvement, thyroid infiltration leading to hypothyroidism, and carpal tunnel syndrome.

Laboratory abnormalities occur, but are inconsistent, and include a raised erythrocyte sedimentation rate, abnormal liver function tests, and elevated creatine phosphokinase. Hyperlipidaemia is seen in about 40 per cent of cases. Paraproteinaemia of γ heavy-chain type has been encountered but serological tests for such as rheumatoid factor are otherwise usually normal.

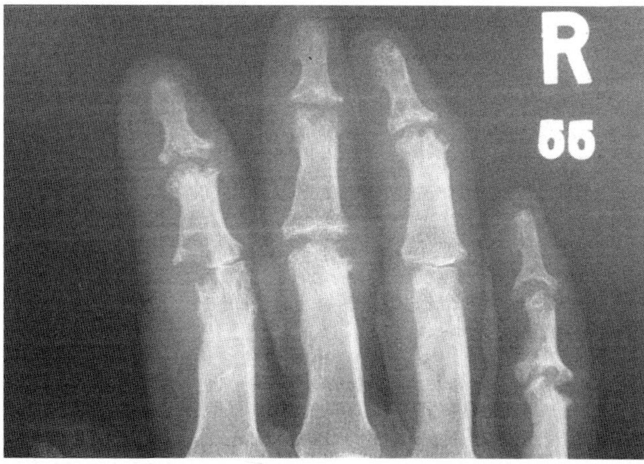

Fig. 1 Radiograph of the hand in multicentric reticulohistiocytosis.

Gallium scintiscans have been used to evaluate multicentric reticulohistiocytosis but the abnormalities are non-specific.

Approximately 30 per cent of patients with multicentric reticulohistiocytosis have been reported to have malignant disease (Snow and Muller 1995). Associations have mostly been with internal carcinomas of the colon, breast, bronchus, cervix, ovary, and stomach. Cases have also been associated with sarcomas and lymphomas. Patients with malignant melanoma and pleural mesothelioma have also been reported. In one review of the literature (Nunnink et al. 1985), the onset of both diseases occurred in several patients within 1 year. The onset of multicentric reticulohistiocytosis in adulthood necessitates, therefore, a thorough clinical examination, including a chest radiograph, to look for signs of malignant disease. It is not necessary, however, to embark on invasive procedures to look for occult neoplasms. It should be borne in mind that there may be a bias towards reporting cases with underlying malignancy, especially previously unreported tumours, and some of the associations may be purely coincidental.

Pathology

Histologically, the nodular infiltrates, which have a granular or ground-glass appearance, consist of multinucleate (up to 20 nuclei) giant cells of the foreign-body type and histiocytes of the monocyte–macrophage lineage admixed with small numbers of CD4+ lymphocytes and B cells. Histochemically, the cytoplasm of the giant cells contains diastase-resistant, periodic acid–Schiff-positive material thought to be glycoprotein, neutral fats, phospholipids, and iron. Immunohistochemical studies have yielded conflicting findings with some supporting either a lymphocyte or dermal dendrocyte origin. However, the finding of most studies is that giant cells and mononuclear histiocytes express the surface markers of the monocyte–macrophage lineage such as HAM56, CD68, Mac387, α1-antitrypsin, CD11b and c, CD14, and CD15 (Gorman et al. 2000). Furthermore, cytokines produced by activated macrophages such as tumour necrosis factor (TNF) and interleukin-1 (IL-1), have been identified and may have a role in the pathogenesis of, for example, bone and cartilage destruction.

Diagnosis

The diagnosis is confirmed by skin or synovial biopsy. Solitary reticulohistiocytomas have identical histological findings but there is no evidence of systemic disease (Zegler et al. 1994).

Diseases that may possibly be confused with multicentric reticulohistiocytosis on the basis of clinical or histological findings are:

1. Rheumatoid or psoriatic arthritis; chronic gout;
2. Sarcoid dactylitis—associated with discrete tubercles that lack foam cells or giant cells typical of multicentric reticulohistiocytosis;
3. Xanthomas;
4. Fibroxanthoma;
5. Histiocytosis X—usually presents in childhood and proliferating cells are epidermotropic Langerhans cells rather than of true monocyte–macrophage lineage;
6. Generalized eruptive histiocytoma—not associated with arthritis and lesions do not exhibit the typical multinucleate giant cells;
7. Tendon sheath giant-cell tumours—solitary, well-circumscribed nodules in the hands;
8. Farber's disease—lipogranulomatosis, usually fatal in infancy.

Treatment and course

The disease often runs a waxing and waning course and sometimes it stabilizes. It is difficult to predict the course in the individual case but as a rule the disease 'burns out' after 5–8 years, with regression of the cutaneous nodules, leaving the patient with severe joint deformities. Occasionally, systemic involvement can be severe enough to be life threatening but otherwise the prognosis is dominated by whether or not there is an associated malignancy.

Various drug treatments have been proposed to suppress the condition, including corticosteroids, adrenocorticotrophic hormone, salicylates, antimalarials, cytotoxic agents and, more recently, methotrexate and cyclosporin A. There are no controlled trials, as the condition is so rare, and therefore reports of efficacy should be interpreted with caution.

Corticosteroids are of limited use. Skin infiltration does not usually respond, although there may be relief of troublesome pruritus. Joint symptoms sometimes improve (Davies et al. 1968).

There are several reports of improvement in skin, joint, and systemic disease with alkylating agents and patients with long-lasting remission after therapy with cyclophosphamide or chlorambucil have been reported (Doherty et al. 1984; Ginsburg et al. 1989; Kenik et al. 1990). For a while these agents were considered to be the treatment of choice. More recently, there has been success with less toxic agents. Methotrexate has been used in multicentric reticulohistiocytosis since 1991 (Gourmelen et al. 1991) and since then suppression of both the skin disease and arthritis has been reported with this agent (Cash et al. 1997; Rentsch et al. 1998). Similarly, cyclosporin A has been reported to induce complete remission in this condition (Saito et al. 2001). The success of a sequential approach to the drug treatment of multicentric reticulohistiocytosis has been reported (Liang and Granston 1996), starting with methotrexate and involving alkylating agents only if there is a lack of response. Based on the experience reported so far, Fig. 2 shows an algorithm for treating multicentric reticulohistiocytosis. In view of the possible role of macrophage-derived cytokines such as TNF and IL-1, specific anticytokine reagents may prove to be effective in treating refractory cases of the disease.

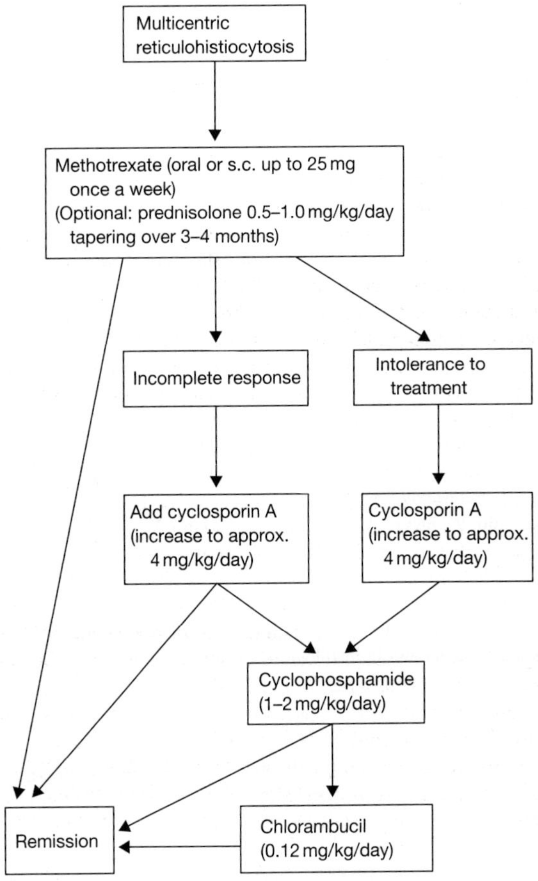

Fig. 2 An algorithm for treating multicentric reticulohistiocytosis.

References

Barrow, M.V. and Holubar, K. (1969). Multicentric reticulohistiocytosis: a review of 33 patients. *Medicine (Baltimore)* **48**, 287–305.

Campbell, D.A. and Edwards, N.L. (1991). Multicentric reticulohistiocytosis: systemic macrophage disorder. *Baillières Clinical Rheumatology* **5**, 301–19.

Cash, J.M., Tyree, J., and Recht, M. (1997). Severe multicentric reticulohistiocytosis: disease stabilization achieved with methotrexate and hydroxychloroquine. *Journal of Rheumatology* **24**, 2250–3.

Davies, M.E., Roenigk, H.H., Hawk, W.A., and O'Duffy, J.D. (1968). Multicentric reticulohistiocytosis: report of a case with histochemical studies. *Archives of Dermatology* **97**, 543–7.

Doherty, M., Martin, M.F., and Dieppe, P.A. (1984). Multicentric reticulohistiocytosis associated with primary biliary cirrhosis: successful treatment with cytotoxic agents. *Arthritis and Rheumatism* **27**, 844–8.

Fortier-Beaulieu, M., Thomine, E., Boullie, M.C., Le Loet, X., Lauret, P., and Hemet, J. (1993). New electron microscopic findings in a case of multicentric reticulohistiocytosis. Long spacing collagen inclusions. *American Journal of Dermatopathology* **15**, 587–9.

Ginsburg, W.W., O'Duffy, J.D., and Morris, J.L. (1989). Multicentric reticulohistiocytosis: response to alkylating agents in six patients. *Annals of Internal Medicine* **111**, 384–8.

Gold, R.H., Metzger, A.L., and Mirra, J.M. (1975). Multicentric reticulohistiocytosis (lipoid dermato-arthritis): an erosive polyarthritis and distinctive clinical, roentgenographic and pathological features. *American Journal of Roentgenology, Radiation Therapy and Nuclear Medicine* **124**, 610–24.

Goltz, R.W. and Layman, C.W. (1954). Multicentric reticulohistiocytosis of the skin and synovia. *Archives of Dermatology and Syphilology* **69**, 717–22.

Gorman, J.D., Danning, C., Schumacher, H.R., Klippel, J.H., and Davis, J.C., Jr. (2000). Multicentric reticulohistiocytosis: case report with immunohistochemical analysis and literature review. *Arthritis and Rheumatism* **43**, 930–8.

Gourmelen, O. et al. (1991). Methotrexate treatment for multicentric reticulohistiocytosis. *Journal of Rheumatology* **18**, 627–8.

Katz, R.W. and Anderson, K.F. (1988). Multicentric reticulohistiocytosis. *Oral Surgery, Oral Medicine, Oral Pathology* **65**, 721–5.

Kenik, J.G., Fok, F., Huerter, C.J., Hurley, J.A., and Stanoshek, J.F. (1990). Multicentric reticulohistiocytosis in a patient with malignant melanoma: a response to cyclophosphamide and a unique cutaneous feature. *Arthritis and Rheumatism* **33**, 1047–51.

Liang, G.C. and Granston, A.S. (1996). Complete remission of multicentric reticulohistiocytosis with combination therapy of steroid, cyclophosphamide, and low-dose pulse methotrexate. Case report, review of the literature, and proposal for treatment. *Arthritis and Rheumatism* **39**, 171–4.

Nunnick, J.C., Krusinski, P.A., and Yates, J.W. (1985). Multicentric reticulohistiocytosis and cancer: a case report and review of the literature. *Medical Pediatric Oncology* **13**, 273–9.

Raphael, S.A., Cowdery, S.L., Faerber, E.N., Lischner, H.W., Shumacher, R., and Tourtellotte, C.D. (1989). Multicentric reticulohistiocytosis in a child. *Journal of Paediatrics* **114**, 266–9.

Rentsch, J.L., Martin, E.M., Harrison, L.C., and Wicks, I.P. (1998). Prolonged response of multicentric reticulohistiocytosis to low dose methotrexate. *Journal of Rheumatology* **25**, 1012–15.

Saito, K., Fujii, K., Awazu, Y., Nakayamada, S., Fujii, Y., Ota, T., and Tanaka, Y. (2001). A case of systemic lupus erythematosus complicated with multicentric reticulohistiocytosis (MRH): successful treatment of MRH and lupus nephritis with cyclosporin A. *Lupus* **10**, 129–32.

Snow, J.L. and Muller, S.A. (1995). Malignancy-associated multicentric reticulohistiocytosis: a clinical, histological and immunophenotypic study. *British Journal of Dermatology* **133**, 71–6.

Zayid, I. and Farraj, F. (1973). Familial histiocytic dermatitis: a new syndrome. *American Journal of Medicine* **54**, 793–800.

Zegler, B., Soyer, H.P., Misch, K., Orchard, G., and Wilson-Jones, E. (1994). Reticulohistiocytoma and multicentric reticulohistiocytosis. Histopathologic and immunophenotypic distinct entities. *American Journal of Dermatopathology* **16**, 577–84.

6.12.10 Hyperlipidaemias

Keng Hong Leong, J.P.D. Reckless, and Neil John McHugh

Introduction

The relationship of lipid disorders to rheumatic diseases is multifaceted. Several abnormalities in the lipid and lipoprotein profile (or dyslipidaemia) have been documented in various forms of chronic arthritis. The dyslipidaemia may depend on the type or activity of the joint disease, treatment and other factors. It may influence disease outcome by accelerating atheroma, although the contribution of dyslipidaemia to the increased mortality from vascular disease observed in several rheumatic disorders is uncertain.

Potentially toxic lipid particles, such as oxidized low density lipoprotein (LDL), may accumulate within joints (Winyard et al. 1993). Oxidized LDL may be a target for pathogenic autoantibodies that cross react with phospholipids (Vaarala et al. 1993). Dietary modification of lipid intake may have beneficial effects and supplementation with polyunsaturated fatty acids of the omega 3 and omega 6 series may be effective, as in animal models of inflammatory arthritis.

Lipid metabolism

Lipid composition

Lipoproteins are complex particles that transport lipids through the plasma. Each particle is composed of a non-polar core containing variable proportions of hydrophobic lipids (triglycerides and cholesterol ester) surrounded by a polar coat of phospholipids and free cholesterol, containing various apolipoproteins. This outer coat allows the particle to be soluble in aqueous plasma. The apolipoproteins have structural roles in the lipoproteins and functional roles as enzyme activators, or as ligands with high affinity for specific tissue-cell receptors. There are five main types of lipoprotein, defined by their relative density. They differ in composition of lipid and type of apolipoprotein (Table 1). Apolipoprotein A (apoA) is the major apolipoprotein in high density lipoprotein (HDL) and apolipoprotein B (apoB) is the major structural apolipoprotein of the other lipoproteins, chylomicrons, very low dense lipoprotein (VLDL), intermediate density lipoprotein (IDL), and LDL. The full apoB (apoB100) is found in VLDL, IDL, and LDL, with structural and functional components, but a truncated form, apoB48, with only the structural role, is present in chylomicrons made by gut cells. The main cholesterol-carrying lipoproteins are LDL and HDL, while the main triglyceride-carrying lipoproteins are chylomicrons and VLDL. As VLDL is catabolized, remnants are formed known as IDL, normally rapidly removed from the liver, or converted to LDL.

Lipid sub-classes

The major lipoproteins are heterogeneous and sub-classes can be detected by methods such as precipitation, or ultracentrifugation. HDL can be

Table 1 The major classes of lipoproteins

Lipoprotein	Major lipids	Major lipoproteins
Chylomicrons and remnants	Dietary triglycerides	AI, AII, B48, CI, CII, CIII, E
VLDL	Endogenous triglycerides	B48, CI, CII, CIII, E
IDL	Cholesteryl esters, triglycerides	B100, CIII, E
LDL	Cholesteryl esters	B100
HDL	Cholesteryl esters	AI, AII

HDL2 or HDL3. HDL3 accepts cholesterol from cholesterol-replete tissues, converts to larger HDL2, which delivers cholesterol to the liver, or other lipoproteins. LDL can be LDL1, LDL2, and LDL3 separated by cumulative flotation ultracentrifugation. The normal LDL pattern is predominantly LDL2 with some LDL1 and less LDL3. This pattern can shift towards smaller particles with a predominance of small, dense LDL3, which is cholesterol depleted and triglyceride rich. LDL3 is less readily recognized by normal LDL receptors and more readily recognized by macrophages in the arterial subintimal space, which form the foam cells of the fatty streak of early atheroma (Campos et al. 1992). VLDL can be VLDL1, VLDL2, and VLDL3. The larger, more buoyant, triglyceride-rich VLDL1 particles, formed especially when there is increased hepatic triglyceride synthesis, are more likely to be precursors for LDL3. Small VLDL particles favour generation of the larger LDL sub-classes. Changes in the proportion of lipoprotein sub-classes are not apparent in basic lipid screening, yet this has an important bearing on the risk of atherosclerosis and may be influenced by metabolic and systemic alterations accompanying chronic rheumatic disorders.

Exogenous pathway of lipid transport

Chylomicrons carry dietary triglycerides and cholesterol from the intestine to adipose tissue and skeletal muscle. Lipoprotein lipase liberates free fatty acid and monoglycerides, which cross the endothelium to the peripheral tissue for further metabolism. The chylomicron remnant is removed by the liver.

Endogenous pathway of lipid transport

Triglycerides are synthesized in the liver and incorporated into VLDL particles in peripheral tissue, where triglycerides are hydrolyzed. VLDL becomes IDL, which is either taken back up by the liver, or loses further triglyceride and apolipoproteins and becomes cholesterol-rich LDL. Both the liver and extrahepatic tissues that utilize cholesterol recognize LDL via receptor-mediated pathways. Otherwise, a variable amount of LDL is scavenged by the reticuloendothelial system, particularly macrophages. HDL can accept cholesterol from cholesterol-replete tissues. Cholesterol is esterified on the surface of HDL by the enzyme lecithin, cholesterol acyltransferase, to become a HDL core cholesterol ester that can be exchanged with VLDL and LDL through the action of cholesterol ester transfer protein. HDL-cholesterol can be returned to the liver.

Lipoprotein (a)

ApoA is a complex protein with a protease domain and multiple repeats, called kringles, which have considerable homology with plasminogen. It is linked by a single disulfide bridge to the apoB of a LDL molecule to give lipoprotein (a). The apoA gene is highly polymorphic and lipoprotein (a) levels are mainly genetically determined. Lipoprotein (a) has been associated with coronary heart disease (Terres et al. 1995). The risk of atherosclerosis may be greater when high levels of lipoprotein (a) are associated with concomitant elevation in LDL-cholesterol levels (Maher and Brown 1995) but may not be as good a predictor of atheroma in the long term. Recent work in transgenic mice suggests that lipoprotein (a) inhibits plasminogen activation, leading to reduced activation of transforming growth factor-β and adverse effects on vessel wall function (Grainger et al. 1994).

Lipids and inflammation

Essential fatty acids and inflammatory mediators

In addition to being core components of complex lipids, fatty acids are also incorporated into cell membranes, or serve as precursors for biologically active metabolites. Essential fatty acids cannot be synthesized by mammals and are required in the diet. Polyunsaturated fatty acids contain at least two double bonds in their carbon backbone.

Omega-3 fatty acids are essential polyunsaturated fatty acids found in fish oils and include eicosapentaenoic acid. They are precursors of the 3-series prostanoids and the 5-series leukotrienes that inhibit formation of proinflammatory eicosanoids derived from arachidonic acid. Evening primrose oil contains gammalinoleic acid, a precursor of prostaglandin E1 and 15-OH-dihomo-gammalinoleic acid. Prostaglandin E1 has anti-inflammatory effects and 15-OH-dihomo-gammalinoleic acid inhibits both 5-and 12-lipoxygenases, which generate proinflammatory eicosanoids.

Lipid peroxidation and antioxidants

Polyunsaturated fatty acids are the main target for lipoperoxidative injury by oxygen free radicals. Polyunsaturated fatty acids and their attached phospholipid in plasma LDL can be oxidized by endothelial cells and macrophages. Oxidized LDL may exert several proinflammatory effects by virtue of its chemotactic, cytotoxic, and immunogenic properties. LDL is modified by close contact with endothelial cells and becomes a much more ready substrate for scavenger uptake by subintimal macrophages. LDL3 in particular is more likely to be oxidized, immunogenic, poorly recognized by the LDL receptor and more readily taken up by the scavenger pathway. Therefore, the generation of oxidized LDL may be an important factor in atherosclerosis. Certain micronutrients act as antioxidants that may have relevance to the susceptibility of LDL to oxidation (Fox 1996).

Types of hyperlipidaemia

Various patterns of elevated lipoproteins have been recognized (Table 2). Most patterns can be either caused by several different genetic disorders, or secondary to other metabolic disturbances. A framework to classify the primary inherited hyperlipidaemias is shown in Table 3, together with what is known about their genetic basis. Many hyperlipidaemias are the result of environmental factors exacerbating an underlying hyperlipidaemic tendency or background.

Several drugs used in the treatment of hyperlipidaemia are known to give rise to rheumatic complaints, although this is extremely rare. Myopathy has been described in patients treated with statins, fibrates, or nicotinic acid and rhabdomyolysis is possible (Goldman et al. 1989; Ross Peirce et al. 1990; Zuckner 1990; Hino et al. 1996). Recently, the Committee on the Safety of Medicines have calculated that the statin or fibrate use risk of serious myositis is less than one per 100 000 patient years exposure. There are case reports of drug-induced lupus caused by lovostatin and clofibrate (Howard and Brown 1973; Ahmad 1991).

Musculoskeletal manifestations of primary hyperlipidaemia

Musculoskeletal symptoms may be the first manifestation of a hyperlipidaemia. A transient polyarthritis is common in patients with familial hypercholesterolaemia (Khadchadurian 1968). Oligoarthritis and periarticular hyperaesthesia have been described in patients with type 4 hyperlipidaemia (Goldman et al. 1972; Buckingham et al. 1975). Recurrent tendinitis

Table 2 Patterns of dyslipidaemia

Lipoprotein pattern	Lipoprotein	Lipid
Type 1	Chylomicrons	Triglycerides
Type 2a	LDL	Cholesterol
Type 2b	LDL and some VLDL	Cholesterol and triglycerides
Type 3	Chylomicron remnants and IDL	Triglycerides and cholesterol
Type 4	VLDL	Triglycerides
Type 5	VLDL and chylomicrons	Triglycerides (and some cholesterol)

Table 3 Primary hyperlipidaemias

Genetic disorder	Biochemical defect	Lipoproteins elevated (pattern)	Clinical findings
Lipoprotein lipase deficiency	Lipoprotein lipase deficiency	Chylomicrons (1)	Pancreatitis, eruptive xanthomata
Apoprotein CII deficiency	Apoprotein CII deficiency	Chylomicrons and VLDL (1 or 5)	Pancreatitis
Familial type 4 hyperlipoproteinaemia	Abnormal apoprotein E	Chylomicron remnants and IDL (3)	Palmar and tuberous xanthomata, premature atherosclerosis
Familial hypercholesterolaemia	LDL receptor deficiency	LDL (2A)	Tendon xanthomata, premature atherosclerosis
Familial hypertriglyceridaemia	Unknown	VLDL (4)	Eruptive xanthomata
Familial combined hyperlipidaemia	Unknown	LDL and VLDL (2a, 2b, 4)	

is also common in patients with familial hypercholesterolaemia. Tendinous, tuberous, or periosteal xanthomata may also be present. Sometimes, tenosynovitis may occur without obvious xanthomata. Tendinitis may occur during the early weeks of statin use, usually in patients with very high cholesterol levels. Palmar xanthomata are typically seen in type III, remnant lipidaemia (familial dysbetalipoproteinaemia). Types I, V, and severe IV hyperlipoproteinaemias may be associated with eruptive xanthomatas. In a recent study of 80 patients with hyperlipidaemia, tendon xanthomatas, particularly of the tendo-Achillis, were found in approximately 50 per cent of patients, often with an associated tendinitis. The manifestations improved with lipid-lowering therapy (Klemp et al. 1993).

For primary hypercholesterolaemia requiring drug therapy, statins (3-hydroxy-3-methylglutaryl coenzyme A, HMG Co-A, reductase inhibitors) are the agents of choice, with or without resins where tolerated. For mixed lipidaemia, fibrate drugs (fenofibrate, ciprofibrate, bezafibrate, or gemfibrozil) are first choice. Most cases of acute arthropathy associated with hyperlipidaemia resolve spontaneously. The synovial fluid is usually non-inflammatory.

Lipids in joints

Lipid microspherules have been found in the joints of patients with rheumatoid arthritis. The mean levels of apoAI, apoB, and cholesterol levels were significantly higher in the synovial fluid of 12 patients with untreated rheumatoid arthritis than in eight patients with degenerative joint disease (Ananth et al. 1993). A likely explanation is the increased permeability for these lipoprotein constituents across inflamed synovial membranes. Concomitant systemic lipid abnormalities and antilipoprotein antibodies were not found in such patients (Lazarevic et al. 1993a).

Whether synovial lipoproteins are involved in the pathogenesis of rheumatoid arthritis is unclear. Synovial membrane of rheumatoid arthritis patients has been reported with positive immunostaining for oxidized LDL (Winyard et al. 1993). Peroxidation products have been detected in synovial fluid (Selley et al. 1992). Reduced levels of the lipid soluble antioxidant α-tocopherol, which terminates the process of lipid peroxidation, may point to increased oxidative activity (Fairburn et al. 1992).

The pattern of dyslipidaemia in rheumatic disorders

Low levels of HDL have been found in several chronic inflammatory disorders and seem related to disease activity. The mean HDL-cholesterol and apoAI were markedly lower in untreated and clinically active systemic lupus erythematosus (SLE) patients compared to controls. Levels of HDL-cholesterol and apoAI returned to normal as the SLE became less active (Ilowite et al. 1988). In our own patients, low levels of HDL were found with SLE and psoriatic arthritis, most noticeably in active disease (Jones et al. 1994; Leong et al. 1995). In rheumatoid arthritis, low levels of HDL-cholesterol have been found, which return to normal with treatment (Svenson et al. 1987a,b; Lazarevic et al. 1992).

Low levels of HDL are associated with high triglycerides epidemiologically. However, there are conflicting results for levels of other lipoprotein components in rheumatic disorders, which may be explained by corticosteroid treatment, renal disease, and altered catabolic states. Increased levels of total triglycerides and VLDL-cholesterol have been found in children with SLE (Ilowite et al. 1988). SLE patients, selected for absence of renal disease or corticosteroid treatment, had lower levels of total cholesterol, triglycerides, and total LDL (although LDL3 was increased), but VLDL was unchanged (Leong et al. 1995). A similar pattern was seen in patients with psoriatic arthritis (Jones et al. 1994). In a study of 48 patients with untreated rheumatoid arthritis and 21 with seronegative spondyloarthropathy, the patients with active rheumatic disease had lower levels of VLDL-cholesterol and VLDL-triglyceride, as well as lower HDL-triglyceride and HDL-cholesterol, compared to healthy controls (Svenson et al. 1987a). Low levels of LDL-cholesterol were also found in patients with active rheumatoid or psoriatic arthritis (Lazarevic et al. 1992).

In individuals without rheumatic disorders, the usual effect of endogenous steroids, or exogenous steroid therapy, is to increase serum cholesterol. There is often increased triglycerides and HDL-cholesterol may rise with prednisolone treatment (Havel et al. 1980; Zimmerman et al. 1984).

Corticosteroids, or nephrotic syndrome, contribute to a type 2b hyperlipidaemia. SLE patients had higher levels of total cholesterol, total triglyceride, and LDL-cholesterol than controls (Ettinger et al. 1987; Ettinger and Hazzard 1988). Those who were not on steroids had levels similar to controls, apart from a lower HDL-cholesterol. Similar results were found in a study of 100 Chinese patients with SLE (Leong et al. 1994). In the latter study, the type 2b pattern was associated with renal involvement and the use of corticosteroids. Raised concentrations of triglyceride and apoB have been found in SLE patients treated with corticosteroids (MacGregor et al. 1992).

Evidence for increased mortality from atherosclerosis in rheumatic disorders

Rheumatoid arthritis is associated with an increased mortality. Mortality is higher in those with more severe disease (Prior et al. 1984; Wolfe et al. 1994; Callahan and Pincus 1995).

A bimodal pattern of mortality in SLE with early deaths due to active disease or infections and late events related to atherosclerotic complications has been recognized (Urowitz et al. 1976; Abu-Shakra et al. 1995). Atherosclerosis is a major cause of death and morbidity in patients with SLE. It is not clear whether the late cardiovascular disease is related to corticosteroid treatment or other manifestations of the disease. Risk factors for coronary artery disease include age at SLE diagnosis, duration of corticosteroid use, requirement for antihypertensive treatment, maximum cholesterol level, and obesity (Petri et al. 1992). Women with SLE between ages 18 and 44 were more likely to have myocardial infarction, congestive heart failure, and stroke compared to age matched controls (Ward 1999).

Many studies have shown premature coronary atherosclerosis and myocardial infarction in relatively young patients with SLE. Subepicardial and myocardial fat was increased in SLE patients on corticosteroids compared to patients not on corticosteroids. In 42 per cent of the 18 patients who received corticosteroids for more than 1 year, the lumen of at least one of the three major coronary arteries was narrowed by more than 50 per cent by atherosclerotic plaques. None of the 17 patients who received corticosteroids for less than 1 year had such findings. Systemic hypertension was twice as common in patients who received corticosteroids for longer than 1 year (Buckley and Roberts 1975).

Conditions thought to have a better outlook, such as ankylosing spondylitis, may also have an excess death rate (Radford et al. 1977). As our ability to manage patients improves due to our increasing knowledge, survival of patients will be prolonged, as has already happened with SLE.

Mechanisms for dyslipidaemia

Several mechanisms may account for the dyslipidaemia associated with chronic inflammatory disorders. Lipoprotein lipase is a membrane-bound enzyme responsible for liberation of fatty acids from VLDL, resulting in formation of LDL. Reduced mass, or inhibition of activity of lipoprotein lipase, is an attractive hypothesis accounting for reduced clearance of VLDL-triglyceride and associated rises in plasma triglycerides. Normal or slightly low, LDL-cholesterol would be expected as a result of lower precursor input into LDL and LDL concentrations in plasma would tend to fall. HDL levels would also fall, because of slower reduction in VLDL size and less VLDL surface coat given up to provide HDL.

Lipoprotein lipase activity is inhibited by several regulatory cytokines (Querfeld et al. 1990). Furthermore, tumour necrosis factor-α is associated with a decrease in serum cholesterol and HDL levels (Spriggs et al. 1988). Cytokines may also stimulate hepatic lipid secretion and increase de novo fatty acid synthesis (Feingold and Grunfeld 1992). Lipoprotein lipase is also an insulin-dependent enzyme and its synthesis in adipose and muscle is increased by insulin treatment. Whether the dyslipidaemia in active rheumatic disease may be due to a form of insulin resistance is not known.

An increased production, by the liver, of acute phase proteins in inflammation may occur at the expense of lipoprotein production. Also, acute phase reactants may interfere with HDL metabolism. In patients with rheumatic disease, total HDL-cholesterol is lower than in normal subjects and inversely correlated with plasma concentrations of serum amyloid A protein (Kumon et al. 1993). Serum amyloid A protein may displace apoA-I and apoA-II on HDL particles, especially HDL3.

Antilipoprotein antibodies against VLDL and LDL were found in one-third of patients with active rheumatoid arthritis, but not in patients with osteoarthritis, psoriatic arthritis, or healthy blood donors (Lazarevic et al. 1993b). Autoantibodies against LDL have been demonstrated in diabetes mellitus. Anti-apoAI antibodies have been described in SLE (Merrill et al. 1995). Antibodies against apoC-II may be associated with severe hypertriglyceridaemia, due to myeloma and clonal production of the antibody.

Corticosteroids cause increased hepatic production of VLDL, resulting in elevated plasma cholesterol, plasma triglyceride, HDL-C, VLDL-C, and LDL-C. Proteinuria leads to increased generalized hepatic protein synthesis and lipoprotein synthesis, which may also be driven by urinary loss of apoA of HDL. Conversely, control of hyperlipidaemia may retard the development of glomerulosclerosis (Kasiske et al. 1988).

Rheumatic disorders

Systemic lupus erythematosus

Mechanisms accounting for vasculopathy

Factors to account for the increase in vascular disease in SLE include corticosteroid treatment, renal disease, dyslipidaemia, an underlying coagulopathy, vasculitis, and, possibly, antibody or immune-complex mediated injury (Kabakov et al. 1992).

Lipoprotein (a)

There are conflicting findings concerning the levels of lipoprotein (a) in SLE and the risk of thrombosis, myocardial infarction, and cerebral infarction (Takegoshi et al. 1990; Borba et al. 1994; Matsuda et al. 1994; Kawai et al. 1995).

Lipids and antiphospholipid antibodies

A plasma cofactor which forms part of the antigenic complex recognized by antiphospholipid antibodies has been identified as β_2-glycoprotein I, or apoH. Whether lipoproteins other than β_2-glycoprotein I, are involved in the pathogenesis of the antiphospholipid syndrome is unknown. There may be an additive risk of thrombotic clinical events if both antiphospholipid antibodies and hyperlipidaemia are present together (Garrido et al. 1994). Anticardiolipin antibodies are associated with low levels of HDL and apoAI, although cholesterol levels are also low in these patients (Lahita et al. 1993).

Antibodies to oxidized LDL have been described in patients with SLE (Vaarala et al. 1993). Monoclonal antibodies to cardiolipin have been derived from a mouse model of the antiphospholipid syndrome that have reactivity against β_2-glycoprotein and cross react with oxidized LDL (Mizutani et al. 1995). In a prospective study of middle-aged dyslipidaemic men, there was a correlation between anticardiolipin levels and antibodies to oxidized LDL and the presence of both had an additive risk for myocardial infarction (Vaarala et al. 1995).

Rheumatoid arthritis

Studies have shown that patients with rheumatoid arthritis have a lipid profile increasing the risk of atherosclerosis, especially during active phases of the disease (Svenson 1987a,b; Lazarevic et al. 1992). The most consistent abnormality is a reduction in HDL. Dyslipidaemia associated with active rheumatoid arthritis needs to be considered as a contributing factor to the death rate.

Psoriatic arthritis

Patients with psoriatic arthritis have a similar pattern of dyslipidaemia to rheumatoid arthritis (Lazarevic et al. 1992; Jones et al. 1994). Elevated LDL3 may be particularly important as it is much more likely to be taken up by macrophages in the arterial subintimal space (Campos et al. 1992). There may also be an imbalance in fatty acids and antioxidants (Azzini et al. 1995).

Systemic sclerosis

Vascular impairment, secondary to reperfusion injury and the formation of free radicals, are postulated as disease mechanisms in scleroderma. LDL in patients with systemic sclerosis are more susceptible to oxidation (Bruckdorfer et al. 1995). In addition to its toxic effects on endothelium, oxidized LDL may contribute to increased matrix synthesis in systemic sclerosis, by upregulating adhesion molecules and growth factors.

Gout

There is a clear association between gout and type 4 hyperlipidaemia (Matsubara et al. 1989). The association is unlikely to be causal as patients with gout often have other predisposing factors for hyperlipidaemia, such as obesity, increased alcohol consumption, and altered nutritional habit. Hyperlipidaemia may also be more directly associated with decreased renal excretion of uric acid (Tinahones et al. 1995).

Management

The use of essential fatty acids in the treatment of rheumatic diseases

The use of essential fatty acids to treat inflammation is supported by *in vivo* and biochemical studies, although the clinical efficacy and cost-effectiveness of such treatment in man remains uncertain. In animal models, marine oils have been effective in suppressing inflammation. Eicosapentaenoic acid supplementation prevented renal disease from developing in NZB/NZW mice (Prickett et al. 1981). A fish oil diet had a beneficial effect on the severity of collagen-induced arthritis (Cathcart and Gonnerman 1991) and on lupus-like features in MRL-*lpr* mice (Robinson et al. 1986).

The addition of omega 3 or omega 6 polyunsaturated fatty acids to the diet may shift the balance of prostaglandin metabolism towards substances that have less of a proinflammatory action. The two most extensively studied therapies have been fish oils and evening primrose oil.

Several studies in rheumatoid arthritis have shown beneficial effects of diets containing essential fatty acids in fish oils, such as a reduced requirement for non-steroidal anti-inflammatory drugs (NSAIDs) (Lau et al. 1993; Leventhal et al. 1993; Geusens et al. 1994). It is worth mentioning that olive oil may also have some active beneficial effects as it contains mainly unsaturated fats.

There is some evidence that fish oils may be beneficial in other conditions such as psoriasis (Bittiner et al. 1988), but findings are not universal (Walton et al. 1991; Veale et al. 1994). Another benefit of a fish oil diet is an alteration of the thromboxane/prostacyclin ratio towards substantially less thrombotic thromboxane and a substantially more antithrombotic prostacyclin.

It is important to note that the amount of essential fatty acids needed to produce clinical effects are often in excess of the dose available in commercial preparation. Also, it may be difficult to achieve such doses by ingestion of natural food substances. The therapeutic dose in many studies, 7.5 g of fish oil, is the equivalent of 700 g of fish and carries a 70 calorie load (Fahrer et al. 1991).

Longer-term studies with larger numbers of patients are required to clarify the therapeutic role of essential fatty acids. It is possible that essential fatty acid supplementation may be a reasonable alternative to NSAIDs when the latter are contraindicated. Fish oils can improve moderate to marked hypertriglyceridaemia in some individuals, but do not alter LDL–cholesterol much.

Rationale for lipid-lowering treatment

Rheumatic diseases may carry an increased risk of morbidity and mortality from premature atherosclerosis, although more evidence is needed. Abnormalities in the LDL sub-fraction are present in patients on long-term corticosteroid treatment (Ettinger et al. 1987; Ettinger and Hazzard 1988; MacGregor et al. 1992). Risk of myocardial infarction is associated with higher levels of LDL-cholesterol and inversely associated with HDL levels (Castelli et al. 1986; Neaton et al. 1992).

Treatment of lipid abnormalities influences outcome, with reduced coronary heart disease deaths and events (Lipid Research Clinics Program 1984; Frick et al. 1987). More recently, the more potent statins have shown reduction in coronary heart disease deaths and events, coronary artery surgery requirements, and total mortality (Scandinavian Simvastatin Survival Study 1994; Shepherd et al. 1995). Many studies have shown slowing of progression and some regression of atheroma in patients actively treated for hyperlipidaemia after coronary artery graft surgery (Blankenhorn et al. 1987).

Serum C-reactive protein level has been shown to be a significant independent predictor of coronary artery disease, peripheral arterial disease, and ischaemic stroke (Kervinen et al. 2001; Napoli et al. 2001; Ridker et al. 2001). Statin therapy has been shown to lower the rate of coronary events, post-myocardial infarction, in patients who have average levels of serum cholesterol and elevated C-reactive protein (Sacks et al. 1996).

Approach to treatment

Risk factors for hyperlipidaemia need to be assessed for the individual patient. A basic fasting lipid profile may be appropriate on any patient with a chronic inflammatory rheumatic disease, although subtle changes in lipid subfraction composition may be missed. Other associated risk factors, such as hypertension, are important and need to be fully discussed with the patient and managed.

Dietary intervention plays a major role in the management of hyperlipidaemia. While dietary change may produce only modest change in lipid levels, it may be sufficient in moderate hyperlipidaemia. Target levels for treatment of dyslipidaemia have been set in national and international guidelines (National Cholesterol Education Program 1994; Pyorala et al. 1994). In SLE, benefit of dietary change at 6 months has been shown in patients receiving corticosteroids (Hearth-Holmes et al. 1995). In adolescents with SLE, dietary modification with fish oil supplementation improved the lipid profile (Ilowite et al. 1995). However, a significant number of SLE patients require further pharmacological therapy for persistent dyslipidaemia.

The role of hydroxychloroquine

Hydroxychloroquine is often used in the treatment of mild SLE and rheumatoid arthritis. Besides its immunomodulatory properties, hydroxychloroquine may have a protective role against hyperlipidaemia induced by corticosteroids (Hodis et al. 1993) and is associated with low levels of cholesterol, triglycerides, and LDL-cholesterol regardless of concomitant corticosteroid use (Wallace et al. 1990). In a cohort longitudinal study involving SLE patients using a regression model for steroid use, a change in prednisolone dose of 10 mg was associated with a change in cholesterol level of 7.5 mg ($\pm$1.46 SD) and a weight gain of 2.5 kg ($\pm$0.6 SD). On the other hand, hydroxychloroquine at 200 or 400 mg/day was associated with lower serum cholesterol (Petri et al. 1994). No prospective randomized study of hydroxychloroquine on lipoprotein and lipid levels has been carried out.

Conclusions

Lipid metabolism is altered in chronic rheumatic diseases and may promote accelerated atherosclerosis. Further long-term studies are needed to determine the risk more precisely and the contribution of treatments, such as corticosteroids. Dietary intervention is a sensible first treatment step, but lipid lowering agents may be required, appropriate target levels being cholesterol less than 5.0 mmol/l, triglyceride less than 2 mmol/l, and LDL-cholesterol less than 3.5 mmol/l. A low-fat high-fibre diet, partly supplemented by mono- and polyunsaturated fatty acids, should be encouraged. Whether dietary supplementation with marine oils has a place in reducing requirements for anti-inflammatory agents is uncertain and the dose of fat supplement may be unacceptable.

Lipid peroxidation products, such as oxidized LDL, may play an important role in promoting endothelial and synovial injury in addition to atheroma and warrant further study, together with the possible protective role of antioxidants. Where patients have risk factors for coronary heart disease, in addition to those from the rheumatic disease itself, attention to all possible risk factors may be necessary to help prevent coronary heart disease. Treatment of risk factors is essential in patients who have manifested macrovascular disease.

References

Abu-Shakra, M., Urowitz, M.B., Gladman, D.D., and Gough, J. (1995). Mortality studies in systemic lupus erythematosus. Results from a single centre. 1. Causes of death. *Journal of Rheumatology* **22**, 1259–64.

Ahmad, S. (1991). Lovastatin-induced lupus erythematosus. *Archives of Internal Medicine* **151**, 1667–8.

Ward, M.M. (1999). Premature morbidity from cardiovascular and cerebrovascular diseases in women with SLE. *Arthritis and Rheumatism* **42**, 338–46.

Winyard, P.G., Tatzber, F., Esterbauer, H., Kus, M.L., Blake, D.R., and Morris, C.J. (1993). Presence of foam cells containing oxidised low density lipoprotein in the synovial membrane from patients with rheumatoid arthritis. *Annals of the Rheumatic Diseases* **52**, 677–80.

Wolfe, F., Mitchell, D.M., and Sibley, J.T. (1994). The mortality of rheumatoid arthritis. *Arthritis and Rheumatism* **37**, 481–94.

Zimmerman, J., Fainaru, M., and Eisenberg, S. (1984). The effects of prednisone therapy on plasma lipoproteins and apolipoproteins. A prospective study. *Metabolism* **33**, 521–6.

Zuckner, J. (1990). Drug-induced myopathies. *Seminars in Arthritis and Rheumatism* **19**, 259–68.

6.13 Soft-tissue rheumatism

6.13.1 Fibromyalgia and diffuse pain syndromes—adult onset

Johannes W.G. Jacobs, Rinie Geenen, and Johannes W.J. Bijlsma

Introduction, the development of the concept of fibromyalgia

Fibromyalgia is a clinical syndrome, characterized by chronic, generalized pain in joints, muscles, and the spine. Although pain is felt in joints, there is no arthritis; the pain originates from muscles and other so-called soft tissues. Therefore, fibromyalgia is commonly classified as soft tissue rheumatism. The pain is often accompanied by several non-specific symptoms, such as fatigue, depressive mood, and sleep disturbance, hence the term syndrome. The Mexican painter Frida Kahlo beautifully depicted her fibromyalgia in a self-portrait named 'The broken column', expressing generalized peripheral and axial pain, tender points, headache, depression, and social isolation. Most patients experience early morning stiffness, but there are no signs of inflammation. At physical examination tender points are found, that is, soft tissues are painful on pressure. Laboratory investigations give normal results. The old synonym fibrositis, suggesting inflammation, is misleading and obsolete. Damage to joints or other tissues does not occur.

Although the demanding modern Western society might be seen as a risk factor for development of musculoskeletal complaints, chronic musculoskeletal pain has been described frequently over the past centuries. All kinds of abnormalities in muscle tissue were thought to be the cause of pain. However, currently the hypothesis that muscle abnormalities play a primary or key role in the pathophysiology of fibromyalgia has been rejected (Simms 1998). Another hypothesis for the cause of chronic musculoskeletal pain was expressed by the label 'psychogenic rheumatism', as it was thought to be the musculoskeletal expression of psychoneurosis. From the 1970s onward, the multidimensional concept of the chronic generalized musculoskeletal pain state now termed 'fibromyalgia' really developed. Milestones were investigations into sleep disturbances (Moldofsky et al. 1975), extensive description of the clinical picture and development of diagnostic features (Yunus et al. 1981), development of classification criteria (Wolfe et al. 1990), and research into neurohormonal dysregulation (Griep et al. 1993) and aberrant central pain processing.

In this chapter, the focus will be on fibromyalgia. Other diffuse pain syndromes will be discussed in the context of fibromyalgia. Many of the mechanisms described in fibromyalgia also apply to other chronic pain disorders.

Epidemiology

Estimations of prevalence of fibromyalgia differ, because prevalence depends on the population that is investigated and the methods of case-finding. In the general population, prevalence was 2 per cent, 3.4 per cent for women, and 0.5 per cent for men (Wolfe et al. 1995), but lower prevalences of 0.7–1.3 per cent have also been reported. Fibromyalgia occurs in children and adolescents, but the prevalence increases with age, with highest values between 55 and 65 years (Wolfe et al. 1995). For chronic widespread pain in the general adult population, a prevalence as high as 11 per cent was found (Bergman et al. 2001).

Of consecutive new referrals to a general rheumatology clinic, 10 per cent had fibromyalgia in one (Reilly and Littlejohn 1992), and 4 per cent in another study (Wolfe and Cathey 1983).

Female sex, middle age, lower household income, being disabled, divorced or separated, and lower educational status are factors associated with fibromyalgia and chronic generalized pain in general (Wolfe et al. 1995).

No clear genetic predisposition exists, but in families with many fibromyalgia cases, a weak genetic predisposition might play a role (Yunus et al. 1999).

Clinical picture

Symptoms, pain-modulating factors

In addition to generalized pain, patients with fibromyalgia report manifold non-specific symptoms (see Table 1) (Yunus et al. 1981; Campbell et al. 1983; Quimby et al. 1988; Straus 1988; Wolfe et al. 1990; Jacobs et al. 1996). These, together with chronic generalized pain characterize fibromyalgia. Patients with fibromyalgia use more adjectives to describe their pain than patients with rheumatoid arthritis or osteoarthritis. Another characteristic of fibromyalgia is that pain, in contrast to articular rheumatic conditions, does not respond well to pain medication. Commonly, symptoms are reported to be increased by exposure to noise and light or stress, posture, pregnancy (especially the last trimester); the pre-menstrual period and weather may also exacerbate symptoms. However, in quantitative research no relation between the severity of complaints and meteorological factors was found (de Blecourt et al. 1993), nor did hormonal changes connected with abortion, breast feeding or the use of hormonal contraceptives modulate symptom severity (Ostensen et al. 1997).

Signs, tender points

On physical examination, multiple painful spots on pressure are evident, especially over bony prominences, localized in muscle, ligaments, bursae, fat pads, muscle–tendon junctions, and tendon-insertions: *tender points.* Test–retest stability and interobserver agreement of tender point scores at manual palpation or using a pressure algometer is moderate to high (Cott et al. 1992; Jacobs et al. 1995; Tunks et al. 1995), but manual palpation and pressure algometer scores are not equivalent (Cott et al. 1992). Tender points are not specific of fibromyalgia. Healthy adults often have some tender points, but it is the number and severity that is characteristic of fibromyalgia (Wolfe 1997). Among patients with fibromyalgia, tender point scores show a lack of correlation with most of the typical symptoms of fibromyalgia (Jacobs et al. 1996; Wolfe 1997).

Some locations have been defined as non-tender or control points, for example, the forehead, forearm (ulna mid-shaft), the thumb, hyopthenar, and shin (mid-tibia, anteromedial surface) (Campbell et al. 1983). The utility of control points is low; control points are less tender than tender points in

Table 1 Prevalences of symptoms (%) among patients with fibromyalgia in secondary referral centres, in comparison with prevalence of symptoms among patients with chronic fatigue syndrome (in italic)

	Yunus et al. (1981)	Campbell et al. (1983)	Quimby et al. (1988)	Wolfe et al. (1990)	Jacobs et al. (1996)	*Straus (1988)*
Pain in muscles	100	100	100	100	100	*80*
Morning stiffness	72	91	86	76	85	
Fatigue	92	100	91	78	83	*100*
Sleep disturbance	56	68	79	76	71	*70*
Paraesthesia	58			67	60	
Headache	44	55	63	54	56	*90*
Psychiatric symptoms	70		56	45	47	*65*
Irritable bowel	34	50	37	36	29	*40*

fibromyalgia patients (Campbell et al. 1983; Smythe et al. 1992), and not (Campbell et al. 1983) or somewhat (Smythe et al. 1992) more tender than in control patients. Possibly, control points are a reflection of the pain threshold and tender points of distress, pain behaviour, and coping (Wolfe 1997). Less frequently, *trigger points* are encountered: painful, sometimes palpable taut bands of muscle fibres that trigger pain in a referred area on pressure, but trigger points are more characteristic of myofascial pain syndrome (regional pain syndromes). Swelling of joints often reported by patients cannot be objectified. In the older literature subcutaneous 'fibrositic nodules' are mentioned, but this is an occasional and non-specific finding.

Classification criteria

In 1990, classification criteria for fibromyalgia were published (Wolfe et al. 1990). To develop the criteria, patients in whom the participating treating rheumatologist had made the clinical diagnosis fibromyalgia and control patients were studied. Widespread pain (axial plus upper and lower segment plus left- and right-sided pain) was found in 98 per cent of all patients with fibromyalgia and in 69 per cent of all control patients. The combination of widespread pain and pain at 11 or more of 18 specific tender point sites yielded a sensitivity of 88 per cent and a specificity of 81 per cent for fibromyalgia. On the basis of these results, criteria for the classification of fibromyalgia are (i) widespread pain (Table 2) in combination with (ii) pain at 11 or more of the 18 specific tender point sites (Fig. 1). As the criteria performed equally well in primary (no underlying disease, as is most frequently the case) and secondary or concomitant fibromyalgia (associated with a disease), no exclusions are made for the presence of concomitant radiographic or laboratory abnormalities or for underlying conditions (Wolfe et al. 1990). In the absence of a gold standard, the diagnosis fibromyalgia in the classification study was made on clinical grounds, including generalized pain and tender points. It is thus not surprising that generalized pain and tender points are included as classification criteria (Quinter and Cohen 1999). Fibromyalgia is clearly a descriptive diagnosis: fibromyalgia does not cause pain, it *is* pain.

Classification criteria are used for discrimination of groups of patients, for example, to include or exclude patients for studies. At the individual patient level, classification criteria for fibromyalgia are not intended for use as diagnostic criteria. Sometimes, the diagnosis is made in a patient who does not meet the classification criteria.

A source of confusion is that in the ACR-criteria 'tender points' that are only tender, do not fulfil the definition of tender point: tender points have to be painful. In this sense, pain points would have been a more appropriate term. Patients with fibromyalgia can have many more than 18 tender points; the ones selected in the ACR criteria performed best.

Table 2 The American College of Rheumatology 1990 criteria for classification of fibromyalgia[a]

A. History of widespread pain for at least three months. Pain is considered widespread when it is present at all of the following sites:[b]
—The left side of the body
—The right side of the body
—Above the waist
—Below the waist
—In the axial skeletal (cervical spine or anterior chest or thoracic spine or low back)

B. Pain on digital palpation in at least 11 of the following 18 tender point sites; all sites bilateral (see Fig. 1):[c]
1. Occiput: at the suboccipital muscle insertion
2. Low cervical: at the anterior aspect of the intertransverse spaces at C5–7
3. Trapezius: at the midpoint of the upper border
4. Supraspinatus: at the origin, above the scapular spine near the medial border
5. Second rib: at the second costochondral junction, just lateral to the junction on the upper surface
6. Lateral epicondyle: 2 cm distal to the epicondyle
7. Gluteal: in the upper outer quadrant of the buttock in the anterior fold of muscle
8. Greater trochanter: posterior to the trochanteric prominence
9. Knee: at the medial fat pad proximal to the joint line

[a] For purposes of classification, patients will be said to have fibromyalgia if both criteria A and B are satisfied. The presence of a second clinical disorder does not exclude the classification of fibromyalgia (Wolfe et al. 1990).

[b] Pain in a patient in for instance the left shoulder, right buttock, and cervical spine is generalized, according to these criteria.

[c] Digital palpation should be performed with an approximate force of 4 kg. For a tender point to be considered positive, the palpation has to be painful. 'Tender points' that are only tender are not tender points.

Why classification as soft-tissue rheumatism?

Being a non-articular, non-inflammatory condition, fibromyalgia is a somewhat atypical entity in the field of rheumatology, a medical specialty dealing typically with articular, inflammatory diseases. Muscle abnormalities do not play a key role in the pathophysiology; at the level of joint pathology and impairment there are no serious problems, in contrast to the degree of problems on the level of handicap. In this respect, fibromyalgia differs from an inflammatory joint disease such as rheumatoid arthritis (see Table 3). So why do we still classify fibromyalgia as soft-tissue rheumatism or as a rheumatic condition? Our answer is that rheumatologists are the specialists best able to discriminate this condition from other causes of pain in and around joints and spine, and to look for an underlying condition.

Diagnosis and differential diagnosis

Diagnosis is based on pattern recognition of the above mentioned, characteristic set of symptoms and presence of tender points. Fibromyalgia does

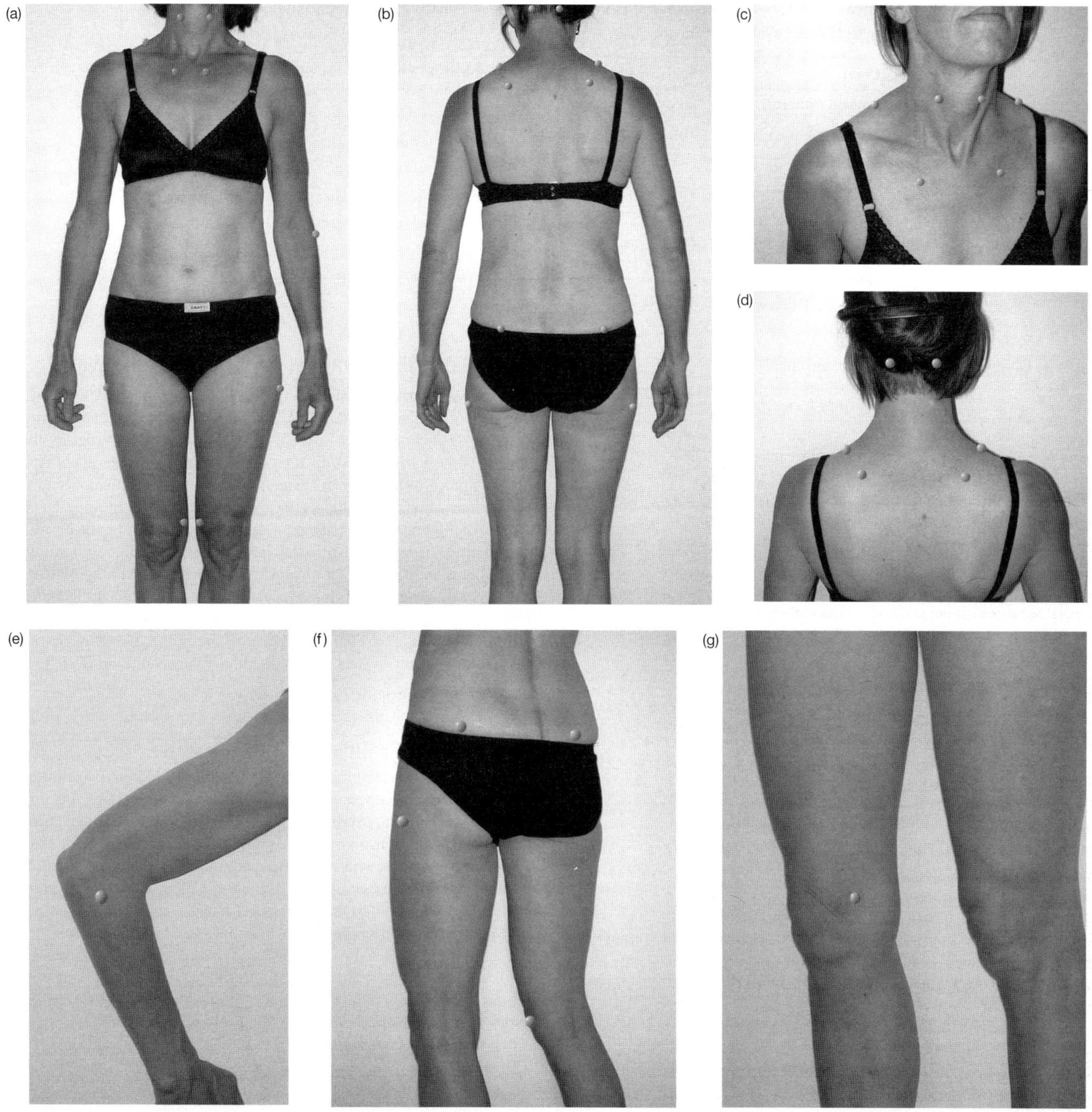

Fig. 1 Localization of tender points (a) 2, 3, 5, 6, 8, and 9; (b) 1, 3, 4, 7, and 8; (c) 2, 3, and 5; (d) 1, 3, and 4; (e) 6; (f) 7–9; and (g) 9 (see Table 2).

not seem to be a distinct disease entity in the sense that only patients have the symptoms and tender points and controls do not (Croft et al. 1994; Wolfe et al. 1995). For pain and tender points, fibromyalgia appears to be the extreme of the normal population distribution. In that respect, it resembles conditions like osteoarthritis and osteoporosis.

Sometimes, a patient reports such a wide range of somatic symptoms that the diagnosis is not easy to make. Fibromyalgia is a descriptive diagnosis; the physician should always look for an underlying condition. However, when the diagnosis of primary fibromyalgia can be made, only rarely an underlying somatic disease is present (Ledingham et al. 1993). In general, a patient with long-standing (years) symptoms suggestive of fibromyalgia has much less risk of an underlying disorder if it is clinically not evident than a similar patient with complaints for only some months. In all patients, a full physical examination should be done. In patients with recent or atypical features for fibromyalgia, a careful diagnostic process particularly is warranted. 'Red flags' are a history of unexplained weight loss and fever. Signs, such as muscle atrophy, arthritis, or myxoedema must be looked for.

Laboratory and other tests should be guided by the clinical picture of each individual patient. Overinvestigation must be avoided because it can cause or consolidate illness behaviour. Routine testing with tests like rheumatoid and antinuclear factor and serology for viruses and Lyme disease is not adequate, because these tests lack specificity.

Table 3 Differences between the biomedical disease rheumatoid arthritis and the dysfunctional syndrome fibromyalgia

Level	Signs, symptoms	Rheumatoid arthritis	Fibromyalgia
Synovial pathology	Effusion, warmth	+++	−
Impairment	Stiff, painful knee, with limited flexion	+++	+
Disability	Cannot walk	+++	++
Handicap	Cannot do shopping	+++	+++
Additional symptoms	Fatigue, headache, sleep disturbance	+++	++++

Table 4 Differential diagnosis of fibromyalgia[a]

Disease	Key investigation[b]
Inflammatory rheumatic diseases	
Sjögren's syndrome	Ophthalmologic, ESR, ENA
Polymyalgia rheumatica	ESR
Myopathy, myositis	Serum creatine kinase
Early rheumatoid arthritis	(ESR, rheumatoid factor)
Systemic lupus erythematosus	(ESR, full blood count, antinuclear factor)
Systemic vasculitis	ESR
Non-inflammatory rheumatic diseases	
Generalized osteoarthritis	(Joint X-rays)
Hypermobility	Beighton's clinical score
Endocrine disorders	
Hypothyroidism	Thyroid function
Hyperparathyroidism	Serum calcium and alkaline phosphatase
Hypovitaminosis D, osteomalacia	Serum 25-hydroxy-vitamin D
Chronic Infections	
Hepatitis C virus infection	Serology, liver enzyme tests
Malignancy	
Disseminated malignancy	Bone scintigraphy
Myeloma	Plasma and urine paraproteins
Adverse-effect of medication	
Glucocorticoid withdrawal	Medical history
Post-chemotherapy arthralgia	Medical history
Eosinophilia–myalgia syndrome	Check of medication (L-tryptophan?)
HMG-CoA reductases (statins)	Check of medication

[a] If a patient with one of these conditions also fulfils the fibromyalgia classification criteria, secondary or concomitant fibromyalgia is diagnosed.

[b] Key investigation: additional to full physical investigation. ESR, erythrocyte sedimentation rate; ENA, extractable nuclear antigens. Between brackets are investigations with low diagnostic value for the given situation, e.g. in case of early rheumatoid arthritis, the ESR is often normal and rheumatoid factor not present; for systemic lupus erythematosus, antinuclear factor is a sensitive, but not a specific test.

In Table 4, differential diagnoses for fibromyalgia and investigations, to discriminate each condition from fibromyalgia are listed. Often myofascial pain syndrome is mentioned in the list of differential diagnoses of fibromyalgia, but the former is a regional and the latter a generalized pain syndrome.

Some physicians worry about the diagnostic label 'fibromyalgia', and argue against using it. However, in case of long-standing severe unexplained symptoms, the diagnosis fibromyalgia can be a relief for the patient. A long hunt for a diagnosis can be harmful to a patient's health, because the next step cannot be taken, which is acceptance and dealing as best as possible with the situation. One has to avoid that a diagnostic label causes a patient to remain sick, though. The diagnosis should be presented with adequate patient information and education.

Secondary fibromyalgia; is it clinically relevant?

In the publication of the American College of Rheumatology 1990 classification criteria for fibromyalgia, it is stated that *on the diagnostic or classification level*, the distinction between primary and secondary fibromyalgia is abandoned (Wolfe et al. 1990). This does not mean that the clinical entity secondary fibromyalgia has been abandoned. Among new patients seen in an outpatient rheumatology clinic, secondary or concomitant fibromyalgia was diagnosed in 12 per cent of patients with rheumatoid arthritis and 7 per cent of patients with osteoarthritis (Wolfe and Cathey 1983). In a study of 100 patients with subclinical or biochemical primary hypothyroidism, in 5 per cent the diagnosis of fibromyalgia was made (Carette and Lefrancois 1988). Other underlying or concomitant conditions are for instance ankylosing spondylitis, and Sjögren's syndrome. Secondary fibromyalgia could respond beneficially to treatment of the underlying condition (Carette and Lefrancois 1988).

Overlapping dysfunctional syndromes

Fibromyalgia shares symptoms and neuroendocrine dysfunction with other common disorders without obvious organ pathology, called by many different names: functional, psychosomatic, somatization, stress-related, affective spectrum, central sensitivity, and dysfunctional syndromes or disorders. Symptoms of patients with fibromyalgia and those of patients with chronic fatigue syndrome show clear overlap (Table 1) (Yunus et al. 1981; Campbell et al. 1983; Quimby et al. 1988; Straus 1988; Wolfe et al. 1990; Jacobs et al. 1996). Dysfunctional syndromes, which have key overlapping symptoms with fibromyalgia, are shown in Table 5. Overlap can exist for symptoms only or for whole syndromes. The classification criteria for the chronic fatigue syndrome (Table 6) resemble those of fibromyalgia (Fukuda et al. 1994). In a study, among females, 58 per cent of fibromyalgia cases met the full criteria for chronic fatigue syndrome, compared to 26 and 13 per cent of controls with widespread and localized pain, respectively. Male percentages were 80, 22, and 0 per cent, respectively (White et al. 2000). Because of the overlap, one could hypothese that fibromyalgia and related syndromes are not separate diagnostic entities, but overlapping manifestations of one single dysfunctional syndrome. The existence of separate diagnoses could be an artifact, because medical specialities focus on symptoms pertinent to their specialty. However, the reported overlap of fibromyalgia and related syndromes in research at secondary or tertiary care settings is probably an overestimate. In a community-based sample, patients showed less overlap (Jason et al. 2000). Moreover, there are differences in pathophysiological mechanisms and findings between fibromyalgia and related syndromes. Patients with fibromyalgia are already a heterogeneous group with respect to psychosocial and behavioural characteristics as well as response to pharmacological treatment.

Discrimination of dysfunctional syndromes enables the specialist (e.g. the rheumatologist in case of pain in muscles and joints) to distinguish the alleged dysfunctional syndrome from other, somatic disorders, to find specific therapeutic modalities and to give adequate advise. These aims are not served by grouping all dysfunctional syndromes together.

Table 5 Dysfunctional syndromes that overlap with fibromyalgia[a]

Syndrome	Key overlapping symptoms
Chronic fatigue syndrome	Fatigue, generalized pain
Myalgic encephalomyelitis	Fatigue, cognitive dysfunction
Post-traumatic stress syndrome, Persian Gulf syndrome	Fatigue, depression, pain
Temporomandibular dysfunction	Facial pain
Irritable bowel syndrome	Abdominal cramps and pain
Tension headache	Headache, psychological stress
Restless legs syndrome	Muscle cramps, paraesthesia
Depression and anxiety disorders	Depression, anxiety, psychological stress
Primary dysmenorrhoea	Abdominal cramps and pain
Multiple chemical sensitivity	Autonomic dysfunction

[a] This is not a complete list. Overlap can exist for symptoms only or for whole syndromes: e.g. if a patient meets both the classification criteria for fibromyalgia and chronic fatigue syndrome, both syndromes are supposed to be present.

Table 6 Revised Centers for Disease Control criteria for chronic fatigue syndrome[a]

A case of chronic fatigue syndrome is defined by the presence of:

1. Clinically evaluated, ***unexplained, persistent, or relapsing fatigue*** that is of new or definite onset; is not the result of ongoing exertion; is not alleviated by rest; and results in substantial reduction of previous levels of occupational, educational, social, or personal activities; and
2. Four or more of the following symptoms that persist or recur during six or more consecutive months of illness and that do not predate the fatigue:
   Muscle pain
   Multijoint pain without redness or swelling
   Unrefreshing sleep
   Headaches of a new pattern or severity
   Self-reported impairment in short-term memory or concentration
   Sore throat
   Tender cervical or axillary nodes
   Post-exertional malaise lasting at least 24 h

[a] Bold and italic symptoms overlap with those of fibromyalgia.

Psychiatric disorders in fibromyalgia

Psychiatric disorders that have been most frequently reported in association with fibromyalgia are depression and anxiety or panic disorders. These problems clearly occur more often in fibromyalgia than in the general population (Epstein et al. 1999), although it can be argued that the psychological and psychiatric studies of patients with fibromyalgia have utilized instruments that do not control for pain and therefore may be falsely interpreted (Goldenberg 1989). Difficult questions are whether psychiatric disorders or symptoms occur more frequently in fibromyalgia than in rheumatic diseases, for example, rheumatoid arthritis [no (Clark et al. 1985; Goldenberg 1989), yes (Walker et al. 1997a)], and whether psychiatric disorders are the cause of fibromyalgia, or vice versa. The finding of an increased rate of somatoform disorders in patients with fibromyalgia with psychological questionnaires is virtually identical to the clinical finding of manifold somatic symptom reporting in fibromyalgia and does not answer the question of cause or consequence. Other hypotheses are that there is a coexistence of fibromyalgia and psychiatric symptoms or disorders because of common pathophysiological mechanisms and that the finding of concomitant psychiatric disorders is related to health care-seeking behaviour associated with these disorders. In pain patients, concurrent psychological factors are predictive of persistence of the symptoms (McBeth et al. 2001). Similarly, in pain patients, concurrent manifold symptoms, including psychiatric problems, were associated with subsequent development of fibromyalgia in a longitudinal population study (Forseth et al. 1999). However, this temporal relationship between manifold symptoms and development of chronic pain may not be a causal one.

Pathophysiological mechanisms

Theories about the pathogenesis of fibromyalgia have shifted over time from peripheral pathology (muscles) to central pathology (pain processing) and from unicausal to multicausal hypotheses. Some hypotheses have been abandoned, for example, that the primary cause is localized in muscles. Associations of development of fibromyalgia with infections in the past seem coincidental, not causal. However, there may be a relationship between hepatitis C virus infection and fibromyalgia symptoms (Rivera et al. 1997). Other hypotheses, for instance about psychogenic factors and sleep disturbances still play a role, but only as one of many aspects of fibromyalgia. We will first discuss separate mechanisms in fibromyalgia and thereafter integrate these mechanisms in a model.

Chronic psychosocial stress

A current hypothesis is that fibromyalgia is a stress related, neuroendocrine disorder. In acute stress, pain is inhibited via central pain modulation called stress-induced analgesia, but chronic stress could have the opposite effect. Humans today have the same neuroendocrine and pain regulatory systems as our caveman forebears. The environment of humans however has changed: acute physical stress encountering predators has changed into chronic daily psychological stress of the modern society. Instead of running or fighting we try to cope with situations, which are for a major part beyond our direct control. This chronic stress could via its influence on central mechanisms lead to symptoms, like pain. Patients with fibromyalgia report more stressful live events in the past as well as more daily stressful 'hassles' than patients with rheumatoid arthritis or pain-free healthy controls. A higher frequency of sexual abuse in childhood has also been reported (Boisset-Pioro et al. 1995; Walker et al. 1997). It should be borne in mind however that persons who currently experience psychological stress are likely to report more adverse events in the past (McBeth and Silman 2001). Probably also recall bias can play a role in the reporting of virus infections and traumata preceding fibromyalgia. Work related psychological factors, such as work demands, job control, and social support and psychological distress are associated with reporting of musculoskeletal pain, especially when pain is reported at multiple sites (Bergman et al. 2001).

Sleep disturbance

Studies on sleep in patients with fibromyalgia reported alpha–delta sleep anomaly in the electroencephalogram during non-rapid eye movement (non-REM) sleep, reflecting light, unrefreshing sleep. The hypothesis of sleep disturbance as the cause of fibromyalgia was attractive, because it would explain many of the problems of patients with fibromyalgia, such as unrefreshed awakening with pain and stiffness, fatigue, headache, and in addition to these somatic features of malaise also psychic malaise. However, sleep disturbance proved to be not specific for fibromyalgia: it was also found in patients with rheumatoid arthritis, osteoarthritis, Sjögren's syndrome, chronic fatigue syndrome and in normal controls when deep pain was induced during sleep. Moreover, different sleep anomalies have been described in different studies and only some fibromyalgia patients have sleep disturbances. Thus, sleep disturbances are neither uniform nor specific for fibromyalgia. Sleep anomalies could cause disturbance in nocturnal metabolic and endocrine functions, such as growth hormone secretion in non-REM sleep (Spiegel et al. 1999). For the development and persistence of fibromyalgia, sleep disturbance seems to be a non-specific risk factor.

Neuroendocrine dysregulation

Neuroendocrine dysfunction found in fibromyalgia can be divided into alterations of the two major stress systems, the hypothalamic–pituitary–adrenal (HPA) axis and the autonomous nervous system.

HPA-related functioning

In fibromyalgia, almost all hormonal feedback mechanisms controlled by the hypothalamus are dysfunctional. After stimulation of the HPA axis with exogenous corticotropin-releasing hormone (CRH) or by insulin induced hypoglycaemia, exaggerated pituitary adrenocorticotropin hormone (ACTH) release has been observed, with (given this ACTH hyper-responsiveness) adrenal hyporesponsiveness (Griep et al. 1993; Crofford et al. 1994) (see Fig. 2). Moreover, indications for sub-normal basal levels of serum growth hormone have been found consistently (Dinser et al. 2000). Serum thyroid hormone levels are normal, but after intravenous injection of 400 μg thyrotropin-releasing hormone, patients with primary fibromyalgia responded with a significantly lower secretion of thyrotropin and thyroid hormones within a 2 h observation period (Neeck and Riedel 1992). How should these data be interpreted? HPA axis studies could be seen as being indicative of HPA hypofunction, but also has been attributed to hyperactivity of CRH neurons. The latter hypothesis seems compatible with the hypothesis that fibromyalgia is a stress-related, neuroendocrine disorder, but not with some hypotheses on serotonin metabolism in fibromyalgia.

Autonomic nervous system

In several studies, altered autonomic nervous system activity has been observed in fibromyalgia, but the results are difficult to interpret. Most studies did not control for physical activity levels of participants (Petzke and Clauw 2000), but if effects of physical activity are taken into account, results might be interpreted as being indicative of tonic sympathetic hyperactivity in a subset of patients. This observation is consistent with the hypothesis of hyperactivity of CRH neurons. With respect to autonomic nervous system reactivity, aggregate data suggest a somewhat blunted stress response (Petzke and Clauw 2000).

The finding of neuroendocrine dysregulations does not mean that they have a causal relation to the development and persistence of fibromyalgia. They could be secondary to pain mechanisms or merely be epiphenomena. Furthermore, at the group level, neuroendocrine functioning of fibromyalgia patients tends to deviate from norm reference groups, but apparently only sub-groups of patients suffer from clinical significant altered autonomic nervous system activity, HPA axis perturbations, or subnormal growth hormone secretion. It could well be that individual patients differ in the spectrum of dysregulations.

In other dysfunctional syndromes, dysregulation of the HPA axis and of the autonomous nervous system have also been described. However, there are differences, for instance between fibromyalgia and chronic fatigue syndrome, with respect to HPA axis dysregulation (Crofford and Demitrack 1996), autonomic nervous system dysfunctioning (Naschitz et al. 2001), and growth hormone metabolism (Buchwald et al. 1996).

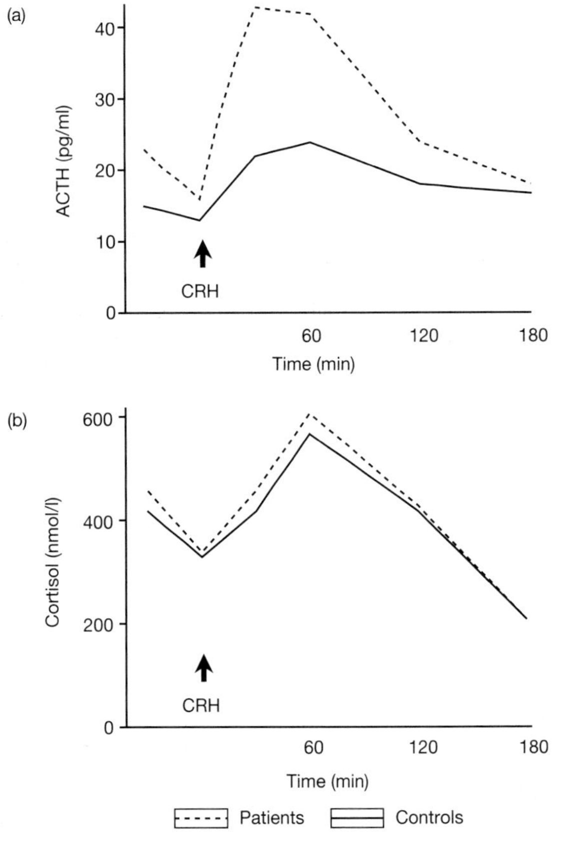

Fig. 2 Responses of (a) ACTH and (b) cortisol to injection with CRH in patients with fibromyalgia and controls (Griep et al. 1993).

Disturbed pain modulation

Pain has biophysiological and psychological aspects. Initially, the hypothesis was that psychological aspects dominated the pain in fibromyalgia, hence the label 'psychogenic rheumatism'. In recent years, the role of abnormal sensory processing in fibromyalgia has become clear. Patients with fibromyalgia often have *allodynia*, the perception of pain in response to stimuli that are normally not painful, such as touch, moderate heat or cold, electrical stimulation, and proprioceptive input. In addition, pain has exaggerated intensity and duration: *hyperalgesia*. Mechanisms of abnormal sensory processing in fibromyalgia can be divided into increased activity in pain-facilitating (pronociceptive) mechanisms and reduced pain-inhibiting (antinociceptive) mechanisms on the spinal and cerebral level.

Enhanced pain-facilitating mechanisms

Sensitization of nociceptive neurons in the spinal dorsal horn by hyperexcitable receptors, such as the glutamate receptor *N*-methyl-D-asparate (NMDA), could be one of the mechanisms responsible for pain in fibromyalgia. In animal and human studies, NMDA antagonists like ketamine seem to inhibit pain-facilitating mechanisms, but whether this is specific for patients with fibromyalgia or a general phenomena in painful musculoskeletal disorders is not known. The NMDA hypothesis is compatible with correlation of intensity of pain in fibromyalgia and levels in the cerebrospinal fluid of amino acids, which appear to modulate NMDA receptors (Larson et al. 2000).

Pain regulation by supraspinal centres is poorly understood. Fibromyalgia shares increased reactivity to various stimuli (sensitization) with several other syndromes such as multiple chemical sensitivity and irritable bowel syndrome. This suggests that shared stimulus-facilitating pathways are involved in these syndromes. The limbic system has been hypothesized to play a role in sensory gating, and may contribute to the increased 'weight' that is given to various sensations. An abnormality that is consistent with the conception of fibromyalgia as a central pain amplification syndrome, is the repeated observation of elevated cerebrospinal fluid concentrations of several chemical pain mediators including substance P (Russell 1998). Levels of substance P in cerebrospinal fluid in patients with chronic fatigue syndrome are normal (Evengard et al. 1998).

Decreased pain-inhibiting mechanisms

From the brain stem as well as from the thalamus, hypothalamus, limbic system, and cortex originate multiple descending, pain-inhibitory pathways, modulating the activity of spinal nociceptive neurons. Patients with fibromyalgia as well as other chronic pain patients have low levels of regional cerebral blood flow in the caudate nucleus and thalamus, possibly indicating decreased descending, pain-inhibitory activity. Serotonin is one of the neurochemical modulators of the descending inhibitory pathways; the finding of low concentrations of serotonin in serum and cerebrospinal fluid of patients with fibromyalgia in several studies might indicate decreased pain-inhibiting mechanisms. However, the role of serotonin in the pathophysiology of fibromyalgia is not clear.

Physical deconditioning

Neuroendocrine dysfunction, for example, via altered growth hormone metabolism, sleep disturbances, and avoidance of physical activities because of pain may all cause physical deconditioning in patients with fibromyalgia. Abnormalities found in muscle biopsies are a non-specific result of this deconditioning. Physical deconditioning will lead to more stiffness, fatigue, and pain at physical activities, causing a vicious circle or downward spiral.

Biopsychosocial model

Based on the increasing knowledge about pathophysiological mechanisms in fibromyalgia, a biopsychosocial model can be developed as a functional framework, integrating mechanisms of persistence of symptoms (Fig. 3). The model is functional, not anatomical. Some relations described in the model are more hypothetical than others; not all vicious circles described are equivalent in their (supposed) effect.

Recurrent psychological stress is associated with chronic sleep disturbance, which directly results in decreased physical fitness. The poorly rested muscles 'protest' by causing symptoms of pain, stiffness, and fatigue. Sleep anomalies also contribute to neuroendocrine dysregulation. An example is growth hormone, as about 80 per cent of this hormone is secreted (in pulses) during this phase of sleep. Susceptibility to muscle deconditioning could be increased as a result of dysregulation of growth hormone as it has an anabolic function. Compatible with this hypothesis is the finding that levels of the collagen precursor serum procollagen III—that is, growth hormone dependent—were related to the amount of symptoms and tender points in fibromyalgia patients (Jacobsen et al. 1990). Apart from these mechanisms via sleep disturbances, stress in general can lead to altered pituitary–adrenal and autonomic responses (Heim et al. 2000). So also indirectly, via neuroendocrine disturbances physical fitness may be lowered by chronic sleep disturbances and psychological stress. Chronic neuroendocrine disturbances could by sensitizing the central nervous system by neuropeptides and other regulatory mechanisms change the processing of sensory input and ultimately lead to pain. The model also shows the detrimental role of decreased physical activity and deconditioning. Physical inactivity might also facilitate pain perception by incomplete extinguishing of a neurophysiological 'pain memory' (Harvey 1990).

Using Fig. 3 as a hypothetical model, the clinical relevance of pathophysiological mechanisms, their interplay with symptoms and the mode of action of therapeutic interventions can be better placed into perspective.

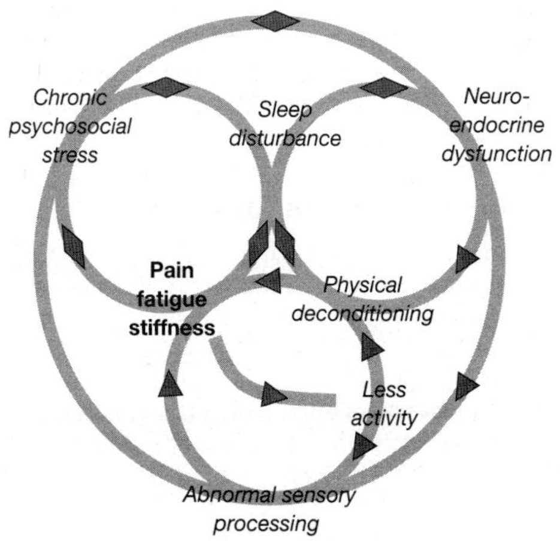

Fig. 3 Vicious circles with pathophysiological mechanisms (in italic) and ensuing symptoms (in bold), with uni- and bi-directional influences: shaded triangles and diamonds, respectively. Neuroendocrine dysfunction, due to psychosocial stress and sleep disturbances causes physical deconditioning and disturbed pain modulation. Disturbed pain modulation, together with physical deconditioning, psychosocial stress, and sleep disturbances causes the symptoms pain, fatigue, and stiffness.

Management

Patient information

The first step in management of diseases, illnesses, ailments, and afflictions is patient information and education. Patients should be informed that the symptoms they experience are real and severe and that the physician takes the patient seriously, but that fibromyalgia can be better described as an ailment or condition than as a disease. To convey this message properly, the physician should realize that the contradiction between the patients' perception of disease and the lack of objective findings is stressful: patients may feel rejected, misunderstood, and disbelieved, which prevents them from dealing with their situation constructively. The patient should be informed that the condition is neither crippling nor deforming, and does not have to be treated aggressively with drugs. This is the positive side of the coin. The other, negative side is that symptoms may wax and wane, but that they do not disappear for the majority of patients with long-standing fibromyalgia. It can be explained that it is not exactly known how fibromyalgia develops, but that some mechanisms of how symptoms persist, are known.

Patient education and principles of management

The message that fibromyalgia cannot be cured is an important aspect of patient education. It must be made clear that the primary aim in the management of fibromyalgia is enhancement of functional capacity and quality of life and that an active role of the patient is essential. The role of the physician is more supportive than therapeutic in character. From a clinical and behavioural point of view, it must be avoided that pain gets a central place in management. Pain is very hard to treat in fibromyalgia. A poor or at best a moderate response to analgesics and non-steroidal anti-inflammatory drugs is a characteristic of fibromyalgia, it is almost a diagnostic feature. The same holds true for other pain treating modalities. To enhance patient's self-management and to induce adherence to physical exercise, it is necessary to tackle possible wrong attributions the patient has about the origin of the complaints. A simple question that the physician could ask is: 'what do you think is the cause of the symptoms?' Often, patients think physical activities and exercise should be avoided to prevent damage to joints. A key principle of management is to tailor the therapy to the needs of the individual patient. Problems due to fibromyalgia and causes of stress should be identified and discussed with each patient, and help should be provided on how to cope with these problems. The intention should be to omit long-lasting drug-therapy; for instance sleep disturbances could be tackled with sleep 'hygiene' principles.

Physical exercises

Graded daily physical exercise seems to be the key therapy for patients with fibromyalgia to prevent progression of physical deconditioning and to enhance functional capacities; it may also improve fibromyalgia symptoms. Physical fitness training seems feasible and beneficial (Martin et al. 1996; Gowans et al. 1999), but long-term effects of exercise require further evaluation. Not all studies on physical fitness training report positive results. Exercise should initially be of a low-impact type and gradually intensified. Some patients benefit from additional regular stretching and relaxation exercises. Exercises in warm water and balneotherapy may give additional symptomatic relief. Patients often argue that they are busy the whole day and that exercises are not necessary. It should be explained that activities in daily life are essentially different from whole body exercises. Adherence to physical exercise will be improved if this treatment is embedded in an educational package aimed at tackling incorrect notions (e.g. that exercise will worsen the condition), at enhancing coping skills and increasing motivation.

To explain the negative downward spiral or vicious circle of pain at physical activity → avoidance of physical activities → deconditioning → more pain at physical activities, Fig. 4 can be used.

Another often-heard objection against physical exercise is that it is not possible to perform them because they will increase pain. It should be made clear that exercises start off at a very low-level, and that in general there is and should be no increase in pain following an adequate scheme. Overdoing exercise should be avoided, because as a consequence of increased pain, motivation could be lost. In clinical practice, it is helpful to ask a physiotherapist to plan and demonstrate slowly intensifying exercise to the patient, to encourage adherence to the programme and, if necessary, to adapt the exercise-programme in follow-up contacts. Though there is no evidence-based, long-term programme for physical exercises for patients with fibromyalgia, patients who perform physical exercise of the whole body, for example, during 20 min a day, are likely to benefit. A slowly progressive scheme should be tailored to the needs and possibilities of the individual patient.

Other non-pharmacological therapies, psychobehavioural management

The effect of biofeedback, hypnotherapy, relaxation response training, and many other complementary and non-pharmacological therapies has not been properly investigated (Simms 1994). The multifaceted nature of problems in fibromyalgia with its profound influence on physical, psychological, and social aspects of quality of life, warrant a multidisciplinary team approach, including cognitive–behavioural intervention. The aim is to help patients manage symptoms and consequences of fibromyalgia and assist them in realizing individualized realistic goals in life and in defining the steps that have to be taken to achieve these goals. If treatment is tailored to individual patients' psychosocial needs, patients are likely to benefit in the short run (Turk et al. 1998), but long-term benefits of cognitive–behavioural interventions are not proven (Rossy et al. 1999). Patients with concomitant psychiatric illness or severe psychological disorders need to be treated by a psychiatrist or clinical psychologist.

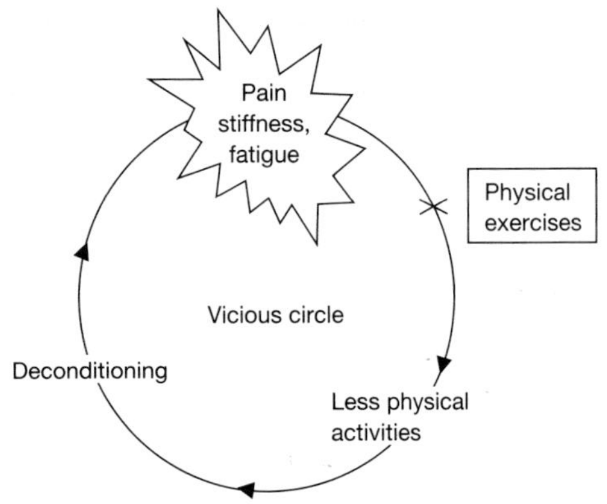

Fig. 4 Simple model to educate patients and motivate them for daily physical exercises. The physician can draw this model in front of the patient on a piece of paper and illustrate it with a little story about the different chances a triathlon athlete and a lazy princess have of pain in muscles after the same physical activity, solely based on the different levels of conditioning, fitness of muscles. The negative vicious circle of pain at physical activities, therefore less activities followed by deconditioning and thus more pain at physical activities can be broken by daily physical exercises.

Pharmacological treatment

Drug treatment should be part of a therapeutic strategy encompassing education and physical exercises. In a meta-analysis the latter treatment appeared to be at least as efficacious as pharmacological treatment alone in improving fibromyalgia symptoms (Rossy et al. 1999).

Analgesics like tramadol and non-steroidal anti-inflammatory drugs only partially improve symptoms. Two weeks after local injection therapy with 0.5 per cent xylocaine of trigger points in the upper trapezius muscle in patients with fibromyalgia, there was improvement in pain and range of motion, but at the expense of significant post-injection soreness (Hong and Hsueh 1996). Glucocorticoids should not be used in patients with fibromyalgia.

The effect of antidepressants, particularly tricyclics such as amitriptyline, has been studied frequently in patients with fibromyalgia. Most tricyclics have a mean moderately beneficial effect (Arnold et al. 2000), but many patients do not respond: the percentage of responders ranges from 25 to 37 (Arnold et al. 2000). It is not possible to predict the response to antidepressants in individual patients. Long-term effectiveness has not been proven: in the only study with a follow-up longer than 3 months, the percentage of patients clinically responding at 6 months in the amitriptyline group did not differ significantly from the percentage in the placebo group (Carette et al. 1994). Whether the beneficial effect is independent of depression needs further study, but response to some antidepressants in patients with fibromyalgia, for instance amitriptyline, occurs at doses lower than those used in major depression, suggesting an independent mode of action. Another argument for this hypothesis is that not all antidepressants are equally helpful in patients with fibromyalgia, for instance moclobemide lacks the beneficial effect of amitriptyline (Hannonen et al. 1998). A third argument is the finding that fluoxetine decreased depression scores, but not fibromyalgia symptoms (Wolfe et al. 1994).

Based on the hypotheses of pathophysiological mechanisms discussed above, antidepressants and other drugs with specific and theoretically appropriate modes of action have been tested in fibromyalgia, showing for most drugs disappointing results. The conclusion is that as adjunct to education and physical exercise, drug treatment may have a place in the management of fibromyalgia, but that it is only a modest place. Analgesics and non-steroidal anti-inflammatory drugs can be tried to diminish pain, if necessary with pain modulating drugs such as the tricyclic agents amitryptyline (start 25 mg at bedtime, if ineffective after 6 weeks 50 mg, maximally 75 mg) or cyclobenzaprine (10 mg at bedtime). Adverse effects of tricyclic agents are dry mouth and drowsiness. Not all patients respond; medication that is not effective should be stopped.

Directions for further clinical trials

Because of the multidimensional nature of fibromyalgia, is not to be expected that cure will be found in the near future. Pharmacological therapy should preferably be investigated for its additional effect to the basic, non-pharmacological therapy. To determine which (sub-groups of) patients benefit from adjunctive therapy and whether the effect can be predicted merits future investigation. The Fibromyalgia Impact Questionnaire is a responsive measure to assess perceived clinical improvement and its inclusion as a primary endpoint in clinical trials is recommended (Dunkl et al. 2000).

Prognosis, social consequences, cost

In the long-term, most patients have a poor prognosis regarding morbidity. After a mean follow-up of 4 years following diagnosis, 97 per cent of 72 patients still had symptoms typical of fibromyalgia (Ledingham et al. 1993). In another study, after 5 years, 50 per cent of 56 patients with fibromyalgia reported that pain, fatigue, and sleep problems had increased, less than 20 per cent reported improvement, and in more than 30 per cent there was no change (Henriksson 1994). Patients followed for as long as 7 years showed that their high scores for pain, functional disability, fatigue, sleep disturbance, and psychological status did not change substantially over time.

Fibromyalgia also has negative social–economic consequences. In a multicentre survey in 1988 in the United States, more than 16 per cent of patients with fibromyalgia reported receiving social security disability payments (highest centre rate 36 per cent; lowest 6 per cent) compared to 2.2 per cent of the US population and 29 per cent of patients with rheumatoid arthritis seen at one centre. Overall, 27 per cent reported receiving at least one form of disability payment (Wolfe et al. 1997a). In Brazil, there was a decrease in family income for 65 per cent of 44 female patients with fibromyalgia and for 75 per cent of 41 patients with rheumatoid arthritis. Fifty-five per cent of patients with fibromyalgia and 67 per cent of those with rheumatoid arthritis received social security aid (Martinez et al. 1995). Thus, work disability is a serious problem, but most patients with fibromyalgia can work, if adaptations are made.

In the United States, the hospitalization rate for patients with fibromyalgia was 1 every 3 years and almost half of admissions was related to fibromyalgia-associated symptoms. In addition, patients had more surgical interventions in their medical history compared with patients with other rheumatic disorders. The mean yearly per-patient cost of fibromyalgia in 1996 was US$ 2274. Some patients with high costs skewed results; many patients used few services and had limited costs. Total costs and utilization were associated independently with the number of self-reported comorbid or associated conditions, functional disability, and global disease severity (Wolfe et al. 1997b). In Canada, direct health care cost associated with fibromyalgia within a representative community sample was estimated to be Canadian $493 yearly per patient (White et al. 1999).

Litigation, medicolegal aspects

Because of its perceived subjective nature and the absence of well-defined criteria for diagnosis and severity of the condition, fibromyalgia creates problems in litigation, and the determination of rehabilitation costs and disability payments. For a rheumatic disease like rheumatoid arthritis, in most cases the diagnosis is indisputable; in case of litigation, the issue is disability. In fibromyalgia, key litigation issues are the diagnosis, is the claimant faking or exaggerating pain, and the grade of disability. Among subjects giving true responses or deliberately exaggerating pain at assessment of tender points (fakers), exaggeration was difficult to detect but accurate discrimination of fakers was possible. The detection of fakers was improved by also assessing pain behaviour (Smythe 1997). In a similar study, fakers could not be discriminated on the basis of tenderness at 'control points'. Using the classification criteria for fibromyalgia and bedside observations, fakers were misidentified as fibromyalgia patients in 1/3 of judgements, and fibromyalgia patients as simulators in 1/5 of judgements (Khostanteen et al. 2000).

A diagnosis neither reflects the degree of disability nor the severity of the condition. Verifying the diagnosis would be less important, if disability could be objectively assessed. For fibromyalgia this would require detailed observation in the non-clinical setting, conversations with family and co-workers and psychological and comprehensive physical testing. In most cases, this is not feasible. Frank malingering is probably rare. Litigation can be a major source of stress in fibromyalgia and other pain patients, rarely aggravating symptoms, though.

Conclusions

Fibromyalgia is a common, chronic generalized musculoskeletal pain syndrome, characterized by multiple symptoms and tender points, that has a severe impact on the daily life of the patients. The origin of the syndrome probably is multidimensional. For groups of patients, several dysfunctional central neurohormonal and pain processing systems are found, but at an individual patient level, there is no diagnostic laboratory test. Research findings have broadened our insight into the mechanisms of fibromyalgia, but have not led to an effective therapy. Because of its multidimensional nature, effective pharmacological therapy is unlikely to be available in the near future. Management of the syndrome needs to be tailored to the individual patient's symptoms and needs. Therapy, which always should include education and physical exercises, is only symptomatic.

References

Arnold, L.M., Keck-PE, J., and Welge, J.A. (2000). Antidepressant treatment of fibromyalgia. A meta-analysis and review. *Psychosomatics* **41**, 104–13.

Bergman, S., Herrstrom, P., Hogstrom, K., Petersson, I.F., Svensson, B., and Jacobsson, L.T.H. (2001). Chronic musculoskeletal pain, prevalence rates, and sociodemographic associations in a Swedish population study. *Journal of Rheumatology* **28**, 1369–77.

Boisset-Pioro, M.H., Esdaile, J.M., and Fitzcharles, M.A. (1995). Sexual and physical abuse in women with fibromyalgia syndrome. *Arthritis and Rheumatism* **38**, 235–41.

Buchwald, D., Umali, J., and Stene, M. (1996). Insulin-like growth factor-I (somatomedin C) levels in chronic fatigue syndrome and fibromyalgia. *Journal of Rheumatology* **23**, 739–42.

Campbell, S.M., Clark, S., Tindall, E.A., Forehand, M.E., and Bennett, R.M. (1983). Clinical characteristics of fibrositis. I. A 'blinded', controlled study of symptoms and tender points. *Arthritis and Rheumatism* **26**, 817–24.

Carette, S. and Lefrancois, L. (1988). Fibrositis and primary hypothyroidism. *Journal of Rheumatology* **15**, 1418–21.

Carette, S. et al. (1994). Comparison of amitriptyline, cyclobenzaprine, and placebo in the treatment of fibromyalgia. A randomized, double-blind clinical trial. *Arthritis and Rheumatism* **37**, 32–40.

Clark, S., Campbell, S.M., Forehand, M.E., Tindall, E.A., and Bennett, R.M. (1985). Clinical characteristics of fibrositis. II. A 'blinded', controlled study using standard psychological tests. *Arthritis and Rheumatism* **28**, 132–7.

Cott, A. et al. (1992). Interrater reliability of the tender point criterion for fibromyalgia. *Journal of Rheumatology* **19**, 1955–9.

Crofford, L.J. and Demitrack, M.A. (1996). Evidence that abnormalities of central neurohormonal systems are key to understanding fibromyalgia and chronic fatigue syndrome. *Rheumatic Diseases Clinics of North America* **22**, 267–84.

Crofford, L.J. et al. (1994). Hypothalamic–pituitary–adrenal axis perturbations in patients with fibromyalgia. *Arthritis and Rheumatism* **37**, 1583–92.

Croft, P., Schollum, J., and Silman, A. (1994). Population study of tender point counts and pain as evidence of fibromyalgia. *British Medical Journal* **309**, 696–9.

de Blecourt, A.C., Knipping, A.A., de Voogd, N., and van Rijswijk, M.H. (1993). Weather conditions and complaints in fibromyalgia. *Journal of Rheumatology* **20**, 1932–4.

Dinser, R., Halama, T., and Hoffmann, A. (2000). Stringent endocrinological testing reveals subnormal growth hormone secretion in some patients with fibromyalgia syndrome but rarely severe growth hormone deficiency. *Journal of Rheumatology* **27**, 2482–8.

Dunkl, P.R., Taylor, A.G., McConnell, G.G., Alfano, A.P., and Conaway, M.R. (2000). Responsiveness of fibromyalgia clinical trial outcome measures. *Journal of Rheumatology* **27**, 2683–91.

Epstein, S.A. et al. (1999). Psychiatric disorders in patients with fibromyalgia. A multicenter investigation. *Psychosomatics* **40**, 57–63.

Evengard, B. et al. (1998). Chronic fatigue syndrome differs from fibromyalgia. No evidence for elevated substance P levels in cerebrospinal fluid of patients with chronic fatigue syndrome. *Pain* **78**, 153–5.

Forseth, K.O., Husby, G., Gran, J.T., and Forre, O. (1999). Prognostic factors for the development of fibromyalgia in women with self-reported musculoskeletal pain. A prospective study. *Journal of Rheumatology* **26**, 2458–67.

Fukuda, K., Straus, S.E., Hickie, I., Sharpe, M.C., Dobbins, J.G., and Komaroff, A. (1994). The chronic fatigue syndrome: a comprehensive approach to its definition and study. International Chronic Fatigue Syndrome Study Group. *Annals of Internal Medicine* **121**, 953–9.

Goldenberg, D.L. (1989). Psychological symptoms and psychiatric diagnosis in patients with fibromyalgia. *Journal of Rheumatology* **19** (Suppl.), 127–30.

Gowans, S.E., de Hueck, A., Voss, S., and Richardson, M. (1999). A randomized, controlled trial of exercise and education for individuals with fibromyalgia. *Arthritis Care and Research* **12**, 120–8.

Griep, E.N., Boersma, J.W., and de Kloet, E.R. (1993). Altered reactivity of the hypothalamic–pituitary–adrenal axis in the primary fibromyalgia syndrome. *Journal of Rheumatology* **20**, 469–74.

Hannonen, P., Malminiemi, K., Yli, K.U., Isomeri, R., and Roponen, P. (1998). A randomized, double-blind, placebo-controlled study of moclobemide and amitriptyline in the treatment of fibromyalgia in females without psychiatric disorder. *British Journal of Rheumatology* **37**, 1279–86.

Harvey, A.R. (1990). A neurogenic model for soft-tissue rheumatism and its implications for management. *Journal of Orthopaedic Rheumatology* **3**, 231–42.

Heim, C. et al. (2000). Pituitary–adrenal and autonomic responses to stress in women after sexual and physical abuse in childhood. *Journal of the American Medical Association* **284**, 592–7.

Henriksson, C.M. (1994). Longterm effects of fibromyalgia on everyday life. A study of 56 patients. *Scandinavian Journal of Rheumatology* **23**, 36–41.

Hong, C.Z. and Hsueh, T.C. (1996). Difference in pain relief after trigger point injections in myofascial pain patients with and without fibromyalgia. *Archives of Physical and Medical Rehabilitation* **77**, 1161–6.

Jacobs, J.W., Geenen, R., van der, H.A., Rasker, J.J., and Bijlsma, J.W. (1995). Are tender point scores assessed by manual palpation in fibromyalgia reliable? An investigation into the variance of tender point scores. *Scandinavian Journal of Rheumatology* **24**, 243–7.

Jacobs, J.W. et al. (1996). Lack of correlation between the mean tender point score and self-reported pain in fibromyalgia. *Arthritis Care and Research* **9**, 105–11.

Jacobsen, S., Jensen, L.T., Foldager, M., and Danneskiold, S.B. (1990). Primary fibromyalgia: clinical parameters in relation to serum procollagen type III aminoterminal peptide. *British Journal of Rheumatology* **29**, 174–7.

Jason, L.A., Taylor, R.R., and Kennedy, C.L. (2000). Chronic fatigue syndrome, fibromyalgia, and multiple chemical sensitivities in a community-based sample of persons with chronic fatigue syndrome-like symptoms. *Psychosomatic Medicine* **62**, 655–63.

Khostanteen, I., Tunks, E.R., Goldsmith, C.H., and Ennis, J. (2000). Fibromyalgia: can one distinguish it from simulation? An observer-blind controlled study. *Journal of Rheumatology* **27**, 2671–6.

Larson, A.A., Giovengo, S.L., Russell, I.J., and Michalek, J.E. (2000). Changes in the concentrations of amino acids in the cerebrospinal fluid that correlate with pain in patients with fibromyalgia: implications for nitric oxide pathways. *Pain* **87**, 201–11.

Ledingham, J., Doherty, S., and Doherty, M. (1993). Primary fibromyalgia syndrome—an outcome study. *British Journal of Rheumatology* **32**, 139–42.

Martin, L., Nutting, A., MacIntosh, B.R., Edworthy, S.M., Butterwick, D., and Cook, J. (1996). An exercise program in the treatment of fibromyalgia. *Journal of Rheumatology* **23**, 1050–3.

Martinez, J.E., Ferraz, M.B., Sato, E.I., and Atra, E. (1995). Fibromyalgia versus rheumatoid arthritis: a longitudinal comparison of the quality of life. *Journal of Rheumatology* **22**, 270–4.

McBeth, J. and Silman, A.J. (2001). The role of psychiatric disorders in fibromyalgia. *Current Rheumatological Reports* **3**, 157–64.

McBeth, J., Macfarlane, G.J., Hunt, I.M., and Silman, A.J. (2001). Risk factors for persistent chronic widespread pain: a community-based study. *Rheumatology* **40**, 95–101.

Moldofsky, H., Scarisbrick, P., England, R., and Smythe, H.A. (1975). Musculoskeletal symptoms and non-REM sleep disturbance in patients with 'fibrositis syndrome' and healthy subjects. *Psychosomatic Medicine* **37**, 341–55.

Naschitz, J.E. et al. (2001). Cardiovascular response to upright tilt in fibromyalgia differs from that in chronic fatigue syndrome. *Journal of Rheumatology* **28**, 1356–60.

Neeck, G. and Riedel, W. (1992). Thyroid function in patients with fibromyalgia syndrome. *Journal of Rheumatology* **19**, 1120–2.

Ostensen, M., Rugelsjoen, A., and Wigers, S.H. (1997). The effect of reproductive events and alterations of sex hormone levels on the symptoms of fibromyalgia. *Scandinavian Journal of Rheumatology* **26**, 355–60.

Petzke, F. and Clauw, D.J. (2000). Sympathetic nervous system function in fibromyalgia. *Current Rheumatological Reports* **2**, 116–23.

Quimby, L.G., Block, S.R., and Gratwick, G.M. (1988). Fibromyalgia: generalized pain intolerance and manifold symptom reporting. *Journal of Rheumatology* **15**, 1264–70.

Quintner, J.L. and Cohen, M.L. (1999). Fibromyalgia falls foul of a fallacy. *Lancet* **353**, 1092–4.

Reilly, P.A. and Littlejohn, G.O. (1992). Peripheral arthralgic presentation of fibrositis/fibromyalgia syndrome. *Journal of Rheumatology* **19**, 281–3.

Rivera, J., de Diego, A., Trinchet, M., and Garcia, M.A. (1997). Fibromyalgia-associated hepatitis C virus infection. *British Journal of Rheumatology* **36**, 981–5.

Rossy, L.A. et al. (1999). A meta-analysis of fibromyalgia treatment interventions. *Annals of Behavioural Medicine* **21**, 180–91.

Russell, I.J. (1998). Advances in fibromyalgia: possible role for central neurochemicals. *American Journal of Medical Sciences* **315**, 377–84.

Simms, R.W. (1994). Controlled trials of therapy in fibromyalgia syndrome. *Baillieres Clinical Rheumatology* **8**, 917–34.

Simms, R.W. (1998). Fibromyalgia is not a muscle disorder. *American Journal of the Medical Sciences* **315**, 346–50.

Smythe, H. (1997). Strategies for assessing pain and pain exaggeration: controlled studies. *Journal of Rheumatology* **24**, 1622–9.

Smythe, H.A., Gladman, A., Dagenais, P., Kraishi, M., and Blake, R. (1992). Relation between fibrositic and control site tenderness; effects of dolorimeter scale length and footplate size. *Journal of Rheumatology* **19**, 284–9.

Spiegel, K., Leproult, R., and Van Cauter, E. (1999). Impact of sleep debt on metabolic and endocrine function. *Lancet* **354**, 1435–9.

Straus, S.E. (1988). The chronic mononucleosis syndrome. *Journal of Infectious Diseases* **157**, 404–12.

Tunks, E. et al. (1995). The reliability of examination for tenderness in patients with myofascial pain, chronic fibromyalgia and controls. *Journal of Rheumatology* **22**, 944–52.

Turk, D.C., Okifuji, A., Sinclair, J.D., and Starz, T.W. (1998). Differential responses by psychosocial subgroups of fibromyalgia syndrome patients to an interdisciplinary treatment. *Arthritis Care and Research* **11**, 397–404.

Walker, E.A., Keegan, D., Gardner, G., Sullivan, M., Katon, W.J., and Bernstein, D. (1997a). Psychosocial factors in fibromyalgia compared with rheumatoid arthritis: I. Psychiatric diagnoses and functional disability. *Psychosomatic Medicine* **59**, 565–71.

Walker, E.A., Keegan, D., Gardner, G., Sullivan, M., Bernstein, D., and Katon, W.J. (1997b). Psychosocial factors in fibromyalgia compared with rheumatoid arthritis: II. Sexual, physical, and emotional abuse and neglect. *Psychosomatic Medicine* **59**, 572–7.

White, K.P., Speechley, M., Harth, M., and Ostbye, T. (1999). The London Fibromyalgia Epidemiology Study: direct health care costs of fibromyalgia syndrome in London, Canada. *Journal of Rheumatology* **26**, 885–9.

White, K.P., Speechley, M., Harth, M., and Ostbye, T. (2000). Co-existence of chronic fatigue syndrome with fibromyalgia syndrome in the general population. A controlled study. *Scandinavian Journal of Rheumatology* **29**, 44–51.

Wolfe, F. (1997). The relation between tender points and fibromyalgia symptom variables: evidence that fibromyalgia is not a discrete disorder in the clinic. *Annals of the Rheumatic Diseases* **56**, 268–71.

Wolfe, F. and Cathey, M.A. (1983). Prevalence of primary and secondary fibrositis. *Journal of Rheumatology* **10**, 965–8.

Wolfe, F. et al. (1990). The American College of Rheumatology 1990 criteria for the classification of fibromyalgia. Report of the Multicenter Criteria Committee. *Arthritis and Rheumatism* **33**, 160–72.

Wolfe, F., Cathey, M.A., and Hawley, D.J. (1994). A double-blind placebo controlled trial of fluoxetine in fibromyalgia. *Scandinavian Journal of Rheumatology* **23**, 255–9.

Wolfe, F., Ross, K., Anderson, J., Russell, I.J., and Hebert, L. (1995). The prevalence and characteristics of fibromyalgia in the general population. *Arthritis and Rheumatism* **38**, 19–28.

Wolfe, F. et al. (1997a). Work and disability status of persons with fibromyalgia. *Journal of Rheumatology* **24**, 1171–8.

Wolfe, F. et al. (1997b). A prospective, longitudinal, multicenter study of service utilization and costs in fibromyalgia. *Arthritis and Rheumatism* **40**, 1560–70.

Yunus, M., Masi, A.T., Calabro, J.J., Miller, K.A., and Feigenbaum, S.L. (1981). Primary fibromyalgia (fibrositis): clinical study of 50 patients with matched normal controls. *Seminars in Arthritis and Rheumatism* **11**, 151–71.

Yunus, M.B., Khan, M.A., Rawlings, K.K., Green, J.R., Olson, J.M., and Shah, S. (1999). Genetic linkage analysis of multicase families with fibromyalgia syndrome. *Journal of Rheumatology* **26**, 408–12.

6.13.2 Local pain syndromes—adult onset

Michael Shipley

Pain in one part of the body is common. It can arise from joints, muscles, tendons, ligaments, or any combination, or may be referred from a more proximal structure. It may be due to an injury, to unaccustomed use, or to overuse, for example, gardening, a change in technique for a sportsperson or musician, or a change in working practice for a keyboard worker. Repetitive wrist movements, psychological distress, and illness behaviour increase the risk of developing, for example, forearm pain. Job dissatisfaction is also a risk factor. Although many such episodes are short-lived and recover, short-term recovery, with or without treatment is often followed by further episodes of pain in the same place (Mcfarlane et al. 2000) or elsewhere.

There may be minimal or no intervention from a doctor or a physical therapist. Thus, only 34 per cent of a general practice population who reported having had forearm pain in the previous 2 years had reported it to a doctor. Although intuitively it seems appropriate, there is little evidence that earlier intervention is helpful in the longer term. Nonetheless, one in four patients with shoulder pain responds well to early treatment by a general practitioner with a non-steroidal anti-inflammatory drug (NSAID) (Winters et al. 1999).

Some conditions are well defined by their symptoms and physical findings, others less easy to define. Shoulder pain is subject to a wide variation of specific diagnoses even amongst specialists (Bamji et al. 1996). An evidence base for the treatment of many regional pain syndromes is lacking or inadequate. This does not mean that treatments do not work, merely that acceptable studies have not yet been undertaken (Green et al. 1998). Simple pain control and the passage of time, with a brief period of rest often suffice. Rehabilitation, learning new work or sport techniques, postural improvements, and simple exercise help to avoid recurrences.

An individual with a more generalized condition may present initially with localized pain. For example, carpal tunnel syndrome as the first sign of rheumatoid arthritis, or shoulder pains in an older patient as the initial symptom of polymyalgia rheumatica. An individual complaining of localized shoulder, forearm, or spinal pain may do so in the context of chronic generalized pain or fibromyalgia. Treatment should always be approached in the context of an appropriate medical history and a screening musculoskeletal examination (Doherty et al. 1992). Any ill health, weight loss, or fever should trigger a search for a more serious underlying cause.

This chapter will take an anatomical approach to the main sites of pain and a practical approach to their diagnosis and management. It is important to understand, however, that pain syndromes often overlap several anatomical sites.

Regional pain syndromes in the neck, shoulder, and arm

Pain in the arm may arise locally, be referred from the neck, or be part of a generalized condition. Neck pain is common and is discussed in greater detail elsewhere. Pain in the arm may be referred from the neck, usually when there is nerve root impingement due to a disc prolapse, spondylosis with osteophytes causing root canal narrowing, a cervical rib, or thoracic outlet syndrome. Nerve pain is burning and usually associated with other abnormal sensory symptoms and loss of power or reflexes. A disc prolapse makes the neck acutely painful and stiff but the neck symptoms in spondylotic root impingement or with a cervical rib are minimal. A whiplash injury produces vague and non-specific arm symptoms. An intensely painful shoulder or arm causes secondary muscle spasm in the trapezius and paracervical muscles.

Pain in the whole arm may be central, for example, thalamic pain, or due to chronic regional pain syndrome type I—Sudek's atrophy.

Pain in the shoulder and neck—shoulder girdle pain

The exact site of shoulder pain is defined by asking the patient to point to it—'shoulder' in English is atomically imprecise. Shoulder girdle pain or muscular pattern neck pain is common, usually diffuse and unilateral or bilateral. The patient describes burning discomfort in the trapezius muscle, neck, and occiput. Neck movements are restricted and trigger point tenderness develops. Tension-type headaches also occur. Unaccustomed use of a computer, sleeping awkwardly, or an injury may trigger such pain. Shoulder girdle pain also may be secondary to protective muscle spasm with a severely painful shoulder. Whatever the cause, it is often short-lived and best treated with simple analgesia and occasionally a soft collar. A recent review of the conservative management of mechanical neck pain concludes that, although many treatments are applied, there is little evidence from well-structured trials to support or refute their use (Aker et al. 1996). There is some evidence that manipulative treatment is more effective than simple physiotherapy (Winters et al. 1999). Acupuncture may also help when it has become chronic (Irnich et al. 2001). Early treatment after a whiplash injury and an explanation that it will persist for several weeks or months helps reduce the risk of its becoming chronic. Evidence suggests the best indicator that it will become chronic after an injury is the severity of the injury itself (Cassidy et al. 2000).

Pain in the shoulder

Shoulder pain has an annual incidence of around 1 per cent in those over 45 years of age. Pain arising from an acromioclavicular or sternoclavicular joint localizes to the affected joint. Pain arising from the rotator cuff is felt in the upper, outer arm and is severe at night. Adhesive capsulitis produces diffuse, intense aching shoulder pain, and severe loss of all shoulder movements. The shoulder is examined for deformity and palpated for tenderness, swelling, or instability. Its full active and passive ranges and loss of power in specific resisted movements are recorded (Dalton).

Differential diagnosis of shoulder pain (Table 1)

Disorders of the rotator cuff—tendinitis

The rotator cuff is a common source of pain and shoulder stiffness. It is usually unilateral and occasionally follows direct trauma. The diagnosis can be made from the history and physical findings. Pain is felt in the deltoid and upper arm and is characteristically worse at night. It is increased by abduction and elevation of the arm, particularly in the mid range. Full elevation, when possible, reduces the pain as the painful part of the tendon moves proximal to the acromion and coracoacromial ligament. Shoulder movements are limited, particularly elevation and reaching behind the back and neck. Passive elevation reduces impingement and is less painful. Examined from behind, the normal scapulothoracic rhythm is lost and the scapula rotates earlier during elevation. Severe pain from the rotator cuff virtually immobilizes the shoulder, although some rotation is retained with the arm by the side. This distinguishes a rotator cuff lesion from adhesive capsulitis or glenohumeral arthritis, in which rotation may be completely lost. A painful shoulder often produces painful trapezius muscle spasm and this causes diagnostic confusion with pain originating from the neck. Shoulder

Table 1 Differential diagnosis of shoulder pain

Shoulder girdle (muscular) pain and whiplash injury
Disorders of the rotator cuff mechanism Rotator cuff tendinitis Subacromial bursitis Impingement syndrome Rotator cuff tears Calcific tendinitis and subacromial bursitis
Adhesive capsulitis (true frozen shoulder)
Acromioclavicular syndromes
Proximal bicipital tendinitis
Glenohumeral instability
Brachial neuralgia (neuralgic amyotrophy)
Inflammatory arthritis
Polymyalgia rheumatica (usually bilateral)
Osteoarthritis
Crystal synovitis
Infective arthritis

problems produce restriction of shoulder movements whereas neck problems allow normal shoulder movements but the neck is restricted. Dynamic high-resolution ultrasound examination demonstrates the cause and helps devise a rational treatment plan (Roberts et al. 2001). The rotator cuff impinges on the acromion during normal movement, especially under loading. Tendinitis usually affects a relatively avascular region of the cuff about 1 cm proximal to the greater tuberosity. Initially oedema and haemorrhage develop, then fibrosis and inflammation in the tendon and adjacent bursa. Later, tendon degeneration, tears, and secondary changes in the humeral head and acromion may develop. The acromion varies from virtually horizontal to steeply angled, and this contributes to impingement, as does acromial or acromioclavicular joint osteophytosis.

Analgesics or NSAIDs help mild pain but many rheumatologists advise a corticosteroid injection as a safe and effective means of controlling pain (Green et al. 1998). The evidence-base for treatment is poor, largely because of difficulties defining the exact underlying diagnosis. A plain X-ray is usually normal. Dynamic ultrasound demonstrates subacromial bursitis, inflammation, or a full or partial tear of the rotator cuff, impingement and bunching of the rotator cuff during elevation, acromioclavicular joint instability or a joint effusion (Farin et al. 1990). Ultrasound guided is more logical than 'blind' injection although impractical until rheumatologists are trained to use diagnostic ultrasound. MRI images the rotator cuff and the associated structures.

Shoulder impingement syndrome

In addition to typical rotator cuff-derived pain there is crepitus on abduction and rotation of the arm at 90° of abduction. Impingement and rotator cuff dysfunction may be an element of all rotator cuff problems. Bony change in the greater tuberosity and inferior acromion on X-ray and acromioclavicular joint instability or osteoarthritis cause more marked impingement. There may be a partial or complete tear of the rotator cuff. A local injection helps some. Increasingly arthroscopic trimming of the acromion and of osteophytes and repair of the rotator cuff are used for recurrent or persistent impingement pain. Outcomes are good in specialist hands although the evidence base is poor. Intensive physiotherapy and graded exercises for several months are essential post-operatively (Tytherleigh-Strong et al. 2001).

Torn rotator cuff

Trauma at any age is a cause but it occurs spontaneously in the elderly and in rheumatoid arthritis. Partial tears are managed conservatively. A full tear prevents active abduction of the arm although passive elevation is full if the patient can relax sufficiently. Once elevated, the arm can be held in place by deltoid. In chronic, full thickness tears patients learn to initiate elevation using their other arm but it is disabling, especially when also painful.

It is not clear if local corticosteroids can be used safely but they are best avoided in the first few weeks after an injury. In younger people, the tear is repaired surgically. In the elderly, a conservative approach is tried first, although surgical repair is possible if undertaken before the muscles retract and fibrose. Repair of friable tissue in rheumatoid arthritis is rarely possible. If the tear is chronic or the patient too frail for surgery, occasional local steroid injections may control pain.

Calcific tendinitis and bursitis

Around 5 per cent of painful shoulders show calcium pyrophosphate tendon deposits. They are not always symptomatic, and may be bilateral. The pathogenesis is unclear, although it affects the avascular part of the tendon. It is rare before the age of 40. It causes acute pain and restriction of movement or chronic recurrent shoulder pain and a catching sensation as the arm is lowered. The calcification is visible radiologically on anteroposterior view. Asymptomatic calcification is left untreated. NSAIDs help in mild pain but a local corticosteroid injection helps, although it may delay resorption of the deposit. Extracorporeal sock wave therapy is being studied as a means to resolve the calcification (Charrin and Noel 2001). Aspiration of the deposit under X-ray or ultrasound control may be required for persistent or recurrent pain. Rarely, surgical removal is necessary.

Shedding of crystals into the subacromial bursa causes severe pain and shoulder restriction. The shoulder becomes hot and swollen, and there is diffuse opacity in the bursa on X-ray. The differential diagnosis is gout, pseudogout, or septic arthritis. Aspiration and injection with corticosteroid helps once infection has been excluded.

Adhesive capsulitis—frozen shoulder

Definition of this uncommon condition is unsatisfactory. It is difficult to treat and causes intense, diffuse shoulder pain. Within a few weeks, the joint stiffens with complete loss of all movements, including rotation. It may follow a rotator cuff tendinitis, a myocardial infarction, a stroke, or an injury, or develop spontaneously. It is rare before the age of 40, is more common men and affects poorly controlled insulin-dependent diabetics. The cause is unknown. The joint capsule fibroses but no synovial inflammation or acute phase response occurs. The pain resolves in a few months but the stiffness persists much longer. The degree of eventual recovery is variable. Adhesions form in the joint and the capsule contracts during the stiff phase. Joint arthrography shows the normally lax axillary capsule extension, needed for movement, is obliterated—an essential diagnostic feature of adhesive capsulitis. Capsulitis is poorly visualized on MRI.

High doses of NSAIDs and analgesics help but the pain is difficult to control initially. The early use of oral corticosteroids reduces pain but does not alter the natural history. The role of intra-articular injections of corticosteroids combined with upto 10 ml of local anaesthetic to distend the joint is unclear. The shoulder must be mobilized, with the help of a physiotherapist, once the pain reduces. A manipulation under anaesthetic during the fibrotic phase helps restore movement but capsule or rotator cuff tears are a risk in the elderly. Untreated, it recovers in 1–2 years (Warner 1997).

Acromioclavicular and sternoclavicular syndromes

Pain is localized at the acromioclavicular joint. Lifting the arm fully and reaching far behind the back or across the chest reproduces the pain. Trauma is a common cause in sports people, producing short-term pain but predisposing to long-term instability and secondary osteoarthritis. The joint is locally tended and displacement is visible and instability palpable. X-rays show displacement or instability when the arm is loaded, then relaxed. Occasionally, osteolysis of the distal clavicle develops. Secondary osteoarthritis causes inferior osteophyte formation and rotator cuff impingement. Pain control and rest in a sling help, as may a local steroid injection. Rest should not be prolonged and should be followed by an exercise programme. Rarely, a surgical opinion should be sought. Inflammatory arthritis or infection of the joint is rare.

Sternoclavicular joint pain radiates into the upper anterior chest wall and is worse when the shoulder is loaded or when lying on the affected side. It may be dislocated, affected by inflammatory arthritis or osteoarthritis, and is rarely the site of a septic arthritis.

Proximal bicipital tendinitis

This is rare in isolation, usually occurring with rotator cuff tendinitis or impingement. Alone, it may arise from weight lifting or repetitive unaccustomed carrying. It causes anterior shoulder pain, worsened by flexion and supination of the elbow against resistance. Rest, analgesia, NSAIDs, and rehabilitation help, as may a corticosteroid injection, inserted alongside the tendon in its groove.

Rupture of the tendon is usually preceded by recurrent shoulder problems but may occur spontaneously in older patients who develop sudden shoulder pain and swelling and upper arm bruising. Contracting biceps causes bunching of the muscle. Although rarely necessary, MRI demonstrates abnormalities of the extra- and intra-articular portions of the tendon and fluid in the bicipital groove. Tears are treated conservatively and cause little disability once the pain has settled. In young athletes surgical advice is needed.

Gleno-humeral instability

Young people occasionally develop recurrent shoulder dislocations after an injury. This may mimic a rotator cuff syndrome. It requires specialist management, especially in young athletes.

Brachial neuralgia

This uncommon problem causes severe, diffuse burning pain in the trapezius region and upper arm when the upper brachial plexus is involved. The lower plexus is less often affected. Muscle wasting develops as the pain decreases. Upper plexus lesions may be confused with a rotator cuff problem before the weakness and wasting develop or if they are not noticed. Involvement of the suprascapular nerve leads to wasting of supraspinatus and infraspinatus. Winging of the scapula develops if the scapulothoracic nerve is affected. This is best seen from behind with the patient holding the arms held forwards and pressed palm to palm. Weakness of shoulder elevation also results. The cause is unknown. It is more common in men than women and may follow an infective illness. The nerves are demyelinated and nerve conduction studies are diagnostic and may demonstrate re-nervation, an indicator of recovery. Weakness persists for several months after the pain has settled but usually recovers. Some recommend a short course of oral steroid early in the painful phase and rest in a sling.

Elbow pain

Pain in the elbow is usually periarticular but is occasionally referred from the neck or due to arthritis.

Differential diagnosis of elbow pain (Table 2)

Medial and lateral epicondylitis

Pain at the insertion of the common extensor tendon at the lateral epicondyle ('tennis elbow') is more common than pain from the common flexor tendon at the medial epicondyle ('golfer's elbow'). They occur typically in the middle aged, less fit person. Age-related changes in collagen probably increase the risk. Pain is worst at the epicondyle but radiates into the forearm. Gripping hard or holding a heavy bag worsens lateral epicondylitis and resisted dorsiflexion of the wrist or middle finger with the elbow extended reproduces the pain of lateral epicondylitis and is a useful test. Holding a heavy object with the hands and forearms supinated worsens the pain of medial epicondylitis and resisted flexion of the wrist with the elbow straight reproduces the pain. Pain may occur at rest. The affected epicondyle is tender. Investigations are rarely justified because the clinical diagnosis is clear-cut. X-rays are usually normal but rarely show microcalcification. The lesion is visible on ultrasound or MRI. Radial tunnel syndrome or compression of the posterior interosseus nerve as it passes through the supinator muscle occasionally mimics lateral epicondylitis.

Table 2 Differential diagnosis of elbow pain

Lateral epicondylitis (wrist extensor enthesitis)
Medial epicondylitis (wrist flexor enthesitis)
Olecranon bursitis
Distal biceps enthesitis
Triceps enthesitis
Inflammatory arthritis
Osteoarthritis
Crystal arthritis
Infective arthritis

Lateral and medial epicondylitis are frequently self-limiting and rarely disabling so conservative treatment is appropriate—rest, locally applied NSAID gels, and physiotherapy. There is no evidence base for these treatments. Studies do not support the use of laser treatment. The value of splints and bands is limited but they remind the patient to rest the arm. If the pain is severe, disabling, or persists despite rest, local injection of corticosteroid at the most tender point is more effective than oral NSAIDs (Hay et al. 1999). Occasionally, patients develop intense pain after the injection so all should be warned. The ulnar nerve must be identified when injecting medial epicondylitis. One repeat injection is sometimes needed but repeated injections are best avoided. The superficial nature of the lesion increases the risk of local subcutaneous fat atrophy and skin depigmentation with long-acting corticosteroids. Most individuals recover even if untreated—a few who respond successfully to treatment will have a recurrence by 6 months. Surgical procedures are rarely needed.

Pain occurs at two other muscle insertions around the elbow. The distal biceps inserts into the radial tuberosity and causes pain in the antecubital fossa when the elbow is flexed and supinated against resistance. Triceps inserts into the posterior olecranon and produces pain on resisted elbow extension.

Olecranon bursitis

The olecranon bursa is a common site of trauma or repetitive friction—student's elbow. Bursitis causes swelling, pain, and tenderness. Elbow movements are full but flexion is uncomfortable. Traumatic bursitis produces minimal inflammation. The fluid is clear or blood stained. In inflammatory arthritis, the fluid is cloudy. The bursa may contain rheumatoid nodules. Gout causes very marked pain and swelling and surrounding urate cellulitis. The fluid is highly cellular and contains urate crystals. Infective olecranon bursitis from local bacterial penetration through damaged skin also causes pain, swelling, and cellulitis. The fluid is purulent and the patient may have lymphadenitis.

Aspiration of the fluid relieves the pain. Cloudy fluid is examined by polarized light microscopy for urate crystals, and Gram staining and culture for infection. Infective bursitis requires antibiotics; otherwise a local corticosteroid injection helps. A recurrently inflamed bursa can be removed surgically.

Forearm pain

Pain in the forearm may radiate from structures around the elbow, arise from tendons or muscles in the forearm itself or be due to carpal tunnel syndrome, one of the few causes of pain that radiates proximally. Median nerve compression at the elbow (pronator teres syndrome) is rare. Severe shoulder pain radiates to the radial side of the forearm. Forearm pain of neurological origin arises from the lower brachial plexus (thoracic outlet syndrome or Pancoast's tumour) or the cervical spine.

Differential diagnosis of forearm pain (Table 3)

Entrapment syndromes: if the posterior interosseous nerve is entrapped just distal to the elbow, it produces forearm aching and mimics medial epicondylitis but the tenderness is distal to the epicondyle. If the anterior interosseous nerve is entrapped proximal to pronator teres, it produces forearm aching and weakness of pronation and wrist flexion.

Median nerve entrapment in the elbow (pronator teres syndrome) produces forearm aching and the symptoms of carpal tunnel syndrome but a wrist splint relieves them. Forearm pain is a common complaint of keyboard workers, sometimes in isolation or as part of more generalized pain. The aetiology of work-related upper limb pain is controversial (Helliwell 1999) and its management is complex. Early diagnosis and treatment of localizable problems such as epicondylitis, carpal tunnel syndrome, or tenosynovitis is essential. Affected individuals may suffer high levels of psychological distress and other somatic disorders or show illness behaviour. Work-related pain often develops after a sudden increase in workload or changed working practices. A combination of work-related mechanical causes and psychosocial factors is involved. Workplace disharmony or dissatisfaction with levels of support from colleagues or middle managers is common. Affected individuals, their managers, and the occupational health team all become anxious and more workers in the office are affected. Litigation or threats of it, and worries about loss of employment all add to the stress and it risks becomes self-perpetuating. Ergonomic assessment of the workplace and of the individual's working posture helps but it is often necessary to address office stresses and working practices also. Changing work practices and methods of compensation and less publicity all combined to reduce the high incidence of this problem in Australian industries (Feuerstein et al. 1998). Studies have indicated similar risk factors in other regional pain syndromes (Macfarlane 1999).

Differential diagnosis of wrist pain (Table 4)

Flexor tenosynovitis and carpal tunnel syndrome

The tendons of the finger flexors run through the carpal tunnel in a synovial sheath. This is a common site of inflammation. Unaccustomed overuse or repetitive use is often the cause, particularly do-it-yourself activities. Flexor tenosynovitis produces palmar swelling and tenderness just proximal and distal to the wrist. Finger flexor tenosynovitis in the palm may also be present. The fingers and wrist feel stiff, swollen, and painful. This may be part of an inflammatory arthritis.

Table 3 Differential diagnosis of forearm pain

Posterior interosseous syndrome
Anterior interosseous syndrome
Pronator teres syndrome
Non-specific (work-related) forearm pain
Pain radiating from the elbow or shoulder
Cervical nerve root impingement
Thoracic outlet syndrome
Compartment syndrome

Table 4 Differential diagnosis of wrist pain

Flexor tenosynovitis and carpal tunnel syndrome
De Quervain's tenosynovitis
Extensor tenosynovitis
Ganglion
Scaphoid fracture
Osteonecrosis of lunate (Kienboeck's disease)
Pseudogout gout
Inflammatory arthritis
Osteoarthritis
Hypertrophic pulmonary osteoarthropathy

Carpal tunnel syndrome is the most commonest of the peripheral nerve entrapment lesions. It occurs with flexor tenosynovitis and during the later stages of pregnancy, probably due to increased weight and fluid retention. Wrist arthritis, a ganglion, amyloidosis, or myxoedema may also cause it. Repetitive handwork may cause carpal tunnel syndrome although its status as a work injury is controversial (Yagev et al. 2001).

The patient complains of any combination of pain, tingling, and numbness, or of the fingers feeling swollen even when no swelling is apparent. The hand symptoms are restricted to the distribution of the median nerve and the little finger and the ulnar side of the ring finger is spared. They typically waken the patient or are present on wakening. Shaking the hand and holding it down out of bed help. The patient often volunteers this information. When it is severe, all the fingers feel affected: the patient may need to record the distribution on a hand outline. Intense aching of the forearm is common. Rarely proximal, the median nerve is compressed in the forearm by pronator teres. Holding a book or newspaper may cause the symptoms. The patient's description is often diagnostic. Clinical tests that precipitate the symptoms include: Tinel's sign—tapping the median nerve in the carpal tunnel, or Phalen's test—holding the wrist is forced dorsiflexion. Untreated, the numbness may become permanent and wasting of the thenar eminence muscles (flexor pollicis and opponens pollicis) develops. The hand feels clumsy and weak. Resisted abduction of the dorsal phalanx of the thumb with the thumb adducted towards the fifth digit is weak. Ultrasound imaging demonstrates any abnormality in the carpal tunnel and reduction of the normal movement of the median nerve during flexion and extension.

A dorsiflexion wrist support worn at night regularly for several weeks often relieves or reduces the symptoms. This response is diagnostic and often therapeutic. A more proximal cause of the symptoms is unlikely.

If the symptoms recur or if there is permanent numbness or weakness, nerve conduction studies are obligatory. They demonstrate slower median nerve conduction across the wrist when compared with conduction proximal to the wrist or in ulnar nerve across the wrist. The action potential may be reduced or absent if nerve damage is severe. Needle electromyography is unpleasant but detects denervation. Significant nerve damage warrants surgical decompression. Some surgeons advocate endoscopic surgery. Post-operatively, the pins and needles may worsen briefly as the nerve recovers. Recovery of sensation and/or strength is limited if the damage is longstanding.

The role of carpal tunnel corticosteroid injection is controversial although many patients experience relief. The procedure can be undertaken in the consulting room. The controversy surrounds possible damage which might be caused by the injection itself or by the crystalline nature of some steroid preparations which remain in situ for prolonged periods. Careful positioning of the needle is essential. Hydrocortisone acetate 25 mg is effective and non-toxic (Wong et al. 2001). Local ultrasound is more effective than sham ultrasound but has not been compared with injection.

De Quervain's tenosynovitis

De Quervain's stenosing tenosynovitis causes pain and swelling at the radial styloid and is due to inflammation of the synovial sheath of the abductor policis longus and extensor policis brevis tendons as they pass under the retaining retinaculum. There is local tenderness and swelling. Tendon swelling and stenosis of the tunnel cause crepitus and occasionally thumb triggering. The pain is worsened by passively flexing the thumb into the palm—Finkelstein's test. This also worsens first carpometacarpal osteoarthritis but then the pain is at the base of the thumb and the joint is tender. Resting the thumb and wrist and avoiding thumb extension and pinching movements help. Immobilization splints are cumbersome. Therapeutic ultrasound or local NSAID gels may help but corticosteroid injected alongside the tendon under low pressure brings rapid relief. A second injection or surgery is sometimes necessary.

Extensor tenosynovitis

Inflammation of the common extensor (fourth) compartment causes well-defined swelling on the back of the hand and distal forearm. Constriction by the extensor retinaculum causes an 'hour-glass' swelling. In contrast, synovitis of the wrist joint causes diffuse swelling distal to the radius and ulna. Extensor tenosynovitis is caused by repetitive wrist movements and is a cause of forearm pain in keyboard workers who hold their wrists in excessive extension. It is also common in rheumatoid arthritis. It is important to look at work practices. Keyboard and mouse wrist supports help avoid recurrences. If rest does not help, a corticosteroid injection into the tendon sheath does.

Ganglion

A ganglion is a cystic swelling in continuity with a joint or tendon sheath through a fault in the capsule and filled with clear, thick, hyaluronan-rich fluid. Ganglia are common around the wrist. They are often painless and resolve spontaneously. A wrist splint relieves pain. Injection is popular but rarely effective and surgical excision is best if the ganglion is symptomatic.

Scaphoid fracture

This causes pain in the anatomical snuffbox after a fall onto the outstretched hand. Immediate X-rays may not be diagnostic, so any severe wrist injury is managed as a potential scaphoid fracture and plaster is applied. The patient is X-rayed again in 3 weeks. Unrecognized scaphoid fractures eventually cause pain because of failed union, osteonecrosis of the proximal third of the bone, and secondary osteoarthritis.

Osteonecrosis

Kienboeck disease causes wrist pain after a dorsiflexion injury. It occurs in heavy labourers. It leads to fragmentation and collapse of the lunate and carpal shortening. The radiological changes of osteonecrosis take upto 18 months to appear. Eventually, secondary osteoarthritis of the wrist develops.

Differential diagnosis of pain in the hand and fingers (Table 5)

Trauma, sometimes unnoticed, is the most common cause of hand pain. A careful history and examination are essential to an accurate differential diagnosis. Synovitis produces 'boggy' swelling around affected joints or tendon sheaths. The flexor tendons may be thickened or nodular. Skin changes occur in scleroderma and in diabetes. There may be signs of vasculitis. X-Rays are helpful if there is a history of trauma to rule out a fracture and are important in the differential diagnosis of inflammatory arthritis—periarticular osteoporosis, juxta-articular erosions, and joint space narrowing are diagnostic of rheumatoid arthritis. Typical appearances appear in psoriatic arthritis and tophaceous gout. The acute phase reactants are usually raised in inflammatory polyarthritis. The presence of joint space loss and periarticular osteophytes on X-rays at the IP joints or at the base of the thumb is typical of nodal osteoarthritis.

Table 5 Differential diagnosis of pain in the hand

Trauma
Finger flexor tenosynovitis and trigger finger
Thumb flexor tenosynovitis and trigger thumb
Nodal and first carpometacarpal osteoarthritis
Diabetic stiff hand
Carpal tunnel syndrome (pronator teres syndrome)
Ulnar nerve compression syndromes
Inflammatory arthritis and dactylitis
Writer's cramp
Dupuytren's contracture

Finger flexor tenosynovitis and trigger finger

Flexor tendinitis occurs individually or affects several fingers. Excessive gripping and hard manual work cause palpable tendon thickening and nodularity. This is not always symptomatic. Finger stiffness in the morning may be prolonged and pain is felt in the palm or along the dorsum of the finger. Flexor tenosynovitis is common in rheumatoid and is part of dactylitis in seronegative arthritis. Nodular flexor tenosynovitis is more common in diabetic than in non-diabetic people and less responsive to treatment (Stahl et al. 1997). Excessive nodularity or thickening may lead to catching of the nodule at the pulley that overlies the proximal MCP joint in the palm, thereby causing a 'trigger' finger. The primary lesion is tenosynovitis causing fibrosis and constriction of the tendon sheath. The patient wakes with the finger flexed into the palm and has to forcibly extend it with a sudden painless or painful click. This also occurs during tight gripping and becomes disabling. There is a tender, palpable nodule and the 'catch' in the movement is felt in the palm although the patient often feels pain along the whole finger. The pain is reproduced by passive extension of the affected finger. A corticosteroid injection alongside the tendon nodule in the palm under low pressure helps (Rankin and Rankin 1998). If persistent or recurrent, surgical release is indicated.

Thumb flexor tenosynovitis and trigger thumb

Overuse or local trauma, for example, opening a tight jar, is the most commonest cause. The interphalangeal joint either sticks in flexion but snaps straight or cannot be flexed or fully extended. There is local tenderness over the sesamoid bone in the flexor pollicis brevis tendon over the volar aspect of the first MCP joint. A local corticosteroid injection at the site of maximal tenderness adjacent to the sesamoid bone helps.

Nodal and first carpometacarpal osteoarthritis

Nodal osteoarthritis of the DIP joints is common and usually familial. Initially, the joint is swollen, inflamed, and painful. The pain subsides over a period of weeks or months leaving bony swelling (Heberden's nodes). They are usually of little long-term consequence unless instability develops, when surgical fixation in slight flexion improves hand function. Most patients manage with local analgesic applications or no treatment once they are reassured about the good outcome. Involvement of the PIPs is less frequent but more troublesome because, although the pain settles, stiffness of the proximal joints impairs hand function. Bony swellings of the PIP joints are called Bouchard's nodes. When PIP involvement occurs without Heberden's nodes, it may be mistaken for early rheumatoid arthritis. Pain at the base of the thumb develops in the early phase of first carpometacarpal osteoarthritis. Initially disabling, with time the joint stiffens and adducts, and pain and disability reduce. Conservative management is preferable although a local corticosteroid injection helps severe pain. The outcome of replacement surgery is good in the small number for whom it is warranted.

Diabetic stiff hand (cheiroarthropathy—limited joint mobility syndrome)

Between 5 and 10 per cent of type I diabetic patients develop stiff hands. It is more common when diabetic control is poor. The skin is waxy and tight and they complain of mild pain and paraesthesia. It is associated with limited shoulder mobility, diabetic nephropathy, and retinopathy. Limited joint mobility in diabetes is often multifactorial and there may be flexor tenosynovitis, Dupuytren's contracture, and nodal osteoarthritis (Griggs et al. 1995). Good diabetic control is essential and it is helpful to inject symptomatic flexor tenosynovitis but there is no specific treatment for the skin changes.

Writer's cramp

This is the most common dystonia. It occurs during writing or other complex hand functions such as playing a musical instrument and is most common in professional writers or musicians. They complain of clumsiness and painful tightness in the hand and forearm whilst writing or playing. Abnormal tension and strange posturing of the hand and arm develop during the precipitating activity. Locally injected botulinum toxin produces temporary relief. Behavioural training and learning new techniques may help but the outlook is poor and some musicians give up their careers.

Dupuytren's contracture

This is a relatively common and painless condition. Palpable fibrosis develops in the palmar aponeurosis, usually in the palm, occasionally at the base of a digit. Painless contraction of the aponeurosis draws the digit(s) into flexion. An early sign is skin pitting or puckering. Later a tight band which does not move with the underlying tendons is palpable and visible. The ring finger is most commonly affected. It runs a variable course and often causes no disability. Progressive tightness and flexion is disabling and is more common in familial disease. Histologically fibroblasts proliferate in the superficial fascia initially but later invade the dermis. It is more common in males, Caucasians, heavy drinkers, and smokers and in diabetes mellitus. It is familial tendency, suggesting a genetic factor. The exact aetiology is unknown although repeated trauma may be important. Other types of nodular fibromatosis such as nodular plantar fibromatosis and knuckle pads (Garrod's pads) and with Peyronie's disease of the penis may coexist.

MRI scanning assesses its extent. The role of local corticosteroid injections early in the condition is unclear (Ketchum and Donahue 2000). Radiotherapy in early disease has been shown to produce good results at 12 months (Seegenschmiedt et al. 2001). Surgical excision is frequently used and probably helpful but recurrence is common and there are no controlled studies.

Cubital tunnel syndrome

Ulnar nerve compression at the elbow by direct pressure, for example, leaning on the elbow, or stretched when the elbow is held in prolonged flexion, for example, holding a telephone causes pins and needles in the lateral hand. Prolonged entrapment causes hypothenar wasting and weakness of the hand intrinsic muscles. The nerve is tender and sensitive and Tinel's sign is positive. Conservative treatment, avoiding direct pressure and stretching the nerve, and occasionally splinting the elbow at night at 40° of flexion all help. Nerve conduction studies are normal in around 50 per cent—severe changes may warrant surgical anterior transposition of the nerve. The ulnar nerve is occasionally compressed in Guyon's canal at the wrist.

Pain in the back and leg

Pain in the leg arises locally, is referred from the back, or is part of a generalized condition—rheumatoid arthritis, polymyalgia rheumatica, or a chronic pain syndrome. Spinal pain is common and is discussed elsewhere. Pain in the leg due to nerve root impingement from a disc prolapse, from spondylosis casing root or spinal canal narrowing, or from a spondylolisthesis, is sharp or burning and usually associated with other sensory symptoms and loss of power or reflexes. It may worsen with walking—spinal claudication. When caused by a disc prolapse, the back is acutely painful and stiff and there is often a scoliosis. Facet joint osteoarthritis produces pain which radiates from the buttock to the posterior thigh and is made worse by back extension. There may be a short or long history of back pain. These features are important in sorting out the differential diagnosis of pain in the leg.

Pain in the hip

Great care is needed to identify the site and origin of pain around the hip. Hip pain is divided into anterior groin pain, lateral trochanteric pain, or posterior buttock pain. Hip joint pain is usually diffuse. Primarily felt in the anterior groin, it radiates to the anterolateral thigh, buttock, or anterior knee, rarely to the shin or trochanteric region. It worsens with weight bearing. Osteoarthritis is the most common cause of arthritis in adults. Inflammatory arthritis is less common but occurs in younger people with seronegative arthritis. Sacroiliitis produces pain deep in the buttock and radiates to the posterior thigh. Periarticular causes of pain are important and cause localized tenderness. Trochanteric pain arises from the trochanteric bursa, local muscle insertions, or the thoraco-lumbar spine, less commonly from the hip joint. It may be due to a disc prolapses at L1/2 or L2/3. Buttock pain may be referred from the lumbar spine, arise from the sacroiliac or hip joint or the ischiogluteal bursa or be due to vascular insufficiency. Where pain is persistent, and in elite athletes, there is an argument for using MRI to establish an accurate diagnosis (De Paulis et al. 1998).

Differential diagnosis of hip pain (Table 6)

Lateral trochanteric pain

Trochanteric bursitis and greater trochanteric pain syndrome

Direct local trauma or unaccustomed walking or weight bearing exercise causes trochanteric bursitis. It is also associated with ipsilateral hip arthritis, pain or obesity, and rheumatoid arthritis. A tight iliotibial band crossing the greater trochanter causes a painful 'snapping' hip. The deep, aching pain radiates from the trochanter to the lateral thigh. It worsens when walking, squatting, going down stairs, sitting with the affected leg crossed, or lying on the affected side. There is local tenderness and resisted hip abduction is painful. Hip movements are unaffected unless the pain is severe. Rest is helpful and milder cases settle spontaneously or with NSAIDs. A local corticosteroid injection onto the trochanter at the point of maximum tenderness helps although pain may recur, especially in the physically active middle aged patient (Shbeed et al. 1996). Stretching exercises for the iliotibial band help to reduce recurrence. If the response is poor or the symptoms atypical ultrasound or MRI are warranted to see if the gluteus tendon is torn or inflamed.

Table 6 Differential diagnosis of hip pain

	Main site of pain
Lateral trochanteric pain	
Trochanteric bursitis	Lateral thigh to knee (locally tender over trochanter)
Meralgia paraesthetica	Anterolateral thigh to knee + dysaesthesia
Anterior groin pain	
Osteoarthritis of hip	Groin, buttock, anterior thigh to knee
Fracture of femur	Groin and anterior upper thigh
Adductor tendinitis	Medial groin and upper medial thigh
Pubic symphysitis	Midline and medial groin
Rectus abdominis enthesitis	Groin
Iliopsoas bursitis	Groin and upper anterior thigh
Rectus femoris enthesitis	Lateral groin (anterior superior iliac spine)
Inguinal or femoral hernia	Groin
Inflammatory arthritis	Groin, buttock, anterior thigh to knee
Osteonecrosis	Groin
Hip dysplasia and labral tear	Groin
Referred from retroperitoneal structures	Groin and anterior thigh
Posterior buttock pain	
Referred from back	Buttock ± lateral thigh (T12 and L1) or groin (L2–4)
Fibrositic nodulosis	Upper buttock
Ischiogluteal bursitis	Lower buttock
Sacroiliitis (AS)	Buttock(s) and back
Polymyalgia rheumatica	Buttocks and posterior thighs (+shoulders) >55 years
Vascular insufficiency	Buttock, thigh, and leg

The best predictor of a tear is a positive Trendelenberg sign—the affected hip drops during affected leg standing rather than the normal rise. MRI is essential before surgery, particularly if there is a positive Trendelenberg sign (Bird et al. 2001). A persistently painful bursa can be excised.

Meralgia paraesthetica

This symptom complex is caused by entrapment of the lateral femoral cutaneous nerve (LFCN) and comprises severe burning pain, dysaesthesia, and numbness of the anterolateral thigh from the trochanter to just above the knee. The dysaesthesia distinguish it from trochanteric bursitis, and it is not usually painful to lie on the affected side. The pain worsens when sitting, with sudden weight increase or wearing tight clothing. There is no loss of power or muscle wasting. It may develop after pelvic or inguinal surgery, prone positioning for surgery, or a direct injury. The LFCN usually runs under the lateral inguinal ligament close to the anterior superior iliac spine and superficial to sartorius but may lie superficial to the anterior iliac wing or pass through the sartorius muscle where it can be compressed. Compression also occurs as it emerges through the fascia lata about 10 cm distal to the anterior superior iliac spine. A lateral L2/3 disc compressing the L3 nerve root mimics the syndrome, although there is usually also back pain and may be wasting of vastus lateralis. Local anaesthetic injection at any point of tenderness, usually at the point where the nerve exits the pelvis helps diagnosis. Electrostimulation localizes the nerve precisely prior to injection of corticosteroid. Avoidance of local pressure, and rest are also helpful. Patients often live with it, especially when numbness is the only symptom. Pain is rarely intractable but surgical neurolysis may be needed (Grossman et al. 2001).

Anterior groin pain

Adductor tendinitis

Groin injuries are common in soccer, horse riding, and gymnastics. Adductor enthesopathy produces medial groin pain. Tears at the tendon insertion into the pubic tubercle or about 1 cm distally cause tenderness. Pain is worsened by abduction and resisted adduction of the hip. Intercourse is uncomfortable for a woman. Rest, ultrasound, and NSAIDs are all used. A corticosteroid injection is helpful in refractory cases.

Rectus abdominis enthesitis

This variant of groin strain in athletes is seen after repeated sit-ups and in throwers. The pain localizes to the upper pubic ramus and lower abdomen. Inflammation is clearly seen on MRI. Conservative measures and rest are appropriate. The tendon rarely ruptures close to its insertion and requires surgical repair.

Iliopsoas bursitis

The iliopsoas tendon runs under the inguinal ligament to the lesser trochanter. It flexes the hip. The tendon is separated from the hip joint by a bursa which may communicate with the joint, especially in inflammatory arthritis. Iliopsoas bursitis is underdiagnosed. It presents as a painful mass lateral to the neurovascular bundle in the groin. The pain is worsened by hip hyperextension and resisted flexion. It is clearly seen on MRI and can be injected with corticosteroid under ultrasound guidance.

Pubic symphysitis (osteitis pubis)

This uncommon inflammatory condition may be septic osteomyelitis following pelvic surgery but it is more commonly sterile. It occurs after childbirth, pelvic surgery, or athletic trauma. The cause is unknown but is possibly a form of algodystrophy. Pain and tenderness develop over the symphysis and pain is worsened during the stance phase of walking. X-Rays show widening of the symphysis and lysis of the bony surfaces. Aspiration and culture are essential to exclude infection. Most settle with rest and NSAIDs. A local corticosteroid injection is occasionally tried.

Rectus femoris enthesitis

Rectus femoris flexes the hip and extends the knee and is injured during sprint starts and blocked kicks. Damage just distal to its insertion into the anterior superior iliac spine causes pain and local tenderness. The pain is worsened by resisted hip flexion.

Hip dysplasia and labral tears

Congenital dislocation and severe hip dysplasia are usually noticed in infancy or childhood. Minor dysplasia causes hip pain and sudden painful giving way in young physically active adults and predisposes to osteoarthritis. The normally horizontal upper acetabulum slopes up and laterally and the femoral head is less well covered than usual, leading to increased stress on the upper outer portion of the acetabulum. The adjacent labrum is stressed and may tear. MRI arthrography demonstrates ganglion formation in the bone or adjacent soft tissue and any labral damage. Osteotomy is advocated to prevent pain and early onset of osteoarthritis.

Osteonecrosis of the femoral head

The common femoral artery supplies the femoral neck and most of the head. It can be damaged by femoral neck fracture leading to osteonecrosis although anastamoses with arteries in the ligamentum teres exist in some. Femoral head osteonecrosis also occurs in adults on corticosteroids, alcoholics, deep-sea divers, and tunellers. It causes severe hip pain. Initially X-rays are normal. MRI is the best early non-invasive diagnostic technique (Wu et al. 1998). Surgical core decompression is used before the femoral head has collapsed although the benefit is not clear (Simank et al. 2001). Later, femoral head replacement is necessary.

Pain in the buttock

Fibrositic nodulosis

Fibro-fatty nodules ('back mice') in the upper buttock, around the iliac crest are of no significance unless tender and associated with buttock and posterior thigh pain. There is no evidence to support local corticosteroid injections but they seem to help.

Ischiogluteal bursitis

The ischiogluteal bursa is covered by gluteus maximus when standing but is subcutaneous and exposed when sitting. Bursitis is due to direct trauma or repeated friction to the ischium while sitting (weaver's bottom). Sitting or lying on it worsens the pain. The ischial tuberosity is tender. Avoiding direct pressure helps and a corticosteroid injection helps if the pain is persistent. The injection is safest with the patient lying on the other side with the affected hip flexed. The sciatic nerve lies just lateral to the bursa. Enthesitis occurs in seronegative arthritis and produces a similar syndrome.

Pain in the knee

Knee pain in the adult arises from periarticular soft tissue lesions, intra-articular mechanical derangements, or arthritis. The hip must be examined as a potential source of referred pain. Injury is the most common cause in a young adult. With increasing age the prevalence of radiological osteoarthritis increases but is not always the cause of pain. Obesity, poor quadriceps muscle tone, and clinical depression all contribute to worsening knee osteoarthritis (Doherty 2001).

Differential diagnosis of knee pain (Table 7)

Periarticular anterior knee pain

Bursitis: anterior knee pain may be due to prepatellar bursitis following trauma or due to inflammatory synovitis. The swelling is superficial to the patella and fluctuant. There may be marked inflammation. Aspiration and injection of a corticosteroid helps if infection has been ruled out. The deep infrapatellar bursa lies between the patellar tendon and the tibia and is locally tender when inflamed. It is difficult to feel, especially in fat patients. Ultrasound guided aspiration and corticosteroid injection helps. The superficial infrapatellar bursa lies over the patellar tendon at its insertion into the tibial tubercle.

Patellar mal-tracking presents in adolescence or early adult life and is associated with a valgus knee deformity (increased Q-angle—the angle between a . . .), lateral displacement of the patella, and a tendency to lateral

Table 7 Differential diagnosis of knee pain

Trauma and overuse
Periarticular problems
Anterior knee pain
Pre and infrapatellar bursitis
Patellar tendinitis (jumper's knee)
Patellar tracking problems
Medial knee pain
Medial collateral ligament strain
Pellegrini–Stieda disease
Anserine buristis/pes anserinus tendinitis
Lateral knee pain
Lateral collateral ligament strain
Iliotibial band friction syndrome (runner's knee)
Posterior knee pain
Popliteal (baker's) cyst
Ruptured popliteal cyst
Osteoarthritis
Inflammatory arthritis
Acute monoarthritis (Pseudogout, gout, septic arthritis)
Pauciarticular (<5 joints) (seronegative spondarthritis, atypical rheumatoid arthritis)
Polyarticular (rheumatoid arthritis)
Osteochondritis dissecans
Pigmented villonodular synovitis
Hypermobility and dysplasia
Referred from the hip joint

dislocation. The patella may lie higher than usual (patella alta) and on skyline X-rays in 30–40° of flexion the patella rides high on the lateral femoral condyle. Quadriceps strengthening, especially of vastus medialis helps some. The role of surgery to loosen the patella laterally is unproven.

Anterior knee pain syndrome without a specific cause is often bilateral and occurs in young women, causing peripatellar pain during sports and at night. Walking in high heels causes knee flexion and increases the strain exerted through the patella. Avoiding high heels and isometric quadriceps exercises help.

Chondromalacia patellae is an arthroscopic diagnosis, with fibrillation and thinning of patellar cartilage often in association with a mal-tracking patella. Diagnosed early, patellar realignment may help but otherwise quadriceps strengthening and hamstring stretches are recommended.

Pain may arise at the insertion of quadriceps into the proximal patella or of the patellar tendon proximally or distally due to overuse. Tenderness and swelling are highly localized to the enthesis.

Plica syndrome arises from a congenital abnormality of the knee internally. Incomplete separation of the membrane which initially separates the suprapatellar bursa from the knee joint causes anteromedial knee pain, a sense of snapping followed by pain and localized swelling. It is an arthroscopic diagnosis and removal of the plica may help.

Periarticular medial knee pain

The medial ligament becomes painful at its insertion into the medial tibial plateau after a valgus injury and in older overweight women with fat thighs and valgus knees. There is local tenderness. Exerting a valgus stress on the knee increases pain. It is difficult to distinguish from anserine bursitis or pain at the insertion of the pes anserinus although the latter produces tenderness more distally. Rest helps, as does a local corticosteroid injection.

Injuring the medial ligament at its insertion into the medial femoral condyle causes Pellegrini–Stiega disease and produces local pain and tenderness. Linear calcification, probably in a haematoma, forms overlying the medial aspect of the medial femoral condyle. Rest helps, as does occasionally a local corticosteroid injection.

Periarticular lateral knee pain

The lateral collateral ligament may cause pain at its insertion into the fibula. Iliotibial band friction syndrome is the most common cause of overuse knee pain in younger runners and cyclists. The lateral femoral condyle is painful and tender. As the knee flexes the iliotibial band crosses the lateral collateral ligament and femoral epicondyle and friction occurs. Pressure is greatest at about 30° of flexion. The lateral synovial recess may be inflamed and form a bursa as part of the syndrome. MRI is the investigation of choice. Rest followed by retraining is effective for most.

Periarticular posterior knee pain

A communicating semi-membranosus bursa can become distended by a knee effusion when there is a valve like opening which allows fluid into the cyst but not out. Pressure increases during walking, standing from sitting, and stair climbing. Rupture of the cyst results in sudden pain behind the knee and in the upper calf, upper calf tenderness and swelling, and ankle oedema. Rupture temporarily reduces the knee effusion, so it is important to ask about prior knee pain and swelling when a patient presents with calf pain. It is often acutely painful. Although it mimics a deep venous thrombosis (DVT) superficially, the latter causes pain and tenderness lower in the calf. Doppler ultrasound examination confirms the diagnosis and excludes a DVT. The affected leg is rested NSAIDs help but anticoagulation is contraindicated. Aspiration and injection of the knee is necessary if there is an inflammatory arthritis. Occasionally a slow leak of fluid from a ruptured popliteal cyst causes a painless calf cyst.

Meniscal tears

The medial and lateral menisci are fibrocartilagenous structures. In the young they are resilient but can be damaged by twisting injuries with the knee partly flexed. The menisci stiffen with age and are prone to degeneration which predisposes to osteoarthritis. Meniscal injuries occur during sport and cause severe pain, initially at the medial or lateral side of the joint, followed rapidly by generalized pain and swelling. It is painful to bear weight and fully extend the knee. There is localized joint line tenderness and an effusion. After the acute episode the knee may settle, become unstable, be liable to catching or locking, or may swell episodically. MRI is the non-invasive investigation of choice and clearly demonstrates the lesions. There is often an associated cruciate injury. Arthroscopic trimming or repair if the vascularized part of the meniscus is affected is worthwhile in the young. This will reduce the symptomatic episodes but may not prevent later development of osteoarthritis in the affected compartment (Englund et al. 2001).

In the older patient, tears occur but the more diffuse damage is seen on MRI. The value of arthroscopy is less clear although often undertaken. There is often associated osteoarthritis.

Cruciate ligament tears

Cruciate ligament tear is the commonest cause of a knee haemarthrosis in the young. There may be rotatory or anteroposterior instability causing unsteadiness and pain or the knee may become symptom free once the acute episode has settled. Chronic anteroposterior instability is demonstrated with the knee in 45° of flexion with the foot fixed and then applying anteroposterior pressure to the lower leg. The anterior cruciate is more commonly torn. This allows the knee to hyperextend and the tibia can be drawn forwards abnormally. The tear is seen on MRI. Treatment for cruciate ligament tears is controversial and best managed by a specialist knee surgeon.

Osteochondritis dissecans

The medial aspect of the lateral femoral condyle is a common site of this lesion in young adults. A fragment of bone and overlying cartilage detach and may remain in situ or become a loose body. It presents with pain and swelling, occasionally locking or giving way. The cause is unknown but it is familial. The pathology is that of osteonecrosis. The lesion can be seen best on a tunnel anteroposterior X-ray or MRI. Loose fragments can be reattached or removed but recovery is best in the adolescent. In older patients, a similar lesion develops as part of osteoarthritis.

Pigmented villonodular synovitis (Durr et al. 2001)

This unusual condition occurs most commonly at the knee. Initially a localized proliferative synovitis, it becomes nodular and brown because of haemosiderin deposition. Typically the effusion is also deep brown. The lesion is locally invasive in some patients, causing bone damage. The cause is unknown. The patient complains of pain and swelling. The diagnosis is usually made on MRI or arthroscopy. Arthroscopic excision is best, sometimes followed by radiotherapy.

Differential diagnosis of lower leg pain (Table 8)

Compartment syndromes (Mubarak et al. 1989)

These arise from increased pressure in confined anatomic compartments and are due to ischaemia of the muscles and nerves. Unrelieved, they cause muscle necrosis and permanent nerve damage. The most common is anterior compartment syndrome of the leg, affecting tibialis anterior, extensor digitorum longus and extensor hallucis longus muscles, the deep peroneal nerve, and the anterior tibial artery and vein. Exertional compartment syndrome occurs during or after exercise and causes diffuse cramp-like pain which resolves with rest but recurs with further exertion. The compartment is swollen and is tender. The diagnosis is easily overlooked but is important in the differential diagnosis of exertion-related leg pain. It may resolve with rest. Intracompartmental pressures are measured before and after exercise prior to surgical decompression. Acute compartment syndrome is a surgical emergency and follows trauma. Unrecognized, the pressure causes permanent muscle damage and disability. Compartment syndromes also occur in the other compartments of the leg and in the volar compartment of the forearm.

Stress fracture

These are caused by fatigue failure in normal bone in dancers, runners, and jumpers, and occur spontaneously in older people with osteoporosis. Women athletes with amenorrhoea are particularly at risk. The pain worsens with exercise and there is local tenderness and swelling. Common sites are the fibula and tibia and the second metatarsal. Initially, X-rays are normal although a technetium bone scan is diagnostic. Early recognition, rest for upto 6 weeks, and exercise in water help maintain fitness in elite athletes and others. Assessment for osteoporosis is obligatory.

Fibular tunnel syndrome

Compression of the lateral popliteal nerve as it rounds the fibula occurs after fracture, compression by a walking cast, or sitting cross-legged. The patient complains of pins and needles or numbness of the lateral calf and foot. Rarely, a foot drop develops. The lesion can be localized by nerve conduction studies.

Table 8 Differential diagnosis of lower leg pain

Compartment syndromes
Ruptured popliteal cyst
Deep venous thrombosis
Stress fracture
Fibular tunnel syndrome
Tibialis anterior tenovaginitis
Low lumbar disc prolapse

Differential diagnosis of ankle and foot pain (Table 9)

Arch disorders and foot pain (flat or pronated—high arched or supinated)

Flattening of the foot's longitudinal arch is often asymptomatic but may produce midtarsal pain or muscular aching. The foot normally flattens and everts as it enters the stance phase of walking with weight borne mainly along the lateral border of the foot. The foot then inverts as weight is taken onto the metatarsal heads during heel raise and prior to toe off. Flat foot may be congenital or acquired and reversible or irreversible. Congenital flat foot is more common and may be rigid or reversible and associated with hypermobility. Congenital flat foot is often familial and asymptomatic until adolescence or adulthood. The rigid flat foot is associated with bridging between talus and calcaneous or navicula and calcaneous (tarsal coalition), causing permanent loss of the medial longitudinal arch; the navicular and talus become weight bearing. Acquired flat foot may be flexible, rigid (common in rheumatoid arthritis), or due to peroneal muscle spasm. The latter produces aching in the peroneal muscles and tendons. Arch supports and inversion exercises help the painful but still mobile flat foot. Untreated it leads to a spastic flat foot and painful peroneal muscle spasm. Chronic flat foot may be associated with inflammation or rupture of the tibialis posterior tendon. The end stage flat foot is rigid. A molded semi-rigid insole offers some pain relief.

A high arched foot (pes cavus) is associated with toe clawing and is usually congenital and hereditary. It causes pain due to poor shock absorption because eversion of the foot during the stance phase is lost. Shoes with high arch supports and metatarsal pads help.

Pain around the medial ankle

Tibialis posterior tendinitis

The tibialis posterior muscle is a dynamic stabilizer of the hind foot and limits eversion. It is under greatest tension when the foot is flat and during

Table 9 Differential diagnosis of foot and ankle pain

Trauma	
Arch disorders (flat—pronated; high arched—supinated)	
Pain around the medial ankle	
Tibialis posterior tendinitis	
Tarsal tunnel syndrome	
Pain around the lateral ankle	
Peroneus longus and brevis tendinitis	
Pain at the front of the ankle	
Dorsal (extensor) tendinitis	
Tibialis anterior tendinitis	
Heel pain	
Plantar fasciitis	Below heel
Plantar spur or bursitis	Below heel
Painful calcaneal fat pad	Below heel
Achilles tendinopathy/bursitis	Behind heel
Pain in the mid and forefoot	
Stress or march fracture	
Hallux valgus/rigidus (±OA)	
Metatarsalgia and Morton's neuroma	
Sesamitis	
Inflammatory arthritis	
Acute, monoarticular—gout, infection	
Chronic, pauciarticular—seronegative spondarthritis	
Chronic, polyarticular—rheumatoid arthritis	
Bone disorders	
Osteoarthritis	

running and dancing. The tendon develops longitudinal splits (tendinopathy) and may tear. There may be an associated or independent synovitis of the tendon sheath near the medial malleolus. This is common in rheumatoid arthritis. Rest helps, sometimes in a plaster or boot. An associated inversion deformity requires an insole. After an ultrasound examination to exclude longitudinal tendon splitting and a potential tear, a corticosteroid injection into the tendon sheath helps inflammation. If there is severe hindfoot instability, a triple arthrodesis reduces pain and disability.

Tarsal tunnel syndrome

This is underdiagnosed as a cause of foot pain. The posterior tibial nerve and the flexor hallucis and digitorum longus tendons pass under the retinaculum around the medial malleolus. Bony deformity after an ankle fracture, a flat foot, inflammation of the tendons, or an ankle synovial cyst can compress the nerve, causing burning pain and pins and needles in the toes, sole, and heel and an aching calf at night. Plantar branch compression weakens toe flexion. There is swelling and tenderness around the medial malleolus and Tinel's sign is positive. If there is doubt, nerve conduction studies are diagnostic. Treatment of any local cause for compression is appropriate. Occasionally, surgical section of the retinaculum is necessary.

Pain around the lateral ankle

Peroneus longus and brevis tendinitis

The peroneus muscles evert the foot and stabilize the arch during toe off. The tendons and their sheath lie in a tunnel under the superior peroneal retinaculum and behind the lateral malleolus. The longus tendon runs around the calcaneum, under the cuboid, and crosses the sole to insert into base of the first metatarsal bone. The brevis tendon inserts into the base of the fifth metatarsal. Pain and tenderness are caused at the lateral malleolus by tendinitis and at the base of the fifth metatarsal by tendinitis. Rest and occasionally a corticosteroid injection help.

Pain at the front of the ankle

Tibialis anterior lies in the anterior compartment and, with extensor digitorum longus and extensor hallucis longus, is the main foot dorsiflexor. Tibialis anterior tenovaginitis produces pain and crepitus in front of the ankle and proximal to it where the tendon runs under the extensor retinacula. Dorsal or extensor tendinitis causes pain, a longitudinal swelling, and crepitus over the dorsum of the foot. The swelling of tenosynovitis at the ankle extends across the joint, while synovitis of the ankle joint bulges to either side of the extensor tendons. It arises from unaccustomed walking, or running, or tight shoes. Rest, looser shoes, and occasionally a corticosteroid help.

Pain around the heel

Plantar fasciitis is a common cause of heel pain and is due to an acute or recurrent injury to the origin of the plantar fascia causing enthesitis at the anterior calcaneum. It is seen in sports involving a heavy heel strike and in the overweight and middle aged. Tautness of the fascia, biomechanical problems of the foot, or scarring also contribute. Standing pain occurs under the heel, particularly when getting up from bed or chair, then eases initially when walking but limits long distance walking. Tenderness is localized to the anterior calcaneum. There is no palpable swelling. A bony spur at the origin of the plantar fascia is seen on X-ray in around 30 per cent of patients with heel pain but these may be asymptomatic and bilateral. A spur probably increases the risk of injury. Subcalcaneal bursitis produces swelling but is difficult to distinguish clinically from fasciitis. In older patients, the calcaneal fat pad becomes painful as its normal fibrous septa, packed with fat, rupture after direct trauma and in the obese. The pain and tenderness of bursitis or a painful heel pad are more diffuse than that of plantar fasciitis. Occasionally, MRI is warranted to differentiate the lesions. Plantar fascia enthesitis may occur in seronegative arthritis. Treatment is controversial. Reduced weight bearing, shock absorbing heel cushions help. Stretching exercises reduce shortening of the plantar fascia and some advise nocturnal dorsiflexion splinting. An associated flat foot is treated with an arch support. Injections of local anaesthetic and corticosteroid are commonly employed and are helpful although they can cause damage. The evidence base for such these treatments is weak (Crawford et al. 2000). No published trial indicates that extracorporeal shockwave therapy helps plantar fasciitis, but if its efficacy can be proven it is a potentially attractive non-invasive alternative to injections or surgery.

Achilles tendinopathy and bursitis

The Achilles tendon is the body's strongest tendon but prone to injury during sports or when changing from heeled shoes to walking barefoot. The most common lesion is an overuse tendinopathy, with incomplete repair of tendon microtrauma, causing pain and diffuse tendon swelling or peritendinitis just proximal to the calcaneal insertion. Rest and a heel raise are usually sufficient, with stretching exercises to prevent a recurrence. Recovery and a return to sport occur in 75–85 per cent. Local corticosteroid injections are best avoided as they may precipitate tendon rupture. Rupture occurs in the middle aged or older patient during sports. In the younger, active patient, the tear is repaired surgically but in the older patient, conservative management in a plaster cast is usual (Jarvinen et al. 2001).

Pain at the insertion of the tendon itself is due to overuse or occasionally a seronegative arthritis. Rest, a heel raise, and NSAIDs help but an adjacent low-pressure corticosteroid injection may be appropriate. In chronic inflammatory Achilles enthesitis, radiotherapy is effective.

Retrocalcaneal bursitis is less common. The pain is anterior to the tendon and there is diffuse swelling between the Achilles tendon and the ankle joint. It occurs in dancers, runners, and inflammatory arthritis and can be safely injected with corticosteroid. High-backed training shoes cause a painful subcutaneous bursa superficial to the Achilles tendon.

Pain in the mid- and forefoot

Stress or march fracture

The neck or shaft of the second metatarsal is most commonly affected. Fracture is due to unaccustomed walking or osteoporosis. The pain starts suddenly, tenderness is localized, and dorsal swelling develops. X-Rays are usually normal for several weeks but an isotope bone scan or MRI show the fracture clearly. Rest and cushioned shoes help. The pain settles over 6–8 weeks.

Hallux valgus/rigidus (+/− OA)

A combination of medial splaying of the first metatarsal (metatarsus primus varus) and lateral displacement of the great toe is common and may be familial, or due to footwear. It is common in rheumatoid arthritis. Initially hallux valgus is painless but pressure from the shoe and high heels cause pain at the first MTP joint and an adventitious bursa (bunion) forms. Greater displacement leads the second toe to hammer. Eventually the first toe may over- or underlie the second. Painful callosities form under the second MTP joint. Surgical realignment helps severe pain.

Osteoarthritis of the great toe MTP joint causes stiffening and pain. Marginal osteophytes are palpable around the joint and, with loss of joint space, are seen on X-ray. It causes pain during the toe-off phase of walking, relieved by flexing the lateral toes, externally rotating the leg, and rolling into eversion during walking. A shoe with a longitudinally rounded sole helps. Some need surgical fusion in dorsiflexion. Arthroplasty is sometimes successful.

Metatarsalgia and Morton's 'neuroma'

The first and fifth metatarsal heads are the main weight bearing structures of the forefoot when standing and during the heel-off phase of walking and running. Pressure on the middle three metatarsal heads is reduced during toe-off by toe flexion. Claw toes or flexor weakness cause painful callous formation under the metatarsal heads. Short-lived metatarsalgia is common in normal feet after a change of shoes or unaccustomed exercise and when using high heels. It usually settles spontaneously with rest and thick-soled shoes. A metatarsal support carries weight behind the exposed metatarsal heads and helps persistent pain. Callouses over the claw-toe

PIP joints are help by padding and a deep toe box. These deformities are common in rheumatoid arthritis and may require a forefoot arthroplasty. Morton's interdigital 'neuroma' is due to too tight and/or high heeled shoes. It also occurs with pes planus and cavus and in rheumatoid arthritis. It causes lancinating toe pain, pins and needles, and numbness of adjacent surfaces of two toes, commonly the third and fourth. Removing the shoe relieves the pain. An interdigital bursa or synovial cyst which may be palpable and tender compresses the interdigital nerve. Occasionally, there is a true neuroma. Wide shoes and lower heels usually suffice. A dorsal interdigital corticosteroid injection helps. MRI delineates the problem if surgery is being contemplated.

Inflammation of the sesamoid bones in the bipartite flexor hallucis brevis tendon occasionally causes pain under the first MTP joint. Running and dancing cause it. Rest and padding are helpful. These sesamoid bones may be bipartite but a fracture is rare.

References

Aker, P.D., Gross, A.R., Goldsmith, C.H., and Peloso, P. (1996). Conservative management of mechanical neck pain: systematic review and meta-analysis. *British Medical Journal* **313**, 1291–6.

Bamji, A.N., Erhardt, C.C., Price, T.R., and Williams, P.L. (1996). The painful shoulder: can consultants agree? *British Journal of Rheumatology* **35**, 1172–4.

Bird, P.A., Oakley, S.P., Shnier, R., and Kirkham, B.W. (2001). Prospective evaluation of magnetic resonance imaging and physical examination findings in patients with greater trochanteric pain syndrome. *Arthritis and Rheumatism* **44**, 2138–45.

Cassidy, J.D., Carroll, L.J., Cote, P., Lernstra, M., Berglund, A., and Nygren, A. (2000). Effects of eliminating compensation for pain and suffering on the outcome of insurance claims for whiplash. *New England Journal of Medicine* **342**, 1179–86.

Charrin, J.E. and Noel, E.R. (2001). Shockwave therapy under ultrasonographic guidance in rotator cuff tendinitis. *Joint Bone and Spine* **68**, 241–4.

Crawford, F., Atkins, D., and Edwards, J. (2000). Interventions for heel pain (Cochrane review). *Cochrane Database System Review* CD000416.

Dalton, S. (1993). The shoulder. In *Rheumatology* 2nd edn. (ed. J.H. Klippel and P.A. Dieppe), pp. 7.1–7.13. London: Mosby.

De Paulis, F., Cacchio, A., Michelini, O., Damiani, A., and Saggini, R. (1998). Sports injuries in the pelvis: diagnostic imaging. *European Journal of Radiology* (Suppl. 1), S49–59.

Doherty, M., Dacre, J., Dieppe, P., and Snaith, M. (1992). The 'GALS' locomotor screen. *Annals of the Rheumatic Diseases* **51**, 1165–9.

Doherty, M. (2001). Risk factors for progression of knee osteoarthritis. *Lancet* **358** (9284), 775–6.

Durr, H.R., Stabler, A., Maier, M., and Refior, H.J. (2001). Pigmented villonodular synovitis. Review of 20 cases. *Journal of Rheumatology* **28**, 1620–30.

Englund, M., Roos, E.M., Roos, H.P., and Lohmander, L.S. (2001). Patient-relevant outcomes fourteen years after meniscectomy: influence of type of meniscal tear and size of resection. *Rheumatology* **40**, 631–9.

Farin, P.U., Jaroma, H., Hanju, A., and Soimakallio, S. (1990). Shoulder impingement syndrome: sonographic evaluation. *Radiology* **176**, 845–9.

Feuerstein, M., Miller, V.L., Burrell, L.M., and Berger, R. (1998). Occupational upper extremity disorders in the federal workforce. *Journal of Occupational and Environmental Medicine* **40**, 546–55.

Green, S., Buchbinder, R., Glazier, R., and Forbes, A. (1998). Systematic review of randomised controlled trials of interventions for painful shoulder: selection criteria, outcome and assessment. *British Medical Journal* **316**, 354–60.

Griggs, S.M., Weiss, A.P., Lane, L.B., Schwenker, C., Akelman, E., and Sachar, K. (1995). Treatment of trigger finger in patients with diabetes mellitus. *Journal of Hand Surgery (America)* **20**, 787–9.

Grossman, M.G., Ducey, S.A., Nadler, S.S., and Levy, A.S. (2001). Meralgia paraesthetica: diagnosis and treatment. *Journal of the American Academy of Orthopaedic Surgery* **9**, 334–6.

Hay, E.M., Paterson, S.M., Lewis, M., Hosie, G., and Croft, P. (1999). Pragmatic randomised controlled trial of local corticosteroid injection and naproxen for treatment of lateral epicondylitis of elbow in primary care. *British Medical Journal* **319**, 964–8.

Helliwell, P. (1999). The elbow, forearm, wrist and hand. In *Clinical Rheumatology: Regional Musculoskeletal Pain* (ed. P. Croft and P.M. Brooks), pp. 311–28. London: Balliere Tindall.

Irnich, D., Behrens, N., Molzen, H., Konig, A., Krauass, M., Natalis, M., Beyer, A., and Schops, P. (2001). Randomised trial of acupuncture compared with 'sham' laser and acupuncture for treatment of neck pain. *British Medical Journal* **322**, 1574.

Jarvinen, T.A.H., Kannus, P., Paavola, M., Jarvinen, T.L.N., Jozsa, L., and Jarvinen, M. (2001). Achilles tendon injuries. *Current Opinion in Rheumatology* **13**, 150–5.

Ketchum, L.D. and Donahue, T.K. (2000). The injection of nodules of Dupuytren's disease with triamcinolone acetonide. *Journal of Hand Surgery (America)* **25**, 1157–62.

Macfarlane, G.J., Hunt, M.H., and Silman, A.J. (2000). Role of mechanical and psychological factors in the onset of forearm pain: prospective population based study. *British Medical Journal* **321**, 676–9.

Macfarlane, G.J. (1999). Generalised pain, fibromyalgia and regional pain: an epidemiological view. *Baillière's Clinical Rheumatology* **13**, 403–14.

Mubarak, S.J., Pedowitz, R.A., and Hargens, A.R. (1989). Compartment syndromes. *Current Orthopaedics* **3**, 36–40.

Rankin, M.E. and Rankin, E.A. (1998). Injection therapy for management of stenosing tenosynovitis (de Quervain's disease) of the wrist. *Journal of the National Medical Association* **90**, 474–6.

Roberts, C.S., Walker, J.A., II, and Seligson, D. (2001). Diagnostic capabilities of shoulder ultrasonography in the detection of complete and partial rotator cuff tears. *American Journal of Orthopaedics* **30**, 159–62.

Seegenschmiedt, M.H., Olschewski, T., and Guntrum, F. (2001). Radiotherapy optimization in early-stage Dupuytren's contracture; results of a randomized study. *International Journal of Radiation Oncology, Biology, and Physics* **49**, 785–98.

Shbeed, M.I., O'Duffy, J.D., Michet, C.J., Jr., O'Fallon, W.M., and Matteson, E.L. (1996). Evaluation of glucocorticosteroid injection for the treatment of trochanteric bursitis. *Journal of Rheumatology* **23**, 2104–6.

Simank, H.G., Brocai, D.R., Brill, C., and Lukoschek, M. (2001). Comparison of results of core decompression and intertrochanteric osteotomy for non-traumatic osteonecrosis of the femoral had using Cox regression and survivorship analysis. *Journal of Arthroplasty* **16**, 790–4.

Stahl, S., Kanter, Y., and Karnelli, E. (1997). Outcome of trigger finger treatment in diabetes. *Journal of Rheumatology* **24**, 931–6.

Tytherleigh-Strong, G., Hiahara, A., and Miniaci, A. (2001). Rotator cuff disease. *Current Opinion in Rheumatology* **13**, 135–45.

Warner, J.J. (1997). Frozen shoulder; diagnosis and management. *Journal of the American Academy of Orthopaedic Surgeons* **5**, 130–40.

Winters, J.C., Jorritsma, W., Groenier, C.H., Sobel, J.S., Meyboom-de Jong, B., and Arendzen, H.J. (1999). Treatment of shoulder complaints in general practice: long term results of a randomised, single blind study comparing physiotherapy, manipulation, and corticosteroid injection. *British Medical Journal* **318**,1395–6.

Wong, S. M., Hui, A.C.F., O'Gradaigh, D., and Merry, P. (2001). Corticosteroid injection for the treatment of carpal tunnel syndrome. *Annals of the Rheumatic Diseases* **60**, 897.

Wu, Z., Yan, X., Liu, Z., Pan, S., and Cao, X. (1998). Avascular necrosis of the femoral head: MR imaging with radiological and histological correlation. *Chinese Medical Journal (English)* **111**, 599–602.

Yagev, Y., Carel, R.S., and Yagev, R. (2001). Assessment of work-related risk factors for carpal tunnel syndrome. *Israel Medical Association Journal* **3**, 569–71.

6.13.3 Pain syndromes—childhood onset

Kevin J. Murray

Introduction

Chronic musculoskeletal pain syndromes (CPS) represent an important case burden for most paediatric rheumatology clinics. The term CPS is usually applied to conditions where chronic pain is complained of in tissues related to the musculoskeletal system that have no obvious other definable specific medical disorder to account for the pain. Implied in the term is pain which is ongoing (usually >3 months) beyond what might be considered reasonable for any initiating event. Clinical descriptions of patient populations with onset in childhood or adolescence has lagged behind those of adults and only come to prominence in the last two decades (Sherry 2000; Malleson et al. 2001). It is likely this reflects the development of paediatric rheumatic and musculoskeletal medicine, as specific referral centres became available. Doubtless, more defined criteria for grouping and description of similar patients has influenced apparent prevalence rates. It may be that corresponding rises in psychological and somatization disorders in western societies may be influencing the frequency of diagnosis of these disorders in less explicit ways.

This chapter describes the discrete disorders or syndromes as they occur in childhood. It focuses on the unique spectrum of clinical features seen in childhood, the influence upon the developing child, and the impact of child development upon the expression of the disorders. Given the imprecise nature of diagnostic criteria, and overlapping features of these disorders, it is not surprising that numerous classification systems have arisen. Some authors use terms such as 'psychosomatic musculoskeletal pain disorders' (Sherry et al. 1991) to encompass the whole group reflecting a central role for psychological issues. Others suggest use of the phrase 'idiopathic pain syndromes' perhaps to avoid the implication of definite psychological aetiology for all cases (Malleson et al. 1992). The use of more general terminology reflects that children often do not fulfil all the diagnostic criteria for the specific disorders, as defined for adults, and would be considered as having incomplete syndromes or *form fruste* versions of the disorders.

Background

Discrete musculoskeletal pain disorders of non-inflammatory origin in childhood have been recognized for a many decades now. 'Growing pains' or benign paroxysmal nocturnal leg pains, have been described from early last century, and are said to occur in upto 20 per cent of school children (Peterson 1986). Report of ongoing non-traumatic musculoskeletal pain in childhood is said to occur in up to 30 per cent of children surveyed in the non-clinic setting (Goodman and McGrath 1991) as well as between 1 and 2 per cent of all paediatric accident and emergency attendances (Allen 1993). It was Apley (1976) who first drew attention to these conditions in childhood, linking them with non-organic abdominal pain and headaches. At the same time the first desciptions of reflex sympathetic dystrophy (RSD) in children were being reported.

With the development of paediatric rheumatology as a sub-specialty larger populations of such patients were recognized and common patterns of presentation, and approach to treatment began to be described (Sherry and Weisman 1988; Malleson et al. 1992). While most conditions have their reflection in similar disorders in the adult population, unique issues arise when they occur in childhood and adolescence. Involvement of the family in the diagnostic and therapeutic process is integral, and treatment of the child may mandate treatment of family members (usually a parent) before major progress can be made. While conditions such as Munchausens syndrome (by proxy) are rare, they point to the often critical expression of parental influences in their dependant offspring. This may be as either as a primary or perpetuating factor.

Conceptual developments in pain research have aided the understanding and treatment of chronic pain disorders of childhood. The International Association for the Study of Pain has defined pain as 'An unpleasant sensory and emotional experience associated with actual or potential tissue damage, or described in terms of such damage'. They go further to distinguish pain from physiological activity in the nocioceptor or related neurones induced by a noxious stimulus. The former being an emotional state and the latter a neurological process, which may or may not be accompanied by the subjective perceptual phenomenon we know as pain. This allows departure from the dualistic philosophy of pain being either organic or psychogenic in origin.

Specific chronic pain syndromes

Grouping patients into individual categories is recognized as relatively arbitrary, but felt to be useful to develop management strategies, and certainly favoured when sharing information with patients and families.

Reflex sympathetic dystrophy

The term RSD is used in preference here, to localized idiopathic pain syndrome, or chronic regional pain syndrome type I (CRPS I). This reflects that it remains the most recognized descriptive term still in widespread usage. Controversy exists regarding the pathogenesis of RSD with many authors feeling abnormalities or the sympathetic nervous system have no primary aetiological role, and evidence of true 'reflexive' mechanisms is lacking (Ochoa 1999). This disagreement leads to the use of various terms such as algo-(neuro)-dystrophy and causalgia, or terms such as localized idiopathic pain syndrome (Malleson et al. 1992). Development of the term CRPS to some degree reflects this also (Stanton-Hicks et al. 1995).

Diagnosis

Discrete reports of RSD in childhood date from the 1970s onward, though it seems likely the condition has existed perhaps unrecognized for much longer. Early reports appeared to indicate the extreme rarity of this condition but more recent case series tell us it is a considerable fraction of the case-load of paediatric rheumatology and orthopaedic centres (Wilder et al. 1992; Stanton et al. 1993; Sherry 1999; Murray et al. 2000).

The criteria used to classify or diagnose RSD in childhood are similar to those in adults whilst recognizing that the features are more variable, and modifications are often employed. Table 1 lists the commonly used criteria for diagnosis emphasizing the presence of chronic spontaneous pain associated with dysfunction of the limb and variable presence of autonomic signs.

No accurate estimates exist of the incidence or prevalence of RSD in childhood. This is not surprising given the difficulty of case definition, referral of patients to multiple sub-specialities, and relatively poor recognition at the primary care level. In general, CPS represents approximately upto 10–15 per cent of new referrals to paediatric rheumatology units (Cicuttini and Littlejohn 1989; Gedalia et al. 2000).

RSD has virtually never been reported before 5 years of age, and is reported with increasing frequency into teenage years. Such estimates are

Table 1 Criteria for diagnosis of RSD (chronic regional pain syndrome I)

1. The presence of an initiating noxious event, or a cause of immobilization
2. Continuing pain allodynia or hyperalgesia with which the pain is disproportionate to any inciting event
3. Evidence at some time of oedema, changes in skin blood flow, or abnormal sudomotor activity in the region of the pain
4. This diagnosis is excluded by the presence of conditions that would otherwise account for the degree of pain and dysfunction

Note: Criteria 2–4 must be satisfied.

Source: Sherry (1999).

inherently biased as most reports come from defined paediatric rheumatology or orthopaedic units, where adolescents from 14 years onwards are often referred to adult units. Thus, the peak age of onset quoted between 10 and 13 years of age in most reports probably does not wane but may well continue at that level at least into early adult years.

Clinical features

The usual presentation of RSD is of a previously physically well child, who reports after some minor trauma that the limb becomes painful, worse with use and weight bearing, and there is a rapid loss of function. Dysaesthesia then supervenes with the pain occurring spontaneously, often changing in character to a continuous 'burning, stabbing, or stinging' sensation. Light touch is felt intensely (hyperaesthesia) and usually produces the experience of pain (allodynia). Some patients report that even the sensation of a breeze is intensely discomforting. Sensory abnormalities can also include hypoaesthesia (tactile stimuli) and hypothermaesthesia (thermal stimuli) in some individuals. At this stage most will have been seen by a medical practitioner and, if appropriate therapy is not instituted, or in relatively unresponsive cases, progression of the signs may occur. This includes colour changes in the affected limb usually dusky or cyanotic in appearance. The so-called erythematous (early) phase reported in adults is rarely reported in children. Often the limb or area will be cool to touch, compared with the contralateral side or limb. Hyperhidrosis occurs in some cases but not nearly as frequently as reported in adults. These colour and temperature changes are often worse when the limb is held dependent or after immersion in water. Mild to moderate diffuse oedema of the affected area is often appreciated at this time. Effectively the limb behaves at this stage as a pseudo-paralysis marked reduction of spontaneous movement. Considerable variability in many of these manifestations can be seen day-to-day in patients. With chronicity it is recognized potentially irreversible tissue damage occurs with atrophic changes such as hair loss or hypertrichosis, altered nail growth, subcutaneous and muscle tissue atrophy, contracture formation, and eventually loss of limb growth, and osteopaenia with fracture risk. These latter changes are much less common in childhood as compared to adults possibly related to the overall better prognosis of the condition in young people (Kavanagh et al. 1995). Most studies report a relative predominance of females being diagnosed with this condition (Table 2), the ratio of male to female being on average about 4–5 : 1.

A number of reports allude to three separate phases of the condition existing possibly along a spectrum with pain, warmth of the area and minimal vasomotor/sympathetic changes initially (2–3 months). Subsequently more profound temperature changes and colour changes along with increased severity of pain (3–6 months) and finally an atrophic cold phase with permanent tissue damage occurs. Others have debated the existence of such a separation and feel that separate sub-types may exist explaining the variability (Veldman et al. 1993; Bruehl et al. 2002). Most childhood onset cases of RSD start with a 'cold' extremity (Bernstein et al. 1978; Goldsmith et al. 1989). As illustrated in Table 2, lower limb involvement predominates in most childhood series, as compared to adult series where upper and lower limb involvement is relatively equal (Veldman et al. 1993). The distal part of the extremity is often involved in a 'glove or stocking' distribution but localization to the knee or elbow and adjacent soft tissues can be seen as well as occasional hip or hindquarter involvement. In a number of patients, the whole of the limb can be affected. Rarely two limbs or areas can be affected at once (see Plate 180), but certainly multiple sites may be affected over time, or there is recurrence in the same site. This recurrence of RSD seems more frequent in younger patients (Veldman and Goris 1996). In many patients, physical symptoms from other body areas are reported (Sherry et al. 1991). RSD can also occur at the site of active or previous pathology or rheumatic disease, such as with coexisting inflammatory arthritis.

Investigations

There are no specific diagnostic tests for RSD, and it remains largely a clinical diagnosis. Investigations have often been performed when the diagnosis is uncertain, but none are particularly useful or necessary to establish the diagnosis. Laboratory parameters are usually normal including acute phase reactants such as ESR, CRP, and blood counts. Antinuclear antibodies have been seen in some but usually of low titre and perhaps no more frequent than is seen coincidentally in any childhood or clinic population. Initial plain radiographs are usually normal, unless showing minor evidence of some previous trauma. In the author's experience a number of patients are referred with reports of abnormal radiographs, which on further review usually reveal normal variants in developing musculoskeletal system that may have been misinterpreted as 'possible' osteochondritis, stress fracture, or even infection. With time or chronicity some radiographs can show osteopaenia, which is perhaps not unexpected considering the disuse associated with RSD. Interestingly nucleotide bone scans when done are often abnormal in established RSD, but in contrast to most adult series they usually show reduced uptake in the blood and bone phases in children (Laxer et al. 1985; Goldsmith et al. 1989). This is not absolute and occasional reports of increased uptake have been published (Silber and Majd 1988). Thermography has been reported to be of use in one study in children with reduced skin temperature in RSD limbs, but it is doubtful whether it contributes much more than good clinical examination, though it may help delineate the total area involved and demonstrate its improvement over time (Lightman et al. 1987).

Table 2 Published case series (10 or more patients) of RSD/chronic regional pain syndrome type I with onset in childhood

Study/author (year of publication)	No. of patients (episodes)	Sex ratio (F : M)	Mean age at onset (range)	Limb/body areas (LE : UE)
Bernstein et al. (1978)	23 (24)	18 : 5	12.4 (9–16)	20 : 4
Laxer et al. (1985)	11 (15)	6 : 5	11.4 (9.4–17.2)[a]	10 : 5
Kesler et al. (1988)	10	9 : 1	12.9 (8–18)	5 : 5
Silber and Majd (1988)	18	11 : 7	14 (9–19)[a]	11 : 7
Goldsmith et al. (1989)	15	12 : 3	11.6 (9–18)[a]	12 : 3
Wesdock et al. (1991)	36 (49)	24 : 12	13.4	30 : 10
Malleson et al. (1992)	41[b]	38 : 3	10.8 (9–15)	30 : 11
Wilder et al. (1992)	70	59 : 11	12.5	61 : 9
Barbieri (1999)	10	9 : 1	11 (5–16)	N/R
Sherry (1999)	103	87 : 16	13.0	83 : 11
Murray et al. (2000)	46	35 : 11	12.0[c] (8–15.2)	31 : 15

[a] Age at diagnosis.

[b] Only 24/41 patients fulfilled all criteria for RSD.

[c] Median age at diagnosis.

Note: LE, lower; and UE, upper extremity.

Pathogenesis

While there is clear evidence of altered activity of various components of the peripheral nervous system, evidence for direct or aetiological involvement of the sympathetic components is weak at best (Ochoa 1999). Vasomotor changes are well described, but these are also seen in other conditions of immobility in childhood, such as cerebral palsy, and neuro-degenerative disorders, though not usually associated with pain. Similarly direct involvement of the sympathetic nervous system in the pain is lacking (Ochoa 1999). Few biopsy studies are reported, with no pathognomonic changes seen. Some argue, as did Sudeck, that RSD may represent an aggravated inflammatory response to minor trauma (Veldman et al. 1993) but most consider tissue changes secondary to immobilization or other idiopathic events.

Psychological studies of children with RSD reveal high levels of distress during episodes, and there is evidence that psychological factors may play an aetiological role (Sherry and Weisman 1988; Sherry et al. 1991; Malleson et al. 1992). Patient profiles have not been as well studied in children as they have in adults, but evidence indicates that inherent coping strategies influence either the occurrence of RSD, or the chronicity and perhaps response to treatment (see below). From a practical point of view the patient population varies greatly on the degree of the symptomatology, physical findings, and the level of psychological distress or psychosocial disorder within the families. Inherent in this is, however, an implication that investigation or documentation of family structure and current issues is mandatory when treating children with RSD or any similar chronic condition. A number of studies have demonstrated the existence of chronic pain models in the family, including close relatives with RSD-like conditions, physical injury, disease affecting a limb (Sherry et al. 1991; Malleson et al. 1992), or a high level of chronic ill health (including psychiatric) in family members. Prior emotional, physical, and sexual abuse of some RSD patients has been reported but not uniformly (Sherry et al. 1991; Wesdock et al. 1991). Interestingly, in studies of adults with CPS (especially fibromyalgia, or FM) increased frequency of such abuse in childhood has been reported (Alexander et al. 1998).

No single or specific aetiological explanation has been elucidated for RSD. It seems the patient group is a heterogeneous one, and the condition in a sense blurs the lines between what might be considered abnormal physiology (and perhaps psychology) as a response to immobility and the development of visible permanent pathology or damage. No specific genetic studies have been done in RSD in childhood, but RSD has been reported along with conversion disorder at the same time in both of identical twin siblings (Jaworowski et al. 1998). No true multiplex family studies have been reported. The predisposition appears complex, with both inherent physical and psychological factors, and shared environment, rather than any specific Mendelian inheritance. Physical predispositions include levels of physical fitness, inherent pain threshold, and at least one report suggests underlying hypermobility and ligamentous laxity in a substantial number of cases (Francis et al. 1987).

Management

Making the diagnosis, and explaining the underlying mechanism or nature of the condition to families, is perhaps as important as any future therapeutic endeavour. Considerable time is required to engage with these families, who have often seen a large number of both medical and allied health professionals. Many of them have sensed an implication that the symptoms are factitious in nature or 'all in my child's head'. Detailed age appropriate explanation of the interdependency of physical and psychological features in RSD is useful.

Attitudes or management styles from health professionals are felt to be potential iatrogenic contributors to the maintenance of CPS in both children and adults. It is likely that health professionals unwittingly contribute to chronicity and pathology in various ways. Examples of this are giving in to pressure to perform unnecessary investigations, prescribing medications of doubtful value, or adherence to short-term cure type strategies rather than chronic pain models with focus on functional goals and self-management.

Many smaller studies quote the use of specific modalities (such as TENS machines), and techniques such as regional anaesthetic or sympathetic blocks (ganglion or epidural space), in children with RSD, though none of them have been randomized or blinded studies (Lloyd-Thomas and Lauder 1995; Kesler et al. 1998). The use of such techniques is possibly more common in clinics supported by specific pain services (Chalkiadis 2001) or orthopaedic surgical services, which may tend to be more interventional. Similarly the use of medications including NSAIDs, analgesics (both narcotic and non-narcotic), antidepressants, antiepileptics, ('antineurogenic'), and vasodilators have all been quoted as useful in uncontrolled studies. Similarly, use of bisphosphonates has been reported in uncontrolled case series of adult patients with RSD (and anecdotal reports in children) based upon the premise that the osteopaenia may be in some way linked to ongoing pain (Cortet et al. 1997).

The larger series of paediatric RSD patients report successful outcome with minimal use of such agents. Where clinical depression exists unequivocally it makes sense to consider appropriate use of antidepressants, with the support of a psychiatrist if possible. Low doses of antidepressant-type medicines, such as amitryptyline, may be useful where sleep disturbance is significant. There appears to be little benefit in pursuing the use of multiple medications or changes in medications in an effort to ablate pain before any other treatment is undertaken.

Virtually all reports emphasize the effectiveness of physical therapies in treatment of RSD in children. The physical therapies reported to be useful are directed towards remobilization and desensitization of the affected limb. In children hydrotherapy is often used as an initial treatment because of the potential ability to gain movement more easily with buoyancy as well as the 'play' or game aspects which can be introduced for children who are fearful of moving the limb. Dry land stretching movements both passive and active are pursued at the same time as well as well as involvement in functional tasks, and aerobic exercise training. Desensitization can take many forms including towel rubbing, textured fabric rubs and hot and cold contrast baths, deep tissue massage, and progression to children engaging in their own sensitization techniques. Focussing on functional tasks including taking shoes and socks on and off or playing football games are often very useful. Involvement of an occupational or similar therapist in guiding such treatment is very useful (Oerlermans et al. 2000).

One particular group reported success with large numbers of RSD patients and advocated intensive daily (5–6 h) therapy for all children for up to 2 weeks as the initial treatment period (Sherry et al. 1999). In this cohort, a 92 per cent success rate was reported with 88 per cent remaining symptom free for upto 2 years after the initial episode. In this group, the majority also had a full psychological assessment and referral for specific counselling for pain management in all, and family or cognitive behavioural therapy in many.

Outcome

The majority of reports emphasize the relatively good prognosis of RSD in childhood, with between 75 and 95 per cent of episodes resolving in most series. The length of time to recovery is quite variable ranging from weeks to months and even years, with the rare patient appearing to enter an irreversible chronic phase. The length of time or 'delay' to diagnosis seems important in prognosis. Recurrence can occur in the same limb or area in up to 10–45 per cent of cases in different studies (Tong and Nelson 2000).

It seems likely that use of specific medications or procedures in the absence of multidisciplinary team input as described is associated with a poorer outcome and that the use of invasive procedure should be restricted to particularly resistant cases to provide a possible window of opportunity for 'hands on' input. Emphasis should be on functional rehabilitation and self management where responsibility lies with the child and family for progress through the physiotherapeutic algorithm, as has been emphasized by a recent consensus report (Stanton-Hicks et al. 1998).

Fibromyalgia

Much like RSD the use of the term or the existence of the condition fibromyalgia (FM) as a discrete medical entity has been recently challenged. There is great variation in the frequency with which this diagnosis is made and many authors prefer use of the more inclusive, but less specific term 'chronic widespread pain'. This allows for inclusion of patients who do not completely satisfy the classification criteria for FM. This may be particularly relevant for adolescents or children with FM-like conditions who fail to have as many definable tender points, for example, and lower rates of sleep disturbance. In the United Kingdom, in particular, and other parts of Europe, the terms myalgic encephalomyelitis (ME) (and chronic fatigue syndrome) have been used to describe what appears to be overlapping groups of patients (Buskila 2001). There is now an increase in frequency of diagnosis or use of the term FM in apparent parallel to a fall in the numbers being diagnosed with ME. Similar overlaps appear to exist between FM and chronic fatigue syndrome. Many authors support the concept that such diagnoses or categorization are influenced by cultural expression or expectations which perhaps provides a mould into which CPS express themselves. Malleson and others (1992) prefer the term diffuse idiopathic pain syndrome to encompass this group of patients, recognizing the inherent variability in modes of presentation in childhood and adolescence. This approach to such clinical grouping is illustrated in Table 3.

A definable group of patients does exist with onset under 16 years who suffer chronic widespread soft tissue or musculoskeletal pain, with variable amounts of non-restorative sleep, fatigue, tender points, and other associated symptoms, with relatively high levels of disability. The usual classification criteria used to establish the formal diagnosis of juvenile fibromyalgia (JFM) are listed in Table 4 (Yunus and Masi 1985).

The incidence and prevalence of FM with onset under 16 years is uncertain, but a number of studies have recently approached this question in various ways. Several studies report the caseload burden in paediatric rheumatology clinics, varying from 10 to 30 per cent of diagnoses made (Cicuttini and Littlejohn 1989; Siegel et al. 1998; Gedalia et al. 2000). Several population studies looked at the prevalence of JFM. Buskila et al. (1993) found a prevalence of 6.2 per cent in 3338 schoolchildren in the United States, Mikkelsson (1999), widespread pain in 7.5 per cent of 1756 Finnish school students, only 1.3 per cent of the total student group satisfying criteria for JFM. Clark et al. (1998) found a frequency of 1.2 per cent in 548 Mexican children, and Sardini et al. (1996) in 1.2 per cent of 2408 Italian students, of JFM. The onset age ranged from 8 to 16 years, the majority being 11–12 years or older at diagnosis (Yunus and Masi 1985; Malleson et al. 1992; Gedalia et al. 2000). The average onset of symptoms however may be up to 1–2 years earlier (Table 5).

Clinical features

Table 4 lists criteria commonly used to diagnose JFM. Pain occurs spontaneously in the soft tissues, muscles, or joints, and is exacerbated by physical activity. Daytime fatigue is prominent and progressive disturbance of sleep pattern occurs. This includes difficulty getting off to sleep, as well as a perception of sleep disturbed by pain (though not always corroborated by parent report). Difficulty or symptomatic complaints upon rising from sleep is also common. This may be due to a combination of hypersomnolence (after non-restorative sleep), pain avoidance behaviour, and even school avoidance. The last is a common issue in children with pain syndromes in general, and in some cases the child may have lost up to between 6 and 12 months of schooling prior to referral to specialist units. Periodic limb movements in sleep were significantly increased in JFM, and associated with prolonged sleep latency, shortened total sleep time, increased wakefulness (Tayag-Kier et al. 2000). Parents (usually the mother) have become involved in the illness process and express high levels of anxiety or distress regarding the child's condition, and may often appear to be enmeshed. This parent or other close family member may suffer from a CPS or other medical disability themselves.

Physical examination is variable, but evidence of poor physical conditioning, lowered muscle tone or mass with generalized tenderness or tender points being typical. During the examination many children protest strongly at the discomfort induced but are quite distractible from this. This is in contrast to the appearance on history taking where the patient may have an almost '*la belle* indifference' whilst expressing ongoing pain levels of an extreme nature. Many have very poor endurance and overall fitness levels when full physiotherapy led assessments are made, and some may have hypermobility.

Pathogenesis

No single definable or specific aetiology of this condition has been elucidated in children much as for adults. There is a familial predisposition, with mother/daughter pairs in particular being seen (Buskila et al. 1996; Roizenblatt et al. 1997) with actual FM diagnosis or sleep patterns. A study of 11-year-old Finnish twins indicated that approximately 10 per cent had widespread chronic pain, and the majority concordant for pain, were non-identical (Mikkelsson et al. 2001). The majority of liability to chronic widespread pain was deemed due to environmental factors in this study.

Many studies have been performed in adult groups of patients attempting to show a unifying basis for this disorder, none of which has specifically included paediatric onset patients. Two somewhat polarized groups argue as to whether FM has an as yet undefined biological basis, or whether it is predominantly a psychosomatic or somatization type of disorder

Table 3 Classification of amplified or idiopathic pain syndromes according to Malleson et al. (1992)

Syndrome classification	Criteria
Diffuse idiopathic pain syndromes With tender points Without tender points	1. Pain present in at least three areas of the body for at least 3 months and no identifiable physical cause 2. Exclusion of disorders that would reasonably explain the symptoms Both 1 and 2 must be satisfied
Localized idiopathic pain syndromes With overt autonomic signs Without overt autonomic signs	1. Pain localizing to one limb persisting (a) One week with medically directed treatment or (b) One month without medically directed treatment 2. Absence of prior trauma that could reasonably explain the symptoms 3. Exclusion of diseases that could reasonably explain the pain Criteria for classification require all 3

Table 4 Criteria for the diagnosis of juvenile fibromyalgia syndrome

Musculoskeletal aching at three or more sites for 3 or more months in the absence of an underlying condition plus
Five or more tender points
Upper border of trapezius
Lower part of sterno-cleido-mastoid
Lateral part of pectoralis major
Mid-supraspinatus
Lateral aspect of elbow
Upper outer quadrant of gluteal region
Greater trochanter
Medial fat pad of the knee
Three or more of the following
Chronic anxiety or tension
Fatigue
Poor sleep
Chronic headache
Irritable bowel
Subjective soft-tissue swelling
Numbness
Pain modulation by physical activity
Pain modulation by weather
Pain modulation by anxiety and stress

Source: Yunus and Masi (1985) with permission.

Table 5 Published case series (more than 10 patients) of fibromyalgia/widespread chronic pain

Author	No. of patients	Sex distribution	Mean age of diagnosis	Mean age at onset (range)	Outcome
Yunus et al. (1985)	33	31:2	14.7	11.7	18.8 (average) months F/U: generally improved; 5% mild, 45% moderate, 50% severe symptoms
Romano (1991)	15	10:5	13	N/R	N/R
Malleson et al. (1992)	35 (40)[a]	39:1	N/R	11.5	N/R
Buskila et al. (1995)	21	14:7	N/R		30 months F/U (15/22 patients): 27% still had full JFM
Roizenblatt et al. (1997)	34	22:12	10.9	8.9	N/R
Flato et al. (1997)	26	21:5	N/R	9.7	9 years F/U (15/26 patients): generalized pain in 4, localized pain in 4, 7 no pain
Siegel et al. (1998)	45	41:4	N/R	9.8	2–3 years F/U: most improved, reduction of 4.8/10 on severity scale
Schanberg et al. (1998)	21	18:3	N/R	N/R	N/R
Mikkelsson (1999)	20	19:3	10.8	N/R	1 year F/U: (16/22 patients) 25% had persistent FM
Gedalia et al. (2000)	59	47:12	15.5	13.7	1 year F/U: (50/59 patients) 60% had improved, 36% unchanged 4% worse

[a] Defined as diffuse idiopathic pain syndrome in this study with 35 fulfilling criteria for JFM.

Note: N/R = not reported.

(Breau et al. 1999; McBeth et al. 2001). Most likely it is mutifactorial in origin encompassing inherent or physiological risk factors, with contibuting psychological and family predisposing factors. Some studies show strong evidence of psychological and psychosocial factors either in the causation or at least perpetuation of symptoms (Vandvik and Forseth 1994; Aasland et al. 1997; Mikkelsson 1997, 1999). Family environment and parental pain factors have been felt to be important in how children coped with JFM in one major study (Schanberg et al. 1996, 1998). In another study disability among children with FM was felt to be a function of the children's psychological adjustment and physical state, and of the parents' physical state and method of coping with pain rather, than primarily a psychogenic condition (Reid et al. 1997).

Treatment

Intensive treatment regimes are favoured, either outpatient or inpatient based. Physiotherapy, occupational therapy, and psychology input as part of a multidisciplinary team provides the most successful approach. Improvement in sleep patterns by behavioural means or use of low doses of antidepressant type medications may be helpful (Siegel et al. 1998). Graduated approaches to improved fitness with focus on functional tasks of relevance to home and school are important. OT assessment is important in planning graded reintroduction to those environments. Cognitive behavioural therapy is used in some institutions with success in JFM (Walco and Ilowite 1992; Brown et al. 2001). Other elements may include distraction therapy, relaxation therapy, guided imagery, and art therapy, much as with RSD.

Outcome

Most evidence indicates that the outcome of JFM patients is probably better than that of their adult FM counterparts (see Table 5), and some even appear 'cured' in short- to medium-term follow-up. Though considerably improved symptomatically, many still have considerable levels of pain and dysfunction at follow-up.

Hypermobility and chronic pain

Ligamentous laxity or 'benign joint hypermobility' (BJH) is associated with arthralgias or musculoskeletal pain, and other disorders in a 'significant' number of young people (Hudson et al. 1998; Grahame 2000; Murray and Woo 2001). Individuals with BJH appear prone to recurrent sprain/strain type injuries, and have or develop relative muscle weakness (at least of those muscle groups supporting joints) and impaired proprioception. Subsequent loss of function and inactivity or loss of physical conditioning appears to predispose to further injury, and possibly lowered pain thresholds, leading to a chronic pain cycle in some. Not all children with hypermobility develop chronic pain, but they appear to be at some risk of developing an FM-like pain disorder (Gedalia et al. 1993). The aetiology is likely to be multifactorial based upon the severity of the ligamentous laxity (often accompanied by easy bruising and overly elastic skin), other inherent personal factors (including pain threshold), or factors such as chronic pain models in the family. One study of Finnish schoolchildren, however, failed to find a specific association between hypermobility and musculoskeletal pain in pre-adolescents (Mikkelsson et al. 1996). Treatment usually focuses on strengthening core trunk muscles and muscles that stabilize joints, with the approach used for rehabilitation in markedly disabled children, similar to that used for CPS.

Auto-erythrocyte sensitization disorder (psychogenic purpura)

This rare disorder, also known as Diamond Gardner syndrome has been reported in children (Campbell et al. 1983; Sorensen et al. 1985). It presents as gradual onset of painful swelling and bruising of a limb or body area in response to minor trauma. This becomes more severe over days with larger tissue areas involved far beyond the anatomical area of injury, associated with marked loss of function. Severe disability may occur for weeks to months but physical recovery from each episode is usually complete. Multiple areas of the body may be involved and recurrences may occur over years. Interestingly, subcutaneous injection of the person's red blood cells can incite lesions to occur in areas visible to the patient, with some evidence of immune sensitization to red cell constituents. Major psychosocial or traumatic events are reported as common antecedents, and psychosocial interventions are an essential part of therapy, along with physical rehabilitation much as for RSD.

Back pain

Upto 40 per cent of schoolchildren report recent musculoskeletal pain on epidemiological questionnaire-based surveys, and a smaller number report it on a recurrent basis, including back pain (Wedderkopp et al. 2001; Widhe 2001). Reports of back pain may be developmentally related with the frequency increasing from 7 per cent in early childhood to more than 50 per cent by the third decade of life (LeBouef-Yde and Kyvik 1998). Persistent severe back pain should be assessed promptly in young children because serious organic causes such as infection and malignancy are more frequent than in adult cohorts. Structural abnormalities of the spine and osteochondritides (such as Scheurmanns disease) can be a source of chronic or recurrent back pain, as can be juvenile ankylosing spondylitis and other inflammatory disorders.

Some children, particularly adolescents, present with chronic back pain where no obvious rheumatic or structural organic cause is evident. In a number of these 'BJH' or ligamentous can be identified. There is usually a history of remarkable spinal mobility for much of childhood (e.g. being able to place hands flat on the floor with forward bending). Such patients often have a moderate hyperlordosis and increased thoracic curvature, giving the typical 'round shouldered posture'. In some individuals excessive weight gain may be a precipitant of the chronic pain. Back pain is felt to be due to recurrent sprain/strain injuries and may be localized to one spinal segment. Occasionally, spondylolysis/listhesis is seen. Whether this represents a true antecedent to adult chronic back pain, is unknown but if such a physiological predisposition does exist then preventative strategies in childhood may well affect the outcome of a major public health problem in the adult years (Smedbraten et al. 1998). Interestingly reports of back pain in a group of Swiss schoolchildren indicated strong familial tendencies and association with psychological factors, indicating again potential overlap with CPS in children (Balague et al. 1995).

Chronic fatigue syndrome

Chronic fatigue syndrome (CFS) is discussed in brief because of its relationship to CPS. From the descriptions of young patients, they have much in common with CPS (Bell et al. 1994; Breau et al. 1999; Buskila 2001). Pain is a frequent complaint in those with CFS, and fatigue is a major issue in generalized forms of CPS. Preceding viral type infections are often regarded as precipitants of CFS and it is well recognized that in many CPS patients (particularly adolescents) that such illness are associated with flares in symptomatology and deterioration in functional level. In both groups non-restorative or poor quality sleep is seen, and is felt to be a major factor driving symptomatology, and treatment of this improves the outcome of patient directly. Similarly the psychological profile of the patient groups share many characteristics.

As to whether a patient ends up being diagnosed with CFS or a CPS (such as FM) may depend much upon the specialty to which the patient is referred, and which symptomatology is considered by the patient, family, or health professionals as most important.

Myalgic encephalomyelitis

Again this condition will not be described in detail as it is an infrequent diagnosis made in paediatric rheumatology practice. As described, ME comprises a patient population who develop a constellation of chronic symptoms (often after a viral infection), comprising muscle pain, severe headaches, subjective CNS dysfunction symptoms, sleep disturbance, and usually profound fatigue. Clearly, it has much in common with CFS, and has been a term in relatively common usage in European centres, but uncommonly used in North American literature at least. High levels of dysfunction are experienced with individuals often unable to attend school, participate in physical activities such as sports, and often becoming socially withdrawn. Non-restorative sleep and psychosocial issues are felt by many to be key factors much as with CFS and CPS. Epidemiological studies suggest it is not uncommon for ME to have its onset in childhood, and that the symptom complex is similar to adults though perhaps with a better overall outcome.

Somatization and the somatoform pain disorder

This phenomenon or disorder relates to the concept of a patient who experiences and communicates emotional distress or arousal primarily in the form of physical symptoms. As a disorder defined by Diagnostic and Statistical Manual of Mental Disorders (DSM-IV) this condition requires the presence of a history of complaints (of pain in this context) in multiple organ systems or body areas with no observable organic cause or disporortionate to the physical findings, together with a preoccupation with the symptoms for at least 6 months. Many have recognized that the phenomenon or process of somatization may be an element of some, if not most, CPS patients (McBeth et al. 2001), but that it is not pathognomonic and may be present in patients suffering from a pain producing organic pathology. In this latter case, the patient is likely to exhibit more conspicuous pain behaviour and disability than the tissue damage would warrant. In a similar way, others have argued that CPS in childhood have much overlap in clinical characteristics and management of the conversion disorders (Brazier and Venning 1997).

Differential diagnosis

There are important differential diagnoses to be considered in patients who present with either localized or widespread pain disorders. Detailed history taking and examination will help to exclude most. Infections which may mimic a generalized CPS include viral infections such as Epstein–Barr virus (infectious mononucleosis) which may produce a prolonged illness with musculoskeletal pain and fatigue in some teenagers. Lyme disease has been reported to be associated with widespread influenza like symptoms and joint complaints which can be persistent in some patients. History of the typical rash and evidence of frank arthritis associated with specific positive serology usually helps to identify the correct diagnosis. So does knowledge of whether patients have resided in a risk area where there is the tick and spirochaete. Some patients may have been mislabelled chronic Lyme disease when they present with atypical symptoms and non-specific positive serology, and others may subsequently develop a CPS after the original infection been treated (Sigal and Patella 1992).

Occult malignancy in childhood can masquerade as either widespread or localized pain disorders. Neuroblastomas, lymphomas, and leukaemia can all present with chronic musculoskeletal pain. Usually true bony tenderness, evidence of weight loss, and abnormalities of laboratory parameters point to the diagnosis, but investigations such as bone scan may be useful to help make the diagnosis. Occasional benign bone tumours such as osteoid osteoma can masquerade as localized pain syndromes. The presence of night pain which, with exquisite sensitivity to NSAIDs, helps define the disorder along with diagnostic imaging. Occasionally endocrine disorders may present with widespread chronic pain in childhood, including hyper- or hypothyroidism, hyperparathyroidism, and vitamin D resistant and deficient rickets. Appropriate radiology and biochemical studies usually help to make these diagnoses.

Conclusions

All of the conditions discussed here have many management strategies in common. Establishment of the specific diagnosis allowing initiation of a definitive treatment plan is essential. When the diagnosis is expressed with confidence by the caring physician, the family are far more likely to engage with the therapeutic programme. Critical to the process is agreement that further medical investigations are inappropriate, to allow full engagement with the intense multidisciplinary programme which is required.

Detailed assessment by a physiotherapist and occupational therapist may reveal valuable clues as to the complex issues occurring in such patient and families. A full psychological assessment is valuable to identify specific issues which may be playing either an aetiological role or a perpetuating role in the pain and disability. Careful explanation of the integral role of the psychologist in the team approach for all patients as a routine often makes this more acceptable.

An intense period of rehabilitation is required for most patients particularly if family dynamics are considered to be detrimental to progress, such as parental enmeshment. Drug treatment and procedures may be useful in selected cases but are not a substitute for the multidisciplinary team to which most young people will respond if seen early.

References

Aasland, A., Flato, B., and Vandvik, I.H. (1997). Psychosocial factors in children with idiopathic musculoskeletal pain: a prospective, longitudinal study. *Acta Paediatrica* **86**, 740–6.

Alexander, R.W. et al. (1998). Sexual and physical abuse in women with fibromyalgia: association with outpatient health care utilization and pain medication usage. *Arthritis Care and Research* **11**, 102–15.

Allen, R. (1993). Differential diagnosis of arthritis in childhood. *Baillière's Clinical Paediatrics* **1**, 665–94.

Apley, J. (1976). Limb pains with no organic disease. *Clinics in Rheumatic Disease* **2**, 487–91.

Balague, F. et al. (1995). Low back pain in schoolchildren. A study of familial and psychological factors. *Spine* **20**, 1265–70.

Barbier, O., Allington, N., and Rombouts, J.J. (1999). Reflex sympathetic dystrophy in children: review of a clinical series and description of the particularities in children. *Acta Orthopaedica Belgica* **65** (1), 91–7.

Bell, D.S., Bell, K.M., and Cheney, P.R. (1994). Primary juvenile fibromyalgia syndrome and chronic fatigue syndrome in adolescents. *Clinical Infectious Diseases* **18** (Suppl. 1), S21–3.

Bernstein, B.H. et al. (1978). Reflex neurovascular dystrophy in childhood. *Journal of Pediatrics* **93**, 211–15.

Brazier, D.K. and Venning, H.E. (1997). Conversion disorders in adolescents: a practical approach to rehabilitation. *British Journal of Rheumatology* **36**, 594–8.

Breau, L.M., McGrath, P.J., and Ju, L.H. (1999). Review of juvenile primary fibromyalgia and chronic fatigue syndrome. *Journal of Developmental Behavioral Pediatrics* **20**, 278–88.

Brown, G.T. et al. (2001). Juvenile fibromyalgia syndrome: proposed management using a cognitive-behavioral approach. *Physical and Occupational Therapy in Pediatrics* **21**, 19–36.

Bruehl, S. et al. (2002). Complex regional pain syndrome: are there distinct subtypes and sequential stages of the syndrome? *Pain* **95**, 119–24.

Buskila, D. (2001). Fibromyalgia, chronic fatigue syndrome, and myofascial pain syndrome. *Current Opinion in Rheumatology* **13**, 117–27.

Buskila, D. et al. (1993). Assessment of nonarticular tenderness and prevalence of fibromyalgia in children. *Journal of Rheumatology* **20**, 368–70.

Buskila, D. et al. (1995). Fibromyalgia syndrome in children—an outcome study. *Journal of Rheumatology* **22**, 525–8.

Buskila, D. et al. (1996). Familial aggregation in the fibromyalgia syndrome. *Seminars in Arthritis and Rheumatism* **26**, 605–11.

Campbell, A.N., Freedman, M.H., and McClure, P.D. (1983). Autoerythrocyte sensitization. *Journal of Pediatrics* **103**, 157–60.

Chalkiadis, G.A. (2001). Management of chronic pain in children. *Medical Journal of Australia* **175**, 476–9.

Cicuttini, F. and Littlejohn, G.O. (1989). Female adolescent rheumatological presentations: the importance of chronic pain syndromes. *Australian Paediatric Journal* **25**, 21–4.

Clark, P. et al. (1998). Prevalence of fibromyalgia in children: a clinical study of Mexican children. *Journal of Rheumatology* **25**, 2009–14.

Cortet, B. et al. (1997). Treatment of severe, recalcitrant reflex sympathetic dystrophy: assessment of efficacy and safety of the second generation bisphosphonate pamidronate. *Clinical Rheumatology* **16**, 51–6.

Flato, B. et al. (1997). Outcome and predictive factors in children with chronic idiopathic musculoskeletal pain. *Clinical and Experimental Rheumatology* **15**, 569–77.

Francis, H. et al. (1987). Benign joint hypermobility with neuropathy: documentation and mechanism of tarsal tunnel syndrome. *Journal of Rheumatology* **14**, 577–81.

Gedalia, A. et al. (1993). Joint hypermobility and fibromyalgia in schoolchildren. *Annals of the Rheumatic Diseases* **52**, 494–6.

Gedalia, A. et al. (2000). Fibromyalgia syndrome: experience in a pediatric rheumatology clinic. *Clinical and Experimental Rheumatology* **18**, 415–19.

Goldsmith, D.P. et al. (1989). Nuclear imaging and clinical features of childhood reflex neurovascular dystrophy: comparison with adults. *Arthritis and Rheumatism* **32**, 480–5.

Goodman, J.E. and McGrath, P.J. (1991). The epidemiology of pain in children and adolescents: a review. *Pain* **46**, 247–64.

Grahame, R. (2000). Pain, distress and joint hyperlaxity. *Joint Bone Spine* **67**, 157–63.

Hudson, N. et al. (1998). The association of soft-tissue rheumatism and hypermobility. *British Journal of Rheumatology* **37**, 382–6.

Jaworowski, S., Allen, R.C., and Finklestein, E. (1998). Reflex sympathetic dystrophy in a 12 year old twin with comorbid conversion disorder in both twins. *Journal of Paediatrics and Child Health* **34**, 581–3.

Kavanagh, R. et al. (1995). Reflex sympathetic dystrophy in children. Dystrophic changes are less likely. *British Medical Journal* **311** (7018), 1503.

Kesler, R.W. et al. (1988). Reflex sympathetic dystrophy in children: treatment with transcutaneous electric nerve stimulation. *Pediatrics* **82**, 728–32.

Laxer, R.M. et al. (1985). Technetium 99m-methylene diphosphonate bone scans in children with reflex neurovascular dystrophy. *Journal of Pediatrics* **106**, 437–40.

Leboeuf-Yde, C. and Kyvik, K.O. (1998). At what age does low back pain become a common problem? A study of 29 424 individuals aged 12–41 years. *Spine* **23**, 228–34.

Lightman, H.I. et al. (1987). Thermography in childhood reflex sympathetic dystrophy. *Journal of Pediatrics* **111**, 551–5.

Lloyd-Thomas, A.R. and Lauder, G. (1995). Lesson of the week. Reflex sympathetic dystrophy in children. *British Medical Journal* **310** (6995), 1648–9.

Malleson, P.N., al-Matar, M., and Petty, R.E. (1992). Idiopathic musculoskeletal pain syndromes in children. *Journal of Rheumatology* **19**, 1786–9.

Malleson, P.N. et al. (2001). Chronic musculoskeletal and other idiopathic pain syndromes. *Archives of Diseases of Childhood* **84**, 189–92.

McBeth, J. et al. (2001). Features of somatization predict the onset of chronic widespread pain: results of a large population-based study. *Arthritis and Rheumatism* **44**, 940–6.

Mikkelsson, M. (1999). One year outcome of preadolescents with fibromyalgia. *Journal of Rheumatology* **26**, 674–82.

Mikkelsson, M., Salminen, J.J., and Kautiainen, H. (1996). Joint hypermobility is not a contributing factor to musculoskeletal pain in pre-adolescents. *Journal of Rheumatology* **23**, 1963–7.

Mikkelsson, M., Sourander, A., Piha, J., and Salminen, J.J. (1997). Psychiatric symptoms in preadolescents with musculoskeletal pain and fibromyalgia. *Pediatrics* **100**, 220–7.

Mikkelsson, M. et al. (2001). Widespread pain among 11-year-old Finnish twin pairs. *Arthritis and Rheumatism* **44**, 481–5.

Murray, C.S. et al. (2000). Morbidity in reflex sympathetic dystrophy. *Archives of Diseases in Childhood* **82**, 231–3.

Murray, K.J. and Woo, P. (2001). Benign joint hypermobility in childhood. *Rheumatology* **40**, 489–91.

Ochoa, J.L. (1999). Truths, errors, and lies around 'reflex sympathetic dystrophy' and 'complex regional pain syndrome'. *Journal of Neurology* **246**, 875–9.

Oerlemans, H.M. et al. (2000). Adjuvant physical therapy versus occupational therapy in patients with reflex sympathetic dystrophy/complex regional pain syndrome type I. *Archives of Physical Medicine and Rehabilitation* **81**, 49–56.

Peterson, H. (1986). Growing pains. *Pediatric Clinics of North America* **33**, 1365–72.

Reid, G.J., Lang, B.A., and McGrath, P.J. (1997). Primary juvenile fibromyalgia: psychological adjustment, family functioning, coping, and functional disability. *Arthritis and Rheumatism* **40**, 752–60.

Roizenblatt, S. et al. (1997). Juvenile fibromyalgia: clinical and polysomnographic aspects. *Journal of Rheumatology* **24**, 579–85.

Romano, T.J. (1991). Fibromyalgia in children; diagnosis and treatment. *West Virginia Medical Journal* **87**, 112–14.

Sardini, S. et al. (1996). Epidemiological study of a primary fibromyalgia in pediatric age. *Minerva Pediatrics* **48**, 543–50.

Schanberg, L.E. et al. (1996). Pain coping strategies in children with juvenile primary fibromyalgia syndrome: correlation with pain, physical function, and psychological distress. *Arthritis Care and Research* **9**, 89–96.

Schanberg, L.E. et al. (1998). Social context of pain in children with juvenile primary fibromyalgia syndrome: parental pain history and family environment. *Clinical Journal of Pain* **14**, 107–15.

Sherry, D. (1999). Pain syndromes. In *Adolescent Rheumatology* (ed. D.A. Isenberg and J.J. Miller), pp. 197–223. London: Martin-Dunitz.

Sherry, D.D. (2000). Pain syndromes in children. *Current Rheumatology Report* **2**, 337–42.

Sherry, D.D. and Weisman, R. (1988). Psychologic aspects of childhood reflex neurovascular dystrophy. *Pediatrics* **81**, 572–8.

Sherry, D.D. et al. (1991). Psychosomatic musculoskeletal pain in childhood: clinical and psychological analyses of 100 children. *Pediatrics* **88**, 1093–9.

Sherry, D.D. et al. (1999). Short- and long-term outcomes of children with complex regional pain syndrome type I treated with exercise therapy. *Clinical Journal of Pain* **15**, 218–23.

Siegel, D.M., Janeway, D., and Baum, J. (1998). Fibromyalgia syndrome in children and adolescents: clinical features at and status at follow-up. *Pediatrics* **101** (3 Pt 1), 377–82.

Sigal, L.H. and Patella, S.J. (1992). Lyme arthritis as the incorrect diagnosis in pediatric and adolescent fibromyalgia. *Pediatrics* **90**, 523–8.

Silber, T.J. and Majd, M. (1988). Reflex sympathetic dystrophy syndrome in children and adolescents. Report of 18 cases and review of the literature. *American Journal of Diseases of Childhood* **142**, 1325–30.

Smedbraten, B.K. et al. (1998). Self-reported bodily pain in schoolchildren. *Scandinavian Journal of Rheumatology* **27**, 273–6.

Sorensen, R.U., Newman, A.J., and Gordon, E.M. (1985). Psychogenic purpura in adolescent patients. *Clinical Pediatrics* **24**, 700–4.

Stanton, R.P. et al. (1993). Reflex sympathetic dystrophy in children: an orthopedic perspective. *Orthopedics* **16**, 773–9.

Stanton-Hicks, M. et al. (1995). Reflex sympathetic dystrophy: changing concepts and taxonomy. *Pain* **63**, 127–33.

Stanton-Hicks, M. et al. (1998). Complex regional pain syndromes: guidelines for therapy. *Clinical Journal of Pain* **14**, 155–66.

Tayag-Kier, C.E. et al. (2000). Sleep and periodic limb movement in sleep in juvenile fibromyalgia. *Pediatrics* **106**, E70.

Tong, H.C. and Nelson, V.S. (2000). Recurrent and migratory reflex sympathetic dystrophy in children. *Pediatric Rehabilitation* **4**, 87–9.

Vandvik, I.H. and Forseth, K.O. (1994). A bio-psychosocial evaluation of ten adolescents with fibromyalgia. *Acta Paediatrica* **83**, 766–71.

Veldman, P.H. and Goris, R.J. (1996). Multiple reflex sympathetic dystrophy. Which patients are at risk for developing a recurrence of reflex sympathetic dystrophy in the same or another limb? *Pain* **64**, 463–6.

Veldman, P.H. et al. (1993). Signs and symptoms of reflex sympathetic dystrophy: prospective study of 829 patients. *Lancet* **342**, 1012–16.

Walco, G.A. and Ilowite, N.T. (1992). Cognitive-behavioral intervention for juvenile primary fibromyalgia syndrome. *Journal of Rheumatology* **19**, 1617–19.

Wedderkopp, N. et al. (2001). Back pain reporting pattern in a Danish population-based sample of children and adolescents. *Spine* **26** (17), 1879–83.

Wesdock, K.A., Stanton, R.P., and Singsen, B.H. (1991). Reflex sympathetic dystrophy in children. A physical therapy approach. *Arthritis Care and Research* **4**, 32–8.

Widhe, T. (2001). Spine: posture, mobility and pain. A longitudinal study from childhood to adolescence. *European Journal of Spine* **10**, 118–23.

Wilder, R.T. et al. (1992). Reflex sympathetic dystrophy in children. Clinical characteristics and follow-up of seventy patients. *Journal of Bone and Joint Surgery* **74**, 910–19.

Yunus, M.B. and Masi, A.T. (1985). Juvenile primary fibromyalgia syndrome. A clinical study of thirty-three patients and matched normal controls. *Arthritis and Rheumatism* **28**, 138–45.

6.14 Osteoarthritis

Michael Doherty, Adrian Jones, and Tim Cawston

Introduction

Osteoarthritis is the most common disease of synovial joints and a major cause of locomotor pain. It results in a significant public health problem with major resource implications (Badley et al. 1994). It has been estimated that 15 per cent of the UK population who are aged greater than 55 years have symptomatic knee osteoarthritis (McAlindon et al. 1992) (Fig. 1). It is the major indication for joint replacement surgery and as a result has increasingly become a focus for clinical, biochemical, epidemiological, genetic, and pharmacological research. Previously considered a boring 'wear and tear', 'degenerative' disease that must be accepted as the inevitable consequence of trauma and ageing, osteoarthritis is now viewed as a dynamic, essentially reparative process with a marked genetic predisposition. In view of the huge population burden of osteoarthritis, there is massive potential for prevention and health intervention.

Historical perspective

At the turn of the century, pathologists and radiologists differentiated two main categories of chronic arthritis—atrophic and hypertrophic. The former was characterized by synovial inflammation with erosion or atrophy of cartilage and bone; it was subsequently found to encompass several disease entities including rheumatoid arthritis. Hypertrophic arthritis, by contrast, was characterized by more focal cartilage loss, minimal evidence of inflammation, and by hypertrophy of adjacent bone and soft tissues; this group became synonymous with osteoarthritis (Goldthwaite 1904) (Fig. 2). Since associations with ageing and previous joint trauma are readily recognized, this led to ready acceptance of the alternative term 'degenerative joint disease'. With the major rheumatological interest focusing on inflammatory arthropathies, osteoarthritis was often used as a 'non-inflammatory' control disease, or even as a surrogate for normal joint tissue, in clinical and laboratory research. The alternative term 'osteoarthrosis' was often used to emphasize the absence of overt inflammation.

Advances in cartilage biochemistry and the recognition of calcium crystal-associated disease subsets proved important factors in renewing interest in this condition. Although clinical and histological inflammation is not as florid as in rheumatoid arthritis or seronegative spondyloarthropathies, it is an undoubted component in many cases. Thus the term osteoarthritis is now generally preferred.

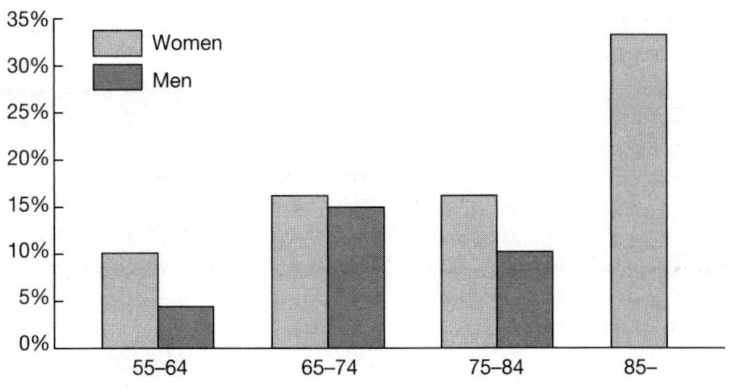

Fig. 1 Prevalence of symptomatic knee osteoarthritis by age group and gender in a UK community population. Derived from McAlindon et al. (1992).

Definition of osteoarthritis

The definition of osteoarthritis depends on the clinical circumstances and the research question being asked. At a clinical level osteoarthritis is characterized by: involvement of synovial joints, cartilage loss (chondropathy), and evidence of accompanying periarticular bone response. All these features are usually detected by radiography.

The drawbacks of this clinical definition both for patient care and research include:

- The difficulty of identifying joints with early, pre-radiographic (initial) change, when studies on aetiopathogenesis and prevention may be most fruitful;

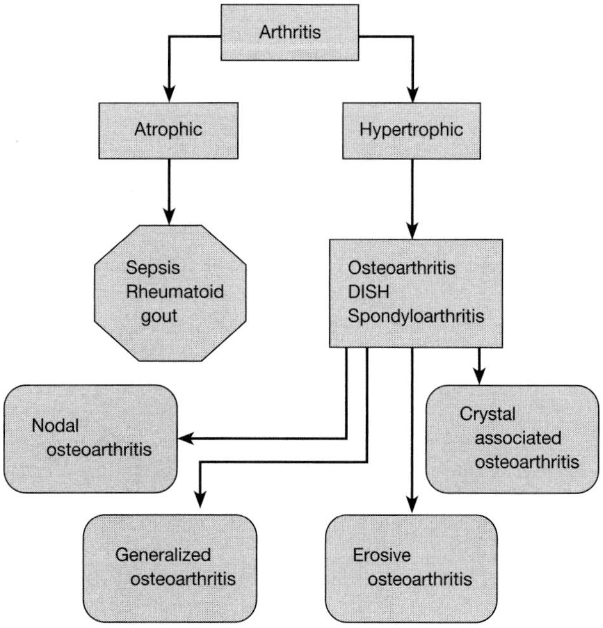

Fig. 2 The increasing differentiation of arthritis subtypes.

- an overemphasis on cartilage and bone even though all joint components (synovium, capsule, entheses, muscle) are involved and may be more amenable to intervention (Fig. 3);
- an emphasis on structure rather than function;
- lack of appreciation of the effects on the whole person.

For the purposes of clinical trial work the American College of Rheumatology has devised criteria for classification of symptomatic osteoarthritis of the knee (Altman et al. 1986) (Fig. 4), hand (Altman et al. 1990), and hip (Altman et al. 1991). These use clinical, laboratory, and/or radiological features and can be applied in various ways using either a traditional checklist approach or a decision making 'tree' format. These criteria are useful in distinguishing osteoarthritis from other painful joint conditions for the purposes of clinical trials but are not diagnostic criteria. They are insensitive for use in epidemiological and genetic studies since they only identify symptomatic rather than structural osteoarthritis.

For population studies a number of definitions have been proposed based on either:

—the association of specific structural features with symptoms (e.g. osteophytosis with knee pain (Spector et al. 1993), joint space narrowing with hip pain (Croft et al. 1990));

—or the association of physical signs with structural (radiographic) features (e.g. restriction of hip range of internal rotation with radiographic joint space narrowing) (Birrell et al. 2001).

The lack of an absolute gold standard means that the definitions must be tailored to the research question. A knee pain questionnaire might be the best way to start to identify a primary care sample of symptomatic knee osteoarthritis whereas a radiographic definition may be more appropriate for a genetic study.

Epidemiology

Current epidemiological data in osteoarthritis is beset by the issues of definition discussed above and histopathological changes are clearly not appropriate for living subjects.

As a result most epidemiological data have relied on a combination of radiographic features and pain for case-definition. Grading or measurement

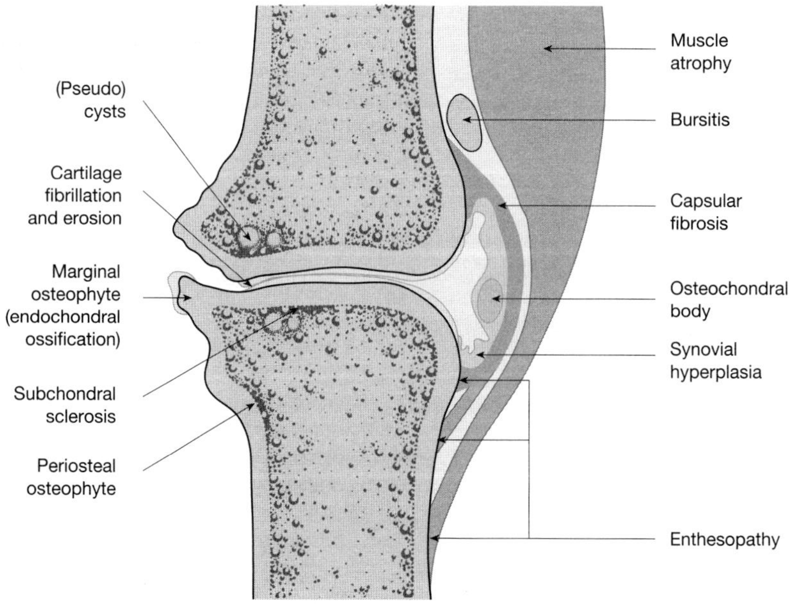

Fig. 3 Joint tissues affected in osteoarthritis. Redrawing from Doherty (ed.). Colour Atlas and Text of Osteoarthritis. Wolfe, London. (Sokoloff 1994.)

of radiological features has also been used to assess 'disease severity'. Of the various radiographic criteria, the most widely employed have been those of Kellgren and Lawrence (1957). Although differing in detail by joint site and by publication, these grade osteoarthritis into four categories depending on the presence and degree of various features (Fig. 5). Although there are problems with this definition it has allowed comparison between data sets.

As a result of these difficulties attempts have been made to:

- improve radiographic imaging by utilizing better defined, more reproducible protocols, multiple views and/or magnification techniques;
- assess individual features of osteoarthritis separately using either atlases or measurement of joint space;

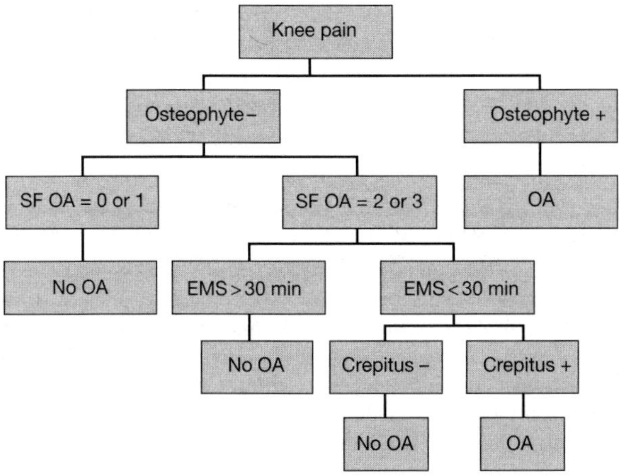

Fig. 4 Decision tree based classification of knee osteoarthritis according to the American College of Rheumatology classification criteria. Derived from Altman et al. (1986).

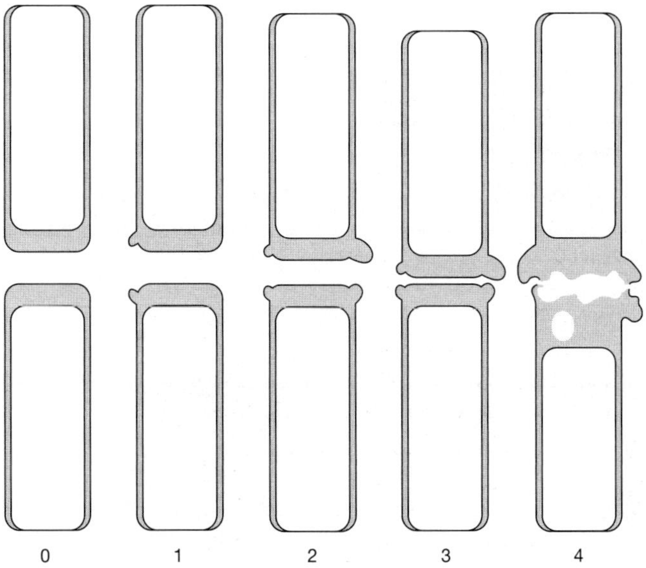

Fig. 5 Basis of Kellgren and Lawrence grading scheme. Grade 0, normal; Grade 1, minimal osteophyte, normal joint space; Grade 2, definite osteophyte, possible joint space narrowing; Grade 3, definite osteophyte and joint space narrowing; Grade 4, definite osteophyte and joint space narrowing with sclerosis and abnormal joint contour.

- concentrate on those features that best seem to define osteoarthritis at a particular site (e.g. osteophyte at the knee, joint space narrowing at the hip).

The radiographic/clinical correlates are tabulated (Table 1).

Clinical definitions of osteoarthritis have also been developed. These rely principally on pain in an at-risk population or on clinical signs such as Heberden's nodes or clinical examination (Claessens et al. 1990; Altman 1991; Hart et al. 1991; Birrell et al. 2001).

Such problems in the definition of osteoarthritis, radiograph interpretation, and clinical measurement make the epidemiology of osteoarthritis difficult to analyse but several conclusions can be drawn.

Descriptive studies

Autopsy studies suggest that the majority of subjects over age 65 have evidence of osteoarthritis in at least one joint site at the time of death. Prevalence estimates from such studies tend to be higher than those from radiographic surveys, perhaps because the whole joint surface is available for study.

Radiographic studies also report high prevalence in the middle-aged and elderly. This prevalence varies according to joint site and age. For example, hand interphalangeal joints and first metatarsophalangeal joints are commonly affected and at a relatively young age, whereas glenohumeral joints are less commonly involved and principally in the elderly. From large radiographic studies (Mikkelson et al. 1970; Lawrence 1977; Felson 1988; van Saase et al. 1989) the following generalizations can be made.

Age

This is a major determinant of prevalence at all sites. Prevalence is low in those aged less than 45 years and when it occurs it is almost invariably monoarticular possibly reflecting a traumatic aetiology. Prevalence increases up to age 65, when there is involvement of at least one joint group in at least 50 per cent of the population. Continuing increase in prevalence in those over age 65 is less clear-cut, indeed a plateauing out of prevalence in the very old has been suggested (Bagge et al. 1992) (Plate 181).

Gender

This is important at some, but not all, joint sites. Although there is little or no gender difference in the prevalence of mild osteoarthritis, a female preponderance becomes more apparent:

- for severe grades of osteoarthritis;
- in older age groups;
- for osteoarthritis of the hands and knees.

There is also a polyarticular form of hand osteoarthritis that has a predilection for peri-menopausal women often termed nodal generalized osteoarthritis. This is discussed further below.

Table 1 Radiographic–pathologic correlates in osteoarthritis

Pathological change	Radiographic abnormality
Cartilage fibrillation, erosion	Decrease in interosseous distance (localized)
Subchondral new bone formation	Sclerosis
New cartilage formation and endochondral ossification	Osteophyte
Fibrous-walled pseudocysts resulting from fluid intrusion or myxoid degeneration	Subchondral cysts
Trabecular compression	Bone collapse/attrition
Fragmentation of osteochondral surface; cartilage and bone metaphasia in synovium	Osseous ('loose') bodies

Ethnic group

Given the difficulties of representative sampling and reproducible assessments, comparison between populations shows surprising similarity in age-specific prevalence by joint site (van Saase et al. 1989). Possible exceptions are:

- hip osteoarthritis (lower prevalence among Black and Oriental populations compared to Whites);
- polyarticular hand osteoarthritis (less common in African and Malaysian populations);
- knee osteoarthritis [commoner in Chinese populations (Zhang et al. 2001)].

Geographic variation—'endemic osteoarthritis'

Several forms of disabling polyarticular 'osteoarthritis' occur with high frequency in certain geographical locations. The best described are Kashin–Beck disease (south-eastern Siberia, northern China, North Korea) and Mselini disease (limited to the Zulu and Tonga tribes people of south-east Africa). Other forms of endemic osteoarthritis occur in Malnad and elsewhere in India. These conditions share in common:

- onset during the first or second decade;
- variable growth restriction;
- characteristics of acquired rather than inherited disease (at a young age movement out of the area eliminates its development, whereas movement into the area affords an acquired risk of the disease);
- involvement of impoverished rural communities.

The conditions radiographically most closely resemble those of spondylo-epiphyseal dysplasia, and histologically show chondronecrosis as a likely initial event. The cause(s) of the endemic osteoarthritides remains largely unknown although some progress is now being made. For example, Kashin–Beck disease is now thought to be due to a combination of both hypothyroidism and selenium deficiency (Moreno-Reyes et al. 1998).

Analytical studies

Individual risk factors for osteoarthritis may conveniently be viewed as:

- those influencing or marking a generalized predisposition to the condition;
- those resulting in abnormal biomechanical loading at specific sites (Fig. 6).

Generalized susceptibility

Obesity

This is closely associated with knee osteoarthritis with an odds ratio for those 50 per cent above ideal body weight (compared to those with ideal body weight) of 4.5 for men and 9.0 for women (Lawrence et al. 1990).

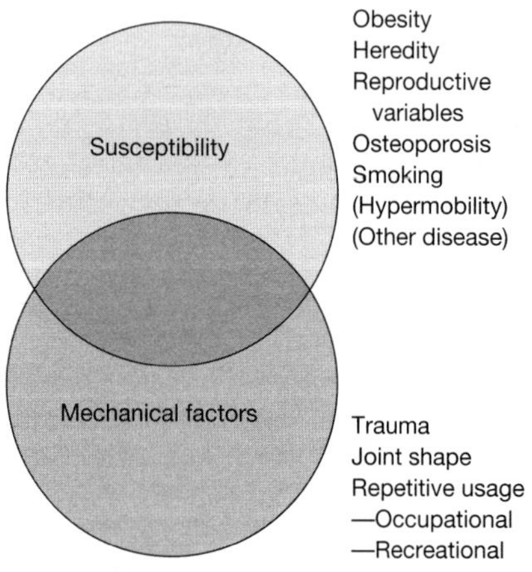

Fig. 6 Susceptibility to osteoarthritis: interaction between generalized and local factors.

Interestingly obesity does not seem to be such a strong risk factor at the hip. At the knee, obesity precedes rather than follows knee osteoarthritis and indeed weight loss may prevent the development of knee osteoarthritis (Felson et al. 1992) (Fig. 7). It is associated with radiographic change irrespective of whether symptoms are present or not, arguing against painful knees leading to obesity due to an enforced sedentary lifestyle. Obesity also increases the risk of knee pain for a given degree of structural change. The mechanism relating obesity and osteoarthritis remains speculative. An interrelationship with varus/valgus knee alignment has been noted. It is suggested that obesity results in a major increased risk of structural change only when knee alignment is suboptimal (Sharma et al. 2000).

Genetic factors

A strong familial tendency is recognized for many forms of osteoarthritis:

- nodal generalized osteoarthritis is a polyarticular form of osteoarthritis characterized by Heberden's nodes occurring mainly in women of peri-menopausal age. Heberden's nodes appear to be inherited independently as an autosomal dominant trait with greater penetrance in women.
- hip osteoarthritis has a significant genetic component (age adjusted relative risk to siblings of >5) (Lanyon et al. 2000).
- Classic twin studies also suggest a major genetic contribution to development of knee, hand and hip osteoarthritis and possibly spinal disc degeneration (Spector et al. 1996).

The nature of the genetic abnormality remains unclear. Initial reports suggested an association of the COL2A1 gene with rare hereditary forms of premature polyarticular osteoarthritis with mild dysplasia (Knowlton et al. 1990). Similar genetic changes have been found in some, but not all, forms of hereditary osteo-opthalmoarthropathy (Stickler's syndrome) which is characterized by variable ocular and mid-facial abnormalities and a premature osteoarthritis-like syndrome (Williams and Jimenez 1993). It is apparent, however, that common knee and hip osteoarthritis and nodal generalized osteoarthritis are not monogenic conditions. Several or many genes are likely to confer genetic predisposition and gene–gene and gene–environmental/constitutional interactions will be important in determining phenotypic expression and outcome. Association studies have identified a number of potential sites, especially on chromosomes 2, 4, 6, 7, 11, 12, and 16, that may be involved (Loughlin 2001). COL2A1 and vitamin D receptor gene polymorphisms may also be included within the genetic risk profile (Uitterlinden et al. 2000).

Reproductive variables

Polyarticular osteoarthritis has:

- a strong female predominance
- a frequent onset around the menopause
- an association with previous hysterectomy and gynaecological surgery
- and a possible association with altered levels of sex hormone binding globulin.

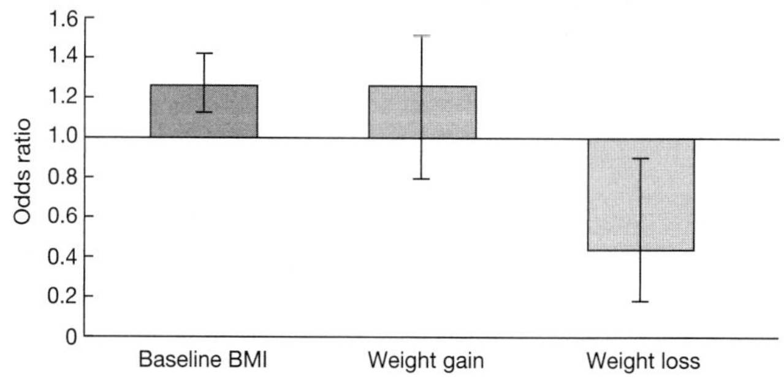

Fig. 7 Risk of symptomatic knee osteoarthritis per 2 units of body mass index (BMI) expressed as odds ratio and 95 per cent confidence interval. Derived from Felson et al. (1992).

This has led to the suggestion that hormonal factors are important in this subgroup (Spector and Campion 1989). Manipulation of sex hormones in animal models of 'osteoarthritis' and identification of oestrogen receptors on chondrocytes also lend support to a role for hormonal modulation. In a prospective cohort study, use of oestrogen replacement therapy did seem to be associated with a reduced rate of progression of knee osteoarthritis (Zhang et al. 1998). In a large randomized controlled trial, however, no benefits for knee pain or disability were obtained in postmenopausal women from 4 years treatment with oestrogen plus progestin (Nevitt et al. 2001). As yet oestrogen replacement therapy has no established place in the management of osteoarthritis.

Bone density

A negative association has been reported between osteoporosis and osteoarthritis at certain sites particularly the hip (Lane and Nevitt 1994). The negative association is weak and in the clinical setting the two conditions often occur together and may cause difficulty with for example arthroplasty. One possible explanation for this relationship may be that weak bone could absorb excessive impact loading and thus protect hyaline cartilage from damage and subsequent osteoarthritis. In the converse rare situation of osteopetrosis, where the skeleton is diffusely sclerotic, a high incidence of premature polyarticular osteoarthritis is reported. Alteration in bone density in osteoarthritis may, however, not simply reflect a generalized osteopaenia. High resolution studies of subchondral bone has suggested that there may be alterations in this strata with reduced bone density resulting in subchondral fracture and deformity. This may in turn alter cartilage loading thus predisposing to joint failure. The difference between the role of osteoporosis in these two strata is a little difficult to resolve and is discussed further below.

Cigarette smoking

A protective influence of smoking on knee osteoarthritis has been reported from several studies including the Framingham study (Felson 1988). The mechanism is unclear but smoking is a risk factor for osteoporosis, is associated with an increased body mass index in women, has antioestrogenic properties, and has many effects on cell function. It is unclear which, if any, of these is important.

Other suggested factors

Less definite associations are reported with diabetes, hypertension, and hyperuricaemia, which are independent of obesity. Clearer associations with acromegaly and haemochromatosis are evident. An increased frequency of osteoarthritis in subjects with generalized hypermobility has also been suggested but rigorous epidemiological support for this is still required. An increased risk of first carpometacarpal, but reduced risk of distal interphalangeal osteoarthritis in those with joint laxity of the hand, however, is reported from Iceland (Jonsson and Valtysdottir 1995). There are scant data on the possible role of nutrition, though low intake of antioxidant vitamins (A, C, E) and vitamin D may be associated with increased risk of progression of established knee osteoarthritis (McAlindon and Felson 1997), and reduced levels of vitamin D with increased risk of incident hip osteoarthritis (Lane et al. 1999). Such interesting observations with obvious public health implications require further study although a recent 6-month trial of vitamin E failed to demonstrate any benefit in symptom relief over placebo (Brand et al. 2001).

Local mechanical factors

Trauma

Major direct injury, particularly if resulting in a fracture of the articular surface is considered as a cause of osteoarthritis (Wright 1990) although evidence for this is retrospective and uncontrolled. Major injury, particularly fracture, may also predispose to osteoarthritis at distant sites by altering mechanical loading of the joint. Examples of this include fractures of the femoral shaft (hip osteoarthritis) (Fig. 8), scaphoid (wrist osteoarthritis), tibia (ankle osteoarthritis), or humerus (shoulder osteoarthritis). The role of less severe trauma has, until recently, been unclear but a recent prospective study in college students suggests that significant trauma during college years is associated with a subsequent increased incidence of osteoarthritis in later years (Gelber et al. 2000). Although the site of osteoarthritis may be determined by trauma it is unclear whether it affects the lifetime prevalence of osteoarthritis. For example, knee osteoarthritis does not develop in all patients following total meniscectomy and appears to occur only in those subjects with evidence of a generalized predisposition to osteoarthritis (i.e. those with distal interphalangeal joint osteoarthritis) (Doherty et al. 1983). However, the finding that trauma in college years (mean age 22) increases the subsequent prevalence of osteoarthritis in subjects in their 60s, does suggest that measures to reduce trauma, particularly that related to sport, may be important in reducing clinical osteoarthritis amongst workers (Gelber et al. 2000).

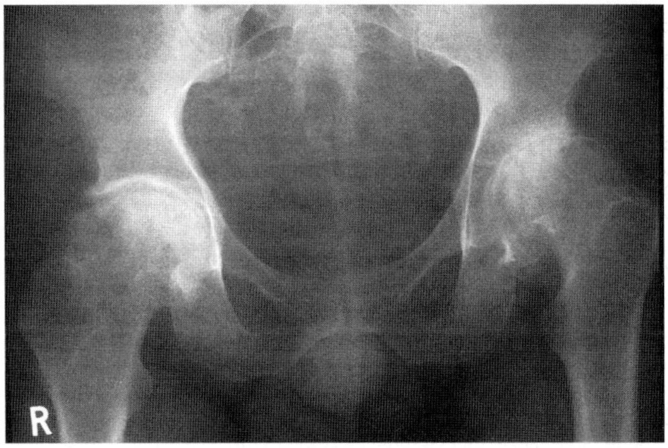

Fig. 8 Asymmetric hip osteoarthritis following previous trauma on the right side in a patient (Ledingham et al. 1992).

Joint shape

Abnormalities of articular contour which lead to abnormal load transmission across the joint have been suggested to predispose to osteoarthritis at the hip and knee. Although childhood hip disorders such as Perthe's disease, slipped capital epiphysis, and congenital dislocation lead to premature hip osteoarthritis, the role of lesser degrees of acetabular dysplasia is unclear and probably responsible for little if any excess in hip osteoarthritis (Croft et al. 1991). The role of unrecognized, dysplasia of the femoral condyles similarly predisposing to knee osteoarthritis is even less clear.

Occupational and recreational activities

Repetitive impact loading and trauma have been implicated in reported increased frequencies of osteoarthritis in miners (knees, spine), cotton workers (distal interphalangeal joints), and pneumatic drillers (elbows). As discussed above trauma in teenage years is also associated with osteoarthritis at the knee and much of this is sport related. At the knee repetitive occupational knee bending carrying weights greater than 20 kg is associated with osteoarthritis with an odds ratio greater than 2 (Felson et al. 1991).

At the hip, several studies have shown a convincing increased incidence of osteoarthritis in farmers such that hip osteoarthritis in farmers can now be considered an industrial disease. The mechanism underlying this association remains unclear. Certain sports played at professional or elite amateur level may be a risk factor for osteoarthritis. Professional soccer, for example, may increase the risk of knee osteoarthritis even after adjusting for sports-associated traumatic injury. Moderate sports activity that does not cause joint injury, however, is unlikely to be an important risk factor, the benefits of aerobic activity possibly outweighing any detrimental effects of prolonged repetitive loading.

Reduced muscle strength and proprioception

Apart from effecting movement, muscle performs important sensorimotor functions that may influence joint health and function. Knee osteoarthritis, for example, is associated with reduced quadriceps strength, reduced knee proprioception, and impairment of standing balance. Such factors may predispose to development of knee pain and reduced function, and possibly precede rather than follow development of structural osteoarthritis (Slemenda et al. 1998). They may also relate to the increased risk of falls in subjects with knee osteoarthritis.

Clinical features

Symptoms and impact of osteoarthritis

The principal clinical features of osteoarthritis are:

- symptoms (pain, stiffness),
- functional impairment,
- signs (primarily anatomical change).

Though interrelated, there is often marked discordance between these three.

Symptoms

Although pain is the chief complaint its origin is not always clear. Hyaline cartilage is aneural and this means that metabolic or structural alteration in this tissue is unlikely to be directly perceived as painful. Several other mechanisms of symptom production have been suggested (Fig. 9). These include:

- stimulation of capsular pain fibres and mechanoreceptors by raised intra-articular pressure due to synovial hypertrophy, increased fluid production, and decreased joint compliance;
- inflammatory mediators stimulating pain fibres in the synovium and capsule;
- stimulation of periosteal nerve fibres by intraosseous hypertension accompanying osteoarthritis;
- perception of subchondral microfractures;
- painful periarticular structures such as entheses and bursae possibly resulting from abnormal biomechanics and/or muscle weakness;
- adaptive changes in the spinal cord (central sensitization, 'wind-up') and brain (disinhibition, impairment of the Diffuse Noxious Inhibitory Control system) leading to persistent pain perception.

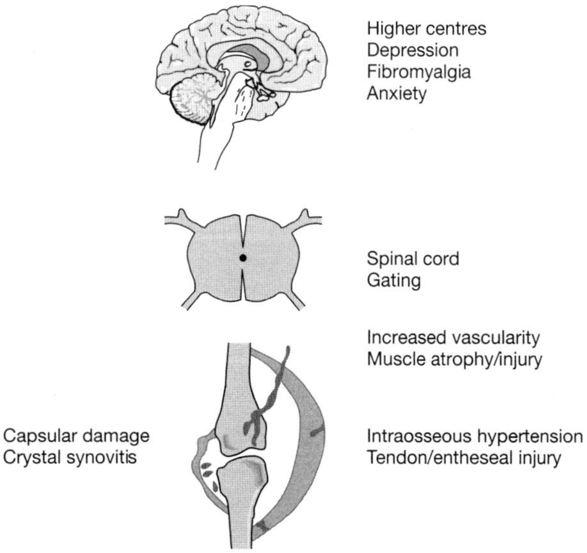

Fig. 9 Potential sites of pain perception and/or modification in osteoarthritis. Redrawn from Jones and Doherty (1992).

It has been suggested that these different mechanisms may produce different pain characteristics but studies exploring this are scanty (Creamer et al. 1998). It is suggested that pain:

- on usage is principally due to mechanical or entheseal problems;
- after rest is inflammatory in origin;
- at night is due to intraosseous hypertension.

The last of these, night pain, may be a particularly poor prognostic factor, indicating severe damage. It may, however, also predict a better response to non-steroidal anti-inflammatory drugs. Pain in osteoarthritis may be a transient feature and can be absent in spite of severe joint damage (Fig. 10). Correlation between pain and radiographic change varies according to site. It is best at the hip and then knee, with the poorest correlation occurring in the hands and inter-vertebral facet joints. Joints with more severe radiographic change are more likely to be symptomatic than those with mild change (Fig. 11) but in general other factors are more important. Several recent studies have demonstrated that psychological factors may be a more important correlate with disability than radiographic change. Indeed factors associated with radiographic outcome may be independent from, and distinct from those associated with knee pain and disability (Davis et al. 1992). Recent community-based studies have therefore addressed the burden of knee pain in the community rather than radiographically defined knee osteoarthritis.

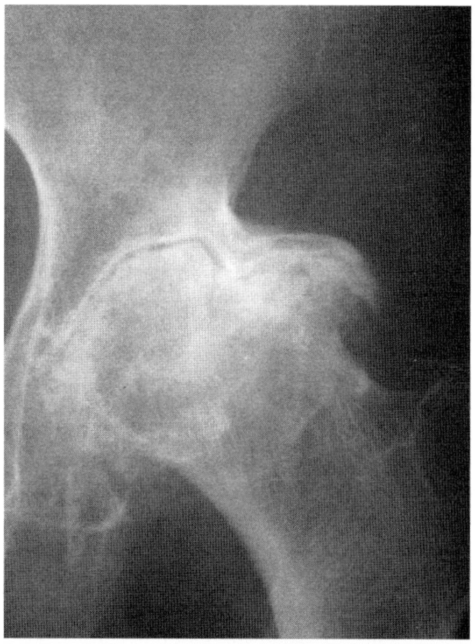

Fig. 10 Radiograph of an asymptomatic individual with severe radiographic osteoarthritis change.

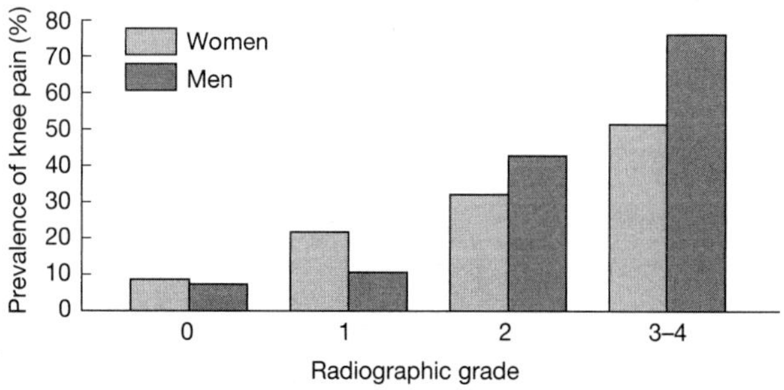

Fig. 11 Prevalence of knee pain by radiographic grade and gender in a US community population. Derived from Davis et al. (1992).

It may be that the lack of association is spurious and related to the relatively poor sensitivity and specificity of current radiographic techniques. More sensitive imaging techniques such as MRI may give better associations with pain. A recent MRI study of the knee, for example, showed that bone changes that may reflect intraosseous oedema ('bruising') is common in osteoarthritis and is associated with the severity of reported pain (Felson et al. 2001).

Stiffness is the other chief complaint. This is often described as 'gelling' of the joint after inactivity with difficulty in initiating movement. Prolonged morning or inactivity stiffness, often taken as a reflection of inflammation, is uncommon but may occur.

Some patients may complain of joint swelling and deformity (particularly of hands), and coarse crepitus, even in the absence of other symptoms. At the knee associated meniscal damage or loose body formation may result in other mechanical symptoms such as 'locking'.

Functional impairment

Disability is principally associated with pain. However, psychological factors and muscle weakness are also important and in most cases more important than radiographic change (Davis et al. 1992; O'Reilly et al. 1998; Creamer et al. 2000). For an individual patient reduced range of movement (e.g. at the hip) may be associated with specific functional limitations, for example, during sexual intercourse or getting out of a car.

Mortality

In addition to morbidity, cumulative mortality rates among subjects aged 55–74 in the National Health and Nutrition Examination Survey (NHANES-I) were significantly greater (relative risk 1.1) for women but not men with knee osteoarthritis (Lawrence et al. 1990). An increased mortality has also been associated with knee osteoarthritis in Sweden (Danielsson and Hernborg 1970). The mechanisms underlying this are unclear but may include:

- the toxic effects of drugs, principally non-steroidal anti-inflammatory drugs
- increased cardiovascular morbidity due to either co-morbidities (e.g. obesity) or lack of aerobic fitness.

Signs

Several features reflecting altered joint structure and function may be present. These include:

- coarse crepitus, thought to be due to irregularity of the articular surface;
- bony enlargement, due to remodelling and osteophyte formation;
- deformity;
- instability;
- restricted movement;
- stress pain.

Varying degrees of synovitis (warmth, effusion, synovial thickening) may also be present and there may be joint line tenderness. Signs of associated meniscal damage and 'loose body' formation can occur and periarticular sources of pain, demonstrated by point tenderness away from the joint line and by stress testing, are commonly seen. Muscle wasting and weakness around an affected joint may also be observed and are associated with reduced joint proprioception and balance on loading.

Osteoarthritis 'subsets'

Since osteoarthritis is a process that can potentially be triggered by diverse constitutional and environmental factors, a wide spectrum of clinical expression and outcome should be expected. It is possible to look at osteoarthritis as a single entity or to try to classify sub-groups of patients with osteoarthritis. Both strategies are fraught with difficulties.

Osteoarthritis was initially classified as primary (no cause identified) or secondary (an obvious cause identified, such as trauma or dysplasia). Indeed such a distinction is still retained in the American College of Rheumatology criteria (Altman et al. 1991). Such artificial separation has often proved unsatisfactory due to:

- frequent lack of an identifiable cause, resulting in a large heterogeneous primary group;
- overlap between subsets, as shown, for example, by the influence of predisposition to 'primary' generalized osteoarthritis in determining development of post-meniscectomy 'secondary' osteoarthritis (Doherty et al. 1983);
- lack of evidence to suggest that the underlying pathological features and processes differ.

Other more objective features have therefore often been used to define subsets:

- joint site involved (e.g. hip, knee, hand);
- site within a joint (e.g. at the knee medial tibiofemoral, lateral tibiofemoral, patellofemoral);
- number of joints involved (e.g. one, few, many);
- presence of associated calcium crystal deposition;
- presence of marked clinical inflammation;
- radiographic bone response (e.g. atrophic, hypertrophic);
- age of onset (e.g. premature osteoarthritis under age 45);
- syndromal features (e.g. Stickler's syndrome or hereditary arthro-ophthalmopathy).

Although a number of 'subsets' have emerged it is important to note that sharp distinctions between subsets do not exist and many of the above characteristics represent different aspects of the osteoarthritis process (e.g. the balance between damage and repair, the number of joints involved), and different characteristics may dominate the clinical picture at just one phase in the evolution of the condition. One 'subset' may thus evolve into another, and different 'subsets' may exist at different sites within the same individual. The partitioning of osteoarthritis may be revolutionized by the genetics of osteoarthritis if specific genotypic sub-setting becomes possible.

Nodal generalized osteoarthritis

This is the best recognized subset and is characterized by:

- polyarticular finger interphalangeal joint involvement;
- Heberden's and Bouchard's nodes;
- female preponderance;
- peak onset around the menopause;
- predisposition to osteoarthritis of the knee, hip, spine, and thumb base;
- marked familial predisposition.

The typical patient is a woman aged 40–60 who develops discomfort followed by swelling of a single finger interphalangeal joint. A few months later another interphalangeal joint becomes painful, then another, producing a 'stuttering' onset polyarthritis of distal and proximal interphalangeal joints. Affected interphalangeal joints may feel very stiff, be tender, and show tight posterolateral swelling with overlying erythema. Aspiration of such swellings may reveal viscous, clear, hyaluronate-rich 'jelly': these cysts are thought to represent mucoid transformation of periarticular fibroadipose and may communicate with the joint. Each interphalangeal joint tends to go through a symptomatic phase while swelling and deformity become established, resulting in perhaps 1–3 years of episodic discomfort and stiffness. In almost all cases symptoms then subside, leaving the patient with:

- typical posterolateral firm Heberden's (distal interphalangeal joint) and Bouchard's (proximal interphalangeal joint) nodes;
- characteristic lateral subluxations of interphalangeal joints (Plate 182);
- and radiographic evidence of osteoarthritis (Fig. 12).

In addition to finger interphalangeal joints, the first carpometacarpal, metacarpophalangeal, and interphalangeal joints of the thumb are

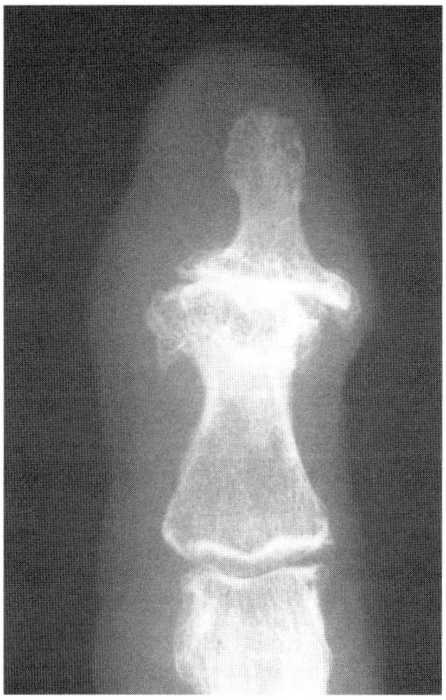

Fig. 12 Radiograph of distal interphalangeal joint showing many of the typical radiographic features of osteoarthritis (joint space narrowing, sclerosis, osteophyte).

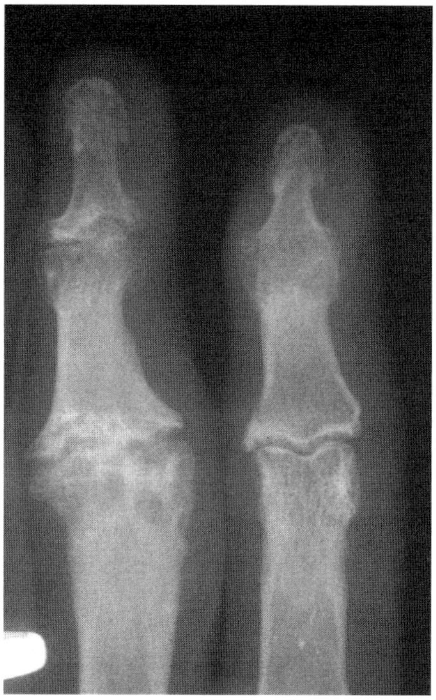

Fig. 13 Subchondral erosive change in erosive osteoarthritis.

commonly affected. Other joint involvement in the hand and wrist is usually restricted to the index and middle metacarpophalangeal, scaphotrapezoid, and pisiform-triquetral articulations. The functional prognosis for the hand seems to be good.

Nodal generalized hand osteoarthritis is associated with an increased frequency of osteoarthritis at other sites, particularly knees, hips, first metatarsophalangeal joints, and cervical and lumbar apophyseal joints (Kellgren and Moore 1952). This concept of 'generalized osteoarthritis', with hand involvement as the marker for predisposition, was first described by Haygarth in 1805 and is supported by several studies. One such survey (Acheson and Collart 1975) suggests division into two groups (although such distinction is not supported by others):

- nodal generalized osteoarthritis;
  - nodes
  - distal interphalangeal joint involved more than proximal interphalangeal joint
  - marked female preponderance
  - familial aggregation
- non-nodal generalized osteoarthritis;
  - proximal interphalangeal joint involved more than distal interphalangeal joint
  - more equal sex distribution.

The inevitable problem that arises is that in the elderly one or just a few Heberden's nodes and limited interphalangeal joint osteoarthritis are common often asymptomatic findings. It is not always clear, therefore when should the title 'nodal generalized osteoarthritis' be applied. Although criteria for this have not been defined, some studies suggest that involvement of even a single interphalangeal joint may be important (Croft et al. 1992).

Erosive ('inflammatory') osteoarthritis

This relatively uncommon condition is characterized by:

- hand interphalangeal joint involvement;
- often florid inflammation;
- radiographic subchondral erosive change;
- tendency to interphalangeal joint ankylosis.

The condition clinically resembles nodal generalized osteoarthritis in beginning as an additive polyarthritis of finger joints. Inflammatory symptoms and signs are often marked although episodic. Unlike nodal generalized osteoarthritis, proximal and distal interphalangeal joints are equally involved. Less frequently, index and middle metacarpophalangeal joints are also involved. Interphalangeal joint instability, which is rare in nodal generalized osteoarthritis, is common and, since there is also occasional spontaneous ankylosis of one or a few interphalangeal joints, the prognosis for hand function is less favourable than for nodal generalized osteoarthritis (Pattrick et al. 1989). The hallmark feature of this condition is the presence of subchondral erosive change (Fig. 13) which may lead to a 'gull's wing' appearance as remodelling occurs (Fig. 14). Early, florid subchondral erosive change is easily recognized, but lesser degrees of erosion, particularly in established cases, may prove difficult to distinguish from the cysts and subchondral bony change of nodal generalized osteoarthritis. It is unclear whether erosive osteoarthritis is a distinct subset or one end of a spectrum of change (Cobby et al. 1991).

Microscopically the synovium is infiltrated with lymphocytes and monocytes, and pannus may be seen. The nature of this inflammatory, destructive condition is unknown although it is of interest that similar hand changes may occur in some patients with Sjögren's syndrome. Of note, perhaps, is that 15 per cent of patients presenting with Sjögren's syndrome and erosive osteoarthritis subsequently developed seropositive rheumatoid arthritis (Ehlich 1975).

Large joint osteoarthritis

Knee osteoarthritis

The knee is commonly affected by osteoarthritis. Involvement is usually bilateral unless there is predisposing trauma. Although osteoarthritis may affect the knee as a mono- or pauciarticular problem it often occurs in association with hand osteoarthritis, especially in women (Kellgren and Moore 1952;

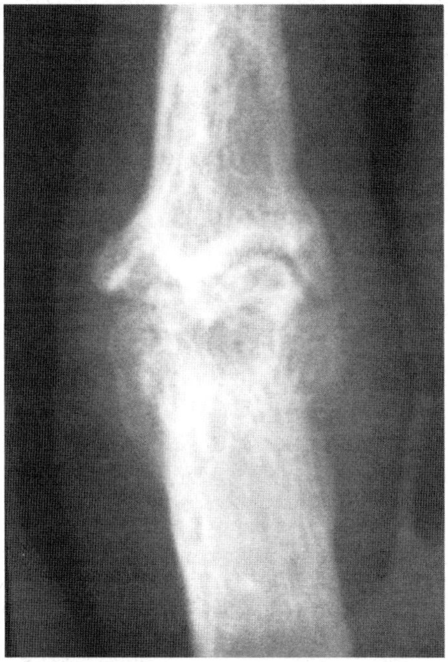

Fig. 14 'Gull's wing' deformity in erosive osteoarthritis.

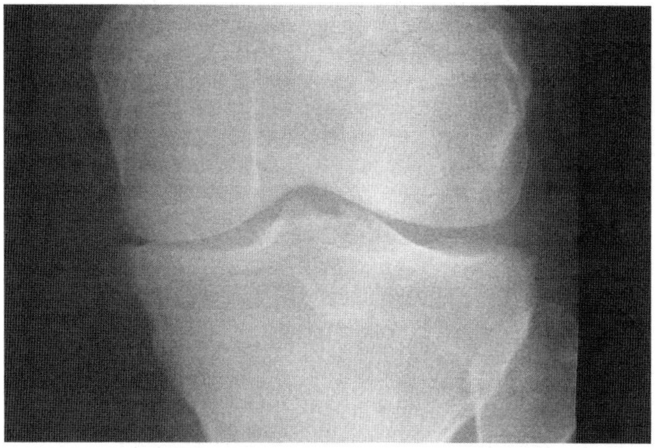

Fig. 15 Predominant medial compartment osteoarthritis at the knee (standing anterioposterior radiograph).

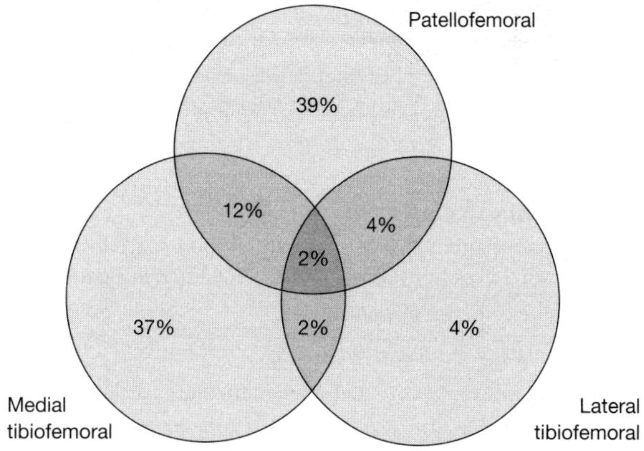

Fig. 16 Sites of radiographic involvement of knee osteoarthritis in patients with radiographic change in a community survey in the United Kingdom. Derived from McAlindon et al. (1992).

Acheson and Collart 1975). Involvement at the knee is often focal with the principal sites involved being the:

- medial tibiofemoral compartment (Fig. 15), with severe bone and cartilage attrition at this site resulting in a characteristic varus deformity (Plate 183);
- patellofemoral compartment (lateral more than medial), which because of its intimate relationship with the quadriceps mechanism is possibly associated with greater functional impairment (McAlindon et al. 1992) (Fig. 16).

Risk factors for development of knee osteoarthritis are discussed above. Whether differing risk factors are important at different compartmental sites is unclear but some studies do suggest that this may be the case. For example tibiofemoral disease may be more strongly associated with trauma whereas patellofemoral disease may be associated with the presence of pyrophosphate crystals and female gender.

Hip osteoarthritis

Study of this joint has been hampered by a lack of a consistent definition and classification of pattern of involvement. Two main patterns of migration of the femoral head have been emphasized:

Superior pole osteoarthritis

This is the commonest pattern, characterized by focal cartilage loss in the superior part of the joint (Fig. 17). Osteophyte formation is most prominent at the lateral acetabular and medial femoral margins, often in combination with thickening (buttressing) of the cortex of the medial femoral neck by periosteal osteophyte (Fig. 18). Subchondral sclerosis and cyst formation on both sides of the narrowed joint may be marked. Originally it was suggested that this pattern is:

- relatively more common in men;
- mainly unilateral at presentation;
- likely to progress, with superolateral (Fig. 18) or superomedial femoral migration;
- commonly secondary to local structural abnormality.

More recent studies have questioned whether there is often an underlying structural abnormality (Croft et al. 1991). In a hospital based population, progression has been confirmed to be more likely than in other patterns (Ledingham et al. 1993).

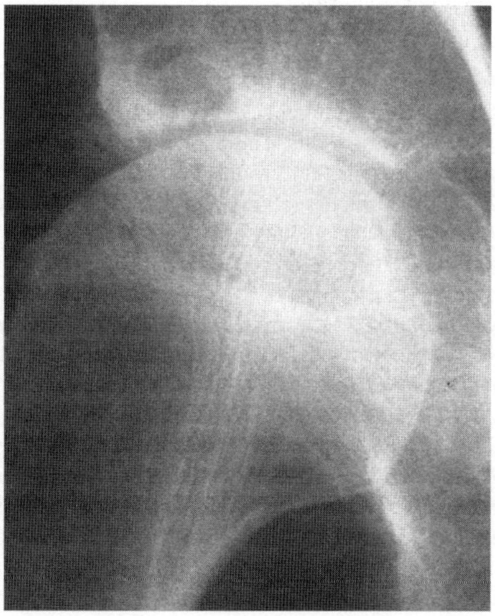

Fig. 17 Superior pole pattern of hip osteoarthritis (early) showing localized reduction in interosseous distance with focal sclerosis at the superior part of the joint, minor femoral osteophyte, and acetabular roof cyst.

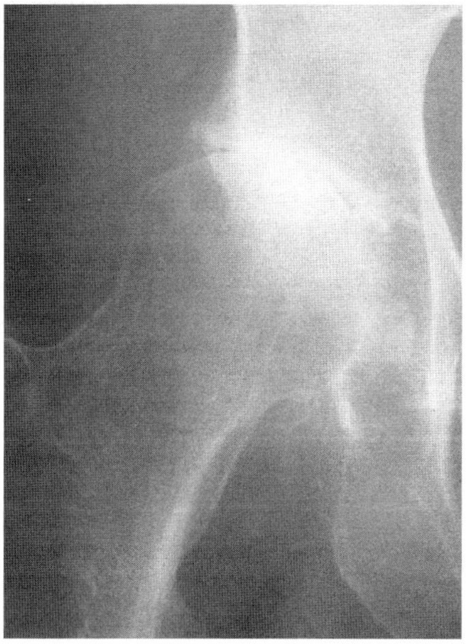

Fig. 18 Superior pole osteoarthritis (late) showing superolateral femoral head migration, bone attrition, and 'buttressing' medial periosteal osteophyte of the femoral neck.

Central (medial) osteoarthritis

This less common pattern shows more central joint space loss, with less prominent femoral neck buttressing. It is suggested that this pattern is:

- relatively more common in women;
- commonly bilateral at presentation;
- more strongly associated with nodal generalized osteoarthritis;
- less likely to progress and when it does it is with axial or medial migration (Fig. 19).

Other patterns are described (e.g. concentric) and many patients have 'indeterminate' radiographic patterns. Most disease is symmetrical unless there is a structural alteration in joint loading (Fig. 9) (Ledingham et al. 1992). Differentiation of these patterns does appear warranted since there may be differences in the association with hand osteoarthritis (Marks et al. 1979), and in prognosis (Danielsson 1964; Ledingham et al. 1992).

Crystal-associated subsets

A number of particles are commonly identified in synovial fluid and other tissues from osteoarthritic joints. These include calcium pyrophosphate dihydrate crystals and apatite (i.e. carbonate substituted hydroxyapatite and other basic calcium phosphates) (Plate 184). The origin and role of such particles in osteoarthritis remain unknown (Dieppe et al. 1988). By analogy with monosodium urate monohydrate crystals in gout, it was initially assumed that such crystals were always pathogenic and the cause of specific 'crystal deposition disease' (McCarty 1976). Calcium pyrophosphate dihydrate and apatite are certainly phlogistic agents and can cause acute synovitis. In addition being particulate they might also act as wear particles on the joint surface. However, the not uncommon occurrence of these crystals in asymptomatic, otherwise normal joints, the lack of association with specific locomotor disease, and the variable prevalence of crystals depending on technique and experience used in crystal identification (Swan et al. 1994) has questioned such a direct pathogenic role. It currently seems that calcium pyrophosphate dihydrate and apatite, in the context of osteoarthritis are epiphenomenona possibly reflecting the underlying physiological processes of osteoarthritis. Apart from alerting the clinician to an underlying metabolic or genetic predisposition their value in a clinical setting is unclear.

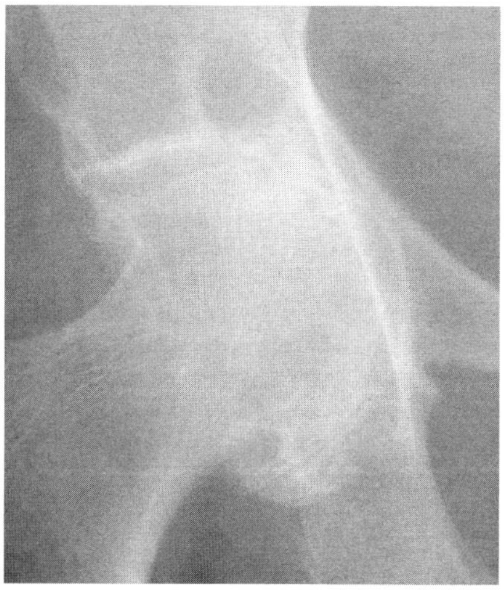

Fig. 19 Medial pole osteoarthritis, showing progression to a protrusio acetabulae deformity.

Pyrophosphate arthropathy

In its chronic form calcium pyrophosphate dihydrate crystals are associated with a form of osteoarthritis that perhaps has several distinct features compared to common osteoarthritis. These include:

- predominance in elderly females;
- an often florid inflammatory component possibly with superimposed acute attacks;
- particular involvement of the knee;
- frequent involvement of joints and joint compartments uncommonly affected by 'sporadic osteoarthritis' (e.g. glenohumeral, mid-tarsal, metacarpophalangeal);
- frequent 'hypertrophic' radiographic appearance;
- calcification of articular structures;
- synovial fluid calcium pyrophosphate dihydrate crystals.

Large and medium sized joints are principally involved, with the knees being the most usual and severely affected site, followed by wrists, shoulders, elbows, hips, and mid-tarsal joints. In the hand, metacarpophalangeal joints (particularly index and middle) are often affected. Symptoms are usually restricted to just a few joints, though single or multiple joint involvement also occurs. Acute attacks may be superimposed upon chronic symptoms. Affected joints show signs of osteoarthritis (bony swelling, crepitus, restricted movement) and varying degrees of inflammation. Synovitis may be marked and is usually most evident at the knee, radiocarpal, or glenohumeral joints. Knees typically demonstrate bi- or tricompartmental involvement, with marked, usually predominant patellofemoral disease. In severe cases fixed flexion with either valgus or varus deformity may occur. Examination often reveals more widespread but asymptomatic joint abnormality; nodal generalized osteoarthritis, for example, is a common accompaniment.

The radiographic changes of this arthropathy are basically those of osteoarthritis but characteristics which may suggest pyrophosphate arthropathy are:

- atypical joint and compartmental involvement;
- often prominent, exuberant osteophyte and cyst formation (particularly at the knee).

These features combine to produce a distinctive 'hypertrophic' appearance and distribution which suggests calcium pyrophosphate dihydrate arthropathy even in the absence of radiographic chondrocalcinosis (Fig. 20). Many cases of pyrophosphate arthropathy, however, appear not dissimilar

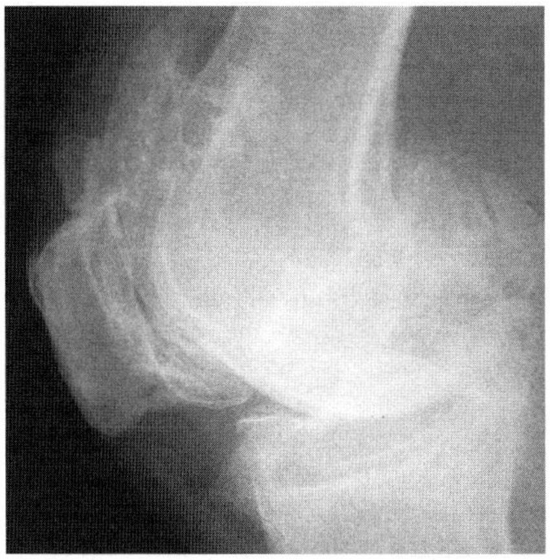

Fig. 20 Exuberant osteophytosis in patellofemoral compartment in pyrophosphate arthropathy.

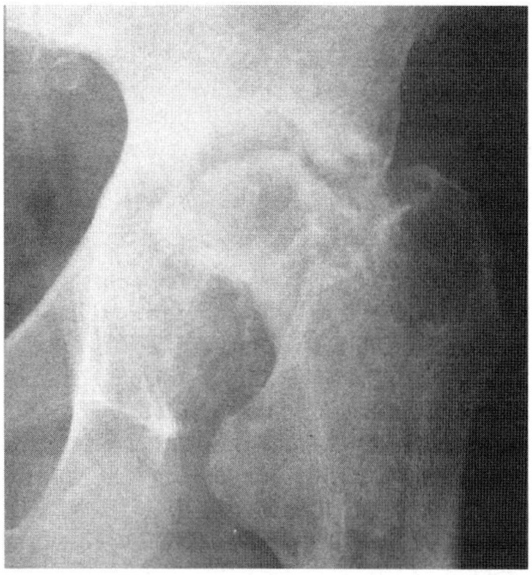

Fig. 21 Radiograph of apatite associated destructive arthritis of the hip, showing apparent increase in joint space (non-loaded film), marked loss of bone (femoral and acetabular components), and minimal bone response.

to 'uncomplicated' osteoarthritis. Furthermore, since nodal generalized osteoarthritis often coexists it is common to find otherwise typical osteoarthritis changes in some joints, with more distinctive changes of pyrophosphate arthropathy at others. It is probable, therefore, that pyrophosphate arthropathy is part of the spectrum of osteoarthritis rather than a truly distinct entity. As discussed further below the presence of crystals may tell us something about the underlying pathophysiological processes at work in the joint.

Apatite associated arthropathy

This uncommon condition usually is:

- confined to the elderly particularly women;
- localized to large joints;
- associated with rapid progression with resultant joint instability;
- associated with marked attrition of cartilage and bone;
- characterized by abundant apatite deposition in synovial fluid and synovium.

This condition has a number of synonyms, including 'Milwaukee shoulder', and 'basic calcium phosphate deposition disease'. Typical patients are elderly women with rapidly progressive arthropathy of the hip, shoulder, or knee. Usually only one or a few joints are affected. Onset is often quite sudden and within a few weeks or months the patient has severe rest and night pain, and the joint has a large, cool effusion, with gross instability. Aspirated synovial fluid is often blood-stained, highly viscous but with only a modest increased cellularity. Alazarin red S staining at acidic pH shows multiple calcium containing aggregates (Plate 184) which can be identified as apatite, most commonly carbonate substituted hydroxyapatite, by more definitive means. The principal radiographic features are marked attrition of cartilage and bone, with a paucity of osteophyte and sclerosis, that is, a markedly 'atrophic' appearance (Fig. 21). The differential diagnosis includes sepsis, an atrophic neuropathic joint, and late avascular necrosis.

The pathogenesis of this condition, particularly as regards the role of the apatite aggregates, is controversial (Halverson and McCarty 1988). McCarty and colleagues have emphasized the presence of activated collagenase in synovial fluid, a proliferative response to crystals in the synovium, and the frequency of accompanying periarticular calcification. They therefore suggest that apatite that has been deposited in capsule and periarticular structures is enzymatically 'strip-mined', the free apatite then interacting with synoviocytes, resulting in further collagenase release, further strip-mining, and progression of arthropathy and instability via an 'amplification loop'. Others, however, have not confirmed an increase in collagenase activities, and suggest that the apatite primarily originates from subchondral and marginal bone. The non-specific finding of apatite in varying quantities in other arthropathies, and even in small amounts in normal joints, is consistent with the latter interpretation. The speed of onset and progression, lack of overt inflammation, marked bone loss, specificity to certain anatomic sites, radiographic similarity to late avascular necrosis, and neuropathic joints support the contention that this arthropathy reflects a widespread nutritional catastrophe for the joint, possibly initiated by age-related compromise of subchondral bone blood flow. The large amount of observed apatite may thus simply reflect the rapidity of bone damage. Other hypotheses seem less plausible; for example that the condition results from non-steroidal anti-inflammatory drug usage and is a specific 'iatrogenic Charcot arthropathy'.

Mixed crystal deposition

Comparison of clinical and radiographic features of typical calcium pyrophosphate dihydrate and apatite associated arthropathies shows marked contrasts, though each clearly falls within the spectrum of 'osteoarthritis'. The finding of both calcium pyrophosphate dihydrate and apatite in the joints of some patients is common although there is little evidence that their combined presence is associated with particular clinical or radiographic characteristics.

Osteoarthritis at other joint sites

Selection of osteoarthritis for certain joint sites is striking. For example, compared to osteoarthritis of interphalangeal joints, hips, or knees, involvement of the elbow, glenohumeral joint, or ankle is relatively unusual and principally confined to the elderly.

Osteoarthritis of spinal apophyseal joints (particularly lower cervical and lower lumbar segments), first carpometacarpal, and/or first metatarsophalangeal joints is common and may occur as part of a pattern of generalized osteoarthritis (nodal or non-nodal) or as an isolated feature. In addition to nodal generalized osteoarthritis and trauma, suggested associations include:

- metatarsus primus varus and the first metatarsophalangeal joint;
- intervertebral disc degeneration and subsequent apophyseal joint osteoarthrosis;

As with other arthropathies, the predilection of osteoarthritis for certain sites remains unexplained. One intriguing, unifying hypothesis is that in all species the joints most commonly affected by osteoarthritis are in general those that have undergone the most rapid and recent evolutionary change.

In man these are the joints associated with bipedal locomotion and oppositional grip (Hutton 1987). Such joints may not have had sufficient evolutionary time to fully adapt to the tasks demanded of them. They therefore have insufficient mechanical reserve, and thus fatigue and 'fail' more commonly than joints that have had longer to adapt to their new function.

Osteoarthritis as part of other disease

If osteoarthritis represents the inherent repair process of synovial joints, then it would be expected to occur during certain phases of other defined arthropathies. For example, in rheumatoid arthritis, osteophytosis, sclerosis, and remodelling often occurs as a late feature in established disease. In such instances 'osteoarthritis' can be viewed as an accompanying process of tissue response/repair rather than an acquired second condition.

The same considerations pertain to other inflammatory, metabolic, or structural arthropathies. Ochronosis and spondylo-epiphyseal dysplasia, for example, are sometimes included within the umbrella of osteoarthritis since many of their radiographic features are typical of osteoarthritis but of course many are not and are very distinctive. Similarly, endemic forms of osteoarthritis need consideration in their own right. For clinical purposes, however, it may still be useful to consider together conditions that may result in a non-inflammatory arthropathy with radiographic changes predominantly of osteoarthritis (Table 2) and an atypical presentation should lead one to search for a defined, possibly treatable underlying cause. In patients with 'osteoarthritis' one should consider specific predisposing factors when there is:

- premature onset osteoarthritis, that is, less than 45 years;
- an atypical joint distribution, for example, prominent metacarpophalangeal and radiocarpal involvement in haemochromatosis;
- premature onset of chondrocalcinosis, that is, less than 55 years;
- florid polyarticular chondrocalcinosis at any age.

Investigations

Osteoarthritis is a diagnosis made on clinical and radiological grounds. To date there are no satisfactory diagnostic criteria or specific laboratory tests. Radiographic changes of osteoarthritis may often be asymptomatic and thus the problem is that even if osteoarthritis is present radiographically it may not be the cause of current symptoms. Investigations play little part in this decision, which should be made by thorough clinical assessment. Some investigations may be necessary to exclude alternative diagnoses or predisposing disease.

Osteoarthritis is not associated with extra-articular disease, synovitis is usually only mild or moderate, and overt immunological abnormality is not a feature. Changes reflecting an acute phase response [anaemia, thrombocytosis, elevated erythrocyte sedimentation rate, and/or C-reactive protein (CRP)] or overt immunological abnormality (autoantibodies, complement breakdown products) are therefore usually absent. However, evidence of a marked acute phase response occurs with pseudogout, and modest elevation of erythrocyte sedimentation rate and CRP may occur in the 'inflammatory' subsets of osteoarthritis, particularly chronic pyrophosphate arthropathy. A high normal range CRP measured using a highly sensitive assay may also be associated with an increased subsequent risk of disease progression. A search for predisposing metabolic or endocrine disease may be undertaken in selected patients with:

- atypical joint distribution;
- premature-onset of osteoarthritis;
- atypical radiographic features;
- early-onset or polyarticular chondrocalcinosis.

Such patients often have other clinical or radiographic clues as to an underlying diagnosis.

Imaging may be useful in determining the degree of structural change and may also identify chondrocalcinosis. Other techniques such as synovial fluid analysis and biochemical markers are of uncertain value in routine clinical practice.

Table 2 Principal conditions with presentations and radiographic changes that may simulate osteoarthritis

Generalized 'osteoarthritis'	(Spondylo-)epiphyseal dysplasia Ochronosis Haemochromatosis Wilson's disease Endemic osteoarthritis (e.g. Kashin–Beck disease)
Pauciarticular, large joint 'osteoarthritis'	Neuropathic joints syringomyelia—shoulders, wrists, elbows diabetes—hindfoot, midfoot tabes—knees, spine Acromegaly Avascular necrosis (mainly proximal and distal femur, proximal humerus)

Imaging

Imaging is used to establish the diagnosis and as an aid in planning the appropriateness and extent of surgical intervention. It may also be useful in excluding alternative diagnoses particularly if there is a sudden change in the character or severity of the pain. Methods include plain radiographs, magnetic resonance imaging, and possibly radioisotope scanning. The objective of the user determines the most appropriate modality. Generally techniques that demonstrate structural change do so at the expense of demonstrating current biochemical/physiological activity and vice versa. As discussed below, a possible exception to this may be magnetic resonance imaging.

Plain films

Radiographs give an anatomical picture, that is they demonstrate past structural change rather than current 'disease activity'. Bony structures are well defined but soft tissue imaging is uncertain. Cartilage is not directly visualized and its thickness has to be inferred by assuming that it comprises the vast majority of the interosseous distance between two articulating bones. Focal cartilage loss is very difficult to detect and the bony changes reflect relatively late pathological abnormalities. Nevertheless, the availability of plain radiographs and their widespread current and historical use in studying osteoarthritis make them still the principal imaging modality for diagnosis.

Joint space narrowing, osteophyte, sclerosis, and subchondral radiolucencies are the hallmark radiological signs of osteoarthritis (Fig. 22). A spectrum of changes exist for each of these features and there is no fixed correlation between one sign and another. Although no one feature has really been shown to have particular discriminatory value at all sites, osteophyte at the knee (Spector et al. 1993) and joint space narrowing at the hip (Croft et al. 1990) may be the best predictors of pain in population surveys. Additional features and complications may also be visualized including:

- effusions
- the osseous component of osteochondral ('loose') bodies
- joint alignment
- subluxations
- chondrocalcinosis
- collapse due to avascular necrosis

Absence of features of other arthritides is expected although the radiographic diagnosis of osteoarthritis does not exclude other coexisting disease.

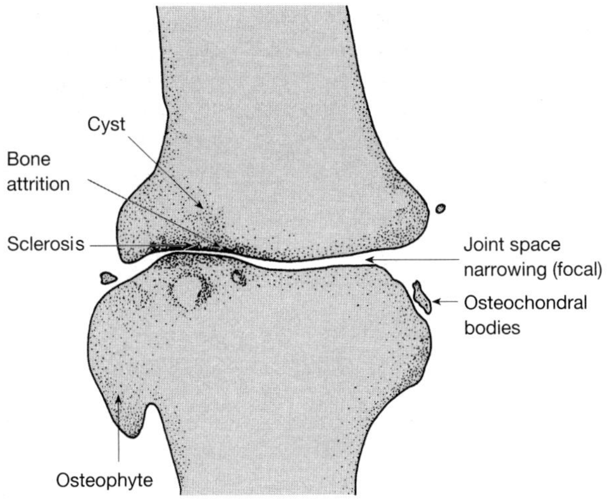

Fig. 22 Major radiographic features of osteoarthritis.

Plain radiography of specific joints

Hand

The pattern of involvement of the interphalangeal joints helps to distinguish osteoarthritis and erosive osteoarthritis from rheumatoid and psoriatic arthropathy. For this purpose a single posteroanterior view of the hand is usually satisfactory. The distinctive changes are (Fig. 23):

osteoarthritis: bone sclerosis, focal narrowing, and lateral subluxation unaccompanied by erosion;

erosive osteoarthritis: changes of osteoarthritis plus erosion through the subchondral bone plate, 'gull's wing' appearance;

rheumatoid arthritis: marginal 'bare area' erosions without bone proliferation ('non-proliferative erosions'); juxta-articular and generalized osteopaenia;

psoriatic arthritis: marginal erosions associated with bone/periosteal response ('proliferative erosions'); retained, or even locally increased, bone density.

Knee

Weight-bearing films of the knee show the more functional position of the limb and allow more precise information on the extent of joint space narrowing. However, the changes of fibrillation, cartilage narrowing, and cratering are focal. The use of semi-flexed ('Schuss') as opposed to extended standing views may better detect early narrowing which initially often occurs in a more posterior part of the femoral condyle. For serial measurements the problem of reproducible patient positioning, without resorting to fluoroscopy, may in part be overcome by careful positioning of the first metatarsophalangeal joints (Buckland-Wright et al. 1999). Patellofemoral joint views are also required and for diagnostic purposes either a lateral or skyline view may be taken. The 'skyline' view may be preferable if joint space progression needs to be assessed (Lanyon et al. 1996) although in routine clinical practice this is rarely required.

Hip

A single non-weight-bearing anteroposterior view of the pelvis is usually satisfactory and has the advantage of incorporating both hips on the same radiograph. Although gonadal dosage may be a problem with this view shielding can be used.

Sacroiliac joints

In the sacroiliac joints, osteophyte and joint space loss may need to be distinguished from inflammatory sacroiliitis. The latter gives erosion and intra-articular ankylosis, whereas osteoarthritis gives more focal joint space narrowing and focal sclerosis with overlying osteophytes. These are usually anterosuperior or inferior, and may be identified by discontinuity of trabecular lines across the joint in contrast to the continuous lines of ankylosis (Fig. 24). Although a coned posteroanterior view of the sacroiliac joints may be more sensitive than a single anteroposterior pelvis view the differentiation of these two clinical scenarios is usually made on clinical grounds.

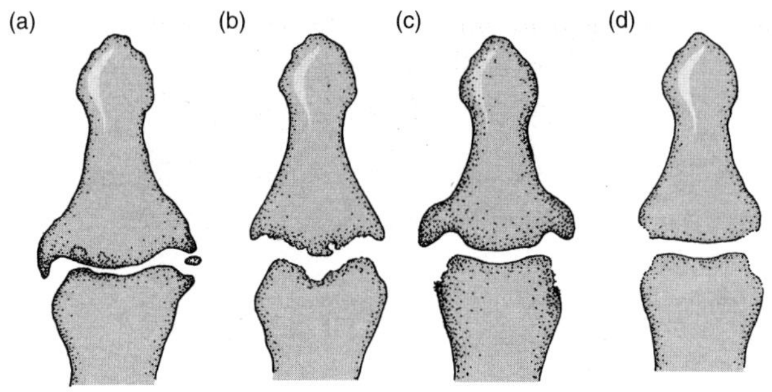

Fig. 23 The radiographic differences between (a) osteoarthritis, (b) erosive osteoarthritis, (c) psoriatic arthritis, and (d) rheumatoid arthritis.

Foot

As a common site of osteoarthritis a single posteroanterior radiograph of the foot is probably the simplest method required to demonstrate involvement of the first metatarsophalangeal joint. Specialized views are required to demonstrate involvement of mid-tarsal and ankle joints.

Spine

This can be a difficult area to assess for osteoarthritis. Changes suggestive of osteoarthritis (i.e. sclerosis, joint space narrowing, and osteophyte) are virtually universal in middle-aged and elderly adults. These are particularly evident in the lower cervical and lower lumbar spine and may involve the facet joints and in the cervical region the uncovertebral joints (the joints of Luschka). The precise views necessary to detect spinal osteoarthritis are not clear but lateral and anteroposterior lumbosacral and cervical views are probably the most appropriate.

Disease of the spine, particularly if it involves the facet joints with subsequent osteophytosis, may result in either foraminal compression of the nerve roots or canal stenosis. Although plain views, particularly if oblique foraminal views are taken, may demonstrate narrowing (Fig. 25), more specialized techniques such as magnetic resonance imaging or computed axial tomography ± myelography are usually required.

Standardization of the assessment of plain radiographs

Attempts to standardize and quantitate radiographic image analysis have utilized two approaches. The first is to compare study films against atlases of standard films (Kellgren and Lawrence 1957), and the second is to assess radiographic features, especially narrowing, using semi-automated and automated measurements. Using an atlas, two further approaches have been employed.

The first has attempted to produce a single a grade of osteoarthritis from a combination of different radiographic features. The use of such a 'global osteoarthritis' grade is attractive since it simplifies statistical analysis and means a joint is assigned to only one of a few radiographic grades. There are dangers with such an approach as already discussed above.

The alternative approach which has gained increasing favour is to grade for individual features of osteoarthritis such as osteophyte, joint space narrowing, cysts, and sclerosis. This has the advantage of not assuming a particular hierarchy of change or inter-relationship of features. However, a large amount of descriptive data is generated for each joint which is difficult to combine and can be problematic to analyse. Simply summating scores for each feature is probably not valid. No consensus has been reached as to which approach is preferable.

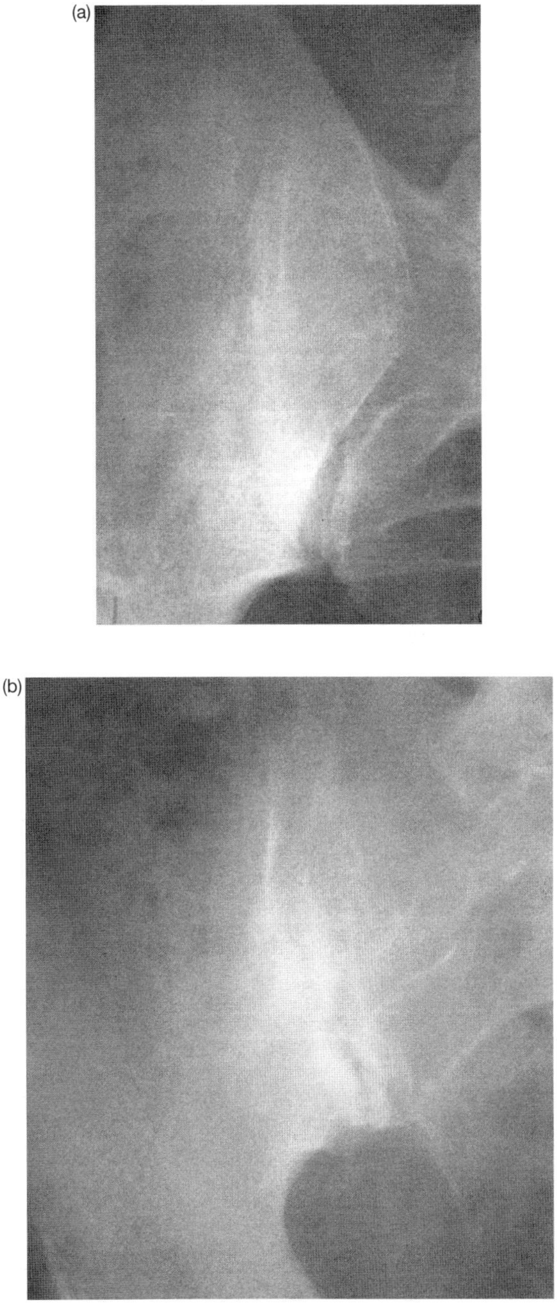

Fig. 24 (a) Sacroiliitis compared to (b) sacroiliac osteoarthritis.

In an attempt to reduce inter-observer error, various manual and semi-automated methods have been evaluated particularly in the measurement of joint space. For an individual radiograph such an approach may be very reproducible particularly if an automated computerized method is used. Problems still remain regarding the obtaining of reproducible radiographs upon which to make the measurements.

Modified radiographic techniques

Microfocal radiography is a magnification technique that allows higher resolution imaging, with the possibility of stereoscopic reconstruction. This technique appears particularly useful in showing early subchondral bone abnormalities and demonstrating small changes in joint space width over short periods of time (Buckland-Wright et al. 1990). Requirements of relatively long exposures and special equipment confine this method to a research tool but one which has particular potential in longitudinal studies.

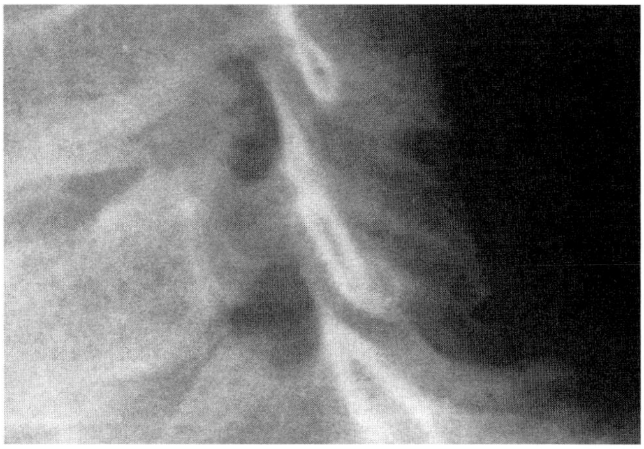

Fig. 25 Foraminal osteophytic encroachment in the neck of a patient who presented complaining of intermittent numbness and paraesthesia of the right arm.

Some of the limitations of plain films can be overcome by computed axial tomography which produces cross-sectional images and avoids the problems of interpreting overlying structures. Radiation exposure is, however, increased.

Magnetic resonance imaging

This method uses the properties of hydrogen ions, principally those in water. Since cartilage contains a high proportion of water, it can allow cartilage to be imaged. The potential and limitations of this modality in respect to osteoarthritis are still being explored (Burgkart et al. 2001) but many of the previous limitations are being overcome such as:

- resolution issues by using more powerful magnets and surface coils;
- the differentiation of cartilage, synovial fluid and synovium by using specialized sequences and contrast agents;
- claustrophobia by using peripheral or open scanners;
- lengthy scanning times by shortening image acquisition time by using more powerful magnets or better sequencing protocols.

In addition magnetic resonance imaging enables the imaging of soft-tissue structures such as menisci that may be invaluable in differentiating the causes of knee pain. However, cost and the access to scanning time remains a problem in many health care systems.

Radionuclide studies

Isotope bone scans give information on perfusion and bone synthetic activity. The mechanism of bone uptake is non-specific, but is more sensitive than radiographs at identifying involvement. It may detect abnormalities before radiographic signs are identified, and identify patients with 'active' disease who may go on to show progression (Dieppe et al. 1993). Its role in the clinical management of patients has not yet been established.

Potential markers of tissue destruction, inflammation, and repair in osteoarthritis

There is continuing interest in measuring biochemical markers in synovial fluid or serum to:

- allow the diagnosis of diseases
- follow progression of disease

- determine response to treatment
- determine disease prognosis and mechanism.

Although there are no clearly identified markers that definitively allow any of these parameters to be followed recent progress has allowed the contribution of individual tissues to be monitored (Garnero et al. 2000). Osteoarthritis involves active cellular processes of biosynthetic activity and matrix turnover and measurement of different markers from the synovium, cartilage or bone could allow these processes to be monitored. Such studies are based on two assumptions:

- When cartilage or bone is damaged there is a loss of matrix components, cytokines, or proteinases into synovial fluid, the lymphatic system, serum, and urine.
- This loss is quantitative, with changes in concentration reflecting changes in rates of turnover.

The first of these assumptions is proven but data to support the second are confounded by unknown physiological variables. For example, the concentration of fragments in synovial fluid depends not only on the rate of release from cartilage, but also on the volume and turnover of joint fluid and the speed of lymphatic drainage (all difficult to quantify). Similar problems apply to measurements in serum or urine. Although they are more readily accessible compartments, the concentrations in them reflect release from all joints (normal and abnormal) and from other cartilage sites. Selective, rapid elimination by the lymph nodes or liver, and the possible influence of renal and liver disease further complicate interpretation (see Fig. 26). Finally, it is essential to know what a 'marker' signifies in terms of joint physiology: a reduction in the concentration of a cartilage marker after an intervention may be interpreted as reduced cartilage breakdown, it may signify inhibition of matrix synthesis or reflect the absence of any remaining cartilage within the joint.

A variety of markers have been measured in osteoarthritic patients and these include cytokines, proteoglycan and glycosaminoglycan fragments, collagen fragments or crosslinks, and proteinases and inhibitors. The origin of these components and the way in which they can be processed in different body compartments (e.g. joint fluid, lymphatics, serum, and urine) is illustrated in Fig. 26. Some markers can be specific for different tissues within the joint such as synovium, cartilage or bone and examples of different markers and the tissues that produce them are listed in Table 3.

Although many biochemical products have been investigated (Table 4) none is yet of proven value in clinical practice.

Diagnosis

The diagnosis of osteoarthritis is essentially clinical and many comments regarding this have already been made in the section on investigations. There are several different clinical problems.

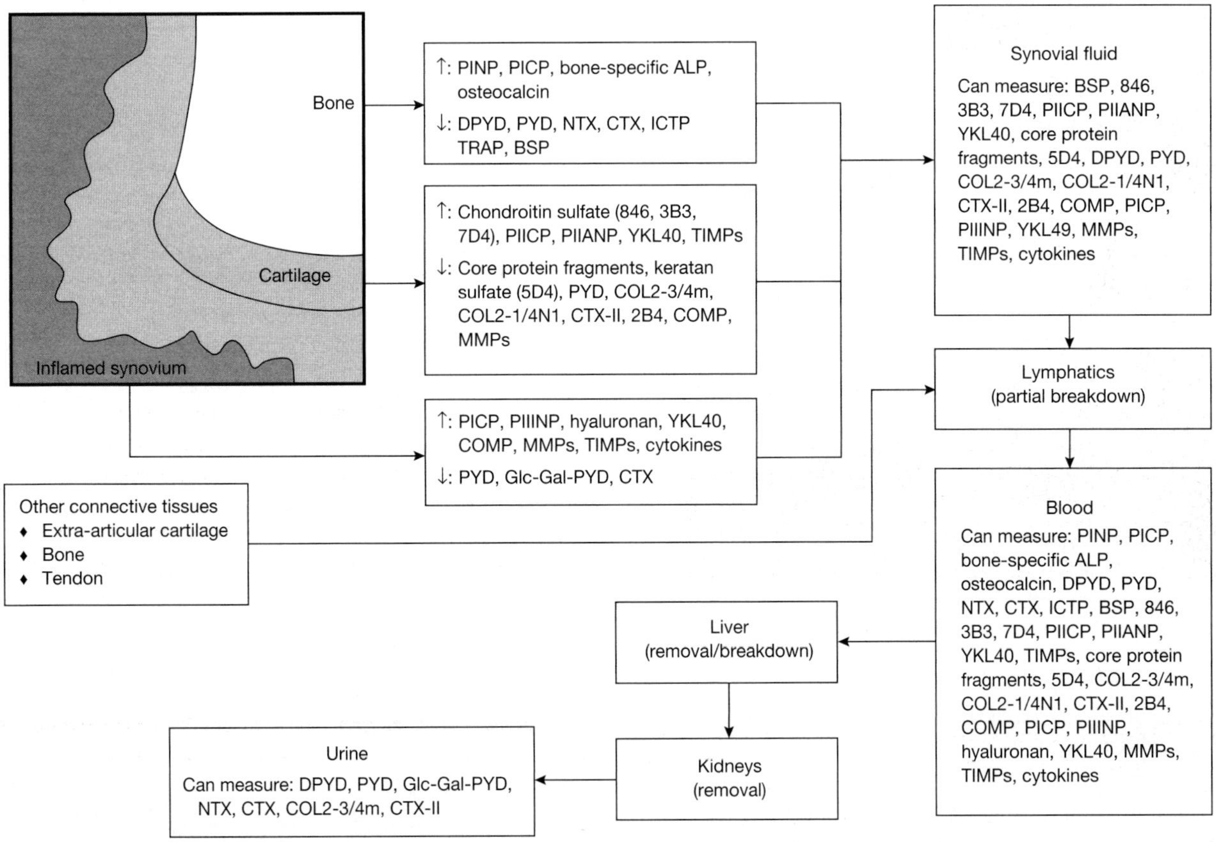

Fig. 26 Potential 'markers' of the osteoarthritic process. (PINP = amino-terminal type I procollagen propeptide; PICP = carboxy-terminal type I procollagen propeptide; bone-specific ALP = bone-specific alkaline phosphatase; DPYD = deoxypyridinoline; PYD = pyridinoline; Glc-Gal-PYD = glucosyl-galactosyl-pyridinoline; NTX = type I collagen *N*-terminal telopeptide; CTX = type I collagen *C*-terminal telopeptide-2; ICTP = type I collagen *C*-terminal telopeptide-1; TRAP = plasma tartrate resistant acid phosphatase; BSP = bone sialoprotein; 846, 3B3, and 7D4 = chondroitin sulfate epitopes; PIICP = carboxy-terminal type II procollagen propeptide; PIIANP = amino-terminal type IIA procollagen propeptide; 5D4 and AN9P1 = keratan sulfate epitopes; COL2-3/4m and COL2-1/4N1 = collagen type II neoepitopes; CTX-II = type II collagen *C*-terminal telopeptide; COMP = cartilage oligomeric protein; MMPs = matrix metalloproteinases; TIMP = tissue inhibitor of metalloproteinases; PIIINP = amino-terminal type III procollagen propeptides.)

Table 3 Physiological correlates of matrix markers of tissue destruction, inflammation, and repair in osteoarthritis and rheumatoid arthritis

Matrix component	Marker	Synthesis	Breakdown
Synovium	Types I and III collagen	Procollagen peptides PICP, PIIIANP	PYD GLc-Gal-PYD CTX
	Non-collagen protein	Hyaluronan YKL-40 COMP MMP-1, 2, 3, 9 TIMP-1, -2	
Cartilage	Aggrecan	Chondroitin sulfate 846, 3B3, 7D4	Core protein fragments Keratan sulfate 5D4, AN9P1
	Type II collagen	Procollagen propeptides PIICP, PIIANP	Crosslinks PYD Collagenase epitopes COL2-3/4m COL2-1/4N1 Collagen II telopeptides CTX-II
	Other proteins	YKL-40	Compaq
Bone	Type I collagen	Procollagen peptides PINP, PICP	Crosslinks DPYD, PYD Telopeptides NTX, CTX, ICTP
	Non-collagenous proteins	Bone-specific ALP Osteocalcin	TRAP BSP

Table 4 Measurement of matrix markers of tissue destruction, inflammation, and repair

Assay	Advantages	Disadvantages
Where?		
Serum	Easy collection All patients with consent	Dilution of marker Contribution from other tissues
Synovial fluid	Local to inflamed joint Reflect changes in single joint	Infrequent aspiration Small proportion of patients Low levels may result when large volumes of fluid produced
Urine		Difficult to collect 24 h urine Final level depends on clearance rate in other compartments May not reflect overall disease activity
How?		
Immunoassay	Measurement of total level	Also measures non-functional proteins
Activity assay	Measures 'active' protein	Inhibitors often also present; sample may require further fractionation
Fluorescent assay	Measure activity in serum even when complexed to α2M (Beekman et al. 1996)	Will not be specific for individual enzymes

Note: Low levels may result when most of the cartilage tissue has been destroyed.

The patient with pain

This is the commonest clinical situation. The priorities in this situation are to determine whether:

- 'osteoarthritis' is the cause of the symptoms;
- there is an articular or periarticular cause for the pain;
- there are predisposing or adverse factors for the development or progression of osteoarthritis;
- there is another underlying arthropathy;
- there are other factors that are modifying the pain experience (e.g. psychological factors, social issues).

Resolving these difficulties depends on a careful clinical history and examination; radiography and laboratory investigations play a relatively minor role. The examination aims to:

- localize the site of the pain—joint line or periarticular;
- detect the presence of clinical signs of osteoarthritis—crepitus, bony swelling, restricted range of motion;
- define any adverse features—obesity, malalignment, reduced strength, abnormal usage (occupational or habitual);
- rule out features of other arthropathy—rheumatoid arthritis, gout, seronegative arthropathy;
- determine factors which might be affecting recovery—coexistent fibromyalgia, depression, sleep disturbance.

The radiograph merely helps to confirm the presence of the structural change but since the radiograph is relatively insensitive, particularly in early disease, a normal radiograph does not rule out a diagnosis of osteoarthritis. Conversely, as has already been discussed, an abnormal radiograph is not necessarily the cause of symptoms.

The radiographic findings

It is not uncommon for patients to have radiographs taken following an acute episode of pain or trauma, particularly of the spine, and for osteoarthritic changes to be discovered. The difficulty then lies in knowing what, if anything to do regarding these findings. Undue emphasis on the structural changes can result in patients being unduly alarmed and adopting inappropriate illness behaviour. Again a careful clinical history and examination is necessary to determine the association between the current clinical problem and any structural change with accurate and effective communication necessary to prevent misinterpretation of the situation.

Neurological findings

Neurological finding are important, particularly in the lumbar and cervical spine where osteophytosis of the facet or apophyseal joint may lead to foraminal encroachment and subsequent nerve root compression. Peripheral nerve entrapment may also occur as a result of osteophytosis or synovitis of peripheral joints. Possible sites for this are the ulnar nerve at the ulnar groove and the median nerve in the carpal tunnel. In such a situation, particularly in the spine, magnetic resonance imaging and/or nerve conduction studies are required to fully elucidate the nature, site, and presence of nerve compression.

As well as direct pressure on a nerve, vascular claudication may also occur, particularly in the lumbar spine. In this situation, exercise results in neurological symptoms and signs in the legs. The diagnosis is essentially based on the history but evidence of canal and/or foraminal stenosis is sought, usually with magnetic resonance imaging.

In all situations, particularly in the spine, it is essential to ensure that there is a good match between clinical findings and demonstrated structural abnormalities.

Pathogenesis

The nature of osteoarthritis

It has been widely suggested that osteoarthritis is a process, rather than a disease, that shows variability in outcome. Support for this comes from several considerations:

- osteoarthritis has accompanied man throughout his evolutionary history;
- a similar process occurs in other animals that have fused epiphyses in the adult;
- radiographic osteoarthritis is very common in adults, showing increased frequency with age;
- in most instances osteoarthritis occurs without symptoms or disability, and its radiographic presence is not necessarily the explanation of locomotor pain;
- symptoms relating to osteoarthritis are often phasic and may not necessarily be associated with a poor prognosis.

Such phylogenetic preservation, discordance between symptoms and structural change, and generally good outcome suggest that osteoarthritis reflects the inherent repair process of synovial joints (Fig. 27). In most cases this metabolically active process keeps pace with a variety of triggering insults and is non-progressive. In some, however, it fails to compensate, resulting in 'joint failure' (decompensated osteoarthritis) with perceived symptoms and disability. This interpretation partly explains the marked heterogeneity of osteoarthritis. A wide variety of 'insults' can trigger a repair reaction but each results in a different pattern of involvement.

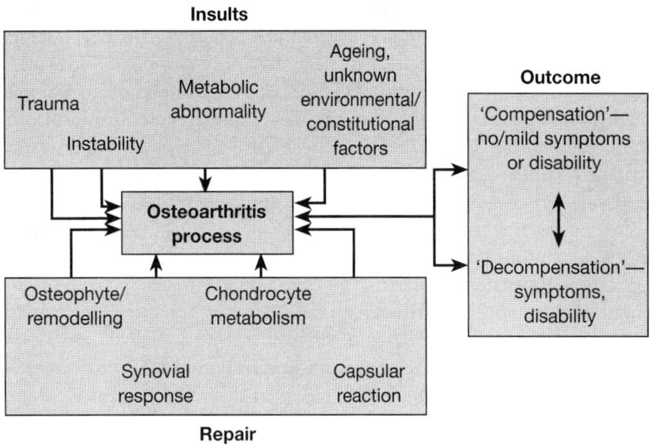

Fig. 27 Diagrammatic representation of osteoarthritis as the inherent repair process of synovial joints.

As with any biological process, multiple constitutional and environmental factors may further modify the response, leading to variable outcome.

The mechanical, genetic, and metabolic factors that may 'insult' the joint and thus trigger the osteoarthritis process have been discussed above. Indeed most evidence regarding the initiation of osteoarthritis in man derives from such studies since diagnosis of the early stages of sporadic osteoarthritis *in vivo* is currently not possible. The response of the joint to these insults has been studied by a variety of methods including *in vivo* animal models, *ex vivo* studies on tissue explants, and from pathological human tissue. The results from such studies and the insights which they give into the nature of osteoarthritis are discussed below.

Structure and metabolism of osteoarthritic tissues

Investigation of human osteoarthritis tissue is problematic: pathological studies often focus on surgical specimens of late 'end-stage' osteoarthritis, whilst cadaveric studies examining 'early' osteoarthritis lack clinical correlates. All such studies are confounded by the heterogeneity of osteoarthritis and by restriction to single time point examination. Much work on pathophysiology therefore derives from animal models and *in vitro* experiments. Animal models often employ small quadrupeds, utilize invasive mechanical or chemical insult to stimulate joint response, or investigate hereditary forms of premature joint failure. The time scale is often short and immature rather than mature animals may be used. Although some models (e.g. cruciate section in the adult dog) appear closer to human osteoarthritis than others their relevance is still disputed. Rather than exact models of osteoarthritis, they are probably best viewed as a means of studying, in a well defined and controlled situation, dynamic biochemical and structural events at the earliest stages of joint insult. Thus, while animal models and human studies *in vitro* provide useful insights, caution is required in drawing together the available disparate data to develop a more complete understanding of pathophysiology relevant to human osteoarthritis.

Structural changes

The histological changes characteristic of osteoarthritis cartilage from humans and animal models are well described and include:

- reduction in stainable proteoglycan
- fibrillation
- collagen crimping
- chondrocyte multiplication or migration (cloning)
- loss of cartilage (Plate 185)

Initially, localized areas of softening present a pebbled texture at the surface, followed by disruption along collagen fibre planes (tangential 'flaking', vertical 'fibrillation'). At the earliest stage of surface erosion and irregularity cartilage appears moderately hypercellular with alteration in staining quality of the matrix; the tide-mark may also show irregularities and violation by blood vessels. As increasingly deep clefts form in cartilage, nearby matrix is depleted of metachromatic material indicating loss of proteoglycans. Microscopic changes are also apparent in cells, and necrosis ('ghosting') is often present. More common, however, is focal proliferation producing clumps ('clones') of chondrocytes, often surrounded by intense metachromatic material indicating increased proteoglycan. Such cell proliferation and metabolic activity represents attempted 'intrinsic' repair. With continuing movement fibrillated cartilage in habitually loaded areas may abrade to expose underlying bone, with progression to variable degrees of structural damage. It is noteworthy, however, that fibrillation itself is not necessarily progressive. Indeed, it is a normal finding in adult human joints (e.g. hip, knee, humeroradial joint) in areas of cartilage that are habitually unloaded.

In addition to intrinsic repair, 'extrinsic' repair commonly occurs by formation of new cartilage at the joint margin or in subchondral bone; such cartilage is generally more cellular than pre-existing hyaline cartilage and the chondrocytes are evenly distributed throughout the matrix. Extrinsic repair is with fibrocartilage, containing predominently type I collagen. Proliferating nodules of fibrocartilage arising from underlying marrow spaces may protrude through defects in the bone surface, occasionally coalescing to form a near continuous layer of replacement tissue.

In parallel with the cartilage changes, new bone formation occurs in subchondral bone and at the joint margins (central and marginal osteophyte), and occasionally beneath adjacent periosteum (e.g. femoral neck 'buttressing'—periosteal osteophyte). Osteophyte forms through the process of endochondral ossification, either by vascular penetration of existing cartilage or from marginal foci of cartilaginous metaplasia, particularly at capsular and ligamentous insertion sites. The location of osteophyte is characteristic for individual joints. Proliferation of subchondral bone is most apparent beneath areas of cartilage erosion and fibrillation. In such areas the tidemark is generally more irregular, thickened, and reduplicated (showing often three or more parallel tidemarks); new bone and thickening of existing trabeculas gives rise to sclerosis seen radiographically. With gross cartilage loss repeated motion may polish the bone ('eburnation') and, as a result of increased local stress, surface bone additionally may undergo focal pressure necrosis.

Subarticular cysts (more correctly 'pseudocysts') predominate where overlying cartilage is thinned or absent. Pathologically, cysts show features of bone necrosis (loss of trabeculae, fibromyxomatous degeneration of marrow), frequently contain dead bone, cartilage, and amorphous material, and are surrounded by a rim of reactive new bone and fibrous tissue. They are thought to result from high intra-articular pressure transmitted through defects (microfractures) in the overlying cortex, or from intraosseous hypertension generated through abnormal loading and force transmission in the mechanically altered joint. As with fibrillation, both marginal osteophyte and cysts may occur in the absence of other features of osteoarthritis, reflecting bone response to mechanical stimulation.

Separated fragments of cartilage and bone may form 'loose bodies', undergo dissolution, or become incorporated into the synovium and proliferate locally. As they grow, their centres necrose and calcify, and periodic extensions give rise to a concentric ringed appearance: endochondral ossification of these bodies may follow vascular invasion. Osteochondral bodies may also arise in synovium by chondroid metaplasia of fibroblastic cells.

The synovium becomes both hypertrophic and hyperplastic, and the capsule thickens and contracts. In the synovium lymphoid follicles, as well as more diffuse infiltration by T and B lymphocytes and macrophages (DR positive), may be identified (Revell et al. 1988), often with accompanying diffuse and perivascular fibrosis. Synovial extension onto the articular surface (i.e. pannus) is common, particularly at the hip, but both synovitis and pannus are less extensive and aggressive than in rheumatoid arthritis, synovitis usually being confined to synovium rimming the cartilage. Haemosiderin staining of synovium, reflecting previous intra-articular bleeding, is common in large joints, and occasionally is marked. The role of particulate debris (osteochondral fragments, calcium crystals) in producing chronic inflammation is uncertain but, in general, synovitis is regarded more as a secondary, usually late phenomenon than a primary, early event in osteoarthritis.

Calcification is an integral part of new bone formation, and many osteoarthritis joints show evidence of calcium crystal deposition in cartilage, with presumed secondary uptake in synovium. Carbonate-substituted hydroxyapatite is the commonest particulate identified, particularly adjacent to hypertrophic and degenerating chondrocytes (Ohira and Ishikawa 1987). Calcium pyrophosphate dihydrate crystal deposition is also associated with osteoarthritis at certain sites, particularly in the elderly. The precise relationship between calcium crystal formation and osteoarthritis is unclear (see earlier).

Despite loss of bone and cartilage in some parts of the joint, the net effect of new cartilage and bone formation is an increase in joint size and remodelling of shape. The balance between degradative and reparative features is variable and leads to varying consequences with respect to joint congruity, stability, and load transmission. Associated periarticular abnormalities (muscle atrophy, bursitis, enthesitis) are a common accompaniment to established osteoarthritis. The radiographical–pathological correlations seen in osteoarthritis are outlined in Table 1.

Metabolic changes

Though changes occur in all joint tissues in osteoarthritis, most experimental work has investigated cartilage. The extracellular matrix of cartilage is complex, and its composition and turnover vary:

- in different joints;
- at different locations within the same joint;
- through the depth of the tissue.

The initiating insult (e.g. mechanical, metabolic) also varies and age-related changes occur. It is sometimes, therefore, difficult to identify common events in osteoarthritis (Table 5).

Analytical studies

The changes in composition of osteoarthritis cartilage, which are markedly different from those due to ageing, include:

- an increase in water content;
- a loosening of the 'collagen network' with a reduction in collagen fibre size, though the collagen concentration and phenotypes appear normal;
- a reduction in proteoglycan concentration with a smaller proportion of total proteoglycan in aggregates, and alteration in proteoglycan structure.

Whereas ageing human cartilage undergoes some degree of dehydration, osteoarthritis cartilage has an increased water content. This increase is one of the earliest changes detected in animal models, initially within loaded regions but eventually involving all of the cartilage. This change probably reflects a defect in the arrangement of collagen fibres that allows proteoglycans to swell. The marked swelling of osteoarthritic cartilage when placed in hypotonic solutions *in vitro* is consistent with a loosening of the collagen network, and ultrastructural studies using animal models confirm early loss of orientation among superficial collagen fibrils, with individual fibrils being more widely spaced than normal. This basic structural change may arise in type II collagen fibres themselves (Maroudas et al. 1986), or more likely in cross-link molecules such as type IX collagen, a decrease of which (with little change in production) is reported in the rabbit postmeniscectomy model and in human osteoarthritis. This increase in swelling can be mimicked by treatment of cartilage with stromelysin indicating that proteolytic attack within the telopeptide regions may account for the changes in the collagen fibril that allows the proteoglycan to swell (Bonassar et al. 1995).

Table 5 Metabolic changes in osteoarthritic cartilage

General	Increased hydration Increased swelling Loss of tensile strength Increased biosynthesis of proteoglycan and collagen in early disease and decreased in late disease Increased rates of matrix turnover with net loss of proteoglycan and collagen
Specific collagens	Initial swelling of collagen fibrillar network Net loss of type II collagen Specific cleavage of collagen by collagenases Loss of tensile strength Type III and X collagen can be synthesized Increased content collagen type IV
Proteoglycans	Increased extractability Decreased monomer size Specific cleavages produced early by aggrecanases and later by MMPs Diminished/normal aggregation Increased rate of maturation of hyaluronate-binding region Loss of decorin from surface layers
Cytokines, proteinases, and inhibitors	Increase in proinflammatory cytokines Increase in aggrecanases, MMPs, and cathepsins Decrease in overall inhibitor levels

A decrease in proteoglycan content is the most consistent feature found in all studies of osteoarthritis. The main finding for glycosaminoglycans in human osteoarthritic cartilage is a decrease in keratan sulfate content. This is a real event, not merely reflecting a decrease in cartilage thickness (the deeper layers of normal cartilage are richer in keratan sulfate than the surface zones). The concomitant decrease in chondroitin-6-sulfate relative to chondroitin-4-sulfate gives an overall composition akin to that of immature cartilage, suggesting that, in osteoarthritis, chondrocytes revert to a chondroblastic state and synthesize foetal-like, immature proteoglycan. Because of the uncertainty over the production of the proteoglycan, however, it remains unclear in established human osteoarthritis if such changes are biosynthetic or arise primarily from catabolic events.

Changes in keratan sulfate : chondroitin-6/-4-sulfate ratios are an inconsistent finding in animal models, and such changes may principally occur late in the pathogenesis. Specific modifications in the sulfation of chondroitin sulfate chains, however, appear early in animal models (at 3 months in Pond–Nuki model) and may relate to larger chain size. In addition, proteoglycans from cartilage with activated chondrocytes react with monoclonal antibodies to novel sequences of sulfation on chondroitin sulfate chains with similar epitopes being detected in proteoglycan from human osteoarthritis and normal immature cartilage. The significance of these structural changes in chondroitin sulfate is unknown, though one function may be to increase matrix binding of growth factors, thereby increasing the local pool of these agents.

There is little evidence from animal or human studies to suggest that proteoglycan is lost from the matrix through any abnormalities in its ability to aggregate. Aggregation of proteoglycan appears to be normal, and although the hyaluronan content of osteoarthritic cartilage is reportedly low, there appears sufficient to accommodate the reduced concentration of proteoglycan (Brocklehurst et al. 1984). The hyaluronan-binding regions of most proteoglycan monomers in osteoarthritic cartilage appear fully functional. In most animal models this also applies to newly synthesized proteoglycans, even though they are often larger than normal. In cartilage from late-stage human osteoarthritis, the assembly of newly synthesized proteoglycans into aggregates in the extracellular matrix appears faster than in normal adult joints, and more similar to that in immature cartilage. This aspect of proteoglycan structure could profoundly affect turnover rates and complicate further our understanding of mechanisms of cartilage repair.

Growth factors and cytokines

Matrix synthesis

Within arthritic tissues there are areas of cartilage where synthesis of new matrix takes place and areas where net loss of the extracellular matrix occurs. A variety of growth factors and cytokines act on chondrocytes to alter the rate of proliferation and either the synthesis or degradation of matrix components (van den Berg 1999; Goldring 2000). A number of cytokines and growth factors are listed together with the possible effect on matrix metabolism (Table 6). Many of these agents act together to alter the composition of the matrix in osteoarthritic cartilage and recent data suggest that they play an active role in altering the balance between matrix synthesis and degradation.

Cartilage metabolism may be influenced by effects on cellular proliferation, migration or differentiation and the control of individual genes. The effect of any particular growth factor will also depend on the state of differentiation of the cell. Other local conditions will affect the response of the tissues such as mechanical loading, oxygen tension, and the presence of other stimulating factors.

TGF-β increases the synthesis of matrix components by chondrocytes (Blumenfeld and Livne 1999) and TGF-β can down-regulate the production of matrix-degrading proteinases and up-regulate proteinase inhibitors such as TIMP-1 or plasminogen activator inhibitor. This suggests that this may prevent cartilage destruction by both stimulating synthesis and blocking breakdown pathways. This growth factor is locally synthesized by chondrocytes. IGF-1 mimics many of the actions of TGF-β and has a significant effect on matrix synthesis. Within the cartilage, TGF-β and IGF-1 are stored in considerable quantity bound to different matrix components. Thus the source of these growth factors will vary. They can be produced by cells outside the cartilage and diffuse in, they can be produced locally by the chondrocytes or released from the matrix as it is degraded. The control mechanisms are complex. Growth factors also exist in a latent form and other proteins may be present, such as binding proteins, that sequester the factors and prevent them from binding to cellular receptors.

Growth factors are recognized as protective to cartilage, stimulating matrix synthesis and blocking the effects of the proinflammatory cytokines. All these growth factors (Table 6) are likely to stimulate repair within cartilage and many do not act alone but rather act synergistically to promote new matrix synthesis.

Table 6 Effect of cytokines and growth factors on chondrocyte metabolism

Growth factor	Major function in cartilage metabolism
Anabolic	
TGFβ (β1, β2, β3)	Chondrocyte proliferation, matrix synthesis, modulates effect of IL-1 Increases proteinase inhibitors
FGF (2, 4, 8)	Proliferation and differentiation of chondrocytes MMP production
PDGF	Proliferation of chondrocytes
Bone morphogenetic proteins (2, 4, 6, 7, 9, 13)	Increase matrix synthesis
IGF-1	Increases GAG and collagen synthesis Protects cartilage from effects of proinflammatory cytokines
Catabolic	
IL-1	Increases MMPs, PGE2, and other cytokines Inhibits GAG synthesis
TNFα	Similar catabolic effects to IL-1
Oncostatin M	Combines with IL-1 and TNFα to promote matrix breakdown Increases matrix synthesis and proteinase inhibitors Can increase MMPs
IL-17	Stimulates GAG and collagen release, increases MMPs Increases expression of IL-1β and IL-6
IL-18	Increases expression of IL-1β and IL-6, increases MMPs
Regulatory	
IL-6	Increases proteinase inhibitor production and proliferation of chondrocytes Acts on chondrocytes when soluble receptor is present
IL-4, IL-13	Oppose effects of proinflammatory cytokines
IL-1 receptor antagonist	Blocks effects of IL-1
Interferon γ	Opposes effects of proinflammatory cytokines

Chondrocytes can increase their biosynthesis to counteract increased loss, particularly early rather than late in the process. For example in the Pond–Nuki model (section of the anterior cruciate ligament in the mature canine stifle joint), chondrocytes from macroscopically normal cartilage show increased incorporation of ^{35}S-sulfate as an early feature that predates fibrillation, and other areas of cartilage that do not proceed to fibrillation may also show this change. In other models early hypermetabolic activity cannot be demonstrated.

In established human osteoarthritis, the variability in proteoglycan synthesis reported from different centres (i.e. increased or normal) may reflect sampling differences as much as variability of osteoarthritis itself. For example in reports of increased ^{35}S-sulfate incorporation by human osteoarthritic cartilage, with correlation between synthetic activity and histological grading (Ryu et al. 1984), the high-scoring samples could be mainly mid- and deep-zone cartilage, which in normal tissue contains cells with higher synthetic rates. After 'correcting' for topographical and zonal sampling, no difference in proteoglycan synthesis was apparent between osteoarthritic and normal, age-matched cartilage at the hip or knee (Brocklehurst et al. 1984).

Chondrocytes show an increased rate of synthesis of type II collagen early in animal models. The long turnover time of type II collagen in adult cartilage might suggest that mature chondrocytes have little chance of even minimal repair of defective collagen network. Nevertheless, an increase in collagen synthesis in human osteoarthritic cartilage has been demonstrated. When type II collagen fibrils form in the extracellular matrix, the N- and C-propeptides (CP-II) are removed by specific proteases and are lost from the matrix: increased CP-II is found in human osteoarthritic compared to normal cartilage, mainly in the lower mid- and deep zones rather than the surface and upper mid zones where collagen degradation is more prevalent (Dodge and Poole 1989). There may thus be the potential for limited repair in deep zones, but an effective response in late osteoarthritis, when major disruption in collagen architecture has occurred, seems less likely.

Type X collagen, with its presumed role in mineralization, is regarded as a unique marker for hypertrophic chondrocytes, which are also rich in alkaline phosphatase activity. In osteoarthritic cartilage the alkaline phosphatase activity is very high, not just in the deep but also in the mid-zones (Plate 186), and deposition of type X collagen once again becomes evident. Such characteristics are reminiscent of immature cartilage, and suggest that chondrocytes throughout the cartilage are resuming their potential to mineralize. Other genes associated with the growth plate and endochondral ossification are also upregulated in osteoarthritic tissues.

Matrix degradation

Just as anabolic growth factors can influence matrix synthesis, the proinflammatory cytokines can increase matrix degradation. Both interleukin 1 and tumour necrosis factor are present in osteoarthritic joints in which the extracellular matrix is degraded (see Table 6) (Hamerman 1989; Goldring 2000). These cytokines when added to cartilage rapidly cause the release of proteoglycan with the later release of collagen fragments (Ellis et al. 1994) and at the same time the synthesis of matrix components is also down regulated. The release of matrix fragments is accelerated when cytokines are combined; oncostatin M is especially effective in combination with the proinflammatory cytokines (Cawston et al. 1998).

Extracellular matrix proteins are broken down by different proteolytic pathways. There are four main classes of proteinases, cysteine, serine, aspartate, and metallo- which are classified according to the chemical group which participates in the hydrolysis of peptide bonds. The pathway that predominates will vary with different resorptive situations and often a complex interplay between different cell types is involved (e.g. bone resorption) that use different classes of proteinases. In osteoarthritis the proteinases produced by chondrocytes are thought to be most important in cartilage breakdown with some contribution from synovial cells.

Collagen release

The proteinases responsible for the release of collagen are the matrix metalloproteinases (MMPs) (Brinkerhoff et al. 1991). Levels of this enzyme family are increased in response to proinflammatory cytokines (Murphy et al. 1991) and they are present in diseased synovial fluids (Cawston et al. 1983).

Cartilage collagen breakdown can be blocked by tissue inhibitors of metalloproteinases (TIMPs). MMPs are a family of zinc and calcium dependant proteinases that degrade the proteins of the extracellular matrix at neutral pH and are divided into four main groups—the collagenases, the stromelysins, the gelatinases, and the membrane-type MMPs (MT-MMPs) (Plate 187) (Vincenti et al. 1994; Nagase and Woessner 1999). These enzymes contain common sequences of amino acids. The N-terminal domain contains a characteristic sequence of zinc-binding histidines and contains the catalytic zinc whilst the C-terminal domain binds to different ECM components and determines the differences in substrate specificity. The MMPs are potent enzymes and so are controlled at different points (Plate 188) which include the stimulation of synthesis and secretion by cytokines, activation of proenzyme forms, and the inhibition by specific inhibitors called TIMPs (Cawston 1996; Brew et al. 2000). The collagenases MMP-1, -8, and -13 can all cleave collagen at the $\frac{3}{4}/\frac{1}{4}$ position but differ in their ability to cleave different types of collagen. As MMP-13 is most efficient at degrading type II collagen and specific inhibitors block the release of collagen from osteoarthritic cartilage this enzyme is thought to be important in collagen breakdown in osteoarthritic cartilage (Dahlberg et al. 2000). However all three collagenases are present in osteoarthritic cartilage (Shlopov et al. 1997; Tetlow et al. 2001) and all probably contribute to cartilage breakdown. In addition to MMPs being present in osteoarthritic cartilage and synovial fluid, osteoarthritic cartilage is deficient in endogenous protease inhibitors such as the TIMPs (Dean et al. 1989). This imbalance between matrix metalloproteinases and their inhibitors is likely to play a part in the accelerated breakdown of the matrix (Dean et al. 1989; Hamerman 1989). Specific inhibitors of matrix metalloproteinases prevent collagen release from resorbing cartilage *in vitro* and in animal models (Andrews et al. 1992; Cawston et al. 1994). Other proteinases that belong to the cysteine proteinase family are also implicated in the destruction of cartilage collagen in osteoarthritis (Buttle et al. 1993). A recent study by Keyszer et al. suggested that the production of mRNA for the cysteine proteinases cathepsin B and L was less pronounced compared to that for the MMPs in osteoarthritic synovial tissue as compared to rheumatoid synovial tissue (Keyszer et al. 1998). The cysteine proteinase, cathepsin K, is produced by osteoclasts and responsible for much of the collagen I cleavage during the turnover of bone matrix. No conclusive studies have been published that demonstrate a role for this enzyme in osteoarthritic bone although there is clear evidence for a role for cathepsin K in rheumatoid arthritis (Hummel et al. 1998).

Proteoglycan turnover

Recent studies have shown that a proteinase family, closely related to the MMPs, is also implicated in cartilage biology and in the turnover of the matrix particularly in relation to proteoglycan turnover. ADAMs (*a disintegrin and metalloproteinase*) are usually membrane anchored, multi-domain proteinases that are associated with cell–cell fusion and with the shedding of cell surface proteins when a metalloproteinase domain is present. The enzymes responsible for proteoglycan turnover belong to the ADAM-ts (*a disintegrin and metalloproteinase with thrombospondin domains*) family (Tang 2001) and members are distinguished from other ADAMs in that they have additional thrombospondin-1 domains (which can number up to 13) predominantly at the *C*-terminus which are thought to mediate interactions with the extracellular matrix. ADAM-ts4 and ADAM-ts5 were recently described (Tortorella et al. 2001) as aggrecanases and these enzymes are thought to be responsible for cleavage of proteoglycan. Both of these enzymes can cleave cartilage proteoglycan at the specific site within the interglobular region to release the same epitopes that are found *in vivo* (Sandy et al. 1992). Other members of this family (e.g. ADAM-ts1) can also cleave at this same site and an enzyme is present on the surface of chondrocytes that also cleaves aggrecan. It is not clear if this represents an ADAM-ts member tightly bound to the cell surface or a distinct enzyme (Billington et al. 1998). Many of the ADAM-ts family are inhibited by TIMP-3. ADAM-ts1 is upregulated by IL-1 but there is conflicting data for ADAM-ts4 and -5. It could be that the correct arrangement and activation of pre-existing enzymes at the cell surface, following cytokine stimulation, is the critical step that initiates proteoglycan turnover.

Recently, the analysis of the fragments released from resorbing cartilage have been studied in order to determine degradative mechanisms. A unique epitope hidden in native collagen but exposed by proteolytic cleavage has been successfully used to follow collagen turnover. In osteoarthritis, cartilage collagen cleavage can be shown by immunohistochemistry in both the superficial and intermediate zones (Poole 1993; Hollander et al. 1994). Studies have shown that the early lesion in osteoarthritic cartilage in terms of collagen cleavage occurs at the surface of the cartilage and then proceeds to the deeper layers (Hollander et al. 1994).

Debate still continues over the relative importance of cartilage and bone changes in the initiation and progression of osteoarthritis (Burr 1998). It is recognized that physiology and structure are intimately linked and that all joint tissues (including synovium, capsule, and periarticular tissues) interact together. Thus 'weakening' of cartilage and surrounding tissues and 'stiffening' of subchondral bone will each be deleterious in all tissues. All locomotor tissues require continuing physical stimulation to sustain normal development, nutrition, and adaptation. Interestingly, many of the metabolic and structural responses of cartilage and bone seen in animal models only develop if joint loading continues, suggesting that the potential repair process of joints is similarly driven by this physiological need. A more pressing question, of course, is what stops all joints progressing once cartilage loss and altered biomechanics have occurred. Articular cartilage has only a limited ability to 'repair' whereas bone is able to remodel and readily adapt to changing biochemical requirements. With respect to progression or non-progression in osteoarthritis, it may be that bone response (Burr 1998) and less investigated aspects (e.g. neuromuscular control, capsular fibrosis) will also prove to be important. With regard to bone it appears that it is the subchondral component that is altered at an early phase of osteoarthritis. The net effect of the changes observed are to make the bone stiffer and less able to 'protect' the overlying cartilage by acting as a shock absorber (Li and Aspden 1997a,b).

Management

There is no proven, effective treatment for the osteoarthritis process. Nevertheless, considerable benefit to the patient can be achieved by often very simple interventions, and surgery for severe 'end stage', particularly large joint, osteoarthritis is excellent. Although a number of guidelines have been produced to inform the rational management of osteoarthritis, the quality of evidence underlying their development and interpretation is variable. The principal goals of management are:

- education of the patient about osteoarthritis
- pain relief
- achieving and maintaining optimal joint and limb function
- reducing adverse factors to beneficially modify the osteoarthritis process and its outcome.

A wide variety of modalities are available to realize these goals (Table 7), and an approach to management is outlined in the 'Management summary' (Box 1). As with any branch of medicine, an 'holistic' approach is appropriate and more likely to succeed. The frequent discordance between structural change, symptoms, and function is pertinent; since pain and physical handicap are the main clinical problems arising from osteoarthritis, their causes and treatment usually need consideration as independent issues.

General approach

Successful management centres on careful questioning and examination of the patient. The history should yield clear information particularly about:

- symptoms and their impact on the patients life
- functional disability
- functional requirements and thus the level of handicap
- patient expectations both from osteoarthritis and its treatment
- psychological factors including specific concerns and depression.

Table 7 Current management of osteoarthritis

Goals of management
Education
Relief of symptoms
Optimization of function
Available modalities
Counselling
Educational literature
Physical therapy
Occupational therapy
Drugs
Complementary medicine
Coping strategies
Surgery

Box 1 Management summary

Education concerning osteoarthritis
Protect compromised joints from excessive loading, e.g.
- Reduce obesity
- Modifying inappropriate daily/occupational activities especially knee-lifts
- Use a walking stick
- Shock-absorbing footwear
- Correct leg length discrepancy
- Consider wedge insoles

Maintain function
- Maintain aerobic fitness, e.g. with swimming and walking
- Maintain joint motion and stability
- Muscle strengthening exercises/physiotherapy
- Regular activity

Reduce pain and stiffness
- Analgesics
- Intermittent/regular analgesics (acetaminophen)
- Consider Topical NSAIDs
- Consider topical capsaicin
- Consider oral NSAIDs
- Consider oral glucosamine sulfate
- Consider peri- and intra-articular corticosteroid injection
- Consider hyaluronic acid injection
- Consider TENS and nerve blocks for severe pain

Reduce impact of pain and disability
- Treat depression, anxiety, fibromyalgia
- Consider coping strategies
- Modify patient environment to reduce handicap

Consider surgery for
- Persistent severe pain
- Disability

Careful examination should determine the:
- extent of locomotor abnormality
- origin of current pain, either articular and/or periarticular
- degree of accompanying synovitis
- presence of instability
- local and general muscle condition
- evidence of accompanying fibromyalgia, neurological, or other relevant medical disease.

Thus an accurate diagnosis can be made, the extent of the problems assessed, and any associated factors identified. An individual management programme can then be constructed with the patient. The results of such interventions need to be reviewed and the programme modified as the patient's characteristics and requirements change. As symptomatic osteoarthritis is a potentially complex problem, it often requires a multidisciplinary, co-ordinated approach.

Helping the patient understand osteoarthritis

The myth that osteoarthritis is an inevitable, progressive wear and tear disease of old age persists. This leads to negative attitudes in both patients and doctors and may encourage inappropriate action, for example reduced activity for fear of 'wearing the joints out'. It is important that all those involved in patient management have similar concepts so that conflicting information is avoided. It is also important to address the questions that the patient wants answered, and to respond in a manner understandable to the patient. For example, most patients want to know about diet, exercise, and factors in their life that may have brought on their arthritis; explanation of cartilage and bone changes may have little relevance for them. Although the natural history of osteoarthritis is poorly documented, available data suggests that it is often considerably better than patients expect. This is not only true for hand involvement in nodal generalized osteoarthritis but also at the hip and knee. A reasonably optimistic, though not unrealistic, approach is therefore justified. There is good evidence to support the use of educational programmes that help patients understand and develop their own self-management strategies such as the 'Challenging Arthritis' programme.

Addressing mechanical factors

Protecting compromised osteoarthritis joints from excessive or unusual loading often reduces pain. Obesity increases joint loading throughout the body and obese patients are best advised to lose weight. This may also prevent or retard the development and progression of osteoarthritis (Felson et al. 1991). A low fat, complex carbohydrate rich, reduced calorie 'healthy' diet should therefore be encouraged. Appropriate use of a walking stick for hip or knee osteoarthritis will help reduce loading through the affected joint, and shock-absorbing footwear (e.g. 'trainers') may reduce impact; both manoeuvres may benefit symptoms. Altered mechanics due to leg length discrepancy may produce pain which is commonly periarticular and correction with a heel raise may be helpful. Some evidence is emerging that a loose knee support (e.g. tubular bandaging) may improve symptoms possibly by altering proprioception.

Modification of both workplace and home activities should be considered if appropriate. Appropriate advice regarding sexual activity may also be helpful, particularly for patients and their partners with hip osteoarthritis.

The integrity of articular tissues is maintained, and repair of damaged cartilage facilitated, by normal movement and loading of the joint. Patients should therefore be advised to keep active. Aerobic exercise should be encouraged since this has been demonstrated to be of symptomatic benefit in osteoarthritis (Kovar et al. 1992). In addition there is evidence at the knee that specific strengthening exercises aid functional restoration and reduce pain (van Baar et al. 1998; van Baar et al. 1999). Increasing evidence suggests that this can be provided in a primary care setting although the persistence of any benefit seen is unclear (O'Reilly et al. 1999; van Baar et al. 2001). It is important, however, to use a paced goal setting approach to limit activity cycling, that is, overactivity on good days leading to prolonged periods of increased pain and reduced activity.

Direct attempts to relieve symptoms

A variety of physical measures, such as local heat, cold, massage, or hydrotherapy, may give temporary pain relief. Such modalities are usually administered initially by physiotherapists, and there is considerable inter-patient variability as to which may help.

Simple analgesics and non-steroidal anti-inflammatory drugs are commonly used with good benefit. They should be regarded as an adjunct, rather than substitute, for other treatments. Comparative studies suggest that non-steroidal anti-inflammatory drugs are only marginally more effective than analgesics (Bradley et al. 1991; Pincus et al. 2001) but are associated with a significant number of side-effects, particularly in the elderly. There is some evidence, however, of greater efficacy in those patients with night or rest pain. Simple analgesics should therefore be tried first, including a trial at maximal regular dosage. If unsuccessful, sequential trials of several non-steroidal anti-inflammatory drugs may be considered. There is currently no convincing evidence that one non-steroidal anti-inflammatory drug is superior to another in the symptomatic relief of osteoarthritis. There are, however, emerging differences in the side-effect profiles of different non-steroidal anti-inflammatory drugs (see Chapter 4.5.1). It would therefore seem prudent to begin with a drug with a lower incidence of gastrointestinal side-effects such as ibuprofen or nabumetone before using alternative agents. The role of the newer Cox-1 protective agents is currently under review but they may be advantageous in patients at increased risk of peptic ulceration (Bradley 2001; Francois 2001). The patient should be made aware that the aim of these drugs is to reduce, rather than abolish, pain and that they may be taken on an as required basis. Symptoms in osteoarthritis are often phasic: repeat prescribing is to be avoided, and if a patient is taking an non-steroidal anti-inflammatory drug with apparent benefit they should still regularly experiment by stopping the drug to see whether it is still needed. It is possible that some non-steroidal anti-inflammatory drugs may adversely affect the osteoarthritis process (e.g. indomethacin) (Huskisson et al. 1995).

Topically applied non-steroidal anti-inflammatory drugs offer advantages over oral preparations in terms of reduced side-effects but their use when compared to simpler rubefacients remains controversial. We feel that they have a role in the symptomatic relief of osteoarthritis and encourage patient self-management. Topical capsaicin, a substance P depleting agent also has a role in the symptomatic relief of osteoarthritis pain but patients need to be warned of the stinging and burning that may occur when first using these preparations and the latency of onset of action (Zhang and Po 1994).

If pain is thought to be predominantly periarticular in origin (e.g. due to enthesopathy or bursitis), then local injection of corticosteroid, possibly with local anaesthetic to the tender site, may prove helpful and allow participation in other aspects of the management programme (e.g. exercise).

In patients with symptoms unresponsive to other measures, local injection with corticosteroid may produce temporary benefit, permitting involvement in physiotherapy and exercise, or allowing the patient to undertake a 'special event', for example a holiday or a family occasion. The effect is short-lived, probably lasting less than 6 weeks but individual patients, often those too infirm or otherwise unsuitable for alternative approaches, may derive benefit from occasional injection.

Patients with chronic synovitis may gain more prolonged control of synovitis and symptoms from intra-articular radiocolloid although in osteoarthritis the results are often disappointing (Taylor et al. 1997).

Intra-articular hyaluronate preparations are now available and they may provide relatively long-term (6 month) symptomatic benefit. The size of this effect is, however, comparable to that seen with non-steroidal anti-inflammatory drugs (Altman et al. 1998) and their cost in terms of direct drug costs and operator time (multiple intra-articular injections) remains an issue. Although putative disease modifying effects have been demonstrated *in vitro* this has not yet been convincingly demonstrated in humans. They may prove a useful adjunct in those unfit or not yet suitable for surgery especially if the patient is intolerant of other pain relieving strategies, for example, oral non-steroidal anti-inflammatory drugs.

The oral agent glucosamine sulfate also appears to have a slow onset prolonged symptomatic benefit in osteoarthritis (McAlindon et al. 2000; Reginster et al. 2001). Since it is licensed as a pharmaceutical agent in some parts of the world (e.g. Italy) but a health food product in others (e.g. UK, USA) there remain issues regarding funding and quality assurance. Many other similar agents are under investigation, for example, chondroitin sulfate. This group of drugs has been termed symptomatic slow acting drugs in osteoarthritis (SYSADOAs).

For patients with troublesome knee synovitis joint lavage with saline either arthroscopically or via percutaneous irrigation may offer benefit, sometimes for several months. The mechanism of this non-specific treatment is unclear.

Local nerve blocks, particularly suprascapular and obturator blocks for glenohumeral and hip osteoarthritis, are also worthy of consideration. These have less side-effects, and are generally more effective than major, centrally acting analgesics. A word of caution has been raised by retrospective studies that have suggested more rapid deterioration in patients treated in this manner. Since these procedures are usually used in patients unfit for or awaiting replacement arthroplasty this fear may be unwarranted.

Surgery

The biggest revolution in the therapy of osteoarthritis has been the treatment of severe disease by surgery. The two principal surgical interventions for hips and knees are arthroplasty and arthroscopy.

The overt success of arthroplasty has encouraged widespread use of this procedure at the hip and knee and now increasingly also at the shoulder, elbow, and thumb base. There are still unresolved issues regarding the funding and equity of access to arthroplasty surgery in many parts of the world. In addition, the unpredictable natural history of large joint osteoarthritis and considerations of cost-benefit for different care strategies mean that there are still major uncertainties regarding the indications for and timing of such surgery. Furthermore, surgeons now face the growing epidemic of revision surgery. As new medical interventions and data regarding arthroplasty outcome and cost-benefit become available the role of surgery will need to be rigourously appraised.

Arthroscopy is increasingly used for osteoarthritis. It allows direct inspection of the articular surface enabling the detection and assessment of minor degrees of articular cartilage damage. It also allows visualization and surgical correction of ligamentous and meniscal injury. These are increasingly being recognized as important accompaniments and possibly even initiating factors in osteoarthritis. Finally it is also a means whereby joint lavage and removal of 'loose bodies' can be performed. The precise role of arthroscopy in the management of osteoarthritis is still uncertain.

Can we modify osteoarthritis?

The possibility of therapeutic manipulation of the osteoarthritic process has gained acceptance though concrete examples in man are not yet established. In preparation for these perceived advances a new class of osteoarthritis drugs with potentially disease modifying properties has been defined, the disease modifying osteoarthritis drugs (DMOADs). Available compounds such as non-steroidal anti-inflammatory drugs, hyaluronate, sulfated glycosaminoglycans and glucosamine sulfate have so far been examined in this regard and agents under current study include oral tetracycline, metalloproteinase inhibitors, and bisphosphonates.

Unfortunately there is concern that some existing agents may have detrimental rather than beneficial DMOAD properties. For example, there is considerable *in vitro* and *in vivo* evidence that different non-steroidal anti-inflammatory drugs may:

- variably influence several aspects of cartilage metabolism;
- show either detrimental or protective effects in spontaneous or induced animal models of 'osteoarthritis';
- affect radiographic loss of joint space in man (Huskisson et al. 1995).

The mechanisms of such actions remain unexplained but appear largely independent of prostaglandin inhibition. Interestingly, susceptibility to influence by non-steroidal anti-inflammatory drugs appears greater for osteoarthritic than for normal cartilage. This could relate to:

- increased drug delivery from the hypervascular synovium and breaching of the calcified zone by subchondral vessels;
- enhanced drug penetration due to the increased surface area of fissured cartilage and its altered charge characteristics;
- increased susceptibility of stimulated chondrocytes.

It is apparent that many non-steroidal anti-inflammatory drugs have suppressive effects on proteoglycan synthesis and other aspects of cartilage metabolism that may be considered potentially detrimental; conversely, others have little or no suppressive effects at concentrations usually attained in man, and may be beneficial to compromised cartilage. Such observations cannot be directly extrapolated to the clinical situation of human osteoarthritis and there are few studies to date that have directly addressed whether non-steroidal anti-inflammatory drugs influence structural osteoarthritis in man. The most rigourous study is that of (Huskisson et al. 1995). In a parallel group study patients with knee osteoarthritis receiving indomethacin developed significantly more rapid joint space loss at the knee than those receiving placebo. No significant effect was seen in a group receiving tiaprofenic acid compared to placebo though it should be noted that a statistically non-significant trend to more rapid joint space loss was seen in the tiaprofenic acid group.

One 3 year randomized controlled trial (Reginster et al. 2001) has reported both symptom benefit and slowing of radiographic medial tibiofemoral narrowing from daily oral glucosamine sulfate (1500 mg/day). In contrast in a 3 year study of the interleukin 1-β inhibitor diacerein although a reduction in joint space loss at the hip was observed, compared to placebo, no corresponding improvement in symptoms was seen (Dougados et al. 2001).

Some recent progress has been made with the design of low molecular weight inhibitors of the MMPs that have been shown to be effective *in vitro* and in animal models *in vivo* at preventing cartilage breakdown (Cawston 1995). Such compounds remain under development and are being tested in man to determine if cartilage and bone can be protected from degradative enzymes without resulting adverse effects on other tissues such as tendon (Vincenti et al. 1994). There is a substantial body of evidence to support the concept that tetracycline might slow cartilage loss and the results of an ongoing US randomized controlled trial are awaited with interest.

The problem remains that, because of the heterogeneity of osteoarthritis, the chronicity of the condition, the discordance between anatomical, functional, and symptomatic manifestations, and unresolved difficulties of assessment, studies seeking to demonstrate even marked differences between drugs prove difficult and expensive to organize. Advances in imaging techniques and the appropriate selection of the clinical model (e.g. studying patients after a defined trauma to the joint, studying the rate of accrual of new interphalangeal joint involvement in patients with nodal osteoarthritis) may allow considerable reduction in sample size. Furthermore, although cartilage may be the best understood component and the usual focus of interest, other joint tissues (bone, capsule, synovium, muscle) may also influence the outcome of osteoarthritis. Therapeutic modifications (good or bad) of all joint tissues requires consideration.

Prognosis

For such a common disease, the prognosis of osteoarthritis is largely unknown. From the data that is available one can be relatively optimistic about outcome for most patients.

Knee

Hernborg and Nilsson observed clinical and radiographic deterioration in the majority of cases of knee osteoarthritis followed for 10–18 years. Predictors of poor outcome were varus deformity, earlier age of onset, and female gender (Hernborg and Nilsson 1977). Isolated osteophytosis alone in this study did not lead subsequent development of osteoarthritic change. In a long-term (12-year) study investigating cartilage loss in the general population (Schouten et al. 1992) obesity, presence of generalized osteoarthritis, age and varus/valgus knee deformity were all associated with progressive loss of cartilage. Varus or valgus malalignment has recently been confirmed as an important risk factor for progression of both radiographic tibiofemoral joint space narrowing and functional deterioration (Sharma et al. 2001). In a study of hospital-referred patients, only the presence of inflammation and calcium pyrophosphate deposition was associated with progression (Ledingham et al. 1995). In addition to increased morbidity, knee osteoarthritis is associated with increased mortality (Danielsson and Hernborg 1970; Lawrence et al. 1990).

Hip

Again the prognosis may be reasonably optimistic. Over a 10-year period, Danielsson found a deterioration in symptoms in only 17 per cent of hip osteoarthritis subjects with symptoms improving in 59 per cent, and completely resolving in 12 per cent. Radiographic progression similarly occurred in only a minority of cases, principally those with an initial superolateral pattern of joint space loss (Danielsson 1964). Occasional patients with apparently progressive osteoarthritis which improve with spontaneous 'healing' on radiographs (remodelling and partial restoration of joint space) are well described if uncommon (Perry et al. 1972). Possible risk factors for progression of hip joint osteoarthritis include: superior pole pattern (Danielsson 1964); obesity (Watson 1976); and presence of chondrocalcinosis at other sites (Menkes et al. 1985).

Hand

The prognosis for hand osteoarthritis is generally good. Symptoms and hand function of patients with nodal generalized osteoarthritis examined two or more decades after onset is no worse than that of similarly aged subjects with no hand osteoarthritis. In contrast, in erosive osteoarthritis, in which bony ankylosis and instability is more common, long-term functional outcome may be worse (Pattrick et al. 1989).

Functional outcome for thumb base involvement, carpo-metacarpophalangeal joint, and scaphotrapezoid disease is less clear-cut but may also be relatively poor.

Spine

Prognosis for osteoarthritis of the spine is unclear. This is largely because of the difficulty of correlating symptoms with structural change. In cases of either cord or nerve root compression prognosis is unclear deterioration is often slow unless there is additional disc protrusion, vascular insult or trauma.

Chronic pyrophosphate arthropathy

The natural history of chronic pyrophosphate arthropathy is poorly documented. Despite often severe symptoms and structural change at presentation, one 5-year, hospital-based, prospective study suggests that most patients run a benign course. Symptomatic deterioration occurred mainly in large lower limb joints that is, knees and hips, but even in severely affected knees, two-thirds of patients showed stabilization or improvement of symptoms. The commonest radiographic change is an increase in osteophyte with bone remodelling, rather than progressive cartilage and bone attrition. Nevertheless, severe, progressive 'destructive pyrophosphate arthropathy' may occasionally occur, particularly at the knee, shoulder, and hip. This is virtually confined to elderly women or in association with haemochromatosis and may cause problematic recurrent haemarthroses and a radiographic appearance of marked destruction resembling a Charcot or neuropathic joint.

Apatite associated destructive arthropathy

The prognosis of this form is seemingly poor with the majority having marked joint destruction requiring joint replacement.

References

Acheson, R.M. and Collart, A.B. (1975). New Haven Survey of joint diseases. XVII. Relationships between some systemic characteristics and osteoarthrosis in a general population. *Annals of the Rheumatic Diseases* **34**, 379–87.

Altman, R.D. (1991). Criteria for classification of clinical osteoarthritis. *Journal of Rheumatology* **18** (Suppl. 27), 10–12.

Altman, R. et al. (1986). Development of criteria for the classification and reporting of osteoarthritis: classification of osteoarthritis of the knee. *Arthritis and Rheumatism* **29**, 1039–49.

Altman, R. et al. (1990). The American College of Rheumatology criteria for the classification and reporting of osteoarthritis of the hand. *Arthritis and Rheumatism* **33**, 1601–10.

Altman, R. et al. (1991). The American College of Rheumatology criteria for the classification and reporting of osteoarthritis of the hip. *Arthritis and Rheumatism* **34**, 505–14.

Altman, R.D., Moskowitz, R., and the Hyalgan Study Group (1998). Intraarticular hyaluronate (Hyalgan) in the treatment of patients with osteoarthritis of the knee: a randomised clinical trial. *Journal of Rheumatology* **25**, 2203–12.

Andrews, H.J., Plumpton, T.A., Harper, G.P., and Cawston, T.E. (1992). A synthetic peptide metalloproteinase inhibitor, but not TIMP, prevents the breakdown of proteoglycan within articular cartilage *in vitro*. *Agents and Actions* **37**, 147–54.

Badley, E.M., Rasooly, I., and Webster, G.K. (1994). Relative importance of musculoskeletal disorders as a cause of chronic health problems, disability, and health care utilisation: findings from the 1990 Ontario Health Survey. *Journal of Rheumatology* **21**, 505–14.

Bagge, E., Bjelle, A., and Svanborg, A. (1992). Radiographic osteoarthritis in the elderly. A cohort comparison and a longitudinal study of the '70-year old people in Göteborg'. *Clinical Rheumatology* **11**, 486–91.

van Baar, M.E. et al. (1998). The effectiveness of exercise therapy in patients with osteoarthritis of hip or knee: a randomised clinical trial. *Journal of Rheumatology* **25**, 2432–9.

van Baar, M.E., Asendelft, W.J.J., Dekker, J., Oostendorp, R.A.B., and Bijlsma, J.W.J. (1999). Effectiveness of exercise therapy in patients with osteoarthritis of the hip or knee. *Arthritis and Rheumatism* **42**, 1361–9.

van Baar, M.E., Dekker, J., Oostendorp, R.A.B., Bijl, D., Voorn, T.B., and Bijlsma, J.W.J. (2001). Effectiveness of exercise in patients with osteoarthritis of hip or knee: nine months follow up. *Annals of the Rheumatic Diseases* **60**, 1123–30.

Beekman, B., Drijfhout, J.W., Bloemhoff, W., Ronday, H.K., Tak, P.P., and Koppele, J.M. (1996). Convenient flourometric assay for metalloproteinase activity and its application in biological media. *FEBS Letters* **390**, 221–5.

van den Berg, W.B. (1999). The role of cytokines and growth factors in cartilage destruction: osteoarthritis and rheumatoid arthritis. *Zeitschrift fur Rheumatologie* **58**, 136–41.

Billington, C.J., Clark, I.M., and Cawston, T.E. (1998). An aggrecan degrading activity associated with chondrocyte membranes. *Biochemical Journal* **336**, 207–12.

Birrell, F., Croft, P., Cooper, C., Hosie, G., Macfarlane, G., Silman, A., and the P.C.R. hip study group (2001). Predicting radiographic hip osteoarthritis from range of movement. *Rheumatology* **40**, 506–12.

Blumenfeld, I. and Livne, E. (1999). The role of transforming growth factor beta, insulin like-growth factor-1 in osteoarthritis and aging of joints. *Experimental Gerontology* **34**, 821–9.

Bonassar, L.J., Frank, E.H., Murray, J.C., Paguio, C.G., Moore, V.L., Lark, M.W., Sandy, J.D., Wu, J.-J., Eyre, D.R., and Grodzinsky, A.J. (1995). Changes in cartilage composition and physical properties due to stromelysin degradation. *Arthritis and Rheumatism* **38**, 173–83.

Bradley J.D. (2001). Celecoxib and rofecoxib: a distinction with a difference. *Journal of Clinical Rheumatology* **7**, 137–8.

Bradley, J.D., Brandt, K.D., Katz, B.P., Kalasinski, L.A., and Ryan, S.I. (1991). Comparison of an anti-inflammatory dose of ibuprofen, an analgesic dose of ibuprofen, and acetaminophen in the treatment of patients with osteoarthritis of the knee. *New England Journal of Medicine* **325**, 87–91.

Brand, C., Snaddon, J., Bailey, M., and Cicuttini, F. (2001). Vitamin E is ineffective for symptomatic relief in knee osteoarthritis: a six month double blind, randomised, placebo-controlled study. *Annals of the Rheumatic Diseases* **60**, 946–9.

Brew, K., Dinakarpandian, D., and Nagase, H. (2000). Tissue inhibitors of metalloproteinases: evolution, structure and function. *Biochimica et Biophysica Acta* **1477**, 267–83.

Brinkerhoff, C.E. (1991). Joint destruction in arthritis: metalloproteinases in the spotlight. *Arthritis and Rheumatism* **34**, 1073–5.

Brocklehurst, R., Bayliss, M.T., Maroudas, A., Coysh, H.L., Freeman, M.A.R., Revell, P.A., and Ali, S.Y. (1984). The composition of normal and osteoarthritic articular cartilage from human knee joints. *Journal of Bone and Joint Surgery (America)* **66A**, 95–106.

Buckland-Wright, J.C., MacFarlane, D.G., Lynch, J.A., and Clark, B. (1990). Quantitative microfocal radiographic assessment of progression in osteoarthritis of the hand. *Arthritis and Rheumatism* **33**, 57–65.

Buckland-Wright, J.C., Wolfe, F., Ward, R.J., Flowers, N., and Hayne, C. (1999). Substantial superiority of semiflexed (MTP) views in knee osteoarthritis: a comparative radiographic study, without fluoroscopy, of standing extended, semiflexed (MTP), and Schuss views. *Journal of Rheumatology* **26**, 2664–74.

Burgkart, R., Glaser, C., Hyhlik-Dürr, A., Englmeier, K.-H., Reiser, M., and Eckstein, F. (2001). Magnetic resonance imaging-based assessment of cartilage loss in severe osteoarthritis. *Arthritis and Rheumatism* **44**, 2072–7.

Burr, D.B. (1998). The importance of subchondral bone in osteoarthritis. *Current Opinion in Rheumatology* **10**, 256–62.

Buttle, D.J., Handley, C.J., Ilic, M.Z., Saklatvala, J., Murata, M., and Barrett, A.J. (1993). Inhibition of cartilage proteoglycan release by a specific inactivator of cathepsin B and an inhibitor of matrix metalloproteinases; evidence for two converging pathways of chondrocyte-mediated proteoglycan degradation. *Arthritis and Rheumatism* **36**, 1709–17.

Cawston, T.E. (1995). Proteinases and connective tissue breakdown. In *Mechanisms and Models in Rheumatoid Arthritis* (ed. B. Henderson, J.C.W. Edwards, and E.P. Pettipher), pp. 333–. San Diego CA: Academic Press.

Cawston, T.E. (1996). Metalloproteinase inhibitors and the prevention of connective tissue breakdown. *Pharmacology Therapy* **3**, 163–82.

Cawston, T.E., Mercer, E., De Silva, M., and Hazleman, B.L. (1983). Metalloproteinases and collagenase inhibitors in rheumatoid synovial fluid. *Arthritis and Rheumatism* **27**, 641–6.

Cawston, T.E., Plumpton, T.A., Curry, V.A., Ellis, A., and Powell, L. (1994). The role of TIMP and MMP inhibition in preventing connective tissue breakdown. *Annals of the New York Academy of Science* **732**, 75–83.

Cawston, T.E., Curry, V.A., Summers, C.A., Clark, I.M., Riley, G.P., Life, P.F., Spaull, J.R., Goldring, M.B., Koshy, P.J.T., Rowan, A.D., and Shingleton, W.D. (1998). The role of oncostatin M in animal and human connective tissue collagen turnover and its localization within the rheumatoid joint. *Arthritis and Rheumatism* **41**, 1760–71.

Claessens, A., Schouten, J., van den Ouweland, F., and Valkenburg, H. (1990). Do clinical findings associate with radiographic osteoarthritis of the knee? *Annals of the Rheumatic Diseases* **49**, 771–4.

Cobby, M., Cushnaghan, J., Creamer, P., Dieppe, P., and Watt, I. (1990). Erosive osteoarthritis: is it a separate disease entity? *Clinical Radiology* **42**, 258–63.

Creamer, P., Lethbridge-Cejku, M., and Hochberg, M.C. (1998). Where does it hurt? Pain localisation in osteoarthritis of the knee. *Osteoarthritis and Cartilage* **6**, 318–23.

Creamer, P., Lethbridge-Cejku, M., and Hochberg, M.C. (2000). Factors associated with functional impairment in symptomatic knee osteoarthritis. *Rheumatology* **39**, 490–6.

Croft, P., Cooper, C., Wickham, C., and Coggon, D. (1990). Defining osteoarthritis of the hip for epidemiologic studies. *American Journal of Epidemiology* **132**, 514–522.

Croft, P., Cooper, C., Wickham, C., and Coggon, D. (1991). Osteoarthritis of the hip and acetabular dysplasia. *Annals of the Rheumatic Diseases* **50**, 308–10.

Croft, P., Cooper, C., Wickham, C., and Coggon, D. (1992). Is the Hip involved in generalized osteoarthritis? *British Journal of Rheumatology* **31**, 325–8.

Dahlberg, L., Billinghurst, R.C., Manner, P., Nelson, F., Webb, G., Ionescu, M., Reiner, A., Tanzer, M., Zukor, D., Chen, J., van Wart, H.E., and Poole, A.R. (2000). Selective enhancement of collagenase-mediated cleavage of a resident

Type II collagen in cultured osteoarthritic cartilage and arrest with a synthetic inhibitor that spares collagenase 1 (matrix metalloproteinase-1). *Arthritis and Rheumatism* **43**, 673–82.

Danielsson, L.G. (1964). Incidence and prognosis of coxarthrosis. *Acta Orthopaedica Scandinavica* **66** (Suppl.), 1–114.

Danielsson, L.G. and Hernborg, J. (1970). Morbidity and mortality of osteoarthritis of the knee (gonarthrosis) in Malmo, Sweden. *Clinical Orthopaedics and Related Research* **69**, 224–6.

Davis, M.A., Ettinger, W.H., Neuhaus, J.M., Barclay, J.D., and Segal, M.R. (1992). Correlates of knee pain amongst US adults with and without radiographic knee osteoarthritis. *Journal of Rheumatology* **19**, 1943–9.

Dean, D.D., Martel-Pelletier, J., Pelletier, J.P., Howell, D.S., and Woessner, J.F. (1989). Evidence for metalloproteinase and metalloproteinase inhibitor imbalance in human osteoarthritic cartilage. *Journal of Clinical Investigation* **84**, 678–85.

Dieppe, P.A., Campion, G., and Doherty, M. (1988). Mixed crystal deposition. *Rheumatology Diseases Clinics of North America* **14**, 415–26.

Dieppe, P., Cushnaghan, J., Young, P., and Kirwan, J. (1993). Prediction of the progression of joint space narrowing in osteoarthritis of the knee by bone scintigraphy. *Annals of the Rheumatic Diseases* **52**, 557–63.

Dodge, G.R. and Poole, A.R. (1989). Immunohistochemical detection and immunochemical analysis of type II collagen degradation in human normal, rheumatoid and osteoarthritic articular cartilages and in explants of bovine articular cartilage cultured with interleukin 1. *Journal of Clinical Investigation* **83**, 647–61.

Doherty, M., Watt, I., and Dieppe, P. (1983). Influence of primary generalised osteoarthritis on development of secondary osteoarthritis. *Lancet* **ii**, 8–11.

Dougados, M., Nguyen, M., Berdah, L., Mazieres, B., Vignon, E., and Lesquesne, M. for the ECHODIAH investigators study group. (2001). Evaluation of the structure-modifying effects of diacerein in hip osteoarthritis. *Arthritis and Rheumatism* **44**, 2539–47.

Ehlich, G.E. (1975). Osteoarthritis beginning with inflammation. Definitions and correlations. *Journal of the American Medical Association* **232**, 157–9.

Ellis, A.J., Curry, V.A., Powell, E.K., and Cawston, T.E. (1994). The prevention of collagen breakdown in bovine nasal cartilage by TIMP, TIMP-2 and a low molecular weight synthetic inhibitor. *Biochemical Biophysical Research Communications* **201**, 94–101.

Felson, D.T. (1988). Epidemiology of hip and knee osteoarthritis. *Epidemiologic Reviews* **10**, 1–28.

Felson, D.T., Hannan, M.T., Naimark, A., Berkely, J., Gordon, G., Wilson, P.W.F., and Anderson, J. (1991). Occupational physical demands, knee bending, and knee osteoarthritis: results from the Framingham study. *Journal of Rheumatology* **18**, 1587–92.

Felson, D.T., Ahange, Y., Anthony, J.M., Naimark, A., and Anderson, J.J. (1992). Weight loss reduces the risk for symptomatic knee osteoarthritis in women. *Annals of Internal Medicine* **116**, 535–9.

Felson, D.T., Chaisson, C.E., Hill, C.L., Totterman, S.M.S., Gale, E., Skinner, K.M., Kazis, L., and Gale, D.R. (2001). The association of bone marrow lesions with pain in knee osteoarthritis. *Annals of Internal Medicine* **134**, 541–9.

Francois, D. (2001). Spin doctors. *Journal of Clinical Rheumatology* **7**, 139–41.

Garnero, P., Rousseau, J.-C., and Delmas, P.D. (2000). Molecular basis and clinical use of biochemical markers of bone cartilage and synovium in joint diseases. *Arthritis and Rheumatism* **43**, 953–68.

Gelber, A.C., Hochberg, M.C., Mead, L.A., Wang, N.-Y., Wigley, F.M., and Klag, M.J. (2000). Joint injury in young adults and risk for subsequent knee and hip osteoarthritis. *Annals of Internal Medicine* **133**, 321–8.

Goldring, M.B. (2000). The role of the chondrocyte in osteoarthritis. *Arthritis and Rheumatism* **43**, 1916–26.

Goldthwaite, J.E. (1904). The differential diagnosis and treatment of so-called rheumatoid diseases. *Boston Medical Surgery Journal* **151**, 529–34.

Halverson, P.B. and McCarty, D.J. (1988). Clinical aspects of basic calcium phosphate crystal deposition. *Rheumatology Diseases Clinics of North America* **14**, 427–39.

Hamerman, D. (1989). The biology of osteoarthritis. *New England Journal of Medicine* **320**, 1322–30.

Hart, D.J., Spector, T.D., Brown, P., Wilson, P., Doyle, D.V., and Silman, A.J. (1991). Clinical signs of early osteoarthritis: reproducibility and relation to X-ray changes in 541 women in the general population. *Annals of the Rheumatic Diseases* **50**, 467–700.

Hernborg, J.S. and Nilsson, B.E. (1977). The natural course of untreated osteoarthritis of the knee. *Clinical Orthopaedics and Related Research* **123**, 130–7.

Hollander, A.P., Heathfield, T.F., Webber, C., Iwata, Y., Bourne, R., Rorabeck, C., and Poole, A.R. (1994). Increased damage to type II collagen in osteoarthritic articular cartilage detected by a new immunoassay. *Journal of Clinical Investigation* **93**, 1722–32.

Hummel, K.M., Petrow, P.K., Franz, J.K., Muller-Ladner, U., Aicher, W.K., Gay, R.E., Bromme, D., and Gay, S. (1998). Cysteine proteinase cathepsin K mRNA is expressed in synovium of patients with rheumatoid arthritis and is detected at sites of synovial bone destruction. *Journal of Rheumatology* **25**, 1887–94.

Huskisson, E.C., Berry, H., Gishen, P., Jubb, R.W., and Whitehead, J., on behalf of the LINK study group (1995). Effects of antiinflammatory drugs on the progression of osteoarthritis of the knee. *Journal of Rheumatology* **22**, 1941–6.

Hutton, C. (1987). Generalised osteoarthritis: an evolutionary problem? *Lancet* **1**, 1463–5.

Jones, A.C. and Doherty, M. (1992). *British Journal of Clinical Pharmacology* **33**, 357–62.

Jonsson, H. and Valtysdottir, S.T. (1995). Hypermobility features in patients with hand osteoarthritis. *Osteoarthritis and Cartilage* **3**, 1–5.

Kellgren, J.H. and Moore, R. (1952). Generalised osteoarthritis and Heberden's nodes. *British Medical Journal* **1**, 181–7.

Kellgren, J.H. and Lawrence, J.S. (1957). Radiological assessment of osteoarthritis. *Annals of the Rheumatic Diseases* **16**, 494–502.

Keyszer, G., Redlich, A., Haupl, T., Zacher, J., Sparmann, M., Ungethum, U., Gay, S., and Burmester, G.R. (1998). Differential expression of cathepsins B and L compared with matrix metalloproteinases and their respective inhibitors in rheumatoid arthritis and osteoarthritis. *Arthritis and Rheumatism* **41**, 1378–87.

Knowlton, R.G., Katzenstein, P.L., Moskowitz, R.W., Weaver, E.J., Malemud, C., Pathria, M., Jimenez, S., and Prockop, D.J. (1990). Demonstration of genetic linkage of a polymorphism in the type II procollagen gene (Col2A1) to primary osteoarthritis associated with mild chondrodysplasia. *New England Journal of Medicine* **322**, 526–30.

Kovar, P.A., Allegrante, J.P., MacKenzie, C.R., Peterson, M.G.E., Gutin, B., and Charlson, M.E. (1992). Supervised fitness walking in patients with osteoarthritis of the knee. *Annals of Internal Medicine* **116**, 529–34.

Lane, N.E. and Nevitt, M.C. (1994). Osteoarthritis and bone mass. *Journal of Rheumatology* **21**, 1393–6.

Lane, N.E., Gore, R., Cummings, S.R., Hochberg, M.C., Scott, J.C., Williams, E.N., and Nevitt, M.C. (1999). Serum vitamin D levels and incident changes of radiographic hip osteoarthritis. *Arthritis and Rheumatism* **42**, 854–60.

Lanyon, P., Jones, A., and Doherty, M. (1996). Assessing progression of patellofemoral osteoarthritis: a comparison between two radiographic methods. *Annals of the Rheumatic Diseases* **55**, 875–9.

Lanyon, P., Muir, K., Doherty, S., and Doherty, M. (2000). Assessment of a genetic contribution to osteoarthritis of the hip: sibling study. *British Medical Journal* **321**, 1179–83.

Lawrence, J.S. *Rheumatism in Populations.* London: Heinemann Medical Books, 1977.

Lawrence, R.C., Everett, D., and Hochberg, M.C. (1990). Arthritis. In *Health Status and Well-being of the Elderly: National Health and Nutrition Examination-I Epidemiologic Followup Survey* (ed. R. Huntley and J. Cornoni-Huntley), pp. 136–51. New York: Oxford University Press.

Ledingham, J., Dawson, S., Preston, B., Milligan, G., and Doherty, M. (1992). Radiographic patterns and associations of osteoarthritis of the hip. *Annals of the Rheumatic Diseases* **51**, 1111–16.

Ledingham, J., Dawson, S., Preston, B., Milligan, G., and Doherty, M. (1993). Radiographic progression of hospital referred osteoarthritis of the hip. *Annals of the Rheumatic Diseases* **52**, 263–7.

Ledingham, J., Regan, M., Jones, A., and Doherty, M. (1995). Factors affecting radiographic progression of knee osteoarthritis. *Annals of the Rheumatic Diseases* **54**, 53–8.

Li, B. and Aspden, R.M. (1997a). Mechanical and material properties of the subchondral bone plate from the femoral head of patients with osteoarthritis or osteoporosis. *Annals of the Rheumatic Diseases* **56**, 247–54.

Li, B. and Aspden, R.M. (1997b). Composition and mechanical properties of cancellous bone from the femoral head of patients with osteoporosis and osteoarthritis. *Journal of Bone and Mineral Research* **512**, 641–51.

Loughlin, J. (2001). Genetic epidemiology of primary osteoarthritis. *Current Opinion in Rheumatology* **13**, 111–16.

Marks, J.S., Stewart, I.M., and Hardinge, K. (1979). Primary osteoarthrosis of the hip and Heberden's nodes. *Annals of the Rheumatic Diseases* **38**, 107–11.

Maroudas, A. et al. (1986). Physiochemical properties and functional behaviour of normal and osteoarthritic human cartilage. In *Articular Cartilage Biochemistry* (ed. K.E. Kuettner, R. Schleyerbach, and V. Hascall), pp. 311–30. New York: Raven Press.

McAlindon, T.E. and Felson, D.T. (1997). Nutrition: risk factors for osteoarthritis. *Annals of the Rheumatic Diseases* **56**, 397–402.

McAlindon, T.E., Snow, S., Cooper, C., and Dieppe, P.A. (1992). Radiographic patterns of osteoarthritis of the knee joint in the community: the importance of the patellofemoral joint. *Annals of the Rheumatic Diseases* **51**, 844–9.

McAlindon, T.E., LaValley, M.P., Gulin, J.P., and Felson, D.T. (2000). Glucosamine and chondroitin for treatment of osteoarthritis: a systematic quality assessment and meta-analysis. *Journal of the American Medical Association* **283**, 1469–75.

McCarty, D.J. (1976). Calcium pyrophosphate dihydrate crystal deposition disease 1975. *Arthritis and Rheumatism* **19** (Suppl.), 275–86.

Menkes, C.-J., Decraemere, W., Postel, M., and Forest, M. (1985). Chondrocalcinosis and rapid destruction of the hip. *Journal of Rheumatology* **12**, 130–3.

Mikkelsen, W.M., Duff, I.F., and Dodge, H.J. (1970). Age, sex specific prevalence of radiographic abnormalities of the joints of the hands, wrists, and cervical spine of adult residents of the Tecumseh, Michigan community health study area, 1962–1965. *Journal of Chronic Diseases* **23**, 151–9.

Moreno-Reyes, R., Snettons, C., Mathieu, F., Begaux, F., Zhu, D., Rivera, M.T., Boelaert, M., Neve, J., Perlmutter, N., and Vanderpas, J. (1998). Kashin-Beck osteoarthropathy in rural Tibet in relation to selenium and iodine status. *New England Journal of Medicine* **339**, 1112–20.

Murphy, G., Docherty, A.J.P., Hembry, R.M., and Reynolds, J.J. (1991). Metalloproteinases and tissue damage. *British Journal of Rheumatology* **30**, 25–31.

Nagase, H. and Woessner, J.F. (1999). Matrix metalloproteinases. *Journal of Biological Chemistry* **274**, 21491–4.

Nevitt, M.C., Felson, D.T., Williams, E.N., and Grady, D. (2001). The effect of estrogen plus progestin on knee symptoms and related disability in post-menopausal women. *Arthritis and Rheumatism* **44**, 811–18.

Ohira, T. and Ishikawa, K. (1987). Hydroxyapatite deposition in osteoarthritic articular cartilage of the proximal femoral head. *Arthritis and Rheumatism* **30**, 651–60.

O'Reilly, S.C., Jones, A., Muir, K.R., and Doherty, M. (1998). Quadriceps weakness in knee osteoarthritis: the effect on pain and disability. *Annals of the Rheumatic Diseases* **57**, 588–94.

O'Reilly, S.C., Muir, K.R., and Doherty, M. (1999). Effectiveness of home exercise on pain and disability from osteoarthritis of the knee: a randomised controlled trial. *Annals of the Rheumatic Diseases* **58**, 15–19.

Pattrick, M., Aldridge, S., Hamilton, E., Manhire, A., and Doherty, M. (1989). A controlled study of hand function in nodal and erosive osteoarthritis. *Annals of the Rheumatic Diseases* **48**, 978–82.

Perry, G.H., Smith, M.J.G., and Whiteside, C.G. (1972). Spontaneous recovery of the joint space in degenerative hip disease. *Annals of the Rheumatic Diseases* **31**, 440–8.

Pincus, T. et al. (2001). A randomised, double-blind, crossover clinical trial of diclofenac plus misoprostol versus acetaminophen in patients with osteoarthritis of the hip or knee. *Arthritis and Rheumatism* **44**, 1587–98.

Poole, R.A. (1993). Immunochemical markers of joint inflammation, skeletal and repair. Where are we now? *Annals of the Rheumatic Diseases* **53**, 305.

Reginster, J.Y., Deroisy, R., Rovati, L.C., Lee, R.L., Lejeune, E., Bruyere, O., Giacovelli, G., Henrotin, Y., Dacre, J.E., and Gossett, C. (2001). Long-term effects of glucosamine sulphate on osteoarthritis progression: a randomised, placebo-controlled clinical trial. *Lancet* **357**, 251–6.

Revell, P.A., Mayston, V., Lalor, P., and Mapp, P. (1988). The synovial membrane in osteoarthritis: a histological study including the characterisation of the cellular infiltrate present in inflammatory osteoarthritis using monoclonal antibodies. *Annals of the Rheumatic Diseases* **47**, 300–7.

Ryu, J., Treadwell, B.V., and Mankin, H.J. (1984). Biochemical and metabolic abnormalities in normal and osteoarthritic human articular cartilage. *Arthritis and Rheumatism* **27**, 49–56.

van Saase, J.L.C.M., Van Romunde, L.K.J., Cats, A., Vandenbrouke, J.P., and Valkenburg, H.A. (1989). Epidemiology of osteoarthritis: Zoetermeer survey. Comparison of radiological osteoarthritis in a Dutch population with that in 10 other populations. *Annals of the Rheumatic Diseases* **48**, 271–80.

Sandy, J.D., Flannery, C.R., Neame, P.J., and Lohmander, L.S. (1992). The structure of aggrecan fragments in human synovial fluid: Evidence for the involvement in osteoarthritis of a novel proteinase. *Journal of Clinical Investigation* **89**, 1512–16.

Sharma, L., Song, J., Felson, D.T., Cahue, S., Shamiyeh, E., and Dunlop, D.D. (2001). The role of knee alignment in disease progression and functional decline in knee osteoarthritis. *Journal of the American Medical Association* **286**, 188–95.

Schouten, J.S.A.G., van den Ouweland, F.A., and Valkenburg, H.A. (1992). A 12 year follow up study in the general population on prognostic factors of cartilage loss in osteoarthritis of the knee. *Annals of the Rheumatic Diseases* **51**, 932–7.

Shlopov, B.V., Lie, W.-R., Mainardie, C.L., Cole, A.A., Chubinskaya, S., and Hasty, K.A. (1997). Osteoarthritic lesions: Involvement of three different collagenases. *Arthritis and Rheumatism* **40**, 2065–74.

Slemenda, C., Heilman, D.K., Brandt, K.D., Katz, B.P., Mazucca, S.A., Braunstein, E.M., and Bird, D. (1998). Reduced quadriceps strength relative to body weight. A risk factor for knee osteoarthritis in women? *Arthritis and Rheumatism* **41**, 1951–9.

Sokoloff. *Color Atlas and Text of Osteoarthritis* (ed. M. Doherty). London: Wolfe, 1994.

Spector, T.D. and Campion, G.D. (1989). Generalised osteoarthritis: a hormonally mediated disease. *Annals of the Rheumatic Diseases* **48**, 523–7.

Spector, T.D., Hart, D.J., Byrne, J., Harris, P.A., Dacre, J.E., and Doyle, D.V. (1993). Definition of osteoarthritis of the knee for epidemiological studies. *Annals of the Rheumatic Diseases* **52**, 790–4.

Spector, T.D., Cicuttini, F., Baker, J., Loughlin, J., and Hart, D. (1996). Genetic influences on osteoarthritis in women: a twin study. *British Medical Journal* **312**, 940–4.

Swan, A., Chapman, B., Heap, P., Seward, H., and Dieppe, P. (1994). Submicroscopic crystals in osteoarthritic synovial fluids. *Annals of the Rheumatic Diseases* **53**, 467–70.

Tang, B.L. (2001). ADAMTS: a novel family of extracellular matrix proteinases. *International Journal of Biochemistry and Cell Biology* **33**, 33–44.

Taylor, W.J., Corkill, M.M., and Rajapaske, C.N.A. (1997). A retrospective review of Yttrium-90 synovectomy in the treatment of knee arthritis. *British Journal of Rheumatology* **36**, 1100–5.

Tetlow, L.C., Adlam, D.J., and Woolley, D.E. (2001). Matrix metalloproteinases and proinflammatory cytokine production by chondrocytes of human osteoarthritic cartilage: Association with degenerative changes. *Arthritis and Rheumatism* **44**, 585–94.

Tortorella, M.D., Malfait, A.M., Deccico, C., and Arner, E. (2001). The role of ADAM-TS4 (aggrecanase-1) and ADAM-TS5 (aggrecanase-2) in a model of cartilage degradation. *Osteoarthritis and Cartilage* **9**, 539–52.

Uitterlinden, A.G., Burger, H., van Duijn, C.M., Huang, Q., Hofman, A., Birkenhager, J.C., van Leewen, J.P.T.M., and Pols, H.A.P. (2000). Adjacent genes, for COl2A1 and the vitamin D receptor, are associated with separate features of radiographic osteoarthritis of the knee. *Arthritis and Rheumatism* **43**, 1456–64.

Vincenti, M.P., Clark, I.M., and Brinkerhoff, C.E. (1994). Using inhibitors of metalloproteinases to treat arthritis. Easier said than done? *Arthritis and Rheumatism* **37**, 1115–26.

Watson, M. (1976). Femoral head height loss: a study of the relative significance of some of its determinants in hip degeneration. *Rheumatology Rehabilitation* 15, 264–9.

Williams, C.J. and Jimenez, S.A. (1993). Heriditary, genes and osteoarthritis. *Rheumatology Disease Clinics of North America* 19, 523–43.

Wright, V. (1990). Post-traumatic osteoarthritis—a medico-legal minefield. *British Journal of Rheumatology* 29, 474–8.

Zhang, W.Y. and Po, A.L.W. (1994). The effectiveness of topically applied capsaicin. *European Journal of Clinical Pharmacology* 46, 517–22.

Zhang, Y., McAlindon, T.E., Hannan, M.T., Chaisson, C.E., Klein, R., Wilson, P.W.F., and Felson, D.T. (1998). Estrogen replacement therapy and worsening of radiographic knee osteoarthritis. *Arthritis and Rheumatism* 41, 1867–73.

Zhang, Y., Xu, L., Nevitt, M.C., Aliabadi, P., Yu, W., Qin, M., Lui, L.-Y., and Felson, D.T. (2001). Comparison of the prevalence of knee osteoarthritis between the elderly Chinese population in Beijing and whites in the United States. *Arthritis and Rheumatism* 44, 2065–71.

6.15 Crystal arthropathies

Ann K. Rosenthal

The crystal arthropathies include gout, calcium pyrophosphate dihydrate (CPPD) deposition disease, the basic calcium phosphate (BCP)-associated syndromes, and calcium oxalate arthritis. The most common forms of crystal-associated arthritis are readily diagnosed at the bedside, and yet continue to present many challenges to the clinician.

Gout

History

Gout is one of the oldest known forms of arthritis, and holds a unique place in the history of medicine. Hippocrates and Syndenham made observations about gout which remain true centuries later. Gout has served as a paradigm for the study of other types of crystal-associated arthritis and as a prime example of the way in which understanding the pathophysiology of a disease leads to the development of effective therapy (Copeman 1964).

Definition

The term gout is derived from the latin word 'guta' meaning a drop, and originally may have referred to a drop of poison or evil humour. Gout remains poorly defined as a clinical descriptor (Simkin 1993). In its most general sense, it is a group of diseases characterized by hyperuricaemia and uric acid crystal formation. These clinical syndromes include gouty arthritis, tophaceous gout, uric acid nephrolithiasis, and gouty nephropathy. In its more narrow and perhaps more commonly used definition, gout refers to arthritis caused by uric acid crystals.

Epidemiology

Gout is not an uncommon disease. Recent statistics from the United States show a self-reported prevalence of 13.6 per 1000 persons in adult males and 6.4 per 1000 persons for females (Collins 1988). With an estimated prevalence of 1 per cent among adults in the United States, gout is the most common cause of inflammatory arthritis in men. Average uric acid levels have been slowly rising over the last two decades (Gresser et al. 1990). Self-reported prevalence studies also show a parallel increase in the prevalence of gout (Lawrence et al. 1989). Despite effective therapy, it is estimated that 37 million working days per year in the United States have been lost to gout (Hochberg 1991).

Incidence rates for gout are more difficult to ascertain. A longitudinal study of American medical students showed an incidence of 1.7 cases per 1000 person-years of follow-up (Roubenoff et al. 1991).

The known risk factors for gout are well characterized and mirror risk factors for hyperuricaemia (Table 1). Gout is clearly more common in men and is rare in women prior to menopause. Mean serum urate levels rise at puberty in boys and remain 1–2 mg/dl higher in men than women until menopause, when gender differences in uric acid levels diminish. Serum urate levels increase with age in both men and women (Becker 1988). The peak incidence of gout in men is between the fourth and sixth decades. In women, it is between the sixth and seventh decades (Puig et al. 1991).

Primary gout is associated with a variety of medical conditions. Some such as obesity, renal insufficiency, and diuretic use clearly cause hyperuricaemia, which is the strongest risk factor for the development of gout (Lin et al. 2000). Serum urate levels are directly correlated with body weight (Roubenoff et al. 1991). Similarly, alcohol use increases uric acid levels by providing a dietary source of purines, increasing lactic acidaemia thus interfering with uric acid excretion, and inducing adenine nucleotide catabolism via acetate intermediaries (Puig and Fox 1984). Between 6 and 18 per cent of gout patients will have a family history of gout.

Other risk factors for gout such as hypertension, hyperlipidaemia, and coronary artery disease may not be causally associated with high uric acid levels, but simply target similar populations. Hypertension occurs in 25–50 per cent of gout patients, and a similar percentage of untreated hypertensives will have hyperuricaemia (Wyngaarden and Kelley 1976). Gout is also associated with hypertriglyceridaemia. The association between gout and coronary artery disease is somewhat controversial. Gout may be associated with atherosclerosis because of the high prevalence of obesity and hypertension in gout patients.

Risk factors for gout in women are not as clearly defined as those for men. As in men, age, renal insufficiency, and diuretic use are certainly linked with gout in women. However, other male risk factors such as body weight and alcohol intake may not play as important a role in gout in women (Puig et al. 1991).

Pathophysiology

Delineating the pathophysiology of gout requires an understanding of purine metabolism, as uric acid is an end product of purine biosynthesis. Hyperuricaemia is a necessary but not a sufficient condition for the development of gout; and although the mechanisms of excess uric acid accumulation are well defined, the subsequent phases of crystal formation and release into tissues remain less well characterized.

Purine metabolism

Purines are derived from two sources. They are ingested in food or are generated via a complex de novo synthetic pathway (Wyngaarden and Kelley 1976). The synthetic pathway is outlined in Fig. 1. Components of the purine ring are complexed to the donor substrate phosphoribosylpyrophosphate

Table 1 Risk factors for primary gout

Male gender
Age >40 years
Obesity
Family history
Alcohol use
Renal insufficiency
Hypertension

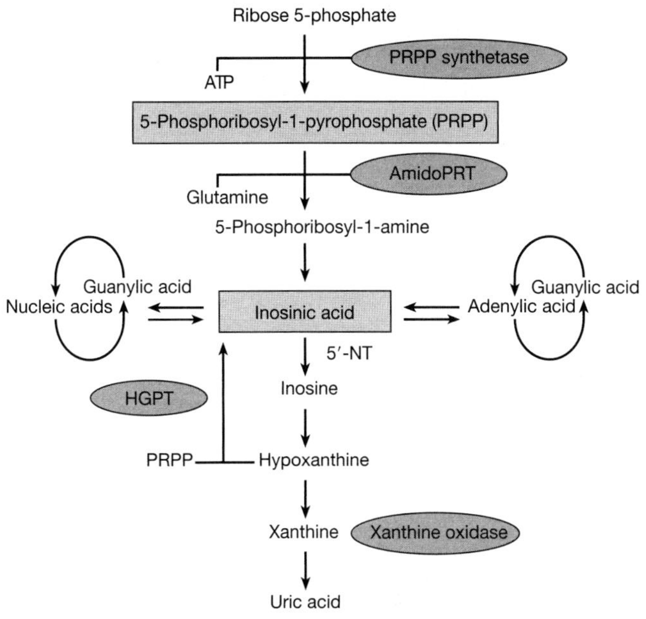

Fig. 1 Simplified scheme of normal purine metabolism in man. PRPP synthetase, phosphoribosylpyrophosphate synthetase; amidoPRT, amidophosphoribosyl transferase; HGPT, hypoxanthine guanine phosphoribosyl transferase; 5′-NT, 5′-nucleotidase.

(PRPP). These are then taken through a 10-step process culminating in purine nucleotide formation. PRPP is also used as a substrate for pyrimidine and pyridine synthesis. Thus, the first committed step in purine synthesis is catalysed by the enzyme amidophosphoribosyl transferase (amidoPRT). The de novo synthetic pathway requires heavy energy consumption in the form of ATP. Consequently, numerous enzymes for salvaging and interconverting premade purines exist to recycle these energy-rich compounds. Two salvage enzymes are particularly important in gout. These are hypoxanthine guanine phosphoribosyl transferase (HPRT) and adenine phosphoribosyl transferase (APRT).

Control of normal purine metabolism in man is well understood. The first committed step in purine biosynthesis is rate limiting. AmidoPRT is allosterically activated by its substrate PRPP and inhibited by purine nucleotides, its end products. The enzyme PRPP synthetase is similarly regulated, but is less sensitive to small changes in end-product concentrations. Thus, control of purine metabolism is negatively affected by purines themselves and positively influenced by PRPP (Becker and Kim 1987).

Uric acid metabolism

Uric acid is ultimately formed from purine nucleotides through the intermediate compounds xanthine, hypoxanthine, and guanine by the enzyme xanthine oxidase. It is a terminal product as no mammalian uricase exists. Uric acid is made primarily in the liver. The average pool size is 1200 mg in men and 600 mg in women. In both men and women, about two-thirds of the total uric acid pool is turned over each day. Uric acid pools in patients with gout are always larger than normal, usually in the range of 2000–4000 mg. In patients with tophi, uric acid burdens can be as high as 30 000 mg (Wyngaarden and Kelley 1985).

Two-thirds of uric acid is renally excreted (Wyngaarden and Kelley 1976). The remainder is degraded by gut bacteria via the process of 'intestinal uricolysis'. The renal handling of uric acid is complex and not fully understood. It entails a four-step process beginning with glomerular filtration, followed by active reabsorption in the proximal tubule, tubular secretion at some distal site, and ending with post-secretory tubular reabsorption (Levinson and Sorenson 1980) (Fig. 2).

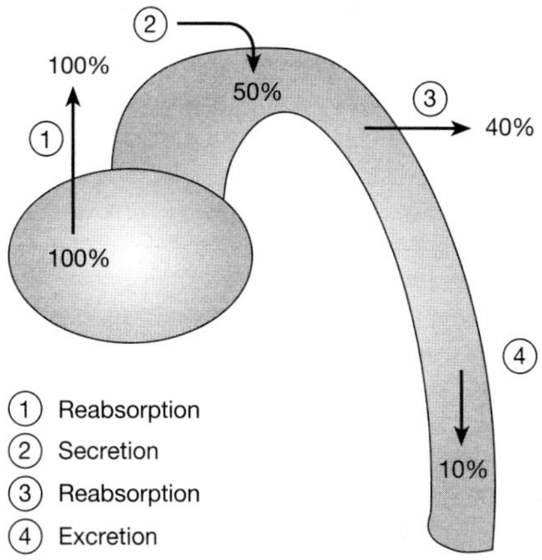

Fig. 2 Simplified scheme of renal excretion of urate: (1) Reabsorption after filtration, (2) secretion in the proximal tubule, (3) reabsorption at some distal site, and (4) excretion in the urine.

For the sake of discussion, we will divide the known metabolic causes of hyperuricaemia associated with gout into three categories: causes of primary gout, defined inborn errors of metabolism, and aetiologies of secondary gout.

Mechanisms of hyperuricaemia in primary gout

Primary gout is simply defined by the absence of any identifiable underlying disease causing hyperuricaemia. This criterion defines the largest group of patients with gout. Most of these patients are older men and 80–85 per cent are hyperuricaemic on the basis of underexcretion of uric acid. There is no difference in rates of intestinal uricolysis in patients with primary gout compared with controls. Thus, the site of the abnormality in patients with primary gout who underexcrete is most likely to be at the kidney. Simkin (1977b) has shown that most patients with primary gout have low fractional uric acid excretion rates. The mechanism of underexcretion remains to be elucidated but is most likely a defect in secretion or reabsorption rather than in filtration (Wyngaarden and Kelley 1985).

A minority of patients with primary gout have high urinary uric acid levels and excessive de novo purine synthesis. The best evidence to date supports a role for increased PRPP availability or decreased purine nucleotide concentrations (thus diminishing feedback inhibition of the synthetic enzymes) in patients with primary gout who overproduce uric acid (Levinson and Becker 1993).

Inborn errors of metabolism causing hyperuricaemia

The enzyme defects associated with gout often present as precocious gout in childhood or early adulthood in the setting of a strong family history of gout. There are three well-characterized enzyme defects causing hyperuricaemia. Together these account for less than 5 per cent of cases of gout. These are summarized in Table 2 and include HPRT deficiency, PRPP synthetase superactivity, and glucose 6-phosphatase (G6P) deficiency.

HPRT deficiency produces hyperuricaemia by increasing de novo synthesis of purine nucleotides through increased availability of the substrate PRPP, which stimulates synthesis (Wyngaarden and Kelley 1985). In its most complete form, HPRT deficiency results in the Lesch–Nyhan syndrome. This syndrome presents in early childhood with severe mental retardation, self-mutilation, choreoathetosis, spasticity, hyperuricaemia, and premature gout. Although it is linked to the X chromosome, there are two reported cases in girls (Yukawa et al. 1992). Partial defects of HPRT result in hyperuricaemia alone without the severe neurological consequences of complete HRPT deficiency. The diagnosis of HPRT deficiency can be made by documenting low HPRT activity in erythrocytes. Numerous different genetic mutations have been described in HPRT deficiency (Jinnah et al. 2000).

Increased PRPP synthetase activity was described by Sperling et al. (1972). Overactivity of this enzyme results in increased PRPP levels and

Table 2 Inherited metabolic disorders causing gout

Syndrome	Pattern of inheritance	Mechanism of hyperuricaemia
HPRT deficiency (Lesch–Nyhan)	X-linked	HPRT deficiency increases PRPP
Increased PRPP synthetase	X-linked	Overactivity of PRPP synthetase
von Gierke's disease (G6P deficiency)	Autosomal recessive	Increased activity of amidoPRT, decreased renal excretion to acidaemia

Table 3 Drugs associated with hyperuricaemia and gout

Drugs causing overproduction	Drugs causing underexcretion
Ethanol	Ethanol
Fructose	Salicylates (<2 g/day)
Cytotoxic drugs	Cyclosporin
Vitamin B_{12}	Diuretics
Warfarin	Ethambutol
	Pyrazinamide
	Levodopa
	Angiotensin
	Vasopressin
	Laxatives
	Nicotinic acid
	Nitroglycerin
	Methoxyflurane

causes profound premature hyperuricaemia. The trait is inherited as an X-linked dominant condition. Three kindreds each with a different genetic mutation have been well characterized. Gout and renal stones develop in the second and third decades in affected males.

The third well-characterized enzyme defect associated with gout is G6P deficiency (Alepa et al. 1967). This is also known as glycogen storage disease type I, or von Gierke's disease. It presents in childhood with short stature, hepatomegaly, and recurrent hypoglycaemia. A bleeding diathesis may also accompany the syndrome. Affected patients cannot release glucose from premade glycogen stores. Subsequent hypoglycaemia results in ATP catabolism, lactic acidaemia, and elevated levels of free fatty acids, pyruvate, and triglycerides. Hyperuricaemia in this syndrome is due to two effects. Renal excretion of uric acid is diminished because other organic anions compete for transport in the kidney. Overproduction via the de novo synthetic pathway due to decreased feedback inhibition of amidoPRT also occurs. Hyperuricaemia is often present from infancy, with gout occurring as early as 10 years of age. In its classic form, it is inherited as an autosomal recessive disorder. Some forms of partial enzyme deficiency have been described.

Causes of secondary gout

The causes of secondary gout are well defined. Some cause hyperuricaemia on the basis of overproduction of uric acid, such as tumour lysis syndrome, myeloproliferative disease, haemolytic anaemia, and psoriasis. All of these conditions are characterized by increased cell turnover with a subsequent increase in purine synthesis and catabolism.

Alternatively, conditions such as renal failure and many drugs produce hyperuricaemia and gout by promoting undersecretion of uric acid. Although mild renal insufficiency from any cause is a risk factor for gout, certain forms of kidney disease such as autosomal dominant polycystic kidney disease may be preferentially associated with gout (Mejias et al. 1989). Interestingly, end-stage renal disease often produces hyperuricaemia, but these patients rarely develop gout (Schreiner et al. 2000).

Lead exposure is a cause of secondary gout. Saternine gout, which is associated with heavy lead exposures (often from the ingestion of lead-laden whisky), is rare today. Lead interferes with renal excretion of uric acid by altering the tubular transport of urate. It affects purine metabolism by altering purine nucleotide turnover. Lead levels are increased in gout patients. However, the clinical association between low level lead exposure and gout remains unclear (Shadick et al. 2000).

Drugs commonly associated with hyperuricaemia are listed in Table 3.

Urate crystal formation (Fig. 3)

Because the vast majority of patients with hyperuricaemia never develop gout, the processes of crystal formation and release define clinical gout. Yet, we know suprisingly little about why uric acid crystals form *in vivo*.

Our current understanding of urate crystal formation is based on knowledge of the biochemistry of urate, *in vitro* studies of crystallogenesis, and the histopathology of gout. Urate is present in two forms in the body. At neutral and alkaline pH, the monosodium salt (MSU) predominates. At acidic pH, such as in urine, the primary form is uric acid. Both forms are relatively insoluble, although uric acid is less soluble than its salt. A solution is supersaturated with monosodium urate at 37°C at concentrations greater

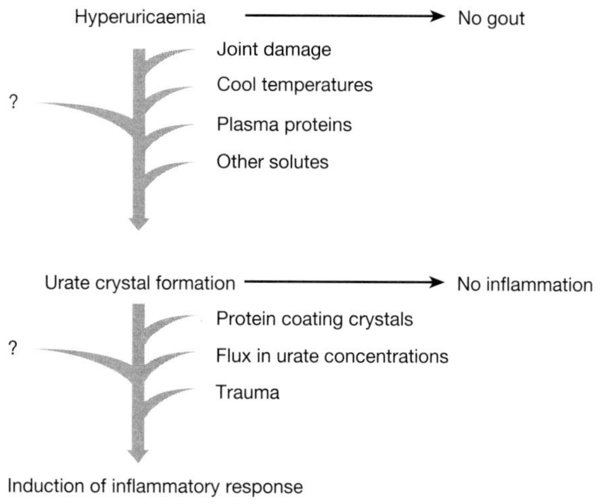

Fig. 3 Overview of factors influencing the development of gouty arthritis.

than 6.4 mg/dl. Cooler temperatures decrease urate solubility, thus predicting the predilection of gout for distal joints.

In vitro studies of crystallogenesis have yielded conflicting results in regard to the influences of serum, synovial fluid, and many individual plasma proteins, including albumin and proteoglycans, on crystal formation (McGill and Dieppe 1991b). In addition, urate crystals themselves initiate further crystal formation (McGill and Dieppe 1991a).

Urate crystals have a unique distribution in the body. They prefer sites rich in connective tissue, such as synovium, cartilage, tendon, skin, and the renal interstitium. Gouty arthritis often develops in previously damaged joints. Disturbances of proteoglycan metabolism or collagen structure may promote crystal formation and release. Joint effusions may also affect urate crystal formation. Because the diffusion of urate through the synovial membrane is less than that of water (Simkin 1977a), resorption of water in a joint with an effusion during recumbency would increase the effective urate concentration and promote crystal formation. This observation may explain the predilection of gout attacks for late night or early morning hours.

Pathogenesis of the acute attack (Fig. 4)

Once MSU crystals form in the joint, they may induce an acute attack of gouty arthritis. Urate crystals clearly cause inflammation; yet we are unable to explain why they are present in synovial fluids from asymptomatic uninflamed joints (Pascual 1991). The type and quantity of protein coating the

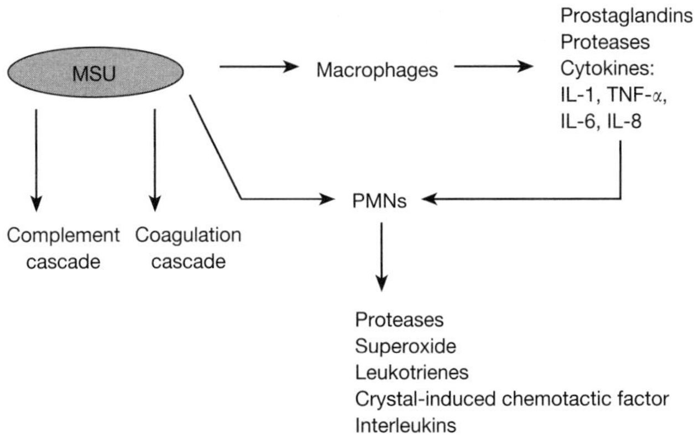

Fig. 4 The mechanisms through which MSU crystals cause inflammation in the joint.

crystals may affect their ability to induce inflammation. IgG is found in association with MSU crystals and increases cell activation (Russell et al. 1983). Terkeltaub et al. (1991) demonstrated a role for the lipoprotein apoE in inhibiting crystal-induced inflammation.

The effects of uncoated MSU crystals on articular and inflammatory cells are well characterized (McColl and Naccache 2000). The cells that urate crystals first encounter in the joint are most probably macrophage-like synovial cells. Here they induce the release of vasoactive prostaglandins, proteases, and proinflammatory cytokines including interleukin-1 (IL-1), IL-6, and IL-8, which initiate a vigorous inflammatory response. Recruited polymorphonuclear leucocytes release proteases, superoxides, leukotrienes, and interleukins when exposed to MSU crystals. MSU crystals activate complement via the classical pathway. They also promote the release of Hageman factor and the subsequent activation of bradykinin, kallikrein, and other coagulation factors.

The mechanisms through which they stimulate these cells remain to be elucidated. Certainly, some crystals are phagocytosed and cause lysis of the phagolysosome, release of its toxic contents, and death of the cell. Other effects may be mediated through cell membrane perturbations. The highly charged surfaces of MSU crystals may bind to and cross-link membrane receptors, thus mediating some of the crystals' immediate effects.

The factors that terminate an acute attack remain unclear. One hypothesis suggests changes in crystal size and protein coating render the crystals less inflammatory. These changes may be mediated through generation of oxygen free radicals by polymorphonuclear leucocytes (Marcalongo et al. 1988).

Tophus formation

Tophi are soft tissue deposits of urate. We know little about how and why they form. Palmer et al. (1989) proposed that tophi are urate-lowering organs. Based on histological studies, they proposed that acini of macrophages develop in areas of high local urate concentrations. These organized cells actively transport urate from the interstitial fluid to the centre of the acinus. They grow to a certain size and then fuse with other acini, eventually forming tophi. Further work is necessary to confirm this theory.

Clinical features

Articular gout is often divided into four clinical stages. The first stage is defined by asymptomatic hyperuricaemia. This is followed by acute gouty arthritis and then by another asymptomatic phase termed intercritical gout. When allowed to proceed untreated, some patients will go on to develop chronic tophaceous gout.

Acute gout

The first clinical symptom of gout is usually an acute, self-limited, monoarticular inflammatory arthritis affecting the joints of the lower extremities. Gout has a predilection for the first metatarsophalangeal joint. As many as 50–70 per cent of first gout attacks occur in the big toe. Other frequently involved joints include those of the foot, ankle, knee, wrist, elbow, and the small joints of the hands. The large axial joints and those of the spine are uncommon sites for early acute gout attacks.

The onset of an attack occurs suddenly and often late at night or early in the morning. Patients will describe very severe pain, associated with swelling, extreme tenderness, and redness overlying the joint. Without intervention, the attack will usually subside within 5–7 days. Low-grade fever, malaise, and anorexia may occur. The attack may be preceded by brief twinges of pain (petit attacks) in the affected joint.

Common precipitants of acute attacks include excess alcohol intake, intercurrent illness, surgery, starvation, trauma, and the initiation of drugs that alter urate metabolism. All of these precipitants alter serum urate levels.

Physical examination shows signs of inflammation with erythema, warmth, and swelling over the joint, often extending to the overlying skin. There is exquisite tenderness over the affected joint. Not infrequently, an overlying cellulitis or accompanying tenosynovitis occurs. The skin may desquamate in the later days of an attack. Acute gout can also occur in bursas, and gout is a common cause of acute inflammatory olecranon bursitis.

After the attack resolves, the patient will be completely asymptomatic. This phase is referred to as intercritical gout. Most patients will go on to have an additional attack within 2 years of the first attack. In one study, 78 per cent had recurrent attacks within 2 years, and after 10 years, 93 per cent had had more than one attack (Gutman 1973). Untreated, the intercritical phases become shorter. Interestingly, they still present an opportunity for diagnosis, as many joints will still have urate crystals in the synovial fluid during the intercritical phase if they were involved in a previous attack, and urate-lowering therapy has not been initiated (Pascual 1991).

Chronic tophaceous gout

In the later stages of untreated disease, clinical manifestations characteristically change. Acute attacks are more often polyarticular. The intercritical stage shortens, and repeated joint damage results in permanent deformities, loss of motion, chronic pain, and tophi.

Polyarticular gout occurs in late-stage disease, although some patients present earlier with polyarticular attacks. Intercritical stages are short or non-existent and involvement of atypical sites including the upper extremities, the spine, and axial joints may ensue. After repeated attacks in a single joint, deformity and loss of motion may occur.

Tophi are deposits of urate embedded in a matrix composed of amorphous urates, lipids, proteins, and calcific debris (Fig. 5). Tophi are usually subcutaneous, but they rarely occur in bone and other organs including the heart valves and the eye. Classic sites include the pinna of the ear, bursas around elbows and knees, the dorsal surfaces of the metacarpophalangeal joints, and the Achilles tendon. Tophi are not distinguishable on physical examination from rheumatoid nodules or other subcutaneous nodules. There is no accompanying inflammation and they are usually painless. The overlying skin may be taut and shiny. A thick white or whitish-yellow exudate is seen if the skin integrity is compromised.

Tophi or chronic polyarthritis may occur as early as 3 years or as late as 42 years after the first acute attack. In the pre-treatment era, 50 per cent of patients with gout had tophi after 10 years of disease (Gutman 1973). Currently, about 5 per cent of patients with gout will have tophi (O'Duffy et al. 1975). Their occurrence is directly correlated with serum urate levels, and they identify a group of patients with severe and prolonged hyperuricaemia. Another group at risk of developing tophi and polyarticular gout are elderly women with primary nodal osteoarthritis on diuretic therapy (Macfarlane and Dieppe 1985).

Other articular manifestations of gout

Gout has been variably associated with avascular necrosis of the femoral head and chondrocalcinosis (Stockman et al. 1980).

Renal disease and gout

The relationship between kidney dysfunction and gout remains complex and confusing. Three renal syndromes are associated with gout. Urate

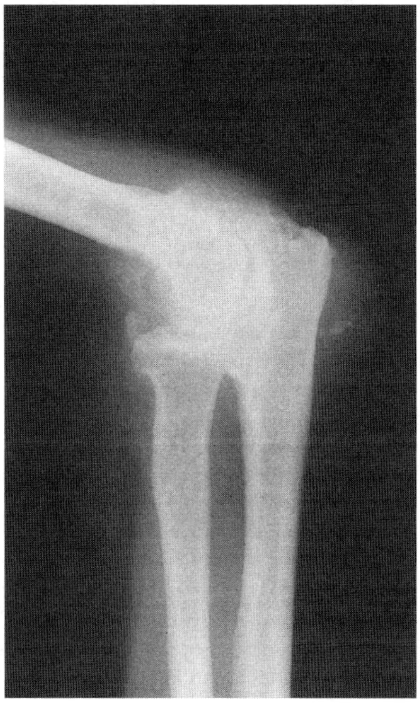

Fig. 5 A tophus in the olecranon bursa appears as a typical soft tissue density with a small amount of calcification.

crystals can form in the renal interstitium causing urate nephropathy. Uric acid can acutely precipitate in the collecting tubules resulting in acute uric acid nephropathy. Lastly, uric acid nephrolithiasis may occur.

Urate nephropathy

The pathological changes that define urate nephropathy are common. MSU crystals in the renal medulla are associated with a giant-cell inflammatory reaction. The clinical significance of these pathological findings, however, remains unclear. Renal insufficiency is unequivocally common in patients with gout, but controversy exists as to the aetiology of this renal dysfunction. Current dogma states that urate crystals themselves produce only a minor amount of renal damage. Most of the renal disease associated with gout is secondary to inadequately controlled hypertension, non-steroidal anti-inflammatory drug (NSAID) use, and other comorbidities (Perez-Ruiz et al. 2000).

Acute uric acid nephropathy

Excluding nephrolithiasis, the renal syndrome most often associated with uric acid today is acute uric acid nephropathy. This often occurs in an acutely ill, dehydrated patient treated with cytotoxic drugs for a lymphoproliferative disorder. An acute obstructive uropathy ensues with oliguric renal failure. Uric acid crystals form in the collecting tubules and are found in the urine. Uric acid/creatinine ratios are often greater than 1.0. This complication can be avoided with adequate hydration and the prophylactic administration of allopurinol prior to initiating chemotherapy.

Uric acid nephrolithiasis

The association between gout and nephrolithiasis is well established. Prevalence figures for renal stones vary between 10 and 42 per cent of patients with gout. Of these stones, 84 per cent are uric acid stones. Risk factors for developing uric acid stones include elevated urinary uric acid levels, and low urine pH (Yu 1981). Half the patients excreting greater than 1100 mg uric acid per day will have stones. Interestingly, however, only 20 per cent of patients with uric acid stones are hyperuricaemic (Talbott 1957). Patients with gout also are at a higher risk for non-urate stones. Of the 16 per cent of stones in patients with gout that do not contain uric acid, 8 per cent are calcium oxalate, 4 per cent are calcium phosphates, and 4 per cent are mixed stones. It is postulated that uric acid serves as a nidus for calcium oxalate crystal growth. Alternatively, or in addition, levels of inhibitors of calcium oxalate stone formation may be decreased in the urine of patients with gout.

Laboratory investigation

Investigation of the patient with an acute attack

Synovial fluid analysis remains the single most important diagnostic study in the patient with suspected gout. Synovial fluid is usually easily obtained from a large joint, while often only a drop of fluid or blood from the joint or adjacent tissues is necessary to provide a sample for definitive diagnosis of gout in a small joint. Synovial fluid is typically inflammatory with a mean white cell count of 20 000 cells/mm^3. Most cells are polymorphonuclear leucocytes. Viscosity is often poor. A definite diagnosis can be made if typical, negatively birefringent, needle-shaped crystals are seen in the fluid with a polarizing light microscope (Plate 189). They may be extra- or intracellular. Rarely one may see spherules of uric acid in acute gout.

Few other laboratory studies are of significant clinical utility in diagnosing acute gout. Serum uric acid levels during the acute attack may not reflect pre-attack levels and cannot be used to make a diagnosis of gout in the absence of urate crystals in the synovial fluid. One may see a peripheral leucocytosis, an elevated erythrocyte sedimentation rate, and increased levels of other acute-phase reactants during an acute attack. Synovial fluid cultures and Gram stains may help rule out concurrent infection. Radiographs are often normal during early episodes of gout. They may be useful to differentiate other problems such as fracture or infection from acute gout. Often, soft tissue swelling is the sole radiographic finding in early gout.

Evaluation of the patient with recurrent attacks

Serum uric acid levels and 24-h urine collections for creatinine and uric acid may be helpful in evaluating the patient once the acute attack has subsided. Serum urate levels over 7 mg/dl define hyperuricaemia in most laboratories. Values of urinary uric acid over 1000 mg/day on an unrestricted diet define patients that overproduce, and may influence the choice of therapy. Patients suspected of a primary metabolic disorder should have a 24-h urine sample tested for creatinine, protein, and uric acid and a careful family history taken. If urinary uric acid levels are high, levels of enzyme activity for HPRT, PRPP synthetase, and G6P can be measured in specialist laboratories.

In later disease, gout has a typical radiographic appearance (Barthelemy et al. 1984). The hallmarks of radiographic gout are due to the presence of tophi in or near the joint. In the soft tissues, tophi appear eccentric and nodular (Fig. 5). A small percentage of them calcify. Tophi may occur in or near a joint or distant from periarticular tissues. As a soft tissue tophus enlarges, it may encroach on the adjacent bone and produce a cortical erosion with focal periosteal new bone formation. This occurrence results in an erosion with a typical overhanging margin, present in 40 per cent of gouty erosions (Fig. 6). When in the joint, tophi produce marginal erosions with a characteristic 'punched out' or sclerotic border (Fig. 7). Erosions are particularly common on the medial and dorsal portions of the first metatarsal head. Similar changes can affect the digits of the hand. Bony abnormalities of the periosteum may occur in association with tophus formation. Specifically, a 'lace pattern' of finely striated periosteal reaction may develop adjacent to a tophus (Fig. 8). Rarely, bony proliferation may occur at the ends or shafts of long bones (mushrooming). Diaphyseal thickening may also occur. The joint space is characteristically well preserved until late in the disease. When joint space narrowing does occur it affects all joint compartments symmetrically, similar to other inflammatory joint disorders (Fig. 9). Bones may be osteopaenic from disuse, but are usually well mineralized.

Diagnosis

A definitive diagnosis of gout can only be made by the identification of urate crystals in the synovial fluid of an affected joint. Identification of urate crystals in tophi also allows a definitive diagnosis to be made. In the absence

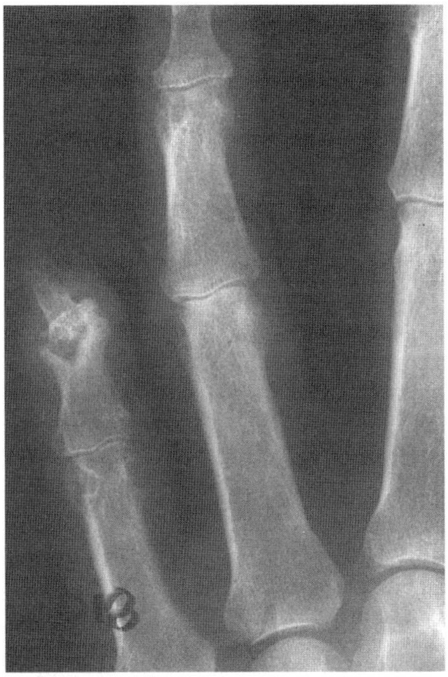

Fig. 6 A typical gouty erosion with overhanging margins is seen on the medial aspect of the proximal interphalangeal joint in this radiograph.

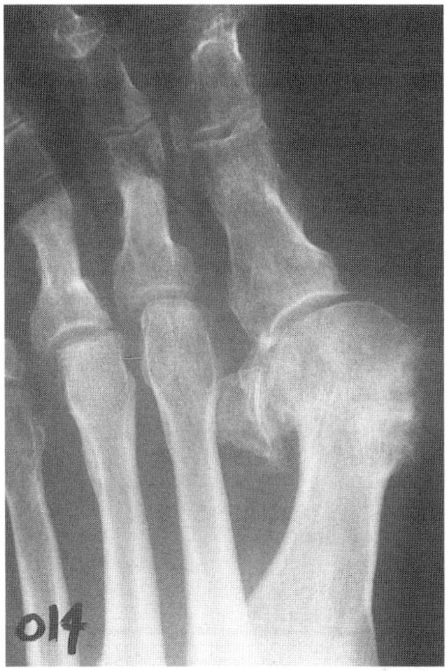

Fig. 8 On the lateral aspect of the distal metatarsal joint, a lace-like periosteal reaction adjacent to a tophus can be seen.

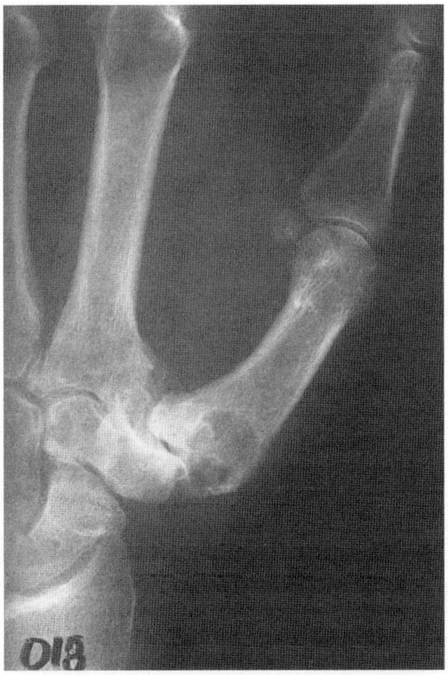

Fig. 7 An interosseus tophus appears as a 'punched out' or sclerotic erosion at the base of the proximal phalanx of the thumb.

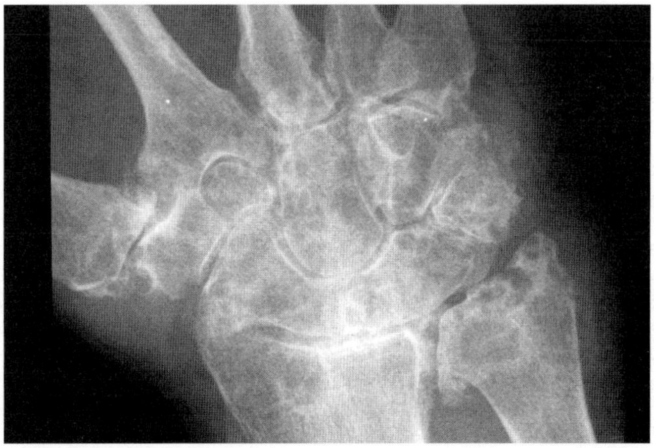

Fig. 9 Extensive bony destruction and deformities are seen with far-advanced gouty arthritis of the wrist.

of these findings, other clinical criteria may be used to make a putative diagnosis of gout (Wallace et al. 1977). As crystals may be present in the intercritical phase, one may aspirate an asymptomatic but previously affected joint to establish a definite diagnosis.

Many clinical conditions can mimic acute gout (Table 4). These include infectious arthritis, other crystal-associated arthropathies such as pseudogout or BCP-associated periarthritis, or trauma. Patients with palindromic rheumatism may give a similar history of self-limited monoarticular attacks associated with exquisite pain, tenderness, and erythema near the affected joint. Rarely, other causes of polyarticular inflammatory arthritis, particularly psoriatic arthritis or Reiter's syndrome, may present with monoarticular self-limited attacks of the lower extremities that may be confused with gout. Once tophi and deformities occur, gout can be misdiagnosed as rheumatoid arthritis. As many as 30 per cent of patients with gout will have positive serum rheumatoid factors (Kozin and McCarty 1977).

Management of gouty arthritis

Management of gouty arthritis can be divided into three phases: treatment of acute gout, treatment of chronic or tophaceous gout, and preventive measures. Despite our extensive understanding of gout and its causes, diagnosis and treatment are often not optimal (Pal et al. 2000).

Preventive measures

Gout is a significant public health problem despite our excellent therapy. Hochberg (1991) suggests that we may be able to decrease the incidence of gout with preventive measures such as avoiding excess weight gain, reducing risks for hypertension, avoiding diuretic therapy, controlling alcohol intake, and minimizing occupational lead exposures. The efficacy of such interventions remains to be proven.

Management of acute gout

Traditional therapies for acute gout include NSAIDs, colchicine, and steroids. Rest and splinting of the affected joint may be helpful adjuncts to any pharmacological therapy. The management of acute gout is summarized in Box 1.

NSAIDs

NSAIDs have replaced colchicine as the most commonly used drugs in the treatment of acute gout (Stuart et al. 1991). They interfere with the inflammation induced by MSU crystals. Traditionally, indomethacin has been the NSAID of choice in acute gout, but probably has no advantage over other NSAIDs (Sterling 1991). Sulindac may be better tolerated in those patients at high risk of renal side-effects from NSAIDs. In general, drugs with shorter half-lives achieve quicker therapeutic plasma levels and faster relief of pain. With treatment, symptoms should subside within 3–5 days. NSAIDs are contraindicated in patients with significant renal insufficiency, peptic ulcer disease, concurrent warfarin therapy, or liver disease.

Table 4 Clinical conditions that mimic gouty arthritis

CPPD disease (pseudogout)
BCP arthritis
Cellulitis
Erythema nodosum arthritis
Trauma
Palindromic rheumatism
Reiter's syndrome
Psoriatic arthritis
Rheumatoid arthritis

Colchicine

Colchicine is the oldest drug for gout, but its safety remains controversial. When used correctly, it can be very effective with a rapid onset of action. Colchicine tends to be much more effective in the early hours of an attack and loses efficacy with time. The mechanism of action of colchicine is unknown. It inhibits polymorphonuclear leucocyte function through its action on microtubules, but may also have very specific effects on crystal-induced inflammation (McColl and Naccache 2000). Colchicine can be given in intravenous and oral forms.

Current recommendations for intravenous use are cautious (Moreland and Ball 1991) (Table 5). A dose of 1–3 mg diluted in 20 ml of normal saline can be slowly instilled into a large vein. Another 1-mg dose can be given 6 h later if the clinical response is incomplete. The maximum dose is 4 mg in 24 h. No additional doses should be given for 7 days after the initial dose. Intravenous colchicine is particularly useful for patients unable to take oral medications. Now that parenteral forms of NSAIDs are available, its use may decline further. Absolute contraindications to the use of intravenous colchicine include significant renal or hepatic compromise, bone marrow suppression, or sepsis. It should be used with great caution in patients with mild renal or hepatic disease, or those on daily oral colchicine prophylaxis. Side-effects range from venous sclerosis or tissue damage from extravasation of colchicine, to fatal bone marrow failure. Other side-effects include renal or hepatic failure, disseminated intravascular coagulation, and neuromuscular toxicity. Deaths from misuse of intravenous colchicine have been reported (Roberts et al. 1987).

Colchicine is currently used more frequently in the oral than in the intravenous form. It is given as an initial 0.5–0.6 mg dose, which is repeated

Box 1 Management of acute gout

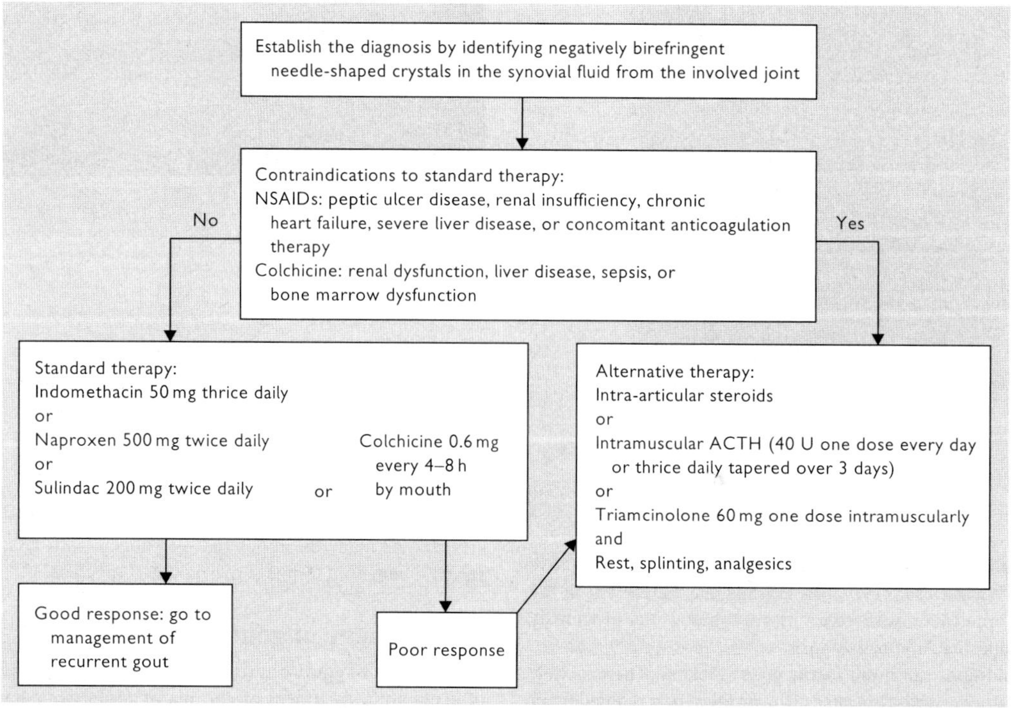

Table 5 Recommendations for the use of colchicine

Intravenous colchicine should not be given in patients with Creatinine clearance <10 ml/min Significant active liver disease or extrahepatic biliary obstruction Sepsis Bone marrow depression
Intravenous colchicine should be used cautiously in patients on oral colchicine prophylaxis, with poor venous access, or with any degree of hepatic or renal compromise
Recommended doses should not exceed 3 mg intravenous per 24 h or 5 mg orally per 24 h

Table 6 Regimens for use of corticosteroids in acute gouty arthritis

Drug	Dose	Route of administration	Length of use
Triamcinolone acetonide	60 mg	Intramuscular	Give once, repeat in 48 h if needed
Prednisone	20–50 mg with daily taper	Oral	3–20 days (mean 10 days)
ACTH	40 IU	Intramuscular	Give once
ACTH	40–80 IU	Intramuscular, intravenous, or subcutaneous	Every 8 h, then every 12 h, then each day on three successive days

every 1–2 h until gastrointestinal symptoms ensue or pain resolves. Doses should not exceed 5 mg in 24 h. Similar side-effects are reported for oral and intravenous forms. Oral colchicine, however, has a higher incidence of gastrointestinal side-effects and a lower incidence of major toxicities, probably because the tolerated dose is lower.

Corticosteroids

Corticosteroid use in gout has endured much ebb and flow in popularity during recent years. Although ACTH has been used for many years to treat gout, textbooks of the last two decades cautioned against systemic steroids because of concerns about rebound symptoms and inconsistent results. More recently, there has been a resurgence of interest in their use in gout. Regimens for acute gout include intramuscular ACTH, intramuscular triamcinolone, and oral steroids (Groff et al. 1990) (Table 6). These regimens are safe and well tolerated. Their efficacy remains to be proven. They may be particularly useful for patients in whom NSAIDs and colchicine are contraindicated. The use of intra-articular steroids is less controversial. Although no studies of the efficacy of intra-articular steroids have been published, they remain a mainstay of therapy in patients unable to tolerate more traditional therapies.

Prophylactic therapy

Drugs that reduce serum uric acid levels such as allopurinol and probenecid are the standard therapies available for prophylaxis of gout attacks. Colchicine and NSAIDs are less commonly used as prophylactic drugs, but may also decrease attack frequency and severity when used alone or in combination with other therapies. Indications for the use of prophylactic drugs include recurrent attacks, tophi, severe or polyarticular disease, renal disease, or an inborn error of metabolism causing gout. Urate-lowering therapies are traditionally not started during an acute attack and are initiated concurrently with a 2-week course of low-dose colchicine or an NSAID. This regimen may avoid the risk of precipitating an acute attack by rapidly lowering uric acid levels. Goals of therapy are to decrease attack frequency, dissolve tophi, and maintain serum uric acid levels in the normal range. The management of recurrent gout is summarized in Box 2.

Allopurinol

Allopurinol is the drug most commonly used for the prevention of acute gout and the treatment of chronic tophaceous gout (Stuart et al. 1991). It is a xanthine oxidase inhibitor and thus decreases uric acid production. It may also have other actions (Adriani and Naraghi 1985). It is very effective in lowering serum uric acid levels and is the drug of choice for patients with renal insufficiency, a history of nephrolithiasis, or tophi. It is also indicated in patients who clearly overproduce uric acid such as those with tumour lysis syndrome or primary metabolic defects. Allopurinol is usually given as a once daily dose of 300 mg. The dose should be adjusted downward in the presence of significant renal compromise. Occasionally, doses as high as 900 mg/day are necessary to achieve normal uric acid levels. The onset of action is rapid and effects can be seen as early as 4 days to 2 weeks. Allopurinol interferes with the metabolism of azathioprine, potentiating its marrow-suppressive effects, and may augment anticoagulant effects of warfarin. In general, the incidence of side-effects with allopurinol is low (less than 2 per cent). The most common side-effects include a hypersensitivity syndrome of rash and fever. Life-threatening reactions, including fulminant hepatitis, interstitial nephritis, and toxic epidermal necrolysis, are even more unusual. Patients with renal disease may have a greater incidence of drug allergy. Allopurinol can be given cautiously to an allergic patient using available desensitization regimens (Fam et al. 1992).

Uricosurics

Probenecid and sulfinpyrazone are the most commonly used uricosuric drugs. They interfere with the renal handling of urate by altering organic anion transport, thus increasing urate excretion. Usual doses of probenecid are 0.5–2 g given in twice daily doses. Sulfinpyrazone is given in doses of 300–400 mg/day. Both drugs are well tolerated and effective. Maximum doses of 3 g/day of probenecid and 800 mg/day of sulfinpyrazone are occasionally necessary to maintain normal serum uric acid levels. Uricosurics are contraindicated in patients with nephrolithiasis and ineffective in patients with significant renal compromise, or those using acetylsalicylates. Side-effects include rare hypersensitivity reactions, rashes, gastrointestinal complaints, and nephrotic syndrome.

Benzbromarone is a uricosuric drug available in Europe. Unlike other commonly used uricosuric drugs, it is effective in patients with renal insufficiency (Perez-Ruiz et al. 1998). At doses of 25–125 mg/day, it may lower serum uric acid values in patients with serum creatinine levels as high as 2.0 mg/dl.

Colchicine

In patients who are unable to take allopurinol or a uricosuric drug, daily low-dose oral colchicine may be useful in preventing further attacks of gout. It is given in doses of 0.5–1.2 mg/day. Unfortunately, serious side-effects have occurred even on this low-dose regimen in patients with renal insufficiency or liver disease.

Drug combinations and other therapies

Patients who continue to have gout attacks on a single prophylactic drug can be treated with a combination of medications (Rosenthal and Ryan 1995). The combination of probenecid and colchicine is more effective than probenecid alone. Small numbers of patients have been reported to respond to a combination of allopurinol and a uricosuric when either one alone was ineffective. Other measures such as eliminating the concurrent use of urate-elevating drugs, decreasing alcohol intake, weight reduction, and improving medication compliance may also help achieve control of uric acid levels in refractory patients. Rarely, patients with long-standing uncontrolled disease have permanent joint dysfunction which is best treated surgically. Tophi may occasionally require surgical removal with a low incidence of recurrence.

Uricase has been used as a novel approach to gout therapy. This enzyme dissolves uric acid crystals and has been used successfully in a small number

Box 2 Management of recurrent gout

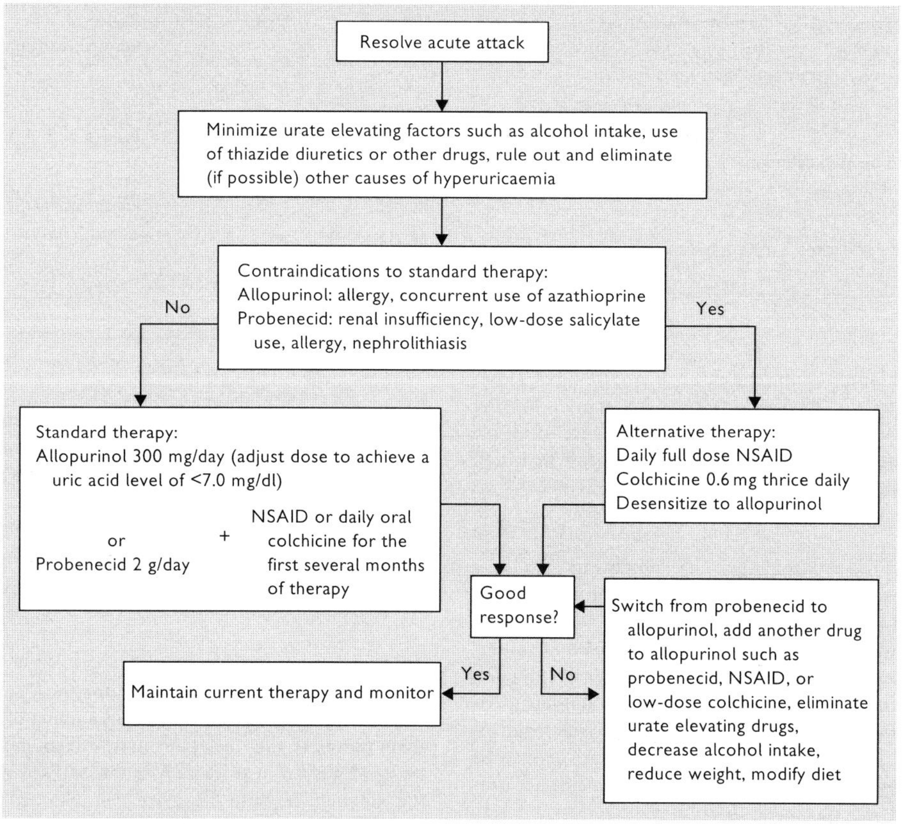

of patients. In some cases, polyethylene glycol treatment of the uricase was used to reduce its immunogenicity (Rosenthal and Ryan 1995).

Management of nephrolithiasis

Patients with uric acid stones are best managed with adequate hydration, urinary alkalinization (with bicarbonate or acetozolamide), and allopurinol. Potassium citrate may be used in place of allopurinol if necessary (Pak et al. 1986). This regimen is also effective in preventing calcium oxalate stones in patients with hyperuricaemia.

Gout in the transplant recipient

In the late 1980s, it was noted that an unusually large number of cases of gout were occurring in renal transplant patients. This coincided with the popular use of cyclosporin as an immunosuppressant. Hyperuricaemia occurs in 30–84 per cent and gout in 7–9 per cent of patients with renal transplants who are treated with cyclosporin (Lin et al. 1989). The incidence of gout in patients with heart and lung transplants on cyclosporin is also significantly increased (Burak et al. 1992). Gout in these patients is often more severe than primary gout. Polyarticular and tophaceous gout occurs earlier in cyclosporin-induced gout than in primary gout. Post-transplant patients can be particularly difficult to treat because of contraindications to the use of NSAIDs and colchicine, resistance to systemic steroids that they take chronically, and concerns about interactions between allopurinol and azathioprine. These patients are frequently on diuretics, and their risk of infection is high because of their compromised immune status. In the acute management of gout in the transplant patient, an arthrocentesis is usually warranted to eliminate the possibility of infection. Once a diagnosis is established, intra-articular steroids and systemic pain medications may be helpful. Chronically, some of these patients may be treated with uricosurics. If allopurinol is indicated, azathioprine can be reduced to one-third of its usual dose and 50–100 mg of allopurinol can be added. Blood counts should be carefully monitored during the initiation of allopurinol therapy.

Prognosis

In the era of antihyperuricaemic therapy, the prognosis for patients with gouty arthritis is excellent. Moreover, despite the association of hyperuricaemia with heart disease, hypertension, and renal insufficiency, there is no evidence that patients with gout have decreased longevity compared with controls who do not have gout.

Calcium pyrophospate dihydrate disease

CPPD disease is the second most common form of the crystal-associated arthritides. Unlike gout, the pathophysiology of CPPD disease remains poorly understood, and consequently no specific therapies for this arthropathy exist.

History

CPPD disease was initially described by McCarty et al. (1962) in the early 1960s. While studying crystals from synovial fluid of patients with presumed gout, it was noted that some crystals were resistant to dissolution by uricase. On further characterization, these crystals were composed of CPPD. Similar crystals were subsequently identified in the synovial fluid from patients with both acute and chronic arthritis. They were noted to be associated with advanced age, radiographic chondrocalcinosis, and a characteristic pattern of severe joint degeneration. Our understanding of the pathophysiology of CPPD crystal formation remains rudimentary.

Definition

No concensus as to the proper nomenclature of CPPD disease exists. CPPD disease or CPPD deposition disease are the terms most commonly used to refer to the arthritis caused by CPPD crystals. Other terms used similarly include CPDD disease and pyrophosphate arthropathy. The acute form of CPPD disease is commonly referred to as pseudogout. Chondrocalcinosis, a frequent associated finding, is defined by the radiographic presence of finely stippled calcification in articular hyaline and fibrocartilage. Although these deposits are usually composed of CPPD crystals, other mineral forms have been identified in pathological specimens with chondrocalcinosis (Marcos et al. 1981).

Epidemiology

Because the clinical syndromes associated with CPPD crystals are heterogeneous and may mimic other rheumatic diseases, the prevalence and incidence of CPPD deposition disease is difficult to define. Small studies have suggested a prevalence rate as high as 0.9 per 1000 (O'Duffy 1976), a figure about half that of gouty arthritis. Gender predominance varies from study to study, but symptomatic CPPD disease may be more common in women (Felson et al. 1989). The average age in the largest collection of symptomatic patients with definite or probable CPPD disease is 72 years (Rosenthal and Ryan 2001).

Most studies on prevalence have relied on autopsy data or are based on radiographic chondrocalcinosis. These studies clearly demonstrate that CPPD crystal deposition increases with age. Autopsy studies show prevalence rates of 20 per cent in knee joints from patients over the age of 60 years (Mitrovic et al. 1988). CPPD crystals are unusual in joints of patients under the age of 60, and may be present in about 50 per cent of nonagenarians (Mitrovic et al. 1988). Radiographic studies confirm this pattern. An overall prevalence of chondrocalcinosis of 8.1 per cent in the population between the ages of 63 and 93 was noted in Framingham, Massachusetts. Age-specific rates rose from 3.2 per cent in the 65–69 year age group to 27.1 per cent in patients over the age of 85 years (Felson et al. 1989).

CPPD disease usually occurs sporadically. However, familial cases in the Chiloean Islands of South America, France, Spain, Mexico, and Canada have been well characterized. Familial CPPD occurs prematurely and is often associated with very severe arthritis presenting in the second and third decades. Although the genetics of these kindreds are variable, most show an autosomal dominant pattern of inheritance. The genetic abnormality in some kindreds has been mapped to the short arm of chromosome 5p (Reginato et al. 1999).

Like gout, CPPD disease is associated with a variety of other medical conditions (Jones et al. 1992). Unlike gout, the pathophysiological connections between CPPD disease and these disorders is not always apparent. Associated conditions can be divided into definite and possible associations. Definite associations include hypomagnesaemia, hypophosphatasia, haemochromatosis Wilson's disease, and hyperparathyroidism. Possible associations include gout, ochronosis, familial hypocalciuric hypercalcaemia, and perhaps other causes of sustained hypercalcaemia, diabetes mellitus, and X-linked hypophosphataemic rickets. An association with hypothyroidism is controversial (Jones et al. 1992).

Clinical features

CPPD disease is a clinically heterogeneous disorder causing both acute and chronic arthritis. Its presentations have been separated into seven syndromes based on clinical features (Rosenthal and Ryan 2001) (Table 7).

The most commonly recognized form of CPPD disease is the acute arthritis known as pseudogout (or CPPD disease type A). Pseudogout is often clinically indistinguishable from gout, hence its name. It is characterized by the acute onset of pain, warmth, erythema, and swelling usually affecting a single joint. The knee is most commonly involved. Other large joints such as shoulders, wrists, elbows, and ankles may also be affected. Pseudogout occurs only rarely in small joints. Attacks are variable in duration, lasting from 2 to 108 days. Few other signs or symptoms are present. Precipitants of acute attacks include intercurrent illnesses, stroke, trauma, surgery (particularly parathyroidectomy), rapid diuresis, and drugs such as tacrolimus, granulocyte–macrophage colony stimulating factor, and possibly intra-articular hyaluronic acid injections (Rosenthal and Ryan 2001).

Table 7 Clinical presentations of CPPD disease

Type	Clinical description	Frequency (%)
A	Pseudogout/acute inflammatory monoarthritis	25
B	Pseudorheumatoid/polyarthritis with synovitis	5
C and D	Pseudo-osteoarthritis/joint degeneration with (type C) or without (type D) acute attacks	50
E	Lanthanic/asymptomatic	?
F	Pseudoneurotrophic/severe joint destruction with or without neuropathy	Rare
Others	Tophaceous CPPD deposits Spinal CPPD deposition Crowned dens syndrome Spinal stenosis	Rare

In the extremely elderly or ill patient, acute pseudogout may have a dramatic presentation. High fever, hypotension, and delerium may mimic sepsis or other systemic diseases (Bong and Bennett 1981).

CPPD disease may have a rheumatoid-like (type B) presentation. This form of CPPD disease accounts for less than 5 per cent of patients with CPPD disease. Symptoms include generalized joint pain and stiffness. The large joints such as knees, wrists, and elbows are commonly involved. Morning stiffness may be prolonged. Synovitis is noted on physical examination. Features that distinguish CPPD disease from rheumatoid arthritis include the absence of small joint involvement, negative serum rheumatoid factor, and the presence of CPPD crystals in the synovial fluid of the involved joints. In addition, patients with rheumatoid arthritis have polyarthritis, which flares in phase, while the patients with pseudorheumatoid disease will have joint flares out of phase with one another (Rosenthal and Ryan 2001).

More than 50 per cent of patients with CPPD disease present with an osteoarthritis-like syndrome. These patients are classified as having the type C and type D forms of the disease. They have pain, stiffness, and limited range of motion of the affected joints. Joints not commonly involved in osteoarthritis may be affected, such as shoulders, elbows, and wrists. Examination shows little or no synovitis. Radiographs may show severe degenerative joint disease. Patients with the type C disease differ from those with type D in that they have acute attacks superimposed on chronic symptoms. Patients with the type D disease do not have acute attacks.

CPPD disease type E is clinically silent. It is also referred to as lanthanic CPPD disease. It is picked up incidently as radiographic chondrocalcinosis. This may be the most common type of CPPD disease.

Type F (or neuropathic) CPPD disease remains controversial and is rare; although described in patients with tertiary syphilis and severe neurotrophic arthritis. A similar clinical picture can be seen even in the absence of significant neuropathy (Menkes et al. 1976).

Although this classification scheme is helpful in describing patients with CPPD disease, not all cases are easily catagorized. The scheme does serve to emphasize the clinical heterogeneity of this disorder and the fact that CPPD disease must be considered as a cause of acute and chronic, inflammatory and non-inflammatory arthritis.

Tophaceous deposits of CPPD crystals have been described, but are not commonly seen. In the wrist they can cause median nerve compression. In the spine, they may involve the ligamentum flavum and have been reported to produce symptoms of central canal stenosis as well as cervical myelopathy (Rosenthal and Ryan 2001). The crowned dens syndrome involves the deposition of CPPD (or BCP) crystals around the atlantoaxial joint and is a cause of acute neck pain (Bouvet et al. 1985). CPPD deposits rarely occur in tendons, bursas, and bone.

Laboratory investigation

CPPD disease is most carefully defined by the presence of CPPD crystals in the synovial fluid of affected joints. Synovial fluids should be collected in heparin-containing tubes and carefully examined under polarized-light microscopy for the weakly-positively birefringent rhomboidal crystals of CPPD (Plate 190). Even in the best of hands, many cases of CPPD deposition disease are missed because of inaccurate crystal identification (Segal and Albert 1999). These crystals may be sparse or abundant and can be either intra- or extracellular. Their number is not correlated with the degree of inflammation in the joint (Rosenthal and Ryan 2001). Synovial fluid from patients with acute pseudogout may have cell counts as low as 500 cells/mm^3 or as high as 50 000 cells/mm^3. The mean cell counts are similar to those of acute gout (20 000 cells/mm^3) with greater than 90 per cent polymorphonuclear leucocytes (Rosenthal and Ryan 2001). Fluid may be haemorrhagic, particularly early in an attack. Many synovial fluids will also contain BCP crystals (Dieppe et al. 1977). During the acute attack, serum levels of acute-phase reactants may be elevated (Rosenthal and Ryan 2001).

Radiographs of the affected joint may not be helpful in establishing a diagnosis acutely. However, the presence of chondrocalcinosis increases the likelihood of CPPD disease. Chondrocalcinosis is found in both fibrocartilage and hyaline articular cartilage. Common sites for chondrocalcinosis are the menisci of the knee (Fig. 10), the triangular cartilage of the wrist (Fig. 11), and the symphysis pubis (Fig. 12) (Rosenthal and Ryan 2001). Other radiographic changes may provide helpful supportive data. Typical findings include eburnation, joint space narrowing, and sub-chondral cyst formation (Resnick et al. 1977). Osteophyte formation is variable, but may be less common than in osteoarthritis. Progressive destruction of the joint with bony collapse and loose body formation occurs frequently in CPPD disease.

The distribution and pattern of radiographic involvement may be helpful in differentiating CPPD disease from osteoarthritis. CPPD disease affects joints not commonly involved in osteoarthritis. Axial involvement with intervertebral disc calcification, sacroiliac erosions, and sub-chondral cysts of the facet joints occur with CPPD disease. In the knee, tricompartmental involvement or isolated patellofemoral abnormalities are seen with CPPD disease more commonly than with osteoarthritis. Cortical erosions on the femur superior to the patella and osteonecrosis of the medial femoral condyle may also be diagnostic clues to CPPD disease (Watt and Dieppe 1983).

Patients with CPPD disease should be screened for one of the unusual metabolic disorders that promotes premature CPPD deposition. Laboratory evaluation should include serum levels of calcium, magnesium, phosphate, iron, and measurement of iron-binding capacity, and alkaline phosphatase.

Diagnosis

A definite diagnosis of CPPD disease can only be made when typical crystals are seen in synovial fluid with polarized-light miscroscopy. Phase-contrast microscopy may be a useful adjunct in detecting crystals. Radiographic changes can be used to establish a probable diagnosis. Diagnostic criteria based on crystal identification and radiological findings have been proposed (Rosenthal and Ryan 2001).

The differential diagnosis of pseudogout is much the same as that of gout. Infectious, arthritis, trauma, and other crystal-associated arthropathies are the conditions that are most often mistaken for pseudogout. The chronic arthritis of CPPD disease can be mistaken for osteoarthritis, any one of the seronegative spondyloarthropathies, rheumatoid arthritis, or neurotrophic arthritis.

Pathogenesis (Fig. 13)

The pathogenesis of CPPD disease remains obscure. Conceptually, CPPD crystal deposition, like gout, can be divided into phases of crystal formation,

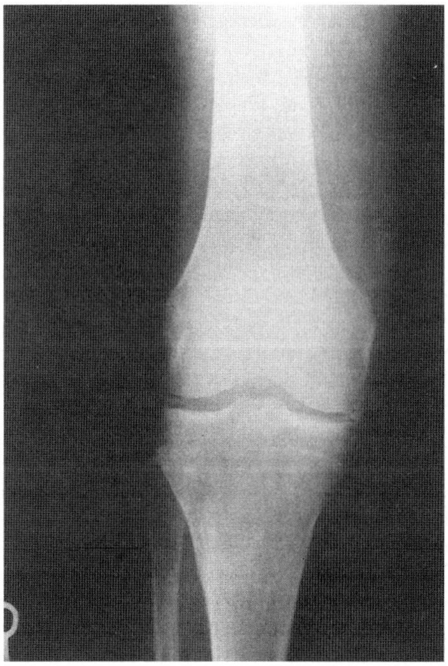

Fig. 10 Chondrocalcinosis is seen as finely stippled calcification of the cartilage in the knee.

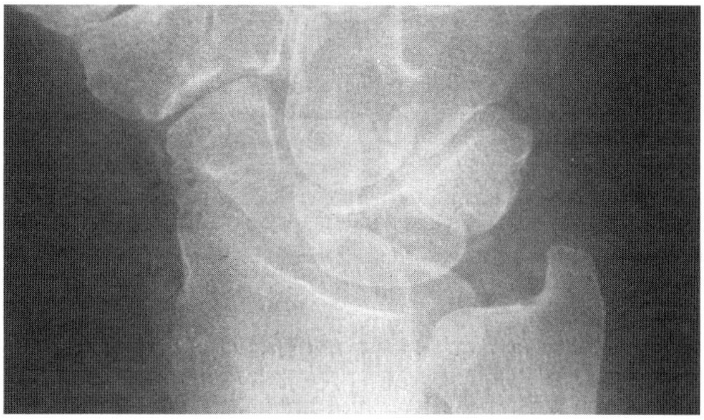

Fig. 11 Chondrocalcinosis is seen in the triangular cartilage of the wrist.

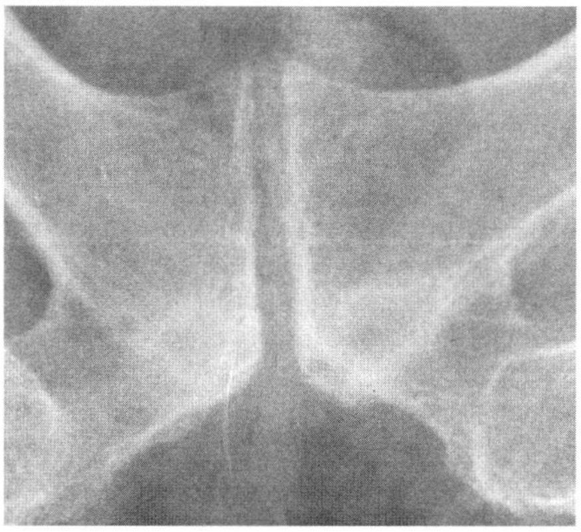

Fig. 12 Chondrocalcinosis is seen in the pubic symphysis.

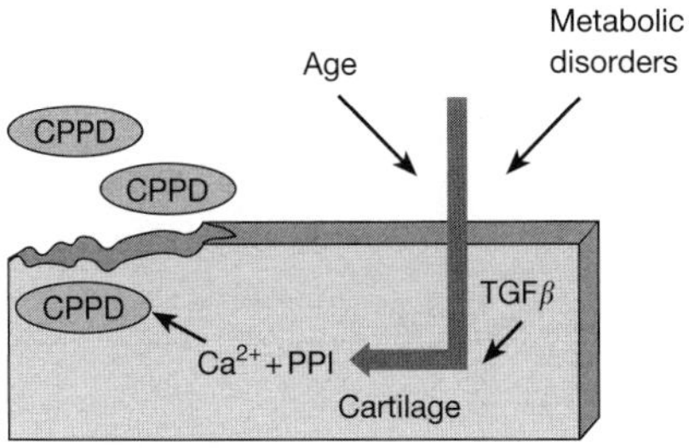

Fig. 13 Scheme of the pathogenesis of CPPD crystal deposition.

crystal release, and the induction and cessation of an inflammatory response. Using gout as a paradigm, much of the work on the pathophysiology of CPPD deposition rests on the theory that various metabolic abnormalities lead via a final common pathway to CPPD crystal formation. Unlike gout, the nature of this final common pathway remains unclear. Both radiological and histological studies of affected joints implicate cartilage as the primary site of CPPD crystal deposition. Crystals form in both fibrocartilage and the mid-zone of hyaline articular cartilage. The smallest and presumably the earliest crystals are found adjacent to chondrocytes or may replace the chondron (Pritzker et al. 1988). Crystals occur less commonly in synovium and tendon and may form in areas of chondroid metaplasia in these tissues (Beutler et al. 1993).

In cartilage, crystals are associated with large or 'hypertrophic' chondrocytes that contain unusual inclusions. These are not seen in osteoarthritic cartilage. Fragmented collagen fibres and histochemical markers associated with degenerated cartilage such as type I collagen, S-100 protein, and the proteoglycan, dermatan sulfate, have been identified near crystal deposits (Masuda et al. 1989).

Theoretically, three components influence CPPD crystal formation (Rosenthal 2001). Changes in local concentrations of calcium and pyrophosphate as well as alterations of cartilage matrix might favour crystallogenesis. Despite the association between sustained hypercalcaemia and CPPD disease, no consistent changes in local calcium concentrations in affected joints have been documented. Moreover, treatment of hyperparathyroidism, for example, does not usually ameliorate the arthritis. Studies of crystal formation in gels implicate a role for the matrix in influencing crystal formation, but in general the influence of the matrix changes has been difficult to approach in the laboratory. For these and other reasons, much of the work on CPPD crystal formation has concentrated on pyrophosphate metabolism.

Pyrophosphate levels are elevated in the synovial fluids of patients with CPPD disease when compared with patients with other types of arthritis. Moreover, skin fibroblasts from patients with familial CPPD disease have higher levels of pyrophosphate than those from normal controls. *In vitro*, normal hyaline and fibrocartilage elaborate extracellular pyrophosphate while other joint tissues do not (Rosenthal 2001).

Thus, disordered pyrophosphate metabolism appears to have a crucial role in CPPD crystal formation. Whether pyrophosphate is generated extracellularly through the activity of the family of ectoenzymes known as nucleoside triphosphate pyrophosphohydrolases or is made inside the chondrocyte remains unclear. A role for transforming growth factor-β, a cartilage growth factor involved in repair, is supported by its unique ability to stimulate pyrophosphate elaboration by cartilage.

Understanding pyrophosphate metabolism may aid in determining the link between CPPD disease and its associated metabolic disorders. For example, magnesium is a cofactor of pyrophosphatase, which hydrolyzes pyrophosphate to phospate. Thus, low magnesium would prevent action of this enzyme and favour elevated pyrophosphate concentrations in the joint. Similarly, hypophosphatasia which is characterized by low alkaline phosphatase activity could cause elevation of pyrophosphate levels by decreasing pyrophosphate hydrolysis. Interestingly, increased levels of parathyroid hormone fragments are also found in patients with haemochromatosis, suggesting a link between these two diseases and a possible role for parathyroid hormone fragments in CPPD crystal formation (Pawlotsky et al. 1999).

When concentrations of pyrophosphate and calcium as well as matrix conditions are favourable, CPPD crystals form. Acute clinical symptoms arise when crystals are released into the synovial space. The mechanisms through which crystals are released into the joint space remain unknown. It has been postulated that trauma or sudden changes in crystal solubility may induce crystal release. Like MSU crystals, CPPD crystals are phlogistic and initiate an inflammatory response similar to that initiated by gout crystals (Malawista et al. 1985). The smallest crystals may be the most inflammatory (Ishikawa et al. 1987). Like gout, the factors terminating an acute attack remain speculative.

Management

Because our understanding of the pathophysiology of CPPD disease is inadequate, we have no specific treatments for this disorder. Standard therapies include NSAIDs, intra-articular corticosteroids, and colchicine. The management of acute and chronic CPPD deposition disease is summarized in Boxes 3 and 4.

NSAIDs are the most commonly used therapy for CPPD disease. There are no controlled trials of their efficacy and no single NSAID is preferable over others. Sulindac may be renal sparing, and may be safer than other NSAIDs in this elderly population.

Joint aspiration with intra-articular instillation of corticosteroids remains a mainstay of therapy for patients with pseudogout. Although no prospective trials of intra-articular corticosteroids in CPPD exist, two retrospective studies support the their effectiveness in shortening the duration of an acute attack (O'Duffy 1976; Masuda and Ishikawa 1987). The use of parenteral corticosteroids for acute pseudogout is controversial (Rosenthal and Ryan 1995).

Intravenous colchicine is of proven efficacy in acute pseudogout (Spilberg et al. 1980). However, the age and comorbidities of patients with CPPD disease often preclude its use. Low-dose oral colchicine may be useful prophylactically. At doses of 1 mg/day, it reduced the frequency of acute attacks of pseudogout in one small study (Avarellos and Spilberg 1986).

Other less traditional treatments for CPPD disease have been proposed (Rosenthal and Ryan 1995). Magnesium carbonate increases the solubility of CPPD crystals and acts as a cofactor for pyrophosphatases. At a dosage of 10 mEq thrice daily, magnesium carbonate decreased the severity of symptoms in patients with chronic CPPD deposition disease. Intra-articular hyaluronon preparations have been reported to both ameliorate and exacerbate CPPD arthritis. Intramuscular gold and hydroxychlorquine have been used in patients with a pseudorheumatoid presentation with reportedly good results. Rest, pain medications, and splinting may be helpful adjunctive measures. Ultimately, joint replacement surgery may be warranted.

Prognosis

The prognosis for CPPD disease patients is not known. Most cases of acute pseudogout are alleviated with standard therapy. However, as no good prophylactic treatment exists, and the disease often coexists with severe joint degeneration, many patients have unrelenting symptoms from CPPD disease.

The basic calcium phosphate associated syndromes

BCP crystals include hydroxyapatite, octacalcium phosphate, and tricalcium phosphate. These crystals are often (less accurately) referred to as apatite or hydroxyapatite crystals. They are associated with a wide variety

Box 3 Management of acute CPPD deposition disease

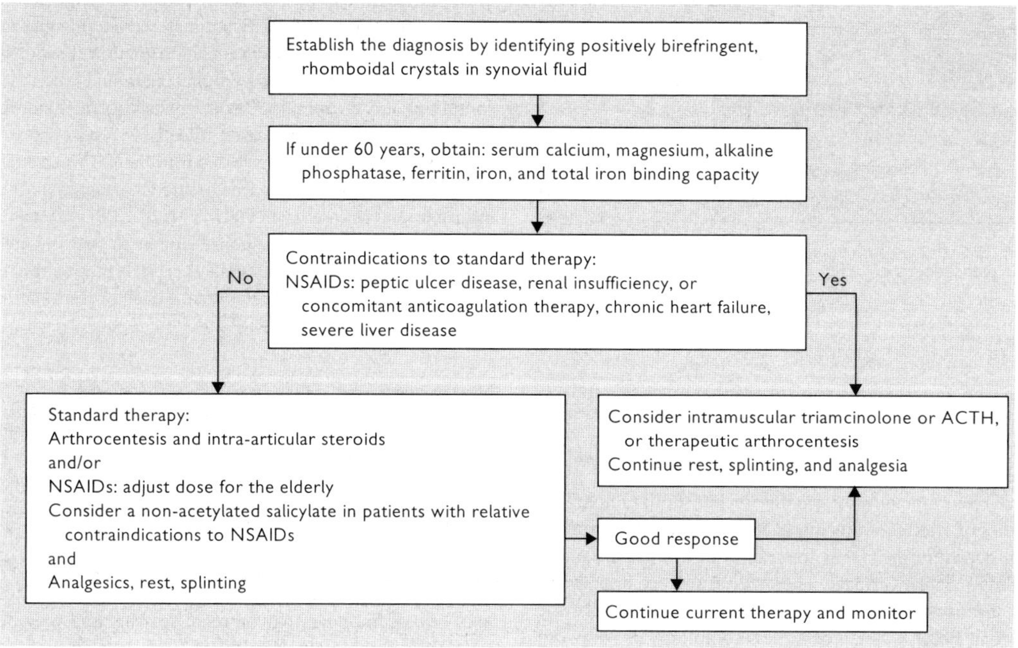

Box 4 Management of chronic CPPD deposition disease

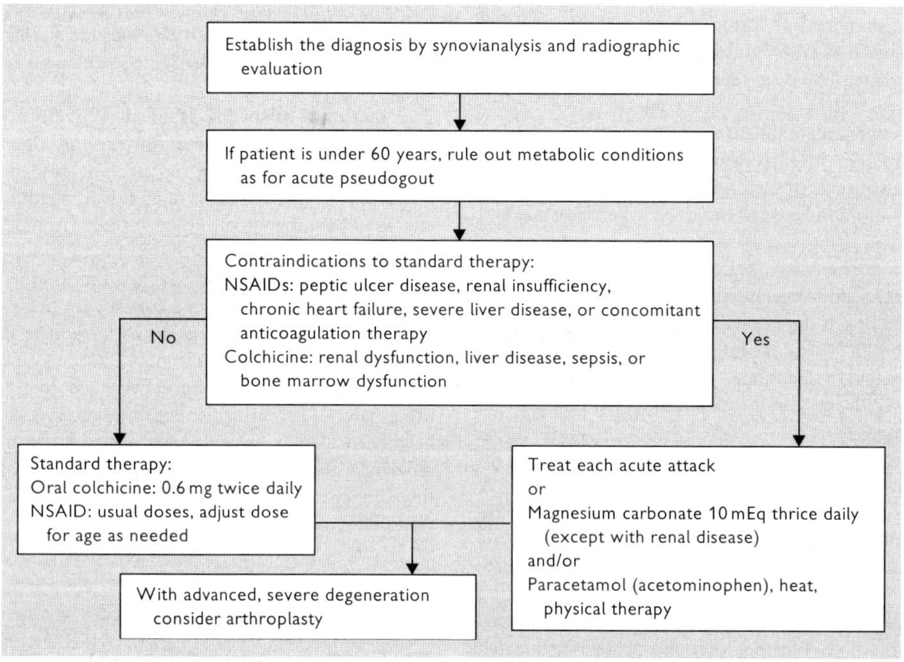

of clinical syndromes as illustrated in Table 8. The management of BCP crystal diseases is summarized in Box 5.

History

Calcific periarthritis and tendinitis have been recognized for many years, and a clinical syndrome similar to Milwaukee shoulder syndrome was described by Robert Adams in 1857 (McCarty 1989). With the identification of BCP crystals in the synovial fluid of patients with arthritis (Dieppe et al. 1976), interest in these crystals and their biological effects grew. Although several BCP-associated syndromes have recently been characterized, there is still much to learn about the significance and distribution of BCP crystals.

Arthritis associated with BCP crystals

Milwaukee shoulder syndrome

This unusual form of arthritis is one of the better defined of the BCP crystal-associated syndromes. Milwaukee shoulder syndrome was initially described in 1981 as a severe shoulder arthropathy of elderly women (McCarty 1982).

Thirty patients with Milwaukee shoulder syndrome have been carefully described. (Halverson et al. 1990). The syndrome is more common in women than men. Patients describe a gradual onset of mild to moderate shoulder pain that is often bilateral and worse at night. Symptoms are more severe on the dominant side. Knee pain, stiffness, and swelling may also occur. Instability, large effusions, and loose bodies are noted on examination of the shoulder. A history of trauma or overuse may antedate the development of this syndrome. Renal disease may also be a predisposing factor.

Radiographs show exaggerated joint degeneration (Fig. 14). Glenohumeral joint space narrowing, deformities of the humeral head with focal osteoporosis, small osteophytes, loose bodies, and calcifications are particularly characteristic. Large and extensive rotator cuff tears are commonly seen on arthrograms. Knee involvement is common and differs from primary osteoarthritis in that the lateral compartment is often predominantly involved. Synovial fluids have low white blood-cell counts (less than 500 cells/mm^3). Particulate collagens and variable levels of active proteases have been identified in effusions from patients with Milwaukee shoulder syndrome. CPPD crystals are present in one-third of patients. There is currently no widely available method for detecting or quantifying BCP crystals. They can not be reliably identified with conventional or polarized-light microscopy. Stains such as Alizarin red are sensitive but not specific for BCP crystals. Characteristic crystals can be seen under electron microscopy. At certain centres, a semi-quantitative radiometric assay based on diphosphonate binding is in use (Halverson and McCarty 1979).

The pathogenesis of Milwaukee shoulder syndrome remains an area of active research. BCP crystals are mitogenic and induce the elaboration of collagenase and other proteases from articular cells (Cheung and Ryan 1995). These proteases may be responsible for the extensive destruction of joint structures seen in this syndrome.

Table 8 Rheumatic syndromes associated with BCP crystals

In joints
Milwaukee shoulder syndrome
Osteoarthritis
Erosive arthritis
Acute inflammatory arthritis
Mixed crystal deposition
Near joints
Periarthritis
Shoulder
Upper extremity in women
Pseudopodagra
Calcific tendinitis and bursitis

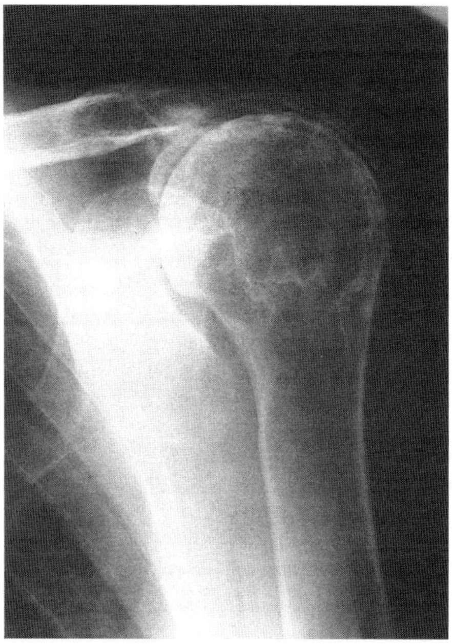

Fig. 14 This radiograph illustrates typical findings in Milwaukee shoulder syndrome. Note the abnormally high position of the humeral head.

Box 5 Management of BCP crystal disease

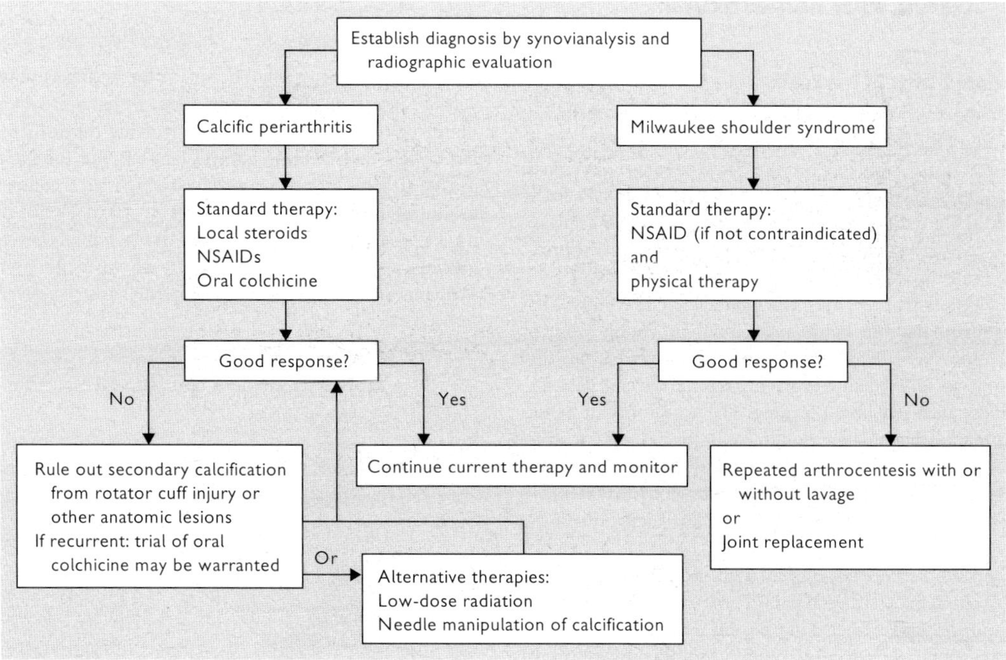

No specific therapy is available for Milwaukee shoulder syndrome. Some patients may respond to conservative treatment with analgesics such as NSAIDs and repeated joint aspirations. The utility of intra-articular corticosteroid injections remains unclear. With far-advanced disease or collapse of the humeral head, shoulder arthroplasties may be indicated.

The prognosis for recovery of motion and decreased pain in patients with far-advanced joint degeneration is not good.

BCP crystals in osteoarthritis

BCP crystals are found in 30–60 per cent of synovial fluids from patients with osteoarthritis using widely available detection techniques (Gibilisco et al. 1985). Small or sparse submicroscopic crystals may be found in even higher percentages of osteoarthritic synovial fluids when carefully examined (Swan et al. 1994). The quantity of BCP crystal present correlates with the degree of radiographic degeneration. There is no association between synovial fluid cell count or the pattern of radiographic appearance and BCP crystals. Thus, the significance of these crystals is unclear.

Erosive arthritis associated with BCP crystals

Several patients with erosive arthritis associated with BCP crystals have been described (Schumacher et al. 1981; Zwillich et al. 1988). These patients have peripheral or axial arthritis with acute attacks. Pre-existing renal disease, chronic arthritis, and tophus-like subcutaneous nodules have also been described. Radiographs show bony erosions and calcifications. ACTH and colchicine improve symptoms in some patients.

Acute arthritis associated with BCP crystals

A small number of patients with an acute gout-like syndrome associated with BCP crystals in the synovial fluid have been reported (Schumacher et al. 1977). These patients have elevated synovial fluid cell counts and normal radiographs. They may represent an early stage of the erosive arthritis described above.

Mixed crystal deposition

BCP and CPPD crystals frequently coexist in a single joint (Dieppe et al. 1977). It is more common to see these crystals together than to identify either one alone. No clear radiographic or clinical syndromes have been characterized on the basis of the coexistence of these two crystals.

Syndromes associated with non-articular BCP crystals

Periarthritis associated with BCP crystals

BCP crystals often cause periarthritis (Swannell et al. 1970). BCP periarthritis occurs most often around the shoulder joint of people between the ages of 30 and 60 years. Familial forms, involving multiple sites, have been described (Marcos et al. 1981). Renal failure may predispose to BCP deposition. Patients usually present with acute pain, warmth, erythema, and swelling in the affected area lasting for several weeks. The diagnosis is suggested by the presence of extra-articular calcium deposits on radiographs.

Two variants of BCP periarthritis have been characterized recently. The first is periarthritis involving the hand and elbow in young women (Yosipovitch and Yosipovitch 1993). This occurs in otherwise healthy young women without an antecedent history of trauma. Several patients had recently given birth and were breast feeding. The symptoms are acute and severe and are often misdiagnosed as gout or cellulitis. Sites of involvement include the lateral epicondyle of the elbow, the wrist, and the finger joints. Symptoms respond dramatically to intralesional corticosteroids. Follow-up radiographs demonstrate resolution of the calcific deposits within 7–36 days.

The term hydroxyapatite pseudopodagra has been used to refer to BCP periarthritis of the first metatarsophalangeal joint. These patients present with acute pain, swelling, warmth, and erythema of this joint (Fam and Rubenstein 1989). It often occurs in young women and is clinically indistinguishable from gout. Radiographs show amorphous periarticular calcifications. No patients had metabolic abnormalities, although pseudopodagra has been reported in pregnancy. Attacks are self-limited, lasting 1–3 weeks, and respond to conservative treatment with NSAIDs. Intralesional corticosteroids have also been used with good success.

Calcific tendinitis and bursitis

This syndrome frequently involves the shoulder. It is often clinically indistinguishable from traumatic tendinitis or bursitis. Patients present with acute onset of severe pain in the affected area lasting several weeks. The radiographic presence of amorphous calcific deposits and the absence of antecedent trauma suggest this diagnosis. Calcific deposits in the shoulder may also occur with chronic rotator cuff injuries. These deposits occur at the insertion site of the rotator cuff on the humerus and are not reabsorbed with time. In contrast, the calcifications of calcific tendinitis occur in metaplastic fibrocartilage within the rotator cuff and disappear with time (Sakar and Uhthoff 1984). The pathophysiology of calcific tendinitis is unknown. Treatment with NSAIDs and intralesional corticosteroids usually results in rapid improvement.

Calcium oxalate arthritis

Calcium oxalate crystals produce an unusual form of arthritis. Although seen most commonly in patients with renal failure on dialysis, calcium oxalate arthritis has also been described in patients with bowel disease and primary oxalosis, a rare inborn error of metabolism.

Epidemiology

There are no good studies of the incidence or prevalence of calcium oxalate arthritis in susceptible populations. Primary oxalosis is quite rare. In contrast, 90 per cent of patients on long-term haemodialysis have pathological evidence of calcium oxalate deposition in kidney and bone tissue (Fayemi et al. 1977).

Ascorbic acid supplementation is an added risk factor in patients on dialysis (Balcke et al. 1984), although oxalate arthritis has been reported in patients on dialysis who did not receive ascorbic acid supplements (Rosenthal et al. 1988). Other risk factors include short bowel syndrome from bowel bypass surgery or inflammatory bowel disease, dietary excesses of unusual foods such as rhubarb, and thiamine and pyridoxine deficiencies (Table 9).

Clinical features

Oxalate arthritis most often occurs in the setting of renal failure. No large-scale studies of affected patients exist. Patients usually present with acute mono- or oligoarticular arthritis involving the small joints of the hands, particularly the proximal interphalangeals and the metacarpophalangeals. Oxalate arthritis may be symmetric, and is often accompanied by tenosynovitis. Bursal involvement has also been described. Unlike gout, initial episodes may be prolonged and chronic arthritis may rapidly develop.

Primary oxalosis results from one of two defined enzyme deficiencies (Williams and Smith 1968). It is inherited as a recessive trait. Patients with

Table 9 Conditions associated with calcium oxalate arthritis

End-stage renal disease on dialysis
Short bowel syndrome
Unusual diets rich in rhubarb, spinach, or ascorbic acid
Thiamine deficiency
Pyridoxine deficiency
Primary oxalosis

primary oxalosis succumb to endstage renal disease in their early twenties. They have diffuse oxalate deposits at autopsy which may also involve articular tissues. Acute and chronic arthritis as well as tenosynovitis have been described in these patients, but identification of crystals in affected joints has been difficult.

Diagnosis

The diagnosis of calcium oxalate arthritis is made by identifying characteristic crystals in synovial fluid from affected joints. Calcium oxalate crystals may be of two morphologies (Reginato et al. 1986). The more commonly identified type is weddelite or calcium oxalate dihydrate. This is a positively birefringent bipyramidal crystal (Plate 191). Less commonly, calcium oxalate monohydrate (whewellite) occurs. Whewellite is polymorphic and may be seen as chunks, rods, ovals, or microspherules. Scanning electron microscopy and X-ray diffraction are often necessary to confirm the identities of these crystals.

Synovianalysis usually shows clear or bloody fluid with normal viscosity. Cell counts are typically low and often neutrophils predominate, although large mononuclear cells have also been described.

Radiographs are not diagnostic but may be helpful. Miliary calcific deposits in the soft tissue can be seen. Similarly, vascular calcification is a common finding. Less commonly, bony abnormalities such as localized or metaphyseal sclerosis, pseudoarthroses, and pathological fractures can be seen (Nartijn and Thijn 1982).

Pathophysiology

Oxalic acid is a metabolic end-product of amino acid synthesis and ascorbic acid metabolism. It is well absorbed from the gut and is renally excreted. Hence, oxalate may accumulate in tissues from excess absorption, overproduction, or underexcretion. Renal failure causes underexcretion of oxalate and levels are high in patients on dialysis. Neither haemo- nor peritoneal dialysis adequately clears oxalate from tissues. Causes of overproduction include the enzyme defects of primary oxalosis, and thiamine and pyridoxine deficiencies. Dietary excesses of spinach, rhubarb, and ascorbic acid supplements may also raise oxalate levels. Excess intestinal absorption may be due to short bowel syndrome from any causes. The most common associated bowel disorders are bowel bypass syndrome from obesity surgery and inflammatory bowel disease.

Once oxalate crystals form in articular tissues, they are released by unknown mechanisms and initiate an inflammatory response.

Management

We have no specific treatment for calcium oxalate arthritis. In general, response to conventional therapies including NSAIDs, intra-articular corticosteroids, colchicine, and increased dialysis are poor. The grim outlook for patients with primary oxalosis may be brightened by early liver transplantation before renal failure has developed (Watts et al. 1991).

Table 10 Other crystals found in synovial fluid

Crystal	Morphology	Setting	Significance
Lipid	Round	Trauma	Uncertain
Cholesterol	Plate-like	Unclear	Uncertain
Steroids	Any shape, very bright	After injection	Recent steroid injection
Cryoglobulin	Polygonal, positively birefringent	Cryoglobulinaemia	
Charcot–Leyden	Bipyramidal or hexagonal	Hypereosinophilia	
Cystine	Hexahedral, weak or bright	Cystinosis	
Xanthine	Rhomboidal or plate-like	Xanthinuria	

Other crystals

Other types of crystals can be identified in synovial fluid. These crystals are listed in Table 10. Commonly seen crystals are illustrated in Plates 192–194.

References

Adriani, J. and Naraghi, M. (1985). Allopurinol: actions, adverse reaction and drug interactions. *Internal Medicine* **6**, 114–23.

Alepa, F.P. et al. (1967). Relationship between glycogen storage disease and tophaceous gout. *American Journal of Medicine* **42**, 58–63.

Avarellos, A. and Spilberg, I. (1986). Colchicine prophylaxis in pseudogout. *Journal of Rheumatology* **13**, 804–6.

Balcke, P. et al. (1984). Ascorbic acid aggravates secondary hyperoxalemia in patients on chronic hemodialysis. *Annals of Internal Medicine* **10**, 344–5.

Barthelemy, C.R. et al. (1984). Gouty arthritis: a prospective radiographic evaluation of sixty patients. *Skeletal Radiology* **11**, 1–8.

Becker, M.A. (1988). Clincial aspects of monosodium urate monohydrate crystal deposition disease (gout). *Rheumatic Diseases Clinics of North America* **14**, 377–94.

Becker, M.A. and Kim, M. (1987). Regulation of purine synthesis de novo in human fibroblasts by purine nucleotides and phosphoribosylpyrophosphate. *Journal of Biological Chemistry* **262**, 14531–5.

Beutler, A., Rothfuss, S., Clayburne, G., Sieck, M., and Schumacher, H.R. (1993). Calcium pyrophosphate dihydrate crystal deposition in synovium: relationship to collagen fibers and chondrometaplasia. *Arthritis and Rheumatism* **36**, 704–15.

Bong, D. and Bennett, R. (1981). Pseudogout mimicking systemic disease. *Journal of the American Medical Association* **246**, 1438–40.

Bouvet, J. et al. (1985). Acute neck pain due to calcifications surrounding the odontoid process: the crowned dens syndrome. *Arthritis and Rheumatism* **22**, 928–32.

Burak, D.A., Griffith, B.P., Thompson, M.E., and Kahl, L.E. (1992). Hyperuricemia and gout among heart transplant recipients receiving cyclosporine. *American Journal of Medicine* **92**, 141–6.

Cheung, H.S. and Ryan, L.M. (1995). Role of crystal deposition in matrix degradation. In *Joint Cartilage Degradation: Basic and Clinical Aspects* (ed. F.J. Woessner and D.S. Howell), pp. 209–21. New York: Marcel Dekker.

Collins, J.G. (1988). *Prevalence of Selected Chronic Conditions, United States 1983–85.* Advance data from Vital and Health Statistics of the National Center for Health Statistics, No. 155, USDHHS, Washington DC.

Copeman, W.C.S. *A Short History of the Gout.* Los Angeles CA: University of California Press, 1964.

Dieppe, P.A. et al. (1976). Apatite deposition disease. A new arthropathy. *Lancet* **7**, 266–76.

Dieppe, P.A. et al. (1977). Mixed crystal deposition disease and osteoarthritis. *British Medical Journal* **1**, 150–60.

Fam, A.G. and Rubenstein, J. (1989). Hydroxyapatite pseudopodagra: a syndrome of young women. *Arthritis and Rheumatism* **32**, 741–7.

Fam, A.G., Lewtas, J., Stein, J., and Paton, T.W. (1992). Desensitization to allopurinol in patients with gout and cutaneous reactions. *American Journal of Medicine* **93**, 299–302.

Fayemi, A.O., Ali, M., and Braun E.V. (1977). Oxalosis in hemodialysis patients. A pathologic study of 80 cases. *Archives of Pathology and Laboratory Medicine* **103**, 58–62.

Felson, D.T., Anderson, J.J., Naimark, A., Kannel, W., and Meenan, R.F. (1989). The prevalence of chondrocalcinosis in the elderly and its association with knee osteoarthritis: the Framingham study. *Journal of Rheumatology* **16**, 1241–5.

Gibilisco, P.A. et al. (1985). Synovial fluid crystals in osteoarthritis. *Arthritis and Rheumatism* **28**, 511–15.

Gresser, U., Gathof, B., and Zollner, N. (1990). Uric acid levels in southern Germany in 1989, a comparison with studies from 1962, 1971, and 1984. *Klinische Wochenschrift* **68**, 1222–8.

Groff, G.D., Franck, W.A., and Raddatz, D.A. (1990). Systemic steroid therapy for acute gout: a clinical trial and review of the literature. *Seminars in Arthritis and Rheumatism* **19**, 329–36.

Gutman, A.B. (1973). The past four decades of progress in the knowledge of gout with an assessment of the present status. *Arthritis and Rheumatism* **16**, 431–45.

Halverson, P.B. and McCarty, D.J. (1979). Identification of hydroxyapatite crystals in synovial fluid. *Arthritis and Rheumatism* **22**, 389–95.

Halverson, P.B., Carrera, G.F., and McCarty, D.J. (1990). Milwaukee shoulder syndrome: fifteen additional cases and a description of contributing factors. *Archives of Internal Medicine* **150**, 677–82.

Hochberg, M.C. (1991). Opportunities for the primary and secondary prevention of gout. *Mediguide to Inflammatory Diseases* **10**, 1–5.

Ishikawa, H., Ueba, Y., Isobe, T., and Hirohata, K. (1987). Interaction of polymorphonuclear leukocytes with calcium pyrophosphate dihydrate crystals deposited in chondrocalcinosis cartilage. *Rheumatology International* **7**, 217–21.

Jinnah, H.A., DeGregorio, L., Harris, J.C., Nyhan, W.L., and O'Neill, J.P. (2000). The spectrum of inherited mutations causing HPRT deficiency: 75 new cases and a review of 196 previously reported cases. *Mutation Research* **463**, 309–26.

Jones, A.C., Chuck, A.J., Arie, E.A., Green, D.J., and Doherty, M. (1992). Diseases associated with calcium pyrophosphate deposition disease. *Seminars in Arthritis and Rheumatism* **22**, 188–202.

Kozin, F. and McCarty, D.J. (1977). Rheumatoid factors in the serum of gouty patients. *Arthritis and Rheumatism* **18**, 49–58.

Lawrence, R.C. et al. (1989). Estimates of the prevalence of selected arthritic and musculoskeletal diseases in the United States. *Journal of Rheumatology* **16**, 427–41.

Levinson, D.J. and Sorenson, L.B. (1980). Renal handling of uric acid in normal and gouty subjects: evidence for a 4-component system. *Annals of the Rheumatic Diseases* **39**, 173–9.

Levinson, D.J. and Becker, M.A. (1993). Clinical gout and the pathogenesis of hyperuricemia. In *Arthritis and Allied Conditions* 12th edn. (ed. D.J. McCarty and W.J. Koopman), pp. 1773–805. Philadelphia PA: Lea and Febiger.

Lin, H.-Y., Rocher, L.L., McQuillan, M.A., Schmaltz, S., Palella, T.D., and Fox, I.H. (1989). Cyclosporine induced hyperuricemia and gout. *New England Journal of Medicine* **321**, 287–92.

Lin, K.C., Lin, H.-Y., and Chou, P. (2000). The interaction between uric acid level and other risk factors on the development of gout among asymptomatic hyperuricemic men in a prospective study. *Journal of Rheumatology* **27**, 1501–5.

Macfarlane, D.G. and Dieppe, P.A. (1985). Diuretic induced gout in elderly women. *British Journal of Rheumatology* **24**, 155–7.

Malawista, S.E. et al. (1985). Crystal-induced endogenous pyrogen production. A further look at gouty inflammation. *Arthritis and Rheumatism* **28**, 1039–46.

Marcalongo, R., Calabria, A.A., Lalumera, M., Gerli, R., Alessandrini, C., and Cavallo, G. (1988). The 'switch-off' mechanism of spontaneous resolution of acute gout attack. *Journal of Rheumatology* **15**, 101–9.

Marcos, J.C. et al. (1981). Idiopathic familial chondrocalcinosis due to apatite crystal deposition. *American Journal of Medicine* **71**, 557–563.

Masuda, I. and Ishikawa, K. (1987). Clincial features of pseudogout attack: a survey of 50 cases. *Clinical Orthopaedics and Related Research* **229**, 173–9.

Masuda, I., Ishikawa, K., and Usuku, G. (1989). A histologic and immunohistologic study of calcium pyrophosphate dihydrate crystal deposition disease. *Clinical Orthopaedics and Related Research* **263**, 272–87.

McCarty, D.J. (1982). The Hebreden Oration. Crystals, joints and consternation. *Annals of the Rheumatic Diseases* **42**, 243–53.

McCarty, D.J. (1989). Robert Adams' rheumatic arthritis of the shoulder: Milwaukee shoulder syndrome revisited. *Journal of Rheumatology* **16**, 668–70.

McCarty, D.J., Kohn, N.N., and Faires, J.S. (1962). The significance of calcium phosphate crystals in the synovial fluid of arthritis patients: the 'pseudogout syndrome' I. Clinical aspects. *Annals of Internal Medicine* **56**, 711–37.

McColl, S.R. and Naccache, P.H. (2000). Crystal-induced arthropathies. In *Inflammation: Basic Principles and Clinical Correlates* 3rd edn. (ed. J.I. Gallin and R. Snyderman), pp. 1039–46. Baltimore MD: Lippincott Williams & Wilkins.

McGill, N.W. and Dieppe, P.A. (1991a). Evidence for a promotor of urate crystal formation in gouty synovial fluid. *Annals of the Rheumatic Diseases* **50**, 558–61.

McGill, N.W. and Dieppe, P.A. (1991b). The role of serum and synovial fluid components in the promotion of urate crystal formation. *Journal of Rheumatology* **18**, 1042–5.

Mejias, E., Lluberes, R., and Martinez-Maldanado, M. (1989). Hyperuricemia, gout, and autosomal dominant polycystic kidney disease. *American Journal of the Medical Sciences* **297**, 145–8.

Menkes, C.J., Simon, F., Delrieu, F., Forest, M., and Delbarre, F. (1976). Destructive arthropathy in chondrocalcinosis articularis. *Arthritis and Rheumatism* **19**, 329–48.

Mitrovic, D.R. et al. (1988). The prevalence of chondrocalcinosis in the human knee joint: an autopsy survey. *Journal of Rheumatology* **15**, 633–41.

Moreland, L.W. and Ball, G.V. (1991). Colchicine and gout. *Arthritis and Rheumatism* **34**, 782–6.

Nartijn, A. and Thijn, C.J.P. (1982). Radiologic findings in primary oxaluria. *Skeletal Radiology* **8**, 21–4.

O'Duffy, J.D. (1976). Clinical studies of acute pseudogout attacks. Comments on prevelance, predispositions and treatment. *Arthritis and Rheumatism* **19** (Suppl.), 349.

O'Duffy, J.D., Hunter, G.G., and Kelly, P.J. (1975). Decreasing prevalence of tophaceous gout. *Mayo Clinic Proceedings* **50**, 227–8.

Pak, C.Y.C., Sakhaee, K., and Fuller, C. (1986). Successful management of uric acid nephrolithiasis with potassium citrate. *Kidney International* **30**, 422–8.

Pal, B., Foxall, M., Dysart, T., Carey, F., and Whittaker, M. (2000). How is gout managed in primary care? A review of current practice and proposed guidelines. *Clinical Rheumatology* **19**, 21–5.

Palmer, D.G., Highton, J., and Hessian, P.A. (1989). Development of the gout tophus: a hypothesis. *American Journal of Clinical Pathology* **91**, 190–5.

Pascual, E. (1991). Persistence of monosodium urate crystals and low-grade inflammation in the synovial fluid of patients with untreated gout. *Arthritis and Rheumatism* **34**, 141–5.

Pawlotsky, Y., Le Dantec, P., Moirand, R., Guggenbuhl, P., Jouanolle, A.M., Catheline, M., Meadeb, J., Brissot, P., Deugnier, Y., and Chales, G. (1999). Elevated parathyroid hormone 44-68 and osteoarticular changes in patients with genetic hemochromatosis. *Arthritis and Rheumatism* **42**, 799–806.

Perez-Ruiz, F., Alonso-Ruiz, A., Calabozo, M., Herrero-Beites, A., Garcia-Erauskin, G., and Ruiz-Lucea, E. (1998). Efficacy of allopurinol and benzbromarone for the control of hyperuricemia. A pathogenic approach to the treatment of primary chronic gout. *Annals of the Rheumatic Diseases* **57**, 545–9.

Perez-Ruiz, F., Calabozo, M., Herroro-Beites, A.M., Garcia-Erauskin, G., and Pijoan, J.I. (2000). Improvement of renal function in patients with chronic gout after proper control of hyperuricemia and gouty bouts. *Nephron* **86**, 287–91.

Pritzker, K.P.H., Cheng, P.T., and Renlund, R.C. (1988). Calcium pyrophosphate crystal deposition in hyaline cartilage. Ultrastructural analysis and implications for pathogenesis. *Journal of Rheumatology* **15**, 828–35.

Puig, J.G. and Fox, I.H. (1984). Ethanol-induced activation of adenine nucleotide turnover. Evidence for a role for acetate. *Journal of Clinical Investigation* **74**, 936–41.

Puig, J.G. et al. (1991). Female gout: clinical spectrum and uric acid metabolism. *Archives of Internal Medicine* **151**, 726–32.

Reginato, A.J. et al. (1986). Arthropathy and cutaneous calcinosis in hemodialysis oxalosis. *Arthritis and Rheumatism* **29**, 1387–96.

Reginato, A.J., Tamesis, E., and Netter, P. (1999). Familial and clinical aspects of calcium pyrophosphate deposition disease. *Current Rheumatology Reports* **1**, 112–20.

Resnick, D. et al. (1977). Clinical, radiologic, and pathologic abnormalities in calcium pyrophosphate dihydrate deposition disease (CPPD) pseudogout. *Diagnostic Radiology* **122**, 1–15.

Roberts, W.M., Liang, M.H., and Stern, S.H. (1987). Colchicine in acute gout. *Journal of the American Medical Association* **257**, 1920–1.

Rosenthal, A.K. (2001). Pathogenesis of calcium pyrophosphate crystal deposition disease. *Current Rheumatology Reports* **3**, 17–23.

Rosenthal, A.K. and Ryan, L.M. (1995). Treatment of refractory crystal related arthritis. *Rheumatic Disease Clinics of North America* **21**, 151–62.

Rosenthal, A.K. and Ryan, L.M. (2001). Calcium pyrophosphate crystal deposition disease; pseudogout; articular chondrocalcinosis. In *Arthritis and Allied Conditions* 14th edn. (ed. W.J. Koopman), pp. 2348–71. Philadelphia PA: Lea and Febiger.

Rosenthal, A.K., Ryan, L.M., and McCarty, D.J. (1988). Arthritis associated with calcium oxalate crystals in an anephric patient treated with peritoneal dialysis. *Journal of the American Medical Association* **260**, 1290–2.

Roubenoff, R., Klag, M.J., Mead, L.A., Liang, K.-Y., Seidler, A.J., and Hochberg, M.C. (1991). Incidence and risk factors for gout in white men. *Journal of the American Medical Association* **266**, 3004–7.

Russell, I.J. et al. (1983). Effects of IgG and C-reactive protein on complement depletion by monosodium urate crystals. *Journal of Rheumatology* **10**, 425–33.

Sakar, K. and Uhthoff, H.K. (1984). Rotator cuff tendinopathies with calcification. In *Calcium in Biological Systems* (ed. R.P. Rubin, G. Weiss, and J.W. Putney), pp. 725–30. New York: Plenum.

Schreiner, O., Wandel, E., Himmelsbach, F., Galle, P.R., and Marker-Hermann, E. (2000). Reduced secretion of proinflammatory cytokines of monosodium urate crystal-stimulated monocytes in chronic renal failure: an explanation for infrequent gout episodes in chronic renal failure patients? *Nephrology, Dialysis, Transplantation* **15**, 644–9.

Schumacher, H.R. et al. (1977). Arthritis associated with apatite crystals. *Annals of Internal Medicine* **87**, 411–16.

Schumacher, H.R., Miller, J.L., Ludivico, C., and Jessar, R.A. (1981). Erosive arthritis associated with apatite crystal deposition. *Arthritis and Rheumatism* **24**, 31–7.

Segal, J.B. and Albert, D. (1999). Diagnosis of cyrstal-induced arthritis by synovial fluid examination for crystals: lesson from an imperfect test. *Arthritis Care and Research* **12**, 376–80.

Shadick, N.A., Kim, R., Weiss, S., Liang, M.H., Sparrow, D., and Hu, H. (2000). Effect of low level lead exposure on hyperuricemia and gout among middle aged and elderly men: the normative aging study. *Journal of Rheumatology* **27**, 1708–12.

Simkin, P.A. (1977a). The pathogenesis of podagra. *Annals of Internal Medicine* **86**, 230–3.

Simkin, P.A. (1977b). Urate excretion in normal and gouty men. *Developmental and Experimental Medicine and Biology* **76B**, 41–5.

Simkin, P.A. (1993). Towards a coherent terminology of gout. *Annals of the Rheumatic Diseases* **52**, 693–4.

Sperling, O. et al. (1972). Accelerated erythrocyte 5′-phosphoribosyl-1-pyrophosphate synthesis. A familial abnormality associated with excessive uric acid production and gout. *Biochemical Medicine* **6**, 310–16.

Spilberg, I. et al. (1980). Colchicine and pseudogout. *Arthritis and Rheumatism* **23**, 1062–3.

Sterling, L.P. (1991). The clinical management of gout. *American Pharmacy (NS)* **31**, 368–74.

Stockman, A., Darlington, L.G., and Scottt, J.T. (1980). Frequency of chondrocalcinosis of the knee and avascular necrosis of the femoral head in gout. *Annals of the Rheumatic Diseases* **39**, 7–11.

Stuart, R.A., Gow, P.J., Bellamy, N., Campbell, J., and Grigor, R. (1991). A survey of current prescribing practices of antiinflammatory and urate-lowering drugs in gouty arthritis. *New Zealand Medical Journal* **104**, 115–17.

Swan, A., Chapman, B., Heap, P., Seward, H., and Dieppe, P. (1994). Submicroscopic crystals in osteoarthritic synovial fluids. *Annals of the Rheumatic Diseases* **53**, 467–70.

Swannell, A.J., Underweeo, F.A., and Dixon, A.S. (1970). Periarticular calcific deposits mimicking acute arthritis. *Annals of the Rheumatic Diseases* **29**, 380–5.

Talbott, J.S. *Gout.* New York: Grune and Stratton, 1957.

Terkeltaub, R.A. et al. (1991). Apolipoprotein E inhibits the capacity of monosodium urate crystals to stimulate neutrophils. *Journal of Clinical Investigation* **87**, 20–6.

Wallace, S.L. (1977). The treatment of the acute attack of gout. *Clinics in the Rheumatic Diseases* **3**, 133–43.

Watt, I. and Dieppe, P. (1983). Medial femoral condyle necrosis and chondrocalcinosis; a causal relationship. *British Journal of Radiology* **56**, 7–22.

Watts, W.E. et al. (1991). Combined hepatic and renal transplantation in primary hyperoxaluria type I: clinical report of 9 cases. *American Journal of Medicine* **90**, 179–87.

Williams, H.E. and Smith, H.E. (1968). Disorders of oxalate metabolism. *American Journal of Medicine* **45**, 715–35.

Wyngaarden, J.B. and Kelley, W.N. *Gout and Hyperuricemia.* New York: Grune and Sratton, 1976.

Wyngaarden, J.B. and Kelley, W.N. (1985). Gout. In *The Metabolic Basis of Inherited Disease* 5th edn. (ed. J.B. Stanbury et al.), pp. 1043–114. New York: McGraw-Hill.

Yosipovitch, G. and Yosipovitch, Z. (1993). Acute calcific periarthritis of the hand and elbows in women. A study and review of the literature. *Journal of Rheumatology* **20**, 1533–8.

Yu, T.-F. (1981). Urolithiasis in hyperuricemia and gout. *Journal of Urology* **126**, 424–30.

Yukawa, T., Akazawa, H., Miyake, Y., Takahashi, Y., Nagao, H., and Takeda, E. (1992). A female patient with Lesch–Nyhan syndrome. *Developmental Medicine and Child Neurology* **34**, 543–6.

Zwillich, S.H., Schumacher, H.R., Jr., Hoyt, T.S., Luger, A.M., Morrison, G., and Walder, S.E. (1988). Universal spondylodiscitis in a patient with erosive peripheral arthritis and apatite crystal deposition. *Journal of Rheumatology* **15**, 123–8.

6.16 Diseases of bone and cartilage

6.16.1 Osteoporosis and osteomalacia

David M. Reid

Osteoporosis

Osteoporosis has been consistently defined at Consensus Conferences as 'a systemic bone disease characterized by reduction in bone mineral content (BMC) accompanied by architectural deterioration of bone leading to enhanced fragility and a consequent increase in fracture risk' (Anonymous 1987; Consensus Development Conference 1993; Consensus Development Panel 2001). While fractures of the vertebral body, distal forearm (Colles), and proximal femur are considered to be characteristic it is important to realize that not all fractures of these bone sites are due to osteoporosis and *low trauma* fractures of most skeletal sites, except arguably the ankle (Ingle and Eastell 2002), can be associated with low bone mass.

As not *all* fractures of even classical sites are associated with low bone mass it is important to have a practical definition which can be used *in vivo.* Architectural features of bone can be only assessed *in vitro* by three-dimensional (3D) computed tomography (CT) techniques and by scanning electronic micrographs which demonstrate marked differences in the trabecular structure of cancellous bone in normal and osteoporotic subjects (Fig. 1).

However, such 3D techniques cannot be used *in vivo* and accordingly a working group of the World Health Organization (WHO) has defined osteopaenia/osteoporosis according to what can be measured, that is, BMC or bone mineral density (BMD) (Table 1) (Anonymous 1994).

Use of this definition has allowed the prevalence of osteoporosis at different skeletal sites to be determined for women in the Western world (Table 2).

The term 'osteopaenia' as used by the WHO can be confused with radiological osteopaenia, that is, bones which appear demineralized on X-ray. As the BMC/BMD term 'osteopaenia' has not subsequently been found to have clinical relevance it has been largely ignored of late. The WHO definition only applies to women although recent reviews have suggested that applying the same definition to men, based on a male normative range would have the same utility (Kanis et al. 2001a) although this is not universally accepted (Melton et al. 2001).

Epidemiology of fracture

The prevalence of the most common osteoporosis related fractures in the United Kingdom compared to the United States are shown in Table 3.

It will be noted that approximately the same number of women over the age of 50 will be found to have osteoporosis at the hip (16 per cent) as suffer a hip fracture at least in the United States. Comparison with other countries indicate that Colles and clinical vertebral rates are higher in Scandinavia and the United States but much lower in African countries (Walker-Bone et al. 2001). Although UK rates for clinical vertebral fractures are lower than some other countries these findings may be confounded by counting statistics and definition. A clinical vertebral fracture, by definition, is one which comes to medical attention but it is recognized that many are asymptomatic. Accordingly it can be of little surprise that a radiologically defined vertebral deformities diagnosed semi-morphometrically by an experienced

(a)

(b)

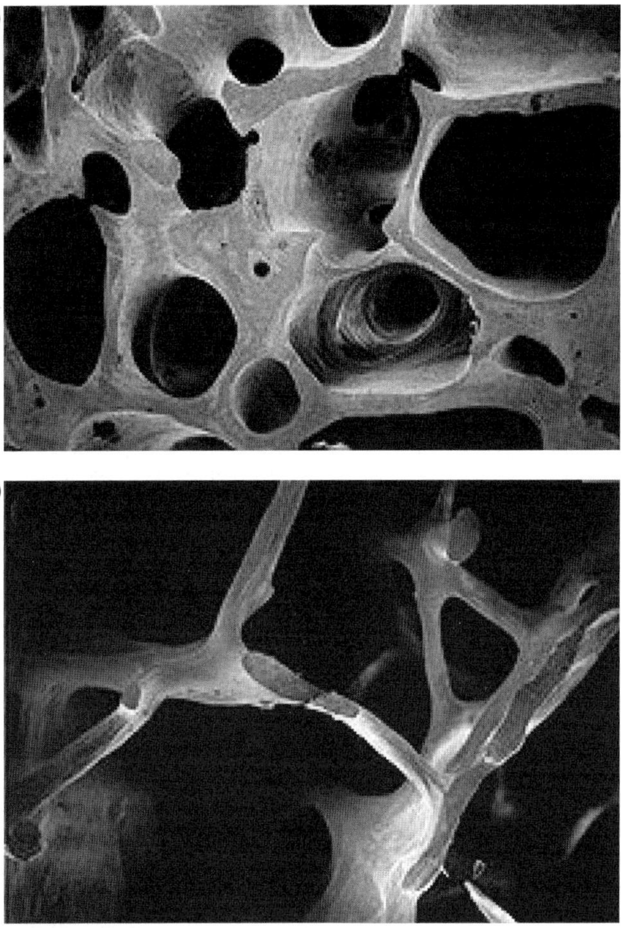

Fig. 1 Scanning electron micrograph of the trabecular structure of cancellous bone from a (a) normal subject and a patient with osteoporosis (b). [Reproduced from *Journal of Bone and Mineral Research* (2000), **15**, 20–4 with permission of the American Society for Bone and Mineral Research.]

Table 1 The definition of osteoporosis as suggested by a Working Group of the World Health Organization (Anonymous 1994)

Normal
Women with BMC or BMD greater than 1 standard below the young normal mean (*T*-score)
Osteopaenia
Women with BMC or BMD less than 1 SD and more than 2.5 SD below the young normal mean (*T*-score)
Osteoporosis
Women with BMC or BMD more than 2.5 SD below the young normal mean (*T*-score)
Severe (established) osteoporosis
Women with BMC or BMD more than 2.5 SD below the young normal mean and previous fragility fractures.

Table 2 Prevalence of osteoporosis in Western women (World Health Organization 1994; Anonymous 1994)

Age range	Osteoporosis at any site (%)	Osteoporosis at hip (%)
30–49	0	0
50–59	14.8	3.9
60–69	21.6	8.0
70–79	38.5	24.5
80+	70.0	47.6
50+	30.3	16.2

Table 3 Life time risk of symptomatic fractures of the major 'osteoporotic sites' in the United Kingdom and the United States

	Males			Females		
	Forearm (%)	Vertebrae (%)	Femoral neck (%)	Forearm (%)	Vertebrae (%)	Femoral neck (%)
UK (van Staa et al. 2001)	2.9	1.2	3.1	16.6	3.1	11.4
USA			5.0	14.4	15.0	14.3

radiologist are more common and in the United Kingdom suggest incidence rates of 6.8 per 1000 patient-years in men and 12.1 per cent in women (EPOS 2002) with the rates being higher in Scandinavia.

Until recently, there were few data on the relative prevalence of Colles fracture rates across centres in the United Kingdom, perhaps largely due to inadequate recording systems in Accident and Emergency departments. However, a detailed audit carried out in five centres across the United Kingdom in 1998 showed that the Colles fracture incidence rates in women varied between 6.1 and 11.9 per 10 000 patient years, although the rates did not follow exactly a decrease from northern to southern centres (O'Neill et al. 2001).

Hip fracture prevalence rates too vary considerably in countries around the world. Unlike Colles and vertebral fracture rates, which largely follow international BMD levels, there are some major discrepancies between levels of hip BMD and fracture rates. For example, peak BMD levels in Japanese and Chinese women are lower than Caucasian women and yet their hip fracture rates are also lower. The fact that age adjustment does not correct the anomaly indicates that reduced life expectancy is not the sole reason for the finding. One possible explanation is differences in the shape of the proximal femur, including a shorter femoral neck length, a factor that is found to be a significant predictor of hip fracture even after correction for BMD values.

Another bone factor that seems to convey excess risk of fracture, specifically at the hip is the rate of bone turnover as measured by biochemical markers especially those indicating higher levels of bone resorption (Delmas 1998). Hence, although BMD is used as the main indicator of fracture there are a number of other bone related factors that are predictive of hip fracture and in part are independent of BMD.

Fracture rates at all of the common sites tend to increase with age from around the age of 50 in both sexes. However, the pattern varies considerably between men and women [Fig. 2(a) and (b)]. Colles fractures are rare in men and show little evidence of an increased prevalence with age. In women, Colles fractures are much more common and, although North American data [Fig. 2(a)] suggest that there is little, if any, increase with age after 60, the recent data from the United Kingdom suggest a modest linear increase from 50 to 80 (O'Neill et al. 2001).

Clinical vertebral fractures were considered to increase in a gradual linear fashion with age in both men and women. However, when fractures are defined by semi-morphometric techniques by measurement of vertebral body height, 'fractures' are apparently much more common in men than had been previously recognized. The relationship with exercise varies considerably with deformities in men being much more related to heavy physical labour. The prevalence rates also increase much less steeply in men. Part of the conundrum probably relates to the fact that many of the vertebral deformities that meet the criteria for a fracture in men are due to changes in vertebral shape due to osteophytes associated with degenerative change, a hypothesis supported by the finding that men with such deformities do not generally have reduced bone mass (Stewart et al. 1995). In women, however, the rates of morphometric deformities rise rapidly with age, in keeping with most of these being due to osteoporosis.

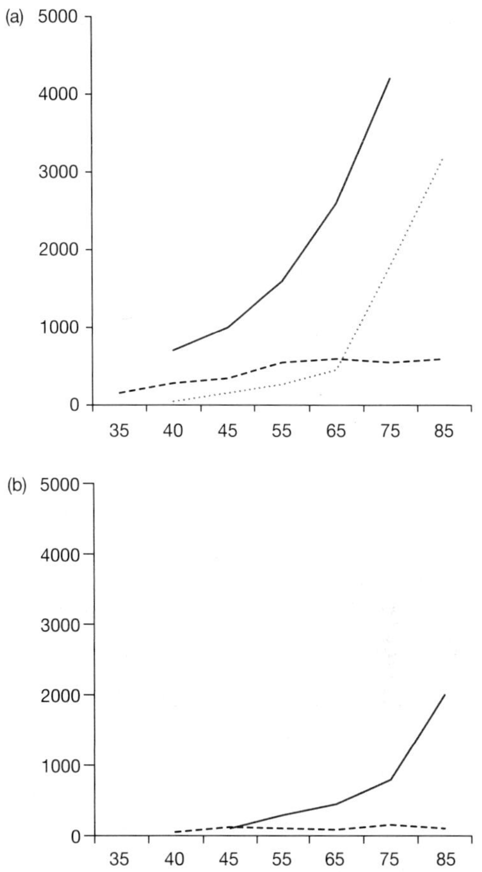

Fig. 2 Fracture rates per 100 000 patient-years: (a) for women; and (b) for men. Solid line, Vertebral fractures; Dashed line, Colles fractures; Dotted line, Hip fractures.

Measurement of bone mass

In the last four decades, there has been increasing interest in capturing numerically the obvious appearance of demineralization, which may be an inevitable accompaniment of ageing of the skeleton (Genant et al. 1996). This interest was initially spurned by the observation that there could be upto 30 per cent reduction in bone mass before it became radiologically evident. This headlong rush to develop new techniques has been given impetus by the decision by the WHO working group to define osteoporosis by BMC or BMD (see above). The various techniques, which are still in use in some guise in the new millennium, are summarized in Table 4.

Initially, techniques used simple measures of cortical thickness (radiogrammetry) measured laboriously and imprecisely from radiographs using a ruler and Vernier calipers. However, the field was revolutionized in the 1960s when Sorenson and Cameron first described the use of photon absorptiometry to measure BMC of the forearm. The physics of the various techniques described since the initial observations are beyond the scope of this chapter but photon absorptiometry has become the standard technique of assessment today with the initial radioisotope sources used to produce photons being replaced with much more stable and reproducible X-ray sources. Peripheral BMC, usually assessed at the radius or os calcis was measured initially using the absorption of transmitted photons from a single energy iodine source (SPA). However, use of a single photon source required the measurement to be carried out while the limb was immersed in water, which acted as a soft tissue equivalent thus allowing the transmission profile of water/soft tissue to be compared with significantly more dense bone.

The use of a water bath is somewhat inconvenient for peripheral bone sites and impossible for axial sites hence encouraging the development of 'dry systems', which now all use a two photon energy system replacing the original isotope photon source with X-rays, namely, dual energy X-ray absorptiometry (DEXA or DXA). This has become the standard clinical methodology for peripheral and axial measurements allowing assessment of area/BMD (BMC corrected for the assessed bone area) at sites of importance for fracture, including the forearm, lumbar spine, and both proximal femurs (Fig. 3).

The DEXA techniques thus allow a measurement of the mineral content of bone partially corrected for skeletal size, albeit only in two dimensions. While assessment of true volumetric bone density is possible using CT technology, this technique has the disadvantage of requiring very expensive CT scanners and also involving high radiation exposure at least when used at axial sites. However, it has the advantage of being able to assess both

Table 4 Advantages and disadvantages of bone measurement techniques

Technique	Site	Advantages	Disadvantages
Peripheral	Heel, forearm	Generally reasonably inexpensive Fairly portable	Measure relatively metabolically inactive bone sites Limited value in monitoring treatment effects or bone loss
Single energy X-ray absorptiometry (pSEXA)	Radius, os calci	Relatively inexpensive	Requires a water bath Has radiation source
Dual energy X-ray absorptiometry (pDEXA)	Radius, os calcis	Does not require a water bath Precise	Has radiation source
Computed tomography (pQCT)	Radius, tibia	Measures *true* bone density	Relatively expensive Precision less than pDEXA
Digital radiogrammetry	Metacarpals, radius	Well tried technique based on digitized radiographs Precise Inexpensive	Measures only cortical bone
Transmission quantitative ultrasound (QUS)	Os calcis	Inexpensive Portable May give data on bone structure Easy to use	Does not measure bone density directly
Reflectance quantitative ultrasound	Radius, phalanx, tibia, metatarsal	Multisite option with some machines	Primarily a measurement of cortical bone Needs training to give good precision
Axial	Spine, hip	Measures areas adjacent to sites of osteoporotic fracture	Not easily portable Needs extensive operator training and interpretation skills
Dual energy X-ray absorptiometry (DEXA)	Lumbar spine, proximal femur, total body, peripheral sites	'Gold' standard technique Multidetector scanners give reasonable image quality Good precision	Measures area/BMD alone Difficult to interpret spine scans in the elderly
Computed tomography (QCT)	Lumbar spine, proximal femur	Measures true bone density	High radiation dose Very expensive and heavily used equipment
Magnetic resonance imaging	Spine, hip, forearm	May give bone quality data	Does not measure bone density Not yet a standard technique

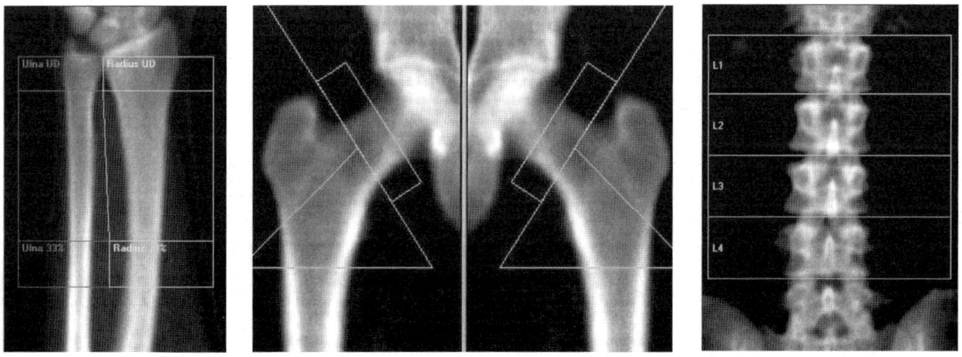

Fig. 3 Images from a Lunar Prodigy®, GE Medical Systems LUNAR, Madison, WI, USA (www.gemedicalsystems.com).

Table 5 Clinical uses of BMD measurements

Reason for use	QUS	Peripheral DEXA	Radiogrammetry	Peripheral QCT	Axial QCT	Axial DEXA
Diagnosis of osteoporosis	No	Yes	Possibly	Yes	Yes	Yes
Prediction of fracture	Yes	Yes	Yes	Yes	Yes	Yes
Targeting patients for axial DEXA	Yes	Possibly	Possibly	?	?	Not relevant
Target therapy	?	?	?	?	?	Yes
Monitoring response to therapy	Probably not	Probably not	Probably not	Possibly	Yes but high radiation	Yes but see text

cortical and trabecular bones either at peripheral sites, usually the radius, or at the important axial sites, most commonly the vertebral bodies.

For peripheral bone measurements a new development has been the use of a non-ionizing radiation method, quantitative ultrasound (QUS). As can be seen from Table 4, this uses either transmission of propagated ultrasound through a peripheral bone or reflection of the ultrasound wave from primarily cortical bone. Transmission QUS allows measurements of attenuation of the broad-band ultrasound beam (BUA) and the speed of passage of the sound-wave across the bone (SOS) along with manufacturer specific combined indices such as the inappropriately named 'stiffness' which is little to do with the elasticity of bone. Such indices correlate rather poorly *in vivo* with site-specific and distant-site BMD measurements, implying that the measurement is assessing other bone parameters as well as BMC and BMD. As QUS techniques do not measure bone density directly, they cannot be used to diagnose osteoporosis as the definition of the condition is firmly dependent on assessment of BMC or BMD. They do, however, predict those patients who subsequently fracture almost as well as BMD measurements and may give additional data on bone structure, a parameter poorly captured by current methods of BMD measurement.

Magnetic resonance imaging (MRI) may be a future way of capturing more on bone quality including internal structure (Hans et al. 1997) but more data are needed and the time to undertake a scan needs to be addressed before it could be a useful clinical tool.

After this brief description of the techniques available it is now important to examine how we can use the techniques in clinical practice. Measurement of bone mass can be used theoretically to address the questions laid out in Table 5.

The requirement to use the various techniques for diagnosing osteoporosis based on BMC or BMD clearly rules out use of QUS or possibly radiogrammetry as potential *diagnostic* tools but the more important question is whether the techniques predict future fracture. If, as seems likely, the diagnosis of osteoporosis in future becomes more allied to lifetime or 10-year fracture risk (Kanis et al. 2001b), then clearly as all techniques predict fracture, all will have future utility in diagnostic terms. It does not seem to matter at which site bone mass is assessed in terms of fracture prediction although site-specific assessment does show a slightly improved relative risk of future fracture compared with distant site assessment (Marshall et al. 1996) (Table 6).

Until intervention thresholds based on absolute fracture risk equations are developed, the over-riding question is whether intervening at a particular bone threshold, for example, a *T*-score of less than -2.5, measured at a specific site, such as the total femur will be associated with fracture reduction. This has only been demonstrated with axial BMD (Table 5) and then only with the bisphosphonates (infra vide). Until such data becomes available with other intervention thresholds it is dangerous to assume that treating women with low QUS scores, for example, will necessarily translate into absolute fracture reduction. For that, if no other reason, current guidelines have suggested that two-site axial DEXA (usually spine and hip) is the current method of choice for diagnosis. The agreed indications for assessment by axial DEXA as published in recent guidelines are shown in Table 7.

Table 6 Relative risks of fracture for each standard deviation reduction in age-standardized BMD

Site of measurement	Forearm fracture	Hip fracture	Vertebral fracture	All fractures
Distal radius	1.7 (1.4–2.0)	1.8 (1.4–2.2)	1.7 (1.4–2.1)	1.4 (1.3–1.6)
Hip	1.4 (1.4–1.6)	2.6 (2.0–3.5)	1.8 (1.1–1.7)	1.6 (1.4–1.8)
Lumbar spine	1.5 (1.3–1.8)	1.6 (1.2–2.2)	2.3 (1.9–2.8)	1.5 (1.4–1.7)

Many of these risk factors are historical and not necessarily evidence based but act as the best decision process available for case finding. As yet there are no cost-effectiveness data available which would argue in favour of population screening at any age, although guidelines in the United States (Eddy et al. 1998) do consider that assessment and treatment of all women over the age of 60 could be cost-effective if a cost per quality associated life year of \$30 000 is accepted. As the costs of the management of current fractures in the United Kingdom has been estimated at £1.7 billion per annum (Torgerson et al. 2001), the potential saving that could be induced by a population-based approach to fracture reduction including targeted assessment of bone mass is likely to be considered in future years.

Risk factors for fracture

Traditionally, the factors associated with risk of future fracture have been considered separately for post-menopausal women and for men. However, the risk factors leading to hip and other fractures are very similar, perhaps with the exception of clear hormonal specific effects such as hypogonadism. Further risk factors for low bone mass have also been considered separately but as these factors drive the indications for bone mass assessment (Table 7) it is sufficient to examine at this juncture those factors which may lead to fracture partly independent of bone density. This approach allows the option of including secondary causes (other diseases or treatments associated with fracture) in a discussion of risk factors.

Risk factors can then be considered as those which primarily effect bone directly and those which are associated with falls as well as a group of fractures which may be associated with risk due to a combination of falls and low bone mass. This approach is illustrated in Table 8 where risk factors for hip fracture in women are listed.

As recognized in a recent Consensus statement (Consensus Development Panel 2001), risk factors for low bone density and fractures, while overlapping, are not identical and this is partly because some of the bone factors listed in Table 8, such as bone turnover and bone geometry and turnover are not captured by BMD measurements while bone architecture cannot be assessed *in vivo* except by MRI or possibly QUS.

It is beyond the scope of this chapter to discuss falls and fall prevention strategies in detail, but clearly the factors listed under this category are not specifically associated with low BMD or other bone disorders. However, in the ageing skeleton increasing fall incidence is an independent risk factor for fracture. Targeting osteoporosis drug treatment at this group of individuals is unlikely to produce a fall in fracture rates, and elderly men and women with excess fracture risk due to falls should rather be subject to fall prevention strategies and perhaps use of hip protectors to limit their chance of future hip fracture in particular (Scottish Integrated Guideline Network 2002). It is therefore in the middle group where excess fracture risk may be in part related to bone and part related to fall risk that is worthwhile examining risk factors in more detail.

Age

As indicated, fractures increase in incidence with age across both sexes with the risk gradient being steeper in women than in men, especially for Colles and vertebral fractures. Recent studies have demonstrated that age is an independent risk factor for fracture even after allowing for the associated fall in BMD. For this reason, the absolute risk of fracture increases with age indicating, that for cost-effective intervention, treatment should be targeted at those men and women closest to the time when fracture is likely to occur.

Genetic factors

It has been estimated that upto 70 per cent of peak bone mass is related to genotypic rather than phenotypic factors. In the last decade numerous candidate genes have been explored to determine their relationship to osteoporosis. The first of these to be described were polymorphisms in the vitamin D receptor, but subsequently a large number of potential functional genes have been explored (Table 9).

With the exception of the COL1A1 gene, these genetic traits have been shown to reflect BMD more than fracture. On the contrary, polymorphisms in the COL1A1 gene have been shown to reflect fracture risk to a greater extent than BMD and are known to produce functional abnormalities in the triple helix molecule, which may partly explain the subsequent bone fragility.

While studies with many candidate genes have shown that they are related to BMD or fracture risk, it is clear that the currently identified genes even when examined together in the same population only explain a modicum of the apparent genetic risk influence on BMD which has been calculated from twin studies. Further, there is clear evidence that maternal history of hip fracture in particular defines increased risk of fracture in her offspring not explained by BMD alone. The reasons for this finding have yet to be fully explored but may reflect familial relationships in bone geometry, microarchitecture or turnover, or potentially even a familial tendency to falls.

Previous fracture

A previous low-trauma or fragility fracture at the forearm or hip increases risk of a further a non-vertebral fracture at the same or distant site by at least 50 per cent in most studies and this seems to apply to both men and women (Eastell et al. 2001). A previous vertebral fracture increases risk of subsequent vertebral deformity by perhaps as much as a factor of 10 times or more. Further, a prevalent vertebral deformity also increases risk of hip fracture, at least in women, by a factor of 4–5 (Ismail et al. 2001). Identification of those men and women who have sustained a low-trauma fracture is therefore a very important requirement to allow targeting of treatment with potential rapid benefit in reducing fracture rates (Eastell et al. 2001).

Weight

Body weight and body mass index are very important determinants of peak bone mass and also fracture risk. Hip fractures in particular are much more common in those with low BMI than those with average or increased BMI. While this finding is undoubtedly in part due to co-morbidities, it does appear that low body weight even in those otherwise healthy leads to excess

Table 7 Risk factors providing indications for the diagnostic use of bone densitometry

1. Presence of strong risk factors
   - Oestrogen deficiency
     - Premature menopause (age <45 years)
     - Prolonged secondary amenorrhoea
     - Primary hypogonadism
   - Corticosteroid therapy
     - Prednisolone >7.5 mg/day for 1 year or more
   - Maternal family history of hip fracture
   - Low body mass index (<19 kg/m^2)
   - Other disorders associated with osteoporosis
     - Anorexia nervosa
     - Malabsorption syndromes
     - Primary hyperparathyroidism
     - Post-transplantation
     - Chronic renal failure
     - Hyperthyroidism
     - Prolonged immobilization
     - Cushing's syndrome
2. Radiographic evidence of osteopaenia and/or vertebral deformity
3. Previous fragility fracture, particularly of the hip, spine, or wrist
4. Loss of height, thoracic kyphosis (after radiographic confirmation of vertebral deformities)

Table 8 Bone- and fall-related factors associated with hip fracture in women

Bone-related	Bone- and fall-related	Fall-related
Low bone mass	Increasing age	Neuromuscular function
Bone geometry such as long femoral neck	Genetic factors including maternal hip fracture	Cognitive impairment
High bone turnover	Previous fracture	Visual acuity
Disturbed microarchitecture	Low body weight	Drug therapy
	Immobility	Fall mechanics
	Smoking	
	Excess alcohol	
	Poor nutrition	
	Endocrine factors	
	Inflammatory arthritis	

Table 9 Candidate genes for osteoporosis

Apolipoprotein E	Galanin receptor 3	PTH
Calcitonin receptor	IGF-1	Peroxisome proliferator- activated receptor (*PPARγ*)
Calcium-sensing receptor	IL-1 receptor antagonist	Transforming growth factor-β1
Collagen type I alpha 1	IL-6	Vitamin D binding protein
Collagenase	MTHFR	Vitamin D receptor
Oestrogen receptor	Osteocalcin	

Source: Adapted from Hobson and Ralston (2001).

fracture risk. In post-menopausal women, there are a number of possible reasons for this finding:

- Oestrogen is metabolized in the post-menopausal women in the subcutaneous fat and thin women will have subsequently lower oestrogen levels than overweight women.
- Excess body weight is likely to induce impact loading on the skeleton more than low body weight leading to increased osteogenic activity.
- Among women who fall, those with less subcutaneous fat will have less natural 'cushioning' than the obese and will therefore suffer greater stress direct to the underlying bone.

Immobility

Medical conditions associated with immobility, such as stroke or paralysis, are associated with profound site-specific bone loss and it is of no surprise therefore that exercise levels in most studies are a determinant of BMD. This is not universal, however, and the effect does appear to be relatively weak, explaining no more than 1–2 per cent of peak bone mass, for example. In terms of the relationship with fracture, the data are even more confusing especially in the elderly. While the more active elderly have better BMD this might not translate into fracture reduction if they were more prone to falls.

It is clear that increasing exercise has a positive, but site-specific benefit on bone mass which seems to be related to the level of 'strain' on the bone. Exercise must be weight bearing to induce benefits. Thus, tennis players may have upto a 30 per cent increased BMD in their dominant arm, rowers have better than expected bone density at the spine and arms, runners have better BMD at the hips, while competitive swimmers do not benefit from their sport in terms of improved BMD.

The implications of this summary on the population fracture risk is that weight-bearing exercise is likely to be of benefit in terms of improving BMD and, although not proven, will probably have a positive effect on fractures. Further muscle strengthening exercises do seem to have a beneficial effect in the elderly on fall rates and are therefore likely to be associated with reduced fracture rates (Scottish Integrated Guideline Network 2002).

Smoking

While smoking is not identified as a risk factor for low BMD, in all epidemiological studies the balance of evidence is in favour of it having a mild detrimental effect on bone mass, which in older women, may in part be due to the observation that smokers tend to go through the menopause at a slightly earlier age.

Excess alcohol

While it is recognized that excessive alcohol, especially in males, is associated with reduced bone mass and an excess fracture risk, it is also clear that moderate alcohol consumption, perhaps within the government 'safe intake' guidelines, will be associated with dose-dependent increases in BMD. Men and women at risk of osteoporosis therefore are advised not to consume excess alcohol but are not inhibited from moderate intakes.

Poor nutrition

A common indication for osteoporosis assessment in which extreme alterations in nutrition will have occurred is anorexia nervosa. However, this risk is not just due to poor nutrition but also to low body weight and irregular menses with hormonal abnormalities. Malabsorption syndromes are also associated with reduced bone mass and excess fracture risk such as is seen in Coeliac disease. While nutritional influences are considered to be primarily due to calcium, there is increasing evidence that other micro- and macronutrients, such as magnesium, potassium, and vitamin D, as well as food groups, such as fruit and vegetables may be beneficial to bone health (Reid and Macdonald 2001).

Endocrine factors

The main endocrine factor associated with osteoporosis risk is premature menopause and low oestrogen levels throughout the pre-menopausal years, as indicated by irregular or absent menses. However, other rather less common endocrine abnormalities are clearly associated with reduced bone mass and excess fracture risk. Prominent amongst these is primary hyperparathyroidism, which causes persistent high bone turnover and excess risk of fracture. While it is clear that excess thyroid hormone is also associated with reduction in bone mass, it is not yet clear whether, in those with persistently over-replaced with thyroxine when being treated for hypothyroidism, are at excess risk of osteoporosis. Other endocrine abnormalities with excess risk are hyperprolactinaemia and low testosterone in males, including that induced by therapies for prostatic hyperplasia.

The main exogenous endocrine abnormality associated with osteoporosis is the use of mainly oral corticosteroids but endogenous Cushing's syndrome is also a well-recognized cause of fractures and low bone mass.

Inflammatory arthritis

While inflammatory arthritis is not always considered to be a major risk factor for osteoporosis there is no doubt that patients with rheumatoid arthritis have reduced bone mass (Reid et al. 1982) and are at increased risk of vertebral and hip fracture. While the pathogenesis of local bone loss may be in part due to the cytokines interleukin (IL)-1β and TNF-α, inducible nitric oxide may also have a role in both peri-articular and generalized bone loss (Armour et al. 2001). Taken together, these associates of osteoporosis drive the advised investigations that are considered valuable to detect secondary osteoporosis in those subjects presenting with low trauma fractures, especially when those involve the hip or vertebrae or in those with unexpectedly low BMD (Table 10).

Pathogenesis of osteoporosis

Post-menopausal osteoporosis

Much is made of there being two different pathogenetic mechanisms, the first accounting for the rapid loss of bone seen at trabecular bone sites after the menopause (Type I) and the second the more gradual loss of both cortical and trabecular bone (Type II) that occur in both sexes from the fifth or sixth decade onwards. The clinical value of this distinction is not obvious save that it implies that fractures of primarily trabecular bone sites (vertebrae and forearm) will commence soon after the menopause. There is also controversy as to whether significant bone loss occurs before the menopause but again the clinical consequences on therapy decisions are not clear. What is clear is that the loss of the protective effect of oestrogen in

Table 10 Investigations for detection of secondary osteoporosis in patients with low trauma fracture or very low BMD

Investigation	Secondary cause
Elevated ESR or C-reactive protein	Multiple myeloma Secondary carcinoma
Full blood count	Multiple myeloma (*anaemia*) Secondary carcinoma (*anaemia*)
Serum calcium, low serum phosphate	Hyperparathyroidism (*hypercalcaemia*) Osteomalacia (*hypocalcaemia, hypophosphataemia*)
Elevated serum alkaline phosphatase	Secondary carcinoma Paget's disease
Elevated serum creatinine	Renal failure
Serum TSH	Hyperthyroidism Over-replacement of hypothyroidism
Serum paraproteinaemia and/or urinary Bence Jones proteins	Multiple myeloma
Serum FSH, LH, testosterone	Detection of hypogonadism
Urinary free cortisol	Detection of Cushing's syndrome

women leads to an increase in osteoclast activity and possibly a slight diminution in osteoblast activity leading to rapid bone loss. Apoptosis of osteoblasts, loss of inhibition of osteoclasts (Weinstein and Manolagas 2000), and reduced sensitivity to endothelial nitric oxide synthase may play a role in this process (Armour et al. 2001).

Corticosteroid-induced osteoporosis (CIOP)

The association between osteoporosis and exogenous glucocorticoid therapy was made shortly after the drugs were first introduced in the 1950s. However, it was not until relatively recently that the frequency of fracture associated with their use was appreciated. In a retrospective cohort study comparing 244 235 oral glucocorticoid users and an equal number of age- and sex-matched controls, the relative risk of any non-vertebral fracture during oral glucocorticoid treatment was 1.33 (95 per cent CI 1.29–1.38), that of hip fracture was 1.61 (1.47–1.76) with evidence of dose-dependency. Increased vertebral fracture became statistically significant with doses in excess of 2.5 mg prednisolone per day while excess hip fracture risk was noted at doses of 7.5 mg or greater (van Staa et al. 2000).

The effects of corticosteroids are dependent on the dose, duration, and steroid type. Although there are theoretical effects which might lead to an increase in bone resorption primarily due to increased urinary calcium loss the major effects on the on the skeleton are due to a reduction of bone turnover by means of suppression of bone formation (Eastell et al. 1998b), the mechanism for which are summarized in Plate 195. Within the various mechanisms increased osteoblast and osteocyte apopotosis is a major factor, an effect which interestingly is reversed by co-prescription of bisphosphonates.

Corticosteroids also influence the synthesis and activity of many locally acting factors that affect osteoblasts, including the cytokines IL-1 and IL-6 and insulin-like growth factors and IGF-binding proteins, effects that may contribute to retarded skeletal growth in children treated with glucocorticoids. Interestingly bisphosphonates can reverse the pro-apoptotic effects of glucocorticoids on osteoblasts and osteocytes, which may contribute to their efficacy in preventing glucocorticoid-induced bone loss.

Osteoporosis in males

As indicated above, there is increasing recognition that bone loss is significant in men and that this phenomenon is associated with an increasing incidence of age-associated low trauma fractures [Fig. 2(b)]. Colles fractures occur relatively infrequently in males but there is increasing awareness of the problem of hip fractures in men. Vertebral deformities as assessed morphometrically are almost as frequent in men as in women, and while some of these are likely to be related to degenerative back disorders, the recognition of symptomatic vertebral fractures in primary or secondary care in men is even less likely than in women.

The pathogenesis and management of idiopathic osteoporosis in men has received scant attention (Eastell et al. 1998a) save to indicate the frequency of secondary causes, which may account for upto 50 per cent of vertebral fractures cases with corticosteroid use being the most prominent followed by anticonvulsant use, hypogonadism, and alcohol abuse (Scane et al. 1999). While androgen levels may be important in modulating bone mass in idiopathic male osteoporosis, there have been recent suggestions that oestrogen may even play a dominant role in men as well as in women (Orwoll 2001).

Management of osteoporosis

Treatment of the osteoporotic fractures themselves are out of the scope of this chapter but the management of acute vertebral fractures includes a brief period of bed rest followed by mobilization physiotherapy and potentially use of transcutaneous electrical nerve stimulator (TENS). While repair of the defect by kyphoplasty or vertebroplasty has been described there are no controlled trials of such therapy at present and such treatment must therefore be considered to be experimental. Early surgical repair of hip fractures is recommended and fall prevention advice or programmes are also of paramount importance (Scottish Integrated Guideline Network 2002).

Non-pharmacological therapy

Good nutrition is a prerequisite to good bone health. While calcium is considered to be the most important mineral for the developing skeleton and is clearly important in later life along with vitamin D (infra vide), there is still controversy as to the required dose for good skeletal health. The recent COMA report in the United Kingdom (DoH 1998) suggested that 800 mg/day (just greater than the amount of calcium present in a pint of milk) is all that is required for good bone health but it is recognized that in those with established osteoporosis receiving therapy with other bone active agents, a higher daily dose may be required to ensure adequate bone mineralization. Increased dietary vitamin D, or supplementation, is also required in the frail elderly and those unable to receive sufficient sunlight exposure.

Physical activity in childhood and early adult life contributes to the final achievement of peak bone mass. Generally, studies suggest, in older individuals, impact exercise to be beneficial and specific exercise programmes can produce small increases in site-specific bone density. Exercise programmes are also successful in preventing falls but it is not yet proven in randomized controlled trials (RCTs) that such programmes reduce fracture rates. Protection from the effect of falls by, for example, improved floor coverings with more absorbency may be useful and there can be little doubt that hip protectors, while not preventing all hip fractures even when worn, do reduce the risk of fracture in high-risk groups (Scottish Integrated Guideline Network 2002).

Drug therapy

An artificial divide between therapies for prevention and treatment is sometimes introduced by 'bone specialities' and drug licensing authorities which confuses the non-specialist. If a decision to treat a woman who has no pre-existing fractures is taken on the basis of a bone density definition of osteoporosis, is this prevention of fracture or treatment of low bone mass? No distinction will be made in this chapter. Once a decision to treat a woman has been taken, a treatment regimen should be determined for each individual patient using the knowledge of each patient's own history, lifestyle, and problems, along with the knowledge of the benefits and side-effect profiles of each of the therapies available.

Hormone replacement therapy

Hormone replacement therapy (HRT), in all its varieties, is still considered to be the drug of choice in the prevention and treatment of osteoporosis in the early post-menopausal years. While use of therapy undoubtedly increases BMD throughout the skeleton evidence for its efficacy in preventing hip and other non-spine fractures is mainly derived from cohort studies. In an oft quoted, small, RCT transdermal oestrogen use was associated with a remarkable 60 per cent reduction in vertebral fracture incidence in only 1 year (Lufkin et al. 1992). The results from recent meta-analyses confirm an overall antivertebral fracture efficacy of 33 per cent and non-spine antifracture efficacy of 27 per cent but the latter positive results were mainly seen in younger post-menopausal women and suggested a waning of the benefit after the age of 65 (Torgerson and Bell-Syer 2001).

It would appear therefore that HRT might be the first line of therapy, at least in the younger post-menopausal women and this would be especially the case if it had cardiovascular benefit. The publication of a negative RCT examining HRT as a tool for the secondary prevention of cardiovascular events (Hulley et al. 1998), coupled with the evidence of a slight excess of breast cancer risk after 5–10 years of therapy (Anonymous 1997), has raised questions as to the long-term use of HRT. When considering the cost-effectiveness of treatment a decision to commence treatment can be made in a more rational manner by the use of bone density measurements if an expensive form of HRT is to be used. This use of BMD to target treatment with HRT is likely to be considered even more efficient by the observation from cohort studies that women with breast cancer have a tendency to higher BMD values. Hence, targeting long-term HRT use at those with low BMD may be extremely cost-effective as the risk of breast cancer in this group may be limited.

How long the effect of HRT lasts after discontinuation is controversial, with most studies suggesting a rapid loss of bone and waning of the antifracture efficacy. However, targeting on those with low BMD may allow HRT use, even in the elderly, without inducing an acceptably high risk of breast cancer. It may well be necessary to supplement older women and those with dietary deficiency with calcium and vitamin D as a recent meta-analysis concluded that the effect of estrogen treatment on BMD was significantly greater if calcium intake was high (mean of 1183 mg/day) compared to where it was lower (mean of 563 mg/day) (Nieves et al. 1998).

Adverse effects of HRT include nausea, breast tenderness, and more seriously a significant increase in venous thrombo-embolism strongly implying that a women with a previous history of such disorders should not receive HRT.

Selective oestrogen receptor modulators

Selective oestrogen receptor modulators (SERMs) are tissue specific oestrogenic agents with agonist and anatagonist porperties. The only such agent currently available for use in the osteoporosis field is raloxifene although tamoxifen is also a SERM. Raloxifene prevents bone loss but does not stimulate breast or uterine tissues.

The efficacy of raloxifene in the prevention of vertebral fractures has recently been reported in the MORE trial. The chosen marketed dose (60 mg/day) reduced vertebral fracture by 50 per cent in those with BMD defined osteoporosis but without pre-existing fractures and 30 per cent in those with vertebral fractures at baseline, giving numbers needed treat of 46 and 10, respectively (Ettinger et al. 1999). Regretfully there was no evidence in this study of antifracture efficacy at non-spine sites.

Raloxifene is generally well tolerated with few upper gastrointestinal symptoms. It lowers serum LDL cholesterol by 8–10 per cent, but unlike oestrogen does not raise HDL cholesterol or triglyceride implying that it might have additional cardiovascular benefits. However, like oestrogen it does appear to have procoagulant effects with an elevation in thromboembolic events. However, breast cancer was reduced by over 75 per cent in the MORE trial where the effect was assessed as a safety end-point, with the effect only being significant in those with oestrogen receptor positive breast cancer (Cummings et al. 1999).

While raloxifene is effective in maintaining bone density and demonstrating small increases at both spine and hip, the effects are insufficiently large to allow efficacy to be proven by repeated BMD measurements in less than 3 or 4 years and the apparent lack of non-vertebral fracture efficacy is a significant disadvantage.

Bisphosphonates

These drugs have made a major impact in recent years, and will continue to contribute strongly to the management of osteoporosis. Working as specific antiresorptive drugs they have been used extensively in the management of Paget's disease of bone and tumour related hypercalcaemia. Although a number of bisphosphonates have been studied only three are licensed in the United Kingdom for use in the management of osteoporosis. Although the clinical effects on bone are similar it appears that they suppress osteoclasts by inducing apotosis in different ways with etidronate interfering with ATP pathways and alendronate and risedronate inhibiting enzymes in the mevulonate pathway (Russell and Rogers 1999).

Disodium etidronate (Didronel PMO®) for the prevention and treatment of osteoporosis, is taken as a 14-day pulse of oral etidronate followed by 76 days of calcium supplementation. The cycle is then repeated. Its license was granted on the basis of what would now be considered inadequately powered Phase III clinical trials where vertebral fracture rates were reduced over 2–3 years of treatment but the effect was only seen over a 3–4 year follow-up in those with the most severe baseline disease (Harris et al. 1993). Although originally only licensed for 3 years continuous use it now holds an open-ended license unlimited by time, with data from 7 years use being available. Although it is considered to have primarily antivertebral fracture efficacy, a recent cohort study using a clinical practice database has suggested efficacy in the prevention of hip fractures (van Staa et al. 1998).

Alendronate (Fosamax®) is licensed for the treatment of osteoporosis in post-menopausal women and is taken as a single tablet, once daily, continuously. If additional calcium supplementation is required it must be taken at a different time of the day to the bisphosphonate. It has been very widely studied. In an initial Phase III trial in patients with BMD-defined osteoporosis, a reduction in vertebral fractures of 48 per cent was seen, a figure almost identical to that seen in a second trial undertaken in subjects with pre-existing vertebral fractures—the fracture arm of the Fracture Intervention Trial (FIT) (Sharpe et al. 2001). The antifracture efficacy seemed therefore to be similar to the much smaller etidronate trials but the increase in spine and hip bone mass was rather greater, especially at the femoral neck. Care should be exercised, however, in interpreting differences between fracture rates in different clinical trials because of differences in study design and fracture definition. This caution is borne out by the results of a second arm of the FIT trial (Cummings et al. 1998). In this study patients with low BMD but who did not have vertebral fractures at baseline were randomized to alendronate or placebo and, as in the fracture arm, received 5 mg alendronate for the first 2 years and 10 mg thereafter, in this case for a further 2 years. Although broadly similar increases in BMD were noted in all sub-groups regardless of the baseline values, it was only in those with BMD in the WHO-defined osteoporosis range that a 36 per cent reduction in non-vertebral fractures was noted. The licensed dose for those who already have osteoporosis is 10 mg daily or 70 mg weekly (infra vide).

Risedronate (Actonel®) has also undergone extensive Phase III clinical trials in the prevention and treatment of post-menopausal and corticosteroid induced osteoporosis. In a major North American trial including 2458 post-menopausal women with at least one vertebral fracture, risedronate 5 mg/day reduced the risk of new vertebral fractures by 41 per cent ($p = 0.003$) over the 3 years of the study, although fracture reduction (65 per cent) was noted as early as 1 year after initiation of therapy (Genant et al. 1996). As expected BMD increased significantly compared with the placebo group, who received 1000 mg of supplemental calcium plus vitamin D if not replete. The increases in BMD at the lumbar spine (5.4 per cent) and femoral neck (1.6 per cent) were slightly less than those seen in phase III trials with alendronate but the study design was different and as yet no direct efficacy comparison study has been reported. Further trials in Europe confirmed the benefit on vertebral and non-vertebral fractures. A subsequent large RCT carried out in over 9000 elderly women was undertaken specifically to investigate the value of risedronate in the prevention of hip fractures. In women aged between 70 and 79 with a diagnosis of osteoporosis based on very low BMD (T-score <-3.0), there was a significant reduction of hip fractures (40 per cent) in the active compared to the placebo group who received calcium and vitamin D alone (McClung et al. 2001). In those with low BMD and a prevalent vertebral fracture, the reduction in hip fracture risk with risedronate was 60 per cent. In women over the age of 80 recruited on the basis of clinical risk factors for hip fracture mainly related to an increased risk of falls, there was no reduction in the rate of hip fractures. This study underlined the importance of targeting the bisphosphonates, alendronate and risedronate to those women that have osteoporosis as defined by BMD measurement if non-spine fracture reduction is desired.

Other bisphosphonates have been shown to be effective in post-menopausal osteoporosis although they do not carry a prevention or treatment licence. One, intravenous pamidronate, produces an increase in BMD when used 3-monthly by intravenous infusion and as such has value in those unable to take oral therapy, albeit prescribed off-label. Another two agents are being developed for intravenous use, either in a 2–3 monthly bolus injection (ibandronate) or as an annual infusion (zoledronate) (Reid et al. 2002).

The major difficulty with oral preparation of these drugs is their poor absorption from the gastrointestinal tract and hence the need for specific and often complex dosing instructions. All oral bisphosphonates require to be taken on an empty stomach, with water, with the additional need for alendronate and risedronate to be taken in an upright position to reduce the chance of upper gastrointestinal dyspepsia including oesophagitis. Less frequent dosing is popular with patients and produces similar benefits on bone density. Weekly oral alendronate (70 mg) is currently marketed and a weekly preparation of risedronate is likely to follow soon. The arrival of injectable preparations on the market is likely to increase the dosing interval.

Calcium and vitamin D preparations

There remains some controversy as to the need for added *calcium* or its use alone in the management of low bone mass or established osteoporosis. However, it has been shown that calcium supplementation can slow the rate of bone loss in post-menopausal women with a borderline reduction of symptomatic fractures. It should be used therefore for all women who have a low natural intake of 800 mg/day or less.

Calcitriol (1,25 dihydroxyvitamin D_3 Rocaltrol®) in a dose of 250 ng BD has been promoted as a treatment for established post-menopausal osteoporosis and has been shown to reduce vertebral fractures compared with placebo calcium in a study where remarkably the fracture rate in the placebo group rose compared to baseline. Although the medication has a licence, it has little of the market in the United Kingdom, perhaps especially as it use requires regular monitoring of serum calcium because of the rare occurrence of hypercalcaemia.

Calcium and vitamin D supplementation has been shown to reduce the rate of bone loss in post-menopausal women and in those over the age of 65. Calcium (1200 mg/day) and vitamin D (800 IU/day) supplementation is particularly important in the elderly where an RCT, carried out in women living in institutions in France, has shown effectiveness in preventing hip fractures by approximately 30 per cent (Chapuy et al. 1994). Whether calcium, vitamin D, or the combination is the effect agent is unclear. A large Medical Research Council funded study is underway in the United Kingdom to give an answer as to which should be used in the secondary prevention of fracture in those who have sustained a fracture at baseline.

Calcitonin

This drug has been in and out of favour as a treatment for osteoporosis over the years. In its marketed form in the United Kingdom its main drawback is that has to be given parentally by subcutaneous injection, although a nasal preparation is available in many European countries. A large 5-year RCT showed a reduction in vertebral fractures by around one-third compared with placebo but only with 200 IU/day and no significant effects was seen with 100 or 400 IU/day doses (Chesnut et al. 2000). A high incidence of systemic reactions to the parenteral therapy, local irritation with the intranasal preparation and expense may limit its widespread use, although in the United States nasal calcitonin is priced at the same level as alendronate. However, as it does appear to have some analgesic effects, it retains an occasional role in the management of intractable pain after vertebral fracture.

As indicated in a recent elegant review of available therapies (Delmas 2002), there are no stimulators of bone formation available for prescription at present in most countries. Sodium fluoride is one such agent should have a role to play in osteoporosis management; however, although it substantially increases bone mass at the lumbar spine, concerns continue regarding the relative dose required for antifracture efficacy despite the use of low-dose therapy. An exciting recent development has been the publication of data on the use of intermittent *1-34 parathyroid hormone* (PTH). While continuous high levels of PTH (such as occur in hyperparathyroidism) are associated with significant loss of bone, intermittent synthetic PTH substantially increases bone mass at the lumbar spine and hip by stimulating bone formation and its use has been associated with reductions of upto 70 per cent relative to placebo in vertebral fracture risk (Neer et al. 2001).

Strontium ranelate is both a resorption inhibitor and a formation stimulator with significant benefits on bone mass in animal models. It is currently undergoing a Phase III clinical trial programme and is one of a series of potential new anabolic agents, which might include statins, undergoing investigation (Mundy 2002).

Prescription of specific drug therapy

Currently prescription decisions in the United Kingdom are driven by the Royal College of Physicians' guidelines which were published in 1999 (Royal College of Physicians 1999), with a management update in 2000 (Royal College of Physicians 2000). These guidelines are based on the relative effectiveness of the various treatments as described above and summarized in Table 11.

Special situations

There are far fewer RCTs of the effects of prevention and treatment of corticosteroid-induced osteoporosis and of osteoporosis in males. Provisional guidelines have been described based on a panel of UK experts (Eastell et al. 1998b) and these have been updated recently following a systematic literature review. The best evidence for efficacy, including antifracture efficacy, is with the bisphosphonates etidronate, alendronate, and risedronate whether used for primary prevention or after corticosteroids have been used for some time. The schema as published in recent Royal College of Physicians Glucocorticoid Induced Osteoporosis Guidelines is shown in Fig. 4 (Anonymous 2002).

For males while there is evidence of efficacy of testosterone on increasing BMD both in hypogonadal and eugonadal men there remains concern about long-term safety. The only drug with a licence for prevention and treatment of osteoporosis in men is alendronate where a small but well-conducted RCT showed efficacy in increasing BMD and reducing vertebral fracture rates (Orwoll et al. 2000).

Duration of treatment

It is not clear how long therapy should be continued. Most Phase III trials are limited to a maximum of 3–5 years for post-menopausal HRT and 1–2 years for CIOP. The effect of HRT on bone loss seems to be fairly soon

Table 11 Effectiveness of intervention on prevention or reduction of bone loss and antifracture efficacy in post-menopausal osteoporosis: grade of evidence

	Antifracture effect			
	Effect on bone loss	Spine	Non-vertebral	Hip
Alendronate	A	A	A	A
Calcitonin	A	A	B	B
Calcitriol	A	A	A	nd
Calcium	A	A	B	B
Calcium and vitamin D	A	nd	A	A
Cessation of smoking	B	—	—	—
Cyclic etidronate	A	A	B	B
Hip protectors	—	—	—	A
HRT	A	A	A	B
Physical exercise	A	nd	B	B
Raloxifene	A	A	nd	nd
Reduced alcohol	C	—	—	—
Risedronate	A	A	A	A
Tibolone	A	nd	nd	nd

Note: Grade A, meta-analysis or at least one RCT or well-controlled study without randomization; Grade B, at least one other type of quasi-experimental study or from well-designed comparative or case–control studies; Grade C, expert committee reports or opinions.

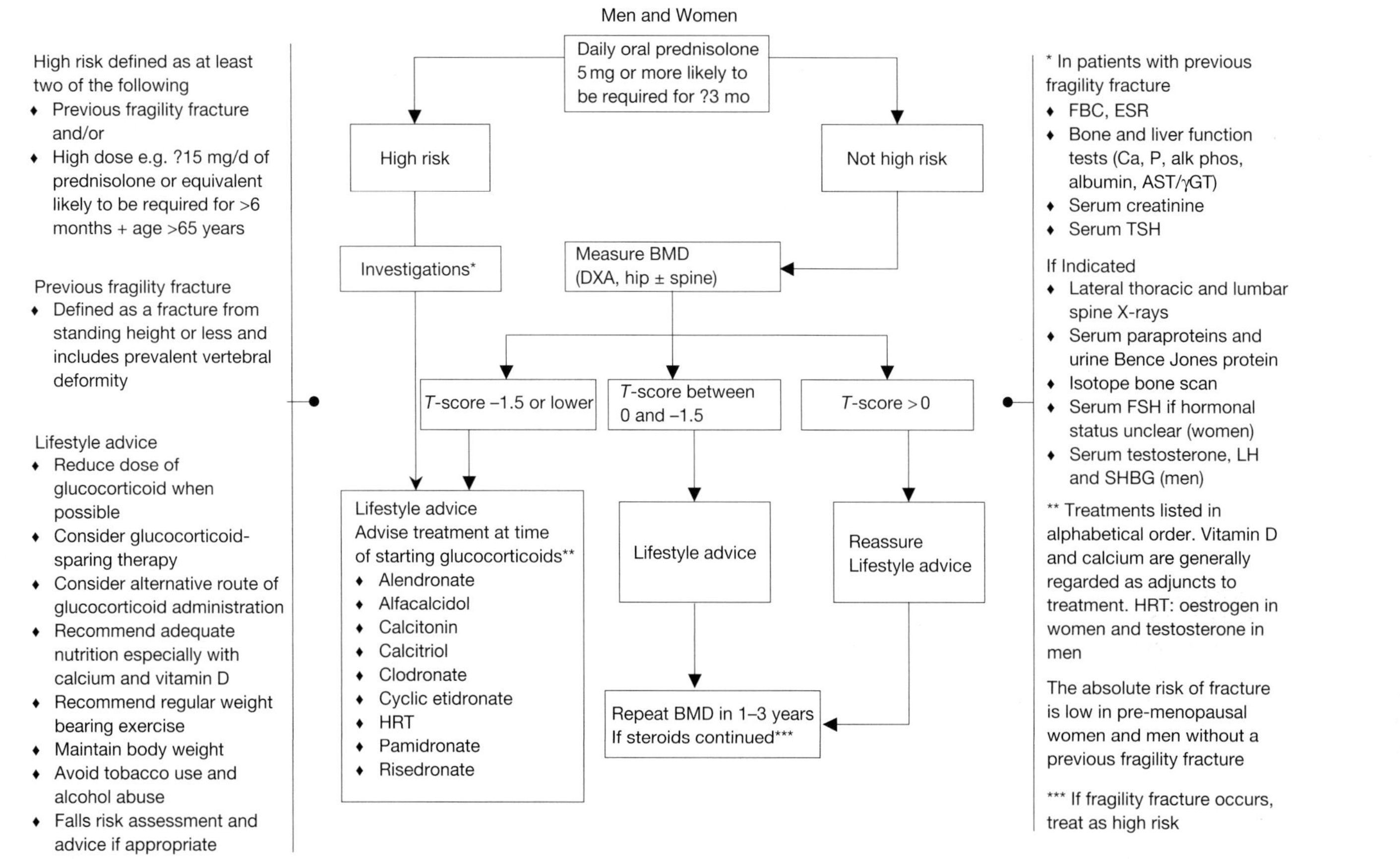
Men and Women
Daily oral prednisolone 5 mg or more likely to be required for ?3 mo
High risk
Not high risk
Investigations*
Measure BMD (DXA, hip ± spine)
T-score −1.5 or lower
T-score between 0 and −1.5
T-score > 0
Lifestyle advice
Advise treatment at time of starting glucocorticoids**
♦ Alendronate
♦ Alfacalcidol
♦ Calcitonin
♦ Calcitriol
♦ Clodronate
♦ Cyclic etidronate
♦ HRT
♦ Pamidronate
♦ Risedronate
Lifestyle advice
Reassure
Lifestyle advice
Repeat BMD in 1–3 years
If steroids continued***
High risk defined as at least two of the following
♦ Previous fragility fracture and/or
♦ High dose e.g. ?15 mg/d of prednisolone or equivalent likely to be required for >6 months + age >65 years
Previous fragility fracture
♦ Defined as a fracture from standing height or less and includes prevalent vertebral deformity
Lifestyle advice
♦ Reduce dose of glucocorticoid when possible
♦ Consider glucocorticoid-sparing therapy
♦ Consider alternative route of glucocorticoid administration
♦ Recommend adequate nutrition especially with calcium and vitamin D
♦ Recommend regular weight bearing exercise
♦ Maintain body weight
♦ Avoid tobacco use and alcohol abuse
♦ Falls risk assessment and advice if appropriate
* In patients with previous fragility fracture
♦ FBC, ESR
♦ Bone and liver function tests (Ca, P, alk phos, albumin, AST/γGT)
♦ Serum creatinine
♦ Serum TSH
If Indicated
♦ Lateral thoracic and lumbar spine X-rays
♦ Serum paraproteins and urine Bence Jones protein
♦ Isotope bone scan
♦ Serum FSH if hormonal status unclear (women)
♦ Serum testosterone, LH and SHBG (men)
** Treatments listed in alphabetical order. Vitamin D and calcium are generally regarded as adjuncts to treatment. HRT: oestrogen in women and testosterone in men
The absolute risk of fracture is low in pre-menopausal women and men without a previous fragility fracture
*** If fragility fracture occurs, treat as high risk

Fig. 4 Algorithm for the prevention and treatment of CIOP in men and women (Anonymous 2002).

after therapy is withdrawn and the antifracture efficacy may well wear off after 3–5 years For bisphosphonates there is some evidence, especially with alendronate, that there is a carry over effect on bone loss rates which may last upto 2 years. Long-term safety of the bisphosphonates after 7–10 years has not been established but it is currently unclear whether treatment should be withdrawn after that period of time at least for a year or two. Pending further information such a course of action may be sound. In CIOP, it is generally advised that therapy should continue as long as the corticosteroids are required for management of the underlying condition.

Monitoring of therapy

Current advice, which takes into account the relative effects of treatments on site specific bone density and the measurable least significant change based on the precision of the measurement tool and bone site (Table 4), is *not* to repeat BMD less than 2 years and then to use lumbar spine DXA. There is potential value of using bone turnover markers as indicators of effectiveness of treatment as these could be demonstrate significant changes in an individual patient, with possible benefit on compliance rates, with a 3–6-month period.

Summary

Clearly, osteoporosis is a major scourge of Western society but interest in the condition has risen exponentially in the last decade partly because of advances in our understanding of the disease process, the ability to predict its onset, measure its progression, and especially the availability of powerful preventative therapies. Further therapeutic advances are likely and the challenge will be how to best target our improved therapies at the expanding elderly population to reduce the impact and costs of fracture and to address the as yet hardly touched concept in this field of compliance with prescribed therapy.

Osteomalacia

Osteomalacia, and its sister condition occurring in the growing skeleton, rickets, can most easily be distinguished from osteoporosis by reference to a simple diagram (Fig. 5).

Here, it can be seen that in the normal state cancellous (trabecular) bone is 80 per cent calcified and 20 per cent uncalcified at any one time. In osteoporosis there is simply too little bone volume tissue present within the anatomical bone structure but that which is present is normally calcified. In osteomalacia, on the other hand, there is sufficient bone volume but the bone has reduced calcification. This rather simplistic way of considering the difference between the two conditions allows understanding of some of the biochemical abnormalities that occur in osteomalacia (Table 12).

For clarity, these abnormalities have been compared with those that occur in primary hyperparathyroidism and the near normal status in osteoporosis. As can be seen in osteomalacia while serum biochemistry can be normal there is frequently a reduction in serum calcium, reduced serum phosphate, and/or an elevation in serum alkaline phosphatase. It is only after a fracture that any such abnormalities occur in osteoporosis and then only an elevation in serum alkaline phosphatase.

Aetiopathogenesis

To understand the aetiology of osteomalacia a rudimentary understanding of the metabolism of vitamin D and its effects on calcium status is required (Fig. 6).

The parent form of vitamin D_3 (cholecalciferol) is a fat soluble vitamin which in humans is derived from two sources (i) the diet, and (ii) metabolism in the skin (from 7-dehydrocholesterol) under the influence of sunlight. For most individuals, metabolism in the skin is the most important source of vitamin D but for those who expose little skin to the influences of the sun for geographical, racial, or religious reasons, the dietary source (ergocalciferol) becomes increasingly important. Dietary sources of vitamin D are supplemented dairy products and margarines, although meat may also be a good source of metabolically available vitamin D. It has also recently become clear that vitamin D is only metabolized from its inactive precursors in the skin after exposure to certain wavelengths of sunlight which only occur in Northern latitudes in the summer months (DOH 1998). Conversion of naturally sourced vitamin D to the metabolically active $25(OH)D_3$ and $1,25(OH)_2D_3$ take place in the liver and kidney, respectively. The conversion mechanisms become less effective in the elderly leading to secondary hyperparathyroidism, bone loss, and consequent risk of osteoporosis (Strause et al. 1994).

Many cases of osteomalacia are due to secondary disorders as shown in Table 13.

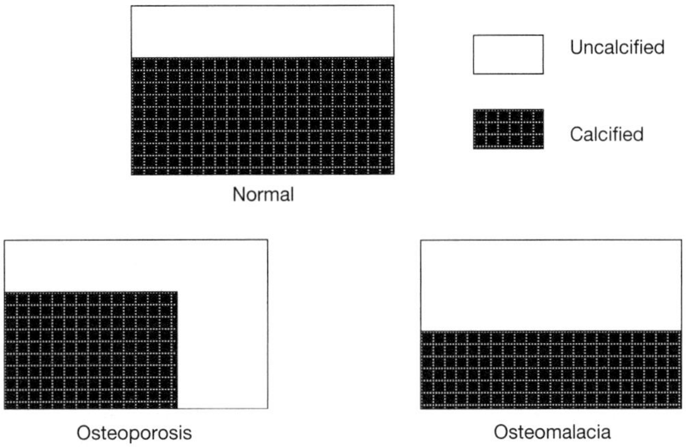

Fig. 5 Proportions of calcified and uncalcified bone in normal, osteoporosis, and osteomalacia.

Table 12 Serum and urinary abnormalities in osteoporosis, osteomalacia, and hyperparathyroidism

	Osteoporosis	Osteomalacia	Primary hyperparathyroidism
Serum calcium	Normal	Low or normal	Elevated
Serum phosphate	Normal	Low or normal	Normal or low
Serum alkaline phospatase	Normal but elevated after fracture	Normal or elevated	Normal or elevated
Serum 25(OH)D	Normal or low	Usually low	Low normal

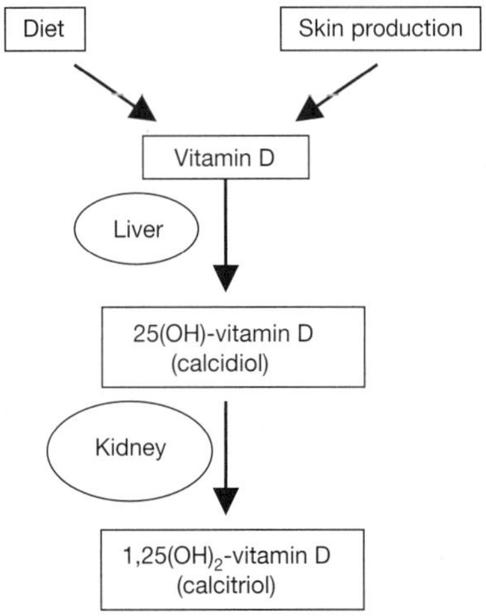

Fig. 6 Metabolism of vitamin D in humans.

Clinical features and investigations

The principal symptoms of osteomalacia are bone pain and tenderness, skeletal deformity, especially in childhood rickets, muscle weakness, and occasional signs of tetany from the associated hypocalcaemia. Bone pain characteristically affects the axial skeleton but localized pain in the groin can occur in the presence of a Looser's zone (infra vide). Muscle weakness is usually proximal and often associated with a characteristic waddling gait and by difficulty in rising from a chair without the aid of the arms.

Investigation is undertaken in the presence of clinical suspicion of disease and particularly if one of the underlying diseases or disorders associated with the condition is present. Hypocalcaemia is usually present but it may be quite mild and may or may not be associated with hypophosphataemia. Serum alkaline phosphatase is usually elevated and in most varieties 25(OH) vitamin D levels are low. Parathyroid hormone levels can be elevated due to secondary hyperparathyroidism.

Radiographs can be diagnostic if the aptly named Looser's zones are present, with the these sites of pseudofracture characteristically occurring in the pubic and ischial rmai, the medial border of the scapula and the medial cortex of the femur. Intervertebral discs may compress the vertebral endplates producing biconcave or 'cod-fish' vertebrae which may be mistaken for osteoporotic fractures. Isotope bone scans may wish show a diffuse increased uptake in bone but this is non-specific.

The definitive investigation is the transiliac bone biopsy preferably after double-labelling with two 3-day courses of oral tetracycline given 2 weeks apart. In osteomalacia the biopsy reveals increased osteoid surfaces but no characteristic separation of the fluorescene labels which would normally be produced by continuing mineralization of new osteoid.

Table 13 Causes of osteomalacia

Primary (nutritional) vitamin D deficiency	Secondary causes
Classic deficiency such as Asian immigrants, elderly, housebound and institutionalized food faddists	Vitamin D deficiency
	Partial gastrectomy
	Small bowel malabsorption
	Hepatobiliary disease
	Pancreatic insufficiency
	Chronic renal failure
	Metabolic acidosis
	Drugs and toxins
	Anticonvulsants
	Aluminium toxicity
	Prolonged etidronate therapy
	Fluoride
	Miscellaneous
	Calcium depletion
	Phosphate depletion
	Magnesium depletion
	Primary hyperparathyroidism
	Hereditary forms [see Scheinman et al. (1999)]

Management principles

The most important aim in adult osteomalacia is to relieve bone pain and to allow muscle strength to recover. The primary pathological process should be treated if possible but the initial aim is to restore serum calcium levels to normal by replacement of vitamin D.

Confusingly, there are five preparations available. Use of calcitriol in a dose of upto 1 μg daily given as a capsule, liquid, or injection has the advantage of a rapid onset of action (usually within a week) and rapid loss of effect after cessation. On the other hand, calciferol, either given as cholecalciferol or ergocalciferol takes 2–3 months to produce a maximum effect and persist for upto 6 months after cessation. Additional mineral supplementation with calcium salts is usually co-prescribed but careful monitoring of serum calcium, phosphate, alkaline phosphate, serum 25(OH) vitamin, and sometimes PTH should be considered.

References

Anonymous (1987). Consensus development conference: prophylaxis and treatment of osteoporosis. *British Medical Journal* **295** (6603), 914–15 (review).

Anonymous (1994). Assessment of fracture risk and its application to screening for postmenopausal osteoporosis. Report of a WHO Study Group. *World Health Organization Technical Report Series* **843**, 1–129 (review with 466 references).

Anonymous (1997). Breast cancer and hormone replacement therapy: collaborative reanalysis of data from 51 epidemiological studies of 52 705 women with breast cancer and 108 411 women without breast cancer. Collaborative Group on Hormonal Factors in Breast Cancer. *Lancet* **350** (9084), 1047–59 (see comments; erratum appears in *Lancet* 1997; **350** (9089), 1484).

Anonymous. *Glucocorticoid Induced Osteoporosis: Guidelines for Prevention and Treatment.* London: Royal College of Physicians, 2002.

Armour, K.E. et al. (2001). Defective bone formation and anabolic response to exogenous estrogen in mice with targeted disruption of endothelial nitric oxide synthase. *Endocrinology* **142** (2), 760–6.

Armour, K.J. et al. (2001). Activation of the inducible nitric oxide synthase pathway contributes to inflammation-induced osteoporosis by suppressing bone formation and causing osteoblast apoptosis. *Arthritis and Rheumatism* **44**(12), 2790–6.

Chapuy, M.C., Arlot, M.E., Delmas, P.D., and Meunier, P.J. (1994). Effect of calcium and cholecalciferol treatment for three years on hip fractures in elderly women. *British Medical Journal* **308** (6936), 1081–2 (see comments).

Chesnut, C.H., III et al. (2000). A randomized trial of nasal spray salmon calcitonin in postmenopausal women with established osteoporosis: the prevent recurrence of osteoporotic fractures study. PROOF Study Group. *American Journal of Medicine* **109** (4), 267–76 (see comments).

Consensus Development Conference (1993). Diagnosis, prophylaxis, and treatment of osteoporosis. *American Journal of Medicine* **94** (6), 646–50 (review).

Consensus Development Panel on Osteoporosis Prevention DaT (2001). Osteoporosis prevention, diagnosis and therapy. *Journal of the American Medical Association* **285** (6), 785–95.

Cummings, S.R. et al. (1998). Effect of alendronate on risk of fracture in women with low bone density but without vertebral fractures: results from the Fracture Intervention Trial. *Journal of the American Medical Association* **280** (24), 2077–82.

Cummings, S.R. et al. (1999). The effect of raloxifene on risk of breast cancer in postmenopausal women: results from the MORE randomized trial. Multiple Outcomes of Raloxifene Evaluation. *Journal of the American Medical Association* **281** (23), 2189–97 (see comments; erratum appears in *Journal of the American Medical Association* **282** (22), 2124).

Delmas, P.D. (1998). The role of markers of bone turnover in the assessment of fracture risk in postmenopausal women. *Osteoporosis International* **8** (Suppl. 1), S32–6.

Delmas, P.D. (2002). Treatment of postmenopausal osteoporosis. *Lancet* **359**, 2018–26.

Dempster, D.W. (2000). The contribution of trabecular architecture to cancellous bone quality. *Journal of Bone and Mineral Research* **15** (1), 20–4.

Department of Health. *Nutrition and Bone Health: With Particular Reference to Calcium and Vitamin D.* London: HMSO, 1998. (Report on Health and Social Subjects; 49.)

Eastell, R. et al. (1998a). Management of male osteoporosis: report of the UK Consensus Group. *Quarterly Journal of Medicine* **91** (2), 71–92.

Eastell, R. et al. (1998b). A UK Consensus Group on management of glucocorticoid-induced osteoporosis: an update. *Journal of Internal Medicine* **244** (4), 271–92.

Eastell, R. et al. (2001). Secondary prevention of osteoporosis: when should a non-vertebral fracture be a trigger for action? *Quarterly Journal of Medicine* **94** (11), 575–97.

Eddy, D.M. et al. (1998). Osteoporosis: review of the evidence for prevention, diagnosis, and treatment and cost-effectiveness analysis. Status report. *Osteoporosis International* **8** (Suppl. 4), 1–82.

Ettinger, B. et al. (1999). Reduction of vertebral fracture risk in postmenopausal women with osteoporosis treated with raloxifene: results from a 3-year randomized clinical trial. Multiple Outcomes of Raloxifene Evaluation (MORE) Investigators. *Journal of the American Medical Association* **282** (7), 637–45 (see comments; erratum appears in *Journal of the American Medical Association* 1999; **282** (22), 2124).

Genant, H.K. et al. (1996). Noninvasive assessment of bone mineral and structure: state of the art. *Journal of Bone and Mineral Research* **11** (6), 707–30.

Hans, D. et al. (1997). How can we measure bone quality? *Baillière's Clinical Rheumatology* **11** (3), 495–515.

Harris, S.T. et al. (1993). Four-year study of intermittent cyclic etidronate treatment of postmenopausal osteoporosis: three years of blinded therapy followed by one year of open therapy. *American Journal of Medicine* **95** (6), 557–67.

Hobson, E.E. and Ralston, S.H. (2001). Role of genetic factors in the pathophysiology and management of osteoporosis. *Clinical Endocrinology* **54** (1), 1–9 (review with 102 references).

Hulley, S. et al. (1998). Randomized trial of estrogen plus progestin for secondary prevention of coronary heart disease in postmenopausal women. Heart and Estrogen/progestin Replacement Study (HERS) Research Group. *Journal of the American Medical Association* **280** (7), 605–13 (see comments).

Ingle, B.M. and Eastell, R. (2002). Site-specific bone measurements in patients with ankle fracture. *Osteoporosis International* **13** (4), 342–7.

Ismail, A.A. et al. (2001). Prevalent vertebral deformity predicts incident hip though not distal forearm fracture: results from the European Prospective Osteoporosis Study. *Osteoporosis International* **12** (2), 85–90.

Kanis, J.A., Johnell, O., Oden, A., De Laet, C., and Mellstrom, D. (2001a). Diagnosis of osteoporosis and fracture threshold in men. *Calcified Tissue International* **69** (4), 218–21 (review with 21 references).

Kanis, J.A., Oden, A., Johnell, O., Jonsson, B., de Laet, C., and Dawson, A. (2001b). The burden of osteoporotic fractures: a method for setting intervention thresholds. *Osteoporosis International* **12** (5), 417–27.

Lufkin, E.G. et al. (1992). Treatment of postmenopausal osteoporosis with transdermal estrogen. *Annals of Internal Medicine* **117** (1), 1–9 (see comments).

Marshall, D., Johnell, O., and Wedel, H. (1996). Meta-analysis of how well measures of bone mineral density predict occurrence of osteoporotic fractures. *British Medical Journal* **312** (7041), 1254–9.

McClung, M.R. et al. (2001). Effect of risedronate on the risk of hip fracture in elderly women. Hip Intervention Program Study Group. *New England Journal of Medicine* **344** (5), 333–40.

Melton, L.J., III, Orwoll, E.S., and Wasnich, R.D. (2001). Does bone density predict fractures comparably in men and women? *Osteoporosis International* **12** (9), 707–9.

Mundy, G.R. (2002). Directions of drug discovery in osteoporosis. *Annual Review of Medicine* **53**, 337–54 (review with 70 references).

Neer, R.M. et al. (2001). Effect of parathyroid hormone (1–34) on fractures and bone mineral density in postmenopausal women with osteoporosis. *New England Journal of Medicine* **344** (19), 1434–41 (see comments).

Nieves, J.W., Komar, L., Cosman, F., and Lindsay, R. (1998). Calcium potentiates the effect of estrogen and calcitonin on bone mass: review and analysis. *American Journal of Clinical Nutrition* **67** (1), 18–24 (see comments; review with 50 references).

O'Neill, T.W. et al. (2001). Incidence of distal forearm fracture in British men and women. *Osteoporosis International* **12** (7), 555–8.

Orwoll, E. et al. (2000). Alendronate for the treatment of osteoporosis in men. *New England Journal of Medicine* **343** (9), 604–10.

Orwoll, E.S. (2001). Androgens: basic biology and clinical implication. *Calcified Tissue International* **69** (4), 185–8 (review with 30 references).

Reid, D.M., Kennedy, N.S., Smith, M.A., Tothill, P., and Nuki, G. (1982). Total body calcium in rheumatoid arthritis: effects of disease activity and corticosteroid treatment. *British Medical Journal (Clinical Research Edition)* **285** (6338), 330–2.

Reid, D.M. and Macdonald, H.M. (2001). Nutrition and bone: is there more to it than just calcium and vitamin D? *Quarterly Journal of Medicine* **94** (2), 53–6.

Reid, I.R. et al. (2002). Intravenous zoledronic acid in postmenopausal women with low bone mineral density. *New England Journal of Medicine* **346** (9), 653–61 (see comments).

Royal College of Physicians. *Osteoporosis: Clinical Guidelines for Prevention and Treatment.* London: Royal College of Physicians, 1999.

Royal College of Physicians. *Osteoporosis Clinical Guidelines for Prevention and Treatment. Update on Pharmacological Interventions and an Algorithm for Management.* London: Royal College of Physicians, 2000.

Russell, R.G. and Rogers, M.J. (1999). Bisphosphonates: from the laboratory to the clinic and back again. *Bone* **25** (1), 97–106 (review with 106 references).

Scane, A.C., Francis, R.M., Sutcliffe, A.M., Francis, M.J., Rawlings, D.J., and Chapple, C.L. (1999). Case–control study of the pathogenesis and sequelae of symptomatic vertebral fractures in men. *Osteoporosis International* **9** (1), 91–7.

Scheinman, S.J., Guay-Woodford, L.M., Thakker, R.V., and Warnock, D.G. (1999). Genetic disorders of renal electrolyte transport. *New England Journal of Medicine* **340** (15), 1177–87 (review with 66 references).

Scottish Integrated Guideline Network. *Prevention and Management of Hip Fracture in Older People* Vol. 56. Edinburgh: Royal College of Physicians, 2002.

Sharpe, M., Noble, S., and Spencer, C.M. (2001). Alendronate: an update of its use in osteoporosis. *Drugs* **61** (7), 999–1039 (review with 207 references).

van Staa, T.P., Abenhaim, L., and Cooper, C. (1998). Use of cyclical etidronate and prevention of non-vertebral fractures. *British Journal of Rheumatology* **37** (1), 87–94 (see comments).

van Staa, T.P., Leufkens, H.G., Abenhaim, L., Zhang, B., and Cooper, C. (2000). Use of oral corticosteroids and risk of fractures. *Journal of Bone and Mineral Research* **15** (6), 993–1000 (see comments; review with 43 references).

van Staa, T.P., Dennison, E.M., Leufkens, H.G., and Cooper, C. (2001). Epidemiology of fractures in England and Wales. *Bone* **29** (6), 517–22.

Stewart, A., Felsenberg, D., Kalidis, L., and Reid, D.M. (1995). Vertebral fractures in men and women: how discriminative are bone mass measurements? *British Journal of Radiology* **68** (810), 614–20.

Strause, L., Saltman, P., Smith, K.T., Bracker, M., and Andon, M.B. (1994). Spinal bone loss in postmenopausal women supplemented with calcium and trace minerals. *Journal of Nutrition* **124** (7), 1060–4.

The European Prospective Osteoporosis Study Group (2002). Incidence of vertebral fracture in Europe: results from the European Prospective Osteoporosis Study (EPOS). *Journal of Bone and Mineral Research* **17** (4), 716–24.

Torgerson, D.J. and Bell-Syer, S.E. (2001). Hormone replacement therapy and prevention of nonvertebral fractures: a meta-analysis of randomized trials. *Journal of the American Medical Association* **285** (22), 2891–7.

Torgerson, D.J., Iglesias, C.P., and Reid, D.M. (2001). The economics of fracture prevention. In *The Effective Management of Osteoporosis* (ed. D. H. Barlow, R. M. Francis, and A. Miles), pp. 111–21. London: Aesculapius Medical Press.

Walker-Bone, K., Dennison, E., and Cooper, C. (2001). Epidemiology of osteoporosis. *Rheumatic Disease Clinics of North America* **27** (1), 1–18.

Weinstein, R.S. and Manolagas, S.C. (2000). Apoptosis and osteoporosis. *American Journal of Medicine* **108** (2), 153–64.

6.16.2 Paget's disease of bone

S.E. Papapoulos

In 1876 Sir James Paget presented to the Royal Medical and Chirurgical Society of London an account of his experience with a previously unrecognized disease of the skeleton which he termed osteitis deformans and which bears his names since. Paget's disease of bone is a focal skeletal disorder that progresses slowly and leads to changes in the shape and size of affected bones and to skeletal, articular, and vascular complications. In some parts of the world it is the second most common bone disorder after osteoporosis. The disease is easily diagnosed and effectively treated but its aetiology and natural history remain largely unknown (Harinck et al. 1986; Delmas and Meunier 1997; Papapoulos 1997; Kanis 1998; Singer and Krane 1998; Siris 1999; Lyles et al. 2001).

Epidemiology

Paget's disease affects typically the elderly, slightly more men than women, and seldom presents before the age of 35 years. The median age of referral to our unit was 63 years for men and 67 years for women and the median duration of symptoms was 5 years. It is noteworthy that one-third of these patients were working full time at the time of presentation and nearly half of them had to retire prematurely because of the disability caused by the disease. There is a distinct geographical distribution; the disease is common in central, western, and parts of southern Europe, the United States of America, Australia, New Zealand, and some countries of South America while it is uncommon in Scandinavia, Asia, and Africa. Its prevalence increases with age and it affects 2–5 per cent of those above 50 years of age. In a recent population survey in the United States the prevalence of radiographically detected pelvic disease was between 1.6 and 3.4 per cent in individuals older than 65 years (Altman et al. 2000). There may be also variations within the same country. For example, in northeast United States the prevalence is about 5-fold higher than in south United States. In parts of northwest England in 1974 the age- and gender-standardized prevalence rate was 8.3 per cent compared to 4.6 per cent in southern towns and cities (Barker et al. 1977). Interestingly, a new radiographic survey in the same centres with identical methodology, reported a decline in the overall prevalence compared to 1974 suggesting that environmental factors may be involved in the pathogenesis of the disease (Cooper et al. 1999). Reports from New Zealand, Great Britain, and Spain suggested, in addition, that the disease may be becoming milder in recent years (Cundy et al. 1997). Despite some methodological limitations, these combined observations, if confirmed by other studies, may provide clues to the aetiology of Paget's disease.

Pathogenesis

Normal bone metabolism

The skeleton is continuously renewed throughout life. In the adult, old bone is replaced by new in the same location, a process termed bone remodelling. Bone is removed by the osteoclasts whereas new bone is formed by the osteoblasts. This occurs in an orderly fashion through temporary anatomic structures called basic multicellular units (BMUs). A BMU comprises a team of osteoclasts in the front and a team of osteoblasts in the back supported by blood vessels, nerves, and loose connective tissue. Osteoclasts resorb bone while osteoblasts move to the resorbed area and lay down new bone matrix which subsequently mineralizes. This sequence is known as coupling. Osteoclasts and osteoblasts are derived from different precursors in the bone marrow. Osteoclasts originate from haematopoietic precursors of the monocyte/macrophage lineage while osteoblasts originate from multipotent mesenchymal stem cells that give also rise to bone marrow stromal cells, chondrocytes, adipocytes, and muscle cells. The signals that determine coupling are not yet fully known but the mediators of the action of bone resorbing factors have been identified. These mediators belong to a ligand/receptor/soluble (decoy) receptor system involving proteins of the TNF receptor superfamily (Suda et al. 1999). These are RANK-ligand, RANK, and OPG. (RANK-ligand is the the receptor activator of NF-κB ligand; other names in the literature are osteoprotegerin ligand, osteoclast differentiation factor, and TRANCE (TNF-related activation-induced cytokine). OPG is osteoprotegerin.) RANK-ligand is expressed by osteoblastic/stromal cells, reacts with RANK, which is localized in haematopoietic osteoclast precursors, and stimulates the formation of osteoclasts. These two factors together with M-CSF are currently thought to be necessary and sufficient for osteoclastogenesis. Bone resorbing factors upregulate the expression of RANK-ligand and thereby of osteoclastogenesis. On the other hand, OPG is a soluble receptor which counteracts the biological effects of RANK-ligand preventing its binding to RANK and thereby suppressing bone resorption.

Pathology

Paget's disease of bone is a focal disorder of bone remodelling characterized by an increase in the number and size of osteoclasts in affected sites while the rest of the skeleton remains normal. The typically large osteoclasts, that may contain up to 100 nuclei per cell, induce excessive bone resorption which is associated with an increased recruitment of osteoblasts to the remodelling sites resulting in increased bone formation and, hence, an overall increase in the rate of bone turnover. The increase in bone formation is thought to be secondary to the increased rate of bone resorption due to the coupling of the two processes. Some recent evidence, however, suggests that osteoblastic/stromal cells may also be primarily affected in Paget's disease (Gehron-Robey and Bianco 1999). The accelerated rate of bone turnover is responsible for the deposition of bone with disorganized architecture and structural weakness. The bone packets lose their lamellar structure and are replaced by woven bone with a characteristic mosaic pattern while bone marrow is infiltrated by fibrous tissue and blood vessels.

Cell biology

In clinical studies the likelihood of a bone being affected by Paget's disease was related to the amount of bone marrow present in that bone leading to the postulation that the development of bone lesions may be related to specific properties of Pagetic bone marrow (Harinck et al. 1986). In bone marrow cultures from patients with Paget's disease the rate of formation of osteoclasts and their number is markedly increased suggesting that intrinsic abnormalities of the bone marrow microenvironment and/or of osteoclast precursors may contribute to the upregulation of osteoclastogenesis (Kukita et al. 1990; Reddy et al. 1999). A number of studies supported these notions and documented two major abnormalities (Fig. 1). First, Pagetic osteoclasts and their precursors express high levels of osteotropic factors such as, for example, IL-6 a bone resorbing cytokine which has been proposed as a possible paracrine/autocrine factor contributing to the pathogenesis of the disease (Roodman et al. 1992; Hoyland et al. 1994). In addition, enhanced expression of RANK-ligand was detected in bone marrow stromal cells from patients with Paget's disease and may contribute to the increased number of osteoclasts (Menaa et al. 2000b; Ross 2000). Second, compared to controls, bone marrow and peripheral cells from patients are hypersensitive to the action of calcitriol, the active metabolite of vitamin D (Menaa et al. 2000a; Neale et al. 2000). Thus, while the cellular and molecular basis of the disease is being currently understood, the precice mechanism(s) that trigger these changes remain to be elucidated.

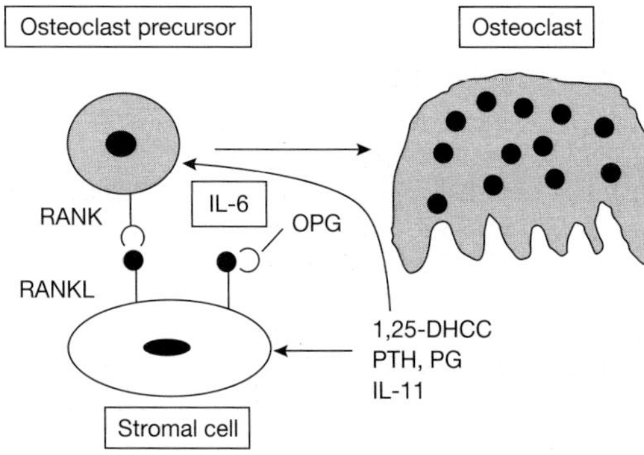

Fig. 1 Schematic presentation of the changes in the bone/bone marrow microenvironment that lead to upregulation of osteoclastogenesis in Paget's disease (see text for details).

Aetiology

Several, not mutually exclusive, hypotheses have been proposed to explain the pathology of the disease, the most relevant being the viral and the genetic. Studies of the distribution of bone lesions in patients with Paget's disease showed that the probability of a bone being affected is very similar to the probability of a bone being affected with haematogenous osteomyelitis suggesting that the disease may be caused by a circulating infectious agent (Harinck et al. 1986). An infection by a slow virus of the paramyxovirus family (measles virus, respiratory syncytial virus, canine distemper virus) was supported by the detection of nuclear and cytoplasmic inclusions resembling paramyxoviral nucleocapsids in osteoclasts and of measles virus nucleocapsid transcripts in bone marrow and peripheral blood monocytes from patients with the disease (Singer 1999). However, paramyxoviral-like structures were also found in specimens from patients with other bone diseases such as familial expansile osteolysis, giant cell tumour of bone, pycnodystostosis, osteopetrosis, and osteosclerosis questioning the specificity of this finding. In addition, further search for viral mRNA sequences with various techniques provided conflicting results and up until now no virus has been isolated from Pagetic bone, a full length viral gene has not been cloned from such material and no suitable animal model of the disease is available. Recently, however, Reddy et al. (2001) reported that measles viral infection of osteoclast precursors of transgenic mice resulted in the formation of osteoclasts that had many features of Pagetic osteoclasts. The potential role of paramyxoviruses as causative agents of Paget's disease remains, therefore, currently open.

In familial aggregation studies in the United States of America the risk of first degree relatives of patients with Paget's disease to develop the disorder was seven times greater than the risk of individuals without such relatives (Siris et al. 1991). This is very similar to our estimate of risk in a Dutch population using the same methodological approach as the American study. Furthermore, a positive family history has been reported in up to 25 per cent of patients and a small but detailed study from Spain revealed that 40 per cent of 35 patients with Paget's disease had at least one affected first degree relative (Morales-Piga et al. 1995). Familial Paget's disease is inherited as an autosomal dominant trait and genetic analysis showed evidence of linkage to chromosome 18q21-22 in some families (Haslam et al. 1998; Hocking et al. 2000). This chromosome contains also the locus of the rare disease familial expansile osteolysis (FEO) which resembles Paget's disease and was found to be associated with activating mutations in the gene encoding RANK (Hughes et al. 2000). This mutation was also found in affected members of a rather unrepresentative family with Paget's disease. Subsequent studies, however, in patients with familial as well as sporadic Paget's disease failed to detect such mutations. Furthermore, analysis of many other families identified possible loci in other chromosomes such as 19, 6, 5, and 1 indicating genetic heterogeneity (Hocking et al. 2000; Laurin et al. 2001). A preliminary report from a genome-wide search for Paget's disease in 327 individuals from 65 kindreds with familial disease identified several candidate loci and confirmed the genetic heterogeneity of the disease (Hocking et al. 2001). It should be also noted that in the region of chromosome 18 which harbours the locus of Paget's disease in some at least families, there is also the putative locus of an osteosarcoma tumour-suppressor gene, a rare malignant tumour, which is the most serious complication of Paget's disease (Nellissery et al. 1998). Available data favour, thus, the hypothesis of the involvement of genetic factors in the pathogenesis of the disease. Identification of such factors will not only help understand the pathogenesis of Paget's disease but may also provide new insights into the modulation of osteoclast formation and function.

Clinical manifestations

The most commonly affected bones are the pelvis (in about two-thirds of patients), the spine, the femora, and the skull but practically any bone of the skeleton may be affected and there is remarkable similarity in the frequency of affected bones in large series of patients from different countries (Meunier et al. 1987; Papapoulos 1997; Kanis 1998). About one-third of patients have only one lesion but the frequency of single lesions varies among series reflecting probably referral patterns and is higher in asymptomatic patients. The anatomical spread of the disease is not related to age or gender, shows no particular symmetry in the body and remains largely unchanged throughout life. The disease progresses slowly within the affected bone but does not generally appear in other bones. Patients with limited bone involvement should, therefore, be reassured that the disease will not progress to other bones with time.

The majority of patients are asymptomatic and the disease may be diagnosed incidentally during investigation of an unrelated complaint by skeletal radiographs or by the finding of an unexplained elevation of serum alkaline phosphatase activity. About 5–10 per cent of affected patients have symptoms. Skeletal morbidity in Paget's disease is determined by the damage caused and the progression of the disease in affected sites as well as by the number and the localization of the lesions. Extensive disease, as originally described by Sir James Paget, occurs in about 5 per cent of symptomatic patients. This is in agreement with the limited chance of an individual to develop extensive disease, as predicted by the distribution of lesions, but changing patterns of the disease to milder forms may also contribute to that.

The symptoms and complications of Paget's disease, summarized in Table 1, can have a great impact on the quality of life of affected individuals (Gold et al. 1996). In the majority of patients the presenting complaint is pain. This is related to the extent and site of the disease, it is usually persistent and present at rest, but is not specific. Pain due to secondary osteoarthritis is common and may hamper assessment of the relative contribution of bone and joint pains to the patient's disability. The origin of such pain can be assessed only retrospectively after treatment which reduces mainly the disease-related pain having a rather limited effect on the arthritic pain. Deformities are present in about 15 per cent of patients at the time of diagnosis and affect mainly weight bearing bones, the most common deformity being bowing of the lower limbs. About 9 per cent of patients present with fractures that can be complete or fissure (incomplete) fractures (Fig. 2). The latter occur more frequently, can be multiple, can cause pain and may develop to complete fractures. Fractures heal generally well although in an older, large series of 182 fractures of the femur the incidence of non-union was 40 per cent (Dove 1980). The skin overlying an affected bone may be warm as a result of increased blood flow and bone turnover locally and hypervascularity of affected bones may cause ischaemia of adjacent structures (steal syndrome). Irreversible hearing loss is the most common neurological complication occurring in about one-third of patients with skull involvement. This is currently thought to be related to structural and/or density changes in the cochlear capsule bone (Monsell et al. 1999). Malignant transformation of Pagetic bone and development of osteosarcoma is a rare (<1 per cent) but extremely serious complication.

Table 1 Symptoms and complications of Paget's disease of bone (from Lyles 2001)

System	Complication
Musculoskeletal	Bone pain Bone deformity Osteoarthritis of adjacent joints Acetabular protrusion Fractures Spinal stenosis
Neurological	Hearing loss Cranial nerve deficits (rare) Basilar impression Increased CSF pressure Spinal stenosis Vascular steal syndrome
Cardiovascular	Congestive heart failure and angina Increased cardiac output Aortic stenosis Generalized atherosclerosis Endocardial calcification
Metabolic	Immobilization hypercalcaemia Hypercalciuria Hyperuricaemia Nephrolithiasis
Neoplasia	Sarcoma (osteosarcoma, chondrosarcoma, and fibrosarcoma) Giant cell tumour

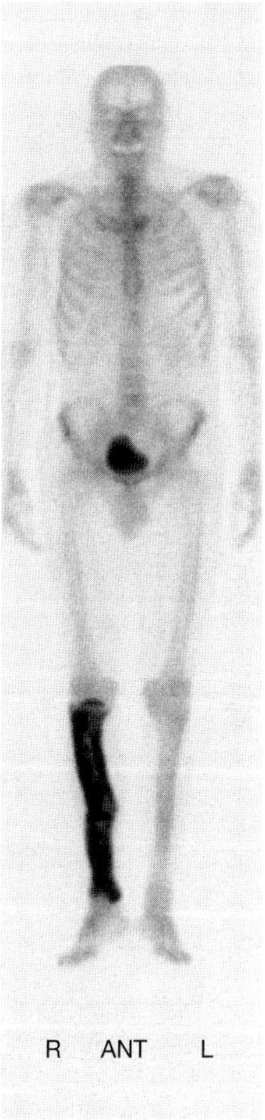

Fig. 2 Bone scan of a 53-year-old man with Paget's disease of the tibia illustrating the deformity and a fracture.

Investigations

Radiographic changes are characteristic of the disease. Increased bone resorption may be detected as a decrease in the density of affected bones; sometimes a wedge- or flame-segment of bone resorption may be seen in long bones and extensive osteolytic areas in the skull (osteoporosis circumscripta). The osteolytic changes in long bones progress at a rate of about 1 cm/year. Older lesions usually have a mixed sclerotic and lytic appearance and in the last stage of the disease sclerotic lesions predominate (Fig. 3). The involved parts of the skeleton are enlarged and deformed and the cortex can be thickened and dense. The radiological changes can be considered pathognomonic but in some cases differential diagnosis may include fibrous dysplasia and bone metastases, particularly from prostate cancer. Bone scintigraphy is used to assess the extent of the disease. It is not specific but it is more sensitive than plain radiographs; upto 15 per cent of lesions detected by bone scintigraphy may have normal radiographic appearance. Bone scintigraphy should always be included in the investigation of patients with Paget's disease and plain radiographs of the areas of increased radioisotope uptake should be subsequently made to confirm the diagnosis.

The pathology of Paget's disease is reflected in the proportional increase in biochemical indices of bone turnover (Alvarez et al. 1997). Classically urinary hydroxyproline excretion is used as an index of bone resorption and serum total alkaline phosphatase activity as an index of bone formation. These can be markedly increased in patients with extensive disease but can be also found within the reference range in patients with limited bone involvement. Patients with skull disease tend to have the highest values of serum alkaline phosphatase activity. More specific and sensitive biochemical indices of bone formation include the bone-specific isoenzyme of alkaline phosphatase and the aminoterminal extention peptide of collagen type I (procollagen I *N*-terminal peptide or PINP). Serum osteocalcin concentrations are within the normal range in about half of the patients with elevated serum alkaline phosphatase values and should not be used in the management of patients with Paget's disease. Urinary hydroxyproline is neither specific nor sensitive enough and its determination depends on specific dietary advice. Of the newer biochemical indices of bone resorption, deoxypyridinoline and peptides of the cross-linking domains of collagen type I, such as the *N*-telopeptide (NTX) or the *C*-telopeptide (CTX), measured in urine or serum are the most sensitive. Impaired isomerization of CTX has been reported in patients with Paget's disease but not in patients with increased bone turnover from other causes, that led to the postulation that this abnormality may reflect the defect in bone structure (Garnero et al. 1997). Degradation products of collagen type II are not increased in urines of patients (Christgau et al. 2001).

In Paget's disease despite the marked changes in the rate of bone and calcium turnover, extracellular calcium homeostasis is generally maintained but some disturbances may occur. Hypercalcaemia may develop in immobilized patients with active, extensive disease or may be due to concurrent primary hyperparathyroidism, the incidence of which is thought to be higher in Paget's disease compared to the general population. Secondary hyperparathyroidism is present in about 20 per cent of patients while serum concentrations of calcitriol are generally normal. Hypercalciuria and renal stone disease occur also more frequently in patients with Paget's disease.

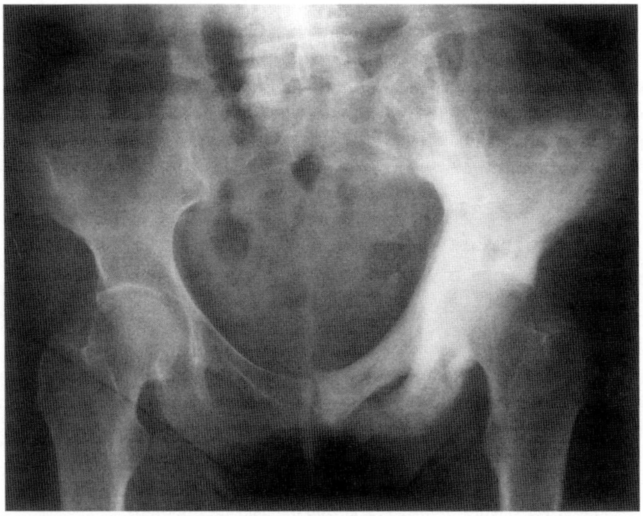

Fig. 3 Radiograph of the pelvis of a 75-year-old woman with Paget's disease with typical changes and destruction of the left hip joint.

Management

During the past 30 years the management of patients with Paget's disease has changed dramatically due to the discovery of the therapeutic potential of the calcitonins and later of the bisphosphonates. Other less frequently used treatments are plicamycin (mithramycin) and gallium nitrate. Bisphosphonates are the preferred treatment of Paget's disease.

Aims and indications of treatment

Classically treatment is given to patients with Paget's disease to relieve symptoms and improve their quality of life. The disease, however, is progressive and patients with symptoms were previously asymptomatic (Fig. 4).

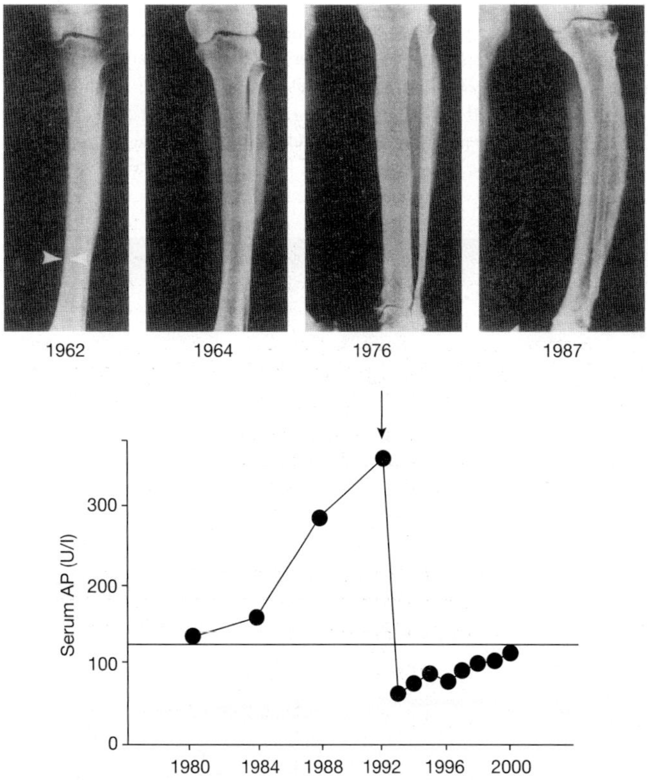

Fig. 4 (Upper panel) Serial radiographs (anteroposterior view) of the tibia of an untreated 68-year-old man with Paget's disease illustrating the progression of the disease (from Siris and Feldman 1997, with permission).
(Lower panel) Sequential measurements of serum alkaline phosphatase (AP) activity over 20 years in a 51-year-old woman with Paget's disease of the pelvis. Note the progressive 3-fold increase in serum AP activity on no treatment. Arrow indicates treatment with oral olpadronate 200 mg/day for 1 month inducing complete, long-lasting remission. Horizontal line represents the upper limit of the normal range.

It is currently impossible to identify patients who will develop symptoms and complications and no way to quantify the risk of complications in an individual. Treatment with potent bisphosphonates does not only relieve symptoms but restores also bone quality and improves or even normalizes radiological appearances (Fig. 5). Moreover, the bulk of evidence obtained with bisphosphonates strongly suggests that complications can be prevented if bone turnover is adequately suppressed whereas there are indications that the contrary is true if bone turnover does not normalize (Meunier and Vignot 1995). Firm evidence, however, from prospective randomized controlled trials is lacking. The following treatment indications are currently recommended: (i) symptomatic disease, (ii) preoperative treatment in preparation for an orthopaedic procedure on Pagetic bone to reduce the increased blood flow and excessive bleeding, (iii) treatment of asymptomatic patients with skeletal localizations at higher risk of future complications such as localizations adjucent to large joints, in the skull, the spine and the weight bearing bones, (iv) young patients (Papapoulos 1997; Christgau et al. 2001; Lyles et al. 2001). The goal of treatment should be to normalize bone turnover, suppress serum alkaline phosphatase activity well within the normal range, and keep it adequately suppressed, if necessary with additional courses of treatment. Retreatment is generally advocated when a previously normal value of serum alkaline activity exceeds the upper limit of normal or when it increases by 20–25 per cent above its nadir value.

Bisphosphonates

Pharmacology

The following properties render bisphosphonates as ideal agents for the treatment of Paget's disease: Selective uptake at active skeletal sites; specific inhibition of bone resorption; short plasma half-life and lack of circulating metabolites; persistence of the effect after stopping treatment. The general structure of the molecule of geminal bisphosphonates allows numerous substitutions that led to the synthesis of a variety of compounds with considerable differences in potency, activity to toxicity ratio and mechanism of action (Fleisch 1998; Russell et al. 1999). Bisphosphonates are divided into two groups according to the presence or not of a nitrogen function in the bioactive moeity of their molecule. The nitrogen increases the potency of the bisphosphonates and determines their mechanism of action. Compounds without a nitrogen function in the side chain are etidronate, clodronate, and tiludronate. Nitrogen-containing bisphosphonates include alendronate, ibandronate, incandronate, neridronate, olpadronate, pamidronate, risedronate, and zolendronate. Practically every bisphosphonate either approved or in clinical development has been used in the treatment of Paget's disease that in turn has served as a human model for investigating the pharmacological properties of these agents (Papapoulos et al. 1989). The bisphosphonates approved around the world for the treatment of the disease are listed in Table 2.

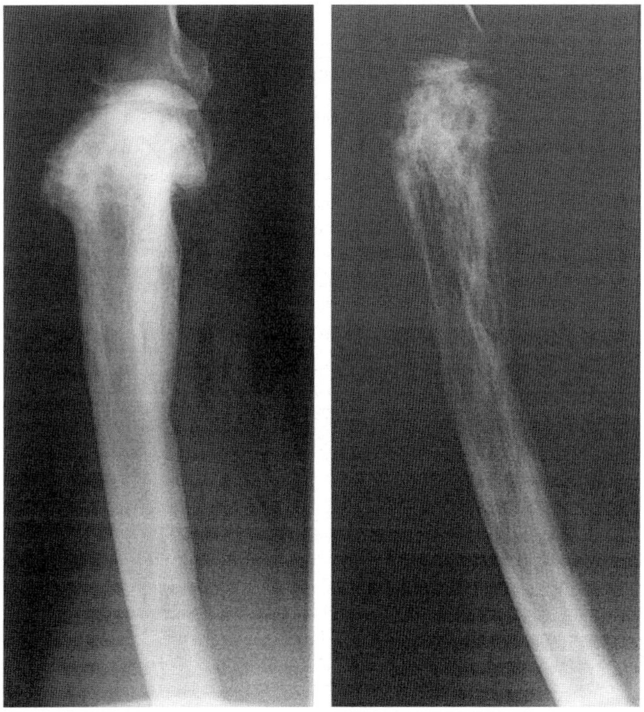

Fig. 5 Radiographs of the distal femur of a 46-year-old man with extensive Paget's disease before (left) and 1 year after (right) treatment with oral olpadronate.

Non-nitrogen containing bisphosphonates inhibit bone resorption by inhibiting osteoclast activity through the intracellular formation of ATP metabolites which are toxic for the cell. Nitrogen-containing bisphosphonates concentrate primarily at sites of increased bone resorption, are released from bone by the decrease in local pH which occurs under the osteoclasts during resorption, are taken up by the osteoclasts, and induce changes in their cytoskeleton, such as loss of the ruffled border. As a result, osteoclasts become inactive and undergo apoptosis. Recent evidence indicated that this action is due to inhibition of farnesyl pyrophosphate synthase, an enzyme of the metabolic pathway of mevalonic acid (Van Beek et al. 1999b; Bergstrom et al. 2000; Fisher et al. 2000). This leads to inhibition of the synthesis of the isoprenoid geranylgeranyl pyrophosphate, which is responsible for the prenylation of small GTP-binding proteins like Ras, Rho, and Rac which are essential for cytoskeletal integrity and intracellular signalling (Fisher et al. 1999; Van Beek et al. 1999a; Coxon et al. 2000). The possible significance of these well documented differences in the mechanism of action of bisphosphonates for their *in vivo* action is currently unknown.

Pharmacodynamics

For the design of optimal therapeutic strategies with bisphosphonates their pharmacodynamic properties need to be considered (Papapoulos 1995). First, when a potent bisphosphonate is given to a patient with Paget's disease, the first measurable effect is the suppression of bone resorption. This occurs within a few days of starting treatment. During this initial period bone formation does not change. This will decrease secondarily, at a slower rate, due to the coupling of bone resorption to bone formation so that a new equilibrium will be reached after 3–6 months (Fig. 6). Thus, adequate suppression of bone resorption will be predictably followed by an adequate suppression of bone formation. Suppression of biochemical indices of bone resorption early during the course of treatment provides, therefore, an indication of the pharmacological efficacy of the bisphosphonate and can subsequently determine the length of treatment (Papapoulos and Frölich 1996). Because of the predictable changes in bone remodelling that follow bisphosphonate therapy in Paget's disease, it is not necessary to prolong treatment until the lowest level of serum alkaline phosphatase is reached and short courses may be sufficient to achieve remissions. Second, the

Table 2 Bisphosphonates approved for the treatment of Paget's disease

Generic name	Dose
Alendronate	Oral, 40 mg daily for 6 months
Clodronate	Oral, 1600 mg daily for 3–6 months
Etidronate	Oral, 400 mg daily for 6 months
Pamidronate	Intravenous, 30–60 mg daily for 3 days[a]
Risedronate	Oral, 30 mg daily for 2 months
Tiludronate	Oral, 400 mg daily for 3 months

[a] Lower dose recommended by the pharmaceutical industry, higher dose recommended by investigators.

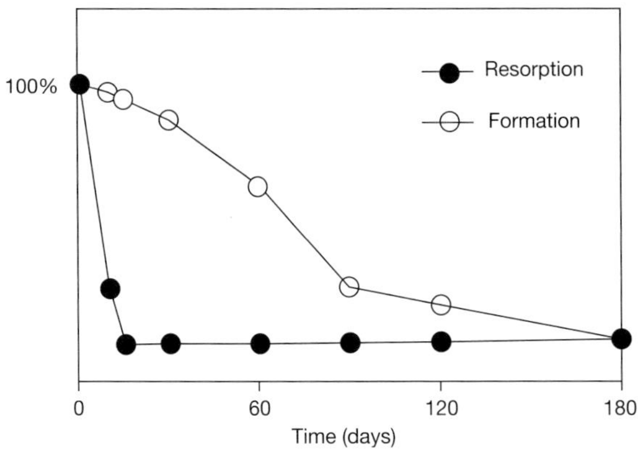

Fig. 6 Schematic presentation of the changes in biochemical indices of bone resorption and bone formation following bisphosphonate treatment of Paget's disease.

concentration of bisphosphonate presented to the bone surface rather than the total dose of the drug is more important for the suppression of the increased rate of bone turnover. Therefore, in Paget's disease bisphosphonate doses should be much higher than those used in the treatment of patients with osteoporosis. Third, the retention of bisphosphonate in the skeleton is proportional to disease activity and inversely proportional to renal function. Therefore, dose adjustments may be required in patients with impaired renal function but no specific studies have addressed this issue. These pharmacodynamic principles and the wide variation of disease activity strongly suggest that treatment needs to be individualized.

The long-term efficacy of treatment is best assessed by measuring biochemical indices of bone formation, serum alkaline phosphatase activity being the most commonly used. In the past, the efficacy of treatment was evaluated by its ability to decrease serum alkaline phosphatase activity by more than 50 per cent of its initial value. With the available potent bisphosphonates, this is not any more appropriate and treatment efficacy should be assessed by its ability to suppress serum alkaline phosphatase values to the normal range (remission). In clinical practice there is no need to measure serum alkaline phosphatase activity earlier than 3 months after the start of treatment, 6 months being the optimal time.

During the initial phase of bisphosphonate treatment, when bone resorption and bone formation are still dissociated, the increased retention of calcium in the skeleton leads to changes in calcium metabolism. There is a fall in serum calcium concentration that stimulates the secretion of parathyroid hormone secretion and consequently the renal production of calcitriol. These hormones, in turn, increase the renal tubular reabsorption of calcium (parathyroid hormone) and its intestinal absorption (calcitriol). The result is a marked, but transient, increase in calcium balance. The concomitant decrease in serum phosphate concentrations is due to the renal action of parathyroid hormone. Such responses are not observed during etidronate treatment that has a weak action on bone metabolism. With the attainment of the new equilibrium of bone remodelling, calcium balance returns towards pretreatment levels and the values of the biochemical indices of calcium metabolism normalize. The adaptive changes of calcium metabolism to the marked alterations in bone remodelling, prevent the development of symptomatic hypocalcaemia in calcium-replete patients. However, elderly patients have frequently calcium-deficient diets and some investigators advocate the use of calcium supplements during treatment of Paget's disease with potent bisphosphonates, especially if these are given intravenously or the disease is very active (Delmas and Meunier 1997; Lyles et al. 2001). Support for this logical assumption by clinical trials is, however, limited.

Treatment responses

Clinical responses to treatment include the disappearance or clear improvement of pain in more than 80 per cent of treated patients, when this is due to the activity of the disease. A decrease in bone pain is generally observed 1–3 months after the start of treatment and the effect is maximal after 6 months and is maintained for as long as biochemical indices of bone turnover remain within the normal range. Soon after the start of therapy with a potent bisphosphonate, particularly if given intravenously, there may be a transient increase in pain at affected sites and patients should be reassured. Pain due to osteoarthritis is unresponsive to treatment in about 75 per cent of patients; NSAIDs can then be used. If the hip joint is affected, hip arthroplasty may be required to control the symptoms. Back pain resulting from involvement of lumbar vertebrae is frequently not relieved by treatment. About half of the patients with pain associated with deformity of the femur or the tibia will respond favourably to bisphosphonate therapy but pain may persist and a corrective osteotomy may be necessary. Deafness is usually not affected but its progression is arrested. There have been also reports of improvement of spinal cord compression with bisphosphonate therapy. Fracture frequency appears to decrease with treatment but data from prospective controlled studies are not available.

Improvement in bone histology and formation of bone with normal lamellar structure and no evidence of a mineralization defect has been reported with alendronate, clodronate, pamidronate, risedronate, and tiludronate. These findings indicate improvement in bone quality. Radiologically, an arrest of the progression of the disease is usually seen. Radiological improvement can be, however, dramatic if lesions are lytic and are localized in long bones or in the skull. In other areas improvement is slow and sometimes difficult to demonstrate by non-experienced radiologists. Treatment induces an exponential decrease in isotope uptake on bone scans. However, even with normalization of disease activity, only about 10–30 per cent of lesions normalize completely and residual uptake (up to 20 per cent of the original) is detected (Vellenga 1995). It has been suggested that the residual uptake is caused by persistent structural abnormality of the lesion rather than by locally increased metabolic activity. The possible relation of these scintigraphic changes to future recurrences has not been adequately studied but some investigators advocate normalization of bone scans as one of the aims of treatment.

These clinical, histological, and radiological observations emphasize the need for an intervention with a bisphosphonate early in the course of the disease and before the development of complications.

All bisphosphonates given to patients with Paget's disease significantly decrease biochemical indices of bone turnover (Fig. 7). Considerable differences exist, however, in their ability to induce remissions. Generally, potent bisphosphonates induce better responses (Harinck et al. 1987; Schweitzer et al. 1993; Roux et al. 1995; Reid et al. 1996; Siris et al. 1996, 1998; Chakravarty and Crisp 1998; Miller et al. 1999; Brown et al. 2000). Head to head clinical trials have been performed only with etidronate 400 mg daily for 6 months as comparator. In all these clinical trials, etidronate was less effective. The limited efficacy, relative to other bisphosphonates, together with the increased risk of osteomalacia, have made etidronate a treatment of the past. Normalization of serum alkaline phosphatase activity has been reported with tiludronate 400 mg daily for 3 months (35 per cent), clodronate 1600 mg daily for 6 months (up to 70 per cent), alendronate 40 mg daily for 6 months (63 per cent), risedronate 30 mg daily for 2 months (up to 70 per cent), and pamidronate, intravenously or orally in variable regimens (up to 90 per cent). It should be noted that comparison of results obtained in different studies is not appropriate due to different selection criteria and disease activity of treated patients. The results of these studies show in addition that despite the availability of effective and convenient treatment regimens with bisphosphonates, there is still need for further improvement.

Follow-up of patients in remission is indicated every 6–12 months. Remissions, estimated from the time of normalization of serum alkaline phosphatase activity, can be long, for example, 27 months in 50 per cent of patients treated with olpadronate (Schweitzer et al. 1993). Remissions can last longer than 10 years and may then be considered cure of the disease. We have observed, however, recurrences occurring 12 or 13 years after induction of complete biochemical remission which illustrates the need for continuous follow-up. The duration of remission is determined by the degree

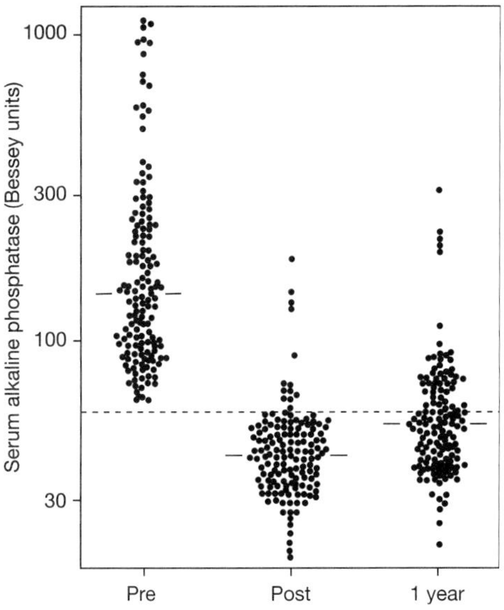

Fig. 7 Serum alkaline phosphatase activity (logarithmic scale) of patients with Paget's disease treated with various regimens of oral or intravenous pamidronate (from Harinck et al. 1987, with permission). Pre, before treatment; Post, at the end of treatment; 1 year, 1 year later without any treatment. Interrupted line represents the upper limit of the normal range.

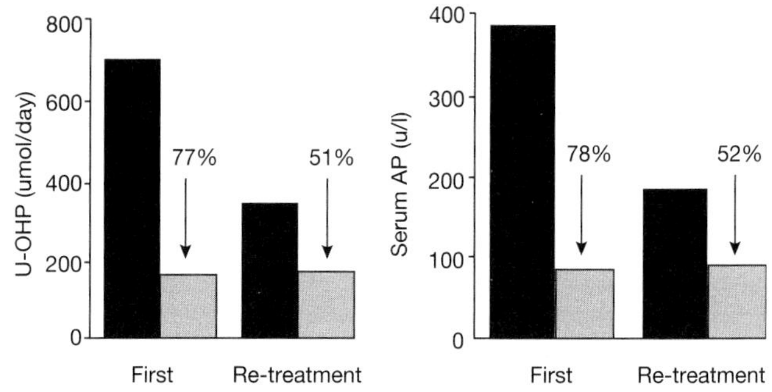

Fig. 8 Apparent resistance to bisphosphonate therapy in Paget's disease. Absolute and per cent changes of urinary hydroxyproline excretion (U-OHP) and serum alkaline phosphatase (AP) activity after first treatment with pamidronate or re-treatment with the same bisphosphonate for a recurrence of the disease (modified from Harinck et al. 1987).

of suppression of serum alkaline phosphatase activity and is not related to the length or to the mode of treatment (oral or intravenous) as long as a potent, efficacious bisphosphonate is given (Harinck et al. 1987; Schweitzer et al. 1993). The lower the serum alkaline phosphatase activity reached with treatment, the longer the period of remission. Suppression of serum alkaline phosphatase activity well within the normal range is a prerequisite for long-term remissions and should be part of treatment strategies.

Resistance to bisphosphonate treatment

Development of resistance to repeated courses of bisphosphonate therapy has been reported for etidronate and more recently for pamidronate (Cutteridge et al. 1999) but the underlying mechanism is not known and it is important to differentiate between real and apparent resistance. Some patients may not respond to oral bisphosphonate but may show a prompt response to the same compound given intravenously (Papapoulos 1997). In such cases factors interfering with the already low intestinal absorption of the drug are most likely responsible for the impaired response to oral treatment. Patients retreated with the same bisphosphonate during a recurrence of their disease can show a reduced fractional decrease in biochemical indices of bone turnover compared to earlier treatments. Some consider this response compatible with development of resistance to therapy. This is, however, wrong because the actual level, rather than the fractional decrease of biochemical indices of bone turnover following every treatment should be compared to those obtained after the initial therapy (Fig. 8). Finally, in patients with concurrent hyperparathyroidism completeness of response is generally less and recurrences occur quicker which might be considered reduced responsiveness. In our studies the probability of remission and recurrence-free periods did not differ between patients treated for the first time and those retreated with a nitrogen-containing bisphosphonate (mostly pamidronate or olpadronate).

Adverse effects

All bisphosphonates, given at very high doses can impair the mineralization of newly formed bone and induce osteomalacia. In clinical practice this is, however, relevant only for etidronate. Doses of potent nitrogen-containing bisphosphonates required to induce osteomalacia exceed by many orders of magnitude those required for effective suppression of bone turnover. Consequently in all reported controlled studies no adverse effects on bone mineralization have been observed. Only in a few patients treated with intravenous pamidronate at doses higher than those recommended, impaired mineralization has been reported. Histological osteomalacia induced by either etidronate or pamidronate is reversible.

In some patients treated for the first time with nitrogen-containing bisphosphonates there is a rise in body temperature and flu-like symptoms during the first 3 days of treatment. These symptoms are transient and subside with no specific measures even when treatment is continued (Adami and Zamberlan 1996). This response is dose-dependent, is associated more frequently with intravenous treatment and does not occur in patients receiving lower oral doses of the bisphosphonates, such as in osteoporosis. Moreover, it does not reccur upon re-treatment, though there are some reports of recurrence during subsequent treatment with i.v. pamidronate but the response is then of lower intensity. Previous exposure to another nitrogen-containing bisphosphonate, but not to etidronate, precludes the development of an acute phase reaction. Laboratory findings are consistent with an acute phase reaction (Schweitzer et al. 1995). There is a transient decrease in blood lymphocytes and a transient increase in serum C-reactive protein possibly due to increases in proinflammatory cytokines, such as IL-6 and TNF-α. Rarely, high doses of nitrogen-containing bisphosphonates may induce opthalmic reactions such as conjunctivitis, iritis or uveitis. There are single reports of ototoxicity and central nervous toxicity after intravenous pamidronate. Allergic skin reactions have been occasionally observed with most of the bisphosphonates.

Mild gastrointestinal complaints occur with low frequency with the use of all bisphosphonates. Some nitrogen-containing bisphosphonates can induce more severe symptoms such as heartburn, nausea, and vomiting in a few patients associated with oesophagitis or gastritis (Adami and Zamberlan 1996). The use of oral alendronate 40 mg daily was associated with higher frequency of epigastric complaints in an open but not in a controlled study and the latter was also the case with oral risedronate 30 mg daily. In a comparative study of alendronate 40 mg/day and risedronate 30 mg/day gastric ulcers and/or large numbers of gastric erosions were detected endoscopically in approximately 3 per cent of patients and their occurrence was comparable with both bisphosphonates (Lanza et al. 2000). The mechanism underlying GI toxicity is not known but evidence from an *in vitro* model of epithelial oesophageal cells indicated that alendronate and risedronate inhibit the same enzymes of the mevalonic acid pathway as in osteoclasts. Nitrogen-containing bisphosphonates should be administered orally with one full glass of water and the patient should remain in an upright position for one half hour to allow quick passage through the oesophagus and to avoid oesophageal irritation. Rapid intravenous injection of bisphosphonates may chelate calcium in the circulation and form complexes which can be nephrotoxic. Bisphosphonates should, therefore, be given by slow infusion. New very potent bisphosphonates such as ibandronate or zolendronate may be given by intravenous injections because of their very low effective doses. More data are needed, however, to show whether doses that can safely be given by intravenous injection can also effectively suppress bone turnover in Paget's disease. Clodronate has been given intramuscularly. Aminobisphosphonates should not be injected intramuscularly because they can cause severe local irritation and necrosis.

References

Adami, S. and Zamberlan, N. (1996). Adverse effects of bisphosphonates. *Drug Safety* **14**, 158–70.

Altman, R.D., Bloch, D.A., Hochberg, M.C., and Murphy, W.A. (2000). Prevalence of pelvic Paget's disease of bone in the United States. *Journal of Bone and Mineral Research* **15**, 461–5.

Alvarez, L. et al. (1997). Relationship between biochemical markers of bone turnover and bone scintigraphy indices in assessment of Paget's disease activity. *Arthritis and Rheumatism* **40**, 461–8.

Barker, D.J.P., Clough, P.W.L., Guyer, P.B., and Gardner, M.J. (1977). Paget's disease of bone in 14 British towns. *British Medical Journal* **1**, 1181–3.

Bergstrom, J.D., Bostedor, R.G., Masarachia, P.J., Reszka, A.A., and Rodan, G. (2000). Alendronate is a specific, nanomolar inhibitor of farnesyl diphosphate synthase. *Archives in Biochemistry and Biophysics* **373**, 231–41.

Brown, J.P., Chines, A.A., Myers, W.R., Eusebio, R.A., Ritter-Hrncirik, C., and Hays, C.W. (2000). Improvement of pagetic bone lesions with risedronate treatment: a radiologic study. *Bone* **26**, 263–7.

Chakravarty, K. and Crisp, A. (1998). Pamidronate disodium in Paget's disease of bone. *Review of Contemporary Pharmacotherapy* **9**, 165–81.

Christgau, S. et al. (2001). Collagen type II C-telopeptide fragments as an index of cartilage degradation. *Bone* **29**, 209–15.

Cooper, C., Schafheutle, K., Dennison, E., Kellingray, S., Guyer, P., and Barker, D. (1999). The epidemiology of Paget's disease in Britain: is the prevalence decreasing? *Journal of Bone and Mineral Research* **14**, 192–7.

Coxon, F.P. et al. (2000). Protein geranylation is required for osteoclast formation, function and survival: inhibition by bisphosphonates and GGTI-298. *Journal of Bone and Mineral Research* **15**, 1467–76.

Cundy, T., McAnulty, K., Wattie, D., Gamble, G., Rutland, M., and Ibbertson, H.K. (1997). Evidence for secular change in Paget's disease of bone. *Bone* **20**, 69–71.

Cutteridge, D.H. et al. (1999). Paget's disease: acquired resistance to one aminobisphosphonate with retained response to another. *Journal of Bone and Mineral Research* **14** (Suppl. 2), 79–84.

Delmas, P.D. and Meunier, P.J. (1997). The management of Paget's disease of bone. *New England Journal of Medicine* **336**, 558–66.

Dove, J. (1980). Complete fractures of the femur in Paget's disease of bone. *Journal of Bone and Joint Surgery (British)* **62-B**, 12–7.

Fisher, J.E. et al. (1999). Alendronate mechanism of action: geranylgeraniol, an intermediate in the mevalonate pathway, prevents inhibition of osteoclast formation, bone resorption and kinase activation *in vitro*. *Proceedings of the National Academy of Science (USA)* **96**, 133–8.

Fisher, J.E., Rodan, G.A., and Reszka, A.A. (2000). *In vivo* effects of bisphosphonates on the osteoclasts mevalonate pathway. *Endocrinology* **141**, 4793–6.

Fleisch, H. (1998). Bisphosphonates: mechanisms of action. *Endocrine Reviews* **19**, 80–100.

Garnero, P., Fledelius, C., Gineyts, E., Serre, C.M., Vignot, E., and Delmas, P.D. (1997). Decreased β-isomerization of C-telopeptides of $\alpha 1$ chain of type I collagen in Paget's disease of bone. *Journal of Bone and Mineral Research* **12**, 1407–15.

Gehron-Robey, P. and Bianco, P. (1999). The role of osteogenic cells in the pathophysiology of Paget's disease. *Journal of Bone Mineral Research* **14** (Suppl. 2), 9–16.

Gold, D.T., Boisture, J., Shipp, K.M., Pieper, C.F., and Lyles, K.W. (1996). Paget's disease of bone and quality of life. *Journal of Bone and Mineral Research* **11**, 1897–904.

Harinck, H.I.J., Bijvoet, O.L.M., Vellenga, C.J.L.R., Blanksma, H.J., and Frijlink, W.B. (1986). Relation between signs and symptoms in Paget's disease of bone. *Quarterly Journal of Medicine* **58**, 133–51.

Harinck, H.I.J., Papapoulos, S.E., Blanksma, H.J., Moolenaar, A.J., Vermeij, P., and Bijvoet, O.L.M. (1987). Paget's disease of bone; early and late responses to three different modes of treatment with aminohydroxypropylidene bisphosphonate. *British Medical Journal* **295**, 1301–5.

Haslam, S.I. et al. (1998). Paget's disease of bone: evidence for a susceptibility locus on chromosome 18q and for genetic heterogeneity. *Journal of Bone and Mineral Research* **13**, 911–17.

Hocking, L., Slee, F., Haslam, S.I., Cundy, T., Nicholson, G., van Hul, W., and Ralston, S.H. (2000). Familial Paget's disease of bone: patterns of inheritance and frequency of linkage to chromosome 18q. *Bone* **26**, 1095–103.

Hocking, L.J. et al. (2001). A genome-wide search in familial Paget's disease of bone. *Bone* **28** (Suppl.), S82.

Hoyland, J.A., Freemont, A.J., and Sharpe, P.T. (1994). Interleukin-6, IL-6 receptor, and IL-6 nuclear factor gene expression in Paget's disease. *Journal of Bone and Mineral Research* **9**, 75–80.

Hughes, A.E. et al. (2000). Mutations in TNFRSF11A, affecting the signal peptide of RANK, cause familial expansile osteolysis. *Nature Genetics* **24**, 45–8.

Kanis, J.A. *Pathophysiology and Treatment of Paget's Disease of Bone* 2nd edn. London: Dunitz, 1998.

Kukita, A., Chenu, C., McManus, L.M., Mundy, G.R., and Roodman, G.D. (1990). Atypical multinucleated cells form in long-term marrow cultures from patients with Paget's disease. *Journal of Clinical Investigation* **85**, 1280–6.

Lanza, F. et al. (2000). Comparison of the effects of alendronate and risedronate on upper gastrointestinal mucosae. *American Journal of Gastroenterology* **95**, 3112–17.

Laurin, N. et al. (2001). Paget's disease of bone: mapping of two loci at 5q35-qter and 5q31. *American Journal of Human Genetics* **69**, 528–43.

Lyles, K.W., Siris, E.S., Singer, F.R., and Meunier, P.J. (2001). A clinical approach to diagnosis and management of Paget's disease of bone. *Journal of Bone and Mineral Research* **16**, 1379–87.

Menaa, C. et al. (2000a). 1,25-dihydroxyvitamin D3 hypersensitivity of osteoclast precursors from patients with Paget's disease. *Journal of Bone and Mineral Research* **15**, 228–34.

Menaa, C. et al. (2000b). Enhanced RANK ligand expression and responsivity of bone marrow cells in Paget's disease of bone. *Journal of Clinical Investigation* **105**, 1833–8.

Meunier, P.J. and Vignot, E. (1995). Therapeutic strategies in Paget's disease of bone. *Bone* **17** (Suppl. 5), 489S–91S.

Meunier, P.J. et al. (1987). Skeletal distribution and biochemical parameters of Paget's disease. *Clinical Orthopaedics* **217**, 37–44.

Miller, P.D., Brown, J.P., Siris, E.S., Hoseyni, M.S., Axelrod, D.W., and Bekker, P.J. (1999). A randomized, double-blind comparison of risedronate and etidronate in the management of Paget's disease of bone. *American Journal of Medicine* **106**, 513–20.

Monsell, E.M., Cody, D.D., Bone, H.G., and Divine, G.W. (1999). Hearing loss as a complication of Paget's disease of bone. *Journal of Bone and Mineral Research* **14** (Suppl. 2), 92–5.

Morales-Piga, A.A., Rey-Rey, J.S., Corres-Gonzales, J., Garcia-Sagredo, J.M., and Lopez-Abente, G. (1995). Frequency and characteristics of familial aggregation of Paget's disease of bone. *Journal of Bone and Mineral Research* **10**, 663–70.

Neale, S.D., Smith, R., Wass, J.A., and Athanasou, N.A. (2000). Osteoclast differentiation from circulating mononuclear precursors in Paget's disease is hypersensitive to 1,25-dihydroxyvitamin D3 and RANKL. *Bone* **27**, 409–16.

Nellissery, M.J. et al. (1998). Evidence for a novel osteosarcoma tumor-suppressor gene in the chromosome 18 region genetically linked with Paget's disease of bone. *American Journal of Human Genetics* **63**, 817–24.

Papapoulos, S.E. (1995). Pharmacodynamics of bisphosphonates in man; implications for treatment. In *Bisphosphonates on Bones* (ed. O.L.M. Bijvoet, H.A. Fleisch, R.E. Canfield, and R.G.G. Russell), pp. 231–63. Amsterdam: Elsevier.

Papapoulos, S.E. (1997). Paget's disease of bone: clinical, pathogenetic and therapeutic aspects. *Baillière's Clinical Endocrinology and Metabolism* **11**, 117–43.

Papapoulos, S.E. and Frölich, M. (1996). Prediction of the outcome of treatment of Paget's disease of bone with bisphosphonates from short-term changes in the rate of bone resorption. *Journal of Clinical Endocrinology and Metabolism* **81**, 3993–7.

Papapoulos, S.E., Hoekman, K., Löwik, C.W.G.M., Vermeij, P., and Bijvoet, O.L.M. (1989). Application of an *in vitro* model and a clinical protocol in the assessment of the potency of a new bisphosphonate. *Journal of Bone and Mineral Research* **4**, 775–81.

Reddy, S.V., Menaa, S., Singer, F.R., Demulder, A., and Roodman, G.D. (1999). Cell biology of Paget's disease. *Journal of Bone and Mineral Research* **14** (Suppl. 2), 3–8.

Reddy, S.V. et al. (2001). Osteoclasts formed by measles virus-infected osteoclast precursors from hCD46 transgenic mice express characteristics of Pagetic osteoclasts. *Endocrinology* **142**, 2898–905.

Reid, I.R. et al. (1996). Biochemical and radiological imrovement in Paget's disease of bone treated with alendronate: a randomized, placebo-controlled trial. *American Journal of Medicine*, 341–7.

Roodman, G.D. et al. (1992). Interleukin-6: a potential autocrine/paracrine factor in Paget's disease of bone. *Journal of Clinical Investigation* **89**, 46–52.

Ross, F.P. (2000). RANKing the importance of measles virus in Paget's disease. *Journal of Clinical Investigation* **105**, 555–8.

Roux, C. et al. (1995). Comparative prospective, double-blind, multicenter study of the efficacy of tiludronate and etidronate in the treatment of Paget's disease of bone. *Arthritis and Rheumatism* **6**, 851–8.

Russell, R.G.G. et al. (1999). The pharmacology of bisphosphonates and new insights into their mechanism of action. *Journal of Bone and Mineral Research* **14** (Suppl. 2), 53–65.

Schweitzer, D.H., Zwinderman, A.H., Vermeij, P., Bijvoet, O.L.M., and Papapoulos, S.E. (1993). Improved treatment of Paget's disease with dimethylaminohydroxypropylidene bisphosphonate. *Journal of Bone and Mineral Research* **8**, 175–82.

Schweitzer, D.H., Oostendorp-van de Ruit, M., van der Pluijm, G., Löwik, C.W.G.M., and Papapoulos, S. (1995). Interleukin-6 and the acute phase reaction during treatment of patients with Paget's disease with the nitrogen-containing bisphosphonate dimethylaminohydroxypro-pylidene bisphosphonate. *Journal of Bone and Mineral Research* **10**, 956–62.

Singer, F.R. (1999). Update on the viral etiology of Paget's disease of bone. *Journal of Bone and Mineral Rresearch* **14** (Suppl. 2), 29–33.

Singer, F.R. and Krane, S.M. (1998). Paget's disease of bone. In *Metabolic Bone Disease and Clinically Related Disorders* 3rd edn. (ed. L.V. Avioli, and S.M. Krane), pp. 545–605. San Diego CA: Academic Press.

Siris, E.S. (1999). Paget's disease of bone. In *Primer on Metabolic Bone Disease and Disorders of Mineral Metabolism* 4th edn. (ed. M.J. Favus), pp. 415–25. Philadelphia PA: Lippincott Williams and Wilkins.

Siris, E.S., Ottman, R., Flaster, E., and Kelsey, J.L. (1991). Familial aggregation of Paget's disease of bone. *Journal of Bone and Mineral Research* **6**, 495–500.

Siris, E. et al. (1996). Comparative study of alendronate versus etidronate for the treatment of Paget's disease of bone. *Journal of Clinical Endocrinology and Metabolism* **81**, 961–7.

Siris, E.S. et al. (1998). Risedronate on the treatment of Paget's disease of bone; an open label, multicenter study. *Journal of Bone and Mineral Research* **13**, 1032–8.

Suda, T., Takahashi, N., Udagawa, N., Jimi, E., Gillespie, M.T., and Martin, T.J. (1999). Modulation of osteoclast differentiation and function by the new members of the tumor necrosis factor receptor and ligand families. *Endocrine Reviews* **20**, 345–57.

Van Beek, E., Löwik, C., van der Pluijm, G., and Papapoulos, S. (1999a). The role of geranylgeranylation on bone resorption and its suppression by bisphosphonates in fetal bone explants; a clue to the mechanism of action of nitrogen-containing bisphosphonates. *Journal of Bone and Mineral Research* **14**, 722–9.

Van Beek, E., Pieterman, E., Cohen, L., Löwik, C., and Papapoulos, S. (1999b). Farnesyl pyrophosphate synthase is the molecular target of nitrogen-containing bisphosphonates. *Biochemical and Biophysical Research Communications* **264**, 108–11.

Vellenga, C.J.L.R. (1995). Quantitative bone scintigraphy in the evaluation of Paget's disease of bone. In *Bisphosphonates on Bones* (ed. O.L.M. Bijvoet, H.A. Fleisch, R.E. Canfield, and R.G.G. Russell), pp. 279–91. Amsterdam: Elsevier.

6.16.3 Miscellaneous disorders of bone, cartilage, and synovium

Peter J. Maddison

In this chapter, a miscellaneous group of disorders affecting components of the joint and periarticular structures is described. They can present a challenge to the clinician in diagnosis and management. There is often a delay in diagnosis causing pain and disability. Frequently, this is due to insufficient clinical suspicion, partly because of the rarity of most of these conditions. Their diagnosis generally depends on recognizing a combination of clinical, laboratory, and histological features, but the advent of techniques such as magnetic resonance imaging (MRI) facilitates earlier diagnosis. This is particularly important for conditions such as osteonecrosis where the institution of treatment at an earlier stage in the course of the process may prevent joint destruction.

Osteoid osteoma

Skeletal neoplasms are discussed in Chapter 1.3.9. Only rarely do they cause problems for the experienced clinician in being mistaken for systemic rheumatic diseases. An exception is hypertrophic osteoarthropathy (Chapter 1.3.9); another is osteoid osteoma. This is a benign osteoid-forming tumour, which can be an elusive cause of bone pain, 'radiculopathy', or 'arthritis' in children and young adults, depending on its site. It is uncommon and accounts for 10–12 per cent of benign bone neoplasms.

The maximum age incidence is in the second and third decades, but this tumour can occur in all age groups, and is two or three times more common in boys than girls. More than two-thirds of the lesions occur in long bones, mostly in the lower extremity and especially involving the femur and tibia. The neck of the femur and the intertrochanteric region are a particularly characteristic location in the femur.

The lesion consists of a small core or nidus of cellular, highly vascularized tissue, with an interlacing network of immature bone and osteoid in varying proportions. The nidus is surrounded by a zone of reactive bone, especially in cortical bone. Very rarely, the osteoid osteoma is multifocal with more than one nidus. High levels of prostaglandins are produced within the lesions. Intra-articular lesions, which are rare and arise at the end of a long bone within the insertion of the joint capsule, are accompanied by a synovitis characterized by a hyperplastic synovium and a prominent lymphocytic infiltrate.

Clinical features

Almost without exception the initial symptom is pain. This may be vague and intermittent at first but becomes increasingly intense. Often, though not invariably, it is worse at night, and typically it is relieved by aspirin and other non-steroidal anti-inflammatory drugs. Although pain is usually felt in the region of the bone lesion, the presentation can be much less characteristic and the diagnosis is often delayed for many months. For example, pain can sometimes be referred or radicular, accompanied by muscle atrophy and diminished or absent tendon reflexes in the affected limb, thus mimicking a spinal lesion (Kiers et al. 1990). Intra-articular lesions can also present a confusing picture, with joint pain, stiffness, effusion, muscle atrophy, and loss of function. Osteoid osteomas that arise in the posterior elements of the spine can present with scoliosis or torticollis.

Diagnosis

A typical lesion [Plate 196(a)] in the cortex of a long bone is seen on a plain radiograph as a well-defined area of sclerosis, 0.5–1.0 cm in diameter, surrounding a radiolucent nidus, which may contain speckled areas of calcification. However, lesions in cancellous bone and neural arch and intra-articular lesions are often difficult to locate with plain radiographs.

A bone scan using $^{99}Tc^{m}$ hydroxymethylene diphosphonate is a highly sensitive technique to screen for an osteoid osteoma, as these lesions avidly accumulate isotope [Plate 196(b)]. Helms et al. (1984) have described the 'double density sign' as characteristic for osteoid osteoma but it is often not seen and the bone scan is then non-specific for differentiating an osteoid osteoma from lesions such as a stress fracture, synovitis, and a Brodie's abscess. Computed tomography (CT) is also valuable for imaging lesions difficult to locate on plain radiographs, especially those in the spine and proximal femur, and for precisely locating the nidus before surgical resection. MRI effectively demonstrates the associated intramedullary and soft tissue changes but the resulting image can lead to diagnostic confusion and CT is generally considered to be the better imaging modality for the diagnosis of osteoid osteoma (Assoun et al. 1994).

Treatment

Surgery is curative, provided the nidus is excised completely. If this is not achieved, the osteoid osteoma may recur, upto 10 years afterwards. Many surgeons use an *en bloc* excision but some use CT- or radioisotope-guided excision of osteomas, mainly of those located in the extremities. Radiofrequency ablation or thermocoagulation have been reported as promising and less invasive alternatives to surgery in selected patients (Campanacci et al. 1999).

Synovial chondromatosis

This is a disorder of unknown aetiology that affects synovium-lined joints, tendon sheaths, and bursas. It is characterized by chondrometaplasia of the subsynovial connective-tissue cells. The joint cavity becomes filled with a thickened synovium containing pearly-white to blue nodules. Some of these lie free in the joint as loose bodies. The histological appearance is of double-nucleated chondrocytes exhibiting moderate hyperchromasia, arranged in clusters with abundant intervening matrix.

The disorder is uncommon and generally occurs in middle-aged men. It has never been reported before puberty. Most commonly it affects the knee (one-half of cases) or hip, but can also involve other large joints such as the elbow, shoulder, and wrist. Extra-articular involvement of tendons occurs, predominantly in the hands and feet.

Clinically, it resembles pigmented villonodular synovitis (see below). The presenting symptoms are mild, but progressive, pain and locking. Aspirated joint fluid is always yellow or straw-coloured. Plain radiographs (Plate 197) show small, punctate calcifications outlining the joint margin and sometimes bony erosions due to raised intra-articular pressure. Large osteochondral fragments can be seen but this is not a specific feature. Loss of articular cartilage does not occur. If the cartilaginous nodules are not calcified or ossified, the diagnosis can only be confirmed by arthroscopy.

This is a benign condition. During the active phase it is very slowly progressive but it becomes self-limiting and regression can be observed. In rare cases, there is transformation to chondrosarcoma.

Treatment is surgical and most authorities suggest that this should consist of removal of loose bodies and excision of the synovial membrane, which can be done via the arthroscope. Removal of loose bodies without an extensive synovectomy has been reported to give similar results (Shpitzer et al. 1990).

Pigmented villonodular synovitis

The term pigmented villonodular synovitis was first coined by Jaffe et al. in 1941 to encompass a group of conditions, previously known by a variety of other terms, characterized by exuberant proliferation of synovial cells and mesenchymal supporting tissue affecting joints, tendons, and bursas. In their seminal paper, Jaffe and colleagues emphasized the villous and nodular proliferation, the deposition of iron and fat, and the non-malignant nature of these conditions. The terminology subsequently was expanded to distinguish localized lesions (sharply localized or pedunculated lesions involving tendon sheaths or part of the joint lining) from diffuse lesions of the joint synovial membrane, which, although similar histologically, are more progressive and tend to recur after treatment.

Aetiological factors

The aetiology is unknown and there are still various hypotheses based on different interpretations of the histological changes (Perka et al. 2000). There is some evidence supporting a neoplastic process especially in the diffuse disease including malignant transformation and, rarely, metastasis (Choong et al. 1995). This view is also supported by some cytogenetic evidence of clonality (Sciot et al. 1999). Most favour a non-neoplastic aetiology; suggestions include a response to blood and blood products from trauma. An epidemiological study (Myers et al. 1980), while showing no evidence for a genetic basis for pigmented villonodular synovitis, demonstrated a history of chronic repetitive trauma and repeated haemarthroses in approximately 50 per cent of cases. However, there has been a general failure to reproduce typical histological changes in experimental models with injection of various substances from whole blood to colloidal iron. Furthermore, clinical experience from haemophiliacs and others with bleeding disorders points away from a reaction to trauma and haemorrhage per se.

Pathology

The striking pathological feature is the proliferation of synovial lining cells at the surface and invading the subsynovial stroma. The result in diffuse pigmented villonodular synovitis is a greatly thickened synovial membrane bristling with big, long villi, which may be interspersed with nodules of various size. The tissue is often stained red-brown from repeated haemorrhage, with mottled areas of yellow-orange from lipid deposition. Histologically, there is marked proliferation of surface lining cells, together with an invasion of the subsynovial stroma by large epithelioid histiocytic cells that electron-microscopic studies show to be a mixture of proliferating synovial fibroblasts and type B synovial lining cells. The stroma also contains multinucleate giant cells and lipid-laden macrophages. In addition, there are a few lymphocytes and plasma cells. Capillary hyperplasia resulting in numerous thin-walled vascular channels is another characteristic feature. Haemosiderin is deposited in the lining and epithelioid cells, and in the stroma. Another typical feature is the ability of pigmented villonodular synovitis to invade subchondral bone. Demonstration of an osteoclast phenotype of giant cells in villonodular synovitis explains the potential for bone destruction (Darling et al. 1997).

Clinical features

Pigmented villonodular synovitis is rare, with an estimated annual incidence of around 1.8 cases/million population (Myers et al. 1980). Typically it affects adults of both sexes in their third or fourth decade, but there is a wide age range and cases have been reported in children and even infants. Classically, it presents as a monoarthritis. In 80 per cent of cases, the knee is involved, followed in order by the hip, ankle, and shoulder; very rarely, multiple joints are involved and there are occasional reports of involvement at sites such as the spine and temporomandibular joint. The onset is usually insidious, with pain the most common complaint; this is mild at first but progressive. Rarely, there may be sudden exacerbation of pain due to torsion or infarction of a nodule of abnormal tissue. Sometimes there are features of internal derangement, such as locking, especially with localized forms of pigmented villonodular synovitis. Occasionally, an affected knee joint becomes unstable. On examination, there is often swelling and sometimes one or more palpable masses of synovium. There may be local warmth and points of tenderness.

Joint aspiration gives fluid that ranges in colour from yellow or straw, with deep xanthochromia from previous haemorrhage, to brown-stained or frankly bloody. Reports of synovial fluid analysis are sparse but findings point to inflammation and include a slight elevation of protein, reduced glucose, and a low to moderate leucocyte count. The results of other laboratory tests are otherwise normal.

Plain radiographs may be normal or only show the soft tissue outline of synovial swelling, which is made more radiodense by haemosiderin deposition. However, calcification, which occurs in malignant lesions such as synovial sarcoma, is absent. In approximately 50 per cent there are osteoarticular changes corresponding to invasion of bone by the lesion. These include multiple subchondral cysts, which can occur on non-weight-bearing surfaces, and well-demarcated erosions due to increased intra-articular pressure. These changes occur earlier in joints with a tight articular capsule, such as the hip, than in the knee in which a more distensible capsule accommodates a greater degree of soft tissue proliferation. In the knee, bony lesions often develop first in the patellofemoral compartment, where intra-articular soft tissue is more likely to be entrapped. Preservation of joint space is reported to be a typical feature of pigmented villonodular synovitis, but, in fact, loss of joint space can occur as a late feature. Juxta-articular osteoporosis and osteophyte formation are not seen. MRI is very characteristic if there is sufficient haemosiderin and fat deposition in the lesion. Haemosiderin deposition produces a low signal intensity on T_1-weighted images, which decreases even further on T_2-weighted images. In contrast, areas with high fat content have high signal intensity. Consequently, an MRI study demonstrating a multinodular intra-articular lesion with patchy areas having characteristics of fat and haemosiderin deposition is highly suggestive of pigmented villonodular synovitis. However, in practice both false positives and false negatives occur. Techniques such as arthrography and arteriography have been used, but the results are rather non-specific.

Diagnosis

The diagnosis is based on a combination of clinical, radiological, and histological findings and the gross appearance of the lesion (Bhimani et al. 2001). The presence of serosanguinous synovial fluid in a young adult in the absence of a history of recent trauma is highly suggestive of the diagnosis of pigmented villonodular synovitis. The definitive diagnosis, however, often rests on the interpretation of a synovial biopsy. Histological criteria for the diagnosis have not been defined. Although features such as epithelioid cells, multinucleate giant cells, and deposition of fat and haemosiderin are highly characteristic, interpretation of the histological features by a specialist in osteoarticular pathology is required.

Conditions to be considered in the differential diagnosis of pigmented villonodular synovitis include:

1. malignant synovioma,
2. synovial haemangioma,
3. synovial chondromatosis,
4. tuberculous arthritis,
5. amyloidosis,
6. haemophilia,
7. lipoma arborescens.

Treatment

Localized forms of pigmented villonodular synovitis are treated by marginal excision of the lesion and have a good prognosis. The diffuse form, however, tends to be progressive and recurrence is not uncommon. Treatment suggestions are largely based on anecdotal experience, the published series are small, and post-treatment follow-up is limited. A range of techniques, which include radiation, wide synovectomy, synovectomy combined with radiation, arthrodesis, bone grafting, primary arthroplasty, and radiation synovectomy, has been used. No single method has a uniformly high proportion of good results.

The most commonly reported treatment is surgical synovectomy. There are recent reports of good results (Durr et al. 2001), although in previous series there have been a high percentage of recurrences, with persistent joint pain and stiffness as common sequelae. The use of radiation therapy as an adjunct does not improve the outcome. Radiation synovectomy using intra-articular yttrium-90 silicate has been reported, with promising results (Franssen et al. 1989). There are several advantages over surgical synovectomy including technical simplicity and fewer complications. There is limited experience, however, and not much long-term follow-up. In advanced cases with joint destruction (especially in the hip), it may be necessary to resort to a total arthroplasty.

Chronic focal osteomyelitis (Brodie's abscess)

This usually follows an acute haematogenous infection in an adolescent male. Three-fourths of Brodie's abscesses develop in the lower extremity, most often in the tibia. The acute episode of infection may have been successfully treated with antibiotics from a clinical point of view, only to be followed by a focus of chronic infection that can persist for years if not surgically drained.

Typically, the infection occurs in the metaphyseal side of the growth plate, where it remains localized. In rare cases, the infection extends through the growth plate into the epiphysis. Usually it is unifocal but multiple abscesses have been reported. Approximately 80 per cent involve *Staphylococcus aureus*, although almost any organism can be implicated.

Pain is the main complaint, described as aching or boring, and may have been present for months or even years. This is accompanied by localized tenderness and sometimes swelling. Occasionally, the abscess dissects through spongy bone and erodes through the cortex to drain into a joint, or through a sinus to the skin surface. The symptoms and signs of systemic illness that generally accompany acute osteomyelitis are conspicuously absent. Laboratory tests may also be normal, although there can be slight leucocytosis or elevation of the erythrocyte sedimentation rate. Radiographs show a sharply demarcated and irregular area of bone destruction surrounded by sclerosis. Cultures from the abscess are positive in 50–80 per cent of cases.

Treatment is by surgical drainage and appropriate antibiotics. The prognosis is good.

Osteonecrosis

Osteonecrosis is a major reason for orthopaedic surgery to the hip, particularly in younger patients. There are several synonyms: avascular necrosis, aseptic necrosis, ischaemic necrosis, steroid necrosis, segmental subchondral infarction. Osteonecrosis at certain sites is associated with eponyms such as Legg–Perthes' disease (hip), Freiberg's disease (metatarsal), and Kienboch's disease (lunate). Occasionally, it is multifocal (Mont et al. 1999).

In 1860, James Paget described the gross appearance of osteonecrosis in his lectures on surgical pathology (Bullough and DiCarlo 1990). Necrosis of the femoral head was associated with Caisson's disease in 1888, with corticosteroids in 1957 (Pietrogrande and Mastromarino 1957), and the association with systemic lupus erythematosus was reported in 1960 (Dubois and Cozen 1960). Before the 1960s, most reported cases were associated with fracture. The current prevalence of osteonecrosis is difficult to assess because many cases are clinically silent. Different forms of osteonecrosis affect children, young adults, or elderly people. However, most of those with atraumatic osteonecrosis are relatively young, with a peak incidence in the fifth decade of life. One group reports that about 18 per cent of femoral heads removed in total hip-replacement procedures for non-traumatic causes show evidence of osteonecrosis (Bullough and DiCarlo 1990). Approximately 60 per cent are bilateral, women are slightly more affected (1.2 : 1), and the mean age of presentation is 55 years compared with 67 years for patients with primary osteoarthritis.

Osteonecrosis, like infarction anywhere, results from a reduction or the obliteration of the blood supply to the affected area. Subchondral bone has a limited collateral circulation and the perfusion pressure and blood flow of epiphyses and fatty marrow is low compared with red diaphyseal marrow. Therefore, ends of bones such as the femoral head are more susceptible to ischaemia. Various mechanisms have been implicated (Mankin 1992):

1. interruption of extraosseous arterial blood supply (e.g. trauma, vasculitis);
2. interruption of intraosseous sinusoidal circulation (e.g. nitrogen bubbles, sickled erythrocytes, thrombi, fat emboli);
3. extravascular compression of sinusoidal circulation (e.g. nitrogen bubbles, intramedullary lipocyte hypertrophy, accumulation of Gaucher's or malignant cells).

Often a combination of factors is involved. A final common pathway appears to be increased bone-marrow pressure, which can be demonstrated in the very earliest stages of the process and which further contributes to the impaired intraosseous microcirculation and progression of necrosis.

The pathology of osteonecrosis is well defined. The first phase is necrosis of bone and bone marrow. A cut section of bone shows a wedge-shaped necrotic zone in the subchondral region, which is demarcated from the normal bone marrow by a hyperaemic border. Granulation tissue develops and then advances from the margin of the infarct and necrotic bone is resorbed. Behind this, a second front of osteoblasts lays down new bone. If articular stress exceeds the structural integrity of the altered bone, there will be collapse of the articular surface and disruption of the joint.

Aetiological factors (Mankin 1992; Chang et al. 1993)

Some of the causes of osteonecrosis are:

1. trauma,
2. sepsis,
3. radiation, thermal, and electrical injury,
4. Caisson's disease,
5. haemoglobinopathies,
6. haemophilia,
7. coagulopathies,
8. Gaucher's disease,
9. alcoholism,
10. Cushing's syndrome,
11. corticosteroid usage,
12. systemic lupus erythematosus,
13. rheumatoid arthritis,
14. systemic sclerosis,
15. vasculitis,
16. organ transplantation (kidney, heart, marrow),
17. chronic dialysis,
18. human immunodeficiency virus infection,
19. pancreatitis,
20. chronic liver disease,
21. hypertriglyceridaemia,
22. pregnancy (especially in the third trimester),
23. idiopathic.

The major cause is a fracture that interferes with the blood supply to areas such as the femoral or humeral head, talus, and scaphoid. Osteonecrosis is a major complication of intracapsular fracture of the femoral neck, which is accompanied by disruption of the circulation in approximately 20 per cent of cases. Osteonecrosis occurs in 18 per cent of compressed-air workers and 4 per cent of divers; it appears to be the result of the development of intravascular and extravascular nitrogen gas bubbles during decompression, effectively occluding the circulation to sites such as the femoral and humeral heads. Lesions are frequently multiple and bilateral; involvement of the humeral heads is particularly characteristic. In Caisson's disease, for some reason, the subchondral bone of the knee and the ankle are not involved.

Depending on the genotype, sickle cell haemoglobinopathies have a 5–14 per cent prevalence of radiographically detectable osteonecrosis. As in Caisson's disease, the femoral and humeral heads are involved.

The two most common causes of non-traumatic osteonecrosis are alcoholism and hypercortisolism, which account for two-thirds of the cases. A feature they have in common is alteration in systemic fat metabolism. Osteonecrosis may be produced as a result of fatty emboli, or of intramedullary lipocyte hypertrophy and consequent intraosseous sinusoidal compression. Osteonecrosis in rheumatoid arthritis and systemic lupus is mostly associated with corticosteroid treatment. However, as in systemic lupus (see below), osteonecrosis is described as a complication of rheumatoid arthritis in the absence of steroids, although there is little information about the prevalence of this. Osteonecrosis has been reported after repeated intra-articular injections of long-acting corticosteroids (Laroche et al. 1990).

Osteonecrosis in systemic lupus

This is a relatively common and disabling complication of lupus. The prevalence of symptomatic, radiographic lesions in 744 adults with systemic lupus was 12.8 per cent (Gladman et al. 2001a). However, asymptomatic lesions detected by MRI are more common and present in up to 35 per cent (Nagasawa et al. 1994). Although some become apparent on plain radiographs, present in up to 25 per cent of adult systemic lupus erythematosus patients and possibly in even more children, in only a minority of lesions is the necrosis extensive enough to cause clinical problems. The major risk factor for osteonecrosis is corticosteroid therapy (Gladman et al. 2001b), but there are reports of the complication before the steroid era (Leventhal and Dorfman 1974). Additional risk factors suggested by some studies, but not others, include younger age, vasculitis, Raynaud's phenomenon, and leucopaenia. Osteonecrosis has been reported in association with antiphospholipid antibodies in patients with the 'primary antiphospholipid syndrome' but others (Migliaresi et al. 1994) have found no correlation between anticardiolipin antibodies and osteonecrosis in their lupus population. It appears that it is the use of large doses of corticosteroids (e.g. prednisolone, 60 mg daily), sustained over a period of months, that is important for the development of osteonecrosis, rather than the duration of corticosteroids or the accumulative dose per se. Giving pulses of megadose corticosteroids either once or repeated after intervals of several weeks does not independently predispose to osteonecrosis. A meta-analysis reported by Felson and Anderson (1987) suggests that this relationship to dose and duration of corticosteroids applies to patients with a variety of clinical conditions. It is worth remembering that a number of malpractice suits have been brought against physicians for failing to inform patients of this complication of corticosteroids.

The onset of localized pain, particularly in a weight-bearing joint, should give rise to a high index of suspicion. The femoral head is most commonly involved, but other sites include the femoral condyle, tibial plateau, humeral head, talus, scaphoid, and lunate. Simultaneous involvement of multiple sites is not infrequent.

Diagnosis

Pain is the principal symptom. In about two-thirds of the patients it occurs at rest and may be troublesome at night (due to increased intraosseous pressure). It is well established that once radiographic changes occur in osteonecrosis the natural history is generally subchondral bone collapse and severe disability. The Ficat and Arlet classification of osteonecrosis is based on the plain radiographic appearance (Ficat and Arlet 1980), as follows:

Stage I: normal appearance;

Stage II: early changes consisting of diffuse osteoporosis, sclerosis, and cyst formation producing a mottled appearance [Plate 198(a)];

Stage III: subchondral bone collapse (crescent sign) with normal joint space;

Stage IV: abnormal contour of bone with joint-space loss.

This has been extended by Steinberg et al. (1984) to provide a more sensitive method of following the progress of osteonecrosis in the femoral and humeral heads.

In early stages the plain radiograph is normal. The imaging technique currently combining the greatest sensitivity and specificity for the diagnosis of early cases is MRI [Plate 198(b) and (c)]. The presence of a low intensity band on T_1-weighted images is an early specific finding of osteonecrosis and MRI has the advantage of identifying early changes in necrotic bone marrow before other changes in bone have taken place. If MRI is not available, an isotope bone scan with $^{99}Tc^{m}$ diphosphonate is indicated. This is also helpful in early diagnosis but it is less specific, anatomical resolution is often poor, and false negatives commonly occur, especially when there is bilateral disease. Other methods used for early diagnosis have included CT with multiplanar reconstruction. This is reported to be more sensitive than bone scan but the significant radiation exposure makes MRI a more attractive option. Bone biopsy of the affected site is sometimes necessary, as local infection can be associated with osteonecrosis.

Osteonecrosis at specific sites

Vertebral

This is uncommon but compared with compression fractures of osteoporosis is more often associated with neurological complications. This mainly happens in elderly people; the lesions are usually single, and at the thoracolumbar junction. It is not usually associated with malignancy and MRI is helpful in early diagnosis. The intravertebral vacuum cleft is the characteristic feature on the plain radiography.

Keinbock's disease

This describes osteonecrosis of the lunate. It may occur after a fracture but in most cases there is no specific history of this. Often it happens in the dominant hand and is thought to be the result of chronic repetitive trauma. It is associated with a short ulna, which probably reinforces the effects of repeated trauma.

Preiser's disease

This is spontaneous osteonecrosis of the scaphoid, usually affecting the proximal pole. Involvement of the scaphoid is usually post-traumatic and in idiopathic cases the trauma may have been minor and unrecognized.

Hegemann's disease

This describes osteonecrosis of the humeral trochlear. This is rare and happens mainly in pre-adolescent and adolescent boys, who present with a swollen elbow; this has reduced movement but is not particularly painful. Usually it resolves spontaneously.

Legg–Perthes' disease

This is osteonecrosis of the femoral head, which occurs in children between the age of 4 and 12 years and affects one or both hips. The aetiology is unknown but the condition is associated with increased intraosseous pressure and venous hypertension. There may be spontaneous resolution, especially in younger patients, in whom conservative management is indicated.

Osteonecrosis of the femoral condyle

This occurs spontaneously in older people, predominantly affecting the medial condyle.

Kohler's disease

This is the rare involvement of the tarsal navicular, which primarily occurs in male children between the ages of 4 and 10 years. It is usually self-limiting.

Freiberg's disease

This is osteonecrosis of the metatarsal head, usually the second. It mainly affects adolescent females and is usually self-limiting.

Treatment

Advanced osteonecrosis of weight-bearing surfaces, such as the femoral head, leads to secondary osteoarthritis and severe disability. Total joint replacement may be the only solution in such cases. The results are satisfactory, giving a long period of good function. However, one still hesitates to recommend total joint replacement in young people and the failure rate may be higher in operations for osteonecrosis, especially when associated with corticosteroids, than in arthroplasties for other conditions. Attempts have therefore been made to treat the condition at an earlier stage in order to preserve the integrity of affected bone.

Osteonecrosis of the femoral condyle in elderly people can often be treated conservatively with initial limitation of weight-bearing, non-steroidal anti-inflammatory drugs, hydrotherapy, and muscle strengthening exercises.

There is little evidence from retrospective studies that bed rest, modified weight bearing, analgesics, or non-steroidal anti-inflammatory drugs are of much benefit in other cases, at least for osteonecrosis of the hip in adults. Because increased intraosseous pressure is a common feature in early stages, core decompression has been recommended. Encouraging results with prevention of progression in early stages of osteonecrosis of the hip (Steinberg et al. 2001) and the shoulder (Mont et al. 1993) have been reported by some groups. However, this is a controversial topic and not all studies have been so encouraging (Learmonth et al. 1990). The use of MRI to assess the extent of osteonecrosis may be a way of selecting those most likely to respond to this procedure (Holman et al. 1995).

Other ways of preserving the femoral head include bone grafting using a variety of procedures (Rosenwasser et al. 1994; Urbaniak et al. 1995), the use of electrical stimulation, and sometimes a combination of these (Steinberg et al. 1985). In addition, various techniques of osteotomy, such as the transtrochanteric osteotomy of the femoral head, have been used to alter the weight-bearing surface away from the involved area. These techniques are still being refined and evaluated.

Osteochondritis dissecans

Osteochondritis dissecans is usually a solitary lesion of the medial femoral condyle in which a fragment composed of articular cartilage and subchondral bone becomes demarcated from the surrounding bone and cartilage and may form an intra-articular loose body. Occasionally, it may involve the elbow, hip, and talus. The aetiology is unknown but anomalies of ossification and low-grade trauma appear to be important.

It predominantly affects adolescent males and should be suspected in a child or teenager who, after minor trauma, develops a relatively sudden onset of knee pain followed by mechanical dysfunction. There may be a hereditary component and familial occurrence has been reported (Paes 1989). This is characterized by multiple articular lesions, particularly affecting the hips and knees, and an autosomal dominant inheritance. Sometimes there is associated dwarfism and a generalized epiphyseal abnormality.

Symptoms are mainly pain, reduced joint movement, effusion, and limp. A plain radiograph shows a well-circumscribed, sclerotic lesion demarcated by a radiolucent line from surrounding bone (Plate 199).

In young patients before skeletal maturity there is a good chance of healing, and treatment is consequently conservative. Once the epiphyses have closed, osteochondritis dissecans is more likely to cause intra-articular loose bodies and subsequent symptoms of internal derangement, and eventually secondary osteoarthritis. Arthroscopy can be helpful in assessing the extent of the lesion. A variety of surgical procedures have been recommended, from drilling of the lesion to promote ingrowth of fibrocartilage to replacement of a large deficit with an osteochondral allograft.

Relapsing polychondritis

This is an uncommon, multisystem disorder of unknown aetiology characterized by episodic and sometimes progressive inflammation of cartilaginous structures and tissues rich in glycosoaminoglycans. The characteristic clinical syndrome, with involvement of the pinna of the ears, nose, larynx and upper airways, joints, heart, blood vessels, inner ear, cornea, and sclera, was first described by Jaksch-Wartenhorse (1923). In about 30 per cent of cases, it is associated with other systemic rheumatic or autoimmune diseases such as systemic vasculitis, rheumatoid arthritis, systemic lupus, Sjögren's syndrome, thyroiditis, ulcerative colitis, psoriasis, and Behçet's syndrome (Molina and Espinoza 2000).

Table 1 Extent of organ involvement in relapsing polychondritis

Organ	Percentage involvement
External ear	85
Arthritis	75
Nose	60
Eye	50
Respiratory tract	50
Internal ear	40
Skin	25
Kidney	20
Heart	10
Blood vessels	8
Central nervous system	Rare

Aetiology and pathogenesis

The most specific lesion is inflammation of cartilage. The lesion is characterized by a dense inflammatory infiltrate of neutrophils, lymphocytes, macrophages, and plasma cells. Initially this involves the perichondral region. There is loss of proteoglycans, destruction of the collagen matrix, and chondrocyte death. Destroyed cartilage is replaced by granulation tissue and there is subsequent fibrosis. The cause is unknown but, on the basis of circumstantial evidence, there may be an autoimmune pathogenesis.

Antibodies, predominantly IgG, which react specifically with collagen types II, IX, and XI (forming the major fibrillar scaffold in cartilage), can be detected in some but not all patients with relapsing polychondritis. The highest titres are found in the early phase of the disease and the titre may relate to disease activity. These antibodies are not disease specific and occur, for example, in rheumatoid arthritis, although possibly they are directed to different epitopes on the collagen molecule (Terato et al. 1990). The possibility that humoral factors are involved in the pathogenesis is suggested by the report of polychondritis occurring in the newborn infant of an affected mother and the subsequent recovery of the baby (Arundell and Haserick 1960). Granular deposits of immunoglobulin and complement have been observed at the chondrofibral junction in biopsies from affected ears (Valenzuela et al. 1980), suggesting the involvement of immune complexes. Thus, there is evidence for humoral immune mechanisms being involved in cartilage injury. In addition, earlier reports of cellular immune reactions to proteoglycan and other matrix components have been supported by the more recent demonstration of cell-mediated immunity to collagen types II, IX, and XI paralleling the humoral response to these structural proteins (Alsalameh et al. 1993). More recently, an immune response (both humoral and cell-mediated) has been demonstrated to matrilin-1, a cartilage matrix protein found uniquely in tracheal, auricular, and nasal cartilage (Buckner et al. 2000).

A significant increase in DR4 antigen frequency has been found (Zeuner et al. 1997) but, in contrast to rheumatoid arthritis, there is no predominance of any DR4 sub-type.

Clinical features

The disease predominantly affects middle-aged White subjects, with a peak incidence in the fourth to fifth decades, although it has been reported in all races and age groups. The patient typically presents with recurrent swelling and pain of the external ear and/or nose, or with uveitis, or with an arthropathy. The cumulative involvement of various organ systems is summarized in Table 1.

Episodes of inflammation of the cartilaginous portion of one or both ears and the nose are often sudden and last several days. Repeated episodes of protracted inflammation, leading to cartilage destruction, produce deformity such as saddle nose [Plate 200(a) and (b)].

Joint involvement is also common and occurs independently of other manifestations. The typical clinical picture is episodic, asymmetrical inflammation of both large and small joints, including the parasternal and sacroiliac joints, lasting several days to weeks. Generally it is non-deforming, non-erosive, and seronegative for rheumatoid factor (Balsa et al. 1995). In contrast to the 'pure' polyarthritis of relapsing polychondritis, the condition can develop against the background of a well-defined, erosive polyarthritis such as rheumatoid arthritis.

A wide range of rather non-specific ocular manifestations occur in relapsing polychondritis. The most common is episcleritis but more severe involvement includes scleritis and peripheral corneal thinning, both of which can lead to perforation, uveitis, retinal vasculitis, and optic neuritis, any of which can lead to blindness. Also reported are palsy of ocular muscles, orbital inflammation, and papilloedema.

The disease affects the respiratory tract in at least one-half of the patients and is the main cause of death. This can lead to the breakdown of tracheal and bronchial cartilage, with resulting airway collapse during the respiratory cycle (Crockford and Kerr 1988). The larynx and upper trachea are frequently involved first, and symmetrical subglottic narrowing is a common finding. Eventually the process can involve the distal trachea and main bronchi. Symptoms of respiratory tract involvement include dysphonia, cough, stridor, and dyspnoea; this involvement can dominate the clinical picture. During the active phase there may be tenderness over the thyroid cartilage and trachea.

Involvement of the inner ear tends to occur later in the course of the disease and leads to vestibular and auditory dysfunction. A wide range of non-specific skin lesions has been reported, including erythema nodosum and leucocytoclastic vasculitis. The MAGIC (mouth and genital ulcers with inflamed cartilage) syndrome describes an overlap with Behçet's syndrome characterized by prominent orogenital ulceration. Renal manifestations have been reported in as many as 20 per cent of cases (Chang-Miller et al. 1987). On renal biopsy, the predominant lesions are reported to be mesangial proliferation and segmental, necrotizing glomerulonephritis with crescents. Immunofluorescence and electron-microscopic studies show faint deposition of immunoglobulin and complement, and small amounts of electron-dense deposits, respectively, mainly in the mesangium. Patients with renal involvement tend to have more severe disease with extrarenal vasculitis and worse prognosis.

The heart is involved in about 10 per cent of patients. Aortic incompetence, either from dilatation of the aortic root or valvular destruction, is the most common manifestation. It is often severe, progressing even when other aspects of the disease are in remission, and requires valve replacement in at least a third. Even when valve replacement is successful, there is the possibility of future dehiscence of the prosthetic valve because of continuing inflammation of perivalvular tissues (Lang-Lazdunski et al. 1995). Other cardiovascular manifestations include pericarditis, myocarditis, heart block, coronary vasculitis leading to myocardial infarction, and aneurysms of the aorta and other large arteries. Vasculitis involving large- and medium-sized arteries may occur independently of cardiac involvement and often carries a poor prognosis.

Meningioencephalitis has been reported in association with polychondritis but central nervous system involvement is rare.

Laboratory abnormalities are non-specific and for the most part reflect chronic inflammation. Common features are an acute-phase response, anaemia of chronic disease, and thrombocytosis. There may be a moderate leucocytosis. The development of a myelodysplastic syndrome has been reported (Diebold et al. 1995). Serological tests demonstrate anti-type II collagen antibodies in up to one-half of patients, circulating immune complexes in the majority, and antinuclear antibodies in approximately 20 per cent. ANCA have been reported in 24 per cent of patients with polychondritis, mainly during the acute phase of the disease, and in some patients in association with vasculitis (Handrock and Gross 1993). Imaging techniques are essential for assessing respiratory complications of the disease. CT scanning is an accurate method for assessing the upper and lower airways (Davis et al. 1989). MRI, however, is superceding this technique, having the advantage of distinguishing inflammation from fibrosis (Heman-Ackah et al. 1999).

The clinical course of this disease is highly variable. It is probable that the literature emphasizes the worst end of the spectrum and that many milder cases go unrecognized. It has been suggested that the 5- and 10-year survival after diagnosis are 74 and 55 per cent, respectively (Michet et al. 1986). However, the prognosis is better in more recent studies (Trentham and Le 1998). The most common causes of death are infection, cardiac and respiratory involvement, and systemic vasculitis.

Diagnosis

Early diagnosis is important in an attempt to prevent potentially life-threatening complications. There are no universally accepted diagnostic criteria but McAdam et al. (1976) proposed that the presence of three of the six following clinical features should be diagnostic:

1. recurrent chondritis of both auricles;
2. non-erosive polyarthritis;
3. chondritis of the nasal cartilage;
4. ocular inflammation including conjunctivitis, keratitis, scleritis/episcleritis, uveitis;
5. involvement of laryngeal and/or tracheal cartilage;
6. cochlear and/or vestibular involvement.

These were modified slightly by Damiani and Levine (1979) to include:

1. three or more of the above criteria;
2. at least one clinical criterion plus histological confirmation;
3. chondritis in two or more separate anatomical locations with a response to treatment.

Treatment

The rarity of relapsing polychondritis, the diversity of its presentation, and the unpredictability of recurrences make it difficult to recommend a particular treatment protocol. There are no controlled trials therefore the following is based on anecdotal experience.

Mild symptoms of joint involvement and inflammation of ear and nose cartilages can sometimes be controlled by non-steroidal anti-inflammatory drugs alone. Dapsone has been reported to be effective for systemic manifestations not controlled with symptomatic treatment alone. Corticosteroids can be effective in suppressing acute, severe manifestations. Often high doses (at least 1 mg/kg/day of prednisolone or equivalent) are required. Alternate-day regimens are not recommended but there are reports of bolus parenteral methylprednisolone being effective for manifestations such as acute airways' obstruction (Lipnick and Fink 1991). It appears that corticosteroids are more effective in treating disease in cartilage of the respiratory tract than, for example, involvement of the joints and eyes. Also, there is no evidence that corticosteroids influence long-term outcome, and in some patients the disease undoubtedly progresses despite giving corticosteroids.

In severe cases, when there is airways and/or other organ involvement, the addition of an immunosuppressive agent is required to control disease activity and to be steroid sparing. Successful responses have been reported using agents such as azathioprine, cyclophosphamide, methotrexate, and cyclosporine A. Cyclophosphamide is the drug of choice for features such as necrotizing scleritis and systemic vasculitis. In refractory cases there have been anecdotal reports of success with monoclonal antibodies to CD4 (Van der Lubbe et al. 1991) and autologous stem cell transplantation (Rosen et al. 2000).

Additional supportive measures may be needed for those with severe respiratory, cardiac, and renal complications. For example, whereas only 14 per cent of patients with this disease present initially with respiratory tract involvement, 80 per cent of these will require tracheostomy. Initially, this is usually for glottic, laryngeal, and subglottic inflammation and oedema producing airways' obstruction. Later, the indication for tracheostomy is often the collapse of laryngeal or tracheal cartilages. The recent introduction of expandable metal stents represents an important development in managing patients with major airway stenosis and collapse (Sarodia et al. 1999).

References

Alsalameh, S., Mollenhauer, J., Scheuplein, F., Stoss, H., Kalden, J.R., Burkhardt, H., and Burmester, G.R. (1993). Preferential cellular and humoral immune reactivities to native and denatured collagen types IX and XI in a patient with fatal relapsing polychondritis. *Journal of Rheumatology* **20**, 1419–24.

Arundell, F.W. and Haserick, J.R. (1960). Familial chronic atrophic polychondritis. *Archives of Dermatology* **82**, 439–41.

Assoun, J., Richardi, G., Railhac, J.J., Baunin, C., Fajadet, P., Giron, J., Maquin, P., Haddad, J., and Bonnevialle, P. (1994). Osteoid osteoma: MR imaging versus CT. *Radiology* **191**, 217–23.

Balsa, A., Espinosa, A., Cuesta, M., MacLeod, T.I., Gijon-Banos, J., and Maddison, P.J. (1995). Joint symptoms in relapsing polychondritis. *Clinical and Experimental Rheumatology* **13**, 425–30.

Bhimani, M.A., Wenz, J.F., and Frassica, F.J. (2001). Pigmented villonodular synovitis: keys to early diagnosis. *Clinical Orthopaedics* **386**, 197–202.

Buckner, J.H., Wu, J.J., Reife, R.A., Terato, K., and Eyre, D.R. (2000). Autoreactivity against matrilin-1 in a patient with relapsing polychondritis. *Arthritis and Rheumatism* **43**, 939–43.

Bullough, P.G. and DiCarlo, E.F. (1990). Subchondral avascular necrosis: a common cause of arthritis. *Annals of the Rheumatic Diseases* **49**, 412–20.

Campanacci, M., Ruggieri, P., Gasbarrini, A., Ferraro, A., and Campanacci, L. (1999). Osteoid osteoma. Direct visual identification and intralesional excision of the nidus with minimal removal of bone. *Journal of Bone and Joint Surgery (British Volume)* **81**, 814–20.

Chang-Miller, A. et al. (1987). Renal involvement in relapsing polychondritis. *Medicine (Baltimore)* **66**, 202–17.

Chang, C.C., Greenspan, A., and Gershwin, M.E. (1993). Osteonecrosis: current perspectives on pathogenesis and treatment. *Seminars in Arthritis and Rheumatism* **23**, 47–69.

Choong, P.F. et al. (1995). Pigmented villonodular synovitis. Monoclonality and metastasis—a case for neoplastic origin? *Acta Orthopaedica Scandinavica* **66**, 64–8.

Crockford, M.P. and Kerr, I.H. (1988). Relapsing polychondritis. *Clinical Radiology* **39**, 386–90.

Damiani, J.M. and Levine, H.L. (1979). Relapsing polychondritis: report of ten cases. *Laryngoscope* **89**, 929–44.

Darling, J.M., Goldring, S.R., Harada, Y., Handel, M.L., Glowacki, J., and Gravallese, E.M. (1997). Multinucleated cells in pigmented villonodular synovitis and giant cell tumour of tendon sheath express features of osteoclasts. *American Journal of Pathology* **150**, 1383–93.

Diebold, L., Rauh, G., Jager, K., and Lohrs, U. (1995). Bone marrow pathology in relapsing polychondritis: high frequency of myelodysplastic syndromes. *British Journal of Haematology* **89**, 820–30.

Dubois, E.L. and Cozen, L. (1960). Avascular (aseptic) bone necrosis associated with systemic lupus erythematosus. *Journal of the American Medical Association* **174**, 966–84.

Durr, H.R., Stabler, A., Maier, M., and Refior, H.J. (2001). Pigmented villonodular synovitis. Review of 20 cases. *Journal of Rheumatology* **28**, 1620–30.

Felson, D.T. and Anderson, J.J. (1987). A cross-study evaluation of association between steroid dose and bolus steroids and avascular necrosis of bone. *Lancet* **i**, 902–5.

Ficat, R.P. and Arlet, J. *Ischaemia and Necrosis of Bone*. Baltimore MD: Williams and Wilkins, 1980.

Franssen, M.J.A.M., Boerbooms, A.M.Th., Karthaus, R.P., Buijs, W.C.A.M., and van de Putte, L.B.A. (1989). Treatment of pigmented villonodular synovitis of the knee with yttrium-90 silicate: prospective evaluations by arthroscopy, histology, and ^{99}mTc pertechnetate uptake measurements. *Annals of the Rheumatic Diseases* **48**, 1007–13.

Gladman, D.D., Urowitz, M.B., Chaudhry-Ahluwalia, V., Hallet, D.C., and Cook, R.J. (2001a). Predictive factors for symptomatic osteonecrosis in patients with systemic lupus erythematosus. *Journal of Rheumatology* **28**, 761–5.

Gladman, D.D., Chaudhry-Ahluwalia, V., Ibanez, D., Bogoch, E., and Urowitz, M.B. (2001b). Outcomes of symptomatic osteonecrosis in 95 patients with systemic lupus erythematosus. *Journal of Rheumatology* **28**, 2226–9.

Handrock, K. and Gross, W.L. (1993). Relapsing polychondritis as a secondary phenomenon of primary systemic vasculitis. *Annals of the Rheumatic Diseases* **52**, 895–6.

Helms, C.A., Hattner, R.S., and Vogler, J.B. (1984). Osteoid osteoma: radionuclide diagnosis. *Radiology* **151**, 779–84.

Heman-Ackah, Y.D., Remley, K.B., and Goding, G.S., Jr. (1999). A new role for magnetic resonance imaging in the diagnosis of laryngeal relapsing polychondritis. *Head and Neck* **21**, 484–9.

Holman, A.J., Gardner, G.C., Richardson, M.L., and Simkin, P.A. (1995). Quantitative magnetic resonance imaging predicts clinical outcome of core decompression for osteonecrosis of the femoral head. *Journal of Rheumatology* **22**, 1929–33.

Jaffe, H.L., Lichtenstein, L., and Sutro, C.J. (1941). Pigmented villonodular synovitis, bursitis and tenosynovitis. *Archives of Pathology* **31**, 731–65.

Jaksch-Wartenhorse, R. (1923). Polychondropathia. *Wiener Archiv für Innere Medizin* **6**, 93–4.

Kiers, L., Shield, L.K., and Cole, W.G. (1990). Neurological manifestations of osteoid osteoma. *Archives of Disease in Childhood* **65**, 851–5.

Lang-Lazdunski, L., Hvass, U., Paillole, C., Pansard, Y., and Langlois, J. (1995). Cardiac valve replacement in relapsing polychondritis. A review. *Journal of Heart Valve Disease* **4**, 227–35.

Laroche, M., Arlet, J., and Mazieres, B. (1990). Osteonecrosis of the femoral and humeral heads after intraarticular corticosteroid injection. *Journal of Rheumatology* **17**, 549–51.

Learmonth, I.D., Maloon, S., and Dall, G. (1990). Core decompression for early atraumatic osteonecrosis of the femoral head. *Journal of Bone and Joint Surgery (British Volume)* **72**, 387–90.

Leventhal, G.H. and Dorfman, H.D. (1974). Aseptic necrosis of bone in systemic lupus erythematosus. *Seminars in Arthritis and Rheumatism* **4**, 73–93.

Lipnick, R.N. and Fink, C.W. (1991). Acute airway obstruction in relapsing polychondritis: treatment with pulse methylprednisolone. *Journal of Rheumatology* **18**, 98–9.

McAdam, L.P., O'Hanlan, M.A., Bluestone, R., and Pearson, C.M. (1976). Relapsing polychondritis: prospective review of 23 patients and review of the literature. *Medicine (Baltimore)* **55**, 193–215.

Mankin, H.J. (1992). Nontraumatic necrosis of bone (osteonecrosis). *New England Journal of Medicine* **326**, 1473–9.

Michet, C.J., Jr., McKenna, C.H., Luthra, H.S., and O'Fallen, W.M. (1986). Relapsing polychondritis: survival and predictive roles of early disease manifestations. *Annals of Internal Medicine* **104**, 74–8.

Migliaresi, S., Picillo, U., Ambrosone, L., Di Palma, G., Mallozzi, M., Tesone, E.R., and Tirri, G. (1994). Avascular osteonecrosis in patients with SLE: relation to corticosteroid therapy and anticardiolipin antibodies. *Lupus* **3**, 37–41.

Molina, J.F. and Espinoza, L.R. (2000). Relapsing polychondritis. *Clinical Rheumatology* **14**, 97–109.

Mont, M.A., Maar, D.C., Urquhart, M.W., Lennox, D., and Hungerford, D.S. (1993). Avascular necrosis of the humeral head treated by core compression. A retrospective review. *Journal of Bone and Joint Surgery (British Volume)* **75**, 785–8.

Mont, M.A., Jones, L.C., and LaPorte, D.M. (1999). Symptomatic multifocal osteonecrosis. *Clinical Orthopaedics and Related Research* **369**, 312–25.

Myers B.W., Masi, A.T., and Feigenbaum, S.L. (1980). Pigmented villonodular synovitis and tenosynovitis. A clinical epidemiologic study of 166 cases and literature review. *Medicine* **59**, 223–38.

Nagasawa, K., Tsukamoto, H., Tada, Y., Mayumi, T., Satoh, H., Onitsuka, H., Kuwabara, Y., and Niho, Y. (1994). Imaging study on the mode of development and changes in avascular necrosis of the femoral head in systemic lupus erythematosus: long-term observations. *British Journal of Rheumatology* **33**, 343–7.

Paes, R.A. (1989). Familial osteochondritis dissecans. *Clinical Radiology* **40**, 501–4.

Perka, C., Labs, K., Zippel, H., and Buttgerit, F. (2000). Localized pigmented villonodular synovitis of the knee joint: neoplasm or reactive granuloma? A review of 18 cases. *Rheumatology* **39**, 172–8.

Pietrogrande, V. and Mastromarino, R. (1957). Osteopat da prolongata trattamento cortisonico. *Ortopedia e Traumatologia dell' Apparato Matore* **25**, 791–810.

Rosen, O., Thiel, A., Massenkeil, G., Hiepe, F., Haupl, T., Radtke, H., Burmester, G.R., Gromnica-Ihle, E., Radbruch, A., and Arnold, R. (2000). Autologous stem-cell transplantation in refractory autoimmune diseases after *in vivo* immunoablation and *ex vivo* depletion of mononuclear cells. *Arthritis Research* **2**, 327–36.

Rosenwasser, M.P., Garino, J.P., Kiernan, H.A., and Michelsen, C.B. (1994). Long-term followup of thorough debridement and cancellous bone grafting of the femoral head for avascular necrosis. *Clinical Orthopaedics and Related Research* **306**, 17–27.

Sarodia, B.D., Dasgupta, A., and Mehta, A.C. (1999). Management of airway manifestations of relapsing polychondritis. *Chest* **116**, 1669–75.

Sciot, R. et al. (1999). Analysis of 35 cases of localized and diffuse tenosynovial giant cell tumour: a report from the chromosomes and morphology (CHAMP) study group. *Modern Pathology* **12**, 576–9.

Shpitzer, T., Ganel, A., and Engelberg, S. (1990). Surgery for synovial chondromatosis: 26 cases followed up for 6 years. *Acta Orthopaedica Scandinavica* **61**, 567–9.

Steinberg, M.E., Hayken, G.D., and Steinberg, D.R. (1984). A new method for evaluation and staging of avascular necrosis of the femoral head. In *Bone Circulation* (ed. J. Arlet, R.P. Ficat, and D.S. Hungerford), pp. 398–403. Baltimore MD: Williams and Wilkins.

Steinberg, M.E., Brighton, C.T., Hayken, G.D., Tooze, S.E., and Steinberg, D.R. (1985). Electrical stimulation in the treatment of osteonecrosis of the femoral head. *Orthopedic Clinics of North America* **16**, 747–56.

Steinberg, M.E., Larcom, P.G., Streaaford, B., Hosick, W.B., Corces, A., Bands, R.E., and Hartman, K.E. (2001). Core decompression with bone grafting for osteonecrosis of the femeoral head. *Clinical Orthopaedics and Related Research* **386**, 71–8.

Terato, K. et al. (1990). Specificity of antibodies to type II collagen in rheumatoid arthritis. *Arthritis and Rheumatism* **33**, 1493–500.

Trentham, D.E. and Le, C.H. (1998). Relapsing polychondritis. *Annals of Internal Medicine* **129**, 114–22.

Urbaniak, J.R., Coogan, P.G., Gunneson, E.B., and Nunley, J.A. (1995). Treatment of osteonecrosis of the femoral head with free vascularized fibular grafting. A long-term follow-up study of one hundred and three hips. *Journal of Bone and Joint Surgery (American Volume)* **77**, 681–94.

Valenzuela, R., Cooperrider, P.A., Gogate, P., Deodhar, S.D., and Berfeld, W.F. (1980). Relapsing polychondritis: immunomicroscopic findings in cartilage of ear biopsy specimens. *Human Pathology* **11**, 19–24.

Van der Lubbe, P.A., Multenberg, A.M., and Breedveld, F.C. (1991). Anti-CD4 monoclonal antibody for relapsing polychondritis. *Lancet* **337**, 1349.

Zeuner, M., Straub, R.H., Rauh, G., Albert, E.D., Scholmerich, J., and Lang, B. (1997). Relapsing polychondritis: clinical and immunogenetic analysis of 62 patients. *Journal of Rheumatology* **24**, 96–101.

6.16.4 Diseases of bone and cartilage in children

Christine Hall and Patricia Woo

Definitions

Skeletal dysplasias or osteochondrodysplasias are generalized disorders of bone and cartilage growth and development. They are genetically determined and in many instances the chromosome locus has been identified. The gene product continues to exert its influence on each individual condition throughout the lifespan of an affected individual. The latest International Nosology and Classification of Constitutional Disorders of Bone (2001) identifies about 265 dysplasias, which have been divided into 33 groups. The groups reflect either the common genetic defect (such as a Type I or Type II collagen abnormality) or the similar combinations of clinical and radiological features (such as increased bone density with predominant metaphyseal involvement) (Table 1).

The individual skeletal dysplasias are rare; for example, the commonest surviving condition is achondroplasia with a prevalence of between 40 and 60 per million population. The overall group, however, is significant with a prevalence of between 250 and 350 per million population. This compares, for example, with a prevalence of 20 per million population of combined benign and malignant bone tumours. Also included in the latest classification are the dysostoses, which are conditions with localized or more generalized skeletal malformations. Many of these are also genetically determined. Malformations occur early during blastogenesis in the first 8 weeks of embryonic life. The gene product does not continue to exert its influence throughout life and malformations remain static. The dysostoses have been included in the classification because there is often clinical overlap with the skeletal dysplasias leading to diagnostic confusion. The classification identifies three major groups of dysostoses, those with predominant facial and cranial disorders, those with predominant axial involvement, and those with predominant involvement of the extremities.

Malformation syndromes are conditions in which multiple systems are affected and this may include the skeletal system. Several thousand malformation syndromes are currently recognized and some may also cause problems with precise diagnostic evaluation.

Diagnosis

The diagnosis is established from the history, clinical examination, and evaluation of the radiographic skeletal survey. Important points in the clinical evaluation include:

- Family history—other affected family members,
- Stature,
- Body proportions—short trunk, short limbs,
- Limb segment shortening—rhizomelic, mesomelic, acromelic,
- Facial features—dysmorphology,
- Malformations—cleft palate, heart defects,
- Other features—deafness, myopia, mental retardation, skin changes.

The radiographic skeletal survey should include:

- Skull, antero-posterior and lateral,
- Cervical spine; lateral,
- Thoraco-lumbar spine; antero-posterior and lateral,
- Thorax; antero-posterior,
- One upper limb; antero-posterior (include the hand),
- One lower limb; antero-posterior,
- Pelvis; antero-posterior.

Other images may be required; for example, both sides should be imaged if there is clinical asymmetry and computed tomography and magnetic resonance imaging for detailed evaluation of specific skeletal and systemic malformations.

Patients will generally present to rheumatology clinics during childhood or adolescence and it is important that the skeletal survey is undertaken on presentation. Many diagnostic features are no longer apparent in the mature skeleton following closure of the epiphyseal plates making a firm diagnosis difficult to establish. A diagnosis may be made following identification of the major areas of bone abnormality. A useful approach includes examination for the following criteria:

- Location within the limb—rhizomelic, mesomelic, acromelic;
- Location within the long bone—epiphysis, metaphysis, diaphysis;
- Spine involvement—generalized, localized;
- Skull involvement—vault, base;
- Bone density—decreased, increased;
- Bone shape

  Long bones—dumbell, undertubulated, overtubulated, bowed,

  Pelvis, iliac wings—square, flared, tall, crescentic,

  Pelvis, acetabula—sloping, trident,

  Pelvis, iliac crests—lace-like,

  Spine, vertebral bodies—bullet, hooked, scalloped, beaked, wafer;
- Other patterns—striations, stippling;
- Characteristic bone features—exostoses, enchondromata, dislocations, overgrowth, pseudarthroses, short ribs, clubfeet.

The final diagnosis will include a combination of findings and the name often incorporates the major areas affected—for example, 'craniodiaphyseal dysplasia', 'spondyloepiphyseal dysplasia', or 'acromesomelic dysplasia'.

The importance of establishing an accurate diagnosis cannot be overemphasized. Only then can the prognosis be predicted and potential complications indicated from a knowledge of the natural history of the disorder. With an accurate diagnosis, planned management can be introduced to include appropriate investigations and treatment when possible. Treatment may be preventative, curative, or cosmetic. With an accurate diagnosis genetic counselling can be offered to both the patient and to the family. In the context of patients presenting for rheumatological assessment in childhood and adolescence, the clinical features are likely to include a combination of joint problems (pain, stiffness, deformity, swelling, contractures, laxity, dislocations), spinal problems (pain, stiffness, deformity), and systemic problems (autoimmune, skin, eyes). This limits the diagnostic possibilities and based on the international classification, only 11 of the 33 groups (Table 1) merit detailed consideration. In general, joint problcms indicate a major abnormality of epiphyseal growth and development.

Only a few dysplasias will be considered in some detail and the reader is referred to the 'Further reading' section at the end of the chapter for further information.

Group 6

Diastrophic dysplasia

This condition, inherited in an autosomal recessive manner, presents at birth with short stature, severe talipes equinovarus deformities, thickening of the pinnae, short, proximally placed thumbs due to short first metacarpals giving a characteristic 'hitch hiker' appearance, and sometimes a cleft palate. The chromosome locus is at 5q22-q23; the gene is a sulfate transporter gene.

Table 1 Table from the international nomenclature classification including conditions that may present with joint problems

Group Number	Group heading	Diagnoses
6	Diastrophic dysplasia group	Diastrophic dysplasia Multiple epiphyseal dysplasia AR type
8	Type II collagenopathies	Spondyloepiphyseal dysplasia (SED) Congenita Spondyloepimetaphyseal dysplasia (SEMD) Strudwick type Kniest dysplasia SED Namaqualand type Spondyloperipheral dysplasia Mild SED with premature onset Arthrosis
9	Type XI collagenopathies	Stickler dysplasia type I Stickler dysplasia type II Stickler dysplasia type III Marshall syndrome Otospondylomegaepiphyseal dysplasia (OSMED)
10	Other spondyloepi-(meta)-physeal [SE(M)D] dysplasias	X-linked SED tarda SEMD Handigodu type Progressive pseudorheumatoid dysplasia Dyggve–Melchior–Clausen dysplasia Wolcott–Rallison dysplasia Immuno-osseous dysplasia (Schimke) Schwartz–Jampel syndrome SEMD with joint laxity (SEMDJL) SEMD with multiple dislocations (Hall) SPONASTRIME dysplasia SEMD short limb-abnormal Calcification type SEMD Pakistani type Anauxetic dysplasia
11	Multiple epiphyseal dysplasia and pseudoachondroplasia	Pseudoachondroplasia Multiple epiphyseal dysplasia (MED) Familial hip dysplasia (Beukes)
14	Spondylometaphyseal dysplasias	Spondylometaphyseal dysplasia (SMD) Koslowski type SMD Sutcliffe/corner fracture type SMD with severe genu valgum
15	Brachyolmia spondylodysplasias	Hobaek type Maroteaux type Autosomal dominant type
21	Multiple dislocations with dysplasias	Larsen syndrome Larsen-like syndromes
22	Dysostosis multiplex group	Mucopolysaccharidosis (MPS) IH MPS IS MPS II MPS IIIA MPS IIIB MPS IIIC MPS IIID MPS IVA MPS IVB MPS VI MPS VII Fucosidosis a-Mannosidosis b-Mannosidosis Aspartylglucosaminuria GM1 gangliosidosis Sialidosis Sialic acid storage disease Galactosialidosis Multiple sulfatase deficiency Mucolipidosis II Mucolipidosis III
32	Osteolyses	Multicentric carpal–tarsal osteolysis with and without nephropathy Winchester syndrome Torg syndrome Hadju–Cheney syndrome Mandibuloacral syndrome Familial expansile osteolysis Juvenile hyaline fibromatosis (including systemic juvenile hyalinosis)

Radiology:

- Abnormal epiphyses give rise to joint problems;
- Mild platyspondyly which progresses to kyphoscoliosis.

Multiple epiphyseal dysplasia autosomal recessive type

This condition is located at the same chromosome locus as diastrophic dysplasia, presents in childhood, and has mild epiphyseal abnormalities predominantly involving the hips and hands [Fig. 1(a–c)].

Group 8

All the conditions in this group have abnormalities of Type II collagen as a result of mutations in the COL2AI gene on chromosome 12q13.1–q13.3. Type II collagen is found in cartilage, the vitreous of the eye and the inner ear and the conditions all have multiple joint and spine involvement of varying severity. Many also have mid-face hypoplasia, a cleft palate, myopia leading to retinal detachment, and deafness.

Spondyloepiphyseal dysplasia (SED) congenita

This autosomal dominant condition presents at birth with short stature, a flat face, and sometimes with a cleft palate. Myopia develops. There is a waddling gait. Management includes early cleft palate repair. Regular orthopaedic review should be undertaken for coxa vara, posterior hip dislocation, lumbar lordosis, kyphoscoliosis, cervical spine instability, genu valgum, and premature osteoarthritis. Limb lengthening procedures are not usually recommended in this condition. Ophthalmological review will evaluate myopia and prevent retinal detachment.

Radiology:

- Delayed epiphyseal ossification of capital femoral epiphyses; epiphyses at the knees; pubic rami;
- Progressive, severe coxa vara deformity and high-riding greater trochanters leading to a waddling gait;
- Horizontal acetabular roofs;

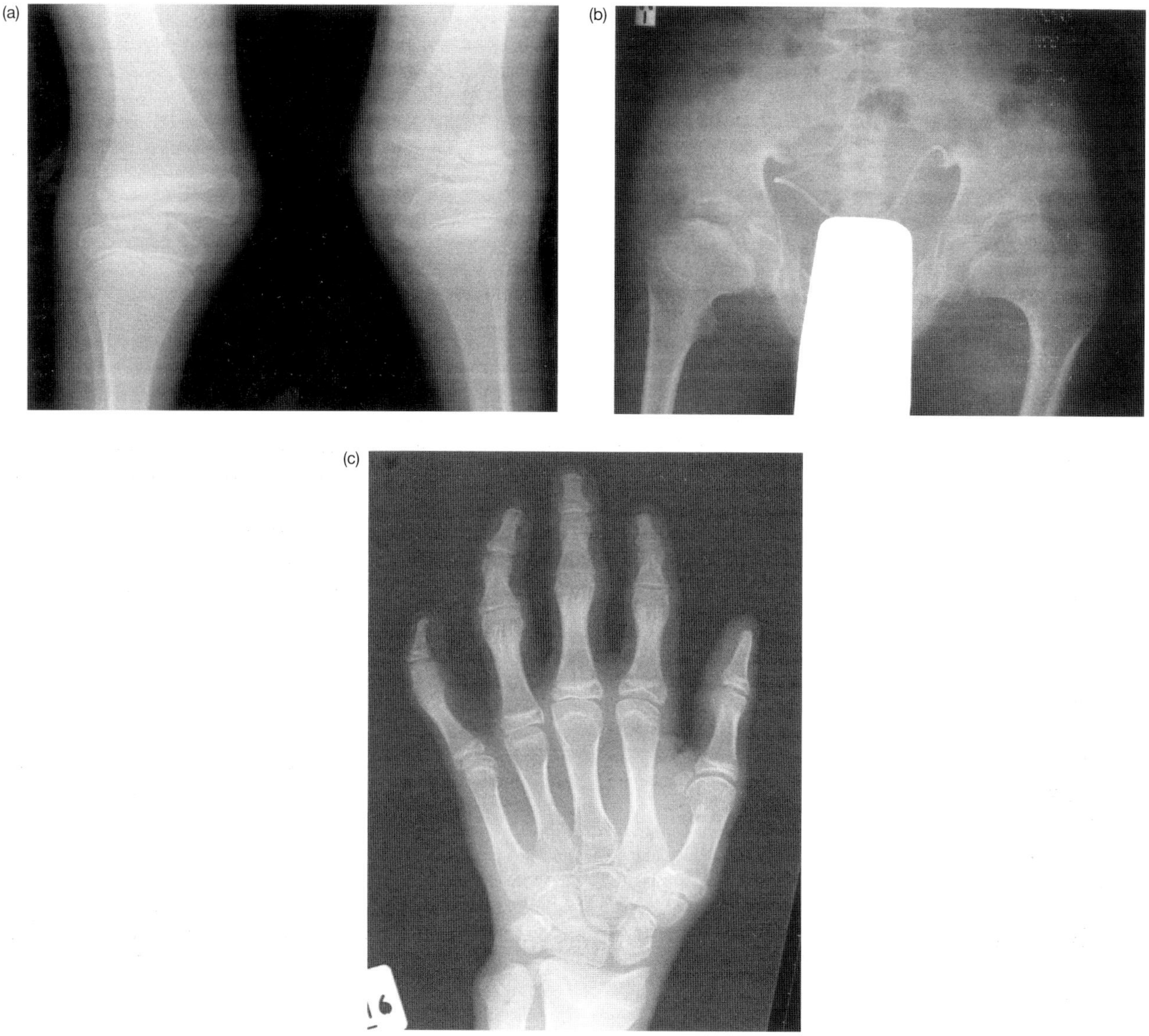

Fig. 1 (a) Multiple epiphyseal dysplasia autosomal recessive type, age 9 years. The antero-posterior view of the knees shows flared metaphyses, flattened epiphyses, joint space narrowing and subluxation. (b) Multiple epiphyseal dysplasia autosomal recessive type, age 12 years. The antero-posterior view of the pelvis shows severe flattening of the capital femoral epiphyses, short, broad femoral necks in various position and irregular, sloping acetabula. (c) Multiple epiphyseal dysplasia autosomal recessive type, age 14 years. The postero-anterior radiograph of the hand shows mild flexion deformities of the fingers with prominent joints and narrow joint spaces with wide metaphyses and flattened, angular epiphyses. There is a radial slope of the epiphysis of the second metacarpal and 'chevron' deformities or large cone-shaped epiphyses of the distal radius and ulna, all features of classic diastrophic dysplasia.

- Generalized platyspondyly
  - Infancy—anisospondyly with L1 being larger than L5. Oval vertebral bodies,
  - Childhood—pear-shaped vertebral bodies with mild posterior constriction and rounded anteriorly. Kyphoscoliosis; cervical kyphosis; cervical instability;
- Short ribs; small thoracic cage;
- Short long-bones and short or even absent femoral necks;
- Normal hands and feet.

Spondyloepimetaphyseal dysplasia (SEMD) type Strudwick

SEMD type Strudwick was identified as a specific variant form of SED congenita in 1982 by several authors (Anderson et al. 1982; Bartsocas et al. 1982), although Spranger and Maroteaux (1982, 1983) questioned whether it should be considered a separate entity. Both conditions represent Type II collagenopathies and are inherited in an autosomal dominant manner. Reports of affected siblings appear to represent parental mosaicism rather than an autosomal recessive inheritance. (Anderson et al. 1982). The gene is linked to chromosome 12q13 and mutations in the COL2A1 chains have been demonstrated (Murray et al. 1989; Vikkula et al. 1993; Tiller et al. 1995; Kaitilla et al. 1996). At birth, the patients are noted to have short limbs and a short trunk, with a cleft palate, small chest, and protuberant abdomen. Respiratory distress may be present. Later myopia develops and this may progress to retinal detachment. There is mild dysmorphism with a flat face and hypertelorism. Stature is significantly reduced and a waddling gait, genu valgum (or varum), and pronounced lumbar lordosis develop. The hands and feet are relatively normal. Intelligence and life expectancy are normal, although lung function may be compromised.

Radiology:

- Infancy—identical to SED congenita;
- Childhood—metaphyses expanded; striking flocculated, dappled fragmentation; islands of relative sclerosis. Initially apparent in the proximal femora. Ulna and fibula more severely affected than radius and tibia;
- Rarely, deforming pseudarthroses cause humerus varus or tibia recurvatum.

Stickler syndrome

This autosomal dominant condition may present at birth with the Pierre-Robin sequence of micrognathia and cleft palate. Stature is usually normal but there is mid-face hypoplasia, severe myopia, and deafness. Some patients with Stickler syndrome do not have mutations in the COL2AI gene, but in the COL11A1 gene located on chromosome 1p21. They have the same phenotype and presentation but most do not have the ocular involvement.

Radiology:

- Early childhood—flattening of capital femoral epiphyses develops leading to hip pain and premature osteoarthritis;
- Localized or generalized platyspondyly resulting in kyphoscoliosis;
- Premature osteoarthritis.

Group 9

The dysplasias in this group have mutations of Type XI collagen and many have Stickler syndrome.

Otospondylomegaepiphyseal dysplasia (OSMED)

This may have autosomal dominant or recessive inheritance and presents at birth with short stature. Deafness develops.

Radiology:

- Generalized platyspondyly;
- Short long bones; large epiphyses; flared metaphyses causing prominent joints.

Group 10

X-linked spondyloepiphyseal dysplasia tarda

This X-linked dominant condition results from a mutation of the SEDLIN gene and is located at Xp22.2–p22.1. Patients present in late childhood with a stiff, painful back and a stocky build with a disproportionately short trunk.

Radiology:

- Spine—characteristic dense mounds of bone on posterior two-thirds of upper and lower vertebral endplates (Fig. 2);
- Mild flattening of capital femoral epiphyses causing premature osteoarthritis.

Autosomal dominant and recessive forms of spondyloepiphyseal dysplasia tarda (SEDT) have been described. It is not possible to differentiate between them on clinical or radiological grounds. They both show severe generalized platyspondyly with narrow disc spaces and an increase in the antero-posterior diameters of the vertebral bodies.

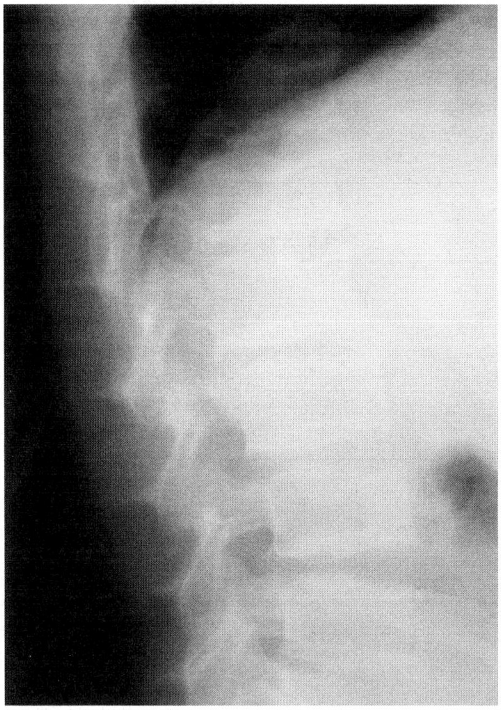

Fig. 2 X-linked SEDT, age 21 years. The lateral radiograph shows platyspondyly with dense mounds of bone on the posterior two-thirds of the vertebral end-plates, a diagnostic feature.

SED Handigodu type

This condition is thought to be the same as Mselini joint disease and to be inherited in an autosomal dominant manner. There is a chronic polyarthritis, presenting in childhood with limitation of movement affecting hips, knees, and ankles. There is mild short stature (Lockitch et al. 1973).

Radiology:

- Irregular, flattened epiphyses causing premature osteoarthritis;
- Protrusio acetabulae;
- Short, deformed distal ends of ulnae;
- Short metacarpals.

Progressive pseudorheumatoid dysplasia

This was first described by Wynne-Davies et al. (1982) as SED tarda with progressive arthropathy, and further delineated by Spranger et al. (1983). Inheritance is autosomal recessive and appears to be more common in Asians. Presentation is between the ages of 5 and 10 years with short stature, a painful stiff back, painful swollen fingers, and painful hips and knees. Acute flare-ups occur and the clinical picture is highly reminiscent of chronic juvenile arthritis (Lewkonia and Beck-Hansen 1992). All the acute phase reactants are normal, as is the blood count, and there are no immune complexes present. Rheumatoid factor, antinuclear antibodies, and DNA are negative. Progressive bony enlargement with limitation of function occurs, affecting the proximal interphalangeal joints in particular. Spinal stenosis may occur as a complication. Odontoid hypoplasia may be present. Premature osteoarthritis requires early hip replacements and pseudogout is a recognized complication (Bradley 1987).

Radiology:

- Large, mildly irregular epiphyses;
- Generalized osteopaenia;
- Flexion of the fingers; expanded distal ends of proximal phalanges;
- Generalized platyspondyly;
- Vertebral bodies increased AP diameter, vertebral end plates irregular, disc spaces narrow, pedicles short [Fig. 3(a)–(c)].

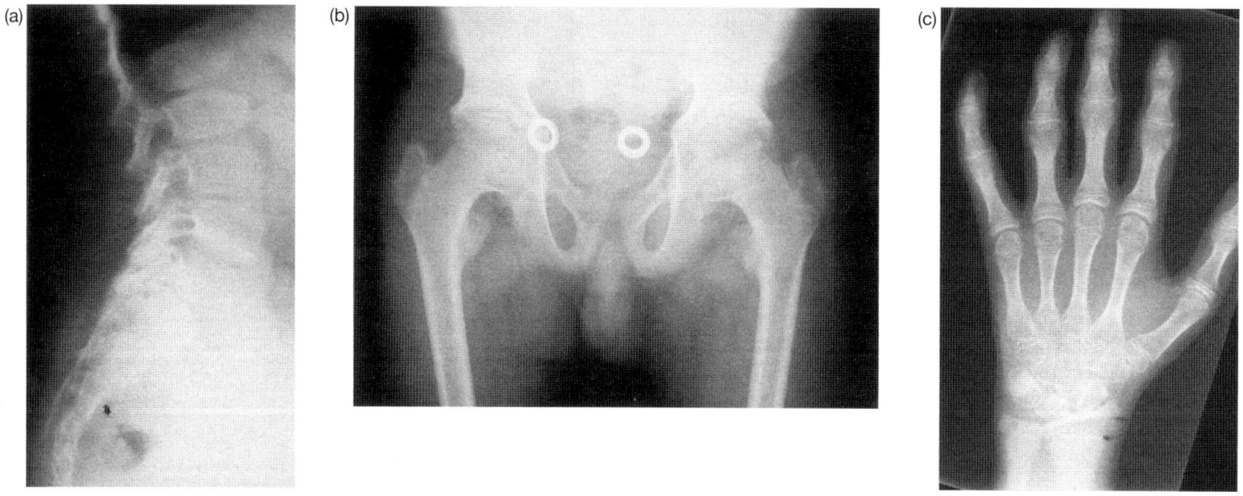

Fig. 3 (a) The lateral radiograph of the spine of an 11-year-old with pseudorheumatoid SEDT shows platyspondyly with some anterior wedging and narrow disc spaces. The lumbar pedicles are short and there is some posterior scalloping. (b) Pseudorheumatoid SEDT in an 11-year-old. His 6-year-old brother was similarly affected. The antero-posterior view of the pelvis shows deep acetabula, relatively large but irregular capital femoral epiphyses and coxa vara. (c) Pseudorheumatoid SEDT in an 11-year-old. The postero-anterior view of the hand shows mild flexion deformities of the fingers, large proximal interphalangeal joints due to expansion of the distal ends of the proximal phalanges, some joint space narrowing, and periarticular osteoporosis. The distal radial and ulnar epiphyses are relatively large.

Dyggve–Melchior–Clausen disease

This condition may be autosomal recessive or X-linked recessive and was first described in 1962 by Dyggve et al. The patients present in early childhood with short stature, coarse facies, a short barrel-shaped thorax, and a significant number have microcephaly with severe mental retardation. The X-linked pedigrees are more likely to have normal intelligence (Yunis et al. 1980). There is a stiff back, restriction of movement of joints, and contractures. Odontoid hypoplasia leads to instability and cord compression if unrecognized (Naffah and Taleb 1974). Progressive dislocation of the capital femoral epiphyses may occur [Fig. 4(a) and (b)].

Radiology:

- Generalized platyspondyly. Central notch on upper and lower vertebral end plates;
- Small, irregular epiphyses;
- Irregular metaphyses;
- Iliac crests irregular (lace-like);
- Inferior angles of scapulae irregular.

Spondyloepimetaphyseal dysplasia

This is a descriptive term of major radiological abnormalities of the spine, epiphyses, and metaphyses of a disparate group of disorders with differing phenotypes, modes of inheritance, and detailed radiographic abnormalities. Several clearly delineated types are recognized but the term SEMD is often used as a general purely descriptive or generic term when a precise diagnosis is not known and does not constitute a definite diagnostic label. In this latter situation it is not possible to predict the evolution of the changes, the mode of inheritance or the complications, except that in general patients with a predominant epiphyseal component as part of a skeletal dysplasia will develop premature osteoarthritis especially of the weight bearing large joints.

SEMD with joint laxity

Torrington and Beighton (1991) identified two Afrikaans-speaking women as the progenitors of this condition in South Africa in the seventeenth century. SEMD with joint laxity was first described by Beighton and Kozlowski (1980). Although the vast majority of patients have been identified in South Africa, other cases have been described in North and South America and Europe (Bradburn and Hall 1995; Pia-Neto et al. 1996). Inheritance is autosomal recessive.

At birth there is short stature and joint and ligamentous laxity with hip dislocation in about one-fourth of patients and dislocation of the radial heads. Kyphoscoliosis is present and is rapidly progressive, in severe cases leading to paraplegia or early death in mid childhood from cor pulmonale. A mobile talipes equino-varus deformity is present. The face is oval with a long philtrum and prominent eyes with variably blue sclerae and hyperelastic, soft skin. Almost half the patients have a cleft or high arched palate. Congenital cardiac anomalies, predominantly septal defects, may be present. Other reported findings include mental retardation, myopia, lens dislocation, and Hirschprung's disease. Differentiation is required from other SEMDs, diastrophic dysplasia, Larsen syndrome, and the mucopolysaccharidoses.

Radiology:

- Severe and progressive kyphoscoliosis;
- Platyspondyly; biconvex vertebral bodies; irregular endplates;
- Iliac wings flared, sacro-sciatic notches short;
- Epiphyseal ossification delayed, metaphyses wide and irregular, trabecular pattern coarse;
- Coxa valga, hip dislocation, dislocation of radial heads;
- Distal radius and ulna expanded;
- Traction exostoses;
- Tubular bones of hands and feet short.

SEMD with multiple dislocations (type Hall)

Langer et al. (1997) initially identified this as a distinct entity and illustrated one case included in a paper on SPONASTRIME dysplasia. They identified a further case in a paper on SPONASTRIME dysplasia by Camera et al. (1994). Hall et al. (1998) described three further unrelated cases and used the term SEMD with multiple dislocations to differentiate it from the group known as SEMD with joint laxity. There is an equal gender distribution and inheritance is autosomal dominant. Presentation is at birth with marked hypotonia, short stature, and some facial dysmorphism with midface hypoplasia and a depressed nasal bridge. None of the patients has had a cleft palate. Intelligence is normal. There is progressive joint laxity with hip dislocation

(a)

(b)

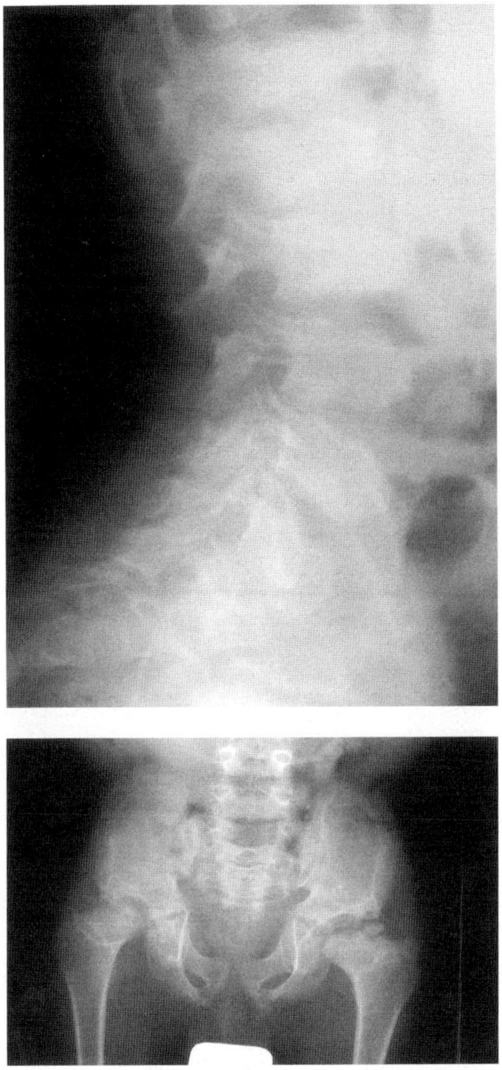

Fig. 4 (a) A 10-year-old boy with Dyggve–Melchior–Clausen disease. His 7-year-old brother was also affected. The lateral radiograph of the spine shows platyspondyly with relatively wide intervertebral spaces and the characteristic central notches on the vertebral end-plates. There is some posterior scalloping of the vertebral bodies. (b) The antero-posterior radiograph of the pelvis of a 10-year-old with Dyggve–Melchior–Clausen disease. The iliac wings are small and show the 'lace-like' irregular ossification of the iliac crests. The capital femoral epiphyses are small, fragmented, laterally placed, and subluxed. The femoral necks are short and in varus.

and genu valgum and dislocations at the knees with weight bearing. A mild scoliosis develops during childhood. Management is aimed at maintaining mobility and preventing dislocations. Knee braces have helped the severe joint laxity here. The major differentiation is from SPONASTRIME dysplasia. This is inherited in an autosomal recessive manner. Radiologically, there is severe platyspondyly in infancy and early childhood. The characteristic sclerotic metaphyseal striations do not become apparent until mid childhood. Apart from a delay of bone maturation, modelling of the tubular bones in the hands is normal.

Radiology:

- Epiphyses delayed ossification, small, flattened, irregular;
- Metaphyses irregular, longitudinal sclerotic striations;
- Femoral necks narrow, curved, and tapered;
- Knees, progressive subluxation through childhood;
- Spine, mild platyspondyly, minor irregularity of vertebral endplates, interpedicular distances fail to widen in the normal manner, sacral spinal dysraphism, thoracic vertebral bodies pear-shaped with mild posterior constriction; adult vertebral bodies biconcave;
- Hands, small epiphyses and carpal bones, overall reduction in size of carpus, gracile metacarpals, squared distal ends of middle phalanges [Fig. 5(a)–(d)].

SEMD Iraqi type or type Sohat

Sohat et al. (1993) reported three affected individuals in a large Iraqi Jewish family and Figuera et al. (1994) reported a further case from Mexico. Presentation is at birth and inheritance autosomal recessive. Clinically, there is short stature because of limb shortening, a protuberant abdomen and hepatosplenomegaly, lumbar lordosis, a short neck, joint laxity, and genu varum deformity. The face is described as being round with thin lips.

Radiology:

- Tubular bones short, irregular, flared metaphyses, delayed epiphyseal ossification;
- Short tubular bones of hands, metaphyseal cupping;
- Coxa vara, short femoral necks;
- Genu varum, long fibula;
- Spine, platyspondyly, central notches of superior and inferior vertebral end plates, narrow interpedicular distances;
- Pelvis, iliac bones short, wide, acetabular roofs horizontal;
- Thorax, short, mildly narrow. Ribs, pronounced cupping of anterior ends;
- Skull, multiple wormian bones.

SEMD Irapa type

This autosomal recessive condition was first described by Arias et al. (1976) in the Irapa Indians of Venezuela and later in a Mexican family by Hernandez et al. (1980). Clinical presentation is about the age of 5 years with rhizomelic shortening, walking difficulty, and joint pains. The joints are enlarged with a reduced range of movement and premature osteoarthritis develops. There is brachydactyly but the index fingers and second toes are relatively long.

Radiology:

- Spine, generalized platyspondyly, vertebral end-plate irregularity;
- Tubular bones short; wide irregular metaphyses of proximal femora and distal humeri, epiphyses delayed ossification;
- Coxa vara;
- Hands; carpal bones small, irregular; carpal fusions; 3rd–5th metacarpals short and wide distally;
- Pelvis; iliac bones short, acetabula dysplastic, symphysis pubis irregular;
- Ribs; anterior ends expanded with irregular ossification;
- Generalized osteoporosis.

SEMD short limb-abnormal calcification type

This autosomal recessive disorder was first described by Borochowitz et al. (1993) and eight further cases by Langer et al. (1993). Presentation is at birth with severe limb shortening, short hands and feet, and a relatively long trunk. There is some joint laxity. Kyphoscoliosis subsequently develops leading to a short trunk. The thorax is narrow. There is facial dysmorphism with a relatively large head and a prominent forehead with midface hypoplasia, a broad, depressed nasal bridge, short, upturned nose, hypertelorism, and prominent eyes. The philtrum is long and there is micrognathia.

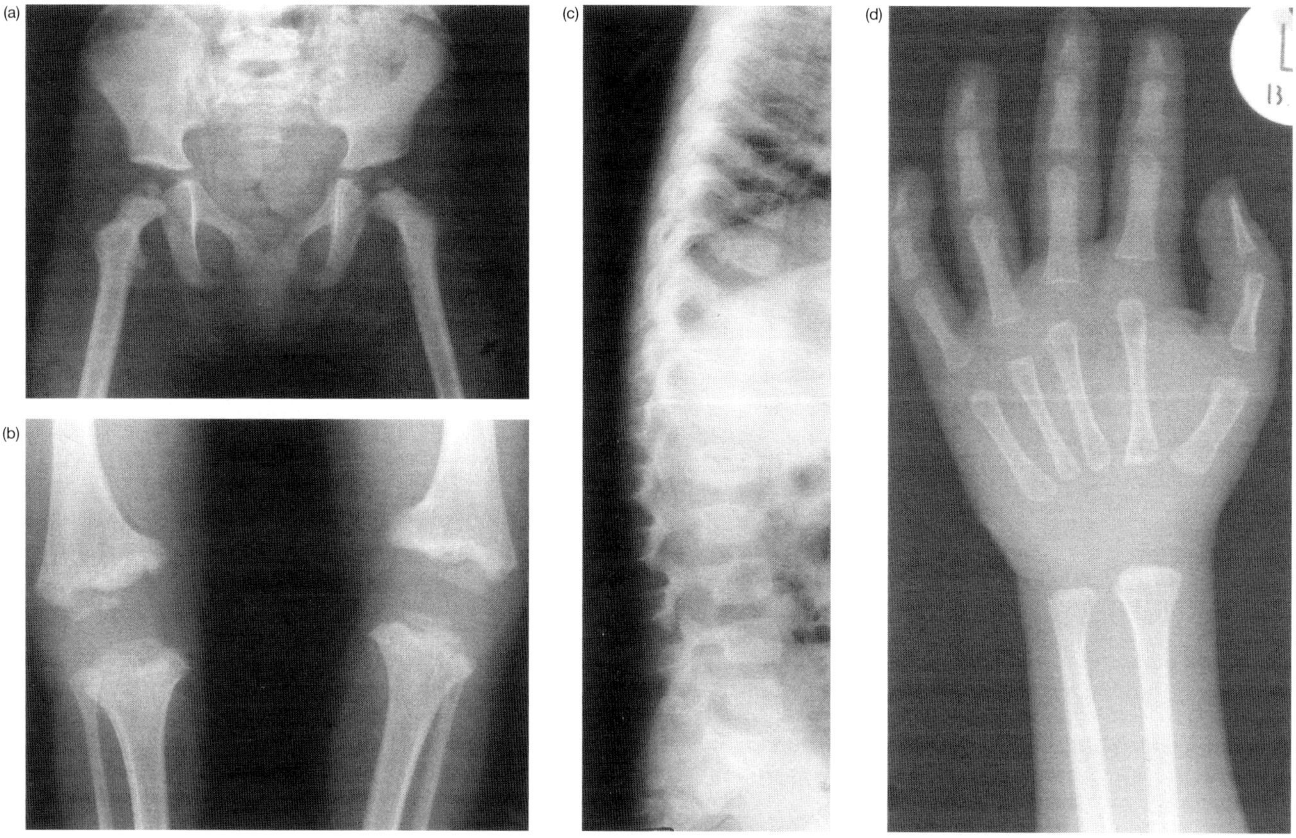

Fig. 5 (a) SEMD with multiple dislocations, type Hall, in a 3-year-old. The antero-posterior view of the pelvis shows long, slender femoral necks and small irregular capital femoral epiphyses. (b) The antero-posterior view of the knees in a 3-year-old with SEMD with multiple dislocations showing bilateral subluxations, small flattened epiphyses, and irregular slightly sclerotic metaphyses. (c) SEMD with multiple dislocations at 3 years. The lateral radiograph of the spine shows mild vertebral end-plate irregularity. In the thoracic region, the vertebrae are 'pear' shaped and in the lumbar spine there is posterior scalloping. (d) The postero-anterior view of the hand shows significant delay in carpal and epiphyseal ossification at the age of 3 years. The metacarpals are unusually slender. Early longitudinal sclerotic striations are present at the distal radial metaphysis.

Complications include cervical cord compression from odontoid hypoplasia and ligamentous laxity, with subluxation of C1 and C2; cor pulmonale as a result of a small thorax and progressive kyphoscoliosis and optic atrophy. Ultrasound can identify the short limbs *in utero*, but the diagnosis can only be confirmed if there have been previously affected sibs or after radiographic evaluation.

In infancy, the premature stippling requires differentiation from chondrodysplasia punctata. The dumbell appearance of the long bones, narrow thorax, and progressive kyphoscoliosis may resemble metatropic dysplasia. Other SEMDs require consideration, particularly SEMD metatropic type and SEMD Strudwick type both of which have an autosomal dominant inheritance. The expanded metaphyses with flocculated ossification and the changes in the spine may be confused with metaphyseal dysplasia type Jansen.

Radiology:

- Infancy; premature stippled calcification of epiphyses, laryngeal cartilages, tracheal and bronchial cartilage, and costochondral junctions;
- Advanced ossification of carpal centres and iliac crest apophyses;
- Long bones short, metaphyses wide and flared. Stippled areas and adjacent metaphyses progress to larger flocculated areas interspersed with lucent areas;
- Tubular bones of hands and feet short with triangular distal phalanges. Calcanea small and stippled;
- Ribs short with cupped anterior and posterior ends. Clavicles relatively long;
- Spine; mild, generalized platyspondyly, wide intervertebral spaces. Vertebral bodies pear-shaped or rounded, deficient ossification posteriorly, mild anterior tonguing. Poor ossification of vertebral bodies in cervical spine. Atlanto-axial subluxation.

SPONASTRIME dysplasia

This autosomal recessive condition was first described by Fanconi et al. (1983) who described four sisters. The term 'SPONASTRIME' is an acronym derived from SPOndylar, NAsal anomalies, and STRIation of MEtaphyses. The dysmorphic features include a depressed nasal bridge, short nose, frontal bossing, and a relatively large head. Camera et al. (1993) and Verloes et al. (1995) described a sub-group with microcephaly and mental retardation. Short stature becomes apparent from birth. A progressive kyphoscoliosis and lumbar lordosis develop. The skeletal changes may be more severe in affected males. Management is largely concerned with dislocations and joint laxity.

Differentiation is required from other forms of SEMD and in particular from SEMD with multiple dislocations. The metaphyseal striations are similar to osteopathia striata but there are no changes in the spine in this condition.

Radiology:

- Spine; marked platyspondyly at birth, wide intervertebral spaces, mild posterior constriction of vertebral bodies with rounded or tongued anterior borders. Increasing height of biconcave vertebral bodies during early childhood;

- Proximal femora, characteristic 'spanner-like' appearance with prominent lesser trochanters and short curved tapered femoral necks;
- Hip dislocation;
- Infancy and early childhood, metaphyses and epiphyses mildly irregular. From 4 years, irregular longitudinal metaphyseal sclerotic striations.

Group 11

Multiple epiphyseal dysplasia

This is one of the more common skeletal dysplasias and patients present in childhood with mild short stature and painful, stiff hips or knees. The fingers may be short. Inheritance is autosomal dominant and there may be a family history. Complications include contractures and premature osteoarthritis, which often results in early hip replacement. Some families have been mapped to 1p32–p33 (Briggs et al. 1994) which is close to the COL9A2 gene and other families map to 19q13 (Oehlmann et al. 1994) with mutations in the cartilage oligomeric matrix protein (COMP) gene (Briggs et al. 1995).

Radiology:

- Epiphyses (commonly capital femoral epiphyses) flattened, irregular, fragmented, sclerotic;
- Hands; delayed bone maturation, epiphyses angular, cone-shaped (causing premature fusion and short phalanges and metacarpals;
- Spine; vertebral end-plate irregularity at thoraco-lumbar junction.

Pseudoachondroplasia

This condition presents at about the age of two with short stature and a waddling gait. Inheritance is autosomal dominant and recurrence in sibs has been shown to be the result of gonadal mosaicism in a parent (Hall et al. 1988). Small irregular epiphyses lead to joint problems with premature osteoarthritis. Dominant pedigrees have been mapped to 19q13 (Briggs et al. 1993; Hecht et al. 1993) and mutations have been demonstrated in the COMP gene by Briggs et al. (1995) and Hecht et al. (1995).

Radiology:

- Epiphyses, small irregular, delayed ossification;
- Metaphyses, flared irregular;
- Spine, in childhood mild platyspondyly, vertebral bodies biconvex with anterior tongues and long pedicles.

Group 22: the dysostosis multiplex group

Mucopolysaccharidoses

These conditions are due to deficiency of enzymes involved in the metabolism of glycosaminoglycans. There is variable severity within the group with some such as the Hurler type (MPS IH) and Maroteaux–Lamy type (MPS VI), presenting in infancy or early childhood with progressive coarsening of the facies, short stature, hepatosplenomegaly, cardiovascular problems, mental retardation, and corneal clouding and others such as types Scheie (MPS IS) or Sanfilippo (MPS III) presenting later with more normal stature with progressive stiffening and contractures of the joints of the hands, elbows, and knees. Intelligence is normal in Scheie and in Morquio disease (MPS IV) and behavioural difficulties occur in Sanfilippo. Inheritance is autosomal recessive in all these conditions except for Hunter (MPS II) which is X-linked recessive. Differentiation between the types relies on laboratory analysis, particularly of urine, leucocytes, and fibroblast culture. Certain radiological findings are common to all this group (dysostosis multiplex) with variable expression of severity, with the exception of Morquio disease.

There is flaring of the iliac wings with shallow, sloping acetabula and small, flattened capital femoral epiphyses. There is a generalized epiphyseal abnormality with mild irregularity of the adjacent metaphyses. The ribs and clavicles are wide and the long bones undermodelled. In the hands there is proximal pointing of the metacarpals and the carpal bones are small

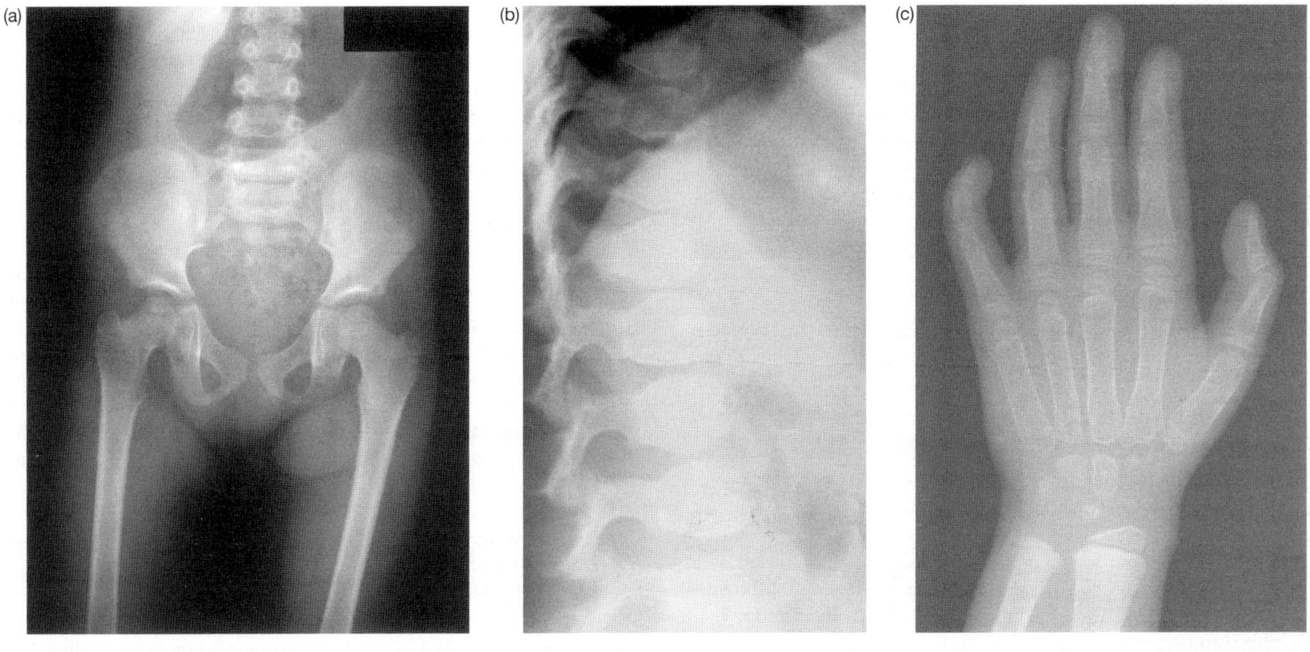

Fig. 6 (a) MPS Scheie (I-S) at the age of 9 years. The antero-posterior view of the pelvis shows flared iliac wings, small capital femoral epiphyses, and short, broad femoral necks. (b) MPS Scheie (I-S) at the age of 9 years. The lateral view of the spine shows rounded vertebral bodies and anterior disc herniation with end-plate irregularity and disc space narrowing at the D11–D12 level. (c) MPS Scheie (I-S). The postero-anterior view of the hand at the age of 9 years shows mild flexion deformities of the fingers and delayed ossification of the carpal centres. The short tubular bones are undermodelled with relatively wide diaphyses.

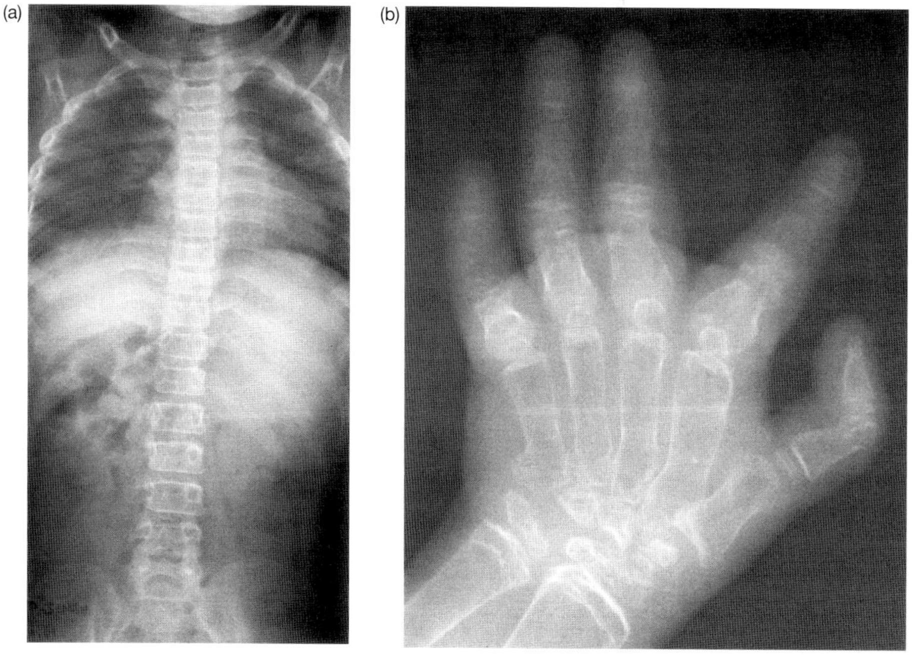

Fig. 7 (a) Winchester syndrome in a 7-year-old. The antero-posterior view of the spine shows severe osteoporosis and wide clavicles and ribs. (b) Winchester syndrome in a 7-year-old. The postero-anterior view of the hand shows osteoporosis and osteolysis and destruction of the carpal bones. The phalanges and metacarpals are wide and there is subluxation of the small joints in the hand.

and irregular. The changes in the spine are variable, ranging from 'hook-shaped' vertebral bodies to wedged or oval. The height of the vertebral bodies is quite well preserved. There may be hypoplasia of the odontoid peg but this is generally not clinically significant. The skull vault may be large with a homogeneous 'ground-glass' opacity. The pituitary fossa is elongated or J-shaped and the mastoid air cells fail to pneumatize. In the mandible the coronoid and condylar processes are tapered and short and the roots of the lower teeth may protrude through the inferior bony cortex [Fig. 6(a)–(c)].

Morquio disease can be differentiated by a normal skull, significant platyspondyly with anterior tongues of the vertebral bodies. The odontoid peg is absent and this combined with ligamentous laxity leads to subluxation, which can progress to cord compression unless stabilized early. The capital femoral epiphyses are initially well developed at the age of 2, but then gradually resorb and have completely disappeared by the age of 10. Hip dislocation may develop. From about the age of 4, there is progressive stiffening and joint enlargement with genu valgum deformity. A kyphosis develops and there is sternal protrusion. Additional complications include carpal tunnel syndrome and deafness.

Group 32: osteolyses

Winchester syndrome

Winchester syndrome was first described by Winchester et al. (1969) in two siblings whose parents were first cousins. Presentation is usually in infancy with symmetrical, painful swelling of the hands, fingers, wrists, and ankles. Intermittent polyarthralgia results in progressive joint contractures. Corneal clouding and coarsening of the face develop. Oval or linear raised areas of thickened skin develop over the back, flank and lateral aspects of the arms. Growth is retarded. Increased urinary oligosaccharide excretion may be present (Lambert et al. 1989; Winter 1989).

Radiology:

- Generalized osteopaenia;
- Carpal and tarsal bones, progressive osteolysis;
- Destruction of small joints of hands and feet [Fig. 7(a) and (b)].

References

Agarwal, S.S. et al. (1997). Mseleni and Handigodu familial osteoarthropathies: syndromic identity? *American Journal of Medical Genetics* **72** (4), 435–9.

Al-Gazali, L.I., Bakalinova, D., and Sztriha, L. (1996). Spondylo-meta-epiphyseal dysplasia, short limb, abnormal calcification type. *Clinical Dysmorphology* **5**, 197–206.

Anderson, C.E. et al. (1982). Spondylometepiphyseal dysplasia, Strudwick type. *American Journal of Medical Genetics* **13**, 243–56.

Arias, S., Mota, M., and Pinto-Cisternas, J. (1976). L'osteochondrodysplasie spondylo-epiphyso-metaphysaire type Irapa. Nouveau nanisme avec rachis et metatarsiens courts. *Nouvelle Presse Medicine* **5**, 319–23.

Arias, S. (1981). Osteochondrodysplasia Irapa type: an ethnic marker gene in two subcontinents. *American Journal of Medical Genetics* **8**, 251–3.

Bartsocas, C.S. et al. (1982). A variant of spondyloepiphyseal dysplasia congenita. *Progress in Clinical Biological Research* **104**, 163.

Beighton, P. and Kozlowski, K. (1980). Spondylo-epi-metaphyseal dysplasia with joint laxity and severe, progressive kyphoscoliosis. *Skeletal Radiology* **5**, 205–12.

Borochowitz, Z. et al. (1993). Spondylo-meta-epiphyseal dysplasia (SMED), short limb-hand type: a congenital familial skeletal dysplasia with distinctive features and histopathology. *American Journal of Medical Genetics* **45**, 320–6.

Bradburn, J.M. and Hall, B.D. (1995). Spondyloepimetaphyseal dysplasia with joint laxity (SEMDJL): clinical and radiological findings in a Guatemalan patient. *American Journal of Medical Genetics* **59**, 234–7.

Bradley, J.D. (1987). Pseudo gout in progressive pseudo-rhumatoid arthritis. *Annals of the Rheumatic Diseases* **46**, 709–12.

Briggs, M.D. et al. (1993). Genetic linkage of mild pseudoachondroplasia (PSACH) to markers in the pericentromeric region of chromosome 19. *Geneomics* **18**, 656–60.

Briggs, M.D. et al. (1994). Genetic mapping of a locus for multiple epiphyseal dysplasia (EDM2) to a region of chromosome 1 containing a type IX collagen gene. *American Journal of Human Genetics* **55**, 678–84.

Briggs, M.D. et al. (1995). Pseudoachondroplasia and multiple epiphyseal dysplasia due to mutations in the cartilage oligomeric matrix protein gene. *Nature Genetics* **10**, 330–6.

Camera, G. et al. (1993). Sponastrime dysplasia: report on two siblings with mental retardation. *Pediatric Radiology* **23**, 611–14.

Camera, G. et al. (1994). Sponastrime dysplasia report on a male patient. *Pediatric Radiology* **24**, 322–4.

Fanconi, S. et al. (1983). The SPONASTRIME dysplasia: familial short-limb dwarfism with saddle nose, spinal alterations and metaphyseal striations. *Helvetica Paediatric Acta* **38**, 267–80.

Figuera, L.E. et al. (1994). Spondyloepimetaphyseal dysplasia (SEMD) Sohat type. *American Journal of Medical Genetics* **51**, 213–15.

Hall, C.M., Elcioglu, N., and Shaw, D.G. (1998). A distinct form of spondyloepimetaphyseal dysplasia with multiple dislocations. *Journal of Medical Genetics* **35**, 566–72.

Hecht, J.T. et al. (1993). Linkage of typical pseudoachondroplasia to chromosome 19. *Genomics* **18**, 661–6.

Hecht, J.T. et al. (1995). Mutations in exon 17B of cartilage oligomeric matrix protein (COMP) cause pseudoachondroplasia. *Nature Genetics* **10**, 325–9.

Hernandez, A., Ramirez, M.L., and Nazara, Z. (1980). Autosomal recessive spondylo-epi-metaphyseal dysplasia (Irapa type) in a Mexican family: delineation of the syndrome. *American Journal of Medical Genetics* **5**, 179–88.

Horn, D. et al. (2001). Anauxetic dysplasia, a spondylometaepiphyseal dysplasia with extreme dwarfism. *Journal of Medical Genetics* **38** (4), 262–5.

Kaitilla, I. et al. (1996). Phenotypic expressions of a Gly154Arg mutation in type II collagen in two unrelated patients with spondyloepimetaphyseal dysplasia (SEMD). *American Journal of Medical Genetics* **63**, 111–22.

Lambert, J.C. et al. (1989). Biochemical and ultrastructural studies of two familial cases of Winchester syndrome. *Journal de Genetique Humaine* **37**, 231–6.

Langer, L.O., Jr. et al. (1993). Further delineation of spondylo-meta-epiphyseal dysplasia, short limb-abnormal calcification type, with emphasis on diagnostic features. *American Journal of Medical Genetics* **45**, 488–500.

Langer, L.O., Jr. et al. (1996). Sponastrime dysplasia: five new cases and review of nine previously published cases. *American Journal of Medical Genetics* **63**, 20–7.

Langer, L.O., Jr., Beals, R.K., and Scott, C.I., Jr. (1997). Sponastrime dysplasia: diagnostic criteria based on five new and six previously published cases. *Pediatric Radiology* **27**, 409–14.

Lockitch, G. et al. (1973). Mseleni joint disease: a pilot study. *South African Medical Journal* **1**, 2283–93.

Lewkonia, R.M. and Beck-Hansen, N.T. (1992). Spondylo-epiphyseal dysplasia tarda simulating juvenile arthritis: clinical and molecular genetic observations. *Clinical and Experimental Rheumatology* **10**, 411–14.

Martignetti, J.A. et al. (2001). Mutation of the matrix metalloproteinase 2 gene (MMP2) causes a multicentric osteolysis and arthritis syndrome. *Nature Genetics* **28**, 261–5.

Murray, L.W. et al. (1989). Type II collagen defects in the chondrodysplasias. 1. Spondyloepiphyseal dysplasias. *American Journal of Human Genetics* **45**, 5–15.

Nicole, S. et al. (2000). Perlecan, the major proteoglycan of basement membranes, is altered in Schwartz–Jampel syndrome (chondrodystrophic myotonia). *Nature Genetics* **26** (4), 480–3.

Oehlmann, R. et al. (1994). Genetic linkage mapping of multiple epiphyseal dysplasia to the pericentromeric region of chromosome 19. *American Journal of Human Genetics* **54**, 3–10.

Pia-Neto, J.M. et al. (1996). Spondyloepimetaphyseal dysplasia with joint laxity (SEMDJL): a Brazilian case. *American Journal of Medical Genetics* **61**, 131–3.

Roby, P. et al. (1999). Autosomal dominant (Beukes) premature degenerative osteoarthropathy of the hip joint maps to an 11cM region on chromosome 4q35. *American Journal of Human Genetics* **64**, 904–8.

Sohat, M. et al. (1993). New form of spondyloepimetaphyseal dysplasia (SEMD) in Jewish family of Iraqi origin. *American Journal of Medical Genetics* **46**, 358–62.

Spranger, J.W. and Maroteaux, P. (1982). Editorial comment: genetic heterogeneity of spondyloepiphyseal dysplasia congenita. *American Journal of Medical Genetics* **13**, 241.

Spranger, J.W. and Maroteaux, P. (1983). Genetic heterogeneity of spondyloepiphyseal dysplasia congenita? *American Journal of Medical Genetics* **14**, 601–2.

Spranger, J. et al. (1983). Progressive pseudo-rheumatoid arthropathy of childhood. A hereditary disorder simulating juvenile rheumatoid arthritis. *European Journal of Paediatrics* **140**, 34–40.

Tiller, G.E. et al. (1995). Dominant mutations in the type II collagen gene, COL2A1, produce spondyloepimetaphyseal dysplasia, Strudwick type. *Nature Genetics* **11**, 87–9 (letter).

Torrington, M. and Beighton, P. (1991). The ancestry of spondyloepimetaphyseal dysplasia with joint laxity (SEMDJL) in South Africa. *Clinical Genetics* **39**, 210–13.

Verloes, A. et al. (1995). Heterogeneity of SPONASTRIME dysplasia: delineation of a variant form with severe mental retardation. *Clinical Dysmorphology* **4**, 208–15.

Vikkula, M. et al. (1993). A mutation in the amino-terminal end of the triple helix of type II collagen causing severe osteochondrodysplasia. *Genomics* **16**, 282–5.

Winchester, P.H. et al. (1989). A new acid mucopolysaccharidosis with skeletal deformities simulating rheumatoid arthritis. *American Journal of Roentgenology* **106**, 121–8.

Winter, R.M. (1989). Syndrome of the month—Winchester's syndrome. *Journal of Medical Genetics* **26**, 772–5.

Wynne-Davies, R., Hall, C., and Ansell, B.M. (1982). Spondylo-epiphyseal dysplasia tarda with progressive arthropathy. *Journal of Bone and Joint Surgery* **64B**, 442–5.

Further reading

Canepa, G., Maroteaux, P., and Pietrogrande, V. *Dysmorphic Syndromes and Constitutional Diseases of the Skeleton.* Padova: Piccin Nuova Libraria S.p.A., 2001.

Hall, C.M. and Washbrook, J. *Radiological Electronic Atlas of Malformation Syndromes and Skeletal Dysplasias.* Oxford: Oxford University Press, 2000.

Hall, C.M. Spondyloepimetaphyseal dysplasia. *Orphanet Encyclopedia*, September 2001, http://orphanet.infobiogen.fr.

Taybi, H. and Lachman, R.S. *Radiology of Syndromes, Metabolic Disorders, and Skeletal Dysplasias.* St Louis MO: Mosby-Year Book Inc., 1996.

Winter, R.M. and Baraitser, M. *London Dysmorphology Database.* Oxford: Oxford University Press, 2001.

6.17 Disorders of the spine

6.17.1 Intervertebral disc disease and other mechanical disorders of the back

Malcolm I.V. Jayson

Introduction

The primary roles of the human spine are to bear the weight of the upper structures of the body, provide flexibility for movements, and protect the vital structures—in particular the spinal cord and the nerves that emerge through the intervertebral foramina. The stresses associated with a lifetime of use, combined with ageing and degenerative changes, and the effects of individual and repeated traumatic episodes are commonly associated with mechanical problems so that degenerative change in the spine is almost a universal experience. Although mechanical and degenerative changes in the lumbar spine are common, the correlation with back pain is weak (Lawrence 1977). Some patients have minor evidence of damage to the spine yet experience major symptoms; others may show advanced degenerative changes and yet be symptom free. Moreover, structural changes in the spine are permanent but the symptoms of back pain are commonly transient. Acute episodes of pain are separated by periods in which symptoms are minimal or absent. We now know that psycho-social factors play a major role in the perception of pain and disability and in particular in the development of chronicity. This complicates our understanding of the pathogenesis of back problems and emphasizes the need for controlled studies of various treatment programmes.

Epidemiology

Back pain is extremely common. Population studies in Britain show a point prevalence of 14 per cent at any one time (Mason 1994), 39 per cent in the last month (Papageorgiou et al. 1995), 37 per cent in the last year (Mason 1994), and a lifetime prevalence of between 58 per cent (Croft and Jayson 1994) and 80 per cent (Waddell 1987). The peak prevalence is between 45 and 59 years although it is common in the young and in the elderly (Papageorgiou et al. 1995). True sciatica appears to be much less frequent. Using strict diagnostic criteria the overall prevalence in the studies by Heliovaara et al. (1987) was estimated to be 5.3 per cent in men and 3.7 per cent in women.

There has been a dramatic increase in the level of disability due to back problem in recent years (Clinical Standards Advisory Group 1994) despite a lack of evidence of any increase in the numbers of back related injuries. Linton et al. (1998) found the prevalence of spinal pain during the past year was 66.3 per cent with 25 per cent having a substantial degree of disability. Thirty-four per cent had reported absenteeism from work. In Britain, in 1993, the total work loss was estimated as approximately 150 000 000 days (Clinical Standards Advisory Group 1994). The prevalence of back disability is increasing rapidly with the numbers of working days lost running at some four times the figures for 20 years ago. Similar changes are found in most countries. There have, however, recently been some signs of improvement (Murphy and Violinn 1999) and there is hope that there is a levelling off or possibly even a decrease in the current levels of back disability. However, this may be due to many cases being classified as stress related injury. Despite these dramatic changes in the morbidity associated with back problems there does not seem to be any change in the nature of back injuries. It seems likely that social, psychological, and employment problems are playing the major role in the dramatic increase in disability.

The costs of back problems are huge. In Britain, the Clinical Standards Advisory Group (1994) estimated that in 1993 the total cost was some £6.5 billion. Cats-Baril and Frymoyer (1991) estimated the cost in the United States to be between $25 and $100 billion in 1990.

There is little difference in the prevalence of back pain and disability between men and women. There is an increased prevalence of low back pain and disability with lower social class; the relationship being stronger in males than females (Walsh et al. 1992; Mason 1994). Many patients report the development of back problems in relation to an accident or injury although this is commonly difficult to evaluate (Mason 1994). Work-related injuries are common (Health and Safety Executive 1993) and the highest incidence appears in the construction industry, the agricultural sector, and in health care workers. Luoma et al. (2000) found an increased risk of low back pain in relationship to signs of disc degeneration but occupational factors played major roles in emphasizing this relationship. There is an association of disc degeneration with heavy manual work (Videman et al. 1990) but this association appears modest. A number of studies have shown an increased lifetime prevalence of back problems in those involved in heavy occupations as compared to light work (Biering-Sorenson 1985; Rihimaki et al. 1989) but it is difficult to know whether this is due to the direct effects of overloading the spine, or repeated minor trauma, or simply because workers with comparable degrees of degenerative change would be unable to perform heavy manual work but could cope with a sedentary job. Mitchell (1985) found that people performing heavy manual work had no increase in the numbers of spells off work with back pain but they were of increased duration.

There is an association between back pain and long-term exposure to driving and vibration (Hulshof and van Zanten 1987) but Drerup (1999) did not find any differences in quantitative analyses of disc structure between workers exposed to long-term whole body vibration and control subjects.

There is also evidence that repeated flexion and rotation of the trunk and lifting at work are moderate risk factors for low back pain especially at great levels of exposure (Hoogendoorn et al. 2000) although again it can be difficult to determine whether the physical activities were causative of the back problem or simply associated with inability to undertake these activities.

Battie et al. (1995) and Sambrook et al. (1999) identified genetic factors as playing an important role in predicting the development of disc degeneration. However, both authors have emphasized that environmental factors are also directly relevant. There are associations of back pain with neck pain (Porter and Hibbert 1983; Papageorgiou et al. 1996) chronic and widespread musculoskeletal pain (Makela 1993; Papageorgiou et al. 1996) and between cigarette smoking and back pain (Goldberg et al. 2000). Possible explanations about smoking include vascular damage and ischaemia leading to degeneration in the spine, an association between smoking and osteoporosis and smoking being associated with psychological distress which also accompanies back pain. There is supportive evidence of the importance of vascular damage (Kurunlahti et al. 2000) when an association between atheromatous lesions in the abdominal aorta and the segmental arteries and low back pain was demonstrated.

Obesity is often blamed as causative of back problems. However, a systematic literature review (Leboeuf-Yde 2000) only found weak evidence supporting this association.

Many patients report their symptoms are worse in cold and damp weather. A prospective study only found a minor evidence of association suggesting that weather conditions may influence subjective reporting of low back pain but the effects are small in magnitude (McGorry et al. 1998).

Psychological distress is common in particular in patients with chronic pain and disability (Vlaeyen and Linton 2000). In a prospective study of a back pain free population, Croft et al. (1996) symptoms of psychological distress predicted the future development of new episodes of low back pain. Indeed it was estimated that the proportion of new episodes of new back pain attributable to psychological factors in the general population is 16 per cent. The whole is aggravated by compensation factors (Rainville et al. 1997) and there is little doubt that patients involved in medico-legal claims of one sort or another report more pain, depression, and disability than patients without compensation involvement.

Back pain in children

Although it receives little attention, back pain is common in young people. Gunzburg et al. (1999) reported 36 per cent of children having suffered at least one episode of low back pain and 23 per cent had required some form of medical help. Harreby et al. (1999) found in a group of 13–16-year-old Danish schoolchildren a lifetime prevalence of 58.9 per cent and a 1 year prevalence of 50.8 per cent. Recurrent or continuous low back pain in a moderate to severe degree was recorded in 19.4 per cent.

Structure and function of the lumbo-sacral spine

The five lumbar and first sacral vertebrae form the principal load carrying structure for the back. Each pair of vertebrae is joined by the intervertebral disc anteriorly and the two apophyseal joints posteriorly. These joints cannot move in isolation and all movements between vertebrae necessarily affect all three. For this reason, each pair of vertebrae and the connecting three joints are known as a spinal unit.

The intervertebral disc in the adult consists of a central gelatinous nucleus pulposus surrounded by the tough fibres of the annulus fibrosus. The annular fibres spiral obliquely in fascicles between the vertebral rims lying at about 60° to the spinal axis and interdigitating with each other (Fig. 1). This arrangement makes the intervertebral disc an effective shock absorber which accommodates vertical loads by slight squashing of the disc and bulging of the peripherae and flexion, extension and lateral flexion movements by alteration of the angles of the crossing fascicles. However, torsion of the lumbar spine is less readily accommodated as twisting one vertebra on that below means that some collagen fibres of the annulus will be stretched. This is one of the reasons why twisting movements of the lumbar spine are more likely to be associated with annular damage.

There is a lumbar lordosis that is most marked at L4/5 and L5/S1. The associated increase in pressures in the posterior part of the disc, together with the lower lumbar discs carrying higher loads than the upper discs account for the greater prevalence of lumbar problems at these sites.

The gel-like nucleus of the normal disc consists of a matrix of water and glycosaminoglycan in a random meshwork of Type II collagen fibres (McDevitt 1988). With ageing and disc degeneration there is alteration of the glycosaminoglycan with a reduction of its molecular size (Adams and Muir 1976) and the nucleus becomes more fibrous. There is loss of water content and the gel-like character of the nucleus is lost. As a result, it is no longer able to redistribute pressures in an isotropic fashion. Localized areas of pressure concentration appear and may be associated with focal damage and an increase in the proportion of the body load is borne by the annulus fibrosus. The normal annulus consists of Type I collagen fibres at its outer periphery but with a gradual change to Type II fibres at its inner margin with the nucleus (Eyre and Muir 1976). Type I collagen is characteristic of the collagens involved in resisting tensile loads which is the primary function of the outer annulus, whereas the inner annular and nuclear Type II collagen is more typical of cartilage collagen and has to withstand compressive loads. There is clearly an appropriate functional adaptation of collagen structure within the disc. In degenerative disease this pattern is lost. There is an excess of Type I collagen in both the annulus and the nucleus (Herbert et al. 1975) interfering with the biomechanical efficiency of the disc. There are alterations in the patterns of degradative enzymes with disc degeneration and herniation (Ng et al. 1986) but it is not clear whether these changes play a fundamental role in degeneration of the disc or are secondary to disc damage. Experimental induction of disc prolapse shows that extensive vascular ingrowth is followed by more florid evidence of internal disc disruption (Vernon Roberts 1992). Angiogenic factors associated with the proliferation of new blood vessels are capable of activating degradative enzymes (Weiss and McLaughlin 1993) so providing a possible mechanism for the initiation of disc degeneration.

Measurements of pressures within the intervertebral disc show the increase associated with the upright posture and load bearing (Nachemson 1992). The load on the lumbar spine, is increased by contraction of the paravertebral muscles, which stabilize the spine, and reduced by the lumbar lordosis. The design of car seats is largely related to information about stresses on the disc with varying degrees of lumbar support and back-rest inclination.

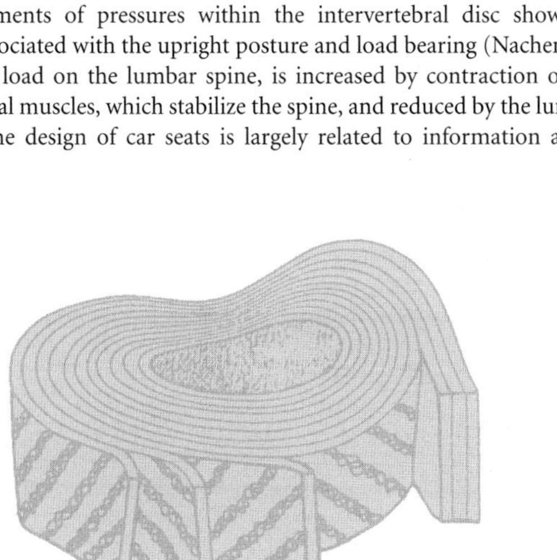

Fig. 1 The collagen fibres of the annulus fibrosus spiralling obliquely around the margins of the intervertebral disc. (By courtesy of Dr J.B. Weiss.)

The vertebral end-plates provide the interface between the intervertebral discs and the vertebral bodies. Diffusion across the end-plate is critical for disc nutrition and vascular channels and nerve fibres may grow into and across the vertebral end-plate. The end-plate is susceptible to mechanical failure. Schmorl's nodes may develop due to trauma (Fahey et al. 1998) or some congenital weakness. Moore (2000) reviewed the structure and function of the vertebral end-plate and emphasized its importance in maintaining the health of the intervertebral disc.

Pain commonly experienced in the back and lower limbs

It may arise from stimulation of the nerve roots or nociceptive receptors (Wyke 1987). They are distributed in:

1. the skin and subcutaneous tissues,
2. the fibrous capsules of the apophyseal and sacro-iliac joints,
3. the outer layers of the annulus fibrosus,
4. the longitudinal ligaments of the spine and in particular the posterior longitudinal ligaments,
5. the periostium and attached fasciae, aponeuroses, and tendons,
6. walls of blood vessels in and around the spine,
7. the dura mata and epidural adipose tissues.

There is a complex anastomatic network of sensory fibres around the vertebral column and in particular around the margin of the intervertebral disc penetrating the outer annulus fibrosis and the encircling blood vessels (Ashton et al. 1994). When there is degeneration there is nerve growth deeper into the diseased intervertebral disc. These nerve fibres express substance P and there is an association with pain (Freemont et al. 1997).

Recent work suggests central mechanisms by which the perception of pain is modulated. Following nociceptive damage neuro-morphological and neuro-chemical changes occur within the dorsal horn. These may be long lasting so the sensation of pain may persist despite the lack of minimal peripheral cause. The cells may be sensitized with increased sensitivity to minor stimulation and the message may spread within the spinal cord so that symptoms are perceived over a wide area (Dubner and Basbaum 1994).

The sympathetic chains run alongside the vertebral column with multiple anastamosing sympathetic fibres and the peripheral sympathetic system accompanies blood vessels extending into the lower limbs. Many patients with chronic low limb pain show evidence of a sympathetic dysfunction syndrome. Most often this follows surgery to the lumbar spine but it can occur in association with mechanical problems (Sachs et al. 1993).

Pathological changes in the spine

Herniated intervertebral disc

Nuclear material can burst through the annulus fibrosus displacing and damaging the surrounding structures. Most often this occurs at the level of the L4/5 and L5/S1 intervertebral discs. The prolapse is usually in the postero-lateral direction although sometimes it can be much nearer or in the mid line. As a result the prolapse may directly damage nerve roots in addition to ligaments, periosteum, blood vessels, dura, and other tissues. The degrees of herniation are known as protrusion, extrusion and, sequestration according to their extent and whether the herniated material retains contact with the disc. Herniation often develops after heavy load bearing with the spine in a flexed and twisted position. However, there is evidence that compression of a healthy disc will usually cause the vertebral end-plate fracture and that posterior and postero-lateral herniation only occur when there is previous disc degeneration and a fissure producing weakening of the annulus fibrosus (Jayson et al. 1973). The particular stress may have acted as the final precipitating cause for this problem.

Adams et al. (2000) suggested that repetitive loading of the spine can lead to end-plate damage and this could be followed by progressive disruption of the intervertebral disc.

The herniated material is often surrounded by an area of erythema and oedema. Usually, it will gradually heal with fibrosis and shrinkage so that eventually the symptoms will remit. However, the disc is already degenerated and the annulus is damaged and there is a considerable risk of further disc herniation and further secondary degenerative changes. The herniated material may press directly on nerves or compress the epidural veins producing venous obstruction and ischaemia of the relevant nerve. It may be complicated by ischaemia of the neural sheaths with both peri- and intraneural fibrosis and followed by neuronal atrophy (Hoyland et al. 1989).

The herniated disc can cause direct nerve root and blood vessel compression. Commonly however, there is surrounding inflammation and this can be the cause of nerve root damage. Experimental application of autologous nucleus pulposus induces histological and neurophysiological changes in porcine nerve roots (Olmarker et al 1993). The discal cells express TNF-alpha and when applied to nerve roots mimic the effects of nucleus pulposus (Igarashi et al. 2000). These observations have lead to trials of TNF-alpha blockade in sciatica. Preliminary results look promising (Karppinen et al. 2003).

A more central posterior prolapse can damage the posterior longitudinal ligament which is innervated by the sinuvertebral nerve and produce central back pain. A large central posterior prolapse can compress the cauda equina leading to multiple nerve damage in the lower limbs and sphincter disturbance.

There appears to be some predisposition towards the development of disc herniation. Pathological studies in cadavers (Jayson and Barks 1973) and magnetic resonance imaging (MRI) in life (Powell et al. 1986) show that when disc degeneration is present there is an increased risk of changes at multiple levels. There may be familial factors predisposing towards the development of prolapse although no specific immunogenetic pattern has been identified (Postacchini et al. 1988). In MRI scans in monozygotic and dizygotic twins, Sambrook et al. (1999) identified important genetic influences in the variation in intervertebral disc degeneration. Environmental factors also clearly play a part. Moderate amounts of physical activity are good for the back but lack of exercise and excessive physical loads are both associated with increased risks of back pain, degenerative disease and disc herniation (Videman et al. 1990; Battie et al. 1995).

The classical presentation of a herniated intervertebral disc is the acute onset of back pain followed by radicular pain, numbness and paraesthesiae in one or other lower limbs. The problem may develop after some stress and in particular bending, twisting and lifting which when combined seem to produce the greatest risk. Most patients, however, will give a history of some preceding history of stiffness in the back over the previous few days.

Clinical pattern

Direct damage to the nerve root will produce pain, numbness, and paraesthesiae as shown in Table 1. A small lateral herniation of the L4/5 disc will commonly affect the L5 root and herniation of the L5/S1 disc will affect the S1 root. However, a large prolapse, particularly if it is more central, may affect several nerve roots with widespread neurological symptoms and signs and perhaps sphincter disturbance. There is considerable overlap in the distributions of the various nerve roots and the symptoms and physical signs only act as approximate guides to which disc has been damaged. In addition, pressure on ligaments and other soft tissues will produce referred pain felt in the buttock and lower limb. This is often confused with radicular symptoms due to nerve root damage. Referred pain is poorly defined and patients commonly have difficulty in describing its distribution. The symptoms of disc herniation are made worse by spinal movements and also by Valsalva manoeuvres such as coughing, sneezing, micturition, and defaecation which raise the cerebrospinal fluid pressure. Examination may show a sciatic scoliosis due to the unilateral spasm of the para-spinal muscles. There may be severe limitation of spine movements, but often in only one or two directions and in particular movements including flexion. Palpation of the spine may show local areas of tenderness over the spine or sometimes elsewhere such as in the sacro-iliac joints. Straight leg raising is limited with a positive Lasegue's test. The specific neurological signs of nerve root damage should be sought (Table 1).

Investigations

The blood sedimentation rate, plasma viscosity, and routine haematological and biochemical parameters are normal. The cerebrospinal fluid obtained by lumbar puncture is usually normal but when there is a large prolapse with a spinal block, the protein level may be elevated.

Imaging techniques commonly used are:

Plain radiography

In an acute prolapse, the spine is normal except perhaps for a scoliosis. When followed over several years disc narrowing may develop and later on there may be secondary spondylotic changes.

Radiculography

Water-soluble radio opaque dye is injected into the subarachnoid space at lumbar puncture. The dye penetrates along the nerve roots and obstruction to flow produced by a prolapse can be clearly identified (Fig. 2).

Table 1 Principal changes used for identifying the sites of lumbar nerve root lesions

Root	Superficial paraesthesiae and sensory change	Muscle weakness	Tendon reflex changes
L2	Upper thigh: anterior, medial, and lateral surfaces	Flexion and adduction of hip	None
L3	Anterior surface of lower thigh Anterior and medial surfaces of knee	Adduction of hip; extension of knee	Knee jerk possibly decreased
L4	Anteromedial surface of leg	Extension of knee; dorsiflexion and inversion of foot	Knee jerk decreased
L5	Anterolateral surface of leg, dorsum and medial surface of foot, especially dorsal surface of hallux	Extension and abduction of hip Flexion of knee; dorsiflexion of foot and toes, especially hallux	None
S1	Lateral border and sole of foot, back of heel, and lower calf	Flexion of knee; plantar flexion and eversion of foot	Ankle jerk decreased

Note: This table does not list the total distribution of each root.

Discography

Direct injections may be made into an intervertebral disc. A normal healthy disc will accept about 0.5 ml of fluid without producing significant symptoms. Larger volumes will be accepted by herniated discs with reproduction of symptoms. The pain may be relieved by injection of local anaesthetic. The radiographic appearances of disc herniation may be identified (Fig. 3).

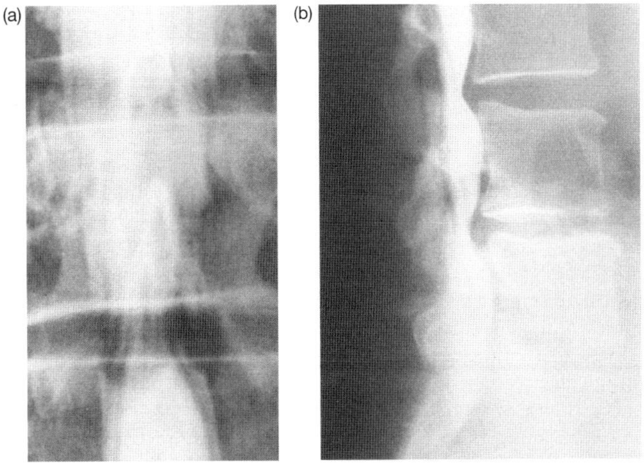

Fig. 2 Radiculogram showing (a) left sided L4/5 disc herniation and (b) smaller disc protrusion at L3/4.

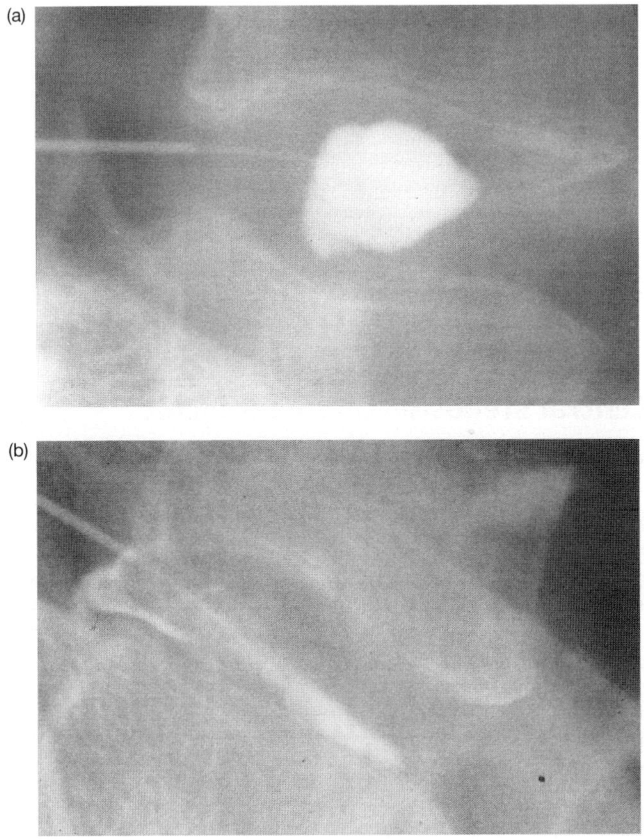

Fig. 3 Discography: (a) normal and (b) disc degeneration with leakage of the dye into the epidural space.

Computered axial tomographic (CAT) scan

Herniation of a disc and the size and extent of nerve root involvement can be determined. This technique is sometimes used to complement radiculography when details of nerve root damage may be clarified.

Magnetic resonance imaging scan

This technique has become the investigation of choice. It has the advantage of avoiding the use of X-rays. It will demonstrate the size and extent of disc herniation as well as degenerative change in the disc by loss of signal on the T_2 image and reduction of disc height (Fig. 4). A focal area of high intensity is sometimes observed in the posterior annulus. This is thought to represent a fissure. There is an association of pain with the presence of the high intensity zone (Aprill and Bogduk 1992) although this appearance can also be found in asymptomatic subjects (Carragee et al. 2000).

Lumbar spondylosis

Degenerative changes in the spine are common. Pathological studies show they start to appear around 25 years of age and are almost universal in older people. Although patients with severe degrees of spondylosis more commonly develop back pain than those with pristine spines, the correlation between back pain and radiographic evidence of lumbar spondylosis (Lawrence 1977) and MRI evidence of disc bulging and protrusion (Jensen et al. 1994) is poor. Because they are so common it is better to call these appearances 'ageing change' rather than 'degenerative change' as the latter term conveys a perjorative image to patients with an implication of long-term problems which is frequently not the case.

There is disorganization of the internal structure of the disc with loss of the clear distinction between the nucleous pulposis and the annulus fibrosis. Cleft formation within the disc is common. In the normal disc nerve fibres are confined to the outer third of the annulus fibrosis. However, in degenerative discs in patients with chronic low back pain, Freemont et al. (1997) showed that there was proliferation of nerve fibres extending into the inner one-third of the annulus fibrosus and into the nucleus pulposus and that this was accompanied by expression of substance P deep within the diseased

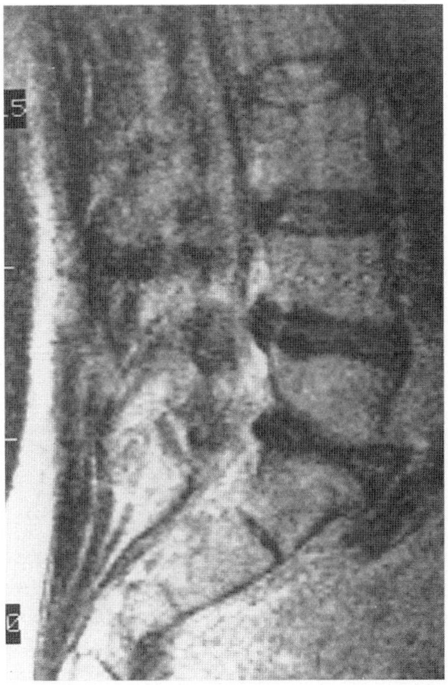

Fig. 4 MRI scan, vertical reconstruction. There is loss of signal at the L3/4, L4/5, and L5/S1 discs indicating disc degeneration with herniation at L4/5 and L5/S1.

intervertebral discs. The disc becomes narrowed with osteophytosis around the vertebral margins. Osteoarthritic changes may also develop in the apophyseal joints and it is commonly not clear whether such changes precede or follow degeneration of the disc. Lumbar spondylosis with osteophytes and often minor degrees of disc herniation can directly impinge upon nerve roots and other structures. More commonly, however, they may contribute towards obstruction of vascular flow and be associated with periintraneural fibrosis and neural atrophy (Hoyland et al. 1989).

There is no defined clinical pattern associated with lumbar spondylosis. Some patients only suffer postural backache with pain associated with prolonged sitting or standing in a poor posture or aggravated by heavy manual work. Others suffer more severe episodes often provoked by trivial stress. These acute episodes usually will resolve within a few days but the patient is always at risk of further episodes. The pain may be felt across the back but often spreads into the buttock and lower limb. If there is nerve root entrapment there may be specific radicular symptoms and signs (Table 1). Soft tissue damage can produce referred pain spreading to the limb which is often not in a well-defined distribution.

Radiographic changes include narrowing of disc space, gas in the disc, sclerosis of the vertebral end-plates, and marginal osteophytosis (Fig. 5). It is important to remember that these changes are common in the symptom-free population particularly in older subjects. Their presence therefore does not mean they are the source of the symptoms and careful evaluation is always required to ensure there is no other problem in any individual patient.

Internal disc disruption

After trauma, and, in particular, compressive loads on the spine perhaps associated with vertebral end-plate fracture, there may be degradation of the nucleus spreading outwards to involve the annulus fibrosis. This may irritate the nerve endings in the outer border of the annulus and lead to the development of pain. Loss of disc height may contribute towards venous obstruction and tissue ischaemia (Crock 1992).

In some patients a focal area of high signal may be detected in the posterior annulus. This has been called a 'tear' although a fissure is a better term. Aprill and Bogduk (1992) reported a strong correlation between the presence of annular high intensity zones and provocative discography in patients with low back pain but Carragaee et al. (2000) found this lesion to be not uncommon in asymptomatic individuals although greater in symptomatic patients. There is therefore some indication that the high intensity zone indicates a pain producing lesion but doubt still exists.

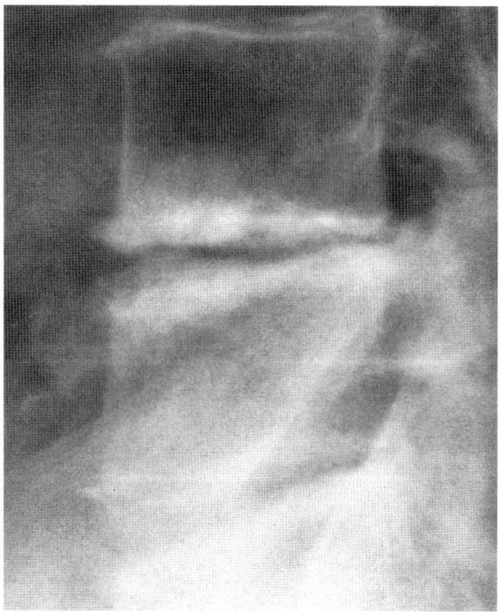

Fig. 5 Lumbar spondylosis at L4/5 and L5/S1.

Symptoms arising as a result of internal disc disruption or a fissure are felt in the back or referred into the buttock or lower limb. They are aggravated by movements. However, the nerve root may not be affected, in which case there are no specific neurological signs. In the early stages, plain radiographs appear normal, but later there may be progressive narrowing of the disc space. Likewise, the myelogram and CT scan may be normal although the MRI scan may show loss of signal and the high intensity zone. Discography, perhaps supplemented by a CT scan, may show characteristic morphological changes. Reproduction of the pain by raising the pressure within the individual disc and relief by local anaesthetic is a valuable indication that a particular disc is responsible for the clinical problem.

Facet joint syndromes

The apophyseal joints are true synovial joints and commonly develop osteoarthritic changes. Patients may experience pain that arises from the apophyseal joints. The typical picture is of pain in the back spreading into one or other buttock or into the back of the thigh. It is aggravated by extension and on palpation there is marked tenderness over the facet joints. However, each facet joint has a nerve supply arising from several levels and, as a result, the pain often has a widespread distribution making it difficult to identify which specific joint is the source of the symptoms.

Facet joint arthrography may be helpful as it may demonstrate osteoarthritic change. In particular, if injection of the joint aggravates the symptoms and local anaesthetic provides relief, this strongly suggests that the joint is responsible for the development of pain (Fairbank et al. 1981). However, the diagnosis is controversial as the correlation between the response to interventional procedures and clinical findings is poor and it remains possible that when symptoms are relieved by anaesthetic it has leaked out of the joint and provided symptomatic relief simply by affecting nerve endings in a widespread distribution.

Spinal stenosis

There is considerable variation in the size and shape of the vertebral canal. In particular, some patients have a canal with a small diameter and a trefoil shape due to osteoarthritic hypertrophy of the apophyseal joints. The nerve roots may be tightly packed. As a result, there is an increased rate of back problems following any further intrusion into the canal. It is known that patients developing symptoms from a disc protrusion have significantly smaller canal measurements than the normal population (Porter et al. 1980). Symptoms due to spinal stenosis may develop in later life as a result of osteophytosis, disc bulging, and ligament thickening intruding into a tight canal space.

There are two principal syndromes associated with spinal stenosis—central stenosis and foraminal stenosis.

Central stenosis—and neurogenic claudication

On walking, the patients progressively develop discomfort, numbness, paraesthesiae, heaviness, and a dead feeling in the lower limbs that will eventually make them stop. On resting the symptoms gradually ease over a period of 5–10 minutes and the patient may start walking again. The problem is frequently confused with claudication due to a poor arterial supply in the lower limbs. As the patients are frequently elderly and may also have an arteriopathy, the differential diagnosis may sometimes be difficult. The vertebral canal has slightly greater dimensions when the spine is flexed and many patients describe bending forwards to relieve their pain. Likewise they may find it easier to walk uphill when they lean forwards than downhill when they lean back.

On examination, they may stand with the spine, hips, and knees slightly flexed. They can usually bend forwards without problem but extension is limited. Neurological examination is unhelpful.

Plain radiographs may show the evidence of degenerative change but it is difficult to determine the dimensions of the vertebral canal. Myelography

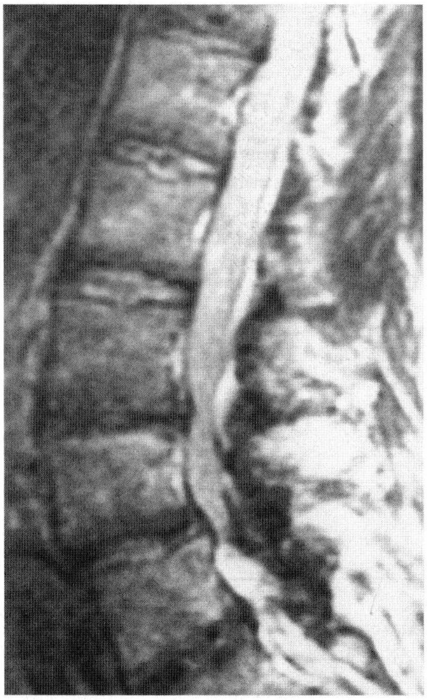

ig. 6 MRI scan showing spinal stenosis, most marked at L3/4 and L4/5, with egenerative disc disease.

an be technically difficult because of the crowding of the nerve roots. CT nd MRI scans are most helpful for determining the extent and severity of ne stenosis and measurement of the vertebral canal dimensions may be nade (Fig. 6).

oraminal stenosis (root entrapment yndrome)

larrowing of the intervertebral foramen with nerve root entrapment can ive rise to a specific pattern of radicular pain in the lower limb (Porter 992). This narrowing may be due to bony osteophytosis from the apo-hyseal joints, postero-lateral osteophytes on the vertebral bodies, ossifica-on and hypertrophy of the posterior spinous ligaments, and fibrous roliferation of the nerve root sheaths.

The patient develops a pattern of radicular pain distinct from that of prolapsed intervertebral disc. In particular, the pain is often severe and nremitting, being present at rest in bed as well as on exercise although it nay be aggravated by physical activity. Back movements may be full and nany patients do not show restriction of straight leg raising.

CT (Fig. 7) and MRI scans are most helpful for demonstrating foraminal tenosis. Nerve root injection with local anaesthetic can also be helpful for lentifying the site of the pain producing lesion (Dooley et al. 1988).

pondylolysis and spondylolisthesis

)efects in the pars interarticularis (spondylolysis) are common and usually ot of significance. Spondylolisthesis refers to slipping, usually forward but ccasionally backwards, on the vertebra below. Spondylolisthesis has been lassified by Wiltse and Rothman (1990) as follows:

. congenital;

. isthmic;

(a) lytic—stress failure of the pars interarticularis,

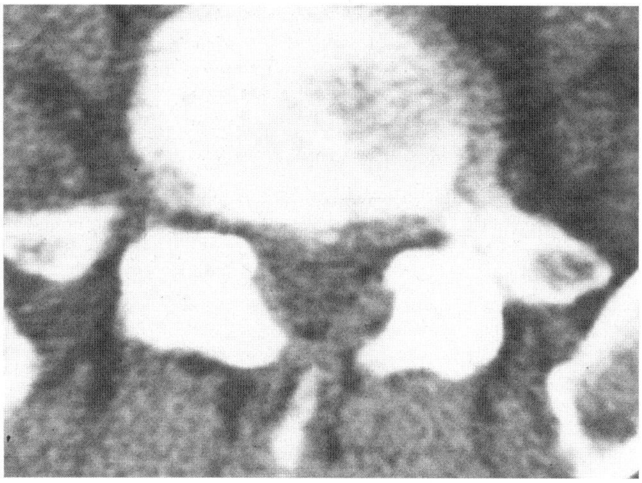

Fig. 7 CT scan showing foraminal stenosis.

(b) an elongated but intact pars secondary to a healed stress fracture,

(c) fracture.

3. degenerative;
4. post-traumatic;
5. pathological—due to destruction of the posterior elements;
6. surgical.

Patients may develop pain in the back and in the lower limb, aggravated by standing and walking, and relieved by rest. Narrowing of the vertebral canal can cause symptoms suggestive of spinal stenosis. The physical findings will depend on the degree of slip and extent of neurological damage. It may be possible to palpate a step in the spine on forward flexion in gross cases.

Post-surgical back pain

Many patients undergo surgery for spinal disorders. A significant proportion fail to respond or develop recurrent back problems. Careful assessment is required to determine the cause of the problem in each individual case. Problems that may be identified are as follows:

1. the operation was undertaken at the incorrect level,
2. inadequate surgery perhaps with failure to adequately decompress a nerve root or excise a disc herniation,
3. recurrent disc herniation at the same or another level,
4. secondary or degenerative change perhaps associated with extensive removal of bone,
5. peri-neural fibrosis and arachnoiditis (see below),
6. sympathetic dysfunction syndromes (Sachs et al. 1993),
7. psychological factors,
8. unrelated pathology.

Peri-neural fibrosis and arachnoiditis

Abnormal fibrosis may develop in the peri-radicular tissues (peri-neural fibrosis) or within the dural sac (arachnoiditis). The former develops most commonly in a florid form in patients who have undergone spine surgery and may be due to retained cotton debris from the surgical swabs and patties (Hoyland et al. 1988). However, minor degrees of peri-radicular fibrosis are common in association with lumbar spondylosis. It is frequently difficult to correlate the presence of epidural fibrosis and the development of back and nerve root symptoms (Cooper et al. 1991).

Arachnoiditis

Arachnoiditis was first described following meningitis. It can develop following surgery but it is then restricted to the level of the operation. The most widespread forms of arachnoiditis are found in those patients who have in the past undergone myelography using oil based myelographic media. There is inflammation around the nerve roots followed by fibrosis and adhesions. The pathological changes and pathological features of arachnoiditis have been described by Burton (1990). Radiculograms will show a grossly distorted thecal sac (Fig. 8). High-resolution MRI scans are most helpful for demonstrating the presence of arachnoiditis (Fig. 9).

Non-specific back pain

In many patients, it is difficult to define a precise cause for the symptoms. They suffer persistent or recurrent episodes of back pain. Examination may reveal limitation of spine movements but without neurological signs. Radiographs may show varying degrees of lumbar spondylosis but it is difficult to determine their significance.

Within this group many will have areas of localized tenderness over the spine or the sacro-iliac joints. Pressure on these areas may reproduce the patients symptoms and they are sometimes called areas of subluxation or dysfunction by osteopaths and chiropractors although there is no pathological basis for these terms. Collee et al. (1990) described ileo-lumbar and greater trochanteric pain syndromes occurring in patients with chronic low back pain. However, no specific pathology has been demonstrated and the cause of the symptoms remain uncertain.

Hypermobile patients often suffer recurrent back pain. Radiographs show marked evidence of degenerative change yet these subjects retain a remarkably good range of back movements. It is believed that injury of the ligaments and joint capsules, perhaps associated with small fractures may be the source of pain in these circumstances.

The fibromyalgia syndrome is also a source of confusion. These patients have multiple tender and painful trigger points particularly around the neck, the shoulder, and hip girdles and is commonly associated with a poor sleep pattern. Many are depressed and there is an association with migraine and an irritable bowel syndrome. In fibromyalgia, patients have an amplified perception of the severity of physical problems with the result that they

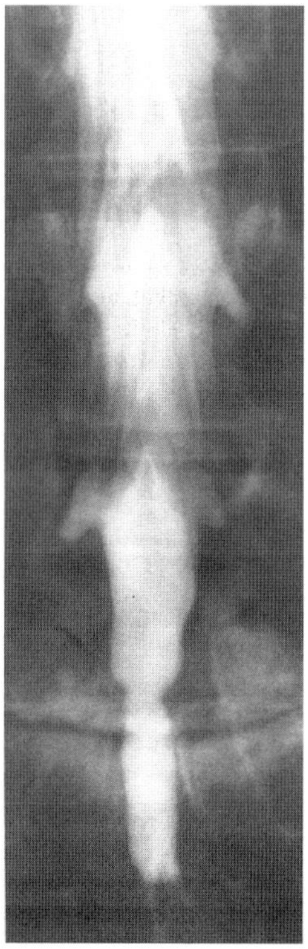

Fig. 8 Radiculogram in a patient with arachnoiditis showing gross distortion of the thecal sac.

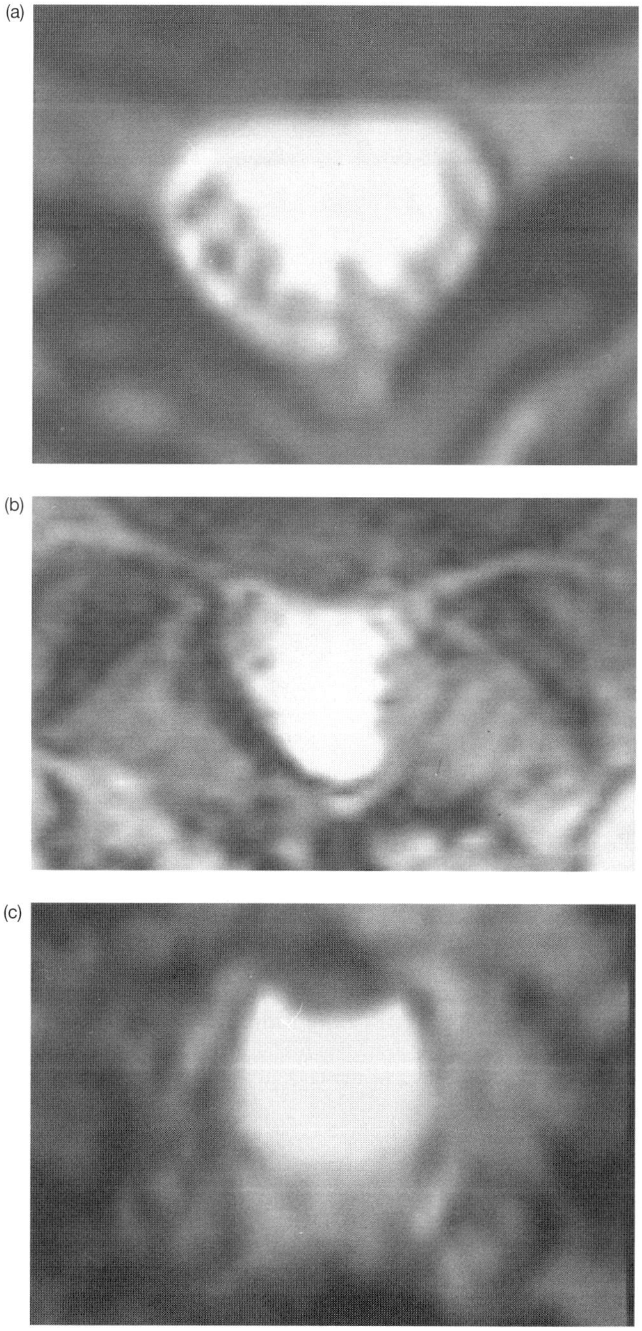

Fig. 9 High resolution MRI scans showing the nerve roots (a) normal, (b) arachnoiditis. The nerve roots are adherent to each other, atrophic, and stuck to the wall of the thecal sac. (c) The nerve roots have atrophied completely and can no longer be seen. Residual Myodil is still present anteriorly.

apparently experience severe symptoms in relationship to minor degrees of degenerative change. There is no evidence of a specific back pathology in fibromyalgia although the patient with the fibromyalgia syndrome can experience widespread back pain (see Chapter 6.13.1).

The prevention of back pain

Although enormous effort has been expended on developing and providing interventions aimed at preventing the development of back problems, the results have been a disappointment. Back care education programmes have not been effective in preventing work associated low back injury (Daltroy et al. 1997; Van Poppel et al. 1997). A systematic review of the prophylactic use of lumbar supports (Jellema et al. 2001) suggested that lumbar supports were not effective for prevention of back pain although the quality of trials was generally poor. Exercise and physical fitness seem to help although most studies were methodologically flawed and the effects were only weak (Linton and von Tulder 2001). The Faculty of Occupational Medicine (Carter and Birrell 2000) summarized the evidence and concluded that high job satisfaction and good industrial relations are the most important organizational characteristics associated with low disability and sickness absence rates attributed to back pain.

Management

Each patient will require individual assessment. In particular, it is important to distinguish patients with acute, recurrent, and chronic mechanical pain syndromes.

Acute back pain

Most acute back problems are seen in primary care. Many patients do not seek medical advice and a high proportion will be treated by a physiotherapist, osteopath, or chiropractor.

It is generally believed that about 90 per cent of acute episodes settle within 6 weeks (Waddell 1987). However, these estimates may be over-optimistic. Croft et al. (1998) pointed out that although the majority of patients fail to consult after a period of about 3 months, nevertheless most have continued back problems when re-assessed 1 year later.

In acute back pain, the patients should be triaged into those with simple backache, nerve root pain, and possible serious spinal pathology. Remarkably similar guidelines for classifying these three groups have been published in the United Kingdom by The Clinical Standards Advisory Group (1994), The Royal College of General Practitioners (1999), and The Faculty of Occupational Medicine (Carter and Birrell 2000). Similar guidelines exist for other countries.

Simple backache

Clinical criteria

- Patient aged 20–55 years;
- Pain in the lumbo-sacral region, buttocks, and thighs;
- Pain mechanical in nature varies with physical activity and with time;
- Patient is well.

Blood tests and radiographs of the lumbar spine are not indicated unless there is doubt about the diagnostic triage. Kendrick et al. (2001) did not find any clinical improvements associated with radiographs of the lumbar spine in patients with low back pain of at least 6 weeks duration although there was improved patient satisfaction.

Patients with simple back pain should be managed with simple analgesics such as paracetamol (aminocetophen). Alternatives are anti-inflammatory drugs. A systemic review (Van Tulder et al. 2000) showed that non-steroidal anti-inflammatory drugs are effective for providing short-term symptomatic relief in acute back pain. There is no evidence that any specific types of anti-inflammatory drugs are better than others. Narcotics should be avoided and never given for more than a couple of weeks.

Bed rest should only be prescribed if essential and then normally for only 1–3 days. This produces less disability than prolonged periods of bed rest (Deyo et al. 1986).

It is always important to provide ergonomic advice on posture while standing, working, sitting, and lifting in order to protect the back against excessive loads.

Early physical activity is encouraged and reduces pain. Indeed, ordinary activities whenever possible seem to produce the best outcome (Malmivaara et al. 1995). Patients should be advised that exercise is not harmful and reduces pain, and that physical fitness is beneficial. A randomized controlled trial of an exercise programme (Moffett et al. 1999) showed this was more effective than traditional general practitioner management. The patient should be encouraged to return to work as soon as possible and it is not necessary for symptoms to have cleared completely before returning to work although care should be taken to avoid over stressing the back. With a regimen such as this most patients will return to normal function rapidly.

The role of the therapist is restoration of function and encouraging the patient to be mobile. Physical exercise has an important role. The actual type of exercise is relatively unimportant. The benefits seem to lie in the quantity of exercise rather than its specific nature. A positive attitude and encouragement to return to work as soon as possible is all important.

In order to remobilize the patient, there is a wide variety of forms of physiotherapy and manual treatments. There is no evidence that heat, cold, ultrasound, or massage provide any benefit other than comfort at the time they are administered. Exercise and physical fitness are important and an incremental aerobic fitness programme of physical reconditioning is advised.

With this programme, the vast majority of acute episodes recover within 6 weeks. If the pain still persists, the diagnostic triage should be reviewed and investigations such as the erythrocyte sedimentation rate and radiographs of the lumbar spine should be requested if specifically indicated.

Early identification of psycho-social problems is important as they predict the risk of acute back pain becoming chronic (Burton et al. 1995). Kendall et al. (1997) on behalf of the Accident Rehabilitation and Compensation Insurance Corporation and the National Health Committee in New Zealand produced guidelines for the assessment of psycho-social yellow flags predictive of risks of chronicity of a back problem. They included attitudes and belief about pain, abnormal behaviours, compensation issues, diagnosis and treatment issues, emotions, family problems, and work problems.

For the patient with persistent backache, an active physical rehabilitation may be necessary and consideration given to these psycho-social issues. At this stage, referral may be required for a second opinion, additional assessment, rehabilitation, pain management, and occasionally surgery.

Manipulation is practised by physiotherapists, osteopaths, chiropractors, physicians, and surgeons. Although there has been some conflicting evidence from various trials, overall it appears that manipulation accelerates the rate of recovery in recent onset back pain although not making any long-term difference to the outcome (Twomey and Taylor 1995). A comparison of overall outcomes by patients receiving care from primary care practitioners, chiropractors, or orthopaedic surgeons (Carey et al. 1995) suggested similar outcomes. Manipulation can cause a temporary exacerbation of pain but generally this resolves (Barrett and Breen 2000). There is no evidence to distinguish the effects of manipulation by the various types of practitioner except that manipulation of the lumbar spine under general anaesthesia carries a significant risk of neurological damage to the cauda equina (Haldeman and Rubinstein 1992).

Nerve root pain (clinical criteria)

- Unilateral leg pain worse than low back pain;
- Pain generally radiates to the foot or toes;
- Numbness and paraesthesiae in the same distribution;
- Nerve irritation signs with reduced straight leg raising;
- Motor sensory or reflex change limited to one nerve root.

The management of such patients is similar to simple backache but undertaken more slowly. The recovery rate is not as good and only 50 per cent recover from the acute attack within 6 weeks.

If a patient fails to improve by this time he or she may need more detailed assessment. Such patients may require scans and be considered for possible surgery.

Possible serious spinal pathology—red flags

Factors which give rise to concern are:

- Age of onset less than 20 or greater than 55 years;
- Violent trauma;
- Constant progressive non-mechanical back pain;
- Gradual onset with morning stiffness, limitation of movements in all directions, peripheral joint involvement and other features suggesting ankylosing spondylitis or related disorders;
- Systemically unwell, weight loss;
- Widespread neurology;
- Significant medical history such as previous carcinoma, steroid therapy, etc.

In such circumstances, the patient will require intensive and appropriate investigations.

Recurrent back pain

Many patients experience recurrent episodes of back pain which may be precipitated by lifting, twisting, and bending. A detailed understanding of the structure and function of the spine and the appropriate way to protect it in a variety of physical activities combined with simple exercises to increase physical fitness and strengthen the abdominal and spinal muscles seem helpful in preventing further recurrences of back problems. The role of the physiotherapist in back education and the training may be formalized as a series of lessons in a 'Back School' (Andersson 1992). The results of such training programmes are at least as good and probably better than conventional physiotherapy programmes.

Chronic back pain

Many patients suffer persistent pain in the back which may spread into the lower limbs. They become severely and permanently disabled. Many have undergone one or more spinal operations. Detailed assessments are required to elucidate the pathogenesis of the pain in individual subjects and to plan a treatment programme.

We now know that chronic back pain is not the same as acute back pain lasting longer (Jayson 1997). It is common for secondary factors to play significant roles in perpetuation of symptoms.

Chronic back pain may be due to:

1. Chronic disc herniation with persistent nerve root damage.
2. Severe degenerative change in the intervertebral discs.
3. Non-mechanical pathologies such as inflammatory spondyloarthropathies, neoplasms, infections, Paget's disease, etc.
4. Incomplete discectomy or nerve decompression.
5. Recurrent or new disc prolapse.
6. Scar tissue forming around the nerves perhaps as a reaction to surgery; retained microscopic dust from the swabs, patties used in operations may be of direct relevance here (Hoyland et al. 1988).
7. Arachnoiditis due to previous oil based myelography (Fig. 8).
8. Sympathetic syndromes with referred symptoms felt in the lower limb (Sachs et al. 1993).
9. Fibromyalgia.
10. Psychological factors—these play an important part in many patients perpetuating the chronic nature of back pain. They include depression, anxiety, and compensation factors. Operant conditioning refers to the psychological reinforcement of pain behaviour and may include not only financial benefits but sympathy, concern, and over-protection by relatives, friends, medical, and paramedical staff. Fear avoidance of activity is common in chronic back pain syndromes and may further exacerbate disability (Vlaeyn and Linton 2000).
11. Central nervous system modulation with imprinting of the pain memory within the brain and spinal cord.

Assessment of the chronic back pain patient requires a very careful history and examination. The findings suggestive of a substantial non-organic component to the problem (Waddell et al. 1980) include:

(i) Pain behaviour.

(ii) Pain production on simulated stress of the spine such as pressure on the skull and rotation of the pelvis.

(iii) Restricted straight leg raising on formal testing but unrestricted distracted straight leg raising such as being able to sit upright with the lower limbs extended.

(iv) Regional weakness or sensory disturbance in a non-neurological distribution.

(v) Widespread superficial tenderness over the back.

Adequate management can only be undertaken after a thorough evaluation of each individual patient. This should include a very careful review of the medical history together with physical and psychological assessments. When specific pathologies can be identified they may be amenable to appropriate therapy. For many patients this is not possible. Forms of treatment which may be beneficial include:

1. *The use of appropriate medication.* Pure analgesics such as paracetamol or perhaps codeine or its derivatives or dextropropoxyphene are adequate for most patients. For some, particularly if there is a pain pattern suggestive of secondary/fibrotic/inflammatory element with pain aggravated by rest, the non-steroidal drugs seem particularly helpful. Muscle relaxants such as chlormezanone and baclofen may be helpful when there is a major element of muscle spasm. Some patients describe a neuralgic element to the pain with electric shock sensations radiating down the lower limbs. This may be relieved by antiepileptic drugs such as carbamazepamine or sodium valporate. Others have widespread superficial paraesthesiae and tenderness and features suggestive of fibromyalgia and may respond to tricyclic antidepressant drugs such as amitriptyline. In the spinal stenosis syndrome, there is some uncertain evidence (Porter and Hibbert 1983) that calcitonin may provide relief perhaps by altering blood flow dynamics within the vertebral column.
2. *Physiotherapy and ergonomic advice.* This teaches the patient how to perform tasks within their physical capabilities and helps to give them confidence.
3. *Local injections may be helpful for some people.* They include:
   (a) Trigger point and local injections of steroid and anaesthetic: although commonly used the evidence for their value is in doubt.
   (b) Facet joint injections: although often used their value remains in doubt (Garvey et al. 1989).
   (c) Epidural injections: there have been a number of controlled studies with conflicting results (Moskovich 1998). Overall, it is thought the technique is of value for the patient with radicular pain which has failed to resolve completely. Major adverse effects are rare and are principally associated with dural puncture and intrathecal injection (Bogduk 1995).
   (d) Acupuncture: although some studies suggest that needling has advantages over controlled treatment all have major methodological flaws. There do not appear to be any differences in outcome comparing needling in the Chinese meridians and misplaced needling. TENS machines are an alternative method of providing acupuncture.

4. *Patient education.* Failure to provide an adequate explanation of the problems leads to patient dissatisfaction (Deyo and Diehl 1986). A back education programme, perhaps structured as a back school, is appreciated by patient although the specific value with regard to outcome remains in doubt.
5. *Lumbar corsets and belts.* The evidence for the efficacy is confused. In a systematic review, Jellema et al. (2001) found limited evidence that lumbar supports led to improvement in symptoms and function in patients with chronic back problems. Many patients come to depend on their corsets and may develop severe restriction of spine movements. My own view is that they should not be in general use.
6. *Activity modification.* Bed rest should be avoided in chronic back pain. Patients should be encouraged to remain active and undertake regular exercise programmes to improve physical fitness (Frost et al. 1995).
7. *Surgery and chemonucleolysis.* Procedures available include discectomy, decompression, and fusion of the lumbar spine. In the patient with persistent sciatic pain with clear neurological signs and confirmation by appropriate imaging, there is now strong evidence that discectomy is effective and produces better long-term results than conservative treatment (Gibson et al. 1999). Surgical discectomy is more effective than chemical discectomy. The results of surgical procedures for patients with degenerative lumbar spondylosis, however, are not as good and the overall review of the evidence did not find that surgical decompression or fusion was effective compared with the natural history, placebo, or conservative management (Gibson et al. 1999). The results of second and subsequent operations tend to be poor. Further surgery should only be contemplated in patients for whom there is a very clearly defined lesion causing symptoms and for which there is an adequate surgical solution.
8. *Multidisciplinary functional restoration programmes.* Detailed assessments including physical, vocational, and psychological factors are an essential preliminary. The patient must accept that no further specific investigations will help. They then enter a programme combining intensive physical activation, counselling for the understand of pain and related problems, reducing the use of medication health care, dealing with depressive symptoms and anxiety, relaxation therapy, and cognitive therapy together with encouragement to return to normal activities. These programmes are time-consuming and expensive but are effective in improving function, return to work rates, and work retention (Mayer et al. 1987; Burke et al. 1994).

Conclusion

In recent years there has been a major increase of interest in the back pain problem. With careful scientific study, new imaging procedures, and psychological assessments we now have a much better understanding of the mechanisms of pathogenesis of various back pain syndromes and the reasons why the problems may persist and become chronic. With this better understanding targeted therapy appears effective and lends hope of providing better control of this problem in the future.

References

Adams, P. and Muir, H. (1976). Qualitative changes with age of proteoglycans of human lumbar discs. *Annals of the Rheumatic Diseases* **35**, 289–96.

Adams, M.A., Freeman, B.J.C., Morrison, H.P., Nelson, I.W., and Doland, P. (2000). Mechanical initiation of intervertebral disc degeneration. *Spine* **25**, 1625–36.

Andersson, G.B.G. (1992). Back schools. In *The Lumbar Spine and Back Pain* 4th edn. (ed. M.I.V. Jayson), pp. 409–16. Edinburgh: Churchill Livingstone.

Aprill, C. and Bogduk, N. (1992). High intensity zone: a diagnostic sign of painful lumbar disc on magnetic resonance imaging. *British Journal of Radiology* **65**, 361–9.

Ashton, I.K. et al. (1994). Neuropeptides in the human intervertebral disc. *Journal of Orthopaedic Research* **12**, 186–92.

Barrett, A.J. and Breen, A.C. (2000). Adverse effects of spinal manipulation. *Journal of the Royal Society of Medicine* **93**, 258–9

Battie, M.C., Videman, T., Gibbons, L.E., Fisher, L.D., Manninem, H., and Gill, K. (1995). Determinants of lumbar disc degeneration. A study relating lifetime exposures and magnetic resonance imaging findings in identical twins. *Spine* **20**, 2601–12.

Biering-Sorenson, F. (1985). Risk of back trouble in individual occupations in Denmark. *Ergonomics* **28**, 51–60.

Bogduk, N. (1995). Epidural steroids. *Spine* **20**, 845–8.

Burke, S.A., Harms-Constas, C.K., and Aden, P.S. (1994). Return to work/work retention outcomes of a functional restoration programme. A multi-centre prospective study with a comparison group. *Spine* **19**, 1880–6.

Burton, C.V. (1990). Adhesive arachnoiditis. In *Neurological Surgery III* Vol. II (ed. Youmans), pp. 2856–63. Philadelphia PA: W.B. Saunders.

Burton, A.K., Tillotson, K.M., Main, C.J., and Hollis, S. (1995). Psychosocial predictors of outcome in acute and subacute low back trouble. *Spine* **20**, 722–8.

Carey, T.S., Garrett, G., Jackman, A., McLaughlin, C., Fryer, J., Smucker, D.R., and the North Carolina Pain Project (1995). *New England Journal of Medicine* **333**, 913–17.

Carragee, E.J., Paragioudakis, S.J., and Khurani, S. (2000). Lumbar high intensity zone and discography in subjects without low back problems. *Spine* **23**, 2987–92.

Carter, J.T. and Birrell, L.N., ed. Occupational Health Guidelines for the management of low back pain at work—principal recommendations. London: Faculty of Occupational Medicine, 2000.

Cats-Baril, W.L. and Frymoyer, J.W. (1991). The economics of spinal disorders. In *The Adult Spine: Principles and Practice* (ed. W. Frymoyer), pp. 85–105. New York: Raven Press.

Clinical Standards Advisory Group. *Back Pain.* London: HMSO, 1994.

Collee, G., Dijkmans, B.A.C., Vanderbrouke, J.P., Rouzing, P.M., and Cats, A. (1990). A clinical epidemiological study in low back pain: description of two clinical syndromes. *British Journal of Rheumatology* **29**, 354–7.

Cooper, R.G., Mitchell, W.S., Illingworth, K., St Clair Forbes, W., Gillespie, J.E., and Jayson, M.I.V. (1991). Role of epidural fibrosis and defective fibrinolysis in the persistence of post-laminectomy back pain. *Spine* **16**, 1044–8.

Crock, H.V. (1992). Isolated disc resorption. In *The Lumbar Spine and Back Pain* 4th edn. (ed. M.I.V. Jayson), pp. 307–12. Edinburgh: Churchill Livingstone.

Croft, P. and Jayson, M.I.V. Low back pain in the community and in hospitals. A report to the Clinical Standards Advisory Group of the Department of Health. Prepared by the Arthritis and Rheumatism Council, Epidemiology Research Unit, Manchester, 1994.

Croft, P.R., Papageorgiou, A.C., Ferry, S., Thomas, E., Jayson, M.I.V., and Silman, A.J. (1996). Psychological distress and low back pain. Evidence from a prospective study in the general population. *Spine* **20**, 2731–7.

Croft, P.R., Macfarlane, G.I., Papageorgiou, A.C., Thomas, E., and Silman, A.J. (1998). Outcome of low back pain in general practice: a prospective study. *British Medical Journal* **316**, 1356–9.

Daltroy, L.H., Iverson, M.D., Larson, Lew, R., Wright, E., Ryan, J., Zwerling, C., Fossel, A.H., and Liang, M.H. (1997). A controlled trial of an educational programme to prevent low back injuries. *New England Journal of Medicine* **337**, 322–8.

Deyo, R.A. and Diehl, A.K. (1986). Patient satisfaction with medical care for low-back pain. *Spine* **11**, 28–30.

Deyo, R.A., Diehl, A.K., and Rosenthal, M. (1986). How many days rest for acute low back pain? A randomised clinical trial. *New England Journal of Medicine* **315**, 1064–70.

Dooley, J.F., McBroom, R.J., Taguchi, T., and MacNab, I. (1988). Nerve root infiltration in the diagnosis of radicular pain. *Spine* **13**, 79–83.

Drerup, B. (1999). Assessment of disc injury in subjects exposed to long-term whole body vibration. *European Spine Journal* **8**, 458–67.

Dubner, R. and Basbaum, A.I. (1994). Spinal dorsal horn plasticity following tissue or nerve injury. In *Textbook of Pain* (ed. P.D. Wall and R. Melzak), pp. 225–41. Edinburgh: Churchill Livingstone.

Eyre, D.R. and Muir, H. (1976). Types I and II collagens in intervertebral discs. *Biochemical Journal* **157**, 267–70.

Fairbank, J.L.T., Park, W.M., McCall, I.W., and O'Brien, J.P. (1981). Apophyseal injection of local anaesthetic as a diagnostic aid in low back syndromes. *Spine* **6**, 598–605.

Fahey, V., Opeskin, K., Silberstein, M., Anderson, R., and Briggs, C. (1998). The pathogenesis of Schmorl's nodes in relation to acute trauma. *Spine* **23**, 2272–5.

Freemont, A.J., Peacock, J.E., Goupille, P., Hoyland, J.A., O'Brien, J., and Jayson, M.I.V. (1997). Nerve ingrowth into diseased intervertebral discs in chronic back pain. *Lancet* **350**, 178–81.

Frost, H., Klaber Moffett, J.L., Moser, J.S., and Fairbanks, J.C.T. (1995). Randomised controlled clinical trial for patients with chronic low back pain. *British Medical Journal* **310**, 151–4.

Garvey, T.A., Marks, M.R., and Wiesel, S.E. (1989). A prospective, randomised double-blind evaluation of trigger-point injection therapy for low-back pain. *Spine* **14**, 962–4.

Gibson, J.N.A., Grant, I.C., and Waddell, G. (1999). The Cochrane review of surgery for lumbar disc prolapse and lumbar spondylosis. *Spine* **24**, 1820–32.

Goldberg, M.S., Scott, S.C., and Mayo, N.E. (2000). A review of the association between cigarette smoking and the development of non-specific back pain and related outcomes. *Spine* **25**, 995–1014.

Gunzberg, R., Balagué, F., Nordin, M., Szpalski, M., Duyck, D., Bull, D., and Mélot, C. (1999). Low back pain in a population of school children. *European Spine Journal* **8**, 439–43.

Haldeman, S. and Rubinstein, S.M. (1992). Cauda equina syndrome in patients undergoing manipulation of the lumbar spine. *Spine* **17**, 1469–73.

Harreby, M., Nygaard, B., Jessen, T., Larsen, E., Storr-Paulsen, A., Lindahl, A., Fisker, I., and Laegaard, E. (1999). Risk factors for low back pain in a cohort of 1387 Danish school children: an epidemiologic study. *European Spine Journal* **8**, 444–50.

Health and Safety Executive (1993). Key fact sheet on back injuries to employees between 1987/88 and 90/91. Health and Safety Executive, Statistical Services Unit.

Heliovaara, M. et al. (1987). Incidence and risk factors of herniated lumbar intervertebral disc or sciatica leading to hospitalisation. *Journal of Chronic Diseases* **40**, 251–8.

Herbert, C.M., Lindberg, K.A., Jayson, M.I.V., and Bailey, A.J. (1975). Changes in the collagen of human intervertebral discs during ageing and degenerative disc disease. *Journal of Molecular Medicine* **1**, 79–91.

Hoogendoorn, W.E., Bongers, P.E., de Vet, H.C.W., Douwes, M., Koes, B.W., Miedema, M.C., Airens, G.A.M., and Bouter, L.M. (2000). Flexion and rotation of the trunk and lifting at work are risk factors for low back pain. *Spine* **25**, 3087–92.

Hoyland, J.A., Freemont, A.J., and Jayson, M.I.V. (1988). Retained surgical debris in post laminectomy arachnoiditis. *Journal of Bone and Joint Surgery* **70B**, 659–62.

Hoyland, J.A., Freemont, A.J., and Jayson, M.I.V. (1989). Intervertebral foramen venous obstruction—a cause of peri-radicular fibrosis. *Spine* **14**, 558–68.

Hulshof, C. and van Zanten, B.V. (1987). Whole body vibration and back pain. *Archives of Occupational and Environmental Health* **59**, 205–20.

Igarashi, T., Kikuchi, S., Shubayev, V., and Myers, R.R. (2000). Exogenous tumour necrosis factor-alpha mimics nucleus pulposus induced neuropathology. *Spine* **25**, 2975–80.

Jayson, M.I.V. (1997). Why does acute back pain become chronic? Chronic back pain is not the same as acute back pain lasting longer. *British Medical Journal* **314**, 1639–40.

Jayson, M.I.V. and Barks, J.J. (1973). Structural changes in the intervertebral discs. *Annals of the Rheumatic Diseases* **32**, 10–15.

Jayson, M.I.V., Herbert, C.M., and Barks, J.S. (1973). Intervertebral discs, nuclear morphology and bursting pressures. *Annals of the Rheumatic Diseases* **32**, 308–15.

Jellema, P., van Tulder, M.W., van Poppe, M.N.M., Nachemson, A.L., and Bouter, L.M. (2001). Lumbar supports for prevention and treatment of low back pain. *Spine* **26**, 377–86.

Jensen, M.C., Brant-Zawadzki, M.N., Obuchowski, N., Modic, M.T., Malkaisian, D., and Ross, J.S. (1994). Magnetic resonance imaging of the lumbar spine in people without back pain. *New England Journal of Medicine* **331**, 69–73.

Karppinen, J. et al. (2003). Tumour necrosis factor-alpha monoclonal antibody, Infliximab used to manage severe sciatica. *Spine* **28**, 750–3.

Kendall, N.A.S., Linton, S.J., and Main, C.J. Guide to assessing psychosocial yellow flags in acute low back pain: risk factors for long-term disability and work loss. Accident rehabilitation and compensation. Wellington NZ: Insurance Corporation of New Zealand and the National Health Committee, 1997.

Kendrick, D., Fielding, K., Bentley, E., Kerslake, R., Miller, P., and Pringle, M. (2001). Radiography of the lumbar spine in primary care patients with low back pain: randomised controlled trial. *British Medical Journal* **322**, 440–5.

Kurunlahti, M., Tervoren, O., Vanharenta, H., Ilkko, E., and Suramo, I. (2000). Association of atherosclerosis with low back pain and the degree of disc degeneration. *Spine* **24**, 2080–4.

Lawrence, J.S. (1977). Disc disorders. In *Rheumatism in Populations*, pp. 68–97. London: Heinemann.

Lebouef-Yde, C. (2000). Body weight and low back pain. A systematic literature review of 56 journal articles reporting on 65 epidemiologic studies. *Spine* **25**, 226–37.

Linton, S.J. and von Tulder, M.W. (2001). Preventive interventions for back and neck problems. *Spine* **26**, 778–87.

Linton, S.J., Hellsing, A.L., and Hallden, K. (1998). A population based study of spinal pain among 35–45 year old individuals. Prevalence, sick leave, and health care use. *Spine* **23**, 1457–63.

Luoma, K., Rihimaki, H., Luukonen, R., Raininko, R., Viikari-Juntari, E., and Lamminen, A. (2000). Low back pain in relation to disc degeneration. *Spine* **25**, 487–92.

Makela, M. *Publications of the Social Insurance Institution.* Helsinki: The Research and Development Unit, 1993.

Malmivaara, A., Hakkinen, U., Aro, T., Heinrichs, M.-L., Koskenniemi, L., Kuosma, E., Lappi, S., Paloheimo, R., Servo, C., Vaaranen, V., and Hemberg, S. (1995). The treatment of acute low back pain—bed rest, exercises or ordinary activity? *New England Journal of Medicine* **332**, 351–5.

Mason, V. *The Prevalence of Back Pain in Great Britain.* (A report prepared for the Department of Health by the Office of Population Censuses and Surveys, Social Survey Division based on the Omnibus Survey March, April, June 1993.) London: HMSO, 1994.

Mayer, T.G., Gatchel, R.J., Mayer, H., Kishino, N.D., Keeley, J., and Mooney, V. (1987). A prospective two-year study of functional restoration in industrial low back injury. *Journal of the American Medical Association* **258**, 1763–7.

McDevitt, C.R. (1988). Proteoglycans of the intervertebral disc. In *Biology of the Intervertebral Disc* (ed. P. Ghosh), pp. 151–70. New York: CRC Press.

McGorry, R.W., Hsiang, S.M., Snook, S.H., Clancy, E.A., and Young, S.L. (1998). Meteorological conditions and self report of low back pain. *Spine* **23**, 2096–102.

Mitchell, J.N. (1985). Low back pain and the prospects for employment. *Journal of Social and Occupational Medicine* **35**, 91–4.

Moffett, J.K., Torgerson, D., Bell-Syer, S., Jackson, D., Llewelin-Philips, H., Farrin, A., and Barber, J. (1999). Randomised controlled trial of exercise for low back pain: clinical outcomes, costs and preferences. *British Medical Journal* **319**, 279–83.

Moore, R.J. (2000). The vertebral end-plate: what do we know? *European Spine Journal* **9**, 92–6.

Moskovich, R. (1996). Epidural injection for the treatment of low back pain. *Bulletin Hospital for Joint Diseases* **55**, 178–84.

Murphy, P.L. and Violinn, E. (1999). Is occupational low back pain on the rise. *Spine* **24**, 692–7.

Nachemson, A. (1992). Lumbar mechanics as revealed by lumbar intra-discal measurements. In *The Lumbar Spine and Back Pain* (ed. M.I.V. Jayson), pp. 157–71. Edinburgh: Churchill Livingstone.

Ng, S.C.S., Weiss, J.B., Quinnel, R., and Jayson, M.I.V. (1986). Abnormal connective tissue degrading enzyme patterns in prolapsed intervertebral disc. *Spine* **11**, 695–701.

Olmarker, K., Rydevik, B., and Nordborg, C. (1993). Autologous nucleus pulposus induces neurophysiologic and histologic changes in porcine cauda equina nerve roots. *Spine* **18**, 1425–32.

Papageorgiou, A., Croft, P., Jayson, M.I.V., and Silman, A. (1995). Estimating the prevalence of low back pain in the general population. Evidence from the South Manchester back pain survey. *Spine* **20**, 1889–94.

Papageorgiou, A.C., Croft, P.R., Thomas, E., Ferry, S., Jayson, M.I.V., and Silman, A.J. (1996). Influence of previous pain experience on the episodic incidence of low back pain: results from the South Manchester Back pain Study. *Pain* **66**, 181–5.

Porter, R.W. (1992). Spinal stenosis of the central and root canal. In *The Lumbar Spine and Back Pain* (ed. M.I.V. Jayson), pp. 313–32. Edinburgh: Churchill Livingstone.

Porter, R.W. and Hibbert, C. (1983). Calcitonin treatment for neurogenic claudication. *Spine* **8**, 585–92.

Porter, R.W., Hibbert, C., and Wellman, P. (1980). Backache and the lumbar spinal canal. *Spine* **5**, 99–105.

Postacchini, F., Lami, R., and Pugliese, O. (1988). Familial predisposition to discogenic low back pain. *Spine* **12**, 1403–6.

Powell, M.C., Wilson, M., Szypryt, P., Symonds, E.M., and Worthington, B.S. (1986). Prevalence of lumbar disc degeneration observed by magnetic resonance in symptomless women. *Lancet* **ii**, 1366–7.

Rainville, J., Sobel, J.B., Hartigan, C., and Wright, A. (1997). The effect of compensation involvement on the reporting of pain and disability by patients referred for rehabilitation of chronic low back pain. *Spine* **22**, 2016–24.

Rihimaki, H., Tola, S., Videman, T., and Hannin, K. (1989). Low back pain and occupation. *Spine* **14**, 204–9.

Royal College of General Practitioners. *Clinical Guidelines for the Management of Acute Low Back Pain.* London: Royal College of General Practitioners, 1999.

Sachs, B.T., Zindrick, M.R., and Beasley, R.D. (1993). Reflex sympathetic dystrophy after operative procedures on the lumbar spine. *Journal of Bone and Joint Surgery* **75A**, 721–5.

Sambrook, P.N., MacGregor, A.J., and Spector, T.D. (1999). Genetic influences on cervical and lumbar disc degeneration. *Arthritis and Rheumatism* **42**, 366–72.

Twomey, L. and Taylor, J. (1995). Exercise and manipulation in the treatment of low back pain. *Spine* **20**, 615–19.

Van Poppell, M.N.M., Koes, B.W., Smid, T., and Bouter, L.M. (1997). A systematic review of controlled clinical trials on the prevention of back pain in industry. *Occupational and Environmental Medicine* **54**, 841–7.

Van Tulder, M.W., Schloten, R.J.P.M., Koes, B.W., and Deyo, R.A. (2000). Nonsteroidal anti-inflammatory drugs for low back pain. *Spine* **25**, 2501–13.

Vernon Roberts, B. (1992). Age related and degenerative pathology of the intervertebral disc and apophyseal joints. In *The Lumbar Spine and Back Pain* 4th edn. (ed. M.I.V. Jayson), pp. 17–41. Edinburgh: Churchill Livingstone.

Videman, T., Nurminen, M., and Troup, J.D.G. (1990). Lumbar spinal pathology in cadaveric material in relation to history of back pain, occupation and physical loading. *Spine* **15**, 728–40.

Vlaeyen, J.W.S. and Linton, S.J. (2000). Fear-avoidance and its consequences on chronic musculo-skeletal pain: a state of the art. *Pain* **85**, 317–32.

Waddell, G. (1987). A new clinical model for the treatment of low back pain. *Spine* **12**, 632–44.

Waddell, G., McCullough, J.A., Kummel, E., and Venner, R.M. (1980). Non organic physical signs in low back pain. *Spine* **5**, 117–25.

Walsh, K. et al. (1992). Low back pain in eight areas of Britain. *Journal of Epidemiology and Community Health* **26**, 227–30.

Weiss, J.B. and McLaughlin, B. (1993). Activation of gelatinase-A and reactivation of the gelatinase-A inhibitor complex by endothelial cell stimulating angiogenesis factor. *Journal of Physiology* **456**, 49.

Wiltse, L.L. and Rothman, S.L.G. (1990). Lumbar and lumbosacral spondylolisthesis: classification, diagnosis and natural history. In *The Lumbar Spine* (ed. J.N. Weinstein and S.W. Weisel), pp. 471–99. Philadelphia PA: Saunders.

Wyke, B. (1987). The neurology of low back pain. In *The Lumbar Spine and Back Pain* 3rd edn. (ed. M.I.V. Jayson), pp. 56–99. Edinburgh: Churchill Livingstone.

6.17.2 Cervical pain syndromes

Allan I. Binder

Introduction

The vast majority of patients with neck pain have degenerative or mechanical lesions. 'Cervical spondylosis' is often used to describe neck pain of a mechanical nature, but the term is variably applied to include soft tissue, disc, and degenerative bony lesions. Furthermore, the boundary between 'normal' ageing and disease is unclear. The pathology of cervical spondylosis is assumed to be similar to lumbar spondylosis, but this has been questioned (Bland and Boushey 1990). Less research has been performed into cervical than lumbar pain, as severe disability is less common with cervical disease.

This chapter will concentrate on the common mechanical and degenerative pain syndromes that predominantly affect the cervical spine and the principles of their treatment. Other conditions that can cause neck pain will be considered in more detail in the relevant chapters devoted to the particular diseases.

Epidemiology

About two-thirds of people will experience neck pain at some time in their lives (Mäkelä et al. 1991; Cote et al. 1998), with prevalence being highest in middle age. In the United Kingdom, about 15 per cent of hospital-based physiotherapy (Hackett et al. 1987), and in Canada 30 per cent of chiropractic referrals (Waalen et al. 1994) are for neck pain. While the prevalence of neck pain is similar to that of low back pain, it is unusual to lose time from work, and under 1 per cent of patients develop neurological deficit. As many patients with neck pain never seek medical care, the true prevalence of chronic disease is uncertain.

Functional anatomy of the cervical spine

The cervical spine is the most mobile and least stable part of the human spine, consisting of seven vertebrae connected by five intervertebral discs. There are 37 separate articulations (Bland and Boushey 1990), and a complex system of ligaments and muscles, which with the varying shapes of individual vertebrae, and different methods of articulation, are responsible for the complexity of movements possible for the head and neck. Any of these structures can be the source of pain.

The vertebral arteries pass close to the zygapophyseal joints, immediately anterior to the emerging cervical nerve roots. The pre-ganglionic sympathetic nerve fibres run closely adherent to the carotid and vertebral vessels, to synapse with the stellate, middle, and superior cervical ganglia. The post-ganglionic sympathetic fibres then separate into three directions: some fibres go to the upper limbs to provide autonomic control of circulation, sweating, and proprioception; some fibres re-enter the spinal cord via the intervertebral foramina to synapse in the vestibular apparatus, cerebellum, thalamus, and hypothalamus; and some fibres pass upward with the vertebral and carotid arteries to the brain (Bland and Boushey 1990). Involvement of the vertebral arteries and sympathetic nerves in the degenerative process may explain many of the unusual features associated with disease of the cervical spine.

The lack of room in the spinal canal between C4 and T2 is due to the enlargement of the cord in this region. As degenerative changes are also most frequent and severe between C5 and T1 (Hayashi et al. 1988), compression of the cord usually develops at this site. Inflammatory arthropathies, in contrast, have a predilection for involvement of the atlantoaxial and upper cervical spine. Minor congenital spinal abnormalities increase the risk of degenerative change, and there is a remarkable similarity in the pattern of degenerative disease in monozygous twins (Palmer et al. 1984), possibly reflecting the similarity in the shape of their vertebrae.

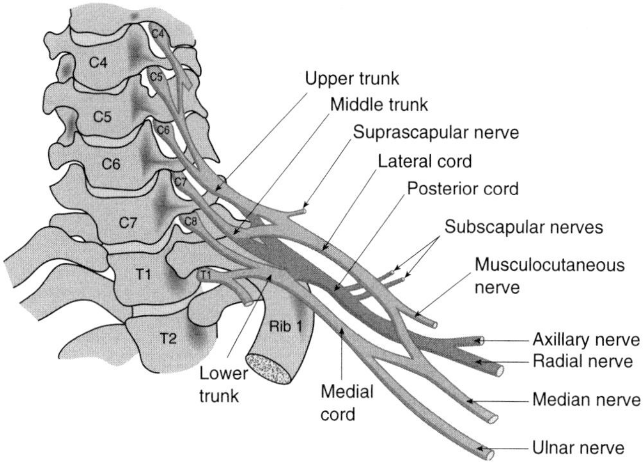

Fig. 1 Diagram showing the nerve roots (C4 to T1) forming the brachial plexus, with the peripheral nerves that arise from the plexus.

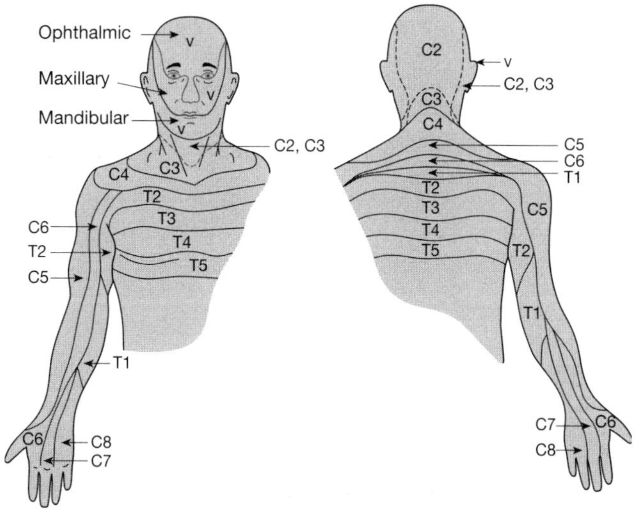

Fig. 2 Dermatomal distribution of the cervical and upper thoracic nerves that reflect the radicular pattern of nerve root lesions.

The anterior and posterior nerve roots from C4 to T1 exit through the dural root sleeves, and traverse the intervertebral foramina. They then merge to form the brachial plexus (Fig. 1), which lies between the clavicle and first rib, in close proximity to the subclavian vessels. The neurovascular bundle is susceptible to compression at various sites in the thoracic outlet, which lies between the neck and axilla. Cervical nerves have a dermatomal representation (Fig. 2), which explains the radicular pattern of symptoms in the upper limbs caused by impingement on nerve roots.

Aetiology of neck pain

Although 'cervical spondylosis' accounts for most cases of neck pain, there are many other causes of pain which need to be excluded (Table 1). The cervical spine is frequently involved in polymyalgia rheumatica, rheumatoid arthritis, and other arthropathies, and neck pain can result from serious local pathology, such as infection or malignancy. It is also often the site of referral of pain from distant sources (Table 2).

Table 1 Causes of neck pain

Soft tissue lesions
Acute neck strain
Posture-related neck pain
Psychogenic—'tension', anxiety, depression
Occupation and sport-related neck pain
'Fibrositis/fibromyalgia' and pain-amplification syndromes
Torticollis and wry-neck
Trauma—musculoligamentous injury, 'whiplash' syndrome
Degenerative and mechanical lesions
Cervical spondylosis
Cervical disc prolapse
Diffuse idiopathic skeletal hyperostosis (DISH) and ossification of the posterior longitudinal ligament (see text)
Inflammatory arthropathies
Rheumatoid arthritis
Ankylosing spondylitis and spondarthropathies
Juvenile chronic arthropathy
Polymyalgia rheumatica
Other arthropathies
Metabolic bone disease
Paget's disease, osteoporosis, osteomalacia
Crystal arthropathies—gout, pseudogout
Fibrous dysplasia
Infection
Osteomyelitis of cervical vertebra
Tuberculosis
Malignancy
Primary tumours
Secondary tumours and pathological fracture
Myeloma, lymphoma, blood dyscrasias
Brachial plexus lesions
Idiopathic cryptogenic brachial neuropathy
Thoracic-outlet syndromes—e.g. cervical rib
Trauma—motor cycle injury
Referred pain (see Table 2)

Table 2 Sites of referred pain to the neck

Acromioclavicular joint, temporomandibular joint, teeth
Heart—angina pectoris, myocardial infarction
Aorta—aneurysm
Pharynx—infection, tumour
Lung—bronchogenic carcinoma, Pancoast tumour, apical lesion
Abdomen—disease of the gallbladder, stomach, oesophagus (including hiatus hernia), and pancreas
Diaphragm—subphrenic abscess
Central nervous system—migraine, 'tension' headache, tumour, posterior fossa lesion, meningitis, arachnoiditis
Lymph node—cervical lymphadenitis
Shoulder—frozen shoulder, reflex sympathetic dystrophy

Cervical spondylosis

Pathology

With ageing, degenerative change develops in the cervical spine, and is apparent on radiographs of most adults over the age of 30 years. The term 'cervical spondylosis' refers to this progressive degenerative process, which affects all levels of the cervical spine, but with more severe changes at the lower levels (Hayashi et al. 1988). There is a sequential change in the intervertebral discs, with osteophytosis of the vertebral bodies and changes in the facet joints and laminal arches. There is a continuum from 'normal' ageing to the overtly pathological state, and a poor correlation between the degree of radiological change and the presence and severity of pain (Van der Donk et al. 1991).

With increasing age, there is a steady decrease in the degree of hydration of the intervertebral discs, and radiolucent nitrogen-filled spaces (vacuum disc phenomenon) may form within the disc, confirming the degenerative nature of the process. Other changes associated with the ageing process are loss of disc height, osteophytosis, and degenerative changes (osteoarthritis) in the nearby zygapophyseal joints and other articulating surfaces. Involvement of the spinal ligaments in the degenerative process can lead to a loss of stability, which is an important factor in causing myelopathy in elderly patients.

Clinical assessment

Detailed history and examination will usually confirm the degenerative nature of the condition or alert one to a need to exclude more serious pathology. Assessment of the shoulder joints is also necessary to determine if there is coexisting shoulder pathology, although cervical pathology itself frequently causes painful limitation in the range of shoulder flexion and abduction above the horizontal.

Symptoms

Pain

This is the most common symptom of cervical pathology, and is usually poorly localized to the neck and shoulders when arising from deep structures, such as ligaments, muscles, joints, discs, or bone. The pain can, however, be clearly defined and in a dermatomal distribution when caused by irritation of the nerve roots (Fig. 2). Pain arising from structures of the cervical spine is characteristically altered (aggravated or relieved) by their movement. The causes of neck pain are shown in Table 1.

Pain is most often referred to the occiput, nuchal muscles, and superior aspect of the shoulders. Heaviness or aching of the upper limbs also reflects cervical origin, and the pain can closely mimic soft tissue lesions of the shoulder, elbow, and wrist (Murray-Leslie and Wright 1976). Retro-orbital and temporal pain suggest referral from the upper cervical levels (C1 to C3), and temporal pain when associated with tenderness can be misinterpreted as evidence of giant-cell arteritis. Pain can also be referred to the upper thoracic spine and interscapular areas. Some patients, especially with lesions of C6 and C7 complain of anterior chest pain, which closely mimics coronary ischaemia (Brodsky 1985). Pseudoangina of this type is sometimes associated with local tenderness of the chest wall. There is particular diagnostic difficulty in patients with a combination of both coronary insufficiency and cervical spondylosis, as anginal pain is more likely to radiate to the neck in patients with symptomatic cervical spondylosis. Coronary angiography is the key investigation in the assessment of the severity of the cardiac lesion in these cases. Occipital headache is a common manifestation of cervical degenerative disease, especially when the disease affects the upper cervical levels, but occipital neuralgia will need to be excluded in these cases.

Stiffness

This is a common accompaniment of ageing, degeneration, and most vertebral diseases. It may or may not be associated with pain and may be reversible or irreversible.

Dizziness

This may occur as a result of involvement of the vertebral arteries, especially in the presence of severe degenerative spinal disease. Atheroma and disturbance of flow in the vertebral vessels may contribute to the development of dizziness in older patients. Vertigo and faintness caused by vertebrobasilar disease is nearly always accompanied by other focal symptoms of transient ischaemia of the brainstem or occipital lobes. In some patients with cervical pathology, tinnitus and gait disturbance (Sudarsky and Ronthal 1983) can occur as a result of irritation of the sympathetic nerves.

Paraesthesia and sensory loss

Numbness and tingling is usually vague and ill-defined in cervical spondylosis, but can be precise, following the clear segmental dermatomal distribution of nerve entrapment (see 'Radiculopathy' below). The symptoms are often affected by neck movement, or are postural, being worse at night or with specific activities. Lesions of C1 to C3 can cause paraesthesia affecting the face, head, and tongue. Involvement of the C4 root gives symptoms referred to the superior aspect of the shoulder, and C5 to T1 lesions give numbness in the upper limb (see Fig. 2).

Weakness

Mechanical disease of the cervical spine most typically gives a subjective feeling of heaviness or weakness, especially affecting the hands, but without true weakness on formal testing. Objective muscle weakness, wasting, and fasciculation in the absence of systemic upset suggests a radiculopathy, thoracic-outlet syndrome, or neuropathy of the brachial plexus. Abnormality of gait due to spasticity of the lower limbs suggests myelopathy.

Rare manifestations

Unusual features sometimes resulting from pathology of the cervical spine are shown in Table 3. Most of these symptoms result from irritation of the sympathetic nerves, but the clue to their vertebral origin is reproducibility with neck movement.

Signs

Tenderness

When due to degenerative disease, tenderness is poorly localized and of variable severity. It is usually worse in the lower cervical region, and may be associated with muscle spasm. Tender myofascial trigger points are a characteristic feature of the 'fibrositis/fibromyalgia' syndrome (Smythe 1986), but also occur with disease of the facet joints. Exquisite localized tenderness over a vertebral body may suggest osteomyelitis or malignancy, particularly if the patient has features of systemic upset or abnormality of blood tests such as full blood count, erythrocyte sedimentation rate, C-reactive protein, or protein electrophoresis.

Limitation of movement

This is a feature of ageing and degeneration and may be otherwise asymptomatic or accompanied by pain. Severe irreversible loss of range particularly on lateral flexion and rotation occurs with cervical spondylosis, but is more characteristic of the spondarthropathies and diffuse idiopathic skeletal hyperostosis (DISH). Reversible stiffness, worse in the early morning, is more suggestive of polymyalgia rheumatica or an inflammatory arthropathy than of a degenerative lesion.

Neurological deficit

Neurological abnormalities are characteristic of myelopathy, radiculopathy, but also occurs in thoracic-outlet syndromes and neuropathy of the brachial plexus (see below).

Table 3 Rarer symptoms arising from cervical spine pathology

Visual—blurring, diplopia, retro-orbital pain
Auditory—tinnitus, nerve deafness, earache, poor balance
Intestinal—dysphagia, nausea, vomiting, diarrhoea
Cardiac—'pseudoangina', dyspnoea, palpitations
Respiratory—cough, dyspnoea, sneezing
Central nervous system—syncope, 'drop attacks', vertebro-basilar insufficiency, speech disturbance, migraine

Radiological assessment

Routine radiographs of the anteroposterior and lateral spine are sufficient to indicate the severity of bone and disc pathology, but correlates very poorly with symptoms. A through-mouth view to outline the odontoid peg, when combined with flexion/extension radiographs, will demonstrate existing subluxation. Oblique views of the cervical spine may demonstrate intervertebral foraminal narrowing, and are useful in patients suspected of having a radiculopathy (Fig. 3). Loss of cervical lordosis on the lateral radiograph in patients with neck pain is usually ascribed to muscle spasm, but this association has been questioned (Helliwell et al. 1994).

Magnetic resonance imaging (MRI) is the radiological investigation of choice, giving detailed information about the spinal cord, bones, discs, and soft tissue structures (Figs 4 and 5). MRI is particularly valuable in demonstrating congenital abnormalities, cord tumours, demyelination, and disc lesions. Degenerative vertebral changes are well demonstrated, but as they occur normally with ageing, they need to be interpreted with care. Asymptomatic people often show important pathological lesions, such as narrowing of the disc space, osteophytosis, or even compression of the spinal cord (Boden et al. 1990), and the frequency of abnormal scans in asymptomatic people increases with age. Decisions about surgery should be based on clinical indications with the support of the MR findings, and not on radiological data alone. Similar false-positive studies have been described with plain radiography, computed tomography (CT), and other radiological techniques.

CT, myelography, and CT–myelography, are useful alternative radiological modalities to MRI for the assessment of cervical disease especially at the upper cervical levels, which are hard to visualize on routine radiographs. However, investigations that include myelography are considerably more invasive.

Electrodiagnostic studies

Electromyography, nerve conduction studies, and somatosensory evoked potentials may help in the elucidation of the diagnosis, especially where primary neurological disease or polymyositis need to be differentiated from radiculopathy or myelopathy secondary to degenerative vertebral disease (Dvorak et al. 1990). Specific neurophysiological findings have been described in cervical spondylosis associated with myelopathy or radiculopathy, but are unreliable, particularly in uncomplicated cervical spondylosis.

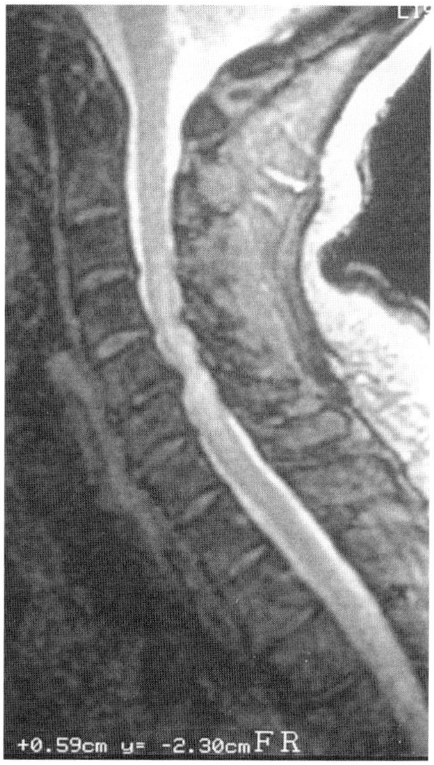

Fig. 4 MRI scan showing loss of height and signal affecting several discs, with multisegmental spondylotic bars. Compression of the cord is noted by protrusion of the C5/6 disc with myelopathic changes in the cord.

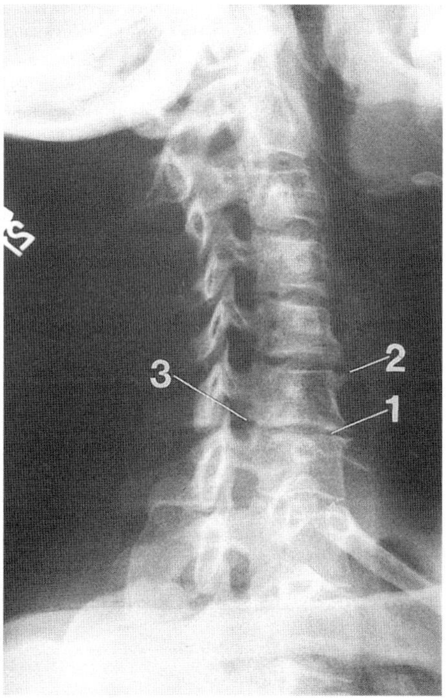

Fig. 3 Oblique radiograph of the cervical spine in a patient with cervical spondylosis, showing the loss of disc height (1), anterior osteophytosis (2), and foraminal narrowing (3).

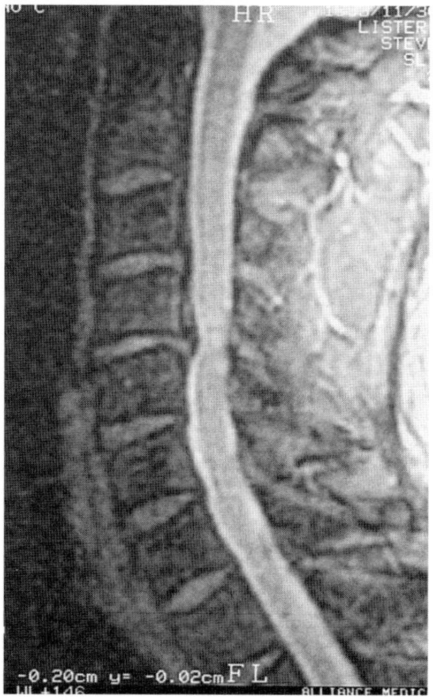

Fig. 5 MRI scan showing a cervical disc prolapse at C4/5 with impingement upon the cervical cord and secondary myelopathic changes in the cord itself.

Other tests

Other tests such as full blood count, erythrocyte sedimentation rate, C-reactive protein, protein electrophoresis, liver function tests, urate, rheumatoid factor, and bone scan may be necessary to exclude other causes of neck pain (Tables 1 and 2).

Complications of cervical spondylosis

While cervical myelopathy and radiculopathy often result from progressive degeneration of the cervical spine, the other important causes in the differential diagnosis also need to be considered.

Cervical myelopathy

The relatively tight fit of the spinal cord in the lower cervical region, as a result of the natural expansion of the cervical cord, accounts for an increased risk of development of a myelopathy at this site.

Myelopathy can develop de novo, or can occur in patients with known cervical spondylosis, particularly in the presence of a congenitally narrow spinal canal. With progressive degeneration and resulting osteophytosis and instability, pressure on the spinal cord can develop.

In elderly patients, myelopathy can result from compression of the spinal cord, disturbed blood supply, or a combination of both factors. Disc protrusion, posterior osteophyte formation, and retrolisthesis (posterior slide) due to ligamentous laxity, contribute to age-related spondylotic spinal compression (Hayashi et al. 1988). Even when the static spinal canal diameter is adequate, many elderly patients show significant and progressive 'dynamic' spinal stenosis (Hayashi et al. 1988), which can be demonstrated by a comparison of flexion and extension on CT or MRI scans.

In young patients, a sudden onset of myelopathy or radiculopathy suggests cervical disc prolapse (see below). Cervical myelopathy can also result from vertebral diseases such as osteomyelitis, malignancy, and crystal arthropathy, and intramedullary disease can present with similar symptoms (Table 4).

Cervical myelopathy typically presents with a slowly progressive disability over a period of weeks or months, although the onset can be sudden, especially when caused by trauma or central disc prolapse. The most common, early manifestations of myelopathy are clumsiness, weakness, or dysaesthesia of the hands, or gait disturbance due to upper motor-neurone abnormality in the lower limbs.

Numbness or tingling in the hands is poorly localized, unless radiculopathy is also present. There is usually no gross sensory deficit, but blunting of light touch, pin-prick, and temperature sensation can occur. Stereoanaesthesia, and isolated loss of position sense in the hands, is also sometimes seen, particularly in high cervical lesions. Clumsiness or weakness of the hands may rarely be associated with variable degrees of wasting and evidence of lower motor-neurone abnormality at the level of the lesion. Characteristic features in the legs are of a spastic paraparesis, and in elderly patients, undiagnosed cervical myelopathy is an important case of gait disturbance (Sudarsky and Ronthal 1983).

Tendon reflexes are often reduced in the arms and increased in the legs with up-going plantar responses and ankle clonus, although the balance is dependent on the level of the lesion. Inversion of the supinator jerk (reduced or absent supinator reflex with brisk finger flexion when tapping over the lower radius), with a brisk triceps jerk, suggests involvement of the spinal cord at the C5/6 level. A brisk finger-flexion reflex (on tapping the examiner's own fingers when placed over the flexor surface of the terminal phalanges) and a positive Hoffman's sign (brisk thumb flexion when the distal phalanx of the middle finger is flicked into extension) also suggests hyperreflexia. Sphincter control is usually well maintained in cervical myelopathy complicating cervical spondylosis.

Neck pain may not be a prominent feature of myelopathy, and when present, its mechanism of production is complex and poorly understood. The cervical lesion is often multisegmental (Fig. 4), and in some cases there is a large discrepancy between the sensory level on clinical examination and the true level of cord compression (Simmons et al. 1986).

Table 4 Differential diagnosis of cervical myelopathy

Cervical spondylotic myelopathy
Other causes of compressive cervical myelopathy
Central disc prolapse
Congenital spinal canal stenosis
Inflammatory arthropathy, especially rheumatoid arthritis
DISH and ossification of the posterior longitudinal ligament (see text)
Crystal diseases—gout, pseudogout
Paget's disease
Haematoma, trauma
Infection—tuberculosis, spinal epidural abscess
Tumour—meningioma, neurofibroma, lymphoma, leukaemia, myeloma, secondaries, pathological fracture
Radiation myelopathy
Primary spinal cord disease
Spinal multiple sclerosis
Subacute combined degeneration of the cord
Motor neurone disease (amyotrophic lateral sclerosis)
Hereditary spastic paraplegia and other genetic disorders
Infective or inflammatory myelitis, e.g. sarcoid, systemic lupus, and HIV infection
Syringomyelia
Parasagittal cranial meningioma
Anterior spinal artery syndrome (onset usually sudden)

Shooting electric pain down the spine, arms, or legs, or temporary neurological deficit when the head is flexed (Lhermitte phenomenon) may be mentioned by the patient. Great caution (and prior radiography) is necessary when attempting to confirm the presence of this sign, as permanent deterioration in the neurological condition may follow its performance. Lhermitte phenomenon is usually a sign of cervical myelopathy of an inflammatory type (typically multiple sclerosis), but can be due to compressive, or rarely other (e.g. vitamin B_{12} deficiency) causes.

MRI (Fig. 4) is the investigation of choice in patients with suspected myelopathy, although CT–myelography can also be used. The anteroposterior or sagittal diameter of the canal on radiological investigation is a useful indicator of possible myelopathy, and compression of the cord is likely if the diameter at any level is 10 mm or less (Murone 1974). With a diameter above 13 mm, compressive symptoms rarely occur solely on the basis of degenerative disease. Atrophy of the spinal cord on CT–myelography, or intrinsic spinal cord damage on MRI (Fig. 4), especially after myelopathic decompression, are associated with a less favourable outcome.

Cervical radiculopathy

Nerve root compression as a result of cervical spondylosis usually occurs at the C5 to C7 level with lesions being single or multiple, and uni- or bilateral.

Acute radiculopathy in the young usually follows trauma or lateral prolapse of a cervical disc. In middle-aged and elderly patients, asymptomatic osteophytic encroachment gradually narrows the nerve root foramina until trivial trauma is sufficient to precipitate acute or subacute radiculopathy. Chronic radiculopathy may arise insidiously, or may follow the more acute syndromes. As chronic radicular syndromes are usually due to degenerative disease, they can be associated with myelopathy.

Neurological features follow a segmental distribution in the upper limb (see Fig. 2). Sensory symptoms such as shooting pain, paraesthesia, and hyperaesthesia are more common than motor weakness or a change in the reflexes. Arm weakness, when present, is of a lower motor-neurone type, and may be accompanied by a loss of reflex (biceps and supinator jerk in C5/6 lesions; triceps jerk in C7 lesions).

Radicular pain can be exacerbated by manoeuvres that stretch the affected root, or by an increase in intrathoracic or intra-abdominal pressure, as occurs with coughing, sneezing, or the Valsalva manoeuvre. If sustained shoulder abduction induces a temporary relief in radicular pain, a C6 lesion can be

Table 5 Differential diagnosis of cervical radiculopathy

Cervical spondylotic radiculopathy
Other causes of compressive cervical radiculopathy Lateral disc prolapse Inflammatory arthropathy, e.g. rheumatoid arthritis Trauma, haematoma Arachnoiditis Infection DISH and ossification of the posterior longitudinal ligament (see text) Tumour—primary, secondary, Pancoast tumour of lung
Brachial plexus and thoracic-outlet syndromes
Peripheral nerve and 'double-crush' syndromes
Complete rotator-cuff tear and reflex sympathetic dystrophy
Motor neurone disease and other primary spinal cord diseases (see Table 4)

expected (Fast et al. 1989). This test has value both diagnostically and as part of a conservative treatment regimen (Farmer and Wisneski 1994).

Oblique cervical radiographs often demonstrate narrowing of the nerve root foramina (Fig. 3) in patients with radiculopathy, but this is better demonstrated by MRI. Electromyography may show abnormalities in patients with clinical signs of root compression, and additional information can sometimes be obtained from studying superficial radial sensory-evoked potentials. However, these techniques are of limited value where symptoms of radiculopathy occur without objective signs.

Cervical radiculopathy (Table 5) can rarely be caused by malignant tumours, such as Pancoast tumour, or nasopharyngeal malignancies, particularly when accompanied by bony infiltration. There is often difficulty in differentiating cervical spondylosis with myelopathy or radiculopathy from primary neurological diseases, such as syringomyelia, motor neurone disease (amyotrophic lateral sclerosis), or tumour, particularly when unrelated osteoarthrosis of the cervical spine coexists (see Tables 4 and 5). MRI is the investigation of choice in these patients.

Other important mechanical pain syndromes

Cervical disc prolapse

Herniation of a cervical disc is a common cause of neck, shoulder, and arm pain in the younger patient. It typically presents as a sudden onset of neck pain with associated muscle spasm, followed by radicular symptoms and signs in the upper limb. It may follow trivial trauma or awkward movements of the neck, but in many cases there is no obvious cause. Some patients give a history of preceding mechanical cervical pain, and manipulation or chiropractic therapy can rarely precipitate the acute disc prolapse. The lesions almost always affect the lower cervical levels.

Lateral disc protrusion, which is more common, results in radiculopathy affecting the C7 root in 70 per cent of cases, the C6 root in 20 per cent, and the C5 or C8 root in the remaining 10 per cent of cases. The site of pain and the neurological features depend on the level of the lesion (Smythe 1994; Nakajima and Hirayama 1995), but the syndromes are often incomplete. Limitation of cervical range is usual, and pain can be aggravated by movement (especially hyperextension), coughing, and sneezing, and relieved by traction on the neck.

Central disc prolapse, if large, causes myelopathy (Fig. 5), and when painless may simulate degenerative syndromes of the spinal cord, such as motor neurone disease or multiple sclerosis (see Table 4). MRI or CT–myelography are essential to differentiate disc prolapse or other causes of compressive myelopathy from intrinsic disease of the spinal cord, even when the latter is considered more likely.

Disc prolapse is much less common in the thoracic spine and is difficult to diagnose clinically, unless myelopathy or radiculopathy intervene.

Diffuse idiopathic skeletal hyperostosis (DISH, Forestier's disease, ankylosing hyperostosis)

This common disorder of unknown aetiology is most often diagnosed in middle-aged or elderly white males, who show an ossifying diathesis. Patients develop flowing ossification along the anterior and lateral aspects of the spine, bridging between vertebrae, but with preservation of normal disc heights. The condition affects the thoracic spine most severely, but can also occur in the cervical and lumbar regions. The lesions start at the ligamentous insertions (entheses), with progressive ossification along the ligaments. Similar changes can occur at entheses along the pelvis and other parts of the skeleton.

Severe limitation of cervical spine movement usually develops without any other symptoms. However, some patients present with pain, myelopathy, and less commonly, radiculopathy. Large anterior osteophytes in the cervical region can also cause dysphagia due to oesophageal obstruction. If anterior osteophytes as a result of cervical spondylosis or DISH are suspected as the cause of the dysphagia, barium swallow is the preferred method of assessment, as endoscopy carries some risk of inadvertent oesophageal perforation.

Ossification of the posterior longitudinal ligament

This is probably a variant of DISH (Hukuda et al. 1983), or is closely associated with it. It is most frequently found in Japanese or other Asian patients, but can affect all ethnic groups. Like DISH, it occurs most often in middle-aged and elderly males, with a majority of cases producing no symptoms. However, in association with congenital and degenerative vertebral abnormalities, even trivial trauma can precipitate cervical myelopathy or radiculopathy. The ossification can be difficult to detect on plain radiographs, and both MRI and CT scanning have value where the diagnosis is suspected. Calcification of the ligamentum flavum and posterior longitudinal ligament can also result from calcium pyrophosphate crystal deposition (pseudogout), confirmed on biopsy in patients having surgery for compressive myelopathy (Baba et al. 1993).

Soft tissue syndromes considered to be 'mechanical'

Spasm, postural, and anxiety/tension-related neck pain

Most adults suffer transient neck pain and stiffness, which is attributed to awkward posture of the neck, especially during sleep. The pathology is uncertain and the condition is self-limiting within days. Occupations and hobbies that involve heavy lifting or unusual positions of the neck are a cause of recurrent pain of this type. Anxiety and tension can manifest as episodic or chronic neck pain in susceptible individuals. Poor posture of the cervical and thoracic spine, which can cause muscle spasm, and hence traction on the nerve roots, may explain these symptoms. The interaction between cervical spondylosis, tension, and the fibrositis/pain-amplification syndrome needs further clarification.

'Fibrositis/fibromyalgia' and pain-amplification syndrome

'Fibrositis' is a term that has been used for many decades to describe non-specific neck pain. Smythe (1986) defined the diagnosis more precisely, describing a pain-amplification syndrome associated with localized points of myofascial tenderness. This can be confined to the cervical spine (fibrositis), or can be more generalized (fibromyalgia), with the tender points concentrated around the entheses. Patients localize the pain to the posterior and lateral regions of the neck with associated stiffness. Tenderness is noted most specifically anterior to the transverse processes in the lower cervical spine. Sleep disturbance and fatiguability have been described in some cases. There is greater agreement on diagnostic features with the adoption of the American College of Rheumatology Fibromyalgia Classification Criteria (Wolfe et al. 1990).

Neck pain associated with tender trigger points is also found as a stress-related phenomenon (Croft et al. 1994; Wolfe et al. 1995). Poor posture, underlying vertebral degeneration, especially of the facet joints, sleep disturbance, and pain amplification may be important elements contributing to the severity of pain in these cases. Pain amplification may also explain the disproportionately severe pain in some patients with rheumatoid arthritis and other inflammatory arthropathies. Treatment of fibromyalgia is disappointing, and the level of disability is often similar to rheumatoid arthritis (Martinez et al. 1995).

Whiplash-associated disorder

Flexion–extension injuries, typically as a result of rear-end impact automobile accidents, can cause acute neck pain (Whiplash-Associated Disorder, WAD), even in the absence of bone damage. A systematic review by Spitzer et al. (1995), highlighted the paucity of good data on this condition, but suggested the Quebec Classification of WAD (Table 6) with possible prognostic significance and to act as a framework for prospective study. The current discussion is limited to Grades 1–3 of their classification. While symptoms are usually self-limited in days or weeks, many patients develop persistent disability. The marked variation in the frequency of chronic disability between countries or even different regions in the same country remains unexplained (Ferrari and Russell 1999), and WAD has become an international medicolegal and social minefield with regard to diagnosis and optimal treatment.

WAD usually presents with severe cervical pain, spasm, loss of range, and occipital headache, starting within 24 h of a neck injury. Many patients also complain of widely radiating pain, headache, vertigo, memory loss, poor concentration, fatigue, or neurological symptoms in the upper limbs (Radanov et al. 1992).

The pathology of the condition is unclear, but soft tissue damage, bleeding into the muscles, and zygapophysial joint injury (Barnsley et al. 1995) may explain the acute pain and spasm. Traction and microinjury of the cord, and acceleration/deceleration injury to the brain may be responsible for some of the other symptoms. The presence of cervical spondylosis adds to the risks of damage to the spinal cord or emerging nerve roots. Despite the frequency of whiplash injury, there is no objective investigation, which, if carried out early on, can define the site and severity of the damage and so predict outcome. Scintigraphy, CT, and MRI are useful in excluding other pathology, but rarely correlate with clinical symptoms and signs of whiplash.

The management of acute whiplash remains controversial, but there is increasing evidence that resumption of normal activities (Borchgrevink et al. 1998) and early mobilization (Bonk et al. 2000; Rosenfeld et al. 2000) are associated with a better outcome than inactivity and a collar. This emphasis on early active treatment and maintenance of normal activities may help prevent prolonged disability.

Factors associated with a poor outcome are uncertain, but include older age, neck stiffness, referred symptoms, abnormal neurological signs, degenerative changes on radiographs, and symptoms persisting for more than 2 months. Psychosocial factors and personality traits were less important than the physical factors (reflecting severity) mentioned above, in predicting outcome (Radanov et al. 1994), and the settlement of litigation was not always associated with recovery (Parmar and Raymakers 1993). The risk of persistent symptoms at 6 months has also been found to correlate with the severity grade on the Quebec Classification at presentation (Hartling et al. 2001). It is uncertain if whiplash injury accelerates the progression of degenerative change in affected patients.

Once whiplash symptoms become established and have proven unresponsive to physical therapies, the prognosis for recovery is poor. More detailed study of the psychological and medicolegal aspects of WAD, and factors that influence regional variations in incidence of chronic disease is necessary.

Table 6 The Quebec classification of whiplash-associated disorders (Spitzer et al. 1995)

Grade	Clinical presentation
0	No complaint about neck, no physical signs
1	Neck complaint (pain, stiffness, or tenderness) No physical signs
2	Neck complaint and musculoskeletal signs (↓ range, tenderness)
3	Neck complaint and neurological signs (↓ reflexes, weakness, sensory loss)
4	Neck complaint and fracture or dislocation

Treatment of mechanical cervical disease

Most mechanical neck pain is responsive to conservative therapeutic measures, but few therapies currently used have been studied in sufficient detail to confirm their efficacy (Binder 2003). Box 1 summarizes the principles of therapy and timing of MRI scanning in patients with uncomplicated acute and chronic mechanical cervical syndromes and those with neurological complications.

Physical therapies

There is some evidence of efficacy for active exercise regimes that emphasize improvement in muscle strength, mobility, and proprioceptive control (Jordan et al. 1998; Taimela et al. 2000), but very little evidence for physical therapies such as heat, cold, acupuncture, laser, and electrotherapy (Gross et al. 1999; Binder 2003). However, all these modalities may provide symptomatic relief to some patients, especially where more active therapies are contraindicated. Dizziness, when due to cervical causes, usually proves unresponsive to physiotherapy and is often a limiting factor to this type of treatment.

Manual therapies

Manual therapies are increasingly used to treat spinal conditions, and are the treatments of choice for many patients with chronic neck pain. *Mobilization* (any manual treatment to improve joint function that does not involve high- velocity movement, anaesthesia, or instrumentation) is usually provided by physiotherapists, and *manipulation* (short- or long-lever high-velocity thrusts directed at one or more of the cervical spine joints that does not involve anaesthesia or instrumentation) is carried out by a variety of therapists such as osteopaths and chiropractors. A systematic review of manual therapies found them superior to a variety of less active therapies (Hurwitz et al. 1996), although the long-term benefits are rarely documented. Furthermore, Jordan et al. (1998) did not find any difference in outcome between mobilization, manipulation, and an intensive exercise regime.

The only adverse effect associated with *mobilization* has been an occasional increase in pain. *Manipulation* has been reported to cause rare but serious adverse events including death and serious disability caused by vertebrobasilar and other strokes, dissection of the vertebral arteries, disc herniation, and other neurological complications. The estimated risk from case reports of cerebrovascular accident is 1–3 per million manipulations, which is considerably less than for non-steroidal anti-inflammatory drugs (Dabbs and Lauretti 1995).

Box 1 Principles of treatment of mechanical cervical syndromes and timing of MRI scanning

Mechanical cervical spine lesions			
No neurological signs		**With neurological signs**	
Chronic or recurrent	**Acute**	**Myelopathy**	**Radiculopathy**
First			
Mobilization/manipulation Other physio—traction, hydro Postural advice and home exercise Cervical pillow Pain control* Intermittent soft collar	Pain control* Gentle physiotherapy Muscle relaxant Soft collar Tricyclic agent nocte ? Rest or bedrest	Collar—firm or soft Pain control* Muscle relaxant ? Rest or bedrest Muscle relaxant URGENT MRI SCAN	Collar—firm or soft Pain control* Muscle relaxant Tricyclic agent nocte ? Rest or bedrest
Then			
Tricyclic agent nocte Inject 'trigger' points Acupuncture	Gentle mobilization	Scan abnormal— neurosurgical referral *or* review diagnosis Scan normal—review diagnosis Walking aid	Gentle traction MRI scan Scan normal—further traction and/or epidural injection Scan abnormal—neurosurgical referral *or* review diagnosis
If no better			
MRI scan Scan normal—epidural injection Scan abnormal—neurosurgical referral *or* review diagnosis	MRI scan Scan normal—epidural injection Scan abnormal— neurosurgical referral *or* review diagnosis	Pain clinic	Pain clinic
If still no better			
Pain clinic	Pain clinic		

* Simple analgesics and/or anti-inflammatory drugs.

Soft collar and cervical or soft pillow

A soft collar can be worn during periods of increased pain, and is especially valuable to facilitate sleep when this is disturbed by pain. Special pillows can also provide support for the neck during sleep, although some clinicians prefer to recommend a soft pillow that can be moulded into the appropriate shape to support the neck. Patients should be discouraged from using more than one or two pillows, to prevent undue angulation of the neck, which can precipitate symptoms at night and on waking. Use of a collar combined with inactivity after acute whiplash may slow recovery and increase the risk of chronic disability.

Advice and home exercise

Advice on posture and relaxation (such as the Alexander technique), weight reduction, and a home exercise programme are also likely to be beneficial. The avoidance of awkward head positions and lifting heavy weights, especially in occupational or recreational activities, may also prove of value.

Rest or bedrest

Bedrest is only justified for acute neck lesions, such as a prolapsed cervical disc, trauma, or when there is a suspicion of infection or malignancy, especially when accompanied by a neurological deficit. A hard collar is advisable in these cases, and patients should be watched carefully for a deterioration in neurological status, when urgent neurosurgical intervention may be necessary.

Drug therapy

Analgesic tablets can be used during periods of increased pain, but anti-inflammatory and muscle relaxant drugs are only required in acute situations where pain is particularly severe. Low-dose amitryptiline (10–30 mg at night) may alter the pain amplification cycle noted in some patients. However, there are no studies of efficacy for any of these therapies in mechanical neck pain (Binder 2003).

Cervical epidural injection

The injection of depot steroids into the cervical epidural space can maximize pain control in patients in whom serious underlying pathology, such as infection or tumour, or gross neurological deficit have been excluded (Bush and Hillier 1996). While epidural injections appear to produce long-lasting improvement in some patients with intractable neck pain or radicular symptoms, there are no controlled studies of this therapy. The injection of local steroid alone, or in combination with local anaesthetic agents, into painful 'trigger' points or near painful facet joints or impinged nerve roots, may also relieve pain and spasm in some cases.

Surgery

Neurosurgical intervention is only necessary in patients with progressive cervical myelopathy, or rarely with radiculopathy or intractable pain. Even with a prolapsed cervical disc, most patients will recover spontaneously or with conservative measures. Compared to prolapse of a lumbar disc, herniation of a cervical disc is associated with a slower rate of recovery—over weeks or months. Conservative therapy should be continued for longer in patients who are neurologically stable, as the result of decompressive surgery is often disappointing in patients with cervical myelopathy due to degenerative disease. While the rate of progression of the neurological deficit may be slowed by the surgery, the lost function may not recover. This poor outcome reflects the irreversible nature of the damage to the spinal cord (see Figs 4 and 5) and also the compromised vascular supply to the cord in some cases. Some patients show a good initial recovery following surgery, but with relapse some time later. This relapse may reflect recurrence of the original pathology, or scar tissue developing at the site of the initial operation. The likely benefits of further surgery are based on detailed reinvestigation by MRI and other means.

In principle, surgical intervention can be achieved via the anterior and/or posterior routes, with the operative procedure being individually selected on the basis of detailed clinical and radiological assessment. In cases of myelopathy, a multisegmental operation is often necessary to obtain satisfactory results. This multisegmental approach is particularly important where neurological abnormality is associated with DISH or ossification of the posterior longitudinal ligament that have been unresponsive to conservative therapy.

Although many operations using the anterior or posterior approach have been advocated for cervical myelopathy, they are all based on the principles of fusion to prevent excessive motion (especially if only one or two levels are involved), and decompression by laminectomy, laminoplasty, or discectomy.

Surgery is less often necessary for cervical radiculopathy. The principles of treatment are similar to those for myelopathy, but decompression can be achieved by foraminotomy and/or partial discectomy. High-risk patients with radiculopathy may be successfully treated conservatively with physiotherapy and a collar (Persson et al. 1997), even when due to cervical disc prolapse (Saal et al. 1996).

Pain clinic

Where physical approaches to therapy have been exhausted, the multidisciplinary approach of the pain clinic may assist the patient in learning to cope with the chronic pain. This approach is more often required for low-back-pain syndromes, where prolonged disability is more likely.

Neck pain, shoulder pain, and soft tissue lesions in the upper limb

Patients with cervical spondylosis often complain of shoulder pain, and it is important to differentiate neck pain referred to the shoulder (usually the superior aspect) from primary conditions of the shoulder. Many patients have features that suggest both cervical and shoulder lesions, and these can be difficult to separate. Treatment may need to be directed at both sites.

The 'double-crush' syndrome refers to a combination of both cervical radiculopathy and a peripheral nerve entrapment lesion. The most common peripheral lesion is carpal tunnel syndrome, although the ulnar and radial nerves can also be affected. Elucidation of the peripheral lesion is usually possible using electromyography and nerve conduction studies. Somatosensory evoked potentials and electromyographic sampling of the more proximal muscles may provide evidence of cervical radiculopathy or plexus lesions in addition to the peripheral lesion. In double-crush lesions, surgical intervention should be directed at the peripheral entrapment before the cervical lesion.

Cervical spondylosis can also mimic epicondylitis and other localized soft tissue lesions in the upper limbs, and there is a well-documented association between cervical spondylosis and these soft tissue lesions (Murray-Leslie and Wright 1976).

Referred pain syndromes

Where appropriate, assessment for polymyalgia rheumatica, reflex sympathetic dystrophy, inflammatory arthropathy, infection, malignancy, and even crystal arthropathies may be necessary. Table 2 shows the sites of origin, and the more common causes of pain referred to the cervical region.

Brachial plexus lesions

Pain of brachial plexus origin is felt in the neck, shoulder, forearm, or hand. Supraclavicular pain is common and may be accompanied by local tenderness, and bony (cervical rib), or pulsatile (aneurysm) swelling at this site. The pain can often be induced by certain manoeuvres or changes in the position of the arm (see below). Table 7 shows the causes of brachial plexus injury.

Thoracic-outlet obstruction

Compression of the distal nerve roots, brachial plexus, subclavian vessels, or the combined neurovascular bundle can occur at various sites between the neck and the axilla (the thoracic-outlet). Possible contributing factors are shown in Table 8. 'Cervical ribs', which vary from simple exostoses of the transverse processes of C7 to fully formed extra ribs, are the most common cause of the thoracic-outlet syndrome. As 0.5 per cent of the population have bilateral cervical ribs yet less than 10 per cent ever get symptoms, other factors must also be important in symptomatic patients. Poor posture and sagging or droopy shoulders (Swift and Nichols 1984) have been identified as important factors in the development of symptoms, especially in females of early or middle age, in whom the syndrome is most often diagnosed.

The typical symptoms of thoracic-outlet obstruction vary according to the site of compression of the neurovascular bundle (Novak et al. 1993). Pain is usually present in the neck, shoulder, or upper arm. Vasomotor abnormalities such as numbness, paraesthesia, coldness, colour change, or Raynaud's phenomenon are characteristic of the lesion and may dominate the picture. Compression of the lower levels of the brachial plexus result in neurological features such as sensory loss in the C8 and T1 dermatomes, with paraesthesia, or weakness in the hand. Some patients show well-defined syndromes due to selective compression of the subclavian vein, artery, or brachial plexus (Wilbourn 1993).

Obliteration of the radial or brachial pulse may be noted, either when the patient takes and holds a full breath with the head tilted back or rotated laterally (Adson test), or when the arm is abducted and externally rotated

Table 7 Causes of brachial plexus lesions

Trauma—birth and motor cycle injury, surgery, cannulae or needles
Thoracic-outlet syndrome—e.g. cervical rib
Traction—surgery, e.g. medial sternotomy, rucksack palsy, post-anaesthesia
Brachial plexus neuropathy (brachial neuritis)
Infection—viral, bacterial
Toxins—heroin
Injection of foreign serum or vaccine
Systemic illness—lupus, vasculitis, Hodgkin's disease
Familial brachial plexus neuropathy
Idiopathic
Radiotherapy
Tumour—especially Pancoast tumour of lung, breast
Lightening, electric shock

Table 8 Contributing factors to thoracic-outlet syndrome

Cervical rib
Congenital fibromuscular bands
Congenital abnormality of clavicle or first rib
Interscalenus muscle hypertrophy
Clavipectoral lesions—the 'hyperabduction syndrome'
Old fracture of the first rib or clavicle
Vascular disorders and hyperviscosity syndromes
External compression, e.g. heavy weights, rucksack lesions
Poor posture, sagging, or droopy shoulders
Excessive muscle development around shoulders

while the shoulders are braced (Wrights manoeuvre). Both tests can be noted with thoracic-outlet syndrome, but are not reliable indicators of this condition.

Ten per cent of patients develop serious vascular complications, which can be venous or arterial. Thrombosis of the axillosubclavian vein can present acutely or chronically, sometimes following prolonged exercise. Typical features are pain and swelling of the arm aggravated by exercise, with the diagnosis being confirmed by venography. Compression of the subclavian artery can be followed by post-stenotic dilatation, aneurysm formation, and retrograde thromboembolic phenomena. Claudication, vasomotor phenomena, digital gangrene, and acute limb-threatening ischaemia can occur. Arteriography and in some cases Doppler ultrasonography are necessary to confirm the arterial abnormality.

Thoracic-outlet syndrome may be difficult to show objectively (Novak et al. 1993), and few patients have the diagnosis confirmed (Wilbourn 1993). Radiographs of the cervical spine may demonstrate cervical ribs, congenital bony abnormalities, or old fractures. MRI can also define soft tissue bands and other lesions causing distortion or deviation of nerves and blood vessels in the thoracic-outlet. Electromyography and somatosensory evoked potentials may offer some supportive evidence to confirm the diagnosis, or exclude lesions such as cervical radiculopathy, carpal tunnel syndrome, or ulnar neuropathy, which can closely mimic this syndrome. Arteriography and venography are necessary in difficult cases, especially with vascular complications.

Conservative treatment with shoulder-girdle exercises and improved posture often fails to remove all the symptoms, but is all that should be advocated for most cases, especially where the diagnosis remains in doubt.

Surgical intervention is often unsuccessful, carries considerable risks, and should be avoided, except in patients with serious vascular or other complications, or in severe cases of proven thoracic-outlet syndrome. In these patients neurosurgical or vascular surgical advise should be sought.

Cryptogenic brachial plexus neuropathy (brachial neuritis, neuralgic amyotrophy)

This condition usually develops acutely in healthy adults aged between 25 and 65 years. Some cases follow viral or other infection, injection of serum or vaccine, heroin use, or strenuous exercise. Rare cases are familial. An ache first develops around the shoulder or neck with increasing severity over 1–2 weeks. As the acute pain starts to settle, there is rapid onset of weakness and wasting of the shoulder and upper limb muscles. The distribution of wasting depends on the pattern of injury of the brachial plexus nerves. Sensory loss, paraesthesia, hyperaesthesia, and hyporeflexia may also occur. The pain is exacerbated by use of the affected muscles, which may become totally paralyzed. The lesion can be bilateral, and in some cases, is associated with involvement of the phrenic nerve or other peripheral and even cranial nerves. Electromyography of the affected muscles reveals fibrillation potentials and positive waves, in a pattern characteristic of combined damage to nerve roots and peripheral nerves. The electromyographic abnormality is often bilateral, even where this is not clinically apparent.

Brachial plexus neuropathy needs to be differentiated from acute poliomyelitis, rotator cuff tears, extradural malignancy, Pancoast tumour of the lung, thoracic-outlet syndrome, and cervical radiculopathy. Although the course is variable, the prognosis for recovery is good. Most recover within 6 months, with 90 per cent showing a complete recovery within 3 years. Recurrences do occur, but are rare.

Conclusion

Degenerative lesions in the cervical region cause many varied symptoms, which are not always recognized to be from this source. 'Cervical spondylosis', which is a vague term used to describe a whole range of degenerative and mechanical lesions, causes less disability than similar lesions affecting the lumbar spine, and has therefore been the subject of less study. The more common mechanical syndromes and associated complications and their treatment have been discussed, with consideration being given to other causes of neck pain and neurological deficit in the upper limbs.

References

Baba, H., Maezawa, Y., Kawahara, N., Tomita, K., Furusawa, N., and Imura, S. (1993). Calcium crystal deposition in the ligamentum flavum of the cervical spine. *Spine* **18**, 2174–81.

Barnsley, L., Lord, S.M., Wallis, B.J., and Bogduk, N. (1995). The prevalence of chronic cervical zygapophysial joint pain after whiplash. *Spine* **20**, 20–6.

Binder, A.I. (2003). Neck pain. In *Clinical Evidence* (concise) Vol. 10, pp. 262–4. London: BMJ Publishing Group.

Bland, J.H. and Boushey, D.R. (1990). Anatomy and physiology of the cervical spine. *Seminars in Arthritis and Rheumatism* **20**, 1–20.

Boden, S.D., McCowin, P.R., Davis, D.O., Dina, T.S., Mark, A.S., and Wiesel, S. (1990). Abnormal magnetic-resonance scans of the cervical spine in asymptomatic subject. A prospective investigation. *Journal of Bone and Joint Surgery* **72A**, 1178–84.

Bonk, A.D., Ferrari, R., Giebel, G.D., Edelmann, M., and Huser, R. (2000). Prospective, randomized, controlled study of activity versus collar, and the natural history for whiplash injury, in Germany. *Journal of Musculoskeletal Pain* **8**, 123–32.

Borchgrevink, G.E., Kaasa, A., McDonagh, D., Stiles, T.C., Haraldseth, O., and Lereim, I. (1998). Acute treatment of whiplash neck sprain injuries: a randomised trial of treatment during the first 14 days after a car accident. *Spine* **23**, 25–31.

Brodsky, A.E. (1985). Cervical angina. A correlative study with emphasis on the use of coronary arteriography. *Spine* **10**, 699–709.

Bush, K. and Hillier, S. (1996). Outcome of cervical radiculopathy treated with periradicular/epidural corticosteroid injections: a prospective study with independent clinical review. *European Spine Journal* **5**, 319–25.

Cote, P., Cassidy, D., and Carroll, L. (1998). The Saskatchewan health and back pain survey: the prevalence of neck pain and related disability in Saskatchewan adults. *Spine* **23**, 1689–98.

Croft, P., Schollum, J., and Silman, A. (1994). Population study of tender point counts and pain as evidence of fibromyalgia. *British Medical Journal* **309**, 696–9.

Dabbs, V. and Lauretti, W.J. (1995). A risk assessment of cervical manipulation versus NSAIDS for the treatment of neck pain. *Journal of Manipulative Physiology and Therapy* **18**, 530–6.

Dvorak, J., Janssen, B., and Grob, D. (1990). The neurologic workup in patients with cervical spine disorders. *Spine* **15**, 1017–22.

Farmer, J.C. and Wisneski, R.J. (1994). Cervical spine nerve root compression. An analysis of neuroforaminal pressures with varying head and arm positions. *Spine* **19**, 1850–5.

Fast, A., Parikh, S., and Marin, E.L. (1989). The shoulder abduction relief sign in cervical radiculopathy. *Archives of Physical Medicine and Rehabilitation* **70**, 402–3.

Ferrari, R. and Russell, A.S. (1999). Epidemiology of whiplash: an international dilemma. *Annals of the Rheumatic Diseases* **58**, 1–5.

Gross, A.R., Aker, P.D., Goldsmith, C.H., and Peloso, P. (1999). Physical medicine modalities for mechanical neck disorders. In *The Cochrane Library* Issue 2. Oxford: Update Software.

Hackett, G.I. et al. (1987). Evaluation of the efficacy and acceptability to patients of a physiotherapist working in a health centre. *British Medical Journal* **294**, 24–6.

Hartling, L., Brison, R.J., Arden, C., and Pickett, W. (2001). Prognostic value of the Quebec Classification of whiplash-associated disorders. *Spine* **26**, 36–41.

Hayashi, H., Okada, K., Hashimoto, J., Tada, K., and Ueno, R. (1988). Cervical spondylotic myelopathy in the aged patient. A radiographic evaluation of the aging changes in the cervical spine and etiologic factors of myelopathy. *Spine* **13**, 618–25.

Helliwell, P.S., Evans, P.F., and Wright, V. (1994). The straight cervical spine: does it indicate muscle spasm? *Journal of Bone and Joint Surgery* **76B**, 103–6.

Hukuda, S., Mochizuki, T., Ogata, M., and Shichikawa, K. (1983). The pattern of spinal and extraspinal hyperostosis in patients with ossification of the posterior longitudinal ligament and the ligamentum flavum causing myelopathy. *Skeletal Radiology* **10**, 79–85.

Hurwitz, E.L., Aker, P.D., Adams, A.H., Meeker, W.C., and Shekelle, P.G. (1996). Manipulation and mobilization of the cervical spine: a systematic review of the literature. *Spine* **21**, 1746–60.

Jordan, A., Bendix, T., Nielsen, H., Hansen, F.R., Host, D., and Winkel, A. (1998). Intensive training, physiotherapy, or manipulation for patients with chronic neck pain. A prospective, single-blinded, randomized clinical trial. *Spine* **23**, 311–19.

Mäkelä, M., Heliövaara, M., Sievers, K., Impivaara, O., Knekt, P., and Aromaa, A. (1991). Prevalence, determinants, and consequences of chronic neck pain in Finland. *American Journal of Epidemiology* **134**, 1356–67.

Martinez, J.E., Ferraz, M.B., Sato, E.I., and Atra, E. (1995). Fibromyalgia versus rheumatoid arthritis: a longitudinal comparison of the quality of life. *Journal of Rheumatology* **22**, 270–4.

Murone, I. (1974). The importance of the sagittal diameters of the cervical spine canal in relation to spondylosis and myelopathy. *Journal of Bone and Joint Surgery* **56B**, 30–6.

Murray-Leslie, C.F. and Wright, V. (1976). Carpal tunnel syndrome, humeral epicondylitis, and the cervical spine: a study of clinical and dimensional relations. *British Medical Journal* **1**, 1439–42.

Nakajima, M. and Hirayama, K. (1995). Midcervical central cord syndrome: numb and clumsy hands due to midline cervical disc protrusion at the C3–4 intervertebral level. *Journal of Neurology, Neurosurgery and Psychiatry* **58**, 607–13.

Novak, C.B., Mackinnon, S.E., and Patterson, G.A. (1993). Evaluation of patients with thoracic-outlet syndrome. *Journal of Hand Surgery* **18A**, 292–9.

Palmer, P.E., Stadalnick, R., and Arnon, S. (1984). The genetic factor in cervical spondylosis. *Skeletal Radiology* **11**, 178–82.

Parmar, H.V. and Raymakers, R. (1993). Neck injuries from rear impact road traffic accidents: prognosis in persons seeking compensation. *Injury* **24**, 75–8.

Persson, L.C., Carlsson, C.A., and Carlsson, J.Y. (1997). Long-lasting cervical radicular pain managed with surgery, physiotherapy, or a cervical collar: a prospective randomised study. *Spine* **22**, 751–8.

Radanov, B.P., Dvorak, J., and Valach, L. (1992). Cognitive deficits in patients after soft tissue injury of the cervical spine. *Spine* **17**, 127–31.

Radanov, B.P., Sturzenegger, M., Di Stefano, G., and Schnidrig, A. (1994). Relationship between early somatic, radiological, cognitive and psychosocial findings and outcome during a one year follow-up of 117 patients suffering from common whiplash. *British Journal of Rheumatology* **33**, 442–8.

Rosenfeld, M., Gunnarsson, R., and Borenstein, P. (2000). Early intervention in whiplash-associated disorders: a comparison of two treatment protocols. *Spine* **25**, 1782–7.

Saal, J.S., Saal, J.A., and Yurth, E.F. (1996). Nonoperative management of herniated cervical intervertebral disc with radiculopathy. *Spine* **16**, 1877–83.

Simmons, Z., Biller, J., Beck, D.W., and Keyes, W. (1986). Painless compressive cervical myelopathy with false localizing sensory findings. *Spine* **11**, 869–72.

Smythe, H.A. (1986). Referred pain and tender points. *American Journal of Medicine* **81** (Suppl. 3A), 90–2.

Smythe, H.A. (1994). The C6–7 syndrome: clinical features and treatment response. *Journal of Rheumatology* **21**, 1520–6.

Spitzer, W.O. et al. (1995). Scientific monograph of the Quebec Task Force on whiplash-associated disorders: redefining 'whiplash' and its management. *Spine* **20** (Suppl. 8), 1–73.

Sudarsky, L. and Ronthal, M. (1983). Gait disorders among elderly patients. A survey study of 50 patients. *Archives of Neurology* **40**, 740–3.

Swift, T.R. and Nichols, F.T. (1984). The droopy shoulder syndrome. *Neurology* **34**, 212–15.

Taimela, S., Takala, E.P., Asklof, T., Seppala, K., and Parviainen, S. (2000). Active treatment of chronic neck pain: a prospective randomized intervention *Spine* **25**, 1021–7.

Van der Donk, J., Schouten, J.S., Passchier, J., van Romunde, L.K., and Valkenburg, H.A. (1991). The associations of neck pain with radiological abnormalities of the cervical spine and personality traits in a general population. *Journal of Rheumatology* **18**, 1884–9.

Waalen, D., White, P., and Waalen, J. (1994). Demographic and clinical characteristics of chiropractic patients: a 5-year study of patients treated at the Canadian Memorial Chiropractic College. *Journal of Canadian Chiropractice Association* **38**, 75–82.

Wilbourn, A.J. (1993). Brachial plexus disorders. In *Peripheral Neuropathy* Vol. 2, 3rd edn. (ed. P.J. Dyck and P.K. Thomas), pp. 911–51. Philadelphia PA: W.B. Saunders.

Wolfe, F. et al. (1990). The American College of Rheumatology 1990 criteria for the classification of fibromyalgia. Report of the Multicenter Criteria Committee. *Arthritis and Rheumatism* **33**, 160–72.

Wolfe, F., Ross, K., Anderson, J., and Russell, I.J. (1995). Aspects of fibromyalgia in the general population: sex, pain, threshold, and fibromyalgia symptoms. *Journal of Rheumatology* **22**, 151–6.

6.18 Miscellaneous abnormalities of connective tissue

6.18.1 Complex regional pain syndrome (algodystrophy/reflex sympathetic dystrophy syndrome)

Geoffrey O. Littlejohn

Introduction

Complex regional pain syndrome (CRPS) is characterized by regional dysfunction of the pain system with secondary effects on musculoskeletal, skin, and vascular systems. The syndrome may be severe and prolonged resulting in significant disability and profound psychosocial effects. It is important to recognize the syndrome in the early or incomplete phase if currently available therapeutic approaches are to be most effective.

Nomenclature

The distinctive but varied clinical features of CRPS have provided classic clinical descriptions for over 100 years. There are a large number of synonyms for CRPS, including reflex sympathetic dystrophy syndrome, algodystrophy, causalgia, and Sudeck's atrophy, among others. The role of the sympathetic nervous system, depending on response to sympathetic blockade, has been incorporated through use of the terms sympathetic-maintained (or mediated) pain and sympathetically-independent pain (Roberts 1986; Campbell et al. 1992).

Epidemiology

CRPS occurs in either sex and all ages, races, and geographical regions. The 'classical case' is easily recognized but minor variants are more common. In some instances, minor CRPS following trauma may be regarded as a part of the normal response to injury. The true prevalence of CRPS is thus unclear.

Following specific trauma, between 1 in 200 and 1 in 20 will develop CRPS (Kozin 1994). Of 109 unselected patients with Colles' fracture, 25 per cent had two or more features of CRPS at 9 weeks, and 62 per cent showed some residual abnormalities at 6 months (Atkins et al. 1989). CRPS should be anticipated where there are triggering events known to be associated with the syndrome.

Clinical features

The pain may be spontaneous or easily provoked by otherwise innocuous stimuli (allodynia). In addition, there is increased pain perception to a given painful stimulus (hyperalgesia) and hyperpathia, where there is delayed overreaction particularly to a normal repetitive cutaneous stimulus, may also be present. The pain will usually occur some days to weeks after a triggering factor, if present, and will generally be constant, but usually varies in intensity. Although burning pain is characteristic, more commonly the pain is described as a deep, dull aching sensation. Paroxysms of pain may occur, lasting for seconds. The pain may disturb sleep and slight movement that mechanically stimulates the sensitized region will worsen the pain. The patient may report the use of cold, wet compresses to relieve the discomfort.

Typically, CRPS involves the distal part of a limb; for instance, a hand and lower forearm region (Fig. 1) or a foot and lower leg.

Significant proximal extension often occurs, with tenderness and muscle co-contraction present at the root of the limb, such that spinal movements become stiff (Maleki et al. 2000). In the majority, the same abnormal clinical features occur in the opposite limb over time, but these are usually subtler (Hooshmand and Hashmi 1999). The syndrome may involve one digit or rarely all four limbs. Shortly after the onset of pain, swelling, the second most common feature, occurs (Blumberg et al. 1994). This may initially be intermittent and associated with a change in the texture of the overlying skin, producing a reticular or lividoid appearance. Palmar erythema may be noted. Early in the course the involved region is warmer than the surrounding region. Varying degrees of sweating may occur and there may be piloerection.

Examination confirms a decreased pain threshold, particularly to mechanical stimuli, leading to abnormal tenderness that is the principal clinical finding. Early in the course this allodynia tends to be periarticular, but later regions well away from joints and particularly those over bone also become exquisitely tender. This distribution is non-(neuro-)anatomical and found over a wide region of the involved parts. For instance, if the principal involvement were in the mid-tarsal region of the foot, one would usually find tenderness on palpation of a meta-tarsophalangeal joint and regions of the lower leg, as well as in intervening areas. Mild oedema may be noted, either pitting or not. Early on, joint movement in the region will be restricted by pain but with care it be demonstrated that the range of motion is often near normal. There may be a prominent motor component with tremor, weakness, muscle tightness, or occasionally involuntary movements, including dystonia.

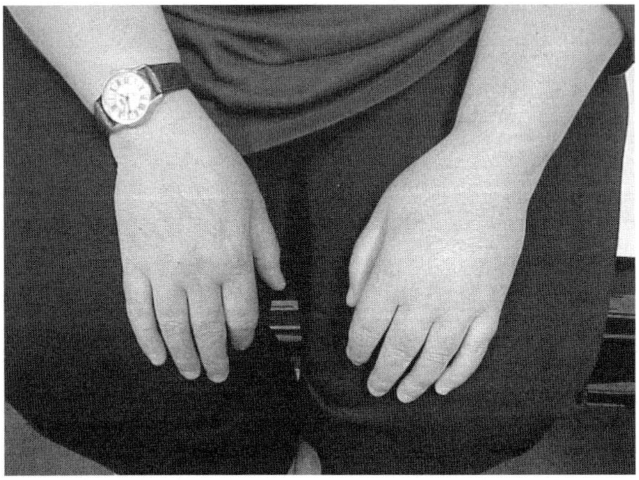

Fig. 1 Left forearm/hand swelling, pain, and allodynia in a 32-year-old female 4 months after simple work-related soft-tissue injury (since resolved) to extensor aspect of wrist.

Triggering events

Trauma, particularly fracture, is a trigger in around half of subjects (Doury 1988; Kozin 1994). However, even apparently trivial sprains, strains, contusions, or jarring injuries, particularly to the distal part of the limbs, especially to joints, may trigger CRPS. Surgical procedures, including arthroscopy, peripheral burns, and frostbite can all induce CRPS. The subsequent development of CRPS affects less than 1 per cent of all community traumatic events. Perhaps a common thread among injuries that result in CRPS is the individual's reaction to pain and the frightening nature of the injury, be it major or apparently trivial.

About 25 per cent of cases relate to various causes. Neurological triggers include conditions resulting in hemiplegia, cerebral tumour, meningitis and syringomyelia, among others. Peripheral nerve injury may include trauma, *herpes zoster*, nerve-root impingement, or peripheral neuropathy. Pain arising from a visceral or deep somatic structure, such as myocardial ischaemia in the former instance and mechanical spinal pain in the latter, or from inflammatory arthritis or after deep venous thrombosis, may provoke CRPS. Certain medications, particularly barbiturates and isoniazid, have been reported as triggers. Other linked conditions include pregnancy (with particular involvement of the hip), metastatic tumours, acrodermatitis continua, and prolonged immobilization of a peripheral limb (Schwartzman and McLellan 1987).

At least 25 per cent of cases have no easily identifiable trigger. Here the search for central factors or psychological distress is often made. In children, it is common to find an unresolved stress or an unsatisfactory psychosocial state in the background (Sherry and Weisman 1988). In adults, this is more difficult to identify. A small percentage of patients will have a defined psychiatric condition, such as depression or anxiety, but many more are likely to have excessive reactions to psychosocial stressors. There is often a strong clinical impression that such factors play an important part in expression of the syndrome. However, in many patients, no such factors can be identified. There is no evidence that particular personality traits predispose a person to develop CRPS (Bruehl and Carlson 1992; Lynch 1992).

Course

In most instances, the above clinical features persist, fluctuate, or gradually resolve according to the natural history or treatment intervention, without further sequelae. In some patients there is a dystrophic phase, usually some months after the start of the problem. Here the limb becomes cool, and cutaneous pallor or cyanosis replaces the previous erythema. There is decreased growth of dermal appendages, such as hair, and the nails become brittle. Skin and subcutaneous tissues may atrophy. Increased sweating becomes more prominent and the pain persists and often worsens. There may be dysaesthesia (painful, abnormal skin sensation) in a non-anatomical distribution. Radiological evaluation will show change in the mineral content of bone in the area. Joints become tighter, this time due to contracture of surrounding structures (Plate 201).

After several months there may be an atrophic phase. Pain usually decreases at this stage but can remain intractable in some. There may be marked atrophy of subcutaneous tissue, such as to cause tapering of digits, and flexion contractures of peripheral joints become prominent. The limb is characterized by vasoconstriction and coolness and the skin is cyanotic, smooth, and glossy. Hair growth can be increased or decreased.

Variants of CRPS are particularly common in children where the painful limb is usually cool and slightly swollen from the outset and the syndrome does not tend to go through the 'classical' phases, often resolving much more quickly than in an adult.

Traditionally, the disorder has been staged according to observations by Steinbrocker and Argyros (1958), where stage 1 comprises the 'acute' clinical features with predominant pain, tenderness, swelling, and vasomotor and pseudomotor changes with stage 2 dominated by dystrophic features, lasting several months and stage 3 comprising longer lasting atrophic changes. In extreme cases this classification is of use but in the average situation most patients do not progress beyond stage 1 or early stage 2.

Classification

There is no validated classification for diagnosis in the clinical setting or for research purposes. The classification of Kozin et al. (1981) defines *definite* CRPS when there is pain, tenderness, swelling, vasomotor, or pseudomotor changes of an extremity. Dystrophic change may be present. *Probable* CRPS consists of pain and tenderness, together with vasomotor and pseudomotor changes or swelling; *possible* CRPS comprises vasomotor or pseudomotor changes; and *doubtful* CRPS is considered where there is pain and tenderness out of keeping with any preceding injury or other organic disease process. The International Association for Study of Pain criteria (Merskey and Bogduk 1994) suggested the need for an inciting event, which is not always present, and further diagnostic guidelines have been proposed (Stanton-Hicks et al. 1998). Table 1 presents further refinements to this process (Harden et al. 1999); however, no criteria have been well validated. No criteria attempt to accommodate psychological perspectives.

Regions involved

The arm may be involved in a unipolar fashion, with either shoulder (frozen shoulder) or hand being affected. Involvement of the shoulder is associated with marked retraction of the joint capsule, restricted range of motion, and pain persisting for several months. On resolution of the syndrome, loss of range of motion of the shoulder is common, although usually not clinically significant. Peripheral involvement may include a single digit, a few metacarpal rays or more typically the whole hand and lower forearm may be involved. Bipolar forms include the shoulder–hand syndrome. Up to 25 per cent of upper-limb involvement is bilateral, the changes in the opposite side often being more evident after investigation (Kozin et al. 1976; Maleki et al. 2000).

Table 1 Modified diagnostic criteria for complex regional pain syndrome

1.	Continuing pain which is disproportionate to any inciting event	
2.	At least one symptom in each of the four following categories	
	Sensory	Reports of hyperaesthesia
	Vasomotor	Reports of temperature asymmetry, and/or skin colour changes, and/or skin colour asymmetry
	Sudomotor/oedema	Reports of oedema and/or sweating changes and/or sweating asymmetry
	Motor/trophic	Reports of decreased range of motion, and/or motor dysfunction (weakness, tremor, dystonia), and/or trophic changes (hair, skin, nail)
3.	At least one sign in two of the four following categories	
	Sensory	Evidence of hyperalgesia (to pin prick) and/or allodynia (to light touch)
	Vasomotor	Evidence of temperature asymmetry and/or skin colour changes and/or skin colour asymmetry
	Sudomotor/oedema	Evidence of oedema and/or sweating changes and/or sweating asymmetry
	Motor/trophic	Evidence of decreased range of motion, and/or motor dysfunction (weakness, tremor, dystonia), and/or trophic changes (hair, skin, nail)

Leg involvement, although more common, is less dramatic than that of the arm. Here the features are usually confined to a part of the limb such as the foot, knee, or hip. Bipolar and bilateral involvement is less common than in the arm. Involvement of the knee, either of the whole or of part, including the patella, may occur (Coughlan et al. 1987).

CRPS of the hip is less commonly recognized because the hip joint is deeply positioned and there is a lack of the cutaneous features. The duration of symptoms is shorter, possibly because early mobilization is easier. Some suggest that this variant is distinct enough to be termed transient regional osteoporosis. Absence of precipitating trauma, good outcome, and a propensity for recurrent episodes and involvement of multiple regions is characteristic of this variant. Signs of cutaneous or vascular change are uncommon. CRPS may also affect the spine and occasionally other areas of the skeleton.

Investigations

Laboratory investigations

There is no abnormality of acute-phase reactants or of standard biochemical markers. In some patients with early disease, 24-h urinary hydroxyproline excretion may be increased, reflecting bone demineralization (Doury 1988).

Imaging

A number of imaging techniques may show characteristic abnormalities. As there is no 'gold standard' for diagnosis it is difficult to establish their clinical usefulness. The main problem arises from the many variations of the syndrome and most studies have considered only severe CRPS, thus producing a distorted view of their clinical utility.

Plain radiographic changes reflect bone demineralization; these may take several weeks to months to appear after the onset of the syndrome. On resolution, these changes persist longer than other clinical features. Some patients never have radiological change, others only subtle ones. It is essential that good technique and meticulous examination of radiographs, with comparison of the affected side to the other side, be performed. Characteristically, children have far less radiological changes than adults, with only the minority showing demineralization. In adults, patchy osteopaenia may be seen in the early stages and diffuse changes characterize the later stages. Typically in the hip or knee, changes are most obvious in the subchondral region where there is loss of subchondral bone and preservation of subchondral plate. Severe juxta-articular changes might include erosions; however, the joint space is never affected. The sensitivity and specificity of radiological appearances are around 70 per cent for well-defined CRPS (Kozin et al. 1981). Plain radiography is an essential investigation but has only moderate predictive value for diagnosis. Fine-detailed radiography better shows the demineralization, which is accentuated around epiphyseal regions, reflecting hyperaemia at this site. Subperiosteal, endosteal, and intracortical bone resorption together with juxta-articular and subchondral erosions, are observed frequently with this technique (Genant et al. 1975).

Magnetic resonance imaging (MRI) may also show changes characteristic of bone loss. For instance, in the hip, low intensity signal on T_1-weighted images and high intensity on T_2-weighted images may be seen. The clinical usefulness of this technique and absorptiometry, which also may reflect bone loss, is yet to be established.

Scintigraphic studies using technetium have a high specificity but a similar sensitivity to that of plain radiographs. Typically a three-phase study (Kozin et al. 1976) is made, with the early phase showing regional blood flow over the first 2–3 min, the second phase showing the blood-pool image, and the third phase (some 2–4 h later) showing the standard bone-uptake findings. While any of these three phases may be abnormal it is more common to find increased flow (early phase) and uptake (late phase) in around 80 per cent of abnormal studies. Diminished flow and uptake are more commonly seen in children and adolescents than in adults (Goldsmith et al. 1989). Scintigraphy appears more accurate if symptoms have been present for less than 6 months or if the patient is older than 50 years (Werner et al. 1989). Multiple investigations are often needed.

Thermography may show changes in regional cutaneous temperatures compared with the unaffected side (Perelman et al. 1987). Typically there is an early increased or, particularly in children, decreased cutaneous heat emission. Critical evaluation of this technique is required before it can be usefully applied clinically.

Histopathological changes

Synovial biopsies of joints in the region of CRPS will often show low-grade synovitis characterized by proliferation of synovial cells and small blood vessels, together with a mild chronic perivascular infiltrate. There have only been limited studies on the bone demineralization, periarticular fibrosis, and dermal atrophy (Arlet et al. 1978; Doury et al. 1981).

Diagnosis

The diagnosis of CRPS is based on the clinical features. A high degree of clinical suspicion is required, particularly in early diagnosis. Focal disease may mimic inflammatory or infectious arthritis or bone disease, trauma, or osteonecrosis. Characteristic clinical features, elimination of other causes for such symptoms, and appropriate imaging will usually allow for a clinically robust diagnosis. The most important thing in diagnosis is to think of the possibility of CRPS.

Pathophysiology

CRPS is caused by a regional change in function of the pain system. This involves both peripheral and central mechanisms in a complex manner.

Table 2 summarizes the principal clinical characteristics of the syndrome and possible causative mechanisms. Input from two afferent fibre types, the small diameter, non-myelinated C-fibres and the large, myelinated A-β-fibres, together with change in function of sympathetic efferents, appear the likely mediators of many of the peripheral features. Sympathetic activity, through release of noradrenaline, and inflammatory prostaglandins, may sensitize peripheral nociceptors, thus decreasing threshold to peripheral mechanical and chemical stimuli. It has been suggested that α_1-adrenergic receptors may become expressed on such nociceptors, particularly in a post-injury situation, and that these receptors will respond to sympathetic fibre release of noradrenaline (Campbell et al. 1988). Subsequent release of proinflammatory neuropeptides, such as substance P, by activated C-fibres would contribute to regional neurogenic inflammation with increase in blood flow and oedema. The associated synovitis may be due to this mechanism. Periarticular osteoporosis may relate to the hyperaemia in the epiphyseal vessels in particular, or to neuropeptide effects on bone mineral metabolism. Allodynia is likely to reflect abnormality within the large myelinated afferent fibre system, as blocking these fibres by local anaesthetics will abolish this finding in other situations (Meyer et al. 1972; Roberts 1986).

Table 2 Pathophysiological mechanisms in CRPS

Characteristic	Mechanism
Pain	
Spontaneous	Sensitized peripheral/central nociceptors
Allodynia	Large myelinated fibre input to sensitized dorsal horn transmission neurones
Hyperalgesia	C-fibre sensitization of periphery + sensitized 2nd order neurones
Movement pain	Large myelinated fibre input to sensitized dorsal horn transmission neurones
Swelling	Neuropeptides from C-fibres; sympathetic effects on post-capillary venules
Bone change	Hyperaemia secondary to neuropeptide release; sympathetic effects
Synovitis	Neuropeptides—substance P, calcitonin gene-related peptide
Dystrophy	Unknown neurological mechanism; mechanical effects

In sophisticated tests, sympathetic efferents can be shown to have abnormal activity in the majority of patients with this syndrome. However, most patients do not get complete response to sympathetic blockade. The interaction between the products of the sympathetic nervous system and the peripheral nociceptors is supported by the knowledge that injection of noradrenaline will exacerbate pain and this is blocked by intravenous administration of the α_1-adrenergic antagonist, phentolamine. The phentolamine test can be used diagnostically to help predict patients who have a large sympathetically maintained component to their syndrome and those who are likely to benefit from sympathetic blockade (Arner 1991; Campbell et al. 1992).

The cause for these functional changes in the peripheral pain system is still unclear. Livingston (1943) suggested that there was a persisting peripheral afferent stimulus that led to abnormal activation of internuncial neurones situated in the dorsal horn at the relevant level. Efferent sympathetic activity was felt to follow that stimulus. The realization that the majority of patients with CRPS do not have an identifiable persisting afferent stimulus in the region of pain, has led to an appreciation that a functional change within the dorsal horn itself is the most important cause for the syndrome. This functional dorsal horn abnormality is usually triggered by minor trauma, often in an emotional context. This was accounted for by Lankford and Thompson's (1977) theory.

Roberts (1986) has suggested that initial activation of the unmyelinated C-fibre nociceptors, through unknown mechanisms, leads to sensitization of wide dynamic range neurones in the dorsal horn. Such neurones receive not only nociceptive input but input from other sources, including low-threshold, large myelinated afferents that otherwise serve functions such as proprioception. Input from these fibres resulting, say, from change in joint position or movement will impinge on the sensitized wide dynamic range neurone in the dorsal horn and this input will be perceived as pain (allodynia). Central sensitization mechanisms mediated by excitatory amino acids and their interaction with the *N*-methyl-D-aspartate receptor, as well as the neuropeptides, are relevant to this process (Schwartzman 1993).

With activation of the pain system, automatic reflex changes at a segmental level lead to both muscle change and stimulation of the sympathetic system. The former may result in various neuromuscular features that can accompany CRPS, such as dystonia or other movement disorders (Schwartzman and Kerrigan 1990). The latter will affect functions in peripheral tissues and may result in a number of the dystrophic features of the syndrome. In addition, the cycle is completed if sympathetic efferent activity maintains peripheral fibre sensitization, which in turn feeds back into the dorsal horn system initiating further sympathetic activity. Such neurogenic reflexes are usually bilaterally represented, explaining the bilateral findings in many patients with CRPS.

The reason for change in function of these interactions in the dorsal horn is unclear. It seems naive to explain such intense pain syndromes on purely segmental and peripheral pathophysiological changes. The complex and hierarchical nature of the pain system includes essential connections to the higher centres including the cortex. Important descending influences from higher centres impinge on the dorsal horn and modulate many components of the pain system. Thus central events that might include a variety of cortical and psychological factors may further influence this system. These might include the stress of pain itself and its effects on the central nervous system and the hypothalamic–pituitary axis, the patient's beliefs, mood, emotions, and even their quality of sleep. A change in any of these factors may affect the homeostatic mechanisms involved in pain control and sensitization phenomena in the dorsal horn. It is through such mechanisms that the emotional and affective components of the painful stimulus modify the peripheral reception and processing of further information relating to pain (Harvey 1987).

CRPS shares many features with fibromyalgia syndrome, another common chronic pain syndrome (Petzke and Clauw 2000). The overlap of clinical features between different pain syndromes emphasizes more the difficulties with nomenclature and classification than the essential nature of the 'different' pain syndromes.

Other factors that may be important in the pathophysiology have been variously reviewed (Fields 1987; Kozin 1994; Janig 1996; Schwartzman and Popescu 2002).

Management

It is essential to treat the whole patient and not just the abnormal area of pain complaint in order to provide effective treatment.

Preventive strategies include the recognition of situations that are likely to provoke the syndrome. Thus early mobilization after myocardial infarction, cerebrovascular accident, hand surgery, or mild peripheral injury is essential. Appropriate reassurance and direction in the handling of patients in any post-traumatic setting, particularly in emotionally charged, work-related events is essential.

Many authorities indicate that prognosis for full recovery relates inversely to the duration of symptoms before the onset of treatment; however, others feel that the syndrome can reverse, to a large extent, at any time.

In milder forms, the principles of management (Table 3) include adequate pain relief, reassurance, and explanation. A positive approach in regard to outcome is appropriate and necessary. Careful explanation is required to ensure that the patient, according to their level of understanding, understands the holistic concept of a chronic pain state. This is essential; it leads to a cooperative management plan that has the patient as the key person in the team. This syndrome is not well served by the adoption of the 'injury' model where a powerful external 'treater' is required to give the 'curative' treatment. Such well-intentioned approaches often lead to a denser ingraining of the syndrome, probably through blocking of positive benefits that would come from modulation of the central pathways on to the dorsal horn. Similarly, certain systems of compensation and other medicolegal events appear to inhibit early resolution of the syndrome, likely through modulation of central psychological processes which impact on pain control systems.

Counselling the patient, attending to the associated anxiety, and correcting any sleep disturbance, often through the use of low-dose tricyclic medication, are beneficial and prevent further amplification of the syndrome.

Essential treatments in milder CRPS, particularly in children, are exercise programmes that might include hydrotherapy. Activation of muscles and mechanoreceptors probably inhibits the activated dorsal-horn pain system on a local, segmental basis.

Table 3 Principles of management of CRPS

Accurate, early diagnosis
Explanation, reassurance
Adequate analgesia (medication, transcutaneous electrical stimulation)
Prevention of dystrophic change—exercise, movement
Attention to sleep disturbance
Attend to pain behaviour, psychosocial stresses, including compensation, litigation issues
Transient interruption of sympathetic activity
Skilled pain management/psychological counselling
Other

Numerous other treatment programmes have been suggested for the more severe or persistent types of CRPS; however, there is no robust evidence-based systematic review on which to draw.

Analgesia may need to include long-acting opioid medication in order to initiate and maintain sustained exercise of the affected limb. Membrane stabilizing drugs, such as carbamazepine, sodium valproate, or gabapentin lead to variable improvement. Topical capsaicin, through temporary disablement of nociceptors may help but may need to be given at doses that might require regional anaesthesia in order to tolerate the induced burning discomfort. Oral or topical local anaesthetics have been tried in some, again with unpredictable results.

Some find systemic corticosteroids to be beneficial, even when the syndrome has been long-lasting (Kozin et al. 1981). A typical course might commence at around 50 mg of prednisolone a day in divided doses and decrease to zero over 3–4 weeks. Subsequent courses may be needed. Some have advocated calcitonin, for example, 100–160 IU/day over 10–14 days, which has been shown to have benefits over placebo (Gobelet et al. 1992). Clondronate has shown similar effects (Varenna et al. 2000).

Interruption of the sympathetic efferent system to the region through various techniques has been used for some time and may help some patients. Phentolamine (non-specific α_1/α_2 antagonist) infusion will assess the degree of sympathetic nervous system involvement. If the patient responds favourably then subsequently a regional sympathetic ganglion block is given, using up to five short-acting sympathetic blocks, on a daily or alternate-day basis. If pain relief results, the patient is started on a more vigorous physiotherapy or exercise programme. Such approaches may result in 40 per cent of patients having a better result after 3-year follow-up; however, the majority have a less useful outcome (Wang et al. 1985).

Regional sympathetic blocks compare favourably with ganglion blockade (Bonnelli et al. 1983). These may be achieved using the Bier technique, whereby occlusion of venous outflow to the region, usually the lower arm or leg, is followed by intravenous installation of guanethidine or another similar agent. The exact mechanism of action of sympathetic modulation is unclear.

Peripheral nerve blocks in the axilla will also modify afferent nerve transmission and may be useful. Again these procedures often need to be repeated to achieve sustained results (Schwartzman and McLellan 1987). The exact role of these approaches is not established and Schott (1998) has concluded, 'there is little if any evidence that interrupting the sympathetic supply is more effective than placebo in alleviating the pain of causalgia and reflex sympathetic dystrophy'.

Surgical sympathectomy is only done if there is definite, but short-lived, improvement with the previous procedures.

Many other approaches have been used; these range from epidural opioids to cutaneous clonidine patches. Attempts to modulate the NMDA receptor include use of amantadine, dihydrodexmorphine, or ketamine. Controlled studies are lacking for most of these approaches (Dotson 1993). The large variety of therapies emphasizes the difficulty in treating established CRPS.

Psychological support or behavioural therapy should be considered in all cases (Stanton-Hicks et al. 1998).

My approach to management is as follows:

1. Young patient, any severity, any duration:

Always

(a) accurate diagnosis, explanation, reassurance as to expected good outcome;

(b) identification and management of psychosocial stressors especially family, school, or other;

(c) establishment of a regular activity programme—walking, bicycle riding, swimming, etc.;

(d) resumption of all previous activities, especially those related to school;

(e) careful supervision of programme and close liaison with parents, especially the mother if a female patient.

Often

(a) transcutaneous nerve stimulation to help pain control and allow entry into activity programme;

(b) hydrotherapy if limb sensitivity to movement is extreme. An empathetic physiotherapist is often the most powerful tool in this programme.

Sometimes

(a) tricyclic medication to correct sleep disturbance and increase the pain threshold;

(b) a clinical psychologist to help manage pain and consider psychosocial background dynamics;

(c) regional temporary sympathetic/ganglion blocks;

(d) other approaches.

2. Adult patient, mild severity, and duration:

Always

(a) accurate diagnosis, explanation, reassurance as to probable good outcome;

(b) identification and management of any obvious psychosocial stressors including work-related or legal issues: aim to resolve these quickly;

(c) adequate analgesia;

(d) establishment of regular activity programme using involved limb;

(e) planned return to all previous activities currently abandoned due to pain;

(f) careful supervision of the programme with attention to the 'blocks' to progress that often occur.

Often

(a) supervision of the physical programme by a physiotherapist with use of transcutaneous nerve stimulation, hydrotherapy, and similar tactics to control pain and encourage activity;

(b) short-term use of tricyclic medication.

Sometimes

(a) pain-management counselling by clinical psychologist or similar skilled person;

(b) regional temporary sympathetic/ganglion blocks;

(c) other approaches, such as short-course corticosteroids.

3. Adult patient, moderate/severe, prolonged duration:

Always

(a) use all the above approaches, sometimes sequentially and sometimes concomitantly;

(b) put emphasis on pain-management counselling early in programme, with frequent use of interventions to block efferent sympathetic outflow; consider medications such as corticosteroids or NMDA antagonists, such as ketamine, carefully;

(c) stay with the patient—sub-optimal therapeutic responses require longer-term support.

Prognosis

The outcome for patients with CRPS is quite varied. Minor forms seem to have an excellent outcome and children with the condition are expected to regain normal function and lose their pain. Some adults with severe forms of the condition may have protracted chronic pain states, significant dystrophic tissue change and longer-term disability. Pain usually eases over time even in those patients.

Summary

Complex regional pain syndrome is a common and significant musculoskeletal condition that results from a multifaceted neurophysiological change in the pain transmission pathways. The syndrome is characteristic and reproducible but many variants occur clinically. The best treatment is through early recognition and management along principles used in other chronic pain syndromes, but with added attention to the potential role of the sympathetic nervous system.

References

Arlet, J., Ficat, P., Durroux, R., Theallie, J.P., Mazieres, B., and Bouteiller, G. (1978). Histopathologie des lesions osseuses dans 9 cas d'algodystrophie de la hanche. *Revue de Rhumatisme et des Maladies Osteoarticulaires* **45**, 691–8.

Arner, S. (1991). Intravenous phentolamine test: diagnostic and prognostic use in reflex sympathetic dystrophy. *Pain* **46**, 17–22.

Atkins, R.M., Duckworth, T., and Kanis, J.A. (1989). Algodystrophy following Colles' fracture. *Journal of Hand Surgery* **14**, 161–4.

Blumberg, H., Hoffman, U., Mohadjer, M., and Scheremet, R. (1994). Clinical phenomenology and mechanisms of reflex sympathetic dystrophy: emphasis on edema. In *Proceedings of the 7th World Congress on Pain. Progress in Pain Research and Management* Vol. 2 (ed. G.F. Gebhart, D.L. Hammond, and T.S. Jensen), pp. 455–81. Seattle WA: IASP Press.

Bonnelli, S., Conoscente, F., and Movilia, P.G. (1983). Regional intravenous guanethidine vs stellate ganglion block in reflex sympathetic dystrophies; a randomized trial. *Pain* **16**, 297–307.

Bruehl, S. and Carlson, C.R. (1992). Predisposing psychological factors in the development of reflex sympathetic dystrophy. *Clinical Journal of Pain* **8**, 287–99.

Campbell, J.N., Raja, S.N., and Meyer, R.A. (1988). Painful sequelae of nerve injury. In *Proceedings of the 5th World Congress on Pain* (ed. R. Dubner, G.F. Gebhart, and M.R. Bond), pp. 135–43. Amsterdam: Elsevier.

Campbell, J.N., Meyer, R.A., and Raja, S.N. (1992). Is nociceptor activation by alpha-1 adrenoreceptors the culprit in sympathetically maintained pain. *American Pain Society Journal* **1**, 3–11.

Carlson, T. and Jacobs, A.M. (1986). Reflex sympathetic dystrophy syndrome. *Journal of Foot Surgery* **25**, 149–53.

Coughlan, F.J., Hazleman, B.L., and Page-Thomas, D.P. (1987). Algodystrophy: a common unrecognized cause of chronic knee pain. *British Journal of Rheumatology* **26**, 270–4.

Dotson, R.M. (1993). Causalgia—reflex sympathetic dystrophy—sympathetically maintained pain: myth and reality. *Muscle and Nerve* **16**, 1049–55.

Doury, P. (1988). Algodystrophy: reflex sympathetic dystrophy syndrome. *Clinical Rheumatology* **7**, 173–80.

Fields, H.L. (1987). Efferent activity and pain: the reflex sympathetic dystrophy syndrome. In *Pain*, pp. 145–55. New York: McGraw-Hill.

Genant, H.K., Kozin, F., Bekerman, C., McCarty, D.J., and Sims, J. (1975). The reflex sympathetic dystrophy syndrome: a comprehensive analysis using fine-detail radiography, photon absorptiometry, and bone and joint scintigraphy. *Radiography* **117**, 21–32.

Gobelet, C., Waldburger, M., and Meier, J.L. (1992). The effect of adding calcitonin to physical treatment on reflex sympathetic dystrophy. *Pain* **48**, 171–5.

Goldsmith, D.P., Vivino, F.B., Eichenfield, A.H., Athreya, B.H., and Heyman, S. (1989). Nuclear imaging and clinical features of childhood reflex neurovascular dystrophy: comparison with adults. *Arthritis and Rheumatism* **32**, 480–5.

Harden, R.N., Breuhl, S., Galer, B.S., Saltz, S., Bertram, M., Backonja, M., Gayles, R., Rudin, N., Bhugra, M.K., and Stanton-Hicks, M. (1999). Complex regional pain syndrome: are the IASP diagnostic criteria valid and sufficiently comprehensive? *Pain* **83**, 211–19.

Harvey, A.R. (1987). Neurophysiology of rheumatic pain. *Clinical Rheumatology* **1**, 1–26.

Hooshmand, H. and Hashmi, M. (1999). Complex regional pain syndrome (reflex sympathetic dystrophy syndrome): diagnosis and therapy—a review of 824 patients. *Pain Digest* **9**, 1–24.

Janig, W. (1996). The puzzle of 'reflex sympathetic dystrophy': mechanisms, hypotheses, open questions. In *Reflex Sympathetic Dystrophy: A Reappraisal* (ed. W. Janig and M. Stanton-Wicks), pp. 1–24. Seattle WA: IASP Press.

Kozin, F. (1994). Reflex sympathetic dystrophy syndrome. *Current Opinions in Rheumatology* **6**, 210–16.

Kozin, F., McCarty, D.J., Sims, J., and Genant, J. (1976). The reflex sympathetic dystrophy syndrome. I. Clinical and histologic studies: evidence for bilaterality, response to corticosteroids, and articular involvement. *American Journal of Medicine* **60**, 321–31.

Kozin, F., Fyan, L.M., Carrera, G.F., Soin, J.S., and Wortmann, F.L. (1981). The reflex sympathetic dystrophy syndrome. III. Scintigraphic studies, further evidence for the therapeutic efficacy of systemic corticosteroids and proposed diagnostic criteria. *American Journal of Medicine* **70**, 23–30.

Lankford, L. and Thompson, J. (1977). Reflex sympathetic dystrophy, upper and lower extremity: diagnosis and management. *American Academy of Orthopaedic Surgeons Instructional Course Lectures* Vol. 26, pp. 163–78. St Louis MO: Mosby.

Livingston, W.K. *Pain Mechanisms: A Physiologic Interpretation of Causalgia and its Related States.* New York: Macmillan, 1943.

Lynch, M.E. (1992). Psychological aspects of reflex sympathetic dystrophy: a review of the adult and paediatric literature. *Pain* **49**, 337–47.

Maleki, J., LeBel, A.A., Bennett, G.J., and Schwartman, R.J. (2000). Patterns of spread in complex regional pain syndrome, Type 1 (reflex dystrophy syndrome). *Pain* **88**, 259–66.

Merskey, H. and Bogduk, N. *Classification of Chronic Pain: Descriptions of Chronic Pain Syndromes and Definition of Pain Terms* 2nd edn. Seattle WA: IASP Press, 1994.

Meyer, R.A., Campbell, J.N., and Raja, S. (1972). Peripheral neural mechanisms of cutaneous hyperalgesia. *Advances in Pain Research and Therapeutics* **9**, 53–71.

Perelman, R.B., Adler, D., and Humphreys, M. (1987). Reflex sympathetic dystrophy: electronic thermography as an aid in diagnosis. *Orthopaedic Review* **16**, 561–6.

Petzke, F. and Clauw, D.J. (2000). Sympathetic nervous system function in fibromyalgia. *Current Rheumatology Reports* **2**, 116–23.

Roberts, W.J. (1986). An hypothesis on the physiological basis for causalgia and related pains. *Pain* **24**, 297–311.

Schott, G.D. (1998). Interrupting the sympathetic outflow in causalgia and reflex sympathetic dystrophy: a futile procedure for many patients. *British Medical Journal* **316**, 792–3.

Schwartzman, R.J. (1993). Reflex sympathetic dystrophy. *Current Opinions in Neurology and Neurosurgery* **6**, 531–6.

Schwartzman, R.J. and McLellan, T.L. (1987). Reflex sympathetic dystrophy: a review. *Archives of Neurology* **44**, 555–61.

Schwartzman, R.J. and Kerrigan, J. (1990). The movement disorder of reflex sympathetic dystrophy. *Neurology* **40**, 57–61.

Schwartzman, R.J. and Popescu, A. (2002). Reflex sympathetic dystrophy. *Current Rheumatology Reports* **4**, 165–9.

Sherry, D.D. and Weisman, M.A. (1988). Psychologic aspects of childhood reflex neurovascular dystrophy. *Paediatrics* **81**, 572–8.

Small, N.C. (1993). Complications in arthroscopic surgery of the knee and shoulder. *Orthopedics* **16**, 985–8.

Stanton-Hicks, M., Baron, R., Boas, R., Gordh, T., Harden, N., Hendler, N., Kolzenburg, M., Raj, P., and Wilder, R. (1998). Consensus report: complex regional pain syndromes: guidelines for therapy. *Clinical Journal of Pain* **14**, 155–66.

Steinbrocker, O. and Argyros, T.G. (1958). The shoulder–hand syndrome: present status as a diagnostic and therapeutic entity. *Medical Clinics of North America* **42**, 1538–53.

Varenna, M., Zucchi, F., Ghiringhelli, D., Binelli, L., Bevilacqua, M., Bettica, P., and Sinigaglia, L. (2000). Intravenous clodronate in reflex sympathetic dystrophy syndrome. A randomised double-blind controlled study. *Journal of Rheumatology* **27**, 1477–83.

Wang, J.K., Johnson, K.A., and Ilstrup, D.M. (1985). Sympathetic blocks for reflex sympathetic dystrophy. *Pain* **23**, 13–17.

Werner, R., Davidoff, G., Jackson, D., Cremer, S., Ventocilla, C., and Wolf, L. (1989). Factors affecting the sensitivity and specificity of the three-phase technetium bone scan in the diagnosis of reflex sympathetic dystrophy syndrome in the upper extremity. *Journal of Hand Surgery* **14A**, 520–3.

6.18.2 Rheumatic complications of drugs and toxins

Robert M. Bernstein

Congratulations if you have reached this chapter or happened upon it by chance. The author felt obliged to meet you here, because Francis Bacon held 'every man a debtor to his profession'. Bacon was also of the opinion that 'books must follow sciences, and not sciences books', but often books follow books: they contain not truth but copies of bad maps, so it is up to the student to read the scientific literature directly as well as learn by exploration and experience.

This chapter deals briefly with rheumatological presentations of adverse drug reactions and poisoning; more extensive reviews are available (Shoenfeld and Isenberg 1990; Kahn 1991). With so much public whim and paranoia it is easy to close our minds in defence of what we do, particularly when it comes to prescribing strange chemicals or eating them. Assessment of a potential reaction should involve clinical observation during therapy, after withdrawal of the drug, and, if possible, upon rechallenge; where the reaction is subjective rechallenge should be blinded.

Immunological reactions

A long list of drugs can trigger autoimmune diseases in many ways similar to their idiopathic counterparts (Table 1). These serve as important models for the study of idiopathic disease. Apart from anaphylaxis, which is immediate, and rashes, which often occur early in treatment, most of these reactions develop gradually after an appreciable exposure to the drug (Perry 1973). Some reactions are rare, but others may affect over 10 per cent of patients with sufficient drug exposure. Factors influencing susceptibility include cumulative dose, renal and hepatic function, genetic polymorphisms influencing drug metabolism (particularly acetylation and sulfoxidation), sex, and immunological response (HLA–DR type and complement null alleles). Grounds for imputing an immunological mechanism include infiltration with lymphocytes (hepatitis, myositis) and the presence of autoantibodies (haemolytic anaemia, myasthenia gravis, lupus, Goodpasture's syndrome, pemphigus). The autoantibodies are usually similar to those arising in the relevant idiopathic autoimmune condition (Table 1), but generally occur much more frequently than any clinical expression of disease. Thus, hydralazine induces antinuclear antibodies in upto 60 per cent of patients but the lupus syndrome in only 2–10 per cent, and Coombs' antibody need not cause haemolysis.

Drug-induced lupus

Starting with observations by Perry in the 1950s on a late toxic reaction to hydralazine therapy (Perry 1973) and then similar observations with procainamide, many drugs have been reported to induce systemic lupus erythematosus (SLE) or a lupus-like syndrome (Table 2). To implicate a drug with certainty the syndrome should remit after drug withdrawal

Table 1 Drug-induced autoimmune syndromes and autoantibodies

Syndrome	Autoantibody specificity
Lupus	Histones Single-stranded DNA Poly(ADP-ribose) Mitochondria (venocuran-induced) Myeloperoxidase
Myositis	Nuclear
Myasthenia gravis	Acetylcholine receptor
Scleroderma	None recognized[a]
Haemolytic anaemia	I antigen of red cell
Thrombocytopaenia	Platelet membrane
Pemphigus	Skin basement membrane
Goodpasture's syndrome	Kidney basement membrane

[a] Topoisomerase I in silica miners.

Table 2 Drugs reported to induce a lupus syndrome

Definite	*Probable*
Hydralazine	Penicillamine
Isoniazid	Sulfasalazine
Procainamide	Acebutalol
Minocycline	Labetalol
	Methyldopa
	Captopril
	Phenytoin
	Carbamazepine
	Chlorpromazine
	Lithium
	Propylthiouracyl
	Quinidine
	Psoralen/ultraviolet A (PUVA)
	Venocuran

Note: For a more comprehensive list see Solinger (1988).

and recur on rechallenge. However, some drugs have been implicated by rather few case reports and rechallenge is rarely attempted.

Case reports have to be studied cautiously because idiopathic lupus may have been developing at the time. There may be only an association by chance but oestrogens and sulfonamides can exacerbate or bring on idiopathic SLE, and hair dyes containing aromatic amines have been implicated in a cluster of cases of SLE and scleroderma in a small town in Georgia (Freni-Titulaer et al. 1988). Statin therapy may very rarely cause drug-induced lupus, but one case report concerning fluvastatin is probably better explained as the onset of idiopathic lupus (Sridhar and Abdulla 1998).

Surveys of patients with rheumatoid arthritis or Crohn's disease receiving therapy to inhibit tumour necrosis factor (blocking TNF) have confirmed the development of autoantibodies in less than one-tenth of cases and a fully reversible lupus syndrome in less than 1 per cent (Schaible 2000).

Minocycline, a semisynthetic tetracycline used over prolonged periods for the treatment of acne vulgaris and rosacea, is now probably the commonest cause of reversible drug-induced lupus (Schlienger et al. 2000). Minocycline can also induce an autoimmune hepatitis, which also resolves after drug withdrawal. The only other tetracycline derivative implicated in drug-induced lupus-like syndrome is an experimental anticancer agent with antiangiogenic activity, COL-3 (Ghate et al. 2001).

Clinical features

The clinical features of drug-induced lupus are shown in Table 3, with data on idiopathic SLE for comparison. Common, early manifestations (after several

Table 3 Clinical and laboratory manifestations of idiopathic SLE and drug-induced lupus

Manifestations	Proportion positive (%)		
	SLE	Hydralazine lupus	Procainamide lupus
Arthralgia	90	90	90
Arthritis	90	50	18
Fever	84	50	45
Rash	72	25	5–18
Lymphadenopathy	59	14	0–9
Myalgia	48	2–34	20–50
Pleurisy	45		
Pleural effusion	33	25–30	33
Pulmonary infiltrate	8		30
Pericarditis	31	2	16
Hepatosplenomegaly	5–10	~10	20–33
CNS/seizures	16–25	0	1
Raynaud's phenomenon	23	Rare	5
Joint deformities	10–26	0	0
Renal involvement	46	2–20	0–5
Anaemia (Hb $<$11.5 g/dl)	57	30	9–21
Leucopaenia ($<4 \times 10^9$/l)	43	26	2–32
LE cells	76	66	76
Antinuclear antibody	95	100	100
Rheumatoid factor	50	22	32–50
False positive test for syphilis	11	5–18	Rare
Coombs' test	25	Rare	33
Antinative DNA antibody	~60	Rare	Rare
Antipoly(ADP-ribose) antibody	~60	~100	Not known
Antihistone antibody	~60	~100	~100

Source: Adapted from a review of several series by Harmon and Portanova (1982).

months of drug exposure) are arthralgia, aching, malaise, and elevated erythrocyte sedimentation rate. Arthritis, rash, lymphadenopathy, pleurisy and pleural effusion, pericardial effusion, and hepatosplenomegaly occur less often, and Raynaud's phenomenon, central nervous system involvement, and renal disease are rare.

Drug-induced lupus is clearly distinguished from idiopathic SLE by the dearth of renal, central nervous system, and Raynaud's involvement, the lower frequency of rash, a narrower autoantibody profile, the rarity of hypocomplementaemia, and a different HLA background (Tables 3 and 4). However, these are not all necessarily fundamental differences, since drug-induced lupus is usually curtailed within the first couple of years of clinical expression by withdrawal of the drug or (if misdiagnosed) by treatment with corticosteroid. A few cases do go on to cutaneous vasculitis (Bernstein et al. 1980) and may progress to glomerulonephritis. After stopping the drug, clinical features generally improve within days or weeks and resolve within months of stopping the offending drug; the antinuclear antibody titre wanes over a year or two (Mansilla-Tinoco et al. 1982).

Antibody profile

The antinuclear antibody profile in drug-induced lupus is much narrower than in idiopathic SLE. Antibodies to extractable nuclear antigens are rare,

Table 4 Risk factors for hydralazine lupus

	Hydralazine-treated controls	Hydralazine lupus	Odds ratio
Mean hydralazine intake	65 g	150 g	
Female	31%	81%	9.9
White	63%	96%	8.2
Slow acetylator	55	96	8.2
HLA–DR4	25%	73%	8.1
C4 null	43%[a]	76%	4.3

[a] Healthy controls not treated with hydralazine.

Source: Based on Batchelor et al. (1980), Mansilla-Tinoco et al. (1982), and Speirs et al. (1989).

and to cardiolipin and native DNA uncommon. The characteristic antinuclear antibody is of homogenous pattern and high titre—the sort producing the LE cell phenomenon (Schett et al. 2000). The specificity of these antibodies is for histones and poly(ADP-ribose), sometimes for single-stranded DNA, but only rarely for native double-stranded DNA (Hobbs et al. 1987). Serial measurement of DNA binding may show a slight rise and then a fall on drug withdrawal but this usually remains within the normal range of DNA binding (which laboratories set quite high to exclude the modest levels of anti-DNA antibody seen in quite a wide range of autoimmune conditions). Antihistone antibody titres rise much higher in drug-induced lupus than in idiopathic SLE, whereas levels of antibody to poly(ADP-ribose) are similar. Antibodies to myeloperoxidase (anti-MPO), giving a pANCA pattern of immunofluorescence on alcohol-fixed neutrophils, have also been reported in drug-induced lupus (Nässberger et al. 1990). The presence of autoantibodies is not per se a reason to discontinue treatment.

Risk factors

Dose and metabolism

The risk factors for developing hydralazine-induced lupus are fairly clear (Table 4). A modest dose must be taken for a year or two or a large dose for several months, and almost always the patient is a 'slow acetylator'. Drug acetylation occurs immediately after absorption on first pass through the liver, and we know that administration of acetylprocainamide (itself an effective antiarrhythmic drug) never leads to the lupus syndrome even though a little of the dose is deacetylated (Woosley et al. 1978). The antinuclear antibody frequency rises faster in slow than fast acetylators. Indeed, it was thought for a time that acetylation of dietary toxins might be relevant to the genesis of idiopathic SLE but this is not the case.

Sex and race

As in idiopathic SLE, females are more at risk than men (though drugs like hydralazine and procainamide are used more often in men), but, in contrast to idiopathic SLE, Perry observed that black patients are highly resistant to the development of hydralazine lupus.

Major histocompatibility complex

Hydralazine lupus is associated with HLA–DR4 (Batchelor et al. 1980) and with null alleles of the complement component C4 (Speirs et al. 1989). HLA–DR4 and C4B null are known to be in linkage disequilibrium, just as in idiopathic SLE the HLA–DR2 and –DR3 associations may reflect the frequency of haplotypes containing C4A null alleles together with these DR antigens.

Pathogenesis

Drug-induced lupus is an autoimmune condition, but this is not to say it is a hypersensitivity reaction to traces of a chemical immunogen. Rather, the drugs causing the disease are acting at pharmacological concentrations and by one or more pharmacological mechanisms (Reidenberg 1981). Recent experimental work has given new insights.

Modulation of lymphocyte function

Drugs inducing autoimmune disease have a pharmacological action on lymphocyte function. Recent studies have built on the observation that T lymphocytes from patients treated with methyldopa show reduced suppression of lymphocyte responsiveness to phytohaemagglutinin and of immunoglobulin synthesis. Rubin and his colleagues have studied 10 drugs capable of inducing the lupus syndrome and have implicated reactive drug metabolites rather than the parent drugs (Rubin 1999). Oxidative transformation mediated by activated neutrophils (a process involving free radicals and enzymes such as myeloperoxidase) yields drug metabolites capable of causing local tissue damage. What might 'stimulate the phagocytes' is not clear, but the site of the action appears to be the thymus gland. This is the organ that controls T lymphocyte maturation and self-tolerance, and it also happens to be a tissue made up mostly of chromatin. When a reactive metabolite such as procainamide hydroxylamine is injected directly into the thymus gland of mice, an autoimmune response builds up producing chromatin-reactive T lymphocytes within the gland and circulating antinuclear antibodies directed at chromatin (Rubin and Kretz-Rommel 1999; Kretz-Rommel and Rubin 2000).

Autoantibody targets: The fine specificity of autoantibodies in drug-induced lupus is in keeping with this model. Histones and poly(ADP-ribose) are components of the nucleosome (unit of chromatin structure) and the histone epitopes recognized are those exposed on the surface of the nucleosome (Craft et al. 1987). This pattern of immune response can be imitated by immunization of rabbits with whole nucleosomes, whereas naked histones induce antibodies to epitopes that are normally buried. One wonders whether antibodies to myeloperoxidase reflect the postulated activation of neutrophils within the thymus.

Role of autoantibodies: The development of autoantibodies is necessary but not sufficient for the clinical expression of drug-induced lupus. In the lupus syndrome the antinuclear antibody is usually present at high titre, of both IgG and IgM classes, and able to fix complement, but these characteristics still need not lead to disease. Additional factors must be involved, amongst which are the genetic background (such as HLA) and possibly pharmacological effects on apoptosis (Hieronymus et al. 2000) and the function of complement.

Complement dysfunction induced by drugs

Serum complement levels are usually normal in drug-induced lupus, but the drug may interfere with complement function. In immune complex disease, complement is important in the solubilization of immune complexes and in their removal on the CR1 receptor of red cells (Schifferli et al. 1986). Most patients with idiopathic SLE have a null allele of C4 or occasionally C2, and homozygous deficiency of any of the early components of complement often leads to SLE. One pharmacological property of several lupus-inducing drugs is the ability to block the transient activated form of C4. Inhibition of C4 activity has been demonstrated *in vitro* with hydralazine, isoniazid, penicillamine and the hydroxylamine form of procainamide, but not acetylprocainamide (Sim et al. 1984). It is rather disappointing, however, for this line of reasoning that hydralazine does not exacerbate idiopathic SLE *in vivo*.

Drug-induced myositis

Toxic myopathies occur occasionally with various drugs including statins, clofibrate, emetine, chloroquine, ε-aminocaproic acid, vincristine, lithium, amphotericin B, salbutamol, colchicine, and nitroxoline (Le Quintrec and Le Quintrec 1991). A true drug-induced myositis is seen occasionally with D-penicillamine and also reported with penicillin, sulfonamides, procainamide, hydralazine, phenytoin, propylthiouracil, phenylbutazone, cimetidine, and tamoxifen. Statin therapy may exacerbate idiopathic myositis. In penicillamine therapy for rheumatoid arthritis, the frequency of myositis is 0.2–1.2 per cent rather than the expected coincidence of less than 0.001 per cent. Most cases of drug-induced myositis are antinuclear-antibody positive, and there seems to be a high frequency of dysphagia and muscle weakness but little myalgia. Myositis is mediated mainly by T cells, and in a case associated with cimetidine therapy there was a marked increase in the proportion of cytotoxic/suppressor T cells in the peripheral blood similar to the inflammatory infiltrate in muscle.

Drug-induced myasthenia gravis

Rheumatoid arthritis and idiopathic myasthenia gravis are weakly associated, but in 1975 Bucknall et al. described four cases of myasthenia gravis developing during penicillamine therapy and remitting after treatment was discontinued (Bucknall et al. 1975). This reaction may occur in upto 1 per cent of rheumatoid arthritis patients after several months of penicillamine therapy at daily doses of 500 mg or more. Antibodies to the acetylcholine receptor are found in all cases but their specificity is restricted to the human receptor. HLA typing shows more BW35 and DR1 and less B8 and DR3 than in idiopathic myasthenia gravis, and less DR4 than in rheumatoid arthritis controls (Dawkins et al. 1981).

Drug-induced scleroderma

Scleroderma-like disease with the typical microvascular and fibrotic changes can follow exposure to a variety of drugs and chemicals. The drugs include bleomycin, 5-hydroxytryptophan, carbidopa, pentazocine, penicillamine, phytonadione, diethyopropion, and mazindol (appetite suppressants), and intravenous cocaine abuse. In bleomycin-induced scleroderma, there is increased collagen synthesis by dermal fibroblasts *in vitro* and administration of bleomycin to rats produces skin thickening with increased collagen synthesis (Rush et al. 1984; Bourgeois and Aeschlimann 1991).

Chemicals inducing scleroderma-like disease

Just as there are chemical causes of cirrhosis and pulmonary fibrosis, there are chemicals other than drugs that induce a scleroderma-like disease. These include vinyl chloride and the outbreak of 'Spanish oil disease'. Fears about silicone implants have proven unfounded, but there are still concerns that systemic sclerosis may be triggered by exposure to various organic chemicals (Mayes 1999). The evidence for what would have to be a rare and idiosyncratic response comes from a few case reports of scleroderma developing soon after excessive or accidental exposure to organic solvents such as carbon tetrachloride, and the observation that cases of systemic sclerosis tend to cluster under the flight approaches to airports.

Silicone implants

Silicones are polymers mainly of dimethylsiloxane (chains of alternating silicon and oxygen atoms with two methyl groups attached to each Si atom). The silicone forms a liquid, gel, or rubber-like material (elastomer) depending on the number of cross-links between the polymer chains. Being fairly inert within the body, silicone is used to lubricate syringes and has been incorporated in intraoccular lenses, ventriculoperitoneal shunts, and heart valves, as well as forming breast implants and artificial testicles.

Anecdotal reports of rheumatic symptoms arising after silicone injection or implantation have been published since the 1960s (Kamugai et al. 1984) and in a welter since medicolegal interest arose (Sanchez-Guerrero et al. 1994).

There is good epidemiological evidence against any increased frequency of connective tissue diseases in relation to silicone although the overall community prevalence of scleroderma may have increased in the past 50 years (Sanchez-Guerrero et al. 1994).

An independent review group with expertise in epidemiology, immunology, rheumatology, and pathology came to reassuring conclusions in their advice to the British Government. Yet, despite the lack of scientific evidence, some patients may wish to have their implants removed for peace of mind. If the manufacturers survive bankruptcy, their settlement offer may reward those with common complaints like fatigue, widespread aching, paraesthesia, and the like. We must guard against this windfall making our patients feel worse.

Vinyl chloride disease

Workers exposed to vinyl chloride for prolonged periods in the manufacture of polyvinylchloride may develop an illness characterized by breathlessness, Raynaud's phenomenon, and contracture of the hands with thickening of the skin. Deposits of complement and fibrinogen are present in blood vessel walls (emphasizing that, like systemic sclerosis, this is a disease of the microvasculature as well as fibrosis), but anticentromere and anti-Scl-70 antibodies are not found. It is suggested that HLA–DR5 influences susceptibility and DR3 influences the severity of vinyl chloride disease (Black et al. 1983).

Spanish oil disease

The sale of contaminated rape-seed oil as cooking oil to about 20 000 people in the Madrid area led to a 'toxic oil syndrome' with an initial acute phase of fever, rash, gastrointestinal upset, neurological disturbance, acute interstitial pneumonia, and sometimes death. Many recovered, but several hundreds went on to develop hardened, thickened skin, Raynaud's phenomenon, dysphagia, pulmonary hypertension, alopecia, dry eyes, dry mouth, arthritis, and flexion contractures. Autoantibodies were not a feature, but there was microvascular damage with endothelial proliferation and infiltration of vessel walls by lymphocytes and macrophages (Spurzem and Lockey 1984).

Eosinophilia–myalgia syndrome

First reported to the Centers for Disease Control in November 1989, almost 1500 cases had been notified 4 months later and it was clear that the ingestion of tryptophan as a health-food supplement was responsible. The amino acid all came from one manufacturer and a contaminant in the manufacturing process has been implicated. Long-term follow-up is underway but new cases have ceased occurring. The syndrome is characterized by the abrupt onset of malaise, myalgia, weakness, contractures, induration of fascia, morphoea-like lesions, and blood eosinophilia ($1–30 \times 10^9$/l). Neuromyopathy is frequent and cardiac abnormalities have been seen, with some deaths. The histological findings resemble eosinophilic fascitis with an interstitial and perivascular inflammatory infiltrate (Le Quintrec and Le Quintrec 1991).

Serum sickness and hypersensitivity vasculitis

Serum sickness is an immune-complex disease. First seen following the injection of antiserum for the treatment of bacterial infections such as diphtheria and tetanus, it now occurs rarely with some drugs, particularly penicillin, sulfonamides, penicillamine, and thiouracil. The first indication is usually fever, appearing 7–12 days after the beginning of treatment, followed by urticaria, joint pains, and occasionally glomerulonephritis or myocarditis (Rich 1942); this may progress to vasculitis.

Hypersensitivity or leucocytoclastic vasculitis is characterized by an infiltrate of dead or dying polymorphonuclear white cells in the walls of small blood vessels. There is often no obvious cause but in some cases drugs have been implicated, particularly sulfonamides, penicillin, thiouracil, iodides, organic arsenicals, oestrogens, and hydantoins (Dubost et al. 1991). For more on vasculitis see Chapters 6.10.1–6.10.9.

Food and arthritis

Despite much folklore and several books, there is little convincing evidence that immune reactions to what we eat have any bearing on the pathogenesis of arthritis or the connective tissue diseases (Walport et al. 1982). Anecdotal reports of food allergy have involved foods such as wheat, eggs, beef, and pork, and one diet recommends avoiding 'acidic' foods. Features often associated with arthritis in 'allergic' cases are migraine headaches, rhinitis, and gastrointestinal symptoms. After 50 years of open study, double-blind trials of diet are now in progress. It is possible that a diet of fish oil alters prostaglandin synthesis in a way that reduces the intensity of inflammation.

Specific syndromes occasionally associated with food allergy include palindromic rheumatism (reports of provocation by nitrates and menthol), vasculitis (various foodstuffs and in one case a particular brand of beer), hydrarthrosis of the knees (a case induced by English walnuts), and seronegative rheumatoid arthritis (a case exacerbated by milk and cheese). Most of these studies involved withdrawal of the foodstuff and rechallenge in open fashion.

Could rheumatoid arthritis be caused or exacerbated by absorption of antigens from the bowel? Pigs develop arthritis and nodules if fed a diet high in fish protein, and the onset of arthritis is associated with increased isolation of *Clostridium perfringens* from the gut flora. Arthritis is commoner in people with selective IgA deficiency, again highlighting mucosal defence. After intestinal bypass (once in favour as a treatment for morbid obesity), arthritis, often accompanied by features of Behçet's syndrome, may develop, and radiolabelled fragments of *E. coli* administered by mouth have been demonstrated in joints.

Metabolic reactions to drugs and toxins

Drugs and toxins causing gout

The relationship of alcohol to gout is complex in that many who drink well also eat well (with a high intake of purines), but it does seem that a high alcohol intake stimulates endogenous urate synthesis while high doses of alcohol temporarily reduce urate excretion (Scott 1991).

Lead rather than alcohol may have been responsible for the frequency of 'saturnine' gout in Georgian times when pewter was in fashion (lead-induced renal tubular damage leading to reduced excretion of uric acid). Nowadays, thiazide and loop diuretics are a common cause of hyperuricaemia, and gout is well recognized not just in bucolic men but also in elderly women; the average increase in serum urate is about 70 μmol/l.

Salicylates have a uricosuric effect at higher doses but at low dose (with a low urine salicylate concentration) the excretion of uric acid is actually inhibited. Even the uricosuric agent probenecid has this paradoxical effect if given at a tiny dose. Among non-steroidal anti-inflammatory drugs, azapropazone has the most clinically useful uricosuric effect.

Hyperuricaemia, through an effect on the kidney, can also occur with pyrazinamide, ethambutol, and cyclosporin. Increased production of urate is caused by nicotinic acid and various cytotoxic agents, including vincristine, busulfan, thiotepa, cytarabine, 6-mercaptopurine, chlorambucil, cyclophosphamide, and the like. Increased tissue destruction leads to the release of purines and their metabolism to uric acid; this pathway can be blocked by the xanthine oxidase inhibitor allopurinol but with the warning that allopurinol increases the bioavailability of the azathioprine metabolite 6-mercaptopurine.

Fluoride and bone pain

In certain areas of India very high levels of fluoride in water lead to increased bone density and hyperostosis that goes on to cause widespread nerve root entrapment. Ingestion of moderate amounts of fluoride, as sometimes used in the treatment of osteoporosis, can cause severe pain in the legs, felt mainly around the joints. This lower limb pain occurs in upto 25 per cent of patients and remits when fluoride therapy is stopped or the dose reduced (Reeve 1990); microfractures may be the cause (Laroche and Mazieres 1991; Rooney et al. 1991).

Rheumatological effects of retinoids, quinolones, and proton pump inhibitors

Retinoids are derivatives of vitamin A used in the treatment of severe acne. Chronic administration whether as a food fad or as dermatological treatment can cause arthralgias, arthritis, bone pain, hypercalcaemia, and periosteal new bone formation. Hyperostosis of the appendicular skeleton can occur, especially in children, and premature closure of the epiphyses has been reported (Kaplan and Haettich 1991).

Quinoline antibiotics include nalidixic acid and ciprofloxacin. Very rarely these cause arthralgias and tenosynovitis in children, while puppies and the young of other susceptible species show surface blistering of the articular cartilage (Ribard and Kahn 1991). Case reports of Achilles tendon rupture have not been substantiated by larger surveys of ciprofloxacin use.

Omeprazole and lansoprazole may cause arthralgias in occasional patients.

Transplant arthropathy

A painful, self-limiting, pseudoinflammatory arthropathy of lower limb joints can occur a few months after organ transplantation. There are clinical, radiological, and scintigraphic similarities to reflex sympathetic dystrophy. Knees or ankles are affected most often, but hip and wrist involvement has been seen. The clinical features are joint pain and tenderness and there may be effusion, periarticular oedema, and erythema. Blood tests for inflammation and autoantibodies are unhelpful; joint fluid cytology is non-inflammatory and does not reveal crystals. Radiographs show no specific abnormality, but isotope bone scans show greatly increased uptake on both sides of the joint (as well as in clinically unaffected joints sometimes). Avascular necrosis does not develop and spontaneous resolution after several months is the rule. This arthropathy has been recognized since the widespread adoption of cyclosporin for immunosuppression in organ transplantation. Cyclosporin levels have often been high when the arthropathy began and resolution tends to follow a reduction in cyclosporin levels. For instance, in our series of eight cases, mean cyclosporin levels were 458 mg/l at onset and 175 mg/l at resolution (Jones and Bernstein 1994). Tacrolimus, which like cyclosporin, is an inhibitor of calcineurin, and has also caused this syndrome of non-inflammatory joint pain with 'hot' isotope bone scan. It has been suggested that calcineurin inhibition itself may be responsible for the condition and that calcium-channel blockers may be useful in treatment (O'Neill and Sloan 1998).

Toxicity of antirheumatic treatment

Simple analgesics

Simple analgesics such as phenacetin, though probably not paracetamol, can cause renal papillary necrosis; this is commoner in hot climates where the urine is likely to be concentrated. Analgesics have a narrow safety range: eight tablets of paracetamol daily are safe, yet 30 tablets can ruin the liver.

Non-steroidal anti-inflammatory drugs

Gastrointestinal damage

Non-steroidal anti-inflammatory drugs commonly irritate the gastrointestinal tract (Henry et al. 1996), possibly through inhibition of prostaglandins, which are important in protecting the mucosa and in the cellular mechanism for mending mucosal breaches. Endoscopy studies have shown that upto 20 per cent of patients have ulcers and a further 30 per cent minor gastroduodenal lesions at any one time, and the risk of an acute bleed, perforation, or death rises from under 0.1 per cent in middle life to about 2.5 per cent in the elderly (Beardon et al. 1989). There are arguments that the presence of *Helicobacter pylori* may be protective rather than harmful in these circumstances. Proton pump inhibitors and the synthetic prostaglandin E_1 misoprostol reduce the risk of non-steroidal anti-inflammatory-induced damage in the stomach and duodenum by about half, whereas H_2-antagonists are protective only in the duodenum. Selective inhibitors of the inducible cyclooxygenase (COX-2) are proving to have no more effect on the stomach than placebo, but some of this benefit is lost when aspirin is coprescribed.

Renal, haematological, and skin reactions

Non-steroidal anti-inflammatory drugs and COX-2 inhibitors (coxibs) can reduce renal blood flow causing a tendency to hypertension and renal insufficiency (especially in the presence of hypovolaemia or pre-existing renal damage). Only sulindac is said to spare the kidneys. Other complications of non-steroidal anti-inflammatory drugs therapy include thrombocytopaenia caused by increased platelet destruction, aplastic anaemia, and thrombocytopaenia with phenylbutazone (now restricted in the United Kingdom to the hospital treatment of ankylosing spondylitis). Rashes are uncommon and occur most often with fenbufen.

Effects on cartilage

Shortly after the introduction of indomethacin there were reports of accelerated osteoarthritis of the hip, and in a clinical study of osteoarthritis of the hip, deterioration to the end-point of joint replacement was rather faster in patients treated with a strong inhibitor of prostaglandin synthesis (indomethacin) than with a weak inhibitor (azapropazone) (Rashad et al. 1989). Experimental data suggest various ways in which non-steroidal anti-inflammatory drugs might damage or even protect articular cartilage, and new chondroprotective agents are being sought by the pharmaceutical industry.

Disease modifying, second-line therapy

Ocular toxicity from the deposition of antimalarial drugs such as chloroquine is well known. Rashes are common with most of the second-line drugs but with gold and penicillamine there is a particular risk of exfoliative dermatitis. Gold and penicillamine also cause membranous glomerulonephritis with nephrotic syndrome and, rarely, renal failure, while bone marrow toxicity with leucopaenia, thrombocytopaenia, or occasionally aplastic anaemia can occur with gold, penicillamine, sulfasalazine, and cytotoxic agents such as methotrexate, azathioprine, and cyclophosphamide; though onset can be abrupt, it is often gradual, so regular monitoring of the blood count and urine is recommended. Gold can also cause, rarely, pneumonitis and, not uncommonly, a 'post-injection flare' of arthritis (Rooney et al. 1991).

Penicillamine

Penicillamine used in the treatment of rheumatoid arthritis and Wilson's disease can trigger the whole range of drug-induced autoimmune reactions (membranous glomerulonephritis presenting as nephrotic syndrome, Goodpasture's syndrome, myasthenia gravis, polymyositis, pemphigus, lupus, and scleroderma), accompanied by the appropriate autoantibody (to kidney or skin basement membrane, acetylcholine receptor, double-stranded DNA, etc.). Susceptibility to at least some of these reactions is increased by the HLA antigen DR3 and by slow sulfoxidation of penicillamine (Emery et al. 1984).

Corticosteroids

Corticosteroid therapy (Geusens and Dequeker 1991) reduces resistance to infection whether administration is systemic or intra-articular, and this must be borne in mind in all sick patients on steroids. A hot, red joint following a steroid injection may be infected or (more often, one hopes) a gout-like reaction to particles in the steroid preparation responsive to non-steroidal anti-inflammatory drug therapy. Repeated steroid injections can lead to avascular necrosis. In the shoulder there is the added risk of rotator cuff degeneration, so injections there should be limited to a few.

Osteonecrosis (avascular necrosis) is also a serious complication of systemic steroid therapy, affecting usually one or both hips but sometimes other joints such as knees and shoulders. It may occur in 5 per cent or more of patients on long-term steroid therapy, and there is a particular risk with high-dose intravenous steroids used in the treatment of transplant rejection and sometimes for connective tissue diseases.

Osteoporosis is a concern with systemic corticosteroid therapy. In younger women treated with prednisolone at doses of 5–7.5 mg/day there was no bone loss detectable by dual photon absorptiometry over a 1-year period, but exacerbation of bone loss after the menopause is more of a problem. Preventitive therapy with a bisphosphonate (and adequate calcium intake) should be considered in all patients when the daily dose of corticosteroid is equivalent to prednisolone 7.5 mg or more.

References

Batchelor, J.R. et al. (1980). Hydralazine-induced systemic lupus erythematosus: the influence of HLA–DR and sex upon susceptibility. *Lancet* **i**, 1107–9.

Beardon, P.H.G., Brown, S.V., and McDevitt, D.G. (1989). Gastrointestinal events in patients prescribed non-steroidal anti-inflammatory drugs: a controlled study using record linkage in Tayside. *Quarterly Journal of Medicine* **71**, 497–505.

Bernstein, R.M., Egerton-Vernon, J., and Webster, J. (1980). Hydralazine induced cutaneous vasculitis. *British Medical Journal* **1**, 156–7.

Black, C.M., Walker, A.E., Welsh, K.I., Bernstein, R.M., Catoggio, L.J. McGregor, A.R., and Lloyd-Jones, J.K. (1983). Genetic susceptibility to scleroderma-like disease induced by vinyl chloride. *Lancet* **i**, 53–5.

Bluestein, H.G., Zvaifler, N.J., Weisman, M.H., and Shapiro, R.F. (1979). Lymphocyte alteration by procainamide: relation to drug-induced lupus erythematosus syndrome. *Lancet* **ii**, 816–19.

Bourgeois, P. and Aeschlimann, A. (1991). Drug-induced scleroderma. *Clinical Rheumatology* **5**, 13–20.

Bucknall, R.C. et al. (1975). Myasthenia gravis associated with penicillamine treatment for rheumatoid arthritis. *British Medical Journal* **1**, 600–2.

Craft, J.E., Radding, J.A., Harding, M.W., Bernstein, R.M., and Hardin, J.A. (1987). Autoantigenic histone epitopes: a comparison between procainamide- and hydralazine-induced lupus. *Arthritis and Rheumatism* **30**, 689–94.

Dawkins, R.L. et al. (1981). Immunobiology of D-penicillamine. *Journal of Rheumatology* **7**, 56–61.

Dubost, J.-J., Souteyrand, P., and Sauvezie, B. (1991). Drug-induced vasculitides. *Clinical Rheumatology* **5**, 119–38.

Emery, P., Panayi, G.S., Huston, G., Welsh, K.I., Mitchell, S.C., Idle, J.K., Smith, R.L., and Waring, R.H. (1984). D-Penicillamine toxicity in rheumatoid arthritis. The role of sulphoxidation status and HLA–DR3. *Journal of Rheumatology* **11**, 626–32.

Freni-Titulaer, L.W.J., Kelley, D.B., Grow, A.C., Hochberg, M.C., and Arnett, F.C. (1988). Clustering of connective tissue diseases in a small Georgia community. III. A search for environmental factors. *Arthritis and Rheumatism* **31**, s75.

Ghate, J.V. et al. (2001). Drug-induced lupus associated with COL-3: report of 3 cases. *Archives of Dermatology* **137**, 471–4.

Geusens, P. and Dequeker, J. (1991). Locomotor side-effects of corticosteroids. *Clinical Rheumatology* **5**, 99–118.

Goldstein, J.L. et al. (2000). Reduced risk of upper gastrointestinal ulcer complications with celecoxib, a novel COX-2 inhibitor. *American Journal of Gastroenterology* **95**, 1681–90.

Gough, A., Chapman, S., Wagstaff, K., Emery, P., and Elias, E. (1996). Minocycline induced autoimmune hepatitis and systemic lupus erythematosus-like syndrome. *British Medical Journal* **312**, 169–72.

Harmon, C.E. and Portanova, J.P. (1982). Drug-induced lupus. *Clinics in Rheumatic Disease* **8**, 121–35.

Henry, D. et al. (1996). Variability in risk of gastrointestinal complications with individual non-steroidal anti-inflammatory drugs: results of a collaborative meta-analysis. *British Medical Journal* **312**, 1563–6.

Hieronymus, T. et al. (2000). Chlorpromazine induces apoptosis in activated human lymphoblasts: a mechanism supporting the induction of drug-induced lupus erythematosus? *Arthritis and Rheumatism* **43**, 1994–2004.

Hobbs, R.N., Clayton, A.-L., and Bernstein, R.M. (1987). Antibodies to the five histones and poly(adenosine diphosphate-ribose) in drug induced lupus: implications for pathogenesis. *Annals of the Rheumatic Diseases* **46**, 408–16.

Jones, P.B.B. and Bernstein, R.M. (1994). Joint pain after organ transplantation. *Arthritis and Rheumatism* **37**, S273.

Kahn, M.-F., ed. (1991). Drug-induced rheumatic diseases. *Clinical Rheumatology* **5**, 1–196.

Kamugai, Y. et al. (1984). Clinical spectrum of connective tissue disease after cosmetic surgery. Observations on eighteen cases and a review of the Japanese literature. *Seminars in Arthritis and Rheumatism* **27**, 1–12.

Kaplan, G. and Haettich, B. (1991). Rheumatological symptoms due to retinoids. *Clinical Rheumatology* **5**, 77–97.

Kretz-Rommel, A. and Rubin, R.L. (2000). Disruption of positive selection of thymocytes causes autoimmunity. *Nature Medicine* **6**, 298–305.

Laroche, M. and Mazieres, B. (1991). Side-effects of fluoride therapy. *Clinical Rheumatology* **5**, 61–76.

Le Quintrec, J.-S. and Le Quintrec, J.-L. (1991). Drug-induced myopathies. *Clinical Rheumatology* **5**, 21–38.

Mansilla-Tinoco, R. et al. (1982). Hydralazine, antinuclear antibodies and the lupus syndrome. *British Medical Journal* **284**, 936–9.

Mayes, M.D. (1999). Epidemiological studies of environmental agents and systemic autoimmune diseases. *Environmental Health Perspectives* **107** (Suppl. 5), 743–8.

Nässberger, L., Sjöholm, A.G., Jonsson, H., Sturfelt, G., and Åkesson, A. (1990). Autoantibodies against neutrophil cytoplasm components in systemic lupus erythematosus and in hydralazine induced lupus. *Clinical and Experimental Immunology* **81**, 380–3.

O'Neill, E.A. and Sloan, V.S. (1998). A potential mechanism of cyclosporine-associated bone pain. *Arthritis and Rheumatism* **41**, 585–6.

Perry, H.M. (1973). Late toxicity to hydralazine resembling systemic lupus erythematosus or rheumatoid arthritis. *American Journal of Medicine* **54**, 58–72.

Rashad, S., Hemmingway, A., Rainsford, K., Revell, P., Low, F., and Walker, F. (1989). Effect of non-steroidal anti-inflammatory drugs on the course of osteoarthritis. *Lancet* **ii**, 519–22.

Reeve, J. (1990). Restoring trabecular bone mass in established osteoporosis. In *Osteoporosis 1990* (ed. R. Smith), pp. 143–55. London: RCP Publications.

Reidenberg, M.M. (1981). Clinical induction of SLE and lupus like illness. *Arthritis and Rheumatism* **24**, 1004–9.

Ribard, P. and Kahn, M.-F. (1991). Rheumatological side-effects of quinolones. *Clinical Rheumatology* **5**, 175–92.

Rich, A.R. (1942). The role of hypersensitivity in periarteritis nodosa: as indicated by seven cases developing during serum sickness and sulphonamide therapy. *Bulletin of the Johns Hopkins Hospital* **71**, 123–40.

Rooney, P.J., Balint, G.P., Szebenyi, B., and Petrou, P. (1991). Rheumatic syndromes caused by antirheumatic drugs. *Clinical Rheumatology* **5**, 139–73.

Rubin, R.L. (1999). Etiology and mechanisms of drug-induced lupus. *Current Opinion in Rheumatology* **11**, 357–63.

Rubin, R.L. and Kretz-Rommel, A. (1999). Initiation of autoimmunity by a reactive metabolite of a lupus-inducing drug in the thymus. *Environmental Health Perspectives* **107** (Suppl. 5), 803–6.

Rush, P.J., Bell, M.J., and Fam, A.G. (1984). Toxic oil syndrome (Spanish oil disease) and chemically induced scleroderma-like conditions. *Journal of Rheumatology* **11**, 262–4.

Sanchez-Guerrero, J., Schur, P.H., Sergent, J.S., and Liang, M.H. (1994). Silicone breast implants and rheumatic disease: clinical, immunologic and epidemiologic studies. *Arthritis and Rheumatism* **37**, 158–68.

Schaible, T.F. (2000). Long term safety of infliximab. *Canadian Journal of Gastroenterology* **14** (Suppl. C), 29c–32c.

Schett, G. et al. (2000). The lupus erythematosus cell phenomenon: comparative analysis of antichromatin antibody specificity in lupus erythematosus cell-positive and -negative sera. *Arthritis and Rheumatism* **43**, 420–8.

Schifferli, J.A., Ng., Y.C., and Peters, D.K. (1986). The role of complement and its receptor in the elimination of immune complexes. *New England Journal of Medicine* **315**, 488–95.

Schlienger, R.G., Bircher, A.J., and Meier, C.R. (2000). Minocycline-induced lupus. A systematic review. *Dermatology* **200**, 223–31.

Scott, J.T. (1991). Drug-induced gout. *Clinical Rheumatology* **5**, 39–60.

Shoenfeld, Y. and Isenberg, D. *The Mosaic of Autoimmunity*, pp. 321–43 and 397–400. Amsterdam: Elsevier, 1990.

Sim, E., Gill, E.W., and Sim, R.B. (1984). Drugs that induce systemic lupus erythematosus inhibit complement component C4. *Lancet* **ii**, 422–4.

Solinger, A.M. (1988). Drug-related lupus. *Clinics in Rheumatic Disease* **14**, 187–202.

Speirs, C., Fielder, A.H.L., Chapel, H., Davey, N.J., and Batchelor, J.R. (1989). Complement system protein C4 and susceptibility to hydrazaline-induced systemic lupus erythematosus. *Lancet* **i**, 922–4.

Spurzem, J.R. and Lockey, J.E. (1984). Toxic oil syndrome. *Archives of Internal Medicine* **144**, 249–50.

Sridhar, M.K. and Abdulla, A. (1998). Fatal lupus-like syndrome and ARDS induced by fluvastatin. *Lancet* **352**, 114.

Walport, M.J., Parke, A.L., and Hughes, G.R.V. (1982). Food and the connective tissue diseases. *Clinics in Immunology and Allergy* **2**, 113–20.

Woosley, R.L., Drayer, D.E., Reidenberg, M.M., Nies, A.S., Carr, K., and Oates, J.A. (1978). Effects of acetylator phenotype on the rate at which procainamide induces antinuclear antibodies and the lupus syndrome. *New England Journal of Medicine* **298**, 1157–60.

7

Surgical intervention and sports medicine

7 Surgical intervention and sports medicine

7.1 Surgery in adults

Justin P. Cobb and C.B.D. Lavy

Introduction

The surgeon is an indispensable member of the team involved in the treatment of a patient with arthritis. He or she should be available not only as a technician to perform operations but ideally should also be involved in the decision making processes in the management of the patient, such as the timing of surgery, the order in which affected joints should be treated, and of course the procedures undertaken. Most large units have combined clinics where the experience of rheumatologist, surgeon, physiotherapist, occupational therapist, and patient can be shared. In patients with polyarthritis, where several joints are likely to need surgery, a valuable relationship between patient and surgeon can be developed—a relationship which gives the patient trust and confidence and gives the surgeon a greater understanding of the patient's specific needs than can be gained by a single meeting.

This chapter will first list the options available to the surgeon dealing with rheumatic disease. Second, it will cover specific pre- and post-operative considerations that must be addressed by the surgeon. The third and largest part of the chapter will focus on specific anatomical regions in detail, outlining the procedures most commonly used. Operating theatre technique will not be covered. For this, the reader is referred to specific operative texts, some of which are included in the references.

Surgical technique

The armamentarium of surgical treatment of arthritis includes the following procedures:

1. arthroscopy and arthroscopic debridement;
2. synovectomy;
3. soft tissue release, realignment, or repair;
4. tendon transfer;
5. osteotomy;
6. excision arthroplasty;
7. prosthetic arthroplasty;
8. arthrodesis and stabilization.

Not all the above are relevant in every anatomical region but they are listed here for completeness. The particular techniques that are commonly used will be outlined under individual joints and regions below.

Special considerations in planning surgery in rheumatic diseases

When to operate

It is difficult to give specific guidelines as to when surgery should be considered for a particular joint as no joint can be considered in isolation from the other joints in the limb or the other limbs, the patient, his or her position in the family and community. However, with all the above in mind, the two factors that most affect the decision to proceed with surgery are pain and loss of function. If the patient's pain cannot be adequately controlled by conservative means and their life, or more particularly their sleep, is being affected then surgery should be considered (Seyfer 1993). Similarly, if the patient's function is being significantly impaired by joint destruction or deformity then surgery to reconstruct or replace the joint should be considered.

Prophylactic surgery has a limited place in the treatment of rheumatic diseases. Synovectomy is certainly of use in incipient tendon rupture. It has also been performed in an effort to prevent deterioration of inflammatory arthritis; however, no long-term study has shown significant slowing of joint destruction. Prophylactic surgery also has a role in stabilizing the potentially unstable spine.

Which joint to operate on first

The order of surgery in patients who have several joints that will benefit from surgery is a common problem in polyarthritic conditions such as rheumatoid arthritis. In deciding which joints to start with there are no hard and fast rules but there are several considerations that must be taken into account. First, when surgery to upper and lower limbs is being considered the lower limb is usually done first as this restores important independent mobility. Rehabilitation following such surgery, however, often requires the use of crutches and if the arm function is so poor that even gutter crutches cannot be used, then surgery to the upper limb may have to precede that to the lower limb. Second, when two joints in a limb are equally affected it is usual to operate on the proximal joint before the distal joint. This helps to reduce pain and improve the proximal stability in the limb before surgery to the distal joint. Where two joints in a limb are both equally affected, for example, the hip and the knee, it may be found that surgery to the hip so improves lower limb function that surgery to the knee is no longer needed. Similarly, surgery to the shoulder may dramatically reduce pain and functional demand on the elbow so that pain is improved and surgery to the elbow is not needed. In other patients, the opposite may be found—surgery is so successful in relieving pain in the most painful joint that the patient's attention now turns to a less affected joint, one that previously had not troubled them much which now becomes the focus of their attention. Sequential surgery does not carry undue risk, however, and has been described with good long-term follow-up (Gill et al. 1999).

The final consideration in the order of surgery is the concept of surgical success. When a number of procedures are likely to be necessary it is often helpful to the patient's morale to start with a procedure that carries a high statistical likelihood of success. An example of this is excision of the distal ulna and synovectomy of the wrist.

Patient's consent and preparation

The Patient's consent must be sought for surgery. This includes not only understanding the operation and its important complications but also the nature of the rehabilitation process involved which may be long. It is helpful if the physiotherapist and occupational therapist both meet the patient beforehand. It can also be of help for the patient to meet others who have had similar surgery.

Anaesthetic considerations

Patients with rheumatic diseases often have associated medical conditions that must be considered during surgery (Skues and Welchew 1993). For example, in rheumatoid arthritis, cervical spine instability means that great care must be taken with endotrachial incubation and, if in doubt, fibreoptic intubation used. With some rheumatic diseases temporomandibular joint function is also limited and cricoarytenoid cartilages can be involved—both also causing airway difficulties. Patients with chronic inflammatory disorders are also often anaemic and some require pre-operative transfusion. Pulmonary, cardiovascular, and renal complications in rheumatic diseases can also affect anaesthesia. These are discussed elsewhere.

Drugs affecting surgery

Patients who have been on steroids or antimetabolic drugs may have thin, delicate skin that tears or bruises easily. Great care must therefore be taken during surgery and in positioning and handling the anaesthetized patient. Skin may also be sensitive to the adhesive compound used in some dressings. Steroids and antimetabolic drugs may also reduce the patient's response to infection and also delay wound healing, although they are not in themselves contradictions to surgery. Specific medical complication to steroids and other disease-modifying agents will be considered elsewhere.

Positioning the patient

Often joint stiffness and restriction of movement will not allow normal positioning to be used. For example, shoulder and elbow stiffness may not allow the hand to be flat on a table beside the patient. A degree of flexibility on the part of the surgeon is therefore needed. Great care must always be taken of the anaesthetized patient to ensure that joints are not over stressed. This is especially the case with rheumatoid arthritis where the soft tissues and bones are fragile. Care must also be taken at pressure points to avoid skin necrosis, bruising, and damage to peripheral nerves.

Surgical treatment in specific anatomical regions

Shoulder

The shoulder is commonly involved in inflammatory arthritis with clinical features of pain in 47 per cent (Laine et al. 1954). Petersson (1986) reports radiographic changes in the shoulders in 83 per cent of patients with rheumatoid arthritis. There is, however, little correlation between clinical signs and symptoms and radiographic appearance and it is not uncommon for a grossly destroyed shoulder joint to present with few symptoms.

The shoulder comprises four main anatomical areas; the sternoclavicular joint, the acromioclavicular joint, the subacromial region, and the glenohumeral joint. Pain arising from the sternoclavicular joint is usually easy to diagnose as it is localized to the sternoclavicular region. However, it is more difficult to be specific about the anatomical origin of pain and tenderness in the area around the shoulder itself. Physical signs can point to one of the three sites as the origin of the pain but most surgeons rely on the additional diagnostic information given by local anaesthetic tests. One per cent lignocaine is injected sequentially into the subacromial space, the acromioclavicular joint, the region of the biceps tendon, and the glenohumeral joint until the pain is abolished. Many patients will have some involvement at more than one, or indeed all, of these sites (Kelly 1990).

Sternoclavicular joint

If conservative measures such as injection of steroids cannot control the pain arising from this joint then synovectomy can be considered or a limited excision of the medial end of the clavicle can be performed, keeping the excision medial to the costoclavicular ligaments. Care must be taken to avoid instability by preserving as much of the capsule as possible. The surgeon should also be cautious as the immediate posterior relation of the left joint is the innominate vein.

Acromioclavicular joint

This joint is involved in 70 per cent of rheumatoid shoulders (Crossan 1980). If pain becomes severe and cannot be controlled by conservative treatment or injection, the distal end can be excised lateral to the coracoclavicular ligaments which provide stability.

Subacromial region

Pain commonly arises from this region due to subacromial impingement which may be associated with inflammation in the subacromial bursa or a partial or complete rotator cuff tear. If pain from this area is abolished by local anaesthetic injection yet not controlled by steroid injection, then a subacromial decompression can be performed. This can be done as an open operation or, where the expertise exists, as an arthroscopic procedure using a powered burr. Rotator cuff repair is usually unrewarding in late rheumatoid arthritis because of the atrophied nature of the supraspinatus tendon.

Glenohumeral joint

This is involved in more than two-thirds of patients with rheumatoid arthritis (Ennevarra 1967). In early cases synovectomy can be performed either as an open procedure or arthroscopically (Bennett and Gerber 1994). Ogilvie-Harris and Wiley (1986) had good results in nine out of 11 patients who had this procedure arthroscopically. In moderate to severe bony destruction, a double osteotomy, as described by Benjamin, can be performed (Benjamin et al. 1979). This comprises an osteotomy of the humerus at the surgical neck and a similar osteotomy of the scapula at the glenoid neck. The mechanism of action of this procedure is poorly understood but it has been shown to have good results in terms of pain relief and increased movement in 25 out of 29 patients in Benjamin's series and in 29 out of 32 patients in Jaffe and Learmonth's series (Benjamin 1987; Jaffe and Learmonth 1989).

Joint replacement

Arthroplasty of the shoulder has not been as successful as in the knee or the hip in terms of pain relief or restoration of range of movement. This has been due to poor bone stock in which to anchor prostheses and poor quality soft tissues, especially the rotator cuff. Despite these difficulties, shoulder replacement is a useful therapeutic tool in rheumatoid arthritis giving pain relief in over 90 per cent of patients (Friedman et al. 1989). Later results as expected, show proximal migration of the humeral component with eccentric loading of the glenoid and inevitable loosening, but with few serious symptoms or complications (Sojbjerg et al. 1999).

Early shoulder replacements were constrained, for example, the Stanmore shoulder, which had a plastic glenoid cup holding a humeral head fully captive (Lettin et al. 1982), or the Kessel shoulder which had the ball joint the other way around (Kessel and Bayley 1982). More recent total shoulder replacements such as the Neer (Neer et al. 1982), the Global, or the Copeland have an anatomically shaped humeral head that can articulate with the patient's own glenoid if this is not severely damaged, or with a prosthetic glenoid which is usually cemented in place. The range of movement following total shoulder replacement depends largely on the state of the rotator cuff.

Where the rotator cuff is intact the reconstruction of the anatomical contours of the shoulder joint following arthroplasty can give a very good range of movement with abduction to over 90°. In severe bony destruction, however, there is often virtually no rotator cuff remaining and range of movement is minimally increased by surgery. Indeed the main benefit of the procedure is pain relief. Fixation may be obtained without cement using the Copeland prosthesis, and there is some evidence that this method of fixation, where possible, will avoid loosening for longer (Levy and Copeland 2001).

Arthrodesis

The success of arthroplasty means that arthrodesis is hardly ever indicated in rheumatic diseases. Even in rare cases where because of infection total shoulder replacements need to be removed a stable fibrous pseudoarthrosis usually gives a better functional result than an arthrodesis.

Elbow

Extra-articular procedures commonly performed around the elbow in rheumatoid arthritis include removal of nodules and transposition of the ulnar nerve. Rheumatoid nodules are common around the elbow and they may become painful, unsightly, or ulcerated. Ulnar nerve dysfunction may be motor or sensory and can result both from mechanical and pressure factors due to the presence of swollen and inflamed synovium and a deforming joint. Ischaemic factors also have a role. Ulnar nerve function may be improved by a simple release or, if it is clearly tight, then transposition anterior to the medial epicondyle is recommended.

Synovectomy

Synovectomy of the elbow joint itself is difficult as surgical access to all parts of the intact joint requires several incisions; however, it gives some benefit at least in the short-term when there is gross swelling. Porter et al. (1974) reported relief of pain and return of function in 12 out of 16 patients over a 5-year period. Arthroscopic synovectomy is a new tool that has to be performed with care as the radial and median nerves are closely related to the anterior capsule.

Excision of radial head

When the radial side of the joint is giving rise to the majority of symptoms, excision of the radial head can be performed at the same time as synovectomy (Copeland and Taylor 1979). This is an excellent procedure in terms of pain relief. Stability of the joint should be considered but is seldom significantly compromised in low demand patients. Silastic replacement of the radial head has not proved universally successful.

Arthroplasty

When there is severe pain in the presence of destructive changes in the elbow joint, both in rheumatoid arthritis and in osteoarthritis, arthroplasty can be performed. The simplest and oldest comprises excision arthroplasty which relieves pain but has unreliable stability. Inter position arthroplasty using silicon or metal had limited popularity (Coates et al. 1991) but most surgeons now use a form of total joint replacement. The older fully constrained hinges such as the Stanmore mark 1 replacement have been superceded by semiconstrained hinges such as the GSB (Fig. 1), or a minimally constrained surface replacement such as the Souter (Souter 1990; Pritchard 1991) or Roper–Tuke (Yanni et al. 2000). Long-term survival is good, comparable with hip and knee arthroplasty figures. The Souter has 87 per cent surviving to 13 years (Shah et al. 2000), the Kudo with 90 per cent survival at 16 years (Tanaka et al. 2001), and the GSB with 88 per cent survival at 13 years (Geschwend et al. 1999).

(a)
(b)
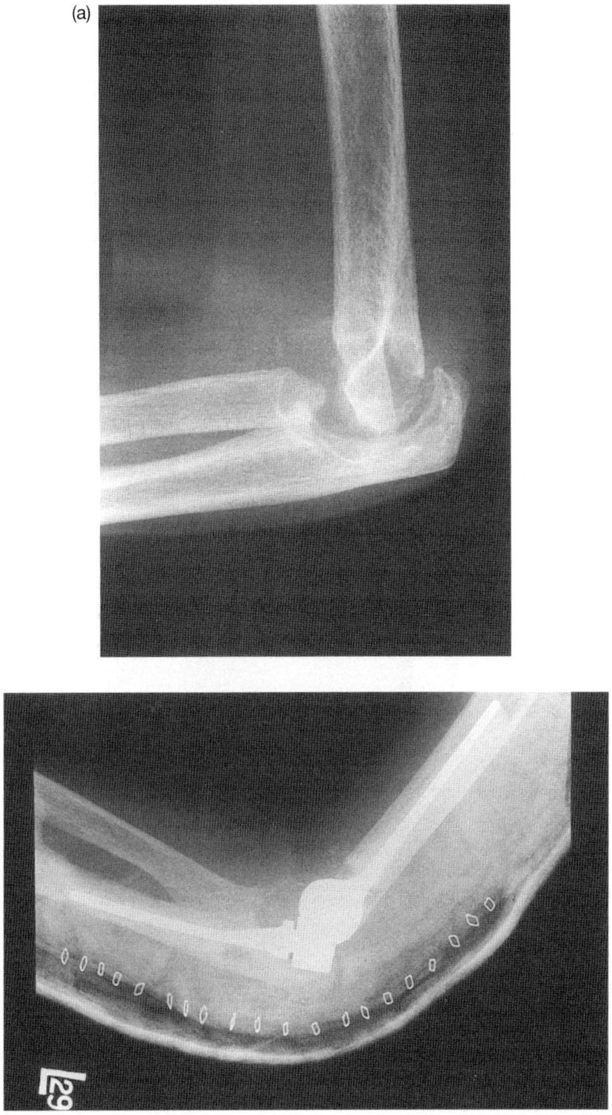

Fig. 1 Rheumatoid elbow (a) pre- and (b) post-arthroplasty using a GSB semiconstrained hinge prosthesis.

Wrist

Osteoarthritis

Osteoarthritis of the wrist is not common and is usually post-traumatic, following either fracture of the distal radius or carpal bones, especially the scaphoid. When pain cannot be controlled, conservatively surgery should be considered. Joint replacement, as described below for rheumatoid arthritis, is an option in very low demand patients. Excision of the proximal carpal row can be performed where the disease is confined to this region. The space previously occupied by the excised proximal row becomes a pseudoarthrosis, relieving pain at the expense of some stability. Limited carpal fusions can also be performed particularly when the osteoarthritis is confined to the radial side of the wrist. This procedure does not have a high rate of success but if pain persists or recurs it can be revised to a complete wrist fusion.

Rheumatoid arthritis

Rheumatoid arthritis can affect the wrist joint as well as the flexor and extensor tendons and surgery to the tendons, such as synovectomy or transfer of the extensor tendons, is often combined with surgery to the wrist; however, in this text we will consider them separately. Rheumatoid arthritis can affect the radioulnar as well as the radiocarpal joints and often it is this joint that gives much of the pain, both from instability and from impingement on the carpus. Treatment by excision of distal 10–15 mm of the ulnar

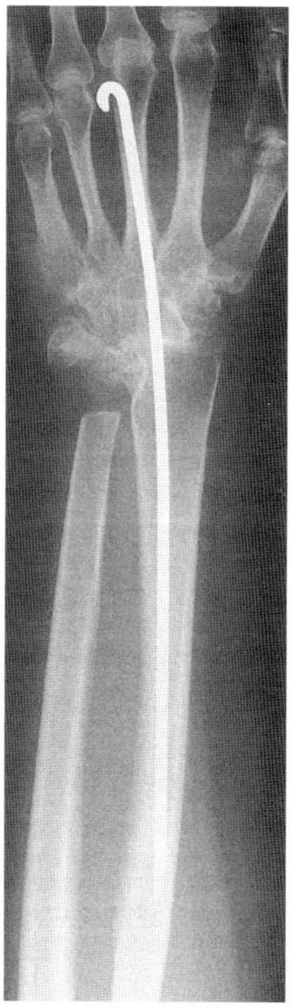

Fig. 2 Rheumatoid wrist following fusion using an intramedullary Rush pin.

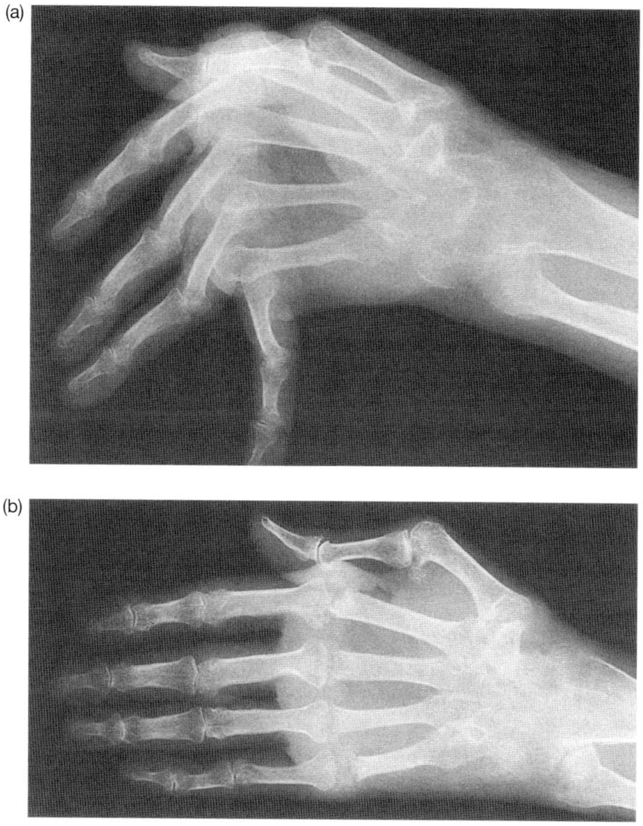

Fig. 3 Rheumatoid hand (a) before and (b) after silastic metacarpophalangeal joint replacements.

is very effective in terms of relief of pain and also removes an unsightly lump (Clawson and Stern 1991; Posner and Ambrose 1991). When the pain is also arising from the radiocarpal joint, the surgical options are fusion or arthroplasty. Limited wrist fusion such as the Chamay technique (Chamay et al. 1983), which uses graft from the distal ulnar to fuse the radius to the lunate, are of use when there is good bone stock remaining but in most late cases there is such distortion of the normal anatomy that complete arthrodesis is performed.

The commonest method used involves insertion of a Rush pin (Fig. 2) or a Steinmann pin down the third metacarpal and across the wrist. This can be supplemented with a staple to improve stability. The position of stabilization is slight radial deviation and dorsiflexion. However, if both wrists are to be fused then perineal toilet is often improved if one is fused in slight flexion. This can safely be achieved percutaneously (Christodoulou et al. 1999) but requires a plaster cast. Alternatively, the use of a specific titanium plate allows the wrist to be managed without cast support (Houshian and Schroder 2001).

Joint replacement

The Swanson design silastic prosthesis is the most popular form of arthroplasty in Britain (Fig. 3). The proximal carpal row is excised and the prosthesis fills the gap with one stem that fits into the distal radius and one that fits into a hole made through the capitate into the third metacarpal. Metal grommets can be used to protect the prosthesis from the sharp edges of the bone. This procedure gives good results in terms of relief of pain in low demand patients (Jolly et al. 1992) but range of movement is usually limited to an arc of 40–50°. There are other designs of wrist replacement, such as the Meuli ball and socket joint which is popular in continental Europe. Where both wrists are involved in rheumatoid arthritis, many surgeons fuse the dominant wrist which is likely to take more force and confine arthroplasty to the non-dominant side. Uncemented joint replacement has some promising early results and is now a conservative option, allowing bone stock to be preserved so that a later arthrodesis would not be compromised (Radmer et al. 1999).

Surgery to extensor tendons

In early disease, synovectomy of the extensor tendons is often combined with surgery to the wrist. The tendons are exposed by reflecting a flap of the dorsal extensor retinaculum, then after synovectomy the flap is replaced deep to the extensor tendons thus protecting them from the wrist joint. Synovectomy relieves pain and swelling and also reduces the risk of rupture.

The most common tendons to be ruptured are the extensor pollicis longus and the extensor digiti minima. The former is commonly treated by transfer of the extensor indicis proprius tendon from the index finger, which conveniently has two extensor tendons, and the remaining extensor indicis communes is adequate to extend the index. Treatment of rupture of extensor digiti minimi is usually by joining the distal end of the tendon to the extensor tendon of the ring finger. Realignment of the extensor tendons can be performed in rheumatoid arthritis. This commonly occurs at the level of the metacarpophalangeal joints where all the tendons tend to shift in an ulnar direction but also at the wrist where the extensor carpi ulnaris can migrate in a volar direction around the ulnar head.

Surgery to the flexor tendons

Synovitis also occurs around the flexor tendon in the synovial sheaths at the wrist and the fingers. When this interferes with function because of pain or by restricting flexion, synovectomy can be performed to improve movement and reduce the risk of rupture. In late cases rupture can occur. Surgical treatment of such rupture is complex and involves tendon grafting, often with a staged procedure. In mild cases of synovitis, triggering can occur around the neck of the flexor sheath. This is treated by simple division of the tight neck of the sheath. A limited synovectomy can also be performed.

Carpal tunnel syndrome

Median nerve compression is common in rheumatoid arthritis and can be relieved by carpal tunnel release. This is easily performed as a day case procedure under local anaesthetic. Endoscopic carpal tunnel release is popular in Europe and in the United States but because of early reports of nerve injury it has had a cautious reception so far in the United Kingdom.

Hand

Surgery to the fingers in rheumatoid arthritis

Boutonnière or Swan neck deformity can be corrected surgically by soft tissue procedures provided the joints are passively mobile. Once fixed deformity of the PIP joints occurs, correction is much harder and surgical improvement may only be achieved by fusion in a position of function or arthroplasty using a silastic replacement joint. The position of fusion is usually 45–90° of flexion but depends on the range of movement at the metacarpophalangeal joints.

Surgery to the thumb in rheumatoid arthritis

Rheumatoid arthritis commonly causes a Z-deformity of the thumb and can cause instability of either the metacarpophalangeal or interphalangeal joint. Such instabilities are seldom helped by soft tissue procedures and a fusion is usually necessary (Toledano et al. 1992).

Surgery to the metacarpophalangeal joints

When rheumatoid arthritis involves the metacarpophalangeal joint there is often a tendency to subluxation of these joints in an ulnar and volar direction. In early cases, this can be treated with synovectomy and soft tissue realignment (Wynn Parry and Stanley 1993). This does slightly decrease range of movement but improves function because of decreased pain and increased power. In late cases where there is bony destruction of the metacarpal head, metacarpophalangeal joint replacement using Swanson silastic prostheses may be necessary. This is always performed in conjunction with soft tissue release and realignment. Such reconstructive surgery, however, should only be done in order to improve function in the hand and should not be performed purely to improve the cosmetic appearance of a deformed rheumatoid hand. The post-operative care of metacarpophalangeal joint replacement and soft tissue realignment is extensive and involves the close cooperation of a hand therapist with experience in splinting as well as physical exercise techniques (Stanley 1992). As in other joints, the longer term is yielding problems of loosening, with bone loss and secondary instability. Newer prostheses are encouraging (Moller et al. 1999), but silastic is not the perfect material for durability, so more progress is needed in this area.

Cervical spine

Rheumatoid arthritis can affect all the synovial joints in the cervical spine including the bursa between the odontoid process and the transverse ligament. This can result not only in destruction of joints but also in attenuation of ligaments and consequent instability of the cervical spine (Heywood et al. 1988). The commonest sites for involvement in the cervical spine were reported recently in a Swedish national survey (Christensson et al. 2000):

1. atlantoaxial subluxation or anterior subluxation of C1 on C2: 66/82;
2. atlantoaccipital impaction, also known as cranial settling: 10/82;
3. subaxial subluxation of the cervical vertebrae: 27/82.

Surgery is not indicated in all cases of cervical instability but it is very important that instability is fully investigated with flexion and extension radiographs, a full neurological examination, and, where there are any neurological signs, a magnetic resonance imaging scan. Neurological impairment can be caused not only by the mechanical effect of the instability but also by pressure from proliferation of soft tissues.

The nature of surgery indicated depends on the pathology demonstrated. If there is progressive instability then prophylactic stabilization can be performed to prevent later deterioration. There are several methods of stabilization of the cervical spine including bone grafting and fixation with plates or preformed wire rectangles or loops (Ranawat et al. 1979; Ransford et al. 1986). Stabilization is also indicated when there is intermittent or persistent neurological deficit. In these cases it may also be necessary to decompress the spinal cord or nerve roots (Johnston and Kelly 1990). This decompressive and stabilizing surgery in a group of ill patients with poor prognoses is still very rewarding when performed in specialist centres (Moskovich et al. 2000), where excellent results can be obtained or many, but with a mortality of 10 per cent at 1 month that is proportional to the co-morbidity in this group.

Foot and ankle

In the foot, as in other areas, meticulous attention to the history and clinical signs is essential. Pain may arise from impingement or entrapment of tendons or nerves, or from joints that are unstable not just destroyed. The judicious use of soft tissue procedures, selective arthrodeses, and joint arthroplasty may maintain fore- and hindfoot function for some years. When destruction and deformity have progressed, it is still usually possible to salvage a painless, albeit flat, foot by forefoot arthroplasty, and triple arthrodesis of the hindfoot.

Synovectomy and soft tissue procedures

While little is published regarding synovectomy alone in the foot, there is some evidence that early synovectomy may delay deterioration in the ankle as in other joints (Hecker et al. 1982; Mohing et al. 1982; Kvien et al. 1987). Pain around the lateral malleolus in the valgus hindfoot may be due to impingement of the lateral malleolus, or to peroneal tendon entrapment. Injection of the tendon sheath is a simple diagnostic and therapeutic procedure that may give relief for some years. A conservative approach to the foot and ankle may also include early decompression of the tibialis posterior tendon and other medial structures to prevent rupture and subsequent deformity (Cracchiolo 1984).

Excision arthroplasty

Damage to the foot, and especially the forefoot, occurs very early in rheumatoid arthritis. A painful and deformed forefoot with hallux valgus, dorsal dislocation of the lesser metatarsophalangeal joints together with significant synovitis is the rule. The buttonholing of the metatarsal heads through the plantar fascia makes walking exquisitely painful. The surgical goal is a foot that is comfortable for slow pedestrian life, as part of the management of a systemic condition. Forefoot arthroplasty is the procedure of choice: the metatarsal heads are resected, allowing the hammering toes to drop down into the plane of the foot. The hallux valgus may be corrected by excising the metatarsal head or the base of the proximal phalanx (Fowler 1959; Kates et al. 1967; Gainor et al. 1988).

Arthrodesis

Isolated painful destruction of the ankle joint in rheumatoid arthritis is best treated by arthrodesis (Fig. 4). Several methods of internal fixation are available (Iwata et al. 1980; Holt et al. 1991; Moran et al. 1991; Dent et al. 1993). These have a lower complication rate and are better tolerated than the traditional method using Charnley external fixation clamps which have a significant infection rate (Moeckel et al. 1991).

More commonly, the significant valgus deformity of the hindfoot is accompanied by pantalar arthritis. In these circumstances, triple or pantalar arthrodesis is the treatment of choice (Vahvanen 1967). In the badly damaged hindfoot, a nail may be inserted from the sole up into the tibia, with or without the use of bone graft. A painless ankylosis can usually be obtained (Stone and Helal 1991). Talonavicular joint destruction with

(a)

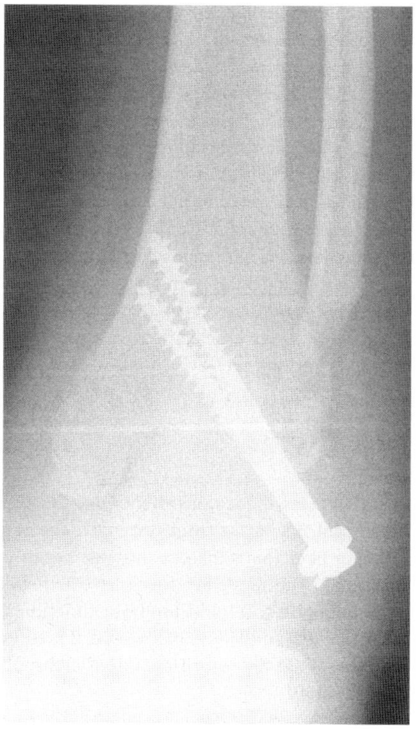

(b)

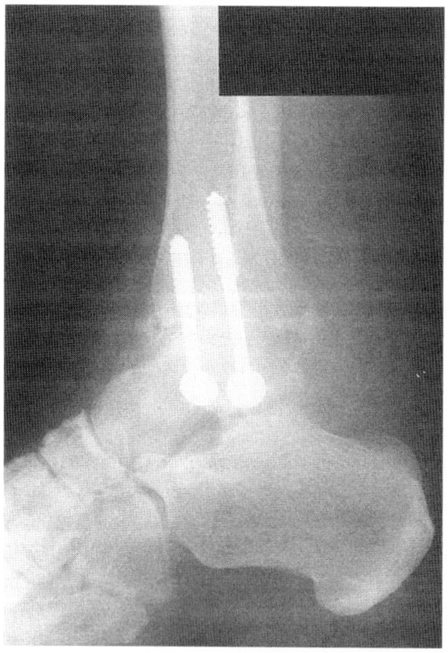

Fig. 4 Anterioposterior (a) and lateral (b) radiographs showing an ankle joint arthrodesed using parallel screws. The subtalar joint is normal.

valgus deformity should also be corrected early and before the forefoot, if symptomatic: it may reduce symptoms in the foot by reducing the valgus shearing forces (Cracchiolo 1984). Fusion and relief of symptoms can be expected in over 90 per cent of cases, but the more severe the deformity, the higher the risk of complications, and failure to correct the deformity fully will probably lead to failure of the arthrodesis (Maenpaa et al. 2001).

Joint replacement

While ankle joint replacement is technically possible, the clinical results are disappointing compared to fusion (Stauffer 1977; Wagner 1982; Jensen and Kroner 1992). It may offer some early advantage in elderly patients with low physical demands, but these benefits are outweighed by the complication rate and difficulty in salvage (McGuire et al. 1988).

Prosthetic replacement of the first metatarsophalangeal joint has its advocates but the long-term results are not good enough to justify the additional complications (Hasselo et al. 1987).

Knee

Synovectomy

Arthroscopic synovectomy can effectively abolish the pain and stiffness in knees with a florid synovitis that is refractory to conservative measures (Ogilvie-Harris and Basinski 1991). It has considerable advantages over open synovectomy, in terms of hospital stay and morbidity, while the results of the two methods appear comparable with both groups regaining an average of 75° of movement (Matsui et al. 1989). This improvement is maintained for about 5 years although in that time the radiographic appearances continue to deteriorate (Paus and Dale 1993), but even at 14 years 67 per cent have remained in remission from the inflammatory element of their condition (Ishikawa et al. 1986). Simpler arthroscopic lavage and debridement may provide temporary relief but nothing more than this.

Joint replacement

The stiff and painful knees of the inflammatory arthropathies are best treated by total knee replacement. Double osteotomies were used in the past with varying effects, but excision of the entire articular surface and a thorough synovectomy is possible during total knee replacement reducing the rate of reactivation following the operation (Low et al. 1994). There is a considerable biological advantage to this removal of all antigenic stimulation as well as the great advantage of excellent mechanical function.

Prosthetic design

The current designs allow only the joint to be resurfaced with a minimum of bone resected. The great advantage this has over the hinge replacements, such as the Stanmore, is that of bone stock preservation. By resecting as little bone as possible, the prosthesis loads the juxta-articular cancellous bone, preventing stress shilding and bone loss. Ligaments may be spared if present. In rheumatoid arthritis where they are often absent, their absence may be accommodated by constraining the knee with a moulded polyethylene insert (Fig. 5). This will give the stability needed for a normal gait without the problems of loosening, fracture, and massive loss of bone stock encountered by the hinge knees of the 1970s and 1980s.

The present condylar-type knee replacements have had significant problems with excessive wear of the tibial and patellar insert followed by secondary loosening. Many prostheses have been withdrawn from use following relatively unsuccessful trials (Kim and Oh 1995) and their failure rates vary considerably (Knutson et al. 1994).

Cemented or uncemented

There is little to choose between cemented and uncemented in total knee replacement at present although loosening seems slightly less in the tibial component if cemented (Knutson et al. 1994).

Outcome studies

Total knee replacement has evolved over the last three decades into a procedure that rivals total hip replacement for reliability and safety. In the Swedish knee arthroplasty register, which holds the records of over 30 000 knee replacements since 1976, the revision rate at 5 years has fallen from 10 to 3 per cent (Knutson et al. 1994). Despite the softened bone and often deformed joints, the success rate in rheumatoid arthritis is just as gratifying as in osteoarthritis, with no significant difference in outcome (Briggs and Augenstein 1995; Hsu et al. 1995).

Complications

Aseptic loosening This remains the principal problem in the long-term. Poor surgical technique resulting in malalignment of the prosthesis is a significant cause of early loosening (Harvey et al. 1995).

(a)

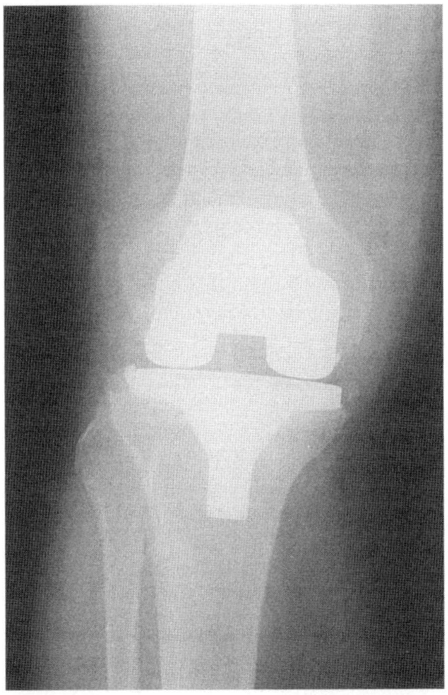

(b)

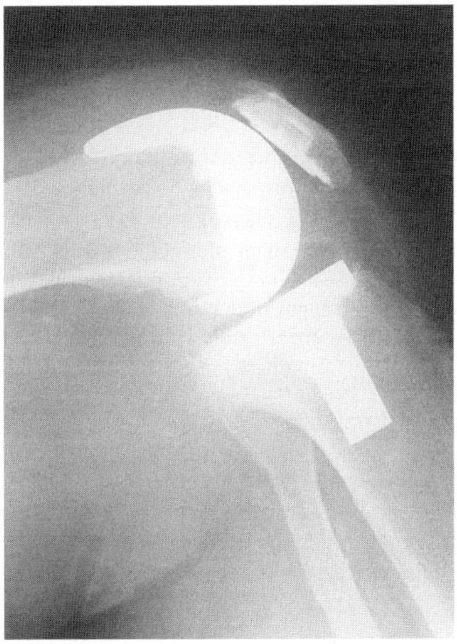

Fig. 5 Anterioposterior (a) and lateral (b) radiographs showing a cemented total condylar knee replacement. The patella has been resurfaced.

Other knees loosen after excessive wear of the tibial insert. This leads to eccentric movement and abnormal loading. Early designs of replacement prevented normal joint motion and the constraints themselves caused the abnormal loads and early failure (Rickhuss et al. 1994). All knee replacements now allow some rotation as well as unlimited flexion, and this freedom from constraints has been a major factor in preventing early failure. The results of revision knee replacements were very disappointing when the initial prosthesis was a hinge-type joint. The huge loss of bone stock led to rapid loosening once again, and many patients in the end faced excision arthroplasty or amputation (Ahlberg and Lunden 1981). Today, the more conservative joint resurfacing procedures have a lower revision rate and last longer so while the annual revision rate is still rising, the percentage of operations that are revisions has actually fallen over the last decade. The osteoporotic bone of rheumatoids, thought to be a poor prognostic factor, is not shown to be one, with loosening being shown to be completely independent of osteoporosis (Sugita et al. 1999).

Arthrodesis

Joint replacement has a good track record now and the operation of knee fusion is only indicated as a salvage procedure in osteoarthritis affecting few joints. If properly performed, the mechanical function of the individual can be excellent (Behr et al. 1985; Figgie et al. 1987). If many joints are affected, the impact of knee fusion is so mechanically serious that this should not be considered.

Excision arthroplasty

Failed revision arthroplasty may occasionally result in a flail leg without a functioning joint but with so little bone stock that an arthrodesis would be difficult or impossible. This is a procedure for a very low level of activity and only really appropriate if many other joints are involved and repeated infection or poor soft tissue cover cause revision surgery to fail (Adam et al. 1994).

Hip

When the hip has been damaged by an inflammatory arthropathy, the principal surgical intervention is joint replacement. Arthroscopy and arthroscopically assisted synovectomy are technically difficult and of limited benefit. Corrective osteotomies around the hip are rarely appropriate, as the primary pathology is not mechanical. The possible beneficial effects of osteotomy in IA, which are poorly understood and inconsistent, been superseded by the more reliable effects of joint replacement.

Synovectomy

Synovitis in the hip although present in upto 40 per cent of patients as shown on ultrasound, does not correlate well with clinical findings. Many of the joint with florid synovitis on ultrasound will have few hip symptoms while other symptomatic hips have little synovial thickening (Eberhardt et al. 1995). The hip itself is not simply accessible for open surgery and carries with it a high risk of avascular necrosis of the femoral head. Open synovectomy requiring hip dislocation has been reported in younger patients with some success (Albright et al. 1975) but is not common practice. Arthroscopically assisted synovectomy has also been reported (Gondolph-Zink et al. 1988) but this is a difficult procedure with limited application.

Joint replacement

Total hip replacement has specific problems related to each of the IAs, and their biological manifestations. Ankylosing spondylitis causes progressive ankylosis that may continue after the operation, while rheumatoid arthritis sufferers will usually have very poor bone stock and may have eroded the acetabulum. While these specific problems may make the technical aspects of the replacement demanding, the procedure is as successful for patients with rheumatoid arthritis as those with osteoarthritis. Despite being a major operation, involving pain and 10 days in hospital, joint replacement remains the most important intervention in a rheumatoid patient's disease process and, by their perception, well ahead of methotrexate and early aggressive management (Fries 1988).

Prosthetic design

Numerous designs of prosthesis exist, with little to recommend one over another. None has performed as well as John Charnley's original design (Wroblewski 1986) but several others have a proven record such as the Exeter (Fowler et al. 1988).

Cemented or uncemented?

Aseptic loosening remains the major cause of failure in total hip replacement. Improvements in cementing technique have reduced the rate at which early signs of loosening now appear, but the erosion of bone by the loosening process remains a concern. Various surface treatments have been used to attempt to stabilize the prosthesis–bone interface without the use of poly(methylmethacrylate). Extensive use of porous surfaces coating the prostheses have failed to demonstrate any advantage over cement in terms of overall survival and symptom control. There may, however, be some improvement in bone stock, with less loss of bone mass owing to stress shielding. Hydroxyapatite coating has been available since 1988 years and seems very promising (Fig. 6). There may be a significant improvement in bone mass in the uncemented hydroxyapatite coated group, making the revision a more successful operation, but this is not yet proven. The uses of a cemented stem and an uncemented cup, a 'hybrid' hip replacement, is another acceptable compromise.

Biomaterials

Polyethylene wear particles from the artificial joint have been implicated in the loosening process. Small particles excite an inflammatory reaction causing erosion of bone, visible on radiographs as radiolucent lines. Improvements in the density of the polyethylene and the smoothness of the cobalt–chrome alloy femoral head have reduced this. Ceramic bearings have theoretically superior wear characteristics and should further reduce the volume of particulate debris. Long-term clinical results are not available.

Outcome

Rheumatoid arthritis sufferers consider joint replacement to be the most successful and significant intervention in their disease, being rated above any of the pharmacological therapies. Total hip replacements is certainly reliable and durable; 96 per cent of Charnley cemented total hip replacements were reported as being good to excellent at 15–21 years (Wroblewski 1986) in Charnley's own unit, while at the Mayo clinic 79 per cent were good or excellent at 15 years (Kavanagh et al. 1989). The Exeter hip has also a good record with 5.5 per cent needing revision at 13.5 years (Fowler et al. 1988).

In rheumatoid arthritis, the reduction in bone density seems to be offset by the low level of exercise and most authors find the outlook worse for those patients with rheumatoid arthritis. One single-arm study showed a 91 per cent chance of the hip still functioning well at 11 years in rheumatoid arthritis (Severt et al. 1991). In another series of over 1000 rheumatoids, all receiving Charnley cemented hip replacements in Finland, 90 per cent were unrevised at 15 years (Lehtimaki et al. 1999).

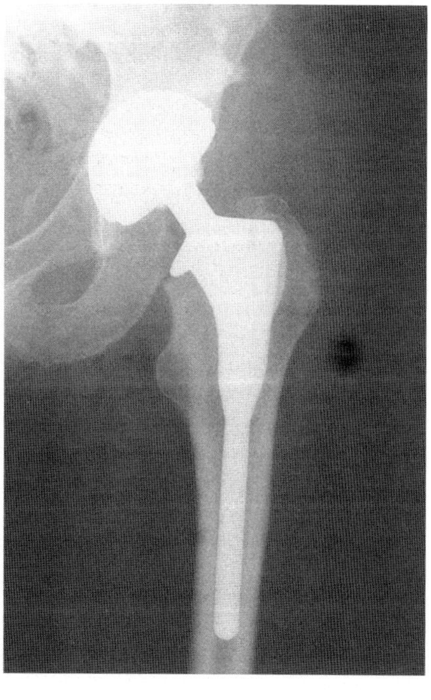

Fig. 6 A hip 1 year after hydroxyapatite-coated, uncemented total hip replacement. Radiolucent lines are not visible indicating solid fixation.

Complications of total hip replacement

Infection The systemic administration of prophylactic antibiotics, together with ultraclean air theatres have made the infection rate in primary hip replacement very low with figures of less than 1 per cent. However, in rheumatoid arthritis the rate is higher, at around 3 per cent (Severt et al. 1991), owing to immunocompromise and poor skin healing. The infected total hip replacement can often be salvaged by extensive debridement, and one or two stage revision followed by long-term antibiotics. In the long-term however, repeated infection will lead to an excision arthroplasty.

Aseptic loosening Hips may loosen for a number of reasons:

1. excessive wear leading to eccentric motion of the head and thus high peakloads;
2. stress shielding of the bone leading to resorption of the proximal bone and loss of bone stiffness;
3. faulty technique;
4. aggressive granulomatous reaction.

If the interface between the implant and bone is not solid, progressive motion will cause slow resorption of bone and an increasing zone of soft tissue between the implant and the bone. The painful total hip replacement should be revised early rather than left for as long as possible, as the enlarging radiolucent line around a prosthesis on radiographs represents resorption of bone and thus progressive weakening of the remaining bone stock. The results of revision surgery are fair: most people are helped considerably but the life expectancy of the revised hip is less than for the primary total hip replacement. A 10 per cent failure rate at 5 years would be average (Lord et al. 1988).

For this reason, cementless revisions with porous ingrowth or hydroxyapatite coating is being tried in many centres with results that are comparable with cemented implants (Jana et al. 2001; Keisu et al. 2001). Bone graft may be needed, either in the shape of cancellous chips from the pelvis or allograft from femoral heads harvested during primary total hip replacements. These are used to augment the failing bone stock of either proximal femur or acetabulum, in conjunction with metal reinforcement cages to prevent the acetabulum from migrating into the pelvis. If there is pelvic discontinuity, then even structural allograft may not be sufficient to prevent failure (Berry et al. 1999). Inevitably, if the process of joint replacement is started young, and the patient has an oligoarthropathy, with a relatively active lifestyle, then repeated revisions will culminate in excision arthroplasty. Without a hip joint, an otherwise fit person will walk with two sticks, but a typical polyarthritic rheumatoid arthritis sufferer will become comfortable but wheelchair bound.

Arthrodesis

Arthrodesis of the hip is the operation of choice in active young people with a single very painful and stiff joint. It will give good service for 20 years and may be revised safely. It does not have a role in polyarticular disease, where the change in biomechanics increases the stress to the knee joint unacceptably.

Excision arthroplasty

Excision arthroplasty of the hip is not necessary in uncomplicated rheumatoid arthritis. While it will give considerable relief of pain and will not deteriorate, it is only indicated where infection or very poor bone stock make further reconstructive attempts unwise. While the range of motion is excellent, the power is minimal. Walking without sticks is possible for otherwise fit people, and this is an acceptable solution following failed arthroplasty in those circumstances (Renvall and Einola 1990). For someone with rheumatoid arthritis however, this is not acceptable, and the excision of the hip joint, while pain relieving, is considered a failure by most surgeons as the function of the limb is effectively completely lost, rendering the patient wheelchair bound.

References

Adam, R.F., Watson, S.B., Jarratt, J.W., Noble, J., and Watson, J.S. (1994). Outcome after flap cover for exposed total knee arthroplasties. A report of 25 cases. *Journal of Bone and Joint Surgery* **76**, 750–3.

Ahlberg, A. and Lunden, A. (1981). Secondary operations after knee joint replacement. *Clinical Orthopaedics and Related Research*, 1704.

Albright, J.A., Albright, J.P., and Ogden, J.A. (1975). Synovectomy of the hip in juvenile rheumatoid arthritis. *Clinical Orthopaedics and Related Research*, 48–55.

Behr, J.T., Chmell, S.J., and Schwartz, C.M. (1985). Knee arthrodesis for failed total knee arthroplasty. *Archives of Surgery* **120**, 350–4.

Benjamin, A. (1987). Double osteotomy of the shoulder. *Scandinavian Journal of Rheumatology* **3**, 65.

Benjamin, A., Hirschowitz, D., and Arden, G.P. (1979). The treatment of arthritis of the shoulder. *International Orthopaedics* **3**, 211–16.

Bennett, W.F. and Gerber, C. (1994). Operative treatment of the rheumatoid shoulder. *Current Opinion in Rheumatology* **6**, 177–82.

Berry, D.J. et al. (1999). Pelvic discontinuity in revision total hip arthroplasty. *Journal of Bone and Joint Surgery* **81A**, 1692–702.

Briggs, J.R. and Augenstein, J.S. (1995). Tricon hybrid total knee arthroplasty: a review of 81 knees followed for 2 to 4 years. *Orthopedics* **18**, 341–6.

Chamay, A., Delia Santa, D., and Vilaseca, A. (1983). Radiolunate arthrodesis; a factor of stability for the rheumatoid wrist. *Annales de Chirugie de la Main* **2**, 5–17.

Christensson, D., Saveland, H., and Rydholm, U. (2000). Cervical spine surgery in rheumatoid arthritis. A Swedish nation-wide registration of 83 patients. *Scandinavian Journal of Rheumatology* **29**, 314–19.

Christodoulou L., Patwardhan, M.S., and Burke, F.D. (1999). Open and closed arthrodesis of the rheumatoid wrist using a modified (Stanley) Steinmann pin. *Journal of Hand Surgery* **24**, 662–6.

Clawson, M.C. and Stern, P.J. (1991). The distal radioulnar joint complex in rheumatoid arthritis: an interview. *Hand Clinics* **7**, 373–81.

Coates, C.J., Bolton-Maggs, B.G., and Helal, B.H. (1991). Interpositional arthroplasty in the management of rheumatoid arthritis of the elbow. In *Rheumatoid Arthritis Surgery of the Elbow* (ed. M. Hämälainen and F.W. Hagena), pp. 52–9. Basel: Karger.

Copeland, S.A. and Taylor, J.G. (1979). Synovectomy of the elbow in rheumatoid arthritis. The place of excision of the head of the radius. *Journal of Bone and Joint Surgery* **61B**, 69–73.

Cracchiolo, A., III (1984). Foot abnormalities in rheumatoid arthritis. *Instructional Course Lectures* **33**, 386–404.

Dent, C.M., Patil, M., and Fairclough, J.A. (1993). Arthroscopic ankle arthrodesis. *Journal of Bone and Joint Surgery* **75**, 830–2.

Eberhardt, K., Fex, E., Johnsson, K., and Geborek, P. (1995). Hip involvement in early rheumatoid arthritis. *Annals of the Rheumatic Diseases* **54**, 45–8.

Ennevaara, K. (1967). Painful shoulder joint in rheumatoid. *Acta Rheumatologica Scandinavica* **11**, 1–116.

Figgie, H.E.D., Brody, G.A., Inglis, A.E., Sculco, T.P., Goldberg, V.M., and Figgie, M.P. (1987). Knee arthrodesis following total knee arthroplasty in rheumatoid arthritis. *Clinical Orthopaedics and Related Research*, 237–43.

Fowler, A.W. (1959). A method of forefoot reconstruction. *Journal of Bone and Joint Surgery* **41B**, 507–13.

Fowler, J.L. et al. (1988). Experience with the Exeter total hip replacement since 1970. *Orthopedic Clinics of North America* **19**, 477–89.

Friedman, R.J., Thornhill, T.S., Thomas, W.H., and Sledge, C.B. (1989). Non-constrained total shoulder replacement in patients who have rheumatoid arthritis and class 4 function. *Journal of Bone and Joint Surgery* **71A**, 494–8.

Fries, J.F. (1988). Milestones in rhematologic care (1965–1985). In *Milestones in Management: Rheumatoid Arthritis* (ed. J.F. Fries). Puerto Rico: Syntex.

Gainor, B.J. et al. (1988). Metatarsal head resection for rheumatoid deformities of the forefoot. *Clinical Orthopaedics and Related Research* **230**, 207–13.

Geschwend, N. (1991). The case for a linked elbow prosthesis. In *Rheumatoid Arthritis Surgery of the Elbow* Vol. 15 (ed. M. Hämälainen and F.W. Hagena), pp. 98–112. Basel: Karger.

Geschwend, N., Scheier, N.H., and Baehler, A.R. (1999). Long-term results of the GSB III elbow arthroplasty. *Journal of Bone and Joint Surgery* **81B**, 1005–12.

Gill, D.R., Cofield, R.H., and Morrey, B.F. (1999). Ipsilateral total shoulder and elbow arthroplasties in patients who have rheumatoid arthritis. *Journal of Bone and Joint Surgery* **81A**, 1128–37.

Gondolph-Zink, B., Puhl, W., and Noack, W. (1988). Semiarthroscopic synovectomy of the hip. *International Orthopedics* **12**, 31–5.

Grossman, J.F. and Valance, R. (1980). Clinical and radiological features of the shoulder joint in rheumatoid arthritis. *Journal of Bone and Joint Surgery* **62B**, 116.

Harvey, I.A., Manning, M.P., Sampath, S.A., Johnson, R., and Elloy, M.A. (1995). Alignment of total knee arthroplasty: the relationship to radiolucency around the tibial component. *Medical Engineering and Physics* **17**, 182–7.

Hasselo, L.G. et al. (1987). Forefoot surgery in rheumatoid arthritis: subjective assessment of outcome. *Foot and Ankle* **8**, 148–51.

Hecker, R.L., Furness, I.C., and Gostich, C.M. (1982). Ankle synovectomy: an approach to the rheumatoid ankle. *Journal of Foot Surgery* **21**, 4–6.

Heywood, A.W., Learmonth, I.D., and Thomas, M. (1988). Cervical spine instability in rheumatoid arthritis. *Journal of Bone and Joint Surgery* **70A**, 702–7.

Holt, E.S., Hansen, S.T., Mayo, K.A., and Sangeorzan, B.J. (1991). Ankle arthrodesis using internal screw fixation. *Clinical Orthopaedics and Related Research*, 21–8.

Houshian, S. and Schroder, H.A. (2001). Wrist arthrodesis with the AO titanium wrist fusion plate: a consecutive series of 42 cases. *Journal of Hand Surgery* **26**, 355–9.

Hsu, R.W., Fan, G.F., and Ho, W.P. (1995). A follow-up study of porous-coated anatomic knee arthroplasty. *Journal of Arthroplasty* **10**, 29–36.

Ishikawa, H., Ohno, O., and Hirohata, K. (1986). Long-term results of synovectomy in rheumatoid patients. *Journal of Bone and Joint Surgery* **68A**, 198–205.

Iwata, H., Yasuhara, N., Kawashima, K., Kaneko, M., Sugiura, Y., and Nakagawa, M. (1980). Arthrodesis of the ankle joint with rheumatoid arthritis: experience with the transfibular approach. *Clinical Orthopaedics and Related Research*, 189–93.

Jaffe, R. and Learmonth, I.D. (1989). Benjamin double osteotomy for arthritis of the glenohumeral joint. *Rheumatology* **12**, 52.

Jana, A.K. et al. (2001). Total hip arthroplasty using porous-coated femoral components in patients with rheumatoid arthritis. *Journal of Bone and Joint Surgery* **83B**, 686–90.

Jensen, N.C. and Kroner, K. (1992). Total ankle joint replacement: a clinical follow up. *Orthopedics* **15**, 236–9.

Johnston, R.A. and Kelly, I.G. (1990). Surgery of the rheumatoid cervical spine. *Annals of the Rheumatic Diseases* **49** (Suppl. 2), 845–50.

Jolly, S.L., Ferlic, D.C., Clayton, M.L., Dennis, D.A., and Stringer, E.A. (1992). Swanson silicone arthroplasty of the wrist in rheumatoid arthritis: a long-term follow-up. *Journal of Hand Surgery—American Volume* **17**, 142–9.

Kates, A., Kessel, L., and Kay, A. (1967). Arthroplasty of the forefoot. *Journal of Bone and Joint Surgery* **49B**, 552–7.

Kavanagh, B.F., Dewitz, M.A., Ilstrup, D.M., Stauffer, R.N., and Coventry, M.B. (1989). Charnley total hip arthroplasty with cement. Fifteen-year results. *Journal of Bone and Joint Surgery* **71A**, 1496–503.

Keisu, K.S. et al. (2001). Cementless femoral fixation in the rheumatoid patient undergoing total hip arthroplasty: minimum 5-year results. *Journal of Arthroplasty* **16**, 415–21.

Kessel, L. and Bayley, I. (1982). Prosthetic replacement of the shoulder joint. *Journal of the Royal Society of Medicine* **72**, 748–52.

Kim, Y.H. and Oh, J.H. (1995). Evaluation of the anatomic patellar prosthesis in uncemented porous-coated total knee arthroplasty: seven-year results. *American Journal of Orthopedics* **24**, 412–19.

Knutson, K., Lewold, S., Robertsson, O., and Lidgren, L. (1994). The Swedish knee arthroplasty register. A nation-wide study of 30 003 knees 1976–1992. *Acta Orthopaedica Scandinavica* **65**, 375–86.

Kvien, T.K., Pahle, J.A., Hoyeraal, H.M., and Sandstad, B. (1987). Comparison of synovectomy and no synovectomy in patients with juvenile rheumatoid arthritis. A 24-month controlled study. *Scandinavian Journal of Rheumatology* **16**, 81–91.

Laine, V.A.I., Vainio, K.J., and Pekanmaki, K. (1954). Shoulder affections in rheumatoid arthritis. *Annals of the Rheumatic Diseases* **13**, 157–60.

Lehtimaki, M.Y. et al (1999). Charnley low-friction arthroplasty in rheumatoid patients: a survival study up to 20 years. *Journal of Arthroplasty* **14**, 657–61.

Lettin, A.W.F., Copeland, S.A., and Scales, J.T. (1982). The Stanmore total shoulder replacement. *Journal of Bone and Joint Surgery* **64B**, 47–51.

Levy, O. and Copeland, S.A. (2001). Cementless surface replacement arthroplasty of the shoulder. 5- to 10-year results with the Copeland mark-2 prosthesis. *Journal of Bone and Joint Surgery* **83B**, 213–21.

Lord, G., Marotife, J.-H., Guillamon, J.-L., and Blanchard, J.-P. (1988). Cementless revisions of failed aseptic cemented and cementless total hip arthroplasties. *Clinical Orthopaedics and Related Research,* 67–74.

Low, C.K., Tan, S.K., Satku, K., and Kumar, V.P. (1994). Reactivation of rheumatoid arthritis in knees following total knee replacement. *Annals of Academic Medicine, Singapore* **23**, 887–90.

Maenpaa, H., Lehto, M.U., and Belt, E.A. (2001). What went wrong in triple arthrodesis? An analysis of failures in 21 patients. *Clinical Orthopaedics and Related Research,* 218–23.

Matsui, N., Taneda, Y., Ohta, H., Itch, T., and Tsuboguchi, S. (1989). Arthroscopic versus open synovectomy in the rheumatoid knee. *International Orthopaedics* **13**, 17–20.

McGuire, M.R., Kyle, R.F., Gustilo, R.B., and Premer, R.F. (1988). Comparative analysis of ankle arthroplasty versus ankle arthrodesis. *Clinical Orthopaedics and Related Research,* 174–81.

Moeckel, B.H., Patterson, B.M., Inglis, A.E., and Sculco, T.P. (1991). Ankle arthrodesis. A comparison of internal and external fixation. *Clinical Orthopaedics and Related Research,* 78–83.

Mohing, W., Kohler, G., and Coldewey, J. (1982). Synovectomy of the ankle joint. *International Orthopaedics* **6**, 117–21.

Moller, K. et al. (1999). Early results with osseointegrated proximal interphalangeal joint prostheses. *Journal of Hand Surgery* **24**, 267–74.

Moran, C.G., Pinder, I.M., and Smith, S.R. (1991). Ankle arthrodesis in rheumatoid arthritis. 30 cases followed for 5 years. *Acta Orthopaedica Scandinavica* **62**, 538–43.

Moskovich, R. et al. (2000). Occipitocervical stabilization for myelopathy in patients with rheumatoid arthritis. Implications of not bone-grafting. *Journal of Bone and Joint Surgery* **82B**, 349–65.

Neer, C.S., II, Watson, K.C., and Stanton, F.J. (1982). Recent experience in total shoulder replacement. *Journal of Bone and Joint Surgery* **64A**, 319–37.

Ogilvie-Harris, D.J. and Wiley, A.M. (1986). Arthroscopic surgery of the shoulder. *Journal of Bone and Joint Surgery* **68B**, 201–7.

Ogilvie-Harris, D.J. and Basinski, A. (1991). Arthroscopic synovectomy of the knee for rheumatoid arthritis. *Arthroscopy* **7**, 91–7.

Paus, A.C. and Dale, K. (1993). Arthroscopic and radiographic examination of patients with juvenile rheumatoid arthritis before and after open synovectomy of the knee joint. A prospective study with a 5-year follow-up. *Annales Chirurgiae et Gynaecologie Fenniae* **82**, 55–61.

Petersson, C.J. (1986). Painful shoulders in patients with rheumatoid arthritis. *Scandinavian Journal of Rheumatology* **15**, 275–9.

Porter, B.B., Richardson, C., and Vianio, K. (1974). Rheumatoid arthritis of the elbow: the results of synovectomy. *Journal of Bone and Joint Surgery* **56B**, 427–37.

Posner, M.A. and Ambrose, L. (1991). Excision of the distal ulnar in rheumatoid arthritis. *Hand Clinics* **7**, 383–90.

Pritchard, R.W. (1991). Total elbow joint arthroplasty in patients with rheumatoid arthritis. *Seminars in Arthritis and Rheumatism* **21**, 24–9.

Radmer, S., Andresen, R., and Sparmann, M. (1999). Wrist arthroplasty with a new generation of prostheses in patients with rheumatoid arthritis. *Journal of Hand Surgery* **24**, 935–43.

Ranawat, C.S. et al. (1979). Cervical spine fusion in rheumatoid arthritis. *Journal of Bone and Joint Surgery* **61A**, 1003.

Ransford, A.O. et al. (1986). Craniocervical instability treated by contoured loop fixation. *Journal of Bone and Joint Surgery* **68B**, 173–7.

Renvall, S. and Einola, S. (1990). Girdlestone operation. An acceptable alternative in the case of unreconstructable hip arthroplasty. *Annals Chirugiae Gynaecologiae* **79**, 165–7.

Rickhuss, P.K., Gray, A.J., and Rowley, D.I. (1994). A 5–10 year follow-up of the Sheehan total knee endoprosthesis in Tayside. *Journal of the Royal College of Surgeons, Edinburgh* **39**, 326–8.

Severt, R., Wood, R., Cracchiolo, A., and Amstutz, H.C. (1991). Long-term follow-up of cemented total hip arthroplasty in rheumatoid arthritis. *Clinics in Orthopedics* **265**, 129–36.

Seyfer, A.E. (1993). Indications for upper extremity surgery in rheumatoid arthritis patients. *Seminars in Arthritis and Rheumatism* **23**, 125–34.

Shah, B.M. et al. (2000). The effect of epidemiologic and intraoperative factors on survival of the standard Souter–Strathclyde total elbow arthroplasty. *Journal of Arthroplasty* **15**, 994–8.

Skues, M.A. and Welchew, E.A. (1993). Anaesthesia and rheumatoid arthritis. *Anaesthesia* **48**, 989–97.

Sojbjerg, J.O. et al. (1999). Late results of total shoulder replacement in patients with rheumatoid arthritis. *Clinical Orthopaedics and Related Research,* 39–45.

Souter, W.A. (1990). Surgery of the rheumatoid arthritis. *Annals of the Rheumatic Diseases* **49** (Suppl. 2), 871–82.

Stanley, J.K. (1992). Conservative surgery in the management of rheumatoid disease of the hand and wrist. *Journal of Hand Surgery—British Volume* **17**, 339–42.

Stauffer, R.N. (1977). Total ankle joint replacement. *Archives of Surgery* **112**, 1105–9.

Stone, K.H. and Helal, B. (1991). A method of ankle stabilization. *Clinical Orthopaedics and Related Research,* 102–6.

Sugita, T. et al. (1999). Influence of tibial bone quality on loosening of the tibial component in total knee arthroplasty for rheumatoid arthritis: long-term results. *Orthopedics* **22**, 213–15.

Tanaka, N. et al. (2001). Kudo total elbow arthroplasty in patients with rheumatoid arthritis: a long-term follow-up study. *Journal of Bone and Joint Surgery* **83A**, 1506–13.

Toledano, B., Terrono, A.L., and Millender, L.H. (1992). Reconstruction of the rheumatoid thumb. *Hand Clinics* **8**, 121–9.

Vahvanen, V.A. (1967). Rheumatoid arthritis in the pantalar joints. A follow-up study of triple arthrodesis on 292 adult feet. *Acta Orthopaedica Scandinavica* (Suppl. 107), 3.

Wagner, F.W., Jr. (1982). Ankle fusion for degenerative arthritis secondary to the collagen diseases. *Foot and Ankle* **3**, 24–31.

Wroblewski, B.M. (1986). Fifteen to twenty-one year results of the Charnley low friction arthroplasty. *Clinics in Orthopedics* **211**, 30–5.

Wynn Parry, C.B. and Stanley, J.K. (1993). Synovectomy of the hand. *British Journal of Rheumatology* **32**, 1089–95 (review).

Yanni, O.N. et al. (2000). The Roper–Tuke total elbow arthroplasty. 4- to 10-year results of an unconstrained prosthesis. *Journal of Bone and Joint Surgery* **82B**, 705–10.

7.2 Surgery in children

Johann Delf Witt and Malcolm Swann

Introduction

Surgery now has a firmly established place in the management of juvenile idiopathic arthritis and in the rheumatic diseases of childhood (Arden and Ansell 1978; Swann 1983; Rydholm 1990). This chapter is principally concerned with surgery of juvenile idiopathic arthritis and includes the scope and indications, problems, and outcome. Experience drawn from the Medical Research Council unit at the Canadian Red Cross Hospital at Taplow and at Wexham Park Hospital, Slough (England), forms the basis for the conclusion drawn here (Ansell and Swann 1983). There are some 5000 patients with juvenile idiopathic arthritis on the records and of these

10 per cent have had a surgical procedure and many of them multiple procedures. In this surgically treated group, half have seropositive arthritis.

Surgery should be seen as complementing the other forms of treatment. Thus, all the patients must have full exposure to conservative treatment including medication, physiotherapy, and splintage. At some stage it may become evident that these methods are failing and that further help must be sought. There are no markers to indicate when the disease will undergo remission or finally burn out. The problem is compounded by the unpredictable response to medication, which in itself may have side-effects; by physiotherapy, which can be painful if inappropriate; and by structural changes, which cannot be overcome by conservative means. For instance, splints need to be moulded, comfortable, and changed frequently if there is any alteration in a position. Thus, in our present state of knowledge, some problems cannot be surmounted by conservative means alone and surgical intervention will be required. Surgical help may be required in such cases in order to recover lost ground. There can be no doubt that the management of juvenile idiopathic arthritis is best supervised in special centres (Woo et al. 1990).

The hip

Causes of deformity

Involvement of the hip occurs in 30–63.5 per cent of patients with juvenile idiopathic arthritis according to various reports in the literature (Jacqueline et al. 1961; Isdale 1970), and this is the most common cause of limited mobility (Ansell 1978). Inflammatory synovitis leads to pain and muscle spasm with the inevitable development of joint contractures if this cycle is not broken. The tendency to contracture is greater in seronegative patients, often with minimal effusion, whereas seropositive patients tend to experience a proliferative synovitis more like their adult counterparts.

An effusion in the joint will cause pain, and the tendency will be for the joint to be held in the position in which the capsule has the maximum capacity thereby reducing the pressure within the joint. In the hip this position is in neutral rotation with about 45° of flexion (Rydholm et al. 1986a–c). In time, with the persistence of an inflammatory synovitis and pannus formation, the articular cartilage degenerates. This is exacerbated by the stiff, contracted nature of the joint that impairs the normal mechanisms of cartilage nutrition (Ekholm and Norback 1951; Salter and Field 1960). In addition, peri-articular inflammation induces regional osteopaenia, which is compounded by the muscle weakness and relative immobility of these patients.

A combination of regional hyperaemia and abnormal mechanical forces on the hip induces growth abnormalities and a failure of the normal remodelling process of the proximal femur. The exact pattern of the deformity is related to the age of onset and the duration of the disease (Rombouts and Rombouts-Lindemans 1971). Children below the age of 9 tend to develop coxa magna where the femoral head is enlarged, and there is an elongated valgus femoral neck with marked anteversion, and an acetabulum that appears dysplastic. In children over the age of 9, coxa magna often occurs, but frequently with premature fusion of the growth plate of the femoral head producing a short and varus femoral neck. Continued growth of the trochanteric epiphysis contributes to the varus deformity. A protrusio pattern of deformity is another feature that may develop in the older child.

In time, narrowing and irregularity of the joint space occurs, with bone erosions, destruction, and sometimes subluxation of the femoral head. In a proportion of cases there is evidence of avascular necrosis of the head. This was seen in 10 of 72 hips in 36 children with hip disease, and a further 20 showed suspected late sequelae of the ischaemic process (Kabayakawa et al. 1989). This is thought to occur secondary to a tamponade of the joint resulting from the synovitis and effusion as the nutrient vessels to the capital epiphysis are largely intra-capsular.

The typical deformity of the affected hip that ultimately develops is one of fixed flexion, adduction, and internal rotation (McCullough 1994). Both hips are not necessarily involved to the same extent, but a fixed flexion deformity in one hip will tend to induce the same in the other. As a consequence of the hip deformity, the patients develop an excessive lumbar lordosis and also a tendency towards fixed flexion deformities of the knees. The fixed adduction at the hip leads to the development of a genu valgum deformity, and this combined with internal rotation may lead to external tibial torsion.

Surgical management

Intra-articular steroid

In the early stages of hip involvement, patients may present with acute irritability of the hip but without changes on X-ray. Examination will reveal a flexion deformity and adductor spasm. Some cases may respond to appropriate analgesics and anti-inflammatory medication combined with a physical therapy programme including traction, aimed at preventing fixed deformities.

In those that do not respond, it is worthwhile performing a gentle examination under anaesthetic. In these circumstances it is possible to determine if a fixed deformity has developed, but often the deformity disappears and there is no limitation of movement. A steroid injection can then be performed. In our practice, confirmation of localization of the hip joint is made by performing an arthrogram at the time. Post-operatively traction should be continued while the irritability persists, interspersed with physiotherapy. Prone lying is encouraged for part of each day to help overcome the fixed flexion deformity. In the meantime the other involved joints should continue to be treated.

Synovectomy and soft tissue release

The role of synovectomy of the hip by itself is not clear as usually it is combined with some sort of soft tissue release procedure. There is evidence that it is effective in reducing pain but possibly at the expense of some range of motion (Mogensen et al. 1982). A soft tissue release procedure is used in established flexion contracture with limitation of range of motion and where a joint space can still be demonstrated.

The majority of cases can be managed with a release of the tight adductors and the psoas through a small incision in the groin. Swann and Ansell (1986) reported an improvement in the flexion contracture from an average of 26° before surgery to 9° at 1 year and this was maintained in 46 of 89 hips at 3 years. In addition, this was associated with marked pain relief that is probably due to decompression of the joint (Soto-Hall et al. 1964). However, the longer-term improvement is likely to reflect changes in disease activity. For patients with more severe fixed flexion deformities a more extensive release procedure has been described (Witt and McCullough 1994) where the muscles are stripped from their attachments to the ilium and which is also combined with a partial synovectomy. Using this procedure the average pre-operative flexion contracture in 31 hips was reduced from 35 to 9.5° at 1 year and at 3 years it was 18°. In some cases it was noted that there was an improvement in the appearance of the hip on X-ray with a reduction in the degree of porosis, a clearer definition of the joint line, and a widening of the joint space.

The post-operative management is extremely important in order to maintain the improved range of motion. Traction with the hips in abduction is commenced together with a range of motion exercises immediately post-operatively, and hydrotherapy once the wounds have healed. As the hips become more comfortable the patients are mobilized with traction continued at night.

Osteotomy

Theoretically, osteotomy would be indicated in cases where there is marked femoral neck valgus associated with a dysplastic acetabulum and subluxation of the hip. However, owing to the porotic bone and restricted range of motion usually present it is rarely appropriate. It may occasionally be used in a patient whose disease is no longer active and who still has a good range of motion with a preserved joint space.

Total hip replacement

Pain in patients with severely destroyed joints is the main indication for total hip replacement. Less commonly the indication may be for ankylosis in a poor position leading to functional impairment and secondary deformity of other joints. The results in a number of series have demonstrated a marked reduction in pain and a major improvement in functional ability. However, of concern is the rate of loosening and the subsequent problems associated with revision hip surgery. Witt et al. (1991) in a study on 92 hip replacements in patients with juvenile chronic arthritis found that 25 per cent of hips had been revised after an average follow-up of 11.5 years. Chmell et al. (1997) reviewed 66 hips and found that 15 per cent of femoral components and 35 per cent of acetabular components required revision for aseptic loosening after an average follow-up of 12 years.

There are significant technical problems associated with total hip replacement in this group of patients. The bones may be extremely porotic, and with considerable proximal femoral deformity, insertion of standard components may not be possible. The disappointing medium-term results in terms of loosening rates in cemented hip replacements has led to the use of uncemented implants. These may need to be custom made for the individual specialized modular implants are also available. The implants have a porous coating applied to them to allow bone ingrowth to occur, or may have an hydroxyapatite coating that is able to bond directly to bone. Although there is limited follow-up on this type of implant, the early clinical and radiographic results are encouraging (Fig. 1).

Of equal or greater importance than the mode of fixation of the implant to the bone is the bearing surface used. Traditional surfaces have been a cobaltchrome femoral head articulating with an ultra-high molecular weight polyethylene acetabular component. Advances in ceramic and metal-on-metal articulations raises the possibility of reduced wear debris around the hip in the longer term, which we now know is the major cause of component loosening.

Some of the more recent advances in hip replacement implants are not applicable in patients with juvenile arthritis. In particular, surface replacement options where the femoral head is not resected but is resurfaced with a thin metal shell and allows conservation of bone stock is not possible because the femoral head is too deformed and the bone too osteoporotic to support the implant.

The knee

The knee is commonly involved in all subgroups of juvenile idiopathic arthritis. Inflammation results in the joint being held in a position of flexion and hamstring spasm will prevent straightening. In time-resistant flexion contractures may develop as the periarticular structures undergo fibrosis and extra-articular adhesions as well as intra-articular adhesions progressively limit joint movement. It is important to identify factors that may exacerbate the deformity such as ipsilateral hip involvement and contralateral knee involvement. Because the knee's two epiphyseal growth plates account for 70 per cent of lower extremity growth, it is not surprising that involvement leads to growth abnormalities. Simon et al. (1981) published a detailed study of leg-length discrepancies and reported 100 cases of monoarticular disease in juvenile chronic arthritis. It was noted that if the disease began before the age of 9 years, the involved side was always the longer one and the final discrepancy was rarely more than 3 cm. None of the patients with disease beginning before the age of 9 years had premature epiphyseal closure. If the disease had its onset after that, rapid premature growth-plate closure was evident and leg-length differences of up to 5.9 cm were observed. The medial side of the growth-plate seems to have the propensity to be stimulated to a greater extent and this is one of the causes of a valgus deformity.

Surgical treatment

Steroid injection and synovectomy

Physiotherapy and rest splints are indicated in the early stages of the disease. If the flexed position is resistant to treatment with a vigorous conservative programme including reversed dynamic traction, then an examination under anaesthetic and intra-articular steroid injection is valuable. If a fixed flexion deformity persists, then a programme of serial plastering is started to gradually correct this.

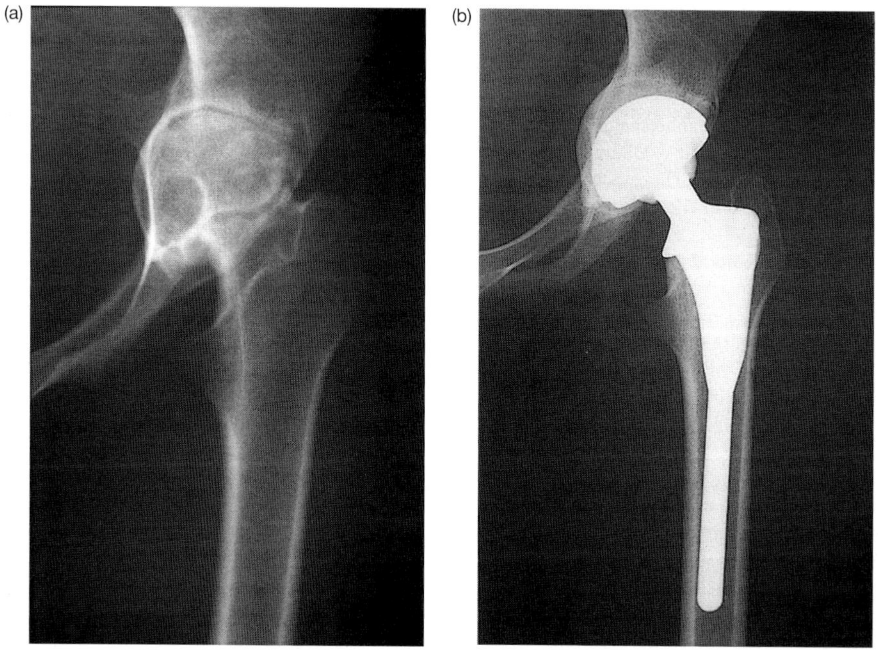

Fig. 1 (a) Sixteen-year-old girl with juvenile idiopathic arthritis showing a severe protrusio deformity. (b) Treatment with an hydroxyapatite coated cementless hip replacement.

The role of synovectomy in the management of symptoms, the most appropriate timing for the procedure, and the influence on disease progression have not been determined. Because of the thick articular cartilage in children, subchondral cysts and erosions are late to appear on radiographs and cartilage destruction seen at operation often far exceeds that seen on radiographs. In general, better results are likely in patients with oligo-articular or monoarticular disease (Kampner and Ferguson 1972; Rydholm et al. 1986a–c).

Soft tissue release

In instances where a fixed flexion deformity persists and has been resistant to serial casts, it may be necessary to release the contracted tissues surgically. To perform a release, posteromedial and posterolateral incisions are needed. The hamstring tendons are lengthened and the posterior capsule of the knee joint is exposed by blunt dissection. Taking care to protect the neurovascular bundle, the posterior capsule is incised transversely so that the joint is entered. Post-operatively patients are maintained in a cast for 2–3 days. This is then bivalved and motion exercises are commenced.

In one series of 31 knees (19 patients), a mean fixed flexion deformity of 38° was reduced to 12° at the 6-month follow-up. This correction was maintained until the 3-year follow-up and then tended to deteriorate (Moreno Alvarez et al. 1992). Rydholm et al. (1986a–c) reported on 29 releases in 23 children, with 21 knees having a flexion contracture greater than 15°. At a mean follow-up of 3.9 years only eight knees had a flexion deformity exceeding 15°.

Osteotomy

In those cases in which the deformity is fixed and associated with more advanced joint destruction it may be appropriate to perform a supracondylar extension osteotomy and any valgus deformity can be corrected at the same time. This creates a second deformity that masks the first. Because of the porosity of the bone, stable internal fixation is not usually possible; therefore, these patients require a cast post-operatively. This is removed as early as possible to try and avoid too much stiffness, usually at about 4 weeks, and motion exercises are commenced.

Forty knee osteotomies in 24 patients, aged 16 or less, resulted in the satisfactory correction of the deformity and bone union in all cases (Swann 1987). Relapse of the deformity occurred in five patients and osteotomies had to be repeated in three. Four knees lost movement following surgery.

Although there clearly is a place for osteotomy, this should be reserved for the younger child and in the older child should perhaps only be performed when a reasonable joint surface remains and where the disease is less active. The reason for this is that performing an osteotomy makes the subsequent operation of a knee replacement much more difficult because of the distorted anatomy. The results of current design total knee replacements are extremely good, and, therefore, if it can be predicted that a patient will end up requiring a knee replacement, an osteotomy should probably be avoided if at all possible.

Epiphyseodesis

Epiphyseodesis has been used to correct valgus deformity and leg length discrepancy (Rydholm et al. 1987). Its use is probably best confined to monoarticular disease in juvenile chronic arthritis. Simon et al. (1981) reported on the results in 15 patients out of 35 followed to skeletal maturity and showed satisfactory results.

Total knee replacement

The indication for total knee replacement is primarily pain but this is often associated with significant deformity resulting in major functional incapacity. Skeletal immaturity is not necessarily a contraindication to surgery. Considerable pre-operative planning is required because of the small sizes of the knees in many cases and because of the distorted local anatomy. A further concern is the degree of osteoporosis that is present and great care has to be taken when operating, to release the fibrous intra- and extra-articular adhesions in order to expose the joint without fracturing the bone.

The results of current designs of condylar resurfacing total knee replacements in adults with rheumatoid arthritis are extremely good with a predicted survival rate of 91 per cent at 15 years (Rodriguez et al. 1996). Early results of total knee arthroplasty in juvenile idiopathic arthritis are also very encouraging (Fig. 2). Sarokhan et al. (1983) reported results in 29 knees in 17 patients with an average age of 23 years and a follow-up of 2–11 years (average 5 years). Pain relief was present in all cases, there was one late deep infection but no patients required revision for aseptic loosening. Carmichael and Chaplin (1986) reported on 21 total knee replacements in 11 patients with an average age of 20.1 years. At a mean follow-up of 61 months no revisions were required, and no infections or loosenings occurred. Others have reported similar results (Stuart and Rand 1988) and also using uncemented implants in very selected cases (Boublik et al. 1993).

The foot and ankle

Virtually any conceivable combination of deformities can occur in juvenile chronic arthritis (Rana 1982). Pronation of the foot with the valgus of the heel is a frequent finding. Clawing of the toes is common with or without a cavus deformity of the forefoot. A varus hindfoot, hallux valgus, and hammertoe deformities also occur. Tarsal joint involvement is common with a tendency to early ankylosis. The key to the management of these problems is to try to prevent fixed deformities from developing and to preserve as much range of motion as possible. Most important is to try and preserve neutral alignment of the foot and ankle. In children with more proximal joints involved and who may be partly wheelchair bound there is a tendency for the ankle and foot to drift into equinus due to gravity.

Non-operative treatment

The arthritic foot should be well supported most of the time. Careful attention to footwear with prescription of appropriate heels, sole wedges, lasts, arch supports, and metatarsal weight relieving inserts are important. Deformity of the foot and ankle should be corrected by serial plastering and maintained subsequently with the use of orthotic devices at night. Intra-articular injections of steroids may also help control active synovitis.

Operative treatment

Soft tissue release

Resistant equinus of the ankle may be corrected by tendo achilles lengthening and capsulotomies of the ankle and subtalar joints. Varus deformity of the hindfoot can be corrected by performing a posteromedial release similar to the procedures developed for clubfoot. Similarly, a variety of release procedures may allow correction of a cavus foot or claw toes.

Osteotomies

Occasionally, a calcaneal osteotomy may allow correction of fixed hindfoot varus while retaining movement in the adjacent joints. Midtarsal osteotomies usually combined with a dorsal wedge resection allow correction of equinus at the midtarsal joints where these have ankylosed (Fig. 3). First metatarsal osteotomies for hallux valgus are sometimes appropriate, although if there are severe lesser toe deformities with dorsal and lateral subluxation then arthrodesis is often a better alternative.

Arthrodesis

Once children reach the age of 12–14, fixed deformities of the hindfoot may be best corrected by performing a triple arthrodesis, although if the subtalar joint alone is involved then a subtalar fusion may be sufficient. Occasionally, an isolated talo-navicular joint fusion may be appropriate where this joint is painful, and conversion to a triple arthrodesis is possible should this be required. If the ankle joint is painful and clinically and radiographically deformed then an ankle fusion is the recommended procedure. Ankle arthroplasty is an alternative in selected patients. The results of ankle arthroplasty in the long-term remain to be determined. Results from

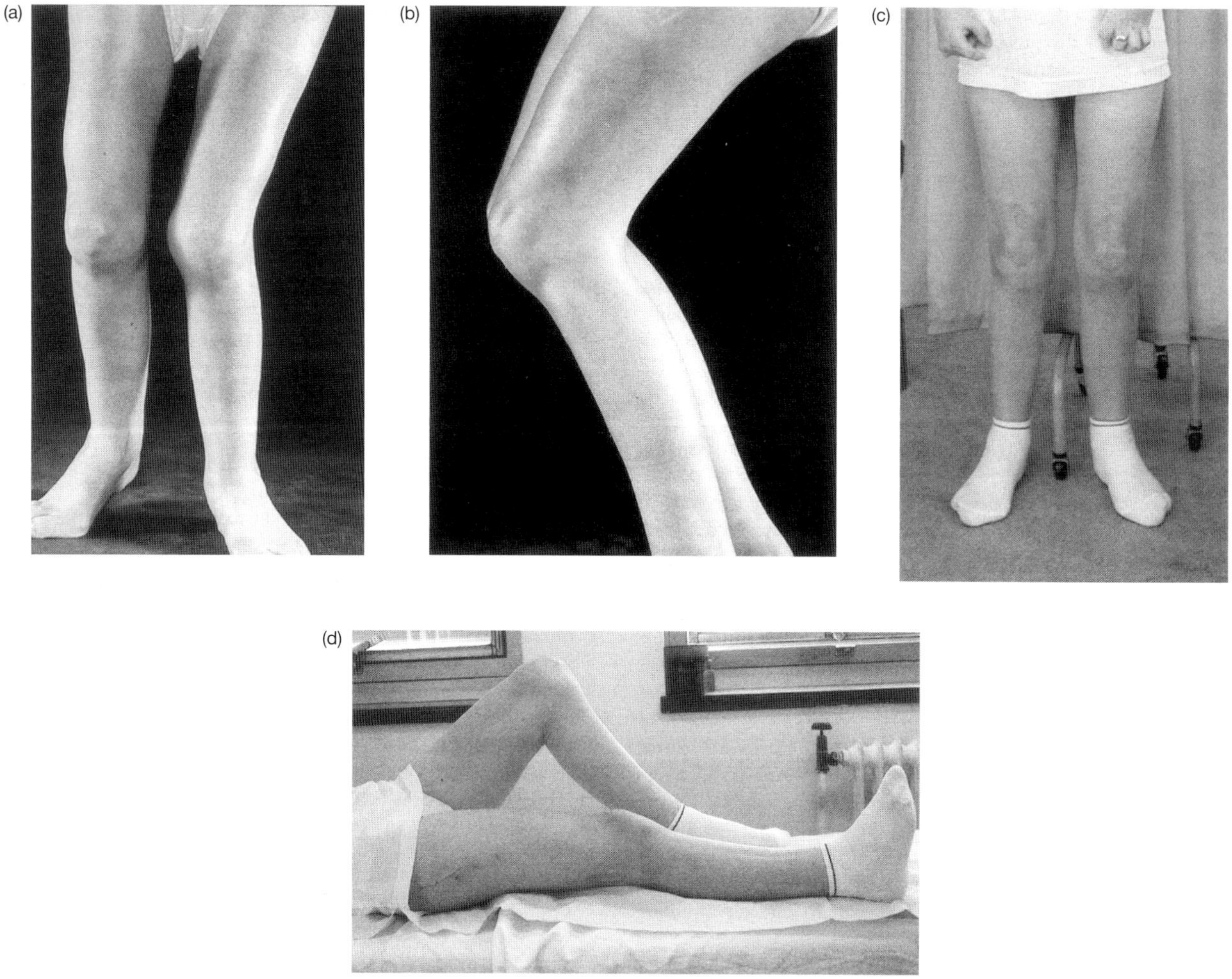

Fig. 2 (a, b) Nineteen-year-old girl with polyarticular juvenile idiopathic arthritis showing severe fixed flexion deformities of both knees. (c, d) Appearance following treatment wtih staged bilateral posterior soft tissue release procedures, followed by bilateral total knee replacements.

earlier designs have shown failure rates of 30–70 per cent after 5 years. More recent designs with an unconstrained meniscal bearing seem to show more promise with better survival rates beyond 5 years (Kofoed and Sorensen 1998). There are no reports of ankle arthroplasty specifically in patients with juvenile arthritis. The difficulties of replacement in this group of patients stem largely from the poor bone quality and from the associated deformites and malalignment of the ankle and subtalar joints.

Resection arthroplasty

In the majority of cases, subluxation and dislocation of the metatarsophalangeal joints can be managed with suitable footwear. Once all the epiphyses around the metatarsals and phalanges have fused excision arthroplasty can be considered. The long-term results of these procedures are disappointing (Tillman 1997) with recurrence of deformity in 8–10 years and so are best put off for as long as possible.

Upper limb

The most common problems that need to be considered by the surgeon in juvenile idiopathic arthritis are those in the lower limb; however, timely intervention for damaged joints in the upper limb can help maintain and maximize function.

The shoulder

The incidence of shoulder involvement varies according to the type of arthritis. It is the least frequently involved major joint overall and in cases of pauciarticular onset disease is virtually absent. However, the incidence in polyarticular onset disease is 50 per cent and this rises to 80 per cent in patients with systemic onset disease (Libby et al. 1991). In 95 per cent of cases where there is shoulder involvement this is bilateral. The synovitis may not only involve the glenohumeral joint but also the acromioclavicular joint, the subacromial bursa, and the rotator cuff tendons.

The onset is often insidious and symptoms may first come to light when crutches are required to aid mobility. The characteristics of shoulder involvement are pain and limitation of movement most commonly affecting internal rotation followed by abduction. A painful arc and positive impingement signs signify involvement of the rotator cuff and subacromial bursa.

Management of the shoulder initially involves physiotherapy with daily range-of-motion exercises to preserve muscle strength and function and in particular to avoid the development of contractures. In the early phase of the disease, local injections of corticosteroid into the glenohumeral joint or subacromial bursa may be very helpful.

Synovectomy

The indications for synovectomy would be a painful joint with little in the way of erosive changes on X-ray, no joint contracture, and not responsive to local

(a)
(b)
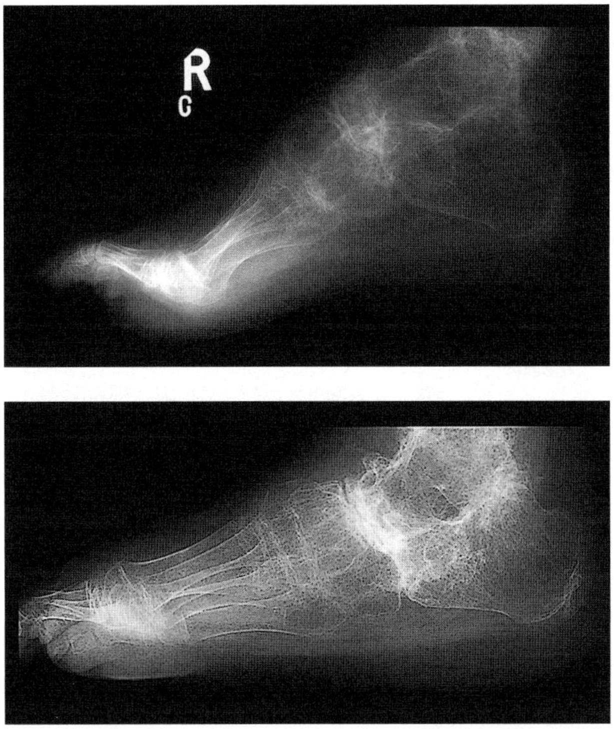

Fig. 3 (a) Equinus deformity at the midtarsal joint of a 15-year-old boy with juvenile idiopathic arthritis. (b) Appearance following corrective midtarsal osteotomy.

steroid injection. It is likely that the results will be similar to that in other major joints but there are little data available on its use in the shoulder.

Osteotomy

The results in terms of pain relief for an osteotomy around the shoulder are reported as good (Benjamin 1987); however, in general, this does not improve range of movement. This technique has become generally less popular as experience with shoulder arthroplasty increases.

Total shoulder replacement

This is rarely indicated in the younger patient in whom the epiphyses have not yet fused. It is indicated for pain resistant to other modalities of treatment and for poor function as a result of this. The results in terms of gain in range of movement are often rather disappointing and are less good than in patients with osteoarthritis who undergo this procedure. This is because of the associated rotator cuff pathology that is commonly present.

There are no reported results to date in patients specifically with juvenile idiopathic arthritis. However, in adult patients with rheumatoid arthritis (including some patients with juvenile arthritis) good or excellent pain relief can be achieved in 80–90 per cent with an improvement in abduction of 20° and with over 90 per cent implant survival at 11 years (Thomas et al. 1990; Stewart and Kelly 1997).

The elbow

The elbow is more frequently involved than the shoulder in juvenile arthritis with 45 per cent of patients having problems at 15 years follow-up. One of the earliest signs of involvement of the elbow joint is loss of full extension that may occur before significant pain or external evidence of swelling.

Early management is concentrated on controlling synovitis with medical management and intra-articular steroids. Night splints may be useful in controlling the progression of fixed flexion deformities.

Synovectomy ± radial head excision

Recurrent attacks of pain and swelling may derive benefit from synovectomy; if the radial head is damaged and growth has reached maturity this can also be excised. There are little data to indicate the overall efficacy of this procedure in patients with juvenile arthritis. Ovregard et al. (1990) in their series of 394 joint synovectomies in this group of patients documented only 15 carried out at the elbow. Reports in adults with rheumatoid arthritis generally show improvement in terms of pain in the short term; however, the results in terms of range of movement are more variable (Gendi et al. 1997). In the long-term, the results are less favourable with 50–67 per cent of patients having satisfactory results at 6 years (Tulp and Winia 1989).

The results of arthroscopic synovectomy of the elbow have also been reported in a small series by Lee and Morrey (1997), in which 93 per cent achieved a good or excellent result in the short-term but with only 57 per cent maintaining this rating at an average on 42 months.

Elbow reconstruction

Interposition arthroplasty

This procedure involves re-lining the joint with either strips of fascia or skin and is indicated in patients with severe pain and stiffness. It maybe indicated in the younger patient where there is greater concern regarding the later development of prosthetic loosening. There are no reports of results in patients with juvenile arthritis but good relief of pain and improved range of movement in both rheumatoid arthritis and post-traumatic arthritis have been reported (Froimsen et al. 1976; Vainio 1976).

Prosthetic replacement

Total elbow replacement may be indicated in a proportion of patients with severe pain. The procedure is difficult to perform because of the contracture of soft tissues and the extremely small bones and intramedullary cavities. A report by Connor and Morrey (1998) on 24 elbows in 19 patients showed that the average arc of flexion improved from 63° pre-operatively to 90° post-operatively. At an average follow-up of 7.4 years, 52 per cent had an excellent result, 35 per cent good, and 13 per cent poor. Late complications (aseptic loosening, instability, and worn bushings) led to three poor results. None of the 18 semiconstrained prostheses had radiographic evidence of loosening.

The wrist

The wrist is one of the most commonly affected joints in juvenile idiopathic arthritis. Involvement leads to loss of extension of the wrist and in severe cases a fixed flexion deformity develops. In cases of progressive synovitis, the distal radius develops a volar tilt and the carpus subluxates in a volar and ulnar direction. Early closure of the ulna growth plate contributes to the ulna shortening and ulna drift of the carpus.

Early management is directed at controlling synovitis with the aid of local corticosteroid injections and splints to help realign the carpus and prevent the development of fixed flexion deformities which are so debilitating (Evans et al. 1991).

Synovectomy

This procedure is indicated where there is no contracture and minimal or no erosive changes seen on radiographs. Tenosynovectomy is frequently performed as part of the procedure. Kvien et al. (1987) compared synovectomy with no synovectomy in patients with juvenile idiopathic arthritis over a 2-year period. The synovectomy group showed decreased pain and swelling compared to the non-synovectomy group and this improvement was maintained for at least 2 years.

Hanff et al. (1990) reported the results of synovectomy in 20 wrist joints of patients with juvenile idiopathic arthritis and at 3 years, 60 per cent noted improvement in terms of pain and grip strength, although the range of movement had decreased. Overall, 20 per cent of patients went on to require arthrodesis.

Excison of the distal ulna (Darrach procedure)

This is indicated in patients with significant disease affecting the ulna styloid and distal radio-ulna joint causing ulnar–carpal impingement together with pain and restriction of forearm rotation. The ulna should not be excised unless the growth plate has closed. The results in patients with rheumatoid arthritis are very good and the procedure may be combined with synovectomy and tendon reconstruction.

Arthroplasty

Arthroplasty may be indicated in severe wrist joint disease with intact flexor and extensor tendons. Some feel that it is only indicated in bilateral disease where a fusion has been performed on one side and an arthroplasty performed on the other. The most frequently used implant has been the Swanson prosthesis, which is a stemmed silicone elastomer spacer. A limited range of motion in the region of 40–60° is generally achieved with this procedure. Results in adults are quite good with Fatti et al. (1991) reporting 75 per cent of wrists with good pain relief at 2.5 years. Concern remains with regard to use of this prosthesis in younger patients because of the problems associated with implant loosening, migration, fracture, and silicone synovitis.

Arthrodesis

Spontaneous fusion of the wrist occurs in a significant proportion of patients with juvenile idiopathic arthritis. As there is always a possibility of this occurring in patients with severe wrist disease, maintaining the carpus in good alignment, and avoiding a fixed flexion deformity is very important. Once the carpus starts to drift into ulnar deviation, corrective ostetomies about the radius or ulna are not usually of help because of the associated involvement of the distal radio-ulnar and radio-carpal joints. Correction or deformity is best achieved at the time of wrist fusion.

Arthrodesis remains the procedure of choice in those with disabling wrist pain and severe destructive changes seen on X-ray. A variety of techniques can be used to achieve a fusion; most commonly either an intramedullary pin passing from the third metacarpal shaft into the radius or a dorsally applied plate and screws. The results in general are very satisfactory. Kobus and Turner reported on 87 wrist fusions after an average follow-up period of 6 years and showed that 97 per cent had good or excellent relief of pain following the procedure.

The hand

Hand involvement in juvenile idiopathic arthritis is common and may follow a somewhat different pattern than in the adult. At onset there is progressive stiffness of the metacarpo-phalangeal joints (MCP) and proximal interphalangeal joints (PIP). In contrast to adults the child may develop ulnar deviation of the metacarpals and radial deviation of the fingers. At the MCP joints loss of flexion without loss of extension may be seen. Boutonniere deformities are common as are fixed flexion deformities of the interphalangeal joints. Swan-neck deformities are seen less commonly than in adults.

Treatment of the hand is focused on prevention of functional deficits. Early splinting with static and dynamic splints is essential together with physiotherapy and hydrotherapy. Steroid injections into tendon sheaths and finger joints are also helpful. Surgery is indicated in the presence of established deformity associated with poor function and is directed at the soft tissues where the deformities are passively correctable, but in the presence of a fixed deformity, arthrodesis or arthroplasty is required.

Tenosynovectomy

In the presence of bulging synovium over tendons or joints, tenosynovectomy is indicated, in particular, to help prevent tendon rupture. This is frequently combined with removal of bony spurs and prominences. Trigger fingers can generally be successfully managed by steroid injection into the tendon sheath and is effective in about 60 per cent of patients (Anderson and Kaye 1991).

Synovectomy

Synovectomy of the MCP and PIP joints may be of use in certain cases but the loss of movement associated with the procedure may lead to poor results. In the series by Ovregard et al. (1990) results in 107 synovectomies of MCP and PIP joints were good for 3 years and then steadily declined.

Arthroplasty

MCP joint arthroplasty is indicated when there is severe pain and deformity associated with bone destruction. It is not indicated before skeletal maturity. The most frequently used prosthesis is the Swanson silastic flexible interposition implant. Good results can be achieved in terms of pain relief and active finger flexion to about 60° can be expected (Beckenbaugh 1983).

Arthrodesis

Arthrodesis is the treatment of choice for severely affected PIP joints. The joint is fused in a position of approximately 40° of flexion and is considered a reliable procedure in terms of pain relief and function.

The spine

The cervical spine is affected in both seropositive and seronegative juvenile arthritis (Swann 1983), the dorsal spine exhibits crush fractures when steroids have been exhibited, and the lumbar spine takes the brunt of ankylosing spondylitis.

Patients with seronegative juvenile chronic arthritis may present with a painful torticollis and if this is neglected the patient will be left with a permanent disability with the head tilted rigidly on one side. These patients should be given a general anaesthetic, if necessary, in order to relieve the spasm, and whilst the head and neck are held straight a firm collar is applied. This is taken off for daily exercise and then reapplied, for although it will not prevent fusion occurring it does permit it to take place in a more satisfactory position. Seropositive arthritis, on the other hand, leads to instability and it is particularly at the atlantoaxial level where the subluxation or dislocation may occur. There is an absolute indication for surgical fusion at this level if there is a neurological involvement or severe pain or both.

It is of particular importance that the anaesthetist should be aware of these problems in the cervical spine in both types of disease (see also Chapter 1.3.11). The rigidity of the neck, associated with a small airway, may make intubation difficult or impossible by conventional means. Subluxation or dislocation at the atlantoaxial level will equally be a hazard because attempts at intubation may lead to cord damage. It is essential that an up-to-date radiograph should be available immediately before the patient is given a general anaesthetic. The use of the fibreoptic laryngoscope and other airway techniques have obviated the worries that existed previously; many patients who are having lower limb surgery can be managed well with spinal or epidural anaesthesia (Smith 1990).

Scoliosis

Structural scoliosis occurs more commonly in patients with juvenile chronic arthritis than in the normal population (Ross et al. 1987). This may arise from the postural curves associated with asymmetrical involvement of the lower limb joints causing pelvic tilting. Timely surgical relief of the primary cause in the lower limbs has led to a lessening of the spinal curve. Asymmetrical involvement of the apophyseal joints may also contribute to this problem. In patients with scoliosis, careful appraisal of the underlying pathology should be made, but if there is a need, conventional methods of correction and stabilization can be used.

Fractures

The limited activity of these patients and their inability to participate in sport protects them largely from this problem. Nevertheless, they are prone to pathological fractures because of their osteoporosis and the stiffness of their joints. This is particularly so with supracondylar fractures of the knee and underlines the inadvisability of manipulating the joints under anaesthesia. Examination under anaesthesia is permissible but must be attended with utmost care.

After fractures, immobilization in a cast must be maintained for the minimal time consistent with union to prevent additional stiffness of the adjacent joint. The degree of osteoporosis usually precludes internal fixation of the fragments.

A number of patients have suffered crush fractures of the spine, particularly if they are on corticosteroids. No special treatment is indicated and recovery with remarkable reformation of the vertebrae can be expected.

Summary

All synovial joints are vulnerable to the deformity and functional loss that can occur in juvenile idiopathic arthritis. The principles outlined in this chapter should be applied intensively in this polyarthritic condition. The prognosis in terms of complete remission for many sufferers makes the treatment all the more demanding and worthwhile so that they may grow into physically functional adults.

References

Anderson, B. and Kaye, S. (1991). Treatment of flexor tenosynovitis of the hand ('Trigger finger') with corticosteroids: a prospective study of the response to local injection. *Archives of Internal Medicine* **151**, 153–6.

Ansell, B.M. (1978). Heberden Oration 1977. Chronic arthritis in childhood. *Annals of the Rheumatic Diseases* **37**, 107–20.

Ansell, B.M. and Swann, M. (1983). The management of chronic arthritis of children. *Journal of Bone and Joint Surgery* **65B**, 536–43.

Arden, G. and Ansell, B.M., ed. *Surgical Management of Juvenile Chronic Arthritis.* London: Academic Press, 1978.

Beckenbaugh, R.D. (1983). Implant arthroplasty in the rheumatoid hand and wrist. *Journal of Hand Surgery* **8**, 675–8.

Benjamin, A. (1987). Double osteotomy of the shoulder. *Scandinavian Journal of Rheumatology* **3**, 65–70.

Boublik, M., Tsahakis, P.J., and Scott, R.D. (1993). Cementless total knee arthroplasty in juvenile onset rheumatoid arthritis. *Clinical Orthopaedics* **286**, 88–93.

Carmichael, E. and Chaplin, D.M. (1986). Total knee arthroplasty in juvenile rheumatoid arthritis. A seven-year follow-up study. *Clinical Orthopaedics* **210**, 192–200.

Chmell, M.J., Scott, R.D., Thomas, W.H., and Sledge, C.B. (1997). Total hip arthroplasty with cement for juvenile rheumatoid arthritis. Results at a minimum of ten years in patients less than thirty years old. *Journal of Bone and Joint Surgery* **79-A**, 44–52.

Connor, P.M. and Morrey, B.F. (1998). Total elbow arthroplasty in patients who have juvenile rheumatoid arthritis. *Journal of Bone and Joint Surgery* **80-A**, 678–88.

Ekholm, R. and Norback, B. (1951). On the relationship between articular changes and function. *Acta Orthopaedica Scandinavica* **21**, 81–98.

Evans, D.M., Ansell, B.M., and Hall, M.A. (1991). The wrist in juvenile rheumatoid arthritis. *Journal of Hand Surgery (Scotland)* **16**, 293–304.

Fatti, J.F. et al. (1991). Long term results of Swanson interpositional wrist arthroplasty II. *Journal of Hand Surgery* **16**, 432–7.

Froimsen, A., Silva, J.E., and Richley, W.G. (1976). Cutis arthroplasty of the elbow joint. *Journal of Bone and Joint Surgery* **58-A**, 863–5.

Gendi, N.S.T., Axon, J.M.C., Carr, A.J., Pile, K.D., Burge, P.D., and Mowat, A.G. (1997). Synovectomy of the elbow and radial head excision in rheumatoid arthritis. *Journal of Bone and Joint Surgery* **79-B**, 918–23.

Hanff, G., Sollerman, C., Elborogh, R., and Pettersson, H. (1990). Wrist synovectomy in juvenile chronic arthritis. *Scandinavian Journal of Rheumatology* **19**, 280–4.

Isdale, I.C. (1970). Hip disease in juvenile rheumatoid arthritis. *Annals of the Rheumatic Diseases* **29**, 603–8.

Jacqueline, F., Boujot, A., and Canet, L. (1961). Involvement of the hips in juvenile rheumatoid arthritis. *Arthritis and Rheumatism* **4**, 500–13.

Kabayakawa, M., Rydholm, G., Wingstrand, H., Pettersson, H., and Lindgren, L. (1989). Femoral head necrosis in juvenile chronic arthritis. *Acta Orthopaedica Scandinavica* **60**, 164–9.

Kampner, S. and Ferguson, A.B. (1972). Efficacy of synovectomy in juvenile rheumatoid arthritis. *Clinical Orthopaedics* **88**, 94–109.

Kobus, R.J. and Turner, R.H. (1990). Wrist arthrodesis for treatment of rheumatoid arthritis. *Journal of Hand Surgery* **15**, 541–6.

Kofoed, H. and Sorensen, S. (1998). Ankle arthroplasty for rheumatoid arthritis and osteoarthritis. Prospective long-term study of cemented replacements. *Journal of Bone and Joint Surgery* **80-B**, 328–32.

Kvien, T.K., Pahle, J.A., Hoyeraal, H.M., and Sandstad, B. (1987). Comparison of synovectomy and no synovectomy in patients with juvenile rheumatoid arthritis. *Scandinavian Journal of Rheumatology* **16**, 81–91.

Lee, B.P.H. and Morrey, B.F. (1997). Arthroscopic synovectomy of the elbow for rheumatoid arthritis. *Journal of Bone and Joint Surgery* **79B**, 770–2.

Libby, A.K., Sherry, D.D., and Dudgeon, B.J. (1991). Shoulder limitation in juvenile rheumatoid arthritis. *Archives of Physical Medicine Rehabilitation* **72**, 382–4.

McCullough, C.J. (1994). Surgical management of the hip in juvenile chronic arthritis. *British Journal of Rheumatology* **33**, 178–83.

Mogensen, B., Brattstrom, H., Ekelund, L., Svantesson, H., and Lidgren, L. (1982). Synovectomy of the hip in juvenile chronic arthritis. *Journal of Bone and Joint Surgery (Britain)* **64-B**, 295–9.

Moreno Alvarez, M.J., Espada, G., Maldonado-Cocco, J.A., and Gagliardi, S.A. (1992). Longterm follow-up of hip and knee soft tissue release in juvenile chronic arthritis. *Journal of Rheumatology* **19**, 1608–10.

Ovregard, T., Hoyeraal, H.M., Pahle, J.A., and Larsen, S. (1990). A 3 year retrospective study of synovectomies in children. *Clinical Orthopaedics* **259**, 76–82.

Rana, N.A. (1982). Juvenile rheumatoid arthritis of the foot. *Foot and Ankle* **3**, 2–11.

Rodriguez, J.A., Saddler, S., Edelman, S., and Ranawat, C.S. (1996). Long-term results of total knee arthroplasty in class 3 and 4 rheumatoid arthritis. *Journal of Arthroplasty* **11**, 141–5.

Rombouts, J.J. and Rombouts-Lindemans, C. (1971). Involvement of the hip in juvenile rheumatoid arthritis. *Acta Rheumatologica Scandinavica* **17**, 248–67.

Ross, A.C., Edgar, M.A., Swann, M., and Ansell, B.M. (1987). Scoliosis in juvenile chronic arthritis. *Journal of Bone and Joint Surgery* **69-B**, 175–8.

Rydholm, U., ed. *Surgery for Juvenile Chronic Arthritis.* Lund: Ortolani, 1990.

Rydholm, U. et al. (1986a). Sonography, arthroscopy, and intracapsular pressure in juvenile chronic arthritis of the hip. *Acta Orthopaedica Scandinavica* **57**, 295–8.

Rydholm, U., Elborgh, R., Ranstam, J., Schroder, A., Svantesson, H., and Lidgren, L. (1986b). Synovectomy of the knee in juvenile chronic arthritis. A retrospective, consecutive follow-up study. *Journal of Bone and Joint Surgery (Britain)* **68-B**, 223–8.

Rydholm, U., Brattstrom, H., and Lidgren, L. (1986c). Soft tissue release for knee flexion contracture in juvenile chronic arthritis. *Journal of Pediatric Orthopaedics* **6**, 448–51.

Rydholm, U., Brattstrom, H., Bylander, B., and Lidgren, L. (1987). Stapling of the knee in juvenile chronic arthritis. *Journal of Pediatric Orthopaedics* **7**, 63–8.

Salter, R.B. and Field, P. (1960). The effects of continous compression on living articular cartilage: an experimental investigation. *Journal of Bone and Joint Surgery (America)* **42-A**, 31–49.

Sarokhan, A.J., Scott, R.D., Thomas, W.H., Sledge, C.B., Ewald, F.C., and Cloos, D.W. (1983). Total knee arthroplasty in juvenile rheumatoid arthritis. *Journal of Bone and Joint Surgery (America)* **65**, 1071–80.

Simon, S., Whiffen, J., and Shapiro, F. (1981). Leg-length descrepancies in monoarticular and pauciarticular juvenile rheumatoid arthritis. *Journal of Bone and Joint Surgery* **63-A**, 209–15.

Smith, B.L. (1990). Anaesthesia in paediatric rheumatology. In *Pediatric Rheumatology Update* (ed. P. Woo, P.H. White, and B.M. Ansell), pp. 124–30. New York: Oxford University Press.

Soto-Hall, R., Johnson, L.H., and Johnson, R.A. (1964). Variations in the intra-articular pressure of the hip joint in injury and disease: a probable factor in avascular necrosis. *Journal of Bone and Joint Surgery (America)* **46-A**, 509–16.

Stewart, M.P.M. and Kelly, I.G. (1997). Total shoulder replacement in rheumatoid disease. *Journal of Bone and Joint Surgery* **79-B**, 68–76.

Stuart, M.J. and Rand, J.A. (1988). Total knee arthroplasty in young adults who have rheumatoid arthritis. *Journal of Bone and Joint Surgery* **70-A**, 84–7.

Swann, M. (1983). Juvenile chronic arthritis: surgical aspects. In *Clinical Orthopedics* (ed. N.H. Harris), pp. 249–67. Bristol: Wright PSG.

Swann, M. and Ansell, B.M. (1986). Soft-tissue release of the hips in children with juvenile chronic arthritis. *Journal of Bone and Joint Surgery (Britain)* **68-B**, 404–8.

Tillman, K. (1997). Surgery of the rheumatoid forefoot with special reference to the plantar approach. *Clinical Orthopaedics* **340**, 39–47.

Thomas, B.J., Amstutz, H.C., and Cracchiolo, A. (1990). Shoulder arthroplasty for rheumatoid arthritis. *Clinical Orthopaedics* **265**, 125–8.

Tulp, N.J. and Winia, W.P. (1989). Synovectomy of the elbow in rheumatoid arthritis: long term results. *Journal of Bone and Joint Surgery* **71-B**, 664–6.

Vainio, K. (1976). Arthroplasty of the elbow and hand in rheumatoid arthritis. In *Synovectomy and Arthroplasty in Rheumatoid Arthritis* (ed. G. Chapchal), pp. 66–70. Stuttgart: Thieme Verlag.

Witt, J.D. and McCullough, C.J. (1994). Anterior soft tissue release of the hip in juvenile chronic arthritis. *Journal of Bone and Joint Surgery* **76-B**, 267–70.

Witt, J.D., Swann, M., and Ansell, B.M. (1991). Total hip replacement for juvenile chronic arthritis. *Journal of Bone and Joint Surgery (Britain)* **73-B**, 770–3.

Woo, P., White, P.H., and Ansell, B.M., ed. *Pediatric Rheumatology Update.* New York: Oxford University Press, 1990.

7.3 Corticosteroid injection therapy

Allan I. Binder

Introduction

The injection of local anaesthetic and corticosteroid agents into joints or soft tissue structures constitutes one of the most effective therapeutic options for the treatment of localized painful lesions of articular and soft tissue structures. The value of this form of treatment is widely appreciated, but there is some concern with regard to the adequacy of the skills and experience of general practitioners and other healthcare workers (Phelan et al. 1992) who increasingly perform these injections.

This chapter will outline the basic principles of steroid injection therapy, with the technique and special considerations for the more common conditions where it is employed. Sports-related and spinal use is more specialized and will not be considered in detail. The majority of injections can be performed in the clinic, ward, or, if necessary, in the patient's home, using an aseptic no-touch technique.

Effect of steroid on joints and soft tissue structures

Systemic corticosteroid agents have potent anti-inflammatory effects which result in an improvement in pain, stiffness, and systemic symptoms of active inflammatory arthropathy. They may also reduce the rate of joint damage in early rheumatoid arthritis. However, the limiting factor for long-term steroid therapy is the considerable risk of side-effects such as osteoporosis, reduced resistance to infection, deficient wound healing, accelerated atherosclerosis, and the suppressive effect on the hypothalamic–pituitary–adrenal axis, which can persist for up to a year after steroids have been withdrawn. Atlantoaxial subluxation and early death are also more common in rheumatoid patients treated with systemic steroids.

Local steroid injected into a joint aims to achieve a sustained concentration of the drug in the synovial fluid and to provide the maximum anti-inflammatory effect locally whilst minimizing absorption into the plasma with its attendant risk of systemic side-effects.

There are many steroid agents available and the localized effects depend on the potency, solubility, and dose of the particular agent used. Hydrocortisone acetate is short acting, has a weak anti-inflammatory effect, is fairly soluble, and is completely absorbed from the joint within hours. The synthetic corticosteroids, such as methylprednisolone acetate, prednisolone acetate, and triamcinolone acetonide, are much more potent and less soluble and remain localized in the joint for much longer.

The systemic absorption of corticosteroid after local joint injection, may be sufficient to reduce inflammation in non-injected joints, and suppress the hypothalamic–pituitary–adrenal axis for several weeks after a single dose of a long-acting steroid. However, serious systemic side-effects are rare after a single injection, except in patients with brittle diabetes or infection.

Outside the joints, local steroid injection may benefit many acute or chronic soft tissue lesions. There is little data on the absorption of steroid from tendon sheaths, bursae, or other soft tissue structures, although methylprednisolone has been shown to produce measurable plasma levels for a mean of 16 days after soft tissue injection (Mattila 1983). Not all the effects of local steroid on soft tissue structures are beneficial, with impairment in the healing of damaged ligaments, and atrophy of up to 40 per cent of skin and subcutaneous tissue thickness, following a single injection of steroid.

Indications for local steroid injection

Joint puncture permits the aspiration of fluid for microbiological, crystal, and, occasionally, biochemical assessment, and should always precede steroid injection where infection, haemarthrosis, or crystal arthropathy is suspected. The colour, smell, turbidity, and viscosity of the aspirated fluid may help differentiate inflammatory arthropathy from crystal-related or non-inflammatory disease, but a heavy concentration of polymorphs (pyoarthrosis) is equally likely with acute rheumatoid, infection, or gout. Conventional light and polarized microscopy and, in some cases, microbiological culture of the synovial fluid may be necessary before steroid can be safely injected. Soft tissue lesions, such as olecranon bursitis, are also amenable to aspiration, with fluid from these lesions being subjected to analysis similar to synovial fluid, before steroid is injected.

The injection of local anaesthetic with steroid also has value as a diagnostic tool where the source of the pain is uncertain. For example, the abolition of a 'painful arc' on abduction, as a result of local anaesthetic injected with the steroid, confirms the diagnosis of rotator cuff impingement (tendinitis). High-resolution ultrasound may also assist in diagnosis and facilitate aspiration and/or steroid injection.

However, the main use of local steroid injection is for treatment of inflammatory and non-inflammatory conditions of joints or soft tissues. Even acute gout and pseudogout will respond to steroid injection, although this therapy is not always feasible. The result of steroid injection of osteoarthritic joints is unpredictable, but more likely to be beneficial in the presence of an effusion.

Contraindications to local injection

There are some absolute and other relative contraindications to steroid injection therapy as shown in Table 1. Any suspicion of sepsis within the affected joint, on the same limb, or systemically, precludes steroid injection until infection has been excluded or adequately treated. Steroid injection is best avoided in joints previously affected by septic arthritis, as local defence mechanisms within the joint are suspect. Monoarthritis of unknown cause

Table 1 Contraindications to local steroid injection

Absolute contraindication
Septic arthritis, septicaemia, active sepsis in locality, tuberculosis
Febrile patient, cause unknown
Serious allergy to local anaesthetic, steroid, or previous local injection
Relative contraindication
Monoarthritis of unknown type
Neutropaenia, thrombocytopaenia
Anticoagulants or bleeding diathesis

should always be regarded with suspicion and steroid injection delayed, until infection has been excluded.

Septic arthritis is particularly easy to overlook in rheumatoid patients who are frail and elderly or being treated with systemic steroid or immunosuppressive drugs. In these patients infection is often polyarticular, mimicking an exacerbation of the inflammatory disease. Although *Staphylococcus aureus* is the most common infecting organism, patients may not present with fever, weight loss, or other features associated with systemic infection. A mild rise in neutrophil count and a high sedimentation rate may also fail to differentiate infective from inflammatory causes, although an exceptionally high C-reactive protein level is more suggestive of infection. While systemic ill health can be a prominent feature in septic arthritis, it can also occur in rheumatoid patients without infection (systemic rheumatoid), and steroids should not be given by any route until infection, including tuberculosis, has been sought and if necessary treated.

Patients need to be asked about previous allergic reactions to local anaesthetic agents (e.g. with dental treatment), steroids, or local injections. An exacerbation of the pain for 24–48 h following a previous steroid injection does not suggest allergy, but rather a crystal-related phenomenon (Berger and Yount 1990). Neutropaenia, thrombocytopaenia, and clotting abnormalities constitute relative contraindications to local steroid injection. If patients are on anticoagulants, these should be stopped for at least 24 h before the steroid injection. With other clotting abnormalities or blood dyscrasias, haematological advice should be sought, and appropriate preparations made to reduce the risk of bleeding following the injection. While haemophilic arthropathy has been successfully treated with cautious steroid injection (Shupak et al. 1988), this therapy should be avoided in sickle cell disease (Gladman and Bombardier 1987) as a sickle crisis may be precipitated by the procedure.

Potential dangers and side-effects

Local steroid injections are extremely safe, provided that the indication is appropriate, there are no contraindications, and a careful aseptic technique is used. Some side-effects apply to all injections (Table 2), while others are site-specific, and will be discussed below. While the exacerbation of pain for up to 48 h following the injection suggests a crystal-related phenomenon (Berger and Yount 1990), pain persisting beyond this time requires assessment for infection or other complications. Infection following steroid injection constitutes the most important adverse event, but it is very rare, with an estimated sepsis rate of 1 in 14 000–50 000 injections. Chronic debilitating illness such as severe diabetes or rheumatoid and factors such as drug abuse and alcoholism (Haslock et al. 1995), which suppress general immunity can predispose patients to infection. Post-injection sepsis may result from contamination of the injection equipment or skin, haematogenous spread, or reactivation of a previous infection. Accelerated joint destruction will also follow the injection of steroid into an undiagnosed septic joint.

Subcutaneous tissue atrophy (Plate 202) or depigmentation (Plate 203) are more likely if large or repeated doses of long-acting steroid are given. While tendon rupture (Fig. 1) or facial flushing is encountered fairly frequently, other side-effects (Table 2) are rare. The importance of local steroid injection in the development of avascular necrosis or a Charcot joint remains uncertain.

Table 2 Side-effects attributed to local steroid injection

Exacerbation of pain for 24–48 h (crystal related)
Septic arthritis
Accelerated destruction of an unsuspected septic joint
Subcutaneous tissue atrophy
Depigmentation
Transient facial flushing
Anaphylaxis
Peripheral nerve injury
Tendon rupture
Avascular necrosis, Charcot joint
Loss of diabetic control
Reactivation of tuberculosis
Cartilage damage
Soft tissue calcification

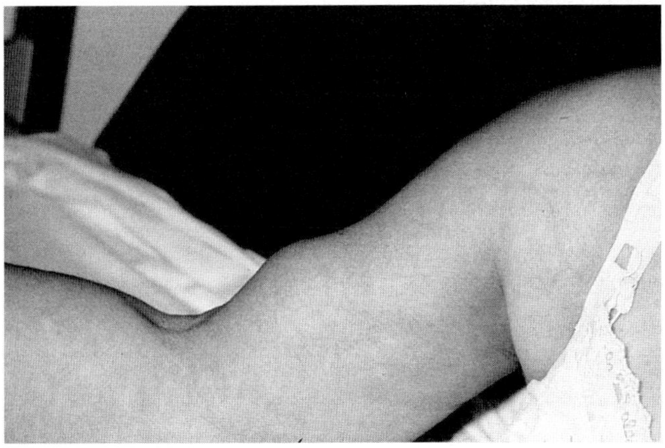

Fig. 1 Rupture of the long head of the biceps tendon following anterior shoulder injection.

Method of steroid injection

The method of injection of local steroid into painful joints and soft tissue structures is similar, although the exact technique may depend on the local anatomy, the size, and depth of the lesion concerned, and the need to aspirate fluid before injection. With deeper joints like the hip, radiological screening may be necessary. The broad principles of injection therapy will be outlined with locally determined modification in techniques being considered under the individual conditions.

As the success of local injection therapy depends on the accurate placement of the injected steroid, knowledge of the anatomy at the site of injection is important. Consistency in the choice of equipment (needles and syringes) and adequacy of relaxation of the patient, and especially of the limb to be injected, further improve feel and reliability. While the injection of large fluid-filled joints is relatively easy, other injections may require considerable skill and experience.

There is no single 'correct' method of performing steroid injection and most skilled operators develop their own unique style (Haslock et al. 1995), based on training, experience, and the equipment available. Irrespective of the individual variation in method, this should always be based on a consistent, safe, aseptic, 'no-touch' technique. The method presented reflects the author's own practice.

Equipment

Table 3 summarizes the equipment needed for routine steroid injection. Single-dose ampoules of steroid and local anaesthetic agents should always be used to eliminate any possibility of cross infection.

Steroid agents

Hydrocortisone acetate is short-acting with limited use for superficial lesions, where there is a risk of subcutaneous atrophy or depigmentation, or in lesions (such as Achilles tendinitis) where tendon rupture may occur. Although there are many long-acting steroid agents available (Table 3), familiarity with one or two agents is adequate, as the differences between agents is not great. Methylprednisolone acetate and triamcinolone acetonide are most widely used and are superior to hydrocortisone in most circumstances (Blyth et al. 1994).

The dosage of steroid used varies according to the lesion injected. For most joint and soft tissue lesions, 25 mg of hydrocortisone, 40 mg of methylprednisolone or triamcinolone acetonide is adequate. Large joints, like the knee and ankle may require double and very small joints or lesions half this dose.

Local anaesthesia

Local anaesthesia of the skin can be achieved by the use of a refrigerant spray such as ethyl chloride and is especially useful in the hand and other sensitive parts of the body. The skin is sprayed only until it turns white to achieve anaesthesia without a painful burn.

Lignocaine 1 per cent can be introduced in combination with the steroid, but where the injection is technically difficult or fluid aspiration is to precede injection, the lignocaine is introduced first. The volume of local anaesthetic agent injected will vary according to the size of the joint or lesion being injected. While the use of lignocaine may reduce the immediate post-injection pain in tennis elbow or other soft tissue lesions (Haslock et al. 1995), the rationale for routine use in large joint injection is less clear cut.

Other equipment

Sealed isopropyl alcohol swabs or other alcohol-based agents provide a safe and cost-effective method of achieving skin cleansing. While a 2 or 5 ml sterile syringe is adequate for most steroid injections, 10 and 20 ml syringes are required for fluid aspiration. The choice of needle for any given site is also important. Most medium-sized joints and soft tissue lesions can be injected with a 23G (blue) needle. A larger 21G (green) needle is used for larger joints, especially where aspiration is required, and for deep soft tissue lesions such as those round the buttocks and thighs. Where the synovial effusion is large or the fluid is thick, fibrinous, or purulent, a 19G (white) needle may be needed for successful aspiration. Small hand and foot joints and superficial soft tissue lesions are best injected with a fine 25G (orange) needle.

Table 3 Equipment required for local steroid injection

Steroid preparations (individual ampoules) Short acting hydrocortisone acetate 25 mg/ml Long acting methylprednisolone acetate 40 mg/ml methylprednisolone acetate 40 mg/ml, lignocaine 10 mg/ml triamcinolone hexacetonide 20 mg/ml triamcinolone acetonide 40 mg/ml
Single-dose 1% lignocaine ampoules for injection
Refrigerant spray
Sealed isopropyl alcohol swabs
Other Sealed single-use needles—25G, 23G, 21G, and 19G Single-use syringes Sterile cottonwool Elastoplast, crepe bandages

Preparation

The method of preparation for joint aspiration and steroid injection is shown in Table 4.

The patient must be as relaxed as possible, as tension in surrounding muscles can make the injection difficult or even impossible. Where patient anxiety is a concern, most injections can be carried out with the patient lying supine with the head comfortably supported on pillows. This position facilitates the treatment of vasovagal attacks if they occur. The presence of a nurse helps to reassure and position the patient but the nurse must be dissuaded from drawing up the drugs or shaking them out onto a tray or table before the operator is ready. The procedure should be described to the patient in detail before starting the injection, to reduce the risk of airborne infection. At the same time, the patient can be assessed for sepsis, allergy, or other contraindications to the injection.

Simple hand washing (or use of an alcohol rinse) is adequate for the procedure if a no-touch technique is to be employed, and should precede preparation of the injection. Careful hand drying will prevent water running down the needle. While gloves have been recommended for joint aspiration, most rheumatologists (Haslock et al. 1995) currently do not heed this advice. The injection is prepared with a combination of steroid and local anaesthetic in the same syringe in most cases. Where the injection is likely to be difficult or where aspiration is to precede injection, the two agents are drawn up separately, the lignocaine being in a larger syringe. As steroid preparations are crystalline, they need to be thoroughly mixed before being drawn up and again before injection. The needle should ideally be changed following preparation to maintain sharpness, and must remain covered until the injection is given to reduce the risk of infection.

Injection technique

A method for aspiration and/or steroid injection is summarized in Table 5 , with talking being kept to a minimum during the procedure. The exact site for injection is carefully marked with a blunt-pointed object such as a ball-point pen with the point retracted. This mark should only be made once careful positioning of the patient has been achieved, and needs to remain visible even after skin cleansing to permit a no-touch aseptic technique to be used.

Only one or two joints should be injected per session, with the same joint being injected no more than three or four times a year. Where large effusions exist, they should be aspirated fully before steroid injection (Weitoft and Uddenfeld 2000). Patients should be warned of possible side-effects such as a temporary exacerbation of pain or destabilization of diabetic control following the injection. The patients should also be told about

Table 4 Preparation for steroid injection

Exclude contraindications or allergy
Explain procedure before starting
Position patient so patient and limb are relaxed
Wash hands and dry carefully
Prepare injection immediately before use To aspirate: lignocaine and steroid separate To inject only: lignocaine and steroid mixture
Mix steroid thoroughly before preparation and before injection
Use single-dose ampoules
Draw up the drugs yourself!
Change needle before injecting
Keep needle covered before use

Table 5 Technique for steroid injection

Mark exact point of needle insertion with a blunt object
Use no-touch technique
Cleanse injection site with two to three alcohol swabs
Spray refrigerant spray for skin anaesthesia
Reswab injection site
Insert needle without touching the metal
For aspiration: hold needle stationary as fluid is tapped, then change syringe and inject steroid
For injection: pull back plunger before injecting
Remove needle carefully and check for bleeding
Use elastoplast if not allergic; crepe bandage after aspirating knee
Dispose of all needles and syringes safely to avoid needle-stick injury
Rest or splint joint after injection if possible
Re-emphasize possible side-effects and benefits

ıe possible beneficial effects of the absorbed steroid on systemic symptoms r other inflamed joints.

ᵉost-injection

'he injected part should, where possible, be rested for 24–48 h after injec-on, although admission for absolute bed rest is neither cost-effective nor ractical. Splinting the injected joint may also prolong the duration that the teroid remains localized at that site. Where a large effusion has been rained, as from a knee, a crepe bandage should be firmly applied to pro-ide support and take up the slack in the tissues stretched by the effusion. 'he maximum improvement usually develops in 2–4 weeks, and may last ıany months.

oint and soft tissue lesions

'he most common lesions amenable to steroid injection will be considered n a regional basis.

'he painful shoulder

houlder pain usually arises from soft tissue lesions, although arthropathies ffecting the glenohumeral, acromioclavicular, and sternoclavicular joints lso occur, with most lesions being amenable to steroid injection.

Injection therapy is more effective than physiotherapy for most shoulder :sions but the site of steroid injection needs to be based on anatomical athology rather than the localization of tender or trigger points.

ılenohumeral joint

'his joint communicates with the tendon sheath of the long head of the iceps tendon, but not with the subacromial bursa unless rupture of the otator cuff has occurred. Aspiration and or injection of the glenohumeral ɔint can be achieved using the anterior or posterior route, as both provide ood access to the joint, although the posterior route is technically easier.

ınterior route

'his route gives more reliable access in patients with frozen shoulder (adhes-ve capsulitis), and is better suited for aspiration of large shoulder effusions. Vith the patient lying supine, the arm is rotated to identify the coracoid rocess and joint line anteriorly, and acromium posteriorly. Laying the arm cross the abdomen to result in partial internal rotation of the shoulder, the ıjection is made just lateral to the coracoid in the line of the joint margin, vith the needle directed towards the acromium. If correctly sited, the injec-ion can be given without resistance.

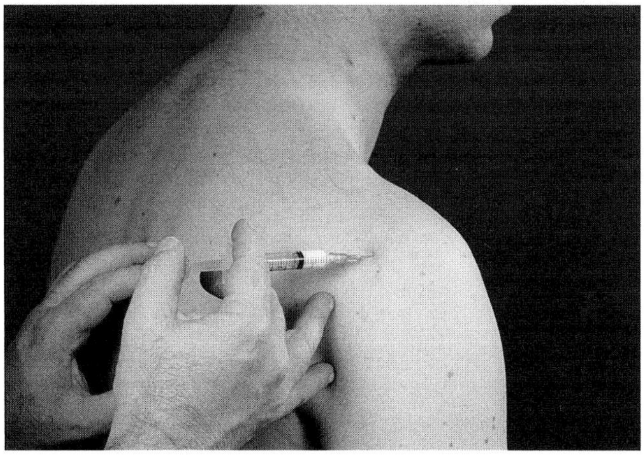

Fig. 2 Injection of the shoulder joint via the posterior route.

Posterior route (Fig. 2)

This is especially useful where the cause of the pain is uncertain or the operator lacks skill in injection procedures. With the patient seated across the couch and approached from behind, the thumb is used to identify the spine of the scapula which is followed laterally until it bends forward as the acromium. The point just below the acromium is marked. The forefinger is then used to palpate the coracoid process in front, rotating the shoulder if necessary to locate it. The needle is inserted under the acromium and gently advanced without resistance with the needle pointing towards the outer side of the coracoid process. More superficial injection is used to treat cuff lesions.

Subacromial bursa—lateral approach

Injection into the bursa is particularly useful for rotator cuff lesions, especially when accompanied by a painful arc on abduction. Although subacromial bursitis is rarely a primary diagnosis, it is frequently secondarily affected by pathological processes arising in the rotator cuff and surrounding structures. The subacromial space is very large, being in continuity with the subdeltoid space and also, with cuff rupture, the glenohumeral joint.

To inject the subacromial space, the patient should be seated and approached from the lateral aspect with the arm hanging vertically down, to use gravity to enlarge the gap between the acromium above and the humeral head below. This gap is palpated, marked, and the needle advanced into the space, directed medially and slightly posteriorly. A relatively large volume of local anaesthetic (2–10 ml) is mixed with the steroid in view of the large capacity of the space being injected. The local anaesthetic rapidly abolishes the 'painful arc', which both helps confirm the diagnosis of a rotator cuff lesion and the correct siting of the injection. The benefit of this injection is particularly dramatic in patients with acute calcific tendinitis, where the pain is so acute that patients often present as an emergency.

While steroid injection to the glenohumeral joint or subacromial bursa often ameliorates the pain associated with frozen shoulder, it has less effect on the recovery of range of movement. Arthrographic capsular distension, which ruptures the capsule, when combined with steroid injection, may lead to earlier recovery in range (Rizk et al. 1994) in frozen shoulder. However, a home exercise regimen which encourages hourly wall climbing to increase abduction and forward flexion, achieves a satisfactory rate of recovery in most patients with frozen shoulder.

Individual rotator cuff tendons

The individual rotator cuff tendons can also be injected with appropriate expertise, but ultrasound guidance permits more accurate identification and injection of these lesions. Bicipital tendinitis is difficult to distinguish from rotator cuff tendinitis, but often coexists with it. While steroid injection via the anterior route may reduce pain from this source, rupture of the long head of biceps may follow the injection (Fig. 1).

Acromioclavicular joint

The acromioclavicular joint, which is on the anterosuperior aspect of the shoulder, is located by following the clavicle laterally until the joint is reached. Local tenderness confirms joint involvement. The joint is injected from the anterior or superior route, but only accepts 0.5 ml of fluid. Care is necessary to avoid deep injection as a pneumothorax can result from apical lung penetration.

Elbow

Elbow pain is extremely common and usually results from epicondylitis. Care is necessary to exclude pain referred from the cervical spine, brachial plexus, or shoulder, which can closely mimic primary elbow pathology. Most elbow lesions are injected from the lateral side, with the patient sitting in a relaxed manner and with the elbow resting on the examination table at an angle of 90°. Medial epicondylitis and ulnar entrapment neuropathy require a greater angle and appropriate positioning to permit access to the medial aspect of the elbow.

Epicondylitis

Lateral epicondylitis (tennis elbow) (Fig. 3)

In tennis elbow, localized tenderness is found either just distal to the lateral epicondyle or over the radial head. Pain is exacerbated by wrist dorsiflexion against resistance, especially when the elbow is extended and the hand prone. Grip strength is also reduced with the arm held in a similar position.

Local steroid injection is directed to the site of maximum tenderness, with the injection aimed at 45°, to end near the insertion of the common extensor tendon to bone. A fair amount of pressure is needed to inject at this site, so care should be taken to ensure the needle is firmly attached to the syringe.

Medial epicondylitis (golfer's elbow)

Golfer's elbow causes tenderness very similar to tennis elbow but it is localized to the region of the medial epicondyle.

Injection is again directed at the site of maximum tenderness, near the insertion of the common flexor tendon to bone. Care is necessary to keep anterior to the medial epicondyle to avoid injury to the ulnar nerve which lies in a groove just behind the medial epicondyle.

Methylprednisolone should be used as it is more effective than hydrocortisone and causes less atrophy of the subcutaneous tissue than triamcinolone. Temporary post-injection exacerbation of pain and early relapse of symptoms are common following the injection, but injection should be limited to no more than three, to avoid long-lasting or irreversible atrophy.

Elbow joint

The elbow joint is commonly involved in inflammatory arthropathies and can be injected using either the posterior or anterolateral route.

Posterior approach (Fig. 4)

The posterior joint line can be identified by placement of the thumb on the lateral epicondyle and third finger on the olecranon. The paraolecranon groove between the two fingers identifies the joint line, which runs between the two heads of the triceps tendon. Injection into the joint is just above and slightly lateral to the olecranon, where a bulge can be felt in the presence of a joint effusion.

Olecranon bursitis

Olecranon bursitis can result from infection, trauma, rheumatoid arthritis, or gout. Once infection has been excluded, the bursa can be aspirated and injected with steroid, but secondary infection, chronic local pain, fistula formation, or skin atrophy may follow the injection and surgical removal of the bursa may be necessary.

Ulnar nerve entrapment

The ulnar nerve lies in the groove just behind the medial epicondyle, and can be impinged on by local pressure, trauma, or inflamed synovial tissue. Patients present with pain on the medial side of the elbow, paraesthesia of the ulnar digits, and occasionally sensory or motor abnormalities in the hand. A positive Tinel sign, elicited by local percussion over the nerve behind the medial epicondyle, suggests the diagnosis, which can be confirmed by electromyography. Steroid injection at this site may reduce the symptoms, especially when the lesion has an inflammatory cause, but care is necessary to avoid injury to the nerve during the procedure.

Wrist

Although the wrist and surrounding structures are often involved in the inflammatory arthropathies, there are many other non-inflammatory wrist lesions which are amenable to steroid injection therapy.

Wrist joint (Fig. 5)

Wrist injection is carried out with the patient seated, and with the limb resting on the examination couch with the hand held palm down and the joint opened up by palmar flexion over a pillow or similar object. The joint margin is felt as a triangular gap between the lower end of the radius and the

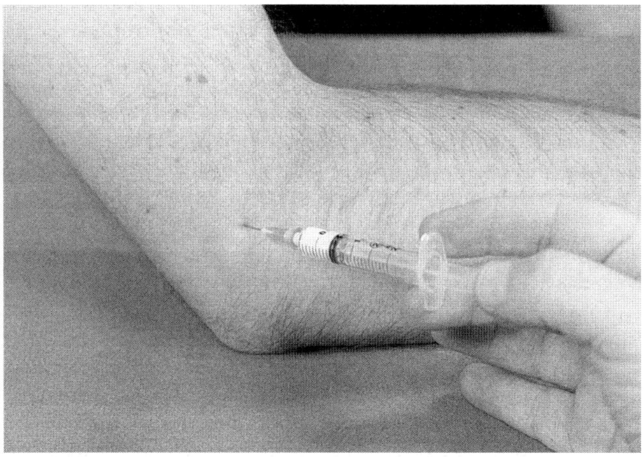

Fig. 3 Injection of a tennis elbow lesion.

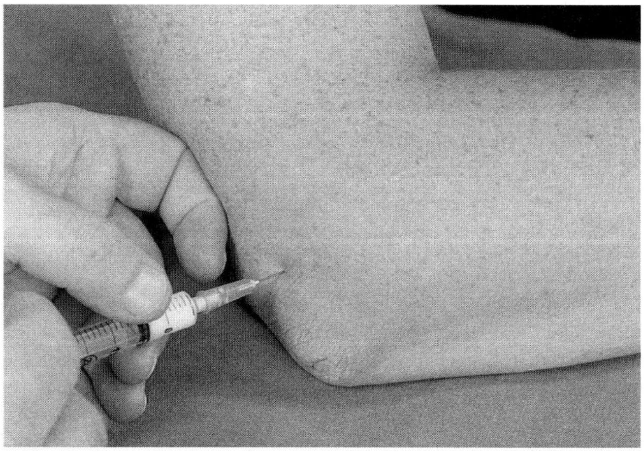

Fig. 4 Injection of the elbow joint via the posterior approach.

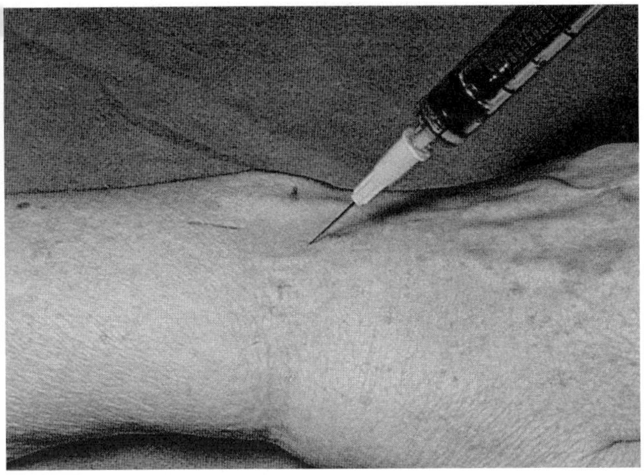

Fig. 5 Injection of the wrist joint.

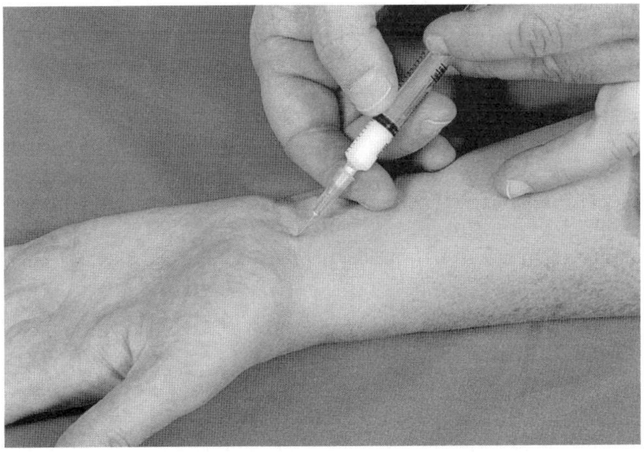

Fig. 6 Injection of carpal tunnel syndrome to the ulnar side of the palmaris longus tendon.

lunate and scaphoid bones. The needle is inserted into the joint pointing in a proximal direction at an angle of about 60°. Immobilization of the wrist may prolong the beneficial effects of the injection.

Carpal tunnel syndrome (Fig. 6)

Carpal tunnel syndrome results from median nerve compression in the carpal tunnel of the wrist and can be mimicked by cervical spine or brachial plexus lesions, and electromyography, although not infallible, may assist diagnosis in difficult cases.

The injection is carried out just medial (ulnar) to the midline of the ventral aspect of the wrist, in the first crease, at the junction to the hand. If the palmaris longus tendon is present, it overlies the median nerve and injection using a long-acting steroid preparation should be just medial and parallel to it. A fine 25G needle is inserted, just medial to the midline or palmaris longus tendon, to a depth of 1 cm, directing the needle towards the palm. If the needle is correctly positioned, there should be no resistance, pain, or paraesthesia during the procedure.

Care is necessary to avoid damage to the nerve, which can cause persistent pain and paraesthesia. A wrist splint, especially if used at night, may also hasten recovery. In idiopathic lesions, especially affecting women under the age of 40 years, steroid injection is less likely to be successful, and early surgery should be considered. The presence of thenar muscle wasting, persistent sensory loss, or a lack of response to steroid injection, is associated with a less favourable outcome even following surgical decompression.

De Quervain's tenosynovitis

Stenosing tenovaginitis of the extensor pollicus brevis and abductor pollicus longus (De Quervain's tenosynovitis) is common and often occupational or due to repeated minor trauma. It causes pain on gripping especially with use of the thumb. Tenderness is noted in the 'snuffbox' area of the wrist where palpable crepitus may be found. Pain can be increased by ulnar deviation of the wrist against resistance after placing the patients thumb in the palm (Finkelstein's test), with the arm held in the midprone position.

The injection for this lesion is given at the point of maximum tenderness, using a fine-bore needle which is inserted tangentially along the tendon sheath. When correctly sited, the injection can be given without resistance. Local steroid injections should be combined with a thumb pillar splint and modification of the activities which caused the lesion. Although long-acting steroids are more effective, hydrocortisone is less likely to cause complications such as subcutaneous atrophy or depigmentation (Plates 202 and 203), especially after repeated injection. Dark skinned patients need to be warned that these cosmetic complications may follow the injection.

Hand

The small joints in the hands

These joints are frequently involved in inflammatory arthropathies and are all amenable to steroid injection to reduce pain and swelling. However, the injections are painful and it is only possible to inject one or two joints per session, unless general or regional anaesthesia is used. The presence of a joint effusion simplifies the procedure and distortion of the normal anatomy makes it considerably more difficult.

The technique of steroid injection is similar for all the small hand joints and can be performed with the patient seated with the hand palm down across the table or examination bench. The joint margin on the lateral or medial side of the joint is identified by gently flexing and extending the digit. The superior part of the joint line is marked, with the joint flexed to an angle of 45°. By distracting the finger with one hand, it is injected with the other hand, using the superolateral or superomedial approach to avoid injury to the neurovascular structures. The joint will only accept 0.5–1 ml of injected fluid, which should contain a combination of long-acting steroid and local anaesthetic. Splintage of the joint may prolong the effect of the injection.

Metacarpophalangeal joint (Fig. 7)

The joint line, which is located about 1 cm distal to, and not at, the crest of the knuckle, is identified by passive movement of the finger. After marking the joint line, the patients finger is distracted as the joint is injected, tangentially under the extensor expansion.

Proximal and distal interphalangeal joint

Injection is also carried out by distracting the joint as the steroid is injected tangentially under the extensor expansion. The distal joints are technically more difficult to inject unless an effusion is present.

First carpometacarpal joint

This joint is characteristically affected in primary generalized osteoarthritis and non-inflammatory arthropathies. For injection, the hand is rested on the couch in the midprone position, with the joint line being identified laterally. By applying pressure on the thumb the joint can be distracted, and the injection facilitated. The patient needs to relax the thumb as the needle is angled slightly distally to enter the joint. Different approaches to the joint may be necessary once gross distortion of the joint has occurred. The Patient should also be provided with a thumb pillar splint to protect the joint against further damage.

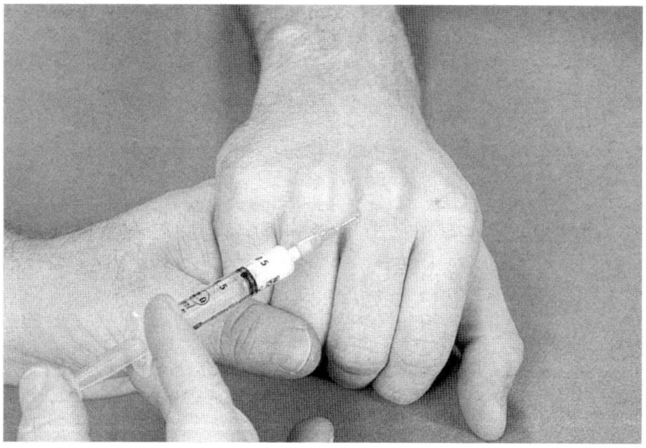

Fig. 7 Injection of the metacarpophalangeal joint.

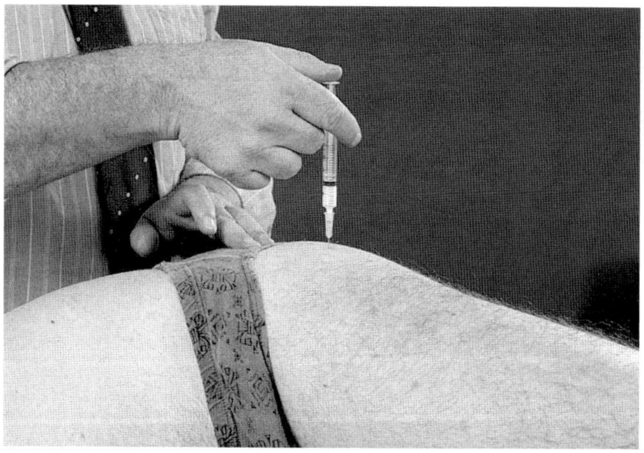

Fig. 8 Injection of trochanteric bursitis.

Flexor tenosynovitis and 'trigger' fingers

Flexor tenosynovitis is a common cause of poor hand function in inflammatory arthropathies, lupus, or diabetes mellitus but can also result from trauma or be idiopathic. Nodules may form within the tendon sheathes, making it difficult for the tendon to move freely past the anatomical constrictions, thus leading to 'triggering' of the digit. The nodules can be palpated either attached to the tendon in the pad of tissue adjacent to the proximal phalanx or in the palm opposite the distal palmar crease. They can also occur at the base of the thumb.

The affected tendon sheath is injected with the patient seated with the hand resting palm up on the couch. The needle is advanced tangentially along the tendon sheath in a proximal direction, using a fine-bore needle. Similar injection is possible for thumb tendon nodules.

Steroid injection improves over two-thirds of patients with flexor tenosynovitis, and the success rate rivals surgical intervention. Rupture of tendons may rarely follow steroid injection at this site.

Hip region

Although hip pathology is common, many patients referred with hip problems have pain arising from soft tissue lesions around the hip. The extreme depth of the hip joint and technical difficulty associated with anatomical derangement or osteophyte formation, preclude hip injection as a routine outpatient procedure. Aspiration and, if appropriate, steroid injection, needs to be carried out by an orthopaedic surgeon in theatre or, better, by a radiologist under suitable radiological screening. Although the hip joint itself is not routinely injected, many soft tissue lesions around the hip are amenable to steroid injection in an outpatient setting.

Trochanteric bursa (Fig. 8)

Patients presenting with trochanteric bursitis have pain and local tenderness maximally around the greater trochanter of the femur.

To inject the lesion, the patient is positioned with the painful thigh uppermost and flexed, and the lower leg kept extended. By rotating the affected hip, the prominence of the greater trochanter with its associated tenderness is located, marked, and injected at right angles to the skin. The injection site can be very deep seated in patients with obese thighs, and a longer (5.08 cm) 21G needle may be needed to reach the bursa. While steroid injection therapy has a high success rate in both inflammatory and mechanical lesions, postural advice and review of gait by a physiotherapist is necessary to prevent recurrence of the lesion.

Meralgia paraesthetica

This lesion is an entrapment neuropathy of the lateral cutaneous nerve of the thigh as it traverses the deep fascia, about 10 cm below and medial to the anterior superior iliac spine. Clearly demarcated blunting of pinprick or hyperaesthesia may be found over the anterolateral aspect of the thigh, with tenderness localized to the point where the nerve penetrates the fascia (10 cm below the anterior superior iliac spine). If this point is found, infiltration with steroid and local anaesthetic may abolish the symptoms.

Ischial tuberosity

The ischial tuberosities, located deep in the medial side of the buttocks, have overlying bursas which can become inflamed and cause pain on sitting, especially on a bicycle seat. These lesions are amenable to infiltration of steroid and local anaesthetic with the patient lying on the lateral side facing away from the examiner. The tender point is identified and injected using a long 21G needle.

Knee

Knee joint

A knee effusion is a common finding and—where the cause is uncertain—aspiration of synovial fluid for microbiological and crystal assessment should precede steroid injection.

The most common technique for knee aspiration and injection is to use the retropatellar route, via either the medial or lateral approaches. With the patient lying supine, the knee should be extended and the quadriceps muscle relaxed. In the presence of fixed flexion contracture of the knee, support under the knee is necessary to encourage quadriceps relaxation.

Lateral retropatellar approach (Fig. 9)

The joint line is marked between the upper and middle third of the patella, with the needle advanced tangentially between the patella and femoral condyle. By pushing on the medial aspect of the patella, the gap between the patella and femur can be increased, facilitating joint penetration. Aspiration as the needle is inserted, will reveal fluid as soon as the joint capsule is entered, so reducing the risk of cartilage injury.

Medial retropatellar approach

The site of joint entry is just below the midline of the patella, with the needle advanced tangentially towards the suprapatellar pouch.

Irrespective of the approach, a 21G or larger-bore needle is used, to remove as much of the inflammatory fluid and debris as possible (Weitoft and Uddenfeldt 2000), before steroid is injected. The fluid should also be viewed and, if purulent, examined in the laboratory to exclude infection before steroid is injected.

Long-acting steroid agents are more effective than hydrocortisone (Blyth et al. 1994), with a relatively large dose of steroid being necessary. Significant absorption of steroid into the circulation can be anticipated and patients need to be informed of both potential benefits to other inflamed

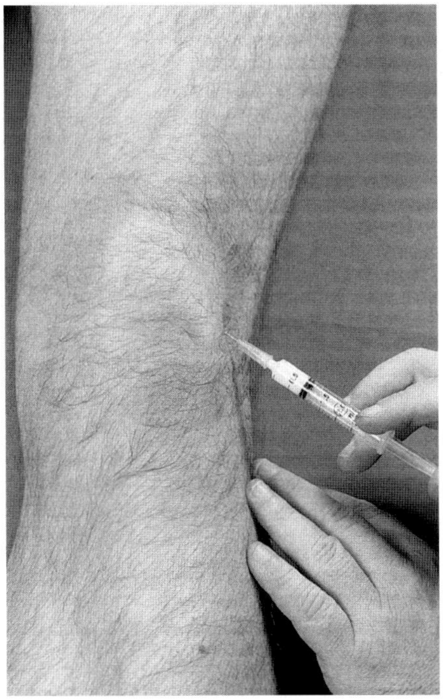

Fig. 9 Injection of the knee joint via the lateral retropatellar approach.

joints and possible risks, such as destabilization of diabetic control, following the injection.

A bandage should be firmly applied to support the knee following injection if a large effusion is drained. Rest for 24 h following the injection prolongs the beneficial effects.

Popliteal (Baker's) cyst

Patients with a knee effusion may develop a popliteal (Baker's) cyst as a result of a one-way valve between the knee joint and semimembranosus or gastrocnemius bursa.

If a Baker's cyst requires treatment, the knee joint proper should be aspirated and injected as described above. Attempts to inject the cyst directly could result in damage to the neurovascular structures at the back of the knee. For a ruptured Baker's cyst, a below knee support stocking should be used to facilitate sealing of the capsular rupture, following steroid injection into the knee joint proper.

Other knee lesions

Non-infected prepatellar bursitis, painful collateral ligaments, and other painful trigger spots around the knee may be amenable to local steroid injection, which is given at the point of maximum tenderness. If an infected prepatellar or other superficial bursa is aspirated, care is necessary to avoid entry into the knee joint as septic arthritis may ensue.

Ankle and hindfoot

The tendon sheathes around the ankle often communicate with the ankle joint and can be involved in inflammatory or other pathological processes. Most ankle and hindfoot lesions can be injected with the patient lying supine on the couch.

Ankle joint (Fig. 10)

The ankle joint is located by dorsiflexing the foot to stretch the tibialis anterior ligament and so make it visible. The joint margin which lies between the tibia and talus is then palpated just lateral to the tendon. After marking the injection site, the needle is inserted almost horizontal to the foot,

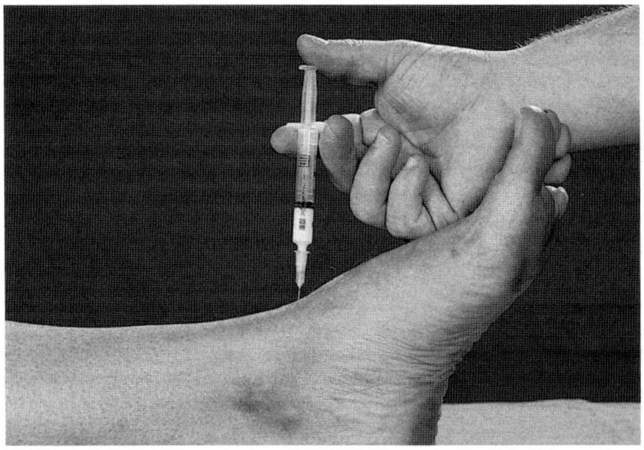

Fig. 10 Injection of the ankle joint.

curving over the talus. If an effusion is present, the joint can be aspirated before steroid is injected.

Tendon sheaths

Injection of steroid along swollen and inflamed tendon sheathes is possible behind the medial malleolus (posterior tibial tendon), or lateral malleolus (peroneal tendon), with improvement in pain and swelling following successful injection.

Tarsal tunnel syndrome

Entrapment of the posterior tibial nerve by the flexor retinaculum can occur behind and below the medial malleolus. Patients present with burning, tingling, and numbness in the distribution of the nerve, most prominently in the toes and distal part of the sole. Tenderness with a positive Tinel sign elicited by percussion over the nerve near the medial malleolus will confirm the diagnosis. Injection under the flexor retinaculum between the calcaneum and medial malleolus may relieve the symptoms.

Posterior heel pain

Many lesions can affect the Achilles tendon, and partial tendon rupture or core necrosis cannot be clinically distinguished from Achilles tendinitis.

While steroid injection is feasible with peritendinitis or bursitis, it is not always successful, and is only justified once partial tendon rupture has been excluded using ultrasound or other radiological investigations. Even if partial tendon rupture is not found, patients need to be warned of the risk of tendon rupture following steroid injection. Short-acting steroid agents lessen the risk of rupture, especially if patients avoid exercise for a few weeks following the injection.

Inferior heel pain

Pain under the heel can result from a plantar (calcaneal) spur, or can be associated with more diffuse pain radiating up the arch of the foot (plantar fasciitis), especially in patients with loss of the longitudinal arch of the foot.

Plantar fasciitis and pain under the heel and can usually be improved by the use of a cushioned insole, although a local steroid injection under the heel may be indicated for resistant cases. If an injection is needed, the thick skin of the sole should be avoided, with injection being made from the medial side after careful localization of the point of maximum tenderness. The needle is inserted tangentially through the softer skin, so the point of the needle is under the point of maximum tenderness near the bony spur. A cushioned insole should also be provided following injection but recurrence of pain is common. Rupture of the calcaneal origin of the plantar fascia may follow steroid injection.

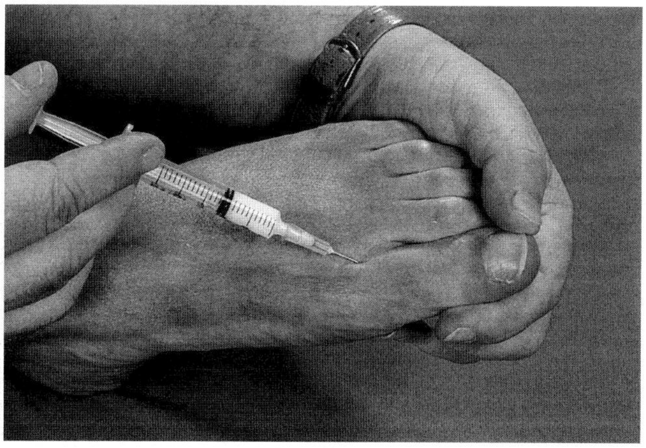

Fig. 11 Injection of the first metatarsophalangeal joint.

Forefoot

Metatarsophalangeal joints (Fig. 11)

Forefoot pain is extremely common, and steroid injection therapy is often very effective in reducing pain especially in the period before serious deformity has developed. The lateral metatarsophalangeal joints are located by moving the toe between thumb and forefinger. Once the joint line is found and marked, the joint is injected using a dorsal approach with the needle entering tangentially from the lateral side, passing under the extensor tendon which overlies the dorsum of the joint. The first metatarsophalangeal joint is sometimes easier to enter from the medial side, using a similar technique to the other joints. The foot joints need to be injected with particular care, as the risk of infection is greater than at other sites.

Conclusion

Local steroid injection is one of the most useful therapeutic modalities for the amelioration of pain arising from joint and soft tissue structures. While considerable latitude exists with regard to the precise technique employed, the method must be based on a safe and accurate aseptic no-touch technique. A method of joint injection has been outlined with consideration of the most frequently used injections.

References

Berger, R.G. and Yount, W.J. (1990). Immediate 'steroid flare' from intraarticular triamcinolone hexacetonide injection: case report and review of the literature. *Arthritis and Rheumatism* **33**, 1284–6.

Blyth, T., Hunter, J.A., and Stirling, A. (1994). Pain relief in the rheumatoid knee after steroid injection: a single-blind comparison of hydrocortisone succinate, and triamcinalone acetonide or hexacetonide. *British Journal of Rheumatology* **33**, 461–3.

Gladman, D.D. and Bombardier, C. (1987). Sickle cell crisis following intra-articular steroid therapy for rheumatoid arthritis. *Arthritis and Rheumatism* **30**, 1065–8.

Haslock, I., MacFarlane, D., and Speed, C. (1995). Intra-articular and soft tissue injections: a survey of current practice. *British Journal of Rheumatology* **34**, 449–52.

Mattila, J. (1983). Prolonged action and sustained serum levels of methylprednisolone after a local injection of methylprednisolone acetate. *Clinical Trials Journal* **20**, 18–23.

Phelan, M.J., Byrne, J., Campbell, A., and Lynch, M.P. (1992). A profile of the rheumatology nurse specialist in the United Kingdom. *British Journal of Rheumatology* **31**, 858–9.

Rizk, T.E., Gavant, M.L., and Pinals, R.S. (1994). Treatment of adhesive capsulitis (frozen shoulder) with arthroscopic capsular distension and rupture. *Archives of Physical Medical Rehabilitation* **75**, 803–7.

Shupak, R., Teitel, J., Garvey, M.B., and Freedman, J. (1988). Intraarticular methylprednisolone therapy in haemophilic arthropathy. *American Journal of Hematology* **27**, 26–9.

Weitoft, T. and Uddenfeldt, P. (2000). Importance of synovial fluid aspiration when injecting intra-articular corticosteroids. *Annals of the Rheumatic Diseases* **59**, 233–5.

7.4 Sports medicine

Mark Harries

Fundamentals of exercise physiology

Energy production

ATP synthesis

The energy for all biological processes derives from the hydrolysis of adenosine triphosphate (ATP) to form adenosine diphosphate (ADP) and inorganic phosphate (Pi), yielding 7.6 kcal/mol. Elucidation of the tertiary structure of ATP synthase, the enzyme that drives the reverse reaction, and the discovery of its remarkable rotating action, is a fairly recent event and one for which the Nobel Prize in chemistry was awarded in 1997. Perhaps more remarkable still is the realization that this enzyme is common to all species, mammals, birds, reptiles, plants, and fungi. In plants this process is called photophosphorylation, but the term reserved to describe respiration in animals is oxidative phosphorylation. These findings have been as revolutionary to exercise physiology, as the first description of the double helix must have been for geneticists. The Royal Swedish Academy of Sciences has likened the mechanism of action of ATP synthase to that of a water hammer minting coins, 'three coins of ATP currency minted with each turn of the wheel' (Fig. 1). And it has been estimated that an active young person will generate his or her own body weight in ATP each day!

At the root of modern understanding of energy transfer is the chemiosmotic theory first proposed by Mitchell (1977). It describes the electrochemical gradient across the cell membrane created by protons generated during respiration and explains how this provides the motive force that turns the ATP synthase molecule. Manufacture of ATP from ADP and Pi by the F1 particle requires three protons, with an additional proton to export it to the cytosol. And so a total of four protons are needed to generate one molecule of ATP. Mitchell's theory won him the Nobel Prize in chemistry in 1978. It has resulted in a re-evaluation of the long-accepted estimate figure for the number of moles of ATP generated from each mole of substrate oxidized, from 38 to 31 for glucose, and 129 to 102 moles for palmitate.

Role of mitochondria

When considering the beginnings of life on Earth, it is believed that for the first billion years or so all organisms were anaerobic, protected from the ultraviolet rays of the sun by seawater. The evolution of photosynthesis by specific membrane-enclosed organelles known as chloroplasts, resulted in pollution of the environment with oxygen. Other life forms then had to adapt to existence in an oxidizing atmosphere. This was made possible with the appearance of similar structures, also membrane-enclosed, known as mitochondria.

Their origins are a mystery. But recent evidence describes a complete set of genes encoding components of the tricarboxylic acid (Kreb's) cycle and

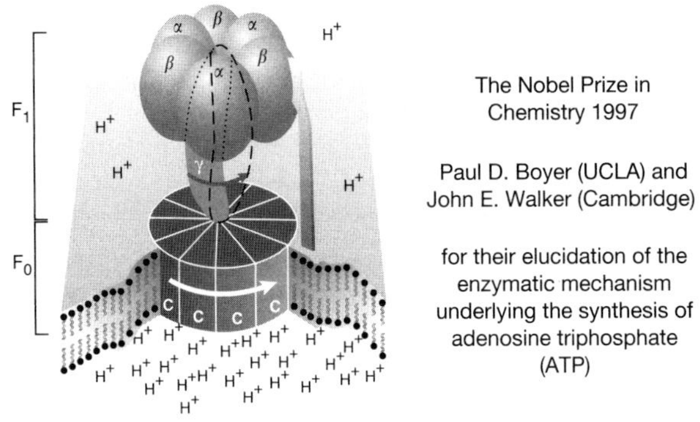

F_1
F_0
The Nobel Prize in Chemistry 1997
Paul D. Boyer (UCLA) and John E. Walker (Cambridge)
for their elucidation of the enzymatic mechanism underlying the synthesis of adenosine triphosphate (ATP)

Fig. 1 ATP synthase: likened to a water hammer minting coins of ATP, the common currency of all energy systems. One mole of ADP is crushed with Pi within each of the three pairs of sub-units (α and β) forming ATP. Each turn of the wheel demands the transfer of 12 protons three for each mole of ATP liberated and an additional proton for each mole exported to the cytosol. (Reproduced with permission, Royal Swedish Academy of Sciences.)

the respiratory-chain complex present in *Rickettsia prowazekii*, the causative agent of epidemic typhus (Andersson et al. 1998). This has led to the astonishing conclusion that our entire terrestrial existence may be attributable to a chance symbiosis with genes of bacterial origin that 'infected' the stem cell early in our evolution and that like bacteria, mitochondria reproduce by binary fission! What is more, it is now known that all mitochondrial DNA is of maternal origin, the paternal contribution is destroyed on conception. Mitochondria contain their own messenger RNA, and so are largely independent of the host nucleus, a further example of their symbiotic existence.

Waste disposal

Coping with acid production

Oxidation reactions involving glycogen and fatty acids generate protons (acid) and bicarbonate ions, the dissociation products of carbon dioxide in water. They also create oxygen singlets and triplets collectively known as super-oxides. These are highly reactive but are neutralized in the mitochondria. It is the resulting flow of protons that spin ATP synthase. Surges in pH caused by rapid addition of protons during physical activity are 'buffered' by plasma proteins and other systems, of which bicarbonate is the most readily accessible for measurement. Normal plasma bicarbonate settles at around 24 mmol/l. The extent to which the buffer is indented and bicarbonate falls below normal, known as the base deficit, provides an indication of the number of protons added. Most laboratories can now measure proton numbers directly in plasma, providing a clearer appreciation of the severity of the acidosis than does pH alone. The kidney voids surplus protons.

Voiding carbon dioxide

The high solubility of CO_2 and the abundance of carbonic anhydrase, ensure that bicarbonate can always be absorbed in the tissues and voided from the lungs regardless of the rate of production. Indeed, such is the capacity of the lungs to liberate CO_2, that hyperventilation is deployed as the chief mechanism used to compensate partially the acidosis created acutely by lactate accumulation, and by more chronic metabolic states such as keto-acidosis or renal failure. Arterial CO_2 should never rise even during all-out exercise and in metabolic acidosis typically it falls.

How muscle uses its fuel

Respiratory exchange ratio

Ability of mitochondria to utilize fat in addition to glycogen is what gives motile creatures their endurance capacity. The rate at which ATP is produced during anaerobic combustion is almost 10 times that generated by aerobic processes. But glycogen is in short supply and without replenishment, stores can be exhausted in less than 2 h.

The relative use of fat (for endurance performance) or glucose (for power) is indicated by the ratio of the volume of carbon dioxide evolved to the volume of oxygen consumed. At the tissue level this is known as the respiratory quotient (RQ), whereas when pulmonary measurements are made, the term respiratory exchange ratio (RER) is used.

One mole of glucose requires six moles of oxygen for complete oxidation, yielding six moles of carbon dioxide. Thus, when glucose is the principal fuel, RER = 1 (i.e. 6/6). Combustion of fat demands a relatively larger volume of oxygen and RER falls below unity. During low intensity steady-state exercise RER is around 0.85, indicating that 50 per cent of the energy derives from fat. But when the work rate is near maximal, almost all the energy comes from glucose. Trained endurance athletes are able to use a higher proportion of fat than the untrained, thereby conserving their glycogen. However, modern views recognize that it is the rate of demand for energy by the active muscle tissue that dictates where the fuel comes from (Holloszy and Coyle 1984). And it is the rate of demand for ATP to fuel movement in combination with the redox state of the metabolic pathway that determines whether energy comes predominantly from one source or another. That is, from glucose or long-chain fatty acids.

Maximal oxygen consumption ($\dot{V}O_2$ max)

The rate at which these oxidation reactions proceed ($\dot{V}O_2$ l/min) is expressed as the product of cardiac output and the difference between arterial and venous oxygen content. However, on the assumption that the alveolar-capillary membrane is perfectly permeable to gas, using the product of minute ventilation and the inspired/expired oxygen difference can make a less invasive estimate. During peak exercise, sedentary young men typically consume around 40 ml of oxygen/kg body weight/min, but are only able to sustain about 60 per cent of this maximum (i.e. of their $\dot{V}O_2$ max). Fitter individuals reach 60 $ml.kg.min^{-1}$ but elite endurance athletes may consume in excess of 90 $ml.kg.min^{-1}$ and can sustain a higher fraction of this rate for longer.

Lactate inflection point

When the demand for ATP can no longer be met rapidly enough, more intensive activity is still possible with the degradation of glycogen to form lactate. During exercise of moderate to high intensity, a substantial amount of the lactate produced is then oxidized for use as an energy substrate by diffusion into neighbouring muscle fibres. The concentration of lactate in the blood during steady-state exercise reflects a balance between production and removal. At rest blood lactate is around 1.0 mmol/l, a reflection of the obligatory glycolytic activity of the erythrocytes (which have no mitochondria), but as exercise intensity increases, production exceeds removal and lactate accumulates in blood.

The steep rise in blood lactate occurring during exercise of increasing intensity is known as the lactate inflection point. It is training at this intensity that most improves endurance performance. Plasma lactate at the inflection point shows considerable individual variation ranging from less than 2 to 6 mmol/l so the term 'anaerobic threshold' is no longer favoured. In essence, the objective of endurance training is to achieve a higher power output (or velocity) at the inflection point and consequently to be able to work at a higher percentage of $\dot{V}O_2$ max.

Disorders of glycogen storage

Glycogen is a polymer of glucose and as such, is insoluble in water. It is stored in granular form in liver and muscle where it lies in very close proximity to the mitochondria. Errors of carbohydrate assimilation that result from inborn enzyme deficiencies in the glycolytic pathway, are relatively rare but of interest because of the insight into muscle physiology that they provide. Glycogen is unavailable and accumulates upstream causing enlargement of the liver and spleen, affording the term glycogen storage diseases. These share an autosomally recessive mode of inheritance and so there is evidence of consanguinity. None is sex-linked, but all are more common in males.

McArdle's syndrome and Tarui's disease

When myophosphorylase is deficient, type V storage disease or McArdle's syndrome (Chen and Burchell 1995), only peripheral blood glucose is available for glycolysis and so anaerobic power is limited. But a deficiency of phospho-fructokinase (type V11 storage or Tarui's disease) results in a complete inability to utilize glucose (Haller and Lewis 1991). Fat then becomes the only source of energy and physical activity is severely curtailed due to the slower energy yield. Other defects are rarer still and include type 11 disease (a deficiency of α 1-glucosidase deficiency, variously known as acid maltase deficiency or Pompe's disease), and type 111 disease (a deficiency of the enzyme that de-branches glycogen).

The age of presentation varies from childhood to late forties. Often, there is an associated neuropathy. Myopathic signs include muscle pain on exercise, high plasma creatine kinase and bilirubin, and sometimes myoglobinuria. The diagnosis was originally made on periodic acid-Schiff staining of the muscle biopsy, which shows massive accumulations of glycogen, but is now established with genetic screening finding the R49X or R50X mutation (Andreu et al. 1998). Some of these conditions are fatal, presenting with respiratory failure later in life due to a myopathy of the diaphragm.

Physiological adaptation to exercise

Adaptations of muscle to aerobic exercise

Oxidative potential and fibre mix

Biopsy samples taken from the same individual comparing the untrained and trained state show a striking increase in the numbers of both mitochondria and capillaries. The result is an increase in the oxidative potential of muscle, evidenced by an increase in $\dot{V}O_2$ max, in the order of 20–25 per cent. Human limb muscle contains only three myosin-heavy-chain isoforms: 1, 11a, and 11b. Endurance activities tend to utilize the slow-twitch or type 1 fibres, while 11a and 11b are fast-twitch fibres and provide explosive force. Their relative distribution varies with soleus richer in slow-twitch fibres than biceps. There are also racial differences, and although the fibre mix is genetically controlled, it is possible to train one group in favour of the other. What is more, there is now evidence that with endurance training, type 11 fibres may revert to type 1 activity (Lavine et al. 1997; Dudley 1982).

Pulmonary adaptations to exercise

Flow volume loop spirometry and minute ventilation

Gas flow in the lungs is limited by the width of the air passages through which it must pass. Forced expiration followed by maximum effort inspiration describes the limits of flow. Flow limitation is always greater on expiration than inspiration. For normal subjects during exercise, the timing of the two phases is roughly equal (i.e., a ratio of 0.5). And so provided that fall in airflow is linear, breathing capacity can be estimated at any point on the flow loop thus:

$$\text{Minute ventilation (MV l/min)} = \text{FEF \%VC (l/s)} \times 60 \times 0.5,$$

where FEF is the forced expiratory flow at the selected percentage of vital capacity, and 0.5 is the inspiratory/expiratory ratio.

Vital capacity and minute ventilation

Generating adequate ventilation is a trade off between the work of breathing at very high frequency close to residual volume, or at a lower frequency close to forced vital capacity. If minute ventilation during exercise is known, MV/30 can be plotted on the expiratory loop, to show what percentage of vital capacity the subject is using to breathe. During sustained exercise, such as marathon running, athletes elect to breathe at around 50 per cent of their vital capacity. But over short periods of time, say 10 s, most subjects can increase their respiratory capacity to reach maximum voluntary ventilation (MVV) by breathing at 80 per cent of vital capacity or higher (Freedman 1970). This observation is singled out as evidence that the lungs do not normally limit exercise capability. However, many elite performers during all-out exercise breathe very close to MVV, and some can achieve a higher minute ventilation during their chosen sport than with voluntary effort while at rest (Plate 204).

The effects of airways obstruction

This model may be applied to reveal strategies adopted by those for whom breathing difficulties have been created by obstructive disease of the airways. Here the added effort of breathing out raises intrathoracic pressure causing small airways collapse. Expiratory flow is no longer linear, with a more rapid fall in flow rate than is normal initially. Airways collapse is exacerbated by the loss of elastic tissue, as in emphysema. Adequate minute ventilation can only be achieved by shortening the inspiratory phase, raising airways pressure by pursing the lips and by breathing at a higher percentage of vital capacity, that is, closer to total lung capacity (Babb 1999). If airways obstruction is chronic, these adaptations must be sustained. The result is a gradual rise in total lung capacity due to increased residual volume, and a switch in fibre mix in the diaphragm from fast to slow twitch, that is, from type 11b to type 1 (Lavine et al. 1997).

Cardiac adaptations to exercise

Dilatation and hypertrophy

There is a fairly reliable dictum that states cardiac failure does not occur with a normal sized heart. But in athletes, the cardiac silhouette frequently exceeds half that of the transverse diameter of the chest. What is more, left ventricular wall thickness may often measure beyond 12 mm. Sixteen millimetres is now considered by most to represent the upper limit of normal (Pelliccia et al. 1991). Left ventricular dilatation and hypertrophy frequently coexist, but not necessarily in equal measure. Power athletes such as weight lifters show more hypertrophy than dilatation, with the reverse seen in marathon runners. But the athletes who show both hypertrophy and dilatation to the greatest extent are those who require endurance and power. These are rowers, cross-country skiers, and cyclists.

Abnormalities of rhythm and ECG

Training may increase cardiac output by over 20 per cent, largely due to an increase in stroke volume and ejection fraction. This means that adequate tissue perfusion can be achieved with a relatively lower heart rate. Resting heart rate may fall below 40 beats a minute in the highly trained. The electrocardiogram may show sino-atrial block, especially when recorded at night (Ector et al. 1984). Abnormalities of re-polarization characterized by T-wave inversion in the lateral chest leads are common. Coupled with the rise in CK following exercise, these appearances can mimic acute myocardial infarction, but without the Q-wave. Nodal ectopic beats occur frequently and clear on exercise, but ventricular ectopic beats, particularly occurring in couplets or triplets are abnormal. Runs of ventricular ectopics indicate serious myocardial disease and the subject must stop exercising (Plate 205).

Skeletal adaptations to exercise

Bone density increases in response to exercise in all subjects except amenorrhoeal women. Rise in mineral content is greatest in bone subject to the most stress, such as the femur of runners, the lumbar spine of rowers, and the radius of gymnasts and racket players (Wolman et al. 1990). Women who train intensively develop amenorrhoea. The result is a loss in bone density exactly analogous to that which occurs following the menopause. The earliest changes are seen in bone with the highest rate of turnover, and appear first in the trabecular bone of the lumbar spine. Bone loss is detectable after as few as 6 months of amenorrhoea. Losses great enough to result in pathological fracture are usually only seen in women with an associated eating disorder such as anorexia nervosa. Treatment is with oestrogen in the form of hormone replacement therapy (Drinkwater et al. 1984; Tomkinson et al. 2003).

Clinical syndromes associated with exercise

Introduction

The health benefits of taking regular exercise are beyond dispute. The risk of osteoporotic fracture later in life is reduced (Heinonen et al. 1996). Furthermore, there is now direct evidence of a reduced risk of acute myocardial infarction in men and exercise is a major factor in controlling obesity and diabetes (Helmrich et al. 1991; Lakke et al. 1994), although evidence that exercise benefits hypertension is less strong (Blumenthal et al. 1991). Nevertheless, in the United States of America it is recommended that 'every adult should accumulate 30 min or more of moderate-intensity physical activity on most, preferably all, days of the week' (Pollock et al. 1998).

Sudden death

Although rare, sudden death is almost always due to a cardiac cause. It is assumed that the terminal event is ventricular fibrillation, and limited forensic evidence often reveals an underlying abnormality, such as coronary atheroma or a congenital abnormality, the most common of which appears to be hypertrophic cardiomyopathy, accounting for 50 per cent of sudden cardiac deaths in the USA. Even moderate levels of exercise have been implicated; for instance, 12 deaths occurred over 6 years among the joggers of Rhode Island, all but one of these were found to be due to coronary artery disease, with the mortality estimated to be seven times the expected mortality in a sedentary population (Thompson et al. 1992). With the rising popularity of veteran events, it is clear that coronary artery disease in sport is going to pose an ever-increasing problem.

Cardiomyopathy

Obstructive cardiomyopathy, also know as muscular subaortic stenosis, is an absolute contraindication to strenuous dynamic or static activity, because it is a condition that may lead to sudden unexpected death from ventricular fibrillation at a young age. The outflow tract of the left ventricle becomes obstructed in systole by the interventricular septum, which is disproportionately hypertrophied with respect to the ventricular wall. The ratio of the thickness of the septum to the ventricular wall, which is normally 1.3 : 1, exceeds 1.5 : 1 (Fagard et al. 1984). Death occurs, often in the second decade of life, during the course of vigorous physical activity. Faintness or syncope associated with exercise is one of the few symptoms, providing an early indication for urgent investigation. The electrocardiogram is unhelpful because T-wave changes suggesting left ventricular hypertrophy are often seen in normal highly trained individuals. The diagnosis is made by echocardiography (Hillis et al. 1994).

The condition is inherited as an autosomal dominant, so all first-degree relatives should be screened. In a large study of athletes only 7 out of 4500 echocardiograms performed showed obstructive cardiomyopathy (Spirito 1994). There was once a vogue for treatment with surgery which involved shaving the septum, but medical treatment aimed at suppressing the ventricular arrhythmias is now more established. The drug of choice has been amiodorone, though inhibitors of angiotensin-converting enzyme are currently being assessed.

Both aortic and pulmonary stenosis also cause outflow tract obstruction which may have the same effects as hypertrophic obstructive cardiomyopathy during vigorous exertion. On the other hand, tricuspid and pulmonary regurgitation are very common in the highly trained athlete, occurring in over 90 per cent. The murmurs produced may be difficult to distinguish clinically and expert advice should be sought.

Heat stroke

During extremes of exercise, rectal temperature may reach 41°C. Heat loss by radiation through peripheral vasodilatation is limited and further losses can only be achieved by evaporating sweat. Once these homeostatic mechanisms are rendered ineffective, such as in a very humid environment or with sweat failure, core temperature rises unchecked. Heat stroke is rare amongst experienced athletes except where there has been stimulant abuse. The usual clinical setting is one of an undertrained individual, competing for the first time and with inadequate fluid intake (Clowes and O'Donnell 1974). A similar picture is also seen in people who have taken amphetamine (speed) or MDMA (Ecstasy) tablets and who have been dancing to exhaustion.

Confusion or coma is the rule with a clinical presentation very similar to septicaemic shock. The skin may be clammy and cold, contrasting with the high rectal temperature. Grand mal seizures occur with decerebrate posturing. Rhabdomyolysis develops early with the creatine kinase often reaching over 100 000 U/l. Paradoxically in the face of dehydration, serum sodium may be low, sometimes below 110 mmol/l. Disseminated intravascular coagulation, renal failure, and liver failure may occur within 24 h (Sutton 1994). Rapid intravenous infusion can be life saving with an initial infusion of 4 l of saline given in the first hour. Broad-spectrum antibiotics effective against Gram-negative organisms should also be given.

Immune deficiency

There is some evidence that those suffering fatigue syndrome due to overtraining seem to develop frequent infections of the upper respiratory tract. Furthermore, the infecting agent occasionally proves to be unusual (such as *Toxoplasma gondii*). These and other observations have led to the suggestion that overtraining leads to an immunosuppressed state (Khansari et al. 1990). Some support for this concept is obtained from studies of plasma glutamine levels. Glutamine is an essential fuel for lymphocytes: it is synthesized by muscle and is found to be low in chronic fatigue states (Newsholme et al. 1991).

Drugs to avoid

Amphetamine-like substances and drugs with α-adrenergic (stimulant) actions are all banned. These include isoprenaline, adrenaline, noradrenaline, and phenylpropanolamine. For example, adrenaline may not be given by local injection mixed with an analgesic such as lignocaine. Over-the-counter cold cures often contain one, or more, of these agents. Corticosteroids may not be given by parenteral injection, which effectively outlaws all depot preparations, but hydrocortisone may be given by intra-articular injection or into soft tissue injuries such as a tennis elbow. At the time of writing, the position of systemically acting corticosteroids is under review by the IOC's Medical Commission.

References

Andersson, S.G.E. et al. (1998). The genome sequence or *Rickettsia prowazekii* and the origin of mitochondria. *Nature* **396**, 133–40.

Andreu, A.L. et al. (1998). Molecular genetic analysis of McArdle's disease in Spanish patients. *Neurology* **51**, 260–2.

Babb, T. (1999). Machanical ventilatory constraints in ageing, lung disease, and obesity: perspectives and a brief review. *Medicine and Science in Sports and Exercise* **31**, S12–22.

Boyer, P.D. (1997). The ATP synthase—a splendid molecular machine. *Annual Review of Biochemistry* **66**, 717–49.

Blumenthal, J., Siegel, W., and Applebaum, M. (1991). Failure of exercise to reduce blood pressure in patients with mild hypertension: results of a randomized controlled trial. *Journal of the American Medical Association* **266**, 2098–104.

Chen, Y.-T. and Burchell, A. (1995). Glycogen storage diseases. In *The Metabolic and Molecular Basis of Inherited Disease* 7th edn. (ed. C.R. Scriver, A.L. Beaudet, M.S. Sly, and D. Valle), pp. 935–65. New York: McGraw-Hill.

Clowes, G. and O'Donnell, T. (1974). Heat stroke. *New England Journal of Medicine* **291**, 564–7.

Drinkwater, B., Nilson, K., Chestnut, C., Bremner, W., Shainholtz, S., and Southworth, M. (1984). Bone mineral content of amenorrhoeic and eumenorrhoeic athletes. *New England Journal of Medicine* **311**, 277–81.

Dudley, G., Araham, W., and Terjung, R. (1982). Influence of exercise intensity and duration on biochemical adaptations in skeletal muscle. *Journal of Applied Physiology* **53**, 844–50.

Ector, H. et al. (1984). Bradycardia, ventricular pauses, syncope, and sports. *Lancet* **ii**, 591–4.

Fagard, R., Aubert, A., Staessen, J., Vanden Eynde, E., Vanchees, L., and Amery, A. (1984). Cardiac structure and function in cyclists and runners. Comparative echocardiographic study. *British Heart Journal* **52**, 124–9.

Freedman, S. (1970). Sustained maximal voluntary ventilation. *Respiration Physiology* **8**, 230–44.

Haller, R. and Lewis, S. (1991). Glucose-induced exertional fatigue in muscle phosphofructokinase deficiency. *New England Journal of Medicine* **324**, 364–9.

Heinonen, A. et al. (1996). Randomized controlled trial of effect of high-impact exercise on selected risk factors for osteoporotic fractures. *Lancet* **348**, 1343–7.

Helmrich, S., Ragland, P., Leung, R., and Paffenbarger, R. (1991). Physical activity and reduced occurrence of non-insulin-dependent diabetes mellitus. *New England Journal of Medicine* **325**, 147–52.

Hillis, S.W., MacIntyre, P., Maclean, J., Goodwin, J., and McKenna, W. (1994). Sudden death in sport. *British Medical Journal* **309**, 657–60.

Holloszy, J.O. and Coyle, E.F. (1984). Adaptations of skeletal muscle to endurance exercise and their metabolic conequences. *Journal of Applied Physiology* **56** (4), 831–8.

Khansari, D., Murgo, A., and Faith, R. (1990). Effects of stress on the immune system. *Immunology Today* **11**, 170–4.

Lakke, T., Venalainen, J., Rauramaa, R., Salonen, R., Tuomilehto, J., and Salonen, J. (1994). Relation of leisure-time physical activity and cardiorespiratory fitness to the risk of acute myocardial infarction in men. *New England Journal of Medicine* **330**, 1549–54.

Lavine, S. et al. (1997). Cellular adaptations in the diaphragm in chronic obstructive pulmonary disease. *New England Journal of Medicine* **337**, 1799–806.

Mitchell, P. (1977). Vectorial chemiosmotic processes. *Annual Review of Biochemistry* **46**, 996–1005.

Newsholme, E., Parry-Billings, M., McAndrew, N., and Budgett, R. (1991). A biochemical mechanism to explain some characteristics of overtraining. In *Advances in Nutrition and Top Sport* Vol. 32 (ed. F. Brouns), pp. 79–93. Basel: Medical Sports Science.

Pelliccia, A., Maron, B., Spataro, A., Proschan, M., and Spirito, P. (1991). The upper limit of physiological cardiac hypertrophy in highly trained elite athletes. *New England Journal of Medicine* **324**, 292–302.

Spirito, P. (1994). Morphology of the 'athlete's heart' assessed by echo-cardiography in 947 elite athletes representing 27 sports. *American Journal of Cardiology* **74**, 802–6.

Sutton, J. (1994). Physiological and clinical consequences of exercise in heat and humidity. In *Oxford Textbook of Sports Medicine* (ed. M. Harries et al.), pp. 231–8. Oxford: Oxford University Press.

Thompson, P., Funk, E., Carleton, R., and Stumer, W. (1992). Incidence of death during jogging in Rhode Island from 1975 through 1980. *Journal of the American Medical Association* **247**, 1535–8.

Tomkinson, A., Gibson, J.H., Lunt, M., Harries, M., and Reeve, J. (2003). Changes in bone mineral density in the hip and spine before, during, and after the menopause in elite runners. *Osteoporosis International* **14**, 462–8.

Wolman, R., Clark, P., McNally, E., Harries, M., and Reeve, J. (1990). Menstrual state and exercise as determinants of spinal trabecular bone density in female athletes. *British Medical Journal* **301**, 516–18.

7.5 Sports injuries

J.R. Jenner and M. Shirley Emerson

Introduction

Regular aerobic exercise has been shown to have a beneficial effect on several aspects of health including:

1. reducing the risk of cardiovascular disease, particularly coronary artery disease and hypertension (Kohl 2001; Wagner et al. 2002);
2. reducing the incidence of osteoporosis (Bonaiuti et al. 2002);
3. helping with weight loss by increasing the metabolic rate;
4. inducing a feeling of general well-being and reducing depression (Royal College of Physicians 1991; Dimeo et al. 2001).

As a result of these findings, the government has actively encouraged the general population to participate in sporting activities. Unfortunately, one side-effect of sport is injury. If these injuries are not treated promptly and appropriately, the injury may become recurrent or chronic.

Different sports have different rates of injury and different injury profiles (Plate 206) but the fundamental principles underlying the treatment of acute injuries, as well as their rehabilitation, apply across sports. The major cause of injury in sport is acute trauma to soft tissues such as muscle, tendon, or ligaments. Chronic sporting injuries result from either adverse body mechanics, resulting in excess strain, or overuse, leading to fatigue. Children and teenagers with immature or rapidly growing musculoskeletal systems are prone to injuries not encountered in the adult and these injuries deserve special mention.

Injury prevention

Prevention of injury involves several strategies.

Modification of the environment

Many accidents are due to poor surfaces and inadequate equipment. Uneven pitches, collapsing gymnastic equipment, and worn landing mats have all been shown to contribute to injury. These injuries are definitely preventable. Up to 10 per cent of sports injuries in the United Kingdom are due to collisions with the 'furniture' of the playing field or pitch (Nicholl et al. 1991), but other environmental conditions such as weather are probably more important risk factors for injury than the state of the playing surface (Lee and Garraway 2000).

Education and behaviour modification

1. Changes in the rules of some games may be necessary to reduce injury levels. Banning the dangerous practices of 'spearing' in American football has resulted in a reduction in the number of injuries producing permanent cervical quadriplegia (Torg et al. 1985).
2. Good referees are needed to prevent deliberate fouls, which often lead to injury.
3. Continuing player education is also important to persuade players to obey the rules and not to indulge in 'sport rage'.
4. Trained coaches should have a good knowledge of exercise physiology and be able to advise on good techniques, diet, and to help players avoid overuse injuries through improved training techniques.
5. Matching of young players in team games should be done by size and not by age.
6. Relevant protective equipment should be used. Mouth guards have been shown to reduce the number of dental and oral injuries but many players do not like using them (Jennings 1990).

Personal strategies

1. *Training to build up muscle strength and endurance.* Many injuries occur during the second half of a game, when fatigued muscles do not respond quickly to new situations. This is seen particularly in weekend athletes who do no other training.
2. *Warm up and cool down.* There are differing opinions on the benefit of warm ups and cool downs but the majority of athletes and coaches are in favour of some mobility exercises and gentle exercise to raise the heart rate and body temperature. After an intense effort, continuing light exercise does seem to allow an enhanced rate of removal of lactic acid and also prevents blood 'pooling' in the lower limbs. Stretching to improve flexibility both before and after exercises is popular but there is little hard evidence that it reduces injuries (Pope et al. 2000).
3. *Diet.* There is overwhelming evidence as to the importance of adequate carbohydrate intake while competing and training to maintain and replace muscle glycogen. Carbohydrate should provide 50–60 per cent of the calorie intake and the athlete may need to take some of this as a carbohydrate drink (Costill and Hargreaves 1992). Cyclists on the *Tour de France* need to consume about 7000 calories/day and this would be impossible to eat as solid food.
4. *Hydration.* Most athletes are now aware of the importance of adequate rehydration but children need to be encouraged to drink as part of the game. Immediate post-exercise replacement of fluid and carbohydrate, within the first hour, has been shown to restore rapidly muscle glycogen. Reduced glycogen levels lead to muscle fatigue and injury, and reduced muscle glycogen is associated with a reduction in muscle and plasma glutamine levels.
5. *Avoiding overtraining.* Many athletes and sports players are convinced that 'more is better' and are not prepared to incorporate rest and recovery into their schedule. The overtraining syndrome produces symptoms of fatigue, sleeplessness, and loss of appetite (Budgett 1999). Intense and prolonged exercise has also been shown to produce immune system depression for 6–20 h after exercise (Newsholme 1994). This may explain why an athlete is more susceptible to injury and illness, including opportunistic infections such as toxoplasmosis and why injuries may take longer to heal.

Acute injuries

Acute management

Trauma results in bleeding. Blood in the extra vascular space is an extreme irritant causing an acute inflammatory response with swelling, an increase in pressure, and, if this pressure becomes great enough, tissue necrosis occurs. Acute treatment of soft tissue trauma is aimed at limiting the bleeding and its subsequent deleterious affect (Fig. 1). This is achieved by rest, ice, compression, elevation, and non-steroidal anti-inflammatory agent. This treatment is often given the mnemonic of RICE or NICER.

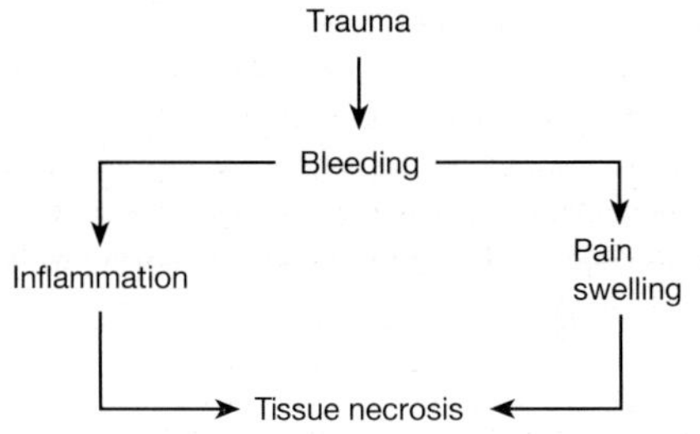

Fig. 1 Flow chart for the treatment of soft tissue injuries after acute injury.

RICE is an attempt to apply basic principles to limit bleeding. Leaving the field of play immediately after an injury together with compression and elevation of the injured part is common sense. Research into the efficacy of this algorithm has not been done and the added value of ice and non-steroidals remains controversial.

Haematomas

Muscle haematoma may be due to either extrinsic or intrinsic injury. After injury, there is disruption of the muscle fibres and capillaries with associated bleeding. The torn ends retract from the injury leaving it filled with blood.

An intact muscle sheath results in an intramuscular haematoma—a swelling within the muscle—causing pain and a considerable amount of disability that resolves slowly over many weeks. An intermuscular haematoma results when there is a tear in the fascial sheath or there is a tearing of vessels between the muscle fascicles. In this situation the blood disperses by gravity, to some distance away from the injury and the appearance can be quite spectacular with considerable bruising.

Symptoms depend to some degree on the type of injury. Extrinsic or compression injuries are common in contact sports such as a rugby tackle, when the quadriceps muscle is compressed against the femur, the bleeding may be slow allowing the player to continue and only after the game does the increased swelling and accompanying pain and disability become apparent. An overstretching injury as in sprinting is sudden and acutely painful immediately. The commonest presentation is seen in sprinters who overstretch suddenly against resistance and tear hamstring muscles. Here, the sudden acute pain feels like a blow on the back of the leg and may be severe enough for the athlete to fall to the ground. Patients with a severe intramuscular haematoma of the hamstrings often present with a flexion deformity. The diagnosis can be confirmed and treatment monitored by ultrasound.

Rehabilitation

Except in the most severe haematomas, early mobilization is indicated as it:

1. speeds the return of muscle strength;
2. improves the orientation of regenerating muscle fibres;
3. encourages recapillarization;
4. prevents disuse atrophy.

After 24–48 h of rest and ice, a rehabilitation programme should begin. This should initially consist of gentle stretching with the aim of restoring a full range of joint movement. The physiotherapist may also use various modalities of electrotherapy to assist healing and relieve pain. Stretching and strengthening programmes for all the muscle groups of the involved limb are essential, as some injuries may be due to a pre-existing lack of elasticity either in the injured muscle or its antagonist. The importance of balance between the muscle groups in the prevention of injury has been recognized and may be measured using an isokinetic machine, both for assessment and muscle retraining.

Cardiovascular fitness can be maintained by cycling (real bike or exercise bike), swimming, and running in water using a specially designed 'wet vest' to keep the athlete upright. Apart from the physical benefits of this exercise, being active in this way helps to maintain the sanity of the injured athlete. Many committed athletes become anxious and even depressed if exercise is not permitted.

Return to sport

A muscle haematoma can be considered to be completely healed when there is full and pain free muscle contraction. An intermuscular haematoma will usually resolve in 2–4 weeks. An intramuscular haematoma may take 8 weeks or more to completely heal, but there is a great variation depending on the site and severity of the injury. Before returning to competition, a further programme of sport-specific training must be carried out. This includes sprints, rapid deceleration, twists, and sharp turns. Co-ordination and proprioception are impaired by injury and the athlete must relearn specific techniques with the help of a coach.

Myositis ossificans

A severe crush injury may be followed by the development of heterotopic ossification or myositis ossificans. This is more likely to occur if the injury is aggravated by continuing activity and further bruising. Applications of heat and vigorous massage may further exacerbate the problem, although the exact cause of the calcification is not clear. Suspicions are raised if the patient is unable to achieve full contraction of the affected muscle. The calcification may be seen on radiographs or ultrasound.

Various treatments apart from rest have been used, including high doses of indomethacin, diphosphonates, and the calcium channel blocker, diltiazem, but their efficacy remains doubtful. Although the calcification may persist radiologically, intervention is rarely required as functional impairment related to the calcification is extrememly rare.

Muscle ruptures

Muscles may rupture and, although the defects look dramatic, they rarely need surgical repair unless the rupture is complete.

Chronic injuries

The vast majority of chronic sports injuries are to the lower limb, predominantly affecting the knee. A description of the majority of these injuries and their treatment can be found in other sections of this book, particularly the section on soft tissue rheumatism (Chapter 6.13). In this section, a few of the commonest problems encountered in a sports injury clinic are described—further information can be found in specialist textbooks (Harries et al. 1998; Peterson and Renstrom 2001). A full and detailed history is important for diagnosis, particularly to ascertain if there has been overuse or a sudden unaccustomed use of the lower limbs.

Examination must always start with the spine and include the whole upper or lower limb. Leg length inequality of more than 2 cm should be noted. Chronic lower limb sporting injuries are frequently associated with the 'malicious malalignment syndrome' with a broad pelvis, patellas that look towards each other, internal tibial torsion, and flat or hyperpronated feet. Examination should include the joints, soft tissues, and neurological system as well as skin and circulation. The examination is completed by inspecting the running shoes for signs of wear.

Correcting leg length inequality of 2 cm or more with a simple insole may resolve back problems. Simple shock absorbing insoles may also help many chronic overuse problems. The use of more elaborate insoles to correct hyperpronation and other foot problems are also popular but their success is unpredictable.

Stress fractures

Stress fractures can occur in any loaded bone and are seen most commonly in lower limbs, particularly in the tibia and metatarsals but they also occur in the upper limb girdle, such as in the ribs of rowers and the arms of gymnasts (Karlson 1998). Approximately 55 per cent over the tibia, 23 per cent metatarsal, 14 per cent in the fibula, 4 per cent in the femoral neck, and 2 per cent each in femoral shaft and pubic arch.

Stress fractures occur when bone fails to adapt to new or unusual loading. Normally, microdamage stimulates new bone where needed. When microdamage outpaces the development of new bone, a stress fracture results. Foot biomechanics may influence the development of stress fractures, such as rigid, poorly adapting feet or conversely hypermobile feet. Running on hard surfaces using 'collapsed' running shoes or racing flats certainly has an influence. Women appear to be at greater risk of developing a stress fracture. In a survey of 218 consecutive patients presenting with a stress fracture to our sports injury clinic almost half were women, although women only accounted for one-fourth of all the patients seen in the clinic (Fig. 2). Some of the fractures may be due to an inadequate calorie and calcium intake in sports where leanness is favoured, especially if low food intake results in amenorrhoea and secondary osteoporosis. These factors do not entirely account for the high incidences in women.

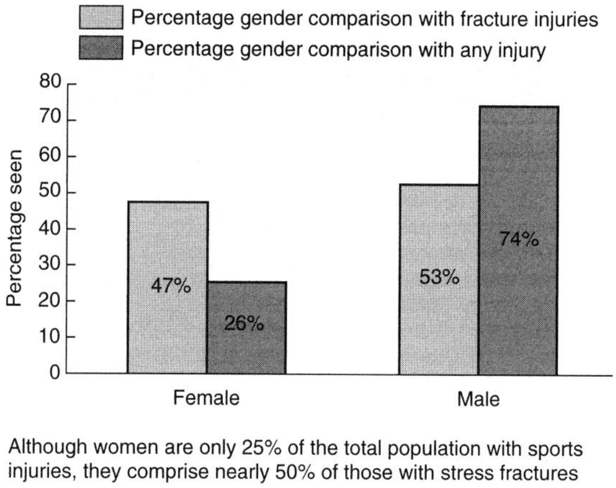

Fig. 2 Comparison of the incidence of stress fractures and all injuries between females and males attending a sports injury clinic.

Clinical features

In vigorous sports, such as high jumping and gymnastics, the onset of pain is sudden and acute, completely preventing the continuation of the activity. In other less-explosive sports, such as long distance running, the onset may be insidious over several days or even weeks, with pain present at first only during exercise and weight bearing but eventually aching at rest and during the night. The site of the pain is very localized and local pressure produces exquisite pain over the fracture, causing the patient rapidly to pull the injured limb away. A stress fracture may be diagnosed on these clinical grounds, but in order to persuade an exercise-addicted athlete to rest there is frequently a need for some corroboration.

Radiographs are not very helpful as they do not show the injury until it is healing and may be not even then. Bone scans are extremely sensitive and can differentiate between osteitis of the tibia and a stress fracture. Although not absolutely necessary for diagnosis, a positive scan does help to convince the athlete of the nature of his problem and need for rest (Fig. 3).

Although the majority of stress fractures respond to conservative measures, stress fractures of the femoral neck have the potential for serious complications, including avascular necrosis and persistent non-union, and may need a surgical assessment (Clough 2002). These present with vague groin pain, pain in the anterior thigh and the knee, and are most commonly seen in long distance runners.

Management

Reduction of weight bearing is essential, usually with the help of elbow crutches. Modification of activity should continue until symptoms are absent. During this time the athlete can do some form of non- or partial-weight-bearing exercise. Sport can be resumed when there is no pain on weight bearing and must be gradually increased.

Using this regime, the majority of athletes will be able to return to sport in 6–8 weeks. Problems arise when the athlete is not prepared to rest. Under these circumstances the fracture can continue to cause problems for several months and sometime the only way to prevent continuing disability is to apply a plaster of Paris case and insist on no weight bearing. If not properly dealt with, a stress fracture can persist for 6 months or more.

Anterior knee pain

A patient presenting with poorly localized anterior knee pain, without any history of trauma, is a very common occurrence in a sports injury clinic.

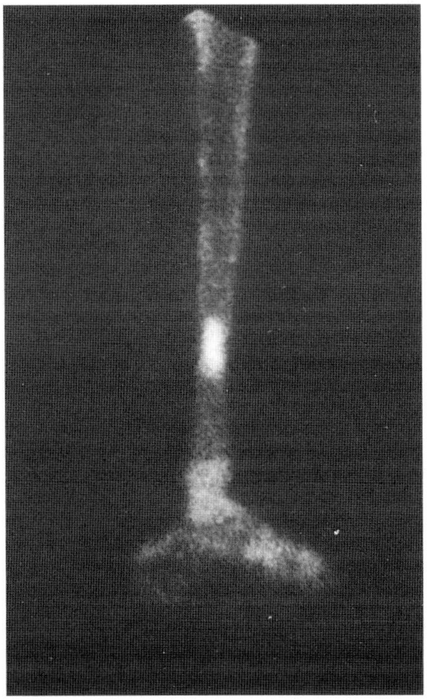

Fig. 3 Tc-99m bone scan showing high focal uptake typical of a stress fracture of the tibia.

The patient is often teenaged and a sports enthusiast, playing or training on a daily basis. However, older patients responding to advice to increase their exercise also present with this problem.

Aetiology

Patellofemoral joint stability depends on many factors:

- torsional deformities of tibia/femur (winking or frog eye patella);
- high or lateral patella;
- weak or absent vastus medialis obliquus;
- tight muscles on the lateral aspect—vastus lateralis and iliotibial band;
- increased quadriceps angle;
- excessive foot pronation;
- weak ankle dorsiflexors;
- reduced range of motion at the ankle;
- tight hamstrings.

Any of these factors can cause an imbalance of the patellofemoral joint. It has long been assumed that patellofemoral pain was caused by abnormal patella tracking but all of these anatomical variations are common in the general population and only cause problems when the patellofemoral joint is subjected to chronic overload by repetitive overuse and excessive eccentric muscle contraction as in deep squats. Risk factors associated with the development of anterior knee pain include shortened quadriceps, a hypermobile patella, and decreased explosive strength (Witrouw et al. 2000).

Clinical features

The patient complains of generalized anterior knee pain. There is no history of trauma but more of a gradual increase in pain over several weeks, often affecting both knees. The pain is made worse by activity, either during sport or going up and down stairs. The knee may feel unstable or 'give way'; this is due to reflex quadriceps inhibition rather than a true instability. Clicking and crepitus is common. There is pain and sometimes crepitus if the patella is compressed against the femur and the leg flexed and extended. There is usually some tenderness on the posterior surface of the patella.

Patella subluxation, which can present with similar symptoms, is excluded by the patella apprehension test. The patella is usually very mobile and pushing it sideways produces great anxiety.

Management

The patient, and often relatives, need to be reassured that this complaint is common and does not mean indefinite incapacity. Radiographs may be required to exclude any more serious pathology, especially if the problem affects one knee only. In mild cases, some reduction of the level of activity is all that is necessary—the patient decides what is tolerable. Activities not causing pain, such as swimming, can be substituted to maintain fitness. Local applications of ice after exercise and a course of non-steroidal anti-inflammatory drugs can hasten recovery.

Rehabilitation

When the acute symptoms have settled, a strengthening and stretching programme involving hamstring and quadriceps is begun under the care of a sports-orientated physiotherapist. The treatment involves selectively strengthening the vastus medialis obliquus, while at the same time reducing the pull of the vastus lateralis. Muscle re-education using biofeedback techniques or isokinetics during various exercises can be used. In addition to muscle strengthening, corrective foot orthoses and a progressive resistance brace have been found helpful but patellofemoral orthoses, patellar mobilizations, and patella taping lack evidence to support their use (Crossly et al. 2001).

Although the vast majority of patients will improve using these measures, it is important that they understand this is not a cure. Adolescent sufferers may well improve with the passage of time, as some of the imbalance may be associated with growth spurts. If there are persistent anatomical features, the patient will have to be prepared to continue the muscle strengthening exercises indefinitely in order to control their pain. Ten per cent of patients do not improve with the above measures; some may be prepared to modify their lifestyles but others may request surgery. Various surgical options are available, the most common being lateral release, again with little evidence of long term benefit.

Anterior shin pain induced by exercise ('shin splints')

Chronic pain in the shins induced by exercise (commonly known as 'shin splints') is a frequent occurrence in sportsmen and women but is rarely seen in any other group of patients. This syndrome embraces a variety of conditions:

1. stress fracture of the tibia or fibula;
2. fasciitis of tibialis posterior;
3. compartment syndrome;
4. popliteal artery stenosis;
5. referred pain from the spine (cord claudication);
6. peripheral vascular disease (intermittent claudication).

Fasciitis of tibialis posterior

Hyperpronation of the feet puts extra stress on the tibialis posterior muscle, which inserts onto the posterior aspect of the tibia and fibula. The tendon of the muscle runs behind the medial malleolus and in association with a flat hyperpronated foot is easily overstretched by repetitive activity resulting in a traction injury at the fascial insertion along the posterior border of the tibia.

Patients complain of pain in the shins, which starts after starting to run. They can run through the pain only for it to return with great severity on ceasing activity. The pain often takes days to wear off. Examination reveals diffuse tenderness along the medial border of the tibia. The diagnosis may be confirmed with a bone scan that will also exclude the diagnosis a stress fracture.

Treatment is difficult. Rest is vital and is followed by a gradual return to sport with appropriate footwear. Orthotic supports to correct the hyperpronation and to provide shock absorption can be tried.

Compartment syndrome

Acute swelling of muscles within a muscle compartment leading to muscle ischaemia and even necrosis is a well-recognized complication of acute trauma. The chronic form of this condition is less well known and occurs almost exclusively in endurance sports such as long distance running. As the muscles are exercised they swell within a tight fascial compartment raising the pressure sufficiently to reduce tissue perfusion. There are four separate compartments in the lower limb: anterior (tibialis anterior), posterior (gastrocnemius/soleus), deep posterior (tibialis posterior), and lateral (peroneii). Compartment syndrome commonly follows a sudden increase in training. Symptoms are absent at rest but pain in the shin commences at a variable time after the onset of exercise and invariably increases until exercise is stopped or moderated. In contrast to patients with tibialis fasciitis, if the limb is rested the pain usually wears off quite quickly within a few hours. Examination is often unremarkable although highly developed calf muscles that feel tense at rest may be noted. A Tc-99 bone scan will exclude a stress fracture or fasciitis. Pressure studies can be performed by inserting catheters into each compartment and measuring the pressure rises. This is an invasive investigation and only available at specialist centres. If the symptoms do not settle with rest, the appropriate compartments can be released by a surgical fasciotomy.

Popliteal artery entrapment

Rarely, similar symptoms can be caused by entrapment of the popliteal artery by a fibrous band or hypertrophied head of gastrocnemius. Arteriography may be required to confirm the diagnosis.

Children and sport

Children are prone to similar injuries to adults but should not be regarded as 'little adults' as their physiology and anatomy are very different, resulting in injuries not encountered in the adult:

1. They take shorter, more shallow breaths and need more oxygen for their activity than an adult;
2. They also have lower glycogen levels and essential muscle enzymes and waste more energy;
3. Children perceive exercises as less fatiguing than adults and can almost exercise to destruction, but they also have the capacity to recover very quickly;
4. Muscle, tendon, and ligaments are stronger than bone until bony maturity is reached at 18–21 years;
5. Bones are still growing with active apophyses and epiphyses that can be the site of pathology;
6. Growth occurs in spurts, resulting in tight muscles and loss of flexibility making adolescents particularly prone to injury.

Avulsion fractures

Tendons, ligaments, and muscles, especially trained muscles, are stronger than bone and more so at the epiphyseal junctions. Sudden, intense loading of a muscle does not produce a muscle tear as in an adult but is more likely to cause an avulsion fracture where the bony attachment of the muscle or ligament is torn away. Common sites for avulsion fractures are the growth zones around the pelvis, including the attachments at the ischial tuberosity and the attachments of rectus femoris and sartorius. The less severe injuries can sometimes present only as a pain in the groin, with loss of function of the appropriate muscle. These injuries do not show up on radiographs and a bone scan is necessary. The usual treatment is rest followed by physiotherapy treatment, with an emphasis on restoring strength to the injured muscle. Healing may take up to 6 months.

Overuse injuries of the apophysis

In children and adolescents the muscle tendon attachment to bone or the apophysis presents as a 'high-risk' area for overuse. Overuse caused a traction apophysitis and occurs at various sites:

- tibial tubercle (Osgood–Schlatters);
- lower pole of patella (Sinding–Larsen, Johannason);
- achilles tendon attachment to calcaneum (Severs disease).

Osgood–Schlatter disease follows overloading of the patellar tendon at its attachment to the tibial tubercle. Very active boys, between the ages of 14 and 16 years, and girls at a slightly younger age, present with swelling, pain, and acute tenderness over the tibial tubercle. The treatment of all the apophyseal overuse injuries is by modifying activity, playing only to a bearable level of discomfort, and using ice before and after exercise. Most respond to this regime but this may take several months and some persist until growing has ceased.

Osteochondritis

This is a collection of conditions affecting various sites of uncertain aetiology and is thought to be due to avascular necrosis of bone and subsequent flattening of the affected bones. Examples include: Perthes' disease (hip), Scheuermann's disease (vertebral ring epiphysis), Kohler's disease (navicular bone), Freiburg's disease (second or third metatarsal), and Panner's disease (elbow capitellum).

Perthes' disease and the potentially disastrous unrelated hip problem of slipped femoral epiphysis may present with a limp and a painful knee. This can cause diagnostic problems as the child may present following an injury, drawing attention away from the real source of the problem. When faced with this history a radiograph is mandatory, as both conditions require urgent orthopaedic referral.

Scheuermann's disease mainly affects the thoracic vertebrae and because the anterior border of the vertebrae are subjected to deforming forces a kyphosis may occur. Often this is asymptomatic, although some discomfort after hard exercise does occur. Reduction of exercise to a pain-free zone with flexibility exercises for the hip flexors and hamstrings and abdominal strengthening are sufficient until the disease spontaneously ends.

Osteochondritis dissecans

Osteochondritis dissecans is a disease of unknown aetiology, occurring in young people between the ages of 12 and 16 years. There is destruction and subsequent disintegration of cartilage and bone. Popular theories are trauma or continuous repetitive damage (Fairbanks 1993), ischaemia, and genetic factors. In the United States, the condition is seen as one of the entities in 'little league elbow', seen in young baseball pitchers.

The knee is a common presenting site and the history is of a diffuse knee ache, made worse by activity and accompanied by occasional effusion. When a fragment of bone becomes loose in the joint the patient may present with an episode of locking and effusion. The diagnosis can be confirmed by radiography. Surgical replacement of the loose fragment can give excellent results.

References

Boanaituti, A. et al. (2002). Exercise for preventing and treating osteoporosis in postmenopausal women. *Cochrane Database Systems Review* Issue 3, CD000333.

Budgett, R. *The Overtraining Syndrome. ABC Sports Medicine* 2nd edn. London: British Medical Journal Publications, 1999.

Clough, T.M. (2002). Femoral neck strees fractures: the importance of clinical suspicion and early review. *British Journal of Sports Medicine* **36** (4), 308–9.

Costill, D.L. and Hargreaves, M. (1992). Carbohydrate nutrition and fatigue. *Sports Medicine* **12**, 86–92.

Crossly, K. et al. (2001). A systematic review of physical interventions for paellofemoral pain syndrome. *Clinical Journal of Sports Medicine* **11** (2), 103–10.

Dimeo, F. et al. (2001). Aerobic exercise improves mood in patients with major depression. *British Journal of Sports Medicine* **35** (2), 114–17.

Fairbanks, H.A.T. (1993). Osteochondritis dissecans. *British Journal of Surgery* **21**, 67.

Harries, M., Williams, C., and Stanish, W., ed. *Oxford Textbook of Sports Medicine* 2nd edn. Oxford: Oxford University Press, 1998.

Jennings, D.C. (1990). Injuries sustained by users and non users of gum shields in local rugby union players. *British Journal of Sports Medicine* **24**, 159–65.

Karlson, K.A. (1998). Rib stress fractures in elite rowers. A case series and proposed mechanisms. *American Journal of Sports Medicine* **26** (4), 516–19.

Kohl, H.W. (2001). Physical activity and cardiovascular disease: evidence for a dose response. *Medicine and Science in Sports and Exercise* **33** (Suppl. 6), S472–83.

Lee, A.J. and Garraway, W.M. (2000). The influence of environmental factors on rugby football injuries. *Journal of Sports Science* **18** (2), 91–5.

Newsholme, E.A. (1994). Biochemical mechanisms to explain immunosuppression in well-trained and overtrained athletes. *International Journal of Sports Medicine* **15** (Suppl. 3), 5142–7.

Nicholl, J.P., Coleman, P., and Williams, B.T. *Injuries in Sport and Exercise.* London: London Sports Council, 1991.

Peterson, L. and Renstrom, P.A.F.H. *Sports Injuries: Their Presentation and Treatment* 3rd edn. Human Kinetics, 2001.

Pope, R.P. et al. (2000). A randomized trial of pre-exercise stretching for prevention of lower limb injury. *Medicine and Science in Sports and Exercise* **32** (8), 271–7.

Royal College of Physicians. *Medical Aspects of Exercise. Benefits and Risks.* London: Royal College of Physicians of London, 1991.

Torg, J.S. et al. (1985). The national football head and neck injury registry. *Journal of the American Medical Association* **254**, 3439–43.

Wagner, A. et al. (2002). Physical activity and coronary event incidence in Northern Ireland and France: the Prospective Epidemiological Study of Myocardial Infarction (PRIME). *Circulation* **105** (19), 247–52.

Witrvouw, E., Lysens, R., Bellermans, J., Cambier D., and Vanderstraeten, G. (2000). Intrinsic risk factors for the development of anterior knee pain in an athletic population. A two-year prospective study. *American Journal of Sports Medicine* **28** (4), 480–9.

Index

Main index entries are given in **bold.**
Page numbers in *italics* refer to tables.